Textbook of

PEDIATRIC INTENSIVE CARE

Textbook of
PEDIATRIC INTENSIVE CARE

Third Edition

Editor

Mark C. Rogers
Vice Chancellor for Health Affairs
Chief Executive Officer of Duke University
Hospital and Health System
Distinguished Professor of Pediatrics and Anesthesiology

Associate Editor

David G. Nichols
Director of Pediatric Intensive Care Unit
Johns Hopkins Hospital

Section Editors

Alice D. Ackerman
J. Michael Dean
William J. Greeley
James J. Fackler
Randall C. Wetzel

SANS TACHE

Williams & Wilkins
A WAVERLY COMPANY

BALTIMORE • PHILADELPHIA • LONDON • PARIS • BANGKOK
BUENOS AIRES • HONG KONG • MUNICH • SYDNEY • TOKYO • WROCLAW

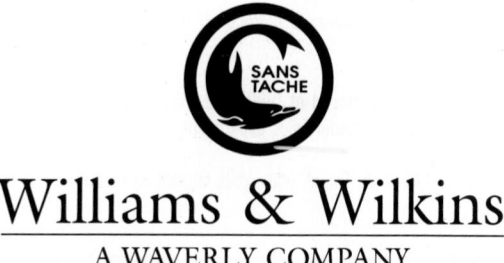

Editor: Carroll Cann
Managing Editor: Tanya Lazar
Development Editor: Joanne Husovski
Production Coordinator: Peter J. Carley
Copy Editor: Susan Rockwell
Designer: Nancy Hagan Abbott
Illustration Planner: Peter J. Carley
Cover Designer: Nancy Hagan Abbott
Typesetter: Clarinda Composition
Printer: R.R. Donnelley
Digitized Illustrations: Clarinda Composition
Binder: R.R. Donnelley

351 West Camden Street
Baltimore, Maryland 21201-2436 USA

Rose Tree Corporate Center
1400 North Providence Road
Building II, Suite 5025
Media, Pennsylvania 19063-2043 USA

Printed in the United States of America

Third Edition

Library of Congress Cataloging-in-Publication Data

Textbook of pediatric intensive care / editor, Mark C. Rogers ;
associate editor, David G. Nichols.--3rd ed.
p. cm.
Includes bibliographical references and index.
ISBN 0-683-18034-7
1. Pediatric intensive care. I. Rogers, Mark C. II. Nichols,
David G. (David Gregory), 1951- .
[DNLM: 1. Intensive Care--in infancy & childhood. WS 366 T3555
1996]
RJ370.T49 1996
618.92'0028--dc20
DNLM/DLC
for Library of Congress

ISBN 0-683-18034-7

9 780683 180343

96-14624
CIP

To purchase additional copies of this book, call our customer service department at (800) 638-0672 or fax orders to (800) 447-8438. For other book services, including chapter reprints and large quantity sales, ask for the Special Sales department.

Canadian customers should call (800) 268-4178, or fax (905) 470-6780. For all other calls originating outside of the United States, please call (410) 528-4223 or fax us at (410) 528-8550.

Visit Williams & Wilkins on the Internet: http://www.wwilkins.com or contact our customer service department at custserv@wwilkins.com. Williams & Wilkins customer service representatives are available from 8:30 am to 6:00 pm, EST, Monday through Friday, for telephone access.

97 98 99
2 3 4 5 6 7 8 9 10

Dedication

This book is dedicated to the many young trainees in the field of pediatric intensive care who are assuming responsibility for the awesome task of making life and death decisions on critically ill children. This book is written for them and for the children whom they serve.

Preface

This is now the third edition of the Textbook of Pediatric Intensive Care. As we have traveled throughout the world, it has been very gratifying to see the book on the shelves of pediatric intensive care units and libraries in sophisticated medical centers and in rural pediatric intensive care units. We have tried very hard to continue the tradition that this is the most comprehensive review of the subject and the one most likely to contain the information necessary for the pediatric intensive care specialist to best be able to make a proper diagnosis or develop a proper treatment plan.

The book continued to grow more sophisticated and complex even as its presentation is trying to be made more user friendly and the length of the book is kept constant. This is a reflection on the growth of the sophistication of the specialty and of the people who practice the wonderful medical art of pediatric intensive care.

Publisher's Foreword

We have made a significant change in the third edition of this TEXTBOOK OF PEDIATRIC INTENSIVE CARE, one that will be immediately evident to users of the previous editions. The textbook is now *one volume,* instead of two. Still, its goals remain the same—to be the most comprehensive review of the subject and to provide all of the information necessary for the care of critically ill children.

First published in 1988, this book became the standard reference source for pediatric critical care medicine. Created by one of the founders of the specialty (Dr. Rogers), it defined the field by encompassing all areas of clinical care relevant to the pediatric intensive care unit. The elements that set it apart from other texts in the field are as much a part of this new third edition as they were with the first edition. The editors have maintained the organ system organization, with each topic covering basic pathophysiology, patient management guidelines, and treatment protocols.

Several timely additions can also be found in the new edition. A new section has been added on PICU administration, including quality assurance, ethical issues, and outcomes analysis. This edition provides expanded coverage of neonatology to reflect recent changes in research, and greater coverage of molecular biology. It also contains more current material on emergency management of the upper airway. As before, diagrams and tables appear throughout the book to aid its practical value; 445 new illustrations have also been added to this edition. Finally, the authoritative authorship is a key to this book and now Dr. Nichols has joined Dr. Rogers as associate editor, with Drs. Ackerman, Dean, Greeley, Fackler, and Wetzel serving as section editors, to assure that the book maintains the balanced scientific and practical approach that won it praise in previous editions.

Our major contribution, as publishers, is in design and packaging. Without sacrificing content or quality, we have been able to publish the third edition in one volume. This change has been made possible through technological advances in printing and binding. The book that has been called the "bible" in its field *now contains 50 chapters, still has 10 sections, and is still over 1700 pages in length.* But now readers will not have to wonder which volume they need to open to find the information they need—it's all here in one handy resource. Another advantage of the new format is that it will allow us to lower the selling price of the book, making it affordable for a greater number of people who will need to rely on it for daily reference. We hope that the enhanced content and design benefit practitioners and patients around the world, and set new standards for future works.

The Publisher,
Williams & Wilkins

Acknowledgement

The authors would like to acknowledge the support that their spouses and children have provided in allowing and encouraging the enormous effort required to put together such a massive work. In addition, they would like to thank Ms. Gail McLamb for her dedication and effort in the production of this book.

Contributors

Alice D. Ackerman, M.D., F.A.A.P., F.C.C.M.
Department of Pediatrics
University of Maryland School of Medicine
Baltimore, Maryland

Elizabeth Allen, M.D.
Division of Pediatric Critical Care
University of Utah School of Medicine
Primary Children's Medical Center
Salt Lake City, Utah

John Arnold, M.D.
Multidisciplinary Intensive Care Unit
Children's Hospital
Boston, Massachusetts

Jolene D. Bean
Scott & White Hospital
Department of Anesthesiology
Temple, Texas

Elizabeth A. Bello, M.D.
Duke University Medical Center
Durham, North Carolina

A. Resai Bengur, M.D.
Division of Pediatric Cardiology
Duke University Medical Center
Durham, North Carolina

Frank E. Berkowitz, M.B., B.Ch., F.C.P. (PAED) (SA)
Department of Pediatrics
Emory University School of Medicine
Atlanta, Georgia

Ivor D. Berkowitz, M.B., B.Ch.
Department of Anesthesiology, Critical Care Medicine & Pediatrics
The Johns Hopkins Hospital
Baltimore, Maryland

Mark Bernstein, M.D.
Department of Hematology
Montreal Children's Hospital
Montreal, Quebec

Richard S. Boyer, M.D.
Department of Pediatric Radiology
University of Utah
Salt Lake City, Utah

Susan L. Bratton, M.D.
Department of Anesthesia and Critical Care
Children's Hospital and Medical Center
Seattle, Washington

Mark C. Bugnitz, M.D.
Department of Pediatrics—Critical Care Medicine
LeBonheur Children's Medical Center
Memphis, Tenessee

Jeffrey Burns, M.D., M.P.H.
Division of Pediatric Critical Care
Children's Hospital
Harvard Medical School
Boston, Massachusetts

G. Patricia Cantwell, M.D.
Medical Training & Simulation Laboratory
University of Miami School of Medicine
Miami, Florida

Ira Cheifetz, M.D.
Pediatric Critical Care Medicine
Duke University Medical Center
Durham, North Carolina

W. Bruce Cherny, M.D.
Division of Pediatric Neurosurgery
University of Utah
Primary Children's Medical Center
Salt Lake City, Utah

David W. Christensen, M.D.
Department of Pediatrics/PICU
Loma Linda University Medical Center
Loma Linda, California

Bonnie Clay, M.S., P.N.P., C.C.R.N.
Division of Pediatric Intensive Care
Primary Children's Medical Center
Salt Lake City, Utah

J. Michael Dean, M.D.
University of Utah
Primary Children's Medical Center
Salt Lake City, Utah

Jayant K. Deshpande, M.D.
Department of Pediatric Critical Care Medicine
Vanderbilt University Medical Center
Nashville, Tennessee

Clifford S. Deutschman, M.S., M.D.
Department of Anesthesiology
University Hospital of Pennsylvania
Philadelphia, Pennsylvania

Robert Englander, M.D.
Department of Pediatrics, Division of Critical Care
University of Maryland School of Medicine
Baltimore, Maryland

Allen E. Eskenazi, M.D.
Division of Pediatric Hematology/Oncology
University of Maryland School of Medicine
Baltimore, Maryland

James C. Fackler, M.D.
Multidisciplinary ICU
Children's Hospital
Boston, Massachusetts

John J. Farley, M.D.
Department of Pediatric Immunology
University of Maryland School of Medicine
Baltimore, Maryland

Francis M. Filloux, M.D.
Department of Neurology
University Neuropsychiatric Institute
Salt Lake City, Utah

Debra Fiser, M.D.
Department Pediatric Critical Care
Arkansas Children's Hospital
Little Rock, Arkansas

Glenn Furuta, M.D.
Division of Gastroenterology
Children's Hospital
Boston, Massachusetts

John B. Gordon, M.D., C.M., F.R.C.P.(C)
Department of Pediatrics and Critical Care Medicine
University of Maryland School of Medicine
Baltimore, Maryland

Mary Jo Grant, M.S., P.N.P., C.C.R.N.
Pediatric Intensive Care Unit
Primary Children's Medical Center
Salt Lake City, Utah

Eva Nozik Grayck, M.D.
Division of Pediatric Critical Care Medicine
Duke University Medical Center
Durham, North Carolina

William J. Greeley, M.D.
Department of Anesthesiology and Pediatric Critical Care
Duke University Medical Center
Durham, North Carolina

Michael Green, M.D., M.P.H.
Department of Pediatrics and Surgery
Pittsburgh University School of Medicine
Pittsburgh Children's Hospital
Pittsburgh, Pennsylvania

Robert S. Greenberg, M.D.
Department of Anesthesiology
Johns Hopkins Medical Institute
Baltimore, Maryland

Barbara A. Haber, M.D.
GI Nutrition Division
Children's Hospital of Philadelphia
University of Pennsylvania
Philadelphia, Pensylvania

Matthew Hand, D.O.
Division of Nephrology
Children's Hospital
Boston, Massachusetts

William Harmon, M.D.
Division of Nephrology
Children's Hospital Boston
Boston, Massachusetts

A. Marc Harrison, M.D.
University of Utah
Primary Children's Medical Center
Salt Lake City, Utah

Steven E. Haun, M.D.
Department of Critical Care Medicine
Children's Hospital, Inc.
Columbus, Ohio

William R. Hayden, M.D.
Department of Critical Care Pediatrics
Rush Medical College
Chicago, Illinois

Eugenie S. Heitmiller, M.D.
Department of Anesthesiology
The Johns Hopkins University Medical Center
Baltimore, Maryland

Mark A. Helfaer, M.D.
Division of Pediatric Anesthesiology
The Johns Hopskins Hospital
Baltimore, Maryland

Frank H. Kern, M.D.
Department of Anesthesiology and Pediatrics
Duke University Medical Center
Durham, North Carolina

Jeffrey R. Kirsch, M.D.
Department of Anesthesiology and Critical Care Medicine
The Johns Hopkins Hospital
Baltimore, Maryland

Daniel S. Kohane, M.D., Ph.D.
Department of Anesthesia
Children's Hospital
Boston, Massachusetts

Isaac S. Kohane, M.D., Ph.D.
Division of Endocrinology
Children's Hospital
Boston, Massachusetts

John W. Kuluz, M.D.
Division of Critical Care Medicine
Department of Pediatrics
University of Miami School of Medicine
Miami, Florida

Dorothy G. Lappe, R.N., M.S.
Baltimore, Maryland

Gitte Y. Larsen, M.D.
Division of Critical Care
University of Utah
Primary Children's Medical Center
Salt Lake City, Utah

Allen Leichtner
Department of Gastro-Interology
Children's Hospital
Boston, Massachusetts

Erica Liebelt, M.D.
Yale-New Haven Hospital
New Haven, Connecticut

Lynn D. Martin, M.D.
Department of Anesthesiology and Critical Care Medicine
University o Washington School of Medicine
Children's Hospital and Medical Center
Seattle, Washington

Karin A. McCloskey, M.D.
Department of Pediatrics
Children's Medical Center
Dallas, Texas

Gwenn McLaughlin, M.D.
Department of Pediatrics
University of Miami School of Medicine
Miami, Florida

Michael McManus, M.D.
Department of Anesthesia and Pediatrics
Children's Hospital
Boston, Massachusetts

Jon N. Meliones, M.D.
Department of Critical Care, Pediatrics
Duke University Medical Center
Durham, North Carolina

James D. Mellema, M.D.
Department of Anesthesiology and Critical Care Medicine
University of Washington School of Medicine
Children's Hospital and Medical Center
Seattle, Washington

William T. Merritt, M.D.
Department of Anesthesiology and Critical Care Medicine
The Johns Hopkins Hospital
Baltimore, Maryland

Karen J. Miller, M.D.
Department of Pediatrics
University of Maryland School of Medicine
Baltimore, Maryland

Mark J. Mogul, M.D.
Emory University School of Medicine
Atlanta, Georgia

Joshua P. Needleman, M.D.
Pediatric Pulmonology
St. Christopher's Hospital for Children
Philadelphia, Pennsylvania

Charles Newton, MB, ChB, MD, MRCP (UK)
Johns Hopkins University Medical School
Baltimore, Maryland

David G. Nichols, M.D.
Department of Anesthesia and Critical Care Medicine
The Johns Hopkins Hospital
Baltimore, Maryland

Richard A. Orr, M.D.
Pediatric Critical Care Medicine
Children's Hospital of Pittsburgh
Pittsburgh, Pennsylvania

Jurgen Peters, M.D.
Institut fur Klinische Anasthesiologie
Universitat of Dusseldorf
Dusseldorf, Germany

W. Bradley Poss, M.D.
Department of Pediatrics
Naval Medical Center
San Diego, California

Gail E. Rasmussen, M.D.
Department of Anesthesiology and Pediatrics
Divisio of Pediatric Critical Care and Anesthesia
Vanderbilt University Medical Center
Nashville, Tennessee

James L. Robotham, M.D.
Department of Anesthesiology/CCM
The Johns Hopkins Hospital
Baltimore, Maryland

Elizabeth L. Rogers, M.D.
Duke University Medical Center
Durham, North Carolina

Mark C. Rogers, M.D.
Duke University Medical Center
Durham, North Carolina

Mark E. Rowin, M.D.
Department of Pediatrics/Critical Care Medicine
University of Utah Primary Children's Medical Center
Salt Lake City, Utah

Charles L. Schleien, M.D.
Department of Pediatrics
University of Miami School of Medicine
Miami, Florida

Scott R. Schulman, M.D.
Division of Pediatric Cardiac Anesthesia and Critical Care Medicine
Duke University Medical Center
Durham, North Carolina

Deborah Schwengel, M.D.
Department of Anesthesiology and Critical Care Medicine
Johns Hopkins University School of Medicine
Baltimore, Maryland

Nancy A. Setzer, M.D.
University of Florida College of Medicine
Gainesville, Florida

Donald H. Shaffner, M.D.
Departments of Anesthesiology and Critical Care Medicine
The Johns Hopkins University Hospital
Baltimore, Maryland

Robert M. Spear, M.D.
Departments of Anesthesiology and Critical Care Medicine
Children's Hospital and Health Center
San Diego, California

Gregory Stidham, M.D.
Division of Critical Care Medicine
LeBonheur Children's Medical Center
Memphis, Tennessee

Vera Fan Tait, M.D.
Department of Pediatrics and Pediatric Neurology
Primary Children's Medical Center
University of Utah
Salt Lake City, Utah

Masao Takata, M.D.
Pathophysiology Research Laboratory
Children's Medical Research Center
Tokyo, Japan

Robert C. Tasker, M.D., B.S., M.R.C.P. (UK)
Hospital for Sick Children
London, England

Joseph Tobias, M.D.
Department of Anesthesia and Critical Care Medicine
Vanderbilt University Medical Center
Nashville, Tennessee

Joseph R. Tobin, M.D.
Department of Anesthesia
Bowman Grey School of Medicine
Winston-Salem, North Carolina

Randall L. Tressler, M.D.
Department of Pediatrics
University of Maryland School of Medicine
Baltimore, Maryland

Robert Truog, M.D.
Children's Hospital
Boston, Massachusetts

Andreas Tzakis, M.D.
Department of Surgery
University of Miami Medical School
Miami, Florida

Donald D. Vernon, M.D.
Primary Children's Medical Center
Salt Lake City, Utah

Peter E. Vink, M.D.
Department of Pediatrics
University of Maryland School of Medicine
Baltimore, Maryland

L. Kyle Walker, M.D.
Department of Anesthesiology and Critical Care Medicine
The Johns Hopkins Hospital
Baltimore, Maryland

Katherine A. Welkie, R.N., B.S.N.
Pediatric Critical Care Services
Primary Children's Medical Center
Salt Lake City, Utah

Randall C. Wetzel, M.D., B.S., F.C.C.M.
The Johns Hopkins Hospital
Baltimore, Maryland

Rodney E. Willoughby, M.D.
Department of Pediatrics
Johns Hopkins School of Medicine
Baltimore, Maryland

Barbara G. Wilson
Pediatric Critical Care Medicine
Duke University Medical Center
Durham, North Carolina

Madolin K. Witte, M.D.
Department of Pediatrics and Critical Care Medicine
University of Utah
Salt Lake City, Utah

Alan Woolf, M.D., M.P.H.
Department of Pediatrics
Massachusetts Poison Control Center
Boston, Massachusetts

Myron Yaster, M.D.
Department of Anesthesia and Critical Care Medicine
The Johns Hopkins Hospital
Baltimore, Maryland

Andrew Yeager, M.D.
Department of Pediatrics
Emory University School of Medicine
Atlanta, Georgia

Aaron Zuckerberg
Department of Pediatrics
Sinai Hospital
Baltimore, Maryland

Contents

Section X
PICU ADMINISTRATION

Emergency Resuscitation and Acute Airway Management

Section One

Section Editor

David G. Nichols

Cardiopulmonary Resuscitation 1

Charles L. Schleien
John W. Kuluz
D. Hal Shaffner
Mark C. Rogers

INTRODUCTION

Cardiopulmonary arrest is the final common pathway for many life-threatening diseases. Although cardiopulmonary resuscitation (CPR) was once thought to be a miracle cure for patients suffering a cardiac arrest, outcome studies indicate otherwise. These studies show that the survival rate after CPR is less than 50%, and, in many cases, even less than 15%. Because of the low survival rate there are many that claim that CPR is ineffective. What many forget, however, is that without receiving basic CPR, survival after a cardiac arrest is rare. Today many patients continue to lead highly functioning lives after a cardiac arrest as a result of the timely application of CPR.

Controversies abound regarding principles of the basic physiology of blood flow during CPR and indications for many of the drugs used in advanced life support. These controversies, including differences between the adult and pediatric patient, will be discussed within this chapter. The incidence of in-hospital pediatric cardiac arrests has risen with the increased length of survival of children with serious illnesses such as congenital heart disease, renal insufficiency, metabolic disorders, malignancy, and immunodeficiency states. Thus it is critical for all physicians caring for children in the hospital to understand the pathophysiology of cardiopulmonary arrest and the mechanisms involved in the mechanical and pharmacologic aspects of CPR.

HISTORICAL PERSPECTIVE

The first recorded description of a pediatric resuscitation exists in the Book of Kings; the prophet Elisha revived a child by putting his mouth on his mouth, his eyes upon his eyes and his hands upon his hands; and as he pressed upon him the child's body grew warm. Elisha got up and walked once up and down the room; then, getting onto the bed again, he pressed upon him and he breathed into him seven times; and the boy opened his eyes[(1)].

About 177 AD, Galen used a bellows to inflate the lungs of a dead animal[(2)]. In the 16th century Vesalius described a technique of breathing into a reed that had been placed into an animal's trachea in order to observe the living thoracic contents in vivo[(3)]. In 1744, Tossack described the first successful use of mouth-to-mouth resuscitation in humans[(4)]. Even though this method was successful, it was not accepted for another 200 years.

In 1783, DeHaen described a "manual," chest-pressure arm-lift method of resuscitation[(2)]. About this time, Hosack recommended inserting a tube connected to a bellows into the trachea, which had to be removed after each inflation[(5)]. In 1809, Burns of Glasgow preached inflating the lungs and shocking the chest to resuscitate "the recently dead[(6)]." Because of other historical developments, such as the introduction of anesthesia in 1842, there was impetus for research into methods to restart the heart after iatrogenic cardiac arrest.

Although unsuccessful in restoring the circulation, in 1847, Schiff performed the first open-chest cardiac massage in dogs in order to provide circulation after arrest. In 1878, Bochin performed closed-chest cardiac massage in cats[(7)]. In 1880, Neihaus, although unsuccessful, first attempted closed-chest cardiac massage in humans[(8)]. Over the next 10 years, Koenig and Maass described eight cases of successful closed-chest cardiac massage in humans[(9)]. Despite their reports, open-chest CPR remained the method of choice for the next 60 years.

In 1892, Bazy was the first to attempt open-chest cardiac massage in humans, and in 1898, Tuffier and Hallian reported the first successful resuscitation using this method[(8)]. Crile published his success with closed-chest cardiac massage in dogs and humans[(8)]. In addition, he described the use of saline and epinephrine during a cardiac arrest, and first described the "MAST" suit[(8)]. Guthrie, after the electrocution of his brother, was also a forerunner in the early 1900s in the use of epinephrine for cardiac arrest. With this interest, he later developed a sternal compressor, a forerunner of the mechanical compressor devices presently used[(10)].

Up until the mid 1950s these manual methods were still in use. Successful mouth-to-mouth resuscitation had actually been reported in 1744 by Tossack, who rescued an apneic, pulseless, coal miner who had been trapped in a burning coal mine[(4)]. In the late 1700s, William Hunter used mouth-to-mouth resuscitation in stillborn children, and it was this use in newborns that kept the practice alive[(4)]. In 1958, Safar et al., published their studies establishing the superiority of mouth-to-mouth ventilation over the manual

Table 1.1. Etiology of Pediatric Cardiopulmonary Arrest

Causes of Cardiac Arrest	*Eisenberg (12)*	*Lewis (13)*	*O'Rourke (14)*
SIDS	32	11	24
Drowning	22		21
Respiratory/airway	11	14	10
Congenital cardiac	4	30	
Neurologic	4		
Cancer	3		
Miscellaneous cardiac	3		
Drug overdose	3		
Anaphylaxis	2		
Endocrine	1		
Infection		16	10
Trauma/abuse			34
Miscellaneous	15	29	

methods. Mouth-to-mouth ventilation has subsequently become the standard method of artificial respiration[11].

In 1960, Kouwenhoven et al., working at Johns Hopkins Hospital, published their classic study on resuscitation utilizing closed-chest cardiac massage with mouth-to-nose ventilation and defibrillation[7]. Because of their successes, these methods have been used and incorporated into every resuscitation training program over the past 35 years.

ETIOLOGY OF CARDIOPULMONARY ARREST

The etiology of cardiopulmonary arrest in children is different from that in adults. Eisenberg et al. reviewed the causes of cardiac arrest in 119 patients younger than 18 years of age[12]. The most common presentation was associated with SIDS (32%). The second most common cause was drowning (22%), followed by other respiratory causes (9%), congenital cardiac problems (4%), neurological problems (4%), cancer (3%), other cardiac causes (3%), drug overdose (3%), smoke inhalation (2%), anaphylaxis (2%), and endocrinopathies (2%). Forty-five percent of the patients were less than one year of age, 64% less than three years of age. Lewis et al. reported on the etiology of arrest in pediatric patients[13]. Children with congenital heart disease, including postoperative death, accounted for the largest group of these patients (30%), followed by infection (including neonatal) (16%), airway problems (14%), and SIDS (11%). Other causes of cardiac arrest were neurologic problems, drowning, trauma, postoperative death after airway surgery, drug overdose, and miscellaneous cardiac problems. O'Rourke reviewed the outcome and etiology of out-of-hospital pediatric arrests[14]. The causes cited for cardiac arrest in this study were SIDS (24%), drowning (21%), trauma (24%), upper airway obstruction (10%), infection (10%), and child abuse (10%). Thus, the cause of arrest is dependent on the patient population studied. In most out-of-hospital arrests, respiratory causes or SIDS are prevalent. This may be the reason that the majority of children who suffer an arrest present with asystole or a bradyarrhythmia. In-hospital data may reflect only the most frequent diagnosis cared for in that particular setting **(Table 1.1).**

BASIC LIFE SUPPORT—RESPIRATION

The use of basic life support is intended to externally support the circulation and ventilation of a patient who has suffered either a respiratory or cardiorespiratory arrest **(Table 1.2).** The objective from a physiologic standpoint of performing CPR is to provide oxygen to the vital organs, the heart and brain, until normal circulation is restored. Management of the critically ill or injured child should be approached in a systematic fashion and should begin with the primary survey. The child is assessed and priorities of treatment and diagnosis are established on the basis of existing and potentially life-threatening problems, as well as on the stability of the child's vital signs. The steps in the primary survey are: A) Airway, B) Breathing and ventilation, and C) Circulation and hemorrhage.

Beginning CPR

The beginning steps of CPR include establishing the unresponsiveness of the patient by gently shaking, tapping, and shouting at him or her. The bystander or physician should then provide approximately 1 minute of basic life support before activating emergency medical services. Care should be taken not to aggravate a spinal cord injury or over-jostle a head-injured patient.

If the patient is unresponsive, the absence of adequate ventilation and circulation should be determined immediately. If ventilation alone is absent or inadequate, opening the airway, rescue breathing, or both may be all that is necessary. If the circulation is inadequate, artificial circulation should also be started at this time.

In the following section, based on the Standards and Guidelines for CPR and Emergency Cardiac Care (ECC)[15], methods of recognizing the adequacy or absence of breathing and circulation, and the recommended techniques for performing artificial ventilation and circulation both in and out of the hospital will be discussed.

Opening the Airway

The first step in basic CPR is to open the airway and restore breathing. Methods for opening the airway of an unconscious patient are directed at relieving obstruction which

Table 1.2. Airway and Breathing

Airway	*Breathing*
Determine unresponsiveness	2 initial slow breaths (1–1.5 sec/breath)
Begin BLS for 1 minute	
Call for help (activate EMS system)	
Supine position	
Head-tilt/chin lift or jaw thrust	20 Breaths/min

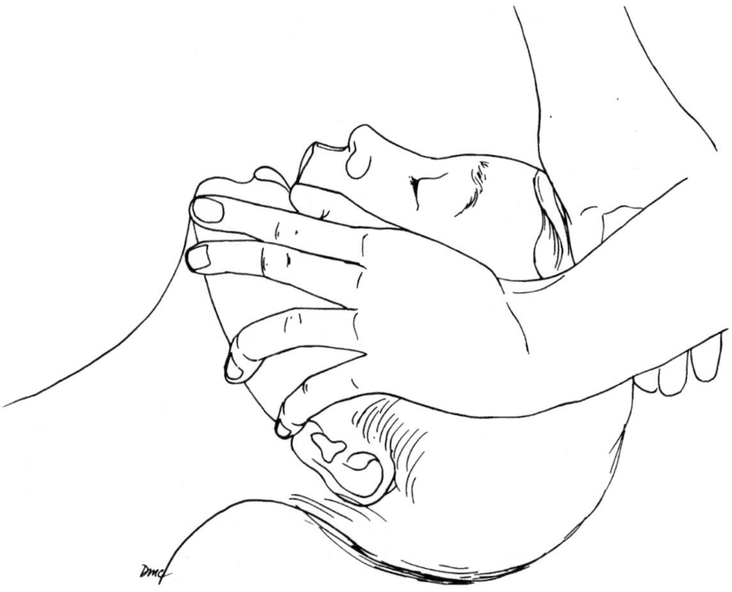

Figure 1.1. Head tilt-chin lift airway position. The rescuer places one hand on the forehead, with other hand supporting the angle of the mandible while pulling the chin upward.

is usually caused by the tongue. Since the tongue is attached to the mandible, moving the mandible forward will lift the tongue away from the back of the throat, thus clearing the airway. If there is enough tone in the muscles of the jaw, tilting the head back will cause the mandible to move forward and open the airway. In the absence of sufficient muscular tone, which is often the case in an unconscious patient, a head tilt alone may be insufficient to open the airway. Frequently, the tongue occludes the airway during an active inspiration when negative pressure is generated. When this is the case, the mandible may need active physical support, including the head-tilt/chin-lift or jaw thrust to provide a sufficient airway (Fig. 1.1). The head-tilt/chin-lift is the initial step in opening the airway unless neck trauma is suspected. The rescuer's hand is placed on the patient's forehead and with gentle backward pressure the head is brought into the sniffing position. The head should not be overextended especially in the infant since this may result in airway obstruction. Additional assistance in opening the airway is then performed using the chin-lift method. The head tilt/chin-lift method is performed by placing the fingertips of one hand under the mandible near the protuberance of the chin, bringing the chin forward and supporting the jaw, which results in tilting the head back. Care should be taken not to compress the soft tissues of the chin, which might obstruct the patient's airway, especially in the infant. The rescuer's other hand continues to press on the patient's forehead in order to tilt the head back. The chin is lifted so that the teeth are nearly brought together, without completely closing the mouth. Only rarely should the thumb be used when lifting the chin, and then only to slightly depress the lower lip so that the mouth remains partially open.

Additional forward movement of the jaw may be needed if the head-tilt/chin-lift is unsuccessful in opening the airway (Fig. 1.2). To perform a jaw thrust, the rescuer grabs the angles of the mandible and lifts with both hands, one on each side, displacing the mandible forward while tilting the head backward. If the lips close, the lower lip is retracted by the rescuer's thumbs. Jaw thrust without head-tilt is the safest technique in opening the airway of the patient with a suspected neck injury, because it is accomplished without extending the neck. The head should be carefully supported without turning it from side to side or extending. If this maneuver is unsuccessful, the head may be extended slightly and another attempt made to ventilate.

An infant or child who is struggling to breathe but is acyanotic and has an adequate airway, is best treated by immediate transportation to a hospital or assessment in the

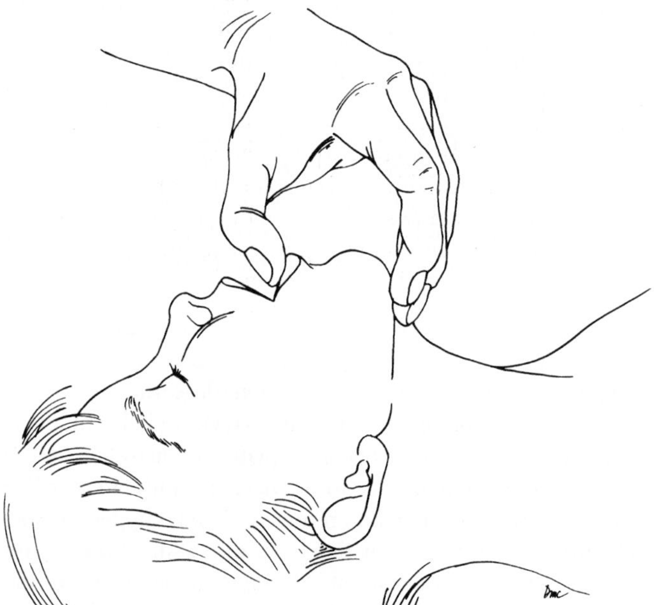

Figure 1.2. Jaw thrust airway position. The rescuer grasps and pulls forward the patient's jaw with thumb in mouth and other fingers under the chin.

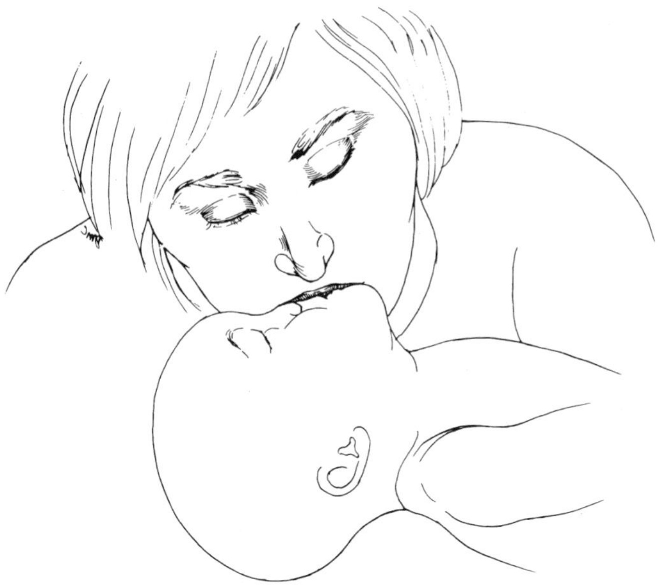

Figure 1.3. Artificial ventilation in infants. The rescuer places patient's head in sniffing position and places his or her mouth over both mouth and nose, making a tight seal.

present hospital by the most experienced person trained in airway management. If the infant or child is unconscious, is cyanotic, or experiencing bradycardia, the airway should be opened.

Establishing Breathlessness

After the airway is opened, the rescuer should again check whether the patient is breathing effectively. This is done by placing the ear over the victim's mouth and nose, and viewing the patient's chest and abdomen. If the chest and abdomen fall, and the rescuer feels air from the mouth and nose and hears air during exhalation, then the patient is ventilating. If the patient has respiratory efforts without air exhalation, then the airway is obstructed. Frequently, opening the airway and maintaining airway support is all that the patient needs in order to breathe effectively. If the patient is not ventilating then rescue breathing is begun. If after opening the airway, the patient is gasping or struggling to breathe, the decision to begin rescue breathing depends on the presence or absence of cyanosis.

Initiating Rescue Breathing

Rescue breathing is initiated once breathlessness is established. In the infant, the rescuer makes a tight seal covering the infant's mouth and nose with his mouth (Fig. 1.3). In the older child the nose is pinched, and the mouth of the patient is covered by the rescuer's mouth (Fig. 1.4).

When an airtight seal has been established by either of the above methods, two slow breaths are delivered, 1.0 to 1.5 seconds per breath with a pause between to allow for a rescuer's breath. An appropriate tidal volume is one that allows the patient's chest to rise and fall. Patency of the airway should be ascertained if air does not enter freely. An obstruction should be suspected if after adjusting support, the chest still does not rise. During one or two-rescuer CPR, one breath is administered at the end of every fifth compression. If breathing is absent but a pulse is present, breathing should be provided at a rate of 20 breaths per minute.

In some cases, mouth-to-nose ventilation is more effective than mouth-to-mouth ventilation. Mouth-to-nose ventilation is recommended when it is impossible to ventilate through the mouth because of a facial injury or anatomic abnormality, or when it is difficult to achieve a tight seal around the mouth. To perform this maneuver, the rescuer maintains the head tilt while lifting the mandible to close the mouth if it is open. During exhalation, with this technique, it may be necessary to open the patient's mouth or separate his lips to allow the air to escape.

When a patient has a tracheostomy in place, mouth-to-stoma artificial ventilation should be used. If during this technique, a leak exists through the mouth or nose, the rescuer should seal the mouth and nose with his hand. This problem usually does not occur if the tracheostomy tube has an inflatable cuff.

Cricoid pressure should be used during resuscitation to prevent regurgitation and possible aspiration. The technique consists of applying backward pressure on the cricoid cartilage against the cervical vertebra[16]. Pressure is released once an endotracheal tube is successfully placed confirmed by auscultation of bilateral breath sounds. Cricoid pressure is effective in preventing regurgitation against an esophageal pressure of up to 100 cm H_2O.

The effects of ventilation and oxygenation have been studied during external cardiac massage. Severe hypocapnia may occur during CPR[17]. Adding 5% CO_2 to the gas mixture during CPR, may prevent complications as a result

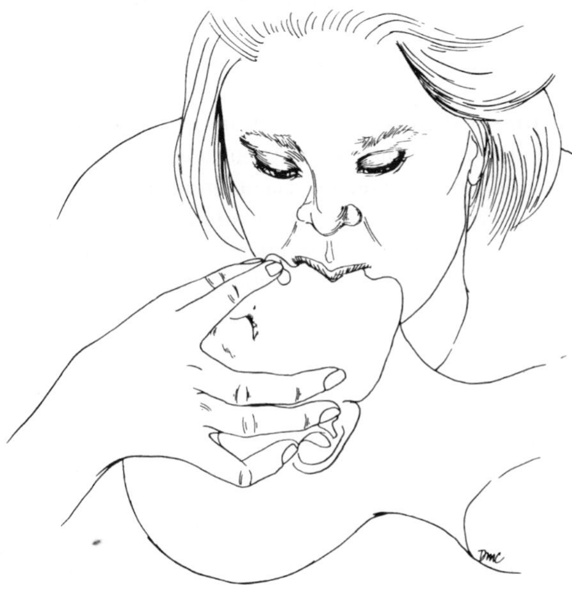

Figure 1.4. Mouth-to-mouth ventilation. The rescuer places the patient's head in the sniffing position, pinches off the nose, takes a deep breath, and exhales into the patient's mouth.

of hypocapnia and alkalemia which include ionized hypocalcemia and precipitation of ventricular fibrillation. The P_aO_2 remained above 63 mmHg in patients ventilated with expired air for 1 hour of CPR in that study.

Because of the risk of transmission of infection during mouth-to-mouth resuscitation, and the lack of negative effects of hypercapnia on success of resuscitation, many have questioned whether ventilation is necessary during bystander CPR. In dogs, chest compression alone can produce enough pulmonary gas exchange to maintain arterial oxygen saturation greater than 90% for 4 minutes[(18)], while insufflation with 100% O_2 without active ventilation maintained resuscitability in rats after 6 min of CPR[(19)]. However, the limit of viability without ventilation is probably surpassed after longer arrest times or CPR duration[(20)].

Gastric Distention

Gastric distention occurring during artificial ventilation interferes with ventilation by elevating the diaphragm, resulting in a decreased lung volume. It occurs more frequently in children, and is minimized by limiting the tidal volume to that which raises the chest. This maneuver may avoid exceeding the esophageal opening pressure. Gastric distention also commonly occurs when the airway is partially or completely obstructed. Attempts at relieving gastric distention during CPR by pressure on the abdomen should not be performed because of the high risk of inducing emesis and causing aspiration of gastric contents into the lungs. If ventilation becomes ineffective because of gastric distention, then gastric decompression should be attempted by using an oro- or nasogastric tube, or by turning the patient to the side and applying pressure to the epigastrium, in the out-of-hospital setting.

FOREIGN BODY AIRWAY OBSTRUCTION

Infants

Cardiac arrest usually occurs secondary to airway obstruction in pediatric patients. Airway obstruction is most commonly caused by an infectious or allergic process which causes swelling of the airway, or by a foreign body. Differentiating between airway obstruction as a result of a foreign body or that because of infection is important. If infection is present, maneuvers to dislodge a foreign body are dangerous and may result in an inappropriate delay in transporting or treating the patient.

A foreign body may cause partial or complete obstruction of the airway. The acyanotic patient with adequate air exchange should be allowed and encouraged to continue to cough and breathe spontaneously without interference.

Clinical signs of poor air exchange include an inefficient cough, increased respiratory difficulty with retractions, nasal flaring, an increased work of breathing, high-pitched noises during inhalation, stridor, and cyanosis of the lips, nails, and skin. Relief of airway obstruction by a foreign body depends on the age of the patient. In the infant less than one year of age, a combination of back blows and chest thrusts is performed **(Table 1.3)**. Abdominal thrusts are not recommended in this age group because of the potential danger of injury to the abdominal organs, especially the liver.

An infant with foreign body airway obstruction is straddled over the arm of the rescuer with the head lower than the trunk. The infant's head is supported with the rescuer's hand around the jaw and chest. When support is adequate, five back blows are rapidly delivered with the heel of the hand between the shoulder blades (Figure 1.5). The infant is then turned, with her back placed on the rescuer's thigh, head lower than the body. Five chest thrusts are delivered in the same manner as external chest compressions are performed (using the two- or three-finger method) at a slower rate (Fig. 1.5). If the child is too large to straddle the rescuer's forearm, the rescuer should kneel on the floor and place the child across his thighs, keeping the head lower than the trunk. With greater force than that used in the infant, five back blows are delivered. With the head and back supported, the child is then rolled onto the floor and five chest thrusts are given.

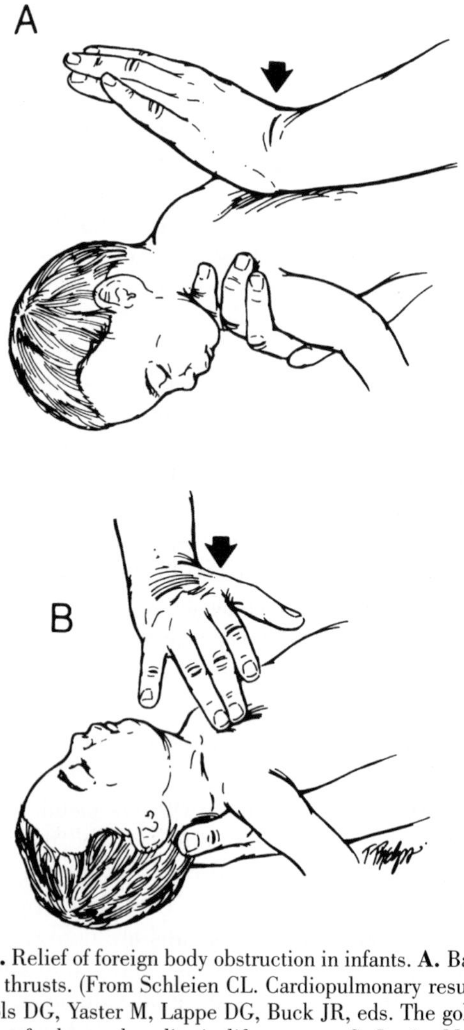

Figure 1.5. Relief of foreign body obstruction in infants. **A.** Backblows. **B.** Chest thrusts. (From Schleien CL. Cardiopulmonary resuscitation. In: Nichols DG, Yaster M, Lappe DG, Buck JR, eds. The golden hour handbook of advanced pediatric life support. St Louis: Mosby-Year Book, 1991:113.)

Back blows are recommended because they produce an artificial cough. This increases pressure in the distally blocked respiratory passages, which may result in partial or complete dislodgement of the foreign body[21]. However, back blows can cause an upward acceleration of the neck and upper back of more than three times the force of gravity, causing propulsion of a supraglottic foreign body toward the glottis, thus converting partial airway obstruction into complete airway blockage[22].

After maneuvers to relieve an airway obstruction, the airway is opened by the head-tilt/chin-lift method, and if spontaneous breathing is absent, rescue breathing is performed. If the chest does not rise, and after repositioning of the head the airway is still obstructed, then the maneuvers to relieve a foreign body obstruction are repeated.

Children and Adults

In children and adults, the Heimlich maneuver, a series of subdiaphragmatic thrusts, is recommended for foreign body airway obstruction. First described by Heimlich in 1974, manual thrusts have become the mainstay in relieving foreign body obstruction of the airway[23]. Manual thrusts consist of thrusts to the upper abdomen in order to force air out of the lungs, creating an artificial cough. The rescuer stands behind the patient and wraps his hands around the patient's waist, grasping one fist with the other hand and placing the thumb side of this fist against the patient's abdomen, between the waist and the rib cage. To avoid injury, the rescuer's hands should never be placed on the xiphoid process or on the lower margins of the rib cage. The rescuer then presses his fist five times into the patient's abdomen with a quick inward and upward thrust[24] (Fig. 1.6).

To perform this maneuver on an unconscious or supine patient, the rescuer should face the patient kneeling astride his hips. With one of the rescuer's hands on top of the other, manual thrusts are applied as described above. Manual thrusts may be self-administered by forcing the clasped hand into the substernal region[25].

Chest thrusts rather than abdominal thrusts are now only recommended for adults and children in special circumstances such as late pregnancy or marked obesity. Chest thrusts are applied by the rescuer standing behind the patient, with his or her arms directly under the patient's axillae, and encircling the patient's chest. The rescuer places the thumb side of his or her fist into the mid-sternal area of the patient, avoiding the xiphoid process or the margins of the rib cage. The rescuer grabs his or her fist with his or her other hand, and four backward thrusts are applied. Each thrust is administered with the intention of relieving the airway obstruction without necessarily completing the full series.

Table 1.3. Foreign Body Airway Obstruction

INFANT	Chest thrusts (5 times) Back blows (5 times)
CHILD	Heimlich maneuver (5 times)
ADULT	Heimlich maneuver (5 times)

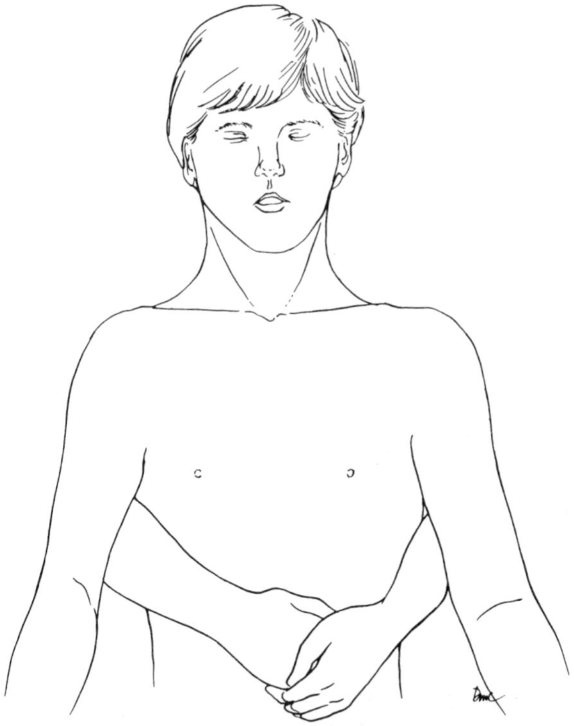

Figure 1.6. Foreign body obstruction—manual thrusts with the patient standing and the rescuer behind the patient. The rescuer places hands and clasps them in the midabdominal area below the xiphoid and exerts a rapid inward thrust on the abdomen.

Abdominal and chest thrusts may cause complications to internal organs, such as rupture or laceration of abdominal or thoracic viscera[26,27]. In addition, regurgitation of gastric contents may occur as a result of an abdominal thrust.

During an abdominal thrust, one liter of air is expelled with an average pressure at the proximal airway of 31 mmHg[24]. Back blows may actually be superior in generating a higher airway pressure[28]. Centrifugation has been used in children with foreign body airway obstruction to achieve the same effect[29].

Finger Sweeps

Blind finger sweeps are generally avoided in infants and children, as they may force a foreign body deeper into the airway. In the unconscious adult patient, the finger sweep is performed by opening the mouth by grasping the tongue and mandible between the thumb and fingers and lifting. This maneuver alone may relieve the obstruction by inserting the index finger of the free hand down along the inside of the cheek and deeply into the throat down to the base of the tongue. A hooking action should be used to dislodge the foreign body. Care should be taken not to force the foreign body deeper into the airway. The finger sweep should not be used in the conscious patient. If a foreign body is visualized it may be removed with the use of a Kelly clamp or Magill forceps.

Table 1.4. Causes of Difficult Airway

Foreign body obstruction
Trauma:
- larynx
- trachea
- facial structures

Edema of upper airway:
- infection (i.e. epiglottitis, croup)
- burn
- allergic reaction

Tumor:
- oro- or nasopharynx
- larynx
- extrinsic compression of trachea

Cervical spine injury (patient in halo)
Anatomic abnormality:
- macroglossia (mucopolysaccharidoses, hypothryoidism)
- micrognathia (Pierre-Robin syndrome, Treacher-Collins syndrome)
- midface hypoplasia (Apert syndrome, Goldenhar syndrome)
- short/rigid neck (patient in halo, rheumatoid arthritis, Klippel-Feil Syndrome)

Cricothyrotomy

Emergency cricothyrotomy is a procedure which is worthwhile to know, since it may be the last access to the airway for the intensivist when faced with a patient in whom he/she is unable to intubate the trachea. Inability to intubate the trachea could be because of an anatomic deformity (including oropharyngeal edema secondary to a burn, allergy or infection), a foreign body causing obstruction, trauma to the face or larynx causing distortion or obstruction, or cervical spine injury impeding adequate positioning **(Table 1.4).**

Performing a cricothyrotomy is simple and necessitates equipment which is readily available to the intensivist. A 14- or 16-gauge angiocath (18-gauge in smaller children) is passed through the cricothyroid membrane, located between the inferior edge of the thyroid cartilage and the upper edge of the cricoid cartilage. The larynx is stabilized with the fingers while palpating the cricothyroid membrane. The angiocath is placed at a caudad angle (approximately 30° from the skin) in the midline of the neck into the trachea in order to avoid injury to the larynx. This is done while aspirating gently on an attached syringe in order to determine when the trachea is successfully entered. Once air is aspirated, the plastic catheter is advanced into the trachea. The connector from a 3.0 endotracheal tube fits snugly onto the angiocath (Fig. 1.7). Alternatively, the barrel of a 3 ml syringe will also fit into the angiocath which can then be attached to a 7.0 mm endotracheal tube connector. This setup allows attachment of an ambu bag or other source of oxygen. It is prudent to have this attachment readily available on an arrest crash cart **(Table 1.5).**

Complications secondary to cricothyrotomy include difficulty in palpating landmarks in infants and young children, formation of a false passage, subcutaneous or mediastinal emphysema, injury to vascular, neural, or pulmonary structures of the neck, infection, fistula formation, or laryngeal edema **(Table 1.6).**

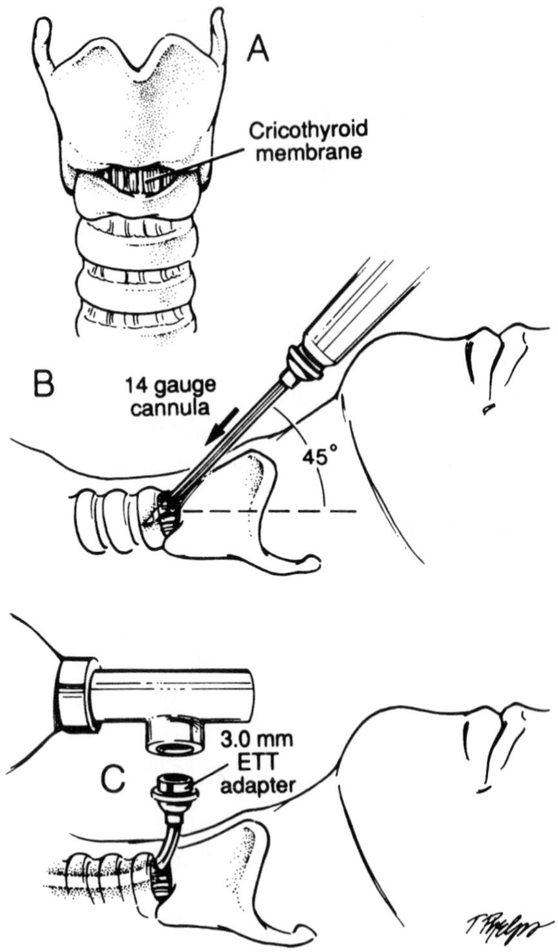

Figure 1.7. Cricothyrotomy. **A.** anatomical view. **B.** Insertion of 14-gauge intravenous cannula. **C.** Bag attached to 3.0-mm endotracheal tube (*ETT*) adaptor connected to intravenous cannula. (From Yaster M. Airway management. In: Nichols DG, Yaster M, Lappe DG, Buck JR, eds. The golden hour handbook of advanced pediatric life support. St. Louis: Mosby-Year Book, 1991:46.)

The technique, first described in 1956 by Jacoby et al., was designed to deliver oxygen to the patient without concern for adequate ventilation[30]. Based on the Venturi principle for oxygen delivery, jet ventilation was first used in 1967 during bronchoscopy[31]. Spoerel et al., using wall oxygen (50 psi) and a gas flow of 500 ml/sec, could maintain adequate blood gas values in patients with normally compliant lungs[32]. In 1972, Jacobs described the first use of emergency cricothyrotomy, delivering oxygen through a 14-gauge catheter in arrested patients[33]. This technique has

Table 1.5. Cricothyrotomy Set-up

INFANTS	18-gauge intravenous cannula 3.0-mm endotracheal tube connector Ambu Bag
OTHER CHILD	14- or 16-gauge intravenous cannula 3-ml syringe barrel 7.0-mm endotracheal tube connector Ambu bag

Table 1.6. Complications of Cricothyrotomy

Inability to place catheter
Trauma to trachea
Obesity
Subcutaneous or mediastinal emphysema
Trauma to:
Vascular structures
Nerves
Airway
False passage
Fistula formation
Infection
Laryngeal edema

been used in arrested pediatric patients[34]. When percutaneous transtracheal jet ventilation was compared with endotracheal high frequency jet ventilation and IPPV, oxygenation was adequate with both techniques[35]. Although ventilation was inadequate with transtracheal jet ventilation, adequate oxygenation was achieved with 100% oxygen[36].

Advantages of the cricothyroidotomy include its ease of placement in adult patients, the capability of continuing cardiac massage during placement of a tracheal catheter, and the ability to suction the pharynx if needed. In addition, the use of jet ventilation in this manner has been shown to have the capability of dislodging a foreign body in the trachea by increasing intrapulmonary pressure[37].

BASIC LIFE SUPPORT—CIRCULATION

Assessing Pulse

Once the airway has been opened adequately and two breaths delivered, it must be determined whether only breathing has stopped or whether a cardiac arrest has occurred simultaneously. Absence of a pulse in the large arteries in an unconscious victim who is not breathing defines a cardiac arrest.

As in the adult, the pulse of a child can be felt over the carotid artery. While maintaining the head-tilt, the carotid pulse is palpated between the tracheal cartilage and the neck muscles. The artery should be palpated gently so as not to lose the pulsation. Palpation of the carotid pulse is recommended in adults and children because of ready accessibility to the rescuer while performing artificial ventilation without the need to remove any clothing. In addition, the carotid arteries can frequently still be felt when peripheral pulses, such as the radial artery, are no longer palpable in the shock state (Fig. 1.8).

Palpation of the carotid pulse in an infant is difficult because of the infant's short, fat neck. Precordial activity in the infant is unreliable because it represents an impulse rather than a pulse. Some infants with good cardiac activity may have a quiet precordium, leading to the erroneous diagnosis of cardiac arrest. Thus, it is recommended that the brachial pulse be palpated in infants for the presence or absence or a cardiac arrest. The brachial pulse can be located on the inside of the upper arm, midway between the elbow and shoulder, while pressing lightly toward the humerus (Fig. 1.9).

When there is a pulse but no effective ventilation, then

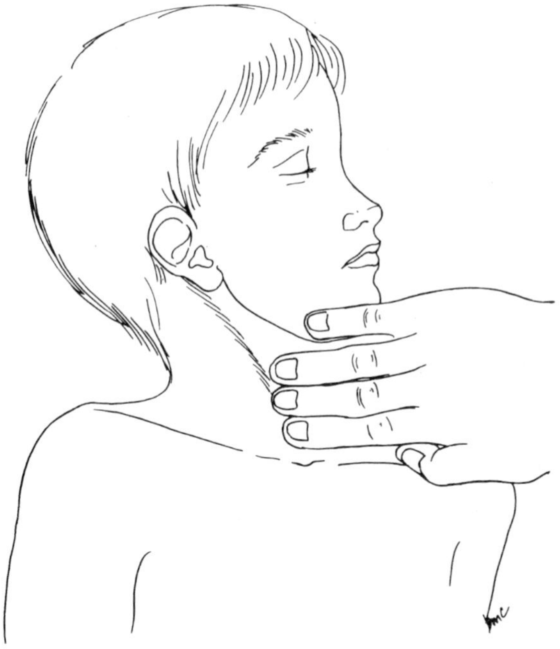

Figure 1.8. Feeling the carotid pulse. The fingers are placed laterally into the groove between the trachea and the sternocleidomastoid muscle.

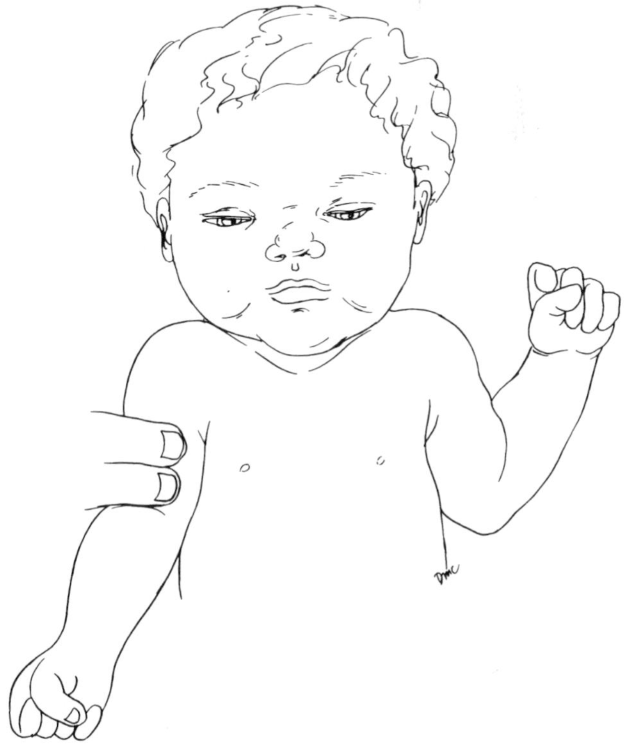

Figure 1.9. Feeling the brachial pulse. The brachial pulse is palpated with two fingers along the medial aspect of the upper arm above the antecubital region.

Table 1.7. Chest Compressions in Infants and Children

	Compressions/Method	*Hand Position*	*Sternal Depression (Inches)*	*Compressions/Min*
INFANT	Encircling or 2 finger	1 finger breadth below intermammary line	0.5–1	≥100
TODDLER	One hand	Lower Third of sternum	1–1½	100
LARGE CHILD	Two hands	Lower Third of sternum	1½–2	100

only breathing has arrested, and rescue breathing should be continued. Absence or questionable presence of a pulse is the indication for starting artificial circulation by means of external chest compression. Chest compression should never be performed without rescue breathing.

Chest Compression—Children and Adults

In order to perform external chest compressions, the patient must be in the supine position. It is also imperative, because of the effects of gravity, not to have the head above the level of the heart. For external chest compressions to be fully effective, the patient should be on a firm surface, a hard board, the ground, or the floor. A board, preferably the full width of the bed, should be placed under the patient if the patient is in bed. However, chest compressions should not be delayed while waiting for a bed board[15].

The rescuer should position herself close to the side of the patient. The lower margin of the patient's rib cage on the side next to the rescuer should then be located with the middle and index fingers. The fingers are run up along the rib cage to the notch where the ribs join the sternum in the center of the lower part of the chest. One finger is then left on that notch, with the other finger placed next to the first finger on the lower level of the sternum. The location of the xiphoid process is irrelevant when utilizing this technique. The heel of the hand closest to the head is then placed next to the index finger of the first hand, which locates the notch on the long axis of the sternum. This maneuver keeps the force of compression on the sternum and decreases the chance of a rib fracture. The first hand is then placed on top of the other hand so that the heels of both hands are parallel with the fingers directed away from the rescuer. The fingers may be extended or interlaced but must be kept off the chest.

Another position that can be used is to grasp the wrist of the hand on the chest with the other hand. This technique is useful for rescuers with arthritic problems of the hand or wrist. The elbows are then straightened with the rescuer's shoulders directly over the hands so that the thrust for chest compression is straight down.

In a normal-sized child, the sternum should be depressed 1 to 1½ inches and 1½ to 2 inches in adults. Between compressions, pressure should be released completely in order to allow return of blood to the chest. The time allowed for release should be equal to the time required for compression. Compressions should be uninterrupted, regular, and smooth. The hands of the rescuer should not be lifted off the chest or changed in position because correct hand position may be lost in that instance. The compression rate should be 100/min. Periodically, the pulse should be palpated for effectiveness of chest compressions or the return of a spontaneous pulse. This should be performed after 1 minute of CPR and every few minutes thereafter.

In one-rescuer CPR, both artificial ventilation and circulation are performed using a 15 to 2 chest compression to ventilation ratio at a rate of 80 to 100 compressions per minute. After four cycles of compressions are delivered, the patient should be reevaluated for return of breathing and pulse.

Chest Compression—Infants

The recommended area of chest compression is one finger width below the intersection of the intermammary line and the sternum **(Table 1.7).** Two techniques to perform external chest compressions in the infant include placement of two or three fingers on the sternum (Fig. 1.10), or to encircle the chest of the infant, forming a rigid surface on the back, using the thumbs to deliver compressions (Fig. 1.11)[38]. The encircling method may generate higher arterial and coronary perfusion pressures[39].

The infant's sternum should be compressed approximately 20% of the anteroposterior width of the chest, ½ to

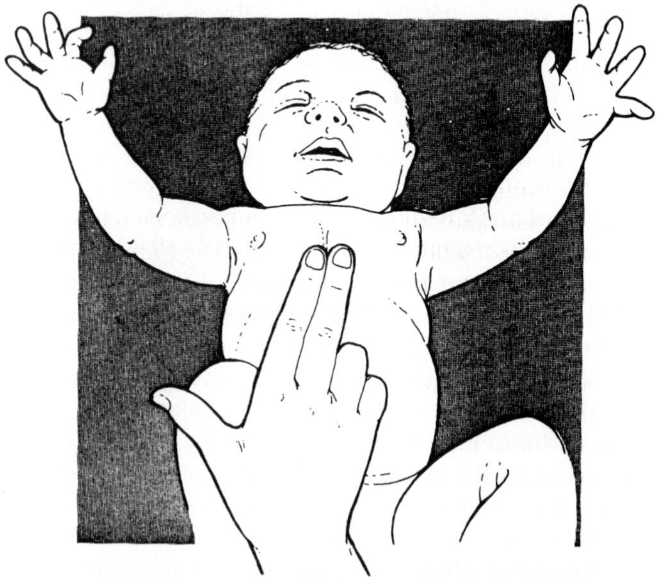

Figure 1.10. Two-finger method of external chest compression in infants. The rescuer places two fingers on the sternum 1 finger width below the line intersecting the nipples and compresses ½ to 1 inch at a rate of 100 compressions/min. Ventilation is not shown for the sake of clarity. (From Schleien CL. Recent advances in pediatric CPR. Anesthesiol Rep 1988;1:6.)

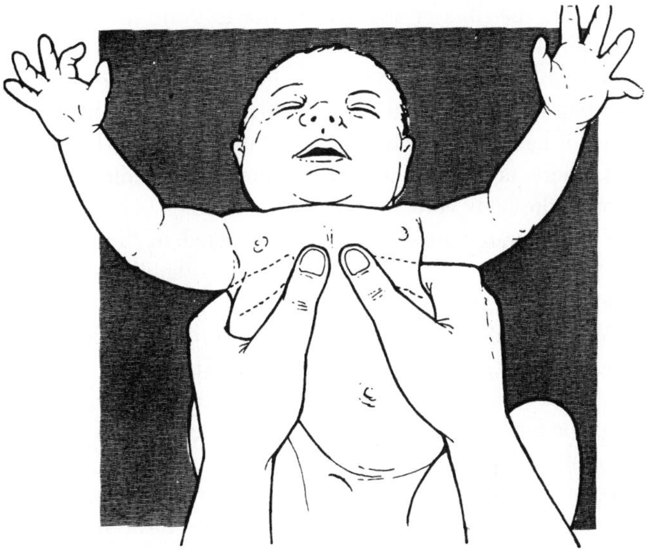

Figure 1.11. Encircling method of external chest compression in infants. Place thumbs over sternum 1 finger width below the line intersecting the nipples. Rescuer clasps hands behind infant's back. (From Schleien CL. Recent advances in pediatric CPR. Anesthesiol Rep 1988;1:6.)

1 inch in the infant. When the infant becomes large enough so that three fingers cannot adequately depress the sternum or the rescuer's hands cannot reach around the infant's chest, the heel of one hand should be used. As in the adult, the rescuer's fingers should be kept off the chest. If the patient is large enough to require the heel of the hand for com pression, the depth of the compression is increased to 1 to 1½ inches (Fig. 1.12).

The compression rate for external chest CPR in infants is at least 100 per minute. The ratio of compressions to breaths is 5 to 1 for one or two rescuers. See below for a further discussion of rate and duty cycle requirements.

Precordial Thump

The precordial thump is used in order to convert asystole to a life-sustaining rhythm(40,41). It has also been shown to restore a sinus rhythm when delivered early after the onset of ventricular tachycardia or fibrillation(42). The precordial thump is thought to be effective by establishing a low energy current through electromechanical transduction which depolarizes a reentry pathway and terminates the arrhythmia.

The precordial thump should never be used in the pediatric patient. It is no longer recommended as a routine procedure in adults because it may precipitate ventricular fibrillation or asystole when used to treat ventricular tachycardia. The precordial thump now is only recommended in the following situations:

1. When a patient is being monitored by an electrocardiogram, it may be administered after recognition of ventricular tachycardia or ventricular fibrillation.
2. When the patient is monitored, it may be administered immediately after the onset of asystole caused by heart block, where repetitive thumps produce QRS complexes and an associated pulse, and may thus sustain the circulation until a pacemaker can be inserted. If an effective cardiac output is not maintained, CPR should be initiated.

The precordial thump is delivered by a sharp, quick, single blow over the midportion of the sternum, with the bottom of the fist starting from 20 to 30 cm above the chest. After thumping, the ECG and pulse should immediately be checked. If there is ventricular fibrillation or ventricular tachycardia without a pulse, countershock is performed as soon as possible and CPR is begun.

ADVANCED CPR

Vascular Access and Fluid Administration

One of the key aspects of successful CPR is the early establishment of an intravascular line for the administration of fluids and medications. If an IV line cannot be established rapidly because of technical difficulties, common with a chubby, clamped-down infant, then one of the other alternatives, intraosseous or endotracheal access, can be used.

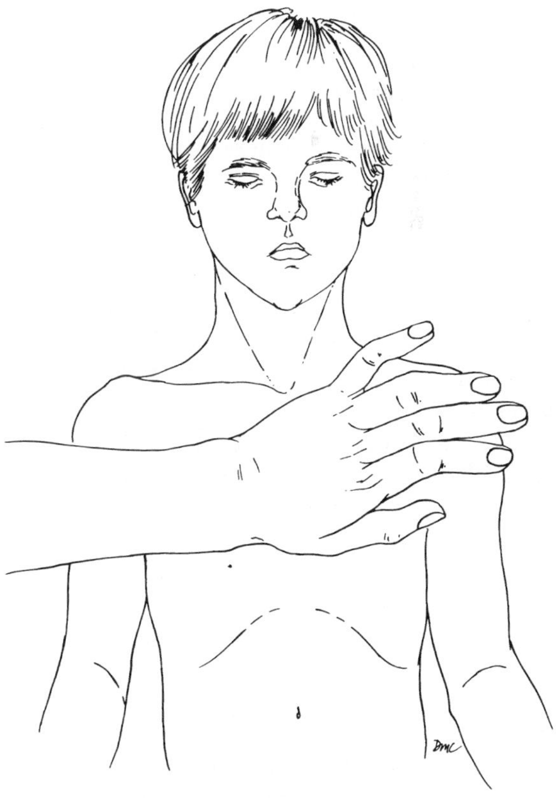

Figure 1.12. External chest compression in the young child. The heel of the hand is placed 2 finger widths above the bottom of the sternum for compression. In the older child, the two-hand compression is used as in adults.

Table 1.8. Intravenous Access

Children	(younger than 5 years old)
	First attempt - peripheral line (including antecubital vein)
	After 90 seconds (if unsuccessful) - intraosseous line
	Later: saphenous vein cutdown or central line placement - (femoral, subclavian, external or internal jugular vein)
Children	(older than 5 years old)
	First attempt - peripheral line
	Second attempt - saphenous vein cutdown or central line placement

IV Access

During CPR, the rapid establishment of IV access is critical. Whenever possible, central venous access is preferable to peripheral venous or other modes of fluid and drug administration. In children less than five years old, a brief attempt is made to start a peripheral IV line. If no access is achieved after 90 seconds, then an intraosseous needle should be placed for vascular access[43]. A large peripheral vein such as the antecubital vein could be used. Attempts at either the jugular or subclavian vein frequently interfere with bag-mask ventilation during CPR. When additional assistance is present then attempts at central venous cannulation should be attempted. Possible approaches to the circulation via the central venous system include the internal and external jugular vein, subclavian vein, femoral vein, saphenous vein via cutdown, or axillary veins. External and internal jugular or subclavian venous cannulation are more easily performed once the trachea is intubated **(Table 1.8).**

In the older child, peripheral venous access generally is easier than in the younger patient. If peripheral IV placement fails, then a saphenous venous cutdown or other central venous line should be placed. The placement of an intraosseous needle in the older child is difficult because of the thick bony cortex.

There may be a significant delay in the circulation time of drugs administered from a peripheral site compared to a central site during CPR[44,45], although levels may be equal[46,47].

Intraosseous Access

The intraosseous route of fluid and medication administration, described originally in 1934[48], is an important adjunct to the arrest protocol. All medications used during CPR and fluids, including whole blood, have been given by the intraosseous route. This technique should be considered a temporary measure during emergencies when other vascular sites are not available. In the young child this route should be used after approximately 90 seconds of attempting peripheral venous access.

The technique of placing an intraosseous line is straightforward. A standard 16- or 18- gauge needle, spinal needle with stylet, or bone marrow needle, is inserted into the anterior surface of the tibia, 1 to 3 cm below the tibial tuberosity. The needle is directed in a 90° angle to the medial surface of the tibia or slightly inferior to avoid the epiphyseal plate (Fig. 1.13). The infusion is successful if the needle is in the marrow cavity as evidenced by the needle standing upright without support. It loses the upright position if it has slipped into the subcutaneous tissue. In addition, there is loss of resistance after the needle passes through the bony cortex of the tibia. At times bone marrow can be aspirated into a syringe connected to the needle. Free flow of the drug or fluid infusion without significant subcutaneous infiltration also should be demonstrated[49].

Meola, in 1944 reported 326 successful intraosseous infusions with only one complication[50]. Heinild et al., reported the results of 984 infusions in which five children developed osteomyelitis without any other complications[51]. Orlowski et al. revealed a high rate of occurrence of fat and bone marrow embolism after the administration of both fluids and medications by this route. Despite these findings, there were no significant alterations in PaO_2 or intrapulmonary shunt[52]. Large amounts of isotonic fluid have been successfully administered to reverse hemorrhagic shock in

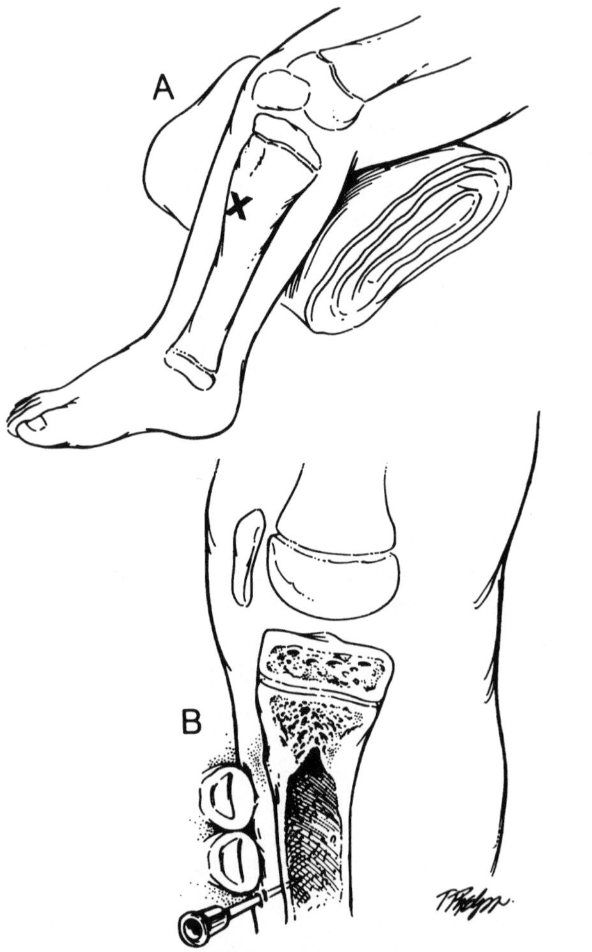

Figure 1.13. Intraosseous needle placement. Insert the needle at a level of tibial tubercle on the medial portion of the tibia. The needle is aimed caudally and laterally. (From Schleien CL. Cardiopulmonary resuscitation. In: Nichols DG, Yaster M, Lappe DG, Buck JR, eds. The golden hour handbook of advanced pediatric life support. St Louis: Mosby-Year Book, 1991:121.)

Table 1.9. Endotracheal Administration of Drug

Epinephrine
Atropine
Naloxone
Lidocaine

a rabbit model[53]. Blood pH was raised equally by the administration of sodium bicarbonate through a central IV or intraosseous line[54]. The hemodynamic response, time of onset, and the time to peak effect were similar when comparing epinephrine administration by these two routes[55].

Endotracheal Access

During CPR, the rapid establishment of an IV line can be difficult. This is especially true in the obese patient, infant and small child. In these cases, drugs including lidocaine, atropine, naloxone, and epinephrine can be given through the endotracheal tube **(Table 1.9).** The use of ionized medications such as sodium bicarbonate or calcium chloride is not recommended by the endotracheal route. The rate of absorption and physiologic effects of lidocaine, epinephrine and atropine administered via the endotracheal route compare favorably to the IV route in most studies[56–58]. The peak level of epinephrine or lidocaine administered via the endotracheal route may be lower compared to the intraosseous route. There is inconsistency in obtaining therapeutic levels of lidocaine when administered by the endotracheal route to humans during CPR[59]. The peak drug concentration of epinephrine was one-tenth after endotracheal administration compared to IV administration in anesthetized dogs. The endotracheal dose of epinephrine producing a 50% success of resuscitation was 130 mcg/kg[60]. Thus, the effective dose of epinephrine by the endotracheal route may be much larger than presently recommended. **The recommended dose of endotracheal epinephrine is now ten times the IV/IO dose: 0.1 mg/kg for bradycardia or pulseless arrest.**

The volume and the diluent in which the medications are administered may play a role in the success of this technique. When large volumes of fluid are used, pulmonary surfactant may be altered or destroyed, resulting in atelectasis. The total volume of fluid delivered into the trachea should not exceed 10 ml in the adult or 5 ml in the infant[61]. The use of normal saline may have the least detrimental effects on lung mechanics[61] and may be important for the absorption of medication from the bronchial tree[62]. Absorption into the systemic circulation may be enhanced by deep intrapulmonary administration. This is performed by passing a Swan-Ganz catheter or suction catheter to a wedged position deep into the bronchial tree[63]. **Current recommendation is to dilute drugs given by this route into 1 to 2 ml of normal or half-normal saline.**

The risk associated with the endotracheal route of administration is the formation of an intrapulmonary depot of drug, which may prolong the drugs' effect. This could result in post-resuscitation hypertension or the recurrence of fibrillation after normal circulation is restored.

Types of Fluids

Fluid management during CPR remains an ubiquitous part of the resuscitation process. As in other types of shock, colloid does not offer any proven advantage over crystalloid with respect to outcome. After head injury and hemorrhagic shock, there may be an advantage in using a hypertonic solution instead of an isotonic crystalloid solution. This benefit may be related to a combination of volume expansion[64], enhanced cardiac performance[64–68], vasodilation of systemic arterioles[69–72], or by decreasing ICP and cerebral edema after head injury and hemorrhagic shock[73–76].

Volume loading increases arterial blood pressure, carotid blood flow, and cardiac output during CPR[77–79]. Despite this, perfusion pressures to the heart and brain are lower when volume loading occurs on the venous side of the circulation[77,79,80]. Thus, there may be an advantage to volume loading on the arterial side of the circulation. Dextrose-containing solutions should be avoided during CPR because of the possible detrimental effects of hyperglycemia. **(See glucose section).**

Monitoring during CPR

Assessment of the patient during CPR is similar to other clinical situations **(Table 1.10).** A basic clinical examination adhering to basic principles including inspection, palpation, and auscultation of the patient is performed. The chest is carefully observed for adequacy of chest expansion with artificial ventilation and for equal and normal breath sounds. In addition, one should constantly reevaluate the depth of compression and the position of the rescuer's hands in performing chest compressions. Palpation is essential in establishing pulselessness, in assessing the adequacy of blood flow during chest compressions, and in locating landmarks. Simply palpating the peripheral pulses may not allow for an accurate assessment of blood flow during CPR. This is a result of the intense vasoconstriction that occurs with the use of epinephrine or other α-adrenergic agonist drugs.

Adequacy of vital organ blood flow or function may not be well assessed by the clinical examination. An indwelling arterial catheter, when available, is an invaluable moni-

Table 1.10. Patient Assessment During CPR

Inspection
Chest excursion
Depth of compression
Position of rescuer's hands
Palpation
Establish pulselessness
Peripheral pulses
Landmarks (central line placement)
Auscultation
Breath sounds
Heart sounds

tor in assessing the arterial blood pressure. The effects of volume expansion and drugs on arterial blood pressure is critical. Aortic diastolic pressure relates directly to adequacy of coronary perfusion during CPR. In addition, an arterial line allows frequent blood sampling, particularly for measurement of arterial pH, $PaCO_2$, PaO_2 and base excess. An arterial line may be placed into the radial artery by percutaneous placement or cutdown, the femoral artery by the Seldinger technique, the axillary artery, dorsalis pedis, or posterior tibial artery. The state of oxygen delivery can also be determined by transcutaneous monitoring of PO_2 or by pulse oximetry. Pulse oximetry can be used during CPR to determine not only the oxygen saturation but also the level of cardiac output, as reflected in the plethysmograph[81,82].

Vital organ function should be repeatedly assessed during and after CPR. The 12-lead electrocardiogram is an integral part of the monitoring protocol during CPR. The ECG can reflect the adequacy of myocardial blood flow, reveal metabolic imbalances that could affect the resuscitation, and show electrical disturbances that require rapid changes in therapy. Cardiac output is often too low to be measured during CPR[83,84], however, end-tidal CO_2 concentration has been shown to correlate well with pulmonary blood flow and, thus cardiac output[85,86]. Disposable colorimetric $P_{ET}CO_2$ analyzers can reliably differentiate between a tracheal and esophageal intubation in infants and children[87–89]. End-tidal CO_2 has been correlated with the coronary perfusion pressure[86], which is the critical parameter for resuscitation of the heart. With epinephrine administration, the end-tidal CO_2 may not be an accurate indicator of blood flow as it may result in increased intrapulmonary shunting[90–92]. A low $P_{ET}CO_2$ ($<1\%$) may also be related to airway obstruction, tension pneumothorax, pericardial tamponade, pulmonary embolism, or hypothermia.

The neurologic examination, although routinely performed during CPR, should not be used as a predictor of outcome[93]. Use of the electroencephalogram has been shown to be a poor predictor of survival during CPR[94–96]. Somatosensory evoked potentials (SSEP) have been used as a monitor of adequacy of cerebral blood flow and function during and after CPR in animals[97,98]. Recent clinical studies have indicated that the bilateral absence of cortical SSEP portends a poor neurologic outcome[99].

Temperature should be monitored routinely during CPR as it may vary widely during the resuscitation or at presentation to the hospital. The resuscitation of the patient with hypothermia as the cause of cardiac arrest must be continued until the patient's core temperature has risen above 35°. (See special resuscitation situations.) Repeated measurements of core body temperature should be made at several sites (rectal, bladder, esophageal, axillary, tympanic membrane) if possible to avoid misleading temperature readings from a single site, which might be affected by the alterations in regional blood flow during CPR. Use of a glass bulb thermometer allows measurement of temperature to much more precise levels. Temperature can affect the success of resuscitation, the short-term neurological status and the eventual neurological outcome. External rewarming should be done carefully to avoid overheating the patient once spontaneous circulation has been restored. The therapeutic use of hypothermia may be applied eventually to improve outcome from resuscitation **(Table 1.11).**

Table 1.11. Monitoring During CPR

Electrocardiogram (ECG)
Noninvasive BP
End-tidal CO_2
Arterial pressure (when line obtained)
Central venous pressure (when line obtained)
Pulse oximeter
Temperature
EEG (if available)
Evoked potentials (experimental)

Adjuncts for Airway and Ventilation

Oxygen

In patients with cardiac arrest, numerous factors contribute to hypoxemia and inadequate oxygen delivery to tissues. One hundred percent oxygen must be administered in a cardiorespiratory arrest, as soon as possible. Expired air given during mouth-to-mouth resuscitation provides approximately 16% oxygen concentration, and provides less than 80 torr of alveolar oxygen tension. Oxygen toxicity occurs during prolonged mechanical ventilatory support using high oxygen concentrations. However, the short term use of 100% oxygen is not currently considered to be harmful and should always be used until adequate arterial oxygenation can be ascertained.

Suction

Portable and installed suction equipment should be available, if possible, for resuscitative emergencies. The portable unit should provide vacuum and flow adequate for oropharyngeal suction. The unit should be fitted with a large bore, nonkinking suction tubing and a tonsil suction tip. In the emergency room setting, two suction devices should be available at the bedside. In addition, appropriate sized suction catheters for the endotracheal tube or tracheostomy, a nonbreakable collection bottle, and a supply of sterile water for clearing tubes and catheters should be available.

Deep suctioning of the airway can incite bronchospasm, worsen pulmonary hypertension, reduce functional residual capacity, cause tracheal hemorrhage and increase ICP. For these reasons, the suction catheter should be inserted only to the tip of the endotracheal tube. An installed suction unit should have the capability of providing an air flow of more than 30 liters per minute at the end of the delivery tube and a vacuum of greater than 300 mmHg when the tube is clamped. Variable suction should be available for use on infants and small children.

Oropharyngeal Airway

Oropharyngeal airways should only be used when the patient is unconscious. When introduced into the conscious or stuporous patient, laryngospasm or vomiting may be induced. Proper placement of the oral airway, utilizing a tongue depressor and guiding the airway over the tongue is critical. Improperly placed oral airways displace the tongue posteriorly and usually worsen the degree of airway obstruction. Oropharyngeal airways should be available in different sizes at the bedside.

Masks

In the hospital setting, and more frequently in the public setting, ventilation is performed using a mask with a bag-valve-mask system. The mask should be tight-fitting and reach from the midportion of the bridge of the nose to the protuberance of the chin without extending over the end of the chin. A variety of mask sizes should always be available during an in-hospital arrest.

Endotracheal Intubation

Endotracheal intubation is the preferred technique for acquiring access to the airway and requires skilled, experienced personnel. Endotracheal intubation during CPR is performed for a variety of reasons. The endotracheal tube is used to protect the airway from gastric contents, to keep the trachea patent, and to deliver high concentrations of oxygen to the lungs. In the emergency situation, the trachea is intubated by the oral route. The patient should be preoxygenated first with 3 to 4 breaths of 100% oxygen. Cardiac compressions should not be interrupted for more than 15 seconds during the tracheal intubation procedure.

The equipment necessary for emergency tracheal intubation, and for possible extraction of a foreign body, are two laryngoscopes with functioning bulbs, several different laryngoscope blades (preferably straight blades for children), and an assortment of endotracheal tubes (uncuffed tubes should be used in children under 8 years of age), a syringe for cuff inflation, a variety of oral airways, a stylet, a tonsil suction catheter with adequate suction, tape, benzoin, and a Kelly clamp or Magill forceps for foreign body extraction.

During the emergency tracheal intubation, cricoid pressure should be administered at the point that anesthetic drugs are given or during the CPR procedure if the patient is unconscious. Originally described by Sellick in 1961[16], cricoid pressure is applied by an assistant by palpating the cricoid cartilage between the thumb and second finger and exerting downward pressure so that the esophagus is occluded between the trachea and bodies of the cervical vertebrae. Cricoid pressure is released when the cuff of the endotracheal tube is inflated or an uncuffed endotracheal tube is in place in the trachea and breath sounds are heard over the lung fields bilaterally.

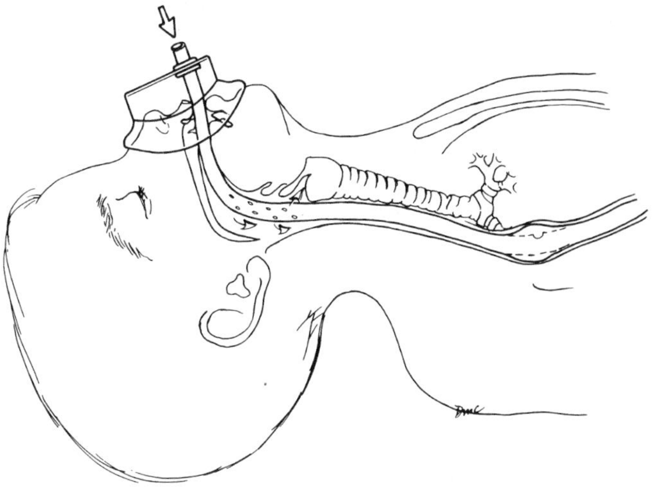

Figure 1.14. Esophageal obturator airway. The airway is shown in place, with the cuff inflated in the esophagus. *Arrows* show the direction of oxygen into the trachea.

Laryngeal Mask Airway

The recently developed laryngeal mask airway, is a device that can be used to manage the airway of infants and children. It consists of a mask (an inflatable silicon cuff that seals the perimeter of the larynx) and a wide bore tube that connects to an ambu bag or anesthesia circuit[100]. The device has been used successfully during CPR[101].

Esophageal Obturator Airway

The esophageal obturator airway (EOA) was developed to overcome the need for technical expertise in placing an endotracheal tube[102]. The EOA is a curved plastic tube similar in shape to an endotracheal tube mounted on a cuffed mask with an inflatable balloon at the distal end of the tube. The tube is passed blindly into the esophagus, the mask is seated on the face, and the balloon is inflated. (Fig. 1.14)

The EOA has been used successfully in oxygenating and ventilating the pre-hospital patient suffering a cardiac arrest. However, it may be difficult to place and to oxygenate the patient effectively[103]. The EOA is recommended for use in adult patients only. Development of a pediatric EOA has been difficult because of the need for tubes of variable lengths[104]. Complications of its use include esophageal rupture and tracheal intubation[28,105,106].

Mechanical Chest Compressors

Mechanical devices that compress the chest have been used extensively in adults, but not in children. Like any other technical device it must be used by trained personnel. This device was developed in order to optimize chest compression and to reduce rescuer fatigue in prolonged resuscitative efforts. The device consists of a mounted plunger powered by compressed gas. It may be adjusted to vary the depth of chest compression. The device is sometimes equipped with the capability to ventilate the patient. Problems related to its use include sternal fractures, poor positioning resulting in inadequate compressions, and mechanical failure[15]. The device has been used extensively in the laboratory to deliver simultaneous compression-ventilation CPR and has been used on infant-sized animals (i.e. piglets)[107].

Special Resuscitation Situations

Near Drowning

Resuscitation procedures after a near-drowning episode are similar to those presented above. Rescue breathing should be initiated as quickly as possible even before the patient is moved out of the water, as hypoxemia is the most important consequence of a near drowning episode. If neck injury is suspected, as in all diving accidents, the victim's neck should be supported in the neutral position and the victim should be floated onto a back support before being extracted from the water. Airway support with a jaw thrust should be used. Since aspiration is usually minimal, efforts to clear the airway of water should be avoided unless the rescuer suspects that foreign matter is obstructing the airway or ventilation is inadequate. In those cases the Heimlich maneuver can be applied with the victim supine but with the head to the side. External chest compressions should not be attempted in deep water because of the inability to maintain the patient in the horizontal position and the head above the water. Efforts at resuscitation should be initiated despite prolonged submersion, especially in cold water, because of reports of successful outcomes after submersion of 30 min or longer[108,109]. For a further discussion of near drowning, see Chapter 14.

Accident Cases

Treatment of the patient who develops cardiac arrest after trauma is based on the cause of the arrest which may alter the prognosis and treatment plan. The initial approach to the injured patient in cardiac arrest should include an attempt to resuscitate the patient by applying the standard ABCs and other algorithms of CPR. Resuscitation should not be attempted in patients with obvious severe blunt trauma with or without vital signs, pupillary response, or an organized or shockable cardiac rhythm at the scene. In patients for whom resuscitative efforts are attempted, rapid extrication should occur with preparation for rapid evacuation. During all procedures, but specifically including airway procedures, in-line stabilization of the neck by an assistant should be performed to avoid inflicting further injury by turning or tilting the head. A cervical fracture should be expected in any patient with head trauma or other injury above the clavicles resulting in altered consciousness or with the mechanism of injury that may have subjected the spine to sudden acceleration or deceleration associated with a motor vehicle, fall or diving accident. The jaw thrust should be used to open the airway in those situations. Typically, unless other circumstances prohibit immediate evacuation, IV line placement should not be attempted until the patient is en route to a Trauma Center. Early evacuation of a tension pneumothorax should be performed. Signs suggestive of a tension pneumothorax include asymmetry of breath sounds or chest movement or an acute increase of airway resistance. In addition, in the patient with ventricular fibrillation, defibrillation should be attempted immediately, even before chest compressions are begun in the prehospital setting.

Hypothermia

Hypothermia exists in the presence of an internal core temperature of 35°C (95°F) or less. Severe hypothermia exists when the core temperature falls below 32°C. At this level of body temperature, sinus bradycardia usually intervenes, leading to T wave inversion, prolongation of the QT interval, acute elevation of the QRS-ST segment junction, and ultimately leading to ventricular ectopy and ventricular fibrillation. Even when bradycardia is present, peripheral pulses may be difficult to detect because of severe peripheral vasoconstriction. The neurologic examination may be consistent with clinical brain death as a result of the marked depression of cerebral blood flow and cerebral metabolism that exist under this condition. Thus, hypothermic patients who appear to be dead should be resuscitated aggressively.

Hypothermia occurs most commonly in three specific groups of patients. The first group consists of accident patients, particularly the very old, the very young, near drowning patients, and those suffering an accident coincident with inebriation. Infants are particularly prone to hypothermia because of their large surface area relative to volume which allows more rapid heat loss, less subcutaneous tissue and thinner skin than exist in the older child or adult, and the inability to shiver to produce heat. The second group consists of patients with chronic illness including hypothyroidism, pituitary insufficiency, Addison's disease, pancreatitis, stroke, and cirrhosis. The third group consists of patients with acute illness, including shock, some intoxications, sepsis, hypoglycemia, acute respiratory failure, and congestive heart failure. In addition, a person who suffers a cardiac arrest while normothermic will quickly begin to cool, especially when in a cold environment. If the arrest was unwitnessed, rescuers will not know if the arrest was because of hypothermia or if hypothermia was a sequel to the arrest. Physicians must use clinical judgement to proceed with resuscitative efforts in the hypothermic patient.

If the hypothermic patient is not breathing, rescue breathing should be initiated. Chest compressions are indicated in the pulseless, unmonitored patient. ECG monitoring is critical because of the difficulty in palpating a peripheral pulse. Airway management and transport should be performed as gently as possible to avoid precipitating ven-

Table 1.12. Treatment of Hypothermic Arrest

Begin CPR
Transport to warm environment
Begin monitoring (including core temperature)
External rewarming
Remove wet clothes
Wrap patient in warm blankets
Radiant warmer
Warmed humidified O_2
Warmed IV fluids
Internal warming (for temperature <32°C)
Intubation-ventilation with warmed, humidified O_2
Gastric irrigation with warmed saline
Thoracotomy and cardiac irrigation with warmed saline
Cardiopulmonary bypass
If asystole or ventricular fibrillation occur
Continue CPR until either
Temperature >32°C and there is no improvement
or
Adequate blood pressure and rhythm are reached

tricular fibrillation. During transport, further heat loss should be prevented by removing wet clothing, and by insulating the patient and adding heat by external means if available. These include warmed, humidified oxygen, warmed IV fluids, and a radiant warmer. In the emergency department, invasive measures to rewarm include endotracheal intubation and assisted ventilation with heated and humidified gases, peritoneal lavage with warm dialysate, thoracotomy and irrigation of the mediastinum with warmed fluids, and extracorporeal blood warming with partial bypass. If ventricular fibrillation is detected, three shocks should be delivered. Defibrillation is typically impossible until the patient is warmed to a temperature of 32°C. If CPR is initiated, it should be continued until the patient has remained unresponsive to CPR efforts despite being rewarmed to a temperature greater than 32°C. The use of central venous or pulmonary artery lines during rewarming is discouraged because of the possible induction of ventricular fibrillation. When the resuscitation effort is successful, the patient should be closely monitored including blood pressure, ECG, central venous pressure, temperature, arterial blood gases, electrolytes, and glucose **(Table 1.12).**

Electric Shock and Lightning Strike

Electric shock injuries result from the direct effects of current on cell membranes and vàscular smooth muscle. In addition, the production of heat energy as it is converted from electrical energy causes injury as current passes through body tissues. The factors that determine the severity of electric shock include the voltage, magnitude of energy, resistance of skin, type of current, duration of current, and the pathway taken through the body. Alternating current is often worse, because it results in tetanic muscle contraction, which prevents the victim from releasing the source of the electricity, leading to a prolonged duration of exposure.

Ventricular tachycardia, fibrillation and asystole occur as a result of electric shock. The frequency of alternating current increases the likelihood of exposure of the myocardium during the vulnerable period of the cardiac cycle, which may precipitate ventricular fibrillation[110]. Transthoracic current flow (i.e. hand-to-hand) is more often fatal than a vertical (i.e. hand-to-foot) or foot-to-foot current path as a result of its path through the heart. Respiratory arrest secondary to electric shock is because of direct electrical damage to the medullary respiratory center, tetanic contraction of the diaphragm and intercostal muscles, or prolonged paralysis of the respiratory muscles after electric shock.

After electrocution, vigorous resuscitative measures are indicated because of unknown factors of the shock (such as duration of arrest) and the usual pre-existing good health of victims who are shocked. After the rescuer assures himself that he or she is not in danger of electric shock, basic life support techniques should be initiated. In addition, smoldering clothing should be removed from the patient to prevent further thermal damage. Endotracheal intubation should be performed early if any soft tissue swelling of the face is present as facial or airway swelling worsens rapidly. Arrhythmias should be treated as described previously. Hypovolemia is common so rapid IV fluid administration is indicated to treat shock, correct ongoing fluid losses, and maintain a diuresis to avoid renal shutdown as a result of myoglobinuria secondary to tissue breakdown.

Lightning strike, which causes 200 to 300 fatalities per year in the United States, has a 30% mortality rate and a 70% rate of significant morbidity[111]. Primary cause of death as a result of lightning strike is cardiac arrest associated with ventricular fibrillation or asystole[112]. The lightning strike itself acts as a massive direct current countershock depolarizing the entire myocardium resulting in asystole. Frequently, sinus rhythm returns spontaneously, however, concomitant respiratory arrest as a result of thoracic muscle spasm or suppression of the brainstem respiratory center may cause a cardiac arrest secondary to hypoxia.

After a lightning strike, triage for multiple victims is reversed from the usual triage procedure. Highest priority should be given to patients in respiratory or cardiac arrest with usual basic and advance life support measures. This is because most patients who die from lightning strikes are those who suffer an immediate cardiac or respiratory arrest. Patients who do not have a cardiac arrest typically have an excellent chance of recovery.

PHARMACOLOGY

Adrenergic Agonists

The use of adrenergic agonists during CPR was first described by Redding and Pearson in 1963, three years after the original description of closed-chest CPR[113]. These authors subsequently showed that early administration of epinephrine in a canine model of cardiac arrest improved the success rate of CPR. They later demonstrated that the in-

Table 1.13. α- versus β-Adrenergic Agonist Effects

α-adrenergic effects
Vasoconstrict peripheral vessels
Maintain aortic diastolic pressure
Improve coronary blood flow
No metabolic stimulatory effect
β-adrenergic effects
Vasodilate peripheral vessels
Decrease aortic diastolic pressure
Increase cellular metabolic rate
Positive inotrope
Increase intensity of ventricular fibrillation
Increase heart rate and/or arrhythmias following resuscitation

crease in diastolic aortic pressure generated by the administration of adrenergic agonist drugs was responsible for the success of resuscitation[(114)]. They theorized that vasopressors such as epinephrine were of value because the drug increased peripheral vascular tone.

Yakaitis et al. investigated the relative importance of α- and β-adrenergic agonist actions during resuscitation[(115)]. Only 27% of dogs that received both an α-adrenergic receptor antagonist and a β-adrenergic receptor agonist, such as isoproterenol, were resuscitated successfully. In contrast, all of the dogs that received an α-adrenergic agonist drug with a β-adrenergic antagonist drug were resuscitated successfully. These data suggested that the α-adrenergic agonist receptor action of epinephrine is responsible for successful resuscitation **(Table 1.13).**

More recent studies have reinforced this concept. Michael et al. demonstrated that the effects of epinephrine during CPR were mediated by the selective vasoconstriction of peripheral vessels except those supplying the brain and heart. During an epinephrine infusion, higher aortic pressures were maintained resulting in higher perfusion pressures to the heart and brain[(116)]. Despite the increase in aortic pressure, flow to other organs such as the kidneys and small intestine were decreased significantly, as a result of the intense vasoconstriction of the vessels supplying those organs[(107,116,117)].

Coronary Blood Flow

The increase in aortic diastolic pressure associated with epinephrine administration during CPR is critical for maintaining coronary blood flow and enhancing the success of resuscitation. In the beating heart, the contractile state of the myocardium is increased by β-adrenergic agonism. During CPR, β-adrenergic agonism may stimulate spontaneous myocardial contractions and increase the intensity of ventricular fibrillation. In contrast, the inotropic effect of β-adrenergic agonists might actually be deleterious to the fibrillating heart by increasing intramyocardial wall pressure and hence the downstream pressure for coronary perfusion[(118)]. This results in a decreased coronary perfusion pressure and decreased subendocardial blood flow. In addition, β-adrenergic stimulation might also increase the myocardial oxygen demand superimposed on the low coronary blood flow available during CPR. In normally beating hearts, subendocardial blood flow occurs almost entirely during diastole. Ventricular fibrillation has been shown to simulate a period of sustained contraction[(119)]. This leads to higher intramyocardial wall pressure during fibrillation, resulting in a decrease in myocardial perfusion pressure and coronary blood flow. The combination of increased oxygen demand by the β-agonist action[(120)] and decreased oxygen supply by the decrease in coronary blood flow may cause further damage to an already ischemic heart.

Other adrenergic agonist drugs, some with pure α-adrenergic actions have been used successfully during CPR. These drugs, such as phenylephrine and methoxamine, cause peripheral vasoconstriction during CPR, increasing aortic diastolic pressure. Moreover, they do not increase myocardial oxygen demand because of the absence of β-adrenergic stimulation. This results in a higher oxygen supply to demand ratio in the ischemic heart.

These agonists as well as other vasopressors (i.e. vasopressin)[(121)] have been used successfully for resuscitation[(97,113–115)]. These drugs maintain myocardial blood flow as well as epinephrine during CPR[(115)]. Schleien et al. found that high aortic pressures can be sustained for 60 minutes in a canine model of CPR with phenylephrine[(97)]. Myocardial perfusion pressure and coronary blood flow were not different in dogs treated with phenylephrine or epinephrine during CPR. This resulted in a resuscitation rate of 75% with the use of either drug. In that study, phenylephrine did not alter the distribution of blood flow within the myocardium compared to epinephrine as the ratio of endocardial to epicardial blood flow was the same in both groups. Debate continues, however, about the merits of pure α-adrenergic agonist drugs for resuscitation[(122–124)].

Cerebral Blood Flow

Cerebral blood flow during CPR, like coronary blood flow, depends on the vasoconstriction of peripheral vessels and is enhanced by the use of α-adrenergic agonists. Epinephrine and other α-agonists produce selective vasoconstriction of noncerebral peripheral vessels to areas of the head and scalp (i.e., tongue, facial muscle and skin) without causing cerebral vasoconstriction in adult[(63,116)] and infant models of CPR[(107)]. Phenylephrine is as effective as epinephrine in generating and sustaining cerebral blood flow during CPR in adult dogs[(97)] and in infant piglets[(125)]. When epinephrine or phenylephrine was administered nine minutes after ventricular fibrillation in dogs, one group of investigators failed to detect differences in neurological deficits 24 hours later[(126)]. Other investigators, though, have found that the use of epinephrine during CPR results in higher vital organ blood flow compared to pure α-agonists[(122,123,127)]. This may have been because of the use of dosages of drugs that were not equally potent in increasing vascular pressure and subsequent blood flow.

Cerebral oxygen uptake may be increased by a central β-adrenoceptor effect if a sufficient amount of epinephrine crosses the blood-brain barrier during or after resuscitation[128,129]. In addition, epinephrine may vasoconstrict or vasodilate cerebral vessels depending on the balance between α- and β-adrenergic actions[130]. When cerebral ischemia is brief, epinephrine and phenylephrine have similar effects on cerebral blood flow and metabolism. Cerebral oxygen uptake during 20 minutes of CPR was maintained at prearrest levels in both epinephrine and phenylephrine treated dogs, implying that cerebral blood flow was higher than is necessary to maintain adequate cerebral metabolism and that β-receptor stimulation does not increase cerebral oxygen metabolism[97]. In this situation, the blood-brain barrier is most likely undisrupted[97]. Catecholamines may cross the barrier when mechanical disruption or when enzymatic barriers to vasopressors (i.e., monoamine oxidase inhibitors) are overwhelmed during tissue hypoxia[131,132].

During CPR the blood-brain barrier may be disrupted by the large fluctuations of cerebral venous and arterial pressures during chest compressions[133]. The permeability of the barrier may also increase during the large increase in cerebral blood flow that may occur in a maximally dilated vascular bed after resuscitation, particularly when systemic hypertension occurs[134]. An increase in cerebral oxygen demand when flow is limited could affect cerebral recovery adversely. Using a small neutral amino acid, α-aminoisobutyric acid (AIB) as a marker of blood-brain barrier permeability in adult dogs, Schleien et al. found that after 8 minutes of cardiac arrest the blood-brain barrier was not disrupted during CPR, immediately after or four hours after resuscitation[134]. However, in young piglets after eight minutes of cardiac arrest, the blood-brain barrier was permeable to AIB four hours after return to spontaneous circulation[135]. These investigators later showed the increase in blood-brain barrier permeability could be prevented by prearrest administration of conjugated superoxide dismutase and catalase[136], indicating a role for oxygen free radicals in the pathogenesis of the injury to the blood-brain barrier. Ultrastructural examination of the piglet brain after 8 minutes of cardiac arrest revealed endothelial membrane abnormalities which included luminal membrane disruption, membrane bleb formation and swelling of perivascular astrocytic end feet, occasionally associated with extravasation of the larger molecular weight protein horseradish peroxidase (MW 40,000) through the blood-brain barrier[137].

Dosage

The correct dose of epinephrine during CPR remains controversial. The dose currently recommended in the American Heart Association's Guidelines for CPR and Emergency Cardiac Care has been modified because of the research suggesting increased survival when doses larger than previously recommended are administered after cardiac arrest in children[15]. Several recent clinical studies, however, have not demonstrated any effect of higher doses of epinephrine on short or long term survival after cardiac arrest.

The physiologic responses of animals and humans to higher doses of epinephrine have been studied. Cerebral blood flow increases further in response to administration of larger doses of epinephrine[126,138–139]. In animals, several investigators have shown that high-dose epinephrine increases myocardial and subendocardial blood flow, improves oxygen delivery over oxygen consumption[140–144], is associated with less depletion of myocardial ATP stores and more rapid repletion of phosphocreatine[145]. In neonatal lambs after asphyxia-induced bradycardia, high dose epinephrine resulted in a higher heart rate, but lower stroke volume and cardiac output[146]. However, increased myocardial oxygen consumption and decreased left ventricular subendocardial blood flow with epinephrine administration have been demonstrated in fibrillating animal models[118,147,148]. In a swine model, high-dose epinephrine produced lower levels of myocardial blood flow than achieved with lower doses of epinephrine[138].

Studies in humans have been contradictory regarding survival of patients who were given high-dose epinephrine after cardiac arrest. In earlier studies, investigators were optimistic that higher doses of epinephrine would increase aortic diastolic pressure and therefore improve the return to spontaneous circulation compared with standard epinephrine doses. Gonzalez et al. demonstrated a dose-dependent increase in aortic blood pressure in patients who failed to respond to prolonged resuscitation efforts[149,150]. Also, Paradis et al. showed that high dose epinephrine increased aortic diastolic pressure and improved the rate successful resuscitation in patients who failed ACLS protocols[151]. They also reported on seven pediatric patients treated successfully with 0.2 mg/kg of epinephrine[152]. Others reported on four other children treated successfully with the use of higher than standard doses of epinephrine[153]. Other investigators have also reported higher aortic diastolic pressures and an increase in the rate of return of spontaneous circulation[151,154,155]. In these nonrandomized, unblinded studies there were few survivors, although three patients survived in the pediatric study cited above.

Even more recently, three large multicenter studies were published which dampened the enthusiasm for the use of high dose epinephrine. Stiell et al. reported on 650 adult patients who suffered cardiac arrest, randomly assigned to either a standard or a high-dose (7 mg) epinephrine protocol. High-dose epinephrine did not improve survival (18% versus 23% 1-hour survival; 3% versus 5% hospital discharge) or alter neurologic outcome[156]. In a multicenter prospective study, Brown et al. reported on 1,280 adult patients who received either standard (0.02 mg/kg) or high-dose (0.2 mg/kg) epinephrine after cardiac arrest. Again, differences were not seen in either the return to spontaneous circulation, survival to hospital discharge, or neurologic outcome between these two groups of patients[157]. In the report by Callaham et al, in 816 adult patients, high-dose epinephrine did improve the rate of return of spontaneous circulation but did not alter the hospital discharge rate or survival of these patients(158). This type of study in children has not been performed to date.

High doses of epinephrine may account for some of the adverse effects that occur after resuscitation(159). High doses may worsen myocardial ischemia and result in tachyarrhythmias, hypertensive crisis, pulmonary edema, digitalis toxicity, hypoxemia, and cardiac arrest.(49,135,160,161) The use of β-adrenergic blockers after the return of spontaneous circulation has been suggested to attenuate these deleterious effects of epinephrine(98,162,163). Epinephrine induced a decrease in PaO_2 and an increase in alveolar dead space ventilation, thought to be a result of redistribution of pulmonary blood flow, compared with a pure α-adrenergic agonist(164,165). High doses of epinephrine (greater than 15 mg) given to adults during CPR resulted in lower cardiac index, systemic oxygen consumption, and systemic oxygen delivery during the first six hours after resuscitation(159).

The differences in the results of these studies account for the ambivalence in recommendations from the 1992 American Heart Association Standards and Guidelines for CPR and ECC(15). To treat a pulseless arrest in children, the first IV or intraosseous (IO) dose is 0.01 mg/kg. All endotracheal (ET) doses are ten times this dose or 0.1 mg/kg; second and subsequent IV/IO/ET doses are 0.1 mg/kg administered every 3 to 5 minutes during arrest. The present guidelines recommend shortening the epinephrine dosing interval for adult patients from 5 minutes to 3 to 5 minutes. Higher-dose epinephrine can be neither recommended nor discouraged. An intermediate dose of 2 to 5 mg IV, escalating doses from 1 to 3 to 5 mg, and a high dose of 0.1 mg/kg IV are all possible regimens in adults.

Sodium Bicarbonate

Clinical Effects

The use of sodium bicarbonate during CPR remains a controversial issue. This stems from the drug's potential side effects and the paucity of evidence to show that either laboratory animals or humans actually benefit from receiving bicarbonate during CPR(167–169).

Administration of sodium bicarbonate results in an acid-base reaction in which bicarbonate combines with hydrogen to form water and CO_2, thereby elevating blood pH.

$$HCO^-_3 + H^+ \rightarrow H_2CO_3 \rightarrow H_2O + CO_2$$

Since carbon dioxide is generated from bicarbonate, adequate alveolar ventilation must be present prior to its administration.

Indications

Sodium bicarbonate is indicated for correction of significant metabolic acidosis, especially when there are signs of cardiovascular compromise. Acidosis depresses myocardial function by prolonging diastolic depolarization, depressing spontaneous cardiac activity, decreasing the electrical threshold for ventricular fibrillation, lowering the inotropic state of the myocardium and reducing the cardiac response to catecholamines(170–172). Acidosis also decreases systemic vascular resistance and blunts the vasoconstrictor response of peripheral vessels to catecholamines(173). This is contrary to the desired effect during CPR **(Table 1.14)**. In addition, the vascular resistance of the pulmonary circulation increases with a decreasing pH. Rudolph et al.(174) observed a two-fold increase in pulmonary vascular resistance in calves when pH was lowered from 7.40 to 7.20 under normoxic conditions. Therefore, correction of even mild acidosis may be helpful in resuscitating patients who have the potential for right-to-left shunting through a cardiac septal defect, a patent ductus arteriosus, or a synthetic central shunt. As a result of the adverse effects of bicarbonate listed below, the indications for its use are limited to cardiac arrest associated with hyperkalemia, patients with pre-existing metabolic acidosis and after approximately 10 minutes into the routine cardiac arrest sequence **(Table 1.15)**.

Table 1.14. Adverse Effects of Acidosis

Cardiac:	
	Impair sinus node function
	Decrease contractility
	Depress diastolic depolarization
	Lower threshold for ventricular fibrillation
	Decrease responsiveness to catecholamines
Vascular:	
	Decrease systemic vascular resistance
	Decrease systemic vascular responsiveness to catecholamines
	Increase pulmonary vascular resistance

Dosage

When the $PaCO_2$ and pH are known, the dose of bicarbonate to correct the pH to 7.40 can be calculated using the following formula:

$$0.3 \times \text{weight (kg)} \times \text{base deficit} = \text{mEq bicarbonate}$$

Because of the possible side effect of bicarbonate and the large arterial-venous CO_2 gradient that develops during CPR, we recommend giving half the dose based on a volume of distribution of 0.6. If blood gases are not available, the initial dose is 1 mEq/kg followed by 0.5 mEq/kg every 10 minutes of ongoing arrest(175). Again, the importance of alveolar ventilation cannot be overemphasized, as well as the need for repeated arterial blood gas analysis.

Table 1.15. Indications for Sodium Bicarbonate

Pre-existing metabolic acidosis
Prolonged CPR (after 10 minutes)
Pulmonary hypertensive crisis
Hyperkalemia

Table 1.16. Adverse Effects of Sodium Bicarbonate

Hypercapnia
Hypernatremia
Hyperosmolality
Paradoxical intracellular acidosis
Decrease myocardial contractility
Leftward shift of oxyhemoglobin dissociation curve, decreasing release of oxygen from hemoglobin

Side Effects

The side effects of bicarbonate administration include metabolic alkalosis, hypercapnia, hypernatremia and hyperosmolality[176], all of which are associated with a high mortality rate **(Table 1.16)**. Metabolic alkalosis causes a leftward shift of the oxyhemoglobin dissociation curve and so impairs release of oxygen from hemoglobin to tissues[177]. Hypernatremia and hyperosmolality may decrease organ perfusion by increasing interstitial edema in microvascular beds. Bicarbonate administration may produce a paradoxical intracellular acidosis because of the rapid entry of carbon dioxide into cells with a slower egress of hydrogen ion out of cells. A marked hypercapnic acidosis in both systemic venous, cerebral venous and coronary sinus blood develops during cardiac arrest and CPR, and may be worsened by administration of bicarbonate[178,179]. Myocardial hypercapnic acidosis is associated with decreased myocardial contractility[170,171]. Falk et al.[180] found that the venoarterial difference in PCO_2 was 24 ± 15 mm Hg in five patients during CPR. In one patient this difference increased from 16 to 69 mm Hg after the administration of bicarbonate. In another study of 16 patients during CPR the mean difference between the $PaCO_2$ and $PvCO_2$ was 42 mm Hg[179]. In the central nervous system, however, paradoxical intracellular acidosis probably does not occur unless overcorrection of the pH occurs. Sessler et al. demonstrated that after two 5 mEq/kg doses of bicarbonate to neonatal rabbits recovering from hypoxic acidosis, the arterial pH increased to 7.41 and intracellular brain pH measured by nuclear magnetic resonance (NMR) spectroscopy increased to its pre-hypoxia level[181]. They did not observe paradoxical intracellular cerebral acidosis. The belief that respiratory acidosis is injurious to the central nervous system has recently been challenged by Cohen et al. who showed that the intracellular brain ATP concentration did not change when extreme hypercarbia was produced for 70 minutes in rats even though the intracellular brain pH fell to 6.5[182]. After hypercarbia these animals could not be distinguished from normal controls and their brains were not histologically different from controls. Using NMR spectroscopy of the brain in dogs during CPR and cardiac arrest, Eleff et al. showed that after 6 minutes of cardiac arrest, intracellular brain pH decreased to 6.29 and ATP concentration approached zero. After 6 minutes of effective CPR, ATP level was 86% of pre-arrest control and by 35 minutes of CPR, brain pH returned to normal, despite ongoing peripheral arterial acidosis[183].

Other Alkalinizing Agents

Several other alkalinizing agents have been used experimentally in animals and humans to avoid the side effects of sodium bicarbonate. Unfortunately, none have demonstrated any real advantage over sodium bicarbonate. Carbicarb, a solution of equimolar amounts of sodium bicarbonate and sodium carbonate, may prove to be useful in correcting metabolic acidosis during CPR without many of the side effects of sodium bicarbonate[184]. Sodium carbonate consumes CO_2 and generates bicarbonate as illustrated in the following equation:

$$Na_2CO_3 + CO_2 + H_2O \rightarrow 2\ HCO^-_3 + 2\ Na^+$$

In animal models of CPR, Carbicarb administration resulted in a greater increase in arterial pH, and smaller increases in $PaCO_2$, lactate, and serum osmolality[184–186]. However, Carbicarb was not better than bicarbonate during hypovolemic shock in rats[187].

Dichloroacetate (DCA), another new alkalinizing agent, increases the activity of pyruvate dehydrogenase, which facilitates the conversion of lactate to pyruvate[188]. When administered to adult and pediatric patients with lactic acidosis, DCA decreased lactate concentration by 50% and increased bicarbonate concentration and pH[189]. DCA has been shown to improve cardiac output, possibly by enhancing myocardial metabolism of lactate and carbohydrate[190,191]. Unfortunately, in a multicenter trial of patients with lactic acidosis, DCA did not improve outcome compared with standard alkalinizing agents[192].

Tromethamine (THAM, tris-[hydroxymethyl]aminomethane), is an organic amine that attracts and combines with hydrogen ions. It is available as a 0.3M solution adjusted to a pH of 8.6. A dose of 3 ml/kilogram should raise the bicarbonate concentration by 3 mEq/liter. Side effects of this drug include hyperkalemia, hypoglycemia, acute hypocarbia, and apnea. In addition, peripheral vasodilation may occur when administered during CPR. THAM is contraindicated in patients with renal failure.

Calcium

The recommendations for the use of calcium during CPR have been restricted to a few specific situations, namely, hypocalcemia, hyperkalemia, hypermagnesemia and calcium channel blocker overdose. These restrictions are based on the possibility that exogenously administered calcium may worsen ischemia-reperfusion injury. Intracellular calcium overload occurs in many pathologic conditions, including ischemia, and appears to play an important role in the process of cell death[193,194]. Calcium channel blockers have been shown to improve blood flow and function after ischemia to the heart[195], kidney[196], and brain[197]. These studies suggest that intracellular calcium overload may contribute to the development of post-ischemic hypoperfusion. Calcium channel blockers also raise the threshold of the ischemic heart to ventricu-

Table 1.17. Adverse Effects of Hypocalcemia

Decrease myocardial contractility
Decrease systemic vascular resistance
Decrease catecholamine release
Decrease cardiovascular response to catecholamines

lar fibrillation[198]. For these reasons, it appears that the recommended restrictions for the use of calcium during CPR are well founded. On the other hand, no studies have shown that the transient elevation of plasma calcium concentration, which occurs after the administration of calcium, worsens outcome from cardiac arrest. Since the normal ratio of extracellular to intracellular calcium is on the order of 1,000:1 to 10,000:1, it seems unlikely that the rate of influx of calcium into cells would be influenced by a relatively small increase in its extracellular concentration.

The calcium ion is essential in myocardial excitation-contraction coupling, in increasing ventricular contractility, and in enhancing ventricular automaticity during asystole[199]. Ionized hypocalcemia leads, therefore, to decreased ventricular performance, peripheral vasodilation and blunting of the hemodynamic response to catecholamines[200–202] **(Table 1.17).** In addition, severe ionized hypocalcemia (mean 0.67 mmole/L) has been documented in adult patients suffering from out-of-hospital cardiac arrest[203] or sepsis[204], and in animals during prolonged CPR[205]. Because of these well established facts, physicians engaged in CPR must identify patients at risk for ionized hypocalcemia, determine if it is present, and treat it as expeditiously as possible.

Indications

Hypocalcemia occurs in patients with conditions predisposing to low total body calcium stores such as hypoparathyroidism, Di George syndrome, renal failure, pancreatitis and long-term use of loop diuretics. Ionized calcium concentration can be low in the presence of a normal total calcium. This can occur with severe alkalosis during iatrogenic hyperventilation and after the use of alkalinizing agents. Ionized hypocalcemia also occurs after massive or rapid transfusion of citrated blood products. The degree of hypocalcemia caused by citrated blood products depends on the rate of administration, the total dose, and the hepatic and renal function of the patient. Administration of 2 ml/kg/min of citrated whole blood causes a significant decrease in ionized calcium concentration in anesthetized patients **(Table 1.18).**

Table 1.18. Indications for Calcium

Hypocalcemia (total or ionized)
Hyperkalemia
Hypermagnesemia
Calcium channel blocker overdose

Table 1.19. Indications for Atropine

Bradycardia
Heart block (second- or third-degree)
Slow idioventricular rhythm
Asystole
Pulseless electrical activity

Dosage

The pediatric dose of calcium chloride is 20 mg/kg. The adult dose is 200 mg, or 2 ml of the 10 percent solution. Calcium gluconate is as effective as calcium chloride in raising ionized calcium concentration during CPR[206]. Calcium gluconate can be given at a dose of 30 to 100 mg/kg, with a maximum dose of 2 g in pediatric patients. Calcium should be given slowly through a large bore, free-flowing IV line, preferably a central venous line. Severe tissue necrosis occurs when calcium infiltrates into subcutaneous tissue. When administered too rapidly, calcium may cause severe bradycardia, heart block or ventricular standstill.

Atropine

Clinical Effects

Atropine is a parasympatholytic agent that acts by blocking cholinergic stimulation of the muscarinic receptors of the heart[207] This usually results in an increase in the sinus rate and shortening of atrio-ventricular node conduction time[208]. Atropine may activate latent ectopic pacemakers. Atropine has little effect on systemic vascular resistance, myocardial perfusion pressure or myocardial contractility[209].

Indications

Atropine is indicated for treatment of asystole, pulseless electrical activity (PEA), bradycardia associated with hypotension[210] second- and third-degree heart block, and slow idioventricular rhythms[211] **(Table 1.19).** In children who present in cardiac arrest, sinus bradycardia or asystole is commonly the initial rhythm and atropine is therefore useful as a first-line drug. Atropine is typically used in clinical conditions associated with excessive parasympathetic tone.

Dosage

The recommended pediatric dose of atropine is 0.02 mg/kg with a minimum dose of 0.15 mg and a maximum dose of 2.0 mg. A minimum dose is used because of the occurrence of paradoxical bradycardia resulting from a central stimulating effect on the medullary vagal nuclei[212]. Atropine may be given by any route including IV, endotracheal, intraosseous, intramuscular, or subcutaneous. Its onset of action occurs within thirty seconds and its peak effect occurs between 1 and 2 minutes after an IV dose. The recommended adult dose of atropine is 0.5 mg IV every 5 minutes until the desired heart rate is obtained, up to a maximum of 2.0 mg. For asystole, 1.0 mg IV is given and repeated in 5 minutes if asystole persists. Full vagal blockade is usually obtained with a dose of 2.0 mg.

Side Effects

Atropine should not be used in patients in whom tachycardia is undesirable. In patients after myocardial infarction or ischemia with persistent bradycardia, atropine should be used in the lowest dose possible to increase the heart rate. Tachycardia, which increases myocardial oxygen consumption and can lead to ventricular fibrillation, is common after large doses of atropine in these patients. In patients with pulmonary or systemic outflow tract obstruction or idiopathic hypertrophic subaortic stenosis, tachycardia can decrease ventricular filling and lower cardiac output.

Glucose

The administration of glucose during CPR should be restricted to patients with documented hypoglycemia because of the possible detrimental effects of hyperglycemia on the brain during ischemia. Myers et al. were the first to hypothesize that hyperglycemia worsens neurologic outcome after cardiac arrest[(213)]. He found that infant monkeys that received glucose before cardiac arrest were more likely to develop seizures, prolonged coma, brain death or cerebral necrosis than those that received saline. Siemkowicz and Hansen confirmed this finding when they demonstrated that after 10 minutes of global brain ischemia the neurologic recovery of hyperglycemic rats was worse then that of normoglycemic controls[(214)]. The mechanism by which hyperglycemia exacerbates ischemic neurologic injury may be a result of an increased production of lactic acid in the brain by anaerobic metabolism. During ischemia under normoglycemic conditions, brain lactate concentration reaches a plateau, whereas in a hyperglycemia milieu, brain lactate concentration continues to rise for the duration of the ischemic period[(215)]. The severity of intracellular acidosis during brain ischemia is directly proportional to the pre-ischemic glucose concentration[(216)]. The deleterious effect of hyperglycemia during brain ischemia appears to require a "trickle" of blood flow, as Prado et al. showed that collaterally perfused but not end-arterial brain tissue had greater neuronal damage during hyperglycemic ischemia[(217)].

Clinical studies have shown a direct correlation between the initial serum glucose concentration and poor neurologic outcome[(218–221)]. Longstreth et al. have suggested that a higher admission glucose concentration may be an endogenous response to severe stress and thus is a marker and not the cause of the more severe brain injury[(222)]. In a recent study of infant piglets, post-ischemic administration of glucose did not worsen neurologic outcome after global hypoxia-ischemia[(223)]. However, given the likelihood of additional ischemic and hypoxic events in the post-resuscitation period it seems prudent to maintain serum glucose in the normal range. Voll and Ames have shown that the administration of insulin to hyperglycemic rats after global brain ischemia improved neurologic outcome[(224)]. Interestingly, the effect of insulin may be independent of its ability to lower blood glucose since these investigators later showed that normoglycemic insulin-treated rats had less brain injury than placebo-treated controls[(225)]. Additional studies need to be done to determine if the benefit from tight control of serum glucose after cardiac arrest outweighs the risk of iatrogenic hypoglycemia.

Infants, particularly prematures and debilitated patients with low endogenous glycogen stores are prone to developing hypoglycemia during and after a physiologic stress (i.e. surgery)[(226)]. In these patients, bedside monitoring of serum glucose is critical and allows intervention before the critical point of substrate delivery has been reached. The dose of glucose needed to correct hypoglycemia is 0.5 to 1.0 g/kg given as 50% dextrose in adults and children, and as 10% dextrose in infants (the osmolarity of 50% dextrose is approximately 2700 osm/L and may cause intraventricular hemorrhage in neonates and infants).

Oxygen

Patients in cardiac arrest or low cardiac output states should receive 100% oxygen as soon as possible regardless of the etiology of the arrest. Oxygen increases arterial oxygen tension, hemoglobin saturation and arterial oxygen content if ventilation is maintained. A higher PaO_2 lowers pulmonary vascular resistance and decreases right ventricular stroke work index. One hundred percent oxygen should not be withheld from patients in cardiac arrest who have bronchopulmonary dysplasia or chronic obstructive pulmonary disease.

Newer and Experimental Drug Therapies

In the field of brain resuscitation, many investigators have laid claim to miracle drugs which improve neurologic outcome. To date, none of these drugs have actually been shown to improve neurologic outcome after global brain ischemia in humans. The list of pharmacologic and other therapeutic maneuvers to enhance cardiac or cerebral recovery after cardiac arrest or other global ischemic events continues to grow in length and variety. It remains to be seen whether these therapeutic modalities will ever become part of resuscitation protocols **(Table 1.20).**

THERAPY FOR VENTRICULAR FIBRILLATION

Electric Countershock

History

In 1775, Squires described a possible cardiac arrest and successful electrical defibrillation of a 3 year-old child who had fallen out of an upper story window[(6)]. Hosack, in the early 1790s, wrote about the use of electricity in resuscita-

Table 1.20. Experimental Therapies

Calcium channel blockers
Glutamate receptor antagonists
Opiate receptor antagonists
Central alpha-2 receptor antagonists
Beta receptor antagonists
Oxygen radical scavengers
Iron chelators
Xanthine oxidase inhibitors
Inhibitors of arachidonic acid metabolism
Thrombolytic agents
Corticosteroids
21-aminosteroids
Magnesium
Cerebral vasodilators
Metabolic activators
Hypothermia

tion. The Humane Society of New York called electricity at that time, "a most powerful agent, a very proper remedy". The Society outlined a procedure for defibrillation whereby the patient was electrified for 4 to 5 minutes in order to excite the heart to action[5].

In 1899, Prevost and Batelli reported the first documented use of alternating current (AC) to defibrillate an open dog heart[227]. The electric utility companies actually funded much of the early research in defibrillation hoping to reverse the high number of electric shock fatalities in their workers[228,229]. In 1933, Hooker and coworkers[230] at Johns Hopkins University again described successful open-heart defibrillation in dogs. In 1939, the Soviets, Furvich and Yuniev[3] described the first successful external defibrillation in dogs. In 1947, Beck performed the first successful open-chest defibrillation of an operating room patient[231]. Zoll, in 1956, performed the first documented successful external defibrillation in humans[232].

Physiology of Ventricular Fibrillation

Ventricular fibrillation is a sustained burst of multiple, uncoordinated regional ventricular depolarizations and contractions which are associated with an absent cardiac output and no myocardial blood flow. The rhythm is maintained by re-entrant impulses generated within the ventricles with multiple, shifting circuits. Conditions which lower the threshold for ventricular fibrillation include hypoxemia, hypercapnia, myocardial ischemia, hypothermia, metabolic acidosis, and electrolyte disturbances including Na^+, K^+, Ca^{++}, and Mg^{++} **(Table 1.21).**

Ventricular fibrillation and ventricular tachycardia are uncommon rhythms during cardiac arrest in children. Walsh and Krongrad examined the terminal electrocardiograms in 100 in-hospital pediatric arrest patients and found that in over 90% of cases the initial electrical disturbance was a bradyarrhythmia which progressed to asystole, without any evidence for ventricular ectopy. Children with congenital heart disease, a history of cardiac surgery, severe electrolyte disturbance, toxic ingestion or infiltrative disease of the heart are at increased risk for ventricular fibrillation.

Physiology of Electric Countershock

Electric countershock is the treatment of choice for ventricular fibrillation and ventricular tachycardia when a pulse is not present or when the patient is comatose as a result of the arrhythmia. Drug treatment by itself cannot be relied upon to terminate ventricular fibrillation in these instances. Antiarrhythmic agents such as lidocaine are known cardiac depressants and may transform ventricular fibrillation into intractable asystole[231,232]. High-voltage electric shock, when properly applied, sends more than 2 amperes through the heart. Ventricular fibrillation is terminated by simultaneously depolarizing and causing a sustained contraction of the entire myocardium which allows return of spontaneous coordinated cardiac contractions, assuming the myocardium is well oxygenated and the acid-base status is normal.

Modern day defibrillators deliver only direct current (DC) shocks. Alternating current (AC) countershock is no longer used because it is hazardous to both the patient and the operator. Furthermore, DC defibrillators are portable, while AC defibrillators depend on wall current. The type of wave form of current may influence the amount of energy needed to defibrillate the heart. Most defibrillators use a dampened sine wave form although some use a trapezoidal wave form.

Higher energy levels cause a greater amount of myocardial damage[233,234]. Moreover, as the energy dose increases, the incidence of post-defibrillation arrhythmias increases[235]. Frequent, concentrated high-density electrical currents can damage the myocardium, decrease the likelihood of successful defibrillation and lead to post-defibrillation arrhythmias[236]. These arrhythmias are thought to be associated with prolonged depolarization of the myocardial cell membrane, which increases with the intensity of the stimulus and provides an ideal setting for re-entrant arrhythmias[237]. High dose defibrillation causes a transient electromechanical deformation of the cell membrane[237]. In humans after synchronized defibrillation, the frequency of arrhythmias and the amount of ST segment displacement are directly related to the energy level used[198]. Two low-energy shocks may cause more damage than a single shock of identical total energy so an adequate energy level should be used. However, myocardial damage was greater when one dose was given compared to the same total energy delivered in two doses in another study[238].

In the majority of adult cases, energy levels of 100 to

Table 1.21. Conditions That Lower the Threshold for Ventricular Fibrillation

Hypoxemia
Hypercapnia
Metabolic acidosis
Myocardial ischemia
Hypothermia
Electrolyte disturbances (Na^+, K^+, Ca^{++}, Mg^{++})

Table 1.22. Defibrillation

	Dose–1st Attempt	Dose–2nd Attempt	Dose–3rd and Subsequent	Paddle Size	
				External	Internal
Infant	2J/kg	4J/kg	4J/kg	4.5cm	2cm
Child	2J/kg	4J/kg	4J/kg	8cm	4cm
Adult	200J	200J	400J	13cm	6cm

300 J are successful when shocks are delivered with minimal delay. The claim that larger patients require higher voltage (500–1000 J) has been refuted by a number of investigators[(236,239)]. In one study reviewing 233 episodes of ventricular fibrillation in an in-hospital group of adults, 95% were successfully defibrillated with 200 J stored energy, even in patients weighing more than 100 kg[(239)]. Another group compared the use of 175 and 320 J shocks in 249 adult patients with ventricular fibrillation. Survival was unrelated to the energy level used for defibrillation or the weight of the patient, which ranged up to 102 kg[(236)]. Studies supporting the need for very high energy levels for defibrillation, especially in larger patients, were based on retrospective clinical data and on experimental studies comparing different species of animals[(240)]. Others have reaffirmed the successful use of low-energy shocks for defibrillation, even in large patients[(241,242)], and one study showed no differences in heart weight or energy per gram of heart weight to defibrillate in patients who ultimately had an autopsy[(243)]. The goal of defibrillation is to deliver a minimum of electrical energy to a critical mass of ventricular muscle while avoiding high current that could further damage the heart.

Zipes et al. found that a critical amount of myocardial tissue must be depolarized to terminate ventricular fibrillation[(244)]. However, depolarization of every myocardial cell is not necessary to terminate fibrillation of the heart. Electric shocks terminate ventricular fibrillation most often when the shocks are delivered between electrodes located at the apex of the right ventricle and the posterior base of the left ventricle, and least often when the shock is delivered between two right ventricular electrodes.

Several clinical factors affect the efficacy of ventricular defibrillation in humans. The most reliable predictor of success of defibrillation is the duration of fibrillation prior to the first countershock[(243)]. The success of defibrillation decreases with an increased duration of fibrillation. Defibrillatory attempts were successful in patients who were shocked before 8 minutes elapsed after the onset of ventricular fibrillation, whereas attempts were unsuccessful in patients shocked with a mean of 17 minutes after the onset of fibrillation[(243)]. Acidosis and hypoxia also decrease the success of defibrillation[(243)]. The temperature of the patient does not alter the energy dose required for successful defibrillation[(245)]. Patients with terminal illness are more resistent to successful defibrillation[(246)], as are those who fibrillate later in the course of their myocardial infarction.

Table 1.23. Reevaluation if Defibrillation is Unsuccessful

Oxygenation
Ventilation
Acid-base status
Mechanical problem
Pneumothorax
Inadequate paddle/chest wall interface
Excessive distance between paddles
Inadequate paddle pressure on chest
Poor paddle position

Clinical Aspects of Pediatric Defibrillation

For the first defibrillatory attempt, 200 to 300 J delivered energy should be administered to adults and 2 J/kg to children **(Table 1.22).** If this attempt is unsuccessful, a second and third attempt are made immediately, using the same energy dose in adults and 4 J/kg in children. If these attempts are unsuccessful, then basic life support is continued, epinephrine is administered, and sodium bicarbonate is given if metabolic acidosis is documented or if the duration of cardiac arrest warrants its administration **(Table 1.23).** A fourth defibrillatory attempt is then made at a setting that does not exceed 360 J of delivered energy or 4 J/kilogram in children. If ventricular fibrillation recurs frequently, lidocaine, bretylium, or procainamide may be used. It is not necessary to increase the energy dose on each successive shock during defibrillation. On the contrary, the threshold for ventricular fibrillation often increases after CPR and resuscitation drugs are administered **(Table 1.24).**

The dose of 2 J/kg is based on 71 defibrillatory attempts in 27 children. Fifty seven shocks were within 10 J above or below an energy dose of 2 J/kg of body weight. Ninety-one percent of these shocks were effective[(247)].

Correct paddle size and position are critical to the success of defibrillation. Three paddle sizes are used to defibrillate externally: 13 cm in diameter for adults, 8 cm for older children, and 4.5 cm for infants. The largest paddle size appropriate for the patient should be used because a larger size reduces the density of current flow, which in turn reduces myocardial damage. If the entire paddle does not rest firmly on the chest wall a current of high density will be delivered to a small contact point. The paddles should be positioned on the chest wall so that a majority of myocardium lies directly between them. One paddle is placed to the right of the upper sternum below the clavicle, the other positioned just below and to the left of the left nipple. For patients with dextrocardia, the position of the paddles should be a mirror image. An alternative approach is to place one paddle anteriorly over the left precordium and the other paddle posteriorly between the scapulae.

Table 1.24. Algorithm for Treatment of Ventricular Fibrillation

Begin CPR (Airway, Breathing, Circulation)		
1st defibrillate	(2J/kg)	
2nd defibrillate	(4J/kg)	
3rd defibrillate	(4J/kg)	
1st epinephrine	(10 µg/kg) IV/IO 100 µg/kg-ETT	Subsequent doses of epinephrine every 3–5 mins: 100 µg/kg - IV/IO/ETT
1st lidocaine	(1 mg/kg) IV/IO/ETT	
4th defibrillate	(4 J/kg)	
2nd epinephrine	(see sidebar)	
2nd lidocaine	(1 mg/kg)	
1st bretylium	(5 mg/kg)	
5th defibrillate	(4J/kg)	
2nd bretylium	(10 mg/kg)	

The interface between the paddle and chest wall can be electrode cream, paste, saline, soap, or moist gauze pads. The electrode cream produces lower impedance than the paste. Electric current follows the path of least resistance, so care should be taken that the substance from one paddle does not touch that of the other paddle. This is especially important in infants, where the distance between paddles is short. If the gel is continuous between paddles, a short circuit is created, and an insufficient amount of current will cross the heart.

If the duration of ventricular fibrillation is less than 2 minutes, then a defibrillatory attempt should be administered as soon as possible. If ventricular fibrillation has been present for longer than 2 minutes or for an undetermined period of time, then basic life support should be initiated for at least 2 minutes before attempting defibrillation in order to improve myocardial oxygenation and acid-base status(248).

Open-Chest Defibrillation

If the chest is already opened, ventricular fibrillation should be treated with open-chest defibrillation, using internal paddles applied directly to the heart. These should have a diameter of 6 cm for adults, 4 cm for children, and 2 cm for infants. Handles should be insulated. Saline-soaked pads or gauzes should be placed between the paddles and the heart. One electrode is placed behind the left ventricle and the other over the right ventricle on the anterior surface of the heart. The dosage used should begin at 5 J in infants and 20 J in adults.

Lidocaine

Chemistry

Lidocaine is a class IB anti-arrhythmic. The chemical structure of lidocaine is an aromatic group—2 to 6 xylidine coupled to diethylglycine via an amide bond. It is a weak base with a pKa of 7.85.

Electrophysiology

Lidocaine causes a decrease in automaticity and in spontaneous phase 4 depolarization of pacemaker tissue. Lidocaine increases the ventricular fibrillatory threshold, and slightly increases or has no effect on the ventricular diastolic threshold for depolarization. The duration of action potential of Purkinje fibers and ventricular muscle is decreased, while the effective refractory period of these fibers is increased. Lidocaine has no effect on conduction times through the AV node or on intraventricular conduction time.

By decreasing automaticity, lidocaine prevents or terminates ventricular arrhythmias because of accelerated ectopic foci. Lidocaine abolishes re-entrant ventricular arrhythmias by decreasing the action potential duration and the conduction time of Purkinje fibers, and increases the effective refractory period of Purkinje fibers, reducing the nonuniformity of contraction. Because the microcirculation of ischemic myocardium may differ greatly from that of normal tissue, and since ventricular arrhythmias are thought to originate from ischemic areas of myocardium, lidocaine concentration as well as oxygen content may be much lower in ischemic zones than in the usual in vitro preparations(249).

Lidocaine has been shown to be effective in terminating ventricular premature beats (VPBs) and ventricular tachycardia in humans during general surgery, before or after cardiac surgery, after an acute myocardial infarction, and in patients with digitalis intoxication. Treatment of VPBs after myocardial infarction is indicated if they occur at a rate of more than 5 per minute of unifocal origin, on a normal T-wave, with multifocal VPBs or with ventricular tachycardia. Lidocaine is also effective in preventing and treating ventricular arrhythmias during cardiac catheterization. It is indicated after cardioversion from ventricular fibrillation especially with recurrent ventricular fibrillation or tachycardia. Lidocaine has not been found to be effective in the treatment of atrial or AV junctional arrhythmias.

Hemodynamic Effects

In dogs, when lidocaine is given by a rapid IV bolus, there is a transient decrease in stroke work, blood pressure, systemic vascular resistance(250), and left ventricular contractility(251), and a slight increase in the heart rate. In healthy adults, no change in heart rate or blood pressure occurs with lidocaine administration(252). In patients with cardiac disease, there is only a slight or no decrease in ventricular function when a lidocaine bolus is administered intravenously(252). In patients with cardiac disease, especially in those with acute myocardial infarction, excessive doses of lidocaine given by rapid infusion may lead to a decrease in cardiac function. Therefore, slow IV administration, no greater than 50 to 100 mg/minute in adults, is recommended(249).

Pharmacokinetics and Pharmacodynamics

Lidocaine is metabolized mainly in the liver by the microsomal enzyme system[249]. Its major degradative pathway is by oxidative N-de-ethylation, followed by hydrolysis to 2 to 6 xylidine. Its minor degradative pathway is by hydroxylation of its aromatic nitrogen. Normally up to 10% of the dose is excreted unchanged in the urine, however, this fraction is increased when the urine is acidic. There is no biliary excretion and no intestinal absorption in humans.

After an IV dose of lidocaine is given, or after discontinuing a constant infusion, the changes in plasma concentration follow a biphasic curve. The early, rapid fall in concentration, the α, has an average half-life of 8 to 17 minutes. It exists as a result of changes in distribution of lidocaine within two compartments: the central compartment containing the intravascular space, and the peripheral compartment, which includes hepatic metabolism of the drug in the central compartment. In patients with normal liver function, the hepatic extraction ratio for lidocaine is approximately 70%. The β region, during which there is a slower decrease in serum concentration and an average half-life of 87 to 108 minutes, is a result of transfer of drug from the larger, peripheral compartment to the smaller, central compartment.

To achieve and maintain therapeutic levels of the drug, a bolus dose of lidocaine should be given at the same time that a constant infusion is initiated. Without an initial bolus, approximately five half-lives are required to approach plateau concentration of an infused drug[249]. With a half-life of 108 minutes, a 9 hour infusion of lidocaine would be required to reach a plateau concentration. Ventricular arrhythmias often return within 15 to 20 minutes after an IV bolus as a result of rapid clearance from the central compartment[252].

Lidocaine toxicity occurs when the serum concentration exceeds 7 to 8 μg/ml, and occurs most commonly in patients with severe hepatic disease or severe congestive heart failure. Lidocaine clearance decreases during low cardiac output states because of the concomitant fall of hepatic blood flow. During CPR, lidocaine clearance is decreased because of the inherent decrease in cardiac output. In dogs, with use of conventional CPR to attain a blood pressure of 20% of control, a bolus of lidocaine of 2 mg/kilogram IV resulted in very elevated blood and tissue concentrations compared to control animals, distribution of the drug, as measured by tissue extraction, was complete in 20 minutes. Also, lidocaine clearance and distribution may be altered because of changes in protein binding and metabolism during CPR[253]. In humans, high peak blood and tissue concentrations of lidocaine are observed during CPR, with a delay in the time to the peak concentration of the drug[254].

Dosage

In patients with normal cardiac and hepatic function, an initial IV bolus of 1.5 to 2 mg/kg of lidocaine is given followed by a constant IV infusion at a rate of 55 μg/kg/minute. If the arrhythmia recurs, a second IV bolus at the same dose can be given[199]. The eventual steady state plasma concentration of the drug is not affected by this dose. Patients with a moderate decrease in cardiac output or those suffering an acute myocardial infarction should receive only 1 to 1.5 mg/kg IV bolus, with an infusion rate of 30 μg/kg/minute. In patients with severe diminution of cardiac output, a bolus of no greater than 0.75 mg/kg is administered, followed by an infusion at the rate of 10 to 20 μg/kg/minute. In patients with hepatic disease, dosages should be decreased to 50% of normal. Patients with chronic renal disease on hemodialysis have normal lidocaine pharmacokinetics. However, toxic metabolites may accumulate in patients receiving infusions over a long period of time. Thus, caution should be used in these patients. In patients with hypoproteinemia, the dose of lidocaine should also be lowered, owing to the increase in free fraction of drug. Measurement of steady-state lidocaine concentration is useful in achieving the therapeutic effects of lidocaine while avoiding its side effects.

Drug interactions with lidocaine are common. Phenobarbital increases lidocaine metabolism, so higher doses of lidocaine are needed. Isoniazid and chloramphenicol decrease lidocaine metabolism, so lower doses should be used with those drugs. Propranolol increases the serum concentration by decreasing cardiac output, while isoproterenol decreases the serum concentration by increasing cardiac output.

Side Effects

Toxic effects of lidocaine are seen when the serum concentration of free drug exceeds 7 μg/ml and usually involve the central nervous system. The central nervous symptoms of lidocaine toxicity include seizures, psychosis, drowsiness, paresthesias, disorientation, agitation, tinnitus, muscle spasms, and respiratory arrest. Treatment of choice for lidocaine-induced seizures is phenobarbital or a benzodiazapene (i.e. midazolam). Barbiturates may be the better choice since they also increase the hepatic metabolism of lidocaine. True allergic reactions to lidocaine are rare. Cardiovascular side effects, as discussed above, are usually seen when large IV boluses are given rapidly to patients with decreased myocardial function. Conversion of second-degree heart block to complete heart block has been described[255], as well as severe sinus bradycardia. These effects appear to be infrequent and occur when large doses are administered. These potential side effects do not prohibit the cautious use of lidocaine **(Table 1.25)**.

Bretylium

Chemistry

Bretylium, a class III anti-arrhythmic, is a bromobenzyl quaternary ammonia compound and is not structurally related to lidocaine.

Pharmacokinetics

The half-life of bretylium gradually increases over time, with a mean elimination half-life of 9.8 hours[256]. The drug

Table 1.25. Characteristics of Lidocaine and Bretylium

	Lidocaine	*Bretylium*
Chemical Structure	Aromatic 2–6 xylidine coupled to diethylglycine	Bromobenzyl quaternary ammonia compound
Metabolism	Liver 10% unchanged in urine	>90% unchanged in urine
Electrophysiology	↓Automaticity of pacemaker tissue ↑Ventricular fibrillatory threshold ↓Action potential duration in ventricle ↑Effective refractory period of ventricle AV node–no effect	Initial release of norepinephrine followed by a blockade of release of norepinephrine ↑Action potential duration in ventricle ↑Effective refractory period in ventricle ↑Ventricle fibrillatory threshold
Clinical antiarrhythmic effects	Frequent ventricular premature beats (VPB) (>6/min) Coupled VPBs Multiform tachycardia Ventricular tachycardia Prophylaxis during cardiac catheterization Prophylaxis following resuscitation	Treat ventricular tachycardia when first line treatment fails
Half-life	~90 min	~10 hours
Dosage	1 mg/kg bolus, IV If arrhythmia recurs, give second bolus; decrease dose if there is coexisting decrease in cardiac output or hepatic disease	5–10 mg/kg IV over 10 min
Side Effects	CNS–seizures, psychosis, drowsiness, paresthesias, disorientation, muscle twitching, agitation, respiratory arrest; CV–slight decrease in cardiac function in patients with pre-existing heart disease	Nausea and vomiting Initial increase in blood pressure and heart rate followed by a decrease in blood pressure Increased sensitivity to dopamine, epinephrine, and norepinephrine Parotid swelling

is 80% excreted unchanged in the urine over the first 24 hours. An additional 10% of the drug is excreted in the urine over the next 72 hours[(257)].

Mechanism of Action

The mechanism of action of bretylium appears to be by adrenergic stimulation. There is an initial release of norepinephrine from adrenergic nerve endings, with subsequent inhibition of release of norepinephrine[(258)]. The drug also blocks the reuptake of norepinephrine and epinephrine into these adrenergic nerve endings, thereby potentiating the action of these agonists on adrenal receptors.

Bretylium appears to have direct cardiac effects, which are not abolished by β-adrenergic blockade[(259)], nor prevented by pretreatment with reserpine or denervation of the heart[(260)]. Bretylium increases the action potential duration of cardiac muscle and the effective refractory period of Purkinje and ventricular muscle fibers. In dogs, bretylium decreases the disparity in action potential duration between normal and infarcted areas of the heart. This is the most plausible explanation for its antiarrhythmic actions[(260)]. Bretylium also increases the electrical threshold for ventricular fibrillation in normal and infarcted hearts. Bretylium has been noted to defibrillate a heart without electric countershock[(261)]. It may be more effective in raising the ventricular fibrillatory threshold than lidocaine, phenytoin, procainamide, propranolol, or quinidine.

Clinical Effects

Many studies have found bretylium to be effective in suppressing ventricular arrhythmias when other antiarrhythmics have not, including ventricular fibrillation resistant to electric countershock[(262)]. It is presently indicated for the treatment of life-threatening ventricular arrhythmias, principally ventricular fibrillation and ventricular tachycardia, that have failed to respond to adequate doses of the first-line antiarrhythmic agents, lidocaine or procainamide. Of course, electrical cardioversion in still the first line of treatment for the above problems. The drug is not used to suppress asymptomatic VPBs, nor is the drug used to treat atrial arrhythmias.

When lidocaine and bretylium were compared as the initial treatment for 146 patients suffering from out-of-hospital ventricular fibrillation, there was no difference in the number of patients achieving a stable rhythm, the time needed to achieve a stable rhythm, the number of defibrillation shocks required, or the number of patients discharged from the hospital[(263)].

Dosage

The dose of bretylium is 5 to 10 mg/kg given by rapid IV bolus to treat ventricular fibrillation. If the drug can be given less urgently, 500 mg should be diluted in no less than 50 ml of fluid. It should be given over 10 minutes, which decreases the severity of orthostatic hypotension in the awake patient. Its onset of action in suppressing ventricular fibrillation and facilitating electrical conversion is within minutes, although it can be delayed up to 10 to 15 minutes. After an intramuscular injection, the drug is not effective for 20 to 60 minutes. Its duration of action is 6 to 12 hours[(262)].

After an IV bolus of bretylium is given, an electric countershock should be administered. If the arrhythmia persists, the drug can be repeated every 15 to 30 minutes, up to a total dose of 30 mg/kg. If the arrhythmia is eradicated, a

Table 1.26. Causes of Pulseless Electrical Activity

Cardiac–Primary
Depletion of myocardial energy stores
Non-Cardiac Secondary
Hypovolemia
Pericardial tamponade
Tension pneumothorax
Pulmonary embolism

maintenance dose, the same as the initial dose, can then be given every 6 to 8 hours. If ventricular tachycardia is being treated, the second dose should be repeated in 1 to 2 hours and then every 6 to 8 hours for maintenance. The drug can also be given by constant infusion at 1 to 2 mg/minute in adults.

Side Effects

When bretylium is given, an initial increase in blood pressure, as a result of norepinephrine release, is often seen[(258)]. A slight increase in heart rate, cardiac output and an increase in the frequency of VPBs may also be seen. After administration of bretylium, 50 to 75% of patients subsequently show a mild decrease in blood pressure as a result of the adrenergic blocking effects of bretylium[(262)]. If hypotension is severe, fluids and vasopressors should be given. After receiving bretylium, there may be an exaggerated response to dopamine, norepinephrine, and epinephrine because of the impaired reuptake of these drugs. On maintenance doses, patients become tolerant within a few days to its hypotensive effect. With a rapid infusion of the drug, nausea and vomiting are common. Parotid swelling and pain have been seen with oral bretylium use[(262)] **(Table 1.25).**

PULSELESS ELECTRICAL ACTIVITY

Pulseless electrical activity (PEA), formerly known as electromechanical dissociation (EMD) is defined as organized ECG activity, excluding ventricular tachycardia and fibrillation, without clinical evidence of a palpable pulse or myocardial contractions. It may occur spontaneously after cardiac arrest or as an intervening rhythm associated with treatment for cardiac arrest. The etiology of PEA is divided into primary (cardiac) and secondary (non-cardiac) causes **(Table 1.26)**. Primary PEA, associated with cardiac arrest, is a result of depletion of myocardial energy stores and, as such, responds poorly to therapy. Drugs used for primary PEA include epinephrine, atropine, calcium and sodium bicarbonate. The causes of secondary PEA include hypovolemia, tension pneumothorax, pericardial tamponade, pulmonary embolism, and sympathetic nervous system failure[(264)]. In secondary PEA, intervention is directed at the underlying disorder and usually results in a successful resuscitation. In contrast, patients with primary PEA are difficult to resuscitate. When the cause of PEA is unknown and the patient does not respond to medical intervention one should consider giving a fluid bolus and inserting needles into the pleural and pericardial spaces. In a study of 503 adults with PEA, patients who were successfully resuscitated more commonly had normal QRS and QT intervals, tachycardia, presence of P waves and return of P waves after pharmacologic intervention, compared to those not resuscitated from PEA[(265)]. Resuscitation, but not survival, of patients with PEA was improved with the use of cardiopulmonary bypass and epinephrine[(266)].

Table 1.27. Open-chest CPR–Indications

Operating Room
Cardiac arrest secondary to:
Cardiac tamponade
Critical aortic stenosis
Hypothermia
Ruptured aortic aneurysm
Chest already opened during surgery
Non-Operating Room
Penetrating chest trauma
Crushed chest injury
Anatomic chest wall abnormalities
Failure of closed-chest CPR

OPEN-CHEST CPR

The use of open-chest cardiac massage has generally been replaced by closed-chest CPR[(7)]. Compared to closed-chest CPR, open-chest CPR generates higher cardiac output and vital organ blood flow. During open-chest CPR there is much less elevation of intrathoracic, right atrial or intracranial pressure. This results in higher coronary and cerebral perfusion pressure and higher myocardial and cerebral blood flow[(267–269)].

Open-chest CPR is obviously not a technique that can be applied by most health care personnel. In the operating room, critical care units and emergency departments equipped with the necessary surgical and technical expertise, open-chest CPR is indicated for cardiac arrests secondary to cardiac tamponade, hypothermia, critical aortic stenosis, and ruptured aortic aneurysm. Other indications for open-chest CPR include cardiac arrest secondary to penetrating or crushed chest wall injuries and chest wall abnormalities that make closed-chest CPR impossible or ineffective[(15)]. Open-chest CPR is indicated for selected patients when closed-chest CPR has failed, although exactly which patients should receive this method of resuscitationis controversial. When initiated early after failure of closed-chest CPR, open-chest CPR may improve outcome[(270,271)]. When performed after 15 minutes of closed-chest CPR, open-chest CPR significantly improves coronary perfusion pressure and the rate of successful resuscitation[(272)] **(Table 1.27).**

TRANSCUTANEOUS CARDIAC PACING

Transcutaneous cardiac pacing (TCP) is used as a method of noninvasive pacing of the ventricles for a relatively short

Table 1.28. Indications for Temporary Pacing

Symptomatic bradycardia
Heart block with slow ventricular rate

period of time. Emergency cardiac pacing is successful in resuscitation only if it is initiated soon after the onset of the arrest. In the absence of in situ pacing wires or an indwelling transvenous or esophageal pacing catheter, transcutaneous cardiac pacing is the preferred method for temporary electrical cardiac pacing. The 1992 American Heart Association's ACLS guidelines recommends early use of an external pacemaker in patients with symptomatic bradycardia and suggested its use for patients in asystole[(15)].

Zoll established TCP in 1952 as a clinically useful method of pacing adult patients during ventricular standstill (Stokes-Adams attacks) and bradycardia-associated hypotension[(272a)]. Since that time, numerous anecdotal reports have appeared supporting the use of TCP in bradycardia or asystolic arrests[(273)]. Zoll et al. reported successful in-hospital resuscitation of 12 of 16 patients with hypotensive bradycardia or asystole if TCP was initiated within 5 minutes of the arrest. In contrast, if TCP was begun between 5 and 30 minutes after the arrest, only 8 of 44 patients with these rhythms could be resuscitated[(274)]. In two controlled clinical trials of pre-hospital TCP there were no differences in the survival rate or success of resuscitation in paced and non-paced patients who had asystole or PEA[(275,276)]. In patients with symptomatic bradycardia, the use of TCP resulted in a higher incidence of return of palpable pulses and ultimate survival[(277)].

To date there have been no studies of the efficacy of TCP in pediatric resuscitation. Beland et al. showed that effective transcutaneous cardiac pacing could be achieved in hemodynamically stable children during induction of anesthesia for heart surgery. They were successful in 53 of 56 pacing trials and their patients suffered no complications[(278)].

TCP is indicated for patients whose primary problem is impulse formation or conduction, with preserved myocardial function. TCP is most effective in patients with sinus bradycardia or high-grade AV block with slow ventricular response who also have a stroke volume sufficient to generate a pulse. At this time, TCP is not indicated for patients in prolonged arrest, as this most likely would result in electrical but not mechanical cardiac capture and may delay or interfere with other resuscitative efforts **(Table 1.28).**

TCP involves placing two stimulating electrodes on the thorax, one placed anteriorly at the left sternal border and the other posteriorly just below the left scapula. Smaller pediatric electrodes are available for infants and children; adult size electrodes can be used in children over 15 kg[(278)]. ECG leads should be connected to the pacemaker, the demand, or asynchronous mode selected, and an age-appropriate heart rate used. The stimulus output should be set at zero when the pacemaker is turned on and then increased gradually until electrical capture is seen on the monitor. The output required for hemodynamically unstable rhythms is higher than that for hemodynamically stable rhythms in children in whom the mean stimulus required for capture was between 51 and 65 mA[(256)]. After electrical capture is achieved, one must ascertain whether effective arterial pulses are generated. If pulses are not adequate, other resuscitative efforts should be employed.

The most serious complication of TCP is the induction of ventricular arrhythmias[(279)]. Fortunately, this is rare and may be prevented by pacing only in the demand mode. Mild transient erythema beneath the electrodes is common. Skeletal muscle contraction can be minimized by using large electrodes, a 40 ms pulse duration and the smallest stimulus required for capture. Sedatives or analgesics may be necessary in the awake patient. If defibrillation or cardioversion is necessary, one must allow a distance of 2 to 3 cm between the electrode and paddles to prevent arcing of the current.

SUPRAVENTRICULAR TACHYCARDIA

Supraventricular tachycardia (SVT) is a common arrhythmia which may be associated with severe circulatory compromise or even cardiac arrest. Therapy for this arrhythmia should be based on the child's hemodynamic status. SVT associated with poor circulation including poor peripheral perfusion, hypotension, or a depressed level of consciousness should be immediately treated with synchronized cardioversion beginning at a dose of 0.5 J/kg. If IV access is available, adenosine can be used as cardioversion is being prepared, however cardioversion should not be delayed while IV access is being achieved.

Adenosine is the medical treatment of choice for SVT. The underlying mechanism in children is usually a re-entry circuit involving the atrio-ventricular (AV) node. Adenosine is an endogenous nucleoside that causes a temporary block in the AV node and interrupts this re-entry circuit. It is rapidly and highly effective with minimal side effects[(280)]. It has been used in a variety of settings including during general anesthesia[(281)], open heart surgery[(282)], and in the ICU[(283)]. The initial dose is 0.1 mg/kg given as a rapid IV bolus. Central venous administration is preferable since the drug is rapidly metabolized by red blood cell adenosine deaminase and thus has a half-life of only ten seconds; higher doses may be necessary when the drug is given peripherally. If there is no interruption in the re-entry circuit, successive doses should be doubled up to a maximum single dose of 12 mg until the arrhythmia is broken. In neonates, a smaller initial dose of 0.05 mg/kg is given and increased by 0.05 mg/kg/dose until termination of the arrhythmia up to a maximum of 0.25 mg/kg is suggested[(284)]. When SVT appears without any circulatory compromise, conversion of the arrhythmia may be first attempted with a vagal maneuver such as ice water to the face. If ineffective, then adenosine should be used as the first line drug. Digoxin is often ineffective and may have substantial side effects. Verapamil should be avoided in infants because of its association with congestive heart failure and cardiac arrest as a result of its negative inotropic effects[285]. Its use in older children is also discouraged. Other therapies include β-adrenergic blockers, edrophonium and β-agonists. If SVT persists despite medical therapy and the patient progresses to circulatory instability, electrical cardioversion should proceed immediately.

Algorithms for CPR Situations

(Tables 1.24, 1.29, 1.30, 1.31.)

Table 1.29. Treatment of Asystole

Begin CPR (Airway, Breathing, Circulation)
↓
↓
IV or intraosseous access
↓
↓
Epinephrine–1st dose: 10 μg/kg - IV/IO; 100μg/kg - ETT
↓
↓
↓
Epinephrine–2nd dose: 100μg/kg - IV/IO/ETT; -repeat every 3–5 min
↓
↓
Consider Atropine, Sodium bicarbonate, Calcium chloride

COMPLICATIONS OF CPR

Complications of CPR can affect every organ system, and at times make for an interesting reading of the literature. These have even included rescuer complications, such as the occurrence of a Spigelian hernia while training in a CPR course[286]. The potpourri of reported complications in the arrest victim include mechanical injuries to the neck, larynx, thorax, and abdomen, bone marrow and air emboli, pulmonary aspiration, and electrolyte imbalances.

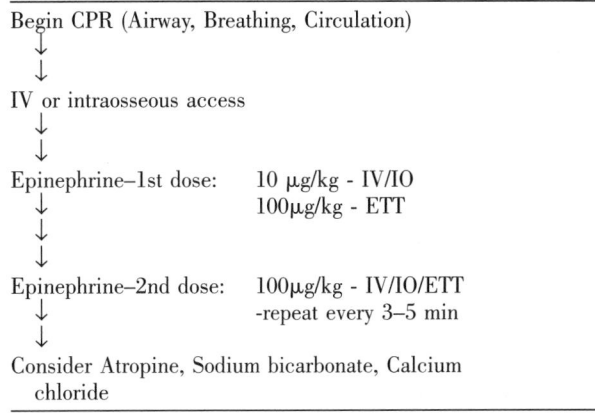

Complications involving the thoracic cavity make up the largest percentage of all complications during CPR. In one study, thoracic complications were observed in 43% of cases. A total of 32% of patients had rib fractures, 21% had sternal fractures, and 18% were reported as having an anterior mediastinal hemorrhage. In addition, 20% of cases had an upper airway complication, 31% had abdominal visceral complications, and 13% had pulmonary complications not related to the chest wall[287]. Pulmonary edema during CPR is common and has multiple causes[287,288] **(Table 1.32).** Pulmonary hemorrhage, cardiac contusion, laceration, or rupture are also seen. Esophageal intubation occurred in 4% of adult patients who were intubated in the prehospital setting[289]. The incidence of esophageal intubation in children is probably much higher because of unfamiliarity of the rescuer with the pediatric airway. Trauma to the neck can involve damage to the hyoid bone and to the thyroid cartilage[290].

Electrolyte disturbances frequently occur during CPR because of the large changes of intravascular volume, severe swings in serum pH, and the administration of many drugs which increase the load of a particular electrolyte. Although hyperkalemia has been associated with CPR[291], hypokalemia is the more common abnormality in the postresuscitation period[292]. Hypokalemia may be a result of a rapid shift of potassium into the intracellular compartment by pH change or by exogenous epinephrine, or endogenous hormonal release of epinephrine, insulin or others.

The incidence of infection spread to the rescuer continues to receive a lot of attention. This includes transmission of the hepatitis B virus (HBV) and the human immunodeficiency virus (HIV)[293,294]. Performance of mouth-to-mouth resuscitation or any invasive procedure can result in exchange of blood or other body fluids between victim and rescuer, especially if either has breaks in the skin, on or around the lips, or soft tissues of the oral cavity mucosa. Thus, there is a real risk of transmitting infections to the rescuer during mouth-to-mouth resuscitation. The position statement of the American Heart Association states that the risk of infection is

Table 1.30. Drug Therapy for Asystole/Ventricular Fibrillation

Drug	*Route of Administration*	*Dosage*	*How Supplied*
Epinephrine	IV (intraosseous) endotracheal	10 μg/kg (100 μg/kg on subsequent doses)	1:10,000 1:1,000 should be used for 100 μg/kg dose
Atropine	IV (intraosseous) endotracheal subcutaneous	0.1 mg/kg minimum dose=0.15 mg	0.1 mg/ml or 1.0 mg/ml
Sodium bicarbonate	IV (intraosseous)	1 mEq/kg/dose or 0.3 × wgt (kg) × base deficit	1 mEq/ml
Calcium chloride	IV (intraosseous)	20 mg/kg 0.2 ml/kg	10% solution (100 mg/ml)
Lidocaine	IV (intraosseous) endotracheal	1 mg/kg	1%, 2%, 4% solution
Bretylium	IV (intraosseous)	5 mg/kg; 1st dose 10 mg/kg; 2nd dose (up to 30 mg/kg)	

Table 1.31. CPR Card

Pt wt. ______________________ kg

Drug	*Concentration*	*Dose*	*ml/kg*	*Final dose*
Epinephrine 1:10,000	0.1 mg/ml	0.1	x	ml EPI
Epinephrine 1:1,000	1 mg/ml	0.1	x	
$NaHCO_3$	1 mEq/ml	1.0	x	ml $NaHCO_3$
Atropine	0.1 mg/ml	0.1	x	ml ATRO
$CaCl_3$ 10%	100 mg/ml	0.2	x	ml Ca Cl_3
Calcium gluconate 10%	100 mg/ml	0.3	x	ml Ca GLU
Lidocaine 1%	10 mg/ml	0.1	x	ml LIDO
Naloxone	20 mg/ml	0.025	x	ml NARC
	0.4 mg/ml	0.025	x	ml NARC
Defibrillation	2 watts–sec/kg		x	
	4 wall–sec/kg		x	

Signed: ______________________ R.N.
______________________ M.D.

Drugs	Pt. wt.	Drips Final dose (mg/100 ml D5W)		
Dopamine Dobutamine	$6 \times \frac{2}{1} \times$ ______	= ______	mg → 1 ml = 2 μg/kg/min	
Epinephrine Isoproterenol	$6 \times \frac{0.05}{1} \times$ ______	= ______	mg → 1 ml = 0.05 μg/kg/min	
Nipride Nitroglycerin	$6 \times \frac{0.5}{1} \times$ ______	= ______	mg → 1 ml = 0.5 μg/kg/min	
Lidocaine	$6 \times \frac{10}{1} \times$ ______	= ______	mg → 1 ml = 10 μg/kg/min	

greater for salivary or aerosol transmission of herpes simplex virus, Neisseria meningitides, tuberculosis, and other respiratory infections[15]. The transmission of hepatitis B virus or HIV during mouth-to-mouth resuscitation has not been documented. However, to minimize this risk, ventilation using barrier devices should be accessible to all health care workers[294] **(Table 1.33).** These barrier devices include masks with one-way valves and plastic mouth and nose covers. The decision not to perform mouth-to-mouth ventilation on an unknown victim when these devices are not available should be guided by one's moral and ethical values of preserving life and assisting those in distress balanced against the risk that may exist in those situations[15]. The decision not to perform mouth-to-mouth ventilation has not been challenged in courts.

Table 1.32. Causes of Pulmonary Edema During CPR

- Airway Obstruction
  - Development of large negative intrathoracic pressure
- Acute development of negative intrathoracic pressure
  - On resumption of spontaneous respiration
- Aspiration
- Overhydration
  - Increased hydrostatic pressure
  - Decreased plasma colloid osmotic pressure
- α-adrenergic agonists
  - Increased central blood volume
- Leaky capillary syndrome
  - Due to hypoxic and/or ischemic injury
- Left ventricular failure
- Decreased lymph flow during CPR
- Neurogenic pulmonary edema

PHYSIOLOGY OF CPR

History

Kouwenhoven's original work on CPR[7] proposed that blood flow during closed-chest compressions resulted from the heart being squeezed between the sternum and the vertebral column. The assumption that there is direct compression of the heart led to what is known as the cardiac pump mechanism of blood flow during CPR. The cardiac pump mechanism implies that ventricular compression causes closure of the atrioventricular valves and that the ejection of blood reduces ventricular volume. During chest relaxation, ventricular pressures fall below atrial pressure, allowing the atrioventricular valves to open and the ventricles to fill. This sequence of events resembles the normal cardiac cycle and occurs during cardiac compression when open-chest CPR is used.

Several observations of the hemodynamics during CPR are inconsistent with the cardiac pump mechanism. Closed-chest CPR produces similar elevations in arterial and venous intravascular pressures, possibly because of a generalized increase in intrathoracic pressure[306]. Reconstructing the integrity of the thorax with flail sternum improves blood pressure during CPR[307]. This is surprising, since a flail sternum should allow direct cardiac compression during closed-chest CPR. In 1976, Criley made the dramatic observation that several patients who developed ventricular fibrillation during cardiac catheterization produced enough blood flow to maintain consciousness by repetitive coughing[308] (Fig. 1.15). The production of blood flow by increasing intrathoracic pressure without direct car-

Table 1.33. Complications of CPR

		References
Neck:	Endotracheal tube placement in esophagus	289
	Esophageal tear	295
	Trauma to hyoid bone	290
	Trauma to thyroid cartilage	290
Thorax:	Rib fracture	287, 289, 290
	Sternal fracture	287, 289, 290
	Hemopericardium	287
	Ventricular contusion	289
	Cardiac laceration	296
	Cardiac rupture	297
	Pulmonary edema	287–289
Abdomen:	Gastric distention	295, 298
	Liver rupture	287, 289, 299, 300
	Splenic rupture	299
	Pneumoperitoneum	301
	Aspiration	289
Vascular:	Fat emboli	302
	Bone marrow emboli	290, 302
	Disseminated intravascular coagulopathy (DIC)	303
	Thrombosis	304
Electrolytes:	Hypokalemia	292
	Hyperkalemia	291
	Hypocalcemia	292
	Hypomagnesemia	292
Rescuer associated:	Infection (bacteria, TB, HIV, hepatitis)	293, 294, 305
	Physical stress	286

diac compression describes the intrathoracic pump mechanism of blood flow during CPR. Much of the subsequent research regarding CPR has addressed the relative importance of the cardiac and thoracic pump mechanisms of blood flow during CPR.

Thoracic Pump Mechanism

Chest compression during CPR generates almost equal pressures in the left ventricle, aorta, right atrium, pulmonary artery and the esophagus (Fig. 1.16)[307]. Since all

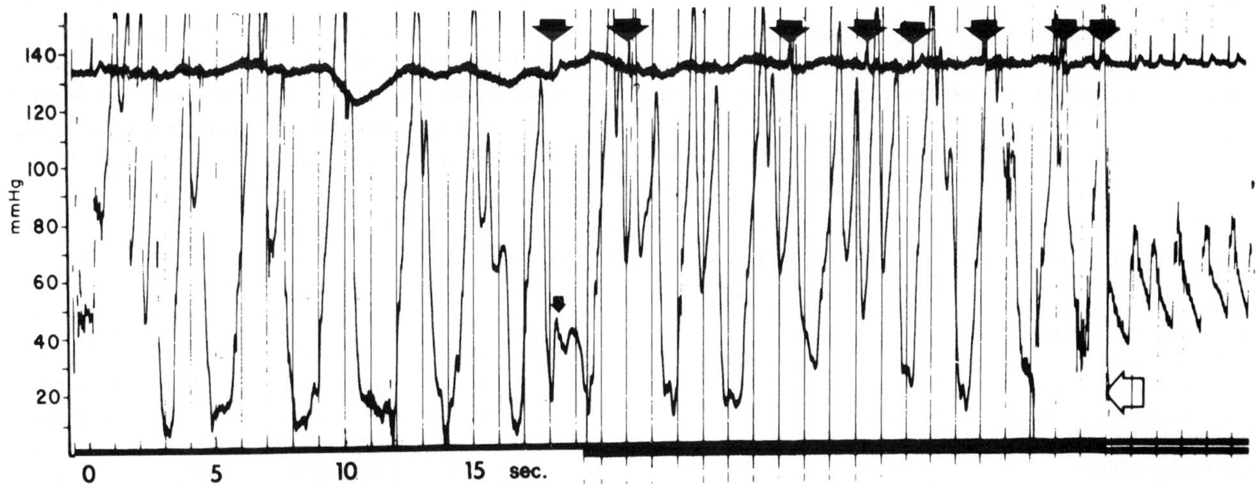

Figure 1.15. Cough-CPR during prolonged ventricular asystole after coronary arteriographic injection. An 18-second period of asystole after a right coronary arteriographic injection is depicted. During this period, the patient coughed every 2 seconds, generating peak aortic pressures of over 140 mm Hg. *Large arrows* mark the intrinsic QRS complexes after the 18-second period of asystole, and the *small arrow* marks the resultant aortic pressure from the first intrinsic beat. The patient continued to cough until the cardiac rhythm stabilized 40 seconds later. (From Niemann JT, Rosborough J, Hausknecht M, Brown D, Criley JM. Cough-CPR. Documentation of systemic perfusion in man and in an experimental model: A "window" to the mechanism of blood flow in external CPR. Crit Care Med 1980;8:143.)

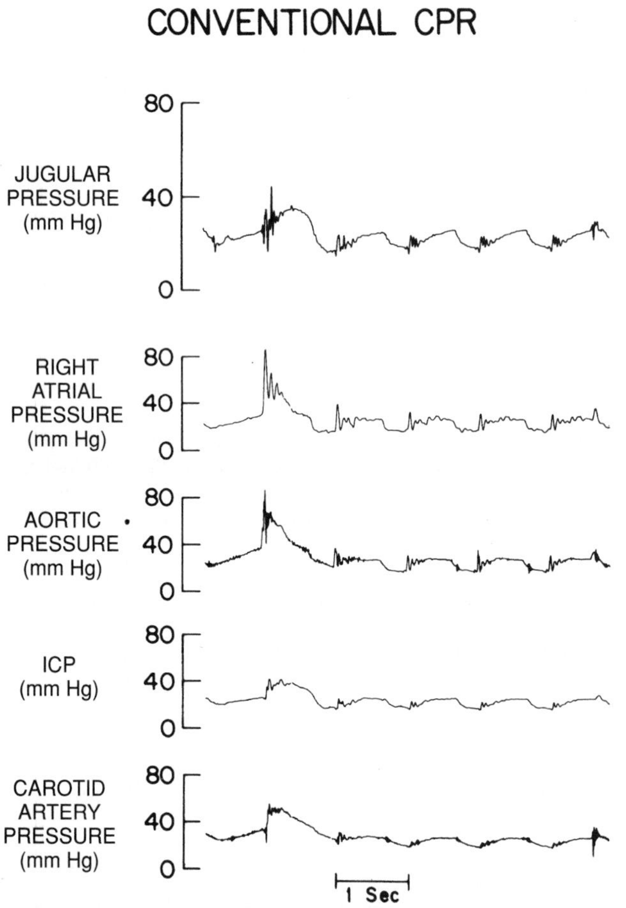

Figure 1.16. Original record during conventional CPR. The first compression for conventional CPR follows the lung inflation that occurred during the previous release phase. Notice increase in pressure on this compression. (From Koehler RC, Chandra N, Guerci AD, Tsitlik J, Traystman RJ, Rogers MC, Weisfeldt ML. Augmentation of cerebral perfusion by simultaneous chest compression and lung inflation with abdominal binding after cardiac arrest in dogs. Circulation 1983;67:271.)

intrathoracic vascular pressures are equal, the suprathoracic arterial pressures must be higher than the suprathoracic venous pressures for blood flow to exist. The direct transmission of positive intrathoracic pressure to the suprathoracic veins is prevented by anatomic venous valves. The presence of these jugular venous valves has been demonstrated in animals[307,309,310] and humans[311–313] undergoing CPR. This unequal transmission of intrathoracic pressure to the suprathoracic vasculature establishes the gradient necessary for blood to flow with this mechanism of CPR.

During normal cardiac function the lowest pressure in the vascular circuit occurs on the atrial side of the atrioventricular valves. This low pressure compartment is the downstream pressure for the systemic circulation which allows venous return to the pump. Angiographic studies show blood passing from the vena cavae through the right heart to the pulmonary artery and from the pulmonary veins through the left heart to the aorta during a single chest compression[312,314]. Echocardiographic studies have shown that, unlike normal cardiac activity or during open-chest CPR, during closed-chest CPR in both dogs[312] and humans[315,316] the atrioventricular valves are open during blood ejection and aortic diameter decreases rather than increases during blood ejection[312,316]. These findings during closed-chest CPR support the thoracic pump theory and demonstrate that the heart is a passive conduit for blood flow **(Table 1.34).**

Cardiac Pump Mechanism

There appear to be specific situations when the cardiac pump predominates during closed chest CPR. When more force is applied during chest compressions, the likelihood of direct cardiac compression increases. In animals undergoing CPR, increasing the force of chest compressions increases the chance of closing the atrioventricular valves, implying direct cardiac compression[317]. A smaller chest size may allow for more direct cardiac compression. Adult dogs with small chests have better hemodynamics during closed-chest CPR than dogs with large chests[318]. Third, the infant chest is more compliant and may permit more direct cardiac compression. Blood flow during closed-chest CPR in a piglet model is superior when compared to most adult models[97]. Unlike the adult model, the addition of simultaneous compression with ventilation (SCV-CPR) does not augment the flow produced during piglet CPR[319]. The lack of contribution of SCV-CPR in the infant implies that excellent compression occurs with conventional CPR, and that additional intrathoracic pressure is of no benefit.

Table 1.34. Comparison of Mechanisms of Blood Flow During Closed Chest Cardiac Massage

	Cardiac Pump	*Thoracic Pump*
Proposed Mechanism:	Heart compressed between sternum and spine	Generalized increase in intrathoracic pressure
Findings during compression:		
Atrioventricular valves:	Closed	Open
Aortic diameter:	Increased	Decreased
Blood movement:	Left ventricle to aorta	Pulmonary veins to aorta
Ventricular volume:	Decreased	Little change
Compression rate:	Dependent	Little effect
Duty cycle:	Little effect	Dependent
Compression force:	Increased role	Decreased role
Clinical Situations:	Small chest	Large chest
	High compliance	Low compliance

Rate and duty cycle

In 1986 and reiterated in 1992, the American Heart Association, in the Guidelines for CPR and ECC, increased the recommended rate of chest compressions from 60 to 80 to 100 per minute[(15)]. This change represented a compromise between advocates of the thoracic pump mechanism and the cardiac pump mechanism[(15)]. Duty cycle is defined as the ratio of the duration of the compression phase to the entire compression-relaxation cycle expressed as a percentage. For example, at a rate of 30 compressions per minute, a 1.2 second compression time produces a 60% duty cycle. If blood flow is generated by direct cardiac compression, then the stroke volume is determined by the force of compression. Prolonging the compression (increasing the duty cycle) beyond the time necessary for full ventricular ejection should have no additional effect on stroke volume. Increasing the rate of compressions increases cardiac output, since a fixed, relatively small, blood volume is ejected with each cardiac compression. In contrast, if blood flow is produced by the thoracic pump, the reservoir of blood to be ejected comes from the large capacitance of the thoracic vasculature. With the thoracic pump mechanism, flow is enhanced by increasing either the force of compression or the duty cycle, but is not affected by changes in compression rate over a wide range of rates[(311)]. Mathematical models of the cardiovascular system have confirmed that blood flow is determined by both the applied force and the compression duration with the thoracic pump mechanism[(320,321)]. It appears from experimental animal data that both the thoracic pump and cardiac pump mechanisms can effectively generate blood flow during closed-chest CPR. Differences between various investigators may be attributed to differences in CPR models or compression techniques. These differences may involve issues of chest compliance and geometry, maturity of different animal species, or chest compression techniques. For example, in an infant with a very compliant chest wall, either mechanism of blood flow may come into play. Differences in techniques may include the magnitude of sternal displacement, compression force, momentum of chest compression, compression rate, and duty cycle.

Results of several studies in dogs have demonstrated a benefit of a compression rate of 120/min compared to slower rates during conventional CPR[(322–325)]. In studies in piglets[(326)], puppies[(327)], and humans[(311,328)] no difference was found in the effectiveness of conventional CPR at various rates. In a study on piglet CPR, duty cycle was the major determinant of cerebral perfusion pressure. The duty cycle at which venous return became limited varied with age. Increasing duty cycle was more effective in the younger piglets[(326)].

The discrepancy between the importance of rate and duty cycle in various models by different investigators generates confusion. However, increasing the rate of compressions during conventional CPR to 100 per minute satisfies both those who prefer the faster rates and those who support a

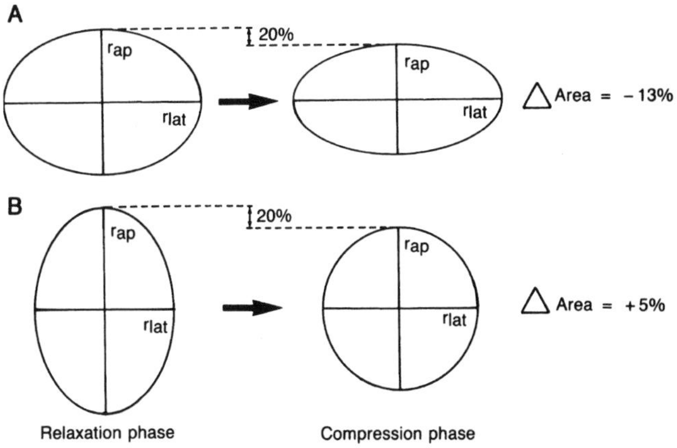

Figure 1.17. Changes in area of ellipses with constant circumference. Each ellipse is labeled with anteroposterior radius (r_{ap}) and lateral radius (r_{lat}), and a 20% anteroposterior compression is applied. Indicated change in areas equals relaxed area minus compressed area. **A.** Initial anteroposterior-to-lateral ratio, 0.7; and compression leads to position ejection because relaxed area minus compressed area is negative. **B.** Initial anteroposterior-to-lateral ratio, 1.4; and compression toward a circular shape results in an increase in area. (From Dean JM, Koehler RC, Schleien CL, et al. Age-related changes in chest geometry during cardiopulmonary resuscitation. J Appl Physiol 1987;62:2212.)

longer duty cycle. This is true because it is easier to produce a longer duty cycle at a faster rate[(322)].

Chest geometry

Chest geometry plays an important role in the ability of extrathoracic compressions to generate intrathoracic pressure. Shape, compliance, and deformability are the chest characteristics which have the greatest impact during CPR, and these differ with age.

The change in cross-sectional area of the chest during anterior to posterior delivered compressions is related to its shape[(329)] (Fig. 1.17). The ratio of the chest anteroposterior diameter to the lateral diameter is referred to as the thoracic index. A keel-shaped chest, as in an adult dog, has a greater anteroposterior diameter and thus a thoracic index greater than one. A flat chest, as in a thin human, has a greater lateral diameter and thus a thoracic index of less than one. A circular chest has a thoracic index of one. A circle has a larger cross-sectional area than either of these elliptical chests. As the anteroposterior compression flattens a circle it decreases the cross sectional area and compresses the contents. In contrast, as an anteroposterior compression is applied to the keel-shaped chest the cross-sectional area increases as a circular shape is approached. The cross-sectional area of the keel-shaped chest does not decrease until the chest compression continues past the circular shape to flatten the chest. This implies a threshold past which the compression must proceed before intrathoracic contents are decreased and squeezed[(329)]. Thus the rounder, flatter chests of small dogs and pigs may require less chest displacement than the keel-shaped chests of adult dogs to

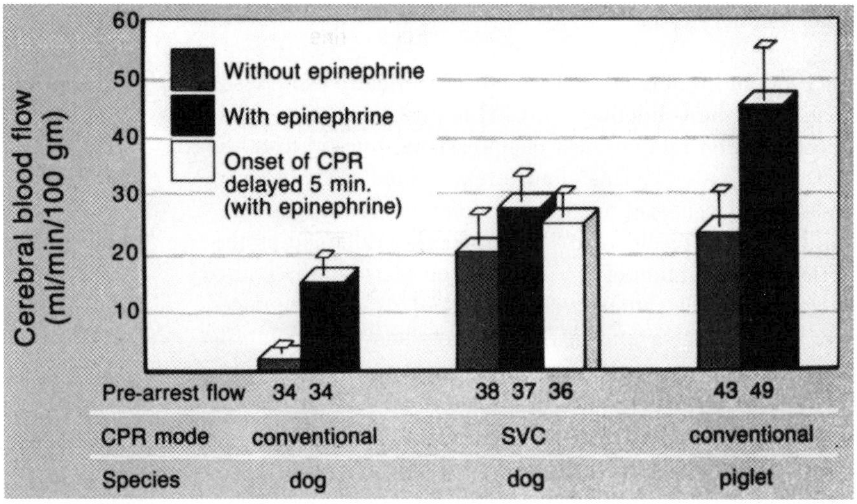

Figure 1.18. Cerebral blood flow (mean and SE) during CPR with and without continuous epinephrine infusion. Mean prearrest flows are indicated under *bars* for each group. (From Koehler RC, Michael JR, Guerci AD, et al. Beneficial effect of epinephrine infusion on cerebral and myocardial blood flows during CPR. Ann Emerg Med 1985;14:744.)

generate thoracic ejection of blood. This has been demonstrated in small dogs with round chests compared to adult dogs with keel-shaped chests[318].

As humans age, chest cartilage calcifies, causing decreased chest wall compliance. Older patients may require greater compression force to generate the same anteroposterior displacement. A three month old piglet requires much greater chest force for anteroposterior displacement than their one month old counterparts[329]. The compliance of the chest not only effects the degree of chest displacement but also what structures becomes compressed. Direct cardiac compression is more likely to occur in the more compliant chest of a younger animal. Production of cerebral and myocardial blood flow in an infant piglet model of external CPR was much greater than expected when compared to adults[107] (Figs. 1.18, 1.19). Thus the more compliant chest of the infant may allow for more direct cardiac compression to occur. This may account for the high organ blood flow which resembles that produced by open-chest cardiac massage.

Chest deformation occurs as CPR is prolonged[107] (Fig. 1.20). The chest assumes a flatter shape producing a larger percent decrease in cross-sectional area at the same absolute chest displacement. Progressive deformation may be beneficial if it leads to more direct cardiac compression. Unfortunately too much deformation may decrease the recoil of the chest wall during the relaxation phase. Decreased chest recoil with progressive deformation limits displacement and renders compressions less effective. A progressive decrease in the effectiveness of chest compressions to produce blood flow is seen in a pediatric model of conventional CPR[107]. The permanent deformation of the chest in this model approaches 30% of the original anteroposterior diameter. Attempting to limit deformation by increasing intrathoracic pressure from within during CPR with simultaneous compression-ventilation CPR was ineffective[319]. Neither the amount of deformation nor the time to deterioration of flows was different. Using a thoracic vest to limit deformation when performing CPR greatly decreased the permanent chest deformation (3% vs. 30%)[330]. Unfortunately this did not attenuate the deterioration of blood flow with time.

The characteristics of chest geometry of animals may relate to humans. Body weight, surface area, chest circumfer-

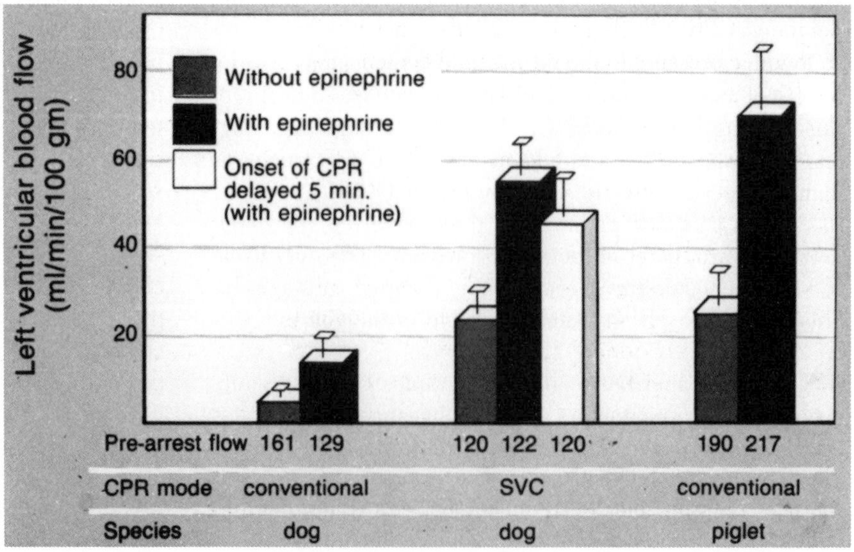

Figure 1.19. Left ventricular blood flow (mean and SE) during CPR with and without continuous epinephrine infusion. Mean prearrest flows are indicated under *bars* for each group. (From Koehler RC, Michael JR, Guerci AD, et al. Beneficial effect of epinephrine infusion on cerebral and myocardial blood flows during CPR. Ann Emerg Med 1985;14:744.)

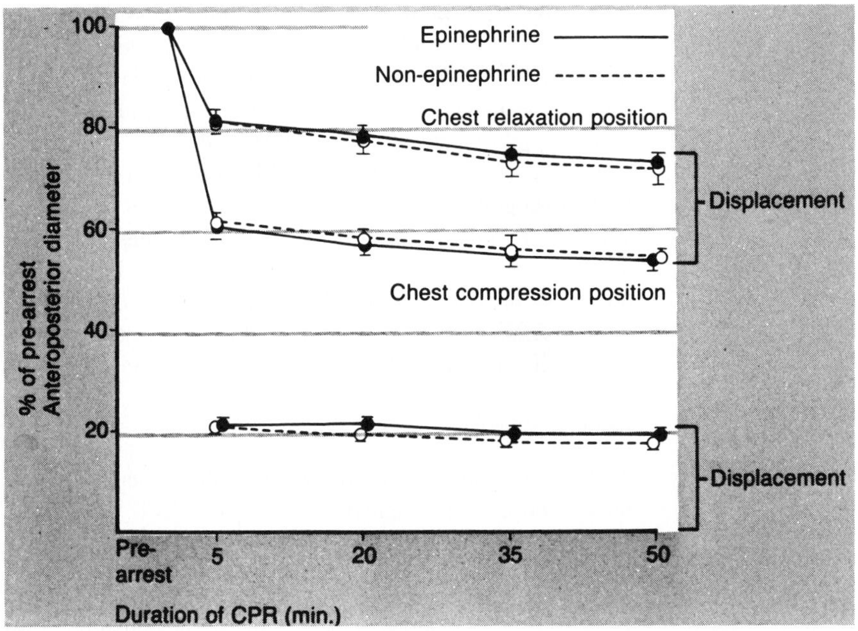

Figure 1.20. Piston position during chest compression and relaxation phases of the cycle, and net piston displacement expressed as a percent of prearrest anteroposterior chest diameter (12.0 ± 0.3 cm). Note that displacement was essentially unchanged over the 50-minute duration but that marked deformation occurred during the relaxation phase by 5 minutes and continued to deform over the 50-minute period in both the epinephrine (*solid line*) and no epinephrine (*dashed line*) groups. (From Schleien CL, Dean JM, Koehler RC, et al. Effect of epinephrine on cerebral and myocardial perfusion in an infant animal preparation of cardiopulmonary resuscitation. Circulation 1986;73:809.)

ence and diameter did not correlate with the magnitude of aortic pressure produced during CPR in a study of nine adults already declared dead[(331)]. A direct comparison of adult and pediatric human CPR has not been done. The increased compliance and deformability of the infant chest make it likely that pediatric CPR would be more effective in increasing intravascular pressure and flow than in adults.

Effects of CPR on ICP

The difference between the mean intrathoracic aortic pressure, the upstream pressure for cerebral blood flow, and the mean intracranial pressure (ICP), the downstream pressure, is the cerebral perfusion pressure. During external chest compression, increases in intrathoracic pressure are transmitted through the venous system of the head and neck to the intracranial vault to increase ICP. Large swings in ICP corresponding to chest compressions occur in children undergoing CPR[(332)] (Fig. 1.21). This transmission of intrathoracic pressure to the intracranial contents accounts for the low cerebral perfusion pressure and cerebral blood flow during closed chest CPR[(333)].

Transmission of intrathoracic pressure to the intracranial space occurs via the vertebral veins and the cerebrospinal fluid during CPR in dogs[(334)]. Balloon occlusion of the ascending aorta does not decrease the transmission of intrathoracic pressure during CPR[(334)]. The jugular venous system has valves that prevent the transmission of pressure retrograde to the intracranial contents[(334)]. These valves have been mapped anatomically in humans during CPR and are located below the clavicle near the angle of Louis[(311)]. They appear to be functional during CPR whether the chest is opened or closed[(310)]. The transmission of intrathoracic pressure can be reduced by ligating the cervical spinal cord in the dog. Further reduction in the transmission of pressure occurs if the vertebral veins are also tied off[(334)].

The relationship of ICP to intrathoracic pressure during CPR is linear. In dogs receiving conventional CPR, ICP increased by one-third of the rise of intrathoracic pressure from 10 to 90 mm Hg[(334)]. This linear relationship allows one to predict the rise in ICP.

However, some modes of CPR change the intrathoracic to ICP relationship. In dogs, abdominal binding increases the transmission of pressure to the intracranial space to 50% of the rise of intrathoracic pressure[(335)]. SCV-CPR, a mode of CPR designed to generate higher intrathoracic pressures, is similar to conventional CPR in its transmission of pressure to the cranium[(334)]. Open-chest CPR decreases the transmission of pressure and improves cerebral perfusion pressure compared to conventional CPR[(336)]. These findings increase the concern that new modes of CPR designed to increase intrathoracic pressure may not effectively improve cerebral perfusion pressure.

An increased baseline ICP impairs the generation of cerebral perfusion pressure during CPR. In dogs raising the baseline ICP to 22 to 30 mm Hg by increasing cerebrospinal fluid volume changed the relationship of pressure transmission. In this case, 75% of the intrathoracic pressure was transmitted to the intracranial space[(334)]. This implies that performing CPR when the ICP is already increased will be much less effective at generating a sufficient cerebral perfusion pressure.

NEWER CPR TECHNIQUES

Simultaneous Compression-Ventilation CPR

Simultaneous compression-ventilation CPR (SCV-CPR) represents a CPR model that augments conventional CPR by

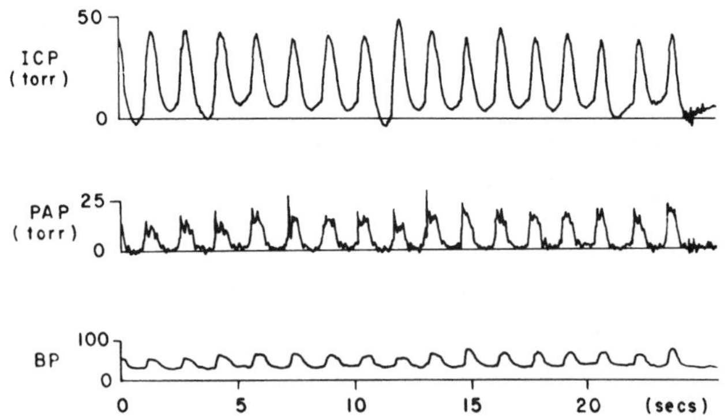

Figure 1.21. Relationship of intracranial pressure, pulmonary artery pressure, and arterial blood pressure during closed-chest cardiac massage. Note that each chest compression is accompanied not only by a rise in arterial and pulmonary artery pressure but also by a sharp rise in intracranial pressure. (From Rogers MC, Nugent SK, Stidham GL. Effects of closed-chest cardiac massage on intracranial pressure. Crit Care Med 1979;7:455.)

increasing the thoracic pump mechanism contribution to blood flow. Delivering ventilation simultaneously with every compression, (instead of after every fifth compression), increases intrathoracic pressure and augments blood flow produced by closed-chest CPR.

Hemodynamic data indicate that SCV-CPR increases the carotid blood flow when compared with conventional CPR[318,336–339]. Subsequent studies have confirmed physiologic advantages of SCV-CPR in canine models[340,341]. However, in infant pigs[319] and small dogs[318,342,343], SCV-CPR offered no advantage over conventional CPR. In these small animals, the compliance and geometry of the chest may allow more direct cardiac compression. Thus, higher intrathoracic pressure may be achieved with conventional CPR[107,326,339]. Coronary perfusion pressure was either only minimally increased[339] or even decreased in humans when comparing SCV to conventional-CPR. Survival was significantly worse in both animals[342] and humans[344] when SCV-CPR was used when compared to those who received conventional CPR. No study has shown an increased survival with this technique of CPR.

Vest CPR

Vest CPR employs an inflatable bladder, resembling a blood pressure cuff, wrapped circumferentially around the chest. It is inflated physically to deliver chest compressions by diffuse application of pressure. Chest dimensions are changed minimally and so direct cardiac compression is unlikely. In addition, the even distribution of pressure decreases the likelihood of trauma.

Improvement of cerebral and myocardial blood flows[341,345,346] and survival[346,347] with vest CPR compared to conventional CPR has been shown in dogs. In a pediatric piglet model only a 3% permanent chest deformation was seen after 50 minutes of vest CPR[330], compared with an almost 30% deformation produced during an equivalent period of conventional CPR[107]. In a human study, vest CPR increased aortic systolic pressure but had little effect on diastolic pressure when compared to conventional CPR[331]. Despite its late application, vest CPR improved the hemodynamics and return to spontaneous circulation in adult patients in another study[348]. The lack of metallic parts has allowed vest CPR to be used experimentally during nuclear magnetic resonance spectroscopy to study brain intracellular pH[183]. The vest has also been used as an external cardiac assist device in nonarrested dogs with heart failure[349]. Clinically, the use of vest CPR depends on sophisticated equipment and it remains experimental at this time.

Abdominal binding

Abdominal binders and military antishock trousers (MAST) have been used to augment closed-chest CPR (Fig. 1.22). Both methods apply continuous compression circumferentially below the diaphragm. Three mechanisms have been proposed for the augmentation of CPR by these binders. First, binding the abdomen decreases the compliance of the diaphragm and raises intrathoracic pressure. Second, blood may be moved out of the intrathoracic structures to increase circulating blood volume. Third, applying pressure to the subdiaphragmatic vasculature and increasing resistance may increase suprathoracic blood flow. These effects increase aortic pressure and carotid blood flow in both animals[299,340,350] and humans[351]. Unfortunately, as aortic pressure increases, the downstream component of coronary perfusion pressure increases to an even greater extent, resulting in a decrease in coronary perfusion pressure[342,350] and myocardial blood flow[350]. These techniques also lower the cerebral perfusion pressure. The transmission of intrathoracic pressure to the intracranial vault raises the ICP (the downstream component of the cerebral perfusion pressure), resulting in decrease in the cerebral perfusion pressure[334]. Clinical studies have failed to shown an increase in survival when an abdominal binder or MAST suit is used to augment CPR[342,352].

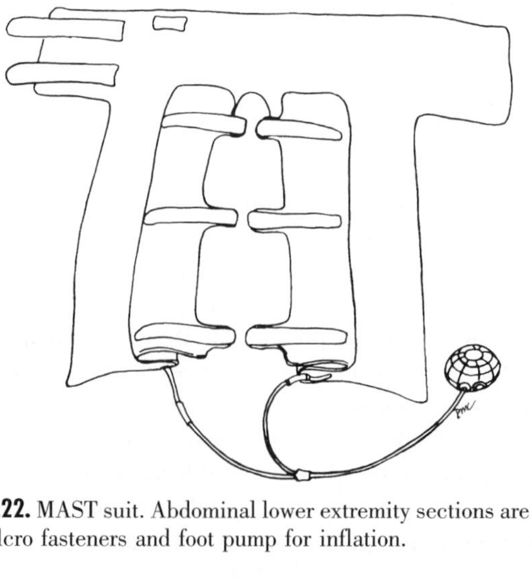

Figure 1.22. MAST suit. Abdominal lower extremity sections are shown with Velcro fasteners and foot pump for inflation.

Abdominal Compression

Interposed abdominal compression CPR (IAC-CPR) represents the delivery of an abdominal compression during the relaxation phase of chest compression. IAC-CPR may augment conventional CPR in several ways. First IAC-CPR may return venous blood to the chest during chest relaxation.[353,354] Second, IAC-CPR increases intrathoracic pressure and augments the duty cycle of chest compression[355]. Third, IAC-CPR may compress the aorta and return blood retrograde to the carotid or coronary arteries[354].

Hemodynamic improvements secondary to IAC-CPR have been shown in several studies. In animal experiments, cardiac output, and cerebral and coronary blood flow were improved when IAC-CPR was compared with conventional CPR[353,355–358] but not in an infant model[359]. Human studies also demonstrated an increase in aortic pressure and coronary perfusion pressure during IAC-CPR compared to conventional CPR[311,360–363]. Clinically IAC-CPR requires additional manpower and equipment and remains experimental until additional outcome studies prove its superiority over conventional techniques of CPR.

Active Compression-Decompression CPR

A newer technique, active compression-decompression (ACD) CPR uses a negative pressure "pull" on the thorax during the release phase of chest compression using a handheld suction device[364]. This technique has been shown to improve vascular pressures and minute ventilation[365] during CPR in animals[366,367] and humans[368,369]. The mechanism of benefit is typically attributed to enhanced venous return related to active decompression. However, its benefit may actually result from the greater chest expansion and filling with air between compressions, thus when this technique is used with impedance to inspiratory gas exchange vascular pressures and flow increase further[370]. This results in a greater rise in intrathoracic pressure and vascular flows as occurs with vest CPR. Preliminary results show an increased survival of adults with the use of this new technique[364,371].

Cardiopulmonary Bypass

Cardiopulmonary bypass (CPB) represents one of the most effective ways to restore circulation after cardiac arrest. Animal studies show that CPB increases the survival at 72 hours, recovery of consciousness, and preserves the myocardium better than conventional CPR[372]. In dogs CPB resulted in better neurologic outcome than conventional CPR after a 4 minute ischemic period, but neurologic outcome was dismal in both groups when the ischemic period lasted 12 minutes[372]. Twenty-four hour survival was seen for 90% of dogs after 15 or 20 minutes of cardiac arrest, but only 10% survived with 30 minutes of arrest time when CPB was used for stabilization during defibrillation[373]. CPB decreased myocardial infarct size in a model involving coronary artery occlusion when compared to conventional CPR[374]. In all animal models, CPB improves the success of resuscitation when compared to conventional CPR.

Human experience with CPB for cardiac arrest outside the operating room is minimal. Percutaneous femoral artery to vein bypass was successful in resuscitating five patients with "refractory" cardiac arrest[375]. Two patients in that study died and the neurologic status of the three survivors was not reported. In a separate study, one of six patients resuscitated with CPB for cardiac arrest survived and is neurologically normal[376]. Two recent, larger studies have been reported in humans. In one, 29 patients with cardiac arrest were placed on CPB[377]. Unfortunately, 22 of 29 could not be weaned from CPB. Only one of the seven patients who were weaned survived and was able to leave the hospital. In the second of these studies, 36 patients with cardiac arrest were placed on CPB. Eighteen patients were able to be weaned from CPB and six survived to discharge[378]. No studies of CPB have been done in pediatric arrest victims.

CPB requires a great deal of technical support and sophistication. It can be implemented quickly in systems set up to do so[375,377]. Despite rapid availability and restoration of circulation, the lack of effective resuscitation prior to institution of CPB limits the ability to preserve neurologic or cardiac function. Because of these limitations, CPB is not recommended for patients who suffer out-of-hospital cardiac arrest or more than 30 minutes of conventional CPR in any setting[377].

INDICATIONS FOR TERMINATION OF RESUSCITATION

The decision to undertake CPR should always be performed on patients unless a specific order not to resuscitate is on the medical record or a physician familiar with the patient's medical history has been communicated with. The decision to forego CPR is predicated by a number of concerns including the possible outcome of the resuscitative attempt based on the patient's medical history, the potential quality of life, the legal rights of the patient including living wills and advanced directives (in adults), and patient rights regarding their understanding of the disease process, the treatment options, risks and benefits of therapy, and prognosis.

Once CPR is initiated, the decision to terminate efforts to resuscitate is based on a number of factors. Further history gathering during the resuscitative effort may affect the decision to continue with CPR. In addition, the severity of anatomic or metabolic derangements and other coexisting factors such as age, duration of CPR, and presenting cardiac rhythm, will help the physician determine the course of CPR. Absence of neurologic function should not be used as a criterion to cease CPR efforts as it is unreliable as a prognostic sign. Brain death is not a valid diagnosis during the CPR effort and only after cardiovascular function is reestablished should neurological status be determined in order to consider withdrawal of life support. Rigid criteria to stop CPR efforts have been advocated by some, but the uncertainties regarding etiology, duration of arrest, metabolic and biochemical aberrations, and young age all play a role in determining the eventual course of the resuscitation effort.

OUTCOME

With the development of basic CPR in the early 1960s, skilled resuscitation teams, both in and out of the hospital, were developed. This led to saved lives when previously every victim of cardiac arrest had died. Soon thereafter, successful resuscitation of patients by basic life support measures, defibrillation, and medications became common after even as long as five hours after the commencement of CPR[(383)].

However, more recent data have shown that the success of CPR is dependent on many factors, although its immediate use is a key reason for a successful resuscitation. Other pre-existing factors which play a role in the success of CPR include patient age, prior medical condition, presenting cardiac rhythm, and the mechanism of cardiac arrest. Eisenberg et al. have published a series of articles that confirm that survival from cardiac arrest is determined by the interplay of all of these factors[(379–382)].

Many clinical studies have reviewed out-of-hospital survival after CPR. In King County, Washington, the survival rate for bystander-initiated CPR after a witnessed arrest was 32%, compared with a survival rate of 3% for unwitnessed cardiac arrests without bystander CPR[(384)]. The benefit of a witnessed arrest is that the bystander may sooner notify the emergency medical system and have nothing at all to do with the early initiation of basic CPR measures. Studies from Milwaukee demonstrate that with a brief interval between a witnessed arrest and the arrival of emergency personnel, that bystander CPR contributes little to the success of resuscitation. When the arrest time is very short it is the early application of defibrillation which appears to be the critical element in the success of resuscitation[(385,386)].

Outcome of patients after CPR in the hospital is not very different from those suffering an out-of-hospital arrest. A heterogenous array of in-hospital studies show resuscitation rates ranging from 13 to 52% in this group. Long term survival rates for these patients are lower, ranging from 5 to 27%. Recent criticism of CPR methods because of these low rates of survival may be unfair owing to the fact that without the use of CPR, survival would most likely be much lower[(387–393)].

The success rate for return of spontaneous circulation of infants and children is similar to that seen in adult patients. In one study of out-of-hospital pediatric arrests, only 28% of these children survived to hospital discharge. All of these eight survivors suffered a severe neurologic insult and all were discharged to a chronic care facility[(14)]. Survival rates among patients who suffer out-of-hospital arrest range from 15%[(12)] to 57%[(387)].

The low resuscitation rate in children, even when the patient does not suffer from pre-existing disease, is probably because of the high incidence of asystole as the presenting rhythm. Asystole was the presenting rhythm in 77% of the children suffering out-of-hospital cardiac arrest. Eleven percent presented in an idioventricular rhythm and only 9% of the patients presented with ventricular fibrillation[(12)]. Asystole is a more common presenting rhythm in children as a result of airway obstruction or other causes of respiratory arrest resulting in hypoxemia. Adults who present in asystole have a higher mortality rate than those who present with other rhythms.

As the use of medical resources plays a more important role, predicting survival after cardiac arrest will play an increasingly important role. The Glasgow coma score over the first post-resuscitation week may be helpful in predicting outcome[(388)], although only the absence of spontaneous breathing on admission to the hospital after cardiac arrest was predictive of an unfavorable neurologic outcome in another study[(13)]. The use of CPR in patients at the extremes of age has been questioned. There were no survivors among 38 infants less than 1500 g who received CPR in the first 3 days of life. The resuscitation rate was 36% in those infants receiving CPR after the third day of life[(389)]. These authors felt that CPR may not be warranted in small premature patients. The study was flawed, however, in that many of the patients did not receive chest compressions, infants who were successfully resuscitated in the delivery room were omitted from the results, and the medical interventions were heterogenous and poorly defined.

The effectiveness of CPR in critically ill children in the ICU depends on the balance between the negative factors intrinsic to the underlying disease(s) of the patient versus the rapid response time and enhanced resuscitative skills of the ICU personnel. The implication from recent published data is that for many individuals, basic and advanced life support, as we presently practice it, may not provide sufficient blood flow to maintain the viability of critical organs for prolonged periods of times. Compared to the pre-1960 era however, CPR is a miracle cure for those still alive after suffering a cardiac arrest. Thus, basic scientific as well as clinical research remains to be done to improve our understanding of the pathophysiology of cardiac arrest and vital organ ischemia in order to improve the quality of survival of more patients receiving CPR.

References

1. Kings II: 4:34–35 (KGV).
2. Baker AB: Artificial respiration: The history of an idea. Med Hist 15:336, 1971.
3. DeBard ML: The history of cardiopulmonary resuscitation. Ann Emerg Med 9:273, 1980.
4. Elam JO, Brown ES, Elder JD Jr: Artificial respiration by mouth-to-mask methods: Study of respiratory gas exchange of paralyzed patients ventilated by operator's expired air. N Engl J Med 250:749, 1954.

5. Bartecchi CE: Cardiopulmonary resuscitation–An element of sophistication in the 18th century. Am Heart J 100:580, 1980.
6. Julian DG: Cardiac resuscitation in the eighteenth century. Heart Lung 4:46, 1975.
7. Kouwenhoven WB, Ing DR, Jude JR, Knickerbocker GG: Closed-chest cardiac massage. JAMA 173:94, 1960.
8. Jude JR, Kouwenhoven WB, Knickerbocker GG: Cardiac arrest. JAMA 128:1063, 1961.
9. Jude JR, Kouwenhoven WB, Ing DR, Knickerbocker GG: External cardiac resuscitation. Monogr Surg Sci 1:59, 1964.
10. Stephenson HE Jr: Charles Claude Guthrie's contribution to cardiac resuscitation. Crit Care Med 9:428, 1981.
11. Safar P, Lourdes EA, Elam JO: A comparison of the mouth-to-mouth and mouth-to-airway methods of artificial respiration with the chest-pressure arm-lift methods. N Engl J Med 258:671, 1958.
12. Eisenberg M, Bergner L, Hallstrom A: Epidemiology of cardiac arrest and resuscitation in children. Ann Emerg Med 12:672, 1983.
13. Lewis JK, Minter MG, Eshelman SJ, Witte MK: Outcome of pediatric resuscitation. Ann Emerg Med 12:297, 1983.
14. O'Rourke PP: Out-of-hospital cardiac arrest in pediatric patients: Outcome. Crit Care Med 12:283, 1984.
15. Standards and guidelines for cardiopulmonary resuscitation (CPR) and emergency cardiac care (ECC). JAMA 268:2171, 1992.
16. Sellick BA: Cricoid pressure to control regurgitation of stomach contents during induction of anesthesia. Lancet 2:404, 1982.
17. Lee WR, Baillie HD, Clarke AD, Levy LS, Zoledziowski S, Massoud AAE: An experimental comparison in dogs of expired air and oxygen ventilation during external cardiac massage. Br J Anaesth 43:38, 1971.
18. Chandra NC, Gruben KG, Tsitlik JE, Brower R, Guerci AD, Halperin HH, Weisfeldt ML, Permutt S: Observation of ventilation during resuscitation in a canine model. Circulation 90:3070, 1994.
19. Tang W, Weil MH, Sun S, Kette D, Kette F, Gazmuri RJ, O'Connell F, Bisera J: Cardiopulmonary resuscitation by precordial compression but without mechanical ventilation. Am J Resp Crit Care Med 150:1709, 1994.
20. Idris AH, Becker LB, Fuerst RS, Wenzel V, Rush WJ, Melker RJ, Orban DJ: Effect of ventilation on resuscitation in an animal model of cardiac arrest. Circulation 90:3063, 1994.
21. Greensher J, Mofenson HC: Emergency treatment of the choking child. Pediatrics 70:110, 1982.
22. Day RL, Crelin ES, DuBois AB: Choking. The Heimlich abdominal thrust vs back blows: An approach to measurement of inertial and aerodynamic forces. Pediatrics 70:113, 1982.
23. Heimlich HJ: Pop goes the cafe coronary. Emerg Med 6:154, 1974.
24. Heimlich HJ, Hoffmann KA, Canestri FR: Food-choking and drowning deaths prevented by external subdiaphragmatic compression. Ann Thorac Surg 20:188, 1975.
25. Carlile T: Self-administered Heimlich maneuver. JAMA 249:3175, 1983.
26. Visintine RE, Baick CH: Ruptured stomach after Heimlich maneuver. JAMA 234:415, 1975.
27. Palmer E: The Heimlich maneuver misused. Curr Prescrip 5:45, 1979.
28. Guildner CW, Williams D, Subitch T: Airway obstructed by foreign material: The Heimlich maneuver. JACEP 5:675, 1976.
29. Katsilabros L: Centrifugal force as a life-saving manoeuvre for choking on food. Lancet 1:874, 1980.
30. Jacoby JJ, Hamelberg W, Ziegler CH, Flory FA: Transtracheal resuscitation. JAMA 162:625, 1965.
31. Sanders RD: Two ventilating attachments for bronchoscopes. Del Med J 39:170, 1967.
32. Spoerel WE, Narayanan PS, Singh NP: Transtracheal ventilation. Br J Anaesth 43:932, 1985.
33. Jacobs HB: Emergency percutaneous transtracheal catheter and ventilator. J Trauma 12:50, 1972.
34. Smith RB, Myers EN, Sherman H: Transtracheal ventilation in pediatric patients. Br J Anaesth 46:313, 1974.
35. Swartzman, Pfister RC, Van Sonnenberg E: Percutaneous transtracheal jet ventilation for cardiopulmonary resuscitation: Evaluation of a new jet ventilator. Crit Care Med 12:8, 1984.
36. Neff CC, Pfister RC, Van Sonnenberg E: Percutaneous transtracheal ventilation: Experimental and practical aspects. J Trauma 23:84, 1983.
37. Rock JJ, Pfaeffle H, Smith RB: High pressure jet insufflation used to prevent aspirations and its effect in the tracheal mucosal wall. Crit Care Med 4:135, 1976.
38. Rogers MC, Nugent SK, Stidham GL: Effects of closed-chest cardiac massage on intracranial pressure. Crit Care Med 7:454, 1979.
39. Menegazzi JJ, Auble TE, Nicklas KA, Hosack GM, Rack L, Goode JS: Two-thumb versus two-finger chest compression during CPR in a swine infant model of cardiac arrest: Ann Emerg Med 22:240, 1993.
40. Michael TAD: Precordial percussion in cardiac resuscitation. Am Heart J 69:721, 1965.
41. Scherf D, Bornemann C: Thumping of the precordium in ventricular standstill. Am J Cardiol 5:30, 1960.
42. Pennington JE, Taylor J, Lown B: Chest thump for reverting ventricular tachycardia. N Engl J Med 283:1192, 1970.
43. Schleien CL: Cardiopulmonary Resuscitation: *Golden Hour Handbook of Advanced Pediatric Life Support.* Edited by Nichols DG, Yaster M, Lappe DG, Buck JR. pgs 105–136, Mosby Year Book, Baltimore, 1991.
44. Hedges JR, Barsan WB, Doan LA, et al.: Central versus peripheral intravenous routes in cardiopulmonary resuscitation. Am J Emerg Med 2:385, 1984.
45. Kuhn GH, White BC, Swetnam RE, et al.: Peripheral vs central circulation times during CPR: A pilot study. Ann Emerg Med 10:417, 1981.
46. Barson WG, Levy RC, Weir H: Lidocaine levels during CPR: Differences after peripheral venous, central venous, and intracardiac injections. Ann Emerg Med 10:73, 1981.
47. Emerman CL, Pinchak AC, Hancock D, Hagen JF: Effect of injection site on circulation times during cardiac arrest. Crit Care Med 16:1138, 1988.
48. Josefson LM: A new method of treatment-intraossal injections. Acta Medica Scand 81:550, 1934.
49. Berg RA: Emergency infusion of catecholamines into bone marrow. Am J Dis Child 138:810, 1984.
50. Meola F: Bone marrow infusions as routine procedure in children. J Pediatr 25:13, 1944.
51. Heinild S, Sondergaard T, Tudvad F: Bone marrow infusion in childhood: Experiences from 1,000 infusions. J Pediatr 30:400, 1947.
52. Orlowski JP, Julius CJ, Petras RE, Porembka DT, Gallagher JM: The safety of intraosseous infusions: Risks of fat and bone marrow emboli to the lungs. Ann Emerg Med 18:1062, 1989.
53. Morris RE, Schonfeld N, Haftel AS: Treatment of hemorrhagic shock with intraosseous administration of crystalloid fluid in the rabbit model. Ann Emerg Med 16:1321 1987.
54. Spivey WH, Lathers CM, Malone DR, et al.: Comparison of intraosseous, central, and peripheral routes of sodium bicarbonate administration during CPR in pigs. Ann Emerg Med 14:1135, 1985.
55. Andropoulos DB, Soifer SJ, Schreiber MD: Plasma epinephrine concentrations after intraosseous and central venous injection during cardiopulmonary resuscitation in the lamb. J Pediatr 116:312, 1990.
56. Hornchen U, Schuttler J, Stoeckel H, Eichelkraut W, Hahn N: Endobronchial instillation of epinephrine during cardiopulmonary resuscitation. Crit Care Med 15:1037, 1987.
57. Roberts J, Greenberg M, Knaub M: Comparison of the pharmacological effects of epinephrine administered by the intravenous and endotracheal routes. JACEP 7:260, 1978.
58. Roberts J, Greenberg M, Knaub M: Blood levels following intravenous and endotracheal epinephrine administration. JACEP 8:53, 1979.
59. McDonald JL: Serum lidocaine levels during cardiopulmonary resuscitation after intravenous and endotracheal administration. Crit Care Med 13:914, 1985.
60. Ralston SH, Tacker WA, Showen L, Carter A, Babbs CF: Endotracheal versus intravenous epinephrine during electromechanical dissociation with CPR in dogs. Ann Emerg Med 14:1044, 1985.
61. Greenberg MI, Roberts JR, Baskin SI: Use of endotracheally administered epinephrine in a pediatric patient. Am J Dis Child 135:767, 1981.
62. Redding JS, Asuncion JS, Pearson JW: Effective routes of drug administration during cardiac arrest. Anesth Analg 46:253, 1967.
63. Ralston SH, Voorhees WD, Babbs CF: Intrapulmonary epinephrine during prolonged cardiopulmonary resuscitation: Improved regional blood flow and resuscitation in dogs. Ann Emerg Med 13:79, 1984.
64. Nakayama S, Sibley L, Gunther RA, Holcroft JW, Kramer GC: Small-volume resuscitation with hypertonic saline (2,400 mOsm/liter) during hemorrhagic shock. Circ Shock 13:149, 1984.
65. Rowe GG, McKenna DH, Corliss RJ, Sialer S: Hemodynamic effects of hypertonic sodium chloride. J Appl Physiol 32:182, 1972.
66. Traverso LW, Bellamy RF, Hollenbach SJ, Witcher LD: Hypertonic sodium chloride solutions: Effect on hemodynamics and survival after hemorrhage in swine. J Trauma 27:32, 1987.
67. Velasco IT, Pontieri V, Silva RE Jr, Lopes OU: Hyperosmotic NaCl and severe hemorrhagic shock. Am J Physiol, 239:H664, 1980.
68. Wildenthal K, Skelton CL, Coleman HN: Cardiac muscle mechanics in hyperosmotic solutions. Am J Physiol 217:302, 1969.

69. Gazitua S, Scott JB, Swindall B, Haddy FJ: Resistance responses to local changes in plasma osmolality in three vascular beds. Am J Physiol 220:384, 1971.
70. Maningas PA: Resuscitation with 7.5% NaCl in 6% dextran-70 during hemorrhagic shock in swine: Effects on organ blood flow. Crit Care Med 15:1121, 1987.
71. Nerlich M, Gunther R, Demling RH: Resuscitation from hemorrhagic shock with hypertonic saline or lactated Ringer's (effect on the pulmonary and systemic microcirculations). Cir Shock 10:179, 1983.
72. Read RC, Johnson JA, Vick JA, Meyer MW: Vascular effects of hypertonic solutions. Circ Res 8:538, 1960.
73. Gunnar WP, Merlotti GJ, Barrett J, Jonasson O: Elevated intracranial pressure and hemorrhagic shock: Beneficial effects of hypertonic saline resuscitation in an experimental model. Fed Proc 46:805, 1987.
74. Gunnar WP, Jonasson O, Merlotti G, Stone J, Barrett J: Head injury and hemorrhagic shock: Studies of the blood brain barrier and intracranial pressure after resuscitation with normal saline solution, 3% saline solution, and dextran-40. Surgery 103:398, 1988.
75. Prough DS, Johnson JC, Poole GV Jr, Stullken EH, Johnston WE Jr: Effects on intracranial pressure of resuscitation from hemorrhagic shock with hypertonic saline versus lactated Ringer's solution. Crit Care Med 13:407, 1985.
76. Prough DS, Johnson JC, Stump DA, Stullken EH, Poole GV Jr, Howard G: Effects of hypertonic saline versus lactated Ringer's solution on cerebral oxygen transport during resuscitation from hemorrhagic shock. J Neurosurg 64:627, 1986.
77. Ditchey RV, Lindenfeld J: Potential adverse effects of volume loading on perfusion of vital organs during closed-chest resuscitation. Circulation 69:181, 1984.
78. Harris LC, Kirimli B, Safar P: Augmentation of artificial circulation during cardiopulmonary resuscitation. Anesthesiology 28:730, 1967.
79. Voorhees WD, Ralston SH, Kougia C, Schmitz PMW: Fluid loading with whole blood or Ringer's lactate during CPR in dogs. Resuscitation 15:113, 1987.
80. Tomaszemski CA, Meador SA: Theoretical effects of fluid infusions during cardiopulmonary resuscitation as demonstrated in a computer model circulation. Resuscitation 15:97, 1987.
81. Narang VPS: Utility of the pulse oximeter during cardiopulmonary resuscitation. Anesthesiology 65:239, 1986.
82. Waxman K: Noninvasive monitoring in emergency resuscitation. Ann Emerg Med 15:1434, 1986.
83. DelGuercio LRM, Coomaraswamy RP, State S: Cardiac output and other hemodynamic variables during external cardiac massage in man. N Engl J Med 269:1398, 1963.
84. Silver DI, Murphy RJ, Babbs CF, Geddes LA: Cardiac output during CPR: A comparison of two methods. Crit Care Med 9:419, 1981.
85. Gudipati CV, Weil MH, Bisera J, Deshmukh HG, Rackow EC: Expired carbon dioxide: A noninvasive monitor of cardiopulmonary resuscitation. Circulation 77:234, 1988.
86. Sanders AB, Kern KB, Otto CW, Milander MM, Ewy GA: End-tidal carbon dioxide monitoring during cardiopulmonary resuscitation: A prognostic indicator for survival. JAMA 262:1347, 1989.
87. Bhende MS, Thompson AE, Orr RA: Utility of an end-tidal carbon dioxide detector during stabilization and transport of critically ill children. Pediatr 89:1042, 1992.
88. Bhende MS, Thompson AE, Cook DR, et al.: Validity of a disposable end-tidal CO_2 detector in verifying endotracheal tube placement in infants and children. Ann Emerg Med 21:142, 1992.
89. O'Flaherty D, Adams AP: The end-tidal carbon dioxide detector. Assessment of a new method to distinguish oesophageal from tracheal intubation. Anaesthesia 45:653, 1990.
90. Martin GB, Gentile NT, Paradis NA, Moeggenberg J, Appleton TJ, Nowak RM: Effect of epinephrine on end-tidal carbon dioxide monitoring during CPR. Ann Emerg Med 19:396, 1990.
91. Cantineau JP, Merck P, Lambert Y, et al.: Effect of epinephrine on end-tidal carbon dioxide pressure during prehospital cardiopulmonary resuscitation. Am J Emerg Med 12:267, 1994.
92. Tang W, Weil MH, Gazmuri RJ, et al.: Pulmonary ventilation/perfusion defects induced by epinephrine during cardiopulmonary resuscitation. Circulation 84:2101, 1991.
93. Jorgensen EO, Malchow-Moller A: Cerebral prognostic signs during cardiopulmonary resuscitation. Resuscitation 6:217, 1979.
94. Morillo LE, Tulloch JW, Gumnit RJ, Snyder BD: Compressed spectral array patterns following cardiopulmonary arrest. A preliminary report. Arch Neurol 40:287, 1983.
95. Moss J, Rockoff M: EEG monitoring during cardiac arrest and resuscitation. JAMA 244:2750, 1980.
96. Young WL, Ornstein E: Compressed spectral array EEG during cardiac arrest and resuscitation. Anesthesiology 62:535, 1985.
97. Schleien CL, Koehler RC, Gervais H, et al.: Organ blood flow and somatosensory evoked potentials during and after cardiopulmonary resuscitation with epinephrine and phenylephrine. Circulation 79:1332, 1989.
98. Gervais HW, Schleien CL, Koehler RC, Berkowitz ID, Rogers MC, Traystman RJ: Effect of adrenergic drugs on cerebral blood flow, metabolism and evoked potentials after delayed onset of CPR in dogs. Stroke 22:1554–1561, 1991.
99. Goodwin SR, Friedman WA, Bellefleur M: Is it time to use evoked potentials to predict outcome in comatose children and adults? Crit Care Med 19:518, 1991.
100. Brain AI: The laryngeal mask - a new concept in airway management. Br J Anaesth 55:801, 1983.
101. Kokkinis K: The use of the laryngeal mask airway in CPR. Resuscitation 27:9, 1994.
102. Michael TAD, Lambert EH: Mouth-to-lung airway for cardiac resuscitation. Lancet 2:1329, 1968.
103. Smith JP, Bodai BI, Seifkin A, Palder S, Thomas V: The esophageal obturator airway. JAMA 250:1081, 1983.
104. Melker R, Cavallaro D, Krischer J: A pediatric gastric tube airway. Crit Care Med 9:426, 1981.
105. Pilcher DB, DeMeules JE: Esophageal perforation following use of esophageal airway. Chest 69:377, 1976.
106. Micheal TAD, Gordon AS: The esophageal obturator airway: A new device in emergency cardiopulmonary resuscitation. Br Med J 281:1531, 1980.
107. Schleien CL, Dean MJ, Koehler RC, et al.: Effect of epinephrine on cerebral and myocardial perfusion in an infant animal preparation of cardiopulmonary resuscitation. Circulation 77:809, 1986.
108. Nugent SK, Rogers MC: Resuscitation and intensive care monitoring following hypothermia. J Trauma 20:814, 1980.
109. Rod HST, Lind HBB: Survival after 40 minutes submersion without cerebral sequelae. Lancet 1:1275, 1975.
110. Geddes LA, Bourland JD, Ford G: The mechanism underlying sudden death from electric shock. Med Instrum 20:303–315, 1986.
111. Cooper MA: Lightning injuries: prognostic signs for death. Ann Emerg Med 9:134–138, 1980.
112. Kleiner JP, Wilkin JH: Cardiac effects of lightning strike. JAMA 240:2757–2759, 1978.
113. Redding JS, Pearson JW: Evaluation for drugs for cardiac resuscitation. Anesthesiology 24:203, 1963.
114. Pearson JW, Redding JS: Influence of peripheral vascular tone on resuscitation. Anesth Analg 44:746, 1965.
115. Yakaitis RW, Otto CW, Blitt CD: Relative importance of α and β adrenergic receptors during resuscitation. Crit Care Med 7:293, 1979.
116. Michael JR, Guerci AD, Koehler RC, et al.: Mechanisms by which epinephrine augments cerebral and myocardial perfusion during cardiopulmonary resuscitation in dogs. Circulation 69:822, 1984.
117. Koehler RC, Michael JR: Cardiopulmonary resuscitation, brain blood flow, and neurologic recovery. Crit Care Cl 1:205, 1985.
118. Livesay JJ, Follette DM, Fey KH, et al.: Optimizing myocardial supply/demand balance with a-adrenergic drugs during cardiopulmonary resuscitation. J Thorac Cardiovasc Surg 76:244, 1978.
119. Downey J, Chagrasulis RW, Hemphill V: Quantitative study of intramyocardial compression in the fibrillating heart. Am J Physiol 237:H191, 1979.
120. Ditchey RV, Goto Y, Lindenfeld J: Myocardial oxygen requirements during experimental cardiopulmonary resuscitation. Cardiovasc Res 26:791–797, 1992
121. Lindner KH, Prengel AW, Pfenninger EG, Linder IM, Strohmenger HU, Georgieff M, Lurie KG: Vasopressin improves vital organ blood flow during closed-chest cardiopulmonary resuscitation in pigs. Circulation 91:215, 1995.
122. Brown CG, Werman HA, Davis EA, Katz S, Hamlin RL: The effect of high-dose phenylephrine versus epinephrine on regional cerebral blood flow during CPR. Ann Emerg Med 16:743, 1987.
123. Brown CG, Davis EA, Werman RL: Methoxamine versus epinephrine on regional cerebral blood flow during cardiopulmonary resuscitation. Crit Care Med 15:682, 1987.
124. Holmes HR, Babbs CF, Voorhees WD, Tacker WA, DeGaravilla B: Influence of adrenergic drugs upon vital organ perfusion during CPR. Crit Care Med 8:137, 1980.
125. Schleien CL, Koehler RC, Berkowitz ID, et al.: Effect of phenylephrine on cerebral and myocardial perfusion during CPR in a swine model. Anesthesiology 65:A76 [Abstract], 1986.

126. Brillman JA, Sanders AB, Otto CW, Fahmy H, Bragg S, Ewy GA: Outcome of resuscitation from fibrillatory arrest using epinephrine and phenylephrine in dogs. Crit Care Med 13:912, 1985.
127. Brown CG, Birinyi F, Werman HA, Davis EA, Hamlin RL: The comparative effects of epinephrine versus phenylephrine on regional cerebral blood flow during cardiopulmonary resuscitation. Resuscitation 14:171, 1986.
128. Carlsson C, Hagerdal M, Kaasid AE, Siesjo BK: A catecholamine-mediated increased in cerebral oxygen uptake during immobilization stress in rats. Brain Res 119:223, 1977.
129. MacKenzie ET, McCulloch J, O'Keane M, Pickard JD, Harper AM: Cerebral circulation and norepinephrine: Relevance of the blood-brain barrier. Am J Physiol 231:483, 1976.
130. Winquist RJ, Webb RC, Bohr OF: Relaxation to transmural nerve stimulation and exogenously added norepinephrine in porcine vessels. A study utilizing cerebrovascular intrinsic tone. Circ Res 51:769, 1982.
131. Edvinsson L, Hardebo JE, MacKenzie ET, Owman C: Effect of endogenous noradrenaline on local cerebral blood flow after osmotic opening of the blood-brain barrier in the rat. J Physiol (Lond) 274:149, 1978.
132. Lasbennes F, Sercombe R, Seylaz J: Monoamine oxidase activity in brain microvessels determined using natural and artificial substances: Relevance to the blood-brain barrier. J Cereb Blood Flow Metab 3:521, 1983.
133. Arai T, Watanabe T, Nagaro T, Matsuo S: Blood-brain barrier impairment after cardiac resuscitation. Crit Care Med 9:444, 1981.
134. Schleien CL, Koehler RC, Shaffner DH, Traystman RJ: Blood-brain barrier integrity during cardiopulmonary resuscitation in dogs. Stroke 21:1185, 1990.
135. Schleien CL, Koehler RC, Shaffner DH, Eberle B, Traystman RJ: Blood-brain barrier disruption after cardiopulmonary resuscitation in immature swine. Stroke 22:477, 1991.
136. Schleien CL, Eberle B, Schaffner DH, Koehler RC, Traystman RJ: Reduced blood-brain barrier permeability after cardiac arrest by conjugated superoxide dismutase and catalase in piglets. Stroke 25:1830–1834, 1994.
137. Caceres MJ, Schleien CL, Kuluz JW, Gelman B, Dietrich WD: Early endothelial damage and leukocyte accumulation in piglet brains following cardiac arrest. (In Press, Acta Neuropathological)
138. Berkowitz ID, Gervais H, Schleien CL, et al.: Epinephrine dosage effects on cerebral and myocardial blood flow in an infant swine model of cardiopulmonary resuscitation. Anesthesiology 75:1041, 1991.
139. Brown CG, Werman HA, Davis EA, et al.: Comparative effects of graded doses of epinephrine on regional brain blood flow during CPR in a swine model. Ann Emerg Med 15:1138, 1986.
140. Brown CG, Werman HA, Davis EA, et al.: The effects of graded doses of epinephrine on regional myocardial blood flow during cardiopulmonary resuscitation in swine. Circulation 75:491, 1987.
141. Brown CG, Taylor RB, Werman HA, et al.: Myocardial oxygen delivery/consumption during cardiopulmonary resuscitation: a comparison of epinephrine and phenylephrine. Ann Emerg Med 17:332, 1988.
142. Brown CG, Taylor RB, Werman HA, et al.: Effect of standard doses of epinephrine on myocardial oxygen delivery and utilization during cardiopulmonary resuscitation. Crit Care Med 16:536, 1988.
143. Chase PB, Kern KB, Sanders AB, et al.: Effects of graded doses of epinephrine on both noninvasive and invasive measures of myocardial perfusion and blood flow during cardiopulmonary resuscitation. Crit Care Med 21:413, 1993.
144. Jackson RE, Joyce K, Danosi SF, et al.: Blood flow in the cerebral cortex during cardiac resuscitation in dogs. Ann Emerg Med 13:657, 1984.
145. Hoekstra JW, Griffith R, Kelley R, et al.: Effect of standard-dose versus high-dose epinephrine on myocardial high-energy phosphates during ventricular fibrillation and closed-chest CPR. Ann Emerg Med 22:1385, 1993.
146. Burchfield DJ, Preziosi MP, Lucas VW, et al.: Effects of graded doses of epinephrine during asphyxia-induced bradycardia in newborn lambs. Resuscitation 25:235, 1993.
147. Berg RA, Otto CW, Kern KB, et al.: High-dose epinephrine results in greater early mortality after resuscitation from prolonged cardiac arrest in pigs: a prospective, randomized study. Crit Care Med 22:282, 1994.
148. Ditchey RV, Lindenfeld J: Failure of epinephrine to improve the balance between myocardial oxygen supply and demand during closed chest resuscitation in dogs. Circulation 78:382, 1988.
149. Gonzalez ER, Ornato JP, Levine RL: Vasopressor effect of epinephrine with and without dopamine during cardiopulmonary resuscitation. Drug Intell Clin Pharm 22:868, 1988.
150. Gonzalez ER, Ornato JP, Garnett AR, et al.: Dose-dependent vasopressor response to epinephrine durig CPR in human beings. Ann Emerg Med 18:920, 1989.
151. Paradis NA, Martin GB, Rivers EP, et al.: Coronary perfusion pressure and the return of spontaneous circulation in human cardiopulmonary resuscitation. JAMA 263:1106, 1990.
152. Goetting MG, Paradis NA: High dose epinephrine in refractory pediatric cardiac arrest. Crit Care Med 17:1258, 1989.
153. Polin K, Leikin JB: High-dose epinephrine in cardiopulmonary resuscitation. JAMA 269:1383, 1993.
154. Cipolotti G, Paccagnella A, Simini G: Successful cardiopulmonary resuscitation using high doses of epinephrine. Int J Cardiol 33:430, 1991.
155. Martin D, Werman HA, Brown CG: Four case studies: high dose epinephrine in cardiac arrest. Ann Emerg Med 19:322, 1990.
156. Stiell IG, Hebert PC, Weitzman BN, et al.: High-dose epinephrine in adult cardiac arrest. N Engl J Med 327:1045, 1992.
157. Brown CG, Martin DR, Pepe PE, et al.: A comparison a standard-dose and high-dose epinephrine in cardiac arrest outside the hospital. N Engl J Med 327:1051, 1992.
158. Callaham M, Madsen C, Barton CW, et al.: A randomized clinical trial of high-dose epinephrine vs standard-dose epinephine in prehospital cardiac arrest. JAMA 268:19, 1992.
159. Rivers EP, Wortsman J, Rady MY, Blake HC, McGeorge FT, Buderer NM: The effect of the total cumulative epinephrine dose adminstered during human CPR on hemodynamic, oxygen transport, and utilization variables in the postresuscitation period. Chest 106:1499–1507, 1994.
160. Deleted
161. Angelos MG, Ward KR, Beckley PD: Norepinephrine-induced hypertension following cardiac arrest: effects on myocardial oxygen use in a swine model. Ann Emerg Med 24:907–914, 1994
162. Ditchey RV, Slinker BK: Phenylephrine plus propranolol improves the balance between myocardial oxygen supply and demand during experimental cardiopulmonary resuscitation. Am Heart J 127:324, 1994.
163. Ditchey RV, Rubio-Perez A, Slinker BK: Beta-adrenergic blockade reduces myocardial injury during experimental cardiopulmonary resuscitation. J Am College Cardiol 24:804–812, 1994.
164. Tang W, Weil MH, Gazmuri RJ, et al.: Pulmonary ventilation/perfusion defects induced by epinephrine during cardiopulmonary resuscitation. Circulation 84:2101, 1991.
165. Von Planta I, Wagner O, Von Planta M, et al.: Coronary perfusion pressure, end-tidal CO_2 and adrenergic agents in haemodynamic stable rats. Resuscitation 25:203, 1993.
166. Deleted
167. Stacpoole PW: Lactic acidosis: The case against bicarbonate therapy. Ann Intern Med 105:276, 1986.
168. Guerci AD, Chandra N, Johnson E, et al.: Failure of sodium bicarbonate to improve resuscitation from ventricular fibrillation in dogs. Circulation 74:IV75, 1986.
169. Graf H, Leach W, Arieff AI: Evidence for a detrimental effect of bicarbonate therapy in hypoxic lactic acidosis. Science 227:754, 1985.
170. Cingolani HE, Mattiazi AR, Blesa ES: Contractility in isolated mammalian heart muscle after acid-base changes. Circ Res 26:269, 1970.
171. Pannier JL, Leusen I: Contraction characteristics of papillary muscle during changes in acid-base composition of the bathing fluid. Arch Int Physiol Biochem 76:624, 1968.
172. Steinhart CR, Permutt S, Gurtner GH, Traystman RJ: b-adrenergic activity and cardiovascular response to severe respiratory acidosis. Am J Physiol 244:H46, 1983.
173. Wood WB, Manley Jr ES, Woodbury RA: The effects of CO_2 induced respiratory acidosis on the depressor and pressor components of the dog's blood pressure to epinephrine. J Pharmacol Exp Ther 139:238, 1963.
174. Rudolph AM, Yuan S: Response of the pulmonary vasculature to hypoxia and hydrogen ion concentration changes. J Clin Invest 45:399, 1966.
175. Martinez LR, Holland S, Fitzgerald J, Kountz S: pH homeostasis during cardiopulmonary resuscitation in critically ill patients. Resuscitation 1979;7:109.
176. Mattar JA, Weil MH, Shubin H, Stein L: Cardiac arrest in the critically ill: II. Hyperosmolal states following cardiac arrest. Am J Med 56:162, 1974.
177. Bishop RL, Weisfeldt ML: Sodium bicarbonate administration during cardiac arrest: Effect on arterial pH, pCO_2, and osmolality. JAMA 235:506, 1976.
178. Grundler W, Weil MH, Rackow EC: Arteriovenous carbon dioxide and pH gradients during cardiac arrest. Circulation 77:234, 1988.

179. Weil MH, Rackow EC, Trevino R, Grundler W, Falk JL, Griffel MI: Differences in acid-base state between venous and arterial blood during cardiopulmonary resuscitation. N Engl J Med 315:153, 1986.
180. Falk JL, Rackow EC, Weil MH: End-tidal carbon dioxide concentration during cardiopulmonary resuscitation. N Engl J Med 318:607, 1988.
181. Sessler D, Mills P, Gregory G, Litt L, James T: Effects of bicarbonate on arterial and brain intracellular pH in neonatal rabbits recovering from hypoxic lactic acidosis. J Pediatr 111:817, 1987.
182. Cohen Y, Chang LH, Litt L, et al.: Stability of brain intracellular pH during prolonged hypercapnia in rats. J Cere Blood Flow Metab 10:277, 1990.
183. Eleff SM, Schleien CL, Koehler RC, et al.: Brain-bioenergetics during cardiopulmonary resuscitation. Anesthesiology 76:77–84, 1992.
184. Gazmuri RJ, Planta M, Weil MH, Rackow EC: Cardiac effects of carbon dioxide-consuming and carbon dioxide-generating buffers during cardiopulmonary resuscitation. JACC 15:482, 1990.
185. Sun JH, Filley GF, Hord K, Kindig NB, Bartle EJ: Carbicarb: An effective substitute for $NaHCO_3$ for the treatment of acidosis. Surgery 102:835–839, 1987.
186. Bersin RM, Arieff AI: Improved hemodynamic function during hypoxia with Carbicarb, a new agent for the management of acidosis. Circulation 77:227, 1988.
187. Beech JS, Nolan KM, Iles RA, Cohen RD, Williams SC, Evans SJ: The effects of sodium bicarbonate and a mixture of sodium bicarbonate and carbonate ("Carbicarb") on skeletal muscle pH and hemodynamic status in rats with hypovolemic shock. Cl Exp 43:518, 1994.
188. Stacpoole PW: The pharmacology of dichloroacetate. Metabolism: Clinical & Experimental 38:1124, 1989.
189. Stacpoole PW, Lorenz AC, Thomas RG, Harman EM: Dichloroacetate in the treatment of lactic acidosis. Annals of Internal Med 108:58, 1988.
190. Wargovich TJ, MacDonald RG, Hill JA, Feldman RL, Stacpoole PW, Pepine CJ: Myocardial metabolic and hemodynamic effects of dichloroacetate in coronary artery disease. Am J Cardiology 61:65, 1988.
191. Stacpoole PW, Gonzalez MG, Vlasak J, Oshiro Y, Bodor N: Dichloroacetate derivatives. Metabolic effects and pharmacodynamics in normal rats. Life Sciences 41:2167, 1987.
192. Stacpoole PW, Wright EC, Baumgartner TG, Bersin RM, Buchalter S, Curry SH, Duncan CA, Harman EM, Henderson GN, Jenkinson S, et al.: A controlled clinical trial of dichloroacetate for treatment of lactic acidosis in adults. The Dichloroacetate-Lactic Acidosis Study Group. N Engl J Med 327:1564, 1992.
193. Katz AM, Reuter M: Cellular calcium and cardiac cell death. Am J Cardiol 44:188, 1979.
194. White BC, Winegar CD, Wilson RF, Hoehner PJ, Trombley JH: Possible role of calcium blockers in cerebral resuscitation: A review of the literature and synthesis for future studies. Crit Care Med 11:202, 1983.
195. Clark RE, Kristlieb IY, Henry PD: Nifedipine: A myocardial protective agent. Am J Cardiol 44:825, 1979.
196. Burke TJ, Arnold PE, Gordon JA, Bulger RE, Dobyan DC, Schrier RW: Protective effect of intrarenal calcium membrane blockers before or after renal ischemia: functional, morphological, and mitochondrial studies. J Clin Invest 74:1830, 1984.
197. Holthoff V, Beil C, Hartmann-Klosterk:otter U, et al.: Effect of nimodipine on glucose metabolism in stroke patients. Stroke 21(12 Suppl):IV95, 1990.
198. Resnekov L: Calcium antagonist drugs - Myocardial preservation and reduced vulnerability to ventricular fibrillation during CPR. Crit Care Med 9:360, 1981.
199. Greenblatt DJ, Gross PL, Bolognini V: Pharmacotherapy of cardiopulmonary arrest. Am J Hosp Pharm 33:379, 1976.
200. Bristow MR, Schwartz HD, Binetti G, Harrison DC, Daniels JR: Ionized calcium and the heart. Elucidation of in vivo concentration-response relationships in the open chest dog. Circ Res 41:565, 1977.
201. Drop LJ, Scheidegger D: Plasma ionized calcium concentration: important determinant of the hemodynamic response to calcium infusion. J Thorac Cardiovasc Surg 79:425, 1980.
202. Urban P, Scheidegger D, Buchmann B, Skarvan K: The hemodynamic effects of heparin and their relation to ionized calcium levels. J Thorac Cardiovasc Surg 91:303, 1986.
203. Urban P, Scheidegger D, Buchmann B, Barth D: Cardiac arrest and blood ionized calcium levels. Ann Int Med 109:110, 1988.
204. Burchard KW, Simms HH, Robinson A, DiAmico R, Gann DS: Hypocalcemia during sepsis: Relationship to resuscitation and hemodynamics. Arch Surg 127:265–272, 1992.
205. Cairns CB, Niemann JT, Pelikan PC, Sharma J: Ionized hypocalcemia during prolonged cardiac arrest and closed-chest CPR in a canine model. Ann Emerg Med 20:1178–1182, 1991.
206. Heining MPD, Band DM, Linton RAF: Choice of calcium salt: A comparison of the effects of calcium chloride and gluconate on plasma ionized calcium. Anaesthesia 39:1079, 1984.
207. Dhingia R, Amat-y-Leon F, Wyndham C: Electrophysiologic effects of atropine on human sinus node and atrium. Am J Med 38:492, 1976.
208. Gillette PC, Garson A: *Pediatric Cardiac Dysrhythmias.* Grune and Stratton, Inc. New York, NY, 1981.
209. Gilman AG, Rall TW, Nies AS, Taylor P: *Goodman and Gilman's The Pharmacological Basis of Therapeutics,* 8th edition. Pergamon Press, Inc. Elmsford, New York, 1990.
210. Goldberg AH: Cardiopulmonary arrest. N Engl J Med 290:381, 1974.
211. Scheinman MM, Thorburn D, Abbott JA: Use of atropine in patients with acute myocardial infarction and sinus bradycardia. Circulation 52:627, 1975.
212. Kottmeier CA, Gravenstein JS: The parasympathomimetic activity of atropine and atropine methylbromide. Anesthesiology 29:1125, 1968.
213. Myers R: Lactic acid accumulation as a cause of brain edema and cerebral necrosis resulting from oxygen deprivation. In: *Advances in Perinatal Neurology.* Edited by Korbin R, Gilleminault C, New York, Spectrum, pp.84–114, 1979.
214. Siemkowicz E, Hansen AJ: Clinical restitution following cerebral ischemia in hypo-, normo- and hyperglycemic rats. Acta Neurol Scandinav 58:1, 1978.
215. Siesjo, BK: Cerebral circulation and metabolism. Neurosurg 60:883, 1984.
216. Chopp M, Welch KMA, Tidwell CD, Helpern JA: Global cerebral ischemia and intracellular pH during hyperglycemia and hypoglycemia in cats. Stroke 19:1383, 1988.
217. Prado R, Ginsberg MD, Dietrich WD, Watson BD, Busto R: Hyperglycemia increases infarct size in collaterally perfused but not end-arterial vascular territories. J Cereb Blood Flow Metab 8:186,1988.
218. Pulsinelli WA, Levy DE, Sigsbee B, Scherer P, Plum F: Increased damage after ischemic stroke in patients with hyperglycemia with or without established diabetes mellitus. Am J Med 74:540, 1983.
219. Longstreth WT, Inui TS: High blood glucose level on hospital admission and poor neurological recovery after cardiac arrest. Ann Neurol 15:59, 1984.
220. Ashwal S, Schneider S, Tomasi L, Thompson J: Prognostic implications of hyperglycemia and reduced cerebral blood flow in childhood near-drowning. Neurology 40:820, 1990.
221. Woo E, Chan YW, Yu YL, Huang CY: Admission glucose level in relation to mortality and morbidity outcome in 252 stroke patients. Stroke 19:185, 1988.
222. Longstreth WT, Diehr P, Cobb LA, Hanson RW, Blair AD: Neurologic outcome and blood glucose levels during out-of-hospital cardiopulmonary resuscitation. Neurology 36:1186, 1986.
223. LeBlanc MH, Huang M, Patel D, et al.: Glucose given after hypoxic ischmia does not affect brain injury in piglets. Stroke 245:1443, 1995.
224. Voll CL, Auer RN: The effect of postischemic blood glucose levels on ischemic brain damage in the rat. Ann Neurol 24:638, 1988.
225. Voll CL, Auer RN: Insulin attenuates ischmic brain damage independent of its hypoglycemic effect. J Cereb Blood Fl Metab 11:1006, 1991.
226. Auer RN: Progress review: Hypoglycemic brain damage. Stroke 17:699, 1986.
227. Kouwenhoven WB, Ing DR, Milnor WR, Knickerbocker GG, Chestnut WR: Closed chest defibrillation of the heart. Surgery 42:550, 1957.
228. Kouwenhoven WB, Langworthy OR: Cardiopulmonary resuscitation of an account of forty-five years of research. Hopkins Med J 132:186, 1973.
229. Roth N: Electroresuscitation and the occult. Med Instr 14:120, 1980.
230. Hooker DR, Kouwenhoven WB, Langworthy OR: The effect of alternating electrical currents on the heart. Am J Physiol 103:444, 1933.
231. Beck CS, Pritchard WH, Feil HS: Ventricular fibrillation of long duration abolished by electric shock. JAMA 135:985, 1947.
232. Zoll PM, Linenthal AJ, Gibson W, Paul MH, Normal LR: N Engl J Med 254:727, 1956.
233. Dahl CF, Ewy GA, Warner ED, Thomas ED: Myocardial necrosis from direct current countershock: Effect of paddle electrode size and time interval between discharges. Circulation 50:956, 1974.
234. DiCola VC, Freedman GS, Downing SE, Zaret BL: Myocardial uptake of technetium-99m stannous pyrophosphate following direct current transthoracic countershock. Circulation 54:980, 1976.
235. Peleska B: Cardiac arrhythmias following condenser discharges and

their dependence upon strength of current and phase of cardiac cycle. Circ Res 13:21, 1963.
236. Weaver WD, Cobb LA, Copass MK, Hallstrom AP: Ventricular defibrillation - A comparative trial using 175-J and 320-J shocks. N Engl J Med 307:1101, 1982.
237. Jones JL, Lepeschkin E, Jones RE, Rush S: Response of cultured myocardial cells to countershock-type electrical field stimulation. Am J Physiol 235:H214, 1978.
238. Adgey AAJ, Patton JN, Campbell NPS, Webb SW: Ventricular defibrillation: Appropriate energy levels. Circulation 60:219 [Editorial], 1979.
239. Campbell NPS, Webb SW, Adgey AA, Pantridge JF: Transthoracic ventricular defibrillation in adults. Br Med J 2:1379, 1977.
240. Tacker WA Jr, Ewy GA: Emergency defibrillation dose: Recommendations and rationale. Circulation 60:223, 1979.
241. Gascho JA, Crampton RS, Sipes JN, Cherwek ML, Hunter FP, O'Brien WM: Energy levels and patient weight in ventricular fibrillation. JAMA 242:1380, 1979.
242. DeSilva RA, Lown B: Energy requirement for defibrillation of a markedly overweight patient. Circulation 57:827, 1978.
243. Kerber RE, Sarnat W: Factors influencing the success of ventricular defibrillation in man. Circulation 60:226, 1979.
244. Zipes DP, Fischer J, King RM, Nicoll A, Jolly WW: Termination of ventricular fibrillation in dogs by depolarizing a critical amount of myocardium. Am J Cardiol 36:37, 1975.
245. Tacker Jr WA, Babbs CF, Abendschein DR, Geddes LA: Transchest defibrillation under conditions of hypothermia. Crit Care Med 9:390, 1981.
246. Gascho JA, Crampton RS, Cherwek ML, Sipes JN, Hunter FP, O'Brien WM: Determinants of ventricular defibrillation in adults. Circulation 60:231, 1979.
247. Gutgesell HP, Tacker WA, Geddes LA, Davis JS, Lie JT, McNamara DG: Energy dose for ventricular defibrillation of children. Pediatrics 58:898, 1976.
248. Niemann JT, Cairns CB, Sharma J, Lewis RJ: Treatment of prolonged ventricular fibrillation: Immediate countershock versus high-dose epinephrine and CPR preceding countershock. Circulation 85:281–287, 1992.
249. Collingsworth KA, Kalman SM, Harrison DC: The clinical pharmacology of lidocaine as an antiarrhythmic drug. Circulation 50:1217, 1974.
250. Constantino RT, Crockett SE, Vasko JS: Cardiovascular effects and dose response relationships of lidocaine. Circulation 36(Suppl II):89, 1967.
251. Austen WG, Moran JM: Cardiac and peripheral vascular effects of lidocaine and procainalol. Am J Cardiol 16:701, 1965.
252. Jewitt DE, Kishow Y, Thomas M: Lidocaine in the management of arrhythmias after myocardial infarction. Circulation 37:965, 1968.
253. Chow MSS, Ronfeld RA, Hamilton RA, Helmink R, Fieldman A: Effect of external cardiopulmonary resuscitation on lidocaine pharmacokinetics in dogs. J Pharmacol Exp Ther 224:531, 1983.
254. Chow MSS, Ronfeld RA, Ruffett D, Fieldman A: Lidocaine pharmacokinetics during cardiac arrest and external cardiopulmonary resuscitation. Am Heart J 102:799, 1981.
255. Lichstein E, Chadda KD, Gupta PK: Atrioventricular block with lidocaine therapy. Am J Cardiol 31:277, 1973.
256. Romhilt DW, Bloodfield SS, Lipicky RJ: Evalution of bretylium tosylate for the treatment of premature ventricular contractions. Circulation 45:800, 1972.
257. Kuntzman R, Tsai I, Chang R: Disposition of bretylium in man and rat: A sensitive chemical method for its estimation in plasma and urine. Clin Pharmacol Ther 11:829, 1970.
258. Markis JE, Koch-Weser J: Characterizations and mechanisms of inotropic and chronotropic actions of bretylium tosylate. J Pharmacol Exp Ther 178:94, 1971.
259. Bigger JT Jr, Jaffe CC: The effect of bretylium tosylate on the electrophysiologic properties of ventricular muscle and Purkinje fibers. Am J Cardiol 27:82, 1971.
260. Chatterjee K, Mandel WJ, Vyden JK, Parmley WW, Forrester JS: Cardiovascular effects of bretylium tosylate in acute myocardial infarction. JAMA 223:757, 1973.
261. Bacaner MB: Bretylum tosylate for suppression of induced ventricular fibrillation. Am J Cardiol 17:528, 1966.
262. Koch-Weser J: Drug therapy-bretylium. N Engl J Med 300:473, 1979.
263. Haynes RE, Chinn TL, Copass MK, Cobb LA: Comparison of bretylium tosylate and lidocaine in management of out-of-hospital ventricular fibrillation: A randomized clinical trial. Am J Cardiol 48:353, 1981.
264. Chin DT, Vincent R, Bagg RL: Adrenaline-responsive electromechanical dissociation. Resuscitation 27:215, 1994.
265. Vanags B, Thakur RK, Stueven HA, Aufderheide T, Tresch DD: Interventions in the therapy of electromechanical dissociation. Resuscitation 17:163, 1989.
266. DeBehnke DJ, Angelos MG, Leasure JE: Use of cardiopulmonary bypass, high-dose epinephrine, and standard-dose epinephrine in resuscitation from post-countershock electromechanical dissociation. Ann Emerg Med 21:1051, 1992.
267. Bircher N, Safar P, Stewart R: A comparison of standard, "MAST"-augmented, and open-chest CPR in dogs: A preliminary investigation. Crit Care Med 8:147, 1980.
268. DelGuercio LRM, Feins NR, Cohn JD, Coomaraswamy RP, Wollman SB, State D: Comparison of blood flow during external and internal cardiac massage in man. Circulation 3[Suppl 1]:I171, 1965.
269. Weiser FM, Adler LN, Kuhn LA: Hemodynamic effects of closed and open-chest cardiac resuscitation in normal dogs and those with acute myocardial infarction. Am J Cardiol 10:555, 1962.
270. Kern KB, Sanders AB, Ewy GA: Open-chest cardiac massage after closed-chest compression in a canine model: When to intervene. Resuscitation 15:51, 1987.
271. Sanders AB, Kern KB, Atlas M, Bragg S, Ewy GA: Importance of the duration of inadequate coronary perfusion pressure on resuscitation from cardiac coronary arrest. J Am Coll Cardiol 6:113, 1985.
272. Sanders AB, Kern KB, Ewy GA, Atlas Bailey L: Improved resuscitation from cardiac arrest with open-chest massage. Ann Emerg Med 13:67, 1984.
272a. Zoll PM: Resuscitation of the heart in ventricular standstill by external electrical stimulation. N Engl J Med 247:768, 1952.
273. Falk FH, Jacobs L, Sinclair A, Madigan-McNeil C: External noninvasive cardiac pacing in out-of-hospital cardiac arrest. Crit Care Med 11:779, 1983.
274. Zoll PM, Zoll RH, Falk RH, Clinton JE, Eitel DR, Antman EM: External noninvasive temporary cardiac pacing: Clinical trials. Circulation 71:937, 1985.
275. Barthell E, Troiano P, Olson D, Stueven HA, Hendley G: Prehospital external cardiac pacing: a prospective, controlled clinical trial. Ann Emerg Med 17:1221, 1988.
276. Hedges JR, Syverud SA, Dalsey WC, Feero S, Easter R, Shultz B: Prehospital trial of emergency transcutaneous cardiac pacing. Circulation 76:1337, 1987.
277. Hedges JR, Feero S, Shultz B, Easter R, Syverud SA, Dalsey WC: Prehospital transcutaneous cardiac pacing for symptomatic bradycardia. Pacing Cl Electrophysiol 14:1473, 1991.
278. Beland MJ, Hesslein PS, Finlay CD, Faerron-Angel JE, Williams WG, Rowe RD: Noninvasive transcutaneous cardiac pacing in children. PACE 10:1262, 1987.
279. Beland MJ, Hesslein PS, Rowe RD: Ventricular tachycardia related to transcutaneous pacing. Ann Emerg Med 17:279, 1988.
280. Ralston MA, Knilans TK, Hannon DW, et al.: Use of adenosine for diagnosis and treatment of tachyarrhythmias in pediatric patients. J Pediatr 124:139, 1994.
281. Litman RS, Keon TP, Campbell FW: Termination of supraventricular tachycardia with adenosine in a healthy child undergoing anesthesia. Anesth Analg 73:665, 1991.
282. Stemp LI, ROy WL: Adenosine for the cardioversion of supraventricular tachycardia during general anesthesia and open heart surgery. Anesthesiology 76:849, 1992.
283. Dimich I, Singh PP, Herschman Z, et al.: Role of adenosine in the diagnosis and treatment of postoperative supraventricular tachyarrhythmias. J Clin Anesthesia 5:325, 1993.
284. Green AP, Giattina KH: Adenosine administration for neonatal VT. Neo Net 12:15, 1993.
285. Epstein ML, Kiel EA, Victorica BE: Cardiac decompensation following verapamil therapy in infants with supraventricular tachycardia. Pediatrics 75:737, 1985.
286. Brockman GF, Rodman GH: Acute Spigelian hernia, an unusual complication of cardiopulmonary resuscitation. J Ky Med Assoc 77:511, 1979.
287. Krischer JP, Fine EG, Davis JH, Nagel EL: Complications of cardiac resuscitation. Chest 92:287, 1987.
288. Dohi S: Postcardiopulmonary resuscitation pulmonary edema. Crit Care Med 11:434, 1983.
289. Nagel EL, Fine EG, Krischer JP, Davis JH: Complications of CPR. Crit Care Med 9:424, 1981.
290. Powner DJ, Holcombe PA, Mello LA: Cardiopulmonary resuscitation-related injuries. Crit Care Med 12:54, 1984.
291. Powner DJ: Blood potassium measurements during CPR. Chest 69:371 [Editorial], 1981.

292. Salerno DM, lsperger KJ, Helseth P, Murakami M, Chepuri V: Serum potassium, calcium and magnesium after resuscitation from ventricular fibrillation: A canine study. J Am Coll Cardiol 10:178, 1987.
293. JAMA - Infection Control Guidelines for CPR Providers. JAMA 262:2732, 1989.
294. JAMA - Risk of Infection During CPR Training and Rescue: Supplemental Guidelines. JAMA 262:2714, 1989.
295. McGrath RB: Gastroesophageal lacerations: A fatal complication of closed chest cardiopulmonary resuscitation. Chest 83:571, 1983.
296. Wild LM, Lajos TZ, Lee AB, Wright J: Left ventricular laceration due to stented prosthesis. Chest 77:216, 1980.
297. Baldwin JJ, Edwards JE: Rupture of right ventricle complicating closed chest cardiac massage. Circulation 53:562, 1976.
298. Aguilar JC: Fatal gastric hemorrhage: A complication of cardiorespiratory resuscitation. J Trauma 21:573, 1981.
299. Lee HR, Wilder RJ, Downs P, Massion W, Blank WF: MAST augmentation of external cardiac compression: Role of changing intrapleural pressure. Ann Emerg Med 10:560, 1981.
300. Morgan RR: Laceration of the liver from closed-chest cardiac massage. N Engl J Med 265:82, 1961.
301. Clinch SL, Thompson JS, Edney JA: Pneumoperitoneum after cardiopulmonary resuscitation: A therapeutic dilemma. J Trauma 23:428, 1983.
302. Vagn-Hansen PL: Complications following external cardiac massage with special emphasis on cerebral embolism. Acta Pathol Microbiol Scand 79[Sect A]:505, 1971.
303. Mehta B, Briggs DK, Sommers SC, Karpatkin M: Disseminated intravascular coagulation following cardiac arrest: A study of 15 patients. Am J Med Sci 264:353, 1972.
304. Hay E, Cohen H, Pasik S: Acute thrombosis of subclavian artery during CPR. Ann Emerg Med 16:447, 1987.
305. Achong MR: Infectious hazards of mouth-to-mouth resuscitation. Am Heart J 100:759, 1980.
306. Weale FE, Lond MS, Rothwell-Jackson RL: The efficiency of cardiac massage. Lancet 1:990, 1962.
307. Rudikoff MT, Maughan WL, Effron M, Freund P, Weisfeldt ML: Mechanisms of blood flow during cardiopulmonary resuscitation. Circulation 61:345, 1980.
308. Criley JM, Blaufuss AJ, Kissel G: Cough-induced cardiac compression. JAMA 263:1246, 1976.
309. Fisher J, Vaghaiwalla BS, Tsitlik J, et al.: Determinants and clinical significance of jugular venous valve competence. Circulation 65:188, 1982.
310. Gudipati CV, Weil MH, Deshmukah HG, Rackow EC, Bisera J, Holst M: Right atrial-jugular venous pressure gradients during experimental CPR. Chest 89:443S, 1986.
311. Chandra NC, Tsitlik JE, Halperin HR, Guerci AD, Weisfeldt ML: Observations of hemodynamics during human cardiopulmonary resuscitation. Crit Care Med 18:929, 1990.
312. Niemann JT, Rosborough JP, Hausknecht M, Garner D, Criley JM: Pressure-synchronized cineangiography during experimental cardiopulmonary resuscitation. Circulation 64:985, 1981.
313. Paradis NA, Martin GB, Goetting MG, et al.: Simultaneous aortic, jugular bulb, and right atrial pressures during cardiopulmonary resuscitation in humans: Insights into mechanisms. Circulation 80:361, 1989.
314. Cohen JM, Chandra N, Alderson PO, VanAswegen A, Tsitlik JE, Weisfeldt ML: Timing of pulmonary and systemic blood flow during intermittent high intrathoracic pressure cardiopulmonary resuscitation of the dog. Am J Card 49:1883, 1982.
315. Rich S, Wix HL, Shapiro EP: Clinical assessment of heart chamber size and valve motion during cardiopulmonary resuscitation by two-dimensional echocardiography. Am Heart J 102:368, 1981.
316. Werner JA, Greene HL, Janko CL, Cobb LA: Visualization of cardiac valve motion in man during external chest compression using two-dimensional echocardiography. Circulation 63:1417, 1981.
317. Feneley MP, Maier GW, Gaynor JW, et al.: Sequence of mitral valve motion and transmitral blood flow during manual cardiopulmonary resuscitation in dogs. Circulation 76:363, 1987.
318. Babbs CF, Tacker WA, Paris RL, Murphy RJ, Davis RW: CPR with simultaneous compression and ventilation at high airway pressure in 4 animal models. Crit Care Med 10:501, 1982.
319. Berkowitz ID, Chantarojanasiri T, Koehler RC, et al.: Blood flow during cardiopulmonary resuscitation with simultaneous compression and ventilation in infant pigs. Pediatr Res 26:558, 1989.
320. Beyar R, Kishon Y, Sideman S, Dinnar U: Computer studies of systemic and regional blood flow mechanisms during cardiopulmonary resuscitation. Med Biol Eng 22:499, 1984.
321. Halperin HR, Tsitlik JE, Beyar R, Chandra N, Guerci AD: Intrathoracic pressure fluctuations move blood during CPR: Comparison of hemodynamic data with predictions from a mathematical mode. Ann Biomed Eng 15:385, 1987.
322. Maier GW, Tyson GS, Olsen CO, et al.: The physiology of external cardiac massage: High-impulse cardiopulmonary resuscitation. Circulation 70:86, 1984.
323. Fitzgerald KR, Babbs CF, Frisora HA, Davis RW, Silver DI: Cardiac output during cardiopulmonary resuscitation at various compression rates and durations. Am J Physiol 241:H442, 1981.
324. Feneley MP, Maier GW, Kern KB, et al.: Influence of compression rate on initial success of resuscitation and 24 hour survival after prolonged manual cardiopulmonary resuscitation in dogs. Circulation 77:240, 1988.
325. Sanders AB, Kern KB, Fonken S, Otto CW, Ewy GA: The role of bicarbonate and fluid loading in improving resuscitation from prolonged cardiac arrest with rapid manual chest compression CPR. Ann Emerg Med 19:1, 1990.
326. Dean JM, Koehler RC, Schleien CL, et al.: Age-related effects of compression rate and duration in cardiopulmonary resuscitation. J Appl Physiol 68:554, 1990.
327. Fleisher G, Delgado-Paredes C, Heyman S: Slow versus rapid closed-chest cardiac compression during cardiopulmonary resuscitation in puppies. Crit Care Med 15:939, 1987.
328. Ornato JP, Gonzales ER, Garrett AR, Levine RL, McClung BK: Effect of cardiopulmonary resuscitation compression rate on end-tidal carbon dioxide concentration and arterial pressure in man. Crit Care Med 16:241, 1988.
329. Dean JM, Koehler RC, Schleien CL, et al.: Age-related changes in chest geometry during cardiopulmonary resuscitation. J Appl Physiol 62:2212, 1987.
330. Shaffner DH, Schleien CL, Koehler RC, Eberle B, Rogers MC, Traystman R: Cerebral and coronary perfusion with vest cardiopulmonary resuscitation in piglets. Crit Care Med 22:1817, 1994.
331. Swenson RD, Weaver WD, Niskanen RA, Martin J, Dahlberg S: Hemodynamics in humans during conventional and experimental methods of cardiopulmonary resuscitation. Circulation 78:630, 1988.
332. Rogers MC, Nugent SK, Stidham GL: Effects of closed-chest cardiac massage on intracranial pressure. Crit Care Med 7:454, 1979.
333. Rogers MC, Weisfeldt ML, Traystman RJ: Cerebral blood flow during cardiopulmonary resuscitation. Anesth Analg 60:73, 1981.
334. Guerci AD, Shi A, Levin H, Tsitlik J, Weisfeldt ML, Chandra N: Transmission of intrathoracic pressure to the intracranial space during cardiopulmonary resuscitation in dogs. Circ Res 56:20, 1985.
335. Neimann JT, Rosborough JP, Pelikan PC: Hemodynamic determinants of subdiaphragmatic venous return during closed-chest CPR in a canine cardiac arrest model. Ann Emerg Med 19:1232, 1990.
336. Bircher N, Safar P: Comparison of standard and "new" closed-chest CPR and open-chest CPR in dogs. Crit Care Med 9:384, 1981.
337. Chandra N, Rudikoff M, Weisfeldt ML: Simultaneous chest compression and ventilation at high airway pressure during cardiopulmonary resuscitation. Lancet 1:175, 1980.
338. Chandra N, Weisfeldt ML, Tsitlik J, et al.: Augmentation of carotid flow during cardiopulmonary resuscitation by ventilation at high airway pressure simultaneous with chest compression. Am J Card 48:1053, 1981.
339. Harris L, Kirimli B, Safar P: Ventilation - cardiac compression rates and ratios in cardiopulmonary resuscitation. Anesthesiology 28:806, 1967.
340. Koehler RC, Chandra N, Guerci AD, et al.: Augmentation of cerebral perfusion by simultaneous lung inflation with abdominal binding after cardiac arrest in dogs. Circulation 67:266, 1983.
341. Luce JM, Ross BK, O'Quinn RJ, et al.: Regional blood flow during cardiopulmonary resuscitation in dogs using simultaneous and nonsimultaneous compression and ventilation. Circulation 67:258, 1983.
342. Sanders AB, Ewy GA, Alferness CA, Taft T, Zimmerman M: Failure of one method of simultaneous chest compression, ventilation, and abdominal binding during CPR. Crit Care Med 10:509, 1982.
343. Babbs CF, Fitzgerald KR, Voorhees WD, Murphy TJ: High-pressure ventilation during CPR with 95% O_2: 5% CO_2. Crit Care Med 10:505, 1982.
344. Krischer JP, Fine EG, Weisfeldt ML, Guerci AD, Nagel E, Chandra N: Comparison of prehospital conventional and simultaneous compression-ventilation cardiopulmonary resuscitation. Crit Care Med 17:1263, 1989.
345. Halperin H, Tsitlik J, Guerci AD, et al.: Determinants of blood flow to vital organs during cardiopulmonary resuscitation in dogs. Circulation 73:539, 1986.

346. Halperin HR, Guerci AD, Chandra N, et al.: Vest inflation without simultaneous ventilation during cardiac arrest in dogs: improved survival from prolonged cardiopulmonary resuscitation. Circulation 74:1407, 1986.
347. Criley JM, Niemann JT, Rosborough JP, Hausknecht M: Modifications of cardiopulmonary resuscitation based on the cough. Circulation 74:IV42, 1986.
348. Halperin HR, Tsitlik JE, Gelfand M, et al.: A preliminary study of cardiopulmonary resuscitation by circumferential compression of the chest with use of a penumatic vest. N Engl J Med 329:762, 1993.
349. Beyar R, Halperin HR, Tsitlik JE, et al.: Circulatory assistance by intrathoracic pressure variations: optimization and mechanisms studied by a mathematical model in relation to experimental data. Circ Res 64:703, 1989.
350. Niemann T, Rosborough JP, Ung S, Criley JM: Hemodynamic effects of continuous abdominal binding during cardiac arrest and resuscitation. Am J Card 53:269, 1984.
351. Chandra N, Snyder LD, Weisfeldt ML: Abdominal binding during cardiopulmonary resuscitation in man. JAMA 246:351, 1981.
352. Mahoney BD, Mirick MJ: Pneumatic trousers in refractory cardiopulmonary arrest. Ann Emerg Med 13:410, 1984.
353. Ralston SH, Babbs CF, Niebauer MJ: Cardiopulmonary resuscitation with interposed abdominal compression in dogs. Anesth Analg 61:645, 1982.
354. Hoekstra OS, Van Lambalgen AA, Groeneveld AB, Van Den Bos GC, Thijs LG: Abdominal compressions increase vital organ perfusion during CPR in gods: relation with efficacy of thoracic compressions. Ann Emerg Med 25:375–385, 1995
355. Einagle V, Bertrand F, Wise RA, Rousos C, Magder S: Interposed abdominal compressions and carotid blood flow during cardiopulmonary resuscitation: Support for a thoracoabdominal unit. Chest 93:1206, 1988.
356. Voorhees WD, Babbs CF, Niebauer MJ: Improved oxygen delivery during cardiopulmonary resuscitation with interposed abdominal compressions. Ann Emerg Med 12:128, 1983.
357. Voorhees WD, Ralston SH, Babbs CF: Regional blood flow during cardiopulmonary resuscitation with abdominal counterpulsation in dogs. Am J Emerg Med 2:123, 1983.
358. Waller JW, Bruestle JC, White BC, Evans AT, Indreri R, Bialeh H: Perfusion of the cerebral cortex by use of abdominal counterpulsation during cardiopulmonary resuscitation. Am J Emerg Med 2:391, 1984.
359. Eberle B, Schleien CL, Shaffner DH, Koehler RC, Traystman RJ: Effects of three models of abdominal compression on vital organ blood flow in piglet CPR model. Anesthesiology 73:A300, 1990.
360. Berryman CR, Phillips GM: Interposed abdominal compression - CPR in human subjects. Ann Emerg Med 13:226, 1984.
361. Howard M, Carruba C, Foss F, Janiak B, Hogan B, Guiness M: Interposed abdominal compression-CPR: its effects on parameters of coronary perfusion in human subjects. Ann Emerg Med 16:253, 1987.
362. Ward KR, Sullivan RS, Zelenak RR, Summer WR: A comparison of interposed abdominal compression CPR and standard CPR by monitoring end-tidal pCO_2. Ann Emerg Med 18:831, 1989.
363. Barranco F, Lesmes A, Irles JA, Blasco J, Leal J, Rodrigues J, Leon C: Cardiopulmonary resuscitation with simultaneous chest and abdominal compression: Comparative study in humans. Resuscitation 20:67, 1990.
364. Lurie KG, Shultz JJ, Callaham ML, et al.: Evaluation of active compression-decompression CPR in victims of out-of-hospital cardiac arrest. JAMA 271:1405, 1994.
365. Tucker JK, Khan JH, Savitt MA: Active compression-decompression resuscitation: effects on pulmonary ventilation. Resuscitation 26:125, 1993.
366. Cohen TJ, Tucker KJ, Lurie KG, et al.: Active compression-decompression: A new method of cardiopulmonary resuscitation. JAMA 267:2916, 1992.
367. Lindner KH, Pfenninger EG, Lurie KG, et al.: Effects of active compression-decompression resuscitation on myocardial and cerebral blood flow in pigs. Circulation 88:1254, 1993.
368. Cohen TJ, Tucker KJ, Redberg RF, et al.: Active compression-decompression resuscitation: a novel method of cardiopulmonary resuscitation. Am Heart J 124:1145, 1992.
369. Shultz JJ, Coffeen P, Sweeney M, et al.: Evaluation of standard and active compression-decompression CPR in an acute human model of ventricular fibrillation. Circulation 89:684, 1994.
370. Lurie KG, Coffeen P, Shultz J, McKnite S, Detloff B, Mulligan K: Improving active compression-decompression cardiopulmonary resuscitation with an inspiratory impedance valve. Circulation 91:1629–1932, 1995.
371. Cohen TJ, Goldner BG, Maccaro PC, et al.: A comparison of active compression-decompression cardiopulmonary resuscitation with standard cardiopulmonary resuscitation for cardiac arrests occurring in the hospital. N Engl J Med 329:1918, 1993.
372. Levine R, Gorayeb M, Safar P, Abramson N, Stezoski W, Kelsey S: Cardiopulmonary bypass after cardiac arrest and prolonged closed-chest CPR in dogs. Ann Emerg Med 16:620, 1987.
373. Reich H, Angelos MG, Safar P, Sterz F, Leonov Y: Cardiac resuscitability with cardiopulmonary bypass after increasing ventricular fibrillation times in dogs. Ann Emerg Med 19:887, 1990.
374. Angelos MG, Gaddis M, Gaddis G, Leasure JE: Cardiopulmonary bypass in a model of acute myocardial infarction and cardiac arrest. Ann Emerg Med 19:874, 1990.
375. Phillips SJ, Ballantine B, Slonine D, et al.: Percutaneous initiation of cardiopulmonary bypass. Ann Thorac Surg 36:223, 1983.
376. Mattox KL, Beall AC: Resuscitation of the moribund patient using portable cardiopulmonary bypass. Ann Thorac Surg 22:436, 1976.
377. Hartz R, LoCicero J, Sanders JH, Frederikson JW, Joob AW, Michaelis LL: Clinical experience with portable cardiopulmonary bypass in cardiac arrest patients. Ann Thorac Surg 50:437, 1990.
378. Reichman RT, Joyo CL, Dembitsky WP, et al.: Improved patient survival after cardiac arrest using a cardiopulmonary support system. Ann Thorac Surg 49:101, 1990.
379. Eisenberg MS, Bergner L, Hallstrom A: Paramedic programs and out-of-hospital cardiac arrest. I. Factors associated with successful resuscitation. Am J Public Health 69:30, 1979.
380. Eisenberg MS, Copass MK, Hallstrom A, Cobb LA, Bergner L: Management of out-of-hospital cardiac arrest: failure of basic emergency medical technician services. JAMA 243:1049, 1980.
381. Eisenberg MS, Bergner L, Hallstrom A: Out-of-hospital cardiac arrest: improved survival with paramedic services. Lancet II:812, 1980.
382. Eisenberg MS, Bergner L, Hallstrom AP, Cummins RO: Sudden cardiac death. Scientific American 254:37, 1986.
383. Ramsay ID: Survival after imipramine poisoning. Lancet II:1308, 1967.
384. Cummins RO, Eisenberg MS, Hallstrom AP, Litwin PE: Survival of out-of-hospital cardiac arrest with early initiation of cardiopulmonary resuscitation. Am J Emerg Med 3:114, 1985.
385. Stueven H, Troiano P, Thompson B, et al.: Bystander/first responder CPR: ten years experience in a paramedic system. Ann Emerg Med 15:707, 1986.
386. Thompson BM, Stueven HA, Mateer JR, Aprhamian CC, Tucker JF: Comparison of clinical CPR studies in Milwaukee and elsewhere in the United States. Ann Emerg Med 14:750, 1985.
387. Nichols DG, Kettrick RG, Swedlow DB, Lee S, Passman R, Ludwig S: Factors influencing outcome of cardiopulmonary arrest in children. Pediatr Emerg Care 2:1, 1986.
388. Mullie A, Verstringe P, Buylaert W, et al.: Predictive value of Glasgow Coma Score for awakening after out-of-hospital cardiac arrest. Lancet I:23, 1988.
389. Bedel SE, Delbanco TL, Cook EF, Epstein FH: Survival after cardiopulmonary resuscitation in the hospital. N Engl J Med 309:569, 1983.
390. DeBard ML: Cardiopulmonary resuscitation: analysis of six years' experience and review of the literature. Ann Emerg Med 10:408, 1981.
391. Fusgen I, Summa JK: How much sense is there in an attempt to resuscitate an aged person? Gerontology 24:37, 1978.
392. George AL, Folkin BP, Crecelius PL, Campbell WB: Pre-arrest morbidity and other correlates of survival after in-hospital cardiopulmonary arrest. Am J Med 87:28, 1989.
393. Hahn RG, Hutchinson JC, Conte JE: Cardiopulmonary resuscitation in a university hospital. An analysis of the cost and survival. West J Med 131:344, 1979.
394. McGrath RB: In-house cardiopulmonary resuscitation - after a quarter of a century. Ann Emerg Med 16:1365, 1987.
395. Rozenbaum EA, Shenkman L: Predicting outcome of in-hospital cardiopulmonary resuscitation. Crit Care Med 16:583, 1988.
396. Taffet G, Teasdale TA, Luchi RJ: In-hospital cardiopulmonary resuscitation. JAMA 260:2069, 1988.

Airway Management in Pediatric Critical Care 2

Aaron L. Zuckerberg
David G. Nichols

INTRODUCTION

Management of the airway is an integral component in the overall care of a critically ill child. Children can present with a critical airway for a variety of reasons that depend on the underlying critical illness. For instance, partial upper airway obstruction may be a consequence of an altered level of consciousness (trauma or a postictal state), or from airway edema (infection or traumatic injury). The former may be managed adequately with the establishment of a patent airway, oxygen administration, secretion removal, and bag mask ventilation. The latter often require expeditious endotracheal intubation and represent a challenge for even the most experienced laryngoscopist. Endotracheal intubation is life saving. However, the technique requires skill and familiarity with hypnotic and neuromuscular blocking agents. Inexperience or injudicious drug therapy may exacerbate the patient's condition.

This chapter reviews the anatomy and evaluation of the pediatric airway and basic airway management. Emphasis will be placed on recognition of the difficult airway, pharmacological management and techniques for securing an airway when endotracheal intubation is not possible. The management of specific pediatric airway situations will be reviewed as well.

THE ANATOMY OF THE AIRWAY

The larynx is made up of a group of nine cartilages—the thyroid, cricoid epiglottis corniculate[2], cuneiform[2] and arytenoid[2]—which are covered by folds of mucosa, con-

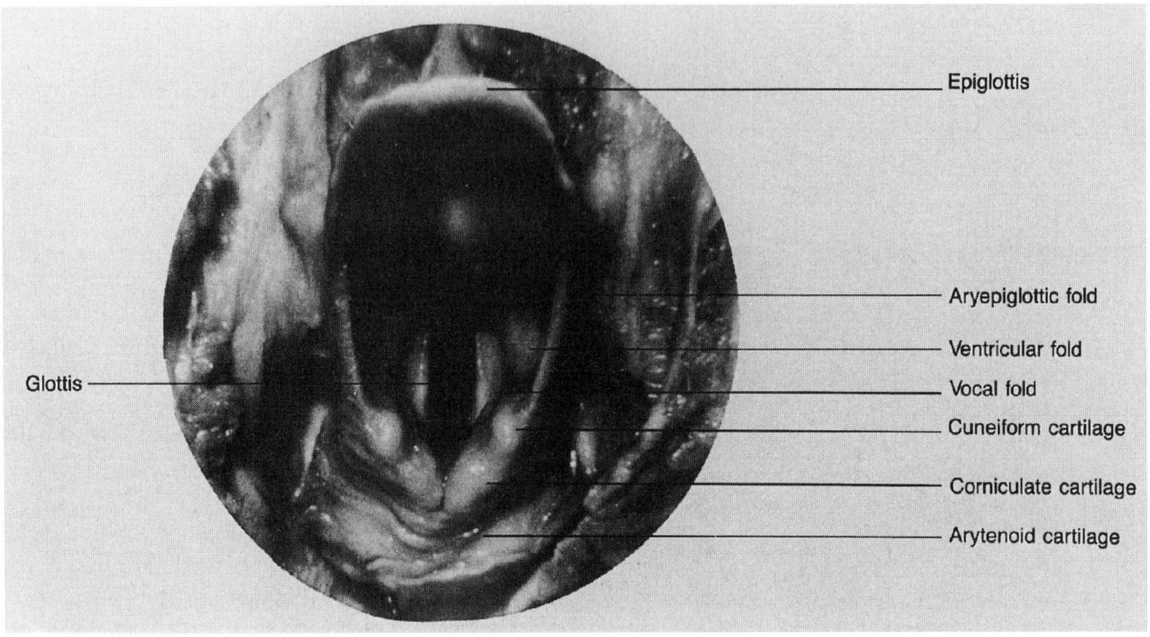

Figure 2.1. Anatomy of the larynx. (From Barash PG, Cullen BF, Stoelting RK Clinical Anesthesia 2nd Edition.)

nective tissue and muscle. There are important laryngeal tissue folds which define the glottis (Fig. 2.1 and **Table 2.1**).

The innervation of the larynx is through the superior and recurrent laryngeal nerves. Supraglottic sensation is mediated by the superior laryngeal nerve, while the infraglottic region is innervated by the inferior laryngeal nerve. The motor innervation of the larynx is primarily through the recurrent laryngeal nerves. Only the cricothyroid muscle is innervated by a branch of the superior laryngeal nerve.

The mucosa lining the airway contains ciliated and squamous epithelium, is highly vascular and overlies a rich network of submucosal lymphatic vessels. The airway mucosa and submucosa are loosely connected to the underlying structures except in the areas of the vocal cords and the laryngeal surface of the epiglottis. This has tremendous clinical implications. Subglottic inflammation is usually limited to the loosely adherent mucosa below the vocal cords and rarely spreads to the supraglottic structures. Similarly, most supraglottic inflammatory processes are limited by the barrier of firmly adherent mucosa at the level of the vocal cords and will not spread to the subglottic region[1]. This region's tight adherence with limited capacitance to accommodate edema and inflammatory changes is seen most dramatically in epiglottitis, in which modest edema leads to a gross distortion of tissue planes and anatomical positions.

Table 2.1. The Components of the Glottis

- Paired aryepiglottic folds extend from the epiglottis to the superior surface of the arytenoids.
- Paired vestibular cords, the false cords, extend from the posterior surface of the thyroid cartilage to the superior aspects of the arytenoids.
- Paired vocal folds, the true vocal cords, extend from the posterior surface of the thyroid cartilage to the anterior projections of the arytenoids.
- A single intra-arytenoid fold bridges the arytenoid cartilages.
- A single thyrohyoid fold extends anteriorly from the hyoid bone to the thyroid cartilage.

Oral intubation requires the establishment of a line of vision from the incisor teeth to the larynx. This path has three axes: the oral axis, the pharyngeal axis and the laryngeal axis (Fig. 2.2). Normally the oral axis is perpendicular to the laryngeal axis, and the pharyngeal axis forms a 45 degree angle with the laryngeal axis. Positioning of the patient with modest neck flexion (the "sniffing position") and atlanto-occipital joint extension superimposes these axes. A cushion or folded towel placed under the occiput will adequately flex the neck on the body. Failure to position the patient correctly is a common error and frequently results in an unnecessarily difficult or impossible intubation.

The line of vision necessary for intubation requires deflection of the tongue and soft tissues out of the oro-pharyngeal-laryngeal path. These structures are displaced into a potential space, defined by the anterior and lateral rami of the mandible and the hyoid bone (Fig. 2.3)[2]. Alteration in the anatomic structures of this area, such as in the mandibular dysplasias, will decrease the space in which the soft tissue can be displaced with the laryngoscope and making laryngoscopy and intubation difficult. An increase in the amount of soft tissue in the tongue, floor of the mouth or submandibular space has the same effect (e.g. mucopolysaccharidoses). Although neuromuscular blockade will maximize the potential displacement

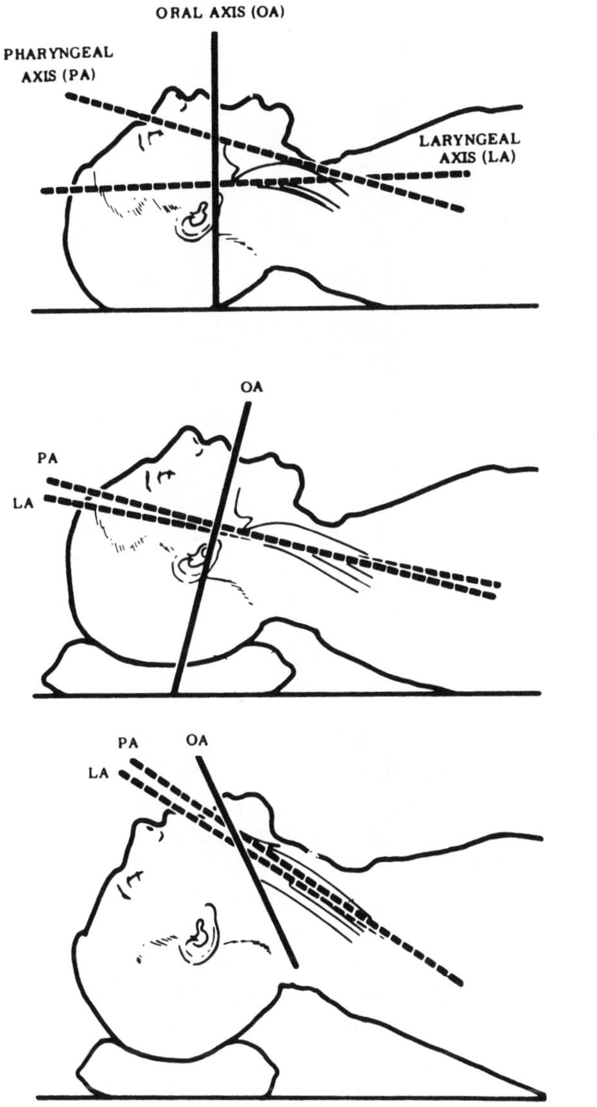

Figure 2.2. The three airway axes. With proper head extension and neck flexion these axes are superimposed to establish the necessary line of vision. (From Berry FA, Anesthetic Management of Difficult and Routine Pediatric Patients, 2nd edition, Churchill Livingstone, 1990, p 172.)

space, no amount of drug will relax bony abnormalities or tense tissue infiltration from either mass or edema.

DEVELOPMENTAL AIRWAY CONSIDERATIONS

The infant's airway differs in many respects from that of the adult. The differences that are critical for airway management are outlined in **Table 2.2** and depicted in Fig. 2.4.

The infant's tongue is large in proportion to the rest of the oral cavity and is closer to the palate, thus more easily obstructing the airway. Laryngoscopic stabilization of the tongue is more difficult. The rostral position of the larynx functionally shortens the distance in which the three axes need to be superimposed. As a result the larynx appears "very anterior" and may be difficult to visualize. The epiglottis is omega shaped, short, stiff and not amenable to displacement by vallecular suspension. Rather, suspension of the epiglottis leads to a clear view of the glottal structures. The adult vocal cords lie perpendicular to the laryngeal axis. However, in a child, the anterior attachment of the vocal cords is more inferior than the posterior attachment, producing an antero-caudal angulation (Fig. 2.5). This feature can lead to the endotracheal tube becoming caught on the anterior commissure when passing through the larynx. Simple rotation of the tube to the right or left allows the tube to slip off and pass. Finally, the protuberant occiput can result in excessive neck flexion. Occipital elevation in the infant is therefore not necessary.

There are maturational differences in the subglottic region as well. The narrowest portion of the infant's airway is at the level of the cricoid ring, producing a funnel shape to the laryngeal complex. In contrast, the narrowest aspect of the adult larynx is the opening between the vocal cords, creating a cylindrical shape (Fig. 2.6). This difference impacts on the size of an endotracheal tube that will fit in younger patients. In children less than the age of 8 years, an endotracheal tube may pass through the vocal cords but be unable to traverse the region of the cricoid ring. An excessively large endotracheal tube compresses the tracheal mucosa leading to the development of subglottic edema and post-extubation croup[3].

The length of the trachea also changes with development. The distance from the glottis to the carina in the newborn is 4 cm. Over the first 12 months of life the trachea grows to 7 cm. In a child the trachea is 8 cm long. By adulthood, the trachea is 12 cm long[4,5]. In some patients precise mid-tracheal positioning of the tip of the endotracheal tube may be difficult, (e.g. tracheo-esophageal fistula). After deliberate endobronchial intubation, the endotracheal tube is withdrawn until bilateral breath sounds are just appreciated. At this point the tube is withdrawn an additional 2 cm. The endotracheal tube will be mid-tracheal in virtually all situations.

THE DIFFICULT AIRWAY: ASSESSMENT AND PHYSIOLOGY

The ability to recognize a difficult airway is imperative in individuals responsible for airway management. In the adult population, moderately difficult intubations are relatively common, occurring in 1 to 18% of patients[6,7]. A definite

Table 2.2. Distinctive Characteristics of the Infant Airway

- Relatively large tongue.
- Higher position of the larynx (C3–4 vs C4–5).
- Laryngeal configuration.
- A protuberant occiput.

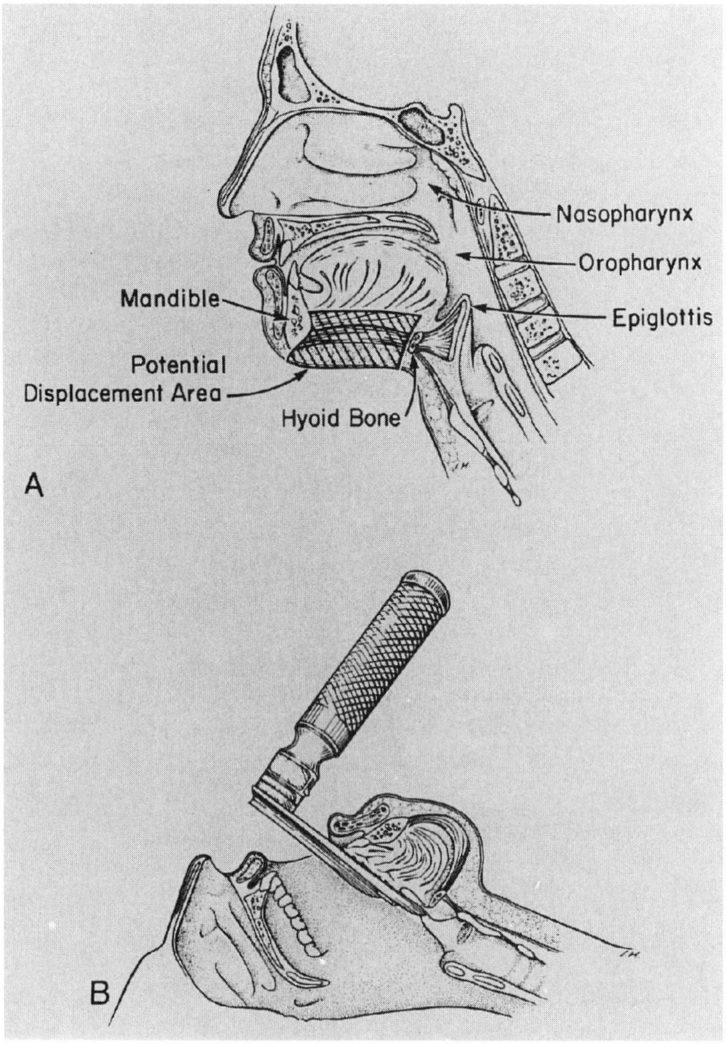

Figure 2.3. The potential displacement area is the region that is translocated during laryngoscopy. (A) demonstrates the anatomical structures that make up the displacement area. (B) demonstrates the translocation of these structures at the time of laryngoscopy. (From Berry FA, Anesthetic Management of Difficult and Routine Pediatric Patients, 2nd edition, Churchill Livingstone, 1990, p 173.)

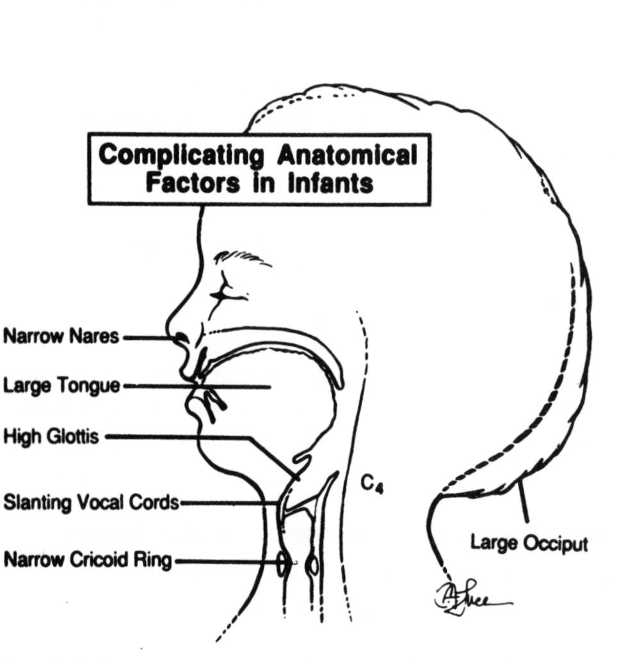

Figure 2.4. The specific anatomic characteristics of an infant's airway. (Berry and Yemen, Pediatr Clin NA 1994;41:153.)

failure of intubation occurs in 0.35% of adults. Ten percent of these patients could neither be ventilated nor intubated[8]. In the absence of an obvious airway abnormality or specific syndrome, most difficult airways can be recognized by performing the three maneuvers outlined in **Table 2.3.**

The Oropharyngeal Examination

The oropharyngeal examination is performed by having the patient open her mouth to the widest extent with maximal tongue protrusion. The range of motion at the temporomandibular joint and the size of the tongue relative to the size of the oral cavity are documented. Mallampatti has classified the degree of airway difficulty based on the ability to visualize the faucial pillars, soft palate and uvula (Fig. 2.7). Intubation is successful >99% of the time in patients with a class I airway, in whom all three structures are visualized. Patients with a class IV airway, in whom none of the pharyngeal structures are visible, suffer a failed intubation 1 to 4% of the time[9]. A highly arched palate also increases the difficulty of intubation.

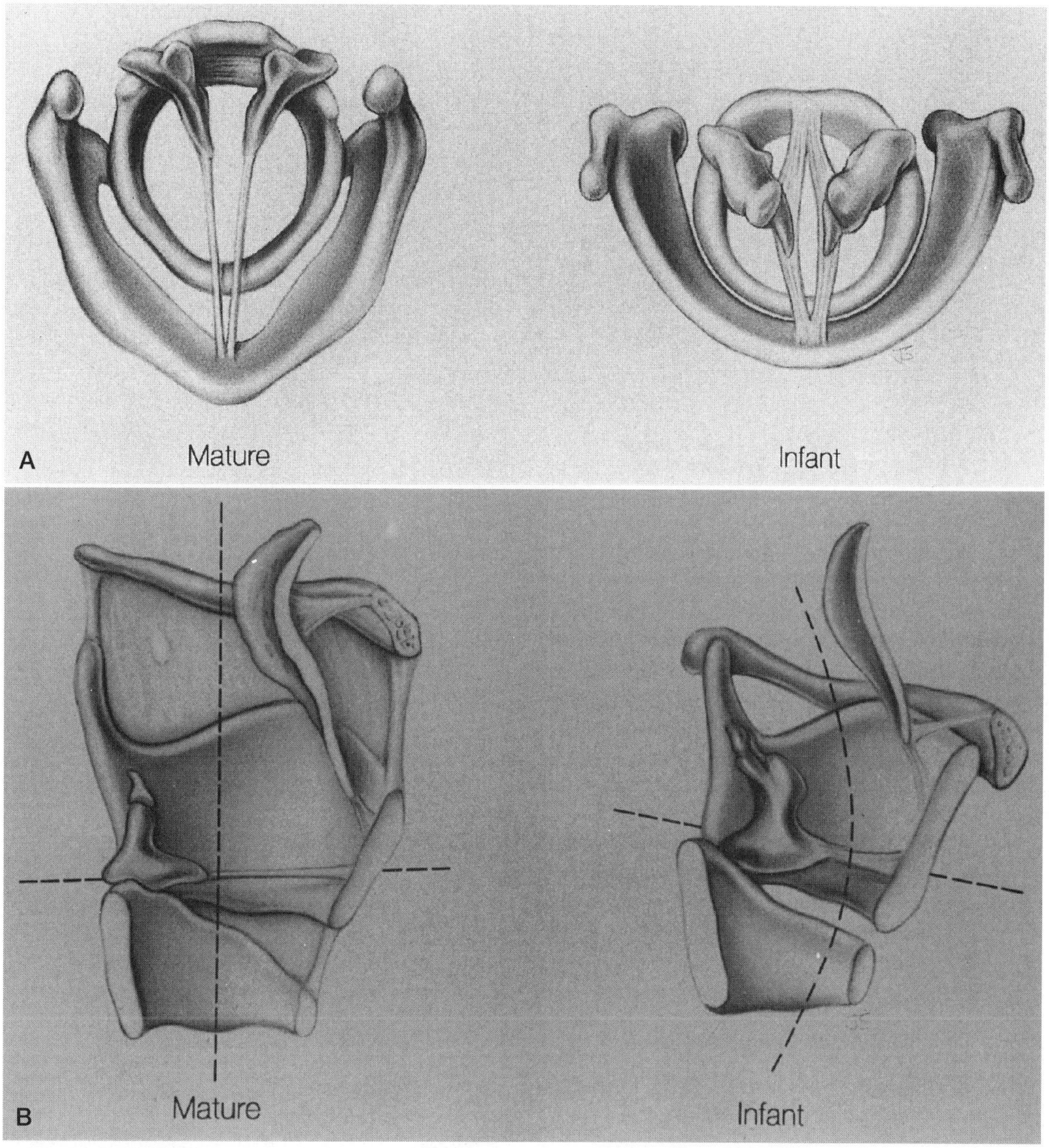

Figure 2.5. The internal laryngeal anatomy. (A) The adult's vocal cords are perpendicular to the laryngeal axis. In contrast, the infant's cords are rotated such that the anterior attachments are more inferior, producing an antero-caudal angulation. (B) Note the differences in the shape and positioning of the intrinsic laryngeal cartilages. (From Norton, Brown. Difficult Airway Atlas with Diagnostic & Management Criteria. Mosby-Year Book, 1991.)

Atlanto-occipital Joint Extension

Reduction in the range of motion at the atlanto-occipital joint will clearly affect the ability to establish a line of sight to the glottic structures. Normally, 35 degrees of extension is possible. Excessive reduction in this range of motion will lead to increasing difficulties with laryngoscopy[10].

Table 2.3. The Three Components of the Airway Exam

- An oropharyngeal exam.
- Evaluation of range of motion at the atlanto-occipital joint.
- Measurement of the potential displacement area.

The Potential Displacement Area

The mandibular space is important for 2 reasons. If the thyromental distance is short, then the pharyngeal axis will make a more acute angle with the laryngeal axis and it will be more difficult for atlanto-occipital extension to superimpose the three airway axes into a line of sight. In the adult with atlanto-occipital extension, a thyromental distance of 6 cm is associated with an easy laryngoscopy. If the mandibular space is small, the tongue and soft tissues must be compressed into a much smaller compartment, making laryngoscopy much more difficult. In a child, if 2 fingers can be placed between the anterior ramus of the mandible and

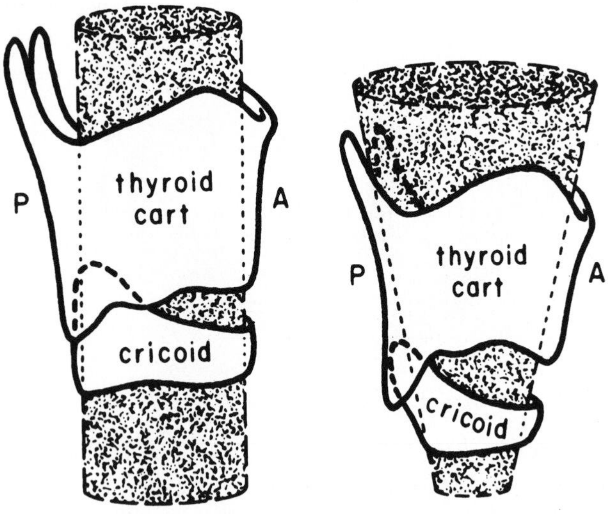

Figure 2.6. The infant's larynx is funnel shaped as compared to the adult's cylindrical larynx. (From Cote CJ, Ryan JF, Todres DI, A practice of anesthesia for infants and children. Philadelphia, WB Saunders 1993, p 61.)

the hyoid bone, the potential displacement area is adequate[11]. For a normal airway, with the head in a neutral position, the minimum distance from the hyoid to the mentum is 3 cm (2 finger breadths) in adults and 1.5 cm in infants[12]. The result of a decreased displacement space is an increased difficulty in visualizing the glottis. This is often referred to as an anterior larynx. As Berry points out, the larynx is not any more anterior than in any one else. Rather, since the laryngoscopy remains in a posterior position, the larynx appears to be anterior to the line of vision. These three tests in combination have a 100% predictive value in recognizing the difficult airway in adults[13].

Unfortunately, many take for granted that patients with difficult airways can still be managed by bag mask ventilation. This is not the case. The anatomic and pathophysiological situations that contribute to the difficult airway can also produce a physiologic milieu in which bag mask ventilation will be unsuccessful. This can be illustrated by the examples of edema, inflammatory or infiltrative processes, or localized lesions in the hypopharyngeal-supraglottic region. Any of these processes increase the resistance to airflow through the upper airway. The greater the resistance to airflow, the greater the driving force needed to maintain the required tidal volume. During spontaneous respiration, a larger negative pressure must be generated, which will increase the tendency for the upper airway to collapse.

Further airway obstruction is the result of the Bernoulli principle. This principle states that the total energy—kinetic and potential—will be constant during fluid flow. Because the volume of flow is constant, when air passes through a narrowing the velocity and therefore its kinetic energy will increase. Since total energy is constant, the potential energy must decrease. This loss of potential energy results in a fall in pressure at the level of the constriction, producing further airway collapse. Positive pressure venti-

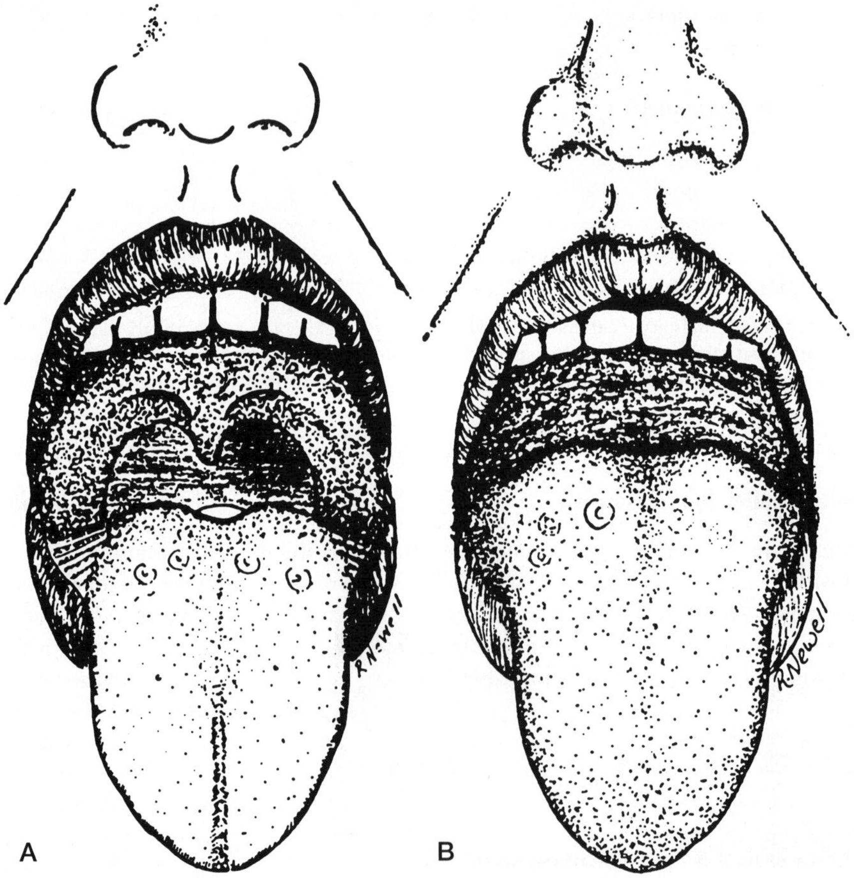

Figure 2.7. (A) Patient in whom the tonsillar pillars, soft palate and uvula are visualized. A class 1 airway. (B) Patient in whom none of the pharyngeal structures are visualized. A Class IV airway. (From Mallampati et al.)[9]

lation in this situation only worsens the degree of airway obstruction by filling the piriform sinuses and increasing external pressure on the airway at the level of the vestibular and true cords[14–16].

Although this Bernoulli biophysical argument was applied to a supraglottic lesion, abnormalities in the relationships of the oropharyngeal soft tissues (e.g., micrognathia) will be affected in a similar fashion. *Never assume successful bag/mask ventilation in a patient in whom a difficult intubation is anticipated.*

THE DIFFICULT PEDIATRIC AIRWAY

Airway symptoms or anatomic features usually point to the child with a difficult airway. Nevertheless, there are children in whom a difficult airway is appreciated only at the time of intubation. For this reason, every ICU must practice recognition and have a management strategy for the difficult airway. The syndromes associated with airway difficulties may be categorized by the principal airway anomaly.

Micrognathia

Micrognathia is the most difficult of the airway abnormalities primarily because of its effects on the insertion of the tongue, the soft tissues and the suspension of the larynx.These structures lie more cephalad in relation to the mandible, often perceived as "very anterior." Visualization of the glottis can be extremely difficult if not impossible. Classic examples include the Pierre Robin and Treacher Collins syndromes.

Cervical Spine Abnormalities

Cervical spine abnormalities limit the establishment of the line of sight to the glottis structures. Goldenhar and Klippel-Fiel syndromes exemplify the congenital syndromes associated with cervical spine abnormalities. Disease processes with significant cervical spine abnormalities include juvenile rheumatoid arthritis[17], and the neuromuscular scolioses. Atlanto-occipital instability represents a different form of cervical spine abnormality and is most commonly considered in patients with trisomy 21. Atlanto-occipital instability is assumed in neck trauma.

Macroglossia and Glossoptosis

Macroglossia and glossoptosis clearly affect visualization of the larynx. Macroglossia is an enlargement of the tongue and is seen in patients with Beckwith-Wiedemann syndrome and Trisomy 21. Glossoptosis is the downward and backward displacement of the tongue which is commonly seen in achondroplasia.

Infiltration of the Soft Tissues

Infiltration of the soft tissues in the potential displacement area will affect laryngscopy. Not only will visualization be-difficult, but severe anatomic distortion of the laryngeal complex should be expected. Examples include submandibular masses such as cystic hygroma, edema and cellulitic involvement secondary to oro-pharyngeal processes such as Ludwig's angina, and epiglottitis. Epidermolysis bullosa should be included in this category, as 25% of patients with epidermolysis bullosa have difficult oral intubations, requiring alternative approaches such as blind nasal or fiberoptic intubations[18].

The Morbidly Obese Patient

The morbidly obese patient has a short thick neck with a limited range of motion and a large tongue. Excessive chest wall soft tissue further complicates laryngoscopy by its sheer mass, and physical obstruction to airway instrumentation.

The Mucopolysaccharidoses and Musculoskeletal Syndromes

In a study of 34 children undergoing 89 intubations, the overall incidence of difficult intubation is 25% and failed intubation is 8%. Children with Hurler's syndrome are the most difficult with a failed intubation rate of 23%[19]. Arthrogryposis multiplex congenita (AMC) is a rare musculoskeletal disorder defined by multiple fixed joints in the upper and lower extremities (Fig. 2.8). Abnormalities in

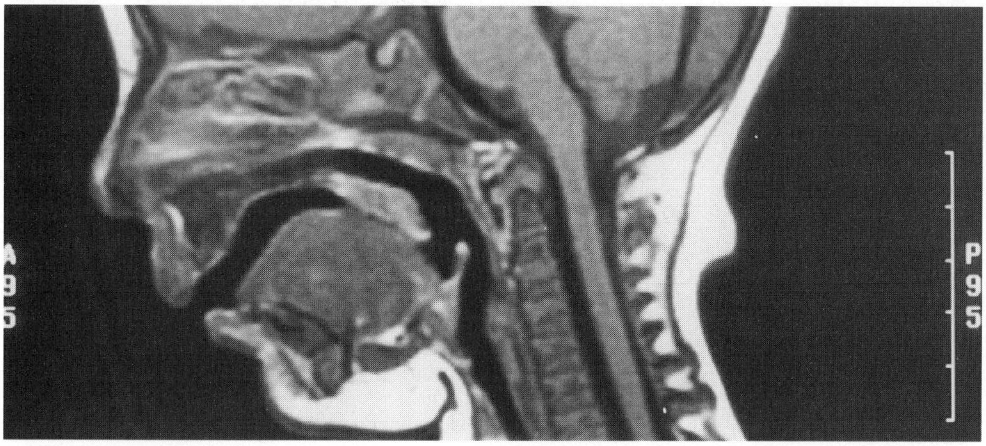

Figure 2.8. MRI of a patient with arthrogryposis multiplex congenita demonstrating the marked micrognathia and high arched palate. The age-appropriate characteristic subglottic narrowing is seen well in this image.

AMC that impact on airway management can include: micrognathia, a high arched palate, and an omega-shaped epiglottis, but otherwise normal larynx, and trachea. Achalasia, and multiple aspiration pneumonias can further complicate an affected child's management[20].

BASIC AIRWAY MANAGEMENT

Basic airway management skills should be familiar to all pediatric critical care providers. Airway patency is maintained with proper head positioning and secretion removal. The tongue is the principal cause of airway obstruction in most situations. With atlanto-occipital extension, the space between the base of the tongue and the posterior pharynx is increased[21]. Airway patency is frequently re-established with a chin lift and jaw thrust. Airway adjuncts such as an oropharyngeal airway or a nasopharyngeal airway function by further separating the tongue from the soft tissues of the posterior pharynx (Figs. 2.9, 2.10). The complications of airway trauma, worsening airway obstruction, laryngospasm, and epistaxis are frequently related to the selection of an inappropriately sized airway. Nasopharyngeal instrumentation is contraindicated in patients with basilar skull fractures, cerebrospinal fluid leaks, and patients who are anti-coagulated.

Once airway patency is assured, oxygen can be administered through a variety of devices. The exact concentration of oxygen being administered to the patient is dependent on the oxygen flow rate, as well as the patient's minute ventilation and inspiratory flow rate, which will dictate the amount of diluent room air inspired. Since oxygen therapy is titrated to the adequacy of the patients oxygen saturation or oxygen tension, the exact FiO_2 is unimportant. However, when determining the patient's alveolar-arterial (Aa) gradient or PaO_2/FiO_2 index, a precise delivery of oxygen concentration is desired. In these circumstances, the preferred delivery device is a non-rebreathing oxygen mask attached to a venturi system or a gas blender.

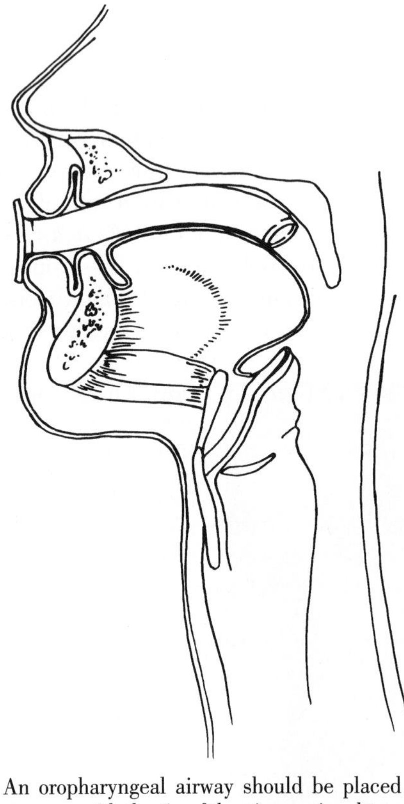

Figure 2.9. An oropharyngeal airway should be placed to follow the curve of the tongue, with the tip of the airway aimed toward the larynx.

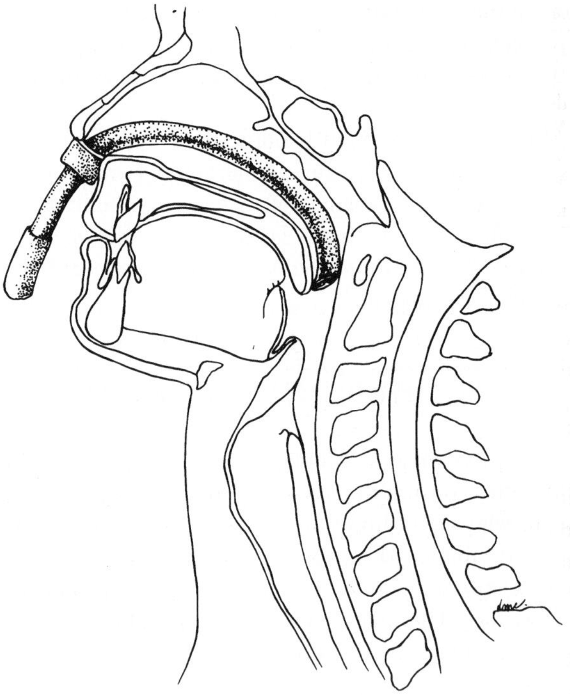

Figure 2.10. A soft nasopharyngeal airway is placed in line with the nose to follow the natural curve of the nasal cavity.

Positive Pressure Ventilation

The Full Stomach Quagmire

The conventional anesthetic wisdom is that all acutely injured patients have full stomachs until proven otherwise. Patients with full stomachs, defined as a gastric residual volume in excess of 0.4 mL/kg and a pH less than 2.5 are at risk of acid aspiration during positive pressure ventilation and induction of anesthesia before intubation[22]. Children appear to be at least as susceptible to regurgitation and aspiration as adults **(Table 2.4)**[23].

In this situation, pediatric anesthesiologists have luxuries available to them that are not afforded to the pediatric

Table 2.4. Factors that Contribute to the Child's Increased Risk of Pulmonary Aspiration

- Excessive aerophagia during crying.
- Strenuous diaphragmatic activity during airway obstruction.
- A shorter esophagus.
- A smaller hydrostatic gradient betwen the stomach and the larynx.

Table 2.5. Approach to the Patient with a Full Stomach

- Decompress the stomach if possible (in the awake patient).
- Denitrogenate and preoxygenate to minimize the ensuing oxygen desaturation.
- Minimize the period of time between the onset of apnea and ideal intubating conditions (The Rapid Sequence).
- Minimize the amount of air entering the stomach during bag mask ventilation.

intensivist. On many occasions the anesthesiologist is able to delay a procedure to allow for adequate gastric emptying and for gastroprophylactic drugs to take effect. This is certainly inconceivable in a patient with status asthmaticus, epiglottitis or a central nervous system injury.

Aspiration pneumonitis is the result of inhalation of acidic fluid, leading to damage of the pulmonary capillary endothelium and inhibition of surfactant production. Bronchospasm and acute pulmonary vasoconstriction may develop. Atelectasis, interstitial pulmonary edema and significant hypoxemia follow. Changes in the chest radiograph occur 6 to 12 hours after the injury(24). At present, although there are no data regarding the incidence of aspiration pneumonitis during resuscitative airway maneuvers, the anesthetic experience demands that we be more vigilant in minimizing this complication. Specifically, the aspiration syndrome is responsible for 19% of all deaths attributed to anesthesia(25). Therefore it is appropriate that pediatric intensivists adopt the tenets of the anesthetic approach to the patient with a full stomach **(Table 2.5).**

If a non-depolarizing muscle relaxant is used to facilitate intubation, the child should receive (specifically, virtually all children encountered in a critical setting should receive) bag-mask ventilation through applied cricoid pressure to prevent regurgitation of stomach contents(26). The absolute minimum amount of positive inspiratory pressure that is sufficient to cause chest wall excursion should be used. Cricoid pressure is removed only after the restoration of the patient's airway reflexes, or placement of an endotracheal intubation which is confirmed by bilateral breath sounds and end-tidal CO_2 demonstration.

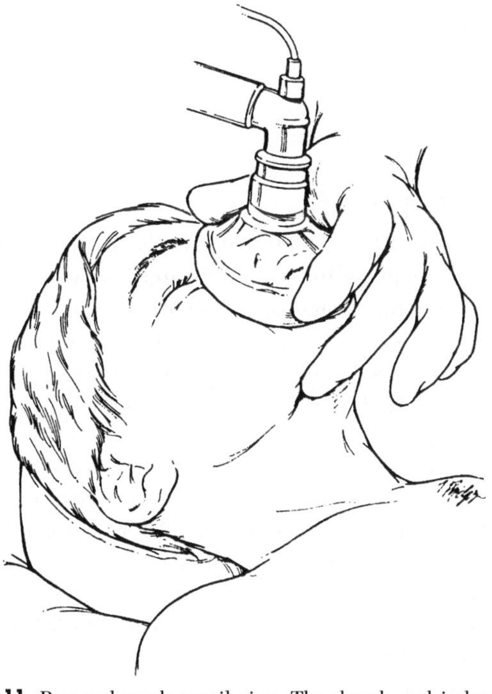

Figure 2.11. Bag and mask ventilation. The thumb and index fingers produce the seal and the middle finger lies on the mandible to lift the jaw upward. (From the Golden Hour 2nd edition edited by Nichols DG et al. Mosby, 1995.)

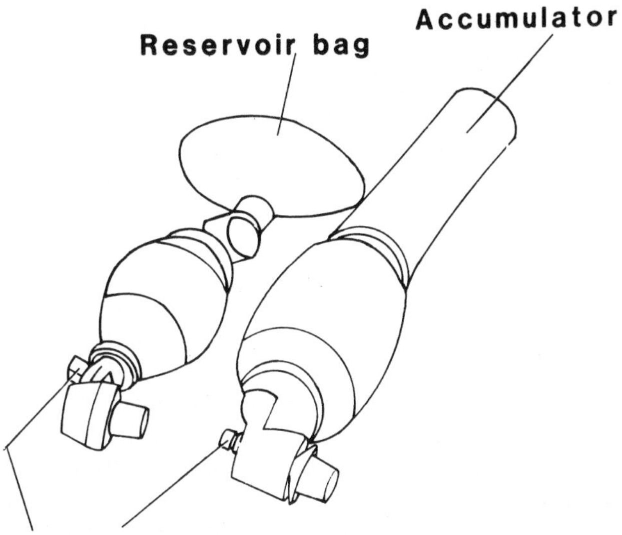

Figure 2.12. Self-inflating resuscitation bags. Reservoir bag on distal end and accumulator allow delivery of 100% oxygen with high flow rates.

Equipment and Technique

In the setting of inadequate breathing, the patient's ventilation is assisted after the establishment of airway patency. Positive pressure breaths can be given by mouth-mask-mouth ventilation, or by bag-mask ventilation. A secure mask fit is necessary to ventilate the patient reliably. The face mask should be held firmly on the face with 90% of the effort directed towards bringing the face into the mask and only 10% directed towards pushing the mask down on the child's face. In larger children and adults, the resuscitator uses the thumb and index finger for downward pressure on the mask. The remainder of the fingers are placed on the ramus of the mandible to position the neck and bring the face into the mask (Fig. 2.11).

In smaller children, finger misplacement leads to inadvertent compression of the submandibular soft tissues and airway obstruction. Infants in particular are susceptible to this iatrogenic airway obstruction. For this reason we alter the mask grip in infants and children. The thumb and index finger completely encircle the stem of the mask, while the middle finger lies along the mandible, extending from the midposition on the left side of the mandible to the midposition of the right. The middle finger is used to provide the necessary chin lift, and head position. The remaining 2 fingers are held extended, not touching any part of the infant's face. The other hand is used to squeeze the bag. Mask repositioning, additional padding, and on occasion 2 hands on the mask are necessary to compensate for abnormalities in mandibular contour and mask leaks.

A wide variety of ventilating bags are available for use in infants and children. They can be categorized as self-inflating bags and anesthesia-type bags. The self-inflating bags are easy to use in that they do not require an optimal mask seal in order to function. The drawback of a self-inflating bag is that the bag will continue to fill even in the face of a disconnection from an oxygen source. Two bags in this category are the Puritan manual resuscitator (PMR) and the Laerdal resuscitator bags (Figs. 2.12 and 2.13). Both of these bags allow for oxygen administration during spontaneous ventilation. The PMR bag can supply an FiO_2 of 1.0 using high flow oxygen source. The child PMR2 bag has a volume of 870 mL and a pressure-relief (pop-off) valve that opens at 45 cm H_2O. The Laerdal bag can deliver a 100% FiO_2 only if a reservoir bag is used. The infant Laerdal resuscitator bag has a 240 mL volume while the child bag has a 500 mL bag. The Laerdal pop-off valve opens at 35 cm H_2O. The airway pressure generated from a bag deflation is determined by the effectiveness of the squeeze, the adequacy of the mask seal, airway resistance and the pop-off value. In the setting of poor pulmonary or chest wall compliance, the pressure relief valve should be sealed in order to provide effective ventilation[28].

Anesthesia bag systems offer the advantages of identifying an immediate disconnection from the oxygen source and being light in weight. These systems have no inspiratory valves and allow for spontaneous inspiration. Because these systems require an optimal mask seal, they are more difficult for the inexperienced user. A Mapelson D and modified Mapelson C circuit are useful in the PICU and transport setting. Both bags supply fresh gas flow close to the face mask. The Mapelson C has a pop-off valve and reservoir bag a short distance away from the mask. During expiration, alveolar gas and fresh gas flow into the reservoir bag and out the pop-off valve. The modified Mapelson D circuit differs only in that a length of tubing is placed between the mask and the pop-off reservoir complex. At end exhalation, fresh gas flow drives the expiratory gas toward the pop-off valve and reservoir bag (Fig. 2.14).

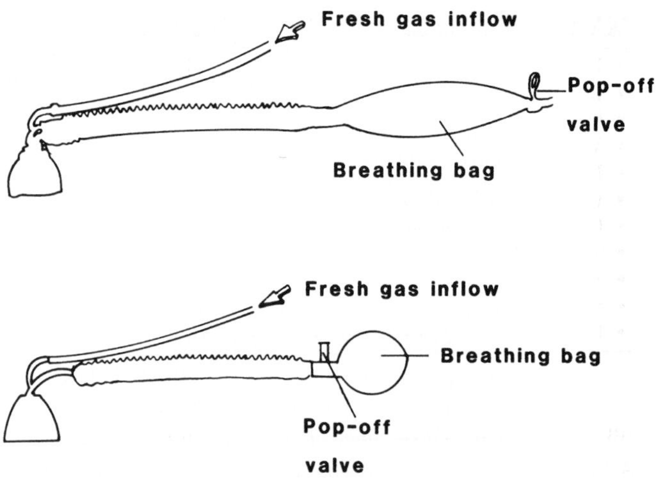

Figure 2.14. Schematic representation of conventional anesthesia bags with fresh gas inflow *(arrow)*, pop-off valve, and reservoir bag available in a range of sizes. *Top:* Jackson Rees system. *Bottom:* Mapelson D system.

In both Mapelson systems, the exact composition of inspired gas will depend on the amount of expiratory gas that is rebreathed. Mapelson C systems are more likely to dilute the fresh gas with expired gas. During spontaneous respirations, a large minute ventilation gas can be attained from the reservoir bag and corrugated tubing. High flow rates of oxygen ($>$ 4 L/minute) are required to minimize rebreathing. During controlled ventilation, expired gas is usually pushed out the pop-off valve and almost pure fresh gas is delivered to the patient.

The choice of the ideal resuscitation bag remains controversial. In light of the almost universal use of pulse oximetry and the variable experience amongst those who need to respond to pediatric airway emergencies, most institutions utilize a self-inflating bag.

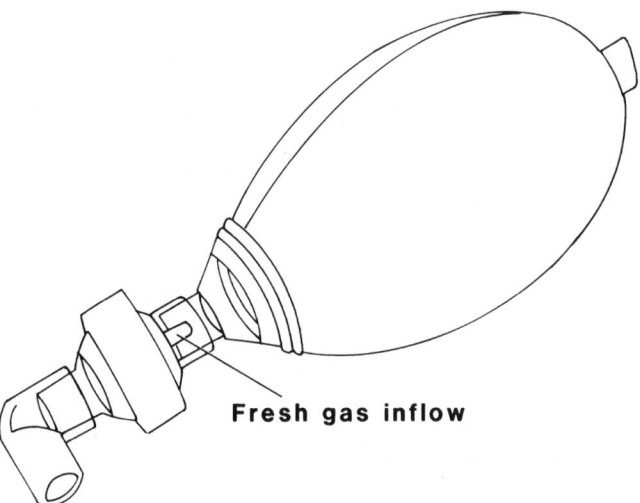

Figure 2.13. Manual resuscitator bag without reservoir system or capability of delivering high concentrations of oxygen.

ENDOTRACHEAL INTUBATION

The indications for endotracheal intubation are respiratory failure, airway protection and the relief of airway obstruction. The equipment necessary for endotracheal intubation is listed in **Table 2.6.** Availability of suction apparatus is essential during intubation. Oxygen is administered before laryngoscopy and intubation to provide a reservoir of oxygen for the apnea period, especially for infants whose resting oxygen consumption is high. Adequate oxygen reserves may be provided by preoxygenation with 100% oxygen for 4 to 5 minutes prior to paralysis, laryngoscopy, and

Table 2.6. Equipment Needed for the "Rapid Sequence Intubation"

- Large suction catheter "Yankauer" and reliable suction.
- Bag and mask.
- Oxygen source.
- Ventilation system.
- Endotracheal tubes.
- Laryngoscopes and handles.
- Oropharyngeal airways.
- Tongue blade.
- Tape.
- Stylet.
- Expired carbon dioxide detection device.

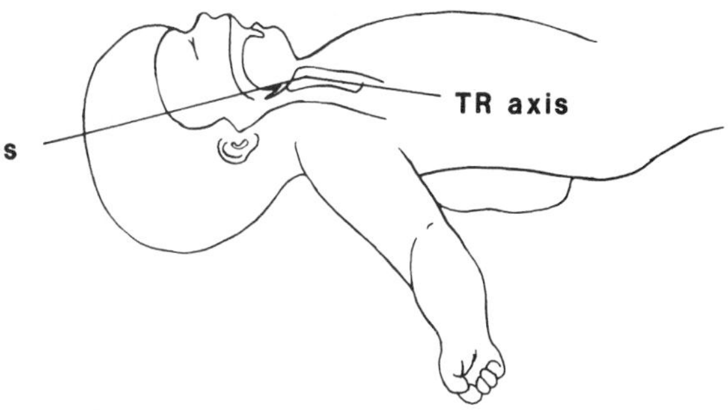

Figure 2.16. Without elevation of the occiput, neck extension results in a separate plane for the tracheal axis (TR) and pharyngeal axis (PH).

intubation or by three vital capacity breaths of 100% oxygen[27–30].

The technique for endotracheal intubation depends on the indication for airway placement and the clinical condition of the patient. Only clinical experience in controlled settings will prepare one for management of an airway in difficult circumstances.

The infant's head is placed in a neutral position. For the older child, if the head is extended at the atlanto-occipital joint and the occiput is elevated to the "sniffing" position, the oropharyngolaryngeal axes are aligned (Fig. 2.15). Extension of the head without elevation of the occiput rotates the larynx anteriorly (Fig. 2.16). The mouth is opened by pressure on the mandible. The laryngoscope is held in the left hand, inserted into the right side of the mouth, the tongue on the left side of the blade. The tongue is moved to the left side of the mouth as the laryngoscope is moved to the midline. The blade is then advanced slowly over the tongue. The choice of straight versus curved blade is largely dictated by the age of the patient as well as the preference and experience of the physician (Fig. 2.17). Straight blades are by and large used in infants, small children and patients with "anterior " laryngeal placement. It is easier to lift the base of the tongue and fix an infants epiglottis with a straight blade. *The channel of the straight blade is the intubators visual path, not the endotracheal tube insertion guide.* Curved blades are used primarily in those older than 2 to 3 years of age. The advantages of a curved blade include a large flange which provides better control of the tongue, less perceived need to lever on the upper teeth and

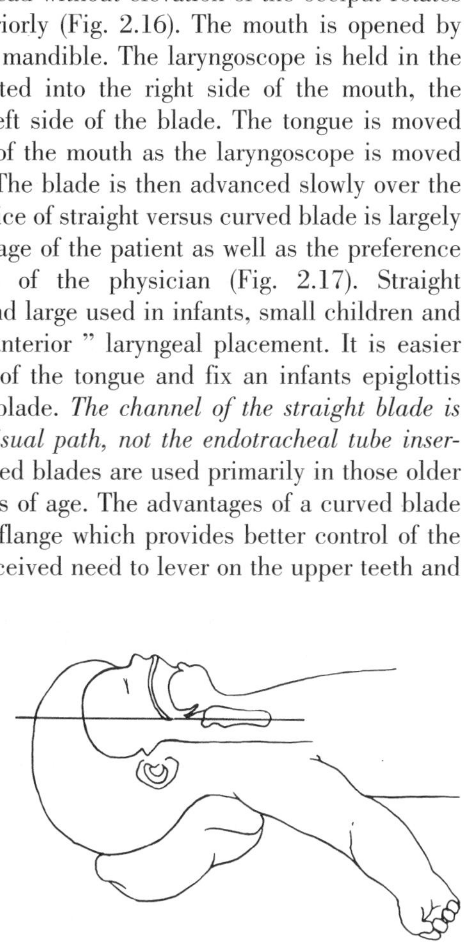

Figure 2.15. Placement of the head in "sniffing" position aligns the pharyngeal and laryngotracheal axes (combined PH-LTR axis).

therefore less potential dental damage and more available oropharyngeal space.

With a straight blade (Miller, Wisconsin, Wis-Hippel), the tip is moved under the laryngeal side of the epiglottis, and with an upward pull along the axis of the handle, the epiglottis and the base of the tongue are raised to expose the glottis (Fig. 2.18). If the larynx is not easily visualized, external pressure on the larynx may help bring the glottis into view. If the blade has been advanced too deeply in to the esophagus, the blade is withdrawn until the glottis is visualized. With a curved blade (Macintosh), the laryngoscope blade is advanced from the right side of the mouth into the valleculae (Fig. 2.19). With an upward pull along the axis of the laryngoscope handle, the glottis is visualized. The tongue is more easily controlled with the curved blade.

The most common errors the novice makes are:

1. Levering on the upper incisors instead of lifting the axis of the laryngoscope handle at a 45° angle, thus pulling the tongue away from the upper incisors;
2. Allowing the tongue to slip back into the path of vision when it protrudes over the right side of the laryngoscope blade;
3. Trapping the lips between the laryngoscope blade and the teeth.

The endotracheal tube is advanced from the right side of the mouth with the curve aimed anteriorly. Polyvinylchloride tubes, which are inert, soft, and molded at body temperature to the shape of the airway, are recommended. These tubes have either 1 or three markings at the distal end, to guide appropriate depth of placement. The criteria considered in the selection of the size of endotracheal tubes in children is discussed in several reviews[31–34].

The appropriate size of endotracheal tube can be estimated by the size of the child's little finger or by the equation:

$$\frac{16 + \text{age(yrs)}}{4}$$

Age is a more reliable determinant of endotracheal tube size than is height. *In children with congenital anomalies a*

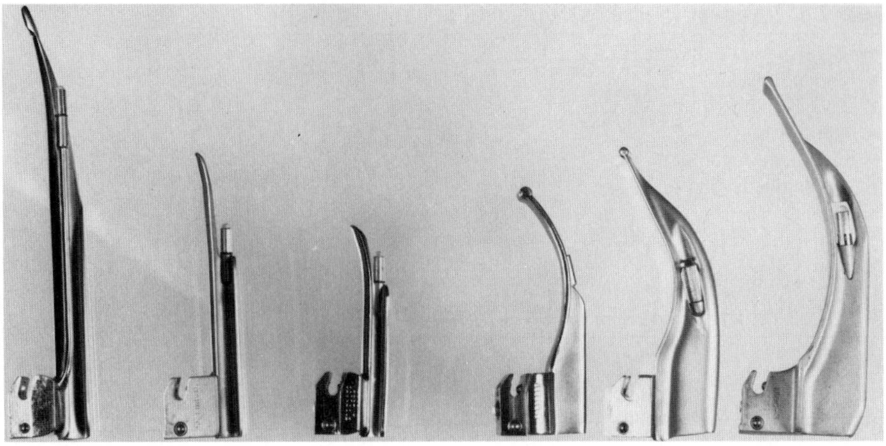

Figure 2.17. Straight and curved laryngoscope blades are available in varying sizes suitable for children.

half-size smaller endotracheal tube is usually appropriate. **Table 2.7** lists appropriate endotracheal tubes for age. A variety of tube sizes should be available at the time of intubation including the appropriate size, a size larger, and a size smaller.

The appropriate size endotracheal tube is important, as a very small tube will decrease the cross-sectional area of the airway and result in both an increased resistance to flow and work of breathing. With a stethoscope placed on the anterior neck overlying the trachea and an aneroid manometer connected to the breathing system, the inspiratory pressure at which the gas "leaks" around the endotracheal tube can be monitored. If testing is done with a neutral head position in the presence of neuromuscular blockade, the leak can be measured reliably(35). The leak pressure has been suggested as an indication of fit between the endotracheal tube and the size of the trachea(36). It has been recommended that the leak be less than 20–25 cm H_2O to reduce post-extubation stridor(37).

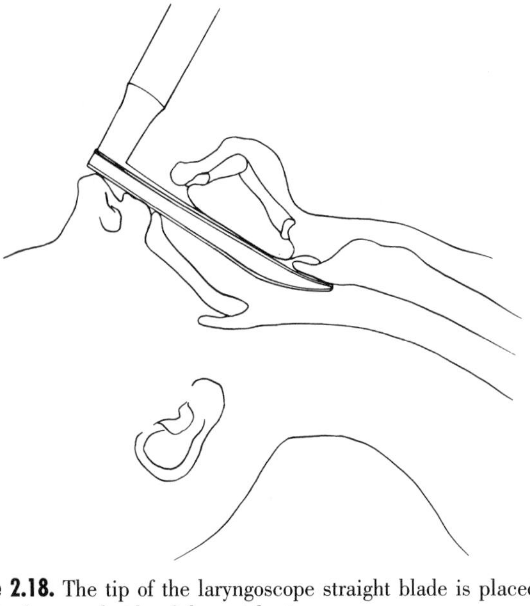

Figure 2.18. The tip of the laryngoscope straight blade is placed under the laryngeal side of the epiglottis.

The appropriate distance for endotracheal tube insertion also varies with age, as is expected based on the pattern of tracheal growth described. By convention the distance is recorded as the position of the endotracheal tube at the gum or incisor. Insertion nomograms have been devised to estimate the appropriate length for tracheal intubation(32). In addition to age, weight has been used; 7 cm for the 1 kg infant, 8 cm for the 2 kg infant, and 9 cm for the 3 kg infant(38). For children over 3 years of age the formula for depth of insertion to the incisors is(39):

$$\text{Depth of insertion (cm)} = (\text{age}/2) + 12$$

A useful rule of thumb for the depth of insertion is three times the size (internal diameter) of the endotracheal tube. Head position will affect endotracheal tube position. With neck flexion, the tip of the tube will move closer to the carina, possibly causing an endobronchial intubation. Neck extension results in withdrawal of the tube towards the glottis(40). *The change in the position of the tube mimics the change in position of the patients nose.*

The intubator should watch as the tracheal tube passes through the vocal cords to ensure **endotracheal** placement. The endotracheal tube should be positioned so that either the single line, the middle line or the cuff is just below the level of the vocal cords.

Table 2.7. Suggested Endotracheal Tube Size

Age	Internal Diameter (ID)
Premature infant	2.5–3.0
Newborn	3.0
Newborn–6 month	3.5
6m–12m	3.5–4.0
12m–2y	4.0–4.5
3–4y	4.5–5.0
5–6y	5.0–5.5
7–8y	5.5–6.0
9–10y	6.0–6.5
11–12y	6.5–7.0
13–14y	7.0–7.5

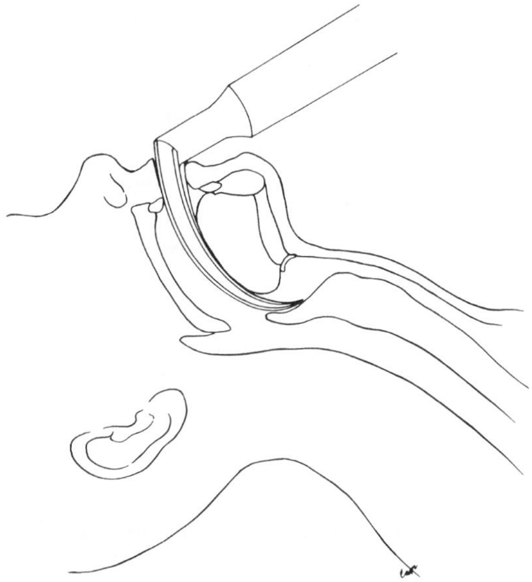

Figure 2.19. The tip of the laryngoscope curved blade is placed anterior to the epiglottis into the vallecula.

At this stage novices commonly make these mistakes:

1. Poor visualization of the glottic structures prior to endotracheal tube placement.
2. Poor visualization of passage of the endotracheal tube because of inadequate tongue displacement to the left.

Endotracheal intubation must be confirmed. Although mist in the tube, auscultation of bilaterally equal breath sounds and the absence of air entry during epigastrium auscultation are traditional confirmatory findings, they can be misleading. *The detection of expired carbon dioxide with a capnograph or mass spectrometer is the most reliable evidence of tracheal rather than esophageal intubation*[41–44]. Mid-tracheal position is then confirmed by auscultation of bilateral breath sounds, by palpation of the tube tip at the suprasternal notch, chest radiograph or by bronchoscopy[45,46].

For children over 8 years of age, cuffed tubes are usually used. Traditionally, the endotracheal tubes used in infants and young children have usually been uncuffed because of the concern for the development of subglottic damage. Because the narrow segment of the infant's airway lumen is the cricoid ring, any excessive pressure in this area was thought to result in postextubation stridor. As the infant's airway is in a conical configuration, a circular endotracheal tube will be sufficient to prevent an excessive air leak. In 1984 Finholt suggested the use of an air leak of 15 to 25 cm H_2O as a sign of a safe endotracheal tube fit[47]. The dramatic decrease in the incidence of post-extubation croup in the past decade has been attributed to the incorporation of the "safe" air leak into pediatric anesthesia practice[48].

Presently, many practitioners are reevaluating this practice now that high volume-low pressure cuffs are available. The safe use of cuffed endotracheal tubes would prevent the need for multiple tube changes in the search of the "perfect leak". In addition, children in the PICU frequently have significant abnormalities in pulmonary compliance necessitating mechanical ventilation at peak inspiratory pressures in excess of 25 cm H_2O, surpassing the safe leak zone. There are preliminary data to suggest that there is no difference in the development of post-extubation stridor in children who were intubated with cuffed tubes as compared to those who received uncuffed ones[49].

Cuffed endotracheal tubes should be considered in children with marked alterations in pulmonary compliance, such as ARDS. The cuff should be inflated to the minimal pressure required to seal an air leak and allow effective ventilation. Cuff filling is confirmed by distention of the pilot balloon. Cuff pressure should be monitored: it is recommended to keep the pressure less than 20 mm Hg[50]. As pressure equilibrates across the cuff wall, the intracuff pressure approximates that of the lateral tracheal wall. This cuff pressure should be checked every 8 hours to avoid the development of an excessive cuff seal. Problems arise because prestretched cuffs may not inflate symmetrically, temperature changes may change cuff pressure[51] and the cuff can herniate over the end of the tube, causing partial obstruction. Further data are needed before we can advocate a *universal* change to the use of cuffed endotracheal tubes in children.

A stylet is used to change the position of the tip of the tube for patients with anatomic abnormalities. The stylet is only rarely necessary. Its use is usually necessitated by poor technique rather than airway abnormalities. Unfortunately, the stylet may traumatize the airway if not used properly (there is the potential for trauma from the stylet itself or from stiffening the tube). The intubator must be certain that the stylet does not protrude from the end of the endotracheal tube and is well lubricated to ensure easy removal once the tube is in.

The Pharmacological Management of Endotracheal Intubation

The technique for endotracheal intubation depends on the indication for airway placement and the clinical condition of the patient. The flaccid child in cardiopulmonary arrest requires no pharmacological intervention. Bag-mask ventilation through cricoid pressure, laryngoscopy and intubation are usually accomplished without difficulty. Conversely, a combative child with a rapidly declining neurological status resulting from head trauma requires a rapid, smooth anesthetic induction and intubation which limits the intracranial pressure response as well as the risks of pulmonary aspiration. Before committing to a specific technique, the intensivist must assess the child's airway anatomy and intravascular status.

Novices commonly err in the choice of intubation technique as a result of:

1. Underappreciation of the airway anomalies.
2. Underappreciation of the hemodynamic derangement of the patient and the further deleterious effects the pharmacologic agents will have.
3. Underappreciation of the risk of pulmonary aspiration.

Table 2.8. Dosing Guidelines for Induction Agents

Sodium pentothal	4–6 mg/kg IV 2–3 mg/kg IV if unstable
Ketamine	2 mg/kg IV
Lidocaine	1.5 mg/kg IV
Midazolam	0.05–0.1 mg/kg IV
Diazepam	0.1–0.2 mg/kg IV

The airway must be secured in the **safest manner possible.** Intubation can be accomplished under three conditions: awake, sedated and anesthetized.There are situations in which, even in the most experienced of hands, the safest technique is that in which the patient is intubated awake, without drugs.

Awake Intubation

There are no absolute indications for " awake" (no pharmacological adjuncts) intubation of the trachea, with the exception of the patient in cardiopulmonary arrest. The intensivist must weigh the risks of a biting, struggling child who will recall intubation against the benefits of maintaining a spontaneously breathing child with a protected airway in the event intubation is difficult. An awake intubation is often necessary in patients with airway anomalies, upper gastrointestinal hemorrhage, cervical spine abnormalities, and in patients with facial trauma. Patients who are already hypoxemic may not tolerate even the shortest apneic period, and are therefore excellent candidates for an awake intubation.

Viscous or aerosolized lidocaine may be used to topicalize the tongue and decrease gagging during laryngoscopy. This is often the only suitable pharmacological adjunct for the child in shock. The use of superior laryngeal and translaryngeal nerve blocks are contra-indicated in the management of patients at risk for pulmonary aspiration.

Sedated Intubation

A carefully titrated sedation is a useful approach to the patient with an uncertain airway or who has lung disease with a moderate O_2 requirement. The goal is to increase the patient's cooperation and ease of intubation without excessively depressing the patient's airway reflexes and spontaneous respiratory drive. This technique is usually more successful in older children than in infants, in whom this "perfect" plan of sedation may be difficult to achieve. Drugs such as the benzodiazepines and ketamine are used for the sedated intubation. The dosing guidelines are found in **Table 2.8.** Benzodiazepines provide amnesia and some sedation for laryngoscopy. The initial recommended dose should be decreased by 50 to 75% in the setting of hypovolemia or poor cardiac function. Once the cardiovascular effects of the drug have been determined, additional drug may be given, titrating to the desired sedation plane.

Ketamine is a dissociative anesthetic with minimal respiratory effects. Ketamine rarely causes apnea and leaves the laryngeal reflexes intact. It also relieves coughing and laryngospasm and has bronchodilatory properties[52–54]. Ketamine is a potent sialogogue and requires the coadministration of a muscarinic antagonist, atropine or glycopyrrolate, to decrease airway secretions. It has indirect sympathomimetic properties, and as a result will preserve blood pressure and cardiac output in acutely hypovolemic patients. However, in the setting of a prolonged shock state, with endogenous catecholamine depletion, ketamine is a primary myocardial depressant and peripheral vasodilator. Ketamine does increase EEG activity and intracranial pressure and therefore is contraindicated in patients with intracranial pathology[55]. Co-administration of a small amount of benzodiazepine has been effective at decreasing the hallucinations seen with ketamine administration.

Anesthetized Intubation

Complete pharmacological control with an anesthetic intubation provides optimal intubating conditions. This technique not only provides amnesia, sedation and muscle paralysis but it also blunts the various physiological responses to intubation that may exacerbate a patient's underlying pathophysiological process. A child with severe head trauma and intracranial hypertension is an optimal candidate for an anesthetized intubation. Laryngoscopy and endotracheal intubation are extremely potent intracranial hypertensive stimuli. Unblunted in a patient with poor intracranial compliance, this response can severely compromise cerebral perfusion and worsen the ultimate neurological outcome. The components of an anesthetic induction include a hypnotic such as thiopental or ketamine, a neuromuscular blocker and drugs to modulate the physiologic responses to intubation. This latter group of drugs will be dictated by the child's co-existing disease; bronchodilators for asthma, beta blockade for essential hypertension, lidocaine for intracranial hypertension, sodium nitroprusside for an intracerebral aneurysm. Since virtually all patients requiring airway management in the pediatric intensive care setting are at significant risk for pulmonary aspiration of gastric contents, this approach is summarized in the rapid sequence intubation section.

Airway safety should not be jeopardized for the sake of pharmacological intervention.

Neuromuscular Blockade

Neuromuscular blockade facilitates laryngoscopy and endotracheal intubation, as well as controlled ventilation. However, muscle relaxants are contraindicated if there is any doubt about the success of endotracheal intubation. Loss of airway reflexes and spontaneous respiration is disastrous, especially when bag-mask ventilation is unreliable. Therefore the principles of the use of neuromuscular blockade in acute airway management include an adequate airway assessment and the utilization of short onset, short duration drugs to minimize such problems in the event intubation is unsuccessful.

A review of neuromuscular transmission is provided by Nugent et al.[56] and Standaert[57]. Briefly, acetylcholine is released into the synaptic cleft between the terminal axoplasmic membrane and the postsynaptic membrane receptors in response to the transmission of a nerve impulse. As acetylcholine combines with postsynaptic endplate receptor sites, depolarization of the muscle endplate results. At a "critical threshold" of endplate potential, an action potential and subsequent depolarization continue over the entire muscle membrane, resulting in contraction. Acetylcholine action is terminated by hydrolysis by cholinesterase in the junctional cleft. *Depolarizing* neuromuscular blocking agents are quaternary ammonium moieties that closely resemble acetylcholine and bind to the endplate receptor. Through this *non-competitive* binding mechanism the depolarizing drug causes a persistent depolarization of the postjunctional membrane, resulting in transient muscle fasciculation with subsequent paralysis. There are no antagonists of this action. *Nondepolarizing agents compete with the acetylcholine for the receptor sites,* and as such, the action of the acetylcholine is blocked. A cholinesterase inhibitor that slows the rate of hydrolysis of the acetyl-choline makes more acetylcholine available to compete for receptor sites at the neuromuscular junction. Neostigmine and the other cholinesterase inhibitors (in conjunction with atropine or glycopyrrolate) are therefore useful in reversing the effects of a non-depolarizing neuromuscular blocker.

Succinylcholine

Succinylcholine is the only depolarizing neuromuscular blocking agent available. Complete airway relaxation is achieved within 30 to 60 seconds. Rapid redistribution away from the neuromuscular junction results in a short duration of action, 3 to 5 minutes[58]. Succinylcholine is hydrolyzed by plasma cholinesterase produced by the liver. The action of succinylcholine is prolonged by a decreased or atypical plasma cholinesterase, liver disease, malnutrition, hypothermia, magnesium sulfate administration, extracellular hyperkalemia, and alkalosis. The duration of action is less in the setting of acidosis, decreased cardiac output (limiting distribution of the drug to the neuromuscular junction) and extracellular hypokalemia[56]. The recommended intravenous dose of succinylcholine is 2 mg per kilogram for infants and 1 to 1.5 mg per kilogram for older children and adults.

Succinylcholine has many of the characteristics of an ideal muscle relaxant: quick onset, superb intubating conditions, and brief duration of action. However, succinylcholine has a myriad of non-paralytic effects, many of which are exaggerated in the pediatric population. **Table 2.9** lists these effects and **Table 2.10** lists the contraindications to succinylcholine[59,60].

In normal patients, succinylcholine increases plasma levels of potassium by 0.3 to 0.5 mEq/liter, reaching a peak at 5 minutes. Life-threatening levels of hyperkalemia, as high as 13 mEq/liter, have been reported when succinylcholine has been given to patients with progressive neurological disease, spinal cord injury, cerebrovascular accidents, and those who had recent burn or major muscle trauma. The exact etiology for the hyperkalemic response is unclear, however, the common pathway appears to be the presence of a large mass of denervated muscle. Although the data would suggest that the susceptibility of burn and trauma patients to this hyperkalemic response exists only between 7 and 60 days[61–63], *our practice is to avoid succinylcholine from 72 hours after the injury, to 6 months–1 year.* Cerebral palsy is not a contraindication to succinylcholine. Prolonged severe intraabdominal infections (>1 week) have also been associated with a hyperkalemic response to succinylcholine administration[64].

Succinylcholine appears to increase intragastric, intracranial and intraocular pressure. These effects are related to the intensity of muscle fasciculations. Pretreatment with a small dose (10% of intubating dose) of a nondepolarizing muscle relaxant prevents muscle fasciculations by partially blocking depolarization by succinylcholine. With regard to increases in intragastric pressure, children have a much lower increase in intragastric pressure after succinylcholine administration than adults. Succinylcholine can increase cerebral blood flow and intracranial pressure in patients with decreased intracranial compliance. This effect is blunted by an adequate sedation and a defasciculating dose of a nondepolarizing muscle relaxant[65]. In a similar fashion the adverse effects of succinylcholine may successfully be managed with careful pretreatment with a defasciculating dose of a non-depolarizing drug and an induction dose of sodium pentothal. This is dramatically substantiated by a study by Libonati in which patients

Table 2.9. The Non-paralytic Effects of Succinylcholine

Sinus bradycardia in infants and small children
Nodal rhythms
Hyperkalemia after:
burn, trauma
spinal cord injury
progressive neurologic disease (e.g., multiple sclerosis)
recent stroke
Masseter spasm
0.06% incidence in children
50% of those will have a positive halothane contracture test for malignant hyperthermia
Increased intracranial/ocular pressure (effects mitigated by adequate sedation)

Table 2.10. Contraindications to Succinylcholine

Hyperkalemia	K > 5.5 mEq/L
Burn	3days–6months after injury
Trauma	3days–1year after injury
Paraplegia	3days–1year after injury
Duchenne's Muscular Dystrophy	
Myotonic Dystrophy	
Amyotrophic Lateral Sclerosis	
Multiple Sclerosis	
Friedreich's Ataxia	
Guillain Barre Syndrome	
Parkinson's Disease	
Progressive neuromuscular diseases	

with intraocular injuries who underwent a pretreatment-barbiturate-succinylcholine induction had no loss of intraocular contents[66].

Succinylcholine, especially with the co-administration of a halogenated vapor anesthetic such as halothane, is a trigger agent for malignant hyperthermia. Malignant hyperthermia is a hypermetabolic response to a trigger agent characterized by increased CO_2 production and oxygen consumption. Fever, tachycardia, tachypnea, acidosis, hyperkalemia, ventricular dysrhythmias, and rhabdomyolysis result. The mortality rate in fulminant malignant hyperthermia is 10%. Malignant hyperthermia is autosomal dominant in humans, and most cases seem to affect children and young adults. In addition to a positive family history, Duchenne muscular dystrophy and the uncommon myopathies of central core disease, myotonia congenita and King-Denborough syndrome are thought to be risk factors for the development of malignant hyperthermia.

An occasional patient may develop masseter spasm (a tight jaw), after the administration of succinylcholine. Masseter spasm may be the only initial manifestation of a malignant hyperthermic response. The incidence of masseter spasm in otherwise healthy children is 0.06%[67]. Evaluation of these patients suggests that about 50% are at risk for the development of malignant hyperthermia. Often premature attempts at laryngoscopy, before the drug has taken effect, will be mistaken as masseter spasm[68].

These side-effects have led many practitioners to avoid succinylcholine in children. Nevertheless, in the appropriate patient, when immediate airway control is necessary, succinylcholine has no peer.

Until recently there were no nondepolarizing relaxants that compared to succinylcholine for rapidity of onset and brief duration of action. Mivacurium is a short-acting nondepolarizing blocker which is rapidly metabolized by plasma cholinesterase at 70% of the rate at which succinylcholine is metabolized[69]. After a dose of 0.25 to 0.3 mg/kg, mivacurium provides good intubation conditions within 90 seconds, lasting about 10 minutes. Complete spontaneous recovery of neuromuscular function occurs by 13 minutes[70]. If a "priming dose" of 0.02 mg/kg is administered 2 minutes before intubation, the onset of action is decreased to 75 seconds, but the duration is increased to 15 to 20 minutes. Similarly, rocuronium may produce paralysis within 60 to 75 seconds if given in high doses (0.6–1.0 mg/kg). When mivacurium is administered in large doses ($\geq$ 0.3 mg/kg) or by rapid injection, histamine release can produce cutaneous flushing and a transient decrease in blood pressure[71–73].

The remainder of the nondepolarizing neuromuscular blockers may be divided into intermediate and long-acting agents. The intermediate acting drugs vecuronium and atracurium have an onset of 90 to 200 seconds which can be shortened either by the use of larger intubating doses, or priming, as summarized in **Table 2.11.** Unfortunately, these modifications result in a significant extension of the duration of blockade.

Table 2.11. Dosage for Priming or Intubation to Decrease Onset Time

	Prime (mg/kg)	*Intubating Dose (mg/kg)*	*Onset (sec)*	*Duration (min)*
Succinylcholine		1.0–1.5	60	5–8
Mivacurium		0.25	90	10–12
Mivacurium	0.02	0.25	90	12–18
Mivacurium	0.02	0.3	75	15–20
Rocuronium		0.6	90	30–45
Rocuronium		0.8	75	45–70
Atracurium		0.6	90	30–45
Vecuronium	0.01	0.25	90	70–120
Pancuronium		0.1–0.15	90–120	45–60

Mivacurium is the only drug that compares favorably to succinylcholine regarding its latency to onset and its brief duration. Once the airway is secured any of the nondepolarizers can be used to maintain neuromuscular blockade. The specific choice of drug should be dictated by the metabolic profile of the individual drugs. Pancuronium is excreted by the kidneys, although there is a minor hepatobiliary component. Vecuronium relies principally on hepatic excretion. Rocuronium is not metabolized but is excreted unchanged in the urine and bile. Atracurium is inactivated by a non-specific ester hydrolysis and Hoffman degradation. Therefore, atracurium is an excellent choice in the setting of significant hepato-renal disease, if a short well defined period of paralysis is planned. Alternatively, any of the longer acting drugs may be used, if they are titrated to the desired effect (e.g., toe movement).

RAPID SEQUENCE INTUBATION

A vast majority of patients that the pediatric intensivist is called upon to intubate are at risk for pulmonary aspiration. Patients considered to have a full stomach are listed in **Table 2.12.**

Intubation is accomplished in these situations under "awake" conditions to preserve pharyngolaryngeal reflexes as described above or by a rapid sequence infusion of medications and utilizing cricoid pressure. The "rapid sequence" refers to the brief period of time between infusion of medicines, loss of airway reflexes and ideal intubating conditions. The risk of passive regurgitation of gastric contents

Table 2.12. Risk factors for Pulmonary Aspiration Syndrome

Recent oral intake.
Delayed gastric emptying from pain, ascites, peritonitis, diabetes mellitus.
Swallowed blood from oro-facial trauma.
Increased intra-abdominal pressure from abdominal mass.
Abnormal lower esophageal tone: pregnancy, connective tissue diseases.
Gastro-esophageal reflux.
Altered level of consciousness.

can be significantly reduced with the application of cricoid pressure[26]. Cricoid pressure has been shown to occlude effectively the esophagus in infant cadavers, even with the presence of a nasogastric tube in the esophageal lumen[74]. Strict adherence to all the steps in the rapid sequence induction, as well as a running intravenous line and the availability of an assistant are mandatory. All equipment must be within an arms reach, and checked (again) just prior to the induction. Two suction set ups must be available and set to maximal settings. A pulse oximeter is invaluable during a rapid sequence intubation.

The patient is preoxygenated, actually denitrogenated, for 2 to 3 minutes, breathing 100% oxygen through a tight fitting mask. The head is placed in the optimal sniffing position. Cricoid pressure is applied by the assistant. A defasciculating dose of a nondepolarizer may be administered; it is our practice to only use a defasciculating dose in patients with intracranial hypertension or a ruptured globe. If there is any question regarding the intravascular status of the child, a bolus of isotonic fluid is administered at this time. An assistant then administers the medications listed. If rapid oxygen desaturation occurs while awaiting for complete relaxation, **gentle** bag-mask ventilation through cricoid may be used. Once adequate relaxation is achieved, laryngoscopy and intubation are performed. Cricoid pressure is released only after a successful endotracheal intubation is confirmed by the presence of expired CO_2 gas and bilateral breath sounds. A nasogastric or orogastric tube should be placed at this point to decompress the stomach.

Infrequently, intubation after the rapid sequence induction of anesthesia is unsuccessful. The approach in this situation is dictated in large part by the clinical status of the patient. If intubation is unsuccessful, but bag-mask ventilation and oxygenation (pulse oximeter > 90%) are effective, the intensivist can reevaluate the patients airway position, need for alternative laryngoscopic blades and determine why intubation was unsuccessful. The use of shortacting agents affords the ability to bag-mask ventilate until spontaneous respirations resume.

If bag-mask ventilation is difficult and the patient is rapidly desaturating, the intensivist may have to proceed to the emergency establishment of an artificial airway. Exactly when this path should be taken depends in large part on the experience of the intensivist. The less experienced the intubator, the sooner one should consider establishing an emergent airway by needle cricothyrotomy in order to maintain oxygenation.

The properties of ketamine have already been discussed. Short-acting barbiturates produce a rapid loss of consciousness. They would provide suitable amnesia for intubation although myocardial depression and hypotension may result if the patient is hypovolemic or has poor myocardial function. Thiopental lowers both cerebral blood flow and the cerebral metabolic rate for oxygen ($CMRO_2$) and, therefore, is a useful agent for intubation of patients with elevated intracranial pressure.

Reversal of Neuromuscular Blockade

Reversal of nondepolarizing neuromuscular blocking agents is faster if fewer receptors are blocked when the reversal agents are given. Agents suitable for reversal include the anticholinesterase drugs neostigmine (0.07 mg/kg, maximum 5 mg) or pyridostigmine (0.2 mg/kg, maximum 10 mg). In addition, an anticholinergic drug is given to prevent the muscarinic effects of the anti-cholinesterase agents. Frequently used anticholinergic drugs include atropine 0.02 mg/kg or glycopyrrolate 0.01 mg/kg. The maximum dose given at one time is usually 1 mg for atropine and 10 mg for pyridostigmine. Antagonism of neuromuscular blockade is more likely to be successful if some return of neuromuscular function is evident in spontaneous movement or movement elicited by a nerve stimulator prior to injection of the reversal agents. There are several measures of adequate antagonism including sustained tetanus during nerve stimulation at 50 Hz, an inspiratory force greater than–25 cm H_2O, flexion of the arms and legs, or the ability to lift the head for 5 seconds. Neuromuscular block may be prolonged by hypothermia, magnesium, which prohibits prejunctional release of acetylcholine; the streptomycin/neomycin group of antibiotics, which inhibit prejunctional release of acetylcholine and decrease the postjunctional sensitivity to acetylcholine; as well as polymyxin, tetracycline, and lincomycin antibiotics by an unknown action[75].

Nasotracheal Intubation

Nasotracheal intubation provides a more secure airway for a critically ill patient and may be more comfortable. The tape is less prone to disturbance from oral secretions, and the tube is less susceptible to damage and dislodgement. Nevertheless nasotracheal tube placement is less time efficient and a technically more difficult skill.

Nasotracheal intubation may be performed without the aid of laryngoscopy ("blindly") with the patient breathing spontaneously, preferably sitting straight up in bed. During preoxygenation the patency of the individual nares is assessed. The most patent nare is anesthetized with a slurry of 3 ml 4% lidocaine and 1 ml of phenylephrine, 10 mg/ml. The nare is then dilated by inserting progressively larger nasopharyngeal airways which have been well lubricated with lidocaine jelly. Once adequate dilatation is achieved, the endotracheal tube is inserted through the nares to the ramus of the mandible. At this point the patient is instructed to take a deep breath in and a deep breath out. These instructions are repeated twice more. During the 3rd cycle, the endotracheal tube is rapidly advanced during inspiration, while listening for loud breath sounds at the 15 mm adapter end of the endotracheal tube.

Alternatively, nasotracheal intubation can be accomplished using direct laryngoscopy to visualize the glottis and allow the tube to be guided under direct vision. The tube is advanced by pushing at the nasal end and directing the tip with intubating forceps. The forceps should be used only

Table 2.13. Drugs for Rapid Sequence Induction

Defasciculating dose:	Pancuronium 0.01 mg/kg	
Induction agent:		
Isovolemic	Thiopental	5–7 mg/kg
Head trauma	Thiopental	5–7 mg/kg
Hypovolemia+head trauma	Thiopental	2–3 mg/kg
Asthma	Ketamine	2 mg/kg
Hypovolemia	Ketamine	2 mg/kg
Shock	Ketamine	0.5–1 mg/kg

for directing, and not for pushing the tube through the vocal cords.

Complications associated with a nasotracheal tube include epistaxis, trauma to the adenoids, pressure necrosis of the nares, trauma to the mucosa, and posterior dissection of the posterior pharyngeal wall at the area of the sphenoid prominence,[76] obstruction of the Eustachian tube, and possible otitis media or maxillary sinusitis if long-term intubation is used. The overall complication rate from nasotracheal intubation is 8%[77]. Nasal deformities secondary to nasotracheal intubation are more common in very low birth weight infants (less than 1000 g) and with prolonged intubation of longer than 5 days' duration[78].

Contraindications to nasal intubation include a:

1. Fracture of the cribriform plate with cerebro-spinal fluid leak, because of the risk of infection and meningitis or intracranial passage of the tube;
2. Bleeding disorders or the use of anticoagulants, because of the risk of active hemorrhage necessitating nasal packing; or
3. Deformity of the nose obstructing passage of the tube.

Special Situations Requiring Intubation

The Child with an Open Globe Injury

With penetrating injuries to the eye, vitreous humor can leak from the open globe if intraocular pressure increases, as may occur with coughing, struggling during laryngoscopy, or intubation. For patients with an open globe and who need to have an airway established, it is imperative that laryngoscopy and intubation are performed under ideal pharmacological control. In the absence of a full stomach and the risks of pulmonary aspiration syndrome, a recommended sequence for intubation would include preoxygenation with 100% oxygen, followed by thiopental and mivacurium **(Table 2.13).** The ocular hypertensive response to laryngoscopy and intubation may be blunted by using lidocaine 1.5–2.0 mg/kg i.v.[79]. Unfortunately, most of these children have a "full stomach." In this circumstance, a rapid sequence induction with either succinylcholine or a mivacurium (0.25–0.3) mg/kg should be employed. Succinylcholine's increase in intraocular pressure appears to be mitigated by adequate doses of an anesthetic agent and a defasciculating dose of a nondepolarizer. Results of a recent retrospective evaluation indicated no problems when using pretreatment with a nondepolarizing agent, followed by a barbiturate and succinylcholine for rapid sequence induction. In any case, the primary concern is the airway. Once intubated, the child should continue to receive sedation to avoid straining against the endotracheal tube when paralysis is no longer present.

The Child with Elevated Intracranial Pressure

Children with head injuries frequently require establishment of an artificial airway as protection from aspiration if the level of consciousness is decreased or if the protective cough and gag reflexes are decreased. In children with intracranial hypertension, elective intubation and controlled ventilation are necessary to control arterial PO_2 and PCO_2. Intubation may be difficult. Often, cervical spine or facial injuries may be present. It is important to evaluate the mouth for loose teeth, blood, and debris and to avoid manipulation of the cervical spine until x-ray evaluation has been completed. If intubation is necessary before x-ray completion, axial in-line traction should be applied to stabilize the neck. Laryngoscopy and intubation have been associated with an increase in intracranial pressure, even in the anesthetized patient. Awake intubation in a conscious or semiconscious child may aggravate an already elevated intracranial pressure with struggling and coughing. Nasotracheal intubation may be contraindicated if basilar skull fracture or nasopharyngeal bleeding is present. If the child has a normal hemodynamic status, sedation and relaxation can be achieved with thiopental and either mivacurium or succinylcholine, after pretreatment with a defasciculating dose of a nondepolarizing muscle relaxant (pancuronium 0.01 mg/kg i.v.) **(Table 2.13).** If hypovolemia is present or the vital signs are unstable, a smaller dose of thiopental (1–2 mg/kg i.v.) is sufficient. Intravenous lidocaine at 1.5 mg/kg may be used to prevent elevations of intracranial pressure with laryngoscopy and intubation[80]. If the airway anatomy is obscured by orofacial trauma or difficulty with laryngoscopy is anticipated, fiberoptic intubation, a retrograde catheter, or a cricothyrotomy airway as described in the section on the difficult airway, may be required.

The Child with Hypovolemia

Children with airway embarrassment frequently have coexisting hemodynamic instability either from hypovolemia or cardiac dysfunction secondary to traumatic injury. The intravascular status of the child can be rapidly assessed by performing a "tilt test". While monitoring heart rate and blood pressure, reposition the patient successively in the trendelenburg, neutral and then reverse trendelenburg positions. If the heart rate increase is greater than 10 to 15 bpm, hypovolemia is reasonably assured. If possible, fluid therapy to replenish the intravascular volume should begin immediately, coincident with efforts to establish a secure airway.

Preoxygenation with 100% oxygen is important in patients with hypovolemia and marginal cardiac output. The minimal doses of drugs should be used to achieve adequate intubating conditions without precipitating cardiovascular collapse. If hypovolemia has not been adequately corrected, ketamine followed by a muscle relaxant would be the technique of choice. In the presence of a full stomach as a result of recent oral intake, swallowed blood, ascites, or increased abdominal pressure from intra-abdominal bleeding, a rapid sequence technique utilizing cricoid pressure should be used. *Nevertheless, there are certain instances in which the child is so unstable that the only safe approach is to intubate the child without pharmacological adjuncts.* Care should be taken to avoid the cardiovascular collapse that can be precipitated by the use of excessive airway pressures in the hypovolemic patient.

The Child with Epiglottitis, Other Forms of Upper Airway Obstruction or Tracheal Injury

Acute epiglottitis is a life threatening acute inflammation of the entire supraglottic region with an extremely rapid clinical course. Typically, the affected child was well until hours before the onset of fever, stridor and a very painful dysphagia. The child often assumes the classic tripod position: sitting up and forward with the mouth open, drooling. Although some data suggest that the patient with epiglottitis is most likely to be between 2 and 4 years of age, up to 33% of patients may be less than 2 years of age[81–84].

Prior to 1987, the predominant cause (> 98%) of epiglottitis was a systemic Haemophilus influenzae type B infection. With licensure of the first polysaccharide-protein conjugate vaccines, the prevalence of epiglottitis has decreased dramatically. Nevertheless, of the cases reported by Valdepena, 75% were still attributable to Haemophilus Influenzae type B. The remaining patients had Staphylococcus aureus, Klebsiella or Candida Albicans. Of those children infected with Haemophilus Influenzae type B, 50% had not been immunized[85].

Despite the decrease in the prevalence of epiglottitis in the current era, the lessons learned in the airway management of this disease are valuable and generally applicable to the management of any difficult pediatric airway. Ideally, the child suspected of having acute epiglottitis must be managed in a collaborative fashion by an experienced otolaryngologist, anesthesiologist and pediatric intensivist. Most clinicians believe that there is no place for radiographs in the evaluation of a patient with epiglottitis. The role of miniflexible nasopharyngoscopy in the Emergency Department evaluation of these patients remains unclear.

It is our practice to bring the child to the operating room as soon as possible. The child is maintained in a calm atmosphere and upright position during evaluation and transport. Laying the child down to do unnecessary procedures may result in complete and irreversible airway obstruction. Oxygen administration and pulse-oximetry monitoring are sufficient until the child arrives in the operating room accompanied by all the resources needed to establish a surgical airway should airway obstruction occur.

There are several approaches to the anesthetic technique depending on the clinical experience of the physicians in attendance. It must be emphasized that the most experienced individuals available should be directing the management of these difficult patients[86]. The principal considerations in the approach to these patients are outlined in **Table 2.14**.

Table 2.14. Potential Problems in a Patient with an Airway Obstruction

- Airway edema
- Secretions
- Distorted anatomy
- Hypoxia
- Decreased functional residual capacity
- Dehydration
- Fatigue
- Metabolic Acidosis
- Sepsis: increased oxygen demand, decreased level of consciousness

The anatomy may be so distorted from inflammation and edema that the glottic structures will be unidentifiable. If the child is breathing spontaneously, air bubbles during exhalation will define the glottis and an endotracheal tube can be introduced through this area. As a result of this extensive edema the glottis will be much smaller than normal, and therefore a wide selection of endotracheal tubes with a small diameter (3.0–4.5 mm i.d.), but sufficient length (28 cm) must be available.

For these reasons, it is the predominant practice in our institution to proceed with a slow inhalational induction of anesthesia, initially with the child in the upright position. The ideal moment to place an intravenous (IV) catheter continues to be hotly debated. One school of thought maintains that IV placement before induction of anesthesia in a child with a critical airway is worth the risk of upsetting the child, but that further airway compromise would be unlikely, as long as the child is maintained upright. Another school strongly argues that there is sufficient time to place an intravenous catheter once the child is sufficiently anesthetized.

Once sufficiently anesthetized, and a bolus of isotonic fluid is administered, direct laryngoscopy is performed. If the laryngoscopist can identify the glottic structures, the endotracheal tube is placed, cultures are obtained, and antibiotics are administered. If glottic structures are not identified, and the patient is well saturated, the otolaryngologist can attempt to place a ventilating bronchoscope and establish control of the airway. If this proves impossible, or if severe oxygen desaturation intervenes, the otolaryngologist proceeds with an emergency cricothyrotomy or tracheostomy.

After successful airway management, the child is admitted to the PICU. Timing of extubation of the child with epiglottitis is another controversial area. One school of thought maintains that revisualization of the supraglottic structures is necessary prior to extubation. Our approach is to reevaluate the clinical status of the patient. On return to the

PICU these patients are kept sedated with a minimum amount of benzodiazepine, without neuromuscular blockade. Once the child's fever has decreased, evidence for toxicity has abated, intravascular volume has been repleted and a leak around the endotracheal tube is present, extubation is contemplated. This usually takes between 12 to 24 hours. Extubation should be performed only when the personnel and equipment are available should acute airway obstruction occur. Approximately 10% of children have some post-extubation stridor attributable to the trauma of intubation which is treated with racemic epinephrine and continued corticosteroids[87].

Acute pulmonary edema has been described in children with the relief of airway obstruction, such as secondary to an obstructed endotracheal tube, croup, epiglottitis, or laryngospasm[88–92]. Usually, this post-obstructive pulmonary edema, manifests itself immediately or within a few hours of the relief of obstruction. Several mechanisms have been proposed, including an increased left ventricular transmural pressure gradient from the negative pleural pressure generated against the airway obstruction as well as right heart failure and leftward displacement of the intraventricular septum secondary to pulmonary vasoconstriction because of alveolar hypoxia[93]. Systemic vasoconstriction as a result of hypoxemia may also result in an increase in blood distributed to the pulmonary circulation[94]. Negative intrathoracic pressure may also cause left ventricular dysfunction[95]. Treatment involves airway support, oxygen administration, and continuous positive airway pressure or positive end-expiratory pressure. Diuretics may be needed, depending on the clinical condition and fluid status. The acute pulmonary edema usually resolves within 24 hours.

The Child with a Cervical Spine Injury

Trauma patients with probable cervical spine injuries represent another group of patients with potentially difficult airways. In this situation, conventional management includes oral intubation after the application of cricoid pressure and manual in-line stabilization. The concern with this approach has been the potential for further exacerbation of the neurological injury during laryngoscopy. Criswell reviewed the 73 patients with traumatic cervical spine injury who were managed using this approach within 30 minutes of presentation. No further neurological injury was attributed to airway management[96]. Alternative approaches include fiberoptic bronchoscopic intubation, retrograde intubation and tracheostomy.

The Child with Down Syndrome

Atlanto-occipital instability occurs in 10% to 20% of patients with Down syndrome who are at risk for atlantoaxial subluxation. To identify patients who are at risk for atlantoaxial subluxation, guidelines have been adapted from the recommendations of the American Academy of Pediatrics and the Special Olympics Inc. which include preoperative neurologic assessments and cervical roentgenograms in the neutral, flexion, and extension positions. Children with an atlantodental interval of greater than 4.5 mm or with peripheral neurologic findings should have further evaluation[97]. In the face of uncertainty and impending airway compromise, it is prudent to treat all children with Trisomy 21 as if they do in fact have atlanto-occipital instability. Our approach to these patients is identical to those with cervical spine injuries.

THE DIFFICULT AIRWAY

Fiberoptic Laryngoscopy

Fiberoptic laryngoscopy is an alternative method for obtaining a secure airway. The fiberoptic laryngoscope is flexible with a mobile tip and is useful in allowing visualization of the glottis in patients with limited neck and temporomandibular joints motion. Topical anesthesia is useful in decreasing the vagal stimulation and the risk of laryngospasm from stimulation of the epiglottis and posterior pharyngeal wall. Fiberoptic bronchoscopy has been used to evaluate the larynx in infants and prematures without sedation[98]. Evaluation in the awake patient allows observation of the functioning airway, including vocal cord movement. Pediatric scopes are available to allow evaluation through endotracheal tubes as small as 3.5 mm in internal diameter. The larger fiberoptic bronchoscopes also have a suction channel to clear secretions for better visualization. The fiberoptic scope is lubricated and passed through an endotracheal tube which has been placed in a nare in preparation for nasotracheal intubation. Local anesthetic is injected through the working channel of the scope when vocal cords are visualized.

Once adequate airway anesthesia is obtained, the scope is then maneuvered gently but swiftly through the vocal cords down to just above the carina. At this point the endotracheal tube is advanced over the bronchoscope and then secured in place. Unsuccessful attempts at intubation using the fiberoptic bronchoscope may be encountered with inadequate airway anesthesia, bleeding, edema, fogging of the scope, a failed light source, or inappropriate positioning and a failure to keep the scope in the midline.

In addition to airway access, the fiberoptic bronchoscope has a number of therapeutic roles in the PICU setting including relief of atelectasis, hemoptysis, evaluation of the immunocompromised host and the safe exchange of endotracheal tubes[99]. One of the principal causes of acute lobar collapse and massive atelectasis is mucous plugging. Utilizing fiberoptic bronchoscopy and selective intrabronchial air insufflation, Haenel and associates have safely demonstrated dramatic clinical improvements as measured by radiographic changes and PaO_2/FiO_2 in patients with critical hypoxemia or persistent massive atelectasis[100]. The therapeutic success of bronchoscopic intervention appears to be limited to those with lobar collapse but not in those with mild atelectasis or pulmonary infiltrates on radiographs taken within 24 hours[101]. The bronchoscope may also be useful in evaluating the airway before and after extubation and prior to reintubation if necessary[102,103].

Retrograde Catheter

Another technique for intubation of patients with a difficult airway involves the use of a retrograde catheter[104–108]. A Tuohy needle is used for puncture of the cricothyroid membrane. An epidural catheter with stylet is then advanced through the needle and rotated to pass through the pharynx and out the mouth. Lidocaine injected through the cricothyroid membrane prior to catheter insertion may lessen the risk of laryngospasm from catheter stimulation. Forceps may be used to pull the catheter out the mouth. If a nasotracheal intubation is planned, a suction catheter may be passed through the nose and out the mouth; this is tied to the epidural catheter, which is then pulled out the nose. Once the catheter is in place, the Tuohy needle and stylet are removed. The endotracheal tube is then advanced over the catheter, which should be kept tight because loops may form in the pharynx and then be pushed into the esophagus with the endotracheal tube[108]. When the position of the endotracheal tube is confirmed, the epidural catheter is cut at the neck and pulled out the nose or mouth. The retrograde catheter technique is less practical in small infants because it is difficult to locate the cricothyroid membrane. Nevertheless it has been successfully reported in a 30-month-old child[109].

Emergency Establishment Of An Artificial Airway

Emergency Management of the Difficult Airway

Airway obstruction and rapid desaturation can occur frightfully fast in children with difficult airways. The choice of an emergency artificial airway is dependent on the clinical scenario and the intensivist's experience. Orotracheal intubation is the fastest, yet it is not always possible based on the preceding discussion. Rather than continuing to perform unsuccessful airway techniques, the intensivist must establish an alternative airway and reverse the developing hypoxia. Needle cricothyrotomy is the most rapid and reliable method available for oxygenating this group of patients.

Cricothyrotomy

When intubation is not possible or is contraindicated, surgical establishment of an airway is indicated. A cricothyrotomy is fast and requires fewer instruments and less skill than an emergency tracheostomy. This procedure is indicated if intubation is not possible because of anatomic difficulties, airway obstruction, severe oropharyngeal edema or cervical spine injury limiting laryngoscopic visualization.

Needle Cricothyrotomy

The cricothyroid membrane is located between the inferior edge of the thyroid cartilage and the upper edge of the cri-

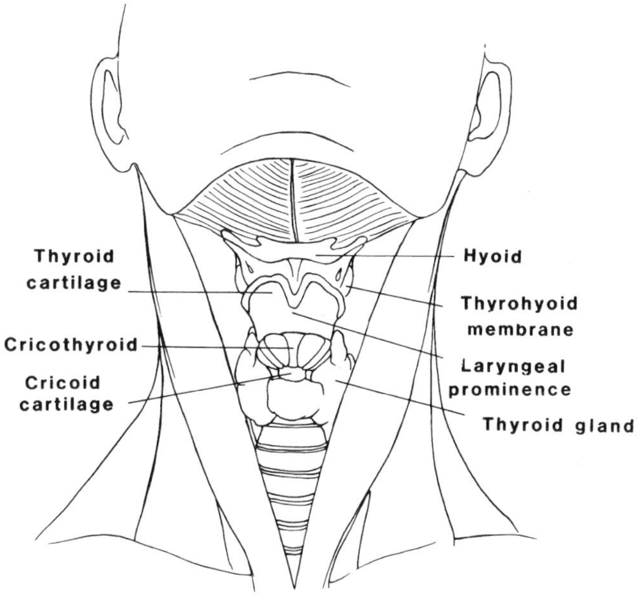

Figure 2.20. Establishment of an airway by cricothyrotomy may be accomplished by puncture of the cricothyroid membrane in the anterior midline of the neck.

coid cartilage (Fig. 2.20). If there is no injury to the cervical spine, the head may be tilted back and the larynx stabilized with the fingers while the cricothyroid membrane is palpated. The membrane can be punctured in the anterior midline of the neck. A 14-gauge intravenous catheter is suitable for this technique. The catheter should be inserted at a caudad angle to avoid injury to the vocal cords, which are located cephalad. It will be necessary to penetrate skin, subcutaneous tissue, cervical fascia, and then the cricothyroid membrane.

Air aspirated through the catheter confirms its tracheal placement. If a 1 4-gauge intravenous catheter is used, an adaptor from a 3.0 mm ID endotracheal tube can be used to connect to a resuscitation bag.

Cricothyrotomy by Seldinger Technique

Although oxygenation is assured, the limitation of the needle cricothyrotomy is its inability to reliably ventilate the patient[110]. Recently, using modifications of the Seldinger technology, a cricothyrotomy catheter set has become available. Utilizing the procedure outlined above, once needle access to the trachea is assured, a wire guide is advanced through the needle. The needle is removed and an airway catheter/dilator assembly is then advanced over the wire guide. Once secured, the wire and internal dilator are removed leaving a cricotracheostomy tube of sufficient size for *reliable oxygenation and ventilation.* Clearly if this type of kit is available it is the preferable device.

Problems encountered with the cricothyrotomy techniques include difficulty in palpating landmarks in infants and young children, bleeding, formation of a false passage, subcutaneous or mediastinal emphysema, and injury to vascular, neural, or pulmonary structures of the neck[111]. Complications can be prevented with careful needle placement and confirmation of location, observation of airway pressure, and attention to inspiratory time. The needle cricothyrotomy should be thought of as a life saving technique,which will provide adequate oxygenation and ventilation until a secure airway can be established.

Tracheostomy

Indications for tracheostomy include subglottic stenosis, bilateral vocal cord paralysis, congenital airway malformations, airway tumors, and a requirement for prolonged ventilator therapy(112,113). A tracheostomy performed in a child has a complication rate ranging from 10% to 33%, and a mortality rate of 1 to 3%. The mortality has been significantly reduced as a result of the advancements in the postoperative critical care management of these children(113,114). Young children have the highest complication rate(114–117). Immediate complications of the procedure include subcutaneous emphysema of the neck and face, pneumothorax pneumomediastinum, poor positioning of the tube, postoperative bleeding, self-extubation, and thyroid injury(118–122). Immediate postoperative care of the child with a new tracheostomy involves evaluation of a chest x-ray for air accumulation and tube position. The tracheostomy tube should be tied securely around the neck and the neck protected from irritation. As the normal humidifying mechanisms of the mouth and nose are bypassed, humidified oxygen should be supplied. Airway secretions are frequently increased for 24 to 48 hours, necessitating intensive pulmonary supportive care. Tracheostomy tube obstruction is a life-threatening complication in the postoperative period. *Suction equipment, scissors, tracheal dilators, and replacement tracheostomy tubes should be available at the bedside.* Multiple sizes and types of tubes should be available to ensure a tube of the appropriate diameter and length for each patient. **Table 2.15** shows suggested sizes for plastic tracheostomy tubes.

If tachypnea, respiratory distress, cyanosis or decreased breath sounds are observed in a child with a tracheostomy, the tracheostomy tube is assumed to be obstructed until proven to be patent. This obstruction is common because of increased secretions(123). The child should be ventilated with 100% oxygen, the head and neck extended to expose the tracheostomy site, and the suction catheter passed. If the suction catheter will not pass, a new tracheostomy tube is inserted through the tract to allow ventilation. If the tract narrows, a smaller cannula or endotracheal tube may be necessary to allow ventilation. Within the first week of tracheostomy creation, the tract has not had an opportunity to epithelize. As such, this tract may not be readily identifiable, making reintubation through the stoma difficult. It is for this reason that otolaryngologists place tracheal sutures, to assist in re-exposing the actual orifice. Have an assistant firmly but gently pull these tracheostomy sutures up and away from the midline, re-exposing the stoma. If either an endotracheal tube or a new tracheostomy tube will not pass, an oxygen catheter with a high flow should be passed into the tract to allow oxygenation in the spontaneously breathing patient. If assisted ventilation is needed for a child on ventilator support, the stoma should be covered with a gauze pad, and the patient ventilated by the face mask. As the tracheostomy tract matures later in the first postoperative week, the first tracheostomy tube change is usually performed by the otolaryngologist in the intensive care unit. Other equipment necessary for tracheostomy tube change is noted in **Table 2.16.**

Late complications of tracheostomy include tracheitis, skin ulceration, wound infection, aspiration, accidental decannulation, and tracheal granulations(123,124). Innominate artery erosion secondary to the tip of the tracheostomy tube may also occur(115). If sudden, rapid bleeding from the lumen of the tracheostomy tube occurs, a cuffed tube should be passed beyond the vessel erosion and the cuff inflated to prevent blood aspiration to the remainder of the tracheobronchial tree.

Table 2.15. Suggested Tracheostomy Tube Size

Age		*Shiley Tube*	*Internal Diameter (mm)*	*Length (mm)*
Premature infant	Neonatal	00	3.1	30
	Pediatric	00	3.1	3.9
Newborn	Neonatal	0	3.4	32
	Pediatric	0	3.4	40
Newborn–6 months		1	3.7	41
6–12 months		1–2	3.7–4.1	41–42
12 months–2 years		3	4.8	44
3–6 years		4	5.0	46
7–10 years		4	5.0	46
10–12 years		6 (single cannula tube)	7.0	67

Table 2.16. Equipment Available for Tracheostomy Tube Change

Suction–source, catheters
Oxygen–source, bag
Tracheostomy tubes–appropriate sizes
Laryngoscope–blade, handle, bulb, battery
Endotracheal tubes–appropriate sizes
Tracheal dilator and wound retractors
Ties–to secure tube
Mask–for ventilation with stoma covered if unable to replace tracheostomy tube

SUPPORT OF THE PATIENT WITH AN ARTIFICIAL AIRWAY

Endotracheal intubation bypasses several functions of the upper airway, including warming and humidification. These functions are replaced by warming and humidifying the oxygen supplied to the artificial airway. As the artificial airway also interferes with ciliary action and tracheal mucous flow, it is important to change the child's position to mobilize secretions and to suction frequently for secretions. Saline instillation may be necessary to suspend secretions.

COMPLICATIONS FROM ENDOTRACHEAL INTUBATION

Complications from endotracheal intubation are variable. Immediate complications include the hemodynamic responses to laryngoscopy, such as bradycardia, dysrhythmias, hypertension as well as apnea, coughing and upper airway spasm[125,126]. Aspiration may occur after vomiting or regurgitation. Subluxation of the cervical spine may occur with head positioning in patients with congenital deformity or previous abnormality of the cervical spine. Manipulation of the laryngoscope may cause loss of the teeth, especially in the child 4 to 11 years of age with loose deciduous teeth. Similarly, the laryngoscope may cause injury to lips or gingivae, and ulceration of the posterior pharyngeal wall, epiglottis, aryepiglottic folds, and arytenoids. Hypoxemia may occur with prolonged attempts at intubation or in a patient with decreased oxygen reserves.

Early complications of intubation may involve laceration or hematoma of the vocal cords and erosions of the posterior cords and around the tracheal cuff site, as a result of pressure necrosis and mechanical trauma. Sore throat is frequently noted in patients after intubation. Self-extubation may also occur. Accidental extubation appears to be more common in infants under 1 year of age than in older children. Bronchial intubation and atelectasis, especially of the right upper lobe, are common complications of intubation[127].

For cuffed tubes, an increased air leak may be noted. Treatment may involve checking the location of the tube by laryngoscopy to confirm that the cuff is not above the vocal cords, packing the oropharynx, increasing fresh gas flow to compensate for the air leak, adding air to the cuff to compensate for the leak, removal of the endotracheal tube, and reintubation if needed. Other complications from the endotracheal tube include ulcers, usually seen on the medial vocal processes of the arytenoid cartilage, posterior vocal cords, dorsolateral subglottic area, anterior tracheal wall, epiglottis, site of the tip of the tube, and cuff site. Symptoms of ulcers include pain and hoarseness. Mucosal lesions also involve hemorrhage and focal abrasions[128].

Clinical symptoms of aspiration while the patient is intubated are uncommon. In a prospective study of pediatric patients, it was noted that an uncuffed tube can effectively protect from aspiration, with evidence of dye placed on the tongue appearing in tracheal aspirates of 16% of patients with no significant clinical symptoms[129]. Some institutions use food coloring added to feedings to monitor for a change in the color of the pulmonary secretions.

The most serious of the late complications of intubation is acquired subglottic stenosis which has been reported to occur in 2–6% of pediatric patients[130,131]. The pathology of changes caused by endotracheal intubation have been described as initial hyperemia, edema, exudate, and mucosal hemorrhage. These changes have been noted after only 24 hours of intubation. After 6 days, ulceration and erosion have been noted[132]. After 7 days of intubation with uncuffed endotracheal tubes, reversible lesions involving ulcers and inflammation have been reported in puppies[133]. Stenosis with a 40 to 50% decrease in luminal size has been reported in puppies intubated with uncuffed endotracheal tubes for 14 or more days. These lesions are usually noted at the cricoid area, since it is the narrowest portion of the child's airway and the complete cartilage ring prevents outward expansion with edema and trauma. The lesions may be a web, band, or circumferential narrowing. Symptoms of airway obstruction from subglottic stenosis are usually seen 2 to 6 weeks after extubation. Diagnosis is confirmed by endoscopy. Treatment for subglottic stenosis involves anterior cricoid split or tracheostomy[134–136].

EXTUBATION

Extubation is attempted when the indications for intubation have resolved. In anticipation, feedings are withheld, and sedation is weaned, so that the risks of pulmonary aspiration and upper airway obstruction are minimized. The criteria for extubation include an intact cough and gag, a negative inspiratory force of 25–50 cm H_2O, a forced vital capacity breath in excess of 15 ml/kg, an air leak around the tube at inflating pressures < 25 cm H_2O as well as the maintenance of acceptable oxygenation and ventilation on minimal ventilatory support. The adequate antagonism of neuromuscular blockade is demonstrated by either a sustained head lift or, in an infant, leg lift. During the final preparation for extubation the FiO_2 should be increased to 1.00 to minimize the risk of post-extubation hypoxemia. All personnel and equipment necessary for reintubation are immediately available at the bedside should the child's airway compromise recur.

The oropharynx should be suctioned and cleared of secretions. If a cuffed endotracheal tube is present, the cuff is deflated, as indicated by collapse of the pilot balloon. Oxygen is applied by mask or hood after extubation. Chest physical therapy is continued because ciliary function is often ineffective secondary to the mucosal changes resulting from intubation[137].

The immediate complications after extubation include pulmonary aspiration, laryngospasm, bronchospasm and post-extubation croup. These sequelae should be anticipated and the appropriate therapies be immediately available. Laryngospasm results from the stimulus of extubation or residual secretions draining onto the epiglottis and vocal cords. Most commonly, laryngospasm occurs in patients who are in a "light stage" of sedation and is usually characterized by high pitched sounds ("crowing"). The incidence of laryngospasm is reduced by ensuring the adequate recovery of upper airway reflexes, and minimizing the presence of oral secretions at the moment of extubation. Under most circumstances laryngospasm can be successfully treated with gentle PEEP of 5 to 10 cm H_2O delivered by bag-mask ventilation. Should precipitous desaturations occur, succinylcholine is given to facilitate effective bag-mask ventilation. Aspiration may also occur because of ineffective cough and upper airway reflexes.

Post-extubation croup occurs in 1 to 6% of pediatric patients, more commonly in children between 1 to 4 years of age. The symptoms of hoarseness, stridor, and croupy cough, with or without inspiratory retraction, begin immediately to 3 hours after extubation, and peak at 8 hours. These symptoms usually resolve by 24 hours, although residual hoarseness may persist for up to 72 hours. Children are at an increased risk for the development of postextubation croup if there is an excessive air leak ($>$ 30 cm H_2O), excessive movement and coughing with an endotracheal tube in place, and after neck surgery. No relationship has been noted between the occurrence of postextubation croup and the use of lubricant on the tube, tracheal analgesic spray, humidification, or a history of upper respiratory infection[138].

Treatment of post-extubation croup includes cool mist or humidified oxygen, racemic epinephrine and corticosteroids[139]. The action of racemic epinephrine is unclear but may be related to topical vasoconstriction. The efficacy of corticosteroids in the prevention and treatment of postextubation croup has not been resolved. Edema owing to endotracheal intubation in animals has been reported to decrease after dexamethasone[140]. It has also been suggested that clinical improvement occurs in children treated with steroids[139]. However, prophylactic use of corticosteroids in intubated patients has not reduced the incidence of stridor after extubation[141]. Use of a helium-oxygen gas mixture by mask or headbox may also allow decreased respiratory work, as the low-density helium allows increased airflow through the narrowed airway[142]. This may provide additional time for resolution of edema without requiring replacement of an artificial airway for respiratory distress.

References

1. Ballinger JJ. Anatomy of the Larynx. IN Diseases of the Nose, Throat, and Ear, 12th edition. J Ballinger (ed), Lea & Febiger, Philadelphia, 1977, pp 330–336.
2. Berry FA. Anesthesia for the Child with a Difficult Airway. IN Anesthetic Management of Difficult and Routine Pediatric Patients, 2nd Edition, Churchill Livingstone, New York, 1990, pp 167–198.
3. Koka BV, Jeon IS, Andre JM, MacKay I, Smith RM. Postintubation croup in children. Anesth Analg 1977; 56:501.
4. Morgan GAR, Steward DJ. Linear dimensions in children: including those with cleft palate. Can Anaesth Soc J 1982; 29:1.
5. Fearon B, Whalen JS. Tracheal dimensions in the living infant. Ann Otol 1967; 76:964.
6. Deller A, Schreiber MN, Gromer J, Ahenfeld FW. Difficult intubation: incidence and predictability: A prospective study of 82,484 adult patients. Anesthesiology 1990; 73:A1054.
7. Hirsch IA, Reagan JO, Sullivan N. Complications of direct laryngoscopy: A prospective analysis. Anesthesiology Review 1990; 17:34–40.
8. Glassenburg R, Vaisrub N, Albright G. The incidence of failed intubation in obstetrics–is there a irreducible minimum? Anesthesiology 1990; 73:A1061.
9. Mallampati SR, Gatt SP, Gugino LD, Desa SP, Waraksa B, Feiberger D, Liu PL. A clinical sign to predict difficult tracheal intubation: a prospective study. Canadian Anaesth Soc J 1985; 32:429–434.
10. Brechner VL. Unusual problems in the management of airways. Flexion-extension mobility of the cervical spine. Anesth Analg 1968; 47:362–373.
11. Berry FA, Yemen TA. Pediatric airway in health and disease. Ped Clin N Am 1994; 41:153–180.
12. Berry FA. Anesthesia for the child with a difficult airway. IN Anesthetic Management of Difficult and Routine Pediatric Patients, 2nd Edition, Churchill Livingstone, New York, 1990, pp 167–198.
13. Belihouse CP, Dpre C. Criteria for estimating the difficulty of endotracheal intubation: MacIntosh laryngoscope. Anaes Inten Care 1988; 16:329–337.
14. Fink BR, Demarest RJ. Laryngeal Biomechanics, Cambridge, MA, Harvard University Press, 1978.
15. Sukerman S, Healy GB. Sleep apnea syndrome associated with upper airway obstruction. Laryngoscope 1979; 6:878–884.
16. Norton ML. Physiology and Variations of the Difficult Airway. IN Atlas of the Difficult Airway: A Source Book. Norton ML, Brown ACD (ed), Mosby Year Book, St. Louis, MO, 1991, pp 83–86.
17. Vetter TR. Acute airway obstruction due to arytenoiditis in a child with juvenile rheumatoid arthritis. Anesth Analg 1994; 79:1198–1200.
18. Mayou BJ. The anaesthetic management of patients with dystrophic epidermolysis bullosa. A review of 44 patients over a 10 year period. Anaesthesia 1993; 48:810–815.
19. Morris P, Wraith JE: Anaesthesia and mucopolysaccharidoses. A review of airway problems in children. Anaesthesia 1994; 49:1078–1084.
20. Laureano AN, Rybak LP. Severe otolaryngologic manifestations of arthrogryposis multiplex congenita. Ann Otol Rhinol Laryngol 1990; 99:94–97.
21. Morikawa S, Safar P, DeCarlo J. Influence of the head and jaw position upon upper airway patency. Anesthesiology 1961; 22:265.
22. Cote CJ, Goudsouzian NG, Liu LMP. Assessment of risk factors related to the acid aspiration syndrome in pediatric patients, gastric pH and residual volume. Anesthesiology 1982; 56:70–72.
23. Salem MR, Wong AY, Collins VJ. The pediatric patient with a full stomach. Anesthesiology 1973; 39:435.
24. Browne CH, Chew HER, Clarke E. The management of pulmonary aspiration syndrome. Intensive Care Med 1977; 3:257–266.
25. Nimmo WS. Aspiration of gastric contents. Br J Hosp Med 1985; 34:176–179.
26. Sellick BA. Cricoid pressure to control the regurgitation of stomach contents during induction of anaesthesia. Lancet 1961; 2:204.
27. Bertholid M, Read DH, Norma J. Preoxygenate–How long? Anaesthesia 1983; 38:96.
28. Gold MI, Muravchick S. Arterial oxygenation during laryngoscopy and intubation. Anesth Analg 1981; 60:316.
29. Drummond GB, Parik GR. Arterial oxygen saturation before intubation of the trachea. Br J Anaesth 1984; 56:987.
30. Cole WL, Stoelting VK. Blood gases during intubation following two types of oxygenation. Anesth Analg 1971; 50:68.
31. Wittenborg MH, Gyepes MT, Crocker D. Tracheal dynamics in infants with respiratory distress, stridor, and collapsing trachea. Radiology 1967; 88:653.
32. Keep PJ, Manford MLM. Endotracheal tube sizes for children. Anaesthesia 1974; 29:181.
33. Chodoff P, Helrich M. Factors affecting pediatric endotracheal tube size. A statistical analysis. Anesthesiology 1967; 28:779.
34. Dorsch JA, Dorsch SE. Understanding Anesthesia Equipment: Construction, Care and Complications. Williams & Wilkins, Baltimore, MD, 1980, pp 253–258.
35. Finholt DA, Henry DB, Raphaely RC. Factors affecting leak around tracheal tubes in children. Can Anaesth Soc J 1985; 32:326.
36. Finholt DA, Audenaert SM, Stirt JA, Marcella KL, Frierson HF, Suddarth LT, Raphaely RC. Endotracheal tube leak pressure and tracheal lumen size in swine. Anesth Analg 1986; 65:667.
37. Koka BV, Jeon IS, Andre JM, MacKay I, Smith RM. Postintubation croup in children. Anesth Analg 1977; 56:501.
38. Tochen ML. Orotracheal intubation in the newborn infant: a method for determining depth of tube insertion. J Pediatr 1979; 9;5:1050.
39. Morgan GAR, Steward DJ. Linear airway dimensions in children: including those with cleft palate. Can Anaesth Soc J 1982; 29:1.
40. Kuhns LR, Poznanski AK. Endotracheal tube position in the infant. J Pediatr 1971; 78:991.
41. Standards for basic intraoperative monitoring. ASA Newsletter 1990; 54:18.

42. Cote CJ, Liu MP, Szyfelbein SK, Firestone S, Goudsouzian NG, Welch JF, Daniels AL. Intraoperative events diagnosed by expired carbon dioxide monitoring in children. Can Anaesth Soc J 1986; 33:315–320.
43. Tinker JH, Dull DL, Caplan RA, Ward RJ, Cheney FW. Role of monitoring devices in prevention of anesthetic mishaps: a closed claims analysis. Anesthesiology 1989; 71:541–546.
44. Caplan RA, Posner KL, Ward RJ, Cheney FW. Adverse respiratory events in anesthesia: a closed claims analysis. Anesthesiology 1990; 72:828–833.
45. Pollard RJ, Lobata EB. Endotracheal tube location verified reliably by cuff palpation. Anesth Analg 1995; 81:135–138.
46. Bednarek FJ, Kuhns LR. Endotracheal tube placement in infants determined by suprasternal palliation: a new technique. Pediatrics 1974; 56:224.
47. Finholt DA, Henry DB, Raphaely RC. The "leak" test: A standard method for assessing tracheal tube fit in pediatric patients. Anesthesiology 1984; 61:A450.
48. Berry FA. Miscellaneous Potholes. IN Anesthetic Management of Difficult and Routine Pediatric Patients, 2nd Edition, Churchill Livingstone, New York, 1990, pp 411–432.
49. Deakers TW, Reynolds G, Stretton M, Newth CJ. Cuffed endotracheal tubes in pediatric intensive care. J Pediatr 1994; 125:57–62.
50. Stenquist O, Bagge U. Cuff pressure and microvascular occlusion in the tracheal mucosa. Acta Otolaryngol 1979; 88:451.
51. Blanc VF, Tremblay NA. The complications of tracheal intubation: A new complication with a review of the literature. Anesth Analg 1974; 53:202.
52. Corssen G, Gutierrez J, Reves JG. Ketamine in the anesthetic management of asthmatic patients. Anesth Analg 1972; 51:588.
53. White PF, Way WI, Trevor AJ. Ketamine- its pharmacology and therapeutic uses. Anesthesiology 1982; 56:119.
54. Soliman MG, Brinale GF, Kuski G. Response to hypercapnia under ketamine anaesthesia. Can Anaesth Soc J 1975; 22:486.
55. Silvay G. Ketamine. Mt. Sinai J Med 1983; 50:300.
56. Nugent SK, Laravuso R, Rogers MC. Pharmacology and use of muscle relaxants in infants and children. J Pediatr 1979; 94:481.
57. Standaert FG. Release of transmitter at the neuromuscular junction. Br J Anaesth 1982; 54:131.
58. Cook DR. Muscle relaxants in infants and children. Anesth Analg 1981; 60:335.
59. Korde M, Waud BE. Serum potassium concentrations after succinylcholine in patients with renal failure. Anesthesiology 1972; 36:142.
60. John DA, Tobey RE, Homer LD, Rice CL. Onset of succinylcholine-induced hyperkalemia following denervation. Anesthesiology 1976; 45:294–299.
61. Schaner PJ, Brown RL, Kirksey TD. Succinylcholine-induced hyperkalemia in burned patients. Anesthesiology 1969; 27:494.
62. Belin KP, Carleen CI. Cardiac arrest in the burned patient following succinylcholine administration. Anesthesiology 1966; 27:516.
63. Bisch AA, Mitchell GD, Playford GA. Changes in serum potassium response to succinylcholine following trauma. JAMA 1969; 210:490.
64. Kohlschutter B, Baur H, Roth F. Suxamethonium induced hyperkalemia in patients with severe intra-abdominal infections. Br J Anaesth 1976; 48:557.
65. Minton MD, Grosslight K, Stirt JA. Increases in intracranial pressure from succinylcholine: prevention by prior nondepolarizing blockade. Anesthesiology 1986; 65:165.
66. Libonati MM, Leahy JJ, Ellison N. The use of succinylcholine in open eye surgery. Anesthesiology 1985; 62:637.
67. Lerman J, Burrows FA, Creighton RE. The incidence of masseter muscle rigidity after succinylcholine in infants and children. Can J Anaesth 1994; 41:475–479.
68. Rosenberg H, Fletcher JE. Masseter muscle rigidity and malignant hyperthermia susceptibility. Anesth Analg 1986; 65:161–164.
69. Fox MH, Hunt PC. Prolonged neuromuscular block associated with mivacurium. Br J Anaesth 1995; 74:237–238.
70. Ali HH, Saverese JJ, Embree PB. Clinical pharmacology of mivacurium chloride infusion: comparison with vecuronium and atracurium. Br J Anaesth 1988; 61:541–546.
71. Goudsouzian NG, Alifimoff JK, Eberly C. Neuromuscular and cardiovascular effects of mivacurium in children. Anesthesiology 1989; 70:237–242.
72. Sarner JB, Brandom BW, Woelfel SK, Dong ML, Horn MC, Cook DR, McNulty BF, Foster VJ. Clinical pharmacology of mivacurium chloride (BW B1090U) in children during nitrous oxide-halothane and nitrous oxide-narcotic anesthesia. Anesth Analg 1989; 68:116–121.
73. Ali HH, Brull SJ, Witkowski T, Kopman A, Silverman DG, Goudsouzian NG, Bartkowski R, Weakley JN. Efficacy and safety of divided-dose administration of mivacurium for rapid tracheal intubation. Anesthesiology 1993; 79:A934.
74. Salem MR, Wong AY, Fizzotti GF. Efficacy of cricoid pressure in preventing aspiration of gastric contents in paediatric patients. Br J Anaesth 1972; 44:401.
75. Pittinger C, Adamson R. Antibiotic blockade of neuromuscular function. Ann Rev Pharmacol 1972; 12:169.
76. Ament R. A systemic approach to the difficult intubation. Anesthesiol Rev 1978; 5:12.
77. Black AE, Hatch DJ, Nauth-Misir N. Complications of nasotracheal intubation in neonates, infants and children: A review of 4 years' experience in a children's hospital. Br J Anaesth 1990; 65:461–467.
78. Gowder K, Bull MJ, Schreiner KL, Lemons JA, Gresham EL. Nasal deformities in neonates. Their occurrence in those treated with nasal continuous positive airway pressure and nasal endotracheal tubes. Am J Dis Child 1980; 134:954.
79. Lerman J, Kidkid AA. Lidocaine attenuates the intraoccular pressure response to rapid intubation in children. Can Anaesth Soc J 1985; 32:339.
80. Hamill JF, Bedford RF, Weaver DC, Colohan AR. Lidocaine before endotracheal intubation: intravenous or laryngotracheal? Anesthesiology 1981; 55:578.
81. Crysdale WS, Sendi K. Evolution in the management of acute epiglottitis: a 10 year experience with 242 children. Anesthesiol Clin 1988; 1:32–38.
82. Emmerson SGP, Richman B, Spahn T. Changing patterns of epiglottitis in children. Otolaryngol Head Neck Surg 1991; 104:287.
83. Losek JD, Dewitz-Zink BA, Meizer-Lange M, Havens PL. Epiglottitis: comparison of and symptoms in children less than 2 years old and older. Ann Emerg Med 1990; 58.
84. Walker P, Crysdale WS. Croup, epiglottitis, retropharyngeal abscess and bacterial tracheitis: evolving patterns of occurrence and care. Int Anesthesiology Clinics 1992; 30:57–70.
85. Valdepena HG, Wald ER, Rose E, Ungkamomot K, Casselbrant ML. Epiglottitis and Haemophilus influenza immunization: The Pittsburgh experience–a five year review. Pediatrics 1995; 96:424–427.
86. Berry FA. Anesthesia for the child with a difficult airway. IN Anesthetic Management of Difficult and Routine Pediatric Patients, 2nd edition. Churchill Livingstone, New York, 1990, pp 167–198.
87. Butt W, Shann F, Walder C. Acute epiglottitis: A different approach to management. Crit Care Med 1988; 16:43.
88. Barin ES, Stevenson IF, Donnelly GL. Pulmonary oedema following acute upper airway obstruction. Anaesth Intensive Care 1986; 14:54.
89. Sofer Bar-Ziv J, Scharf SM. Pulmonary edema following relief of upper airway obstruction. Chest 1984; 86:401.
90. Warner LO, Beach TP, Martino JD. Negative pressure pulmonary oedema secondary to airway obstruction in an intubated infant. Can J Anaesth 1988; 35:507.
91. Kanter RK, Watchko JF. Pulmonary edema associated with upper airway obstruction. Am J Dis Child 1984; 38:356.
92. Galvis AG, Stool SE, Bluestone CD. Pulmonary edema following relief of acute upper airway obstruction. Ann Otol 1980; 80:124.
93. Travis KW, Todres ID, Shannon DC. Pulmonary edema associated with croup and epiglottitis. Pediatrics 1977; 59:695.
94. Theodore J, Robin ED. Pathogenesis of neurogenic pulmonary edema. Lancet 1975; 2:749.
95. Robotham JL, Liffeld W, Holland L. Effects of respiration on cardiac performance. J Appl Physiol 1978; 44:703.
96. Criswell JC, Parr MJ, Nolan JP. Emergency airway management in patients with cervical spine injuries. Anaesthesia 1994; 49:900–903.
97. Harley EH, Collins MD. Neurologic sequelae secondary to atlantoaxial instability in Down syndrome. Implications in otolaryngologic surgery. Arch Otolaryngol Head Neck Surg 1994; 120:159–165.
98. Fan LL, Flynn JW. Laryngoscopy in neonates and infants: experience with the flexible fiberoptic bronchoscope 1981; 91:451.
99. Turner JS, Wilcox PA, Hayhurst MD. Potgieter PD. Fiberoptic bronchoscopy in the intensive care unit–a prospective study of 147 procedures in 107 patients. Crit Care Med 1994; 22:259–264.
100. Haenel JB, Moore FA, Moore EE, Read RA. Efficacy of selective intrabronchial air insufflation in acute lobar collapse. Am J Surg 1992; 164:501–505.
101. Snow, N, Lucas AE. Bronchoscopy in the critically ill surgical patient. Am Surg 1984; 50:441–445.

102. Watson CB. Fiberoptic bronchoscopy for anesthesia. Anesthesiol Rev 1982; 9:17.
103. Fan LL, Sparks LM, Fix EJ. Flexible fiberoptic endoscopy for airway problems in a pediatric intensive care unit. Chest 1988; 93:556.
104. Borland LM, Swan DM, Leff S. Difficult pediatric endotracheal intubation: a new approach to the retrograde technique. Anesthesiology 1981; 55:577.
105. Bourke D, Levesque PR. Modification of retrograde guide for endotracheal intubation. Anesth Analg 1974; 53:1013.
106. Perkin RM. Retrograde intubation difficulty in an 18-year old muscular dystrophy patient. Am J Emerg Med 1995; 13:100–101.
107. Jagtap SR, Malde AD, Pantvaidya SH. Anaesthetic considerations in a patient with Fraser syndrome. Anaesthesia 1995; 50:39–41.
108. Waters DJ. Guided blind endotracheal intubation for patients with deformities of the upper airway. Anaesthesia 1963; 18:158.
109. Borland LM, Swan DM, Leff S. Difficult pediatric endotracheal intubation: a new approach to the retrograde technique. Anesthesiology 1981; 55:577.
110. Attia RR, Battit GE, Murphy JD. Transtracheal ventilation. JAMA 1975; 234:1152.
111. Kress TD, Balasubramaniam S. Cricothyroidotomy. Ann Emerg Med 1982; 11:197.
112. Filston HC, Johnson DG, Crumrine RS. Infant tracheostomy: a new look with a solution to the difficult cannulation problem. Am J Dis Child 1978; 132:1172.
113. Simma B, Spehler D, Burger R, Uehlinger J, Ghelfi D, Dangel P, Hof E, Fanconi S. Tracheostomy in children. Eur J Pediatr 1994; 153:291–296.
114. Zeitouni A, Manoukian J. Tracheotomy in the first year of life. J Otolaryngol 1993; 22:431–434.
115. Crysdale WS, Feldman RI, Naito K. Tracheostomies: a 10-year experience in 319 children. Ann Otol Rhinol Laryngol 1988; 97:439.
116. Gaudet PT, Peerless A, Sasaki CT, Kirchner JA. Pediatric tracheostomy and associated complications. Laryngoscope 1978; 88:1633.
117. Okafor BC. Tracheostomy in the management of pediatric airway problems. Ear Nose Throat J 1983; 62:50.
118. Allen TH, Steven IM. Prolonged endotracheal intubation in infants and children. Br J Anaesth 1965; 37:566.
119. Carter P, Benjamin B. Ten-year review of pediatric tracheotomy. Ann Otol Rhinol Laryngol 1983; 92:398.
120. Gilmore BB, Michelson SA. Pediatric tracheotomy–controversies in management. Otolaryngol Clin No Am 1986; 19:141.
121. Ameye F, Mattelin W, Ingels K, Bradwell R. Bilateral pneumothorax after emergency tracheotomy: two case reports and a review of the literature. J Laryngol Otol 1994; 108:69–70.
122. Tepas JJ III, Heroy JH, Shermeta DW, Haller JA. Tracheostomy in neonates and small infants: problems and pitfalls. Surgery 1981; 89:635.
123. Friedberg J, Morrison MD. Paediatric tracheotomy. Can J Otolaryngol 1974; 32:147.
124. Gilmore BB, Mickelson SA. Pediatric tracheotomy–controversies in management. Otolaryngol Clin No Am 1986; 19:141.
125. Marshall TA, Deeder R, Pai S, Berkowitz GP, Austin TL. Physiologic changes associated with endotracheal intubation in preterm infants. Crit Care Med 1984; 12:501.
126. Blanc VF, Tremblay NA. The complications of tracheal intubation: a new complication with a review of the literature. Anesth Analg 1974; 53:202.
127. Dumas C, Patriquin HB, Pare L, Tetreault L. Latrogenic lesions of the upper airway in the newborn. J Can Assoc Radiol 1983; 34:3.
128. Liu AT, Tamura Y, Koobs DH. The pathology of laryngotracheal complications. Arch Otolaryngol 1961; 74:1052.
129. Goitein KJ, Rein AJ-JT, Gornstein A. Incidence of aspiration in endotracheally intubated infants and children. Crit Care Med 1984; 12:19.
130. Mattila MAK, Suntarinen T, Sulamaa M. Prolonged endotracheal intubation or tracheostomy in infants and children. J Pediatr Surg 1969; 4:674.
131. Parkin JL, Stevens MH, Jung AL. Acquired and congenital subglottic stenosis in the infant. Ann Otol 1976; 85:673.
132. Strome M, Ferguson CF. Multiple post-intubation complications. Ann Otol 1974; 83:432.
133. Suprance JS, Reilly JS, Doyle WJ, Bluestone CD, Hubbard J. Acquired subglottic stenosis following prolonged endotracheal intubation. Arch Otolaryngol 1982; 108:727.
134. Palasti S, Respler DS, Fieldman RJ, Levitt J. Anterior cricoid split for subglottic stenosis: experience at the Children's Hospital of New Jersey. Laryngoscope 1992; 102:997–1000.
135. Tavin E, Singer L, Bassila M. Problems in postoperative management after anterior cricoid split. Arch Otolaryngol Head Neck Surg 1994; 120:823–826.
136. Balakrishnan A. The cricoid split: an alternative to paediatric tracheostomy. Ann Acad Med Singapore 1991; 20:700–703.
137. Paegle RD, Syres SM, Davis S. Rapid tracheal injury by cuffed airways and healing with loss of ciliated epithelium. Arch Surg 1973; 106:31.
138. Kemper KJ, Benson MS, Bishop MJ. Predictors of post-extubation stridor in pediatric trauma patients. Crit Care Med 1991; 19:352.
139. Jordan WS, Graves CL, Elwyn RA. New therapy for post-intubation laryngeal edema and tracheitis in children. JAMA 1970; 212:585.
140. Postma DS, Prazma J, Woods CL, Sidman J, Pillsbury HC. Use of steroids and a long-acting vasoconstrictor in the treatment of post-intubation croup. A ferret model. Arch Otolaryngol Head Neck Surg 1987; 113:844–849.
141. Tellez DW, Galvis AG, Storgion SA, Amer HN, Hoseyni M, Deakers TW. Dexamethasone in the prevention of post-extubation stridor in children. J Pediatr 1991; 118:289–294.
142. Skrinskas GJ, Hyland RH, Hutcheon MA. Using helium-oxygen mixtures in the management of acute upper airway obstruction. Can Med Assoc J 1983; 128:555.

Transportation of Critically Ill Children 3

Karin A. McCloskey
Richard Orr

INTRODUCTION

The sophisticated medical care available in pediatric intensive care units (PICUs) has lowered morbidity and mortality rates for many devastating illnesses and injuries[1]. The regionalization of PICUs and the fact that most pediatric illnesses and injuries do not occur near a tertiary care center means that critically ill or injured children frequently travel long distances to reach definitive care. However, appropriate initial stabilization followed by appropriate mechanism of transport should result in decreased rates of morbidity and mortality.

This chapter reviews the development of pediatric transportation both between and within hospitals and discusses guidelines necessary for the safe and effective transportation of critically ill children. The underlying principle is that intensive care can be delivered to the patient at the referring institution via the transport team and continued en route to the PICU.

HISTORY

The concept of emergency transport of the ill or injured is not new. An early example comes from St. Luke 10:33 to 4, "A certain Samaritan . . . went to him and bound up his wounds, pouring oil and wine, and set him on his own beast, and brought him to an inn, and took care of him." Since that time we have witnessed dramatic changes in health care delivery. Military victims began to receive better care during the 18th century when, in the Battle of Blenheim, the Duke of Marlborough took care that the wounded were transported to the hospital by "all available wagons from the surrounding countryside"[2,3]. In the 18th century, regionalization of care appeared in London as hospitals were built in locations designed to reduce the travel time required to obtain assistance.

Air transportation was introduced in 1870 during the Franco-Prussian War when 160 casualties were evacuated from the siege of Paris by hot-air balloons just before Bismarck's defeat of Napoleon's armies[2,3]. Air transport became increasingly sophisticated during the numerous military conflicts of the twentieth century, with the greatest impact coming from the rapid evacuation of the injured from the battlefield to mobile surgical hospitals by helicopter during the wars in Southeast Asia.

This experience benefitted civilian transport, leading to the development in the late 1960s and early 1970s of transport systems for critical victims of multiple trauma and for neonates. Critical care centers were regionalized to manage the complex illnesses of many of these patients more easily. Trauma and neonatal services were asked to transport critically ill pediatric patients to pediatric tertiary care centers. From these, a large network of pediatric emergency transport systems has developed throughout the country.

The organization of emergency medical services has improved the development of transport systems as well. The National Highway Safety Act of 1966 led to better trained emergency medical technicians (EMTs) and paramedics[4]. Technological improvements have made it possible to extend intensive care to patients before they reach the intensive care units (ICUs). Mobile monitors, ventilators, automated blood pressure devices, oximeters, end tidal CO_2 monitors, portable blood gas analysis, and dipstick-type chemical analysis have enabled the extension of sophisticated intensive care to the field[5–7].

Regional neonatal centers have been developed to treat the large numbers of ill infants born in outlying hospitals. The transport systems that emerged as a result of regionalization have demonstrated that acutely ill infants can be evacuated by helicopters, fixed-wing aircraft, and ambulances with great safety, as long as appropriate care is given[8].

Smaller community hospitals may lack funding and personnel to care adequately for critically ill children because the number of pediatric patients is generally lower than that of adult patients, and therefore, pediatric care is more expensive. As pediatric intensive care[1] and pediatric surgical capabilities improved in the major medical centers, young patients were moved to more sophisticated units.

The primary goal for an interhospital transport program is to provide excellent medical care during transit that, as much as is possible, resembles the care given in the receiving institution. Thus, intensive care is extended via the transport team and via communication with the referring hospital (where comprehensive intensive care is not available) and is continued en route to the receiving institution.

TRANSPORT GUIDELINES

In November, 1986 the American Academy of Pediatrics (AAP) Committee on Hospital Care published Guidelines for Air and Ground Transportation of Pediatric Patients[9]. In 1993 the AAP Task Force on Interhospital Transport updated the Guidelines as a 150 page manual to be promoted and distributed more widely than the original article[10].

The Task Force included representatives from the fields of Pediatric Critical Care, Emergency Medicine, Surgery and Anesthesiology as well as Perinatology and the major all-age transport organization, the Association for Air Medical Services (AAMS). The manual addressed the organization of a pediatric interfacility transport service; communications and the dispatch center; administrative issues, transport system personnel; team composition, selection and training; quality improvement; safety; vehicles; equipment and medications; outreach education; the transport data base; and air medical physiology. The manual's mission statement indicated that the AAP, as advocates for children, provided guidelines and education for pediatricians and other professionals who make decisions about the interhospital transport of children.

The Guidelines manual was specifically written to all providers of pediatric critical care transport, not just the members of teams which only transport children. The premise for this focus was that anyone agreeing to take responsibility for the life of a child should meet certain basic criteria which should not be set at different levels for different types of teams. It is recommended that if a system does not transport enough children to support specific pediatric training and equipment, then it should work in conjunction with other local systems to regionalize pediatric transports.

WHO IS TRANSPORTED?

Not all patients undergoing interhospital transfer need a critical care transport team. The severity of illness, the capabilities of the referring hospital, and the goals and training of the transport team will all affect the decision to use a specialized team. Initially, teams transporting patients of all ages cared primarily for trauma victims and adult patients with cardiac problems[14,15]. Neonatal teams care primarily for patients with respiratory distress, prematurity, and congenital heart disease. Several published reports describe the range of illnesses in patients transported by individual systems[2,11–20]. Thus, teams transporting pediatric patients must care for a wider range of illnesses **(Table 3.1)**. Differences in the types of illnesses handled between

Table 3.1. Diagnostic Categories of Transported Children[a]

Diagnostic Category	*Black (9)*	*McCloskey (10)*	*Dobrin (11)*	*Goldstein (16)*	*Britten (17)*	*Smith (18)*	*Frankel (12)*	*Avg %*
Neurologic	22	11		12	12	52	49	26
Respiratory	19	25	30	36	20	28	30	27
Cardiovascular	5	12	7	12	2	12	11	9
Trauma–head	14		46	6	17	21		
–multiple	5	6		6	26			11
Other	28	46	17	28	23	8	10	22
Total Number	747	341	125	122	121	115		

[a] *Percent of total transports.*

systems are related to geography, the capabilities of the referral hospital, the pediatric training and experience of the transport team and vehicle availability. For example, teams that use rotorcraft are more likely to transport a high percentage of trauma patients than are teams that travel only by ground. Teams which transport patients of all ages may or may not offer the same level of pediatric critical care as teams which are dedicated only to transporting children.

TRIAGE

Because transport team resources are limited, and because not every patient transferred between hospitals needs the sophisticated services of a critical care transport team, the decision to use one must be made prudently. Judging the patient's status over the telephone, especially when the referring physician may have little experience with critically ill children is difficult. The experienced transport physician often finds his or her initial perception of the patient's status different from that encountered upon assumption of patient care[21].

Goals for using a transport team may differ among hospitals. In some cases, the team is designed to transport all incoming patients, whereas in others, only critically ill patients are transported. Triage decisions will depend on each system's philosophy, as well as on geographical considerations, weather and vehicle and team availability. Teams that transport most incoming patients (e.g., neonatal teams) have less difficult triage decisions to make than do teams that strive to transport only patients with a high potential for instability. For this reason, discussion will focus on triage of transport resources to only the sickest patients.

Widely used objective triage systems have been shown to be ineffective for pediatric critical care transport. A single numerical scoring index is unlikely to be developed for all transport systems because of differences in geography, vehicle use, the capabilities of the referring hospital, and the types of illness. Research to devise triage tools for transport allocation has been limited in the past but has become an important issue in transport medicine.

Attempts have been made, with limited success, to apply established severity of illness indices to transport triage[13,22–24]. Such indices are sometimes used because their components are easily obtained or seem "reasonable" for determining severity of illness. Attempts to validate the function of these systems have emphasized primarily their ability to predict only mortality, not morbidity[25,26]. Severity-of-illness indices that have been validated for determination of in-hospital mortality risk must be used cautiously in transport settings. Many of the physiologic variables that these indices require for scoring may be unavailable at the time of transport or may have been normalized by medical intervention (e.g., intubation, mechanical ventilation), and thus the degree of physiologic instability and need for continuing intensive therapy may be underestimated. However, other variables that indicate a greater mortality risk (e.g., elevated serum bilirubin) may not necessarily indicate the need for a highly skilled transport team. The use of the Pediatric Risk of Mortality (PRISM) score[27] is a primary example. A patient with a treatable respiratory illness and a subsequently low PRISM score may have a low risk of mortality when properly treated in a PICU, but a high risk of morbidity or mortality if not appropriately treated during transport. For example, a five-year-old patient brought to a local emergency department with cyanosis, gasping respirations (rate 60), and a heart rate of 150 will generate a PRISM score of only 1, or perhaps 4 (both a calculated risk of mortality of $<5\%$), provided blood gas measurements are available during the transport process. In contrast, a five-year-old patient with end-stage liver disease who is being transported for a transplant evaluation might have a PRISM score as high as 23 (risk of mortality, 45%) and can be brought safely to the hospital from home by the parents. Risk of morbidity should be the focus during transport[28–30].

Other scores which have been used for transport triage include the Physiologic Stability Index (PSI)[31], Glasgow Coma Scale (GCS), Modified Injury Severity Score (MISS)[32], Therapeutic Intervention Scoring System[33] and Pediatric Trauma Score (PTS)[34]. The PSI requires many components that are not available in the pretransport setting and was developed and validated only for a PICU setting. The GCS, MISS, and PTS may prove useful for certain categories of patients, such as those with multiple trauma or neurologic disease.

Orr et al. in a study of 2288 transported patients have defined four simple variables, available prior to transport, which predict in hospital mortality. The variables, abnormal blood pressure, abnormal respiratory rate altered level of consciousness and oxygen requirement also predicted need for major interventions by the transport team. Probabilities of mortality and need for interventions can be developed by examining the four variables. This data is the first step toward developing an objective transport specific, triage scoring tool[35].

When developing triage tools for pediatric transport, several questions need to be answered[36]. First, does every patient transferred between hospitals need a critical care transport team? If not, is it possible to determine in advance when a critical care transport team will be needed? If so, how can that determination be made?

Intuitively, many transferred patients do not need a transport team. Kanter and Tompkins[23], in a study of 117 patients, suggested that low-risk patients as determined by a PRISM score of 10 or less, could be safely transported by the referring hospital personnel with little deterioration en route. However, Orr et al.[24] showed that a low pretransport PRISM score often is an insensitive indicator of physiologic instability and that some patients with low scores are so physiologically unstable as to require major life-saving intervention. They concluded that a PRISM score is neither useful nor appropriate for assessing pretransport severity of illness. One must be careful in interpreting data implying a low risk. In most transports, there is little deterioration if the patient is well stabilized before departure. The transport team is needed to provide intervention if needed. For example, a 5% rate of dislodged endotracheal tubes may appear to present a "low risk." However, if available personnel are not experienced in pediatric intubation, a 5% rate failure would be unacceptable.

Few studies have defined objective criteria that predict need for a transport team. McCloskey et al.[37] have reported an increased probability of needing 1) a major procedure, 2) major pharmacologic intervention, or 3) on subjective retrospection a physician during transport of patients who, at the time of the initial call, are intubated or are younger than one year with unstable vital signs.

McCloskey and Johnston[21] in a study of 167 patients, showed that it was possible to predict accurately the need for a physician (and, in that particular system, the need for a team) 72% of the time. Need was overestimated 25% of the time and underestimated 3% of the time.

Several transport triage systems are in current use, until one or more validated objective scores can be developed. Elements of such a scoring system might include 1) the judgment of any physician, including house officers, who accepts patients in transfer; 2) the judgment of an experienced attending physician who knows the capabilities of the area's referring hospitals and physicians; 3) a classification system of patient status; 4) use of a "common sense" approach; and 5) use of existing objective data on certain clinical variables.

The first system is not desirable, as experience and consistency may be lacking. The second may be useful if the information given over the telephone is complete and accurate.

The third system, status classification, evaluates patients according to severity of illness and level of intervention [11,38]. Examples of clinical and interventional variables used to determine patient status using a range of severity from category 1 (normal) to 5 (critical) are as follows. Oxygen requirement: a patient requiring no supplemental oxygen (category 1); one requiring a low level of oxygen (category 2); one requiring a high level of oxygen by mask (category 3); one requiring ventilatory support with a high level of oxygen (category 4); and one meeting category 4 criteria but with a low arterial oxygen saturation (category 5). Respiratory distress: a patient with no respiratory distress (category 1); one with tachypnea (category 2); one with respiratory distress as indicated by grunting, flaring, and retractions (category 3); one with apnea or respiratory failure (category 4); and one with respiratory arrest (category 5). Neurologic evaluation may range from normal (category 1) to a GCS of 3 (category 5). Cardiovascular function may range from normal (category 1) to asystolic (category 5). Medications may range from none (category 1) to antibiotics (category 2) to aerosolized bronchodilators (category 3), to IV anticonvulsants (category 4) to multiple, complex medications, including vasopressors and neuromuscular blockade (category 5). Requirement of a transport team, as well as team composition (use of a respiratory therapist, physician, second nurse, or other specialists) is then determined based on the patient's highest category.

The fourth system, the "common sense" approach determines the need for a special transport team according to whether the patient 1) will be admitted to an ICU, (based on the principle that if that level of care is required on arrival at the tertiary care center, it will be required en route); 2) has potential for significant respiratory, cardiovascular, or neurologic deterioration during transport (e.g., a patient with bronchospasm or croup who is too sick to be cared for in a community hospital); 3) has multiple trauma and has not yet been stabilized in a trauma center; or 4) required resuscitation from a life-threatening event which could reoccur (e.g., seizure with apnea, shock, cardiopulmonary arrest). Children meeting these criteria should always be accompanied by a specialized transport team, because several studies have shown that the routine training received by ambulance crews is often inadequate for pediatric patients [15,39–41].

Multiple simultaneous transport requests can present another triage problem. Some systems are designed to handle only one transport at a time, others more than one, but all teams will eventually reach a limit. How a transport system will manage multiple requests should be planned in advance. In general, the sickest patients should take priority when there are more requests than available teams. However, distance and knowledge of the referring institution may be taken into consideration. If the sickest patient is in a hospital that is capable of managing the condition, while another patient is in a hospital with minimal pediatric resources, the second patient should take priority. Similarly, if one patient is three hours away while the other is 20 minutes away, transporting the second patient first may be most efficient. Determination of which patient is "sickest" can be difficult if one must rely on assessments from physicians who may not be experienced in the care of children. If transport is not available within the usual mobilization time and another qualified transport team is available in the same region, the referring hospital should be offered the opportunity to use the alternative.

If transport is deferred, because of the lack of an available team or because of another factor such as weather, the receiving hospital must maintain communication and recommend appropriate care. An estimated time of the team's arrival should be provided and updated as appropriate. Telephone calls should be made periodically to check on the patient's clinical status and offer additional advice as needed.

INITIAL COMMUNICATION, ASSESSMENT, AND STABILIZATION

The referring institution has the initial role of immediate resuscitation and care, with telephone assistance from the PICU consultant staff as needed. On arrival, the transport team will assume care from the referring physicians, reassess the patient, stabilize the patient as needed for the transport environment and continue care until it is assumed by the receiving physician. The success of the transfer of the patient will depend on the adequacy of the communication between hospitals, the initial and subsequent assessments, stabilization, and preparation of the patient for transport. Advance preparation is vital to the success of any pediatric transport.

The referring hospital should prepare for transport before a critically ill or injured child actually arrives for care. The Joint Commission on Accreditation of Healthcare Organizations (JCAHO) mandates that a hospital agreeing to accept all patients be prepared to care for those patients until appropriate transport can be provided[42]. To achieve this, the hospital can take several steps to prepare for transport and to appropriately manage the patient before a team arrives. As part of its community outreach program, the tertiary care center can assist referring hospitals to prepare in advance for transport.

Transport preparation should start with a list of receiving hospitals and their telephone numbers attached to or near the emergency department telephone. If transport systems from other than those hospitals might be used, numbers for those transport teams should be included on the list. Pediatric resuscitation cards and weight-for-age charts should be kept in a designated location or posted nearby. A pediatric equipment pack or pediatric resuscitation room should be stocked and easily accessible at all times. Advance preparation can also include pediatric resuscitation courses such as the Pediatric Advanced Life Support, Neonatal Resuscitation Program, or Advanced Pediatric Life Support for emergency department personnel. In addition, if administrative details of transfer may present a problem (e.g., in transfers of unfunded patients or those crossing state lines), protocols or contracts should be developed in advance to expedite the referral process.

The referring physician is responsible for direct verbal contact with the receiving physician. The referring hospital is responsible for providing reasonable and accurate information about the patient's clinical status, including all vital signs, mental status, an assessment of perfusion, respiratory status, and details of significant injuries **(Table 3.2).** Information on interventions and response, laboratory and x-ray data, and current management (ventilation, medications, etc.) should also be provided. Advice received should be documented. If suggested interventions are impossible or are considered unnecessary, the reasons should be documented.

The receiving hospital provides medical advice according to the information received, which can be difficult without a hands-on assessment. At the time of the initial call, a brief history is obtained, advice on basic stabilization is offered, if needed, and then the transport team is dispatched before more detailed information and recommendations are exchanged. The referring hospital can be called back when additional communication is necessary.

Table 3.2. Pretransport Information

Referring physician, hospital, city, telephone number
Patient name, age, weight
Prehospital history
Clinical status at presentation
Interventions performed
Current medications
Current problem list
Current clinical status

When providing medical advice, the reasonable capabilities of the referring hospital should be kept in mind. The basics of resuscitation (airway, breathing, circulation) should be emphasized, as they are often overlooked in the panic that may ensue when a critically ill child arrives at a facility that cares primarily for adults. When suggesting medications, it is helpful to include doses as a matter of routine. If intravenous access is difficult, intraosseous infusion can be suggested if appropriate. Even if intraosseous infusion has never been performed, it can be easily described by telephone and rapidly implemented.

When giving advice on stabilization, prior measures taken by the referring hospital should never be criticized. It must be assumed that the referring staff has acted to the best of its abilities and in the best interest of the patient. Criticism will demoralize and, perhaps, lead to inappropriate transport decisions for future patients. If management by the referring hospital has to be altered, a diplomatic attitude ('there is more than one right way to do things, and we've found that this way works well for us' or 'our transport protocols require that we do this') is most helpful.

The referring hospital should be informed in advance of paperwork the team will need. This includes copies of records and x-rays, consent to transport, and any administrative contracts that have been negotiated. When the transport team has been dispatched, the referring hospital should be apprised of the estimated time of arrival. The patient's condition can be reevaluated during this call, and can be adjusted accordingly. Again, all communications between the hospitals should be well documented, especially with regard to the time of call, the information received, and the advice given.

Preparations made by the referring hospital can expedite turnaround time for the transport team **(Table 3.2).** Records and x-rays can be copied in advance, and written consent for transport can be obtained from the parents. Consent should include both the name of the receiving hospital and the mode of transport. Some pediatric teams ask that the parents remain at the referring hospital until the team arrives. The team can then establish a relationship with the parents and obtain additional information that may be needed upon arrival at the receiving hospital. This is especially important if the parents will arrive at the receiving hospital significantly later than the transport team and there is a need for an immediate surgical procedure. The referring hospital can also obtain any blood products that might be needed during the transport and provide a telephone number to call for any laboratory data pending at the time of transfer. If appropriate, the cervical spine and any fractures can be stabilized for transport.

Vascular access and endotracheal tubes should also be secured for transport. The movement of the transport environment makes it difficult to maintain these items that otherwise may be secure in the stable environment of the emergency department or the ICU. The transport environment necessitates use of plastic IV catheters rather than metal or butterfly type ones. The team will have to be able to assure function of any lines prior to transport. Transport team members should be capable of replacing an intravenous catheter or a dislodged endotracheal tube, although most teams would prefer not to have to do so in a moving vehicle. All of these preparations can assist in shortening the time the transport team must spend at the scene.

Before departure the team should also consider what medical interventions may be needed during transport. For example, if the patient is intubated and requires neuromuscular blockade, the team should have the following items ready: a bag-valve-mask, an endotracheal tube and laryngoscope of appropriate size, suction apparatus equipment for the initial treatment of a pneumothorax, and additional doses of sedatives and neuromuscular blockers.

En route to the referring hospital, the transport team can make preparations that will also minimize the time needed for stabilization upon arrival. Doses of medications can be calculated and intravenous infusions that may be needed can be prepared. A plan of action must be devised in case the patient's condition deteriorates. Certain parts of the transport paperwork can be completed. A team that arrives at the referring hospital prepared with a plan of action will be efficient and appear professional.

Upon arrival, stabilization efforts by the transport team should be efficient but thorough. Appropriate attention should be given to stabilizing vital signs and neurologic status, assuring adequate oxygenation and ventilation, administering necessary medications, securing of intravenous catheters and endotracheal tubes, and communicating a complete report to the receiving unit. Again, while these actions should be performed efficiently, quality of stabilization to improve or preserve the patient's status during transport is much more important than speed of departure from the referring hospital.

ADMINISTRATIVE DESIGN

Responsibilities of the Pediatric Tertiary Care Facility

The chief responsibility of the pediatric tertiary care facility is to provide access to care within the referral community. Commitment to a formal structure is essential to the success of a pediatric transport system. The essential components that ensure the success of a transport program include the administrative staff, medical control, well-trained transport team members, the communications center, reliable equipment, and safety.

Administrative Staff

The hospital administrative staff should play a key role in the organization of a transport system and its ongoing function. There are substantial costs involved in setting up a transport system, including equipment, vehicles, personnel, public relations and operating expenses. Well-organized transport systems are often effective marketing tools, and demands on them often may exceed the capacity to respond to the referral community during the start-up phase. Consequently, careful planning should include continued upgrading to meet these demands in order to avoid losing referrals.

Medical Director

The Medical Director acts in conjunction with an administrative Program Director (in fairly small programs, the Medical and Program Directors may be the same individual) and a nursing Transport Coordinator to oversee the development and function of the entire transport system. According to the 1993 AAP Transport Guidelines[10], the Medical Director for pediatric transports should be a specialist in pediatric emergency medicine, pediatric critical care, or neonatology. Teams transporting children with multiple trauma or surgical emergencies need a Medical Director input from a pediatric surgeon. Systems which transport both adult and children need a Pediatric Medical Director to act in conjunction with an adult specialist, in order to develop appropriate training, equipment and triage and management protocols for pediatric patients. The Medical Director should be clearly designated an appropriate physician for alternate coverage. The Pediatric Medical Director may act at times as the Pediatric Medical Control Physician.

Medical Control

Medical control is essential to maintain the organization of a transport system and ensure optimal pediatric management in the field. The American Academy of Pediatrics (AAP) recommends that the medical director be a physician in either pediatric emergency medicine or critical care medicine[9,10]. This physician must be experienced in fielding transport calls and in suggesting treatment for the patient until the arrival of the transport team. The medical control physician must also have the authority to accept transferred patients without further consultation (after being informed of the availability of resources such as beds and team members). He or she functions as a consultant to the transport team, provides training programs for team members, establishes patient care protocols, assures quality of care, and serves as a liaison to the referral community through personal contact and outreach education. The medical control physician should provide referring physicians and hospitals with follow-up on the patient's diagno-

Table 3.3. Equipment and Supplies for Transport

Respiratory	Pressure
Oxygen tanks (twice amount expected for transport)	Arterial, venous
Oxygen hood	Transducers
Bag-valve-masks for age	Defibrillator
Pressure manometer	Pediatric Paddles
Intubation equipment	Pulse oximeter
Endotracheal Tubes	Stethoscope
(uncuffed, 2.0–6.5)	Blood pressure cuffs (all sizes)
(cuffed, 5.0–8.0)	**Procedure packs**
Oral airways	Cutdown kit
Laryngoscopes (assorted blades, extra bulbs)	Thoracostomy kit
Magill forceps	Venous catheterization kits
Ventilator (battery- or pressure-driven with PEEP[a] capability and apnea/disconnect alarms)	**Fluids, infusion devices**
Nebulizer for aerosols	5% dextrose in water, 0.9% saline, 5% albumin, Lactated Ringer's solution
Suction equipment	Infusion pumps
Monitors (with spare battery)	Intravenous catheters and accessories
ECG	**Miscellaneous**
Respiratory	Skin preparation solutions
Temperature	
Tape	
Electrodes	

[a] *Positive end-expiratory pressure.*

sis, therapy, and clinical condition at appropriate intervals, or facilitate this communication between the referring and receiving physicians. Ideally, a transport team coordinator (either a nurse or a paramedic) should assist the medical control physician with transport team functions. If possible, either the medical control physician or the coordinator should participate in patient transport to maintain perspective.

Communications Center

The success of the transfer will depend on the adequacy of the communication between hospitals, the initial and subsequent assessments, and the stabilization and preparation of the patient for transport. An easily accessible emergency medical communications system is required so that contact between the referring health care team, the transport coordinator, the medical transport team, and the surface or air ambulance carrier can be maintained. The communications system should be staffed round-the-clock by full-time dispatchers who are trained in handling emergency calls and who have no other distracting duties that would delay a response. These individuals should always know if the hospital and ICU have beds available and if the transport team is available. Information received and advice given are documented on a standardized form, which serves as both a reminder of all necessary questions and a legal record. Telephone calls that come through the hospital's general operators, the emergency department, or a unit clerk within a patient care area, have the potential to be misdirected. Such calls should be 1) avoided, by provision of a transport "hot line" and 2) transferred immediately to that hot line if received elsewhere. The line should record calls on tape for later review and documentation. A critical element in communications is locating and informing the transport personnel when a request has been received. Dispatchers should be trained to arrange all aspects of the transport so that both the referring physician and the team can attend to mobilization and patient care rather than waste valuable time on the telephone. Additional components of the communication system should include a reference source for regional hospital and emergency medical systems information, transport protocol documents, and a means of recording all transport transactions. The reference source should have regional information on community hospitals that is pertinent to medical transport, on ambulance carriers, airports, ground distances, and transport times between facilities according to type of carrier. Equipment for direct contact with the communications center should be available in every transport vehicle.

Equipment

Pediatric patients are transferred for a wide range of illnesses and injuries therefore, a comprehensive variety of equipment and medications should be included on all transports. Equipment taken on transport should be complete and adequate to provide continuing intensive care throughout the trip **(Tables 3.3** and **3.4).** The operation and maintenance of the equipment should be the sole responsibility of the transport team. Transport isolettes should be capable of providing a neutral thermal environment for infants at all times. Portable monitoring equipment should be capable of measuring heart rate (ECG display), respiratory rate, blood pressure (at least one channel for intravascular monitoring), arterial saturation (pulse oximetry), temperature, and for premature infants, transcutaneous tissue oxygenation. End tidal CO_2 monitoring is rapidly becoming standard. Transport monitoring equipment should be battery-powered and capable of functioning independently of the

Table 3.4. Medications for Transport

Resuscitation	**Pulmonary**
Epinephrine	Aminophylline
Sodium bicarbonate	Terbutaline/albuterol
Atropine	Racemic epinephrine
Glucose	Methylprednisolone
Naloxone	**Sedation/Analgesia**
Lidocaine/bretylium	Morphine
Isoproterenol	Midazolam
Cardiovascular	Fentanyl
Digoxin	**Antibiotics**
Dopamine/dobutamine	Ampicillin/nafcillin
Prostaglandin E_1	Cefotaxime/ceftriaxone
Furosemide	Aminoglycoside
Nitroprusside	Clindamycin
Hydralazine	**Muscle Relaxants**
Phenylephrine	Pancuronium/vecuronium
Central Nervous System	Succinylcholine
Phenobarbital	**Miscellaneous**
Phenytoin	Potassium chloride
Diazepam/lorazepam	Calcium chloride
Thiopental	Heparin
Dexamethasone	Charcoal
Insulin	

electrical supply of both surface and air carriers for at least twice the anticipated transport time. It should also be light weight and relatively free of movement artifact.

Respiratory problems are common in transported pediatric patients. Oxygen requirements should be calculated for each patient transported, and the on-board supply should be at least twice the amount needed for the expected duration of the trip (in case of delays, patient deterioration, or equipment malfunction). An oxygen analyzer should be available to assess the fraction of inspired oxygen (FiO_2). Particularly in preterm infants, compressed air may be mixed with oxygen to provide a precise range of FiO_2 (0.21 to 1.00). For full-term infants and children, oxygen alone is appropriate. Transport teams should also be equipped to provide mechanical ventilation within appropriate parameters for the individual patient (e.g., pressure, volume, high frequency). If possible, ventilators should be electrically operated to conserve gas supply. If a transport vehicle cannot supply enough power, a pressure-driven (fluidic) ventilator can be used. The ventilator should allow a variety of ventilatory techniques, including positive end-expiratory pressure (PEEP) and continuous positive airway pressure, with appropriate alarms for pressures, volumes, and flows. If the equipment requires a 50 psi oxygen source, then it must connect directly to the ambulance oxygen supply with standard connecting devices. If a 50 psi oxygen source is not needed, then the ambulance must have a standard oxygen flow meter capable of delivering up to 15 liters per minute.

Transport equipment must be able to withstand the stress of the transport environment and be easily loaded into transport vehicles by two individuals. It must also be secured to maintain physical and functional integrity when subjected to an impact deceleration, and it must meet all applicable federal and state regulations, including Federal Aviation Regulation (FAR) requirements for air-medical transports. It must be compatible for use with all types of ambulance oxygen and power supplies (surface vehicle, fixed-wing aircraft, and rotorcraft). The transport team should have information concerning the ability of the medical supplies and equipment to function throughout the entire range of temperatures and barometric pressures anticipated during transport. Portable, compartmentalized equipment packs must be designed for easy access. Most important, the transport team should be self-sufficient and not dependent on the referring hospital for supplies. All equipment should be routinely checked and maintained after transport by a team member dedicated to that task.

Safety

Safety should be a high priority in any transport program. First, the referring and receiving physicians must agree that the patient has been sufficiently stabilized for transport, and that it is safe to transport the patient under the circumstances. Second, the safety of the health care worker must also be considered. Emergency vehicle operation involves substantial risks, not only to the crew and patient, but also to others in its vicinity. The medical director ultimately is responsible for maintaining a safe environment for crew members and the patient. Transport team members should be required to have specific training in transport medicine, including air-medical and surface transport safety and orientation, communication skills, choice of appropriate attire, survival techniques, and fitness and health.

Air-Medical Transport

Training, teamwork, and coordination are essential for safe air-medical transport. Air-medical crew members can contribute significantly to the safe performance of the mission. In systems with flexible team composition, pediatric specialty team members who accompany a full-time air-medical crew must conform to the safety standards as outlined by the air-medical profession to the extent that these standards allow them to perform their specialty. Medical Directors of specialty teams should have a specific understanding of the vendors and aircraft used for air-medical missions. They should also be certain that all air-medical equipment is certified for air taxi use and that pilots are airline transport rated. Some services that advertise as air taxi or air ambulance operators are not qualified.

Weather is the leading cause of air-medical accidents, followed by engine malfunction, collision with an obstacle, and loss of control [43]. Cloud ceiling or visibility limitations, ambient temperature, icing conditions, and wind are all part of the weather equation and may prohibit safe aircraft operation. It is important that individuals in the critical care continuum (emergency medical services, emergency department physicians, intensivists, and surgeons) respect the decisions made by pilots regarding flight conditions. They should never use the patient's condition to seek an alternate air-medical service or try to influence the pilot's decision to fly. Air-medical crew members and specialty team members should conduct themselves as safety role models in the referral community.

While some teams (all-age or pediatric only) use the same team composition for all transports, many will vary crew configuration by using "specialty teams" for pediatric or neonatal patients. The individuals who comprise the "specialty" component of the team may not be fulltime transport team members and thus may have a lower level of training and experience in aircraft operations.

Altitude limitations should also be appreciated. The Federal Aviation Administration (FAA) requires that supplemental oxygen be used by both the pilot and passengers in an unpressurized cabin when cruising at 10,000 feet or more above sea level. Aircraft performance is also affected by an increase in altitude, and combined weight of crew members and equipment in the aircraft may have to be decreased for high-altitude operations.

Transport team members who participate in air-medical transport should be familiar with pertinent Federal Aviation Regulations[(44)]. FAR Part 91 governs all general operations and flight rules. FAR Part 135 contains flight rules for air taxi and commercial operations that are pertinent to most air-medical operations. The ultimate responsibility rests with the pilot for safe operation of the aircraft. Passengers and crew members must function entirely at the pilot's discretion.

Important aspects of normal operating procedures must be observed by specialty team members. Lights should never be shined toward the aircraft during landing or take-off, in order to prevent accidental blinding of the pilot. Landing zones should not be marked with loose articles. People and equipment should not be allowed within 100 feet of the landing perimeter. No one should approach an aircraft until signaled to do so by a crew member. Rotorcraft should be approached from the downhill side and never from the rear near the tail rotor. Loading and unloading of equipment and patients should be directed by the flight crew at all times. All passengers, including the patient, must be restrained with FAA-approved restraining devices for all take-offs and landings, and they should remain restrained throughout the flight. Crew members should be in a position to render patient care without having to remove restraining devices. All loose articles and equipment, especially any sharp objects, must be secured before take-off and landing. Transport isolettes should be equipped with internal padding to protect infants from rapid accelerating and decelerating forces. Portable oxygen cylinders may remain on board if they are a component of an isolette transport system and are locked in a secure position. Otherwise, only on-board oxygen should be used. After landing, passengers must observe similar safety precautions upon leaving the aircraft. Team members must remain clear of flight controls, radios, and switches, and should inform the pilot when any distracting medical equipment will be in use. They should also adhere to protocols involving night-lighting in the cabin: red or amber is preferred, and lights should be dimmed or turned off during night approaches. Passengers should not disembark until instructed by the pilot or a crew member.

Air-medical crew members and specialty teams should be familiar with emergency procedures in the event of an off-airport landing. Emergency training should include ap propriate topics found in FAR Part 135.331, and these rules should be reviewed regularly by both crew members and specialty teams through in-service meetings as outlined by the local air-medical provider. Crew members and specialty care providers should be prepared to deal with in-flight emergencies such as engine or electrical failure, fire, and emergency aircraft shutdown. One should know the location of fire extinguishers, exits, fuel shutoff valves (rotorcraft), oxygen shutoff valves, and the emergency locator transmitter. Stabilization of the electrical system is at the pilot's discretion and usually consists of disconnecting the aircraft batteries. It is important to follow all pilot directives.

Surface Transport

An essential component of pediatric interhospital referrals is surface transport, and safety precautions similar to those used in air-medical transport should be practiced. The medical director is responsible for thoroughly researching vendors of ground transport services in the areas of maintenance, safety records, experience of drivers, and reliability of equipment. Written contracts between the institution and the vendor should include specific details on insurance. Unfamiliar ground services should not be used. Ambulance drivers should be discouraged from exceeding the speed limit, as there is no evidence that this has any positive effect on patient outcome. All vehicles should meet the safety inspection criteria for their particular region, including appropriate restraint devices for patient, crew, and equipment.

Communication

Effective communication is vital to the safe and efficient operation of a transport system, providing an important link between transport team members and the medical control facilities. In order to effect safe operation, crew members, specialty team members, and dispatchers should understand the basic skills for effective communication. Any confusion created through communication may adversely affect patient outcome or be potentially harmful to transport personnel. It is important to keep non-essential conversation to a minimum during the critical phases of flight, and to use proper terminology to avoid confusion. For air-medical transports, one should maintain communication with the pilot, providing necessary information on air traffic, obstructions during take-off and landing, use of distracting equipment, and the needs of the patient.

Proper use of the microphone should be taught to all users. Important pieces of information are often lost when one improperly transmits through a voice-activated system. One should organize thoughts before transmission and then speak clearly at a normal rate and volume. One should avoid slang and dialect because there may be others listening on the same frequency. A communications specialist (dispatcher) should assist in tracking the team (flight following), know the capabilities of the communications center, and record the conversation for medicolegal purposes.

Appropriate Attire

The selection of a standard uniform will vary with each transport program according to that program's mission, and local climate and terrain. Uniforms should be selected with the following factors in mind: safety, efficiency, comfort, and appearance. It has been suggested that the ideal uniform in the air-medical profession be a flight suit that offers protection from heat and flame (with multiple layers and a quarter-inch air space), leather high-top boots, and flight helmets. Until such issues are strictly regulated, common sense still plays the more important role in choosing appropriate attire. Specialty teams rarely perform "scene runs," so leather high-top boots are probably unnecessary in most of their transports. Uniforms should be long-sleeved, loose-fitting, flame retardant, and free from any synthetic fibers which might melt in the event of a fire. Shoes should be sturdy, with closed toes and low heels. Teams who transport in winter climates should always dress for cold weather (hats, gloves, extra socks, boots with good traction) in case the aircraft or ground unit is temporarily diverted and shut down because of bad weather, or even more important, in case an unplanned off-site landing or vehicle breakdown occurs. Jewelry should be avoided because it can aggravate or cause injury and may get caught on doors or equipment.

Survival Techniques

Every transport team should have training in survival techniques appropriate to their region. Team members should have a basic understanding of the pathophysiology, signs, symptoms, and treatment of hypothermia and hyperthermia. "Crash survival" procedures increase the chance of survival when an aircraft crashes. "Wilderness survival" procedures are used when environmental conditions are such that body temperature is either raised or lowered beyond survivable limits. Each transport vehicle or aircraft should be equipped with a survival kit. By preparing for the extremes involved in crash survival and wilderness survival, a team will be able to handle minor critical situations effectively.

Fitness and Health

Fitness plays an integral role in the ability of transport team members to carry out and complete patient care within the transport environment. A physically and mentally fit team member is able to maintain a safe environment while performing patient care according to performance expectations. Policies regarding crew fitness vary among programs and should reflect the specific mission requirements of each program. Employee health, human resources, and risk management programs all can provide needed guidance during the development of specific policy requirements to ensure that they are reasonable and nondiscriminatory. Physical limitations, weight restrictions, and potentially disqualifying physical and mental conditions should be clearly outlined.

Transport team members are expected to load and unload patients and equipment and to carry loads over various types of terrain. Therefore, a physical examination (including visual and auditory acuity) should be part of the pre-employment screening and should be repeated annually. Each transport program should establish medical standards categories that will qualify or disqualify a candidate from performing transport team functions. Pre-employment and annual screenings should be performed to ensure that the team member is free from contagious diseases (rubella, tuberculosis, human immunodeficiency virus, hepatitis). The applicant's permission must be obtained before these tests. Positive tests for certain diseases do not automatically exclude otherwise healthy team members from practice, but appropriate precautions must be used to avoid transmission of contagious diseases.

Alert and well-rested crew and specialty team members are essential for the transport missions, so a built-in mechanism must be provided to protect individuals in this capacity. Specialty team members should not be sent out on transport after being on-call for more than a single shift for in-house responsibilities. Transport team personnel should not donate blood within 72 hours of the beginning of a shift of duty, and no medication should be consumed within eight hours of the start of duty if it either produces drowsiness or impairs judgment. Alcohol should not be consumed within a minimum of 8 hours of the start of a shift.

Medical personnel in emergency department and ICU setting have been shown to experience unusually high levels of stress[45]. Psychological, social and physical conditions include but are not limited to cardiovascular and GI tract diseases, suicide, drug abuse, psychiatric disorders and marital disharmony. In addition to the stressors encountered in certain in-hospital environments, transport team members are subject to:

1. The potential for vehicular accidents and concerns for personal safety.
2. Having to practice medicine in an unfamiliar environment, often without access to many resources available in the usual hospital setting.
3. The sense of being isolated as possibly the only one who can make certain decisions or perform life-saving procedures.
4. Erratic work schedules (e.g., when on call one must be prepared to leave rapidly to care for a patient with numerous possible problems, or the team member may stay on alert for the entire shift without going anywhere, or may end up on a long transport that goes well beyond the scheduled end of a shift.)

5. Pressure to work when off duty because of personnel shortages during periods of increased activity.
6. Equipment management.
7. Lack of understanding by nontransport colleagues of "downtime" responsibilities.
8. The need for diplomatic, calm, effective communication with colleagues, referring and receiving hospital personnel, the patient, and the patient's parents.
9. Limited resources requiring clinical skills and judgements unnecessary in hospital setting.
10. The potential for having to work "alone out there" with other team members in whom one may not have total confidence.
11. Feeling of lack of control over many situations (vehicle or equipment breakdowns, physician noninvolvement or over involvement at the referring hospital, etc.) for the team members who are not primarily pediatric.
12. The physical stress of working in a moving, vibrating, noisy environment (including motion sickness, sleep and food deprivation, etc.).
13. The additional emotions and fears involved in being responsible for a very sick child.

As a result of the substantial stressors in the transport setting, all teams should offer members 1) access to stress management programs and 2) a formal Critical Incident Stress Debriefing (CISD) system. Appropriate *recognition* of prevention and development of protective mechanisms against stress related symptoms can lead to a higher perception of quality of life as well as a decrease in staff burnout, disability, excessive absenteeism, and premature retirement.

Responsibilities of the Referring Hospital

Referring hospitals should operate within the boundaries established by their level of commitment to emergency care[(40)]. A hospital may choose not to accept children younger than a certain age, to examine and treat children with only certain categories of non-urgent conditions, or to examine and treat all pediatric patients, including those with critical conditions[(46)]. Some argue that perhaps all critically ill and injured patients in the prehospital setting should be transported only to designated critical care facilities and trauma centers that are able to provide optimal care[(47–49)]. Hospitals that choose to examine and treat all patients with critical conditions should follow standard guidelines for pediatric resuscitation and be equipped to provide intensive care for several hours, if necessary, until specialized transport services are available, especially when circumstance (e.g., inclement weather) may preclude a rapid response by such services.

It is important that a referring physician contact the regional center *before* transfer to avoid abandonment of the patient. Abandonment is defined as "the unilateral termination of a physician-patient relationship by the physician, without the patient's consent and without giving the patient sufficient opportunity to secure the services of another competent physician"[(50)]. Under federal law, the Consolidated Omnibus Budget Reconciliation Act (COBRA)[(51)] and the Omnibus Reconciliation Act [(52)], legal liability has been expanded beyond the previous standard for transfers. COBRA now requires the transferring hospital to assume responsibility for the medical integrity of the receiving hospital, as well as for the appropriateness of the patient's transfer. COBRA also requires hospitals to examine all patients who present to the emergency department and to provide all medical care necessary for stabilization **(Table 3.5).** Patients are not to be transferred until they are stabilized, and the referring physician must certify that the need to transfer to another medical facility for additional treatment will outweigh the potential risk of the transfer. The referring hospital will be held accountable for using the most suitable type of transport for the patient's condition and must ensure that the ambulance or aircraft has appropriate equipment and medical personnel to provide any necessary therapy during transfer[(53,54)]. JCAHO also mandates that a hospital be "capable of instituting essential lifesaving measures and implementing emergency procedures that will minimize further compromise of the condition of any infant, child, or adult being transported"[(42)]. It is the authors' experience that referring hospitals often are uncomfortable with providing initial stabilization to pediatric patients and would prefer to transfer critically ill children before they have received appropriate therapy. This apparent preference for getting the child to the tertiary center "as quickly as possible" with any available means (rather than ensuring that the transporting personnel are qualified and adept at pediatric resuscitation) might save time, but it may subject the critically ill child to a less-sophisticated level of care between hospitals. A number of studies[(40,49,53,55–60)] suggest that 24% to 70% of transferred patients are inadequately stabilized before and during the transfer. One should not assume that everyone on board a medical transport is adequately trained and adept at pediatric resuscitation[(17,61,62)].

Table 3.5. Preparations by Referring Hospital for Transport Team

Copy all records and x-rays.
Record telephone number for pending laboratory data.
Obtain consent to transport–include receiving hospital and type of transport team.
Prepare blood products for transport, if needed.
Stabilize all intravenous access and endotracheal tube for transport.

PHILOSOPHY OF TRANSPORT AND ANTICIPATED PROBLEMS

The initiation and completion of the transport process is complex. Unexpected events occur with regularity. Various problems might be expected during the initial request for transfer, during the transport itself, and on arrival, especially when the transport crew is not provided by the receiving institution.

Regional flight teams and emergency medical services are focused essentially on the adult population and have been developed to deal primarily with myocardial infarction and trauma, the major causes of morbidity in adults[(63)]. These teams are trained for rapid response and are expected to keep the time at the scene to a minimum. This is generally appropriate for prehospital scene runs, where the environment can be precarious and resources are extremely limited. However, for most interhospital transfers, the time taken for transport to the regional center is not so important to patient outcome as is the time taken for delivery of the center's expert care to the patient[(64)]. An exception would be the subset of patients with life-threatening injuries (less than 5% of all trauma victims), where the definitive care could be rendered only in a Level I pediatric trauma center[(65)]. Therefore, the "scoop and run" philosophy probably does not influence outcome in most patients being transported. In the authors' experience, pediatric patients have been particular victims of this philosophy, especially when they are transported by teams that are not specially trained in pediatrics, often arriving at our hospital in full arrest from airway obstruction and without having received appropriate resuscitation. Children differ from adults in both anatomic and physiologic aspects and, when in critical condition, often require more extensive care before arrival at the destination hospital. Therefore, the time the transport team spends with the patient before transport should be determined by the medical circumstances and not by precipitous haste.

Regional flight teams are often asked to document or to offer a formal explanation to their medical director for any transport that exceeds the flight program's "acceptable standard" for ground time. The "golden hour" of trauma is often incorrectly applied to the entire spectrum of pediatric illness. The air-medical profession often is perceived by many in the field as an "industry". Anything that prolongs scene time (patient stabilization) could result in fewer flights and missed transports. As a result, team members may feel pressured to leave the scene before adequate resuscitation measures have been carried out. In addition, the referring physician may pressure the team to evacuate the patient from the emergency department quickly because of his or her discomfort over pediatric emergencies. Referring physicians must understand that resuscitation is more easily handled in the emergency department than in a crowded, moving vehicle.

The goal of any transport team, whether at the scene of an accident or in the emergency department of a referring hospital, should be to provide treatment at a juncture that is critical to the patient's survival. If they are only minutes away from the regional center, the transport team may elect to minimize scene time and postpone necessary procedures until arrival at the regional center. On the other hand, if they are to embark on a long-distance transport, they may elect to spend more time on the ground stabilizing the patient.

The procedures performed on the prehospital scene should be limited to the basics of resuscitation, the maintenance of adequate oxygen delivery, and the preservation of cerebral function. At one extreme, this may involve simply placing an oxygen mask on the patient, obtaining a quick report, and departing within minutes. At the other extreme, this may involve a substantial amount of time spent performing a controlled endotracheal intubation while restoring blood pressure in an attempt to protect cerebral circulation. In addition, the decision as to when to move the patient is often influenced by extraneous factors such as weather, additional calls, and surrounding conditions.

The level of stabilizing care that should be provided to victims of life-threatening injuries is controversial. Several studies of the management of life-threatening injuries in the field have revealed that precious time often is wasted in unsuccessful attempts to secure vascular access, when the ultimate treatment for such injuries is prompt delivery of the patient to the surgical suite at the regional center[(66–71)]. Cowley et al.[(72)] defined the golden hour as the period immediately after injury that determines survival. If the patient arrives at the definitive care facility within the "golden hour," survival can be expected. The golden hour concept was implemented 22 years ago, when medical personnel rarely performed endotracheal intubation and vascular access at the scene as they do today. Without performing these procedures, it only makes sense that transport time to the receiving facility probably did influence outcome. However, one must question whether this is true for the 1990s. In addition, the study was performed on adult trauma victims and cannot be arbitrarily applied to pediatric patients or to those with life threatening medical illnesses. Perhaps most pediatric scene transports would fare even better if personnel would focus more on the ABCs of pediatric resuscitation and less on the "critical ten minutes" at the scene or on the golden hour!

Another set of problems occurs when the responsibility for patient care is transferred. The transport team should consider themselves responsible for the patient from the time they arrive to assist until the patient is admitted to the receiving institution after appropriate evaluation. One fundamental problem may be a major change in care, especially when the referring physicians are unfamiliar with pediatric illnesses, resuscitation, and general care. Common problems in care include hypothermia and inappropriate intravenous fluid administration. Infants may have been exposed for examination in an air-conditioned environment and may develop hypothermia. Fluid resuscitation may be inadequate because of the fear of overloading infants, or it may be excessive through rapid intravenous infusions with adult-sized devices for intravenous administration. Medications may be appropriate in choice, but not in dose. Ventilatory parameters may need to be adjusted, and respiratory and airway management may need to be changed quickly. It remains the responsibility of the referring center to assess the need for such specific care, but it becomes the responsibility of the transport team to begin optimal management on arrival while being supportive when discussing appropriate changes in the care of the patient. Some problems may be avoided by offering specific advice during the initial telephone contact. If there is a disagreement between the transport team members and the referring physician over patient management, it is important to have the medical control physician or the attending physician for the transport communicate with the referring physician to agree on a plan.

MODE SELECTION

Critical care transport systems use some combination of ground ambulances, rotorcraft, and fixed-wing aircraft. Factors considered in choosing a transport vehicle include available space, distance, facilities for monitoring and resuscitation, cost, speed, and vehicle availability.

Ground-Based Transport Vehicles

The ambulance is the most frequently used vehicle for all interhospital transports. Many critical care transport teams, especially neonatal teams and those in large cities, use specially equipped ambulances as mobile ICUs. The advantages of ground transport for children include cost, the relatively large interior working space, and, most importantly, the ability to easily stop the vehicle to assess clinical parameters or to perform procedures. In addition, personnel who drive ambulances are often trained in emergency medical services and can provide additional assistance during a medical crisis.

The disadvantages of ambulance transport include the time involved in round-trip travel and, in cities, the difficulty of navigating through heavy traffic. Fear may be instilled in the patients because of the sirens and the movement required to maneuver in traffic. Motion sickness can also be a problem during rapid ground-based transport.

Rotorcraft

Medical transport via rotorcraft was initially used to evacuate battlefield casualties during the Korean and Vietnam wars. Civilian, hospital-based transport services were developed in the early 1970s initially to transport trauma victims and later to transport adult cardiac patients needing rapid thrombolytic therapy. For these purposes, speed of arrival at the tertiary care center, within the golden hour for trauma or as fast as possible for a patient with an acute myocardial infarction, was the major priority. Attempts to apply that philosophy to transport of pediatric patients have raised some problems.

One advantage of rotorcraft transport for children is the rapidity of deployment and return. When a hospital provides a rotorcraft program, it also makes a commitment to have a team available for rapid mobilization to expedite this process. In urban areas, rotorcraft can provide additional speed by passing over traffic congestion.

There are several disadvantages of rotorcraft transport for the pediatric patient. The noise and vibrations interfere with clinical assessment and monitoring, making the performance of procedures difficult on an adult, but even more so on the much smaller "target" of a child. Assessment of breath sounds, crucial to the evaluation of respiratory status in a patient, can be impossible in a helicopter[73]. Hypothermia is always a risk in winter conditions. Rotorcraft are not pressurized and often have a very small cabin space in which to work. Operation costs are high compared with ground transport. The national average charge for a 100-mile round-trip rotorcraft transport is $2,500–$3,000, with some being much higher. This includes the base or lift-off fee, the per-mile or hourly fee, and the medical team charges[74]. If there is no appropriate landing site next to the hospital, the patient must undergo multiple transfers between ambulances and the rotorcraft. Depending on the region, rotorcraft are out of service as much as 10% to 20% of the time because of weather conditions. This presents an additional hazard to children who arrive at emergency departments that may be inadequately prepared to care for children and that routinely depend on rotorcraft for quick retrieval.

One model, while expensive, has been used successfully in some programs. It involves using a rotorcraft to deliver the team to a patient and an ambulance to return the team and the patient to the tertiary care center. This system delivers a high level of care quickly and keeps the rotorcraft available to serve other patients. Simultaneously, it allows a larger, less noisy working area, which can be stopped, if necessary, to assess the patient more carefully and to perform procedures.

Fixed-Wing Aircraft

Fixed-wing aircraft are useful for pediatric transport, but only for distances of about 150 miles or greater. The working environment is often larger than that of rotorcraft, with less noise and vibration. Fixed-wing aircraft also can be flown by instrument under weather conditions that prevent the use of rotorcraft. If the patient's condition might be worsened by an increase in altitude, airplane cabins can be pressurized to sea level, even when flying at an altitude of 20,000 feet.

The disadvantages of fixed-wing transport include the high cost, the need for airports in reasonable proximity to both hospitals, and the need for multiple transfers of the patient between the aircraft and ambulances. Another apparent disadvantage is the length of time required for preflight planning, which includes filing a flight plan, fueling the aircraft, and checking the weather. This usually requires about one hour from the time of notification until departure. Generally this time is made up by the speed of travel during flight.

In summary, each of the three modes of travel has its advantages and disadvantages. The choice of which to use or on which to base a referral system is determined by geography, the financial feasibility based on frequency and distance of transports, and the proximity of heliports and airports. However, the most important consideration is not necessarily the type of vehicle chosen for transport, but rather the capability of the team traveling in that vehicle to care for the child. Therefore, the mode of transport should not be chosen solely on the basis of speed, but also on the quality of the attending team.

AIR-MEDICAL PHYSIOLOGY

Transport team members must be able to function in the air-medical environment. Changes in altitude may have adverse effects on both the patient and the team member, so it is important for the transport team member to have at least a basic understanding of altitude physiology.

The sum of the partial pressures of individual gases in the atmosphere defines the barometric pressure. An inverse relationship exists between altitude and barometric pressure **(Table 3.6)**. Dalton's law states that the sum of the partial pressures of individual gases in a mixture is equal to the total pressure of that mixture. Therefore, the partial pressure of oxygen (PO_2) at any altitude, given that it comprises 21% of the atmosphere, may be calculated as follows:

$$\text{sea level: } 760 \text{ torr} \times 0.21 = 160 \text{ torr}$$
$$8{,}000 \text{ feet: } 565 \text{ torr} \times 0.21 = 119 \text{ torr}$$

The expected PO_2 in arterial blood (PaO_2) can then be determined from the simplified alveolar gas equation. When there is no significant intrapulmonary shunting, alveolar PO_2 (PAO_2) should approximate PaO_2.

Table 3.6. The Relationship Between Altitude and Barometric Pressure

Altitude (ft)	*Barometric Pressure (mm Hg)*
Sea level	760 mm Hg
2000	706 mm Hg
5000	632 mm Hg
8000	565 mm Hg
18,000	379 mm Hg

Table 3.7. Ratio of Gas Volume to Atmospheric Pressure at Various Altitudes

	Altitude (ft)	*Atmosphere*	*Gas Volume*
Sea level	1.00	1.00	
	5,000	0.83	1.20
	8,000	0.77	1.33
	18,000	0.50	2.00

$$PAO_2 = PIO_2 - \frac{PACO_2}{R} = (PB\text{–}47) \times FiO_2 - \frac{PCO_2}{0.8}$$

where PIO_2 is the partial pressure of inspired oxygen as determined by the difference of barometric pressure and partial pressure H_2O at 37° C times the FiO_2, $PACO_2$ is the alveolar partial pressure of carbon dioxide (use $PaCO_2$), R is the respiratory quotient (generally 0.8), PB is the barometric pressure, and PCO_2 is the partial pressure of carbon dioxide. Therefore, if one is traveling in an aircraft with a cabin altitude of 8000 feet, and breathing room air, the resultant PaO_2 would be calculated as follows, assuming a partial pressure of carbon dioxide in arterial blood ($PaCO_2$) of 40 torr:

$$PAO_2 = PIO_2 - \frac{PACO_2}{R} = (565 - 47) \times 0.21 - \frac{40}{0.8}$$
$$PAO_2 = 518 \times 0.21 - 50$$
$$PAO_2 = 58 \text{ torr}$$

Therefore, as altitude increases, the resultant decrease in barometric pressure will result in alveolar hypoxemia and increased pulmonary vascular resistance unless the FiO_2 is adjusted to compensate for the change.

Those disturbances in the body (except hypoxia) that result from a difference between ambient pressure and the pressure of gases within body cavities, tissues, and fluids are known as dysbarisms. Boyle's law states that at constant temperature, the volume of a gas varies inversely with the pressure **(Table 3.7)**. Accordingly, the volume of gas within a closed space will change with changes in barometric pressure (e.g., a balloon will double in volume from sea level to 18,000 feet). Clinical parallels must be appreciated and would include pneumothorax, bowel obstruction, endotracheal tube cuffs, air splints, military anti-shock trousers, and the like.

Cabin pressurization reduces the effects of altitude by maintaining a preset barometric pressure within the cabin. A cabin altitude of 8,000 feet simply means that the barometric pressure within the cabin is equivalent to that at 8,000 feet above sea level, regardless of the actual altitude of the aircraft. Cabin pressure can be maintained by the flight crew. If the cabin is equipped with an altimeter, it should be set before departure to match the field elevation. The in-flight indication on the altimeter will be the cabin altitude.

Rapid decompression is a threat to both patient and crew

while traveling in a pressurized aircraft. The risk is higher in small cabins when the volume of the cabin relative to the surface area of a decompression orifice is small. If a child is not intubated, the airway is usually open and respiratory gases can escape. Patients who are intubated may suffer from the rapid expansion of pulmonary gases, resulting in pneumothorax or air emboli. A slow ascent is always recommended to decrease the risk of sudden pressure changes. In the unlikely event of a sudden decompression at altitude, it may be necessary to quickly and briefly disconnect the endotracheal tube from the ventilator in order to allow gas escape.

Crew members should understand that high-altitude conditions will potentiate the effects of medications, sleep deprivation, fatigue, and eating habits (hypoglycemia). As a result, it is inappropriate for any person to act or attempt to act as a crew member within eight hours after consuming any alcoholic beverage or while using any drug that affects the faculties in any way that would compromise safety(75). Night vision is impaired at cabin altitudes above 5,000 feet. Vibration and noise will enhance fatigue, so it is important to use headsets when feasible, even though it may seem inconvenient. Changes in gravitational forces during ascent, descent, and banking may produce vertigo. Humidity is generally low during in-flight conditions, therefore insensible water loss can be substantial in both the crew member and the patient.

TEAM COMPOSITION

The members of a pediatric transport team collectively must possess the skill and knowledge to provide a level of care commensurate with the current and anticipated needs of the patient and similar to that rendered in the PICU. The team should be composed of at least two individuals, and they should have 1) the ability to function in complex environments with limited resources, 2) specific training in transport medicine and in pediatrics, and 3) a fundamental knowledge of field priorities. Team members should perform within their capability and scope of employment. For example, the medical control physician should never allow an individual to assist in a pediatric transport if that individual is inexperienced in handling pediatric emergencies within the institution. An interhospital transport team is usually an extension of a regional center and, therefore, is medicolegally protected as an agent of that institution provided it conforms to the standard of care defined by the institution. Each team member must carefully follow standard resuscitation guidelines and protocols approved by the medical control physician.

Decisions about team composition currently are some of the most difficult in pediatric transport. Limited resources, legal considerations, difficulty in assessing patients by telephone, concerns for optimal patient care, and lack of conclusive research into team composition all complicate the decision. Additional considerations include geography and team goals (e.g., whether to transport only critically ill patients).

A 1988 study of pediatric training centers showed that 100% of the teams used a physician, although 72% included second-year pediatric residents against the advice of the 1986 AAP guidelines. The survey, however, did not include the growing number of pediatric centers that successfully transport children without physicians. In 1995, many pediatric training centers use physicians for only a portion of transports. In addition, the 1988 study reported that 100% of the teams included a nurse, and 50% included a respiratory therapist(76).

It is widely accepted that adult and neonatal transport teams do not always require a physician as part of the team, although some systems use physicians anyway, believing that they provide a higher level of care. While little objective data exists on need for a physician in pediatric transport, more pediatric teams than adult or neonatal teams currently include one. Pediatric transport differs from adult and neonatal transport in several respects. These differences make it difficult for some teams to provide nonphysicians who are appropriately qualified to lead a pediatric team.

Both adult and neonatal teams transport patients with a relatively narrow range of sizes and diagnoses. Adult transports primarily serve cardiac patients or victims of multiple trauma. Neonatal transports usually serve patients with respiratory distress, congenital heart disease, or surgical emergencies. In contrast, pediatric transports must serve a broad range of illness and trauma—the two-week-old patient with heart disease, the three-month-old survivor of sudden infant death syndrome, the year-old patient resuscitated from a submersion accident, the two-year-old with epiglottitis, the five-year-old with meningitis, the eleven-year-old with multiple trauma, and everything in between.

Other problems in pediatric transport include the fact that few hospitals train nonphysician personnel in pediatric procedures, and that many broad-based teams transport too few children to develop or maintain critical skills. Additional expertise is needed when performing invasive procedures in children because of their smaller size and anatomical differences. Procedures are further complicated when they are performed on a small, often uncooperative child in a moving environment.

The 1993 AAP Guidelines specifically address the issue of team composition by acknowledging the differences in team goals, available personnel and local non-physician practice parameters(10). Recommendations focus on skill levels rather than on educational degrees of team members. Skills defined in detail as necessary to transport pediatric patients include cognitive skills, procedural skills, communication skills and "other" skills.

Several studies have attempted to answer whether physicians are needed for pediatric transport. McCloskey et al. surveyed 191 transports with regard to procedures performed, medications used, and a subjective assessment of the attending physician, and concluded that a physician was not always necessary[36]. How to predict which transports will need a physician remains unanswered. This study was performed in a center where only physicians could perform certain procedures and make decisions regarding medication.

Routine training for the EMTs, paramedics, and nurses who are often used in regional transport systems is usually deficient in pediatric medicine[16,17,39,40]. McNab[41] reviewed the charts of 130 seriously ill or injured children transported to a tertiary level ICU to determine the incidence of secondary insults incurred as a result of insufficient training of the transport personnel. In this study, 72% of all insults occurred with escorts (EMTs, paramedics, flight nurses) who had not received specialized training in pediatric transport; 20% occurred with escorts who had received an intensive 18-month training course in pediatric transport with ongoing recertification; and 8% occurred with escorts who specialized in pediatric transport, and who were accompanied by a pediatric intensive care physician. Although the escorts who had received pediatric training performed much better than those with no formal pediatric training, the combination of a critical care physician and escorts who had pediatric training was associated with even fewer insults in this particular study.

Rubenstein et al. reported a prospective assessment of need for a physician in 129 consecutive transports of infants and children. Admission to the pediatric ICU was considered to indicate need for a physician. 39% of the transported patients required either what was considered in their system to be physician-only procedural or medical interventions or admission to the PICU. It is noted that not every system considers PICU admission as criteria for needing a physician on transport and that some interventions considered physician-only are performed by other medical professionals in some other transport systems. The authors demonstrated that certain objective information obtained during the transport request was reliable. They also concluded that at the time of request for transfer, subjective judgement, PRISM score, and the presence of tachycardia did not predict the need for physician presence during transport[24].

Optimal care during pediatric transport requires individuals who are not only adept at procedural skills, but who also have a thorough understanding of pediatric pathophysiology when they encounter various crises. This is best accomplished by using individuals who have *ongoing* exposure to the pediatric critical care environment. Pediatric critical care physicians are not always an available resource in many transport programs. Therefore, an increasing number of programs are exploring the possibility of using nonphysician transport teams to transport critically ill pediatric patients. This may be appropriate as long as patient morbidity from secondary insults (e.g., airway complications) is equal to or less than that which is acceptable within the PICU.

In summary, decisions about team composition will depend on the type of transport and the skills of available personnel, and must be made primarily with optimal care of the individual patient in mind. The ultimate answer may well be that the educational degrees of the individuals will not be as important as the ability to recognize and competently manage the range of potential crises that can occur during transport, while maintaining morbidity and mortality rates within the range considered acceptable by the critical care areas of the institution. The optimal team composition for a pediatric transport should be a combination of medical professionals who are trained and experienced in the type of diagnosis and treatment most likely to be required for each patient's condition. The goal of a successful pediatric transport is to deliver the patient in the best possible condition. Accordingly, team composition should be determined in the patient's best interest, and not on a financial or administrative basis.

INTRAHOSPITAL TRANSPORT

Despite the focus of transport on prehospital and interhospital settings, intrahospital transport from the intensive care unit to the operating room, the radiology department etc. can be almost as dangerous to the patient. Nonportable diagnostic tests that aid physicians in diagnosing complex problems are becoming increasingly sophisticated, and require the transport of critically ill patients from the ICU for prolonged periods. Intrahospital transports are common and require the same meticulous care and attendance as do interhospital transports. Patients undergoing procedures, especially radiologic procedures, are often moved great distances, both horizontally and vertically, through the hospital into potentially adverse environments. For example, patients with head injuries are often moved to the computed tomography (CT) scanner during the initial resuscitation phase of their management, already potentially the most hazardous part of their hospitalization. CT scanning areas are kept at low temperatures and require personnel to be separated from the patient for protection from repeated exposure to radiation. Therefore, it is important to ensure optimal patient assessment through both visible and audible monitoring devices.

The process of transfer of critically ill patients to another hospital location should be treated, as in interhospital transport, as an extension of the intensive care unit. Personnel, equipment, and monitoring should be appropriate for the occasion and should not result in a degradation of care. Therefore, adequate medical supervision should be provided during the entire intrahospital transfer. There is a tendency to believe that patients will probably remain stable, that the hospital's tertiary care center's sophisticated services are readily available everywhere, or to send the most expendable and usually therefore the least-experienced individuals on a transfer. It is easier to not consider the unlikely events, such as broken elevators, malfunctioning equipment, fire alarms or patient deterioration which could be hazardous to the patient who is sent with inappropriate/incomplete equipment or personnel. The attending physician from the ICU ultimately is responsible for all that occurs during the transport and, therefore, should be aware of all in-house transports and be ready to respond to an emergency.

The supplies required for the transport may vary with the illness of the patient, but basic resuscitative and therapeutic equipment and medications are always necessary. This portable system should include everything normally found on a "crash cart:" an "airway compartment" with suction apparatus, laryngoscopes, endotracheal tubes, bag-valve-mask sets, and medication for "crash" induction of anesthesia. All items should be checked for completeness and proper function after each use and at each change of shift. Prior to transport, supplies should be double checked for the specific sizes and doses needed for the individual patient. Most importantly, the team should not rely on the equipment supply of other departments.

Monitoring should include the cardiorespiratory system (ECG, impedance pneumography) at the least, pulse oximetry for patients in whom oxygen delivery is a potential concern, and the addition of capnography for patients who require mechanical ventilation. Any other continuous monitoring (intravascular, intracranial pressure, etc. should also be continued. It is important to use monitors with reliable batteries, in the event of power loss or unexpected delays.

Little has been written about intrahospital patient transport. Insel et al.[77] reported a 13% morbidity rate in patients transferred from the operating room to the ICU and significant increases in both heart rate and systolic blood pressure. Indeck et al.[78] reported a very high incidence (68%) of significant physiologic changes during the time away from the ICU. Waddell[79] demonstrated that critically ill patients developed life-threatening complications, such as arrhythmias and systemic hypotension, during 20% of intrahospital moves.

SUMMARY

The function of pediatric transport is to deliver timely, high quality intensive care to the critically ill child. This begins with immediate consultation over the radio or by telephone while the transport team and vehicles are being mobilized. Adequate communication between facilities is essential. Consultants must be available to assist in handling transport requests, and to offer assistance with patient stabilization. A trained transport team is needed to further stabilize, treat, and move the patient in as expeditious a manner as possible. Various transport modalities are needed in accordance with the geography, the frequency of calls, and the severity of clinical condition of the patients. The process of transfer of critically ill or injured children requires a great deal of cooperation and expertise to function well.

Transport is clearly a challenge to the pediatric intensivist or other referring and receiving physicians, who often must make difficult choices in a complex treatment environment. The risk/benefit ratio should always be examined, with specific attention paid to the risk of transport versus the risk of not performing the transfer or procedure. Pediatric intensivists, emergency medicine specialists, surgeons or neonatologists must be actively involved in the planning, maintenance, and quality assurance of transport if optimal care is to be expected. Required principles include: ensuring patient and personnel safety, keeping transport time to a minimum, providing constant optimal care, and having an accountable physician in charge at all times.

References

1. Pollack MM, Alexander SR, Clarke N, Ruttimann UE, Tesselaar HM, Bachulis AC: Improved outcomes from tertiary center pediatric intensive care: a statewide comparison of tertiary and nontertiary care facilities. Crit Care Med 1991;19:150–159.
2. Harris BH, Orr RE, Boles ET Jr: Aeromedical transportation for infants and children. J Pediatr Surg 1975;10:719–724.
3. Hart HW: The conveyance of patients to and from hospital, 1720–1850. Med His 1978;22:397–407.
4. Sadler AM, Sadler BF, Webb SB: Emergency Medical Care: The Neglected Public Service. Cambridge, MA, Ballinger Publishing Company, 1977:29.
5. Clarke TA, Zmora He, Chen JH, Ready G, Merritt A: Transcutaneous oxygen monitoring during neonatal transport. Pediatrics 1980;65:884–886.
6. Hanning CD, Gilmour DG, Hothersall AP, Aitkenhead AR, Venner RM, Ledingham IM: Movement of the critically ill within hospital. Intensive Care Med 1978;4:137–143.
7. Park GR, Johnson S: A ventilator for use during mobile intensive care and total intravenous anesthesia: The Drager Oxylog. Anaesthesia 1982;37:1204–1208.
8. Sumners JS, Harris HB, Jones B, Cassidy G, Wirtschafter DD: Regional neonatal transport: Impact of an integrated community center system. Pediatrics 1980;65:910–916.
9. American Academy of Pediatrics Committee on Hospital Care: Guidelines for air and ground transportation of pediatric patients. Pediatrics 1986;78:943–950.
10. American Academy of Pediatrics Committee on Interhospital Transport: Guidelines for air and ground transport or neonatal and pediatric patients. Pediatrics 1993;4:30–31
11. Black RE, Mayer T, Walker ML, et al.: Air transport of pediatric emergency cases. N Engl J Med 1978;307:1465–1468.
12. McCloskey KA: Letter to the Editor. Pediat Emerg Care 1988;4:230.
13. Dobrin RS, Block B, Gilman JI, Massaro TA: The development of a pediatric emergency transport system. Pediatr Clin North Am 1980; 27:633–640.
14. Frankel LR: The evaluation, stabilization and transport of the critically ill child. Int Anesthesiol Clin 1987;25:77–103.
15. Kissoon N, Frewen TC, Kronick JB, Mohammed A: The child requiring transport: Lessons and implications for the pediatric emergency physician. Pediatr Emerg Care 1988;4:1–4.

16. Seidel JS, Hornbein M, Yoshiyama K, Kuznets D, Finklestein JZ, St. Geme JW: Emergency medical services and the pediatric patient: Are the needs being met? Pediatrics 1984;73:769–772.
17. Seidel JS: Emergency medical services and the pediatric patient: Are the needs being met? II. Training and equipping emergency medical services providers for pediatric emergencies. Pediatrics 1986;78:808–812.
18. Goldstein B, Cardenas N, McDonald T, Todres ID: Emergency transport of pediatric trauma patients [Abstract]. Pediatr Emerg Care 1988;4:160.
19. Orr RA, McCloskey KA, Britten AG: Transportation of critically ill children. In: Rogers MC, ed. Textbook of pediatric intensive care. Baltimore: Williams & Wilkins, 1989:1571–1587.
20. Smith DF, Hackel A: Selection criteria for pediatric critical care transport teams. Crit Care Med 1983;11:10–12.
21. McCloskey KA, Johnston C: Critical care interhospital transports: Predictability of the need for a pediatrician. Pediatr Emerg Care 1990;6:89–92.
22. Bion JF, Edlin SA, Ramsay G, McCabe S, Ledingham IM: Validation of a prognostic score in critically ill patients undergoing transport. Br Med J 1985;291:432–434.
23. Kanter RK, Tompkins JM: Adverse events during interhospital transport: Physiologic deterioration associated with pretransport severity of illness. Pediatrics 1989;84:43–48.
24. Orr RA, Venkataraman ST, Singleton CA: Pediatric Risk of Mortality Score (PRISM): A poor predictor in triage of patients for pediatric transport. Crit Care Med, 1994; 22:1:101–107.
25. Baxt WG, Moody P: The impact of a physician as part of the aeromedical rehospital team in patients with blunt trauma. JAMA 1987; 257:3246–3250.
26. Snow N, Hull C, Severns J: Physician presence on a helicopter emergency medical service: Necessary or desirable? Aviat Space Environ Med 1986;57:1176–1178.
27. Pollack MM, Ruttimann UE, Getson PR: The pediatric risk of mortality (PRISM) score. Crit Care Med 1988;16:1110–1116.
28. Rubenstein JS, Gomez MA, Rybicki, L, Zehave LN: Can the need for a physician's part for the pediatric transport team be predicted? A prospective study: Crit Care Med 1992; 20:1657–1661
29. Kanter RK, Boeing NM, Hannan WP, Kanter DL: Excess morbidity associated with interhospital transport. [Abstract] Pediatric 1992; 90:893–898
30. Orr RA, Karr VA, Assessing severity of illness before transport. Pediatric Transport Medicine 1995; 14:123–131
31. Yeh TS, Pollack MM, Ruttiman UE, Holbrook PR, Fields AI: Validation of physiologic stability index for use in critically ill infants and children. Pediatr Res 1984;18:445–451.
32. Walker ML, Storrs BB, Mayer T: Factors affecting outcome in the pediatric patient with multiple trauma. Childs Brain 1984;11:387–397.
33. Cullen DJ, Civetta JM, Briggs BA, Ferrara LC: Therapeutic Intervention Scoring System: a method for quantitative comparison of patient care. Crit Care Med 1974;2:57–60.
34. Tepas JJ, Mollitt DL, Talbert JL, Bryant M: The Pediatric Trauma Score as a predictor of injury severity in the injured child. J Pediatr Surg 1987;22:14–18.
35. Orr RV, Venkataraman S, McCloskey K, Brandestein M, Jonosky J: Four simple pre transport variables accurately predict in-hospital mortality. Crit Care Med 1995; 23:224.
36. McCloskey KA, King WD, Byron L: Pediatric critical care transport: Is a physician always needed on the team? Ann Emerg Med 1989;18:247–249.
37. McCloskey K, Faries G, King W, Orr R, Plouff R: Variables predicting the need for major interventions during pediatric critical care transport. Pediatr Emerg Med, Feb 1992;8:1:1–3.
38. Day S, McCloskey K, Orr R, Notterman D, Hackel A: Pediatric interhospital critical care transport: Consensus of a national leadership conference. Pediatrics, Oct 1991;88:4:696–704.
39. Aijian P, Tsai A, Knopp R, Kallsen GW: Endotracheal intubation of pediatric patients by paramedics. Ann Emerg Med 1989;18:489–494.
40. Seidel JS: A needs assessment of advanced life support and emergency medical services in pediatric patient: State of the art. Circulation 1986;74:129–133.
41. McNab AJ: Optimal escort for interhospital transport of pediatric emergencies. J Trauma 1991;31:205–209.
42. Joint Commission for the Accreditation of Healthcare Organizations: Accreditation manual for hospitals, Chicago: 1991:33.
43. Collett HM: Accident trends for air medical helicopters Hosp Aviation 1989;8:6.
44. Federal Aviation Regulations/Airman's Information Manual. Renton, Washington: Aviation Supplies and Academics, 1991.
45. Myers DV: Stress and the transport team. Pediatric Transport Medicine 1995; 39:532–541
46. Bushore M: Emergency care of the child. Pediatrics 1987;79:572–575.
47. Cales RH: Trauma mortality on Orange County: The effect of implementation of a regional trauma system. Ann Emerg Med 1984;13:1–10.
48. Trunkey DD: Towards optimal trauma care. Am Coll Surg Bull 1984;69:2.
49. West JG, Trunkey DD, Lim RC: Systems of trauma care. A study of two counties. Arch Surg 1979;114:455–460.
50. Youngberg BJ: Legal issues related to transport. Pediatric Transport Medicine 1995;36:504–516
51. PL 99–272, US Government Printing Office, 42 US Code Service, 1395 dd. Washington, DC: Lawyer Cooperative Publishing Company, 1986.
52. Omnibus Budget Reconciliation Act of 1989, Sec. 6018 42 USC § 1395cc (West Supp. 1990).
53. Annas GJ: Your money or your life: "Dumping" uninsured patients from hospital emergency wards. Am J Public Health 1986;76:74–77.
54. Youngberg BJ: Legal issues related to transport. Pediatric Transport Medicine 1995;36:504–516.
55. Galbraith S: Misdiagnosis and delayed diagnosis in traumatic intracranial haematoma. Br Med J 1976;1:1438–1439.
56. Greenburg DS: Health-care thrift spurs patient-dumping. Los Angeles Times, November 12, 1984; Part II:5.
57. Himmelstein DU, Woolhandler S, Harnly M, et al.: Patient transfers: Medical practice as social triage. Am J Public Health 1984;74:494–497.
58. Mayer TA, Walker ML: Severity of illness and injury in pediatric air transport. Ann Emerg Med 1984;13:108–111.
59. Olson CM, Jastremski MS, Vilogi JP, Madden CM, Beney KM: Stabilization of patients prior to interhospital transfer. Am J Emerg Med 1987;5:33–39.
60. Spitz L, Wallis M, Graves HF: Transport of the surgical neonate. Arch Dis Child 1984;59:284–288.
61. Chance GW, Matthew JD, Gash J, Williams G, Cunningham K: Neonatal transport: A controlled study of skilled assistance. J Pediatr 1978;93:662–666.
62. Hood JL, Cross A, Hulka B, Lawson EE: Effectiveness of the neonatal transport team. Crit Care Med 1983;11:419–423.
63. Ehrenwerth J, Sorbo S, Hackel A: Transport of critically ill adults. Crit Care Med 1986;14:543–547.
64. Black RE, Mayer T, Walker ML et al.: Air transport of pediatric emergency cases. N Engl J Med 1982;307:1465–1468.
65. Birnbaum ML: Prehospital and interhospital transport of adults. In: Shoemaker WC, Ayers S, Grenvik A, et al. (eds). Textbook of critical care. 4th ed. Philadelphia: W. B. Saunders Company, 1989: 69–82.
66. Smith JP, Bodai BI, Hill AS, et al.: Prehospital stabilization of critically injured patients: A failed concept. J Trauma 1985;25:65–70.
67. Eggold R: Trauma care regionalization: A necessity. J Trauma 1983; 23:260–262.
68. Von Wagoner FH: Died in-hospital: A three year study of deaths following trauma. J Trauma 1961;1:401.
69. Ramenofsky ML, Luterman A, Quindlen E, Riddick L, Curreri PW: Maximum survival in pediatric trauma: The ideal system. J Trauma 1984;24:818–823.
70. West JG, Cales RH, Gazzangia AB: Impact of regionalization: The Orange County experience. Arch Surg 1983;118:740–744.
71. Ramenofsky ML, Luterman A, Curreri PW, Talley MA: EMS for pediatrics: Optimum treatment or unnecessary delay? J Pediatr Surg 1983;18:498–504.
72. Cowley RS, Hudson F, Scanlan E, et al.: An economical and proved helicopter program for transporting the emergency critically ill and injured patient in Maryland. J Trauma 1973;13:1029–1038.
73. Hunt RC, Bryan DM, Brinkley VS, Whitley TW, Benson NH: Inability

to assess breath sounds during air medical transport by helicopter. JAMA 1991;265:1982–1984.
74. Collett H: 1991 transport charge survey. The Journal of Air Medical Transport 1991:17.
75. Federal Aviation Regulations/Airman's Information Manual: Part 91.17. Renton, Washington: Aviation Supplies and Academics, 1991:19.
76. McCloskey KA, Johnston C: Pediatric critical care transport survey: Team composition and training, mobilization time, and mode of transportation. Pediatr Emerg Care 1990;6:1–3.
77. Insel J, Weissman C, Kemper M, Askanazi J, Hyman AI: Cardiovascular changes during transport of critically ill and postoperative patients. Crit Care Med 1986;14:539–542.
78. Indeck M, Peterson S, Smith J, Brotman S: Risk, cost, and benefit of transporting ICU patients for special studies. J Trauma 1988;28:1020–1025.
79. Waddell G: Movement of critically ill patients within hospital. Br Med J 1975;2:417–419.

Developmental Physiology of the Respiratory System

4

Mark A. Helfaer
David G. Nichols
Mark C. Rogers

GENERAL CONSIDERATIONS

Introduction

Respiratory failure accounts for 50% of intensive care unit admissions for children[1]. Since the precise incidence of respiratory failure in infants and children is unknown, the magnitude of this problem can be inferred only by examining death rates for those diseases associated with respiratory failure. Data from the National Center for Health Statistics show that all respiratory disorders are the second most common cause of death in infants with congenital anomalies[2]. The third most common cause of infant mortality is sudden infant death syndrome. Close inspection of the subcategories of other causes of death reveal that many of the fatalities probably were caused by major injury to the respiratory system, such as burns, drowning, and suffocation[2]. Thus, the management of respiratory failure is likely to remain a great challenge for the pediatric intensivist both because of the large numbers of patients involved and because of the wide array of diseases that may lead to respiratory failure. It is necessary for the clinician to identify those elements of the respiratory system that have become dysfunctional, leading to respiratory failure in the patient. The clinician caring for children must also appreciate the many developmental changes occurring in the respiratory system of the infant and child. A more specific therapeutic regimen may then be chosen based on the knowledge of respiratory physiology and of the developmental stage of the patient. Therefore, this chapter discusses respiratory physiology with particular emphasis on those developmental changes that put the pediatric patient at risk for respiratory failure.

Definition of Respiratory Failure

Whatever the cause, the final common pathway in respiratory failure is the inability of the respiratory system to meet the metabolic demands of the body for oxygenation and carbon dioxide excretion. Although signs and symptoms of respiratory distress often accompany respiratory failure, this is not invariably so, and arterial blood gas measurement is required to verify inadequate oxygenation and carbon dioxide excretion. For instance, patients with respiratory center depression from drug overdose may present with few clinical signs of respiratory distress but significant laboratory evidence of hypoxemia, hypercarbia, and acidosis.

There are instances in which only clinical observation over a period of time, coupled with serial blood gas measurements, will adequately define respiratory failure. The asthmatic patient with large alveolar dead space is an example. Such a patient might present with moderate respiratory distress, markedly increased minute ventilation, and hypocapnia. With time, respiratory distress may worsen; however, minute ventilation cannot be increased further, and PCO_2 rises. In this context, a "normal" PCO_2 would be considered evidence of impending respiratory failure.

Disturbance in acid-base homeostasis is one of the consequences of inadequate oxygenation and/or carbon dioxide excretion. Although the presence of acidosis is not essential for the fulfillment of respiratory failure criteria, acid-base determinations will assist in defining the duration, cause, and therapy of respiratory failure.

Complete characterization of an acid-base disorder includes a notation of *(a)* its separate components (respiratory and metabolic), *(b)* the degree of compensation (pH in the normal range), and *(c)* whether the process is acute or chronic. Normal blood gas and acid-base values are given in **Table 4.1.** Based on this notation, most cases of untreated respiratory failure with an acid-base disorder fall into one of three categories: acute uncompensated respiratory acidosis, chronic (partially) compensated respiratory acidosis, and acute mixed (respiratory and metabolic) uncompensated acidosis. The patient with a pH less than 7.35 to 7.40 due exclusively to an elevated PCO_2 has an acute uncompensated respiratory acidosis. Conversely, chronic hypoventilation may be inferred if time has allowed renal compensatory mechanisms to raise serum bicarbonate concentration, thus restoring pH close to normal in spite of persistently elevated PCO_2. An acute uncompensated mixed acidosis is present in the respiratory failure patient with hypercapnia and a deficit in buffer base (mainly bicarbonate) in the blood. The base deficit usually results from inadequate oxygen delivery to peripheral tissues, with resultant anaerobic metabolism and lactic acid production.

Classification of Respiratory Failure

Respiratory failure is classified according to both anatomic and physiologic considerations **(Table 4.2).** The anatomic elements that make up the respiratory system fall into two broad categories: the lungs and the "respiratory pump," consisting of the nervous system, respiratory muscles, and thorax.

The lungs are made up of conducting airways, alveoli, and pulmonary circulation; and their principal function is to exchange oxygen (O_2) and carbon dioxide (CO_2) across the alveolar-capillary membrane. Therefore, whenever lung disease leads to respiratory failure, gas exchange has been disturbed in some way. In the great majority of patients, this disturbance in gas exchange involves an alteration in the normal distribution of ventilation ($\dot{V}$) and perfusion ($\dot{Q}$) in the lung. All such patients are hypoxic, while PCO_2 remains normal or low initially. The pathophysiologic mechanisms responsible for $\dot{V}/\dot{Q}$ mismatching and intrapulmonary shunting of blood are discussed below in the subsections on alveolar ventilation, pulmonary circulation, and matching of ventilation to perfusion. Once pulmonary capillary blood has successfully been oxygenated, it must be transported to peripheral tissues to support tissue respiration. These issues are discussed in the subsections on transport of oxygen in blood and tissue respiration.

The respiratory pump consists of the nervous system, respiratory muscles, and thorax. The purpose of the pump is to ventilate the lungs. In response to chemical (rising PCO_2 and falling PO_2) and reflex stimuli, the respiratory centers in the brainstem signal the respiratory muscles to contract. Phrenic and intercostal nerves convey this signal from the central nervous system to the respiratory muscles. Contraction of respiratory muscles enlarges the thorax and thereby lowers pleural pressure, resulting in a pressure gradient favoring gas flow into the lungs. Exhalation occurs

Table 4.1. Normal Mean Arterial Blood Gas Values at 37°C[a]

	Newborn (age 24 hr)	*Infant (1–24 mo)*	*Child (7–19 yr)*	*Adult*
pH	7.37	7.40	7.39	7.40
P_aO_2	70	90	96	100
P_aCO_2	33	34	37	40
BE (mEq/liter)	−6.0	−3.0	−2.0	0.0
HCO_3 (mEq/liter)	20	20	22	24

[a] Data are combined from:
Koch G, Wendel H. Biol Neonate 1968;12:136.
Albert MS, Winters RW. Pediatrics 1966;37:728.
Levison H, Featherby EA, Weng TR. Am Rev Respir Dis 1970;101:972.
Comroe JH. Physiology of respiration. 2nd ed. Chicago: Year Book Medical Publishers, 1974.
Downes JJ. Unpublished data.

passively through elastic recoil. Any dysfunction in elements of the respiratory pump leads to hypoventilation and hypercarbia, which is the hallmark of respiratory failure from pump dysfunction. Hypoxia is usually also present because increased alveolar CO_2 dilutes available O_2 in the lungs. These issues are discussed in the subsection on the respiratory pump.

GAS EXCHANGE

Introduction

The purpose of the lung is to exchange O_2 and CO_2 across the alveolar-capillary membrane. Inspired gas containing O_2 must reach individual alveoli in quantities that match the volume of blood being distributed to pulmonary capillaries. Finally, the alveolar-capillary membrane must permit the transfer of gases while restricting the movement of fluid from pulmonary vasculature to alveoli. The developmental anatomy and physiology of these processes are detailed.

Table 4.2. Classification of Respiratory Failure

Site of abnormality	*Representative diseases*
Lung	
Central airway obstruction	Tracheomalacia
	Subglottic stenosis
	Epiglottis
	Croup
	Vocal cord paralysis
	Foreign body aspiration
	Vascular ring
	Adenotonsillar hypertrophy
	Near-strangulation
Peripheral airway obstruction	Bronchiolitis
	Asthma
	Aspiration
	Cystic fibrosis
	Bronchomalacia
Diffuse alveolar damage (adult respiratory distress syndrome)	Sepsis
	Pneumonia
	Pulmonary edema
	Near-drowning
	Pulmonary embolism
	Lung contusion
	Shock
Respiratory pump	
Chest wall deformity	Kyphoscoliosis
	Diaphragmatic hernia
	Flail chest
	Eventration of diaphragm
	Prune belly syndrome
Brainstem	Sleep apnea
	Poisoning
	Trauma
	Central nervous system infection
Spinal cord	Trauma
	Poliomyelitis
	Werdnig-Hoffmann disease
Phrenic/intercostal nerve palsy	Postoperative nerve injury
	Birth trauma
	Infantile botulism

Alveolar Ventilation

Developmental Anatomy

Conducting airways make up that portion of the lung that is lined by ciliated epithelium. During the embryonic period of intrauterine growth, the airways first appear as an outpouching of the ventral surface of the primitive foregut. Ultimately, the conducting airways extend from the trachea to the respiratory bronchiole, which opens up into the gas-exchanging region of the lung lined by alveolar-type epithelium. Analysis of the structural and functional properties of the airway is of great clinical importance because peripheral airway disease represents a common form of respiratory illness in infancy[3]. The branching of the conducting airway system occurs during the pseudoglandular stage of lung development, between the 4th and 16th week of gestation[4]. Intrauterine growth of the conducting airways may be inhibited by a diaphragmatic hernia. The resulting lung hypoplasia leads to severe respiratory distress at birth[5]. Even after successful repair of the diaphragmatic hernia at birth, prognosis for survival remains grave because postnatal branching of the airways cannot occur, and lung hypoplasia remains irreversible.

The airway enlarges in diameter and length with age[6]. However, it appears that growth of the distal airway lags behind that of the proximal airway during the first 5 years of life[7]. The relatively narrow distal airway until age 5 years presumably accounts for the high peripheral airway resistance in this age group. Resistance to flow is inversely related to the fourth power of the radius (Poiseuille's law): therefore, a small decrement in caliber of the infant's airway from inflammation or edema may lead to a very large increase in peripheral airway resistance. This phenomenon explains why viral infections of the lower airway pose a greater threat to infants and young children[7].

Cartilaginous support is essential for the stability of conducting airways from the trachea down to the level of segmental bronchi. Cartilage will have spread to its most distal point, the segmental bronchus, by the 12th week of gestation[8]. After birth, cartilage increases in number until 2 months of age and then increases in total area throughout the remainder of childhood[6, 9]. The relative weakness of cartilaginous support in infants compared with that in adults may lead to dynamic compression of the trachea in situations associated with high expiratory flow rates and increased airway resistance, such as bronchiolitis, asthma, or even crying. The transmural pressure of the intrathoracic trachea decreases during forced expiration and is the principal cause of the observed dynamic compression[10] (see subsection on sites of increased airway resistance).

After birth, there is a dramatic increase in the number of alveoli[11]. The future generations of alveoli develop from the 20 million alveolar saccules present at birth[12]. By age

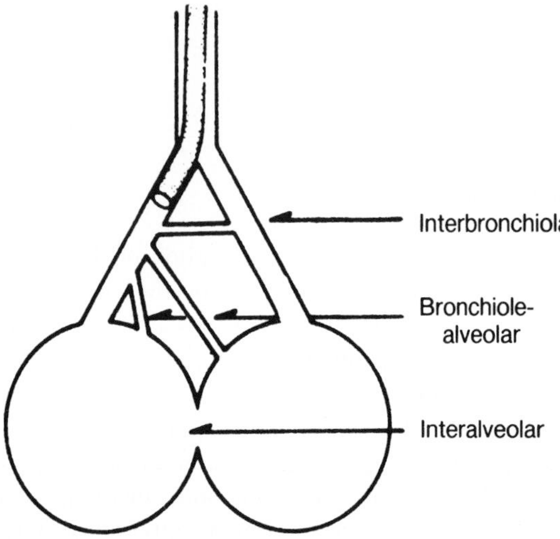

Figure 4.1. Pathways for collateral ventilation. Anatomic evidence of collateral ventilation is not found until after infancy. (From Menkes HA, Traystman RJ. Collateral ventilation. Am Rev Respir Dis 1977;116:287.)

8 years, 300 million alveoli have developed[11]. It remains unclear whether alveolar multiplication continues beyond that age or whether further lung growth is solely due to enlarged alveolar size[13].

Although alveolar multiplication is the predominant mechanism for lung growth, increases in the size of individual alveoli are also a contributing factor. The average diameter of an alveolus is 150–180 μm at age 2 months. By adulthood, the average diameter of the alveolus has enlarged to 250–300 μm[11]. The smaller alveolar size of the infant is a liability because it predisposes the infant to alveolar collapse (see subsection on alveolar elasticity and surfactant).

The tremendous expansion in alveolar number and dimensions results in a steady increase in alveolar surface area during childhood. At birth, the alveolar surface area is 2.8 m^2[11]. By 8 years of age, the child has an alveolar surface area of 32 m^2, whereas the adult alveolar surface area is 75 m^2[11]. Although surface area is only one of several factors that determine diffusing capacity of O_2 across the alveolar-capillary membrane, it is noteworthy that the infant's diffusing capacity is only one-third to one-half that of the adult's, even when normalized to body surface area[14].

The adult lung contains anatomic channels that allow ventilation distal to an obstructed airway or "collateral ventilation." Three types of pathways have been described (Fig. 4.1): *(a)* interalveolar (pores of Kohn), *(b)* bronchiole-alveolar (Lambert's channel), and *(c)* interbronchiolar. Although collateral ventilation in newborns has been suggested based on roentgenographic evidence[15], no anatomic pathways for collateral ventilation have been identified in histologic sectioning of an infant lung. Therefore, it is generally assumed that collateral ventilation does not develop until after infancy. The pores of Kohn appear as holes in alveolar walls, thus allowing interalveolar communication. They first appear sometime between the first and second years of life[16]. Lambert's channels provide communication between bronchiole and adjacent alveolus beginning at age 6 years[17]. Interbronchiolar channels have not been found in healthy human lungs; however, they may develop during disease[16]. Without pathways for collateral ventilation, the infant and young child are presumably at increased risk for atelectasis or emphysematous changes and consequent ventilation/perfusion mismatching.

During the stage of development of the airways and alveoli, the infant respiratory system is handicapped in many ways; nevertheless, there is a distinct advantage in continued alveolar development. Should a disease process result in destruction of a portion of the infant's lung, its surface area will expand for gas exchange with time. Comparable lung destruction in the adult is unlikely to lead to as much compensatory growth as is found in the infant[18].

Distribution of Inspired Gas

This subsection outlines the factors governing distribution of inspired gas so as to understand how deviation from the ideal matching of ventilation to pulmonary perfusion occurs. The first part of this discussion is a review of the fact that a variable portion of each breath never reaches the gas-exchanging units of the lung. This volume of gas is, therefore, "wasted" or considered dead space ventilation.

Dead Space Ventilation

Dead space ($\dot{V}_D$) is partitioned into two components: anatomic dead space and alveolar dead space. Anatomic dead space represents that volume of gas within the conducting airways, which by definition cannot participate in gas exchange. In the normal lung, the anatomic dead space is approximately 1 ml per pound of body weight. The volume of the anatomic dead space may also be calculated if the concentrations of alveolar (end-expiratory or end-tidal) CO_2 (F_ACO_2) and mixed expired CO_2 (F_ECO_2) are measured and the concentration of CO_2 in dead space (F_DCO_2) is assumed to be zero. By employing the argument originally developed by Bohr, the total volume of CO_2 expired equals the sum of the volume of CO_2 in the dead space and the alveoli, or

$$F_ECO_2\,\dot{V}_E = F_DCO_2\,\dot{V}_D + F_ACO_2\,\dot{V}_A \quad \text{(Eq. 4.1)}$$

where $\dot{V}_E$ is the expired minute ventilation and $\dot{V}_A$ is the alveolar ventilation. Since $F_DCO_2\,\dot{V}_D$ equals zero and $\dot{V}_A$ equals $\dot{V}_E$ minus $\dot{V}_D$, then

$$F_ECO_2\,\dot{V}_E = F_ACO_2\,(\dot{V}_E - \dot{V}_D) \quad \text{(Eq. 4.1}A\text{)}$$
$$F_ACO_2\,\dot{V}_D = (F_ACO_2 - F_ECO_2)\dot{V}_E \quad \text{(Eq. 4.1}B\text{)}$$

solving for the dead space ventilation:

$$\dot{V}_D = (F_ACO_2 - F_ECO_2)\,\dot{V}_E/F_ACO_2 \quad \text{(Eq. 4.2)}$$

The alveolar dead space is that volume of inspired gas that passes through the conducting airways to reach alveoli but does not participate in gas exchange because of inadequate perfusion to the involved alveoli. The mechanisms governing pulmonary perfusion are discussed in greater detail in the subsection on pulmonary circulation. The major causes of inadequate pulmonary perfusion are hypotension, decreased cardiac output, obliteration of pulmonary vasculature in certain lung diseases, and pulmonary embolus.

The volume of the alveolar dead space gas can be estimated by comparing arterial PCO_2 (P_aCO_2) and end-tidal (end-expiratory) PCO_2. The following assumptions are made [19]. After exhalation of apparatus and anatomic dead space gas, the final portion of the expirate consists of a mixture of "ideal" alveolar gas, which has participated in gas exchange, and alveolar dead space gas, which has not. The PCO_2 of the "ideal" alveolar gas will be lowered whenever it is diluted with alveolar dead space gas containing virtually no CO_2. The PCO_2 of "ideal" alveolar gas is assumed to be the same as P_aCO_2 because there is no gradient between alveolar PCO_2 and pulmonary capillary PCO_2. Furthermore, pulmonary capillary PCO_2 is the same as P_aCO_2 because the gradient between mixed venous PCO_2 (P_vCO_2) and P_aCO_2 (46–40 mm Hg) is so small that any venous admixture would have only a negligible effect. If, for instance, the P_aCO_2 is 40 mm Hg and the end-tidal PCO_2 is 20 mm Hg, the "ideal" alveolar gas in the expirate has been diluted by an equal volume of alveolar dead space gas.

The total (anatomic and alveolar) dead space is also termed physiologic dead space. The Bohr equation (Eq. 4.2) may be used to calculate the physiologic dead space by simply substituting P_aCO_2 for the end-expired values. As noted above, the discrepancy between P_aCO_2 and end-expired CO_2 occurs only if alveolar dead space gas is present in addition to anatomic dead space gas. Therefore,

$$\dot{V}_D \text{ (physiologic)} = (P_aCO_2 - P_ECO_2)\dot{V}_E/P_aCO_2 \quad \text{(Eq. 4.3)}$$

The alveolar dead space may then be calculated, since

$$V_D \text{ (alveolar)} = V_D \text{ (physiologic)} - V_D \text{ (anatomic)} \quad \text{(Eq. 4.4)}$$

Similarly, $V_D/V_T = 1 - P_E\ CO_2/P_A\ CO_2$

It is customary to express V_D (physiologic) as a fraction of the tidal volume (V_T) or V_D/V_T. The normal V_D/V_T ratio is approximately 0.3 in infants and adults[20]. Patients with respiratory failure have elevated V_D/V_T ratios, which leads to hypoxia and hypercarbia unless counteracted by an increased $\dot{V}_E$. This concept is considered again in the subsections on matching of ventilation to perfusion and respiratory pump, effects of hypoventilation.

Effect of Pleural Pressure on Gas Distribution

Among the factors that govern the distribution of inspired gas, changes in pleural pressure are paramount. During spontaneous breathing, a greater proportion of gas is directed to dependent regions of the lung[21]. Although the precise mechanisms are unclear, it is assumed that gravitational force creates a less subatmospheric (negative) intrapleural pressure (P_{pl}) at the base than at the apex of the lung. Alveolar pressure (P_A) remains constant in all lung regions. Therefore, the transpulmonary distending pressure ($P_A - P_{pl}$) is reduced in dependent portions of the lung. A reduced transpulmonary distending pressure implies a reduced lung volume for these dependent regions. These smaller alveoli in dependent portions of the lung lie on a steeper part of the curve relating transpulmonary pressure to lung volume, and a given transpulmonary pressure change results in a greater change in alveolar volume (Fig. 4.2). Consequently, a greater portion of the tidal volume goes to dependent alveoli during normal breathing, with inspiration beginning at functional residual capacity (FRC). This is fortunate because the greater portion of pulmonary blood flow also goes to dependent lung regions. Thus, ventilation and perfusion are matched more closely.

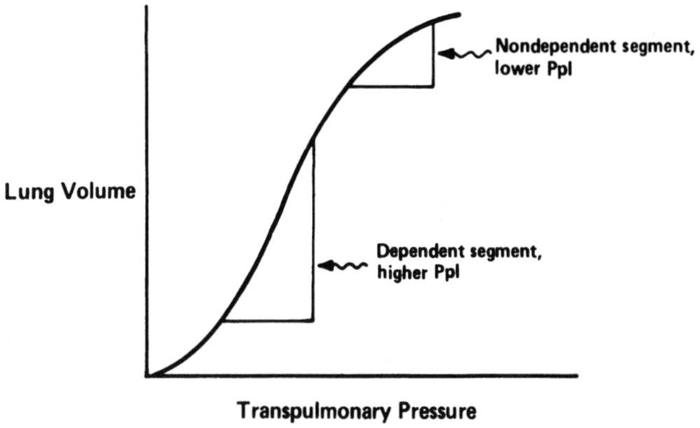

Figure 4.2. Effect of changes in pleural pressure from the apex to the base of the lung. Pleural pressure increases from the apex to the base of the lung. With the increase in pleural pressure, alveoli become smaller at the base. Smaller alveoli are on the steep portion of the pressure-volume (compliance) curve, and thus a given change in transpulmonary pressure produces a greater increase in volume in the smaller alveoli. (Modified from Benumof J. Respiratory physiology and respiratory function during anesthesia. In: Miller RD, ed. Anesthesia. New York: Churchill Livingstone, 1981:683.)

However, it is possible for lung volumes to be so reduced below FRC that small alveoli and airways in dependent regions of the lung are "closed." The lung volume at which this occurs has been termed "closing capacity." The relationship between FRC and closing capacity determines to a large extent the matching of ventilation to perfusion and, thus, the P_aO_2[22]. It is important to examine this relationship because much of pediatric respiratory disease may be viewed as an alteration of FRC, closing capacity, or both.

FRC represents the volume of gas remaining in the normal lung at the end of expiration during tidal breathing. It is also the sum of expiratory reserve volume and residual volume (Fig. 4.3). The FRC serves as a source of oxygen during expiration until the lungs can be reinflated with the next breath. Therefore, major changes in alveolar PO_2 are buffered. FRC is a physiologic capacity. In normal lung it is the same as end expiratory lung volume (EELV). In diseased lung EELV is greater or less than FRC. When we say "FRC is increased" we mean EELV is greater than FRC. When EELV is greater or less than FRC compliance, elasticity and PVR are abnormal. In lung diseases (e.g., ARDS), when EELV is less than FRC, intrapulmonary shunt is increased and compliance decreased. In the extreme example, if the lungs were so severely damaged that EELV approaches zero, alveolar PO_2 would approach the mixed venous PO_2.

The closing capacity is defined as the sum of closing volume and residual volume (Fig. 4.3). The significance of the closing volume is appreciated by reviewing how this measurement is obtained.

Through inhalation of a tracer gas (e.g., xenon) or dilution of a resident gas (e.g., nitrogen), it is possible to label nondependent regions of the lung(23). After expiration to residual volume, airways to dependent lobes tend to close because gravitational forces produce a higher pressure surrounding those lobes. Pressure surrounding airways is approximated closely by the intrapleural pressure. The raised Ppl in dependent areas of the lung leads to a lower airway transmural pressure (transmural pressure equals pressure within airways minus pressure surrounding airways). With inspiration from residual volume during the next breath, gas containing the tracer travels first to the only open alveoli, namely those in nondependent regions. With full inspiration from residual volume, gas in nondependent lobes have a higher tracer concentration than gas in dependent parts of the lung. Finally, the patient is asked to expire from total lung capacity. When the dependent airways begin to close during this expiration, there is a sudden increase in concentration of tracer emanating from open nondependent lung segments. The absolute volume above residual volume at which tracer concentration suddenly increases (phase IV) is the closing volume (Fig. 4.4).

When closing capacity exceeds FRC, some lung segments are closed during a portion of tidal breathing. As a result, the ventilation/perfusion ratio decreases such that hypoxia may ensue. When closing capacity exceeds FRC and tidal volume, those lung segments will be closed dur-

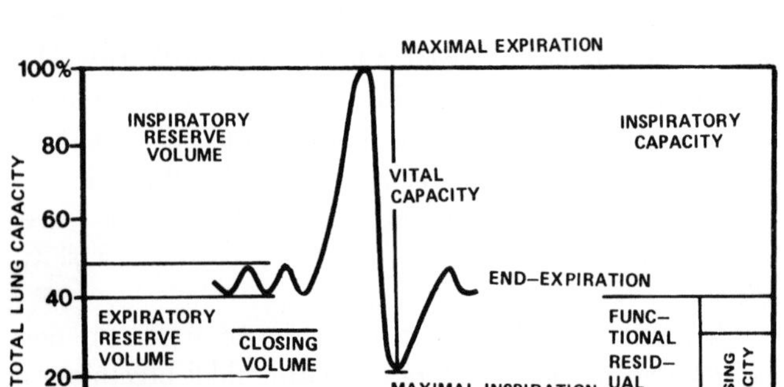

Figure 4.3. Typical spirogram showing tidal breathing followed by maximal inspiration and then maximal expiration. Standard lung volumes are shown. (From Smith CA, Nelson NM. The physiology of the newborn infant. Springfield, Illinois: Charles C Thomas Publishers, 1976:206.)

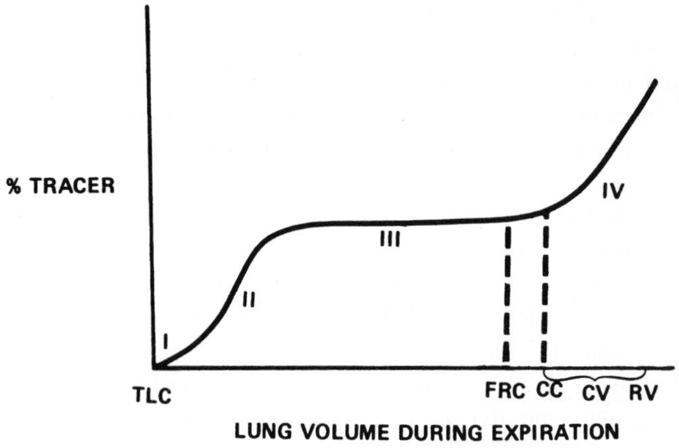

Figure 4.4. Demonstration of closing volume by recording change in concentration of exhaled tracer gas. The subject inhales tracer gas from residual volume *(RV)*, which preferentially goes to nondependent lung segments. During expiration from total lung capacity *(TLC)*, tracer concentration suddenly rises (phase IV) when dependent airways close at closing volume *(CV)*. Note that closing capacity *(CC)* equals closing volume plus residual volume.

ing both inspiration and expiration of tidal breathing. This represents complete atelectasis and shunt. The use of end-expiratory pressure, whether positive end-expiratory pressure (PEEP) or continuous positive airway pressure (CPAP), increases EELV above closing capacity in diseases associated with alveolar collapse. Shunt is decreased and compliance improved.

Children younger than 6 years and adults older than 40 years have a closing capacity greater than FRC when they are in the supine position(24). Zapletal et al.(25) suggested that the relatively high closing capacity in these two age groups is due to reduced elastic recoil of the lung. Elastic recoil is that property of the lung that causes it to retract away from the chest wall, creating a subatmospheric pressure in the intrapleural space. When elastic recoil is reduced, the subatmospheric pressure in the intrapleural space is raised, leading to airway closure in dependent regions of the lung. Developmental changes in elastic tissue may explain the differences in elastic recoil with age. Since elastic tissue increases with age(26), it is not surprising that elastic recoil of the lung should also increase with age.

Since the chest wall of the newborn is very compliant, lung volume in the completely relaxed state (allowing full passive recoil of the respiratory system) is 10–15% of the total lung capacity as compared with that of the adult, which is 30–35% of total lung capacity. The FRC of full-term infants, however, is maintained at a higher lung volume by a mechanism known as expiratory braking. This expiratory braking mechanism is an active process whereby upper airway resistance is increased during expiration, thus increasing end-expiratory lung volumes(27). These mechanisms are arousal and age dependent. Premature infants may lack this mechanism, and they may further diminish expiratory braking during active sleep(28). This may exaggerate the loss of O_2 stores during apnea, which can, in turn, increase the degree of desaturation associated with expiratory apnea of the newborn. These mechanisms are also bypassed when anesthesia is induced and FRC is decreased (which can be reversed by the administration of PEEP). By the use of a single breath washout technique, FRC in anesthetized children has been related to weight and height:

$$\text{FRC (ml)} = .00175 \times \text{height (cm)}^{2.66}$$

or

$$\text{FRC (ml)} = 9.51 \times \text{weight (kg)}^{1.31}$$

The FRC was 17 ± 1.4 ml/kg in infants less than 1 year of age and 24 ± 1.6 ml/kg in children more than 1 year of age. These results were not different from children with cardiac anomalies[(29)].

In addition to expiratory abnormalities in the immature, inspiratory pathology is also evident. During partial obstruction to inspiration, there is an inward distortion of the compliant newborn chest with an outward movement of the abdomen. This thoracoabdominal asynchrony can cause a decrease in tidal volume and minute ventilation. The severity of this pathology can be quantitated and can be used to monitor infants in the PICU[(30)].

Mechanical Properties of the Respiratory System

During breathing, the transpulmonary pressure must be generated in order to overcome the opposing forces of elastic recoil of the lungs as well as the force due to frictional resistance to gas flow. The inertial force of the respiratory system is negligible under normal circumstances and is not discussed further. The pressure gradient necessary to overcome the elastic recoil depends on tidal volume (V_T) and lung "stiffness" or compliance (C_L), while the pressure gradient required to overcome frictional forces is a function of airway resistance (R) and gas flow rate ($\dot{V}$):

$$P_{TP} = V_T/C_L + R\dot{V} \qquad \text{(Eq. 4.5)}$$

COMPLIANCE. The preceding section alluded to the relationship of changes in pressure and volume in the lung as a factor that influences distribution of inspired gas. The change in volume per unit change in pressure is termed compliance.

For gas to flow into or out of the lung, a pressure gradient must exist between the atmosphere and the alveoli. Inspiration occurs when the external force of respiratory muscle contraction enlarges the thorax and thus stretches the attached lung. As the respiratory muscles cease to contract and the external force is removed, the lung recoils to its rest position. Since the lung is an elastic tissue, it obeys Hooke's law such that a force (or pressure change) produces a proportional change in distance (or volume). Compliance refers to the proportionality constant of the pressure-volume relationship:

$$\Delta V/\Delta P = \text{compliance} \qquad \text{(Eq. 4.6)}$$

In practice, lung compliance is measured under static conditions (i.e., zero airflow) by determining intrapleural pressure via an esophageal balloon at the end of an inspiration of a preset volume. The procedure is repeated at different inspired volumes. Thus a curve may be constructed relating lung volume (V) to the change in the alveolar-to-intrapleural pressure gradient (i.e., the transpulmonary pressure, P_{TP}). The slope of that curve is the lung compliance (Fig. 4.5). The flatter the curve becomes, the "stiffer" is the lung

$$\text{Lung compliance} = \Delta V/\Delta P_{TP} \qquad \text{(Eq. 4.6}A\text{)}$$

Lung compliance depends not only on the elasticity of lung tissue but also on the initial lung volume before inflation. Greater pressure gradients must be generated in order to inflate a lung from a very low lung volume. Therefore, a comparison of lung compliance in different age groups requires that compliance be referenced to a specific lung volume. The specific compliance is lung compliance divided by FRC. Values for newborn and adult specific compliances are in close agreement[(14)].

In addition to lung compliance, chest wall compliance (C_{CW}) and total respiratory system compliance (C_T) may be determined by inserting the appropriate transmural pressure gradient into the denominator of Equation 4.5 (Fig. 4.5) such that

$$C_{CW} = V/(P_{ambient} - P_{pl}) \qquad \text{(Eq. 4.7)}$$

and

$$C_T = V/(P_A - P_{ambient}) \qquad \text{(Eq. 4.8)}$$

Since the reciprocals of compliance are additive according to the equation,

$$1/C_T = 1/C_{CW} + 1/C_L \qquad \text{(Eq. 4.9)}$$

chest wall compliance can also be derived by subtracting lung compliance from total compliance. The important developmental aspects of chest wall mechanics are discussed in the subsection on chest wall mechanics and respiratory muscle function.

RESISTANCE TO GAS FLOW. Changes in airway resistance play a major role in many pediatric pulmonary diseases, such as croup, bronchiolitis, and asthma. It is therefore necessary to understand the laws governing resistance to flow of gas through airways.

Gas flows through a tube from a point of higher pressure to a point of lower pressure. The magnitude of the pressure drop and its relationship to the gas flow rate ($\dot{V}$) depend on the pattern of flow. Two flow patterns have been recognized: laminar and turbulent.

When gas progresses down a tube in parallel, concentric layers at less than a certain critical velocity, the pattern is called laminar. The pressure drop (P) required to produce laminar flow is given by the Hagen-Poiseuille equation,

$$P = \dot{V}8nl/\pi r^4 \qquad \text{(Eq. 4.10)}$$

where l is the length of the tube, n is a viscosity coefficient of the gas, $\dot{V}$ is the gas flow rate, and r is the radius of the

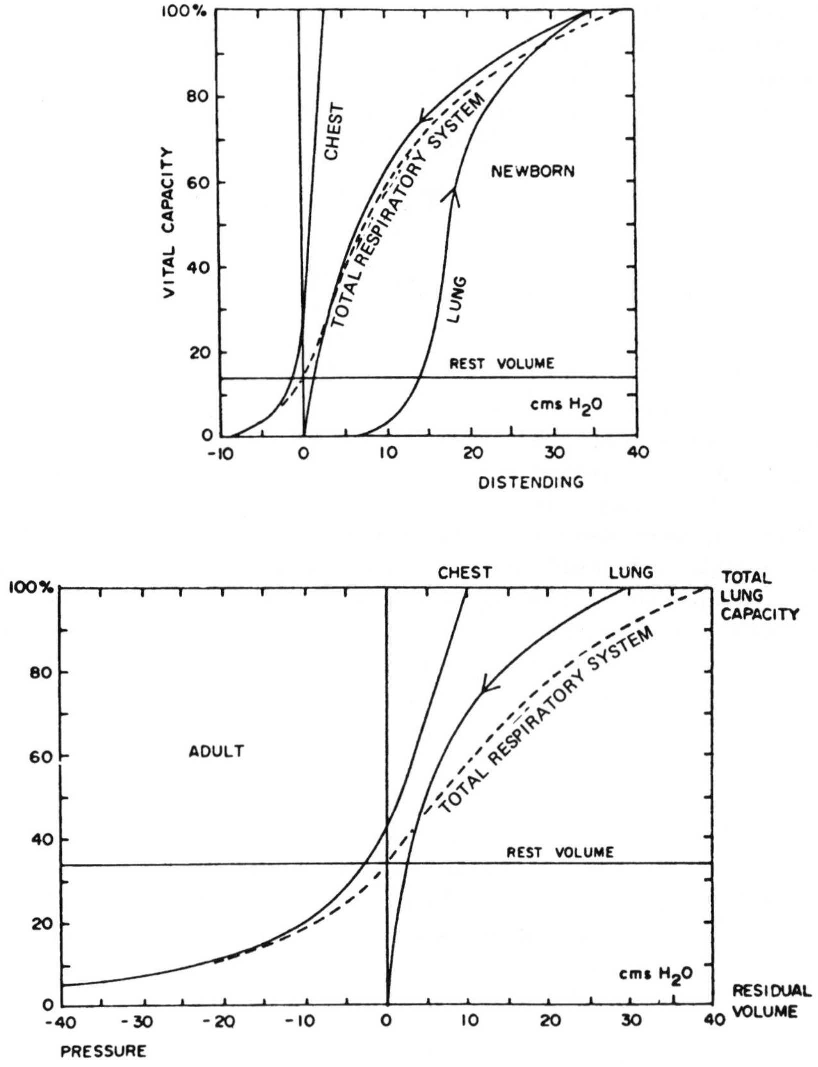

Figure 4.5. Static pressure-volume (compliance) curves of the newborn and the adult. (From Smith CA, Nelson NM. The physiology of the newborn infant. Springfield, Illinois: Charles C Thomas Publishers, 1976:205.)

tube. By rearranging terms, it can be seen that resistance is primarily determined by the radius of the tube during laminar flow:

$$\text{Resistance} = P/\dot{V} = 8nl/\pi r^4 \qquad \text{(Eq. 4.11)}$$

Laminar flow ceases and becomes turbulent when the gas flow rate rises excessively or when the angle or diameter of the tube changes abruptly, such as at branch points. Turbulent flow differs from laminar flow in that the pressure drop required to maintain turbulent air flow is proportional to the square of the gas flow rate and to the density of the gas instead of the viscosity. In such diseases as croup, a turbulent airflow pattern occurs because of the sudden constriction of the airway at the subglottis. According to Poiseuille's law, the same degree of subglottic narrowing in the infant as in the adult results in a much greater increase in the infant's airway resistance in absolute terms. Attempts have been made to take advantage of the proportionality between gas density and resistance in turbulent flow by allowing patients with croup to breathe a helium-oxygen mixture that has a lower density than air-oxygen[31].

Although the infant's resistance to airflow is much higher in absolute terms than that of the adult, the infant is required to move less gas at lower velocities. The ease of gas flow is expressed as the reciprocal of resistance and is termed conductance. Conductance referenced to lung volume is "specific" conductance, which is quite similar in adults and infants[32].

SITES OF INCREASED AIRWAY RESISTANCE. Adults differ from children in the site of the major contribution to the total airflow resistance. The upper airway, particularly the nose, accounts for the major portion of total resistance in the adult. Conversely, Hogg et al.[33] showed that peripheral airway resistance in children younger than 5 years is approximately four times higher than in adults or older children. Presumably, this observation explains the high incidence of lower airway obstructive disease in young children. Similar degrees of lower airway inflammation would not be sufficient to produce symptoms in the adult because normal peripheral airway resistance is much lower in the adult.

In pathologic states, airway resistance is elevated either by obstruction from within the lumen or by external com-

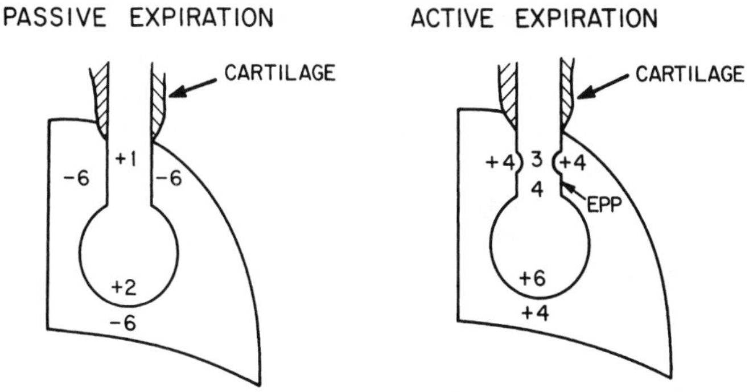

Figure 4.6. Dynamic compression of airways during forced expiration. Intrapleural pressure becomes positive during forced expiration. At the equal pressure point *(EPP)*, the transmural pressure gradient across the airway is zero.

pression or contraction of the walls of the airway. Collapse of the airway during forced expiration is an example of dynamic compression produced by an external force. Peripheral airways are held open by the tethering action of the three-dimensional elastic mesh of the pulmonary parenchyma and by the transmural pressure gradient in which the intraluminal airway pressure is greater than the intrapleural pressure. The patency of larger intrathoracic airways is again secured by a favorable transmural pressure gradient and, in addition, by cartilaginous support. During forced expiration, the favorable transmural pressure gradient is lost, and airway collapse occurs through the following mechanism (Fig. 4.6). Even normal expiration is associated with a pressure drop from alveolus to mouth in order for airflow to take place. However, as intraluminal pressure falls, it still remains higher than the normally subatmospheric pressure surrounding the airway (i.e., intrapleural pressure). Therefore, a distending transmural pressure is maintained during normal expiration. Conversely, forced expiration significantly raises intrapleural pressure, which is transmitted to the alveoli. Elastic recoil pressure from the pulmonary parenchyma raises alveolar pressure even further, so that the transmural pressure across the alveoli and distal airways is favorable initially. However, because an intraluminal pressure drop must again occur from alveolus to mouth, a point along the airway will be reached where intraluminal pressure just equals intrapleural pressure. This point is called the equal pressure point. As gas moves further toward the mouth, the forces favoring airway patency (tethering action of parenchyma and rigidity of cartilage) are overwhelmed by the now unfavorable transmural pressure gradient. Thus, the airway will collapse. Airway collapse is even more likely to occur if the elastic meshwork of the pulmonary parenchyma is destroyed, as in bronchopulmonary dysplasia[34] and α_1-antitrypsin deficiency[35], or if the cartilaginous support is relatively weak, as in tracheomalacia.

TIME CONSTANTS—COMBINED EFFECT OF RESISTANCE AND COMPLIANCE. The time needed for a lung unit to fill is given by the product of resistance (R) and compliance (C) and is called the time constant (TC):

$$\text{TC (sec)} = \text{R } H_2O/(l/sec) \cdot \text{C } (l/cm\ H_2O) \quad \text{(Eq. 4.12)}$$

The time constant is the time needed for the lung unit to reach 63% of its final volume. Alveoli with shorter time constants fill faster than those with longer ones. The concept of the time constant illuminates the effect of varying resistances and compliances on the distribution of inspired gas.

If R and C are identical in two adjacent lung units, then the time constant will be the same, and no gas will be redistributed from one lung unit to the other (Fig. 4.7). Suppose the time constant of lung unit A is now lengthened by doubling its resistance relative to lung unit B. As the compliances in A and B are equal, they will ultimately attain the same volume. However, it will take lung unit A much longer to do so because its resistance is higher. Lung unit A is, therefore, a "slow" unit. If inflation of A and B were interrupted prematurely, the fast lung unit B would already have a greater volume than A. The higher volume in B than A for equivalent compliances implies that intraluminal pressure in B is also higher (P = V/C). Therefore, gas from

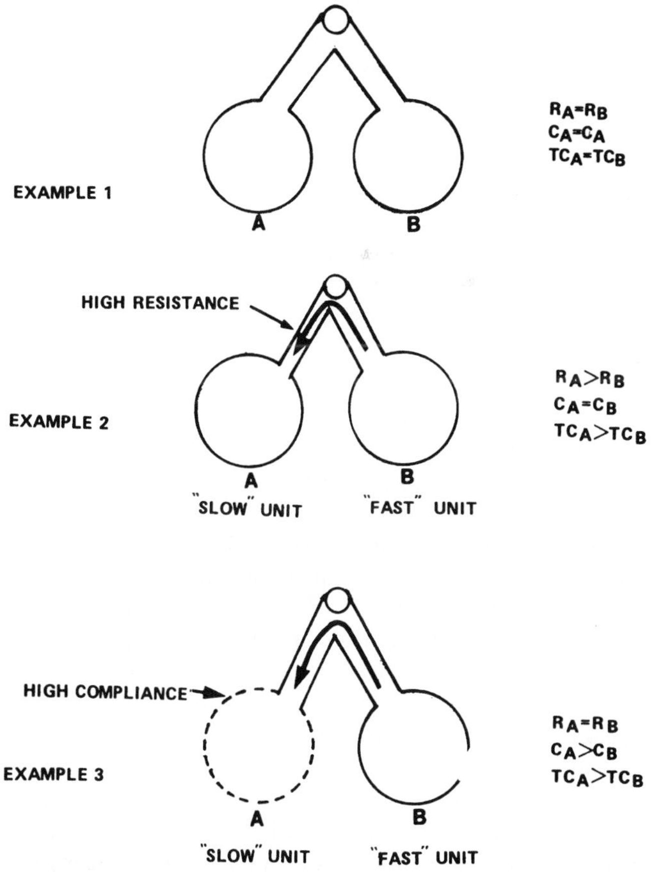

Figure 4.7. Effect of changes in resistance and compliance on distribution of gas between *lung units A* and *B*. In *example 1*, the resistances *(R)* and compliances *(C)*, and thus the time constants *(TC)* of *A* and *B*, are equal, and no redistribution of gas occurs if inspiration ends before the lung units are filled to maximal capacity. In *examples 2* and *3*, *lung unit B* has a shorter time constant. If inspiration ends prematurely, gas will be redistributed from *B* to *A (arrows)*.

B will be redistributed to A. A third example: imagine that the time constant of A is lengthened by increasing its compliance relative to B, while the resistances remained equal. Now, A is again a "slow" lung unit and B a "fast" one. The less compliant lung unit B will never inflate to as great a volume as A. If inflation is again interrupted prematurely, the pressure within the less compliant (but faster) lung unit B will exceed that of A, and gas will be redistributed to A.

ALVEOLAR ELASTICITY AND SURFACTANT. Although the time dependence of elastic properties of the lung does allow for some redistribution of gas between alveoli, this effect is not predominant. In fact, normal lung units are relatively stable and do not change much in size. This observation was somewhat paradoxical because alveoli were known to have a certain surface tension in which intermolecular forces align to create the smallest possible surface area at the gas-liquid interface, just as in a bubble. The Laplace equation gives the relationship between distending pressure (P), surface tension (T), and radius (r):

$$P = 2T/r \qquad \text{(Eq. 4.13)}$$

This equation predicts that small alveoli empty into larger ones, resulting in the ultimate collapse of small alveoli and the overdistention of large alveoli. The paradox was resolved with the discovery of a surface-active material (surfactant)[36]. Surfactant lines the walls of alveoli and promotes alveolar stability by varying surface tension. When alveoli are decreased in size, surface tension falls so that the distending pressure P required to maintain patency is also reduced. The primary chemical constituent of surfactant is a phospholipid, dipalmitoyl lecithin, which is produced by type II alveolar pneumocytes where it is stored within lamellated bodies. It is first detectable at approximately the 21st week of gestation. Phosphatidylcholine content of the surfactant increases, and an increasing proportion of the phosphatidylcholine becomes saturated with more than 60% being saturated at full term[37]. The mature lung contains more phoshatidylglycerol and less phosphatidylinositol[38]. Surfactant protein mRNA levels for surfactant protein (SP) increase throughout development. Specifically, SP-A increases late in gestation, though little is known about SP-B and SP-C[39]. When separating the surfactant from the alveolar space ultraheavy, heavy, and light subtypes can be fractionated by sucrose density gradients. The heavy subtype contains the greatest quantity of the surfactant proteins. The light subtype does not function as surfactant and is contained in small vesicles[40]. The quantity of surfactant increases with age in response to plasma beta agonists and stretch[41]. At birth, all of the surfactant in the airways is the heavy-subtype, which converts into the light-subtype. This conversion plateaus at 7 hours of life when the mature ratios exist (60% heavy-subtype and 40% light-subtype)[42]. Alveolar collapse occurs in a number of lung diseases, resulting at least in part from surfactant deficiency. The classic example of such a disease is respiratory distress syndrome of the newborn[43], which occurs in about 1% of deliveries annually. As expected for a developmental abnormality, the incidence of respiratory distress syndrome is dependent on gestational age. At 28 weeks gestation, the incidence is 50–60%, whereas respiratory distress syndrome rarely occurs at term. In the preterm lung there not only is a decreased pool of surfactant, but there is also diminished function of the heavy-subtype. Further, there is an increase in the conversion of the heavy-subtype to the inactive light-subtype[44]. All of these factors contribute to the respiratory distress of the preterm child.

Surfactant synthesis also depends on normal pH and pulmonary perfusion; therefore, it is not surprising that other diseases may exhibit surfactant deficiency. Examples include hemorrhagic shock[45] and pulmonary edema[46].

Exogenous surfactant replacement has proved effective in preventing or ameliorating respiratory distress syndrome in the premature infant[47]. In contrast, the adult respiratory distress syndrome (ARDS), which may be associated with permeability pulmonary edema and hemorrhagic shock, cannot be cured with surfactant replacement therapy, in part because surfactant is inactivated by plasma proteins, all membrane lipids, and hemoglobin (see Chapter 9 on the adult respiratory distress syndrome)[48, 49].

Other aspects of developmental physiology besides surfactant have been postulated to contribute to the greater susceptibility of newborn lungs. Specifically, newborn lungs have less catalase activity which implies that a greater amount of hydrogen peroxide is not scavenged and can cause greater tissue damage (in the presence of oxygen) compared with older lungs [50].

Pulmonary Circulation

Just as alveolar ventilation depends on the development and function of airways and alveoli, the developmental anatomy and physiology of the pulmonary circulation have important consequences on gas exchange. In fact, lung growth is determined in large measure by adequate blood flow to the lungs[51].

Developmental Anatomy

The developmental features of the pulmonary circulation have been described by Reid[52] and Hislop and Reid[53]. Two main themes emerge from their studies:

1. Development of pulmonary vasculature closely follows development of airways and alveoli.
2. During development, there is remodeling of the muscular wall of the pulmonary arterial tree.

Preacinar arteries develop in utero along with conducting airways. Restriction of thoracic space from congenital diaphragmatic hernia not only leads to alveolar and airway hypoplasia but also limits pulmonary vascular development and contributes to pulmonary hypertension[5].

In addition to preacinar arteries, which branch along with airways, the preacinar region also contains many extra arteries that do not travel with airways. These "supernumerary" arteries reach the pulmonary capillary bed via a more direct route than preacinar arteries. Their probable function is to provide a "collateral" circulation analogous to collateral ventilation in the airways.

The arterial tree undergoes complex remodeling changes in the more peripheral regions of the pulmonary circulation. This fetal remodeling of the pulmonary vasculature follows changes in wall stress[54]. Proper description of these processes requires that they be considered in terms both of changing wall thickness of the artery and of the position of the muscular artery in relation to the acinus.

Muscular arteries extend all the way out to the pleural surface in the adult. This is not the case in the fetus and newborn (Fig. 4.8), in whom muscular arteries end at the level of the terminal bronchiole and thus are removed from the gas-exchanging unit. During childhood, muscular arteries gradually extend to reach the alveolar level. The change from muscular to nonmuscular arteries is not consistently related to the size of the artery. Although the pulmonary arteries of the newborn and the adult have approximately the same muscle content for a given size, much larger arteries are devoid of muscle in the child. It was once thought that insoluble elastin, once laid down in its extracellular, cross-linked form, turns over very slowly. For instance, the half-life of aortic elastin has been postulated to be measured in years. On the contrary, the efficiency of incorporation of newly synthesized elastin and collagen in growing animals may be underestimated. Therefore, remodeling may take place and affect the final pathologic processes in lung[55].

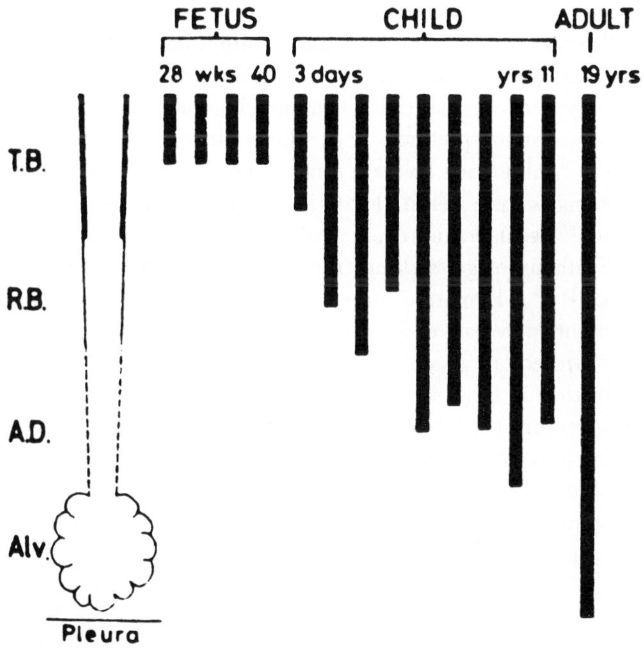

Figure 4.8. Age-related distribution of muscular pulmonary arteries. With advancing age, muscular pulmonary arteries extend further toward the alveolus. *T.B.*, terminal bronchiole; *R.B.*, respiratory bronchiole; *A.D.*, alveolar duct; *Alv.*, alveolus. (From Reid LM. The pulmonary circulation: remodeling in growth and disease. Am Rev Respir Dis 1979;119:531.)

Pulmonary vascular muscle thickness seems to be a function of gestational age and blood flow. Children with long-standing pulmonary hypertension from congenital heart disease will have a significant increase in smooth muscles in their pulmonary arteries[56]. Prematurely born infants have less well-developed vascular smooth muscle, which regresses more quickly after birth than that of the term infant. Incomplete development and earlier regression of pulmonary arterial smooth muscle produces an earlier drop in pulmonary vascular resistance (PVR) in the premature infant after birth. Consequently, onset of congestive heart failure from a left-to-right shunting can be expected earlier in the premature than the term infant.

Pulmonary Blood Volume

The lungs receive the entire cardiac output, which is appropriate for an organ involved in gas exchange. In addition to the blood volume ejected by the right ventricle into the pulmonary artery, blood flows through the bronchial circulation (approximately 1% of cardiac output), which starts at the arch of the aorta and supplies the pulmonary parenchyma with oxygenated blood. Anastomoses exist between the bronchial and pulmonary circulations[57]. Under conditions of decreased pulmonary artery perfusion, bronchial anastomoses dilate and accept a greater fraction of the cardiac output.

Posture is the major determinant of pulmonary blood volume. Pulmonary blood volume is increased in the supine position, presumably because of a shift of blood from dependent portions of the body to the central circulation. The blood volume shift may be transient, so that during prolonged recumbency the pulmonary blood volume returns to normal or even below-normal levels[58].

Pulmonary Vascular Pressures and Resistance

Three different types of pressures are associated with pulmonary circulation, and precision is necessary in defining which pulmonary vascular pressure applies.

Intravascular Pressure

Intravascular pressure is measured by placing a catheter in the pulmonary artery and measuring pressure referenced to atmospheric pressure at heart level. Systolic, diastolic, and mean arterial pressures are obtained and are analogous to blood pressure measured in the systemic circulation. Immediately after birth, pulmonary artery pressure falls as the lungs are inflated[59]. Within the first few months of life, average adult values for pulmonary artery pressure of 22/8/15 mm Hg (systolic/diastolic/mean) are found.

The driving or perfusion pressure is the pressure gradient between a point upstream in the circulation and a point downstream in the circulation. This pressure gradient is necessary for blood to flow. In the pulmonary circulation, the pressure gradient is usually measured between pulmonary artery (P_{PA}) and left atrium (P_{LA}). Therefore,

$$\text{Driving pressure} = P_{PA} - P_{LA} \quad \text{(Eq. 4.14)}$$

A balloon-tipped catheter (e.g., Swan-Ganz) may be wedged in a pulmonary artery branch, and the pulmonary capillary wedge pressure can be used as an approximation of left atrial pressure, provided there is no pulmonary venous obstruction. There are situations in which left atrial pressure does not represent the true downstream pressure. Apical (nondependent) lung regions may experience an alveolar pressure (P_A) that is greater than P_{LA} (particularly during positive pressure ventilation). Under these circumstances,

$$\text{Driving pressure} = P_{PA} - P_A \quad \text{(Eq. 4.15)}$$

The effects of such changes in downstream pressure on distribution of pulmonary blood flow are discussed below in the subsection on normal distribution of pulmonary blood flow.

The PVR is the driving pressure divided by the pulmonary blood flow ($\dot{Q}$), or

$$\text{PVR} = (\text{mean } P_{PA} - \text{mean } P_{LA})/\dot{Q} \quad \text{(Eq. 4.16)}$$

An increase in pulmonary blood flow (as with exercise or inotropic drugs) produces a drop in the calculated resistance across pulmonary circulation, as shown in the above equation. Such a fall in PVR is due to the recruitment of additional, previously closed pulmonary capillaries, such that the total cross-sectional area of the pulmonary circulation is increased.

The transmural pressure (P_{TM}) is the pressure inside the vessel minus the pressure outside the vessel or, in the case of pulmonary arteries, the gradient between pulmonary artery pressure and pleural pressure:

$$P_{TM} = P_{PA} - P_{PL} \quad \text{(Eq. 4.17)}$$

The pressure outside of pulmonary capillaries is more difficult to define and probably lies between the pleural pressure and alveolar pressure. The larger the transmural pressure, the more distended is the vessel, and therefore, the greater will be the flow. The capillary transmural pressure gradient supplies the hydrostatic force, which would tend to drive fluid into the pulmonary interstitium were it not opposed by the oncotic pressure (see below).

Normal Distribution of Pulmonary Blood Flow

Appreciation of these different pulmonary vascular pressures allows an understanding of how pulmonary blood flow is distributed. Pulmonary perfusion is distributed according to gravitational forces, such that the most blood travels to dependent regions of the lung (Fig. 4.9). The vertical hydrostatic gradient in the lung requires the expenditure of kinetic energy from the right ventricle for blood to flow up to the pulmonary artery. At some point within the apex of the lung, the alveolar pressure (P_A) is greater than the pulmonary artery pressure (P_{PA}) and much greater than the pulmonary venous pressure (P_V). The pulmonary vessels collapse; pulmonary blood flow and, consequently, gas exchange cease. Ventilation to this region is "wasted." West et al.[60] termed this region "zone 1."

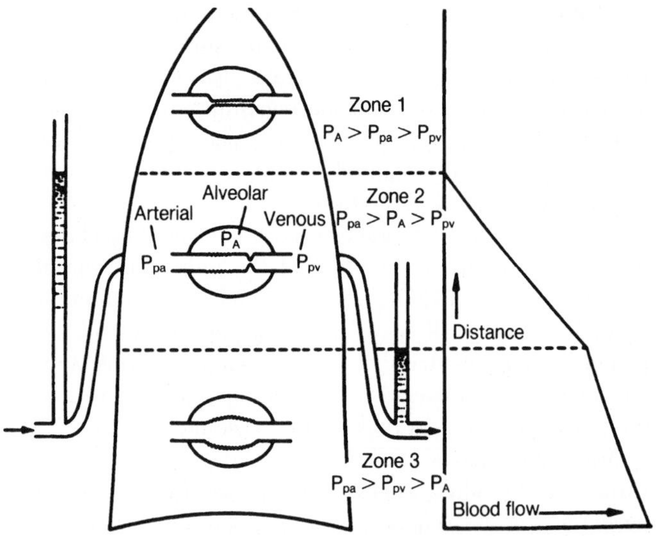

Figure 4.9. Normal distribution of pulmonary blood flow. Gravitational force makes flow greatest in the base. At the apex *(zone 1)*, there is no flow because alveolar pressure *(P_A)* exceeds pulmonary arterial *(P_{PA})* and venous *(P_V)* pressures. Flow begins in *zone 2* and is determined by the *P_{PA}-P_A* driving pressure gradient. In *zone 3*, vessels dilate because of an increased transmural pressure *(P_{PA}-P_{PL}* and *P_V-P_{PL})*. Therefore, flow increases even though driving pressure *(P_{PA}-P_V)* is constant throughout *zone 3*. (From West JB, Dollery CT, Naimark A. Distribution of blood flow in isolated lung: relation to vascular and alveolar pressures. J Appl Physiol 1964;19:713.)

Further down the lung (zone 2), blood flows once P_{PA} exceeds P_A. Flow rate increases linearly as the $P_{PA} - P_A$ gradient increases down the lung, until pulmonary venous pressure equals alveolar pressure.

In zone 3, P_{PA} and P_V are both greater than P_A. The driving pressure ($P_{PA} - P_V$) is constant throughout zone 3 because gravity produces equal increases in P_{PA} and P_V in the more dependent regions of zone 3. However, pleural pressure does not increase as much as either P_{PA} or P_V, moving further down the lung in zone 3. Therefore, the transmural pressures ($P_{PA} - P_{PL}$ and $P_V - P_{PL}$) are increased in the more dependent regions of the lung. With increased transmural pressures, vessels are dilated and flow increases in the more dependent regions of zone 3, even though driving pressure remains constant.

The above model of zones of the lung is based on the study of adults in the upright position. Although the distribution of pulmonary perfusion in infants lying supine has not been studied, it is reasonable to assume that the general features of gravity-dependent distribution of flow still apply. However, because the height of the lung is reduced in the supine position, gravity-related differences in distribution of flow are probably less pronounced. It is doubtful that the infant lying supine experiences regions of the lung that are truly unperfused (zone 1).

Abnormal Distribution of Pulmonary Blood Flow

A number of factors cause the pattern of pulmonary perfusion to deviate from the normal pattern given by West's zones of the lung. Hypoxia, age, sex, certain diseases, and various chemical mediators may all alter the pattern of pulmonary perfusion.

Alveolar hypoxia causes pulmonary vasoconstriction, called hypoxic pulmonary vasoconstriction (HPV)[61, 62]. HPV may involve the entire lung or only localized regions of the lung, depending on whether there is diffuse or regional alveolar hypoxia[63]. Inhalation of a hypoxic gas mixture produces whole-lung HPV and an increase in intravascular pulmonary artery pressure. Reduction of PVR with the onset of breathing allows pulmonary blood to flow through a previously underperfused lung. This is mediated by a stimulation of pulmonary vascular prostacyclin synthesis[64]. This physiologic mechanism is age dependent, and indomethacin reverses the age-dependent attenuation of hypoxic vasoconstriction in neonatal lambs[65]. HPV increases as a function of postnatal age in infants, and the infant HPV response is more dramatic than the adult response[61, 66]. If the newborn's circulation is still in a transitional state, the elevated pulmonary artery pressure may produce right-to-left shunting through a patent ductus arteriosus or foramen ovale with resultant severe arterial desaturation.

Driving (perfusion) pressure increases much more than flow in whole-lung HPV: therefore, pulmonary vascular resistance must rise significantly. The right heart must work harder to overcome this increase in resistance. The anatomic changes that result are again exaggerated in the newborn and infant. Newborns who live at high altitudes and, therefore, are chronically hypoxic have persistent right ventricular hypertrophy. By 1 month of age, the walls of pulmonary arteries have thickened abnormally, and muscle has extended into smaller vessels[67]. Animal studies have shown that after the hypoxic environment is removed, the immature animal is left with greater residual pulmonary hypertension than is the adult animal[68]. These experimental results are consistent with the finding of pulmonary hypertension and right heart failure in infants with severe bronchopulmonary dysplasia who are chronically hypoxic [69–71].

Regional HPV from localized alveolar hypoxia usually does not raise pulmonary artery pressure. Rather, the localized vasoconstriction redistributes blood to normoxic areas of the lung with lower vascular resistance. Thus, regional HPV represents a protective mechanism that favors better matching of ventilation to perfusion.

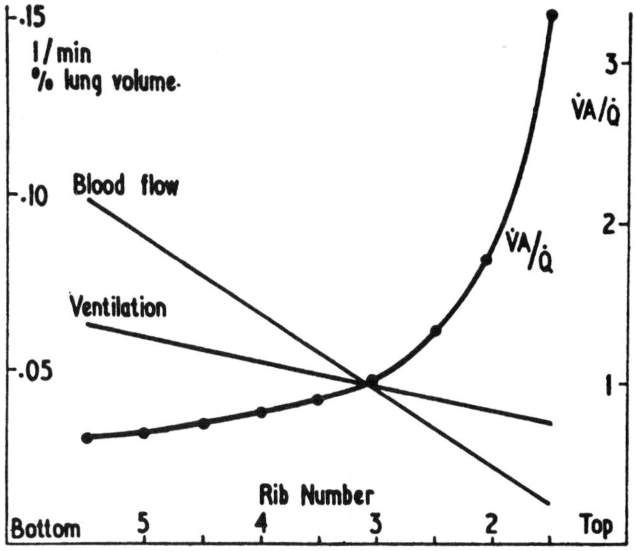

Figure 4.10. Distribution of ventilation, pulmonary blood flow, and ventilation/perfusion ratio according to location between apex and base within the upright lung. (From West JB. Ventilation/blood flow and gas exchange. 2nd ed. Oxford: Blackwell Scientific, 1970:33.)

Matching of Ventilation ($\dot{V}$) to Perfusion ($\dot{Q}$)

Concept of $\dot{V}/\dot{Q}$ Ratio

Matching of ventilation to perfusion depends to a large extent on gravity. Ventilation and perfusion both rise with increasing distance down the lung; however, perfusion increases more than ventilation (Fig. 4.10). Thus, apical regions of the lung are underperfused ($\dot{V}/\dot{Q}$ = 3), while basal regions are somewhat underventilated in relation to perfusion ($\dot{V}/\dot{Q}$ = 0.6).

Effect of $\dot{V}/\dot{Q}$ Mismatching on O_2

Definitions

In the discussion that follows, the terms *venous admixture* and *shunt* are used. Confusion is avoided by adhering to strict definitions of these terms.

Shunt (also called anatomic shunt) refers to venous blood that has traveled from the right side of the circulation to the left side without coming in contact with the ventilated lung. Therefore, the $\dot{V}/\dot{Q}$ ratio for a shunt is zero. Examples of shunt include the normal bronchial and Thebesian circulations, blood flow through completely atelectatic lung segments, and cyanotic congenital heart disease with blood flow directly from the right side of the heart to the left side.

Venous admixture is the amount of venous blood that would have to be added to arterial (actually pulmonary end-capillary) blood to produce the observed arterial oxygen content. Venous admixture does not imply any anatomic pathway of the circulation; rather, it is strictly a calculated value. The actual anatomic pathways leading to the deposition of desaturated blood into the arterial side of the cir-

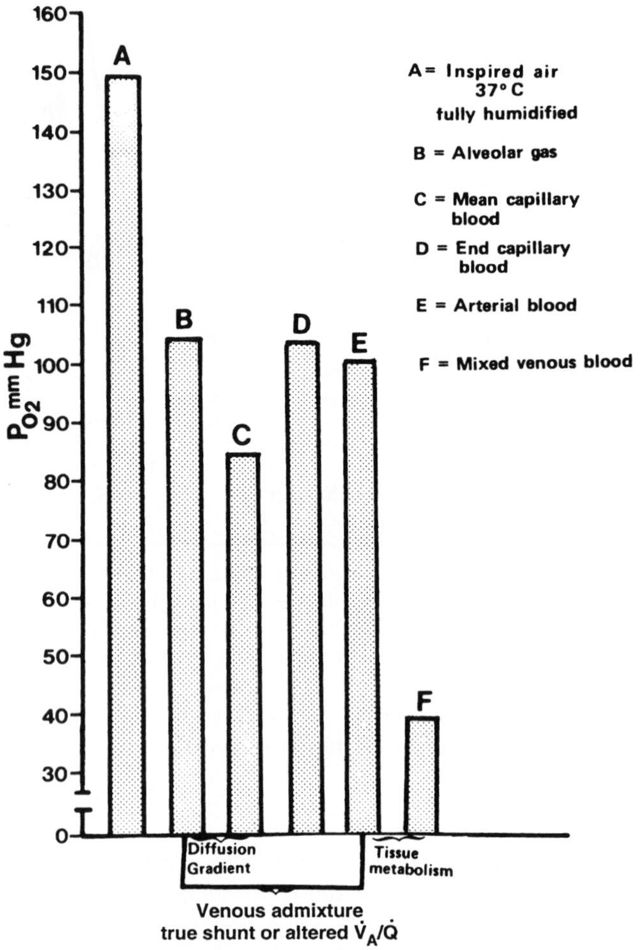

Figure 4.11. Oxygen cascade showing PO_2 at different sites in the lung, blood, and peripheral tissue. (Modified from O'Brodovich HM, Chernick V. The functional basis of respiratory pathology. In: Kendig EL, Chernick V, eds. Disorders of the respiratory tract in children. Philadelphia: WB Saunders, 1983:25.)

culation may include true anatomic shunts and/or blood flow through areas of the lung with low but finite $\dot{V}/\dot{Q}$ ratios.

Oxygen Cascade

There is a normal stepwise decrease in oxygen tension from the level of inspired gas to the level of the arterial circulation (Fig. 4.11). The changes in oxygen tension between inspired gas and alveolar gas are predicted by Dalton's law, which states that the total pressure exerted by a gas mixture is equal to the sum of the pressures of the individual gases. The total pressure of the gas mixture is the barometric pressure (P_B, approximately 760 mm Hg). The partial pressure of inspired O_2 is the product of the fractional concentration of O_2 (F_IO_2) and P_B. Since the inspired gas is diluted with water vapor in the upper airway and with CO_2 in the alveoli, the alveolar PO_2 is reduced by the amounts of the partial pressures of water vapor and CO_2. The final step in deriving the alveolar air equation takes into account that usually more O_2 is consumed than CO_2 is produced. Therefore, the alveolar CO_2 is corrected by the respiratory exchange ratio (R), where

$$R = CO_2 \text{ production}/O_2 \text{ consumption} \qquad (\text{Eq. } 4.17A)$$

Thus, the alveolar air equation may be written as

$$P_AO_2 = P_IO_2 - (P_aCO_2/R) \qquad (\text{Eq. } 4.18)$$

where P_AO_2 is the alveolar PO_2, P_IO_2 is the inspired PO_2, P_aCO_2 is the arterial PCO_2, and R is the respiratory quotient. This simplified form of the alveolar air equation makes two assumptions:

1. There are no differences in inspired and expired gas volumes, which is true only if R equals 1.
2. There is no inert gas exchange.

A more general form of the alveolar air equation that does not depend on these assumptions may be written as follows:

$$P_AO_2 = P_IO_2 - P_aCO_2\,(P_IO_2\text{-}P_EO_2/P_ECO_2) \qquad (\text{Eq. } 4.19)$$

where P_EO_2 is the end-expiratory PO_2.

Once the factors that influence the alveolar PO_2 have been established, it is apparent that the arterial PO_2 is always lower than the corresponding alveolar value. This alveolar-arterial PO_2 difference ($AaDO_2$) is due to imperfect matching of ventilation to perfusion, i.e., venous admixture. Under normal circumstances, the relatively small $AaDO_2$ is due to an anatomic shunt through bronchial and Thebesian circulations. The hypoxemic patient may have additional anatomic shunts (cyanotic congenital heart disease) or increased $\dot{V}/\dot{Q}$ mismatching, leading to increased venous admixture.

It is intuitively obvious that the addition of mixed venous blood to pulmonary end-capillary blood through anatomic shunts lowers the arterial PO_2 and therefore widens the $AaDO_2$. $\dot{V}/\dot{Q}$ mismatching also lowers arterial PO_2 for two reasons: First, more blood flows through low $\dot{V}/\dot{Q}$ segments than through high $\dot{V}/\dot{Q}$ segments; therefore, the mixture of blood emerging in the pulmonary veins contains a larger fraction of relatively desaturated blood. Second, the sigmoidal shape of the oxyhemoglobin dissociation curve implies that alveolar PO_2 is not proportional to oxygen content or saturation (see subsection on oxyhemoglobin dissociation curve). If there is a scatter in alveolar PO_2 values around that PO_2 value at which the bend in the oxyhemoglobin dissociation curve occurs, then those low $\dot{V}/\dot{Q}$ segments with lower alveolar PO_2 values will demonstrate a proportionately greater drop in oxygen content, because they lie on the steep portion of the curve. Conversely, those high $\dot{V}/\dot{Q}$ segments with higher alveolar PO_2 values will not exhibit a commensurate increase in oxygen content, because they lie on the flat portion of the curve where changes in PO_2 have very little effect on oxygen content or saturation (Fig. 4.12). The net effect is that slightly higher oxygen contents from high $\dot{V}/\dot{Q}$ segments are unable to compensate for the significantly lower oxygen contents from low $\dot{V}/\dot{Q}$ segments, and arterial desaturation results.

The precise contribution of $\dot{V}/\dot{Q}$ mismatching to arterial desaturation is difficult to measure. Therefore, the concept of venous admixture is a convenient way to quantify the amount of mixed venous blood that would have to be added to pulmonary end-capillary blood to produce the observed arterial oxygen content. It makes the assumption that pulmonary end-capillary blood originated from two sources only: *(a)* the functioning alveoli with the same $\dot{V}/\dot{Q}$ ratio, and *(b)* the shunt. Venous admixture may then be expressed as the ratio of shunted blood ($\dot{Q}_S$) to total pulmonary blood flow ($\dot{Q}_T$). The $\dot{Q}_S/\dot{Q}_T$ ratio thus becomes a measure of the efficiency of oxygenation in the lung.

The formula for $\dot{Q}_S/\dot{Q}_T$ is derived from the law of conservation of mass. The total cardiac output is composed of shunted blood and pulmonary capillary blood flow ($\dot{Q}_c$), or

$$\dot{Q}_T = \dot{Q}_S + \dot{Q}_c \qquad \text{(Eq. 4.20)}$$

Furthermore, the total amount of oxygen ejected from the left heart each minute ($\dot{Q}_T \cdot C_aO_2$) comes from oxygen carried in pulmonary capillary blood ($\dot{Q}_c \cdot C_cO_2$) and mixed venous oxygen carried in shunted blood ($\dot{Q}_S \cdot C_vO_2$), or

$$\dot{Q}_T \cdot C_aO_2 = \dot{Q}_S \cdot C_vO_2 + \dot{Q}_c \cdot C_cO_2 \qquad \text{(Eq. 4.21)}$$

The shunt equation is arrived at by solving for $\dot{Q}_S/\dot{Q}_T$:

$$\dot{Q}_S/\dot{Q}_T = (C_cO_2 - C_aO_2)/(C_cO_2 - C_vO_2) \qquad \text{(Eq. 4.22)}$$

where C_cO_2, C_aO_2, and C_vO_2 are the pulmonary capillary, arterial, and mixed venous O_2 contents, respectively. C_aO_2

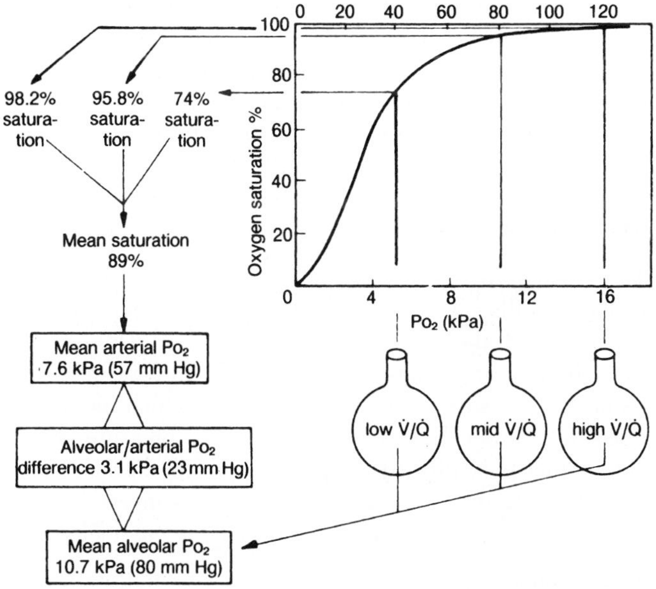

Figure 4.12. Effect of $\dot{V}/\dot{Q}$ scatter on arterial PO_2 and saturation. Three lung units with low, mid, and high $\dot{V}/\dot{Q}$ ratios and alveolar PO_2s of 40, 80, and 120 mm Hg, respectively, are depicted. Because of the shape of the oxyhemoglobin dissociation curve, the mean arterial PO_2 is only 57 mm Hg, and the mean O_2 saturation is only 89%. (From Nunn JF. Applied respiratory physiology. 2nd ed. London: Butterworths, 1977:284.)

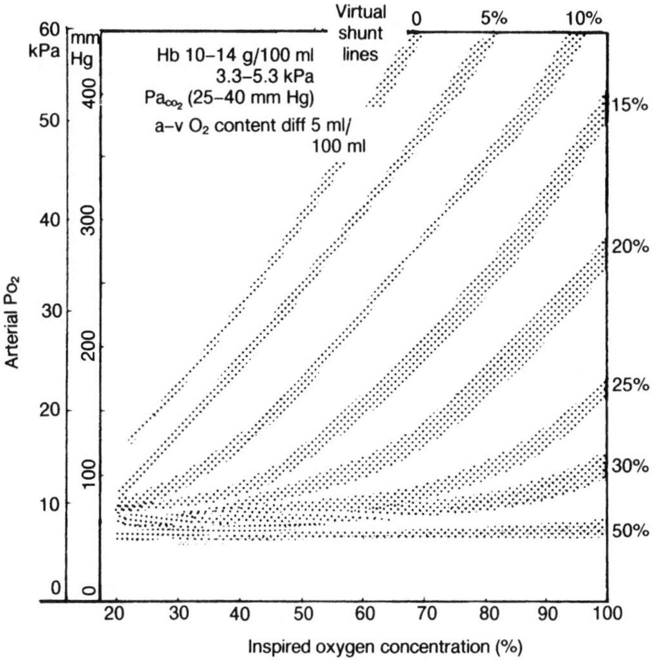

Figure 4.13. Isoshunt diagram showing the effect of F_IO_2 on arterial PO_2 for increasing fractions of shunted mixed venous blood ($\dot{Q}_S/\dot{Q}_T$). (From Benatar SR, Hewlett AM, Nunn JF. The use of isoshunt lines for control of oxygen therapy. Br J Anaesth 1973;45:711.)

and C_vO_2 are measured directly or calculated according to the formula,

$$O_2 \text{ content} = (SO_2 \cdot Hb \cdot 1.34) + (0.003 \cdot P_aO_2) \qquad \text{(Eq. 4.23)}$$

where SO_2 is the percent saturation of hemoglobin with O_2, and Hb is the hemoglobin concentration. C_cO_2 cannot be measured directly; however, it may be calculated by assuming that the pulmonary capillary PO_2 is equivalent to the alveolar PO_2.

The magnitude of $\dot{Q}_S/\dot{Q}_T$ determines in part what effect increasing F_IO_2 will have on P_aO_2 (Fig. 4.13). The isoshunt diagram reveals that if $\dot{Q}_S/\dot{Q}_T$ is 0%, the increase in F_IO_2 produces a linear increase P_aO_2. At the other extreme, an increase in F_IO_2 will have no effect on P_aO_2, with $\dot{Q}_S/\dot{Q}_T$ of 50%.

It is important to consider not only the magnitude of $\dot{Q}_S/\dot{Q}_T$ but also the O_2 content of the blood flowing through the shunt, i.e., C_vO_2. For any given $\dot{Q}_S/\dot{Q}_T$, C_aO_2 will fall if the shunted blood has become more desaturated. C_vO_2 depends primarily on oxygen consumption ($\dot{V}O_2$) and $\dot{Q}_T$, as given by the Fick equation:

$$\dot{V}O_2 = \dot{Q}_T\,(C_aO_2 - C_vO_2) \qquad \text{(Eq. 4.24)}$$

If $\dot{Q}_T$ falls while $\dot{V}O_2$ remains constant, C_vO_2 must fall. Similarly, if $\dot{V}O_2$ rises for a constant $\dot{Q}_T$, C_vO_2 will fall.

These concepts are discussed in greater detail in the sections on transport of oxygen in blood and tissue respiration.

Effect of $\dot{V}/\dot{Q}$ Mismatching on CO_2

As noted in the subsection on alveolar ventilation, P_aCO_2 is determined mainly by the degree of alveolar ventilation ($\dot{V}_A$) in relation to the patient's CO_2 production ($\dot{V}CO_2$):

$$P_aCO_2 = k(\dot{V}_A/\dot{V}CO_2) \qquad \text{(Eq. 4.25)}$$

$\dot{V}_A$ is lowered by increased alveolar dead space, which occurs when alveoli are ventilated but unperfused. This circumstance is reflected in a measured gradient between end-expiratory PCO_2 (P_ECO_2) and (mixed) alveolar PCO_2 (P_ACO_2). P_ECO_2 is lower than P_ACO_2 because of the addition of alveolar dead space gas, which does not contain CO_2.

P_ACO_2 is difficult to measure directly, and the assumption is made that P_ACO_2 is equal to P_aCO_2. This assumption is valid for the following reasons: CO_2 is quite diffusible across the alveolar-capillary membrane, such that alveolar PCO_2 and pulmonary capillary PCO_2 quickly reach equilibrium. The difference between mixed venous PCO_2 (46 mm Hg) and pulmonary end-capillary PCO_2 (40 mm Hg) is small. Consequently, even a large admixture of venous blood to the pulmonary end-capillary would produce only a small increase in arterial PCO_2. The small change in CO_2 tension occurs because in the normal range of PCO_2 values, the CO_2 dissociation curve is linear and relatively steep. Therefore, changes in CO_2 content lead to only small changes in CO_2 tension.

Developmental Differences in $\dot{V}/\dot{Q}$ Matching

The normal-term newborn exhibits a significantly lower P_aO_2 than the adult **(Table 4.1)**. This widened gradient between alveolar PO_2 and arterial PO_2 reflects increased venous admixture in the newborn, which probably arises mainly from a combination of right-to-left shunting through persistent fetal vascular channels and atelectatic areas of the lung[59, 60]. Venous admixture from low but finite $\dot{V}/\dot{Q}$ segments plays a less important role in the newborn than it does in the normal adult in whom the major component of venous admixture is due to maldistribution of ventilation and not shunt. The healthy premature infant is at even greater risk for venous admixture than the term newborn. Sometime during late infancy and early childhood, venous admixture falls to adult levels. Beyond the age of 7 years, P_aO_2 does not vary with age and remains constant at the adult value of approximately 95–100 mm Hg[72].

Alveolar-Capillary Membrane

The alveolar-capillary membrane is the physical barrier that separates alveolar gas from pulmonary capillary blood. Gases move from one side to the other through the process of diffusion. Under normal circumstances, this barrier helps prevent liquid movement from the circulation into the alveolus, thereby avoiding alveolar flooding and collapse. The purpose of this subsection is to analyze the features of the alveolar-capillary membrane as a gaseous diffusion barrier and as a fluid transfer barrier. From the clinical standpoint, "diffusion block" is rarely if ever the sole cause of significant hypoxemia. However, transudation of fluid across the alveolar-capillary membrane, with resultant pulmonary, interstitial and alveolar edema, is a major cause of respiratory failure.

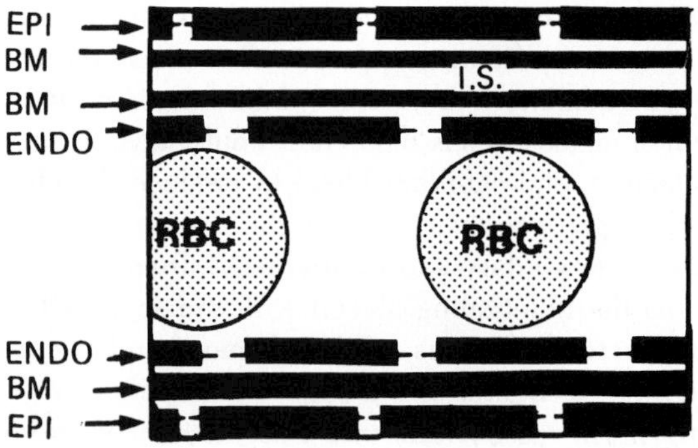

Figure 4.14. Schematic diagram of the alveolar-capillary membrane. *EPI,* epithelium; *BM,* basement membrane; *ENDO,* endothelium; *IS,* interstitial space; *RBC,* red blood cell. (From Fishman AP. Pulmonary edema: the water exchanging function of the lung. Circulation 1972;46:390.)

Schematically, the alveolar-capillary membrane consists of a thick side and a thin side (Fig. 4.14)[73]. On the thick side, the inner part of the alveolar wall is bounded by alveolar epithelial cells separated by relatively tight junctions. Immediately adjacent lies the epithelial basement membrane. Between the epithelial and endothelial basement membranes lies a widened interstitial space that contains connective tissue and lymphatic channels. The pulmonary capillary endothelium completes the alveolar-capillary membrane. Junctions between individual endothelial cells are not as tight as those between epithelial cells. The thin side of the alveolar-capillary membrane differs because of the absence of the widened interstitial space and an intimately fused common endothelial/epithelial basement membrane.

Gaseous Diffusion Barrier

The actual movement of oxygen from the alveolus to the pulmonary capillary and of CO_2 in the opposite direction proceeds through the passive process of diffusion. Diffusion is defined as the net transfer of a gas from an area in which its partial pressure is higher to an area in which its partial pressure is lower. In addition to the partial pressure gradient, diffusion is directly proportional to the surface area available and the solubility of the gas; it is inversely proportional to the length of the path that the gas molecules must traverse.

In practice, diffusion is measured by the diffusing capacity (D_L), which is analogous to conductance (reciprocal of resistance) in an electric circuit. In other words, diffusing capacity equals flow divided by driving pressure. Therefore, the diffusing capacity for oxygen (D_{LO2}) is:

$$D_{LO2} = \dot{V}O_2/(P_AO_2 - P_cO_2) \qquad \text{(Eq. 4.26)}$$

Diffusing capacity for oxygen is influenced to a large extent by the time it takes for oxygen to combine chemically with hemoglobin. This problem and a variety of technical problems are overcome by using the diffusing capacity for carbon monoxide (D_{LCO}) as a measure of alveolar-capillary membrane conductance.

Comparison of D_{LCO} in infants and children and with that in adults is complex. The differences in D_{LCO} in the various age groups primarily reflect differences in the surface area available for diffusion, which in turn is a function of the amount of ventilated and perfused lung. Results vary depending on how the quantity of ventilated and perfused lung is measured. D_{LCO} increases with age, height, and body surface area, reflecting the increase in diffusing capacity with increasing total surface area available for diffusion[74]. However, different results become evident if D_{LCO} is referenced to $\dot{V}_A$, such that

$$K_{CO} = D_{LCO}/\dot{V}_A \qquad \text{(Eq. 4.27)}$$

where K_{CO} is called the transfer factor or diffusion constant for carbon monoxide. K_{CO} decreases with age and height[75]. O'Brodovich et al.[75] reasoned that with growth, the vertical distance between the apex and base of the lung increases, thereby leading to a greater proportion of unperfused alveoli in apical lung segments (zone 1) in the upright position. Reduced capillary volume in apical regions results in diminished regional carbon monoxide uptake, which in turn lowers the overall diffusion constant for carbon monoxide.

Fluid Transfer Barrier

The pulmonary capillary membrane serves as a semipermeable barrier to retard the movement of fluid from the pulmonary capillary to the pulmonary interstitium. The rate of flow of fluid depends on the filtering properties of the membrane and on the balance of hydrostatic and oncotic pressures in the pulmonary capillary and interstitium:

$$\dot{Q} = K[(P_c - P_{is}) - (\pi_{pl} - \pi_{is})] \qquad \text{(Eq. 4.28)}$$

where $\dot{Q}$ is the filtration rate across the capillary membrane, K is the filtration coefficient that is dependent on the permeability of the membrane and its surface area, P_c and P_{is} are the capillary and interstitial hydrostatic pressures, and π_{pl} and π_{is} are the plasma and the interstitial oncotic pressure, respectively.

The hydrostatic gradient (P_c–P_{is}) tends to drive fluid into the interstitium. P_c is not amenable to direct measurement; however, its value lies in between pulmonary artery pressure and left atrial pressure. Thus, P_c can be increased by either increasing left atrial pressure (e.g., as occurs in congestive heart failure) or by increasing pulmonary artery pressure (e.g., increased pulmonary blood flow from a large left-to-right shunt). Pulmonary edema does not develop until P_c, as measured by left atrial pressure, exceeds 20 to 24 mm Hg in dogs with normal oncotic pressures[76]. Hydrostatic pressure in the interstitial space is believed to be subatmospheric under normal circumstances[77].

Fluid movement out of the pulmonary capillary into the interstitium is opposed by the force of the osmotic pressure gradient because the plasma protein concentration is greater than the interstitial protein concentration. This osmotic gradient is maintained as long as the pulmonary capillary membrane is intact and plasma protein concentration is normal. Several types of insults may disrupt alveolar-capillary membrane integrity, and the resultant pulmonary edema in the face of (initially) normal hydrostatic pressures is called "adult respiratory distress syndrome" (see Chapter 9). Hypoproteinemia alone is unlikely to cause pulmonary edema as long as the alveolar-capillary membrane is intact; however, hypoproteinemia lowers the hydrostatic pressure gradient necessary for transudation of fluid into the pulmonary interstitium.

There is some evidence for developmental differences in alveolar-capillary membrane permeability. Levine et al.[78] have shown in the dog model that more fluid accumulates in the immature lung than in the adult lung for equivalent hydrostatic filtration pressures. However, Brigham et al.[79] could not confirm these results in the sheep model. Lymphatic channels in the interstitial space clear excess interstitial fluid and protein. When this important safety mechanism is overwhelmed, edema fluid first collects in the alveolar septae and as cuffs around bronchi and pulmonary arteries[80]. Subsequently, fluid may collect in the corners of individual alveoli where curvature and surface tension are greatest (Fig. 4.15)[80].

Finally, fluid may flood an alveolus in an all-or-none manner, since microscopic observation shows completely fluid-filled alveoli adjacent to normal gas-filled alveoli or alveoli with only small amounts of fluid in the corners of their polyhedral structure. Once a small amount of fluid in the corners has decreased the radius, according to the Laplace equation, a critical surface tension will be reached at which the transpulmonary pressure is inadequate to maintain a stable and patent alveolus. The alveolus rapidly collapses to a smaller volume filled with fluid.

TRANSPORT OF OXYGEN IN BLOOD

Introduction

Oxygen reaches peripheral tissues through transport in the blood. Most oxygen in the blood is chemically combined with hemoglobin. When blood is fully saturated, 1 g of hemoglobin carries 1.34 ml of O_2, compared with only 0.003 ml per mm Hg of O_2, which can be carried as dissolved O_2 in 100 ml of plasma. It is apparent that without the affinity of O_2 for hemoglobin, cardiac output would have to increase tremendously in order to deliver sufficient quantities of O_2 to meet peripheral tissue needs.

Oxyhemoglobin Dissociation Curve

The affinity of O_2 for the hemoglobin molecule commonly is discussed in the context of the oxyhemoglobin dissociation curve, which relates oxygen tension to the percentage of hemoglobin saturation or oxygen content (Fig. 4.16). Two aspects of the dissociation curve are of interest: its shape and its position (i.e., displacement to the right or to the left).

The dissociation curve is sigmoidal in shape. At higher levels of PO_2 (greater than 50–60 mm Hg), the curve flattens and increasing PO_2 produces very little increase in saturation of hemoglobin. This upper flat portion of the curve encompasses the PO_2 range, in which O_2 binds to hemoglobin in the lungs. It is fortunate that when hemoglobin is exposed to normal alveolar PO_2 of about 100 mm Hg at sea level, it becomes 97% saturated with O_2. Even individuals living at a high altitude with an alveolar PO_2, for example, of 70 mm Hg will still achieve 94% saturation.

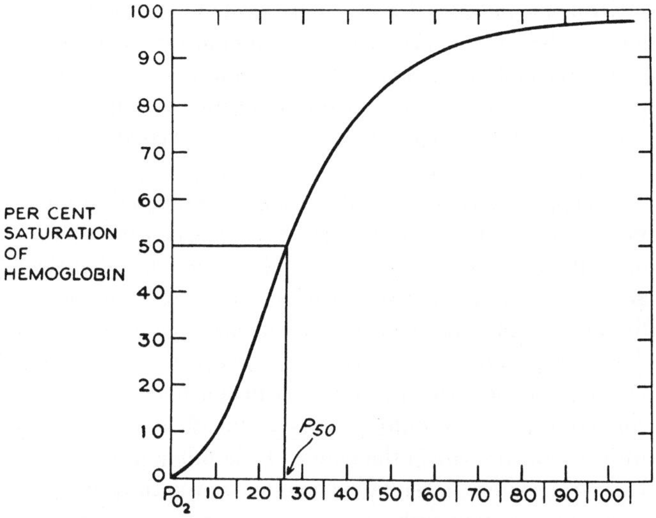

Figure 4.16. Oxyhemoglobin dissociation curve. (Modified from Comroe JC. Physiology of respiration. 2nd ed. Chicago: Year Book Medical Publishers, 1974:184.)

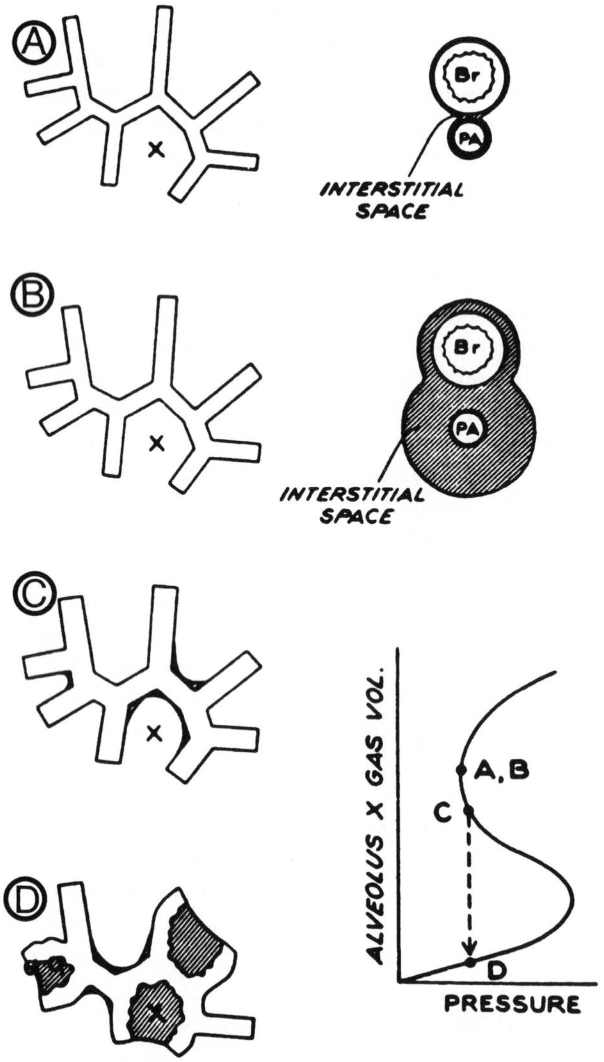

Figure 4.15. Sequence of fluid accumulation during acute pulmonary edema. **A.** Normal alveolar walls and no excess fluid in perivascular connective tissue space. **B.** Initial fluid leak with fluid cuffs in the interstitial space around vessels and bronchi. **C.** Tissue space is filled, alveolar wall edema increases, and fluid overflows into alveoli at the corners where curvature is great. **D.** Quantal filling. Individual alveoli reach critical configuration at which existing inflation pressure can no longer maintain stability. Alveolar gas volume passes to a new configuration with much reduced curvature *(inset graph)*. The volume deficit is absorbed by either fluid filling or alveolar collapse. (From Staub NC, Nagano H, Pearce ML. Pulmonary edema in dogs, especially the sequence of fluid accumulation in lungs. J Appl Physiol 1967;22:227.)

At low PO_2, the curve is steep, and small changes in PO_2 result in large changes in hemoglobin saturation. This steep lower portion of the curve encompasses the PO_2 range of tissue PO_2 (10–40 mm Hg), in which O_2 must be unloaded from hemoglobin. Because of the shape of the dissociation curve, a small drop in PO_2 allows a large quantity of O_2 to be unloaded to peripheral tissue.

The the dissociation curve may shift to the right or to the left, depending on the affinity of oxygen for the hemoglobin molecule. The PO_2 at which the hemoglobin molecule is 50% saturated (P_{50}) is used as an index of the relative position of the dissociation curve. A shift to the right of the curve (increased P_{50}) implies a lowered affinity of O_2 for hemoglobin. Conversely, a shift to the left (decreased P_{50}) means O_2 is more tightly bound to hemoglobin.

The quaternary structure of the hemoglobin molecule regulates its affinity for oxygen. Several factors may change the quaternary structure of hemoglobin and thus shift the position of the dissociation curve. These factors include primarily pH, PCO_2, and temperature.

Increased hydrogen-ion concentration shifts the dissociation curve to the right—a phenomenon known as the Bohr effect (Fig. 4.17). Elevations of temperature and PCO_2 also shift the curve to the right, such that saturation is decreased at any given PO_2. Because of the sigmoidal shape of the curve, a shift in position has little effect on saturation when the PO_2 is in the normal arterial range of 95–100 mm Hg. However, when the PO_2 is in the normal venous range of approximately 40 mm Hg, a rightward shift of the curve leads to a significantly greater decrease in saturation. Thus, unloading of O_2 to tissues occurs much more readily, while only slightly less O_2 can be loaded onto hemoglobin in the lungs. Assuming that other factors remain constant and, in particular, that a constant volume of O_2 is extracted in tissues, a rightward shift in the dissociation curve produces an increase in venous PO_2 (Fig. 4.17). Since venous PO_2 reflects tissue capillary PO_2, the net effect of the rightward shift of the curve is to improve tissue oxygenation. It is important to realize that such factors as cardiac output and O_2 consumption usually do not remain constant because pH, PCO_2, and temperature affect them at the same time that they produce a shift in the dissociation curve. Thus, in the clinical situation, the position of the dissociation curve must be considered in the context of simultaneously occurring changes in cardiac output and O_2 consumption.

Dissociation curve position also depends on hemoglobin type. Hemoglobin A, the usual adult type, consists of two α-chains and two β-chains, each of which contains a heme group with iron. Hemoglobin F is fetal hemoglobin and differs from hemoglobin A in that the two β-chains of hemoglobin A have been replaced by two γ-chains. This substitution alters the affinity of O_2 for the hemoglobin molecule. Benesch and Benesch[81] and Chanutin and Curnish[82] noted that the organic phosphate 2,3-diphospho-glycerate (DPG) regulates O_2 affinity for hemoglobin. DPG lowers hemoglobin O_2 affinity by binding either to β-chains of hemoglobin A or to γ-chains of hemoglobin F. However, the interaction of DPG and γ-chains does not lower O_2 affinity to as great an extent as the interaction of DPG with β-chains. Therefore, the fetal hemoglobin dissociation curve lies to the left of the hemoglobin A dissociation curve. The

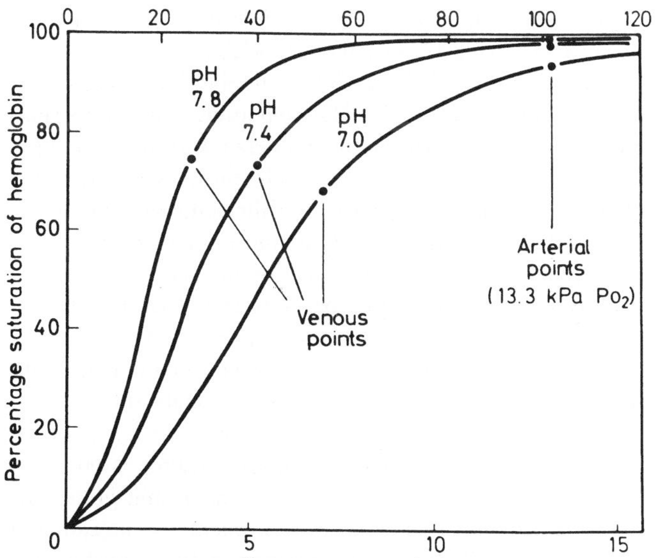

Figure 4.17. Bohr effect on oxyhemoglobin dissociation curve position. Acidosis causes a rightward shift, while alkalosis causes a leftward shift in position of the dissociation curve. (From Nunn JF. Applied respiratory physiology. 2nd ed. London: Butterworths, 1977:406.)

P_{50} of hemoglobin F is 19 mm Hg, compared with a P_{50} of 27 mm Hg for hemoglobin A. The hemoglobin F curve position is appropriate for the lower PO_2 ranges encountered in utero.

The relative amounts of fetal and adult hemoglobin types change during the latter half of gestation and the first 6 months of life. At the 24th week of gestation, hemoglobin F is by far the predominant hemoglobin type, accounting for 90% of total hemoglobin. Thereafter, F levels gradually decline, such that term newborns have 70% hemoglobin F and 30% hemoglobin A. By the end of the first 6 months of life, hemoglobin A has virtually replaced hemoglobin F, and only trace levels of F are detectable.

Sickle-cell anemia is a genetic disease caused by the presence of an abnormal hemoglobin (S), which differs from hemoglobin A by the substitution of valine for glutamic acid at position 6 of the amino acid sequence of the chain. Hemoglobin S has a lower P_{50}, and O_2 is not as readily unloaded in peripheral tissues. Furthermore, in the deoxygenated state, the hemoglobin S molecule goes through a conformational change, which distorts the red cell membrane and ultimately leads to sickling.

Methemoglobin is a hemoglobin molecule in which iron is in its oxidized or ferric (Fe^{3+}) form. Methemoglobin is functionally useless because it is unable to bind oxygen. In the presence of significant quantities of methemoglobin (greater than 30–40%), symptoms of decreased O_2 delivery to tissues become evident.

Methemoglobinemia is a group of disorders characterized by elevated levels of methemoglobin in the red cell. Acquired and congenital forms of methemoglobinemia exist. In the acquired form, the delicate balance between oxidation of hemoglobin to methemoglobin and reduction of methemoglobin by the enzyme methemoglobin reductase is upset. In the presence of certain chemicals (nitrates) or drugs, the oxidation process is accelerated beyond the capacity of methemoglobin reductase to remove the rising concentrations of methemoglobin. Newborns are particularly susceptible because the iron in hemoglobin F is oxidized more readily[83] and because newborns and young infants are relatively deficient in methemoglobin reductase[84]. Cyanosis and symptoms of decreased O_2 transport are noted when methemoglobin levels exceed 30–40% of total hemoglobin. Such patients may be treated with 1 mg per kilogram of 1% methylene blue solution. Congenital methemoglobinemia is caused either by a hereditary hemoglobinopathy, in which hemoglobin M is produced instead of hemoglobin A, or by the hereditary deficiency of methemoglobin reductase. These forms of methemoglobinemia are comparatively rare.

Carbon monoxide poisoning illustrates another clinical condition in which O_2 transport is impaired. Carbon monoxide gas is produced in virtually every fire. Its affinity for the hemoglobin molecule is 210 times greater than the affinity of O_2 for hemoglobin. Thus, a very small inhaled concentration of carbon monoxide will lead to a significant carboxyhemoglobin concentration and, consequently, a lowered oxyhemoglobin concentration. If increased affinity for hemoglobin were the only property of carbon monoxide, carbon monoxide poisoning would be analogous to severe anemia—in effect, lowering hemoglobin concentration available for O_2 transport. However, in addition, carbon monoxide increases the affinity of O_2 for hemoglobin and thus shifts the position of the oxyhemoglobin dissociation curve to the left[85]. Hemoglobin cannot readily unload the remaining O_2 bound to it in tissue capillaries. For instance, if peripheral tissues extract 25% of available O_2, the patient with carbon monoxide poisoning and a leftward shifted dissociation curve must attain significantly lower tissue (and venous) PO_2 values than the normal individual in order to achieve the same 25% extraction of available O_2. Therefore, carbon monoxide poisoning is more deleterious than severe anemia because not only is the available O_2 content reduced, the remaining O_2 bound to hemoglobin cannot readily be unloaded to supply tissue needs.

Oxygen Delivery

The preceding concepts may be summarized by recalling that O_2 content (C_aO_2) in blood consists of a hemoglobin-bound fraction and a small dissolved fraction and is a function of O_2 saturation (SO_2), hemoglobin concentration (Hb), and PO_2, as shown previously in Equation 4.23:

$$C_aO_2\ (\text{ml/dl}) = (SO_2 \cdot Hb \cdot 1.34) + (0.003 \cdot P_aO_2) \qquad (\text{Eq. } 4.28)$$

The volume of oxygen delivered to peripheral tissues per unit time is the oxygen delivery (DO_2) (also called oxygen transport or oxygen availability) and is simply the product of C_aO_2 and cardiac output ($\dot{Q}$):

$$DO_2\ (\text{ml/min}) = C_aO_2 \cdot \dot{Q} \qquad (\text{Eq. } 4.29)$$

Based on these relationships, Barcroft[86] recognized that the causes of inadequate oxygen delivery could be divided into three groups, which he labeled anoxic anoxemia, anemic anoxemia, and stagnant anoxemia. Anoxic anoxemia exists when the arterial oxygen saturation has been lowered significantly. Its most common cause in a pediatric intensive care unit is lung disease with $\dot{V}/\dot{Q}$ mismatching. Anemic anoxemia refers to any condition in which the hemoglobin concentration available to carry oxygen has been reduced significantly. Examples include hemorrhage, methemoglobinemia, and carboxyhemoglobinemia. (As noted above, carboxyhemoglobin also interferes with unloading of oxygen from hemoglobin.) Stagnant anoxemia occurs in the presence of significantly reduced cardiac output or shock that is typically septic, cardiogenic, or hemorrhagic in origin.

It is important to appreciate that the variables governing oxygen delivery are interdependent and that the same clinical condition may affect oxygen delivery in several ways. For instance, the reduced oxygen delivery in anemia may be offset by the associated increase in cardiac output, which is secondary to reduced blood viscosity[76]. Conversely, severe lung disease may lead to a reduced arterial oxygen saturation (anoxic anoxemia), which, if severe enough, will be further exacerbated by anoxic myocardial depression (stagnant anoxemia).

Consumable Oxygen

For tissues to use the oxygen delivered to them, the tissue capillary PO_2 probably must be greater than 20 mm Hg. This conclusion was reached based on the observation that a jugular venous oxygen saturation of less than 24% is associated with unconsciousness, suggesting that intraneuronal PO_2 has dropped below a level that can be used by the cell[87, 88]. Furthermore, a dramatic rise in serum lactate concentration occurs when the mixed venous PO_2 is less than 20 mm Hg. This fact has led to an expansion of the concept of oxygen delivery to include the concept of "consumable oxygen," first introduced by Bryan-Brown et al.[89]. The consumable oxygen is the volume of oxygen delivered at a PO_2 greater than 20 mm Hg, or

$$\text{Consumable } O_2 = (C_aO_2 \cdot \dot{Q}) - (S_{20v}O_2 \cdot 1.34 \cdot Hb + 0.003 \cdot PaO_2) \cdot \dot{Q} \qquad (\text{Eq. } 4.30)$$

where $S_{20v}O_2$ is the derived oxygen saturation for mixed venous blood with a PO_2 of 20 mm Hg.

TISSUE RESPIRATION

Role of Oxygen in Cell

The ultimate purpose of oxygenation in the lungs and oxygen transport in the blood is to provide oxygen for consumption by all tissues in the body and thus allow aerobic metabolism. This confers a great advantage on the organism, because almost 20 times more energy is made available when substrate is metabolized aerobically rather than anaerobically (Fig. 4.18). The important steps of aerobic metabolism occur within the mitochondrion in a process called oxidative phosphorylation. In this process, a series of electron-carrier enzymes (pyridine-linked dehydrogenases, flavoproteins, and cytochromes) deliver electrons from substrate oxidation to the terminal electron acceptor (oxidant), namely, molecular oxygen. At certain steps in this chain of electron-carrier enzymes, electron transfer is coupled with the production of high-energy phosphate bonds in the form of adenosine triphosphate from adenosine diphosphate.

Electron transfer and thus aerobic energy production cease if the carrier enzymes are inhibited or if mitochondrial PO_2 falls below a critical level. Cyanide is an example of a compound that can disrupt the electron transfer process by inhibiting the cytochrome a/a_3 complex. In the presence of cyanide, cellular oxygen cannot accept electrons, and aerobic metabolism ceases. Electron transfer requires

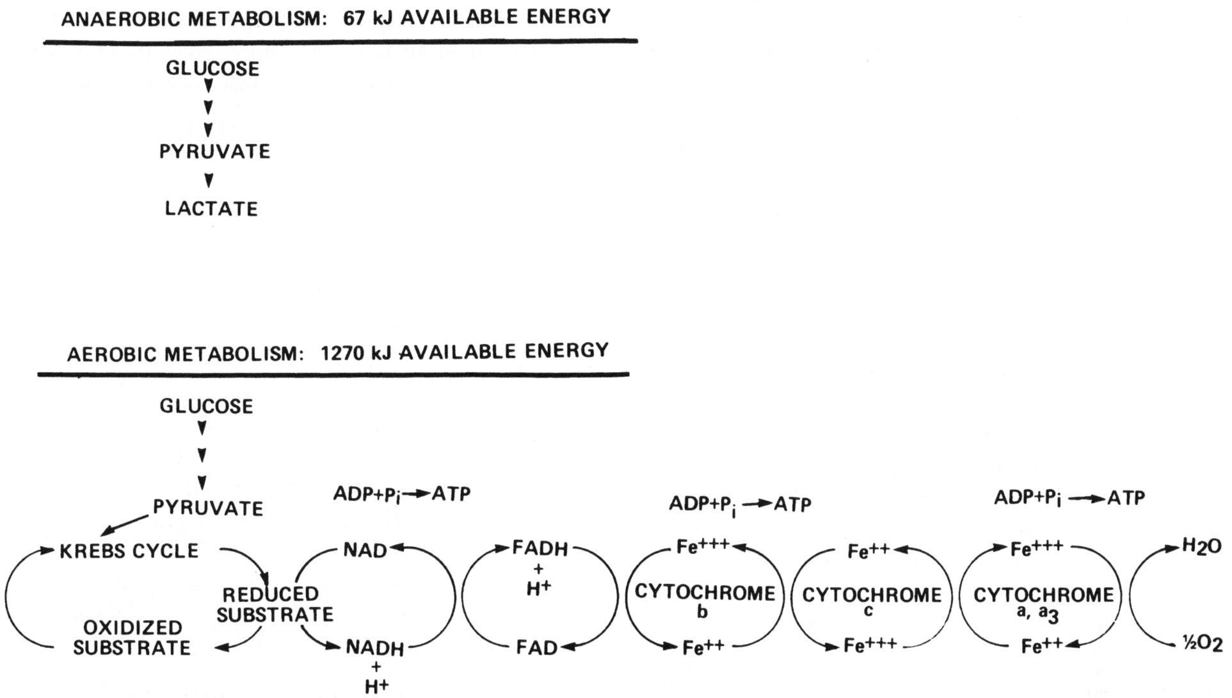

Figure 4.18. Simplified comparison of aerobic versus anaerobic pathway for ATP production.

a certain minimal mitochondrial oxygen tension. This critical level of mitochondrial PO_2 is thought to be around 1 mm Hg.

Tissue PO_2 Measurement

Some measure of tissue oxygenation is necessary because a normal oxygen delivery ($C_aO_2 \cdot \dot{Q}$) does not guarantee adequate tissue oxygenation. There are two reasons for this:

1. Even though C_aO_2 and $\dot{Q}$ may be normal, this distribution of $\dot{Q}$ through tissue vascular beds may be quite abnormal. In certain disease states (see below), delivered oxygen is shunted away from tissue capillaries.
2. Tissue oxygenation occurs through diffusion of O_2 from capillary to mitochondrion.

As seen in Figure 4.19, equivalent quantities of O_2 may be delivered to tissue at very different partial pressures[90]. For instance, two individuals, A and B, can have the same normal O_2 delivery of 1000 mL/min. However, B accomplishes this by doubling his or her cardiac output ($\dot{Q}$) from 5 to 10 L/min and halving his or her arterial O_2 content (C_aO_2) from 20 to 10 ml/dl. Even though A and B deliver identical quantities of O_2 to the capillary, B is left with a substantially lower partial pressure gradient for O_2 diffusion from capillary to mitochondrion because of the sigmoid shape of the oxyhemoglobin dissociation curve.

Ensuring the adequacy of tissue PO_2 levels is a prime objective of intensive care medicine; therefore, it is extremely helpful to measure tissue PO_2. Unfortunately, it is impossible to measure tissue PO_2 directly in the clinical setting. The physician must resort to examining various indirect measures of tissue oxygenation, such as regional or mixed venous PO_2, O_2 consumption, and O_2 extraction.

Using a model developed by Krogh[91], Tenney[92] provided a theoretical analysis supporting the notion that venous PO_2 is a good approximation of tissue PO_2 under normal circumstances. There is also clinical evidence that supports the correlation between tissue and venous PO_2. As noted above, a jugular venous oxygen saturation of less than 24% results in unconsciousness, implying that intraneuronal PO_2 has fallen below a critical level[88].

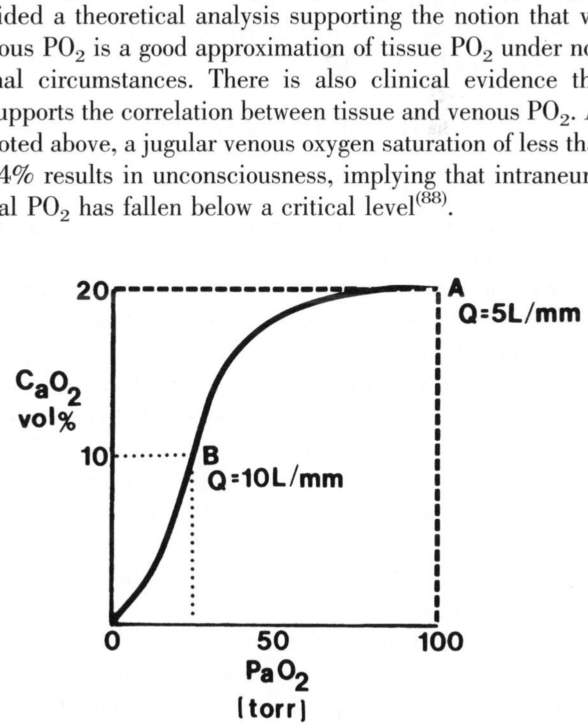

Figure 4.19. Equivalent oxygen delivery at two points on the oxyhemoglobin dissociation curve. (From Miller MJ. Tissue oxygenation in clinical medicine: an historical overview. Anesth Analg 1982; 61:527.)

The venous PO_2 does not correlate with tissue PO_2 when the distribution of flow and capillary density in tissue change. In certain disease states, such as septic shock, the circulation is redistributed through normally closed arteriolar channels[93]. Tissue capillaries are bypassed, and arterial blood is shunted directly into the venous circulation of the tissue. This arterial admixture in peripheral tissues raises venous PO_2 while the tissue is actually deprived of oxygen.

The various regional circulations ultimately mix in the right ventricle, and the PO_2 of blood sampled from the proximal pulmonary artery is called the mixed venous PO_2. The mixed venous PO_2 has been used as an index of overall tissue oxygenation[94]. Mixed venous PO_2 (or oxygen content, C_vO_2) depends on four factors: O_2 delivery, circulatory distribution, P_{50}, and O_2 consumption. Because oxygen is not produced in tissues, it is obvious that a low O_2 delivery will lead to a low venous O_2 content and tissue hypoxia, if it is assumed all other factors remain constant. A normal or high O_2 delivery, with a resultant normal or high mixed venous O_2 content, does not necessarily guarantee adequate tissue oxygenation in that flow may have been distributed away from tissues, as noted above.

P_{50} is an index of the relative position of the oxyhemoglobin dissociation curve. When the P_{50} is high and the dissociation curve is shifted to the right, O_2 is unloaded more readily from hemoglobin, which in turn tends to raise mixed venous PO_2, with all other factors being equal.

According to the Fick principle, the quantity of O_2 consumed ($\dot{V}O_2$) must equal the difference between the quantity of O_2 entering tissue ($C_aO_2 \cdot \dot{Q}$) and the quantity of O_2 leaving tissues ($C_vO_2 \cdot \dot{Q}$):

$$\dot{V}O_2 = (C_aO_2 - C_vO_2) \cdot \dot{Q} \qquad \text{(Eq. 4.31)}$$

When O_2 consumption rises, such as during fever, C_vO_2 is expected to fall, assuming all other factors are unchanged.

Resting O_2 consumption in the newborn is twice that in the adult on a body weight basis (6 versus 3 ml/kg/min). O_2 consumption in the newborn is exquisitely sensitive to environmental temperature. The neutral thermal environment is that environmental temperature (approximately 35°C) at which O_2 consumption is minimal. Even modest lowering of environmental temperature can lead to dramatic increases in the newborn's O_2 consumption. If environmental temperature falls from 33°C to 31°C, O_2 consumption almost doubles[95]. If the baby is unable to increase O_2 delivery to meet these demands, tissue oxygenation and mixed venous PO_2 will fall.

In summary, whenever the mixed venous PO_2 is used, caution must be exercised in considering those factors that affect mixed venous PO_2. A falling mixed venous PO_2 indicates decreased tissue oxygenation if it is assumed that O_2 consumption and circulatory distribution have remained unchanged. A normal mixed venous O_2 does not guarantee adequate tissue oxygenation, since circulatory distribution is usually unknown.

The ratio of oxygen consumption to oxygen delivery is the O_2 extraction ratio (E) and represents that portion of delivered oxygen that actually has been consumed:

$$E = (C_aO_2 - C_vO_2)/C_aO_2 \qquad \text{(Eq. 4.32)}$$

The O_2 extraction ratio provides an index of the efficiency of the O_2 delivery system in meeting metabolic demand for O_2. The normal extraction ratio is 0.25[85]. Extraction ratio increases when O_2 delivery is inadequate to meet metabolic demands. When O_2 extraction is maximal in the face of inadequate O_2 delivery, the organism can no longer consume O_2 and shifts to anaerobic metabolism. Conversely, a low extraction ratio may be indicative of circulatory redistribution with arterial admixture.

RESPIRATORY PUMP

The respiratory pump typifies a feedback loop mechanism consisting of sensors (chemoreceptors and lung and airway receptors), controllers (cerebrum, brainstem, and spinal cord), and effectors (muscles of respiration)[96, 97]. Failure of the respiratory pump leads to hypoventilation and, ultimately, to apnea. In this section, the function of the individual constituents of the respiratory pump is examined with particular emphasis on developmental differences that threaten pump function.

Chemical and Neural Control of Breathing

The chemoreceptors are the principal sensors in this system. The carotid bodies are peripheral chemoreceptors. They are located at the bifurcation of the common carotid arteries and thus lie in a strategic position to monitor PO_2 of blood perfusing the brain. As the carotid bodies sense a

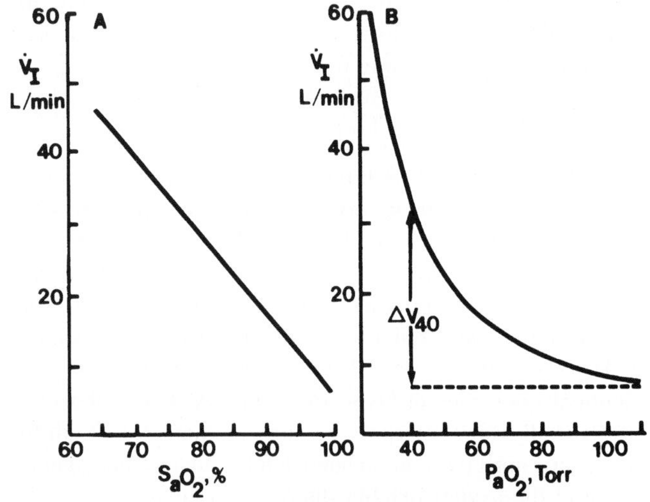

Figure 4.20. Hypoxic ventilatory drive in normal man at sea level and standard constant PCO_2. There is an exponential increase in inspired minute ventilation ($\dot{V}_I$) as P_aO_2 falls. ΔV_{40} is an index of hypoxic sensitivity and represents the increment in ventilation. P_aO_2 is reduced from 150 to 40 mm Hg. (From Berger AJ, Mitchell RA, Severinghaus JW. N Engl J Med 1977;297:194.)

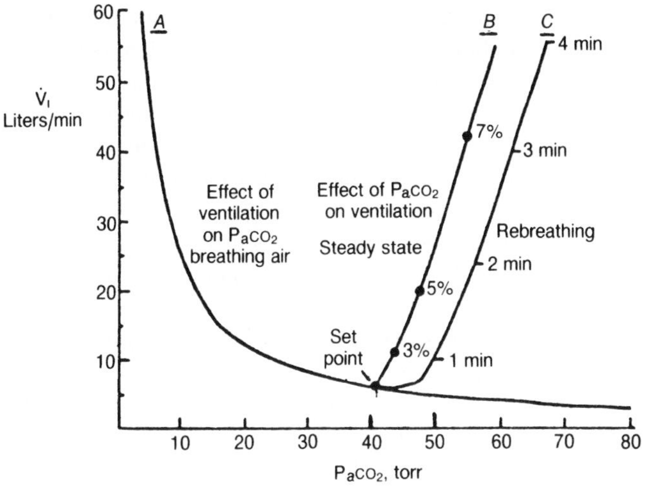

Figure 4.21. Three carbon dioxide response curves showing inspired minute ventilation ($\dot{V}_I$) as a function of P_aCO_2. *Curve A* is the CO_2 excretion hyperbola showing the effect of ventilation on PCO_2. *Curves B* and *C* demonstrate the effect of P_aCO_2 on ventilatory response. *Curve B* is a steady-state response curve obtained by breathing three different CO_2 mixtures. *Curve C* is the rebreathing CO_2 response curve obtained by rebreathing from a bag with 7% CO_2 in 40–93% O_2. (From Berger AJ, Mitchell RA, Severinghaus JW. Regulation of respiration. N Engl J Med 1977;297:194.)

falling P_aO_2 below 500 mm Hg in the adult, they signal the brainstem to increase ventilation gradually. When the P_aO_2 reaches 50 mm Hg, ventilation increases dramatically (Fig. 4.20)[97]. Hypercarbia and acidosis accentuate this response[98].

The central chemoreceptor lies on the ventrolateral surface of the medulla[99]. In response to hypercarbia, the cerebrospinal fluid bathing this chemoreceptor is acidified, and the increased H^+ ion concentration on the chemoreceptor signals the brainstem to increase minute ventilation in a linear fashion (Fig. 4.21). Hypoxia increases the slope of the CO_2 response curve.

A number of pulmonary reflexes modulate breathing[100]. The receptors for these reflex arcs lie in the upper airways or lung. Experimental studies in animals suggest that stimulation of these receptors may lead to apnea. For example, chemical or mechanical stimulation of the oropharynx and nasopharynx leads to apnea and bradycardia. Stimulation of laryngeal receptors produces cough, wheezing, and apnea. Excess interstitial fluid may activate the juxtapulmonary capillary receptor ("J" receptor) in the lung, which results in apnea, bradycardia, and hypotension.

Sensory input from the receptors described above is received by the respiratory controller in the brainstem, which is responsible for initiating automatic respiration[97]. Based on the original work by Lumsden[101, 102], it was found that the brainstem respiratory controller is divided into the pneumotaxic center, the apneustic center, and the medullary center. The pneumotaxic center fine-tunes respiration by switching inspiration to expiration. The apneustic center seems to be responsible for cutting off inspiration. Neither the pneumotaxic center nor the apneustic center (both located in the pons) is essential for rhythmic expiration. However, destruction of the medullary center will lead to apnea. Thus, the medulla is believed to be the site of the basic respiratory rhythm generator. The cerebral cortex connects with the brainstem respiratory centers and with the spinal cord, thus allowing voluntary control of respiration. The spinal cord is the final integrating station of all central nervous system commands before they are relayed to the muscles of respiration via the phrenic and intercostal nerves.

Developmental Differences in Chemical and Neural Control

The respiratory pump of the normal awake newborn and preterm infant lacks many of the defense mechanisms observed in the adult[103]. Most preterm infants breathe periodically, defined as breathing marked by pauses lasting 5 to 10 seconds. The more premature the infant, the higher the incidence of periodic breathing. Even though periodic breathing is thought to be a benign disorder, there is an association between periodic breathing and true apnea, defined as absent airflow for 20 seconds or more. Overall, 25% of preterm infants may develop apnea[104], which can lead to bradycardia and hypoxemia.

Compared with the adult, the normal term newborn must meet higher oxygen demands per unit mass ($\dot{V}O_2$ per kilogram). The normal term newborn adapts in two ways to sustain these higher oxygen demands: *(a)* greater minute ventilation per unit mass ($\dot{V}_E$ per kilogram), and *(b)* the CO_2 response curve displaced to the left (Fig. 4.22). Thus, the term newborn's resting PCO_2 is only 33 mm Hg. The infant with periodic breathing fails to adapt, and his or her CO_2 response curve lies much closer to the adult CO_2 response

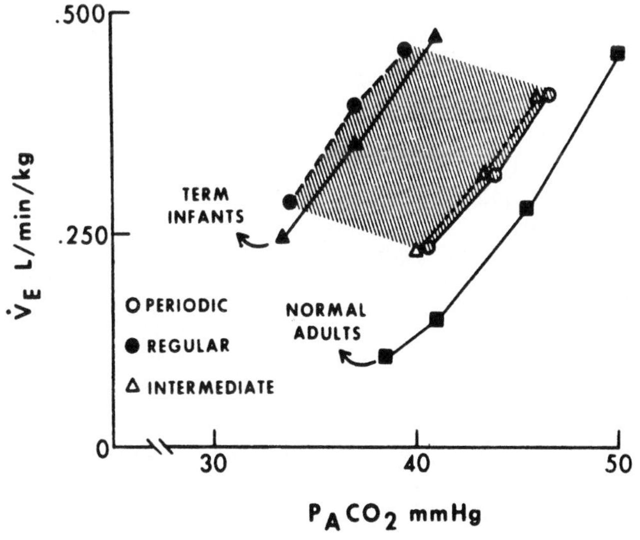

Figure 4.22. Steady-state CO_2 response curves of infants breathing periodically, regularly, and semiperiodically (intermediate) compared with curves of normal term infants and adults. CO_2 response curve of the normal term newborn is shifted to the left of normal adult curve. Infants breathing periodically have a response curve similar to that for the adult. (From Rigatto H. Apnea. Pediatr Clin North Am 1982;29:1105.)

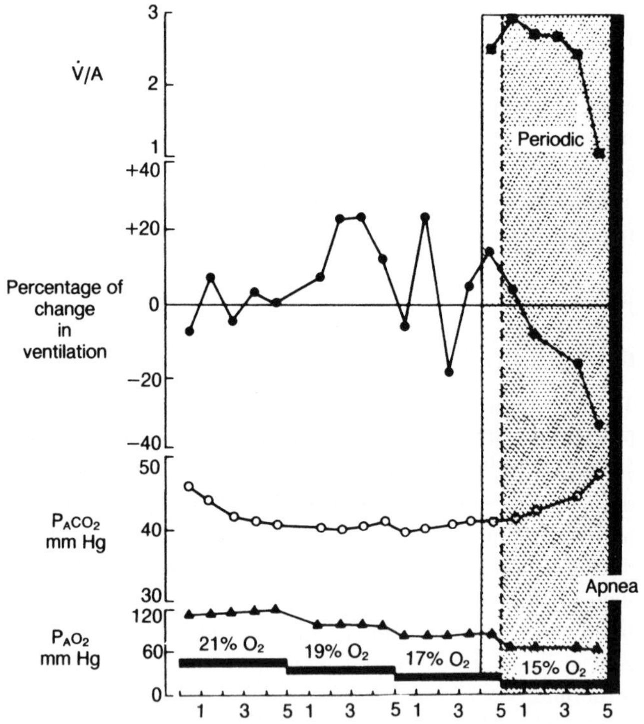

Figure 4.23. Change in ventilation and alveolar gas tensions while breathing a hypoxic gas mixture in a 34-week gestational age infant. Note initial increase followed by a decrease in ventilation with F_IO_2 of 19% and 17%. Periodic breathing (indicated by V̇/A, duration of ventilation/duration of apnea) appears during the last minute of 17% F_IO_2 and during 15% F_IO_2. (From Rigatto H. Apnea. Pediatr Clin North Am 1982;29:1105.)

curve, with a resting PCO_2 of 40 mm Hg (Fig. 4.22). The slope of the CO_2 response curve is a function of gestational age. The more immature the infant, the flatter the CO_2 response curve becomes[103]. This implies that they develop a smaller minute ventilatory response to a given PCO_2 stimulus. Sudden infant death syndrome may represent in part a failure of maturation of ventilatory response to a given CO_2 stimulus[105].

Hypoxia depresses respiration in all newborns[103, 105]. As the infant's F_IO_2 is lowered to 15%, there is an initial 30-second increase in ventilation, followed by a progressive reduction in ventilation with periodic breathing. Apnea may result after 5 minutes of hypoxia (Fig. 4.23)[106]. The biphasic ventilatory response of the hypoxic newborn probably represents intact chemoreceptor activity, which accounts for the initial increase in ventilation followed by centrally mediated respiratory depression or respiratory muscle dysfunction during hypoxia. Intact carotid body chemoreceptor function during hypoxia has been demonstrated in the kitten model[107].

Chest Wall Mechanics and Respiratory Muscle Function

Respiration requires the development of a pressure gradient between mouth and alveoli. During spontaneous breathing, this pressure gradient is achieved by contraction of respiratory muscles that enlarge the thoracic cavity and lower pleural pressure to subatmospheric. Some normal developmental phenomena as well as various diseases may interfere with this process. Therefore, it is necessary to examine the effect of structure of the developing chest wall on its static and dynamic mechanical properties.

The chest wall of the infant and especially of the newborn is cartilaginous, soft, and pliable. It must be so to negotiate passage through the birth canal without multiple rib fractures. With further growth and development, the rib cage ossifies.

The mechanical consequences of the changing chest wall structure are evident from an inspection of the pressure volume curves of the chest wall or the total respiratory system (Figs. 4.5 and 4.24). As noted in the section on mechanical properties of the respiratory system, compliance is the change in volume per unit change in transmural pressure. In the case of chest wall compliance, the relevant transmural pressure gradient is the difference between ambient and pleural pressures. Because of technical difficulties in the measurement of pleural pressures, the compliance curve of the total respiratory system is more frequently obtained, in which the transmural pressure gradient is between alveolar and ambient pressures. Chest wall compliance is then inferred from total respiratory system compliance.

The newborn chest wall is highly compliant; i.e., changes in volume are associated with virtually no change in pressure[108, 109] (Fig. 4.5). With increasing age there is a progressive reduction in chest wall compliance, as inferred from the reduction in compliance of the total respiratory system (Fig. 4.24)[110].

The transmural pressure gradient of the chest wall or the total respiratory system can be thought of as the elastic re-

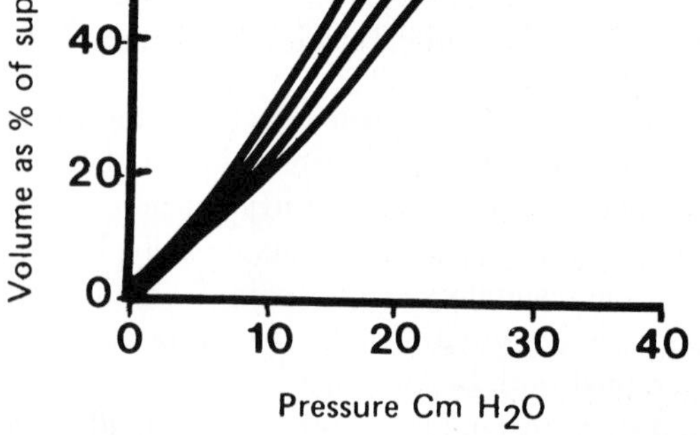

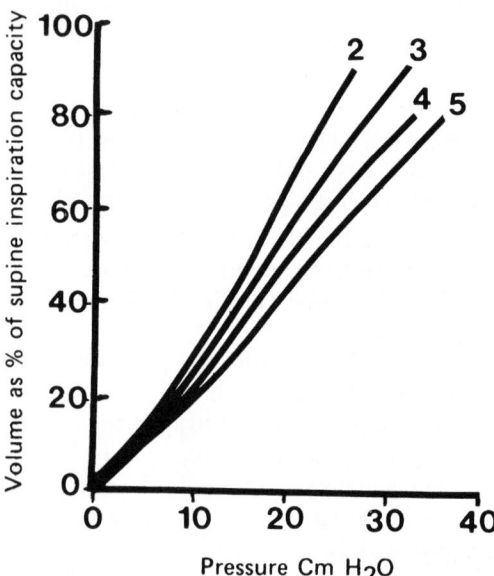

Figure 4.24. Total respiratory system compliance curves at various ages. Note decrease in compliance and increase in elastic recoil pressure with advancing age. Mean ages for *groups 2, 3, 4,* and *5* are 5.0, 8.1, 1, 2.5, and 15.7 years, respectively. (From Sharp JT, et al. Total respiratory compliance in infants and children. J Appl Physiol 1970;29:775.)

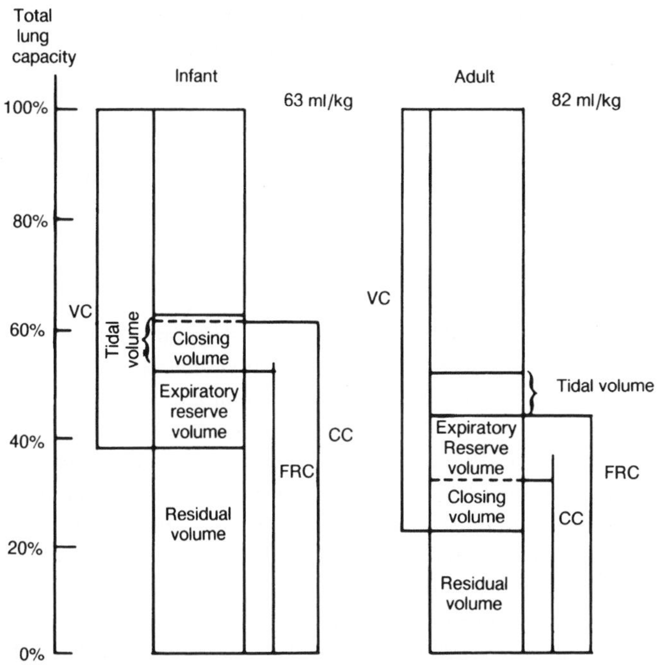

Figure 4.25. Lung volumes in infants and adults. Note that tidal breathing in the infant takes place in the range of the closing capacity *(CC)* of the lung. *VC,* vital capacity; *FRC,* functional residual capacity. (From Smith CA, Nelson NM. The physiology of the newborn infant. Springfield, Illinois: Charles C Thomas Publishers, 1976:207.)

coil pressure of the chest wall or of the total system, respectively. Elastic recoil is that property of an elastic body that causes it to return to its rest position after having been deformed. In the normal adult, the chest wall would tend to recoil outward at FRC were it not restrained by the counterbalancing force of the lung, which tends to collapse to residual volume. As seen in Figure 4.5, the elastic recoil pressure of the newborn chest wall at resting lung volume is close to zero. With increasing age, elastic recoil pressure increases (Fig. 4.24). It is assumed that the increase in recoil pressure results from progressive ossification of the rib cage, improvement in intercostal muscle tone, and the development of a negative pressure on the abdominal side of the diaphragm. Presumably, outward recoil of the chest wall is inhibited in the infant lying supine with a relatively small abdomen. Once the upright posture has been assumed and the abdomen has grown, abdominal contents shift away from the upper abdomen, creating a more negative subdiaphragmatic pressure that favors outward recoil of the chest wall.

There are several clinical implications of these mechanical differences between the developing and mature chest walls. The very low elastic recoil pressure of the newborn chest wall raises the risk of lung collapse. In fact, most tidal breathing in the infant takes place in the range of the closing capacity of the lung (see the section on the effect of pleural pressure on gas distribution and Fig. 4.25).

The highly compliant neonatal chest wall is at a mechanical disadvantage during breathing because the infant must generate greater pressure and perform more work to move the same tidal volume.

This is so because contraction of the diaphragm produces a negative pleural pressure that distorts the highly compliant rib cage in addition to allowing exchange of a tidal volume[(111)]. A portion of the force of contraction of the diaphragm is wasted in distorting the rib cage[(112)]. The chest wall retractions (distortions) noted on physical examination of the infant in respiratory distress occur as the rib cage is sucked inward during forceful diaphragmatic contraction.

Clinicians have frequently noted that when infants are confronted with the need to increase their work of breathing because of lung disease, a certain percentage of them will fatigue and ultimately stop breathing[(113)]. The clinical impression of diaphragmatic fatigue has been confirmed by noting the characteristic electromyographic frequency spectrum of fatiguing skeletal muscle in the diaphragms of those babies who show clinical deterioration and become apneic in the face of increased work of breathing from lung disease or even active (rapid-eye movement) sleep[(114)].

Respiratory Muscle Histology and Function

The cellular basis of diaphragmatic fatigue in infants is not completely clear. Keens et al.[(115)] initially suggested that diaphragmatic fatigue may be due to incomplete development of slow-twitch, highly oxidative, fatigue-resistant muscle fibers of the diaphragm in young infants. Maxwell et al.[(116)] disputed this conclusion, based on their work in the premature baboon model. They did not find a paucity of highly oxidative muscle fibers in the newborn of that species. Instead, they noted that the latent period and the contraction and relaxation times were longer in the premature muscle than in the adult respiratory muscle. The lack of sarcoplasmic reticulum observed in electron micrographs of fetal diaphragmatic muscle supported the observation of long contraction and relaxation times in this type of muscle. It might be expected that respiratory muscle with sparse sarcoplasmic reticulum would take longer to initiate as well as to terminate a contraction. These data suggest that the long contraction-relaxation times observed in premature respiratory muscle may result in respiratory muscle ischemia at high respiratory rates. Fatigue might then occur as a result of inadequate substrate supply.

Intercostal Muscles

The intercostal muscles serve two important purposes on inspiration. First, contraction of the intercostal muscles elevates the anterior end of each rib, thereby increasing thoracic volume on inspiration. Second, intercostal muscle contraction tenses the intercostal space, thereby stabilizing the rib cage during diaphragmatic descent.

In the face of diaphragmatic fatigue, some infants are unable to recruit intercostal muscle activity[(117)]. This group of infants falls into a vicious cycle in which contractions of the fatiguing diaphragm produce ever more chest wall distortion because of the infant's inability to recruit intercostal muscle activity. As more and more energy is wasted in distorting the chest wall, diaphragmatic fatigue worsens, ultimately leading to apnea.

Reflex mechanisms mediated through intercostal muscle spindles may also play a role in neonatal apnea. Knill and Bryan[(118)] demonstrated that rapid chest wall distortion prematurely terminates inspiration. Distortion of the rib cage stretches the affected intercostal muscles and activates their spindles. It is hypothesized that intercostal muscle spindle activation inhibits central inspiratory drive through unknown mechanisms. This inhibitory reflex may explain the inability of the infant to compensate for an inspiratory load during active rapid eye movement sleep[(119)]. The normal adult experiences an initial fall in tidal volume if forced to breathe against a respiratory load. However, tidal volume promptly returns to control during subsequent breaths (i.e., load compensation occurs). The young infant cannot compensate for respiratory loads during active sleep. It is believed that tonic inhibition of intercostal muscles is present during active sleep, which allows rib cage distortion during inspiration. Distortion of the rib cage rapidly changes intercostal muscle spindle length and prematurely terminates inspiration through an unknown reflex mechanism, thus preventing load compensation from taking place. This is a serious handicap because premature infants may spend up to 50% of their time in active sleep and during that period are unable to defend themselves against an increased respiratory load[(120)].

Apnea

The causes of apnea can be considered as *(a)* central, without any initiation of breathing, or *(b)* obstructive, with the upper airway providing sufficient resistance to airflow to stop ventilation despite diaphragmatic movement and respiratory effort. Most apneas are mixed and have components of both. Pathophysiologically, a link between the two types of apnea can be made by understanding that obstructive apnea can cause brainstem hypoxia that can inhibit the respiratory center, leading to central apnea. Brainstem hypoxia can also diminish the neural traffic to the muscles of the upper airway, thus decreasing tone during inspiration and worsening the apnea. This spiral can be worsened in a multitude of disease processes. Infants often have an acute life-threatening event (ALTE) characterized by cyanosis, floppiness, unconsciousness, and/or apnea. A surgical or medical cause can be identified in 61% of such cases[(121)]. These patients have a greater degree of both obstructive and mixed apneas[(122, 123)]. In adults with obstructive sleep apnea, the site of obstruction is likely to be the oropharynx[(124)], but in infants with ALTE, the site of obstruction may be at another level, such as the larynx[(125)]. In any case, without intervention, these infants are at risk for a repeat episode and possible death. It is not clear how to identify which infants are particularly at risk, but a polysomnograph is oftentimes helpful in identifying reversible pathology.

The relationship between sudden infant death syndrome and the control of breathing (especially sleep apnea) is not well established. Whenever a child with an apnea spell is admitted to the pediatric intensive care unit, an underlying diagnosis should be sought from history and physical findings. The differential diagnosis includes underlying disorders such as prematurity, cardiac or pulmonary diseases, infections, suffocation[(126)], and drug ingestions.

Obstructive sleep apnea in infants and children may be due to tonsillar and/or adenoidal hypertrophy that is amenable to surgical correction[(127)]. These patients may come to the pediatric intensive care unit postoperatively because of worsening airway obstruction from edema or diminished central ventilatory drive after anesthesia and surgery. Their disease process may also have progressed, with chronic severe hypoxemia that leads to pulmonary hypertension, which, in turn, leads to right heart failure[(128)]. The central control mechanism in these patients may well be deranged and may be related to increased opioid activity found in their cerebral spinal fluid[(129)].

Gastroesophageal reflux (GER) may be related to apnea (often obstructive) and can be documented by analysis of esophageal pH during a sleep study. The casual relationship between these two entities has not been established, but the association is accepted. GER is amenable to surgical (i.e., Nissen fundoplication) or medical (i.e., H_2-blockers, antacids) therapy[(130)].

Respiratory syncytial virus (RSV) infection in infants is associated with apnea in 16% of RSV-infected hospitalized infants. This apnea is central, and the mechanism or mechanisms are unknown[(131)].

Central apnea may be unmasked by anesthesia in the infant. Premature children of less than 60 weeks conceptual age (the sum of intrauterine age and postnatal age) may exhibit life-threatening apnea postoperatively and should therefore have cardiopulmonary monitoring for 12–24 hours after anesthesia[(132, 133)]. Spinal anesthesia with sedation (ketamine) confers no advantage over general anesthesia in this regard, although spinal anesthesia with no other medications may decrease the incidence of postoperative apnea[(134)]. There have been case reports of full-term infants having postoperative apnea[(135, 136)], but the implications of this on clinical care remain unclear.

When a child with apnea is evaluated, underlying causes should be sought to guide appropriate therapy (either medical or surgical). Specific therapy is controversial. Generation of a metabolic acidosis with acetazolamide may have unpredictable effects on ventilation[(137)]. Aminophylline, on the other hand, will reliably increase breathing without changing the pH or CO_2 tension surrounding the respiratory center[(138)].

Increased Chest Wall Compliance from Neurologic Diseases

There are a number of diseases leading to respiratory failure peculiar to infants that follow from the chest wall mechanics of the infant described above. Phrenic nerve palsy with resultant hemidiaphragmatic paralysis is a life-

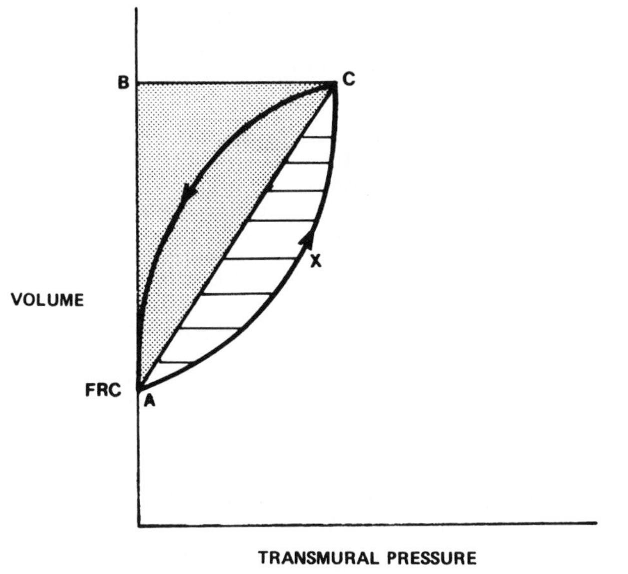

Figure 4.26. Pressure-volume curve of a single breath. Work needed to overcome tissue elastic resistance is equal to the area contained in *ACB (stippled area).* Work needed to overcome frictional airway resistance is equal to the area contained in *AXCA (crosshatched area).* Total work is given by *AXCBA (stippled plus crosshatched areas).*

threatening event in infants, while adults remain virtually asymptomatic. The difference lies in the excessive compliance of the rib cage and the ineffective stabilizing properties of the intercostal muscles in infants. When the contralateral normal hemidiaphragm contracts, creating a negative intrapleural pressure, the compliant rib cage, intercostal muscles, and paralyzed ipsilateral diaphragm are all sucked into the chest[(139)]. Thus, hemidiaphragmatic paralysis in the infant is equivalent to a massive flail chest.

Cervical spine injury below the C5 level may result in respiratory compromise, even though function of the diaphragm remains intact. Paralysis of the intercostal muscles deprives the compliant infant chest wall of a potential stabilizing force. Therefore, each contraction of the diaphragm is accompanied by chest wall retraction. Abdominal muscle paralysis prevents the infant from generating an effective cough. Respiratory failure may follow from the loss of lung volumes secondary to chest wall retraction and mucous plugging of the airway as well as from the increased work of breathing with chest wall distortion.

Work of Breathing

Although "work of breathing" has been referred to in previous sections and its meaning is intuitively apparent, it is now appropriate to define the concept of work in respiratory physiology more precisely. Work is defined as the product of force and distance. During spontaneous breathing, work is the pressure (P) generated by the respiratory muscles to move a volume (V) of gas.

$$\text{Work} = P \cdot V \qquad \text{(Eq. 4.33)}$$

Respiratory muscles perform approximately half of their work during inspiration to move the tidal volume. The remainder of the inspiratory work is stored as potential energy in the tissues, which have been stretched from their rest positions. Thus, expiration is normally passive as potential energy is released when tissues recoil to their rest position.

There are two major sources of resistance to breathing that the work from respiratory muscle contraction must overcome during each breath. The first source is the tissue elastic resistance that is generated by the displacement of lung and chest wall from their rest positions. If change in volume is plotted as a function of change in pressure during a single breath as in Figure 4.26, the work required to overcome tissue elastic resistance is given by the *stippled area* of *triangle ACB.* Note that the pressure volume curve *(line AC)* is the hypotenuse of a triangle and represents the compliance of the system.

The second major source of resistance stems from the friction generated by gas molecules flowing through the airway. Thus work is also necessary to overcome airway resistance. This additional work is described by the *crosshatched area AXC* in Figure 4.26. Thus, the total work needed to overcome tissue elastic resistance (compliance) and airflow frictional resistance is contained in area *AXCBA.*

The pressure-volume curve in Figure 4.26 is used to describe work performed in a single breath. The rate at which work is performed (work per unit time) is called power. Although firmly entrenched in common usage, the term work of breathing is inaccurate. Power (expressed in joules per second) is the precise term.

Breathing is most efficient when respiratory rate and tidal volume are set to require the minimum expenditure of work. The higher resting respiratory rate of the infant is consistent with this concept. The newborn infant minimizes work when breathing 30–40 times/min[(140)].

Effect of Hypoventilation on Alveolar Gas Tensions

Failure of the respiratory pump leads to hypoventilation, which, in turn, leads to hypercarbia and hypoxia. There is a hyperbolic relationship between alveolar ventilation ($\dot{V}_A$) and P_ACO_2 (or P_aCO_2) (Fig. 4.27) such that

$$P_ACO_2 = \dot{V}CO_2/\dot{V}_A \qquad \text{(Eq. 4.34)}$$

where $\dot{V}CO_2$ is the CO_2 production rate. As alveolar ventilation falls, PCO_2 rises. Conversely, as alveolar ventilation rises, the alveolar CO_2 concentration approaches the inspired CO_2 concentration.

The relationship between alveolar ventilation and alveolar PO_2 is also hyperbolic (Fig. 4.27) and is expressed in the alveolar air equation, which may be written:

$$P_AO_2 = P_IO_2 - (\dot{V}O_2/\dot{V}_A) \qquad \text{(Eq. 4.35)}$$

where P_IO_2 is the inspired partial pressure of oxygen, and $\dot{V}O_2$ is the oxygen consumption rate. It is apparent that P_AO_2 falls at first slowly, then precipitously, as $\dot{V}_A$ falls.

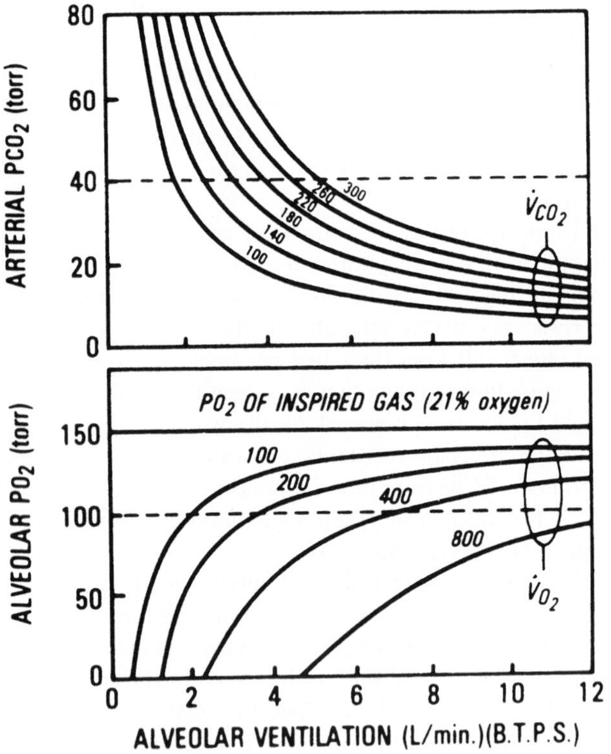

Figure 4.27. Hyperbolic relationship between alveolar ventilation and arterial PCO_2 *(upper graph)* and alveolar PO_2. Position of the curves depends on CO_2 production and O_2 consumption. As alveolar ventilation increases, PO_2 and PCO_2 approach their inspired values. As alveolar ventilation falls, a critical value is reached at which there is a sudden rise in PCO_2 and fall in PO_2. (From Benumof J. Respiratory physiology and respiratory function during anesthesia. In: Miller RD, ed. Anesthesia. New York: Churchill Livingstone, 1981:699.)

Furthermore, with a raised P_IO_2 or a lower $\dot{V}O_2$, even greater degrees of hypoventilation would be needed to produce alveolar hypoxia.

References

1. Gregory GA. Respiratory failure in the child. Clin Crit Care Med 1981;3:7.
2. Wegman ME. Annual summary of vital statistics—1989. Pediatrics 1990;86:835–847.
3. Wohl MEB, Chernick V. Bronchiolitis. Am Rev Respir Dis 1978;118:759.
4. Bucher U, Reid L. Development of the intra-segmental tree: the pattern of branching development of cartilage at various stages of intrauterine life. Thorax 1961;16:207.
5. Kitagawa M, Hislop A, Boyden EA, Reid L. Lung hypoplasia in congenital diaphragmatic hernia. A quantitative study of airway, artery, and alveolar development. Br J Surg 1971;58:342.
6. Thurlbeck WM. Postnatal growth and development of the lung. Am Rev Respir Dis 1975;111:803.
7. Hogg JC, Williams J, Richardson JB, Macklem PT, Thurlbeck WM. Age as a factor in the distribution of lower-airway conductance and in the pathologic anatomy of obstructive lung disease. N Engl J Med 1970;282:1283.
8. Loosli CJ, Hung KS. Development of pulmonary innervation. In: Hodson WA, ed. Development of the lung. New York: Marcel Dekker, 1977:269.
9. Sinclair-Smith CC, Emery JL, Gadson D, Linsdale F, Baddeley J. Cartilage in children's lungs: a quantitative assessment using the right middle lobe. Thorax 1976; 31:40.
10. Wittenborg MH, Gyepes M, Crocker D. Tracheal dynamics in infants with respiratory distress, stridor, and collapsing trachea. Radiology 1967;88:653.
11. Dunnill MS. Postnatal growth of the lung. Thorax 1962;17:329.
12. Boyden EA, Tompsett DH. The changing patterns in the developing lungs of infants. Acta Anat (Basel) 1965;61:164.
13. Thurlbeck WM, Angus GE. Growth and aging of the normal human lung. Chest 1975;67(Suppl):3S.
14. Nelson NM. Respiration and circulation after birth. In: Smith CA, Nelson NM, eds. The physiology of the newborn infant. Springfield, Illinois: Charles C Thomas Publisher, 1976:117.
15. Robotham JL, Menkes HA, Chipps BE, Inners CR, Alderson P, Hutchins GM, Tepas JJ, Haller JA. A physiologic assessment of segmental bronchial atresia. Am Rev Respir Dis 1980;121:533.
16. Macklem PT. Airway obstruction and collateral ventilation. Physiol Rev 1971;51:368.
17. Boyden EA. Development and growth of the airways. In: Hodson WA, ed. Development of the lung. New York: Marcel Dekker, 1977:3.
18. McBride JT, Wohl MEB, Strieder DJ. Lung growth and airway function after lobectomy in infancy for congenital lobar emphysema. J Clin Invest 1980;66:962.
19. Nunn JF. Applied respiratory physiology. London: Butterworths, 1977:213.
20. Polgar G, Weng TR. The functional development of the respiratory system. Am Rev Respir Dis 1979;120:625.
21. Rehder K, Sessler AD, Rodarte JR. Regional intrapulmonary gas distribution in awake and anesthetized-paralyzed man. J Appl Physiol 1977;42:391.
22. Craig DB, Wahba WM, Don HF, Couture JD, Becklake R. Closing volume and its relationship to gas exchange in seated and supine positions. J Appl Physiol 1971;31:717.
23. Dolfuss R, Milic-Emili J, Bates D. Regional ventilation of the lung studied with boluses of 133 Xenon. Respir Physiol 1967;2:232.
24. Mansell A, Bryan C, Levison H. Airway closure in children. J Appl Physiol 1972;33:711.
25. Zapletal A, Paul T, Samanek M. Pulmonary elasticity in children and adolescents. J Appl Physiol 1976;40:953.
26. Pierce JA, Hobcott JB. Studies on the collagen and elastin content of the human lung. J Clin Invest 1960;39:8.
27. Kosch PC, Stark AR. Dynamic maintenance of end-expiratory lung volume in full-term infants. J Appl Physiol 1984;57:1126–1133.
28. Stark AR, Cohlan BA, Waggener TB, Frantz ID III, Kosch PC. Regulation of end-expiratory lung volume during sleep in premature infants. J Appl Physiol 1987; 62:1117–1123.
29. Thorsteinsson A, Jonmarker C, Larsson A, Vilstrup C, Werner O. Functional residual capacity in anesthetized children: normal values and values in children with cardiac anomalies. Anesthesiology 1990;73:876–881.
30. Davis GM, Cooper DM, Mitchell I. The measurement of thoraco-abdmonial asynchrony in infants with severe laryngotracheobronchitis. Chest 1993;103:1842–1848.
31. Duncan PG. Efficacy of helium-oxygen mixtures in the management of severe viral and post-intubation croup. Can Anaesth Soc J 1979;26:206.
32. Phelan PD, Williams HE. Ventilatory studies in healthy infants. Pediatr Res 1969;3:425.
33. Hogg JC, Williams J, Richardson JB, Macklem PT, Thurlbeck WM. Age as factor in the distribution of lower airway conductance and in the pathologic anatomy of obstructive lung disease. N Engl J Med 1970;282:1283.
34. Merritt TA. Oxygen exposure in the newborn guinea pig-lung lavage cell populations, chemotactic and elastase response: a possible relationship to neonatal broncho-pulmonary dysplasia. Pediatr Res 1982;16:798.
35. Houstek J, Copova M, Zapletal A, Tomasova H, Samanek M. Alpha-1 antitrypsin deficiency in a child with chronic lung disease. Chest 1973;64:773.
36. Brown ES, Johnson RP, Clements JA. Pulmonary surface tension. J Appl Physiol 1959;14:717.
37. Post M, Van Golde LMG. Metabolic and developmental aspects of the pulmonary surfactant system. Biochim Biophys Acta 1988;947:249–286.
38. Hallman M, Kulovich M, Kirkpatrick E, Sugarman RG, Gluck L. Phosphatidylinositol and phosphatidylglycerol in amniotic fluid: indices of lung maturity. Am J Obstet Gynecol 1976;125:613–617.
39. Weaver TE, Whitsett JA. Function and regulation of expression of pulmonary surfactant-associated proteins. Biochem J 1991; 273:249–264.
40. Wright JR, Benson BJ, Williams MC, Goerke J, Clements JA. Protein composition of rabbit alveolar surfactant subfractions. Biochim Biophys Acta 1984;791:320–332.

41. Chander A, Fisher AB. Regulation of lung surfactant secretion. Am J Physiol 1990;258:H241–H253.
42. Bruni R, Baritussio A, Quaglino D, Gabelli C, Benevento M, Ronchetti IP. Postnatal transformations of alveolar surfactant in the rabbit: changes in pool size, pool morphology and isoforms of the 32-38 kDa apolipoprotein. Biochim Biophys Acta 1988;958:255–267.
43. Avery ME, Mead J. Surface properties in relation to atelectasis and hyaline membrane disease. Am J Dis Child 1959;97:517.
44. Ueda T, Ikegami M, Jobe AH. Developmental changes of sheep surfactant: in vivo function and in vitro subtype conversion. J Appl Physiol 1994;76:2701–2706.
45. Henry JN. The effect of shock on pulmonary alveolar surfactant. J Trauma 1968;8:756.
46. Said SI, Avery ME, Davis RK, Bannerjee CM, El-Gohary M. Pulmonary surface activity in induced pulmonary edema. J Clin Invest 1965;4:458.
47. Merritt TA, Hallman M, Bloom BT, Berry C, Benirschke K, Sahn D, Key T, Edwards D, Jarvenpaa AL, Pohjavuori M, Kankaanpaa K, Kunnas M, Paatero H, Rapola J, Jaaskelainen J. Prophylactic treatment of very premature infants with human surfactant. N Engl J Med 1986; 315:785–790.
48. Holm BA, Notter RH. Effects of hemoglobin and cell membrane lipids on pulmonary surfactant activity. J Appl Physiol 1987;63:1434–1442.
49. Fuchimukai T, Fujiwara T, Takahashi A, Enhorning G. Artificial pulmonary surfactant inhibited by proteins. J Appl Physiol 1987;62:429–437.
50. Bonuccelli CM, Permutt S, Sylvester JT. Developmental differences in catalase activity and hypoxic-hyperoxic effects on fluid balance in isolated lamb lungs. Pediatr Res 1993;33:519–526.
51. Wallen LD, Perry SF, Alston JT, Maloney JE. Morphometric study of the role of pulmonary artery flow in fetal lung growth in sheep. Pediatr Res 1990;27:12–127.
52. Reid LM. The pulmonary circulation: remodeling in growth and disease. Am Rev Respir Dis 1979;119:531.
53. Hislop A, Reid LM. Pulmonary arterial development during childhood: branching pattern and structure. Thorax 1973;28:129.
54. Belik J, Keeley FW, Baldwin F, Rabinovitch M. Pulmonary hypertension and vascular remodeling in fetal sheep. Am J Physiol 1994;266:H2303–H2309.
55. Johnson DJ, LaBourene J, Rabinovitch M, Keeley FW. Relative efficiency of incorporation of newly synthesized elastin and collagen into aorta, pulmonary artery and pulmonary vein of growing pigs. Connective Tissue Res 1993;29:213–221.
56. Rabinovitch M, Keane JF, Norwood WI, Castaneda AR, Reid L. Vascular structure in lung tissue obtained at biopsy correlated with pulmonary hemodynamic findings after repair of congenital heart defects. Circulation 1984;69:655–667.
57. Deal CW, Louis E, Kerth WJ, Osborne JJ, Gerbode F. Bronchopulmonary precapillary blood flow during cardipulmonary bypass. Am Heart J 1968;75:43.
58. Hirasuna JD, Gorin AB. Effect of prolonged recumbency on pulmonary blood volume in normal humans. J Appl Physiol 1981;50:950.
59. Dawes GS, Mott JL, Widdicombe JG, Wyatt DG. Changes in the lung of the newborn lamb. J Physiol 1953;121:141.
60. West JB, Dollery CT, Naimark A. Distribution of blood flow in isolated lung: relation to vascular and alveolar pressures. J Appl Physiol 1964;19:713.
61. James LS, Rowe RD. The pattern of response of pulmonary and systemic arterial pressures in newborn and older infants to short periods of hypoxia. J Pediatr 1957;51:5.
62. Fishman AP, Fritts HW, Cournand A. Effects of acute hypoxia and exercise on the pulmonary circulation. Circulation 1960;22:204.
63. Marshall BE, Marshall C. Continuity of response to hypoxic pulmonary vasoconstriction. J Appl Physiol 1980;49:189.
64. Leffler CW, Hessler JR, Green RS. The onset of breathing at birth stimulates pulmonary vascular prostacyclin synthesis. Pediatr Res 984;18:938–942.
65. Gordon JB, Tod ML, Wetzel RC, McGeady ML, Adkinson NR, Sylvester JT. Age-dependent effects of indomethacin on hypoxic vasoconstriction in neonatal lamb lungs. Pediatr Res 1988;23:580–584.
66. Fike CD, Hansen TN. Hypoxic vasoconstriction increases with postnatal age in lungs from newborn rabbits. Circ Res 1987;60:297–303.
67. Arias-Stella J, Saldana M. The terminal portion of the pulmonary arterial tree in people native to high altitude. Circulation 1963;28:915.
68. Rabinovitch M, Gamble WJ, Miettinen OS, Reid L. Age and sex influence on pulmonary hypertension of chronic hypoxia and on recovery. Am J Physiol 1981;240:H62.
69. Abman SH, Wolfe RR, Accurso FJ, Koops BL, Bowman M, Wiggins JW. Pulmonary vascular response to oxygen in infants with severe bronchopulmonary dysplasia. Pediatrics 1985;75:80.
70. Koch G, Wendel H. Adjustment of arterial blood gases and acid base balance in the normal newborn infant during the first week of life. Biol Neonate 1968;12:136.
71. Koch G. Alveolar ventilation, diffusing capacity, and $AaPO_2$ difference in the newborn infant. Respir Physiol 1968;4:168.
72. Levison H, Featherby EA, Weng TR. Arterial blood gases, alveolar-arterial oxygen difference, and physiologic deadspace in children and young adults. Am Rev Respir Dis 1970;101:972.
73. Fishman AP. Pulmonary edema: the water exchanging function of the lung. Circulation 1972;46:390.
74. Bucci G, Cook C, Barrie H. Studies of respiratory physiology in children. J Pediatr 1961;58:820.
75. O'Brodovich HM, Mellins RB, Mansell AL. Effects of growth on the diffusion constant for carbon monoxide. Am Rev Respir Dis 1982;125:670.
76. Guyton AC, Lindsey AW. Effect of elevated left atrial pressure and decreased plasma protein concentration on the development of pulmonary edema. Circ Res 1959;1:649.
77. Meyer BJ, Meyer A, Guyton AC. Interstitial fluid pressure. V. Negative pressure in the lungs. Circ Res 1968;22:263.
78. Levine OR, Martinez-Rodriguez F, Mellins RB. Fluid filtration in the lungs of the intact puppy. J Appl Physiol 1973;34:683.
79. Brigham KL, Sundell H, Harris TR, Catterton Z, Kovar I, Stahlman M. Lung water and vascular permeability in sheep. Newborns compared with adults. Circ Res 1978;42:851.
80. Staub NC, Nagano H, Pearce ML. Pulmonary edema in dogs, especially the sequence of fluid accumulation in lungs. J Appl Physiol 1967;22:227.
81. Benesch R, Benesch R. Effect of organic phosphates from human erythrocytes on the allosteric properties of hemoglobin. Biochem Biophys Res Commun 1967;26:162.
82. Chanutin A, Curnish R. Effect of organic and inorganic phosphates on the oxygen equilibrium of human erythrocytes. Arch Biochem Biophys 1967;121:96.
83. Martin H, Huisman THJ. Formation of ferrihemoglobin in isolated human hemoglobin types by sodium nitrite. Nature 1963;200:898.
84. Bartos HR, Desforges JF. Erythrocyte DPNH dependent diaphorase levels in infants. Pediatrics 1966;37:991.
85. Roughton FJW, Darling RC. The effect of carbon monoxide on the oxyhemoglobin dissociation curve. Am J Physiol 1944;141:17.
86. Barcroft J. On anoxaemia. Lancet 1920;2:485.
87. Race D, Dedichen H, Schenk WG. Regional blood flow during dextran-induced normovolemic hemodilution in the dog. J Thorac Cardiovasc Surg 1967;53:578.
88. Lennox W, Gibbs F, Gibbs E. Relationship of unconsciousness to cerebral blood flow and to anoxemia. Arch Neurol Psychiatry 1935; 34:1001.
89. Bryan-Brown CW, Baek SM, Makabali G, Shoemaker WC. Consumable oxygen: availability of oxygen in relation to oxyhemoglobin dissociation. Crit Care Med 1973;1:17.
90. Miller MJ. Tissue oxygenation in clinical medicine: an historical overview. Anesth Analg 1982;61:527.
91. Krogh A. The number and distribution of capillaries in muscles with calculations of the oxygen pressure head necessary for supplying the tissue. J Physiol 1919; 52:409.
92. Tenney SM. A theoretical analysis of the relationship between venous blood and tissue oxygen pressures. Respir Physiol 1974;20:283.
93. Miller M, Cook R, Mithoefer J. Limitations of the use of mixed venous PO_2 as an indicator of tissue hypoxia. Clin Res 1979;27:401A.
94. Lutch JS, Murray JF. Continuous positive pressure ventilation: effects on systemic oxygen transport and tissue oxygenation. Ann Intern Med 1972;76:193.
95. Hill JR, Rahimtulla KA. Heat balance and metabolic rate of newborn babies in relation to environmental temperature, and effect of age and weight on basal metabolic rate. J Physiol 1965;180:239.
96. Grenvik A. Respiratory, circulatory, and metabolic effects of respiratory treatment: a clinical study in post-operative thoracic surgical patients. Acta Anaesthesiol Scand 1966;19:1.
97. Berger AJ, Mitchell RA, Severinghaus JW. Regulation of respiration. N Engl J Med 1977;297:92,138,194.
98. Gabel RA, Weiskopf RB. Ventilatory interaction between hypoxia and H^+ at chemoreceptors of man. J Appl Physiol 1975;39:292.
99. Mitchell RA. Respiratory responses mediated through superficial chemosensitive areas on the medulla. J Appl Physiol 1963;18:523.

100. Paintal AS. Vagal sensory receptors and their reflex effects. Physiol Rev 1973;53:159.
101. Lumsden T. Observation on the respiratory centers in the cat. J Physiol 1923;57:153.
102. Lumsden T. Observations on the respiratory centers. J Physiol 1923;57:354.
103. Rigatto H. Apnea. Pediatr Clin North Am 1982;29:1105.
104. Daily WJR, Klaus M, Mayer HBP. Apnea in premature infants: monitoring, incidence, heart rate change, and effect of environmental temperature. Pediatrics 1972; 50:202.
105. Shannon DC, Kelly DH, O'Connell K. Abnormal regulation of ventilation in infants at risk for sudden infant death syndrome. N Engl J Med 1977;297:747.
106. Rigatto H, Brady JP. Periodic breathing and apnea in preterm infants. II. Hypoxia as a primary event. Pediatrics 1972;50:219.
107. Blanco CE, Hanson MEA, Johnson P, Rigatto H. Breathing pattern of kittens during hypoxia. J Appl Physiol 1984;56:12.
108. Agostini E. Volume-pressure relationships of the thorax and lung in the newborn. J Appl Physiol 1959;14:909.
109. Richards C, Bachman L. Lung and chest wall compliance in apneic paralyzed infants. J Clin Invest 1961;40:273.
110. Sharp M, Druz W, Balagot R, Bandelin V, Danon J. Total respiratory compliance in infants and children. J Appl Physiol 1970;29:775.
111. Bryan AC, Mansell AL, Levison H. Development of the mechanical properties of the respiratory system. In: Hodson WA, ed. Development of the lung. New York: Marcel Dekker, 1976:445.
112. Guslits BG, Gaston SE, Bryan MH, England SJ, Bryan AC. Diaphragmatic work of breathing in premature human infants. J Appl Physiol 1987;62:1410–1415.
113. Muller N, Volgyesi G, Bryan MH, Bryan AC. The consequences of diaphragmatic muscle fatigue in the newborn infant. J Pediatr 1979;95:793.
114. Muller N, Volgyesi G, Calle D, Whitton J, Froese AB, Bryan MH, Bryan AC. Diaphragmatic muscle fatigue in the newborn. J Appl Physiol 1979;46:688.
115. Keens TG, Bryan AC, Levison H, Ianuzzo CD. Developmental patterns of muscle fiber types in human ventilatory muscles. J Appl Physiol 1978;44:909.
116. Maxwell LC, McCarter RJM, Kuehl TJ, Robotham JL. Development of histochemical and functional properties of baboon respiratory muscles. J Appl Physiol 1983;54:551.
117. Lopes JM, Muller NL, Bryan MH, Bryan AC. Synergistic behavior of inspiratory muscles after diaphragmatic fatigue in the newborn. J Appl Physiol 1981;51:547.
118. Knill R, Bryan AC. An intercostal-phrenic inhibitory reflex in human newborn infants. J Appl Physiol 1976;40:352.
119. Knill R, Andrews W, Bryan AC, Bryan MH. Respiratory load compensation in infants. J Appl Physiol 1976; 40:357.
120. Nichols DG. Respiratory muscle performance in infants and children. J Pediatr 1991;118:493–502.
121. Kahn A, Mantauk AL, Blum D. Diagnostic categories in infants referred for an acute event suggesting near-miss sudden infant death syndrome. Eur J Pediatr. 1987;146:458–460.
122. Guilleminault C, Ariagno R, Souquet M, Dement WC. Abnormal polygraphic findings in nearmiss sudden infant death. Lancet 1976;1326–1327.
123. Kahn A, Blum D, Rebuffat E, et al. Polysomnographic studies of infants who subsequently died of sudden death syndrome. Pediatrics 1988;82:721–727.
124. Guilleminault C, Hill WH, Simmons FB, Dement WC. Obstructive sleep apnea: electromyographic and fiberoptic studies. Exp. Neurol. 1978;62: 48–67.
125. Ruggins NR, Milner AD. Site of upper airway obstruction in infants following an acute life-threatening event. Pediatrics 1993; 91:595–601.
126. Meadow R. Suffocation, recurrent apnea, and sudden infant death. J Pediatr 1990;117:351–357.
127. Brouillette RT, Fernbach SK, Hunt CE. Obstructive sleep apnea in infants and children. J Pediatr 1982; 100:31–40.
128. Bradley TD, Rutherford R, Grossman RF, Lue F, Zamel N, Moldofsky H, Phillipson A. Role of daytime hypoxemia in the pathogenesis of right heart failure in the obstructive sleep apnea syndrome. Am Rev Respir Dis 1985; 131:835–839.
129. Gislason T, Almqvist M, Boman G, Lindholm CE, Terenius L. Increased CSF opioid activity in sleep apnea syndrome. Chest 1989;96: 250–254.
130. Walsh JK, Farrell MK, Keenan WJ, Lucas M, Kramer M. Gastroesophageal reflux in infants: relation to apnea. J Pediatr 1981;99:197–201.
131. Anas N, Boettrich C, Hall CB, Brooks JG. The association of apnea and respiratory syncytial virus infection in infants. J Pediatr 1982;101:65–68.
132. Kurth CD, Spitzer AR, Broennle AM, Downes JJ. Postoperative apnea in preterm infants. Anesthesiology 1987;66:483–488.
133. Liu LMP, Cotè CJ, Goudsouzian NG, Ryan JF, Firestone S, Dedrick DF, Liu PL, Todres D. Life-threatening apnea in infants recovering from anesthesia. Anesthesiology 1983;59:506–510.
134. Welborn LG, Rice LJ, Hannallah RS, Broadman LM, Ruttimann UE, Fink R. Post-operative apnea in former preterm infants: prospective comparison of spinal and general anesthesia. Anesthesiology 1990;72:838–842.
135. Cotè CJ, Kelly DH. Postoperative apnea in a full-term infant with a demonstrable respiratory pattern abnormality. Anesthesiology 1990; 72:559–561.
136. Tetzlaff JE, Annand DW, Pudimat MA, Nicodemus HF. Postoperative apnea in a full-term infant. Anesthesiology 1988;69:426–428.
137. Sharp JT, Druz WS, D'Souza V, Diamond E. Effect of metabolic acidosis upon sleep apnea. Chest 1985; 87:619–624.
138. Lavaher S, Evers JAM, Teppema LJ. Increase in ventilation caused by aminophylline in the absence of changes in ventral medullary extracellular fluid pH and carbon dioxide tension. Thorax 1989;44: 121–125.
139. Robotham JL. A physiologic approach to hemidiaphragm paralysis. Crit Care Med 1979;7:563.
140. Cook CD, Sutherland JM, Segal S, Cherry RB, Mead J, McIlroy MB, Smith CA. Studies of respiratory physiology in the newborn infant. III. Measurement of mechanisms of respiration. J Clin Invest 1957;36:440.

Lower Airway Disease: Bronchiolitis and Asthma 5

Mark A. Helfaer
David G. Nichols
Mark C. Rogers

INTRODUCTION

Lower airway disease is a common cause of admission to pediatric intensive care units (PICUs). Lower airway disease includes both bronchiolitis and asthma. Physiologic and clinical approaches of both these entities are discussed in this chapter.

BRONCHIOLITIS

Bronchiolitis is an acute inflammatory disease of the lower respiratory tract, resulting in obstruction of small airways. It commonly is stated that bronchiolitis is the wheezing disease of infants up to 2 years of age, while asthma begins at that age. This approach is too simplistic, however, because infants have been diagnosed with asthma. As a result, this chapter considers bronchiolitis from a pathophysiologic perspective and includes independent discussions on its etiology and management.

Etiology

Many diseases appear as bronchiolitis-like illnesses, with the overwhelming majority of these diseases due to viral causes. A number of different viral pathogens cause bronchiolitis. Respiratory syncytial virus (RSV) accounts for most cases of bronchiolitis in which a specific agent can be identified. It is estimated that in 40% to 75% of infants admitted to hospitals with bronchiolitis, RSV is the cause[1]. Other viruses that cause bronchiolitis are rhinovirus[2], parainfluenza virus type 3[3], adenovirus types 3, 7, and 21[4], influenza virus[2], and occasionally mumps[5]. Although *Mycoplasma pneumoniae* is usually associated with lower respiratory tract disease in older children, it rarely causes bronchiolitis in infants[6].

Abundant evidence indicates that immunologic mechanisms play a role in inciting the lower airway disease seen in RSV bronchiolitis. It has been noted that infants may develop severe RSV bronchiolitis despite prior immunization with a killed RSV vaccine and the subsequent production of high levels of complement-fixing and neutralizing antibody to RSV[7]. Kim et al.[8] have postulated that type IV or cell-mediated immune response to RSV may be responsible for the severe manifestations of bronchiolitis in vaccinated infants.

A type I allergic reaction to RSV mediated by immunoglobulin E (IgE) antibody may account for clinically significant bronchiolitis. RSV-specific IgE antibodies are present in the nasopharyngeal secretions of infants with severe RSV bronchiolitis[9]. In contrast to this, some studies suggest that maternally acquired neutralizing antibody may ameliorate the severity of the disease[10, 11].

An additional protective factor may be found in secretory immunoglobulin A (IgA) antibody. Support for this view comes from the observation that viral shedding ends once specific IgA secretory antibody appears in nasopharyngeal secretions[12]. Also, IgA is secreted in colostrum, and breast-fed babies appear relatively protected from bronchiolitis[13]. Other mediators, such as leukotriene C_4 (LTC_4), have been found in high concentrations in the nasopharynx of infants with bronchiolitis and may play a pathologic role in RSV infections[14].

Epidemiology

Using a broad clinical definition of "wheezing associated with respiratory infection," Henderson et al.[6] noted that the highest incidence of this disease was in the first year of life, with 11.4 cases/100 children/year. The incidence fell to 6/100 children/year during the second year of life. In cases of RSV-induced bronchiolitis that required hospitalization, the incidence was 5/1000 live births/year for infants born to low-income families in Houston[11]. Over 80% of those infants hospitalized were younger than 6 months of age. Therefore, it was concluded that younger infants suffer a more severe form of the disease and require hospitalization. Those young infants who contract severe bronchiolitis may be at higher risk because of low levels of maternally transmitted neutralizing antibody[11].

Among infants and young children, boys are more frequently and more severely affected than girls[2, 11]. Approximately 2 to 5% of hospitalized infants progress to respiratory failure and require mechanical ventilatory support. Of hospitalized infants with culture-proven RSV infection, 18 to 20% may develop apnea[15, 16]. Prematurity and young age predispose those patients with RSV bronchiolitis to apnea. Infants with congenital heart disease represent another high-risk group for RSV infection. The overall mortality rate for hospitalized infants with RSV bronchiolitis is less than 1%, the mortality rate for infants with congenital heart disease and RSV infection is 2.5%[17]. Identification of this high-risk group has led to the effective prophylactic administration of respiratory syncytial virus immune globulin to these patients. The use of this immune globulin is an effective means of preventing lower respiratory tract infection[18].

RSV epidemics occur each winter, while parainfluenza virus outbreaks occur in the fall[2]. The disease is highly contagious. Once the virus is introduced in a day-care setting, virtually all exposed children (98%) become infected[19]. Transmission of RSV within families is also significant, with 46% of the other family members becoming infected once one family member has acquired the disease[20].

The rate of nosocomial spread is also high. During a community outbreak of RSV infections, 45% of previously uninfected hospitalized infants became ill with RSV respiratory disease. The risk of infection increased with length of hospital stay. Hospital staff members are probably the major carrier source during nosocomial spread of RSV infection through contamination with secretions from infected infants. The hospital staff suffers approximately the same attack rate (42%) as do the infants[21].

Clinical Manifestations

The affected infant is typically infected by exposure to an older child or an adult with an upper respiratory infection. Cough, sneeze, and rhinorrhea develop initially. Subsequently, the patient suffers marked respiratory distress characterized by tachypnea, flaring of alae nasi, chest wall retractions, wheezing, and irritability. A low-grade fever may be present, and marked dyspnea can make feeding difficult. During breathing, there is a thoracoabdominal asynchrony that correlates with the degree of airflow obstruction[(22)]. The lungs are hyperinflated, and the liver may be palpable several fingerbreadths below the costal margin. Auscultation of the lungs reveals diffuse wheezes, prolonged expiration, and rales.

Appropriate laboratory tests for the infant with severe bronchiolitis include chest x-ray, complete blood count, arterial blood gases, culture and fluorescent antibody tests for RSV, and bacterial cultures in cases where bacterial pneumonia cannot be ruled out. A very reliable bedside diagnostic tool to identify patients with RSV is likely to be available in the near future[(23)]. Radiologic examination of infants with acute bronchiolitis demonstrates air trapping in most patients (Fig. 5.1). About half the patients will have evidence of peribronchial thickening[(24)]. Consolidation and collapse are seen less commonly on chest x-ray. Bacterial pneumonia cannot be excluded on radiologic grounds alone. The complete blood count is generally normal. RSV may be identified by complement fixation or indirect immunofluorescent antibody testing on nasal wash specimens as well as culture of the organism.

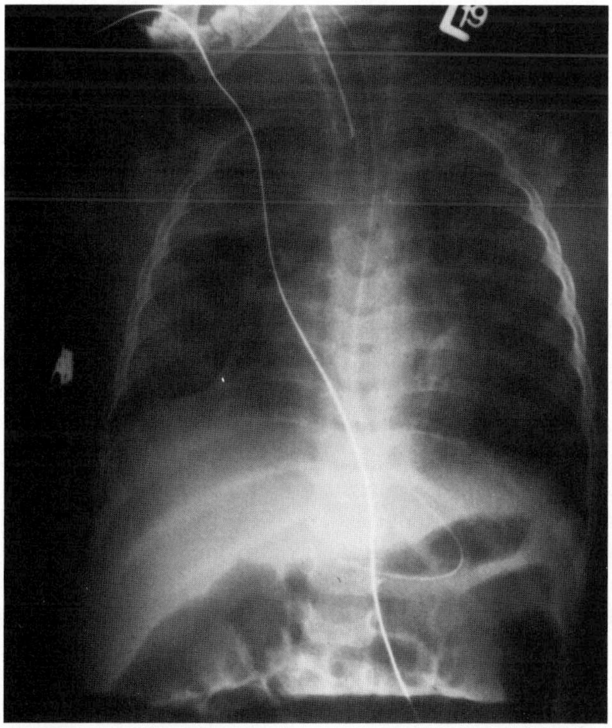

Figure 5.1. Chest x-ray of infant with bronchiolitis and respiratory failure, showing air trapping and peribronchial thickening.

To make the diagnosis of respiratory failure in bronchiolitis, arterial blood gas measurements are necessary. Based on a series of 32 infants with RSV bronchiolitis, Hall et al.[(25)] concluded that all infants were hypoxemic, with a mean oxygen saturation of 87%. Hypoxemia was persistent, lasting 3 to 7 weeks even after clinical improvement had occurred[(25)]. Downes et al.[(26)] studied 30 infants (mean age 5.8 months) who had been admitted to a PICU with bronchiolitis. Among those patients, 96% were hypoxic in room air. Approximately one-third of these patients developed "acute" or "impending" respiratory failure based on a P_aCO_2 of 65 mm Hg or higher. Acid-base analysis revealed a severe uncompensated respiratory acidosis in the group with respiratory failure.

Histology

The histologic hallmark of bronchiolitis is an inflammatory reaction of the respiratory epithelium that physiologically leads to small airway obstruction. After necrosis of ciliated epithelium in small airways occurs, there is proliferation of cuboidal cells without cilia. Adventitia and submucosa of the airway become edematous. Alveolar debris and fibrous strands develop within bronchioles, and the absence of ciliated epithelium prevents adequate mobilization of secretions and debris. Bronchioles become partially or completely obstructed. After 3 to 4 days, recovery begins with a regeneration of basal layers. Cilia regenerate after 15 days. Alveoli may also be involved in the inflammatory process of bronchiolitis. Infiltration with lymphocytes and edema of alveolar lining cells may appear.

Adenovirus has been associated with a particularly severe reaction termed bronchiolitis obliterans[(27)]. In this entity, destruction of respiratory epithelium is extensive, with subsequent proliferation of stratified, undifferentiated epithelium and an intense inflammatory response extending from the peribronchial space to the alveolus. The reparative phase is characterized by fibrosis and obliteration of small airways. Swyer and James[(28)] described a unilateral hyperlucent lung syndrome following adenovirus infection. Pathologic examination of lungs of the patients with this syndrome shows destruction of bronchi and bronchioles, with fibrous tissue occluding the lumen of terminal bronchioles, coupled with decreased pulmonary vasculature on angiogram[(29)].

There has been an attempt to correlate the various radiologic pictures seen in bronchiolitis with pathology. When air spaces in the lungs are opacified, this correlates with *proliferative bronchiolitis* characterized by organizing intraluminal exudate within the airways. When lobular areas of decreased attenuation and airway dilatation are present, these correlate with *constrictive bronchiolitis,* which is characterized by alterations in the walls of membranous and respiratory bronchioles, often without extensive changes in alveolar ducts and alveolar walls[(30)].

Pathophysiology

The results of pulmonary function studies follow predictably from the small airway obstruction and hyperinflation in bronchiolitis. The thoracic volume at end expiration is increased almost twofold above normal[31]. Most studies demonstrate an increase in inspiratory and expiratory resistance[31, 32]. The expiratory resistance is generally increased to a greater extent than the inspiratory resistance.

The hyperresponsiveness of the airways associated with RSV may be related to neural control. In guinea pigs, parainfluenza virus infection damages the inhibitory M_2 muscarinic receptors in the airway smooth muscle. Loss of these inhibitory signals increases the release of acetylcholine and may contribute to the small-airway constriction. It is conceivable that the same pathophysiology applies to RSV-infected humans[33].

The principal abnormality in gas exchange is hypoxemia[34]. Because hypoxemia is typically relieved with a modest amount of supplemental oxygen (40%), Reynolds[35] concluded that ventilation/perfusion mismatching accounts for arterial desaturation. He reasoned that the degree of hypoxemia encountered in his patients should not be responsive to 40% oxygen if it were due to a right-to-left intrapulmonary shunt. Most infants, in spite of an increased physiologic dead space-to-tidal volume ratio (V_D/V_T), are able to maintain normocarbia by increasing minute ventilation (V_E) significantly. Hypercarbia and respiratory failure develop when the infant becomes fatigued and minute V_E falls to predicted basal levels[26]. The high V_E is due mainly to the increased respiratory rate, while tidal volume is unchanged or somewhat lower than normal[36]. Respiratory muscle fatigue is not surprising, considering the infant may increase work of breathing up to sixfold during acute bronchiolitis[36, 37]. Apnea in RSV bronchiolitis is not due to upper airway obstruction but rather to a complete absence of respiratory effort[38].

Management

The infant with acute bronchiolitis and respiratory distress should be hospitalized, particularly if the infant's age is less than 6 months, respiratory rate is elevated, or there is a history of chronic cardiorespiratory disease. Pediatric ICU admission should be considered for younger infants and particularly for those showing signs of impending respiratory failure. If the high risk of nosocomial spread of the disease is taken into consideration, these infants should be cohorted, and staff members involved in their care should employ strict hand-washing procedures[39]. Arterial blood gas analysis should be performed on those patients with respiratory distress and bronchiolitis. Because hypoxemia is the most common abnormality detected, supplemental oxygen administration is the mainstay of therapy[35]. Oxygen may be conveniently administered in a croup tent; however, there is no evidence indicating that a mist tent is more beneficial than normally humidified supplemental oxygen alone.

Because expiratory resistance in particular is increased in bronchiolitis, aerosolized isoproterenol and salbutamol have been tried as bronchodilators[40, 41]. No beneficial effect was demonstrated in these studies. More recently, nebulized albuterol (0.015 mg/kg/dose) resulted in modest symptomatic improvement in infants with bronchiolitis in a double-blind randomized trial in the emergency room[42]. The safety of continuous nebulized albuterol remains controversial despite the widespread use of this practice. In one study in a Pediatric ICU, there were no EKG changes or dysrhythmias during this therapy. However, 3 of the 16 patients demonstrated elevation of creatinine kinase, and two patients demonstrated elevated levels of CPK-MB[43]. Using forced expiratory flows at functional residual capacity a subgroup of patients demonstrated improvement with metaproterenol, which was difficult to identify prospectively[44]. Subcutaneous epinephrine (10 μg/kg) was demonstrated to diminish the signs of respiratory distress in a randomized double-blind outpatient study of wheezing infants less than 2 years of age[45]. In fact, racemic epinephrine (0.1 ml/kg) was found to be superior to salbutamol in the treatment of infants having their first episode of acute bronchiolitis[46]. Even intubated patients with bronchiolitis benefit from aerosolized β_2-agonists[47]. Ipratropium bromide, an aerosolized anticholinergic agent, has not been demonstrated to be of help in the management of the wheezy infant[48]. In summary, even though population statistics fail to demonstrate a uniform compelling effect of bronchodilators, it seems reasonable to administer these agents on a trial basis to individual patients with bronchiolitis and gauge the clinical response.

A large, controlled, multi-institutional study[49] showed corticosteroids to be of no value in the treatment of bronchiolitis. Although of questionable benefit in the acute illness, nebulized beclomethasone may have salutary effects long after an attack of bronchiolitis[50]. Although population statistics demonstrate the lack of efficacy of steroids in bronchiolitis, careful evaluation of the response of individual patients demonstrates that some patients do indeed respond favorably to steroids. It is unclear whether one can predict how to differentiate the responders from the nonresponders, but theoretically, it may be that early institution of steroids, as the edema is forming, may be beneficial. Steroid therapy in adenovirus-induced bronchiolitis obliterans has not been studied. As expected in a viral infection, antibacterial agents are useless[51]. Occasionally, bacterial pneumonia cannot be excluded on clinical or radiologic grounds. In such circumstances, antibiotics may be started until appropriate cultures are negative. In addition, adults with panbronchiolitis have been treated with erythromycin with good response. Data in mice treated with recombinant IL-8 suggest that erythromycin inhibits neurophil chemotaxis. In consequence, erythromycin may diminish pulmonary inflammation by reducing the amount of inflammation contributed by neutrophils[52]. No such study has been conducted in children.

Over the years, antiviral chemotherapy with ribavirin

aerosol, a nucleoside analog, has shown some success in clinical trials[53]. Virus shedding diminishes more rapidly in ribavirin-treated patients. Although upper respiratory tract infection symptoms are not affected by ribavirin, systemic complaints and fever occur less often when bronchiolitic patients receive ribavirin aerosol[54]. These findings have been verified by a 3-year prospective blind multicenter study in which early treatment with ribavirin caused a slightly greater rate of overall clinical improvement, lower oxygen requirements, and fewer desaturations with no other demonstrable effect. It is noteworthy that there was no effect on the length of hospital stay or mortality rate[55]. The findings of this study emphasize that the efficacy of ribavirin documented thus far is small. If the administration of ribavirin is considered, it should be given early in the course of the disease. Ribavirin aerosols have a tendency to crystallize and disrupt ventilator tubes and valves, and because of this, ribavirin has been withheld from infants requiring mechanical ventilation. With proper monitoring and frequent changes of tubing, such infants can be safely treated with ribavirin aerosols[56, 57]. In a recent study, ribavirin decreased the ventilatory support, oxygen requirement, and hospitalization needs of patients compared with controls[58]. Thus, although ribavirin has only modest effects on spontaneously breathing infants, the effects on infants requiring mechanical ventilation (who are presumably sicker) might be salutary. This study has been criticized because the control group received sterile water (which is the vehicle for the ribavirin). In some asthmatics, nebulized sterile water may worsen forced expiratory volume in 1 second (FEV_1)[59] and therefore, if this is also true of the control population in this study, it may make the control group sicker and the treatment group appear better. In more recent studies, although ribavirin has been demonstrated to be safely administered to children on ventilators, the therapy does not affect the immediate clinical outcome[60]. If one decides to use ribavirin, a high-dose, short duration (6 gm/100 ml of water administered for 2 hours three times per day) is equally efficacious to the normal regimen (6 gm/300 ml of water for 18 hours)[61].

The teratogenicity of ribavirin in humans is highly controversial. No studies have demonstrated any damage to health care workers; yet the Centers for Disease Control recommend that health care workers who are or may be pregnant ". . . should be advised of the potential risks of exposure during direct care when patients are receiving ribavirin through oxygen tent or mist mask"[62].

In summary, the place of ribavirin in the therapeutic approach to RSV infection remains controversial. The American Academy of Pediatrics Committee on Infectious Diseases recommends consideration of ribavirin in RSV-infected infants **(Table 5.1)**[63]. Wald and colleagues[64] suggest a very judicious approach to ribavirin until beneficial effects of ribavirin have been clearly demonstrated by objective outcome measures such as mortality or hospital stay.

The use of respiratory syncytial virus immunoglobulin at high doses (500 to 750 mg/kg) has demonstrated promise. It has been used to prevent RSV in patients at risk for this disease. These include premature infants less than 6 months of age with bronchopulmonary dysplasia or congenital heart disease[65]. Use of this aerosolized immunoglobulin has shown promise in the treatment of children with RSV bronchiolitis, yet these are preliminary findings[66].

Prematurely born infants less than 3 months postnatal age are at increased risk for RSV-associated apnea, particularly if they have a history of apnea of prematurity[15, 16]. Therefore, these patients should receive cardiorespiratory monitoring on admission to the hospital. Agitation should alert the clinician to the possibility of hypoxia; an oxygen saturation monitor should also be used, or an arterial blood gas should be obtained. The use of sedation in these infants should be discouraged and reserved for the most difficult cases. Sedation not only will mask the signs of hypoxia, but will also depress respirations and worsen ventilation and oxygenation. Even chloral hydrate, often touted as a drug with minimal respiratory effects, will decrease the oxygen saturations of wheezy infants[67].

When the PCO_2 rises above the normal 40 to 45 torr in a patient with tachypnea and respiratory distress, impending respiratory failure exists. There are no absolute criteria

Table 5.1. American Academy Recommendations for Consideration of Treatment with Ribavirin[a]

The intent of the new recommendation is to allow practitioners to decide whether ribavirin therapy is appropriate by taking into account the particular clinical situation and their own perferences. Recommendations may be modified as new information becomes available. Ribavirin aerosol therapy may be considered in the following list of selected infants and young children at high risk for serious RSV disease.

- Those with complicated congenital heart disease (including pulmonary hypertension) and those with bronchopulmonary dysplasia, cystic fibrosis, and other chronic lung disease. Previously healthy premature infants (<37 weeks' gestational age) and those less than 6 weeks of age are also at greater risk for severe RSV illness, but less so than patients with underlying disease.
- Those with underlying immunosuppressive diseases or therapy (eg, those with acquired immunodeficiency syndrome, severe combined immunodeficiency disease, or organ transplantation) who have high mortality and/or prolonged RSV illness.
- Those who are severely ill with or without mechanical ventilation. Because severity of illness is often difficult to judge clinically in infants with RSV infection, useful guidelines include blood gas measurements and the infant's response to other therapies.
- Hospitalized patients who may be at increased risk of progressing from a mild to a more complicated course because they are younger than 6 weeks or have an underlying condition, such as multiple congenital anomalies or certain neurologic or metabolic diseases (eg, cerebral palsy or myasthenia gravis).

[a]From American Academy of Pediatrics Committee on Infectious Diseases. Reassessment of the indications for ribavirin therapy in respiratory syncytial virus infections. Pediatrics 1996;97(1):137–140.

for endotracheal intubation, and in fact, most infants with bronchiolitis do not require intubation. If endotracheal intubation is necessary, attention should be directed to the size of the endotracheal tube. Many premature infants are at risk for or have preexisting subglottic narrowing that dictates the need for a smaller endotracheal tube than predicted based on age. Symptoms such as lethargy, increasing respiratory distress, apneic spells, or cyanosis all point to the need for mechanical ventilation. In general, when the PCO_2 reaches 60 to 65 torr, frank respiratory failure has occurred and positive pressure ventilation is instituted(26). Although mechanical ventilation remains standard therapy for respiratory failure in most centers, Beasley and Jones(68) reported a series of 23 infants in respiratory failure from bronchiolitis who were managed with continuous positive airway pressure (CPAP). Seventeen of the 23 patients were younger than 2 months old. The majority of patients were successfully managed with CPAP via nasal cannula at 5 cm H_2O pressure. If nasal CPAP failed, the patient was intubated and received CPAP via endotracheal tube. All patients showed immediate clinical improvement, and PCO_2 fell from a mean of 59 mm Hg to 47 mm Hg in the first 4 hours of treatment. The only complication was a small pneumothorax in one patient. These findings were reproduced using nasal CPAP of 6 to 7 cm H_2O(69). These results argue for a trial of nasal CPAP before endotracheal intubation and mechanical ventilation are instituted. Once mechanically ventilated, however, positive-end expiratory pressure (PEEP) (0, 3, 6, or 9 cm H_2O) contributes to air trapping and does not improve pulmonary mechanics(70).

When all conventional treatment modalities have been tried, and significant hypoxemia persists despite maximum therapy, high-frequency oscillatory ventilation can be attempted(71). In addition, extracorporeal membrane oxygenation has been instituted with some degree of success in a small number of patients (7 of 12 survivors)(72). This highly aggressive therapy should be reserved for those patients whose underlying lung disease is mild enough to allow full recovery from their acute bronchiolitic illness. Inhaled nitric oxide has been attempted with some success in improving oxygenation in an infant with RSV(73).

Fluid Administration

Infants with bronchiolitis are in the state of hypervolemia because of elevated antidiuretic hormone (ADH) levels, yet they also have elevated renin levels that lead to secondary hyperaldosteronism(74). As a clinical consequence, these infants typically have weight gain and diminished urine output but a normal urine sodium. The optimal fluid regimen in bronchiolitis has not been studied, yet it seems reasonable to reverse some of the hypervolemia, thus decreasing lung water. This can be accomplished by judicious use of diuretics or careful fluid restriction, once preexisting fluid deficits have been repleted. This is especially important when impending respiratory failure is diagnosed; fluid administration must be tightly controlled in order to ensure euvolemia without risking overhydration. Various investigators(75) have shown that decreased intrapleural pressure in asthmatic patients with severely obstructed airways may favor the development of pulmonary edema. It is reasonable to assume that patients with lower airway obstruction from bronchiolitis are also at risk for pulmonary edema. Furthermore, severe bronchiolitis may include a necrotizing injury to bronchiolar and alveolar walls, which would favor transudation of fluid into air spaces(27).

Monitoring

Respiratory failure from bronchiolitis is usually relatively short lived. Nevertheless, during the period of impending respiratory failure, patients require meticulous surveillance and monitoring in the pediatric ICU. Nursing observations include frequent notation of vital signs, sensorium, breathing pattern, and skin color, as well as fluid intake and output. A continuous record of heart rate and respiratory rate is mandatory, particularly in view of the high incidence of apnea, especially in the very young or prematurely born infant.

Respiratory therapy is guided by an assessment of oxygenation and ventilation. The arterial blood gas remains the standard means of measuring oxygenation and ventilation. However, care of these infants is now facilitated greatly by the noninvasive measurement of cutaneous oxygen saturation (pulse oximetry). Furthermore, in patients who have been intubated, end-tidal CO_2 is measured by placement of an infrared sensor directly between the endotracheal tube and gas delivery tubing or, alternatively, by inserting a catheter proximal to the endotracheal tube that conveys the sampled gas to the analyzer. Accurate measurement requires the absence of leaks from the tubing and endotracheal tube so that the exhaled CO_2 may reach a true plateau at end expiration. If this condition is met and there is normal pulmonary perfusion, the end-tidal CO_2 closely reflects arterial PCO_2. Central venous and pulmonary artery catheter placements are generally unnecessary in these patients with respiratory failure, because the critical phase of the disease is not associated with major hemodynamic changes.

Outcome

Respiratory failure in bronchiolitis generally resolves after 48 to 72 hours(26). However, impaired oxygenation may exist for several weeks after apparent clinical recovery(25). In fact, one long-term follow-up study(76) showed that 75% of asymptomatic children examined 10 years after an acute episode of bronchiolitis had abnormal small airways resistance and arterial PO_2. The relationship between acute bronchiolitis in infancy and the subsequent development of asthma is becoming clearer. Studies have shown that between 5% and 50% of children with acute bronchiolitis in infancy develop recurrent wheezing later in life[77]. This can occur even after 2 to 3 years following bronchiolitis[78]. Infants with poorer lung function before any lower respiratory illness (LRI) are more prone to develop bronchiolitis[79]. After the first episode of wheezing during the first year of life, there is chronic increase in airway resistance[80, 81]. However, the majority of these children have a family history of allergy. It is therefore unclear whether bronchiolitis leads to subsequent development of asthma or whether atopic individuals are predisposed to bronchiolitis.

Bronchiolitis obliterans produces a far more severe acute lung injury and a more debilitating chronic lung disease in survivors. It is caused by a variety of conditions, including infections caused by adenovirus, mycoplasma, influenza, parainfluenza virus type 3, measles, and gastroesophageal reflux[82].

Summary

A life-threatening deterioration in patients with severe bronchiolitis can be managed successfully. The required care relies on the intensivist's understanding of the pathophysiologic derangements involved. The mainstay of pediatric ICU management of this disease is the provision of supplemental oxygen, which may be combined with CPAP or mechanical ventilation in those patients with frank respiratory failure. Other important measures include cardiorespiratory monitoring and close attention to fluid balance. Bronchodilators, steroids, and ribavirin should be considered.

The goal for the future will be to prevent the disease altogether or, at least, to prevent the life-threatening complications associated with it. Improved management will be gained by enhancing insights in the following areas:

1. *Immunopathology.* Prevention of bronchiolitis will depend on the development of an effective vaccine. A great deal of research shows promise in this area[83]. The use of alpha-2A-interferon has been attempted to modulate the response of children with RSV bronchiolitis; the results have been somewhat disappointing[84], yet it has opened the door to an area of research to modulate the immunologic response to the infection.
2. *Antiviral chemotherapy.* Because current antiviral chemotherapy can reduce viral shedding and improve the clinical condition of the sickest infant, the hope is that better agents will be developed with a more remarkable effect on the less severely ill infants.
3. *Infantile apnea.* RSV-induced bronchiolitis is one of the many conditions associated with infantile apnea. Because airway obstruction does not seem to be the cause of apnea in bronchiolitic infants, a disorder in neural regulation of breathing and/or respiratory muscle function is likely. For instance, it is conceivable that apnea in bronchiolitis is caused by excess respiratory muscle oxygen (or nutrient) demand during a period of limited oxygen (or nutrient) supply.

ASTHMA

Definition and Introduction

Asthma is a diffuse, obstructive pulmonary disease characterized by airway inflammation and hyperreactivity manifested by difficulty in breathing resulting from generalized narrowing of the airways. The character of this airway obstruction is intermittent and reversible either spontaneously or as a result of treatment. A history of recurrent attacks with a relatively symptom free period in between is the hallmark of this disease. The pulmonary function studies during asymptomatic periods usually show signs of improvement, although some abnormalities still may persist.

Asthma is the most common chronic disease of childhood; it is a leading cause of school absence, is a common cause for hospital and ICU admission of older infants and children, and is associated with significant morbidity and mortality from the complications of the disease. The asthmatic episodes may be progressive and may result in an impairment of respiratory function ranging from a moderate degree of disability to life-threatening respiratory failure. Asthma is reversible, however, and with an appropriate intensive management, it is possible to minimize morbidity and mortality associated with the disease.

Prevalence

Although it is one of the most common chronic diseases in childhood, the prevalence and the incidence of asthma have not been well defined because of the nonuniformity of acceptable guidelines for the diagnostic criteria and unreliability of the methods that are used in identifying the patients. As a result, there are no reliable population-based figures that have used uniform diagnostic criteria on the incidence or prevalence of asthma in the United States. However, the information available indicates an incidence from 4% to 9% of children in this country[85, 86], and the disease seems to be more frequent in younger males and older females as well as more common in the South than in the other regions of the country. Asthma is disproportionately represented in the black and the poor population. This may be a result of environmental or social situations. Such independent factors associated with childhood asthma include maternal smoking, poverty, large family size, smaller size of home, low birth weight, and maternal age younger than 20 years at the child's birth[87].

It is particularly difficult to document the mortality from asthma. Even with the recent improvements in the treatment of chronic asthma and in intensive therapy during acute attacks, reports of mortalities still occur. The current mortality rate from asthma in the United States is estimated at approximately 1 to 2 deaths/100,000 population/year[88]. This rate may be increasing because of asphyxia rather than cardiac arrhythmias, which implies that many of these deaths could be prevented by aggressive treatment[89]. Fatal asthma may be a distinct entity with unique characteristics. Characteristic factors identifying these patients at risk are young men, severe mixed acidosis with extreme hypercapnia (P_aCO_2 97 ± 31 mm Hg), and a silent chest on admission[(90)]. In children, risk factors include greater frequency of respiratory failure requiring intubation, a decrease in steroid use in the month before the attack, failure to vomit with initial therapy, a history of family disturbances, and abnormal reaction to separation or losses expressed as helplessness and despair[(91)]. Pathophysiologically, this may be due to abnormalities in airway smooth muscle. Bronchial smooth muscle from victims of fatal asthma have a greater maximal response to contractile agonists and an impaired relaxation to β-agonists and theophylline[(92)].

Etiology

The fundamental abnormality in all asthma attacks is the presence of a nonspecific hyperirritability of the tracheobronchial tree, which results in an airway obstruction and clinical signs and symptoms of asthma[(93)]. It can be precipitated by an allergen exposure, infection (especially viral respiratory tract infection), exercise, emotional stress, or administration of drugs **(Table 5.2).** For example, β-blockers and aspirin are known to provoke acute asthmatic attacks in patients with a history of asthma. There may be no single etiologic factor that can explain this clinical syndrome; however, genetic, allergic, and pulmonary factors appear to play important roles.

Genetic Factors

A genetic component to asthma has long been suspected because of the tendency of the children of allergic parents to develop atopic dermatitis in infancy and asthma or allergic rhinitis in later childhood[(94, 95)]. More recently, linkage studies on serum IgE and bronchial hyperresponsiveness as manifestations of the asthmatic phenotype have been per-

Table 5.2. Some Factors That Precipitate Bronchoconstriction in Asthma

Allergy (mediator release)
Histamine
SRS-A
Prostaglandins
Thromboxane
Other
Autonomic imbalance
Excessive cholinergic response
Reduced β-adrenergic responsiveness
Nonspecific irritant
Infections
Viral respiratory tract infection
Pharmacologic agents
β-Adrenergic blockade (propranolol)
Prostaglandin inhibitors (aspirin and nonsteroidal anti-inflammatory drugs)
Exercise induced
Psychogenic

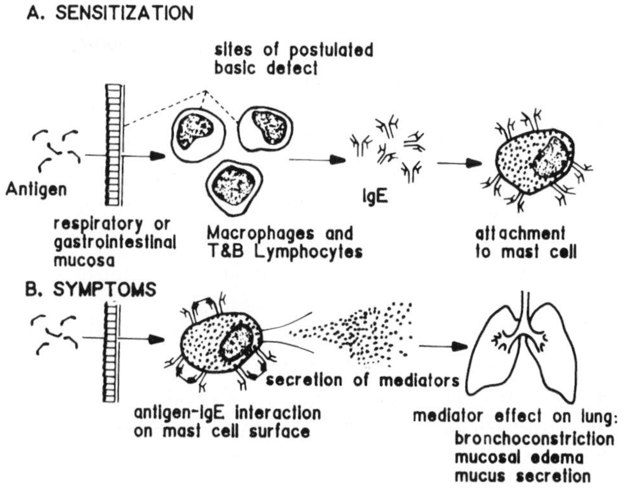

Figure 5.2. Allergic theory of asthma. The pathophysiology may be seen as a two-stage process. **A.** Sensitization of mast cell by an abnormal response to antigens. **B.** Subsequent antigen—IgE interaction causes the release of histamine and other mediators (SRS-A, eosinophil and neutrophil chemotactic factors, prostaglandins, etc.). (From Leffert F. Asthma: a modern perspective. Pediatrics 1978; 62:1062.)

formed. These studies suggest linkage of IgE production and bronchial hyperresponsiveness to polymorphic markers on chromosome 5q[(96)]. A region on the long arm of chromosome 5q is also known to be the site of genes coding for T-lymphocytes derived interleukins. Polymorphisms in the 5′ promoter region of these genes may reflect base exchanges in segments regulating transcriptional dysregulations of T-cell cytokines[(97)].

Allergic Factors

It is believed that allergy plays an important role in "extrinsic" asthma (Fig. 5.2). This is defined as a situation in which a tissue-sensitizing antibody of the IgE type is present in abnormally large amounts and where a significant quantity of antibody specific to the allergen is also present. This IgE binds directly to high-affinity Fc receptors on mast cells in the respiratory tract, and subsequent antigen-IgE interaction causes the release of histamine and other mediators (e.g., slow-reacting substance of anaphylaxis (SRS-A), eosinophil and neutrophil chemotactic factors, and prostaglandins). This causes a direct stimulating effect on the H1 receptor of the airway smooth muscles and causes *bronchoconstriction* (Fig. 5.2)[(98)]. These bronchoconstrictive effects and related mediators from mast cells[(99)] have been divided into three phases (Fig. 5.3)[(100)].

The first phase is described as the *rapid and spasmodic phase.* This bronchoconstrictive effect occurs within 10 to 15 minutes after allergen challenges, and reversibility can occur spontaneously or secondary to treatment. Plasma histamine and neutrophil chemotactic factor of anaphylaxis rise during the same period of increased airway obstruction. Corticosteroid does not inhibit this reaction, whereas

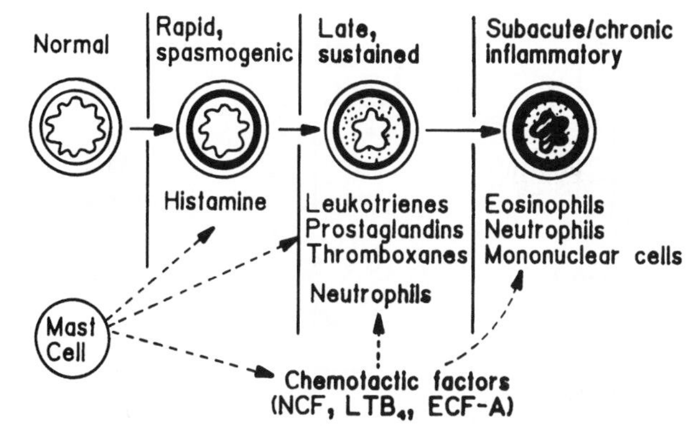

Figure 5.3. Mast cell mediators and phases of airway obstruction in bronchial asthma. (From Kay AB. Basic mechanism of allergic asthma. Eur J Respir Dis (Suppl) 1982;122:13.)

disodium cromoglycate or H_1 and H_2 receptor antagonists can reverse this effect if the drugs are given before the challenge.

The second or *sustained phase* is characterized by a more severe increase in airway obstruction, which occurs maximally in 6 to 8 hours after allergen challenge. Mast cell mediators that are responsible in this phase include leukotrienes, prostaglandins, thromboxanes, and neutrophil chemotactic factor of anaphylaxis. This reaction, which was previously proposed as an example of an Arthus reaction, has been shown to be associated with reactivation of mast cells and to cause submucosal edema accompanied by prolonged contraction of bronchial smooth muscle. Prior administration of corticosteroid inhibits this reaction.

The third or *subacute/chronic inflammatory phase* is a prolonged and resistant phase in bronchoconstriction that is believed to result from substantial inflammation of bronchial submucosa, which is caused by eosinophils and monocytes. Mast cell-derived chemotactic factors, e.g., eosinophil chemotactic factor of anaphylaxis (ECF-A) and LTB_4, induce the mobilization of these cells, and the cytotoxic substances released from eosinophilic granules include major basic protein that contributes to mucosal edema[(101)] and is responsible for the late reaction in airway obstruction of asthmatic patients.

Deranged Autonomic Nervous System

It is well known that airway smooth muscle tone is regulated by the autonomic nervous system **(Table 5.3).** The cholinergic receptor, specifically the M3 muscarinic receptor (Fig. 5.4)[(102)], mediates a potent bronchoconstriction. The M_2 muscarinic receptor serves an inhibitory function, which decreases the cholinergic outflow to the airway smooth muscle[(33)]. The M_2 receptor provides important feedback inhibition to vagally mediated bronchoconstriction. The loss of M_2 receptor function from viral pneumonia or inhalation of ozone leads to unopposed M_3 stimulation and airway hyperresponsiveness[(103)]. The cellular mechanism of cholinergic receptor stimulation is mediated by an increased level of cyclic guanosine monophosphate (cGMP), which in turn causes mast cell degranulation and bronchial smooth muscle contraction. The reflex bronchoconstrictive effect of various mechanical and chemical stimulations of cholinergic receptor can be blocked either by cutting the vagus nerve or by administration of atropine[(104)]. This suggests that histamine and other mast cell mediators cause bronchoconstriction by an indirect vagal reflex via the afferent irritant receptor in the bronchi, and amplification of this impulse in the central nervous system[(105)].

On the other hand, stimulation of β-adrenergic receptors on bronchial smooth muscle (β_2-subtype) causes bronchodilatation. Szentivanyi[(106)] proposed a theory of reduced β-adrenergic responsiveness in asthmatic patients based on animal experiments and other supportive studies[(107–109)] (Fig. 5.5). Contrary to these findings, sympathectomy induced by high thoracic epidural does not decrease resting airway resistance in susceptible individuals, as expected. Furthermore, when these patients were stimulated with in-

Table 5.3. Neurologic Regulation of Airway Smooth Muscle Tone[a]

System	*Effect on airway smooth muscle*	*Airway innervation*	*Humoral receptors*
Sympathetic α_1 and α_2	Constrictor	First six generations not significant without β-blockade	Major resistance airways; significance in distal airway unknown; causes bronchoconstriction after β-blockade
β_2	Dilator	First six generations	All airway smooth muscle; causes substantial bronchodilatation after stimulation
Cholinergic vagus nerve	Constrictor	≤ first nine generations; peripheral airways not innervated	All airways
Histamine	H_1 Constrictor	No direct innervation	Released from mast cells; tissue concentration of histamine increases from trachea to periphery
	H_2	May partially inhibit mast cell release of histamine; may have a dilator effect on human airway smooth muscle	
Nonadrenergic (purinergic) Inhibitory	Dilator	Major resistance	Airway

[a]Adapted from Leff A. Pathophysiology of asthmatic bronchoconstriction. Chest 1982;82:13S.

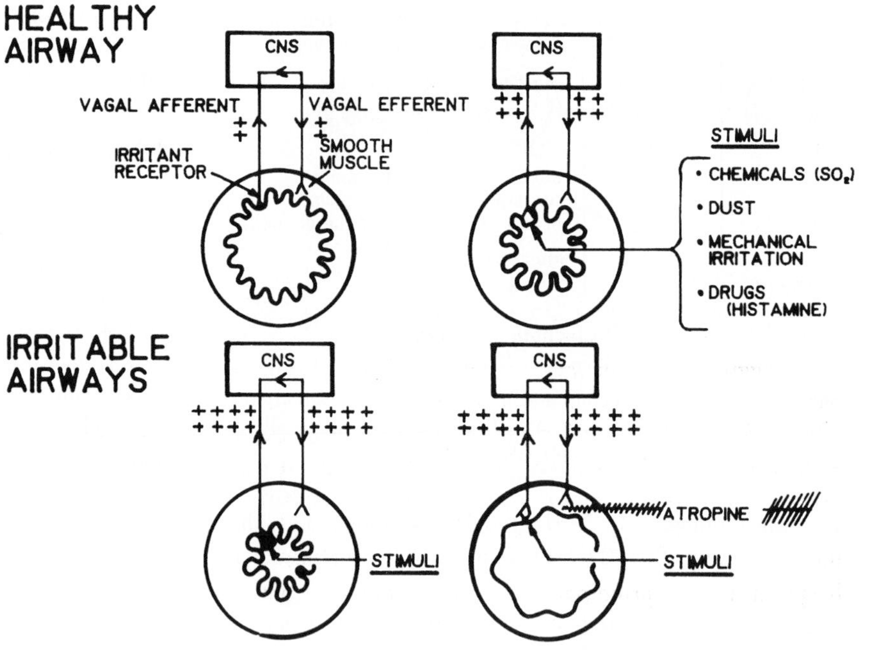

Figure 5.4. Hypothesis of irritant receptor-bronchoconstrictor reflex. Schematic of pathway of vagal reflex from irritant receptor in the airway mucosa to central nervous system (CNS). *Plus signs* relate relative frequency of firing of nerves. *Upper:* Normal control subject—mild bronchoconstriction associated with slight neural activity *(left)* compared with moderate bronchoconstriction during stimulation of irritant receptor and moderate neural activity *(right)*. *Lower:* Patient with irritable airways exposed to same stimuli responds more severely to bronchoconstriction and marked activity of nervous pathway *(left)*. This bronchoconstrictive response can be blocked by atropine *(right)*. (From Nadal JA. Neurophysiologic aspects of asthma. In: Austen KF, Lichtenstein LM, eds. Asthma, physiology, immunopharmacology and treatment. New York: Academic Press, 1973:29.)

haled bronchospasm provocation, they tolerated these provocations better with intravenous local anesthetic as well as epidurally administered local anesthetic. This suggests it is the local anesthetic that attenuates the response rather than the sympathetic blockade[110]. The autonomic imbalance produced by the postulated impairment of β-adrenergic responsiveness, leaving relatively unopposed cholinergic bronchoconstrictive reflexes, could explain the bronchial hyperreactivity that is the feature of this disease.

One of the endothelial derived relaxant factors, nitric oxide, has been evaluated in its role in reversal of bronchospasm. Nitric oxide (as well as atropine) can totally abolish the response to histamine induced bronchoconstriction, with partial reversal of this abolition by methylene blue. On the other hand, nitric oxide only partially reversed methacholine induced bronchoconstriction. This implies that nitric

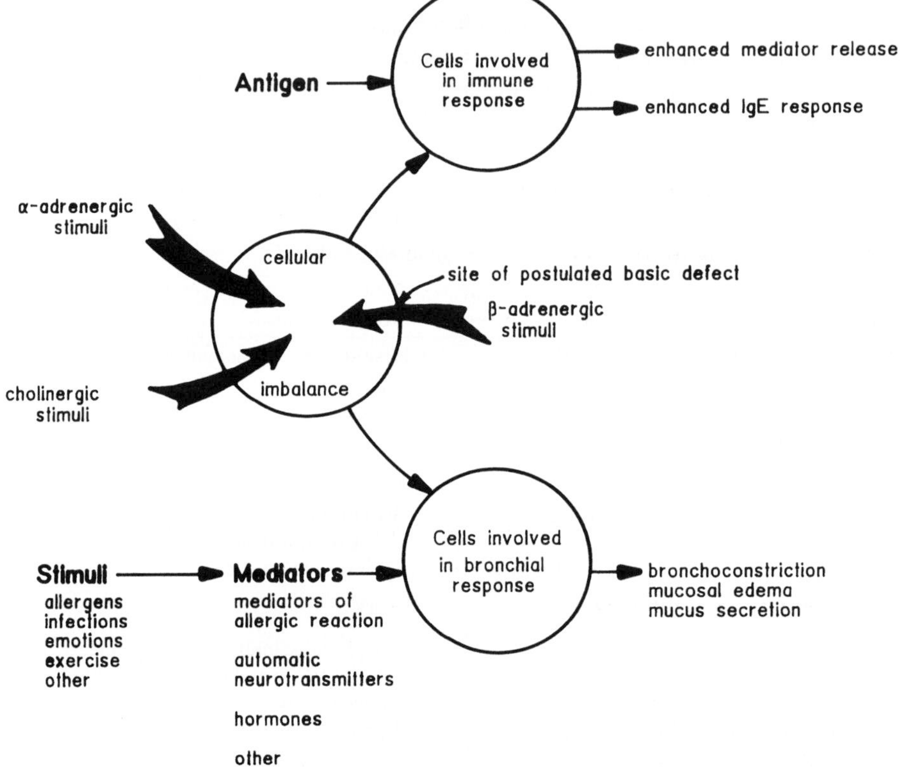

Figure 5.5. β-Adrenergic theory of asthma. The autonomic imbalance produced by reduced β-adrenergic responsiveness causes the hyperresponsiveness of cells involved in both immunologic and bronchial functions. (From Leffert F. Asthma: a modern perspective. Pediatrics 1978;62:1065.)

oxide acts directly upon the smooth airway muscle in much the same way it acts on vascular smooth muscle; that is, to cause an increase in cGMP with consequent smooth muscle dilation. In addition, however, nitric oxide acts in an indirect manner on the smooth muscle of the airways[(111)].

Pathology

The autopsy finding of the patient who dies from status asthmaticus shows not only hypertrophy of smooth muscle in the bronchial wall but also associated inflammation and mucous plugging of the airways. This triad of smooth muscle spasm, mucosal inflammation, and mucous plugging has been known as the major cause of airway obstruction in asthma. The importance of each pathophysiologic feature may vary considerably with the severity and reversibility of the disease[(112)]. The rapid onset and disappearance of the attack after bronchodilator therapy suggests that the bronchospasm is the principal cause of airway obstruction, whereas mucosal inflammation and mucous plugging are likely to be responsible for the more slowly reversible forms of this disease, as found in status asthmaticus patients[(113)].

Smooth Muscle Spasm

The smooth muscle of the tracheobronchial tree in asthmatic patients is believed to function as a single unit that has high resting tone and has more potent and prolonged contraction than the bronchial smooth muscle in a normal person[(114)]. Therefore, smooth muscle constriction alone can be responsible for the airway obstruction in asthma, as shown in experimental animals[(115)]. This is supported by pathohistologic findings of hypertrophied smooth muscle that are found in patients[(116)].

Mucosal Edema

The presence of edema[(117)] and eosinophilic infiltration of mucosa and submucosal tissue are the prominent pathologic features in asthmatic patients. Various nonspecific stimuli e.g., viral infection[(118)], nitrogen dioxide[(119)], ozone[(120)], and cigarette smoke[(86)]—can produce an inflammatory reaction in the airway mucosa. These inflammatory reactions cause an increase in mucosal permeability[(121)] and are associated with a hyperreactivity of the airway to these nonspecific stimuli. The bronchial wall contains increased numbers of activated eosinophils, T-lymphocytes, mast cells, and macrophages[(122)]. Another important histologic feature is a markedly thickened basement membrane[(123)]. This change may be due to the increase in epithelial turnover in the repair period after inflammation, and this theory is supported by the finding of squamous cells and clusters of ciliated columnar cells, known as creola bodies[(124)], in the sputum of these patients. The loss of the mucosal cells leaves large areas of bronchial surface denuded of epithelium and contributes to muscle spasm[(125)] and submucosal edema[(117)] and is also associated with the production of excessive secretions from hypertrophied mucous goblet cells.

Mucosal Plugging of Airways

Segmental and subsegmental atelectasis secondary to tenacious mucous plugging of the airways is a common pathologic feature in patients who die from status asthmaticus[(112)]. These plugs contain mucus, albumin[(126)], large numbers of epithelial cells, and eosinophilic leukocytes. The increase in production of mucus secondary to hypertrophy of bronchial mucous glands[(116)] and goblet cell hyperplasia[(117)] and the decrease in clearance are factors responsible for the plugging. This contributes to airflow obstruction that can be fatal.

Pathophysiology

Although airflow obstruction is a prominent feature of the asthmatic attack, all pulmonary function tests demonstrate abnormalities. These derangements correlate roughly with the severity of the disease.

Airflow Obstruction

Generalized narrowing of the airways with little lung parenchymal involvement is the major pathophysiologic finding in uncomplicated asthma. As a result, airway resistance (R_{aw}) is the important component in lung resistance (lung resistance is composed of airway resistance and tissue resistance) that contributes to airflow obstruction. Measurement of airway resistance can be obtained accurately with a constant-volume, variable-pressure plethysmograph[(127)], which measures R_{aw} at the low flow rates (1 to 1.5 liters/sec) and represents the static or resting airway resistance. This R_{aw} varies inversely with lung volume as well as airway caliber. Both high lung volume (discussed in more detail in next section) and a decrease in airway diameter are found in asthmatic patients. The increase in R_{aw} is related to the severity of the attack and is correlated well with the decrease in large airway diameter but is unrelated to narrowing of the small peripheral airways unless those changes are extensive[(128)]. Another approach for assessing the degree of obstruction is to measure the patient's ventilatory capacity during a forced maximal expiration. The standard indices from this technique are the forced vital capacity (FVC), FEV_1, maximum expiratory flow rate (MEFR), maximum midexpiratory flow rate (MMEFR), and the $FEV_{1.0}$/FVC ratio. The spirogram is sensitive to dynamic events and is influenced by the resistance of the airways, the elasticity of the lungs and chest wall, the absolute volume of the air in the bronchi, and the cooperation of the patient. The types of alterations seen during an acute asthmatic attack are prolonged forced expiratory time, low FVC, marked depression of the $FEV_{1.0}$, and decreased flow

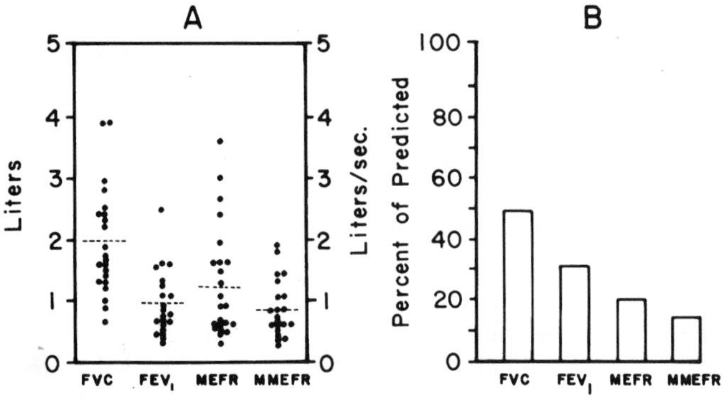

Figure 5.6. Alterations in spirometric measurements seen during acute asthma. **A.** Absolute value. **B.** Pattern obtained using percentages of normal. *FEV_1*, $FEV_{1.0}$. (From McFadden ER Jr. Asthma: airway dynamics, cardiac function and clinical correlates. In: Middleton E Jr, Reed CE, Ellis EF, eds. Allergy: principles and practice. St Louis: CV Mosby, 1983:843.)

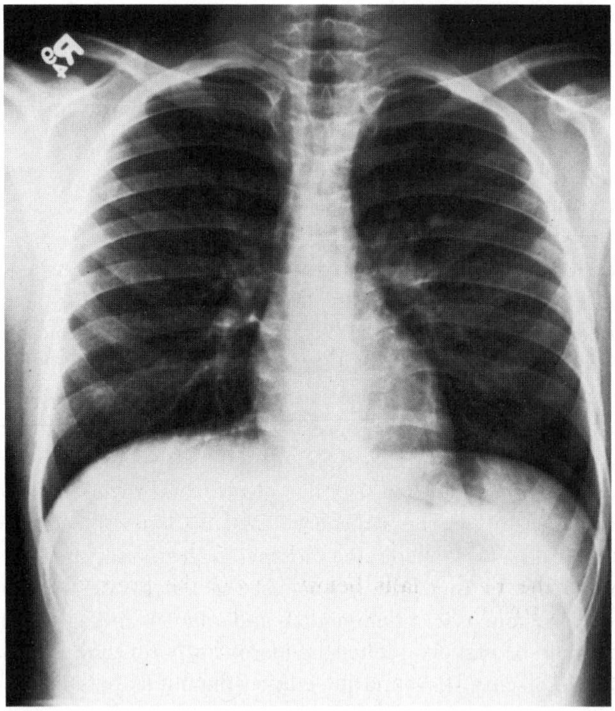

Figure 5.7. Typical chest x-ray of patient with uncomplicated asthma. Hyperaeration of both lung fields is demonstrated.

rate[129–133]. The most important factor in determining the early part of the maximum expiratory flow volume curve is the patency of major airways at or near full lung inflation, whereas the subsequent part of the curve reflects the resistance within the peripheral airway (<2 mm in bronchial diameter). In acute asthma, the MMEFR demonstrates the most severe fall, followed by MEFR, $FEV_{1.0}$, and FVC (Fig. 5.6); after treatment, $FEV_{1.0}$, MEFR, and R_{aw} tend to improve initially, while the MMEFR remains markedly depressed for up to 2 weeks after the onset of acute attack. Portable peak flow meters can be used to easily follow the clinical course of a given asthmatic patient by measuring the peak expiratory flow rate (PEFR). When the PEFR is less than 30 to 50% of predicted or the patient's personal best, a severe asthma attack is present[134]. Extremely dyspneic patients should not be forced to carry out the PEFR maneuver because it may exacerbate bronchospasm in that setting[135]. These findings indicate that the reversibility of airway involvement occurs first in the major airways, followed by improvement of the smaller airways after some period of time.

Lung Volume

Hyperinflation of the lung as seen on physical examination and on x-ray (Fig. 5.7) is a prominent feature of an asthma attack. This change is responsible for the symptoms of respiratory distress in asthma, as described by McFadden and others[136–138]. Residual volume (RV) and functional residual capacity (FRC) are increased during the acute symptoms, with the increase in RV exceeding the change in FRC. Vital capacity, inspiratory capacity, and expiratory reserve volume are all reduced to the same extent. Total lung capacity is variably increased (Fig. 5.8)[139, 140]. Although the mechanisms that are responsible for the change in lung volume are still not known, it is postulated that the decrease in elastic recoil of the lung secondary to airflow obstruction causes more air to be trapped in the alveoli and alveolar ducts and subsequently causes increases in FRC and RV[138, 141–143]. In addition, the premature closure of the airway due to bronchial spasm, mucosal edema, and mucous plugging also results in an increase in air trapped within the lungs. In addition, lung compliance is reduced at high lung volumes. These events cause the asthmatic patient to have to try to overcome the airway obstruction by generating more negative pleural pressures. They also cause the symptoms of respiratory distress and the continued increase in FRC unless the airway obstruction is reversed.

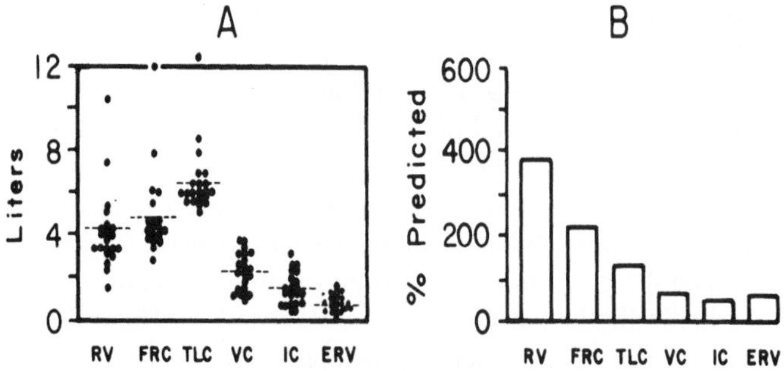

Figure 5.8. Alterations in lung volume seen during acute asthma. **A.** Absolute value. **B.** Pattern obtained using percentages of normal. *ERV,* expiratory reserve volume; *IC,* inspiratory capacity; *TLC,* total lung capacity; *VC,* vital capacity. (From McFadden ER Jr. Asthma: airway dynamics, cardiac function and clinical correlates. In: Middleton E Jr, Reed CE, Ellis EF, eds. Allergy: principles and practice. St Louis: CV Mosby, 1983:843.)

Abnormality in Gas Exchange

Hypoxia, hypocapnia, and respiratory alkalosis are usually seen early in uncomplicated acute asthma attacks[144–146]. The ventilation/perfusion abnormality is associated with nonuniform airway obstruction during an acute asthma attack and accounts for the abnormal gas exchange. Simultaneous changes in pulmonary blood flow result from the high intra-alveolar pressure causing the maldistribution in perfusion. The degree of hypoxemia correlates well with the degree of airway obstruction, as assessed by the reduction in $FEV_{1.0}$[146] (Fig. 5.9). Hypocapnia is caused by alveolar hyperventilation secondary to the activation of pulmonary reflexes and does not seem to be well-correlated with the degree of airway obstruction. A normal level of P_aCO_2 in the presence of respiratory distress indicates severe airway obstruction, with an inability to eliminate CO_2 sufficiently. Elevated P_aCO_2 normally occurs when the $FEV_{1.0}$ falls below 20% of the predicted value (Fig. 5.10)[146]. Some severe asthmatic patients may also exhibit a metabolic acidosis, the etiology of which is unclear[147]. Postulated mechanisms include renal bicarbonate wasting after prolonged respiratory alkalosis, tissue hypoxia, beta adrenergic agonist effects, and increased work of breathing.

Patients with respiratory acidosis with or without metabolic acidosis should be monitored closely in an intensive care unit. Hypercapnia by itself is not necessarily an indication for intubation and mechanical ventilation if the patient is responding to therapy and remains conscious and hemodynamically stable. Conversely, normocapnic patients who are deteriorating rapidly and exhibit hypoxemia, unconsciousness, or hemodynamic instability require immediate intubation and ventilatory support.

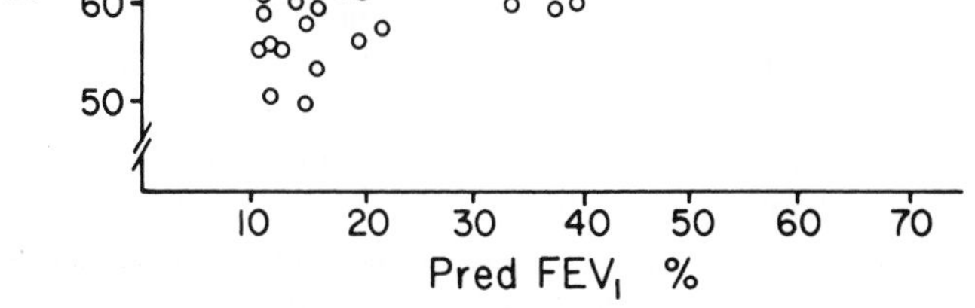

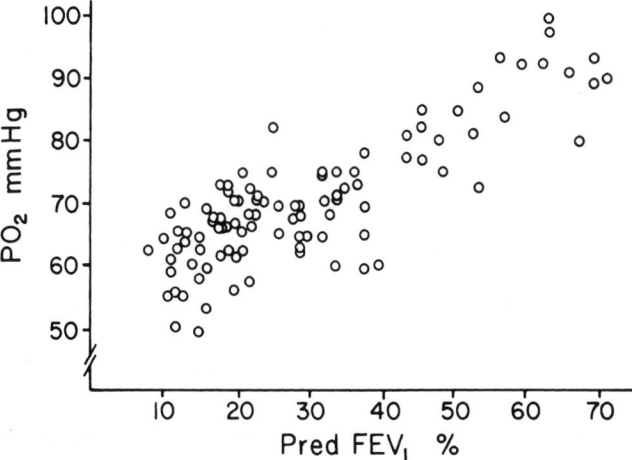

Figure 5.9. Relationship between P_aO_2 and degree of airway obstruction as determined by $FEV_{1.0}$ *(FEV_1)* during acute asthma. (From McFadden ER Jr, Lyons HA. Arterial blood gas tension in asthma. (N Engl J Med 1968;278:1029, reprinted by permission of the *New England Journal of Medicine.*)

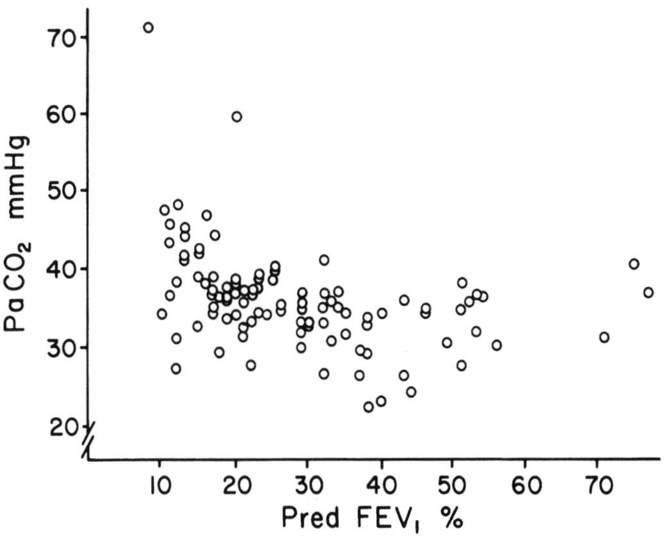

Figure 5.10. Relationships between P_aCO_2 and degree of airway obstruction as determined by $FEV_{1.0}$ *(FEV_1)* during acute asthma. (From McFadden ER Jr, Lyons HA. Arterial blood gas tension in asthma. N Engl J Med 1968;278:1029, reprinted by permission of the *New England Journal of Medicine.*)

Cardiovascular Effects

Many factors can cause abnormal cardiovascular function in an acute asthmatic attack. Small airway obstruction leads to air trapping with hyperinflation, resulting in increasingly negative intrapleural pressures during inspiration[143]. Ventilation/perfusion mismatching results in hypoxemia, and the increased work of breathing can lead to a metabolic acidosis compounded by a respiratory acidosis if respiratory muscle fatigue results in hypoventilation. The strain placed on the right heart is, therefore, the product of hypoxic pulmonary vasoconstriction, acidosis, and an elevated lung volume, each of which contributes to an increased pulmonary vascular resistance[148–150]. The strain placed on the left ventricle results from the increased work required to maintain an elevated cardiac output necessary to deliver oxygen and substrates to the respiratory muscles. This left ventricular strain is exaggerated by the effective increase in afterload imposed with each inspiration by the markedly negative intrathoracic pressures (see Chapter 11). The combination of an inspiratory leftward shift of the interventricular septum and an increased afterload leads to a reduced left ventricular output with each inspiration and a subsequent sharp increase during the ensuing expiration, producing the clinical sign of pulsus paradoxus in the peripheral arterial blood pressure[151–155]. Consistent with these pathophysiologic events, Rebuck and Read[156] studied 76 patients with severe asthma and found that 35 had abnormal electrocardiograms and 34 had pulsus paradoxus. While pulsus paradoxus in an airway obstructive process reflects the size of the pleural pressure swing with respiration, a decrease in pulsus paradoxus may reflect a smaller fall in pleural pressure because the airway obstruction is less or because the patient is fatiguing and in impending respiratory failure. Further discussion of the physiology of cardiorespiratory interactions during airway obstruction can be found in Chapter 11.

Status Asthmaticus

Definition

Status asthmaticus is a life-threatening form of asthma that is defined as a condition in which a progressively worsening attack is unresponsive to usual appropriate therapy with β_2-adrenergic drugs and theophylline and that leads to pulmonary insufficiency. Most attacks can be provoked by the usual causes of asthma and manifested by persistent dyspnea, prolonged expiratory wheezing, tachycardia, use of accessory respiratory muscles, and, in the late stages, cyanosis. The term *status asthmaticus* has been given various definitions by different authors. The definition we use is based on clinical considerations of therapeutic interventions that should alert the physicians who take care of these patients. Failure to respond to one dose of epinephrine followed by three β_2-adrenergic aerosols is a useful definition used at our institution.

Mechanism of Airway Obstruction

The primary mechanical event in status asthmaticus is a progressive increase in airflow resistance(157,158) caused by multiple factors, including bronchial muscle spasm, mucosal edema, and thick mucous secretion. Mucous plugging and mucosal edema or inflammation are the major causes for the delayed response or lack of response to therapy found in patients dying of status asthmaticus(112). As airway obstruction persists, the airflow in expiration as well as in inspiration is impaired, which leads to overinflation of the lungs. Because neither airway obstruction nor perfusion is uniformly distributed, ventilation/perfusion mismatching results(159). This process causes a significant increase in physiologic dead space in overinflated areas and a shunt-like effect in underinflated areas. An increase in minute ventilation by using accessory respiratory muscles occurs in order to compensate for the increase in physiologic dead space and results in a reduction in P_aCO_2 in the initial stages of illness(160). As work of breathing is increased, oxygen consumption and CO_2 production also increase. Hypoxemia results from the uneven distribution of ventilation and perfusion, increased oxygen requirement secondary to increased work of breathing, and perhaps increased interstitial lung fluid associated with the large transpulmonary pressure gradient(41). Hypercapnia begins to develop whenever the compensatory mechanism is exhausted or CO_2 production is greater than the CO_2 elimination. Fluid and nutritional deprivation as well as large doses of exogenous catecholamines during the initial phase of the acute attack contribute to ketonemia and lactic acidosis(160). The combination of hypoxemia, hypercapnia, and acidosis may result in cardiovascular depression and cardiopulmonary arrest. The pathophysiologic events in status asthmaticus are summarized in Figure 5.11.

Diagnosis and Evaluation

Cough, dyspnea, and wheezing are the major clinical features in asthma, but the presentation varies with age. In some children, the presentation is persistent cough at night(161–164) or during exercise. In others, shortness of breath may be the predominant symptom of asthma. In infants, the first asthmatic attack is frequently associated with viral respiratory infection. In older children, attacks are usually preceded by symptoms of upper respiratory tract infection, i.e., runny nose and coughing followed by bronchospasm. Other common precipitating causes include exposure to allergens, cigarette smoke, dust, exercise, and infection. During the acute attack, the cough usually sounds tight and is generally nonproductive. The degree of wheezing does not correlate well with the severity of the attacks(165), but the relative absence of wheezing in the presence of respiratory distress and poor air entry on auscultation of the lungs is indicative of severe obstruction. The use of accessory muscles of respiration(165) and the presence of pulsus paradoxus(156) signify severe compromise of respiratory function.

Laboratory Tests

The *routine complete blood count* is usually normal and is rarely useful in the assessment of acute asthma. The differential white blood cell count usually shows eosinophilia and leukocytosis. The leukocytosis may be induced by adrenaline, corticosteroid administration, or stress. Therefore, elevated white blood cell count alone does not always signify the presence of infection. On many occasions, the initial urinalysis may show high specific gravity with ketonuria, which indicates dehydration and previous poor intake. These abnormalities should disappear as the treatment begins and the attack resolves.

Nasal secretions usually have a great number of eosinophils, which are sometimes confused with the polymorphonuclear cells. The presence of eosinophils in the sputum(166) of a child suggests accompanying nasal allergy, whereas the presence of polymorphonuclear cells and intracellular bacterial organisms suggests associated infection.

Chest x-rays should be obtained in every child admitted to the Pediatric ICU with status asthmaticus to define the extent of the associated parenchymal disease and any complications and to differentiate other disease entities, e.g., foreign bodies. The chest roentgenogram of the child with uncomplicated asthma frequently shows only minor abnormalities(167), including hyperinflation and peribronchial thickening. Right middle lobe atelectasis is common in young children and may cause a recurrent problem. Small segmental areas of atelectasis are frequently observed during the acute attack and may be misinterpreted as pneumonia. A paranasal sinus x-ray is usually indicated in children with suspected sinusitis.

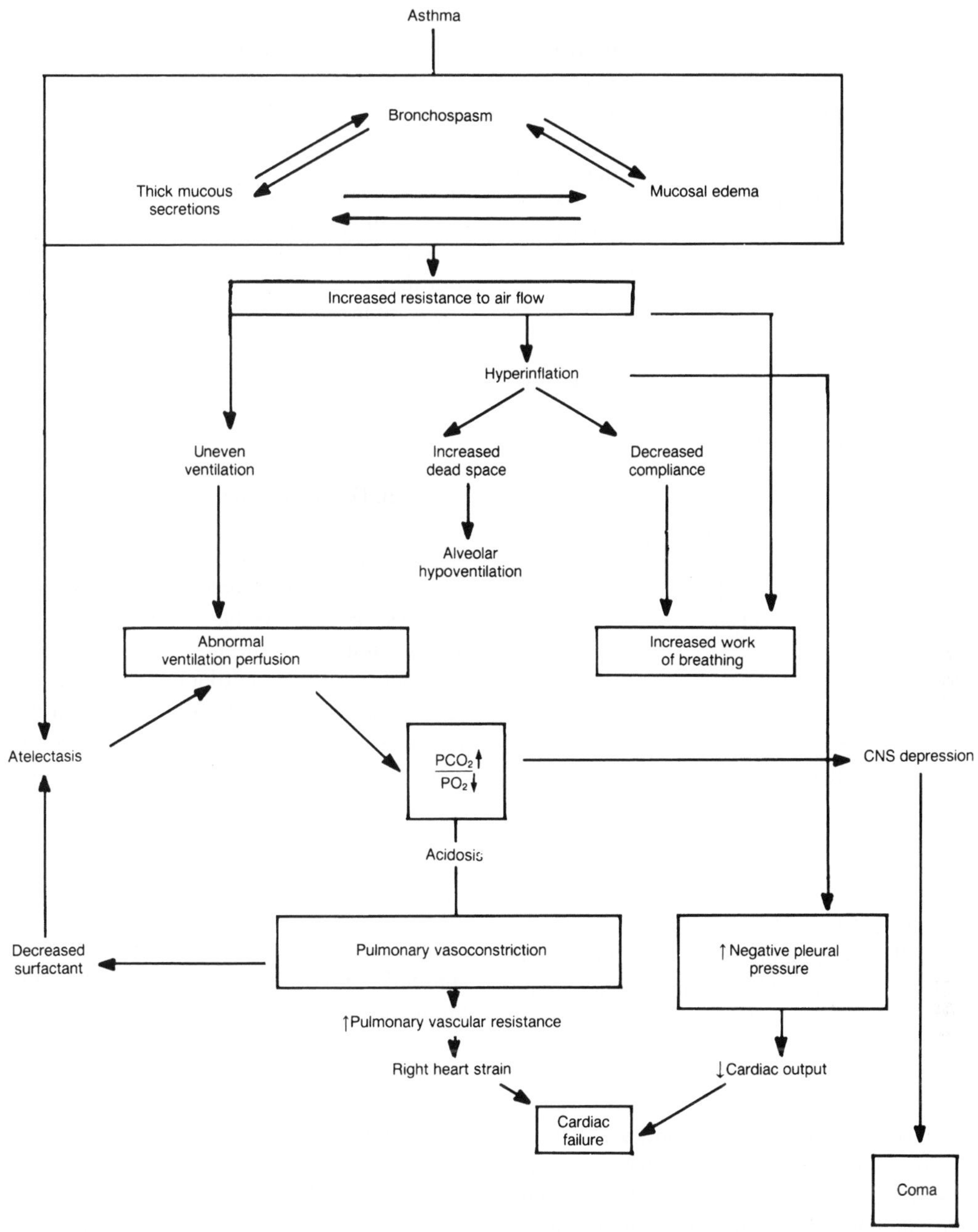

Figure 5.11. Pathophysiologic events in status asthmaticus. *CNS*, central nervous system; *PCO_2*, P_aCO_2; *PO_2*, P_aO_2. (Modified from Siegel SC. Bronchial asthma. In: Kelly C, ed. Practice of pediatrics. Hagerstown, Maryland: Harper & Row, Chap 63, 1974:163.)

Spirometry is a useful pulmonary function test in appropriate clinical settings, but it may not be reliable in very young children and may be too difficult to perform in the older child in severe respiratory distress. The PEFR measured with a small hand held flow meter is easier to obtain and can be used to diagnose the severity of status asthmaticus since the clinical impression alone is frequently misleading. Measurements obtained by spirometry are useful in assessing the degree of airway obstruction and impairment of gas exchange, measuring airway response to allergens and other etiologic agents, quantifying airway hyperreactivity, determining the acute effect of bronchodilator treatment, and evaluating the treatment over the course of the disease[(168)]. Abnormal findings include a decrease in $FEV_{1.0}$, a decrease in FVC[(169)], and an increase in RV and total lung capacity. The fall in $FEV_{1.0}$ has been shown to correlate well with the degree of airway obstruction and hypoxemia[(146)]. An extensive review of spirometry in asthma is covered earlier in this chapter in the section on the pathophysiology of airway obstruction.

It is essential to evaluate the ability of the lung to maintain adequate blood-gas tension. Obtaining arterial blood gas measurement can also help set important guidelines for planning the treatment of the patient. Typical blood gases during an acute uncomplicated asthmatic attack reveal low P_aO_2, low P_aCO_2, and respiratory alkalosis. Hypoxemia is due to ventilation/perfusion mismatching, whereas low P_aCO_2 is secondary to hyperventilation. A progressive increase in P_aCO_2[170] is an early warning sign of severe airway obstruction coupled with fatigue of the patient. Hypercapnia and metabolic acidosis in the presence of aggressive medical treatment correlate well with severity of illness and may indicate a need for artificial airway and mechanical ventilation. This is discussed in the section on criteria for intubation in Chapter 2.

Differential Diagnosis

Although the prominent finding in asthma is wheezing, it is not the pathognomonic sign of this disease. Various respiratory tract infections or obstructions, especially in infants and young children, can cause wheezing that may be confused with asthma. Careful history-taking, thorough physical examination, and some laboratory tests can differentiate asthma from other disease entities. The following conditions must be considered in the differential diagnosis of asthma in infants and young children.

Congenital Malformations

Congenital anomalies of the respiratory, cardiovascular, and gastrointestinal systems can cause varying degrees of airway obstruction that may mimic asthma. Among those common malformations are laryngotracheomalacia, vocal cord paralysis, tracheal or bronchial stenosis, lobar emphysema, lung cysts, vascular ring, and gastroesophageal reflux. These can be differentiated from asthma by history, age of onset, type of clinical presentation, physical findings, and some laboratory tests, e.g., esophagography, angiography, and endoscopy.

Foreign Bodies

Sudden onset of dyspnea, cough, and respiratory distress in previously healthy children without a history of recurrent attack favors the diagnosis of foreign body, in either the trachea or the bronchi. The symptoms of foreign body obstruction vary, depending on the type and location of obstruction. Sometimes, symptoms are not apparent immediately. If the foreign body is not removed, secondary obstruction and inflammation will follow. These lead to persistent atelectasis, pneumonia, lung abscess, and bronchiectasis and can result in chronic irreversible lung disease. Aids to diagnosis include a high degree of suspicion, chest auscultation, chest x-ray in inspiratory, expiratory, and lateral decubitus positions, fluoroscopy, and bronchoscopy.

Infections

Any respiratory tract infection in infants and young children can cause signs and symptoms of either upper or lower airway obstruction. Etiologic agents include viruses, bacteria, and fungi. Viruses are the most common and important cause of many clinical syndromes and can be differentiated from asthma by history and clinical presentation.

Croup

The presence of inspiratory stridor, hoarse voice, and barking cough with a history of upper respiratory infection is the typical clinical manifestation of croup. There is a higher prevalence rate of recurrent croup in children with asthma[171], as well as a high incidence of persistent hyperreactivity of both the upper and the lower respiratory tract in children with recurrent croup[172].

Acute Bronchiolitis

This common viral syndrome, caused by RSV and other respiratory viruses (e.g., parainfluenza, influenza), occurs in infants and young children during the first 2 years of life. The clinical signs of cough, coryza, wheezing, progressive dyspnea, and, in the late stage, respiratory failure, cannot be differentiated from asthma. Chest x-rays can also show evidence of hyperventilation resulting from generalized bronchiolar obstruction. Many investigators have demonstrated a relationship of bronchiolitis in infants with recurrent wheezing in later life[173, 174]. A history of recurrent episodes, an allergic background in the family, and an elevated IgE level are suggestive of asthma.

Bronchitis and Asthmatic Bronchitis

Acute bronchitis usually develops after an acute upper respiratory tract infection. Signs and symptoms of bronchial inflammation include productive cough, rhonchi, and coarse and medium crepitations. Whereas recurrent or chronic bronchitis may be confused with asthma, acute bronchitis can generally be distinguished from asthma. So-called asthmatic bronchitis refers to recurrent attacks of wheezing that only occur in association with respiratory tract infections. Some pediatricians and allergists do not consider asthmatic bronchitis a separate entity. In fact, progression of bronchial obstruction in the acute stages of any respiratory tract infection may be a common precipitating event stimulating an asthmatic attack. Similarly, the changes in $FEV_{1.0}$ may persist long after the respiratory tract infection is resolved[175]. However, long-term follow-up reveals that a significant number of these children have asthma and other allergic problems[176,177].

Evaluation and Prediction of Need for Hospitalization and for Intensive Care

An acute asthmatic attack is an unpredictable, life-threatening condition that needs immediate, continuous, and adequate assessment both in the emergency department and at the office of the private physician. Despite advanced knowledge about its pathophysiology, improved technology, and improved drugs in the treatment of acute severe attacks, asthma still causes considerable morbidity and mortality in children because of failure to recognize the severity of the disease or because of improper management. Certain steps can assist in the early prediction of the need for hospitalization and intensive care admission in children with acute asthma.

History

As in other chronic diseases, the nature of past episodes is one of the most useful pieces of information in assessing the severity of the disease. Knowledge of prior hospitalizations, frequency of attacks, and medication history can help the physician determine which individuals require hospital management. Furthermore, airway obstruction lasting longer than 12 to 24 hours[178] or failure to respond to previously effective therapy are also possible indications for admission.

Physical Signs

Among the clinical manifestations of asthma, the use of accessory respiratory muscles seems to correlate well with the severity of airway obstruction as determined by spirometric measurement; dyspnea and wheezing do not[165]. However, the presence of wheezing followed by a subsequent decrease in wheezing with persistent signs of dyspnea may indicate that the airways are obstructed extensively with very little air passing through to produce the wheezing sound. The pulse and respiratory rates also do not reflect the severity accurately[179], but the presence of pulsus paradoxus (over 10 mm Hg change in systolic blood pressure between inspiration and expiration) correlates well with the severity of the disease. Pulsus paradoxus is present in two-thirds of patients with an $FEV_{1.0}$ less than 40% of their best $FEV_{1.0}$ and in all patients with $FEV_{1.0}$ less than 20% of their best $FEV_{1.0}$ (Fig. 5.12)[148].

Diaphoresis in the adult patient with status asthmaticus is indicative of severe disease that warrants hospital admission[180]. Disturbance in consciousness, fatigue, cyanosis, and other signs of hypoxemia indicate the episode is very severe, but these clinical signs of hypoxemia are usually late[181]. Subcutaneous emphysema indicates the presence of pneumomediastinum or pneumothorax and, therefore, requires immediate investigation[182].

Laboratory Tests

Blood Gases

The most important component of the arterial blood gas that determines the severity of the attack is P_aCO_2[170]. In the early stage, P_aCO_2 is usually low due to the compensatory hyperventilation. It starts to rise to normal or even higher than normal value in more severe airway obstruction, as assessed by $FEV_{1.0}$[146]. A P_aCO_2 of 40 to 45 mm Hg[183] in the presence of dyspnea and wheezing should alert the physician that the patient is fatigued and needs immediate attention. Otherwise, catastrophic consequences will ensue. Hypoxemia in a P_aO_2 range of 60 to 80 mm Hg[145] is frequently found even in moderately severe asthma. However, a P_aO_2 less than 60 mm Hg[183] is an additional danger signal. Arterial pH is the other factor that determines the overall balance between metabolic demand and respiratory compensation. Acidemia in excess of that predicted from the measured P_aCO_2, accompanied by an abnormally large serum anion gap and high plasma lactate level, has been shown to occur in severe asthmatic patients who require intubation[184]. Furthermore, serial measurements of P_aCO_2, P_aO_2, and pH are more useful in assessing the result of the treatment than is a single arterial blood gas.

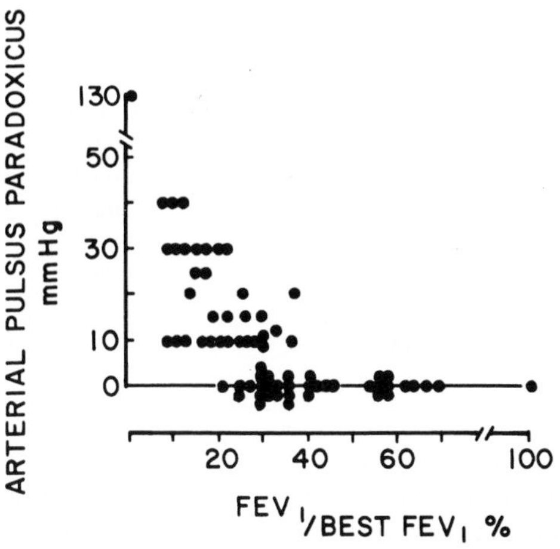

Figure 5.12. Degree of pulsus paradoxus *(pulsus paradoxicus)* plotted against $FEV_{1.0}$ *(FEV_1)*. $FEV_{1.0}$ is expressed as a percentage of the best $FEV_{1.0}$ in each patient. (From Rebuck AS, Read J. Assessment and management of severe asthma. Am J Med 1971;51:788.)

Pulmonary Function

Although the effort-dependent pulmonary function study is often difficult to perform, especially in acutely distressed or very young patients, the simple peak-expiratory flow rate and $FEV_{1.0}$ have been demonstrated to be good indexes for predicting the need for hospitalization[185]. Portable small devices can be used to evaluate peak flow. PEFR values of less than 16% of the predicted value and the failure to increase significantly by more than 16% 15 to 20 minutes after a single subcutaneous dose of epinephrine usually indicate the need for hospitalization[186]. Those who had a $FEV_{1.0}$ less than 20 to 30% of the predicted value and who failed to improve by 35% at the end of 60 minutes of intense treatment have been shown to require admission ultimately for control of the symptoms[185, 187].

Other laboratory findings that may be used as evidence of severe asthmatic episodes include electrocardiographic findings of P pulmonale[148], right ventricular strain, right

Table 5.4. Clinical Asthma Evaluation Score[a]

Variables	*0*	*1*	*2*
P_aO_2	70–100 in air	<70 in air	<70 in 40% O_2
Cyanosis	None	In air	In 40% O_2
Inspiratory breath sounds	Normal	Unequal	Decreased to absent
Accessory muscles used	None	Moderate	Maximal
Expiratory wheezing	None	Moderate	Marked
Cerebral function	Normal	Depressed or agitated	Coma

[a]*Clinical asthma score for children with status asthmaticus score ≤5 equaling impending respiratory failure, score ≤7 equaling plus P_aCO_2, and ≤65 mm Hg equaling existing respiratory failure. (From Wood DW, Downes JJ, Lecks HI. A clinical scoring system for the diagnosis of respiratory failure. Am J Dis Child 1972;123:227.)*

bundle branch block, and right axis deviation[188]. The presence of pneumomediastinum, severe hyperinflation[189], pneumonia, or atelectasis is indicative of severity of disease.

Summary

In summary, the following features of a severe acute attack may indicate the need for hospitalization and intensive care:

1. History of frequent repeated attacks, previous severe asthma that resulted in hospitalization, excessive daily use of bronchodilator and corticosteroids for control of symptoms, and failure to respond to previous effective therapy
2. Use of accessory respiratory muscles
3. Pulsus paradoxus over 18 mm Hg[190] in teenagers and over 10 mm Hg in children
4. Change in consciousness and/or obvious exhaustion
5. Cyanosis
6. Pneumothorax and pneumomediastinum
7. $FEV_{1.0}$ or PEFR less than 20% predicted value, with little or no response to acute therapy
8. Hypoxemia, P_aO_2 less than 60 mm Hg
9. Hypercapnia, P_aCO_2 over 40 mm Hg in the presence of dyspnea and wheezing
10. Metabolic acidosis
11. Electrocardiographic abnormalities

In pediatric patients, Wood et al.[191] developed a clinical scoring system to detect impending or existing respiratory failure in status asthmaticus patients, based on the signs and symptoms of airway obstruction, use of accessory respiratory muscles, oxygenation, and cerebral function. It seems also to be correlated well with both an increase in P_aCO_2 and a decrease in P_aO_2 **(Table 5.4).** Patients who have the following clinical signs and therapeutic requirements that suggest respiratory failure should be admitted to the ICU:

1. Impending and/or existing respiratory failure as assessed by an asthma score higher than 5
2. Isoproterenol infusion
3. Respiratory arrest and/or cardiac arrest
4. Mechanical ventilation
5. Risk for development of theophylline toxicity, i.e., congestive heart failure or hepatic cirrhosis

Treatments Generally Used

Acute bronchial asthma is one of the most common causes of emergency department visits in all hospitals. This condition demands an immediate assessment, including a thorough history of illness and previous medications used. Patients with relatively mild respiratory distress can deteriorate within a few minutes, and those with severe airway obstruction can improve if the proper therapeutic measures are initiated promptly. The primary goal of treatment of the acute asthmatic attack is to provide prompt bronchodilatation and reduce airway reactivity. Aqueous epinephrine (1:1000) solution has been the first-line drug used most commonly as a therapeutic agent for acute asthma in childhood; its rapid onset of action causes the prompt relief of bronchoconstriction in a dose of 0.01 ml/kg administered subcutaneously, with a maximum dose of 0.35 ml every 20 to 30 minutes, given 2 to 3 times, depending on the response of the patient. Because of its cardiovascular side effect and rather short duration of action, the more specific β_2-agonist (e.g., terbutaline) has been used as an alternative to epinephrine. Terbutaline has an equivalent bronchodilatory effect, longer duration of action, and less cardiovascular activity in a dose of 0.01 mg/kg (subcutaneous), with a maximum dose of 0.25 mg every 20 to 30 minutes, for a total of three doses[192–194]. However, the β_2-receptor in skeletal muscle is also stimulated, and terbutaline causes a pronounced tremor in some children.

Aerosolized adrenergic agents have been proven by many investigators[192, 195–197] to be equally effective at lower dosages than required by parenteral injection. Because the cardiovascular side effects of these agents are dose related, many of the undesirable effects of the drugs, as well as the unpleasant feeling of injection, can be avoided by aerosolized treatment. Therefore, aerosolized β_2-agonists have replaced subcutaneous epinephrine as first-line therapy in acute asthma attacks. Examples of these agents are isoproterenol, isoetharine, metaproterenol, terbutaline, albuterol, and salbutamol. These agents are available for self-administration in older children, and even in younger children the drugs can still be nebulized effectively by the use of an oxygen-air-mixture compressor via face mask. Subcutaneous injection of adrenergic agents and the aerosol administration can be used in combination if the patient fails to respond to either method alone. If the patient responds to initial therapy and is ready to be discharged from the emergency department, an injection of sustained-release epinephrine (Sus-Phrine) in a dose of 0.005 ml/kg (maximum 0.15 ml) may be given to maintain bronchodilatation until oral medication becomes fully effective.

In addition to acute medical management, general supportive therapy should be given simultaneously to treat possible dehydration from poor intake and vomiting, as well as hypoxemia from ventilation/perfusion mismatching. Thus, fluid therapy and humidified oxygen administration are indicated as part of the treatment for acute asthmatic attacks. Furthermore, many therapeutic drugs (e.g., epinephrine, isoproterenol, and aminophylline) can reduce the hypoxic pulmonary vasoconstriction and aggravate ventilation/perfusion imbalance, leading to the worsening of hypoxemia[(198–200)]. If the patient fails to respond satisfactorily to treatment with adrenergic drugs, intravenous theophylline and steroids should be started (see section on theophylline). The dose of theophylline is determined with consideration of previous oral theophylline intake and serum theophylline level. Both are necessary for planning further treatment and avoiding toxicity. Corticosteroids should be started early, especially in the patient who has a history of corticosteroid requirement and in status asthmaticus (see section on corticosteroids). The pharmacologic agents for the treatment of acute and severe asthma are summarized in **Table 5.5.** If the above therapeutic measures fail to reduce bronchospasm, the patient should be admitted to the hospital so that more supportive and aggressive treatment can be provided. The aggressiveness of therapy and the location to

Table 5.5. General Pharmacologic Agents for Treatment of Acute and Severe Asthma in Children

Agent	*Parenteral*	*Aerosol inhalation*
Adrenergic drugs		
Epinephrine hydrochloride	Subcutaneous (1:1000) solution, 1 mg/ml, 0.01 ml/kg/dose (maximum 0.5 ml) every 15–20 min; repeat 3 times as necessary	Not indicated
Sus-Phrine	Subcutaneous (1:200) solution, 5 mg/ml, 0.005 ml/kg/dose (maximum 0.15 ml) every 6 hr	Not indicated
Terbutaline	Subcutaneous (0.05%) solution, 0.5 mg/ml, 0.01 mg/kg/dose (maximum 0.25 mg) every 20–30 min for three doses, as necessary	1% solution, 11 mg/ml, 0.03 ml/kg (maximum 1 ml); diluted with 1.5 ml saline every 4–6 hr
Albuterol (salbutamol)	Intravenous (0.1%) solution, 1 mg/ml, 0.2 μg/kg/min (maximum 2 μg/kg/min or 10 μg/kg diluted and given over 10 min)	0.5% solution, 5 mg/ml, 0.01–0.03 ml/kg (maximum 1 ml); diluted with 1.5 ml saline every 4–6 hr
Isoproterenol	Intravenous (0.02%) solution, 0.2 mg/ml, 0.05–0.1 μg/kg/min, increase by 0.05–0.1 μg/kg/min every 15–20 min	0.5% solution, 5 mg/ml, 0.01–0.02 ml/kg (maximum 0.5 ml); diluted with 1.5 ml saline every 2–6 hr
Isoetharine	Not available	1% solution, 10 mg/ml, 0.01 ml/kg (maximum 0.5 ml); diluted with 1.5 ml saline every 2–6 hr
Metaproterenol	Subcutaneous (0.10%) solution, 1.0 mg/ml, 0.01 ml/kg every 20–30 min for three doses, as necessary	5% solution, 50 mg/ml, 0.005–0.010 ml/kg (maximum 0.4 ml); diluted with 1.5 ml saline every 4–6 hr
Theophylline	Intravenous (aminophylline USP 25 mg aminophylline/ml), loading dose 6–7.5 mg/kg over 20 min by constant infusion pump; modifying loading dose on basis of previous medication history or initial serum theophylline level, or 1 mg/kg for each 2 μg/ml, increased if desired in previous serum theophylline level; continuous infusion (monitor serum levels): <10 kg body weight—0.65 mg/kg/hr; <10 kg body weight—0.9 mg/kg/hr	No
Anticholinergic drugs		
Atropine	0.03–0.05 mg/kg nebulized	
Ipratropium bromide	20–40 μg metered dose every 6 hr (>6-yr-old); 250 μg nebulized (<6-yr-old)	
Corticosteroid drugs		
Hydrocortisone	Intravenous loading dose, 5–7 mg/kg; maintenance, 5 mg/kg every 6 hr	No
Methylprednisolone	Intravenous loading dose, 1 mg/kg; maintenance, 0.8 mg/kg every 4–6 hr	No
Beclomethasone dipropionate	No	50–100 μg every 6 hr, inhaler dose; provided 42 μg metered dose
Cromolyn sodium		
(useful for prevention of attacks)	No	1% solution, 10 mg/ml; 2 ml every 6 hr

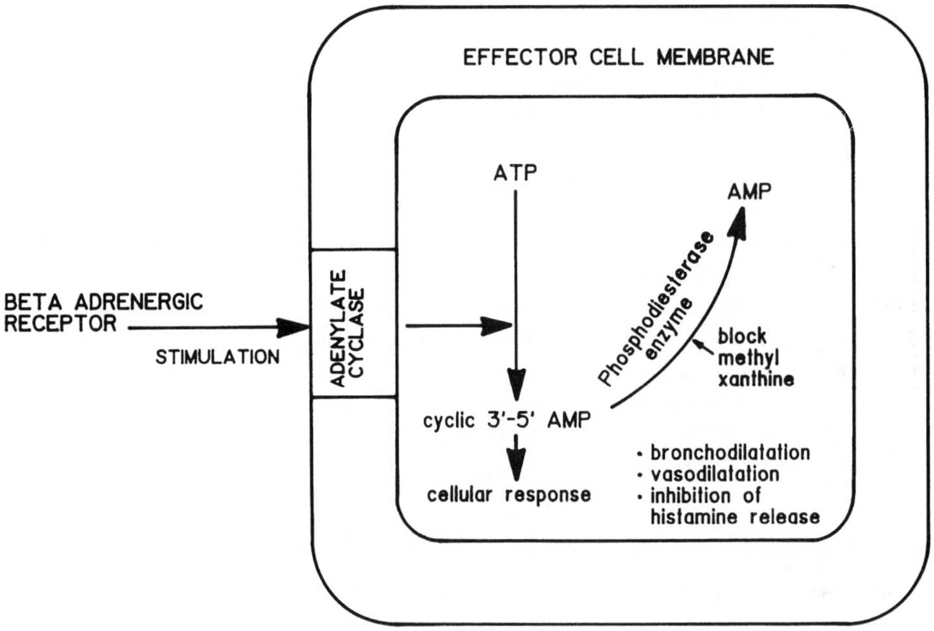

Figure 5.13. Biochemical events in the production and breakdown of cyclic 3′,5′-AMP.

which the patient should be admitted (i.e., general pediatric ward or pediatric ICU) are dictated by the severity of the disease as well as by response to the treatment and the likelihood of complications (see previous section on need for hospitalization).

Sympathomimetic Bronchodilators

β-Adrenergic agonists are the most potent bronchodilators. Bronchodilating effects are believed to be mediated through the β-adrenergic receptor, which has been associated with smooth-muscle relaxation in the bronchial tree, uterus, ciliary muscle, and skeletal muscle blood vessels[(230)]. β-Adrenergic receptors have been subdivided further into two subtypes: β_1 and β_2[(231)]. These subtypes are based on the differences in physiologic response of various target tissues or organs to β-adrenergic agonists and antagonists. Stimulation of β_1-receptors located in the cardiac tissue produces inotropic and chronotropic responses, whereas stimulation of β_2-receptors located in the bronchial and vascular smooth muscle results in bronchodilatation and vasodilatation. This bronchodilating effect occurs in both central and peripheral airways. Furthermore, β_2-stimulation prevents exercise-induced asthma[(232)] and enhances mucociliary clearance in the tracheobronchial lumen[(233)].

Epinephrine

Epinephrine has both β_1-adrenergic and β_2-adrenergic agonist effects, has short action, and is effective when given by either inhalation or subcutaneous injection. It is ineffective when given orally because it is susceptible to inactivation by catechol-*o*-methyltransferase (COMT), an enzyme that is present in the gastrointestinal tract. Because epinephrine affects both β_1-receptors and β_2-receptors, it also affects the cardiovascular system in addition to the pulmonary system. Research showed that drugs that have predominantly β_2 or bronchodilator effects have a longer duration of action and are not susceptible to inactivation by the enzyme COMT, so they can be given by mouth[(234)]. However, epinephrine is rarely given in the ICU to treat bronchospasm.

Isoetharine

Isoetharine (e.g., Bronkometer or Bronkosol) is a bronchoselective catecholamine that has a longer duration of action than epinephrine and is still susceptible to COMT enzymes, so that it is ineffective by mouth. Its peak activity is 15 minutes after inhalation, and the duration of bronchodilatation is less than 2 hours[(235)]. Some cardiovascular side effects do occur.

Metaproterenol

Metaproterenol (e.g., Alupent) is a noncatecholamine adrenergic bronchodilator that is resistant to inactivation by COMT and is effective orally and parenterally as well as by aerosol. It has a longer duration of action and equivalent action to isoproterenol in its relative cardiac and bronchodilator potency[(236)]. Tremor is a common adverse effect of the drug, particularly after oral administration (Fig. 5.13).

Terbutaline and Albuterol

The noncatecholamine β_2-selective adrenergic bronchodilators terbutaline[(234, 237)] and albuterol[(238, 239)] (e.g., salbutamol) have been shown to stimulate β_2-receptors in the bronchial trees more than β_1-receptors in the heart. These drugs are effective when given orally, parenterally (subcutaneously, terbutaline; intravenously, albuterol), as well as by in-

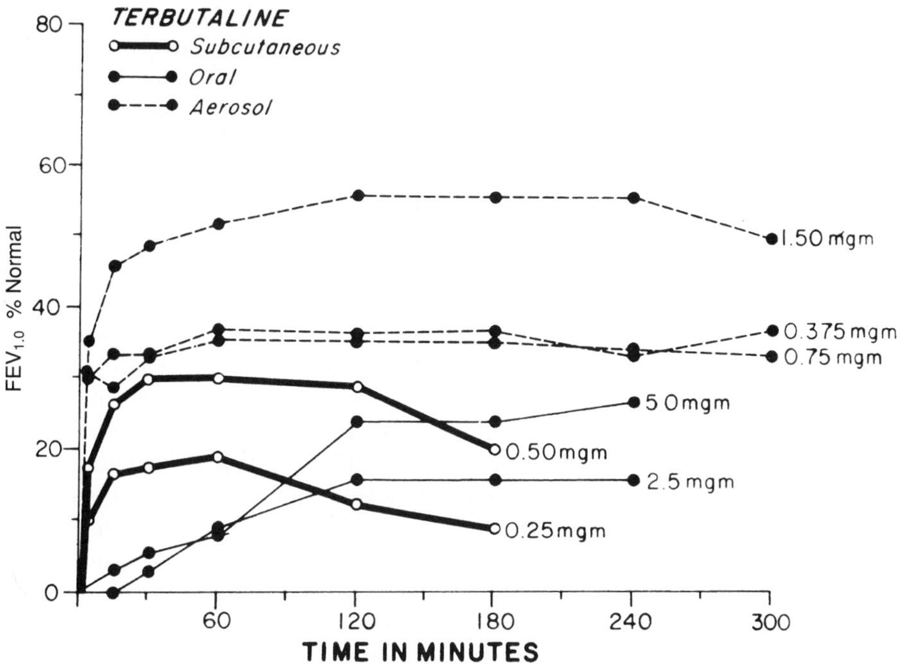

Figure 5.14. Effect of three different routes of administration of terbutaline on $FEV_{1.0}$. (From Dulfano MJ, Glass P. The bronchodilator effects of terbutaline: route of administration and pattern of response. Ann Allergy 1976;37:357.)

halation, and they have a longer duration of action than epinephrine. Both drugs are equally effective when given orally[240, 241] or by aerosol[242] in equivalent doses. Although the bronchodilator response of albuterol given parenterally is no different from that of albuterol given by aerosol, the relief of pulsus paradoxus has been shown to be significantly superior with the aerosol treatment[243]. Subcutaneous administration of terbutaline is widely used as an alternative to epinephrine in the treatment of acute asthmatic attacks. The dose response of terbutaline by various routes of administration has been clearly demonstrated (Fig. 5.14)[244]. Nebulized terbutaline has safely been administered to children with severe asthma (up to 0.4 mg/kg/dose) as well as by continuous nebulization (0.4 mg/kg/hr) with good results[245]. The bronchodilator response of parenteral albuterol seems to be greater than that of parenteral aminophylline, but the differences are not statistically significant, and the side effects of albuterol are less marked[246]. Continuously aerosolized albuterol has been used for severe asthma in children. This modality is gaining widespread acceptance. The combination of β_2-agonists, given either subcutaneously or by aerosol, and aminophylline in the treatment of acute attacks gives a significantly greater improvement in $FEV_{1.0}$ at the end of 1 hour than does epinephrine alone[247]. However, all β_2-agonists share the same limiting adverse effects due to the β_2-stimulation in skeletal muscle (i.e., tremor) and in the cardiovascular system (i.e., tachycardia)[248]. Their relative selectivity for the β_2-receptor, however, mitigates the tachycardia effects of these drugs.

Isoproterenol

Isoproterenol is a nonselective β-adrenergic agonist that has both β_1-receptor and β_2-receptor stimulation. It is one of the most potent bronchodilators when administered by inhalation, with peak bronchodilatation attained within 5 minutes, which progressively declines over 2 hours[249, 250]. Intravenous isoproterenol has been shown to be effective in managing children with respiratory failure and CO_2 retention from asthma. In addition, intravenous isoproterenol has been said to prevent the need for mechanical ventilation in approximately 80 to 90% of these patients[251–255], thereby obviating complications from positive pressure ventilation. All children in those studies had CO_2 retention, despite adequate initial therapy with aqueous epinephrine, humidified oxygen, intravenous fluid for the correction of dehydration, sodium bicarbonate for raising the pH over 7.20, aminophylline infusion with serum concentration in the therapeutic range (10 to 20 μg/ml), adrenergic aerosol, and steroids parenterally. The patients were admitted to the ICU with continuous monitoring of heart rate, respiratory rate, blood pressure, electrocardiographic monitoring, fluid balance, and arterial pressure via arterial line. The isoproterenol infusion was started at a rate of 0.05 to 0.1 μg/kg/min by means of a constant infusion pump and increased every 15 minutes by 0.05 μg/kg/min until the patient responded with a fall in P_aCO_2 or until marked tachycardia (heart rate increased greater than 20% or heart rate over 200/min) or an arrhythmia developed. As the patient improved, the isoproterenol infusion was slowly tapered off.

Whether concomitant aminophylline infusion should be continued with isoproterenol is controversial. Aminophylline was discontinued in the studies by Downes and Heiser[256] because of the potential additive cardiac dysrhythmogenic effect when it is combined with isoproterenol[229, 257]. However, other researchers[204, 254, 255] continued the aminophylline infusion, based on the belief that xanthine and the sympathomimetic bronchodilators act at different sites in the cyclic AMP system. Synergistic effects of isoproterenol and aminophylline might account in part for the demonstrated response to a lower initial isoproterenol dose (0.05 μg/kg/min) as well as the lower mean response time to treatment. Regardless of the controversy, great care must be taken when these drugs are used in combination.

The dose of aminophylline required to maintain a therapeutic level is increased during concomitant isoproterenol therapy because clearance of aminophylline is increased[(204, 205)]. As a result, careful monitoring of serum theophylline level is necessary to maximize the response and minimize the chance of toxicity.

The cardiovascular side effects either of isoproterenol infusion alone or of infusion of isoproterenol with aminophylline include tachyarrhythmias and increased myocardial oxygen consumption. In addition, hypoxemia, hypercapnia, and acidosis characteristic of acute severe asthmatic attacks enhance the cardiotoxicity of isoproterenol, which can lead to myocardial ischemia[(258, 259)] and necrosis[(260)] (see Chapter 12). It seems prudent, if isoproterenol treatment is initiated, for the electrocardiogram and creatine phosphokinase-MB levels to be monitored for evidence of myocardial ischemia[(261)]. However, the safety of this combination therapy can be enhanced by the proper intensive care setting, adequate oxygenation, and continuous monitoring of cardiac rhythm, blood pressure, electrocardiogram, arterial blood gases, and fluid balances[(254, 255, 262)].

Anticholinergic Agents

It is well known that stimulation of cholinergic receptors by various mechanical and chemical stimuli causes reflex bronchoconstriction, which can be blocked either by cutting the vagus nerve or by administering atropine[(263–267)]. The anticholinergic agents are believed to act by blocking the irritant receptors and inhibiting cyclic guanosine monophosphate[(268)] metabolism, which results in bronchodilatation. The anticholinergic agents that are most frequently used and have been extensively studied for bronchodilator effects are atropine sulfate, atropine methonitrate, and the synthetic agent ipratropium bromide.

Atropine

Atropine is the prototype of anticholinergic drugs. It has been used for the treatment of reversible airway obstruction since the beginning of the 19th century[(269)]. It is well absorbed from the gastrointestinal tract as well as the respiratory tract mucosa when administered by inhalation and is distributed throughout the body, crossing the blood-brain barrier. Its serum half-life is approximately 3 hours in young adults and 2 to 3 times longer in elderly patients and children[(270)]. It is mostly excreted in the urine within 24 hours, with one-fourth to one-third of the administered dose remaining in active form. The peak serum concentration of atropine is obtained within 15 to 20 minutes after an intramuscular injection and subsequently declines slowly[(271)]. The bronchodilating response depends on the dose and route of administration. The predominant effect on large and central airways is obtained by aerosol administration[(272–275)], whereas the generalized bronchodilating response occurs after intravenous administration[(273, 274, 276)]. Atropine sulfate inhalation is used at the dose of 0.05 to 0.10 mg/kg, producing maximal bronchodilatation and consistently reducing airflow obstruction[(269, 277–281)]. A dose of 1 to 2 μg of aerosolized atropine is as effective as 100 to 200 μg of salbutamol by inhalation[(282, 283)]. Subcutaneously administered atropine (0.6 mg) was shown to be a significantly less effective bronchodilator than subcutaneous adrenaline (0.5 ml of 1 : 1000 solution) or intravenous aminophylline (500 mg)[(284)] when assessed 20 minutes after administration. Orally administered atropine (1.05 mg) or subcutaneously injected atropine (0.6 mg) is also somewhat less effective than terbutaline (5.0 mg) orally[(285)]. Furthermore, the combination of anticholinergic agents (e.g., atropine and ipratropium bromide) with β-adrenergic agents or theophylline always results in a better bronchodilatation effect than either drug given alone[(282, 286–291)]. Atropine also prevents exercise-induced asthma[(292, 293)]. The systemic side effects of atropine are dose-related and range from dryness of mouth and blurred vision to mental confusion. The effect on bronchial secretion is of special concern because it can cause the drying and inspissation of airway secretion, which can contribute to more severe airway obstruction. In fact, the effect of atropine on mucous viscosity and transportability was found to be minimal[(294–297)]. The side effects of atropine are more common with intravenous administration but may also occur when it is administered by inhalation[(298)]. Green et al.[(299)] found some beneficial effect of inhaled atropine in four of six patients with status asthmaticus who had already received conventional therapy with therapeutic theophylline level, parenteral steroids, and parenteral and inhaled β_2-agonists. However, the current recommendation is to try atropine therapy only in patients who are relatively unresponsive to optimum doses of β-adrenergic agonists and theophylline[(300, 301)]. This mode of treatment seems to be especially useful for patients with bronchospasm associated with chronic bronchitis[(302, 303)]. For the patient with asthma, at least some of the reversible airway obstruction that is mediated through parasympathetic activity is abolished by this adjunct atropine therapy.

Ipratropium Bromide

This compound is a synthetic, quaternary ammonium derivative of atropine. It is poorly absorbed from the intestine and does not cross the blood-brain barrier. When given by inhalation, its peak effect appears 30 minutes later and lasts 4 to 6 hours. The usual dose of 20 to 80 μg, delivered by a metered dose inhaler, has a selective effect on airway smooth muscle[(304)] and has been shown to be an effective bronchodilator in patients with asthma[(290, 305–308)] and chronic obstructive bronchitis. In comparison to aerosolized adrenergic agents, a dose of 40 μg of inhaled ipratropium bromide is equivalent to 100 μg of salbutamol[(283)] but is significantly less effective than 200 μg of inhaled salbutamol[290, 309–311]. The combination with a β-adrenergic drug is significantly more effective than either drug given alone. This is consistent with the evidence that β-adrenergic drugs exert their physiologic effect mainly on small airways, whereas aerosolized anticholinergics show a predominant effect on larger airways. In addition, the combination with corticosteroids, in either aerosolized or oral form, also results in the more effective bronchodilatation than anticholinergic agents alone[312–314]. The side effects of ipratropium bromide seem to be fewer than those of atropine; there is no central nervous system effect because ipratropium bromide does not cross the blood-brain barrier. Also, there is no significant effect on the tracheal mucous transport rate[315], but dryness of the mouth and complaints of a bad taste are occasionally reported. There have been case reports describing the association of administration by nebulizer and face mask and acute angle-closure glaucoma as well as unilateral fixed dilated pupil. In a double blind, randomized crossover study, no changes in intraocular pressure, pupillary size or pupillary response were documented with nebulized ipratropium in children[316]. Ipratropium may cause paradoxical bronchoconstriction by preferentially blocking the M_2 muscarinic receptor. This latter receptor usually inhibits the M_3 receptor in the airway. By inhibiting this inhibitory fiber, vagal tone, and hence bronchoconstriction, will increase[317]. The role of ipratropium bromide in antiasthmatic therapy is evolving. It may be a useful adjunct or alternative to β-adrenergic agents in patients who suffer from tachycardia or marked tremor in response to usual doses of those agents. The beneficial effect in older patients who have nonatopic disease or psychogenic asthma has also been described[300].

Corticosteroids

There is general agreement that corticosteroids are of great value in reducing morbidity in acute severe asthmatic attacks that are refractory to standard bronchodilator therapy. However, the precise mechanisms are still uncertain. The most likely explanations are:

1. They inhibit the synthesis and release of chemical mediators, including histamine, SRS-A, ECF-A, bradykinin, and prostaglandins. Some of these mediators (e.g., SRS-A and histamine) have a direct bronchospastic property. Furthermore, SRS-A may be responsible for the pathophysiologic events of relatively refractory airway obstruction in asthma, including the excessive production and viscosity of sputum as well as the cellular infiltration and edema of the bronchial mucosa[318, 319].
2. They inhibit the cholinergic mechanism and probably act through the change in level of cyclic-adenosine monophosphate (AMP) and cyclic guanosine monophosphate in the tissue[320, 321], in which corticosteroids may potentiate the action of cyclic AMP[322, 323] and inhibit the formation of cyclic guanosine monophosphate[324].
3. They directly effect smooth muscle relaxation[325].
4. They suppress immune mechanisms and/or mediators of inflammation by preventing the release of arachidonic acid from membrane phospholipids. The so-called macrocortin[326] and lipomodulin[327] proteins are synthesized by steroid-sensitive tissue, including neutrophils. These proteins inhibit the activity of phospholipase A[327–330] and prevent the formation of leukotrienes and prostaglandins, which are the potent mediators for airway smooth muscle contraction and increased vascular permeability.
5. They enhance the response to catecholamines by increasing synthesis and restoring β-adrenergic receptors[331, 332]. Some investigators have also suggested that corticosteroids potentiate the catecholamine effect on cyclic AMP synthesis[331, 333, 334] and may inhibit the cyclic AMP phosphodiesterase enzyme[335].

The guidelines for initiating steroid therapy in asthma depend on the severity of the disease, the history of the patient's requirement for glucocorticoid, and his or her response to previous therapy. It is recommended for every child hospitalized with acute severe asthma, especially with life-threatening status asthmaticus. However, it was suggested that patients with severe airflow obstruction whose $FEV_{1.0}$ is less than 40% of normal after intensive therapy may be the group of high-risk patients[185] who benefit most from a prompt administration of steroids[336]. When steroids are given to patients with asthma, a period of time is required before the effects of steroid are apparent clinically. The initial improvement usually occurs within 6 hours after steroid administration[337, 338], and a longer time is usually required for the effect of steroids to become fully manifest in more severe cases. The recommended dose of steroids varies, and it has been suggested that plasma steroid concentration be maintained in a range of 100 to 150 μg cortisol/dl[339, 340]. This can be achieved by giving 4 to 8 mg of hydrocortisone hemisuccinate per kilogram intravenously or an equivalent every 4 to 6 hours[339] or 2 to 3 mg of methylprednisolone per kilogram per day in four divided doses, which produces less sodium retention than hydrocortisone. In a double-blind trial of asthmatics between the ages of 6 and 60 months, 4 mg of methylprednisolone per kilogram given intramuscularly in addition to β-agonists reduced the hospital admission rate of those treated with β-agonists alone[341]. This may be tapered after 48 hours as the patient improves. However, in less severe cases, oral prednisolone, 1 to 2 mg/kg/day, is also effective in controlling the symptoms. The aerosolized steroids are useful only in chronic maintenance therapy and are not recommended in the treatment of acute asthma. The side effects of long-term steroid therapy include increased susceptibility to infection, hypothalamic-pituitary-adrenal axis suppression, Cushing's appearance, growth retardation, bone demineralization, hyperglycemia and glycosuria, myopathy, sodium retention, and secondary hypertension. However, there is no evidence that a short period of therapy (less than 2 weeks) is associated with a significant risk of serious adverse reactions. In addition, steroids may help to reverse a potentially life-threatening episode of severe asthma.

Theophylline

Theophylline is a xanthine derivative that has a structure similar to caffeine. It has been used widely for more than 50 years for acute exacerbation of asthma. The mechanism of action was previously thought to be the inhibition of phosphodiesterase enzymes[(342)], which degrade the cyclic 3′,5′-adenosine monophosphate (AMP) to AMP. Cyclic AMP was believed to mediate the cellular responses, resulting in bronchodilatation, vasodilatation, and inhibition of histamine release[(343)]. However, this mechanism has been questioned because other phosphodiesterase inhibitors are not bronchodilators[(344)], and the degree of inhibition of this enzyme is minimal at therapeutic concentrations of theophylline[(28)]. It has been suggested that the bronchodilating effect of theophylline may occur by one or more of the following mechanisms: prostaglandin antagonism[(345)], increased binding of cyclic AMP to cyclic AMP-binding protein[(346)], adenosine receptor antagonism[(347)], inhibition of cyclic guanosine monophosphate metabolism[(348)], stimulation of endogenous catecholamine release[(349)], and β-adrenergic agonism[(350)]. None of these proposed mechanisms has clearly been proven. However, they may play a contributory role in the explanation of the bronchodilating effect by theophylline.

It has recently been proposed that aminophylline (equivalent to anhydrous theophylline) will augment diaphragmatic contractility[(351, 352)] and protect against diaphragmatic fatigue[(353)]. Thus, reversal of respiratory failure with theophylline in patients with obstructive lung disease results from both its beneficial effect on respiratory muscle function and its bronchodilator action. Furthermore, there are other pharmacologic effects of theophylline, some of which may contribute to the side effects during initiation of therapy. These include a transient diuretic effect[(354)], central nervous system stimulation[(355)], cerebral vasoconstriction[(356)], and cardiovascular effects such as decreased left ventricular ejection time in normal persons[(357)] and increased right ventricular ejection fractions in patients with chronic obstructive pulmonary disease[(358)].

The use of theophylline is falling out of favor because of the efficacy of many other agents such as β_2-agonists in the face of a high incidence of side effects associated with theophylline. With proper monitoring of blood levels and clinical condition, theophylline may still have a role in patients with respiratory failure secondary to status asthmaticus[(359, 360)].

Pharmacokinetic and Clinical Implications

Theophylline is distributed throughout the body water, predominantly in extracellular fluid, with 60% bound to plasma protein[(361)]. Theophylline passes freely into breast milk[(362)] and crosses the placenta[(363)] and the blood-brain barrier[(364)]. Salivary concentration appears about 60% of serum level[(365, 366)]. Theophylline is eliminated from the body by biotransformation in the liver, and less than 15% is excreted by the kidney unchanged. The rate of elimination varies among individuals[(367)]; for example, there is a decrease in theophylline clearance in neonates[(368)].

Table 5.6. Guidelines for Continuous Infusion Rate of Theophylline after Loading Dose for Target Concentration of Theophylline of 10 μg/ml[a]

Patient	*Theophylline (mg/kg/hr)*	*Aminophylline[b] (mg/kg/hr)*
Neonates	0.13	0.16
Infant	0.4	0.5
Infants 6–11 mo	0.7	0.85
Children 1–9 yr	0.8	1.0
Children over 9 yr and otherwise healthy adults who smoke	0.6	0.75
Otherwise healthy nonsmoking adults	0.4	0.5
Cardiac decompensation and liver dysfunction	0.2	0.25

[a]*Modified from Weinberger M, Hendeles L, Ahrens R. Clinical pharmacology of drugs used for asthma. Pediatr Clin North Am 1983;28:47.*
[b]*Aminophylline equals theophylline dose/0.8.*

The bronchodilator effect of theophylline is well correlated with increasing serum concentration within the range of 5 to 20 μg/ml[(369, 370)], whereas the optimal response usually occurs at a serum concentration over 10 μg/ml[(371–373)]. Because of the wide variations in elimination and the narrow effective therapeutic range, the efficacy and toxicity of theophylline are correlated more closely with serum level than with the administered dosage[(374)]. The serum theophylline level can be used as a good therapeutic guideline for dosage and dosing interval, but it cannot normally be obtained soon enough to guide therapy in the emergency situation. By using knowledge of the pharmacology of the drug and careful history-taking of previous medication intake, an appropriate intravenous loading dose is derived[(375)]. If the patient has not received a theophylline preparation within the previous 24 hours, the loading dose of 5 to 10 mg/kg should be given slowly over 20 minutes, followed by a continuous infusion dose that depends on the age and other underlying diseases of the patient **(Table 5.6).** If the patient has taken theophylline recently, a serum theophylline level should be obtained. Clinical evidence of theophylline toxicity must be excluded before the lower loading dose of 2.5 mg/kg is administered and followed by the same continuous infusion dose as above. Further adjustment of the theophylline infusion rate depends on the clinical response and serum theophylline concentration.

If the serum concentration of theophylline, obtained 30 minutes after the loading dose, ranges from 10 to 20 μg/ml, the same infusion dose should be continued. If the serum concentration of theophylline is less than 10 μg/ml, an additional loading dose can be given at 1 mg/kg for each 2 μg/ml desired increase in serum concentration. In contrast, if the serum concentration of theophylline is over 25 μg/ml, a level associated with a high degree of toxicity,

Table 5.7. Medications That Alter Theophylline Clearance

Increased theophylline metabolism	
Barbiturate	Increased theophylline clearance by 25% on average when phenobarbital was used for at least 1 month and had a serum concentration over 10 μg/ml
Phenytoin	Increased theophylline clearance by 75% on average when phenytoin was used for more than 10 days and serum levels of phenytoin ranged between 10 and 20 μg/ml; phenytoin level was also reduced
Isoproterenol	Increased theophylline clearance by 15–20% during the concomitant intravenous therapy; clearance resumed to previous level after cessation of isoproterenol infusion
Decreased theophylline metabolism	
Allopurinol	Decreased theophylline clearance by 25% on average when allopurinol was administered in high dose (600 mg/day); theophylline clearance decreased after 2 weeks of therapy
Cimetidine	Decreased theophylline clearance ranged from 23% to 100% and caused serum theophylline concentration increase by twofold to threefold
Erythromycin (base and salts)	Decreased theophylline clearance by 25% on average; effect appeared after 7–10 days of erythromycin therapy and was dose-related; erythromycin level also was reduced
Troleandomycin	Decreased theophylline clearance by 50%; serum theophylline concentraton increased twofold
Propranolol	Decreased theophylline clearance by 40% in cigarette smokers and 20% in nonsmokers
Oral contraceptives	Decreased theophylline clearance by 34% in chronic contraceptive users for 6 months or longer

the infusion should be discontinued until the serum concentration of theophylline falls below 20 μg/ml. A subsequent theophylline level should be obtained 4 to 6 hours later, and the infusion dose should be adjusted, using the same guidelines given. After the steady state is obtained, the serum theophylline level should be drawn daily or as dictated by clinical evidence of toxicity.

Pharmacodynamic and Clinical Implications

DRUG INTERACTIONS. Aside from individual variation in elimination of theophylline from the body, many drugs that have been given concomitantly in the asthmatic patient can alter the theophylline metabolism[201–221]. These are summarized in **Table 5.7.**

The complications of theophylline therapy are related closely to the serum concentration of the drug[222]. Minor side effects, including nausea, vomiting, diarrhea, irritability, and insomnia, are usually associated with a serum theophylline level over 25 μg/ml. The more severe adverse effects, such as cardiac arrhythmias[223,224], hypotension, sudden cardiac arrest[225], and seizures[226,227], are usually associated with a serum concentration over 35 μg/ml and rapid intravenous administration, particularly through a central venous catheter[228]. This serious complication has frequently been reported in patients with congestive heart failure, hepatic cirrhosis[228], and respiratory failure[229] in whom the usual intravenous dosage of theophylline has been given. Cardiac decompensation and liver disease cause a decrease in theophylline clearance[224], whereas hypoxemia, hypercapnia, and acidosis result in a decrease in the threshold for ventricular fibrillation and enhance the cardiotoxic effect of the drug[229]. These life-threatening complications can be prevented by careful monitoring of serum theophylline concentration and modifying the intravenous doses on the basis of the underlying diseases or conditions that may alter the clearance of the drug. (The treatment of theophylline toxicity is discussed in detail in Chapter 32.)

Antibiotic Therapy

Because autopsy findings have shown evidence of pneumonitis in asthma[376, 377], antibiotics are frequently recommended for treating status asthmaticus despite the absence of clinical evidence of bacterial involvement[378–381]. Although respiratory tract infections are an important precipitant of asthmatic attacks, most of these infections are caused by viruses (e.g., RSV, parainfluenza virus, and adenovirus)[382, 383], and no specific therapy is available. In recent studies, investigators have concluded that the routine use of antibiotics in status asthmaticus is not advantageous[384–386]. However, antibiotic therapy should be reserved for asthmatic patients who have signs and symptoms suggesting bacterial infection[387], which can be assessed by correlating clinical and laboratory findings, including fever, leukocytosis, and intracellular bacterial organisms on Gram's stain of sputum. Furthermore, the presence of lobular infiltration on a chest x-ray and evidence of sinusitis[388] by physical or radiographic examination all support the diagnosis of bacterial infection. An appropriate antibiotic should be initiated promptly in these children to eliminate the source that precipitates bronchospasm and therefore reduce the morbidity from asthma.

Hydration and Correction of Acidosis

Decreased fluid intake and increased insensible loss of water from hyperventilation, vomiting, and diuretic effect of aminophylline are thought to be important causes of dehydration in patients with status asthmaticus. As a result, secretions become viscid and contribute to a worsening degree of airway obstruction. The correction of dehydration, if present, is the rule for treatment of children with status asthmaticus. Once adequate urinary output is established, careful monitoring of fluid intake, urine output, serum electrolytes, and osmolarity are necessary to prevent excessive fluid administration and allow early detection of hyponatremia and evidence of water intoxication due to an increase in antidiuretic hormone secretion[389]. Furthermore, the more negative intrapleural pressure during severe asthmatic attacks favors fluid accumulation in the interstitial space[75] around the bronchiole. This effect, if combined with the overhydration, can facilitate the development of pulmonary edema. Hence, the guideline for hydration in asthmatic patients is to maintain the patient at near-normal water balance and avoid excessive fluid administration.

Metabolic acidosis and ketonemia are also found in over 75% of children under 4 years of age with status asthmaticus[390]. This acidosis can cause depression of the catecholamine response and can result in refractory airway obstruction[391,392].

Frequent monitoring of serum electrolytes, arterial blood gases, and pH are mandatory in order to optimize the treatment and prevent complications (i.e., hypernatremia, hypokalemia, and hypercapnia) that can accompany sodium bicarbonate therapy. Furthermore, excessive $NaHCO_3$ therapy in the absence of adequate ventilation can result in an adverse increase in P_aCO_2[393].

Mechanical Ventilation

Despite the understanding of pathophysiologic consequences of acute severe asthmatic attacks and recent advances in the pharmacologic management of status asthmaticus with isoproterenol infusion or continuous albuterol nebulization, a small number of children still develop rapidly progressive respiratory failure, leading to coma and death. The most effective treatment of respiratory failure in these children is mechanical ventilation to reduce the work of breathing and allow bronchodilator drugs to reverse the basic pathophysiology of status asthmaticus[394]. Mechanical ventilation should be used only when bronchodilator therapy alone has failed to prevent worsening hypercapnia. Mechanical ventilation remains a source of iatrogenic morbidity and mortality. Usually, careful monitoring and appropriate therapeutic maneuvers can obviate the need for mechanical ventilation[395].

There are no absolute guidelines for initiating mechanical ventilation in status asthmaticus patients, except in cases of cardiopulmonary arrest and coma; however, the following criteria should be considered:

1. Intubation
2. A decrease in respiratory effort due to progressive exhaustion[396, 397]
3. Deterioration in mental status[396, 398]
4. Absence of breath sounds and wheezing[399]
5. Cyanosis in 40% oxygen
6. Hypoxemia with P_aO_2 less than 60 torr on 6 liters O_2/min [399, 400]
7. Hypercapnia with P_aCO_2 over 65 torr and increasing by more than 5 torr/hr[399]

Choice of Ventilator

Successful mechanical ventilation for patients with status asthmaticus depends less on the type of ventilator or even on the ventilatory mode, but rather on the incorporation of principles that enhance patient safety, principally limiting the risk of lung hyperinflation (volutrauma) and barotrauma. The appropriate respiratory rate depends on the patient's age and usually ranges from 10/min to 20/min with an inspiratory/expiratory ratio of 1:2 to 1:6. This longer expiratory time usually allows adequate time for expiration and reduces further air trapping in an already hyperinflated lung. An appropriate initial tidal volume is approximately 10 to 15 ml/kg. Subsequent adjustment should be done on the basis of clinical adequacy of ventilation by chest auscultation and arterial blood gases. An indwelling arterial catheter is essential for frequent blood samples and continuous arterial pressure monitoring[401]. The appropriate bronchodilators and steroids should be continued. Chest physical therapy and frequent suctioning are necessary to keep the airway patent. This procedure can increase bronchospasm, but gentle manipulation and intratracheal administration of 1 mg/kg of lidocaine in 5 to 10 ml of normal saline 5 minutes before suctioning can diminish this bronchospastic response[402, 403]. The principle of ventilator management is permissive hypercarbia, which is also used in the ventilatory management of adult respiratory distress syndrome. In an effort to minimize barotrauma, the peak pressures are minimized by accepting a range of P_aCO_2 in the high 60s[404]. In addition, the goals include maintenance of pH >7.2 and inflation pressures less than 30 cm H_2O. A sedative and/or a muscle relaxant is required for the frightened and uncooperative patient to promote synchronization of breathing with the ventilator, which will ultimately result in decreased oxygen consumption and less barotrauma. Choice of sedative varies; intravenous diazepam (0.2 to 0.3 mg/kg) is preferred because of its anxiolytic, hypnotic, and amnestic properties. Even though morphine (0.1 to 0.3 mg/kg) is frequently used[256, 378, 405], it must be administered with caution because of the possibility of worsening bronchospasm from morphine-induced histamine release. The neuromuscular blocker, pancuronium bromide (0.1 mg/kg)[406], is favored over *d*-tubocurarine because the latter also causes histamine release[407] and may aggravate the bronchospasm. The patient should receive controlled ventilation initially. Subsequent changes can be made based on physiologic and clinical criteria that signify the reversal of bronchospasm. At that point, the volume-cycled respirator can be placed on the intermittent mandatory ventilation modes or pressure support, which facilitates weaning from the respirator. Most children require mechanical ventilation for approximately 24 to 48 hours[398].

The use of PEEP is generally not recommended in mechanically ventilated patients with asthma. However, one study[408] showed that PEEP of up to 25 cm H_2O can combat air trapping. PEEP increases intraluminal pressure more than intrapleural pressure during respiration; hence, the transmural bronchiolar pressure is increased, which prevents small airway collapse during increased expiratory effort. Although PEEP can slightly increase P_aO_2, it is at the expense of decreased oxygen delivery, detrimental effects of lung volumes, and circulatory parameters[409]. Another study reported the use of CPAP in acute severe asthma and concluded that CPAP up to 10 cm H_2O reduces the work of breathing and decreases the energy requirement of inspiratory muscle, thereby improving ventilation and ultimately resulting in a decrease in P_aCO_2[410, 411]. However, the reliability and safety of CPAP and PEEP in severe asthma still need further studies before they can be recommended.

Experience with more aggressive forms of support for severe asthma has been limited. The role of high-frequency oscillatory ventilation has not been established for pediatric asthma patients, and although mean airway pressures may increase on institution of this form of ventilation, the peak pressures will often decrease[71]. If maximal medical therapy has failed, it is an unproven but a rational approach for the patient to consider the use of extracorporeal membrane oxygenation to support the patient through this period of reversible lung disease.

Monitoring

The continuous monitoring of patients during mechanical ventilation is required for assessment of the patients' condition and early detection of complications. Monitoring should include the following:

1. Continuous arterial pressure measurement via an indwelling catheter, which permits determination of arterial blood gases and the degree of pulsus paradoxus
2. Electrocardiogram, which is of help in the early detection of cardiotoxic effects of theophylline and isoproterenol (such as ST-T-wave changes)
3. Chest x-ray after intubation and then daily, and as determined by the clinician when complications are suspected
4. Peak inspiratory pressure, which is directly related to increased airway resistance and to the risk of pneumothorax
5. Hourly intake and output to keep the patient at near-normal water balance and not overhydrated
6. Serum electrolytes, especially in patients receiving steroids

Criteria used for weaning status asthmaticus patients from mechanical ventilation should be based on reliable physiologic data and evidence of clinical improvement of reversible airway obstruction. These include:

1. Decreased bronchospasm
2. Normal arterial blood gases in 40% oxygen
3. Inspiratory pressure of less than 30 cm H_2O
4. Pulsus paradoxus of less than 10 mm Hg
5. Chest x-ray showing reduced hyperaeration with minimal or no atelectasis

When these conditions are present, the effects of sedatives and muscle relaxants are reversed and the patient may be weaned. Extubation can be considered if the arterial blood gases remain stable, the tidal volume is greater than 5 ml/kg, vital capacity is more than 15 ml/kg, and negative inspiratory pressure is more than -25 cm H_2O. In addition, the patient should be alert with a good cough and gag reflex, which can be determined during endotracheal suction or stimulation. The patient should stay in the ICU for at least 24 hours after extubation. If the condition remains stable, the patient can be weaned gradually from the isoproterenol infusion, or the nebulized bronchodilator administration, and the arterial line may be withdrawn.

Complications

The complications associated with the use of positive pressure ventilators in status asthmatic children include pneumothorax, pneumomediastinum, and subcutaneous emphysema, which is found in 10 to 15% of cases[398, 405]. Such barotrauma is related to the use of high peak inspiratory pressures. The incidence of subglottic stenosis or granulation is approximately 10%[398], compared with an incidence of postextubation subglottic stenosis of 3 to 5% in children who have been intubated because of other diseases[412, 413]. The mortality rate is approximately 10%[401] and ranges from 0% to 30%, depending on the period of study[89, 378, 414–416].

Unusual Forms of Treatment

Anesthetics

Historically, inhalation anesthetic agents such as diethyl ether and cyclopropane have been used in the operating room as therapeutic bronchodilators in severe asthma[417]. More recently, halothane has been described as a useful bronchodilator in pediatric and adult patients with status asthmaticus[418–420]. The mechanism by which halothane dilates baseline airways (as measured by high resolution computed tomography) is through an inhibition of vagal tone[421]. Halothane concentrations of 0.5 to 1.5% and oxygen may produce prompt bronchodilator response, with the rapid improvement in P_aCO_2 and pH within 15 to 20 minutes in patients who had failed other forms of aggressive medical therapy. The duration of treatment with halothane depends on clinical response and P_aCO_2. Once the P_aCO_2 is stabilized and clinical airway obstruction is diminished, as indicated by decreased peak inspiratory pressure or decreased wheezing, halothane inhalation can be discontinued. Halothane has been shown to antagonize the bronchoconstriction effect of histamine and cholinergic agents in experimental animal models[422–424].

An effect similar to β_2-receptor stimulation has also been proposed[425]. The bronchodilator effect of halothane remains active, even in the severely acidotic patient. However, halothane has several adverse effects that must be considered before this agent is used. These side effects include myocardial depression[426], and arrhythmia[427]. The hypotensive effect (secondary to the depression in myocardial function) can contribute to the fall in blood pressure and cause an increase in ventilation/perfusion mismatching secondary to inhibition of hypoxic pulmonary vasoconstriction[428]. In addition, impairment of macrophage and ciliary function in the bronchial tree has been described recently(429), but this seems to be related to the dose and is reversible after cessation of this therapy. As a result, the decision to use halothane should be based on the risks and benefits of this mode of therapy in patients with severe status asthmaticus who are not responding well despite mechanical ventilation and aggressive medical treatment. The failure of aggressive medical treatment necessitating halothane is very rare. The presence of a person who is experienced with halothane administration as well as continuous monitoring of blood pressure, electrocardiogram, and arterial blood gases are mandatory for the success and safety of this mode of treatment.

The bronchodilatory effects of other inhalational anesthetics has been investigated in the laboratory. Isoflurane has been the focus of many of these investigations. Halothane at doses less than 1.2%—i.e., 1.7 times the minimum alveolar concentration (MAC)—is a more effective bronchodilator than isoflurane at 1.9% (also 1.7 times MAC). At doses greater than this, both drugs are at least equipotent(430).

For these and other reasons, isoflurane has been used for the same purpose. Although less is published about the clinical use of isoflurane for this indication, it remains quite effective. The most concerning adverse effect of the drug is hypotension, which, unlike halothane, is mediated by vasodilatation. This is treated with intravenous fluids and phenylephrine infusions. Neither the isoflurane nor the phenylephrine is arrhythmogenic, so that particular side effect (of halothane) is obviated. Isoflurane has also been studied for its saltatory effects on oxygen supply and demand in a compromised myocardium. Although this question has not been evaluated in an asthma model, it seems reasonable that isoflurane would be superior to halothane in its propensity to contribute to or reverse myocardial ischemia. Newer inhalational anesthetics such as sevoflurane may share some of these bronchodilatory effects(431).

Ketamine by continuous infusion (40 μg/kg/min) has been reported to sedate children in the PICU and contribute favorably to the successful treatment of bronchospasm(432).

Local Anesthetics

Local anesthetics can largely block the reflexes that would otherwise stimulate bronchospasm. This has been examined in the trachea(402), which has prompted many to administer lidocaine prior to suctioning a patient who is endotracheally intubated to prevent bronchospasm. Blocking these irritant receptors in the airway has also been evaluated with mexiletin, a longer-acting, orally active anesthetic. At doses comparable to those used to treat dysrhythmias, this agent, which is chemically related to lidocaine, can block vagally mediated bronchospasm(433). Although it should never be used clinically, intravenous bupivacaine has been demonstrated to attenuate bronchospastic provocations(110). Although bupivacaine is not a good intravenous agent because of a narrow therapeutic margin, intravenous lidocaine is an agent with which we have a great deal of experience. Sometimes an intravenous infusion of lidocaine can be used to treat bronchospasm.

Helium

Helium (60%) in 40% oxygen has been reported to decrease airway pressures and CO_2 retention in intubated asthmatic patients. The efficacy of this therapeutic maneuver is based on the fact that reduction of gas density leads to less resistance to airflow(434).

Magnesium

Intravenous magnesium sulfate (0.615 mmol/min for 20 min) in addition to conventional therapy (β-agonists and theophylline) has been reported to improve $FEV_{1.0}$ more than conventional therapy alone in adult asthmatics(435). The role of magnesium in the treatment of asthmatic children remains to be seen.

Future Directions

Calcium Antagonists

This new concept in the treatment of asthma is involved in the prevention of pathophysiologic events that occur during the disease processes, although the use of these agents is not in clinical practice at this time. The pathophysiologic features of allergic bronchial asthma and hyperactive airway disease, including mediator release from sensitized mast cells, smooth muscle spasm, and mucous hypersecretion, are all calcium-dependent phenomena(436). Therefore, calcium antagonists such as verapamil and nifedipine, which interfere with calcium transport across the cell membrane(437), may be useful in both the prevention and treatment of asthmatic attacks.

Verapamil and nifedipine have been studied for their effects in preventing bronchospasm in both humans(438–443) and experimental animals(440, 444–446). However, the results of all studies reported to date are conflicting. Nifedipine was shown to inhibit the effect of histamine-induced bronchospasm in guinea pigs and human airway smooth muscle(440, 441, 444). In addition, the inhibiting actions on acetylcholine-induced and histamine-induced bronchoconstriction as well as exercise-induced asthma have also been demonstrated(439, 440, 447). Nifedipine and verapamil inhibit the grass pollen extract-induced bronchoconstriction(440, 448), whereas both nifedipine and verapamil were shown to have no effect on *Dermatophagoides pteronyssinus*-induced asthma(442). These inconsistent results may have been caused by differences in the dosage of drugs used, the interindividual variability in the degree of protection, and the heterogenicity of the mast cell in various organs and species(449).

The beneficial effects of calcium antagonists in preventing spontaneously occurring asthmatic attacks are not yet established. Although not routinely used in the clinical care of patients in status asthmaticus, absence of adverse effects of calcium antagonists on resting airway tone[440, 450–452] make the concept of calcium channel blockade an important investigative avenue for the development of newer drugs that will have more specific effects on airway smooth muscle tone and mast cell secretion.

Arachidonic Acid Pathway Mediators

Prostaglandins and thromboxanes are oxidative metabolites of arachidonic acid via the cyclo-oxygenase pathway. These arachidonic acids are derived from membrane phospholipids by the activity of phospholipase enzymes, which can be blocked by corticosteroids. Moreover, SRS-A is a potent mediator that can cause an asthmatic attack. This substance has also been shown to be a family of arachidonic acid metabolites formed through the lipoxygenase pathway and is now known to consist of leukotrienes (Fig. 5.15)[453].

The effects of these arachidonic acid metabolites on bronchial smooth muscles, airway mucosa, and mucous secretion are well described[454–458]. Prostaglandin F_2 (PGF_2), thromboxane A_2, and SRS-A (e.g., LTC_4, LTD_4, and LTE_4) are bronchoconstrictors, whereas PGE_2 and PGI_2 are bronchodilators. Asthmatic individuals are especially sensitive to LTE_4, compared with nonasthmatic individuals[459]. This relationship can provide a possible explanation of how aspirin and other prostaglandin inhibitors induce asthmatic attacks[453]. Shunting the arachidonic acid metabolism from the cyclo-oxygenase pathway toward the lipoxygenase pathway, with increases in leukotriene synthesis, ultimately results in bronchospasm, mucosal edema, and mucous secretion. The bronchodilator mechanism of PGE_2 and PGI_2 are believed to be mediated through increases in cyclic AMP in most tissues. The bronchoconstrictive effects of the three components of SRS-A are not the same. The LTC_4 and LTD_4 have much greater bronchospastic potency and greater selectivity for peripheral airways in comparison to LTE_4[460, 461]. Furthermore, LTC_4 and LTD_4 have been shown to have approximately 4000 times more potent bronchoconstrictive properties than histamine[462, 463].

This recent knowledge in regard to arachidonic metabolism and leukotriene biosynthesis may lead to a new therapeutic approach in this disease. Intravenous or aerosolized PGE_2 has been shown to block the bronchoconstrictive effects of acetylcholine, histamine, serotonin, and bradykinin[464, 465]. Even aerosolized PGE_1 and PGE_2 are 10 times more potent bronchodilators than isoproterenol, but the response is slower, and the duration of action is only 30 minutes[466, 467]. Furthermore, the aerosol preparation of PGE_1 and PGE_2 cause bronchial irritation. However, diethylcarbamazine[468], an enzyme inhibitor in the lipoxygenase pathway of leukotriene biosynthesis, has been developed, and the agents that can block the leukotriene effect at the level of the end-organ receptor response[469, 470] are still under investigation. This may contribute to the development of important therapeutic agents for the patient with asthma and other allergic diseases.

Inhibition of the LTD_4 receptor by the drug MK571 attenuates the bronchospasm associated with exercise-induced bronchoconstriction[470]. Likewise, the asthmatic response to cold air is ameliorated by blocking the production of these leukotrienes through inhibition of the enzyme 5′-lipoxygenase (with the drug A-64077)[471]. The therapeutic manipulation of the mediators within the arachidonic acid pathway may be the future approach to asthma treatment.

Nitric Oxide

Because of the laboratory evidence in support of nitric oxide[110], this modality has been studied in adult humans. At a dose of 80 ppm, nitric oxide did not affect airway tone in healthy individuals, but was a weak bronchodilator in patients suffering from bronchial asthma[472]. Furthermore, it modulated the bronchoconstrictive response to inhaled methacholine with an exaggerated saltatory effect when a beta-2 agonists. There was no effect of nitric oxide in adults with chronic obstructive pulmonary disease[472].

SUMMARY

The care of children with lower airway diseases is one of the most common problems encountered by the pediatric

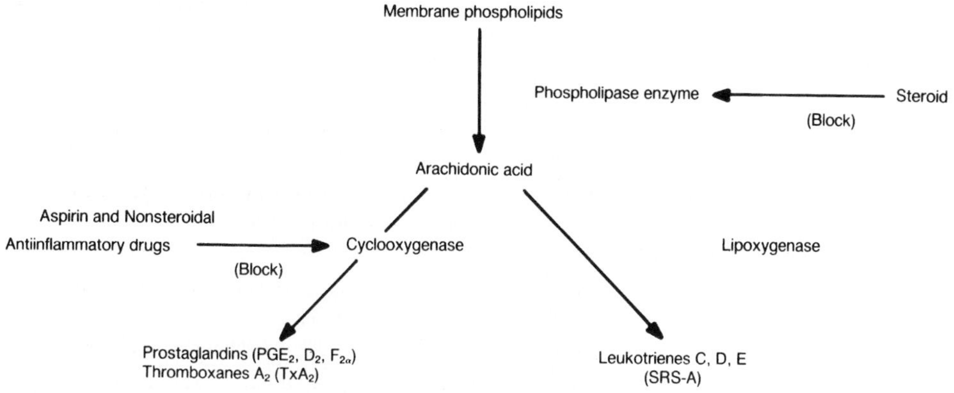

Figure 5.15. Prostaglandin, thromboxane, and leukotriene biosynthesis from metabolite products of arachidonic acid.

intensivist. Bronchiolitis and asthma are frequent reasons for admission to the pediatric ICU. The role of the intensivist in the management of asthma has become more important in recent years with the rising incidence of near-fatal asthma attacks. At the same time the use of continuously nebulized β-agonists has added a powerful new convenient tool in the care of children with severe status asthmaticus. Furthermore, ribavirin has proven itself to be of help in the sickest of RSV-infected infants. Future research directed at the subcellular regulation of bronchial tone should produce further refinements in the therapy available for these patients.

References

1. Carlsen KH, Orstavik I, Halvorsen K. Viral infections of the respiratory tract in hospitalized children. Acta Pediatr Scand 1983;72:52.
2. Glezen WP, Loda FA, Clyde WA, Senior RJ, Sheaffer CI, Conley WG, Denney FW. Epidemiologic patterns of acute lower respiratory disease of children in a pediatric group practice. J Pediatr 1971;78:397.
3. Downham MAPS, McQuillin J, Gardner PS. Diagnosis and clinical significance of parainfluenza virus infections in children. Arch Dis Child 1974;49:8.
4. Clarke SKR, Corner BD, Gambier DM, Macrae J, Peacock DB. Viruses associated with acute respiratory infections. Br Med J 1964;1:1536.
5. Foy HM, Cooney MK, Hall CE, Bor E, Maletzky AJ. Isolation of mumps virus from children with acute lower respiratory tract disease. Am J Epidemiol 1971;94:467.
6. Henderson FW, Clyde WA, Collier AM, Denney FW. The etiologic and epidemiologic spectrum of bronchiolitis in pediatric practice. J Pediatr 1979;95:183.
7. Kapikian AZ, Mitchell RH, Chanock RM, Shvedoff RA, Stewart CE. An epidemiologic study of altered clinical reactivity to respiratory syncytial (RS) virus infection in children previously vaccinated with an inactivated RS virus vaccine. Am J Epidemiol 1968;89:405.
8. Kim HW, Leikin SL, Arrobio J, Brandt CD, Chanock RM, Parrott RH. Cell mediated immunity to respiratory syncytial virus induced by inactivated vaccine or by infection. Pediatr Res 1967;10:75.
9. Welliver RC, Wong DT, Sun M, Middleton E, Vaughan R, Ogra P. The development of respiratory syncytial virus-specific IgE and the release of histamine in nasopharyngeal secretions. N Engl J Med 1981;305:841.
10. Lamprecht CL, Krause HE, Mufson MA. Role of maternal antibody in pneumonia and bronchiolitis due to respiratory syncytial virus. J Infect Dis 1976;134:211.
11. Glezen WP, Paredes A, Allison JE, Taber LH, Frank AL. Risk of respiratory syncytial virus infection for infants from low income families in relationship to age, sex, ethnic group, and maternal antibody level. J Pediatr 1981;98:708.
12. McIntosh K, McQuillin J, Gardner PS. Cell free and cell bound antibody in nasal secretions from infants with respiratory syncytial virus infection. Infect Immun 1979;23:276.
13. Downham MAPS, Scott R, Sims DG, Webb JKG, Gardner PS. Breast feeding protects against respiratory syncytial virus infections. Br Med J 1976;2:274.
14. Volovitz B, Welliver RC, DeCastro G, Krystofik DA, Ogra PL. The release of leukotrienes in the respiratory tract during infection with respiratory syncytial virus: role of obstructive airway disease. Pediatr Res 1988;24: 504–507.
15. Burhn FW, Mohrohisky ST, McIntosh K. Apnea associated with respiratory syncytial virus infection in young infants. J Pediatr 1977;90:382.
16. Church NR, Anas NG, Hall CB, Brooks JG. Respiratory syncytial virus related apnea in infants. Am J Dis Child 1984;138:247.
17. Moler FW, Khan AS, Meliones JN, Custer JR, Palmisano J, Shope, TC. Respiratory syncytial virus morbidity and mortality estimates in congenital heart disease patients: A recent experience. Crit Care Med 1992;20:1406–1413.
18. Groothuis JR, Simoes EAF. Levin MJ, Hall CB, Long CE, Rodriguez WJ, Arrobio J, Meissner HC, Fulton DR, Welliver RC, Tristram DA, Siber GR, Prince GA, Raden MV, Hemming VG. Prophylactic administration of respiratory syncytial virus immune globulin to high-risk infants and young children. N Engl J Med 1993;329:1524–1530.
19. Henderson FW, Collier AM, Clyde WA Jr, Denney FW. Respiratory syncytial virus infections, reinfections, and immunity. N Engl J Med 1979;300:530.
20. Hall CB, Geiman JM, Biggar R, Kotok DI, Hogan PM, Douglas RG. Respiratory syncytial virus infection within families. N Engl J Med 1976;294:414.
21. Hall CB, Douglas RG, Geiman JM, Messner MK. Nosocomial respiratory syncytial virus infections. N Engl J Med 1975;293:1343.
22. Allen JL, Wolfson MR, McDowell K, Shaffer TH. Thoracoabdominal asynchrony in infants with airflow obstruction. Am Rev Respir Dis 1990;141:337–342.
23. Krilov LR, Lipson SM, Barone SR, Kaplan MH, Ciamician Z, Harkness SH. Evaluation of a rapid diagnostic test for respiratory syncytial virus (RSV): Potential for bedside diagnosis. Pediatrics 1994;93:903–906.
24. Simpson W, Hacking PM, Court SDM, Gardner PS. The radiologic findings in respiratory syncytial infections in children. I. Definitions and interobserver variations in the assessment of abnormalities on the chest x-ray. Pediatr Radiol 1974;2:97.
25. Hall CB, Hall J, Speers DM. Clinical and physiological manifestations of bronchiolitis and pneumonia. Am J Dis Child 1979;133:798.
26. Downes JJ, Wood DW, Striker TW, Haddad C. Acute respiratory failure in infants with bronchiolitis. Anesthesiology 1968;29:426.
27. Becroft DMO. Bronchiolitis obliterans, bronchiectasis, and other sequelae of adenovirus type 21 infection in young children. J Clin Pathol 1971;24:72.
28. Swyer P, James G. Case of unilateral pulmonary emphysema. Thorax 1953;8:133.
29. Cumming GR, MacPherson RK, Chernik V. Unilateral hyperlucent lung syndrome in children. J Pediatr 1971;78:250.
30. Garg K, Lynch DA, Newell JD, King TE: Proliferative and constrictive bronchiolitis: classification and radiologic features. AJR 1994;162:803–808.
31. Phelan PPD, Williams HE, Freeman M. The disturbance of ventilation in acute viral bronchiolitis. Aust Pediatr J 1968;4:96.
32. Wohl MEB, Stiegol LC, Mead J. Resistance of the total respiratory system in healthy infants and infants with bronchiolitis. Pediatrics 1969;43:494.
33. Fryer AD, Jacoby DB. Parainfluenza virus infection damages inhibitory M_2 muscarinic receptors on pulmonary parasympathetic nerves in the guinea-pig. Br J Pharmacol 1991;102(1):267–271.
34. Reynolds EOR. Arterial blood gas tensions in acute disease of lower respiratory tract in infancy. Br Med J 1963;1:1192.
35. Reynolds EOR. The effect of breathing 40 per cent oxygen on the arterial blood gas tensions of babies with bronchiolitis. J Pediatr 1963;63:1135.
36. Krieger I. Mechanics of respiration in bronchiolitis. Pediatrics 1964;33:45.
37. Muller N, Gulston G, Cade D, Whitton J, Froese AB, Bryan MH, Bryan AC. Diaphragmatic muscle fatigue in the newborn. J Appl Physiol 1979;46:688.
38. Anas N, Boettrich C, Hall CB, Brooks JG. The association of apnea and respiratory syncytial virus infection in infants. J Pediatr 1982;101:65.
39. Hall CB, Geiman JM, Douglas RG, Meager MD. Control of nosocomial respiratory syncytial virus infections. Pediatrics 1978;62:728.
40. Phelan PD, Williams HE. Sympathetic drugs in acute viral bronchiolitis. Pediatrics 1969;44:493.
41. Rutter N, Milner AD, Hiller J. Effects of bronchodilators on respiratory resistance in infants and young children with bronchiolitis and wheezy bronchitis. Arch Dis Child 1975;50:719.
42. Schuh S, Canny G, Reisman JJ, Kerem E, Bentur L, Petric M, Levison H. Nebulized albuterol in acute bronchiolitis. J Pediatr 1990;117:633–637.
43. Katz RW, Kelly HW, Crowley MR, Grad R, McWilliams BC, Murphy SJ. Safety of continuous nebulized albuterol for bronchospasm in infants and children. Pediatrics 1993;92:666–669.
44. Tepper RS, Rosenberg D, Eigen H, Reister T. Bronchodilator responsiveness in infants with bronchiolitis. Pediatr Pulmonol 1994;17:81–85.
45. Lowell DI, Lister G, VonKoss H, McCarthy P. Wheezing in infants: the response to epinephrine. Pediatrics 1987; 79(6):939–945.
46. Sanchez I, De Koster J, Powell RE, Wolstein R, Chernick V. Effect of racemic epinephrine and salbutamol on clinical score and pulmonary mechanics in infants with broncholitis. J Pediatr 1993;122:145–151.
47. Mallory GB, Motoyama EK, Koumbourlis AC, Mutich RL, Nakayama DK. Bronchial reactivity in infants in acute respiratory failure with viral bronchiolitis. Pediatr Pulmonol 1989;6:253–259.
48. Prendiville A, Green S, Silverman M. Ipratropium bromide and airways function in wheezy infants. Arch Dis Child 1987;62:397–400.

49. Leer JA, Bloomfield NJ, Green JL, Heimlich EM, Hyde JS, Moffet HL, Young GA, Barron BA. Corticosteroid treatment in bronchiolitis: a controlled collaborative study in 297 infants and children. Am J Dis Child 1969;117:495.
50. Carlsen KH, Leegaard J, Larsen S, Orstavik I. Nebulised beclomethasone dipropionate in recurrent obstructive episodes after acute bronchiolitis. Arch Dis Child 1988; 63:1428–1433.
51. Field CMB, Connolly JH, Murtabh G, Slattery CM, Turkington EE. Antibiotic treatment of epidemic bronchiolitis—a double blind trial. Br Med J 1966;1:83.
52. Kadota J-I, Sakito O, Kohno S, Sawa H, Mukae H, Oda H, Kawakami K, Fukushima K, Hiratani K, Hara K. A mechanism of erythromycin treatment in patients with diffuse panbronchiolitis. Am Rev Respir Dis 1993;147:153–159.
53. Taber LH, Knight V, Gilbert BE, McClung HW, Wilson SZ, Norton HJ, Thurson JM, Gordon WH, Atmar RL, Schlaudt WR. Ribavirin aerosol treatment of bronchiolitis associated with respiratory syncytial virus infections in infants. Pediatrics 1983;72:613.
54. Hall CB, Walsh EE, Hruska JF, Betts RF, Hall WJ. Ribavirin treatment of experimental respiratory syncytial viral infection. A controlled double-blind study in young adults. JAMA 1983;249:2666.
55. Groothuis JR, Woodin KA, Katz R, Robertson AD, McBride JT, Hall CB, McWilliams BC, Lauer BA. Early ribavirin treatment of respiratory syncytial viral infection in high-risk children. J Pediatr 1990; 117:792–798.
56. Outwater KM, Meissner HC, Peterson MB. Ribavirin administration to infants receiving mechanical ventilation. Am J Dis Child 1988; 142:512–515.
57. Frankel LR, Wilson CW, Demers RR, Parker JR, Lewiston NJ, Stevenson DK, Smith DW. A technique for the administration of ribavirin to mechanically ventilated infants with severe respiratory syncytial virus infection. Crit Care Med 1987;15(11):1051–1054.
58. Smith DW, Frankel LR, Mathers LH, Tang ATS, Ariagno RL, Prober CG. A controlled trial of aerosolized ribavirin in infants receiving mechanical ventilation for severe respiratory syncytial virus infection. N Engl J Med 1991;325:24–29.
59. Obata T, Iikura Y. Comparison of bronchial reactivity to ultrasonically nebulized distilled water, exercise and methacholine challenge test in asthmatic children. Annals of Allergy 1994;167–172.
60. Meert KL, Sarnaik AP, Gelmini MJ, Lieh-Lai MW. Aerosolized ribavirin in mechanically ventilated children with respiratory syncytial virus lower respiratory tract disease: A prospective, double-blind, randomized trial. Crit Care Med 1994;22:566–572.
61. Englund JA, Piedra PA, Ahn Y-M, Gilbert BE, Hiatt P. High-dose, short-duration ribavirin aerosol therapy compared with standard ribavirin therapy in children with suspected respiratory syncytial virus infection. J Pediatr 1994;125:635–641.
62. Assessing exposure of health-care personnel to aerosols of ribavirin-California. Leads from the MMWR. JAMA 1988;260:1844–1845.
63. Ribavirin therapy of respiratory syncytial virus. Committee of Infectious Diseases. Pediatrics 1987;79:475–478.
64. Wald ER, Dashefsky B, Green M. In re ribavirin: a case of premature adjudication? J Pediatr 1988;112:154–158.
65. Groothuis JR. Role of antibody and the use of respiratory syncytial virus immunoglobulin in the prevention of respiratory syncytial virus disease in preterm infants with and without bronchopulmonary dysplasia. Pediatr Infect Dis J 1994;13:454–458.
66. Rimensberger PC, Schaad UB. Clinical experience with aerosolized immunoglobulin treatment of respiratory syncytial virus infection in infants. Pediatr Infect Dis J 1994:13:328–330.
67. Mallol J, Sly PD. Effect of chloral hydrate on arterial oxygen saturation in wheezy infants. Pediatr Pulmonol 1988;5:96–99.
68. Beasley JM, Jones SEF. Continuous positive airway pressure in bronchiolitis. Br Med J 1981;283:1506.
69. Soong W-J, Hwang B, Tang R-B. Continuous positive airway pressure by nasal prongs in bronchiolitis. Pediatr Pulmonol 1993;16:163–166.
70. Smith PG, El-Khatib MF, Carlo WA. PEEP does not improve pulmonary mechanics in infants with bronchiolitis. Am Rev Respir Dis 1993;147:1295–1298.
71. Arnold JH, Hanson JH, Toro-Figuero LO, Gutierrez J, Berens RJ, Anglin DL. Prospective, randomized comparison of high-frequency oscillatory ventilation and conventional mechanical ventilation in pediatric respiratory failure. Crit Care Med 1994;22:1530–1539.
72. Steinhorn RH, Green TP. Use of extracorporeal membrane oxygenation in the treatment of respiratory syncytial virus bronchiolitis: the national experience, 1983 to 1988. J Pediatr 1990;116:338–342.
73. Leclerc F, Riou Y, Martinot A, Storme L, Hue V, Flurin V, Deschildre A, Sadik A. Inhaled nitric oxide for a severe respiratory syncytial virus infection in an infant with bronchopulmonary dysplasia. Intensive Care Med 1994;20:511–512.
74. Gozal D, Colin AA, Jaffe M, Hochberg Z. Water, electrolyte, and endocrine homeostasis in infants with bronchiolitis. Pediatr Res 1990;27:204–209.
75. Stalcup SA, Mellins RB. Mechanical forces producing pulmonary edema and acute asthma. N Engl J Med 1977;197:592.
76. Kattan M, Keens TG, Lapierre JG, Levison H, Bryan AC, Reilly BJ. Pulmonary function abnormalities in symptom-free children after bronchiolitis. Pediatrics 1977;59:683.
77. Wittig HJ, Cranford NJ, Glaser J. The relationship between bronchiolitis and childhood asthma. J Allergy 1959;30:19.
78. Korppi M, Reijonen T, Poysa L, Juntunen-Backman K. A 2- to 3-year outcome after bronchiolitis. AJDC 1993;147:628–631.
79. Martinez FD, Morgan WJ, Wright AL, Holberg CJ, Taussig LM, GMHA Personnel. Diminished lung function as a predisposing factor for wheezing respiratory illness in infants. N Engl J Med 1988;319: 1112–1117.
80. Martinez FD, Morgan WJ, Wright AL, Holberg C, Taussig LM, the Group Health Medical Associates. Am Rev Respir Dis 1991;143:312–316.
81. Weiss ST, Tager IB, Muñoz A, Speizer FE. The relationship of respiratory infections in early childhood to the occurrence of increased levels of bronchial responsiveness and atopy. Am Rev Respir Dis 1985;131:573–578.
82. Hardy KA, Schidlow DV, Zaeri N. Obliterative bronchiolitis in children. Chest 1988;93(3):460–466.
83. Homa FL, Brideau RJ, Lehman DJ, Thomsen DR, Olmsted RA, Wathen MW. Development of a novel subunit vaccine that protects cotton rats against both human respiratory syncytial virus and human parainfluenza virus type 3. J Gen Virol 1993;74:1995–1999.
84. Chipps BE, Sullivan WF, Portnoy JM. Alpha-2A-interferon for treatment of bronchiolitis caused by respiratory syncytial virus. Pediatr Infect Dis J 1993;12:653–658.
85. Dodge RR, Burrows B. The prevalence and incidence of asthma and asthma-like symptoms in a general population sample. Am Rev Respir Dis 1980;122:567.
86. Smith JM. Incidence of atopic disease. Med Clin North Am 1974;58:3.
87. Weitzman M, Gortmaker S, Sobol A. Racial, social, and environmental risks for childhood asthma. Am J Dis Child 1990;144:1189–1194.
88. National Center for Health Statistics. Vital statistics of the United States, 1971 mortality. Rockville, Maryland: U S Department of Health, Education and Welfare, 1974:2.
89. Molfino NA, Nannini LJ, Martelli AN, Slutsky AS. Respiratory arrest in near-fatal asthma. N Engl J Med 1991;324:285–288.
90. Wasserfallen JB, Schaller MD, Feihl F, Perret CH. Sudden asphyxic asthma: a distinct entity? Am Rev Respir Dis 1990;142:108–111.
91. Miller BD, Strunk RC. Circumstances surrounding the deaths of children due to asthma. Am J Dis Child 1989;143:1294–1299.
92. Bai TR. Abnormalities in airway smooth muscle in fatal asthma. Am Rev Respir Dis 1990;141:552–557.
93. Reed CE. The pathogenesis of asthma. Med Clin North Am 1974;58:55.
94. Rowntree S, Cogswell JJ, Platts-Mills TAE, Mitchell EB. Development of IgE and IgG antibodies to food and inhalant allergens in children at risk of allergic disease. Archives of Disease in Childhood 1985;60:727–735.
95. Buffum WP, Settipane GA. Prognosis of Asthma in Childhood. Amer J Dis Child 1966;112:214–217.
96. Meyers DA, Postma DS, Panhuysen CIM, Xu J, Amelung PJ, Levitt RC, Bleecker ER. Evidence for a locus regulating total serum IgE levels Mapping to chromosome 5. Genomics 1994;23:464–470.
97. Borish L, Mascali JJ, Klinnert M, Leppert M, Rosenwasser LJ. SSC polymorphisms in interleukin genes. Human Molecular Genetics 1994; 3:1710.
98. Leffert F. Asthma: a modern perspective. Pediatrics 1978;62:1061.
99. Casale TB, Marom Z. Mast cell and asthma. The role of mast cell mediators in the pathogenesis of allergic asthma. Ann Allergy 1983;1:2.
100. Kay AB. Basic mechanism in allergic asthma. Eur J Respir Dis (Suppl) 1982;122:9.
101. Gleich GJ, Frigas E, Loegering D, Wassom DL, Steinmuller D. Cytotoxic properties of the eosinophil major basic protein. J Immunol 1979;123:2925.
102. Barnes PT, Minette P, Maclagan J. Muscarinic receptor subtypes in airways. Trends Pharmacol Sci 1988; 9:412–416.
103. Schultheis AH, Bassett DJP, Fryer AD. Ozone-induced airway hyperresponsiveness and loss of neuronal M_2 muscarinic receptor function. J Appl Physiol 1994;76:1088–1097.

104. Nadel JA, Widdicombe JG. Reflex effects of upper airway irritation on total lung resistance and blood pressure. J Appl Physiol 1962;17:861.
105. Nadel JA. Neurophysiologic aspects of asthma. In: Austen KF, Lichtenstein LM, eds. Asthma, physiology, immunopharmacology, and treatment. New York: Academic Press, 1973:29.
106. Szentivanyi A. The beta-adrenergic theory of the atopic abnormality in bronchial asthma. J Allergy 1968;42:203.
107. Brooks SM, McGowan K, Bernstein JL, Altenau P, Peagler J. Relationship between numbers of beta adrenergic receptors in lymphocytes and disease severity in asthma. J Allergy Clin Immunol 1979;63:401.
108. Nelson HS, Block JW, Branch LB. Subsensitivity to epinephrine following the administration of epinephrine and ephedrine to normal individuals. J Allergy Clin Immunol 1975;55:299.
109. Galant SR, Durisetti L, Underwood S, Allred S, Insel PA. Beta adrenergic receptors of polymorphonuclear particulates in bronchial asthma. J Clin Invest 1980;65:577.
110. Groeben H, Schwalen A, Irsfeld S, Tarnow J, Lipfert P, Hopf, H-B. High thoracic epidural anesthesia does not alter airway resistance and attenuates the response to an inhalational provocation test in patients with bronchial hyperreactivity. Anesthesiology 1994;81:868–874.
111. Brown RH, Zerhouni EA, Hirshman CA. Reversal of bronchoconstriction by inhaled nitric oxide: histamine versus methacholine. Am J Respir Crit Care Med 1994;150:233–237.
112. Hogg JC. The pathophysiology of asthma. Chest (Suppl) 1982;82:8S.
113. Dunnill MS. Pathology of asthma. Ciba Found Symp 1971;38:35.
114. Daniel EE, Davis C, Jones T. Control of airway smooth muscle. In: Hargreave E, ed. Airway hyperreactivity, mechanisms and clinical relevance. Proceedings of a symposium, McMaster University, Hamilton, Ontario, Canada. Astra Pharmaceuticals, 1975:June.
115. Jeffries E, Pare PD, Hogg JC. Measurements of airway edema in allergic bronchoconstriction in the guinea pig. Am Rev Respir Dis 1981;123:687.
116. Dunnills MS, Massarella GR, Anderson JA. A comparison of the quantitative anatomy of the bronchi in normal subjects, in status asthmaticus, in chronic bronchitis and in emphysema. Thorax 1969;24:176.
117. Dunnill MS. The pathology of asthma, with special reference to change in the bronchial mucosa. J Clin Pathol 1960;13:27.
118. Empey DW, Laitinen LA, Jacobs L. Mechanisms of bronchial hyperreactivity in normal subjects after upper respiratory tract infection. Am Rev Respir Dis 1976;113:131.
119. Orehek J, Masari JP, Gayrard P, Grimaud C, Charpin J. The effect of short-term low-level nitrogen dioxide exposure on bronchial sensitivity in asthmatic patients. J Clin Invest 1976;57:301.
120. Golden JA, Nadel JA, Boushey HA. Bronchial hyperirritability in healthy subjects after exposure to ozone. Am Rev Respir Dis 1978;118:287.
121. Boucher RC, Johnson J, Inoue S, Hubert W, Hogg JC. The effect of cigarette smoke on the permeability of guinea pig airways. Lab Invest 1980;43:94.
122. Bousquet J, Chanez P, Lacoste JY, White R, Vic P, Godard P, Michel FB. Asthma: a disease remodeling the airways. 1992;47:3–11.
123. Hulbert WC, Walker DC, Jackson A, Hogg JC. Airway permeability to horseradish peroxidase in guinea pigs: the repair phase after injury by cigarette smoke. Am Rev Respir Dis 1981;123:320.
124. Naylor B. The shedding of the mucosa of the bronchial tree in man. Thorax 1962;17:69.
125. Houston JC, deNaevasqez S, Trounce JR. A clinical and pathological study of fatal cases of status asthmaticus. Thorax 1953;8:207.
126. Sanerkin NG, Evans DM. The sputum in bronchial asthma pathopneumonic pattern. J Pathol 1965;89:535.
127. DuBois AB, Botelho SY, Comroe JH Jr. A new method for measuring airway resistance in man using a body plethysmograph: values in normal subjects and in patients with respiratory disease. J Clin Invest 1956;35:327.
128. Macklem PT, Mead J. Resistance of central and peripheral airway measured by a retrograde catheter. J Appl Physiol 1967;22:395.
129. Campbell EJM. Mechanisms of airway obstruction in emphysema and asthma. Proc R Soc Med 1958;51:108.
130. McFadden ER Jr, Lyons HA. Serial studies of factors influencing airway dynamics during recovery from acute asthma attacks. J Appl Physiol 1969;27:452.
131. Ruth WE, Andrews CE. Airway resistance studies in bronchial asthma. J Lab Clin Med 1959;54:889.
132. Mellins RB, Lord GP, Fishman AP. Dynamic behavior of the lung in acute asthma. Med Thorac 1967;24:81.
133. Well RR Jr. Mechanics of respiration in bronchial asthma. Am J Med 1959;26:384.
134. Lenfant C. I. Definition and diagnosis. The Journal of Allergy and Clinical Immunology. 1991;88:425–438.
135. Lim TK, Ang SM, Rossing TH, Ingenito EP, Ingram RH. The effects of deep inhalation of maximal expiratory flow during intensive treatment of spontaneous asthmatic episodes. Am Rev Respir Dis 1989;140:340–343.
136. Woolcock AJ, Read J. Lung volumes in exacerbation of asthma. Am J Med 1966;41:259.
137. Freedman S, Tattersfield AE, Pride NB. Changes in lung mechanics during asthma induced by exercise. J Appl Physiol 1975;38:974.
138. McFadden ER Jr, Ingram RH Jr. Spirometry, lung volumes and distribution of ventilation in asthma. In: Segal MS, Weiss EB, eds. Bronchial asthma: mechanisms and therapeutics. Boston: Little, Brown, 1976:279.
139. Mayfield JD, Paez PN, Nicholson DP. Static and dynamic lung volume and ventilation perfusion abnormalities in adult asthma. Thorax 1971;26:591.
140. Otis AB, McKerrow CB, Bartlett RA, Mead J, McIlroy MB. Selverstone NJ, Radford EP. Mechanical factors in distribution of pulmonary ventilation. J Appl Physiol 1956;8:427.
141. Leith DE, Mead J. Mechanism determining residual volume of the lung in normal subjects. J Appl Physiol 1967;23:221.
142. McCarthy D, Millic-Emili, J. Closing volume in asymptomatic asthma. Am Rev Respir Dis 1973;107:559.
143. Permutt S. Physiologic changes in the acute asthmatic attack. In: Austin KF, Lichtenstein LM, eds. Asthma, physiology, immunopharmacology, and treatment. New York: Academic Press, 1973:15.
144. Tai E, Read J. Blood gas tension in bronchial asthma. Lancet 1967;1:644.
145. Weng TR, Langer HM, Featherby EA, Levison H. Arterial blood gas tensions and acid-base balance in symptomatic and asymptomatic asthma in childhood. Am Rev Respir Dis 1970;101:274.
146. McFadden ER Jr, Lyons HA. Arterial blood gas tensions in asthma. N Engl J Med 1968;278:1027.
147. Mountain RD, Heffner JE, Brackett NC, Sahn SA. Acid-base disturbances in acute asthma. Chest 1990;98:651–655.
148. Pierson RN Jr, Grieco MH. Pulmonary blood volume in asthma. J Appl Physiol 1972;32:391.
149. Simmons DH, Linde LM, Miller JH, O'Reilly RJ. Relation between lung volume and pulmonary vascular resistance. Circ Res 1961;9:465.
150. Williams MH Jr, Zohman LR. Cardiopulmonary function in bronchial asthma: a comparison with chronic pulmonary emphysema. Am Rev Respir Dis 1960;81:173.
151. Buda AJ, Pinsky MR, Ingels NB Jr, Daughters GT II, Stinson EB, Alderman EL. Effect of intrathoracic pressure on left ventricular performance. N Engl J Med 1979;301:453.
152. Knowles GK, Clark TJH. Pulsus paradoxus as a valuable sign indicating severity of asthma. Lancet 1973;2:1356.
153. McGregor M. Pulsus paradoxus. N Engl J Med 1979;301:480.
154. Rebuck AS, Pengelly LD. Development of pulsus paradoxicus in the presence of airways obstruction. N Engl J Med 1973;288:66.
155. Shim C, Williams MH Jr. Pulsus paradoxicus in asthma. Lancet 1978;1:530.
156. Rebuck AS, Read J. Assessment and management of severe asthma. Am J Med Levi;1971;51:788.
157. Levison H, Collins-Williams C, Bryan AC, Reilly BJ, Orange RP. Asthma, current concepts. Pediatr Clin North Am 1974;21:951.
158. Siegel SC, Heimlich EM, Richards WS. Bronchial asthma. In: Kelly VC, ed. Practice of pediatrics. Hagerstown, Maryland: Harper & Row, 1974, Ch 63.
159. Ledbetter MK, Bruck E, Farhi LE. Perfusion of the under ventilated compartment of the lungs in asthmatic children. J Clin Invest 1964;43:2233.
160. Downes JJ, Wood DW, Striker TW, Pittman JC. Arterial blood gas and acid base disorders in infants and children with status asthmaticus. Pediatrics 1968;42:238.
161. Cloutier MM, Loughlin GM. Chronic cough in children: a manifestation of airway hypersensitivity. Pediatrics 1981;67:6.
162. Corrao WM, Braman SS, Irwin RS. Chronic cough as the sole manifestation of bronchial asthma. N Engl J Med 1979;300:633.
163. Konig P. Hidden asthma in childhood. Am J Dis Child 1981;135:1053.
164. Hannaway PJ, Hopper DK. Cough variant asthma in children. JAMA 1982;247:206.
165. McFadden ER Jr, Kiser R, DeGroot W. Acute bronchial asthma: Relations between clinical and physiologic manifestations. N Engl J Med 1973;288:221.
166. Mullarky MF, Hill JS, Webb DR. Allergic and nonallergic rhinitis: their

characterization with attention to the meaning of nasal eosinophilia. J Allergy Clin Immunol 1980;65:122.
167. Eggleston PA, Ward BH, Pierson WE, Bierman CW. Radiographic abnormalities in acute asthma in children. Pediatrics 1974;54:442.
168. Bouhuys A. Breathing, physiology, environment and lung diseases. New York: Grune & Stratton, 1974.
169. Weng TR, Levison H. Pulmonary function in children with asthma at acute attack and symptom-free status. Am Rev Respir Dis 1969;99:719.
170. Weiss EB, Faling LJ. Clinical significance of $PaCO_2$ during status asthma. The cross-over point. Ann Allergy 1968;26:545.
171. Konig P. The relationship between croup and asthma. Ann Allergy 1978;41:227.
172. Zach MS, Schnall RP, Landua LI. Upper and lower airway hyperreactivity in recurrent croup. Am Rev Respir Dis 1980;121:979.
173. McIntosh K. Bronchiolitis and asthma: possible common pathogenetic pathways. J Allergy Clin Immunol 1976;57:595.
174. Welliver RC, Wong PT, Sun M, Middleton E Jr, Vaughan RS, Ogra PL. The development of respiratory syncytial virus-specific IgE and the release of histamine in nasopharyngeal secretions after infection. N Engl J Med 1981;305:841.
175. Kondo S, Ito M, Saito M, Sugimori M, Watanabe H. Progressive bronchial obstruction during the acute stage of respiratory tract infection in asthmatic children. Chest 1994;106:100–104.
176. Freeman GL, Todd RH. The role of allergy in viral respiratory tract infections. Am J Dis Child 1962;104:330.
177. Foucard T. A follow-up study of children with asthmatoid bronchitis. I. Skin test reaction and IgE antibodies to common allergens. Acta Pediatr Scand 1973;62:633.
178. Lulla S, Newcomb RW. Emergency management of asthma in children. J Pediatr 1980;97:346.
179. Carden DL, Nowak RM, Sarkar D, Tomlanovich MC. Vital signs including pulsus paradoxus in the assessment of acute bronchial asthma. Ann Emerg Med 1983;12:80.
180. Brenner BE, Abraham E, Simon RR. Position and diaphoresis in acute asthma. Am J Med 1983;74:1005.
181. Rees HA, Millar JS, Donald KW. A study of the clinical course and arterial blood gas tension of patients in status asthmaticus. Q J Med 1968;37:541.
182. Hiller FC, Wilson FJ Jr. Evaluation and management of acute asthma. Med Clin North Am 1983;67:669.
183. Nowak RM, Tomlanovich MC, Sarkar DD, Kvale PA, Anderson JA. Arterial blood gases and pulmonary function testing in acute bronchial asthma. JAMA 1983;249:2043.
184. Appel D, Rubenstein R, Schrager K, Williams MH. Lactic acidosis in severe asthma. Am J Med 1983;75:580.
185. Fanta CH, Rossing TH, McFadden ER Jr. Emergency room treatment of asthma. Am J Med 1982;72:416.
186. Banner AS, Shah RS, Addington WW. Rapid prediction of need for hospitalization in acute asthma. JAMA 1976;235:1337.
187. Silver RB, Ginsburg CM. Early prediction of the need for hospitalization in children with acute asthma. Clin Pediatr 1984;23:81.
188. Siegler D. Reversible electrocardiographic changes in severe acute asthma. Thorax 1977;32:328.
189. Ellis EF. Asthma in childhood. J Allergy Clin Immunol 1983;72:526.
190. Fischl MA, Pitchenik A, Gardner LB. An index predicting relapse and need for hospitalization in patients with acute bronchial asthma. N Engl J Med 1981;305:783.
191. Wood DW, Downes JJ, Lecks HI. A clinical scoring system for the diagnosis of respiratory failure. Am J Dis Child 1972;123:227.
192. Schwartz AL, Lipton JM, Warburton D, Johnson LB, Twarong FJ. Management of acute asthma in childhood. Am J Dis Child 1980;134:474.
193. Simons FER, Gillies JD. Dose response of subcutaneous turbutaline and epinephrine in children with acute asthma. Am J Dis Child 1981;135:214.
194. Sly RM, Badiei B, Faciane J. Comparison of subcutaneous terbutaline with epinephrine in the treatment of asthma in children. J Allergy Clin Immunol 1977;59:128.
195. Ben-Zvi Z, Lam C, Hoffman J, Teets-Grimm KC, Kattan M. An evaluation of the initial treatment of acute asthma. Pediatrics 1982;70:348.
196. Becker AB, Nelson NA, Simons FER. Inhaled salbutamol (albuterol) vs injected epinephrine in the treatment of acute asthma in children. J Pediatr 1983;102:465.
197. Smith PR, Heurich AE, Leffler CT, Henis MM, Lyons HA. A comparative study of subcutaneously administered terbutaline and epinephrine in the treatment of acute bronchial asthma. Chest 1977;71:129.
198. Tai E, Read J. Response of blood gas tension to aminophylline and isoproterenol in patients with asthma. Thorax 1967;22:563.
199. Gazioglu K, Condemi JJ, Hyde RW, Kaltreider NL. Effect of isoproterenol on gas exchange during air and oxygen breathing in patients with asthma. Am J Med 1971;50:185.
200. Hales CA, Kazemi H. Hypoxic vascular response of the lung. Effect of aminophylline and epinephrine. Am Rev Respir Dis 1974;110:126.
201. Piafsky KM, Sitar DS, Ogilvie RI. Effect of phenobarbital on the disposition of intravenous theophylline. Clin Pharmacol Ther 1977; 22:336.
202. Landay RA, Gonzalez MA, Taylor JC. Effect of phenobarbital on theophylline disposition. J Allergy Clin Immunol 1978;62:27.
203. Marquis JF, Carruthers SG, Spence JD, Brownstone YS, Toogood JH. Phenytoin-theophylline interaction. N Engl J Med 1982;307:1189.
204. O'Rourke PP, Crone RK. Effect of isoproterenol on measured theophylline levels. Crit Care Med 1984;12:373.
205. Hemstreet MP, Miles MV, Rutland RO. Effect of intravenous isoproterenol on theophylline kinetics. J Allergy Clin Immunol 1982;69:360.
206. Manfredi R, Vesell ES. Inhibition of theophylline metabolism by long-term allopurinol administration. Clin Pharmacol Ther 1981;29:224.
207. Jackson JE, Powell JR, Wandell M, Bentley J, Dorr R. Cimetidine decreases theophylline clearance. Am Rev Respir Dis 1981;123:615.
208. Reitberg DP, Bernhard H, Schentag JJ. Alteration of theophylline clearance and half-life by cimetidine in normal volunteers. Ann Intern Med 1981;95:582.
209. Roberts RK, Grice J, Wood L, Petroff V, McGuffie C. Cimetidine impairs the elimination of theophylline and antipyrine. Gastroenterology 1981;81:19.
210. Weinberger M, Smith G, Milavetz G, Hendeles L. Decreased theophylline clearance due to cimetidine. N Engl J Med 1981;304:672.
211. May DC, Jarboe CH, Ellenburg CJ, Roe EJ, Karibo J. The effects of erythromycin on theophylline elimination in normal males. Clin Pharmacol 1982;22:125.
212. Renton KW, Gray JD, Hung OR. Depression of theophylline elimination by erythromycin. Clin Pharmacol Ther 1981;30:422.
213. Zarowitz BJM, Szefler SJ, Lasezkay GM. Effect of erythromycin base on theophylline kinetics. Clin Pharmacol Ther 1981;29:601.
214. Kozak PP, Cummins LJ, Gillman SH. Administration of erythromycin to patients on theophylline [Letter]. J Allergy Clin Immunol 1977;60:149.
215. Reisz G, Pingleton SK, Melethil S, Ryan PB. The effect of erythromycin on theophylline pharmacokinetics in chronic bronchitis. Am Rev Respir Dis 1983;127:581.
216. Richer C, Mathieu M, Bah H, Thuillez C, Duroux P, Giudicelli JF. Theophylline kinetics and ventilatory flow in bronchial asthma and chronic airflow obstruction: influence of erythromycin. Clin Pharmacol Ther 1981;31:579.
217. Iliopoulou A, Aldhous ME, Johnston A, Turner P. Pharmacokinetic interaction between theophylline and erythromycin. Br J Clin Pharmacol 1982;14:495.
218. Weinberger M, Hudgel D, Spector S, Chidsey C. Inhibition of theophylline clearance by troleandomycin. J Allergy Clin Immunol 1977; 59:228.
219. Conrad KA, Nyman DW. Effects of metoprolol and propranolol on theophylline elimination. Clin Pharmacol Ther 1980;28:463.
220. Jusko WJ, Gardner MJ, Mangione A, Schentag JJ, Koup JR, Vance JW. Factors affecting theophylline clearance: age, tobacco, marijuana, cirrhosis, congestive heart failure, obesity, oral contraceptives, benzodiazepines, barbiturates, and ethanol. J Pharm Sci 1979;68:1358.
221. Tornatore KM, Kanarkowski R, McCarthy TL, Gardner MJ, Yurchak AM, Jusko WJ. Effect of chronic oral contraceptive steroids on theophylline disposition. Eur J Clin Pharmacol 1982;23:129.
222. Jacobs MH, Senior RM, Kessler G. Clinical experience with theophylline: relationship between dosage, serum concentration and toxicity. JAMA 1976;235:1983.
223. Helliwell M, Berry D. Theophylline poisoning in adults. Br Med J 1979;2:1114.
224. Hendeles L, Bighley L, Richardson RM, Hepler CD, Carmichael J. Frequent toxicity from IV aminophylline infusions in critically ill patients. Drug Intell Clin Pharm 1977;11:12.
225. Camarata SJ, Weil MH, Hanashiro PK, Shubin H. Cardiac arrest in the critically ill. I. A study of predisposing causes in 132 patients. Circulation 1971;44:688.
226. Zwillich CW, Sutton FD, Neff TA, Cohn WM, Matthay RA, Weinberger MM. Theophylline induced seizures in adults: correlation with serum concentrations. Ann Intern Med 1975;82:784.
227. Culberson CG, Langston JW, Herrick M. Aminophylline encephalopathy: a clinical, electroencephalographic and neuropathological analysis. Trans Am Neurol Assoc 1979;104:224.

228. Jacobs MH, Senior RM. Theophylline toxicity due to impaired theophylline degradation. Am Rev Respir Dis 1974;110:342.
229. Horowitz LN, Spear JF, Moore EN, Rogers R. Effects of aminophylline on the threshold for initiating ventricular fibrillation during respiratory failure. Am J Cardiol 1975;35:376.
230. Ahlquist RP. A study of the adrenotropic receptors. Am J Pharm 1948;153:586.
231. Lands AM, Arnold A, McAuliff JP, Luduena FP, Brown TG Jr. Differentiation of receptor systems activated by sympathomimetic amines. Nature 1967;216:597.
232. Bourne HR, Lichtenstein LM, Melmon KL, Henney GS, Weinstein Y, Shearer GM. Modulation of inflammation and immunity by cyclic AMP. Science 1974;184:19.
233. Wanner A. Clinical aspects of mucociliary transport. Am Rev Respir Dis 1977;116:73.
234. Carlstrom S, ed. Studies on terbutaline, a new selective bronchodilating agent. Acta Med Scand (Suppl) 1970;512:7.
235. Riker JB, Cacace LG. Double-blind comparison of metaproterenol and isoetharine-phenylephrine solutions in intermittent positive pressure breathing in bronchospastic condition. Chest 1980;78:723.
236. McEvoy JDS, Vall-Spinosa A, Paterson JW. Assessment of orciprenaline and isoproterenol infusions in asthmatic patients. Am Rev Respir Dis 1973;108:490.
237. Westling H. Circulatory effects of 2 receptor agonists in man. Acta Pharmacol Toxicol (Copenh) 1979;44(Suppl II):36.
238. Jack D. An introduction to salbutamol and other modern beta-adrenoreceptor stimulants. Postgrad Med J (Suppl) 1971;47:8.
239. Paterson JW, Evans RJ, Prime FJ. Selectivity of bronchodilator action of salbutamol in asthmatic patients. Br J Dis Chest 1971;65:21.
240. Legge JS, Gaddie J, Palmer KNV. Comparison of two oral selective beta-2 adrenergic stimulant drugs in bronchial asthma. Br Med J 1971;1:637.
241. Cochrane GM, Clark TJ, Hanan ME. The role of oral bronchodilator therapy as shown by a comparison between salbutamol and terbutaline. Curr Med Res Opin 1973;1:517.
242. Gaddie J, Legge JS, Palmer RNV. Aerosols of salbutamol, terbutaline and isoprenaline/phenylephrine asthma. Br J Dis Chest 1973;67:215.
243. Bloomfield P, Carmichael J, Petrie GR, Jewell NP, Crompton GK. Comparison of salbutamol given intravenously and by intermittent positive pressure breathing in life threatening asthma. Br Med J 1979;1:848.
244. Dulfano MJ, Glass P. The bronchodilator effects of terbutaline: route of administration and patterns of response. Ann Allergy 1976;37:357.
245. Kelly HW, McWilliams BC, Katz R, Murphy S. Safety of frequent high dose nebulized terbutaline in children with acute severe asthma. Ann Allergy 1990;64:229–233.
246. Williams SJ, Parrish RW, Seaton A. Comparison of intravenous aminophylline and salbutamol in severe asthma. Br Med J 1975;4:685.
247. Rossing TH, Fanta CH, McFadden ER Jr. A controlled trial of the use of single versus combined drug therapy in the treatment of acute episodes of asthma. Am Rev Respir Dis 1981;123:190.
248. Thiringer G, Svedmyr N. Comparison of infused and inhaled terbutaline in patients with asthma. Scand J Respir Dis 1977;57:17.
249. Bachus BF, Snider GL. The bronchodilator effects of aerosolized terbutaline: a controlled, double-blind study. JAMA 1977;238:2277.
250. Choo-Kang YFJ, Simpson WT, Grant IWB. Controlled comparison of the bronchodilator effect of three β-adrenergic stimulant drugs administered by inhalation to patients with asthma. Br Med J 1969;2:287.
251. Wood DW, Downes JJ, Scheinkopf H, Lecks HI. Intravenous isoproterenol in the management of respiratory failure in childhood status asthmaticus. J Allergy Clin Immunol 1972;50:75.
252. Downes JJ, Wood DW, Harwood I, Sheinkopf HN, Raphaely RC. Intravenous isoproterenol infusion in children with severe hypercapnia due to status asthmaticus. Crit Care Med 1973;1:63.
253. Cotton EK, Parry W. Treatment of status asthmaticus and respiratory failure. Pediatr Clin North Am 1975;22:163.
254. Parry WH, Martorano F, Cotton EK. Management of life-threatening asthma with intravenous isoproterenol infusions. Am J Dis Child 1976;130:39.
255. Herman JJ, Noah ZL, Moody RR. Use of intravenous isoproterenol for status asthmaticus in children. Crit Care Med 1983;11:716.
256. Downes JJ, Heiser MS. Status asthmaticus in children. In: Gregory GA, ed. Respiratory failure in the child. New York: Churchill Livingstone, 1981:107.
257. Urthaler F, James TN. Both direct and neurally mediated components of the chronotropic actions of aminophylline. Chest 1976;70:24.
258. Winsor T, Mills B, Winbury MM, Howe BB, Berger HJ. Intramyocardial diversion of coronary blood flow: effects of isoproterenol-induced subendocardial ischemia. Microvasc Res 1975;9:261.
259. Matson JR, Loughlin GM, Strunk RC. Myocardial ischemia complicating the use of isoproterenol in asthmatic children. J Pediatr 1978; 92:776.
260. Kurland G, Williams J, Lewiston NJ. Fatal myocardial toxicity during continuous infusion intravenous isoproterenol therapy of asthma. J Allergy Clin Immunol 1979;63:407.
261. Maguire JF, Geha RS, Umetsu DT. Myocardial specific creatine phosphokinase isoenzyme elevation in children with asthma treated with intravenous isoproterenol. J Allergy Clin Immunol 1986;78:631–636.
262. Klaustermeyer WB, Di Bernardo RL, Hale FC. Intravenous isoproterenol: rationale for bronchial asthma. J Allergy Clin Immunol 1975; 55:325.
263. Colebatch HJH, Halmagyi DFJ. Effect of vagotomy and vagal stimulation on lung mechanics and circulation. J Appl Physiol 1963;18:881.
264. Olsen CR, Colebatch HJH, Mebel PE, Nadel JA, Staub NC. Motor control of pulmonary airways studied by nerve stimulation. J Appl Physiol 1965;20:202.
265. Karczewski W, Widdicombe JG. The effect of vagotomy, vagal cooling and efferent vagal stimulation on breathing and lung mechanics of rabbits. J Physiol (Lond) 1969;201:259.
266. Martinez J, de Letona J, Castro de la Mata R, Aviado DM. Local and reflex effects of bronchial arterial injection of drugs. J Pharmacol Exp Ther 1961;133:295.
267. Nadel JA, Widdicombe JG. Reflex control of airway size. Ann N Y Acad Sci 1963;108:712.
268. Goldberg ND. Cyclic GMP and cyclic AMP in biological regulation: the yin yang hypothesis. In: Stein M, ed. New directions in asthma. Park Ridge, Illinois, American College of Chest Physicians, 1975:123.
269. Klock LE, Miller TD, Morris AH, Watanabe S, Dickman M. A comparative study of atropine sulfate and isoproterenol hydrochloride in chronic bronchitis. Am Rev Respir Dis 1975;112:371.
270. Virtanen R, Kanto J, Iisalo E, Salo M, Sjovell S. Pharmacokinetic studies on atropine with special reference to age. Acta Anaesthesiol Scand 1982;26:297.
271. Kalser SC. The fate of atropine in man. Ann NY Acad Sci 1971;179:667.
272. Weiss JW, McFadden ER Jr, Ingram RH Jr. Parenteral vs inhaled atropine: density dependence of maximal expiratory flow. J Appl Physiol 1982;53:392.
273. Holtzman MJ, McNamara MP, Sheppard D, Fabbri LM, Hahn HL, Graf PD, Nadel JA. Intravenous versus inhaled atropine for inhibiting bronchoconstrictor responses in dogs. J Appl Physiol 1983;54:134.
274. De Troyer A, Yernault J-C, Rodenstein D. Effects of vagal blockade on lung mechanics in normal man. J Appl Physiol 1979;46:217.
275. Hensley MJ, O'Cain CF, McFadden ER Jr, Ingram RH Jr. Distribution of bronchodilatation in normal subjects: beta agonist versus atropine. J Appl Physiol 1978;45:778.
276. Woolcock AJ, Macklem PT, Hogg JC, Wilson NJ. Influence of autonomic nervous system on airway resistance and elastic recoil. J Appl Physiol 1969;26:814.
277. Cavanaugh MJ, Cooper DM. Inhaled atropine sulfate: dose response characteristics. Am Rev Respir Dis 1976;114:517.
278. Altounyan RE. Variation of drug action on airway obstruction in man. Thorax 1964;19:406.
279. Dautrebande L, Lovejoy FW Jr, McCredie RM. New studies on aerosols. XVIII. Effects of atropine micro-aerosols on the airway resistance in man. Arch Int Pharmacodyn Ther 1962;139:198.
280. Cropp GJA. The role of the parasympathetic nervous system in the maintenance of chronic airway obstruction in asthmatic children. Am Rev Respir Dis 1975;112:599.
281. Larsen GL, Barron RJ, Cotton EK, Brooks JG. A comparative study of inhaled atropine sulfate and isoproterenol hydrochloride in cystic fibrosis. Am Rev Respir Dis 1979;119:399.
282. Pierce RJ, Allen CJ, Campbell AH. A comparative study of atropine methonitrate, salbutamol and their combination in airway obstruction. Thorax 1979;34:45.
283. Firstater E, Mizrachi E, Topilky M. The effect of vagolytic drugs on airway obstruction in patients with bronchial asthma. Ann Allergy 1981;46:332.
284. Crompton GK. A comparison of responses to bronchodilator drugs in chronic bronchitis and chronic asthma. Thorax 1968;23:46.
285. Chick TW, Janne JW. Comparative bronchodilator response to atropine and terbutaline in asthma and chronic bronchitis. Chest 1977; 72:719.

286. Bruderman I, Cohen-Aronovski R, Smorzik J. A comparative study of various combinations of ipratropium bromide and metaproterenol in allergic asthmatic patients. Chest 1983;83:208.
287. Elwood RK, Abboud RJ. The short-term bronchodilator effects of fenoterol and ipratropium in asthma. J Allergy Clin Immunol 1982;69:467.
288. Ruffin RE, McIntyre E, Crockett AJ, Zeilonka K, Alpers JH. Combination bronchodilator therapy in asthma. J Allergy Clin Immunol 1982;69:60.
289. Lefcoe NM, Toogood JH, Blennerhassett G, Baskerville J, Patterson NAM. The addition of an aerosol anticholinergic to an oral beta agonist plus theophylline in asthma and bronchitis. Chest 1982;82:300.
290. Petrie GR, Palmer KNV. Comparison of aerosol ipratropium bromide and salbutamol in chronic bronchitis and asthma. Br Med J 1975;1:430.
291. Herzog H. Comparison of anticholinergic agents other than bronchodilators and the effect of combining these drugs. Postgrad Med J (Suppl) 1975;51:146.
292. Deal EC Jr, McFadden ER Jr, Ingram RH Jr, Haeger JJ. Effects of atropine on potentiation of exercise-induced bronchospasm by cold air. J Appl Physiol 1978;45:238.
293. Tinkleman DG, Cavanaugh MJ, Cooper DM. Inhibition of exercise-induced bronchospasm by atropine. Am Rev Respir Dis 1976;114:87.
294. Blanshard G. Sputum viscosity and postoperative pulmonary atelectasis. Dis Chest 1960;37:75.
295. Lopez-Vidriero MT, Costello J, Clark TJH, Das I, Keal EE, Reid L. Effect of atropine on sputum production. Thorax 1975;30:543.
296. Costello JF, Lopez-Vidriero MT, Charman J, Das I, Keal EE, Reid L. The effect of atropine sulfate on sputum production [Abstract]. Postgrad Med J 1975;51(Suppl 7):107.
297. King M, Cohen C, Viires N. Influence of vagal tone on rheology and transportability of canine tracheal mucus. Am Rev Respir Dis 1979;120:1215.
298. Kradjan WA, Lakshminarayan S, Hayden PW, Larson SW, Marini JJ. Serum atropine concentrations after inhalation of atropine sulfate [Note]. Am Rev Respir Dis 1981;123:471.
299. Green AW, Stoklosa J, Middleton Jr E. Inhaled atropine sulfate in status asthmaticus. J Allergy Clin Immunol 1978;61:149.
300. Rebuck AS, Chapman KR, Braude AC. Anticholinergic therapy of asthma. Chest (Suppl) 1982;82:55S.
301. George RB, Payne DK. Anticholinergics, cromolyn and other occasionally useful drugs. Clin Chest Med 1984;5:685.
302. Marini JJ, Lakshminarayan S. The effect of atropine inhalation in "irreversible" chronic bronchitis. Chest 1980;77:591.
303. Marini JJ, Lakshminarayan S, Kradjan WA. Atropine and terbutaline aerosols in chronic bronchitis. Efficacy and sites of action. Chest 1981;80:285.
304. Englehardt A, Klupp H. The pharmacology and toxicology of a new tropane alkaloid derivative. Postgrad Med J 1975;51(Suppl 7):82.
305. Baigelman W, Chodosh S. Bronchodilator action of the cholinergic drug, ipratropium bromide (Sch 1000), as an aerosol in chronic bronchitis and asthma. Chest 1977;71:324.
306. Poppius H, Salorinne Y. Comparative trial of a new anticholinergic bronchodilator, Sch 1000, and salbutamol in chronic bronchitis. Br Med J 1973;4:134.
307. Poppius H, Salorinne Y, Viljanen AA. Inhalation of a new anticholinergic drug, Sch 1000, in asthma and chronic bronchitis: effect on airway resistance, thoracic gas volume, blood gases and exercise-induced asthma. Bull Physiopathol Respir 1972;8:643.
308. Storms WW, DoPico GA, Reed CE. Aerosol Sch 1000: an anticholinergic bronchodilator. Am Rev Respir Dis 1975;111:419.
309. Ullah MI, Newman GB, Saunders KB. Influence of age on response to ipratropium and salbutamol in asthma. Thorax 1981;36:523.
310. Ruffin RE, Fitzgerald JD, Rebuck AS. A comparison of the bronchodilator activity of Sch 1000 and salbutamol. J Allergy Clin Immunol 1977;59:136.
311. Thiessen B, Pederson OF. A double blind cross-over study of maximal expiratory flows and arterial blood gas tensions in normals, asthmatics and bronchitics after salbutamol and ipratropium. Scand J Respir Dis (Suppl) 1979;103:170.
312. Lin MT, Lee-Hong E, Collins-William C. A clinical trial of the bronchodilator effect of Sch 1000 aerosol in asthmatic children. Ann Allergy 1978;40:326.
313. Lightbody IM, Ingram CG, Legge JS, Johnston RW. Ipratropium bromide, salbutamol and prednisolone in bronchial asthma and chronic bronchitis. Br J Dis Chest 1978;72:181.
314. Jolobe OMP, Lane DJ. Atropine responsiveness in asthma in relation to steroid aerosol therapy. Br J Dis Chest 1981;75:413.
315. Pavia D, Bateman JRM, Sheahan NF, Clarke SW. Effect of ipratropium bromide on mucociliary clearance and pulmonary function in reversible airway obstruction. Thorax 1979;34:501.
316. Watson WTA, Shuckett EP, Becker AB, Simons FER. Effect of Nebulized ipratropium bromide on intraocular pressures in children. Chest 1994;105:1439–1441.
317. Brown, RH, Groeben H. Ipratropium causes paradoxical bronchoconstriction by preferential M_2 muscarinic blockade. AJRCCM 1995; 151:A222.
318. Orange RP. Immunopharmacological aspects of bronchial asthma. Clin Allergy (Suppl) 1973;3:521.
319. Piper PJ, Samhoun MN, Tippins JR. Pharmacological studies on pure SRS-A and synthetic leukotrienes C_4 and D_4. In: Piper PJ: ed. SRS-A and leukotrienes. Chichester, England: John Wiley & Sons, 1980:19.
320. Koopman WJ, Orange RP, Austen KF. Immunochemical and biologic properties of rat IgE. III. Modulation of the IgE-mediated release of slow reacting substance of anaphylaxis by agents influencing the level of cyclic 3′, 5′ adenosine monophosphate. J Immunol 1970;105:1096.
321. Lichtenstein LM, Margolis S. Histamine release in vitro: inhibition by catecholamines and methylxanthines. Science 1968;161:902.
322. Liu AY, Greengard P. Regulation by steroid hormones of phosphorylation of specific protein common to several target organs. Proc Natl Acad Sci U S A 1976;73:568.
323. Liu AY, Walter U, Greengard P. Steroid hormones may regulate autophosphorylation of adenosine-3′, 5′ monophosphate dependent protein kinase in target tissues. Eur J Biochem 1981;114:539.
324. Ignarro LJ, Cech SY. Lysosomal enzyme secretion from human neutrophils mediated by cyclic GMP: inhibition of cyclic GMP accumulation and neutrophil function by glucocorticosteroids. J Cycl Nucleotide Res 1975;1:283.
325. Spector SL. The use of corticosteroids in the treatment of asthma. Chest (Suppl) 1985;87:73S.
326. Blackwell GJ, Carnuccio R, DiRosa M, Flower RJ, Parenta L. Persico P. Macrocortin: a polypeptide causing the anti-phospholipase effect of glucocorticoids. Nature 1980; 287:147.
327. Hirata F, Schiffmann E, Venkatasubramanian K, Salomon D, Axelrod J. A phospholipase A_2 inhibitory protein in rabbit neutrophils induced by glucocorticoids. Proc Natl Acad Sci U S A 1980;77:2533.
328. Flower RJ, Blackwell GJ. Anti-inflammatory steroids induce biosynthesis of a phospholipase A_2 inhibitor which prevents prostaglandin generation. Nature 1979; 278:456.
329. Hong SL, Levine L. Inhibition of arachidonic acid release from cells as the biochemical action of anti-inflammatory corticosteroids. Proc Natl Acad Sci U S A 1976;73:1730.
330. Lewis GP, Piper PJ. Inhibition of release of prostaglandins as an explanation of some of the actions of anti-inflammatory corticosteroids. Nature 1975;254:308.
331. Davies AO, Lefkowitz RJ. Corticosteroid-induced differential regulation of beta-adrenergic receptors in circulating human polymorphonuclear leukocytes and mononuclear leukocytes. J Clin Endocrinol Metab 1980;51:599.
332. Fraser CM, Venter JC. The synthesis of beta-adrenergic receptors in cultured human lung cells: induction by glucocorticoids. Biochem Biophys Res Commun 1980; 94:390.
333. Logsdon PJ, Middleton E Jr, Coffey RG. Stimulation of leukocyte adenyl cyclase by hydrocortisone and isoproterenol in asthmatic and nonasthmatic subjects. J Allergy Clin Immunol 1972;50:45.
334. Parker CW, Huber MG, Baumann ML. Alterations in cyclic AMP metabolism in human bronchial asthma. III. Leukocyte and lymphocyte responses to steroids. J Clin Invest 1973;52:1342.
335. Manganiello V, Vaughan M. An effect of dexamethasone on adenosine 3′, 5′-monophosphate content and adenosine 3′, 5′-monophosphate phosphodiesterase activity of cultured hepatoma cells. J Clin Invest 1972;51:2763.
336. Fanta CH, Rossing TH, McFadden EF Jr. Glucocorticoids in acute asthma: a critical controlled trial. Am J Med 1983;74:845.
337. Pierson WE, Bierman CW, Kelley VC. A double-blind trial of corticosteroid therapy in status asthmaticus. Pediatrics 1974;54:282.
338. Shenfield GM, Hodson ME, Clark SW, Paterson JW. Interaction of corticosteroids and catecholamines in the treatment of asthma. Thorax 1975;30:430.
339. Collins JV, Clark TJ, Harris PW, Townsend J. Intravenous corticosteroids in the treatment of acute bronchial asthma. Lancet 1970; 2:1047.
340. Dwyer J, Lazarus L, Hickie JB. A study of cortisol metabolism in patients with chronic asthma. Aust Ann Med 1967;16:297.

341. Tal A, Levy N, Bearman JE. Methylprednisolone therapy for acute asthma in infants and toddlers: a controlled clinical trial. Pediatrics 1990;86(3):350–355.
342. Bergstrand H. Phosphodiesterase inhibition and theophylline. Eur J Respir Dis 1980;61(Suppl 109):37.
343. Walker SR. Recent advances in drug therapy. In: Kuzemko JA, ed. Asthma in children. Baltimore: University Park Press, 1976:78.
344. Sheppard H. Phosphodiesterase inhibitors and analogs of cyclic AMP as potential agents for the treatment of asthma. In: Austin KF, Lichtenstein LM, eds. Asthma, physiology, immunopharmacology, and treatment. New York: Academic Press, 1973:235.
345. Horrobin DF, Manku MS, Franks DJ, Hamet P. Methylxanthine phosphodiesterase inhibitors behave as prostaglandin antagonists in a perfused rat mesenteric artery preparation. Prostaglandins 1977;13:33.
346. Miech RP, Niedzwicki JG, Smith TR. Effect of theophylline on the binding of cAMP to soluble protein from tracheal smooth muscle. Biochem Pharmacol 1979;28:3687.
347. Fredholm BB. Theophylline actions on adenosine receptors. Eur J Respir Dis (Suppl) 1980;109:29.
348. Fenger M, Erikson PB, Andersen O, Nielsen MK, Knudsen PJ. Plasma concentrations of the cyclic nucleotides, adenosine 3',5'-monophosphate and guanosine 3',5'-monophosphate in healthy adults treated with theophylline. Pharmacology 1982;24:215.
349. Higbie MD, Kumar M, Galant SP. Stimulation of endogenous catecholamine release by theophylline. A proposed additional mechanism of action for theophylline effects. J Allergy Clin Immunol 1982;70:377.
350. Mackay AD, Baldwin CJ, Tattersfield AE. Action of intravenously administered aminophylline on normal airways. Am Rev Respir Dis 1983;127:609.
351. Aubier M, DeTroyer A, Sampson M, Macklem PT, Roussos C. Aminophylline improves diaphragmatic contractility. N Engl J Med 1981;305:249.
352. Aubier M. Murciano D, Viires N, Lecocguic V, Palacios S, Pariente R. Increased ventilation caused by improved diaphragmatic efficiency during aminophylline infusion. Am Rev Respir Dis 1983;127:148.
353. Viires N, Aubier M, Murciano D, Fleury B, Talamo C, Pariente R. Effects of aminophylline on diaphragmatic fatigue during acute respiratory failure. Am Rev Respir Dis 1984;129:396.
354. Truitt EB Jr, McKusick VA, Krantz JC. Theophylline blood levels after oral, rectal and intravenous administration and correlation with diuretic action. J Pharmacol Exp Ther 1950;100:309.
355. Andersson KE, Persson CG. Extrapulmonary effects of theophylline. Eur J Respir Dis 1980;61(Suppl 109):17.
356. Weschsler RL, Kleiss LM, Kety SS. The effects of intravenously administered aminophylline on cerebral circulation and metabolism in man. J Clin Invest 1950;29:28.
357. Ogilvie RI, Fernandez PG, Winsberg F. Cardiovascular response to increasing theophylline concentrations. Eur J Clin Pharmacol 1977;12:409.
358. Matthay RA, Berger HJ, Loke J, Gottschalk A, Zaret BL. Effects of aminophylline upon right and left ventricular performance in chronic obstructive pulmonary disease: noninvasive assessment by radionuclide angiocardiography. Am J Med 1978;65:903.
359. Rooklin A. Priority on pediatric asthma. J Pediatr 1989;115:841-846.
360. Szefler SJ, Bender BG, Jusko WJ, Lanier BQ, Lemanski Jr, RF, Skoner DP, Stempel DA. Evolving role of theophylline for treatment of chronic childhood asthma. J Pediatr 1995;127:176-185.
361. Lesko LJ, Tabor KJ, Johnson BF. Theophylline serum protein binding in obstructive airway disease. Clin Pharmacol Ther 1981;29:776.
362. Yurchak AM, Jusko WJ. Theophylline secretion into breast milk. Pediatrics 1976;57:518.
363. Arwood LL, Dasta JF, Friedman C. Placental transfer of theophylline: two case reports. Pediatrics 1979;63:844.
364. Somani SM, Khanna NN, Bada HS. Caffeine and theophylline: serum/CSF correlation in premature infants. J Pediatr 1980;96:1091.
365. Koysooko R, Ellis EF, Levy G. Relationship between theophylline concentration in plasma and saliva of man. Clin Pharmacol Ther 1974;15:454.
366. Levy G, Ellis EF, Koysooko R. Indirect plasma-theophylline monitoring in asthmatic children by determination of theophylline concentration in saliva. Pediatrics 1974;53:87.
367. Ginchansky E, Weinberger M. Relationship of theophylline clearance to oral dosage in children with chronic asthma. J Pediatr 1977;91:655.
368. Aranda JV, Sitar DS, Parsons WD, Loughman PM, Neims AH. Pharmacokinetic aspects of theophylline in premature newborns. N Engl J Med 1976;295:413.
369. Mitenko PA, Ogilvie RI. Rational intravenous doses of theophylline. N Engl J Med 1973;289:600.
370. Levy G, Koysooko R. Pharmacokinetic analysis of the effect of theophylline on pulmonary function in asthmatic children. J Pediatr 1975;86:789.
371. Jackson RH, McHenry JI, Moreland FB, Raymer WJ, Etter RL. Clinical evaluation of elixophyllin with correlation of pulmonary function studies and theophylline serum levels in acute and chronic asthmatic patients. Dis Chest 1964;45:75.
372. Jenne JW, Wyze E, Rood FS, McDonald FM. Pharmacokinetics of theophylline: application to adjustment of the clinical dose of aminophylline. Clin Pharmacol Ther 1972;13:349.
373. Nicholson DP, Chick TW. A re-evaluation of parenteral aminophylline. Am Rev Respir Dis 1973;108:241.
374. Piafsky KM, Ogilvie RI. Dosage of theophylline in bronchial asthma. N Engl J Med 1975;292:1218.
375. Weinberger M, Hendeles L, Ahrens R. Clinical pharmacology of drugs used for asthma. Pediatr Clin North Am 1981;28:47.
376. Richards W, Patrick JR. Death from asthma in children. Am J Dis Child 1965;110:4.
377. Bullen SS. Correlation of clinical and autopsy findings in 176 cases of asthma. J Allergy 1952;23:193.
378. Sheehy AF, Di Benedetto R, LeFrak S, Lyons HA. Treatment of status asthmaticus. A report of 70 episodes. Arch Intern Med 1972;130:37.
379. Richards W, Siegel SC, Strauss J, Leigh MD. Status asthmaticus in children. JAMA 1967;201:75.
380. Bocles JS. Status asthmaticus. Med Clin North Am 1970;54:493.
381. Pierson WE, Bierman CW, Stamm SJ, Van Arsdel PP Jr. Double-blind trial of aminophylline in status asthmaticus. Pediatrics 1971; 48:642.
382. McIntosh K, Ellis EF, Hoffman LS, Lybass TG, Eller JJ, Fulginiti VA. The association of viral and bacterial respiratory infections with exacerbations of wheezing in young asthmatic children. J Pediatr 1973;82:578.
383. Minor TE, Baker JW, Dick EC, DeMeo AN, Ouellette JJ, Cohen M, Reed CE. Greater frequency of viral respiratory infections in asthmatic children as compared with their nonasthmatic siblings. J Pediatr 1974;84:472.
384. Shapiro GG, Eggleston PA, Pierson WE, Ray CG, Bierman CW. Double-blind study of the effectiveness of a broad spectrum antibiotic in status asthmaticus. Pediatrics 1974;53:867.
385. Berman SZ, Mathison DA, Stevenson DD, Tan EM, Vaughan JH. Transtracheal aspiration studies in asthmatic patients in relapse with "infective" asthma and in subjects without respiratory disease. J Allergy Clin Immunol 1975;56:206.
386. Graham VAL, Milton AF, Knowles GK, Davies RJ. Routine antibiotics in hospital management of acute asthma. Lancet 1982;20:418.
387. DeBlic J, Scheinmann P, Dhont P, Pfister A, Paupe J, Dalage C. Deciding on need for antibiotics in children with acute asthma. Lancet 1982;13:629.
388. Faling LJ. The role of antibiotics in status asthmaticus. In: Weiss EB, ed. Status asthmaticus. Baltimore: University Park Press, 1978:255.
389. Baker JW, Yerger S, Segar WE. Elevated plasma anti-diuretic hormone levels in status asthmaticus. Mayo Clin Proc 1976;51:31.
390. Downes JJ, Wood DW, Striker TW, Lecks HI. Diagnosis and treatment: advances in the management of status asthmaticus in children. Pediatrics 1966;38:286.
391. Blumenthal JS, Brown EB, Campbell GS. Molar sodium lactate in acute epinephrine-fast asthmatic patients. Ann Allergy 1956;14:506.
392. Mithoefer JC, Runser RH, Karetzky MS. The use of sodium bicarbonate in the treatment of acute bronchial asthma. N Engl J Med 1965;272:1200.
393. Ostrea EM, Odell GB. The influence of bicarbonate administration on blood pH in a "closed system": clinical implications. J Pediatr 1972;80:671.
394. Misuraca L. Mechanical ventilation in status asthmaticus. N Engl J Med 1966;275:318.
395. Braman SS, Kaemmerlen JT. Intensive care of status asthmaticus. JAMA 1990;264:366–368.
396. Stempel DA, Mellon M. Management of acute severe asthma. Pediatr Clin North Am 1984;31:879.
397. Bierman CW, Pierson WE, Shapiro GG. Treatment of status asthmaticus in children. South Med J 1975;68:1556.
398. Wood DW, Downes JJ, Lecks HI. The management of respiratory failure in childhood status asthmaticus. Experience with 30 episodes and evolution of a technique. J Allergy 1968;42:261.

399. Schulaner FA, Mattikoiw MS. Treatment of status asthmaticus: bronchial asthma. Part III. J Med Soc N J 1980;77:501.
400. Petty TL. Oxygen and mechanical ventilation in status asthmaticus. In: Weiss EB, ed. Status asthmaticus. Baltimore: University Park Press, 1978:285.
401. Dales RE, Munt PW. Use of mechanical ventilation in adults with severe asthma. Can Med Assoc J 1984;130:391.
402. Weiss EB, Anderson WJ, O'Brien KP. The effect of a local anesthetic, lidocaine, on guinea pig trachealis muscle in vitro. Am Rev Respir Dis 1975;112:393.
403. Weiss EB, Hargraves WA, Viswanath SG. The inhibitory action of lidocaine in anaphylaxis. Am Rev Respir Dis 1978;117:859.
404. Hickling KG, Walsh J, Henderson S, Jackson R. Low mortality rate in adult respiratory distress syndrome using low-volume, pressure-limited ventilation with permissive hypercapnia: A prospective study. Crit Care Med 1994;22:1568–1578.
405. Simons FER, Pierson WE, Bierman CW. Respiratory failure in childhood status asthmaticus. Am J Dis Child 1977;131:1097.
406. Levin N, Dillon JB. Status asthmaticus and pancuronium bromide. JAMA 1972;222:1265.
407. Salem MR, Kim Y, El Etr AA. Histamine release following intravenous injection of *d*-tubocurarine. Anesthesiology 1968;29:380.
408. Qvist J, Anderson JB, Pemberton M, Bennike KA. High-level PEEP in severe asthma. N Engl J Med 1982;307:1347.
409. Tuxen DV. Detrimental effects of positive end-expiratory pressure during controlled mechanical ventilation of patients with severe airflow obstruction. Am Rev Respir Dis 1989;140:5–9.
410. Martin JG, Shore S, Engel LA. Effect of continuous positive airway pressure on respiratory mechanics and pattern of breathing in induced asthma. Am Rev Respir Dis 1982;126:812.
411. Tenaillon A, Salmona J-P, Burdin M. Continuous positive airway pressure in asthma [Letter]. Am Rev Respir Dis 1983;127:658.
412. Hatch DJ. Prolonged nasotracheal intubation in infants and children. Lancet 1968;1:1272.
413. Stiker T, Stool S, Downes JJ. Prolonged nasotracheal intubation in infants and children. Arch Otolaryngol 1967;85:210.
414. Picado C, Montserrat JM, Roca J, Rodriquez-Roisin R, Estopa R, Xaubet A, Marin A, Agusti-Vidal A. Mechanical ventilation in severe exacerbation of asthma. Study of 26 cases with six deaths. Eur J Respir Dis 1983;64:102.
415. James OF, Mills RM. Allen KM. Severe bronchial asthma: factors influencing intensive care management and outcome. Anaesth Intensive Care 1977;5:11.
416. Petty TL. Status asthmaticus in adults. In: Middleton E Jr, Reed CE, Ellis EF, eds. Allergy: principles and practice. St Louis: CV Mosby, 1983:987.
417. Shnider SM, Papper EM. Anesthesia for the asthmatic patient. Anesthesiology 1961;22:886.
418. Gold MI, Helrich M. Pulmonary mechanics during general anesthesia. V. Status asthmaticus. Anesthesiology 1970;32:422.
419. O'Rourke PP, Crone RK. Halothane in status asthmaticus. Crit Care Med 1982;10:341.
420. Schwartz SH. Treatment of status asthmaticus with halothane. JAMA 1984;251:2688.
421. Brown RH, Mitzner W, Zerhouni E, Hirshman CA. Direct in vivo visualization of bronchodilation induced by inhalational anesthesia using high resolution computed tomography. Anesthesiology 1993;78:295-300.
422. Fletcher SW, Flacke W, Alper MH. The actions of general anesthetic agents on tracheal smooth muscle. Anesthesiology 1968;29:517.
423. Hirshman CA, Bergman NA. Halothane and enflurane protect against bronchospasm in an asthma dog model. Anesth Analg 1978;57:629.
424. Hickey RF, Graf PD, Nadel JA, Larson Jr CP. The effects of halothane and cyclopropane on total pulmonary resistance in the dog. Anesthesiology 1969;31:334.
425. Klide AM, Aviado CM. Mechanism for the reduction in pulmonary resistance induced by halothane. J Pharmacol Exp Ther 1967;158:28.
426. Merin RG, Kumazawa T, Luka NL. Myocardial function and metabolism in the conscious dog and during halothane anesthesia. Anesthesiology 1976;44:402.
427. Zink J, Sasyniuk BI, Dresel PE. Halothane-epinephrine-induced cardiac arrhythmias and the role of heart rate. Anesthesiology 1975;43:548.
428. Stone JG, Sullivan SF. Halothane anesthesia and pulmonary shunting. Anesthesiology 1972;37:582.
429. Manawadu BR, LaForce FM. Impairment of pulmonary antibacterial defense mechanisms by halothane anesthesia. Chest 1979;75(Suppl 2):242.
430. Brown RH, Zerhouni EA, Hirshman CA. Comparison of low concentration of halothane and isoflurane as bronchodilators. Anesthesiology 1993;78:1097–1101.
431. Mitsuhata H, Saitoh J, Shimizu R, Takeuchi H, Hasome N, Horiguchi Y. Sevoflurane and isoflurane protect against bronchospasm in dogs. Anesthesiology 1994;81:1230–1234.
432. Strube PJ, Hallam PL. Ketamine by continuous infusion in status asthmaticus. Anaesthesia 1986;41:1017–1019.
433. Brown RH, Robbins W, Staats P, Hirshman C. Prevention of bronchoconstriction by an orally active local anesthetic.
434. Gluck EH, Onorato DG, Castriotta R. Helium-oxygen mixtures in intubated patients with status asthmaticus and respiratory acidosis. Chest 1990;98:693–698.
435. Noppen M, Vanmaele L, Impens N, Schandevyl W. Bronchodilating effect of intravenous magnesium sulfate in acute severe bronchial asthma. Chest 1990;97:373–376.
436. Middleton E Jr. Antiasthmatic drug therapy and calcium ions: review of pathogenesis and role of calcium. J Pharm Sci 1980;69:243.
437. Ellrodt G, Chew CYC, Singh BN. Therapeutic implications of slow-channel blockade in cardiocirculatory disorders. Circulation 1980; 62:669.
438. Ringqvist T. Effect of verapamil in obstructive airway disease. Eur J Pharmacol 1974;7:61.
439. Cerrina J, Denjean A, Alexandre G, Lockhart A, Duroux P. Inhibition of exercise-induced asthma by a calcium antagonist, nifedipine. Am Rev Respir Dis 1981;123:156.
440. Henderson AF, Heaton RW, Dunlop LS, Costello JF. Effects of nifedipine on antigen-induced bronchoconstriction. Am Rev Respir Dis 1983;127:549.
441. Drazen JM, Fanta CH, Lacouture PG. Effect of nifedipine on constriction of human tracheal strips in vitro. Br J Pharmacol 1983;78:687.
442. So SY, Lam WK, Yu DYC. Effect of calcium antagonists on allergen-induced asthma. Clin Allergy 1982;12:595.
443. Patel KR, Alshama MR, Kerr JW. The effect of inhaled verapamil on allergen-induced bronchoconstriction. Clin Allergy 1983;13:119.
444. Fanta CH, Venugopalan CD, Lacouture PG, Drazen JM. Inhibition of bronchoconstriction in the guinea pig by a calcium channel blocker, nifedipine. Am Rev Respir Dis 1982;125:61.
445. Weiss EB, Markowicz J, Barbero L. Effect of calcium antagonists in experimental asthma. Allergy 1982;37:513.
446. Brugman TM, Darnell ML, Hirshman CA. Nifedipine aerosol attenuates airway constriction in dogs with hyperreactive airways. Am Rev Respir Dis 1983;127:14.
447. Corris PA, Nariman S, Gibson GJ. Nifedipine in the prevention of asthma induced by exercise and histamine. Am Rev Respir Dis 1983;128:991.
448. Miadonna A, Tedeschi A, Leggieri E, Cottini M, Restuccia M, Bianchini C. Effect of verapamil on allergen-induced asthma in patients with respiratory allergy. Ann Allergy 1983;51:201.
449. Russi EW, Ahmed T. Calcium and calcium antagonists in airway disease. A review. Chest 1984;86:475.
450. Williams DO, Barnes PJ, Vickers HP, Rudolf M. Effect of nifedipine on bronchomotor tone and histamine reactivity in asthma. Br Med J 1981;283:348.
451. Hills EA. Improveratril and bronchial asthma. Br J Clin Pract 1970;24:116.
452. Patakas D, Vlachoianni E, Tsara V, Louridas G, Argiropoulou P. Nifedipine in bronchial asthma. J Allergy Clin Immunol 1983;72:269.
453. Weissman G. The eicosanoids of asthma. N Engl J Med 1983; 308:454.
454. Kaliner M. Mast cell mediators in asthma. Chest 1985;87(Suppl 1):2S.
455. Lewis RA. Leukotrienes and other lipid mediators of asthma. Chest 1985;87(Suppl 1):5S.
456. Spannhake EW, Leman RJ, Wegmann MJ, Hyman AL, Kadowitz PJ. Effects of arachidonic acid and prostaglandins on lung function in the intact dog. J Appl Physiol 1978;44:397.
457. Sweatman WJ, Collier HO. Effects of prostaglandins on human bronchial muscle. Nature 1968;217:69.
458. Stenson WF, Snider DE, Parker CW. Prostaglandins and other arachidonic metabolites. In: Middleton E Jr, Reed CE, Ellis EF, eds. Allergy: principles and practice. St Louis: CV Mosby, 1983:653.
459. Arm JP, O'Hickey SP, Hawksworth RJ, Fong CY, Crea AEG, Spur BW, Lee TH. Asthmatic airways have a disproportionate hyperresponsiveness to LTE_4, as compared with normal airways, but not to LTC_4, LTD_4,

methacholine, and histamine. Am Rev Respir Dis 1990; 142: 1112–1118.
460. Drazen JM, Austen KF, Lewis RA, Clark DA, Goto G, Marfat A, Corey EJ. Comparative airway and vascular activities of leukotrienes C-1 and D in vivo and in vitro. Proc Natl Acad Sci U S A 1980; 77:4354.
461. Drazen JM, Venugopalan CS, Austen KF, Brion F, Corey EJ. Effects of leukotriene E on pulmonary mechanics in the guinea pig. Am Rev Respir Dis 1982;125:290.
462. Weiss JW, Drazen JM, Coles N, McFadden ER Jr, Weller PF, Corey EJ, et al. Bronchoconstrictor effects of leukotriene C in humans. Science 1982;216:196.
463. Weiss JW, Drazen JM, McFadden ER Jr, Weller PF, Corey EJ, Lewis RA, Austen F. Airway constriction in normal humans produced by inhalation of leukotriene D: potency, time course, and effect of aspirin therapy. JAMA 1983;249:2814.
464. Rosenthal ME, Dervinis A, Kassarich J. Bronchodilator activity of the prostaglandins E_1 and E_2. J Pharmacol Exp Ther 1971;178:541.
465. Rosenthal ME, Dervinis A, Strike D. Actions of prostaglandins on the respiratory tract of animals. Adv Prostaglandin Thromboxane Res 1976;1:477.
466. Cuthbert MF. Effect on airways resistance of prostaglandin E_1 given by aerosol to healthy and asthmatic volunteers. Br Med J 1969;4:723.
467. Mathe AA, Hedqvist P. Effects of prostaglandins F_2 and E_2 on airway conductance in healthy subjects and asthmatic patients. Am Rev Respir Dis 1975;111:313.
468. Razin E, Romeo LC, Krilis S, Liu FT, Lewis RA, Corey EJ, Austen F. An analysis of the relationship between 5-lipoxygenase product generation and the secretion of preformed mediators from mouse bone marrow-derived mast cells. J Immunol 1984;133:938.
469. Krilis S, Lewis RA, Corey EJ, Austen KF. Specific receptors for leukotriene C_4 on a smooth muscle cell line. J Clin Invest 1983;72:1516.
470. Manning PJ, Watson RM, Margolskee DJ, Williams VC, Schwartz JI, O'Byrne PM. Inhibition of exercise-induced bronchoconstriction by MK-571, a potent leukotriene D_4-receptor antagonist. N Engl J Med 1990;323:1736–1739.
471. Israel E, Dermakarian R, Rosenberg M, Sperling R, Taylor G, Rubin P, Drazen JM. The effects of a 5-lipoxygease inhibitor as asthma induced by cold, dry air. N Engl J Med 1990;323:1740–1744.
472. Hogman M, Frostell CG, Hedenstrom H, Hedenstierna G. Inhalation of nitric oxide modulates adult human bronchial tone. Am Rev Respir Dis 1993;148:1474–1478.

Chronic Lung Disease in Infants and Children 6

James D. Mellema
Lynn D. Martin

INTRODUCTION

Chronic respiratory insufficiency in the infant emerged in the 1980s as a major problem for all health care workers involved in the care of critically ill children. Because of the more aggressive and successful management of neonates with acute respiratory failure, many more infants have survived today than otherwise would have survived without aggressive neonatal respiratory support. Unfortunately, along with improved survival came the sequelae of their modern therapy: chronic respiratory insufficiency. The clinical spectrum of the chronic lung disease (CLD) may range from mild, asymptomatic disease to crippling cardiopulmonary dysfunction with significant morbidity and mortality. CLD of infancy as a result of neonatal lung disease is commonly called bronchopulmonary dysplasia (BPD).

Although BPD accounts for the majority of cases of chronic respiratory insufficiency in childhood, a heterogeneous set of rare diseases can also produce respiratory compromise that requires admission to the pediatric intensive care unit (PICU). These unusual ailments can be broadly grouped into genetic (cystic fibrosis, dyskinetic cilia syndrome) or acquired (pulmonary hemosiderosis, interstitial lung disease, bronchiectasis) categories. These disorders continue to carry a high morbidity and mortality rate and may result in frequent PICU visits.

Infants and children with chronic pulmonary dysfunction may require admission to the PICU for many reasons, including long-term ventilatory management, acute decompensation of their chronic pulmonary insufficiency, or postoperative management. With an ever-growing number of infants with residual pulmonary dysfunction and disease, it is likely that pediatric critical care physicians will continue to encounter this complex population of patients for years to come. This review encompasses a discussion of the epidemiology of CLD of infancy, the chronic multisystem pathophysiology of chronic pulmonary dysfunction in infants, and the therapeutic approaches to management of these infants in the PICU. Finally, a brief discussion of a few of the more common causes of chronic respiratory insufficiency in childhood that require admission to the PICU is presented.

CLD IN INFANTS

The syndrome of BPD has evolved since the initial description by Northway et al. in 1967[1]. In today's literature, the diagnosis of BPD implies significant respiratory and medical problems, frequent hospitalizations, and continuing psychosocial and financial drain on the family. Although most cases follow respiratory distress syndrome (RDS) in premature infants, identical respiratory dysfunction may occur in term babies or infants requiring mechanical ventilation for a variety of conditions, including meconium aspiration[2], persistent pulmonary hypertension[3], pulmonary hypoplasia[4], and major anomalies (i.e., congenital diaphragmatic hernia, tracheoesophageal fistula)[5]. In addition, chronic aspiration[6] and congenital or neonatal infections[7] may also result in chronic pulmonary dysfunction in a neonate.

EPIDEMIOLOGY

Diagnostic criteria for CLD of the newborn are not well established. Historically, Wilson-Mikity syndrome[8] and BPD have been clearly delineated. The former has been exclusively limited to CLD of prematurity prior to neonatal intensive care and mechanical ventilation, while the latter has been associated with neonates receiving mechanical ventilation. Another term not widely adopted, chronic pulmonary insufficiency of prematurity[9], probably represents the less severe end of the spectrum of Wilson-Mikity syndrome. These distinctions may be arbitrary; all of these syndromes may represent unique clinical presentations of the same disease.

Wilson-Mikity syndrome is characterized by the insidious onset of tachypnea and progressive dyspnea in premature infants without RDS. Radiographic and pathologic findings are very similar to those reported for BPD. The findings include foci of atelectasis and hyperinflation, with emphysematous cysts and pulmonary fibrosis in the later stages. The disease is usually self-limited, reaching clinical and radiologic peaks weeks to months after birth. This is followed by a gradual resolution. The pathogenesis of Wilson-Mikity syndrome remains unclear. A recent prospective study demonstrated a clear association between chorioamnionitis and elevated serum immunoglobulin M (IgM) levels with the subsequent development of the disease[10]. Perhaps the intrauterine infection associated with a fetal immunologic response (elevated serum IgM levels) results in an inflammatory response with neutrophil migration and elaboration of elastase into the lung. This could then overwhelm the fetal antiproteinase activity, leading to the development of the pulmonary changes days to weeks postnatally.

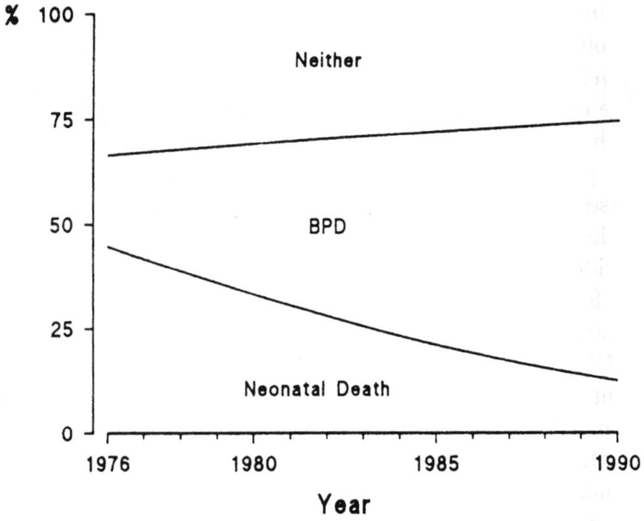

Figure 6.1. Predicted probability of neonatal death and bronchopulmonary dysplasia for a 29-week gestational age, 1000-g, male, white, inborn neonate, with 5-minute Apgar score of 6 and diagnosis of hyaline membrane disease. (From Parker RA, Lindstrom DP, Cotton RB. Improved survival accounts for most, but not all of the increase in bronchopulmonary dysplasia. Pediatrics 1992;90:663).

Since the original description[1], the typical sequence of change from severe RDS to severe chronic obstructive lung disease is much less commonly seen in today's neonatal intensive care unit. BPD is now recognized as a clinical spectrum of disease much broader than the severe cystic emphysema originally described[1]. BPD has been characterized by respiratory distress and a requirement for supplemental oxygen persisting beyond 1 month of age after oxygen and mechanical ventilation therapy in the newborn period[11]. More recently, oxygen dependence at 28 days was not found to be a useful indicator of CLD in infants who were born prior to 30 weeks gestational age[12]. However, oxygen requirement at 36 weeks corrected postgestational age was found to be an excellent predictor of chronic pulmonary dysfunction[12]. Furthermore, gas exchange and sequential pulmonary mechanics testing revealed similar pulmonary development in infants with and without oxygen requirements at 4 weeks of age, calling into question the rationale for defining BPD at 4 weeks of age[13,14].

The incidence of BPD in infants requiring mechanical ventilation for RDS varies widely. It may be as low as 10% or as high as 38% in infants under 1500 g[5,11]. It appears to be increasing at a rate that cannot solely be accounted for by the increased survival of the micropremie[15] (Fig. 6.1). The incidence is dependent on birth weight, exceeding 50% in infants less than 750 g and 40% for infants between 750 and 1000 g[5,11,16]. In addition, male sex and white race are independent risk factors for the development of BPD. Increased duration of hospital stay has been associated with higher mortality rates in BPD patients, a survival rate of 47% and 17% was seen when the patient remained hospitalized at 3 and 5 months respectively[17]. Another study suggests that lower-birth-weight-infants can develop BPD with little or no RDS[18]. The development of late episodes of patent ductus arteriosus usually associated with nosocomial infection appeared to play a key role in the pathogenesis of CLD. A multicenter retrospective study raised the possibility that improved ventilator management of low-birth-weight infants may significantly decrease the incidence of BPD[16]. A multicenter, historical-cohort analysis found that mechanical ventilation management, as demonstrated by higher ventilator rates at 96 hours and a lower P_aCO_2 at 48 hours, is a predictor of CLD[19]. A more recent European multicenter analysis showed that the duration of $FiO_2 > 0.6$, peak inspiratory pressure (PIP) >25 cm H_2O, PDA, bacteremia, and pneumothorax were all independent predictors of development of BPD[20]. The results of these studies suggest that ventilator management in the neonatal period is a significant factor in the pathogenesis of CLD.

Early evaluation of the data regarding the prophylactic use of exogenous surfactant in premature infants showed no significant decline in the incidence of BPD[21–24]. However, more recent work involving several doses of exogenous surfactant has shown a significant decrease in the incidence of BPD[25,26]. Additionally, the use of surfactant has been associated with a significant financial saving per preemie survivor (approximately $5800 or roughly $200 million dollars per year in the United States)[24]. Despite the widespread introduction of surfactant therapy into newborn ICUs and these recent promising results, it is clear that many infants will continue to require mechanical ventilation and develop BPD in the future.

In an attempt to improve enrollment criteria in clinical trials for the prevention or treatment of BPD, formulas have been developed to predict the approximate risk of BPD developing in an individual neonate[27,28]. Unfortunately, both studies are hampered by the fact that BPD was defined by supplemental oxygen requirement at 28 days of age[29]. As stated earlier, low-birth-weight neonates requiring supplemental oxygen at 28 days of age have only a 37% probability of abnormal pulmonary outcome. Adjusting for gestational age, specifically oxygen requirement at 36 weeks postgestational age, leads to a 63% probability of abnormal pulmonary outcome[12].

PATHOGENESIS

The pathogenesis of CLD in infants is complex, multifactorial, and incompletely understood. As originally proposed by O'Brodovich and Mellins[30], BPD is the result of unresolved neonatal acute lung injury. Four central elements (host susceptibility, primary and secondary lung injury, and altered lung repair) have been recognized as key factors in the pathogenesis of BPD[31] **(Table 6.1).** In addition, many individual factors are associated with each central element. These individual factors also have multiple, complex interactions with other factors involved in the pathogenesis of BPD. Therefore, it is unlikely that any single therapy aimed at a single factor will have a significant impact on the incidence of BPD in infants. Only multiple therapeutic interventions aimed at several factors in the pathogenesis of BPD will likely have a beneficial response.

Host Susceptibility

Immaturity

Clearly, the major susceptibility factor for CLD in infants is lung immaturity associated with premature birth[1,5,16,32]. Both structural and biochemical immaturity may be involved in the pathogenesis. Decreased alveolar and airway number as well as increased distensibility of the tracheobronchiolar tree predisposes premature infants to barotrauma during mechanical ventilation[33,34]. Saccular time constant variability results in a pattern of alternating atelectasis and overdistension. A different pattern of diffuse alveolar injury is seen in premature versus adult animals with comparable lung injury[35]. Immaturity that leads to surfactant deficiency was found to be the significant factor in infants dying from RDS[36]. Immaturity is also associated with a deficiency in the antioxidant defense system that leaves premature infants susceptible to oxidant injury[37,38]. For example, antioxidant enzyme levels (superoxide dismutase and glutathione peroxidase) increase 110% in the last 3 to 5 days before birth[39]. Intrauterine and neonatal nutritional deficiencies may play a role in further compromising the antioxidant defense system[40,41]. Vitamin A deficiency has been demonstrated in premature infants who develop

Table 6.1. Proposed Pathogenesis and Potential Therapies for Bronchopulmonary Dysplasia

Central Elements	*Factors Involved*	*Potential Therapies*
Host Susceptability	Prematurity Genetic predisposition Fetal asphyxia Fetal infection	Prenatal care Antenatal care Intrapartum care
Primary Lung Injury	Structural immaturity Surfactant deficiency Antioxidant deficiency Pulmonary edema Infection	Gentle ventilation Surfactant replacement Antioxidants Fluid restriction Antibiotics
Secondary Lung Injury	Surfactant dysfunction Barotrauma Infection Oxygen toxicity Inflammatory Mediators	Surfactant replacement Gentle ventilation Antibiotics Antioxidants Anti-inflammatory agents Antiproteases
Abnormal Lung Repair	Hyperoxia/hypoxia Hypercapnia Abnormal fibrosis Oxygen toxicity Malnutrition	Monitor oxygenation Monitor ventilation Antifibrotic agents Antioxidants Nutritional support

BPD[42,43]. Deficiency of vitamin A results initially in basal cell layer proliferation of the conducting airway epithelium followed by necrosis of ciliated and nonciliated epithelial cells[44]. These cells slough and undergo squamous metaplasia, which results in increased permeability and mucociliary dysfunction[44], a sequence of changes similar to those seen in neonates with BPD[45]. Furthermore, vitamin A supplementation has been shown to reduce oxygen and mechanical ventilatory requirements, decrease the incidence of BPD, and shorten intensive care stays[45]. Finally, maternal medications to inhibit preterm labor have been implicated the pathogenesis of BPD. In a randomized trial of a β-agonist versus indomethacin for preterm labor, indomethacin was shown to significantly increase incidence of BPD in those infants who were born prematurely[46].

Fetal Conditions

Fetal conditions are also involved in the pathogenesis of BPD. As described earlier, fetal infections (as demonstrated by chorioamnionitis) and hypoxemia have been related to pathologic findings in infants who develop Wilson-Mikity syndrome[10]. Fetal asphyxia results in accumulation of hypoxanthine in blood and tissue, leading to oxygen radical generation by xanthine oxidase during oxygen therapy, which results in secondary lung injury[47–49].

Genetic Predisposition

Some infants may be genetically predisposed to the development of BPD. The finding of an increased incidence of airway hyperactivity in infants who develop BPD and their relatives has led to the concern that some infants may be genetically predisposed to pulmonary dysfunction and CLD[50,51]. Furthermore, a prospective study has also revealed an association between HLA-A2 antigen and the susceptibility to CLD in newborns, adding further weight to the theory of genetic predisposition for at least a portion of the population of infants who acquire BPD[52].

Primary Lung Injury

Surfactant Dysfunction

Both surfactant deficiency and surfactant dysfunction play a major role in the initial and ongoing lung injury. Traditionally, study has focused on quantitative rather than qualitative abnormalities in surfactant[53]. Little data support the hypothesis that quantitative surfactant deficiency is responsible for continuing lung injury; however, evidence indicates that both infants and adults with acute lung injury have significant qualitative surfactant dysfunction[54,55]. Alveolar edema fluid affects the surface tension characteristics in the lungs[56,57]. A plasma protein has been identified that inhibits surfactant in a dose-dependent fashion[57]. In addition, this protein has been identified in the airway fluid from premature lambs and neonates with RDS[57,58]. (SP-A) has been shown to reduce the effects of plasma proteins on the surface tension lowering properties of pulmonary surfactant in vitro[59]. Levels of SP-A have been found to be depressed initially and remain depressed in the bronchoalveolar lavage (BAL) fluid in a primate model of BPD[59]. A quantitative surfactant protein A (SP-A) deficiency in BPD patients is feasible, alveolar type II cells containing SP-A are present only at term and not before[59]. A more recent study also demonstrated that SP-A mRNA expression was deficient in preterm primates and persisted in BPD but not control animals[60]. The recent demonstration that SP-A enhances in vitro alveolar macrophage function[61,62] suggests that SP-A deficiency may be a plausible factor in the persistent inflammation and subsequent development of BPD.

Surfactant deficiency or dysfunction promotes edema fluid formation within the lungs by increasing surface tension[63,64]. This increased permeability has been seen in both premature animals and infants with RDS[65,66]. The increased surface tension has been shown experimentally to promote collapse of alveoli, with dilatation of alveolar ducts[67]. These data suggest a possible explanation for the decreased lung compliance, alveolar edema, and atelectasis that are commonly seen with acute lung injury. Any further insult results in increased permeability and pulmonary edema formation, with the resultant protein-rich alveolar fluid inhibiting the function of surfactant, leading to a cycle of further decreases in lung compliance, more edema fluid, atelectasis, and lung injury.

Pulmonary Edema

There are three methods of increasing transvascular fluid flux into the interstitium of the lung: increased transvascular pressure, increased microvascular surface area (recruitment), and increased microvascular permeability. Once the transvascular fluid flux exceeds the lymphatic fluid clearance rate, the edema fluid will exceed the capacity of the bronchovascular interstitial space and flood into the alveolar space. Alveolar edema fluid has been widely recognized in RDS[66,68,69]. The transvascular pressure gradient appears to be significantly elevated in infants with RDS[63–65]. Increased surface tension or more negative pleural pressures result in a more negative interstitial (perimicrovascular) pressure in the lung[64,70], thus increasing transvascular hydrostatic pressure and promoting edema formation. In addition, neonates have decreased total protein concentrations with decreasing gestational age, which correlates with the increasing incidence of RDS[71]. The resultant colloid oncotic pressure is lower, further exacerbating edema fluid formation. Recruitment via increased pulmonary blood flow during exercise has been shown to increase lung water and lymph flow[72]. This may explain why factors associated with an increase in pulmonary blood flow (i.e., patent ductus arteriosus) lead to a higher incidence of BPD[73] and the improvement seen in infants receiving early treatment (ligation of a patent ductus arteriosus) for these conditions[74]. A subpopulation of BPD patients have been found to have hypertrophied systemic to pulmonary collaterals, which may further contribute to the formation of alveolar edema fluid[75].

Lung permeability is increased in neonates with RDS[66]. However, recent investigation showed that this increased permeability resolves by 28 days in RDS[76]. In contrast, neonates who go on to develop BPD have a persistent microvascular leak[76,77]. The mechanisms involved in the increased permeability remain incompletely understood and are likely multifactorial. Increased surface tension may directly increase permeability as described above[65,78] or may mechanically damage the alveolar-capillary membrane[79,80]. Neutrophils and elastase of neutrophil origin are present in airway fluids in neonates who develop BPD[81-84] and could potentially induce pulmonary membrane injury via protease and oxygen radical release[85–88]. Premature infants also have decreased levels of all plasma proteinase inhibitors, further increasing the potential for neutrophil-protease-induced lung injury[89]. Inflammatory mediators such as eicosanoids and platelet-activating factor (PAF) have also been implicated in the pathophysiology of the increased permeability pulmonary edema[90,91].

Infection

Neonatal infections (particularly nosocomial infections) have been implicated as factors in the pathogenesis of CLD[18]. Pulmonary bacterial infections result in accumulation of intraparenchymal neutrophils and macrophages that, as described above, can release oxygen radicals and elastolytic enzymes[83,84,92,93]. *Ureaplasma urealyticum* has been reported to produce chorioamnionitis[94] and congenital pneumonia[95] and can be a factor in the pathogenesis of CLD[96,97]. Acquired viral infections, such as cytomegalovirus or respiratory syncytial virus have resulted in CLD in premature infants[7,98,99]. Therefore, neonatal infections from commonly seen pathogens (such as group B streptococcal sepsis to rare organisms such as *Ureaplasma* and the resulting inflammatory response) can produce CLD in infants.

Secondary Lung Injury

Iatrogenic Pulmonary Parenchymal Injury

Evidence suggests that mechanically assisted ventilation in infants with respiratory failure causes progressive lung injury that ultimately leads to BPD[16,19]. Premature infants requiring ventilation for persistent apnea have developed BPD[100]. Airway injury has been described by several investigators as a consequence of intubation and mechanical ventilation[101–103]. This is a prominent feature in the pathologic finding in neonates dying from severe BPD[1,104,105].

Epithelial necrosis can be demonstrated after brief periods of positive pressure ventilation in surfactant-deficient animals[106,107]. Furthermore, ciliary function is severely impaired with mechanical ventilation, slowly regenerating and recovering over a period of months[108]. No direct correlation between PIP and development of BPD has been found, with some neonates developing BPD with PIP never >30 cm H_2O[109]. Pressure-related lesions expose the interstitial space, thus potentially leading to pulmonary interstitial emphysema (PIE)[110]. When air is forced into connective tissue sheaths, compression of the airway occurs, increasing airway resistance and causing hyperinflation[111] as well as impaired lymphatic drainage promoting edema fluid formation[112]. Once extra-alveolar air develops, it may dissect into the mediastinum, peritoneum, pericardium, and pleural or subcutaneous spaces and delay recovery, resulting in a higher incidence of BPD[113].

Ventilatory strategies attempting to limit the amount of alveolar volume the neonatal lung is exposed to have not changed the incidence of BPD or other outcomes[109]. Initial studies using various methods of high-frequency ventilation (oscillatory, flow-interrupter, jet) showed no improvement in outcome[114-116] and were associated with an increase in intracranial hemorrhage[114]. More recently, animal studies using a high-volume strategy and use of high-frequency oscillatory ventilation immediately after an initial surfactant dose have suggested a decrease in alveolar leak [117], improvement in the distribution of surfactant[118], and good outcome in one small series[119]. A delay of even 30 minutes results in less uniform surfactant distribution[120]. The early use of high-frequency oscillatory ventilation is supported by studies showing injury to premature rabbit lungs occurs within minutes[121]. Little data exist regarding deliberate limitation of mechanical ventilation in neonates with RDS leading to hypercapnia. This strategy has the theoretical benefit of decreased volutrauma. This benefit must be weighted against the concerns regarding increased pulmonary vascular resistance and pulmonary hypertension as well as increased antidiuretic hormone secretion associated with hypercapnia.

The use of heliox (helium:oxygen gas mixture) in the ventilation of patients at risk for the development of BPD is limited. In a randomized, controlled, double-blind study of premature infants with RDS, heliox (initial helium concentration of 78%) showed a significant improvement in $PaCO_2$, shorter duration of mechanical ventilation, and lower mean airway pressure to inspired oxygen ratio[122]. There was a trend toward a decreased incidence of BPD. The use of heliox is limited by the hypoxia which is a common manifestation in patients with BPD. It is often necessary to use higher oxygen and lower helium concentrations in the inspired gas. Future studies with larger numbers are needed before this therapy is used routinely.

Oxygen Toxicity

Inhalation of pure normobaric oxygen ($FiO_2 = 1.0$) for prolonged periods leads to the production of toxic oxygen radicals[123] and has been shown to be lethal in laboratory animals[124]. Oxygen toxicity leads to impaired ciliary motility[125], inhibits endothelial cell metabolic functions[126], increases alveolar-capillary membrane permeability[127], causes alterations in subcellular organelles of type II pneumocytes, inactivates surfactant[128], and has been implicated as a major element in the development of BPD[129]. Evidence suggests that premature and term infants are deficient in a major antioxidant enzyme, superoxide dismutase[130]. In fact, bovine superoxide dismutase, when administered in a controlled trial to infants with RDS, resulted in improved radiologic and clinical status but failed to decrease the duration of mechanical ventilation or oxygen therapy required[131]. Neonatal animals survive longer in toxic oxygen environments than do adult animals of the same species[132]. However, prolonged survival does not mean that significant lung injury is not occurring. In human neonates, expression of copper-zinc and manganese superoxide dismutase in lungs was found to be similar to that in adults, casting further doubt on the theory that infants are more susceptible to oxygen injury[133]. Vitamin E, a natural antioxidant, failed to decrease the incidence of BPD in control trials[134] and, in fact, has been associated with decreased neutrophil bactericidal activity and a higher incidence of sepsis and necrotizing enterocolitis[135].

Oxygen toxicity in the neonate may occur indirectly. Infants who progress to BPD produce greater quantities of lipid peroxidation products when exposed to supplementary oxygen than neonates with self-limited RDS[136]. Hydrogen peroxide, a frequent byproduct in oxygen toxicity, stimulates a mitogen-activated protein kinase in bovine myocytes[137] and may be involved in the mechanism of bronchiole smooth muscle hypertrophy seen in BPD. Prolonged supplemental oxygen exposure may act synergistically with other factors (macrophages, neutrophils, etc.) to produce greater quantities of oxygen radicals and appears to have a role in the genesis of continuing lung injury. Hypoxanthine, which accumulates in neonates after stress[47], may promote oxygen radical-induced lung injury[48]. Oxygen-related injury also causes release of other potential mediators of lung injury, such as arachidonic acid metabolites, continuing the cascade of events that promote ongoing lung injury[138,139].

Inflammatory Mediators

During the last decade, a wealth of knowledge has accumulated concerning the role that mediators may play in primary and secondary lung injury, which ultimately culminates in multiple organ system failure[140]. Conclusions regarding putative mediators of secondary lung injury are typically inferred from *(a)* the effect of inhibitors of their synthesis or action, *(b)* correlation between pathophysiologic changes and the levels of the mediators, and *(c)* similarities between the action of the compounds and features of lung injury. Difficulties remain in ascertaining the relative importance of each potential mediator and to what extent each compound is a cause of, rather than a marker for, injury.

The principal humoral mediators of injury are two groups of potent lipids: arachidonic acid and platelet-activating factor (PAF) (Fig. 6.2). Evidence suggests that human neutrophils generate both arachidonic acid metabolites and PAF from a common precursor (arachidonate-containing phosphoglycerides) via phospholipase A_2 activation[141]. Arachidonic acid is then transformed by a host of different cell populations (leukocytes, macrophages, endothelium, and epithelium) into several compounds (eicosanoids) that have multiple, potent actions. Cyclo-oxygenase catalyzes production of multiple eicosanoids; however, the principal products

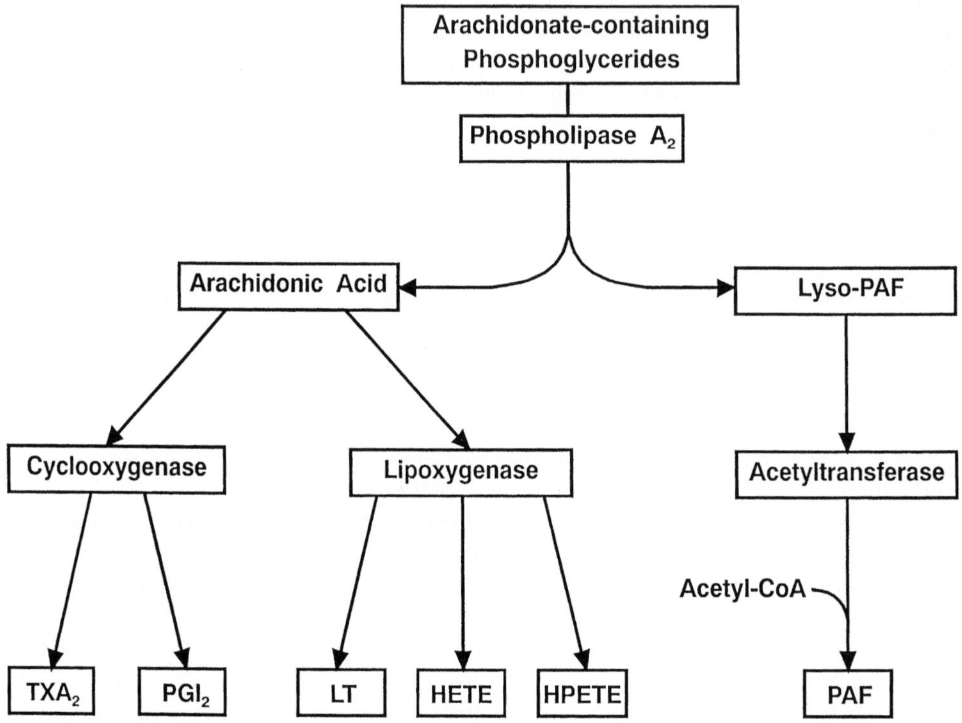

Figure 6.2. Arachidonate-containing phospholipids are the precursor of the common lipid mediators of lung injury and inflammation.

are thromboxane A_2 (TXA_2) and prostacyclin (PGI_2)[142]. Arachidonate is also catalyzed by lipoxygenase to produce leukotrienes (LT), hydroxyeicosatetraenoic acid (HETE), and hydroperoxyeicosatetraenoic acid (HPETE)[143]. Different cells are associated with different patterns of arachidonate metabolism; the endothelium synthesizes predominantly PGI_2, and platelets form chiefly TXA_2, while neutrophils and macrophages produce mainly lipoxygenase products[143].

The two principal arachidonate mediators involved in the pathogenesis of lung injury appear to be TXA_2 and leukotrienes. The principal effects of TXA_2 are bronchoconstriction, vasoconstriction, and platelet aggregation. Pulmonary TXA_2 synthesis is stimulated in experimental lung injury and is believed to contribute to pulmonary hypertension and decreased lung compliance[144–146]. Inhibition of TXA_2 synthesis protects against many of the features of experimental lung injury[145,146].

Leukotrienes also have multiple effects. Formerly known as "slow-reacting substance of anaphylaxis" (SRS-A), leukotrienes LTC_4, LTD_4, and LTE_4 induce bronchial and vascular constriction, increase microvascular permeability, and decrease myocardial contractility[90,143,147]. LTB_4 stimulates leukocyte migration, aggregation, and adherence to endothelium and has been implicated as a significant mediator of secondary lung injury[92,143,146]. Increased leukotriene levels have been found in infants and adults who are at risk or develop severe lung injury[90,91,148]. Although eicosanoids appear to be important mediators of lung injury, in newborn rabbits exposed to hyperoxia, LTD_4 and LTE_4 receptor antagonists were insufficient to decrease hyperoxic lung injury, pulmonary edema, or mortality rate, suggesting leukotrienes play a minor role in the multifactorial etiology of BPD[149].

The second major lipid mediator, PAF, is also derived from arachidonic acid-containing phosphoglycerides, via phospholipase A_2 and acetyltransferase. Synthesized and released by multiple cells (neutrophils, eosinophils, macrophages, platelets, endothelium, etc.), PAF has many biologic effects[150]. In addition to its proinflammatory actions (activation of neutrophils, macrophages, platelets), it stimulates eicosanoid synthesis, superoxide production, chemotaxis, adherence, and release of lysosomal enzymes[150]. The pulmonary responses to PAF include airway constriction and hyperreactivity, pulmonary hypertension, decreased lung compliance, and the development of pulmonary edema[151,152]. PAF has also been identified in neonates with BPD[90].

Many cytokines have been implicated in experimental and clinical examples of acute lung injury[153]. Complement, released by a variety of injury-provoked mechanisms, results in increased microvascular permeability, neutrophil activation, and oxygen radical production[154]. Tumor necrosis factor (TNF) has been shown to increase endothelial membrane permeability directly and lead to pulmonary edema[155–157]. Like TNF, interleukin-1 (IL-1), which is secreted by activated macrophages, is capable of inducing high-membrane permeability edema[158]. Alveolar macrophages from newborn rabbits have upregulated production of IL-1[159]. An infusion of IL-1 in rabbits results in increased alveolar septal wall granulocytes, increased lung wet/dry weight, and extravasation of albumin into alveoli[160]. In BAL fluid of ventilated infants who progressed to BPD, IL-1 levels were elevated by 24 hours of age and were significantly higher at 14 days than in those infants with self-limited RDS[161]. Soluble IL-2 receptors have been identified as markers of lymphocyte activation and have been found to be significantly elevated in patients with evolving or established BPD compared with neonates with self-limited RDS[162]. Serial BAL samples from neonates with evolving BPD show elevated IL-6 activity, compared with matched RDS controls, with no increase in antigen count, suggesting an inhibitor deficiency[163]. The multiple sources, sites of action, and potential interaction make it difficult to elucidate the role each mediator plays in secondary lung injury. Clearly, further work is required, particularly in the area of neonatal lung disease.

Inflammatory cell infiltration into BAL fluid has been used to identify neonates who go on to develop BPD[81,164]. Neutrophil activation is associated with release of multiple lipid and enzyme mediators as well as the generation of oxygen radicals. Proteinase of neutrophil origin could easily overwhelm the immature antiproteinase system of the neonate. BAL fluid from neonates has elevated elastase coupled with low proteinase inhibitor levels[83,84]. Furthermore, this elastase-proteinase inhibitor imbalance has been associated with lung connective tissue destruction and fibrotic changes associated with BPD[165]. This imbalance has been shown to persist in neonates requiring oxygen and mechanical ventilation at 28 days of life [166]. Nosocomial infections played a significant role in the maintenance of this inflammatory state within the lung in this group of susceptible infants[167]. Activated inflammatory cells (macrophages, neutrophils, lymphocytes), by release of a large variety of cytokines, can amplify or modulate the inflammatory response and ultimately have a profound impact on the reparative response of the lung[92,153,167].

The first step in inflammatory cell infiltration is adhesion to the endothelium. This is followed by transendothelial migration to the site of inflammation. Recently identified cell surface molecules are essential to leukocyte adhesion and transendothelial migration. Thus, they play a pivotal part in normal cellular immunity and tissue reparative processes[168–172]. Adhesion molecules consist of three distinct groups: selectins, integrins, and members of the immunoglobulin superfamily (e.g., intracellular adhesion molecule [ICAM], platelet-endothelial adhesion molecule [PECAM]). Selectins are expressed on both leukocytes and endothelial cells and bind to carbohydrate ligands on leukocytes in low-affinity binding called *"rolling"* (Fig. 6.3). L-selectin is expressed constitutively on all leukocytes and is rapidly shed from polymorphonuclear cells (PMNs) by proteolysis upon inflammatory activation. In patients at risk for ARDS, soluble L-selectin was found to be lower in those who progressed to ARDS[173]. This suggests that soluble L-

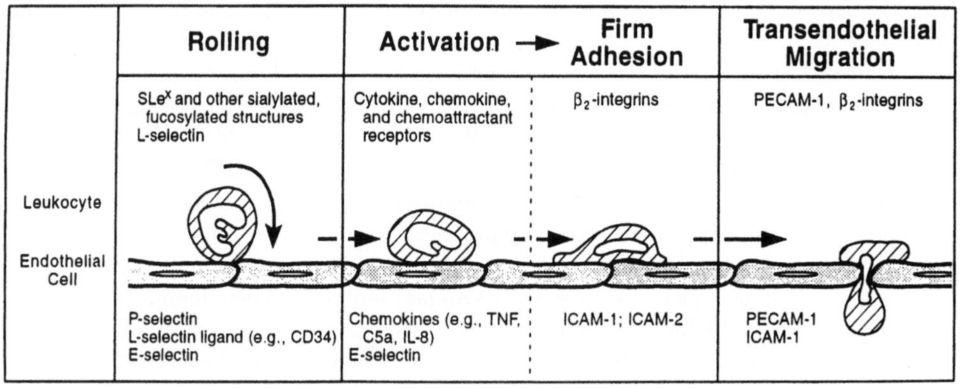

Figure 6.3. The *adhesion cascade.* Selectins mediate early recruitment of polymorphonuclear neutrophils (PMNs) from the peripheral circulation, slowing PMNs to allow firm adhesion that is primarily β_2 integrin-mediated. PECAM, platelet-endothelial cell adhesion molecule; ICAM, intercellular adhesion molecule; IL, interleukin; TNF, tumor necrosis factor. (From Talbott GA, Sharar SR, Harlan JM, Winn RK. Leukocyte-endothelial interactions and organ injury: the role of adhesion molecules. New Horizons 1994;2:545).

selectin may bind to leukocytes and inhibit endothelial binding, thereby modifying the inflammatory response. In an IgG deposition or complement activation model, F(ab′) anti-L-selectin was protective for lung injury[174]. P-selectin is expressed by platelets and endothelial cells in vitro in response to histamine, thrombin, terminal complement components, and TNF. In a cobra venom model, a P-selectin-dependent injury, pretreatment with sialyl Lewis X (oligosaccharide) dramatically reduced neutrophil-dependent acute lung injury in rats[175].

The integrins consist of a common β subunit (CD18) and one of three α subunits. The β integrins are expressed on the surface of leukocytes with CD11b/CD18 (Mac-1) being expressed solely on PMNs, monocytes, and natural killer (NK) cells. The surface expression of Mac-1 is upregulated by many proinflammatory mediators (TNF, granulocyte colony stimulating factor, LTB_4, and $C5_a$) via translocation of intracellular stores. When induced by inflammatory mediators, Mac-1 and other β integrins bind tightly to ICAM-1 and -2 and are essential for *"rolling"* to progress to tight binding with subsequent transendothelial migration of PMNs[172]. The expression of intracellular adhesion molecules (ICAM-1 and -2) is both constitutive and inducible with inflammatory stimuli such as TNFα, IL-1, endotoxin, and interferon γ[176]. Early evidence suggests these cell surface adhesion molecules play a role in the development of BPD. In tracheal aspirates of premature infants, soluble ICAM-1 was significantly elevated at 6 to 7 and 12 to 14 days of age in those patients who went on to develop BPD[177]. Despite limited data, mounting evidence suggests that adhesion molecules are essential in many acute lung injury models[168–172]. Future experimentation with monoclonal F(ab′) and oligosaccharides will be necessary to evaluate their utility in arresting the inflammatory cascade of BPD. However, an area of ongoing concern will be the possible immunosuppression that may be achieved with neutralization of these molecules and the subsequent risk of concomitant nosocomial infections.

The ability of the neonate to modulate the inflammatory response may be involved in the pathogenesis of BPD. A recent prospective study demonstrated decreased cortisol secretion in response to adrenocorticotropic hormone (ACTH) in infants who develop BPD compared with controls recovering without CLD[178]. It appears that some infants may be unable to secrete adequate amounts of cortisol in the setting of increased stress, placing them at risk for continued inflammation and lung injury, ultimately resulting in BPD.

Lung Repair

The principal histologic finding in lungs of neonates with CLD is an extravagant fibroproliferative response far in excess of the needs to repair the damage that occurred[179]. It appears that overgrowth of fibroblasts, smooth muscle, and airway epithelial cells is in response to some poorly understood, nonspecific stimulation of cell proliferation in both neonates and adults[179–181].

Pulmonary Neuroendocrine Cells

Recently, the potential role that pulmonary neuroendocrine cells (PNEC) may play in this pathologic proliferation has been suggested[182] (Fig. 6.4). After epithelial injury, PNEC are among the first cells to differentiate in the regenerating epithelium. Hyperplasia of PNEC, which peaks at 2 months of age, is seen in neonates with CLD[183–185]. The increase in PNEC is associated with a 3-fold increase in gastrin-releasing peptide, a 10-fold increase in calcitonin, and a 34-fold increase in serotonin immunoreactive cells in infants who died of BPD compared with infants who died of noncardiopulmonary disease[184]. The factors associated with this proliferative response are unknown. Elevated levels of the secretory products (potent mitogenic substances) of PNEC, in turn, lead to a nonspecific proliferation of fibroblasts and of airway smooth muscle and epithelial cells. As the histologic changes evolve, the pathophysiologic manifestations of ventilation-perfusion imbalance (hypoxia and hypercapnia) become evident. Airway hypoxia and/or hypercapnia augment the release of the se-

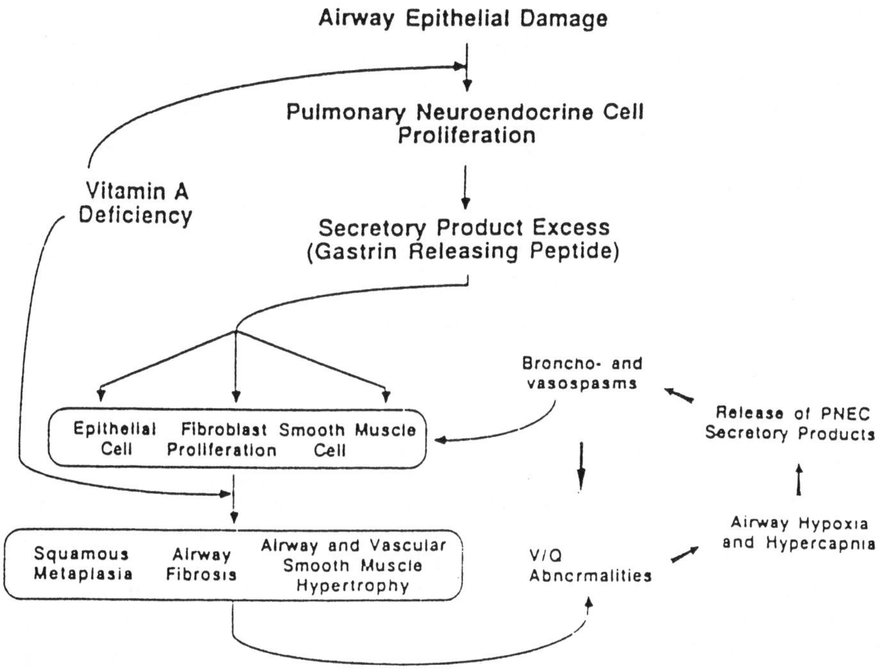

Figure 6.4. Proposed interaction of pulmonary neuroendocrine cell secretory products in the development of the anatomic and pathophysiologic changes observed in bronchopulmonary dysplasia. (From Johnson DA, Georgieff MK. Pulmonary neuroendocrine cells. Their secretory products and their potential roles in health and chronic lung disease in infancy. Am Rev Respir Dis 1989;140:1807.)

cretory products of PNEC via chemoreceptor mechanisms[186,187]. Chemoreceptor stimulation results in bronchospasm and vasospasm, which causes further smooth muscle proliferation.

Histopathologic differences between the chronic stages of infant and adult RDS support a role for PNEC and their secretory products in the pathogenesis of BPD. Despite similarities in both the acute pathophysiologic response to primary injury and risk factors for secondary injury, adolescents and adults rarely develop the same pulmonary fibrosis seen in neonates. These differences may be explained by the far greater absolute number of PNEC present in a newborn[184,185,188,189]. This leads to elevated amounts of growth-promoting secretory products in the airways of infants rather than of older children or adults with similar degrees of lung injury[189]. This may also explain the increased incidence and severity with decreasing gestational age[182].

Malnutrition

Malnutrition, a condition frequently seen in the premature population, has been reported to have profound effects on lung defenses and repair capabilities and may be a key pathogenic factor in the development of BPD[190]. The potential mechanisms by which malnutrition may affect the susceptible infant are numerous **(Table 6.2).** As previously noted, vitamin A deficiency impairs epithelial integrity[31,191] and is associated with BPD[43,44]. Nutritional deprivation limits biosynthetic material for such vital functions as cell replication, protein synthesis (antioxidant and antiproteinase enzymes)[43], and extracellular matrix production[30,190]. Malnutrition is also associated with impaired cellular and humoral defenses against pathogens[190,192].

Other Factors

Other factors may also alter or impair the normal reparative response of the lung to injury. Oxygen toxicity not only produces lung injury but also impairs the response to injury. In neonatal rats, exposure to 100% oxygen for as little as 2 hours leads to a significant decrease in DNA synthesis in the lung[193], while prolonged exposure can arrest DNA synthesis completely[194]. Furthermore, oxygen toxicity can prolong interstitial edema, thus interfering with lung repair[195]. An imbalance of competing activities of coagulation and fibrinolysis may contribute to the premature lungs' response to acute injury. Lung lavage of children with BPD exhibits significantly depressed levels of tissue plasminogen activator with measurable levels of procoagulants (mostly factor VII)[196]. This early imbalance may influence clearance of alveolar fibrinous exudate and promote alveolar septal organization in those infants who progress to BPD.

As can be seen from the preceding discussion, the pathogenesis of CLD in neonates is a complex process. Extensive work by physicians and scientists over several decades has only recently begun to shed light on the interplay between the host factors, injury, and side effects associated

Table 6.2. Nutritional Factors Affecting Lung Repair

	References
Decreased epithelial integrity	43-45, 190
Decreased antioxidant defense system	30, 40, 41, 190
Decreased antiproteinase system	89, 190
Decreased lung biosynthesis (repair of injury)	30, 190
Delayed replication and structural maturation	30, 190
Altered extracellular matrix	30, 181, 190
Increased susceptibility to infection	30, 190

with modern intensive care that culminates in BPD. Clearly, this multifactorial disease will not be prevented or treated with single interventions. Improved prenatal and intrapartum care to decrease host susceptibility, treatment of primary injury such as surfactant replacement, prevention of secondary injury by gentle mechanical ventilation with permissive hypercapnia, and optimal nutritional supportive care all must be combined to have a real impact on the incidence and severity of BPD in the next decade.

Pathology

In 1967, Northway et al.[1] described four distinct stages of pathologic progression of the lung in a child with developing BPD. In stage 1, the classic findings of RDS are seen on chest radiograph: generalized granular pattern, increased pulmonary density consistent with widespread atelectasis, and air bronchograms. Histologically, these neonates' lungs demonstrated hyaline membranes, hyperemia, atelectasis, dilated lymphatics, and necrosis of the bronchiole mucosa. The second stage exhibits nearly complete opacification of the lung fields on chest radiograph, and histologic findings of necrosis and repair of alveolar epithelium, persistent hyaline membranes, and coalescence of alveoli are seen. In the third stage (days 10 to 20 of life) small, round areas of radiolucency are distributed throughout the lungs, fewer hyaline membranes are present, and continued alveolar epithelial damage is observed. Hyperplasia and metaplasia of the bronchial/bronchiolar mucosa are present. In the final stage (IV), the classic cobblestone appearance of the lung is seen, representing areas of alternating atelectasis or marked scarring with hyperinflation. Histologic features of hypertrophied peribronchiolar smooth muscle, squamous metaplasia of all airways, chronic inflammation and edema, and hypertrophy of submucosal glands are present. Morphometric analysis of the BPD lung over different age groups demonstrates severe somatic growth retardation with reduced lung volumes[197]. Bronchiolar density is increased but tends to normalize with advancing age. Hypertrophy of bronchiolar smooth muscle is a constant. In patients with long-standing BPD, alveolar number is severely decreased, with little compensatory alveolar development with increasing age[197]. The acinar structure is simplified with thickened tortuous and irregularly distributed alveolar elastic fibers[197]. The number of small pulmonary arteries is also decreased. It is now recognized that many infants do not exhibit all of the stages as described by Northway et al., and only the radiographic changes of stage IV and a compatible clinical history are necessary to make the diagnosis of BPD[198].

SEQUELAE OF NEONATAL LUNG INJURY

Because of the multifactorial pathogenesis of neonatal lung disease, it should come as no surprise that the sequelae of the injury result in a complex spectrum of pathophysiologic processes that vary widely in severity and typically involve many separate organ systems. Not only are there multiple sequelae, but these sequelae frequently have many complicated and variable interactions. Finally, the pathophysiologic manifestations of these sequelae commonly evolve with time as the injury resolves and the child grows and recovers.

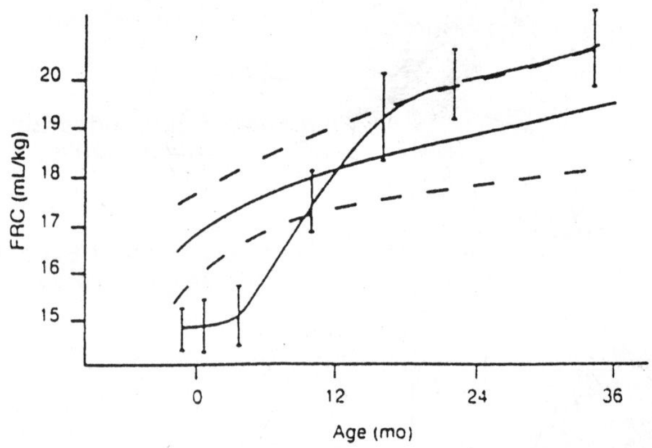

Figure 6.5. Sequential measurements of functional residual capacity (FRC) expressed as FRC per kilogram of body weight (mean +/− SEM) in infants with CLD. For comparison, the curve for normal infants with 95% confidence limits is also shown. (From Fanaroff AA, Martin RJ, Hack M. Long-term outcome of respiratory distress in infants. Respir Care 1991;36:707.)

Respiratory System

A typical clinical manifestation of BPD is chest hyperinflation. Surprisingly, functional residual capacity, as measured by both plethysmography and helium dilution, has been found to be low or normal in patients with CLD in the first 6 months of life[199–202] (Fig. 6.5). Measurements in later childhood can be normal or show the more typical pattern of lung volumes seen in obstructive pulmonary disease (elevated ratio of residual volume to total lung capacity)[203–206]. These findings have recently been shown to persist into adulthood[207].

Increased airway resistance has been clearly demonstrated in infants with CLD[199,200,202,208,209]. In addition, BPD is associated with decreased lung compliance as a result of the widespread fibrosis and decreased number of alveolar units[199–201,208–210]. The decreased lung compliance can be partially corrected with bronchodilating agents consistent with increased airway resistance[211,212]. With time, lung compliance has been shown to improve to near normal levels[208]. Dynamic compliance improves with diuretics[213–215] and following treatment of pulmonary vascular engorgement[73,216–218], suggesting that pulmonary edema may contribute to the decreased airway resistance.

Until recently, it has been impossible to measure maximal inspiratory or expiratory flow rates in uncooperative infants reliably and objectively. Two techniques have been developed that now make these measurements possible. One method applies negative pressure to a maximally inflated lung to generate a maximal expiratory flow-volume maneu-

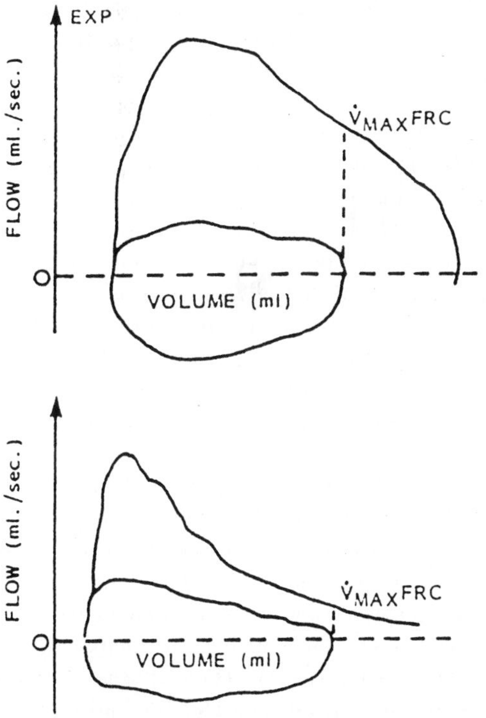

Figure 6.6. Partial expiratory flow volume curves. The smaller inner curve represents tidal breathing, and the larger curve represents maximal expiratory flow generated by rapid compression technique. Maximal expiratory flow at functional residual capacity ($V/_{max}FRC$) is indicated by the dashed line. The difference between tidal breathing and maximal expiratory flow represents expiratory flow reserve. Upper curves: Normal control infant has convex to linear maximal expiratory flow volume curve, with large expiratory flow reserve. Lower curves: Infant with BPD has concave flow volume curve, with decreased expiratory flow reserve and $V/_{max}FRC$, compared with the infant represented in the upper curves. (From Tepper RS, Morgan WJ, Cota K, Taussig LM. Expiratory flow limitation in infants with bronchopulmonary dysplasia. J Pediatr 1986;109:1041.)

ver[(219)]. A second method, the partial expiratory flow volume (PEFV) maneuver, uses the application of positive pressure to the chest and abdomen to generate a forced exhalation[(202)]. These maneuvers in infants with BPD have shown that tidal breathing approaches expiratory flow limitation[(202)] (Fig. 6.6). The persistent expiratory flow limitations suggest that distal, small airways are not developing normally and that the decreased expiratory reserve makes these infants more prone to recurrent episodes of acute respiratory failure. The airflow limitation has been shown to persist in many survivors of BPD into adolescence and early adulthood[(203–207)].

It has been suggested that infants are more sensitive to provoked (i.e., reactive) airflow limitation[(220,221)]. However, methodologic problems with these techniques may have led to erroneous conclusions[(222)]. Recent data corrected for these methodologic problems have led to the conclusion that airway reactivity is similar in infants, children, and adults[(223)]. In spite of this controversy, infants with CLD have been shown to have bronchial hyperreactivity that can be rapidly reversed with inhaled β-agonists[(211,212,224,225)]. Bronchial hyperreactivity has been shown to persist through school age and into early adulthood[(203,204,207)]. Unfortunately, no long-term studies are available regarding the efficacy of bronchodilator drugs have in terms of therapy on bronchial hyperreactivity. A study of chronic inhaled β-agonists in rats demonstrated enhanced pulmonary vascular muscle hypertrophy and right ventricular hypertrophy (RVH) in a model of hypoxic pulmonary hypertension compared with hypoxia-only controls, bringing into question the long-term safety of these agents[(226)].

Airflow limitation may also be due to anatomic abnormalities of the airways. Autopsy findings of the airways in infants with severe BPD include airway epithelial necrosis with squamous metaplasia, submucosal necrosis and fibrosis, muscular hyperplasia, and submucosal inflammation, leading to airway narrowing and/or obliteration[(179,227)]. In addition to these pathologic lesions, functional lesions of the airway frequently cause increased resistance to airflow in infants with BPD[(228)]. This has been seen both fiberoptically and with sequential computed tomography (CT) scans of the chest[(228,229)]. In addition, oxygen supplementation has been shown to relieve hypoxic airway constriction, decrease airway resistance, and improve dynamic compliance in infants with BPD[(230)]. Finally, some conditions, such as tracheomalacia and bronchomalacia, may mimic bronchial hyperreactivity and have paradoxical responses to bronchodilators[(231)].

Further down the airways, necrotizing bronchiolitis leading to bronchiolitis obliterans, cystic bronchiolectasis, and interstitial fibrosis is commonly seen[(227,232,233)]. Two distinct morphologic patterns of distal airway anatomy have been described in infants with BPD[(234)]. The most common pattern seen includes various sizes of areas of interstitial fibrosis with distortion of the air spaces, while the second pattern has normal conducting airways with uniform enlargement of distal air spaces and little interstitial fibrosis. Many infants have both patterns coexisting. Marked distortion in alveolar anatomy and a significant decrease in alveolar number are commonly seen in infants with CLD[(234,235)]. Ultimately, cystic dilations of the airways are frequently encountered, with overexpanded regions that are interspersed with dense fibrotic areas. Fortunately, respiratory bronchioles and alveoli continue to increase in number and size throughout early childhood. Therefore, children with BPD, when treated aggressively, tend to improve as they grow and frequently may be successfully weaned from mechanical ventilation.

The profound, diffuse lung damage associated with BPD clearly leads to increased work of breathing. Esophageal pressure swings and calculated work of breathing in infants with BPD were several times higher than those of the preterm or term infant[(236)]. Low-density gas mixtures of helium and oxygen significantly decreased airway resistance and work. Increased work of breathing can be further corroborated by several studies that have demonstrated elevated oxygen consumption (VO_2) rates in these infants compared with controls[237–239]. However, technical difficulties associated with VO_2 measurements, particularly when supplemental oxygen is required, must be considered when these results are interpreted[240]. Furthermore, compared with overall consumption, respiratory muscle energy consumption is small indeed. Improvement in pulmonary mechanics and the work of breathing by theophylline and diuretics did not change the VO_2 in infants with BPD[239].

Because of diffuse lung pathology, the distribution of ventilation is abnormal in infants with BPD[113]. Pulmonary gas exchange is significantly impaired in infants with CLD, resulting in hypoxemia and hypercapnia. These alterations in arterial blood gas tensions can persist into the school years[123,124]. Minute ventilation, as a result of increased dead space ventilation and work of breathing, is persistently elevated throughout the first several years of life[200,201,208]. However, minute ventilation at maximum exercise was significantly lower and was associated with elevations in transcutaneous CO_2 tensions with maximal work in the long-term survivors of BPD[204]. In addition, VO_2 at maximal workload was similar to that of controls, but at the expense of a fall in arterial oxygen saturation.

Despite these abnormalities in gas exchange and blood oxygen and CO_2 tension seen in infants with CLD, little has been reported on the ventilatory response to hypoxemia and hypercapnia in this group of patients. It has been clearly demonstrated that adult patients with chronic obstructive pulmonary disease have a blunted ventilatory response to elevated CO_2 tensions[241]. Frequently, these patients are dependent on the hypoxic stimulation to maintain a normal minute ventilation[242]. In fact, low concentrations of supplemental oxygen have been shown to significantly impede ventilatory drive[243]. Peripheral chemoreceptor function has been shown to be intact in preterm and term neonates[244–246]. However, preterm infants initially hyperventilate in response to hypoxia, followed quickly by hypoventilation, periodic breathing, and finally apnea[244,245]. To date, no studies have been published concerning the relationship between the altered gas exchange (hypoxemia, hypercapnia) associated with BPD, age, and ventilatory drive. Infants with BPD have been reported to have a blunted arousal response to hypoxia[247] that has been implicated in the high incidence of sudden infant death syndrome in this group of patients[248]. However, even in this study[248], end-tidal CO_2 decreased, presumably in response to an increase in minute ventilation, followed by prolonged apnea after the hypoxic stimulus.

Respiratory muscle dysfunction associated with many clinical circumstances may predispose infants and children to respiratory failure[249]. Infants are believed to be more vulnerable to respiratory muscle fatigue than older children or adults, particularly in situations where the workload on the muscles is increased, as in BPD[250]. Obstructive lung diseases may lead to poor diaphragmatic performance because of hyperinflation and shortened fiber length, as well as an unfavorable energy balance secondary to hypoxia and persistent inspiratory activity during expiration[251]. To date, no data are available regarding diaphragmatic performance in patients with BPD. Increased chest wall compliance places infants at a mechanical disadvantage and survivors with BPD can have significantly decreased chest wall anteroposterior diameter[252]. In children with severe BPD, asynchronous chest wall movement occurs during non-REM sleep secondary to loss of intercostal muscle tone and further increase in chest wall compliance[253]. Finally, prolonged mechanical ventilation may lead to the development of disuse atrophy of the respiratory muscles[254]. Thus, improvement in respiratory muscle physiology and resolving dysfunction may play a key role in the improvement with growth.

Infants with BPD are naturally susceptible to routine childhood infections, have less ventilatory reserve, and frequently require hospitalization for acute respiratory distress[202]. Lower respiratory tract infections and hospitalization for respiratory illness were found to be significantly more common in infants with BPD compared to age and weight matched controls[255]. These illnesses occurred most frequently during the first year of life and decreased with increasing age. Not only are respiratory illnesses more common, they are also more severe[256]. In particular, respiratory syncytial virus is a common pathogen that can lead to severe or fatal respiratory disease in these susceptible children[257,258].

Cardiovascular System

Pulmonary hypertension with cor pulmonale is a common complication of severe CLD in infancy. Pulmonary vascular disease has been well described in BPD[105]. Medial hyperplasia and adventitial thickening within the walls of small pulmonary arteries and arterioles is frequently seen[105,229,232,235]. The medial hypertrophy ultimately leads to increases in pulmonary vascular resistance and pulmonary hypertension[259–262]. Pulmonary vascular basal tone is increased, and a heightened response to acute hypoxia has been noted[263]. Additionally, infants with BPD fail to extract circulating norepinephrine, which may lead to myocardial hypertrophy and increased pulmonary vascular resistance[264]. In response to lung injury and an attempt to adapt to the pathophysiologic conditions, systemic-pulmonary anastomoses have occasionally been noted[262,265,266]. Infants with BPD frequently have intrapulmonary shunting that leads to worsening hypoxia and therefore elevates pulmonary pressures and resistances further.

The sustained elevations of pulmonary vascular resistance and pressures result in right ventricular hypertrophy[259–261]. Right ventricular hypertrophy has been documented by electrocardiogram (ECG)[260–262] even up to school age[203] and at autopsy[227,267]. The right ventricular hypertrophy is irregular, with necrotic or fibrotic scars, which are likely the result of ischemic insults[268,269], in-

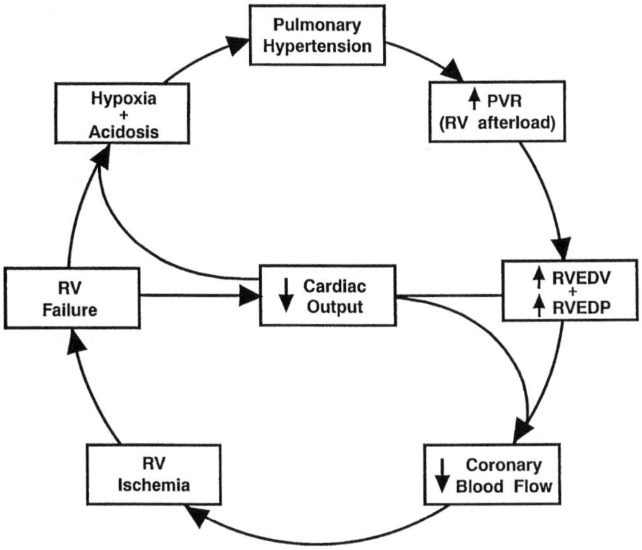

Figure 6.7. Effect of pulmonary hypertension on right ventricular function. RV, right ventricle; RVEDP, right ventricular end-diastolic pressure; RVEDV, right ventricular end-diastolic volume; PVR, pulmonary vascular resistance. (Modified from Perkin RM, Anas NG. Pulmonary hypertension in pediatric patients. J Pediatr 1984; 105:511.)

terspersed with the hypertrophied areas(267). Right ventricular end-diastolic pressures and contractility are normal in some patients with pulmonary hypertension secondary to BPD(259–261). Finally, in response to increasing right ventricular afterload, right ventricular preload (right ventricular end-diastolic volume) is increased (Fig. 6.7). As right ventricular pressure and volume increase, coronary blood flow to the right ventricle, which normally occurs during both systole and diastole, is restricted to diastole only, while wall stress increases. Furthermore, initial hyperplasia of proximal coronary arteries has been seen in infants with BPD(267). Thus, right ventricular myocardial oxygen demand increases while supply is limited, resulting in subendocardial ischemia and right heart failure(270–271). Right ventricular volume overload alters left ventricular geometry, increases left ventricular volume and pressure, and decreases left ventricular volume and compliance (Fig. 6.8). Thus, left ventricular output decreases, leading to decreased tissue oxygen delivery, increased oxygen extraction, decreased venous oxygen saturation, and metabolic acidosis(271). Right or biventricular hypertrophy has been noted frequently at autopsy(227,267) and appears to be an important cause of death in infants with severe BPD(272). As noted previously, chronic β-agonist usage may play a role in the development of RVH and pulmonary hypertension through enhanced pulmonary vascular smooth muscle hypertrophy(226).

Because the sequelae of pulmonary hypertension are cumulative and time dependent, the long-term follow-up of the cardiovascular system in infants at risk for pulmonary hypertension is important. Right ventricular hypertrophy on ECG is a specific but not a sensitive indicator of pulmonary hypertension(273). Patients may have significant pulmonary hypertension before ECG changes are manifested; therefore, echocardiography is the most common method used to assess right ventricular function and pressures in infants with CLD(259,262,272,274,275). In fact, prolongation of the preejection period in relation to the ejection time has been shown to be a prognostic indicator of poor outcome in infants with BPD(272). Radionuclide angiography has also been used to evaluate right ventricular performance in patients with BPD and pulmonary hypertension(276). Using this technique also made it possible to detect an improvement in right ventricular ejection fraction with supplemental oxygen. The most sensitive and specific method of assessing cardiac function remains cardiac catheterization; however, the invasive nature of the procedure limits its clinical utility(259–261). Long-term follow-up with repeated catheterization is rare; however, in severely ill patients, pulmonary artery pressure and resistance did decrease with increasing age but remained above normal age-appropriate values(261). Cardiac catheterization not only is diagnostic but also may be of help in the therapeutic arena. Responses to possible pulmonary vasodilators (oxygen, ventilation, vasodilator) can be objectively assessed(259–262,266,277). Finally, cardiac catheterization may identify previously unrecognized cardiopulmonary abnormalities that may be leading to a failure in the resolution of the signs and symptoms of BPD(278).

Systemic hypertension has also been reported in patients with BPD(279) but appears unlikely to be the cause of left ventricular hypertrophy. Although the exact mechanism pro-

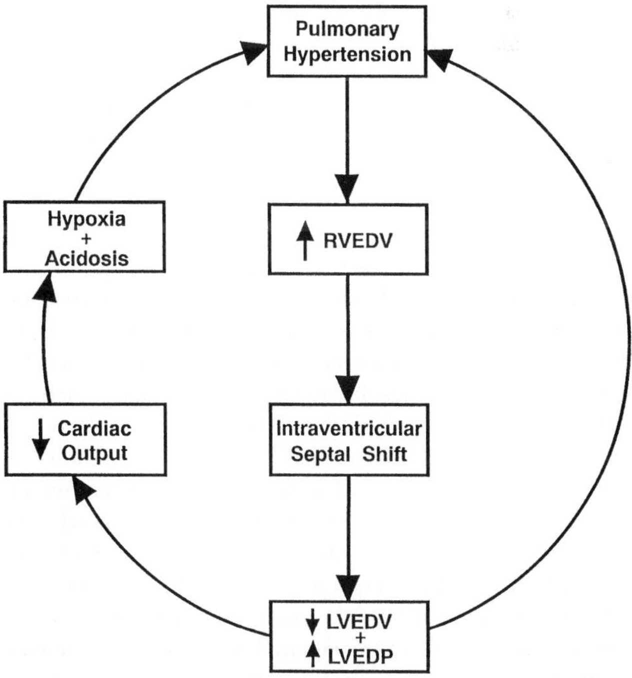

Figure 6.8. Effect of pulmonary hypertension on left ventricular function. RVEDV, right ventricular end-diastolic volume; LVEDV, left ventricular end-diastolic volume; LVEDP, left ventricular end-diastolic pressure. (Modified from Perkin RM, Anas NG. Pulmonary hypertension in pediatric patients. J Pediatr 1984;105:511.)

moting the hypertrophic process in the left ventricle is unknown, the more negative intrathoracic pressures observed in patients with BPD[(236)] increase left ventricular afterload and could certainly contribute to this process. In addition, elevated levels of circulating norepinephrine previously mentioned may also contribute to left ventricular hypertrophy[(264)].

Neurodevelopment

The incidence and the severity of neurologic and developmental deficits in survivors of BPD vary widely. These sequelae may be progressive or nonprogressive and include spastic diplegia and quadriplegia, ataxia, aphasia, hydrocephalus, seizures, hearing loss, vision loss, and developmental delay[(280–282)]. The severity of lung disease (as defined by the duration of mechanical ventilation and supplemental oxygen requirement) has been correlated with the neurologic outcome by some[(283,284)] but not by all investigators[(285)]. When the criteria of Northway et al. are used for the diagnosis of BPD, there is a higher incidence of growth and development delays[(281)]. The incidence of cerebral palsy has ranged from 11 to 24%, with the incidence of neurologic impairment ranging from 17 to 35%[(280–286)].

Dysmaturity of the electroencephalographic (EEG) activity, as demonstrated by the presence at term of EEG activity that normally disappears in premature infants by 36 to 37 weeks conceptual age, has been reported to be a prognostic indicator in infants with BPD of an unfavorable outcome[(287)]. This dysmature EEG pattern also correlated with the severity of lung disease. Thus, it appears that the long-term neurodevelopmental outcome of infants with CLD is clearly dependent on the extent of their initial disease. Newer therapies, such as surfactant treatment, steroids, and nonconventional mechanical ventilation, may profoundly alter the incidence and severity of these well-recognized sequelae in the future.

Nutrition

As described previously (see the section on pathogenesis), malnutrition may have a significant impact on many functions of the respiratory system, including surfactant production, respiratory muscle function, pulmonary defense mechanisms, and synthetic functions[(190–192,249)]. There is a very high incidence of acute and chronic malnutrition in infants with CLD[(190)]. Several studies have shown that infants with BPD are at or below the third percentile for height and weight during the first 2 years of life[(281,284)]. The increased work of breathing has been associated with a higher basal caloric requirement[(237,238)]. Some evidence indicates that children with BPD have impaired fuel usage, as demonstrated by higher oxygen consumption and CO_2 production with intravenous glucose infusion[(288)]. Furthermore, the neurodevelopmental sequelae associated with CLD may impair caloric intake[(281)]. Therefore, the high incidence of malnutrition in this population of patients should not be unexpected.

MANAGEMENT OF BRONCHOPULMONARY DYSPLASIA

The management of the pulmonary and nonpulmonary sequelae that infants with CLD acquire remains one of the predominant health care problems in neonatal and pediatric critical care units. The diverse sequelae involving several organ systems lends itself to a systematic, rational approach in management that frequently requires many individuals with specialized skills and expertise. This systematic team approach to the management of these chronically ill infants can take place in many different environments, such as pediatric and neonatal ICUs, a chronic respiratory unit, a chronic care facility, or, in many cases, the home with specialized equipment and support. Before the details involved in the team management of these patients are discussed, some general principles and therapies required in nearly all patients with BPD are reviewed.

Oxygen Therapy

Although frequently contributing to the pathogenesis of BPD when used in toxic concentrations, oxygen is the single most essential drug for the infant with CLD. Acute, recurrent hypoxia precipitated by such simple things as handling, feedings, or infections[(289–293)] results in a greater tendency toward the development of pulmonary hypertension and may result in a pulmonary vascular crisis or sudden death[(289,292)]. Thus, continuous oxygen therapy to prevent recurrent or chronic hypoxia has many potentially therapeutic effects. Infants with CLD have been shown to have better weight gain and a significant decrease in pulmonary vascular pressure and resistance in response to low-flow oxygen therapy[(260,262,293)]. Inspired oxygen tension sufficient to achieve a P_aO_2 greater than 55 torr or a hemoglobin saturation greater than 90%[(294)] should be sufficient to prevent the deleterious effects of chronic hypoxia, while limits should be maintained to prevent oxygen toxicity. Therefore, it is advisable to continue oxygen therapy until these goals (hemoglobin saturation greater than 90%) are documented while the infant is sleeping and feeding in room air.

A secondary consideration during oxygen therapy should be the promotion of adequate oxygen delivery. Since oxygen delivery is dependent on not only hemoglobin saturation but also hemoglobin concentration, anemia potentially could have adverse effects on oxygen delivery. Anemia has been associated with periodic breathing, apnea, and cyanotic episodes that resolve with correction[(295–298)]. Caloric and nutrient intake should be sufficient so that intrinsic red cell production is not limited. The potential risks (fluid overload, transfusion reaction, infection) need to be taken into consideration prior to each transfusion.

Table 6.3. Inhaled Agents Used in Chronic Lung Disease

Agent	*Dose*	*Interval (hr)*
Isoproterenol	0.01–0.025 ml/kg 0.5% solution (5 mg/kg) (50–100 βg/kg)	2–6
Isoetharine	0.01–0.02 ml/kg 1% solution (10 mg/ml) (100–200 βg/kg)	2–6
Metaproterenol	0.005–0.01 ml/kg 5% solution (50 mg/ml) (250–500 βg/kg)	2–6
Terbutaline	0.01–0.03 ml/kg 1% solution (10 mg/ml) (100–300 βg/kg)	2–6
Albuterol	0.01–0.04 ml/kg 0.5% solution (5 mg/ml) (50–200 βg/kg)	4–6
Atropine	30–50 βg/kg	6
Ipratropium bromide	20–50 βg/kg	6
Cromolyn sodium	20 mg 1% solution (10 mg/ml)	6

Bronchodilator Therapy

Initial descriptions of BPD were noted for the frequent observation that many of these infants had recurrent episodes of bronchospasm, while survivors had bronchial hyperreactivity[11,203]. It has also been demonstrated that infants who died of BPD had hypertrophied peribronchial smooth muscle at an early age[106]. The clinical impressions and pathologic data led to the rational conclusion that bronchodilator therapy would play a primary role in the management of infants with CLD.

Inhaled Agents

Sympathomimetic drugs that stimulate the β_2-receptors, delivered via the inhalation route by nebulizers, have clearly been demonstrated to be effective in infants with CLD. Many different sympathomimetic drugs with varying β_2-receptor selectivity and potency have been used in these patients. General guidelines for dosage and intervals have also been published **(Table 6.3).** The β_2-stimulation activates adenyl cyclase, thereby increasing intracellular cyclic adenosine monophosphate (cAMP), and causes smooth muscle relaxation of the airways and blood vessels. Many of the side effects (tachycardia, arrhythmias, tremor, hypertension, hyperglycemia, hypocalcemia) are related to the nonselective (β_1) stimulation. Therefore, the newer more selective agents (terbutaline, albuterol) tend to have fewer and less severe side effects.

Isoproterenol decreased airway resistance briefly in infants with BPD[211]. The use of this drug is severely hampered by the nonselective β-receptor stimulation and rapid metabolism and, therefore, short duration of action. Isoetharine decreased airway resistance and improved dynamic compliance in infants with developing BPD[225,299]. This agent has intermediate β-receptor selectivity. Metaproterenol also has been shown to result in short-term improvements in pulmonary mechanics in infants with CLD[300,301]. This drug is more resistant to metabolism, leading to a longer half-life. Terbutaline, a more selective β_2-agonist, significantly decreased airway resistance and increased tidal volume in ventilator-dependent infants with evolving BPD[302]. Albuterol, a β_2-specific adrenergic agent, also decreases resistance and improves compliance in short-term (hours) and intermediate-term (days) studies[212,303].

The adrenergic agents can also be administered via other routes. Subcutaneous terbutaline resulted in significant improvements in pulmonary mechanics and clinical status in ventilator-dependent infants in a short-term study[304]. Intravenous salbutamol (albuterol) similarly improved pulmonary mechanics in ventilator-dependent infants[305]. Inhalational administration is the preferred method of delivery for β-agonists[306] because of the more rapid onset, few side effects, and greater bronchoselectivity. Endotracheal tube size, inspiratory flow rate, and aerosol droplet size have a profound impact on the percentage of drug actually delivered to the site of action[307]. Improved mucociliary function is another potentially beneficial effect of β_2-agonist aerosol therapy[308]. Oxygen-induced impairment of mucociliary clearance is decreased by aerosolized racemic epinephrine or isoproterenol[125].

Despite all the short-term benefits of β-agonist administration in this select population of patients, no long-term studies have clearly established their clinical efficacy. Furthermore, not all the effects of bronchodilator agents are beneficial. Airway anomalies, such as bronchial and tracheal malacia, may lead to a paradoxical worsening in airflow limitation after bronchodilator administration, caused by the decrease in airway smooth muscle tone and increased airway compliance and collapsibility[228,229]. Additionally, in a rat model of hypoxia-induced pulmonary hypertension, chronic inhaled β_2 agonist use resulted in increased pulmonary vascular smooth muscle hypertrophy and RVH[226], bringing to question the safety of chronic use of these agents in humans.

Aerosolized muscarinic antagonists have been shown to cause bronchial smooth muscle relaxation[309]. Atropine, a tertiary ammonium compound, although less effective than β-agonists, caused a significant improvement in pulmonary mechanics[301,310]. Ipratropium bromide, a quaternary ammonium compound with greater potency and fewer side effects than atropine, resulted in improvement in compliance and resistance similar to that seen after albuterol[303]. Because of the less effective bronchodilation and systemic absorption and associated side effects, these compounds are frequently added as a second-line medication to potentiate the bronchodilation caused by the β_2-agonists. Indeed, the combination of ipratropium and β_2-agonists appears to be more effective than either drug alone[311]. Again, no long-term studies of efficacy are available.

Cromolyn sodium inhibits mediator release (histamine, leukotrienes) from mast cells in the lungs. Since mediator release (leukotrienes, PAF) into the airways may participate in the pathogenesis of CLD[90,91], cromolyn may be useful as a prophylactic, chronic anti-inflammatory agent in infants with CLD. Preliminary data demonstrated that cromolyn administration decreased leukocyte concentration, and although leukotriene and PAF concentrations were not mentioned, resulted in clinical improvement[312]. However, one recent prospective randomized clinical trial of intubated neonates showed that cromolyn failed to reduce the incidence of BPD or shorten time on the ventilator[313], but these results have not been confirmed[314]. Obviously, more studies regarding the short- and long-term efficacy of this drug are required.

Systemic Agents

The methylxanthines are a group of chemically related alkaloids that have been used extensively in newborns for the treatment of apnea and to facilitate weaning from mechanical ventilation[315,316]. These compounds have several potential therapeutic effects, including increased chemoreceptor sensitivity to CO_2[316,317], improved diaphragmatic contractility[249], anti-inflammatory activities[318], and improved lung compliance and resistance, presumably through bronchodilation and fluid diuresis[319–321]. The molecular mechanisms responsible for its bronchodilatory activity in clinical diseases are ill defined. Several cellular activities probably contribute to this action, including nonspecific cyclic nucleotide phosphodiesterase inhibition[322], adenosine receptor antagonism[323], and stimulation of catecholamine release[324].

Many adverse side effects to methylxanthines have been observed, including gastrointestinal disturbance (vomiting and diarrhea), central nervous system toxicity (agitation, jitters, seizures), cardiovascular toxicity (tachycardia, arrhythmias, hypertension), and metabolic disturbances (fevers, hyperglycemia, hypokalemia), which limit their clinical utility[315]. Unfortunately, the pharmacokinetics of theophylline in infants with BPD vary widely and are altered by changes in clinical status (respiratory illness, cardiac failure)[325]. Furthermore, the therapeutic range (10 to 20 mg/dl) is narrow; thus, careful monitoring of plasma theophylline levels is required.

Diuretic Therapy

Diuretics are commonly used to treat many of the factors in the pathogenesis and sequelae of CLD in infants. Pulmonary interstitial edema is a primary element in the pathophysiology of the primary lung injury[31] and frequently prolongs the duration of mechanical ventilation that is required. In addition, BPD itself, via air-trapping, pulmonary hypovolemia, and decreased left atrial transmural pressure, causes elevated levels of antidiuretic hormone and arginine vasopressin to be secreted[326,327]. Thus, these infants are unable to tolerate normal fluid requirements while excess fluid further worsens pulmonary mechanics.

Both the short- and long-term use of diuretics in infants with CLD have been shown to improve pulmonary mechanics[213–216,320,328,329]. Recently, randomized, controlled trials of the long-term use of diuretics have demonstrated not only improved lung function but also improved survival [330,331]. Furthermore, the beneficial improvement in pulmonary function may not be due only to the diuretic properties[332]. These other properties include vasodilation with reduction in ventricular preload and pulmonary vascular resistance, which ultimately decreases pulmonary transvascular fluid filtration[320,332].

Several diuretics are commonly used in children with CLD **(Table 6.4).** Furosemide, a chloride transport inhibitor in the ascending loop of Henle, is the most commonly used and studied diuretic. Hypovolemia, hypokalemia, hypochloremic metabolic alkalosis, hypercalcinuria, and ototoxicity are recognized complications of long-term therapy[333,334]. Chloride depletion, a common side effect of diuretic use, has been implicated as a factor in poor outcome in infants with BPD[335]. Therefore, potassium chloride supplementation is frequently required to prevent potassium and chloride depletion, while sodium chloride supplementation is avoided because of increased water retention. Furosemide increases urinary calcium excretion and has been associated with renal calcifications[336] and metabolic bone disease in this population[337]. The induced metabolic alkalosis may decrease minute ventilation and lead to elevations in P_aCO_2[338]. Thiazide diuretics alter sodium reabsorption in the ascending loop of Henle and are commonly used for chronic diuretic therapy in infants with CLD. These diuretics do not alter calcium excretion, as does furosemide, because of distal tubule absorption. The side effects of thiazides are similar to those found with furosemide. Spironolactone, a competitive inhibitor of aldosterone, is a potassium-sparing diuretic frequently used in combination with the loop diuretics. Serum potassium levels need to be monitored when this diuretic is used.

In an attempt to avoid the renal and electrolyte complications associated with systemic diuretic use, a study of nebulized lasix in preterm, ventilator-dependent infants was conducted. Nebulized lasix (1 mg/kg of body weight) demonstrated significant improvement in lung compliance, pulmonary resistance, and tidal volume beginning 1 to 2 hours after the dose and lasting up to 6 hours[339]. The nebulized lasix caused no diuresis or electrolyte changes. Other studies have demonstrated that nebulized lasix produces decreased bronchoconstriction and neutrophil chemotactic activity in some asthmatic patients[164,340].

Table 6.4. Diuretic Agents Used in Chronic Lung Disease

Agent	*Dose (mg/kg)*	*Route*	*Interval (hr)*
Furosemide	0.5–2.0	IV, PO	6–12
Chlorothiazide	5–20	IV, PO	12
Hydrochlorothiazide	0.5–1.5	PO	12
Spironolactone	0.5–1.5	PO	12

IV, intravenous; PO, by mouth.

Table 6.5. Infant and Adult Enteral Formulas per Deciliter

Formula	*Kcal/ml*	*g*	*% cal*	*g*	*% cal*	*g*	*% cal*	*Na (mEq)*	*K (mEq)*	*Ca (mg)*	*P (mg)*	*Fe (mg)*	*Solute (mOsm/k)*
Infant													
Enfamil	0.67	1.5	9	6.9	41	3.8	50	0.8	1.9	46	32	0.11	300
Enfamil	0.81	1.8	9	8.3	41	4.6	50	1.0	2.2	55	38	0.13	360
Enfamil	0.67	2.0	12	7.4	44	3.4	44	1.1	1.7	112	56	0.17	260
Enfamil	0.81	2.4	12	9.0	44	4.1	44	1.4	2.1	134	68	0.20	310
Nutramig	0.67	1.9	11	9.1	54	2.6	35	1.4	1.9		43	1.28	320
Portagen	0.67	2.3	14	7.8	46	3.3	40	1.6	2.2	64	48	1.28	230
Pregestl	0.67	1.9	11	6.9	41	3.8	48	1.2	1.9	64	43	1.28	340
Similac	0.67	1.5	9	7.2	43	3.6	48	0.8	1.9	51	39	0.15	300
Similac	0.81	2.2	11	8.5	42	4.3	47	1.2	2.7	73	57	0.18	380
Similac	0.67	1.8	11	7.1	42	3.6	47	1.3	2.2	122	61	0.25	250
Similac	0.81	2.2	11	8.5	42	4.3	47	1.5	2.7	146	73	1.50	300
SMA 20	0.67	1.5	9	7.2	42	3.6	48	0.7	1.4	42	28	0.15	300
SMA	0.81	2.0	10	8.6	42	4.4	48	1.4	1.9	75	40	0.30	300
Adult													
Enrich	1.08	3.9	15	16.0	55	3.7	30	3.6	4.3	71	71	1.28	480
Ensure	1.04	3.7	14	14.3	55	4.7	31	3.6	3.7	52	52	0.94	470
Ensure	1.48	3.7	14	19.7	53	5.3	32	4.9	5.3	70	70	1.25	690
Isocal	1.07	3.4	13	13.3	50	4.4	37	2.3	3.4	63	53	0.50	300
Osmolite	1.04	3.7	14	14.3	55	3.8	31	2.7	2.6	52	52	0.94	300
Pediasur	1.00	3.0	12	11.0	44	5.0	44	1.7	3.3	97	80	1.40	325
Pulmocar	1.50	6.3	17	10.6	28	9.2	55	5.7	4.9	106	106	1.90	520
Sustacal	1.00	6.1	24	14.0	55	2.3	21	4.1	5.4	101	93	1.69	620

Nutritional Therapy

Infants with CLD have increased caloric requirements[237,238], while medical and neurodevelopmental problems[281] frequently impede the intake of adequate calories to sustain adequate growth[281,284]. Provision of sufficient calories can significantly shorten the natural history of the lung injury, repair process, and ultimately the sequelae of BPD. Although there are specific problems of nutritional therapy for infants with CLD, there are also general principles that apply to nearly all critically ill children.

Nutritional therapy should begin as soon as is practical. The gastrointestinal tract is the preferred route of administration; enteral nutrition is more physiologic, efficient, cost-effective, and less invasive. However, prematurity frequently is associated with many gastrointestinal problems. Many commercially available formulas for infants and children are available **(Table 6.5).** As a general principle, infants younger than 12 months should receive infant formulas, while those older than 12 months may be given adult formulas. Frequently, the formulas may be modified with the use of additives such as carbohydrate polymers, medium-chain triglycerides, or corn oil to increase caloric content **(Table 6.6).**

When the enteral route of administration is limited or not available, then parenteral nutrition is indicated. Intravenous glucose-amino acid solutions plus intralipids can provide partial or total caloric requirements but are associated with difficult and risky maintenance of peripheral or central venous access for prolonged periods.

Several problems unique to infants with CLD must be addressed when nutritional support in this population is being planned. Not only are these patients with lung disease vulnerable to fluid overload, but they have increased caloric requirement. Therefore, additives such as carbohy-

Table 6.6. Enteral Nutrition Supplements

Component	*Source*	*Content*	*Calories*
Protein			
Calcium	Calcium caseinate	88 g/100 g powder	370 kcal/100 g
Promod	Whey protein	75 g/100 g powder	425 cal/100 g
Propac	Whey protein	75 g/100 g powder	395 cal/100 g
Carbohydrate			
Moducal	Corn starch hydrolysate	95 g/100 g powder	900 cal/dl
Polycose	Corn starch hydrolysate	50 g/dl liquid	770 cal/dl
		94 g/100 g powder	450 cal/dl
Fat			
Corn oil	Corn oil	100 g/dl	900 cal/dl
Microlipid oil	Coconut oil C_8 and C_{10} Triglycerides	93 g/dl	770 cal/dl
Microlipid	Safflower oil	50 g/dl	450 cal/dl

drate polymers and medium-chain triglycerides are fre quently used to increase caloric density up to 30 cal/oz to maintain adequate caloric intake while limiting total fluid. Up to 140 to 160 cal/kg/day may be required to sustain growth and development[112,341]. Although excessive carbohydrate calories can have adverse effects on critically ill patients with respiratory insufficiency[342], a recent study has shown improved oxygenation and growth in infants with BPD that can augment their minute ventilation in response to the increased CO_2 production[343]. Although it is fairly standard practice to use low-carbohydrate, high-fat formulas or to modify infant formulas with additives, no controlled studies demonstrate the potential benefits of this practice. Osteopenia of prematurity may increase an already-compliant rib cage, further impairing gas exchange. Therefore, close monitoring of serum calcium, phosphate, and vitamin D supplementation are routinely advocated[341]. Vitamin A supplementation in one trial reportedly reduced the incidence of BPD in infants at risk[45]; however, more extensive trials are needed. Finally, gastroesophageal reflux has been noted in infants with BPD and may cause a significant deterioration in pulmonary function[344]. Although the incidence may be low in infants with BPD[345], when it is identified and treated, significant improvements in pulmonary function and clinical status are frequently seen[346]. Furthermore, gastrostomy feedings will eliminate the need for chronic nasogastric tubes and another source of noxious oral stimulation.

Immune Prophylaxis

Children with BPD are at increased risk for developing more severe forms of many childhood diseases[341]. The potential danger of pertussis infection in these patients[347] requires that the infants and their siblings complete their immunizations. In the report from the Committee on Infectious Disease, children with BPD are considered high risk and require additional immune prophylaxis[348]. It has also been recommended that infants and children with CLD receive influenza vaccinations[349]. In fact, these recommendations state not only that children with BPD older than 6 months and younger than 9 years should receive annually the split virus influenza vaccine in two doses 1 month apart, but children older than 9 years require one dose and after 13 years of age may receive the whole virus vaccine[348]. It is recommended that the pneumococcal vaccine be given to any child with significant chronic disease who is older than 2 years. Revaccination 3 to 5 years after the first should be considered if still at high risk.

Premature infants are known to have decreased levels of immunoglobulins secondary to decreased maternal transfer of these proteins, which occurs primarily in the latter half of the third trimester[350]. This hypogammaglobulinemic state, in addition to prolonged hospital exposure to resistant organisms and multiple invasive procedures, predisposes these infants to nosocomial infections. Unfortunately, attempts at immune prophylaxis with intravenous immunoglobulin have failed to reduce the incidence of hospital acquired infection or incidence of BPD[351].

Respiratory syncytial virus (RSV) is the most important cause of lower respiratory tract infection in infants and young children. Additionally, RSV bronchiolitis in the first year of life has been shown to be a significant risk factor for development of asthma and sensitization to common allergens[352]. Recent studies[353,354] have demonstrated the safety and efficacy of RSV-specific immunoglobulin (RSVIG) in decreasing the incidence and severity of lower respiratory tract infection, hospitalizations, and hospital days in children with BPD. The use of high-dose RSVIG (750 mg/kg IV)[354] monthly from December to March or April may be a useful prophylactic measure, although further study is warranted.

Corticosteroid Therapy

Inflammation plays a prominent role in the pathogenesis of CLD in infancy. Corticosteroids, glucocorticoids in particular, are powerful anti-inflammatory compounds that are increasingly being used in the therapy of these patients. Corticosteroids were first used antenatally to promote surfactant production in premature fetuses[355]. Antenatal steroids have been shown to significantly decrease morbidity, including BPD, and mortality in prematurely born infants[356,357].

Dexamethasone, a potent synthetic corticosteroid with a long half-life and minimal mineralocorticoid effect, when administered to ventilator-dependent infants with BPD in multiple controlled studies, has been associated with improvements in clinical status and pulmonary function[358–362]. Results of several studies suggest that while short-term pulmonary function improves, the hospital course and mortality rate are unaffected[361,362]; however, the results of other studies show long-term benefits[360]. The mechanism whereby corticosteroids are effective in BPD is likely multifactorial[363] but includes cell and lysosomal membrane stabilization[300], increased surfactant synthesis[38,355], antioxidant enzyme stimulation[38], eicosanoid synthesis inhibition[364], decreased polymorphonuclear cell recruitment to the lung[365], breakdown of pulmonary microvascular granulocyte aggregates[366], enhanced β-adrenergic receptor activity[367], decreased collagen type I synthesis [368] and diuretic activity with reduction of pulmonary edema fluid[367,369].

The use of inhaled corticosteroids has recently been evaluated. The rapid uptake from epithelial cell surfaces and biotransformation in the liver of any systemically absorbed fluoridated steroids make inhaled corticosteroids an attractive alternative to oral dosing. A trial of nebulized beclomethasone in infants 7 to 18 months of age with steroid-dependent BPD resulted in slow improvement in pulmonary resistance, immunoglobulin levels, linear growth, and weight gain[370]. Several infants were able to stop oral steroids with no noted side effects. Further studies evaluating both the acute and chronic effects of inhaled steroids are needed. The Food and Drug Administration has not yet approved the use of inhaled steroids in neonates.

Corticosteroid use for BPD may be associated with significant side effects. Potential side effects include fluid overload and hypertension from mineralocorticoid stimulation, hyperglycemia, hyperglycemic ketoacidosis, reversible hypertrophic obstructive cardiomyopathy, gastric ulceration, osteoporosis, steroid myopathy, cataracts, and immune suppression. Dexamethasone use for BPD has been associated with prolonged suppression of hypothalamic-pituitary-adrenal axis function[(371)]. Evaluation of this function before discontinuation of prolonged dexamethasone therapy is necessary to ensure adequate adrenal secretory response. It also appears that corticosteroids, when given during a critical window of time, may decrease lung DNA synthesis and alveolarization of the lung[(101)]. Dexamethasone therapy may also be associated with a marked catabolic state[(372)].

In view of the serious side effects, the potential benefits must clearly outweigh the risks of corticosteroid therapy. This therapy should be reserved for ventilator-dependent infants who have failed to wean with more conventional therapy. In addition, the results of this therapy in older ventilator-dependent children in the PICU are unknown. Controlled trials examining this population need to be performed prior to incorporating this therapy into routine clinical practice.

Vasodilator Therapy

The principal vasodilator used for infants with evidence of BPD and pulmonary hypertension is oxygen. As previously described, pulmonary vascular reactivity to oxygen is maintained in this population[(259–262)]. Pharmacologic vasodilation is occasionally attempted in oxygen-dependent infants with CLD and pulmonary hypertension. Vasodilating drugs used with variable results have included hydralazine[(262,373)], calcium channel blockers, diltiazem[(373)], nifedipine[(277,373–375)], and prostacyclin[(266)]. Several studies suggest that vasodilators may lower pulmonary vascular pressure and resistance more than oxygen does[(266,277,375)]. Unfortunately, the vasodilating response is not uniformly found in all patients tested. Enlarged systemic to pulmonary collaterals found in some patients with BPD may explain the occasional paradoxical response to vasodilators[(75)]. Each patient should be evaluated individually for his or her response to each potential vasodilator. Finally, the short- and long-term efficacy and safety of these vasodilators in treating infants with CLD and pulmonary hypertension is yet to be established.

BRONCHOPULMONARY DYSPLASIA IN THE PICU

Pediatric critical care physicians will, with increasing frequency, be faced with the task of caring for infants with BPD. These patients will require admission to the PICU for a variety of reasons, including postoperative care after a surgical procedure, transfer from the neonatal ICU for chronic ventilatory management, and after acute decompensation of their chronic pulmonary disease. The following discussion deals specifically with these latter two instances.

Long-Term Mechanical Ventilation

With our improved understanding of the pathophysiology and treatment of neonatal lung disease, we face an ever-increasing number of infants with chronic respiratory failure who require long-term mechanical ventilation. Up to one-third of the pediatric patients requiring chronic mechanical ventilation are now infants with BPD[(376,377)]. In one study these patients required mechanical support of ventilation for an average of 12 months (range 1 to 47 months)[(377)]. Fortunately, as a result of the continued lung growth with aggressive care, the prognosis for long-term survival without mechanical ventilation remains good.

The chronic, slowly resolving nature of the lung disease is not well suited to the rapidly changing environment of the neonatal or pediatric ICU. Patients with BPD can potentially suffer in the critical care unit. Medical, nursing, and support staff are frequently rotated in the stressful ICU environment, thus potentially leading to differences in philosophies and approaches to therapy that can serve as a source of frustration for the parents and staff. These differences are frequently a major issue when the patient is initially transferred from the acute to the chronic care facility. Therefore, these patients are best served with a systematic team approach with clearly defined primary physicians, nurses, and therapists. The primary care team will facilitate a smooth transition between caretakers and orchestrate the overall care of these patients, which includes regular meetings with the staff to discuss management issues as well as serving as a consistent resource for the staff and family. The frequency and the composition of these meetings are dependent on the needs of each patient and family.

One of the primary issues in dealing with patients with chronic respiratory failure is the provision of access to the airway for a prolonged period. Tracheostomies have several major advantages for patients who require chronic mechanical ventilation. First, tracheostomies allow stable, long-term access to the airway with less of a risk to develop subglottic stenosis. By bypassing the upper airway and shortening the length of the artificial airway, the work of breathing is reduced facilitating weaning of mechanical ventilation. A tracheostomy will allow pleasant oral stimulation, such as nipping. In addition, the tracheostomy allows more mobility and more aggressive physical, occupational, and developmental therapy. Finally, because the patient has a chronically stable airway, he or she may be admitted to an appropriate chronic care facility designed to treat the patient who requires chronic, intensive, supportive care.

In general, the mechanical support of ventilation for these patients can be divided into acute, subacute, and weaning phases[(378)]. The acute phase is typically dealt with in the ICU. The goal of the acute phase is to provide stable oxygen delivery via mechanically supported ventilation and to maintain adequate cardiac output while limiting secondary lung injury (oxygen toxicity, barotrauma, inflammation, infection) as much as possible.

The diffuse lung pathology manifested by decreased lung compliance, increased airway resistance, and altered gas exchange only improve slowly over a prolonged period of time. Therefore, the subacute phase of mechanical ventilation may last months or years in patients with BPD. During this time many of the management issues discussed in the previous section apply. Improvement in pulmonary function and clinical status only occur with lung growth; therefore, the major goal during the subacute phase is to provide sufficient mechanical support of ventilation and nutrition to establish consistent growth and development while minimizing further lung injury.

The final phase of mechanical ventilation, the weaning phase, begins when respiratory stability and weight gain have been achieved. The primary goal throughout this phase of care is maintenance of a consistent weight and length gain. Weaning of mechanical ventilation should be slow, systematic, and stopped at the first sign of intolerance, which frequently is failure to thrive.

The ability to be successfully liberated from mechanical support of ventilation depends on the balance between energy supply and demand to the respiratory muscles **(Table 6.7).** Therapy should be directed toward maximizing respiratory muscle capacity and limiting respiratory muscle demands. Only when respiratory muscle capacity exceeds demands will attempts to wean mechanical ventilation be successful.

Many factors associated with decreased respiratory muscle capacity have been recognized in infants with CLD. Oxygen delivery to the muscles may be compromised by several factors: inadequate arterial hemoglobin quantity and

Table 6.7. Factors That May Contribute to Respiratory Muscle Pump Failure

Decreased respiratory muscle capacity
Decreased oxygen supply
Cardiac failure
Decreased arterial oxygen content
Hyperinflation
Malnutrition
Electrolyte abnormalities
Respiratory acidosis
Respiratory muscle disuse atrophy
Respiratory muscle fatigue
Increased respiratory muscle pump load
Increased ventilatory requirements
Increased dead space ventilation
Increased CO_2 production
Increased work of breathing
Increased resistive load
Increased elastic load
Imposed work
Efficiency of breathing
Increased chest wall compliance
Respiratory pattern

oxygen saturation, decreased myocardial performance, and possibly impaired blood supply to the diaphragm. Diaphragmatic performance is impaired by hyperinflation commonly seen in obstructive lung diseases similar to BPD(249). Electrolyte abnormalities such as hypophosphatemia, hypomagnesemia, hypokalemia, and hypocalcemia may adversely affect respiratory muscle performance(379–381). Respiratory acidosis decreases the contractility and endurance of the diaphragm(382). Prolonged mechanical ventilation in infants has been associated with pathologic evidence of respiratory muscle atrophy(254). Primary respiratory muscle dysfunction has only recently been recognized as a possible cause of failure to wean from mechanical ventilation. Many clinical circumstances predispose infants and children to respiratory muscle dysfunction and respiratory failure(249). Once respiratory muscle dysfunction has resolved, weaning strategies associated with periods of respiratory muscle exercise and periods of rest should be used.

Increases in respiratory muscle load also need to be considered when weaning CLD infants from mechanical ventilation. Increased dead space ventilation is a prominent feature of BPD(200,208), thus attempts to improve the ratio of dead space to tidal volume (tracheostomy, minimizing of positive intrathoracic pressure, optimal pulmonary perfusion) are beneficial. In the setting of elevated dead-space ventilation, small increases in CO_2 production (fever, increased respiratory work, excess carbohydrate load) require large increases in minute ventilation to maintain a stable arterial CO_2 tension. Attempts to reduce the resistive load (tracheostomy, bronchodilators) and elastic load (diuresis, chest physiotherapy) can have profound effects on lung mechanics and decrease the work of breathing. Ventilator circuitry can also impose significant work upon the patient. Two principal types of ventilator circuits are in use clinically: the continuous-flow circuit and the demand-valve circuit(278). Continuous-flow circuits have the least circuit impedance and minimize the work of breathing(383). Newer demand-valve circuits are more efficient and have only slightly higher circuit impedances. These circuits also allow the use of synchronized mechanical ventilation (either volume- or pressure-limited). Modifications to demand-valve circuits (small, noncompliant circuit tubing, proximal airway pressure monitoring, flow triggering) may further improve ventilatory performance and decrease circuit impedance and imposed work of breathing(384). Finally, the highly compliant chest wall and rapid, shallow respiratory pattern of neonates severely decreases ventilatory efficiency and increases the work of breathing.

The ability to liberate the patient successfully from mechanical ventilation depends on improvements in lung mechanics(200,208). A point in the clinical course of these children is reached at which compliance and resistance improve, while minute ventilation and dead-space ventilation remain elevated(385). As the balance between lung mechanics and chest wall strength improve, the efficiency of breathing improves to the point at which the infants are able to sustain the elevated respiratory workload. Attempts to wean before efficiency improves are frequently futile and poorly tolerated by the children.

Many methods of weaning from mechanical support of ventilation have been used in infants and adults with chronic respiratory insufficiency. No single mode of ventilation has been clearly shown to be preferable in comparative trials[386,387]. Although some investigators advocate pressure support ventilation[112], the most commonly used method of weaning infants with BPD from mechanical ventilation is slowly decreasing intermittent mandatory ventilation (IMV) via a continuous-flow circuit[378]. The IMV rate is decreased very slowly (1 breath/min once every several days to weeks). Often, the first signs that the weaning is not tolerated are subtle, such as poor weight gain or irritability, followed by more obvious signs of chronic respiratory failure[111]. Once the IMV rate is decreased to 10 to 15 breaths/min, intermittent continuous positive airway pressure (CPAP) trials during the day are started. These brief periods of CPAP allow training of the diaphragm, interspersed with rest periods to prevent respiratory muscle fatigue. The CPAP trial durations are slowly increased with careful monitoring to the point at which the child is ventilated at night only. Finally, the night ventilation can be withdrawn. It must be emphasized that at any point during the weaning process if the child fails to gain adequate weight, becomes more irritable, shows decreased tolerance for physical activity (feeding, physical and occupational therapy), or shows a worsening in clinical status, the weaning may be progressing too rapidly, or the patient may have developed an intercurrent infection. Weaning must stop, and investigations for infections must be considered. Failure to intervene early frequently results in a significant setback in all aspects of the child's care and delays further weaning for weeks or months.

Infections, particularly respiratory infections, are potentially dangerous or lethal to children with CLD. It is essential that attempts to minimize this risk are used as much as possible[341]. As previously mentioned, RSV is a significant respiratory pathogen with profound consequences in infants with CLD[257,258,388]. Nosocomial spread of RSV infection has been noted in these patients[388]. Ribavirin, a synthetic nucleoside with antiviral activity, has been shown in controlled clinical trials to decrease clinical severity scores and oxygen requirement in normal infants and in those with BPD[389,390]. The clinical improvements were not associated with shorter hospitalization. Many institutions have treated ventilated infants; some recent studies show significant improvement in clinical symptoms and shorter duration of ventilation, oxygen supplementation, and hospitalization[391,392]. Based principally upon this information, the Committee on Infectious Disease recommends the use of ribavirin in children with CLD and documented RSV infection. More recent examination in a blind, placebo, controlled study failed to show any benefit of ribavirin administration[393]. Thus, it appears that the use of ribavirin remains controversial and at the discretion of the individual clinician.

It has been noted that sudden unexpected late deaths contributed significantly to mortality in older infants with severe BPD after prolonged mechanical ventilation[394]. The mechanics underlying the sudden nature of the deaths of these infants remains unclear. Recurrent cyanotic spells and multiple episodes of unexplained fevers were common. Other investigators have also noted the association between poor outcome and recurrent cyanotic spells in infants with BPD who have required intermittent muscle paralysis or long-term sedation[395,396]. Myocardial hypertrophy, polypharmacy with methylxanthines and adrenergic agonists, and hypoxia may have led to an acute pulmonary vascular crisis and sudden death[341]. Recurrent, profound cyanotic episodes and sudden, unexplained death in response to a stimulus such as pain, fear, or anger have recently been shown to be due to right-to-left intrapulmonary shunting in patients without lung disease[292]. This mechanism could also apply to patients with underlying lung disease and preexisting elevations in pulmonary vascular resistance and pressure. Finally, acute bronchospasm leading to life-threatening respiratory acidosis and later sudden death despite advanced cardiopulmonary resuscitation has also been reported[397].

Because of the prolonged complex care these infants require, home discharge must be planned well in advance. Occasionally, circumstances permit discharge while an infant is receiving mechanical ventilation. However, medical stability must be an absolute criterion before contemplating home mechanical ventilation. The very real incidence of sudden death in this patient population makes this recommendation all the more important[398].

Most children are discharged home after having been successfully weaned from mechanical ventilation while still requiring supplemental oxygen. The discharge planning meetings should include the primary physicians, nurses, therapists, social workers, parents, and medical staff who will provide ongoing care on an outpatient basis (primary physician, home nurses). A list of tasks must be prepared prior to discharge **(Table 6.8)**. The care providers must master all aspects of the child's care prior to discharge. Clearly defined lines of communication for routine and emergent problems need to be established. Discharge to home frequently results in considerable savings in health care costs; decreased risk of severe, nosocomial infection; and better infant-parent bonding and therefore should be accomplished as soon as medically feasible.

Acute Decompensation in CLD

Infants with CLD are frequently readmitted to the hospital during the first 2 years of life[255]. Because of the marginal pulmonary reserves in infants with BPD, almost any infection (e.g., otitis media, viral gastroenteritis) may precipitate acute respiratory failure[202]. The most common reason for readmission to the hospital is an acute viral lower respiratory tract illness that frequently leads to acute respiratory failure[205,256,286]. The viral etiology, as mentioned earlier,

Table 6.8. Tasks for Discharge Planning

Training of care providers
Resuscitation
Medical therapy
Nutritional requirement
Medications
Respiratory therapy
Oxygen equipment
Suction
Chest physiotherapy
Physical and occupational therapy
Equipment
Monitors
Oxygen supply
Resource notification
Insurance company (financial assistance)
Fire department (paramedics)
Electric and phone companies
Nearest hospital (emergency department)
Identify ongoing care providers
Community physician
Hospital physician (pulmonologist)
Nursing services
Other services
Follow-up planning
Emergency planning

is commonly RSV; however, influenza, adenovirus, and parainfluenza virus have also been responsible for readmission. Unfortunately, no specific data are available regarding PICU admissions for children with CLD.

The typical clinical presentation of an infant with respiratory distress includes tachypnea, wheezing, retractions, and feeding intolerance. Hypoxemia is common, while in severe cases acute hypercarbia and overt respiratory failure may occur. Because of the chronic nature of their lung disease, initial arterial blood gas and chest radiograph interpretation may be difficult. Significant hypoxia (hemoglobin saturation less than 90%) and acute respiratory acidosis as indicated by hypercapnia with acidosis should be emergently treated with endotracheal intubation and mechanical ventilation.

A detailed description of the acute ventilatory management of the child with respiratory failure is beyond the scope of this discussion (see Chapter 9). Provision of mechanical ventilatory assistance should be accompanied by maintenance of adequate oxygen delivery with as little risk of oxygen toxicity and barotrauma as possible. Meticulous airway management to minimize further potential injury to the airway is essential. Fluid overload and bronchospasm should be aggressively treated as previously outlined. The precipitating infectious agent should be identified and treated as soon as possible.

Readmission to the hospital is commonly associated with many psychosocial concerns. The parents frequently believe that they have failed in their care because their child became ill. Furthermore, the parents may be unfamiliar with the staff, procedures, and routines in the PICU, which may lead to difficulties with interactions between the care providers and parents. Awareness of these problems and a supportive role are key to helping the family through the trying times associated with the acute illness.

Finally, the acute illness may have profound effects on the overall health of the child. Although the sequelae of the acute infectious process may resolve in several days, it is not uncommon for the chronically ill infant to take several weeks to return to his or her pre-illness condition. Attempts to minimize further lung injury while providing adequate nutritional support to maintain lung growth are vital.

FUTURE TRENDS

Biochemists, molecular biologists, and physiologists have greatly expanded our understanding of CLD in infancy. This discussion has shown that this complex, multifactorial disease will not be successfully treated with any single magic bullet such as surfactant replacement[22,23], antioxidants[37,38,131], anti-inflammatory agents[38,356,360], or mode of ventilation[16,114]. Therapeutic interventions must be aimed at preventing (improved prenatal and intrapartum care) or inhibiting (surfactant replacement, anti-inflammatory, antioxidant, antiadhesion molecule, and antiprotease agents) the primary and secondary lung injury while modifying the lung response to injury to promote normal healing. With a better understanding of the pathophysiologic events associated with BPD in infants, our ability to define high-risk populations has improved[27–29], thus facilitating future scientific study in randomized clinical trials of interventions aimed at this disease. Infants with BPD will continue to constitute a significant proportion of children requiring care in the pediatric critical care units well into the next century.

CLD IN CHILDREN

Chronic respiratory disease that develops in childhood is a relatively common cause for admission to the PICU. Most of these admissions are caused by common illnesses discussed in separate chapters in this text (upper airway disease, Chapter 2; lower airway disease, Chapter 5; neuromuscular disease, Chapter 8). Less common diseases can result in CLD developing in childhood and may occasionally lead to respiratory insufficiency or overt failure, requiring admission to the PICU. These rare diseases can be divided into two broad categories: genetic and acquired.

Genetic

Cystic Fibrosis

Cystic fibrosis (CF) is the most common, lethal, hereditary disorder in the United States. The incidence of the disease is roughly 1 in 2,500 live births, and 1 in 20 whites is a heterozygote. Although the genetic basis of CF was discovered in 1989[399], with a single mutation accounting for 60 to 70% of cases, it is now recognized that more than 250 mutations cause CF. The severe pulmonary phenotype does not correlate well with any specific mutation. With the characterization of the cystic fibrosis transmembrane conductance regulator (CF gene product), it has been demonstrated that CF is caused by the defective activation of a cyclic adenosine monophosphate-dependent ion channel. A concomitant increased reabsorption of sodium occurs, with resultant dehydration of intraluminal fluids. The clinical manifestations of CF primarily involve the lung, intestinal tract, pancreas, and liver. Respiratory symptoms predominate, with thick mucus, chronic infections, and inflammation. Absent exocrine function of the pancreas leads to malabsorption, with associated poor somatic growth. Liver failure and diabetes may also occur. The average cost, not including human suffering, for one year of care for a CF patient is more than $27,000.

With the aggressive use of antibiotic and pulmonary toilet, the average life span of a child born with CF has increased to 27 years in the United States. Children born today with CF can expect to live into their 40s. In an attempt to decrease sodium reabsorption, aerosolized amiloride is now in clinical trials[(400)] and appears promising. Dornase Alfa (rhDNase) has been shown to decrease viscoelasticity of inspissated secretions in patients with CF and cause a significant improvement in forced expiratory volume in one second compared with controls in phase III trials[(401)]. Clinical studies are currently underway to evaluate cDNA transfer to pulmonary epithelial cells using recombinant adenovirus. A heart-lung or single/double lung transplantation has been offered to end-stage CF patients with only moderate success. Survival statistics for 1 year are between 40 and 70%[(402–407)], with rejection, infection, and bronchiolitis obliterans accounting for most of the deaths. Children with CF are admitted to the PICU for acute reversible complications of their disease (i.e., pneumothoraces), procedures (i.e., central line placement), or for postoperative care and complications of their heart lung transplant (e.g. pulmonary infection, acute rejection).With the increase in number of these patients receiving lung transplantation, pediatric intensivists may see many more of these patients in the ICU than in the past.

Dyskinetic Cilia Syndrome

Immotile cilia syndrome, or ciliary dyskinesis, is a rare disorder; there are two forms: genetic and acquired. The triad of bronchiectasis, sinusitis, and situs inversus (Kartagener's syndrome) has been long recognized as the genetic form and is associated with symptoms of recurrent pulmonary infection and sinusitis from early age (e.g., 1 month). Those with the acquired form generally become symptomatic at a later age. Pneumonia with associated respiratory failure is the most common cause for admission of these patients to the PICU.

The ciliary defect can be at any part of the microtubular apparatus or may not be evident with electron microscopy (EM) and may involve abnormal flagellar beat frequency. Diagnosis is made by demonstrating abnormal ciliary microtubule ultrastructure on EM or abnormal ciliary wave form from a nasopharyngeal brushing. The mainstay of treatment involves inhaled β-agonists and postural drainage. Aggressive antibiotic use is also critical. Early ear, nose, and throat involvement for myringotomy tubes and sinus windows is controversial. Surgical resection of areas of bronchiectasis is generally contraindicated secondary to the diffuse nature of this disease. Prognosis is generally good, with most patients achieving a normal life span.

Acquired

Pulmonary Hemosiderosis

Pulmonary hemosiderosis (PH) is a rare clinical syndrome characterized by recurrent episodes of respiratory distress and patchy infiltrates on chest radiograph, with concomitant iron deficiency anemia. PH is a diagnosis of exclusion; Goodpasture's syndrome, systemic lupus erythematosus, mixed connective tissue disease, and Wegener's granulomatosis have a similar presentation. The diagnosis is made by finding hemosiderin-laden macrophages on BAL or open lung biopsy. Acute treatment includes bronchodilators, oxygen, and transfusions as necessary. Antibiotic use is frequent secondary to difficulty discerning pneumonia from a new bleeding episode. Acute pulmonary hemorrhage associated with a lower respiratory tract infection and respiratory failure can lead to frequent PICU admissions. Mechanical ventilation with positive-end expiratory pressure is often necessary to treat refractory hypoxemia due to intraalveolar blood. Prognosis is variable, with some patients having one episode and others having recurrent bleeds and subsequent pulmonary fibrosis.

Interstitial Lung Disease

The term *interstitial lung disease* (ILD) describes a heterogeneous group of more than 150 pulmonary disorders in which both the alveolar walls and adjacent interstitial tissue are inflamed and fibrotic. Causes of ILD include infections, environmental exposure, connective-tissue disorders, iatrogenic disorders, cardiopulmonary disease, or disorders associated with a systemic disease **(Table 6.9).** The incidence of ILD in children is unknown but thought to be rare. An injury to the lung leads to chronic inflammation and recruitment of leukocytes, with resultant fibrosis and alteration of pulmonary parenchymal cells. ILD is categorized by histologic criteria based on cellular content and pattern of inflammation (desquamative interstitial pneumonitis [DIP], lymphocytic interstitial pneumonitis [LIP]). Children with ILD can have dyspnea, dry cough, failure to thrive, or tachypnea. Cyanosis is often present at the time of diagnosis. Symptoms are often insidious. A thorough history may give clues to the underlying cause (e.g., toxic exposures). Diagnosis is made by a combination of chest radiograph demonstrating linear or reticular shadows, clinical examination, and history of insidious onset without clear etiology. CT scans of the chest may show a ground-glass appearance (alveolar proteinosis), irregular linear pattern (idiopathic pulmonary fibrosis), cystic pattern (lymphangiomatosis), or a nodular pattern (sarcoidosis, etc). BAL may be of value by demonstrating the presence of *Pneumocystis carinii*, cytomegalovirus, fungi, or *Legionella pneumophila*.

The diagnostic procedure of choice, however, remains the open lung biopsy, with the site of biopsy often guided by results of chest CT scans. A definitive diagnosis is found in >90% of open lung biopsies[408], while clinical criteria alone are correct only 55 to 60% of the time. Treatment of ILD is directed at reducing inflammation and restoring normal gas exchange. Corticosteroids are used in the treatment of DIP and LIP with response rates of approximately 60%[409]. Use of other chemotherapeutic agents (e.g., cyclophosphamide) have occasionally been successful in individual cases. Lung transplantation for these patients is controversial. Children with ILD are often admitted to the PICU for refractory hypoxemia and often require positive-pressure mechanical ventilation. The high mean airway pressure required to maintain adequate arterial oxygen saturation place these patients at extreme risk for development of pneumothoraces and pulmonary interstitial emphysema. Long-term prognosis depends on the underlying cause of the ILD and the extent of lung involvement.

Table 6.9. The Differential Diagnosis of Interstitial Lung Disease in Children

Infections	Oxygen toxicity
Mycobacteria	Radiation fibrosis
Viruses	Drug toxicity
Cytomegalovirus	Chemotherapy
Epstein-Barr virus	Busulfan
Respiratory syncytial virus	Bleomycin
Adenovirus	Cyclophosphamide
Influenza/parainfluenza	Methotrexate
virus	Mitomycin
Pneumocystis carinii	Nitrosourens (BCNU)
Mycoplasma pneumoniae	Procarbazine
Chlamydia trachomatis	Antibiotics
Legionella pneumoniae	Nitrofurantoin Penicillin
Ureaplasma urealyticum	Sulfonamides
Fungi	Others
Coxiella burnetii	Carbamazine
Environmental Causes	Diphenylhydantoin
Organic dusts	Gold salts
Toxic gases (NO_2, SO_2, Br, Cl)	Propranolol
Insecticides	Interstitial Pneumonitis
Connective Tissue Disorders	Usual interstitial pneumonitis
Systemic lupus erythematosus	(UIP)
Rheumatoid arthritis	Desquamative interstitial
Systemic Sclerosis	pneum. (DIP)
Sjogren syndrome	Lymphocytic infiltrative
Ankylosing spondylitis	disorders
(LIP)	Lymphocytic interstitial
Inflammatory bowel disease	pneum.
Cardiopulmonary Disease	Pulmonary lymphoid
Chronic pulmonary emboli	hyperplasia
Chronic pulmonary edema	Nodular lymphoid
Veno-occlusive disease	hyperplasia
Arteriolitis	Follicular bronchiolitis
Congenital anomalies	Idiopathic pulmonary
Anomalous pulm. venous	fibrosis
return	Bronchiolitis obliterans
Pulmonary vein stenosis	Specific Disorders
Nonspecific Disorders	Sarcoidosis
Malignant neoplasms	Amyloidosis
"Allergic" reactions	Alveolar proteinosis
Telangectasia/lymphangiectasia	Pulmonary hemosiderosis
Aspiration syndromes	Wegeners granulomatosis
Immunodeficiency diseases	Goodpasture's syndrome
Histiocytic diseases	Pulmonary
Adverse Response to	Neurocutaneous disorders
Therapy	Idiopathic/unclassified

Bronchiectasis

Bronchiectasis is the result of unresolved acute airway injury, primarily of infectious origin[410]. The injury leads to distortion of the bronchial architecture, with resultant impairment of the mucociliary apparatus. Chronic bacterial infection with low-virulence organisms *(e.g., Pseudomonas)* follows, with destruction of the elastic supporting tissue. Bronchiectasis is characterized by dilated bronchi, with acute and chronic inflammation and associated fibrosis. In the later stages of the disease, multiple microabscesses are seen in peribronchial tissue. Clinical manifestations include cough, dyspnea, hemoptysis, rhonchi, with pulmonary hemorrhage and cyanosis in some patients. Cystic changes and alternating hyperinflation and atelectasis are seen on chest radiograph. Chest CT, bronchoscopy, or a bronchogram demonstrate the dilated bronchi and thickened bronchial walls. Treatment is directed at interrupting the cycle of inflammation and infection. Identification and treatment of the primary disease process (chronic aspiration) is essential. High-dose antibiotics (used to decrease bacterial colonization), bronchodilators, and postural drainage are the mainstay of treatment. Surgical resection of affected areas is generally avoided secondary to the diffuse nature of this disease. Patients with bronchiectasis are seen in the PICU with acute exacerbations of their disease, with purulent material spilling into normal airways, many requiring mechanical ventilation. Prognosis depends on initial cause of the disease (e.g., CF) and the extent of lung involvement.

CONCLUSIONS

The management of CLD in infants and children is both challenging and frustrating to the pediatric intensivist. The frequent admissions during the winter months for acute pulmonary decompensation are often unavoidable and generate a considerable amount of financial and emotional strain on the families of these patients. Some newer therapies on the horizon may lead to fewer of these children requiring intensive care, but at present the trend toward greater resource use by this unfortunate group of pulmonary patients is likely to continue.

References

1. Northway WH Jr, Rosan RC, Porter DY. Pulmonary disease following respirator therapy of hyaline-membrane disease. N Engl J Med 1967;276:357.
2. Swaminathan S, Quinn J, Stabile MW, Bader D, Platzker ACG, Keens TG. Long-term pulmonary sequelae of meconium aspiration syndrome. J Pediatr 1989;114:356.
3. Hageman JR, Adams MA, Gardner TH. Pulmonary complications of hyperventilation therapy for persistent pulmonary hypertension. Crit Care Med 1985;13:1013.
4. Ghutani VK, Abbasi S, Weiner S. Neonatal pulmonary manifestations due to prolonged amniotic leak. Am J Perinatol 1986;3:225.
5. Northway WH Jr. Observations on bronchopulmonary dysplasia. J Pediatr 1979;95:815.
6. Danus O, Casar C, Larrain A, Pope CE. Esophageal reflux—an unrecognized cause of recurrent obstructive bronchitis in children. J Pediatr 1976;89:220.
7. Whitley RJ, Brafsield D, Reynolds DW, Stagno S, Tiller RE, Alford CA. Protracted pneumonitis in young infants associated with perinatally acquired cytomegaloviral infection. J Pediatr 1976;89:16.
8. Wilson M, Mikity VG. A new form of respiratory disease in premature infants. Am J Dis Child 1960;99:489.
9. Krauss AN, Klain DB, Auld PAM. Chronic pulmonary insufficiency of prematurity (CPIP). Pediatrics 1975;55:55.
10. Fujimura M, Takeuchi T, Kitajima H, Nakayama M. Chorioamnionitis and serum IgM in Wilson-Mikity syndrome. Arch Dis Child 1989; 64:1379.
11. Bancalari E, Gerhardt T. Bronchopulmonary dysplasia. Pediatr Clin North Am 1986;33:1.
12. Shennan AT, Dunn MS, Ohlsson A, Lennox K, Hoskins EM. Abnormal pulmonary outcomes in premature infants: prediction from oxygen requirement in the neonatal period. Pediatrics 1988;82:527.
13. Troug WE, Jackson C, Badura RJ, Sorensen GK, Murphy JH, Woodrum DE. Bronchopulmonary dysplasia and pulmonary insufficiency of prematurity. Am J Dis Child 1985;139:351.
14. Greenspan JS, Abbasi S, Bhutani VK. Sequential changes in pulmonary mechanics in the very low birth weight (< 1000 grams) infant. J Pediatr 1988;113:732.
15. Parker RA, Lindstrom DP, Cotton RB. Improved survival accounts for most, but not all of the increase in Bronchopulmonary Dysplasia. Pediatrics 1992;90:663.
16. Avery ME, Tooley WH, Keller JB, Hurd SS, et al. Is chronic lung disease in low birth weight infants preventable? A survey of eight centers. Pediatrics 1987;79:26.
17. Shankaran S, Szego E, Eizert D, Siegel P. Severe Bronchopulmonary Dysplasia: Predictors of survival and Outcome. Chest 1984; 86:607.
18. Rojas MA, Gonzalez A, Bancalari E, Claure N, Poole C, Silva-Neto. Changing trends in the epidemiology and pathogenesis of neonatal chronic lung disease. J Pediatr 1995;126:605.
19. Kraybill EN, Runyan DK, Bose CL, Khan JH. Risk factors for chronic lung disease in infants with birth weights of 751 to 100 grams. J Pediatr 1989;115:115.
20. Corcoran JD, Patterson CC, Thomas PS, Halliday HL. Reduction in the risk of bronchopulmonary dysplasia from 1980-1990: results of multivariate logistic regression analysis. Eur J Pediatr 1993; 152:677.
21. Kendig JW, Notter RH, Cox C, Aschner JL, Benn S, et al. Surfactant replacement therapy at birth: final analysis of a clinical trial and comparisons with similar trials. Pediatrics 1988;82:756.
22. Horbar JD, Soll RF, Sutherland JM, Kotagal U, et al. A multicenter randomized, placebo-controlled trial of surfactant therapy for respiratory distress syndrome. N Engl J Med 1989;320:959.
23. Soll RF, Hoekstra RE, Fangman JJ, Corbet AJ, et al. Multicenter trial of single-dose modified bovine surfactant extract (Survanta) for prevention of respiratory distress syndrome. Pediatrics 1990;85:1092.
24. Schwartz RM, Luby AM, Scanlon JW, Kellogg RJ. Effect of surfactant on morbidity, mortality, and resource use in newborn infants weighing 500 to 1500 g. N Engl J Med 1994;330:1476.
25. Gortner L, Bartmann P, Pohlandt F, et al. Early treatment of respiratory distress syndrome with bovine surfactant in very preterm infants: a multicenter controlled clinical trial. Pediatr Pulmonol 1992,14:4.
26. Egberts J, de Winter JP. Meta-analysis of surfactant and bronchopulmonary dysplasia revisited. Lancet 1994;344:882.
27. Palta M, Gabbert D, Fryback D, Widjaja I, et al. Development and validation of an index for scoring baseline respiratory disease in the very low birth weight neonate. Pediatrics 1990;86:714.
28. Sinkin RA, Cos C, Phelps DL. Predicting risk for bronchopulmonary dysplasia: selection criteria for clinical trials. Pediatrics 1990; 86:728.
29. Dunn MS. Predicting risk for bronchopulmonary dysplasia. Pediatrics 1990;86:788.
30. O'Brodovich HM, Mellins RB. Bronchopulmonary dysplasia. Unresolved neonatal acute lung injury. Am Rev Respir Dis 1985; 132:694.
31. Goetzman BW. Understanding bronchopulmonary dysplasia. Am J Dis Child 1986;140:330.
32. Wung JT, Koons AH, Driscoll JM Jr, James LS. Changing incidence of bronchopulmonary dysplasia. J Pediatr 1979;95:845.
33. Meyrick B, Reid L. Pulmonary arterial and alveolar development in normal postnatal rat lung. Am Rev Respir Dis 1982;125:468.
34. Bhutani VK, Shaffer TH. Time-dependent tracheal deformation in fetal, neonatal, and adult rabbits. Pediatr Res 1982;16:830.
35. Coalson JJ, Kuehl TJ, Prihoda TJ, DeLemos RA. Diffuse alveolar damage in the evolution of bronchopulmonary dysplasia in the baboon. Pediatr Res 1988;24:357.
36. Farrell PM, Avery ME. Hyaline membrane disease. Am Rev Respir Dis 1975;111:657.
37. Frank L, Sosenko IRS. Development of lung antioxidant enzyme system in late gestation: possible implications for the prematurely born infant. J Pediatr 1987;110:9.
38. Frank L, Lewis PL, Sosenko IRS. Dexamethasone stimulation of fetal rat lung antioxidant enzyme activity in parallel with surfactant stimulation. Pediatrics 1985;75:569.
39. Frank L, Groseclose EE. Preparation for birth into an O_2-rich environment: the antioxidant enzymes in the developing rabbit lung. Pediatr Res 1984;18:240.
40. Frank L, Lewis PL, Garcia-Pons T. Intrauterine growth-retarded rat pups show increased susceptibility to pulmonary O_2 toxicity. Pediatr Res 1985;19:281.
41. Frank L, Groseclose E. Oxygen toxicity in newborn rats: the adverse effects of undernutrition. J Appl Physiol 1982;53:1248.
42. Hustead VA, Gutcher GR, Anderson SS, et al. Relationship of vitamin A (retinol) status to lung disease in the preterm infant. J Pediatr 1984;105:610.
43. Shenai JP, Chytil F, Stahlman MT. Vitamin A status of neonates with bronchopulmonary dysplasia. Pediatr Res 1985;19:185.
44. Wong YC, Buck RC. An electron microscopic study of metaplasia of the rat tracheal epithelium in vitamin A deficiency. Lab Invest 1971;24:55.
45. Shenai JP, Kennedy KA, Chytil F, Stahlman MT. Clinical trial of vitamin A supplementation in infants susceptible to bronchopulmonary dysplasia. J Pediatr 1987;111:269.
46. Eronen M, Pesonen E, Kurki T, Teramo K, Ylikorkala O, Hallman M. Increased incidence of bronchopulmonary dysplasia after antenatal administration of indomethacin to prevent preterm labor. J Pediatr 1994,124:782.
47. Saugstad OD, Gluck L. Plasma hypoxanthine levels in newborn infants: a specific indicator of hypoxia. J Perinatol Med 1982;10:266.
48. Saugstad OD, Hallman M, Abraham JL, et al. Hypoxanthine and oxygen-induced lung injury: a possible basic mechanism of tissue damage? Pediatr Res 1984;18:501.
49. McCord JM. Oxygen-derived free radicals in postischemic tissue injury. N Engl J Med 1985;312:159.
50. Nickerson BG, Taussig LM. Family history of asthma in infants with bronchopulmonary dysplasia. Pediatrics 1980;65:1140.
51. Bertrand J-M, Riley P, Popkin J, Coates AL. The long-term pulmonary sequelae of prematurity. The role of familial airway hyperreactivity and the respiratory distress syndrome. N Engl J Med 1985; 312:742.
52. Clark DA, Pincus LG, Oliphant M, Hubbell C, Oates RP, Davey FR. HLA - A2 and chronic lung disease in neonates. JAMA 1982; 248:1868.
53. Notter RH, Findelstein JN. Pulmonary surfactant: an interdisciplinary approach. J Appl Physiol 1984;57:1613.
54. James DK, Chiswick ML, Harkes A, Williams M, Hallworth J. Nonspecificity of surfactant deficiency in neonatal respiratory disorders. Br Med J 1984;288:1635.
55. Hallman M, Spragg R, Harrell JH, Moser KM, Gluck L. Evidence of lung surfactant abnormality in respiratory failure. Study of bronchoal-

veolar lavage phospholipids, surface activity, phospholipase activity, and plasma myoinositol. J Clin Invest 1982;70:673.
56. Said SI, Avery ME, Davis RK, Banerjee CM, El-Gohary M. Pulmonary surface activity in induced pulmonary edema. J Clin Invest 1965;44:458.
57. Ikegami M, Jobe A, Jacobs H, Lam R. A protein from airways of premature lambs that inhibits surfactant function. J Appl Physiol 1984;57:1134.
58. Ikegami M, Jacobs H, Jobe A. Surfactant function in respiratory distress syndrome. J Pediatr 1983;102:443.
59. Yukitake K, Brown C, Schlueter MA, Clements JA, Hawgood S. Surfactant apoprotein A modifies the inhibitory effect of plasma proteins on surfactant activity in vivo. Pediatr Res 1995;37:21.
60. Coalson JJ, King RJ, Yang F, et al. SP-A deficiency in primate model of bronchopulmonary dysplasia with infection. Am J Respir Crit Care Med 1995;151:854.
61. van Iwaarden F, Welmers B, et al. Pulmonary surfactant protein A enhances host-defense mechanism of rate alveolar macrophages. Am J Respir Cell Mol Biol 1990;2:91.
62. Wright JR, Youmans DC. Pulmonary surfactant protein A stimulates chemotaxis of alveolar macrophages. Am J Physiol 1993;264:L338.
63. Albert RK, Lakshminarayan S, Hildebrandt J, Kirk W, Butler J. Increased surface tension favors pulmonary edema formation in anesthetized dogs' lungs. J Clin Invest 1979;63:1015.
64. Beck KC, Lai-Fook SJ. Alveolar liquid pressure in excised edematous dog lung with increased static recoil. J Appl Physiol 1983;55:1277.
65. Jobe A, Ikegami M, Jacobs H, Jones S, Conway D. Permeability of premature lamb lungs to protein and the effect of surfactant on that permeability. J Appl Physiol 1983;55:169.
66. Jefferies AL, Coates G, O'Brodovich H. Pulmonary epithelial permeability in hyaline-membrane disease. N Engl J Med 1984;311:1075.
67. Robertson CH, Hall DL, Hogg JC. A description of lung distortion due to localized pleural stress. J Appl Physiol 1973;34:344.
68. Rudolph AM, Drorbaugh JE, Auld PAM, et al. Studies on the circulation in the neonatal period: the circulation in the respiratory distress syndrome. Pediatrics 1961;27:551.
69. Lauweryns JM. Hyaline membrane disease: a pathological study of 55 infants. Arch Dis Child 1965;40:618.
70. Stalcup SA, Mellins RB. Mechanical forces producing pulmonary edema in acute asthma. N Engl J Med 1977;297:592.
71. Bland RD. Cord-blood total protein level as a screening aid for the idiopathic respiratory distress syndrome. N Engl J Med 1972;287:9.
72. Coates G, O'Brodovich H, Jefferies AL, Gray GW. Effects of exercise on lung lymph flow in sheep and goats during normoxia and hypoxia. J Clin Invest 1984;74:133.
73. Mahony L, Carnero V, Brett C, Hyemann MA, Clyman RI. Prophylactic indomethacin therapy for patent ductus arteriosus in very-low-birth-weight infants. N Engl J Med 1982;306:506.
74. Gay JH, Daily WJ, Meyer BH, Trump DS, Cloud DT, Molthan ME. Ligation of the patent ductus arteriosus in premature infants: report of 45 cases. J Pediatr Surg 1973;8:677.
75. Ascher DP, Rosen P, Null DM, de Lemos AR, Wheller JJ. Systemic to pulmonary collaterals mimicking patent ductus arteriosus in neonates with prolonged ventilatory courses. J Pediatr 1985;107:282.
76. O'Brodovich H, Coates G. Pulmonary clearance of ^{99m}Tc-DTPA in infants who subsequently develop bronchopulmonary dysplasia. Am Rev Respir Dis 1988;137:210.
77. Groneck P, Gotze-Speer B, Oppermann M, Eiffert H, Speer CP. Association of pulmonary inflammation and increased microvascular permeability during the development of bronchopulmonary dysplasia: a sequential analysis of inflammatory mediators in respiratory fluids of high-risk preterm neonates. Pediatrics 1994;93:712.
78. Egan EA, Nelson RM, Beale EF. Lung solute permeability and lung liquid adsorption in premature ventilated fetal goats. Pediatr Res 1980;14:314.
79. DeSa DJ. Pulmonary fluid content in infants with respiratory distress. J Pathol 1969;97:469.
80. Nilsson R, Grossman G, Robertson B. Lung surfactant and the pathogenesis of neonatal bronchiolar lesions induced by artificial ventilation. Pediatr Res 1978;12:249.
81. Merritt TA, Stuard ID, Puccia J, et al. Newborn tracheal aspirate cytology: classification during respiratory distress syndrome and bronchopulmonary dysplasia. J Pediatr 1981;98:949.
82. Bruce M, Boat T, Martin R, Dearborn D, Fanaroff A. Proteinase inhibitors and inhibitor inactivation in neonatal airways secretions. Chest 1982;81(Suppl):44S.
83. Merritt TA, Cochrane CG, Holcomb K, et al. Elastase and α-proteinase inhibitor activity in tracheal aspirates during respiratory distress syndrome: role of inflammation in the pathogenesis of bronchopulmonary dysplasia. J Clin Invest 1983;72:656.
84. Ogden BE, Murphy SA, Saunders GC, Pathak D, Johnson JD. Neonatal lung neutrophils and elastase/proteinase inhibitor imbalance. Am Rev Respir Dis 1984;130:817.
85. Tate RM, Repine JE. Neutrophils and the adult respiratory distress syndrome. Am Rev Respir Dis 1983;128:552.
86. Flick MR, Perell A, Staub NC. Leukocytes are required for increased lung microvascular permeability after microembolization in sheep. Circ Res 1981;48:344.
87. Brigham KL, Meyrick B. Interactions of granulocytes with the lungs. Circ Res 1984;54:623.
88. Martin WJ II. Neutrophils kill pulmonary endothelial cells by a hydrogen-peroxide-dependent pathway: an *in vitro* model neutrophil-mediated lung injury. Am Rev Respir Dis 1984;130:209.
89. Andrew M, Massicotte-Nolan PM, Karpatkin M. Plasma protease inhibitors in premature infants: influence of gestational age, postnatal age and health status. Proc Soc Exp Biol Med 1983;173:495.
90. Stenmark KR, Eyzaguirre M, Westcott JY, Henson PM, Murphy RC. Potential role of eicosanoids and PAF in the pathophysiology of bronchopulmonary dysplasia. Am Rev Resp Dis 1987;136:770.
91. Mirro R, Armstead W, Leffler C. Increased airway leukotriene levels in infants with severe bronchopulmonary dysplasia. Am J Dis Child 1990;144:160.
92. Martin TR, Altman LC, Albert RK, et al. Leukotriene B_4 production by the human alveolar macrophage: a potential mechanism for amplifying inflammation in the lung. Am Rev Respir Dis 1984;129:106.
93. Merritt TA. Oxygen exposure in the newborn guinea pig lung lavage cell populations, chemotactic and elastase response: a possible relationship to neonatal bronchopulmonary dysplasia. Pediatr Res 1982;16:798.
94. Kundsin RB, Driscoll SG, Monson RR, Yeh C, Biano SA, Cochran WD. Association of *Ureaplasma urealyticum* in the placenta with perinatal morbidity and mortality. N Engl J Med 1984;310:941.
95. Quinn PA, Gillan JE, Markestad T, St John MA, et al. Intrauterine infection with *Ureaplasma urealyticum* as a cause of fatal neonatal pneumonia. Pediatr Infect Dis 1985;4:538.
96. Sanchez PJ, Regan JA. *Ureaplasma urealyticum* colonization and chronic lung disease in low birth weight infants. Pediatr Infect Dis J 1988;7:542.
97. Wang EEL, Frayha H, Watts J, Hammerberg O, et al. Role of *Ureaplasma urealyticum* and other pathogens in the development of chronic lung disease in prematurity. Pediatr Infect Dis J 1988;7:547.
98. Sawyer MH, Edwards DK, Spector SA. Cytomegalovirus infection and bronchopulmonary dysplasia in premature infants. Am J Dis Child 1987;141:303.
99. Hall CB, Kopelman AE, Douglas RG Jr, Geiman JM, Meagher MP. Neonatal respiratory syncytial virus infection. N Engl J Med 1979; 300:393.
100. Fitzhardinge PM, Pape P, Arstikaitis M, Boyle M, et al. Mechanical ventilation of infants of less than 1,501 gm birth weight: health, growth, and neurologic sequelae. J Pediatr 1976;88:531.
101. Kirpalani H, Higa T, Perlman M, Friedberg J, Cutz E. Diagnosis and therapy of necrotizing tracheobronchitis in ventilated neonates. Crit Care Med 1985;13:792.
102. Miller RW, Woo P, Kellman RK, Slagle TS. Tracheobronchial abnormalities in infants with bronchopulmonary dysplasia. J Pediatr 1987;111:779.
103. Schellhase DE, Graham LM, Fix EJ, Sparks LM, Fan LL. Diagnosis of tracheal injury in mechanically ventilated premature infants by flexible bronchoscopy. A pilot study. Chest 1990;98:1219.
104. Taghizadeh A, Reynolds OR. Pathogenesis of bronchopulmonary dysplasia following hyaline membrane disease. Am J Pathol 1976;82:241.
105. Bonikos DS, Bensch KG, Northway WH Jr, Edwards DK. Bronchopulmonary dysplasia: the pulmonary pathologic sequel of necrotizing bronchiolitis and pulmonary fibrosis. Hum Pathol 1976;7:643.
106. McAdams AJ, Coen R, Kleinman LI, et al. The experimental production of hyaline membranes in premature rhesus monkeys. Am J Pathol 1973;70:277.
107. Lachman B, Johnson B, Lindroth M, et al. Modes of artificial ventilation in severe respiratory distress syndrome: lung function and morphology in rabbits after wash-out of alveolar surfactant. Crit Care Med 1982;10:724.
108. O'Brodovich H, Forrest JB, Newhouse MT. Ciliary defects associated with the development of bronchopulmonary dysplasia. Am Rev Respir Dis 1984;129:190.

109. Bancalari E, Gerhardt T. Bronchopulmonary dysplasia. Ped Clin North America 1986;33:1.
110. Hansen TN, Gest AL. Oxygen toxicity and other ventilatory complications of treatment of infants with persistent pulmonary hypertension. Clin Perinatol 1984;11:653.
111. Marini JJ. The physiological determinants of ventilator dependence. Respir Care 1986;31:271.
112. Katz R, McWilliams B. Bronchopulmonary dysplasia in the pediatric intensive care unit. Crit Care Clin 1988;4:755.
113. Watts JL, Ariagno RI, Brady JP. Chronic pulmonary disease in neonates after artificial ventilation: distribution of ventilation and pulmonary interstitial emphysema. Pediatrics 1977;60:273.
114. HIFI study group. High-frequency oscillatory ventilation compared with conventional mechanical ventilation in the treatment of respiratory failure in preterm infants. N Engl J Med 1989;320:88.
115. Pardou A, Vermeylen D, Muller MF, Detemmerman D. High-frequency ventilation and conventional mechanical ventilation in newborn babies with respiratory distress syndrome: a prospective randomized trial. Int Care Med 1993;19:406.
116. Ogawa Y, Miyasaka K, Kawano T, et al. A multicenter randomized trial of high frequency oscillatory ventilation as compared with conventional mechanical ventilation in preterm infants with respiratory failure. Early Hum Dev 1993;32:1.
117. Jackson JC, Truog WE, Standaert TA, et al. Reduction in lung injury after combined surfactant and high-frequency ventilation. Am J Respir Crit Care Med 1994;150:534.
118. Dunn MS, Jefferies AL, Young T, et al. The role of high frequency oscillation in surfactant replacement. In Eklund L, Jonson B, eds. Surfactant and the respiratory tract. Amsterdam: Elsevier Science Publishers 1989:233.
119. Claris O, Lapillonne A, Madinier-Chappat N, Miquet D, Salle BL. Ventilation par oscillation a haute frequence (OHF) apres surfactant au cours de la maladie des membranes hyalines. Cahiers d'anesthesiologie 1994;42:325.
120. Walther FJ, Kuipers IM, Gidding CE, Willebrand D, Buchholtz RTF, Bevers EM. A comparison of high-frequency oscillation superimposed onto backup mechanical ventilation and conventional mechanical ventilation on the distribution of exogenous surfactant in premature lambs. Ped Res. 1987;22:725.
121. Robertson B, Grossman G, Jobe A, Idegami M, Pettenazzo A, Seidner S. Vascular to alveolar leak of iron dextran (120 kD) in the immature ventilated rabbit lung. Ped Res 1989;25:130.
122. Elleau C, Galperine RI, Guenard H, Demarquez JL. Helium-oxygen mixture in respiratory distress syndrome: a double-blind study. J Pediatr 199;122:132.
123. Freeman BA, Crapo JD. Biology of disease. Free radicals and tissue injury. Lab Invest 1982;47:412.
124. Lodato RF. Oxygen toxicity. Crit Care Clin 1990;6:749.
125. Laurenzi GA, Yin S, Guarneri JJ. Adverse effect of oxygen on tracheal mucus flow. N Engl J Med 1968;279:333.
126. Krulewitz AH, Fanburg BL. The effect of oxygen tension on the *in vitro* production and release of angiotensin-converting enzyme by bovine pulmonary artery endothelial cells. Am Rev Respir Dis 1984; 130:866.
127. Kistler GS, Caldwell PR, Weibel ER. Development of fine structural damage to alveolar and capillary lining cells in oxygen-poisoned rat lungs. J Cell Biol 1967;32:605.
128. Anderson WR, Engel RR. Cardiopulmonary sequelae of reparative stages of bronchopulmonary dysplasia. Arch Pathol Lab Med 1983;107:603.
129. Delemos RA, Coalson JJ, Gerstmann DR, Kuehl TJ, Null DM Jr. Oxygen toxicity in the premature baboon with hyaline membrane disease. Am Rev Respir Dis 1987;136:677.
130. McCarthy K, Bhogal M, Nardi M, Hart D. Pathogenic factors in bronchopulmonary dysplasia. Pediatr Res 1984;18:483.
131. Rosenfeld W, Evans H, Concepcion L, Jhaveri R, Schaeffer H, Friedman A. Prevention of bronchopulmonary dysplasia by administration of bovine superoxide dismutase in preterm infants with respiratory distress syndrome. J Pediatr 1984;105:781.
132. Frank L, Bucher JR, Roberts RJ. Oxygen toxicity in neonatal and adult animals of various species. J Appl Physiol 1978;45:699.
133. Strange RC, Cotton W, Fryer AA, Jones P, Bell J, Hume R. Lipid peroxidation and expression of copper-zinc and manganese superoxide dismutase in lungs of premature infants with hyaline membrane disease and bronchopulmonary dysplasia. J Clin Lab Med 1990;116:666.
134. Saldanha RL, Cepeda EE, Poland RL. The effect of vitamin E prophylaxis on the incidence of severity of bronchopulmonary dysplasia. J Pediatr 1982;101:89.
135. Johnson L, Bowen RW Jr, Abbasi S, Herrmann N, et al. Relationship of prolonged pharmacologic serum levels of vitamin E to incidence of sepsis and necrotizing enterocolitis in infants with birth weight 1,500 grams or less. Pediatrics 1985;75:619.
136. Schlenzig JS, Bervoets K, von Loewenich V, Bohles H. Urinary malondialdehyde concentration in preterm neonates: is there a relationship to disease entities of neonatal intensive care? Acta Paediatr 1993; 82:202.
137. Abe MK, Chao T-S, Solway J, Rosner MR, Hershenson MB. Hydrogen peroxide stimulates mitogen-activated protein kinase in bovine tracheal myocytes: implications for human airway disease. Am J Respir Cell Mol Biol 1994;11:577.
138. Jackson RM, Chandler DB, Fulmer JD. Production of arachidonic acid metabolites by endothelial cells in hyperoxia. J Appl Physiol 1986;61:584.
139. Sporn PHS, Murphy TM, Peters-Goldman M. Complex effects of *in vitro* hyperoxia on alveolar macrophage arachidonic acid metabolism. Am J Respir Cell Mol Biol 1990;2:81.
140. Said SI, Foda HD. Pharmacologic modulation of lung injury. Am Rev Respir Dis 1989;139:1553.
141. Chilton FH, Murphy RC. Remodeling of arachidonate-containing phosphoglycerides within the human neutrophil. J Biol Chem 1986; 261:7771.
142. Henderson WR Jr. Eicosanoids and lung inflammation. Am Rev Respir Dis 1987;135:1176.
143. Samuelsson B, Dahlern SE, Lindgren JA, Rouzer CA, Serhan CN. Leukotrienes and lipoxins; structures, biosynthesis, and biological effects. Science 1987;237:1171.
144. Demling RH. Role of prostaglandins in acute pulmonary microvascular injury. Ann N Y Acad Sci 1982;384:517.
145. Gee MH, Perkowski SZ, Tahamont MV, Flynn JT. Arachidonate cyclooxygenase metabolites as mediators of complement-initiated lung injury. Fed Proc 1985;44:46.
146. Malik AB, Perlman MB, Cooper JA, Noonan T, Bizios R. Pulmonary microvascular effects of arachidonic acid metabolites and their role in lung vascular injury. Fed Proc 1985;44:36.
147. Voelkel NF, Stenmark KR, Reeves JT, Mathias MM, Murphy RC. Actions of lipoxygenase metabolites in isolated rat lungs. J Appl Physiol 1984;57:860.
148. Stephenson AH, Lonigro AJ, Hyers TM, Webster RO, Fowler AA. Increased concentration of leukotrienes in bronchoalveolar lavage fluid of patients with ARDS or at risk for ARDS. Am Rev Respir Dis 1988;138:714.
149. Kertesz NJ, Holtzman RB, Adler L, Hageman JR. Evaluation of a leukotrie ne receptor antagonist in prevention of hyperoxic lung injury in newborn rabbits. Prost Leuk Essent Fatty Acids 1992;45:159.
150. Braquet P, Touqui L, Shen TY, Vargaftig BB. Perspectives in platelet-activating factor research. Pharm Rev 1987;39:97.
151. Hamasaki H, Mojarad M, Saga S, Tai HH, Said SI. Platelet-activating factors raises airway and vascular pressures and induces edema in lungs perfused with platelet-free solution. Am Rev Respir Dis 1984;129:742.
152. Chang SW, Fedderson CO, Henson PM, Voelkel NF. Platelet-activating factor mediates hemodynamic changes and lung injury in endotoxin-treated rats. J Clin Invest 1987;79:1498.
153. Kelley J. Cytokines of the lung. Am Rev Respir Dis 1990;141:765.
154. Hosea SF, Brown E, Hammer C, Frank M. Role of complement activation in a model of adult respiratory distress syndrome. J Clin Invest 1980;66:375.
155. Goldblum SE, Sun WL. Tumor necrosis factor-α augments pulmonary arterial transendothelial albumin flux in vitro. Am J Physiol 1990;258:L57.
156. Stephens KE, Ishizaka A, Larrick JW, Raffin TA. Tumor necrosis factor causes increased pulmonary permeability and edema. Am Rev Respir Dis 1988;137:1364.
157. Leeper-Woodford SK, Carey PD, Byrne K, Jenkins JK, et al. Tumor necrosis factor. Alpha and beta subtypes appear in circulation during onset of sepsis-induced lung injury. Am Rev Respir Dis 1991; 143:1076.
158. Goldblum SE, Jay M, Yoneda K, Cohen DA, McClain CJ, Gillespie MN. Monokine-induced acute lung injury in rabbits. J Appl Physiol 1987;63:2093.
159. Rozycki HJ. Elevated productions of Interleukin-1-Beta from alveolar macrophages isolated from newborn rabbits. Biol Neonate 1994;66:93.
160. Goldblum SE, Jay M, Yoneda K, Cohen DA, McClain CJ, Gillespie MN.

Monokine-induced acute lung injury in rabbits. J Appl Physiol 1987;63:2093.
161. Rozycki H. Bronchoalveolar interleukin-1-beta in infants on day 1 of life. South Med J 1994;87:991.
162. Stefano JL, Spear ML, Pearlman SA, Fawcett P, Proujansky R. Soluble interleukin-2 receptor levels in infants with bronchopulmonary dysplasia. Pediatr Pulmonol 1992;14:58.
163. Bagchi A, Viscardi RM, Taciak V, Ensor JE, McCrea K, Hasday JD. Increased activity of interleukin-6 but not tumor necrosis factor-β in lung lavage of premature infants is associated with development of bronchopulmonary dysplasia. Pediatr Res 1994;36:244.
164. Ogden BE, Murphy S, Saunders GC, Johnson JD. Lung lavage of newborns with respiratory distress syndrome. Prolonged neutrophil influx is associated with bronchopulmonary dysplasia. Chest 1983; 83(Suppl):31S.
165. Bruce MC, Wedig KE, Jentoft N, et al. Altered urinary excretion of elastin cross-links in premature infants who develop bronchopulmonary dysplasia. Am Rev Respir Dis 1985;131:568.
166. Walti H, Tordet C, Gerbaut L, Saugier P, Moriette G, Relier JP. Persistent elastase/proteinase inhibitor imbalance during prolonged ventilation of infants with bronchopulmonary dysplasia: evidence for the role of nosocomial infections. Pediatr Res 1989;26:351.
167. Fantone JC, Feltner DE, Brieland JK, Ward PA. Phagocytic cell-derived inflammatory mediators and lung disease. Chest 1987;91:428.
168. Bevilacqua MP, Nelson RM, Mannori G, Cecconi O. Endothelial-leukocyte adhesion molecules in human disease. Annu Rev Med 1994;45:361.
169. Wortel CH, Doerschuk. Neutrophils and neutrophil-endothelial cell adhesion in adult respiratory distress syndrome. New Horizons 1993;1:631.
170. Walsh CJ, Leeper-Woodford SK, Carey D, et al. CD18 adhesion receptors, tumor necrosis factor, and neutropenia during septic lung injury. J Surg Res 1991;50:323.
171. Hill PA, Lan HY, Nikolic-Paterson DJ, Atkins RC. Pulmonary expression of ICAM-1 and LFA-1 in experimental Goodpasture's syndrome. Am J Path ol 1994;145:220.
172. Talbott GA, Sharar SR, Harlan JM, Winn RK. Leukocyte-endothelial interactions and organ injury: the role of adhesion molecules. New Horizons 1994;2:545.
173. Donnelly SC, Haslett C, Dransfield I, et al. Role of selectins in development of adult respiratory distress syndrome. Lancet 1994;344:215.
174. Mulligan MS, Miyasaka M, Tamatani T, Jones ML, Ward PA. Requirements for L-selectin in Neutrophil-mediated lung injury in rats. J Immunol 1994;152:832.
175. Mulligan MS, Paulson JC, DeFrees S, Zheng Z, Lowe JB, Ward PA. Protective effects of oligosaccharides in P-selectin-dependent lung injury. Nature 1993;364:149.
176. Carlos TM, Harlan JM. Leukocyte-endothelial adhesion molecules. Blood 1994;84:2068.
177. Kojima T, Sasai M, Kobayashi Y. Increased soluble ICAM-1 in tracheal aspirates of infants with bronchopulmonary dysplasia. Lancet 1993;342:1023.
178. Watterberg KL, Scott SM. Evidence of early adrenal insufficiency in babies who develop bronchopulmonary dysplasia. Pediatrics 1995; 95:120.
179. Anderson WR, Engel RR. Cardiopulmonary sequelae of reparative stages of bronchopulmonary dysplasia. Arch Pathol Lab Med 1983;107:603.
180. Snyder LS, Hertz MI, Harmon KR, Bitterman PB. Failure of lung repair following acute lung injury. Regulation of the fibroproliferative response (part 1). Chest 1990;98:733.
181. Snyder LS, Hertz MI, Harmon KR, Bitterman PB. Failure of lung repair following acute lung injury. Regulation of the fibroproliferative response (part 2). Chest 1990;98:989.
182. Johnson DE, Georgieff MK. Pulmonary neuroendocrine cells. Their secretory products and their potential roles in health and chronic lung disease in infancy. Am Rev Respir Dis 1989;140:1807.
183. Johnson DE, Lock JE, Elde RP, Thompson TR. Pulmonary neuroendocrine cells in hyaline membrane disease and bronchopulmonary dysplasia. Pediatr Res 1982;16:445.
184. Johnson DE, Kulik TJ, Lock JE, Elde RP, Thompson TR. Bombesin-, calcitonin-, and serotonin-immunoreactive pulmonary neuroendocrine cells in acute and chronic neonatal lung disease. Pediatr Pulmonol 1985;1(Suppl):13.
185. Sunday ME, Kaplan LM, Motoyama E, Chin WW, Spindel ER. Gastrin-releasing peptide (mammalian bombesin) gene expression in health and disease. Lab Invest 1988;59:5.
186. Keith IM, Will JA. Dynamics of the neuroendocrine cell-regulatory peptide system in the lung: specific overview and new results. Exp Lung Res 1982;3:387.
187. Lauweryns JM, Van Lommel A. Morphometric analysis of hypoxia-induced synaptic activity in intrapulmonary neuroepithelial bodies. Cell Tissue Res 1982;226:201.
188. Redick ML, Hung K-S. Quantification of pulmonary neuroneutrophil bodies in pre- and postnatal rabbits. Cell Tissue Res 1984;238:583.
189. Johnson DE, Wobken JD, Landrum BG. Change in bombesin, calcitonin and serotonin immunoreactive pulmonary neuroendocrine cells in cystic fibrosis and after prolonged mechanical ventilation. Am Rev Respir Dis 1988;137:123.
190. Frank L, Sosenko IRS. Undernutrition as a major contributing factor in the pathogenesis of bronchopulmonary dysplasia. Am Rev Respir Dis 1988;138:725.
191. Wong YC, Buck RC. An electron microscopic study of metaplasia of the rat tracheal epithelium in vitamin A deficiency. Lab Invest 1971;24:55.
192. Chandra RK. Nutrition, immunity, and infection: present knowledge and future directions. Lancet 1983;1:688.
193. Wood MW, Seidler FJ, Slotkin TA. Immediate decline in DNA synthesis in neonatal rat lung caused by exposure to 100% oxygen. Res Comm Chem Path Pharm 1993;80:323.
194. Evans MJ, Hackney JD, Bils RF. Effects of high concentration of oxygen on cell renewal in the pulmonary alveoli. Aero Med 1969:1365.
195. Cheney FW, Huang TW, Gronka R. The effects of 50% oxygen on the resolution of pulmonary injury. Am Rev Respir Dis 1980;122:373.
196. Viscardi RM, Broderick K, Sun, C, et al. Disordered pathways of fibrin turnover in lung lavage of premature infants with respiratory distress syndrome. Am Rev Respir Dis 1992;146:492.
197. Margraf LR, Tomashefski JF, Bruce MC, Dahms BB. Morphometric analysis of the lung in bronchopulmonary dysplasia. Am Rev Respir Dis 1991;143:391.
198. Bancalari E, Gerhardt T. Bronchopulmonary dysplasia. Ped Clin NA 1986;33:1.
199. Bryan MH, Hardie MJ, Reilly BJ, Swyer PR. Pulmonary function studies during the first year of life in infants recovering from the respiratory distress syndrome. Pediatrics 1973;52:169.
200. Morray JP, Fox WW, Kettrick RG, Downes JJ. Improvement in lung mechanics as a function of age in the infant with severe bronchopulmonary dysplasia. Pediatr Res 1982;16:290.
201. Gerhardt T, Hehre D, Feller R, Reifenberg L, Bancalari E. Serial determination of pulmonary function in infants with chronic lung disease. J Pediatr 1987;110:448.
202. Tepper RS, Morgan WJ, Cota K, Taussig LM. Expiratory flow limitation in infants with bronchopulmonary dysplasia. J Pediatr 1986; 109:1040.
203. Smyth JA, Tabachnik E, Duncan WJ, Reilly BJ, Levison H. Pulmonary function and bronchial hyperreactivity in long-term survivors of bronchopulmonary dysplasia. Pediatrics 1981;68:336.
204. Bader D, Ramos AD, Lew CD, Piatzker ACG, Stabile MW, Keens TG. Childhood sequelae of infant lung disease: exercise and pulmonary function abnormalities after bronchopulmonary dysplasia. J Pediatr 1987;110:693.
205. Hakulinen AL, Heinonen K, Launsimies E, Kiekara O. Pulmonary function and respiratory morbidity in school-age children born prematurely and ventilated for neonatal respiratory insufficiency. Pediatr Pulmonol 1990;8:226.
206. Blayney M, Kerem E, Whyte H, O'Brodovich H. Bronchopulmonary dysplasia: improvement in lung function between 7 and 10 years of age. J Pediatr 1991;118:201.
207. Northway WH Jr, Moss RB, Carlisle KB, Parker BR, et al. Late pulmonary sequelae of bronchopulmonary dysplasia. N Engl J Med 1990;323:1793.
208. Loeber NV, Morray JP, Kettrick RG, Downes JJ. Pulmonary function in chronic respiratory failure of infancy. Crit Care Med 1980;8:596.
209. Goldman SL, Gerhardt T, Sonni R, Feller R, et al. Early prediction of chronic lung disease by pulmonary function testing. J Pediatr 1983;102:613.
210. Tepper RS, Morgan WJ, Cota K, Wright A, Taussig LM. Physiologic growth and development of the lung during the first year of life. Am Rev Respir Dis 1986;134:513.
211. Kao LC, Warburton D, Platzker ACG, Keens TG. Effect of isoproterenol inhalation on airway resistance in chronic bronchopulmonary dysplasia. Pediatrics 1984;73:509.
212. Rotschild A, Solimano A, Puterman M, Smyth J, Sharma A, Albersheim S. Increased compliance in response to salbutamol in premature

infants with developing bronchopulmonary dysplasia. J Pediatr 1989;115:984.
213. Kao LC, Warburton D, Sargent C, Platzker ACG, Keens TG. Furosemide acutely decreases airways resistance in chronic bronchopulmonary dysplasia. J Pediatr 1983;103:624.
214. Kao LC, Warburton D, Cheng MH, Cedea C, Platzker ACG, Keens TG. Effect of oral diuretics on pulmonary mechanics in infants with chronic bronchopulmonary dysplasia: results of a double-blind crossover sequential trial. Pediatrics 1984;74:37.
215. McCann EM, Lewis K, Deming DD, Donovan JM, Brady JP. Controlled trial of furosemide therapy in infants with chronic lung disease. J Pediatr 1985;106:957.
216. Naulty CM, Horn S, Conry J, Avery GB. Improved lung compliance after ligation of patent ductus arteriosus in hyaline membrane disease. J Pediatr 1978;93:682.
217. Yeh TF, Thalji A, Luken L, Lilien L, Carr I, Pildes RS. Improved lung compliance following indomethacin therapy in premature infants with persistent ductus arteriosus. Chest 1981;80:698.
218. Hordof AJ, Mellins RB, Gersony WM, Steeg CN. Reversibility of chronic obstructive lung disease in infants following repair of ventricular septal defect. J Pediatr 1977;90:187.
219. Motoyama EK. Pulmonary mechanics during early postnatal years. Pediatr Res 1977;11:220.
220. LeSouef PN, Geelhoed GC, Turner DJ, Morgan SEG, Landau LI. Response of normal infants to inhaled histamine. Am Rev Respir Dis 1989;129:62.
221. Montgomery GL, Tepper RS. Changes in airway reactivity with age in normal infants and young children. Am Rev Respir Dis 1990;142:1372.
222. Turner DJ, Morgan SEG, Landau LI, LeSouef PN. Methodological aspects of flow-volume studies in infants. Pediatr Pulmonol 1990;8:289.
223. Stick SM, Turnbull S, Chua HL, Landau LI, LeSouef PN. Bronchial responsiveness to histamine in infants and older children. Am Rev Respir Dis 1990;142:1143.
224. Greenspan JS, DeGiulio PA, Bhutani VK. Airway reactivity as determined by a cold air challenge in infants with bronchopulmonary dysplasia. J Pediatr 1989;114:452.
225. Motoyama EK, Fort MD, Klesh KW, Mutich RL, Guthrie RD. Early onset of airway reactivity in premature infants with bronchopulmonary dysplasia. Am Rev Respir Dis 1987;136:50.
226. Winter R, Collins C, Ruddock PE, Rudd RM. the effect of systemic beta-2 agonist therapy on the pulmonary hypertensive response to chronic hypoxia in rats. Am Rev Respir Dis 1986;134:763.
227. Stocker JT. Pathologic features of long-standing "healed" bronchopulmonary dysplasia: a study of 28 3- to 40-month-old infants. Hum Pathol 1986;17:943.
228. McCubbin M, Frey EE, Wagener JS, Tribby R, Smith WL. Large airway collapse in bronchopulmonary dysplasia. J Pediatr 1989;114:304.
229. Miller RW, Woo P, Kellman RK, Slagle TS. Tracheobronchial abnormalities in infants with bronchopulmonary dysplasia. J Pediatr 1987;111:779.
230. Tay-Uyboco JS, Kwiatkowski K, Cates DB, Kavanagh L, Rigatto H. Hypoxic airway constriction in infants of very low birth weight recovering from moderate to severe bronchopulmonary dysplasia. J Pediatr 1989;115:456.
231. Prendiville A, Green S, Silverman M. Paradoxical response to nebulized salbutamol in wheezy infants assessed by partial expiratory flow-volume curves. Thorax 1987;42:86.
232. Travis J. Oxidants and antioxidants in the lung. Am Rev Respir Dis 1987;135:773.
233. Anderson WR. Bronchopulmonary dysplasia: a correlative study by light, scanning, and transmission electron microscopy. Ultrastruct Pathol 1990;14:221.
234. Erickson AM, de la Monte S, Moore GW, Hutchins GM. The progression of morphologic changes in bronchopulmonary dysplasia. Am J Pathol 1987;127:474.
235. Sobonya RE, Logvinoff MM, Taussig LM, Theriault A. Morphometric analysis of the lung in prolonged bronchopulmonary dysplasia. Pediatr Res 1982;16:969.
236. Wolfson MR, Bhutani VK, Shaffer TH, Bowen FW Jr. Mechanics and energetics of breathing helium in infants with bronchopulmonary dysplasia. J Pediatr 1984;104:752.
237. Yunis KA, Oh W. Effects of intravenous glucose loading on oxygen consumption, carbon dioxide production, and resting energy expenditure in infants with bronchopulmonary dysplasia. J Pediatr 1989;115:127.
238. Kurzner SI, Garg M, Bautista DB, Sargent CW, Bowman CM, Keens TG. Growth failure in bronchopulmonary dysplasia: elevated metabolic rates and pulmonary mechanics. J Pediatr 1988;112:73.
239. Kao LC, Durand DJ, Nickerson BG. Improving pulmonary function does not decrease oxygen consumption in infants with bronchopulmonary dysplasia. J Pediatr 1988;112:616.
240. Kalhan SC, Denne SC. Energy consumption in infants with bronchopulmonary dysplasia. J Pediatr 1990;116:662.
241. Fahey PJ, Hyde RW. "Won't breathe" vs "can't breathe". Detection of depressed ventilatory drive in patients with obstructive pulmonary disease. Chest 1983;84:19.
242. Watts JL, Ariagno RL, Brady JP. Chronic pulmonary disease in neonates after artificial ventilation: distribution of ventilation and pulmonary interstitial emphysema. Pediatrics 1977;60:273.
243. Fleetham JA, Bradley CA, Kryger MH, Anthonisen NR. The effect of low flow oxygen therapy on the chemical control of ventilation in patients with hypoxemic COPD. Am Rev Respir Dis 1980;122:833.
244. Rigatto H, Brady JP, de al Torre-Verduzco R. Chemoreceptor reflexes in preterm infants: I. The effect of gestational and postnatal age on the ventilatory response to inhalation of 100% and 15% oxygen. Pediatrics 1975;55:604.
245. Rigatto H, de la Torre-Verduzco R, Gates DB. Effects of O_2 on the ventilatory response to CO_2 in preterm infants. J Appl Physiol 1975; 39:896.
246. Parks YA, Beardsmore CS, MacFadyen UM, Pallot DJ, et al. The effect of a single breath of 100% oxygen on breathing in infants at 1, 2, and 3 months of age. Am Rev Respir Dis 1991;144:141.
247. Garg M, Kurzner SI, Bautista D, Keens TG. Hypoxic arousal responses in infants with bronchopulmonary dysplasia. Pediatrics 1988;82:59.
248. Werthammer J, Brown ER, Neff RK, Taeusch HW Jr. Sudden infant death syndrome in infants with bronchopulmonary dysplasia. Pediatrics 1982;69:301.
249. Nichols DG. Respiratory muscle performance in infants and children. J Pediatr 1991;118:493.
250. Muller N, Gulston G, Cade D, et al. Diaphragmatic muscle fatigue in the newborn. J Appl Physiol 1979;46:688.
251. Weiner P, Suo J, Fernandez E, Cherniack RM. The effect of hyperinflation on respiratory muscle strength and efficiency in healthy subjects and patients with asthma. Am Rev Respir Dis 1990;141:1501.
252. DeBoeck K, Smith J, Van Lierde S, Van Gijsel D, Devlieger H. Flat chest in survivors of bronchopulmonary dysplasia. Pediatr Pulmonol 1994;18:104.
253. Goldman MD., Pagani M, Trang, H, Praud J, Sartene R, Gaultier C. Asynchronous chest wall movements during non-rapid eye movement and rapid eye movement sleep in children with bronchopulmonary dysplasia. Am R ev Respir Dis 1993;147:1175.
254. Knisely AS, Leal SM, Singer DB. Abnormalities of diaphragmatic muscle in neonates with ventilated lungs. J Pediatr 1988;113:1074.
255. McCormick MC, Shapiro S, Starfield BH. Rehospitalization in the first year of life for high-risk survivors. Pediatrics 1980;66:991.
256. Myers MG, McGuinness GA, Lachenbruch PA, Koonts FP, Hollingshead R, Olson DB. Respiratory illnesses in survivors of infant respiratory distress syndrome. Am Rev Respir Dis 1986;133:1011.
257. Groothuis JR, Salbenblatt CK, Lauer BA. Severe respiratory syncytial virus infection in older children. Am J Dis Child 1990;144:346.
258. Groothuis JR, Gutierrez KM, Lauer BA. Respiratory syncytial virus infection in children with bronchopulmonary dysplasia. Pediatrics 1988;82:199.
259. Berman W Jr, Yabek SM, Dillon T, Burstein R, Corlew S. Evaluation of infants with bronchopulmonary dysplasia using cardiac catheterization. Pediatrics 1982;70:708.
260. Abman SH, Wolfe RR, Accurso FJ, Koops BL, Bowman CM, Wiggins JW Jr. Pulmonary vascular response to oxygen in infants with severe bronchopulmonary dysplasia. Pediatrics 1985;75:80.
261. Berman W Jr, Katz R, Yabek SM, Dillon T, Fripp RR, Papile L-A. Long-term follow-up of bronchopulmonary dysplasia. J Pediatr 1986;109:45.
262. Goodman G, Perkin RM, Anas NG, Sperling DR, Hicks DA, Rowen M. Pulmonary hypertension in infants with bronchopulmonary dysplasia. J Pediatr 1988;112:72.
263. Abman SH, Wolfe RR, Accurso FJ, Koops BL, Bowman CM, Wiggins J W. Pulmonary vascular response to oxygen in infants with severe bronchopulmonary dysplasia. Pediatrics 1985;75:80.
264. Abman SH, Schaffer MS, Wiggins J, Washington R, Manco-Johnson M, Wolfe RR. Pulmonary vascular extraction of circulating norepinephrine in infants with bronchopulmonary dysplasia. Pediatr Pulmonol 1987;3:386.
265. Tomashefski JR Jr, Oppermann HC, Vawter GF, et al. Bronchopulmonary dysplasia: a morphometric study with emphasis on the pulmonary vasculature. Pediatr Pathol 1984;2:469.
266. Bush A, Busst CM, Knight WB, Hishop AA, Haworth SG, Shinebourne

EA. Changes in pulmonary circulation in severe bronchopulmonary dysplasia. Arch Dis Child 1990;65:739.
267. DeSa DJ. Myocardial changes in immature infants requiring prolonged ventilation. Arch Dis Child 1977;52:138.
268. Arnold J, O'Brodovich H, Whyte R, Coates G. Pulmonary thromboemboli following neonatal asphyxia. J Pediatr 1985;106:806.
269. Donnelly WH, Bucciarelli RL, Nelson RM. Ischemic papillary muscle necrosis in stressed newborn infants. J Pediatr 1980;96:295.
270. Perkin RM, Anas NG. Pulmonary hypertension in pediatric patients. J Pediatr 1984;105:511.
271. Vlahakes GJ, Turley K, Hoffman JI. The pathophysiology of failure in acute right ventricular hypertension: hemodynamic and biochemical correlations. Circulation 1981;63:87.
272. Fouron J-C, Le Guennec J-C, Villemant D, Bard H, Perreault G, Davignon A. Value of echocardiography in assessing the outcome of bronchopulmonary dysplasia of the newborn. Pediatrics 1980;65:529.
273. Walsh EP, Laney P, Ellison RC, et al. Electrocardiogram of the premature infant at 1 year of age. Pediatrics 1986;77:353.
274. Newth CJ, Gow RM, Rowe RD. The assessment of pulmonary arterial pressures in bronchopulmonary dysplasia by cardiac catheterization and M-mode echocardiography. Pediatr Pulmonol 1985;1:58.
275. Halliday HL, Dumpit FM, Brady JP. Effects of inspired oxygen on echocardiographic assessment of pulmonary vascular resistance and myocardial contractility in bronchopulmonary dysplasia. Pediatrics 1980;65:536.
276. Alpert BE, Cainey MA, Schidlow DV, Capitanio MA. Effect of oxygen on right ventricular performance evaluated by radionuclide angiography in two young patients with chronic lung disease. Pediatr Pulmonol 1987;3:149.
277. Brownlee JR, Beekman RH, Rosenthal A. Acute hemodynamic effects of nifedipine in infants with bronchopulmonary dysplasia and pulmonary hypertension. Pediatr Res 1988;24:186.
278. Abman SH, Accurso FJ, Bowman CM. Unsuspected cardiopulmonary abnormalities complicating bronchopulmonary dysplasia. Arch Dis Child 1984;59:966.
279. Abman SH, Warady BA, Lum GM, Koops BL. Systemic hypertension in infants with bronchopulmonary dysplasia. J Pediatr 1984;104:928.
280. Fanaroff AA, Martin RJ, Hack M. Long-term outcome of respiratory distress in infants. Respir Care 1991;36:707.
281. Vohr BR, Bell EF, Oh W. Infants with bronchopulmonary dysplasia. Am J Dis Child 1982;136:443.
282. Wheater M, Rennie JM. Poor prognosis after prolonged ventilation for bronchopulmonary dysplasia. Arch Dis Child 1994;71:F210.
283. Shankaran S, Szego E, Eizert D, Siegel P. Severe bronchopulmonary dysplasia. Predictors of survival and outcome. Chest 1984;86:607.
284. Davidson S, Schrayer A, Wielunsky E, Krikler R, Lilos P, Reisner SH. Energy intake, growth, and development in ventilated very-low-birthweight infants with and without bronchopulmonary dysplasia. Am J Dis Child 1990;144:553.
285. Luchi JM, Bennett FC, Jackson JC. Predictors of neurodevelopmental outcome following bronchopulmonary dysplasia. Am J Dis Child 1991;145:813.
286. Sauve RS, Singhal N. Long-term morbidity of infants with bronchopulmonary dysplasia. Pediatrics 1985;76:725.
287. Hahn JS, Tharp BR. The dysmature EEG pattern in infants with bronchopulmonary dysplasia and its prognostic implications. Electroencephalogr Clin Neurophysiol 1990;76:106.
288. Yunis KA, Oh W. Effects of intravenous glucose loading on oxygen consumption, carbon dioxide production, and resting energy expenditure in infants with bronchopulmonary dysplasia. J Pediatr 1989; 115:127.
289. Long JG, Philip AG, Lucy JF. Excessive handling as a cause of hypoxemia. Pediatrics 1980;65:203.
290. Garg M, Kurzner SI, Bautista DB, Keens TG. Clinically unsuspected hypoxia during sleep and feeding in infants with bronchopulmonary dysplasia. Pediatrics 1988;81:635.
291. Southall DP, Thomas M, Gurney A, Lambert HP. Prolonged expiratory apnea and respiratory tract infections in infancy. Early Hum Dev 1988;17:91.
292. Southall DP, Samuels MP, Talbert DG. Recurrent cyanotic episodes with severe arterial hypoxaemia and intrapulmonary shunting: a mechanism for sudden death. Arch Dis Child 1990;65:953.
293. Groothuis JR, Rosenberg AA. Home oxygen promotes weight gain in infants with bronchopulmonary dysplasia. Am J Dis Child 1987;141:992.
294. Furfaro S, Prosmanne J, Bard H. Hemoglobin oxygen dissociation (P_{50}) in bronchopulmonary dysplasia. Biol Neonate 1990;57:72.
295. Holowach J, Thurston DL. Breath-holding spells and anemia. N Engl J Med 1963;268:21.
296. DeMaio JG, Harris MC, Deuber C, Spitzer AR. Effect of blood transfusion on apnea frequency in growing premature infants. J Pediatr 1989;114:1039.
297. Joshi A, Gerhardt T, Shandloff P, Bancalari E. Blood transfusion effect on the respiratory pattern of preterm infants. Pediatrics 1987;80:79.
298. Alverson DC, Isken VH, Cohen RS. Effect of booster blood transfusions on oxygen utilization in infants with bronchopulmonary dysplasia. J Pediatr 1988;113:722.
299. Gomez D-RM, Gerhardt T, Hehre D, Feller R, Bancalari E. Effect of a beta-agonist nebulization on lung function in neonates with increased pulmonary resistance. Pediatr Pulmonol 1986;2:287.
300. Cabal LA, Larrazabai C, Ramanathan R, Durand M, et al. Effects of metaproterenol on pulmonary mechanics, oxygenation, and ventilation in infants with chronic lung disease. J Pediatr 1987;110:116.
301. Kao LC, Durand DJ, Nickerson BG. Effects of inhaled metaproterenol and atropine on the pulmonary mechanics of infants with bronchopulmonary dysplasia. Pediatr Pulmonol 1989;6:74.
302. Brudno DS, Parker DH, Slaton G. Response of pulmonary mechanics to terbutaline in patients with bronchopulmonary dysplasia. Am J Med Sci 1989;297:166.
303. Wilkie RA, Bryan MH. Effect of bronchodilators on airway resistance in ventilator-dependent neonates with chronic lung disease. J Pediatr 1987;111:278.
304. Sosulski R, Abbasi S, Bhutani VK, Fox WW. Physiologic effects of terbutaline on pulmonary function of infants with bronchopulmonary dysplasia. Pediatr Pulmonol 1986;2:269.
305. Kirpalani H, Koren G, Schmidt B, Tan Y, Santos R, Soldin S. Respiratory response and pharmacokinetics of intravenous salbutamol in infants with bronchopulmonary dysplasia. Crit Care Med 1990; 18:1374.
306. Shim C, Williams MH. Bronchial response to oral versus aerosol metaproterenol in asthma. Ann Intern Med 1980;93:428.
307. Aherns RC, Ries RA, Popendorf W, et al. The delivery of therapeutic aerosols through endotracheal tubes. Pediatr Pulmonol 1986;2:19.
308. Santa-Cruz R, Landa J, Hirsch J, Sackner MA. Tracheal mucous velocity in normal man and patients with obstructive lung disease: effects of terbutaline. Am Rev Respir Dis 1974;109:458.
309. Gross NJ, Skorodin MS. Anticholinergic, antimuscarinic bronchodilators. Am Rev Respir Dis 1984;129:865.
310. Logvinoff MM, Lemen RJ, Taussig LM, Lamont BA. Bronchodilators and diuretics in children with bronchopulmonary dysplasia. Pediatr Pulmonol 1985;1:198.
311. Brundage KL, Mohsini KG, Froese AB, Fisher JT. Bronchodilator response to ipratropium bromide in infants with bronchopulmonary dysplasia. Am Rev Respir Dis 1990;142:1137.
312. Stenmark KR, Eyzaguirre M, Remigio L, Seccombe J, Henson PM. Recovery of platelet activating factor and leukotrienes from infants with severe bronchopulmonary dysplasia: clinical improvement with cromolyn treatment [Abstract]. Am Rev Respir Dis 1985;131:A236.
313. Watterberg KL, Murphy S. Failure of cromolyn sodium to reduce the incidence of bronchopulmonary dysplasia: a pilot study. Pediatrics 1993;91:803.
314. Yamamoto C, Kojima T, Sasai M. Matsuzaki S, Kobayashi Y. Disodium cromoglycate in the treatment of bronchopulmonary dysplasia. Acta Paediatr Jpn 1992;34:589.
315. Aranda JV, Turmen T. Methylxanthines in apnea of prematurity. Clin Perinatol 1979;6:87.
316. Harris MC, Baumgart S, Rooklin AR, Fox WW. Successful extubation of infants with respiratory distress syndrome using aminophylline. J Pediatr 1983;103:303.
317. Davi MJ, Sankaran K, Simons KJ, Simons FER, Seshia MM, Rigatto H. Physiologic changes induced by theophylline in the treatment of apnea in preterm infants. J Pediatr 1978;92:91.
318. Torphy TJ, Undem BJ. Phosphodiesterase inhibitors: new opportunities for the treatment of asthma. Thorax 1991;46:512.
319. Rooklin AR, Moomjian AS, Shutack JG, Schwartz JG, Fox WW. Theophylline therapy in bronchopulmonary dysplasia. J Pediatr 1979; 95:882.
320. Kao LC, Durand DJ, Phillips BL, Nickerson BG. Oral theophylline and diuretics improve pulmonary mechanics in infants with bronchopulmonary dysplasia. J Pediatr 1987;111:439.
321. Davis JM, Bhutani VK, Stefano JL, Fox WW, Spitzer AR. Changes in pulmonary mechanics following caffeine administration in infants with bronchopulmonary dysplasia. Pediatr Pulmonol 1989;6:49.

322. Beavo JA, Reifsnyder DH. Primary sequence of cyclic nucleotide phosphodiesterase isozymes and the design of selective inhibitors. Trends Pharmacol Sci 1990;11:150.
323. Fredholm BB. Are methylxanthine effects due to antagonism of endogenous adenosine? Trends Pharmacol Sci 1980;1:129.
324. Poisner AM. Direct stimulant effect of aminophylline on catecholamine release from the adrenal medulla. Biochem Pharmacol 1973;22:469.
325. Nahata MC, Serafini D, Edwards R. Theophylline pharmacokinetics in patients with bronchopulmonary dysplasia. J Clin Pharm Ther 1989;14:225.
326. Rao M, Eid N, Herrod L, Parekh A, Steiner P. Antidiuretic hormone response in children with bronchopulmonary dysplasia during episodes of acute respiratory distress. Am J Dis Child 1986;140:825.
327. Kojima T, Fukuda Y, Hirata Y, Matsuzaki S, Kobayashi Y. Changes in vasopressin, atrial natriuretic factor, and water homeostasis in the early stage of bronchopulmonary dysplasia. Pediatr Res 1990;27:260.
328. Engelhardt B, Elliott S, Hazinski TA. Short- and long-term effects of furosemide on lung function in infants with bronchopulmonary dysplasia. J Pediatr 1986;109:1034.
329. Engelhardt B, Blalock WA, DonLevy S, Rush M, Hazinski TA. Effect of spironolactone-hydrochlorothiazide on lung function in infants with chronic bronchopulmonary dysplasia. J Pediatr 1989;114:619.
330. Albersheim SG, Solimano AJ, Sharma AK, Smyth JA, et al. Randomized, double-blind, controlled trial of long-term diuretic therapy for bronchopulmonary dysplasia. J Pediatr 1989;115:615.
331. Rush MG, Engelhardt B, Parker RA, Hazinski TA. Double-blind, placebo-controlled trial of alternate-day furosemide therapy in infants with chronic bronchopulmonary dysplasia. J Pediatr 1990; 117:112.
332. Bland RD, McMillan DD, Bressack MA. Decreased pulmonary transvascular fluid filtration in awake newborn lambs after intravenous furosemide. J Clin Invest 1978;62:601.
333. Koo WW, Guan ZP, Tsang RC, Laskarzewski P, Neumann V. Growth failure and decreased bone mineral of newborn rats with chronic furosemide therapy. Pediatr Res 1986;20:74.
334. Salamy A, Eldredge L, Tooley WH. Neonatal status and hearing loss in high-risk infants. J Pediatr 1989;114:847.
335. Perlman JM, Moore V, Siegel MJ, Dawson J. Is chloride depletion an important contributing cause of death in infants with bronchopulmonary dysplasia? Pediatrics 1986;77:212.
336. Hurnagle KG, Shadid NK, Penn D, et al. Renal calcifications: a complication of long-term furosemide therapy in preterm infants. Pediatrics 1982;70:360.
337. Venkataraman PS, Han BK, Tsang RC, Daugherty CC. Secondary hyperparathyroidism and bone disease in infants receiving long-term furosemide therapy. Am J Dis Child 1983;137:1157.
338. Hazinski TA. Furosemide decreases ventilation in young rabbits. J Pediatr 1985;106:81.
339. Rastogi A. Luayon M, Ajayi O, Pildes RS. Nebulized furosemide in infants with bronchopulmonary dysplasia. J Pediatr 1994;125:976.
340. Clement A, Chadelat K, Sardet A, Grimfeld A, Tourner G. Alveolar macrophage status in bronchopulmonary dysplasia. Pediatr Res 1988; 23:470.
341. Southall DP, Samuels MP. Bronchopulmonary dysplasia: a new look at management. Arch Dis Child 1990;65:1089.
342. Ashkenazi J, Rosenbaum SH, Hyman AI, et al. Respiratory changes induced by the large glucose levels of total parenteral nutrition. JAMA 1980;243:1444.
343. Chessex P, Belanger S, Piedboeuf B, Pineault M. Influence of energy substrate on respiratory gas exchange during conventional mechanical ventilation of preterm infants. J Pediatr 1995;126:619.
344. Ciuffre RM, Rubin S, Mitchell L. Antireflux surgery in infants with bronchopulmonary dysplasia. Am J Dis Child 1987;141:648.
345. Sindel BD, Maisels MJ, Ballantine TVN. Gastroesophageal reflux to the proximal esophagus in infants with bronchopulmonary dysplasia. Am J Dis Child 1989;143:1103.
346. Jolley SG, Halpern CT, Sterling CE, Feldman BH. The relationship of respiratory complications from gastroesophageal reflux to prematurity in infants. J Pediatr Surg 1990;25:755.
347. Southall DP, Thomas MG, Lambert HP. Severe hypoxemia in pertussis. Arch Dis Child 1988;63:598.
348. American Academy of Pediatrics (Section 1) In: Peter G, ed. 1994 Red Book: Report of the Committee on Infectious Diseases. 23rd ed. Elk Grove Village, IL: American Academy of Pediatrics;1994:60,396.
349. Groothuis JR, Levin MJ, Rabalais GP, Meiklejohn G, Lauer BA. Immunization of high-risk infants younger than 18 months of age with split-product influenza vaccine. Pediatrics 1991;87:823.
350. Wilson CB. Immunologic basis for increased susceptibility of the neonate to infection. J Pediatr 1986;108:1.
351. Fanaroff AA, Korones SB, Wright LL, et al. A controlled trial of intravenous immune globulin to reduce nosocomial infections in very-low-birth-weight infants. N Engl J Med 1994;330:1107.
352. Sigurs N, Bjarnason R, Sigurbersson F, Kjellman B Bjorksten B. Asthma and immunoglobulin E antibodies after respiratory syncytial virus bronchiolitis: a prospective cohort study with matched controls. Pediatrics 1995;95:500.
353. Goothuis JR. Role of antibody and the use of respiratory syncytial virus immunoglobulin in the prevention of respiratory syncytial virus disease in preterm infants with and without bronchopulmonary dysplasia. Pediatr Infect Dis J 1994;13:454.
354. Groothuis JR, Simoes EAF, Levin M, et al. Prophylactic administration of respiratory syncytial virus immune globulin to high risk infants and young children. N Engl J Med 1993;329:1524.
355. DeLemos RA, Shermeta DW, Knelson JH, Kotas R, Avery ME. Acceleration of appearance of pulmonary surfactant in the fetal lamb by administration of corticosteroids. Am Rev Respir Dis 1970; 102:459.
356. Doyle LW, Kitchen WH, Ford GW, Rickards AL, Lissenden JV, Ryan MM. Effects of antenatal steroid therapy on mortality and morbidity in very low birth weight infants. J Pediatr 1986;108:287.
357. Van Marter LJ, Leviton A, Kuban KC, Pagano M, Allred EN. Maternal glucocorticoid therapy and reduced risk of bronchopulmonary dysplasia. Pediatrics 1990;86:331.
358. Mammel MC, Green TP, Johnson DE, Thompson TR. Controlled trial of dexamethasone therapy in infants with bronchopulmonary dysplasia. Lancet 1983;1:1356.
359. Avery GB, Fletcher AB, Kaplan M, Brudno S. Controlled trial of dexamethasone in respirator-dependent infants with bronchopulmonary dysplasia. Pediatrics 1985;75:106.
360. Cummings JJ, D'Eugeno DB, Gross SJ. A controlled trial of dexamethasone in preterm infants at high risk for bronchopulmonary dysplasia. N Engl J Med 1989;320:1505.
361. Harkavy KL, Scanlon JW, Chowdhry PK, Grylack LJ. Dexamethasone therapy for chronic lung disease in ventilator- and oxygen-dependent infants: a controlled trial. J Pediatr 1989;115:979.
362. Kazzi NJ, Brans YW, Poland RL. Dexamethasone effects on the hospital course of infants with bronchopulmonary dysplasia who are dependent on artificial ventilation. Pediatrics 1990;86:722.
363. Wilson JW. Treatment of prevention of pulmonary cellular damage with pharmacologic doses of corticosteroid. Surg Gynecol Obstet 1972; 134:675.
364. Hong S-CL, Levine L. Inhibition of arachidonic acid release from cells as the biochemical action of anti-inflammatory corticosteroids. Proc Natl Acad Sci U S A 1976;73:1730.
365. Yoder MC Jr, Chua R, Tepper R. Effect of dexamethasone on pulmonary inflammation and pulmonary function of ventilator-dependent infants with bronchopulmonary dysplasia. Am Rev Respir Dis 1991;143:1044.
366. Skubitz KM, Craddock PR, Hammerschmidt DE, August JT. Corticosteroids block binding of chemotactic peptide to its receptor on granulocytes and cause disaggregation of granulocyte aggregates in vitro. J Clin Invest 1981;68:13.
367. Coffey RG, Logsdon PJ, Middleton E Jr. Leukocyte adenyl cyclase and ATPase in asthma: effect of corticosteroid therapy. Chest 1973; 63(Suppl):2S.
368. Co E, Chari G, McCulloch K, Vidyasagar D. Dexamethasone treatment suppresses collagen synthesis in infants with bronchopulmonary dysplasia. Pediatr Pulmonol 1993;16:36.
369. Gladstone IM, Ehrenkranz RA, Jacobs HC. Pulmonary function tests and fluid balance in neonates with chronic lung disease during dexamethasone treatment. Pediatrics 1989;84:1072.
370. Cloutier MM, McLellan N. Nebulized steroid therapy in bronchopulmonary dysplasia. Pediatr Pulmonology 1993;15:111.
371. Alkalay AL, Pomerance JJ, Puri AR, Lin BJC, Vinstein AL, Neufeld ND, Klein AH. Hypothalamic-pituitary-adrenal axis function in very low birth weight infants treated with dexamethasone. Pediatrics 1990;86:204.
372. MacDonald PD, Galea P, Alroomi LG. A catabolic state in dexamethasone treatment of bronchopulmonary dysplasia. Arch Dis Child 1990;65:560.
373. Kasian GF, Ninan A, Duncan WJ, Bingham WT, et al. Treatment of pulmonary hypertension with diltiazem in a child with bronchopulmonary dysplasia. Can J Cardiol 1988;4:181.
374. Kochanek PM. Zaritsky A. Nifedipine in the treatment of a child with

pulmonary hypertension associated with severe bronchopulmonary dysplasia. Clin Pediatr 1986;25:214.
375. Johnson CE, Beekman RH, Kostyshak DA, Nguyen T, Oh D-M, Amidon GL. Pharmacokinetics and pharmacodynamics of nifedipine in children with bronchopulmonary dysplasia and pulmonary hypertension. Pediatr Res 1991;29:500.
376. Kettrick RG, Donar ME. The ventilator-dependent child: medical and social care. Clin Chest Med 1985;6:F1.
377. Schreiner MS, Downes JJ, Kettrick RG, Ise C, Voit R. Chronic respiratory failure in infants with prolonged ventilator dependency. JAMA 1987;258:3398.
378. McWilliams B. Mechanical ventilation in pediatric patients. Clin Chest Med 1987;8:1.
379. Newman JH, Neff TA, Ziporin P. Acute respiratory failure associated with hypophosphatemia. N Engl J Med 1977;296:1101.
380. Dhingra S, Solven F, Wilson A, McCarthy DS. Hypomagnesemia and respiratory muscle power. Am Rev Respir Dis 1984;129:497.
381. Aubier M, Viires N, Piquet J, Murciano D, et al. Effects of hypocalcemia on diaphragmatic strength generation. J Appl Physiol 1985; 58:2054.
382. Juan G, Calverley P, Talamo C, Schnader J, Roussos C. Effect of carbon dioxide on diaphragmatic function in human beings. N Engl J Med 1984;310:874.
383. Gibney RT, Wilson R, Pontoppidan H. Comparisons of work of breathing in high gas flow and demand valve continuous positive airway pressure ventilation. Chest 1982;82:692.
384. Martin LD, Rafferty JF, Wetzel RC, Gioia FR. Inspiratory work and response times of a modified pediatric volume ventilator during synchronized intermittent mandatory ventilation and pressure support ventilation. Anesthesiology 1989;71:977.
385. Morray JP, Fox WW, Kettrick RG, Downes JJ. Clinical correlates of successful weaning from mechanical ventilation in severe bronchopulmonary dysplasia. Crit Care Med 1981;9:815.
386. Groeger JS, Levinson MR, Carlon GC. Assist control versus synchronized intermittent mandatory ventilation during acute respiratory failure. Crit Care Med 1989;17:607.
387. Tomlinson JR, Miller S, Lorch DG, Smith L, Reines HD, Sahn SA. A prospective comparison of IMV and T-piece weaning from mechanical ventilation. Chest 1989;96:348.
388. Meert K, Heidemann S, Lieh-Lai M, Sarnaik AP. Clinical characteristics of respiratory syncytial virus infections in healthy versus previously compromised host. Pediatr Pulmol 1989;7:167.
389. Hall CM, McBride JT, Walsh EE, et al. Aerosolized ribavirin treatment of infants with respiratory syncytial viral infection. N Engl J Med 1983;208:114.
390. Groothuis JR, Woodin KA, Katz R, Robertson AD, et al. Early ribavirin treatment of respiratory syncytial viral infection in high-risk children. J Pediatr 1990;117:792.
391. Frankel LR, Wilson CW, Demers RR, et al. A technique for the administration of ribavirin to mechanically ventilated infants with severe respiratory syncytial virus infection. Crit Care Med 1987;15:1051.
392. Smith DW, Frankel LR, Mathers LH, Tang AT, Ariagno RL, Prober CG. A controlled trial of aerosolized ribavirin in infants receiving mechanical ventilation for severe respiratory syncytial virus infection. N Engl J Med 1991;325:24.
393. Meert KL, Sarnaik AP, Gelmini MJ, Lieh-Lai MW. Aerosolized ribavirin in mechanically ventilated children with respiratory syncytial virus lower respiratory tract disease: a prospective, double-blind, randomized trial. Crit Care Med 1994;22:566.
394. Abman SH, Burchell MF, Schaffer MS, Rosenberg AA. Late sudden unexpected deaths in hospitalized infants with bronchopulmonary dysplasia. Am J Dis Child 1989;143:815.
395. Nickerson BG. Bronchopulmonary dysplasia. Chronic pulmonary disease following neonatal respiratory failure. Chest 1985;87:528.
396. Gibson RL, Jackson JC, Twiggs GA, Redding GJ, Truog WE. Bronchopulmonary dysplasia. Survival after prolonged mechanical ventilation. Am J Dis Child 1988;142:721.
397. Devaskar UP, Devaskar SU, Keenan WJ. Acute bronchospasm resembling status asthmaticus during the neonatal period. Crit Care Med 1986;14:472.
398. Goldberg AI. Late sudden unexpected deaths in hospitalized infants with bronchopulmonary dysplasia. Am J Dis Child 1990; 144:270.
399. Riordan JR, Rommens JM, Kerem B, et al. Identification of the cystic fibrosis gene: cloning and characterization of complementary DNA. Science 1989;245:1066.
400. Tomkiewicz RP, App EM, Zayas JG, et al. Amiloride inhalation therapy in cystic fibrosis. Am Rev Respir Dis 1993;148:1002.
401. Fuchs HJ, Borowitz DS, Christiansen DH, et al. Effect of aerosolized recombinant human Dnase on exacerbations of respiratory symptoms and on pulmonary function in patients with cystic fibrosis. N Engl J Med 1994;331:637.
402. Armitage JM, Kurland G, Michaels M, et al. Critical issues in pediatric lung transplantation. J Thorac Cardiovasc Surg 1995;109:60.
403. Spray TL, Mallory GB, Canter CB, Huddleston CB. Pediatric lung transplantation. J Thorac Cardiovasc Surg 1994;107:990.
404. Spray TL. Projections for pediatric heart-lung and lung transplantation. J Heart Lung Transplant 1993;12:S337.
405. Armitage JM, Fricker FJ, Kurland G, Michaels M, Griffith BP. Pediatric lung transplantation: expanding indications, 1985-1993. J Heart Lung Transplant 1993;12:S246.
406. Shennib H, adoumie R, Noirclerc M. Current status of lung transplantation for cystic fibrosis. Arch Int Med 1992;152:1585.
407. Metras D, Kreitmann B, Shennib H, Noirclerc M. Lung transplantation in children. J Heart Lung Transplant 1992;11:S282.
408. Early GL, Williams TE, Kilman JW. Open lung biopsy: Its effect on therapy in the pediatric patient. Chest 1985;87:467.
409. Steinkamp G, Muller KM, Schrig E, Von Der Hardt H. Fibrosing alveolitis in childhood. Acta Pediatr Scand 1990;79:823.
410. Barker AF, Bardana EJ. Bronchiectasis: Update on an orphan disease. Am Rev Respir Dis 1988;173:969.

Acute Respiratory Distress Syndrome 7

James C. Fackler
John H. Arnold
David G. Nichols
Mark C. Rogers

GENERAL CONSIDERATIONS

Introduction

Acute respiratory failure after injury to the alveolar capillary unit may occur after a variety of insults in patients with previously healthy lungs. The severity of injury may vary. Acute respiratory distress syndrome (ARDS) is the most severe manifestation of parenchymal injury after any one of the triggering insults. The radiographic and histologic pictures are nonspecific[1]. However, the pathophysiology of the alveolar-capillary injury is similar. It is argued, given these similarities, that the term *acute respiratory distress syndrome* is a convenient heading under which a wide array of insults leading to alveolar damage and acute respiratory failure may be grouped. Such terms as *shock lung, traumatic wet lung,* and *noncardiogenic pulmonary edema* describe a subset of the same pathophysiologic changes. The pathologic changes reflect the limited repertoire of the lung in responding to a variety of insults. On the contrary, grouping such diverse pathophysiologies within the same syndrome makes the study of underlying mechanisms and possible therapies frustrating[2]. Recent work has focused on the mediator cascade and cellular events in ARDS that might permit the development of specific therapy in the future. Although the same insults injure an adult's and a child's lung, far fewer pediatric studies have been published.

Definition

Ashbaugh et al.[3] introduced *acute* respiratory distress in adults with a 1967 report of 12 patients, one of whom was an 11-year-old. The term *adult* respiratory distress syndrome (either conveniently or confusingly also ARDS) was introduced a few years later[4]. At that time, the term *adult respiratory distress syndrome* was chosen to differentiate the syndrome from the recently described respiratory distress syndrome shown to be associated with surfactant deficiency in premature newborns. Diagnosis of the adult respiratory distress syndrome required the following elements:

1. A catastrophic pulmonary or nonpulmonary event in the patient with previously normal lungs
2. Respiratory distress with hypoxemia, decreased pulmonary compliance, and increased shunt (Q_S/Q_T) fraction
3. Radiologic evidence of diffuse pulmonary infiltrates
4. Exclusion of left heart disease and congestive heart failure[5]

In 1988, Murray et al.[6] argued that lumping a diverse set of triggering events and diseases under the term adult respiratory distress syndrome on the basis of the above definition only obscures a more precise understanding of the pathogenesis and prognosis of the syndrome. Their expanded definition of the adult respiratory distress syndrome includes a three-part notation of (a) acute or chronic course, (b) severity of lung injury using lung injury score **(Table 7.1)**, and (c) cause or associated event (e.g., aspiration pneumonitis, sepsis).

The semantic return from *adult* to *acute* in ARDS occurred as a result of a recent American-European Consensus Conference on ARDS[7]. Any definition of ARDS was recognized as arbitrary, but ARDS represents a subset of acute lung injury (ALI). ARDS and ALI both require the following characteristics:

1. Acute onset of respiratory symptoms
2. Frontal chest radiograph with bilateral infiltrates
3. No clinical evidence of left atrial hypertension (or pulmonary artery wedge pressure less than 18 mm Hg)

ALI further requires the following:

$PaO_2/FIO_2 \leq 300$ mm Hg (regardless of the positive end-expiratory pressure [PEEP] level)

ARDS, as a subset of ALI, requires more severe respiratory failure:

$PaO_2/FIO_2 \leq 200$ mm Hg (regardless of the PEEP level)

Although these critiera may appear to describe an only moderately ill population, a 2-year study of 153 adults enrolled

Table 7.1. Components and Individual Values of the Lung Injury Score[a]

		Value
1. Chest roentgenogram score		
No alveolar consolidation		0
Alveolar consolidation confined to 1 quadrant		1
Alveolar consolidation confined to 2 quadrants		2
Alveolar consolidation confined to 3 quadrants		3
Alveolar consolidation in all 4 quadrants		4
2. Hypoxemia score		
P_aO_2/F_IO_2	>300	0
P_aO_2/F_IO_2	225–299	1
P_aO_2/F_IO_2	175–224	2
P_aO_2/F_IO_2	100–174	3
P_aO_2/F_IO_2	<100	4
3. PEEP score (when ventilated)		
PEEP	>5 cm H_2O	0
PEEP	6–8 cm H_2O	1
PEEP	9–11 cm H_2O	2
PEEP	12–14 cm H_2O	3
PEEP	>15 cm H_2O	4
4. Respiratory system compliance score (when available)		
Compliance	>80 ml/cm H_2O	0
Compliance	60–79 ml/cm H_2O	1
Compliance	40–59 ml/cm H_2O	2
Compliance	20–39 ml/cm H_2O	3
Compliance	<19 ml/cm H_2O	4

The final value is obtained by dividing the aggregate sum by the number of components that were used.

	Score
No lung injury	0
Mild-to-moderate lung injury	0.1–2.5
Severe lung injury (ARDS)	>2.5

[a] Abbreviations: P_aO_2/F_IO_2, ratio of arterial oxygen tension to inspired oxygen concentration; PEEP, positive end-expiratory pressure; ARDS, adult respiratory distress syndrome. (From Murray JF, et al. An expanded definition of adult respiratory distress syndrome. Am Rev Respir Dis 1988;138:720–723.)

Table 7.2. Incidence and Case Fatality Rates by Predisposed Group[a]

Risks for predisposition	*Patients at risk*	*Patients with syndrome* *n*	*Incidence rate[b]* (per 100)	*Patients who died*	*Case-fatality rate (per 100)*
Cardiopulmonary bypass	237	4	1.7	2	50.0
Burn	87	2	2.3	1	50.0
Bacteremia	239	9	3.8	7	77.8
Hypertransfusion	197	9	4.6	4	44.4
Fracture	38	2	5.3	0	
Pneumonia in intensive care	84	10	11.9	6	60.0
Disseminated intravascular coagulation	9	2	22.2	1	50.0
Pulmonary aspiration	45	16	35.6	15[c]	93.8
All single-risk patients	936	54	5.8	36	66.7
Multiple-risk patients	57	14	24.6	10	71.4
Total of patients with known risks	993	68	6.8	46	67.6
Other patients with syndrome[d]		20		11	35.0

[a] From Fowler AA, et al. Adult respiratory distress syndrome: risk with common predispositions. Ann Intern Med 1983;98:593–597.
[b] The incidence rates for the eight predisposed groups were significantly different overall (χ square, 110.9; $p > 0.00001$.
[c] Includes two deaths in the 6 months after extubation.
[d] Patients at risk were not prospectively identified.

with $PaO_2/FIO_2 \leq 250$ mm Hg demonstrated all but 2% meeting other published criteria for ARDS (within 7 days of study enrollment)[8]. The American-European Consensus Conference report has many excellent suggestions about the design and conduct of clinical research in the area of ALI and ARDS[7].

Epidemiology

An estimated 150,000 adults per year develop ARDS[9,10]; however, more recent data questions that number[11]. Focusing specifically on patients at risk for ARDS, in a 1-year, prospective, multi-institutional survey, Fowler et al.[12] noted a 6.8% incidence of ARDS in a population of 993 adult patients with one or more ARDS risk factors. The incidence varied widely depending on the nature of the risk factor, with witnessed aspiration syndrome accounting for the highest incidence rate (35.6%) **(Table 7.2).** From a single-institution study of 695 adults who met one criterion for seven risk factors associated with ARDS, a higher overall percentage of patients developed ARDS (26%). The sepsis syndrome was the individual risk factor associated with the highest incidence of ARDS (43%)[13].

The incidence of ARDS in children appears similar to that in adults. ARDS was shown, in a single-institution study, to have a 12% incidence in children admitted with sepsis, viral pneumonia, smoke inhalation, or drowning[14]. ARDS was present in 2.7% of all admissions to the intensive care unit (representing 8% of all patient days).

Examining only patients with ARDS (based on a nonuniform set of criteria), the mortality from ARDS in children was 80% in the mid 1970s and remained as high in the early 1990s[14–25].

The most broad-based description of ARDS in children comes from a 41-institution collaboration sponsored by the Pediatric Critical Care Study Group[26]. Approximately 8000 charts for patients with ARDS during calendar 1991 were reviewed. Patients included in the study were between 2 weeks and 18 years of age who had 12 continuous hours of PEEP of 6 or greater and an F_IO_2 of 0.5. Excluded were patients with intracardiac shunts or operations on the cardiovascular system during the screened admission. Data were analyzed on 679 cases. The median age was 1.88 years. Of total patients, 303 were girls. Overall mortality was 52%. Median length of stay was 26 days for survivors and 13 days for nonsurvivors. Of the 352 deaths, 312 occurred within the first 28 days.

Unlike the published experience in children, Milberg et al.[27] suggest that the mortality of adults with ARDS has diminished over the last decade. They report a single-institution experience with 918 consecutive patients, aged 18 years or older, from 1983 through 1993, who met ARDS criteria. Mortality ranged from 53 to 68% from 1983 to 1987. The overall mortality fell to 36% in 1993. The mortality decline was seen best in patients under age 60 and in patients whose ARDS was associated with sepsis. A similar adult experience is reported by Morris et al.[28] Knaus et al.[29] correctly add to the complexity of understanding mortality prediction by pointing out that even in a population of adults with a $PaO_2/FIO_2 \leq 150$ mm Hg (more severe than the ARDS definition above), the individual risk of mortality, based on the APACHE III, ranged from less than 10% to more than 90%.

Again, unlike the experience of Milberg et al., no reproducible mortality trend has been demonstrated in children.

Causes

Because ARDS is a clinical syndrome for which no specific marker exists, it is unclear whether the precipitating events are truly causative or merely associated phenomena[30]. Shock, sepsis, and drowning are the most common causes in published pediatric series[21,24]. Conditions associated with ARDS are discussed in more detail at the end of the chapter.

PATHOLOGY

On gross inspection, lungs with ARDS appear red, heavy, and airless. Katzenstein et al.[31] coined the term *diffuse alveolar damage,* which emphasizes the site of microscopic injury in ARDS. The various features of this alveolar capillary injury may be separated into three stages: exudative, proliferative, and fibrotic[32,33].

Exudative Stage

The sequence of pathologic events in ARDS begins in the first 6 hours with capillary congestion and intraluminal aggregation of platelets, fibrin, and neutrophils in pulmonary arteries 25 to 250 μm in diameter[34]. At 12 to 24 hours, marked capillary congestion progresses to periarterial and interstitial hemorrhage. Hyaline membranes develop by 72 hours (Fig. 7.1).

Pulmonary capillary endothelial cells undergo swelling and focal necrosis with destruction of mitochondria, endoplasmic reticulum, and ribosomes during the first few hours of ARDS[35]. Intercellular junctions between endothelial cells appear remarkably spared despite the changes in endothelial cell structure. This may be due to the ability of endothelial cell extensions to repair gaps in the endothelial cell layer quickly[36].

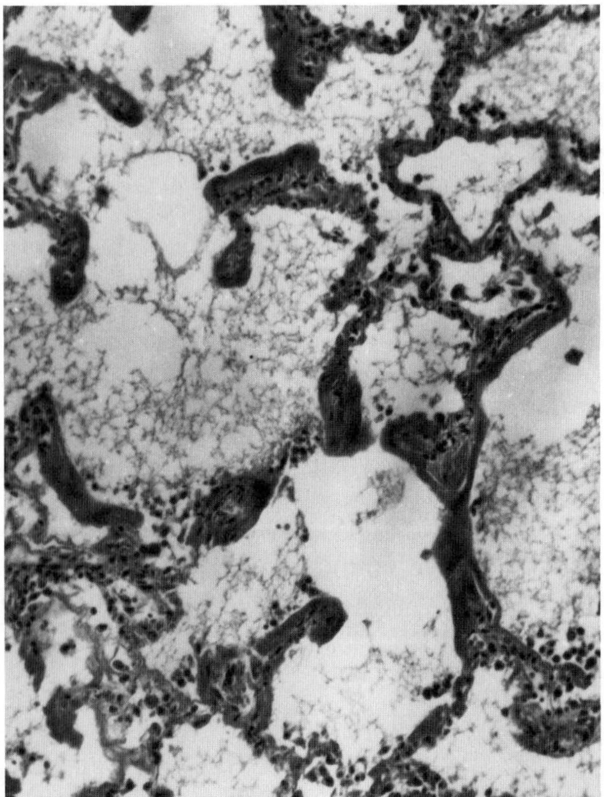

Figure 7.1. Acute pathologic changes in early adult respiratory distress syndrome. Note degeneration of alveolar pneumocytes, neutrophil aggregation, and hemorrhagic fluid in the interstitium.

Several mechanisms have been suggested to explain endothelial cell injury:

1. Neutrophil aggregation and complement release[37,38]
2. Endothelial injury from products of intravascular coagulation[39]
3. Release of inflammatory mediators[40]
4. Activation of other inflammatory cells, such as macrophages[41] and eosinophils[42]

Damage also occurs early on the epithelial side of the capillary-alveolar unit. Normally, type I pneumocytes are connected by tight junctions and thus restrict the passage of fluid and protein across the alveolar wall. Degeneration of alveolar epithelial cells, particularly type I pneumocytes, occurs early in ARDS. These degenerative changes include cytoplasmic swelling, membrane fragmentation, and chromatin clumping[43].

Whatever the mechanism of epithelial and endothelial cell injury, the outcome is clear. The alveolar-capillary membrane is disrupted, and permeability pulmonary edema develops. The subendothelial space between basement membrane and endothelial cell demonstrate trapped fibrous strands. A proteinaceous hemorrhagic fluid first fills the interstitium. The pulmonary lymphatics clear excess fluid from the interstitium[44]. When the lymphatic clearance mechanism is overwhelmed, pulmonary edema fluid develops around bronchi and larger vessels (Fig. 7.1). The thin part of the alveolar wall involving gas exchange and the intra-alveolar space are involved last in permeability pulmonary edema[45]. This proteinaceous fluid may coalesce and adhere to alveolar epithelium, producing hyaline membranes. Typically, these membranes coalesce around the tips of alveoli. Various staining techniques have demonstrated that these membranes are composed of immunoglobulins, fibrinogen, complement, and fibronectin[46].

Pulmonary vascular occlusion is a major component of the pathologic changes in ARDS and accounts, in part, for the pulmonary hypertension that may be seen during the illness. Fibrous clots and microthrombi consisting of red blood cells, platelets, and granulocytes may extend into capillary lumen[43,47].

Proliferative Stage

The proliferative stage occurs between the first and third weeks after lung injury. It is initially characterized by proliferation of type II pneumocytes, fibroblasts, and myofibroblasts. The replication and function of these cells, however, are abnormal. The cuboidal type II pneumocytes contain fewer and poorly developed lamellated bodies, suggesting deficient surfactant production[48]. Only type II pneumocytes appear to function as stem cells capable of mitosis. Subsequently, they are transformed into type I pneumocytes to permit repair of alveolar epithelium[49,50]. Fibroblasts migrate into intra-alveolar spaces and convert the hemorrhagic exudate into cellular granulation tissue and eventually cause fibrosis by deposition of collagen. Interstitial edema and inflammatory cells stimulate the fibroblasts to lay down collagen, which in turn causes widening of alveolar septae (Fig. 7.2).

Fibrotic Stage

If ARDS has persisted for over 3 weeks, the lungs are typically remodeled by collagenous tissue[51]. Bronchoalveolar lavage (BAL) fluid and serum yield metabolites of collagen synthesis in patients with ARDS[52]. BAL fluid can also be assayed for angiogenesis activity and enhanced endothelial cell migration[53]. In tissue culture, mechenymal cell migration is enhanced[54]. The replication of cells and production of collagen lead to destruction of the acinar architecture (Fig. 7.2). Vascular changes continue during the intermediate and late stages of ARDS, with obliteration of small precapillary vessels and an increase in medial thickness of intra-acinar pulmonary arteries[32,55,56]. Macroscopic evaluation of the lungs reveals cystic lesions with areas of fibrotic scarring. This process of fibrosis results in a life-threatening decrease in the surface area available for gas exchange.

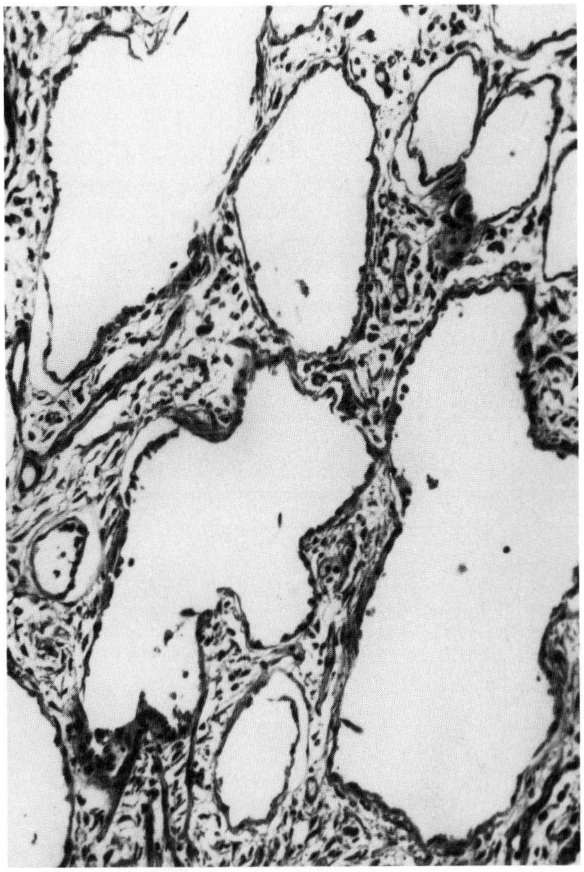

Figure 7.2. Chronic pathologic changes in late adult respiratory distress syndrome. Note proliferating pneumocytes, organization of fibrous tissue, and migration of white blood cells into interstitium. Original acinar architecture is destroyed.

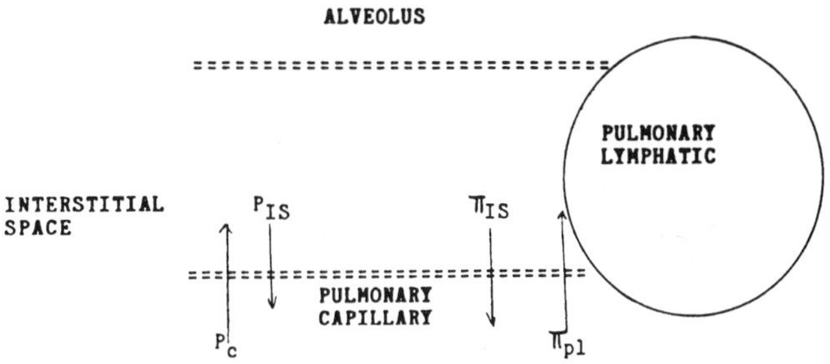

Figure 7.3. Starling forces governing fluid movement across pulmonary capillary into interstitium. P_{is}, interstitial hydrostatic pressure; P_c, capillary hydrostatic pressure; π_{is}, interstitial oncotic pressure; and π_{pi}, capillary oncotic pressure. Interstitial fluid is cleared by the pulmonary lymphatic until lymphatic capacity is overwhelmed, at which point fluid appears in the alveolus.

PATHOPHYSIOLOGY

As might be expected from the severe derangements in lung structure, dysfunction of the cardiorespiratory system is the major pathophysiologic feature of ARDS and is marked by severe arterial hypoxemia. Biochemical and cellular abnormalities lead to the reduction in lung volumes and the disruption of normal gas exchange, factors that culminate in acute respiratory failure and associated cardiovascular disturbances.

Mechanism of Pulmonary Edema

The Starling formula characterizes movement of fluid across the alveolar capillary membrane such that the rate of flow is a function of the filtering properties of the alveolar capillary membrane and the balance of hydrostatic and oncotic forces in pulmonary capillary and interstitium (Fig. 7.3):

$$\dot{Q} = K(P_C - P_{IS}) - \sigma(\pi_{PL} - \pi_{IS}) \qquad \text{(Eq. 7.1)}$$

where $\dot{Q}$ equals filtration rate across capillary membrane, K equals filtration coefficient, P_C equals capillary hydrostatic pressure, P_{IS} equals interstitial hydrostatic pressure, σ equals reflection coefficient, π_{PL} equals plasma oncotic pressure, and π_{IS} equals interstitial oncotic pressure.

Normal pulmonary capillary hydrostatic pressures have been measured in patients in the early stages of ARDS[57]. The later increases in pulmonary capillary hydrostatic pressures are secondary phenomena in ARDS caused by mediator-induced pulmonary vasoconstriction, thromboembolic occlusion of the pulmonary vasculature, and vascular remodeling[47]. Thus Starling's law dictates that the early onset of pulmonary edema must be due to an alteration in capillary permeability and/or oncotic pressure gradient. Ultrastructural evidence cited earlier supports the notion that disruption of the alveolar capillary membrane is responsible for pulmonary edema in ARDS. The normal alveolar capillary membrane restricts transfer of plasma protein into the interstitium. The high protein content of edema fluid in patients with ARDS suggests that the restrictive properties of the membrane have been disrupted(55). In a sheep model developed by Staub (Erdmann et al.[58]), hydrostatic pulmonary edema actually resulted in a decrease in lung lymph protein below control levels. In contrast, the injection of *Pseudomonas* endotoxin leads to a dramatic increase in lung lymph flow of high protein content(59). Permeability pulmonary edema floods the lungs more rapidly than hydrostatic pulmonary edema, as predicted by Starling's equation and confirmed in Staub's studies. This is so because in addition to the increase in capillary permeability, the protective osmotic gradient between capillary and interstitium is lost.

Mediators in ARDS

That mediators are important for the development of ARDS is a concept at least 40 years old(60). An exponentially growing body of literature has since described a vast array of mediators that have complex interactions with various cells in the lung and with each other (Fig. 7.4). Because sepsis is commonly associated with ARDS in adults and children(13,14), the mediators most studied include those produced by inflammatory cells (neutrophils, macrophages, eosinophils, and lymphocytes), complement, endotoxin, cytokines, platelets, products of disseminated intravascular coagulation (DIC), and products of arachidonic acid metabolism (prostaglandins and leukotrienes). Yet, the above is certainly incomplete. For example, a receptor not typically associated with the lung (N-methyl-D-aspartate [NMDA]) has been identified in the pulmonary parenchyma, and activation of NMDA receptors results in (probably neurogenic) tissue injury(61).

A brief description of the major mediators and their putative roles in ARDS is given in the following paragraphs. Definition of individual effects of these mediators in ARDS is difficult because their effects are tightly interwoven. A typical example of the latter is seen in the postulated protective effects of heat shock protein (HSP). HSP protects against oxygen free radical (including nitric oxide) toxicity. HSP also protects against tumor necrosis factor (TNF-α) and interleukin-1 (IL-1)(62). It is fascinating that HSP has been shown to be protective (when induced before intratracheal phospholipase A_2 installation) in a rat

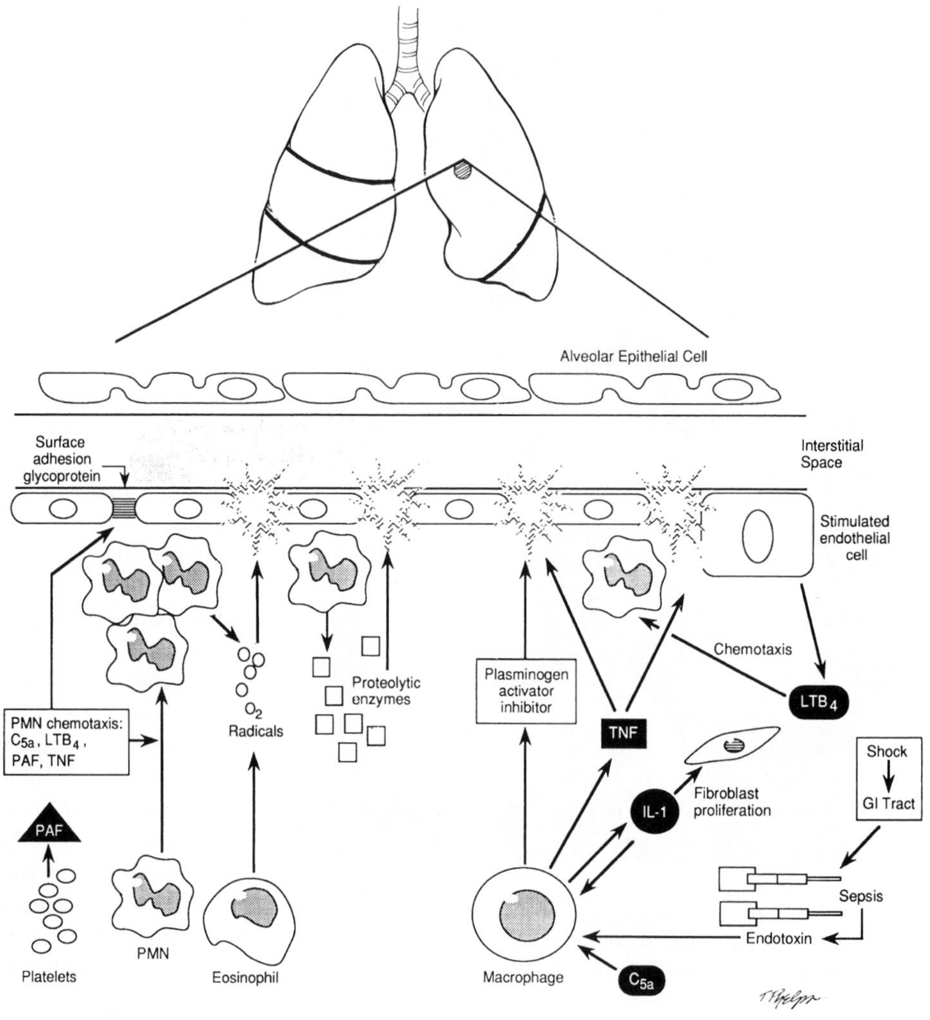

Figure 7.4. Schematic representation of mediators causing alveolar capillary membrane injury. Major events include (a) aggregation and activation (chemotaxis) of polymorphonuclear leukocytes (PMN) mediated by complement C5a (C_{5a}), leukotriene B_4 (LTB_4), platelet-activating factor (PAF), and tumor necrosis factor (TNF); (b) activated neutrophils releasing O_2 radicals and proteolytic enzymes that injure endothelium; and (c) endotoxin stimulating the macrophage to release TNF, interleukin-1 (IL-1), and plasminogen activator inhibitor. GI, gastrointestinal. See text (Mediators in Adult Respiratory Distress Syndrome) for further details.

model of ARDS(63); however, extrapolation of animal data to the bedside is treacherous.

Neutrophils

Sequestration and activation of neutrophils in the pulmonary microvasculature by various mediators appear to be important pathogenic mechanisms in ARDS. In vitro and in vivo experiments demonstrate that complement (C5a), leukotriene B_4 (LTB_4), platelet-activating factor (PAF), TNF-α, and IL-1 are chemotactic agents for neutrophils(64–69). C5a, LTB_4, TNF, and PAF promote adherence of neutrophils by eliciting the expression of surface adhesive glycoproteins(70). Conversely, an antagonist of LTB_4 (LY-306669) diminished migration of neutorphils to the alveolar air spaces, accumulation of extravascular lung water, and systemic arterial hypoxemia and pulmonary hypertension(71). TNF and IL-1 enhance sequestration of neutrophils by inducing the expression of endothelial-leukocyte adhesion molecule 1 (ELAM-1) on the surface of endothelial cells(72).

Endotoxin also appears to mediate adhesion of neutrophils to endothelial cells. Once they are adherent to the endothelial cells, activation of neutrophils by the mediators leads to the production of proteolytic enzymes and oxygen free radicals that subsequently cause endothelial cell damage. BAL fluid from patients with ARDS has been found to contain activity from the proteolytic enzyme elastase elaborated by neutrophils(73). Glutathione is found in the oxidized state and may be indicative of excessive neutrophil-driven oxygen-free-radical toxicity(74). In addition, endogenous inhibitors of proteolytic enzyme activity, such as the α_1-proteinase inhibitor, are inactivated in patients with ARDS(75). Experimental evidence with granulocyte-depleted models of acute lung injury have shown a decrease in pulmonary vascular permeability(76,77).

Although the neutrophil plays a primary role in mediating the inflammatory process associated with ARDS, several clinical studies have demonstrated ARDS in children and adults with neutropenia(78–80). These studies further corroborate the involvement of other mediators in ARDS.

Macrophages

The development of ARDS in neutropenic patients is probably due (at least in part) to the diverse role of macrophages in mediating the associated inflammatory reaction. In most of the described neutropenic patients the cause of ARDS was sepsis. The release of endotoxin into the bloodstream and local tissue beds such as the lung has profound effects on macrophages. This interaction leads to the production of TNF, IL-1, thromboxane, LTB_4, and other chemotactic factors by resident macrophages in the lung(81). Macrophages, like neutrophils, also produce oxygen free radicals. Furthermore, macrophages produce growth factors that modulate the development of fibrosis in ARDS(81).

Eosinophils

Evaluation of BAL fluid from patients with ARDS versus patients after major surgery has demonstrated that patients with ARDS have higher levels of eosinophilic cationic protein (ECP), a major constituent of eosinophil granules that can injure endothelial cells and produce lung edema(82). Experimental evidence from studies using isolated perfused rat lungs shows that activated eosinophils cause increased permeability and morphologic changes in the lungs consistent with ARDS. The acute injury in this model is due in part to the production of free radicals(83).

Endotoxin

Endotoxin from gram-negative organisms has been demonstrated to be a primary mediator in the development of ARDS(84). Numerous in vivo and in vitro studies have demonstrated that bacterial lipopolysaccharide (LPS), an endotoxin, can directly affect the integrity of the intact endothelial monolayer(85). Endotoxin is also the prime effector for stimulating macrophages to produce TNF and IL-1(86,87). Neutrophils are "primed" by LPS for production of free radicals(88). It has been proposed that the continued inflammatory response in ARDS is secondary to endotoxin leaking from the gut and causing activation of inflammatory cells(89).

Complement

In the 1960s, hemodialysis patients were noted to have mild pulmonary dysfunction and transient neutropenia during hemodialysis(90). Further analysis of this phenomenon revealed that the cellophane dialysis membranes were causing complement activation, which led to sequestration of neutrophils in the pulmonary vasculature(91). This observation led many investigators to postulate that the primary cause of intrapulmonary sequestration of neutrophils seen in ARDS was due to complement activation.

Thus, complement levels were measured in patients at risk for ARDS. Conflicting studies showed positive and negative correlations with levels of C5a and C3a; however, there seems to be a good correlation for risk of ARDS when elevated levels of C5a are associated with endotoxemia(64,92–94). Normal C5a levels may still allow significant neutrophil chemotaxis, because patients with ARDS exhibit a functional loss of chemotactic factor inactivator (CFI)(95). The loss of CFI permits increased C5a-directed neutrophil chemotaxis(95). Thus complement, especially C5a, probably plays a significant role in ARDS by causing chemoattraction and activation of neutrophils. Furthermore, C5a can induce the production of TNF and IL-1 from monocytes and/or macrophages(96,97). In a septic primate model, anti-C5a antibodies were able to attenuate the associated lung injury(98).

Tumor Necrosis Factor

TNF is a 17-kD protein product of macrophages and/or monocytes and an important representative of a class of compounds known as cytokines. TNF has been measured in the serum and BAL fluid of patients with ARDS[(99,100)]. Endotoxin and C5a stimulate macrophages and/or monocytes to produce TNF[(81)].

The release of TNF produces cytokine amplification of an ongoing inflammatory response through numerous effects on endothelium, neutrophils, lymphocytes, and monocytes and/or macrophages. The effects on neutrophils, which are seen in ARDS, include chemotaxis with pulmonary leukostasis, increased expression of surface adhesion molecules, degranulation, increased production of oxygen free radicals, and production of PAF[(67,70,101)]. In an in vitro model, TNF caused increased permeability to albumin across an endothelial monolayer[(102)]. Other effects of TNF on pulmonary endothelium include increased production of arachidonate metabolites, increased procoagulant activity, increased expression of ELAM-1, the production of PAF, and the production of other cytokines, such as platelet-derived growth factor (PDGF)[(72,81,101,103,104)]. TNF induces further production of IL-1 from endothelial cells and macrophages[(105)].

Interleukin-1

It was recently shown that adults with high IL-1 beta (and TNF-alpha, IL-6, and IL-8) early in the course of ARDS, also had persistent elevation of these inflammatory cytokines and died[(106)]. Survivors showed lower elevations of plasma cytokines and rapid reduction of IL-1. IL-1 production is induced by the same agents that induce TNF; the two cytokines are present with the development of sepsis. IL-1 has many of the same effects that TNF has on cells and may act synergistically with TNF to damage lung endothelium[(105)]. TNF-stimulated release of IL-1 activates an immunoregulatory cascade that causes activation of B-lymphocytes and the production of other lymphokines from T-lymphocytes, such as IL-2, which has a major effect on the replication and function of other lymphocytes[(105)]. IL-1 may also be more important than TNF in the chronic stages of ARDS, since it causes fibroblast proliferation and stimulates macrophages to produce growth factors[(105)].

Platelet-Activating Factor

Although PAF has not been described in patients with ARDS (presumably because of its short half-life), experimental evidence suggests that it may play a role in mediating ARDS. PAF is a phospholipid metabolite released from the membranes of neutrophils, platelets, and endothelial cells[(101)]. In rabbits, intravenous infusion of PAF causes morphologic changes in the lung tissue that is typically seen in patients with ARDS[(107,108)]. Furthermore, it is similar to TNF in that it can also cause neutrophil chemotaxis and activation, increased endothelial permeability, and production of arachidonic acid metabolites[(109)]. Recent data that PAF may be an important component of the biochemical alterations associated with mechnical ventilation-induced lung injury are discussed below).

Platelets

Microthrombi with platelet plugging is typically found on autopsy in patients with ARDS. Experimental studies have demonstrated that platelets can cause increased permeability, activate neutrophils, and cause pulmonary hypertension; however, the evidence for the role of platelets in human ARDS is scant[(110)]. Platelet-specific α-granule proteins and thrombospondin are elevated in the BAL fluid of patients with ARDS compared with that of control patients[(111)]. Some of these proteins, such as platelet factor 4 and β-thromboglobulin, act as chemotactic agents for monocytes and neutrophils, stimulate leukocyte elastase, and can be chemotactic for fibroblasts[(112–114)]. Conversely, some experimental evidence also suggests that platelets may attenuate oxidant lung injury, since platelets contain an active antioxidant system[(115)].

Disseminated Intravascular Coagulopathy

DIC, with its usual microthrombi composed of platelets and fibrin, along with fibrin degradation product, may be seen in patients with ARDS[(36)]. Several studies have shown that fibrin degradation products can cause increased vascular permeability and affect inflammatory responses[(36,116,117)]. The balance between coagulation and fibrinolysis appears to be shifted toward coagulation in patients with ARDS. One cause of procoagulant activity in ARDS is decreased fibrinolysis secondary to increased plasminogen activator inhibitor production[(118,119)]. A rich source of plasminogen activator inhibitor is the macrophage after stimulation by TNF[(119,120)]. Since the alveolar spaces normally contain little fibrin and active fibrinolytic mechanisms, it has been postulated that the endothelial damage seen in ARDS allows for the passage of fibrin degradation products and plasminogen activator inhibitor into the alveolar spaces[(118)]. The increased fibrin, with decreased turnover secondary to the presence of plasminogen activator inhibitor, can potentially stimulate fibroblast migration and subsequent fibrosis.

Prostaglandins and Leukotrienes

Prostaglandins represent a class of compounds that are released as a result of the enzymatic action of cyclo-oxygenase on arachidonic acid after it is cleaved from the cell membrane by phospholipase. Various experimental models of ARDS have suggested cyclo-oxygenase pathway products may play a role in the pathogenesis of ARDS, in that (a) prostaglandin F_2 (PGF_2) and thromboxane B_2 are found in significantly increased concentrations in lung lymph after endotoxin-induced ARDS and are potent pulmonary vasoconstrictors that may contribute to pulmonary hypertension in ARDS[(121)]; (b) hypoxia potentiates the pressor response of the pulmonary vasculature to PGF_2[122]; (c) the initial rise in pulmonary artery pressure (PAP) in ARDS models can be abolished completely with various cyclo-oxygenase inhibitors, such as meclofenamate and indomethacin[123]; and (d) bronchoconstriction occurs in ARDS models and coincides with a rise in thromboxane A_2 levels that can be blocked by cyclo-oxygenase inhibitors[123]. Despite these experimental data, it is unclear whether cyclo-oxygenase products play a significant role in human ARDS.

There is greater evidence for the role of the lipoxygenase products of arachidonic acid metabolism, leukotrienes, in human ARDS. Elevated levels of leukotriene D_4 (LTD_4) have been isolated from edema fluid in patients with ARDS[124]. Hypoxia does not alter the profile of cyclo-oxygenase products in the lung, whereas the synthesis of LTE_4 and LTB_4 increases tenfold during hypoxia[125]. The effects of leukotrienes on the lung are consistent with pathophysiologic derangements in ARDS. Binding of leukotrienes to receptors on pulmonary veins and arteries leads to profound pulmonary vasoconstriction[126]. Leukotriene B_4 is a powerful chemotactic agent for neutrophils[127] but may also injure the pulmonary endothelium through direct effects[128].

Diminished Surfactant Activity and Airway Collapse

Surfactant is a surface-active material that lines alveoli and promotes alveolar stability. Its primary chemical constituent is a phospholipid, dipalmitoyl lecithin, which is produced by type II alveolar pneumocytes. The physiologic importance of surfactant is appreciated from the Laplace equation:

$$P = 2T/r \qquad \text{(Eq. 7.2)}$$

In the absence of surfactant, the surface tension (T) would remain constant, despite changes in alveolar size. The result would be that alveoli of small radius (r) would require greater transpulmonary pressure (P) to stay open. Small alveoli would regularly empty into larger ones, leading to collapse of the smaller alveoli and overdistention of larger alveoli. This clearly does not happen under normal circumstances because of the presence of surfactant, in which surface tension is proportioned to surface area. Thus, as the alveolus gets smaller, surfactant is concentrated over a smaller area, which results in a decrease in surface tension. The alveolus remains inflated at the same transpulmonary pressure.

In ARDS, alveoli are unstable, functional residual capacity (FRC) is reduced, and lung compliance is diminished in part because of inadequate surfactant activity. Henry et al.[129] and Henry[130] showed that after hemorrhagic shock, phospholipid synthesis in the lung is impaired.

Phospholipid composition of lung tissue in patients with ARDS is abnormal, with low lecithin-to-sphingomyelin ratios[131]. Total phospholipid content of the lung in patients with ARDS may be low, remain unchanged, or even increase compared with patients with normal lungs, yet the phospholipid shows poor surface activity[131–133]. Components of pulmonary edema fluid, including cell membrane lipids, plasma proteins, and hemoglobin, may cause inactivation of the phospholipids of surfactant[134,135].

Lung Volumes and Mechanics

Patients with ARDS consistently exhibit reduced lung volumes, especially a reduction in FRC[136]. The low FRC is associated with a large intrapulmonary shunt fraction ($\dot{Q}_S/\dot{Q}_T$) and hypoxemia. Because raising FRC with PEEP greatly improves arterial oxygen tension, it is assumed that low FRC reflects closure of many terminal gas-exchanging units and is a major cause of hypoxemia in this disease (see section on PEEP). Measurement of low FRC is fully consistent with the histologic appearance of fluid-filled alveoli, acinar destruction, and alveolar collapse, as well as with the impairment of surfactant activity, noted above.

The lowered lung volumes in ARDS imply a change in the mechanical properties of the diseased lung. These mechanical properties are evident in a plot of transpulmonary distending pressure ($P_{airway} - P_{pleural}$) against lung volume. Under static conditions (i.e., no airflow), a curve is produced with an inspiratory limb and an expiratory limb (Fig. 7.5). Compared with normal individuals, patients with ARDS exhibit several abnormalities[137]:

1. The slope of the curve ($\Delta V/\Delta P$) or compliance is flatter, indicating that a greater transpulmonary pressure is required to produce a given lung volume. Patients with ARDS, therefore, have relatively noncompliant, stiff lungs.
2. Marked hysteresis occurs; i.e., during inflation of the lung, a much higher transpulmonary pressure is needed to reach a given lung volume than is needed during expiration.
3. In normal individuals, the inspiratory and expiratory limbs of the pressure-volume (PV) curves are exponen-

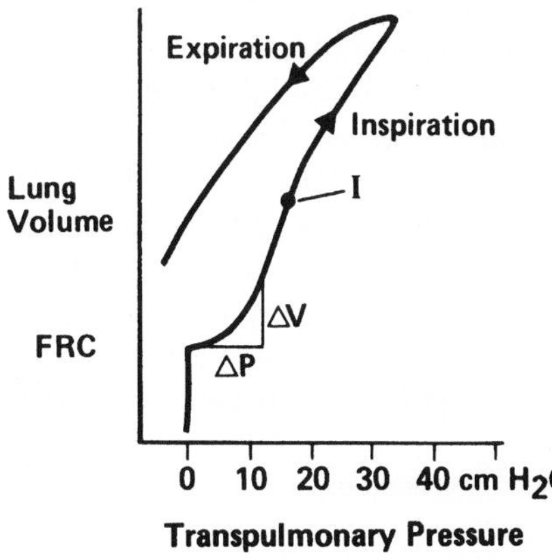

Figure 7.5. Inspiratory and expiratory static pressure (P)-volume (V) curves of the respiratory system in a patient with adult respiratory distress syndrome. Concave portion of the curve lies above the functional residual capacity (FRC); slope of curve ($\Delta V/\Delta P$) is relatively flat at lung volumes in the tidal breathing range. Inflection point (I) is where the PV curve changes from concave to exponential.

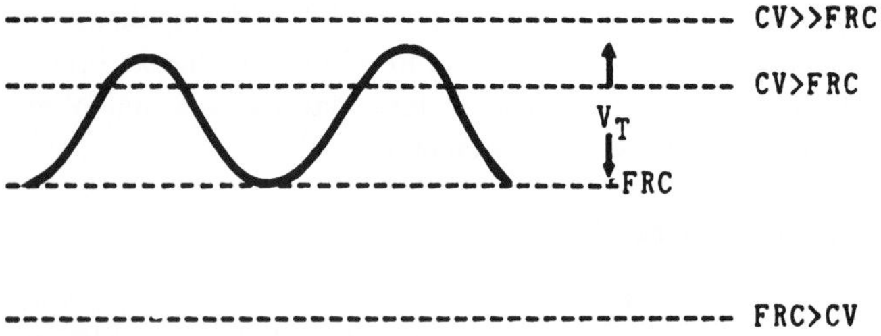

Figure 7.6. Relationship between tidal volumes (V_T), closing volume (CV), and functional residual capacity (FRC) in normal lungs and diseases characterized by low FRC, such as adult respiratory distress syndrome. In normal lungs, FRC is greater than CV. In lungs with low FRC, CV is greater than FRC, corresponding to complete atelectasis.

tial above FRC and concave at lung volumes less than FRC(138). The concavity of the curve below FRC is due to airway closing(138). The point on the PV curve where shape changes from concave to exponential is known as the inflection point (I), and the lung volume at this point virtually coincides with the closing volume as determined by xenon-133 or nitrogen washout curves(138). Patients with ARDS and pulmonary edema differ from normal individuals in that their PV curves are concave above FRC and have an inflection point at lung volumes greater than FRC(139,140).

These data imply that the lung volume at which small dependent airways close (closing volume) is in the range of tidal breathing in ARDS (Fig. 7.6)(141) (see section on PEEP for further discussion of pulmonary mechanics in ARDS).

Total respiratory system resistance ($R_{rs,max}$) and elastance (E_{rs}) have been determined with the end-inflation occlusion method, in which inflation of a relaxed respiratory system is followed by rapid airway occlusion(142). The post-occlusion decline in tracheal pressure until a plateau value is reached allows partitioning of $R_{rs,max}$ into a component caused by airways and tissue-resistance factors ($R_{rs,min}$) and a component caused by mechanical unevenness of the system ($R_{rs,u}$). Patients with ARDS experience increased $R_{rs,max}$ primarily because of increased mechanical unevenness of the respiratory system that reflects a reduction in distal airway caliber presumably secondary to bronchoconstriction, reduced lung volumes, or peribronchiolar edema accumulation. These data suggest that mechanical ventilation with high inspiratory flow rates may allow more uniform gas distribution and improved gas exchange, which in turn may explain the beneficial effects of such techniques as inverse ratio ventilation in patients with ARDS(142,143).

Gas Exchange Abnormalities

Venous Admixture

Arterial hypoxemia with a large venous admixture ($\dot{Q}_S/\dot{Q}_T$) is a consistent finding in ARDS, which could be explained by either $\dot{V}/\dot{Q}$ mismatching or right-to-left intrapulmonary shunting. Standard blood gas analysis is usually inadequate to define precisely the cause of arterial hypoxemia in ARDS, because venous admixture ($\dot{Q}_S/\dot{Q}_T$) measured at an F_IO_2 of less than 1 may be due to either shunt units or low $\dot{V}/\dot{Q}$ units, and 100% O_2 may convert low $\dot{V}/\dot{Q}$ units to shunt through absorption atelectasis. Therefore, more sophisticated techniques are required to study gas exchange in ARDS.

A number of investigators have examined the relative contributions of intrapulmonary right-to-left shunting versus $\dot{V}/\dot{Q}$ mismatching in producing the severe hypoxemia seen in ARDS. The multiple inert gas elimination technique quantifies the fraction of the cardiac output and minute ventilation supplying shunt, low $\dot{V}/\dot{Q}$, normal, and high $\dot{V}/\dot{Q}$ (dead space) units. With this technique, it has become clear in both patients and experimental animals with ARDS that the venous admixture results from distribution of a portion of the pulmonary circulation to both shunt units and low $\dot{V}/\dot{Q}$ units(141,144). Intrapulmonary shunt is clearly the predominant cause of venous admixture, particularly in patients with the most severe ARDS(141). However, some patients also have low $\dot{V}/\dot{Q}$ units. Earlier work had suggested that there was likely to be a contribution of low $\dot{V}/\dot{Q}$ units to venous admixture in this patient population. Markello et al.(145) demonstrated an arterial-alveolar nitrogen gradient ($aADN_2$) in addition to the usual alveolar-arterial oxygen gradient ($AaDO_2$) in intensive care unit patients. Although $\dot{V}/\dot{Q}$ mismatching and intrapulmonary shunt could have accounted for the $AaDO_2$, only $\dot{V}/\dot{Q}$ mismatching with perfusion to low $\dot{V}/\dot{Q}$ units could explain the $aADN_2$. The presence of low $\dot{V}/\dot{Q}$ ratio units is consistent with the observation that an increase in F_IO_2 leads to an increase in PO_2 in some patients with ARDS(146). It is assumed that these $\dot{V}/\dot{Q}$ units, in fact, are fluid-filled alveoli, which become sufficiently inflated during the inspiratory cycle to allow some gas exchange. Because many units with very low $\dot{V}/\dot{Q}$ ratios collapse when high oxygen concentrations are inhaled because of rapid uptake of oxygen, it is assumed that these low $\dot{V}/\dot{Q}$ lung units cannot represent the stable, continuously ventilated alveoli. Histologic studies support this conclusion. Staub et al.(45) noted that pulmonary edema fluid first appeared in the corners of alveoli. This occurs when lymphatic drainage from the pulmonary interstitium is overwhelmed. The appearance of small amounts of edema fluid in the alveolus increases surface forces and leads to an unstable alveolus, which collapses completely. This is an all-or-none phenomenon, with the alveolus either completely filled or completely empty of fluid. Interstitial edema by itself does not affect gas exchange(147,148).

Venous admixture in patients with acute respiratory failure changes as a function of F_IO_2. If the inspired oxygen rises to 40%, venous admixture decreases and remains unchanged until the inspired oxygen is 60%(149). Thereafter, venous admixture increases again as F_IO_2 is raised to 100%(149,150). The initial decrease in venous admixture with F_IO_2 up to 40% occurs because the venous admixture contribution from some lung units with low but finite $\dot{V}/\dot{Q}$ is eliminated as O_2 tension rises within these low $\dot{V}/\dot{Q}$ units.

Venous admixture increases again with inspired oxygen concentrations greater than 60%, presumably because denitrogenation of unstable alveoli results in complete collapse. Inhibition of hypoxic pulmonary vasoconstriction (HPV) is another explanation for the increase in venous admixture with increasing F_IO_2[149]. Regional HPV represents a protective mechanism that directs pulmonary blood away from collapsed or poorly ventilated lung units to well-ventilated lung units and thereby improves $\dot{V}/\dot{Q}$ matching. Raising the P_AO_2 in low $\dot{V}/\dot{Q}$ units inhibits vasoconstriction of arterioles supplying those segments[151]. Therefore, a fraction of the pulmonary blood bypasses better-ventilated segments, and venous admixture increases.

Dead Space in ARDS

Hypercarbia is seldom found early in the course of ARDS. Hypoxemia and pulmonary reflexes stimulate the patient to hyperventilate, so that PCO_2 is normal or low. After days or weeks, fibrosis and pulmonary capillary obliteration may occur[152]. More segments with elevated $\dot{V}/\dot{Q}$ ratio appear, and the V_D/V_T ratio increases. If the patient is unable to hyperventilate sufficiently, arterial PCO_2 will rise.

Cardiovascular Alterations

Pulmonary Hemodynamics

Although the initial derangement in ARDS involves increased permeability of the alveolar capillary membrane, increases in pulmonary artery pressure (PAP) and pulmonary vascular resistance (PVR) may occur even during the early phases of ARDS. The stimuli for pulmonary vasoconstriction during early ARDS include mediator release (serotonin, thromboxane, leukotrienes), alveolar hypoxia, and neural reflexes[153]. Pulmonary vascular resistance is then raised further by endothelial swelling and the development of microthrombi within capillaries[35,47,153]. The extent of pulmonary hypertension correlates with the severity of lung injury and the degree of pulmonary edema[20,154,155]. Katz et al.[20] noted mild pulmonary hypertension, which returned to normal during the convalescent period, in a group of 23 pediatric patients. Mean PAP was 25 mm Hg in this group initially. Among the survivors, PAP gradually decreased to normal during the next 4 days[20].

If pulmonary hypertension results in a rise in pulmonary capillary pressure, pulmonary edema will be aggravated by hydrostatic forces as well as by increased permeability of the alveolar capillary membrane (see section on mechanism of pulmonary edema). Pulmonary capillary pressure cannot be measured directly; however, extrapolation of the slow exponential decay curve of the PAP after transient balloon occlusion allows estimation of pulmonary capillary pressure[156]. With this method the relative contributions of the arterial and venous segments to total PVR can be estimated. Radermacher et al.[157,158] have noted that the arterial and venous segments account for 72 and 28% of total PVR, respectively, within the first 48 hours of mild to moderate ARDS.

In another subset of patients with ARDS, increases in PAP and pulmonary artery resistance become exaggerated and irreversible and are associated with a poor prognosis. Zapol and Snider[152] reported a series of 30 patients with ARDS whose ages ranged from 12 to 60 years. Nonsurvivors had persistent elevation of PVR, PAP, and right ventricular stroke work index. Katz et al.[20] noted a similar relationship between nonsurvival and persistently raised PAP and pulmonary artery resistance in a series of pediatric patients with ARDS. The irreversibility of these hemodynamic derangements suggests a structural basis. In fact, Greene et al.[159] used angiographic techniques to demonstrate pulmonary artery filling defects in patients with ARDS. The presence of filling defects on angiogram correlated significantly with the severity of the disease, fatal outcome, and presence of increased PVR. Examination of the lungs at autopsy has also revealed extensive clot within the pulmonary vasculature as well as remodeling of the pulmonary arteries with medial muscular hypertrophy[32,56,159].

Consequences of Pulmonary Hypertension

Having reviewed the sources of pulmonary hypertension in ARDS, it is then appropriate to trace the effects of these pulmonary hemodynamic derangements on right and left heart performance and, ultimately, on tissue oxygenation. In the normal individual, pulmonary vasculature is quite distensible, and a rise in pulmonary blood flow ($\dot{Q}$) leads to relatively small elevations in PAP. An increase in PVR from active vasoconstriction or thrombosis in ARDS patients results in a rise in PAP in the face of constant pulmonary blood flow. To maintain pulmonary blood flow at constant levels, the work generated by the right ventricle must increase[20,152,160]. There are limits to the ability of the right ventricle to augment its stroke work. Right ventricular output will begin to fall with further increased PVR (afterload) or with venous return (preload) limited (Fig. 7.7). At this point, volume loading may restore cardiac output to normal by increasing right ventricular end-diastolic volume, which in turn leads to an increase in right ventricular stroke volume, even though ejection fraction remains depressed by increased afterload. However, the increase in right ventricular end-diastolic volume is not without cost. As the right ventricle dilates, expansion of its free wall is limited by a noncompliant pericardium. Further right ventricular dilatation requires (leftward) displacement of the interventricular septum. Septal displacement, in turn, decreases the compliance of the left ventricle, so that a given filling pressure corresponds to a smaller "left ventricular" end-diastolic volume. This phenomenon has been called ventricular interdependence[161,162]. Septal displacement may be exaggerated by PEEP therapy. This problem is discussed in the subsection on hemodynamic effects of PEEP. Russell et al.[163] suggested that survivors of ARDS have greater ventricular compliance than nonsurvivors because they exhibit greater end-diastolic volumes, stroke volumes, and cardiac indexes than nonsurvivors despite similar right atrial and pulmonary artery occlusion pressures in the two groups.

CLINICAL MANIFESTATIONS

Physical Findings

The history of the patient with ARDS will vary depending on the inciting event. In some cases, the time of onset and the nature of the previous injury are unknown. Once direct or indirect lung injury takes place, there is usually a latent period in which the patient seems to be in little respiratory distress except for hyperventilation. Auscultation and x-ray of the chest may be normal. During the next several hours to days, hypoxemia gradually progresses, and unequivocal respiratory distress becomes evident. The patient appears cyanotic, dyspneic, and tachypneic. Chest examination reveals diffuse rales. Supplemental oxygen through nasal prongs or mask fails to improve the clinical appearance.

Arterial blood gas measurements reveal profound hypoxemia refractory to the use of supplemental oxygen alone. The PO_2 is less than 50 mm Hg on an F_IO_2 of greater than 0.6. The ratio of P_aO_2 to F_IO_2 (P_aO_2/F_IO_2) is significantly reduced[164]. A P_aO_2/F_IO_2 ratio of less than 200 correlates with a $\dot{Q}_S/\dot{Q}_T$ of greater than 20%[165]. Other physiologic measurements reveal stiff lungs with decreased total compliance.

Imaging Studies

The radiographic picture of ARDS is nonspecific. Immediately after the inciting event, the x-ray may show an entirely normal chest. Subsequently, interstitial and alveolar

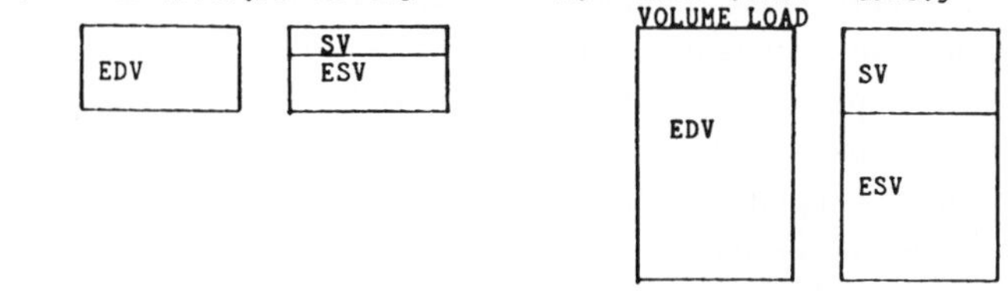

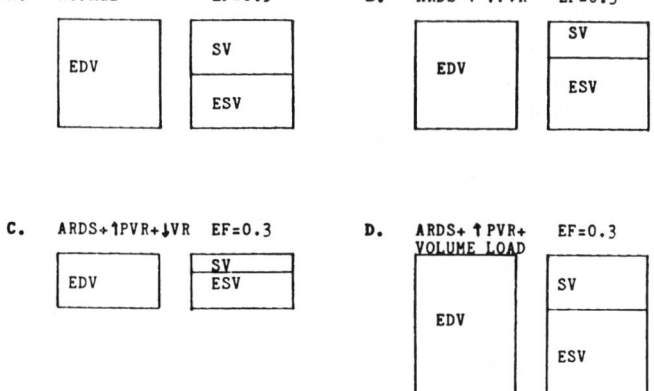

Figure 7.7. Changes in right ventricular end-diastolic volume (EDV) and stroke volume (SV) in normal individuals (A), adult respiratory distress syndrome (ARDS) patients with increasing pulmonary vascular resistance (PVD) (B), ARDS patients with increasing PVR and decreasing venous return (VR) secondary to hypovolemia or positive end-expiratory pressure (PEEP) (C), and ARDS patients with persistently elevated PVR after volume load (D). EF, ejection fraction (SV/EDV); ESV, end-systolic volume. (Modified from Laver MD, Strauss HW, Pohost GM. Right and left ventricular geometry: adjustments during acute respiratory failure. Crit Care Med 1979;7:512.)

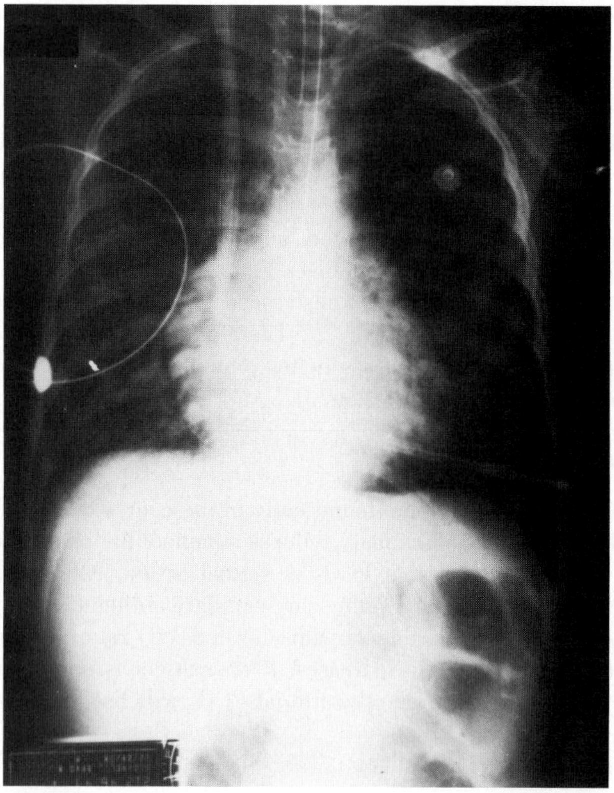

Figure 7.8. Chest x-ray of a patient with early adult respiratory distress syndrome shows mild pulmonary edema with normal heart size.

pulmonary edema without cardiomegaly become apparent (Fig. 7.8)[166]. Although the chest x-ray may suggest diffuse pulmonary infiltrates, computerized tomography (CT) scans of the lungs in early ARDS reveal most of the infiltrates in posterior (dependent) regions of the lung[155]. A picture suggestive of diffuse interstitial fibrosis may develop after several days or weeks (Fig. 7.9)[167]. If the patient survives, the complications of mechanical ventilation may appear on x-ray. These include pulmonary hyperinflation with interstitial gas, pneumothorax, pneumomediastinum, and subcutaneous emphysema (Fig. 7.9)[168,169]. During convalescence, the chest x-ray may return to normal.

MANAGEMENT

Although the inciting event may be specifically treatable, ARDS itself is presently amenable only to supportive care. A major goal of supportive care in ARDS is to deliver sufficient oxygen to satisfy metabolic demands of tissue. The P_aO_2 alone is potentially misleading in determining the adequacy of oxygen delivered to peripheral tissue[170].

Physiologic Concepts Guiding Management

A physiologic approach to the management of ARDS is possible by using the concepts of oxygen delivery ($\dot{D}O_2$), consumption, and extraction (see Chapter 4). DO_2 is the product of cardiac output (Q) and arterial oxygen content (C_aO_2):

$$DO_2 = \dot{Q} \times C_aO_2 \qquad \text{(Eq. 7.3)}$$

From this formula, it is apparent that a major therapeutic goal is to optimize C_aO_2 without depressing $\dot{Q}$, so that DO_2 may supply tissue needs.

Oxygen consumption ($\dot{V}O_2$) is the product of the arterial-venous oxygen content difference ($C_{a-v}O_2$) and cardiac output ($\dot{Q}$):

$$\dot{V}O_2 = C_{a-v}O_2 \times \dot{Q} \qquad \text{(Eq. 7.4)}$$

Shoemaker et al.[171] noted that both very high and very low $\dot{V}O_2$ seem to be associated with poor prognosis. Shoemaker et al. are strongly in support of the position that increasing oxygen delivery (to supraphysiologic levels) decreases mortality[172,173].

The ratio of oxygen consumption to oxygen delivery is the oxygen extraction ratio (E) and represents that portion of delivered oxygen that has actually been consumed:

$$E = C_{a-v}O_2/C_aO_2 \qquad \text{(Eq. 7.5)}$$

The normal extraction ratio is approximately 0.25[174]. The extraction ratio is a measure of circulatory efficiency, since its value increases when delivery of O_2 is inadequate to meet metabolic demand. Conversely, the extraction ratio is decreased when $\dot{V}O_2$ falls in relationship to delivery, such as might be seen with a disturbed microcirculatory pattern in which arterial blood bypasses tissue capillaries while being shunted through normally closed arterial channels.

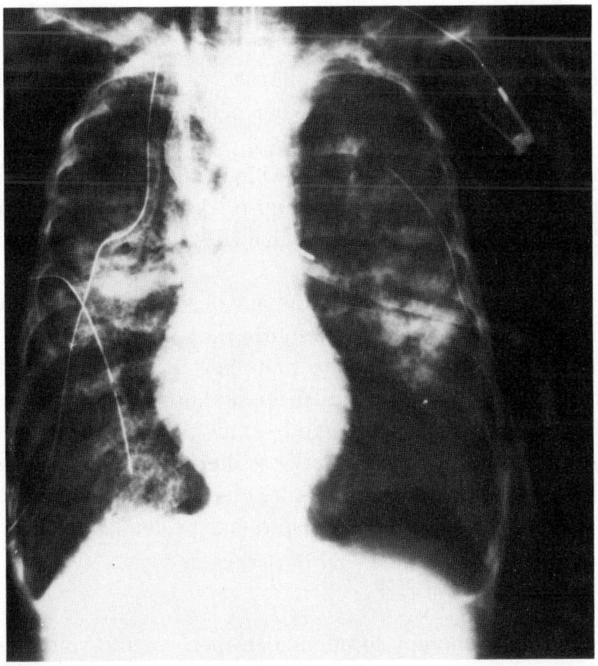

Figure 7.9. Chest x-ray of a patient with late adult respiratory distress syndrome with diffuse interstitial fibrosis and severe barotrauma consisting of pulmonary interstitial emphysema, left pneumothorax, and marked subcutaneous emphysema.

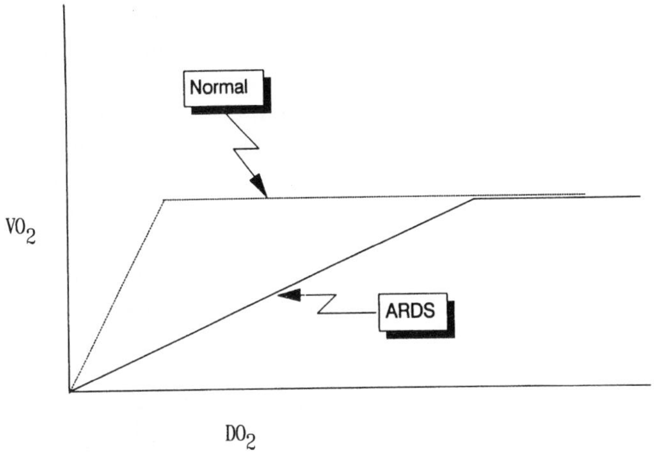

Figure 7.10. Relationship between oxygen delivery (DO_2) and oxygen consumption ($\dot{V}O_2$) in normal individuals and patients with adult respiratory distress syndrome (ARDS). In normal individuals, $\dot{V}O_2$ is constant over a wide range of delivery and is limited only at very low levels of delivery. Conversely, some ARDS patients have delivery-dependent $\dot{V}O_2$, in which a linear relationship exists between delivery and consumption over a wide range of oxygen delivery. Hence, limitation of $\dot{V}O_2$ by inadequate delivery may occur at relatively high levels of delivery.

Oxygen Delivery-Consumption Relationship

In the normal individual, O_2 consumption ($\dot{V}O_2$) does not change over a wide range of O_2 delivery (DO_2)[175]. This independence of $\dot{V}O_2$ from reductions in DO_2 occurs because tissue O_2 extraction is able to rise in the face of falling DO_2, thus maintaining constant $\dot{V}O_2$. If DO_2 falls to critically low values such that O_2 extraction can no longer compensate for the reduced delivery, $\dot{V}O_2$ falls even in the normal individual (Fig. 7.10). This critical oxygen delivery threshold corresponds to DO_2 of 300 to 330 ml/min/m^2 in anesthetized adults[176] and 6 to 10 ml/kg/min in experimental animals[144,145]. Several studies have suggested that O_2 consumption is dependent on O_2 delivery in patients with ARDS over a wide range of cardiac outputs; i.e., the critical oxygen delivery threshold is raised substantially in patients with ARDS[177,178]. Hence, patients with ARDS may have inadequate tissue oxygenation despite apparently adequate arterial O_2 content and cardiac output. Russell et al.[163] demonstrated that ARDS survivors and nonsurvivors alike had delivery-dependent oxygen consumption, but ARDS survivors have greater oxygen consumption than nonsurvivors, which is likely caused by their greater oxygen delivery. Bihari et al.[179] demonstrated delivery-dependent oxygen consumption when oxygen delivery was increased with the vasodilator prostacyclin (PGI_2) in a group of patients with ARDS with sepsis and multiorgan system failure. The patients who died had a significantly greater increase in oxygen consumption after prostacyclin than did the patients who survived. Hence, they concluded that nonsurvivors had already experienced a significant oxygen debt before prostacyclin administration. Management of these patients is complicated because survivors and nonsurvivors could not be distinguished based on illness severity score, baseline oxygen extraction ratios, or mixed venous oxygen tensions. Only prostacyclin administration uncovered the apparent oxygen debt in the nonsurvivor group when oxygen extraction ratios rose after prostacyclin administration[179]. The potential sources of delivery-dependent oxygen consumption are unclear but may include disturbed regional nutrient blood flow secondary to mediator release or microembolization and mitochondrial enzyme dysfunction.

In contrast, several investigators have questioned the linear relationship between oxygen delivery and consumption in ARDS[180–182]. The major theoretical objection to acceptance of data showing delivery-dependent oxygen consumption arises from the fact that all studies showing such a relationship have calculated oxygen consumption as the product of cardiac output and arteriovenous oxygen content difference (Fick equation)[175–178,183–186]. Hence, mathematical coupling of the oxygen delivery and oxygen consumption terms is introduced, because the cardiac output and arterial oxygen content values are used in both the delivery and consumption calculations. Archie[180] suggested that the proposed linear correlation between oxygen delivery and consumption may result from this mathematical coupling, when, in fact, no functional relationship exists. When oxygen consumption was measured independently via mass spectrometry of inspired and expired gases, Annat et al.[181] could not demonstrate a linear relationship between oxygen consumption and delivery. Using simultaneously determined values of oxygen consumption based either on independent measurements of gas exchange or on the Fick equation, Vermeij et al.[182] concluded that consumption measurements based on the Fick equation overestimated the incidence of delivery-dependent oxygen consumption. Nevertheless, 2 of 13 patients in the series had delivery-dependent oxygen consumption confirmed both by independent measurements of consumption and by measurements dependent on determination of cardiac output and arterial oxygen content as determined with the Fick equation. Other theoretical analyses have shown that delivery-dependent oxygen consumption could not be explained solely on the basis of mathematical coupling[187].

Yu et al.[188] reported a randomized trial of supraphysiologic and normal oxygen delivery strategies in adults in the setting of sepsis with or without ARDS. There was no mortality difference between the groups. However, some patients randomized to supraphysiologic oxygen delivery never achieved the target goals. Further, some control patients spontaneously developed supraphysiologic oxygen delivery. Curiously, the group with the lowest mortality was the subgroup that achieved supraphysiologic oxygen delivery either by design (within the experimental group) or spontaneously (within the control group). A recent study also showed no therapeutic benefit of therapy designed to push cardiac index, and hence oxygen delivery, to supranormal levels in critically ill adults[188a,188b].

The conflicting data cited above suggest the following general conclusions:

1. Delivery-dependent oxygen consumption is probably overestimated when the Fick equation is used but does exist in some patients with ARDS.
2. Although no direct proof exists that raising oxygen delivery in patients with delivery-dependent oxygen consumption will improve outcome, the observation that survivors had significantly higher oxygen delivery and consumption within the first 24 hours of ARDS argues for therapeutic attempts at raising delivery.
3. No data on delivery-dependent oxygen consumption have been generated in pediatric ARDS.

Oxygen Therapy

All patients with acute respiratory failure require supplemental oxygen; however, the dose and duration of use of supplemental oxygen must be titrated carefully. Increased inspired concentrations of oxygen denitrogenate the lungs and lead to atelectasis, which in turn worsens right-to-left shunting. This absorption atelectasis cannot be fully prevented by the application of PEP[150]. Furthermore, prolonged exposure to high inspired concentrations of oxygen is directly toxic to lung tissue (see subsection on oxygen toxicity). In the initial stages of the disease process, oxygen may be delivered successfully with nasal prongs or a face mask. However, most patients with ARDS progress rapidly to a stage in which an inspired oxygen concentration of up to 50% delivered by a face mask is no longer sufficient to prevent hypoxemia. At that point, endotracheal intubation is usually required to improve oxygenation by the addition of PEEP without incurring the risks of oxygen toxicity.

Positive End-Expiratory Pressure

No gas exchange occurs in collapsed or fluid-filled alveoli. To achieve and maintain alveolar patency, transpulmonary distending pressure ($P_{airway} - P_{intrapleural}$) must be raised, particularly at end expiration, when transpulmonary pressure is lowest and alveolar collapse is most likely to occur. The concept of PEEP was applied 60 years ago by Barach et al.[189].

A bewildering array of acronyms describing PEEP have found their way into the literature, largely because of the different inspiratory modes that can be combined with PEEP. For the sake of clarity, the authors subscribe to the convention suggested by Shapiro et al.[190], namely, that the unqualified term PEEP describes solely expiration through a threshold resistor or against a column of water, resulting in PEEP without regard to inspiratory mode.

Respiratory Effects of PEEP

It is rational therapy to attempt to increase the volume of ventilated lung, particularly during expiration, in an effort to improve gas exchange in patients with low FRC. Numerous studies have shown that PEEP clearly succeeds in in-

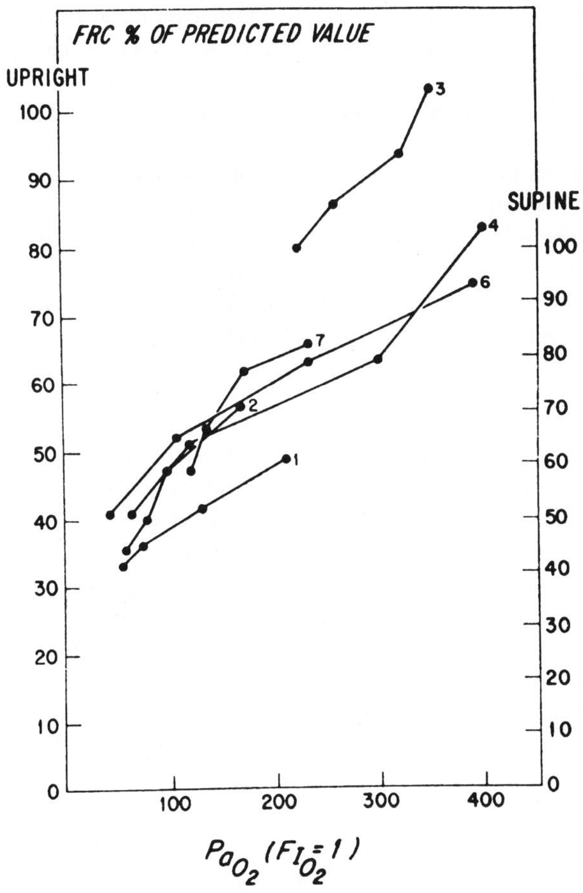

Figure 7.11. Relationship between functional residual capacity (FRC) and partial pressure of oxygen in arterial blood (P_aO_2) at different levels of positive end-expiratory pressure (PEEP): lowest point at 0 PEEP, next point at 5 cm PEEP, etc. (From Falke KJ, Pontoppidan H, Kumar A, Leith DE, Geffin B, Laver MD. Ventilation with end-expiratory pressure in acute lung disease. J Clin Invest 1972;51:2318.)

creasing FRC[136,191]. Falke et al.[136] showed that the relationship between PEEP and FRC was essentially linear over the range of 0 to 15 cm H_20 PEEP in patients with ARDS. Among healthy adult male volunteers, continuous positive airway pressure (CPAP) produced an increase in FRC from 3400 ml at 0 CPAP to 5200 ml at 20 cm H_2O CPAP[191].

Two mechanisms have been proposed to explain the increase in FRC with PEEP: recruitment of previously closed terminal alveoli and overdistention of already-patent alveoli. Although these mechanisms are not mutually exclusive, the weight of the evidence suggests alveolar recruitment as the major mechanism for PEEP-induced increases in FRC. CT studies have shown that stepwise increases in PEEP result in an increased mass of normally inflated lung tissue and progressive clearing of radiographic densities consistent with anatomic alveolar recruitment[155]. The correlation between an increased normally inflated lung mass or FRC and improved oxygenation as measured by increased P_aO_2 or decreased venous admixture further supports the concept of alveolar recruitment by PEEP (Fig. 7.11)[136,140,155]. When PEEP is applied to patients with ARDS, hysteresis of the PV curve is reduced, which implies that the reopening of collapsed units is easier because the transpulmonary pressure at reopening of a collapsed unit is no longer very much greater than transpulmonary pressure at the point of closure of that unit (Fig. 7.5)[192]. The ability of PEEP to prevent inactivation or depletion of surfactant in the lung may facilitate opening terminal air spaces[193,194].

PEEP increases the static compliance of the lung[136,195]. That is, the end-expiratory point is on a steeper portion of the PV curve such that a given transpulmonary pressure change is associated with a larger increment in volume (Fig. 7.12). Greater increases in PEEP level produce greater increases in compliance up to a certain limit, at which point further PEEP increases lead to a fall in compliance[136,195]. Presumably, that limit represents the point at which maximal air space recruitment has been achieved and further increases in PEEP merely overdistend already-open air spaces. In contrast to these findings in patients

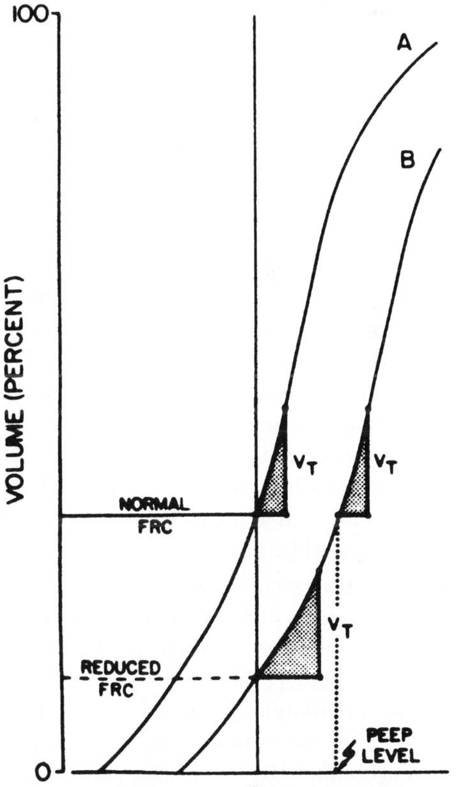

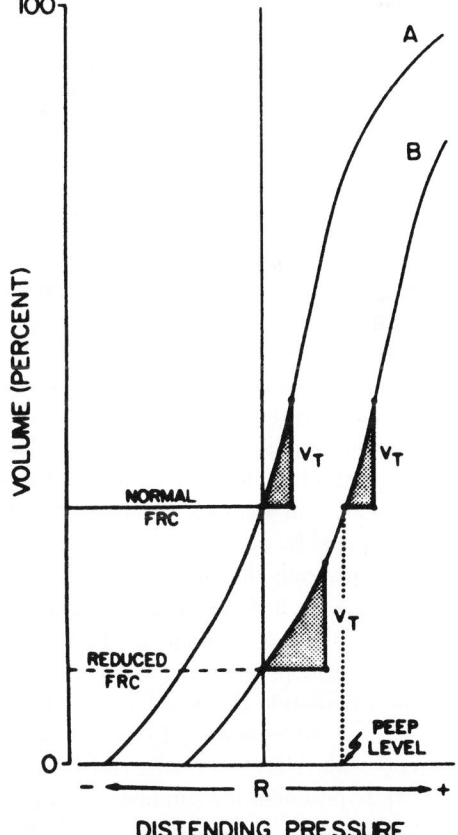

Figure 7.12. Inspiratory static lung compliance curve in normal individuals (A) and patients with adult respiratory distress syndrome (ARDS) (B). PEEP raises the end-expiratory point in ARDS patients to a more favorable position on the compliance curve. V_T, tidal volume. (From Douglas ME, Downs JB. Applied physiology and respiratory care. In: Shoemaker WC, Thompson WL, eds. Critical care state of the art. Fullerton, California: Society of Critical Care Medicine, 1982;3:E15.)

with early ARDS, those with late ARDS (mean duration 31 days) and pulmonary fibrosis do not exhibit an inflection point in their PV curves and do not improve oxygenation with PEEP[140].

In summary, the available evidence indicates that when PEEP is able to lower Q_S/Q_T and increase P_aO_2, it does so by recruiting terminal airways and alveoli, leading to an increase in FRC and compliance. The PEEP level that accomplishes this goal seems to correspond to that transpulmonary pressure that raises the patient's lung volume above closing volume.

CPAP allows an additional mechanical benefit: With increasing CPAP level up to 10 cm and expanding lung volume, the total work of breathing decreases by about half[191]. In contrast, a PEEP system that lacks a high-pressure reservoir bag on the inspiratory limb forces the patient to drop airway pressure below ambient pressure in order to inspire. Predictably, the large pressure gradient required for inspiration during spontaneous breathing with a PEEP system increases the patient's work of breathing[191].

Hemodynamic Effects of PEEP

PEEP improves oxygenation by redistributing pulmonary blood flow to better-ventilated lung units. Because of the pulmonary edema-associated increase in PVR in the gravity-dependent portions of the lung, ARDS causes a redistribution of pulmonary blood flow away from dependent lung regions into nondependent regions[196]. PEEP may lower PVR in the dependent lung and, hence, increase pulmonary blood flow, since increasing lung volume in dependent areas increases the diameter of extra-alveolar vessels. Under these circumstances, PEEP improves $\dot{V}/\dot{Q}$ matching by shifting pulmonary blood flow from nondependent lung regions to dependent regions[141,144,196].

PEEP may also increase lung dead space. The expansion of dead space by high levels of PEEP probably results from an increase in both anatomic dead space and alveolar dead space. Presumably, anatomic dead space enlarges as positive pressure distends the airways. Conversely, alveolar dead space expands as high PEEP levels (greater than 15 cm H_2O) produce alveolar overdistention and raise alveolar pressure to exceed pulmonary capillary pressure such that pulmonary circulation in the affected lung regions is interrupted[144,197]. Nevertheless, hypercarbia is seldom seen in patients with ARDS receiving PEEP early in their course because hypoxemia and pulmonary reflexes stimulate hyperventilation such that the increase in total ventilation exceeds the rise in dead space ventilation. If ARDS progresses to a chronic fibrotic stage, dead space increases significantly because of pulmonary vascular obliteration and obstruction.

The effects of PEEP on right ventricular function have been the subject of conflicting reports for many years. However, there is general agreement that the application of PEEP may result in decreased cardiac output[198–201]. The major source of the reduction in cardiac output is decreased venous return, which has been demonstrated in humans via echocardiography[200] and in experimental animals via end-systolic PV relationships[201] and direct myocardial fiber length measurements with sonomicrometry[202]. Lung expansion by PEEP may lead to compression of the ventricular free wall and restriction of venous return[203].

The effects of PEEP on ventricular contractility are less clear. Several studies have reported decreased ventricular contractility in the presence of PEEP[204–206]. Postulated mechanisms for depression of ventricular contractility by PEEP have included circulating myocardial depressant factors[207], cardiodepressant reflexes induced by pulmonary stretch receptors[208], and coronary hypoperfusion[209]. However, precise interpretation of contractility data requires measurement of contractility at equivalent end-diastolic volumes (preload) on and off PEEP. This requirement is difficult to fulfill, in that PEEP has such a profound effect on preload (see above), and the measurement of filling pressures (atrial or ventricular end-diastolic pressure) as a reflection of preload is subject to error[210]. The filling pressure of the ventricle that determines preload is given by the transmural ventricular end-diastolic pressure, such that

$$RVEDP_{TM} = RVEDP - P_{pl} \qquad \text{(Eq. 7.6)}$$

where $RVEDP_{TM}$ is the transmural right ventricular end-diastolic pressure, RVEDP is the intravascular right ventricular pressure referenced to atmospheric pressure, and P_{pl} is the pleural pressure as measure of intrathoracic pressure. The error is introduced because the clinically useful measures of intrathoracic pressure, such as pleural or esophageal pressure, underestimate juxtacardiac intrathoracic pressure[210]. Determination of ventricular contractility during PEEP via echocardiography or sonomicrometry shows no change in ventricular contractility after the application of PEEP in the absence of underlying heart disease[200,202].

Because PEEP may reduce venous return and hence cardiac output, systemic oxygen delivery may be reduced by this therapy (see Eq. 7.3)[211,212]. After the application of PEEP, cinefluorography and echocardiography have demonstrated a reduction in left ventricular dimensions that may have resulted from lung expansion and extracardiac compression[198,200,213]. The net result is a reduction in left ventricular end-diastolic volume, stroke volume, and cardiac output. The decreased left ventricular end-diastolic volume may be associated with an elevated left ventricular filling pressure, indicating that the left ventricle is more noncompliant in the presence of PEEP[214].

There seems to be a distinct threshold PEEP level of 10 to 12 cm H_2O at which cardiac output falls in adult patients considered euvolemic prior to the application of PEEP[215–217]. In children with ARDS receiving PEEP, systemic oxygen delivery is maximized at PEEP levels ranging from 0 to 15 cm H_2O[218]. At higher PEEP levels, systemic oxygen delivery falls because the fall in cardiac output exceeds any rise in arterial oxygen content. Volume loading restores cardiac output in patients and experimental animals receiving PEEP[180,182,185]. Left ventricular preload is expanded, as measured by an increase in left ventricular end-diastolic area (or volume), despite the presence of PEEP[180].

Jardin et al.[198] suggested that at very high levels of PEEP (30 cm H_2O) the compliance limits of the ventricle may be reached, so that volume expansion becomes ineffective. Others have not encountered this difficulty, using very high PEEP in patients with ARDS. Kirby et al.[219] and Gallagher and Civetta[220] showed that patients with ARDS may tolerate PEEP levels of 40 cm H_2O without a fall in cardiac output, provided additional fluid volume is administered to expand preload. When volume loading alone proved insufficient to maintain cardiac output in the presence of PEEP, inotropic agents were used to restore cardiac output in adults[220] and children[25] with ARDS.

Effect of PEEP on Extravascular Lung Water

When PEEP was first applied to large series of patients with ARDS, it was suggested that one advantage of PEEP was its ability to retard the development of pulmonary edema[221]. Now overwhelming evidence indicates that, in fact, the opposite is true; namely, PEEP favors the development of pulmonary edema[222–225].

The mechanisms by which PEEP influences extravascular lung water (EVLW) are related closely to the effects of PEEP on PAP and interstitial pressure in the lung. The hydrostatic pressure gradient governing transudation of fluid across the alveolar-capillary membrane is the difference between PAP and interstitial pressure. If this hydrostatic pressure gradient increases, EVLW increases. PEEP raises the hydrostatic pressure gradient both by raising PAP and by lowering interstitial pressure. If pulmonary blood flow remains constant, PEEP produces a significant rise in PAP relative to pleural pressure[226]. Conversely, lung inflation has been shown to lower interstitial pressure around small intrapulmonary vessels not directly exposed to alveolar pressure[227]. The net result of these PEEP-induced pressure changes is a rise in EVLW. Nevertheless, the beneficial effects of PEEP on oxygenation clearly outweigh any increase in EVLW, and PEEP should not be withheld from the hypoxemic patient with ARDS because of a fear of increasing EVLW.

Clinical Application of Mechanical Ventilation

The clinician must decide when to intubate the child with ARDS and whether spontaneous ventilation with PEEP (CPAP) or some form of mechanical ventilation with PEEP is indicated in the context of a complete therapeutic plan

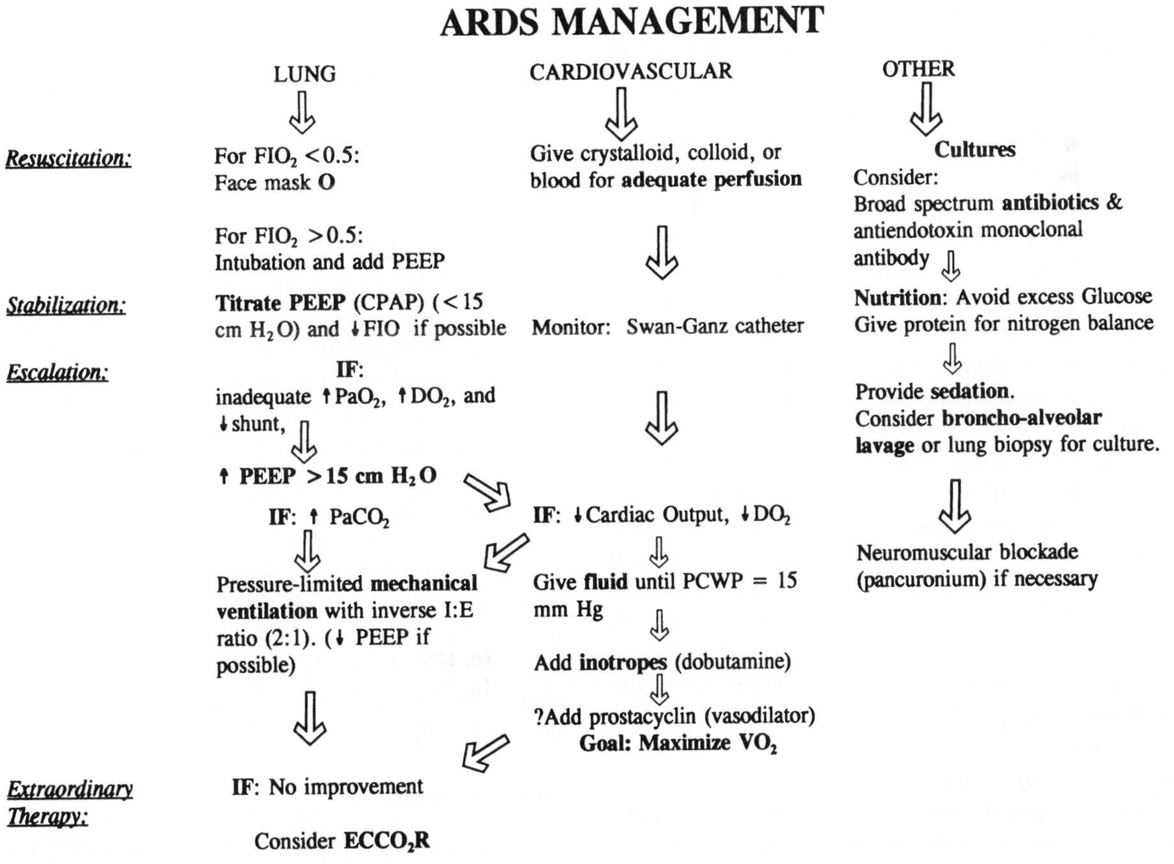

Figure 7.13. Management algorithm for adult respiratory distress syndrome. $ECCO_2R$, extracorporeal CO_2 removal; PCWP, pulmonary capillary wedge pressure; DO_2, oxygen delivery; VO_2, oxygen consumption.

Table 7.3. Guidelines for Determination of Optimal PEEP Level

1. Ensure normal blood volume prior to starting PEEP.[a]
2. Increase PEEP in increments of 3–5 cm H_2O every 3 minutes.
3. Continue PEEP increase until
   OD optimal (usually >650 ml/min/m²)
   $\dot{V}O_2$ optimal (usually >160 ml/min/m²)
4. If decreased cardiac output is encountered, expand volume until wedge pressure equals 18 mm Hg (referenced to atmosphere).
5. Start inotropic agents if cardiac output remains depressed after volume expansion.
6. If cardiac output remains depressed, begin decreasing PEEP in increments until cardiac output is restored.

[a] Abbreviations: PEEP, positive end-expiratory pressure; OD, oxygen delivery; $\dot{V}O_2$, oxygen consumption.

(Fig. 7.13). In either case the optimal PEEP level must be determined.

Pepe et al.[(228)] showed in a well-controlled study that patients at risk for ARDS do not benefit from early or prophylactic application of PEEP. Thus, PEEP must be viewed as valuable supportive therapy, but it will not alter the underlying disease process that led to the development of ARDS[(229)]. In general, endotracheal intubation and application of PEEP are appropriate in the patient with ARDS when the following conditions apply:

1. Clinical and radiographic evidence suggest worsening lung disease.
2. F_IO_2 of 0.5 by face mask is required to prevent hypoxemia.

Considerable debate has focused on the question of how much PEEP to apply. The first goal of PEEP is to improve arterial oxygen content (C_aO_2) and hence raise systemic oxygen delivery while maintaining an inspired oxygen concentration (F_IO_2) of less than 50 to 60% to limit the risk of oxygen toxicity. Through stepwise increases in PEEP, a level should be sought that maintains approximately 90% arterial oxygen saturation (S_aO_2) in the presence of a maximal F_IO_2 of 50 to 60%. Although it has been suggested that PEEP should be increased to lower venous admixture ($\dot{Q}_S/\dot{Q}_T$) to some low target value, maximized oxygen delivery is more important therapeutic goals than an arbitrary $\dot{Q}_S/\dot{Q}_T$ value[(163,217,230,231)]. Carroll et al.[(232)] have shown that adjusting PEEP to achieve P_aO_2 of 60 mm Hg (or approximately 90% S_aO_2) in the presence of 50% F_IO_2 results in fewer episodes of hypotension and pneumothorax than when PEEP is adjusted to decrease $\dot{Q}_S/\dot{Q}_T$ by 50%. If the level of PEEP required to accomplish these goals exceeds 15 cm H_2O, the risk of falling cardiac output and barotrauma must be anticipated[(212,230)]. Several investigators have shown that cardiac output can be preserved despite high PEEP levels (30 to 44 cm H_2O) if circulating volume is expanded[(25,219,220)].

Suter et al.[(233)] argued that the PEEP level, which provided optimal oxygen delivery, also improves lung compliance the most. However, others studies in both children and adults have disputed that finding[(232,234)]. Recommendations for determining optimal PEEP levels are summarized in **Table 7.3.**

CO_2 retention is usually not a problem early in ARDS. However, with decreasing lung compliance and increasing dead space, work of breathing may increase such that respiratory muscles are no longer able to increase minute ventilations sufficiently. At this point, mechanical ventilation becomes necessary.

Various inspiratory modes may be combined with PEEP. For example, the combination of inspiratory positive pressure ventilation (IPPV) and PEEP is termed controlled positive pressure ventilation (CPPV). There are a number of theoretical objections to this mode of ventilation. If the patient's arterial PCO_2 is above apneic threshold, he or she will attempt to breathe spontaneously out of phase with ventilator breaths. This frequently leads to hyperventilation and alkalemia[(235)]. In addition, there seems to be a higher incidence of barotrauma when CPPV is employed[(236)].

Some of these problems may be minimized by use of intermittent mandatory ventilation (IMV) and CPAP. This mode allows the patient to breathe spontaneously through the ventilator circuit. The otherwise spontaneous breathing pattern is interrupted by intermittent mechanical breaths. The use of spontaneous ventilation with this mode allows better distribution of gas, which in turn lowers physiologic dead space, compared with CPPV[(237)]. With this technique it is easier to maintain a normal alveolar ventilation ($\dot{V}_A$) and pH[(237)]. Classically, the frequency of IMV is adjusted such that pH remains between 7.35 and 7.40. The initial tidal volume for IMV may be set at 15 ml/kg (see Permissive Hypercapnea, below).

Pressure Control Inverse Ratio Ventilation

A pressure-controlled mode of ventilation using an inverse ratio of inspiratory-to-expiratory (I/E) time may be more beneficial than conventional volume-controlled IMV in patients with ARDS. Inverse ratio ventilation is instituted by setting a peak inflating pressure limit and lengthening the I/E ratio to 2:1 or 3:1. The inspiratory pattern consists of a square wave pressure pattern with decelerating inspiratory flow[(238)]. Lung compliance may improve within the first several hours of applying pressure control inverse ratio ventilation (PCIRV), which allows peak inflating pressure and PEEP to be lowered in the face of improved P_aO_2 and unchanged CO_2 elimination[(143,239,240)]. The prolonged inspiratory time results in a rise in mean airway pressure that may improve the stability of alveoli in danger of collapse, which in turn results in better compliance and P_aO_2. The hemodynamic effects of inverse ratio ventilation are similar to those of conventional volume-limited IMV with PEEP[(143,240)]. However, Lessard et al.[(241,242)] could not show a benefit of PCIRV in a short-term prospective randomized trial.

Permissive Hypercapnea

Efforts to reduce ventilator-induced lung injury have given rise to a reexamination of the acceptable parameters of minute ventilation. Because systemic oxygen saturations lower than normal can be accepted as long as oxygen delivery is preserved, minute ventilation may be minimized as long as P_aCO_2 is balanced by serum bicarbonate levels such that pH is acceptable (the latter possibly being as low as 7.15)[243]. Hickling et al. have been strong proponents of the approach and reported excellent results in both retrospective and prospective reports[244,245]. Neither study, however, reports having used a control group.

High-Frequency Ventilation

The effects of rapid ventilatory rates on gas exchange was first described in 1915 by Henderson and Chillingworth. Jack Emerson, in 1952, was the first to patent a high-frequency device for clinical use. The theoretical advantages of high-frequency oscillatory ventilation (HFOV) include (a) smaller phasic volume and pressure change, (b) gas exchange at significantly lower airway pressures, and (c) less depression of endogenous surfactant production. The mechanisms of gas exchange involved during high-frequency ventilation have been reviewed in detail elsewhere[246].

Limited published information is available regarding the use of high-frequency ventilation in pediatric patients. Early experience with a variety of high-frequency techniques in adults suggested that although this modality achieves adequate gas exchange, there is no greater improvement in outcome than when conventional ventilation is used[247–250]. More recent experience with HFOV has produced some encouraging results. We described our experience with a small group of children with weights ranging from 3 to 42 kg. An aggressive approach to rapidly attain and maintain optimal lung volume was used. This typically requires an increase of mean airway pressure of 5 to 8 cm H_2O when converting from conventional mechanical ventilation to HFOV. Interestingly, despite significant increases in mean airway pressure, hemodynamic compromise as indicated by cardiac index or oxygen delivery does not appear to be an important problem using this "ideal lung volume" strategy[251]. More recently completed is a prospective, multicenter, randomized clinical study comparing HFOV and conventional mechanical ventilation in pediatric patients with either diffuse alveolar disease or air leak syndrome[252]. These data demonstrate that HFOV offers rapid and sustained improvements in oxygenation without adverse effects on ventilation. The increase in mean airway pressure used during HFOV does not result in an increase in the incidence of barotrauma, and the oxygenation index declines significantly during the first 72 hours of HFOV. Despite the use of higher mean airway pressures, the optimal lung volume strategy used in this study was associated with a lower incidence of barotrauma, as indicated by the requirement for supplemental oxygen at 30 days, and improved outcome compared with conventional mechanical ventilation. In certain circumstances, such as bronchopleural fistula, high-frequency jet ventilation may have distinct advantages over conventional volume-cycled ventilation or HFOV[250].

Weaning from Mechanical Ventilation

The time when a patient moves into a weaning phase of mechanical ventilation is, at best, ill defined. Some parameters to signal that weaning from any mode of respiratory support may be possible may, however, be delineated. The patient should be hemodynamically stable. The effects of narcotics, sedatives, and muscle relaxants should have dissipated. There should be clinical, pulmonary function testing, radiologic, and arterial blood gas evidence of stable or improving lung disease. The weaning process begins with a stepwise reduction in IMV rate while normal arterial pH is maintained. F_IO_2 is decreased to nontoxic levels consistent with adequate oxygen delivery. Finally, PEEP is reduced in small increments (e.g., 2 cm) to prevent sudden decreases in FRC or compliance[253].

The weaning process is beginning to receive scrutiny. Multiple groups have attempted computer-assisted weaning[254–257]. Pressure support ventilation has been compared to intermittent mandatory ventilation; both have been compared to periods of complete spontaneous ventilation[258,259]. The latter study showed that intermittent periods of spontaneous ventilation shortened ventilator hours. Weinberger and Wiess (260) postulated the patients managed in this fashion received more personal attention.

Blood and Fluid Therapy

Patients with ARDS have increased metabolic needs, fluid losses from capillary leak, and decreased venous return from PEEP. Cardiac index and DO_2 must rise in order to meet these needs. Ideal blood and fluid therapy for patients with ARDS would allow optimal tissue perfusion without worsening pulmonary edema and intrapulmonary shunt.

Four types of fluid have been evaluated over the years in ARDS or diseases known to trigger ARDS: (a) crystalloid, (b) colloid, (c) hypertonic crystalloid (with or without colloid), and (d) blood. Most of the clinical studies have examined a variety of outcome variables, including pulmonary morbidity, when these fluid regimens are used in the acute management of shock or trauma. Although some investigators have failed to document an improvement in cardiac output with crystalloid[261,262], most groups have shown that improved cardiac output can be achieved with crystalloid at the expense of a greater tendency toward fluid overload[263], larger fluid volume requirements[264], and prolonged resuscitation times[265] compared with colloid solutions. An unchallenged advantage of crystalloid remains its low cost and ready availability.

Colloidal solutions have the advantage of providing a more sustained increase in plasma volume after administration of a smaller amount of resuscitation solution. It is believed that both colloid and crystalloid may leak into the pulmonary interstitium in ARDS; however, the leakage of colloid may depend on the molecular weight of the colloid. Laboratory studies have suggested that larger molecular weight colloids can limit the movement of water and smaller molecules across capillary walls[266]. Webb et al.[267] showed in an animal model of septic shock that pentastarch, a hydroxyethyl starch of intermediate molecular weight, is associated with decreased interstitial edema compared with hetastarch, a nonhomogeneous synthetic colloid with small, large, and very large molecular weight fractions. The increased pulmonary interstitial edema with hetastarch may result from (a) passage of small molecular weight molecules across the alveolar capillary membrane and (b) obstruction of pulmonary capillaries by very large molecular weight molecules.

Hypertonic (7.5%) saline has been given alone or combined with a colloid solution during resuscitation from endotoxic or hypovolemic shock[268]. Hypertonic solutions have not received widespread acceptance because of conflicting evidence, with some investigators demonstrating beneficial increases in cardiac output sustained for several hours[269] and others showing only transient improvements[270].

While the relative merits of volume expansion with crystalloid versus colloid remain unresolved, volume expansion with blood has clear advantages in patients with ARDS who have incurred blood loss or are anemic. After blood transfusion, DO_2 is improved both by the increased hemoglobin concentration and by the augmented cardiac output. Several lines of evidence suggest that the hematocrit should be maintained between 40 and 49%. DO_2 per unit of cardiac work expended is greatest when hematocrit is kept in this range[271]. Hematocrits in this range may optimize cerebral DO_2[272] and improve ARDS survival rates[273]. Some have questioned whether cellular aggregates and debris in transfused blood lead to ARDS. However, 40-μm micropore filtration of blood products during massive transfusion does not decrease the incidence or severity of ARDS[274].

Because the permeability of the alveolar-capillary membrane is increased in ARDS, some fraction of the administered fluid may leak into pulmonary interstitium and alveoli, ultimately worsening the intrapulmonary shunt. Therefore, cardiac filling pressures should be monitored so that overhydration can be scrupulously avoided. In general, circulating volume is expanded until cardiac output is optimized without exceeding a pulmonary capillary wedge pressure (PCWP) referenced to an atmosphere of 15 to 18 mm Hg[217,220]. The risk of excess water retention is heightened because of mechanical ventilation-stimulated antidiuretic hormone secretion, which leads to reabsorption of water in the distal tubule of the kidney[275].

Monitoring

All patients with acute respiratory failure require meticulous routine care that includes an hourly record of vital signs; frequent observations of sensorium, breathing pattern, and perfusion; and a summary of intake and output after every nursing shift. The patient's weight should be measured daily.

Hemodynamic monitoring requires a continuous record of the electrocardiogram. Arterial lines permit beat-to-beat measurement of blood pressure, which may fluctuate widely, secondary to the underlying disease or PEEP therapy. As suggested previously, knowledge of oxygen delivery and consumption, in addition to Q_S/Q_T and P_aO_2, should guide therapy in ARDS. This requires placement of a pulmonary artery catheter. The information obtained from a pulmonary artery catheter must be interpreted critically. Although determination of cardiac output by thermodilution and mixed venous oxygen content from a pulmonary artery blood sample is likely to be accurate, measurement of PCWP as an indication of left ventricular preload should be approached cautiously. The potential sources of error in using PCWP in patients with ARDS relate to two fundamental assumptions on which PCWP measurements are based. First, left ventricular end-diastolic volume (LVEDV) represents the preload of the left ventricle. As LVEDV is difficult to measure clinically, left ventricular end-diastolic pressure (LVEDP) is used as an approximation of LVEDV. This step assumes that left ventricular compliance is normal. In fact, patients with ARDS, particularly those on PEEP, have decreased left ventricular compliance, so that any given LVEDV is associated with a higher LVEDP[161,162,198,214]. Second, under normal circumstances, it is assumed that PCWP gives an accurate reflection of LVEDP as long as intravascular pressures can be transmitted through a continuous column of blood between the left ventricle and the tip of the pulmonary artery catheter. This assumption allows the pulmonary artery catheter to be zeroed relative to atmospheric pressure at the level of the atrium. PEEP may invalidate this assumption by raising alveolar and pleural pressures so that the pressure on the outside of the pulmonary artery and the heart is no longer atmospheric. In this situation, the effective filling pressure equals the transmural pressure P_{TM}:

$$P_{TM} = PCWP - P_{pl} \qquad \text{(Eq. 7.7)}$$

One approach to this problem is to attempt to measure P_{pl} whenever it is presumed to be significantly greater than atmospheric pressure. Because of the possibility of producing a tension pneumothorax, direct measurement of P_{pl} by placement of a catheter in the pleural space is extremely hazardous in patients on PEEP. Alternatively, esophageal pressure measurement may serve as an approximation of P_{pl}. However, esophageal pressure measurement has its own potential sources of error because of the need to vary the dimensions of the balloon in infants and children of different sizes and because of the unknown weight of the mediastinum in a supine patient[276].

Even though it is recognized that raised P_{pl} may increase LVEDP and left atrial pressure (LAP), it has been clearly demonstrated that PCWP will accurately reflect LAP even in the presence of high PEEP, provided the tip of the catheter lies in dependent regions of the lung (zone 3)[277,278]. In zone 3, distended alveoli do not compress the pulmo-

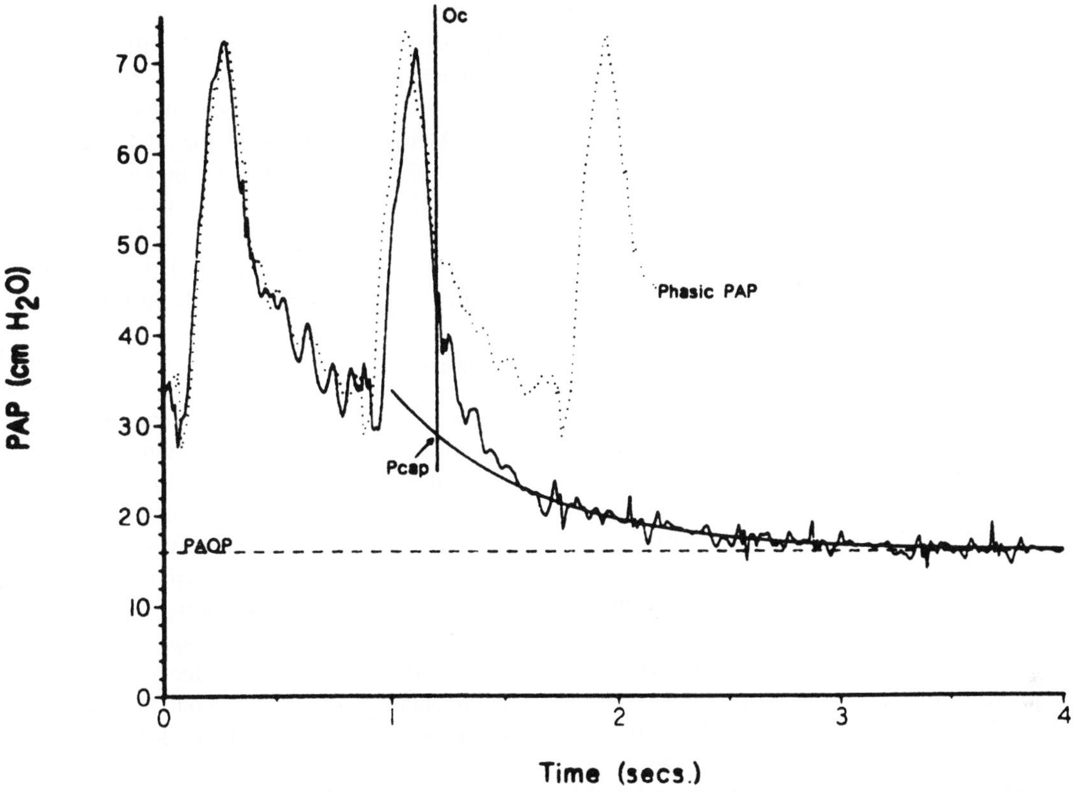

Figure 7.14. Pulmonary capillary pressure (P_{cap}) determination. The time of pulmonary artery (PA) occlusion (i.e., balloon inflation) is indicated by the point at which the phasic PA pressure trace (dotted line) and the PA occlusion pressure (PAOP) trace diverge. Extrapolation of the slow component of the occlusion pressure curve to the time of pulmonary artery occlusion yields P_{cap}. See text for further details. (From Collee GG, et al. Bedside measurement of pulmonary capillary pressure in patients with acute respiratory failure. Anesthesiology 66:614, 1987.)

nary vasculature, and there is a continuous column of blood between the pulmonary artery and the left ventricle. In practice, if the catheter tip lies below the left atrium on lateral chest x-ray, zone 3 conditions have been met even with PEEP up to 30 cm H_2O. If the catheter tip lies above the level of the left atrium, PCWP will overestimate LAP. Wedge pressure measurements should be obtained at end expiration from the screen or a strip chart record, rather than from a digital readout, in order to limit the effects of respiratory variation.

Some investigators have suggested that mathematical analysis of the pressure decay curve after pulmonary artery occlusion may yield a closer estimation of the true filtration pressure into the lung (pulmonary capillary pressure) than PCWP[156,279,280]. With this method, pulmonary capillary pressure is determined by plotting the difference between PAP and PCWP on a semilogarithmic scale as a function of time. The pressure decay after balloon occlusion of the pulmonary artery is biexponential, with an initial rapid component followed by a slow linear component. Extrapolation of the slow linear component of the pressure decay curve to the time of pulmonary artery occlusion yields the pulmonary capillary pressure (Fig. 7.14).

Respiratory monitoring principally involves the evaluation of gas exchange and lung mechanics. The arterial blood gas forms the foundation for monitoring gas exchange. Samples are obtained via an indwelling arterial line. End-tidal CO_2 is analyzed with infrared photometry or mass spectrometry. In the normal lung, end-tidal CO_2 closely approximates arterial PCO_2. When ventilation is poorly matched to perfusion, a gradient develops between end-tidal CO_2 and arterial CO_2. However, end-tidal CO_2 analysis remains useful as a trend monitor and as an additional ventilator disconnect alarm.

The vital capacity and static lung compliance are important measures of mechanics in patients with ARDS. Vital capacity is determined with a hand-held spirometer. A vital capacity of less than 15 ml/kg suggests inadequate strength to cough and defend the airway. A vital capacity of less than 10 ml/kg suggests incipient CO_2 retention.

Because one of the beneficial effects of PEEP is to increase compliance and thereby decrease work of breathing, compliance is a useful measure to follow.

$$\text{Static compliance} = V_T/(\text{PIP} - \text{PEEP}) \qquad \text{(Eq. 7.8)}$$

where V_T is the tidal volume and PIP equals plateau pressure at end inspiration.

A chest x-ray is obtained when there is a sudden change in the patient's clinical status and at least once a day in order to confirm proper position of the endotracheal tube and pulmonary artery catheter as well as to document progression of disease[281]. A chest x-ray is also suggested after endotracheal tube repositioning[282].

Drug Therapy

Steroids

Several large prospective studies have evaluated the use of corticosteroids in ARDS[283,284]. They have shown that steroids do not reverse the pathologic process of ARDS, improve lung function, or increase survival in ARDS. In fact, the use of high-dose steroids for sepsis led to increased mortality in patients with serum creatinine concentrations greater than 2.0 mg/dl[285].

In part because mortality from ARDS is higher when pulmonary fibrosis is present[286], steroids have been employed as therapy for the fibroproliferative response (described above). Meduri and Chinn[287] observed 86% survival in a group of adults with ARDS who responded to steroids. As the authors suggest, a randomized clinical trial is necessary.

Special mention should be made of the 21-amino steroids—so-called *lazaroids*—based on preliminary work in the area of cerebral protection[288,289]. Best described is their antioxidant properties[290]. Specifically, however, 21-amino steroids have been shown to inhibit fibroblast proliferation; their possible use in ARDS is obvious. Recently, it was shown that a particular 21-amino steroid (when given before the insult) could ameliorate cytokine expression in the BAL fluid of rats after an experimental episode of profound shock[291].

Vasodilators

Nonsurvivors in ARDS exhibit the characteristic hemodynamic pattern of increasing PVR, which ultimately may become severe enough to limit cardiac output. For this reason, vasodilators have been tried. Successful pulmonary vasodilator therapy in ARDS would require that PVR be lowered more than systemic vascular resistance and that vasodilation of pulmonary vasculature occur in well-ventilated lung regions in order to improve $\dot{V}/\dot{Q}$ matching.

Most vasodilators, including nitroprusside[292,293], hydralazine[294], the calcium channel blocker diltiazem[295], and nitroglycerin[293,296] do not fulfill these requirements. Nitroglycerin may have some advantage over other vasodilators because systemic vascular resistance is not lowered to a greater extent than pulmonary vasculature resistance[293,296]. However, nitroglycerin shares the drawback common to other vasodilators of worsening $\dot{V}/\dot{Q}$ matching[296]. The calcium blocker nifedipine has been effective in reducing PVR without significantly affecting PO_2 in patients with cystic fibrosis[297] and chronic obstructive pulmonary disease[298]. Nifedipine was considered beneficial in a small adult study[299].

The prostaglandins PGE_1 and PGI_2 are pulmonary vasodilators and have been studied in patients with ARDS. PGE_1 decreases PAP and systemic blood pressure to the same extent and increases cardiac output[300]. However, $\dot{Q}_S/\dot{Q}_T$ also increases, so that P_aO_2 falls and DO_2 is generally unchanged or only marginally improved[300,301]. In a large, multicenter study, long-term outcome was not improved in patients with ARDS receiving PGE_1[242]. PGI_2 (prostacyclin) also decreases PAP and increases cardiac output and $\dot{Q}_S/\dot{Q}_T$. However, the increase in cardiac output (35%) is sufficiently large to raise DO_2 and mixed venous PO_2 and to maintain a constant arterial PO_2[243]. The effect of PGI_2 on survival in ARDS has not been tested.

Inotropic Agents

Increased PVR in ARDS significantly raises the workload placed on the right ventricle. Maintenance of adequate cardiac output depends on the ability of the right ventricle to increase stroke work. When inotropic agents are needed to augment ventricular contractility to maintain cardiac output, dobutamine is the preferred agent because it raises cardiac output without producing significant pulmonary vasoconstriction[302,303]. Amrinone, a phosphodiesterase inhibitor with cardiovascular effects similar to those of dobutamine, may also be useful in patients with ARDS. However, no clinical studies have been performed on its use in ARDS.

Other Experimental Drugs

Because the paragraphs above end with ". . . no clinical studies . . .", ". . . not been tested . . .", and ". . . a randomized clinical trial is necessary . . .", it is reasonable to consider all drugs for ARDS experimental. The drugs discussed below are less routinely used.

Immunotherapy may prove to be a major form of treating ARDS. Monoclonal antibodies have been developed against endotoxin and TNF. Ziegler et al.[304] showed increased survival in septic patients treated with antibody against endotoxin compared with septic patients treated with placebo. However, subsequent trials have failed to confirm improved outcome with antiendotoxin monoclonal antibody therapy. TNF antibodies injected prior to a lethal injection of *Escherichia coli* have been shown to prevent shock and respiratory failure in a primate model[305].

Pentoxifylline, a phosphodiesterase inhibitor, has many effects on the mediators of ARDS[306]. Results of in vitro experiments demonstrated that pentoxifylline decreases neutrophil adhesion and inhibits TNF release from macrophages[67,68]. In vivo experiments with guinea pigs and dogs have shown decreased endotoxin-mediated lung injury with the use of pentoxifylline[307,308]. Human studies are limited[309,310].

Nitric Oxide

As mentioned above (see section on cardiovascular alteration, pulmonary hemodynamics), pulmonary hypertension is often associated with ARDS. Severe pulmonary hypertension has been associated with high mortality[20,152]. It has not been demonstrated that treating the pulmonary hypertension affects the clinical course of ARDS. Certainly, however, until nitric oxide, a selective pulmonary vasodilator has not been available.

Many reports suggest that inhaled nitric oxide, an endothelium-derived relaxant factor (EDRF)[311,312], may effectively lower PAP. Simultaneously, nitric oxide may improve $\dot{Q}_S/\dot{Q}_T$, since this inhaled pulmonary vasodilator is only delivered to well-ventilated parts of the lung[313,314]. Furthermore, nitric oxide is rapidly inactivated by hemoglobin and hence does not cause systemic vasodilation[314]. Nitric oxide, in theory, may be a bronchodilator[315].

Human data describing the use of nitric oxide for ARDS are beginning to emerge[316–318]. Rossaint et al.[319] delivered nitric oxide to 10 young adults with ARDS and, as predicted, showed reductions in PAP and $\dot{Q}_S/\dot{Q}_T$. Similar responses in adults have been described[320]. Seventeen children (10 with ARDS) responded to nitric oxide in a similar fashion[321].

Conversely, nitric oxide overproduction is associated with sepsis—and, of course, sepsis is associated with ARDS[322,323]. It cannot be assumed that inhaled nitric oxide will benefit patients with ARDS.

Surfactant

As noted above (see section on pathophysiology, diminished surfactant activity and airway collapse), surfactant is both quantitatively and qualitatively diminished during ARDS. Alterations in surfactant are an early marker of ARDS in a sheep model of sepsis[324]. Replacement therapy has been considered[325,326].

However, a multi-institutional study of almost 500 adults with ARDS did not show diminished mortality when given aerosolized surfactant for up to 5 days[327]. A randomized trial of surfactant in adults with sepsis-associated ARDS did not affect outcome[328].

Other Supportive Drugs

Depending on the clinical circumstances, various other drugs may be useful for patients with ARDS. Underlying infection should be treated with appropriate antibiotics. If bronchospasm is present, bronchodilators may be tried. Neuromuscular blockade, with a variety of agents, is a common practice and has been used to promote patient-ventilator synchrony. Although it may seem intuitive that pulmonary compliance is enhanced with neuromuscular blockade, in the presence of sedation sufficient to suppress spontaneous ventilation, paralysis may add nothing[329]. Complications, although rare, may be substantial[330,331].

Nutrition

Although nutritional repletion is vital in patients with ARDS just as it is with other critically ill patients, the source of nonprotein calories may have profound effects on respiration. If excessive carbohydrate in the form of hypertonic dextrose is used, CO_2 production may increase dramatically[332]. This occurs because excess glucose is metabolized to fat in the liver. The respiratory quotient for this lipogenesis pathway is 8, leading to large amounts of CO_2 production. Total body respiratory quotient may rise to 7. Patients with respiratory failure may not be able to increase minute ventilation sufficiently to excrete this excess CO_2 load.

Experimental Management

A semantic digression is necessary. In many discussions of therapy for ARDS, therapies that rely on common ventilators (e.g., Servo 900C [Seimens, Danvers Massachusetts] or BIRD VIP [Bird Corporation, Palm Springs, California]) are called conventional therapies. In distinction, more unusual therapies (e.g., HFOV or extracorporeal membrane oxygenation [ECMO]), even with unproved efficacy, are called rescue or bailout therapies. The words *rescue* and *bailout* suggest the possibility of survival. The reason such terms are applied in this domain rests not in data but possibly in an emotional belief that more technology (i.e., more aggressive and invasive therapies) will work. Certainly rescues and bailouts are sometimes unsuccessful. But all true rescues (e.g., pulling a person from a burning building) are proven to improve survival beyond chance. Hence, the term *rescue therapy* has no place in the discussion of novel, experimental approaches to the treatment of ARDS.

Extracorporeal Membrane Oxygenation

An early randomized, controlled trial (in adults) of therapy for ARDS was the study (sponsored by the National Institutes of Health) of ECMO and conventional mechanical ventilation. Although the initial anecdotal experience with ECMO was encouraging[333–335], the data from the randomized trial unequivocally demonstrated no benefit from ECMO[336]. More recently, extracorporeal carbon dioxide removal ($ECCO_2R$) again showed initial promise[337], but its benefit could not be reconfirmed[28]. In fact, the latter authors concluded that ECMO should not be offered (outside a clinical trial) for adult patients with ARDS.

Data are beginning to emerge on the use of ECMO for children with ARDS. Green et al.[337a] examined retrospective multi-institutional data from 1991 of children with ARDS. Excluded from a total of 679 patients were 143 patients who did not have complete data. Patients were more broadly excluded for possible ECMO contraindications and therefore 255 additional patients were also excluded. Consequently, 331 patients from 32 hospitals had complete data for further analysis and had no diagnostic exclusions for ECMO. Thirty-eight patients were treated with ECMO. Fifteen hospitals performed ECMO on one or more patients. The most common diagnoses associated with respiratory failure were bacterial infections, viral infections, trauma (including burns and foreign bodies) and status postsurgical procedures. For 24 ECMO-treated patients, both of the desired two non-ECMO treated case matches were identified. Five ECMO only had one non-ECMO treated case match identified. The remaining nine ECMO-treated patients had no acceptable case match and were therefore excluded from further analysis. Overall, 53 pairs of ECMO- and non-ECMO-treated patients matched for respiratory diagnosis and mortality risk were identified.

Mortality in the ECMO-treated group was 26.3% compared with 49.1% in the non-ECMO-treated controls ($p < .01$). Stratified by risk quartile, ECMO-treated patients in the 50 to 75% mortality risk group had a 28.6% mortality versus 71.4% for the case-matched controls. There were no differences between the ECMO-treated patients and controls in the other three quartiles. However, small sample sizes, particularly in the quartile with more than 75% predicted mortality, limits the power of the comparisons.

ECMO for ARDS within the pediatric population has also been offered sporadically since the first adult cases were attempted. As of January 1995, 883 children have been reported to the Extracorporeal Life Support Organization Registry. The overall survival is 54% (460 of 883). It may be important that survival of patients treated through 1990 was 44%, and survival from 1991 through 1994 was 55%. No effort has been made to standardize diagnoses, procedures, or even indications to initiate ECMO. As is typical of all data in the field, ARDS is classified as "other". Even the diagnostic criteria for viral pneumonia does not demand culture or antigen detection results. For this discussion it is important to reiterate that the aggregate overall survival of children with ARDS treated with conventional mechanical ventilation and treated with ECMO is identical.

Liquid Ventilation

Perfluorocarbon liquids have unique features of high solubility for both oxygen and CO_2, low resistance to gas flow, and significant surface tension-reducing properties. Liquid ventilation using perfluorocarbons has been examined in a number of animal models of lung disease[338] and has been advocated for the treatment of surfactant-deficient lung disease in humans. Perfluorocarbon-associated gas exchange (PAGE) or partial liquid ventilation uses perfluorocarbon to replace the functional residual capacity of the lung. Subsequent gas exchange is provided by the delivery of gas tidal volumes using a conventional ventilator. Leech and colleagues described their experience with perfluorocarbon-associated gas exchange in a premature animal model of respiratory distress syndrome[339]. Dynamic lung compliance increased threefold within 15 minutes of beginning PAGE, and the PO_2 increased from a mean of 59 mm Hg during conventional ventilation to 250 mm Hg during PAGE. Improvements in oxygenation and lung compliance persisted throughout the 60 minutes of study. Also of note was the fact that PCO_2 decreased significantly and pH increased significantly during PAGE compared with values obtained during conventional ventilation. Use of liquid perfluorocarbon with delivery of gas tidal volumes offers a simple technique of supporting gas exchange. It appears to work for the short term in this and other animal models of lung disease. There is also exciting new evidence that liquid ventilation, when compared with conventional mechanical ventilation, decreases the histologic evidence of lung injury in an animal model treated with oleic acid[340]. Appropriate application to older patient populations with acute hypoxia and respiratory failure or syndromes not associated with surfactant deficiency need to be carefully examined.

OUTCOME

Interpretation of mortality rates and clinical status of survivors of ARDS is complicated because of the wide variety of triggering insults, severity of the acute illness, and differences in premorbid pulmonary function. Nevertheless, it is quite apparent that ARDS is associated with a high mortality rate, and preliminary data suggest that pediatric survivors are left with worse pulmonary function than are adults who recover from ARDS. Mortality rates range from 28 to 65% among adult series in which patients received aggressive intensive care, including the use of PEEP[12,28,219,220,341,342].

Death secondary to refractory respiratory failure is relatively rare. Gallagher and Civetta[220] found that in a series of 315 patients with ARDS with 88 deaths, only three deaths could be assigned to refractory respiratory failure. The major cause of death among patients with ARDS is either sepsis or failure of other major organs besides the lung, such as the heart, brain, and liver.

Mortality rates seem to be approximately the same for children and adults; however, the reported series are smaller. The average mortality rate of the five published pediatric series combined is 52%, with a range of 28.5 to 90% **(Table 7.4).** Presumably, better intensive care techniques have led to the gradual reduction in mortality rates, from the initial high of 90% to the more recent mortality rates of 30 to 40% (Table 7.4). Katz et al.[20] attempted to identify those hemodynamic variables that were retrospectively associated with nonsurvival among their patients with ARDS. Increased PVR and PAP characterized the nonsurvivors[20]. Notably, there was no statistically significant difference in P_aO_2, P_aCO_2, or DO_2 between survivors and nonsurvivors after 96 hours of therapy for ARDS, suggesting that refractory respiratory failure is a rare cause of death in children with ARDS.

Adult long-term survivors of ARDS are likely to have normal chest x-rays and minimal respiratory symptoms[343]. However, some pulmonary function tests remain abnormal. In approximately 25% of ARDS survivors, reversible small-airway obstruction develops during the recovery period[344]. By 6 months after the acute illness, lung volumes have been shown to return to normal[345].

Measurements of gas exchange among adult survivors tend to reveal more persistent abnormalities. Carbon monoxide diffusing capacity (DLCO) is decreased in most ARDS survivors[345]. The alveolar-arterial oxygen gradient

($AaDO_2$) is widened during exercise in about one-third of adult ARDS survivors, as opposed to normal individuals who have an unchanged or reduced $AaDO_2$ during exercise[343,345]. These data suggest that the gas-exchanging surface area of the lung is adequate to meet oxygen requirements at rest; however, during exercise, efficient oxygenation is impaired, and P_aO_2 may fall, presumably secondary to residual pulmonary fibrosis.

Only tentative conclusions may be drawn about the clinical status of children who have recovered from ARDS because limited numbers of such patients have been followed. Available data do little to address the outcome variation caused by the myriad of ARDS triggers and responses to therapy. Nevertheless, available information indicates that children are more likely to be left with significant respiratory abnormalities than are adults[346–348]. Potentially because lung growth is not complete until 8 years of age[349,350], the impact of ARDS on the developing lung may be worse than in children and adults. Fanconi et al.[347] examined nine children aged 1 to 4 years after severe ARDS. Three of the nine remained symptomatic, with cough and exertional dyspnea, and two had abnormal chest x-rays. Lung volumes were also abnormal in one-third of the group. Gas exchange was more severely deranged, with uneven distribution of inspired gas in all nine patients and hypoxemia at rest in seven. Ventilation inequalities and hypoxemia correlated with prolonged exposure to F_IO_2 greater than 0.5 and high peak inflating pressures applied during the acute illness. Lyrene and Truog[23] reported one child with obstructive lung disease and another asymptomatic child with an abnormal chest x-ray in a group of six pediatric ARDS survivors. Clearly, more studies with larger numbers of patients are required to delineate the pulmonary abnormalities among children surviving ARDS.

COMPLICATIONS

Oxygen Toxicity

In patients with acute respiratory failure, the histology of O_2 toxicity is difficult to distinguish from that of the underlying disease, and, in fact, release of highly toxic oxygen radicals is part of the pathogenesis of ARDS even in the absence of a hyperoxic environment (see subsection on mediators in ARDS)[351]. However, pulmonary oxygen toxicity is a potential complication in patients receiving respiratory support, and lung function may be affected in several ways. Exposure of monkeys to 100% O_2 produces an acute stage of alveolar septal and capillary endothelial edema as well as an inflammatory cell infiltrate[352]. Inflammatory mediators are present in BAL fluid before chest x-ray findings[353]. Newborn mice breathing 80% O_2 for up to 6 weeks demonstrate only relatively mild acute changes but show chronic changes of peribronchial and parenchymal fibrosis[354]. The ability of alveolar macrophages to trap foreign particles is impaired[355]. Mucociliary clearance is decreased[356]. Normal volunteers first have chest pain, followed by a fall in vital capacity[357]. After 24 hours of hyperoxia, lung compliance decreases and $AaDO_2$ widens[358]. Based on such human volunteer data, it has been concluded that 100% O_2 may be applied for up to 24 hours without risking significant physiologic abnormality or irreversible histologic changes in the lung. Similarly, human volunteers have not exhibited blood gas abnormalities with F_IO_2 up to 50 to 60%, regardless of the duration of the exposure. The safe duration of oxygen exposure in patients with ARDS is unknown.

The mechanism of O_2 toxicity involves the production of highly reactive, unstable intermediate compounds as O_2 is reduced to H_2O. Molecular O_2 is unreactive because of the presence of two unpaired, parallel electronic spins. The direct insertion of a pair of electrons from an organic compound into the half-filled orbitals of O_2 would violate Pauli's exclusion principle, because the same orbital would now contain two electrons of parallel spin[359]. The univalent pathway of O_2 reduction overcomes this so-called spin restriction; however, the intermediate products of the univalent pathway are toxic[360,361]. The univalent reduction pathway involves the stepwise insertion of one electron at a time into oxygen orbitals. Since four electrons must be inserted to reduce molecular O_2 to H_2O, three intermediates are created according to the following formula:

$$O_2 \rightarrow O_2^- \rightarrow H_2O_2 \rightarrow OH \rightarrow H_2O$$

Table 7.4. Mortality Rates for Published Pediatric ARDS Series

Author	*Reference No.*	*Year*	*Location*	*n*	*% mortality*
Holbrook	24	1975–80	Washington	18	90
Lyrene	23	1976–79	Seattle	15	60
Effman	19	1977–83	Durham	9	56
Pfenninger	22	1978–81	Berne	20	40
Katz	20	1979–81	Washington	23	45
Nussbaum	21	1979–82	Long Beach	7	28
Kutting	15	1983–90	Graz	17	59
Rivera	18	1985–88	Australia	42	55
Tamburro	16	1986–90	Memphis	37	45
Timmons	17	1987–90	Salt Lake	44	75
Davis	14	1990–92	Philadelphia	60	62
Timmons	26	1991	41 centers	470	43

in which superoxide anion (O_2^-), hydrogen peroxide (H_2O_2), and hydroxyl radical (OH) appear in succession. Among these reactive intermediates, the hydroxyl radical appears to be the most damaging to cells[362]. It is now believed that most of the toxicity from superoxide anion is mediated through the production of singlet oxygen, the hydroxyl radical, and through the initiation of a lipid peroxidation chain reaction. Singlet oxygen is a highly reactive excited-state oxygen, possibly produced as a byproduct of the dismutation reaction of superoxide anion to hydrogen peroxide or during the next step, in which superoxide anion and hydrogen peroxide react to form the hydroxyl radical[363]. The polyunsaturated fatty acids of cellular membranes undergo lipid peroxidation in the presence of free radicals, such as hydroxyl radical or a previously formed lipid peroxide radical[362]. The peroxidative injury results in the disruption of cell membrane integrity[363].

It is clear that the cell could not tolerate the production of these toxic intermediates. A number of mechanisms have evolved that protect the cell. First, the univalent pathway is not the major pathway for the reduction of oxygen. Most cellular oxygen is reduced by the enzyme cytochrome oxidase without the release of intermediates. Second, scavenging enzymes remove toxic intermediates when they are produced. The first such scavenger is superoxide dismutase, which catalyzes the dismutation reaction of superoxide anion to hydrogen peroxide. Hydrogen peroxide is then reduced to water via catalase and peroxidase reactions. Exposure of an animal to sublethal concentration of O_2 will make the animal tolerant to subsequent exposure to 100% O_2. This tolerance is a function of increased superoxide dismutase activity in the lung[364]. However, investigators have failed in attempts to modify the time course or the extent of pulmonary oxygen toxicity with aerosolized superoxide dismutase in experimental animals[365]. Tolerance is highly species-specific and is more likely to occur in the young of a given species.

Despite this fairly detailed biochemical understanding of pulmonary oxygen toxicity, the clinician has no specific therapy to offer the patient at risk. Therefore, prevention of pulmonary oxygen toxicity is the major goal, and the following guidelines are appropriate:

1. The lowest F_IO_2 consistent with adequate tissue oxygenation should be used.
2. Consider the use of PEEP to permit a lower F_IO_2.
3. Never deny a patient 100% O_2 if this is necessary to prevent hypoxemia.

Mechanical Ventilator-Induced Lung Injury

Clinical Presentation

Pulmonary barotrauma develops in patients with ARDS as a function of both the lung pathology and the therapeutic use of mechanical ventilation. Clinically evident barotrauma occurs after rupture of an overdistended alveolus. With increased transpulmonary pressure exerted by mechanical ventilation, some alveoli become overdistended while the interstitial space is compressed. Partial airway obstruction exaggerates this tendency. Mechanical forces on the alveolar wall produce rupture when a critical traction force is exceeded, particularly in the face of lung tissue that is already damaged and noncompliant. Gas is thought to first enter the perivascular adventitia and then dissect into the pulmonary interstititium, resulting in pulmonary interstititial emphysema. Gas then is thought to dissect the long perivascular sheaths into the mediastinum, producing pneumomediastinum. Accumulation of mediastinal gas often leads to subcutaneous emphysema, or the gas may dissect via the retroperitoneal space into the abdomen. If the mediastinal pressure continues to increase and decompression does not occur via another route, then the mediastinal parietal pleura is violated and a pneumothorax results. Pneumothorax should be suspected whenever the patient with ARDS exhibits an unexplained sudden deterioration in clinical appearance, arterial oxygen tension, or hemodynamic stability. Chest x-ray will confirm the diagnosis. Successful management of the pneumothorax almost always requires closed-chest thoracostomy tube evacuation of air to an underwater seal system, because a continuing leak is virtually inevitable as long as the patient is breathing against positive pressure.

Epidemiology

Pulmonary barotrauma is an ever-present risk in patients with ARDS. In their series of patients with ARDS receiving high PEEP (up to 44 cm H_2O), Kirby et al.[219] noted pneumothoraces in 4 of 28 patients, although subcutaneous emphysema was "a common finding." Pollack et al.[25] found a 42% incidence of pneumothoraces, while Lyrene and Truog[23] reported a 66% incidence. A recent epidemiologic study of adults undergoing mechanical ventilation documented a 13% incidence of barotrauma, defined as the presence of subcutaneous emphysema, pneumothorax, or pneumomediastinum[366]. In this series, the presence of barotrauma was associated with a sixfold increase in mortality and was independently associated with mortality when adjusted for other predicters of poor outcome. It is not clear that barotrauma contributed directly to poor outcome, but it more likely is a marker for the severity of underlying disease. Petersen and Baier[367] examined the relationship between airway pressures and the incidence of extra-alveolar air. Both the level of end expiratory pressure as well as peak inspiratory pressure correlated significantly with an increasing incidence of air leak. The overall frequency of air leak in their study of critically ill adults was 8%. Obviously, extra-alveolar air accumulation represents the most extreme form of pulmonary barotrauma. Clearly, subtler changes occur in the lung, which precede frank extra-alveolar air accumulation; careful attention to factors associated with these subtler changes may lead to improved outcomes.

Pathophysiology

Although much work has been done examining the relationship between airway pressures and barotrauma in both animals and humans, it is clear that the concept of barotrauma and pressure-related lung injury is an oversimplification. Attention to subtler manifestations of ventilator-related lung injury requires a sophisticated understanding of the underlying pathophysiology.

There is an emerging recognition that mechanical ventilation-induced lung injury is related to cyclic volume change. In a classic study, Webb and Tierney[368] showed that ventilating normal rats with peak inspiratory pressures of 45 cm H_2O produced significant perivascular edema and an increase in lung weight. In addition, these investigators showed that an end expiratory pressure of 10 cm H_2O was protective, suggesting that the absolute level of inspiratory pressure is not as important as the volume change the lung undergoes during the duty cycle. It has also been shown in a normal animal that binding of the chest and abdomen, with restriction of chest wall movement, prevented lung injury during ventilation with peak inspiratory pressures of 45 cm H_2O[369]. This study provided important evidence that microvascular permeability is related not to pressure but to volume change. Dreyfuss and colleagues[370] provided similar data in rats, demonstrating that volume is a much more significant contributor to lung injury than is absolute pressure level, and that PEEP may well be protective in an animal model of mechanical ventilator-induced lung injury.

Mathieu-Costello and West[371] showed that high lung volume ventilation is associated with a significant increase in the disruption of the alveolar capillary, and they elegantly documented breaks in the capillary endothelium that are produced by high volume ventilation. Their research convincingly demonstrates that pulmonary edema is an important component of mechanical ventilator-induced lung injury. Fluid and protein in the alveolar space are well-known inhibitors of surfactant function and thereby act synergistically to decrease lung compliance and further the cycle of repetitive cyclic overdistention and further lung injury.

In a series of experiments in a saline-lavaged rabbit model, McCulloch et al.[372] demonstrated that lung-volume maintenance with minimization of alveolar pressure and volume change is associated with the least degree of mechanical ventilator-induced lung injury. They also demonstrated that HFOV, using an optimal-lung-volume strategy designed to reverse atelectasis, resulted in significant improvements in oxygenation and minimized histopathologic evidence of lung injury when compared with a conventionally ventilated group or when compared with animals treated with HFOV and a low-lung-volume strategy. More recently, Sugiura and colleagues[373] showed in the saline-lavaged rabbit that HFOV results in significantly less activation of pulmonary neutrophils, as evidenced by both chemiluminescence and chemotaxis. These findings were confirmed by a separate group of investigators using luminol-dependent chemiluminescence[374]. Furthermore, these investigators have also demonstrated that HFOV prevents the release of thromboxane B_2 and PAF, which are important chemical mediators of inflammatory lung injury[375].

Multiple Organ Failure Syndrome

Multiple organ failure syndrome (MOFS) is not strictly a complication of ARDS. Rather, ARDS occurs as part of MOFS. Lung failure generally precedes failure of other organ systems, such as the kidney, liver, gut, and brain, although subtle signs of liver and kidney injury are already present by the time ARDS develops[376].

The initial injury may be associated with decreased perfusion to several organs and release of mediators known to produce capillary injury. Within 2 to 3 days, capillary leak is evident, and the patient shows signs of hypermetabolism, such as hyperglycemia, hyperlactatemia, increased oxygen consumption, and elevated urinary urea nitrogen excretion[377]. The clinical picture is reminiscent of that seen in patients with fulminant sepsis, although cultures are negative; hence, the term *sepsis syndrome* has been applied. Frank organ system failure may set in over the next 14 to 21 days with encephalopathy, stress ulceration in the gut, ileus, hyperbilirubinemia, reduced hepatic protein synthesis, azotemia, and oliguria. The chances for survival are remote when four or more organs have failed.

CONDITIONS ASSOCIATED WITH ARDS

Drowning

Drowning accounts for 7000 deaths per year in the United States. Toddlers are at greatest risk. Twelve percent of near-drowning victims do not aspirate water because of laryngospasm or breath-holding after submersion[378]. These patients usually do not sustain significant pulmonary injury. The remaining patients aspirate water. The pathophysiology of subsequent lung injury theoretically (but not clinically) depends on whether freshwater or saltwater immersion occurred. Saltwater is hypertonic and draws fluid into alveoli. Pulmonary compliance decreases, and intrapulmonary shunt develops[379]. Although patients sustaining a near-drowning episode in freshwater also have a radiologic picture of pulmonary edema, much of the hypotonic aspirated freshwater diffuses into the circulation, causing a transient hypervolemia. In addition, surfactant is altered so that alveoli become unstable or collapse altogether[380]. Management includes supportive respiratory care as described above. Corticosteroids and prophylactic antibiotics are not indicated in the treatment of respiratory failure after near-drowning[378]. If the patient has aspirated stagnant and contaminated water, the risk of bacterial pneumonia is high. It is prudent to obtain daily tracheal cultures so that specific antibiotic therapy can be started at the first signs of infection. Although application of these therapeutic principles is important for the hospitalized near-drowning victim, prompt resuscitation at the scene of the accident still affords the best chance for survival and prevention of hypoxic brain injury[381].

Pulmonary Infiltrates in the Immunosuppressed Host

Impaired host defenses may disturb lung function in infectious and noninfectious ways. Drugs used in treating patients with compromised host defenses may alter pulmonary function. Corticosteroids are immunosuppressive by virtue of their ability to stabilize lysosomal membranes within phagocytes, promote fungal invasion, and retard leukocyte migration[382]. Prolonged use of the alkylating agent busulfan may produce cough, fever, and a potentially fatal diffuse restrictive lung disease[383]. Cyclophosphamide may be associated with a similar fibrotic reaction in the lung[384]. The antimetabolite methotrexate has led to reversible lung disease characterized by cough, fever, and shortness of breath[385]. Five to ten percent of patients treated with bleomycin sustain acute dyspnea after several weeks of therapy and exhibit a radiologic picture reminiscent of oxygen toxicity[386].

Hematologic malignancy is associated with the greatest risk of respiratory failure among all forms of immunosuppression[387]. This is an ominous problem for children because acute leukemia represents the most common form of childhood cancer. The appearance of fever and pulmonary infiltrates in a patient with leukemia or lymphoma is accompanied by a high mortality rate, and aggressive management is indicated[388]. The pulmonary syndromes in this setting have been divided into three categories on the basis of radiologic appearance: diffuse interstitial disease, localized consolidation, and cavitary disease[389].

Diffuse interstitial lung disease is the most common disease, leading to acute respiratory failure in the immunosuppressed child[390]. Several studies have identified *Pneumocystis carinii,* a protozoan, as the leading infectious cause of this radiographic picture[390–392].

Definitive diagnosis of *P. carinii* requires demonstration of the organisms with methenamine-silver stain on lung fluid or tissue. Open-lung biopsy has the highest yield, although BAL appears to be almost as effective. Effective antibiotic therapy against *P. carinii* is available with trimethoprim (20 mg/kg) and sulfamethoxazole (100 mg/kg) (T/S) combination, divided into four doses daily. This combination is curative in 80% of patients with *P. carinii* and is also effective when given prophylactically[393].

Twenty percent of *P. carinii* patients are resistant to T/S. Pentamidine may be administered to treat *P. carinii* infection when resistance to T/S has been documented. Pentamidine has become a second-line drug against *P. carinii* because of its associated reactions, including nephrotoxicity and hepatotoxicity, hypoglycemia, anemia, hypotension, and thrombocytopenia.

Immunosuppressed patients may sustain a variety of other illnesses that can manifest themselves with diffuse interstitial and alveolar lung disease. Bacterial pneumonia usually appears as localized consolidation or cavitary disease[389]. Because mortality from bacterial pneumonia is high, particularly in granulocytopenic immunosuppressed patients, any febrile immunosuppressed patient with pulmonary symptoms should immediately be given broad-spectrum antibiotics, including coverage of gram-negative bacilli[388]. Although fungal pneumonia typically appears as localized or cavitary disease, 20% of fungal pneumonias have a diffuse interstitial pattern[389]. *Candida* and *Aspergillus* are the most common fungi isolated on lung biopsy. Amphotericin B should be used for antifungal chemotherapy.

Graft-versus-host (GVH) disease occurs when a T-cell-deficient patient receives foreign immunocompetent (killer T-cells), such as during bone marrow transplantation or blood transfusion. GVH is a significant risk factor for the development of interstitial pneumonitis and ARDS after bone marrow transplantation[394]. A variety of infectious agents, including cytomegalovirus, *P. carinii,* herpes simplex virus, *Aspergillus,* and *Candida* have been isolated from the lungs of bone marrow transplantation patients with interstitial pneumonitis. However, most cases do not yield an infectious agent and are classified as idiopathic. The combination of cytomegalovirus infection and GVH may, through unknown mechanisms, lead to severe, diffuse interstitial pneumonitis and acute respiratory failure[395].

Sepsis in the Normal Host

Sepsis is strongly associated with the development of ARDS. In fact, many studies indicate that sepsis is the most frequent event precipitating the development of ARDS[396–398]. Pfenninger et al.[399] examined the causes of ARDS in children aged 2 weeks to 15 years and found that intra-abdominal infection and/or septicemia was the most common cause. Holbrook et al.[24] reported a series of 18 children with ARDS in whom severe infection occurred in 10 patients, with five cases of Gram-negative sepsis, two cases of meningitis, and two cases of gastroenteritis. The nonbacterial pathogens associated with ARDS include rickettsiae, mycoplasma, and such viruses as herpes simplex and measles[22,400–402].

Fat Embolism

Fat embolism is a rare cause of ARDS, occurring after long-bone fracture[403,404]. The classic triad of neurologic dysfunction, respiratory insufficiency, and petechiae after skeletal trauma suggests the diagnosis of fat embolism[405]. This remains a clinical diagnosis of exclusion because no readily available laboratory test is sufficiently sensitive and specific to be of value. In most instances, hypoxemia develops over a 12 to 48-hour period after injury to bone[404]. Other associated laboratory abnormalities in patients with ARDS with fat embolism include isolated thrombocytopenia and disseminated intravascular coagulopathy[404,406].

The pathogenesis of pulmonary injury in fat embolism

seems related to the intravascular release of neutral triglycerides from bone marrow[407,408]. Circulating lipoprotein lipase converts this neural fat into free fatty acids, which in turn injure the pulmonary endothelium. It is believed that the time required for this conversion process accounts for the usual 12- to 48-hour lag time before clinical symptoms appear.

Chest Trauma

ARDS may occur after severe blunt chest trauma and bilateral lung contusion[409,410]. The incidence of acute respiratory failure after chest trauma is 10.7%[346]. Motor vehicle accidents account for the major cause of blunt chest trauma.

Flail chest is the most common associated injury in patients with severe lung contusion. This disruption in chest wall integrity occurs when there are three or more double fractures of adjacent ribs or combined sternum and rib fracture. Lung function is further compromised because the flail segment moves inward with inspiration and outward with expiration. Such ineffective, paradoxical movement leads to atelectasis and V/Q mismatching in lung beneath the flail segment. Respiratory failure after chest trauma is an ominous sign because it is associated with a 32% mortality rate[411].

Head Trauma

Permeability pulmonary edema after head trauma and increased intracranial pressure has been described in children[412]. Most investigators of the mechanism of neurogenic pulmonary edema have focused on the massive sympathetic discharge associated with intracranial hypertension. The sympathetic discharge may be attenuated or blocked by central nervous system depressants or α-adrenergic blockers[413,414]. As a result of this massive sympathetic discharge, intrathoracic vascular pressures rise[415]. Increased pulmonary capillary pressure disrupts pulmonary capillary endothelium, leading to permeability pulmonary edema. Thus, neurogenic pulmonary edema persists, even after vascular pressures have returned to normal. In this setting, PEEP should be applied with caution because increased intrathoracic pressures may decrease cerebral venous return and lead to increased intracranial pressure[416]. However, if PEEP is required to improve oxygenation, it should be used and continuous intracranial pressure monitoring should be considered.

An alternative hypothesis on the generation of neurogenic pulmonary edema has recently been proposed[61]. Best characterized in the central nervous system, NMDA seems to play a central role in neuronal damage after head trauma (and other central nervous system insults). NMDA receptors were recently discovered in the pulmonary parenchyma (but not localized to a particular cell type). NMDA activation triggers acute injury, that is, as in toxicity to central neurons, associated with stimulation of nitric oxide synthesis. The injury can be attenuated by inhibition of nitric oxide synthesis[61].

Smoke Inhalation and Surface Burns

Smoke inhalation and burns may affect the respiratory system in three ways: direct thermal injury, chemical pneumonitis, and carbon monoxide poisoning. Inhalation of hot gases (greater than 300°F) injures the upper respiratory tract. The lower respiratory tract is relatively uninvolved because most heat has been dissipated by the time gas reaches the lower airway[417]. Laryngeal edema and airway obstruction may occur. Steam has a higher heat capacity than hot dry air and therefore produces a more serious burn.

Chemical pneumonitis is caused by the various noxious fumes, gases, and soot in smoke. Cilia are paralyzed and mucosal edema develops[417,418]. By 24 hours after inhalation of smoke, extensive sloughing of necrotic mucosa occurs in the conducting airway[419]. The peribronchial connective tissue space becomes distended with edema fluid. Tracheobronchitis, bronchospasm, and airway compression result[420]. In the Dellwood fire[421], the victims were children who sustained predominantly smoke inhalation injury. At autopsy, the lungs of these children exhibited the extensive injury to conducting airways described previously; in addition, there was prominent intra-alveolar hemorrhage.

When surface burns are added to smoke inhalation, the risk of ARDS is substantially increased[422]. In fact, the combination of smoke inhalation in a closed space and greater than 50% surface burn is most likely to be associated with pulmonary complications and carries a poor prognosis[423]. Pulmonary function tests in patients with surface burns and inhalation injury demonstrate restrictive lung disease 9 hours after the burn, which becomes maximal 58 hours after the burn. Abnormality in pulmonary function has been correlated with the volume of crystalloid fluid received during resuscitation[420]. It is postulated that loss of serum protein through a large burn surface area, coupled with large volumes of crystalloid fluid replacement during resuscitation, may lead to sufficient reduction in colloid oncotic pressure to produce noncardiogenic pulmonary edema. Three to eight days after smoke inhalation, bronchopneumonia poses an additional threat associated with high mortality[423].

Carbon monoxide is a colorless and odorless gas produced by incomplete combustion of organic matter. It is thus found in virtually every fire. Carbon monoxide impairs oxygen delivery by competing with oxygen for hemoglobin-binding sites. Since the affinity of carbon monoxide for hemoglobin is over 200 times that of oxygen, significant carboxyhemoglobin concentrations arise, even when inspired carbon monoxide concentration is low. The normal carboxyhemoglobin concentration is 1%. Smokers may have carboxyhemoglobin concentrations of 5 to 10%, although clinical carbon monoxide poisoning is evident when concentrations greater than 20% develop. Carbon monoxide also causes a shift to the left of the oxyhemoglobin dissociation curve. This higher affinity of oxygen for hemoglobin makes unloading of oxygen at the tissue level more difficult because very low levels of tissue PO_2 must be achieved before appreciable amounts of oxygen are released. P_aO_2 is unchanged in carbon monoxide poisoning even though oxygen content is clearly reduced. The half-life of carboxyhemoglobin is 4 hours during breathing of room air but falls to less than 1 hour during breathing of 100% oxygen. Thus, administration of 100% oxygen is rational therapy for carbon monoxide poisoning.

Acute respiratory failure in the burn victim requires the same supportive respiratory care as in other causes of acute respiratory failure. Endotracheal intubation and application of PEEP may improve oxygenation. In the presence of carbon monoxide poisoning, 100% inspired oxygen concentration should be administered. Overhydration is avoided by monitoring pulmonary artery wedge pressure with a Swan-Ganz catheter. Prophylactic antibiotics may select resistant organisms and are not used. When bronchopneumonia is diagnosed, appropriate antibiotic therapy is immediately begun, pending bacterial culture results. Bronchodilators may be tried if the patient wheezes. Corticosteroids seem to offer no benefit and may, in fact, be detrimental[424].

References

1. Johnson TH, Altman AR, McCaffree RD. Radiologic considerations in adults with respiratory distress syndrome treated with positive end expiratory pressure (PEEP). Clin Chest Med 1982;3:89.
2. Kollef MH, Schuster DP. Medical progress: The acute respiratory distress syndrome. N Engl J Med 1995;332:27.
3. Ashbaugh DG, Bigelow DB, Petty TL, Levine BE. Acute respiratory distress in adults. Lancet 1967;2:319.
4. Petty TL, Ashbaugh DG. The adult respiratory distress syndrome. Clinical features, factors influencing prognosis and principles of management. Chest 1971;60:233.
5. Petty TL. Adult respiratory distress syndrome: definition and historical perspective. Clin Chest Med 1982;3:3.
6. Murray JF, Matthay MA, Luce JM, et al. An expanded definition of the adult respiratory distress syndrome. Am Rev Respir Dis 1988;138:720.
7. Bernard GR, Artigas A, Brigham KL, et al. The American-European Consensus Conference on ARDS. Am J Respir Crit Care Med 1994;149:818.
8. Sloane PJ, Gee MH, Gottlieb JE, et al. A multicenter registry of patients with acute respiratory distress syndrome: Physiology and outcome. American Review of Respiratory Disease 1992;146:419.
9. Hopewell PC, Murray JF. The adult respiratory distress syndrome. Ann Rev Med 1976;27:343.
10. Conference report: Mechanisms of acute respiratory failure. Am Rev Respir Dis 1977;115:1071.
11. Thomsen GE, Morris AH, Danino D, Ellsworth J, Wallace GJ. Incidence of the respiratory distress syndrome in Utah (abstract). Am Rev Respir Dis 1993;147:A347.
12. Fowler AA, Hamman RF, Good JT. Adult respiratory distress syndrome: risk with common predispositions. Ann Intern Med 1983;98:593.
13. Hudson LD, Milberg JA, Anardi D, Maunder RJ. Clinical risks for development of the acute respiratory distress syndrome. Am J Respir Crit Care Med 1995;151:293.
14. Davis SL, Furman DP, Costarino AJ. Adult respiratory distress syndrome in children: Associated disease, clinical course, and predictors of death. J Pediatr 1993;123:35.
15. Kuttnig M, Zobel G, Grubbauer HM, Trop M. [A clinical score system for children with ARDS]. Anaesthesist. 1991;40:282.
16. Tamburro RF, Bugnitz MC, Stidham GL. Alveolar-arterial oxygen gradient as a predictor of outcome in patients with nonneonatal pediatric respiratory failure. J.Pediatr. 1991;119:935.
17. Timmons OD, Dean JM, Vernon DD. Mortality rates and prognostic variables in children with adult respiratory distress syndrome. J Pediatr 1991;119:896.
18. Rivera RA, Butt W, Shann F. Predictors of mortality in children with respiratory failure: possible indications for ECMO. Anaesth Intensive Care 1990;18:385.
19. Effmann EL, Merten DF, Kirks DR, Pratt PC, Spock A. Adult respiratory distress syndrome in children. Radiology 1985;157:69.
20. Katz R, Pollack M, Spady D. Cardiorespiratory abnormalities in severe acute respiratory failure. J Pediatr 1984;104:357.
21. Nussbaum E. Adult-type respiratory distress syndrome in children: experience with seven cases. Clin Pediatr 1983;22:401.
22. Pfenninger J, Zimmerman A. Fatal adult respiratory distress syndrome in a scalded child after immunization with attenuated virus (measles, mumps, rubella). Helv Paediatr Acta 1981;36:371.
23. Lyrene RK, Truog WE. Adult respiratory distress syndrome in a pediatric intensive care unit: predisposing conditions, clinical course, and outcome. Pediatrics 1981;67:790.
24. Holbrook PR, Taylor G, Pollack MM, Fields AI. Adult respiratory distress syndrome in children. Pediatr Clin North Am 1980;27:677.
25. Pollack MM, Fields AI, Holbrook PR. Cardiopulmonary parameters during high PEEP in children. Crit Care Med 1980;8:372.
26. Timmons OD, Havens PL, Fackler JC. Predicting death in pediatric patients with acute respiratory failure. Chest 1995;108:789
27. Milberg JA, Davis DR, Steinberg KP, Hudson LD. Improved survival of patients with acute respiratory distress syndrome (ARDS): 1983-1993. JAMA 1995;273:306.
28. Morris AH, Wallace CJ, Menlove RL, et al. Randomized clinical trial of pressure-controlled inverse ratio ventilation and extracorporeal CO_2 removal for adult respiratory distress syndrome [see comments] [published erratum appears in Am J Respir Crit Care Med 1994 Mar;149(3 Pt 1):838]. American Journal of Respiratory & Critical Care Medicine 1994;149:295.
29. Knaus WA, Sun X, Hakim RB, Wagner DP. Evaluation of definitions for adult respiratory distress syndrome. Am J Respir Crit Care Med 1994;150:311.
30. Hudson LD. Causes of the respiratory distress syndrome—clinical recognition. Clin Chest Med 1982;3:195.
31. Katzenstein ALA, Bloor CM, Liebow AA. Diffuse alveolar damage—the role of oxygen, shock and related factors. Am J Pathol 1976;85:210.
32. Tomashefski JF, Davies P, Boggis C, et al. The pulmonary vascular lesions of adult respiratory distress syndrome. Am J Pathol 1983;112:112.
33. Tomashefski JF. Pulmonary pathology of the adult respiratory distress syndrome. Clin Chest Med 1990;11:593.
34. Blaisdell FW, Lewis FR. Respiratory distress syndrome of shock and trauma: post-traumatic respiratory failure. Philadelphia: WB Saunders, 1977. Major problems of clinical surgery (vol 21).
35. Teplitz C. The core pathobiology and integrated medical science of adult acute respiratory insufficiency. Surg Clin North Am 1976;56:1091.
36. Bachofen M, Weibel ER. Structural alterations of lung parenchyma in the adult respiratory distress syndrome. Clin Chest Med 1982;3:35.
37. Hohn DC, Meyers AJ, Gherini ST, et al. Production of acute pulmonary injury by leukocytes and activated complement. Surgery 1980;88:48.
38. Rinaldo JE, Rogers RM. Adult respiratory distress syndrome: changing concepts of lung injury and repair. N Engl J Med 1982;306:900.
39. Bone RC, Francis PB, Pierce AK. Intravascular coagulation associated with adult respiratory distress syndrome. Am J Med 1976;61:585.
40. Demling RH. The role of mediators in human ARDS. J Crit Care 1988;3:56.
41. Jacobs RF, Kiel DP, Balk RA. Alveolar macrophage function in a canine model of endotoxin-induced lung injury. Am Rev Respir Dis 1986;134:745.
42. Fujimoto K, Parker JC, Kayes SG. Activated eosinophils increase vascular permeability and resistance in isolated perfused rat lungs. Am Rev Respir Dis 1990;142:1414.
43. Bachofen M, Weibel ER. Alterations of the gas exchange apparatus in adult respiratory insufficiency associated with septicemia. Am Rev Respir Dis 1977;116:589.
44. Hurley JV. Current views of the mechanisms of pulmonary edema. J Pathol 1978;125:59.
45. Staub NC, Nagano H, Pearce ML. Pulmonary edema in dogs, especially the sequence of fluid accumulation in lungs. J Appl Physiol 1967;22:227.
46. Fukuda Y, Ishizaki M, Masuda Y, et al. The role of intraalveolar fibrosis in the process of pulmonary structural remodeling in patients with diffuse alveolar damage. Am J Pathol 1987;126:171.
47. Jones R, Reid LM, Kirton OC, et al. Pulmonary vascular pathology. Human and experimental studies. In: Zapol WM, Falke KJ, eds. Acute respiratory failure. New York: Marcel Dekker, 1985:23.
48. Carrington CB, Green TJ. Granular pneumocytes in early repair of diffuse alveolar injury. Arch Intern Med 1970;126:464.

49. Evans MJ, Cabral LJ, Stephens RJ, Freeman G. Renewal of alveolar epithelium in rat following exposure to NO. Am J Pathol 1973;70:175.
50. Kauffman SL, Burri PH, Weibel ER. The postnatal growth of the rat lung. II. Autoradiography. Anat Rec 1974;180:63.
51. Kuhn C, Boldt J, King TE, Jr., et al. An immunohistochemical study of architectural remodeling and connective tissue synthesis in pulmonary fibrosis. Am.Rev Respir.Dis. 1989;140:1693.
52. Farjanel J, Hartmann DJ, Guidet B, Luquel L, Offenstadt G. Four markers of collagen metabolism as possible indicators of disease in the adult respiratory distress syndrome. Am Rev Respir Dis 1993;147:1091.
53. Henke C, Fiegel V, Peterson M, et al. Identification and partial characterization of angiogenesis bioactivity in the lower respiratory tract after acute lung injury. Journal of Clinical Investigation 1991;88:1386.
54. Chen B, Polunovsky V, White J, et al. Mesenchymal cells isolated after acute lung injury manifest an enhanced proliferative phenotype. Journal of Clinical Investigation 1992;90:1778.
55. Riordan JF, Walters G. Pulmonary edema in bacterial shock. Lancet 1968;1:719.
56. Snow RL, Davies P, Pontoppidan H, Zapol WM, Reid L. Pulmonary vascular remodeling in adult respiratory distress syndrome. Am Rev Respir Dis 1982;126:887.
57. Katz S, Aberman A, Frand U, et al. Heroin pulmonary edema: evidence for increased pulmonary capillary permeability. Am Rev Respir Dis 1972;106:472.
58. Erdmann AJ, III, Vaughan TR, Jr., Brigham KL, Woolverton WC, Staub NC. Effect of increased vascular pressure on lung fluid balance in unanesthetized sheep. Circ Res 1975;37:271.
59. Brigham KL, Woolverton WC, Blake LH, Staub NC. Increased sheep lung vascular permeability caused by Pseudomonas bacteremia. J Clin Invest 1974;54:792.
60. Hinshaw LB, Kuida H, Bilbert RP, Visscher MB. Influence of perfusate characteristics on pulmonary vascular response to endotoxin. Am J Physiol 1957;191:293.
61. Said SI, Berisha HI, Pakbaz H. N-methyl-D-aspartate receptors outside the central nervous system: Activation causes acute lung injury that is mediated by nitric oxide synthesis and prevented by vasoactive intestinal peptide. Neuroscience 1995;65:943.
62. Jacquier-Sarlin MR, Fuller K, Dinh-Xuan AT, Richard MJ, Polla BS. Protective effects of hsp70 in inflammation. Experientia 1994;50:1031.
63. Villar J, Edelson JD, Post M, Mullen BM, Slutzky AS. Induction of heat stress proteins is associated with decreased mortality in an animal model of acute lung injury. Am Rev Respir Dis 1993;147:177.
64. Hammerschmidt DE, Weaver LJ, Hudson LD, et al. Association of complement activation and elevated plasma-C5a with adult respiratory distress syndrome. Lancet 1980;947:947.
65. Wedmore CV, Williams TJ. Platelet activating factor, a secretory product of polymorphonuclear leukocytes, increases vascular permeability in rabbit skin. Br J Pharmacol 1981;74.
66. Movat HZ, Rettl C, Burrows CE, Johnston MG. The in vivo effect of leukotriene B4 on polymorphonuclear leukocytes and the microcirculation. Comparison with activated complement (C5a des Arg) and enhancement by prostaglandin E2. Am J Pathol 1984;115:233.
67. Sullivan GW, Carper HT, Novich WJ, et al. Inhibition of the inflammatory action of interleukin-1 and tumor necrosis factor (alpha) on neutrophil function by pentoxifylline. Infect Immun 1988;56:1722.
68. Mandell GL. ARDS, neutrophils, and pentoxifylline. Am Rev Respir Dis 1988;138:1103.
69. Cybulsky MI, McComb DJ, Movat DL. Neutrophil emigration induced by endotoxin. Mediator roles of interleukin-1 and tumor necrosis factor (alpha). J Immunol 1988;140:3144.
70. Tonnesen MG, Anderson DC, Springer TA, et al. Adherence of neutrophils to cultured human microvascular endothelial cells: Stimulation by chemotactic peptides and lipid mediators and dependence upon the Mac-1, LFA-1, P150,95 glycoprotein family. J Clin Invest 1989;83:637.
71. Vandermeer TJ, Menconi MJ, O'Sullivan BP, et al. Acute lung injury in endotoxemic pigs: Role of leukotriene B4. J Appl Physiol 1995;78:1121.
72. Pober JS, Bevilacqua MP, Mendrich DL, et al. Two distinct monokines, interleukin 1 and tumor necrosis factor, each independently induce biosynthesis and transient expression of the same antigen on the surface of cultured human vascular endothelial cells. J Immunol 1986; 136:1680.
73. Lee CT, Fein AM, Lippman M, et al. Elastolytic activity in pulmonary lavage fluid from patients with adult respiratory-distress syndrome. N Engl J Med 1981;304:192.
74. Bunnell E, Pacht ER. Oxidized glutathione is increased in the alveolar fluid of patients with the adult respiratory distress syndrome. Am Rev Respir Dis 1993;148:1174.
75. Johnson D, Travis J. The oxidative inactivation of human α-1 proteinase inhibitor. Further evidence for methionine at the reactive center. J Biol Chem 1981;256:7181.
76. Johnson A, Malik AB. Effect of granulocytopenia on extravascular lung water content after micro-embolization. Am Rev Respir Dis 1980;122:561.
77. Heflin AJ, Brigham KL. Prevention by granulocyte depletion of increased vascular permeability of sheep lung following endotoxemia. J Clin Invest 1981;68:1253.
78. Ognibene FP, Martin SE, Parker MM, et al. Adult respiratory distress syndrome in patients with severe neutropenia. N Engl J Med 1986;315:547.
79. Haufe MD, Simon RH, Fling A, et al. Adult respiratory distress syndrome in neutropenic patients. Am J Med 1986;80:1022.
80. Maunder RJ, Hackman RC, Riff E, et al. Occurrence of the adult respiratory distress syndrome in neutropenic patients. Am Rev Respir Dis 1986;133:313.
81. Sibilla Y, Reynolds HY. Macrophages and polymorphonuclear neutrophils in lung defense and injury. Am Rev Respir Dis 1990;141:471.
82. Modig J, Samuelsson T, Hallgren R. The predictive and discriminative value of biologically active products of eosinophils, neutrophils and complement in bronchoalveolar lavage and blood in patients with adult respiratory distress syndrome. Resuscitation 1986;14:121.
83. Rowen JC, Hyde DM, McDonald RJ. Eosinophils cause acute edematous injury in isolated perfused rat lungs. Am Rev Respir Dis 1990;142:215.
84. Brigham KL, Meyrick B. Endotoxin and lung injury. Am Rev Respir Dis 1986;133:913.
85. Brigham KL, Meyrick B, Berry LC, et al. Antioxidants protect cultured bovine lung endothelial cells from injury by endotoxin. J Appl Physiol 1987;63:840.
86. Dinarello CA. Interleukin-1 and the pathogenesis of the acute phase response. N Engl J Med 1984;311:1413.
87. Beutler B, Krochin N, Milsark IW, et al. Control of cachectin (tumor necrosis factor) synthesis: mechanisms of endotoxin resistance. Science 1986;232:977.
88. Haslett C, Guthrie CLA, Kopaniak MM, et al. Modulation of multiple neutrophil functions by preparative methods or trace concentrations of bacterial lipopolysaccharide. Am J Pathol 1985;119:101.
89. Bersten A, Sibbald WJ. Acute lung injury in septic shock. Crit Care Clin 1989;5:49.
90. Kaplow LS, Goffinet JA. Profound neutropenia during the early phase of hemodialysis. JAMA 1968;203:1135.
91. Craddock PR, Fehr J, Brigham KL, et al. Complement and leukocyte mediated dysfunction in hemodialysis. N Engl J Med 1977;296:769.
92. Duchateau J, Haas M, Schreyen H, et al. Complement activation in patients at risk of developing the adult respiratory distress syndrome. Am Rev Respir Dis 1984;130.
93. Weinberg PF, Matthay MA, Webster RO, et al. Biologically active products of complement and acute lung injury in patients with the sepsis syndrome. Am Rev Respir Dis 1984;130:791.
94. Zilow G, Sturno JA, Rother V, et al. Complement activation and prognostic value of C3a in patients at risk of adult respiratory distress syndrome. J Exp Immunol 1990;79:151.
95. Robbins R, Maunder R, Ossman G, et al. Functional loss of chemotactic factor inactivator in the adult respiratory distress syndrome. Am Rev Respir Dis 1990;141:1463.
96. Okusawa S, Dinarello CA, Yancey KB, et al. C5a induction of human interleukin 1. Synergistic effect with endotoxin or interferon-gamma. J Immunol 1987;139:2635.
97. Okusawa S, Yancey KB, Van DuMeer JWM, et al. C5a stimulates secretion of tumor necrosis factor from human mononuclear cells in vitro comparison with secretion of interleukin 1 beta and interleukin 1 alpha. J Exp Med 1988;168:443.
98. Stevens JH, O'Hanley P, Shapiro JM, et al. Effects of anti-C5a antibodies on the adult respiratory distress syndrome in septic primates. J Clin Invest 1986;77.
99. Millar AB, Singer M, Meagher A, et al. Tumor necrosis factor in bronchopulmonary of patients with adult respiratory distress syndrome. Lancet 1989;2:712.
100. Marks JD, Marks CB, Huce JM, et al. Plasma tumor necrosis factor in patients with septic shock. Mortality rate. Am Rev Respir Dis 1990;141:94.
101. Camussi G, Bussolino F, Salvidio G, et al. Tumor necrosis/cachetin stimulates peritoneal macrophages, polymorphonuclear neutrophils, and vascular endothelial cells to synthesize and release platelet activating factor. J Exp Med 1987;166:1390.

102. Goldblum SE, Sun WL. Tumor necrosis factor alpha augments pulmonary arterial transendothelial flux in vitro. Am J Physiol 1990;258.
103. Clark MA, Chen MJ, Crooke S, et al. Tumor necrosis factor (cachetin) induces phospholipase A2 activity and synthesis of a phospholipase A2-activating protein in endothelial cells. Biochem J 1986;250:125.
104. Bevilacqua MP, Pober JS, Majcau GR, et al. Recombinant tissue necrosis factor induces procoagulant activity in cultured human vascular endothelium: characterization and comparison with the actions of interleukin a. Proc Natl Acad Sci U S A 1986;83:4533.
105. Jacobs RF, Tabor DR. Immune cellular interactions during sepsis and septic injury. Crit Care Clin 1989;5:9.
106. Meduri GU, Headley S, Kohler G, et al. Persistent elevation of inflammatory cytokines predicts a poor outcome in ARDS: Plasma IL-1beta and IL-6 levels are consistent and efficient predictors of outcome over time. Chest 1995;107:1062.
107. McManus LM, Hanahan DJ, Demopoulus CA, et al. Pathobiology of the intravenous infusion of acetyl-glyceryl-ether phosphorylcholine (AGEPC), a synthetic platelet-activating factor (PAF), in the rabbit. J Immunol 1980;124:2919.
108. Worthen GS, Goins AJ, Mitchel BC, et al. Platelet-activating factor causes neutrophil accumulation and edema in rat lungs. Chest 1983;83:135.
109. Henderson WR. Lipid-derived and other chemical mediators of inflammation in the lung. J Allergy Clin Immunol 1987;79:543.
110. Heffner JE, Sahn SA, Repine JE. The role of platelets in the adult respiratory distress syndrome. Am Rev Respir Dis 1987;135:482.
111. Idell SI, Maunder R, Fein AM, et al. Platelet specific alpha-granulate proteins and thrombosponden in bronchoalveolar lavage in the adult respiratory distress syndrome. Chest 1989;96:1125.
112. Lonky SA, Marsh J, Wohl H. Stimulation of human granulocytes with elastase by platelet factor 4 and heparin. Biochem Biophys Res Commun 1978;85:1113.
113. Peurel TF, Senior RM, Chang D, et al. Platelet factor 4 is chemotactic for neutrophil and monocytes. Proc Natl Acad Sci U S A 1981;78:4584.
114. Senior RM, Griffin GL, Huang JS, et al. Chemotactic activity of platelet alpha granule proteins for fibroblasts. J Cell Biol 1983;96:382.
115. Heffner JE, Katz SA, Halushka PV, et al. Human platelets attenuate oxidant injury in isolated rabbit lungs. J Appl Physiol 1988;65:1258.
116. Suciski K, Nanno S, Tanaka K. Permeability enhancing and chemotactic activities of lower weight degradation products of human fibrinogen. Thromb Haemost 1982;45:90.
117. Eddington TS, Curtiss LK, Plow EF. A linkage between the hemostatic and immune systems embodies in the fibrinolytic release of lymphocyte suppressive peptides. J Immunol 1985;134:471.
118. Moalli R, Doyle JM, Tahhan HR, et al. Fibrinolysis in critically ill patients. Am Rev Respir Dis 1989;140:287.
119. Chapman HA, Yang X, Sailor LZ, et al. Developmental expression of plasminogen activator inhibitor type 1 by human alveolar macrophages. J Immunol 1990;145:3398.
120. Chapman HA, Reilly JJ, Kobzik L. Role of plasminogen activator in degradation of extracellular matrix protein by live human alveolar macrophages. Am Rev Respir Dis 1988;137:413.
121. Demling R, Smith M, Gunther R, Flynn JT, Gee MH. Pulmonary injury and prostaglandin production during endotoxemia in conscious sheep. Am J Physiol 1981;240.
122. Lonigro AJ, Dawson CA. Vascular responses to prostaglandin F2 in isolated cat lungs. Circ Res 1975;36:706.
123. Snapper JR, Ogeltree ML, Hutchinson AA, Brigham KL. Meclofenamate prevents increased airway resistance of the lung (RL) following endotoxemia in unanesthetized sheep. Am Rev Respir Dis Suppl 1981;123:200.
124. Matthay MA, Eschenlacher WL, Goetzl EJ. Elevated concentrations of leukotriene D4 in pulmonary edema fluid of patients with adult respiratory distress syndrome. J Clin Immunol 1984;4:479.
125. Ibe BO, Isenberg WB, Raj JU. Endogenous arachidonic acid metabolism by calcium ionophore A23187-stimulated lamb lungs: effect of hypoxia. Am J Respir Cell Mol Biol 1991;4:379.
126. Schellenberg RR, Foster A. Differential activity of leukotrienes upon human pulmonary vein and artery. Prostaglandins 1984;27:475.
127. Thureson-Klein A, Hedqvist P, Lindbom L. Ultrastructure of polymorphonuclear leukocytes in postcapillary venules after exposure to leukotriene B4 in vivo. Acta Physiol Scand 1984;122:221.
128. Malik AB, Noonan TC, Selig WM, Garcia JG. Effects of exogenous leukotrienes on the pulmonary circulation. In: Lefer AM, Gee MH, eds. Leukotrienes in, cardiovascular pulmonary function. New York: Alan R Liss, 1985:221.
129. Henry JN, McArdle AH, Bounous G, et al. The effect of experimental hemorrhagic shock on pulmonary alveolar surfactant. Journal of Trauma 1967;7:691.
130. Henry JN. The effect of shock on pulmonary alveolar surfactant. Its role in refractory respiratory insufficiency of the critically ill or severely injured patient. Journal of Trauma 1968;8:756.
131. Hallman M, Spragg R, Harrell JH, et al. Evidence of lung surfactant abnormality in respiratory failure. J Clin Invest 1982;70:673.
132. Holm BA, Notter RH, Seigle J, et al. Pulmonary physiological and surfactant changes during injury and recovery from hyperoxia. J Appl Physiol 1985;59:1402.
133. Holm BA, Matalon S, Finkelstein JN, et al. Type II pneumocyte changes during hyperoxic lung injury and recovery. J Appl Physiol 1988;65:2672.
134. Holm BA, Notter RH. Effects of hemoglobin and cell membrane lipids on pulmonary surfactant activity. J Appl Physiol 1987;63:1434.
135. Fuchimukai T, Fujiwara T, Takahashi A, et al. Artificial pulmonary surfactant inhibited by proteins. J Appl Physiol 1987;62:429.
136. Falke KJ, Pontoppidan H, Kumar A, et al. Ventilation with end-expiratory pressure in acute lung disease. J Clin Invest 1972;51:2315.
137. Matamis D, Lemaire F, Harf A, et al. Total respiratory pressure-volume curves in the adult respiratory distress syndrome. Chest 1984;86:58.
138. Ingram RH, O'Cain CF, Fridy WW. Simultaneous quasi-static lung pressure-volume curves and "closing volume" measurements. J Appl Physiol 1974;36:135.
139. Lemaire F, Simoneau G, Harf A, et al. Static pulmonary pressure-volume curve. Am Rev Respir Dis Suppl 1979;1119:328.
140. Holzapfel L, Dominique R, Perrin F, et al. Static pressure-volume curves and effect of positive end-expiratory pressure on gas exchange in adult respiratory distress syndrome. Crit Care Med 1983;11:591.
141. Dantzker DR, Brook CJ, Dehart P, Lynch JP, Weg JG. Ventilation-perfusion distributions in the adult respiratory distress syndrome. Am Rev Respir Dis 1979;120:1039.
142. Auler JOC, Saldiva PHN, Martins MA, et al. Flow and volume dependence of respiratory system mechanics during constant flow ventilation in normal subjects and in adults with respiratory distress syndrome. Crit Care Med 1990;18:1080.
143. Tharratt RS, Allen RP, Albertson TE. Pressure controlled inverse ratio ventilation in severe adult respiratory failure. Chest 1988;94:755.
144. Dueck R, Wagner PD, West SB. Effects of positive end-expiratory pressure on gas exchange in dogs with normal and edematous lungs. Anesthesiology 1977;47:359.
145. Markello R, Winter P, Olszowka A. Assessment of ventilation-perfusion inequalities by arterial-alveolar nitrogen differences in intensive care patients. Anesthesiology 1972;37:4.
146. Lamy M, Fallat RJ, Koeniger E, et al. Pathologic features and mechanisms of hypoxemia in adult respiratory distress syndrome. Am Rev Respir Dis 1976;114:267.
147. Muir AL, Hall DL, Despas P, Hogg JC. Distribution of blood flow in the lungs in acute pulmonary edema in dogs. J Appl Physiol 1972;33:763.
148. Noble WH, Kay JC, Obdrzalek J. Lung mechanics in hypovolemic pulmonary edema. J Appl Physiol 1975;38:681.
149. Douglas ME, Downs JB, Dannemiller FJ, Hodges MR, Munson ES. Change in pulmonary venous admixture with varying inspired oxygen. Anesth Analg 1976;55:688.
150. Suter PM, Fairley HB, Schlobohm RM. Shunt, lung volume and perfusion during short periods of ventilation with oxygen. Anesthesiology 1975;43:617.
151. Benumof JL. Mechanism of decreased blood flow to atelectatic lung. J Appl Physiol 1979;46:1047.
152. Zapol WM, Snider MT. Pulmonary hypertension in severe acute respiratory failure. N Engl J Med 1977;296:476.
153. Zapol WM, Jones R. Vascular components of ARDS. Am Rev Respir Dis 1987;136:471.
154. Zapol WM, Snider MT, Rie MA, et al. Pulmonary circulation during adult respiratory distress syndrome. In: Zapol WM, Falke KJ, eds. Acute respiratory failure. New York: Marcel Dekker, 1985:241 .
155. Gattinoni L, Pesenti A, Bombino M, et al. Relationships between lung computer tomographic density, gas exchange and PEEP in acute respiratory failure. Anesthesiology 1988;69:824.
156. Collee GG, Lynch KE, Hill RD, et al. Bedside measurement of pulmonary capillary pressure in patients with acute respiratory failure. Anesthesiology 1987;66:614.
157. Radermacher P, Santak B, Becker H, Falke KJ. Prostaglandin E1 and nitroglycerine reduce pulmonary capillary pressure but worsen VA/Q distributions in patients with ARDS. Anesthesiology 1989;70:601.
158. Radermacher P, Santak B, Wust HJ, et al. Prostacyclin for the treat-

ment of pulmonary hypertension in the adult respiratory distress syndrome: effects on pulmonary capillary pressure and ventilation-perfusion distributions. Anesthesiology 1990;72:238.
159. Greene R, Zapol WM, Snider MT, et al. Early bedside detection of pulmonary vascular occlusion during acute respiratory failure. Am Rev Respir Dis 1981;124:593.
160. Zimmerman GA, Morris AH, Cengiz M. Cardiovascular alterations in the adult respiratory distress syndrome. Am J Med 1982;73:25.
161. Ross J. Editorial: acute displacement of the diastolic pressure-volume curve of the left ventricle: role of the pericardium and the right ventricle. Circulation 1979;59:32.
162. Laver MB, Strauss HW, Pohost GM. Right and left ventricular geometry: adjustments during acute respiratory failure. Crit Care Med 1979;7:509.
163. Russell JA, Ronco JJ, Lockhat D, et al. Oxygen delivery and consumption and ventricular preload are greater in survivors than in nonsurvivors of the adult respiratory distress syndrome. Am Rev Respir Dis 1990;141:659.
164. Horovitz AH, Carrico CJ, Shires GT. Pulmonary response to major injury. Arch Surg 1974;108:349.
165. Covelli AD, Nessan VJ, Tuttle VK. Oxygen derived variables in acute respiratory failure. Crit Care Med 1983;11:646.
166. Ovenfors CO, Hedgcock MW. Intensive care unit radiology: problems in interpretation. Radiol Clin North Am 1978;16:407.
167. Joffe N. The adult respiratory distress syndrome. Am J Roentgenol 1974;122:719.
168. Altman AR, Johnson TH. Roentgenographic findings in PEEP therapy: indicators of pulmonary complications. JAMA 1979;242:727.
169. Johnson TH, Altman AR. Pulmonary interstitial gas: first sign of barotrauma due to PEEP therapy. Crit Care Med 1979;7:532.
170. Barcroft J. On anoxaemia. Lancet 1920;2:485.
171. Shoemaker WC, Montgomery ES, Kaplan E, Elwyn DH. Physiologic patterns in surviving and nonsurviving shock patients. Arch Surg 1973;106:630.
172. Shoemaker WC, Appel PL, Kram HB, Waxman K, Lee TS. Prospective trial of supranormal values of survivors as therapeutic goals in high-risk surgical patients. Chest 1988;94:1176.
173. Shoemaker WC, Patil R, Appel PL, Kram HB. Hemodynamic and oxygen transport patterns for outcome prediction, therapeutic goals, and clinical algorithms to improve outcome; Feasibility of artificial intelligence to customize algorithms. Chest 1992;102 Suppl. 2:617S.
174. Grenvik A. Respiratory, circulatory, and metabolic effects of respiratory treatment: a clinical study in postoperative thoracic surgical patients. Acta Anaesth Scand Suppl 1966;19:1.
175. Cain SM. Assessment of tissue oxygenation. Crit Care Clin 1986;2:537.
176. Shibutani K, Komatsu T, Kubal K, et al. Critical level of oxygen delivery in anesthetized man. Crit Care Med 1983;11:640.
177. Cain SM. Oxygen delivery and uptake in dogs during anemic and hypoxic hypoxia. J Appl Physiol 1977;42:228.
178. Gutierrez G, Warley AR, Dantzker DR. Oxygen delivery and utilization in hypothermic dogs. J Appl Physiol 1986;60:751.
179. Bihari D, Smithies M, Gimson A, Tinker J. The effects of vasodilation with prostacyclin on oxygen delivery and uptake in critically ill patients. N Engl J Med 1987;317:397.
180. Archie JP. Mathematic coupling of data: a common source of error. Ann Surg 1981;193:293.
181. Annat G, Viale JP, Percival C, et al. Oxygen delivery and uptake in adult respiratory distress syndrome. Am Rev Respir Dis 1986;133:999.
182. Vermeij CG, Feenstra BWA, Bruining HA. Oxygen delivery and oxygen uptake in postoperative and septic patients. Chest 1990;98:415.
183. Powers SR, Mannal R, Neclerio M, et al. Physiological consequences of positive end-expiratory pressure (PEEP) ventilation. Ann Surg 1973;178:265.
184. Danek SJ, Lynch JP, Weg JG, Dantzker DR. The dependence of oxygen uptake on delivery in the adult respiratory distress syndrome. Am Rev Respir Dis 1980;122:387.
185. Mohsenifar Z, Goldbach P, Tashkin DP, Campisi DJ. Relationship between O_2 delivery and O_2 consumption in adult respiratory distress syndrome. Chest 1983;84:267.
186. Kariman K, Burns SR. Regulation of tissue oxygen extraction is disturbed in adult respiratory distress syndrome. Am Rev Respir Dis 1985;132:109.
187. Stratton HH, Feustel PJ, Newell JC. Regression of calculated variables in the presence of shared measurement error. J Appl Physiol 1987;62:2083.
188. Yu M, Levy MM, Smith P, et al. Effect of maximizing oxygen delivery on morbidity and mortality rates in critically ill patients: a prospective, randomized, controlled study [see comments]. Crit Care Med 1993;21:830.
188a. Hinds C, Watson D. Manipulating Hemodynamics and oxygen transport in critically patients [editorial; comment]. N Engl J Med 1995;333:1074
188b. Gattinoni L, Brazzi L, Pelosi P, et al. A trial of goal-oriented hemodynamic therapy in critically ill patients. SvO_2 Collaborative Group [see comments]. N Enlg J Med 1995;333:1025.
189. Barach AL, Martin J, Eckman M. Positive pressure respiration and its application to the treatment of acute pulmonary edema. Ann Intern Med 1937;12:754.
190. Shapiro BA, Cane RD, Harrison RA. Positive end-expiratory pressure therapy in adults with special reference to acute lung injury: a review of the literature and suggested clinical correlation. Crit Care Med 1984;12:127.
191. Gherini S, Peters RM, Virgilio RW. Mechanical work on the lungs and work of breathing with positive end-expiratory pressure and continuous positive airway pressure. Chest 1979;76:251.
192. Benito S, Lemaire F. Mechanical ventilation with PEEP improves pulmonary static pressure-volume (P-V) curves in patients with acute respiratory failure (ARF) [Abstract]. Am Rev Respir Dis 1985;131.
193. Wyszogrodski I, Kyei-Aboagye K, Taeusch HW, Avery ME. Surfactant inactivation by hyperventilation: conservation by end-expiratory pressure. J Appl Physiol 1975;38:461.
194. Faridy EE. Effect of ventilation on movement of surfactant in airways. J Appl Physiol 1976;27:323.
195. Suter PM, Fairley HB, Isenberg MD. Effect of tidal volume and positive end-expiratory pressure on compliance during mechanical ventilation. Chest 1978;73:158.
196. Hammon JW, Wolfe WG, Moran JF, Jones RH, Sabiston DC. The effect of positive end-expiratory pressure on regional ventilation and perfusion in the normal and injured primate lung. J Thorac Cardiovasc Surg 1976;72:680.
197. Nieman GF, Paskanik AM, Bredenberg CE. Effect of positive end-expiratory pressure on alveolar capillary perfusion. J Thorac Cardiovasc Surg 1988;95:712.
198. Jardin F, Farcot J, Boisante L, et al. Influence of positive end-expiratory pressure on left ventricular performance. N Engl J Med 1981;304:387.
199. Terai C, Uenishi M, Sugimoto H, et al. Transesophageal echocardiographic dimensional analysis of four cardiac chambers during positive end-expiratory pressure. Anesthesiology 1985;63:640.
200. Mitaka C, Nagura T, Sakanishi N, et al. Two-dimensional echocardiographic evaluation of inferior vena cava, right ventricle, and left ventricle during positive-pressure ventilation with varying levels of positive end-expiratory pressure. Crit Care Med 1989;17:205.
201. Johnston WE, Vinten-Johansen J, Santamore WP, et al. Mechanism of reduced cardiac output during positive end-expiratory pressure in the dog. Am Rev Respir Dis 1989;140:1257.
202. Zwissler B, Forst H, Messmer K. Local and global function of the right ventricle in a canine model of pulmonary microembolism and oleic acid edema: influence of ventilation with PEEP. Anesthesiology 1990; 73:964.
203. Wallis TW, Robotham JL, Compean R, et al. Mechanical heart-lung interaction with positive end-expiratory pressure. J Appl Physiol 1983;54:1039.
204. Cassidy SS, Robertson CH, Pierce AK, Johnson RL. Cardiovascular effects of end-expiratory pressure in dogs. J Appl Physiol 1978;44:743.
205. Culver BH, Marini JJ, Butler J. Lung volume and pleural pressure effects on ventricular function. J Appl Physiol 1981;50:630.
206. Henning RJ. Effects of positive end-expiratory pressure on the right ventricle. J Appl Physiol 1986;61:819.
207. Grindlinger GA, Manny J, Justice R, et al. Presence of negative inotropic agents in canine plasma during positive end-expiratory pressure. Circ Res 1979;45:460.
208. Ashton JH, Cassidy SS. Reflex depression of cardiovascular function during lung inflation. J Appl Physiol 1985;58:137.
209. Jacobs HK, Venus B. Left ventricular regional myocardial blood flows during controlled positive pressure ventilation and positive end-expiratory pressure in dogs. Crit Care Med 1983;11:872.
210. Marini JJ, O'Quin R, Culver BH, Butler J. Estimation of transmural cardiac pressures during ventilation with PEEP. J Appl Physiol 1982;53:384.
211. Gournand A, Motley HL, Werko L, Richard DW. Physiological studies of the effects of intermittent positive pressure breathing on cardiac output in man. Am J Physiol 1948;152:162.
212. Ashbaugh DG, Petty TL. Positive end-expiratory pressure, physiology,

indications and contraindications. J Thorac Cardiovasc Surg 1973; 65:165.
213. Cassidy SS, Mitchell JH, Johnson RL. Dimensional analysis of right and left ventricles during positive pressure ventilation in dogs. Am J Physiol 1982;242.
214. Haynes JB, Carson SD, Whitney WP, et al. Positive end-expiratory pressure shifts left ventricular diastolic pressure-area curves. J Appl Physiol 1980;48:670.
215. Lutch JS, Murray JF. Continuous positive-pressure ventilation: effect on systemic oxygen transport and tissue oxygenation. Ann Intern Med 1972;76:193.
216. Pershau RA, Pepine CJ, Nichols WW, Downs JB. Instantaneous blood flow responses to positive end-expiratory pressure with spontaneous ventilation. Circulation 1979;59:1312.
217. Walkinshaw M, Shoemaker WC. Use of volume loading to obtain preferred levels of PEEP. Crit Care Med 1980;8:81.
218. White MK, Galli SA, Chatburn RL, Blumer JL. Optimal positive end-expiratory pressure therapy in infants and children with acute respiratory failure. Pediatr Res 1988;24:217.
219. Kirby RR, Downs JB, Civetta JM, et al. High level positive end-expiratory pressure (PEEP) in acute respiratory insufficiency. Chest 1975;67:156.
220. Gallagher TJ, Civetta JM. Goal-directed therapy of acute respiratory failure. Anesth Analg 1980;59:831.
221. Ashbaugh DG, Petty TL, Bigelow DB, Harris TM. Continuous positive pressure breathing (CPPB) in adult respiratory distress syndrome. J Thorac Cardiovasc Surg 1969;57:31.
222. Toung TJK, Saharia P, Mitzner WA, Permutt S, Cameron JL. The beneficial and harmful effects of positive end-expiratory pressure. Surg Gynecol Obstet 1978;147:518.
223. Demling RH, Staub NC, Edmunds LH. Effects of end-expiratory pressure on accumulation of extravascular lung water. J Appl Physiol 1975;38:907.
224. Caldini P, Leith JD, Brennan MJ. Effect of continuous positive-pressure ventilation (CPPV) on edema formation in dog lung. J Appl Physiol 1975;39:672.
225. Nieman GF, Bredenberg CE, Paskanik AM. Positive end-expiratory pressure accelerates lung water accumulation in high surface tension edema. Surgery 1990;107:15.
226. Scharf SM, Caldini PB, Ingram RH. Cardiovascular effects of increasing airway pressure in the dog. Am J Physiol 1977;232.
227. Permutt S, Howell JBL, Proctor DF, Riley RL. Effect of lung inflation on static pressure-volume characteristics of pulmonary vessels. J Appl Physiol 1961;16:64.
228. Pepe PE, Hudson LD, Carrico CJ. Early application of positive end-expiratory pressure in patients at risk for the adult respiratory distress syndrome. N Engl J Med 1984;311:281.
229. Rounds S, Brody JS. Putting PEEP in perspective. N Engl J Med 1984;311:323.
230. Kumar A, Falke KJ, Geffin B, et al. Continuous positive pressure ventilation in acute respiratory failure. N Engl J Med 1970;283:1430.
231. Rhodes GR, Newell JC, Shah D, et al. Increased oxygen delivery with hypertonic mannitol in adult respiratory distress syndrome. Surgery 1978;84:490.
232. Carroll GC, Tuman KJ, Braverman B, et al. Minimal positive end-expiratory pressure (PEEP) may be "best" PEEP. Chest 1988;93:1020.
233. Suter PM, Fairley HB, Isenberg MD. Optimum end-expiratory pressure in patients with acute pulmonary failure. N Engl J Med 1975;292:284.
234. Tenaillon A, LaBrousse J, Gateau O, Lissac J. Optimal positive end-expiratory pressure and static lung compliance. N Engl J Med 1978;299:774.
235. Downs JB, Douglas ME, Ruiz BC, Miller NL. Comparison of assisted and controlled mechanical ventilation in anesthetized swine. Crit Care Med 1979;7:5.
236. Mathru M, Rao TLK, Venus B, Jones W. Mode of ventilation and pulmonary barotrauma [Abstract]. Anesthesiology 1979;51.
237. Downs JB, Mitchell LA. Pulmonary effects of ventilatory pattern following cardiopulmonary bypass. Crit Care Med 1976;4:295.
238. Greaves TH, Cramolino GM, Walker DH, et al. Inverse ratio ventilation in a 6 year-old with severe post-traumatic adult respiratory distress syndrome. Crit Care Med 1989;17:588.
239. Lain DC, DiBenedetto R, Morris SL, et al. Pressure control inverse ratio ventilation as a method to reduce peak inspiratory pressure and provide adequate ventilation and oxygenation. Chest 1989;95:1081.
240. Abraham E, Yoshihara G. Cardiorespiratory effects of pressure controlled inverse ratio ventilation in severe respiratory failure. Chest 1989;96:1356.
241. Lessard MR, Guérot E, Lorino H, Lemaire F, Brochard L. Effects of pressure-controlled with different I:E ratios versus volume-controlled ventilation on respiratory mechanics, gas exchange, and hemodynamics in patients with adult respiratory distress syndrome. Anesthesiology 1994;80:983.
242. Marini JJ. Ventilation of the acute respiratory distress syndrome: Looking for Mr. Goodmode. Anesthesiology 1994;80:972.
243. Feihl F, Perret C. Permissive hypercapnia. How permissive should we be? American Journal of Respiratory & Critical Care Medicine 1994;150:1722.
244. Hickling KG, Henderson SJ, Jackson R. Low mortality associated with low volume pressure limited ventilation with permissive hypercapnia in severe adult respiratory distress syndrome. Intensive Care Med 1990;16:372.
245. Hickling KG, Walsh J, Henderson S, Jackson R. Low mortality rate in adult respiratory distress syndrome using low-volume, pressure-limited ventilation with permissive hypercapnia: A prospective study. Crit Care Med 1994;22:1568.
246. Wetzel RC, Gioia FR. High frequency ventilation. Pediatr Clin North Am 1987;34:15.
247. Hurst JM, Branson RD, Davis K, Jr., et al. Comparison of conventional mechanical ventilation and high-frequency ventilation. A prospective, randomized trial in patients with respiratory failure. Ann Surg 1990;211:486.
248. Carlon GC, Guy Y, Groeger JS, Ray C, Howlan S. Early prediction of outcome of respiratory failure. Comparison of high frequency jet ventilation and volume-cycled ventilation. Chest 1984;86:194.
249. Carlon GC, Howlan WS, Ray C, et al. High frequency jet ventilation: a prospective randomized evaluation. Chest 1983;84:551.
250. Derderian SS, Rajagopol KR, Abbrecht PH, et al. High frequency positive pressure jet ventilation in bilateral bronchopleural fistulae. Crit Care Med 1982;10:119.
251. Arnold JH, Truog RD, Thompson JE, Fackler JC. High-frequency oscillatory ventilation in pediatric respiratory failure. Critical Care Medicine 1993;21:272.
252. Arnold JH, Hanson JH, Toro-Figuero LO, et al. Prospective, randomized comparison of high-frequency oscillatory ventilation and conventional mechanical ventilation in pediatric respiratory failure. Crit Care Med 1994;22:1530.
253. Douglas ME, Downs JB. Applied physiology and respiratory care. In: Shoemaker WC, Thompson WL, eds. Critical care state of the art. Fullerton, California: Society of Critical Care Medicine, 1982:1. vol 3).
254. Strickland JH, Hasson JH. A computer-controlled ventilator weaning system. Chest 1991;100:1096.
255. Tong DA. Weaning patients from mechanical ventilation. A knowledge-based system approach. Computer Methods and Programs in Biomedicine 1991;35:267.
256. Dojat M, Brochard L, Lemaire F, Harf A. A knowledge-based system for assisted ventilation of patients in intensive care units. International Journal of Clinical Monitoring and Computing 1992;9:239.
257. Linton DM, Potgieter PD, Davis S, et al. Automatic weaning from mechanical ventilation using an adaptive lung ventilation controller. Chest 1994;106:1843.
258. Esen F, Denkel T, Telci L, et al. Comparison of pressure support ventilation (PSV) and intermittent mandatory ventilation (IMV) during weaning in patients with acute respiratory failure. Advances in Experimental Medicine and Biology 1992;317:371.
259. Esteban A, Frutos F, Tobin MJ, et al. A comparison of four methods of weaning patients from mechanical ventilation. N Engl J Med 1995;332:345.
260. Weinberger SE, Wiess JW. Weaning from ventilatory support (editorial). N Engl J Med 1995;332:388.
261. Hauser CJ, Shoemaker WC, Turpin I, Goldberg SJ. Oxygen transport responses to colloids and crystalloids in critically ill surgical patients. Surg Gynecol Obstet 1980;150:811.
262. Appel PL, Shoemaker WC. Evaluation of fluid therapy in acute respiratory failure. Crit Care Med 1981;8:873.
263. Demling RH, Manohar M, Will JA. Response of the pulmonary microcirculation to fluid loading after haemorrhagic shock and resuscitation. Surgery 1980;87:552.
264. Haupt MT, Rackow EC. Colloid osmotic pressure and fluid resuscitation with hetastarch, albumin, and saline solutions. Crit Care Med 1982;10:159.
265. Shoemaker WC, Schluchter M, Hopkins JA, et al. Fluid therapy in emergency resuscitation: clinical evaluation of colloid and crystalloid regimens. Crit Care Med 1981;9:367.

266. Zikria BA, King TC, Stanford J, et al. A biophysical approach to capillary permeability. Surgery 1989;105:625.
267. Webb AR, Tighe D, Moss RF, et al. Advantages of a narrow range, medium molecular weight hydroxyethyl starch for volume maintenance in a porcine model of fecal peritonitis. Crit Care Med 1991;19:409.
268. Armistead CW, Jr., Vincent JL, Preiser JC, et al. Hypertonic saline solution-hetastarch for fluid resuscitation in experimental septic shock. Anesth Analg 1989;69:714.
269. Velasco IT, Pontieri V, Rocha e Silva MR, Jr., Lopes OU. Hyperosmotic NaCl and hemorrhagic shock. Am J Physiol 1980;239.
270. Prough DS, Johnson JC, Stump DA, et al. Effects of hypertonic saline versus lactated Ringer's solution on cerebral oxygen transport during resuscitation from hemorrhagic shock. J Neurosurg 1986;64:627.
271. Guyton AC, Jones CE, Coleman TG. Circulatory physiology: cardiac output and its regulation. (2 ed.) Philadelphia: WB Saunders, 1973.
272. Humphrey PRD, Marshall J, Russel RWR, et al. Cerebral blood flow and viscosity in relative polycythemia. Lancet 1979;2:873.
273. Asmundson T, Kilburn KH. Survival of acute respiratory failure: a study of 239 episodes. Ann Intern Med 1969;70:471.
274. Durtschi MD, Aisch CE, Reynolds C, et al. Effect of micropore filtration on pulmonary function after massive transfusion. Am J Surg 1979;138:8.
275. Drury DR, Henry JP, Goodman J. The effect of continuous pressure breathing on kidney function. J Clin Invest 1947;26:945.
276. Beardsmore CS, Helms P, Stocks J, Hatch DJ, Silverman M. Improved esophageal balloon technique for use in infants. J Appl Physiol 1980;49:735.
277. Tooker J, Huseby J, Butler J. The effect of Swan-Ganz catheter height on the wedge pressure-left atrial pressure relationship in edema during positive pressure ventilation. Am Rev Respir Dis 1978;117:721.
278. Shasby DM, Dauber IM, Pfister S, et al. Swan-Ganz location and left atrial pressure determine the accuracy of the wedge pressure when positive end-expiratory pressure is used. Chest 1981;80:666.
279. Holloway H, Perry M, Downey J, et al. Estimation of effective pulmonary capillary pressure in intact lungs. J Appl Physiol 1983;54:846.
280. Cope DK, Allison RC, Parmentier JL, et al. Measurement of effective pulmonary capillary pressure using the pressure profile after pulmonary artery occlusion. Crit Care Med 1986;14:16.
281. Hauser GJ, Pollack MM, Sivit CJ, et al. Routine chest radiographs in pediatric intensive care: a prospective study [published erratum appears in Pediatrics 1989 Jul;84(1):17]. Pediatrics 1989;83:465.
282. Levy FH, Bratton SL, Jardine DS. Routine chest radiographs following repositioning of endotracheal tubes are necessary to assess correct position in pediatric patients. Chest 1994;106:1508.
283. Bernard GR, Luce JM, Spring CL, et al. High-dose corticosteroids in patients with the adult respiratory distress syndrome. N Engl J Med 1987;317:1565.
284. Luce JM, Montgomery B, Marks JD, et al. Ineffectiveness of high-dose methylprednisolone in preventing parenchymal lung injury and improving mortality in patients with septic shock. Am Rev Respir Dis 1988;138:62.
285. Bone RC, Fisher CJ, Clemmer TP, et al. A controlled clinical trial of high-dose methylprednisolone in the treatment of severe sepsis and septic shock. N Engl J Med 1987;317:653.
286. Martin C, Papazian L, Payan MJ, Saux P, Gouin F. Pulmonary fibrosis correlates with outcome in adult respiratory distress syndrome: A study in mechanically ventilated patients. Chest 1995;107:196.
287. Meduri GU, Chinn A. Fibroproliferation in late adult respiratory distress syndrome: response to corticosteroid rescue treatment. Chest 1994;105.
288. Singh JP, Bonin PD. Inhibition of proliferation of fibroblasts by lazaroids (21-aminosteroids). Life Sci 1991;49:2053.
289. McIntosh TK, Thomas M, Smith D, Banbury M. The novel 21-aminosteroid U74006F attenuates cerebral edema and improves survival after brain injury in the rat. J Neurotrauma. 1992;9:33.
290. Hall ED, Yonkers PA, Andrus PK, Cox JW, Anderson DK. Biochemistry and pharmacology of lipid antioxidants in acute brain and spinal cord injury. J Neurotrauma. 1992;9 Suppl 2:S425.
291. Shenkar R, Abraham E. Effects of treatment with the 21-aminosteroid, U74389F, on pulmonary cytokine expression following hemorrhage and resuscitation. Crit Care Med 1995;23:132.
292. Prewitt RM, Wood LDH. Effect of sodium nitroprusside on cardiovascular function and pulmonary shunt in canine oleic acid pulmonary edema. Anesthesiology 1981;55:537.
293. Pearl RG, Rosenthal MH, Ashton JPA. Pulmonary vasodilator effects of nitroglycerin and sodium nitroprusside in canine oleic acid-induced pulmonary hypertension. Anesthesiology 1983;58:514.
294. Caplan RA, Bishop MJ, Cheney FW. Effect of hydralazine on cardiac output and venous admixture in experimental lung injury. Am Rev Respir Dis 1984;130:863.
295. Melot C, Naeije R, Mols P, et al. Pulmonary vascular tone improves pulmonary gas exchange in the adult respiratory distress syndrome [Abstract]. Am Rev Respir Dis 1984;129.
296. Colley PS, Chaney FW, Hlastala MP. Pulmonary gas exchange effects of nitroglycerin in canine edematous lungs. Anesthesiology 1981; 55:114.
297. Michael JR, Kennedy TP, Fitzpatrick S, Rosenstein BJ. Nifedepine inhibits hypoxic vasoconstriction during rest and exercise in patients with cystic fibrosis and cor pulmonale. Am Rev Respir Dis 1984;130:516.
298. Simmoneau G, Excourrou P, Duroux P, Lockhart A. Inhibition of hypoxic pulmonary vasoconstriction by nifedipine. N Engl J Med 1981;304:1582.
299. Imhoff M, Hoffmann P. [Therapy of acute lung failure with nifedipine. A study with interventional analysis]. Zeitschrift fur die Gesamte Innere Medizin und Ihre Grenzgebiete 1992;47:452.
300. Melot C, Lejeune P, Leeman M, et al. Prostaglandin E1 in the adult respiratory distress syndrome. Benefit for pulmonary hypertension and cost for pulmonary gas exchange. Am Rev Respir Dis 1989;139:106.
301. Radermacher P, Santak B, Becker H, Falke KJ. Prostaglandin E1 and nitroglycerin reduce pulmonary capillary pressure but worsen ventilation-perfusion distributions in patients with adult respiratory distress syndrome. Anesthesiology 1989;70:601.
302. Regnier B, Safran D, Carlet J, Teisseire B. Comparative haemodynamic effects of dopamine and dobutamine in septic shock. Intensive Care Med 1979;5:115.
303. Schranz D, Stopfkuchen H, Jungst BK, Clemens R, Emmrich P. Hemodynamic effects of dobutamine in children with cardiovascular failure. Eur J Pediatr 1982;139:4.
304. Ziegler EJ, Fisher CJ, Sprung CL, et al. A human monoclonal antibody against endotoxin. N Engl J Med 1991;324:429.
305. Tracey KJ, Fong Y, Hesse DG, et al. Anti-cachectin/TNF monoclonal antibodies prevent septic shock during lethal bacteremia. Nature 1987;330:662.
306. Sullivan GW, Carper HT, Novick WJ, et al. Inhibition of the inflammatory action of IL-1 and TNF on neutrophil function by pentoxifylline. Infect Immun 1988;56:1722.
307. Ishizaka A, Wu Z, Stephens KE, et al. Attenuation of acute lung injury in septic guinea pigs by pentoxifylline. Am Rev Respir Dis 1988;138:376.
308. Welsh CH, Lien D, Worthen GS, et al. Pentoxifylline decreases endotoxin-induced pulmonary neutrophil sequestration and extravascular protein accumulation in the dog. Am Rev Respir Dis 1988;138.
309. Ardizzoia A, Lissoni P, Tancini G, et al. Respiratory distress syndrome in patients with advanced cancer treated with pentoxifylline: a randomized study. Supportive Care in Cancer 1993;1:331.
310. Montravers P, Fagon JY, Gilbert C, et al. Pilot study of cardiopulmonary risk from pentoxifylline in adult respiratory distress syndrome. Chest 1993;103:1017.
311. Higgenbottam T, Pepke-Zaba J, Scott J, et al. Inhaled endothelium derived relaxing factor in primary hypertension. Am Rev Respir Dis 1988;137(suppl):107.
312. Johns RA. EDRF/nitric oxide: The endogenous nitrovasodilator and a new cellular messenger. Anesthesiology 1991;75:927.
313. Falke KJ, Rossaint R, Pison U, et al. Inhaled nitric oxide selectively reduces pulmonary hypertension in severe ARDS and improves gas exchange as well as right heart ejection fraction—a case report. Am Rev Respir Dis 1991;143.
314. Pison U, Lopez F, Heidelmeyer CF, et al. Inhaled nitric oxide selectively reverses hypoxic pulmonary vasoconstriction in a mechanically ventilated sheep model. Am Rev Respir Dis 1991;143.
315. Gaston B, Reilly J, Drazen JM, et al. Endogenous nitrogen oxides and bronchodilator S-nitrosothiols in human airways. Proc Natl Acad Sci USA 1993;90:10957.
316. Zapol WM, Falke KJ, Rossaint R. Inhaled nitric oxide for the adult respiratory distress syndrome. N Engl J Med 1993;329:207.
317. Zapol WM, Hurford WE. Inhaled nitric oxide in adult respiratory distress syndrome and other lung diseases. [Review]. Advances in Pharmacology 1994;31:513.
318. Rossaint R, Gerlach H, Falke KJ. Inhalation of nitric oxide—a new approach in severe ARDS. [Review]. European Journal of Anaesthesiology 1994;11:43.
319. Rossaint R, Falke KJ, López F, et al. Inhaled nitric oxide for the adult respiratory distress syndrome. New England Journal of Medicine 1993;328:399.

320. Bigatello LM, Hurford WE, Kacmarek RM, Roberts JD, Jr., Zapol WM. Prolonged inhalation of low concentrations of nitric oxide in patients with severe adult respiratory distress syndrome. Effects on pulmonary hemodynamics and oxygenation. Anesthesiology 1994;80:761.
321. Abman SH, Griebel JL, Parker DK, et al. Acute effects of inhaled nitric oxide in children with severe hypoxemic respiratory failure. Journal of Pediatrics 1994;124:881.
322. Kilbourn RG, Griffith OW. Overproduction of nitric oxide in cytokine-mediated and septic shock. Journal of the National Cancer Institute 1992;84:827.
323. Smith REA, Radomski MW, Moncada S. Nitric oxide mediates the vascular actions of cytokines in septic shock. European Journal of Clinical Investigation 1992;22:438.
324. Lewis JF, Veldhuizen R, Possmayer F, et al. Altered alveolar surfactant is an early marker of acute lung injury in septic adult sheep. Am J Respir Crit Care Med 1994;150:123.
325. Seeger W, Gunther A, Walmrath HD, Grimminger F, Lasch HG. Alveolar surfactant and adult respiratory distress syndrome. Pathogenetic role and therapeutic prospects. [Review]. Clinical Investigator 1993;71:177.
326. Robertson B. Surfactant inactivation and surfactant replacement in experimental models of ARDS. [Review]. Acta Anaesthesiologica Scandinavica 1991;Supplementum:22.
327. Anzueto A, Baughman R, Guntupalli K, et al. An international randomized placebo-controlled trial evaluating the efficacy of aerosolized surfactant in patients with sepsis-induced ARDS. Am J Respir Crit Care Med 1994;149:A567.
328. Weg JG, Balk RA, Tharratt RS, et al. Safety and potential efficacy of an aerosolized surfactant in human sepsis-induced adult respiratory distress syndrome. JAMA 1994;272:1433.
329. Putensen C, León MA, Putensen-Himmer G. Effect of neuromuscular blockade on the elastic properties of the lungs, thorax, and total respiratory system in anesthetized pigs. Crit Care Med 1994;22:1976.
330. Matsubara S, Okada T, Yoshida M. Mitochondrial changes in acute myopathy after treatment of respiratory failure with mechanical ventilation (acute relaxant-steroid myopathy). Acta Neuropathol (Berl) 1994;88:475.
331. Hansen-Flaschen J, Cowen J, Raps EC. Neuromuscular blockade in the intensive care unit: More than we bargained for. American Review of Respiratory Disease 1993;147:234.
332. Askanazi J, Rosenbaum SH, Hyman AI, et al. Respiratory changes induced by the large glucose loads of total parenteral nutrition. JAMA 1980;243:1444.
333. Kolobow T, Zapol W, Pierce JE, et al. Partial extracorporeal gas exchange in alert newborn lambs with a membrane artificial lung perfused via an A-V shunt for periods up to 96 hours. Trans Am Soc Artif Intern Organs 1968;14:328.
334. Gille JP. World census of long-term perfusion for respiratory support. pp. 525-530. In: Zapol WM, Qvist J, ed. Artificial lungs for acute respiratory failure. New York, Academic Press, 1976.
335. Gille JP, Bagniewski AM. Ten years of use of extracorporeal membrane oxygenation (ECMO) in the treatment of acute respiratory insufficiency (ARI). Trans Am Soc Artif Intern Organs 1976;22:102.
336. Zapol WM, Snider MT, Hill JD, et al. Extracorporeal membrane oxygenation in severe acute respiratory failure. A randomized prospective study. JAMA 1979;242:2193.
337. Gattinoni L, Pesenti A, Mascheroni D, et al. Low frequency positive pressure ventilation with extracorporeal CO_2 removal in severe acute respiratory failure. JAMA 1986;256:881.
337a. Green TP, Timmons OD, Fackler JC, et al. The impact of extracorporeal membrane oxygenation on survival in pediatric patients with acute respiratory failure. Crit Care Med (in press).
338. Fuhrman BP. Perfluorocarbon liquids and respiratory support. Crit Care Med 1993;21:951.
339. Leach CL, Fuhrman BP, Morin III F, Rath MG. Perfluorocarbon-associated gas exchange (partial liquid ventilation) in respiratory distress syndrome: A prospective, randomized, controlled study. Crit Care Med 1993;21:1270.
340. Hirschl RB, Overbeck MC, Parent A. Liquid ventilation provides uniform distribution of perfluorocarbon in the setting of respiratory failure. Surgery 1994;116:159.
341. Venus B, Jacobs HK, Lim L. Treatment of the adult respiratory distress syndrome with continuous positive airway pressure. Chest 1979;76:257.
342. Suchyta MR, Clemmer TP, Orme JF, Jr, Morris AH. Increased survival of ARDS patients with severe hypoxemia (ECMO criteria). Chest 1991;99:951.
343. Elliot CG, Morris AH, Cengiz M. Pulmonary function and exercise gas exchange in survivors of adult respiratory distress syndrome. Am Rev Respir Dis 1981;123:492.
344. Lakshminarayan S, Hudson LD. Pulmonary function following the adult respiratory distress syndrome. Chest 1978;74:489.
345. Yahav J, Lieberman P, Molho M. Pulmonary function following the adult respiratory distress syndrome. Chest 1978;74:247.
346. Klein JJ, Haeringen JR, Slinter HJ, Holloway R, Peset R. Pulmonary function after recovery from adult respiratory distress syndrome. Chest 1976;69:350.
347. Fanconi S, Kraemer R, Weber J, Tschaeppeler H, Pfenninger J. Long term sequelae in children surviving adult respiratory distress syndrome. J Pediatr 1985;106:218.
348. Elliott CG, Rasmusson BY, Crapo RO, Morris AH, Jensen RL. Prediction of pulmonary function abnormalities after adult respiratory distress syndrome (ARDS). Am Rev Respir Dis 1987;135:634.
349. Reid LM. Lung growth in health and disease. Br J Dis Chest 1984;78:113.
350. Reid LM. The pulmonary circulation: remodeling in growth and disease. The 1978 J. Burns Amberson lecture. Am Rev Respir Dis 1979;119:531.
351. Swank DW, Moore SB. Roles of the neutrophil and other mediators in adult respiratory distress syndrome. Mayo Clin Proc 1989;64:1118.
352. Kaplan HP, Robinson FR, Kapanci Y, Weibel ER. Pathogenesis and reversibility of pulmonary lesions of oxygen toxicity in monkeys. I. Clinical and light microscopic studies. Lab Invest 1969;20:94.
353. de los, Santos R, Seidenfeld JJ, et al. One hundred percent oxygen lung injury in adult baboons. Am Rev Respir Dis 1987;136:657.
354. Pappas CTE, Obara H, Bensch KG, Northway WH. Effect of prolonged exposure to 80% oxygen on the lung of the newborn mouse. Lab Invest 1983;48:735.
355. Riffin TA, Simon LM, Braun D, Theodore J, Robin ED. Impairment of phagocytosis by moderate hyperoxia (40 to 60 percent oxygen) in lung macrophages. Lab Invest 1980;42:622.
356. Wolfe WG, Ebert PA, Sabiston DC, Jr. Effects of high oxygen tension on mucociliary function. Surgery 1972;72:246.
357. Jenkinson SF. Pulmonary oxygen toxicity: adult respiratory distress syndrome. Clin Chest Med 1982;3:109.
358. Caldwell PRB, Lee WL, Jr., Schildkraut HS, Archibald ER. Changes in lung volume, diffusing capacity, and blood gases in men breathing oxygen. J Appl Physiol 1966;21:1477.
359. Fridovich I. Hypoxia and oxygen toxicity. Adv Neurol 1979;26:255.
360. McCord JM, Fridovich I. The biology and pathology of oxygen radicals. Ann Intern Med 1978;89:122.
361. Tate RM, Vanbenthuysen KM, Shasby DM, McMurty IF, Repine JE. Oxygen-radical-mediated permeability edema and vasoconstriction in isolated perfused rabbit lungs. Am Rev Respir Dis 1982;126:802.
362. Del Maestro RF. An approach to free radicals in medicine and biology. Acta Physiol Scand Suppl 1980;492:153.
363. Kellogg EW, Fridovich I. Liposome oxidation and erythrocyte lysis by enzymatically generated superoxide and hydrogen peroxide. J Biol Chem 1977;252:6721.
364. Crapo JD, Tierney DF. Superoxide dismutase and pulmonary oxygen toxicity. Am J Physiol 1974;226:1401.
365. Crapo JD, DeLong DM, Sjostrom K, Hasler GR, Drew RT. The failure of aerosolized superoxide dismutase to modify pulmonary oxygen toxicity. Am Rev Respir Dis 1977;115:1027.
366. Schnapp LM, Chin DP, Szaflarski N, Matthay MA. Frequency and importance of barotrauma in 100 patients with acute lung injury. Crit Care Med 1995;23.
367. Petersen GW, Baier H. Incidence of pulmonary barotrauma in a medical ICU. Crit Care Med 1983;1167-69:67.
368. Webb HH, Tierney DF. Experimental pulmonary edema due to intermittent positive pressure ventilation with high inflation pressures: protection by positive end-expiratory pressure. Am Rev Respir Dis 1974;110:556.
369. Hernandez LA, Peevy KJ, Moise AA, Parker JC. Chest wall restriction limits high airway pressure-induced lung injury in young rabbits. Journal of Applied Physiology 1989;66:2364.
370. Dreyfuss D, Soler P, Basset G, Saumon G. High inflation pressure pulmonary edema. Respective effects of high airway pressure, high tidal volume, and positive end-expiratory pressure. American Review of Respiratory Disease 1988;137:1159.
371. Mathieu-Costello OA, West JB. Are pulmonary capillaries susceptible to mechanical stress. 1994 1994;105 Suppl:102S.
372. McCulloch PR, Forkert PG, Froese AB. Lung volume maintenance pre-

vents lung injury during high frequency oscillatory ventilation in surfactant-deficient rabbits. Am Rev Respir Dis 1988;137:1185.
373. Sugiura M, McCulloch PR, Wren S, Dawson RH, Froese AB. Ventilator pattern influences neutrophil influx and activation in atelectasis-prone rabbit lung. J Appl Physiol 1994;77:1355.
374. Matsuoka T, Kawano T, Miyasaka K. Role of high-frequency ventilation in surfactant-depleted lung injury as measured by granulocytes. J Appl Physiol 1994;76:539.
375. Imai Y, Kawano T, Miyasaka K, et al. Inflammatory chemical mediators during conventional ventilation and during high frequency oscillatory ventilation. Am J Respir Crit Care Med 1994;150:1550.
376. Nichols DG, Walker LK, Wingard JR, et al. Predictors of acute respiratory failure after bone marrow transplantation in children. Crit Care Med 1994;22:1485.
377. Barton R, Cerra FB. The hypermetabolism multiple organ failure syndrome. Chest 1989;96:115.
378. Modell JH, Graves SA, Ketover A. Clinical course of 91 consecutive near drowning victims. Chest 1976;70:231.
379. Modell JH, Moya F, Newley EJ, Ruiz BC, Showers AV. The effects of fluid volume in sea water drownings. Ann Intern Med 1967;67:68.
380. Giamona ST, Modell JH. Drowning by total emergence: effects on pulmonary surfactant of distilled water, isotonic saline, and sea water. Am J Dis Child 1967;114:612.
381. Peterson B. Morbidity of childhood near drowning. Pediatrics 1977;59:364.
382. Fenkel JK. Role of corticosteroids as predisposing factors in fungal diseases. Lab Invest 1962;1:1192.
383. Littler WA, Kay JM, Hasleton PS, Health D. Busulfan lung. Thorax 1969;24:639.
384. Rodin AE, Haggard ME, Travis LB. Lung changes and chemotherapeutic agents in childhood, Report of a case associated with cyclophosphamide therapy. Am J Dis Child 1970;120:337.
385. Rosenow EC, III. The spectrum of drug induced pulmonary disease. Ann Intern Med 1972;77:97.
386. Horowitz AL, Friedman M, Smith J, et al. The pulmonary changes of bleomycin toxicity. Radiology 1973;106:65.
387. Snow RM, Miller WC, Rice DL, Ali MK. Respiratory failure in cancer patients. JAMA 1979;241:2039.
388. Sickles EA, Young VM, Greene WH, Wiernik PH. Pneumonia in acute leukemia. Ann Intern Med 1973;79:528.
389. Pennington JE, Feldman NT. Pulmonary infiltrated and fever in patients with hematologic malignancy. Am J Med 1977;62:581.
390. Imoke E, Dudgeon DL, Colombani P, et al. Open lung biopsy in the immunocompromised pediatric patient. J Pediatr Surg 1983;18:816.
391. Goodell B, Jacobs JB, Powell RD, DeVita VT. Pneumocystis carinii: the spectrum of diffuse interstitial pneumonia in patients with neoplastic diseases. Ann Intern Med 1970;72:327.
392. Adeyemi SD, Ein SH, Simpson JS, Turner P. The value of emergency open lung biopsy in infants and children. J Pediatr Surg 1979; 14:426.
393. Hughes WT, Feldman S, Chaudhary S, Ossi MJ, Sanyal K. Comparison of trimethoprim-sulfamethoxazole and pentamidine in the treatment of Pneumocystis carinii pneumonitis [Abstract]. Pediatr Res 1976; 10:399.
394. Weiner RS, Bortin MM, Gale RP, et al. Interstitial pneumonitis after bone marrow transplantation. Ann Intern Med 1986;104:168.
395. Shanley JD, Pomeroy C, Via CS, Shearer GM. Interstitial pneumonitis during murine cytomegalovirus infection and graft-versus-host reaction: effect of ganciclovir. J Infect Dis 1988;158:1391.
396. Fallat RJ, Mielke CH, Rodvien R. Adult respiratory distress syndrome and Gram-negative sepsis. Arch Intern Med 1980;140:612.
397. Browdie DA, Dean R, Shinozaki T, et al. Adult respiratory distress syndrome (ARDS), sepsis and extracorporeal membrane oxygenation (ECMO). J Trauma 1977;17:579.
398. Fulton RL, Jones CE. The cause of the post-traumatic pulmonary insufficiency in man. Surg Gynecol Obstet 1975;140:179.
399. Pfenninger J, Gerber A, Tschaeppeler H, Zimmerman A. Adult respiratory distress syndrome in children. J Pediatr 1982;101:352.
400. Sacks HS, Lyons RW, Lahiri B. Adult respiratory distress syndrome in Rocky Mountain spotted fever. Am Rev Respir Dis 1981;123:547.
401. Dixon C. Mycoplasmal pneumonia and adult respiratory distress syndrome: a complication to be recognized. J Natl Med Assoc 1981;73:549.
402. Tuxen DV, Cade JF, McDonald MI, et al. Herpes simplex virus from the lower respiratory tract in adult respiratory distress syndrome. Am Rev Respir Dis 1982;126:416.
403. Peltier LF. The diagnosis and treatment of fat embolism. J Trauma 1971;11:661.
404. Curtis AM, Knowles GD, Putman CE, et al. The three syndromes of fat embolism: pulmonary manifestations. Yale J Biol Med 1979;52:149.
405. Rokkanen P, Lahdensuu M, Kataja J, Julkunen H. The syndrome of fat embolism: analysis of 30 consecutive cases compared to trauma patients with similar injuries. J Trauma 1970;10:299.
406. Bradford DS, Foster RR, Nossel HL. Coagulation alterations, hypoxemia, and fat embolism in fracture patients. J Trauma 1970;10:307.
407. Whitenack SH, Hausberger FX. Intravasation of fat from bone marrow cavity. Am J Pathol 1971;65:335.
408. Fonte DA, Hausberger FX. Pulmonary free fatty acids in experimental fat embolism. J Trauma 1971;11:668.
409. Wanebo H, Van Dyke J. The high-velocity pulmonary injury: relation to traumatic wet lung syndrome. J Thorac Cardiovasc Surg 1972;64:537.
410. Trinkle JK, Furman RW, Hinshaw MA, Bryant LR, Griffin WO. Pulmonary contusion: pathogenesis and effect of various resuscitation measures. Ann Thorac Surg 1973;16:568.
411. Wilson RF, Gibson DB, Antonenko D. Shock and acute respiratory failure after chest trauma. J Trauma 1977;17:697.
412. Milley JR, Nugent SK, Rogers MC. Neurogenic pulmonary edema in childhood. J Pediatr 1979;94:706.
413. Mackay EM. Experimental pulmonary edema. IV. Pulmonary edema accompanying trauma to the brain. Proc Soc Exp Biol 1950;74:695.
414. Bean JW, Beckman DL. Centrogenic pulmonary pathology in mechanical head injury. J Appl Physiol 1969;27:807.
415. Ducker TB, Simmons RL. Increased intracranial pressure and pulmonary edema. Part 2. The hemodynamic response of dogs and monkeys to increased intracranial pressure. J Neurosurg 1968;28:118.
416. Aidinis SJ, Laferty J, Shapiro HM. Intracranial responses to PEEP. Anesthesiology 1976;45:275.
417. Moritz AR, Henriques FC, McLean R. The effects of inhaled heat on air passages and lungs: an experimental investigation. Am J Pathol 1945;21:311.
418. Trunkey DD. Inhalation injury. Surg Clin North Am 1978;58:1133.
419. Thorning DR, Howard ML, Hudson LD, Schumacher RL. Pulmonary responses to smoke inhalation: morphologic changes in rabbits exposed to pine wood smoke. Hum Pathol 1982;13:355.
420. Whitener DR, Whitener LM, Robertson KJ, Baxter CR, Pierce AK. Pulmonary function measurements in patients with thermal injury and smoke inhalation. Am Rev Respir Dis 1980;122:731.
421. Cox ME, Heslop BF, Kempton JJ, Ratcliff RA. The Dellwood fire. Br Med J 1955;1:942.
422. Nash G, Foley FD, Langlinais PC. Pulmonary interstitial edema and hyaline membrane in adult burn patients: electron microscopic observations. Hum Pathol 1974;5:149.
423. Wroblewski DA, Bower GC. The significance of facial burns in acute smoke inhalation. Crit Care Med 1979;7:335.
424. Moylan JA. Diagnostic techniques and steroids. J Trauma 1979;19:917.

Neuromuscular Disease and Respiratory Failure 8

Donald Shaffner

INTRODUCTION

Although the term *respiratory failure* usually implies pulmonary pathology, it also applies to situations characterized by normal lung parenchyma with impaired respiratory pump function. The respiratory pump is the system that brings external gas (oxygen) into contact with the alveolar membrane for exchange with waste gas (carbon dioxide) through a common intake/exhaust channel. The movement of gas is accomplished by a series of muscles that either participate in gas propulsion or maintain patency of the airway through which the gas moves. The regulation of both sets of muscles is performed by controllers that respond to input from sensors and feedback loops and produce output to the muscles. A graphic representation of this "respiratory pump" is provided (Fig. 8.1). Input pertaining to the systemic P_aCO_2, P_aO_2, and pH from the central and peripheral chemoreceptors, as well as input regarding the presence of airway irritation and the stretch applied to the intercostal muscles, is supplied to the respiratory control centers. The cerebral cortex provides voluntary control while the pons and medulla maintain involuntary regulation of the respiratory rhythm. The output from the respiratory control centers is passed through the cranial and peripheral nerves to the muscles that provide airway patency or produce gas movement.

Disorders that affect the neuromuscular system impact ventilatory gas exchange by impairing the central control of breathing, the patency of the proximal airway, or the effectiveness of the respiratory muscles. Consideration of neuromuscular diseases from an anatomic perspective is useful in developing a therapeutic approach to the respiratory failure associated with these disorders (Fig. 8.2). The brain, spinal cord, peripheral nerves, neuromuscular junction, and muscles are the five anatomic sites of the neuromuscular framework involved. Seizures, central depressant medications, and central hypoventilation syndrome impair ventilatory drive in the brain's respiratory centers and can result in hypoventilation or apnea. Spinal cord trauma, tetanus, and poliomyelitis affect the spinal motor centers, produce primary bulbar and respiratory muscle dysfunction, and result in airway obstruction or hypoventilation. Peripheral neuropathic conditions as a result of systemic processes (e.g., Guillain-Barré syndrome) or as a result of direct injury (e.g., phrenic nerve palsy) produce similar respiratory complications. Myasthenia gravis and botulism, as well as certain types of drug intoxication (e.g., aminoglycoside antibiotics), disrupt transmission at the neuromuscular junction, to produce respiratory muscle weakness. Finally, a number of congenital and acquired diseases of the skeletal muscles lead to severe diaphragmatic and pharyngeal muscle weakness. A summary of the major features of various neuromuscular causes of respiratory failure is provided in **Table 8.1.**

Children with primary neuromuscular disorders frequently suffer respiratory complications requiring intensive care. Although certain principles of respiratory therapy are applicable in all forms of neuromuscular disease, it is important to consider specific aspects of each disorder in order to plan individual therapy and anticipate potential complications.

Recently, appreciation of the role of respiratory muscle fatigue in the pathogenesis of respiratory failure has grown

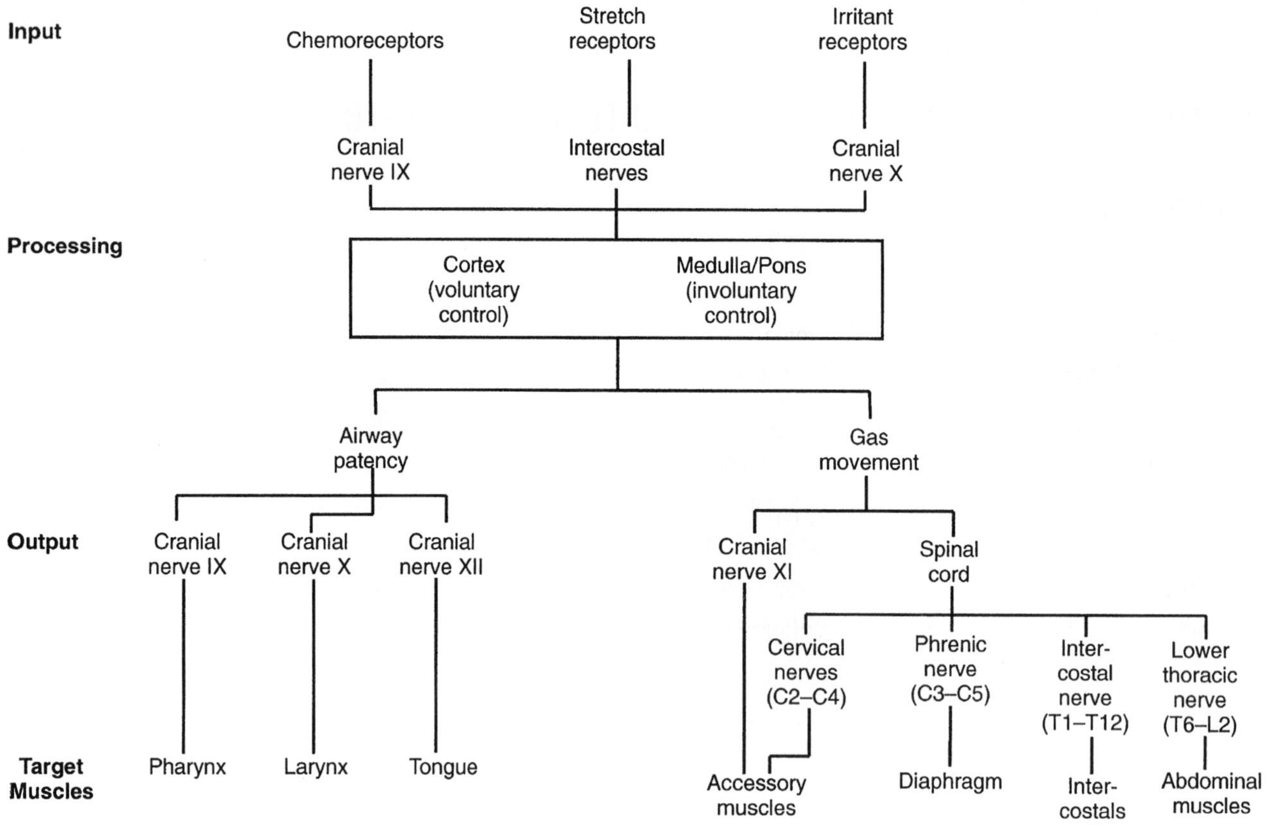

Figure 8.1. Neuromuscular framework of the respiratory system.

substantially. Consequently, the last several years have witnessed a resurgence of interest in the complex role that the neuromuscular system plays in supporting respiratory function[1–7]. Indeed, considerable attention is being directed toward methods of enhancing respiratory muscle function in an effort to offset increases in work of breathing associated with a variety of pulmonary diseases. Therefore, although the following section focuses on neuromuscular diseases associated with primary respiratory muscle dysfunction, respiratory muscle strength is an important consideration in all forms of respiratory failure.

CENTRAL HYPOVENTILATION SYNDROME

Before beginning a discussion of central hypoventilation syndrome, it is important to define the types of apnea encountered in pediatric critical care[8]. Central apnea is a failure of the respiratory control centers to stimulate ventilatory efforts. Obstructive apnea occurs when the airway is blocked and spontaneous respiratory efforts are made that fail to generate respiratory gas flow. Obstructive apnea may be *partial,* with some gas exchange occurring, or *complete,* with no gas exchange occurring. Mixed apnea, as the name implies, has characteristics of central and obstructive apnea. In the case of mixed apnea, a central apneic episode is usually followed by inspiratory efforts that do not generate respiratory gas flow because of superimposed airway obstruction.

Clinical Features

Central hypoventilation syndrome[8–12] is characterized by dysfunction of the respiratory centers responsible for the automatic control of breathing during sleep. Severinghaus and Mitchell (13) labeled the disorder *Ondine's curse* in reference to the tragic hero of German legend whose automatic vital functions, including the unconscious control of breathing, were removed by the water nymph Ondine. As in the legend, patients with central hypoventilation syndrome suffer apnea after they fall asleep and lose voluntary control of respiration.

Central hypoventilation syndrome represents a protracted form of central apnea due to abnormal automatic regulation of breathing at the level of the central nervous system (CNS)[9]. Apnea occurs with quiet, non-rapid eye movement (REM) sleep, and there is little or no ventilatory response to hypercapnia[9–12]. Although ventilation is most depressed during quiet sleep, the respiratory dysrhythmia can progress to hypoventilation during REM sleep and awake states[12]. The respiratory response to hypoxemia in children with central hypoventilation may not be the expected increase in ventilation. Some studies suggest that beyond the newborn period, infants suffering from this disorder become apneic with the administration of oxygen[11].

Central hypoventilation syndrome may be congenital, with onset in the perinatal period, or acquired, associated with any of a variety of diseases. The clinical presentation of congenital central hypoventilation syndrome usually takes the form of cyanosis at birth that responds readily to mechanical ventilatory support[9–12]. Frequently, weaning from respiratory support results in repeated failure. In less severe cases, abnormalities in the respiratory pattern during sleep are noted and lead to a presumptive diagnosis of an acute life-threatening event[14].

In acquired central hypoventilation syndrome, sleep-related respiratory dysrhythmias are seen in association with or following recovery from the underlying disease. Acquired central hypoventilation syndrome can be idiopathic or occur in association with posterior fossa tumors, encephalitis, severe asphyxia, medullary infarction[9], the rare syndrome of idiopathic hypothalamic dysfunction[15], and inborn errors of metabolism, such as pyruvate dehydrogenase deficiency[16].

Structural brain pathology[9] associated with acquired central hypoventilation syndrome is usually related to the underlying CNS disease. On the other hand, the congenital form frequently shows variable degrees of destructive changes in the brainstem that are presumably developmental in origin. In addition, decreased neuronal density in the cerebral cortex, probably secondary to repeated bouts of hypoxemia, have been reported[9].

The abnormal respiratory pattern during sleep, with either congenital or acquired central hypoventilation syndrome, often leads to complaints of diminished school performance, hypersomnolence, or morning headaches. In more severe cases, the abnormal control of breathing can be manifested as prolonged apneic episodes. In all cases of central hypoventilation syndrome, repeated bouts of hypoxemia and acidosis can result in significant pulmonary hypertension and cor pulmonale. Indeed, the cardiovascular complications of this disorder can be the initial symptoms[12,17].

Central hypoventilation syndrome must be differentiated from reversible disorders that can be associated with apnea or hypoventilation[18]. Reversible systemic processes include sepsis, hypothermia, electrolyte abnormalities, hypocalcemia, hypoglycemia, and seizures. Cardiorespiratory disease resulting in severe hypoxemia or respiratory muscle fatigue can culminate in the cessation of breathing. CNS infections, intracranial hemorrhage, acute hydrocephalus, or other conditions associated with acute intracranial hypertension can trigger hypoventilation or apnea. The role of gastroesophageal reflux in the pathogenesis of apnea is controversial[19]. In some cases, reflux may cause stimulation of laryngeal receptors and reflex apnea in infants. These reversible disorders can be differentiated from central hypoventilation syndrome on the basis of the clinical presentation, routine laboratory evaluations, careful neurologic evaluation, and sleep electroencephalogram. Gastroesophageal reflux can be investigated with esophageal manometry and pH monitoring.

In addition to other causes of central apneic episodes, central hypoventilation syndrome must be differentiated from abnormalities that cause blockage of the flow of ventilatory gases in the airway during slumber, i.e., obstructive sleep apnea[8,12]. The presentation of obstructive sleep apnea can be similar to that of central hypoventilation, with sleep-related respiratory irregularity, secondary pulmonary hypertension, cor pulmonale, hypersomnolence, and morning headaches. In adults, this disorder is usually secondary to loss of pharyngeal muscle tone during REM sleep, resulting in functional obstruction of the extrathoracic airway. In contrast, infants and young children with obstructive sleep apnea usually have a fixed anatomic component. The likely causes of obstruction in children include hypertrophy of the tonsils and adenoids, macroglossia (Down's syndrome), micrognathia (Pierre Robin anomalad), other oral or nasal congenital deformities, temporomandibular ankylosis, vascular ring, and paralysis of the vocal cords. Airway obstruction during sleep is also noted periodically after surgical correction of cleft palate deformities. In all of these disorders, treatment is directed at using the safest and most effective method to bypass the obstructive lesion. This

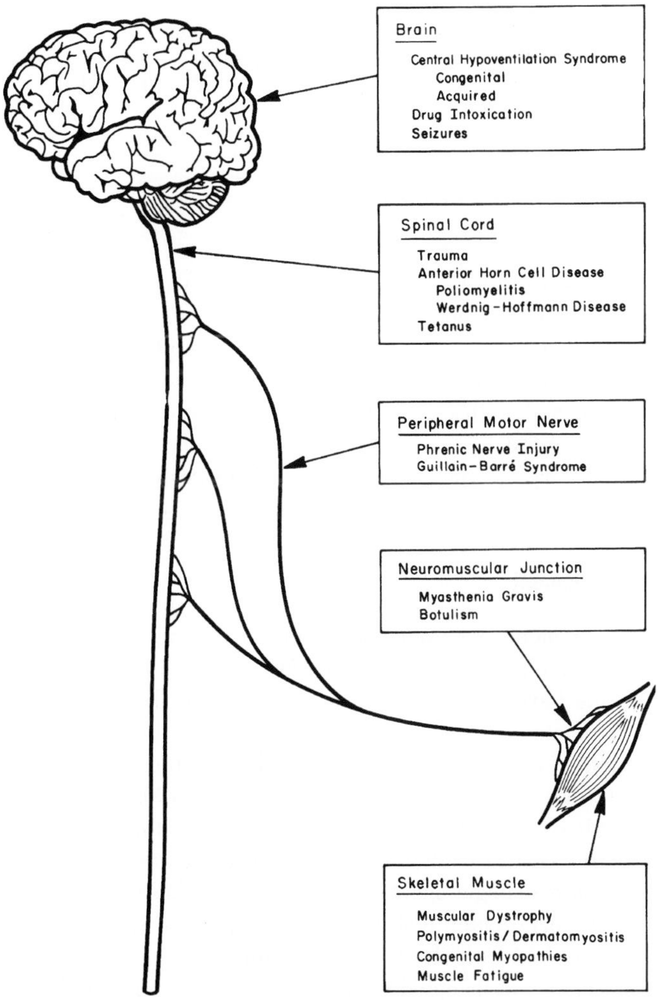

Figure 8.2. Anatomic representation of selected neuromuscular disorders associated with respiratory failure in children.

Table 8.1. Characteristics of Various Neuromuscular Causes of Respiratory Failure[a]

Disease	*Prodrome*	*Onset*	*Presentation*	*DTRs*	*Sensory*	*Autonomic*	*Lab*	*EMG/NCV*
Cortical lesion (UMN)	Mental status change, headache, seizures	Varies	Contralateral hemiplegia, aphasia	↑	Maybe	Variable	CT scan, EEG	Nl
Brainstem lesion (UMN)	Cranial nerve symptoms	Varies	Ipsilateral cranial nerve, contralateral hemiplegia	↑	Maybe	Variable	MR scan	Nl
Spinal cord lesion (UMN)	Trauma, back pain	Varies	Quadriplegia/ paraplegia	↑	Abnl	Variable	X-rays, myelogram	Nl
Tetanus (spinal cord, UMN)	Contaminated wound	3 days–3 wk	Trismus, muscle spasms	↑	Abnl	No	Culture positive in 1/3 of cases	Abnl
Poliomyelitis (anterior horn cell, LMN, bulbar, cortex)	URI or GI symptoms	1–2 wk	Asymmetric paralysis, may involve bulbar muscles	↓	Abnl	Yes	↑ Protein and cells in CSF, virus in stool and oropharynx	Abnl
Guillain-Barré (peripheral nerve, LMN)	URI or GI symptoms, surgery	1–3 wk	Symmetric ascending paralysis, usually proximal	↓	Abnl	Yes	↑ Protein in CSF, Nl CSF cells	Abnl
Infant botulism (NMJ)	Honey, switch from breast-feeding	Days	Ileus, dry mouth, descending paralysis	Nl	Nl	Yes	Neurotoxin in stool and serum	Abnl
Myasthenia gravis (NMJ)	Exacerbations and remissions	Varies	Proximal weakness, ocular findings, fatigability	Nl	Nl	No	Serum antibody, response to edrophonium (Tensilon)	Abnl
Myopathy (muscle)	May be hereditable	Gradual	Symmetric, proximal weakness	Nl	Nl	No	↑ Serum CPK, Nl CSF, abnl biopsy	Abnl

[a]Abbreviations: DTRs, deep tendon reflexes; EMG/NCV, electromyogram/nerve conduction velocity; UMN, upper motor neuron; CT scan, computed tomography scan; EEG, electroencephalogram; Nl, normal; MR scan, magnetic resonance scan; Abnl, abnormal; LMN, lower motor neuron; URI, upper respiratory infection; GI, gastrointestinal; CSF, cerebrospinal fluid; NMJ, neuromuscular junction; and CPK, creatinine phosphokinase.

may require appropriate positioning of the infant, placement of an oropharyngeal or nasopharyngeal airway, or definitive surgery to remove the anatomic obstruction, such as tonsillectomy and/or adenoidectomy or vascular ring release.

It should be noted that mixed apneas occur in several settings, particularly diseases involving the posterior fossa. Arnold-Chiari malformation may be associated with paralysis of the vocal cords due to bulbar palsy as well as hypoventilation secondary to medullary respiratory center compression[(18)]. Also, combined obstructive apnea and central hypoventilation have been noted in infants with achondroplasia due to medullary compression associated with narrowing of the foramen magnum[(20)]. The potential for mixed abnormalities of respiratory rhythm should be anticipated in these disorders. Definitive management may require both surgical decompression of the posterior fossa and relief of upper airway obstruction by tracheostomy.

To evaluate central hypoventilation syndrome, monitoring of respiratory patterns during sleep is necessary[(9–12)]. Continuous recording of the following physiologic variables during a prolonged period of sleep is recommended: (a) heart rate and respiratory rate, (b) chest and/or abdominal excursions with impedance pneumography, (c) arterial oxygenation, using transcutaneous oximetry or comparable monitoring, (d) respiratory gas flow at the airway opening via tidal CO_2 recording, and (e) sleep state, using electroencephalography and/or electronystagmography. In cases of obstructive apnea, respiratory efforts are accompanied by diminished or absent gas flow at the airway opening. In contrast, central hypoventilation reveals total cessation of all respiratory gas flow and of spontaneous respiratory activities.

Management

Management of patients with central hypoventilation syndrome includes several therapeutic options. Pharmacologic agents have been used to try to stimulate the respiratory control centers to prevent hypoventilation. Phrenic nerve stimulation has been attempted to bypass the control centers since the distal neuromuscular framework is intact. Mechanical ventilation produces support without involving the control centers or the neuromuscular framework.

Pharmacologic agents directed at stimulating medullary respiratory center (caffeine, theophylline, amphetamines, progesterone, and doxapram) have mixed results, with salutary effects of theophylline and progesterone reported[(12,21)]. Intravenous doxapram[(22)] has improved respiratory drive in some cases, although severe gastrointestinal side effects have been reported. Generally, drugs that act by increasing the sensitivity of the medullary center (central chemoreceptor) of respiration to the effects of blood carbon dioxide tension have yielded inconsistent results in congenital forms of central hypoventilation. Agents that stimulate peripheral chemoreceptor sensitivity may be more effective[23,24]. Almitrine (stimulates the carotid chemoreceptor) has been employed on a limited basis with some success[23–25]. The role of these agents in the long-term management of central hypoventilation syndrome requires further investigation.

Radiofrequency bilateral phrenic nerve pacing[26–29] has been performed in children suffering from central hypoventilation, including infants with congenital forms of the disorder. In infants, pacing electrodes are generally placed on the phrenic nerve by means of a thoracotomy. An internal radiofrequency receiver, implanted subcutaneously, receives excitation from an external radio signal generator. Candidates for phrenic nerve pacing are evaluated by transcutaneous stimulation under fluoroscopic examination to confirm adequate diaphragmatic contraction with phrenic nerve pacing. In addition, patency of the upper airway and freedom from significant mechanical abnormalities of the respiratory system are operative prerequisites. Recent improvements in phrenic nerve-pacing techniques have allowed the use of continuous pacing without degeneration of the phrenic nerve or diaphragm. Using this technique, several investigators have sustained adequate alveolar ventilation in patients with congenital central hypoventilation syndrome for several years. Alternatively, phrenic nerve pacing has been carried out during daytime activities only, with the patient returning to mechanical ventilatory support during nocturnal sleeping periods. Despite the short-term success of the technique in recent trials, it should be stressed that radiofrequency phrenic nerve pacing currently is a highly specialized procedure that is confined to several centers with expertise in the area.

Chronic mechanical ventilatory support with positive or negative pressure devices has been used successfully in the management of central hypoventilation syndrome. The need for mechanical ventilatory assistance is often permanent in congenital forms of the disease, although recovery of adequate respiratory function has been reported in one instance[9]. Although most patients initially require ventilatory assistance only with sleep, periods of hypoventilation often progress into wakeful states, necessitating the use of continuous ventilatory support. Chronic positive pressure ventilation has been achieved by using a nasal mask as well as the more traditional tracheostomy[30–32]. In older children the nasal mask is well tolerated and may obviate the need for tracheostomy[31,32].

Finally, regardless of the therapeutic approach in central hypoventilation syndrome, particular attention must be directed at the maintenance of adequate oxygenation and carbon dioxide clearance; otherwise, chronic hypoxemia and hypercapnia may lead to severe, irreversible pulmonary hypertension and death[17]. A study of the chronic effects of congenital central hyperventilation syndrome reveals that mortality is low and that the early morbidity (congestive heart failure and hypoxic seizures) is reversible[33].

SPINAL CORD TRAUMA

Fortunately, spinal cord injuries are unusual in children[34–36], representing less than 10% of spinal trauma in the United States. Spinal cord injury is associated with multiple medical complications, and those involving the respiratory system are particularly important. Major respiratory complications, such as acute ventilatory failure, pneumonia, and atelectasis, occur in about one-third of adults with cervical cord injury[37–39] and probably more in children. In infants, pneumonia accounts for most late mortality associated with spinal cord injury[40]. It is not surprising that advances in respiratory intensive care have contributed substantially to recent improvements in the mortality rate associated with spinal injury[41].

Pathogenesis

The pathogenesis of acute respiratory failure associated with spinal cord injury is usually multifactorial. The obvious source of ventilatory dysfunction is the associated respiratory motor deficits. As noted in a review by Luce[42], respiratory motor deficits are directly related to the level of spinal injury. High cervical injuries (C1 to C2) result in apnea and early death. Injury to the middle cervical cord at the level of C3 to C5 occurs in approximately one-third of children with spinal trauma[34]. Injury at this level results in loss of diaphragmatic, intercostal, and abdominal muscle function. Accessory muscles of inspiration in the neck and shoulders remain intact by virtue of their innervation (cranial nerve XI and cervical nerves C2 to C4). Accessory muscles alone are inadequate to maintain gas exchange, resulting in acute hypoventilation shortly after injury, and are even less effective in young children. In an equal number of children, injury is sustained to the lower cervical cord below the origin of the phrenic motor fibers (phrenic arises from C3 to C5). Lesions below C5 result in sparing of the diaphragm, with loss of intercostal and abdominal muscle function. Lack of intercostal muscle function results in chest wall instability, which is magnified in the young child whose chest is more compliant. Thus, diaphragmatic contraction is accompanied by paradoxical chest wall movement with less effective inspiration (normally chest and abdomen expand on inspiration; paradoxical means the chest retracts as the diaphragm pushes abdominal contents out on inspiration). Although older children and adults can frequently maintain alveolar ventilation despite this mechanical disadvantage, ventilatory reserve is significantly diminished, as vital capacity falls to 30% of predicted values [37]. In infants, this level of deficit results in alveolar hypoventilation and respiratory failure. Absence of intercostal muscle function is also associated with decreased functional residual capacity and lung compliance, presumably because of diminished outward recoil of the chest wall[42]. Frequently encountered with this level of spinal injury is ventilation/perfusion mismatching and hypoxemia, despite the maintenance of adequate carbon dioxide elimination. Ledsome and Sharp[37] noted improvement in vital capacity over the course of several weeks in adult patients with lower cervical cord trauma, attributed to the development of intercostal muscle spasticity. Stiffening of the chest wall by intercostal spasticity does not produce a similar improvement in respiratory reserve in children.

The remainder of children with spinal trauma suffer injury at various levels of the thoracolumbar spine[34]. Despite the maintenance of diaphragmatic and intercostal function (muscles of inspiration) with lower thoracic and lumbar injuries, respiratory impairment can arise due to loss of abdominal muscle function (abdominal muscles are responsible for forced expiration). In this setting, patients are incapable of generating intra-abdominal pressures necessary for effective coughing, and vital capacity becomes diminished. Consequently, injuries of this type are complicated by retention of pulmonary secretions, atelectasis, and pneumonia.

Acute respiratory failure can arise during the intensive care course of patients with spinal injury as a result of factors unrelated to respiratory muscle deficits[38,39,41]. Pulmonary edema is noted occasionally and has been attributed to excessive fluid resuscitation of spinal shock or to reactive sympathetic hypertonicity at the time of spinal injury (neurogenic pulmonary edema). Frequently, spinal injuries are associated with severe head or thoracoabdominal injuries that exacerbate hypoventilation or present a source of superimposed pulmonary parenchymal disease. Patients with spinal cord injury are also at high risk of aspiration of gastric contents. Acutely, after spinal injury, gastric and intestinal mobility are decreased and can lead to regurgitation or vomiting. The risk of aspiration is particularly great in patients with associated head trauma and coma. Fat embolization can occur in the presence of associated long-bone fractures, and prolonged immobilization can predispose to deep venous thrombosis and pulmonary emboli. These complications are more frequent in adults.

Management

Despite the relative rarity of spinal cord trauma in children, it should be suspected in all patients with severe trauma, especially those who present with coma, flaccidity, hypotension, or hypoventilation. Spinal cord injury in the newborn usually occurs as a result of birth trauma associated with a breech extraction[40]. In older children, spinal injury is usually associated with major trauma involving motor vehicle accidents or sports injuries[34]. Radiographic examination for spinal osteoarticular abnormalities should be performed routinely in the severely traumatized child. Bony vertebral findings may be absent in as many as 60% of children with spinal cord trauma; therefore, a careful neurologic examination is imperative[35]. When spinal injury is suspected on the basis of the examination, measurement of somatosensory evoked responses may be of help in confirming the clinical impression.

The airway should be secured by endotracheal intubation in cases complicated by coma with diminished airway reflexes, inability to clear pulmonary or pharyngeal secretions, or frank hypoventilation. Intubation should be performed by the most skilled individual available. Although blind nasal intubation is sometimes recommended in the adult, in the younger child this technique is less successful, may induce vomiting, and may cause intracranial perforation with an associated cribriform plate fracture. Therefore, its use in children is discouraged. Orotracheal intubation under direct laryngeal visualization is suggested, with application of direct in-line traction to the head by an assistant. Particular care should be taken to avoid hyperextension. Intubation over a fiberoptic bronchoscope can be considered in the older child, provided equipment and skill with the technique are available. Use of the depolarizing muscle relaxant succinylcholine beyond the first 48 hours of resuscitation can cause severe hyperkalemia and resultant cardiac arrhythmias and should be avoided. After the airway is established, elective tracheostomy is generally recommended for the child with spinal cord injury and respiratory failure because airway control is usually required for extended periods through recovery and rehabilitation. However, in patients requiring anterior cervical fusion for stabilization of the spine, performance of a tracheostomy should be deferred until this procedure has been completed[42].

As noted previously, patients with spinal cord injury frequently suffer from associated ventilation/perfusion mismatching. Therefore, supplemental oxygen is frequently required to avoid hypoxemia. The application of continuous positive airway pressure (CPAP) is helpful in reversing the decrease in functional residual capacity and the associated ventilation/perfusion mismatching. Intermittent positive pressure ventilation should be applied in any patient exhibiting difficulty in maintaining adequate alveolar ventilation and normal P_aCO_2. It should be noted that patients who breathe spontaneously and maintain normal blood gases while awake can develop hypoventilation during sleep, presumably due to abnormalities in central respiratory drive. Under these circumstances, positive pressure ventilatory support is required during periods of sleep.

An aggressive regimen of chest physical therapy is necessary to avoid retention of pulmonary secretions. Position changes can be performed by using a mobile-frame bed. However, placement of the patient in the head-down position may lead to regurgitation and aspiration of stomach contents. Also, if the diaphragm is flaccid, abdominal loading associated with this position may lead to impaired ventilation. Augmentation of the patient's cough with manual abdominal compression (see Chapter 9, Principles and

Practice of Respiratory Support and Mechanical Ventilation) can improve tracheal mucus clearance. Suctioning occasionally induces exaggerated vagal responses, such as bradycardia, in patients with spinal cord trauma and may be prevented by pretreatment with atropine.

Weaning patients with spinal cord trauma from respiratory support depends on the level of respiratory function achieved after the acute posttraumatic period. Patients with incomplete neurologic deficits below the level of spinal cord injury often demonstrate significant recovery of their motor function[34]. On the other hand, patients with complete deficits after stabilization generally do not demonstrate return of motor function. Depending on the degree of involvement of the respiratory muscles, varying amounts of ventilatory assistance are required for indefinite periods of time. The young child with more chest wall compliance suffering from cervical cord injury frequently requires chronic mechanical ventilatory support, with either a positive pressure respirator or a negative pressure tank-type ventilator. Older patients with diaphragmatic function may require less restrictive forms of external mechanical support, such as a pneumobelt, rocking bed, or cuirass ventilator[42,43]. Some patients with cervical injuries have intact phrenic nerve conduction peripherally and may be candidates for radiofrequency electrophrenic pacing[26–29,44] (see Central Hypoventilation Syndrome). Lesions above C3 are amenable to this type of treatment, while lesions at C3 to C5 may have some phrenic nerve cell bodies or lower motor neuron damage[45]. Upper airway occlusion may occur due to asynchronous stimulation of the diaphragm and the upper airway muscles, and these patients require a tracheostomy[43,46]. Phrenic nerve pacing allows some freedom from the ventilator, but there is limited experience in maintaining adequate ventilation in children with this technique beyond a few years. Further experience with this method of ventilatory management is required to identify its precise role in the long-term management of children with respiratory muscle paralysis after spinal cord injury.

TETANUS

Clinical Features

Tetanus is characterized by severe, painful muscle rigidity and spasms caused by the toxic product of the bacterium *Clostridium tetani*. The toxin binds to the presynaptic terminals of inhibitory neurons at the spinal cord level. The toxin interferes with the release of inhibitory transmitters, resulting in the firing of opposing muscle groups simultaneously producing clinical spasms. Involvement of the laryngeal or respiratory muscles can give rise to acute respiratory insufficiency, requiring urgent intervention[47–51]. Indeed, approximately half of the mortality associated with tetanus can be attributed to the respiratory complications of the disease[52–55]. Therefore, survival depends on expert respiratory intensive care. Although the disease is rare in the United States, tetanus remains a major cause of respiratory failure in developing nations[56,57]. The application of modern respiratory intensive care has produced a substantial decrease in the mortality associated with tetanus. Currently, survival rates associated with this self-limited disease range between 80 and 90%[47–50,53,55].

After contamination of a wound, the vegetative form of *C. tetani* elaborates the potent neurotoxin, tetanospasmin, which is responsible for the severe motor manifestations of the disease. Tetanus has been described with virtually every type of wound. In 80% of cases, the site of contamination can be identified by history or examination[47,48]. In newborn infants, tetanus is most frequently linked to contamination of the severed umbilical cord after delivery in the home. Less conspicuous sites of entry for the organism include the tympanic membrane (otitis media), the uterus (septic abortion), and venipuncture sites (illicit drug use)[47,48,56,57].

The incubation period is quite variable, ranging from 3 days to 3 weeks, with an average of 8 days. In the neonate, clinical presentation of tetanus generally occurs at the end of the first week of life[55]. A shorter incubation period may be predictive of more severe disease. Early symptoms are usually attributable to muscle rigidity and spasm. In 50 to 75% of patients, trismus (masseter spasm, lockjaw) is noted at the time of clinical presentation[47,48]. This may be accompanied by nuchal rigidity, generalized body stiffness, irritability, or dysphagia due to pharyngeal and facial muscle dysfunction (risus sardonicus). In the neonate, poor feeding is noted early in the disease, followed by reflex spasm and rigidity that may be interpreted as generalized seizures. Muscle spasms are extremely painful and are frequently provoked by stimulation.

Management

The diagnosis of tetanus is usually made on clinical grounds. Other causes of muscle rigidity and trismus, such as electrolyte disorders, poisoning, and seizures, can usually be excluded on the basis of the clinical picture and appropriate laboratory studies. Wound cultures do not reliably yield the causative organism (less than one-third of cases). Examination of the cerebrospinal fluid (CSF) is characteristically unremarkable, and leukocytosis is an inconsistent finding in the absence of secondary infections. Correct diagnosis can be confounded by the absence of an obvious portal of entry, a situation encountered in approximately 20% of cases[48].

In severe cases of tetanus, life-threatening respiratory and cardiovascular complications can ensue with disturbing rapidity after the initial presentation. However, prediction of eventual disease severity early in the course is difficult. For these reasons, observation in the intensive care unit (ICU) is recommended at least during the early phase of hospitalization. Passive immunization to tetanus toxin, administration of appropriate antibiotics, wound debridement, sedation, muscle relaxation, and control of sympathetic nervous system dysfunction represent critical aspects of specific therapy in tetanus that are discussed in detail elsewhere (see Chapter 33, Specific Infectious Diseases of Interest to the Intensivist).

In addition to acute emergencies arising from sympathetic dysfunction, the major focus of intensive care in tetanus is directed at the management of respiratory complications[47–51]. Several situations that can arise during the course of the disease are associated with respiratory failure. Spasms of the laryngeal muscles can precipitate acute airway obstruction and asphyxia. In addition, muscle spasms of the chest wall and respiratory muscles may interfere with ventilation, either primarily or secondarily, as the result of retained secretions, atelectasis, and pneumonia. Newborn infants afflicted with tetanus seem to be particularly prone to the development of aspiration pneumonitis[54]. The use of sedation in the treatment of tetanic spasms can lead to obtundation and central respiratory depression. Finally, the use of muscle relaxants and controlled positive pressure ventilation (see below) for prolonged periods in the treatment of severe reflex spasms is associated with a particularly high incidence of atelectasis and pneumonia in infants[54,55,58].

Tetanic contractions of the laryngeal muscles can result in acute upper airway obstruction. These so-called respiratory convulsions often arise unexpectedly and may be associated with severe hypoxemia. Episodes of laryngeal spasm require the prompt cessation of muscle contraction. A rapidly acting muscle relaxant is recommended in this setting[47] and should be followed by immediate endotracheal intubation. Continued muscle relaxation after intubation is advised to avoid vocal cord damage from recurrent laryngeal spasms.

Progression of respiratory muscle spasms will interfere with ventilatory gas exchange and should be managed with the administration of a nondepolarizing muscle relaxant and controlled positive pressure ventilation. In series of older children and adults, this approach was required in 80 to 90% of patients admitted to an ICU[48–51]. In neonatal tetanus, the introduction of neuromuscular blockade and mechanical ventilation has been associated with decreased mortality[55]. Several nondepolarizing muscle relaxants have been used in this setting. Duration of mechanical ventilation varies considerably but generally ranges from 3 to 5 weeks. Because this period is complicated by a high incidence of atelectasis and pneumonia[54,55], considerable attention must be directed toward chest physical therapy, frequent postural changes, and tracheal toilet. Although subcutaneous heparin is frequently employed in adults to offset the risk of pulmonary emboli, the usefulness of heparinization in children is questionable, and anticoagulation is not used in neonatal tetanus. Continuation of sedation and analgesia is recommended during the period of ventilatory support.

The approach toward chronic management of the airway in patients with tetanus varies. As noted previously, maintenance of an artificial airway is usually required for a minimum of several weeks. In adults, early tracheostomy has been recommended[49]. In neonates, prolonged nasotracheal intubation compared favorably with tracheostomy in the management of tetanus[58]. Because similar comparisons in older children are lacking, the advantages of prolonged endotracheal intubation outside the newborn period require further clarification.

Weaning from positive pressure ventilatory support is attempted when heavy sedation and muscle relaxants are no longer required to control severe spasms. This generally occurs 2 to 4 weeks after the initiation of mechanical ventilation[50,51,53]. As in other cases of respiratory failure, aggressive weaning should be reserved for patients with minimal requirements for supplemental oxygen and adequate spontaneous ventilatory reserve (see Chapter 9). Weaning should be postponed in the event of recurrent severe spasms. It should be noted that infants with tetanus are particularly prone to laryngeal spasm after extubation[58]. Preparation should be made for rapidly reestablishing the airway in the event of this complication.

Once associated with an average death rate of 45 to 55%, tetanus now carries a fatality rate of 10 to 20%[48,49]. Improved survival in neonatal tetanus is even more striking. At least part of this improvement is attributable to respiratory intensive care practices[54]. The improvement in mortality is particularly gratifying in that long-term complications after acute convalescence are uncommon.

POLIOMYELITIS

Clinical Features

Poliomyelitis represents an acute viral infection of the CNS that, in its severest form, results in widespread muscle paralysis and secondary respiratory failure. As a result of modern immunization practices, poliomyelitis is a rare cause of respiratory failure in industrialized nations, although it continues to plague the childhood population of developing countries[59,60]. Sporadic cases have been reported in the United States in immunocompromised patients exposed to live attenuated virus used for active immunization[61], in unimmunized foreign travelers, and in individuals emigrating from endemic areas.

The clinical expression of the disease is variable. Depending on the location of nervous system involvement, respiratory failure can arise from deficiencies in airway control, clearance of secretions, central control of ventilation, and inspiratory muscle weakness. In acute paralytic poliomyelitis, muscle weakness often progresses with alarming rapidity after the onset of neurologic symptoms. Therefore, patients can come to the ICU with acute respiratory collapse of unknown cause. In addition to the acute disease, the paralytic residua of poliomyelitis can result in chronic respiratory disability.

Poliomyelitis is caused by one of three types of poliovirus (of the enterovirus group) that pass to a susceptible individual by respiratory or fecal-oral contamination. This last portal of entry explains the high association of the disease with poor community sanitation. The virus extends from the gut to the nerves via the bloodstream. The virus spreads along the nerves, causing damage as it progresses. The infecting organism has a predilection for the anterior horn cells of the spinal cord and the cranial nerve nuclei of the brainstem. After inoculation with the organism, an incubation period lasting 1 to 5 weeks ensues. As noted previously, the ultimate clinical expression of the infection varies considerably[(62)]. Fortunately, over 90% of infections are either asymptomatic or result in mild nonparalytic disease; it is estimated that paralytic poliomyelitis occurs in only about 2% of individuals who are actively infected with the virus. In severe forms of poliomyelitis, asymmetrical muscle paralysis ensues. The first expression of disease usually takes the form of a minor febrile illness lasting 1 to 2 days. This prodromal illness generally involves symptoms of an upper respiratory infection or gastroenteritis. Typically, in less than a week after the onset of the prodromal phase, the onset of severe muscle pain occurs, accompanied by fever, headache, irritability, and paresthesia. Patients usually display muscle fasciculations and diminished deep tendon reflexes in affected muscles at the time of presentation. In some cases, this picture progresses to total paralysis in as little as several hours[(63)].

The final distribution and degree of paralysis in poliomyelitis vary. Historically, several forms of disease have been described, which are defined by the regional muscle groups involved[(62)]. In spinal poliomyelitis, asymmetrical flaccid paralysis is noted. Involvement of the lower extremities occurs twice as often as involvement of the upper extremities, and truncal involvement occurs in 25% of cases. There is usually total absence of deep tendon reflexes in the distribution of the involved muscles. Variable degrees of autonomic nervous system involvement, causing abnormal thermoregulation, and systemic blood pressure lability may occur. The clinical manifestations of spinal poliomyelitis are a reflection of the inflammatory damage to the spinal anterior horn cells. Involvement of the motor nuclei of the cranial nerves occurs with bulbar poliomyelitis. This form of the disease is manifested by weakness in the facial, ophthalmic, and pharyngeal muscles. Bulbar involvement occurs in about 15% of cases and is usually associated with disease in the cervical spinal cord. Involvement of other medullary centers results in abnormalities in the central regulation of breathing[(64)] and autonomic tone. Signs of encephalitis are present in about one-third of cases of paralytic poliomyelitis; higher cortical involvement is characterized by changes in level of consciousness. This form of disease can be associated with cerebral edema and intracranial hypertension[(65)].

Several tests are useful in supporting the diagnosis of poliomyelitis. An elevated CSF protein level and a pleocytosis with a predominance of polymorphonuclear leukocytes early in the course of the disease are found. This CSF pleocytosis changes to mononuclear cells as the disease progresses. The causative virus can be isolated from fecal and oropharyngeal specimens. Serologic confirmation of the infection is made by identifying specific antibodies to the poliovirus.

Management

Respiratory failure can arise during the course of paralytic poliomyelitis from several causes. Abnormalities in the control of breathing have been well described during acute paralytic poliomyelitis[(60,64)] and have been incriminated as a cause of sudden infant death syndrome (SIDS) in isolated instances[(66)]. Bulbar palsy can result in loss of airway control as a result of pharyngeal muscle paralysis and can lead to airway obstruction or aspiration of oropharyngeal secretions[(67)]. At a minimum, pharyngeal muscle weakness requires meticulous nursing care and feeding precautions to avoid aspiration. With severe bulbar involvement resulting in loss of airway protective reflexes, endotracheal intubation is required. Also, paralysis of virtually any muscle group involved in normal ventilatory function can occur. Functional loss of the intercostal muscles, diaphragm, or abdominal muscles can occur individually or in combination and can lead to respiratory failure. Intercostal paralysis, particularly in younger children, leads to severe chest wall instability and retractions with diaphragmatic inspiratory motion[(60)]. Frequently, this results in inadequate alveolar ventilation and hypercapnia. Involvement of the cervical cord can lead to diaphragmatic paralysis manifested by acute hypoventilation and diminished respiratory capacity. Loss of abdominal muscle function results in severely impaired coughing, difficulty in clearing the airway, and predilection for pneumonia. All of these respiratory complications require endotracheal intubation, mechanical ventilatory support, and chest physical therapy.

Historically, respiratory support in acute paralytic poliomyelitis was provided with a tank-type respirator, or so-called iron lung. More recently, positive pressure ventilatory techniques have been used[(65)]. Provision of controlled positive pressure ventilatory support should be maintained in any patient displaying hypoventilation from central or peripheral neurologic manifestations of the disease. Despite the customary prolonged need for airway care and positive pressure ventilatory support, some patients with paralytic disease recover rapidly in a few weeks[(62,65)], precluding the need for tracheostomy. Tracheostomy can be performed electively during the course of the disease in more protracted cases. The use of intermittent positive pressure ventilation through a nasal or oral mask has been described in postpoliomyelitis patients[(68)]. This technique avoids the use of a tracheostomy and can be used to free patients from body ventilators.

Recovery of muscle function depends on the severity of involvement of the various motor units[(62,69)]. Usually, strength begins to return within several weeks after the onset of paralysis. Functional recovery occurs in severely flaccid muscle groups in approximately 50% of cases. A 90%

chance of recovery has been reported in groups of muscles that suffer moderate incomplete paralysis. Most recovery occurs in the first year, with little recovery achieved beyond the second year. Of patients who suffered respiratory failure during acute paralytic poliomyelitis, approximately one-third experienced full recovery, one-third were left with mild respiratory disabilities resulting in intermittent bouts of acute pulmonary disease such as pneumonia, and the remaining third had chronic paralysis and respiratory insufficiency requiring variable periods of ventilatory support daily[(70)].

Survival in acute paralytic poliomyelitis is the rule, although mortality in children can surpass 30%[(60)]. Also, as noted previously, persistent residua of the disease can lead to a variety of chronic respiratory difficulties. These include persistent respiratory muscle paralysis, causing variable degrees of respiratory insufficiency[(70,71)]; vocal cord paralysis[(72)]; scoliosis and secondary restrictive lung disease[(73)]; and persistent abnormalities in the central control of breathing, resulting in central hypoventilation[(64,74)]. In addition, an unexplained late-onset form of weakness with respiratory failure has been described in isolated cases[(75)]. Residual respiratory complications of paralytic poliomyelitis require chronic supportive care of the airway and ventilatory assistance[(70,71)] (see Chapter 9).

Although the scope of acute paralytic poliomyelitis has been limited largely to occasional sporadic cases, the disease can be encountered in the pediatric intensive care population. Clearly, selected groups in the United States and other industrialized nations remain susceptible to poliovirus infection, and concern has been expressed over the decreasing prevalence of widespread immunity in certain populations[(65)]. For these reasons, poliomyelitis should be considered in any child with acute onset of respiratory failure associated with bulbar or respiratory muscle weakness.

GUILLAIN-BARRÉ SYNDROME

Clinical Features

Guillain-Barré syndrome, also known as *acute postinfective neuritis* and *acute inflammatory polyradiculoneuropathy*, is an acute, inflammatory peripheral neuropathy that affects both adults and children[(76–78)]. Although associated autonomic nervous dysfunction[(79–81)] can produce life-threatening complications, mortality from Guillain-Barré syndrome is largely attributable to respiratory muscle weakness and secondary respiratory failure[(76,82–84)]. Therefore, careful attention to the progression of respiratory muscle weakness and timely intervention at the first signs of respiratory failure are the cornerstones of management.

The cause of Guillain-Barré syndrome is unknown. Autoimmune mechanisms have been postulated in the disease process, which is characterized by diffuse peripheral nerve demyelination and motor dysfunction. Historical features and clinical presentation of patients with Guillain-Barré syndrome follow a well-described pattern[(76,77)]. Onset of acute neuropathic symptoms is often preceded by a recent viral-type illness, usually an acute upper respiratory infection or gastroenteritis[(85)]. Other infectious prodromal diseases include mononucleosis, scarlet fever, and a variety of exanthemas. The prodromal illness can occur several days to 4 weeks prior to the onset of neurologic symptoms. Clinical disorders similar to Guillain-Barré syndrome have also been described in postsurgical patients approximately 2 to 3 weeks after a variety of operative procedures and/or spinal anesthesia[(78)] and represent a subset of acute inflammatory polyneuropathy.

Classically, the earliest neurologic sign of Guillain-Barré syndrome is weakness in the lower extremities, usually symmetric, involving the distal musculature to a greater degree than the proximal musculature. This is followed by progressive ascending paralysis. Sensory symptoms such as numbness or paresthesias frequently accompany the early onset of weakness and are distributed distally. Owing to these early symptoms, the child comes to medical attention because of nonspecific lethargy and inactivity, loss of previously achieved gross motor functions such as walking or use of the distal extremities, or subjective complaints referable to paresthesias or diminished sensation in the distal extremities.

It should be stressed that deviation from the classic presentation and characteristic ascending progression of weakness is not uncommon[(76–78)]. For example, a well-described variant involves findings dominated by cranial nerve palsies and/or cerebellar ataxia. Also, more than 10% of patients present with weakness predominantly in the upper extremities. In other cases, a form of "descending paralysis" is noted, in which the early dominant symptoms are referable to weakness of ocular, facial, and pharyngeal muscles, with the potential for loss of protective reflexes of the airway. Finally, as many as one-third of patients can present without sensory signs or symptoms. Owing to this array of described presentations of Guillain-Barré syndrome, patients may seek medical attention because of the recent onset of disconjugate gaze, facial weakness, or clumsiness.

Physical findings at presentation include areflexia, muscle weakness in the previously described distribution, and numbness in a stocking-glove distribution pattern. Less frequently, cranial nerve palsies, altered level of consciousness, ataxia, loss of vibratory and/or position sensation, and urinary retention are encountered. After the onset of motor symptoms, weakness generally progresses over a period of several days to 2 weeks. This process culminates in a period of maximal weakness, which is followed by slow remission. Severe respiratory muscle paresis develops during the progressive stage in approximately one-third of patients with Guillain-Barré syndrome[(78,82–84)].

Certain diagnostic studies provide supportive evidence for the diagnosis[(76–78)]. Of particular note is the finding of an elevated CSF protein level (more than 45 mg/dl) in the absence of pleocytosis (the so-called albuminocytologic dissociation). Elevated CSF protein at some point during the course of the disease is encountered in approximately 90% of patients. Although the CSF cell count is generally normal, pleocytosis is encountered in approximately 5% of patients. Abnormalities in electrophysiologic studies become particularly pronounced with progression of the disease. The majority of patients demonstrate delayed nerve conduction 2 to 3 weeks after onset of the disease, and electromyography is consistent with lower motor neuron disease. Although laboratory and electrophysiologic studies can provide additional supportive evidence for the diagnosis, results of these studies may not become positive for several days to weeks after initial presentation. There is no test that is pathognomonic; therefore, the diagnosis of Guillain-Barré syndrome is generally established on the basis of history, clinical presentation, and characteristic disease progression. Other causes of peripheral neuropathy and weakness in childhood, such as heavy-metal poisoning, thiamine deficiency, porphyria, botulism, and poliomyelitis, can usually be differentiated from Guillain-Barré syndrome on the basis of clinical and laboratory findings.

As noted before, the Guillain-Barré syndrome is characterized by variable progression of muscular weakness over the course of days to several weeks, and maximum weakness is generally noted 1 to 2 weeks after the onset of symptoms. During this period, progression of weakness can occur rapidly, necessitating careful patient monitoring and frequent assessment of muscle function and respiratory capacity to avoid the precipitous onset of respiratory failure. Indeed, approximately 20% of patients with Guillain-Barré syndrome undergo progression of the disease to the point of requiring mechanical ventilatory support[(78,83,85)]. Also, dysfunction of the autonomic nervous system during this phase can lead to dangerous cardiac arrhythmias or dramatic swings in systemic arterial pressure (see below).

After maximum muscle weakness is reached, a plateau phase is generally noted that lasts for several days to weeks. The amount of time from maximum muscle weakness to the onset of improvement in motor signs has been related to the achievement of full recovery. Patients experiencing a prolonged plateau phase tend to have residual motor weakness after recovery, a situation encountered in approximately 20% of children[(86)].

Management

It is clear that any child with a clinical picture suggesting Guillain-Barré syndrome requires immediate hospitalization, but specific indications for admission to the ICU in patients without respiratory failure have not been firmly delineated. Inpatient care areas must be capable of providing frequent assessment of respiratory muscle strength, protective airway reflexes, and hemodynamic status. Patients with rapidly progressive weakness or difficulty clearing oral or pulmonary secretions are best observed in an intensive care environment. Obvious indications for admission to the ICU include frank respiratory failure, marginal respiratory muscle reserve (see below), onset of atelectasis or pneumonia, loss of protective reflexes of the airway, and life-threatening signs of autonomic instability, such as arrhythmias or systemic hypotension.

In the ICU, management begins with general supportive care directed at preventing complications of immobilization and decreased motor activity. Second, careful monitoring of the motor weakness progression is imperative, particularly as it affects respiratory muscle function (and appropriate intervention in the event of respiratory failure). Third, observation for other complicating conditions, such as autonomic dysfunction, is required. Finally, consideration should be given to specific therapeutic interventions directed at speeding the onset of recovery and reversing muscle weakness.

The importance of meticulous supportive care cannot be overstated. Significant morbidity and mortality are attributable to aspiration, decubitus ulcers, urinary tract infections, pulmonary emboli, and electrolyte imbalances[(82,83)]. Frequent changes in posture and position are necessary to prevent skin ulceration. In the presence of cranial nerve palsies, clearance of oral secretions and protection from eye desiccation and corneal injury is necessary. Nutrition support in the form of gavage feedings is necessary when pharyngeal weakness causes an insufficient ability to swallow. Fluid retention and hyponatremia, presumably due to increased antidiuretic hormone secretion, have been noted even in patients not needing mechanical ventilatory support[(87)]. This requires frequent monitoring of fluid and electrolyte balance and appropriate adjustment of intravenous fluid therapy. Urinary retention can be encountered, requiring bladder catheterization or manual bladder compression in younger children. While some employ prophylactic subcutaneous heparin for the prevention of deep venous thrombosis in adults[(78,82)], the need for routine anticoagulation in children is unclear.

The care of acute respiratory failure secondary to atelectasis and/or respiratory muscle fatigue is the most important aspect of the intensive care management of patients with Guillain-Barré syndrome. As previously noted, approximately 20% of children with Guillain-Barré syndrome ultimately progress to frank respiratory failure, requiring mechanical ventilatory assistance. Therefore, frequent assessment of respiratory reserve is imperative. In addition to nonspecific clinical signs of respiratory embarrassment, bedside evaluation of indices of respiratory muscle strength can provide early warning of impending respiratory failure. Recommended techniques for the bedside assessment of respiratory muscle strength in children include determination of forced or crying vital capacity and maximum negative inspiratory pressure (see Chapter 9). Although measurement of maximum expiratory pressure is a particularly sensitive index of respiratory muscle weakness and has been widely used in assessing adult patients with neuromuscular disease[(87)], abnormalities in this parameter are not necessarily specific for detecting the onset of acute respiratory failure and alveolar hypoventilation. Assessment of forced or crying vital capacity and maximum negative inspiratory pressure is recommended every 2 to 4 hours, along with generalized neurologic assessment of muscular strength. Provision of mechanical ventilatory assistance should be considered when (a) forced vital capacity falls to less than 15 to 20 ml/kg, (b) maximum negative inspiratory pressure falls to less than 20 to 30 cm H_2O, or (c) alveolar hypoventilation (P_aCO_2 greater than 50 torr) ensues. In addition, endotracheal intubation should be performed whenever there is evidence of retention of pulmonary secretions refractory to chest physical therapy, weakness of protective reflexes of the airway (i.e., cough and gag), or atelectasis.

With appropriate monitoring, indications for endotracheal intubation can be detected early, allowing the elective performance of the procedure. Administration of depolarizing muscle relaxants in cases of chronic or relapsing polyneuropathy has been associated with ventricular arrhythmias; therefore, it is recommended that succinylcholine be avoided when endotracheal intubation is performed in patients with Guillain-Barré syndrome(88). Because of autonomic instability, circulatory responses to intravenous sedatives and anesthetics can be exaggerated, and the administration of these agents for obtundation during intubation should be undertaken with extreme caution.

Previously, tracheostomy was recommended as the preferred method of airway management in patients with acute respiratory failure requiring mechanical ventilatory support. Reports of prolonged nasotracheal intubation in children with Guillain-Barré syndrome(82,89) have suggested that this technique of airway management can be used safely for several weeks. The duration of mechanical support in cases with respiratory failure varies widely, ranging from 2 weeks to 9 months(89,90). Tracheostomy can be avoided completely in selected patients requiring shorter periods of mechanical ventilatory assistance. On the other hand, patients with a lack of protective reflexes of the airway, poor tracheal toilet, or frank respiratory failure for prolonged periods should be considered for tracheostomy. No complications were found in 15 consecutive children who underwent tracheostomy (median duration of tracheostomy 39 days, range 11 to 94 days) for Guillain-Barré syndrome(90).

Mechanical ventilatory support in patients with Guillain-Barré syndrome should be directed at providing adequate alveolar ventilation and oxygenation and at avoiding atelectasis and pneumonia. Initially, complete ventilatory support should be provided, followed by the partial withdrawal of positive pressure support by intermittent mandatory ventilation in patients who can generate effort. Slow weaning from mechanical support is generally required. With the onset of recovery of muscle strength, periods of increasing duration of spontaneous breathing can be attempted, with care taken to avoid precipitating clinical signs of respiratory muscle fatigue. By decreasing the periods of mechanical assistance, support limited to periods of sleep and thus eventual cessation of positive pressure ventilation can be achieved. Alternatively, steady withdrawal of positive pressure breaths can be performed by using intermittent mandatory ventilation techniques(78) (see Chapter 9). Adequate alveolar ventilation is ensured by maintenance of normal P_aCO_2 levels determined by direct measurement during mechanical ventilation (continuous monitoring of end-tidal carbon dioxide tension is also encouraged).

Pneumonia is a complicating factor in two-thirds of patients needing admission to an ICU(82) and requires prompt detection and initiation of antibiotics. Chest physical therapy should be employed to help avoid atelectasis and retention of bronchial secretions. During the period of maximum muscle weakness accompanied by respiratory failure, provision of adequate chest physical therapy assumes added importance. Particular attention should be directed at timely tracheal suctioning.

Given appropriate respiratory intensive care, eventual recovery from respiratory failure associated with Guillain-Barré syndrome is likely. Despite the presence of residual motor deficits in as many as 20% of children with Guillain-Barré syndrome(86), recovery from respiratory insufficiency in survivors of the acute disease is the rule(91).

Certain complications of Guillain-Barré syndrome are attributable to autonomic dysfunction manifested by swings in peripheral vasomotor tone and abnormalities in cardiac rhythm(79–81). In one series(79), specific abnormalities included sinus tachycardia (50%), bradycardia (20%), S-T segment and T-wave abnormalities (64%), hypertension (61%), and postural hypotension (43%). These signs of autonomic dysfunction are usually limited to minor alterations in blood pressure and heart rate. Infrequently, hypotension and severe vasomotor collapse occur, presumably due to lack of sympathetic tone, requiring prompt expansion of intravascular volume(80). Sinus tachycardia, the most common form of cardiac rhythm abnormality, is usually well tolerated in children and requires no specific therapy. In the presence of prolonged and marked tachycardia associated with signs of congestive heart failure, treatment should be considered. However, use of agents acting directly on the autonomic nervous system (e.g., sympathomimetic vasopressors) to offset autonomic abnormalities should be tempered by the fact that these agents have the potential for causing erratic swings in autonomic tone(79).

Specific therapy for Guillain-Barré syndrome remains a topic of controversy. Because of the inflammatory nature of the disease, corticosteroids and adrenal corticotropin have been used in an attempt to improve the clinical course. However, most of these trials have been performed in an uncontrolled fashion, resulting largely in anecdotal reports of improvement (or lack thereof) with corticosteroid therapy. A single prospective randomized trial of prednisolone therapy failed to show beneficial effects from the use of corticosteroids in Guillain-Barré syndrome(92).

Clinical trials have been conducted using plasma exchange techniques in the hopes of removing humoral autoimmune factors involved in the pathogenesis of Guillain-Barré syndrome. Plasmapheresis involves the separation of plasma from cellular components of the blood by centrifugation or filtration. The plasma is replaced with a crystalloid and albumin mixture added to the blood cells and is returned to the body. Early anecdotal reports claimed clinical improvement in motor function with plasmapheresis in acute Guillain-Barré syndrome and chronic relapsing inflammatory neuropathy[93–96]. In one study, patients receiving plasmapheresis required less time on mechanical ventilation and less time in the hospital, compared with a matched, nonconcurrent control group[97]. Isolated and uncontrolled reports of improvement with plasma exchange gave rise to a multicenter evaluation using prospective randomized methodology. In this study, plasmapheresis improved the clinical course of acute Guillain-Barré syndrome as measured by time to recovery of muscle strength and independent ambulation and by outcome at 6 months[98]. Beneficial effects of plasmapheresis were noted, particularly in patients treated within 7 days of the onset of disease and in those who subsequently required mechanical ventilation. It should be noted, however, that children under 12 years of age were excluded from the study. Preliminary reports have suggested that plasmapheresis can be undertaken safely and that instances of hypotension associated with plasma exchange tend to be responsive to intravascular volume expansion. Exchange blood transfusions have been reported as an alternative in an 8-month-old infant in whom plasmapheresis was technically difficult[99].

In a randomized trial, gamma globulin administration was demonstrated to be more effective than plasmapheresis[100]. The plasmapheresis group in this study did worse than groups in other studies. If immunoglobulin administration is effective, the ease of administration may make it preferable to plasma exchange. Despite the promise of these studies directed at developing specific therapy for Guillain-Barré syndrome, the cornerstone of treatment remains supportive. Avoidance of respiratory complications and the provision of mechanical ventilation is crucial. Recovery of adequate respiratory function is the rule, in spite of reports of prolonged respiratory failure in Guillain-Barré syndrome lasting several months, provided life-threatening complications are avoided during the acute phase of the disease.

UNILATERAL DIAPHRAGMATIC PARALYSIS

Clinical Features

Although bilateral weakness of the diaphragm is encountered in a wide range of systemic neuromuscular disorders, unilateral diaphragmatic paralysis in children is most often a result of direct trauma to the phrenic nerve. While uncomplicated loss of hemidiaphragmatic function can be well tolerated in older children and adults, this disorder causes severe respiratory embarrassment in infants[101–105] (see below). Adequate ventilatory exchange can frequently be restored and maintained with CPAP alone[105–107]; however, long-term management may require surgical plication of the affected diaphragm if paralysis persists[107–110].

The degree of functional impairment caused by paralysis of the diaphragm depends on the patient's age. Adults maintain normal arterial oxygenation in the upright position despite the 25% reduction in vital capacity that accompanies unilateral diaphragmatic paralysis[111]. Infants and young children usually display marked abnormalities in gas exchange with hemidiaphragm paralysis.

Several mechanisms explain the exaggerated respiratory dysfunction caused by diaphragmatic paralysis in infants[102,104,105,112]. First, unlike the rigid adult thorax, the highly compliant chest wall of the infant allows significant rib cage distortion during inspiration and fails to anchor the flaccid hemidiaphragm at its skeletal insertions. Second, the horizontal orientation of the rib cage of the infant probably results in less compensatory gas exchange from the "bucket-handle" action of the intact intercostal muscles. Third, infants are usually cared for in the supine position, which exacerbates the restrictive effects of diaphragmatic paralysis on ventilatory capacity in adults[113]. Finally, the frequent association of underlying parenchymal lung disease adds to the mechanical problems arising from the paralyzed diaphragm. For these reasons, children under 3 years of age usually suffer respiratory embarrassment in association with diaphragmatic paralysis[102]; in infants under 6 months of age, this disorder is almost universally accompanied by persistent respiratory insufficiency[101–103].

Most cases of diaphragmatic paralysis occur as a result of birth trauma or injury to the phrenic nerve sustained during cardiothoracic surgical procedures[101–105]. In approximately one-third of phrenic nerve palsy cases, traction injury to the phrenic nerve is sustained during delivery[107]. Simultaneous injury to the brachial plexus, resulting in Erb's palsy, is commonly observed. In the remainder of patients, diaphragmatic paralysis is noted after cardiothoracic surgery, usually for palliation or correction of congenital heart disease. Phrenic nerve injury in this situation can arise from traction, transection, or the application of topical cardiac hypothermia[114–117]. One series has shown a particularly high association with closed-heart surgery, such as aorta-pulmonary shunt procedures, patent ductus ligation or division, and pulmonary artery banding[101], as well as repeated corrective procedures. Half of the cases associated with cardiac surgery are reported after open-heart procedures[102]. Isolated instances of diaphragmatic paralysis have occurred with a variety of procedures, including tracheoesophageal fistula repair[107], radical neck surgery[118], and attempted cannulation of the internal jugular vein[119].

The clinical presentation of diaphragmatic paralysis in children varies widely, depending on age and the presence of underlying lung disease. In uncomplicated cases occurring in older children, signs of diaphragmatic dysfunction are often confined to mild tachypnea and orthopnea. In the newborn infant, the clinical presentation is generally one of severe respiratory distress after a difficult delivery with suspected birth trauma[104]. When diaphragmatic paralysis results from inadvertent phrenic nerve injury during surgical manipulation, the condition often presents as inability to wean from mechanical ventilatory support in the postoperative period[102,103]. Persistent unilateral pleural effusion and basilar atelectasis are common secondary findings. Typically, abnormal elevation of the affected hemidiaphragm is noted on chest radiograph; however, this finding can be obscured in patients receiving positive pressure ventilatory support. For this reason, the disorder is frequently not suspected until unsuccessful attempts have been made to wean the patient from mechanical ventilation. The diagnosis is usually confirmed by fluoroscopic examination of diaphragmatic motion, which demonstrates paradoxical upward movement of the involved hemidiaphragm with inspiration. This upward movement may be accompanied by a concurrent shift of the mediastinal structures toward the contralateral hemithorax.

Several conditions can generate misleading results from fluoroscopic examination[105]. First, performance of the examination during the administration of positive pressure ventilatory support or CPAP may obscure paradoxical diaphragmatic motion; therefore, the examination should be performed with the patient breathing spontaneously without the application of CPAP. Also, particular caution should be taken in interpreting diaphragmatic motion during expiratory grunting that may accompany respiratory distress in infants. During the expiratory grunting maneuver, increased intra-abdominal pressure results in upward motion of the paralyzed hemidiaphragm, followed by descent of the paralyzed diaphragm and outward abdominal motion with relaxation of the abdominal musculature during inspiration. This pattern mimics normal diaphragmatic motion and could confound the interpretation.

Additional supportive evidence of diaphragmatic paralysis can be obtained with transcutaneous phrenic nerve stimulation[120,121]. Stimulation of the phrenic nerve is performed transcutaneously near its cervical origin during simultaneous measurement of diaphragmatic electromyography. Alternatively, evidence of a diaphragmatic motor response to phrenic stimulation is sought by either direct observation or simultaneous fluoroscopic examination[122]. The finding of a brisk response on one side coupled with no response on the contralateral side is strongly suggestive of phrenic nerve injury. In addition to its diagnostic value, transcutaneous phrenic nerve stimulation performed at intervals is advocated by some as a means of assessing reversibility of the phrenic injury (see below). Transcutaneous phrenic stimulation can be particularly helpful in the diagnostic evaluation when ipsilateral pleural effusion or atelectasis obscures the position of the diaphragm radiographically[121].

Management

Acute management of the patient with diaphragmatic paralysis should establish adequate ventilation and oxygenation and then provide treatment of any associated pulmonary disease, such as pneumonia, atelectasis, or pulmonary edema. This usually requires a period of positive pressure ventilation together with positive end-expiratory pressure. After acute stabilization and clearing of associated lung disease, normal gas exchange can usually be sustained with CPAP at 5 to 10 cm H_2O[105–107]. By maintaining ipsilateral lung volume during inspiration, CPAP minimizes the paradoxical motion of the involved hemidiaphragm. In this manner, CPAP provides a form of "internal fixation" of the flaccid diaphragm and compliant chest wall of the infant, thus allowing adequate ventilatory exchange with spontaneous breathing.

Resolution of respiratory failure resulting from diaphragmatic paralysis sometimes requires surgical plication of the diaphragm to offset the paradoxical inspiratory motion. However, surgical plication is usually unnecessary outside the infant age group. In older children, weaning from positive pressure ventilatory support tends to proceed uneventfully, despite persistent diaphragmatic dysfunction. In one series of children with postoperative phrenic nerve palsy, the trachea was successfully extubated within 72 hours in all patients over 18 months of age[101]. Others have reported a maximum duration of intubation of 14 days in postoperative cardiac surgery patients over 3 years of age[102]. Although basilar atelectasis can be a recurrent problem, it usually responds to chest physical therapy.

Long-term management of symptomatic infants with diaphragmatic paralysis, on the other hand, is usually complicated by persistent respiratory failure. Both the role and the timing of surgical plication in this group remain topics of controversy. Some authorities recommend immediate surgical plication of the diaphragm after the diagnosis. Proponents of this approach note that rapid resolution of respiratory failure usually ensues, allowing discontinuation of mechanical ventilatory support and extubation of the trachea[108]. Others suggest a conservative approach, calling for variable periods of continuous positive pressure ventilation or CPAP until the permanency of the diaphragmatic paralysis is more clearly defined[109]. Unfortunately, the period necessary for spontaneous recovery of diaphragmatic function after phrenic nerve injury is extremely variable, ranging from several days to 12 months, during which time infants frequently require positive pressure ventilation support. In infants with postoperative diaphragmatic paralysis, ventilatory assistance is required for an average of 3 weeks, and some patients need positive pressure support for several months[101,103]. Up to 50% of patients demonstrate permanent loss of diaphragmatic function[103]. Recent work suggests that serial evaluation of phrenic nerve conduction with transcutaneous stimulation can assist in predicting the permanency of the phrenic nerve injury[105,120]. The presence of a diaphragmatic response to phrenic stimulation suggests that return of function will occur. The absence of a response is indicative of severe phrenic nerve injury and a prolonged course of paralysis. However, there is no immediately definitive method for determining the ultimate reversibility of diaphragmatic paralysis. As a further consideration, the effects of plication on future diaphragmatic function and lung development have not been clearly defined (105), although return of some diaphragmatic activity after plication has been described in a number of cases[108,110].

Given these considerations, a 2- to 4-week trial of CPAP has been recommended, followed by surgical plication if the infant fails to be weaned from positive pressure support[101,102,107,110,123]. Every effort should be made to resolve any underlying pulmonary parenchymal disease during this period prior to aggressive attempts at weaning from positive pressure support. Patients who fail to improve when placed on CPAP or positive pressure ventilation may have underlying pulmonary parenchymal disease or cardiac disease that needs to be cleared up, or they may not benefit from plication[107,123]. Successful weaning generally eliminates the immediate need for plication. As previously noted, because most older children will tolerate weaning from positive pressure support, even in the absence of diaphragmatic recovery, surgical plication in this group is usually unnecessary. In the older child, recovery without surgical intervention is the rule.

MYASTHENIA GRAVIS

Clinical Features

Classical myasthenia gravis is a chronic disorder characterized by exaggerated fatigability of skeletal muscles, which, in its extreme, can lead to acute respiratory failure[124–127]. The functional deficiency in muscle strength in myasthenia gravis is attributed to immunologic interference, with neuromuscular transmission associated with acetylcholine receptor antibodies. In addition to classic myasthenia gravis, other myasthenic disorders unique to the pediatric age group have been described and can be associated with respiratory failure in infants[128,129]. The intensive care management of myasthenia gravis presents a particular challenge because the disease as well as the medications used to treat it can produce life-threatening respiratory muscle weakness and secondary respiratory failure.

Myasthenia gravis takes several forms in children. Each form is associated with a unique clinical picture, disease course, and pathogenesis[124,128,129]. Classic or juvenile myasthenia gravis represents an extension of the disorder encountered in adults. Onset of disease generally occurs during adolescence, although symptoms have been described in children as young as 2 years of age. The progression of early symptoms is extremely variable but frequently follows an acute viral illness. In this form of the disease, involvement of the muscles in the distribution of the lower cranial nerves is noted earliest; therefore, frequent presenting complaints include ptosis, double vision, and other symptoms attributable to facial weakness. Later, weakness of the extremities can occur, as well as shortness of breath. Approximately half of the patients have clinical remissions during the first several years after the onset of the disease. Weakness can also remain clinically stable for protracted periods in certain patients. Hyperthyroidism and frank thyrotoxicosis have been noted in approximately 10% of patients, and there also seems to be an increased association with collagen vascular disease, particularly systemic lupus erythematosus[124].

In the congenital form of myasthenia gravis, symptoms occur within the first few days of life. Historically, mothers of these patients do not have myasthenia gravis, although a history of the disorder in siblings is common. Extraocular muscle weakness is prominent, as is poor feeding. A prolonged disease course is characterized by persistent and refractory weakness in the involved muscle groups. Fortunately, this results in only mild symptoms, such as persistent ophthalmoplegia. Respiratory failure associated with this form of the disease is unusual.

Neonatal myasthenia gravis, on the other hand, can be associated with severe generalized muscle weakness in two-thirds of patients[128,129]. Muscles in the distribution of the distal cranial nerves are generally involved, resulting in dysphagia and dysphonia that are noted within 24 hours of birth. In this form of childhood myasthenia gravis, involved infants are uniformly born to mothers with myasthenia gravis; indeed, transplacental transmission of antibodies to acetylcholine receptor protein in the neuromuscular junction is believed to account for this disorder[128]. Symptoms usually respond readily to anticholinesterase therapy, and, as anticipated from the pathogenic mechanism, the disorder subsides spontaneously within the first 5 weeks of life.

Familial infantile myasthenia gravis has been described[128,129]. Like congenital myasthenia gravis, patients with this rare disorder are not born to myasthenic mothers but may have a history of sibling involvement. This form of the disease is characterized by marked respiratory depression at birth to the point of apnea. Indeed, familial infantile myasthenia gravis has been incriminated as a rare cause of sudden infant death. Patients are responsive to anticholinesterase therapy, and the disease course, characterized by episodic weakness and apnea during the first 2 years of life, gradually subsides with age.

The different forms of myasthenia gravis encountered in children provide insight into its pathogenesis. In all forms, abnormalities in neuromuscular transmission are found characterized by rapid decay of muscle strength with exercise and amplitude decay of compound muscle action potentials with tetanic stimulation, which are improved or totally reversed with anticholinesterase medication (e.g., edrophonium). An immunologic basis of neonatal and juvenile myasthenia gravis is strongly supported by the presence of an abnormal antibody to acetylcholine receptor protein. This and other autoantibodies have been incriminated in the relative insufficiency of cholinergic activity at the neuromuscular junction found in this disease.

Management

Patients with myasthenia gravis require intensive care under two circumstances. First, after thymectomy as a surgical mode of therapy for juvenile myasthenia gravis, patients may require postoperative intensive care including mechanical ventilatory support. Second, in particularly refractory cases or in cases complicated by progression of muscle weakness of excessive treatment with anticholinesterase therapy, severe respiratory muscle weakness can be encountered, necessitating frequent monitoring of respiratory muscle strength, vigorous chest physical therapy for clearance of pulmonary secretions, or mechanical ventilatory support.

Patients with myasthenia gravis undergoing major surgical procedures usually require intensive care in the immediate postoperative period[130,131]. In addition to general supportive care, approximately one-third of myasthenia patients require mechanical ventilatory support beyond the first several postoperative hours[130–133]. In adult patients undergoing thymectomy, Leventhal et al.[131–133] identified predisposing factors associated with the need for prolonged postoperative ventilatory support. These factors include prolonged duration of disease (more than 6 years), history of respiratory disease, need for high-dose pyridostigmine (more than 750 mg/day) for symptom control, and low preoperative vital capacity (less than 2.9 liters). Although these factors have been useful in predicting postoperative need for mechanical ventilation after thymectomy, they seem to be less useful in predicting postoperative need for mechanical support following other major surgical procedures[130]. Similar predictive indices have not been identified in children; therefore, standard indices of respiratory muscle strength, such as maximum negative inspiratory pressure, forced or crying vital capacity (see Chapter 9), and arterial blood gases, are used to determine the need for mechanical ventilatory support. Combined epidural and general anesthesia during thymectomy has been used to decrease intraoperative muscle relaxant need and facilitate postoperative extubation[134]. Postoperative laryngeal muscle weakness and vocal cord paralysis have been described following anesthesia[135,136] and can be mistaken for postextubation croup. This complicating manifestation of myasthenia gravis should be considered in any patient exhibiting stridor on extubation in the postoperative period.

Respiratory embarrassment due to respiratory muscle weakness is encountered at some point in approximately 10% of adolescent and adult patients with classic myasthenia gravis[126,127]. Respiratory failure in these cases is attributed to respiratory muscle fatigue, leading to alveolar hypoventilation, or to decreased expiratory muscle strength and inadequate cough, causing retained pulmonary secretions and atelectasis or pneumonia. Indeed, approximately 10% of patients requiring mechanical ventilatory assistance ultimately succumb to pulmonary infectious complications[126].

Indications for mechanical ventilatory support in patients with myasthenia gravis include apnea, hypoventilation, or evidence of severe respiratory muscle fatigue. Therefore, frequent assessment of respiratory muscle strength is necessary. Nonspecific indices of respiratory muscle weakness can signal impending respiratory failure; these indices include decreased forced or crying vital capacity (less than 15 mg/kg) and decreased maximum negative inspiratory pressure (less than −20 to −30 cm H_2O) (see Chapter 9). It should be recalled that muscle strength typically deteriorates with repetitive contractions in the myasthenic patient. Therefore, a single, isolated assessment of respiratory muscle strength may not be adequate for detecting impending ventilatory fatigue. Peripheral muscle weakness may be mild in patients with severe respiratory muscle weakness and should not be used as a guide to respiratory muscle strength[137].

Endotracheal intubation is usually required in the presence of acute hypoventilation. This intervention may be necessary for clearance of pulmonary secretions in patients with impaired expiratory muscle function and cough capabilities. Performance of semielective or emergent endotracheal intubation of the myasthenic patient requires attention to several points. Because of the poorly predictable response of myasthenic patients to depolarizing muscle relaxants[135], succinylcholine is not recommended when endotracheal intubation is performed. Also, the underlying abnormality of neuromuscular transmission in myasthenia gravis causes extreme sensitivity to competitive, nondepolarizing neuromuscular blockade; therefore, these agents may be required for intubation but are generally avoided. The rapid recovery of a patient after paralysis with a short-acting nondepolarizing agent administered by continuous infusion has been reported[139]. In patients requiring endotracheal intubation and mechanical ventilatory support, extubation can usually be performed within several weeks, thereby precluding the need for tracheostomy. Nonetheless, the occasional patient requiring prolonged maintenance of an artificial airway due to inadequate muscle function or ongoing need for tracheal toilet should be considered for tracheostomy.

In addition to providing supportive care, management of myasthenia gravis in the ICU should concentrate on specific therapeutic interventions directed at reversing muscle weakness. This is complicated by the fact that respiratory fatigue in the myasthenic patient can be encountered because of excessive or inadequate cholinergic activity at the neuromuscular junction. Specifically, in myasthenic crisis, acute deterioration in muscle strength is attributable to diminished neuromuscular transmission. On the other hand, excessive treatment with anticholinesterase medications can also produce progressive muscle weakness or cholinergic crisis.

Clearly, the management of these two forms of crisis encountered in patients with myasthenia gravis differs markedly. Myasthenic crisis is generally associated with a recent viral illness, surgery, or other systemic stress in a known or previously asymptomatic myasthenic patient. In cases of myasthenic crisis and in newly diagnosed cases of myasthenia gravis, administration of anticholinesterase agents is the primary mode of therapy[124–127]. Use of the short-acting anticholinesterase, edrophonium (Tensilon), is generally reserved for establishing the diagnosis at the time of initial presentation (140). Ongoing therapy with longer-acting anticholinesterases such as neostigmine or pyridostigmine is necessary. Dosage of specific anticholinesterase agents is largely determined by patient response. Administration of an anticholinesterase usually results in prompt improvement in muscle strength and effort-dependent respiratory function[141,142]. Administration of anticholinesterases can be associated with bronchoconstriction[140,143,144], and patients should be monitored carefully for this potential complication.

Cholinergic crisis can usually be differentiated from myasthenic crisis by the presence of signs of excessive parasympathetic activity. These include lacrimation, salivation, diarrhea, and bradycardia. Symptoms attributed to excessive parasympathetic activity are usually responsive to atropine administration. Weakness associated with cholinergic crisis frequently responds to the temporary withdrawal of anticholinesterase medications[124–126].

A variety of drugs commonly used in the critically ill patient can impair neuromuscular transmission[145]. Therefore, the administration of these agents to myasthenic patients poses particular risks of exacerbating or precipitating respiratory failure. In addition to the nondepolarizing muscle relaxants previously discussed, the neuromuscular blocking effects of aminoglycoside antibiotics are exaggerated in myasthenia gravis and may lead to respiratory depression. Therefore, their use should be avoided.

Because of the autoimmune nature of myasthenia gravis, corticosteroids have been used extensively. Studies indicate that prednisone can be a valuable adjunct to anticholinesterase therapy in patients with refractory disease[146,147]. Although specific indications for the use of steroids vary[127], prednisone should be considered in severely affected patients with acute respiratory failure. Exacerbation of muscle weakness upon initiation of steroid therapy is a risk and requires attention. Other immunosuppressants (azathioprine, cyclosporine) are reported to be useful in adults, but pediatric experience is minimal[148,149].

Thymectomy has been performed in cases of juvenile myasthenia gravis with promising results[150–152]. In most reported cases, thymectomy has been followed by progressive improvement over several years in muscle weakness and arrest of disease progression. Development of the transcervical approach for this procedure has decreased the associated complications and simplified the postoperative course.

Plasmapheresis has been used on a limited basis in adult patients with severe refractory respiratory failure[153] or with advanced disease prior to thymectomy[154,155]. Preliminary trials with plasmapheresis indicate that the technique is highly effective in improving muscle strength and decreasing the duration of postoperative mechanical ventilatory support in severely affected patients. The precise role of plasma exchange in the management of myasthenia gravis is unclear, but current applications include presurgical preparation, and exacerbation of disease with respiratory failure or failure to wean from mechanical ventilation.

Although some forms of myasthenia gravis encountered in children can produce life-threatening respiratory muscle weakness, timely intervention with mechanical ventilatory support and chest physical therapy usually results in stabilization. In addition to supportive therapy, proper treatment with anticholinesterase agents and, when indicated, other adjunctive interventions results in control of symptoms and return of adequate respiratory function in the majority of cases.

BOTULISM

Clinical Features

Botulism is an acute paralytic disorder involving disruption of neuromuscular transmission by the neurotoxin of *Clostridium botulinum*[156]. This bacterial toxin causes diffuse muscle weakness that often culminates in loss of protective airway reflexes and respiratory muscle function. Botulism can be encountered in the pediatric population in several settings defined by the specific portal of entry of the *C. botulinum* toxin. A prolonged course of respiratory failure occurs in all forms, requiring mechanical ventilatory support in addition to general supportive care (see also Chapter 33).

C. botulinum is subdivided into seven types, according to the antigenically specific toxin produced. Virtually all human disease is attributable to type A, B, or E organisms. *C. botulinum* toxin is one of the most potent neurotoxins known to humans. After systemic transport, *C. botulinum* toxin binds to presynaptic membranes at ganglionic and postganglionic parasympathetic synapses and at neuromuscular junctions, where it inhibits the release of acetylcholine. Consequently, symptoms of botulism arise from dysfunction of the autonomic nervous system and weakness of skeletal muscles. Binding of *C. botulinum* toxin to its target sites in the peripheral nervous system seems to be irreversible. Recovery depends on the development of new synaptic connections, which at least partially explains its prolonged clinical course.

Botulism is classified clinically into several categories based on the portal of entry of the *C. botulinum* toxin[156,157]. In classic food-borne botulism, preformed toxin is ingested in food that has been contaminated by the organism and processed under anaerobic conditions. In older children and adults, ingestion of the ubiquitous organism itself does not cause disease. Approximately 75% of cases are associated with the ingestion of home-canned foods. Symptoms usually appear within 36 hours of ingestion of the toxin. Anticholinergic effects of the toxin on the gastrointestinal tract account for the early symptoms of nausea, vomiting, colicky abdominal pain, and constipation. Other parasympatholytic effects include decreased salivation and lacrimation. Shortly afterward, motor abnormalities appear in the distribution of the cranial nerves. This early bulbar palsy leads to dysphagia, diplopia, dysarthria and, less commonly, abnormal pupillary reflexes. Generalized motor weakness progresses in a descending, symmetrical fashion, which, in severe cases, ultimately affects the respiratory musculature, resulting in hypoventilation and acute respiratory failure. Despite the severity of peripheral motor weakness, the picture is remarkable for the maintenance of an intact level of consciousness, provided the patient has not incurred secondary neurologic insult from hypoxia. In patients with respiratory failure, the need for mechanical ventilatory support generally lasts from 2 weeks to 3 months. Significantly longer periods are required for total recovery; indeed, motor abnormalities have been reported to persist up to 13 months[158,159].

As the name implies, wound botulism[160–164] is caused by contamination of a wound by clostridial organisms, followed by elaboration of the neurotoxin at the wound site. In this rare form of botulism, toxin is transported to the target sites in the peripheral nervous system from the wound; therefore, early gastrointestinal symptoms are not encountered. The usual incubation period from the time of the initial wound is approximately 7 days but ranges from 4 to 14 days. In this form of botulism, early symptoms arise from bulbar palsy; complaints of diplopia, ptosis, and dysphagia are common. Nearly all cases have been reported after injury to an extremity[160]. Additional aspects of the clinical picture and disease progression are very similar to other forms of botulism. The causative organism is recovered from excised wound or tissue samples in approximately 50% of cases. Circulating toxin in the serum is identified less frequently.

Infant botulism[165–169] represents a unique form of the disease and accounts for the majority of cases reported in children. Initially recognized in 1976, infant botulism has received considerable attention both as a cause of respiratory insufficiency in infants and as a consideration in SIDS[170]. The unique feature of infant botulism is the intestinal portal of entry of the toxin formed in vivo by ingested organisms. Consumption of contaminated honey has been implicated in some cases[171]. Also, a number of breast-fed infants have exhibited the disease after the recent introduction of nonhuman foods into the diet[167]. Soil or dust can act as a vehicle for introduction of organisms into the immediate environment; this explains the association of disease with ground-breaking and construction activities in the vicinity of patients' homes[168].

Reports of infant botulism have been limited to children under 9 months of age. Onset of disease usually occurs between 2 and 4 months of age[165–167]. Constipation caused by the parasympatholytic effects of the toxin is the most frequent early symptom and usually occurs several days after onset. By this time, evidence of neuromuscular dysfunction has characteristically appeared, resulting in poor feeding, lethargy, and generalized hypotonia. In very severe cases, infant botulism can mimic SIDS. In about 25% of patients, decreased lacrimation or salivation has been reported[145]. Severe muscular weakness culminating in respiratory failure is reported in 50 to 90% of afflicted infants[166–168]. Ventilatory support for periods of 2 months or more may be required; in one series, the average duration of assisted ventilation was 2 weeks[167].

The diagnosis of all forms of botulism is based primarily on clinical recognition of the signs and symptoms in conjunction with appropriate confirmatory testing. An acute motor disorder with early bulbar involvement, followed by descending symmetrical muscle weakness, should suggest botulism. Serum electrolytes and CSF examination are typically normal. Electrophysiologic studies can be particularly helpful in diagnosing botulism; electromyography shows the typical pattern of "brief, small-amplitude, overly abundant motor unit action potentials"[166]. Evoked muscle action potentials elicited by rapid repetitive nerve stimulation typically show an incremental response, in contrast to the pattern seen with myasthenia gravis. The finding of normal peripheral nerve conduction velocities differs from the conduction slowing found in Guillain-Barré syndrome. Administration of anticholinesterase agents such as neostigmine or edrophonium does not consistently lead to improvement in muscle strength. Appropriate screening tests and clinical observation usually allow differentiation from other disorders that can be confused initially with botulism, such as organic acidurias, heavy-metal or insecticide intoxication, sepsis, meningitis, primary myopathies, and poliomyelitis.

Management

ICU care includes the careful delivery of general supportive care. Provision of adequate nutrition generally requires the institution of nasogastric or intravenous alimentation because of the frequent swallowing abnormalities encountered due to involvement of the pharyngeal muscles. Oral feedings should be avoided because of the high risk of aspiration pneumonia. This complication has been reported in as many as 25% of infant patients[167]. The anticholinergic effects of *C. botulinum* toxin on the urinary bladder may cause urinary retention and require bladder decompression. At the earliest sign of infectious complications, patients should receive appropriate antibiotic therapy. However, aminoglycoside antibiotics are known to exacerbate the neuromuscular blocking effects of *C. botulinum* toxin and should be avoided. Indeed, the administration of aminoglycosides to infants with botulism has been associated with the precipitation of acute respiratory insufficiency[172] (see Chapter 33).

Recommendations for the treatment of botulism with equine antitoxin vary. In cases of wound and food-borne botulism, administration of trivalent *C. botulinum* antitoxin is usually recommended. However, use of the horse serum antitoxin in infant botulism has been avoided because of its lack of proven efficacy and the relatively high incidence of anaphylactic complications[166]. Other measures occasionally used in botulism include catharsis, enemas, and antibiotics directed at *C. botulinum.* However, the benefits of these measures have not been substantiated. Guanidine has been used on a limited basis in adults because of its theoretical ability to enhance the release of acetylcholine from cholinergic nerve terminals[173]. However, improvements in strength with guanidine have been confined to nonrespiratory muscles and have not altered the course of respiratory failure.

The cornerstone of management in all forms of botulism is timely and expert respiratory care. Respiratory failure in botulism can arise from several processes. First, bulbar palsy is frequently associated with loss of airway protective reflexes as well as the inability to swallow and clear oral secretions. As a result, the risks of aspiration and airway obstruction are high. In addition, descending paralysis frequently progresses to involve the primary muscles of respiration, leading to hypoventilation and respiratory failure. This process can also interfere with the clearance of pulmonary secretions, resulting in secondary respiratory failure from atelectasis or pneumonia. In a series of infants with botulism, maintenance of the airway by endotracheal intubation and ventilatory assistance was required in more than 90% of patients[167]. For this reason, most children with botulism should be cared for in a facility where pediatric intensive care services are readily available.

Because bulbar palsy is a common finding in all forms of botulism, endotracheal intubation is recommended whenever significant depression of the gag reflex is noted. The duration of endotracheal intubation required in patients with botulism is extremely variable. In one series of infants, the median duration of intubation was only 13 days[167]. However, in some cases, an artificial airway was required for several months[174]. Therefore, initial management with nasotracheal intubation is advisable; this can be followed by elective tracheostomy in the event of a more protracted course. Strict guidelines for the performance of a tracheostomy have not been defined.

Indications for mechanical ventilatory support for patients with botulism are the same as for patients with respiratory failure associated with peripheral neuromuscular disease. Specifically, alveolar hypoventilation and hypercarbia are absolute indications for mechanical ventilatory support. Signs of severe third cranial nerve dysfunction have been linked to the eventual development of respiratory muscle failure[175]. In older patients, monitoring of forced vital capacity and maximum negative inspiratory pressure provides a means for assessing respiratory muscle strength at the bedside. Deterioration in these parameters serves as an early indication of impending respiratory failure and the need to institute mechanical ventilatory support (see Chapter 9). In addition, these bedside parameters can be used to track the progress of respiratory muscle recovery[176].

In addition to nonspecific indices of gas exchange and respiratory muscle capacity, the characteristic pattern of muscle function deterioration and recovery in botulism can be used to guide the timing of respiratory therapy interventions. Specifically, the sequence of muscle group recovery in botulism closely approximates the pattern observed after the administration of nondepolarizing muscle relaxants. In both situations, recovery of strength is first noted in the diaphragm, then the peripheral muscles, and, finally, in repetitive-action muscle groups. Demonstration of adequate strength in repetitive-action muscles, such as those responsible for head control, should ensure satisfactory recovery of respiratory muscle functions. Therefore, return of head control can be used in the timing of attempts at aggressive weaning and extubation of the trachea[177].

About 10% of patients with infant botulism have displayed signs of autonomic instability[167]. Signs of autonomic dysfunction in this population include skin flushing, tachycardia or bradycardia, and fluctuations in systemic blood pressure. Aggressive treatment of these fleeting signs of dysautonomia should be tempered by the fact that they frequently resolve spontaneously.

Given appropriate respiratory support, recovery from all forms of botulism is the rule. Mortality in this disease currently stands at less than 10%, largely due to the timely institution and maintenance of appropriate respiratory support. Long-term follow-up suggests that in most patients with types A and B food-borne botulism, physiologic parameters have returned to normal by 12 to 24 months[158,159]. Aggressive physical therapy during the period of support is mandatory to avoid respiratory complications such as atelectasis and pneumonia.

MISCELLANEOUS PERIPHERAL NEUROMUSCULAR DISEASES

Numerous peripheral neuromuscular disorders are complicated by acute respiratory failure[178–181]. Some diseases, such as tick paralysis and dyskalemic periodic paralysis, can be controlled or definitively treated, and respiratory muscle failure is limited in terms of duration and recurrence. Other conditions, such as Duchenne's muscular dystrophy and infantile muscular atrophy (Werdnig-Hoffmann disease type 1), represent progressive degenerative processes culminating in profound, irreversible muscle weakness and chronic respiratory insufficiency. Comparative features of some unusual neuromuscular causes of respiratory failure in children are highlighted in **Table 8.2.** Although each of these disorders represents a distinct pathologic entity, the pathogenesis and management of respiratory failure associated with the various neuromuscular diseases are similar in many respects.

Virtually all forms of motor unit disease encountered in ICUs pose the threat of upper airway obstruction because of involvement of the cranial nerves of pharyngeal muscles primarily[182]. In addition, these bulbar manifestations of neuromuscular disease can produce severe swallowing abnormalities and present the danger of aspiration of oropharyngeal contents. The precise incidence of aspiration pneumonia associated with neuromuscular diseases is unknown. Pulmonary infection is a frequent complication of many of these disorders, particularly in advanced stages of the progressive degenerative types[178,179]. Presumably, at least some of these pneumonic processes are attributable to aspiration of oropharyngeal contents.

At a minimum, bulbar involvement in peripheral neuromuscular diseases calls for strict feeding precautions via the nasogastric route and nursing with the patient in the prone position. If the competency of the gag reflex is in serious question, endotracheal intubation is recommended. The de-

Table 8.2. Neuromuscular Disorders Causing Respiratory Failure[202]

Site	*Course*	*Noted*
Anterior horn cell	Spinal muscular atrophy (Werdnig-Hoffmann disease)[180,203]	Acute Rapidly progressive, fatal Onset <1 year old Proximal muscle preference Intermediate Slowly progressive Autosomal recessive Survival into adulthood Secondary kyphoscoliosis
Peripheral motor nerve	Multiple sclerosis[178,180]	Chronic relapsing Rare in childhood
	Intoxications[180]	Tick paralysis Acute, rapidly progressive Neurotoxin from engorged tick Recovery after tick removal Heavy metal Acute, rapidly progressive Ingestion history Organophosphate Acute, rapidly progressive Salivation, lacrimation
	Uremia[181]	Acute, rapidly progressive Rare
	Acute intermittent porphyria[178]	Acute, fulminant Attacks precipitated by multiple drugs Abdominal pain Recovery over weeks to months
Neuromuscular junction	Antibiotic intoxication[179]	Acute, self-limited Aminoglycosides, polypeptides
	Hypermagnesemia	Acute, self-limited Iatrogenic, cathartic/antacid abuse
Muscle cell	Duchenne's muscular dystrophy[189–191]	Chronic, steadily progressive Sex-linked recessive Respiratory failure Myocardial failure
	Myotonic dystrophy[204,205]	Variable, usually gradual Autosomal dominant Different clinical forms
	Other congenital myopathies[206]	Variable Multiple forms
	Inborn errors	Acid maltase deficiency[207] Rapidly fatal (infant), late-onset respiratory failure (adult) Autosomal recessive Glycogen storage disease Infant, child, and adult types Carnitine deficiency[208] Childhood onset, remitting fatal Autosomal recessive
Electrolyte disorders	Hypokalemia and hyperkalemia[209]	Acute, self-limited Diuretic use Electrocardiogram abnormalities
	Hypophosphatemia[210]	Acute, self-limited Malnutrition Inadequate replacement
	Dermatomyositis/polymyositis[211]	Acute or gradual Proximal weakness Variable progression Therapy: steroids, immunosuppression

cision to perform a tracheostomy depends on factors such as the anticipated duration and course of the underlying disease, the presence of coincidental pulmonary disease, and, to some extent, individual judgment and preference.

Another major concern in the management of peripheral neuromuscular diseases is the presence of respiratory muscle involvement, resulting in loss of bellows function and spontaneous ventilatory capacity[(182–184)]. In the extreme, involvement of the inspiratory muscles results in respiratory paralysis, alveolar hypoventilation, and asphyxia. However, significant abnormalities of respiratory mechanics can arise with less dramatic degrees of weakness. Partial diaphragmatic impairment results in decreased vital capacity by diminishing inspiratory reserve. Furthermore, decreased resting diaphragmatic tone results in a loss of end-expiratory lung volume as the result of the unopposed hydrostatic forces applied by the abdominal contents on the diaphragm. Indeed, diminished functional residual capacity is frequently noted with diaphragmatic involvement in a variety of neuromuscular diseases[(183,184)]. Weakness of the intercostal muscles can lead to instability of the chest wall, particularly in the case of the infant with incomplete development of the bony thorax. Unopposed diaphragmatic inspiratory activity results in inspiratory retractions of the chest wall and decreased ventilatory efficacy.

Involvement of the expiratory muscles is encountered to a greater extent in certain diseases, such as congenital myopathies[(182)], and produces significant respiratory mechanical abnormalities. Functionally, diminished expiratory muscle capacity results in elevation of residual volume and diminished expiratory reserve volume. The expiratory accessory muscles play a critical role in the generation of effective coughing, and their impairment can severely limit the clearance of pulmonary secretions. An extreme example of diminished expiratory muscle function is the congenital absence of the abdominal musculature, also known as the prune-belly syndrome. This congenital abnormality is associated with recurrent pulmonary infections and marginal respiratory reserve.

In most neuromuscular disorders, variable involvement of both inspiratory and expiratory muscles of respiration occurs. Under these circumstances, functional residual capacity, expiratory reserve volume, and inspiratory reserve volume are diminished[(182)]. In addition, decreased lung compliance is a consistent finding in this setting[(183–185)]; although the precise mechanism for this has not been clearly defined, it is probably related to decreased resting lung volume with secondary small airway closure and atelectasis. Even limited respiratory muscle weakness can predispose the patient to atelectasis or pneumonia or both[(185)]. Pulmonary infiltrates consistent with atelectasis are reported in 50% or more of patients requiring intensive care for respiratory failure secondary to neuromuscular disease[(178,179,186)]. In this setting, inability to clear bronchial secretions rapidly leads to infectious complications. For this reason, many patients with degenerative neuromuscular disease initially present with diffuse pneumonia, and the dramatic involvement of the pulmonary parenchyma can divert attention away from the primary neuromuscular disorder. Also, chronic progressive neuromuscular disease is commonly characterized by recurrent bouts of pneumonia that clear with aggressive respiratory support[(180)].

The management of the patient with neuromuscular disease should be anticipatory[(178–180,182)]. Because of the pathogenetic mechanisms discussed previously, acute respiratory failure frequently ensues with extreme rapidity in patients with neuromuscular disease. Therefore, intermittent determination of arterial blood gases is usually inadequate for signaling impending respiratory failure. Early detection of marginal respiratory muscle function is achieved only by appropriate monitoring of bedside indices of respiratory muscle strength[(179,182,187,188)]. Inspiration muscle capacity is evaluated by measuring maximum negative inspiratory airway pressure under static airflow conditions (see Chapter 9). Although normal values for this measurement in infants and young children have not been firmly established, acceptable limits for older children and adults have been identified[(187,188)]. Once this parameter decreases to 50% of its predicted level, further decreases in negative inspiratory pressure are related linearly to arterial PCO_2. Furthermore, inspiratory pressure values less negative than -20 to -30 cm H_2O are generally recognized as a sign of severe inspiratory muscle weakness and impending respiratory failure. Similarly, expiratory muscle function is evaluated by measuring the maximum positive expiratory airway pressure generated at total lung capacity[(187)]. A decreasing trend in this parameter signals a progressive loss of expiratory muscle strength, and a value less than 40 cm H_2O correlates with inability to generate an effective cough for the clearance of secretions[(188)]. Measurement of vital capacity is also valuable in the patient with neuromuscular disease[(179,182)]. Forced vital capacity less than three times the predicted tidal volume is associated with impaired coughing capability and retention of secretions; inability to generate a vital capacity more than two times the predicted tidal volume signals severe impairment in respiratory capacity and impending acute respiratory failure. Furthermore, vital capacity less than 50% of that predicted for the patient's size is associated with alveolar hypoventilation and hypercapnia.

Patients with neuromuscular disease frequently experience respiratory failure precipitated by an acute respiratory complication such as atelectasis or pneumonia. Under these conditions, in addition to limited respiratory capacity and alveolar hypoventilation, some degree of ventilation/perfusion mismatching occurs. Management of these bouts of acute respiratory failure requires aggressive chest physical therapy, appropriate antibiotic treatment, and positive pressure ventilatory support. Intermittent positive pressure breathing treatments alone do not improve lung volumes or pulmonary compliance in patients with respiratory muscle weakness[(183)]. However, intervention with mechanical ventilatory support has been associated with increases in inspiratory and expiratory muscle capacity and maximum voluntary ventilation after several weeks[(182)]. Therefore, "resting" the respiratory muscles in these types of disorders seems to have a rational basis. Weaning from mechanical ventilatory support should be preceded by the provision of adequate nutrition and the correction of any metabolic or electrolyte abnormalities, particularly those associated with decreased respiratory muscle function **(Table 8.2).** In addition, adequate time should be allowed for clearing of any acute coincidental pulmonary parenchymal disease.

Survival after an acute episode of respiratory failure associated with neuromuscular disease is the overwhelming rule, with over 90% of patients recovering from an acute episode[(178–180)]. However, during the course of degenerative neuromuscular diseases, patients ultimately suffer chronic respiratory decompensation characterized by chronic CO_2 retention and recurrent bouts of atelectasis and pneumonia. Others simply may fail to be weaned from positive pressure ventilatory support. At this point, chronic ventilatory assistance is necessary to maintain respiratory stability. All appropriate consultative resources should be made available to the patient and relatives to assist in arriving at a decision to embark on chronic mechanical ventilatory assistance. It should be stressed that patients with chronic degenerative neuromuscular diseases, such as muscular dystrophy, have been maintained for prolonged periods with mechanical support devices designed for home use(189–192). Initially, intermittent use of a negative pressure device, such as the cuirass shell, may be adequate for maintaining respiratory stability without the need for a tracheostomy. Alternatively, an intermittent abdominal pressure respirator (e.g., pneumobelt) or rocking bed can provide ventilatory assistance by alternating compression and decompression of the abdominal contents against the diaphragm[(192)]. Nocturnal nasal bilevel positive airway pressure is often well tolerated and can reverse early hypoventilation/respiratory failure[(193,194)]. Eventually, respiratory muscle insufficiency may progress to the extent that these devices are no longer effective, necessitating the placement of a tracheostomy and initiation of positive pressure ventilatory support with a portable home volume ventilator (see Chapter 9). Via this approach, some patients with muscular dystrophy have enjoyed functional survival for years after the onset of chronic respiratory insufficiency[(192,195)].

NEUROMUSCULAR FAILURE IN THE INTENSIVE CARE UNIT

Respiratory failure resulting from a neuromuscular disorder is the focus of this chapter. However, increasingly reported are critically ill patients who develop a neuromuscular disorder during treatment for respiratory failure. This usually involves patients with sepsis, multisystem organ failure, or status asthmaticus who experience a generalized weakness with respiratory muscle involvement as the primary process is resolving. These patients are slow or unable to be weaned from the ventilator. Weakness and hyporeflexia not previously present are discovered as sedation and paralysis are withdrawn. The list of differential diagnoses for this condition is extensive **(Table 8.3).**

The diagnoses that must be considered include residual neuromuscular junction blockade, metabolites of neuromuscular junction blockers, acquired myopathies, acquired neuropathies, metabolic abnormalities, and unmasking of underlying neuromuscular disease. The differentiation of these processes may require obtaining an appropriate history, physical examination, blood testing, CSF examination, radiographic imaging, electrophysiologic studies, and tissue biopsy. Prevention rather than treatment is preferred and is possible for many of these disorders.

Residual neuromuscular blockade or potentiation of residual neuromuscular junction blockade can be determined by history, physical examination, and electrophysiologic studies. Patients with a history of receiving neuromuscular junction blocking medications can be studied with an electrical nerve (twitch) stimulator to determine the level of residual blockade. Residual blockade persisting after the usual time for resolution implies accumulation of blockers/metabolites (see below) or potentiation by environmental factors or drugs. Environmental factors that potentiate neuromuscular junction blockade include acidosis and hypothermia. Drugs that potentiate neuromuscular junction blockade include aminoglycosides, polymyxins, macrolides, calcium channel blockers, beta-blockers, procainamide, d-penicillamine, and lithium[(196)].

Accumulation of metabolites of neuromuscular junction blockers needs to be considered with prolonged administration of these agents or with liver and kidney failure. Pro-

Table 8.3. Causes of Unanticipated Prolonged Ventilator Dependence

Potentiation of residual neuromuscular junction blockade
Acidosis, respiratory or metabolic
Hypothermia
Aminoglycoside toxicity
Calcium channel blocker toxicity
Metabolites of neuromuscular junction blockade accumulation
Prolonged use
Renal failure
Liver failure
Acquired myopathies
Steroid myopathy
Disuse (immobilization) myopathy
Catabolic (nutritional) myopathy
Septic pyomyositis
Critical illness myopathy
Acquired neuropathies
Guillain Barré polyradiculoneuritis
Critical illness polyneuropathy
Metabolic abnormalities
Hypermagnesemia
Hypophosphatemia
Pancreatic dysfunction
Unmasking of underlying neuromuscular disease
Porphyria
Myasthenia gravis

longed neuromuscular blockade occurs after the termination of long-term treatment with vecuronium despite its intermediate duration of action[197]. Vecuronium and its metabolite 3-desacetyl-vecuronium persist in the blood for weeks after stopping prolonged (15 days) administration in patients with hepatic dysfunction[198]. Vecuronium is 75 to 90% metabolized by the liver but may be more affected by renal failure than liver failure. For vecuronium total dose is not a significant factor, but the presence of renal failure increases risk for prolonged plasma levels[197]. Similar risks occur with most of the neuromuscular junction blocking agents.

Acquired myopathies may develop in patients with respiratory failure during chronic intensive care. Steroid myopathy usually develops after prolonged administration of fluorinated compounds. This may occur with prednisone, methylprednisolone, and dexamethasone even with short durations[199]. Typically this disorder manifests itself as a symmetric weakness involving the proximal limb musculature and spares the respiratory musculature. Creatine kinase is usually not elevated, and the electromyogram shows myopathic changes but no spontaneous activity. Prolonged immobilization may cause a disuse myopathy, and inadequate nutrition will lead to a catabolic myopathy. Septic pyomyositis is seen when organisms and inflammatory cells invade muscles during the course of an infection.

A reversible *critical illness myopathy* of unknown cause occurs in critically ill patients. High doses of steroids and neuromuscular junction blocking agents are often involved. Proximal or generalized weakness (rarely involving the extraocular muscles), respiratory muscle dysfunction, and attenuation of reflexes are present. Creatine kinase is elevated in about half the patients[197]. Nerve conduction is usually normal. Electromyogram shows absent or mildly increased spontaneous activity and early recruitment of short-duration motor-unit potentials. Muscle biopsy shows type 2 fiber atrophy, but muscle necrosis and vacuolization occur. Electron microscopy may show loss of thick (myosin) filaments (a nonspecific finding). This critical illness myopathy usually resolves over weeks to months. There may be a correlation between steroid total dose and duration of the dysfunction[199].

Acquired neuropathies may develop in critically ill patients. Guillain Barré polyradiculoneuritis is discussed earlier in this chapter. The new onset of Guillain Barré in critically ill patients has been associated with fulminant hepatitis and after surgery.

Critical illness polyneuropathy manifests itself as an acute hyporeflexic generalized weakness. This weakness is usually discovered as the critical illness resolves and failure to wean the patient from the ventilator becomes the dominant problem[200]. Distal limb weakness, hyporeflexia, areflexia, and respiratory muscle weakness are noted in patients with sepsis or multiorgan failure. Sensory function is usually much less diminished. Lack of weakness in facial and extraocular muscles is a clue that the neuromuscular junction is involved and critical illness polyneuropathy should be considered[198]. Cerebrospinal fluid is normal. Electrophysiologic studies show motor axonal polyneuropathy, while sensory potentials may vary. Degeneration of motor and sensory axons is seen on pathologic examination[197]. Critical illness polyneuropathy is described in children[201]. The etiology of this process is unknown, but the majority of patients recover from the neuropathy[197].

Metabolic abnormalities may occur in critically ill children and contribute to respiratory muscle weakness. Hypermagnesemia, hypophosphatemia, and pancreatic dysfunction (hypocalcemia) need to be considered. Unmasking of underlying neuromuscular disease may also be a problem. Porphyria or myasthenia gravis are diseases that may go unrecognized until the drugs that impact on these diseases are administered.

Prophylaxis may be easier than treatment, especially for the critical illness neuromuscular disorders. The prophylactic principles are as follows:

1. Keep neuromuscular blocking agents to the lowest possible doses and the shortest possible durations, and use less than a complete blockade.
2. Monitor neuromuscular transmission to keep the myotactic reflex intact.
3. Avoid combining neuromuscular blocking agents and aminoglycoside.
4. Employ extra vigilance when liver or renal failure occurs.
5. Avoid acidosis, hypermagnesemia, and accumulation of metabolites.
6. Use special caution with patients who have had a previous episode of these complications[199].
7. Minimize exposure to and interaction with steroids.

References

1. Braun NMT, Rochester DF. Muscular weakness and respiratory failure. Am Rev Respir Dis 1979;119:123.
2. Faulkner JA, Maxwell LC, Ruff GL, White TP. The diaphragm as a muscle: contractile properties. Am Rev Respir Dis 1979;119:89.
3. Derenne FPH, Macklem PT, Roussos CH. The respiratory muscles: mechanics, control and pathophysiology, I. Am Rev Respir Dis 1978;118:119.
4. Derenne FPH, Macklem PT, Roussos CH. The respiratory muscles: mechanics, control and pathophysiology, II. Am Rev Respir Dis 1978;118:119.
5. Derenne FPH, Macklem PT, Roussos CH. The respiratory muscles: mechanics, control and pathophysiology, III. Am Rev Respir Dis 1978;118:581.
6. Aubier M, DeTroyer A, Sampson M, Macklem PT, Roussos C. Aminophylline improves diaphragmatic contractility. N Engl J Med 1981;305:249.
7. Martin JG, DeTroyer A. The behaviors of the abdominal muscles during inspiratory mechanical loading. Respir Physiol 1982;50:63.
8. Liu HM, Loew JM, Hunt CE. Congenital central hypoventilation syndrome: a pathologic study of the neuromuscular system. Neurology 1978;28:1013.
9. Fleming PJ, Cade D, Bryan MH, Bryan AC. Congenital central hypoventilation and sleep state. Pediatrics 1980;66:425.
10. Shannon DC, Marsland DW, Gould JB, Callahan B, Todres ID, Dennis J. Central hypoventilation during quiet sleep in two infants. Pediatrics 1976;57:342.
11. Hunt CE, Brouillette RT. Abnormalities of breathing control and airway maintenance in infants and children as a cause of cor pulmonale. Pediatr Cardiol 1982;3:249.

12. Chokroverty S, Sharp JT. Primary sleep apnoea syndrome. J Neurol Neurosurg Psychiatry 1981;44:970.
13. Severinghaus JW, Mitchell RA. Ondine's curse failure of respiratory-center automaticity while awake. Clin Res 1962;10:122.
14. Brooks JG. Apnea of infancy and sudden infant death syndrome. Am J Dis Child 1982;136:1012.
15. DuRivage SK, Winter RJ, Brouillette RT, Hunt CE, Noah Z. Idiopathic hypothalamic dysfunction and impaired control of breathing. Pediatrics 1985;75:896.
16. Johnston K, Newth CJ, Sheu KF, Patel MS, Heldt GP, Schmidt KA, Packman S. Central hypoventilation syndrome in pyruvate dehydrogenase complex deficiency. Pediatrics 1984;74:1034.
17. Barlow PB, Barlett D Jr, Hauri P, Hellekson C, Nattie EE, Remmers JE, Schmidt-Nowara WW. Idiopathic hypoventilation syndrome: importance of preventing nocturnal hypoxemia and hypercapnia. Am Rev Respir Dis 1980;121:141.
18. Camfield P, Camfield C, Bagnell P, Rees E. Infant apnea syndrome: a prospective evaluation of etiologies. Clin Pediatr 1982;21:684.
19. Rosen CL, Frost JK Jr, Harrison GM. Infant apnea: polygraphic studies and follow-up monitoring. Pediatrics 1983;71:731.
20. Pauli RM, Scott CI, Wassman ER Jr, Gilbert EF, Leavitt LA, Ver-Hoeve J, Hall JG, Partington MW, Jones KL, Sommer A, et al. Apnea and sudden unexpected death in infants with achondroplasia. J Pediatr 1984;104:342.
21. Milerad J, Lagercrantz H, Lofgren O. Alveolar hypoventilation treated with medroxyprogesterone. Arch Dis Child 1985;60:150.
22. Hunt CE, Inwood RJ, Shannon DC. Respiratory and nonrespiratory effects of doxapram in congenital central hypoventilation syndrome. Am Rev Respir Dis 1979; 119:263.
23. Shannon DC, Sullivan K, Perret L, Kelly DH. Use of almitrine bismesylate to stimulate ventilation in congenital central hypoventilation. Eur J Respir Dis 1983;64(Suppl 126):295.
24. Fleming PJ, Levine MR, Lewis GTR, Pauly N. Almitrine bismesylate in congenital central hypoventilation. Eur J Respir Dis 1983;64(Suppl 126):307.
25. Airlie MAA, Flenley DC, Warren PM. Effect of almitrine on hypoxic ventilatory drive measured by transient and progressive isocapnic hypoxia in normal men. Clin Sci 1989;77:431.
26. Meisner H, Scober JG, Struck E, Lipowski B, Mayser P, Sebening F. Phrenic nerve pacing for the treatment of central hypoventilation syndrome state of the art and case report. Thorac Cardiovasc Surg 1983;31:21.
27. Coleman M, Boros SJ, Huseby TL, Brennom WS. Congenital central hypoventilation syndrome. A report of successful experience with bilateral diaphragmatic pacing. Arch Dis Child 1980;55:901.
28. Ruth V, Pesonen E, Raivio KO. Congenital central hypoventilation syndrome treated with diaphragm pacing. Acta Paediatr Scand 1983;72:295.
29. Brouillette RT, Ilbawi MN, Hunt CE. Phrenic nerve pacing in infants and children: a review of experience and report on the usefulness of phrenic nerve stimulation studies. J Pediatr 1983;102:32.
30. Carroll N, Branthwaite MA. Control of nocturnal hypoventilation by nasal intermittent positive pressure ventilation. Thorax 1988;43:349.
31. Heckmatt JZ, Loh L, Dubowitz V. Night-time nasal ventilation in neuromuscular disease. Lancet 1990;335:579.
32. Ellis ER, Bye PT, Bruderer JW, Sullivan CE. Treatment of respiratory failure during sleep in patients with neuromuscular disease: positive pressure ventilation through a nose mask. Am Rev Respir Dis 1987;135:14.
33. Oren J, Kelly D, Shannon D. Long-term follow-up of children with congenital central hypoventilation syndrome. Pediatrics 1987;80:37.
34. Kewaltramani LS, Tori JA. Spinal cord trauma in children. Neurologic patterns, radiologic features, and pathomechanics of injury. Spine 1980;5:11.
35. Pang D, Wilberger JE Jr. Spinal cord injury without radiographic abnormalities in children. J Neurosurg 1982;57:114.
36. Andrews LG, Jung SK. Spinal cord injuries in children in British Columbia. Paraplegia 1979;17:442.
37. Ledsome JR, Sharp JM. Pulmonary function in acute cervical cord injury. Am Rev Respir Dis 1981;124:41.
38. Sugarman B. Medical complications of spinal cord injury. Q J Med 1985;54:3.
39. Scher AT. The radiology of pulmonary complications associated with acute spinal cord injury. S Afr Med J 1982;62:321.
40. Koch BM, Eng GM. Neonatal spinal cord injury. Arch Phys Med Rehabil 1979;60:378.
41. Tator CH, Rowed DW, Schwartz ML, Gertzbein SD, Bharatwal N, Barkin M, Edmonds VE. Management of acute spinal cord injuries. Can J Surg 1984;27:289.
42. Luce JM. Medical management of spinal cord injury. Crit Care Med 1985;13:126.
43. Mansel JK, Norman JR. Respiratory complications and management of spinal cord injuries. Chest 1990;97:144.
44. Glenn WWL, Hogan JF, Loke JSO, Ciesielski TE, Phelps ML, Rowedder R. Ventilatory support by pacing of the conditioned diaphragm in quadriplegia. N Engl J Med 1984;310:1150.
45. Lee MY, Kirk PM, Yarkony GM. Rehabilitation of quadriplegic patients with phrenic nerve pacers. Arch Phys Rehabil 1989;70:54.
46. Nochomavitz ML, Peterson DK, Stellato TA. Electrical activation of the diaphragm. Clin Chest Med 1988;9:34.
47. Weinstein L. Tetanus. N Engl J Med 1973;289:1293.
48. Alfrey D, Rauscher A. Tetanus: a review. Crit Care Med 1979;7:176.
49. Tetanus United States, 1987 and 1988. JAMA 1990; 263:1192.
50. Trujillo MJ, Castillo A, Espana JV, Guevara P, Eganez H. Tetanus in the adult: intensive care and management experience with 233 cases. Crit Care Med 1980;8:419.
51. Edmondson RS, Flowers MW. Intensive care in tetanus: management, complications and mortality in 100 cases. Br Med J 1979;1:1401.
52. Gleary DT. Management of severe tetanus in a small community hospital. Wis Med J 1984;83:21.
53. Newton-John HF. Tetanus in Victoria, 1957 - 1980. Review of 106 patients managed in one hospital. Med J Aust 1984;140:194.
54. Krishna SR. Neonatal tetanus. Anaesth Intensive Care 1979;7:336.
55. Adams JM, Kenny JD, Rudolph AJ. Modern management of tetanus neonatorum. Pediatrics 1979;64:472.
56. Mahoney JL. Otogenic tetanus in Zaire. Laryngoscope 1980;90:1196.
57. Babajews A, Nicholls MWN. Tetanus associated with dental sepsis. Br J Oral Maxillofac Surg 1985;23:36.
58. Pather M, Hariparsad D, Wesley AG. Nasotracheal intubation versus tracheostomy for intermittent positive pressure ventilation in neonatal tetanus. Intensive Care Med 1985;11:30.
59. Weller TH. Poliomyelitis: its global demise. Pediatrics 1984;74:442.
60. Harries JR. Respiratory paralysis in African children. East Afr Med J 1965;42:479.
61. Feigin RD, Guggenheim MA, Johnsen SD. Vaccine-related paralytic poliomyelitis in an immunodeficient child. J Pediatr 1971;79:642.
62. Weil ML. Infections of the nervous system. In: Menkes JH, ed. Textbook of child neurology. Philadelphia: Lea & Febiger, 1975:213.
63. Auld PAM, Kevy SV, Eley RC. Poliomyelitis in children: experience with 956 cases in the 1955 Massachusetts epidemic. N Engl J Med 1960;263:1093.
64. Plum A, Swanson AG. Abnormalities in central regulation of respiration in acute and convalescent poliomyelitis. Arch Neurol Psychiatry 1958;80:267.
65. Hedley-Whyte J, Burgess GE III, Feeley TW, Miller MG. Respiratory management of peripheral neurologic disease. In: Applied physiology of respiratory care. Boston: Little, Brown, 1976:245.
66. Dunne JW, Harper CG, Hilton JMN. Sudden infant death syndrome caused by poliomyelitis. Arch Neurol 1984;41:775.
67. Walley RV. Control of artificial respiration in poliomyelitis patients with paralysis of swallowing. Lancet 1957;2:1143.
68. Bach JR, Alba AS, Shin D. Management alternatives for post-polio respiratory insufficiency; assisted ventilation by nasal or oral-nasal interface. Am J Phys Med Rehabil 1989;68:264.
69. Bukh N. Muscle recovery in poliomyelitis. Acta Orthop Scand 1968;39:579.
70. Alcock AJW, Hildes JA, Kaufert PA, Kaufert JM, Bickford J. Respiratory poliomyelitis: a follow-up study. Can Med Assoc J 1984;130:1305.
71. Hanninen P, Wendelin H, Rasanen O, Panelius M. Chronic respiratory paralysis. A clinical study of 12 patients in long-term respiratory treatment after poliomyelitis. Acta Paediatr Scand Suppl 1972;228:1.
72. Holinger LD, Holinger PC, Holinger PH. Etiology of bilateral abductor vocal cord paralysis: a review of 389 cases. Ann Otol 1976;85:428.
73. Kafer ER. Respiratory function in paralytic scoliosis. Am Rev Respir Dis 1974;110:450.
74. Hill R, Robbins AW, Messing R, Arora NS. Sleep apnea syndrome after poliomyelitis. Am Rev Respir Dis 1983;127:129.
75. Nichols PJR, Lane DJ, Hamilton EA, Hazelman BL. Late onset of respiratory failure after poliomyelitis. Lancet 1972;2:1320.
76. Loeffel NB, Rossi LN, Mumenthaler M, Lutschg J, Ludin HP. The Landry-Guillain-Barré syndrome. Complications, prognosis and natural history in 123 cases. J Neurol Sci 1977;33:71.

77. Asbury AK. Diagnostic considerations in Guillain-Barré syndrome. Ann Neurol Suppl 1981;9:1.
78. Ropper AH. Management of Guillain-Barré syndrome. In: Ropper AH, Kennedy SK, Zervos NT, eds. Neurological and neurosurgical intensive care. Baltimore: University Park Press, 1983:163.
79. Lichtenfield P. Autonomic dysfunction in the Guillain-Barré syndrome. JAMA 1971;50:772.
80. Weintraub MI. Autonomic failure in Guillain-Barré syndrome: value of Swan-Ganz catheterization. JAMA 1979;242:513.
81. Durocher A, Servais B, Caridroix M, Chopin C, Wattel F. Autonomic dysfunction in the Guillain-Barré syndrome. Hemodynamic and neurobiochemical studies. Intensive Care Med 1980;6:3.
82. Beale EO, Miller MT. The Guillain-Barré syndrome: a review of admissions to an intensive care unit over 8 years. S Afr Med J 1985;67:10.
83. Moore P, James O. Guillain-Barré syndrome: incidence, management and outcome of major complications. Crit Care Med 1981;9:549.
84. Gracey DR, McMichan JC, Divertie MB, Howard FM. Respiratory failure in Guillain-Barré syndrome: a 6-year experience. Mayo Clin Proc 1982;57:742.
85. Kennedy RH, Danielson MA, Mulder DW, Kurland LT. Guillain-Barré syndrome. A 42-year epidemiologic and clinical study. Mayo Clin Proc 1978;53:93.
86. Eberle E, Brink J, Azen S, White D. Early predictors of incomplete recovery in children with Guillain-Barré polyneuritis. J Pediatr 1975;86:356.
87. Griggs RC, Donohoe KM, Utell MJ, Goldblatt D, Moxley RT. Evaluation of pulmonary function in neuromuscular disease. Arch Neurol 1981;38:9.
88. Fergusson RJ, Wright DJ, Wiley RD, Crompton GK, Grant IW. Suxamethonium is dangerous in polyneuropathy. Br Med J 1981;282:298.
89. Newsum JK, Smith RM, Crocker D. Intubation for acute respiratory failure in Guillain-Barré syndrome. JAMA 1979;242:1650.
90. Freezer NJ, Robertson CF. Tracheostomy in children with Guillain-Barré syndrome. Crit Care Med 1990;18:123.
91. Whitehouse AC, Petty TL. Recovery in Landry-Guillain-Barré syndrome after prolonged respiratory support. Lancet 1969;1:1029.
92. Hughes RAC, Newsom-Davis JM, Perkin GD, Pierce JM. Controlled trial of prednisolone in acute polyneuropathy. Lancet 1978;2:750.
93. Brettle RP, Gross M, Legg NJ, Lockwood M, Pallis C. Treatment of acute polyneuropathy by plasma exchange [Letter]. Lancet 1978;2:1100.
94. Ropper AH, Shahani B, Huggins CE. Improvement in four patients with acute Guillain-Barré syndrome after plasma exchange [Abstract]. Neurology 1980;30:361.
95. Valbonesi M, Mosconi L, Garellii S, Zerbi D, Celano I. Successful treatment by plasma exchange in Guillain-Barré syndrome with immune complexes. Vox Sang 1980; 38:181.
96. Server AC, Lefkowith J, Braine H, McKhann GM. Treatment of chronic relapsing inflammatory polyradiculoneuropathy by plasma exchange. Ann Neurol 1979;6:258.
97. Bezwoda WR, Fritz V, Reef HE, Staub H, Derman DP, Lewis M, Kallenbach J, Zaltzman M, Naughton MA. Treatment of acute postinfective polyneuropathy by means of plasma exchange. Acta Neurol Scand 1984;69:112.
98. The Guillain-Barré syndrome study group. Plasmapheresis and acute Guillain-Barré syndrome. Neurology 1985;35:1096.
99. Singh S, Singhi S. Recovery from respiratory paralysis caused by Guillain-Barré syndrome in an infant after repeated exchange transfusions. Clin Pediatr 1989;28:48.
100. van der Meche FGA, Schmitz PIM, Dutch Guillain-Barré Study Group. A randomized trial comparing intravenous immune globulin and plasma exchange in Guillain-Barré syndrome. N Engl J Med 1992; 326:1123
101. Michell JJ, Ob KS, Siewers RD, Galvis AG, Fricker FJ, Matthews RA. Clinical implications of postoperative unilateral phrenic nerve paralysis. J Thorac Cardiovasc Surg 1978;76:297.
102. Lynn AM, Jenkins JG, Edmonds JF, Burns JE. Diaphragmatic paralysis after pediatric cardiac surgery: a retrospective analysis of 34 cases. Crit Care Med 1983;11:280.
103. Hong-Xu Z, D'Agostino RS, Pitlick PT, Shumway NE, Miller DC. Phrenic nerve injury complicating closed cardiovascular surgical procedures for congenital heart disease. Ann Thorac Surg 1985; 39:445.
104. Greene W, L'Heureux P, Hunt CE. Paralysis of the diaphragm. Am J Dis Child 1975;129:1402.
105. Robotham JL. A physiological approach to hemidiaphragm paralysis. Crit Care Med 1979;7:563.
106. Robotham JL, Chipps BE, Shermeta DW. Continuous positive airpressure in hemidiaphragmatic paralysis. Anesthesiology 1980; 52:167.
107. Haller JA Jr, Pickard LR, Tepas JJ, Rogers MC, Robotham JL, Shorter N, Shermeta DW. Management of diaphragmatic paralysis in infants with special emphasis on selection of patients for operative plication. J Pediatr Surg 1979;14:779.
108. Shoemaker R, Palmer G, Brown JW, King H. Aggressive treatment of acquired phrenic nerve paralysis in infants and small children. Ann Thorac Surg 1981;32:251.
109. Bowman ED, Murton LJ. A case of neonatal bilateral diaphragmatic paralysis required surgery. Aust Paediatr J 1984;20:331.
110. Schwartz MZ, Filler RM. Plication of the diaphragm for symptomatic phrenic nerve paralysis. J Pediatr Surg 1978;13:259.
111. Arborelium M Jr, Lilja B, Senyk J. Regional and total lung function studies in patients with hemidiaphragmatic paralysis. Respiration 1975;32:253.
112. Mearns AJ. Iatrogenic injury to the phrenic nerve in infants and young children. Br J Surg 1977;64:558.
113. Gould L, Kaplan S, McElhinney AJ, Stone DJ. A method for the production of hemidiaphragmatic paralysis. Its application to the study of lung function in normal man. Am Rev Respir Dis 1967;96:812.
114. Kohorst WR, Schonfeld SA, Altman M. Bilateral diaphragmatic paralysis following topical cardiac hypothermia. Chest 1984;85:65.
115. Rousou JA, Parker T, Engelman RM, Breyer RH. Phrenic nerve paresis associated with the use of iced slush and the cooling jacket for topical hypothermia. J Thorac Cardiovasc Surg 1985;89:921.
116. Robicsek F, Duncan D, Hawes AC, Rice HE, Harrill S, Robicsek SA. Biological thresholds of cold-induced phrenic nerve injury. J Thorac Cardiovasc Surg 1990;99:16.
117. Curtis JJ, Nawarawong W, Walls JT, Schmaltz RA, Boley T, Madsen R, Anderson SK. Elevated hemidiaphragm after cardiac operations: incidence, prognosis, and relationship to the use of topical ice slush. Ann Thorac Surg 1989;48:76.
118. Moorthy SS, Gibbs PS, Losasso AM, Lingeman RE. Transient paralysis of the diaphragm following radical neck surgery. Laryngoscope 1983;93:642.
119. Hadeed HA, Braun TW. Paralysis of the hemidiaphragm as a complication of internal jugular vein cannulation: report of a case. J Oral Maxillofac Surg 1988;46:40.
120. Moosa A. Phrenic nerve conduction in children. Dev Med Child Neurol 1981;23:434.
121. Moorthy SS, Markand ON, Mahomed Y, Brown JW. Electrophysiologic evaluation of phrenic nerves in severe respiratory insufficiency requiring mechanical ventilation. Chest 1985;88:211.
122. McCauley RGK, Labib KB. Diaphragmatic paralysis evaluated by phrenic nerve stimulation during fluoroscopy or real-time ultrasound. Radiology 1984;153:33.
123. Langer JC, Filler RM, Coles J, Edmonds JF. Plication of the diaphragm for infants and young children with phrenic nerve palsy. J Pediatr Surg 1988;23:74.
124. Menkes JH. Diseases of the motor unit. In: Textbook of child neurology. Philadelphia: Lea & Febiger, 1975:463.
125. Gracey DR, Divertie MB, Howard FM Jr. Mechanical ventilation for respiratory failure in myasthenia gravis. Two-year experience with 22 patients. Mayo Clin Proc 1983;58:597.
126. Ferguson IT, Murphy RP, Lascelles RG. Ventilatory failure in myasthenia gravis. J Neurol Neurosurg Psychiatry 1982;45:217.
127. Drachman DB. Myasthenia gravis. N Engl J Med 1978;298:136, 186.
128. Robertson WC, Chun RW, Korngeth SE. Familial infantile myasthenia. Arch Neurol 1980;37:117.
129. Hutchison AA, Russell G. Respiratory studies in an infant with neonatal myasthenia gravis. Aust Paediatr J 1979;15:44.
130. Grant RP, Jenkins LC. Prediction of the need for postoperative mechanical ventilation in myasthenia gravis: thymectomy compared to other surgical procedures. Can Anaesth Soc J 1982;29:112.
131. Leventhal SR, Orkin FK, Hirsh RA. Prediction of the need for postoperative mechanical ventilation in myasthenia gravis. Anesthesiology 1980;53:26.
132. Gracey DR, Divertie MB, Howard FM Jr, Payne WS. Postoperative respiratory care after transsternal thymectomy in myasthenia gravis. A 3-year experience in 53 patients. Chest 1984;86:67.
133. Younger DS, Braun NM, Jaretzki A III, Penn AB, Lovelace RE. Myasthenia gravis: determinants for independent ventilation after transsternal thymectomy. Neurology 1984;34:336.
134. Gorback MS, Moon RE, Massey JM. Extubation after transternal

thymectomy for myasthenia gravis: A prospective analysis. South Med J 1991;84:702.
135. Florence AM. Anaesthesia for transcervical thymectomy in myasthenia gravis. Ann R Coll Surg Engl 1984;66:309.
136. Colp C, Kriplani L, Nussbaum M. Vocal cord paralysis in myasthenia gravis following anesthesia. Chest 1980; 77:218.
137. Dushay KM, Zibrak JD, Jensen WA. Myasthenia gravis presenting as isolated respiratory failure. Chest 1990;97:232.
138. Mier-Jedrzejowicz AK, Brophy C, Green M. Respiratory muscle function in myasthenia gravis. Am Rev Respir Dis 1988;138:86.
139. Pollard BJ, Harper JN, Doran BRH. Use of continuous prolonged administration of atracurium in the ICU to a patient with myasthenia gravis. Br J Anaesth 1989; 62a:9.
140. Magyar P, Szathmary I, Szobor A. Myasthenia gravis: lung-function studies without and with edrophonium chloride. Eur Neurol 1979;18:59.
141. DeTroyer A, Borenstein S. Acute changes in respiratory mechanics after pyridostigmine injection in patients with myasthenia gravis. Am Rev Respir Dis 1980;121:629.
142. Jain S, Pande JN, Ahuja GK. Pulmonary function studies in myasthenia gravis. Ind J Med Res 1984;79:806.
143. Shale DJ, Lane DJ, Davis CJ. Air-flow limitation in myasthenia gravis. The effect of acetylcholinesterase inhibitor therapy on air-flow limitation. Am Rev Respir Dis 1983;128:618.
144. Szathmary I, Magyar P, Szobor A. Air-flow limitation in myasthenia gravis. The effect of acetylcholinesterase inhibitor therapy on air-flow limitation [Letter]. Am Rev Respir Dis 1984;130:145.
145. Argov Z, Mastaglia FL. Drug therapy: disorders of neuromuscular transmission caused by drugs. N Engl J Med 1979;301:409.
146. Chutorian AM. Corticosteroids and corticotrophin in the treatment of neurologic disorders, with emphasis on neurologic disorders of childhood. Clin Neuropharmacol 1982;5:239.
147. Pascuzzi RM, Coslett HB, Johns TR. Long-term corticosteroid treatment of myasthenia gravis: Report of 116 patients. Ann Neurol 1984; 15:291.
148. Fonesca V, Havard CWH. Long term treatment of myasthenia gravis with azathioprine. Postgrad Med J 1990;66:102.
149. Havard CW. Progress in myasthenia gravis. Br Med J 1977;2:1008.
150. Youssef S. Thymectomy for myasthenia gravis in children. J Pediatr Surg 1983;18:537.
151. Campbell JR, Bisio JM, Harrison MW, Campbell TJ. Surgical treatment of myasthenia gravis in childhood. J Pediatr Surg 1983;18:857.
152. Heiser JC, Rutherford RB, Ringel SP. Thymectomy for myasthenia gravis: a changing perspective. Arch Surg 1982;117:533.
153. Gracey DR, Howard FM Jr, Divertie MB. Plasmapheresis in the treatment of ventilator-dependent myasthenia gravis patients. Report of four cases. Chest 1984;85:739.
154. D'Empaire G, Hoaglin DC, Perlo VP, Pontoppidan H. Effect of prethymectomy plasma exchange on postoperative respiratory function in myasthenia gravis. J Thorac Cardiovasc Surg 1985;89:592.
155. Dau PC, Lindstrom JM, Cassel CK. Plasmapheresis and immunosuppressive drug therapy in myasthenia gravis N Eng J Med 1977;297:1134.
156. Sellin LC. The action of botulism toxin at the neuromuscular junction. Med Biol 1981;59:11.
157. Black RE, Arnon SS. Botulism in the United States, 1976. J Infect Dis 1977;136:829.
158. Wilcox PG, Morrison NJ, Pardy RL. Recovery of the ventilatory and upper airway muscles and exercise performance after type A botulism. Chest 1990;98:62.
159. Wilcox P, Andolfatto G, Fairbarn MS, Pardy RL. Long-term follow-up of symptoms, pulmonary function, respiratory muscle strength, and exercise performance after botulism. Am Rev Respir Dis 1989; 139:15.
160. Hikes DC, Manoli A. Wound botulism. J Trauma 1981;21:68.
161. Keller MA, Miller VH, Berkowitz CD, Yoshimori RN. Wound botulism in pediatrics. Am J Dis Child 1982;136:320.
162. Fullerton P, Gogna NK, Stoddart R. Wound botulism. Med J Aust 1980;1:662.
163. Thorne FL, Kropp RJ. Wound botulism: a life-threatening complication of hand injuries. Plast Reconstr Surg 1983;71:548.
164. Merson MH, Dowell VR Jr. Epidemiologic, clinical and laboratory aspects of wound botulism. N Engl J Med 1973;289:1005.
165. Dowell VR. Infant botulism: new guise for an old disease. Hosp Pract 1978;October.
166. Johnson RO, Clay SA, Arnon SS. Diagnosis and management of infant botulism. Am J Dis Child 1979;133:586.
167. Long SS, Gajewski JL, Brown LW, Gilligan PH. Clinical, laboratory and environmental features of infant botulism in southeastern Pennsylvania. Pediatrics 1985;75:935.
168. Thompson JA, Glasgow LA, Warpinski JR, Olson C. Infant botulism: clinical spectrum and epidemiology. Pediatrics 1980;66:936.
169. Arnon SS, Midura TF, Clay SA, Wood RM, Chin J. Infant botulism. Epidemiological, clinical, and laboratory aspects. JAMA 1977;237:1946.
170. Arnon SS, Damus K, Chin J. Infant botulism: epidemiology and relation to sudden infant death syndrome. Epidemiol Rev 1981;3:45.
171. Arnon SS, Midura TF, Damus K, Thompson B, Wood RM, Chin J. Honey and other environmental risk factors for infant botulism. J Pediatr 1979;94:331.
172. L'Hommedieu CL, Stough R, Brown L, Kettrick R, Polin R. Potentiation of neuromuscular weakness in infant botulism by aminoglycosides. J Pediatr 1979;95:1065.
173. Puggiari M, Cherington M. Botulism and guanidine. Ten years later. JAMA 1978;240:2276.
174. Wolfe JM, Rowe LD. Tracheotomy for infant botulism. Ann Otol 1979;88:861.
175. Terranova W, Palumbo JN, Breman JG. Ocular findings in botulism type B. JAMA 1979;241:475.
176. Lewis SW, Pierson DJ, Cary JM, Hudson LD. Prolonged respiratory paralysis in wound botulism. Chest 1979;75:59.
177. L'Hommedieu C, Polin RA. Progression of clinical signs in severe infant botulism. Clin Pediatr 1981;20:90.
178. Kallenbach J, Lewis M, Zaltzman M, Fritz V, Reef H, Zwi S. Experience with neuromuscular respiratory failure in an intensive care unit. S Afr Med J 1982;61:613.
179. O'Donohue WJ Jr, Baker JP, Bell GM, Muren O, Parker CL, Patterson JL Jr. Respiratory failure in neuromuscular disease: management in a respiratory intensive care unit. JAMA 1976;235:733.
180. Griggs RC, Donohoe KM. The recognition and management of respiratory insufficiency in neuromuscular disease [Editorial]. J Chron Dis 1982;35:497.
181. Brown LW. Differential diagnosis of infant botulism. Rev Infect Dis 1979;1:624.
182. Rochester DF, Arora NS. Respiratory muscle failure. Med Clin North Am 1983;67:573.
183. DeTroyer A, Deisser P. The effects of intermittent positive pressure breathing on patients with respiratory muscle weakness. Am Rev Respir Dis 1981;124:132.
184. Gibson GJ, Pride NB, Davis JN, Loh LC. Pulmonary mechanics in patients with respiratory muscle weakness. Am Rev Respir Dis 1977;115:389.
185. Demedts M, Beckers J, Rochette F, Bulcke J. Pulmonary function in moderate neuromuscular disease without respiratory complaints. Eur J Respir Dis 1982;63:62.
186. Schmidt-Nowara WW, Altman AR. Atelectasis and neuromuscular respiratory failure. Chest 1984;85:792.
187. Black LF, Hyatt RE. Maximal respiratory pressures: normal values and relationship to age and sex. Am Rev Respir Dis 1969;99:696.
188. Black LF, Hyatt RE. Maximal static respiratory pressures in generalized neuromuscular disease. Am Rev Respir Dis 1971;103:641.
189. O'Leary J, King R, Leblanc M, Moss R, Liebhaber M, Lewiston N. Cuirass ventilation in childhood chronic neuromuscular disease. J Pediatr 1979;94:419.
190. Curran FJ. Night ventilation by body respirators for patients in chronic respiratory failure due to late state Duchenne muscular dystrophy. Arch Phys Med Rehabil 1981;62:270.
191. Bach J, Alba A, Pilkington LA, Lee M. Long-term rehabilitation in advanced state of childhood onset, rapidly progressive muscular dystrophy. Arch Phys Med Rehabil 1981;62:328.
192. Alexander MA, Johnson EW, Petty J, Stauch D. Mechanical ventilation of patients with late stage Duchenne muscular dystrophy: management in the home. Arch Phys Med Rehabil 1979;60:289.
193. Padman R, Lawless S, Von Nessen S. Use of BiPAP by nasal mask in the treatment of respiratory insufficiency in pediatric patients: preliminary investigation. Pediatr Pulmonol 1994;17:119.
194. Robertson PL, Roloff DW. Chronic respiratory failure in limb girdle muscular dystrophy: successful long-term therapy with nasal bilevel positive airway pressure. Pediatr Neurol 1994;10:328.
195. Curran FJ, Colbert AP. Ventilator management in Duchenne muscular dystrophy and postpoliomyelitis syndrome: twelve year's experience. Arch Phys Med Rehabil 1989;70:18.
196. Aldrich TK, Prezant DJ. Adverse effects of drugs on the respiratory muscles. Clin in Chest Med 1990;11:177.
197. Segredo V, Caldwell JE, Matthay MA, Sharma ML, Gruenke LD, Miller RD. N Engl J Med 1992;327:524.

198. Barohn RJ, Jackson CE, Rogers SJ, Ridings LW, McVey AL. Prolonged paralysis due to nondepolarizing Neuromuscular blocking agents and corticosteroids. Muscle and Nerve 1994;17:647.
199. Giostra E, Magistris MR, Pizzolato G, Cox J, Chevrolet JC. Neuromuscular disorder in intensive care unit patients treated with pancuronium bromide. Chest 1994;106:210.
200. Gorson KC, Ropper AH. Acute respiratory failure neuropathy: A variant of critical illness polyneuropathy. Crit Care Med 1993;21:267.
201. Sheth RD, Pryse-Phillips WEM, Riggs JE,Bodensteiner JB. Critical illness neuromuscular disease in children manifested as ventilatory dependence. J Pediatr 1995;126:259.
202. Baum GL. Differential diagnosis of chronic respiratory insufficiency. Med Clin North Am 1973;57:623.
203. Richardson RR, Roseman B, Singh N. Diaphragm pacing in spinal muscular atrophy: case report. Neurosurgery 1981;9:317.
204. Sarnat HB, O'Connor T, Byrne PA. Clinical effects of myotonic dystrophy on pregnancy and the neonate. Arch Neurol 1976;33:459.
205. Riley DJ, Santiago TV, Daniele RP, Schall B, Edelman NH. Blunted respiratory drive in congenital myopathy. Am J Med 1977;63:459.
206. McMenamin JB, Curry B, Taylor GP, Becker LE, Murphy EG. Fatal nemaline myopathy in infancy. Can J Neurol Sci 1984;11:305.
207. Rosenow EC III, Engel AG. Acid maltase deficiency in adults presenting as respiratory failure. Am J Med 1978;64:485.
208. Almog C, Fried K, Reif R, Zieghelboim J, Lewinsohn G. Autosomal recessive lipid storage myopathy (probable carnitine deficiency). J Med Genet 1979;16:435.
209. Johnson V, Winternitz WW. Hypokalemic periodic paralysis. South Med J 1984;77:1207.
210. Agusti AGN, Torres A, Estopa R, Agusti-Vidal A. Hypophosphatemia as a cause of failed weaning: the importance of metabolic factors. Crit Care Med 1984;12:142.
211. Braun NMT, Arora NS, Rochester DF. Respiratory muscle and pulmonary function in polymyositis and other proximal myopathies. Thorax 1983;38:616.

Respiratory Failure

Section Two

Section Editor

Randall C. Wetzel

Principles and Practice of Respiratory Support and Mechanical Ventilation

9

Lynn D. Martin
Susan L. Bratton
L. Kyle Walker

Behold, the child was dead . . . and he went up and lay upon the child, put his mouth upon his mouth . . . and the flesh of the child waxed warm. . . .
Kings 4:32-35

INTRODUCTION

Since very early in man's recorded history, the imparting of respiration to an ill, injured, or dying individual has been considered magical or divine in nature. Over the last century, the means of applying this artificial ventilation have evolved from the manual delivery of a breath by an individual to the mechanical application of negative or positive pressure. During the polio epidemics of the 1930's, the use of negative pressure "iron lungs" became widespread throughout the world and led to the development of specialized units for the care of patients with respiratory failure. With the refinement and propagation of the skills necessary for short and long term instrumentation of the airway initially developed in the operating room, the widespread use of positive pressure ventilation became possible in the 1960's. The 1970's were noted for the further improvement in the ability to provide positive pressure ventilation with the introduction of the microprocessor controlled ventilators and the application of positive end-expiratory pressure (PEEP) for acute hypoxemic respiratory failure. The continued increase in morbidity and mortality associated with acute respiratory failure coupled with improved technology, resulted in the development of many experimental forms of mechanical ventilation in the 1980's. Today, the use of mechanical ventilation has become commonplace in the modern intensive care unit of the 1990's. Respiratory therapy is the cornerstone of critical care. Therefore, the delivery of respiratory therapy and mechanical ventilation to acutely ill patients in the intensive care unit requires a thorough understanding of the physiology of ventilation under normal and pathologic conditions, familiarity with the technical aspects of respiratory support modalities, and a clear appreciation for the beneficial and detrimental physiologic consequences that arise from their use. The complexity of respiratory support is further compounded in the pediatric population by the unique needs of the actively growing and developing child. The modern pediatric intensivist is constantly challenged to support ventilatory needs for this population and they must have a meticulous understanding of the principles and practice in the delivery of respiratory support and mechanical ventilation.

The goals of respiratory support in the pediatric intensive care unit (PICU) are a direct extension of the common ventilatory needs of the critically ill as well as the specific requirements of the growing and developing child. Obviously the principal function of the respiratory system (i.e. gas exchange) depends on the provision of a patent airway. Measures to achieve this goal are of primary importance (see chapter 2). Once the security of the airway is assured, attention is directed towards the second goal: maintenance of adequate respiratory gas exchange (oxygen delivery and carbon dioxide clearance from the pulmonary capillaries). Therapy designed to achieve this goal may be as simple as the delivery of supplemental oxygen or as complex as the provision of total ventilatory support by mechanical means that mimic normal respiratory patterns or the use of nonconventional means such as low tidal volume, high frequency ventilation. It must be clearly understood that the maintenance of normal gas exchange is in reality two separate goals (oxygenation and ventilation). Measures designed to increase lung volume and improve oxygenation may be associated with increased deadspace ventilation which decreases alveolar ventilation and carbon dioxide clearance. Third, respiratory management strategies should be designed to preserve normal respiratory mechanics through such interventions as chest physiotherapy and tracheobronchial toilet. Fourth, a goal that is particularly important to children, is to minimize the metabolic expenditures of the respiratory system (i.e. work of breathing). Examples of these objectives in children include infants with chronic respiratory failure (i.e. bronchopulmonary dysplasia) in whom efforts to decrease the work of breathing may redirect caloric intake towards growth and development[1] or in the setting of circulatory shock where decreases in metabolic ex-

TABLE 9.1. Usable Duration Chart for "E" Cylinder Oxygen Source at Various Liter Flows and Internal Pressures

	Internal pressures (psig)[a]										
Liters/min	*2200*	*2000*	*1800*	*1600*	*1400*	*1200*	*1000*	*800*	*600*	*400*	*200*
12	51	46	42	37	32	28	23	18	14	9	4
10	61	56	50	44	39	33	28	22	16	11	5
8	77	70	63	56	49	42	35	28	21	14	7
7	88	80	72	64	56	48	40	32	24	16	8
6	102	93	84	74	65	56	46	37	28	18	9
5	123	112	100	89	78	67	56	44	33	22	11
4	154	140	126	112	98	84	70	56	42	28	14
3	205	186	168	149	130	112	98	74	56	37	18
2	308	280	252	224	196	168	140	112	84	56	28

[a] *To determine the remaining time of use in minutes of an "E" cylinder, locate the column at the top of the table that coincides with cylinder pressure. Follow that column down until it intersects the line that reflects prescribed liter flow. Duration of flow in minutes = [cylinder pressure (psig) = 0.28]/flow (liters/min).*

penditures may allow the shunting of blood to attenuate anoxic injury to vital organs[2]. Lastly, respiratory management can be designed to provide an abnormal ventilatory pattern for therapeutic purposes such as deliberate hyperventilation for pulmonary hypertension[3]. Regardless of the therapeutic objective, these goals of respiratory support must be clearly kept in mind. An understanding of the pathophysiologic process can be used to direct therapy towards interventions designed specifically to circumvent or assuage the specific respiratory impediment.

RESPIRATORY THERAPY

The support of respiratory function in critically ill children involves many modalities besides mechanical ventilation. These include such therapies as medical gas therapy, aerosol administration, and chest physiotherapy. Medical gases (oxygen, air, helium, nitric oxide) are delivered in an attempt to support whole body, organ, and cellular physiology. Medications are administered via aerosol into the respiratory tract to relieve bronchospasm and combat infection. Finally, chest physiotherapy is designed to enhance removal of pulmonary secretions and improve the distribution of gas throughout the lungs.

Medical Gas Therapy

Providing gases of special composition is one of the most frequently used and unappreciated modalities in the modern medical care. This therapy alone or in association with mechanical ventilation is life saving. Three gases (oxygen, air, and helium) comprise the vast majority of medical gas mixtures used in clinical settings, although the therapeutic potential of a fourth (nitric oxide) has only recently been recognized. Since air is used therapeutically only in conjunction with oxygen, only the three remaining gases will be discussed here.

Normobaric Oxygen Therapy

Oxygen therapy is the most common intervention used in the management of respiratory disease. The ubiquitous nature of oxygen therapy in pediatric intensive care tends to foster a casual attitude toward its application. Nevertheless, it must be recalled that the administration of an enriched concentration of oxygen has well-characterized (and potentially catastrophic) toxic effects on the lung and, in the newborn, on the retina. Consequently, oxygen therapy must be administered conscientiously in a manner similar to any other pharmacologic agent.

Technical Aspects of Oxygen Therapy

Medical gas sources for oxygen therapy are of two types[4,5]. *Wall oxygen sources* found in inpatient facilities are supplied by bulk liquid oxygen stores that gradually are warmed and evaporated. Regulations require that wall oxygen sources in the United States provide a working pressure of 50 psi to all outlets in these facilities. This guarantees at least 35 psi driving pressure required by most commercially available mechanical ventilators. Alternatively, *gas cylinders* are used as a source of medical gases. Oxygen cylinders, which operate at internal pressures of 1800-2400 psi, are available in sizes providing 350-7000 liters of gas at room temperature and pressure. The usable duration of a given cylinder is determined by its gas capacity and the rate of gas flow; charts are available that allow the estimation of time to cylinder emptying **(Table 9.1).** The construction, use, and transport of medical gas cylinders in the United States is rigidly controlled by federal and local government statutes[6].

Medical gas sources must be interfaced with administration devices that reduce the system working pressure between the gas source and the patient. In its simplest form, this pressure reducing function is performed by one or more *reducing valves* that drop working pressure from high-pressure gas sources (i.e., cylinder or wall oxygen outlet) to the commonly used medical gas driving pressure of 50 psi. These spring-loaded valves can be placed at single stages in the circuitry or in series with one another to provide multistage reduction in working pressure.

A further drop in system pressure is provided by a *flowmeter;* generally consisting of a needle valve assembly that allows regulation of flow distal to the reducing valve and visualization of the gas flow rate form the system (Fig. 9.1)[4,7]. Manipulation of the flow control allows opening

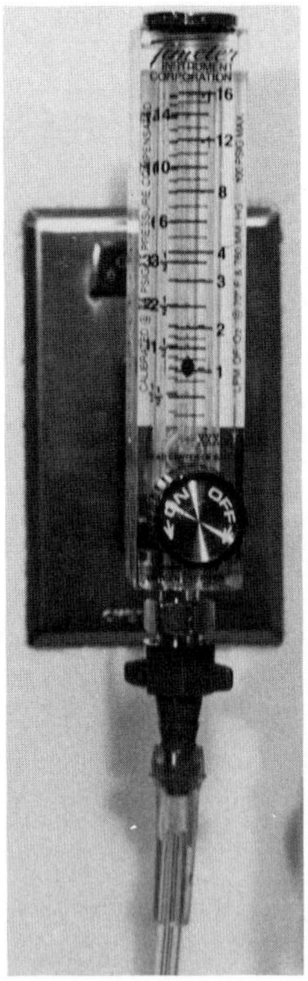

Figure 9.1. Medical gas flowmeter with adjustable flow control and "float-type" flow indicator.

and closing of the valve orifice and adjustment of flow rate. Most commercially available flow meters incorporate "back pressure compensation" so that introduction of flow resistance distal to the needle valve does not result in spuriously elevated flow readings[4,8]. Consequently, impedance to flow in the circuitry distal to the flowmeter is detected by noting a drop in system flow, and this is accurately indicated on the flowmeter (Fig. 9.2).

Devices that combine the functions of a reducing valve (reduction of system working pressure) and a flowmeter (control and measurement of delivered flow) are known as *gas regulators* (Fig. 9.3). Gas regulators usually incorporate a pressure gauge for monitoring system working pressure as well as a downstream needle valve flowmeter for regulation of flow to the patient.

Oxygen Delivery Systems

Oxygen delivery systems may be thought of in two categories: (a) high-flow systems in which the gas flow from the device meets all patient inspiratory requirements; and (b) low-flow systems in which gas flow may be insufficient to meet total patient inspiratory requirements; therefore, room air or gas in the surrounding atmosphere is entrained and mixed with that of the delivery system to provide the inspiratory concentration of oxygen. It should be noted that reference to the system as either high flow or low flow in no way reflects the FiO_2 potential of inspired gases from the delivery device. The decision to employ either a low-flow or high-flow delivery system is determined by consideration of (a) patient comfort, (b) desired FiO_2, (c) need to control the FiO_2, and (d) need for humidification of inspired gases.

Oxygen delivery systems referred to as 'high flow' usually incorporate a Venturi-type device using the Bernoulli principle to entrain atmospheric gases. The result is augmented bulk gas flow. High-flow systems may be used with

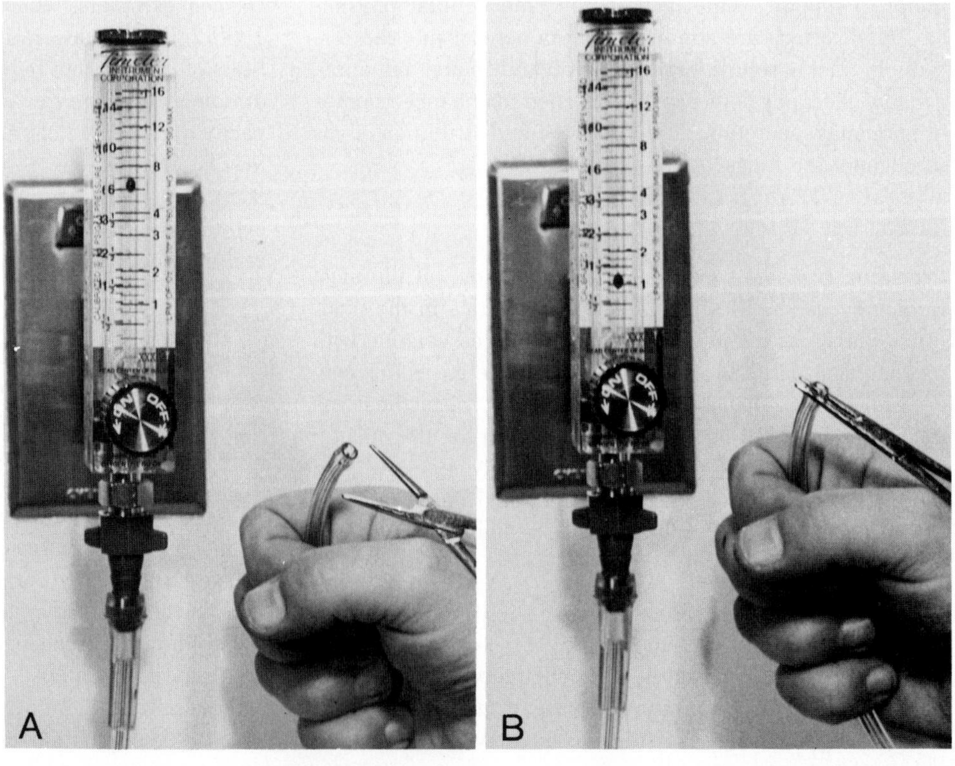

Figure 9.2. Flowmeter back-pressure compensation. A. Flowmeter delivering unimpeded oxygen flow through tubing. B. When gas flow output is decreased by partial occlusion of the delivery tubing, diminished flow output is accurately reflected by the flowmeter.

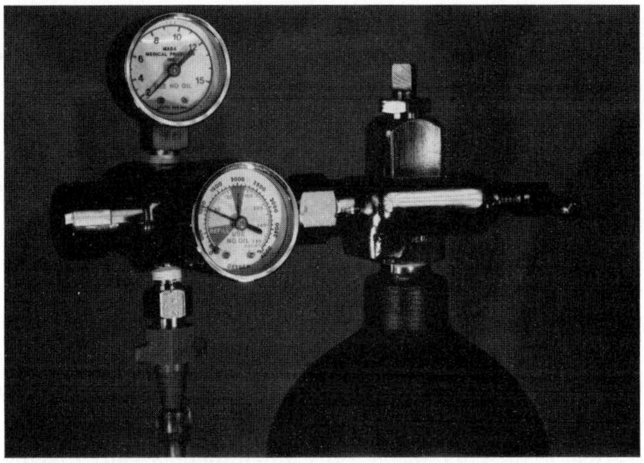

Figure 9.3. Gas regulator mounted to oxygen cylinder.

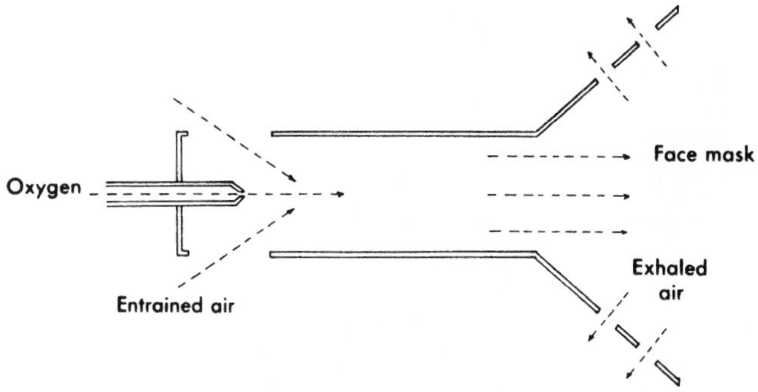

Figure 9.4. Gas delivery system of air entrainment mask. High oxygen flow velocity results in entrainment of air through the entrainment ports, thereby diluting oxygen concentration delivered to the patient. Increasing the velocity of oxygen flow, or increasing the size of the air entrainment ports, results in increased air entrainment and lower inspired oxygen concentration. (From Egan DF. Fundamentals of respiratory therapy. 3rd ed. St. Louis: CV Mosby, 1977:306.)

masks, tracheostomy collars, tents, and hoods. High-flow systems include such devices as oxygen nebulizers used for aerosol generation or simply "Venturi masks" themselves. Venturi masks deliver fixed concentrations at 24%, 28%, 31%, 35%, 40% and 50% oxygen. Nebulizers utilizing the Venturi principle are capable of delivering FiO_2's in the range of 30-100%. Advantages of the high-flow systems are: (a) there is a consistent and accurate FiO_2 delivery independent of changes in the patient's ventilatory pattern; (b) temperature and humidity may be controlled as the total inspired atmosphere is being provided; and (c) FiO_2 is easily and directly measured. Disadvantages of high-flow systems include: (a) augmented gas flow yields is expensive, and (b) high gas flow may be uncomfortable.

Low-flow systems may yield concentrations of oxygen between 25% and 100%. It should be noted that low-flow oxygen delivery devices, in the absence of reservoir capabilities, do not reliably provide a consistent and accurate FiO_2. Low-flow technology includes: (a) nasal cannulae (nasal prongs), (b) simple face masks, and (c) masks with reservoir capabilities (nonrebreather face mask, partial rebreather face mask). Low-flow delivery devices are more economical and enhance patient comfort, but they have a lack of accuracy and dependability.

Oxygen Delivery Equipment

Venturi systems typically operate on the Bernoulli principle. Oxygen is introduced through a "jet" orifice with subsequent entrainment of atmospheric gases through side ports in the device, distal to the strictured orifice (Fig. 9.4). Dependable oxygen concentrations in the range of 24-50% are available by manufacturers of Venturi mask systems (Fig. 9.5) as long as total gas flow exceeds the patient's peak inspiratory flow[4,9]. Because the FiO_2 is dependent on a given oxygen-to-air entrainment ratio, manufacturers usually recommend the operating flow rates. As mentioned earlier, oxygen nebulizers generally used to power aerosol delivery devices also utilize the Venturi adaptation of the Bernoulli principle. In these systems, the FiO_2 is independent of the patient's minute ventilation, provided the patient's inspiratory flow rate does not exceed that of the delivery device. It must be noted that Venturi systems are capable of providing consistent and accurate FiO_2s; however, any degree of distal back pressure will inhibit the entrainment of atmospheric gases and thus elevate FiO_2 for any given flow rate.

Nasal cannulae (nasal prongs) are low-flow oxygen delivery systems operating at flow rates of 0.1-6 liters/min (Fig. 9.6). Most nasal prongs have a curve in the prong design to direct air posteriorly toward the turbinates where the gas will be properly humidified. Nasal cannulae have the advantage of being less restrictive than mask devices and therefore potentially better tolerated by children[4]. The major disadvantage is not being able to measure the FiO_2 clinically[10], but they are generally thought to deliver FiO_2s in the range of 24-50%. FiO_2 delivery is a function of the entrainment of atmospheric gases (occurring with patient inspiratory flow rate and volume) mixing with source gas in the anatomic dead space. Nasal oxygen delivery is not less effective in "mouth breathers." The upper airway is in communication with the remainder of the airway and the deliv-

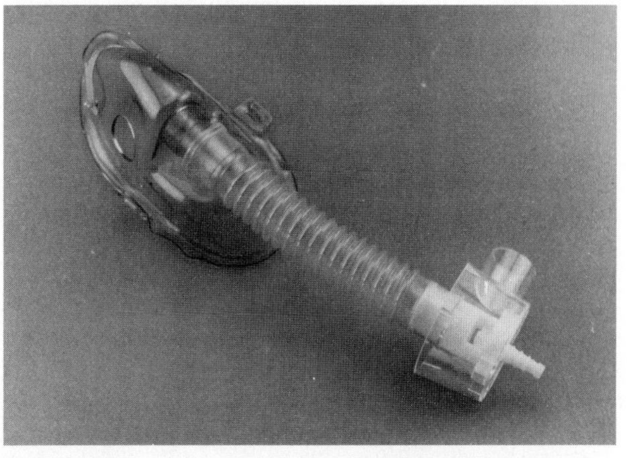

Figure 9.5. Air entrainment (Venturi) mask with adjustable air entrainment system.

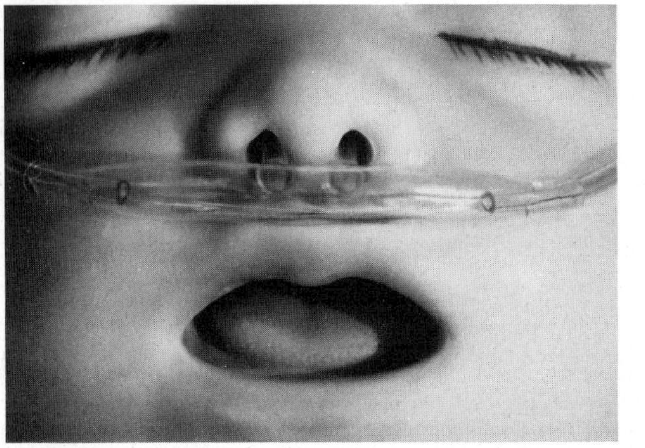

Figure 9.6. Nasal cannula with prongs properly positioned in anterior nares of infant.

ery system is based on the entrainment of atmospheric gases.

Simple face masks were developed in 1789 by Ingenhouse. Today's design is similar and frequently used[11]. Simple face masks are low-flow oxygen delivery systems operating at approximately 6-10 liters/min (Fig. 9.7). The FiO_2 is dependent on the capacity of the oxygen delivery flow rate to flush dead space and the inspiratory flow rate of the patient, but it can approach 35-55%. Typically, the patient's inspiratory flow rate exceeds that of the delivery system with subsequent oxygen dilution by entrainment of atmospheric air through ports in the mask or around the periphery of the mask. Exhalation of gases occurs in the reverse direction.

Nonrebreathing face masks incorporate a reservoir bag with a gas inflow system and a face mask (Fig. 9.8). As the name implies, exhaled gases are eliminated and each patient's inspiratory volume consists of fresh gas. Nonrebreathing face masks typically have a one-way valve between the reservoir bag and the face mask. This allows gas to enter the dead space of the mask, while the presence of this one-way valve prevents exhaled gas from entering the reservoir bag. Another one-way valve is found on the exhalation port of the mask. This one-way valve allows exhalation of gases while preventing entrainment of atmospheric gases. It must be mentioned that the "ideal" nonrebreathing system would be tight fitting with one-way valves on both exhalation ports, thus eliminating any possibility of atmospheric gas entrainment. However, it is common practice to leave one port open in the event that gas flow to the system is interrupted, thereby allowing the patient access to an inspiratory gas source. Nonrebreathing systems are capable of delivery up to 100% oxygen, provided the gas flow to the reservoir system is sufficient to maintain bag distention throughout the respiratory cycle[4,12].

Partial rebreathing masks are similar in design to the nonrebreathing system in that it incorporates a reservoir bag with a gas inflow system and a face mask. The difference lies in the absence of one-way valve mechanisms that provide unidirectional gas flow. As the name implies, part of the patient's exhaled gas or the anatomic dead space gas volume is allowed to reenter the reservoir bag. Since anatomic dead space gas does not participate in gas exchange, it is assumed to be almost entirely source gas (with the exception of a negligible quantity of CO_2). This exhaled gas, combined with the fresh gas, flows into the reservoir bag, forcing the remaining two-thirds of exhaled gas through the exhalation ports in the mask. The danger with partial rebreathing systems is that they are often mistaken for nonrebreathing systems. This could clearly have unfortunate consequences in emergent situations; therefore, some authorities believe there is no place for the partial rebreathing system in the critical care setting. Furthermore, it would simply be more cost effective to remove the valve mechanisms from the nonrebreathing system, should an instance arise where the partial rebreathing system is desired. In this case, should source gas be interrupted, there are two open ports in the partial rebreathing mask structure that allow the patient to draw in atmospheric gases.

Oxygen hoods, generally supplied with source gas from high-flow nebulizer systems incorporating the Venturi adaptation of the Bernoulli principle, provide an unencumbered alternative for gas delivery to the infant (0-6 months) (Fig. 9.9). Hoods, which cover the patient from the neck up, are generally made of plastic, with a removable lid providing easy access to the patient. The trunk and extremities are not involved and, therefore, remain available for ac-

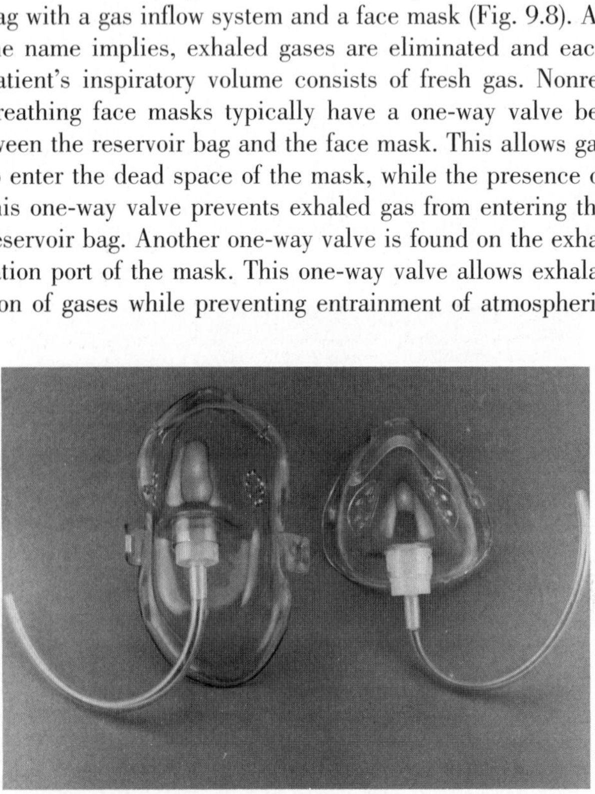

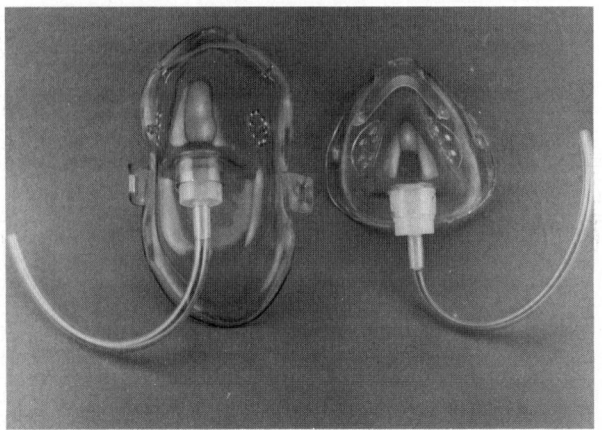

Figure 9.7. Simple oxygen masks, adult and infant sizes.

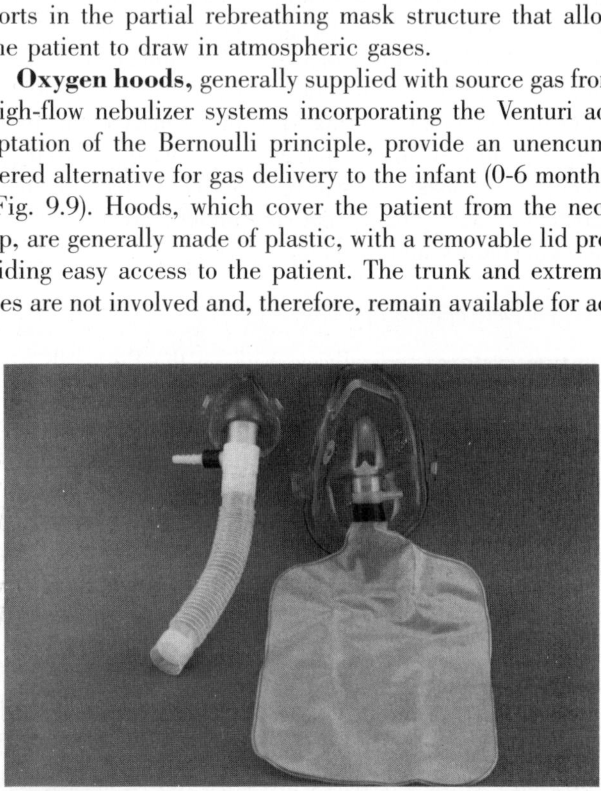

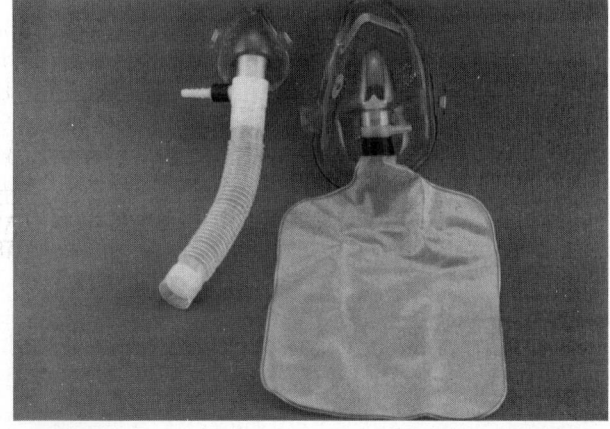

Figure 9.8. Nonrebreathing masks, infant and adult configurations.

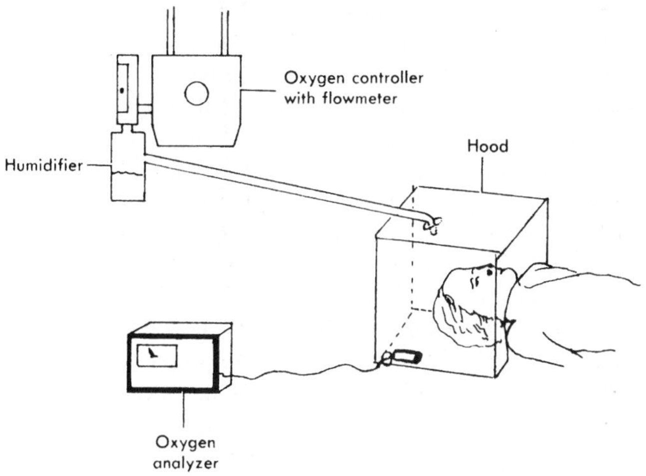

Figure 9.9. Gas delivery system used with oxygen hood. (From McPherson SP. Respiratory therapy equipment. 2nd ed. St Louis: CV Mosby, 1981:98.)

cess and examination. The volume contained within the hood is small enough for quick recovery time of oxygen concentration, yet large enough such that the patient's entire tidal volume may be taken from within the enclosure. Although accurate control of inspired oxygen is possible, it has been shown that oxygen concentration can vary as much as 20% from the top to the bottom of the hood[13]. Therefore, careful analysis of oxygen concentration within the hood is desirable. Another, perhaps intuitive consideration, is that the source gas should be heated to minimize heat loss from the large surface area of the head and face of the infant.

Oxygen tents, historically called "croup tents," were introduced into medical practice in the 1920's but have generally fallen out of vogue. Oxygen tents require high flows of 20-40 L/min to deliver 40-50% oxygen while maintaining CO_2 less than 1%. They are looked on with disdain for four reasons: (a) maintenance of body temperature is difficult; (b) FiO_2 is variable and cannot exceed approximately 50%; (c) access to the patient without removal from the oxygen-rich environment is limited; and (d) observation of the child is compromised.

Hazards of Oxygen Therapy

The administration of oxygen is not without risks. These include physical risks associated with enhanced support for combustion, physiologic changes in response to changes in PaO_2, and cellular toxicity from hyperoxia. Elevation of PaO_2 stimulates reflexes regulating ventilation and perfusion. Ventilatory depression can occur in patients with chronic pulmonary disease who depend on a hypoxic stimulus to breathe. Generally hyperoxia decreases pulmonary vascular resistance, while systemic vascular resistance increases with a resulting drop in cardiac output. Oxygen administration is also known to depress erythropoiesis and cause retinal damage in addition to the well recognized toxicity in the lungs[14].

PHYSIOLOGIC CHANGES IN LUNG FUNCTION. While human volunteers exposed to an FiO_2 of 1.0 for up to 6 hours have no changes in measured lung function, continued exposure is associated with a rapid decline in vital capacity occurring after 60 hours[15]. Initial changes in vital capacity may in part be due to chest pain. Exposure to an FiO_2 of 1.0 after several hours causes pain and cough [16]. The onset of pain coincides with cough and tracheal inflammation. Mucous clearance and ciliary function decrease when exposed to hyperoxia[17]. However, the more important causes of decreased vital capacity as hyperoxic lung injury progresses are capillary leak, decreased surfactant activity and atelectasis[18].

Oxygen therapy causes endothelial cell injury and impairs capillary endothelial integrity. Bronchoalveolar lavage fluid from normal subjects exposed to 95% FiO_2 for 17 hours demonstrated a significant amount of protein leakage [19]. Furthermore, increasing levels of inspired oxygen have been associated with increased protein concentration in the bronchoalveolar fluid[20]. In addition to protein-rich fluid in the alveolar spaces, respiratory compliance is further compromised in hyperoxic injury by decreased surfactant activity. Reports on surfactant synthesis in hyperoxia induced lung injury have varied; however, the majority of studies suggest that surfactant activity is decreased and that treatment with surfactant diminishes lung injury and improves compliance[18,21,22]. Surfactant activity may be decreased from injury to type II pneumocytes, resulting in decreased surfactant production and by surfactant inactivation by intra-alveolar edema[23]. The exact contribution of each mechanism is unclear.

Absorption atelectasis occurs when alveolar gas diffuses into the pulmonary circulation more rapidly than it is replaced by ventilation. The inert gas, nitrogen, which comprises just under 80% of room air, tends to maintain alveolar volume, but replacement of nitrogen with increasing amounts of oxygen which rapidly diffuses, can result in progressive atelectasis. Disease processes that cause poor ventilation of some lung units exacerbate the risk of absorption atelectasis because of increased inspired oxygen concentration[24].

OXYGEN TOXICITY. It would seem ironic that the very existence of humans is fully dependent on a gas that, in excess quantities is toxic and lethal. While it must be understood that oxygen is the mainstay of our clinical inventory to combat hypoxemia, exposure to high concentrations of oxygen will cause pulmonary injury. Although the onset of oxygen toxicity may vary from patient to patient, the contributing elements seem to be constant: (a) the fraction of inspired oxygen, (b) the length of exposure, and (c) the patient's underlying lung disease[25,26]. It is noteworthy that the FiO_2 is probably not the universal factor determining toxicity of oxygen; rather, that factor is the partial pressure of inspired oxygen:

$$PiO_2 = (P_b - P_{H_2O}) \times FiO_2,$$

where P_b is the barometric pressure and P_{H_2O} is the partial pressure of water. At sea level (1 atm) and 37°C, the P_{H_2O}

is 47 torr. The PiO_2 will increase for any FiO_2 as the P_b increases (plunging below sea level) and likewise will decrease if the elevation increases. Hence, while exposure to 21 percent oxygen may cause parenchymal lung injury at 6 atm (PiO_2 = 900 torr), 100% oxygen exposure may have negligible consequences at ⅓ atm (PiO_2 = 235 torr). Oxygen toxicity may also be delayed by interrupting exposures to high concentration for brief periods several times a day[25].

The exact level of oxygen that causes lung disease in humans has not been established. Factors such as age, nutritional status, previous exposure to oxidants, antioxidants and the underlying lung disease may all affect a patient's susceptibility to develop hyperoxic injury. However, at sea level an FiO_2 less than 0.5 can be tolerated for prolonged periods of time without serious effects in normal lungs[27].

Oxygen radicals, which are normal metabolic byproducts, are the major cause of oxygen toxicity. To generate adenosine triphosphate, the electron transport chain of the mitochondria reduces oxygen into two water molecules. During this process, a number of oxygen related products are formed (Fig. 9.10), but are normally bound tightly by cytochrome oxidase. These products include superoxide and hydrogen peroxide which have direct toxic effects, but more importantly in the presence of metals react to produce even more dangerous species: the hydroxyl free radical and singlet oxygen[28]. Hyperoxia provides increased oxygen as a substrate and the concentration of these intracellular reactive products increases[29-31]. They are highly reactive, especially the hydroxyl free radical, and can ultimately cause cellular damage by lipid peroxidation of polyunsaturated fats, depolymerization of mucopolysaccharides, DNA damage, alteration of proteins by sulfhydryl oxidation leading to enzyme inactivation, and activation of arachidonic acids[32,33].

In addition to free radical damage, both the cyclooxygenase and lipoxygenase pathway products have been implicated with hyperoxic lung injury[34-36]. Administration of cyclooxygenase inhibitors, which may be associated with increased lipoxygenase pathway products, has been shown to increase lung injury[35,37]. Administration of a lipoxygenase inhibitor has been shown to attenuate hyperoxic lung injury in rats and decrease leukotriene B_4 concentration[38,39]; however, the exact role of the arachidonic acid metabolites and hyperoxia induced lung injury remains incompletely understood[40].

Tolerance to oxygen toxicity may develop from decreased production of oxygen radicals as a result of decreased cellular respiration, from upregulation of protective enzymes, and by increased vitamin A concentrations which inactivate the free radicals via a nonenzymatic reaction. In addition, the body has three enzyme systems that protect against oxygen radicals: superoxide dismutase, catalase and glutathione peroxidase (Fig. 9.10)[41,42]. Superoxide dismutase accelerates the conversion of superoxide and hydrogen to oxygen and hydrogen peroxide, limiting the production of the more toxic hydroxyl radical or singlet oxygen. The enzyme catalase converts hydrogen peroxide into water and oxygen. Finally, glutathione peroxidase augments the binding of glutathione to oxygen radicals producing lipid hydroxides and water. Glutathione peroxidase is the major enzyme system preventing protein sulfhydryl oxidation which can lead to intracellular enzyme inactivation. Furthermore, glutathione can reverse the oxidation of protein sulfhydryls. Vitamin E (alpha tocopherol) is a nonenyzmatic antioxidant that is lipid soluble and can donate a hydrogen atom, thereby stopping lipid peroxidation, thus making vitamin E a potentially important defender of cell membranes.

Acute hyperoxia lung injury causes increased lung water and protein leak into the interstitial and alveolar spaces. This is because of damage to capillary endothelial and alveolar epithelial cells[41]. Pathologic changes in the lung as a result of oxygen therapy has been extensively studied in animals[43-47]. Injury has been divided into three phases:

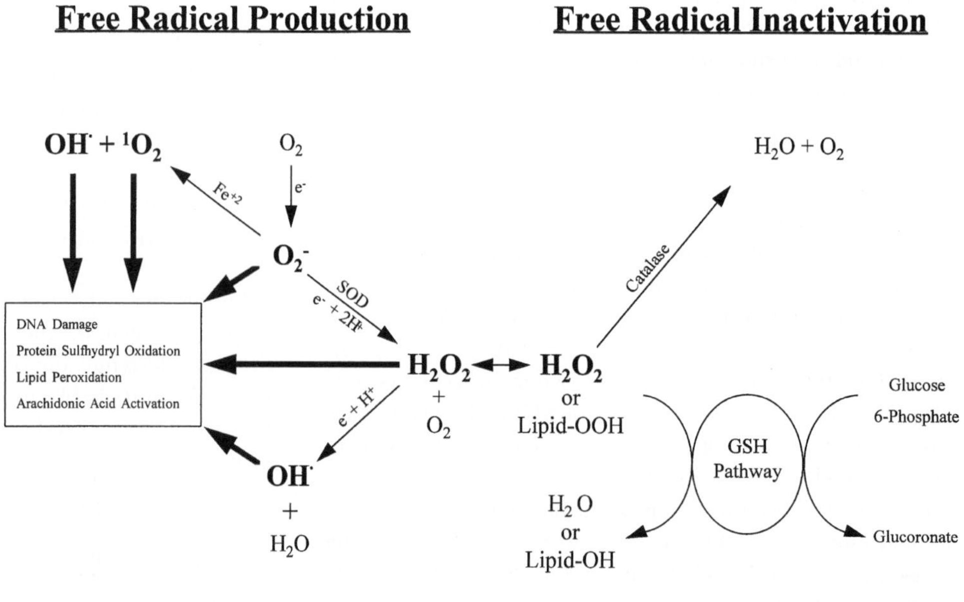

Figure 9.10. The pathogenic mechanisms of oxygen related free radical production and the enzymatic pathways of free radical inactivation which limit oxidative injury to the tissues. Free radical inactivation occurs through three distinct enzymatic reactions: superoxide dismutase (SOD), catalase, and glutathione (GSH) enzymatic pathway. The GSH enzymatic pathway utilizes GSH peroxidase, GSH reductase, and glucose-6-phosphate dehydrogenase generated NADPH to inactivate both hydrogen peroxide and lipid peroxides. O_2 = oxygen, O_2^- = superoxide anion, H_2OO_2 = hydrogen peroxide, OH = hydroxyl radical, $^1O_2$ = singlet excited oxygen.

(1) the latent phase which ranges from 1 to 3 days in animals and is associated with no pathologic changes, (2) the inflammatory phase in which atelectasis, edema and alveolar hemorrhage develop, and (3) the final destructive phase marked by hyaline deposition and proliferation of type II alveolar pneumocytes. During the inflammatory phase, early changes in endothelial cell structure occur, leading to pericapillary fluid accumulation[48] and macrophage, neutrophil and platelet aggregation in the lungs with the release of mediators of inflammation[49,50]. Capillary endothelial cell injury appears to occur earlier than alveolar epithelial cell damage. Endothelial cells are exposed to free radicals and other inflammatory mediators in the serum released from the gathering neutrophils and platelets, while the alveolar epithelial cells are not directly exposed to these products. Moreover, the anti-oxidant defenses of the epithelial and endothelial cells may also differ. The rapidity of disease progression varies by species but is clearly accelerated by increased concentrations of oxygen.

Hyperbaric Oxygen Therapy

Hyperbaric oxygen therapy (HBO) is a highly specialized extension of conventional oxygen therapy directed at achieving one of two therapeutic goals. The first goal is the compression of gasses in isolated body cavities which is the rationale for HBO therapy in decompression sickness and air embolization. The second and more obvious goal is to deliver extremely high partial pressure of oxygen (greater than 760 torr) in the blood and tissues. Under normobaric conditions in room air the partial pressure of oxygen in the alveoli (P_AO_2) is: $P_AO_2 = FiO_2 \times P_b$ $(0.21 \times 760 \text{ torr}) = 159.6$ torr. This value at 2.8 atmospheres (a common treatment pressure) becomes: $0.21 \times (2.8 \times 760 \text{ torr}) = 446.9$ torr. If the fraction of inspired oxygen is increased to 1.0, then the P_AO_2 increases to $1.0 \times (2.8 \times 760 \text{ torr}) = 2128$ torr. Under these circumstances the amount of dissolved oxygen in the plasma becomes a substantial component of blood oxygen content. For example, at 6 atm (the maximal pressure in hyperbaric chambers) the partial pressure of oxygen in arterial blood (PaO_2) approaches 4400 torr. The amount of dissolved oxygen in the plasma would be: $PaO_2 \times 0.003$ vol%/torr $(4400 \text{ torr} \times 0.003 \text{ vol\%/torr}) = 13.2$ vol% or approximately 65% of the arterial oxygen content found in adults under normobaric conditions. The elevation in blood and tissue PO_2 from HBO therapy results in a marked increase in the mass action of oxygen and enhances its activity in cellular chemical reactions.

Unfortunately, the therapeutic potential of HBO is limited by the severity and rapidity of oxygen toxicity. To minimize the risk of this complication, HBO therapy is usually achieved by the intermittent inhalation of enriched oxygen gas mixtures at a pressure greater than sea level (usually 2 to 3 atm). HBO therapy may be done in a multiplace chamber in which the patient breathes an FiO_2 of 1.0 through a mask, head tent or endotracheal tube within the pressurized chamber or in a monochamber where the entire chamber is pressurized with 100% oxygen. One advantage of the multichamber in ICU medicine is that a caregiver can be within the chamber to administer care to a critically ill patient. The utility of HBO therapy is also limited by the requirement for specialized equipment and personnel. Consequently, HBO programs are limited in number and location, further restricting application of the treatment to the critically ill population. Delivery of intensive care therapies within the chamber is technically difficult. No electronic displays are allowed within the chamber while it is pressurized as a result of fire risk in the enriched oxygen environment. Although the ventilator and monitoring devices are pressurized within the multichamber unit, the electrical components of the equipment must be detachable and remain outside the chamber. Ventilators that are approved for use in the pressurized environment are the Siemens Servo 900C and the Oxford Penlon. Monitors and ventilators used with the monochamber are outside the chamber with tubing passing into the chamber. Because of these technical difficulties and limited expertise, many hyperbaric facilities do not provide therapy for children requiring mechanical ventilation.

Approximately 198 hyperbaric centers were in operation in the United States during 1995 and utilization of HBO therapy has increased for diseases in which increased arterial or tissue oxygen offer theoretic advantages. Between 1982 and 1992 approximately 105,000 patients received HBO therapy in the United States and Canada[51]. However, many applications of HBO therapy have not been evaluated by randomized trials and remain of questioned efficacy. Recommendations for the use of HBO therapy are now reviewed by the Undersea and Hyperbaric Medical Society and conditions that are currently approved by the society and for payment by Blue Cross/ Blue Shield funding have been defined **(Table 9.2)**[52,53].

History

HBO was first used by Albert Behnke and the United States Navy for decompression sickness in 1939[54]. Early work on the physiologic effects of HBO was spurred by World War II when the safety limits of oxygen breathing were needed for frogmen. The closed-circuit breathing gear worn

TABLE 9.2. Disorders Approved for Hyperbaric Oxygen Therapy

Decompression illness
Air embolism
Clostridial myonecrosis
Necrotizing soft-tissue infections
Osteomyelitis (refractory)
Acute traumatic ischemias (compartment syndrome)
Skin grafts and flaps (compromised)
Radiation tissue damage
Smoke inhalation
Carbon monoxide poisoning
Cyanide poisoning
Thermal burns
Anemia due to excessive blood loss

by the seamen required pure oxygen to prevent telltale bubbles. At that time, HBO was known to cause seizures in most subjects if administered in excess. Volunteers in naval research units swam at various depths with differing levels of exercise and cold until seizures developed to establish broad safety limits. It is now well established that most subjects will have seizures if exposed to an FiO_2 of 1.0 at 3 atmospheres for greater than 3 hours.

From this and subsequent work, it is known that HBO has potential deleterious effects on various organ systems throughout the body. Decreased lung compliance develops after breathing FiO_2 at 2 atm for approximately 6 hours. However, repeated 1 to 2 hour treatments of FiO_2 at 2 atm do not reduce vital capacity and compliance in humans[(27)]. HBO also alters cardiac function by increasing systemic vascular resistance 30-60% through a reflex vasoconstriction in response to hyperoxia. Cardiac output concurrently decreases 24-35%[(55)]. HBO is also toxic to the eyes and peripheral nerves. Repeated short doses causes progressive myopia which usually resolves after therapy; however, prolonged treatment regimens can lead to cataract formation and neuropathies[(56)].

Contraindications

Absolute contraindications for HBO therapy include: untreated pneumothorax which can progress to a tension pneumothorax while in the chamber and use of certain medications (disulfiran, cis-platinum or adriamycin)[(57,58)]. Hyperoxia appears to increase the toxicity of some chemotherapeutic agents. For example, disulfiran inhibits superoxide dismutase and increases oxygen toxicity.

Several relative contraindications also exist. An upper respiratory tract infection and chronic sinusitis impede equalization of pressure in the middle ear. Myringotomy may be required, especially in infants or children with an endotracheal tube which may further obstruct sinus drainage. Seizures occur in approximately 1.3/10,000 hyperbaric treatments, therefore a seizure disorder *per se* is a mild contraindication[(58)]. Hyperoxia will inhibit the hypoxic drive to breathe in patients with chronic lung disease, and failure to decompress slowly can cause pneumothorax in patients with cystic lung disease. Finally, HBO can cause an acute hemolytic crisis in patients with spherocytosis.

Clinical Uses

DECOMPRESSION SICKNESS AND ARTERIAL AIR EMBOLISM. Decompression sickness (the bends) is caused by excessively rapid decompression when moving from an increased to a decreased ambient pressure. Bubbles and gas containing cavities within the body are subject to the mechanical effects of changing pressure as stated by Boyles Law: PV = nRT, where P is pressure, V is volume, n is number of moles, R is the gas constant and T is temperature. Although decompression illness can be caused by rapid decompression to as little as 20,000 feet above sea level, it typically occurs after rapid decompression from below sea level. High ambient pressure causes nitrogen to become more soluble in the blood; however, after rapid decompression, nitrogen gas is again poorly soluble, resulting in the development of bubbles in the blood stream that subsequently obstruct the microcirculation and cause ischemic injury to the tissues. For this reason, divers are advised to ascend at no greater than 60 feet/minute. Decompression sickness was the first disease treated with HBO therapy[(54)]. HBO therapy is used in decompression sickness associated with signs of central nervous system, bone or joint ischemia or cases with generalized circulatory insufficiency. Air embolism which is usually an iatrogenic complication but which may also occur after penetrating trauma, is also effectively treated with HBO therapy. Procedures with high risk of air embolism include neurosurgical and cardiac surgery, pulmonary needle biopsies and intravascular catheter use.

Repressurization and treatment with HBO therapy not only causes bubble size to decrease but also with elimination of nitrogen from inspired gas will enhance nitrogen removal from the tissues to the blood. Compression of spherical bubbles at 6 atm results in only a 16% decrease in bubble diameter; however, cylindrical shaped bubbles are decreased in length by one third at 3 atm, and decreased to one sixth the original length at 6 atm. Bubbles that are occlusively lodged in blood vessels are distorted by the vessel and may greatly decrease in volume[(60)]. Although treatment regimens are empiric, the success rate for treatment of the bends is about 96%[(54)]. The usual regimen is an initial excursion to 6 atm and FiO_2 0.5 and then treatment at 3.0 atm with an FiO_2 of 1.0 until symptoms improve. Repeat treatments are warranted until the symptoms resolve or no further progress is made[(61)].

CARBON MONOXIDE POISONING. Carbon monoxide (CO) is a common and potentially fatal poisoning. A French study estimated that 17.5/100,000 persons suffer CO poisoning[(62)]. In the United States approximately 3,800 people die annually from CO poisoning; 1,500 are caused by accidents and the remainder as a result of suicide, making CO the most common fatal poisoning in the United States[(63)].

Carbon monoxide is colorless, odorless, tasteless, and non-irritating gas, making detection difficult. It is produced by the incomplete combustion. Carbon monoxide diffuses rapidly across the alveolar-capillary membrane and binds to hemoglobin (Hb) with a 200 fold greater affinity than oxygen[(64)]. The presence of CO shifts the oxyhemoglobin dissociation curve to the left, thereby exacerbating tissue hypoxia. However, CO affects many aspects of metabolism. Carbon monoxide binds to reduced metallic ions and forms weak associations with proteins, allowing it to bind to myoglobin, reduced cytochromes, guanylate cyclase, and nitric oxide synthase[(65-67)].

Carbon monoxide toxicity cannot be attributed solely to COHb mediated hypoxia[(68)], since a poor correlation exists between CO concentration and clinical toxicity[(69,70)]. Furthermore, delayed onset of neurologic deficits are not uncommon in CO poisonings and occurs in the absence of demonstrable COHb levels[71]. Although the exact pathogenesis remains unclear, several mechanisms in addition to tissue hypoxia have been proposed. Carbon monoxide is known to bind to the cytochromes which may impair electron transport and oxidative metabolism[72]. Furthermore, free radicals are generated in the mitochondria after CO poisoning which then may contribute to membrane peroxidation and cellular injury[73]. Unfortunately the myriad of reactions involving CO have prevented elucidation of the exact mechanisms of CO toxicity. The pathologic hallmark of CO intoxication is bilateral necrosis of the globus pallidus; however, other areas of the brain may also be affected including the cerebral cortex, hippocampus, cerebellum and substantia nigra[74].

Acute symptoms of carbon monoxide poisoning include headache, ataxia and dizziness which can progress to seizures and coma. Myocardial dysfunction, which manifests as dysrhythmias and decreased cardiac output, may also occur.[75] In room air, the half-life of COHb is approximately 5 hours and 20 minutes. This is reduced to 90 minutes with an FiO_2 1.0 at 1 atm. At 3 atm, the COHb half life is decreased to 23 minutes[76]. Although hyperbaric oxygen therapy dramatically decreases the half life of COHb, other mechanisms may be important in the treatment of CO poisoning with HBO. HBO had been shown to prevent granulocyte adhesion to integrins, decreasing the inflammatory response[77]. HBO at greater than 2 atm also decreases lipid peroxidation and may affect CO binding to cytochromes[78]; however, the exact means by which HBO therapy alleviates CO toxicity remain poorly understood.

Clinical studies of HBO therapy for CO poisonings have yielded conflicting results. Goulon reported a series of patients treated with HBO using historical controls who received normobaric oxygen[79]. The mortality in the hyperbaric group was 13% compared to 30% in the normobaric group. However, a randomized trial which studied subjects with mild CO intoxication failed to show a difference in neuropsychologic sequelae between the groups[70]. This study was criticized because some subjects had significant delay in HBO treatment. A similar trial of mildly poisoned patients in which all treated subjects received HBO therapy within 6 hours, reported no neuropsychologic deficits in the HBO group of 30 subjects compared to 23% in the normobaric group[80].

Current indications for HBO therapy in CO poisoning are syncope, myocardial ischemia, arrhythmias, severe neurologic symptoms at presentation including coma, focal deficits or seizures, or persistent deficits several hours into 100% oxygen therapy. Usually patients with CO poisonings are treated with one session of HBO therapy. No consensus exists regarding additional treatments for persistent neurologic deficits.

NECROTIZING INFECTIONS. Hyperbaric oxygen therapy has been used in deep seated tissue aerobic and anaerobic infections. The mechanism by which HBO may help treat these surgical lesions is not by inhibition of bacterial growth in a hyperoxic environment, but rather by improvement in local perfusion via compression of tissue bubbles and improving oxygen dependent leukocyte activation[81]. No studies have randomized children with deep seated tissue infections to HBO or normobaric therapy; however, a recent clinical series described 14 children with group A Streptococcal necrotizing fascitis, a severe and rapidly progressive infection associated with significant morbidity and mortality, in which twelve children received HBO in addition to aggressive surgical debridement with limited morbidity and no deaths[82].

Helium

Helium was discovered by Ramsey in 1895, and was introduced into medicine by Barach in 1934 for treatment of airway obstruction[83]. Helium is a biologically inert gas with a low molecular weight that is insoluble in tissue at 1 atm and does not react with biologic membranes. The principal therapeutic property of helium is its low density (0.179 micropoise) compared to air (1.293 micropoise) and oxygen (1.429 micropoise).

Because of its lower density than nitrogen and oxygen, helium would be predicted to improve gas flow through a narrowed orifice. In this situation, gas flow may be turbulent, laminar or a combination of the two. The presence of turbulent flow is predicted by a Reynolds number of greater than 2000. The Reynolds number is a unitless number defined as: $R_e = \rho\ d\ V/\mu$, where ρ is gas density, d is diameter, V is mean linear gas velocity and μ is the gas viscosity. The driving pressure (P) to achieve a given gas flow is proportional to laminar flow and the square of turbulent flow: $P = k_1$ (laminar flow) $+ k_2$ (turbulent flow)^2, where k_1 and k_2 are constants and k_2 depends on the gas density. Helium would be expected to lower resistance to gas flow compared to air or oxygen by increasing the relative proportion of laminar flow and by decreasing the coefficient k_2 which is proportional to density.

Helium can be administered as a gas mixture with oxygen (heliox). The density of the gas is dependent on the relative percentage of helium compared to oxygen. A mixture of 80% helium and 20% oxygen will have the least density and the greatest decrease in airway resistance (oxygen/helium: 20/80 = 0.429 micropoise, 40/60 = 0.678 micropoise, and 80/20 = 1.178 micropoise)[84]. Because heliox is less dense than air, the resulting decrease in the density of the "carrier" gas and decreased resistance to gas flow may result in an increase in bulk gas flow, oxygen flow and decreased work of breathing[85].

The use of heliox is limited in patients who require high inspired oxygen concentrations, since the decrease in density is generally considered clinically insignificant with less than 60% helium[86]. Obviously, helium must never be blended to deliver a hypoxic mixture (less than 20% oxygen). In most clinical settings, heliox with a minimum concentration of oxygen of 20% is blended with pure oxygen to deliver the desired concentrations of oxygen and helium, thereby preventing the accidental delivery of hypoxic gas delivery. An additional safety is the continuous monitoring of the inspired FiO_2.

Laboratory studies suggest that heliox would be beneficial in reducing resistance associated with turbulent gas flow such as the upper airway of a child with croup[87]. Several case series reported relief of airway obstruction with a 20% oxygen and 80% helium blend[88,89]. A more recent crossover randomized controlled study evaluated children with postextubation stridor[90]. In this study, heliox as 30% oxygen and 70% helium significantly decreased stridor symptoms.

Heliox blends may be useful in lower airways diseases. Studies of normal adults breathing heliox demonstrated an increase in FEV_1 and peak inspiratory flow rates[91]. Several reports have evaluated heliox for treatment of severe asthma[84,92,93]. In all of these studies, heliox improved ventilation at lower airway pressures in both intubated and spontaneous breathing subjects.

Heliox can be administered either with a face mask or with a tent. If a patient receives nebulized therapy, the heliox blend can be used as the carrier gas for administering the medication. In fact, asthmatics treated with nebulized therapy with heliox have enhanced distal deposition of aerosolized particles[94]. Caution must be exercised with the use of heliox in children requiring mechanical ventilation. Ventilator blenders are calibrated for air/oxygen so a separate oxygen analyzer is needed. A more notable problem is related to the change in density of the gas and inaccuracy in tidal volume measurement. Most modern microprocessor ventilators utilize pneumotachographs to measure the pressure differential across a resistor to calculate gas flow. The decrease in gas density will result in a smaller pressure differential and thus lead to a falsely low flow and volume reading. Many clinicians may misinterpret the data and inappropriately increase the tidal volume, thereby defeating one of the potential therapeutic advantages of heliox. Ideally, this problem can be overcome by recalibrating the ventilator or defining conversion factors for the specific heliox blend. In the absence of this information, monitoring peak airway pressures and $PaCO_2$ are the only alternative methods of monitoring therapy.

Nitric Oxide

Nitric oxide (NO) has been recognized as an industrial and cigarette pollutant for many years. It is now known to participate as a second messenger in many physiologic reactions throughout the body, including regulation of vasomotor tone, neurotransmission, immune function, and platelet aggregation[95,96]. However, only the effects of NO in the lung will be discussed.

Physiology and Toxicity

Within the lungs, the vascular endothelium as well as inflammatory cells (neutrophils, macrophages), structural cells (fibroblasts, epithelial, vascular and airway smooth muscle), anatomic nerves, and platelets produce NO. A highly lipid soluble molecule, NO diffuses through the pulmonary interstitium and vascular serosa into the vascular smooth muscle. There it binds to the heme iron of guanylate cyclase stimulating the production of cyclic 3,5'-monophosphate (cGMP). Cyclic GMP causes relaxation of vascular and airway smooth muscle through activation of cGMP-dependent protein kinase. As a result of the unstable nature of the compound, NO has a half-life ranging from 0.1 to 5.0 seconds in physiologic systems[95]. Many questions regarding the movement and the numerous cellular reactions of NO remain to be answered.

NO is synthesized from the terminal guanidine nitrogen of L-arginine by the enzyme nitric oxide synthase which has two major components, the reductase and heme domains. The reductase domain provides reducing equivalents from NADPH to the heme domain where oxidation of L-arginine to citrulline occurs with NO as a byproduct[97]. Several different nitric oxide synthase isoforms have been identified and are generally classified as calcium dependent and "constitutive" or calcium independent and "inducible". Calcium/calmodulin regulation of the constitutive form is universal, while the inducible form is regulated by transcription[98].

Methyl and nitro substitution at the guanidine nitrogen of L-arginine results in L-monomethyl arginine (L-NMMA) and L-arginine methyl ester (L-NAME), two of the most commonly used competitive inhibitors of nitric oxide synthase. The constitutive forms of nitric oxide synthase are more sensitive to L-NAME while the inducible forms are more sensitive to L-NMMA[99]. Newly developed inhibitors such as aminoguanidine are reported to be relatively specific for the inducible enzyme[100]. Excess L-arginine reverses the inhibition of these competitive molecules.

The activity of NO is limited by rapid and avid binding to hemoglobin. NO has a 1500 fold greater affinity for hemoglobin than CO, and binds 5 to 20 times more quickly than oxygen[101]. Eighty to ninety percent of inhaled NO reacts with hemoglobin to form nitrosyl-hemoglobin and methemoglobin. Further reactions with oxygen lead to formation of nitrates and nitrites[102]. These are mostly excreted in the urine, but small amounts are excreted in saliva and stool[103].

Nitrogen dioxide and methemoglobinemia are the major *known* toxic byproducts of NO. The rate of conversion of NO to NO_2 is proportional to the square of the NO concentration, the O_2 concentration, and the residence time of NO and O_2. Nitrogen dioxide is a product of grain fermentation and has long been known to cause silo filler's disease, which is a syndrome of pulmonary edema, hemorrhage, and bronchiolitis obliterans[104]. Nitrogen dioxide levels must be monitored continuously during the administration of NO and should be maintained at less than 1 ppm. Nitrogen dioxide can be removed from the breathing circuit with soda lime[97]. Methemoglobin levels must be monitored. Populations with low methemoglobin reductase concentration (neonates and Native Americans) may develop high methemoglobin concentrations during administration of NO. Fifty to sixty percent of inhaled NO_2 is retained in the lung, reacting with water to form nitric and nitrous acids. Although the Occupational Safety and Health Administration has recommended that work safety limits of NO_2 of less than 5 ppm[105], inhalation of 2 ppm is associated with terminal bronchial epithelial hypertrophy and alveolar hyperplasia in rats[106]. Animal studies also demonstrated increased inflammatory cells and increased cytokines with exposures of 1.5 ppm[107,108].

The effects of NO may not be limited to the lungs. NO can bind to other proteins besides hemoglobin and in the presence of superoxide can generate peroxynitrite which causes lipid peroxidation[109]. NO appears to affect the response of alveolar macrophage[110], decreased platelet adhesion[111] and may have neurotoxicity[112]. The toxicity profile of NO in neonates and children is not well described and the long term developmental effects must be followed closely.

Administration

Administration of NO should include: (1) calibrated tanks of NO that do not exceed 1,000 ppm, (2) delivery systems that allow accurate NO delivery with as low as possible O_2 and NO concentrations as well as short residence time of the gases in the circuit and lungs to minimize NO_2 production, (3) minimal contamination of the environment by scavenging exhaust gases, (4) frequent or continuous monitoring of NO and NO_2 concentrations as can be done with chemiluminescence or electrochemical analyzers, (5) periodic measurement of methemoglobin levels, and (6) the lowest effective concentration of NO should be used[97]. Safe and reliable methods of delivery of NO for intubated patients spontaneously or mechanically breathing with various ventilators or in the non-intubated patient have been described[103].

Clinical Uses

Unlike other vasodilators, NO which is delivered as a gas and rapidly bound by hemoglobin, has marked selective pulmonary vascular effects with minimal to no systemic vasodilatation. Because of these selective effects, NO is now used at many centers for treatment of persistent pulmonary hypertension of the newborn[113,114] and primary pulmonary hypertension[115]. NO therapy clearly improves the majority of neonates with severe persistent pulmonary hypertension, avoiding the need for ECMO support. Unfortunately, the criteria for NO therapy are not currently well established[116]. NO is often used diagnostically for patients with primary pulmonary hypertension to evaluate the reactivity of the pulmonary vascular bed. Inhaled NO has also been used in children with elevated pulmonary vascular resistance after cardiac surgery[117]. Cardiopulmonary bypass often exacerbates chronically elevated pulmonary vascular resistance in children because of congenital heart disease. The pathogenesis of this is unclear but appears to be due in part to the effects of cardiopulmonary bypass on the endothelium.

Investigators have also used NO in the treatment of Acute Respiratory Distress Syndrome (ARDS). Inhalation of NO is particularly appealing in this setting because the vasodilatory effects of NO should improve perfusion of only ventilated areas of the lung, creating a diversion of blood flow from poorly ventilated areas, thereby improving matching of ventilation to perfusion. Trials in both adults and children have demonstrated increased oxygenation and decreased pulmonary artery pressure[118,119]. Furthermore, vasodilatation is greatest in patients with severe pulmonary hypertension[120]. Despite these promising improvements in cardiorespiratory function, studies have not yet demonstrated improved long-term survival. Despite the potential therapeutic possibilities for inhaled NO, extensive study regarding the safety with short and long-term administration and controlled clinical trials demonstrating an improvement in outcome (decreased morbidity and/or mortality) are required before the routine clinical use of this gas can be advocated. Until that time, the use of NO should be restricted to controlled trials.

Humidification

Humidity is water vapor in ambient gases, which is essentially invisible moisture. Like any gas component, the content of water vapor in a given mixture of gases can be expressed in terms of its *partial pressure.* Alternatively, the content of water vapor in a given gas can be expressed in terms of the *absolute humidity* or the actual milligrams of water per liter of gas. The physical characteristics of water in the gaseous state dictate the water capacity of gas expressed as the saturated water vapor partial pressure, is related directly to the temperature of the gas in question (increasing with increasing temperature). This provides an additional means of expressing the water vapor content of gases in terms of the ratio of actual water content to the water content capacity at a given temperature *(relative humidity).* For example, at body temperature (37° C), 100% relative humidity (the state at which gas is fully saturated with water vapor) is achieved at a water vapor pressure of 47 mm Hg, representing 43.8 mg of water per liter of gas in terms of absolute humidity[121]. Furthermore, gas at 100% relative humidity at room temperature (22(C) represents less than 40% relative humidity at body temperature (Fig. 9.11).

Normally, inspired gases from the environment contain some degree of humidity. As these gases pass through the upper respiratory system, heating to body temperature and concomitant humidification to 100% relative humidity occur. However, medical gases are virtually dehumidified. In addition, delivery of medical gases to the critically ill patient with an artificial airway involves the bypassing of upper respiratory pathways responsible for heating and humidification during spontaneous breathing. Lack of proper humidification of medical gases under these circumstances presents serious potential complications, such as enhanced respiratory insensible water loss and drying of respiratory secretions, leading to airway obstruction and impaired mu-

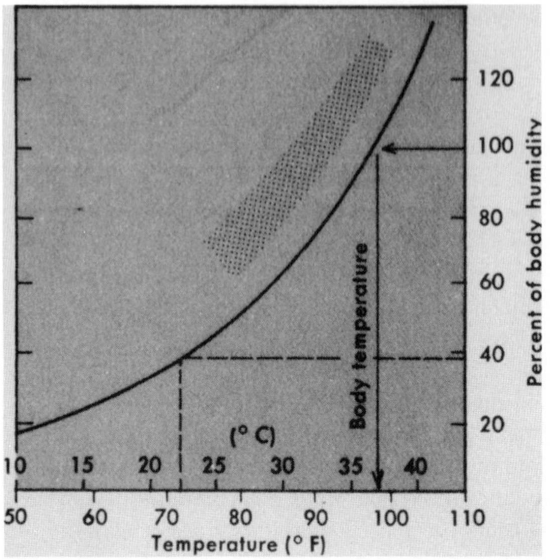

Figure 9.11. Relationship between gas temperature and humidification, as percentage of humidity at body temperature (i.e., percentage of body humidity). *Curve* represents 100% relative humidity at the corresponding temperature. At room temperature (22°C), 100% relative humidity represents less than 40% relative humidity at body temperature (37°C). (From McPherson SP. Respiratory therapy equipment. 2nd ed. St Louis: CV Mosby, 1981:138.)

cociliary function[122]. Adequate humidification of inspired gases must be provided with all forms of respiratory therapy equipment used in the intubated patient. To address the problem of humidification of delivered medical gases, several humidification devices have been developed that can be categorized by the presence or absence of heating elements as well as by the mechanisms of humidification.

Simple Humidifiers

Simple humidifiers are devices that do not use heat and are designed to make gas administration comfortable. These devices achieve 100% relative humidity at room temperature and are generally used with gas delivery systems that do not bypass normal upper airway heating and humidifying structures (e.g., masks and nasal cannula). The gas that enters the patient's airways will undergo normal heating and humidification.

The simplest and most inefficient humidification device is the *passover humidifier.* Gas is directed over a water surface prior to administration to the patient (Fig. 9.12). The *bubble humidifier* directs gas through a water bath where the bubbles interface with the water . The large area of the water-gas interface creates greater humidification (Fig. 9.13). Increased humidification with the bubble humidifier can be achieved by configurations that decrease the size of bubbles injected into the water bath. The *jet humidifier* delivers gas at increased velocity across water droplets, producing an aerosol. Before the gas leaves the humidifier the aerosolized water particles evaporate or condense on system surfaces, thus preventing particulate water from being delivered to the patient. A fourth type of simple humidifier is the underwater jet which incorporates principles of a bubble and jet humidifier[123].

The most commonly used humidification devices presently are bubble-type disposable humidifiers. These humidifiers are generally capable of delivering 100% relative humidity at room temperature. The ability to provide this level of humidification is dependent on the water level of the humidifier, falling off significantly if the water level decreases below a specified level. Therefore, maintenance of proper water levels in bubble humidifiers is essential. In addition to low water levels, excessive gas flow can result in decreased humidification[124].

Heated Humidifiers

Heated humidifiers, as the name implies, are devices that use heating elements to increase temperature as well as humidifying efficiency. Heated humidifiers should be used to supply inspired gas to patients in whom the upper airways have been bypassed. Some heated humidifiers employ bubbling devices that direct gas flow below the level of heated water prior to delivery to the patient (Fig. 9.14). The degree of humidification of delivered gases relative to body temperature depends on the temperature setting, flow rate delivery, water level in the humidifier reservoir, and the length of circuitry tubing from humidifier to patient. *Wick humidifiers* (Fig. 9.15) use a heated paper "wick" through which delivered gases pass, thereby creating a large heated gas-water interface for inspired gases. These humidifiers are used primarily for ventilators. A float in the humidifier reservoir acts to feed the system automatically with additional water when the water level falls, thus maintaining a constant water level in the humidifier. This feature is particularly desirable in humidifiers used with pediatric ventilators, in that low water levels in humidification devices can lead to significant increases in compressible volume of the ventilator circuitry. In addition, digital temperature monitoring accessories are available to monitor inspired gas temperature at the airway opening. Inspired gases are not

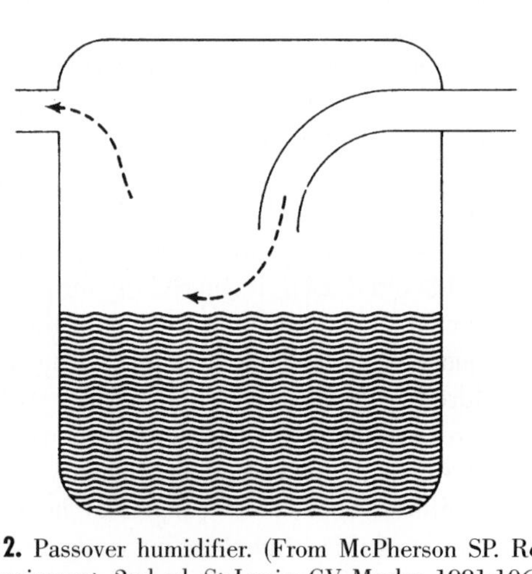

Figure 9.12. Passover humidifier. (From McPherson SP. Respiratory therapy equipment. 2nd ed. St Louis: CV Mosby, 1981:106.)

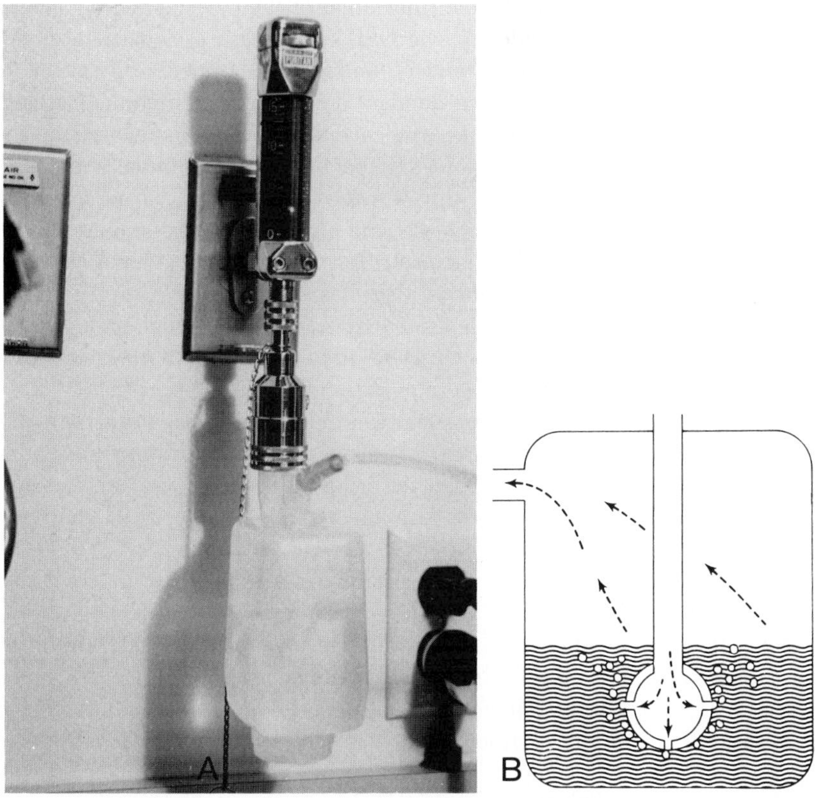

Figure 9.13. Bubble humidifier. A. Bubble humidifier connected to flowmeter and wall oxygen source. B. Schematic diagram of simple bubble humidifier. (From McPherson SP. Respiratory therapy equipment. 2nd ed. St Louis: CV Mosby, 1981:106.)

bubbled through the humidification device; therefore, resistance to spontaneous inspiration is minimal with the wick humidifier, an additional appealing feature in pediatric respiratory therapy. Generally, heated humidifiers are used in high-flow systems (e.g., CPAP circuits) and with mechanical ventilators or other respiratory therapy equipment designed for intubated patients. Temperature monitoring of patient circuits should be incorporated in any heated humidifier system to avoid the serious complication of tracheal burns from excessive inspiratory gas heating[125].

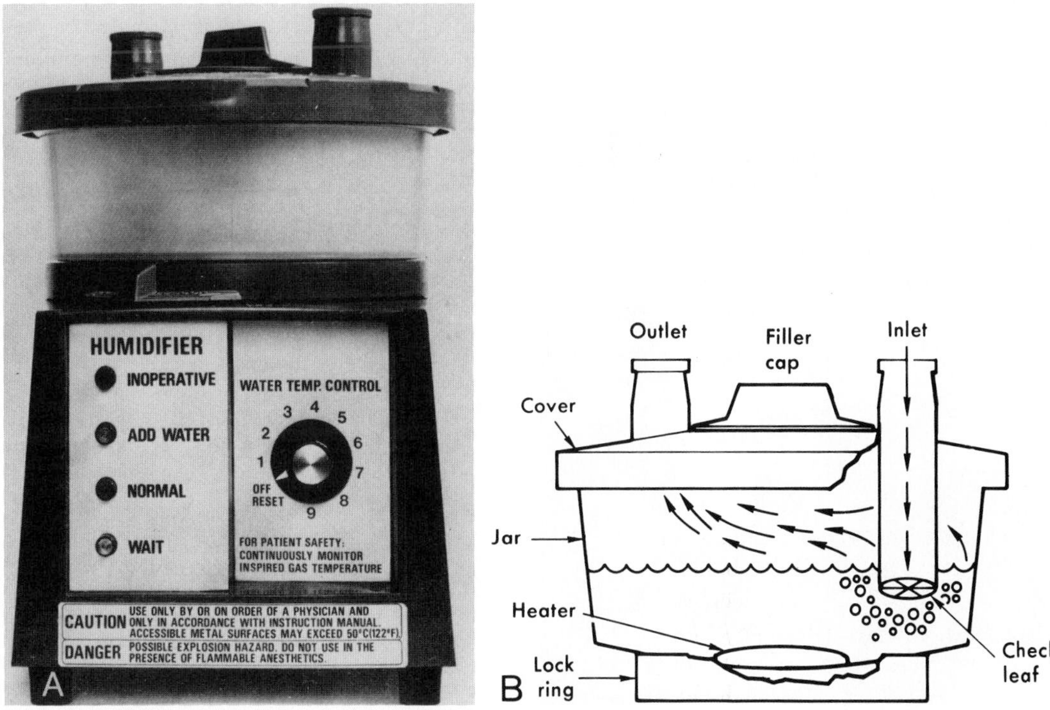

Figure 9.14. A. Heated bubble humidifier. B. Schematic diagram of heated bubble humidifier showing flow of medical gases through humidification system. (Courtesy of Bear Medical Systems, Inc., Riverside, California.)

Heated Wire Circuit

An adjunct to heated humidification in the neonatal and pediatric settings is the introduction of a permanent heated wire circuit. The heated wire maintains the temperature throughout the length of the circuit in an attempt to minimize or eliminate rainout. Several disposable versions have been marketed in which the inspiratory only or both inspiratory and expiratory limbs may be heated. The heated wire controller maintains the temperature in the circuit and controls the temperature in the humidifier so that gas delivered to the patient is at or near the selected temperature. Care must be taken to not allow the wire to melt the circuit.

Aerosol Therapy

Aerosols are used widely in health care, both in diagnosis and therapy. Aerosols have been employed as a means of drug delivery with the theoretical advantage of local delivery of medication in large doses to their site of action with diminished systemic toxicity. Furthermore, aerosols allow delivery of active medication which may not be administered by another route.

All aerosols, whether generated from solutions, suspensions or from a powdered drug, form heterodisperse, nonspherical water droplets. The numerous droplets or particles are irregular in size and shape. These physical properties, as well as parameters of ventilation and airway geometry, determine the degree and site of deposition within the respiratory tree[126]. Aerosol particles are generally described in terms of an aerodynamic diameter which allows description of particles regardless of shape and density to one of equivalent unit density sphere with the same terminal settling velocity in still air. Aerosol particles are characterized by the mass median aerodynamic diameter (MMAD) and the geometric standard deviation of their median aerodynamic diameter (GSD). The GSD is a measure of particle diameter dispersion and is the ratio of the median diameter to the diameter one standard deviation away from the median.

Deposition of particles within the lung is determined by three physical forces: impaction, sedimentation, and diffusion. Particles with MMADs greater than 10 micrometers impact the oropharynx and proximal airways and are eliminated from the aerosol. Respirable particles have MMADs less than 5 microns. Particles ranging from 0.5-1.0 microns are primarily deposited by sedimentation under the influence of gravity[127]. Deposition of still smaller particles will primarily be determined by diffusion. Approximately 80% of the extremely small particles (less than 1 micron) will be expired because the time required to diffuse to an airway is greater than the inspiratory phase of a breath. Particle deposition is also affected by gas velocity. Higher respiratory flow rates increase turbulent gas flow, leading to increased particle deposition in the proximal airways. Airway geometry also alters particle deposition. Numerous bifurcations and narrowing of airways both increase turbulent flow and the likelihood of impaction in the more proximal airways. Higher inspiratory rates and smaller airways of children further impede particle deposition in the lower airways compared to adults.

Therapeutic aerosols are produced by nebulizers and metered-dose inhalers (MDI). Nebulizers utilize air or an enriched oxygen source as the vehicle with aerosolization of drug from a solution. Nebulized aerosols are produced by Venturi-type jet nebulizers or ultrasonic nebulizers. Jet nebulizers use compressed gas to create a jet of fluid carried by the airstream, while ultrasonic nebulizers use a piezoelectric crystal which vibrates at high frequencies, creating waves on the surface of the liquid to produce particle droplets. Although MMADs vary with equipment, jet nebu-

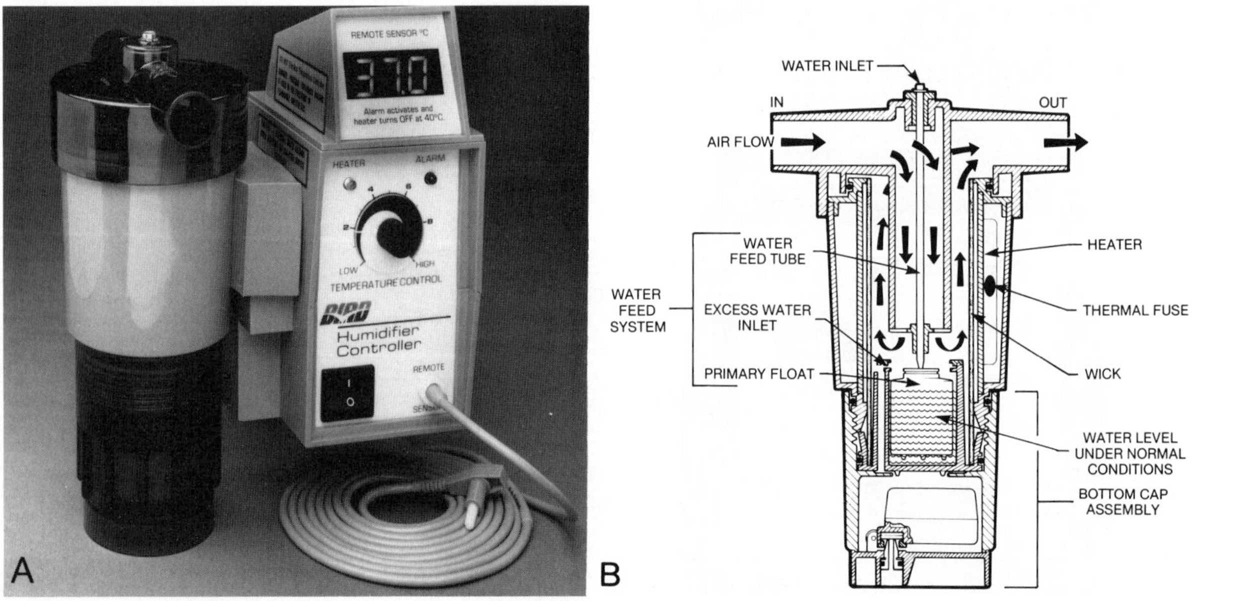

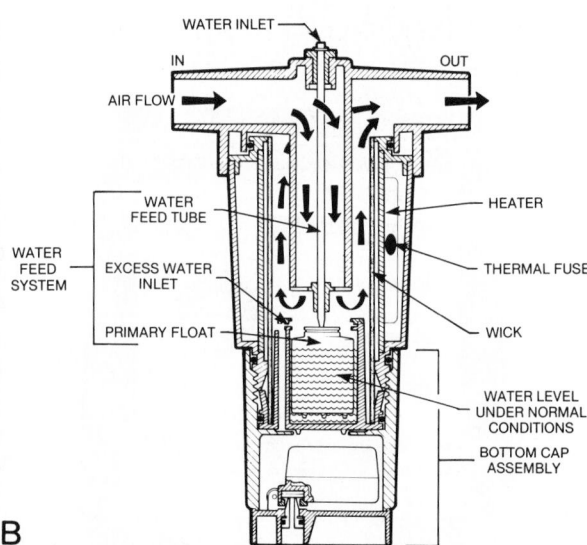

Figure 9.15. Heated wick humidifier. A. Wick humidifier with attached heater control. B. Schematic diagram of wick humidifier showing flow of medical gases through humidification system. (Courtesy of Bird Corp., Palm Springs, California.)

lizers generally produce particles between 2-4 microns while the ultrasonic nebulizers generate slightly larger particles of 4-6 microns. Drug aerosols are generated from MDIs by an artificial surfactant such as soya lecithin, sorbiatan trioleate or oleic acid with a fluorocarbon propellant liquid. MMADs from MDIs range from 1-10 microns.

Aerosol delivery is dramatically altered during mechanical ventilation[(128)]. The endotracheal tube, ventilator circuit, and ventilation parameters all impact aerosol deposition. Early studies demonstrated that delivery of nebulized medication through an adult endotracheal tube was decreased to approximately 3 percent of the original dose[(129)]. Smaller pediatric endotracheal tubes further decreased drug delivery from the endotracheal tube[(130)]. Studies have demonstrated that drug delivery from an MDI into a ventilator is significantly improved by using a spacer with the MDI[(131-134)]. Drug delivery is also improved when the MDI is discharged just prior to inspiration, with low inspiratory flow rates, low respiratory rates, and longer inspiratory times[(135-137)].

Nebulized therapy through a ventilator circuit requires careful adjustment of tidal volumes because of the intermittent addition of the flow from the nebulized gas into the ventilator circuit. Furthermore, filters are required to protect the expiratory valve from crystallization of medication within the ventilator. These factors and cost of administration favor MDI use over nebulized medications in ventilator circuits.

Various medications may be administered in nebulized form. Many of these medications (beta adrenergic agents, anticholinergic agents, steroids, and antibiotics) have been delivered by this method for many years. Others, such as pentamidine, DNAse and ribavirin, have only recently been introduced. Ribavirin, which is a synthetic nucleoside with antiviral properties against both RNA and DNA viruses such as respiratory syncytial virus, has generated a large amount of controversy. It is typically administered with an expensive multi-jet small-particle aerosol generator (SPAG-2) which reliably produces a small aerosol (MMAD 1-2 microns). Ribavirin may be administered safely in mechanically ventilated patients, but requires meticulous attention to prevent occlusion of the endotracheal tube or to the expiratory flow valve by crystallization of medication[(138,139)]. Studies of ribavirin efficacy have yielded conflicting results[(140,141)], although the committee on infectious diseases of the American Academy of Pediatrics has recommended the use of this medication in high risk patients (very young, underlying cardiac or respiratory disease, or immune deficiency).

Chest Physiotherapy

Chest physiotherapy refers to a constellation of maneuvers designed to enhance the removal of pulmonary secretions and improve or maintain distribution of ventilation through the lungs. These maneuvers include *postural drainage, chest percussion, chest vibration,* and *deep breathing exercises.*

Postural Drainage

Postural drainage is a form of chest physiotherapy that, in theory, uses gravitational forces to drain pulmonary secretions from the smaller peripheral airways towards the main bronchi, where expectoration or suctioning can occur[(142)]. Postural drainage requires that the patient be placed in a variety of positions determined by the bronchopulmonary segments of the lungs and airways.

Chest Percussion and Vibration

Chest percussion is performed by striking the chest wall for the purpose of mobilizing secretions from nondependent lung fields to the central conducting airways for expectoration or suctioning. Percussion is thought to transmit forces through the chest to airway secretions, promoting movement centrally in the tracheobronchial tree. This maneuver, in conjunction with postural drainage, is accomplished by rhythmically "clapping" the chest in a forceful but painless fashion with a cupped hand or device. When necessary, a towel can be placed over the chest to increase patient comfort. Chest percussion should not be performed over the clavicles, scapulae, vertebrae, or sternum.

Chest vibration is generated with a battery powered mechanical vibrator placed on the surface of the chest. Like chest percussion, vibration is thought to enhance central movement of secretions. Vibratory therapy is usually administered in conjunction with postural drainage. Vibratory chest physiotherapy is particularly popular in premature newborn, children with rickets and for other patients with fragile chest wall in whom the risk of rib fracture prohibits the use of percussion.

Deep Breathing Exercises

Deep breathing exercises are performed by the cooperative, spontaneously breathing child. Used with positional changes, deep breathing can promote improvement in the mechanics of breathing and the distribution of ventilation[(143)]. Generally, encouragement of deep breathing is all that is required in the cooperative child. As an extension of the concept of biofeedback, various devices have been created for the purpose of semiquantitatively measuring inspiratory flow or exhaled volume at the bedside, providing feedback to the patient on the breath to breath performance of the deep-breathing maneuvers. In this manner, so-called "incentive" spirometry encourages the patient to achieve ventilatory volume-related goals during the deep-breathing exercise sessions. Another adjutant used during deep-breathing exercises involves encouraging the patient to contract muscles of inspiration to enhance the distribution of inspired volume within the lungs. With hands under the lateral costal margins, lateral thoracic expansion can be promoted. Alternatively, with the hands placed anteriorly, anterposterior expansion can be encouraged.

Goals and Efficacy

There are three major goals of chest physiotherapy: (1) clearance of pulmonary secretions[142], (2) avoidance and reversal of alveolar collapse[142,143], and (3) improved matching of ventilation and perfusion[144,145]. Frequent positional changes prevent atelectasis and improve ventilation perfusion matching. Patients receiving mechanical ventilation are frequently positioned supine, for both ease of nursing care and access to intravascular catheters and tubes. Animal studies suggest that prone positioning improves ventilation perfusion matching because transpulmonary pressure then exceeds airway opening pressure to the lower lung segments and prevents preferential atelectasis in these segments[146]. Prone positioning may improve oxygenation in patients with high ventilation perfusion mismatch.

In adults with unilateral lung disease, positioning with the normal lung in the dependent position results in improved oxygenation[147], presumably because ventilation and perfusion is better matched. In small infants with unilateral lung disease, the opposite effect is seen. Decreased oxygenation occurs[148], possibly because of decreased gravitational forces on regional blood flow relative to adults. Another important concept in unilateral lung disease is that progressive hypoxia can occur from overdistention of the better functioning lung which impedes pulmonary perfusion.

The efficacy of chest physiotherapy is not clear[142,149,150], especially in acute lung disease. Chest physiotherapy actually involves several independent interventions. Each component of chest physiotherapy has not been systematically evaluated in critically ill children, either as prophylactic measures or as therapeutic intervention in acute lung disease. Studies of adults with acute respiratory failure have demonstrated that performance of all components of a chest physiotherapy regimen are beneficial in decreasing pulmonary shunt fraction[151], but not in improving oxygenation[152]. Indeed, deterioration in oxygenation has been reported following chest physiotherapy in critically ill newborns[153] and adults[154]. Consideration of the substantial time required of nursing and respiratory therapy personnel in providing various components of chest physiotherapy, and studies evaluating the efficacy of each component are badly needed. In the meantime, children at risk for atelectasis, retained secretions, or suppurative pulmonary complications, and those with preexisting lung disease should receive frequent position changes and deep breathing encouragement at a minimum. The specific aspects of chest physiotherapy regimens should be dictated by the individual needs of the patient.

Possible Complications

Several complications of chest physiotherapy should be considered. Postural changes involving the placement of the head in a dependent position may increase intracranial pressure; therefore, chest physiotherapy, particularly postural drainage should be avoided in suspected or confirmed cases of intracranial hypertension. In addition, chest physiotherapy has been associated with transient decreases in PaO_2 and dyspnea[152,153]. Overzealous chest percussion can cause rib fractures in neonates and in children with bony diseases (e.g. osteogenesis imperfecta, rickets, and osteoporosis). Finally, chest physiotherapy, particularly postural drainage, in the presence of focal suppurative lung disease or lung abscess presents the theoretical risk of contamination of the contralateral lung with the pulmonary pathogens. Strong evidence to support the avoidance of chest physiotherapy in these situations has not been demonstrated.

MECHANICAL VENTILATOR THERAPY

Although the concept of artificial respiration has been recognized throughout nearly all of man's recorded history, it was not until the 20th century that mechanical ventilation has become widely used. Over the last ten years there has been a virtual explosion of new ventilatory techniques that present a confusing array of alternatives for the treatment of patients with respiratory failure. Despite this exponential growth in options for the clinicians, there have been few well-controlled clinical studies defining the role for all of these new techniques. Furthermore, over the last several years our understanding of the potential detrimental effects of mechanical ventilation has also increased. These issues formed the impetus for several international consensus conferences that has been used as a framework for this discussion[154,155].

Physiologic Effects of Mechanical Ventilation

Physicians contemplating the use of mechanical ventilation must keep both the benefits and risks of this medical therapy in mind prior to its utilization. Weighing the beneficial and detrimental physiologic consequences of mechanical ventilation is useful to the clinician to establish a set of goals for mechanical ventilation **(Table 9.3)** and will form the framework for a complete description of the physiologic effects of mechanical ventilation on the growing and developing child.

Maintenance of Oxygenation

The most straightforward means to control oxygenation is achieved by adjusting the inspired oxygen concentration. Despite the simplicity of this system, there is rarely a direct relationship between the fractional inspired oxygen concentration (FiO_2) and arterial oxygen concentration (PaO_2). To gain a better understanding of the physiology of oxygen delivery to the tissues, it is advantageous to start with the calculation of the partial pressure of inspired oxygen (PiO_2):

$$PiO_2 = FiO_2(P_b - P_{H_2}O),$$

TABLE 9.3. Goals and Complications of Assisted Mechanical Ventilation[a]

Goals to Achieve	
	Complications to Avoid
Improve alveolar ventilation and avoid significant hypercapnia and respiratory acidosis	
	Hyperventilation and decreased cerebral blood flow
Reduce V/Q mismatch and maintenance of normal hemoglobin saturation	
	Hypoxemic tissue injury
	Oxygen toxicity to the lungs or other organs
Re-expand atelectatic or collapsed lung segments	
	Alveolar overdistention
	Pulmonary hypoperfusion
	Reduced venous return/cardiac output
	Volutrauma to alveolar structures
Reduce work of breathing and eliminate respiratory muscle fatigue	
	Suppressed ventilatory drive
	Respiratory muscle disuse atrophy
	Increased upper airway resistance (i.e. subglottic edema/stenosis)

[a] *Modified with permission from Chatburn RL. Principles and practice of neonatal and pediatric mechanical ventilation. Respir Care 1991;36:569.*

where P_b is barometric pressure and $P_{H_2}O$ is water vapor pressure. The $P_{H_2}O$ is 47 torr at 37°C. This equation shows that some of the inspired oxygen is displaced by water vapor as the gas traverses the upper airways. Thus, solving the equation for room air at sea level (0.21 × 760 torr − 47 torr) results in a PiO_2 of approximately 150 torr. As the gas continues into the alveolar region of the lungs, more of the oxygen is displaced by carbon dioxide. The partial pressure of oxygen in the alveolus (P_AO_2) is determined by the equation:

$$P_AO_2 = PiO_2 - P_ACO_2,$$

where P_ACO_2 is the alveolar partial pressure of carbon dioxide. For clinical purposes this equation is simplified by the substitution of P_ACO_2 with the arterial partial pressure of carbon dioxide (PaO_2) which can be directly measured and dividing by the respiratory quotient (RQ):

$$P_AO_2 = PiO_2 - PaO_2/RQ.$$

The RQ is determined by the mix of substrates for metabolism (i.e. carbohydrates, proteins, fats) and is generally estimated to be approximately 0.8 in most clinical situations. Thus, using the estimated RQ, 40 torr for the PaO_2 and the 150 torr previously calculated for PiO_2 yields a value of approximately 100 torr for P_AO_2.

The relationship between P_AO_2 and PaO_2 is even further altered by the variations in the overall ventilation-perfusion (V/Q) ratio and the diffusion barrier of the alveolar-capillary membrane. These two factors account for the small difference in the partial pressure of oxygen from the alveolus to artery (approximately 10 torr under normal conditions). One of the primary etiologies of hypoxemia is pulmonary pathology that causes decreased resting lung volume (functional residual capacity, FRC), low lung compliance, and an increased proportion of low V/Q compartments of the lungs[156,157]. The goal of positive pressure support in these settings is to elevate end expiratory volume (EEV) toward physiologic FRC or mean lung volume through the application of continuous distending pressure at the airway opening. The increase in the mean airway pressure ($P_{\overline{aw}}$) serves to recruit atelectatic or poorly ventilated alveolar units, thereby improving V/Q matching and decreasing intrapulmonary right-to-left shunting[158,159]. A useful clinical index of the effect of changes in ventilatory pattern is the $\overline{P}_{aw}$ which reflects the overall changes in ventilation variables such as peak and end-expiratory pressure and the ratio of inspiratory to expiratory time (I:E)[160]. This increase in $\overline{P}_{aw}$ frequently results in a dramatic decrease in the need for supplemental oxygen with maintenance of adequate oxygenation using nontoxic oxygen levels of inspired oxygen. Furthermore, recruitment of collapsed lung units and increased EEV lead to improved lung compliance and decreased work of breathing[158,161]. This may allow the partial or complete withdrawal of positive pressure breaths once adequate levels of continuous positive pressure have been achieved. It has been previously noted that minimal or no intermittent positive pressure breaths associated with adequate $\overline{P}_{aw}$ and partial or complete spontaneous ventilation has several advantages[162]. These included decreased risk of pulmonary barotrauma, improved V/Q matching, and partially reversed adverse circulatory effects of continuous positive pressure ventilation (see below). These beneficial effects on oxygen delivery frequently increase up to the point at which the lung becomes overdistended.

Maintenance of Alveolar Ventilation

A second principal goal of mechanical ventilation is to augment or control alveolar ventilation. In fact, respiratory failure is frequently defined in terms of $PaCO_2$, which is inversely related to alveolar ventilation ($\dot{V}_A$):

$$PaCO_2 \text{ proportional to } \dot{V}_{CO_2}/\dot{V}_A,$$

where $\dot{V}_{CO_2}$ is carbon dioxide production. Alveolar ventilation can be defined (in normal ventilatory frequencies) as:

$$\dot{V}_A = (V_T - V_D)f,$$

where V_T is tidal volume, V_D is dead-space volume, and f is respiratory frequency. Therefore, it is clear that $PaCO_2$ can be altered by regulating V_T and f, which are the components of minute ventilation ($\dot{V}_E$). Most clinicians select typical values for V_T (10-15 mls/kg) and frequencies that they have found through experience result in $PaCO_2$ values within the target range. Subsequent adjustments of $\dot{V}_E$ to alter $PaCO_2$ are again usually made on the basis of experience; however, simplified equations can be used to predict changes in $PaCO_2$ with changes in frequency and constant tidal volume: $n$$PaCO_2$ = $o$$PaCO_2$ × of/nf where n is the new or desired value, o is the old or measured value, $PaCO_2$ is the arterial partial pressure of carbon dioxide, and f is the respiratory frequency.

Unfortunately, the third variable in the equation, dead-space volume (V_D), is not routinely measured, commonly forgotten, and unappreciated. The relationship between the easily and routinely measured clinical variable $\dot{V}_E$ and $PaCO_2$ is:

$$PaCO_2 = 0.863\ \dot{V}_{CO_2}/[\dot{V}_E(1 - V_D/V_T)],$$

where $\dot{V}_{CO_2}$ is the metabolically produced carbon dioxide at standard temperature and pressure. This equation emphasizes the fact that $PaCO_2$ is determined by the relationship between metabolic rate and ventilation, and that not all inspired gas ($\dot{V}_E$) is useful for gas exchange. In normal individuals, most of V_D is a result of the volume of the conducting airways (anatomic V_D). Since this volume is relatively constant with increasing V_T, V_D/V_T tends to decrease and rarely exceeds 0.3. In ventilated patients the configuration of the ventilator circuit (apparatus dead space) can affect V_D, although this is usually a minor consideration. In mechanically ventilated patients with intrinsic lung disease, V_D/V_T has been found to exceed 0.6[163] and is principally related to ventilated but poorly perfused lung regions (alveolar V_D). In this situation, V_D/V_T may not be dramatically decreased by increasing V_T since the higher alveolar pressures required to generate the larger V_T may decrease pulmonary perfusion and increase alveolar V_D. Thus, the quantitative change in $PaCO_2$ as V_T is increased may not be easily predictable. This process can be facilitated by the estimation of V_D/V_T in the clinical setting by measuring end-tidal concentrations of exhaled carbon dioxide and using the following equation:

$$V_D/V_T = (PaCO_2 - P_{et}CO_2)/PaCO_2.$$

The change in $PaCO_2$ in response to alterations in $\dot{V}_E$ may be further confused by the possible effects on the patient's metabolic rate by changes in ventilator settings. For example, the patient may become more relaxed or agitated as ventilator settings are modified. Thus, increases in V_D/V_T and $\dot{V}_{CO_2}$ need to be considered whenever a change in $\dot{V}_E$ does not result in expected change in $PaCO_2$ or when a large $\dot{V}_E$ is required to maintain an acceptable $PaCO_2$.

Mechanics of Ventilation

Pulmonary mechanics are frequently viewed as a simplified single compartment model of the lungs consisting of a single, cylindrical flow-conducting tube (i.e. the conducting airways) connected to a single, spherical elastic compartment (i.e. alveoli) (Fig. 9.16). In this model, the lung is considered a homogeneous assembly of units with uniform pressure-volume (compliance) and pressure-flow (resistance) characteristics derived from this single representative unit. This model provides a means for understanding how the ventilator interacts with the load of the patient's respiratory system. Mathematical derivation of this schematic of the lungs can be used to advance our understanding of the effects of mechanical ventilation on the lungs.

The transrespiratory pressure (P_{tr}) required to achieve inflation is comprised of two components; (1) the transthoracic

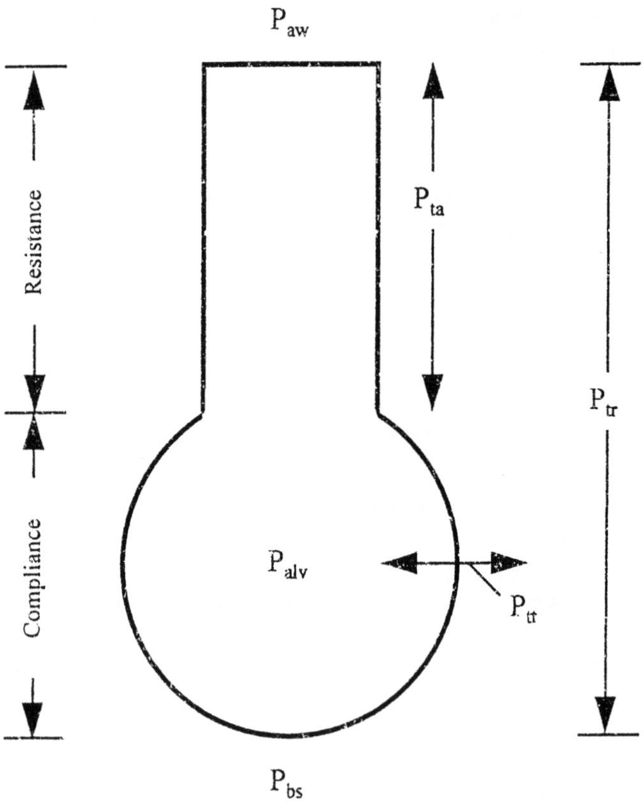

Figure 9.16. The single compartment model of the lungs composed of a flow-resistive element coupled in series with the compliance element. P_{aw} = airway pressure, P_{alv} = alveolar pressure, P_{bs} = body surface (i.e., atmospheric) pressure, P_{ta} = transairway ($P_{aw}-P_{alv}$) pressure, P_{tt} = transthoracic ($P_{alv}-P_{P_{bs}}$) pressure, P_{tr} = transrespiratory ($P_{aw}-P_{bs}$) pressure. The ventilator manometer when measuring airway pressure relative to atmospheric pressure is equivalent to P_{tr}. (Modified from Chatburn RL. Principles and practice of neonatal and pediatric mechanical ventilation. Respir Care 1991;36:569.)

pressure (P_{tt}) which is the pressure required to deliver the tidal volume against elastic recoil and (2) the transairway pressure (P_{ta}) necessary to overcome flow resistance:

$$P_{tr} = P_{tt} + P_{ta},$$

where P_{tr} = airway − body surface pressure, P_{tt} = alveolar − body surface pressure, and P_{ta} = airway − alveolar pressure. The P_{tr} is clinically the difference between the airway pressure at the mouth (or endotracheal tube) and body surface (atmospheric) pressure. The pressure required for inspiration may come from the respiratory muscles (P_{mus}) and/or the ventilator (P_{tr}):

$$P_{mus} + P_{tr} = P_{tt} + P_{ta}.$$

Since the ventilator manometer measures pressure relative to atmospheric pressure, P_{tr} is equal to the airway pressure (P_{aw}) displayed by the ventilator, allowing the substitution of P_{aw} for P_{tr}:

$$P_{mus} + P_{aw} = P_{tt} + P_{ta}.$$

In the single-compartment model of the lungs, the relationships between pressure and volume and between pressure and flow are assumed to be linear. The change in P_{tr} is directly proportional to the corresponding change in lung volume. The constant of proportionality is the slope ($\Delta P/\Delta V$) of the pressure-volume curve (i.e. elastance or the more commonly used reciprocal-compliance). Similarly, the change in P_{ta} is proportional to the change in flowrate and the constant of proportionality ($\Delta P/\Delta \dot{V}$) is resistance. Substituting $\Delta P/\Delta V$ and $\Delta P/\Delta \dot{V}$ for P_{tr} and P_{ta} respectively yields the equation often called the *equation of motion* of the respiratory system for inspiration:

$$P_{mus} + P_{aw} = V/C + (\dot{V})(R)$$

and expiration:

$$V/C = -(\dot{V})(R),$$

where V is the volume inspired or expired, C is the compliance of the respiratory system, $\dot{V}$ is the inspiratory or expiratory flow, and R is the resistance of the respiratory system. Note that during passive exhalation the elastic components of the lungs ($P_{alv} = V/C$) provide the necessary pressure to drive flow. The equation of motion is useful in situations in which the respiratory muscles are relaxed. In this case, measurement of pressure, volume, and flow allows calculation of total respiratory system compliance and resistance. Knowledge of compliance and resistance values allows prediction of the pressure required to deliver a given tidal volume at a set inspiratory flowrate or, conversely, to determine the tidal volume and inspiratory flowrate that will be generated by a given pressure.

The relations represented in the equation of motion can be graphically illustrated (Fig. 9.17). The set of graphs represent airway pressure, lung volume, and air flow for a constant inspiratory flow (left) or constant inspiratory pressure (right). In the former circumstance, the initial rise in pressure is because of resistance and flowrate. The slope of the pressure increase is inversely proportional to compliance, tidal volume, resistance, and inspiratory flowrate. Lung pressure (P_L) and lung volume (V_L) can be expressed as:

$$P_L = (\dot{V})(t)/C,$$
$$V_L = (\dot{V})(t),$$

where t is the inspiratory time. In the latter situation, lung pressure, lung volume, and flowrate during inspiration are exponential functions of time which can be derived from the equation of motion:

$$P_L = \Delta P(1 - e^{-t/\tau}),$$
$$V_L = C(\Delta P)(1 - e^{-t/\tau}),$$
$$\dot{V} = \Delta P/R \times e^{-t/\tau},$$

where ΔP is the change in airway pressure (i.e. peak inspiratory pressure − end-expiratory pressure), t is the inspiratory time, e is the base of the natural logarithm (~ 2.72), and τ is the time constant of the respiratory system. The time constant is the product of resistance (pressure × time/volume) and compliance (volume/pressure) and is measured in seconds. The pressure, volume, and flowrate during passive expiration from any form of

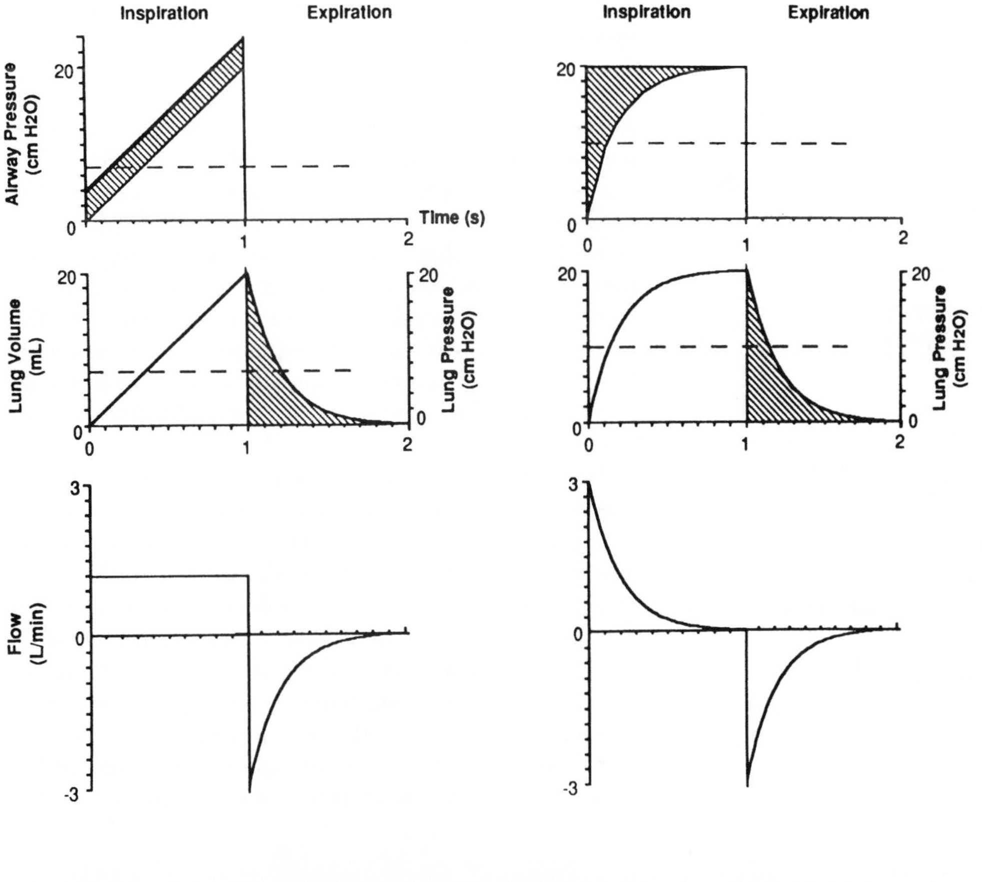

Figure 9.17. Graphical representation of the equation of motion for a constant inspiratory flow (left) and constant inspiratory pressure (right). Pressure, volume, and flow are all measured relative to their respective baseline values at end-expiration. The dotted lines represent mean airway and lung pressures. The shaded sections represent equal geometric areas proportional to the pressure required to overcome resistance while the unshaded areas represent the pressure required to overcome elastic recoil. Note that the constant inspiratory flow pattern is associated with a higher peak airway and lower mean airway pressure than does the constant inspiratory pressure pattern with equal tidal volume and inspiratory flow rate. (From Chatburn RL. Principles and practice of neonatal and pediatric mechanical ventilation. Respir Care 1991;36:569.)

mechanical ventilation can be derived from the equation of motion as:

$$P_L = \Delta P(e^{-t/\tau}),$$
$$V_L = C\,(\Delta P)(e^{-t/\tau}),$$
$$\dot{V} = -\,\Delta P/R \times e^{-t/\tau},$$

where t is the expiratory time. Note that all variables are measured relative to their value at end-expiration. Thus, the lung pressure is actually lung pressure above PEEP and lung volume is the volume above end-expiratory volume.

Assuming that inspiratory and expiratory times are sufficiently long to allow equilibration of airway and lung pressures, several interesting findings become apparent. During inspiration when t is zero, $e^{-t/\tau}$ is 1, lung pressure and volume are zero, and inspiratory flowrate = ΔP/R. When t is infinite, $e^{-t/\tau}$ is zero so that lung pressure is ΔP, tidal volume is ΔP × C, and inspiratory flowrate is zero. Similar results can be derived from the expiratory equations. For inspiratory and expiratory times between zero and infinity, the shapes of the lung-pressure, lung-volume, and flow curves are defined by the time constant. When these variables are plotted against time in units of time constants, useful principles emerge (Fig. 9.18). Regardless of specific values of resistance and compliance, after 1 time constant 63% of lung inflation (inspiratory time constant) or deflation (expiratory time constant) occurs, 95% after three time constants, and for practical purposes complete equilibration after five time constants.

It should be apparent that an increase in either regional resistance or compliance will result in a slowing of the relative pressure-flow dynamics of a given lung compartment, while a decrease in either parameter will have the opposite effect (Fig. 9.19). Most cases of respiratory failure involve widespread abnormalities in regional resistances and compliances with marked inhomogeneity in regional time constants. As a result, with normal tidal breathing, certain compartments fill and empty rapidly (short time constant), while others fill and empty more slowly (long time constant). This gives rise to marked inhomogenieties in the distribution of ventilation and abnormal pulmonary gas exchange. Under these conditions, successful ventilatory support requires the manipulation of inspiratory and expiratory times to allow more uniform distribution of ventilation among the various lung units. This strategy frequently improves ventilation/perfusion matching and decreases intrapulmonary right-to-left shunting.

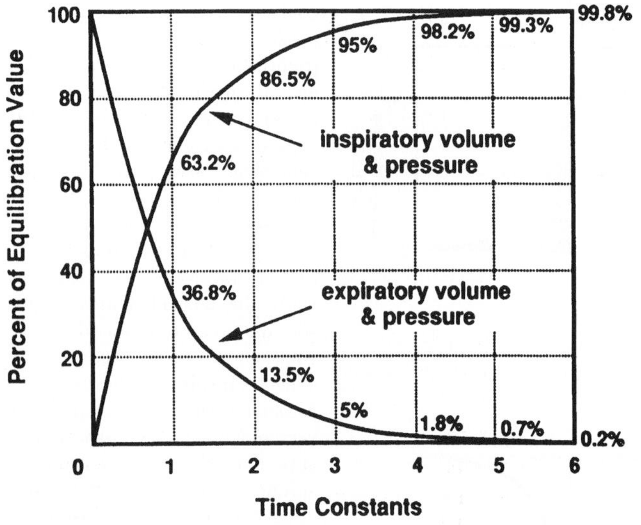

Figure 9.18. Exponential rise and fall of lung pressure and lung volume during inspiration and expiration expressed in terms of time constants. (From Chatburn RL. Principles and practice of neonatal and pediatric mechanical ventilation. Respir Care 1991;36:569.)

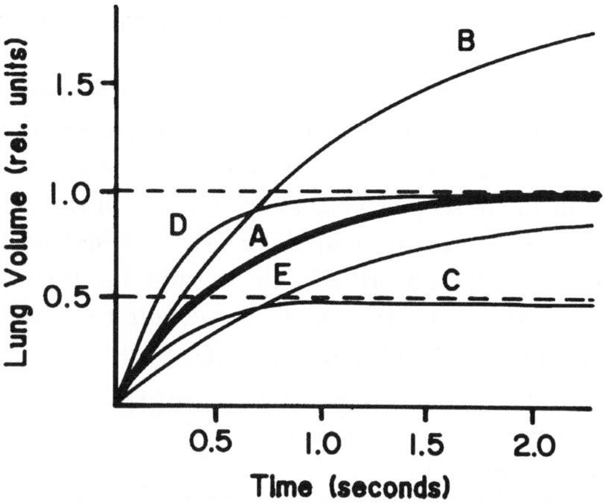

Figure 9.19. Effect of varying time constant on the change in lung volume over time during a positive pressure inflation with the introduction of a constant inflating pressure at the airway opening. *Curve A:* Basic curve under conditions of normal respiratory resistance (R) and compliance (C). Time constant (T) = R × C. Lung volume approaches inspiratory capacity (1.0 relative units) as defined by the elastic properties of the respiratory system. *Curve B:* Respiratory compliance doubled, resulting in doubling of the respiratory time constant (T = R × 2C). Inspiratory capacity has doubled. However, lung volume approaches the inspiratory capacity at one-half the rate of *curve A*. *Curve C:* Compliance halved, resulting in halving of the respiratory time constant (T = R × ½C). Inspiratory capacity of lung volume has been decreased by a factor of 2 (0.5 relative units). However, lung volume approaches the inspiratory capacity at twice the rate of *curve A*. *Curve D:* Resistance halved, resulting in halving of the respiratory time constant (T = ½R × C). Inspiratory capacity has not changed, but lung volume approaches inspiratory capacity at twice the rate of *curve A*. *Curve E:* Resistance doubled, resulting in doubling of the respiratory time constant (T = 2R × C). Inspiratory capacity during positive pressure inflation remains the same, but lung volume approaches inspiratory capacity at one-half the rate of *curve A*. (Modified from Nunn JF. Applied respiratory physiology. 2nd ed. Boston: Butterworths, 1977:148.)

In addition to regional time constant changes, a qualitative knowledge of the respiratory generalized time constant is important in the management of diffuse diseases of the airways or alveoli. For example, diffuse airway obstructive diseases (e.g., asthma or bronchiolitis) are associated with a generalized increase in resistance and prolongation of the time constant, particularly in expiration. The resulting delay in alveolar emptying requires prolonged expiration to minimize alveolar overdistention. During positive pressure ventilation, a low inspiratory-to-expiratory (I/E) ratio with a prolonged expiratory time, is necessary to avoid incomplete alveolar emptying. This problem with alveolar distention, sometimes referred to as "inadvertent PEEP" or "auto-PEEP," can result in marked depression of venous return, decreased cardiac output, decreased pulmonary perfusion, and wasted ventilation because of a secondary increase in physiologic dead space[164,165]. On the other hand, in diseases associated with diffusely decreased compliance (e.g., ARDS, pulmonary edema, and diffuse pneumonia), the time constant of the respiratory system in general is shortened, and less time in expiration is required for alveolar emptying. This allows a more prolonged inspiratory time, which is helpful in recruiting collapsed alveoli. With the return of normal pulmonary compliance, the time allotted for expiration must be reconsidered, and appropriate I/E ratio adjustments must be made to avoid the problems of alveolar overdistention and auto-PEEP associated with the risk of alveolar rupture (i.e., pulmonary barotrauma).

Closer inspection of the equation of motion and the single compartment model of the respiratory system can be used to describe some of the differences between constant flow and constant pressure with a decelerating flow. First, peak airway pressures are higher for the constant-flow pattern compared to the constant-pressure pattern; however, the peak lung pressure is independent of the pattern of inspiratory flow. Peak pressure in the lung depends only on compliance and tidal volume. Second, at each point in time, airway pressure is equal to the volume/compliance plus the resistance/flow. The pressure required to overcome resistance (shaded area of Fig. 9.17.) is constant with the fixed inspiratory flow pattern, while it is greatest initially and decreases exponentially with the decelerating flow pattern. In this example the area is equal for both patterns since tidal volume and inspiratory times are equal. Finally, because of the more rapid approach to the pressure limit, the constant-pressure decelerating flow pattern has a higher mean airway pressure ($\overline{P}_{aw}$) compared to the constant-flow pattern. The $\overline{P}_{aw}$ is derived from the area under the pressure-time curve divided by the time for one ventilatory cycle as:

$$\overline{P}_{aw} = K(\Delta P)(t_i/t_i + t_e) + PEEP,$$

where K is the waveform constant (which ranges between 0.5 to 1.0 depending upon the shape of the waveform), ΔP is the difference between peak and end-expiratory pressures, t_i is the inspiratory time, and t_e is the expiratory time. Notice that $\overline{P}_{aw}$ is independent of ventilator frequency as long as the inspiratory-to-expiratory ratio remains constant. Since all shaded areas are equal (see above), the total area under the airway pressure curve is equal to the total area under the lung pressure curve for each pattern. Thus, the mean airway pressure is the same as the mean lung pressure, which has been verified in animals[166]. Many physicians have come to realize that alterations in $\overline{P}_{aw}$ correspond to similar changes in mean lung volume and are used to manage hypoxemia[167]. In fact, this finding was first reported by neonatologists treating infants with infant respiratory distress syndrome[168].

All of the preceding conclusions are valid if the single-compartment model fits the true behavior of the lungs. This model likely represents a gross simplification of the actual behavior of the lungs. Several examples can readily demonstrate the lack of appreciation for the complexity of the physiology of the lungs. The model assumes equal values for inspiratory and expiratory resistance when in reality expiratory resistance is clearly greater[169]. It also assumes that equilibration is reached at end-inspiration and end-expiration; however, high ventilatory frequencies and/or long time constants would clearly invalidate this assumption. Insufficient inspiratory and expiratory times may result in decreases in delivered tidal volume and increased end-expiratory pressures and volumes, and increased dead space. The limitations associated with conflicts with respiratory time constants and ventilator frequency have been reviewed in detail[170].

One final feature of pulmonary mechanics that needs to be appreciated is the sigmoidal nature of the static pressure-volume (compliance) relationship of the respiratory system. The system's most compliant region is in the mid-volume range, becoming significantly stiffer near the upper (total lung capacity) and lower (residual volume) volume extremes. Tidal ventilation at the upper extremes of lung volume (i.e. near total lung capacity) occurs under two conditions: (1) when total lung volume and/or vital capacity are decreased secondary to intrinsic lung disease and (2) end expiratory volume is decreased. Ventilation at low lung volumes with decreases in compliance also occurs under two different situations: (1) when obesity and/or abdominal distention increase residual volume which encroaches upon the lower range of vital capacity and (2) when intrinsic lung disease results in airway or alveolar closure at end-expiratory volume (i.e. FRC).

It can be seen that the relationship between EEV, the volume from which inspiration occurs, and closing capacity is a critical one. Diseases or conditions that decrease EEC below closing capacity or increase closing capacity above FRC result in maldistribution of ventilation and adversely affect the mechanics of breathing[156] **(Table 9.4).** In the older child and adult, FRC is normally well above closing capacity. However, the relationship seems to be more precarious in the young infant; studies have suggested that closing capacity exceeds FRC, even in normal infants[171]. This observation partially explains the relative frequency of acute respiratory failure in children under 1 year of age[172].

A significant portion of respiratory therapy and support is directed at reestablishing the normal relationship between EEV (FRC) and closing capacity. In situations characterized by EEV less than FRC (e.g., pulmonary edema, interstitial pneumonitis, and adult and infant respiratory distress syndromes), measures such as CPAP or PEEP are used to elevate EEV towards FRC at normal levels. In conditions associated with increased closing capacity (e.g., bronchiolitis and bronchospastic disease), bronchodilators and measures to control pulmonary secretions assist in re-

TABLE 9.4. Conditions Predisposing to Convergence of Closing Capacity and FRC

Elevation of closing capacity
Infancy
Bronchiolitis
Asthma
Bronchopulmonary dysplasia
Smoke inhalation (thermal airway injury)
Cystic fibrosis
Reduction of FRC
Supine position
Abdominal distention
Thoracic or abdominal surgery
Atelectasis
Thoracic trauma
Pulmonary edema
ARDS
Near-drowning
Diffuse pneumonitis
Aspiration
Idiopathic interstitial
Bacterial
Viral
Opportunistic organisms
Radiation

versing the tendency toward airway closure and obstruction.

Work of Breathing

The pressure-volume characteristics (compliance and resistance) of the respiratory system determine the work of breathing, which in reality represents the afterload on the respiratory muscles[173]. The work of breathing overcomes two major sources of impedance: (1) elastic recoil of the lungs and chest wall (Fig. 9.20, *area ADC*), and (2) the frictional resistance to gas flow in the airways (Fig. 9.20, *area ABC*). Total work of breathing (Fig. 9.20, *area ABCD*) is increased either by an increase in resistance properties or by a decrease in respiratory compliance.

If minute volume is constant, the work done against compliance is increased when breathing is deep and slow. Conversely, the work done against airflow resistance is increased when breathing is rapid and shallow. When the two components are summated and the total work is plotted against the respiratory frequency, an optimal respiratory frequency exists which minimizes the total work of breathing (Fig. 9.21). In patients with restrictive lung diseases (low compliance) such as pulmonary edema or ARDS, the optimal respiratory frequency is increased, often leading to rapid, shallow breaths. With obstructive lung diseases (high resistance) such as asthma or bronchiolitis, the optimal strategy is decreased respiratory rate with slow, deep breaths.

Classification of Mechanical Ventilation

Mechanical ventilators are designed to alter, transmit, and directly apply energy in a predetermined way to assist or replace the work of the respiratory muscles and thorax to maintain the gas exchange function of the lungs. Over the last three decades several generations of ventilators with increasing complexity have been developed. By necessity, several generations of classification schemes have also been proposed to assist clinicians' understanding of these devices[174,175]. Unfortunately, many of the classification systems were outdated, vague or frankly contradictory. In an attempt to overcome many of these problems, a more recent classification system has been proposed that is based upon a theoretical framework that can be applied to all ventilators in a consistent manner with specific and appropriate detail[176]. This system provides a common environment for terms and concepts that will facilitate the understanding, interpretation, and assessment of ventilator operating systems and performance characteristics. Although potentially cumbersome to the novice, this system is able to describe clearly, in specific details, all previoús, currently available, and future models of mechanical ventilators. Thus, it should be possible to avoid much confusion in this rapidly developing field. For these reasons, this classification system provides the framework for the ensuing discussion.

The classification system of Chatburn is based upon the physiologic principles of the equation of motion (pressure = volume/compliance + resistance × flow) as described above and utilizes five broad categories to provide a thorough discussion **(Table 9.5)**. This scheme is the first system that can accommodate the differing needs and interests of the intended audiences. For example, administrators may need to know where and what type of ventilator can be used (thus input power and control variable data are necessary), clinicians want to know how the ventilator works (making phase variables and output characteristics impor-

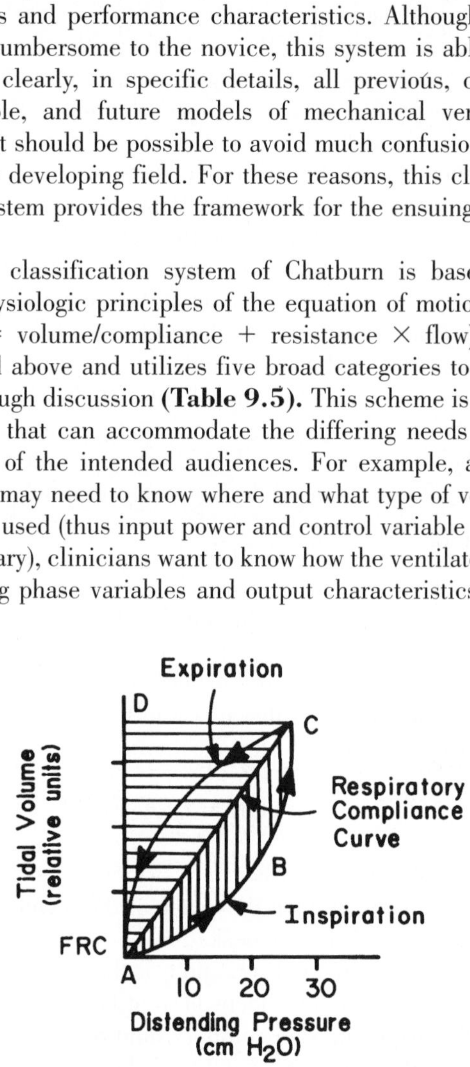

Figure 9.20. Inspiratory/expiratory pressure-volume loop recorded during respiratory cycle. The normal respiratory cycle entails the expenditure of work during inspiration to overcome resistive and elastic impedance to inflation of the lungs. Total work of breathing (pressure × volume) is defined by the sum of resistive work *(area* defined by *ABC)* plus elastic work *(area* defined by *ACD)*. Total work of breathing *(area* defined by *ABCD)* is increased either by an increase in resistive properties of the respiratory system or by a decrease in respiratory compliance *(slope of line* between *A* and *C)*. (Modified from Goldsmith JP, Karotkin EH. Assisted ventilation of the neonate. Philadelphia: WB Saunders, 1981:29.)

tant), researchers need an understanding of the internal workings of the ventilator (knowledge of drive mechanisms, control valves, output waveforms, etc.) while manufacturers should be knowledgeable of all of this information.

Power Input

There are only two sources of power available to provide the energy necessary to assist or replace the work of the respiratory muscles and thorax; either electrical or pneumatic (compressed gas). Electric drive mechanisms may involve either a direct (linear) drive piston or a rotary drive piston. Pneumatic power can be applied at either low or high pressure. Each system has its own inherent liabilities (e.g. loss of gas source with a pneumatic drive machine). For more details, the reader is referred to a more extensive review(175).

Power Transmission

The transmission (or conversion) of power from the original input (electric or pneumatic) to positive pressure gas delivered in a controlled manner is accomplished by the ventilator's drive mechanism(s). These may involve single or double circuits and incorporate either an external or internal compressor and the device's output control systems.

Control Scheme

The ventilator's control scheme may be simple, as in most neonatal ventilators in which only one waveform is available and the pressure is controlled simply by limiting the peak inspiratory pressure. Conversely, the control scheme can be complex as seen on third and fourth generation microprocessor ventilators where the entire shape of the waveform is controlled during inspiration, providing a choice of several different waveforms. Using mathematical terms, it becomes clear that the ventilator is able to control only one variable (the independent or control variable), while the resultant waveform is limited to only one dependent variable. Which variable becomes dependent is determined by selection of the control variable. It should be emphasized that any one of the four variables (pressure, volume, flow, time) can be controlled, making it the independent variable while the others become dependent variables.

Control Variables

The ventilator control variables, as the name implies, are the variables set or controlled by the ventilator to deliver the predetermined energy to the respiratory system. Four possible options for the control variable are available (pressure, volume, flow, time). **Pressure-controllers** are ventilators that control either the airway pressure (increasing it above the ambient pressure for inspiration) or the pressure surrounding the body surface (decreasing it below airway opening pressure for inspiration). This is the basis for classifying ventilators as either positive or negative pressure type ventilators. To be defined as a **volume-controller,** a ventilator must maintain an approximately constant tidal volume regardless of the varying workload (change in compliance and/or resistance) and measure volume to control the waveform. A **flow-controller** also has a constant volume waveform even with alterations in compliance and/or resistance, but volume is not measured or used as a feedback signal to alter flow. If both pressure and volume are affected by changes in lung mechanics, then the only form of control is the timing of inspiration and expiration, thus the only variables controlled are inspiratory and expiratory times and the ventilator is classified as a **time-controller.**

For each control variable, the ventilator manufacturers have established only a few possible waveforms. The most common waveform is rectangular (for pressure and flow control), sinusoidal (for volume and flow control), and accelerating or decelerating (for flow control). For a pressure-controlled ventilator, the tidal volume is a function of time, compliance, resistance, and the amplitude of the pressure (difference in peak and end-expiratory pressure). When volume and/or flow are the controlled variable for the ventilator, the tidal volume may be preset or is simply a function of time and the preset inspiratory-flow pattern.

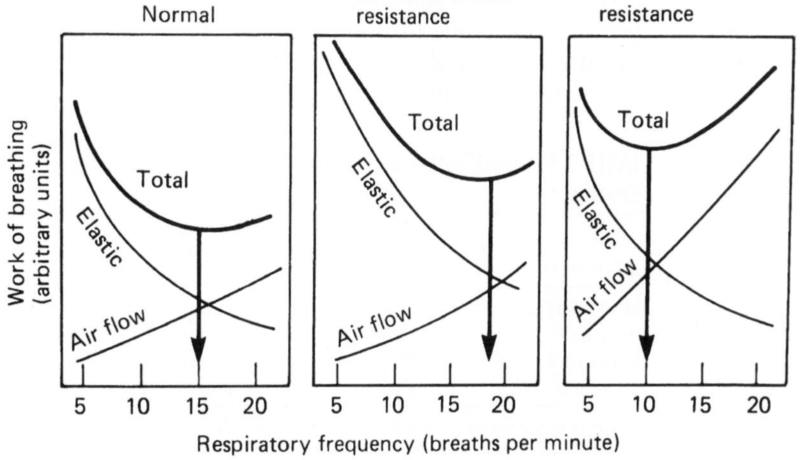

Figure 9.21. Diagrams show the work done against elastic and airflow resistance separately and summated to indicate the total work of breathing at different respiratory frequencies. The total work of breathing has a minimum value at about 15 breaths/min under normal circumstances. For the same minute volume, minimum work is performed at higher frequencies with stiff (less compliant) lungs and at lower frequencies when the airflow resistance is increased. (From Nunn JF. Applied respiratory physiology. 4th ed. Boston: Butterworths, 1993:126.)

TABLE 9.5. Classification Scheme for Mechanical Ventilators

Power Input
Power Transmission
Control Scheme
Control Variable
Phase Variable
Conditional Variable
Output Waveform
Alarms
Input Power Alarms
Control Circuit Alarms
Output Alarms

Phase Variables

Implicit in this classification system is that pressure, volume, and flow are functions of time and the ventilator must control the time intervals for inspiration and expiration. Previous classification systems had introduced the concept of dividing the ventilatory cycle into four phases: (1) the change from the expiratory phase into the inspiratory phase, (2) the inspiratory phase, (3) the change from the inspiratory phase into the expiratory phase, and (4) the expiratory phase[174]. Ventilator design dictates that one or more of the control variables are monitored and when they reach a predetermined value a switch is made from one phase to another. Thus, pressure, volume, flow, and time can be referred to as phase variables. More specifically, four phase-variable categories can be defined: (1) the trigger variable, (2) the limit variable, (3) the cycle variable, and (4) the baseline variable.

All ventilators use one of the four possible variables (pressure, volume, flow, time) to initiate the start of inspiration. The selected variable that initiates or triggers inspiration is called the **trigger variable.** Historically, time was the first trigger variable to be used (i.e. the ventilator initiates a breath according to a set frequency independent of the patient's inspiratory efforts). To allow mechanical ventilation synchronized to the patient's inspiratory efforts, pressure was then and now is commonly used as the trigger variable (i.e. a preset drop in the baseline circuit pressure secondary to the patient's inspiratory effort starts inspiration independent of the set frequency). Recent improvements in ventilator capabilities have led to the development of flow as a trigger variable. In fact, flow triggering is more sensitive and associated with less imposed work for the patient with a standard ventilator circuit than pressure triggering[177]. The sensitivity of the ventilator to the trigger variable and the amount of imposed work for the patient is adjustable by changing the ventilator's sensitivity.

During inspiration, pressure, volume, and flow all increase above their baseline end-expiratory values. One or more of these variables may rise up to a preset limit which is referred to as the **limit variable.** However, to meet the criteria of a true limit variable, inspiration must not be terminated because this variable has achieved its preset limit value as seen with a cycle variable (see below). For consistency, pressure, volume, and flow limits must be specified relative to their end-expiratory values. This is obvious for volume and flow where their end-expiratory values are zero; however, confusion regarding pressure limits can occur. To maintain consistency and avoid any potential confusion, pressure limits must always be measured relative to the end-expiratory pressure (i.e. above PEEP).

Contrast the limit variable to the **cycle variable,** where the specified variable is used to terminate inspiration when a preset value is reached. Clinicians commonly and incorrectly use the terms limit and cycle interchangeably. It must be emphasized that the limit variable attains its peak value *before* end-inspiration, while inspiration is terminated when the cycle variable's preset value is reached. Determining which variable terminates inspiration in a given ventilator can be confusing. Most microprocessor ventilators allow the clinician to set a tidal volume and inspiratory flowrate, leading one to believe that the ventilator is volume-cycled. In fact, these ventilators do not measure volume, instead they set the inspiratory time necessary to achieve the set tidal volume using the set inspiratory flowrate. Thus, the cycle variable is actually time.

During expiration, the ventilator may alter the way the control variables return to their respective baseline values. The variable that is controlled during the expiratory time is the **baseline variable.** Although any of the control variables could theoretically be controlled, pressure is the typical baseline variable in the vast majority of clinical situations. Control of the baseline variable allows the ventilator to control end-expiratory transrespiratory pressure and thus end-expiratory volume. Notice the term transrespiratory rather than airway pressure. This is used to accommodate the situation where a negative pressure ventilator is used to maintain a negative body-surface pressure during expiration or when negative pressure is applied to the airway to facilitate expiration.

Depending upon whether the ventilator or patient controls the triggering, limiting, and cycling variables, four different breath types under two board engineering headings (machine-cycled and patient-cycled) can be described **(Table 9.6).** A **mandatory breath** is triggered, limited, and cycled by the ventilator (i.e. the machine performs all the work). An **assisted breath** is triggered by the patient and limited and cycled by the ventilator (the patient only performs the work to initiate the breath). A **supported breath** is triggered and cycled by the patient and limited by the ventilator (the patient provides the triggering work

TABLE 9.6. Classification of the Available Mechanical Ventilator Breaths[a]

	Phase Variable		
Breath Type	*Trigger*	*Limit*	*Cycle*
Mandatory	Machine	Machine	Machine
Assisted	Patient	Machine	Machine
Supported	Patient	Machine	Patient
Spontaneous	Patient	Patient	Patient

[a]*Modified with permission from Branson RD & Chatburn RL. Technical description and classification of modes of ventilator operation. Respir Care 1992;37:1029.*

and a variable amount of the remaining work depending upon the interaction with the ventilator). A **spontaneous breath** is practically speaking triggered, limited, and cycled by the patient (the patient performs all the work).

Conditional Variables

Modern microprocessor ventilators combine the control and phase variables to deliver the predetermined waveform for each breath. The ventilator may either keep this pattern constant for each breath or it may introduce other patterns (i.e. mandatory and spontaneous breaths, assisted and supported breaths, etc.). Essentially, the ventilator must determine which pattern of control and phase variable to use before each breath, depending upon the value of some preset **conditional variables.** A common example is in the synchronized intermittent mandatory ventilation (SIMV) mode of ventilation. If the ventilator fails to detect a patient's inspiratory effort during a predetermined time (the SIMV window), then a mandatory breath is delivered. If the patient's inspiratory efforts are sensed while the SIMV window is open, then an assisted breath is provided; however, if the patient's inspiratory effort occurs after the SIMV window is closed, then a spontaneous breath is allowed. Under these circumstances, the conditional variables are pressure (or flow) and time.

Output Waveform

The study and understanding of ventilator operation is facilitated by the examination of output waveforms. The obvious output waveforms of interest are the pressure, volume, and flow waveforms used throughout the preceding discussion (Fig. 9.22). The conventional order of presentation corresponds to the mathematical convention used in the equation of motion (i.e. pressure, volume, flow). Convention also dictates that inspiration is depicted by positive (above the horizontal axis) and expiration by negative (below the horizontal axis). The horizontal axis has units of time (seconds) in all three cases. The vertical axes represent the measured variable in its common units of measurement. The specific baseline values are irrelevant for the purpose of identifying the output waveform; what is important is the relative magnitude of each of the variables and how it affects or is affected by the value of the other variables.

Output waveform analysis is a useful tool to examine the characteristics of ventilator operation and provides a graphic display of the various modes of ventilation[178]. It can be used to optimize mechanical ventilatory support and analyze ventilator incidents and alarm conditions. It may also be possible to alter the form of ventilatory support to improve patient-ventilator synchrony, reduce work-of-breathing, and calculate an assortment of physiologic parameters associated with respiratory mechanics. Optimal measurement of these data is obtained when the pressure and flow measuring device is positioned between the patient and the ventilator[178,179]. Measurement of esophageal pressure and integration of the intrapleural pressure en-

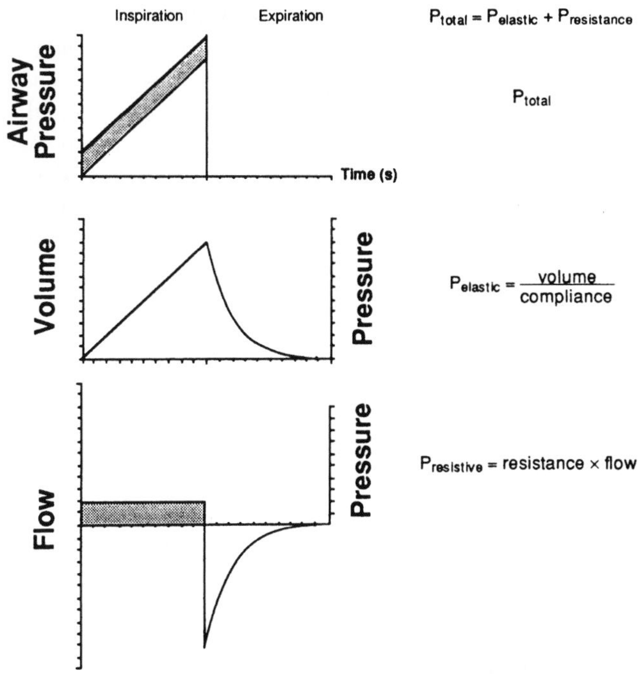

Figure 9.22. The theoretical output waveforms for flow-controlled inspiration presented as specified by equation of motion (pressure-top, volume-middle, flow-bottom). Note that the volume waveform is the same shape as the transthoracic or lung pressure waveform (i.e. pressure is due to elastic recoil) and the flow waveform is the same shape as the transairway pressure waveform (i.e. pressure due to airway resistance). If all the pressure scales are equal, then the height of the airway pressure waveform at any instant in time is the sum of the heights of the two waveforms as indicated by the shaded and unshaded portions of the figure. (From Chatburn RL. Classification of mechanical ventilation. Respir Care 1992;37:1022.)

hances output data analysis and enables measurement of the patient's work-of-breathing[179].

Simultaneously displaying pressure, volume, and flow waveforms over time facilitates the timing sequence of various respiratory events. Patient-ventilator dysynchrony may become evident with delays or distortion of the timing and magnitude of the measured output waveforms. For example, the development of intrinsic PEEP could be detected by the presence of expiratory flow during the initiation of inspiration or the measurement of positive pressure in excess of the desired level at end-expiration.

Alarms

Patient monitoring capabilities have been greatly expanded with the introduction of the microprocessor-based ventilators. Nearly every aspect of the patient's ventilatory pattern can be assessed, monitored, displayed, and alarmed. These alarms may be audible, visual, or both, depending upon the seriousness of the alarm condition. The alarm event may be technical (i.e. inadvertent change in the ventilator's performance) or patient related (i.e. denoting a change in the patient's status as detected by the ventilator).

These improved capabilities are not without fault; the medical staff can easily become overloaded with data, excessive or false positive alarms, which ultimately may impede proper patient management. The false positive and excessive alarms program the medical staff to respond to each alarm slowly, to inactivate the alarm without identifying the cause, or to ignore the alarm altogether. In addition, the accuracy of the monitored data has not been extensively documented. With these limitations in mind, the appropriate selection of alarm parameters should allow safe mechanical support of ventilation with the early identification of potentially serious problems. The types of alarms may be broadly categorized into three groups: input alarms, control alarms, and output alarms.

Input Power Alarms

All ventilators have alarms to notify clinicians of the loss in input power (either electrical or pneumatic). Most ventilators have some sort of battery backup in the case of input power failure to replace the lost electrical power or at least power the alarms to alert the bed-side care providers.

Control Circuit Alarms

Control circuit alarms warn the operator that some aspect of the ventilator self-test has failed or that the selected control-variable parameters are incompatible (e.g. inverse inspiratory/expiratory ratio). In the former case, there is likely something wrong with the ventilator control circuitry itself (i.e. microprocessor failure) and the ventilator would simply report as inoperative.

Output Alarms

Output alarms are defined as an unacceptable state of the ventilator's output. More precisely, an output alarm is activated when the value of a control variable (pressure, volume, flow, or time) exceeds or falls below preset values. Numerous output alarms are routinely used in clinical practice. Examples include: high or low peak, mean, end-expiratory pressure, high or low tidal volume or minute ventilation, and high or low ventilatory frequency (or too long or short of inspiratory or expiratory times). The composition and temperature of the inspiratory and expiratory gases are also be used as output alarms (i.e. high or low FiO_2 or exhaled PCO_2).

Modes of Mechanical Ventilation

Over the last ten to fifteen years there has been a tremendous proliferation of different modes of mechanical ventilation. Each mode has its loyal supporters and its equally determined critics; however, one group frequently does not understand the approach of the other. Furthermore, most clinicians fail to realize that experience and skill with a specific mode are probably the single greatest determinant of success for that mode. Thus, mechanical ventilation could be considered more of a practiced art than a science.

Because of the vast array of choices now available to clinicians, it is easy to become confused by the common clinical descriptions and terminology of many of these modes of ventilation. Using previously described ventilator classification systems classification of modes of mechanical ventilation has been proposed[180]. This system employs the same categories: control variables (pressure, volume, flow, and time), phase variables (trigger, limit, and cycle), and conditional variables. As described earlier **(Table 9.6),** the ventilator may deliver four different types of breaths (mandatory, assisted, supported, or spontaneous). Most of the commonly used modes are in fact a combination of these four types of breaths **(Table 9.7).** This classification system will be used to describe the modes of mechanical ventilation available to the clinician.

Mandatory (Controlled) Ventilation

Mandatory ventilation, known more commonly as controlled ventilation, is a mode of ventilator operation in which all breaths are triggered, limited, and cycled by the ventilator (i.e. the machine performs all the work). Thus, any of the control modes of ventilation are intended for use in patients with limited and/or absent ventilatory drives. In reality, many of the assisted modes of ventilation also become controlled modes when the patient's inspiratory efforts are suppressed (by sedatives, analgesics, or hyperventilation) or otherwise prevented (paralysis).

Volume Control Ventilation

Volume control ventilation (VCV) delivers a preset tidal volume during a set inspiratory time with a set frequency and constant inspiratory flow. This was the only mode of ventilation possible on the first generation of constant-volume ventilators[181]. The ventilator controls all timing parameters of the breath, although modern ventilators will respond to a patient's inspiratory effort (see assisted ventilation below). VCV is typically used only on patients who are apneic from sedation or anesthesia, nervous system injury, drug overdose, neuromuscular blockade, or deliberate mechanical hyperventilation so that the patient's spontaneous ventilator drive is suppressed.

Pressure Control Ventilation

Like the previous mode, pressure control ventilation (PCV) is designed for patients with suppressed ventilatory drive although patient inspiratory efforts will trigger the ventilator to deliver the same pressure-limited breath. In this mode the ventilator delivers positive pressure up to a predetermined pressure limit above PEEP during a selected inspiratory time and at a set frequency. The inspiratory flow depends upon the airway pressure and lung compliance, normally achieving high levels from the beginning of the breath and then decelerating towards zero at the end of inspiration. Since inspiratory pressure is the limiting variable, changes in respiratory system mechanics (i.e. compliance and/or resistance) will result in alteration in the delivered tidal volume and thus minute ventilation. Many of the theoretical advantages and problems related to pressure-limited modes of ventilation have been extensively reviewed[170].

Pressure Regulated Volume Control Ventilation

A new feature of many of the latest generation of microprocessor ventilators combines the characteristics of both volume- and pressure-limited ventilation. One example, marketed by Siemens, is called pressure regulated volume control (PRVC). This mode uses a decelerating inspiratory flow waveform to deliver a set tidal volume during the selected inspiratory time and at a set frequency. The ventilator monitors airway resistance and compliance and uses a predetermined algorithm to deliver the preset tidal volume. Airway pressure is limited below a selected high pressure threshold and may vary by as much as 3 cm H_2O from the previous breath. Thus, the ventilator is continuously adapting the inspiratory pressure to changes in the volume/pressure relationship of the patient's respiratory system.

Assisted Ventilation

Assisted ventilation is essentially identical to the respective controlled modes of ventilation except that patient inspiratory efforts trigger the ventilator to deliver assisted breaths using the preselected limit and cycle variables (i.e. the patient performs only the triggering work while the ventilator completes the remaining work). Assisted ventilation can be provided with either pressure or flow as the limit variable as seen with controlled ventilation. One potential drawback with this class of ventilation revolves around the fact that the inspiratory time is fixed. Rapid respiratory rates with the fixed inspiratory times lead to shorter expiratory times and may result in the delivery of mechanical

TABLE 9.7. Classification System for Common Modes of Mechanical Ventilation.[a]

	Breath Type												
	Mandatory			*Assisted*			*Supported*			*Spontaneous*			
Modes[b]	*trigger*	*limit*	*cycle*	*trigger*	*limit*	*cycle*	*trigger*	*limit*	*cycle*	*trigger*	*limit[c]*	*cycle[c]*	*Conditional Variable*
VCV	time	flow	volume[d]	—	—	—	—	—	—	—	—	—	—
PCV	time	pressure	time	—	—	—	—	—	—	—	—	—	—
PRVC	time	pressure	volume[d]	—	—	—	—	—	—	—	—	—	minute volume
ACV (volume)	time	flow	volume[d]	patient[e]	flow	volume[d]	—	—	—	—	—	—	patient effort or time
ACV (pressure)	time	pressure	time	patient[e]	pressure	time	—	—	—	—	—	—	patient effort or time
IMV (volume)	time	flow	volume[d]	—	—	—	—	—	—	patient[e]	pressure	pressure	—
SIMV (volume)	time	flow	volume[d]	patient[e]	flow	volume[d]	—	—	—	patient[e]	pressure	pressure	patient effort or time
IMV (pressure)	time	pressure	time	—	—	—	—	—	—	patient[e]	pressure	pressure	—
SIMV (pressure)	time	pressure	time	patient[e]	pressure	time	—	—	—	patient[e]	pressure	pressure	patient effort or time
APRV	time	pressure	time	—	—	—	—	—	—	patient[e,f]	pressure	pressure	—
APRV (synch.)	time	pressure	time	patient[e]	pressure	time	—	—	—	patient[e,f]	pressure	pressure	patient effort or time
MMV	time	flow	volume[d]	patient[e]	flow	volume[d]	—	—	—	patient[e]	—	—	minute volume
PSV	—	—	—	—	—	—	patient[e]	press.	flow[g]	—	—	—	—
VSV	—	—	—	—	—	—	patient[e]	press.	flow[g]	—	—	—	minute volume
VAPS	—	—	—	—	—	—	patient[e]	press.	flow[g]	—	—	—	tidal volume
CPAP	—	—	—	—	—	—	—	—	—	patient	pressure	pressure	patient effort

[a]*Modified with permission from Branson RD & Chatburn RL. Technical description and classification of modes of ventilator operation. Respir Care 1992;37:1029.*
[b]*VCV = volume-controlled ventilation, PCV = pressure-controlled ventilation, PRVC = pressure regulated volume control, ACV = assist-control ventilation, IMV = intermittent mandatory ventilation, SIMV = synchronized IMV, APRV = airway pressure release ventilation, MMV = mandatory minute ventilation, PSV = pressure support ventilation, VSV = volume support ventilation, VAPS = volume-assisted pressure support, CPAP = continuous positive airway pressure.*
[c]*Pressure-limited only on demand-valve systems in which the ventilator limits and cycles to maintain constant airway pressures (applies to all modes in this column).*
[d]*Cycling can also be due to set inspiratory time in the setting of a fixed flow.*
[e]*May be either patient generated pressure or flow in the ventilator circuit.*
[f]*Allows spontaneous breaths during both mandatory inspiratory and expiratory time.*
[g]*Flow reflects the interaction of the patient's effort with the respiratory system impedance and ventilator flow rate.*

tidal volumes with inspiratory times in excess of expiratory times (i.e. inverse I/E ratios).

Assist Control Ventilation

Assist-control ventilation (ACV) is a form of mechanical ventilation in which the ventilator provides a pre-set tidal volume (or pressure) in response to every patient-initiated breath. Should the patient fail to initiate a breath within a preselected time, the ventilator will deliver the mechanical tidal volume at a predetermined frequency (i.e. controlled ventilation). In essence, the controlled mode of ventilation on the recent generation of ventilators is ACV when the patient is spontaneously breathing. Since every spontaneous respiratory effort by the patient triggers a mechanical tidal volume, minute ventilation is essentially determined by the patient regardless of the selected ventilator rate (as long as the ventilator rate is lower than the patient's spontaneous rate). When compared to synchronized intermittent mandatory ventilation (SIMV), ACV has been associated with a respiratory alkalosis with equal minute ventilation (presumably secondary to a lower deadspace to tidal volume ventilation ratio) and a higher mean airway pressure and resultant lower cardiac output[182,183]. A perceived problem with a mode of ventilation is the inability to "wean" the mechanical portion of the minute ventilation. Thus, patients are typically extubated from ACV following either a CPAP/t-piece trial or "when they are judged to be ready".

Intermittent Mandatory Ventilation

Introduced into positive pressure ventilatory practice almost two decades ago[184], IMV allows spontaneous breathing between positive pressure breaths with a preset inspiratory time and frequency. The positive pressure breaths may be either pressure or volume limited. Delivery of the mechanical breaths can be triggered at a predetermined time interval (asynchronous IMV) or in response to the patient's spontaneous inspiratory efforts (synchronized IMV). Between the mechanical breaths the patient may breathe spontaneously from either a continuous-gas flow or a demand-flow system[184-186].

IMV was introduced into respiratory care for the purpose of allowing a smooth transition from positive pressure ventilatory support to independent spontaneous breathing (weaning)[184,187]. Theoretically, the gradual decrease in positive pressure ventilatory support and concomitant increase in spontaneous breathing allows smooth, continuous progression from assisted to independent ventilation. Thus, many of the problems with asynchrony between the patient and ventilator are circumvented, decreasing the necessity for sedatives and muscle relaxants in the management of mechanical ventilatory support[188]. In addition, IMV offers the advantage of diminishing the level of positive intrathoracic pressure associated with positive pressure ventilatory support[189]; consequently, it has been suggested that circulatory impairment resulting from impedance to venous return during positive pressure ventilation might be diminished with IMV[190]. Finally, spontaneous breathing is associated with improved distribution of ventilation to dependent lung regions where greater perfusion occurs, while controlled positive pressure ventilation has been found to favor ventilation of nondependent regions (dead space)[191,192]. The fact that (S)IMV allows a certain degree of spontaneous breathing offers the theoretical attraction of improving $\dot{V}/\dot{Q}$ matching in the lungs[193]. For all practical purposes, (S)IMV has become the standard mode of mechanical ventilation in most neonatal and pediatric centers world-wide.

Despite wide-spread use of (S)IMV, clear demonstration of the benefits have been inconsistent. The need for frequent administration of sedatives or muscle relaxants seems to be decreased significantly by using IMV as opposed to controlled mechanical ventilation[194]; however, no comparison studies with AMV are available. Studies focusing on the hemodynamic effects of IMV in comparison to CMV have failed to show consistent improvement in circulatory function with the use of IMV in either clinical[195] or laboratory[196,197] settings; however, others have noted an improvement in cardiac output with IMV mode in association with high levels of PEEP[198].

Airway Pressure Release Ventilation

Airway pressure release ventilation (APRV), as originally described, provides a continuous gas flow circuit to vary the airway pressure between two different CPAP levels (known as CPAP and release pressure) for set periods of time while allowing spontaneous ventilation for the patient at both levels[199]. With this mode of ventilation, airway pressures are intermittently decreased or "released" from the preset CPAP to a lower (release) or ambient pressure. Lung volume transiently decreases, allowing gas to exit the lungs passively, thereby augmenting alveolar ventilation. In principle, APRV was designed to open and stabilize the collapsed alveoli associated with acute lung injury without excessive peak airway pressures, while augmenting spontaneous minute ventilation with the brief, intermittent releases of airway pressure. One of the proposed benefits of APRV, as originally described with the continuous gas flow circuit, is that the patient may breathe spontaneously throughout the ventilatory cycle with minimal imposed work of breathing, and therefore, minimal or no sedation or paralysis is required.

APRV has been incorporated into several ventilators with demand circuits with synchronized patient triggering capabilities[200]. The preset variables that physicians control include the CPAP level, the frequency of the airway pressure releases, the level to which airway pressure is reduced during release, and the duration of airway pressure release. The limit variable is pressure, thus the degree of augmented ventilation is dependent on these variables plus the patient's respiratory system compliance and resistance. Timing (synchronized with the patient's inspiratory efforts) and duration of the release time (as a function of the time constant of the respiratory system) may significantly affect the efficiency of this mode of ventilation[201,202].

Experience with APRV is limited. Laboratory work in dogs before and after induction of acute lung injury with oleic acid demonstrated that APRV maintained oxygenation and decreased physiologic dead space ventilation with similar minute ventilation and thus decreased arterial carbon dioxide, compared with CMV with and without PEEP[203]. In a similar laboratory model, APRV was able to maintain oxygen delivery, while CMV with PEEP resulted in oxygen supply-demand imbalance because of decreased cardiovascular function[204]. Human clinical experience with APRV is limited to two uncontrolled trials[205,206], and two randomized multicenter trials[207,208]. In all cases, APRV resulted in lower peak airway pressures, while mean airway pressures have been lower than[206] or similar to[204] CMV with PEEP. Despite higher $\overline{P}_{aw}$, some investigators have failed to demonstrate improved oxygenation with APRV compared to VCV in humans with acute lung injury[205,206] while others showed significant increases in oxygenation[208]. APRV appears to be more effective than CMV in improving alveolar ventilation in animals[203] and humans[205-207,209].

Pediatric experience with APRV is nonexistent. In a neonatal laboratory model of acute lung injury, APRV provided similar oxygenation and ventilation with lower peak airway pressures and without compromising cardiovascular performance[210]. Much shorter release times than those in adult animals or humans were effective in the same neonatal model[202]. Controlled studies with APRV in adults or children demonstrating improvement in outcome will have to be conducted prior to the widespread clinical application of this mode of mechanical ventilation.

Mandatory Minute Ventilation

A further refinement of ventilatory devices allows the mandatory delivery of a predetermined minute volume in a mode called mandatory minute ventilation (MMV) that is variably distributed between spontaneous and mechanical breaths and depends on the patient's spontaneous ventilation[211]. With MMV, the machine measures the volume of gas breathed spontaneously by the patient over a predetermined time period. If this timed spontaneous volume falls below a preset volume, the machine delivers breaths of either fixed volume or pressure until the preset minute volume is achieved. In this fashion, MMV "guarantees" that a predetermined minute ventilation will be delivered to the patient by either spontaneous or mechanical positive pressure means. This mode of ventilation, employed primarily for the purpose of weaning, has been used infrequently in the United States but has received some attention in Europe[211,212].

Supported Ventilation

Supported ventilation is defined as a breath that is triggered by the patient, limited by the ventilator, and cycled by the patient (i.e. the patient provides the triggering work and interacts with the ventilator to perform a variable amount of the remaining work). Thus, ventilation is spontaneous in nature in that the patient initiates and terminates each breath and is only used in patients with adequate ventilatory drives.

Continuous Positive Airway Pressure

During continuous positive airway pressure (CPAP), the clinician selects a level of pressure which is maintained constant in the ventilator circuit while the patient breathes spontaneously. Care must be taken to avoid confusing CPAP with positive end-expiratory pressure (PEEP). The latter is commonly defined as the elevation in baseline pressure during mechanical ventilation whereas the former is the elevation in baseline pressure during spontaneous ventilation. This definition is limited when IMV is used, because the baseline pressure is elevated after both mandatory and spontaneous breaths. Perhaps the best way to distinguish between the two is that CPAP represents a mode of ventilation, as denoted here, while PEEP is simply the control of the baseline pressure during mechanical ventilation. Although defined as separate entities, both CPAP and PEEP are used for the same purpose, to increase end-expiratory lung volume. Continuous positive airway pressure was introduced into clinical practice in the late 1960's for the treatment of ARDS[213]. Gregory and coworkers[214] described the use of CPAP in premature infants with hyaline membrane disease. Since these early reports, CPAP and PEEP have assumed major roles in the management of acute respiratory failure from a variety of causes[158,159].

Technically, CPAP or PEEP is provided by mechanical ventilatory devices using a modification of standard expiratory valve mechanisms in conjunction with either continuous-flow or inspiratory demand-valve circuitry. Expiratory valves can function either as threshold resistors, which allow unimpeded expiration prior to achieving the preset end-expiratory circuit pressure, or as expiratory flow resistors, which act to impede flow during expiration such that inspiration begins before expiratory airway pressure reaches atmospheric levels (Fig. 9.23). The latter expiratory valve system is undesirable in most clinical settings because it is associated with higher mean intrathoracic pressures, greater circulatory embarrassment, and increased physiologic dead space[215,216].

Pressure Support Ventilation

Pressure support ventilation (PSV) is a mode of positive pressure ventilation in which all of the patient's inspiratory efforts are supported by the ventilator. With PSV, the patient triggers the ventilator to deliver a flow of gas sufficient to meet the patient's inspiratory demands while the exhalation valve closes, thus pressurizing the circuit to a preset pressure limit. Each cycle is terminated when inspiratory flow decreases to a percentage of its initial peak value rather than by volume, pressure, or time. Therefore, the patient retains control of the cycle length as well as its depth and flow characteristics. The patient's effort, the preset positive pressure limit, and the respiratory system impedance determine the delivered tidal volume.

During PSV, the degree of machine support depends on the level of preset pressure. This can range from partial support with low-pressure limits to nearly complete mechanical support with high-pressure limits[217,218]. PSV has been shown to decrease inspiratory work and abolish diaphragmatic muscle fatigue in patients who failed conventional weaning attempts[218]. These changes may be related to the ability to change the pressure-volume characteristics during PSV[219] and enhance the endurance conditioning of the diaphragm[220]. PSV has also been used to compensate for inspiratory work because of endotracheal tube impedance and inspiratory demand valves[221,222]. Recent study has shown that ventilator working pressure is a significant factor in the propagation of airway flow and pressure during PSV which, when excessive, may impede the efficiency of inspiration[223].

PSV may be of help in patients who have been difficult to wean from mechanical ventilation. Two methods of weaning from ventilation with PSV have been advocated[224,225]. In one[224], patients are initially ventilated at PS_{MAX} (defined as the pressure support level required to produce a tidal volume of 10-12 ml/kg). As clinical status dictates, the pressure support level is gradually decreased to a minimal value determined by the diameter of the endotracheal tube, at which time extubation can be performed. The second approach[225], SIMV plus PSV is used when complete machine support is required. "Trials" with PSV can be periodically provided in between periods of SIMV until the patient no longer requires SIMV and the pressure support level is minimal. To date, there are no clinical trials demonstrating that PSV is superior to other methods of weaning from mechanical ventilation.

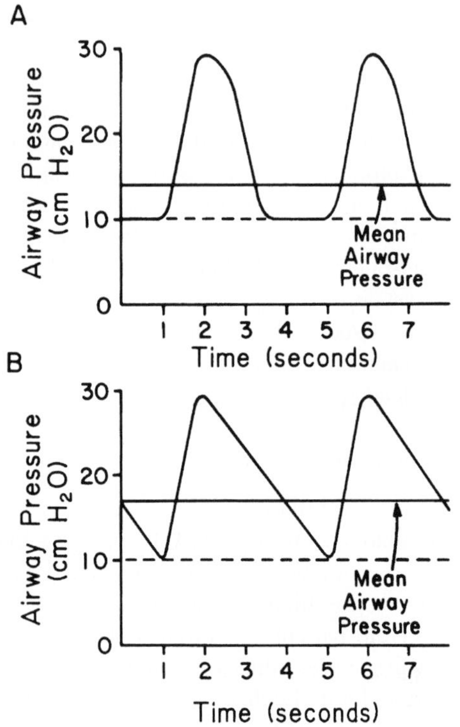

Figure 9.23. Airway pressure pattern during mechanical ventilation with PEEP generated by expiratory threshold value (A) and expiratory flow resistor (B). Both systems generate 10 cm H_2O PEEP. However, the ventilatory pattern generated with the expiratory flow resistor results in increased mean airway pressure.

Clinical experience with PSV in children remains limited. PSV effectively augments spontaneous ventilation and reduces the work of breathing in children[226]. Ventilators specifically designed for children are more efficient than adult ventilators at providing PSV[227]. This latter study clearly demonstrates the importance of trigger sensitivity and the imposed work of breathing in children. Like SIMV, the use of PSV has become widespread in many pediatric critical care centers, particularly with the newer flow-triggering ventilators, without any controlled clinical trials demonstrating improvements in outcome.

Volume Support Ventilation

Several "new" modes have recently been introduced into the support category of breaths by the manufacturers which are dependent upon conditional variables and ventilator logic. Although the manufacturer's names are different (volume support-Siemens vs. volume-assured pressure support-Bird Products), each is similar in that the patient is spontaneously triggering the ventilator to provide a pressure-limited and flow-cycled breath with a conditional "if, then" variable (i.e. minute ventilation-Siemens, tidal volume-Bird Products). Thus, these modes have all the theoretically beneficial characteristics of PSV (the patient controls the inspiratory flow, time, and frequency) with the unique asset of providing a guaranteed minimal minute ventilation. These modes also provide backup mandatory breaths should the patient become apneic. No clinical experience with these theoretically attractive modes of ventilation have been published.

Physiologic Approach to Mechanical Ventilation

The introduction of microprocessors into mechanical ventilators has resulted in a confusing array of products, each with its own unique features and modes of operation. This confusion has been compounded in the medical literature by unproven statements favoring one new device or mode of ventilation over another. Physicians involved in the ventilatory management of patients with respiratory failure should base their approach on physiologic principles, ventilator technology, and an understanding of patient-ventilator interactions.

Indications

Criteria for the application of positive pressure ventilatory support vary according to the clinician's goals. In essence, the desired endpoint of ventilatory support defines the criteria for its use. For example, a progressive increase in activity from rest to heavy exercise is associated with a 100-fold increase in the oxygen cost of breathing[228]. Thus, it is not surprising that several studies have demonstrated the usefulness of positive pressure ventilation in decreasing work of breathing and the oxygen consumption in patients with abnormal pulmonary mechanics. Positive pressure ventilation in these instances has resulted in an average 25% reduction in total oxygen consumption[229,230]. Other investigators have shown that positive pressure ventilation reduces the rate of lactic acid production in animals with circulatory shock[231] and results in the redirection of circulation from respiratory muscles to vital organs[2]. In newborn animals with acute respiratory failure, withdrawal of either positive or negative pressure ventilatory support is associated with a marked rise in cardiac output attributable to the increased work of breathing[232]. In these instances, standard criteria for initiation of mechanical support, based on blood gas indices of pulmonary gas exchange, might be lacking. However, the general benefits of assisted ventilation to the patient may be considerable. This is particularly true in children, who must channel considerable metabolic expenditures toward growth and development. Therefore, positive pressure ventilatory support might prove beneficial—and be indicated—in a number of settings other than acute respiratory failure.

With the above considerations in mind, the most common and obvious indication for mechanical ventilatory support is respiratory failure. This condition can be defined qualitatively as any respiratory condition associated with inadequate alveolar ventilation, failure of arterial oxygenation, or both **(Table 9.8).**

Inadequacy of alveolar ventilation is usually suspected on clinical grounds and documented by measurement of $PaCO_2$; the presence of $PaCO_2$ greater than 50-55 torr in the absence of chronic respiratory disease is generally indicative of inadequate alveolar ventilation and the need for mechanically assisted ventilation. In the presence of diseases associated with abnormal pulmonary mechanics, bedside measurement of vital capacity with a hand-held spirometer can be useful in confirming or predicting hypoventilation; a value less than 15 ml/kg is considered indicative of inadequate respiratory reserve to sustain independent ventilation[233]. However, it is equally important to consider the cause of inadequate alveolar ventilation and its anticipated course when the need for mechanical ventilatory support is being determined. For example, the presence of a progressive neuromuscular disease or pulmonary parenchymal disorder in its early stages would dictate a more immediate approach toward intervention. In contrast, mild hypercapnia in an otherwise healthy, alert adolescent with asthma who has received no prior therapy, often responds to bronchodilators without requiring mechanical ventilatory assistance. It should also be stressed that in all cases, a clinical impression of respiratory failure is just as important as laboratory or pulmonary function testing in evaluating the need for positive pressure support. On the other hand, failure of alveolar ventilation secondary to depression of respiratory drive (e.g., drug overdose, central hypoventilation) is frequently not associated with clinical signs of respiratory distress.

Arterial hypoxemia secondary to $\dot{V}/\dot{Q}$ mismatching and intrapulmonary right-to-left shunt requires consideration of positive pressure support in the form of continuous positive airway pressure. The presence of PaO_2 of less than 70 torr with FiO_2 greater than 0.6 is generally an indication for initiating positive pressure airway support. Other suggested criteria, used mainly in adults, include a calculated alveolar-arterial O_2 tension gradient ($AaDO_2$) greater than 300 torr with FiO_2 equal to 1.0 and a calculated right-to-left shunt fraction ($\dot{Q}_S/\dot{Q}_T$) greater than 15-20%[156,233]. In the presence of normal cardiac output and oxygen consumption, these additional calculated indices of oxygenation add little to the simple measurement of PaO_2 in assessing the degree of abnormal oxygen exchange in the lungs. Therefore, in pediatric practice, these ancillary measurements are usually unnecessary in determining the need for initiating positive pressure support. Once again, the clinical assessment of signs of respiratory failure and fatigue, the anticipated course of the respiratory disease at hand, and its anticipated response to conservative interventions must be considered prior to deciding on positive pressure interventions.

TABLE 9.8. Indications for Initiating Positive Pressure Ventilation, Continuous Distending Pressure, or Both

Absolute
Inadequate alveolar ventilation
Apnea
$PaCO_2 > 50$-55 torr (in the absence of chronic hypercapnia)
Impending hypoventilation
Rising $PaCO_2$
Vital capacity < 15 ml/kg
Dead space/tidal volume ratio > 0.6
Failure of arterial oxygenation
Cyanosis with $FiO_2 \geq 0.6$
$PaO_2 < 70$ torr with $FiO_2 > 0.6$
Other indices of severely impaired oxygenation
$AaDO_2 > 300$ torr with $FiO_2 = 1.0$
$\dot{Q}_S/\dot{Q}_T > 15$-20%
Relative
Secure control of ventilatory pattern and function
Intracranial hypertension
Circulatory insufficiency
Decrease metabolic cost of breathing
Chronic respiratory failure
Circulatory insufficiency

Application of Mechanical Ventilation

Once the decision to initiate ventilatory support has been made, preset mechanical ventilatory parameters should be determined in a systematic fashion **(Table 9.9).** The discussion will be divided into two categories based upon the changes in the respiratory mechanics (normal vs. abnormal).

Normal Respiratory Mechanics

Mechanical ventilation in patients with normal respiratory mechanics should as much as possible attempt to duplicate the normal physiologic state. In cases of hypoventilation, adequate alveolar ventilation should be ensured by initially providing full mechanical support of ventilation. Physiologic standards for respiratory frequency should be employed. However, when the tidal volume is selected, allowances must be made for (1) compressible volume of the ventilator circuit, (2) any associated increase in physiologic dead space as a result of the underlying respiratory disorder, and (3) increased carbon dioxide production, which may accompany acute respiratory failure[234]. Consequently, the preset tidal volume required for normal CO_2 elimination is often significantly greater than that found during spontaneous breathing (i.e., 7-8 ml/kg). As a first approximation, normal levels of $PaCO_2$ are generally achieved with a preset tidal volume of 10-15 ml/kg. Although this serves as a good estimate of tidal volume requirements, ventilation should be assessed clinically at the time positive pressure support is initiated, by noting the adequacy of chest excursions and breath sounds. This should be followed shortly by the determination of $PaCO_2$, and adjustments in tidal volume and ventilatory frequency made accordingly.

Determination of the tidal volume actually delivered to the patient requires assessment of the compressible volume characteristics of the ventilator circuit system. The specific compressible volume of a ventilator and its circuitry is determined by occluding the airway adapter of the circuit during an inspiratory cycle and slowly adjusting the delivered volume until the peak circuit pressure approximates the peak inflating pressure seen when the ventilator is attached to the patient. A hand-held spirometer is placed in line with the exhalation port of the ventilator. Measurement of the "exhaled volume" that is discharged from the ventilator circuit when the exhalation valve opens will be equal to the compressible volume lost in the circuit with each inspiration. This volume must be subtracted from the preset ventilator tidal volume to determine the true delivered tidal volume to the patient with each mechanical breath. Subtraction of the compressible volume from the exhaled volume provides the effective tidal volume (i.e. the volume actually delivered to the lungs for gas exchange). Highly compliant circuits with large compressible volumes have been shown to result in small effective tidal volume and increased dead space ventilation, particularly in neonates[235-237].

As a general rule, deviations from physiologic respiratory patterns with regard to rate and inspiration time are avoided. For example, excessive prolongation of inspiratory time can result in significant elevations in mean airway pressure, decreased venous return and depressed cardiac output[238]. Short inspiratory times and prolonged expiratory times (i.e., low I/E ratio) may be associated with an increased ratio of physiologic dead space and thus hypercapnia[239]. Clearly, the relationship between the inspiratory and expiratory times employed during positive pressure ventilation must be tailored to the patient's underlying physiologic abnormality.

TABLE 9.9. Guidelines for Initiating Positive Pressure Support

Provision of adequate alveolar ventilation

Select rate—physiologic norm for age
Select tidal volume—10-15 ml/kg
Select inspiratory time (I/E ratio)—age-specific norm generally resulting in I/E ratio = 1:2
Obstructive diseases—prolong expiratory time, avoid prolonged inspiratory time
Immediately assess for signs of adequate ventilation (e.g., chest excursion, breath sounds)
Measure $PaCO_2$; adjust SIMV rate and/or tidal volume as needed to maintain level between 35 and 45 torr
Decrease SIMV rate to level tolerated as determined by $PaCO_2$

Maintenance of adequate oxygenation

FiO_2—1.0
PEEP—3 cm H_2O, or higher level if needed, and ability to tolerate hemodynamic effects are anticipated
Immediately assess for signs of adequate oxygenation (e.g., color, pulse oximetry) and circulatory depression (e.g., hypotension, diminished peripheral pulses)
Measure PaO_2
- Decrease FiO_2 maintaining $PaO_2 > 70$ torr
- Restrictive disease (low FRC, low compliance)—increase PEEP as needed to achieve $PaO_2 > 70$ torr at $FiO_2 = 0.4\text{-}0.5$
- Consider direct monitoring of cardiac output if $\bar{P}_{aw} > 25$ cm H_2O; adjust PEEP further to maintain $Q_S/Q_T < 20\%$

Decrease PEEP while maintaining $PaO_2 > 70$ torr

POSTOPERATIVE. The vast majority of patients do not require postoperative mechanical ventilation following surgery. Residual anesthetic effects, usually a result of narcotics and suppression of respiratory drive or neuromuscular blocking agents with respiratory pump failure, may result in the need for mechanical ventilation for a variable period of time in a small portion of patients undergoing operative procedures. Although anesthetic-induced changes in respiratory mechanics have been reported[240,241], in many cases these are of little or no consequence and easily managed. Examples include surgeries involving the face or airway (i.e. craniofacial and tracheal reconstruction, cricoid split, tumors, etc.) in which the patency of the airway is of paramount importance or when deliberate hyperventilation is required for specific therapeutic purposes (i.e. intracranial and pulmonary hypertension). Patients more commonly remain intubated receiving mechanical ventilation postoperatively because of actual or suspected alterations in respiratory mechanics. In this instance, the means and methods of delivery of mechanical ventilation should be adjusted based upon these variations in respiratory mechanics as outlined below.

RESPIRATORY PUMP FAILURE. Patients with respiratory pump failure generally fall into one of the categories of acute (i.e. spinal cord trauma, Guillain-Barré syndrome, botulism, etc.) or chronic (the various muscular dystrophies, myasthenia gravis, polio, etc.) neuromuscular disease. These patients as a general rule have normal ventilatory drives and lung function, while suffering from respiratory muscle weakness making atelectasis and pneumonia common. The maintenance of a patent airway and provision of adequate lung volume are of primary importance for these patients. In fact, there is no evidence to suggest that either positive or negative pressure ventilation is superior in this situation. Further details are provided for this population of patients in chapter 8.

CIRCULATORY PUMP FAILURE. The provision of a patent airway and mechanical ventilation is one of the primary therapeutic interventions for shock. Children with circulatory failure frequently have impaired oxygen delivery from hemodynamic impairment, but also from respiratory muscle dysfunction secondary to hypoxia and acidosis (both metabolic and respiratory in etiology)[242]. Respiratory failure in shock may also be a result of the development of noncardiogenic pulmonary edema as seen in ARDS with its resultant intrapulmonary shunting[243]. Although the increase in intrathoracic pressure during mechanical ventilation is commonly associated with a decrease in venous return and cardiac output, the large negative intrathoracic pressures seen in patients with increased respiratory work leads to increased left ventricular transmural pressure, increased wall stress and afterload with subsequent deleterious effects on myocardial function[244]. In fact, this phenomenon has been documented in critically ill adults[245]. Finally, the reduction in metabolic expenditures and blood flow to the respiratory muscles following initiation of mechanical ventilation in patients with cardiogenic shock may serve to abate further ischemic or anoxic injury to other vital organs[2]. The decision to institute mechanical ventilation for these patients must be tempered by the potential hemodynamic consequences associated with many of the medications used to facilitate airway management and the physiologic changes seen when converting from a largely negative to positive intrathoracic pressure.

NEUROLOGIC INJURY. Mechanical hyperventilation has been the mainstay of therapy for intracranial hypertension for many years. Hypercapnia is the most potent stimulus for cerebral vasodilatation; consequently, one of the most effective means of acutely decreasing intracranial pressure (ICP) is artificially lowering the arterial carbon dioxide tension via hyperventilation. Decreases in ICP do not necessarily reflect increases in cerebral perfusion pressure. While hyperventilation to decrease ICP until other therapies (i.e. diuretics, sedatives, etc.) administered for the same purpose have time to take effect in the acute situation is reasonable, the *chronic* application of prophylactic hyperventilation in patients with head injury without raised ICP has in fact been shown to be detrimental[246]. If the head injured patient has been prophylactically hyperventilated to a $PaCO_2$ 25-30 mm Hg, a dramatic increase in minute ventilation may be required to further decrease $PaCO_2$. The increase in mean airway pressure (and intrathoracic pressure) associated with this increase in minute ventilation may provoke a paradoxical increase in ICP. Thus, stable head-injured patients without elevations in ICP should receive mechanical ventilation sufficient to produce normocapnia while preventing hypoxemia. Care must be exercised when $PaCO_2$ has been lowered for acute ICP management, the return to normocapnia should be gradual so that the ensuing cerebral vasodilation will not increase ICP.

Abnormal Respiratory Mechanics

The vast majority of children who require mechanical ventilation do so because of alterations in their respiratory mechanics which result in hypoxemia and/or hypercapnia. Mechanical ventilation for these children should be tailored to compensate or correct the underlying pulmonary pathophysiology. Because ventilators provide ventilation at nonphysiologic rates, pressures, flow patterns and timing, attempts to "physiologically" ventilate children with lung disease usually fail. The alterations of respiratory mechanics can be divided into two general categories (restrictive vs. obstructive disease). Unfortunately, lung disease commonly involves both airways (obstructive disease) and alveoli (restrictive disease). Historically, lung disease has been considered to be relatively homogenous; however, in reality the changes in respiratory mechanics are usually heterogenous in nature (i.e. areas of abnormally functioning airways and/or alveoli intermixed with areas with relatively normal airways and/or alveolar function). Despite these apparent confounding factors, it is frequently useful from a clinical perspective to categorize the disease processes into the simplified groups based upon the predominate pathophysiology to guide delivery of mechanical ventilation.

RESTRICTIVE LUNG DISEASE. Restrictive lung diseases are characterized by a decrease in lung volume with a proportionate reduction in airflow. Pulmonary function testing demonstrates a low FRC and forced expiratory volume in one second (FEV_1); however, the proportional decrease in expiratory flow would lead to a normal FEV_1/FRC ratio ($\geq$ 80% of the predicted value). Restrictive disease may be a result of abnormalities in either thoracic (obesity, abdominal distention) or lung (alveolar filling or fibrosis) mechanics. As a general rule for this category of diseases, the reduction in compliance will result in a decrease in the time constant of the respiratory system, lower functional residual capacity in conjunction with increased closing volume (defined as the volume at which conducting airways in the dependent regions of the lung begin to collapse), increased $\dot{V}/\dot{Q}$ mismatch and intrapulmonary shunting, and increased work of breathing. For discussion purposes, the provision of mechanical ventilation for patients with acute respiratory distress syndrome (ARDS) will be used as the model for this category of diseases (for more details see chapter 7).

Patients with ARDS exhibit reduced lung volumes (specifically EEV) associated with atelectasis and an elevation in closing volume[247,248]. These changes lead to a generalized decrease in the lungs $\dot{V}/\dot{Q}$ ratio, increased intrapulmonary shunting, and hypoxemia. The reduction in lung volumes cause: (1) decreased lung compliance, (2) alterations in regional resistances secondary to reduction in distal airway caliber by bronchoconstriction, peribronchial edema, and reduced lung volume, and (3) marked hysteresis (i.e. higher transpulmonary pressures are required during inspiration compared to expiration)[144,154,248]. The net result of these alterations in respiratory mechanics is the development of a heterogenous decrease in respiratory system time constant and a significant increase in the transpulmonary pressure (i.e. work of breathing).

The traditional approach to mechanical ventilation of patients with ARDS throughout the 1970s and 1980s was to fully compensate for altered lung function (i.e. normalize arterial blood gases) without inducing oxygen toxicity, barotrauma, or cardiovascular embarrassment. This was achieved principally through the recruitment of collapsed alveoli and improved oxygenation with the use of PEEP and volume-limited, constant flow positive pressure breaths at a frequency to provide normocapnia. Recent insights regarding the role of alveolar distention (i.e. volutrama) in the pathogenesis of ARDS has led to a significant change in the approach to mechanical ventilation in these patients[243,249]. Mechanical ventilation is directed towards the recruitment of as many alveoli as possible while secondarily maintaining transalveolar pressures within a narrow (and ill defined) therapeutic window in an attempt to avoid volutrauma to alveolar tissues (see volutrauma section).

The primary goal of alveolar recruitment is achieved via increases in mean airway pressure ($\overline{P}_{aw}$). It has been shown that $\overline{P}_{aw}$, under passive conditions, correlates closely to the forces holding the lung distended and is associated with the level of oxygenation[167,249]. In clinical practice, $\overline{P}_{aw}$ is manipulated through changes in inspiratory and expiratory pressure and times as well as alteration in inspiratory waveform. While the benefits of alterations in inspiratory waveform (i.e. volume- vs. pressure-limited ventilation) and/or inspiratory/expiratory ratio (i.e. inverse I/E ratio ventilation) remain controversial (see below), the regulation of expiratory and more recently inspiratory pressures appears well established by clinical and experimental evidence.

The first published report of ARDS in 1967 demonstrated the apparent benefit of PEEP[213]. PEEP prevents airway pressure from falling below the alveolar closing pressure, thus maintaining airway patency and alveolar volume throughout the ventilatory cycle. PEEP not only redistributes pulmonary edema fluid from the alveoli to the interstitium, but also may help to maintain surfactant activity by limiting alveolar collapse and concurrent surfactant film collapse[250,251]. This results in improved distribution of ventilation to low $\dot{V}/\dot{Q}$ compartments of the lung and better overall $\dot{V}/\dot{Q}$ matching in the lung[156,157,252,253]. As such, this modality is of primary importance in improving oxygenation, diminishing the necessity for high concentrations of oxygen, increasing EEV, and improving total respiratory compliance in respiratory diseases with decreased resting lung volume and compliance.

Excessive levels of PEEP can be counterproductive in the treatment of acute respiratory failure[254]. High levels of PEEP, even when indicated, can depress cardiac output and oxygen delivery to peripheral organs[161,255,256]. Application of continuous distending pressure beyond its optimal level can lead to increased physiologic dead space and decreased lung compliance as the result of alveolar overdistention[257]. Worsening of oxygenation has also been reported with excessive PEEP[162], presumably because blood flow is shunted to poorly ventilated alveolar units from overdistended regions of the lung. Therefore, selection of the proper level of PEEP is important in achieving optimal results.

Attempts have been made to physiologically define "optimal PEEP" in terms of total oxygen delivery (i.e., arterial O_2 content times cardiac output). Suter and coworkers[161], studying adults with acute respiratory failure, found a specific level of PEEP associated with maximal oxygen delivery. This level of PEEP also coincided with the achievement of maximum total respiratory compliance. Defining optimal levels of PEEP in this manner has been criticized because decreased O_2 delivery secondary to a fall in cardiac output with high levels of PEEP can often be reversed by intravascular volume expansion[258,259] or appropriate inotropic treatment[260]. Further optimization of V/Q matching can frequently be achieved by still higher levels of PEEP[161]. Thus, an alternative definition of optimal PEEP is the level that allows support of oxygenation with nontoxic levels of inspired oxygen without inducing refractory circulatory depression.

More recent investigation has attempted to define "optimal PEEP" in terms of respiratory mechanics (i.e. static pressure-volume curves of the respiratory system). Measurement of static pressure-volume curves in patients in the early stages of ARDS has demonstrated a lower inflection point which disappears later in the disease course[261]. This inflection point appears to represent the alveolar closing pressure; application of PEEP above this threshold is associated with maximal alveolar recruitment and lung compliance while PEEP below this limit allows alveolar collapse and decreased lung compliance. Thus, PEEP at a level just above the inflection point will prevent alveolar collapse and maintain optimal lung volume, compliance, and oxygenation[249]. Unfortunately, the routine measurement of the static pressure-volume curve in most clinical settings is difficult. Thus, clinicians continue to use the lowest amount of PEEP necessary to achieve an easily monitored clinical goal (arterial oxygenation or saturation) with "non-toxic" inspired oxygen concentrations.

Regardless of the means for selecting the level of PEEP, a systematic approach and constant evaluation are most effective and safe for the patient with evolving ARDS. This systematic approach may include the use of "PEEP trials". During the trial, insofar as clinically feasible, the PEEP is the only ventilator variable changed while monitoring oxygenation (PaO_2 or S_pO_2), ventilation ($PaCO_2$, V_D/V_T), compliance, and cardiac output (perfusion, urine output, blood pressure, and occasionally cardiac index/oxygen delivery).

The PEEP levels are instituted at a low level and incrementally increased every 15 minutes while monitoring the defined parameters for improvement or deterioration. These "PEEP trials" may establish the clinically "optimal level of PEEP" for initiating therapy early in the course of ARDS.

When increases in PEEP are indicated, it should be elevated in 2-3 cm H_2O increments with the goal of achieving adequate oxygenation (i.e. arterial hemoglobin saturation $> 90\%$) on non-toxic levels of supplemental oxygen (i.e. $FiO_2 < 0.6$); this usually corresponds roughly to an intrapulmonary shunt $< 20\%$ and an alveolar to arterial partial pressure of oxygen difference of < 250 torr. Because of the risk of circulatory depression, it is recommended that cardiac output monitoring be performed by using a flow-directed, thermodilution pulmonary artery catheter when $\overline{P}_{aw}$ exceeds 25 cm H_2O or when clinical evidence of circulatory compromise is present. As noted above, decreased cardiac output in association with the application of PEEP usually responds to intravascular volume expansion with crystalloid or colloid solution, or to low-dose inotropic support (i.e. dopamine).

The second goal, limiting end-inspiratory alveolar volume, has been derived from a large amount of experimental evidence from multiple investigators in mammalian species in which lung overdistention by mechanical ventilation with high airway pressures produces insidious physiologic and morphologic changes in the lungs (see volutrauma section)[249]. An airway plateau pressure of > 35 cm H_2O may be deleterious to the lung. In clinical conditions associated with decreased chest wall compliance, a plateau pressure threshold somewhat greater than 35 cm H_2O may be acceptable. The clinician may achieve this goal by utilizing either smaller tidal volumes (in volume-limited ventilation) or lower peak airway pressures (in pressure-limited ventilation). This scheme of limiting plateau pressures is frequently responsible for the utilization of small tidal volumes, thus lowering minute and alveolar ventilation and allowing elevations in $PaCO_2$. The term "permissive hypercapnia" has been used to describe this overall strategy of small tidal ventilation with adequate $\overline{P}_{aw}$ to achieve satisfactory oxygenation without toxic inspired oxygen concentrations while allowing $PaCO_2$ to rise if necessary[249,262,263].

The application of permissive hypercapnia is not without adverse side-effects or potential complications. The physiologic effects of hypercapnia include: (1) intracellular acidosis with potential to alter cellular oxidative metabolism, ionic conductances, excitation-contraction coupling, and cell division, (2) increased sympathoadrenergic tone with elevations in heart rate and stroke volume while systemic vascular resistance decreases which lead to an overall increase in cardiac output, (3) cerebral vasodilatation which allows cerebral blood flow to increase, and (4) increased arrhythmias. Many of these adverse effects are minimized by the body's ability to retain bicarbonate and metabolically compensate for a consistent respiratory acidosis. Thus, the only apparent absolute contraindication to permissive hypercapnia appears to be cerebral disorders where increases in blood flow may lead to intracranial hypertension. A review of the physiologic sequelae of alveolar hypoventilation and hypercapnia has recently been published[264].

In summary, the concepts of ventilator induced "volutrauma" and permissive hypercapnia and its associated ventilatory strategies are as yet unproven and require randomized controlled study. Despite these shortcomings, the amount of experimental and clinical evidence has been sufficient for many clinicians to introduce these concepts into clinical practice. Randomized trials comparing the various methods of applying this new ventilatory strategy are needed.

OBSTRUCTIVE LUNG DISEASE. Obstructive lung disease is identified by a reduction in airflow that is greater than any accompanying reduction in forced vital capacity (FVC). Hence the FEV_1 is reduced more than the FVC and the FEV_1/FVC ratio is low. As the disease progresses, a process described as dynamic hyperinflation occurs in which the increased airway resistance causes air trapping and an increase in residual volume (RV), until the elevation in RV begins to encroach upon the vital capacity. Thus, the predominant change in respiratory mechanics is the increase in airway resistance and prolongation of the time constant. The dynamic hyperinflation and increase in RV also causes tidal ventilation to occur on the upper flat portion of the pressure-volume curve of the respiratory system, resulting in decreased compliance. Asthma will be used as the model disease for the discussion of this category of diseases.

Acute respiratory failure in patients with asthma is associated with significant expiratory obstruction and dynamic hyperinflation. Resistance to inspiration and expiration are not only increased by bronchoconstriction but also as a consequence of airway edema and mucous. These patients benefit from mechanical ventilation strategies designed to maximize expiratory time, thereby decreasing end-expiratory lung volume (V_{EE}), intrinsic PEEP, and the risk of cardiovascular compromise[164]. A higher V_{EE}, when utilizing the same tidal volume, will invariably produce a higher end-inspiratory lung volume and a greater risk of volume-related lung injury (volutrauma)[265].

The employment of high inspiratory flow rates will minimize V_{EE}, intrinsic PEEP, and dynamic hyperinflation. However, the effects of turbulence, noncompliant airways, and/or bronchoconstriction may all be sufficient to cause a flow-dependent increase in inspiratory resistance[266]. Furthermore, the increase in inspiratory flow is achieved at the expense of higher peak airway pressures in the conducting airways. Even though the higher airway pressures generated by increased inspiratory flow rate do not strictly correlate with barotrauma or plateau pressure, the amount of central airway pressure that is actually transmitted to the alveoli (the genuine risk factor for volutrama) is difficult to determine. End-inspiratory plateau pressures during mechanical ventilation rise as dynamic hyperinflation increases and may be a better estimate of the risk for volutrama. Therefore, peak inspiratory flow rate should be adjusted to meet the patient's inspiratory demands while providing sufficient time for expiratory flow rate to approach or reach baseline, thereby minimizing the risk of dynamic hyperinflation and volutrauma[(267)].

The second means of minimizing dynamic hyperinflation involves the utilization of the lowest minute ventilation that produces acceptable gas exchange. This strategy of deliberate or controlled hypoventilation for patients with status asthmaticus was first described over ten years ago[(268)] and now has become the standard of care in today's ICUs. To achieve these goals of a diminished minute ventilation and as long as possible expiratory time, most clinicians select a physiologic tidal volume to be delivered at a low frequency. The transmission of the low minute ventilation in combination with the elevation in deadspace ventilation seen with obstructive diseases gives rise to hypercapnia.

Many of the same issues regarding deliberate hypoventilation, hypercapnia, and volutrauma discussed with respect to restrictive lung diseases also apply in this category. Thus, attempts to maintain airway plateau pressures under 35 cm H_2O theoretically should be allied with a decreased risk of volutrauma to the lung. Others suggest that the measurement of dynamic hyperinflation, defined as the failure of the lung volume to return to passive FRC (volume where elastic recoil equals external PEEP) prior to the onset of the next inspiration, may identify patients ventilated for status asthmaticus at risk for morbidity or mortality[(265)]. These same investigators subsequently used this measurement of dynamic hyperinflation to assist with the mechanical ventilation and its weaning in patients with severe asthma[(269)]. The consequences of dynamic hyperinflation include: (1) cycling of tidal volume closer to total lung capacity (where compliance is diminished) making higher airway pressures necessary to deliver the selected tidal volume, (2) interfering with patient efforts to trigger the ventilator in assisted or supported modes of ventilation (i.e. the patient must generate enough pressure to overcome the intrinsic PEEP plus the trigger sensitivity), (3) increasing the work of breathing secondary to both 1 and 2 above, (4) altering cardiovascular function similar to extrinsic PEEP through increases in intrathoracic pressure, and (5) causing overestimation of the pressure difference required for tidal ventilation and underestimation of the true compliance of the respiratory system. In instances when assisted ventilation is used, the application of small amounts of extrinsic PEEP may be advantageous to decrease the work of breathing by improving the patient's ability to trigger the ventilator. Caution must be exercised to limit the application of extrinsic PEEP to a level less than intrinsic PEEP or dramatic increases in FRC and dynamic hyperinflation can occur[(270)]. Regardless of the specific mode of ventilation, careful application with low frequency normal tidal volume ventilation with long expiratory times and the tolerance of hypercapnia has been associated with decreased morbidity and mortality in adults[(271,272)] and children[(273,274)].

FOCAL LUNG DISEASE. Although infrequently encountered, a patient with unilateral lung disease developing respiratory failure necessitating mechanical ventilation presents a significant problem to the bedside clinician. The physiologic change responsible for the initiation of mechanical ventilation is in almost every situation a result of hypoxemia and not hypercapnia. Therapeutic efforts are typically directed towards positional changes of the patient and alterations in inspiratory flow rates in order to improve overall lung function. Simultaneous independent lung ventilation via double-lumen tracheal tubes and differential application of positive airway pressure has been described in both adults[(275)] and children[(276)], but is technically difficult and has not been shown to improve outcome. Therefore, most clinicians continue to use conventional ventilatory techniques. Should difficulties in oxygenation be encountered, a trial of ventilation with the least involved lung in the dependent position is appropriate in larger patients[(147)] and the diseased lung in the dependent position in infants[(148)]. Significant elevations in uniformly applied PEEP is rarely helpful with unilateral disease and clearly places the more compliant, less involved lung at risk for volutrauma. In these instances, attempts directed at reinflating the diseased lung (i.e. flexible fiberoptic bronchoscopy for clearing of involved airways) or other experimental methods of cardiorespiratory support (i.e. independent lung ventilation, high frequency ventilation, extracorporeal life support) may be tried.

Controversies of Mechanical Ventilation

While the method of delivering mechanical ventilation is relatively straightforward in patients with little or no change in respiratory mechanics, the best means of providing mechanical ventilatory assistance in cases of severe alteration of pulmonary function has not been defined. One significant area of controversy involves the relative risks and benefits of volume-limited versus pressure-limited ventilation. A second area of dispute revolves around the use of mechanical ventilation with inspiratory time in excess of expiratory time (inverse ratio ventilation).

Volume-limited vs. Pressure-limited Ventilation

There are unique characteristics for both volume- and pressure-limited ventilation that represent advantages and disadvantages when used in patients with acute lung injury **(Table 9.10).** In traditional flow-limited, volume-cycled ventilation (VCV), the tidal volume, minute ventilation, and inspiratory flow are set by the clinician (Fig. 9.24A). This facilitates the control of alveolar ventilation, and thus $PaCO_2$, while also allowing breath-to-breath monitoring of respiratory impedance (i.e. changes in peak airway pressure will denote alterations in compliance and resistance). The disadvantages of VCV are related to the variable end-inspiratory alveolar volume (increased risk of overdistention) and to the constant inspiratory flow which may be set too low to meet the patient's spontaneous efforts (i.e. flow dyssynchrony and imposed work of breathing). During pressure-controlled, time-cycled ventilation (PCV), a decelerating flow pattern is used to achieve a predetermined upper pressure limit for a set period of time (Fig. 9.24B). By design, the airway pressures are limited so that end-inspiratory alveolar volume is also limited and, in theory, decreases the risk of "volutrauma". The decelerating inspiratory flow has been reported to lead to decreases in peak airway pressures and better distribution of ventilation with a decrease in dead space ventilation in patients with lung injury[(249,277)]. During severe pulmonary dysfunction, recruitment of collapsed distal airways and alveoli requires inspiratory pressures that overcome critical opening pressures for sustained periods of time. This situation appears ideally suited to a pressure-limited mode of ventilation. Unfortunately, because the pressure is set, changes in respiratory impedance may go undetected and will alter delivered tidal volume. Minute ventilation does not increase linearly with frequency but approaches a distinct bounding limit even when applied pressure, resistance, and compliance remain constant, making control of alveolar ventilation and $PaCO_2$ more difficult[(170)].

Two randomized clinical trials comparing VCV and PCV have recently been published[(278,279)]. The former examined the effects on respiratory mechanics, gas exchange, and hemodynamics of short-term applications of VCV compared to PCV with varying inspiratory to expiratory ratios[(278)]. These investigators were unable to demonstrate any improvement in any of the measured parameters with PCV regardless of the I:E ratio. This study may have been limited by the severity of illness of the patients studied (mortality rate of 78%) and the possible progression of their disease prior to study (i.e. the patients had been ventilated for a mean of 7.9 ± 5.1 days prior to the study). Furthermore, the short period of observation (30 minutes) may have prevented the detection of the delayed ability of PCV to recruit atelectatic lung units and improve oxygenation that has been reported by others[(208,280)]. In contrast, the latter study demonstrated a more rapid improvement in static compliance and a shorter duration of mechanical ventilation in patients with severe acute lung injury using PCV when compared to patients randomized to VCV[(279)]. This may support the concept that the early alveolar filling sustains more alveolar tractive force than the constant-flow VCV of similar duration.

TABLE 9.10. Comparative Advantages and Disadvantages of Volume-limited and Pressure-limited Ventilation[a]

Volume-limited	*Pressure-limited*
Advantages	
Guaranteed tidal volume and minute ventilation	
Precise control of flow pattern	
Changes in respiratory system impedance easily detected	
Clinician familiarity	
	Precise control of peak volume (end inspiratory alveolar volume)
	Decelerating flow pattern reported to:
	Improve distribution of ventilation
	Decrease dead space ventilation
	Decrease peak airway pressures
	Increase mean airway pressures
	Higher initial flows more readily match patient's demands
Disadvantages	
Peak airway and alveolar pressure and volumes vary	
Constant flow may not meet patient's initial flow demands (flow dysynchrony)	
	Tidal volume varies with changes in respiratory system impedance
	Changes in respiratory system impedance not easily detected
	Minute ventilation is a complex function of pressure, impedance, and frequency

[a]*Modified from Martin LD. New approaches to ventilation in infants and children. Curr Opin Pediatr 1995;7:253.*

Inverse I/E Ratio Ventilation

Because of the limitation placed on the end-inspiratory alveolar volume (i.e. limited plateau airway pressure) and end-expiratory pressure (i.e. lower inflection point of the pressure-volume curve) during optimal ventilation of patients with acute lung injury, manipulation of mean airway pressure to regulate oxygenation is often accomplished by alteration in the inspiratory to expiratory ratio. The prolongation of the inspiratory phase in excess of the expiratory phase (i.e. inverse ratio ventilation-IRV) during positive pressure ventilation has been used to increase mean airway pressure, FRC, and oxygenation in patients with severe acute lung injury[(280-283)]. The short expiratory time induces intrinsic PEEP[(284)], which promotes alveolar stabilization and prevents alveolar collapse. During IRV, peak airway pressures are lower than with CMV with PEEP[(281,282)]. However, IRV imposes a nonphysiologic breathing pattern with an I/E ratio greater than 1:1; therefore, patients frequently require heavy sedation and/or muscle paralysis.

IRV can be performed by using any of three separate methods: (1) pressure-limited breaths with decelerating inspiratory flow rates and adjustment of the inspiratory time to the desired level; (2) volume-limited breaths with low inspiratory flow rates to achieve the desired inspiratory time; or (3) volume-limited breaths with normal inspiratory flow rates and prolonged inspiratory pause to maintain the prolonged inspiratory phase[(285)]. In practice, pressure-controlled breaths are most commonly used. During pressure-controlled IRV, tidal volume is a function of the airway pressure limit, respiratory system mechanics, the ratio of inspiratory time to total breath cycle, and frequency[(170)]. Thus, for a given respiratory system compliance, resistance, and pressure limit, the higher the I/E ratio and frequency, the smaller the tidal volume will be. Despite the decrease in tidal volume and minute ventilation, alveolar ventilation is usually well maintained[(281,282)], most likely due to a lower dead space to the tidal volume ratio[(283)].

IRV has successfully been used in neonatal[(160,168,286)],

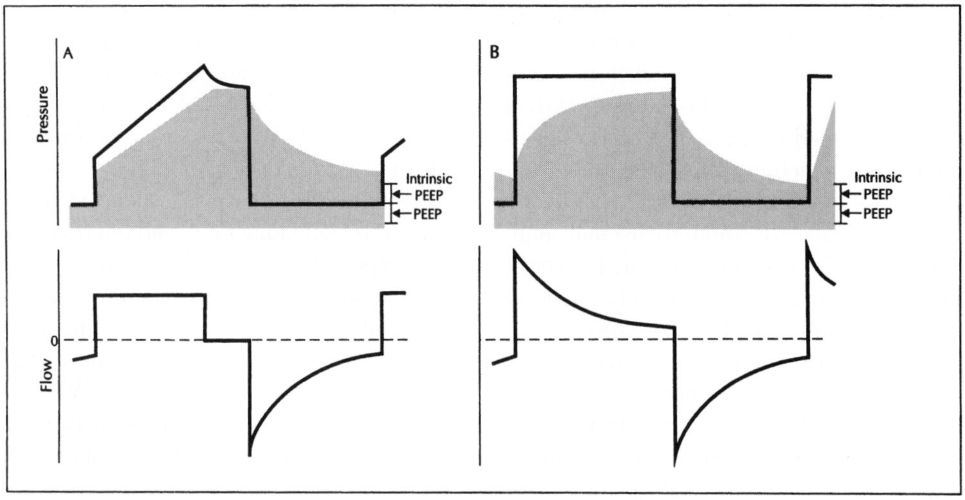

Figure 9.24. Pressure and flow profiles over time during volume-controlled ventilation (A) and pressure-controlled ventilation (B). In both diagrams, there is a discrepancy between alveolar (shaded) and airway pressures and persistent expiratory flows (auto-PEEP). Volume-controlled ventilation is volume-limited and time-cycled while using a constant inspiratory flow (an end-inspiratory pause is included in this example). Note the constant increase in pressure and difference between peak and plateau pressures (reflecting the resistive component of the airway pressure). Mean airway pressure can be increased by: (1) increasing tidal volume; (2) increasing end-expiratory pressure; (3) adding or increasing end-inspiratory pause; (4) or shortening expiratory time with an increase in frequency or decrease in inspiratory flow rate. Pressure-controlled ventilation is pressure-limited and time-cycled but uses a decelerating inspiratory flow which results in a square pressure wave form. Both alveolar pressure and volume increase and decrease exponentially. Mean airway pressure is increased by: (1) increasing peak and/or end-expiratory pressure; (2) lengthening inspiratory time; or (3) increasing frequency (shortening expiratory time). (From Martin LD. New approaches to ventilation in infants and children. Curr Opin Pediatr 1995;7:250.)

pediatric[287], and adult patients[280-283] with severe acute lung injury characterized by low compliance, decreased FRC, and refractory hypoxemia. Although most studies reported improvements in oxygenation with IRV compared to CMV with PEEP[281,282], mortality remained very high. No controlled studies have demonstrated that IRV reduces morbidity or mortality in patients with refractory hypoxemia. This lack of controlled studies showing a benefit with IRV in conjunction with the difficulty in monitoring and regulating the intrinsic or auto-PEEP that can develop, has led others to suggest that IRV is of unproven value in the management of acute lung injury[288].

Another mode of ventilation that combines assets of PCV with IRV while still allowing spontaneous breaths is APRV[203]. In theory, the ability to allow spontaneous unrestricted ventilation throughout the mechanical ventilatory cycle should allow application of this mode with less sedation and avoid altogether the risks of prolonged pharmacologic paralysis. Clinical experience with this method of ventilatory support is still very limited. A prospective, non-randomized crossover trial showed that APRV was equivalent to conventional VCV in adults with moderately severe acute lung injury who were apneic[207]. In a randomized controlled trial comparing VC-IRV with APRV in adults with severe lung injury, APRV was found to have lower peak airway pressures while oxygenation and venous admixture improved over the 24 hour period of observation[208]. As a means of partial ventilatory support, APRV has been shown to be equal to either SIMV or PSV in adults recovering from acute lung injury[289]. However, many patients stated that they were less comfortable with APRV compared to the other more conventional modes

Weaning of Mechanical Ventilation

A small but significant percentage of patients require mechanical ventilation for protracted periods, thereby exposing them to serious hazard and disability at significant costs to the family and society. Greater understanding of respiratory muscle performance in infants and children may improve the decision making during the process of withdrawal (weaning) from mechanical ventilation[290]. The successful weaning of positive pressure support depends on the careful consideration of general patient status, the presence of adequate ventilatory reserve, and the attainment of favorable pulmonary mechanics. The determinants of the ability to resume and sustain spontaneous ventilation are the converse of the indications for mechanical ventilation. Therefore, the pathophysiologic factors that determine ventilator dependence can be divided into hypoxemic failure or hypoventilation.

Physiology

Hypoxemia during a weaning trial may be the result of three separate processes; (1) hypoventilation, (2) impaired pulmonary gas exchange (typically lung volume loss), or (3) decreased mixed venous O_2 content. Impaired gas exchange can be identified by the presence of an elevated alveolar-arterial O_2 tension gradient ($AaDO_2$) that would not be seen during hypoventilation. Should hypoxemia be encountered during the weaning trial, weaning must be stopped until the etiology is identified and rectified (i.e., atelectasis with increased intrapulmonary shunting, anemia with mixed venous desaturation, etc.).

Hypoventilation because of respiratory muscle pump failure is the most common cause of failure to wean from mechanical ventilation. The etiology of respiratory muscle pump failure can be divided into decreased ventilatory capacity or increased respiratory muscle load **(Table 9.11).** Rarely are neurologic causes such as inadequate respiratory center output the cause for the inability to wean from mechanical ventilation, unless pharmacologically active agents (narcotics) are suppressing the output. Hemidiaphragmatic paralysis following phrenic nerve injury in infants is frequently associated with weaning failure because the combination of a compliant chest wall and paralyzed hemidiaphragm leads to massive lung volume loss and atelectasis[(291)]. Mechanical ventilation with PEEP or CPAP is frequently successful in improving gas exchange; however, long-term management may require surgical plication in infants to allow complete weaning of all positive pressure support[(292,293)].

Many diverse conditions may affect respiratory muscle capacity and lead to a failure in weaning from mechanical ventilation. Airway obstruction with lung hyperinflation from diseases such as bronchomalacia, bronchopulmonary dysplasia, or asthma may adversely affect diaphragmatic performance[(294)]. Hyperinflation leads to shortened fiber length, increased radius of curvature causing a decrease in transdiaphragmatic pressure generation, and an inward chest wall recoil leading to an extra elastic load. In addition, tidal breathing occurs at the upper, less compliant portion of the pressure-volume curve of the lung[(295)]. Malnutrition has been shown to impair respiratory muscle performance[(296,297)]. Nutritional support with carbohydrates as the dominant source of calories has been associated with a marked elevation in carbon dioxide production and increased minute ventilation[(298)]. Nutrition management is directed at providing adequate caloric intake to meet ongoing demands with a balanced intake of carbohydrates, proteins, and fats[(299)]. Metabolic derangements such as hypomagnesemia, hypophosphatemia, hypocalcemia, and hypokalemia have been shown to impair respiratory muscle performance and may present as inability to wean from ventilatory support[(300-302)]. Shock, hypoxemia via decreased energy supply, and hypercapnia via impairment of excitation coupling by intracellular acidosis have been shown to diminish diaphragmatic force output[(303-305)]. Disuse atrophy of the respiratory musculature has been demonstrated in premature infants after 12 days of mechanical ventilation and may complicate weaning attempts[(306)]. Respiratory muscle fatigue has been associated with failure to wean from ventilatory support[(307)]. Infants, in particular, with their lack of fatigue-resistant type I fibers may be more susceptible to fatigue than children or adults[(308)].

TABLE 9.11. Etiologies of Respiratory Pump Failure

Decreased ventilatory capacity
Neurologic
Decreased respiratory center output
Cervical spinal cord surgery
Phrenic nerve dysfunction
Respiratory muscle
Hyperinflation
Malnutrition
Metabolic derangements
Decreased oxygen supply
Disuse atrophy
Fatigue
Abdominal wall defects
Increased respiratory muscle load
Increased ventilatory requirements
Increased CO_2 production
Increased dead space ventilation
Inappropriately elevated ventilatory drive
Increased work of breathing
Decreased efficiency of breathing
Increased chest wall compliance
Respiratory pattern

Increased ventilatory requirements may also cause difficulty during attempts to wean from mechanical ventilation. As mentioned earlier, excessive carbohydrate calories during enteral and parenteral nutrition may lead to hypercapnia. In addition, CO_2 production increases with fevers ($\sim$ 10% increase for each 1°C increase) and excessive muscle activity (seizures, shivering, rigor). Diseases that increase the ratio of physiologic dead space to tidal volume, such as asthma, bronchiolitis, and bronchopulmonary dysplasia, require an increase in minute ventilation to maintain normocapnia. Excessive respiratory drive from psychologic stress, neurologic lesions, or pulmonary irritant receptor stimulation may lead to inappropriate hyperventilation and increase respiratory muscle load. Studies in adults have demonstrated high respiratory drives in patients who failed to be successfully weaned from mechanical ventilation[(309)]. Respiratory work, defined as the product of transpulmonary pressure and tidal volume per minute or liter, had to be low before ventilator-dependent adult patients could successfully sustain spontaneous ventilation[(310)]. Finally, the highly compliant chest wall and rapid shallow respiratory pattern of the neonate will significantly decrease ventilatory efficiency and increase the work of breathing.

Predictive Indices

In the adult, objective measures used as criteria for discontinuation of positive pressure ventilation and extubation of the trachea have recently been reviewed[(311)]. The criteria are directed at ensuring adequate gas exchange (oxygenation) and the presence of adequate respiratory reserve (ventilatory pump function). Oxygenation criteria include: (1) PaO_2 greater than or equal to 60 torr with FiO_2 less than or equal to 0.35; (2) $AaDO_2$ less than 350 torr; (3) PaO_2/FiO_2 ratio greater than 200; and (4) $\dot{Q}_S/\dot{Q}_T$ less than 10-

20%. Ventilatory pump criteria are: (1) vital capacity greater than 10-15 ml/kg; (2) maximum negative inspiratory pressure greater than − 30 cm H_2O; (3) minute ventilation less than 10 liters/min; (4) maximum voluntary ventilation greater than or equal to twice resting minute ventilation; (5) thoracic compliance greater than 25 ml/cm H_2O; (6) airway occlusion pressure less than 6 cm H_2O; (7) respiratory frequency less than 25 breaths/min; (8) tidal volume greater than 300 ml; and (9) dead space/tidal volume ratio less than 0.6. Unfortunately, many of the physiologic criteria used to predict outcome of weaning have been shown to have high false positive and false negative rates. Integration of several physiologic indices (frequency/tidal volume) has recently shown promise as a more accurate predictor of success or failure to wean from mechanical ventilation in adults[312].

Specific guidelines for discontinuation of positive pressure support in infants and young children are much less extensive. Several studies have attempted to define more clearly criteria for weaning in younger pediatric patients. Shoults and coworkers[313] were unable to find a correlation between maximum negative inspiratory airway pressure and successful tracheal extubation in a group of neonates. In a group of older infants receiving postoperative positive pressure ventilatory support, the combination of a crying vital capacity greater than 15 ml/kg and a maximum negative inspiratory airway pressure greater than 45 cm H_2O accurately predicted successful discontinuation of ventilatory support[314]. Furthermore, failure to meet these criteria was generally associated with a failure to tolerate withdrawal of positive pressure ventilation and extubation.

Unfortunately, further predictive criteria of successful withdrawal of positive pressure support in infants are not available. Although rigid guidelines do not exist, extubation should be considered in the presence of normal arterial oxygenation and carbon dioxide elimination ($PaCO_2$ less than 45 torr) on minimal positive pressure support (i.e., SIMV less than 4 breaths/min, CPAP or PEEP less than 5 cm H_2O) and nontoxic levels of inspired oxygen (FiO_2 less than 0.4-0.5). Taken together with the previously mentioned indices of respiratory reserve, these criteria should accurately predict the ability to tolerate independent ventilation with acceptable oxygen requirements.

Techniques

Several techniques are used to wean patients from mechanical ventilation. These include T-tube weaning, intermittent mandatory ventilation and, more recently, pressure support ventilation. Despite the wealth of clinical experience with these various techniques, there are no well-controlled clinical trials that demonstrate a clear-cut superiority of one technique over another. In fact, a recent randomized clinical trial demonstrated that a once per day trial of spontaneous breathing via a t-piece led to more rapid weaning of mechanical ventilation than multiple t-piece trials, SIMV, and PSV[315]. Others have shown that PSV appears superior to SIMV or t-piece trials[316]. Despite conflicting data, SIMV has emerged as the standard mode of ventilatory support used for weaning mechanical ventilation in infants and children **(Table 9.12).**

TABLE 9.12. Guidelines for Discontinuing Positive Pressure Support

Weaning
Decrease SIMV rate
Infants—wean to 2-4 breaths/min
Older child—wean to CPAP mode
Decrease continuous distending pressure (CPAP or PEEP)
Infants—wean to 2-3 cm H_2O
Older child—wean to 5 cm H_2O or less
Discontinuing support
Evidence of adequate ventilatory reserve
Infants
Normal $PaCO_2$
Crying vital capacity > 15 ml/kg
Maximum negative inspiratory pressure against occluded airway > 45 cm H_2O
Older child
Normal $PaCO_2$
Vital capacity > 10-15 ml/kg
Maximum negative inspiratory pressure against occluded airway > 20-30 cm H_2O
Ability to double resting minute ventilation
Evidence of adequate oxygenation capability
$PaO_2 > 70$ torr at $FiO_2 \int 0.4$
Ancillary tests
$Aa\dot{D}O_2 < 300$ torr at $FiO_2 = 1.0$
$\dot{Q}_S/\dot{Q}_T < 10\text{-}20\%$
Dead space/tidal volume ratio < 0.6

The use of the SIMV mode allows the withdrawal of a portion of the positive pressure breaths shortly after initiation, and further withdrawal can progress at a pace tailored to the capabilities of the patient. In general, the frequency of positive pressure breaths is decreased in increments of 2-5 breaths/min following the assessment of the patient by using clinical signs and blood gas determination. The appearance of signs of respiratory distress or carbon dioxide retention at any point should temporarily halt attempts to withdraw support. In the older child, the ultimate goal is to withdraw positive pressure ventilation fully, leaving the patient to breathe spontaneously with CPAP. In infants, the presence of an endotracheal tube is associated with increased airways resistance and work of breathing[317,318], which may cause diaphragmatic fatigue with spontaneous breathing alone. Therefore, it is recommended that several mandatory positive pressure breaths (i.e., low IMV or PEEP mode) be maintained during the weaning of positive pressure ventilation in younger children to help offset this mechanical disadvantage.

Others have suggested that PSV either alone or in conjunction with SIMV is the optimal means of gradually withdrawing mechanical ventilation. PSV is particularly appealing because the patient maintains control of the ventilatory frequency and pattern while the degree of machine support depends on the preset pressure[217]. PSV decreases the ventilator imposed work of breathing and relieves diaphragmatic muscle fatigue in patients who fail conventional weaning attempts[218]. These facts may be because of the improved pressure-volume load characteristics and enhanced endurance conditioning of the diaphragm seen with PSV[219,220]. Others use PSV simply to overcome the work imposed by endotracheal tube resistance[221] and gradually decrease the SIMV rate as the means of weaning support. Regardless of the method selected, the clinician must continuously monitor for signs of increased work and halt weaning to avoid respiratory muscle fatigue.

Complications of Mechanical Ventilation

Mechanical ventilation, while frequently lifesaving, is also associated with numerous real and potential complications, some of which are themselves life-threatening[319]. Unfortunately, as is commonly seen throughout medicine, complications with mechanical ventilation have been well recognized in adults, while little work is available in the pediatric literature. Complications include such diverse problems as patient discomfort to unnecessary prolongation of mechanical ventilation with excessive utilization of limited health resources. This discussion is limited to complications related to positive intrathoracic pressure (i.e. pulmonary parenchymal injury-volutrauma, alterations in cardiovascular and other organ functions), required adjunctive therapies (i.e. airway management, sedation, and neuromuscular blockade), and patient-ventilator interactions.

Positive Intrathoracic Pressure

Mechanical ventilation associated with positive intrathoracic pressure alters pulmonary mechanics and affects the function of other organ systems. These alterations in organ function are in reality side effects rather than complications of the continuous positive intrathoracic pressure **(Table 9.13).**

Volutrauma

Over the last decade evidence in mammalian species has been published demonstrating that lung distension by mechanical ventilation with high airway pressures produces insidious physiologic and morphologic changes in previously normal lung. These alterations ultimately produce acute lung injury and can progress to multiple organ failure[249]. Mechanical ventilation with high peak inspiratory pressures and large tidal volumes in normal rats produces pulmonary edema associated with severe permeability alterations, increased filtration, and diffuse alveolar damage[320-322]. It is lung overdistension and not the airway pressure per se which is responsible for these findings. Negative pressure ventilation with large tidal volumes will produce similar injury[323]. This was further demonstrated by the fact that tidal volume limitation via thoracoabdominal binding during high pressure ventilation inhibits the development of permeability changes and edema[323,324]. These experiments led to the evolution of the concept that the mechanism of high pressure pulmonary edema and lung injury from that of "pressure-related" injury (barotrauma) to that of volume-induced injury (volutrauma)[325]. A narrow, ill-defined, therapeutic range exists for the application of positive pressure ventilation for patients with acute lung injury (see restrictive lung disease section).

It is unclear whether a volume threshold exists below which mechanical ventilation will not cause lung damage. What is certain is that many factors are involved in this complex problem. Not only the degree but also the duration of inflation are important determinants of mechanical ventilation-induced lung injury. Mechanical ventilation of sheep with normal lungs using peak airway pressures of 30 cm H_2O, the pressure required to reach total lung capacity, for 48 hours results in significant injury[326]. Several studies show that previously injured lungs are more susceptible to ventilator-induced lung injury[327-329]. Age also appears to be an important factor; young animals appear to be more susceptible to increases in microvascular permeability[330]. Additional work demonstrates: (1) increased tidal volume and resting lung volume (FRC) do individually produce edema but will cause lung injury permeability edema in combination if sufficient pulmonary overinflation occurs; (2) pulmonary edema develops if FRC is sufficiently increased by either positive or negative pressure ventilation, even with normal tidal volume; and (3) the ability of PEEP to decrease edema formation is due at least in part to alteration in hemodynamics (i.e. decreased cardiac output and pulmonary blood flow)[331]. Thus, it appears that end-inspiratory volume is the primary determinant of "volutrauma" and measures to decrease pressure-volume swings and high flow rates may not prove sufficient to protect lungs from ventilator-induced injury.

TABLE 9.13. Adverse Effects That May Be Encountered during the Application of Continuous Distending Pressure (CPAP or PEEP)

Decreased cardiac output
Decreased systemic venous return
Increased pulmonary vascular resistance
Interventricular septal displacement impeding left ventricular filling
Neural and/or humoral depression of left ventricular function
Decreased myocardial blood flow
Decreased cerebral perfusion pressure
Increased intracranial pressure
Systemic hypotension
Altered renal blood flow and/or function
Decreased renal blood flow
Redistribution of renal blood flow
Decreased free water clearance
Decreased creatinine clearance
Decreased sodium excretion
Decreased splanchnic blood flow
Decreased hepatic arterial flow
Decreased intestinal blood flow
Alveolar overdistention
Pneumothorax
Pneumomediastinum
Pneumopericardium
Subcutaneous emphysema
Increased physiologic dead space

Other investigators have established that not only alveolar distention but also cyclic opening and closing of lung units worsens lung injury[332]. Acutely injured lungs exhibit marked heterogeneity in the degree of alterations in alveolar anatomy and physiology which leads to uneven distribution of ventilation. Using computerized tomography, it has been demonstrated that patients with acute lung injury simultaneously have healthy lung tissue, recruitable injured tissue, and lung tissue unresponsive to positive pressure[333]. Healthy lung units may represent as little as 20-30% of the total lung; thus, lungs with acute injury are better thought as "small" rather than "stiff". It is now recognized that with uniformly applied conventional mechanical ventilation (CMV), the bulk of ventilation is directed to the healthy units, causing potentially harmful "volutrauma". Furthermore, the traction exerted on the normally compliant parenchyma surrounding atelectatic areas may also contribute[334]. This led to the hypothesis that the stretch caused by repetitive collapse and reopening of terminal lung units directly damages or worsens previously injured lung[335]. Muscedere et al.[332] showed that lung injury can occur from purely mechanical factors when ventilation results in repeated small airway closure and opening with each respiratory cycle. Furthermore, they demonstrated that the utilization of PEEP to open the airways and alveoli at end-expiration may change the site and severity of lung injury if given in sufficient amounts.

Thus, it appears that not only excessive alveolar distention but also cyclic opening and closing of distal airways and alveoli is associated with progressive injury to the pulmonary parenchyma. These realizations have led to significant changes in the approach to mechanical ventilation (i.e. small tidal volume, permissive hypercapnia) for patients suffering from acute lung injury. Circumstantial evidence suggests that this method of ventilation may be associated with improved outcomes. Hickling et al.[336] reported retrospective data on adults with severe acute lung injury treated with limitation of peak inspiratory pressures to less than 40 cm H_2O at all times and less than 30 cm H_2O when possible using volume-cycled SIMV. Mechanical tidal volumes as low as 5 ml/kg with PEEP as necessary to provide adequate oxygenation (arterial hemoglobin saturation >90%) were used and $PaCO_2$ and spontaneous respiratory rates were allowed to increase. Mortality was significantly lower than that predicted by the Acute Physiology and Chronic Health Evaluation II (APACHE II). This has been subsequently followed by a prospective noncontrolled study by the same investigators in which this same strategy resulted in significantly lower mortality rate than predicted by the APACHE II[337]. This study also showed that the results were not because of regional differences in APACHE II predicted mortality rates (a criticism of the first study). The only randomized, controlled study published to date had a small group of postoperative adult patients at risk for acute lung injury requiring mechanical ventilation randomized to control (12 ml/kg) or small (6 ml/kg) tidal volumes while respiratory rates were adjusted to maintain normocapnia[338]. This small study failed to show a significant reduction in mortality but reported shorter duration of intubation and ICU stay as well as fewer pulmonary infections in the small tidal volume group.

Other Pulmonary Complications

In addition to volutrauma, the use of continuous distending pressure is associated with other pulmonary complications. Extravascular lung water (ELW) has been reported to be increased[339], decreased[323,340], or remain unchanged[341] during CPAP or PEEP. The specific response of ELW to CPAP or PEEP depends on transmural pressure across the pulmonary vasculature and vessel type[342], lymphatic flow[343], and the alteration of alveolar epithelial and pulmonary endothelial permeability[344,345]. Increased transmural pressure of the extravascular vessels with CPAP or PEEP and decreased lymphatic flow will result in increased ELW. Distention of the alveolar epithelium and pulmonary endothelium may increase the permeability to protein and liquid and increase ELW. The clinical significance of the increased ELW in response to CPAP or PEEP is not known.

Barotrauma has become an all-inclusive term describing pathologic changes ranging from pulmonary interstitial emphysema (PIE) to life-threatening events such as tension pneumothorax. The consensus is that the primary offending factor is alveolar overdistention (high peak inflation volume)[346]. High peak inspiratory pressures tend to be encountered in patients who are prone to barotrauma[347]. The area of disruption typically occurs at the border of the alveolar base and the bronchovascular sheath[348]. Once in the interstitium, air dissects toward the hilum and then up and down the mediastinum and into the subcutaneous tissues and pleural and peritoneal spaces. PIE manifests as linear air streaking toward the hilum, perivascular blebs, or subpleural air on radiographic examination and may be an early indicator of barotrauma[349]. PIE, pneumomediastinum, subcutaneous emphysema, and pneumoperitoneum can lead to patient discomfort but rarely are of major clinical significance[350].

Pneumothorax occurs when a communication between the pleural space and the alveolus or atmosphere exists. Air flows down the pressure gradient via the path of least resistance into the pleural space until pressure equalization occurs. The equilibration in transpulmonary pressure in conjunction with the separation of the two pleural membranes causes the lung to recoil inward. Collapse of the lung may be partial or complete, as occurs when transpulmonary pressure equilibrates with atmospheric pressure. The clinical consequences are dependent on the underlying pulmonary function and the degree of collapse, and they range from asymptomatic to severe respiratory distress and death. Tension pneumothorax, a life-threatening complication of barotrauma, is present when interpleural pressure exceeds atmospheric pressure. This occurs when air enters the pleural space during inspiration from the atmosphere or alveolus but cannot escape during expiration. The increasing intrapleural pressure causes progressive ipsilateral lung collapse, shift of the mediastinum with contralateral lung

TABLE 9.14. Conditions Associated with Pulmonary Barotrauma

Impedance to exhalation
Small artificial airway
Ball-valve obstruction of endotracheal tube
Failure to clear tracheobronchial mucus
Intrathoracic obstructive airway diseases
Positive pressure ventilation
Inadequate expiratory time (prolongation of inspiratory time or high ventilatory rate)
Mechanical expiratory retardation
Excessive alveolar volume or pressure
Positive pressure support
High inflating pressure
Prolonged inspiration
Inspiratory pressure hold
High CPAP or PEEP
Patient-ventilator respiratory phase asynchrony
Decreased respiratory compliance
Regional disparities in pulmonary volume distribution
Marked inhomogeneity in regional compliance (focal lung diseases)
Marked inhomogeneity in regional resistance (focal lung diseases)
Mainstem bronchus intubation

compression, and obstruction of venous return to the heart, resulting in compromised cardiac function. The treatment of pneumothorax is evacuation of pleural air via a closed chest thoracotomy tube, but this treatment alone has been shown to complicate patient management and increases morbidity and mortality[347].

Other life-threatening complications of barotrauma have been seen. Pulmonary edema has been noted to occur following rapid reexpansion of a collapsed lung from a pneumothorax because of increased negative interstitial pressure[351]. Pneumopericardium, with the increase in pericardial pressures and impairment of venous return to the heart, is an uncommon but serious complication of barotrauma[352]. Recently, systemic air embolism, with entry of gas into the pulmonary circulation, has been reported following pulmonary barotrauma[353].

The occurrence rate of barotrauma in some form varies between 3% and 65% in patients managed with continuous distending pressure[347,354,355]. Although the use of CPAP or PEEP is associated with increased barotrauma risk, some studies suggest that the use of high positive inflating pressures[356] or prolonged inspiratory time[357] in association with PEEP are more important than PEEP itself in creating increased risk of barotrauma with positive pressure ventilatory support **(Table 9.14).** Also, given the abnormalities in pulmonary mechanics that exist in patients requiring CPAP or PEEP, the risk of barotrauma is increased regardless of the mode of positive pressure support[358]. Therefore, the exact contribution of CPAP or PEEP to the risk of barotrauma is extremely difficult to determine.

Cardiovascular Function

Cardiovascular and peripheral circulatory complications associated with the use of CPAP or PEEP (i.e. elevated mean airway pressure) are well described. Decreased cardiac output accompanies the administration of continuous distending pressure with regularity[359-361]. A variety of mechanisms have been evoked to explain the effects of $\overline{P}_{aw}$ on cardiac output[158]. Decreased cardiac filling associated with increased intrathoracic pressure during positive pressure assistance was documented by the early work of Cournand and associates[362]. Since then, increased intrapleural pressure associated with CPAP or PEEP has been shown to decrease systemic venous return[258,363] and ventricular preload[364]. Increased pulmonary vascular resistance and right ventricular afterload have also been implicated in the depression of cardiac output accompanying PEEP[365]. Studies in adults using high levels of $\overline{P}_{aw}$ (i.e., 30 cm H_2O) have suggested that the associated rise in right ventricular diastolic pressure results in leftward interventricular septal displacement and impedance to left ventricular diastolic filling[366]. Studies in open-chested animals free of mechanical heart-lung interactions have demonstrated decreased cardiac output with the application of PEEP, suggesting that reflex neurohumoral factors contribute to ventricular dysfunction and cardiac output depression[367]. Other investigators have noted a decrease in left ventricular blood flow with the application of PEEP in experimental animals[368], suggesting that continuous distending pressure might lead to left ventricular dysfunction on the basis of ischemia.

Several studies suggest that the adverse hemodynamic effects of continuous airway distending pressure are attenuated if some degree of spontaneous breathing rather than controlled positive pressure ventilation occurs in conjunction with positive expiratory pressure (i.e., using SIMV mode with PEEP or using CPAP). For example, normal antidiuretic hormone activity and sodium excretion have been found when CPAP is substituted for controlled positive pressure ventilation with PEEP[369]. Also, as previously noted, limited laboratory investigation has suggested that cardiac output is maintained more easily when SIMV and PEEP are used rather than controlled continuous positive pressure ventilation[195]. However, most studies comparing the hemodynamic effects of controlled positive pressure ventilation with PEEP and SIMV with PEEP or CPAP have yielded mixed results[158].

Determining precisely what is a hemodynamically "safe" level of $\overline{P}_{aw}$ usually requires individual assessment in each patient. In adults, significant depression of cardiac output has been reported with the use of PEEP at levels as low as 10-15 cm H_2O[161]. On the other hand, application of PEEP in excess of 15 cm H_2O in children with acute respiratory failure has not been associated with significant depression of cardiac output in one series[370]. In any given patient, the effects of elevations in CPAP or PEEP on hemodynamic performance are the end result of many interacting variables, such as intravascular volume status, level of inotropic support, $P_{\overline{aw}}$, and underlying cardiovascular status. Therefore, the most prudent approach when using high levels of continuous distending pressure is to monitor cardiovascular function carefully and intervene with appropriate therapy when indicated. Generally, depression of cardiac output associated with high levels of continuous distending pressure in children can be reversed by basic interventions such as intravascular volume expansion[258] or low-dose dopamine infusion[260].

Other Organ Function

In addition to the adverse effects of elevations in $\bar{P}_{aw}$ on cardiac function, continuous distending pressure is associated with a variety of changes in peripheral organ function that are probably related to changes in perfusion[371]. Decreased urine output[369,372,373], creatinine clearance[369,373], and renal sodium excretion[372,373] have been observed repetitively with the use of PEEP. These effects seem to be a result of decreased renal blood flow, increased antidiuretic hormone levels, and changes in the cortical-medullary distribution of kidney perfusion[373-375]. Laboratory studies in animals have also shown depression of hepatic[376,377], portal venous[376-378], and mesenteric[375] blood flow with continuous positive pressure ventilation. Decreased hepatic perfusion has been noted in adults ventilated at high levels of PEEP (i.e., 20 cm H_2O)[379]. Decreased cerebral perfusion pressure secondary to decreased mean arterial pressure and elevated intracranial pressure has been associated with the use of PEEP in head trauma victims with underlying intracranial hypertension[380]. This implies that PEEP interferes with cerebral venous drainage, thereby producing increased intracerebral blood volume and pressure in susceptible patients.

Required Adjunctive Therapies

Interventions and therapies are frequently required to deliver mechanical positive pressure ventilation to patients with respiratory failure. The single most important intervention associated with mechanical ventilation is airway intubation to assure patency and allow application of positive pressure. Patients with severe alteration in respiratory function may require imposition of an abnormal frequency or pattern of breathing. Nearly every child who receives mechanical ventilatory assistant requires sedation and in some cases neuromuscular blockade to achieve the desired therapeutic goals. Unfortunately, these interventions and therapies are accompanied with their own set of side-effects and complications.

Complications of Airway Intubation

Endotracheal intubation in emergent situations is usually performed via the transoral route; however, when mechanical ventilatory requirements are likely to be present for some period of time, many clinicians utilize the transnasal route (see chapter 2). The nasal route provides a more stable artificial airway and allows mouth closure, improving patient comfort. A nasally placed tube is generally smaller in diameter than its oral counterpart, may generate bleeding during placement, and is associated with the development of sinusitis secondary to ostial occlusion and impeded drainage[381]. Long-term placement of either artificial airway may be associated with glottic edema and/or injury. Although risk factors for tracheal erosion, glottic stenosis, tracheal dilation, and tracheomalacia are not clearly established, endotracheal tube (or cuff) pressures that exceed capillary perfusion pressure (estimated at 25 cm H_2O) appear more likely to cause ischemic injury and advanced mucosal damage[381].

The artificial airway allows pathogens access to the trachea and lower airway from the external environment, increasing the risk of a hospital acquired pneumonia[382]. Nosocomial pneumonias, also defined as ventilator-associated pneumonias, have been identified in 21% of patients ventilated for longer than 48 hours[383]. Host and environmental factors play important roles in the pathogenesis of nosocomial pneumonia[384]. Development of a nosocomial pneumonia is dependent on a source of organisms, frequently Gram-negative bacilli from the patient's own gastrointestinal tract, that colonize the upper respiratory tract and then gain access to the lower respiratory tract through aspiration of hypopharyngeal contents. Retention of gastric acidity while preventing stress ulcer prophylaxis with sucralfate and selective decontamination of the oropharynx and stomach may be beneficial in reducing the incidence of nosocomial pneumonia[385,386]. Guidelines to minimize the risk of nosocomial pneumonia have been published[387].

Sedation and Neuromuscular Blockade

Nearly every child that requires positive pressure mechanical ventilation for cardiorespiratory failure receives sedative and/or analgesic medications in one form or another. Each medication has own potential adverse effects; therefore, the clinician must be familiar with the pharmacokinetics and dynamics of these medications in infants and children (see chapter 46). For example, many of the sedative medications cause systemic vasodilation and may result in profound hypotension in patients with hypovolemia or other disturbances of the cardiovascular system. The chronic administration of these medications is frequently associated with tachyphylaxis and escalating dosage requirements over time and can lead to dependency which necessitates a slow withdrawal[388]. Finally, age-related differences in expression of separation anxiety, number and sensitivity of specific receptors, and pharmacokinetics have been reported to be the possible cause of the increased sedative requirements seen in toddlers compared to infants or adolescents[389]. Clearly, this is an area of clinical practice that demands further investigation.

Perhaps the most widely reported complication of the use of neuromuscular blocking drugs (NMBDs) in the ICU is prolonged muscle weakness. This complication was brought into the spotlight by the report of seven adult ICU patients who developed prolonged paralysis following long-term (2 days) use of NMBDs[390]. The prolonged paralysis in that series appeared to be a result of accumulation of the active 3-desacetyl metabolite of vecuronium in patients with renal failure. This clinical entity has also been commonly associated with the co-administration of aminosteroid NMBDs (pancuronium, vercuronium) and corticosteroids[391,392]. Many have suggested that this combination of medications should not be used in critically ill patients. Others have suggested that atracurium and the other benzylisoquinolinium compounds, which are not steroid-based, may not cause prolonged paresis[393]. Several recent case reports have clearly shown that this hypothesis is not true[394,395]. This complication has also been reported in neonates and children[396-398]. In-depth reviews of prolonged muscle weakness following neuromuscular blockade in the ICU has been recently published[399,400]. Many questions remain to be answered regarding this toxicity of NMBDs in critically ill patients; therefore, the use of this potentially toxic class of medications should be minimized as much as possible.

Patient-Ventilator Interactions

Despite the current availability of sophisticated mechanical ventilatory devices, problems with asynchrony between the child's spontaneous and the mechanical phases of the respiratory cycle are commonly encountered[401]. Spontaneous inspiratory efforts by the distressed infant and child are frequently out of phase with mechanical ventilatory patterns, resulting in the patient "fighting" the ventilator. Ventilator-patient asynchrony has been incriminated in the pathogenesis of pulmonary barotrauma[401] and is frequently associated with deterioration in gas exchange. Specifically, four types of ventilator-patient respiratory cycle interactions have been identified: (1) inspiratory synchrony, (2) initiation of the Hering-Breuer reflex with positive pressure inflation, (3) apnea, and (4) active expiration during the mechanical inspiratory phase[401]. In the latter circumstance, the patient actively exhales during the ventilator inspiratory cycle, a situation associated with an exaggerated rise in alveolar and intrapleural pressures. Other patterns of ventilator-patient interaction are not associated with significant ventilator-patient asynchrony.

Numerous factors increase the breathing workload, augmenting the likelihood of patient-ventilatory asynchrony. These factors include increased endotracheal tube resistance, excessive ventilator trigger threshold and/or response time, insufficient inspiratory flow capacity to meet the patient's peak demands, and the development of dynamic hyperinflation[185,235,236,402-404]. Recent improvements in mechanical ventilator trigger design and function have significantly enhanced the capability of the newest generation of microprocessor ventilators[405]. Specifically, the ability to trigger inspiratory flow by monitoring changes in gas flow rather than circuit pressure have substantially improved the capability of the mechanical ventilator to sense and respond to the patient's inspiratory efforts and reduce the imposed work of breathing[406]. Similar results have been confirmed in laboratory[407] and clinical settings[408,409] by several investigators. This flow-triggering capability has also recently been introduced into the neonatal population and shows promise for providing synchronized ventilatory assistance to the infant recovering from cardiorespiratory failure[410,411].

In circumstances where patient-ventilator asynchrony develop, the use of sedation is helpful in establishing respiratory phase synchronization between the patient and ventilator. In extreme cases of ventilator-patient asynchrony, the use of neuromuscular blockers has been advocated[412]. Clinical trials involving the use of muscle relaxants as an adjunct to ventilatory support in premature infants and young children have produced mixed results with regard to changes in oxygenation. Because a sizable proportion of infants do not experience asynchrony with positive pressure ventilation, benefits from paralysis and controlled ventilatory support would not be expected uniformly. On the other hand, patients displaying an asynchronous pattern of interaction appear to benefit significantly from muscle relaxation. The administration of muscle relaxants has led to a reversal of the tendency toward the development of pneumothorax[413]. Therefore, in cases of ventilator-patient asynchrony, a trial of neuromuscular blockade following appropriate sedation should be considered for its potential salutary effect on oxygenation as well as for its ability to decrease the risks of pulmonary barotrauma. On the other hand, in the absence of significant ventilator-patient asynchrony, the adverse effects of muscle paralysis and controlled positive pressure ventilation on V/Q matching[191-193], along with the potential for prolonged paralysis[399,400] should be considered before neuromuscular blockers are used.

EXPERIMENTAL THERAPY

As it has become apparent that excessive alveolar volume and/or pressure during conventional mechanical ventilation results in iatrogenic lung injury, novel ventilatory techniques have been developed to minimize these problems[414]. These methods of providing ventilatory support represent the next step in management of a patient with respiratory failure. These include non-conventional gas mechanical ventilation such as continuous tracheal gas insufflation and high frequency ventilation as well as other experimental means of cardiorespiratory support like liquid ventilation and extracorporeal life support (ECLS). All use little or no tidal volume to maintain adequate gas exchange in an attempt to minimize iatrogenic lung injury.

Gas Ventilation

Several different forms of experimental gas ventilation are undergoing active investigation for use in patients with severe alterations in pulmonary function. The primary goal for these experimental means of gas ventilation is the use of smaller tidal volumes (often less than dead space) to minimize end-inspiratory alveolar volume, thereby diminishing the potential for volutrauma. One method involves the insufflation of gas into the trachea to decrease the percentage of dead-space ventilation (tracheal gas insufflation). The second encompasses the use of tidal volumes that are less than dead-space volume but delivered at a high respiratory frequency (high frequency ventilation).

Tracheal Gas Insufflation

Tracheal insufflation of gas was an outgrowth of the concept of apneic oxygenation first described in 1944 to provide adequate oxygenation for brief periods of apnea[415]. In 1985, tracheal insufflation of oxygen through a catheter (2-mm internal diameter) placed 1 cm proximal to the carina was shown to produce sufficient gas exchange to support life for prolonged periods in apneic dogs[416]. The apneic, paralyzed dogs had PaO_2 greater than 300 torr, while $PaCO_2$ levels plateaued at approximately 150-200 torr. Turbulence generated by the jet flow and cardiogenic oscillations, as well as diffusion, are the primary mechanisms of gas exchange[417,418]. Recently, tracheal insufflation of oxygen was shown to decrease both $PaCO_2$ and spontaneous minute ventilation in a dog model of severe respiratory failure[419] and in adults with chronic obstructive pulmonary disease[420]. As an extension of this technique, by placing catheters in each mainstem bronchus and using high gas flow rates (1.5-3 liters/min/kg) in apneic animals, investigators have been able to maintain oxygenation and normocarbia[421,422]. A two-zone model involving turbulent flow in zone I and molecular diffusion and cardiogenic oscillations in zone II are the primary gas transport mechanisms[423]; however, collateral ventilation between alveoli also appears to have an important impact on gas exchange[424]. Recently, Kolobow et al.[425] described a modification of this technique called intratracheal pulmonary ventilation (ITPV), where a continuous flow of gas via a specially designed catheter placed at the carina in conjunction with a conventional mechanical ventilator is used to maintain oxygenation and normocarbia with very small tidal volumes (1 ml/kg), higher frequency (120 breaths/min), and lower peak airway pressures (3-4 cm H_2O above PEEP) in an experimental model of acute lung injury. ITPV has also been used to maintain normal gas exchange chronically without evidence of lung injury while only the right upper lobe (12% of lung mass) in lambs is ventilated[426]. Case reports have been published using ITPV for neonates with congenital diaphragmatic hernia following ECMO[427] and a child with acute sickle cell chest syndrome requiring ECMO[428].

These same principles have been applied to adults of respiratory failure. Continuous tracheal gas insufflation combined with pressure-limited mechanical ventilation was shown to augment carbon dioxide elimination by washing out the anatomic dead space[429]. This effect depends on catheter flow rate and to a lesser extent, catheter position (i.e. near the carina) and timing of flow (i.e. continuous > expiratory only > inspiratory only)[430,431]. These effects have subsequently been seen in an acute lung injury laboratory model[432] and in adults recovering from acute respiratory failure[433].

The appealing feature of these techniques is the fact that gas exchange can be maintained with very low tidal volumes in diseased lungs, potentially limiting the amount of iatrogenic lung injury seen with today's conventional therapies. Clearly, what role these constant-flow, low tidal volume methods of ventilatory support may play in the clinical setting is only now becoming apparent. Laboratory investigations should be followed by careful, prospective clinical trials before any of these methods should be introduced into routine clinical practice.

High Frequency Ventilation

Low tidal volume HFV has received considerable attention from both clinical and basic science sectors[434,435]. This technique of mechanical ventilatory support involves the delivery of low tidal volume breaths at frequencies far in excess of physiologic respiratory rates. Conventional positive pressure ventilation stands in marked contrast to HFV in which the usual tidal volume approaches or is less than the dead space volume. In certain settings, HFV has evolved from a laboratory curiosity to an applied clinical tool since its original description in the late 1960s. During this time, considerable progress has been made in elucidating mechanisms of gas exchange during HFV[436-440] as well as secondary effects of the technique on the lung[441-444] and cardiovascular system[445-449]. However, numerous questions remain unanswered, particularly regarding appropriate clinical application of HFV in general and specific categories of acute respiratory failure.

Classification

Many high-frequency ventilators—each with unique and overlapping characteristics—have been developed for clinical use. These characteristics can be used to classify different high-frequency ventilators into broad categories to help clarify and define principal techniques used to deliver HFV **(Table 9.15).** Practitioners must also remember that circuit and delivery system designs may have a major impact on the functioning of high-frequency ventilators.

Originally developed to minimize arterial blood pressure fluctuations with positive pressure ventilation, high-frequency positive pressure ventilation (HFPPV) was also found to be effective in achieving normal blood gas values with reduced airway pressures[450]. HFPPV typically utilizes a standard conventional ventilator with low-compliance tubing, so that adequate tidal volumes can be delivered with very short inspiratory times. This information was then used to develop HFPPV into a clinical modality used intraoperatively[451] and in the intensive care unit[452]. HFPPV uses a pneumatic valve system to deliver compressed gas during inspiration while allowing passive expiration (Fig. 9.25). With HFPPV, the ventilatory frequency is 60-150 breaths/min with tidal volumes of 3-4 ml/kg, while I/E ratios are usually 0.3[453]. Most conventional neonatal ventilators have been modified to include the capacity to deliver rates up to 150/min. Limitations with HF-PPV have been recognized. For example, with increasing

TABLE 9.15. Technical Features of HFV

Feature	*HFPPV*	*HFJV*	*HFFI*[a]	*HFO*
Flow generator	High-pressure gas source	High-pressure gas source	High-pressure gas source	Piston pump acoustic speaker
Fresh gas delivery system	Continuous or valved fresh gas flow	Jet catheter with continuous fresh gas bias flow	Valved flow interruptor	Continuous fresh gas flow
Tidal valve	> dead space	> or < dead space	> or < dead space	< dead space
Expiratory phase	Passive	Passive	Passive	Active
Airway pressure waveform	Variable	Triangular	Triangular	Sine wave
Entrainment	None	Possible	None	None
Frequency (cycles/min)	60-150	60-600	300-1200	60-3600

[a]*HFFI, high-frequency flow interruption.*

frequency, tidal volume delivery may be compromised so that actual alveolar ventilation decreases despite an increase in minute ventilation[454].

A widely used high-frequency ventilatory technique in the United States is high-frequency jet ventilation (HFJV). This technique has undergone considerable clinical and laboratory evaluation since its introduction in 1977[455]. The typical HFJV system uses a high-pressure, air-oxygen gas source to generate flow. A reducing valve allows the adjustment of inspiratory driving pressure from 0 to 50 psi, and a rapidly responding solenoid valve provides timed flow interruption. The flow interrupter can be adjusted to vary the frequency between 60 and 600 insufflations/min (the usual frequency is 100-150/min) with a relatively short inspiratory time (10-50% of the respiratory cycle). Manipulation of the inspiratory driving pressure provides the primary means for regulating tidal volume delivery. Insufflated gases are delivered through a low-volume, noncompliant tubing system connected to a small-diameter (1.0-1.7 mm internal diameter) jet catheter housed within the airway adapter and extending into the endotracheal airway. Alternatively, specially designed endotracheal tubes incorporating a side lumen within the wall of the tube allow the delivery of jet gases into the distal portion of the endotracheal tube.

Inspiratory gases are accelerated as they pass through the jet cannula, and by Bernoulli effect, negative pressure is generated at the airway opening. This results in entrainment of gases along with the delivered volume of the jet ventilator ranging between 5% and 50% of the tidal volume delivered with each jet insufflation[456]. The percentage of entrained gas that supplements the delivered tidal volume is a function of the velocity of jet flow, the jet-velocity profile, and the resistance and compliance of the patient's respiratory system[457,458]. The tidal volume delivered during HFJV is proportional to the driving pressure and inspiratory time and is inversely proportional to ventilator circuit resistance and typically ranges between 2 and 5 ml/kg[457,459]. Entrainment of fresh gas with the appropriate oxygen concentration is ensured by the continuous-flow circuit. Application of appropriate valve devices to the expiratory limb of the circuit allows the provision of PEEP. Finally, insertion of a reservoir bag in the inspiratory limb of the continuous-flow circuit ensures an adequate source of inspired volume in the spontaneously breathing patient. A continuous infusion of sterile saline into the path of the jet gases functions as a source of humidification for insufflated gases with each inspiration; and delivery of dry jet gases has been associated with mucous inspissation, hemorrhagic inflammation of the tracheal mucosa, and retardation of mucociliary function[456]. Passive exhalation occurs around the jet cannula into the continuous-flow circuitry.

The consequences of manipulation of various ventilatory parameters in HFJV have been defined to some degree through laboratory and clinical investigations[460,461]. Elevation of inspiratory driving pressure increases the volume of insufflated gases and enhances carbon dioxide elimination. Carbon dioxide elimination as a function of ventilatory frequency is less predictable. A linear rise in carbon dioxide tension has been demonstrated by using HFJV, with increasing frequency beyond 100 breaths/min[460]. As previously mentioned, this phenomenon has been attributed to expiratory gas trapping, increased physiologic dead space, and a relative decrease in insufflated gas volume with increasing frequency. Positioning of the jet cannula orifice distally in the airway or increasing the internal diameter of the jet cannula has resulted in decreased $PaCO_2$. The response of $PaCO_2$ in different studies to changes in relative inspiratory time (percent inspiration), however, has been erratic[460,461]. Under pathologic conditions, changes in jet ventilation parameters that result in increased mean airway pressure (and mean lung volume) tend to diminish intrapulmonary shunting and improve oxygenation much like CPAP or PEEP in conventional modes of mechanical ventilation[189].

High-frequency flow interrupters (HFFIs) are very similar to jet ventilators. HFFIs provide small tidal volumes (2-5 ml/kg) delivered at high frequency by interrupting a flow or high-pressure source[462]. In contrast to HFJV, no injector jet cannula or gas entrainment is present. Expiration is passive and frequencies are varied between 300 and 1200/min.

High-frequency oscillation (HFO) is unique in that both inspiration and expiration are active; gas is forced into the lungs during inspiration and sucked out of the lungs during expiration[463,464]. HFO uses a reciprocating device (piston pumps, acoustic speaker cones) to produce sinusoi-

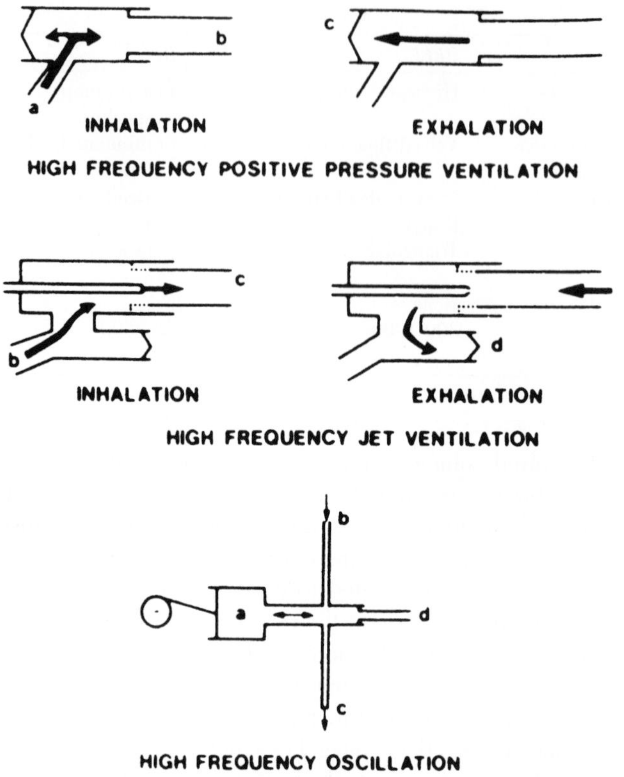

Figure 9.25. Schematic diagrams of HFV circuits. *Top panel:* With HF-PPV, gas is delivered during inhalation from a low compliance ventilator. Exhalation is passive; (a) low compliance circuit; (b) endotracheal tube; (c) one-way valve. *Middle panel:* During HFJV, high-pressure gas enters from a cannula (a) along the endotracheal tube or trachea (c). Additional gas (b) is entrained. Exhalation is passive. *Bottom panel:* During HFO, the piston (a) oscillates while fresh gas (termed the bias flow) enters (b) and exhaust gas exits (c). The bias flow can be positioned anywhere along the airway (d), but gas transport is enhanced as the bias flow is positioned further into the lung. (From Villar J, Winston B, Slutsky AS. Non-conventional techniques of ventilatory support. Crit Care Clin 1990;6:579.)

dal pressure waves at the airway opening at frequencies of 60-3600 cycles/min[436]. A continuous fresh gas (bias flow) is delivered to the proximal airway to supply O_2 and remove CO_2 while tidal volumes are less than dead space volume (1-3 ml/kg)[465]. There are two different types of bias flow (low and high impedance) that have profound impact on the performance of the HFO ventilator[436,464]. The low-impedance flow is more widely used because of safety and simplicity. However, less of the tidal volume is delivered to the patient because some volume is "lost" to the low-impedance bias flow. Because of its greater complexity, high-impedance flow is predominantly used to investigate gas transport mechanisms during HFO. The high-impedance circuit has negligible loss of tidal volume to the bias flow; therefore, it is easier to measure tidal volume.

Mechanics of Gas Exchange

The mechanisms of gas exchange in HFV when tidal volume is < dead space, remain controversial despite the abundance of investigative attention directed to this area. Two fundamental physical processes have been used in proposals to explain gas exchange: *convection* and *molecular diffusion* (Fig 9.26)[414].

Convection is the bulk flow of inspired gas to the level of the alveoli and is the major mechanism of gas transport during conventional mechanical ventilation. Convection also plays a significant role in gas transport during HFV and can be divided into five stages:

1. *Direct alveolar ventilation.* Because of the asymmetry of the bronchial tree, a small percentage of the alveoli will receive bulk flow to inspiratory gas directly[466]. This mechanism becomes less prominent as tidal volume approaches dead space volume.
2. *Asymmetric velocity profile.* Because of viscous shear created by the airways, the inspiratory velocity profile is asymmetric and parabolic. Gas molecules in the center travel faster than those in the periphery. In contrast, expiratory velocity profiles are flat and symmetric. The net result, therefore, is a pattern characterized by the inspiratory gas that moves in the center of the airway towards the alveoli while alveolar gas moves from the alveoli along the periphery of the airway and is called net convective transport[467].
3. *Pendelluft.* Because of differences in regional compliances and resistances (time constants), gas flow into adjacent lung regions may become out of phase, resulting in back-and-forth gas exchange between neighboring units. This intraregional gas mixing is called pendelluft and leads to improved gas mixing and exchange[468].
4. *Augmented dispersion.* Asymmetric velocity profiles result in axial convection. Airway oscillations and bifurcations lead to turbulence, creating eddies and swirling flows in the conducting airways, which result in both laminar and radial (lateral) dispersion of gases, facilitating gas mixing[469].

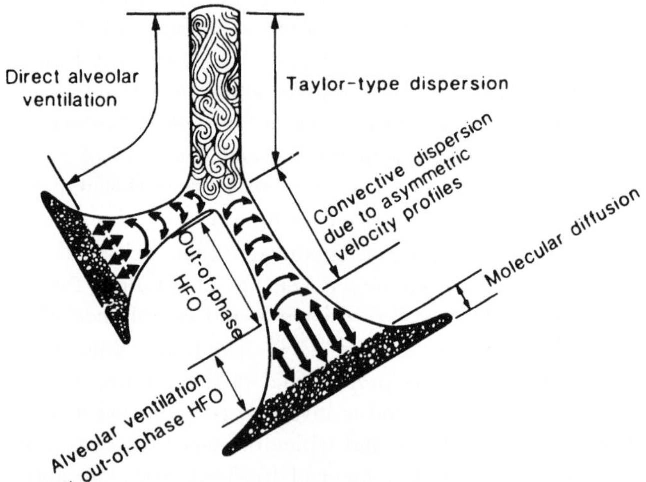

Figure 9.26. Schematic representation of mechanisms of gas transport during HFV. Pendelluft is represented by "alveolar ventilation by out-of-phase HFO". (From Villar J, Winston B, Slutsky AS. Non-conventional techniques of ventilatory support. Crit Care Clin 1990;6:579.)

5. *Cardiogenic oscillations.* Cardiac contractions result in airway oscillations and in increased peripheral gas mixing in the airways[(470)]. This mechanism appears to be of minor importance during HFV[(471)].

Molecular diffusion is the process that accounts for the majority of gas exchange that occurs normally at the alveolar level. Mechanisms that depend on molecular diffusion also have a role during HFV:

1. *Pure molecular diffusion.* During HFV, the amount of time available for equilibration of gas in the alveoli is reduced. If this becomes the rate-limiting step, then the molecular diffusivity of the gas could play an important role in gas exchange during HFV[(417)].
2. *Augmented dispersion.* Radial mixing as previously described occurs also by molecular diffusion and not by convective processes[(469)].

It seems likely that multiple processes are involved in the complex mechanism of gas exchange during HFV. Indeed, it has been suggested that the relative contribution of interregional mixing, turbulence, facilitated dispersion, and convection might differ, depending on the technique of HFV used and the frequency employed[(464)]. Nonetheless, a theoretical basis has been established for explaining the fascinating phenomenon of gas exchange during HFV.

Clinical Applications

Although HFV has been used extensively for intraoperative management during laryngoscopy and bronchoscopy[(434,451)] and with complicated tracheal and bronchial surgery[(472,473)], application of the technique in the management of acute respiratory failure is still in the evaluative stage[(459,474)]. At the present time, most of the theoretical benefits have yet to be demonstrated in clinical settings. The majority of data regarding the use of HFV in the United States has involved one of five high-frequency devices **(Table 9.16).** The principal differences between the various devices are related to the control of mean airway pressure and expiration (both variables directly associated with lung volume and the risk of overdistention). Passive exhalation and indirect control of mean airway pressure potentially complicate the clinician's ability to control intrinsic PEEP and mean lung volume, thereby theoretically increasing the risk of "volutrauma". Use of the Bunnell Life Pulse® jet ventilation device requires the replacement of a conventional endotracheal tube with a specially designed endotracheal tube which allows the high-frequency jets of gas to be delivered directly to the end of the endotracheal tube through a separate lumen. A final problem that complicates the conversion from CMV and application of the various forms of HFV concerns the measurement of proximal airway pressures which may underestimate tracheal and/or alveolar pressures[(475)].

Initial results with various methods of HFV in uncomplicated acute respiratory failure in newborns and adults, have been mixed. Comparison of the results from many clinical studies is complicated by the use of different modes of HFV (i.e., HFPPV, HFJV, HFO). Also, in many clinical trials involving patients with acute respiratory failure, HFV has not been initiated prior to failure of conventional methods. In the only large prospective trial in adults with respiratory failure, no differences in outcome were demonstrated in the 309 patients who were randomly assigned to HFJV or conventional ventilation[(459)]. Several controlled studies comparing HFV to conventional ventilation in infants with respiratory distress syndrome have been published[(476-478)]. In a multicenter, National Institutes of Health (NIH)-sponsored trial (HIFI Study Group) in which 673 preterm infants with respiratory failure at risk for bronchopulmonary dysplasia were randomly assigned to HFO or conventional ventilation[(477)]. Both groups had a similar incidence of bronchopulmonary dysplasia, level of ventilatory support at 28 days of life, and mortality. Furthermore, there was a higher incidence of air leaks, intraventricular hemorrhage, periventricular leukomalacia, and treatment failure in the HFO group. The study design has been criticized for several reasons: (1) delay in institution of HFO, (2) inadequate volume recruitment prior to institution of HFO, and (3) inadequate mean airway pressures in the HFO group[(479,480)]. The use of HFJV in a randomized, controlled study in 42 infants with respiratory failure revealed no differences between the two groups in mortality, air leaks, bronchopulmonary dysplasia, intraventricular hemorrhage, or treatment failure, despite lower mean airway pressures and $PaCO_2$ in the HFJV group[(478)]. In contrast, a multicenter, controlled

TABLE 9.16. Clinical Characteristics of Available High-Frequency Ventilatory Devices[a].

Ventilator	*Type[b]*	*Mean Airway Pressure Control*	*Expiratory Phase*	*Frequency (Hz)*	*Variable Inspiratory Time*
Sensor Medics 3100A	HFO	direct	active	3-15	yes
Senko Med. Instr. Humming II	HFO	direct	active	—	no
Bunnell Life Pulse	HFJV	indirect	passive	4-11	yes
Infrasonics Infant Star HFV	HFFI	indirect	active (venturi)	2-22	no
Bird Space Tech. PVDR-4	HFFI	indirect	passive	2-22	yes

[a]Data with permission from Clarke RH. High-frequency ventilation. J Pediatr 1994; 124-661.
[b]HFO-high frequency oscillator, HFJV-high frequency jet ventilator, HFFI-high frequency flow interrupter.

trial of HFJV in infants with pulmonary interstitial emphysema in the first week of life revealed a higher percentage of patients meeting success criteria in the HFJV group[476]. Despite these observations, morbidity and mortality were similar in both groups.

In contrast to the neonatal and adult experience, recent data on the use of HFV in children has brought what was once thought to be an experimental therapy into the clinical arena. Rosenberg et al.[481] reported the use of both HFO and a high-frequency flow interruption in 12 children with acute lung injury unresponsive to CMV. Both methods of HFV improved oxygenation and ventilation while survivors had more rapid and sustained improvements, as well as shorter duration of conventional ventilation prior to HFV than nonsurvivors. There also appeared to be a difference between the two HFV devices, although this may have been do to the age and duration of prior CMV disparity between the groups (younger age and shorter duration in the HFO group). Smith et al.[482] described their experience with high-frequency jet ventilation (HFJV) in 29 children with acute lung injury complicated by progressive pulmonary barotrauma (extra-alveolar air). Gas exchange in the survivors was maintained with lower airway pressures which may have allowed resolution of the "barotrauma" while minimizing the risk for further "volutrauma". Again, survivors received less CMV prior to HFJV than nonsurvivors, suggesting that early intervention to minimize the progressive development of "volutrauma" is a key factor in survival. The ability to maintain gas exchange at lower mean airway pressure during HFJV[475,482] improves cardiac output in patients recovering from a Fontan procedure who are dependent on the mean central circulatory pressure to mean intrathoracic pressure gradient for systemic blood flow[483]. Preliminary data with the use of the high lung volume strategy with HFPPV in children suffering from severe acute lung injury was correlated with low morbidity and mortality rates[243].

The first prospective, randomized controlled study comparing HFO to CMV in children with acute lung injury was recently published[484]. As stated in the accompanying editorial[485], this study compared the strategy of "ideal lung volume" (HFO) versus "low peak inflating pressure, best PEEP" (CMV). The investigators were able to demonstrate an improvement in oxygenation and ranked outcome (i.e. survival, survival with chronic lung disease, death) with HFO. Pretreatment age and oxygenation index at 24 hours were two independent variables that predicted survival in patients treated with HFO. The lack of improvement at 24 hours (i.e. oxygenation index-42) was suggested by the authors as a means to identify patients who may benefit from alternative forms of therapy early in the course of their disease process where maximal benefit may still be derived.

Newer experimental data continues to support a central role for HFO in patients with acute lung injury. In a rabbit lung lavage model of lung injury, HFO was found to result in fewer granulocytes in bronchoalveolar lavage fluid[486]. The granulocytes recovered from the CMV control group demonstrated oxygen metabolite exhaustion not seen in the HFO group. This lack of oxidative metabolism in a subsequent study with the same model was associated with lower levels of inflammatory mediators (platelet activating factor, thromboxane)[487]. This apparent ability of HFO to mute the inflammatory response may limit further lung injury.

In summary, the data from experimental models and the first controlled study are heartening; however, many questions regarding the role of HFV in patients with acute lung injury remain to be answered by further controlled studies.

Liquid (Perfluorocarbon) Ventilation

In an attempt to eliminate air-fluid interfaces and decrease surface tension, thereby enhancing lung compliance, liquid ventilation utilizing oxygenated perfluorocarbon has been investigated in laboratory and more recently in the clinical arena. Initial attempts were geared towards complete replacement of the gas FRC and tidal ventilation with the oxygenated perfluorocarbon (total liquid ventilation). Recent investigations have been directed towards a liquid FRC while using a conventional mechanical ventilator for gas tidal ventilation (partial liquid ventilation).

Total Liquid Ventilation

Pulmonary gas exchange utilizing perfluorocarbon liquid ventilation has been investigated for over twenty five years[488]. Various studies in premature newborn animals have demonstrated improvements in compliance, gas exchange, and a reduction in airway pressures with total liquid ventilation (TLV) when compared to gas ventilation[489,490]. The development of TLV has been hampered by the specialized equipment necessary to provide tidal liquid ventilation. Despite these difficulties, a short-term trial of TLV has been attempted in extremely premature infants in whom conventional medical therapy had failed and demonstrated significant improvements in compliance[491]. A recent study has disclosed that relatively simple modifications to an existing extracorporeal life-support circuit makes TLV feasible and may allow other centers to apply this new investigational method of ventilation in the laboratory or clinical arena[492]. Before perfluorocarbon TLV assumes a role in clinical practice, safety and effectiveness in a clearly defined population must be demonstrated in a large number of patients in controlled clinical trials with clear advantages over conventional therapy.

Partial Liquid Ventilation

As an attempt to overcome some of the technical difficulties associated with total liquid ventilation, methods have also been developed to apply mechanical gas tidal ventilation with liquid perfluorocarbon filled lungs via conventional instruments (partial liquid ventilation-PLV)[493]. In contrast to total liquid ventilation, PLV has been shown to have few adverse cardiovascular side-effects[494]. Beneficial effects on cardiorespiratory function have been verified in several different laboratory models of lung disease including surfactant deficiency secondary to prematurity[495,496] or saline lavage[497,498] as well as gastric acid aspiration[499]. The improvements in pulmonary function appear to be perfluorocarbon dose-dependent[500] and comparable to administration of exogenous surfactant[501]. Phase I clinical trials of PLV have been completed in neonates, children, and adults with severe acute lung disease unresponsive to conventional medical management and phase II trials are underway. The results of these and other clinical trials will clearly be needed prior to the widespread use of this potentially promising therapeutic modality in routine clinical setting.

Extracorporeal Life Support

The saga behind the development of long-term extracorporeal support is a common one in which a relatively simple concept required multiple technical advancements to make that idea a clinical reality. The term initially used to describe long-term extracorporeal support focused on the function of oxygenation and the type of oxygenator used. Thus, extracorporeal membrane oxygenation (ECMO) became well known in the literature. In some patients, the emphasis shifted to CO_2 removal and extracorporeal CO_2 removal ($ECCO_2R$) was coined to describe the use of extracorporeal circulation and a membrane oxygenator to function primarily for CO_2 removal instead of oxygenation[502]. Extracorporeal support also began to be used for cardiac assist in postoperative cardiac surgical patients[503]. With these different methods of cardiopulmonary support offered by the use of extracorporeal circuitry, a new term, extracorporeal life support (ECLS) has become the standard term to describe this technology[504].

ECLS had its beginnings in the work of Drs. Gibbons and Kirklin, and the development of the "heart-lung machine"[505,506]. This work, which came to fruition between 1953-1955, established the use and utility of extracorporeal circulatory support for the repair of cardiac defects. The early devices were bubble or disk oxygenators with a direct oxygen-blood interface which precluded their use for long-term support because of hemolysis[507,508]. The advent of membrane oxygenators such as that developed by Clowes et al.[509] in 1956, opened the door for prolonged bypass. The 1960's and 1970's were periods of rapid advancement and exploration of the use of prolonged ECLS which proceeded in 3 waves. First, early attempts to use ECLS as an alternative to the then new mechanical ventilator in term and premature infants resulted in periods of successful support, but ultimately death from intracranial hemorrhage[510-512]. Second, support of adults was technically accomplished in the early 1970's with the first reported success in 1972[513]. The subsequent published reports of success[514-516] spurred a rapid increase in use, resulting in the NIH collaborative study begun in 1975[517]. This study was stopped after the entry of 92 of an anticipated 300 patients because survival in both groups was less than 10% and seemed unlikely to change. Adult and pediatric ECLS essentially stopped in the United States after this study was published. Third, in the mid 1970's, there were continued attempts to utilize ECLS support for term infants with the first survivor reported in 1975[518]. Since that time, mushrooming numbers of successfully treated infants with a spectacular difference in expected mortality (> 80% survival in a group with 60-80% expected mortality) have fueled the growth of 109 neonatal ECMO centers[519,520]. There are currently almost 10,000 patients in the international registry maintained by the Extracorporeal Life Support Organization.[520] This success has driven a resurgence of interest in alternative forms of ECLS for adults and older children in the United States.

Classification

The basic classifications of ECLS, venoarterial (VA), venovenous (VV), arteriovenous (AV) are based on the site of blood withdrawal and return, each with distinct advantages and disadvantages **(Table 9.17).** The most common form of support in the past and the most common in neonatal ECLS is VA, where blood is routed from the right atrium through the oxygenator and returned to the arterial circulation, usually into the right common carotid artery (Fig. 9.27). The cannulation is extrathoracic, usually resulting in permanent ligation of the vessels used. This form of ECLS can provide a significant amount of cardiac support as well as pulmonary support and has been used in postoperative cardiac surgery patients with myocardial failure[503]. The benefits of this therapy (cardiac support, excellent oxygenation, relatively low ECLS flows) are associated with significant risks. These include ligation or the need for repair of a large artery, the risks of arterial embolization, and questions concerning the risks/benefits of decreasing pulmonary blood flow[521]. Pulsatility is often decreased for significant periods during the procedure, raising questions about the effects on vascular beds which may depend on pulsatility for autoregulation[522].

During VV-ECLS, venous blood is withdrawn from and

TABLE 9.17. Comparison of Technical and Physiologic Aspects of Venoarterial and Venovenous ECMO Techniques

Venoarterial	Venovenous
Achieves higher PaO_2	Achieves lower PaO_2
Requires lower perfusion rate	Requires higher perfusion rate
Bypasses pulmonary circulation	Maintains pulmonary blood flow
Decreases pulmonary artery pressure	Elevates mixed venous PO_2
Assists systemic circulation	Lacks circulatory assist capability
Requires arterial cannulation	Requires only venous cannulation
Decreases pulmonary blood flow (?)	Presents total venous return to the lungs

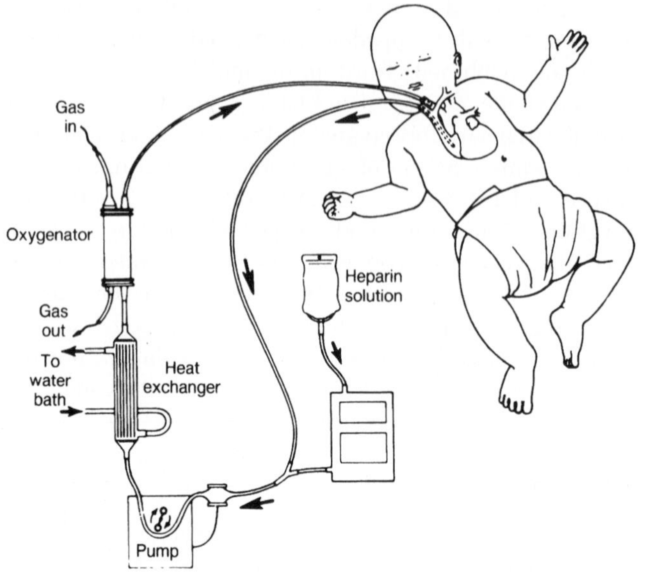

Figure 9.27. Extracorporeal membrane oxygenation perfusion circuit for infant. (From Krummel TM, Greenfield LJ, Kirkpatrick BV, Mueller DG, Ormazabal M, Salzberg AM. Clinical use of an extracorporeal oxygenator in neonatal pulmonary failure. J Pediatr Surg 1982;17:525.)

returned to the venous circulation after oxygenation. This form of ECLS depends on the patient's native cardiac output for oxygen delivery to the periphery. Because there is always a varying rate of "recirculation" of previously oxygenated blood, VV-ECLS requires higher extracorporeal flows, if the pulmonary bed is totally nonfunctional, to maintain adequate oxygenation. The use of VV support does reduce the risk of embolization except in the presence of large right to left shunts and doesn't require sacrifice/repair of a large artery. It maintains well oxygenated pulmonary blood flow which may be of benefit(521) but requires the right ventricle to function in the face of pulmonary hypertension(504).

AV or arteriovenous ECLS is not a clinical entity at present, but has been explored in the lab. It would require an intact cardiovascular system to tolerate the large arteriovenous fistula which would be necessary to achieve gas exchange. Because of the large blood flow requirements for support of gas exchange, its utility may be restricted to partial CO_2 removal(523).

Clinical Applications

Clinically, in this country there is a dichotomous picture, with over 9,000 reported cases of neonatal ECLS and almost 900 pediatric ECLS cases(520,524). This is related to the success rates in neonatal ECMO and pediatric ECMO (80% vs. 50% respectively)(504), the frequency of cases severe enough to warrant support, and the pathophysiology of the disease processes involved. Clearly treatment of PPHN, which is almost always reversible, has been more successful than the treatment of the multifactorial diseases leading to pediatric respiratory failure. This is particularly true if respiratory failure results from severe pulmonary parenchymal disease associated with progressive fibrosis. In addition, pediatric ECLS is technically more difficult than neonatal ECLS(504).

Neonatal ECLS, more commonly referred to as ECMO, was once performed almost exclusively with VA support. The release of a continuous flow, double lumen, 14 French catheter (VVDL, Kendall Healthcare Products Mansfield, MA) has had a major impact in altering that trend. This catheter is designed to be placed in the right internal jugular vein and provide venovenous support. The use of this catheter has escalated rapidly over the past three to four years. In fact, 23% of all neonates reported to the ELSO registry between January 1993 and January 1995 were supported with this catheter(520). Of these 1161 VVDL patients in the registry, 17% were converted to VA support, with a survival of 74%. Randomized studies have shown similar outcomes as judged by survival and neurologic follow-up(523,524). The neurologic follow-up is relatively short term as the bulk of the patients are less than 3 years of age.

The survival rate in neonatal ECMO has remained stable at roughly 80% since 1987 despite dramatic increases in the number of centers (18 to 109)(520). The primary pathophysiologic condition being treated by ECMO, reversible pulmonary hypertension, and its primary diagnoses; meconium aspiration syndrome (MAS), congenital diaphragmatic hernia (CDH), respiratory distress syndrome (RDS), persistent pulmonary hypertension of the neonate (PPHN), and sepsis, have remained the same(519,520). The only diagnosis which has showed a decreased survival has been CDH (70% in 1987 to 60% in 1994)(520). This can be attributed to increasingly aggressive ECMO support of babies with CDH, which now includes patients who have never shown a "honeymoon" and are unable to be safely taken to the operating room for their primary repair because of cardiopulmonary instability. Some of these children would be expected to have fatal pulmonary hypoplasia(525). ECMO does improve survival in critically ill infants with diaphragmatic hernia as described by Van Meurs et al.(525) who showed a survival rate of 67% within a group of infants predicted to have a mortality rate of 100%. The number of patients reported to the ELSO registry has been stable at 1000-1400 per year since 1988, in spite of the development of alternative therapies such as nitric oxide gas administration, high frequency ventilation and surfactant(520). This might change in the next few years as the impact of widespread availability of nitric oxide gas becomes apparent. This therapy appears promising although responses have varied(526,527). There are several large multicenter trials currently in progress which are studying the role of inhaled nitric oxide in the therapy of PPHN.

The clinical status of infants who are placed on ECMO is such that with maximal medical therapy they are felt to have at least an 80% mortality. Although the criteria devised to predict an 80% mortality are based on retrospective reviews(528,529), there have been two prospective studies, both of which showed ECMO to improve survival(530,531). Both studies used adaptive designs to optimize the statistical significance while minimizing the ethical problems of a prospective, randomized study in which death is the end point. This has caused some controversy; however, the study by O'Rourke et al.[531], there can be no question that ECMO improves survival when conventional medical therapy is failing.

Improvement in survival is reasonable only if the majority of patients have a good outcome. Results have been published by several centers showing the majority of patients to be normal on short-term follow-up[532-534]. These results compare favorably with published reports of neonates with severe respiratory failure treated with hyperventilation and tolazoline[535-538]. The most common complication remains a neurologic abnormality on imaging (i.e. cranial ultrasound or CT scan), with 24% of patients showing this finding[534]. Other common complications include hemorrhage, chronic lung disease, and renal insufficiency. Except for hemorrhage, many of these complications can be related to injury suffered secondary to the severity of the illness which necessitated ECLS support[534]. The heparinization, as well as platelet dysfunction seen with ECLS[539], contributes to the bleeding which continues inexorably, thus intracranial hemorrhage early in the course of therapy leads to severe morbidity or mortality.

There were over 300 reported cases of ECMO use in pediatric and adult respiratory failure between 1970 and 1979[504]. Because of the high mortality rate (90%) and the results of the NIH trial, pediatric and adult ECMO stopped in this country in the early 1980's. Drs. Kolobow and Gattinoni subsequently published their laboratory work on the use of ECLS in an alternative fashion for which they coined the term extracorporeal CO_2 removal or $ECCO_2R$[540,541]. $ECCO_2R$ and traditional ECMO utilize the same equipment but differ physiologically in several important aspects. The major focus in $ECCO_2R$ is the use of the circuit and membrane lung to ventilate or remove CO_2 instead of oxygenating the patient. There is some oxygen delivery with this technique, but the primary source of oxygenation is the inflated but apneic lung. Humidified oxygen is insufflated near the carina at a rate equal to the amount of oxygen consumed. The ventilator is set to deliver a low number of pressure limited breaths per minute to avoid atelectasis. Since there is little alveolar ventilation, the alveolar gas composition is determined by the composition and flow of gas ventilating the oxygenator[542,543]. This form of support evolved from the failure of the NIH ECMO trial. In the NIH trial, many patients were maintained on high FiO_2 and ventilatory settings in spite of VA support[544]. Several investigators believe this may have been a factor in the lack of success and emphasized methods to promote lung rest during extracorporeal support[545].

During $ECCO_2R$, peak airway pressures are limited to avoid alveolar overdistention which contributes to ongoing lung injury[545,546]. The maintenance of pulmonary blood flow may also be important in the pathophysiology of ARDS[547]. Hill et al.[513] suggested that the 30% drop in pulmonary blood flow caused by VA bypass was deleterious in a severely damaged lung. In this report, adult patients with pneumonia had large areas of pulmonary infarction which were felt to be a result of the severely damaged lung which were dependent on adequate pulmonary blood flow to maintain viability. Lung infarctions have been demonstrated from tissue alkalosis in areas with ventilation but no perfusion in a lamb model[547]. Although pulmonary blood flow does not decrease during $ECCO_2R$, pulmonary artery pressure usually decreases secondary to a reduction in pulmonary vascular resistance caused by improved oxygenation of the venous blood.

Because of these concerns, work continued on the development of $ECCO_2R$ with successful clinical cases reported as early as 1979[548]. Several uncontrolled series in adults had a 49% survival (expected 10%)[542,543,549]. The centers active in this area claim to be improving their survival as they gain more experience; however, the procedure remains more common in Europe than in the United States. There are currently 171 adult patients in the ELSO registry with a 41% survival rate[550]. The only randomized study that attempted to study efficacy in adults has been performed in the United States and yielded controversial results[551]. Survival in both control and ECLS groups was 40%. This is in contrast to the two years prior to the study when patients with a similar degree of illness had a 10-20% survival. The control group in this study was unique because of the institution of an elaborate computer algorithm control of mechanical ventilation which also improved survival compared to the two previous years[550-553]. The institution which performed the study no longer uses ECLS support for adult respiratory failure, because they found that application of conventional therapy yielded similar survival at lower cost. This computer assisted program is now being piloted in other units. ECLS proponents point to some complicating factors in analyzing the results of the ECLS group in that study. First, the first institutional cases of ECLS support were included in the trial; therefore, raising the question of a learning curve which is significant for this type of support. Second, the length of ECLS support was also limited to 14 days in the first half of the study, prompting many ECLS practitioners to argue that that period of support was too short to declare a treatment failure. Thus, it appears that the controversy continues.

ECLS for children, defined as a term infant greater than two weeks of age with respiratory failure, is ongoing. The ELSO registry contains a total of 884 patients with a cumulative survival of 52%[520]. The number of patients reported to the registry has remained steady at 120-193 per year since 1990. The national experience from 52 centers for pediatric ECLS from 1982-1991 demonstrated a 47% survival for patients with a predicted 85-100% mortality[554]. Moreover, one large center has noted a marked improvement in survival over that time frame (58% survival: 1982-1991 vs. 88% survival: 1991-1993)[555]. These same investigators retrospectively found a 62% survival rate in patients who had an alveolar-arterial oxygenation tension difference ($AaDO_2$) of greater than 400 torr for the 24 hour period prior to initiating ECLS[556]. The $AaDO_2$ of greater than 400 torr has been shown to predict 100% mortality with conventional management in children with severe cardiorespiratory failure[557]. Thus, these investigators suggested that the use of ECLS for this population improved outcome. Further study using multivariate logistic regression suggests improved survival following ECLS in children is associated with several factors prior to initiation of bypass, including patient age (i.e. younger age), duration of mechanical ventilation, peak inspiratory airway pressure, $AaDO_2$, and ECLS administered after 1988[558]. Despite the fact that survival appears to be related to the severity of lung disease and to the occurrence of ECLS complications, recent data establishes that the duration of ECLS is not linked to survival[559]. In fact, ECLS may have been terminated in some patients for pulmonary futility because of the length of bypass at a time when many patients continued on ECLS ultimately survived. Because of these data, interest has remained high and a randomized multicenter clinical trial is currently underway. It is hoped this trial may answer the question of ECMO's utility in children.

For pediatric ECLS, many centers initially continued with VA support and decreased mechanical ventilation in a manner similar to neonatal ECMO[504]. Unfortunately, initiating VV support with the same type of pulmonary management for children, even with high extracorporeal flows, results in arterial saturations in the 85% range. However, as more experience has been gained, a move to support pediatric patients in a fashion closer to $ECCO_2R$ methodology is increasing.

Currently, whether neonatal, pediatric, or adult, ECLS is practiced with some form of "lung rest". In classic neonatal ECMO, the ventilator is decreased to "rest settings" which are typically an FiO_2 of 21-30%, PIP of 15-25 cm H_2O, PEEP of 3-5 cm H_2O, and IMV of 10-15 breaths/min[504,560]. The baby's lungs become totally atelectatic and slowly re-inflate over a period of days[560]. This reinflation has been tied to the reappearance of surfactant protein A and improvement in compliance[561]. Because of these findings, Lotze et al.[562] randomized infants on ECMO to receive surfactant and placebo in a double blinded fashion. While ventilator settings in this study remained at "rest settings", the infants who received surfactant were able to be weaned from bypass 32 hours earlier than control infants. Others have argued that the maintenance of inflation with elevated PEEP will speed recovery by avoiding total atelectasis[563]. Lung inflation is maintained with a PEEP of 12 to 14 cm of H_2O, a rate of 10 breaths per minute, and an inspiratory pressure limit between 20-24 cm H_2O. As the compliance improves and lung expansion increases as measured by chest x-ray, the PEEP is weaned. In a randomized study, bypass time in infants with "high PEEP" was shortened by 34 hours[564]. This method is similar to that used in adult $ECCO_2R$ and thus many centers providing ECLS for pediatric patients and adults use this or a similar method in an attempt to prevent atelectasis.

CONCLUSIONS

The rapid growth of our technical prowess in pediatric respiratory care gives testimony to the creativity and ingenuity of the investigators of the last several decades. Unfortunately, this swift advance in technical capabilities is commonly linked to a dizzying array of buttons, dials, valves, and digital displays that easily confuse the bedside care provider. Despite the temptation to look upon the mechanical tools of respiratory therapy as ends in themselves, it is worth remembering that every contraption gains its worth only to the extent that it achieves therapeutic goals defined by the fundamental principles of respiratory physiology and pathology. As such, no degree of technical lavishness can substitute for respiratory therapy decisions based on a firm understanding of the specific pathophysiologic process at hand. The effectiveness of even the most sophisticated device or method of mechanical ventilation will be limited by the understanding of the pathophysiology of the disease process by the clinician and their capability to integrate this knowledge into the therapeutic application of the device to slow or reverse the pathologic process. Or, as noted by Dr. Thomas Petty twenty years earlier[565],

> IMC [intermittent mandatory cerebration] is . . . the preferred method . . . of mechanical ventilation. Even better, continuous mandatory contemplation (CMC) must emerge as the preferred method . . . used in all forms of respiratory care.

References

1. Schreiner MS, Downes JJ, Kettrick RG, Ise C, Voit R. Chronic respiratory failure in infants with prolonged ventilator dependency. JAMA 1987;258:3398.
2. Viires N, Sillye G, Aubier M, Rassidakis A, Roussos C. Regional blood flow distribution in dog during induced hypotension and low cardiac output: spontaneous breathing versus artificial ventilation. J Clin Invest 1983;72:935.
3. Morray JP, Lynn AM, Mansfield PB. Effect of pH and PCO2 on pulmonary and systemic hemodynamics after surgery in children with congenital heart disease and pulmonary hypertension. J Pediatr 1988;113:474.
4. Egan DF. Gas therapy, In: Fundamentals of respiratory therapy. 3rd ed. St Louis: CV Mosby, 1977:117.
5. McPherson SP. Primary systems: cylinders and piping systems. In: Respiratory therapy equipment. 4th ed. St Louis, CV Mosby 1990:90.
6. McPherson SP. Primary systems: cylinders and piping systems. In: Respiratory therapy equipment. 4th ed. St Louis, CV Mosby 1990:21.
7. McPherson SP. Gas regulation, administration and controlling devices. In: Respiratory therapy equipment. 4th ed. St Louis, CV Mosby 1990:50.
8. McPherson SP. Gas administration devices. In: Respiratory therapy equipment. 2nd ed. St Louis, CV Mosby, 1981:69.
9. Canet J, Sanchis J. Performance of a low flow O2 Venturi mask: diluting effects of the breathing pattern. Eur J Respir Dis 1984;65:68.
10. Schater EN, Littner MR, Luddy P, Beck GJ. Monitoring of oxygen delivery systems in clinical practice. Crit Care Med 1980;8:405.
11. McPherson SP. Gas regulation, administration and controlling devices. In: Respiratory therapy equipment. 4th ed. St Louis, CV Mosby 1990:61.
12. McPherson SP. Gas regulation, administration and controlling devices. In: Respiratory therapy equipment. 4th ed. St Louis, CV Mosby 1990:62.
13. McPherson SP. Gas regulation, administration and controlling devices. In: Respiratory therapy equipment. 4th ed. St Louis, CV Mosby 1990:68.
14. Jenkinson SG. Pulmonary oxygen toxicity. Clin Chest Med 1982;3:109.
15. Caldwell PRB, Weibel ER. Pulmonary oxygen toxicity. In: Fishman AP, ed. Pulmonary diseases and disorders. St Louis, McGraw-Hill 1980:800.

16. Comroe JH, Dripps RD, Dumke, PR, Deming M. Oxygen toxicity. The effect of high concentration of oxygen for twenty-four hours on normal men at sea level and at a simulated altitude of 18,000 feet. JAMA 1945;128:710.
17. Sackner MA, Landa J, Hirsch J, Zapata A. Pulmonary effects of oxygen breathing: a 6 hour study in normal men. Ann Intern Med 1975:82:40.
18. Holm BA, Notter RH, Siegle J, Matalon S. Pulmonary physiological and surfactant changes during injury and recovery from hyperoxia. J Appl Physiol 1985;59:1402.
19. Davis WB, Rennard SI, Bitternab PB, Crystal RG. Pulmonary oxygen toxicity. Early reversible changes in human alveolar structures induced by hyperoxia. N Engl J Med 1983;309:878.
20. Griffith DE, Holden WE, Morris JF, Min LK, Krishnamurthy GT. Effects of common therapeutic concentrations of oxygen on lung clearance of 99 mTc DPTA and bronchoalveolar lavage albumin concentration. Am Rev Respir Dis 1986;134:233.
21. Loewen GM, Bruce AH, Milanowski L, Wild LM, Notter RH, Matalon S. Alveolar hyperoxic injury in rabbits receiving exogenous surfactant. J Appl Physiol 1989;66:1087.
22. Matalon SB, Holm BA, Notter RH. Mitigation of pulmonary hyperoxic injury by administration of exogenous surfactant. J Appl Physiol 1987;62:756.
23. Holm BA, Matalon S, Finkelstein JN, Notter RH. Type II pneumocyte changes during hyperoxic lung injury and recovery. J Appl Physiol 1988;65:2672.
24. Dantzker DR, Wagner PD, West JB. Instability of lung units with low Va/Q ratios during O2 breathing. J Physiol 1975;38:886.
25. Lodato RF. Oxygen toxicity. Crit Care Clin 1990;6:749.
26. Deneke SM, Fanburg BL. Normobaric oxygen toxicity of the lung. N Engl J Med 1980;303:76.
27. Clark JM, Lambertsen CJ. Pulmonary oxygen toxicity: a review. Pharmacol Rev 1971;23:37.
28. Halliwell B, Gutteridge JMC. Oxygen toxicity, oxygen radicals, transition metals and disease. Biochem J. 1984;219:1.
29. Halliwell B. Superoxide and superoxide dependent formation of hydroxyl radicals are important in oxygen toxicity. Trends Biochem Sci 1982;7:270.
30. Fridovich I. The biology of oxygen radicals. Science 1978;201:875.
31. Fridovich I. Chemical aspects of superoxide radical and superoxide dismutases. In: Hayaish O, Asada K, eds. Biochemical and medical aspects of active oxygen. Baltimore, University Press, 1977.
32. Johnson KJ, Fantone JC, Kaplan J, Ward PA. *In vivo* damage of rat lungs by oxygen metabolites. J Clin Invest 1981;67:983.
33. Gurtner GH, Furrukh N, Adkinson NF, et al. The role of arachidonate mediators in peroxide-induced lung injury. Am Rev Respir Dis 1987;136:480.
34. Hageman JR, Babler S, Lee SC, et al. The early involvement of pulmonary prostaglandins in hyperoxic lung injury. Prostaglandins Leukotrienes Med 1986;25:105.
35. Smith LJ, Sommers E, Hunt CE, Pachman L. Hyperoxic lung damage in mice: a possible protective role for prostaglandins. J Lab Clin Med 1986;108:479.
36. Smith LJ, Shamsuddin M, Anderson J, Hsueh W. Hyperoxic lung damage in mice: appearance and bioconversion of peptide leukotrienes. J Appl Physiol 1988;64:944.
37. Klein J, Zijlstra FL, Vincent JE, et al. Cellular and eicosanoid composition of broncho-alveolar lavage fluid in endotoxin protection against pulmonary oxygen toxicity. Crit Care Med 1989;17:247.
38. Taniguchi H, Taki F, Takagi K, et al. The role of leukotriene B^4 in the genesis of oxygen toxicity in the lung. Am Rev Respir Dis 1986;133:805.
39. Burghuber O, Strife R, Zirrolli J, et al. Leukotriene inhibitors attenuate rat injury induced by hydrogen peroxide. Am Rev Respir Dis 1985;131:778.
40. Klein J. Normobaric pulmonary oxygen toxicity. Anesth Analg 1990;70:195.
41. Deneke SM, Fanburg BL. Oxygen toxicity in the lungs: an update. Br J Anaesth 1982;54:737.
42. Jenkinson SG. Oxygen toxicity. New Horizon 1993;1:504.
43. Crapo JD, Barry BE, Foxcue HA, et al. Structure and biochemical changes in rat lungs occurring during exposures to lethal and adaptive doses of oxygen. Am Rev Respir Dis 1980;122:123.
44. Crapo JD, Peters-Golden M, Marsh-Salin J, et al. Pathologic changes in the lungs of oxygen-adapted rats: A morphometric analysis. Lab Invest 1978;39:640.
45. Tierney DF, Ayers L, Kasuyama RS. Altered sensitivity to oxygen therapy. Am Rev Respir Dis 1977;115:59.
46. Massaro D, Massaro GD. Biochemical and anatomical adaptation of the lung to oxygen-induced injury. Fed Proc 1978;37:2485.
47. Hayatdavoudi G, O'Neil JJ, Barry BE, et al. Pulmonary injury in rats following continuous exposure to 60% O2 for 7 days. J Appl Physiol 1981;15:1220.
48. De los Santos R, Seidenfeld JJ, Anzueto A, et al. One hundred percent oxygen lung injury in adult baboons. Am Rev Respir Dis 1987;136:657.
49. Barry BE, Crapo JD. Patterns of accumulation of platelets and neutrophils in rat lungs during exposure to 100% and 86% oxygen. Am Rev Respir Dis 1985;132:548.
50. Fox RB, Hoidal JR, Brown DM, Repine JE. Pulmonary inflammation due to oxygen toxicity: involvement of chemotatic factors and polymorphonuclear leukocytes. Am Rev Respir Dis 1981;123:521.
51. Maryland Institute for Emergency Medical Services System, Hyperbaric Chamber Registry, 1992.
52. Undersea and Hyperbaric Medical Society: Hyperbaric oxygen therapy: A committee report. UHMS Publication 1992;30:1.
53. Kindwall EP. Uses of hyperbaric oxygen therapy in the 1990s. Cleveland Clinic J Med 1992;59:517.
54. Goodman MW, Workman RD. Oxygen-breathing approach to treatment of decompression sickness in divers and aviators. BuShips, Project SF011 06 05, Task 11513-2, Research Report 5-65 US Navy Experimental Diving Unit, 1965.
55. Villanucci S, Marzio D, Scholl M, et al. Cardiovascular changes induced by hyperbaric oxygen therapy. Undersea Biomed Res 1990;17:117.
56. NHLBI Workshop Summary. Hyperbaric oxygenation therapy. Am Rev Respir Dis 1991;144:1414.
57. Heikkila RE, Cabbat FS, Cohen G. *In vivo* inhibition of superoxide dismutase in mice by diethyldithiocarbamate. J Biol Chem 1976;251:2182.
58. Nemiroff PR. Effects of cis-platinum and hyperbaric oxygen on wound healing in mice. Undersea Biomedical Res 1988;40:15.
59. Davis JC, Dunn JM, Heimbach RA. Hyperbaric medicine: Patient selection, treatment procedures, and side-effects. In: Davis JC, Hunt TK eds. Problem Wounds: The Role of Oxygen. Elsevier Science Publishing Co, New York, 1988:233.
60. Hammarlund C. The physiologic effects of hyperbaric oxygen. In: Kindwell E, ed. Hyperbaric Medicine. Best Publishing Co, Flagstaff, Arizona, 1994.
61. Hart GB, Strauss MB, Lennon PA. The treatment of decompression sickness and air embolism in a monoplace chamber. J Hyperbaric Med 1986;1:1.
62. Gajdos P, Conso F, Korach JM, et al. Incidence and causes of carbon monoxide intoxication: results of an epidemiologic survey in a French department. Arch Environ Health 1991;46:373.
63. U.S. Centers for Disease Control. Carbon monoxide intoxication: a preventable environmental health hazard. MMWR 1982;31:529.
64. Rodkey FL, O'Neal JD, Collison HA, Uddin DE. Relative affinity of hemoglobin S and hemoglobin A for CO and O2. Clin Chem 1974;20:83.
65. Brune B, Schmidt KU, Ullrich V. Activation of soluble guanylate cyclase by carbon monoxide and inhibition of superoxide anion. Eur J Biochem 1990;192:683.
66. Chance D, Erecinske M, Wagner M. Mitochondrial responses to carbon monoxide toxicity. Ann NY Acad Sci 1970;174:193.
67. White KA, Marletta MA. Nitric oxide synthase is a cytochrome P-450 type hemoprotein. Biochemistry 1992;31:6627.
68. Raybourn MS, Cork C, Schimmerling W, Tobias CA. An in vitro electrophysiological assessment of the direct cellular toxicity of carbon monoxide. Toxicol Appl Pharmacol 1978:46;769.
69. Raphael JC, Elkharrat D, Jars-Guincestre MC, et al. Trial of normobaric and hyperbaric oxygen for acute carbon monoxide intoxication. Lancet 1989;2:414.
70. Norkool DM, Kirkpatrick JN. Treatment of acute carbon monoxide poisoning with hyperbaric oxygen: a review of 115 cases. Ann Emerg Med 1985;14:1168.
71. Thom SR, Taber RL, Mendiguren II, et al. Delayed neuropsychiatric sequelae following carbon monoxide poisoning and the role of treatment with 100% oxygen or hyperbaric oxygen—a prospective randomized, clinical study. Undersea Biomed Res 1992;19:47.
72. Brown SD, Piantadosi CA. *In vivo* binding of carbon monoxide to cytochrome C oxidase in rat brain. J Appl Physiol 1990;68:604.
73. Zhang J, Piantadosi CA. Mitochondrial oxidase stress after carbon monoxide in the rat brain. J Clin Invest 1991;90:1193.
74. Lapresle J, Fardeau M. The central nervous system and carbon monoxide poisoning: II. Anatomical study of brain lesions following intoxication with carbon monoxide (22 cases). Prog Brain Res 1967;24:31.
75. Tomaszewski CA, Thom SR. Use of hyperbaric oxygen in toxicology. Emerg Med Clinic N Am 1994;12:437.

76. Sasaki T. One-half life clearance of carbon monoxide hemoglobin in blood during hyperbaric oxygen therapy. Bull Tokyo Med Dent Univ 1975:22:63.
77. Thom SR. Functional inhibition of leukocyte B^2 integrins by hyperbaric oxygen in carbon monoxide- mediated brain injury in rats. Toxicol Appl Pharmacol 1993;123:248.
78. Thom SR. Antagonism of carbon monoxide-mediated lipid peroxidation by hyperbaric oxygen. Toxicol Appl Pharmacol 1990;105:340.
79. Goulon M, Barois A, Rapin M, et al. Intoxication oxycarbonee et anoxie aigue par inhalation de gaz de charbon et hydrocarbures. Ann Med Interne 1969;120:335.
80. Thom SR, Taber RL, Mendiguren II, et al. Delayed neuropsychologic sequelae after carbon monoxide poisoning: prevention with hyperbaric oxygen. Ann Emerg Med 1995;25:474.
81. Stevens DL, Bryant AE, Adams K, Mader JT. Evaluation of therapy with hyperbaric oxygen for experimental infections with *Clostridium perfringens.* Clin Infect Dis 1993;17:231.
82. Brogan T, Nizet V, Waldhausen JHT, Rubens CE, Clarke WR. Group A streptococcal necrotizing fascitis complicating primary varicella: a series of fourteen patients. Pediatr Infect Dis J 1995;14:588.
83. Barach AL. Use of helium as a new therapeutic gas. Proc Soc Exp Biol Med 1934;32:462.
84. Gluck EH, Onorato DJ, Castriotta RJ. Helium-oxygen mixtures in intubated patients with status asthmaticus and respiratory acidosis. Chest 1990;98:693.
85. Wolfson MR, Bhutani VK, Shaffer TH, Bowen FW Jr. Mechanics and energetics of breathing helium in infants with bronchopulmonary dysplasia. J Pediatr 1984;104:752.
86. Curtis JL, Mahlmeister M, Fink JB, Lampe G, Matthay MA, Stulbarg MS. Helium-oxygen gas therapy. Use and availability for the emergency treatment of inoperable airway obstruction. Chest 1986;90:455.
87. Barnett TB. Effects of helium and oxygen mixtures on pulmonary mechanics during airway constriction. J Appl Physiol 1967;22:707.
88. Lu TS, Ohmura A, Wong KC, et al. Helium-oxygen in treatment of upper airway obstruction. Anesthesiology 1976;45;678.
89. Jordan WS, Graves CL, Elwyn JF, et al. New therapy for postintubation laryngeal edema and tracheitis in children. JAMA 1970;212:585.
90. Kemper KJ, Ritz RH, Benson MS, Bishop MS. Helium-oxygen mixture in the treatment of postextubation stridor in pediatric trauma patients. Crit Care Med 1991;19:356.
91. Fleming MD, Weigelt JA, Brewer V, McIntire D. Effect of helium and oxygen on airflow in a narrowed airway. Arch Surg 1992;127:956.
92. Manthous CA, Hall JB, Melmed A, et al. Heliox improves pulsus paradoxus and peak expiratory flow in nonintubated patients with severe asthma. Am J Respir Crit Care Med 1995;151;310.
93. Kass JE, Castriotta RJ. Heliox therapy in acute severe asthma. Chest 1995;107:757.
94. Anderson M, Svartengren M, Bylin G, Philipson K, Camner P. Deposition in asthmatics of particles inhaled in air or in helium-oxygen. Am Rev Respir Dis 1993;147:524.
95. Palmer RMJ, Ferrige AC, Moncada S. Nitric oxide release accounts for the biological activity of endothelium-derived relaxing factor. Nature 1987;326:524
96. Moncada S, Palmer RMJ. Biosynthesis and actions of nitric oxide. Semin Perinatology 1991;15:16.
97. Zapol WM, Rimar ST, Gillis N, Marletta M, Bosken CH. NHLBI workshop summary: Nitric oxide and the lung. Am J Respir Crit Care Med 1994;149:1375.
98. Gaston B, Drazen JM, Loscalzo J, Stamler JS. The biology of nitrogen oxides in the airways. Am J Respir Crit Care Med 1994;149:538.
99. Forstermann U, Schmidt HHHW, Pollock JS, et al. Isoforms of nitric oxide synthase: characterization and purification from different cell types. Biochem Pharmacol 1991;42:1849.
100. Corbett JA, Tilton CJ, Chang K, et al. Aminoguanidine, a novel inhibitor of nitric oxide synthase formation, prevents diabetic vascular dysfunction. Diabetes 1992;41:552.
101. Gibson QH, Roughton FJW. The kinetics and equilibria of reactions of nitric oxide and sheep hemoglobin. J Physiol 1957;136:507.
102. Yoshida K, Kasama K. Biotransformation of nitric oxide. Environ Health Perspect 1987;73:201.
103. Wessel DL, Adatia I, Thompson JE, Hickey PR. Delivery and monitoring of inhaled nitric oxide in patients with pulmonary hypertension. Crit Care Med 1994;22:930.
104. Lowry T. "Silo-filler's disease": A syndrome caused by nitrogen dioxide. JAMA 1956;162:205.
105. Centers for Disease Control. Recommendations for occupational safety and health standards. MMWR 1988;37(Suppl):21.
106. Evans MJ, Stephens RJ, Cabral LJ, Freeman G. Cell renewal in the lungs of rats exposed to low levels of NO2. Arch Environ Health 1972;124:180.
107. Williams RA, Rhoades RA, Adams WS. The response of lung tissue and surfactant to nitrogen dioxide exposure. Arch Intern Med 1971;128:101.
108. Maples KR, Sandstrom T, Su Y-F, Henderson RF. The nitric oxide/heme protein complex as a biologic marker of exposure to nitrogen dioxide in humans, rats and in vitro models. Am J Respir Cell Mol Biol 1991;4:538.
109. Stavert DM, Lehnert BE. Nitrogen oxide and nitrogen dioxide as inducers of acute pulmonary injury when inhaled at relatively high concentrations for brief periods. Inhal Toxicol 1990;2:53.
110. Turbow R, Warrarn F, Hallman M, et al. Inflammatory responses and suppressed macrophage function following inhaled nitric oxide. Pediatr Res 1994;35:256.
111. Hogman M, Frostell C, Arnberg H, Hedenstierna G. Bleeding time prolongation and NO inhalation. Lancet 1993;341:1664.
112. Stamler JS, Simon DI, Osborne JA, et al. S-Nitrosylation of proteins with NO: synthesis and characterization of biologically active compounds. Proc Natl Acad Sci USA 1992;89:444.
113. Kinsella JP, Neish SR, Sheffer E, Abram SH. Low-dose inhalation nitric oxide in persistent pulmonary hypertension of the newborn. Lancet 1992;340:819.
114. Roberts JD, Polaner DM, Lang P, Zapol WM. Inhaled nitric oxide in persistent pulmonary hypertension of the newborn. Lancet 1992;340:818.
115. Pepke-Zaba J, Higenbottam TW, Dinh-Xuan AT, Stone D, Wallwork J. Inhaled nitric oxide as a cause of selective pulmonary vasodilatation in pulmonary hypertension. Lancet 1991;338:1173.
116. Kinsella JP, Abman SH. Recent developments in the pathophysiology and treatment of persistent pulmonary hypertension of the newborn. J Pediatr 1995;126:853.
117. Wessel DL, Adatia I, Giglia TM, et al. Inhaled nitric oxide in congenital heart disease. Circulation 1993;87:447.
118. Rossaint R, Falke KJ, Lopez F, et al. Inhaled nitric oxide for the adult respiratory distress syndrome. N Engl J Med 1993;328:399.
119. Abman SH, Griebel JL, Parker DK, Schmidt JM, Swanton D. Acute effects of inhaled nitric oxide in children with severe hypoxemic respiratory failure. J Pediatr 1994;124:881.
120. Bigatello LM, Hurford WE, Kacmarek RM, Roberts JD, Zapol WM. Prolonged inhalation of low concentration of nitric oxide in patients with severe adult respiratory distress syndrome. Anesthesiology 1994;80:761.
121. McPherson SP. Humidifiers and nebulizers. In: Respiratory therapy equipment. 4th ed. St Louis: CV Mosby, 1990:79.
122. Egan DF. Aerosol and humidity therapy. In: Fundamentals of respiratory therapy. 3rd ed. St Louis: CV Mosby, 1977;213.
123. McPherson SP. Humidifiers and nebulizers. In: Respiratory therapy equipment. 4th ed. St Louis: CV Mosby, 1990:82.
124. Dolan GK, Zawadski JJ. Performance characteristics of low-flow humidifiers. Respir Care 1976;21:393.
125. Klein EF Jr, Graves SA. "Hot pot" tracheitis. Chest 1974;65:225.
126. Brain JD, Valberg PA. Deposition of aerosol in the respiratory tract. Am Rev Respir Dis 1979;120:1325.
127. Newhouse M, Dolovich M. Aerosol therapy of asthma: principles and applications. Respiration 1986;50:123.
128. Manthous CA, Hall JB. Administration of therapeutic aerosols to mechanically ventilated patients. Chest 1994;106;560.
129. MacIntyre NR, Silver RM, Miller CW, Schuler F, Coleman RE. Aerosol delivery in intubated, mechanically ventilated patients. Crit Care Med 1985;13:81.
130. Taylor RH, Lerman J. High-efficiency delivery of salbutamol with a metered-dose inhaler in narrow tracheal tubes and catheters. Anesthesiology 1991;74:360.
131. Bishop MJ, Larson RP, Buschman DL. Metered dose inhaler aerosols characteristics are affected by the endotracheal tube actuator/ adapter used. Anesthesiology 1990;73:1263.
132. Rau JL, Harwood RJ, Groff JL. Evaluation of a reservoir device for metered-dose broncho-delivery in intubated adults. Chest 1992; 102:924.
133. Arnon S, Grigg J, Nikander K, Silverman M. Delivery of micronized budesonide suspension by metered dose inhaler and jet nebulizer into a neonatal circuit. Pediatr Pulmonol 1992;13:172.
134. Harvey CJ, O'Doherty MJ, Page CJ, Thomas SHL, Nunam TO, Treacher DF. Effect of a space on pulmonary deposition from a jet nebulizer during mechanical ventilation. Thorax 1995;50:50.

135. Crogan SJ, Bishop MJ. Delivery efficiency of metered dose aerosols given via endotracheal tubes. Anesthesiology 1989;70:1008.
136. O'Doherty MJ, Thomas SHL, Page CG, Treacher DF, Nunan TO. Delivery of a nebulized aerosol to a lung model during mechanical ventilation. Am Rev Respir Dis 1992;146:383.
137. Flavin M, MacDonald M, Dolovich M, Coates G, O'Brodovich H. Aerosol delivery to a rabbit lung with an infant ventilator. Pediatr Pulmonol 1986;2:35.
138. Frankel LR, Wilson CW, Demers RR, et al. A technique for administration of ribavirin to mechanically ventilated infants with severe respiratory syncytial virus infection. Crit Care Med 1987;15:1051.
139. Outwater KM, Meissner HC, Peterson MB. Ribavirin administration to infants receiving mechanical ventilation. Am J Dis Child 1988;142:512.
140. Meert KL, Sarnaik AP, Gelmini MJ, et al. Aerosolized ribavirin in mechanically ventilated children with respiratory syncytial virus lower respiratory tract disease: a prospective, double-blind, randomized trial. Crit Care Med 1994;22:566.
141. Smith DW, Frankel LR, Mathers LH, Tang ATS, Ariagno RL, Prober CG. A controlled trial of aerosolized ribavirin in infants receiving mechanical ventilation for severe respiratory syncytial virus infection. N Engl J Med 1991;325:24.
142. Murray JF. The ketchup-bottle method (editorial). N Engl J Med 1979;300:1155
143. Nunn JF. Mechanisms of pulmonary ventilation. In: Applied respiratory physiology. 2nd ed. Boston: Butterworths, 1977:139.
144. Bryan AC, Bentivoglio LG, Beerel F, MacLeish H, Zidulka A, Bates DV. Factors affecting regional distribution of ventilation and perfusion in the lung. J Appl Physiol 1964;19:395.
145. Kaneko K, Milic-Emili J, Dolovich MB, Dawson A, Bates CV. Regional distribution of ventilation and perfusion as a function of body position. J Appl Physiol 1966;21:767.
146. Lamm WJ, Graham MM, Albert RK. Mechanism by which the prone position improves oxygenation in acute lung injury. Am J Respir Crit Care Med 1994;150:184.
147. Remolina C, Kahn AU, Santigo TV, Edekman NH. Positional hypoxemia in unilateral lung disease. N Engl J Med 1981;304:523.
148. Heaf DP, Helms P, Gordon I, Turner HM. Postural effects on gas exchange in infants. N Engl J Med 1983;308:1505.
149. Belman M, Mittman C. Incentive spirometry: the answer is blowing in the wind. Chest 1981;79:254.
150. Bartlett RH. Postoperative pulmonary prophylaxis: breathe deep and read carefully. Chest 1982;81:1.
151. Mackenzie CF, Shin B. Evaluation of respiratory physical therapy. N Engl J Med 1979;301:665.
152. Mackenzie CF, Shin B, McAslan TC. Chest physiotherapy: the effect on arterial oxygenation. Anesth Analg 1978;57:28.
153. Fox WW, Schwartz JG, Shaffer TH. Pulmonary physiology in neonates: physiologic changes and respiratory management. J Pediatr 1978;92:977.
154. American Association of Respiratory Care. Consensus Statement on the essentials of mechanical ventilators—1992. Respir Care 1992;37:1000.
155. Slutsky AS. Mechanical ventilation. American College of Chest Physicians' consensus conference. Chest 1993;104:1833.
156. Pontoppidan H, Geffin B, Lowenstein E. Acute respiratory failure in the adult. N Engl J Med 1972;287:690,743,799.
157. Dantzker DR, Brook CJ, Dehart P, Lynch JP, Weg JG. Ventilation-perfusion distributions in the adult respiratory distress syndrome. Am Rev Respir Dis 1979;120:1039.
158. Tyler DC. Positive end-expiratory pressure: a review. Crit Care Med 1983;11:300.
159. Weisman IM, Rinaldo JE, Rogers RM. Positive end-expiratory pressure in adult respiratory failure. N Engl J Med 1982;307:1381.
160. Boros SJ, Matalon SV, Ewald R, Leonard AS, Hunt CE. The effect of independent variations in inspiratory-expiratory ratio and end expiratory pressure during mechanical ventilation in hyaline membrane disease: the significance of mean airway pressure. J Pediatr 1977;91:794.
161. Suter PM, Fairley HB, Isenberg MD. Optimum end expiratory airway pressure in patients with acute pulmonary failure. N Engl J Med 1975;292:284.
162. Weisman IM, Rinaldo JE, Rogers RM, Sanders MH. Intermittent mandatory ventilation. Am Rev Respir Dis 1983;127:641.
163. Schuster DP. A physiologic approach to initiating, maintaining, and withdrawing mechanical ventilatory support during acute respiratory failure. Am J Med 1990;88:268.
164. Pepe PE, Marini JJ. Occult positive end-expiratory pressure in mechanically ventilated patients with airflow obstruction. Am Rev Respir Dis 1982;126:166.
165. Simbruner G, Gregory GA. Performance of neonatal ventilators: the effects of changes in resistance and compliance. Crit Care Med 1981;9:509.
166. Fuhrman BP, Smith-Wright DL, Venkataraman S, Orr RA, Howland DF. Proximal mean airway pressure: a good estimator of mean alveolar pressure during continuous positive-pressure breathing. Crit Care Med 1989;17:666.
167. Marini JJ, Ravenscraft SA. Mean airway pressure: physiologic determinants and clinical importance—parts 1 & 2. Crit Care Med 1992;20:1461,1604.
168. Reynolds EOR. Effect of alterations in mechanical ventilator settings on pulmonary gas exchange in hyaline membrane disease. Arch Dis Child 1971;46:152.
169. Perez-Fontan JJ, Heldt GP, Targett RC, Willis MM, Gregory GA. Dynamics of expiration and gas trapping in rabbits during mechanical ventilation at rapid rates. Crit Care Med 1986;14:39.
170. Marini JJ, Crooke PS III, Truwit JD. Determinants and limits of pressure-preset ventilation: a mathematical model of pressure control. J Appl Physiol 1989;67:1081.
171. Mansell A, Bryan C, Levison H. Airway closure in children. J Appl Physiol 1972;33:711.
172. Newth CJL. Recognition and management of respiratory failure. Pediatr Clin North Am 1979;26:617.
173. Banner MJ, Jaeger MJ, Kirby RR. Components of the work of breathing and implications for monitoring ventilator-dependent patients. Crit Care Med 1994;22:515.
174. Mushin WW, Rendell-Baker L, Thompson PW, Mapleson WW. Physical aspects of automatic ventilators: basic principles. In: Automatic ventilation of the lungs. 3rd ed. Oxford: Blackwell Scientific, 1980:62.
175. McPherson SP. Introduction to ventilators. In: Respiratory therapy equipment. 4th ed. St. Louis: CV Mosby, 1990:156.
176. Chatburn RL. Classification of mechanical ventilators. Respir Care 1992;37:1009.
177. Sassoon CS, Giron AE, Ely EA, Light RW. Inspiratory work of breathing on flow-by and demand-flow continuous positive airway pressure. Crit Care Med 1989;17:1108.
178. Tobin MJ. Monitoring of pressure, flow, and volume during mechanical ventilation. Respir Care 1992;37:1081.
179. Branson RD, Campbell RS, Srivastava P, Davis K, Hurst J. Volume monitoring accuracy of four ventilators and the Bicore CP-100 monitor. Respir Care 1991;36:135.
180. Branson RD, Chatburn RL. Technical description and classification of modes of ventilator operation. Respir Care 1992;37:1026.
181. Engstrom CG. The clinical application of prolonged controlled ventilation. Acta Anesthesiol Scand 1963;13(Suppl):1.
182. Hooper RG, Browning M. Acid-base changes and ventilator mode during maintenance ventilation. Crit Care Med 1985;13:44.
183. Groeger JS, Levinson MR, Carlon GC. Assist control versus synchronized intermittent mandatory ventilation during acute respiratory failure. Crit Care Med 1989;17:607.
184. Downs JB, Klein EF Jr, Desautels D, Modell JH, Kirby RR. Intermittent mandatory ventilation: a new approach to weaning patients from mechanical ventilators. Chest 1973;64:331.
185. Hillmann K, Friedlos J, Davey A. A comparison of intermittent mandatory ventilation systems. Crit Care Med 1986;14:499.
186. Christopher KL, Neff TA, Bowman JL, et al. Demand and continuous flow intermittent mandatory ventilation systems. Chest 1985;87:625.
187. Luce JM, Pierson DJ, Hudson LD. Intermittent mandatory ventilation. Chest 1981;79:678.
188. Petty TL. Intermittent mandatory ventilation reconsidered. Crit Care Med 1981;9:620.
189. Kirby RR, Downs JB, Civetta JM, et al. High level positive end-expiratory pressure (PEEP) in acute respiratory insufficiency. Chest 1975;67:156.
190. Downs JB, Douglas ME, Sanfelippo PM, Stanford W, Hodges MR. Ventilatory pattern, intrapleural pressure, cardiac output. Anesth Analg 1977;56:88.
191. Rehder K, Hatch DJ, Sessler AD, Fowler WS. The function of each lung of anesthetized and paralyzed man during mechanical ventilation. Anesthesiology 1972;37:16.
192. Froese AB, Bryan AC. Effects of anesthesia and paralysis on diaphragmatic mechanics in man. Anesthesiology 1974;41:242.
193. Marsh HM, Rehder K, Sessler AD, Fowler WS. Effects of mechanical ventilation, muscle paralysis, and posture on ventilation-perfusion relationships in anesthetized man. Anesthesiology 1973;38:59.
194. Petty TL. In defense of IMV. Respir Care 1976;21:121.
195. Hastings PR, Bushnell LS, Skillman JJ, Weintraub RM, Hedley-Whyte

J. Cardiorespiratory dynamics during weaning with IMV versus spontaneous ventilation in good-risk cardiac-surgery patients. Anesthesiology 1980;53:429.
196. Zarins CK, Bayne CG, Rice CL, Peters RM, Virgilio RW. Does spontaneous ventilation with IMV protect from PEEP-induced cardiac output depression? J Surg Res 1977;22:299.
197. Venus B, Jacobs HK, Mathru M. Hemodynamic responses to different modes of mechanical ventilation in dogs with normal and acid aspirated lungs. Crit Care Med 1980;8:620.
198. Kirby RR, Perry JC, Calderwood HW, Ruiz BC, Lederman DS. Cardiorespiratory effects of high positive end-expiratory pressure. Anesthesiology 1975;43:533.
199. Downs JB, Stock MC. Airway pressure release ventilation: a new concept in ventilatory support. Crit Care Med 1987;15:459.
200. Chiang AA, Steinfeld A, Gropper C, MacIntyre N. Demand-flow airway pressure release ventilation as a partial ventilatory support mode: comparison with synchronized intermittent mandatory ventilation and pressure support ventilation. Crit Care Med 1994;22:1431.
201. Putensen C, Leon MA, Putensen-Himmer G. Timing of pressure release affects power of breathing and minute ventilation during airway pressure release ventilation. Crit Care Med 1994;22:872.
202. Martin LD, Wetzel RC. Optimal release time during airway pressure release ventilation in neonatal sheep. Crit Care Med 1994;22:486.
203. Stock MC, Downs JB, Frolicher DA. Airway pressure release ventilation. Crit Care Med 1987;15:462.
204. Räsänen J, Downs JB, Stock MC. Cardiovascular effect of conventional positive pressure ventilation and airway pressure release ventilation. Chest 1988;93:911.
205. Garner W, Downs JB, Stock MC, et al. Airway pressure release ventilation (APRV). A human trial. Chest 1988;94:779.
206. Cane RD, Peruzzi WT, Shapiro BA. Airway pressure release ventilation in severe acute respiratory failure. Chest 1991;100:460.
207. Räsänen J, Cane RD, Downs JB, et al. Airway pressure release ventilation during acute lung injury: A prospective multicenter trial. Crit Care Med 1991;19:1234.
208. Sydow M, Burchardi H, Ephraim E, Zielmann S, Crozier TA. Long-term effects of two different ventilatory modes on oxygenation in acute lung injury. Am J Respir Crit Care Med 1994,149:1550.
209. Valentine DD, Hammond MD, Downs JB, Sears NJ, Sims WR. Distribution of ventilation and perfusion with different modes of mechanical ventilation. Am Rev Respir Dis 1991;143:1262.
210. Martin LD, Wetzel RC, Bilenki AL. Airway pressure release ventilation in a neonatal lamb model of acute lung injury. Crit Care Med 1991;19:373.
211. Hewlett AM, Plott AS, Terry VG. Mandatory minute volume, a new concept in weaning from mechanical ventilation. Anaesthesia 1977;32:163.
212. Higgs BD, Bevan JC. Use of mandatory minute volume ventilation in the perioperative management of a patient with myasthenia. Br J Anaesth 1979;51:1181.
213. Ashbaugh DG, Bigelow DB, Petty TL, Levine BE. Acute respiratory distress in adults. Lancet 1967;2:319.
214. Gregory GA, Kitterman JA, Phibbs RH, Tooley WH, Hamilton WK. Treatment of the idiopathic respiratory-distress syndrome with continuous positive airway pressure. N Engl J Med 1971;284:1333.
215. Link J. Increase of expiratory resistance by the PEEP-valve of the servoventilator. Intensive Care Med 1983;9:137.
216. Doyle H, Fried J. Reduction of circuit resistance in the Babybird ventilator. Respir Care 1983;28:1143.
217. MacIntyre NR. Respiratory function during pressure support ventilation. Chest 1986;89:677.
218. Brochard L, Harf A, Lorino H, et al. Inspiratory pressure support prevents diaphragmatic fatigue during weaning from mechanical ventilation. Am Rev Respir Dis 1989;139:513.
219. MacIntyre NR, Leatherman NE. Mechanical loads on the ventilatory muscles: a theoretical analysis. Am Rev Respir Dis 1989; 139:968.
220. Leith DE, Bradley M. Ventilatory muscle strength and endurance training. J Appl Physiol 1976;41:508.
221. Fiastro JF, Habib MP, Quan SF. Pressure support compensation for inspiratory work due to endotracheal tubes and demand CPAP. Chest 1988;93:499.
222. Banner MJ, Kirby RR, Blanch PB, Layon AJ. Decreasing imposed work of breathing apparatus to zero using pressure-support ventilation. Crit Care Med 1993;21:1333.
223. Cohen IL, Bilen Z, Krishnamurthy S. The effects of ventilator working pressure during pressure support ventilation. Chest 1993;103:588.
224. MacIntyre NR. Weaning from mechanical ventilatory support: volume-assisting intermittent breaths versus pressure-assisting every breath. Respir Care 1988;33:121.
225. Kacmarek RM. Inspiratory pressure support: does it make a clinical difference? Intensive Care Med 1989;15:337.
226. Tokioka H, Kinjo M, Hirakawa M. The effectiveness of pressure support ventilation for mechanical ventilatory support in children. Anesthesiology 1993;78:880.
227. el-Khatib MF, Chatburn RL, Potts DL, Blumer JL, Smith PG. Mechanical ventilators optimized for pediatric use decrease work of breathing and oxygen consumption during pressure-support ventilation. Crit Care Med 1994;22:1942.
228. Wilson RS. Monitoring the lung: mechanics and volume. Anesthesiology 1976;45:135.
229. Burzstein S, Taitelman U, DeMyttenaere S, et al. Reduced oxygen consumption in catabolic states with mechanical ventilation. Crit Care Med 1978;6:162.
230. Field S, Kelly SM, Macklem PT. The oxygen cost of breathing in patients with cardiorespiratory disease. Am Rev Respir Dis 1982;126:9.
231. Aubier M, Viires N, Syllie G, Mozes R, Roussos C. Respiratory muscle contribution to lactic acidosis in low cardiac output. Am Rev Respir Dis 1982;126:648.
232. Shepard FM, Arango LA, Simmons JG, Berry FA. Hemodynamic effects of mechanical ventilation in normal and distressed newborn lambs: a comparison of negative pressure and positive pressure respirators. Biol Neonate 1971;19:83.
233. Peters RM, Hiberman M, Hogan JS, Crawford DA. Objective indications for respirator therapy in post-trauma and postoperative patients. Am J Surg 1972;124:262.
234. Epstein RA, Hyman AI. Ventilatory requirements of critically ill neonates. Anesthesiology 1980;53:379.
235. Epstein RA. The sensitivities and response times of ventilatory assistors. Anesthesiology 1971;34:321.
236. Martin LD, Rafferty JF, Wetzel RC, Gioia FR. Inspiratory work and response times of a modified pediatric volume ventilator during synchronized intermittent mandatory ventilation and pressure support ventilation. Anesthesiology 1989;71:977.
237. Binda RE Jr, Cook DR, Fischer CG. Advantages of infant ventilators over adapted adult ventilators in pediatrics. Anesth Analg 1976;55:769.
238. Cournand A, Motley HL, Werko L, Richards DW Jr. Physiological studies of the effects of intermittent positive pressure breathing on cardiac output in man. Am J Physiol 1948;152:162.
239. Fairley HB, Blenkarn GD. Effect on pulmonary gas exchange of variations in inspiratory flow rate during intermittent positive pressure ventilation. Br J Anaesth 1966;38:320.
240. Meyers Jr, Lembeck L, O'Kane H, Baue AE. Changes in functional residual capacity of the lung after operation. Arch Surg 1975;110:576.
241. Ali J, Weisel RD, Layug AB, Kripke BJ, Hechtman HB. Consequences of postoperative alterations in respiratory mechanics. Am J Surg 1974;128:376.
242. Ward ME, Roussos C. The respiratory muscles in shock: service or disservice? Intensive Crit Care Dig 1985;4:3.
243. Paulson TE, Spear RM, Peterson BM. New concepts in the treatment of children with acute respiratory distress syndrome. J Pediatr 1995;127:163.
244. Buda AJ, Pinsky MR, Ingels NB Jr, Daughter GT II, Stinson EB, Alderman EL. Effect of intrathoracic pressure on left ventricular performance. N Engl J Med 1979;301:453.
245. Mathru M, Rao TL, el-Etr AA, Pifarre R. Hemodynamic response to changes in ventilatory patterns in patients with normal and poor left ventricular reserve. Crit Care Med 1982;10:423.
246. Muizelaar JP, Marmarou A, Ward JD, et al. Adverse effects of prolonged hyperventilation in patients with severe head injury: a randomized clinical trial. J Neurosurg 1991;75:731.
247. Montgomery AG, Debs RJ, Luce JM, et al. Aerosolized pentamidine as sole therapy for *Pneumocystis carinii* pneumonia in patients with acquired immunodeficiency syndrome. Lancet 1987;2:480.
248. Nunn JF. Mechanisms of pulmonary ventilation. In: Applied respiratory physiology. 2nd ed. Boston: Butterworths, 1977:139.
249. Marini JJ. New options for the ventilatory management of acute lung injury. New Horizons 1993,1:489.
250. Wyszogrodski I, Kyei-Aboagye K, Taeusch HW Jr, Avery ME. Surfactant inactivation by hyperventilation: conservation by end-expiratory pressure. J Appl Physiol 1975;38:461.
251. Notter RH, Taubold R, Mavius RD. Hysteresis in saturated phospholipid films and its potential relevance for lung surfactant function *in vivo*. Exp Lung Res 1982;3:109.

252. Gong H Jr. Positive-pressure ventilation in the adult respiratory distress syndrome. Clin Chest Med 1982;3:69.
253. Hammon JW Jr, Wolfe WG, Moran JF, Jones RH, Sabiston DC Jr. The effect of positive end-expiratory pressure on regional ventilation and perfusion in the normal and injured primate lung. J Thorac Cardiovasc Surg 1976;72:680.
254. Kumar A, Falke KJ, Geffin B, et al. Continuous positive pressure ventilation in acute respiratory failure. Effects on hemodynamics and lung function. N Engl J Med 1970;283:1430.
255. Colgan FJ, Nichols FA, DeWeese JA. Positive end-expiratory pressure, oxygen transport, and the low output state. Anesth Analg 1974;53:538.
256. Kanarek DJ, Shannon DC. Adverse effect of positive end-expiratory pressure on pulmonary perfusion and arterial oxygenation. Am Rev Respir Dis 1975;112:457.
257. Dueck R, Wagner PD, West JB. Effects of positive end-expiratory pressure on gas exchange in dogs with normal and edematous lungs. Anesthesiology 1977;47:359.
258. Zvist J, Pontoppidan H, Wilson RS, Lowenstein E, Laver MB. Hemodynamic responses to mechanical ventilation with PEEP. Anesthesiology 1975;42:45.
259. Venus B, Jacobs HK, Lim L. Treatment of the adult respiratory distress syndrome with continuous positive airway pressure. Chest 1979;76:257.
260. Hemmer M, Suter PM. Treatment of cardiac and renal effects of PEEP with dopamine in patients with acute respiratory failure. Anesthesiology 1979;50:399.
261. Matamis D, Lemaire F, Harf A, Brun-Buisson C, Ansquer JC, Atlan G. Total respiratory pressure-volume curves in the adult respiratory distress syndrome. Chest 1984;86:58.
262. Tuxen DV. Permissive hypercapnic ventilation. Am J Respir Crit Care Med 1994;150:870.
263. Bidani A, Tzouanakis AE, Cardenas VJ Jr, Zwischenberger JB. Permissive hypercapnia in acute respiratory failure. JAMA 1994;272:957.
264. Feihl F, Perret C. Permissive hypercapnia. How permissive should we be? Am J Respir Crit Care Med 1994;150:1722.
265. Williams TJ, Tuxen DV, Scheinkestel CD, Czarny D, Bowes G. Risk factors for morbidity in mechanically ventilated patients with acute severe asthma. Am Rev Respir Dis 1992;146:607.
266. Prezant DJ, Aldrich TK, Karpel JP, Park SS. Inspiratory flow dynamics during mechanical ventilation in patients with respiratory failure. Am Rev Respir Dis 1990;142:1284.
267. Scott LR, Benson MS, Pierson DJ. Effect of inspiratory flowrate and circuit compressible volume on auto-PEEP during mechanical ventilation. Respir Care 1986;31:1075.
268. Darioli R, Perret C. Mechanical controlled hypoventilation in status asthmaticus. Am Rev Respir Dis 1984;129:385.
269. Tuxen DV, Williams TJ, Scheinkestel CD, Czarny D, Bowes G. Use of a measurement of pulmonary hyperinflation to control the level of mechanical ventilation in patients with acute severe asthma. Am Rev Respir Dis 1992;146:1136.
270. Tan IK, Bhatt SB, Tam YH, Oh TE. Effects of PEEP on dynamic hyperinflation in patients with airflow limitation. Br J Anaesth 1993;71:322.
271. Bellomo R, McLaughlin P, Tai E, Parkin G. Asthma requiring mechanical ventilation. A low morbidity approach. Chest 1994;105:891.
272. Corbridge TC, Hall JB. The assessment and management of adults with status asthmaticus. Am J Respir Crit Care Med 1995;151:1296.
273. Dworkin G, Kattan M. Mechanical ventilation for status asthmaticus in children. J Pediatr 1989;114:545.
274. Shugg AW, Kerr S, Butt WW. Mechanical ventilation of paediatric patients with asthma: short and long term outcome. J Paediat Child Health 1990;26:343.
275. Strange C. Double-lumen endotracheal tubes. Clin Chest Med 1991;12:497.
276. Marraro G. Simultaneous independent lung ventilation in pediatric patients. Crit Care Clin 1992;8:131.
277. Al-Saady N, Bennett ED. Decelerating inspiratory flow waveform improves lung mechanics and gas exchange in patients on intermittent positive-pressure ventilation. Inten Care Med 1985,11:68.
278. Lessard MR, Guérot E, Lorino H, Lemaire F, Brochard L. Effects of pressure-controlled ventilation with different I:E ratios versus volume-controlled ventilation on respiratory mechanics, gas exchange, and hemodynamics in patients with adult respiratory distress syndrome. Anesthesiology 1994,80:983.
279. Rappaport SH, Shpiner R, Yoshihara G, Wright J, Chang P, Abraham E. Randomized, prospective trial of pressure-limited versus volume-controlled ventilation in severe respiratory failure. Crit Care Med 1994,24:22.
280. Tharratt RS, Allen RP, Albertson TE. Pressure controlled inverse ratio ventilation in severe adult respiratory failure. Chest 1988, 94:755.
281. Gurevitch MJ, Van Dyke J, Young ES, et al. Improved oxygenation and lower peak airway pressure in severe adult respiratory distress syndrome. Treatment with inverse ratio ventilation. Chest 1986;89:21.
282. Lain DC, DiBenedetto R, Morris SL, et al. Pressure control inverse ratio ventilation as a method to reduce peak inspiratory pressure and provide adequate ventilation and oxygenation. Chest 1989;95:1081.
283. Cole AGH, Weller SF, Sykes MK. Inverse ratio ventilation compared with PEEP in adult respiratory failure. Intensive Care Med 1984;10:227.
284. Anderson JB. Ventilatory strategy in catastrophic lung disease. Inverse ratio ventilation (IRV) and combined high frequency ventilation. Acta Anaesthesiol Scand 1989;90(Suppl):145.
285. Marcy TW, Marini JJ. Inverse Ratio Ventilation in ARDS. Rationale and Implementation. Chest 1991,100:494.
286. Spahr RC, Klein AM, Brown DR, et al. Hyaline membrane disease. A controlled study of inspiratory to expiratory ratio in its management by ventilator. Am J Dis Child 1980;134:373.
287. Greaves TH, Cramolini GM, Walker DH, et al. Inverse ratio ventilation in a 6-year-old girl with severe post-traumatic adult respiratory distress syndrome. Crit Care Med 1989;17:588.
288. Shanholtz C, Brower R. Should inverse ratio ventilation be used in adult respiratory distress syndrome? Am J Respir Crit Care Med 1994, 149:1354.
289. Chiang AA, Steinfeld A, Gropper C, MacIntyre N. Demand-flow airway pressure release ventilation as a partial support mode: Comparison with synchronized intermittent mandatory ventilation and pressure support ventilation. Crit Care Med 1994;22:1431.
290. Nichols DG. Respiratory muscle performance in infants and children. J Pediatr 1991;118:493.
291. Robotham JL. A physiologic approach to hemidiaphragm paralysis. Crit Care Med 1979;7:563.
292. Robotham JL, Chipps BE, Shermeta DW. Continuous positive airway pressure in hemidiaphragmatic paralysis. Anesthesiology 1980;52:167.
293. Haller JA, Pickard LR, Tepas JJ, et al. Management of diaphragmatic paralysis in infants with special emphasis on selection of patients of operative plication. J Pediatr Surg 1979;14:779.
294. Weiner P, Suo J, Fernandez E, Cherniack R. The effect of hyperinflation on respiratory muscle strength and efficiency in healthy subjects and patients with asthma. Am Rev Respir Dis 1990;141:1501.
295. Tobin MJ. Respiratory muscles in disease. Clin Chest Med 1988;9:263.
296. Aurora NS, Rochester DF. Respiratory muscle strength and maximal voluntary ventilation in undernourished patients. Am Rev Respir Dis 1982;126:5.
297. Mansell AL, Anderson JC, Muttart CR, et al. Short-term pulmonary effects of total parenteral nutrition in children with cystic fibrosis. J Pediatr 1984;104:700.
298. Dark DS, Pingleton SK, Kerby GR. Hypercapnia during weaning: a complication of nutritional support. Chest 1985;88:141.
299. Benotti PN, Bistrian B. Metabolic and nutritional aspects of weaning from mechanical ventilation. Crit Care Med 1989;17:181.
300. Molloy DW, Dhingra S, Solven F, Wilson A, McCarthy DS. Hypomagnesemia and respiratory muscle power. Am Rev Respir Dis 1984;129:497.
301. Aubier M, Murciano D, Lecocguic Y, et al. Effect of hypophosphatemia on diaphragmatic contractility in patients with acute respiratory failure. N Engl J Med 1985; 313:420.
302. Aubier M, Viires N, Piquet J, et al. Effects of hypocalcemia on diaphragmatic strength generation. J Appl Physiol 1985;58:2054.
303. Aubier M, Trippenbach T, Roussos C. Respiratory muscle fatigue during cardiogenic shock. J Appl Physiol 1981;51:499.
304. Watchko JF, LaFramboise WA, Standaert TA, Woodrum DE. Diaphragmatic function during hypoxemia: neonatal and developmental aspects. J Appl Physiol 1986;60:1599.
305. Watchko JF, Standaert TA, Woodrum DE. Diaphragmatic function during hypercapnia: neonatal and developmental aspects. J Appl Physiol 1987;62:768.
306. Knisely AS, Leal SM, Singer DB. Abnormalities of diaphragmatic muscle in neonates with ventilated lungs. J Pediatr 1988;113:1074.
307. Cohen CA, Zagelbaum G, Gross D, Roussos C, Macklem P. Clinical manifestations of inspiratory muscle fatigue. Am J Med 1982;73:308.
308. Keens TC, Bryan AC, Levison H, Ionize CD. Developmental patterns of muscle fiber types in human ventilatory muscles. J Apple Physical 1978;44:909.
309. Tobin MJ, Perez W, Guenther SM, et al. The pattern of breathing dur-

ing successful and unsuccessful trials of weaning from mechanical ventilation. Am Rev Respir Dis 1986;134:1111.

310. Fiastro JF, Habib MP, Shon BY, et al. Comparison of standard weaning parameters and mechanical work of breathing in mechanically ventilated patients. Chest 1988;94:232.
311. Tobin MJ, Yang K. Weaning from mechanical ventilation. Crit Care Clin 1990;6:725.
312. Yang KL, Tobin MJ. A prospective study of indexes predicting the outcome of trials of weaning from mechanical ventilation. N Engl J Med 1991;324:1445.
313. Shoults D, Clarke TA, Benumof JL, Manning FL. Maximum inspiratory force in predicting successful neonatal tracheal extubation. Crit Care Med 1979;7:485.
314. Shimada Y, Yoshya I, Tanaka K, Yamazaki T, Kumon K. Crying vital capacity and maximal inspiratory pressure as clinical indicators of readiness for weaning of infants less than a year of age. Anesthesiology 1979;51:456.
315. Esteban A, Frutos F, Tobin MJ, et al. A comparison of four methods of weaning patients from mechanical ventilation. Spanish lung failure collaborative group. N Engl J Med 1995;332:345.
316. Brochard L, Rauss A, Benito S, et al. Comparison of three methods of gradual withdrawal from ventilatory support during weaning from mechanical ventilation. Am J Respir Crit Care Med 1994;150:896.
317. LeSouef PN, England SJ, Bryan AC. Total resistance of the respiratory system in preterm infants with and without an endotracheal tube. J Pediatr 1984;104:108.
318. Wall MA. Infant endotracheal tube resistance: effects of changing length, diameter, and gas density. Crit Care Med 1980;8:38.
319. Zwillich CW, Pierson DJ, Creagh CE, et al. Complications of assisted ventilation: a prospective study of 354 consecutive episodes. Am J Med 1974;57:161.
320. Webb HH, Tierney DF. Experimental pulmonary edema due to intermittent positive pressure ventilation with high inflation pressures. Protection by positive end-expiratory pressure. Am Rev Respir Dis 1974,110:556.
321. Dreyfuss D, Basset G, Soler P, Saumon G. Intermittent positive-pressure hyperventilation with high inflation pressures produces pulmonary microvascular injury in rats. Am Rev Respir Dis 1985,132:880.
322. Parker JC, Hernandez LA, Longnecker GL, Peevy K, Johnson W. Lung edema caused by high peak inspiratory pressures in dogs. Role of increased microvascular filtration pressure and permeability. Am Rev Respir Dis 1990,142:321.
323. Dreyfuss D, Soler P, Basset G, Saumon G. High inflation pressure pulmonary edema. Respective effects of high airway pressure, high tidal volume, and positive end-expiratory pressure. Am Rev Respir Dis 1988,137:1159.
324. Hernandez LA, Peevy KJ, Moise AA, Parker JC. Chest wall restriction limits high airway pressure-induced lung injury in young rabbits. J Appl Physiol, 1989,66:2364.
325. Dreyfuss D, Soler P, Saumon G. Spontaneous resolution of pulmonary edema caused by short periods of cyclic overinflation. J Appl Physiol, 1992,72:2081.
326. Tsuno K, Prato P, Kolobow T. Acute lung injury from mechanical ventilation at moderately high airway pressures. J Appl Physiol, 1990, 69:956.
327. Hernandez LA, Coker PJ, May S, Thompson AL, Parker JC. Mechanical ventilation increases microvascular permeability in oleic acid-injured lungs. J Appl Physiol, 1990,69:2057.
328. Corbridge TC, Wood LDH, Crawford GP, Chudoba MJ, Yanos J, Sznader JI. Adverse effects of large tidal volume and low PEEP in canine acid aspiration. Am Rev Respir Dis, 1990,142:311.
329. Coker PJ, Hernandez LA, Peevy KJ, Adkins K, Parker JC. Increased sensitivity to mechanical ventilation after surfactant inactivation in young rabbit lungs. Crit Care Med 1992,20:635.
330. Adkins WK, Hernandez LA, Coker PJ, Buchanan B, Parker JC. Age affects susceptibility to pulmonary barotrauma in rabbits. Crit Care Med 1991,19:390.
331. Dreyfuss D, Saumon G. Role of tidal volume, FRC, and end-inspiratory volume in the development of pulmonary edema following mechanical ventilation. Am Rev Respir Dis 1993,148:1194.
332. Muscedere JG, Mullen JBM, Slutsky AS. Tidal ventilation at low airway pressures can augment lung injury. Am J Respir Crit Care Med 1994,149:1327.
333. Gattinoni L, Pesenti AN, Avalli L, Rossi F, Bombino M. Pressure-volume curve of total respiratory system in acute respiratory failure. Computed tomographic scan study. Am Rev Respir Dis 1987,136:730.
334. Mead J, Takisima T, Leith D. Stress distribution in lungs: A model of pulmonary elasticity. J Appl Physiol 1970,28:596.
335. Lachmann B. Open the lung and keep the lung open (editorial). Inten Care Med 1992,18:319.
336. Hickling KG, Henderson SJ, Jackson R. Low mortality associated with low volume pressure limited ventilation with permissive hypercapnia in severe adult respiratory distress syndrome. Inten Care Med 1990,16:372.
337. Hickling KG, Walsh J, Henderson S, Jackson R. Low mortality rate in adult respiratory distress syndrome using low-volume, pressure-limited ventilation with permissive hypercapnia: A prospective study. Crit Care Med 1994,22:1568.
338. Lee PC, Helsmoortel CM, Cohn SM, Fink MP. Are low tidal volumes safe? Chest 1990,97:430.
339. Demling RH, Staub NC, Edmunds LH Jr. Effect of end-expiratory airway pressure on accumulation of extravascular lung water. J Appl Physiol 1975;38:907.
340. Bishouty Z, Ali J, Younes M. Effect of tidal volume and PEEP on rate of edema formation in in situ perfused canine lobes. J Appl Physiol 1988;64:1900.
341. Nolop KB, Braude S, Taylor KM, et al. Epithelial and endothelial flux after bypass in dogs: effect of positive end-expiratory pressure. J Appl Physiol 1987;62:1244.
342. Albert RK. Non-respiratory effects of positive end-expiratory pressure. Respir Care 1988;33:464.
343. Van Der Zee H, Cooper JA, Hakim TS, et al. Alterations in pulmonary fluid balance induced by positive end-expiratory pressure. Respir Physiol 1986;64:125.
344. Egan EA. Response of alveolar epithelial solute permeability to changes in lung inflation. J Appl Physiol 1980;49:1032.
345. Egan EA. Lung inflation, lung solute permeability, and alveolar edema. J Appl Physiol 1982;53:121.
346. Pierson DJ. Alveolar rupture during mechanical ventilation: role of PEEP, peak airway pressure, and distending volume. Respir Care 1988;33:472.
347. Haake R, Schlichtig R, Ulstad DR, et al. Barotrauma: pathophysiology, risk factors, and prevention. Chest 1987;91:608.
348. Macklin MT, Macklin CC. Malignant interstitial emphysema of the lungs and mediastinum as an important occult complication in many respiratory diseases and other conditions: an interpretation of the clinical literature in the light of laboratory experiment. Medicine 1944;23:281.
349. Woodring JH. Pulmonary interstitial emphysema in the adult respiratory distress syndrome. Crit Care Med 1985;13:786.
350. Maunder RJ, Pierson DJ, Hudson LD. Subcutaneous and mediastinal emphysema: pathophysiology, diagnosis, and management. Arch Intern Med 1984;144:1447.
351. Trapnell DH, Thurston G. Unilateral pulmonary oedema after pleural aspiration. Lancet 1970;1:1367.
352. Glenski JA, Hall RT. Neonatal pneumopericardium: analysis of ventilatory variables. Crit Care Med 1984;12:439.
353. Marini JJ, Culver BH. Systemic gas embolism complicating mechanical ventilation in the adult respiratory distress syndrome. Ann Intern Med 1989;110:699.
354. Pollack MM, Fields AI, Holbrook PR. Pneumothorax and pneumomediastinum during pediatric mechanical ventilation. Crit Care Med 1979;7:536.
355. Bone RC, Francis PB, Pierce AK. Pulmonary barotrauma complicating positive end-expiratory pressure. Am Rev Respir Dis 1975;111:921.
356. Cohen DJ, Baumgart S, Stephenson LW. Pneumopericardium in neonates: is it PEEP or is it PIP? Ann Thorac Surg 1983;35:179.
357. Primhak RA. Factors associated with pulmonary air leak in premature infants receiving mechanical ventilation. J Pediatr 1983;102:764.
358. Madansky DL, Lawson EE, Chernick V, Taeusch HW Jr. Pneumothorax and other forms of pulmonary air leak in newborns. Am Rev Respir Dis 1979;120:729.
359. Kumar A, Falke KJ, Geffin B, et al. Continuous positive pressure ventilation in acute respiratory failure. Effects on hemodynamics and lung function. N Engl J Med 1970;283:1430.
360. Colgan FJ, Nichols FA, DeWeese JA. Positive end-expiratory pressure, oxygen transport, and the low output state. Anesth Analg 1974;53:538.
361. Biondi JW, Schulman DS, Matthay RA. Effect of mechanical ventilation on right and left ventricular function. Clin Chest Med 1988;9:55.
362. Cournand A, Motley HL, Werko L, Richards DW Jr. Physiological studies of the effects of intermittent positive pressure breathing on cardiac output in man. Am J Physiol 1948;152:162.
363. Hubay CA, Waltz RC, Brecher GA, Praglin J, Hingson RA. Circulatory

dynamics of venous return during positive-negative pressure respiration. Anesthesiology 1954;15:445.
364. Fewell JE, Abendschein DR, Carlson CJ, Murray JF, Rapaport E. Continuous positive-pressure ventilation decreases right and left ventricular end-diastolic volumes in the dog. Circ Res 1980;46:125.
365. Scharff SM, Caldini P, Ingram RH Jr. Cardiovascular effects of increasing airway pressure in the dog. Am J Physiol 1977;232:H35.
366. Jardin F, Farcot JC, Boisante L, Curien N, Margairaz A, Bourdarias JP. Influence of positive end-expiratory pressure on left ventricular performance. N Engl J Med 1981;304:387.
367. Liebman PR, Patton MT, Manny J, Shepro D, Hechtman HB. The mechanism of depressed cardiac output on positive end-expiratory pressure (PEEP). Surgery 1978;83:594.
368. Venus R, Jacobs HK. Alterations in regional myocardial blood flows during different levels of positive end-expiratory pressure. Crit Care Med 1984;12:96.
369. Marquez JM, Douglas ME, Downs JB, et al. Renal function and cardiovascular responses during positive airway pressure. Anesthesiology 1979;50:393.
370. Pollack MM, Fields AL, Holbrook PR. Cardiopulmonary parameters during high PEEP in children. Crit Care Med 1980;8:372.
371. Laver MB. Dr. Starling and the "ventilator" kidney. Anesthesiology 1979;50:383.
372. Baratz RA, Philbin DM, Patterson RW. Plasma antidiuretic hormone and urinary output during continuous positive-pressure breathing in dogs. Anesthesiology 1971;34:510.
373. Hall SV, Johnson EE, Hedley-Whyte J. Renal hemodynamics and function with continuous positive-pressure ventilation in dogs. Anesthesiology 1974;41:452.
374. Gabriele G, Rosenfeld CR, Fixler DE, Wheeler JM. Continuous airway pressure breathing with the head-box in the newborn lamb: effects on regional blood flows. Pediatrics 1977;59:858.
375. Manny J, Justice R, Hechtman HB. Abnormalities in organ blood flow and its distribution during positive end-expiratory pressure. Surgery 1979;85:425.
376. Brienza N, Revelly JP, Ayuse T, Robotham JL. Effects of PEEP on arterial and venous blood flows. Am J Respir Crit Care Med 1995;152:504.
377. Bredenberg CE, Paskanik A. Fromm D. Portal hemodynamics in dogs during mechanical ventilation with positive end-expiratory pressure. Surgery 1981;90:817.
378. Johnson EE, Hedley-Whyte J. Continuous positive-pressure ventilation and portal flow in dogs with pulmonary edema. J Appl Physiol 1972;33:385.
379. Bonnet F, Richard C, Glaser P, Lafay M, Guesde R. Changes in hepatic flow induced by continuous positive pressure ventilation in critically ill patients. Crit Care Med 1982;10:703.
380. Shapiro HM, Marshall LF. Intracranial pressure responses to PEEP in head-injured patients. J Trauma 1978;18:254.
381. Heffner JE. Airway management in the critically ill patient. Crit Care Clin 1990;6:533.
382. Pingleton SK. Complications of acute respiratory failure. Am Rev Respir Dis 1988;137:1463.
383. Craven DE, Make B, McCabe WR, et al. Risk factors for pneumonia in patients receiving continuous mechanical ventilation. Am Rev Respir Dis 1986;133:792.
384. Johanson WG, Pierce AK, Sanford JP. Changing pharyngeal bacterial flora in hospitalized patients: emergence of Gram-negative bacilli. N Engl J Med 1969;281:1137.
385. Driks MR, Craven DE, Celli BR, et al. Nosocomial pneumonia in intubated patients given sucralfate as compared with antacids or histamine type 2 blockers. N Engl J Med 1989;317:1376.
386. Brun-Buisson C, Legrand P, Rauss A, et al. Intestinal decontamination for control of nosocomial multiresistant Gram-negative bacilli. Study of an outbreak of an intensive care unit. Ann Intern Med 1989;110:873.
387. Craven DE, Steger KA. Pathogenesis and prevention of nosocomial pneumonia in the mechanically ventilated patient. Respir Care 1989;34:85.
388. Tobias JD, Schleien CL, Haun SE. Methadone as treatment for iatrogenic narcotic dependency in pediatric intensive care unit patients. Crit Care Med 1990;18:1292.
389. Mickell JJ, Pedigo SA, Lucking SE, Albert MA. Age-related differences in the use of morphine, diazepam, and pancuronium for mechanically ventilated children. Dev Pharmacol Ther 1990;14:20.
390. Segredo V, Caldwell JE, Matthay MA, Sharma ML, Gruenke LD, Miller RD. Persistent paralysis in critically ill patients after long-term administration of vecuronium. N Engl J Med 1992;327:524.
391. Griffin D, Fairman N, Cousin D, Rawsthorne L, Grossman JE. Acute myopathy during treatment of status asthmaticus with corticosteroids and steroidal muscle relaxants. Chest 1992;102:510.
392. Giostra E, Magistris MR, Pizzolato G, Cox J, Chevrolet JC. Neuromuscular disorder in intensive care unit patients treated with pancuronium bromide. Occurrence in a cluster group of seven patients and two sporadic cases, with electrophysiologic and histologic examination. Chest 1994;106:210.
393. Hansen-Flaschen J, Cowen J, Raps EC. Neuromuscular blockade in the intensive care unit. More than we bargained for. Am Rev Respir Dis 1993;147:234.
394. Meyer KC, Prielipp RC, Grossman JE, Coursin DB. Prolonged weakness after infusion of atracurium in two intensive care unit patients. Anesth Analg 1994;78:772.
395. Manthous CA, Chatila W. Prolonged weakness after the withdrawal of atracurium. Am J Respir Crit Care Med 1994;150:1441.
396. Harwood TN, Moorthy SS. Prolonged vecuronium-induced neuromuscular blockade in children. Anesth Analg 1989;68:534.
397. Pascucci RC. Prolonged weakness after extended mechanical ventilation in a child. Crit Care Med 1990;18:1181.
398. Haynes SR, Morton NS. Prolonged neuromuscular blockade with vecuronium in a neonate with renal failure. Anaesthesia 1990;45:743.
399. Raps EC, Bird SJ, Hansen-Flaschen J. Prolonged muscle weakness after neuromuscular blockade in the intensive care unit. Crit Care Clin 1994;10:799.
400. Watling SM, Dasta JF. Prolonged paralysis in intensive care unit patients after the use of neuromuscular blocking agents: a review of the literature. Crit Care Med 1994;22:884.
401. Greenough A, Morley C, Davis J. Interaction of spontaneous respiration with artificial ventilation in preterm babies. J Pediatr 1983;103:769.
402. Gibney RTN, Wilson RS, Pontoppidan H. Comparison of work of breathing on high gas flow and demand valve continuous positive airway pressure systems. Chest 1982;82:692.
403. Viale JP, Annat G, Bertrand O, et al. Additional inspiratory work in intubated patients breathing with continuous positive airway pressure systems. Anesthesiology 1985;63:536.
404. Katz JA, Kraemer RW, Gjerde G. Inspiratory work and airway pressure with continuous positive airway pressure delivery systems. Chest 1985;88:519.
405. Sassoon CSH. Mechanical ventilator design and function: The trigger variable. Respir Care 1992;37:1056.
406. Sassoon CS, Lodia R, Rheeman CH, Kuei JH, Light RW, Mahutte CK. Inspiratory muscle work of breathing during flow-by, demand-flow, and continuous-flow systems in patients with chronic obstructive pulmonary disease. Am Rev Respir Dis 1992;145:1219.
407. Nishimura M, Imanaka H, Yoshiya I, Kacmarek RM. Comparison of inspiratory work of breathing between flow-triggered and pressure-triggered demand flow systems in rabbits. Crit Care Med 1994;22:1002.
408. Sassoon CS, Del-Rosario N, Fei R, Rheeman CH, Gruer SE, Mahutte CK. Influence of pressure- and flow-triggered synchronous intermittent mandatory ventilation on inspiratory muscle work. Crit Care Med 1994;22:1933.
409. Giuliani R, Mascia L, Recchia F, Caracciolo A, Fiore T, Ranieri VM. Patient-ventilator interaction during synchronized intermittent mandatory ventilation. Effects of flow triggering. Am J Respir Crit Care Med 1995;151:1.
410. Bernstein G, Heldt GP, Mannino FL. Increased and more consistent tidal volume during synchronized intermittent mandatory ventilation in newborn infants. Am J Respir Crit Care Med 1994;150:1444.
411. Cleary JP, Bernstein G, Mannino FL, Heldt GP. Improved oxygenation during synchronized intermittent mandatory ventilation in neonates with respiratory distress syndrome: a randomized, crossover study. J Pediatr 1995;126:407.
412. Shepard FM, Arango LA, Simmons JG, Berry FA. Hemodynamic effects of mechanical ventilation in normal and distressed newborn lambs: a comparison of negative pressure and positive pressure respirators. Biol Neonate 1971;19:83.
413. Stark AR, Bascom R, Frantz ID III. Muscle relaxation in mechanically ventilated infants. J Pediatr 1979;94:439.
414. Slutsky AS. Nonconventional methods of ventilation. Am Rev Respir Dis 1988;138:175.
415. Draper WB, Whitehead RW. Diffusion respiration in the dog anesthetized by pentothal sodium. Anesthesiology 1944;5:262.
416. Slutsky AS, Watson J, Leith DE, et al. Tracheal insufflation of O2 (TRIO) at low flow rates sustains life for several hours. Anesthesiology 1985;63:278.

417. Slutsky AS, Khoo MCK, Brown R. Simulation of gas transport due to cardiogenic oscillations. J Appl Physiol 1985;58:1331.
418. Burwen DR, Watson J, Brown R, et al. Effect of cardiogenic oscillations on gas mixing during tracheal insufflation of O2. J Appl Physiol 1986;60:965.
419. Long SE, Menon AS, Kato H, et al. Constant oxygen insufflation (COI) in a ventilatory failure model. Am Rev Respir Dis 1988;138:630.
420. Christopher KL, Spofford BT, Brannin PK, et al. Transtracheal oxygen therapy for refractory hypoxemia. JAMA 1986;256:494.
421. Lehnert BE, Oberdorster G, Slutsky AS. Constant flow ventilation of apneic dogs. J Appl Physiol 1982;53:483.
422. Watson JW, Burwen DR, Kamm RD, et al. Effect of flow rate on blood gases during constant flow ventilation in dogs. Am Rev Respir Dis 1986;133:626.
423. Cybulsky I, Abel J, Menon AS, et al. Contributions of cardiogenic oscillations to gas mixing during constant flow ventilation. J Appl Physiol 1987;63:564.
424. Webster P, Menon AS, Slutsky AS. Constant flow ventilation in pigs. J Appl Physiol 1966;61:2238.
425. Kolobow T, Powers T, Mandava S, et al. Intratracheal pulmonary ventilation (ITPV): control of positive end-expiratory pressure at the level of the carina through the use of a novel ITPV catheter design. Anesth Analg 1994;78:455.
426. Muller EE, Kolobow T, Mandava S, et al. How to ventilate lungs as small as 12.5% of normal: the new technique of intratracheal pulmonary ventilation. Pediatr Res 1993;34:606.
427. Wilson JM, Thompson JR, Schnitzer JJ, et al. Intratracheal pulmonary ventilation and congenital diaphragmatic hernia: a report of two cases. J Pediatr Surg 1993;28:484.
428. Raszynski A, Hultquist KA, Latif H, et al. Rescue from pediatric ECMO with prolonged hybrid intratracheal pulmonary ventilation. A technique for reducing dead space ventilation and preventing ventilator induced lung injury. ASAIO J 1993;39:M681.
429. Nahum A, Burke WC, Ravenscraft SA, et al. Lung mechanics and gas exchange during pressure-control ventilation in dogs. Augmentation of CO2 elimination by an intratracheal catheter. Am Rev Respir Dis 1992;146:965.
430. Nahun A, Ravenscraft SA, Nakos G, et al. Tracheal gas insufflation during pressure-control ventilation. Effect of catheter position, diameter, and flow rate. Am Rev Respir Dis 1992;146:1411.
431. Burke WC, Nahum A, Ravenscraft SA, et al. Modes of tracheal gas insufflation. Comparison of continuous and phase-specific gas injection in normal dogs. Am Rev Respir Dis 1993;148:562.
432. Nahum A, Chandra A, Niknam J, Ravenscraft SA, Adams AB, Marini JJ. Effect of tracheal gas insufflation on gas exchange in canine oleic acid-induced lung injury. Crit Care Med 1995;23:348.
433. Ravenscraft SA, Burke WC, Nahum A, et al. Tracheal gas insufflation augments CO2 clearance during mechanical ventilation. Am Rev Respir Dis 1993;148:345.
434. Sjostrand U. High-frequency positive-pressure ventilation (HFPPV): a review. Crit Care Med 1980;8:345.
435. Wetzel RC, Gioia FR. High frequency ventilation. Pediatr Clin North Am 1987;34:15.
436. Slutsky AS, Drazen JM, Ingram RH, et al. Effective pulmonary ventilation with small-volume oscillations at high frequency. Science 1980;209:609.
437. Slutsky AS, Kamm RD, Drazen JM. A review of experimental and theoretical studies of high frequency ventilation. In: Scheck PA, Sjostrand UH, Smith RB, eds. Perspectives in high frequency ventilation. The Hague: Martinus Nijhoff, 1983:59.
438. Wright K, Lyrene RK, Truog WE, Standaert TA, Murphy J, Woodrum DE. Ventilation by high-frequency oscillation in rabbits with oleic acid lung disease. J Appl Physiol 1981;50:1056.
439. Schmid ER, Knopp TJ, Rehder K. Intrapulmonary gas transport and perfusion during high-frequency oscillation. J Appl Physiol 1981; 51:1507.
440. Robertson HT, Coffey RL, Standaert TA, Truog WE. Respiratory and inert gas exchange during high-frequency ventilation. J Appl Physiol 1982;52:683.
441. Truog WE, Standaert TA, Murphy J, Palmer S, Woodrum DE, Hodson WA. Effect of high-frequency oscillation on gas exchange and pulmonary phospholipids in experimental hyaline membrane disease. Am Rev Respir Dis 1983;127:585.
442. Frantz ID, Stark AR, Davis JM, Davies P, Kitzmiller TJ. High-frequency ventilation does not affect pulmonary surfactant, liquid, or morphologic features in normal cats. Am Rev Respir Dis 1982;126:909.
443. McEvoy RD, Davies NJHK, Hedenstierna G, Hartman MT, Spragg RG, Wagner PD. Lung mucociliary transport during high-frequency ventilation. Am Rev Respir Dis 1982;126:452.
444. Rehder K, Schmid ER, Knopp TJ. Long-term high-frequency ventilation in dogs. Am Rev Respir Dis 1983;128:476.
445. Chakrabarti MK, Sykes MK. Cardiorespiratory effects of high frequency intermittent positive pressure ventilation in the dog. Br J Anaesth 1980;52:475.
446. Thompson WK, Marchak BE, Froese AB, Bryan AC. High-frequency oscillation compared with standard ventilation in pulmonary injury model. J Appl Physiol 1982;52:543.
447. Otto CW, Quan SF, Conahan TJ, Calkins JM, Waterson CK, Hameroff SR. Hemodynamic effects of high-frequency jet ventilation. Anesth Analg 1983;62:298.
448. Gioia FR, Harris AP, Traystman RJ, Rogers MC. Hemodynamic effects of high frequency ventilation. In: Scheck PA, Smith RB, Sjostrand U, eds. Perspectives in high frequency ventilation. The Hague: Martinus Nijhoff, 1982:105.
449. Toutant SM, Todd MM, Drummond JC, Shapiro HM. Cerebral blood flow during high frequency ventilation in cats. Crit Care Med 1983;11:712.
450. Oberg PA, Sjostrand U. Studies of blood pressure regulation. I: common-carotid-artery clamping in studies of the carotid-sinus baroreceptor control of the systemic blood pressure. Acta Physiol Scand 1969;75:276.
451. Heijman K, Heijman L, Jonzon A, Sedin G, Sjostrand U, Widman B. High frequency positive pressure ventilation during anaesthesia and routine surgery in man. Acta Anaesthesiol Scand 1972;16:176.
452. Borg U, Eriksson I, Sjostrand U. High-frequency positive-pressure ventilation (HFPPV): a review based upon its use during bronchoscopy and for laryngoscopy and microlaryngeal surgery under general anesthesia. Anesth Analg 1980;59:594.
453. Sjostrand UH. Review of the physiologic rationale for and development of high frequency positive pressure ventilation—HFPPV. Acta Anaesthesiol Scand 1977;64(Suppl):7.
454. Boros SJ, Bing DR, Mammel MC, Hagen E, Gordon MJ. Using conventional infant ventilators at unconventional rates. Pediatrics 1984; 74:487.
455. Klain M, Smith RB. High frequency percutaneous transtracheal jet ventilation. Crit Care Med 1977;5:280.
456. Carlton GC, Miodownik S, Ray C, Kahn RC. Technical aspects and clinical implications of high frequency jet ventilation with a solenoid valve. Crit Care Med 1981;9:47.
457. Carlton GC, Ray C, Griffin J, et al. Tidal volume and airway pressure on high frequency jet ventilation. Crit Care Med 1983;11:83.
458. Guntapalli, Pinsky MR, Marquez J, et al. Determinants of ventilation during high-frequency jet ventilation. J Crit Care 1987;2:93.
459. Carlton GC, Howland WS, Ray C, et al. High-frequency jet ventilation. A prospective, randomized evaluation. Chest 1983;84:551.
460. Calkins JM, Waterson CK, Quan SF, et al. Effects of high frequency jet ventilation design and operational variables upon arterial blood gas tensions. In: Scheck PA, Sjostrand UH, Smith RB, eds. Perspectives in high frequency ventilation. The Hague: Martinus Nijhoff, 1983:71.
461. Carlon GC, Ray C, Miodownik S, Howland WS, Guy Y, Groeger JS. Physiologic implications of high frequency jet ventilation techniques. Crit Care Med 1983;11:508.
462. Frantz ID III, Werthammer J, Stark AR. High-frequency ventilation in premature infants with lung disease: adequate gas exchange at low tracheal pressures. Pediatrics 1983;71:483.
463. Lunkenheimer PP, Frank I, Rafflenbeul W, Dickhut HH, Keller H, Fuhrmann C. Application of transtracheal pressure oscillations as a modification of "diffusion respiration". Br J Anaesth 1972;44:627.
464. Bohn DJ, Miyasaka K, Marchak BE, Thompson WK, Froese AB, Bryan AC. Ventilation by high-frequency oscillation. J Appl Physiol 1980;48:710.
465. Chang HK. Mechanisms of gas transport during ventilation by high-frequency oscillation. J Appl Physiol 1984;56:553.
466. Froese AB, Bryan AC. High-frequency ventilation. Am Rev Respir Dis 1987;135:1363.
467. Haselton F, Scherer P. Bronchial bifurcations and respiratory mass transport. Science 1980;208:69.
468. Lehr J, Butler J, Westerman P, et al. Photographic measurement of pleural surface motion during lung oscillation. J Appl Physiol 1985;59:623.
469. Fredberg JJ. Augmented diffusion in the airways can support pulmonary gas exchange. J Appl Physiol 1980;49:232.
470. Slutsky AS. Gas mixing by cardiogenic oscillations: a theoretical quantitative analysis. J Appl Physiol 1981;51:1287.

471. Rehder K, Didier EP. Gas transport and pulmonary perfusion during high frequency ventilation in humans. J Appl Physiol 1984;57:1231.
472. Malina JR, Nordstrom SG, Sjostrand UH, Wattwil LM. Clinical evaluation of high-frequency positive-pressure ventilation (HFPPV) in patients scheduled for open-chest surgery. Anesth Analg 1981;60:324.
473. El-Baz N, El-Ganzouri, Ivankovich A. High-frequency positive-pressure ventilation for major airway surgery. In: Scheck PA, Sjostrand UH, Smith RB, eds. Perspectives in high frequency ventilation. The Hague: Martinus Nijhoff, 1983:216.
474. Wattwil LM, Sjostrand UH, Borg UR. Comparative studies of IPPV and HFPPV with PEEP in critical care patients. I. A clinical evaluation. Crit Care Med 1983;11:30.
475. Zobel G, Dacar D, Rödl S: Proximal and tracheal airway pressures during different modes of mechanical ventilation: An animal model study. Pediatr Pulmonol 1994,18:239.
476. Keszler M, Donn SM, Bucciarelli, et al. Multicenter controlled trial comparing high-frequency jet ventilation and conventional mechanical ventilation in newborn infants with pulmonary interstitial emphysema. J Pediatr 1991;119:85.
477. HIFI Study Group. High-frequency oscillatory ventilation compared with conventional mechanical ventilation in the treatment of respiratory failure in preterm infants. N Engl J Med 1989;320:88.
478. Carlo WA, Siner B, Chatburn RL, Robertson S, Martin RJ. Early randomized intervention with high-frequency jet ventilation in respiratory distress syndrome. J Pediatr 1990;117:765.
479. Bryan AC. The use of high-frequency oscillation in hyaline membrane disease. Acta Anaesthesiol Scand 1989;90(Suppl):124.
480. Bohn D. High frequency oscillation. Br J Anaesth 1989;63:16S.
481. Rosenberg RB, Broner CW, Peters KJ, Anglin DL. High-frequency ventilation for acute pediatric respiratory failure. Chest 1993,104:1216.
482. Smith DW, Frankel LR, Derish MT, et al. High-frequency jet ventilation in children with the adult respiratory distress syndrome complicated by pulmonary barotrauma. Pediatr Pulmonol 1993,15:279.
483. Meliones JN, Bove EL, Dekeon MK, et al. High-frequency jet ventilation improves cardiac function after the Fontan procedure. Circulation 1991;84:III-364.
484. Arnold JH, Hanson JH, Toro-Figuero LO, Gutiérrez, J, Berens RJ, Anglin DL. Prospective, randomized comparison of high-frequency oscillatory ventilation and conventional mechanical ventilation in pediatric respiratory failure. Crit Care Med 1994,22:1530.
485. Nichols DG. Taming the technology for adult respiratory distress syndrome in children (editorial). Crit Care Med 1994,22:1521.
486. Matsuoka T, Kawano T, Miyasaka K. Role of high-frequency ventilation in surfactant-depleted lung injury as measured by granulocytes. J Appl Physiol 1994,76:539.
487. Imo Y, Coon T, Miyasak K, Takata M, Imai T, Okuyama K: Inflammatory chemical mediators during conventional ventilation and during high frequency oscillatory ventilation. Am J Respir Crit Care Med 1994,150:1550.
488. Shaffer TH, Wolfson MR, Clark LC Jr. Liquid ventilation. Pediatr Pulmonol 1992;14:102.
489. Wolfson MR, Shaffer TH. Liquid ventilation during early development: theory, physiologic processes and application. J Dev Physiol 1990;13:1.
490. Wolfson MR, Greenspan JS, Deoras KS, Rubenstein SD, Shaffer TH. Comparison of gas and liquid ventilation: clinical, physiological, and histological correlates. J Appl Physiol 1992;72:1024.
491. Greenspan JS, Wolfson MR, Rubenstein SD, Shaffer TH. Liquid ventilation of human preterm neonates. J Pediatr 1990;117:106.
492. Hirschl RB, Merz SI, Montoya JP, et al. Development and application of a simplified liquid ventilator. Crit Care Med 1995;23:157.
493. Fuhrman BP, Paczan PR, DeFrancisis M. Perfluorocarbon-associated gas exchange. Crit Care Med 1991;19:712.
494. Herman LJ, Fuhrman BP, Papo MC, et al. Cardiorespiratory effects of perfluorocarbon-associated gas exchange at reduced oxygen concentrations. Crit Care Med 1995;23:553.
495. Salman Nh, Fuhrman BP, Steinhorn DM, et al. Prolonged studies of perfluorocarbon associated gas exchange and of the resumption of conventional mechanical ventilation. Crit Care Med 1995;23:919.
496. Leach CL, Fuhrman BP, Morin FC III, Rath MG. Perfluorocarbon-associated gas exchange (partial liquid ventilation) in respiratory distress syndrome: a prospective, randomized, controlled study. Crit Care Med 1993;21:1270.
497. Tutuncu AS, Akpir K, Mulder P, Erdmann W, Lachmann B. Intratracheal perfluorocarbon administration as an aid in the ventilatory management of respiratory distress syndrome. Anesthesiology 1993; 79:1083.
498. Tutuncu AS, Faithfull NS, Lachmann B. Comparison of ventilatory support with intratracheal perfluorocarbon administration and conventional mechanical ventilation in animals with acute respiratory failure. Am Rev Respir Dis 1993;148:785.
499. Nesti FD, Fuhrman BP, Steinhorn DM, et al. Perfluorocarbon-associated gas exchange in gastric aspiration. Crit Care Med 1994;22:1445.
500. Tutuncu AS, Faithfull NS, Lachmann B. Intratracheal perfluorocarbon administration combined with mechanical ventilation in experimental respiratory distress syndrome: dose-dependent improvement of gas exchange. Crit Care Med 1993;21:962.
501. Leach CL, Holm B, Morin FC III, et al. Partial liquid ventilation in premature lambs with respiratory distress syndrome: efficacy and compatibility with exogenous surfactant. J Pediatr 1995;126:412.
502. Gattinoni L, Kolobow T, Tomlinson BS, et al. Low-frequency positive pressure ventilation with extracorporeal carbon dioxide removal (LFPPV-ECCO2R): an experimental study. Anesth Analg 1978; 57:470.
503. Kanter KR, Pennington DG, Weber TG, et al. Extracorporeal membrane oxygenation for postoperative cardiac failure in children. J Thorac Cardiovasc Surg 1987;93:27.
504. Bartlett RH. Extracorporeal life support for cardiopulmonary failure. Curr Probl Surg 1990;27:623.
505. Hill JD, John H, Gibbon JR. The development of the first successful heart-lung machine. Part I. Ann Thorac Surg 1982;34:337.
506. Kirklin JW, Donald DE, Harshburger HG, et al. Studies in extracorporeal circulation. Applicability of Gibbon-type pump-oxygenator to human intracardiac surgery: 40 cases. Ann Surg 1956;144:2.
507. Lee WH Jr, Krumhar D, Fonkalsrud EW, et al. Denaturation of plasma proteins as a cause of morbidity and death after intracardiac operations. Surgery 1961;50:29.
508. Dobell ARC, Matri M, Galva R, et al. Biological evaluation of blood after prolonged recirculation through film and membrane oxygenators. Ann Surg 1965;161:617.
509. Clowes GHA Jr, Hopkins AL, Neville WE. An artificial lung dependent upon diffusion of oxygen and carbon dioxide through plastic membranes. J Thorac Surg 1956;32:630.
510. Rashkind WJ, Freeman A, Klein D, Toft RW. Evaluation of a disposable plastic low volume pumpless oxygenator as a lung substitute. J Pediatr 1965;66:94.
511. White JJ, Andrews HG, Risenberg H, et al. Prolonged respiratory support in newborn infants with a membrane oxygenator. Surgery 1971;70:288.
512. Dorson W Jr, Meyer B, Baker E, et al. Response of distressed infants to partial bypass lung assist. ASAIO Trans 1970;16:345.
513. Hill JD, O'Brien TG, Murray JJ, et al. Prolonged extracorporeal oxygenation for acute post-traumatic respiratory failure (shock-lung syndrome): use of the Bramson membrane lung. N Engl J Med 1972;286:629.
514. Soeter JR, Maniya RT, Sprague AY, et al. Prolonged extracorporeal oxygenation for cardiorespiratory failure after tetralogy correction. J Thorac Cardiovasc Surg 1973;66:214.
515. Hiden D, Mielke CH Jr, Rodvien R, et al. Platelets, hemostasis and thromboembolism during treatment of acute respiratory insufficiency with extracorporeal oxygenation: experience with 28 clinical perfusions. J Thorac Cardiovasc Surg 1975;70:644.
516. Bartlett RH, Gazzaniga AB, Fong SW, et al. Extracorporeal membrane oxygenator support for cardiopulmonary failure: experience in 28 cases. J Thorac Cardiovasc Surg 1977;73:375.
517. Zapol WM, Snider MT, Hill JD, et al. Extracorporeal membrane oxygenation in severe acute respiratory failure. JAMA 1979;242:2193.
518. Bartlett RH, Gazzaniger AB, Jeffries R, Huxtable RF, Haiduc N, Fong SW. Extracorporeal membrane oxygenation (ECMO) cardiopulmonary support in infancy. ASAIO Trans 1976;22:80.
519. Stolar CJ, Snedecor SS, Bartlett RH. Extracorporeal membrane oxygenation and neonatal respiratory failure: experience from the extracorporeal life support organization. J Pediatr Surg 1991;26:563.
520. The Neonatal ECMO Registry of the Extracorporeal Life Support Organization, Ann Arbor, MI, July, 1995.
521. Ratliff JL, Hill JD, Fallat RJ, et al. Complications associated with membrane lung support by venoarterial perfusion. Ann Thorac Surg 1975;19:537.
522. Short BL, Walker LK, Gleason CA, et al. Effect of extracorporeal membrane oxygenation on cerebral blood flow and cerebral oxygen consumption in lambs. Pediatr Res 1990;28:50.
523. Schmidt S, Dudenhausen JW, Langner K, et al. A new perfusion circuit for the newborn with lung immaturity: extracorporeal CO2 removal via

an umbilical arterio-venous shunt during apneic 02 diffusion. Int J Artif Organs 1984;8:478.
524. The Pediatric ECMO Registry of the Extracorporeal Life Support Organization, Ann Arbor, MI, July, 1995.
525. Anderson HL, Snedecor SM, Otsu T, Bartlett RH. Multicenter comparison of conventional venoarterial access versus venovenous double-lumen catheter access in newborn infants undergoing extracorporeal membrane oxygenation. J Pediatr Surg 1993;28:530.
526. Van Mears KP, Nguyen HT, Rhine WP, Marks MP, Fleisher BE, Benitz WE. Intracranial abnormalities and neurodevelopmental status after venovenous extracorporeal membrane oxygenation. J Pediatr 1994; 125:304.
527. VanMeurs KP, Newman KD, Anderson KD, et al. Effect of extracorporeal membrane oxygenation on survival of infants with congenital diaphragmatic hernia. J Pediatr 1990;117:954.
528. Finer NN, Etches PC, Kanstra B, Tierney AT, Pliowski A, Ryan CA. Inhaled nitric oxide in infants referred for extracorporeal membrane oxygenation dose response. J Pediatr 1994;124:302.
529. Kinsella JP, Abman SH: Efficacy of inhalational nitric oxide therapy in the clinical management of persistent pulmonary hypertension of the newborn. Chest 1994;105:92S.
530. Krummel TM, Greenfield LJ, Kirkpatrick BV, et al. Alveolar-arterial oxygen gradients versus the neonatal pulmonary insufficiency index for prediction of mortality in ECMO candidates. J Pediatr Surg 1984;19:380.
531. Beck R, Anderson RK, Pearson GD, et al. Criteria for extracorporeal membrane oxygenation in a population of infants with persistent pulmonary hypertension of the newborn. J Pediatr Surg 1986;21:297.
532. Bartlett RH, Roloff DW, Cornell RG, et al. Extracorporeal circulation in neonatal respiratory failure: a prospective randomized study. Pediatrics 1985;76:479.
533. O'Rourke PP, Crone R, Vacanti J, et al. Extracorporeal membrane oxygenation and conventional medical therapy in neonates with persistent pulmonary hypertension of the newborn: a prospective randomized study. Pediatrics 1989;84:957.
534. Krummel TM, Greenfield LJ, Kirkpatrick BV, Mueller PG, et al. The early evaluation of survivors after extracorporeal membrane oxygenation for neonatal pulmonary failure. J Pediatr Surg 1984;19:585.
535. Towne BH, Lott IT, Hicks DA, et al. Long-term follow-up of infants and children treated with extracorporeal membrane oxygenation (ECMO): a preliminary report. J Pediatr Surg 1985;20:410.
536. Glass P, Miller M, Short B. Morbidity for survivors of extracorporeal membrane oxygenation: neurodevelopmental outcome at 1 year of age. Pediatrics 1989;83:72.
537. Adolph V, Ekelund C, Smith C, et al. Developmental outcome of neonates treated with extracorporeal membrane oxygenation. J Pediatr Surg 1990;25:43.
538. Ballard RA, Leonard CH. Developmental follow-up of infants with persistent pulmonary hypertension of the newborn. Clin Perinatol 1984;11:737.
539. Leavitt AM, Watchko JF, Bennett FC, et al. Neurodevelopmental outcome following persistent pulmonary hypertension of the neonate. J Perinatol 1987;7:288.
540. Bifano EM, Pfannenstiel H. Duration of hyperventilation and outcome in infants with persistent pulmonary hypertension. Pediatrics 1988;81:657.
541. Robinson T, Kickler T, Walker LK, Ness P, Bell W. Effect of extracorporeal membrane oxygenation on platelets in newborns. Crit Care Med 1993;21:1029.
542. Kolobow T, Gattinoni L, Tomlinson T, et al. An alternative to breathing. J Thorac Cardiovasc Surg 1978;75:261.
543. Kolobow T, Pesenti A, Solca ME, et al. A new approach to the prevention and treatment of acute pulmonary insufficiency. Int J Artif Organs 1980;3:86.
544. Gattinoni L, Pesenti A, Mascheroni D, et al. Low-frequency positive-pressure ventilation with extracorporeal CO2 removal in severe acute respiratory failure. JAMA 1986;256:881.
545. Knoch M. Treatment of severe ARDS with extracorporeal CO2 removal. In: Gille JP, ed. Neonatal and adult respiratory failure: mechanisms and treatment. Paris: Elsevier, 1989:123.
546. NHLBI-NIH. Extracorporeal support for respiratory insufficiency (DHEW Publication). Bethesda, Maryland: Department of Health, Education and Welfare, 1980.
547. Kolobow T, Solca M, Gattinoni L, et al. Adult respiratory distress syndrome (ARDS): why did ECMO fail? Int J Artif Organs 1981;2:58.
548. Hickling KG. Extracorporeal CO2 removal in severe adult respiratory distress syndrome. Anaesth Intensive Care 1986;14:46.
549. Kolobow T, Spragg R, Pierce J. Massive pulmonary infarction during total cardiopulmonary bypass in unanaesthetized spontaneously breathing lambs. J Artif Organs 1981;42:76.
550. Gattinoni L, Kolobow T, Agostoni A, et al. Clinical application of low-frequency positive-pressure ventilation with extracorporeal CO2 removal (LFPPV-ECCO2R) in the treatment of adult respiratory distress syndrome (ARDS). Int J Artif Organs 1979;2:282.
551. Bindslev L. Extracorporeal circulation using surface heparinized equipment. In: Gille JP, ed. Neonatal and adult respiratory failure: mechanisms and treatment. Paris: Elsevier, 1989:97.
552. The Adult ECMO Registry of the extracorporeal life support organization, Ann Arbor MI, July 1995.
553. Morris AH, Wallace CJ, Menlove AL, et al. Randomized clinical trial of pressure controlled inverse ratio ventilation and extracorporeal CO2 removal for adult respiratory distress syndrome. Am J Respir Crit Care Med 1994;149:295.
554. Morris AH, Menlove RL, Rollins RJ, et al. A controlled clinical trial of a new 3-step therapy that includes extracorporeal CO2 removal for ARDS. ASAIO Trans 1988;34:48.
555. Sittig DF, Gardner RM, Morris AH. Clinical evaluation of computer-based respiratory care algorithms. Int J Clin Monit Comput 1977;7:177.
556. O'Rourke PP, Stolar CJ, Zwischenberger JB, Snedecor SM, Bartlett RH. Extracorporeal membrane oxygenation: support for overwhelming pulmonary failure in the pediatric population. Collective experience from the extracorporeal life support organization. J Pediatr Surg 1993;28:523.
557. Moler FW, Custer JR, Bartlett RH, et al. Extracorporeal life support for severe pediatric respiratory failure: an updated experience 1991-1993, J Pediatr 1994;124:875.
558. Moler FW, Palmisano JM, Caster JR, Meliones JN, Bartlett RH. Alveolar-arterial oxygen gradients before extracorporeal life support for severe pediatric respiratory failure: improved outcome for extracorporeal life support-managed patients? Crit Care Med 1994;22:620.
559. Tambarro RF, Bugnitz MC, Stidham GL. Alveolar-arterial oxygen gradient as a predictor of outcome in patients with non-neonatal pediatric respiratory failure. J Pediatr 1991;119:935.
560. Moler FW, Palmisano J, Custer JR. Extracorporeal life support for pediatric respiratory failure: predictors of survival from 220 patients. Crit Care Med 1993;21:1604.
561. Green TP, Moler FW, Goodman DM. Probability of survival after prolonged extracorporeal membrane oxygenation in pediatric patients with acute respiratory failure. Extracorporeal life support organization. Crit Care Med 1995;23:1132.
562. Short BL, Pearson GD. Neonatal extracorporeal membrane oxygenation: a review. J Intensive Care Med 1986;1:47.
563. Lotze A, Whitsett JA, Kammerman LA, et al. Surfactant protein A concentrations in tracheal aspirate fluid from infants requiring extracorporeal membrane oxygenation. J Pediatr 1990;116:435.
564. Lotze A, Knight GR, Martin GR, et al. Improved pulmonary outcome after exogenous surfactant therapy for respiratory failure in infants requiring extracorporeal membrane oxygenation. J Pediatr 1993;122:261.
565. Keszler M, Subramanian KNS, Smith YA, et al. Pulmonary management during extracorporeal membrane oxygenation. Crit Care Med 1989;17:495.
566. Keszler M, Ryckman FC, McDonald JV, et al. A prospective, multicenter, randomized study of high versus low positive end-expiratory pressure during extracorporeal membrane oxygenation. J Pediatr 1992;120:107.
567. Petty TL. IMV vs IMC. Chest 1975;67:630.

Respiratory Monitoring

10

Jon N. Meliones
Barbara G. Wilson
Ira M. Cheifetz
William R. Hayden
Robert S. Greenberg

INTRODUCTION

Methods for monitoring the respiratory system have rapidly progressed from an early reliance on physical assessment and direct observation to continuous electronic surveillance of a myriad of physiologic parameters. The role of the clinician is also changing to incorporate all facets of respiratory monitoring into a comprehensive, responsive assessment system. Physical examination continues to have great clinical relevance and is often the deciding factor between monitor error and true change in patient status. The role of the physical examination should not be diminished. However, noninvasive techniques to assess gas exchange and pulmonary mechanics supplement physical assessment and provide a continuous data stream, with alarms, to identify changes in patient status and alert caregivers. Appropriate integration and interpretation of all data is essential for efficient, high-quality, cost-effective, pediatric critical care. This chapter addresses the continuum of respiratory monitoring that encompasses physical assessment, continuous noninvasive monitors, and intermittent laboratory assessment. Clinical indications, principles of operation, and functional limitations are discussed.

GUIDELINES AND PRINCIPLES

Tobin[1] has proposed several purposes for monitoring (derived from the Latin word "to warn"): (a) to measure continuously or intermittently key physiologic indices that aid diagnosis and guide management, (b) to provide alarms that notify the caretakers that important changes have occurred in the patient's condition, and (c) to create and evaluate trends that might help the assessment of treatment and prognosis.

When monitoring systems are being selected or developed, several factors become important **(Table 10.1)**[1]. The monitor or monitoring system must be pertinent to patient management and give answers to questions that will guide patient management. The data must be interpretable by the people caring for the patient. The data must be accurate, and the technology must be sensitive enough to detect absolute values and changes in the parameters being measured. The data must be valid and reproducible. The technology must also be practical to use, easy to attach to the patient, function dependably, and occupy as little space as possible. Patient safety should always be the primary goal in the selection of any monitoring system.

Currently, the greatest monitoring question is: What should be monitored? Technology enables us to monitor multiple parameters at various intervals. Just because we can monitor these parameters does not mean we should do so in all patients. Again, the clinician must address what is practical and clinically relevant to the management of each patient, given the pathophysiology and the clinical scenario. Physical assessment and observation should be interposed to assess factors that cannot be electronically monitored. Since the respiratory system provides a means for the body to remove carbon dioxide and transport oxygen to the blood, the technology discussion revolves around monitoring systems that quantify and evaluate these two functions.

The Society of Critical Care Medicine has provided guidelines for the management of patients requiring respiratory support. These guidelines are reproduced in Appendix 10.1.

PHYSICAL EXAMINATION

It is a curious phenomenon of modern intensive care, even to the casual observer, that the basic principles of physical examination are being used with decreasing frequency. Many times the patient is not touched, and the use of the stethoscope is decreasing. It is therefore valuable to review data that support the continued use of physical examination techniques for the evaluation and monitoring of the critically ill.

Table 10.2 presents physical examination findings that give important information regarding the status of a patient's respiratory system. Clinical scoring systems have been developed to evaluate the clinical parameters of skin color, nasal flaring, retractions, accessory muscle use, and the presence and severity of an abnormal sound (wheeze or stridor). Scoring systems generally demonstrate that the more pronounced the abnormality, the worse the prognosis. In one scoring system, to predict criteria for extubation, Pardee et al.[2] studied adults who were breathing spontaneously with an artificial airway just before extubation. A respiratory rate greater than 33/min, heart rate less than 70 or greater than 120 beats/min, palpable recruitment of scalene or expiratory abdominal musculature, and the presence of irregular respiration with apnea predicted failure of extubation and death[2]. If such signs were not present, 90% of the patients remained off the ventilator, and if three or four signs were present, all of the patients required reintubation and 57% later died. These signs were at least as good as and, in many cases, better than measurements of vital capacity, tidal volume, minute volume, maximum inspiratory and expiratory pressures, and tidal volume/vital capacity ratios in predicting successful extubation.

Table 10.1. Criteria of an Ideal Monitoring System[a]

Pertinent to patient management
Interpretable data
High technical accuracy
High sensitivity
Good reproduction
Practical to use
Low risk to the patient
Inexpensive

[a] From Tobin M. Respiratory monitoring in the intensive care unit. Am Rev Respir Dis 1988;138:1625–1642.

Table 10.2. Physical Examination Findings Pertinent to the Examination of the Respiratory System

Observation
Respiratory rate and pattern
Color
Nasal flaring
Retractions
Accessory muscle use
Palpation
Accessory muscle (scalene, abdominal) use
Auscultation
Wheeze
Stridor
Air entry
Crackles (rales)

The phenomenon of noncontinuous advential auscultatory sounds (crackles or rales), first reported by Lae nnec in the 19th century, may have some pathophysiologic correlation also. Siegal et al.[3] found that 10 of 11 adult patients with congestive heart failure and crackles had a reduced capacity for diffusion of carbon monoxide (D_{CO}). Two of 23 with congestive heart failure without crackles had a normal D_{CO}. Clausen[4] commented that the crackles seemed to correlate also with the severity of the decreased total lung capacity (TLC) and believed that this was consistent with a hypothesis that reductions in TLC and vital capacity (VC) related better to lung water quantity than to abnormalities in left ventricular systolic function of the heart. Crackles probably relate to total lung water, which in turn is proportional to mortality in critically ill patients [5].

CONTINUOUS MONITORING

Respiratory Rate and Pattern

Respiratory rate was one of the earliest parameters monitored in the intensive care unit. Although there are several techniques for measuring respiratory movements, impedance pneumography is the method used in most spontaneously breathing patients. This method requires placement of at least three leads over the chest: one over the heart and one each on the opposite sides of the lower lateral thorax. A small current is passed through one pair of electrodes, and the amount of current that passes through the chest is measured by the other electrode pair. The impedance to current flow varies with the fluid content of the chest, which in turn varies with the respiratory cycle, and these differences can be converted by a microprocessor into a waveform that is displayed[6]. Like many other physiologic parameters, respiratory rate and pattern varies **(Table 10.3)**, and each child should be evaluated with reference to the age-adjusted norms and pathophysiologic state.

The discussion of respiratory pattern has generated a great deal of debate in the pediatric literature in the past 10 years, particularly in the definition of respiratory pauses, periodic breathing, and apnea. In general, respiratory pauses occur in children younger than 3 months of age and are of less than 15 seconds duration. Pauses occur in groups of three or more, are separated by less than 20 seconds, and are resolved by 6 months of age(7).

The definition of apnea is even more troublesome because of the role of sudden infant death syndrome in infant mortality, its relation to apnea, and the huge effort under way to prevent this tragic occurrence. A National Institutes of Health Conference consensus statement on infantile apnea defined apnea as cessation of breathing for longer than 20 seconds or any respiratory pause associated with bradycardia, pallor, or cyanosis(8).

Pulse Oximetry

One of the most important advances in the 1980s was the development of pulse oximetry to noninvasively measure percent oxygen saturation of hemoglobin. As a technology, it is relatively inexpensive, safe, accurate, and portable compared with alternative methods.

Pulse oximetry technology has existed since the 1930s. The hardware at that time was bulky, and the tissue bed being tested required heating. The technique did not become widely available until the early to mid-1980s, when several microprocessor developments allowed application in a variety of clinical settings. Advances included light-emitting diodes, microprocessor technology, plethysmography, and spectrophotometry.

A discussion of the physics of pulse oximetry should begin with the Beer-Lambert law, which states that the concentration of an unknown solute in a solvent can be determined by light absorption, or

$$L\ (\text{out}) = L\ (\text{in}) - (DCa) \qquad (\text{Eq. } 10.1)$$

where L is the intensity of light, D is the distance the light travels through a solution, C is the concentration of the solute, and a is the absorption coefficient of the solute (Fig. 10.1).

Table 10.3. Respiratory Rate as a Function of Age[a]

Age (year)	*Mean breaths/min*	*±SD*
2	25	17–33
4	23	18–28
6	21	17–27
8	20	15–26
10	18	15–25
12	18	14–26
14	17	15–23
16	17	12–22

[a] From Iliff A, Lee V. Pulse rate, respiratory rate and body temperature in children between two months and eighteen years of age. Child Dev 1952;23:237.

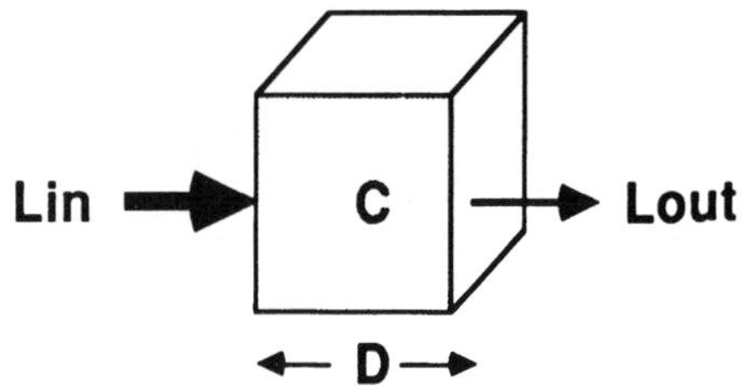

Figure 10.1. Beer-Lambert law. (From Schnapp L, Cohen N. Pulse oximetry: uses and abuses. Chest 1990;98:1244.)

Since we are interested in whether or not oxygen is attached to hemoglobin, the relevant solutes are reduced hemoglobin and oxyhemoglobin and their respective absorption characteristics. Wavelengths of 660 nm (red) and 940 nm (infrared) are used because the absorption characteristics of the two hemoglobins are so different at these two wavelengths (Fig. 10.2).

Beer's spectrophotometric principles are applied through the medium of the light-emitting diode and optical plethysmography. A miniaturized light source is applied to an area of the body that is narrow enough to allow light to traverse a pulsating capillary bed and be sensed by a photo detector (optical plethysmography). Recommended sites include the ear lobe, finger, and toe in adults; the palm in infants; and the arch of the foot in newborns (Fig. 10.3). The nasal septum may be used in low-flow states as the anterior ethmoidal artery flow is maintained(9).

Each heartbeat physiologically produces arterial (oxygen saturated) blood; the increase in oxygen saturation of the hemoglobin results in increased absorption of light. A microprocessor programmed with empirically derived data calculates the amounts of oxyhemoglobin and reduced hemoglobin, and hence the oxygen saturation, by comparing

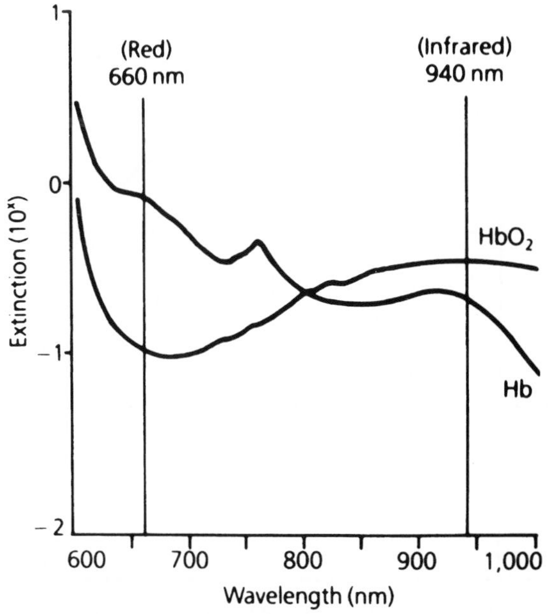

Figure 10.2. Absorption spectrum of reduced hemoglobin (Hb) and oxyhemoglobin (HbO_2). (From McGough EK, Boysen PG. Benefits and limitations of pulse oximetry in the ICU. J Crit Illness 1989;4:23.)

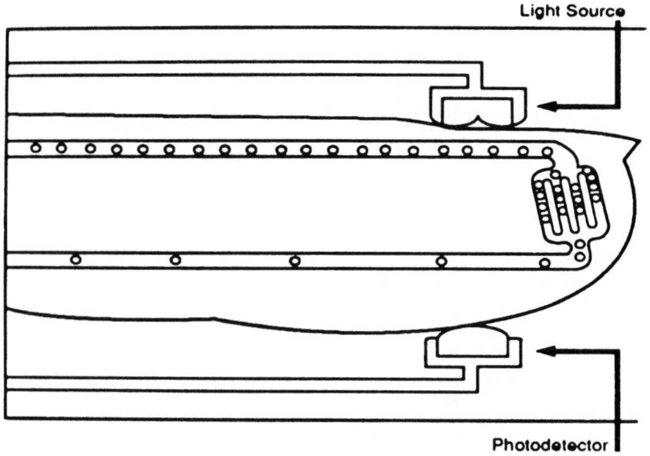

Figure 10.3. Pulse oximetry probe placed across vascular bed of digit. (From Nellcor Incorporated. Principles of pulse oximetry. Hayward, California: Nellcor Incorporated, 1988.)

absorbencies at baseline (BA) and during the peak (PA) of a transmitted pulse at 660 nm (red) and 940 nm (infrared):

$$\text{Red absorbance (R)/infrared absorbance (IR)} = (PA_{660}/BA_{660})/(PA_{940}/BA_{940}) \quad \text{(Eq. 10.2)}$$

The oximetry-determined plethysmographic signal amplitudes at various saturations and the algorithm used by the microprocessor to determine the S_pO_2 by the R/IR ratio are shown in Figures 10.4 and 10.5. By using the two wavelengths of light, the pulse oximeter determines "functional saturation," which is the ratio of oxyhemoglobin to the sum of all functional hemoglobins, i.e., hemoglobin capable of carrying oxygen:

$$\text{Functional } S_pO_2 = HbO_2/(HbO_2 + Hb) \quad \text{(Eq. 10.3)}$$

where HbO_2 is oxygenated hemoglobin and Hb is nonoxygenated hemoglobin. Functional S_pO_2 is contrasted with the fractional S_pO_2 measured by co-oximetry on most blood gas machines, which gives the ratio of oxygenated hemoglobin to the sum of all other hemoglobin types, including carboxyhemoglobin (HbCO) and methemoglobin (Hbmet), which do not carry oxygen:

$$\text{Fractional } S_pO_2 = HbO_2/(HbO_2 + Hb + HbCO + Hbmet) \quad \text{(Eq. 10.4)}$$

The disadvantage of the determination of functional saturation is that other, possibly clinically relevant hemoglobin species such as carboxyhemoglobin and methemoglobin will be missed. This shortcoming can be overcome in ambiguous clinical situations by using periodic co-oximetry for analysis of an arterial blood gas specimen that uses four to six wavelengths to determine the fractional saturation.

It has been demonstrated conclusively that oxygen saturation of normal hemoglobin determined by the pulse oximeter correlates very closely with the oxygen saturation determined by the co-oximeter (correlation coefficient of 0.98) when the saturation is between 70 and 100% in the well-perfused normothermic person[10].

There are only limited data on humans and animals when the saturations are less than 70%, but Severinghaus and Naifeh[11] showed that correlation was good, although there was significant lag time between the central saturation and peripheral sites.

Several clinical studies demonstrate that a fall in S_pO_2 most often precedes any change in other vital signs. Hensley et al.[12] studied 20 patients who were having central line placement prior to major surgery. They had been pre-

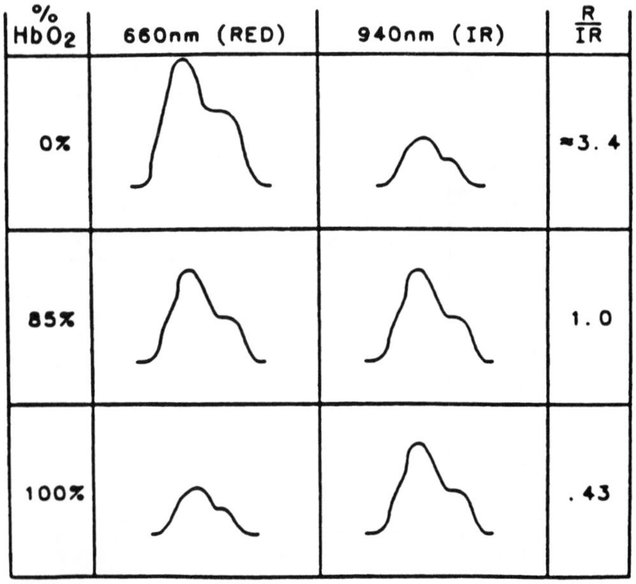

Figure 10.4. Relative plethysmographic (pulse-added) signal amplitudes, assuming the transmission intensities are similar. (From Eisenkraft J. Pulse oximetry desaturation due to methemoglobinemia. Anesthesiology 1988;68:280.)

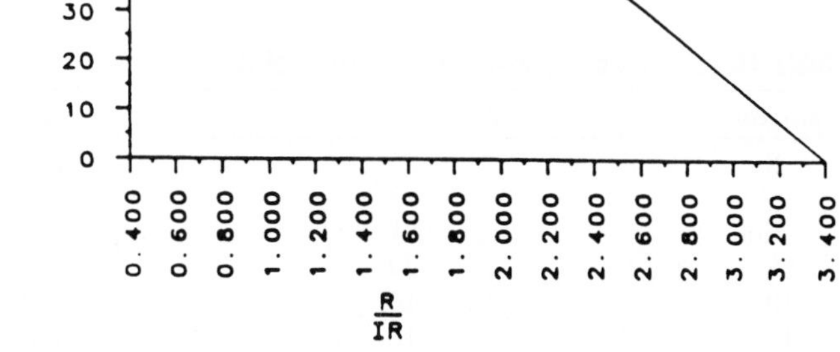

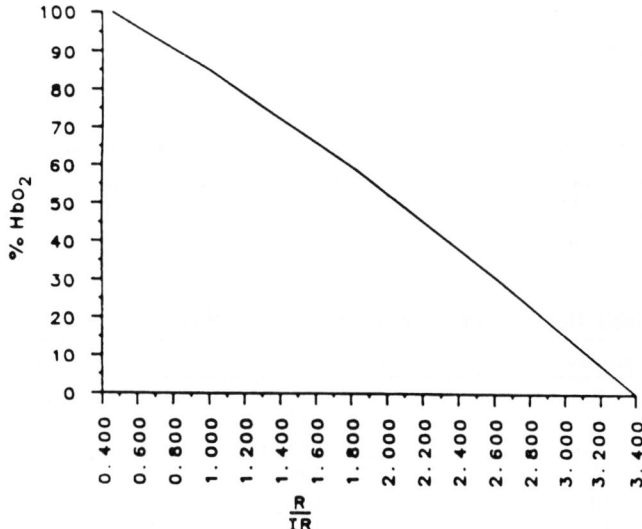

Figure 10.5. Algorithm relating $\%HbO_2$ as *ordinate* to the ratio of the plethysmographic signal amplitudes and R/IR (or 660/940 nm) as *abscissa.* (From Eisenkraft J. Pulse oximetry desaturation due to methemoglobinemia. Anesthesiology 1988;68:280.)

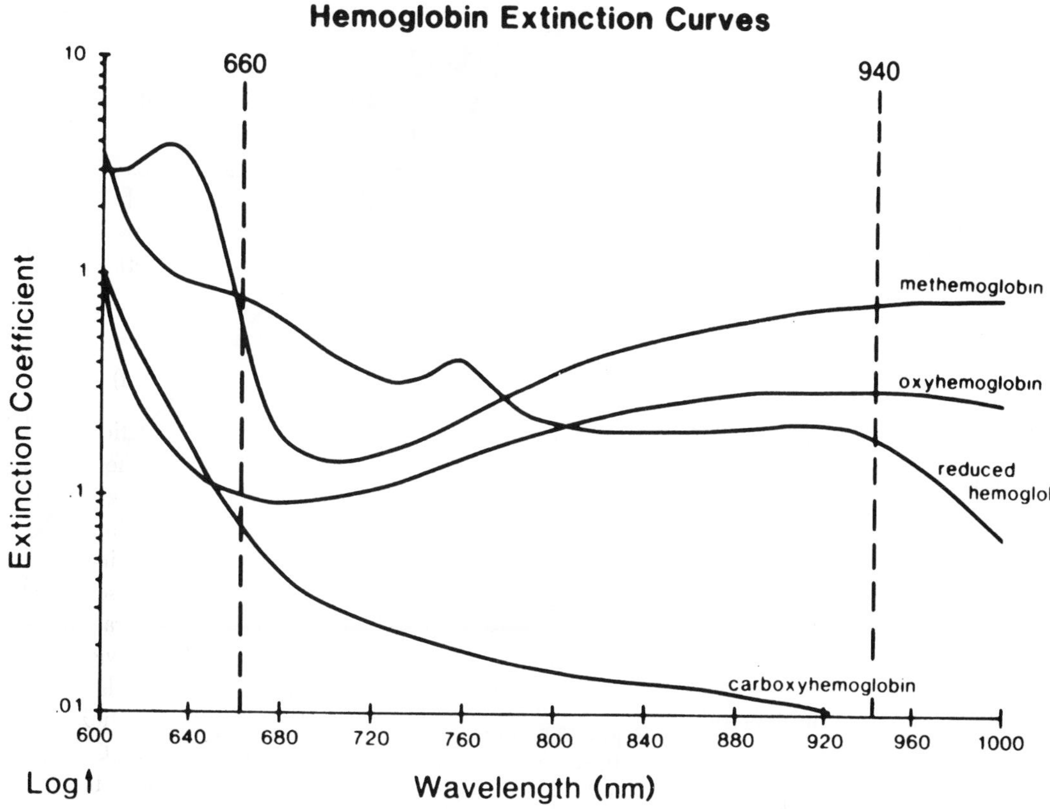

Figure 10.6. Extinction coefficient versus wavelength for the four hemoglobin species: reduced Hb, HbO_2, Hbmet, HbCO. Pulse oximeters use the two wavelengths 660 nm and 940 nm. (From Schnapp L, Cohen N. Pulse oximetry: uses and abuses. Chest 1990; 98:1247.)

medicated, usually with morphine. In 12 of the 20, S_pO_2 dropped to less than 90%, and the likelihood of a drop was related to drugs, Trendelenburg positioning, obesity, smoking, and congestive heart failure. They concluded that patients at risk might have low oxygen saturations not detectable by other means. Careful monitoring and use of oxygen were indicated. However, Cooper et al.[13] demonstrated that the universal use of pulse oximeters in the operating and recovery rooms decreased the frequency of undesirable events (hypotension, hypovolemia, dysrhythmias) without a change in mortality.

Many medical procedures, transfers, and high-risk conditions place patients at risk for oxygen desaturation. These events can be detected early via pulse oximetry, the intervention accomplished, and the morbidity prevented. Tyler et al.[14] discovered that 35% of patients transferred from the operating room to the recovery room had an S_pO_2 less than 90%, and 12% of patients had an S_pO_2 less than 85% when pulse oximetry was used in 95 patients.

Limitations of Pulse Oximetry

Pulse oximetry has several limitations, most of which are predictable and understandable, given the basic physics of oximetry **(Table 10.4):**

Dyshemoglobinemias: The term *dyshemoglobinemia* refers to abnormal species of hemoglobin that result in reduced ability of the hemoglobin molecule to carry oxygen to the tissues because of combination with substances other than oxygen (e.g., carbon monoxide) or molecular alterations that do not allow oxygen to combine with the hemoglobin molecule in a stoichiometrically efficient manner (e.g., methemoglobin and fetal hemoglobin). Figure 10.6 shows the absorption spectra for the dyshemoglobins; note that carboxyhemoglobin and oxyhemoglobin have very similar absorbencies at 660 nm. Carboxyhemoglobin will be interpreted as oxyhemoglobin by the photo detector of the two-light-source pulse oximeter. Thus functional S_pO_2 overestimates the true $\%HbO_2$, but fractional S_pO_2 falls dramatically. A study by Barker and Tremper[15] in dogs (Fig. 10.7) clearly demonstrated that functional S_pO_2 remained elevated in spite of a linear drop in $\%HbO_2$ as the HbCO increased (a fall in fractional S_pO_2). These data and the clinical experience of others make it imperative that co-oximetry be used to determine O_2 saturation in the presence of carboxyhemoglobin, i.e., carbon monoxide poison-

Table 10.4. Factors Contributing to Potential Inaccuracy of Pulse Oximetry[a]

Dyshemoglobinemias
Carbon monoxide
Methemoglobinemia
Fetal hemoglobin
Dyes and pigments
Methylene blue
Indocyanine green
Low perfusion
Increased venous pulsations
Optical interference from external light sources and optical shunt

[a] *From Schnapp L. Pulse oximetry. Chest 1990;98:1244–1250.*

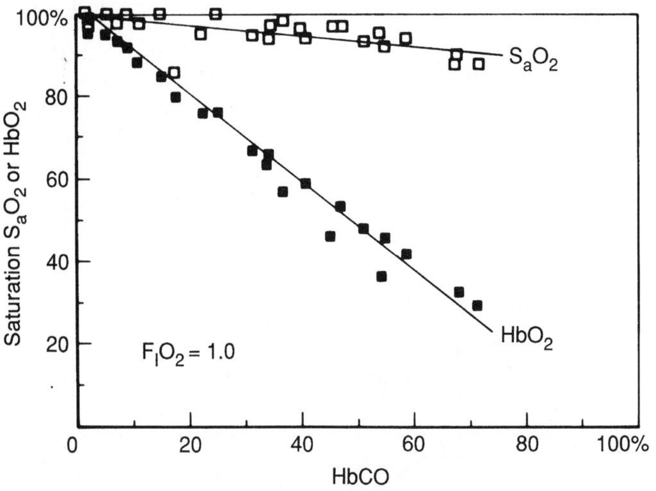

Figure 10.7. S_aO_2 and HbO_2 versus carboxyhemoglobin (HbCO) at F_IO_2 equal to 1.0. S_aO_2 consistently overestimates saturation in the presence of HbCO. At HbCO equal to 70%, S_aO_2 is still roughly 90%, while HbO_2 has fallen to 30%. (From Barker S, Tremper K. The effect of carbon monoxide inhalation on pulse oximetry and transcutaneous PO_2. Anesthesiology 1987;66:678.)

ing, such as smoke inhalation and coma of uncertain cause[16].

Methemoglobin: Eisencraft[17] reported a patient with S_pO_2 of 85–92% with a P_aO_2 of 587 mm Hg. Co-oximetry revealed that the methemoglobin level was 5%. Barker et al.[18] studied a group of dogs with lidocaine-induced methemoglobinemia and showed conclusively that as the methemoglobin level increased to approximately 40%, the S_pO_2 decreased to and plateaued at 85% as the methemoglobin continued to rise (Fig. 10.8). As can be seen in Figure 10.6, this phenomenon is explained by the absorption characteristics of methemoglobin. Methemoglobin absorbs light significantly at both the 660-nm and the 940-nm wavelengths, thereby confusing the oximeter photo detector into believing that both oxyhemoglobin and reduced hemoglobin are increased. This results in increases in both the denominator and numerator of Equation 10.2. The microprocessor-driven algorithm results in the R/IR approaching unity and a S_pO_2 near 85% on the calibration curve (Fig. 10.5).

Dyes and pigments: Methylene blue has maximum absorbance at 668 nm (Fig. 10.9). The oximeter interprets this extra absorbance as reduced hemoglobin and, therefore, a lower S_pO_2. This results in the clinical phenomenon of a sudden (within 30 seconds) drop in saturation when methylene blue is injected for therapeutic or diagnostic purposes, such as testing urinary tract patency[19]. Scheller et al.[20] demonstrated that the S_pO_2 could drop to less than 10% within 30 seconds of an intravenous dose of methylene blue and remain reduced for as long as 2 minutes. Indocyanine green dye used for cardiac output determination can reduce the S_pO_2 mildly (93%) as early as 30 seconds after the injection[20]. The effect may last for a minute or so. Hyperbilirubinemia did not interfere with hemoglobin saturation measured by pulse oximetry when studied in adults with bilirubin levels up to 84.3 mg/dl[21].

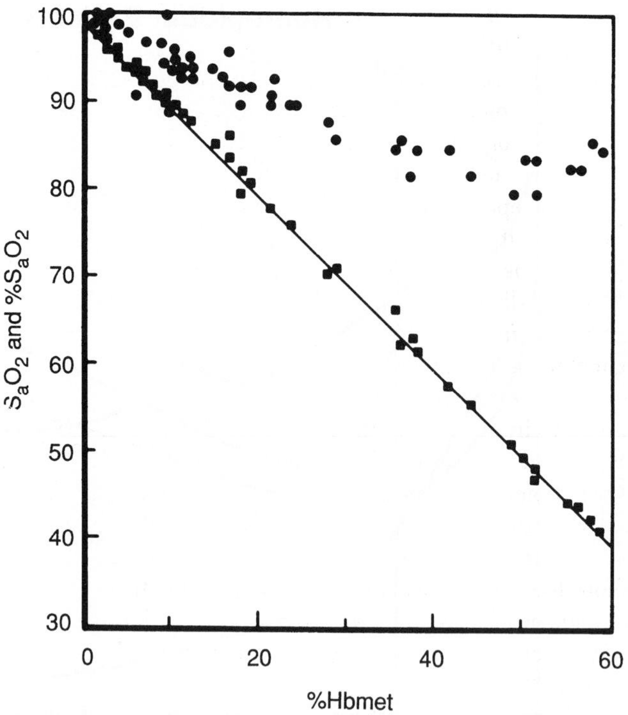

Figure 10.8. Nellcor S_aO_2 and co-oximetry-determined S_aO_2 versus %Hbmet for F_IO_2 equal to 1.0. (From Barker S, Tremper K, Hyatt J. Effects of methemoglobinemia on pulse oximetry and mixed venous oximetry. Anesthesiology 1989;70:113.)

Low perfusion: Since pulse oximetry depends on optical plethysmography, i.e., a pulsatile change in arterial blood, abnormalities in propagation of the pulse to the extremities result in inaccuracy of the pulse oximeter. Shock states, vasopressors, severe edema, and peripheral vascular disease make it difficult for the sensor to distinguish the true signal from background. Placing the sensor on the nasal septum may be of benefit in these low-flow states. Others have recommended warming the extremity and using local vasodilators[22]. Newer models of oximeters have modes that heighten the sensitivity of the probe in low-perfusion states, or link the oximeter to the ECG monitor to improve the cor-

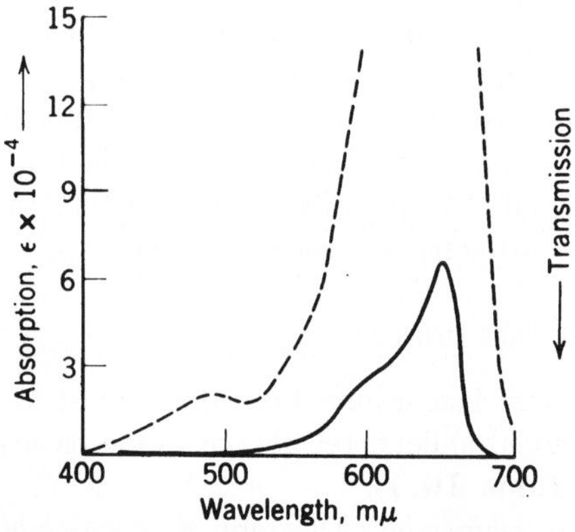

Figure 10.9. Absorption curve of methylene blue dye solution, reflecting maximal absorption at 668 nm at both concentrated *(dashed line)* and dilute *(solid line)* solutions. (From Kessler M, Eide T, Humayun B, Poppers P. Spurious pulse oximeter desaturation with methylene blue injection. Anesthesiology 1986;65:436.)

relation of pulse signals. Each of these methods is helpful for this condition.

Increased venous pulsations: Theoretically, increased venous pulsations could result in errors, since the pulsation would be confused with the arterial pulsations and the amount of unoxygenated hemoglobin overestimated[22]. Mark[23] reported two adults with prominent systolic v-waves in the central venous pressure waveform who had an erroneous S_pO_2 reading from ear oximetry devices and a normal reading from finger probes.

Optical interference and optical shunt: Because pulse oximeters use optical devices, their performance may be affected by external light sources[24]. Light from surgical lamps, bilirubin lamps, fluorescent lights, infrared heating lamps, and direct sunlight can result in inaccurate but apparently normal values. As an example, Hanowell[25] reported an instance in which a pulse oximeter displayed normal values when exposed to bright fluorescent lights alone, before the sensor was applied to the patient. It is therefore recommended that the sensors be covered with opaque material when these light sources might affect oximeter performance[26].

Another source of optical interference is light from the sensor's own light source reaching the sensor without passing through a pulsatile arteriolar bed to the optical shunt ("cross-talk"). This light prevents the oximeter from tracking the pulse and can result in inaccurate measurements. Optical shunting usually occurs as a result of improper positioning of the sensor, incorrect size of the sensor, excessive reuse of disposable sensors, or use of additional tape or a finger cot to secure the sensor after its own adhesive was exhausted[27].

Motion artifact: Excessive motion of the photosensor causes intermittent contact with the skin and mechanically modulates the path length of the transmitted light as well as the amplitude and intensity of the received light. This variance in light transmission and reception through the monitoring site can produce false arterial pulse waveforms that the oximeter may not be able to differentiate from the true arterial waveforms, producing spurious saturation values. Clinicians should verify pulse rate accuracy in the assessment of pulse oximetry values to avoid misinterpretation in the face of motion artifact.

It is important to remember that pulse oximetry in critical care is most beneficial as a continuous monitor. Spot checks provide only intermittent assessment and do not offer the benefits of alarms or trending. Telemetry systems are available that permit continuous centralized monitoring. Computer interfaces allow monitoring and trending of several patients at once with central and local alarms. Pulse oximeter values should be periodically checked against laboratory measurement to assure correlation. These monitors however, can significantly decrease arterial blood gas analysis and facilitate rapid weaning of FiO_2.

Maintenance should follow the manufacturer's recommendations. Clinically, probe sites should be changed every 12 hours to prevent pressure damage to digits. Perfusion distal to the probe attachment should be evaluated to ensure that circulation is not affected. Permanent probes are less expensive, after the initial investment, than disposable probes and lower the cost of providing this technology. Between use on different patients, monitors and probes should be wiped with disinfectant as recommended by the manufacturer.

Transcutaneous Blood Gas Determination

In the late 1970s and early 1980s, professionals in neonatal critical care were highly enthusiastic about transcutaneous blood gas determination ($PTcO_2$ and $PTcCO_2$) using miniaturized Clark PO_2 and Severinghaus PCO_2 electrodes to detect the corresponding values through the skin. In this procedure, the skin is warmed to 41°C to 44°C to facilitate hyperperfusion and allow diffusion of gases through the dermal and epidermal skin layers. Monitors estimate partial pressure of O_2 and CO_2 electrochemically. Electrodes are attached to the skin by adhesive patches to well-perfused, non-bony surfaces. The abdomen, inner thigh, lower back, and chest are desirable sites in neonates; the chest, abdomen, and lower back for larger children and adults[28]. Perhaps the greatest benefit of this technology is continuous monitoring and trending that reduce the frequency of blood gas measurement and hence blood transfusions in small infants.

Transcutaneous monitoring has been limited by the need for frequent calibration of electrodes, cost of supplies, occasional burns induced by the warming component, inaccuracy when the skin is not well perfused, reported inaccuracies in older patients, and the development of pulse oximeter technology. In pediatric patients, the correlation of results with measured blood gas values have been mixed, with transcutaneous monitoring of CO_2 being more accurate than transcutaneous oxygen[29,30]. Skin and capillary bed thickness may play a part in the lack of correlation with older children and adults as compared with neonates. Several studies demonstrated better oxygen correlation with pulse oximetry[31]. As a result, few pediatric critical care units use this technology routinely. A new direction and more accurate data will be necessary before transcutaneous monitoring grows in the pediatric population[28].

Capnography and End-Tidal CO_2

Capnography is defined as the graphic waveform produced by variations in CO_2 concentration throughout the respiratory cycle as a function of time[32]. The two main techniques of capnography measurement are infrared spectroscopy and mass spectrometry. Infrared (wavelengths greater than 1 μ) spectroscopy requires three components: an infrared light source, a gas chamber, and a detector. Its success depends on the fact that each gas has unique absorption characteristics that can be used to quantify the amount (partial pressure) of a particular gas.

Respiratory gases are sampled either from a sidestream catheter or from a chamber attached in-line at the endotra-

Table 10.5. Uses of Capnography[a]

End-tidal CO_2 ($ETCO_2$) determination
Evaluation of respiratory pattern (rate and rhythm)
Dead space determination
Tissue perfusion and cardiac output determination (cardiopulmonary resuscitation prognosis and evaluation)
Endotracheal tube placement
Mechanical ventilator failures
Patient-ventilator sunchrony

[a] *From Snyder J, Elliot L, Grevnik A. Capnography. In: Spence A, ed. Clinics of critical care medicine. Edinburgh: Churchill Livingstone, 1982:100–121.*

cheal tube adaptor. The sidestream sampler aspirates a volume of gas (50 to 200 ml) continuously from the ventilator circuit or at the nares in spontaneously breathing patients. Its disadvantages include the aspiration of mucous and water condensation into the sampling tubing, which blocks the flow of gas, and excess scavenging of the gas flow, which may decrease minute ventilation in very small children. Slow aspiration rates result in significant time delay, and rapid aspiration rates result in aspiration of fresh gas and artifactual lowering of end-tidal CO_2 ($ETCO_2$). Badgwell et al.[33] did show, however, that children less than 8 kg could be monitored if the catheter was placed at a distal end on the endotracheal tube. However, the inspiratory resistance encountered by placing a catheter in a small endotracheal tube precludes this option in infants and small children.

Mainstream capnographs place a light-emitting source and detector on separate sides of an airway adaptor. This equipment does not aspirate gas, but is occasionally susceptible to secretions and humidity covering the light source or detector. Recent technological advances have reduced the weight of these connectors to 18 grams[34] which decreases traction and tension on the endotracheal tube, as previously reported. Deadspace has been reduced to 1.4 ml in the neonatal sensor and no longer poses a re-breathing problem in infants and small children.

Mass spectrometry may be used to measure inspired and expired CO_2, O_2, N_2, as well as anesthetic gases. An aspirated gas sample is ionized by an electronic beam, and charged fragments are accelerated into a dispersion chamber, where they are separated by mass and charge. Detectors then measure and report the component gases. This technology is expensive and does not lend itself to individual patient use. It has been helpful in operating rooms and some intensive care units where a centralized system is assembled to monitor many patients continuously. Capnography can be used for several purposes, as indicated in **Table 10.5.**

$ETCO_2$ is defined as the peak CO_2 value during the expiratory phase of respiration. It is dependent on adequate pulmonary capillary blood flow of CO_2-rich blood to alveoli, which in turn depends on adequate right and left heart function. The normal $ETCO_2$ in healthy subjects is less than 5 mm Hg different from the P_aCO_2; the clinical conditions associated with alterations in $ETCO_2$ are shown in **Table 10.6.**

Practical uses of $ETCO_2$ monitoring in the pediatric intensive care unit include adequacy of alveolar ventilation during mechanical ventilation, respiratory monitoring of spontaneously breathing children, patient-ventilator system function, and endotracheal tube patency. Many institutions use capnography at intubation for rapid assessment of endotracheal tube placement by confirming by the presence of CO_2 in the expired gases[35].

Evaluation of respiratory pattern: Figure 10.10 demonstrates the phasic changes in CO_2 concentration that occur during the respiratory cycle. Evaluation of the respiratory pattern is aided by noting the near-zero end-inspiratory CO_2 ($EICO_2$) value in the normal capnogram, the plateau at end

Table 10.6. Clinical Conditions Associated with Alterations in $ETCO_2$[a]

Increases in $ETCO_2$	
Sudden	Sudden increase in cardiac output
	Sudden release of a tourniquet
	Injection of sodium bicarbonate
Gradual	Hypoventilation
	Increase in carbon dioxide production
Decreases in $ETCO_2$	
Sudden	Sudden hyperventilation
	Sudden decrease in cardiac output
	Massive pulmonary embolism
	Air embolism
	Disconnection of the ventilator
	Obstruction of the endotracheal tube
	Leakage in the circuit
Gradual	Hyperventilation
	Decrease in oxygen consumption
	Decreased pulmonary perfusion
Absent $ETCO_2$	
	Esophageal intubation

[a] *From Tobin M. Respiratory monitoring. JAMA 1990;264:244–251.*

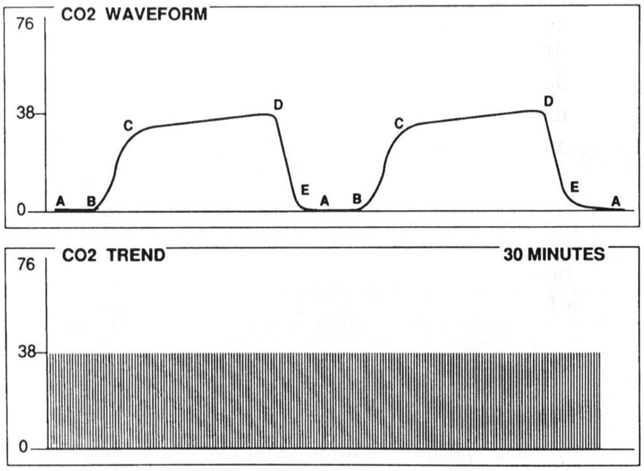

Figure 10.10. Normal capnogram. Exhalation begins at point A. Segment A–B represents tracheal dead space. *Segment B–C* is the early rise in CO_2 concentration as alveolar gas makes its way to the airway. *Segment C–D* is the alveolar plateau. *Point D,* the maximum value in the capnogram, is the end-tidal value of CO_2. Inhalation of CO_2-free gas begins immediately after *point D* and continues to *point E.* The trend display is shown on the *bottom panel.* (From Swedlow D, Irving S. Monitoring and patient safety. In: Blitt C, ed. Monitoring in anesthesia and critical care medicine. New York: Churchill Livingstone, 1990.)

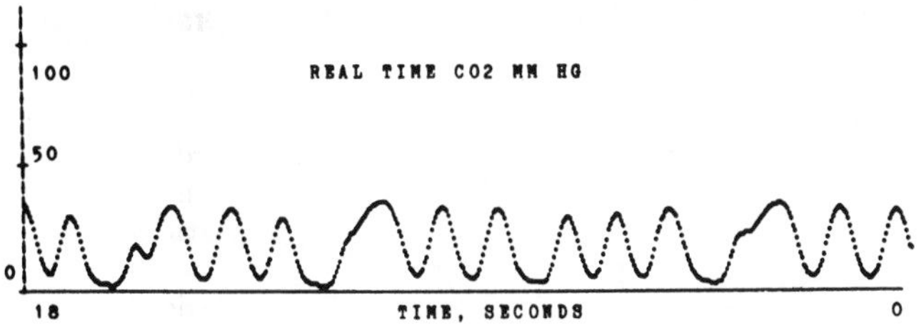

Figure 10.11. Chaotic respiratory pattern in a patient unable to tolerate spontaneous ventilation. (From Carlon G, Ray C, Miodowink S, et al. Capnography in mechanically ventilated patients. Crit Care Med 1988;16:550–556.)

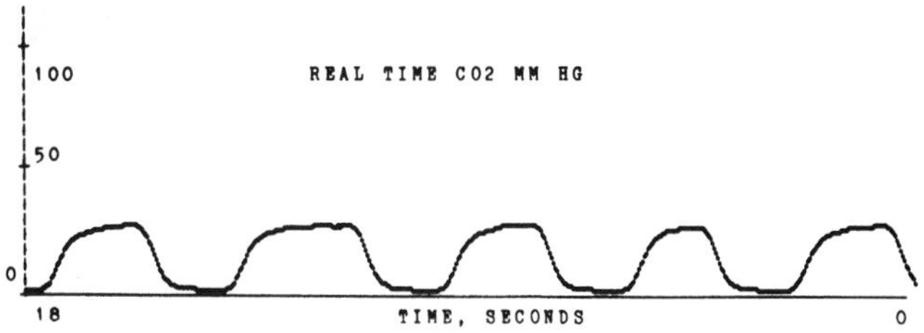

Figure 10.13. Same patient as in Figure 10.12, 15 minutes after addition of 20 cm H_2O pressure support. A normal capnogram and respiratory rate can now be observed. (From Carlon G, Ray C, Miodowink S, et al. Capnography in mechanically ventilated patients. Crit Care Med 1988;16:550–556.)

expiration, and the highest CO_2 recorded ($ETCO_2$). The capnograph converts these phasic values of CO_2 into electrical signals and displays them as respiratory rate, inspiratory CO_2, and $ETCO_2$ either as a waveform and/or digitally. This allows analysis of changes that may take place breath to breath or over longer periods of time.

Capnography can be used to great advantage in mechanically ventilated patients if the waveform is displayed and analyzed along with numeric data. Mechanical failures can be detected, the adequacy of respiratory support can be analyzed, and changes can be made in the mode of ventilation made to maximize the efficiency of ventilation, decrease the patient's work of breathing, and improve patient-ventilator synchrony (Figs. 10.11 to 10.13). Mechanical breaths may be differentiated from spontaneous breathing (Fig. 10.14) at rapid respiratory rates. Mihm et al.[36] applied capnography to the high-frequency jet ventilator and found that the $ETCO_2$ value at the end of one breath of 15 ml/kg interjected into the high-frequency cycle correlated with the P_aCO_2.

Some attention should be given to $EICO_2$ as well as to $ETCO_2$. As noted above, the $EICO_2$ should be near zero. When the $EICO_2$ is greater than zero, the patient is inhaling CO_2-rich gas, usually because previously exhaled gas containing CO_2 is being rebreathed. This may result from spontaneous breathing, in which the fresh gas flow is insufficient to washout CO_2 (Figs. 10.11 and 10.12), inadequate trigger sensitivity to cycle pressure support breaths, or a spontaneous breath occurring during mechanical expiration with the expiratory valve open, thus allowing the patient to inhale CO_2-rich gas (Fig. 10.14). Thus, the tidal CO_2 will not return to baseline, increasing inspired CO_2 above atmospheric CO_2, and therefore pulmonary CO_2 clearance is impaired[37].

Dead Space Determination: Dead space (V_D/V_T) can be determined by a variant of the Bohr equation:

$$V_D/V_T = (P_aCO_2 - ECO_2)/P_aCO_2 \quad \text{(Eq. 10.6A)}$$

or

$$V_D/V_T = 1 - (ECO_2/P_aCO_2) \quad \text{(Eq. 10.6B)}$$

Where ECO_2 = mean expired CO_2

Conditions that cause a significant drop in ECO_2—such as pulmonary embolism, air embolism, or cardiac standstill—increase dead space, impair gas exchange, and alter pulmonary mechanics[38].

Tissue Perfusion and Cardiac Output Determination: Gazmuri et al.[39] studied the dynamics of $ETCO_2$ before, during, and after cardiac arrest in an animal model and demonstrated that there is excellent correlation between $ETCO_2$ and P_aCO_2 when perfusion of the lungs is normal. When the heart stops, however, the relationship is lost (Fig. 10.15).

Gudipati et al.[40] showed that there is a constant relation between $ETCO_2$ and coronary perfusion in experimental animals (Fig. 10.16). The success of resuscitation is proportional to maintaining a coronary perfusion pressure of at least 30 mm Hg during cardiopulmonary resuscitation. Carotid pulse may not be an indicator of adequate resuscitation[41]; $ETCO_2$ monitoring may become important in judging the adequacy of resuscitation. If the $ETCO_2$ does not

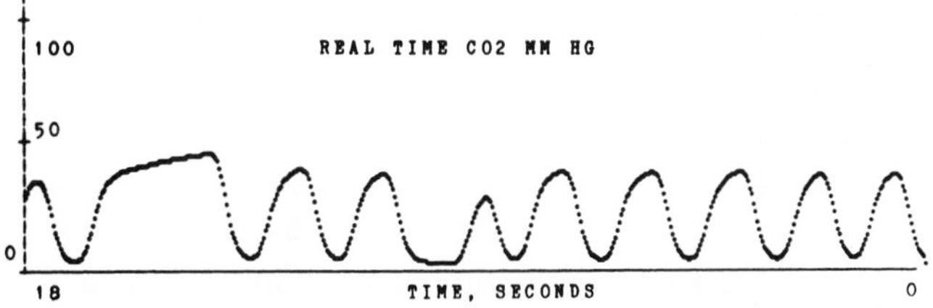

Figure 10.12. Intermittent mandatory ventilation without pressure support. Note irregular respiratory pattern, tachypnea, absence of alveolar plateau, low $ETCO_2$, and high baseline CO_2. (From Carlon G, Ray C, Miodowink S, et al. Capnography in mechanically ventilated patients. Crit Care Med 1988;16:550–556.)

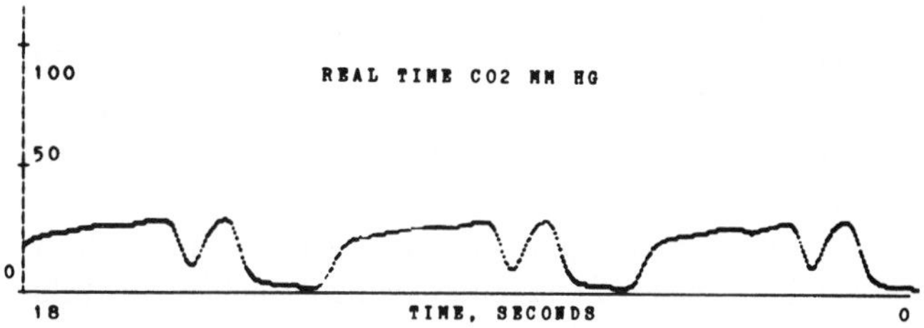

Figure 10.14. Characteristic pattern of a curare cleft indicates spasmodic inspiratory efforts by a diaphragm still mostly paralyzed. (From Carlon G, Ray C, Miodowink S, et al. Capnography in mechanically ventilated patients. Crit Care Med 1988;16:550–556.)

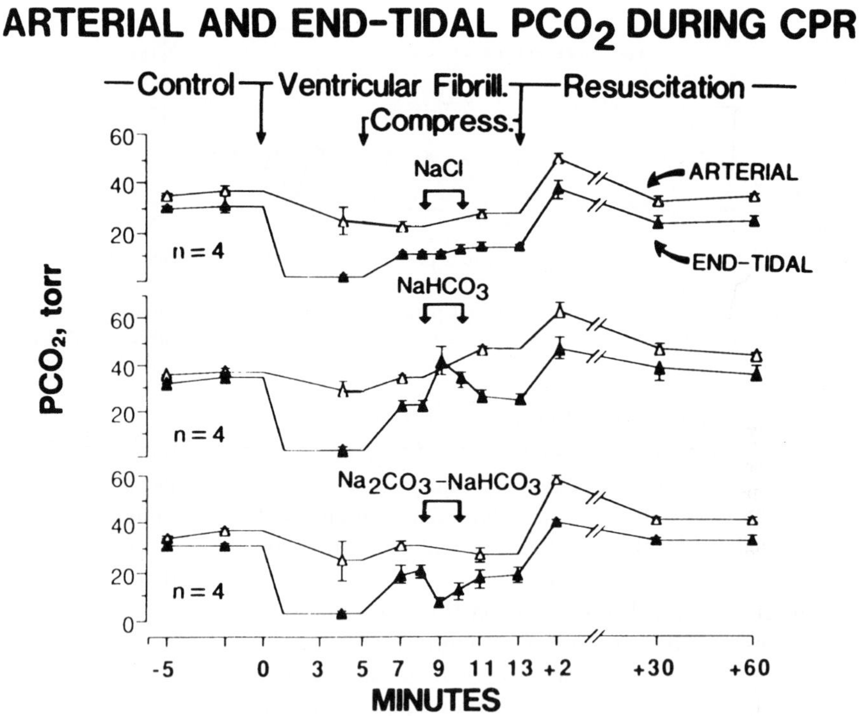

Figure 10.15. P_aCO_2 and $ETCO_2$ changes before, during, and after cardiac arrest in 12 resuscitated pigs. Values are mean ± SEM. (From Gazmuri R, von Planta M, Weil M, Rackow E. Arterial PCO_2 as an indicator of systemic perfusion during cardiopulmonary resuscitation. Crit Care Med 1989;17:239.)

rise to greater than 10 mm Hg, the chances of a successful resuscitation are very poor[42,43].

Monitoring Respiratory Mechanics

Mechanical ventilators deliver gas at a pressure and flow that results in a change in patient lung volume. Before waveform graphics became integral components of ventilator systems, ventilator monitoring was restricted to reading the ventilator's controls, digital monitors, and mechanical gauges as well as physical assessments. Detailed analysis of the patient/ventilator interface was, therefore, impossible. echnological advances now permit continuous respiratory mechanics monitoring, including graphic display of gas flow, tidal volume, and airway pressure. Output waveforms are useful tools with which to study the characteristics of ventilator operation and provide a graphic display of the various modes of ventilation. Waveform analysis can be used to optimize mechanical ventilatory support and to analyze ventilator incidents and alarm conditions. Using this technology, it is now possible to shape the form of ventilatory support to improve patient-ventilator synchrony, reduce work of breathing, and calculate a variety of physiologic parameters related to respiratory mechanics. The goal of this section is to provide a clinical tool that can optimize mechanical ventilation strategy through the use of graphic analysis.

A primary goal of graphic analysis is to rapidly determine the presence of respiratory pathophysiology by evaluating tidal volume, airway pressures, compliance, airways resistance, and pressure/volume and flow/volume relationships. Airway graphic analysis is particularly helpful in determining the effectiveness of various respiratory interventions. Additionally, adverse ventilator effects—including alveolar overdistention, air leak, dynamic hyperexpansion (gas trapping), and patient-ventilator dyssynchrony—can be diagnosed and corrected.

The most commonly reported waveforms are flow, pressure, and volume (y-axis) plotted against time (x-axis). Convention dictates that in these waveforms, positive values correspond to inspiratory events and negative values correspond to expiratory events. The timing sequence of various respiratory events can be determined by these graphics. Comparison of all three waveforms simultaneously facilitates analysis of the patient-ventilator interface. Patient-ventilator dyssynchrony becomes evident when the timing and magnitude of flow, pressure, and volume are dispropor-

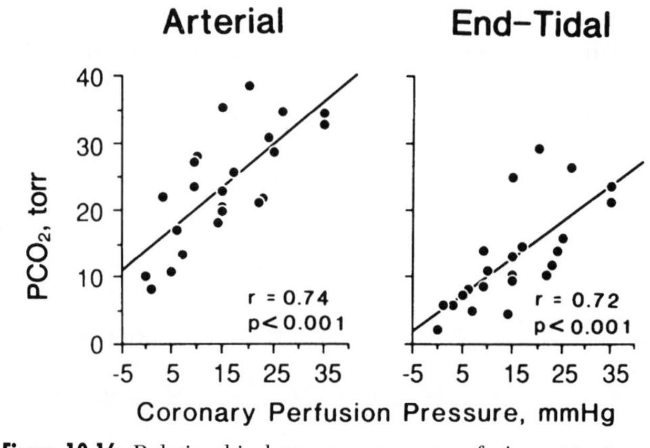

Figure 10.16. Relationship between coronary perfusion pressure and both P_aCO_2 and $ETCO_2$ after 2 minutes of precordial compression in 23 pigs. (From Gudipati C, Weil M, Bisera J, et al. Expired carbon dioxide: a noninvasive monitor of cardiopulmonary resuscitation. Circulation 1988;77:237.)

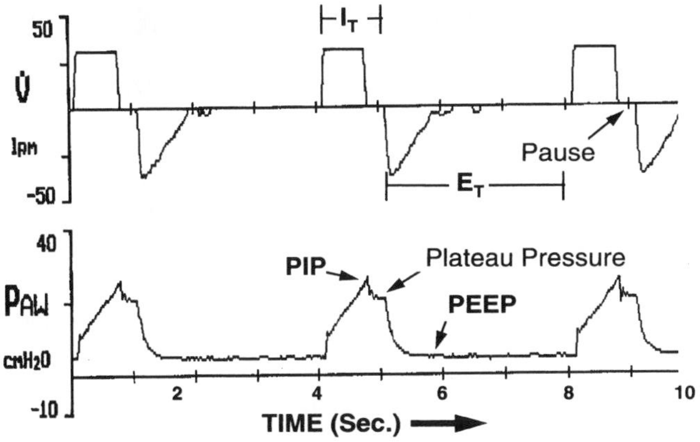

Figure 10.17. Normal scalar display of flow versus time and airway pressure versus time for volume limited ventilation. Paw, airway pressure; PIP, peak inspiratory pressure; PEEP, positive end-expiratory pressure. (Reprinted with permission from Bird Products Corporation, Palm Springs, California.)

tionate or delayed. Additionally, each of these parameters (flow, pressure, and volume) can be plotted against each other. Pressure-volume and flow-volume loops can be particularly helpful in assessing alterations in resistance, compliance, work of breathing, overdistention of the lung, and premature termination of exhalation.

Optimal measurements are obtained when the pressure and flow sensing device (pneumotach) is positioned between the endotracheal tube and the ventilator circuit. Although resistance of the endotracheal tube is a component of the pressure graphic, pressures reported are generally considered to reflect proximal airway pressures. Volume is generally measured by integrating the flow signal over inspiratory time. The upward deflection of the graphic represents the inspiratory volume delivered to the patient, while the downward deflection represents the total expiratory volume. Inspiratory and expiratory volumes should be equal. However, it is not uncommon in children with uncuffed endotracheal tubes or cuffed endotracheal tubes with inadequate cuff inflation, for the expiratory volume to be less than the inspiratory volume. An actual percentage leak can be calculated and may aid in the decision to change the endotracheal tube size or to evaluate the adequacy of cuff inflation.

Scalar Display of Volume Limited Ventilation

A typical airway graphic during time cycled volume limited ventilation is displayed in Figure 10.17. These graphics were recorded in a labortary scenario using a Bird 8400st patient ventilator and graphics monitor (Bird Products Corporation, Palm Springs, California). The top graphic displays flow on the vertical axis and time on the horizontal axis. The bottom graphic displays airway pressure versus time. During volume limited ventilation, the tidal volume is set, and the peak inspiratory pressure (PIP) varies with changes in lung compliance, airways resistance, and delivered flow rate. In this mode of ventilation, inspiration is characterized by a square wave constant flow pattern. This constant flow corresponds to a linear increase in airway pressure until the preset tidal volume is reached. In Figure 10.17, an inspiratory pause is present, represented by the lengthened inspiratory time and the period of zero flow prior to exhalation. Plateau pressure corresponds to this zero flow period during inspiration. The flow returns to zero during expiration, indicating the completion of exhalation. When an unacceptably elevated peak inspiratory pressure occurs during volume limited ventilation, the clinician should consider increasing the inspiratory time, decreasing the inspiratory flow and/or tidal volume, or changing the mode of ventilation.

Scalar Display of Pressure Limited Ventilation

A typical airway graphic taken during pressure limited ventilation with a decelerating inspiratory flow pattern is displayed in Figure 10.18. During pressure limited ventilation with a decelerating flow pattern, the PIP is set, and the tidal volume varies with changes in lung compliance, airways resistance, and delivered flow rate. In the following discussions, PIP refers to the peak inspiratory pressure above zero and not a set inspiratory pressure above the positive end-expiratory pressure (PEEP). The decelerating flow pattern results in a curvilinear increase in airway pressure until the PIP is reached. Note the more rapid increase in pressure during the initial phase of a pressure limited breath versus the linear increase in airway pressure that occurs with a volume limited square wave constant flow pattern breath (Figure 10.17). Due to the length of the inspiratory time, inspiratory flow returns to zero while airway pressure is maintained. During pressure limited ventilation, if delivered tidal volume decreases, the clinician should consider increasing the PIP limit, increasing the inspiratory time, or optimizing the PEEP to improve compliance and improve volume delivery. At a similar tidal volume, the decelerating flow pattern of pressure limited ventilation results in a

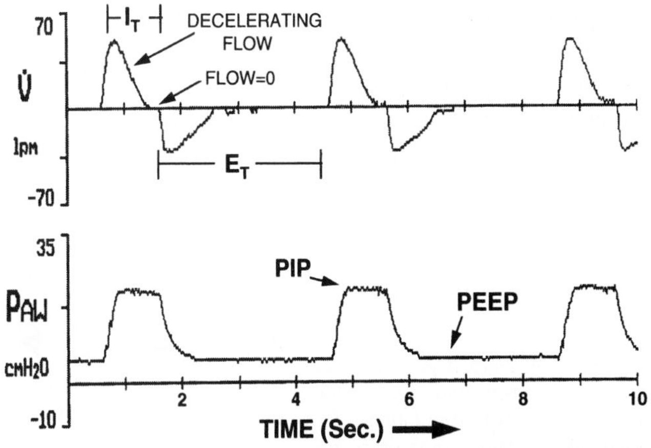

Figure 10.18. Normal scalar display of flow versus time and airway pressure versus time for pressure limited ventilation. Paw, peripheral airways; PIP, peak inspiratory pressure; PEEP, positive end-expiratory pressure. (Reprinted with permission from Bird Products Corporation, Palm Springs, California.)

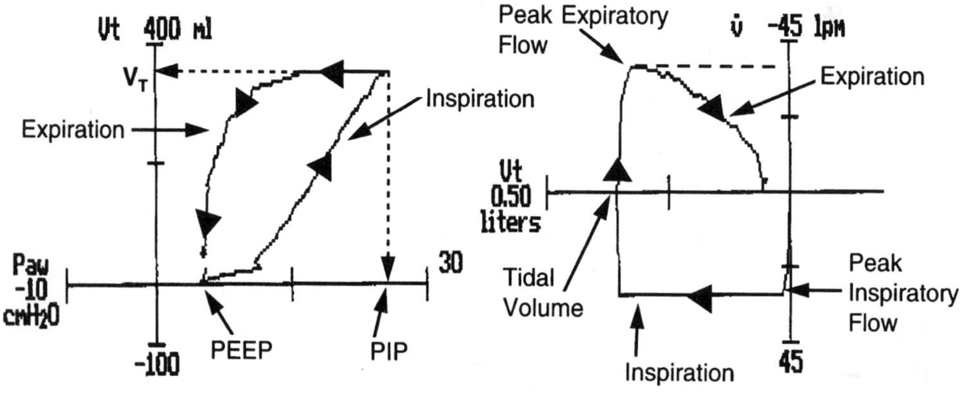

Figure 10.19. Normal pressure/volume and flow/volume loops for volume limited ventilation. Vt, tidal volume; Paw, airway pressure; PEEP, positive end-expiratory pressure; PIP, peak inspiratory pressure. (Reprinted with permission from Bird Products Corporation, Palm Springs, California.)

decrease in PIP and an increase in pulmonary compliance when compared with volume limited ventilation(44,45).

Pressure/Volume and Flow/Volume Loops in Volume limited Ventilation

The typical pressure/volume and flow/volume loops during volume limited ventilation are displayed in Figure 10.19. The pressure/volume graphic displays tidal volume on the vertical axis and airway pressure on the horizontal axis. The flow/volume graphic displays flow on the vertical axis and tidal volume on the horizontal axis. Note that in this flow/volume loop, the delivered inspiratory flow is represented during volume limited ventilation as a square wave below the baseline. These loops provide a graphic display of the pressure/volume and flow/volume relationships, insight into patient pathophysiology, and the response to therapeutic interventions.

As the ventilator delivers gas to the patient, airway pressure increases from the set PEEP level until the set tidal volume is reached and inspiration is terminated. During exhalation there is a reduction of both volume and pressure in the airways until exhaled volume reaches zero, signifying the termination of the breath. Alterations in the shape of the inspiratory limb of the pressure/volume loop provide insight into the compliance of the lung and the presence of various abnormalities, including alveolar atelectasis and overdistention. The tidal volume, PIP, and PEEP can be measured directly from the graphic. The dynamic compliance, which is the slope of the line connecting the PEEP with the PIP, can then be calculated as delivered tidal volume/(PIP to PEEP).

Note in Figure 10.19 that only a small amount of volume is delivered during the initial phase of inspiration. As the inspiratory pressure increases, the critical opening pressure is achieved, and the tidal volume is delivered. Hysteresis, which is a nonlinear change in the pressure/volume relationship over time, is present during both inspiration and expiration. A decrease in compliance results in a flattening of the loop (decreased hysteresis) and a reduction in the slope of the line connecting PEEP with PIP.

The evaluation of inspiratory and expiratory flow patterns can provide important information as to the presence of increased inspiratory or expiratory resistance. In patients with elevated resistance, the response of these abnormalities to various interventions, including suctioning and/or bronchodilator therapy, can then be readily assessed.

Pressure/Volume and Flow/Volume Loops in Pressure Limited Ventilation

The decelerating flow pattern of pressure limited ventilation results in a more rapid rise in airway pressure during the initial phase of the breath versus a volume limited breath. The corresponding pressure/volume loop is demonstrated in Figure 10.20. During the initial phase of inspiration, the airway pressures are higher for a given tidal volume, and the pressure/volume loop demonstrates an initial "scooping." Although the initial airway pressures are higher for a given tidal volume, the tidal volume is delivered at a

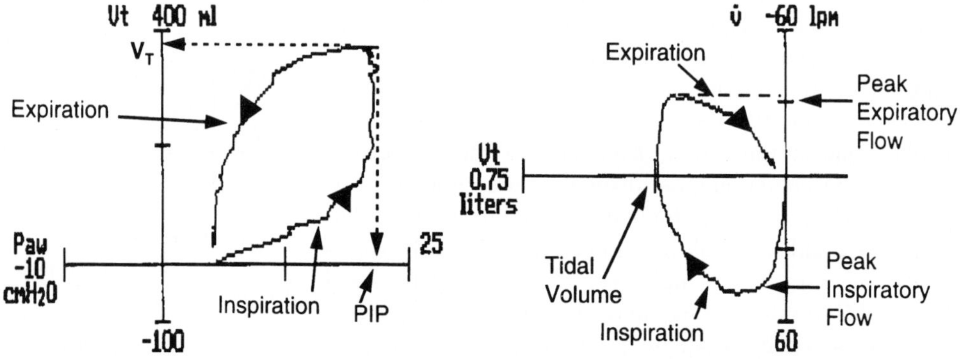

Figure 10.20. Normal pressure/volume and flow/volume loops for pressure limited ventilation. Vt, tidal volume; Paw, airway pressure; PEEP, positive end-expiratory pressure; PIP, peak inspiratory pressure. (Reprinted with permission from Bird Products Corporation, Palm Springs, California.)

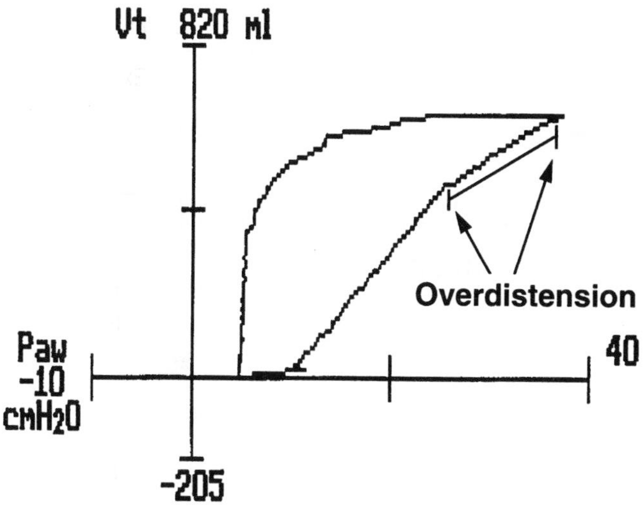

Figure 10.21. Pressure/volume loop demonstrating overdistention. Vt, tidal volume; Paw, airway pressure. (Reprinted with permission from Bird Products Corporation, Palm Springs, California.)

lower PIP, and dynamic compliance improves in this setting[44,45]. This increase in dynamic compliance is demonstrated by the increased slope of the inspiratory loop (line connecting PEEP with PIP).

The decelerating, variable inspiratory flow of pressure limited ventilation is higher than the fixed constant flow of volume limited ventilation. Thus, the peak inspiratory flow generated may better match the inspiratory demands of the patient.

Detection of Overdistention Using Pressure/Volume Loops

Overdistention is defined as an abrupt decrease in compliance at the termination of a breath. This is demonstrated in the pressure/volume loop depicted in Figure 10.21. Overdistention occurs when the volume limit of the lung is approached. As the ventilator attempts to provide gas to the patient, airway pressures increase with little volume being delivered (compliance decreases). This results in a decrease in dynamic compliance, with the inspiratory loop having a reduced slope and terminal "beaking." Overdistention is clinically significant as it can lead to volutrauma/barotrauma and elevation of pulmonary vascular resistance. To eliminate overdistention, one should decrease the PIP in pressure limited ventilation or the tidal volume in volume limited ventilation. Additionally, optimization of the administered PEEP may be beneficial. Excessively high levels of PEEP can lead to overdistention of the more compliant regions of lung[46]. PEEP, therefore, should be titrated carefully as outlined below.

Detection of Air Leak Using Pressure/Volume and Flow/Volume Loops

An air leak is demonstrated in Figure 10.22 by the failure of the expired component of the pressure/volume loop to return to zero volume. Air leak may be secondary to mechanical causes (endotracheal tube/ventilator circuit), patient causes (bronchopleural fistula), or technical causes (pneumotach inaccuracy). The flow/volume loop demonstrates an abnormal expiratory phase. The expiratory flow falls to zero prematurely at a lung volume greater than zero.

Flow/Volume Loops Demonstrating Airway Obstruction

In Figure 10.23A, the delivered inspiratory flow is represented below the baseline as a decelerating wave. During early exhalation there is nearly complete obstruction to flow, resulting in a high expiratory resistance. In Figure 10.23B, the airway obstruction is more severe, and both the inspiratory and expiratory phases are involved. In the inspiratory phase, the decelerating wave form is blunted and approaches a square wave, while in the expiratory phase, the peak flow is limited. Despite an increase in PIP, the tidal volume is reduced as a result of the severity of the obstruction. Both the inspiratory resistance and the expiratory resistance are elevated, indicating a fixed airway obstruction. Abnormalities of inspiratory and expiratory flow patterns can provide important information as to the presence of airway obstruction and the response of the obstruction to various interventions. Expiratory and inspiratory flow abnormalities may be associated with a variety of conditions, including a kinked or blocked endotracheal tube (evaluate endotracheal tube size, position, and need for suctioning), bronchoconstriction (consider bronchodilators and/or steroids), and airway obstruction (anatomic causes).

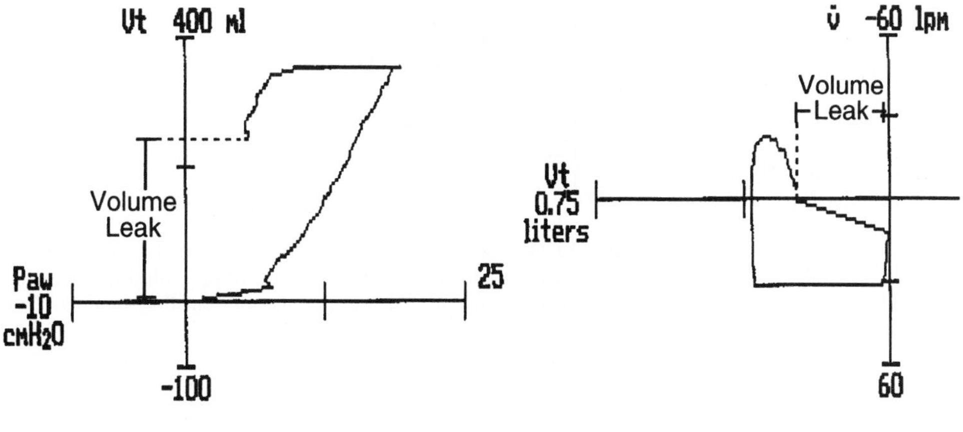

Figure 10.22. Pressure/volume and flow/volume loops demonstrating an air leak. Vt, tidal volume; Paw, airway pressure. A shows mild airway obstruction resulting in a high expiratory resistance. B shows severe airway obstruction involving increased inspiratory and expiratory resistance. (Reprinted with permission from Bird Products Corporation, Palm Springs, California.)

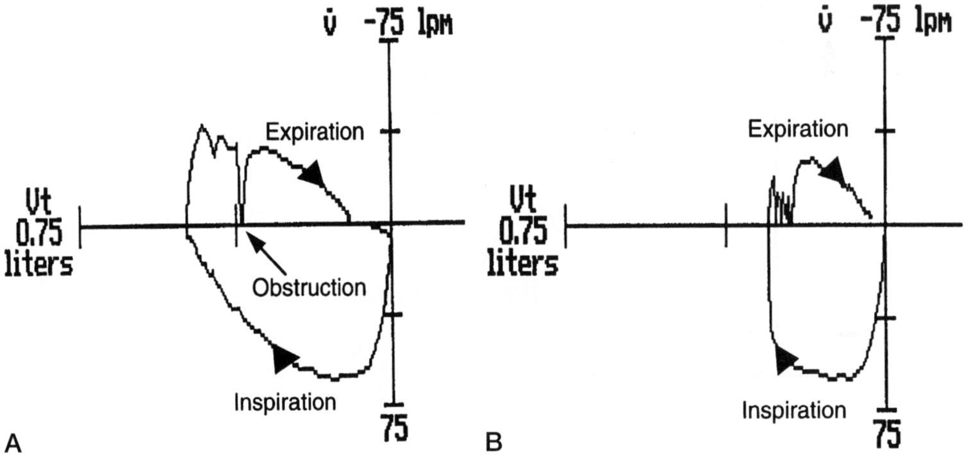

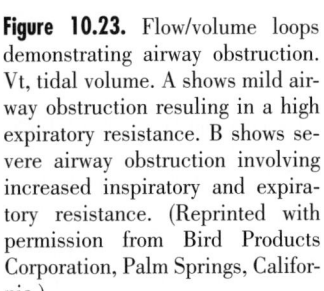

Figure 10.23. Flow/volume loops demonstrating airway obstruction. Vt, tidal volume. A shows mild airway obstruction resuling in a high expiratory resistance. B shows severe airway obstruction involving increased inspiratory and expiratory resistance. (Reprinted with permission from Bird Products Corporation, Palm Springs, California.)

Scalar Display of Volume Limited Ventilation During Adult Respiratory Distress Syndrome

In Figure 10.24, a square wave constant flow pattern during inspiration is again demonstrated (Figure 10.17). However, in adult respiratory distress syndrome (ARDS), if the tidal volume is held constant, a higher PIP is required to generate a similar tidal volume, indicating a decrease in pulmonary compliance. Since the lung compliance has decreased, the PIP, and often the mean airway pressure, must increase to maintain the desired tidal volume. The risk of volutrauma/barotrauma is, therefore, increased[47]. When an excessively elevated PIP develops during volume limited ventilation, the clinician should consider increasing the inspiratory time, decreasing the flow rate, optimizing the PEEP, decreasing the tidal volume (allowing permissive hypercapnia), or changing the mode of ventilation to a decelerating flow, pressure limited approach.

ARDS: Pressure/Volume and Flow/Volume Loops in Volume Limited Ventilation

ARDS causes a reduction in pulmonary compliance (compare Figures 10.19 and 10.25). A decrease in compliance results in elevated airway pressures required to achieve a similar tidal volume. As a result, the pressure/volume loop flattens, and the curvature of the inspiratory and expiratory limbs decreases (decreased hysteresis). Note that during the initial phase of inspiration there is an increase in airway pressure with little gas being delivered to the patient. This is due to alveolar collapse that occurs during expiration. To reexpand the alveoli that are collapsed, the initial phase of inspiration requires an elevation of airway pressure prior to delivering a significant volume of gas. Therefore, the initial phase of the inspiratory limb (reexpansion interval) has a lower slope than the later phase of the inspiratory limb. Subsequently, the PIP may be increased. Increasing the PEEP may maintain alveolar patency during the expiratory phase and minimize this reexpansion interval, as described later.

Scalar Display of Pressure Limited Ventilation During ARDS

As in Figure 10.18, Figure 10.26 demonstrates the decelerating flow pattern during inspiration. However, during ARDS pulmonary compliance is decreased. If the PIP is held constant, the tidal volume will be reduced and gas exchange may be impaired, resulting in a respiratory acidosis. The approach to the loss of tidal volume in this situation should be to allow permissive hypercapnia (tolerating tidal volume reduction) or to increase airway pressures (PIP and/or PEEP) to recruit tidal volume and functional residual capacity. As compared with Figure 10.26, the pressure limit in Figure 10.27 has been increased to achieve a similar delivered tidal volume as in Figure 10.18. As a result, the PIP and mean airway pressure have increased. This recruits tidal volume, improves distribution of ventilation, and increases oxygenation.

In Figure 10.27, note the period of zero flow as a result of a prolonged inspiratory time. The flow is zero; however, the inspiratory pressure remains positive mimicking a pressure-plateau effect and increasing the mean airway

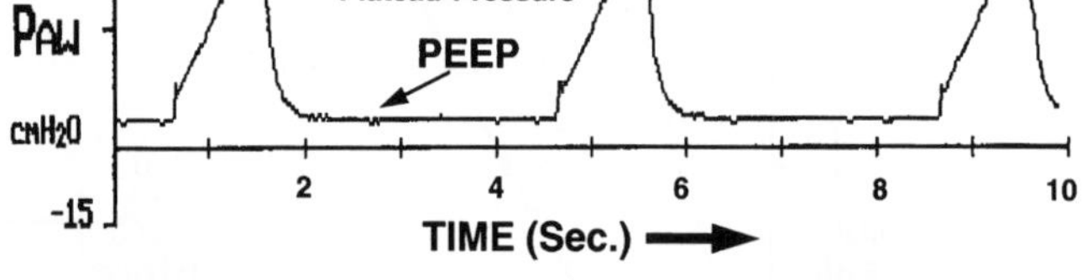

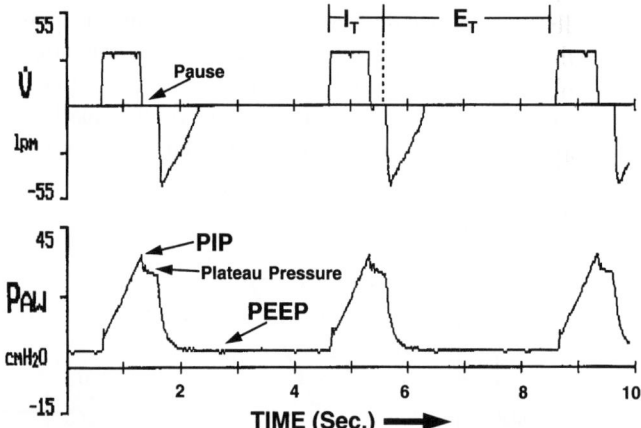

Figure 10.24. Scalar display of flow versus time and airway pressure versus time for volume limited ventilation during adult respiratory distress syndrome. (Reprinted with permission from Bird Products Corporation, Palm Springs, California.)

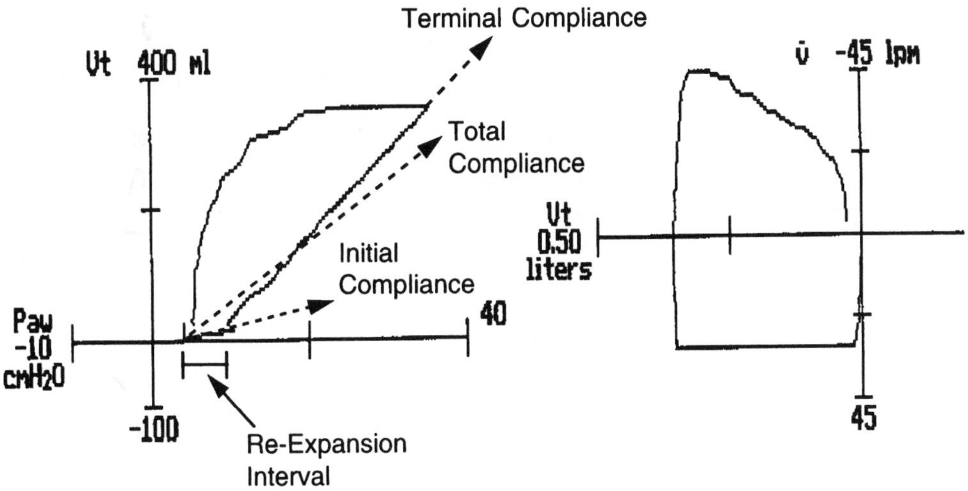

Figure 10.25. Pressure/volume and flow/volume loops for volume limited ventilation during adult respiratory distress syndrome. (Reprinted with permission from Bird Products Corporation, Palm Springs, California.)

pressure. Increasing the airway pressure must be performed cautiously to minimize the risk of volutrauma/barotrauma as well as the detrimental effects of increased mean airway pressure on cardiovascular function[48]. Spontaneously breathing patients may need to be sedated to facilitate this management strategy.

Optimizing PEEP During ARDS

Decreased slope of a pressure/volume loop indicates decreased compliance (Figure 10.28). ARDS causes loss of alveolar stability and diffuse atelectasis. Alveolar collapse and a decrease in end-expiratory lung volume (EELV) may occur during the expiratory phase if the end-expiratory airway pressures are not adequate to maintain alveolar patency[49]. In Figure 10.28A, the PEEP is set at 5 cm H_2O. This is inadequate to maintain alveolar patency as a significant amount of alveolar atelectasis and loss of EELV occurs during the expiratory phase. During the initial phase of inspiration, reexpansion of the collapsed alveoli is necessary, and the inspiratory airway pressures increase dramatically before a volume of gas is delivered to the patient. Once the critical opening volume has been reached, the tidal volume is delivered quickly.

The pressure cost of reexpansion is the amount of inspiratory airway pressure that is necessary to achieve the opening volume. The tidal volume can be delivered only when the critical opening pressure is reached. The development of a significant amount of alveolar atelectasis results in a high pressure cost of reexpansion, elevating the opening pressure as well as the PIP required to deliver the same tidal volume.

Optimizing PEEP is an essential management strategy for patients with acute lung injury[47]. By progressively increasing the PEEP from 5 to 12 cm H_2O (Figure 10.28B), a greater number of alveoli are kept patent during the expiratory phase, and functional residual capacity increases. During the initial phase of inspiration, lower airway pres-

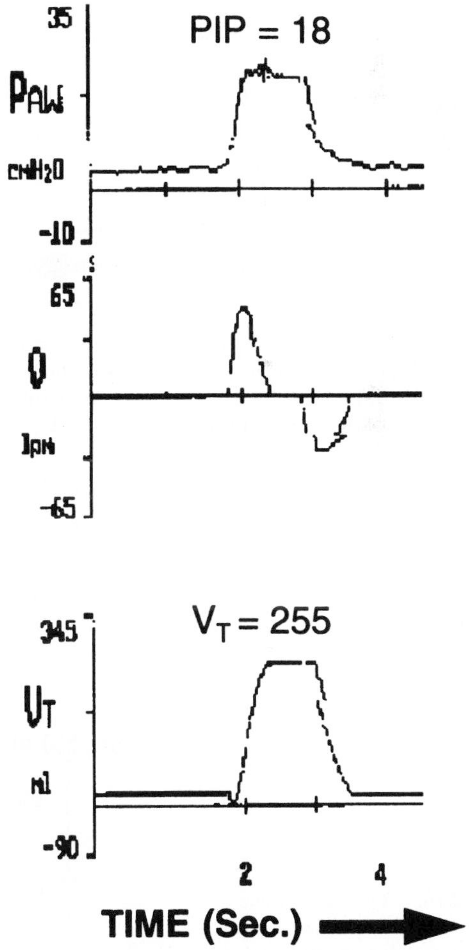

Figure 10.26. Scalar display of flow versus time, airway pressure versus time, and tidal volume versus time for pressure limited ventilation during adult respiratory distress syndrome. A loss of tidal volume occurs when the peak pressure limit is held constant. (Reprinted with permission from Bird Products Corporation, Palm Springs, California.)

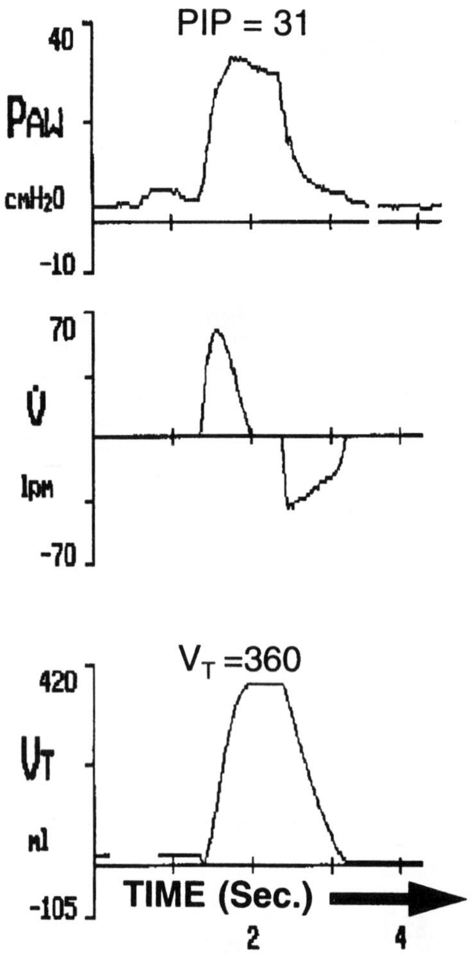

Figure 10.27. Scalar display of flow versus time, airway pressure versus time, and tidal volume versus time for pressure limited ventilation during adult respiratory distress syndrome. Tidal volume is recruited when the peak pressure limit is increased. (Reprinted with permission from Bird Products Corporation, Palm Springs, California.)

sures are required to achieve the opening volume, and the pressure cost of reexpansion (shear stress) is less than in Figure 10.28A. As functional residual capacity is restored by optimizing PEEP, the PIP and shear stress required to deliver the tidal volume may decrease over time. As a result, the tidal volume can be delivered with a smaller change in airway pressure (PIP to PEEP). The result is improved dynamic compliance and a decrease in PIP during volume limited ventilation or a higher tidal volume for a set PIP during pressure limited ventilation. These effects may be more dramatic over time as the increased PEEP continues to recruit collapsed alveoli and further increase EELV and functional residual capacity. Additionally, the risk for volutrauma/barotrauma may decrease as PIPs decrease[47].

Excessive levels of PEEP should be avoided since PEEP can cause detrimental effects on cardiorespiratory function[50]. These effects include (1) a reduction of venous return and cardiac output secondary to increased intrathoracic pressure; (2) increased dead space as pulmonary perfusion decreases, resulting in an increase in $PaCO_2$ for a given minute ventilation; and (3) overdistention of the more normal lung units, with redistribution of blood flow to the more diseased units[46]. To optimize PEEP using graphics, increase the level of PEEP gradually until the best balance is achieved in the following variables: the lowest PIP to deliver the desired tidal volume, the highest compliance, and the best oxygen delivery (requires determination of cardiac output or SVO_2 measurement).

ARDS: Dynamic Hyperexpansion and Inverse Ratio Ventilation

In Figure 10.29, note the square wave constant flow pattern during inspiration as in Figures 10.17 and 10.24. The respiratory rate and inspiratory time have been increased, resulting in a dramatic increase in mean airway pressure. As a result, there is inadequate time to complete exhalation before the next breath is initiated, and dynamic hyperexpansion (gas trapping) occurs[50]. Dynamic hyperexpansion is defined as premature termination of exhalation. Deliberate prolongation of the inspiratory time to a level greater than the expiratory time is referred to as inverse ratio ventilation. Prolongation of the inspiratory time may be beneficial in certain clinical conditions by decreasing PIP

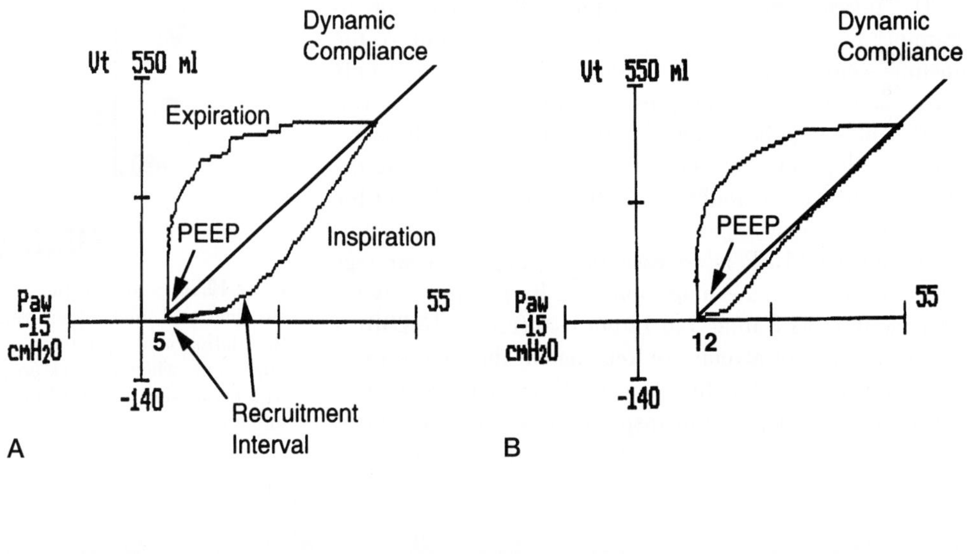

Figure 10.28. Pressure/volume loops indicating the optimization of PEEP during adult respiratory distress syndrome. A represents the compliance at PEEP $+5cmH_2O$. B represents the compliance at PEEP $+12cmH_2O$ (Reprinted with permission from Bird Products Corporation, Palm Springs, California.)

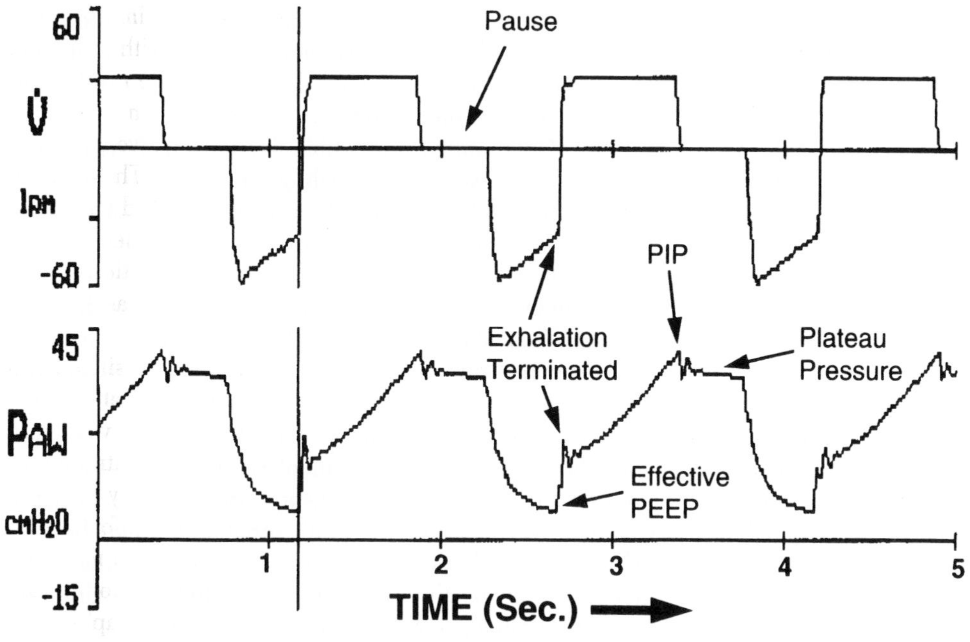

Figure 10.29. Scalar display of flow versus time and airway pressure versus time for volume limited ventilation during adult respiratory distress syndrome. Premature termination of exhalation is shown resulting in dynamic hyperexpansion (gas trapping). (Reprinted with permission from Bird Products Corporation, Palm Springs, California.)

and increasing mean airway pressure. An increase in mean airway pressure would be expected to increase oxygenation; however, an elevation in $PaCO_2$ may occur if enhalation is prematurely terminated.

Dynamic hyperexpansion and inverse ratio ventilation result in *intrinsic PEEP*, which elevates the baseline airway pressure (externally applied PEEP + intrinsic PEEP). However, intrinsic PEEP is relatively uncontrolled as compared with "set" PEEP, which can be more reliably titrated to achieve the desired oxygenation and ventilation end points. The increase in the baseline airway pressure secondary to intrinsic PEEP results in an increase in PIP that is required to maintain the set tidal volume during volume limited ventilation or a decrease in tidal volume during pressure limited ventilation. The combination of an increased PIP and the development of intrinsic PEEP causes the mean airway pressure to rise. Controlled intrinsic PEEP may be desirable in advanced cases of ARDS as it results in improved oxygenation. However, careful monitoring of the amount of intrinsic PEEP is required to limit the development of volutrauma/barotrauma. While prolongation of the inspiratory time may be beneficial, the resulting increase in intrathoracic pressure may compromise cardiac output by limiting venous return. Volume loading and/or the institution of inotropes may limit the effects of dynamic hyperexpansion and inverse ratio ventilation on cardiovascular performance.

Ventilator Dyssynchrony: Inaccurate Sensing of Patient Effort

Spontaneous patient inspiratory effort results in a decrease in airway pressure from baseline as indicated by arrows 1 to 3 in Figure 10.30. A decrease in airway pressure from baseline should result in an assisted breath being delivered in modes using patient-supported ventilation. However, due to inadequate sensitivity the ventilator is unable to determine that a patient effort has occurred in patient breaths 1 to 3. During patient breath 4, the ventilator delivers the preset tidal volume at the preset rate without regard to patient effort. Inadequate sensing of patient effort leads to tachypnea, increased work of breathing, ventilator dyssynchrony,

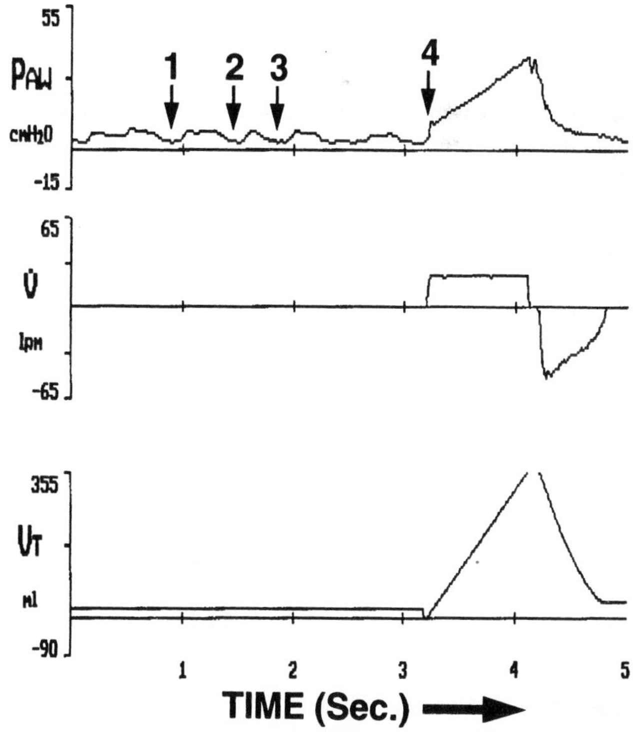

Figure 10.30. Scalar display of flow versus time, airway pressure versus time, and tidal volume versus time, representing patient-ventilator dyssynchrony secondary to inadequate sensing of the patient effort. (Reprinted with permission from Bird Products Corporation, Palm Springs, California.)

and patient discomfort (fighting the ventilator). To improve patient-ventilator synchrony in conditions when the patient effort is not appropriately sensed, the clinician should consider improving the trigger sensitivity by decreasing the trigger pressure to 0 cm H_2O. If this is unsuccessful, changing the pressure trigger to a flow trigger may be beneficial. Flow triggering may be more sensitive in children since a small change in flow requires less inspiratory effort than a small change in pressure. Flow triggering may be especially beneficial in patients with minimal inspiratory effort and small endotracheal tubes. If these interventions are not successful, the clinician should assess the ventilator response time and consider altering the mode of ventilation.

Dyssynchrony may also occur when an air leak leads to the loss of PEEP, resulting in excessive ventilator triggering (auto cycling). This unstable airway pressure baseline may be misinterpreted by the ventilator as a patient effort and result in a mechanical breath being triggered. This abnormality, commonly referred to as autocycling, may lead to frequent ventilator triggering without patient effort. This problem may be resolved by using a minimal leak technique for endotracheal tube cuff inflation or changing to a ventilator which provides additional flow support called leak compensation.

Ventilator Dyssynchrony: Inadequate Ventilatory Support

Figure 10.31 shows a patient effort that results in a decrease in airway pressure (arrows 1 and 2) and triggering of a mechanical breath. However, the inspiratory flow of the delivered mechanical breath is inadequate to meet the patient's inspiratory demands. The patient's effort is not satiated by the inspiratory flow of the mechanical breath, and, as a result, the patient attempts to initiate a spontaneous breath during the mechanical breath (arrow 3). This causes a transient reduction of airway pressure, signified by a decrease in the airway pressure tracing during inspiration (flow dyssynchrony). Inadequate ventilatory support to meet the patient's needs causes tachypnea, increased work of breathing, and patient discomfort.

In volume limited ventilation, a reduction of the inspiratory airway pressure as a result of a patient effort (arrow 3) during the mechanical breath may necessitate an increase in the PIP (arrow 4) required to achieve the set tidal volume. Increasing the flow rate during patient-assisted volume limited ventilation may eliminate flow dyssynchrony. The clinician should titrate the flow rate to reduce the drop in airway pressure (arrow 3) and return the airway pressure tracing to a more normal configuration. When increasing the flow rate is unsuccessful, inadequate ventilatory support may be the cause of the patient-ventilator dyssynchrony. Additionally, decreasing the inspiratory time or changing to another mode of ventilation with variable flow may be beneficial. A variable flow mode may meet the inspiratory demands of the patient. These modes include pressure support ventilation, pressure assist/control ventilation, and volume assured pressure support.

With the technical advances that have occurred in providing mechanical ventilation to patients, clinicians have multiple modes of ventilation and parameters that need to be set and monitored in each patient. The use of airway graphics provides an invaluable tool to help design the most appropriate strategy for each patient. Graphics provide rapid assessment of various parameters, help generate and test hypotheses of patient management, and monitor for the presence of adverse effects of mechanical ventilation.

Mixed Venous Oxygen Saturation

In 1957, Barrett-Boyes and Wood[51] performed cardiac catheterization on 26 healthy adults (22 men and 4 women) and documented the venous oxygen saturation patterns in

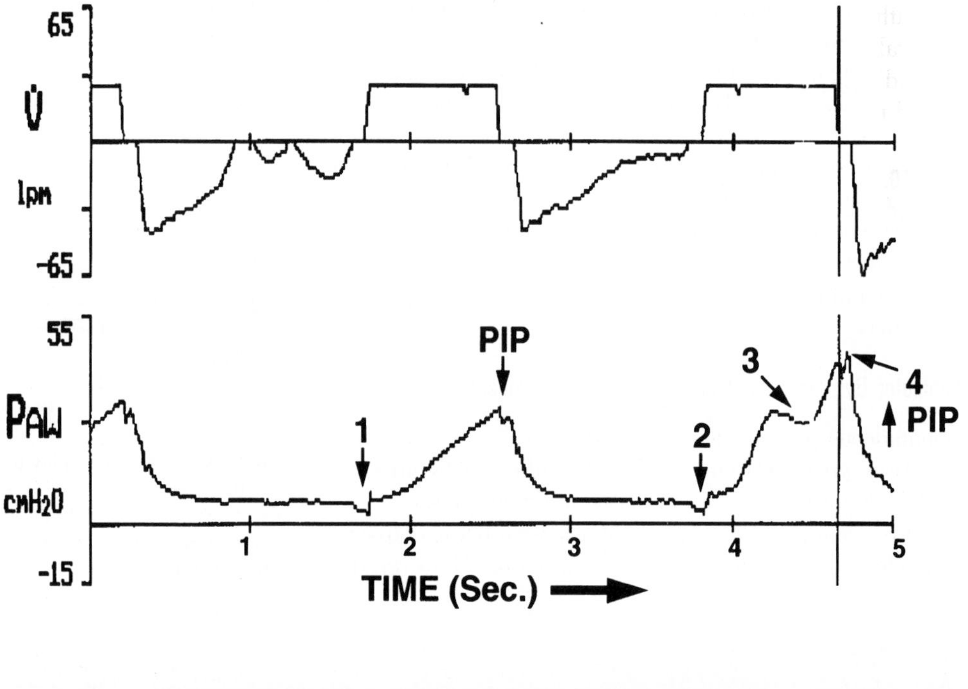

Figure 10.31. Scalar display of flow versus time and airway pressure versus time, representing patient-ventilator dyssynchrony secondary to inadequate ventilatory support. (Reprinted with permission from Bird Products Corporation, Palm Springs, California.)

humans. They demonstrated that the oxygen saturation of hemoglobin did not reach stability until high in the outflow tract of the right ventricle and pulmonary artery because of the differences in saturation from the various venous sources that make up the venous return, i.e., inferior vena cava, superior vena cava, coronary sinus, and Thebesian veins. The normal saturation of hemoglobin in the pulmonary artery (designated the S_vO_2) was determined to be 78.4%, with a range of 73 to 85%.

Rearrangement of the terms of the Fick equation indicates that venous oxygen content (C_vO_2) and hence S_vO_2 are related to oxygen consumption (VO_2) and cardiac output (Q_T) such that increases in oxygen consumption or decreases in cardiac output result in a reduction of S_vO_2 (Eq. 10.5A and 10.5B)[51]:

$$S_vO_2 = \frac{C_vO_2 - \text{dissolved } O_2}{Hb \times 1.36} \quad \text{(Eq. 10.5A)}$$

$$C_vO_2 = C_aO_2 - (VO_2/Q_T) \quad \text{(Eq. 10.5B)}$$

where Hb equals the hemoglobin concentration. **Table 10.7** lists additional causes of changes in the S_vO_2[52].

The data supporting the clinical usefulness of S_vO_2 and P_vO_2 can be illustrated from several sources. For example, Simmons et al.[53] demonstrated that lactate did not accumulate until the P_vO_2 was less than 27 mm Hg in paralyzed animals in which P_aO_2 and cardiac output were varied. Kasnitz et al.[54] demonstrated that when the P_vO_2 was less than 28 mm Hg in adults, all died, and there was a significant correlation with elevated lactate levels. The majority of patients with P_vO_2 greater than 28 mm Hg lived.

Whether continuously monitoring S_vO_2 adds anything to standard monitoring is another issue. Boutros and Lee[55] evaluated a pulmonary artery catheter with a fiberoptic component that displayed S_vO_2 continuously. The display was placed in a "black-box" that the caretakers could not use. They examined the S_vO_2 changes after the pulmonary artery catheter had been removed and concluded that (a) the S_vO_2 value was compatible with findings by present methods and technology and (b) S_vO_2 probably would not have altered management.

Table 10.7. Clinical Conditions Associated with an Alteration in Mixed Venous Oxygen Saturation[a]

Reduction in S_vO_2
Decreased cardiac output
Decreased arterial oxygen saturation
Decreased hemoglobin concentration
Increased oxygen consumption
Increase in S_vO_2
Increased oxygen delivery to the tissues
Decreased oxygen consumption
Decreased oxygen extraction by the tissues
Left-to-right intracardiac shunt
Severe mitral regurgitation
Wedged pulmonary artery catheter
Sepsis

[a] *From Tobin M. Respiratory monitoring. JAMA 1990; 264:244–251.*

Jastremski et al.[56] used a standard pulmonary artery catheter and periodic determination of S_vO_2 in 99 intensive care patients. They demonstrated that (a) a change in condition may not be associated with a change in S_vO_2, (b) most changes in S_vO_2 did not result in changes in care of the patient, (c) hospital costs were higher, and (d) mortality was unchanged.

Therefore, although continuous mixed venous oxygen saturation of hemoglobin is interesting, the technique still seeks clear-cut clinical indications and cost justification. Periodic mixed venous samples drawn from the internal jugular vein with paired arterial blood gas samples facilitate the assessment of $A\text{-}DO_2$ and may be helpful in cardiac output assessment, without the additional cost and morbidity associated with these cathers.

INTERMITTENT MONITORING

Chest X-ray

The chest x-ray is one of the most commonly ordered procedures in the intensive care unit. There has been much debate about the diagnostic, therapeutic, and prognostic usefulness of chest radiographs. The first question concerns the usefulness of a chest x-ray to the clinician's daily evaluation. Strain et al.[57] studied the incidence of unsuspected abnormalities in routine morning x-rays in an intensive care unit and found that 14 to 18% of patients had an unsuspected finding on x-ray that required an intervention. Most, but not all, patients were intubated because of serious pulmonary and cardiovascular disease. There were minimal advantages to routine x-rays in patients with uncomplicated cardiovascular disease and miscellaneous disorders such as diabetic ketoacidosis and meningitis who were not ventilated[57].

Brunel et al.[58] assessed the usefulness of routine x-rays after endotracheal intubation and found that 30 of the 219 endotracheal tubes required repositioning and 10 were in the right mainstem bronchus. In almost all cases, examining the patient and confirming the position of the endotracheal tube on the lip or gum, listening for symmetry of breath sounds in the fourth intercostal space in the midaxillary line, palpating for the cuff in the suprasternal notch, and observing the chest for adequate movement were inadequate means of detecting poor endotracheal tube position in these patients[58].

Hauser et al.[59] compared the physical examination with a chest x-ray in a pediatric intensive care unit and showed that the chest x-ray is much more sensitive than the clinician's examination to detecting significant problems. Twenty-four percent of the routine x-rays showed an abnormality that resulted in a change of management by the caregivers. The abnormalities noted included endotracheal tube and central line malpositions, new or advancing pulmonary infiltrates, and unsuspected pneumothorax. These findings were more common in smaller children. Thirty-five percent of the x-rays done for endotracheal tube placement and 44% of those done for central line placement resulted in repositioning.

Finally, Hall et al.[60] studied the use of only routine morning films in patients being ventilated via endotracheal tube and found that 8% of the x-rays revealed a new, major finding (malposition of an endotracheal tube, nasogastric tube, or central line, or a significant pneumothorax, pulmonary cavitation, or effusion) that resulted in a change in management.

We conclude that x-rays are indicated anytime a patient is intubated or has a central venous line in order to evaluate the position of the tube or line. Daily x-rays are likely to be revealing in patients receiving mechanical ventilation. Stable patients without cardiopulmonary disease are unlikely to benefit from routine x-rays.

Ventilator Monitoring

Ventilator parameters reflect the status of the respiratory system. The prescribed and dynamic values, coupled with physical asssesment, should be included in the respiratory assessment of all mechanically ventilated patients, as changes in ventilator settings demonstrate changes in patient condition. Ventilator parameters should be measured and recorded by trained and experienced personnel at least every 4 to 6 hours.

Spontaneous breathing and ventilator synchrony: Spontaneous tidal volume and respiratory rate are a reflection of lung compliance, respiratory muscle strength, and work of breathing. Synchrony between the ventilator and the patient is essential to minimize work of breathing. Clinicians must balance the patient's work of breathing, sedation, and nutrition to ensure adequate tissue oxygenation and facilitate ventilator weaning. Inspiratory time is important for patient comfort and synchronous breathing during weaning from mechanical ventilation. The patient's age, breathing pattern, and oxygenation are major considerations in the selection of inspiratory time. The inspiratory/expiratory ratio is an expression of the set inspiratory time and the remaining expiratory cycle time. Recommended inspiratory/expiratory ratios vary greatly with ventilator rate. Ratios of 1:2 or 1:3 are most desirable, but usually no lower than 1:1 in assisted ventilation, to allow adequate time for exhalation.

Peak flow is also a major consideration in ventilator synchrony. During volume limited ventilation, with its characteristic fixed flow pattern, peak flow must be titrated to the spontaneous demands of the patient to facilitate synchrony. If peak flow adjustments cannot match inspiratory demands, the patient should be switched to a variable flow mode (i.e., pressure support). Good ventilatory technique achieves a balance of patient comfort and airway pressures. Variable flow modes may improve patient-ventilator synchrony and reduce airway pressures in actively breathing patients and should be considered when peak airway pressures are increased more than PIP 35 cm H_2O in a constant flow mode.

Airway pressures: Peak inspiratory and mean airway pressures are a reflection of the pressure cost of mechanical ventilation. PIPs increase with deterioration in the patient's pulmonary condition. The presence of airway secretions, bronchospasm, tubing kinks, pneumothorax, agitation, and decreased lung compliance increase PIPs for the same tidal volume. Decreases in peak pressures reflect leaks around the endotracheal tube/ventilator circuit and improvement in airway resistance and compliance. Mean airway pressure is an important indicator of the degree of mechanical ventilation required to achieve adequate oxygenation. Shear stress to the lung increases as PIP increases. Ventilatory parameters should be adjusted to provide adequate alveolar ventilation at the lowest mean airway pressure. Mean airway pressures greater than 15 cm H_2O are considered high and should be evaluated for possible reduction via alternative ventilatory modes. Plateau pressure is obtained by recording the pressure after an inspiratory breath-hold maneuver. Plateau pressure (or end-inspiratory plateau) reflects the compliance of the lung during static gas flow and eliminates the airway resistance component. Plateau pressures in excess of 35 cm H_2O have been suggested as an indication for alternate ventilatory strategies[50]. However, these data have yet to be demonstrated in neonatal or pediatric populations.

Fraction of inspired oxygen concentration (FIO_2): FIO_2 should be analyzed continuously with high and low alarm limits set to prevent inadvertent hypoxemia or hyperoxemia. The degree of hypoxemia is directly proportional to the increases in FIO_2. Several measurement methods are available.

Ventilator Alarm Systems: Input power alarms notify clinicians of changes in electrical or pneumatic supplies. Circuit alarms notify the clinician of incompatible parameters or that some aspect of the ventilator self-test has failed. Output alarms indicate unacceptable levels (high and low) of ventilator output: peak airway pressure, mean airway pressure, end-expiratory pressure, total volume, flow, minute ventilation, inspiratory time, expiratory time, gas concentration, and failure of the airway pressure to return to baseline in an acceptable period of time. The limits for these paramters should be adjusted to facilitate close surveillance of the patient-ventilator systm without producing nuisance alarms. Setting ventilator alarms so high that audible and visual alarms are activated late in disease progression defeats the concept of early intervention to reduce patient morbidity. Clinicans must be aware of the dynamic changes in ventilatory status as well as the minimal safety parameter adjustment to ensure patient safety.

Extubation criteria: Several investigators have tried (unsuccessfully) to identify parameters that predict successful extubation in children. Measures of spontaneous breathing effort, maximal inspiratory pressure, vital capacity, and minute ventilation are predictive in adolscent and young adults but not in infants and small children[61–65]. **Table 10.8** summarizies the reliability of respiratory measurements as predictors of weaning from mechanical ventilation. Respiratory assessment prior to extubation should include

Table 10.8. Pulmonary Functions Test as Predictors of Weaning from a Ventilator

Author	*Test*[a]	*Predictive Value*
Sahn (1973)	NIF	<-30 cm H_2O
Tahvanainen	R.Q.	<0.9
(1983)	NIF	<-30 cm H_2O
Montgomery (1987)	P0.1/P0.2H ratio	>1.49
Fiastro (1988)	$\dot{W}$(insp)/min	<1.60 kg·m/min
	$\dot{W}$(insp)/V_E	<0.14 kg·m/liter
Yang (1991)	f/V_T	<105 breaths/min/liter
	CROP index	>13 ml/breath/min

[a] *NIF, negative inspiratory pressure; R.Q., respiratory quotient; P0.1, pressure generated 0.1 second after occluding the airway during a normal inspiration; P0.1H, pressure generated 0.1 second after occluding the airway during a normal inspiration after breathing CO_2 for a short period of time before the test; $\dot{W}$(insp), inspiratory work; f, respiratory rate; V_T, tidal volume; CROP index, C dyn ⋆ P_{imax} ⋆ (P_aO_2/P_AO_2)/f, where P_{imax} equals maximum inspiratory pressure in the 20 seconds after endotracheal tube occlusion during a normal inspiration and C dyn equals dynamic compliance, which equals V_T/peak inspiratory pressure minus PEEP.*

work of breathing, oxygenation versus inspired oxygen concentration, spontaneous tidal volume and respiratory rate, respiratory secretion clearance, level of sedation/alertness, body weight at time of exubation compared with time of intubation, and cardiovascular stability. It has been our experience with infants that increased body weight during the intubation period contributes to increased lung water and decreased compliance. A rule of thumb has been to extubate infants at no more than a 15% increase in body weight from time of intubation.

We have also instituted the use of sedation scales to assist bedside caregivers in determining when to administer sedation/pain relief during weaning from mechanical ventilation **(Table 10.9)**. Physcians prescribe the sedation method and scale value, while the nurses work with the respiratory therapists to continue ventilator and sedation weaning to extubatable ventilator settings (synchronized intermittent mandatory ventilation 5 to 8 beats/min, pressure support 5 to 10 cm H_2O, FIO_2 <0.4, and PEEP ≤5 cm H_2O).

Blood Gases

The physician's order to obtain an areterial blood gas sample may seem quite simple, yet the proper interpretation and response to the results require an understanding of physiology, physics, and chemistry that must be applied to the patient's clinical picture. This section provides an outline of the fundamentals behind blood gas monitoring and the suggestion for a systematic method to approach the results and apply them to the clinical situation.

The history of describing the behavior of pressure and gases has left us with several interchangeable methods of describing force per unit area or pressure. One standard atmosphere (atm) of pressure is defined as 760 mm Hg and corresponds to 1.033 g/cm^2, 1.01325 bar, and 14.7 lb/inch^2. In addition, the kilopascal (kPa) equals 1000 Pa, and by definition, 100 kPa equals 1 bar; hence, 1 atm equals 101.325 kPa. As it happens, the pressure of a gas (in kilopascals) in a mixture at 1 atm is very near the percentage of that gas in the total mixture. For example, oxygen constitutes about 21% of air at sea level and exerts a partial pressure of 21 kPa. In the following discussion we restrict ourselves to the convention of millimeters of mercury (mm Hg) in the description of blood gas interpretations.

Gas laws pertain to the relationships between pressure, volume, and temperature and form the foundation for any consideration of blood gases and physiologic systems[66]. Dalton's law of partial pressure states that in a mixture of gases, each gas exerts the pressure that it would exert if it occupied the volume by itself. This pressure is known as the partial pressure (or tension), and the sum of the partial pressures equals the total pressure of the mixture. Thus, in a mixture of 5% CO_2 in oxygen at a total pressure of 760 mm Hg, the CO_2 partial pressure is:

$$(5/100) \times 760 = 38 \text{ mm Hg}$$

In general terms,

$$P_{GAS} = F_{GAS} \times P_{Barometric} \qquad \text{(Eq. 10.7)}$$

where P_{GAS} is the partial pressure of a gas that contributes F_{GAS} fraction of the total barometric pressure, $P_{Barometric}$. In the alveolar gas at sea level, there is about 6.2% water vapor, which exerts a partial pressure of 47 mm Hg. The available pressure for other gases is, therefore, 713 mm Hg (760 to 47). The partial pressure of each gas that makes up the atmosphere breathed depends on the fraction of the total gases it comprises and the barometric pressure at which it exists. Since much of the physiology we discuss depends on the partial pressure gradient established across membranes, this concept is important.

Much of what happens in physiologic systems occurs in the liquid phase. Henry's law helps us to relate amounts of dissolved gases to partial pressures:

$$n_{GAS} = P_{GAS} \times \lambda_{GAS} \qquad \text{(Eq. 10.8)}$$

where n_{GAS} is the amount of gas determined by P_{GAS}, the partial pressure of the gas, multiplied by the solubility of the gas (λ_{GAS}) in the solution at constant temperature.

Sampling Techniques

In general, the more practical points of actually obtaining a blood gas sample from a patient are best learned through practice and not from a textbook. Nonetheless, key factors in obtaining meaningful data must be discussed.

Proper preparation of materials and documentation of the conditions at the time of sampling are of utmost importance. Effective means for protecting oneself from potential infec-

Table 10.9. Pediatric Sedation Rating Scale[a]

1 =	Barely arousable: asleep; needs shaking or shouting to arouse
2 =	Asleep: eyes closed; arouses with soft voice or light touch
3 =	Sleepy: eyes open, but less active and responsive
4 =	Awake
5 =	Agitated

[a]*As adapted from DUMC Nursing Policy & Procedures.*

tion must be employed when contact with body fluids is possible. Universal precautions include the use of gloves, eye protection, masks, and even gowns to shield one from blood that may spurt from an arterial puncture. The risks associated with exposure to blood are discussed elsewhere in this text (see Chapter 29, The Critically Ill Child with Human Immunodeficiency Virus Infection, and Chapter 33, Specific Infectious Diseases of Interest to the Intensivist).

The patient's condition at the time of the sample must be recorded so that the physician can make an informed interpretation of the results. Current vital signs (heart rate, blood pressure, respiratory rate, and temperature) are recorded, as well as the position of the patient. Ventilatory settings such as mode and rate of ventilation, FIO_2, continuous positive airway pressure (CPAP) or PEEP, and inspiratory time must be recorded. Before obtaining the sample it is important to be reasonably sure that the patient has attained a steady state from the last modification in ventilatory support[(67)]. The clinical state of the patient, including such conditions as cyanosis, coma, or convulsions, is important. Before obtaining the sample one must know whether the patient has any known bleeding abnormalities or disorders that may hinder adequate hemostasis. When possible and reasonable, the procedure should be explained to the patient and/or parent before beginning. This may allow the child to prepare for the procedure[(68,69)]. A few seconds of honest description may make all the difference in being able to obtain a good sample.

Arterial puncture: Several sites are adequate for intermittent arterial sampling. The radial, posterior tibial, and dorsalis pedis arteries are frequently used in children[(70–72)]. Collateral circulation allows tissues downstream from these sites to receive blood from alternative sources, should the procedure cause spasm or thrombosis of the vessel. The femoral or brachial arteries should not be used if alternative sites exist, because these vessels are considered end arteries with inadequate collateral circulation to overcome spasm or thrombosis. The temporal and axillary arteries are also avoided because of the proximity to the central circulation and the attendant risk of retrograde embolization to the brain[(73)].

The area is cleansed with a suitable antiseptic (Betadine or iodine), allowed to dry, and wiped clean with alcohol. This is allowed to dry. Local anesthetic (usually lidocaine 0.5%) may be instilled to create a small anesthetized area. A tuberculin syringe with a short 25-gauge needle works well. A 23-gauge butterfly needle is then attached to a tuberculin syringe that has been prepared with heparin 1000 units/ml. The syringe is prepared by drawing a small amount of heparin into the syringe and moving the plunger in and out to wet the entire inside of the syringe. Excess heparin is then expelled. Some syringes come prepared with dried heparin.

The butterfly needle is inserted into the artery at about a 45-degree angle until blood is seen to pulsate into the syringe; 0.5 to 0.8 ml is withdrawn. The needle is removed, and direct pressure is applied with a sterile gauze pad until the bleeding stops. All air is removed from the syringe, and the sample is immediately capped and placed in ice. Arterial blood sampling is a simple technique that is easy to learn[(74)]. There are, however, risks involved in performing the procedure, which should be recognized[(75–78)]. Close attention to good technique will minimize the frequency of such problems.

Although serious permanent complications are rare, decreased blood flow to the limb distal to the insertion site of the needle is a recognized complication of arterial puncture and cannulation[(79)]. This may result in necrosis or loss of tissue. Thrombosis may also complicate arterial cannulation and may necessitate endarterectomy (especially in the case of femoral cannulae). Administration of heparin (100 units/kg every 4 hours for 48 hours) has been suggested as a method to manage arterial thrombosis with improved results[(80)]. Some have minimized the occurrence of postcannulation radial artery thrombosis in adults by pretreatment with aspirin[(81)]. Various techniques, including Doppler studies, may allow precise identification of collateral flow through, for example, the ulnar artery when the radial artery is to be used for sampling[(79)]. Problems with hemorrhage and hematoma are also recognized, as well as arteriospasm, nerve damage, pain, and vasovagal responses. Finally, infection is always a risk when the skin is pierced and may be minimized by proper antiseptic preparation of the site.

Arterial cannulation: For those children who will require frequent sampling of arterial blood, it may be prudent to insert a cannula into an artery. Although the umbilical artery may be used in neonates[(82)], complications, including thrombosis, organ infarction, infection, and hemorrhage, are well recognized[(83)]. The use of the radial artery has been reported as a reasonable alternative[(70,84,85)]. We have found that the radial, posterior tibial, dorsalis pedis, and femoral arteries are generally suitable for cannulation. Because of the increased incidence of serious complications, including central nervous system embolism[(73)] and thrombosis of a distal portion of a limb[(76)], we refrain from instrumenting the temporal and brachial sites when possible.

When a vessel is catheterized, a continuous infusion of heparinized saline is started, along with continuous monitoring. The site is clearly labeled as arterial, and no other medications, fluids, or blood products are infused via this line.

Capillary samples: In neonates and young children it is often easier to obtain a capillary blood sample than an arterial sample, especially if repeated samples may be necessary, and it is not possible or desirable to place an arterial line. The sample area should be warmed to promote cirulation and arterialize blood prior to the puncture. The sample is usually taken from the heel, finger, or ear lobe. After cleaning the skin with an alcohol preparation, a lancet is used to pierce the skin no deeper than 2 to 3 mm. The first drop of blood is wiped away, and subsequently, free-flowing drops of blood are collected into a heparinized capillary tube. Squeezing the site to encourage flow of blood

Table 10.10. Normal Blood Gas Values (F_IO_2 = 0.21)[a]

	pH	P_aCO_2 (mm Hg)	P_aO_2 (mm Hg)	BE (mEq/liter)	HCO_3^- (mEq/liter)
Umbical vein	7.33	43	28	22	
Capillary infant (1–25 days)	7.40	40	52		
Arterial newborn	1–4 hours	7.30	39	62	19
12–24 hours	7.30	33	68	20	
24–48 hours	7.39	34	63–87	−6	20
96 hours	7.39	36	21		
Arterial infant (1–24 months)	7.40	34	90	−3	20
Arterial child (7–19 years)	7.39	37	96	−2	22
Arterial adult	7.40	40	100	0	24

[a]From Dong SH, et al. Arterialized capillary blood gases and acid-base studies in normal individuals from 29 days to 24 years of age. Am J Dis Child 1985;139:1019. Copyright 1983, American Medical Association.

may distort the results. After an adequate amount of blood has been collected, a gauze is placed over the site, and the tube is sealed on both sides with rubber caps. The blood gas determination is made promptly, as discussed above[86].

The use of capillary samples as a means to estimate arterial blood gas determinations has recently been reviewed[87]. Correlations between arterial and capillary samples vary, but generally they are best for pH, moderate for PCO_2, and worst for PO_2. Normal ranges have been established and are included in **Table 10.10**[88].

Venous samples: The general acid-base status of a patient who is otherwise well perfused may be indicated from a peripheral venous blood sample[89], but because of the differences in perfusion and oxygen use of various organs, assessment of oxygenation is not reliable. Samples from specific venous effluents may indicate uptake and use of oxygen in particular organs, such as the brain, and correlate with outcome[90–92].

Pulmonary artery samples: Mixed venous blood gas samples from the pulmonary artery may be obtained to help evaluate the shunt fraction as well as total body oxygen consumption (see Chapter 4, Developmental Physiology of the Respiratory System). Specimens obtained from the pulmonary artery by gentle withdrawal from the distal port of a Swan-Ganz catheter should be handled in a fashion similar to that used for samples drawn from an artery.

Analyzers

PCO_2 electrode: First introduced by Stowe et al.[93] and later refined by Severinghaus and Astrup[94], the modern PCO_2 electrode incorporates the application of Henry's law into a reliable and efficient device. The blood sample is separated from the measuring half-cell (made of silver-silver chloride) by a silicon elastic membrane, a bicarbonate solution, a nylon spacer, and a pH-sensitive glass. The reference half-cell is also made of silver-silver chloride. The entire electrode is protected by a Lucite jacket and immersed in an electrolyte bath that constantly replenishes the solution at the electrode tip and bridges each half-cell electrically (Fig. 10.32). Carbon dioxide presented to the electrode forces the bicarbonate reaction to form more H^+ as shown below[95]:

$$CO_2 + H_2O \leftrightarrow H_2CO_3 \leftrightarrow H^+ + HCO_3^- \quad \text{(Eq. 10.9)}$$

The change in pH may be used as an indirect measurement of CO_2. Calibration with 5 and 10% known gas mixtures of

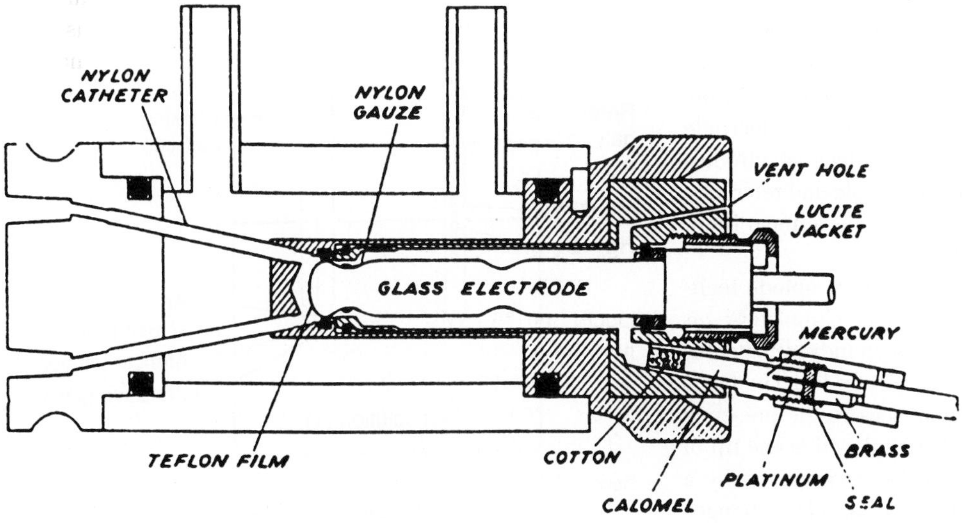

Figure 10.32. Severinghaus CO_2 electrode. (From Severinghaus J. Methods of measurement of blood and gas carbon dioxide during anesthesia. Anesthesiology 1960; 21:717.)

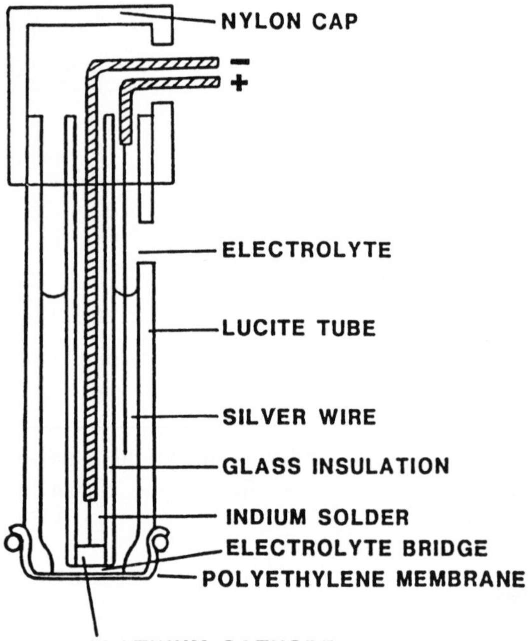

Figure 10.33. Clark O_2 electrode. (From Int Anesth Clin 1987;25(3).)

CO_2 allows definition of a pH slope that is directly proportional to PCO_2.

Clark PO_2 electrode: The polarographic electrode (refined by Clark) is based on the chemical reduction of oxygen at a cathode (Fig. 10.33)[94]. A constant flow of electrons is produced by oxidation when a silver anode is placed in a bath of KCl to form silver chloride. These electrons react with a platinum cathode in the presence of O_2 to form OH, producing a current. The amount of oxygen presented to the cathode is directly proportional to the current produced and can be calibrated by using known oxygen gas mixtures of 0 and 20% to create a slope for comparison.

pH electrode: A glass barrier sensitive to pH generates an electrical potential if placed between solutions of known pH and an unknown sample. This is the principle behind the modern pH electrode. A KCl contact bridge connects a mercury-mercurous chloride electrode (reference electrode) and a silver-silver chloride electrode (measuring electrode) that is embedded within the known pH solution (pH equals 6.840). The sample and known solutions are separated from each other by pH-sensitive glass in the measuring electrode bath (Fig. 10.34). Voltage measured between electrodes, generated from the difference between sample and reference electrodes, can be measured and calibrated as a linear function of the potential difference[94].

Fluorescent optode technology: Fluorescent optode technology affords the ability to monitor various parameters, including blood gases, continuously by using indwelling catheters equipped with miniature optical electrodes. The basis for the technology is a dye that fluoresces in the presence of a particular substance[96]. The dye is placed at the tip of a fiberoptic element separated from the environment by a membrane permeable to the substance to which it changes its fluorescence. Light of appropriate intensity is transmitted along an optical fiber to the dye, which then returns as emitted light energy from the fluorescing dye, thus indicating the presence of membrane-permeable substance. By using specific fluorescent indicators, photometric determination of PO_2, PCO_2, pH, ionic strength, and osmolarity may be measured[97–99].

Potential Sampling Errors

Arterial blood gas sampling errors are summarized in **Table 10.11.**

Air in the sample: Air in the blood sample may cause erroneous results because of equilibration of the sample with a bubble or froth entrapped in the syringe[100]. When a blood sample is placed in a syringe and an air bubble is included, the P_aO_2 of the air (about 158 mm Hg) tends to equilibrate with the blood. Therefore, when a blood sample with a P_aO_2 less than 158 mm Hg is interfaced with a bubble of air, the result will be spuriously higher. In situations in which a high P_aO_2 is expected (as with a healthy patient and a high F_IO_2), the gradient will force O_2 out of the blood and into the bubble, resulting in a lower P_aO_2 being measured. Likewise, because an air bubble has practically no CO_2, a sample will equilibrate and spuriously lower the P_aCO_2. Because of the difference in blood/air solubility coefficients between O_2 and CO_2, the response is more marked with oxygen. As expected, along with decreases in CO_2, the pH will increase. Great care, therefore, must be taken to minimize agitation of a sample that has come into contact with air bubbles. Expelling air from the syringe immediately upon sampling is important and will reduce the occurrence of these errors.

Anticoagulants: Addition of heparin to a blood sample

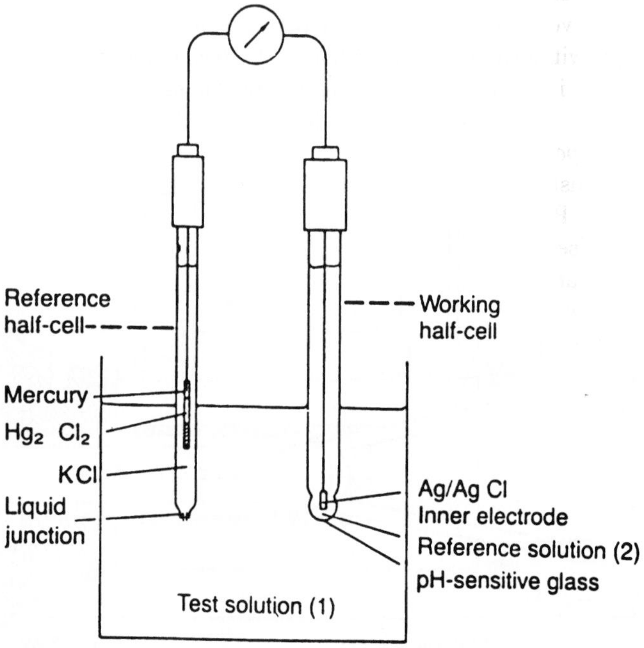

Figure 10.34. Sanz pH electrode. (From Malley WJ. Clinical blood gases. Philadelphia: WB Saunders, 1990:379.)

Table 10.11. Arterial Blood Gas Sampling Errors

	F_IO_2	pH (units)	PCO_2 (mm Hg)	PO_2 (mm Hg)	BE (mEq/liter)	HCO_3^- (mEq/liter)	SO_2 (%)
Normal	0.21	7.40	40	100	0	24	100
Normal	1.0	7.40	40	600	0	24	100
Venous	0.21	7.38	48	40	0	24	75
Air bubble	0.21	7.40	36	138	0	24	100
Air bubble	1.0	7.40	36	260	0	24	100
Heparin	1.0	7.36	36	260	0	24	100
1-hr delay	0.21	7.35	45	68	0	24	92
30°C patient	0.21	7.50	30	54	0	24	100

may dilute the concentrations of gases in the total sample. In contrast to contamination with an air bubble, the major blood gas error associated with excessive heparin is a drop in P_aCO_2. The different solubility coefficients between O_2 and CO_2 (here between blood and heparin) lessen the effects on O_2[101]. The pH of the sample generally does not change because the effects of decreased PCO_2 on pH are canceled by the acidic pH of the heparin solution[102].

As the sample size gets smaller, the relative contribution of the heparin becomes more significant. Newer machines, able to give accurate results with as little as 0.2 ml, may be confounded by up to 40% dilution with anticoagulant in neonatal blood gas samples[103]. Newer syringes prepared with a crystalline heparin may minimize the effects of the dilution. However, it remains important to adhere to proper dilution techniques and to obtain large enough samples to minimize this effect.

Metabolism: Even though the blood sample is placed in a syringe, it remains living tissue. As such, the cellular components (mainly reticulocytes and immature leukocytes) continue to consume oxygen and produce carbon dioxide. This has been recognized to cause a significant effect in patients with severe leukocytosis[104,105]. If the sample is immediately placed in ice, the changes will become very small even over several hours. If a sample cannot be analyzed within 20 minutes, it is appropriate to immerse the syringe in a cup of ice slurry until the sample can be analyzed.

Temperature correction of blood gases: There is a direct relationship between temperature and pressure that causes higher PO_2 and PCO_2 readings at higher temperatures. Likewise, this relationship dictates lower results at lower temperatures. The pH would be expected to follow the changes in PCO_2.

A substantial controversy on temperature correction of blood gases is rooted in the complexities of carbon dioxide and oxygen transport in blood involving both gas solution and chemical reactions that are affected by temperature variation[106,107]. A blood sample from a patient will manifest different gas tensions of O_2 and CO_2 when analyzed at different temperatures.

Blood gases measured in the laboratory at 37°C are called *alpha-stat,* whereas blood gases corrected to the patient's actual temperature are called *pH-stat.* A mechanically ventilated, hypothermic patient with a body temperature of 28°C may have a P_aCO_2 of 40 mm Hg when the blood gas is measured at 37°C. This value would be reported as a P_aCO_2 of 25 mm Hg when corrected for the 28°C. The pH (7.4 at 37°C) of this corrected sample would be 7.52, and the clinician might be inclined to modify therapy to normalize the corrected P_aCO_2 and pH. Animal studies have reported persuasive evidence of the metabolic benefit of increasing alkalosis as temperature decreases if the pH and P_aCO_2 are normal (i.e., 7.4 and 40 mm Hg, respectively) when measured at 37°C (alpha-stat)[108]. Normalization of the corrected (pH-stat) pH and P_aCO_2 in the hypothermic patient would create a relative respiratory acidosis at 28°C, which may be unacceptable.

Evaluation of oxygenation may be significantly affected by the contribution of temperature effect on the arterial blood gas. The oxyhemoglobin dissociation curve will shift to the left with hypothermia, causing C_aO_2 and S_pO_2 to rise for any given P_aO_2 as temperature falls. The measured S_pO_2 (and C_aO_2, if we ignore dissolved O_2) equals the true S_pO_2 in vivo as temperature changes, and thus no correction is needed. Temperature correction for P_aO_2 (particularly if the value at 37°C is borderline hypoxic) may be appropriate, although there are no data on biologic importance of such corrected values.

Unfortunately, a clear understanding of the normal blood gas tensions at various temperatures is still forthcoming. Therefore, it is difficult to suggest what to accept as an adequate P_aCO_2 or P_aO_2 for a child whose core temperature is 30°C or 40°C. At this time we do not believe there are sufficient data to support routine temperature correction of blood gases (pH-stat) obtained in the pediatric intensive care unit, and we use 37°C results (alpha-stat) for patients, regardless of their body temperature, for interpretation of acid-base status **(Table 10.11).**

Interpretation of Clinical Blood Gas Values

Definition of the normal range: The normal mean blood gas values for subjects of different ages are listed in **Table 10.10.** Blood gas values for pH outside of this normal range reflect either acidemia or alkalemia, whereas P_aCO_2 values outside of the normal range reflect either hypoventilation or hyperventilation **(Table 10.12).**

The relationship between P_aO_2 and oxygen saturation (S_pO_2) is a significant determinant of the oxygen content of blood. Therefore, merely knowing the P_aO_2 for a patient does not offer enough information to determine if that par-

Table 10.12. Nomenclature for P_aCO_2 and pH Outside of Acceptable Ranges

pH >7.50
Alkalemia (metabolic and/or respiratory alkalosis)
pH <7.30
Acidemia (metabolic and/or respiratory acidosis)
P_aCO_2 >50 mm Hg
Alveolar hypoventilation (respiratory acidosis)
P_ACO_2 >30 mm Hg
Alveolar hyperventilation (respiratory alkalosis)

ticular patient is "well oxygenated." In the clinical setting, however, at a P_aO_2 above 60 mm Hg, hemoglobin is likely to be more than 90% saturated with O_2, which is adequate to support most patients (see Chapter 4).

Arterial blood gas interpretation: In the approach to any set of blood gases, two basic aspects of breathing are assessed: ventilation (and acid-base balance) and oxygenation. One systematic method of arterial blood gas interpretation of acid-base disorders consists of (a) determining the degree of alveolar ventilation, based on the P_aCO_2; (b) assessing whether the patient's pH can be explained solely on the basis of P_aCO_2 or whether a metabolic component also exists; (c) determining whether the ventilatory or metabolic event was primary or compensatory; and (d) assessing the effectiveness of correction of any hypoxemic state.

Adequacy of alveolar ventilation: Minute ventilation (V_E) is composed of alveolar ventilation (V_A) plus dead space ventilation (V_D):

$$V_E = V_A + V_D \qquad \text{(Eq. 10.10)}$$

In general, the spontaneously ventilating patient is not expected to change dead space ventilation significantly with a change in minute ventilation. Increases in minute ventilation without increases in physiologic dead space lead to decreased P_aCO_2 in patients with adequate cardiopulmonary reserves. One can graph the expected relationship between P_aCO_2 and minute ventilation on the basis of a form of the Bohr equation (Eq. 10.11, Fig. 10.35)[66]. A significant disparity between minute volume and expected P_aCO_2 should alert the physician to the possibility that increased dead space may be present.

It is possible to predict the necessary minute ventilation to effect a desired change in P_aCO_2. Assuming CO_2 output is constant, then

$$V_{A1} \times P_{A1}CO_2 = V_{A2} \times P_{A2}CO_2$$

and rearrangement of the formula yields

$$V_{A2} = (V_{A1} \times P_{A1}CO_2)/P_{A2}CO_2 \qquad \text{(Eq. 10.11)}$$

where $P_{A1}CO_2$ is the present alveolar concentration of CO_2, V_{A1} is the alveolar ventilation that produces $P_{A1}CO_2$, $P_{A2}CO_2$ is the desired alveolar CO_2 concentration, and V_{A2} is the predicted alveolar ventilation to produce this change.

Based on this understanding of the relationship of P_ACO_2 (and P_aCO_2) and minute ventilation, one assesses the adequacy of alveolar ventilation and classifies the blood gas in one of three categories:

1. Respiratory alkalosis (hyperventilation) (P_aCO_2 less than 30 mm Hg)
2. Acceptable alveolar ventilation (P_aCO_2 equal to 30–50 mm Hg)
3. Respiratory acidosis (hypoventilation) (P_aCO_2 more than 50 mm Hg)

Therefore, the first determination during evaluation of the arterial blood gas is the adequacy of alveolar ventilation to eliminate the CO_2 produced by the body. If the P_aCO_2 falls within the range of 30 to 0 mm Hg, alveolar ventilation is in the acceptable range. If, however, P_aCO_2 is below 30 mm Hg or above 50 mm Hg, then hyperventilation or hypoventilation, respectively, is present[95].

Initial assessment of acid-base status: Initial evaluation of the results from a blood gas allows immediate determination of the present acid-base status of the patient. By simply applying the result to the definitions noted earlier **(Table 10.11),** one can identify acidemia (pH less than 7.30), alkalemia (pH more than 7.50), or normal range (pH equal to 7.30 to 7.50)[95].

Just as there is a relationship between minute ventilation and P_aCO_2, there is a predictable relationship that occurs between pH and P_aCO_2 because of chemical reactions involving the plasma bicarbonate-plasma carbonic acid pool. Respiratory acid-base change is thus represented by changes in P_aCO_2 due to variations in alveolar ventilation. Investigation of healthy volunteers has allowed the determination of some of the relationships between pH and carbon dioxide in humans[109,110]. Although the relationship between pH and P_aCO_2 is not precisely linear, within clinical ranges it is adequate to apply a linear model for bedside calculations of acute ventilatory changes. If a starting normal P_aCO_2 of 40 mm Hg is assumed, for every increase

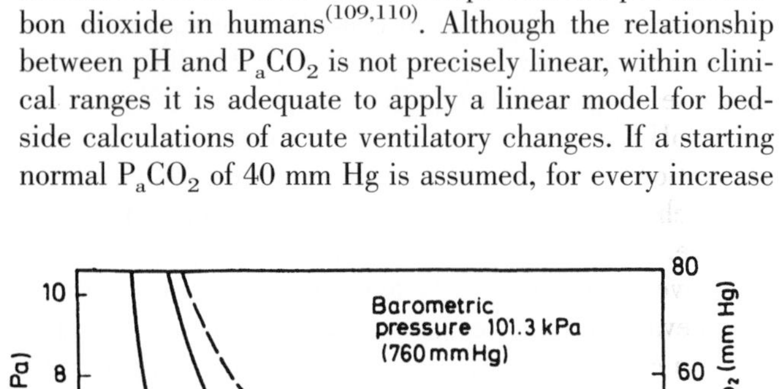

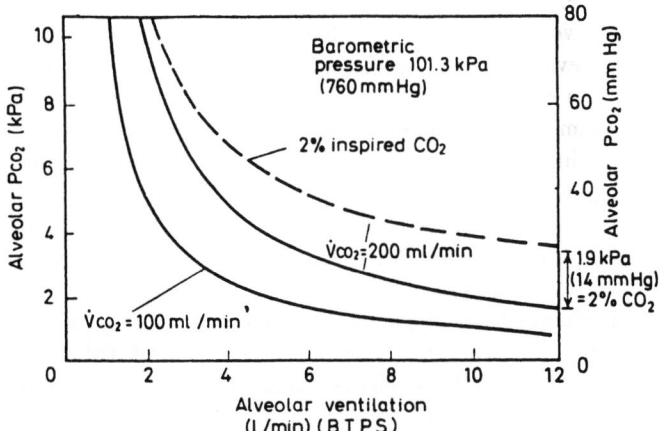

Figure 10.35. Effect of CO_2 output, alveolar ventilation, and inspired CO_2 concentration on alveolar PCO_2. (From Nunn JF. Appendix B. The gas laws. In: Applied respiratory physiology. Boston: Butterworths, 1987:501–504.)

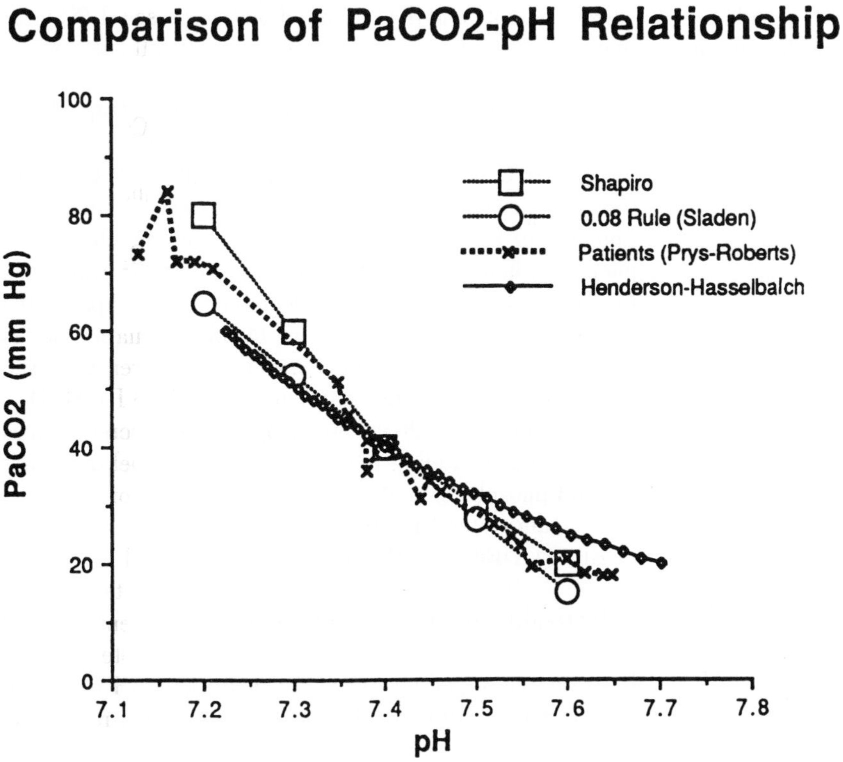

Figure 10.36. $PaCO_2$-pH relationship as determined by three different methods, compared with that found in patients. See text for details.

in P_aCO_2 of 20 mm Hg the pH will decrease by 0.10 unit, and for every decrease in P_aCO_2 of 10 mm Hg the pH will increase by 0.10 unit (Fig. 10.36)[95].

An alternative, simplified method for estimating the relationship between pH and P_aCO_2 is to average the positive and negative inverse relationship to 0.08 pH units for each deviation in P_aCO_2 of 10 mm Hg, in either direction from normal[111].

These two methods of estimating the relationship between pH and P_aCO_2 as well as the data from human investigations are represented in Figure 10.21. To simplify our approach to the interpretation of ventilation and acid-base balance, the "0.08 pH unit method" is used below for illustrative purposes.

By evaluating the relationship between P_aCO_2 and pH, one can determine the extent to which ventilation and metabolism are acutely contributing to the acid-base status. By noting the difference between the expected P_aCO_2 (assumed to be 40 mm Hg) and the result, one can determine the expected pH for that PCO_2, assuming a balanced system. The remaining difference from expected pH determines the contribution from metabolic effects.

For example, a blood gas result has a P_aCO_2 of 60 mm Hg and a pH of 7.24. The difference between the measured P_aCO_2 and the expected P_aCO_2 of 40 mm Hg is 20 mm Hg. For every P_aCO_2 increase of 10 mm Hg above normal, we expect pH to decrease by 0.08 units. Therefore, for this sample with a P_aCO_2 increase of 20 mm Hg, we expect a decrease of 0.16 pH units. Subtracting this from our expected normal pH (7.40 to 0.16) gives a pH of 7.24, which is the sample result. The decrease in pH can be attributed wholly to acute hypoventilation and is termed *respiratory acidosis.*

In another simplified example, a P_aCO_2 of 24 is obtained with a pH of 7.53. The difference between the measured P_aCO_2 and the expected P_aCO_2 of 40 mm Hg is 16 mm Hg. For every P_aCO_2 decrease of 10 mm Hg below normal, we expect pH to increase by 0.08 units. Therefore, for this sample with a P_aCO_2 decrease of 16 mm Hg, we expect an increase in pH of 0.128 units (16/10) × 0.08) to 7.53. This example demonstrates respiratory alkalosis resulting from acute hyperventilation, accounting for the entire change in pH.

Further evaluation must now determine if this state of alveolar ventilation (hyperventilation, normal ventilation, or hypoventilation) is acute or chronic and to what extent it affects any underlying metabolic derangement.

Metabolic acid-base effects: Several attempts have been made to separate the relationship of pH and PCO_2 from the body's metabolic buffer system. Such methods have been described as CO_2-combining power (alkali reserve), standard bicarbonate[112], and base excess[113]. In spite of its inherent inability to take into account the contribution of intracellular and interstitial compartments in the body's response to acid-base disturbances, the base excess system is widely used in clinical medicine. Finally, for some investigators, plasma bicarbonate concentration remains a better alternative as an aid in the assessment of acid-base disturbance[114].

Plasma bicarbonate—HCO_3: The Henderson-

Hasselbalch equation allows us to describe the carbonic acid system with measurable components from the laboratory:

$$pH = pKa + \log(HCO_3^-/\alpha CO_2) \quad \text{(Eq. 10.12)}$$

where pKa is the dissociation constant for the overall reaction shown in Equation 10.9, and α is the solubility coefficient for CO_2 in plasma, with the units in millimoles per liter multiplied by millimeters Hg PCO_2. For plasma at 37°C,

$$pH = 6.1 + \log(HCO_3^-/0.03\ PCO_2) \quad \text{(Eq. 10.13)}$$

with normal values of P_aCO_2 equal to 40 mm Hg and of HCO_3^- equal to 24 mmol/liter. This equation emphasizes the balancing effect on pH that the respiratory system (regulating PCO_2) and the renal system (regulating HCO_3^-) control. Hence, the ultimate pH of the system will reflect the ratio between contributions from each system and thus provide a basis for normal compensatory mechanisms. Compensation is defined as the process of altering the unaffected component in the ratio (HCO_3^- or PCO_2) in an attempt to normalize the overall ratio and attain a normal pH[(101)]. Complicating this relationship is the fact that an alteration in one may have a direct (i.e., not only a compensatory) effect on the other; in general, however, the concept of specific markers for respiratory versus metabolic components of acid-base balance is clinically useful. Finally, knowing two of the three components in the equation allows determination of the third. Substitution in the above equation identifies the normal ratio between HCO_3^- and PCO_2 as

$$\begin{aligned} &\log(HCO_3^-/0.03\ PCO_2) \quad \text{(Eq. 10.14)} \\ &= \log(24/0.03 \times 40) \\ &= \log(24/1.2) \\ &= \log(20/1) \end{aligned}$$

and allows confirmation that normal pH is 6.1 plus log(20) or 7.4. Increases in the ratio from larger amounts of HCO_3^- or smaller values of PCO_2 will produce a higher pH (alkalosis), while decreases will yield a lower pH (acidosis).

Base excess/deficit: A limitation of determining the plasma bicarbonate in clinical situations is that it does not show directly the amount, in milliequivalents of blood, of fixed acid or base causing a change in the base content of a blood sample. This is attributed to the fact that only 75% of the buffer action of blood is due to the carbon dioxide-bicarbonate system[(113)]. The remainder of the buffering system is accounted for by hemoglobin, phosphate, and plasma proteins. Approximations in determining the total base deficit or excess (BE) have used a correction for plasma bicarbonate by multiplying the difference between the normal bicarbonate of 24 and the measured bicarbonate by 1.20, such that

$$BE = -1.2\,(24 - \text{measuredbicarbonate}) \quad \text{(Eq. 10.15)}$$

Exact correction requires knowledge of all buffers in addition to bicarbonate, especially the hemoglobin concentration. Buffer base (BB) defines the amount of buffering capacity in whole blood that includes buffer anions in addition to bicarbonate, especially hemoglobin. BE compares the buffering capacity in the patient's blood with normal and is determined by consultation with the Siggaard-Andersen nomogram (Fig. 10.37). This relates pH, PCO_2, and HCO_3^- while factoring the effects of hemoglobin and other sources of buffering (including plasma and intracellular bicarbonate and phosphates and the plasma proteins).

In acute states an approximation of the effect of change in BE (PIgDBE) on pH can be stated as

$$10\ \text{mEq/liter}\ (\Delta BE) = 0.15\ \text{pH unit}\ (\Delta pH) \quad \text{(Eq. 10.16)}$$

For example, a patient whose BE increases from 0 to +10 after vomiting will raise pH from 7.40 to 7.55 if there is no change in alveolor ventilation. The appeal of the base excess system is that it allows both a qualitative (plus or minus) and quantitative (milliequivalents per liter of blood) determination of buffering capacity. Metabolic alkalosis is associated with a positive base excess, and metabolic acidosis is associated with a negative base excess (base deficit).

Inherent in this system, designed to simplify an extremely complex process, are exceptions and errors. The base excess system may incorrectly quantify the magnitude of a calculated value as well as wrongly identify combined metabolic and respiratory acidosis when a pure respiratory acidosis is present[(101)]. An additional drawback is that this system was designed to diagnose acute disorders and may misclassify chronic conditions. For instance, normal renal compensations for hypoventilation may appear as a metabolic alkalosis complicating respiratory acidosis.

Bicarbonate therapy: An advantage of the base deficit system in the clinical setting is that it allows the calculation of the amount of buffer that can be administered to correct metabolic acidosis. One-third of body weight can be used to estimate extracellular water in calculating total body base deficit:

$$\begin{aligned} &\text{Total body base deficit} = \quad \text{(Eq. 10.17)} \\ &BE \times \text{body weight (kg)}/3 \end{aligned}$$

For example, in a 30-kg patient with a base deficit (i.e., negative base excess) of −10 mEq/liter as determined from the nomogram, one calculates extracellular water to be 10 liters. To correct the total body base deficit, one must add 10 mEq of bicarbonate for each liter of extracellular water, thus 100 mEq total. Most experts would recommend using half of this dose (50 mEq) of bicarbonate and rechecking the result.

Assessment of hypoxemic state: Further evaluation of the arterial blood gas requires assessment of the effectiveness of oxygenation of the blood. Note that this, in and of itself, does not allow evaluation of oxygenation of the patient as a whole. As discussed in Chapter 4, determination of an adequate amount of oxygen delivery may best be related to arterial oxygen content (C_aO_2) and cardiac output. Arterial oxygen content is closely related to hemoglobin saturation, which in turn is related to P_aO_2 by the sigmoid relationship of the oxyhemoglobin dissociation curve. It is with this knowledge that we relate the P_aO_2 to the adequacy of blood oxygenation, with all of its inherent limitations. In general, a patient is considered hypoxemic if the P_aO_2 is less than 60 mm Hg and the oxygen saturation is less than 90%.

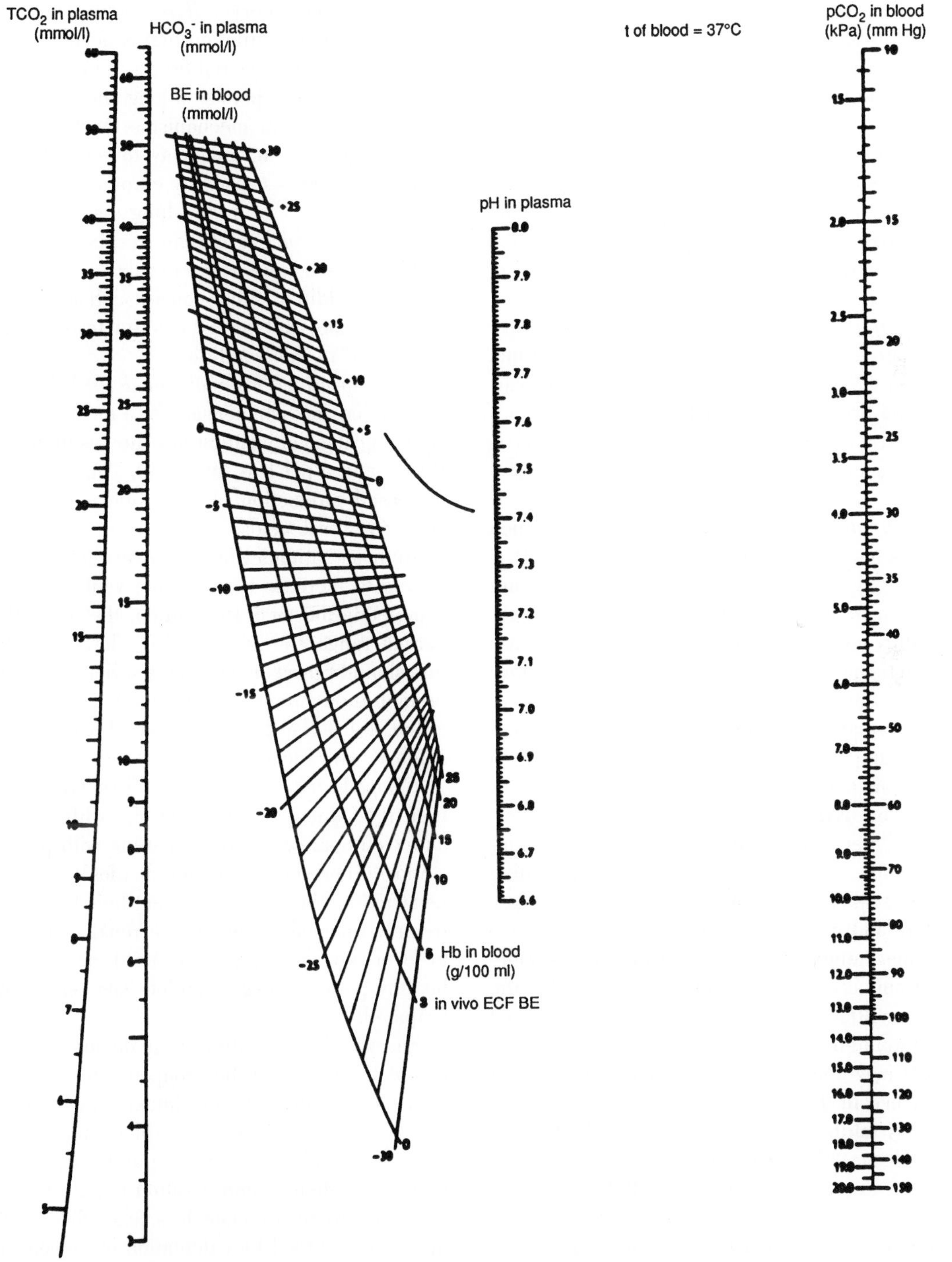

Figure 10.37. Alignment nomogram of Siggaard-Andersen, widely used in teaching and clinical reporting of acid-base balance. TCO_2, total CO_2; *t*, temperature; *BE*, base excess; *Hb*, hemoglobin; *ECF*, extracellular fluid. (From Severinghaus J. Acid-base alignment nomogram: a Boston-Copenhagen dePlaatente. Anesthesiology 1976; 45:539.)

Furthermore, the evaluation of any patient's oxygenation status must be related to the state in which the patient has been studied. For example, even though the blood gas of a patient with a P_aO_2 of 96 mm Hg is not truly hypoxemic, knowing that this sample was obtained while the patient was breathing 100% oxygen allows an interpretation of severe oxygenation deficit. Conversely, if this sample had been obtained while the patient was breathing room air, no hypoxemic state would exist.

Classification of primary acid-base disturbances and compensation: After initial evaluation of a blood gas, it is then convenient to classify acid-base disturbances and compensation as well as the effectiveness of oxygen therapy in order to facilitate communication and monitoring over time. Following is an outline of major disturbances based on the system of evaluation presented above. This should serve as a basis for classifying interpretation from arterial blood gases and allow identification of major abnormalities on the basis of clinical evaluation and a sound understanding of pathophysiology.

Acceptable ventilatory and metabolic acid-base status: The normal situation is represented by a P_aCO_2 of 40 mm Hg and a pH of 7.4. This indicates that the amount of carbon dioxide being produced from metabolism is being adequately cleared by the amount of ventilation. The pH is normal and is not accompanied by an alteration in the PCO_2 or base excess.

Alveolar hyperventilation (respiratory alkalosis): When the P_aCO_2 is less than 30 mm Hg and the change in pH is accounted for entirely by the decrease in P_aCO_2, the compensatory mechanism of the kidneys has not been invoked, and the ventilatory change is recent. Bicarbonate and base excess will be in the normal range because the kidneys have not had adequate time to establish effective compensatory mechanisms. Pain and anxiety are common causes of acute hyperventilation and respiratory alkalosis in children. In addition, hypoxemia may lead to an increase in minute ventilation (to maintain oxygenation) and thus lead to a respiratory alkalosis. Other causes may include overzealous mechanical ventilation, restrictive lung disease (including fibrosis, ascites, scoliosis, pregnancy), and severe congestive heart failure and pulmonary emboli.

Hypoxia or mechanical ventilation longer than 24 hours may lead to chronic alveolar hyperventilation such that the P_aCO_2 is less than 30 mm Hg, but pH is much less elevated (alkalotic) than would be expected on the basis of the P_aCO_2 and, in fact, pH may approach the normal 7.4. Normal pH may be approached in the face of lowered P_aCO_2, because decreased P_aCO_2 inhibits tubular reabsorption of HCO_3^- in the kidney. Hence, plasma HCO_3^- may be reduced by 4–5 mEq/liter for every 10-mm-Hg fall in PCO_2 below 40 mm Hg.

Hypoventilation (respiratory acidosis) and pH: Elevation of the P_aCO_2 above the normal range indicates alveolar hypoventilation and must be further classified as acute, chronic, or partially compensated. Once again, the basis for determination of the resulting state depends on an evaluation of the blood gas in light of the clinical situation.

Acute ventilatory failure (respiratory acidosis): Association of an elevated P_aCO_2 and a low pH represents an acute change in the ventilatory state. Causes include respiratory pathophysiology, drug intoxication (e.g., narcotics, sedatives), residual neuromuscular blockade, or central nervous system disease, such as head trauma.

Chronic ventilatory failure (respiratory acidosis): Inadequate alveolar ventilation that is accompanied by a pH in the acceptable range represents a primary ventilatory abnormality that has persisted long enough for the kidneys to compensate. Renal mechanisms increase the excretion of H^+ within 24 hours and may to some degree correct the resulting acidosis caused by chronic retention of CO_2 (respiratory acid)[115]. Chronic lung disease is the most common cause of such a chronic respiratory acidosis and includes bronchopulmonary dysplasia in the pediatric age group. In addition, other causes such as opiates, neuromuscular disease, and severe electrolyte disturbances may be implicated in this condition.

Uncompensated metabolic acidosis: When the respiratory system does not compensate for a metabolic acidosis by increasing alveolar ventilation, the result will be a normal P_aCO_2 and a pH less than 7.30. This occurs as a result of increased production of metabolic acids and/or failure to eliminate these acids.

In those patients who have overwhelming acidosis or are unable to increase their minute ventilation to compensate completely for such a condition, the pH will not return to normal range and will remain below 7.30. This combination should raise concern that a serious condition exists and prompt intervention is warranted to treat the underlying cause, assist ventilation, and possibly correct the metabolic acidosis with bicarbonate.

Compensated metabolic acidosis: Alveolar hyperventilation (P_aCO_2 less than 30 mm Hg) with a pH of 7.30–7.40 and a clinical scenario compatible with primary metabolic acidosis represents metabolic acidosis that has been compensated by the increase in ventilation. In general, it is extremely unusual for either the renal or respiratory system to overcompensate, but in mild acidoses in otherwise healthy patients, near-complete compensation may be anticipated.

Several clinical entities may demonstrate this acid-base disorder, which may be grouped into categories of (a) increased acid production or intake (e.g., diabetic ketoacidosis or salicylate poisoning), (b) decreased acid excretion (e.g., renal failure), (c) renal tubular dysfunction with impaired bicarbonate conservation (e.g., renal tubular acidosis), and (d) bicarbonate loss (e.g., diarrhea). Differential diagnosis is aided by calculation of unmeasured anions or anion gap:

$$\text{Anion gap} = Na^+ - (Cl^- + HCO_3^-) \qquad \text{(Eq. 10.18)}$$

When the normal anion gap of 12 mEq/liter is exceeded, excess acid production or decreased acid excretion is the likely diagnosis **(Table 10.13).**

In general, patients with chronic metabolic acidosis are unable to hyperventilate sufficiently to lower P_aCO_2 for complete compensation to pH 7.4. This fact, together with the clinical history, serves to distinguish chronic metabolic acidosis from chronic alveolar hyperventilation with compensatory metabolic acidosis, in which complete compensation is more likely to occur.

Uncompensated metabolic alkalosis: Failure of the ventilatory system to compensate for a metabolic alkalosis may be represented by a normal P_aCO_2 associated with a pH greater than 7.50. This failure to compensate may be based on other mechanisms that drive the respiratory centers, such as hypoxemia[(116)]. This condition may be the result of continuous acid removal without the ability to compensate via hypoventilation, as in the continuous nasogastric suctioning of a patient who is mechanically ventilated or in the chronic vomiting of a patient with pyloric stenosis[(115)].

Partially compensated metabolic alkalosis: When a pH more than 7.50 is accompanied by inadequate alveolar ventilation, a primary metabolic alkalosis for which the respiratory system is partially compensating is probably present[(117)]. A child who is losing tremendous amounts of stomach acid through the vomiting associated with pyloric stenosis may compensate for the resulting metabolic alkalosis by retaining CO_2 through hypoventilation. The child's ability to compensate will be limited by hypoxia[(118)].

Uncorrected hypoxemia: If a patient is receiving increased inspired oxygen concentration and arterial blood gas results remain in the hypoxemic range (P_aO_2 less than 60 mm Hg), then attempts at correction have been unsuccessful. The blood gas, therefore, indicates a condition of uncorrected hypoxemia, and other efforts must be implemented to afford adequate oxygenation. Various causes of hypoxemia are identified in Chapter 4.

Corrected hypoxemia: In corrected hypoxemia, oxygen therapy has corrected arterial hypoxemia (which would otherwise be present) to a level within the acceptable range. This designation, in essence, makes two statements: first, that the patient would otherwise be hypoxemic if left to breathe room air, and second, that the selected method of support (increased F_IO_2, PEEP, etc.) was appropriate for the extent of pulmonary deficit.

Excessively corrected hypoxemia: When a patient is receiving more oxygen than is necessary to correct a hypoxemic state, the arterial blood gas may reflect this as a P_aO_2 above the normal range. This may be of concern, especially for infants at risk for retinopathy of prematurity, excessive pulmonary blood flow, and pulmonary oxygen toxicity. Further detailed evaluation may depend on determination of shunt fraction (Qs/Q_T), oxygen delivery and consumption, and alveolar-arterial oxygen gradient (see Chapter 4).

Table 10.13. Classification of Metabolic Acidosis by Anion Gap[a]

Increased anion gap
Ketoacidosis
Lactic acidosis
Toxic ingestion
Renal failure
Glycogen disorders
Normal anion gap
Renal tubular acidosis
Hypoaldosteronism
Potassium-sparing diuretics
Diarrhea
Carbonic anhydrase inhibitors
Acid administration (HCl, NH_4Cl, arginine HCl)
Intravenous hyperalimentation
Sulfamylon, cholestyramine

[a] *Modified from Barash PG, Cullen BF, Stoelting RK. Clinical anesthesia. Philadelphia: JB Lippincott, 1989:697.*

FUTURE CONSIDERATIONS

Future respiratory monitoring systems will incorporate all of the previously described bedside automation with computer feedback systems to close the loop in patient care decision making. In addition, clinical data management systems will allow storage of large volumes of continuously acquired monitoring data. Retrieval and analysis of such data will permit more accurate diagnosis and understanding of the pathophysiology of a variety of respiratory events. However, these systems will be useful only if they increase resource use, decrease cost, and improve patient outcomes.

SUMMARY

Respiratory monitoring has changed dramatically over the last 20 years. Accurate monitoring can now be performed for all patient groups in the critical care unit. Regardless of the method, the goal of intensive care monitoring remains optimization of patient care while minimizing morbidity, mortality, and cost.

References

1. Tobin M. Respiratory monitoring in the intensive care unit. Am Rev Respir Dis 1988;138:1625.
2. Pardee N, Winterbauer R, Allen J. Bedside evaluation of respiratory distress. Chest 1984;85:203.
3. Siegal J, Miller A, Brown L, Teirstein AB. Pulmonary diffusing capacity in left ventricular dysfunction. Chest 1990;98:550.
4. Clausen J. CHF, rales and the D_{CO}. Chest 1990;98:523.
5. Eisenberg P, Hansbrough J, Anderson D, Schuster D. A prospective study of lung water measurements during pulmonary artery catheter management in an intensive care unit. Am Rev Respir Dis 1984;136:662.
6. Truemper E, Vargo T. Principles of pediatric intensive care: monitoring pulmonary function. In: Oski F, ed. Principles and practice of pediatrics. Philadelphia: JB Lippincott, 1990:985.
7. Pasterkamp H. The history and physical examination. In: Chernick V, ed. Kendig's disorders of the respiratory tract in children. Philadelphia: WB Saunders, 1990:59.
8. Little G, ed. Infantile apnea and home monitoring: report of a consensus development conference. Bethesda, Maryland: National Institutes of Health, NIH 87–2905, 1987:3.

9. Scheller J, Loeb R. Respiratory artifact during pulse oximetry in critically ill patients. Anesthesiology 1988;69:602.
10. Yelderman M, New W. Evaluation of pulse oximetry. Anesthesiology 1983;59:349.
11. Severinghaus J, Naifeh K. Accuracy of response of six pulse oximeters to profound hypoxia. Anesthesiology 1987;67:551.
12. Hensley F, Dodson D, Martin D, et al. Oxygen saturation during placement of invasive monitoring in the premedicated, unanesthetized cardiac patient (Abstract). Anesthesiology 1985;65:A22.
13. Cooper J, Cullen D, Nemeskal, et al. Effects of information feedback and pulse oximetry on the incidence of anesthesia complications. Anesthesiology 1987;67:686.
14. Tyler I, Tantisira B, Winter P, Motoyama E. Continuous monitoring of arterial oxygen saturation with pulse oximetry during transfer to the recovery room. Anesth Analg 1985;64:1108.
15. Barker SJ, Tremper K. The effect of carbon monoxide inhalation on pulse oximetry and transcutaneous PO_2. Anesthesiology 1987;66:677.
16. Hampson N. Arterial oxygenation in carbon monoxide poisoning (Letter). Chest 1990;98:1538.
17. Eisencraft J. Pulse oximeter desaturation due to methemoglobinemia. Anesthesiology 1988;68:279.
18. Barker S, Tremper K, Hyatt J. Effects of methemoglobinemia on pulse oximetry and mixed-venous oximetry. Anesthesiology 1989;70:112.
19. Kessler M, Eide R, Humayun B, Poppers P. Spurious pulse oximeter desaturation with methylene blue injection. Anesthesiology 1986;65:435.
20. Scheller M, Unger R, Kelner M. Effects of intravenously administered dyes on pulse oximetry readings. Anesthesiology 1986;65:550.
21. Veyckemans F, Baele P, Guillaume J, et al. Hyperbilirubinemia does not interfere with hemoglobin saturation measured by pulse oximetry. Anesthesiology 1989;70:118.
22. Schnapp L, Cohen N. Pulse oximetry: uses and abuses. Chest 1990;98:1244.
23. Mark J. Systolic venous waves cause spurious signs of arterial desaturation. Anesthesiology 1989;71:158.
24. Brooks D, Paulus D, Winkle W. Infrared heat lamps interfere with pulse oximeters. Anesthesiology 1984;61:630.
25. Hanowell L. Ambient light affects pulse oximeters. Anesthesiology 1987;67:864.
26. Nellcor Incorporated. Controlling external optical interference in pulse oximetry. Pulse Oximetry Note No. 5, 1986.
27. Swedlow D, Running V, Feaster S. Pulse oximetry (Letter). Anesthesiology 1987;67:865.
28. AARC Clinical Practice Guidleines. Transcutaneous Blood Gas Monitoring For Neonates and Pediatric Patients. Resp. Care 1994;39:12: 1176–1179.
29. Hamilton PA, Whitehead MD, Reynolds ER: Underestimation of arterial oxygen tension by transcutaneous electrode with increasing age in infants. Arch Dis Child 1985;60:1162–1165.
30. Rome ES, Stork EK, Carlo WA, et al: Limitations of trancutaneous PO_2 and PCO_2 monitoring in infants with bronchopulmonary dysplasia. Pediatics 1984;74:217–220.
31. Durand M, Ramanathan R: Pulse oximetry for continuous oxygen monitoring in sick newborn infants. J Pediatr 1986; 109:1052–1056.
32. Swedlow D, Irving S. Monitoring and patient safety. In: Blitt C, ed. Monitoring in anesthesia and critical care medicine. New York: Churchill Livingstone, 1990:50.
33. Badgwell J, McLeod M, Lerman J, Creighton R. End-tidal pCO_2 monitoring in infants and children during ventilation with the Air-Shields Ventimeter ventilator (Abstract). Anesthesiology 1986;65:A418.
34. Novametrix CO2SMO Operating Manual, Wallingford, CT, Novametrix Medic al Systems, Inc.
35. Linko K, Paloheimo M, Tammisto T. Capnography for detection of accidental oesophageal intubation. Acta Anaesthesiol Scand 1983;199:2.
36. Mihm F, Feeley T, Rodarte A. Monitoring end-tidal carbon dioxide tensions with high-frequency jet ventilation in dogs with normal lungs. Crit Care Med 1984;12:180.
37. Carlon G, Ray C, Miodowink S, et al. Capnography in mechanically ventilated patients. Crit Care Med 1988; 16:550.
38. Snyder J, Elliot L, Grevnik A. Capnography. In: Spence A, ed. Clinics of critical care medicine. Edinburgh: Churchill Livingstone, 1982:100–121.
39. Gazmuri R, von Planta M, Weil M, Rackow E. Arterial PCO_2 as an indicator of systemic perfusion during cardiopulmonary resuscitation. Crit Care Med 1989;17:237.
40. Gudipati C, Weil M, Bisera J, et al. Expired carbon dioxide: a noninvasive monitor of cardiopulmonary resuscitation. Circulation 1988;77:237.
41. Barton C, Callaham M. Lack of correlation between end-tidal carbon dioxide concentrations and P_aCO_2 in cardiac arrest. Crit Care Med 1991;19:108.
42. Trevino R, Bisera J, Weil M, et al. $ETCO_2$ as a guide to successful cardiopulmonary resuscitation: a preliminary report. Crit Care Med 1985;13:910.
43. Weil M, Bisera J, Trevino R, Rackow E. Cardiac output and $ETCO_2$. Crit Care Med 1985;13:907.
44. Abraham E, Yoshihara G. Cardiorespiratory effects of pressure controlled ventilation in severe respiratory failure. Chest 1990;98:1445.
45. Rappaport SH, Shipner R, Yoshihara G, Wright J, Chang P, Abraham E. Randomized, prospective trial of pressure-limited versus volume limited-ventilation in severe respiratory failure. Crit Care Med 1994;22:22.
46. Gattinoni L, Pesenti A, Bombino M, Baglioni S, Rivolta M, ossi RF, Rossi G, Fumagalli R, Marcolin R, Mascheroni D, Torresin A. Relationships between lung computed tomography density, gas exchange, and PEEP in acute respiratory failure. Anesthesiology 1988;69:831.
47. Slutsky AS. Mechanical Ventilation: ACCP Consensus Conference. Chest 1993;104:1843.
48. Hillman ND, Black DR, Craig DM, Kern FH, Ungerleider RM, Smith PK, Meliones JN. The effect of inspiratory time on cardiopulmonary interactions in a normal and injured lung model. Ped Res 1994;35:53A.
49. Falke KJ, Pontoppidan H, Kumar A, Leithe DE, Geffin B, Laver MB. Ventilation with end-expiratory pressure in acute lung disease. J Clin Invest 1972;51:2315.
50. Slutsky AS. Mechanical Ventilation: ACCP Consensus Conference. Chest 1993;104:1848.
51. Barrett-Boyes B, Wood E. The oxygen saturation of blood in the venae cavae, right-heart chambers, and pulmonary vessels of healthy subjects. J Lab Clin Med 1957;50:93.
52. Tobin M. Respiratory monitoring. JAMA 1990;264:244.
53. Simmons D, Alpas A, Tashkin D, Coulson A. Hyperlactatemia due to arterial hypoxemia or reduced cardiac output or both. J Appl Physiol 1978;45:195.
54. Kasnitz P, Druger G, Yorra F, Simmons P. Mixed venous oxygen tension and hyperlactatemia. JAMA 1976;236:570.
55. Boutros A, Lee C. Value of continuous monitoring of mixed venous blood oxygen saturation in the management of critically ill patients. Crit Care Med 1986;14:132.
56. Jastremski M, Chelluri L, Beney K, Bailly R. Analysis of the effects of continuous on-line monitoring of S_vO_2 on patient outcome and cost effectiveness. Crit Care Med 1989;17:148.
57. Strain D, Kinasewitz G, Vereen L, George R. Value of routine daily chest x-rays in the medical intensive care unit. Crit Care Med 1985;13:534.
58. Brunel W, Coleman D, Schwartz D, et al. Assessment of routine roentgenograms and the physical examination to confirm endotracheal tube position. Chest 1989;96:1043.
59. Hauser G, Pollock M, Sivit C, et al. The routine chest radiographs in pediatric intensive care: a prospective study. Pediatrics 1989;83:465.
60. Hall J, White S, Karrison T. Efficacy of daily routine chest radiographs in intubated, mechanically ventilated patients. Crit Care Med 1991;19:689.
61. Fiastro J, Habib M, Shan B, et al. Comparison of standard weaning parameters and the mechanical work of breathing in mechanically ventilated patients. Chest 1988;94:232.
62. Sahn S, Lakshminarayan S. Bedside criteria for discontinuation of mechanical ventilation. Chest 1973; 63:1002.
63. Tahvanainen J, Salmenpera M. Extubation criteria after weaning from intermittent mandatory ventilation and continuous positive airway pressure. Crit Care Med 1983;11:702.
64. Montgomery A, Halle R, Weagley S, et al. Prediction of successful weaning using airway occlusion pressure and hypercapnic challenge. Chest 1987;91:496.
65. Yang K, Tobin M. A prospective study of indexes predicting the outcome of trials of weaning from mechanical ventilation. N Engl J Med 1991;324:1445–1450.
66. Nunn JF. Appendix B. The gas laws. In: Applied respiratory physiology. Boston: Butterworths, 1987:501–504.
67. Matthews PJ. The validity of P_aO_2 values 3, 6, and 9 minutes after an F_IO_2 change in mechanically ventilated heart-surgery patients. Respir Care 1987;32:1029.
68. Goldberger J, Gaynard L, Wolfer J. Helping children cope with healthcare procedures. Contemp Pediatr 1990;7:141.

69. Wolfer J, Gaynard L, Goldberger J, Laidley LN, Thompson R. An experimental evaluation of a model child life program. CHC 1988; 16:244.
70. Cole FS, Todres ID, Shannon DC. Technique for percutaneous cannulation of the radial artery in the newborn infant. J Pediatr 1978; 92:105.
71. Gregory GA. Monitoring during surgery. New York: Churchill Livingstone, 1989:488.
72. Kisling JA, Schreiner RL. Techniques of obtaining arterial blood from newborn infants. Respir Care 1977;22:513.
73. Simmons MA, Levine RL, Lubchenco LO. Warning: serious sequelae of temporal artery catheterization. J Pediatr 1978;92:284.
74. Petty TL, Bigelow B, Levine BE. The simplicity and safety of arterial puncture. JAMA 1966;195:181.
75. Baker RJ, Chunpraph B, Nylus LN. Severe ischemia of the hand following radial artery catheterization. Surgery 1976;80:449.
76. Eriksen HC, Sorenson HR. Arterial injuries: iatrogenic and noniatrogenic. Acta Chir Scand 1969;135:133.
77. Mathieu A. Expanding aneurysm of the radial artery after frequent puncture. Anesthesiology 1973;38:401.
78. Mortensen JD. Clinical sequelae from arterial needle puncture, cannulation and incision. Circulation 1967; 35:1118.
79. Barnes RW, Hafermann MD, Peterson J, et al. Noninvasive assessment of altered limb hemodynamics and complications of arterial catheterization. Radiology 1973;107:505.
80. Klein MD, Coran AG, Whitehouse WM Jr, et al. Management of iatrogenic arterial injuries in infants and children. J Pediatr Surg 1982;17:933.
81. Bedford RF, Ashford TP. Aspirin pretreatment prevents postcannulation radial artery thrombosis. Anesthesiology 1979;51:176.
82. Symansky MR, Fox HA. Umbilical vessel catheterization. Indications, management, and evaluation of the technique. J Pediatr 1972; 80:820.
83. Cochran WD, Davis HT, Smith CA. Advantages and complications of umbilical artery catheterization in the newborn. Pediatrics 1968;42:769.
84. Adams JM, Rudolph AJ. The use of indwelling radial artery catheters in neonates. Pediatrics 1975;55:261.
85. Todres ID, Rogers MC, Shannon DC, et al. Percutaneous catheterization of the radial artery in the critically ill neonate. J Pediatr 1975;87:273.
86. AARC Clinical Practice Guideline. Capillary Blood Gas Sampling For Neonates and Pediatric Patients. Resp. Care 1994; 39:12:1180–1183.
87. Courtney SE, Weber KR, Breakie LA, et al. Capillary blood gases in the neonate. Am J Dis Child 1990;144:168.
88. Dong SH, Liu HM, Soong GW, et al. Arterialized capillary blood gases and acid-base studies in normal individuals from 29 days to 24 years of age. Am J Dis Child 1985;139:1019.
89. Gambino SR, Thiede WH. Comparisons of pH in human arterial, venous and capillary blood. Am J Clin Pathol 1959;32:298.
90. Frewen TC, Sumabat WO, Del Maestro RF. Cerebral blood flow, metabolic rate, and cross-brain oxygen consumption in brain injury. J Pediatr 1985;107:510.
91. Gayle MO, Frewen TC, Armstrong RF, et al. Regular venous bulb catheterization in infants and children. Crit Care Med 1989;17:385.
92. Robertson CS, Grossman RG, Goodman JC, Narayan RK. The predictive value of cerebral anaerobic metabolism with cerebral infarction after head injury. J Neurosurg 1987;67:361.
93. Stowe RW, Baer RF, Randall BF. Rapid measurement of the tension of carbon dioxide in blood. Arch Phys Med Rehabil 1957;38:646.
94. Severinghaus JW, Astrup P. Carbon dioxide, history of blood gas analysis. Boston: Little, Brown, 1987:224.
95. Shapiro BA, Harrison RA, Cane RD, Kozlowski-Temlin R. Guidelines for obtaining blood gas samples. Chicago: Year Book Medical Publishers, 1989:251.
96. Kavanagh F, Goodwin RO. Fluorescent indicators. Organ Chem Bull 1957;29:1.
97. Gehrich JL, Lubbers DW, Opitz N. Optical fluorescence and its application to an intravascular gas monitoring system. IEEE Trans Biomed Eng 1986;33:117.
98. Opitz N, Lubbers DW. New fluorescence photochemical techniques for simultaneous and continuous measurement of ionic strength and hydrogen ion activities. Sensors Actuators 1983;4:473.
99. Reck B, Himmelspach K, Opitz N, Lubbers DW. Model study with thyroxine on the possibility of continuous hormone measurement in the optode using the principle of homogeneous fluoroimmuno-assays. Pflugers Arch 1985;405:R64.
100. Biswas CK, Ramos JM, Agroyannis B, Kerr DNS. Blood gas analysis: effect of air bubbles in syringe and delay in estimation. Br Med J 1982;282:923–927.
101. Malley WJ. Clinical blood gases. Philadelphia: WB Saunders, 1990:379.
102. Goodwin NM, Schreiber MT. Effects of anticoagulants on acid-base and blood gas estimations. Crit Care Med 1979;7:473.
103. Fan LE, Dellinger KT, Mills AL. Potential errors in neonatal blood gas measurements. J Pediatr 1980; 97:650.
104. Fox MJ, Brody JS, Weintraub LR. Leukocyte larceny: a cause of spurious hypoxemia. Am J Med 1979; 67:742.
105. Shohat M, Schonfeld T, Zaizoz R. Determination of blood gases in children with extreme leukocytosis. Crit Care Med 1988;16:787.
106. Ream AK, Reitz BA, Silverberg G. Temperature correction of PCO_2 and pH in estimating acid-base status: an example of the emperor's new clothes? Anesthesiology 1982;56:41.
107. Rupp SM, Severinghaus JW. Hypothermia. In: Miller RD, ed. Anesthesia. New York: Churchill Livingstone, 1986:1999.
108. Rahn H, Reeves RB, Howell BJ. Hydrogen ion regulation, temperature, and evolution. Am Rev Respir Dis 1975;112:165.
109. Brackett NC, Cohen JJ, Schwartz WB. Carbon dioxide titration curve of normal man. N Engl J Med 1965; 272:6.
110. Prys-Roberts C, Kelman GR, Nunn JF. Determination of the in vivo carbon dioxide titration curve of anesthetized man. Br J Anaesth 1966;38:500.
111. Sladen A. Acid-base balance. In: McIntyre KM, Lewis AJ, eds. Textbook of advanced cardiac life support. Dallas: American Heart Association, 1983:139.
112. Jorgensen K, Astrup P. Standard bicarbonate: its clinical significance and a new method for its determination. Scand J Clin Lab Invest 1957;2:122.
113. Astrup P, Siggaard-Andersen O, Jorgensen K, Engel K. The acid-base metabolism. A new approach. Lancet 1960;1:1035.
114. Schwartz WB, Relman AS. A critique of the parameters used in the evaluation of acid-base disorders. N Engl J Med 1963;268:1382.
115. Finberg L. Water and electrolyte physiology. In: Rudolph AM, Hoffman JI, eds. Pediatrics. Norwalk, Connecticut: Appleton & Lange, 1987:196.
116. Guyton AC. Regulation of respiration. In: Guyton A, ed. Textbook of medical physiology. Philadelphia: WB Saunders, 1981:1074.
117. Stone DJ. Respiration in man during metabolic alkalosis. J Appl Physiol 1962;17:33.
118. Roberts KE, Poppell JW, Vanamee P, et al. Evaluation of respiratory compensation in metabolic alkalosis. J Clin Invest 1956;35:261.
119. Baer D, Belsey R. The evolving regulatory environment and bedside metabolic monitoring of the acute care patient. Chest 1990;97:191S–197S.

Appendix 10.1

Guidelines for Standards of Care for Patients with Acute Respiratory Failure on Mechanical Ventilatory Support

PERSONNEL WHO SHALL BE AVAILABLE

1. Physician
   a. Medical management must be directed or concurrently provided by a physician who possesses credentials granted by the hospital for the management of critically ill patients undergoing mechanical ventilation, who visits the patient at least daily, and is available within 30 minutes, 24 hours/day.
2. Twenty-four hour a day in-house personnel
   a. Personnel with the ability to provide advanced cardiac life support
   b. Personnel with the qualifications and privileges to intubate the trachea
3. Nurse
   a. Minimum 1:2 RN/patient ratio around the clock
   b. Ability to increase to 1:1 ratio around the clock if acuity demands
   c. Special precautions must be maintained for any patient with respiratory paralysis
4. Respiratory therapy
   a. At least one respiratory therapist assigned to the unit at all times
   b. The number of therapists assigned to the unit is based on some measure of acuity

MONITORING THAT SHALL BE AVAILABLE

1. The capability to monitor on a continuous basis
   a. Cardiac rate and rhythm
   b. Oxygen saturation of hemoglobin
   c. End-tidal CO_2
   d. Blood pressure, CVP, and pulmonary artery pressure
   e. Core temperature
2. The capability to monitor on an intermittent basis
   a. Weight of bedridden and ambulating patients
   b. Cardiac output
   c. BP (noninvasively)

SUPPORT SERVICE THAT SHALL BE AVAILABLE

1. Radiographic services
   a. Portable chest radiographic equipment and films available 24 hours/day to unit personnel for immediate review; radiologist available within 30 minutes if consultation is requested
   b. Official chest radiograph interpretation within 24 hours
   c. Pulmonary angiography and lung scans—if not available in-house, transfer arrangements to a facility that has such capability
2. Laboratory services
   a. Available at least daily
      (1) Microbiology laboratory
      (2) Ability to measure PO_4, Ca, and Mg levels
      (3) Ability to measure the following drug levels: theophylline, digoxin, and aminoglycosides
      (4) Cardiac enzymes, including fractionation
   b. Available 24 hours/day; results to be available within 1 hour
      (1) Hemoglobin, hematocrit, and WBC with differential
      (2) Blood glucose, Na, K, Cl, CO_2, BUN, and creatinine
      (3) Prothrombin time, partial thromboplastin time, and platelet count
      (4) Urinalysis
      (5) Arterial blood gas analysis shall be available 24 hours/day; results must be available within 30 minutes unless some form of continuous and alarmed surveillance of patient oxygenation and ventilation is in use for the patient
3. Respiratory services
   a. Diagnostic and therapeutic bronchoscopy as clinically indicated
   b. Twenty-four hour a day availability of measures aimed at pulmonary secretion control, specifically chest physiotherapy and postural drainage, as clinically indicated

EQUIPMENT THAT SHALL BE AVAILABLE

1. Ventilators with the following capabilities
   a. Capability of delivering mechanical breaths via a variety of modalities such as assist control, synchronous intermittent mandatory ventilation, pressure support ventilation, and controlled mechanical ventilation
   b. PEEP
   c. Humidification and warming of gases
   d. Oxygen pressure, volume, and apnea alarms
   e. Capability to manipulate flow rate or inspiration/expiration ratio

2. At each bedside, resuscitation equipment that includes a resuscitation bag and mask of proper size and fit for the patient being ventilated and an oxygen source; resuscitation cart immediately available
3. Portable respirometer
4. Endotracheal tubes and tracheostomy tubes in a wide variety of sizes with high-volume/low-pressure cuffs and uncuffed pediatric tubes
5. Suction equipment at each bedside

GENERAL MANAGEMENT

1. The patient is managed in a unit that meets guidelines for services and personnel and unit design
2. The initial evaluation of the patient shall include the following if indicated by the clinical presentation:
   a. Chest radiograph
   b. ECG (for patients >21 years of age)
   c. Complete blood count
   d. Blood chemistries to include glucose, Na, K, Cl, CO_2, BUN, creatinine, PO_4, Mg
   e. Prothrombin time, partial thromboplastin time, platelet count
   f. Arterial blood gas analysis
   g. Cultures of blood, sputum, and urine
3. Vital signs shall be measured and recorded at least hourly until stable
4. Patients with unstable cardiopulmonary status must have continuous monitoring of their circulation, oxygenation, and ventilation; the use of ECGs, pulse oximeters, and capnographs is encouraged for this purpose
5. Variables that shall be measured and recorded serially at least every 4 hours will relate to the proper functioning of the ventilator and to oxygen delivery (DO_2) or demand and will include
   a. F_IO_2
   b. Minute ventilation
   c. Tidal volume
   d. Peak and mean airway pressures
   e. Temperature of inspired gases
   f. Confirmation that all alarms are set
   g. Oxygen saturation of hemoglobin
   h. Cardiac rate, rhythm, and BP
   i. Temperature
   j. End-exhalation pressure and inspiration/expiration ratio available as needed
6. Intake and output measurements shall be measured and recorded at least every 8 hours
7. The following shall be utilized at intervals to be determined by individual clinical circumstances:
   a. Arterial blood gas analysis
   b. Measurement of vital capacity, negative inspiratory force, and dynamic compliance
   c. Nutritional support—enteral and parenteral
   d. Continuous IV
   e. Objective measurements of nutritional status
   f. Endotracheal tube cuff pressure measurements
   g. Measurements of patient weight
   h. Chest radiographs
8. Consideration should be given to measures aimed at
   a. Stress ulcer prophylaxis
   b. Deep vein thrombosis prophylaxis
   c. Avoidance of nosocomial infection
9. The following therapies or diagnostic modalities shall be available:
   a. Cardiac pacing
   b. Special beds
   c. Temperature control devices
   d. Thoracentesis
   e. Tube thoracotomy
   f. Tracheostomy
   g. Anticoagulation
   h. Dialysis

VENTILATOR MANAGEMENT

Ventilator management must be directed or concurrently provided by a physician with appropriate qualifications. This physician shall be responsible for directing airway management, ventilatory support, and removal from the ventilator. This physician should tailor management to specific circumstances, using the guidelines below when clinically applicable and appropriate.

1. Airway management
   a. The endotracheal tube or tracheostomy tube should be secured safely and comfortably
   b. Attention should be given to the prevention of unplanned extubation, including either physical or medical restraints (sedation or muscle relaxants) when indicated for demented, confused, or agitated patients
   c. Secretions should be suctioned as necessary, using sterile technique
2. Ventilator support
   a. To achieve an adequate level of oxygenation, the patient's oxygen saturation should be maintained at 89%; exceptions can be expected in patients with congenital cyanotic heart disease or far advanced chronic obstructive lung disease
   b. Minute ventilation should be adjusted based on patient comfort, pH, and ventilatory mechanics
   c. To avoid oxygen toxicity and absorption atelectasis, the F_IO_2 should be decreased to <0.5 as soon as possible
   d. To achieve optimal DO_2 to tissues, objective measurements of DO_2 (pH, BP, oxygen saturation, PO_2) should be obtained as dictated by the clinical presentation; assurance of adequacy of DO_2 requires special attention when levels of PEEP >15 cm H_2O are required
   e. The frequency of arterial blood gas analysis should be dictated by the acuity of illness, availability of

noninvasive monitoring, and frequency of ventilator changes

f. To achieve patient comfort, consideration should be given to the use of sedation, if indicated, or an arterial line, if frequent blood testing is required

3. Removal of ventilator support

a. Ventilator weaning should be instituted in a timely manner supported by objective observations of pulmonary mechanics and/or functions and demonstration of improvement or resolution of the problem necessitating ventilation

b. After each substantial change in ventilator support, the patient should be observed for clinical changes; in addition, the need for objective measures of adequacy of DO_2 (measurement of PO_2 or oxygen saturation) should be dictated by clinical circumstances

[a]RN, registered nurse; BP, blood pressure; CVP, central venous pressure; WBC, white blood cell count; BUN, blood urea nitrogen; PEEP, positive end-expiratory pressure; ECG, electrocardiogram; i.v., intravenous infusion. (From Task Force on Guidelines. Guidelines for standards of care for patients with acute respiratory failure on mechanical ventilatory support. Crit Care Med 1991;19:275–278.)

Cardiac and Circulatory Failure

Section Three

Section Editors

Randall C. Wetzel
William J. Greeley

Cardiorespiratory Interactions 11

James L. Robotham
Jurgen Peters
Masao Takata
Randall C. Wetzel

INTRODUCTION

Cardiopulmonary support for critically ill children is a major focus of pediatric intensive care. While the traditional specialties of cardiology and pulmonology concentrate on understanding their respective organ systems, those interested in intensive care must interrelate and integrate the function of both systems. More recently, it has been recognized that ventilatory-induced changes in abdominal pressure can affect venous return to a substantial degree, leading to the appreciation that the thoracoabdominal compartment should be considered as an interactive unit.

A thorough appreciation of the interactions between pulmonary and cardiovascular function is necessary in managing any child with impaired cardiac and or respiratory function. It is clear that the same basic mechanical interactions are common to all modes of ventilation, including spontaneous ventilation with or without airways obstruction, positive pressure ventilation regardless of frequency with or without positive end-expiratory pressure (PEEP), and, finally, cardiopulmonary resuscitation. Understanding any one of these provides the insight necessary to understand them all. Recognition of the cardiopulmonary interactions and their role in the clinical picture is necessary in formulating a complete diagnostic and therapeutic plan. The purpose of this chapter is to establish a physiologic framework for consideration of the individual disease processes discussed throughout this book. This will be done by describing those factors that control systemic venous return, right ventricular (RV) output, pulmonary venous return, and left ventricular (LV) output during changes in intrathoracic or abdominal pressures and lung volume as commonly observed in the intensive care unit (ICU).

INFLUENCE OF RESPIRATION ON CIRCULATION

The recognition of interactions between the circulatory and respiratory systems has been a focus of interest for the physiologist for well over a century[1]. By the turn of the century, observations that were confirmed subsequently had formed the basis for physiologic controversies that continue as central concerns for physicians caring for critically ill patients today. An appreciation of those physiologic variables common to all modes of ventilation allows a cohesive approach to the understanding of the multiple modes of spontaneous and positive pressure ventilation observed in the ICU. The concepts are important to understand the cardiovascular pathophysiology of the respiratory distress syndrome, bronchopulmonary dysplasia, asthma, sleep apnea, upper airway obstruction with croup or epiglottitis, and the effects of intermittent positive-pressure ventilation (IPPV) and PEEP across a spectrum from hypervolemic patients with LV failure to hypovolemic trauma patients.

GENERAL PRINCIPLES OF MECHANICAL INTERACTIONS

Figure 11.1 illustrates a simplified model of a compliant vascular compartment surrounded by a box in which the pressure can be varied. Inflow is generated by a constant pressure source and is proportional to the size of the arrow. The boundaries of the box could represent the thorax, abdomen, or an extremity and illustrate the influence of pressure changes around a compartment, such as a vascular bed or cardiac chamber.

The vascular bed/cardiac chamber inside the box can be given the following characteristics: (a) It will have a pressure-volume relationship (compliance), such that a given volume will exert a given pressure across the wall. This *transmural pressure* is easily calculated as the intravascular minus the surrounding box pressure (Ps). (b) There will be a pressure-flow relationship: resistance. Flow in a steady-state condition is determined by the pressure gradient for perfusion and by the resistance (Q = P/R). The pressure gradient that drives perfusion pressure is the difference between the upstream, inflow pressure and the downstream, outflow or back pressure. This model also allows estimation of an afterload, symbolized by the weight impeding blood flow leaving the compartment. The true calculation of afterload requires knowledge of not only the resistance, but also the compliance of the outflow vessel and inertance of the fluid and vessel wall.

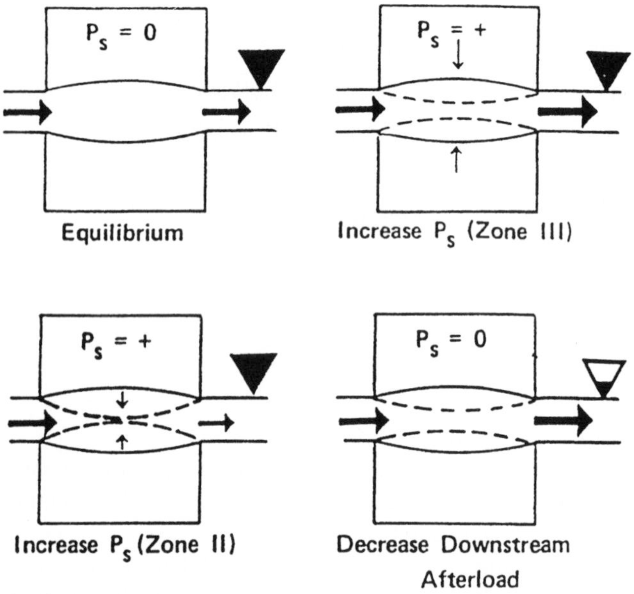

Figure 11.1. Beginning in the *upper left panel* (equilibrium), there is a schematic representation of a vascular compartment (vessel or cardiac chamber) that has a constant pressure source delivering flow *(first arrow).* The vascular chamber is within a compartment surrounded by atmospheric pressures (P_s = 0). Under these steady-state conditions, an equal volume of blood leaves the vascular structure. The *inverted arrowhead* reflects the afterload impeding blood leaving the chamber. This results in some distention of the compliant vessel or chamber within the compartment. In the *upper right panel,* the surrounding pressure within the compartment is increased. This translocates blood out of the vessel or chamber *(reflected by the dashed line);* reducing the volume in the chamber. This models a West zone III lung that, with a moderate increase in pressure, ejects blood out of the alveolar capillary bed. In the *lower left panel,* the surrounding pressure is further increased, emptying the vascular volume within the compartment. Now a predominant resistor function appears. Thus, under zone III conditions an increase in pressure predominantly influences the capacitance effects of the vascular volume, whereas under zone II conditions the additional increase in pressure results in a predominantly resistive function. In the *lower right panel,* a decrease in the downstream afterload, reflected by the half-filled weight-impeding outflow, results in a decreased intravascular volume within the compartment and increased flow out of the compartment. This is precisely the same effect as increasing the surrounding pressure under a zone III condition. Thus, a positive intrathoracic pressure can be equivalent to reducing the afterload on the left ventricle. (From Robotham JL. How respiration affects circulation. The American Society of Anesthesiologists refresher courses in anesthesiology. Philadelphia: JB Lippincott/Harper & Row, 1988; 16:191.)

Given a constant pressure source for inflow, when the surrounding pressure (Ps) is acutely increased, the transmural pressure must decrease. Even if inflow were constant, the outflow from the compliant chamber would transiently increase. This transient increase in outflow as Ps is increased is represented by the large arrow as volume is translocated out of the vascular compartment. Because the inflow is determined by constant pressure and not constant flow, the increase in Ps will reduce the pressure gradient for inflow and thus further reduce the vascular volume in the chamber. Using terminology analogous to West's zones of the pulmonary circulation[2], a zone III condition exists when the outflow, downstream pressure outside the box is higher than the surrounding pressure (e.g., left atrial pressure is higher than alveolar pressure). The steady-state vascular volume (V) of the compartment is related to its compliance (C) and the difference between the inflow and outflow pressures (ΔP), i.e., $V = C \times \Delta P$. A zone II condition exists when Ps is greater than the downstream pressure outside the box, thus reducing the volume in the vascular compartment (e.g., when alveolar pressure with PEEP is much higher than the downstream left atrial pressure). If the box pressure is increased to produce zone II conditions, in which the effective downstream pressure determining flow is Ps, the steady-state effect is to diminish blood flow out of the compartment and reduce inflow. The pressure in the vascular compartment relative to the atmospheric pressure would increase, while the transmural pressure would decrease (because of the increase in Ps). Hence the increase in box pressure (Ps) first acutely diminishes the vascular compartment's volume by increasing outflow. This is effectively equivalent to decreasing vascular compliance. Under these circumstances, increases in both back pressure and resistance diminish inflow and outflow. It is clear that changes in outflow are dependent on the initial vascular volume, whether hypervolemia or hypovolemia. In a fashion analogous to zone III and zone II conditions in the lung, opposite changes in outflow for a given increase in Ps would occur with hypervolemia as compared with hypovolemia.

Finally, in the last panel in Figure 11.1, the effects of afterload are seen. Reducing the afterload causes a decrease

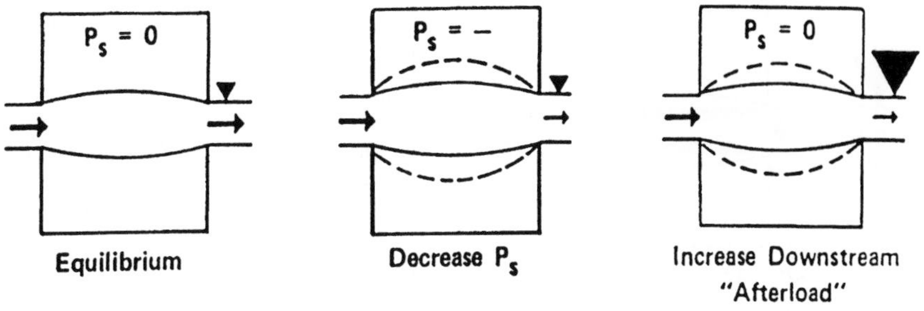

Figure 11.2. *Left panel:* Equilibrium conditions as in Figure 11.1. In the *middle panel,* a negative surrounding pressure is applied that increases intravascular volume and decreases outflow. This is precisely equivalent to increased downstream afterload in the *right panel,* reflected by the increased weight over the outflow vessel. This also increases vascular volume within the compartment and diminishes outflow. Thus, a negative intrathoracic pressure is mechanically equivalent to increasing the afterload outside the compartment on the left ventricle. (From Robotham JL. How respiration affects circulation. The American Society of Anesthesiologists refresher courses in anesthesiology. Philadelphia: JB Lippincott/ Harper & Row, 1988;16:191.)

in vascular volume and an increase in outflow at constant box pressure. It is evident that under these conditions, an increase in Ps, illustrated in the panel immediately above, will have the same results as reducing afterload in terms of the initial effect on chamber volume and outflow. However, while a pure decrease in afterload would enhance the gradient for inflow, an increase in Ps would decrease it. If the box represents the thorax and Ps represents the intrathoracic pressure, with the vascular chamber being the left ventricle (LV), this schema can be applied to understanding clinical cardiorespiratory interactions. In LV failure, increasing intrathoracic pressure would reduce LV preload (decreased inflow) and reduce LV afterload (increased outflow). Thus the steady-state result of increasing intrathoracic pressure, such as by instituting IPPV in spontaneously breathing patients, or adding PEEP in mechanically ventilated patients, could cause either a dominant reduction in preload and reduce the cardiac output, or a dominant reduction in afterload, and increase the cardiac output. Appreciation of these two equally possible but opposite results of applying PEEP in a given patient can account for much of the controversy in the literature concerning what effect positive pressure ventilation has on the circulatory system.

Figure 11.2 schematically uses the same format to illustrate the similarities between decreasing the pressure surrounding a vascular chamber and increasing the afterload. It should not be surprising that a decrease in Ps will increase the volume in the vessel or cardiac chamber and thus decrease outflow. This is equivalent to increasing the afterload, which also results in decreasing outflow and increasing vascular volume. For the LV, a decrease in intrathoracic pressure (more negative) or an increase in afterload are mechanically equivalent. Both maneuvers decrease the amount of blood leaving the thorax. A negative intrathoracic pressure would adversely affect a patient with LV dysfunction by effectively increasing afterload. On the other hand, a negative intrathoracic pressure also increases the gradient for systemic venous return. Thus, the central thoracic compartment (heart and lungs) increases its blood volume as venous return is augmented and arterial outflow is impeded. With a well-functioning heart, the increase in preload would increase cardiac output. Thus, in contrast to a positive intrathoracic pressure, which will decrease LV preload and afterload, a negative intrathoracic pressure should increase LV preload and afterload. While increasing preload and afterload will combine to increase LV volumes, they will have opposite effects on cardiac output. The increased LV volume associated with a negative intrathoracic pressure would cause an increased preload that would tend to increase cardiac output, but an increased afterload would tend to decrease cardiac output. The same analysis can be applied to an increase in intrathoracic pressure. An increased intrathoracic pressure decreases systemic venous return, leading to decreased LV preload and hence decreased cardiac output via the Frank-Starling mechanism. An increase in intrathoracic pressure simultaneously decreases the effective LV afterload, thus decreasing LV volume but increasing cardiac output. This reasoning process should be applicable not only to the normal heart but also to LV failure, and in the extreme to totally absent ventricular function, as during cardiopulmonary resuscitation (CPR).

If changes in intrathoracic pressure only influenced the gradient for systemic venous return to, and arterial egress from the thorax, our understanding of the cardiovascular events would be relatively straightforward. However, as illustrated in Figure 11.3, independent of changes in surrounding pressure, the vascular volume may also be varied by altering the vascular compartment's compliance. With a constant inflow pressure, increasing compliance increases the vascular volume, transiently reduces outflow, and then allows increased inflow and outflow through a lower pressure chamber. With the same constant pressure inflow source, chamber compliance may be diminished by (a) intrinsic stiffening of the chamber walls or (b) extrinsically pushing on the chamber. External compression can occur if the lungs compress the heart, (heart-lung interdependence)[3,4] or may occur because of pericardial constraint of both ventricles. In the condition of pericardial constraint, if the contralateral ventricle fills the intrapericardial space, the septum will shift, thus compressing the contralateral ventricle (ventricular interdependence)[5]. The net effect of any of the above is to raise the chamber pressure, first

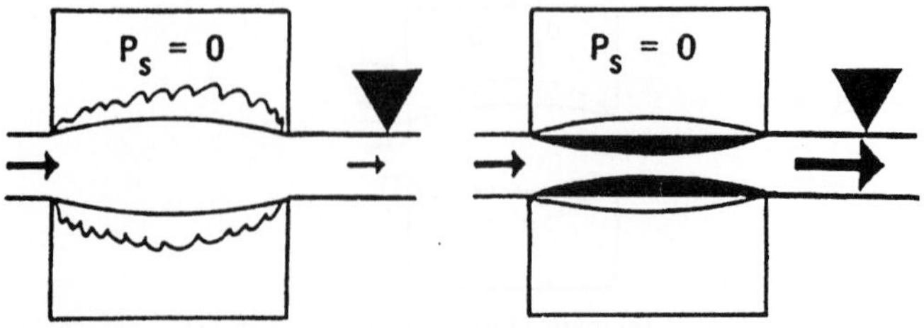

Figure 11.3. Schematic representation of the effect of increasing and decreasing the effective vascular compliance with constant surrounding pressure and constant afterload. In the *left panel,* an acute increase in compliance (represented by the *wavy line* that denotes increased intravascular volume) will at first decrease outflow from the chamber *(smaller arrow);* then, by lowering the intravascular pressure within the compartment, it will increase steady-state outflow equivalent to any increase in steady-state inflow. With a decrease in vascular chamber compliance produced either by an intrinsic stiffening of the walls of the chamber or by extrinsic compression (e.g., a contralateral ventricle or the lungs squeezing the heart), the decrease in chamber volume will first produce a transient increase in outflow (reflected by the *large arrow*) and then diminish inflow. (From Robotham JL. How respiration affects circulation. The American Society of Anesthesiologists refresher courses in anesthesiology. Philadelphia: JB Lippincott/Harper & Row, 1988; 16:191.)

acutely emptying the chamber by increasing outflow and then reducing inflow because of an increased intracavitary downstream pressure. The net effect will be reduced steady-state outflow.

Thus, under conditions of a constant inflow pressure into a vascular compartment, changes in the surrounding pressure, changes in vascular compliance, and changes in afterload may each independently alter outflow. Since the outflow of one vascular compartment is the inflow for the next vascular compartment, analysis of the next compartment must also include this variable inflow. If we then allow vascular compartments to be linked in series, it becomes difficult to predict the net result of a physiologic perturbation that alters inflows, surrounding pressures, compliances, and afterload in multiple compartments. Despite the complexity, if one vascular compartment at a time is considered, there is a logical manner by which to evaluate the whole system.

Cardiorespiratory interactions can influence (a) systemic venous return, (b) RV output, (c) pulmonary venous return, and (d) LV output. By considering events during respiration as composed of these four components, the complex and, at times, opposing effects of multiple variables can be discussed for specific ventilatory modes **(Table 11.1).**

Systemic Venous Return

Despite the emphasis in experimental studies on the effects of respiration on the ventricular performance, the influence of respiration on venous return remains a dominant influence on cardiac output in most circumstances. Given normal ventricular function, with normal pulmonary and systemic vascular resistance, LV output is determined by systemic venous return. The ideal heart will pump all the blood returned to it. The exquisite sensitivity of venous return to respiratory-induced changes has been elegantly described by Guyton et al.[6,7] (Fig. 11.4). Understanding the factors that regulate the venous return curve is essential in understanding cardiorespiratory interaction. The venous return curve is understood by considering the right atrial (RA) pressure (Pra) as the outflow pressure (downstream or back pressure) for venous return. This is the pressure to which the venous capacitance system is "connected" in order to complete the circuit to the heart. The pressure that the venous capacitance bed generates to drive blood back to the RA— i.e., the mean systemic pressure (Pms)—can be measured experimentally by stopping all flow (i.e., Pra when Q = 0) and is equal to the stressed volume ($V - V_0$) in the circuit divided by the mean compliance (C) of the circuit because, by definition, P = V/C. The stressed volume can

Table 11.1. Venous Return—Physiologic Variables During Ventilation

Pleural pressure
Neural reflexes
Extrathoracic perivascular compartment pressures, e.g., abdominal, extremities
Venous blood volume changes—stressed/unstressed
Venous compliance
Venous resistance
Determinants of right atrial pressure
Right and/or left ventricular function
Ventricular compliance
Ventricular interdependence
Heart-lung interdependence

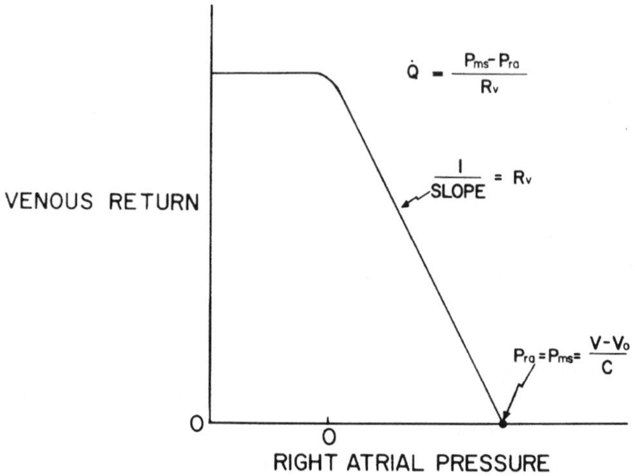

Figure 11.4. Schematic representation of a venous return curve, with a single peripheral venous compartment assumed. Venous return intersects the *abscissa* at the right atrial pressure (Pra) required to stop all venous return, i.e., mean systemic pressure (Pms). The reciprocal of the slope of the venous return curve is equal to the venous resistance (Rv). Maximum venous return occurs with a right atrial pressure of 0, below which further lowering right atrial pressure does not increase venous return because of flow limitation. V equals total venous blood volume, and V_0 equals the unstressed blood volume. The difference between the two ($V - V_0$) equals the stressed volume. (From Sylvester JT, Goldberg HS, Permutt S. The role of the vasculature in the regulation of cardiac output. Clin Chest Med 1983;4:111.)

be defined as the total venous volume (V) minus the volume that could be added to the circuit before the circuit pressure would rise above zero (V_0). Determination of multiple points defines the venous return curve. Its characteristic shape expresses the resistance to venous return as the reciprocal of the slope since $Rv = \Delta Pra/\Delta Q$ and venous return (which equals cardiac output) at a given RA pressure as $Q = (Pms - Pra)/Rv$.

The plateau at Pra = 0 reflects the fact that any further lowering of the RA pressure (below atmospheric) does not increase venous return due to collapse of the highly compliant veins as they enter the thorax. Thus, as intrathoracic pressure falls below zero during spontaneous ventilation, RA intraluminal, or the downstream pressure for venous return, falls below zero, and this is transmitted to the veins as they enter the thorax. At that point, their surrounding pressure changes from intrathoracic pressure to atmospheric or abdominal pressure. Because this surrounding pressure is positive, the vessel will collapse until venous return builds up to increase venous intraluminal pressure above the surrounding pressure, and the vessel reopens. Thus, venous return is limited by this pressure-sensitive resistance. This Starling resistor mechanism explains why venous return does not increase further as Pra pressure falls below zero (atmospheric). This has been experimentally demonstrated by Guyton et al.[(6,7)] and Natori et al.[(8)] using ultrasound in the closed-chest condition to show collapse and flutter of the vena cava just inferior to the diaphragm. This process is analogous to expiratory flow limitation in the bronchial tree during forced expiration. Making the intrathoracic pressure markedly negative will not increase venous return more than when the Pra relative to the periphery is zero. A homeostatic advantage of this is to limit wide swings in venous return when large negative swings in intrathoracic pressure occur with exercise or obstructive airways disease. Similarly, if flow-limiting conditions exist such that the inferior vena cava acts as a Starling resistor at the diaphragm, raising abdominal pressure around the abdominal capacitance bed will not increase flow because there will be an equal increase in pressure in and around the vena cava—i.e., an equal increase in pressure around both the vascular compartment and the outflow does not change the gradient for flow under zone II conditions, in which the effective back pressure is at the exit to the thorax[(9)]. However, if flow limitation is not present (zone III condition), then raising abdominal pressure will increase venous return since the upstream abdominal compartment's venous pressure is raised, but now the effective back pressure to flow is right atrial pressure, which remains constant. This is also relevant to understanding why an increase in intrathoracic pressure around the compliant RA and vena cava will act to transmit this pressure to the intravascular compartment and reduce venous return. Even if the intrathoracic great vessels were completely collapsed, a positive pressure around them would act as the downstream pressure the peripheral venous bed "sees" and must rise above before antegrade flow can occur.

Our understanding of events within specific components of the abdominal compartment have allowed a better understanding of how respiration affects venous return and hence cardiac output, in addition to providing insights into the hemodynamic events in systemic disease processes. Total inferior vena cava (IVC) venous return is composed of regional venous return from the splanchnic and nonsplanchnic circulations. Some investigators have found that inspiration with diaphragmatic descent enhanced splanchnic IVC flow[(10,11)], while others have reported that it reduced the splanchnic IVC flow by increasing transhepatic resistance but enhanced the nonsplanchnic IVC flow[(12,13)]. The splanchnic IVC flow drains blood from the liver and gastrointestinal tract, organ systems that are increasingly being recognized as critical organ beds in the adult respiratory distress syndrome or sepsis[(14,15)]. It could be shown that active diaphragmatic descent and the secondary increases in abdominal pressures produced substantially different changes in both the total and regional IVC venous return under different blood volume conditions[(9,16)]. With hypervolemia in a zone III condition, phrenic nerve stimulation increased the total IVC flow by enhancing the splanchnic IVC flow. With hypovolemia in a zone II condition, phrenic nerve stimulation decreased the total IVC flow by reducing the nonsplanchnic IVC flow and produced a venous pressure gradient in the IVC across the diaphragm. The transient decrease in the nonsplanchnic IVC flow with hypervolemia is likely explained by an increased common downstream pressure to both the splanchnic and nonsplanchnic IVC venous return, produced by the augmented splanchnic IVC flow. The results suggest that regional venous return from the splanchnic and nonsplanchnic IVC circulations may be interdependent via a common downstream venous pressure shared by both circulations and hence homeostatic in allowing both to empty, yet preserving relatively constant flow to the heart.

Phrenic nerve stimulation produces a sustained increase in the splanchnic IVC flow, directly measured with the subhepatic IVC occluded[(16)]. This increase in the splanchnic IVC flow is associated with a substantial increase in focal contact stress over the liver, reflected by an increased local pressure measured over the surface of the liver apposed to the diaphragm[(16)]. With the abdomen widely open and the gut eviscerated, and thus without any increases in general abdominal pressures, the focal contact stress exerted by the descending diaphragm over the liver could discharge blood from the hepatic capacitance bed, thereby enhancing the splanchnic IVC flow. These observations also suggest that with a normal closed abdomen, the focal surface pressure over the liver may increase more than other abdominal pressures during diaphragmatic descent, consistent with the study of Decramer et al.[(17)].

A direct corollary of this finding explains the physiology of Kussmaul's sign, in which a spontaneous inspiration (noted by Kussmaul to be more commonly observed with a deep inspiration) results in an increase in jugular venous pressure rather than the typical inspiratory descent[(18)].

Changes in superior vena cava (SVC) flow and right atrial pressure (which will affect the jugular venous pressure) during respiratory maneuvers are substantially influenced by the blood volume status (hypervolemia versus hypovolemia) and by the degree of diaphragmatic descent and the associated respiratory induced changes in abdominal pressures (airway open to allow diaphragmatic descent, which will increase abdominal pressure versus total airway obstruction with little diaphragmatic movement during a respiratory effort)[19]. Changes in IVC flow are almost identical with the airway open or obstructed in the same blood volume state, but exhibit different flow patterns in the two different volume states. With no pericardial disease or right heart failure present, a Kussmaul's sign can be observed only during inspiration under hypervolemic conditions, with substantial diaphragmatic descent producing substantial increases in abdominal pressures relative to the decreases in intrathoracic pressure. Changes in abdominal pressures modulate the SVC and IVC venous return during respiration, depending on the blood volume status. Normally both show a net increase in flow with a spontaneous inspiration but can become interdependent in a hypervolemic condition—i.e., IVC increases as SVC flow decreases. A respiratory-induced increase in abdominal pressures with diaphragmatic descent, with an increase in IVC flow and decrease in SVC flow, is thus the essential element in the pathogenesis of a Kussmaul's sign[19].

The focal compression of the liver by the diaphragm also occurs with a positive pressure inspiration in which the diaphragmatic motion is passive. The hemodynamic response to PEEP ventilation involves a parallel reduction in cardiac output/venous return[20,21] and total liver blood flow, with reductions in both hepatic arterial and portal venous flows[22]. The reduction in portal venous flow is associated with an increase in the back pressure to flow because of an increase in right atrial pressure as intrathoracic pressure increases and to an increase in resistance to flow across the liver itself, consistent with local diaphragmatic compression[22]. The decrease in portal flow contributes to the reduction in total venous return and may contribute to liver dysfunction associated with PEEP. It may be that the similarities between the mechanisms affecting total IVC and portal flows[20–22] reflect compression of both the intrahepatic IVC and portal venous beds.

It is important to recognize that all the pressures described are measured relative to a simple arbitrary standard—i.e., atmospheric pressure—in order to compare the driving pressures for flow through multiple compartments, each with a different surrounding pressure (e.g., limbs, abdomen, thorax, and head). Although this is the conventional manner in which pressures are measured both experimentally and clinically, it is to be noted carefully that in many of the subsequent discussions, the transmural pressure is considered, i.e., pressure relative to the surrounding pressure. In contrast to flow analysis, which requires a common reference pressure, deductions regarding changes in cardiac chamber pressure-volume characteristics, e.g., contractility or diastolic compliance, require an estimate of the pressure relative to the surrounding pressure. Although an esophageal balloon may serve the clinician well for this purpose, the necessity of a precise surface pressure reference (i.e., over the ventricular wall inside the pericardium) presents major problems for the physiologist. The following examples illustrate the differences between conventional and transmural pressures. With a positive intrathoracic pressure of +5 mm Hg and an intravascular Pra pressure of +6 mm Hg (both relative to atmosphere), the back pressure for venous return from the periphery would be +6 mm Hg; however, the transmural pressure (Pra_{tm}), reflecting the volume status of the RA, would be $+6 - (+5) = +1$ mm Hg. With this understanding, a diminished cardiac output would be predicted based on high Pra limiting venous return and a low Pra_{tm} reflecting a minimal RV preload. Conversely, an elevated cardiac output would be expected with a markedly negative inspiratory intrathoracic pressure of −30 mm Hg and a Pra relative to an atmosphere of −10 mm Hg. Because of maximal venous return based on a low Pra (−10 mm Hg) and a high Pra_{tm} (−10 mm Hg − (−30 mm Hg) = +20 mm Hg), this reflects an elevated RV preload.

Venous return curves were originally produced, with reflex changes blocked[6], to reflect events occurring during the first 7 seconds after an acute perturbation. Therefore, rapidly increasing the downstream RA pressure from 0 to 10 mm Hg stops venous return if all reflexes are blocked. If reflexes are intact, alpha-adrenergic sympathetic activation leads to a compensatory peripheral venoconstriction raising the upstream pressure for venous return (Pms), thus driving blood back to the heart. However, it takes approximately 7 seconds after an acute perturbation for these peripheral compensatory changes to begin. If Pra is increased acutely relative to the peripheral venous bed by increasing intrathoracic pressure, e.g., PEEP, an immediate decrease in venous return is expected. From Figure 11.5 it can be seen that cardiac output will return toward, but often not to, its pre-PEEP values because neural reflexes increase the mean systemic pressure (Pms) so that at the same Pra, venous return is increased. Neurally mediated peripheral venoconstriction increases the stressed volume ($V-V_0$) in the venous bed by reducing its compliance. This effectively increases Pms, i.e., the driving pressure for venous return, by shifting the venous return curve to the right and up. If no venoconstriction occured, i.e., if the unstressed volume remained constant, plasma volume expansion (by increasing total venous volume), and hence the stressed volume, would increase venous return. Thus, an initial PEEP-induced diminution in cardiac output can be compensated by reflex venoconstriction and/or exogenous volume expansion. It is evident that adrenergic blockade[23], venodilation (increasing the unstressed volume at the expense of the stressed volume), or hemorrhage (decreasing the stressed volume) can lead to precipitous falls in venous return when combined with an increased intrathoracic pressure during the institution of mechanical ventilation or the addition of PEEP.

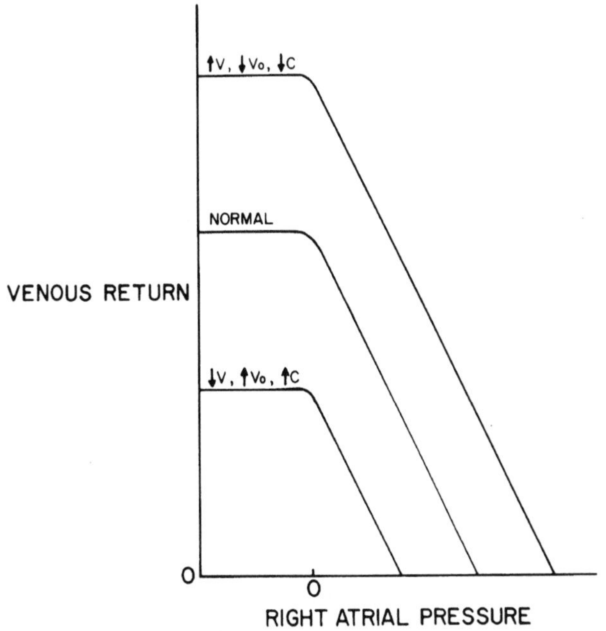

Figure 11.5. Schematic representation of the changes produced in the venous return curve by selectively altering total venous volume (V), unstressed venous volume (V_0), or the compliance of the venous bed {$C = (V - V_0)/P_{ms}$}, where P_{ms} is mean systemic pressure. PEEP will increase right atrial pressure, reducing venous return on the normal curve. Physiologic compensation will include a potential shift of blood volume from the thorax to the peripheral venous bed (≠V), i.e., venoconstriction decreasing the unstressed volume (ϕV_0) by diminishing venous compliance (ϕC). These will shift the curve to the right, tending to compensate for the reduced venous return, despite an elevated right atrial pressure. Plasma volume expansion would increase total venous volume, also contributing to a shift of the curve to the right. All of these would increase P_{ms}, with the assumption for these curves of no change in venous resistance. If venous resistance increases, then, despite an increased P_{ms}, the venous curve would reach its flow-limiting value at a lower maximum venous return, i.e., the slope of the curve shifted down. (From Sylvester JT, Goldberg HS, Permutt S. The role of the vasculature in the regulation of cardiac output. Clin Chest Med 1983;4:111.)

Systemic venous return is the only limiting factor for the control of cardiac output when the heart is a perfect pump that can maintain a Pra of zero at all times, i.e., a ventricular function curve that is perpendicular to the x axis (filling pressure) at 0 mm Hg. Because this is not the case, the ventricular function curve must be integrated with the venous return curve[24]. In Figure 11.6, it is seen that an increase in Pra tends to reduce venous return but increase cardiac output. Because at steady state the same Pra (where $Pra = Pra_{tm}$) acts as the downstream pressure for venous return and as the ventricular filling pressure, there can only be a single point where the two curves intersect, when both systems are in equilibrium (the equilibrium point). The integration of venous return and cardiac performance can therefore be seen to occur at the right atrium. Pathologic processes may alter one or both curves. It is, therefore, important to consider that the many effects of interventions that traditionally have been ascribed to direct effects on ventricular function may have their major effects on venous return, e.g., epinephrine[24,25]. Pharmacologic (epinephrine, nitroprusside), neural (sympathetic tone), mechanical (abdominal pressure), or pathologic (nitric oxide, endothelin) factors that can alter the regional distribution of arterial blood flow will affect venous return by shifting blood flow among beds with different time constants (i.e., different local resistances and compliances), thus affecting the volume of blood that is in the thoracic compartment versus compared with the periphery.

Abdominal Compartment and Venous Return

The same analysis can also be applied to the effects of extravascular pressure applied to veins in the abdomen or limbs. An increase in intra-abdominal pressure should impede blood entering from the legs, yet tends to squeeze venous blood in the abdomen into the thorax. Goldberg et al.[26] demonstrated that positive pressure breathing can translocate sufficient blood volume out of the thorax and into the periphery to increase Pms. This is consistent with the early work of Fenn et al.[27], which showed that positive pressure breathing shifts blood from the upper to the lower body. Military antishock trousers increase the intravascular pressure in both the limbs and abdomen. This increases Pms by reducing the effective venous compliance, thus increasing the stressed volume ($V\text{-}V_0$). A steady-state increase in abdominal pressure (Pab), as seen during abdominal binding or weaning from mechanical ventilation to spontaneous respiration[28,29], would decrease the effective compliance of the abdominal vasculature and shift the ve-

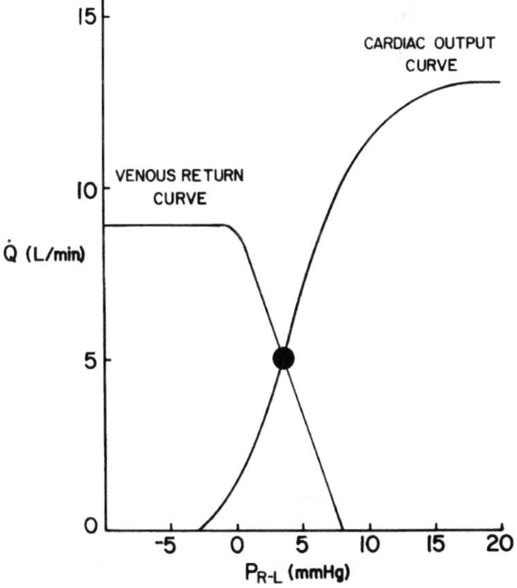

Figure 11.6. Schematic representation of the venous return curve and cardiac output ($\dot{Q}$) curve plotted on the same axis, with the *abscissa* representing the appropriate right or left atrial pressure (PaL) and with the assumption that intrathoracic pressure equals 0, such that the same *abscissa* can be used for both curves. There exists only a single point at the intersection of the two curves that satisfies the conditions for both venous return and cardiac output. (From Sylvester JT, Goldberg HS, Permutt S. The role of the vasculature in the regulation of cardiac output. Clin Chest Med 1983;4:111.)

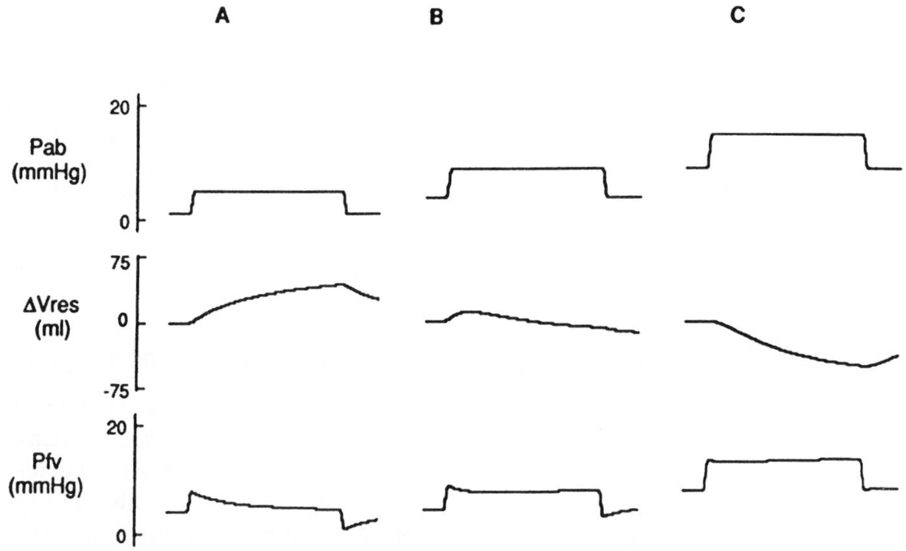

Figure 11.7. A computer simulation of experiments showing changes in abdominal pressure (Pab), reservoir blood volume (ΔVres) that corresponds to inferior vena caval flow (i.e., venous return), and femoral venous pressure (Pfv), the upstream driving pressure for venous return with right atrial pressure maintained constant (see reference 10 for further discussion). The baseline Pab was progressively elevated (*panel A,* 1 mm Hg; *panel B,* 4 mm Hg; and *panel C,* 9 mm Hg), while the baseline right atrial pressure was maintained at 3 mm Hg. The critical closing transmural pressure at the site of the waterfall where the inferior vena cava enters the thorax was −2 mm Hg. *Panel A* represents changes with a pure zone III abdomen (i.e., remaining in zone III before and during the increase in Pab), *panel B* represents changes with a transition from zone III to zone II abdomen as Pab increased, and *panel C* represents changes with a pure zone II abdomen before and during the increase in Pab. The resistance between the downstream abdominal compartment and the measurement site of Pfv was assumed to be minimal. (From Takata M, Wise RA, Robotham JL. Effects of abdominal pressure on venous return: abdominal vascular zone conditions. J Appl Physiol 1990;69:1961.)

nous return curve upward to the right, thereby increasing systemic venous return for a given level of ventricular function. All of these factors must be considered when externally altering intrathoracic, abdominal, or peripheral limb pressures, or when their relationships change, as in instituting positive pressure ventilation or in weaning from mechanical ventilatory support.

Raising abdominal pressure tends to empty the abdominal capacitance bed toward the RA. In the steady state, after the abdominal capacitance bed has been emptied, the increased back pressure to venous return from the extra-abdominal venous bed is still present, thus reducing steady-state venous return. A model explaining the isolated effects of changes in abdominal pressure (regardless of whether produced by ventilation or any other cause) has been developed[9]. Analogous to the description of West et al. of pulmonary vascular zone conditions[2], abdominal vascular zone conditions can also be used to understand the confusing reports that an increase in abdominal pressure can either decrease or increase cardiac output (Fig. 11.7). In a zone III state, the surrounding abdominal pressure at baseline and during an increase is always less than either the upstream femoral venous pressure (Pfv) or the downstream right atrial pressure (Pra), i.e., Pfv>Pra>Pab. This would typically occur with normovolemic or hypervolemic conditions with low abdominal pressures. In this abdominal vascular zone under steady-state conditions, raising Pab shifts blood volume from the abdomen to the thoracic compartment, increasing venous return and cardiac output. While there may be a transient increase in back pressure to venous return from the legs, in the steady state the back pressure returns to baseline, hence only the flow from the abdominal compartment is affected. In an abdominal vascular zone II condition, typically associated with either hypovolemia or markedly elevated abdominal pressures, Pfv > Pab > Pra. As described above, in this condition the effective back pressure IVC venous return is abdominal pressure, right atrial pressure being effectively "disconnected" from the IVC system. Further increases in abdominal pressure can not translocate any blood from the abdominal compartment, but the back pressure for venous return from the extra-abdominal IVC compartment is reduced, hence total venous return/cardiac output decreases. For a complete discussion of these concepts, consideration of the *transition state,* in which the abdomen begins in a zone III state and ends up in a zone II state as abdominal pressure increases, and the specific role of the liver circulation in modulating these events, the reader is referred to references 9, 22, 30, 31.

Other factors that are discussed in detail later but that modulate the variation in venous return during ventilation include the following:

1. Lung inflation in experimental animal studies produces a vagally mediated systemic vasodepressor reflex, which, by causing venodilation, decreases venous return[32]. Although this effect can be elicited with a large tidal volume, its relevance to steady-state quiet ventilation is un-

certain. Indeed, in conscious humans, peripheral venoconstriction can be elicited with hyperinflation[33].

2. Direct compression of the vena cava and right heart by the lungs during inflation (heart-lung interdependence) could contribute to reducing venous return and limiting right heart preload. Brookhart and Boyd[34] in 1947 recognized that the lung can squeeze the heart. More recently, numerous studies[3,4,35–37] have demonstrated with either pericardial surface or isovolumic intraventricular pressures that lung inflation may mechanically compress the heart independently of any change in intrathoracic pressure. Nakhjavan et al.[38] found angiographic evidence of inspiratory reduction in IVC flow at the diaphragm during spontaneous respiration in markedly emphysematous patients. While consistent with lung compression, the latter also raises the additional possibility of diaphragmatic inlet constriction.
3. Right atrial pressure may be influenced significantly by changes in RV and LV function, changes in ventricular compliance via ventricular interdependence, or large increases in pulmonary vascular resistance.

In summary, the great sensitivity of venous return to small changes in pressure make it a major factor in any discussion of cardiorespiratory interactions. The influence of respiration on venous return can be viewed as a group of compartments within compartments, both in series and in parallel. Each compartment has its own volume, compliance, and resistance, modulated by either the active contraction of the respiratory muscles or a mechanical ventilator and any secondary reflex or humoral events. The legs, abdomen, and thorax exist as vascular compartments in series, thus a change in intra-abdominal pressure affects venous flow from the legs and into the thorax. The arms, head, and abdomen exist as vascular compartments in parallel, each returning blood to the thorax, such that a change in intrathoracic pressures may affect the venous returns from each. Whether phasic or steady-state ventilatory changes are considered, the influence of ventilation on venous return must be carefully evaluated before reaching any conclusions about its effect on cardiac function.

Right Ventricular Output

The geometry of the right ventricle is different from that of the left ventricle. The LV can be viewed as an ellipsoid that empties relatively homogeneously during systole[39–41]. Echocardiography, angiography, radiopaque markers, or sonomicrometer crystals to measure LV emptying has enabled satisfactory characterization of the pressure-volume properties of the in vivo LV during both diastole and systole. The RV is a relatively flat, crescent-shaped chamber that can be considered as draped over the septal wall of the LV and contiguous with the free-wall fibers in the LV. This anatomic arrangement of a thin-walled RV applied over the thicker-walled LV could provide a number of the advantages for the RV, but makes assessment of volume changes in the RV very difficult. The continuity of the muscle fibers in both free walls suggests that they may be pulling together toward a common center (as is true with a single ventricle) and thus essentially assisting each other. The septum, serving as a common wall, may be considered under normal conditions as serving four functions: (a) as a mechanical foundation on which the RV free wall anchors for systolic contraction; (b) as a passive structure during diastole that moves according to the relative ventricular diastolic pressures, thus influencing the diastolic compliance of each ventricle; (c) as a systolic contractile component of each ventricle that, depending on its radius of curvature and systolic motion relative to the respective free walls, could assist or hinder ejection from the respective ventricles; and (d) as a transmitter, via the surrounding pericardium, of the intraventricular pressures developed by any septal motion over the entire surface of the heart. There is substantial experimental evidence supporting each of the above complex but nonmutually exclusive roles for the septum[5]. The modulation of the septal contribution to RV function under pathologic conditions has not been well established. Most investigators have considered the septum as a single muscle mass, dominantly related to the LV and indirectly assisting the RV (vide infra). However, research by Hurford et al.[42] suggests that the septum may function mechanically as if it had two parts, a right and a left side[42]. They observed that under the experimental condition of acutely increasing RV afterload by embolizing the pulmonary vascular bed, a marker of metabolic activity was markedly increased in both the RV free wall and the right side of the septum, but not in either the left side of the septum or the LV free wall. If metabolic activity is related to mechanical stress, an assumption on which much of cardiac physiology rests, then the right side of the septum is experiencing a very different load from the left side. Since the same coronary artery supplies the two sides of the septum, this also speaks to the importance of local signals in regulating coronary flow.

The RV functions as a low-pressure pump under normal circumstances. A sphere provides the most efficient means of symmetrically reducing the radius of a chamber to accomplish ejection. Paradoxically, if asymmetric changes are allowed, for a given sarcomere length change, a long, thin chamber may provide a more efficient pump. It seems that under normal circumstances, RV ejection may be assisted substantially by LV ejection. Studies in isolated hearts[43–45] have demonstrated that an increased LV volume increases RV-developed systolic pressure. In both angiographic and echocardiographic studies of either a normal muscular septum or a prosthetic interventricular septum, rightward motion is seen during systole, consistent with a contribution to RV ejection via this septal motion produced by the higher LV systolic pressure[40,46–49].

Both the clinician and the physiologist agree that under normal conditions, the RV functions superbly as a low-pressure volume pump; however, in the presence of a markedly increased afterload, it is intriguing that they may come to different conclusions. Maughan et al.[50] demonstrated in an in vitro system that the RV can function as a pressure pump, generating peak systolic pressures of 80 mm Hg or more for prolonged periods. This, however, must be accomplished at a markedly elevated end-diastolic pressure, which, for the clinician, would be interpreted as RV failure. Thus, the clinician is faced with the situation in which an RV can both acutely and chronically cope with generating an adequate systolic pressure, but at the expense of a diastolic pressure producing peripheral edema, ascites, etc., due to an unacceptably high back pressure for venous return.

An increased pulmonary vascular resistance (PVR) can increase ventricular afterload through alterations in ventricular systolic wall tension. According to the Laplace equation, wall tension will vary directly with the transmural pressure and radius of curvature but inversely with wall thickness. Thus, any physiologic perturbation that changes any of these variables influences the RV afterload. As with the LV, the term afterload is frequently used in two different senses: (a) meaning the peak systolic wall tension and (b) reflecting the impedance of the circuit into which the ventricle ejects. Using the former definition, RV afterload may be reduced by lowering the peak systolic pressure, reducing the radius of curvature, or increasing the wall thickness. The role of changes in both global and regional RV geometry in determining pump performance as distinguished from a pure Frank-Starling mechanism remains to be elucidated. In addition, while enlarging the RV will improve its pumping ability and pressure-generating ability, the potential of pericardial constraint on the RV free wall could limit RV coronary flow[51,52]. Both clinical and experimental studies suggested that RV coronary distribution may be unsuited for long-term support of the chronically hypertensive RV[53,54].

The influence of respiration on RV output **(Table 11.2)** can be considered as an integrated but separate event from respiration's effects on venous return. Because preload is defined as the RV end-diastolic volume, the preceding discussion of systemic venous return must be first included and then expanded.

Particularly pertinent in understanding respiratory variation in RV diastolic performance is the concept of ventricular interdependence, proposed by Dornhorst et al.[55] in 1952. The concept of diastolic interdependence has come to mean the effect of a change in pressure or volume of one side of the heart on the other, having a common septum and a moderate degree of free wall muscle continuity, with all four chambers potentially constrained by the pericardium. Thus, acute volume expansion of one side of the heart, e.g., as occurs with spontaneous inspiration and right heart filling, will affect the filling of the contralateral side by virtue of a septal shift and/or transmission of the increased free wall tension[5,40]. Clearly, the degree of influence of one chamber on the other depends on the relative compliance of the respective free walls and the septum. That is, a thick stiff-walled septum will not be affected nearly as much as a highly compliant thin-walled septum[40]. While the RV, with its much larger respiratory variation in end-diastolic volume, will influence LV compliance, interdependence becomes less important in the hypertrophic RV observed with chronic pulmonary disease or right-sided obstructive congenital heart defects. Diastolic interaction between the ventricles (right influencing left and left influencing right) has been well documented in numerous studies[5]. As total cardiac volume approaches the unstressed volume of the pericardium, the degree of interdependence markedly increases[56]. As importantly, if the total intrapericardial volume remains relatively normal or is diminished, pericardial constraint is minimal and hence interdependence minimal. Therefore, with the spontaneous inspiratory increase in RV volume that increases pericardial constraint, the LV diastolic pressure must increase for a constant LV volume. This will decrease the gradient for pulmonary venous return to the left ventricle and lead to diminished LV inflow. Conversely, during an IPPV inspiration, the increase in intrathoracic pressure, direct heart compression by the lung, and an increase in LV volume secondary to increased pulmonary venous return (which decreases RV compliance) all combine to reduce RV diastolic volume[57].

Table 11.2. Right Ventricular Output—Physiologic Variables During Ventilation

Venous return—preload
Afterload—pulmonary vascular resistance
Fixed anatomic
Variable
Humoral-chemoreceptor
Mechanical
Right ventricular contractility
Left ventricular contractility
Ventricular interdependence
Pericardium
Heart-lung interaction

The role of the pericardium in respiratory-induced acute changes in ventricular loading conditions had not been studied until recently, except with regard to ventricular interdependence. While the pericardium has conventionally been appreciated as limiting large acute changes in preload, in the extreme cardiac tamponade its implicit role in also limiting acute increases in ventricular afterload (defined as peak ventricular wall stress) has rarely been appreciated. Almost a century ago, Yas Kuno, a former student of Starling, recognized that if he markedly increased the afterload in a Starling isolated heart preparation, when the pericardium was acutely removed, the ventricle became hemorrhagic and failed[58]. Takata et al.[59] quantified this concept by measuring the pericardial pressure over each ventricle during acute changes in ventricular loading conditions, including those produced by respiration. They observed that once the elastic limits of the pericardium are reached as a ventricle increases in size, the pericardium produces a proportional increase in pressure over the ventricle. During diastole, this will limit preload increases and reduce venous return. This is an adverse consequence with cardiac tamponade, but a useful consequence in a dilated failing ventricle. As importantly, during systole, the elastic energy stored in the pericardium during diastole as venous pressure distended the ventricle, will assist ventricular ejection. Thus, with either acute increases in diastolic inflow or acute increases in ventricular afterload increasing diastolic ventricular volumes, the pericardium applies a proportional counterforce. This implies that an acute increase in either RV or LV afterload, producing ventricular enlargement and hence elevated pericardial pressure over each ventricle, will attenuate the effects of afterload increase if one considers the respective arterial pressure as an index of impedance. In a simplistic analogy, acutely increasing pulmonary artery by 20 mm Hg will dilate the RV and could raise the pericardial pressure over the ventricle by 5 mm Hg. The effective increase in systolic work the ventricle must perform is related to an increase of 15, not 20, mm Hg in pressure work. This illustrates again the recurring theme that understanding cardiorespiratory interactions requires consideration of the surrounding pressure of each vascular compartment. Thus the pericardium will attenuate large respiratory-induced changes in loading (preload and afterload) for both the RV and LV. Any increase in RV preload should modulate RV systolic afterload via the Laplace relationship—i.e., any thinning of the wall will increase the afterload, while if the RV becomes rounder, the radius of curvature should decrease, diminishing the afterload. Because of the complex geometry of the RV (determined to some degree by the pericardium) and the relatively thin wall, these relationships have not been well studied. The implications this has for understanding biventricular function in postoperative cardiac surgical patients after pericardiotomy have not been fully studied.

However, recent insights into the mechanisms of pericardial-mediated constraint on venous flows and intracardiac pressures in disease states are relevant to the intensivist[60]. If ventricular interdependence is considered as a horizontal pericardially mediated effect, then the influence of pericardial constraint on atrioventricular interactions can be considered as a vertical interaction. The two most prominent pericardial pathologic processes are acute tamponade, in which a fluid (blood, effusion) limits venous return by increasing right and left atrial pressures equally, and the more chronic constrictive pericarditis, typically associated with a thickened adherent pericardium and loculated fluid collections increasing right atrial pressure and reducing venous return, with both pericardial states leading to a hypotensive low output state. However, they exhibit almost diametrically opposite effects on venous flow and pressure wave forms during a cardiac cycle. In acute tamponade, the intrapericardial fluid column that surrounds the heart distributes intrapericardial pressure evenly and immediately over all four chambers, and as such can be conceived as a "coupled" constraint[60]. As the amount of fluid increases, pericardial constraint becomes manifest by increased pressure exerted over each chamber, raising atrial absolute pressures equally and reducing atrial transmural pressures to zero and atrial volumes until all venous return ceases. The only way blood can then return to either atrium is for the ventricles to eject blood during systole, reducing total intrapericardial volume and thus lowering the pressure in the pericardial fluid, which effectively determines the downstream atrial pressure for venous return. Venous flow will then occur until the atria fill to the point at which total intrapericardial volume increases and atrial pressure again precludes further inflow. If the flow is minimal, this process will occur during systole. Thus atrial filling is coupled to ventricular emptying by vertical pericardial constraint. Venous inflow is limited to systole; the decline in atrial pressure allowing filling occurs during systole ("x" descent), and total intrapericardial volume thus remains relatively constant throughout the cardiac cycle. This pattern of flow and pressures can be contrasted to constrictive pericarditis, in which changes in a chamber's volume affect only the local pericardial pressure over the chamber and is thus "uncoupled" from having any effect on the other chambers. In this condition, the pressure exerted by the pericardial constraint over the atrium will only decrease to allow venous inflow when blood moves into the ventricle or when the atrial muscle relaxes after atrial systole. If the increase in pressure produced by the atrial muscle is small compared with the markedly elevated local pericardial pressure, atrial relaxation becomes a minor factor, and hence venous inflow will occur only during ventricular filling (i.e., diastole) when atrial pressure transiently falls ("y" descent). Thus opposite changes in atrial filling occur and the associated differences in atrial and venous pressures can be explained by the effects of coupled versus uncoupled pericardial constraint[60]. Preliminary studies in our laboratory suggest that lung constraint of the heart acts as an uncoupled constraint, and hence analysis of venous pressures and flows may allow monitoring to determine when lung constraint is substantially contributing to reduced venous return with PEEP (unpublished observations).

A significant increase in the PVR will increase RV afterload. Studies on the impedance characteristics of the pulmonary bed suggest that the afterload imposed on the RV for the same pressure may be quite different when created by proximally banding the pulmonary artery as opposed to embolizing multiple small vessels[61]. Thus, the work the RV (or LV) does is influenced not only by the resistance but also by the compliance of the circuit into which it ejects. Therefore, despite the same increase in resistance, a different afterload may be created by lesions in different parts of the pulmonary vascular bed. Fixed arteriolar obstruction can be predicted with primary pulmonary hypertension, chronic hypoxia, chronic high-flow left-to-right shunts, or multiple embolic events. Reversible pulmonary vasoconstriction is most commonly associated with acute or subacute alveolar hypoxia. Changes in lung volume, which by definition means a change in alveolar pressure relative to intrathoracic pressure, have a variable effect on PVR. At minimal lung volume, the PVR is elevated and falls to a minimum near functional residual capacity (FRC), then increases as lung volume increases toward total lung capac-

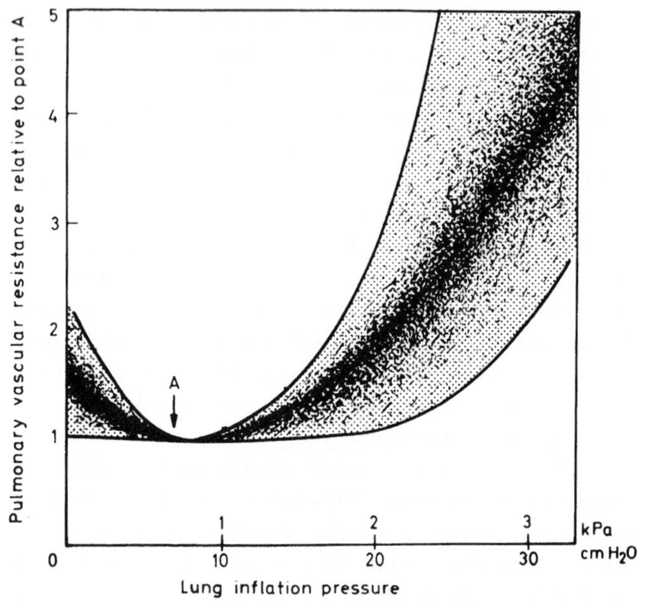

Figure 11.8. Representation of pooled experimental data on the change in pulmonary vascular resistance (PVR) with lung inflation in normal lungs. It is evident that PVR is minimal at *point A*, which corresponds to functional residual capacity (FRC). From that point, with either decreasing or increasing lung inflation, PVR increases. (From Nunn JF. Applied respiratory physiology. London: Butterworths, 1977:259.)

ity[(62)] (Figure 11.8). Thus, from a normal FRC, normal tidal volume inspiration produces inconsequential increases in afterload/impedance[(63,64)]. However, large tidal volumes or tidal volumes superimposed on an elevated lung volume produced by airway obstruction (e.g., small airways obstruction in asthma or PEEP) can significantly increase RV afterload. Thus, a markedly elevated lung volume (i.e., alveolar pressure elevated relative to intrathoracic pressure with either spontaneous or positive pressure ventilation) implies an elevated PVR.

It is easy to understand that the RV afterload is increased with PEEP. As an example, consider a PEEP producing an alveolar pressure of 30 cm H_2O and a pleural pressure (Ppl) of 14 cm H_2O, i.e., a transpulmonary pressure (Ptp) = 16 cm H_2O. The same afterload on the RV would be produced at the end of a spontaneous inspiration, with a Ppl of −16 cm H_2O and an alveolar pressure in equilibrium with the mouth pressure of zero, i.e., Ptp = 16 cm H_2O. If the airway is completely obstructed, a spontaneous inspiratory effort produces an equal fall in pleural and alveolar pressures. In this case, with no change in lung volume and no gradient between the pleural and alveolar space, no increase in RV afterload is produced. Nevertheless, because RV volume increases with the concomitant increased venous return, the RV wall stress would still increase. In addition, any increase in LV afterload, consequent to negative intrathoracic pressure that was transmitted across the pulmonary vascular bed, would also contribute to the RV afterload (vide infra). Under conditions of severe airway obstruction, each spontaneous inspiration would increase the RV afterload by all of the above mechanisms in addition to any increase in PVR with hypoxic pulmonary vasoconstriction due to alveolar hypoxia with hypoventilation.

In a Valsalva's maneuver, in which the intrathoracic pressure around the heart and pulmonary vascular bed increases equally with no change in lung volume (despite the common misinterpretation), the increase in pulmonary artery pressure does not reflect an increase in RV afterload. Indeed, the initial cause for right-to-left shunting with a Valsalva's maneuver must be a reduced LV afterload (vide infra). If the maneuver is prolonged sufficiently to result in alveolar hypoxia, then hypoxic pulmonary vasoconstriction may increase RV afterload.

The influence of the LV on the RV systolic performance via ventricular interdependence is rarely considered. A number of studies have demonstrated that as the LV enlarges, RV systolic pressure increases[(5)]. The mechanism for this is not clearly defined but may reflect some degree of rightward septal shift, which either directly or through modification of RV geometry enhances its pressure-generating capability. At one extreme, the RV free wall can be replaced by a dacron prosthesis and RV performance maintained[(65)]. At the other extreme, the ability of the RV to generate a systolic pressure is compromised markedly by cutting the LV free wall[(45)]. Creation of a prosthetic passive septum results in LV systolic bulging into the RV[(48)]. These experiments raise the critical question of whether optimal LV function is required to maintain RV pump performance in conditions with acute or chronic elevations of PVR. There is little question, based on clinical experience, that LV failure worsens the status of any patient with acute or chronic marked increases in PVR. Such mechanisms almost certainly play a critical role in bronchopulmonary dysplasia and cystic fibrosis and explain why therapy directed at improving LV function may improve the clinical condition of these patients.

Ventricular interdependence also may influence PVR. Experimental and clinical studies have noted that an elevated pulmonary capillary wedge pressure can be observed with severe RV afterloading and dilation, yet a diminutive LV, i.e., LV compliance is decreased[(42,66)]. In zone III conditions (Ppa > Pla > Palv), the left atrial pressure is the downstream pressure for PVR, and thus any increase in Pla would increase PVR. Therefore, not only LV failure or hypervolemia-induced increases in Pla may contribute to PVR, but also any respiratory-induced change in right heart volume will change LV compliance, and hence influence PVR.

In summary, RV performance is still poorly understood when compared with knowledge of LV performance. The right heart, however, forms a critical link in series with the peripheral venous bed, pulmonary vascular bed, and LV and in parallel with the LV, pericardium, and lung parenchyma. In addition, the rapidly emerging body of knowledge of cardiorespiratory interactions at the cellular level responding to the chemical (hypoxia) and mechanical (shear stress) stimuli must now be considered, particularly in pathologic conditions relevant to the ICU.

Table 11.3. Pulmonary Venous Return—Physiologic Variables During Ventilation

Right ventricular output
Lung volume (expiratory/inspiratory)
Alveolar pressure
Alveolar blood volume
Pulmonary arterial and venous extra-alveolar blood volume
Pulmonary arterial pressure
Pulmonary venous (left atrial) pressure
Ventricular interdependence
Heart-lung interaction

Pulmonary Venous Return

The major factors determining pulmonary venous return are listed in **Table 11.3.** In the steady state, it is obvious that pulmonary venous return is equal to pulmonary arterial (RV) input. However, reliable measurement of phasic changes in pulmonary venous return during a respiratory cycle in the intact circulatory system presents major technical problems. Much greater confidence is warranted in experimental data in which isolated lungs or lobes have been studied and the heart essentially eliminated by mechanically setting a downstream left atrial pressure. From these studies[67–69], a number of general principles can be derived. Pulmonary arterial and venous vascular volumes will increase as the respective pressure rises, reaching a limit as the vessels reach the upper limits of their distensibility[70]. Even before the limit of their distensibility is reached, fluid may leak into the interstitium, creating perivascular edema that, if not removed by the lymphatics, will limit intravascular capacitance.

The effect of increasing lung volume is twofold, having opposite effects on the extra-alveolar and intra-alveolar vessels. Extra-alveolar vessels will expand as the lung is inflated, pulled open by the surrounding attached pulmonary parenchyma in a process known as *pulmonary vascular interdependence.* It can be viewed as analogous to stretching a fabric and enlarging the interstices between the threads. If vessels are inside such a "hole," and their sides are attached to the threads creating the hole, the vessels would be pulled open. Indeed, inflating the lung enlarges both pulmonary extra-alveolar arteries and veins by creating a negative pressure around the vessel, thus increasing its local transmural pressure[70,71]. Therefore, if a steady-state pulmonary arterial inflow is created artificially, regardless of the ventilatory mode, lung inflation will produce an increased extra-alveolar vascular volume and take-up volume, transiently reducing pulmonary venous outflow until a steady state again is reached. Conversely, reducing lung volume will diminish extra-alveolar vessel blood volume and tend to produce a transient increase in pulmonary venous outflow.

However, the problem is more complex because the alveolar vascular bed blood volume changes in exactly the opposite direction to the extra-alveolar vessels[68–70] (Figure 11.9). Expanding the alveolar space (whether by spontaneous or a positive pressure) inflation stretches the alveolar capillaries, reducing their capacitance and thus driving blood out of the alveolar compartment into the extra-alveolar compartments. With a pulmonary valve in place, blood squeezed out of the alveolar bed will move antegrade toward the left heart. Combining the above factors, and again assuming constant pulmonary artery inflow, the effects of phasic ventilation on pulmonary venous return can be categorized according to the predominant lung zone. In zone III (Ppa > Pla > Palveolar), particularly with high vascu-

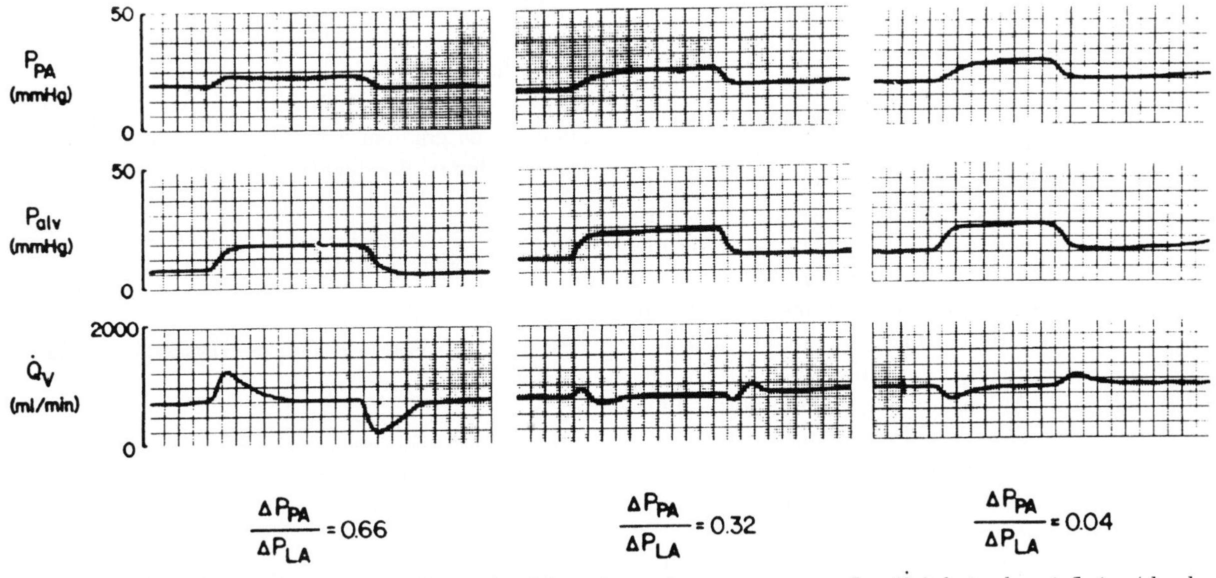

Figure 11.9. Tracings from an isolated constant inflow perfused lung show pulmonary venous outflow ($\dot{Q}v$) during lung inflation (alveolar pressure, P_{alv}, increasing) under different pulmonary vascular lung zones defined by the ratio of ΔPPA to ΔPLA. *Left:* Inflation in zone III results in a transient increase in $\dot{Q}v$. *Right:* Zone II inflation results in a transient decrease in $\dot{Q}v$. *Center:* A biphasic change in $\dot{Q}_v$ is observed when lungs are in transition between zones II and III. PPA, pulmonary arterial pressure; Palv, alveolar pressure; *$\dot{Q}v$,* pulmonary venous flow; Pla, left atrial pressure. (From Brower R, et al. Effect of lung inflation on lung blood volume and pulmonary venous flow. J Appl Physiol 1985;58:954.)

lar pressures expected in hypervolemic or LV failure states, the extravascular vessels, even during expiration, are near their maximum volume. With lung inflation, the dominant effect is antegrade translocation of the alveolar blood volume displaced by alveolar distention. Whatever volume is not taken up by the extra-alveolar venous bed then exits from the lung. The more congested the alveolar vascular bed and the larger the tidal volume, the greater the volume of blood ejected from the lung. In a lung predominantly in zone II (Ppa > Palveolar > Pla), as occurs in hypovolemia or with high PEEP, the alveolar vascular bed is relatively empty during expiration. With a tidal inflation, there is very little blood translocated out of the alveolar bed, while both the pulmonary arterial and venous extra-alveolar vessels will take up volume, dependent on the initial lung volume. Additionally, the inspiratory increase in PVR will further reduce flow across the lung. The net result is a diminution in pulmonary venous outflow, depending on the vascular pressures and lung volumes, as opposing events occur in the alveolar and extra-alveolar beds[(69)].

Extending the above analysis of pulmonary venous return to the intact circulatory systems, two other factors must be considered: (a) ventricular interdependence and (b) variable pulmonary arterial inflow. During respiration, the phasic changes in right heart volume, via ventricular interdependence, influence LV compliance and, therefore, the downstream pressure for pulmonary venous return. An increasing right heart volume tends to reduce pulmonary venous return by this mechanism. However, the influence of the right and left hearts being in parallel with a common wall may be opposed by their relationship in series. For example, a spontaneous inspiration increases right heart volume, which, through interdependence, would reduce pulmonary venous return but, through an increased RV output, increases pulmonary venous return. These two normally opposing factors can work in concert in pathologic conditions to reduce pulmonary venous return. With a very high pulmonary vascular resistance, IPPV and PEEP may increase RV volume during inspiration associated with the expected decrease in systemic venous return and RV output[(72)].

The conclusion that it requires two to three beats for the effects of a change in RV output to traverse the pulmonary vascular bed and influence the LV has been based on the observed "phase lag" in right and left heart outputs[(73,74)]. This conclusion must be contrasted with the work of Maloney et al.[(75)], which indicates that both pressure and flow transmission can occur across the entire pulmonary vascular bed in 400 msec. Although it may require two to three beats for a specific red cell or drop of angiographic contrast material to traverse the pulmonary vascular bed, the fluid column in the pulmonary vessels, which connects the right and left hearts, determines the delay in terms of pressure and flow coupling. In simplistic analogy, a train with a caboose (at the RV) and lead car (at the left atrium) may require a long time for the caboose to reach the left atrium, but a sudden push applied to the caboose is noted very rapidly in the lead car, depending on how tightly the intervening cars are coupled and the degree to which they absorb the "shock" (i.e., depending on the resistance, compliance, and inertance of the pulmonary vascular bed). Thus, if other factors were irrelevant, the series connection between the right and left hearts would dominate. The phasic relationships would demonstrate less than a one-beat phase lag between RV and LV outputs. Because the phase lag between respiratory changes in the RV and LV outputs is usually more than one beat, physiologic factors other than a fluid column connecting the two sides of the heart must be present.

In summary, pulmonary venous return results from modulation of the systemic venous return by RV performance, pulmonary arterial and venous pressures, lung volume, and ventricular interdependence. Similarities of the analysis of systemic venous return with respect to the abdominal compartment and pulmonary venous return with respect to the lung illustrate the usefulness of applying general principles in multiple vascular beds.

Left Ventricular Output

Many of the principles outlined in the discussion of respiratory variation in RV output are also directly applicable to the analysis of LV output **(Table 11.4).** The law of conservation of mass demands that input (pulmonary venous return) and output must be equal. Diastolic modification of the LV preload during ventilation may be influenced significantly by ventricular interdependence, pericardial constraint, heart-lung mechanical interactions (compression), and LV contractility. The two variables that must be considered as affecting LV systolic performance for a given preload are afterload and contractility[(76)].

If the entire circulatory system existed within a single compartment, changes in the pressure surrounding the heart would be irrelevant to analysis of either diastolic or systolic performance because the same pressure changes also would be experienced by the vascular bed. No gradient would be produced to influence systemic venous return, and similarly no gradient would be produced for blood exiting from the thorax. Whether the pressure around the heart were −100, 0, or +100 mm Hg, no effect would be noted. However, the intrathoracic compartment is an area where the pressure around part of the vasculature varies during ven-

Table 11.4. Left Ventricular Output—Physiologic Variables During Ventilation

Pulmonary venous return
Left ventricular end-diastolic pressure-volume relationship
Ventricular interdependence
Pericardial constraint
Heart-lung interaction
Afterload
Systemic arterial resistance and compliance (impedance)
Intrathoracic (pleural) pressure
Abdominal pressure
Left ventricular contractility
Left ventricular end-systolic pressure-volume relationship

tilation. Assuming for the moment that the pressure surrounding the extrathoracic vascular compartment remains constant, then it is easy to understand that increasing intrathoracic pressure would not only reduce venous return, but would also translocate the blood in the thorax out into the extrathoracic compartments. This concept is not new; Visscher et al.[77] in 1924 referred to work by Ludwig in 1847:

> "In considering the peripheral resistance of the flow of blood, it is necessary to consider the fact that the relative pressure against which the heart must work can be altered without changing the condition of the peripheral vessels at all. By lowering the pressure in the thorax and thus in the heart itself, the difference of pressure between the heart and the peripheral arteries is increased. Therefore, the heart must do more work to maintain the arterial pressure at its previous level. This fact was emphasized by Ludwig and it might seem at first thought that it could account for the whole of the respiratory wave in blood pressure." (p 587)

The normal LV is remarkably insensitive to a wide range of acute changes in afterload[78], while the preload is exquisitely sensitive to small changes in pressure. Thus, an afterload effect would not be anticipated to be large under normal physiologic conditions with small changes in intrathoracic pressure during either spontaneous or positive pressure breathing. Rather, preload changes should dominate. However, large changes in afterload, as might be expected with severe airway obstruction, should be evident, even in the normal LV. In contrast, the failing LV is insensitive to preload changes (i.e., functions on the flat portion of the ventricular function curve) but is sensitive to changes in afterload. Therefore, the failing LV is anticipated to be sensitive to ventilation-induced changes in LV afterload, but relatively insensitive to ventilation-induced changes in preload. Just as the effects of such interventions as volume loading or a nitroprusside infusion have different effects on improving LV output in the normal (i.e., preload-sensitive) and failing (i.e., afterload-sensitive) LV, ventilatory effects also may vary according to the underlying conditions.

Our understanding of the ventricular function curve (atrial pressure versus cardiac output) has been extended by studies in which measures of ventricular volume or strain have replaced atrial pressure, affecting the conventional definitions of preload or afterload sensitivity applied to pressure-output relationships. There is substantial evidence that under normal conditions, as right atrial pressure exceeds 3 mm Hg, pericardial constraint increasingly defines the measured right atrial pressure, such that sarcomere length is maintained within a relatively narrow range despite large increases in the absolute atrial pressure[79–82]. In chronically instrumented dogs, it could be demonstrated that the curvilinear flattening of the pressure-output relationship is associated with a straight-line relationship between volume or strain and output. Thus the term *preload insensitive* really reflects pericardial constraint, such that marked increases in atrial pressure, once elevated, produce little, if any, change in sarcomere length and hence minimal change in the Frank-Starling relationship[79].

Regardless of how long the concept has been discussed in the physiology literature, no subject in cardiorespiratory physiology has engendered more discussion and confusion than the effects of respiration on LV performance. The influence of changes in lung volume and intrathoracic pressure of LV performance is critical to understanding hemodynamic events during spontaneous ventilation with or without airway obstruction, during positive pressure ventilation with or without PEEP, and during CPR. Each could be separately and extensively analyzed. However, since the principles involved are the same for all of the above, an evaluation of the factors determining LV output during spontaneous respiration can serve as a basis for consideration of the others. "What causes the inspiratory fall in LV stroke volume (LVSV) during spontaneous ventilation?" can serve as the prototype question. By considering respiration to have both separate and interdependent influences on diastolic and systolic events, much of the confusion surrounding the basic physiologic phenomena during spontaneous and mechanical ventilation can be resolved. Considering the compression phase of a CPR cycle as systole and the relaxation phase as diastole, the same principles can be applied to CPR.

The major hypotheses advanced to account for the inspiratory fall in LV stroke volume (SV) can be divided into two groups, one ascribing the decrease in LVSV to a diminution in ventricular filling (a diastolic event), the second ascribing the decrease in LVSV to an increase in afterload or a decrease in contractility (systolic events)[83]. A primary decrease in preload leads to a decrease in the LV end diastolic volume, which produces a secondary decrease in the LV end systolic volume. An increase in afterload or a decrease in contractility leads first to an increase in the LV end systolic volume and then a secondary increase in the LV end diastolic volume. How to measure ventricular volume changes rapidly and use this information to determine mechanisms has been a major methodologic barrier. Many have used calculated transmural LV pressures, usually referenced to esophageal pressure, assuming a direct relationship between such pressures and LV volume. However, determination of "true" transmural LV pressure is extremely difficult, requiring simultaneous determination of local intrapericardial pressure over the LV and right ventricular pressure "over" the septum, which could then be used in an empirically determined complex weighting ratio[84]. The most direct approach to solving this problem is to determine changes in LV volume directly rather than extrapolating a volume change from a potentially misleading pressure measurement.

Using a variety of methods to measure LV volumes, advocates of a primary decrease in preload have unequivocally demonstrated in human and animal studies that during either a spontaneous inspiration or Müller's maneuver (an inspiratory effort against a completely obstructed airway producing a decrease in intrathoracic pressure with no change in lung volume if gas decompression is ignored), the

LV free wall to septal diameter acutely decreases, and the calculated LV end diastolic volumes diminish accounting for the fall in stroke volume[85–88]. Advocates of an increase in LV afterload causing the fall in SV have similarly presented results in both human and animal studies consistent with increases in LV end systolic volume when intrathoracic pressure decreases during a normal or partially obstructed inspiration[89–91]. The most important conclusion that one can draw from the myriad of well-done studies is that no single mechanism can account for all of the observations.

While the majority of studies lead to the conclusion that a diminished preload is the cause of the inspiratory fall in LV stroke volume, other factors are clearly present. In fact, increased LV volumes may account for the diverse results reported by different groups. Increases in either RV volume (ventricular interdependence) or lung volume (heart-lung interdependence), constraining LV filling, are most commonly believed to be responsible for the inspiratory decrease in LV preload[4,92]. Either an increase in afterload and/or a decrease in contractility could explain increases in LV end systolic and secondarily end diastolic volumes when stroke volume diminishes[32,89].

The phasic change in systemic venous return and RV output with respiration at normal respiratory rates should produce a substantial degree of variation in LV output[93]. While the variation in systemic venous return and hence RV output can account for a great deal of respiratory variation in LV output, it can not explain the observed fall in LV stroke volume with the first inspiratory effort after a prolonged apneic period. Accordingly, it is necessary to evaluate the role of the various potential mechanisms by proving their presence independently from other factors. By investigating the results of changes in intrathoracic pressure and lung volume on diastole alone, and then on systole alone, this becomes possible.

The cardiac cycle can be divided into a diastolic period (ventricular filling, altering preload) and a systolic period (ventricular ejection altered by afterload and contractility). Within each period, further temporal refinement is possible, i.e., early diastole with passive filling and late diastole with active filling associated with atrial contraction. Similarly, systole can be divided into early isovolumic contraction, ejection, and late isovolumic relaxation periods. Since respiration affects ventricular performance, it must affect some or all parts of a cardiac cycle. If ventilation influences only diastole, it could increase or decrease ventricular filling. Assuming a constant preload, if ventilation influenced only systole, the resultant stroke volume could increase, decrease, or be unchanged depending on the relative changes in LV afterload and/or contractility. Apparently contradictory results have served as the fuel for the differing schools of thought, each able to marshal data supporting either a predominant diastolic or systolic event.

Mitral and Aortic Flows During Spontaneous Ventilation

Separation of the diastolic and systolic influences of respiration on cardiac performance can be accomplished by com-

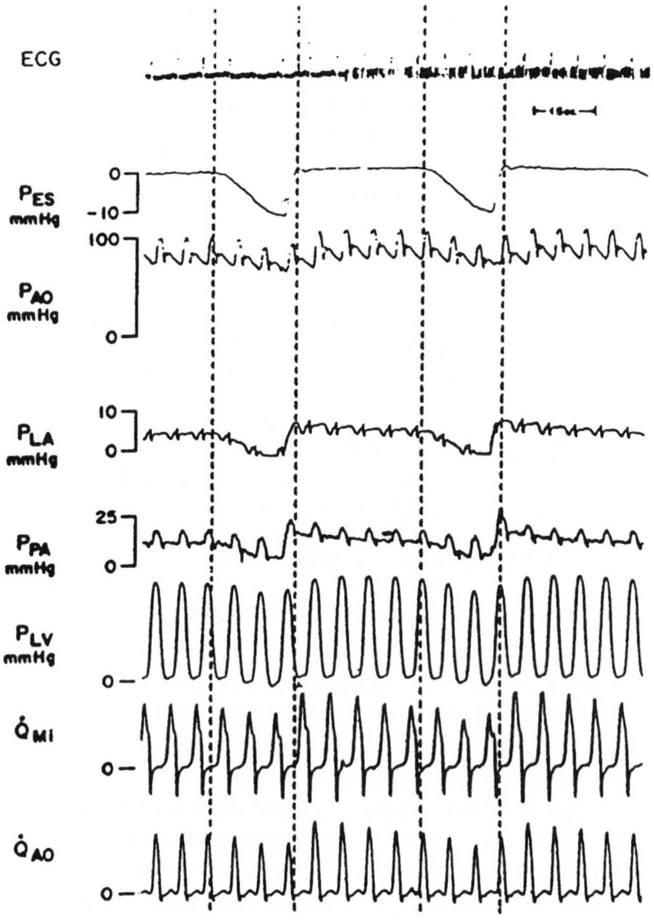

Figure 11.10. Two consecutive respiratory cycles during partial inspiratory airway obstruction in an anesthetized dog postvagotomy. *Vertical dashed lines* demarcate the two periods during which esophageal pressure is reduced during inspiration. Both integrated mitral (Qmi) and ascending aortic (Qao) flows diminish during the inspiration and increase with expiration. There is a large expiratory increase in mitral flow preceding the large increase in aortic flow in both respiratory cycles. Although the rapid increase in esophageal pressure occurs during systole in the second breath, there is little effect on aortic flow. These two respiratory cycles suggest the dominance of mitral flow leading aortic flow during partial inspiratory obstruction with normal left ventricular function. (From Robotham JL, Stuart RS, Doherty K, Borkon MA, Baumgartner W. Mitral and aortic blood flows during spontaneous respiration in dogs. Anesthesiology 1988;69:516.)

parison of changes in the integrated mitral and ascending aortic blood flows allowing assessment of changes in LV end diastolic and end systolic volumes, independent of any assumptions about LV shape. During respiration, variation was evident in both mitral and ascending aortic integrated flows[94,95] (Figure 11.10). However, the cyclical nature of normal spontaneous ventilation and the relatively small changes usually observed between any two cardiac cycles made it difficult to clearly define the events at the beginning of an inspiration as being due to either primary diastolic or primary systolic events. If ventricular interdependence is to account for such rapid changes in LV preload, a phasic relationship between changes in right heart volumes and LV filling must be present. It could be demonstrated that sudden increases in systemic venous return to

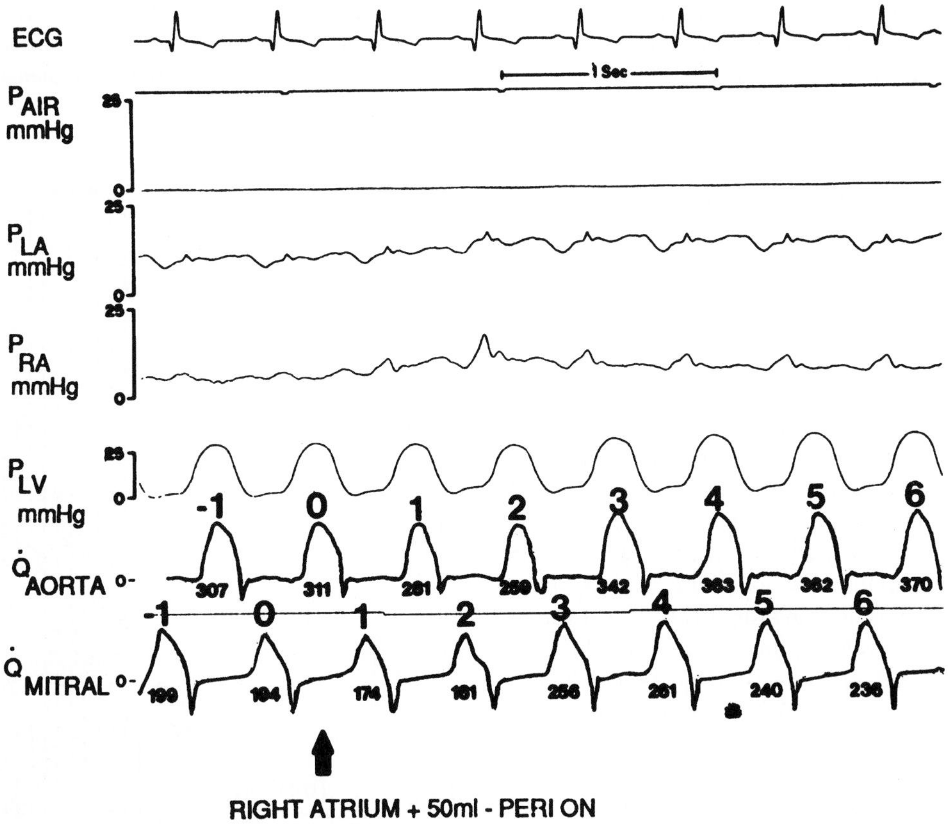

Figure 11.11. Open-chest study in an anesthetized dog during apnea, demonstrating the effects of a rapid infusion of 50 ml of blood into the right atrium with the pericardium present. The rhythm is stable as reflected by electrocardiogram (ECG), and airway pressure (Pair) reflects the apneic state. Left atrial (Pla) and LV (Plv) pressures are measured relative to atmosphere. To facilitate comparisons, flow traces occurring at the experimental perturbation are designated as 0, with negative and positive numbers above each consecutive beat, providing easy reference, with the areas in arbitrary units under each flow trace reflecting the respective volume of mitral inflow and aortic outflow for each cardiac cycle. The beginning of rapid infusion into the right atrium is marked by · and is associated with an immediate fall in the next two mitral flow (Q̇mitral) traces, numbered *1* and *2*, with a subsequent increase over the control period designated by the number 3 (diastolic period). Changes in aortic flow (Q̇aorta) trace follow those in Q̇mitral trace as indicated by numbered beats. Both Pra and Pla increase during infusion into the right atrium and are associated with the initial fall and then increase in Q̇mitral. We interpret this to reflect the right heart, first decreasing LV filling via interdependence and then increasing LV filling as the increased systemic venous return reaches the left side. A lesser effect reducing early Q̇mitral was found when the pericardium was removed. (From Robotham JL, Stuart RS, Borkon MA, Doherty K, Baumgartner W. Effects of changes in left ventricular loading and pleural pressure on mitral flow. J Appl Physiol 1988;65:1662.)

the right heart reduced LV compliance, increasing left heart diastolic pressures and diminishing peak and integrated total mitral flow (Figure 11.11). Consistent with ventricular interdependence mediating this relationship, removal of the pericardium attenuated the decrease in mitral flow[94].

Transient Analysis of a Negative Intrathoracic Pressure

In theory, it should be possible to perturb the ventilatory system in an extremely rapid manner, e.g., such that the separate and independent influences during systole and diastole could be evaluated. Recognition that rapid changes in intrathoracic pressure during spontaneous ventilatory efforts in dogs could produce independent effects on LV filling and emptying[94,95] led to development of a technique to precisely control intrathoracic pressure within specific periods of a cardiac cycle. The use of ECG-triggered bilateral phrenic nerve stimulation for brief periods of time gated to the cardiac cycle produced a rapid decrease of 15 to 25 mm Hg in intrathoracic pressure confined to either systole or diastole. The approach of analyzing rapid transient changes in lung volume and/or intrathoracic pressure becomes a powerful tool to define separate diastolic and systolic events during respiration since the influence of the RV output in series with the LV is eliminated[96]. Similarly, by confining the perturbation to diastole, any influence on the succeeding systole can be evaluated. By confining a perturbation to diastole after the aortic valve has closed, the influence of ventilation on left-sided arterial flow independent of LV function can be evaluated. This information provides insight into a ventilatory perturbation that extends over a complete cardiac cycle. The information gained is equally applicable to understanding all modes of respiration and CPR. Indeed, Pinsky et al.[99] extensively used positive pressure impulses gated to specific portions of the cardiac cycle to evaluate the physiology of cardiorespiratory interactions and apply the principles to the treatment of LV failure.

A series of studies performed in anesthetized dogs allowed ECG-triggered phrenic nerve stimulation while measuring (a) mitral and ascending aortic flow, (b) LV septal to lateral diameter using sonomicrometry, or (c) an ascending aortic flow and intrathoracic aortic diameters just distal to the aortic arch.

Figure 11.12 demonstrates the influence of a phrenic nerve stimulation confined to diastole. When the fall in intrathoracic pressure is confined to diastole, there is a substantial decrease in both the peak mitral flow and the integrated area, reflecting a decrease in LV filling[96]. The subsequent stroke volume when esophageal pressure has returned to baseline is reduced, as would be expected from Starling's law. The subsequent diastolic and systolic periods demonstrate an increase in both the peak and integrated mitral and aortic flows. The reason for the immediate fall in mitral flow is, in all likelihood, not due to a primary pooling of blood in the pulmonary vascular bed since at end-diastole, when esophageal pressure had returned to baseline, both atrial pressures relative to atmosphere were elevated compared with their previous values during apnea, as was the LV end diastolic pressure. Thus, for a diminished LV end diastolic volume, the LV end diastolic pressure was increased, i.e., effective LV diastolic compliance was decreased. Two types of interdependence could account for this, both compatible with the observed increase in right atrial pressure. Heart-lung interdependence, in which the expanding lungs compress the heart, would reduce the effective compliance of both ventricles, reducing biventricular filling[4]. This can not explain the similar findings of decreased mitral inflow and increased LV diastolic pressure when the airway is obstructed completely and the lung volume constant. The dominant mechanism here appears to be ventricular interdependence, in which the sudden increase in right ventricular filling competes with the LV for space within the intrapericardial sac[5]. As a result, LV compliance is diminished as the RV volume rapidly increases, thus reducing mitral flow and the subsequent LV stroke volume. Consistent with this, the LV septal to free lateral wall dimension decreases during a transient diastolic negative intrathoracic pressure[99]. The succeeding diastolic period exhibits a compensatory increase in mitral flow as the blood dammed up during the negative intrathoracic pressure and the increased systemic venous return, contribute to LV filling.

The influence of a fall in intrathoracic pressure confined to systole is illustrated in Figure 11.13. There is an immediate decrease in the peak and total integrated ascending aortic flow. The subsequent mitral flow was decreased, consistent with the presence of an acute increase in the LV end systolic volume. The fall in LV stroke volume during systolic phrenic nerve stimulation proves that a separate systolic mechanism contributes to the inspiratory fall in LV stroke volume. This means either an acute decrease in contractility or an increase in afterload. Since there are no known reflexes that could mediate such a decrease in contractility within 100 ms, a fall in contractility seems unlikely.

To address this issue from another perspective, we measured intrathoracic aortic dimensions in the closed-chest, anesthetized dog during systolic phrenic nerve stimulation. Piezoelectric crystals were placed to measure orthogonal diameters. Qualitative estimates of the true changes in trans-

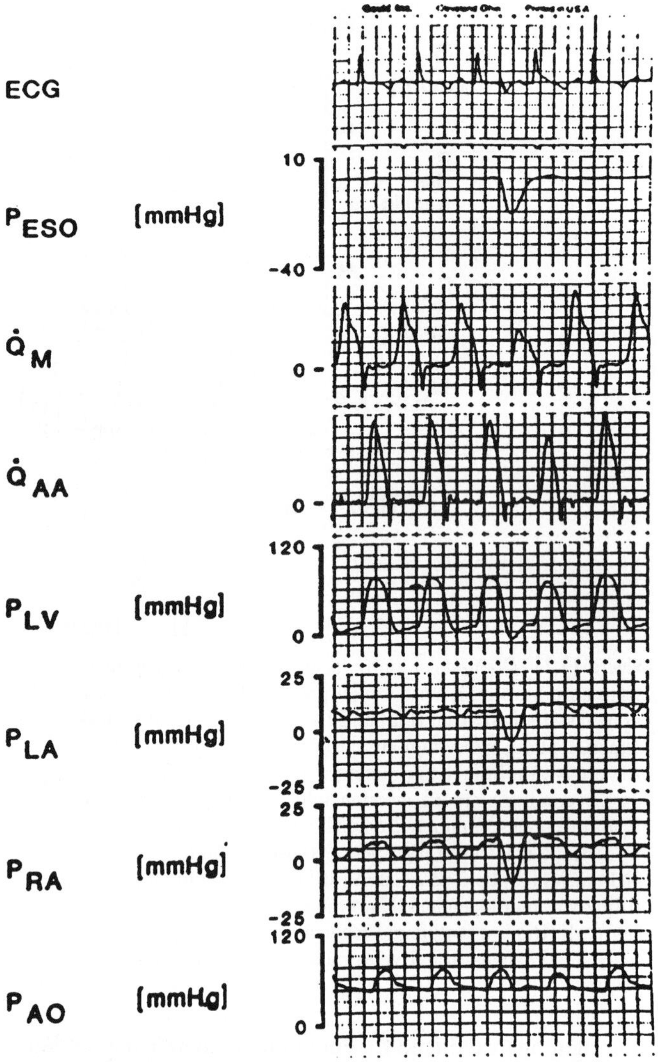

Figure 11.12. Diastolic phrenic nerve stimulation producing a transient decrease in esophageal pressure (Peso) confined to diastole in an acutely instrumented anesthetized dog during phrenic nerve stimulation. Steady-state mitral (QMi) and ascending aortic (QAa) flows are observed prior to the transient fall in intrathoracic pressure. There is an immediate substantial decrease in peak and total mitral flow. The subsequent left ventricular stroke volume (LVSV) is similarly reduced at a time when ITP has returned to its baseline value, such that there could be no effect on LV ejection. The subsequent mitral flow and LVSV demonstrate compensatory increases. Of critical importance, LV end-diastolic pressure (Plv), left atrial pressure (Pla), and right atrial pressure (Pra) are all increased relative to atmospheric pressure at end diastole when esophageal pressure has returned to baseline values. Since LV inflow has diminished, LV end-diastolic volume is reduced, and its pressure is increased, LV effective compliance must be reduced. The increase in right atrial pressure and the pattern of change in mitral flow are consistent with ventricular interdependence being responsible for the reduction in LV preload. (From Robotham JL, Peters J. Cardiorespiratory interactions. In: Zapol W, Lemaire F, eds. Adult respiratory distress syndrome. New York: Marcel Dekker, 1991:223.)

mural intrathoracic aortic pressure were thus possible. The use of the orthogonal diameters, which can be used to calculate the cross-sectional area of an ellipse, allowed an estimate of acute volume changes in the intrathoracic aorta. If anything, an inspiratory effort should increase the length of the intrathoracic aorta. Thus, if the cross-sectional area increases, the intrathoracic aortic volume increases. In effect, the aortic dimensions are used to "transduce" the true aortic transmural pressure. Thus, if a primary decrease in contractility accounts for the fall in LV stroke volume, then with less LV output, the peak systolic aortic volume should

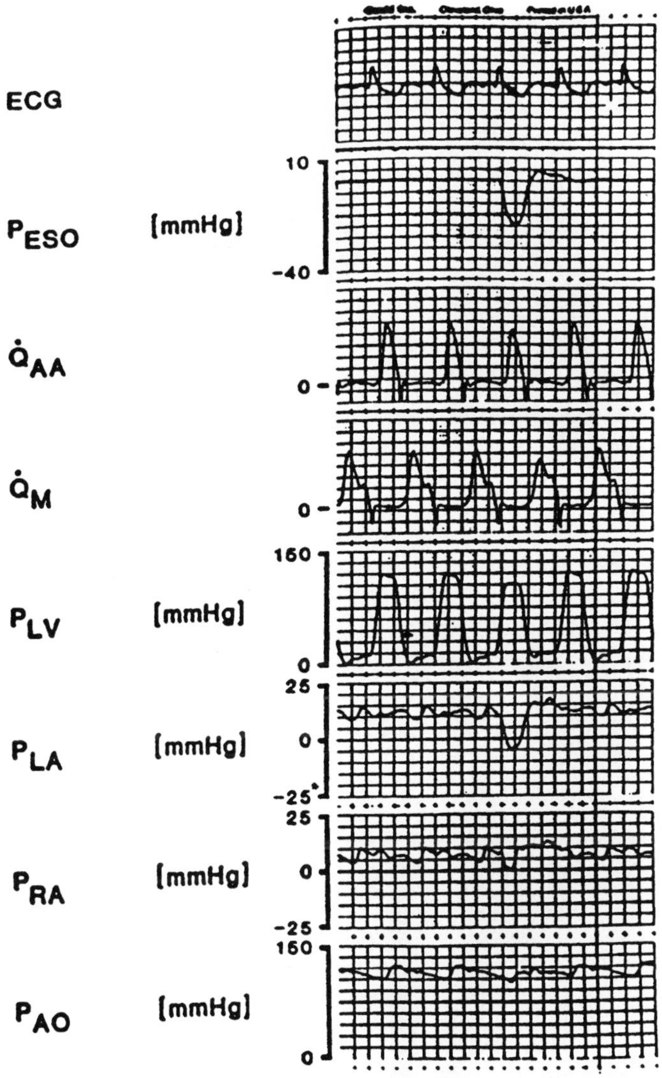

Figure 11.13. Original recording with negative ITP confined to systole and the airway unobstructed, allowing lung volume to increase during phrenic nerve stimulation in an anesthetized dog. The decrease in Peso begins during isovolumic contraction, i.e., after diastolic mitral flow has stopped, and is associated with a fall in ascending aortic flow and LVSV (integrated Q̇Aa). An unchanged LV preload before the systolic negative ITP is indicated by constant Qmi, end-diastolic Plv, and Pla in the immediately preceding beats. Thus, a fall in ITP during systole alone is sufficient to decrease LVSV. (From Peters J, Fraser C, Stuart RS, Baumgartner W, Robotham JL. Negative intrathoracic pressure decreases independently left ventricular filling and emptying. Am J Physiol 1989;257:H120.)

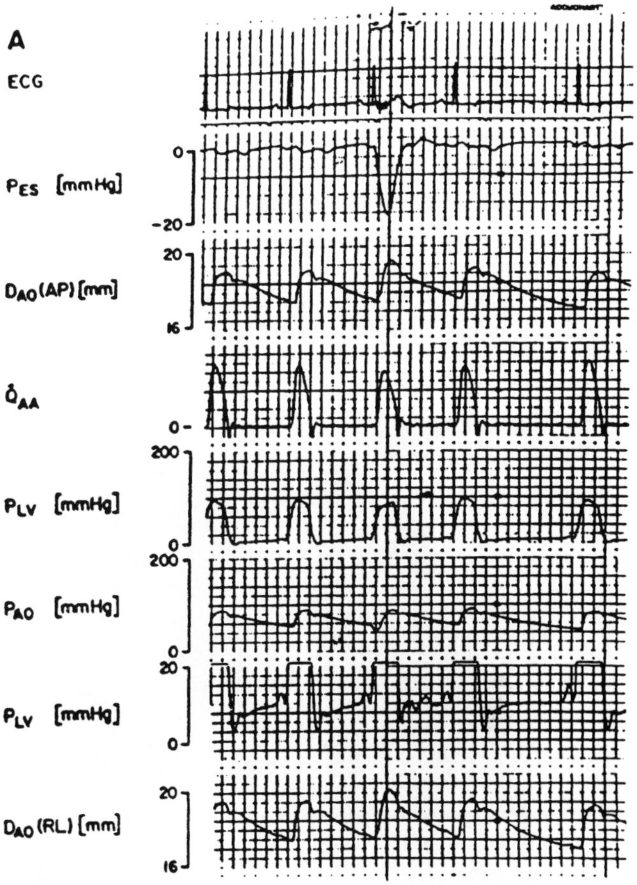

Figure 11.14. Recording with early systolic phrenic nerve stimulation to rapidly decrease intrathoracic pressure in an anesthetized dog. The airway was completely obstructed to keep lung volume constant. The decrease of esophageal pressure (Peso) causes an increase in the systolic anteroposterior intrathoracic aortic diameter (DAo[AP]), but a fall in LVSV derived from the ascending aortic blood flow (Q̇Aa). Both systolic LV (Plv) and aortic pressure (PAo) fall relative to atmospheric pressure. Neither the LV end-diastolic pressure (recorded with a fluid-filled catheter) immediately before phrenic nerve stimulation nor the R-R interval changes compared with the preceding cardiac cycle. Congruent with the increase in systolic DAo(AP), right-to-left aortic diameter (DAo[RL]) also increases. The decrease in LVSV associated with increased DAo (reflecting transmural aortic pressure) is compatible with an increased LV afterload. The same qualitative changes are observed when lung volume is allowed to increase with the fall in esophageal pressure, such that a decrease of ITP alone, with or without a change in lung volume, is sufficient to explain the fall in Q̇Aa and LVSV and the increase in DAo. (From Peters J, Kindred MK, Robotham JL. Transient analysis of cardiopulmonary interactions. II. Systolic events. J Appl Physiol 1988;64:1518.)

decrease. In contrast, if the primary cause of the fall in LVSV was equivalent to an increased afterload imposed at the junction of the intrathoracic and extrathoracic compartments, then the intrathoracic aortic volume/transmural pressure should increase. Figure 11.14 illustrates that with a transient fall in intrathoracic pressure confined to systole, the intrathoracic aortic dimensions increase as the LV stroke volume diminishes. This is consistent with an effective increase in afterload imposed between the intrathoracic and extrathoracic portions of the aorta[100].

In summary, it is clear that as negative intrathoracic

pressure continues for longer than one cardiac cycle, (a) the increased systemic venous return will lead to a gradual increase in LV stroke volume despite an increase in LV afterload; (b) the increased afterload will tend to preserve the end diastolic volume by increasing the end systolic volume; and (c) an increased, decreased, or absent net change in LV volumes could occur during a fall in intrathoracic pressure. Thus, it is not surprising that conflicting and confusing results have been published. Each group of studies reflects the balance of systolic and diastolic influences on LV volumes. It is not until the opposing factors are clearly understood within a single cardiac cycle that the discussions generated by such apparently discordant results can be reconciled.

Applying these principles to spontaneous respiration, it is clear that airway obstruction, either upper or lower, will adversely affect cardiac function and be particularly deleterious to a compromised LV. First, with hypoventilation, carbon dioxide will increase, imposing a respiratory acidosis. Second, the increased alveolar carbon dioxide will limit the partial pressure of oxygen in the alveolar space. Third, the marked increase in respiratory muscle work will pro-

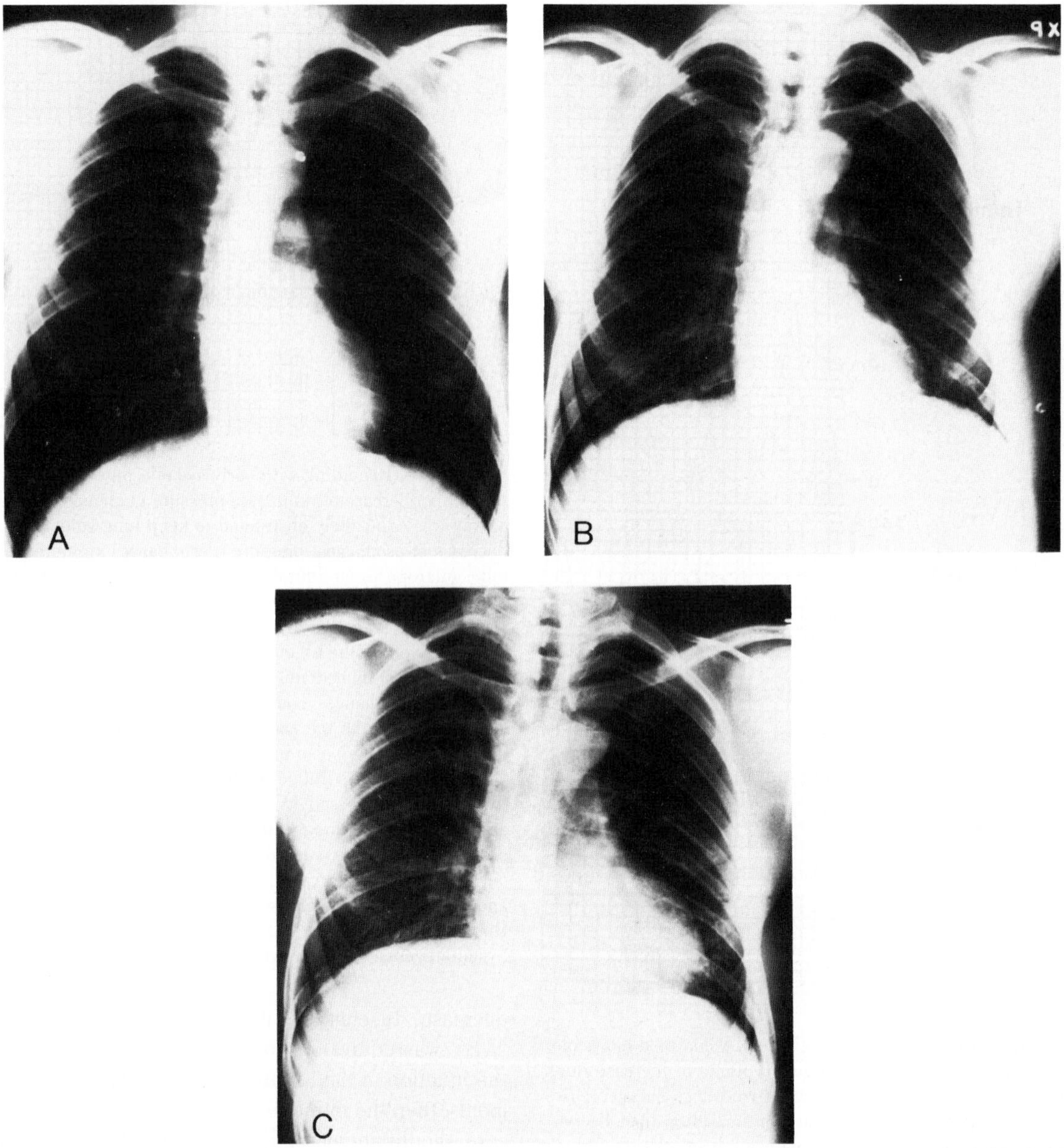

Figure 11.15. Sequential chest x-rays of the same subject. A. Standard posteroanterior film at total lung capacity. The pulmonary vascular markings, cardiac size, and ascending aortic size are all normal. B. The same subject with the film obtained at functional residual capacity to demonstrate "artifactual" increase in pulmonary vascular markings and cardiac and aortic knob size. C. Film taken just before concluding a 10-second vigorous Müller's maneuver, i.e., a maximal inspiratory effort against a closed glottis, producing a markedly negative ITP. There is a dramatic increase in pulmonary vascular markings, cardiomegaly, and dilatation of the ascending aorta, all consistent with a severe acute increase in impedance to LV ejection, as if the aorta had been cross-clamped at the diaphragm. (From Robotham JL. Hemodynamic events: a physiological approach. New York: Churchill Livingstone, 1984:183.)

duce a metabolic load and oxygen deficit as well as increased carbon dioxide and lactate production. This leads to a combined respiratory and metabolic acidosis, which by depressing LV contractility decreases oxygen delivery. If, in addition to these adverse conditions, we impose an increased preload and increased afterload, it is clear that airway obstruction with spontaneous respiration is the worst possible form of ventilation for the patient in LV failure. Any degree of alveolar hypoxemia will lead to hypoxic pulmonary vasoconstriction, increasing right ventricular afterload. If lower airway obstruction is present, lung hyperinflation will increase pulmonary vascular resistance, contributing to a further reduction in RV performance. Thus, not only the left but also the right ventricle will be adversely affected by airway obstruction. Finally, these mechanisms make it clear why acute upper airway obstruction can lead to florid pulmonary edema as the markedly negative intrathoracic pressures increase venous return to, and minimize arterial egress from, the thoracic compartment. This is illustrated in Figures 11.15 and 11.16. In Figure 11.15 a series of chest films demonstrates evidence of cardiomegly, pulmonary venous congestion, and—perhaps most importantly—aortic dilatation at the end of a 10-second Müller's maneuver. All of these findings can be explained by an acute large increase in LV afterload imposedon the aorta at the thoracic exit. Figure 11.16 demonstrates the results of relieving a partial inspiratory airway obstruction in an anesthetized spontaneously breathing dog. The sonomicrometer traces of the three orthogonal axes in the LV demonstrate the reduction in LV size after removal of the airway obstruction, consistent with the acute reduction in both LV preload and afterload.

All of these experiments, from the intact closed-chest circulatory system to isolated heart-lung preparations, force the conclusion that the hemodynamic events during airway obstruction cannot be explained by one or even two simple mechanisms. However, by returning to basic considerations of those factors controlling venous return RV output, pulmonary venous return, and LV output, and then considering events not just within a respiratory cycle but also within the cardiac cycle, a coherent and reasonable understanding is possible. Severe small airways disease with hyperexpansion in bronchopulmonary dysplasia, asthma, or cystic fibrosis have in common pathophysiologic events that influence the hemodynamic events and, hence, the clinical course and therapeutic objectives. An upper airway lesion that produces both inspiratory and expiratory partial obstruction, or an upper airway lesion superimposed on underlying small airway diseases, particularly if hypoxemia occurs concurrently (e.g., subglottic stenosis with bronchopulmonary dysplasia) results in a complicated pathophysi-

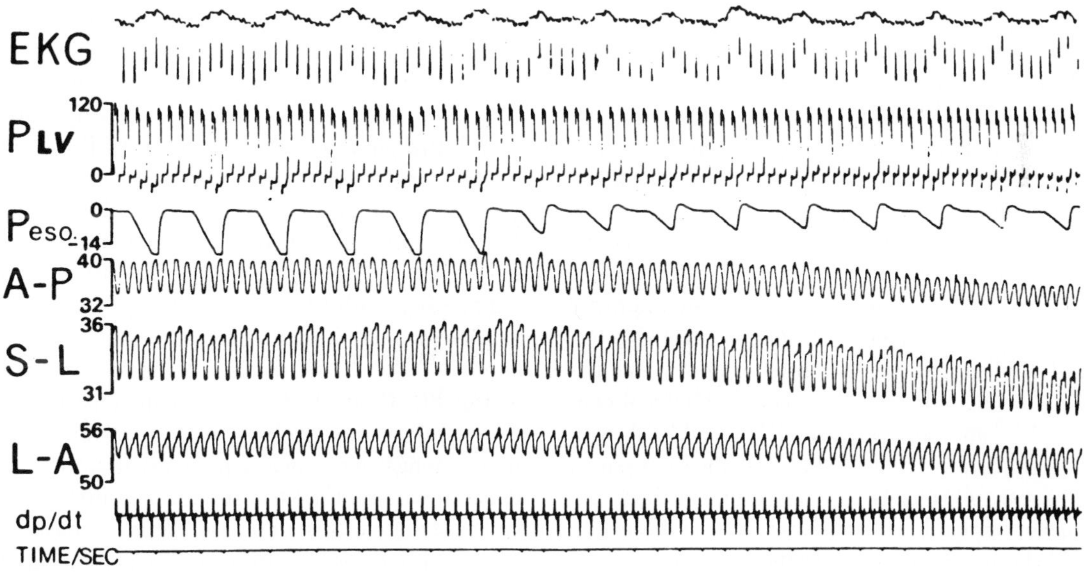

Figure 11.16. Effects of suddenly removing a partial inspiratory obstruction in an anesthetized, chronically instrumented dog breathing an elevated inspired oxygen. The inspiratory port of a one-way valve was partially obstructed, and a steady state was reached over 5 minutes, with negative inspiratory esophageal pressures (Peso) of −15 to −20 mm Hg. The obstruction was then acutely removed, as indicated by the smaller changes in Peso. The electrocardiogram (ECG) demonstrates a stable heart rate, and the LV pressure (Plv) is recorded relative to atmosphere, with the LV dp/dt recorded at the bottom of the tracing (just above the time line), marked every 1 second. The endocardial crystals in the anteroposterior (A-P), septal-to-lateral free wall (S-L), and the apex-base or long axes (L-A) dimensions demonstrate both changes within each respiratory cycle and overall steady-state changes. During each partially obstructed inspiration, there are increases in both end-diastolic and end-systolic dimensions for the A-P and L-A dimensions, while the S-L end-diastolic dimension decreases with little change in the end-systolic dimension. These findings are consistent with the presence of both an increased afterload, increasing the end-systolic volume, and a leftward septal shift and/or lateral lung compression to the heart diminishing the preload and hence the regional ejection fraction in the S-L dimension. Of greater importance is the observation of diminished end-systolic dimensions in all three axes, with relief of the obstruction consistent with removal of a large LV afterload. (From Robotham JL, Scharf SM. The effects of positive and negative pressure ventilation on cardiac performance. Clin Chest Med 1983;4:161.)

ologic process, producing extremely difficult clinical problems. A child with a congenital cardiac defect resulting in a left-to-right shunt and chronic upper airway obstruction (including obstructive sleep apnea) may develop pulmonary vascular disease from either or both processes, e.g., trisomy 21. Both must be recognized and treated. In all of the above examples, recognition of the potential interactions is the first step in approaching bedside diagnostic and therapeutic plans.

POSITIVE PRESSURE VENTILATION

Mechanical ventilatory support is routinely employed in ICUs. Despite numerous papers on the effects of PEEP on the circulatory system, one must first understand the control mode of IPPV[57,101–107]. An understanding of IPPV during both a single respiratory cycle and steady-state conditions offers a physiologic approach to understanding the effects of PEEP by considering PEEP as simply IPPV at an increased lung volume. As was illustrated with an examination of spontaneous ventilation, the array of physiologic variables that are affected by increased lung volume and intrathoracic pressure have, at times, diametrically opposing effects. Thus, baseline conditions may have a profound influence on which factors will play a dominant role. It can be demonstrated that even a question as simple as what effect an increase in intrathoracic pressure has on cardiac output is dependent on baseline conditions.

Despite substantial evidence that with most conditions during IPPV, preload factors dominate in determining respiratory variation in LV output, the question of whether an increase in intrathoracic pressure may reduce LV afterload remains. Criley et al.[108] demonstrated that with no ventricular function, i.e., during ventricular fibrillation, an increase in intrathoracic pressure produced by a cough moves blood out of the thorax. In this extreme example of ventricular failure, the apparent reason for an improved cardiac output was an effective reduction in LV afterload. Clinical studies comparing ventilator-dependent patients—one in moving from spontaneous to mechanical ventilatory support[109] and two comparing IPPV and IPPV with PEEP[110,111]—have all demonstrated that an increase in intrathoracic pressure reduces cardiac output in those patients with low or normal blood volumes, while in those with evidence of LV failure, increased intrathoracic pressure improved their cardiac output. Experimentally, Pinsky et al.[112] demonstrated in a canine model of LV failure that increasing intrathoracic pressure with a combination of PEEP and thoracoabdominal binding can improve cardiac output. Subsequently, Pinsky et al.[113] and Chandra et al.[114] demonstrated that increasing intrathoracic pressure, specifically during systole, maximized the increase in cardiac output. Significantly more work is required to define the physiologic variables producing these findings and the clinical role of afterload reduction with increasing intrathoracic pressure in various clinical states. Negative studies are published less often, but clinical anecdotal experience using modifications of these techniques has not been dramatically successful in the hands of other clinical investigators. This leads one to conclude that very careful attention to details in terms of the baseline cardiac and lung volumes, the amount of pleural pressure, lung volume, or abdominal pressure change are required. If "uncoupled" constraint (vide supra) of the heart by the lungs is present (i.e., venous return is minimal during ventricular systole), then increases in intrathoracic pressure will have little effect on venous return thus optimizing the net result of any effect on reducing LV afterload.

PEEP, in addition to increasing intrathoracic pressure, also increases lung volume, to a degree dependent on total respiratory compliance. If this results in a marked increase in right ventricular pressure, then a further increase in RV volume may be predicted to adversely effect LV compliance via ventricular interdependence. Whether such an increase in RV volume could have an adverse effect on LV systolic performance remains an uncertain factor deserving of study. Importantly, because under most circumstances RV volume diminishes with PEEP, any diminution on LV dimensions cannot be attributed to ventricular interdependence. This raises the question as to whether direct compression of the heart by the lungs may significantly contribute not only to the diminished systemic venous return but also to reduced pulmonary venous return. There are sufficient in vivo and in vitro studies available using either pericardial or intraventricular balloons to clearly document that the surface pressure applied to the ventricles may exceed the intrathoracic pressure generated by lung inflation—i.e., the lungs can squeeze the heart, particularly during inspiration. Initial studies suggesting that PEEP may adversely affect LV performance were likely incorrect because of an overestimation of the transmural LV filling pressure by using an esophageal balloon rather than a the pericardial balloon[115–122]. The apparent increase in transmural LV filling pressure with PEEP was found to occur only when lung volume was allowed to increase without chest wall constraint[118,121,123]. The consensus at this time is that the effect of PEEP on LV diastolic compliance is mediated predominantly, if not exclusively, through direct compression by the lungs, for which a pericardial surface pressure reflects the appropriate transmural pressure[37]. Although vagally mediated, vasodepressor reflexes have been established with PEEP[32]; these reflexes predominantly occur only at high lung volumes, but other phasic reflexes regulating sympathetic tone in regional vascular beds, possibly due to breath to breath changes in chemoreceptor output, may be present and affect venous return. In addition, the mechanical effects of diaphragmatic descent, increasing resistance to blood flow across the liver, with secondary pooling of blood in the gut vasculature, may contribute to the global effects of PEEP on cardiac output[22,124]. The essential conclusions developed above are not altered after vagotomy[125]. With markedly pathologic increases in PVR due to underlying pulmonary disease, the addition of PEEP may in some patients lead to further distention of the RV and hence, via ventricular interdependence, reduce LV preload[66].

Evaluation of the effects of increased intrathoracic pressure on hemodynamic events continues the same pattern developed throughout this chapter. That is, multiple, and at times opposing, factors will interact and variably dominate, depending on the baseline conditions. It should be clear at this point that there is no uniform answer as to what effect PEEP will have on cardiac output. Depending on the circumstances, cardiac output may decrease, show minimal change, or increase. The explanation for the apparently contradictory responses lies in understanding the effects of intrathoracic pressure and lung volume change on venous return, RV output, pulmonary venous return, and LV output.

A similar analysis to that used to evaluate the influence of spontaneous respiration on LV performance should hold for positive pressure ventilation. An increase in intrathoracic pressure, with or without a change in lung volume, will reduce systemic venous return and, if all else remains constant, will reduce LV output[93,105–107,126–130]. This observation is generally accepted as the single most important hemodynamic influence of IPPV, with or without PEEP. Less well recognized is the early inspiratory increase in both arterial pressure and LV output during a positive pressure inspiration[105–107]. This was observed by Lewis in 1908[131] and by Hamilton et al.[130] in the original description of the hemodynamic events associated with Valsalva's maneuver. Little et al.[132] confirmed that a marked increase in intrathoracic pressure in patients with pulmonary congestion does not produce the fall in blood pressure and cardiac output observed in normal patients. Using echocardiographic techniques, Little et al. demonstrated that in congested patients, despite the marked increase in intrathoracic pressure, LV end-diastolic volume did not diminish, and LV stroke volume could increase. Santamore et al.[57], using angiographic techniques in dogs, demonstrated a fall in RV volume but little change in LV volume with a rapid Valsalva's maneuver. In 1946, Carr and Essex[133] postulated that an increase in intrathoracic pressure should expel blood from the intrathoracic to extrathoracic compartments, repeating Donders' conclusions a century earlier[1].

With a positive pressure inflation, in zone III conditions there should be an increase in LV preload and simultaneous decrease in LV afterload. The net result would be an increase in output, with a variable change in LV volumes depending on the dominance of the preload or afterload effect. Studies in anesthetized dogs during IPPV with mitral and aortic flow probes demonstrate that the normal dominant influence on LVSV is the variation in preload resulting from changes in pulmonary venous return as modified by ventricular interdependence. Thus, since a positive pressure inspiration reduced systemic venous return, reducing intrapericardial volume and hence ventricular interdependence, the gradient for blood to move from the lungs to the left heart under zone III conditions is optimized. Mitral flow increased with each inspiration, consistent with the findings of Brower et al.[69] in the isolated lung. The subsequent LV ejection increased, consistent with increased preload. The simultaneous occurrence of increasing preload and decreasing afterload is confirmed by the observation of reduced aortic dimensions despite the increase in stroke volume (unpublished observations). In zone II conditions, despite the reduction in RV volume reducing the influence of ventricular interdependence, mitral flow decreased during a positive pressure inspiration; the LVSV then decreased, following the Frank-Starling law of the heart.

The increased LVSV with an increase in intrathoracic pressure under zone III conditions, which would be expected with LV failure, implies that IPPV in the failing LV should be quite beneficial. First, the work of breathing, which constitutes a significant amount of the increased oxygen consumption, is removed. This will help remedy any degree of metabolic acidosis imposed by the respiratory muscle work if lactate is being produced. Second, by virtue of improving both oxygenation and ventilation, hypoxemia may be relieved and respiratory acidosis corrected. These will both contribute to improved ventricular function. Third, by virtue of a machine-generated change in intrathoracic pressure, the increase in intrathoracic pressure will decrease the average preload of the LV compared with spontaneous ventilation, fill the LV during inspiration (diastole), and assist in emptying the ventricle during inspiration (systole) by effectively reducing its afterload. Thus IPPV, with PEEP as needed, represents a reasonable prescription for helping the failing LV.

CARDIOPULMONARY RESUSCITATION

The fact that an increase in intrathoracic pressure assists LV emptying is most dramatically evident during CPR. With either chest-compression or cough-induced self-administered CPR, increasing intrathoracic pressure drives blood out of the intrathoracic vascular compartments into the systemic circulation[108]. This represents the ultimate example of increased intrathoracic pressure decreasing LV afterload. Studies of CPR using mitral and aortic flow probes have added new insights into the mechanical events producing blood flow during chest compression with or without simultaneous ventilation[134]. It is clear that any mode of CPR that increases intrathoracic pressure around all vascular compartments relative to the extrathoracic compartments will provide a driving force (thoracic pump) to move arterial blood to the periphery and reduce systemic venous return to the thorax. This force is separate from any local compressive forces applied preferentially to the ventricles, e.g., manual open-chest cardiac compression, or with the chest closed, the potential of compressing the heart between the sternum and spine as was originally suggested to occur[135]. Compressing the chest with any external force, local or general, that increases intrathoracic pressure, will produce some element of this thoracic pump mechanism. Other studies have extended our perception of the thoracic pump to hypothesize that changes in alveolar pressure relative to intrathoracic vascular pressures can be both quantitatively different and out of phase due to alveolar gas compression and expansion and lung viscous forces[134]. The essential elements of this concept are related to the work of Brower et al.[69] (Figure 11.9) in that any mechanism that will increase lung volume in a zone III condition will drive blood out of the lung, and, during cardiac arrest, out of the thorax. Lung volume may increase during simultaneous compression and ventilation. However, if only chest compression is occurring, lung volume will decrease because of gas compression. Lung volume increases with release of the chest compression as the alveolar gas decompresses[134]. Thus, the thoracic pump has two components, one related to generalized increase in intrathoracic pressure and a second related to changes in lung volume. These insights into the different mechanisms that drive systemic flow during CPR suggest that the same method of CPR may move blood by different mechanisms during hypovolemia compared with hypervolemia. Future attempts to optimize blood flow may need to tailor the method of CPR to the patient's physiologic status at the time. Thus a different method may be employed initially, but as plasma volume is expanded during resuscitation, another method may be better.

CELLULAR ASPECTS OF CARDIORESPIRATORY INTERACTIONS

Cardiorespiratory interactions are usually ascribed to the effects of intrathoracic pressure, lung volume, and ventilation on cardiovascular events such as venous return, ventricular performance, and arterial outflow. Cardiorespiratory interaction can also occur at both the cellular and molecular levels. The widespread existence of cellular influences on cardiovascular function suggests the possibility that such interactions at the cellular level could mediate cardiorespiratory interactions. Cellular elements that are likely to transduce mechanical and biochemical (blood gas changes) stimuli include vascular and endocardial endothelial, pleural and pericardial cells, and myocytes[136,137].

It is well known that endothelial cells can serve as mechanotransducers. They respond to changes in flow, shear stress, and pressure pulsations by altering vasoactive mediator release[138–140]. It is likely that the increased shear stresses that accompany ventilation-induced alterations in pressure and flow cause the release of nitric oxide and prostacyclin, potent, local and distant vasodilators[141, 142]. Endothelial cells increase the release of prostacyclin in response to hypoxia and can alter nitric oxide release with hypoxia[143,144]. The long-acting vasoconstrictor and potent myocardial inotrope, endothelin, is also influenced by changes in flow and shear stress[145]. Apart from these well-described mediators, a novel mediator released in response to changes in the physical environment by endocardial and vascular endothelial cells, which alters myocardial contractile function, has recently been described[145–147]. Pleural and pericardial mesothelial cells, which are embryologically related to endothelial cells, are also potential sources of vasoactive mediators[148,149]. These mesothelial cells are metabolically active, highly organized structures, with rough endoplasmic reticulum and capable of actively synthesizing and releasing vasoactive mediators[150]. The presence of pericardial mechanoreceptors and the recently demonstrated potential for pericardial cells to respond to flow also support a role for mesothelial cells in these cardiorespiratory interactions[148,151]. Certainly the vast surface areas of pleural and pericardial cells and their close relationship to the cardiovascular structures in the thorax and abdomen present a strategically located potential pathway for mediation of cardiorespiratory interactions.

The interaction between mediator systems such as nitric oxide, prostacyclin and endothelin, with multiple potential feedback pathways, could be important in the response to mechanical and blood gas changes, and in integrating cardiorespiratory function at the cellular level[152,153]. This could occur both acutely and chronically. For example, a ventilation-induced increase in pulmonary vascular resistance could lead to increased right ventricular end-diastolic pressures and alter the flow characteristics of the ventricular endocardium. This in turn would stimulate endocardial endothelial release of nitric oxide and prostaglandin, which could act locally as vasodilators in the subendocardial myocardium. Additionally, the release of prostacyclin could act downstream to dilate the pulmonary circulation in a negative feedback fashion. Acute changes in pulmonary vascular tone, lung inflation, and pulmonary perfusion could alter vascular endothelial prostacyclin production, leading to downstream prostaglandin-mediated direct effects on left ventricular function and coronary circulation, with secondary alterations on myocardial function.

The pericardium is strategically located to act not only as a source of vasoactive mediators, but also as a reservoir to prolong their actions. Alterations in the biochemical milieu of the pericardium have been shown to alter myocardial function and cardiac electrophysiology and to play a role in rhythm regulation[154,155]. Mechanical and biochemical respiratory stimuli transduced by cellular elements with subsequent release of prostaglandins and other factors that alter myocyte function could affect respiratory muscle function. Thus it seems possible that the acute release of mediators from the pulmonary circulation could, by circulation to the diaphragm and other respiratory muscles, acutely alter respiratory muscle function.

Endothelial mediator release can give rise to long-term alterations in cardiorespiratory function. The endothelium and mesothelial cells release a wide variety of factors that affect the growth and development of vascular smooth muscle[155–157]. Chronically, the up-regulation of mediators released by the vascular endothelium by changes in flow and blood-gas tensions could lead to elaboration of growth factors, resulting in vascular as well as myocardial hypertrophy. This may be the basis of long-term cardiorespiratory interaction involved in chronic lung disease. Endothelial elaboration of mitogens and growth factors from the pulmonary circulation could theoretically result in left ventricular hypertrophy. Understanding the molecular basis of these cardiorespiratory interactions at a cellular level could lead to novel therapeutic strategies to ameliorate the adverse cardiac effects of chronic lung disease in children. Thus, although the area of cellular cardiorespiratory interaction is in its infancy, it should be realized that the scope of cardiorespiratory interactions extends beyond the classic mechanical interactions described above.

CONCLUSION

Interactions between the circulatory and respiratory systems continue to challenge the physiologist and present a daily challenge to the intensivist. The next major "black box" in cardiorespiratory interactions to understand is the abdomen. Cardiac output, by definition, must equal venous return. How abdominal organs affect venous return under normal and pathologic conditions remains to be investigated. Except with congenital right heart anomalies, the underlying problem producing right heart dysfunction in the pediatric population continues to be the primary lung disease. Understanding the interaction between respiratory diseases and right heart function and adaptation acutely and chronically to the diseases that increase RV afterload is another major focus for investigation. The appreciation that diastolic and systolic events during respiration will interact in a complex but predictable manner allows reevaluation of previous literature and new insights into numerous clinical occurrences. By concentrating on the changes in lung volume and intrathoracic pressure during systole and diastole, rather than on the traditional focus of spontaneous versus mechanical ventilation, a physiologic framework can be developed that extends our understanding of the hemodynamic events during spontaneous ventilation, mechanical ventilation, and cardiopulmonary resuscitation.

Acknowledgements

To J.B. Lippincott/Harper & Row, Inc., Marcel Dekker, Inc., and B. C. Decker, Inc., respectively, for permission to extensively adapt and modify the following book chapters: Robotham JL: How respiration affects circulation. In: Refesher Courses in Anesthesiology. The American Society of Anesthesiologists Inc. (eds.) PG Barash, S Deutch, J Tinker, 16:191–202, 1988; Robotham JL and Peters J: Cardiorespiratory interactions. In: Adult Respiratory Distress Syndrome. (eds.) W Zapol and F Lemaire, pp. 223–251, 1991; and Robotham JL, Takata M, Peters J: Cardiorespiratory interactions. In: Basic Mechanisms of Pediatric Respiratory Disease: Cellular and Integrative. (eds.) RB Mellins and V Chernick, pp. 256–272, 1991.

To Blackwell Science Ltd. for permission to adapt and modify the following: Robotham JL and Takata M: Mechanical abdomino/heart/lung interaction. Journal of Sleep Research, in press.

The authors wish to express their sincere thanks to Alice Trawinski for her excellent secretarial and editorial assistance. Supported by National Institutes of Health grants: NIH RO1-HL39138–04 and NIH-NHLBI-HL10342.

References

1. Donders FC: Contribution to the mechanism on respiration and circulation in health and disease., Translations in Respiratory Physiology. Edited by West JB. Stroudsburg, Dowden, Hutchinson, and Ross, 1975, pp 291–297.
2. West J, Dollery C, Naimark A: Distribution of blood flow in isolated lung; relation to vascular and alveolar pressures. J Appl Physiol 1964;19:713–724.
3. Lloyd Jr. TC: Respiratory systems compliance as seen from the cardiac fossa. J Appl Physiol 1982;53:57–62.
4. Wallis T, Robotham JL, Compean R, Kindred MK: Mechanical heart-lung interaction with positive end-expiratory pressure. J Appl Physiol 1983;54:1039–1047.
5. Bove AA, Santamore WP: Ventricular interdependence. Prog Cardiovasc Dis 1981;23:365–388.
6. Guyton AC, Lindsey AW, Abernathy B, Richardson T: Venous return at various right atrial pressures and the normal venous return curve. Am J Physiol 1957;189:609–615.
7. Guyton AC, Jones CE, Coleman TG: Effect of right atrial pressure on venous return: The normal venous return curve, In: Circulatory Physiology: Cardiac Output and its Regulation. Edited by Guyton AC, Jones CE, Coleman TG. Philadelphia, Saunders, W.B., 1973, pp 188–204.
8. Natori H, Tamaki S, Dira S: Ultrasonographic evaluation of ventilatory effect on inferior vena caval configuration. Am Rev Respir Dis 1979;120:421–427.
9. Takata M, Wise RA, Robotham JL: Effects of abdominal pressure on venous return: abdominal vascular zone conditions. J Appl Physiol 1990;69:1961–1972.
10. Mixter G: Respiratory augmentation of inferior vena caval flow demonstrated by a low resistance phasic flowmeter. Am J Physiol 1953;172:446–456.
11. Norhagen A: Selective angiography of the hepatic veins. Acta Radiologica 1963;219-222:3–121.
12. Moreno AH, Burchell AR, Van Der WR, Burke JH: Respiratory regulation of splanchnic and systemic venous return. Am J Physiol 1967;213 (2):455–465.
13. Moreno AH, Katz AI, Gold LD: An integrated approach to the study of the venous system with steps toward a detailed model of the dynamics of venous return to the right heart. IEEE Trans Biomed Eng 1969;16:308–324.
14. Matuschak GM, Rinaldo JE: Organ interactions in the adult respiratory distress syndrome during sepsis. Chest 1988;94:400–406.
15. Schwartz DB, Bone RC, Balk RA, Szidon JP: Hepatic dysfunction in the adult respiratory distress syndrome. Chest 1989;95:871–875.
16. Takata M, Robotham JL: Effects of inspiratory diaphragmatic descent on inferior vena caval venous return. J Appl Physiol 1992;72:597–607.
17. Decramer M, De Troyer A, Kelly S, Zocchi L, Macklem PT: Regional differences in abdominal pressure swings in dogs. J Appl Physiol 1984;57:1682–1687.
18. Kussmaul A: Ueber schwielige Mediastino-Pericarditis und den paradoxen Puls. Berliner Klinische Wochenschrift 1873;10:433-435; 445-449;461–465.
19. Takata MD, Beloucif S, Shimada M, Robotham JL: Superior and inferior vena caval flows during respiration: pathogenesis of Kussmaul's sign. Am J Physiol 1992;262:H763–H770.
20. Fessler HE, Brower RG, Wise RA, Permutt S: Effects of positive end-expiratory pressure on the canine venous return curve. Am Rev Respir Dis 1992;146:4–10.
21. Fessler HE, Brower RG, Wise RA, Permutt S: Effects of positive end-expiratory pressure on the gradient for venous return. Am Rev Respir Dis 1991;143:19–24.
22. Brienza N, Revelly JP, Ayuse T, Robotham JL: Effects of PEEP on liver arterial and venous blood flows. Am J Resp Crit Care Med. 1995;152:504–510.
23. Scharf SM, Ingram RH: Influence of abdominal pressure and sympathetic vasoconstriction on the cardiovascular response to positive end-expiratory pressure. Am Rev Respir Dis 1977;116:661–670.
24. Sylvester JT, Goldberg HS, Permutt S: The role of the vasculature in the regulation of cardiac output. Clin Chest Med 1983;4:111–126.

25. Mitzner W, Goldberg H: Effects of epinephrine on resistive and compliant properties of the canine vasculature. J Appl Physiol 1975;39:272–280.
26. Goldberg HS, Mitzner W, Adams K, Menkes H, Lichtenstein S, Permutt S: Effect of intrathoracic pressure on pressure-volume characteristics of the lung in man. J Appl Physiol 1975;38 (3):411–417.
27. Fenn WO, Otis AB, Rahn H, Chadwick LE, Hegnauer AH: Displacement of blood from the lungs by pressure breathing. Am J Physiol 1947;151:258–269.
28. Lemaire F, Teboul JL, Cinotti L, Giotto G, Abrouk F, Steg G, Macquin-Mavier I, Zapol WM: Acute left ventricular dysfunction during unsuccessful weaning from mechanical ventilation. Anesthesiology 1988;69:171–179.
29. Permutt S: Circulatory effects of weaning from mechanical ventilation: The importance of transdiaphragmatic pressure. Anesthesiology 1988;69:157–160.
30. Brienza N, Ayuse T, O'Donnell CP, Permutt S, Robotham JL: Regional control of venous return: liver blood flow. Am. J. Resp. Crit. Care Med. In press
31. Ayuse T, Brienza N, O'Donnell CP, Robotham JL: Pressure-flow analysis of portal vein and hepatic artery interactions in porcine liver. Am. J. Physiol. 1994;267:H1233–H1243.
32. Cassidy SS: Stimulus-response curves of the lung inflation cardiodepressor reflex. Respir Physiol 1984;57:259–268.
33. Browse NL, Hardwick PJ: The deep breath-venoconstriction reflex. Clin Sci 1969;37:125–135.
34. Brookhart JM, Boyd TE: Local differences in intrathoracic pressure and their relation to cardiac filling pressure in the dog. Am J Physiol 1947;148:434–444.
35. Marini JJ, Culver BH, Butler J: Mechanical effect of lung distention with positive pressure on cardiac function. Am Rev Respir Dis 1981;124:382–386.
36. O'Quin RJ, Marini JJ, Culver BH, Butler J: Transmission of airway pressure to pleural space during lung edema and chest wall restriction. J Appl Physiol 1985;59:1171–1177.
37. Takata M, Robotham JL: Ventricular external constraint by the lung and pericardium during positive end-expiratory pressure. Am Rev Respir Dis 1991;143:872–875.
38. Nakhjavan FK, Palmer WH, McGregor M: Influence of respiration on venous return in emphysema. Circulation 1966;33:8–16.
39. Badke FR, Boinay P, Covell JW: Effects of ventricular pacing on regional left ventricular performance in the dog. Am J Physiol 1980;238:H858–H867.
40. Little WC, Badke FR, O'Rourke RA: Effect of right ventricular pressure on the end-diastolic left ventricular pressure-volume relationship before and after right ventricular pressure overload in dogs without pericardia. Circ Res 1984;54:719–730.
41. Walley KR, Grover M, Raff GL et al.: Left ventricular dynamic geometry in the intact and open chest dog. Circ Res 1982;50:573–589.
42. Hurford WE, Barlai-Kovach M, Strauss W, Zapol WM, Lowenstein E: Canine biventricular performance during acute progressive pulmonary microembolization: Regional myocardial perfusion and fatty acid uptake. J Crit Care 1987;2:270–281.
43. Oboler AA, Keefe JR, Gaasch WH, Banas Jr. JS, Levine HJ: Influence of left ventricular isovolumic pressure upon right ventricular pressure transients. Cardiology 1973;58:32–44.
44. Santamore WP, Lynch PR, Heckman JL, Bove AA, Meier GD: Left ventricular effects on right ventricular developed pressure. J Appl Physiol 1976;41:925–930.
45. Santamore WP, Lynch PR, Meier G, Heckman J, Bove AA: Myocardial interaction between the ventricles. J Appl Physiol 1976;4:362–368.
46. Little WC, Reeves RC, Arciniegas J: Mechanism of abnormal interventricular septal motion during delayed left ventricular activation. Circulation 1982;65:1486–1491.
47. Pearlman AS, Clark CE, Henry WL et al.: Determinants of ventricular septal motion. Influence of relative right and left ventricular size. Circulation 1976;54:83–91.
48. Shimazaki Y, Kawashima Y, Mori T et al.: Ventricular function of single ventricle after ventricular septation. Circulation 1980;61:653–660.
49. Weyman AE, Wann S, Feigenbaum H, Dillon JC: Mechanism of abnormal systolic motion in patients with right ventricular volume overload: A cross-sectional echocardiographic study. Circulation 1976;54: 179–186.
50. Maughan WL, Shoukas AA, Sagawa K, Weisfeldt ML: Instantaneous pressure-volume relationship of the canine right ventricle. Circ Res 1979;44:309–315.
51. Jarmakani JM, McHale PA, Greenfield Jr. JC: The effect of cardiac tamponade on coronary haemodynamics in the awake dog. Cardiovas Res 1975;9:112–117.
52. O'Rourke RA, Fischer DP, Escobar EE, Bishop VS, Rapaport E: Effect of acute pericardial tamponade on coronary blood flow. Am J Physiol 1967;212:549–552.
53. Kidd BSL: Complete transposition of the great arteries, Heart Disease in Infancy and Childhood. Edited by Keith J, Roue R, Vald P. New York, Macmillan, 1978, pp 590–611.
54. Vlahakes GJ, Turley K, Hoffman JIE: The pathophysiology of failure in acute right ventricular hypertension: Hemodynamic and biochemical correlations. Circulation 1981;63:87–95.
55. Dornhorst AC, Howard P, Lethart GL: Pulsus paradoxus. Lancet 1952;1:746–748.
56. Robotham JL, Mitzner W: A model of the effects of respiration on left ventricular performance. J Appl Physiol 1979;46:411–418.
57. Santamore WP, Heckman JL, Bove AA: Right and left ventricular pressure-volume response to respiratory maneuvers. J Appl Physiol: Respirat Environ Exercise Physiol 1984;57:1520-1527.
58. Kuno Y: The mechanical effect of fluid in the pericardium on the function of the heart. J Physiol 1917;51:221–234.
59. Takata M, Mitzner W, Robotham JL: Influence of the pericardium on ventricular loading during respiration. J Appl Physiol 1990;68:1640–1650.
60. Beloucif S, Takata M, Shimada M, Robotham JL: Influence of pericardial constraint on atrioventricular interactions. Am J Physiol 1992;263:H125–H134.
61. Calvin JE, Baer RW, Glantz SA: Pulmonary artery constriction produces a greater right ventricular dynamic afterload than lung microvascular injury in the open chest dog. Circ Res 1985;56:40–56.
62. Whittenberger JL, McGregor M, Berglund E, Borst HG: Influence of state of inflation of the lung on pulmonary vascular resistance. J Appl Physiol 1960;15:878–882.
63. Murgo JP, Westerhof N: Input impedance of the pulmonary arterial system in normal man: Effects of respiration and comparison to systemic impedance. Circ Res 1984;54:666–673.
64. Piene H, Hauge A: Influence of moderate vasoconstriction on the wave reflection properties of the pulmonary arterial bed. Acta Physiol Scand 1976;93:37–43.
65. Sawatani S, Mandell G, Kusaba E, Schraut W, Cascade P, Wajszczuk WJ, Kantrowitz A: Ventricular performance following ablation and prosthetic replacement of right ventricular myocardium. Trans Am Soc Artific Intern Organs 1974;20:629–636.
66. Dhainaut JF, Devaux JY, Monsallier JF, Brunet F, Villemant D, Huyghebaert MF: Mechanisms of decreased left ventricular preload during continuous positive pressure ventilation in ARDS. Chest 1986; 90:74–80.
67. Howell JBL, Permutt S, Proctor DF, Riley RL: Effect of inflation of the lung on different parts of pulmonary vascular bed. J Appl Physiol 1961;16:64–70.
68. Permutt S, Howell JBL, Proctor DF, Riley RL: Effect of lung inflation on static pressure-volume characeristics of pulmonary vessels. J Appl Physiol 1961;16:64–70.
69. Brower R, Wise RA, Hassapoyannes C, Bromberger-Barnea B, Permutt S: Effect of lung inflation on lung blood volume and pulmonary venous flow. J Appl Physiol 1985;58:954–963.
70. Smith JC, Mitzner W: Analysis of pulmonary vascular interdependence in excised dog lobes. J Appl Physiol 1980;48:450–467.
71. Lai-Fook SJ, Hyatt RE, Rodarte JR: Effect of parenchymal sheer modulus and lung volume on bronchial pressure-diameter behavior. J Appl Physiol 1978;44:859–968.
72. Jardin F, Delorme G, Hardy A, Auvert B, Beauchet A, Bourdarias JP: Reevaluation of Hemodynamic Consequences of Positive Pressure Ventilation: Emphasis on Cyclic Right Ventricular Afterloading by Mechanical Lung Inflation. Anesthesiology 1990;72:966–970.
73. Morgan BC, Abel FL, Mullins GL, Guntheroth WG: Flow patterns in cavae, pulmonary artery, pulmonary vein, and aorta in intact dogs. Am J Physiol 1966;210:903–909.
74. Franklin DL, Van Citters RL, Rushmer RF: Balance between right and left ventricular output. Circ Res 1962;10:17–26.
75. Maloney JE, Bersel DH, Glazier JB, Hughes JM, West JB: Transmission of pulsatile blood pressure and flow through the isolated lung. Circ Res 1968;23:11–24.
76. Sunagawa K, Maughan WL, Sagawa K: Effect of regional ischemia on the left ventricular end-systolic pressure-volume relationship of isolated canine hearts. Circ Res 1983;52:170–178.

77. Visscher MB, Rupp A, Scott FH: The respiratory wave in arterial blood pressure. Am J Physiol 1924;70:586–606.
78. Bugge-Asperheim B, Kiil B: Cardiac response to increased aortic pressure. Changes in output and left ventricular pressure pattern at various levels of inotropy. Scand J Clin Lab Invest 1969;24:343–360.
79. Glower DD, Spratt JA, Snow ND, Kabas JS, Davis JW, Olsen CO, Tyson GS, Sabiston J D.C., Rankin JS: Linearity of the Frank-Starling relationship in the intact heart: the concept of preload recruitable stroke work. Circulation 1985;71:994–1009.
80. Tyberg JV, Taichman ER, E.R.Smith, Douglas NWS, Smiseth OA, Keon WJ: The relationship between pericardial pressure and right atrial pressure: an intraoperative study. Circulation 1986;73:428–432.
81. Smiseth OA, Frais MA, Kingma I, White AVM, Knudtson ML, Cohen JM, Manyari DE, Smith ER, Tyberg JV: Assessment of pericardial constraint: the relation between right ventricular filling pressure and pericardial pressure measured after pericardiocentesis. J Am Coll Cardiol 1986;7:307–314.
82. Junemann M, Smiseth OA, Refsum H, Sievers R, Lipton MJ, Carlsson E, Tyberg JV: Quantification of effect of pericardium on LV diastolic PV relation in dogs. Am H Physiol (Heart Circ Physiol 21) 1987;252:H963–H968.
83. Robotham JL, Peters J: Mechanical effects of intrathoracic pressure on ventricular performance., Heart/Lung Interactions. Edited by Scharf S, Cassidy S. New York, Marcel Dekker, 1989, pp 251–283.
84. Shabetai R: Pericardial and cardiac pressures. Circulation 1988;77:1–5.
85. Jardin F, Farcot JC, Boisante L, Prost JF, Gueret P, Bourdarias JP: Mechanism of paradoxic pulse in bronchial asthma. Circulation 1982;66:887–894.
86. Rankin JS, Olsen CO, Arentzen CE, Tyson GS, Maier G, Smith PK, Hammon Jr. JW, Davis JW, McHale PA, Anderson RW, Sabiston Jr. DC: The effects of airway pressure on cardiac function in intact dogs and man. Circulation 1982;66:108–120.
87. Robotham JL, Badke FR, Kindred MK, Beaton MK: Regional left ventricular performance during normal and obstructed spontaneous respiration. J Appl Physiol 1983;55:569–577.
88. Brinker JA, Weiss JL, Lappe DL, Rabson JL, Summer WR, Permutt S, Weisfeldt ML: Leftward septal displacement during right ventricular loading in man. Circulation 1980;61:626–633.
89. Summer WR, Permutt S, Sagawa K: Effects of spontaneous respiration on canine left ventricular function. Circ Res 1979;45:719–728.
90. Buda AJ, Pinsky MR, Ingels Jr. NB: Effect of intrathoracic pressure on left ventricular performance. N Engl J Med 1979;301:453–459.
91. Karam M, Wise RA, Natarajan TK, Permutt S, Wagner HN: Mechanism of decreased left ventricular stroke volume during inspiration in man. Circulation 1984;69:866–873.
92. Guz A, Innes JA, Murphy K: Respiratory modulation of left ventricular stroke volume in man measured using pulsed doppler ultrasound. J Physiol 1987;393:499–512.
93. Scharf SM, Brown R, Saunders N, Green LH: Hemodynamic effects of positive pressure inflation. J Appl Physiol 1980;49:124–131.
94. Robotham JL, Stuart RS, Borkon MA, Doherty K, Baumgartner W: Effects of changes in left ventricular loading and pleural pressure on mitral flow. J Appl Physiol 1988;65:1662–1675.
95. Robotham JL, Stuart RS, Doherty K, Borkon MA, Baumgartner W: Mitral and aortic flows during spontaneous respiration in dogs. Anesthesiology 1988;69:516–526.
96. Peters J, Fraser C, Stuart RS, Baumgartner W, Robotham JL: Negative intrathoracic pressure decreases independently left ventricular filling and emptying. Am J Physiol 1989;257:H120–H131.
97. Pinsky MR: Hemodynamic effects of artificial ventilation, In: Textbook of Critical Care. Edited by Shoemaker WC, Ayres S, Grenvick A, Holbrook PR, Thompson WL. Philadelphia, W.B. Saunders, Co., 1989, pp 676–685.
98. Pinsky MR, Matuschak GM, Bernardi L, Klain M: Hemodynamic effects of cardiac cycle-specific increases in intrathoracic pressure. J Appl Physiol 1986;60:604–612.
99. Robotham JL, Peters J: Cardiorespiratory Interactions., Adult Respiratory Distress Syndrome. Edited by Zapol W. New York, Marcel Dekker, 1991, pp 223–251.
100. Peters J, Kindred MK, Robotham JL: Transient analysis of cardiopulmonary interactions. II. Systolic events. J Appl Physiol 1988;64:1518–1526.
101. Pinsky MR: Instantaneous venous return curves in an intact canine preparation. J Appl Physiol: Respirat Environ Exercise Physiol 1984;56:765–771.
102. Pinsky MR: Determinants of pulmonary arterial flow variation during respiration. J Appl Physiol: Respirat Environ Exercise Physiol 1984;56:1237–1245.
103. Cassidy SS, Ramanthan M: Dimensional analysis of the left ventricle during PEEP: Relative septal and lateral wall displacements. Am J Physiol 1984;246:H792–H805.
104. Robotham JL, Cherry D, Mitzner W, Rabson JL, Lixfeld W, Bromberger-Barnea B: A re-evaluation of the hemodynamic consequences of intermittent positive pressure ventilation. Crit Care Med 1983;11:783–793.
105. Morgan BC, Crawford EW, Guntheroth WG: The hemodynamic effects of changes in blood volume during intermittent positive-pressure ventilation. Anesthesiology 1969;30:297–305.
106. Morgan BC, Martin WE, Hornberger JF, Crawford EW, Guntheroth WG: Hemodynamic effects of intermittent positive pressure respiration. Anesthesiology 1966;27:584–590.
107. Morgan BC, Crawford EW, Winterscheid LC, Gunther WG: Circulatory effects of intermittent positive pressure ventilation. Northwest Med 1968;67:149–152.
108. Criley JM, Balfuss AH, Vissel GL: Cough-induced cardiac compression: Self-administered form of cardiopulmonary resuscitation. JAMA 1976;236:1246–1250.
109. Beach T, Millen E, Grenvik A: Hemodynamic response to discontinuance of mechanical ventilation. Crit Care Med 1973;1:85–90.
110. Grace MP, Greenbaum DM: Cardiac performance in response to PEEP in patients with cardiac dysfunction. Crit Care Med 1982;10:358–360.
111. Mathru M, Rao TLK, El-Etr AA, Pifarre R: Hemodynamic response to changes in ventilatory patterns in patients with normal and poor left ventricular reserve. Crit Care Med 1982;10:423–426.
112. Pinsky MR, Summer WR, Wise RA, Permutt S, Bromberger-Barnea B: Augmentation of cardiac function by elevation of intrathoracic pressure. J Appl Physiol 1983;54:950–955.
113. Pinsky MR, Marquez J, Martin D, Klain M: Ventricular assist by cardiac cycle-specific increases in intrathoracic pressure. Chest 1987;91:709–715.
114. Chandra NC, Beyar R, Halperin HR, Tsitlik JE, Wurmb E, B. R, Guerci AD, Weisfeldt ML: Vital organ perfusion during assisted circulation by manipulation of intrathoracic pressure. Circulation 1991;84:279–286.
115. Robotham JL, Lixfeld W, Holland L, MacGregor D, Bromberger-Barnea B, Permutt S, Rabson JL: The effects of PEEP on right and left ventricular performance. Am Rev Respir Dis 1980;121:677–683.
116. Cassidy SS, Eschenbacher WL, Robertson CH, Nixon JV, Blomquist G, Johnson Jr. RL: Cardiovascular effects of positive-pressure ventilation in normal subjects. J Appl Physiol 1979;47:453–461.
117. Cassidy SS, Robertson CH, Pierce AK, Johnson Jr. RL: Cardiovascular effects of positive end-expiratory pressure in dogs. J Appl Physiol 1978;44:743–750.
118. Culver BH, Marini JJ, Butler J: Lung volume and pleural pressure effects on ventricular function. J. Appl. Physiol. 1981;50:630–635.
119. Grindlinger GA, Manny J, Justic R, Dunham B, Shepro D, Hechtman HB: Presence of negative inotropic agents in canine plasma during PEEP. Circ Res 1979;45:460–467.
120. Prewitt RM, Wook LDH: Effect of positive end-expiratory pressure on ventricular function in dogs. Am J Physiol 1979;236:H534–H544.
121. Scharf SM, Caldini P, Ingram RH: Cardiovascular effects of increasing airway pressure in the dog. Am J Physiol 1977;232:H35–H43.
122. Wise RA, Robotham JL, Bromberger-Barnea B, Permutt S: The effect of PEEP on left ventricular function in right heart bypassed dogs. J Appl Physiol 1981;51:541–546.
123. Manny J, Patten MT, Leibman PR, Hechtman HB: The association of lung distention, PEEP and biventricular failure. Ann Surg 1978;187:151–156.
124. Peters J, Hecker B, Neuser D, Schaden W: Regional blood volume distribution during positive and negative airway pressure breathing in supine humans. J Appl Physiol 1993;75:1740–1747.
125. Robotham JL, Scharf SM: The effects of positive and negative pressure ventilation on cardiac performance. In: Clinics in Chest Medicine 1983;4:161–187.
126. Charlier AA, Jaumin PM, Pouleur H: Circulatory effects of deep inspirations, blocked expirations and positive pressure inflatins at equal transpulmonary pressures in conscious dogs. J Physiol 1974;241:589–605.
127. Parisi AF, Harrington JJ, Askenazi J, Pratt RC, McIntyre KM: Echocardiographic evaluation of the Valsalva maneuver in healthy subjects and patients with and without heart failure. Circulation 1976;54:921–927.
128. Brooker JZ, Alderman EL, Harrison DC: Alterations in left ventricular volumes induced by valsalva maneuver. Br Heart J 1974;36:713–718.

129. Korner PI, Tonkin AM, Uther JB: Reflex and mechanical circulatory effects of graded Valsalva maneuvers in normal man. J Appl Physiol 1976;40:434–440.
130. Hamilton WF, Woodbury RA, Harper HT: Physiologic relationships between intrathoracic, intraspinal and arterial pressures. JAMA 1936;107:853–856.
131. Lewis T: Studies of the relationship between respiration and blood-pressure. Part 1. The effect of changes of intra-pericardial pressure on aortic pressure. J Physiol 1908;37:213–232.
132. Little WC, Barr WK, Crawford MH: Altered effect of the Valsalva maneuver on left ventricular volume in patients with cardiomyopathy. Circulation 1985;71:227–233.
133. Carr DT, Essex HE: Certain effects of positive pressure respiration on the circulatory and respiratory systems. Am Heart J 1946;31: 53–73.
134. Beattie C, Guerci AD, Hall T, Borkon MA, Baumgartner W, Stuart RC, Peters J, Halperin H, Robotham JL: Mechanisms of blood flow during pneumatic vest cardiopulmonary resuscitation. J Appl Physiol 1991;70:454–465.
135. Kouwenhoven WB, Jude J, Knickerbocker GC: Closed-chest cardiac massage. J Am Med Assoc 1960;173:1064–1067.
136. Busse R, Trogisch G, Bassenge E: The role of endothelium in the control of vascular tone. Basic Res. Cardiol. 1985;80:475–490.
137. Satoh K, Prescott SM: Culture of mesothelial cells from bovine pericardium and characterization of their arachidonate metabolism. Biochim Biophys Acta 1987;930:283–296.
138. Pohl V, Busse R, Kuon E, Bassenge E: Pulsatile perfusion stimulates the release of endothelial autacoids. J. Appl. Cardiol. 1986;1:215–235.
139. Davies PF: How do vascular endothelial cells respond to flow? News Physiol. Sci. 1989;4:22–25.
140. Mebazaa A, Wetzel R, Cherian M, Abraham M: Comparison between endocardial and great vessel endothelial cells: Morphology, growth and prostaglandin release. Am. J. Physiol. 1995;268:H250–H259.
141. Cannon PJ: Eicosanoids and the blood vessel wall. Circulation 1984;70:523–528.
142. Buga GM, Gold ME, Fukuto JM, Ignarro LJ: Shear stress-induced release of nitric oxide from endothelial cells grown on beads. Hypertension 1991;17:187–193.
143. Martin LD, Barnes SD, Wetzel RC: Acute hypoxia alters eicosanoid production of perfused pulmonary artery endothelial cells in culture. Prostaglandins 1992;43:371–382.
144. Warren JB, Maltby NH, MacCormack D, Barnes PJ: Pulmonary endothelium-derived relaxing factor is impaired in hypoxia. Clin. Sci. 1989;77:671–676.
145. Mebazaa A, Mayoux E, Maeda K, Martin LD, Lakatta EG, Robotham JL, Shah AM: Paracrine effects of endocardial endothelial cells on myocyte contraction mediated via endothelin. Am J Physiol 1993;265:H1841–H1846.
146. Shah AM, Smith JA, Lewis MJ: The role of endocardium in the modulation of contraction of isolated papillary muscles of the ferret. J Cardiovasc Pharmacol 1991;17:S251–S257.
147. Shah AM, Mebazaa A, Wetzel RC, Lakatta EG: Novel cardiac myofilament desensitizing factor released by endocardial and vascular endothelial cells. Circulation 1994;89:2492–2497.
148. Herman AG, Claeys M, Moncada S, Vane JR: Prostacyclin production by rabbit aorta, pericardium, pleura, peritoneum and dura mater. Arch int Pharmacodyn 1978;236:303–304.
149. Chung-Welch N, Patton WF, Yen-Patton GPA, Hechtman HB, Shepro D: Phenotypic comparison between mesothelial and microvascular endothelial cell lineages using conventional endothelial cell markers, cytoskeletal protein markers and in vitro assay of angiogenic potential. Differentiation 1989;42:44–53.
150. Page E, Upshaw-Earley J, Goings G: Permeability of rat atrial endocardium, epicardium, and myocardium to large molecules: Stretch-dependent effects. Circ Res 1992;71:159–173.
151. Kostreva DR, Pontus SP: Pericardial mechanoreceptors with phrenic afferents. Am J Physiol 1993;264:H1836–H1846.
152. Shimokawa H, Flavahan NA, Lorenz RR, Vanhoutte PM: Prostacyclin releases endothelium-derived relaxing factor and potentiates its action in coronary arteries of the pig. Br. J. Pharmacol. 1988;95:1197–1203.
153. Doni MG, Whittle BJR, Palmer RMJ, Moncada S: Actions of nitric oxide on the release of prostacyclin from bovine endothelial cells in culture. Eur J Pharmacol 1988;151:19–25.
154. Miyazaki T, Pride HP, Zipes DP: Prostaglandins in the pericardial fluid modulate neural regulation of cardiac electrophysiological properties. Circulation Res 1990;66:163–175.
155. Eid H, Larson DM, Springhorn JP, Attawia MA, Nayak RC, Smith TW, Kelly RA: Role of epicardial mesothelial cells in the modification of phenotype and function of adult rat ventricular myocytes in primary coculture. Circ Res 1992;71:40–50.
156. Ferrara N, Houck K, Jakeman L, Leung DW: Molecular and biological properties of the vascular endothelial growth factor family of proteins. Endocr. Rev. 1992;13:18–32.
157. Vane JR, Anggard EE, Botting RM: Regulatory functions of the vascular endothelium. N Engl J Med 1990;323:27–36.-

Developmental Cardiac Physiology 12

Frank H. Kern
A. Resai Bengur
Elizabeth A. Bello

INTRODUCTION

The practice of pediatric critical care medicine includes the care of newborns and infants with complex cardiovascular diseases. Newborns, in contrast to older children, respond differently to inotropic and cardiorespiratory support. Normal and abnormal developmental changes in the perinatal and postnatal periods significantly impact upon the ability of these young patients to respond to conventional cardiac support.

Recent advances in our understanding of the development and function of the neonatal and infant myocardium explain why neonatal hearts perform differently than does the more mature myocardium. A reduced response to inotropes, volume loading, and increased sensitivity to afterload can all be explained on developmental differences in the neonatal and infant myocardium. Furthermore, understanding the expected response allows us to more rationally apply therapy and choose approaches with a greater likelihood of being successful.

As pediatric critical care physicians, we are being asked to administer care to newborns and infants with complex cardiac and cardiorespiratory disease in a coordinated venture with cardiologists, surgeons, and nurses. Furthermore, more effective and targeted therapies with proven efficacy and outcome orientation are being required. Newborns and young infants may require therapeutic interventions based on developmental strategies, including prenatal interventional therapies and alternative approaches to cardiac support, which differ from those used for the more mature patient. This chapter will discuss developmental changes that affect the cardiovascular and cardiorespiratory function of the fetus, newborn, and young infant; describe the molecular biology of the heart in the mature and newborn myocardium; and discuss the physiologic responses of the infant heart.

DEVELOPMENTAL CHANGES IN THE ULTRASTRUCTURE OF THE MYOCARDIUM

The Myocyte

The mature myocardial cell consists of mitochondria and highly organized contractile proteins known as filaments. Muscle consists of both thick and thin filaments, which differ in both structure and function. Thick filaments are formed from the protein myosin. Myosin molecules consist of a filamentous tail, which provides structural support, and a "globular" head, which is the biologically active portion of myosin. The conformation of the tail is a "coiled-coil" of two alpha helical heavy chains. Each myosin "head" consists of one heavy chain and a pair of light chains. The light chains combine with two hinge regions to allow flexibility between the head and tail regions[1,2].

Three isoforms of myosin (V_1, V_2, and V_3) have been identified, with the variability occurring within the heavy chains. The composition of the heavy chains determines the amount of adenosine triphosphatase (ATPase) activity within the myosin subunit. ATPase activity reflects muscle-shortening velocities. The V_1 isoform, which consists of two alpha heavy chains, is known as fast myosin because its ATPase activity is high, and it possesses an increased shortening velocity[3,4]. In contrast, the V_3 isoform, or slow myosin, contains two beta heavy chains in the tail region. The beta heavy chains have a much lower ATPase activity level and a reduced shortening velocity. An intermediate myosin isoform, V_2, consists of one alpha and one beta chain and thereby has an intermediate ATPase activity and intermediate shortening velocity. V_1 and V_3 have been found to exist in both ventricles of all animal species, with smaller animals with a higher baseline heart rate having a greater proportion of V_1 and larger animals possessing a higher percentage of the V_3 isoform[5].

Developmentally, the fetal hearts of all mammalian species have a predominance of the V_3 isoform of myosin, which possesses a slow velocity of shortening[6–12]. In certain species, there is a conformational change in the myosin isoform with development. In the rodent, there is a greater proportion of the V_1 isoform during fetal and early neonatal life than is seen in the mature myocardium. The V_1 isoforms plays an important role in maintaining higher heart rates in the fetus and neonate and may play an important role in supporting rate dependency in the neonatal period. During late gestation the composition of myosin changes, and the V_3 isoform predominates.

At birth, human ventricular myosin contains 85 to 100% of the V_3 isoform, which remains relatively constant into adulthood[11,12]. Certain pathophysiologic conditions, however, such as malnutrition, chronic heart failure, and endocrinopathies, cause conformational changes within the heavy chains of myosin. Disease processes that impair contractility or hormonally manipulate the myocardium to attain rapid heart rates develop a relative increase in proportion of the V_1 isoform of myosin. Alterations in myosin may play an important role in the adaptation of the myocardium to various pathologic states in adulthood. The ability to convert to a more immature form of myosin is intriguing in that it suggests that myocytes may be genetically manipulated to express more immature proteins and possibly regain capacity for replication after attaining maturity.

Four individual myosin light chains are identified by the chemicals that remove them from the myosin molecule[13] MLC-1 and MLC-3 are both removed in an alkali pH and are further differentiated by their molecular weight. The other pair (a skeletal and cardiac form) are both designated MLC-2 because they are removed from myosin by ethylenediamene tetra-acetic acid. In skeletal muscle it has been shown that when MLC-2 is phosphorylated, there is an increase in force development in the muscle[14]. Barany et al. found that cardiac MLC-2 can be phosphorylated in a similar manner by a calcium, calmodulin-dependent protein kinase[15]. It is likely that increases in cytosolic calcium during myocardial contraction phosphorylate MLC-2 and amplify force development in cardiac muscle.

In the neonate, the ventricles contain an equal amount of ventricular MLC-1 and MLC-2. From the neonatal period through adolescence, there is an increase in the proportion of MLC-2. This increase in the relative proportion of MLC-2 in the adult myocardium may contribute to an increase in the contractile reserve of mature versus neonatal myocardium.

In muscle, myosin interacts with actin, a small globular protein that forms the backbone of the thin filament. In myocardial cells, actin exists in the F (filamentous) form and is arranged as a double-stranded macromolecular helix, with each strand composed of a chain of actin monomers. Actin has two isoforms: alpha cardiac and alpha skeletal. Human myocardium from the fetal period through adulthood contains predominantly the alpha cardiac isoform, with a small amount of alpha skeletal actin. Actin exhibits two properties that are important in muscle contraction: (1) In vitro activation of myosin ATPase and (2) physiochemical interaction with myosin, thereby both initiating and participating in the act of muscle contraction.

Thin and thick filaments are arranged into sarcomeres, which give muscle its striated appearance. A sarcomere is defined as the region between two Z lines. Thin filaments project from the Z line toward the center of the sarcomere, with thick filaments arranged longitudinally between each thin filament. The A band is the area where thick and thin fibers overlap, whereas the I band consists only of thin filaments. The M line divides the A band. Therefore, each sarcomere consists of a central A band and two adjacent half-I bands (Fig. 12.1).

The interactions between actin and myosin are associated with and regulated by the proteins troponin and tropomyosin. Tropomyosin is made up of two helical peptide chains linked by a disulfide bridge. Two isoforms, alpha and beta tropomyosin, exist, with a greater proportion of alpha tropomyosin in fast muscle. In newborn human atria and ventricles, there are relatively equal amounts of alpha and beta tropomyosin, with the beta form increasing during postnatal life. The concentration of the beta isoform is inversely correlated with heart rate and stages of development[16]. Tropomyosin binds to F-actin and is involved in the regulation of actin and myosin interactions[17].

Troponin also regulates interactions between actin and myosin and is a complex of three distinct proteins: troponin T, troponin I, and troponin C (Fig. 12.2). Troponin T is responsible for binding troponin to tropomyosin, while troponin I inhibits these interactions. Troponin C contains[18] calcium binding sites that regulate muscle contraction. The binding of actin and myosin are dependent on troponin I. When calcium activates troponin C, the bond between troponin I and actin is altered, allowing actin and myosin to interact to generate tension[19]. When troponin C is not ac-

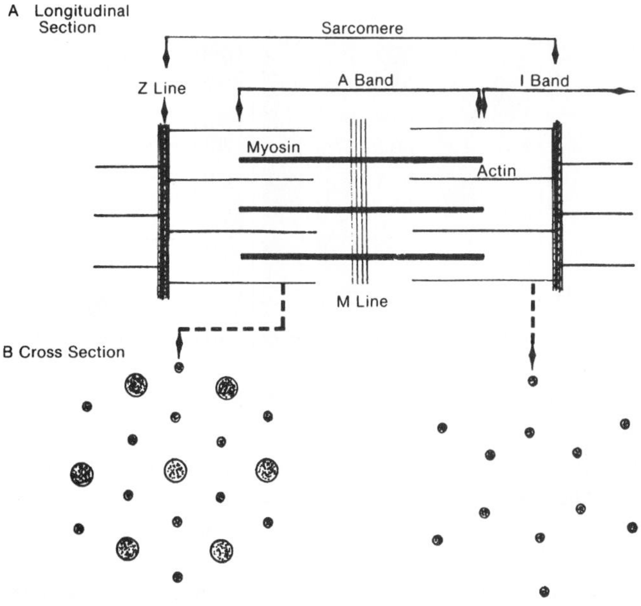

Figure 12.1. The longitudinal section of a sarcomere are represented in **A.** **B** represents the sarcomere in cross-section. (From Garson A, Bricker JT, McNamara DG. The science and practice of pediatric cardiology. Philadelphia, Lea & Febiger, 1990, p. 212.)

tivated by calcium, the affinity between troponin I and actin is high, and myosin binding sites for actin are blocked, thereby inhibiting muscle contraction. Therefore, troponin acts as a calcium-dependent switch that allows a rise in cytosolic calcium to stimulate muscle contraction.

Human fetal myocardium contains two isoforms of troponin I: slow skeletal troponin I (TnIs) and cardiac troponin I (TnIc). The cardiac isoform has an extended N-terminal sequence containing serine residues that are phosphorylated in response to adrenergic stimulation of the heart. Phosphorylation of TnIc increases the affinity of troponin for calcium and therefore increases the contractility of the myocardium[20–22]. Fetal myocardium contains TnIs until birth, when TnIc begins to appear. There is a continued increase in TnIc postnatally, and by 9 months of age TnIc is the only detectable isoform[23] (Fig. 12.3). The expression of TnIs in the neonatal myocardium, characterized by less affinity for calcium in response to adrenergic stimulation, may contribute to the decrease in contractility of the immature myocardium compared to the adult.

Therefore, from birth through adolescence there are changes in the expression of proteins that are integral components of myocardial contraction. The more immature the myocardial protein composition (i.e., more TnIs), the more it favors a response to adrenergic stimulation, a reduced contractile reserve and a depressed contractile response to exogenous adminsitration of catecholamines. These molecular factors will play a pivotal role in the later description of the physiologic differences of the immature myocardium.

Not only are there changes in the muscle protein, but the organization of the neonatal myocyte differs significantly from that of the adult. The ultrastructure of the neonatal myocyte is dominated by organelles (mitochondria, nucleoli, etc.) necessary for cellular synthetic function (Fig. 12.4). The myocyte shape assumes a more globular structure as opposed to the elongated form of the mature myocyte. The total number of myocytes per gram of myocardium is reduced in the neonatal period. The newborn has a 50% reduction in the number of myocytes per gram of myocardium in comparison to the adult heart. In addition, the myocytes are structurally arranged in a nonlinear or chaotic fashion. The nonlinear arrangement impairs contractile efficiency and therefore recruitment of additional myocytes is less effective in augmenting myocardial function. The result is reduced contractility and a reduction in myocardial reserve.

Muscle Contraction

Several hypotheses as to how muscle contracts have been proposed. The sliding filament model, first described by Huxley over 30 years ago, remains the most substantiated[24]. This theory proposes that actin and myosin filaments remain constant in length and slide past each other to produce changes in muscle length during contraction[24–27]. Troponin is activated by calcium and thereby allows actin to stimulate myosin ATPase activity. The energy produced

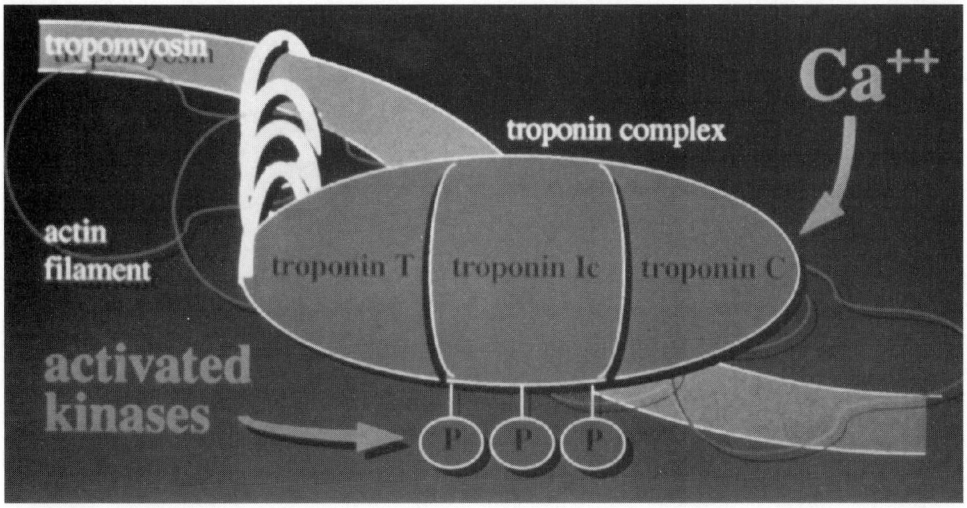

Figure 12.2. The troponin complex is composed of three distinct proteins: troponin T, troponin I, and troponin C. The troponin complex interacts with tropomyosin, Ca++, activated kinase, and actin filaments.

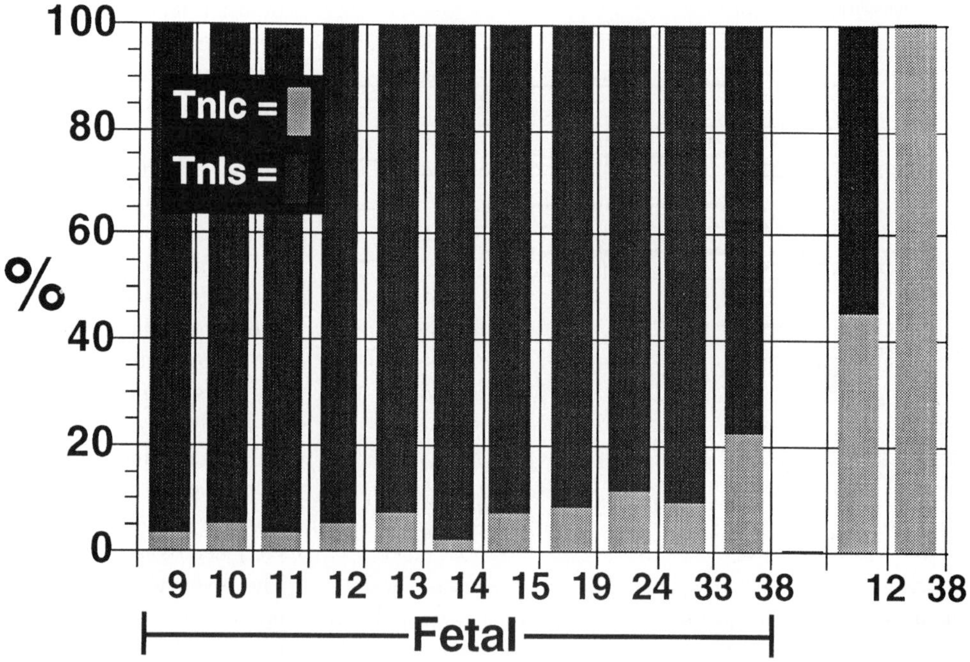

Figure 12.3. Changes in troponin isoforms from the fetal period through postnatal development. Troponin I cardiac (TnIc) is the isoform found in mature cardiac muscle. Troponin I skeletal (TnIs) is the troponin isoform found in skeletal muscle and in the myocardium of the developing fetus. (From Sasse S, Brand NJ, Kyprianou P, et al. Troponin I gene expression during human cardiac development and in end-stage heart failure. Circ Res 1993; 72:932–938.)

allows the myosin head to cyclically attach and detach from the actin filaments, pulling the actin filament toward the center of the A band and causing the muscle to contract. The exact composition of the "cross-bridge" and the precise regulatory control are an area of current research.

The individual sarcomeres formed from actin and myosin are associated with several membrane structures, including the sarcolemma, sarcoplasmic reticulum, and transverse tubules (Fig. 12.5). The sarcolemma surrounds the myocardial cell and functions as a barrier between the intracellular and extracellular space. Transverse tubules invaginate from the sarcolemma toward the center of the myocardial cell. Both the sarcolemma and transverse tubules contain ion pumps, ion channels, and receptors, which establish both chemical and charge gradients across the membrane. The sarcoplasmic reticulum surrounds the contractile proteins and functions primarily to regulate intracellular calcium. Precise control of calcium in the cytoplasm is critical for optimal myocardial contractility. The resting concentration of cytosolic calcium is dependent on the balance be-

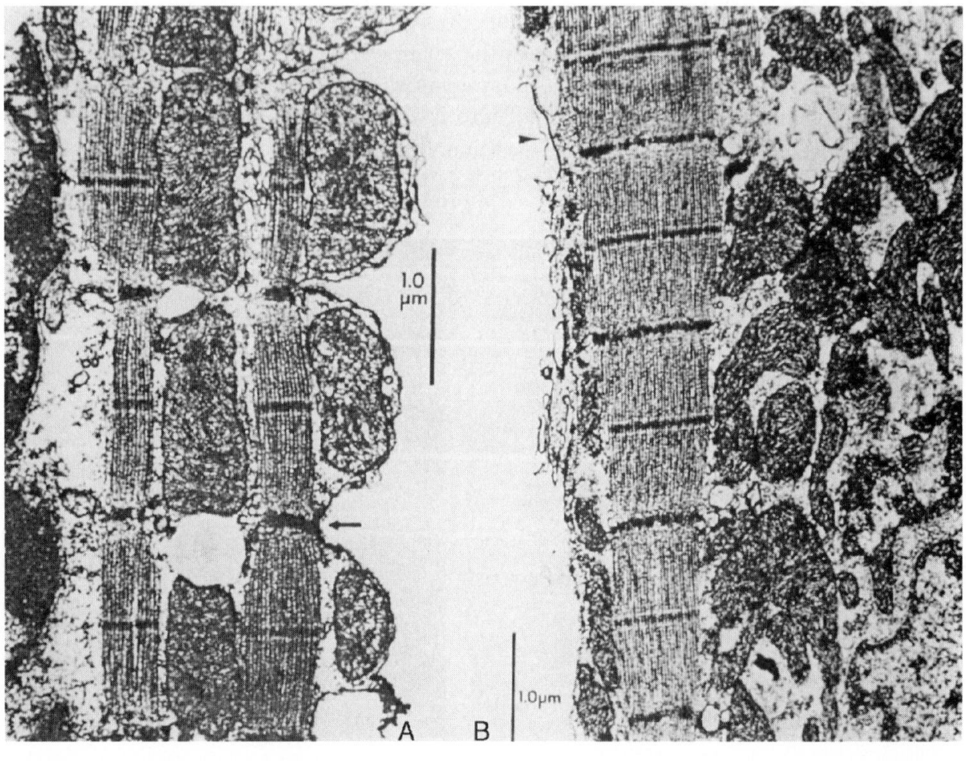

Figure 12.4. Transmission electron micrographs of myocardial cells from postnatal (**A**) and fetal (**B**) myocardium. In the fetal myocardium the mitochondria, golgi apparatus, and sarcoplasmic reticulum are extensive and separated from the myofibrils. In contrast, the postnatal myocardium is well organized, with mitochondria closely associated with each sarcomere. (Nassar R, Reedy MC, Anderson PA. Developmental changes in the ultra structure and sarcomere shortening of the isolated rabbit ventricular myocyte. Circ Res 1987; 3:465–483.)

tween influx and efflux of calcium to the cytoplasm through the membrane.

In the adult, excitation-contraction coupling begins with a small amount of calcium entering the cell across the sarcolemma, which then triggers a substantially larger release of calcium from the sarcoplasmic reticulum. The increase in cytosolic calcium activates the contractile process between actin and myosin. The sarcoplasmic reticulum also removes calcium from the cytoplasm during repolarization.

There is substantial ultrastructural evidence demonstrating a paucity of sarcoplasmic reticulum in the inmature neonatal myocardium[28]. The decrease in sarcoplasmic reticulum makes the neonatal myocardium more dependent upon extracellular calcium, which enters the cytosol through slow calcium channels in the sarcolemma (membrane barrier between the intracellular and extracellular environments). This accounts for the finding that neonatal myocardium is much more sensitive to drugs that block slow calcium channels than is the adult myocardium. The neonatal myocardium is 10 times more sensitive to the calcium channel blockers nifedipine and verapamil than is the adult myocardium[29–31]. Myocardial contractile function in the immature heart is severely impaired when the slow inward calcium current in the sarcolemma is blocked compared with mature myocardium, which contains a more extensive sarcoplasmic reticulum and can rely on intracellular calcium stores for maintaining effective contractility[29–34]. Similarly, blocking intracellular calcium flux has minimal effect on neonatal myocardium, whereas a much greater effect on myocardial contractility can be demonstrated in the adult heart. These studies support the dependency of the neonatal heart on extracellular calcium as the primary source of cytoplasmic free calcium and therefore for optimal myocardial contractility.

Although calcium has fallen in to some disfavor because of concerns over reperfusion injury, calcium supplementation remains an important therapy in the neonate with myocardial dysfunction due to the underdeveloped calcium transport system[29]. Since intracellular calcium concentrations play a central role in myocardial contractility, normal or even elevated plasma levels of ionized calcium may be necessary to augment stroke volume[32]. Hypocalcemia remains an important cause for myocardial dysfunction in the newborn. Calcium therapy, however, must be used with caution because it can induce sinus bradycardia. This can be problematic in the vagotonic newborn.

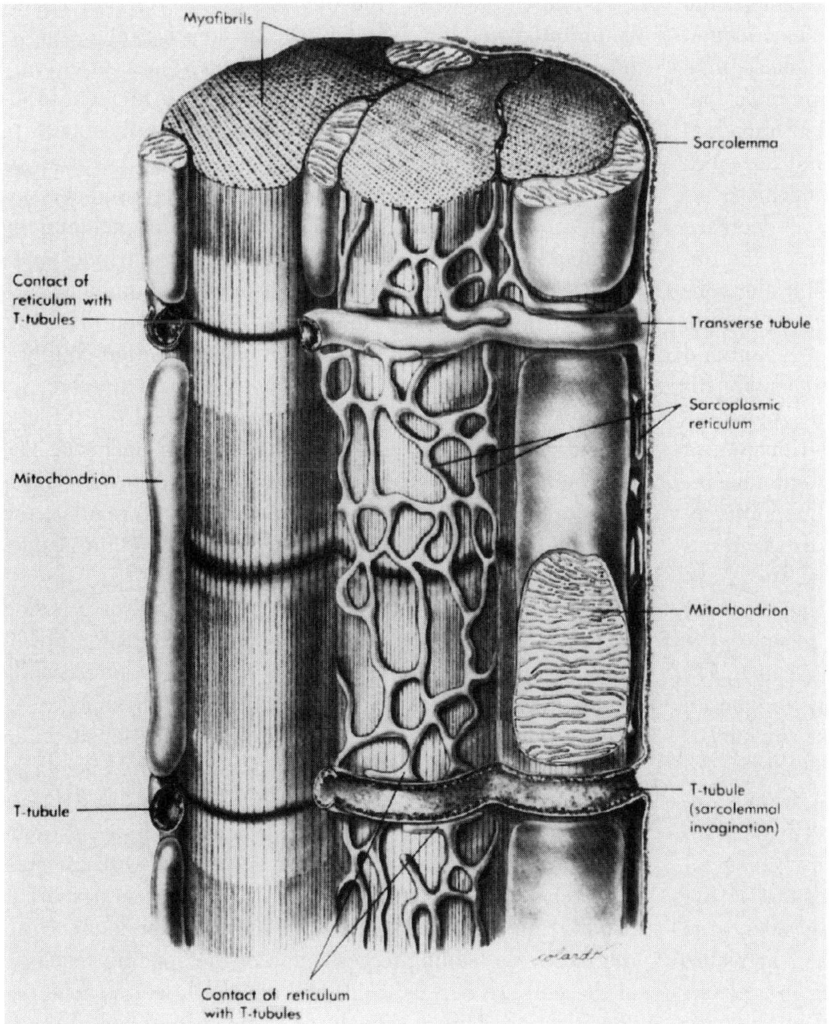

Figure 12.5. Normal mature cardiac fibril.

Myocardial relaxation occurs because of a decrease in the intracellular calcium concentration. The change in concentration is controlled by intracellular storage of calcium and through the extrusion of calcium from the cell by a transmembrane Na-Ca exchange. Hoerter[35] and Caroni[36] found that the myocardial relaxation time constant is not significantly different between the immature and mature myocardium. This suggests that the sarcoplasmic reticulum is not solely responsible for calcium removal during the relaxation phase. Other systems, such as mitochondrial[37] or sarcolemmal Ca ATPase[36], have also been proposed to be involved in relaxation. In neonatal myocardium, the decrease in sarcoplasmic reticulum does not seem to alter the ability of the immature myocardial cell to enter the relaxation phase as quickly as adult myocardium. This suggests an important role for the sarcolemma and mitochondria.

While the neonatal heart is anatomically similar to the adult heart, differences in contractile protein isoforms and the paucity of sarcoplasmic reticulum with the dependence on extracellular calcium for optimal contractility make the immature myocardium functionally unique.

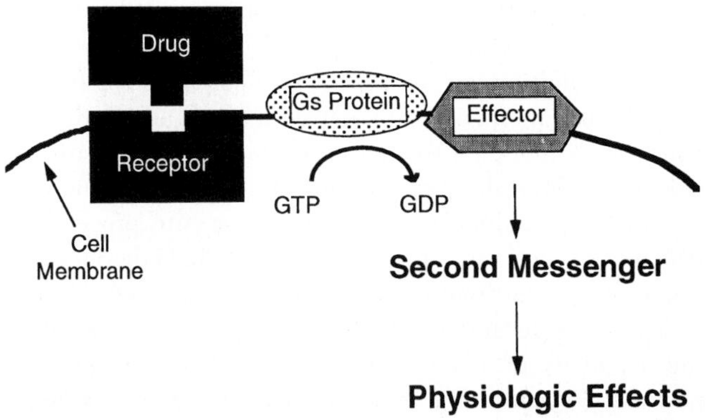

Figure 12.6. Schematic of the G-protein coupled receptors. Gs represents a stimulatory G-protein receptor. Activation results in second messenger generation and a positive physiologic effect. (From Greeley WJ, Kern: FH: Pediatric cardiovascular anesthesia, Smith's Pediatric Anesthesia, Davis P, Motoyama EK (eds). Chicago: Mosby Yearbook, 1995.

Myocardial Receptor Physiology

Myocardial contraction occurs when calcium enters the myocardial cell and initiates the interaction of actin and myosin. This influx of calcium occurs in response to a stimulus acting on a receptor. Receptors are proteins that are responsible for recognizing a signal and then transducing the message to the cell. Molecules that bind to receptors are called ligands. Ligands, which act as agonists, increase receptor activity, whereas antagonists decrease activity. Antagonists may be competitive, in which the decreased response may be overcome by increasing the concentration of the agonist, or act in a noncompetitive fashion where the ligand binds irreversibly to the receptor and blocks the agonist from binding. Myocardial receptors include adrenergic and muscarinic cholinergic receptors.

These receptors fall under the broader classification of G-protein coupled receptors (Fig. 12.6). The G-protein receptor is composed of seven transmembrane lipophilic regions, an extracellular amino terminus, three extracellular loops, and an intracellular carboxyl terminus. The third, fourth, and seventh intracellular regions are important for ligand binding. Once the ligand binds to the receptor, the coupled G protein hydrolyses guanasine triphosphate (GTP) to guanasine diphosphate (GDP). This energy initiates a cascade of second messengers, which results in a physiologic effect depending on the specific receptor and cell involved. There are three different G proteins: Gs, Gi and Gq, each with a specific cellular effect. Gs and Gi are both coupled to the same second messenger pathway, which involves adenyl cyclase. Gs stimulates adenyl cyclase to hydrolyze adenosine triphosphate (ATP) to cyclic adenosine monophosphate (cAMP). Protein kinase is then activated and phosphorylates cellular enzymes, resulting in a physiologic response. Gi uses the same pathway but inhibits adenyl cyclase and therefore blocks phosphorylation. Beta 1 and beta 2 receptors are associated with Gs, whereby alpha 2 and cholinergic receptors are coupled to Gi. For example, when epinephrine stimulates a beta 2 receptor on the myocardium, the final effect is an increase in intracellular calcium and an increase in contractility of the myocardial cell.

When a cholinergic receptor is stimulated, this pathway is inhibited, and intracellular calcium does not increase. Alpha 1 receptors are coupled to Gq, which uses an entirely different second messenger pathway. Gq activates phospholipase C, which converts phosphoinositol diphosphate to diacylglycerol and inositol triphosphate (Fig. 12.7). Diacylglycerol activates protein kinase C, which phosphorylates cellular enzymes and increases intracellular calcium by opening ion channels. Simultaneously, inositol triphosphate releases calcium from the sarcoplasmic reticulum and contributes to an increase in intracellular calcium. This increase in calcium activates excitation-contraction coupling and therefore initiates muscle contraction. Therefore, an alpha-1 agonist also causes muscle contraction but through an entirely different pathway than do beta agonists. The G-protein family coupled to the multitude of second messengers provides researchers an opportunity to regulate the cardiac response at various levels in the second messenger pathway.

When a receptor is stimulated by a ligand for a period of time, receptor regulation may occur. Receptor down-regulation refers to the loss of cell surface receptors, while desensitization refers to a reduction in the physiologic response during continued agonist exposure. Desensitization may occur at the receptor, the G protein, or the effector or by other mechanisms that increase the rate of cAMP degradation. Homologous desensitization is the loss of stimulatory activity in the pathway that is involved with the specific receptor being stimulated. This decrease in activity is usually through modifications in the receptor itself. If all the pathways leading to activation of the specific response of the cell are desensitized, this is called heterologous desensitization. This is thought to occur at the level of the G protein or the effector enzyme itself.

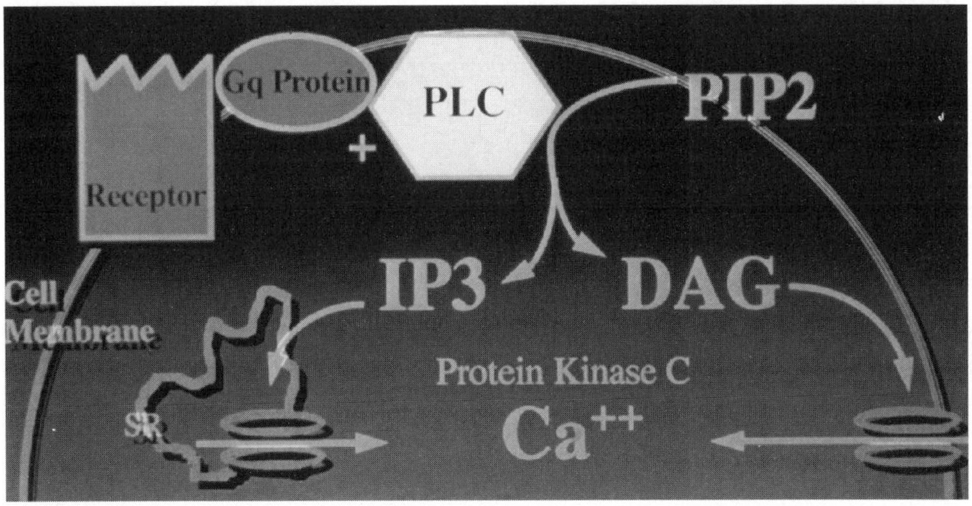

Figure 12.7. Schematic of the second messenger pathway of the G-protein receptors. The Gq protein subunit stimulates phospholipase C (PLC), which converts phosphoinositol diphosphate into diacylglycerol (DAG) and inositol triphosphate (IP3). DAG increases intracellular calcium by opening plasma membrane calcium ion channels. IP3 increases calcium release from the sarcoplasmic reticulum (SR).

When an agonist binds to a receptor, homologous desensitization of the signaling pathway begins. Phosphorylation of the receptor occurs within minutes and uncouples the G protein from the receptor, thereby preventing any further stimulation of the pathway. If the agonist remains bound to the receptor over a period of hours, sequestering occurs where the receptor is removed from the cell surface into the cytoplasm. At this point, the cell can either recycle the receptor back to the cell surface or degrade the receptor completely. A new protein must then be synthesized to form a new functional receptor (Fig. 12.8).

Myocardial receptors, primarily adrenergic receptors, have been studied extensively in the adult. In normal adult myocardium, the ratio of beta-1 to beta-2 receptors have been shown to be 70:30 in the atria and 80:20 in the ventricles. This ratio is not static and has been found to change in response to various stimuli or pathologic conditions. When normal myocardium is exposed to isoproterenol for a short period, the number of beta-2 receptors decreases significantly. However, in adults with congestive heart failure incurring long-term endogenous catecholamine exposure, studies have shown a 50 to 60% decrease in the total number of beta receptors, with beta-1 substantially decreased relative to beta-2[38]. Bristow showed that beta-2 receptors remain the same in number, but that uncoupling of the beta-2 receptor from the G protein may occur[39]. This down-regulation of beta receptors in the failing heart may be responsible for the inability of the myocardium to respond maximally to inotropic agents in the intensive care unit. The response of beta receptors in patients undergoing cardiopulmonary bypass (CPB) has also been studied in adults, with data suggesting that myocardial beta-receptor desensitization occurs during CPB and then reverses after the discontinuation of CPB[40]. These studies showing the changes that occur in beta-receptor subtypes in response to a variety of stimuli and physiologic conditions have potentially important implications for patient management.

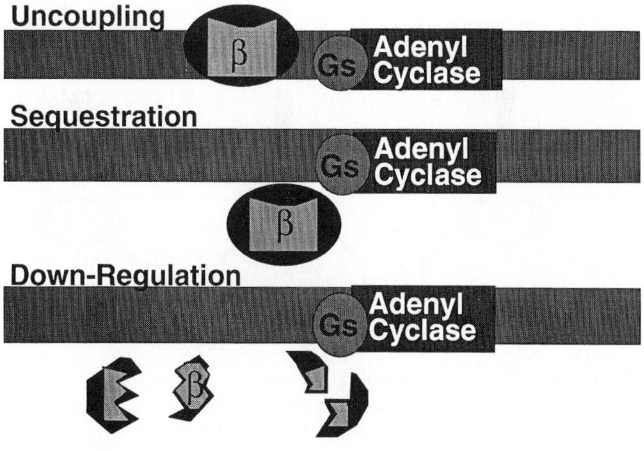

Figure 12.8. The three phases of receptor desensitization (uncoupling, sequestration, and down-regulation). Gs represents a stimulatory G-protein receptor.

While there are multiple studies of myocardial receptors in adults, the data available on infants and children is still limited. Studies of right atrial tissue from infants and children with congenital heart disease who were undergoing cardiac surgery found that children with severe acyanotic or cyanotic heart disease had a significant decrease in the number of beta receptors[41]. As in adults, the down-regulation of beta receptors was beta-1 subtype selective in most cases. However, in infants with transposition of the great vessels and those patients with critical aortic stenosis, there was also a significant reduction in the number of beta-2 receptors. Schranz et al. studied children undergoing CPB with circulatory arrest and demonstrated desensitization in beta receptors without a change in total receptor number[42]. These changes in beta receptors that occur may affect our ability to obtain a maximal response to inotropic agents in patients with congenital heart disease. Hausdorf et al. examined this by administering a phosphodiesterase inhibitor to a group of 16 newborns with postoperative catecholamine-refractory, low-cardiac outputs[43]. Hemodynamic measures improved in 12 of these infants. These studies support the treatment of patients who are unresponsive to catecholamines with agents having a different mechanism of action than that of the myocardial adrenergic receptor. Phosphodiesterase inhibitors provide such an approach.

Table 12–1. Contractility Demonstrated with Different Doses of Dobutamine and Propranol

Intervention	*Index of Inotropy* E_{ES} ($K_{pa}mL^{-1}$)
Control	4.63
Dobutamine—low dose	4.43
—mid dose	4.98
—high dose	4.65
Propranolol	3.51

Table 12–2. Relative Inotropic Effects of G Protein Coupled Receptors

Receptor	*Percent Inotropic Effect*	*Tissue Sample*
β1 + β2	100%	LV, RV
H2	30–40%	LV, RV
5-HT	50–60%	RA
VIP	40%	RV
α1	10–15%	LV
Ang II	30–50%	RA
ET	34%	RA
PGE1	?	

The response of normal neonatal myocardium to catecholamines has not been studied in humans. In rabbits, there is data to suggest that although adult myocardium exposed to isoproterenol results in desensitization of beta receptors, this uncoupling process does not occur in the neonate[44]. Experiments in newborn lambs show only a modest increase in preload independent measures of contractility at dobutamine doses of 8 to 10 μg/kg/min, whereas a moderately severe reduction in contractility has been demonstrated with a 0.5-mg/kg dose of propranolol[45] **(Table 12–1).** This suggests a reduced response to beta specific agonists in the newborn period.

Newborn animals have a reduced number of beta receptors, have high circulating catecholamine levels, and do not desensitize to exogenous catecholamines, suggesting that normal neonates are "functionally desensitized" at birth[46,47]. Further increases in contractility will require more potent inotropic support with higher doses of potent agents such as dopamine and epinephrine than is commonly used in older patients[43,48,49]. This is particularly true with procedures requiring CPB when postoperative left ventricular dysfunction is present. Drugs such as dobutamine increase cardiac output through increases in heart rate but appear to have minimal effects on contractility and therefore may not improve oxygen delivery while increasing myocardial oxygen consumption[48–50]. In patients with bradycardia or heart block, augmentation of heart rate with chronotropic agents or pacing may be beneficial.

Additional consideration must be given to evidence suggesting that myocardial G-protein coupled receptors, which mediate contractility, mature at different rates. For example, in the neonatal rodent the number of beta-adrenergic receptors is significantly less than in mature animals. Alpha receptors are increased in the newborn[51]. Angiotensin II receptors, which are minimally present in adult myocardium, are relatively abundant at birth and mediate an increase in myocardial contractility equal to 30 to 50% of beta receptors[52] **(Table 12–2).** Alternative approaches to inotropic support have been limited by drugs that are nonselective and therefore have additional untoward systemic effects, e.g., angiotensin II.

In addition to conventional inotropic agents, clinical trials are under way with unconventional inotropic agents such as thyroxin, which works by several noncatecholamine mechanisms to augment contractility. Still more theoretical are selective angiotensin-II agonists, which may provide an alternative approach to enhancing myocardial contractility in the neonate. In total, there are 12 known membrane receptors located on myocytes that possess inotropic properties (Fig. 12.9). Current therapeutic approaches use only the bAR (beta-adrenergic receptor) membrane receptor pharmacologically to augment inotropy. It is possible that a more potent combination of receptor system based therapy and cardiotonic agents may be beneficial for the treatment of low cardiac output syndromes in the neonate. Research in this area is in its infancy.

EMBRYOLOGY AND DEVELOPMENT OF THE HEART

The development of the fetal heart is characterized by two phases that determine the anatomic structure and physiologic function of the newborn myocardium. The first phase determines the anatomic relationships of the atria, ventricles, great vessels, and systemic and pulmonary venous return. These relationships are determined very early in gestation and are virtually complete by the first 8 weeks after conception. Once these relationships are established, a second developmental phase, characterized by physical growth of these structures, predominates. Abnormalities in chamber and great vessel size play an important role in the development of hypoplasia of the right or left ventricle and severe cardiac defects such as pulmonary atresia and hypoplastic left heart syndrome. Clinical assessment using fe-

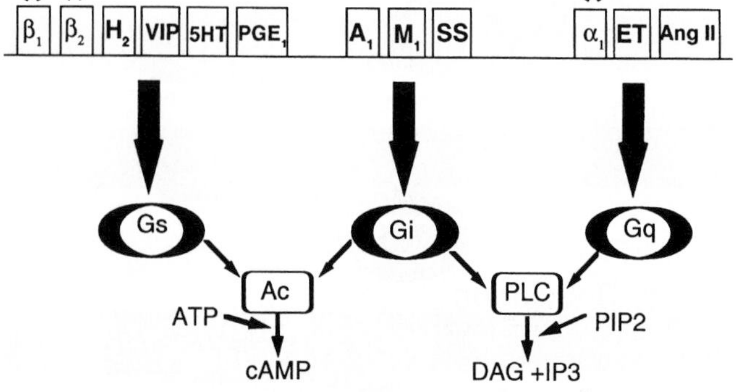

Figure 12.9. The various membrane receptors that are located on myocytes. The asterisks represent the only receptors we currently manipulate pharmacologically. (From Greeley WJ, Kern, FH: Pediatric cardiovascular anesthesia. In: Smith's Pediatric Anesthesia, Davis P, Motoyama EK (eds.). Chicago: Mosby Yearbook, 1995.

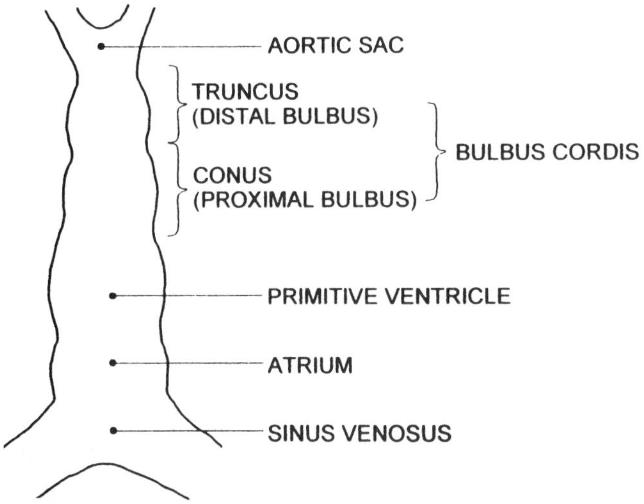

Figure 12.10. The primitive straight heart tube showing the segmental orientation. (From Emmanouilides GW, Allen HD, Riemenschneider TA, Gutgesell HP, eds. Heart disease in infants, children, and adolescence. 5th ed. Philadelphia: Williams & Wilkins, 1995:7.)

tal echocardiography has demonstrated that growth abnormalities can continue throughout late gestation, and the severity of the cardiac defect may continue to develop and progress during the last 20 weeks of gestation. As an example, tetralogy of Fallot can progress to pulmonary atresia, and a normal left ventricle at 20 weeks of gestation will be hypoplastic at birth if no interval growth occurs between the 20th week and term.

Phase 1: Anatomic Development of Cardiac Structures

The following discussion of the embryology of the heart is not intended to be inclusive but rather is intended as an overview of how the heart develops. It is often helpful in describing abnormal anatomy to view the heart in a segmental manner, in which the heart is divided into three segments: the atria, the ventricles, and the great vessels. The heart begins as a straight heart tube (Fig. 12.10), with the inlet of the heart located caudally and the outlet of the heart located cephalad; i.e., blood flows from a caudal to cephalad direction. The primitive left ventricle is located caudally and receives the inlet of the heart, while the primitive right ventricle, or bulbus cordis, is located superiorly and gives rise to the outlet of the heart. At this stage of development there is no differentiation of the aorta and pulmonary artery, and the outlet of the heart consists of the conotruncus, which will later divide into the aorta and the pulmonary artery. The heart tube, primarily through differential growth, loops or bends on itself so the bulbus cordis lies either rightward and anterior or leftward and anterior to the primitive left ventricle. This results in what is referred to as a d-loop (dextro) when the loop is to the right, or an l-loop (levo) when the loop is to the left. The looping—that is, whether the right ventricle comes to lie anterior and rightward of the left ventricle (d-loop) or anterior and leftward of the ventricle (l-loop)—is determined during the very early development phase of the heart (Fig. 12.11). At this early stage of development, the outlet of the heart or conotruncus, (primitive aorta, and pulmonary artery) are committed to the bulbus cordis. The inlet of the heart, on the other hand, is committed to the primitive left ventricle. If the development of the heart arrests at this stage, then it is possible to have either a double inlet left ventricle or a double outlet right ventricle[53].

While the primitive ventricles are undergoing looping, the inlet of the heart migrates cephalad and eventually shifts to the right so that it comes to lie over the interventricular foramen and thus becomes committed to both the right and left ventricles. A significant portion of the atrial mass in the adult heart is derived from the venous tributaries. On the systemic venous side this consists of the sinus venosus. The sinus venosus receives the drainage from the cardinal system of veins. The cardinal system is one of a series of venous plexuses that drain the dorsal portion of the embryo. In its earliest form, the cardinal system consists of a paired (right and left) anterior, a paired (right and left) posterior, and a common cardinal system that connects the left and right components to the midline (Fig. 12.12). The innominate vein forms between the left and right anterior cardinal veins. With its appearance, the left anterior cardinal vein

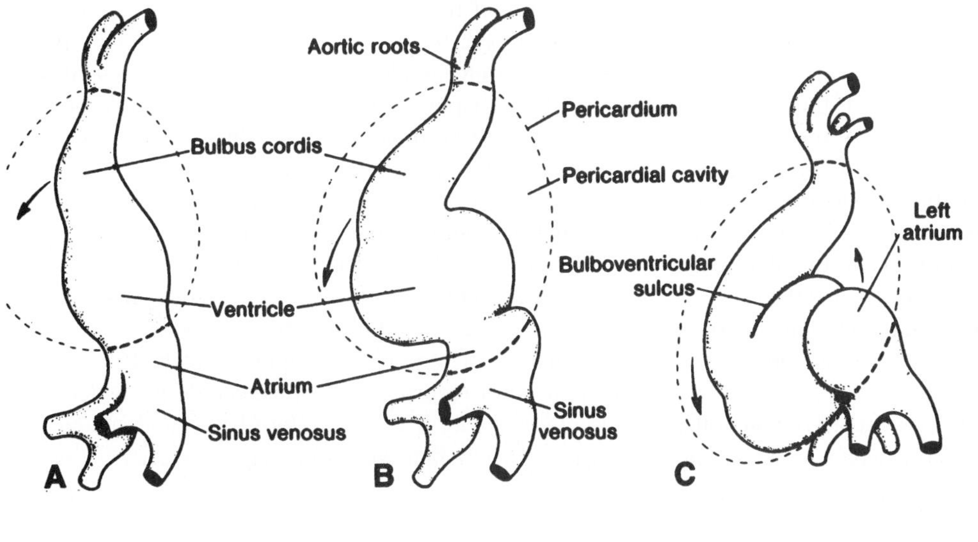

Figure 12.11. The primitive heart tube demonstrating d-looping of the ventricles. Note that the bulbus cordis is to the right of the primitive ventricle after looping occurs. In l-looping the bulbus cordis is to the left after looping occurs. (From Sadler TW. Langman's medical embryology. Philadelphia, Williams & Wilkins, 1990, p. 183.)

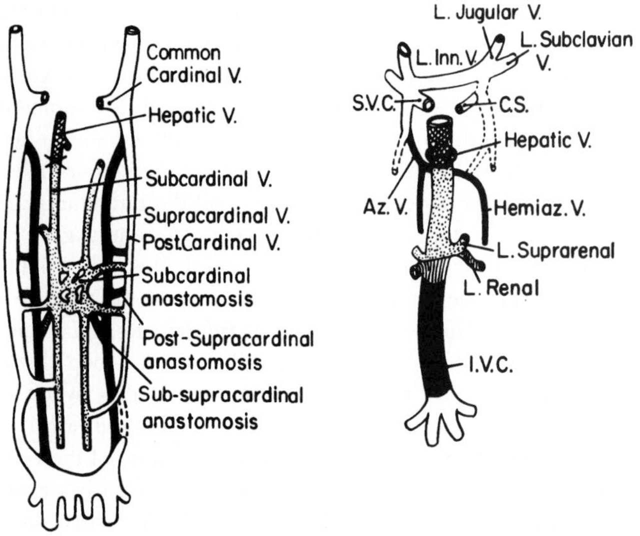

Figure 12.12. Embryologic development of the venous system. There are paired venous systems which, through multiple anastomoses, develop into the normal venous structures seen in the right panel. Note that the inferior vena cava (I.V.C.) in the normal heart comprises the posterior cardinal system (white), supracardinal system (black), renal collar (lines), subcardinal system (stipple) and hepatic veins (cross-hatch). The contributions of the venous drainage to the superior vena cava is described in the text. Az., azygous vein; C.S., coronary sinus, Inn., innominate; Hemiaz., hemiazygos; L., left; V., vein. (From Goor DA, Lilihei CW. Congenital malformations of the heart. Grune & Stratton, 1975; Chapter 2, p. 68.)

obliterates. When the left anterior cardinal vein persists, it becomes a left superior vena cava that drains into the coronary sinus. The great cardiac vein is a remnant of the left posterior cardinal vein. The coronary sinus consists of the left common cardinal vein and a portion of the sinus venosus. On the right, the common cardinal vein forms a portion of the superior vena cava between the azygous vein and the right atrium. The azygous vein is a remnant of the right-sided posterior cardinal system. The right-sided anterior cardinal system becomes the superior vena cava between the innominate vein and the most proximal portion of the superior vena cava. The inferior vena cava at its entry into the right atrium is derived from the hepatocardiac vein and is not a portion of the sinus venosus[53].

A significant portion of the left atrium comprises the entrance of the pulmonary veins. The pulmonary veins arise from the lungs and grow toward the heart. If the pulmonary veins fail to join the left atrium, then they anastomose to systemic venous tributaries, and the result is anomalous pulmonary venous return. Since the anastomosis in total anomalous pulmonary venous return is to systemic venous tributaries, the veins may drain either below the diaphragm into the portal venous system or above the heart to the innominate vein, the superior vena cava, directly into the right atrium, or into the right atrium by way of the coronary sinus.

The aorta and pulmonary artery arise from division of the conotruncus and the aortic sac into separate vessels. The aorta and pulmonary artery arise from septation of the aortic sac by the septum aortopumonale. The conotruncus gives rise to the semilunar valves. While the aorta initially starts out on the right, relative to the pulmonary artery, through rotation the aorta comes to lie over the left ventricle, with the pulmonary artery wrapped around the aorta. Through fusion of the ventricular septum, the heart is divided from a straight tube into two separate flow pathways. It is in this first developmental phase that the major structural abnormalities of the heart form. These include the truncus arteriosus, tetralogy of Fallot, total anomalous pulmonary venous return, double outlet right ventricle and double inlet left ventricle.

Phase 2: Normal and Abnormal Growth of Cardiac Structures

Once the heart has developed in the first 8 weeks of gestation, other significant abnormalities may develop from poor growth of the ventricles, aorta, or pulmonary artery. The development of congenital heart defects because of poor growth has been best delineated through fetal echocardiography, in which serial studies of the fetus can be performed. Generally, these abnormalities do not relate to abnormalities in septation of the atria and ventricles or to the abnormal relationship of cardiac structures. Rather, they relate to reduced blood flow which impairs ventricular and great vessel growth.

Left-Sided Obstructive Lesions

Hornberger and her colleagues have clearly demonstrated through fetal echocardiography that left-sided obstructive lesions may progress during pregnancy[54]. Fetuses with relatively normal-appearing left ventricles at 20 weeks of gestation may develop hypoplastic left heart syndrome if the left ventricle does not grow any further. The reasons for this poor growth are not clear, but it has been postulated that it may relate to reduced blood flow through the ventricles. This hypothesis suggests that cardiac chambers require blood flow in order to grow adequately. If there is premature closure of the foramen ovale, or if there is mitral stenosis or atresia, there will not be adequate blood flow into the left ventricle, and left heart hypoplasia will result. Other causes for hypoplasia of the left ventricle include posterior deviation of the primum septum, which diverts pulmonary venous return to the right ventricle and impairs right-to-left shunting at the atrial level, resulting in reduced left ventricular filling and hypoplasia of the left heart.

Although development of ventricular hypoplasia is primarily flow related, there is also a genetic component. The recurrence of left-sided obstructive lesions in families with a previously affected child is approximately 15%[18]. This compares to a recurrent risk of congenital heart defects as a whole of 2.3%. It may therefore be a combination of in utero blood-flow patterns and a genetic predisposition that may alter ventricular growth and cellular migration on a molecular basis.

Right-Sided Obstructive Lesions

Right-sided obstructive lesions also progress in utero. Serial echocardiography has indicated that fetuses with tetralogy of Fallot have gone on to develop pulmonary atresia at birth[55,56]. In addition, there have been fetuses with pulmonary stenosis in whom the stenosis has become more severe during pregnancy. In some cases fetuses with pulmonary stenosis have gone on to develop complete pulmonary atresia. The postulated mechanism in both cases is diminished flow across the right ventricular outflow tract, resulting in progressive stenosis and atresia.

New Approaches to Congenital Cardiac Anomalies

Congenital cardiac malformations develop as a result of abnormalities in the anatomic relationships of the atria, ventricles, great vessels, systemic and pulmonary veins, and abnormalities in the growth of chambers and great vessels. The knowledge of these developmental concepts are important in the diagnosis and management of the fetus with congenital heart disease. In utero diagnoses currently impact on the anticipated management of the newborn with congenital cardiac disease through perinatal counseling of the parents, transfer of the mother to a high-risk facility with pediatric cardiologists, critical care physicians, and cardiac surgeons committed to early intervention and treatment of newborns with congenital cardiac disease. Recent experimental studies demonstrate that in utero surgical and interventional catheterization procedures can alter intracardiac flow patterns and minimize, or perhaps eliminate, the development of ventricular and great vessel hypoplasia. In utero techniques may provide new clinical approaches to the care of infants with severe forms of ventricular hypoplasia. These approaches could improve the life expectancy and relatively high morbidity associated with conventional univentricular surgical repairs.

TRANSITIONAL CIRCULATION

The cardiovascular system changes markedly at birth due to dramatic alterations in blood-flow patterns (Fig. 12.13)[57]. During fetal life, blood flow returning to the heart bypasses the unventilated fluid-filled lungs. Blood is then preferentially shunted across the patent foramen ovale into the left atrium (LA) or passes from the right ventricle (RV) across the patent ductus arteriosus (PDA) to the systemic circulation. At the time of birth, physiology closure of the PDA and the foramen ovale bring about the normal adult circulatory pattern. The presence of certain congenital heart defects, birth asphyxia, sepsis, or pulmonary disease can disrupt this normal adaptive process, creating persistence of the transitional circulation. Under such circumstances, the continued right-to-left shunting across the foramen ovale or the PDA leads to severe hypoxemia, acidosis, and hemodynamic instability, which is poorly tolerated in the neonate.

Under normal circumstances, the fetal circulation rapidly transitions toward an adult circulation. Cessation of a placental circulation is facilitated by stretching of the umbilical vessels, increased arterial oxygen tension, and eventual clamping of the umbilical cord. The venous return through the inferior vena cava is reduced by approximately 45% when the placenta is removed from the circulation, resulting in a reduction in blood flow through the ductus venosus, facilitating its passive closure[58]. Figure 12.14 displays the volume of blood received from the placenta, lower body, and SVC and the volume of blood ejected by each ventricle.

Pulmonary vascular resistance decreases by approximately 75%, and pulmonary blood flow increases by 450% with the onset of neonatal respiration[59,60]. Several factors contribute to the decrease in pulmonary vascular resistance, including the mechanical expansion of the lungs, increasing alveolar oxygen tension (P_AO_2), and an increase in arterial oxygen tension (PaO_2). Inflation of the lung with 100% nitrogen results in a nearly fourfold increase in pulmonary blood flow[59,61]. Lung expansion reduces pulmonary vascular resistance by increasing the effective cross-sectional area of the pulmonary vasculature. Further increases in pulmonary blood flow augments pulmonary vasodilation by the direct shear forces on the endothelium and through stimulation of biomechanical stretch receptors[61]. Endothelial shear forces stimulate the release of the prostacyclins and enhance the release of nitric oxide, which are primary pulmonary vasodilators[62]. Biomechanical distension of the pulmonary vasculature stimulates the production of bradykinin, which induces the production of prostacyclin and nitric oxide[63,64].

Increases in PaO_2 and (P_AO_2) further augment reduction in pulmonary vascular resistance by the direct effects of oxygen on the pulmonary vasculature and through stimulation of nitric oxide production[65]. Elimination of atelectatic regions of lung result in improvement in P_AO_2. Local increases in PaO_2 reverse hypoxic pulmonary vasoconstriction and therefore enhances and maintains the acute reductions in pulmonary vascular resistance attained through initial lung expansion[66].

As pulmonary blood flow increases, there is an increase in pulmonary venous return, left atrial filling, and left atrial pressure. Concomitantly, the loss of venous return from the placenta results in a reduction in right atrial filling and a right atrial pressure, which favors physiologic closure of the foramen ovale (Fig. 12.14). Prenatal pulmonary artery pressures are approximately 70/45 mm Hg and decrease to 50/30 mm Hg at approximately 24 hours after delivery (Fig. 12.15). Over the ensuing several days pulmonary artery

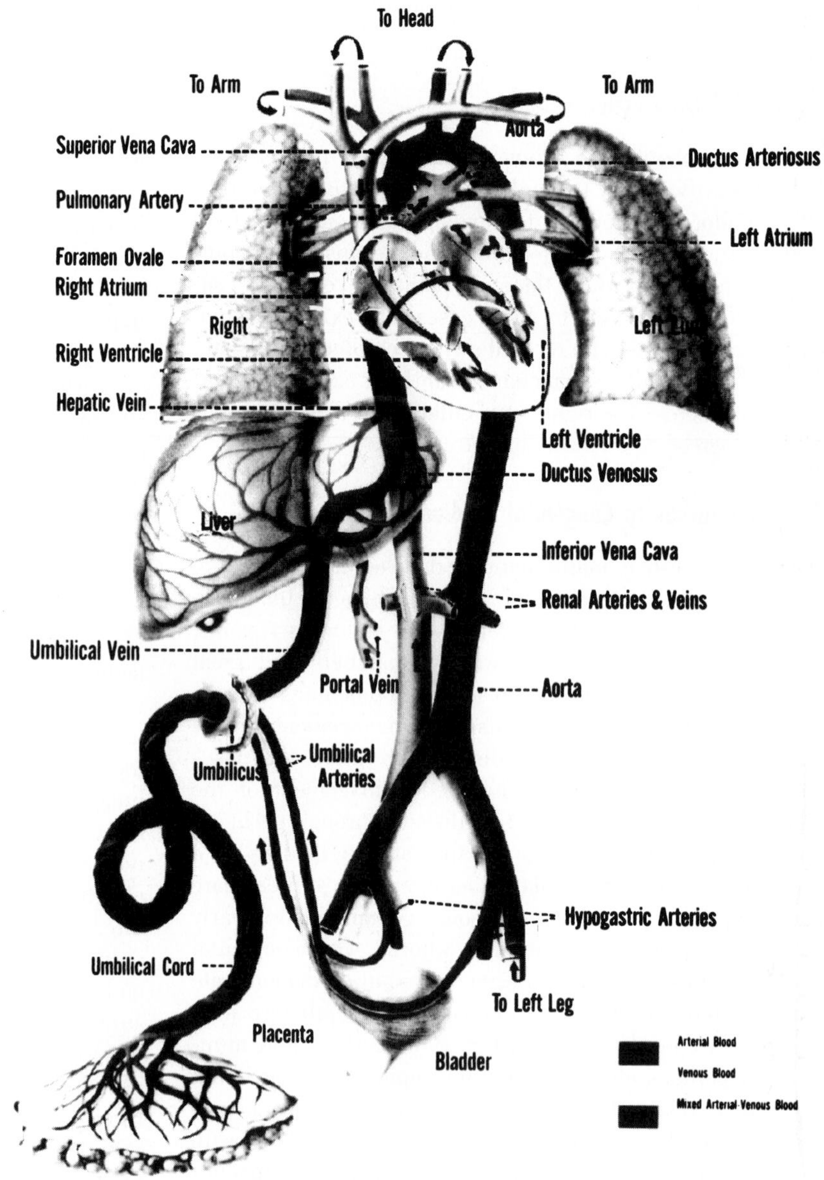

Figure 12.13. The transitional circulation. SVC, superior vena cava; RA, right atrium; LV, left ventricle; PA, Pulmonary artery; IVC, inferior vena cava; LA, left atrium; RV, right ventricle; Ao, aorta. (From Greeley WJ, Kern FH. Anesthesia for pediatric cardiac surgery. Anesthesia. Miller RD (ed.). New York, Churchill Livingston, 1994, p. 1813.)

pressures decrease to approximately 30/12 mm Hg and approach adult levels by 4 weeks of age (Fig. 12.16)[67].

The presence of certain congenital heart defects can disrupt this normal adaptation process, creating a transitional circulation in which right-to-left shunting across the foramen ovale or the PDA persists. When initially treating some forms of cyanotic congenital heart disease, the prolongation of this transitional circulation is actually beneficial, permitting pulmonary blood flow and postnatal viability. Examples include pulmonary atresia, in which pulmonary blood flow is temporarily supplied by the PDA, or hypoplastic left heart syndrome, in which systemic blood flow is temporarily supplied by the PDA from the pulmonary artery to the descending aorta. Closure of the PDA results in absent pulmonary blood flow or systemic blood flow, respectively. In the case of pulmonary atresia, pulmonary blood flow is severely diminished or absent, and severe hypoxemia and death ensue. In hypoplastic left heart syndrome, ductal closure results in minimal or absent systemic blood flow, profound reductions in systemic oxygen delivery, and death without restoration of ductal patency. In both cases, ductal patency can be maintained with the rapid institution of prostaglandin E_1[68].

NEONATAL MYOCARDIAL PERFORMANCE

Birth Cardiac Output

After delivery, there is a rapid increase in left ventricular output. Work by Agata and colleagues have demonstrated a twofold increase in left ventricular cardiac output immediately after birth[69]. Several investigators have suggested that this marked increase in left ventricular output is due to an increase in metabolic demands required by newborns for maintenance of body temperature, work of breathing, feeding, and other changes associated with adaptation to neonatal life[70,71]. More recently it has been suggested that the high cardiac output present in the normal newborn is compensation for left-to-right shunting at the patent ductus arteriosus and for the loss of systemic blood flow supplied by the right ventricular during fetal life[69].

It is the metabolic demands of the tissue that regulate cardiac output and tissue oxygen delivery. Reductions in systemic oxygen delivery and systemic cardiac output from left-to-right shunting at the ductal level must be met by increased cardiac output[59,61,70,72]. Cardiac output will remain elevated until there is physiologic closure of the ductus arteriosus. Reductions in cardiac output occur over the first 24 to 72 hours of life and correlate with reductions in ductal flow; as ductal closure continues, cardiac output decreases to maintain constant tissue oxygen delivery and organ blood flow and to meet tissue metabolic requirements[61].

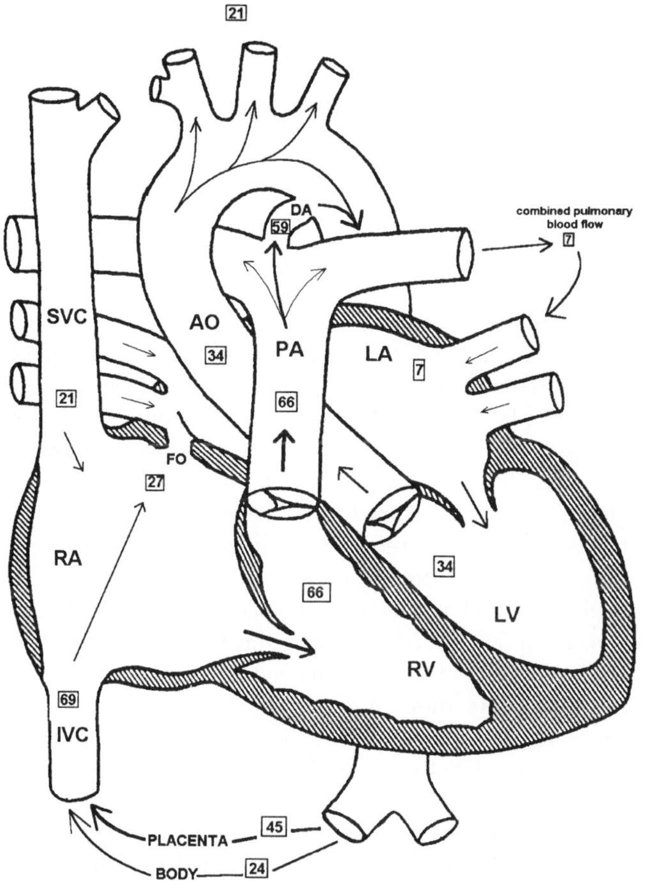

Figure 12.14. Drawing displays the volume of blood received from the placenta, lower body, and superior vena cava (SVC) and the volume of blood ejected by each ventricle in the fetal circulation. The numbers within each square represent oxygen saturations within various chambers of the fetal heart. SVC, superior vena cava; RA, right atrium; LV, left ventricle; PA, Pulmonary artery; IVC, inferior vena cava; LA, left atrium; RV, right ventricle; Ao, aorta. (From Rudolph AM. Congenital diseases of the heart. Chicago, Yearbook Publications, 1974.)

Ventricular Interdependence and the Transitional Circulation

Function of the right and left ventricle are interdependent. In the mature heart, because of the higher pressures created during systole, the ventricular septum is shifted rightward, and the left ventricular cavity assumes a circular configuration[73]. When right and left ventricular pressures are equal, the septum flattens, and left ventricular geometry is altered, reducing left ventricular contractile reserve. With further elevations in right sided pressures the septum shifts in a leftward direction, further disrupting left ventricular geometry, impairing left ventricular ejection and left ventricular shortening fraction[74] (Figs. 17 and 18).

Ventricular interdependence changes during neonatal circulatory transition. Rein and colleagues have demonstrated that systolic right ventricular hypertension at a level sufficient to distort left ventricular configuration is present until day 4 or 5 of life[73]. At end-systole, there is flattening of the intraventricular septum and a reduction in left ventricular shortening fraction. At end-diastole, the left ventricular shape is circular, reflecting a lower end-diastolic right ventricular pressure compared with left ventricular end-diastolic pressure. Therefore, left ventricular systolic function and left ventricular systolic reserve are impaired in early neonatal life. The cause for right ventricular hypertension is elevated pulmonary vascular resistance, which normally falls after birth. If pulmonary vascular resistance remains elevated, however, right ventricular dysfunction may worsen. Right ventricular dysfunction is a common problem in newborns and infants and because of this deserves special consideration.

Right Ventricular Dysfunction in the Newborn and Young Infant

Neonates and young infants usually develop right ventricular dysfunction because of elevated pulmonary vascular resistance (PVR). These patients are quite sensitive to blood volume changes. Elevated pulmonary vascular resistance results in an increased right ventricular afterload. This may result in worsening right ventricular function. Under this circumstance, right ventricular end-systolic and end-diastolic volume and pressure increase, resulting in volume and pressure loading of the right ventricle[57,75,76]. Increases in right ventricular pressure decrease coronary perfusion pressure to the right ventricle, resulting in right ventricular ischemia[77]. In addition, the volume-underloaded left ventricle has decreased filling due to ventricular interdependence discussed above and a septal shift, resulting in decreased left ventricular stroke volume. Systemic perfusion is therefore quite dependent on left atrial preload, which requires a reduction in pulmonary vascular resistance to allow effective filling. Systemic hypotension may further

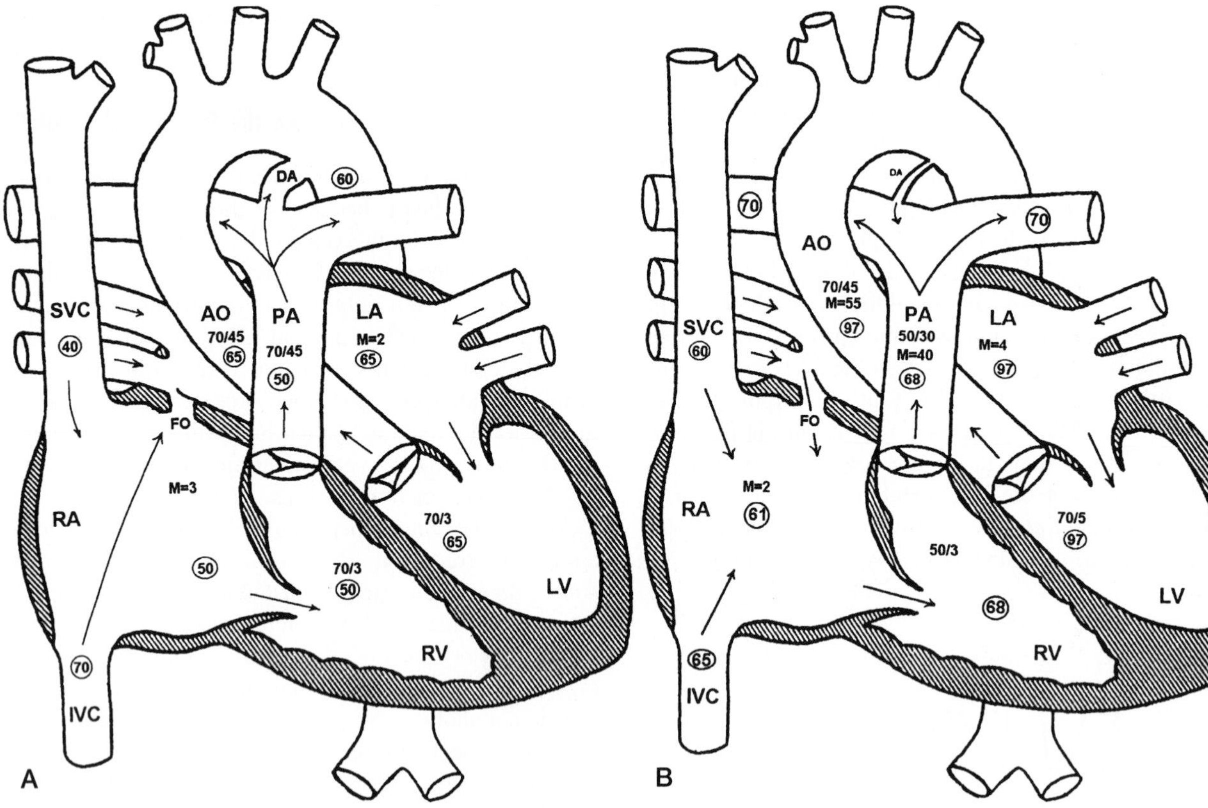

Figure 12.15. The differences in pulmonary artery pressures during the first 24 hours of life are demonstrated. Prenatal pulmonary artery pressures are approximately 70/45 (**A**). At approximately 24 hours after delivery pulmonary artery pressures decrease to 50/30 (**B**). SVC, superior vena cava; RA, right atrium; LV, left ventricle; PA, Pulmonary artery; IVC, inferior vena cava; LA, left atrium; RV, right ventricle; Ao, aorta. (From Rudolph AM. Congenital diseases of the heart. Chicago, Yearbook Publications, 1974.)

affect right ventricular function by reducing coronary perfusion pressure (Fig. 12.19).

Pharmacologic Strategies

Attempts to selectively manipulate pulmonary vascular resistance through pharmacologic interventions has been less than satisfying. Drugs that have shown the greatest promise both clinically and experimentally are the phosphodiesterase inhibitors and nitric oxide. Amrinone, milrinone, and enoximone are phosphodiesterase inhibitors that have been used clinically and experimentally in treating elevations in pulmonary vascular resistance. Phosphodiesterase inhibitors have varying effects on cyclic adenosine monophosphate and cyclic guanosine monophosphate (cGMP). cGMP is a more important mediator of pulmonary vascular smooth muscle. Milrinone and the drug dypyridamole have a predominant effect on cGMP and may be more efficacious in treating pulmonary hypertension than amrinone. These variations, in effect, suggest that receptor subtypes may exist for phosphodiesterase type III inhibitors similar to G-protein receptors discussed above.

Nitric oxide (NO) is an endothelium-derived vasodilator of smooth muscle[78]. The enzyme, NO synthase, converts L-arginine into NO and citrulline. NO diffuses across the endothelial cell to the adjacent smooth muscle, where it activates guanylate cyclase. The enzyme guanylate cyclase increases the production of cyclic GMP. cGMP causes smooth muscle relaxation by preventing the release of calcium from the sarcoplasmic reticulum, thereby inhibiting muscle contraction. When NO diffuses into the intravascular space, it immediately binds with hemoglobin to form nitrosylhemoglobin, which is oxidized to methemoglobin. Methemoglobin is subsequently reduced to nitrates and nitrites and is excreted in the urine. The clinical importance of NO lies in the fact that it can be administered as an inhaled gas and delivered directly to the pulmonary circulation. The close proximity of the alveolus and the pulmonary vascular smooth muscle allows a direct affect of NO on pulmonary vascular smooth muscle. Because of the rapid binding and inactivation of NO by hemoglobin, minimal or no systemic effects occur. NO has been shown to bind 280 times faster to hemoglobin than carbon monoxide, which may explain why the systemic circulation is protected from its vasodilating properties.

Primary right ventricular dysfunction is a common finding in neonates and infants with or without congenital cardiac disease. The treatment of right ventricular dysfunction consists of increasing coronary perfusion pressure, preload augmentation (while avoiding marked increases in right ventricular end diastolic pressure[79] and inotropic support with dopamine, epinephrine, and amrinone[76,80,81]. Dobu-

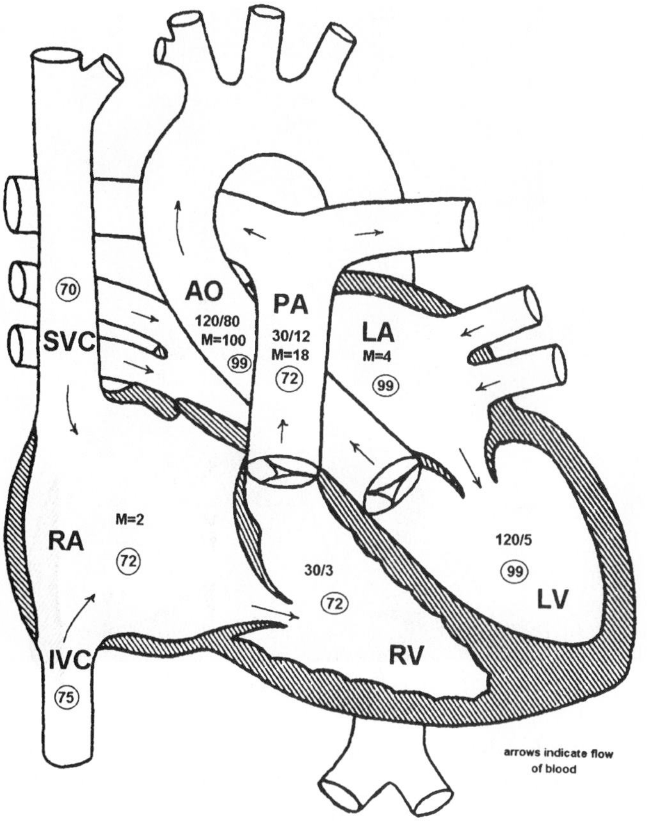

Figure 12.16. Over the ensuing several days pulmonary artery pressures decrease to approximately 30/12 and approach adult levels by 4 weeks of age. (From Rudolph AM. Congenital diseases of the heart. Chicago, Yearbook Publications, 1974.)

tamine may decrease systemic vascular resistance, worsen right ventricular coronary perfusion, and thereby worsen right ventricular function.

Preload, Afterload, and Left Ventricular Function

The newborn heart is both structurally and functionally immature, affecting the response to contractility, preload, and afterload. Friedman studied myocardial contractility in sheep and demonstrated a reduction in active tension by isometric contraction of fetal cardiac muscle as opposed to the adult(79).

The ratio of noncontractile mass (nuclei, mitochondria, and membrane) to contractile mass is 70% in the fetal heart as opposed to 40% in the adult heart. Adult left ventricular muscle can generate more force per unit area versus the neonatal myocardium, which may explain why force generation per gram of tissue in response to an increase in preload is less in the immature heart than in the adult heart. Compliance also differs in the neonatal myocardium. Romero and Friedman(81a) studied isolated intact hearts and found that an increase in left ventricular filling resulted in a disproportionately greater increase in left ventricular wall tension in neonatal hearts. Therefore, in neonates the upper limit of the Frank-Starling curve is reached with a smaller increase in left ventricular filling volume. This stroke volume represents the optimal preload. Further increases in preload do not result in a significant increase in stroke volume; i.e., the Frank-Starling curve is flat. The relative decrease in force generation and ventricular compli-

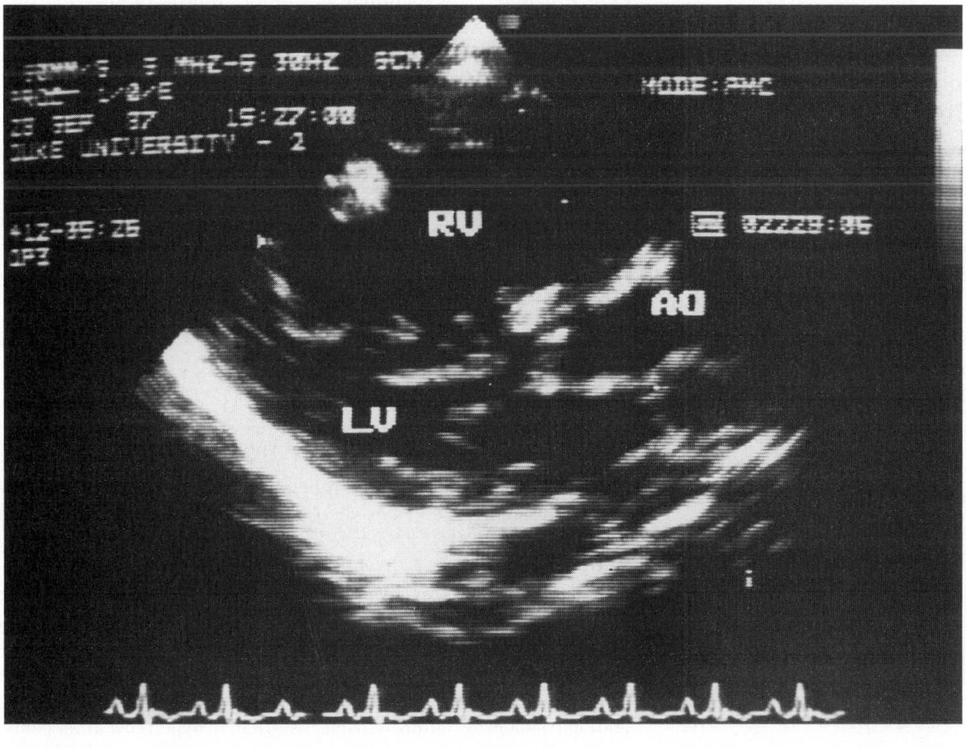

Figure 12.17. Two-dimensional echocardiographic image demonstrating a shift in the septum in a leftward direction, which can impair left ventricular function.

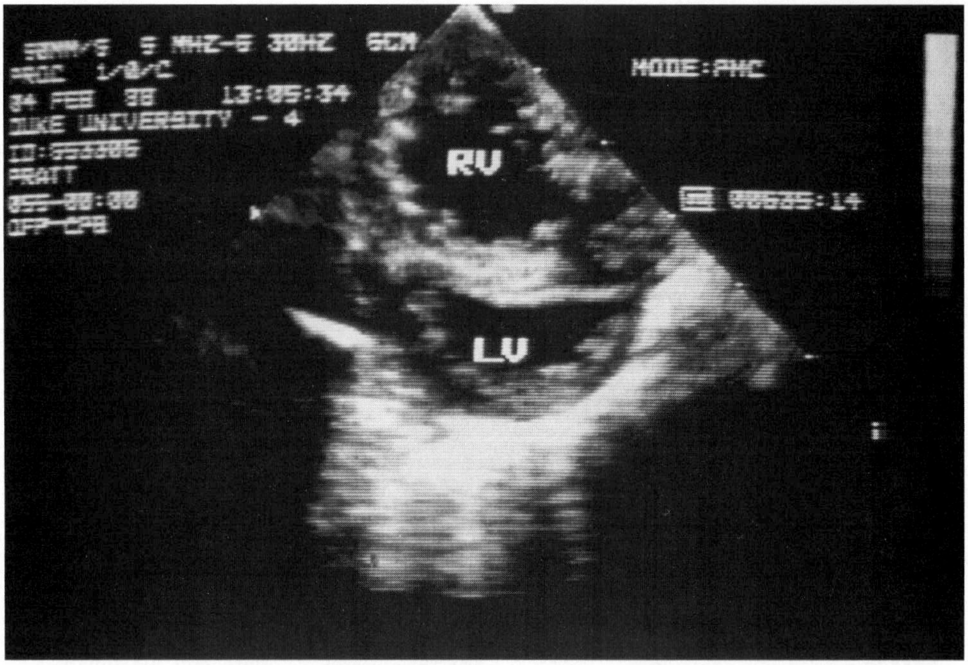

Figure 12.18. Two-dimensional echocardiographic image demonstrating septal flattening, which can impair left ventricular function.

ance and the increase in volume load to the left ventricle that occurs at birth place the newborn at or near the upper limit of the Frank-Starling curve. This has been supported by studies that demonstrate minimal benefit to volume loading beyond a filling pressure of 7 to 12 mm Hg in the newborn. Therefore, in the newborn, left ventricular preload reserve is reduced relative to the adult. It is important to remember, however, in the face of right ventricular dysfunction and elevated pulmonary vascular resistance, that high right-sided filling pressures may not reflect left-sided filling pressures, and under these circumstances left ventricular filling may be impaired.

Increasing afterload in the newborn results in a reduction in stroke volume. The newborn heart is more sensitive to left ventricular afterload than is the adult heart. In fetal sheep, however, a substantial decrease in muscle shortening occurs in response to increasing afterload. Therefore, newborns, and to a greater extent premature infants, demonstrate a reduction in left ventricular stroke volume in response to increased afterload. This means that distinguishing right ventricular from left ventricular dysfunction is essential in the newborn period. Afterload reduction is helpful in left ventricular dysfunction but may further impair right ventricular function by decreasing coronary perfusion and causing right ventricular ischemia.

Heart rate also increases cardiac output. Newborns and premature infants have a high resting heart rate, and further increases in heart rate may be of limited benefit in increasing cardiac output if stroke volume falls. Heart rates much above 180 beats per minute in the newborn may result in reduced cardiac output.

In summary, animal studies demonstrate that under normal circumstances, significant changes in preload, afterload, and heart rate during the newborn period do not dramatically improve cardiac output. In the presence of left ventricular dysfunction afterload reduction, inotropes and mild preload augmentation may be beneficial. Afterload reduction may be harmful, however, when right ventricular dysfunction is the primary pathophysiology in the newborn. There are, however, few studies on human neonatal myocardium.

Myocardial Growth and Development

Gestational and postnatal cardiac growth and development occur primarily in response to hemodynamic factors[82]. Left

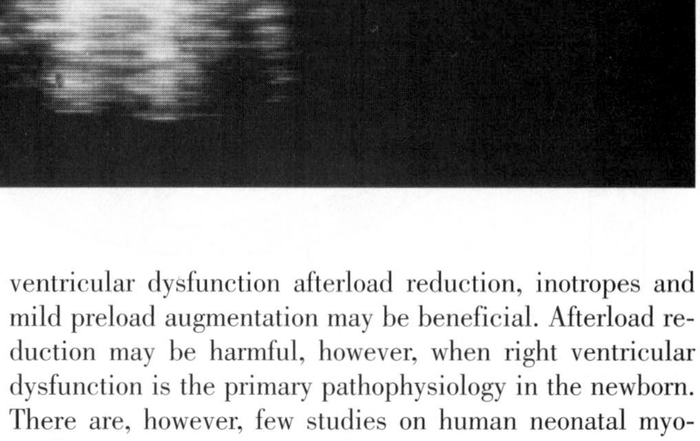

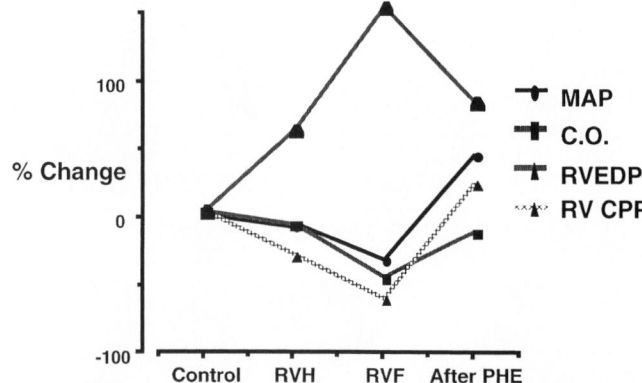

Figure 12.19. Right ventricular function is affected by coronary perfusion pressure. When right ventricular hypertrophy (RVH) or right ventricular failure (RVF) develops, cardiac output (C.O.) and mean aortic pressure (MAP) fall, while right ventricular end-diastolic pressure (RVEDP) rises. Right ventricular coronary perfusion pressure (RVCPP) also decreases. When phenylepinephrine is administered, RVCPP increases, cardiac ouput (C.O.) increases, mean aortic pressure (MAP) increases, and right ventricular end diastolic pressure (RVEDP) decreases. (From Vhalakes GJ, Turley K, Hoffman JIE. The pathophysiology of failure in right ventricular hypertension: hemodynamic and biological correlations. Circulation 1980; 63:87–92.)

ventricular hypoplasia after maneuvers that impair left ventricular filling, and the clinical importance of mitral atresia as an etiology for the development of hypoplastic left heart syndrome, serve as important illustrations of how hemodynamic factors affect fetal cardiac growth(77,83). Ventricular distension and muscle stretch is an important component regulating fetal ventricular growth and development.

Newborns retain the ability of myocyte cell division (hyperplasia) through early neonatal life(84). After birth, myocyte hyperplasia persists through the first month of life and results in a doubling of the number of cardiac myocytes(85). After approximately 3 to 4 weeks of life, however, DNA replication within the myocytes begins to decrease, and an increasing proportion of cardiac growth is accomplished through myocyte hypertrophy. Nonmuscular elements, however, maintain the capacity for cell division for a more prolonged period of time. Hypertrophy is an important part of total myocardial growth in the neonate. During the neonatal period, myocyte volume increases by approximately 30 to 40 times and there is a demonstrable increase in myocyte cytoplasm, and subcellular elements such as mitochondria, nucleoli and myofibrils(85,86). These changes have a direct effect on myocyte function and contractility.

Microvasculature growth, or cardiac angiogenesis, proceeds during early neonatal growth. In rat models the distance between capillaries in the myocardium shortens from about 30 μm at 1 day of age to approximately 17 1/2 μm at 11 days of age, a distance found in adult hearts(87,88). During the hypertrophic phase of myocyte growth, capillaries continue to proliferate in proportion to the increase in myocardial volume. This is necessary to maintain a constant intracapillary distance.

Cardiac hypertrophy develops in response to pressure loading and is an important stimulus for myocardial angiogenesis in newborns and infants(89). The capacity for increased microvascular growth, characteristic of the young developing heart, is lost in more mature hearts. Microvascular proliferation does not accompany pressure overload hypertrophy in the adult myocardium, which develops an increase in intracapillary distance and a predilection for myocardial ischemia(90).

Myocardial angiogenesis is induced by acidic and basic fibroblast growth factor (alpha FGF and beta FGF, respectively)(91). These growth factors are similar in structure to heparin and in fact can be inhibited by the use of the heparin antagonist protamine. In addition to the release of fibroblast growth factors, pressure overload of the left ventricle elicits rapid changes in the expression of other genes, which are important regulators of myocyte hyperplasia and hypertrophy. In mature myocytes, a pressure-overloaded ventricle results in an increase in RNA synthesis, including the genes for fetal protein synthesis and activation of proto-oncogenes(92). Proto-oncogenes are growth-stimulating factors (C-myc and C-fos) that induce mitotic activity in the myocyte.

In the mature rat myocardium, pressure loading of the left ventricle induces the myocardium to synthesize fetal proteins which results in a replacement of the normal adult myosin heavy chains with fetal myosin heavy chains(92). Fetal myosin chains provide less efficient shortening and a reduction in global measures of myocardial contractility and systolic function. This conversion to fetal myosin does not appear to occur in larger animals or humans.

Systolic and Diastolic Function

The traditional approach to myocardial dysfunction in infants and children have emphasized the heart's systolic function by defining heart failure in terms of reduced cardiac output and a decrease in tissue oxygen delivery in relationship to tissue metabolic needs. The heart, however, has both systolic and diastolic function. When myocardial failure exists, the culprit is diastolic dysfunction when there is an inability to fill the ventricle at low pressure. The problem is systolic function when there is an inability to eject blood from the ventricle into the great vessel. Examples of systolic dysfunction, diastolic dysfunction, and mixed systolic and diastolic dysfunction are shown in the pressure volume relationships in Figure 12.20.

Myocardial hypertrophy is a common finding in the right ventricle of normal neonatal hearts and in the left ventricle of newborns with left ventricular outflow tract obstruction. Hypertrophy appears to be a compensatory mechanism to restore wall stress toward normal and improve cardiac performance. An improvement in cardiac performance continues as long as the hypertrophied ventricle does not outstrip its blood supply. Once this occurs, systolic performance, diastolic relaxation, and ventricular distensibility are impaired. In adult animals and humans, hypertrophic changes of the myocardium generally result in normal rest measures of endomyocardial function. However, with increasing demand, as occurs with pacing or exogenous administration of catecholamines, there is a reduction in myocardial contractility in hypertrophied adult hearts. Left ventricular pressure volume loops demonstrate an impairment in diastolic distensibility, as demonstrated by an upward shift in the diastolic pressure volume loop during isovolumic relaxation (Fig. 12.20). This change is not commonly seen with selective coronary occlusion in adult animals, suggesting that hypertrophy results in alterations in microvascular blood flow, and these changes affect both systolic and diastolic function in adult hearts.

In contrast to adult hearts, neonatal hypertrophied hearts have a normal response to exogenous administration of inotropic agents. Hypertrophy in the neonate alters systolic and not diastolic function. Diastolic dysfunction correlates with calcium regulation in the newborn.

In a study designed to evaluate the differences in left ventricular systolic function in response to exogenous administration of catecholamines in both neonatal lambs and adult sheep with experimentally induced left ventricular hypertrophy, systolic function was depressed in the adult sheep but normal in neonatal lambs(93). These results are similar to data obtained in infants with left ventricular hypertrophy caused by congenital aortic stenosis. Neonatal and infant hearts have the ability to maintain normal systolic function despite moderate degrees of left ventricular hypertrophy[94,95]. Although these compensatory changes are apparent in the newborn, over time both systolic and diastolic left ventricular dysfunction occurs if pressure overload persists[95]. Evidence for subendocardial hypoperfusion is found in adult animals with pressure overload hypertrophy induced in the neonatal period. An example is children with tetralogy of Fallot who develop right ventricular hypertrophy and have their surgical repair delayed from 1 to 3 years. These children demonstrate a higher incidence of ventricular arrhythmias and impaired exercise testing when compared with children undergoing earlier repairs[96].

The reason for better systolic performance in neonates with left ventricular hypertrophy may relate to the observation that hypertrophy induced in immature animals is more commensurate with physiologic growth; i.e., angiogenesis accompanies muscle hypertrophy[90]. Angiogenesis factor, a heparin-like substance, can be antagonized by the administration of protamine. Flannagan and colleagues[90] evaluated the effect of left ventricular hypertrophy in lambs receiving protamine to impair microvascular growth. Lambs treated with protamine had a reduction in myocardial capillary density and were not capable of lowering coronary resistance to the same degree as lambs not treated with protamine. The protamine-treated animals demonstrate a myocardial capillary density similar to that of adult sheep with myocardial hypertrophy. Therefore, the preservation of normal systolic function seen in neonates with left ventricular hypertrophy seems to be related to the enhanced vascular supply accompanying hypertrophy in immature animals, a process that does not occur in adult myocardium.

In contrast to systolic function, diastolic function does not appear to be influenced by myocardial capillary density. In studies by Fujii, rapid atrial pacing was used to induce diastolic dysfunction in both lambs and sheep with myocardial hypertrophy[97,98]. Diastolic dysfunction was measured by a prolongation of isovolumic relaxation, initiation of systole prior to complete relaxation, and the presence of elevated left ventricular end-diastolic pressures. Fujii found that diastolic dysfunction during chronotropic stress is greater in the adult sheep with hypertrophy than in lambs with hypertrophy. Lambs treated with the angio-

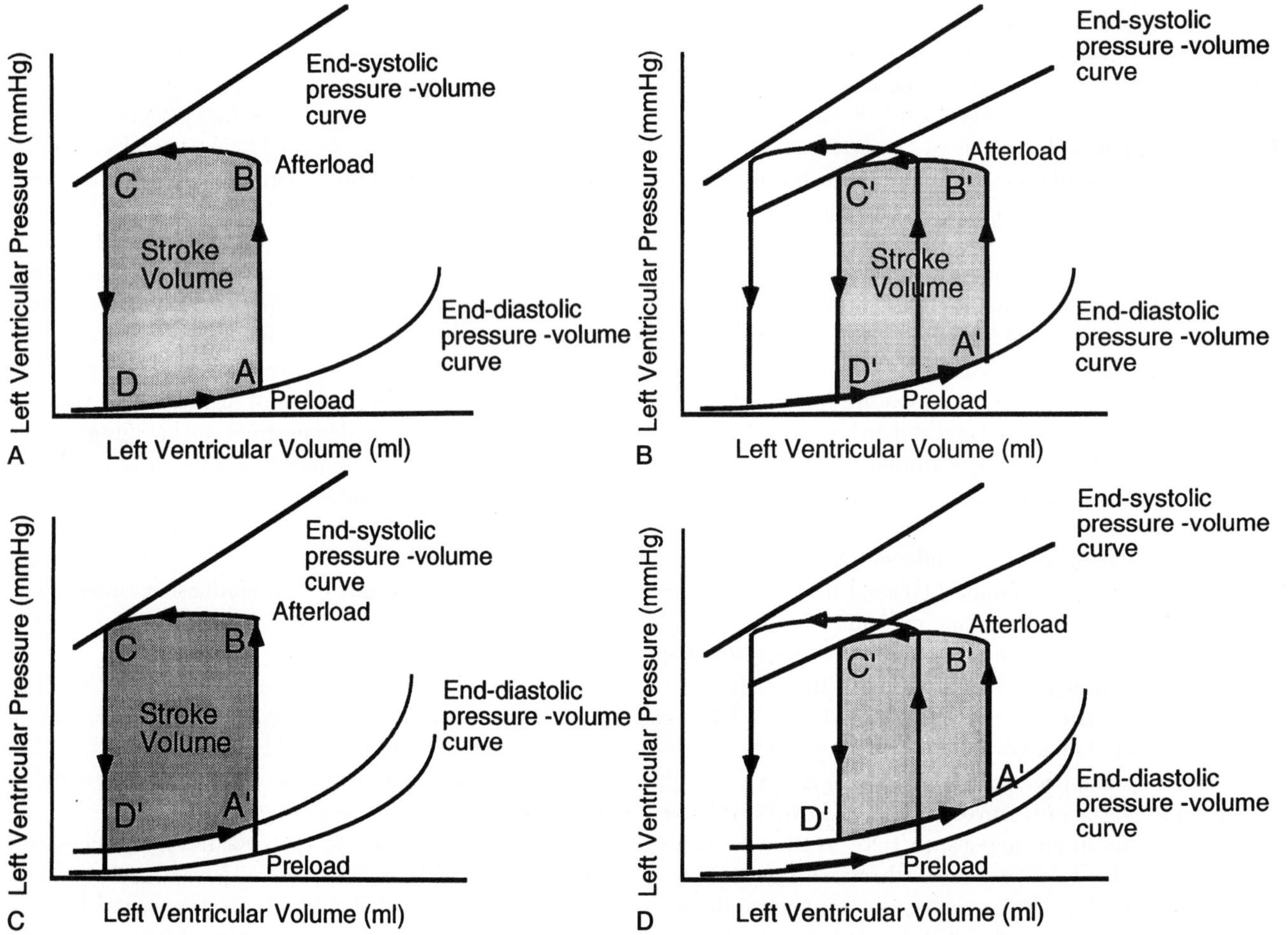

Figure 12.20. Pressure-volume curves show normal (**A**), systolic dysfunction (**B**), diastolic dysfunction (**C**), and systolic and diastolic dysfunction (**D**). The shaded area represents the stroke volume. The end-systolic pressure-volume curve is depressed in pure systolic dysfunction (**B**). Pure diastolic dysfunction is characterized by an increase in resistance to ventricular filling. In (**C**) there is an increase in diastolic pressure at any given volume, while the end-systolic pressure-volume relationship is maintained.

genesis factor inhibitor protamine during the development of hypertrophy demonstrated no difference in the degree of diastolic dysfunction induced by rapid pacing than did lambs with myocardial hypertrophy not receiving protamine. Therefore, other mechanisms appear to be important in the development of diastolic dysfunction in immature animals.

Animals and human studies demonstrate a depression in the sarcoplasmic reticular calcium ATPase and disordered handling of intracellular calcium by the myocyte with diastolic dysfunction. The release of calcium appears to occur normally. The disappearance of calcium appears to be delayed and thus maybe related to the inability of the sarcoplasmic reticulum to efficiently remove calcium from the cytosol. Calcium transport by the sarcoplasmic reticulum is mediated by cyclic adenosine monophosphate (AMP) activation of phospholamban. Phospholamban therefore is an important regulator of diastolic relaxation. Deficiencies of cyclic AMP generation occur in patients with chronic hypertrophy due to the down-regulation of beta receptors, chronic heart failure, and possibly abnormal G-protein expression, specifically an increased production of the inhibitory components of the G-protein complex, which reduces muscle contraction[99,100]. Therefore phosphodiesterase-inhibiting drugs such as milrinone, amrinone, and enoximone, which enhance cyclic AMP levels, may improve diastolic function in patients[101,102]. Several studies have suggested this benefit in adults with diastolic dysfunction and congestive heart failure.

Calcium uptake by the sarcoplasmic reticulum has been measured in adult sheep with myocardial hypertrophy. Adult hypertrophic myocardium has a 79% reduction in calcium ATPase activity and mRNA levels compared with controls[97]. In contrast, lambs with or without myocardial hypertrophy demonstrate calcium ATPase and mRNA levels similar to those in control adult sheep. This suggest that neonates may be more capable of handling and removing high levels of cytosolic calcium in hypertrophied myocardium.

One other factor has been suggested as contributing to diastolic dysfunction in hypertrophied myocardium: the extracellular matrix of the myocardium[103]. In cardiac pressure overload hypertrophy, the amount of collagen relative to muscle increases, and this is accompanied by a change in collagen structure. Renal hypertension in adult monkeys results in an increase in left ventricular collagen concentration, an increase and thickening of collagen strands, an increase in the density of the collagen weave, and, at least early in the phase of hypertrophy, an increase in the deposition of type 3 collagen as compared with type 1 collagen. A functional role for collagen deposition has been demonstrated by Cooper and colleagues, who found an association between collagen deposition and papillary muscle stiffness in pulmonary artery banded kittens[103a]. Caulfield and Borg inhibited the development of the collagen weave network by the administration of beta-amino-proprionitrile in newborn rats[103b]. Inhibition of collagen weave formation resulted in ventricular aneurysms.

Neonates and infants with left ventricular or right ventricular outflow tract obstruction and myocardial hypertrophy have a much greater myocardial reserve than adults. The tolerance of hypertrophic changes in the neonatal and infant myocardium and reduced tolerance later in life is important supportive data for the concept of early neonatal heart repair. The current trends in congenital heart surgery toward early intervention and early complete repair is again supported by the physiologic capacity and tolerance of myocardial hypertrophy in the developing neonate and the fact that delayed repair results in late myocardial dysfunction.

NEONATAL MYOCARDIUM: RESISTANCE TO ISCHEMIC INJURY

The neonatal heart appears to be more resistant to ischemic and reperfusion injury than the normal adult heart. Much of this protection is due to a resistance to calcium influx during and after an ischemic event and larger energy stores in immature myocytes. Calcium influx is reduced by the sarcolemma (cell membrane) of the immature myocyte, which binds calcium more avidly than mature myocardium, thereby reducing calcium entry and calcium-induced cellular injury during ischemia and reperfusion injury[104]. Despite the ability of the immature heart to exclude calcium entry, once calcium has entered the myocyte there is a reduced capacity to extrude calcium from the cell, a function of the sarcoplasmic reticulum, which is underdeveloped in the neonatal heart. Therefore, once calcium entry has occurred, a function of sarcolemma disruption, myocyte damage may be more severe in the neonate.

Additionally, the immature myocardium, by virtue of its growth requirements, has increased glycogen and amino acid stores, which increases cellular anaerobic and aerobic capacity when nutrient delivery is reduced by ischemia[35,105,106]. ATP utilization is reduced in immature hearts due to reduced contractile energy requirements. The neonate maintains ATP-dependent Ca^{++} pumps necessary for calcium removal from the myocyte for a more prolonged period after the initiation of ischemia. Amino acid stores provide a substrate for anaerobic metabolism in the neonatal heart. The neonatal myocyte produces more ATP during anaerobic metabolism than the adult heart. The enhanced ATP production allows for the phosphorylation of glutamate and pyruvate, which undergo anaerobic metabolism to produce additional ATP. Increased production of ATP during anaerobic metabolism maintains cellular integrity and metabolic processes necessary for removing calcium from the cytosol. These factors appear to protect the normal immature myocardium from ischemic injury.

Physiologic studies comparing myocardial recovery in rabbit hearts demonstrated a greater recovery of myocardial function in neonatal hearts than adult hearts. During normothermic ischemia, neonatal rabbit hearts had a 23% greater recovery of left ventricular developed pressure and coronary flow per gram of tissue than adult rabbit hearts.

Under the conditions of hypothermic ischemia, the neonatal myocardium demonstrated a 50 to 55% improvement over the adult myocardium[107].

Although neonatal hearts are more resistant to ischemia, hearts of premature animals and newborns younger than 5 to 7 days of age, may in fact be more susceptible to ischemic injury. In the immediate newborn period, enzymes involved in the production of antioxidants and the synthesis of membrane phospholipids are reduced[105,106,108]. One- to two-day-old neonatal piglets had a much greater production of oxygen free radicals and a reduction in the rate of membrane phospholipid turnover compared with 1-week old piglets. A depressed turnover of membrane phospholipids in the newborn heart may prevent the restoration of intact membrane structures from the phospholipid degradation caused by oxygen free radical damage during ischemia reperfusion. The composition of free fatty acids also changes during the first week of life. A higher proportion of polyunsaturated fats such as linoleic acid are present. Polyunsaturated fatty acids are capable of oxygen radical scavenging and therefore may be protective.

The cyanotic neonate or the neonate who has congestive failure appears to have a myocardial substrate, which is less tolerant of ischemia than the normal neonatal heart[108,109]. Julia and colleagues[108] demonstrated a poor tolerance to ischemia and an impaired functional recovery in immature hearts with a prior exposure to hypoxia. Experimental evidence suggests that this is most likely due to impaired substrate delivery and marginal myocardial energy reserves in both the chronic and acute models of cyanotic heart disease[108,109].

SUMMARY

An optimal physiologic approach to the management of neonates and infants with cardiovascular disease requires an understanding of developmental anatomy, physiology, and molecular biology. Each one of these disciplines explains how myocardial dysfunction develops. Specific congenital cardiac diseases develop in utero, and the more devastating forms, such as pulmonary atresia and hypoplastic left heart syndrome, occur later in development and therefore may be amenable to in utero interventions. Conventional therapies for myocardial dysfunction, such as inotropes, appear to be less effective in neonates. Drugs with primary beta activity, such as dobutamine, may be completely ineffective. Exogenous calcium supplementation, which is quite controversial in the adult population, is clearly indicated in neonates with decreased myocardial function because of limited intracellular calcium stores and a dependence on extracellular calcium for effective myocardial contractility. Reduced intracellular stores of calcium, in contrast, explains why neonates are relatively resistant to ischemic myocardial injury.

Further advances in the care of neonates, children, and adults with cardiovascular disease will undoubtedly be based on a better understanding of molecular regulation of myocardial function and perhaps molecular interventions that may allow new myocardial growth (hyperplasia) and/or vascular growth (angiogenesis) in ischemic myocardium. Understanding developmental biology will undoubtedly be an important component in the future.

References

1. de la Torre JG Bloomfield VA. Confirmation of myosin and diolute solution as estimated from hydrodynamic properties. Biochem 1980; 19:5018–5123.
2. Elliott A, Offen G. Shape and flexibility of the myosin molecule. Mol Bio 1978; 123:505–519.
3. Pope BP, Hoh JFY, Weeds A. The ATPase Activities of rat cardiac myosin isoenzymes. FEBS Letters 1980; 118:205–208.
4. Schwartz K, Lecarpentier Y, Martin JL, et al. Myosin isoenzymic distribution correlates with speed of myocardial contraction. J Mol Cel Cardiol 1981; 13:1071–1075.
5. Cummins PC, Price FM Littler WA. Fetal myosin light chain in human ventricle. J of Muscle Res Cell Motility 1980; 1357–366.
6. Hoh JFY, Yeoh GPS, Thomas MAW, Higginbottom L. Structural differences in the heavy chains of rat ventricular myosin isoenzymes. FEBS Letters 1979; 97(No. 2):330–334.
7. Horn EM, Johnson NJ, Bilezikian JP Rosen MR. Developmental changes in the electrophysiological properties and the β-adrenergic receptor-effector complex in atrial fibers of the canine coronary sinus. Circ Res 1989; 65:325–333.
8. Lompre AM, Mercadier JJ, Wisnewsky C et al. Specie and age dependent changes in the relative amounts of cardiac myosin isoenzymes in mammals. Develop Bio 1981; 84:286–290.
9. Gemelli M, Luca F, Manganaro R, et al. Transient electrocardiographic changes suggesting myocardial ischaemia in newborn infants following tocolysis with beta-sympathomimetics. Eur J Pediatr 1990; 149:730–733.
10. Mercadier JJ, Lompre AM, Wisnewsky C et al. Myosin isoenzymic changes in several models of rat cardiac hypertrophy. Circ Res 1981; 49:525–532.
11. Mercadier JJ, Bouveret P, Gorza L et al. Myosin isoenzymes in normal and hypertrophied human ventricular myocardium. Circ Res 1983; 53:52–62.
12. Schier JJ, Adelstein RS. Structural and enzymatic comparison of human cardiac muscle myosins isolated from infants, adults, and patients with hypertrophic cardiomyopathy. J Clin Invest 1982; 69:816–825.
13. Klotz C, Leger JJ, Elzinga M. Comparative sequence of myosin light chains from normal and hypertrophied human hearts. Circ Res 1982; 50:201–209.
14. Sweeney HL, Stull JT. Alteration of cross-bridge kinetics by myosin light chain phosphorylation in rabbit skeletal muscle: Implications for regulation of actin-myosin interaction. Proc. Natl. Acad. Sci. USA 1990; 87:414–418.
15. Barany K, Barany M, Hager SR, Sayers ST. Myosin light chain and membrane protein phosphorylation in various muscles. Federation Proc. 1983; 42:27–32.
16. Humpherys JE Cummings P. Atrial and ventricular tropomysin and troponin-I in the developing bovine and human heart. J Mol Cell Cardiol 1984; 16:643.
17. Murray JM, Knox MK, Trueblood CE, Weber A. Potentiated state of the tropomyosin actin filament and nucleotide containing myosin subfragment 1. Biochemistry 1982; 21:906–915.
18. Allan LD, Sharland GK, Milburn A, et al. Prospective diagnosis of 1,006 consecutive cases of congenital heart disease in the fetus. JACC 1994; 23:1452–1458.
19. Tao T, Gong BJ, Leavis PC. Calcium-induced movement of troponin-I relative to actin in skeletal muscle thin filaments. Science 1990; 247:1339–1341.
20. Solaro RJ, Moir AJG, Perry SV. Phosphorylation of troponin I and the inotropic effect of adrenaline in the perfused rabbit heart. Nature 1976; 262:615–616.
21. Robertson SP, Johnson JD, Holroyde MJ, et al. The effect of troponin I phosphorylation on the Ca 2+ -binding properties of the Ca 2+ -regulatory site of bovine cardiac troponin. J Bio Chem 1982; 257(1):260–263.
22. Winegrad S. Regulation of cardiac contratile proteins. Circ Res 1984; 55:565–574.
23. Sasse S, Brand NJ, Kyprianou P, et al. Troponin I gene expression dur-

ing human cardiac development and in end-stage heart failure. Circ Res 1993; 72:932–938.
24. Huxley H, H. J. Changes in the cross-striations of muscle during contraction and stretch and their structural interpretation. Nature 1954; 4412:973–976.
25. Huxley AF, Niedergerke R. Structural changes in muscle during contraction. Nature 1954; 4412:971–973.
26. Huxley HE. Structural difference between resting and rigor muscle; evidence from intensity changes in the low-angle equatorial x-ray diagram. J. Mol. Biol 1968; 37:507–520.
27. Huxley HE. Electron microscope studies on the structure of natural and synthetic protein filaments from striated muscle. J. Mol. Biol. 1963;7:281–308.
28. Mahony L Jones LR. Developmental changes in cardiac sarcoplasmic reticulum in sheep. J Biol Chem 1986; 261:15257–15265.
29. Jarmakani JM, Nakanishi T, George BL Bers D. Effect of extracellular calcium on myocardial mechanical function in neonatal rabbit. Dev Pharmacol Ther 1982; 5:1–13.
30. Rebeyka IM, Yeh T Jr, Hanan SA, et al. Altered contractile response in neonatal myocardium to citrate-phophate-dextrose infusion. Circulation 1990; 82:IV–367-IV–370.
31. Boucek RJ, Shelton M, Artman M, et al. Comparative effects of verapamil, nifedipine, and diltiazem on contractile function in the isolated immature and adult rabbit heart. Pediatric Research 1984; 18:948–952.
32. Nakanishi T, Seguchi M Takao A. Intracellular calcium concentrations in the newborn myocardium. Circulation 1987; 76:Suppl IV–455-IV–461.
33. Seguchi M, Jarmakani JM, George BL, Harding J. Effect of CA+2 antagonists on mechanical function in the neonatal heart. Pediatr Res 1986; 20:838–842.
34. Boucek RJ, Shelton ME, Artman M, Landem E. Myocellular calcium regulation by the sarcolemmal membrane in the adult and immature rabbit heart. Basic Res Cardiol 1985; 80.
35. Hoerter J. Changes in the sensitivity to hypoxia and glucose deprivation in the isolated perfused rabbit heart during perinatal development. Pflugers Arch 1976; (303):1–6.
36. Caroni P, Carafoli E. An ATP-dependent Ca2+ -pumping system in dog heart sarcolemma. Nature 1980; 283:765–767.
37. Bygrave FL. Mitochondria and the control of intracellular calcium. Biol Rev Camb Philos Soc 1978; 53(1):43–79.
38. Bristow MR, Ginsburg R, Minobe W, et al. Decreased catecholamine sensitivity and B-adrenergic-receptor density in failing human hearts. N Engl J Med 1982; 307:205–211.
39. Bristow MR, Hershberger RE, Port JD Minobe WR. B1- and B2-adrenergic receptor-mediated adenylate cyclase stimulation in nonfailing and failing human ventricular myocardium. Mol Pharm 1988; 35:295–303.
40. Schwinn DA, Leone BJ, Spahn DR, et al. Desensitization of myocardial β-adrenergic receptors during cardiopulmonary bypass. Circulation 1991; 84:2559–2567.
41. Kozlik-Feldmann R, Kramer HH, Wicht H, Feldmann R R. H&D. Distribution of myocardial β-adrenoceptors subtypes and coupling to the adenylate cyclase in children with congenital heart disease and implications for treatment. J Clin Pharmacol 1993; 33:588–595.
42. Schranz D, Droege A, Broede A, et al. Uncoupling of human cardiac β-adrenoceptors during cardiopulmonary bypass with cardioplegic cardiac arrest. Circulation 1993; 87:422–426.
43. Hausdorf G, Friedel N Berdjis F. Enoximone in newborns with refractory postoperative low-output states (LOS). Eur J Cardiothorac Surg 1992; 6:311–317.
44. Sun LS D. F. Regulation of B Adrenoceptor function differs in adult and neonatal rabbit heart. Circulation in press.
45. Teitel DF, Klautz R, Steendijk P, et al. The end-systolic pressure-volume relationship in the newborn lamb: effects of loading and inotropic interventions. Pediatr Res 1991; 29:473–482.
46. Peterseim DS, Chesnut LC, Meyers CH, et al. Stability of the B-adrenergic receptor/adenylyl cyclase pathway of pediatric myocardium following brain death. Circulation in press.
47. Langercrantz H Slotkin TA. The "stress" of being born. Sci Am 1986; 1:100–107.
48. Bohn DJ, Piorier CS, Edmonds JF, et al. Hemodynamic effects of dobutamine after cardiopulmonary bypass in children. Crit Care Med 1980; 8:367–442.
49. Bohn DJ, Poirer CS Edmonds JF et al. Efficacy of dopamine, dobutamine, and epinephrine during emergence from cardiopulmonary bypass in children. Crit Care Med 1980; 8:367–372.
50. Teitel DF, Dalinghaus M, Cassidy SC, Payne BD Rudolph AM. In utero ventilation augments the left ventricular response to isoproterenol and volume loading in fetal sheep. Pediatr Res 1991; 29:466–472.
51. Han HM, Robinson RB, Bilezikian JP Steinberg SF. Developmental changes in guanine nucleotide regulatory proteins in the rat myocardial a1-adrenergic receptor complex. Circ Res 1989; 65:1763–1773.
52. Urata H, Healy B, Stewart RW, Bumpus FM Husain A. Angiotensin II receptors in normal and failing human hearts. J Clin Endocrinol Metab 1989; 69:54.
53. Goor DA, Lillehei CW. Congenital malformation of the heart: embryology anatomy and operative considerations. Grune & Stratton, Inc. 1975; 38–102.
54. Hornberger LK, Sahn DS, Kleinman CS, Copel JS. NH. Antenatal diagnosis of coarctation of the aorta: a multicenter experience. J. Am Coll Cardiol 1994; 23(2):417–423.
55. Hornberger LK, Sanders SP, Sahn DJ et al. In utero pulmonary artery and aortic growth and potential for progression of pulmonary outflow tract obstruction in Tetralogy of Fallot. JACC 1995; 25:739–745.
56. Hornberger LK, Benacerraf BR, Bromley BS, et al. Prenatal detection of severe right ventricular outflow tract obstruction: pulmonary stenosis and pulmonary atresia. J. Ultrasound in Med. 1994; 13(10):743–750.
57. Rudolph AM. Distribution and regulation of blood flow in the fetal and newborn lamb. Circ Res 1985; 57:811.
58. Pang LM Mellins RB. Neonatal cardiorespiratory physiology. Anesthesiology 1975; 43:171–196.
59. Teitel DF, Iwamoto HS Rudolph AM. Effects of birth-related events on central blood flow patterns. Pediatr Res 1987; 22:557–566.
60. Teitel D Rudolph AM. Perinatal oxygen delivery and cardiac function. Adv Pediatr 1985; 32:321–47.
61. Friedman AH, Fahey JT. The transition from fetal to neonatal circulation: Normal responses and implications for infants with heart disease. Seminars in Perinatology 1993; 17(2):106–121.
62. Heymann MA. Regulation of the pulmonary circulation in the perinatal period and in children. Intensive Care Med 1989; 15:S9–S12.
63. Shimokawa H, Flavahan NA, Lorenz RR, et al. Prostacyclin releases endothelium derived relaxing factor and potentiates its action in coronary arteries of the pig. Br J Pharmacol 1988; 95:1197–1203.
64. Sprague RS, Stephenson AH Lonigro AJ. Prostaglandin I2 supports blood flow to hypoxic alveoli in anesthetized dogs. J Appl Physiol 1984; 56:1246–1251.
65. Shaul PW, Farrar MA Zellers TM. Oxygen modulates endothelium-derived relaxing factor production in fetal pulmonary arteries. Am J Physiol 1992; 262:H355–H364.
66. Cutaia M Rounds S. Hypoxic pulmonary vasoconstriction. Physiologic significance, mechanism and clinical relevance. Chest 1990; 97:706–718.
67. Farooki ZQ, Green EW, Physiology of the circulation, in Pediatric Cardiac Surgery, Arciniegas E, Editor Editors. 1985, Year Book Medical: Chicago. p. 13–18.
68. Lang P, Freed MD, Keane JF et al. The use of prostaglandin E1 in an infant with interruption of the aortic arch. J Pediatr 1977; 91:805–807.
69. Agata Y, Hiraishi S, Misawa H, et al. Regional blood flow distribution and left ventricular output during early neonatal life: A quantitative ultrasonographic assessment. Pediatr Res 1994; 36:805–810.
70. Heyman MA, Iwamoto HS Rudolph AM. Factors affecting changes in the neonatal systemic circulation. Ann Rev Physiol 1981; 43:371–383.
71. Sidi D, Kuipers JRG, Heymann MA Rudolph AM. Effects of ambient temperature on oxygen consumption and the circulation in newborn lambs at rest and during hypoxemia. Pediatric Res 1983; 17:254–8.
72. Wong S-N, Lo RN Hui P-W. Abnormal renal and splanchnic arterial Doppler pattern in premature babies with symptomatic patent ductus arteriosus. J Ultrasound Med 1990; 9:125–130.
73. Rein AJ, Sanders SP, Colan SD, Parness IA, Epstein M. Left ventricular mechanics in the normal newborn. Cirulation 1987; 76(No. 5):1029–1036.
74. Meyer RA, Schwartz DC, Benzing G Kaplan S. Ventricular septum in right ventricular volume overload. Am J Cardiol 1972; 30:349–354.
75. Cullen S, Shore D, Reddington A. Characterization of right ventricular diastolic performance after complete repair of tetralogy of fallot. Restrictive physiology predicts slow postoperative recovery. Circulation 1995; 91:1782–1789.
76. Berner M, Oberhansli I, Rouge JC, Jaccard C et al. Chronotropic and inotropic supports are both required to increase cardiac output early after corrective operations for tetralogy of Fallot. J Thorac Cardiovasc Surg 1989; 97:297–302.
77. Vlahakes GJ, Turley K Hoffman JIE. The pathophysiology of failure in right ventricular hypertension: Hemodynamic and biological correlations. Circulation 1980; 63:87–92.

78. Wessel DL, Adatia I, Giglia TM, Thompson JE Kulik TJ. Use of inhaled nitric oxide and acetylcholine in the evaluation of pulmonary hypertension and endothelial function after cardiopulmonary bypass. Circulation 1993; 88:2128–2138.
79. Friedman WF. The intrinsic properties of the developing heart. Prog Cardiovasc Dis 1972; 15:87–111.
80. Hines R, Barash PG. Right ventricular failure. second ed. Cardiac Anesthesia, ed. eds. Kaplan JA. Vol. 2. 1987, New York: Grune and Stratton.
81. Berner M, Rouge JC Friedli B. The hemodynamic effect of phentolamine and dobutamine after open-heart operations in children: Influence of underlying heart defect. Ann Thorac Surg 1983; 35:643–50.
81a. Romero TE, Friedman WF. Limited left ventricular response to volume overload in the neonatal period: A comparitive study in the adult animal. Pediatr Res 1979;13:910–917.
82. Zak R, Kizu A Bugaisky L. Cardiac hypertrophy: Its çharacteristics as a growth process. Am J Cardiol 1979; 44:941–946.
83. Turley K, Vlahakes GJ Harrison MR. Intrauterine cardiothoracic surgery: The fetal lamb model. Ann Thorac Surg 1982; 34:422–426.
84. Overy HR Priest RE. Mitotic cell division in postnatal cardiac growth. Lab Invest 1966; 15:1100–1103.
85. Oparil S. Pathogenesis of ventricular hypertrophy. J Am Coll Cardiol 1985; 5:57B–65B.
86. Page E, Earley J Power B. Normal growth of ultrastructures in rat left ventrical myocardial cells. Circ Res 1974; 35:12–16.
87. Anversa P, Loud AV Giacomelli F. Absolute morphometric study of myocardial hypertrophy in experimental hypertension. II. Ultrastructure of myocytes and interstitium. Lab Invest 1978; 38:597–609.
88. Olivetti G, Anversa P Loud AV. Morphometric study of early postnatal development in the left and right ventricular myocardium of the rat. II. Tissue composition, capillary growth, and sarcoplasmic alterations. Cir Res 1980; 35:503–512.
89. Dowell RT McManus RE. Pressure induced cardiac enlargement in neonatal and adult rats. Left ventricular functional characteristics and evidence of cardiac muscle cell proliferation in the neonate. Circ Res 1978; 42:303–310.
90. Flanagan MF, Fujii AM Colan SD. Myocardial angiogenesis and coronary perfusion in left ventricular pressure overload hypertrophy in the young lamb: Evidence for inhibition with chronic protamine administration. Circ Res 1991; 68:1458–1470.
91. Abraham JA, Mergia A, Whang JL e. al. Nucleotide sequence of a bovine clone encoding the angiogenic protein, basic fibroblast growth factor. Science 1986; 233:545–548.
92. Mahdavi V, Izumo S Nadal-Ginard B. Developmental and hormonal regulation of sarcomeric myosin heavy chain gene family. Circ Res 1987; 60:804–811.
93. Ayogi T, Mirsky I, Flanagan MF, et al. Myocardial function in immature and mature sheep with pressure overload hypertrophy. Am J Physiol 1992; 31:H1036–H1048.
94. Mirsky I, Aoyagi T, Crocker VM, Colan SD Fujii AM. Load dependence of fiber shortening-rate in left ventricular hypertrophy induced by aortic banding. J Am Coll Cardiol 1990; 15890–899.
95. Borrow KM, Colan SD Neumann A. Altered left ventricular mechanics in patients with valvular aortic stenosis and coarctation of the aorta: Effects on systolic performance and late outcome. Circulation 1985; 72:515–522.
96. Borow KM, Keane JF, Castaneda AR Freed MD. Systemic ventricular function in patients with Tetralogy of Fallot, ventricular septal defect and transposition of the great arteries repaired during infancy. Circulation 1981; 64:878.
97. Fujii AM. Left ventricular function in congenital heart disease. Sem Perinatology 1992; 161:47–54.
98. Fujii AM, Aoyagi T, Flanagan MF, et al. Response of the hypertrophied left ventricle to tachycardia: importance of maturation. Am J Physiol 1993; 264((3 pt 2)):H983–H993.
99. Feldman AM, Cates AE, Veazey WB, et al. Increase of the 40,000-mol wt pertusis toxin substrate (G-protein) in the failing human heart. J Clin Invest 1988; 82:189–197.
100. Feldman MD, Copelas L, Gwarthmey JK, et al. Deficient production of cyclic AMP: Pharmacologic evidence of an important cause of contractile dysfunction in patients with end-stage heart failure. Circulation 1987; 75:331–339.
101. Piscone E, Jaski BE, Wenting GJ Serruys PW. Effect of a single oral dose of milrinone on left ventricular diastolic performance in the failing human heart. J Am Coll Cardiol 1988; 10:1294–1302.
102. Hermann HC, Ruddy TD, Dec GW, et al. Diastolic function in patients with severe heart failure: Comparison of the effects of enoximone and nitroprusside. Circulation 1987; 75:1214–1221.
103. Covell JW. Factors influencing diastolic function possible role of the extracellular matrix. Circulation 1990; 81(Suppl III)III–555-III–158.
103a. Cooper G, Tomanek RJ, Erhardt JC, et al. Chronic progressive pressure overload of the cat right ventricle. Circ Res 1981;48:488–497.
103b. Caulfield JB, Borg TK: The collagen network of the heart. Lab Invest. 1979;40:364–372.
104. Chizzonite RA Zak R. Calcium-induced cell death: Susceptability of cardiac myocytes is age-dependent. Science 1981; (213):508–511.
105. Julia PL, Young HH, Buckberg GD, Kofsky ER Bugyi HI. Studies of myocardial protection in the immature heart.II. Evidence for importance of amino acid metabolism in tolerance to ischemia. J Thorac Cardiovasc Surg 1990; 100:888–895.
106. Julia PL, Kofsky ER, Buckberg GD, Young HH Bugyi HI. Studies of myocardial protection in the immature heart. I. Enhanced tolerance of immature vs adult myocardium to global ischemia with reference to metabolic differences. J Thorac Cardiovasc Surg 1990; (100):879–888.
107. Grice WN, Konishi T, Apstein CS. Resistance of the neonatal myocardium to injury during nomothermic and hypothermic ischemic arrest and reperfusion. Circulation 1987; 76(5):V150–155.
108. Julia PL, Kofsky ER, Buckberg GD, Young HH Bugyi HI. Studies of myocardial protection in the immature heart. III. Models of ischemic and hypoxic/ischemic injury in the immature puppy heart. J Thorac Cardiovasc Surg 1991; 101:14–19.
109. Jarmakani JM, Nagatomo T, Nakazawa M Langer GA. Effect of hypoxia on myocardial high-energy phosphates in the neonatal mammalian heart. Am J Physiol 1978; 235:H475–H481.

Unusual Causes of Myocardial Ischemia, Pulmonary Edema, and Cyanosis

13

Jayant K. Deshpande,
Randall C. Wetzel
Mark C. Rogers

INTRODUCTION

The care of patients with cardiovascular disease in the pediatric intensive care unit (ICU) naturally requires familiarity with the pathophysiology of congenital heart disease. Nevertheless, the authors do not believe it is appropriate to give an abbreviated review of all forms of congenital heart disease. Standard textbooks of pediatric cardiology deal with the various forms of complex congenital heart disease, their individual pathophysiologies, and their treatments. In addition, principles of cardiovascular support are included in the chapters on shock (Chapter 16), dysrhythmias (Chapter 15), and postoperative care (Chapter 14). In this chapter we address the clinical entities that commonly arise in the ICU.

Intensivists are often confronted at presentation with three categories of cardiovascular disease that mimic the symptoms of congenital heart disease and/or respiratory disease—myocardial ischemia, pulmonary edema, and cyanosis—that may not be caused by congenital heart disease. This chapter reviews the pathophysiology and approach to unusual causes of myocardial ischemia, pulmonary edema, and cyanosis likely to confront the intensivist. Although this discussion includes a review of some traditional congenital heart disease syndromes, such as cyanotic spells in the tetralogy of Fallot and myocardial infarction in anomalous left coronary artery, the focus is on more unusual causes of these conditions.

MYOCARDIAL ISCHEMIA IN CHILDREN

Introduction

Classically, the pediatrician tends to ignore myocardial ischemia as a pathophysiologic process in critically ill children. Recently, it has been increasingly recognized that myocardial ischemia, angina, myocardial infarction, and ischemic coronary artery disease occur in children of all ages. Although the leading causes of ischemic heart disease (IHD) in children **(Table 13.1)** are different from that in adults (which is, of course, atherosclerotic coronary artery disease), the physiologic factors underlying myocardial oxygen consumption and oxygen delivery are the same. In addition to diseases in children that are clearly recognized as causing myocardial ischemia, such as anomalous coronary arteries, Kawasaki disease, congenital heart disease, and asphyxia, ischemia may also occur during other generalized disease processes, such as trauma, asthma, cardiac tachydysrhythmias, and shock. For these reasons, it is increasingly important that physicians dealing with critically ill children understand the factors that govern myocardial oxygen consumption ($M\dot{V}O_2$) and myocardial oxygen delivery (MDO_2) and are aware of the disease processes in which myocardial ischemia can occur in children.

Determinants of Myocardial Oxygen Consumption

Hemodynamic performance relies on cardiac output and vascular resistance. Cardiac output, in turn, depends on the product of heart rate and stroke volume, which is determined by preload, afterload, and myocardial contractility. Not surprisingly, all of these determinants of hemodynamic function have distinct effects on $M\dot{V}O_2$. Simplistically, $M\dot{V}O_2$ is determined by the amount of work the myocardium must perform; however, not all myocardial "work" is equally expensive in terms of metabolic demand. Understanding the underlying determinants of $M\dot{V}O_2$ is the basis for avoiding and treating myocardial ischemia.

The heart is an aerobic organ, and as such, substrate oxidation is its major energy source. The myocardium has a very limited ability to acquire an oxygen debt; therefore, under steady state conditions, $M\dot{V}O_2$ accurately reflects total myocardial metabolism. The major portion of MO_2 is used to support myocardial contraction. Indeed, the quiescent heart uses only a portion (approximately 20%) of the contracting heart's $M\dot{V}O_2$[1]. In addition, the fraction of oxygen necessary for electrical activation is a minuscule portion of the total $M\dot{V}O_2$ (less than 1.0%)[2]. The work of myocardial contraction has been divided into internal work, which generates myocardial wall tension, and external work, which can be described as the product of stroke volume and mean aortic pressure ("volume" and "pressure" work)[3].

Wall Tension

As early as 1915, it was known that $M\dot{V}O_2$ and myocardial wall tension were closely related[4]. In the past several years, it has become accepted that wall tension is the major determinant of $M\dot{V}O_2$. Work by Sarnoff and Braunwald

Table 13.1. Causes of Myocardial Ischemia in Childhood

Neonatal ischemic heart disease
Asphyxia neonatorum
Increased demand
Persistent transitional circulation
Pulmonary hypertension, i.e., respiratory distress syndrome, meconium aspiration
Congenital heart disease
Cyanotic heart disease
Total anomalous pulmonary veins
Transposition of great vessels
Obstructive disease
Aortic or pulmonary stenosis
Anomalous coronary arteries
Increased demand
Catecholamine-induced ischemia, i.e., isoproterenol treatment of asthma
Head injury
Vascular disease
Kawasaki disease
Infantile periarteritis nodosa
Embolism
Atheroma (rare)
Trauma
Trauma and head injury

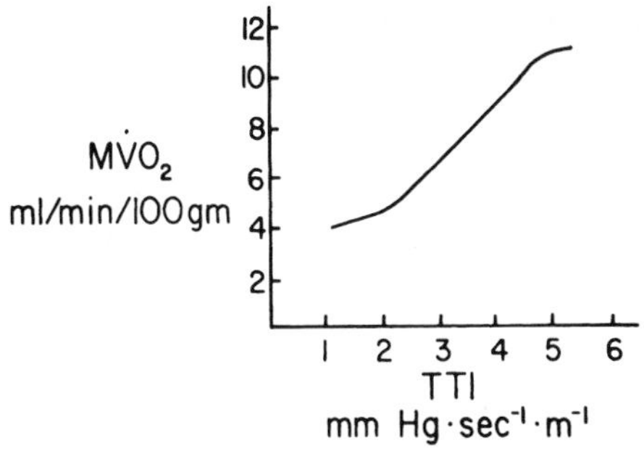

Figure 13.1. Relationship between $M\dot{V}O_2$ and TTI. Note the linear correlation between $M\dot{V}O_2$ and developed tension.

specifically related the tension-time index (TTI) and $M\dot{V}O_2$, demonstrating a very close, nearly 1:1 relationship (Fig. 13.1)[3]. The TTI is described by the area under the left ventricular pressure curve (Fig. 13.2). The Laplace relationship describes myocardial wall tension as directly proportional to intraventricular pressure and intraventricular volume and indirectly related to ventricular wall thickness. Thus, a dilated heart with a large preload and thin left ventricular wall would be expected to have a greater $M\dot{V}_2$ than the small hypertrophied heart. The latter, therefore, would be more efficient at equal stroke volumes. It is also obvious that factors that alter myocardial compliance and thus cause greater ventricular pressures for a given ventricular volume will adversely affect $M\dot{V}O_2$. Poorly compliant hearts, therefore, require increased $M\dot{V}O_2$ and are, thus, less efficient. Ample experimental evidence has subsequently confirmed the importance of myocardial wall tension as a significant determinant of $M\dot{V}O_2$, and because it in turn depends on intraventricular pressure volume (preload) and wall thickness, these factors must be considered when analyzing myocardial oxygen balance[1,3].

Contractility

Another significant determinant of $M\dot{V}O_2$ is the contractile state of the myocardium[3,5]. Studies during isoproterenol administration in humans have revealed poor correlation between $M\dot{V}O_2$ and the TTI, and this suggests that the contractile state of the heart affects $M\dot{V}O_2$, as has been supported by further studies in dogs[6]. Indeed, with use of paired electrical stimulation, $M\dot{V}O_2$ rose sharply while the TTI fell. Using various inotropic stimuli, Sonnenblick and others[7] have demonstrated the role of the contractile state in enhancing $M\dot{V}O_2$. To summarize their work, whereas an 83% increase in wall tension leads to a 50% increase in $M\dot{V}O_2$, at the same wall tension, the same $M\dot{V}O_2$ increase occurs with only a 42% increase in contractility as determined by the velocity of fiber shortening (V_{max})[8]. It can be seen that inotropic stimulation leads to both an increase in wall tension and an increased $M\dot{V}O_2$ at a given wall tension because of enhanced contractility. Although the precise relationship of these two factors in determining $M\dot{V}O_2$ is difficult to define objectively, there is no doubt that the contractile state of the myocardium is a major determinant of $M\dot{V}O_2$. Therefore, it would be expected that in conditions of enhanced contractility, such as occur with sympathetic stimulation or isoproterenol treatment, $M\dot{V}O_2$ would be significantly and, potentially, deleteriously increased.

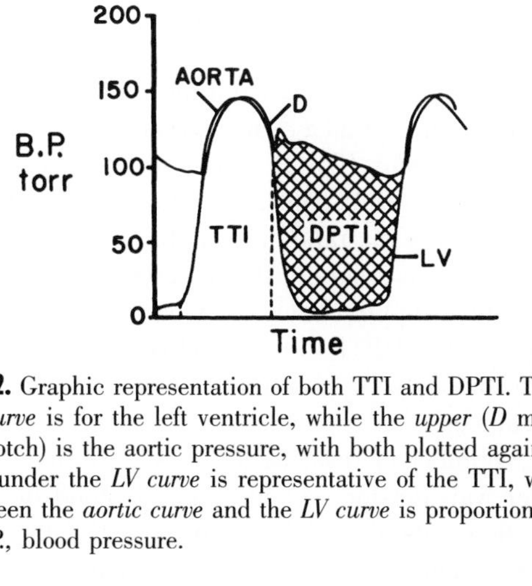

Figure 13.2. Graphic representation of both TTI and DPTI. The *lower pressure curve* is for the left ventricle, while the *upper* (*D* marks the dicrotic notch) is the aortic pressure, with both plotted against time. The *area* under the *LV curve* is representative of the TTI, while the *area* between the *aortic curve* and the *LV curve* is proportional to the DPTI. *B.P.*, blood pressure.

Heart Rate

There is a direct relationship between heart rate and $M\dot{V}O_2$; however, this relationship is a complex one because of alterations in developed tension and the contractile state that occur pari passu with changes in heart rate[1,3,9]. A 50% increase in heart rate is usually associated with a 50% increase in $M\dot{V}O_2$ (Fig. 13.3)[10]. In dogs, when wall stress is constant, $M\dot{V}O_2$ per beat is a function of the reciprocal of heart rate[11]. Unfortunately, it is impossible to separate the effect of changes in contractility and heart rate, per se, on $M\dot{V}O_2$. In the intact adult circulation, as heart rate increases, cardiac output tends to remain constant, and this decrease in stroke volume and end-diastolic volume leads to a decrease in wall tension. The accompanying decrease in $M\dot{V}O_2$ that follows this reduced wall tension tends to offset the increase as a result of increased heart rate in adults, although minute $M\dot{V}O_2$ per beat may be decreased. In infants and small children, the situation may well be differ

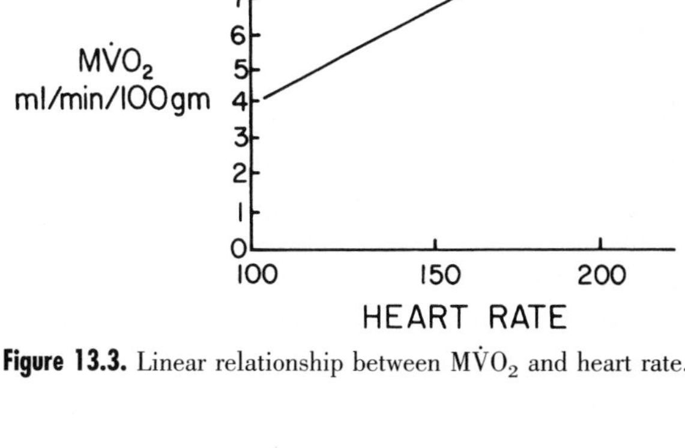

Figure 13.3. Linear relationship between $M\dot{V}O_2$ and heart rate.

ent. The infant has a fairly fixed stroke volume, and as heart rate is increased, cardiac index is increased. As wall tension may be unaltered by this increase in heart rate, the increase in $M\dot{V}O_2$ for a given increase in heart rate may be greater in children than in adults. The relative contribution of the major determinants of $M\dot{V}O_2$ in children may be different from that in adults.

External Work

$M\dot{V}O_2$ is also affected by the amount of external work the heart does[12]. This can be divided simply into the amount of work required to generate aortic pressure (pressure work) and the amount of work required to move the stroke volume (volume work). The early classic work of Evans and Matsuoka[4] noted that increased stroke work (mean aortic pressure times stroke volume) caused by increased aortic pressure increased $M\dot{V}O_2$ much more than an equivalent increase in stroke work caused by increased stroke volume. The oxygen cost of pressure work (isometric contraction) is much greater than volume work (isotonic contraction), and in fact, the amount of oxygen consumption associated with actual fiber shortening is low[13]. Clearly, maintaining blood pressure by increasing stroke volume rather than vasoconstriction is more oxygen efficient. In addition, an increase in cardiac output caused by afterload reduction, which increases stroke volume but decreases pressure, greatly improves the efficiency of the heart and may even decrease $M\dot{V}O_2$. Another clinical example is aortic valve disease. Aortic regurgitation is associated with increased volume work and ischemia is rare, whereas aortic stenosis is associated with increased pressure work and myocardial ischemia frequently occurs.

Several other factors affect $M\dot{V}O_2$. As mentioned, the oxygen cost of excitation and relaxation and basal energy requirements are small[1,3]. In addition, there is evidence that $M\dot{V}O_2$ is related to arterial oxygen content. As O_2 content decreased from normal to 8 vol% (P_aO_2 30 to 35 torr), $M\dot{V}O_2$ increased approximately 20%[14]. Clearly, in children with cyanotic heart disease, the combination of decreased arterial oxygen and the potential for increased $M\dot{V}O_2$ could contribute to myocardial ischemia and explain the chronic ischemic changes often seen in children with such anomalies as transposition of the great vessels.

In summary, the factors that influence $M\dot{V}O_2$ are:

1. Myocardial wall tension
2. Contractile state of the heart
3. Heart rate
4. External workload

Of course, these are interdependent, and alterations in one can have complex effects on overall $M\dot{V}O_2$ by altering the other factors. In children, increased oxygen demand may cause myocardial ischemia, which may be significant, occurring during tachydysrhythmias or increased workload, as in valvular heart disease or pulmonary hypertension. Several of these are discussed below.

Myocardial Oxygen Supply

If myocardial oxygen supply were infinite, increases in $M\dot{V}O_2$ would be irrelevant. Occasionally, even in the infant's and child's heart, myocardial oxygen supply may be compromised or even a normal supply may be inadequate to meet an increased need. To understand oxygen balance, the factors regulating oxygen delivery must be understood. These factors are:

1. Arterial oxygen content
2. Coronary perfusion pressure
3. Coronary artery patency

In any vascular bed, perfusion is determined by perfusion pressure (inflow pressure minus outflow pressure) and vascular resistance. The vascular resistance is, in turn, determined by intrinsic factors (i.e., vascular tone, blood viscosity) and extrinsic factors (i.e., external compression). In the heart, perfusion pressure for the left ventricle is usually defined as aortic pressure minus ventricular pressure. Clearly, both of these pressures vary throughout the cardiac cycle, and thus, phasic flow variation would be expected. The coronary vascular resistance is, as in all vascular beds, autoregulated and subject to metabolic demand but, in addition, is subjected to dramatic external compression as a result of cardiac contraction.

During systole, ventricular pressure rises, the coronary circulation is compressed, the aortic cusps tend to occlude the coronary ostia, and coronary artery inflow pressure tends to be lowered by the Venturi effect[1]. Clearly, coronary blood flow will not be optimal during systole. In diastole, the ventricular pressures are low, the myocardium relaxes, the ostia are unoccluded, and coronary inflow pressure is the same as aortic diastolic pressure. During diastole, then, conditions for coronary perfusion are optimal. Although the factors that regulate coronary blood flow are similar to those in other vascular beds, the marked phasic variability creates significant differences. During asystole, myocardial blood flow increases by upwards of 50%. Left coronary artery flow profiles show the highest flows during diastole. This effect is somewhat less in the adult right coronary artery because the ventricular pressures that are generated are much less in the left ventricle. Clearly, the majority of myocardial perfusion occurs during diastole. In a fashion analogous to the TTI as a descriptor of $M\dot{V}O_2$, the diastolic pressure-time index (DPTI) relates to the myocardial oxygen supply (Fig. 13.2). Thus, the ratio of supply to demand is proportional to the ratio of DPTI to TTI. Factors that decrease diastolic pressure or the duration of diastole will adversely affect supply. Thus, tachycardia and hypotension will lower the DPTI, while tachycardia may increase $M\dot{V}O_2$—obviously, a disadvantageous event under many circumstances[15].

For a number of reasons, the most significant of which is higher wall tension, subendocardial blood flow is more tenuous than subepicardial flow. In general, subendocardial coronary vascular tone is reduced, compared to subepicardial flow, probably owing to a greater wall tension and, therefore, greater metabolic demand(16). Over an average cycle, the ratio of endocardial to epicardial flow is generally 1 : 1, despite many disparities in flow at any given time. However, interventions that adversely affect the ratio of DPTI to TTI tend to reduce endocardial flow preferentially, and this explains the increased susceptibility of subendocardial tissues to ischemia(17).

Clearly, complete coronary artery occlusion, whether it is as a result of thrombosis, embolism, or extrinsic obstruction, will lead to profound myocardial ischemia. If the obstruction is partial, then coronary perfusion pressure will be lower than aortic diastolic pressures distal to the occlusion, and the effective DPTI will obviously be reduced. This will limit the ability of the affected segment to respond to increased needs and, if profound enough, cause ischemia at rest. Although coronary artery disease is uncommon in children, it does occur from many causes, which are discussed below.

The principles of myocardial oxygen balance are important not only when considering primary heart disease but also in circumstances when increased demands may be put on the myocardium or the ability to provide adequate flow is impaired. Their complex interrelationships make other than qualitative assessment very difficult.

Neonatal Ischemic Heart Disease

Previously, myocardial ischemia and infarction were believed to be a rare occurrence in neonates and infants, and then to occur only in those children with congenital heart disease(18). It is now evident that in stressed neonates, even with normal coronary arteries and in the absence of congenital anomalies, myocardial ischemia and necrosis are not uncommon and may even be a significant factor in the mortality of acutely ill infants(19,20). The occurrence of myocardial ischemia and necrosis in these infants is less surprising when the underlying pathophysiology is considered. The unusual stresses imposed on the transitional circulation perinatally can lead to both increased myocardial oxygen demand and impaired oxygen delivery. Superimposition of hypoxia, hypovolemia, sepsis, and respiratory distress during this period can severely impair myocardial perfusion.

That coronary artery occlusion as a result of inflammatory disease, calcification, and thrombosis occurs during the newborn period has long been known(21). In neonatal postmortem examinations, intimal lesions have been reported and even implicated in the pathogenesis of adult atheromatous coronary artery disease(22). There are even reports that document the occurrence of coronary embolism in the fetus and thrombosis in the newborn(23,24). This has been correlated with electrocardiographic evidence of myocardial ischemia, cardiogenic shock, and death. In a series of 856 infant autopsies, coronary embolization had occurred in 28 patients(25). Paradoxical emboli, disseminated intravascular coagulation, and circulatory stasis have all been implicated as causes of coronary thrombosis in the neonatal period(25).

More commonly, myocardial ischemia and infarction occur in neonates and infants as results of abnormal hemodynamic stresses. In 1972, Rowe and Hoffman(26) reported three infants who, after mild hypoxic stress, developed biventricular cardiac failure and electrocardiographic evidence of left ventricular ischemia, which resolved over 2 months. They attributed this clinical picture to transient myocardial ischemia aggravated by an increased pulmonary hypoxic response, right ventricular afterload, and compromised myocardial perfusion. Earlier work showed the occurrence of myocardial necrosis and subendocardial infarction in asphyxiated newborn infants, and subsequent reports have amply confirmed the occurrence of myocardial ischemia after neonatal asphyxia(18–20). This electrocardiographic and postmortem evidence of ischemia has been substantiated by several reports of thallium myocardial imaging demonstrating abnormalities in myocardial perfusion(27). These initial findings have been extended, and it seems that some endocardial ischemia and infarction, especially papillary muscle necrosis, are relatively common in stressed infants(20,28). Although this usually follows asphyxia, other insults including sepsis, respiratory distress syndrome (RDS), and intraventricular hemorrhage apparently cause significant stress, resulting in myocardial necrosis(29). Donnelly et al.(29)reported autopsy findings in 82 infants who died within 7 days and had no evidence of diseases otherwise associated with myocardial necrosis(29). Thirty-one of these infants (38%) demonstrated myocardial ischemic necrosis, with involvement of the papillary muscles occurring in 27. Recent reports substantiate this frequent occurrence of neonatal ischemic heart disease(30–32).

The neonate has a relatively hypertrophied right ventricle and a reactive pulmonary vasculature. In addition, the presence of a ductus arteriosus (especially in asphyxia) lowers the aortic diastolic pressure and presents a potential for a steal phenomenon(32). During asphyxia, pulmonary vascular and systemic vascular resistance increase dramatically, and sympathetic stimulation enhances myocardial heart rate and contractility. All of these factors cause a large increase in $M\dot{V}O_2$. Concurrently, because of increased intracavitary pressures, the possibility of ductal runoff, and variable aortic pressures, perfusion is also impaired. With the addition of global hypoxia and arterial desaturation, it is hardly surprising that myocardial ischemia occurs and can lead to myocardial necrosis in stressed neonates. In addition, a high incidence of right ventricular dysfunction and tricuspid insufficiency would be expected, and this clearly occurs(28). The occurrence of myocardial ischemia in persistent transitional circulation, RDS, and meconium aspiration, as expected, has indeed been documented(33). It is clear that ischemic heart disease should be not only suspected but also sought in ill neonates.

Unfortunately, the clinical picture of IHD in neonates is not sharply delineated from other causes of neonatal respiratory distress. The picture is one of hypoxemia with heart failure characterized by cardiomegaly, tricuspid or mitral insufficiency, and cardiogenic shock(19). Frequently, there is electrocardiographic evidence of ischemia with right ventricular hypertrophy (RVH), S-T segment depression, and T-wave inversion, and even frank myocardial infarction (Fig. 13.4). In addition, creatine phosphokinase (CPK) (CK-MB) may be elevated, although this is a less reliable indicator in children than in adults[30]. The differential diagnosis includes structural heart diseases such as total anomalous pulmonary venous drainage (TAPVD), hypoplastic left heart syndromes, and anomalous origin of the coronary arteries. Angiography and radionuclide imaging may be of help[31].

Therapy is primarily supportive, with increased F_IO_2, ventilatory support, and fluid restriction. Digoxin, diuretics, and inotropic agents have been used beneficially. Therapies that are traditionally used in adults, such as nitroglycerin, β-blockade, and calcium channel blockers have not been reported. The outlook is generally good, and supportive therapy is usually associated with resolution of symptoms in 48 to 72 hours and radiographic and electrocardiographic resolution within 2 weeks[30,31]. Even so, the high incidence of myocardial necrosis at postmortem indicates that this may be an underdiagnosed condition. The long-term prognosis is unknown; it is tempting to speculate that several conditions of unknown cause, such as mitral valve prolapse, idiopathic cardiac dysrhythmias, and cardiomyopathies in older children, may be related to neonatal IHD and unsuspected myocardial infarction.

Myocardial Ischemia Associated with Congenital Heart Disease

It is unusual to consider myocardial ischemia when managing children with congenital heart disease, although logically hypertrophy, cyanosis, increased hematocrit (Hct), and the frequency of the postoperative state would suggest that ischemia would frequently occur. Clearly, coronary artery disease is generally absent from younger children with anatomically normal coronary arteries, and this fact may have led to the lack of emphasis placed on IHD in children with congenital heart disease. Yet, it has long been known that children with congenital heart disease have an increased incidence of abnormal coronary artery changes and that coronary occlusive disease does occur. However, perhaps even more significantly, the classic report of Franciosi and Blanc[18] revealed that myocardial infarction is a frequent complication of congenital heart disease in the absence of anomalous origin of the coronary arteries or other coronary artery disease. They documented both right ventricular and left ventricular infarctions occurring in 33 of 44 hearts examined with total anomalous pulmonary venous drainage, aortic stenosis, pulmonary stenosis, and transposition of the great arteries (TGA). Furthermore, there was evidence of both acute and remote infarction and multiple infarcts of various ages in several hearts, and the incidence seemed unrelated to surgery. The usual site for these infarcts was subendocardial, especially the papillary muscles, with the exact location largely dependent on the particular type of congenital heart disease. These results have been substantiated by Esterly and Oppenheimer from Johns Hopkins[25,34]. Both groups suggested ventricular hypertrophy and relative coronary hypoperfusion as the cause. This is supported by the occurrence of right ventricular infarction in TAPVD, left ventricular infarction in aortic stenosis, and biventricular infarction in TGA. In patients with aortic stenosis and pulmonary stenosis, almost certainly another contributing factor is increased intraventricular pressures and, thus, decreased coronary perfusion pressure. Hyperviscosity and hypoxemia as a result of cyanotic heart disease are also contributing factors. Although electrocardiographic evidence of myocardial infarction is only present in half of the patients, it is clear that significant myocardial ischemia and, possibly, fatal myocardial infarction should be expected in children with certain types of congenital heart disease.

Anomalous Origin of Coronary Arteries from the Pulmonary Artery

One of the most dramatic causes of myocardial ischemia and fatal myocardial infarction in children is the anomalous origin of the left coronary artery from the pulmonary artery[35]. Although rare with a reported incidence of

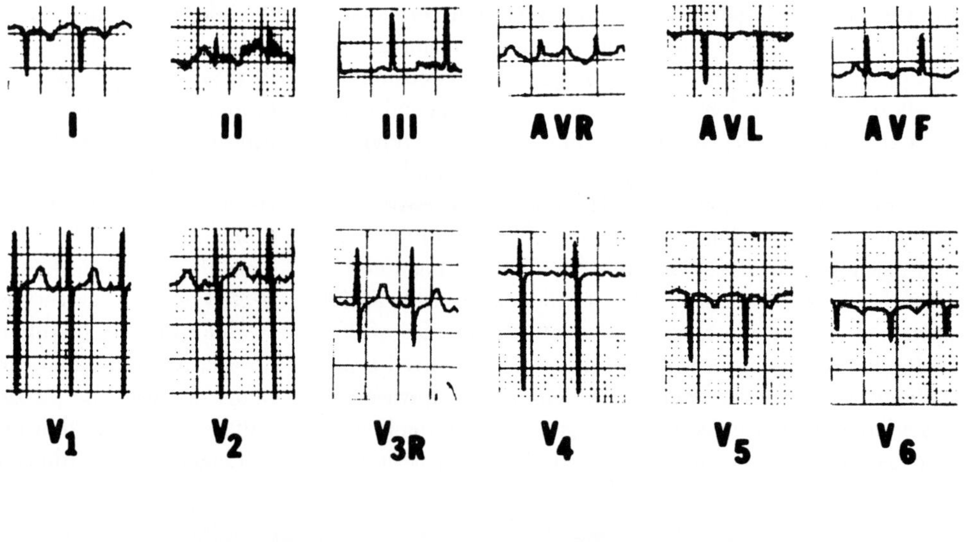

Figure 13.4. ECG of a 13-day-old neonate. Note Qs in I, V_5, V_6, and inverted T-waves in I, II, aV_L, aV_F, V_5, and V_6, which are consistent with inferolateral myocardial infarction. (From Kilbridge H. Myocardial infarction in the neonate with normal heart and coronary arteries. Am J Dis Child 1980;134:759, copyright 1980, American Medical Association.)

0.5%[35a], it is becoming an increasingly recognized condition, and the prospects for successful surgical intervention make early recognition of this lesion worthwhile. This congenital anomaly perhaps most mimics adult coronary artery disease with progressive development of angina, infarction, heart failure, aneurysm formation, and eventual death, although the etiology is very different.

The anomalous origin of a coronary artery results developmentally from abnormal formation of the bulbospiral septum in the truncus arteriosus. The origin of one or both of the coronary arteries may, therefore, be included in the pulmonary artery in approximately 40% of cases, while another 43% arise from an ectopic aortic site[35a]. Anomalous origin of the right coronary artery is generally benign, as the low-pressure right ventricle appears to be adequately supplied by this right coronary artery with additional left coronary artery collaterals. Anomalous origin of both coronary arteries is rare and uniformly rapidly fatal. It is the chance for prolonged survival, surgical correction, and early recognition that focuses the majority of interest on the anomalous origin of the left coronary artery. This lesion is rare, occurring in 1 in 300,000 children and accounts for less than 0.5% of all congenital heart disease[35a]. Although in the past this diagnosis was generally the outcome of a postmortem examination, early recognition of these children has become increasingly common. Several anatomical variants of anomalous origin of the left coronary artery have been described, including left anterior artery descending from the pulmonary artery and left coronary artery originating from the right main pulmonary artery. However, the pathophysiology of these rare anomalies is similar to that of anomalous origin of the left coronary artery[37,38].

The natural history of this disease is determined by cardiovascular developmental changes[35,36]. In utero, both great vessels receive mixed venous, desaturated blood at equal pressures. Therefore, in utero, the origin of the coronary arteries is not significant. After birth, pulmonary artery pressure falls and the aortic outflow is fully saturated. Over the first several weeks, as pulmonary artery pressure falls further, the anomalous left coronary artery, which is first perfused, albeit poorly, with mixed venous blood from the pulmonary artery, eventually undergoes flow reversal. Collateral flow from the right coronary artery leads to high-pressure systemic blood retroperfusing the left coronary artery, which then flows into the pulmonary artery. By 4 months of age, the majority of infants will have developed this flow pattern. This leads to a large left-to-right shunt, which increases myocardial workload at the same time as impairing left ventricular perfusion. Myocardial damage is inevitable, and at least 80% of these children have not survived the first year of life[39]. Several adults have been reported who developed symptoms in middle life or are found to have anomalous arteries at postmortem. Although these are the exception, it should be remembered that in older children with evidence of myocardial ischemia, an anomalous coronary artery must be considered.

Clinical Features

In the first few months of life, the infants seem normal. The symptoms fall into three categories: *(a)* recurrent respiratory infections, *(b)* discomfort, and *(c)* heart failure. Although heart failure may be the first presenting symptom, there is frequently a history of irritability, screaming (especially with feeds), drawing up of the legs, apparent anxiety, pain, pallor, and sweating—all most likely because of anginal symptoms. The most striking symptoms, however, accompany heart failure with dyspnea, tachycardia, wheezing, coughing, and poor perfusion[35,36].

Examination usually reveals an anxious, well-developed, tachypneic, and pale infant. Paroxysmal irritability and crying may occur. In addition, pallor, sweating, and shock similar to symptoms seen in adults with myocardial infarction may be seen. Other findings of failure include edema, hepatomegaly, grunting respirations, and rales. Chest X-ray may reveal cardiomegaly and pulmonary edema with possibly concurrent respiratory tract infection. The most useful diagnostic tool is the electrocardiogram (ECG), which usually reveals a pattern that is consistent with an anterior myocardial infarction pattern characterized by a Q-R pattern and inverted T-waves in I and aVL. Frequently, a left ventricular hypertrophy (LVH) pattern is seen with deep Qs in V_5 and V_6 and S-T changes in the precordial leads. Radionuclide imaging will reveal myocardial hypoperfusion, and angiography will define the anatomy. The differential diagnosis includes defects associated with LVH, such as aortic stenosis, tricuspid atresia, coarctation of the aorta, especially associated with a patent ductus arteriosus, and ventricular septal defects, although these are readily differentiated. More difficult and frequently clinically undiscernible are endomyocardial fibroelastosis and myocarditis, and these can often only be differentiated angiographically, although the presence of Q-waves strongly suggests anomalous coronary arteries.

In addition to this classic presentation, older children may also present to the ICU. The authors have seen several children with acute onset of chest pain (often during exercise), with electrocardiographic evidence of ischemia, who despite no previous symptoms have had an anomalous origin of a coronary artery. In addition, the sudden onset of both supraventricular tachycardia and ventricular tachycardia has occurred as the presenting feature of this disease. This condition must be considered for children with chest pain, ischemia, or infarction and potentially in every child with the acute onset of a dysrhythmia.

Therapy

Medical management directed at initial resuscitation and stabilization traditionally includes oxygen, digoxin, fluids, and diuretics. Logical extension of the therapy for IHD in adults would indicate that optimizing fluid balance, afterload reduction, and antidysrhythmia therapy could be useful. Definitive therapy requires surgical intervention. His-

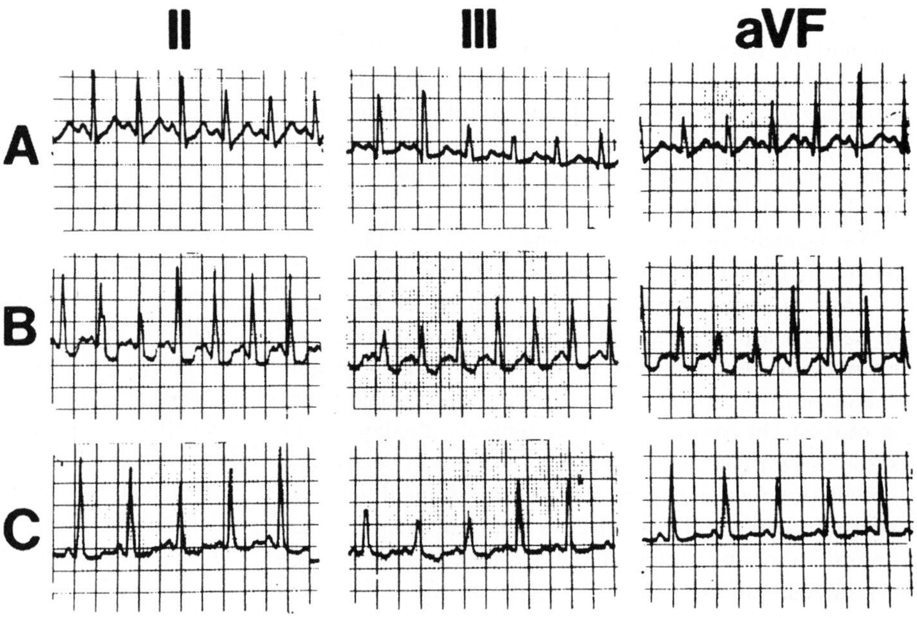

Figure 13.5. Three ECG leads at different times in the child described in the text. A. Before intravenous isoproterenol but 25 minutes after chest pain during isoproterenol aerosol. B. During isoproterenol infusion. C. Twenty minutes after discontinuing infusion. Note profound S-T depression and T-wave changes during isoproterenol administration. (From Matson JR, Loughlin GM, Stunk RC. Myocardial ischemia complicating the use of isoproterenol in asthmatic children. J Pediatr 1978;92:776.)

torically, this has included pulmonary artery banding to reverse flow in the left coronary artery, ligation of the vessel to decrease left-to-right shunting, and grafting of systemic vessels to left coronary artery (e.g., Vineberg, carotid, or subclavian bypass grafting). Recently, efforts have been directed at providing fully oxygenated blood at systemic pressures to the left coronary artery, and this has required either grafting of the saphenous vein from the aorta to the left coronary artery, mobilizing the coronary artery to the aorta, or creation of an aortopulmonary window. These procedures have had mixed results. Presently, several centers favor creation of an aortopulmonary window with a baffle or tunnel through the pulmonary artery to the left coronary artery ostium, thus fashioning a neocoronary artery(40). This procedure offers a potential for growth and eliminates the hazards of mobilizing the left coronary artery while providing systemic pressures and oxygenated blood for left ventricular perfusion.

The prognosis for patients with this condition prior to the advent of surgical repair was very poor. A few adults with hypertrophied right coronary artery, extensive anastomoses, and anginal symptoms have been noted, but survival past childhood was the exception. The long-term prognosis after surgery remains unknown, and the operative mortality remains high. Whether revascularization of previously ischemic myocardium will yield long-term success is questionable. Early surgery before massive infarction and aneurysm formation may be beneficial. Early recognition and correction remains the basis of managing this form of childhood IHD.

Catecholamine-Induced Ischemia

Whereas the previous examples of myocardial ischemia have largely dealt with defects in substrate delivery, theoretically, increased myocardial oxygen demand also could lead to ischemia. In 1978, Matson et al.(41) reported electrocardiographic evidence of myocardial ischemia in a 14-year-old asthmatic who was being treated with intravenous isoproterenol (0.11 μmg/kg/min). After 25 minutes, the child complained of anterior neck pain and S-T-segment depression with T-wave inversion in leads II, III, and aVF was noted (Fig. 13.5). Concurrently, they noticed that the PaO_2 fell from 105 to 77 torr while the heart rate rose from 120 to 160 beats/min and the PCO_2 fell. Although catecholamine-induced ischemia and angina had been reported previously in adults, this constituted the first report of its occurrence in a pediatric patient. They concluded with a warning that "failure to recognize myocardial ischemia could result in myocardial necrosis." In 1979, a report detailed the sudden death from cardiac arrest of an 18-year-old asthmatic treated with a maximum of 0.32 μmg/kg/min of isoproterenol who demonstrated multiple areas of myocardial necrosis at postmortem examination(42). Clinical experience and further reports have supported the existence of myocardial ischemia in asthmatic children receiving isoproterenol(43).

The underlying cause of catecholamine-induced injury is almost certainly multifactorial. In untreated status asthmaticus, desaturation and acidosis occur and may adversely affect myocardial oxygen balance. In addition, negative intrapleural pressures occur and are associated with profound cardiorespiratory interactions (see Chapter 11), the overall effect of which is to increase left ventricular afterload and, thus, oxygen consumption. The addition of isoproterenol to this picture has several effects. Increased heart rate and enhanced myocardial contractility may dramatically increase $\dot{M}V_2$ while compromising delivery by a direct β_2-vascular effect lowering diastolic pressure. The increased heart rate and lowered pressure may significantly decrease the DPTI. In addition, isoproterenol inhibition of hypoxic pulmonary vasomotor responses increases intrapulmonary shunting and regularly decreases PaO_2(44). In children with a chronically stressed heart from chronic lung diseases such as asthma, isoproterenol clearly can present a risk. Experimental evidence exists that demonstrates that subendocardial ischemia occurs during isoproterenol and is part of a coronary artery steal phenomenon, even in animals with normal coronary vessels(45). Isoproterenol myocardial necrosis and catecholamine-induced cardiomyopathies are well-known entities and are probably a result of the combination of factors enumerated previously(46,47). The use of epinephrine and norepinephrine also poses a threat to myocardial oxygen balance. Isoproterenol's marked salutary effects in status asthmaticus need to be balanced against the possibility of induced myocardial ischemia. One further point needs to be made: Theophylline also increases $M\dot{V}O_2$ and, in animals, has led to myocardial necrosis(48). It is conceivable that theophylline and isoproterenol present an additive challenge to the myocardium in these patients. Recently terbutaline has been widely used in the treatment of status asthmaticus. Although it is purported to be more selective for the B_2 receptor, the drug can increase $M\dot{V}O_2$ and exert cardiovascular effects similar to those seen with isoproterenol: significant tachycardia and worsening of the ventilation : perfusion ratio.

Kawasaki Disease

The leading cause of IHD in children is Kawasaki disease(49). This disease was first described by Tomisaku Kawasaki in 1967 as an acute, febrile mucocutaneous lymph node syndrome predominantly affecting infants and small children(50). Although it is a multisystem disease, it has become apparent that the predominant morbidity and mortality of this condition are related to its catastrophic coronary vascular involvement. Twenty percent of children affected by Kawasaki disease develop coronary aneurysm, and 3 to 4% die from myocardial ischemia, usually during the recovery phase of the disease, and these are usually infants(51). Long-term IHD occurs, and the final prognosis regarding myocardial involvement is still not known. Because it is the leading cause of IHD in children, Kawasaki disease is discussed in detail.

Epidemiology

Kawasaki disease, initially reported in Japan, has now been reported in most European countries, Australia, the Middle East, India, Mexico, and Canada and the United States(52). The disease has now become well established and occasionally appears in epidemic proportions; several clusters have now been reported. It is overwhelmingly a disease of young children, with 75% of all deaths occurring in children under 2 years of age and 80% of all cases being reported in children under 4, although sporadic reports of Kawasaki disease in adults exist(53). In addition, it seems that there is an ethnic predisposition, with the highest incidence occurring in children of Japanese descent. Males are more commonly affected than females (1.5 and 1) and demonstrate a higher mortality rate (3 : 1). Although extensive epidemiology studies have been unsuccessful in identifying the cause and relationships of a number of factors in Kawasaki disease, its apparent spread from Japan across the Pacific throughout the United States, its increased frequency in warm weather, its occurrence in clusters, and its clinical symptoms (i.e., fever, leukocytosis, and erythematous rash) indicate an infectious process. However, extensive effort has been unable to demonstrate either a viral, rickettsial, mycoplasmal, bacterial, protozoal, or chlamydial infectious agent(48,52,54). Its similarity to poststreptococcal diseases such as acute glomerulonephritis, scarlet fever, and acute rheumatic fever would suggest an autoimmune cause also; however, investigations of autoimmune phenomena have been consistently negative(48,52). Circulating immune complexes have been identified, but their relationship to the disease process is not clear. It is possible that in genetically predisposed individuals, a wide variety of infectious processes initiate an atypical immune response, which leads to Kawasaki disease.

Clinical Picture

The clinical picture of Kawasaki disease consists of three well-defined phases: *(a)* the acute febrile stage, which usually lasts from 1 to 2 weeks; *(b)* a subacute phase, and *(c)* a convalescent phase, occurring usually after 6 weeks. The diagnosis of Kawasaki disease rests on identification of the following six criteria, at least five of which are required for diagnosis(53–55).

1. A spiking remittent fever of 101 to 104° F, lasting for more than 5 days and usually for approximately 2 weeks.
2. Mucosal changes in the oropharynx, often with bleeding, cracked lips, fissuring, pharyngeal hyperemia, and a strawberry tongue.
3. Cervical lymphadenopathy, with a hard tender lymph node mass greater than 1.5 cm that frequently may be unilateral.
4. Conjunctival involvement with edema and injection of both the bulbar and palpebral conjunctiva.
5. Deep red erythema of the palms and soles, accompanied by induration and edema of the hands and feet, which often limit the ability to walk, and frequently followed by periungual desquamation approximately 2 weeks after the onset of the illness.
6. An erythematous rash that is polymorphous, nonvesiculated, generally pruritic, migratory, occasionally urticarial, and usually truncal.

Other manifestations of Kawasaki disease include aseptic meningitis (25%), diarrhea (40%), meatal ulceration (20%), urethritis (25%), arthralgia (30%), and sporadic central nervous system (CNS) involvement with symptoms of lethargy and emotional irritability. Much more rarely, hydrops of the gallbladder, jaundice, uveitis, hepatitis, pleural and pericardial effusions, and pneumonia occur. In infants (children younger than 6 months of age), the clinical features may be atypical, making diagnosis difficult in this high-risk population[56].

Cardiac Involvement

By far, the most serious feature of Kawasaki disease is myocardial and coronary artery involvement. Although as mentioned above, only 20% of children affected by Kawasaki disease clinically demonstrate cardiac involvement, the heart is affected in at least 40% of all cases, and cardiac involvement is the primary cause of death in 2% of all children with Kawasaki disease. Autopsy studies invariably demonstrate coronary artery involvement. Unfortunately, fatal cardiac complications can arise in patients initially free of clinical cardiac symptomatology. These considerations mandate careful observation and electrocardiographic monitoring, best performed in a pediatric ICU.

Clinically, myocardial involvement may be obvious as patients develop tachycardia and a gallop rhythm. Chest pain is reported to be the most common cardiovascular symptom and may be the sole complaint in some patients. Tachycardia out of proportion to the fever and fatigue and irritability may be the only complaint in other children. More serious arrhythmias and myocardial involvement may occur with pericardial effusion, mitral regurgitation, and heart failure, usually after the ninth day. Electrocardiographic abnormalities are found in 30 to 50% of patients, the most common of which are atrioventricular block, arrhythmias, P-R prolongation, prolonged Q-T interval, and voltage changes compatible with left ventricular strain[57]. Isolated ventricular ectopy without obvious signs of cardiac failure may be the sole manifestation. Pericardial effusions and pericarditis and nonaneurysmal cardiac dilatation have also been reported[58]. Coronary artery aneurysms, with or without thrombosis, and myocardial infarction usually develop in the convalescent period. Aneurysmal coronary artery dilatation has been seen in up to 26% of Kawasaki patients and, when it occurs, is accompanied by biopsy evidence of myocarditis, cellular infiltration, and fibrosis. Coronary artery involvement and cardiac abnormalities are more common in children with Kawasaki disease who are male, are less than 1 year of age, have had a fever for over 2 weeks or have had a recurrent fever, who have a prolonged elevation in the erythrocyte sedimentation rate (ESR) or an ESR greater than 100 mm/hr, or who show significant cardiac involvement in the early stages[58-60]. Recent reports concerning follow-up studies in large numbers of children with Kawasaki disease seem to support the notion that cardiovascular complications are found in over 50% of patients and coronary artery aneurysms are more frequent than hitherto thought[61,62]. In addition, aortic regurgitation caused by myocarditis seems to be a frequent follow-up finding[63]. It should also be emphasized that children can suffer severe and occasionally fatal complications many years after initial involvement with Kawasaki disease[64,65].

Laboratory Findings

There are no specific diagnostic tests for Kawasaki disease; however, several abnormalities have been reported. Leukocytosis with a white count higher than 1500 cells/ml and a leftward shift may persist for several weeks after Kawasaki disease. All acute phase reactants, such as C-reactive protein, α_2-globulin, and ESR, are consistently and dramatically elevated. Thrombocytosis is usually apparent during the second and third weeks, and platelet abnormalities have been detected for months after the acute phase. In addition, it seems that those patients with coagulopathy and platelet activation in Kawasaki syndrome are at a higher risk for the development of coronary artery aneurysms[58,66,67]. Normocytic, normochromic anemia is frequent, and patients may demonstrate hyperbilirubinemia and increased hepatic enzyme levels. The presence of eosinophilia should prompt a search of a parasitic etiology. Proteinuria and pyuria are common; however, marked renal involvement with abnormalities in serum electrolytes is abnormal. Rarely, cerebrospinal fluid (CSF) pleocytosis occurs.

The chest X-ray is frequently normal, although pneumonitis has been reported in a few patients. Cardiomegaly, a result of either left ventricular failure or hypertrophy, and pericardial effusions may occasionally occur during the second or third week. Other noninvasive diagnostic tests specifically designed to detect underlying cardiac abnormalities and an ECG are essential and may show the abnormalities mentioned previously. Echocardiography has been reported to detect a subset of children who develop coronary aneurysms and probably should be serially performed in children with Kawasaki disease. In addition, echocardiographic abnormalities of ventricular wall motion appear to be a sensitive method of detecting cardiac involvement in Kawasaki disease[68]. There has been extensive clinical experience with two-dimensional echocardiography used to demonstrate coronary aneurysms, to follow patients during the recovery phase, and to provide follow-up[69]. It can be expected that over half of these demonstrable coronary aneurysms resolve within the first year[70]. Echocardiographic anomalies alone do not necessarily indicate the need for angiography, and in the absence of clinical findings, serial follow-up would seem the wisest course. A new radionuclide scanning technique using Indium-111 monoclonal antimyosin antibody imaging may prove to be a effective means of accurately diagnosing myocarditis[70A]. More ominous is the development of irritability, pallor, and hypotension during the subacute phase of Kawasaki disease that may herald myocardial infarction. Electrocardiographic monitoring should probably be continued throughout the first 10 days of the illness. The development of Q-waves during electrocardiographic monitoring is an ominous sign associated with full-thickness myocardial infarction in more than 30% of the cases in which it is seen[71,72].

Pathology

The main pathologic feature of Kawasaki disease is a nonspecific panvasculitis[(73)]. Endarteritis of major arteries occurs, especially in the coronary arteries, during the subacute phase and may lead to aneurysms, central destruction, thrombosis, and embolization. With time, these abnormalities are followed by pathologic evidence of ischemia and infarction, aneurysmal rupture, and pancarditis, which may frequently involve the conduction system.

The pathologic evolution of Kawasaki disease seems to undergo four distinct postmortem stages[(73,74)]. Stage 1 (fewer than 10 days) shows a panvasculitis of the microcirculation and includes the coronary arteries. Acute myocarditis, pericarditis, and endocarditis with valvulitis are evident. In stage 2 (11 to 28 days), aneurysm formation and coronary artery stenosis with persistence of pancarditis is found. In stage 3 (28 to 45 days), global evidence of myocardial ischemia with thrombosis and intimal proliferation is obvious. The pancarditis is resolving and the vasculitis is absent. During stage 4 (more than 50 days), resolution of the ravages of the first three stages in the coronary circulation is seen with calcifications, stenosis, scarring, recanalization, and chronic aneurysm formation. Endocardial fibroelastosis and ischemic myocardial changes are prominent. Capillary muscle dysfunction with mitral and tricuspid regurgitation can occur. Although seen throughout the first three stages, ischemia and inflammatory changes in the conducting tissue are generally resolving by the fourth stage. During the first stage, conduction abnormalities in arrhythmias are a common cause of death, whereas myocardial infarction and aneurysm rupture are the predominant causes during stage 2. Ischemic heart disease owing to coronary artery occlusion is the cause of death in stages 3 and 4. Although the natural history of the aneurysms formed during Kawasaki disease is resolution, rupture and sudden death can occur many years later. Aneurysms also occur throughout the circulation and have been found in hepatic, peripheral circulatory, cerebral, iliofemoral, renal, testicular, and splenic vessels. Clinically evident peripheral aneurysms of the brachial, cervical, and femoral arteries should prompt a search for associated central and coronary aneurysms[(75)].

Treatment

Without question, therapy for Kawasaki disease includes prompt treatment at the earliest possible time, with 100 mg/kg/day of aspirin, followed by prolonged treatment with 30 mg/kg/day during the convalescent stage[(76)]. There seems to be ample evidence that this inhibits inflammatory reaction and platelet aggregation; also, therapy seems to be capable of preventing the associated coronary artery disease, coronary thrombosis, and thromboembolism. Although the use of steroids has been recommended in the past, coronary angiography performed in children 2 months after the onset of fever has demonstrated a 65% incidence of aneurysms in those treated with prednisolone, compared with 20% in those treated with antibiotics and only 11% in those treated with aspirin[(77)]. Aspirin should be continued beyond the convalescent stage. Malabsorption of salicylates seems to be a common problem, and therefore, serum levels should be followed in the initial period.

Recently, in a multicenter study[(78)], it was concluded that high-dose intravenous γ-globulin is safe and effective in reducing the prevalence of coronary artery abnormalities when given early in the course of this syndrome[(53,55,65)]. In a second multicenter investigation[(79)], it was found that a single large dose (2 g/kg) of intravenous γ-globulin is even more effective in the treatment of Kawasaki disease than the standard four daily doses[(80)].

The prognosis for children with Kawasaki disease seems to be excellent, with about a 1% mortality[52,56)], down from 3 to 4% in 1975[(49)]. However, the unknown long-term implication of coronary artery disease in children who have suffered from Kawasaki disease is unknown. There has been some early enthusiasm for the correction of coronary artery lesions, and coronary artery bypass grafting has been undertaken, especially in those patients with severe ischemic evidence, such as S-T-wave changes, myocardial infarction, myocardial failure secondary to ischemia, aneurysm rupture, and angina[(75)]. However, the fact that many of the aneurysms apparently resolve and can be followed accurately with two-dimensional echocardiography, coupled with the overall good prognosis of the disease, indicates that conservative management is appropriate, although long-term follow-up is necessary.

Lyme Disease

Lyme disease is a tick borne illness caused by the spirochete *Borrelia burgdorferi* borne by the tick *Ixodes*[(79A).] The illness was first reported in 1975 in Lyme, Connecticut and consists of carditis, arthritis and meningitis[(79B)]. It is now the most common vector borne disease in the United States. It is prevalent in the northeast United States, Minnesota, Wisconsin, and parts of California, Oregon, Texas and Nevada. The vectors in these regions are *Ixodes dominidiae mini* and *I. pacificus.* Cases of Lyme disease have been reported in nearly all 50 states and also in Europe, the former Soviet Union, and Asia. The most common association of Lyme disease in children is the acquisition from deer ticks that have been attached to the human for greater than 48 hours.

Clinical Course

The clinical manifestations of the illness consist of erythema chronicum, migrans, carditis, meningitis and arthritis. Several clinical stages of Lyme disease have been categorized **(Table 13.2).** Localized erythema migrans comprises Stage I which is characterized by an erythematous macula or papule at the site of the bite. Within one to three weeks, the lesion begins to expand with a central clearing. Erythema chronicum migrans may occur at this time and may occur anywhere on the body with the thigh, groin, and axilla most frequently involved. The lesions are usually asymptomatic. Multiple lesions may develop in the first few days. Conjunctivitis and a malar rash may also develop. The patients may have only mild symptoms of lethargy and fatigue, occasional headaches, fevers and chills. Some patients have also been reported to have lymphadenopathy, encephalopathy, splenomegaly and hepatomegaly. The erythrocyte sedimentation rate is elevated in approximately half of the patients and the serum IgM in approximately a third of the patients. Elevated liver enzymes may also be found. The spirochete can be isolated from the skin lesions in this early stage but serologic evidence of infection is rare. This stage usually resolve within the first four weeks with or without treatment.

The stage of disseminated infection (Stage II), can occur in untreated children several weeks to months after tick exposure. The musculoskeletal system is most frequently involved (60%), followed by the central nervous system (10%) and the cardiovascular system (8%). Neurological manifestations may occur as early as 4 weeks into the illness. These include headaches and meningismus, occasionally associated with cranial or peripheral neuropathy. Facial palsies, both unilateral and bilateral, are the most common cranial nerve manifestations. Peripheral neuropathies include motor, sensory and mixed neuropathies. Rarely, Guillain-Barre syndrome, pseudotumor cerebri, cerebellar ataxia, and other manifestations may also occur. Spinal fluid studies have revealed that the spirochetes can be retrieved from the CSF.

Cardiac disease occurs in 4 to 10% of affected children in North America and usually arise by five to six weeks of illness[79C)]. The signs and symptoms include varying conduction abnormalities including first degree AV block, Wenckebach, complete heart block and other sinister conduction abnormalities. Inflammatory heart disease including pericarditis, dilated cardiomyopathy, and a clinical picture mimicking myocardial ischemia may be the primary manifestations. In a review of Lyme carditis by Ciessielski and colleagues[(79D)] from the Center for Disease Control and Prevention, the authors found 19% with conduction abnormalities, 10% with myocarditis and 5% with left ventricular failure. The cardiac manifestations usually resolve by the end of the second month.

Table 13.2. Clinical Stages of Lyme Disease

Stage I	Cutaneous manifestations
	Easy fatigability
	Erythema chronicum migrans
	Malar rash
	Conjunctivitis
	Lymphadenopathy (occasional)
	Elevated Erythrocyte sedimentation rate
	Elevated liver enzymes
Stage II	Disseminated infection
	Myalgias
	Headaches
	Cranial neuropathies (e.g., facial palsies)
	Peripheral neuropathies
	Cardiac involvement (conduction abnormalities, pericarditis, myocarditis)
Stage III	Persistent infection
	Chronic (sometimes progressive) arthritis
	Chronic CNS involvement

Arthritis can occur as early as a week and as late as two years after the onset of the illness. Children who are HLA-DR2 positive manifest a more severe arthritis than those who are not. Most commonly, children present with migratory arthralgias which can progress to arthritis of the larger joints. The signs and symptoms of musculoskeletal involvements may persist for many years or may recur frequently.

Stage III, the stage of persistent infection, occurs rarely in children and only in a minority of adults. The primary morbidity of the chronic stage is progressive arthritis with damage of the joints and disability. Other manifestations may also include chronic central nervous system involvement.

There have been reports of congenital disease in mothers who have had Lyme disease during pregnancy. The neonates have presented with meningoencephalitis and cardiac abnormalities. The patients in these reports have died during infancy. The precise nature of the congenital infections is unknown.

Diagnosis and Treatment

Both diagnosis and treatment rely on a high index of suspicion and recognition of the signs and symptoms of Lyme disease. In addition to the history and findings of erythema chronicum migrans, an elevated sedimentation rate and a positive ELISA for *Ixodes* may be helpful in determining the diagnosis. However, the ELISA test is not yet standardized and false positives and false negatives are common. Serologic tests for Lyme disease are often negative early in the course. Erythema chronicum migrans and other symptoms may resolve with treatment with erythromycin, penicillin, and tetracycline.

The primary treatment for the disease should be prevention by reducing tick exposure, or removing ticks on children as soon as possible. Early medical treatment with tetracycline may prevent subsequent progression and late manifestations of the disease[(80a)]. High dose intravenous penicillin for 2 weeks; tetracycline in doses of 40 mg per kg per 24 hours (maximum 1 g per day) for a 10 to 20 day course; amoxicillin (30 mg per kg per 24 hours) for 10 to 30 days; ceftriaxone 50 mg/kg (maximum 2 g. per day) for 2 to 4 weeks; or, chloramphenicol for two weeks, should effectively treat the borreliosis and produce resolution of most symptoms. Central nervous system involvement and stage II of Lyme disease may require intravenous therapy. Ceftriaxone may provide better therapy than penicillin because of its penetration across the blood brain barrier (2 g IV per day for two weeks). Chronic, persistent infection in stage III requires prolonged therapy with IV penicillin or ceftriaxone, PO tetracycline or amoxicillin. Response to therapy is slow and not completely satisfactory.

Trauma

Another instance where ischemia may result from excessive demand and result in myocardial infarction is that of head injury. Certainly, head injury, subarachnoid hemorrhage, and elevated intracranial pressure have been demonstrated to cause ST-T-wave changes on the ECG that are consistent with myocardial ischemia[81]. It has also been frequently shown that myocardial CPK levels are elevated in children after head injury and cerebral vascular injury, thus indicating myocardial damage in this setting[82,83]. In addition, Wetzel and Rogers[84] in an echocardiographic study in the Johns Hopkins pediatric intensive care unit (PICU) have shown that both left and right ventricular function are impaired significantly in children with isolated head injury. This study showed that the more severe the head injury, the more impaired was ventricular function, as indicated by both shortening fraction and systolic time intervals. Pathologic studies have further confirmed this picture of ischemia, injury, and functional impairment by demonstrating areas of myocardial infarction, especially subendocardially, in patients after head injury as well as in experimental animal models[85,86].

Head injury causes a rather accentuated autonomic response with direct sympathetic cardiac stimulation and enhanced levels of circulating catecholamines[87,88]. One theory concerning the ST-T-wave changes is that they represent abnormalities in ventricular repolarization, not ischemia[89]. Another theory is that these changes are actually caused by ischemic injury[90,91]. In head-injured patients with marked autonomic responses, $M\dot{V}O_2$ would be expected to increase along with elevated heart rate, increased contractility, and increased afterload. This increased demand could lead to relatively insufficient perfusion, if severe enough. As mentioned above, high levels of catecholamines per se seem to lead to myocardial necrosis, possibly through this mechanism[47]. The relationship of this phenomena to neurogenic pulmonary edema is interesting, although poorly delineated. It seems clear that ischemic myocardial injury can occur with head trauma and should be suspected in those children ill enough to require intensive treatment.

Myocardial injury also frequently occurs in the setting of thoracic trauma[92], though the incidence is lower than that in adults[93]. Radionuclide angiography has revealed myocardial dysfunction in 74% of chest trauma victims[94]. This is frequently not accompanied by abnormalities on the ECG (28% abnormal) or an increase in the CK-MB enzyme (8% abnormal)[92,93]. Several forms of injury can accompany chest injuries, including myocardial contusions, myocardial concussion (commotio cordis), valvular damage, rupture, and coronary vascular occlusion, and frequently the diagnosis is missed[92,95,96]. The long-term results include myocardial scarring, arrhythmias, and ventricular aneurysms. Although direct myocardial injury occurs, some have speculated that coronary vascular lesions result in trauma-associated damage[97,98]. Certainly, traumatic coronary artery aneurysm occurs, and the authors have seen acute coronary occlusion after trauma (Fig. 13.6). In the setting of trauma, unexplained hemodynamic compromise should suggest the possibility of myocardial damage or ischemia. Electrocardiography, enzyme tests, and echocardiography may provide useful diagnostic information, but it seems that radionuclide angiography is the most sensitive test to discover traumatic myocardial dysfunction[92,94].

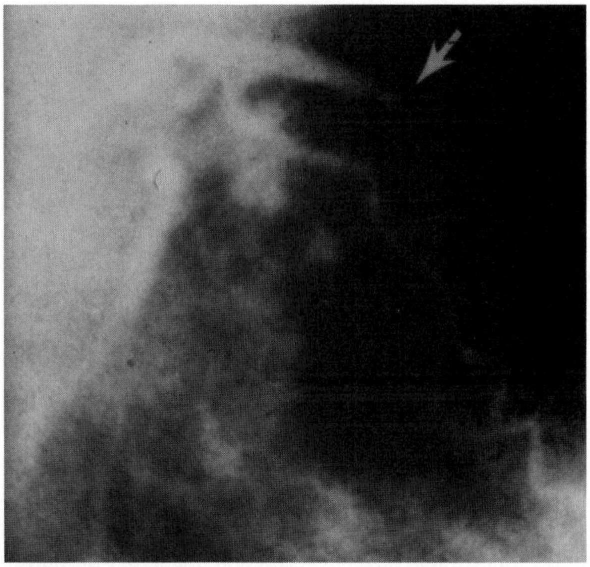

Figure 13.6. Coronary angiogram in a child admitted to the pediatric ICU with hypotension, ECG S-T-wave depression, and chest pain. Note the abrupt occlusion of the left anterior descending coronary artery, which is the branch most commonly occluded. (From Sutherland GR, Calvin JE, Driedger AA, Holliday RL, Sibbald WJ. Anatomic and cardiopulmonary responses to trauma with associated blunt chest injury. J Trauma 1981;21:1.)

Other Causes

Ischemic changes also occur in a host of other pediatric settings but are unusual. In a recent report of 292 autopsies in children from 2 days to 16 years of age, 6 cases of coronary artery disease (2 of children 2 days old and 1 each of children 6 weeks, 3 months, 6 years, and 16 years old) were determined to be a significant cause of death[99]. This coronary artery disease was generally caused by an inflammatory arteritis or coronary thrombosis, which had hitherto been unsuspected in these children and was only diagnosed postmortem. They concluded that 2% of children have significant coronary artery disease, which may indeed lead to death. Coronary vascular disease can be caused by various arteritides, including infantile periarteritis, progeria, lupus erythematosus, diabetes, and idiopathic coronary artery aneurysms. In addition, children with familial hyperlipidemia, especially type II, are at great risk for the early involvement of the coronary arteries by disease[35,100]. Unusual causes of myocardial ischemia continue to be reported. One such case chronicles coronary sinus thrombosis caused by a central hyperalimentation, a complication that leads to myocardial infarction by elevating coronary venous pressures and reducing coronary perfusion[101]. A remaining cause of acute infarction with myocardial ischemia in children may be related to the apparently increasing incidence of atherosclerotic coronary vascular disease in the younger population[35,100].

The occurrence in infancy of fatty streaking and early atheromatous plaques in the aorta, coronary vessels, and carotid is so well documented as to leave little room for doubt. The progression of these early atheromatous lesions seems to be certainly related to the development of atherosclerotic coronary artery disease in later years. In a report of autopsy studies of men who died in accidents, Strong and Magill (1968) stated that all subjects older than 20 years had demonstrable coronary vessel atherosclerosis[102]. Although the fact that atherosclerosis occurs in infants has been known since 1891, what has been less clear is its contribution to morbidity and mortality in children[103]. Numerous reports since then have described teenagers who suffered ischemic cardiac symptoms and died suddenly with advanced coronary atheromatous disease occluding coronary vessels at postmortem and associated with myocardial infarction[103,104]. Although the presentation of children with ischemic heart disease, per se, is extremely uncommon, the presence of significant atheromatous disease should be considered as a compromise of the coronary supply that may be critical to the increased demands of oxygen by the myocardium in critically ill children.

Cocaine and its derivative "crack" are widely used by people of all socioeconomic levels, including intentional or accidental use or exposure by infants and children. Cocaine abuse prenatally by the mother has also been shown to produce cardiovascular problems for the infant[105]. Ventricular hypertrophy (RVH and LVH) occurred in a significant number of these children, who also were at higher risk for having atrial septal defect, patent ductus arteriosus, or ventricular septal defect. Some infants also had conduction or rate disturbances, e.g., sinus tachycardia, ventricular ectopy, ventricular tachycardia, prolonged QT_c interval. In older patients, the persistent sympathomimetic and vasoconstrictive effects of chronic cocaine abuse may induce hypertension or coronary artery spasm, leading to cardiac arrhythmias, myocardial infarction, or sudden death. The pathogenesis of ischemic heart disease may include one or a combination of the following: nonatherosclerotic intimal proliferation of smooth muscle, obstructive platelet thrombosis, or microfocal fibrosis of the myocardium, which have been observed at necropsy[106].

Therapy for Ischemic Heart Disease

Although the management of IHD in children has been reported only rarely, there is no reason to suspect that the recommended therapy would differ from that of adults. Routinely increasing inspired oxygen content and improving the respiratory status are indicated. Hct and volume status should be optimized to ensure adequate oxygen delivery, blood viscosity, and the optimal balance between patients who are "too dry" and therefore have increased systemic vascular resistance and patients who are "too wet" and therefore have increased left ventricular end-diastolic pressures and volumes with a consequent increase in $M\dot{V}O_2$. Arrhythmias should be controlled because of their deleterious effect on both myocardial oxygen demand and delivery (see Chapter 15). β-Blockade has been shown to be beneficial in the postinfarction patient and in patients with chronic myocardial ischemia and should be considered. Afterload reduction, by decreasing both systemic and pulmonary vascular pressures, is definitely beneficial and should always be considered in patients with IHD. Not only is cardiac workload decreased, but filling pressures are decreased with a consequent decrease in wall tension. The concomitant increase in cardiac output, which may occur in the face of reduced $M\dot{V}O_2$, may be ideal. Both nitroglycerin and sodium nitroprusside may be beneficial. The added potential for coronary artery dilatation with nitroglycerin bears noting. The use of anticoagulants and lysis of clots where they exist has received much attention and may be of value in acute coronary artery occlusion[107]. In neonates with transient ischemia, conservative therapy is generally successful, although heart failure should be treated[108].

It should be remembered that all inotropic agents increase $M\dot{V}O_2$ and, thus, can potentiate ischemic lesions. Calcium channel blockers (e.g., nifedipine) have been of value in adults with vasospastic disease and intractable angina. These conditions are rare in children, and the indications for calcium channel blockers in children are unclear. Surgical therapy of occlusive coronary artery lesions in children has been reported in Kawasaki disease[81]. Correction of underlying congenital heart diseases from the anomalous origin of the coronary arteries to underlying structural anomalies is obviously required when indicated.

Conclusion

Although IHD remains an uncommon illness in children, we have become increasingly aware of the potential for its occurrence in critically ill children because of a wide number of causes. Consideration of the factors that determine myocardial oxygen balance under both normal and disease conditions will indicate that children are at special risks for developing IHD as well as suggest guidelines for their therapy. Awareness of the possibility of myocardial ischemia and designing therapies guided by these general principles should reduce the likelihood of the critical care physician worsening an already grave situation by impairing myocardial oxygen balance.

PULMONARY EDEMA

Definition

Pulmonary edema may be defined as the accumulation of abnormal amounts of fluid and solute in the extravascular spaces of the lung. This nonspecific statement can be given pecific dimensions by evaluation of patients with pulmonary edema. Fluid studies have been conducted in normal adult humans during life as well as in autopsy specimens from adults either with normal lungs or with pulmonary edema. The normal lung is about 50% blood by weight during life and has one of the highest water contents of any organ (80%)[109]. **Table 13.3** shows that the lungs of patients dying in acute pulmonary edema are more than twice the predicted normal weight and the increase in water content is nearly 300%. The ratio of extravascular water to blood-free dry weight is doubled in comparison to normal weight, and the dry weight itself is increased because of protein in edema fluid. The mechanisms by which these changes occur require a review of structure and function in the normal and abnormal lung.

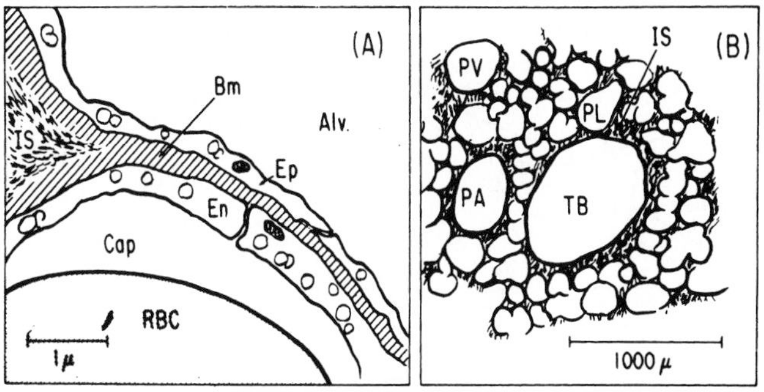

Figure 13.7. Anatomy of water and solute exchange in terminal lung units. In A, abbreviations are: *Alv,* alveolus; *Bm,* basement membrane; *Cap,* capillary; *En,* endothelium; *Ep,* epithelium; *IS,* interstitial space; and *RBC,* red blood cells. In B, abbreviations are: *IS,* interstitial space; *PA,* pulmonary artery branch; *PL,* pulmonary lymphatic; *PV,* pulmonary vein branch; and *TB,* terminal bronchiole. (From Robin ED, Cross CE, Zelis R. Pulmonary edema. N Engl J Med 1973;288:239, 292 (2 parts).)

Anatomy

The movement of fluid from the vascular bed to the alveolus is not the simple transfer between two compartments. There are at least four anatomic compartments: (a) the vascular compartment, (b) the interstitial compartment, (c) the alveolar compartment, and (d) the pulmonary lymphatic compartment (Fig. 13.7)[110].

The vascular compartment not only includes pulmonary capillaries but also includes small pulmonary arterioles and veins[111,112]. The vascular compartment is bound by the endothelial cells of the capillaries, which have a basement membrane separating it from the interstitial connective tissue. The capillary endothelium is relatively permeable to water and small ions, compared with alveolar epithelium.

The interstitial compartment can be thought of as both a defined space and a potential space. The defined space is proximal to alveolar ducts and contains small discrete structures, such as pulmonary arterioles, veins, airways, and lymphatics. As pointed out by Robin et al.[110], a "potential" space also exists if there is separation of the epithelium of the alveolar pulmonary capillaries from the basement membrane to which they are normally attached. As an example, pulmonary edema fluid can cause a separation between the epithelium and the basement membrane and can accumulate in this "potential" space.

In the alveolar compartment, the alveolus has a wall composed of alveolar epithelial cells that separate the air space from the lung interstitium. This wall is largely composed of an epithelium of type I cells. In addition, type II cells, considered responsible for surfactant production, are found in areas of juncture of alveolar septa. The alveolar epithelium itself is lined by a lipoprotein layer of surfactant. Characteristically, the alveolar epithelium is relatively impermeable to fluids and solutes, even those of relatively low molecular weight.

The pulmonary lymphatic compartment represents the extensive lymphatic drainage system of the lungs that exists largely in the connective tissue surrounding the capillaries. When abnormal amounts of fluid accumulate in the alveolar spaces or in the interstitium, they can be drained by these small lymphatic channels into larger pulmonary lymphatic channels that are distant from the alveolar space.

Table 13.3. Human Lung Tissue and Fluid Compartments[a]

	Normal		
Compartment	*Postmortem*	*In life*	*Acute pulmonary edema*
Total wet lung weight (g)	672	977	1642
Total dry lung weight (g)	129	188	216
Lung wet weight/lung dry weight	5.2	7.6	
Blood content (g)	195	500	342
Blood-free wet lung weight (g)	477	477	1300
Blood-free dry lung weight (g)	94	154	
Extravascular water content (g)	383	1145	
Extravascular water/blood-free dry lung weight	4.0	7.4	

[a] *Adapted from Staub NC. Pulmonary edema. Physiol Rev 1974;54:678.*

Physiology

Although the 1970s and 1980s saw the development of progressively more complex models of water and solute movement across the lung, the traditional principles of Starling[113] are still a good place to begin the discussion of the physical factors determining fluid accumulation in pulmonary edema:

$$\dot{Q} = K_f[(P_c - P_i) - \sigma(\pi_c - \pi_i)] \quad \text{(Eq. 13.1)}$$

where $\dot{Q}$ is the net rate of flow across the surface area of capillary, K_f is the capillary filtration coefficient, P_c is the hydrostatic pressure in the capillary, P_i is the hydrostatic pressure in the interstitium, π_c is the oncotic pressure in the plasma, π_i is the oncotic pressure in the interstitium,

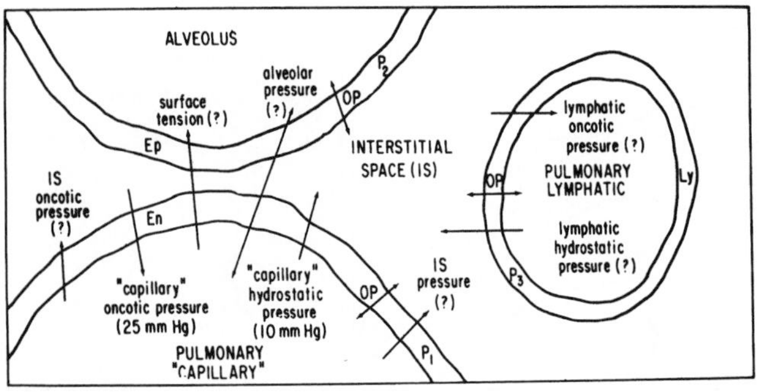

Figure 13.8. Physical forces of liquid exchange in terminal lung exchange unit. P_1, P_2, and P_3 refer to permeability of the indicated cellular membranes to water and solutes; *OP* refers to osmotic pressure across the indicated layer; and *En, Ep,* and *Ly* refer to capillary endothelial, alveolar epithelial, and lymphatic endothelial cellular layers, respectively. *Arrows* show the vectorial direction of the indicated forces. (From Robin ED, Cross CE, Zelis R. Pulmonary edema. N Engl J Med 1973;288:239, 292 (2 parts).)

and σ is the reflection coefficient, which is a measure of the ability of the pulmonary capillary to prevent protein from the plasma crossing the capillary endothelium such that if it equals 0, there is no restriction, and if it equals 1, restriction is absolute.

In normal patients, the hydrostatic pressure in the pulmonary capillary (P_c) is gravity dependent and, when measured with a pulmonary artery catheter, ranges from 8 to 12 torr[114]. The hydrostatic pressure in the interstitium (P_i) is estimated as −10 torr[115]. The colloid oncotic pressure in the plasma (c) is normally 25 torr and, in the interstitial fluid (i), 10 to 15 torr. As a result, this balance of forces in the steady state means that there is continuous filtration of a relatively small amount of fluid out of the vascular space. Because of the relatively low rate of formation of this fluid and the relatively impermeable nature of the alveolar epithelium, this fluid does not enter the alveolar space but is drained from the interstitial space by the lymphatics. A summary of the dynamics involved in this process is shown in Figure 13.8. Note, however, that in this figure there are several additional forces noted beyond those identified in the traditional Starling's equation. Pleural pressure is identified because it fluctuates during respiration and can be significantly subatmospheric during inspiration, particularly in the face of upper airway obstruction (as is discussed in the section), Croup, Epiglottitis, and Pulmonary Reexpansion. Surface-tension forces are also a theoretical influence on pulmonary edema formation because this force could result in fluid flow from the vascular bed directly into the alveolar space. Finally, lymphatic oncotic and lymphatic hydrostatic pressure may also be important. This is a complex area under active investigation since the 1980s, and it is not possible to give a brief summary of this work. Nevertheless, it is clear that there is, even in normal circumstances, a continuing drainage of lymph and that pulmonary edema occurs when the capacity for adequate lymph drainage is exceeded.

Sequence of Formation

The sequence of formation of pulmonary edema conceptualized as the progress from interstitial edema to alveolar flooding is shown[116] in Figure 13.9. It is clear from this picture that as the rate of accumulation of fluid in the interstitium exceeds the capacity of the lymph to remove it, perivascular and peribronchial edema causes swelling of the interstitial space. This is followed by the gradual accumulation of edema fluid around the alveolus, which characteristically begins in alveolar septal angles. Finally, frank alveolar fluid and florid pulmonary edema fill the alveolus, resulting in marked disturbances of the alveolar pressure-volume relationship. This, in turn, results in loss of alveoli volume, atelectasis, and increased pulmonary shunting. It is important to recognize, however, that because the hydrostatic pressure varies in different portions of the lung as a result of gravity, the patient may have portions of the lung with edema and other portions relatively normal. If the patient develops tachypnea, it is possible to have increased alveolar ventilation in normal lung units so that early in the process, pulmonary edema can cause hypoxemia with normocarbia and even hypocarbia.

A simple analysis of the Starling's equation approach to pulmonary edema would suggest that there are only two

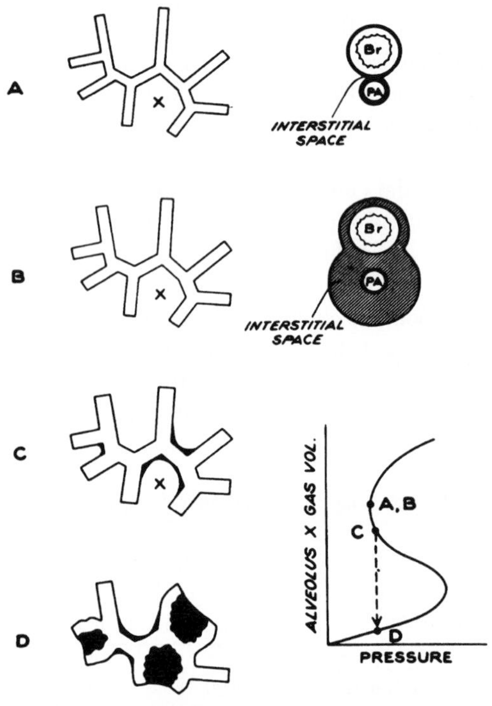

Figure 13.9. Sequence of fluid accumulation in pulmonary edema. A. Normal lung. B. Interstitial edema with fluid accumulation in the perivascular, peribronchial interstitial space. C. Early alveolar edema, which begins in alveolar "corners" and follows filling of the interstitial space. D. Alveolar flooding with a critical change in the pressure-volume relationship of some alveoli and a loss of alveolar volume. (From Staub NC, Nagano H, Pearce ML. Pulmonary edema in dogs, especially the sequence of fluid accumulation in the lungs. J Appl Physiol 1967;22:227.)

kinds of pulmonary edema: *(a)* cardiogenic-hydrostatic edema, which develops due to heart failure and increased pressure in the pulmonary capillaries; and *(b)* noncardiac edema, caused by increased permeability of the pulmonary capillaries. In traditional hydrostatic edema, the time course of fluid accumulation described above is generally slow and is related to the increased hydrostatic pressure in the capillaries. The fluid itself is traditionally thought of as low in protein[117]. On the other hand, when there is capillary endothelial injury and increased permeability, the onset of edema can be very rapid, even in the face of normal hydrostatic pressure. Naturally, the increased capillary permeability allows the leakage of large-molecular-weight compounds, and protein concentration is increased in the fluid of noncardiac edema compared with cardiogenic-hydrostatic edema. These two mechanism approaches to pulmonary edema are useful but are physiologically simplistic, as research in the field has proven. A more comprehensive approach, modified from Robin et al.[110], is shown in **Table 13.4.**

Increased Pulmonary Capillary Pressure

Increased pulmonary capillary pressure is largely produced by cardiac disease and is understandable from an etiologic viewpoint as a series of diseases that impair left atrial or left ventricular filling, left atrial or left ventricular emptying, and left ventricular muscle function. A short list of these causes is included in **Table 13.4.** The role of anthracycline toxicity-induced heart failure and pulmonary edema is discussed later in this chapter. It is also important to recognize noncardiac causes of increased capillary wedge pressure. These include occlusive lesions of the pulmonary veins from fibrosis of multiple etiologies[118–120] and from mediastinal masses, which obstruct pulmonary venous return.

Altered Permeability

The causes of altered permeability of the lung that produce pulmonary edema range from the common to the obscure. One of the most common is associated with infections such as common pneumococcal pneumonia[121] and viral influenza pneumonia[122]. These conditions result in a protein exudate in the interstitial and alveolar spaces of the lung. Recently acute respiratory failure associated with severe pulmonary edema has been reported with an outbreak of hantavirus infections in the Southwest United States. The patients developed a severe endothelial leak syndrome resulting in interstitial pulmonary edema, respiratory failure and death in approximately 40% of patients[122A]. Similar injury results from toxic inhalants such as phosgene[123], ozone [124], oxides of nitrogen[125], and prolonged high-level oxygen exposure. The relationship of oxygen exposure, the hydroxyl radical, superoxide dismutase, and arachidonic acid metabolites has been of intense interest in the 1980s and is covered independently in the next section. Circulating toxins given systematically or resulting from infections can also produce capillary leakage, and these include relatively common toxins, such as endotoxin[126], and relatively rare ones, such as scorpion venom[126A] and coral snake venom[127]. The specific relationship of direct injury, metabolic interruption, and activation of vasoactive substance remains unclear. Fat injury, ranging from experimental oleic acid administration to fat embolism, may also produce capillary leakage.

Our understanding of the role of vasoactive substances ranging from histamine to leukotrienes in the production of pulmonary edema is growing rapidly. Large numbers of disease entities, such as anaphylaxis, are now understood to involve vasoactive substances. Most current theories implicate the role of the endothelium in the production of edema[128,129;129A]. Multiple vasoactive substances produce endothelial damage that actuates activation of actin and

Table 13.4. Causes of Pulmonary Edema Based on Mechanisms[a]

Increased pulmonary capillary pressure
Systemic hypertension, aortic coarctation
Left ventricular outflow obstruction
Myocardial failure secondary to ischemia, myocarditis, high output, shunt, valvular regurgitation or obstruction, toxic antimetabolites (anthracycline)
Cortriatriatum, obstruction to or high resistance in pulmonary veins
Noncardiogenic pulmonary venous disease, such as secondary to mediastinal tumors
Altered permeability
Infectious bacterial and viral pneumonia
Inhaled toxic agents, such as phosgene, ozone, and oxides of nitrogen, and prolonged high-concentration oxygen administration
Circulating toxins, such as alloxan, snake venom, and α-naphthylthiourea
Vasoactive substances, such as histamine, kinins, and arachidonic acid metabolites, such as leukotrienes
Diffuse capillary leak syndrome, such as endotoxemia
Immunologic reactions, drug reactions, including salicylate pulmonary edema, allergic alveolitis, leukocyte sensitivity states, and blood transfusion reactions
Smoke inhalation and associated thermal injury
Disseminated intravascular coagulation
Near-drowning
Aspiration, including acid pneumonitis
Radiation pneumonia
Adult respiratory distress syndrome
Uremia
Decreased oncotic pressure
Hypoalbuminemia secondary to renal or hepatic disease, protein-losing enteropathy, or malnutrition
Lymphatic insufficiency
Congenital or acquired
Increased negative interstitial pressure
High negative pressure—croup or epiglottitis, reexpansion pulmonary edema
Mixed or unknown mechanisms
Neurogenic pulmonary edema
Heroin (narcotic) pulmonary edema
High-altitude pulmonary edema
Pulmonary embolism
Eclampsia
Hypoglycemia
Pancreatitis

[a] *Modified from Robin ED, Cross CE, Zelis R. Pulmonary edema. N Engl J Med 1973;288:239, 292 (2 parts).*

myosin filaments in capillary cells. Tumor necrosis factor (TNF) is one such substance and is a monokine produced by macrophages and monocytes. TNF exerts a variety of effects that can produce the syndrome of septic shock. Stephens and colleagues[130] recently reported that TNF significantly increased pulmonary permeability and lung edema in a guinea pig model of acute lung injury. The precise role of TNF and other specific factors such as interleukins is still being as actively debated today as it was when proposed 15 years ago. However, the net result of the action of these substances is that vasoactive endothelial contraction produces gaps and holes in the endothelial wall through which fluid and protein leak.

Specific subsets of this capillary leak pulmonary edema, such as near-drowning, uremia, aspiration, and acute respiratory distress syndrome (ARDS) are discussed in some detail in the specific chapters dealing with the disease entities producing those conditions. Some of the more important remaining entities, such as oxygen toxicity, pulmonary edema, and aspirin-induced pulmonary edema, are discussed at the end of this section.

Decreased Oncotic Pressure

Capillary oncotic pressure is dependent on plasma protein levels and may be important clinically, even in the face of normal capillary hydrostatic pressures. Patients with protein-losing enteropathies, hepatic failure, starvation, and other forms of malnutrition that produce decreased plasma levels of protein and decreased plasma capillary oncotic pressure are all at risk for developing pulmonary edema.

Lymphatic Insufficiency

The vital role of lymphatic drainage in maintaining fluid balance in the lung makes it immediately apparent that abnormalities in lymphatic drainage dramatically raise the likelihood of pulmonary edema. Experimentally, if the pulmonary lymphatic drainage is obstructed, pulmonary edema does develop[131]. In patients, pulmonary lymphangitis or obstruction may produce a similar picture, and this has been of potential importance in a number of conditions, including lung transplantation[132].

Increased Negative Interstitial Pressure

Increased negative interstitial pressure is a particularly interesting theoretical possibility of significant importance in pediatrics. Travis et al.[133] used this theory to explain the development of pulmonary edema in children with croup and epiglottitis. In Chapter 11 of this book, the influence of pleural pressure on cardiovascular function is reviewed. Specifically, the hemodynamic effects of the Müller maneuver (inspiration against a closed glottis) are discussed, and the implications for epiglottitis and croup are evident [134]. Another variety of this physiology with clinical applications is reexpansion pulmonary edema. In this condition, rapid reexpansion of a lung collapsed with pneumothorax can result in pulmonary edema[135]. Both of these subjects are covered elsewhere in this chapter.

Mixed or Unknown Mechanisms

The variety of conditions associated with pulmonary edema is virtually endless if it is remembered that in the multiple system failure common in seriously ill patients, metabolic, nutritional, cardiac, pulmonary, and infectious complications may all result in pulmonary edema. Nevertheless, there are a number of conditions recognized to be associated with pulmonary edema with interesting postulated mechanisms. A number of these conditions are listed in **Table 13.4**, and some of the specifics of a few of the conditions most important to the intensivist are discussed in the following section.

Important Causes of Heart Failure and/or Pulmonary Edema in the Pediatric Intensive Care Unit

Anthracycline Cardiotoxicity

Of the various causes of heart failure that produce pulmonary edema but that are not related to congenital heart disease, perhaps the most important for the intensivist associated with an institution that has a referral base for children with cancer is anthracycline cardiotoxicity. Anthracycline antimetabolites doxorubicin (adriamycin) and daunomycin are commonly used antitumor agents, and both can cause bone marrow suppression and cardiotoxicity. Early signs of anthracycline cardiotoxicity are generally changes on the ECG that can be transient. On the other hand, cardiomyopathy is a serious, dose-dependent, life-threatening complication[136,137].

Postmortem examination of patients dying in heart failure from anthracycline toxicity reveals a dilated, flabby heart with mild ventricular hypertrophy, without endocarditis or coronary artery disease. The most important findings are microscopic evidence of degeneration characterized by myocardial hypoplasia, myofibrillar damage, interstitial edema, and fibrosis without inflammation. Electron microscopy demonstrates significant focalized degeneration in subcellular mitochondria, sarcoplasmic reticulum, and T-tubules within 4 hours of an initial dose of doxorubicin[138]. The etiology of the cellular damage is not clear. Nevertheless, it has been suggested that doxorubicin enhances lipid peroxidation to generate superoxide radicals, the cardiotoxic effects of which can be prevented by administration of tocopherol. In animals, tocopherol inhibits cardiotoxicity but not DNA binding of doxorubicin[139]. Administration of other chemotherapeutic agents, notably bleomycin and cyclophosphamide, increases the incidence of heart disease resulting from use of anthracycline[140]. Mediastinal radiotherapy also increases the risk of anthracycline cardiotoxicity, heart failure, and pulmonary edema.

The clinical features of anthracycline-induced cardiomyopathy are nonspecific and do not differ from those of other cardiomyopathies. The appearance of heart failure manifested by dyspnea and pulmonary and peripheral edema with tachycardia and cardiomegaly are classic. This is particularly true in a patient who has received more than 500 mg of doxorubicin per square meter. Symptoms may arise at any time, up to years after the last dose of doxorubicin[(141)]. Females are 2 to 3 times more susceptible to doxorubicin induced cardiomyopathy than males[(141A)]. In addition to cardiac failure, the patient may rarely present with actual dysrhythmias, acute hypertension, and a pericarditis-myocarditis syndrome[(137)].

Cumulative dose is important because clinically apparent cardiomyopathy occurs in less than 1% of patients who receive a cumulative dose less than 500 mg/m^2. However, there is a dose-dependent relationship such that of those receiving a total dose of 500 to 600 mg/m^2, 11% develop clinically apparent cardiomyopathy. If the total dose is greater than 600 mg/m^2, this incidence exceeds 30%. Conversely, cardiotoxicity has been associated with anthracycline doses as low as 200 mg/m^2[(138)]. The frequency and rapidity of administration and the use of other chemotherapeutic agents also affect drug tolerance[(141A)]. Acute exposure to anthracyclines can impair cardiac contractility, relaxation, and compliance in isolated heart preparations. The mechanism by which anthracyclines produce myocardial dysfunction is unclear. The agents may disturb mitochondrial and sarcolemmal calcium homeostasis, cause calcium influx in the sarcolemma, and increase cytoplasmic calcium. Calcium overload can pathologically disturb normal cellular and mitochondrial functions and result in free radical generation within the cell. Furthermore, these agents cause increased lipid peroxidation and free radical generation in cardiac tissue. Thus, the myocardial damage may be the direct result of free radical toxicity[(142)]. Long-term effects of toxicity may be very serious and are increasingly recognized[(143)].

If patients with anthracycline toxicity develop pulmonary edema, a mortality rate of at least 50 to 60% can be expected; awaiting development of clinical symptoms is impractical. Diagnostic evaluation with echocardiography, nuclear imaging, and possibly cardiac catheterization may quantify the severity of involvement early in the course and avoid further administration and toxicity. Radionuclide angiography seems to be the best method for predicting clinically significant myocardial impairment in adults[(144,145)]. Its application in children, however, is difficult and therefore of limited use. Using first-pass quantitative angiography, Morgan et al.[(145)] recommended that therapy be discontinued if measured ejection function (EF) decreases more than 14%, if EF falls below 40% in patients with other risk factors, or if EF is less than 35% in patients with no risk factors.

Use of either echocardiographic or angiographic monitoring begins with baseline studies prior to anthracycline therapy and with serial measurements prior to every dose, until the cumulative dose is 250 mg/m^2. If either echocardiographic or angiographic serial measurement of shortening function (SF) is less than 20% or 35%, respectively, cessation of therapy at this point can avoid clinically significant cardiomyopathy and improve the patient's condition[(146)]. It may be possible to continue therapy to cumulative doses greater than 550 mg/m^2 in patients with no evidence of left ventricular dysfunction. Measurements of left ventricular ejection time (LVEP/LVET) are very sensitive but are nonspecific in detecting cardiomyopathy. Cardiac enzyme assays and serial chest X-rays have not been useful in prediction of cardiomyopathy.

Use of monitoring to prevent anthracycline toxicity is preferable to therapy for heart failure and pulmonary edema. Once present, however, fluid and salt restriction, diuretics, and judicious use of digitalis may be all that is required after anthracycline therapy is discontinued. When admission to the pediatric ICU is required, intensive inotropic support with dopamine or dobutamine and forced diuresis can be used. Both acute and chronic afterload reduction can be particularly beneficial. Because anthracycline cardiomyopathy may be reversible in children[(147)], intensive cardiac support including intubation and mechanical ventilation may be warranted to treat an acute episode of pulmonary edema.

Oxygen Toxicity

Although the systemic effects of oxygen toxicity can include a wide variety of physiologic alterations, ranging from paresthesias and seizures to retrolental fibroplasia, in the pediatric ICU setting the most important toxic effects of oxygen involve the lung. In this section, we review generalized lung toxicity to oxygen and oxygen-induced pulmonary edema.

It is now almost a century since Smith[(148)] described oxygen toxicity to the lung. In his original report, he described the effects of oxygen exposure as including an "embarrassment of respiration," which he said was caused by "alveoli [that] were to a great extent filled with exudate." The classic study began a century-long research interest in oxygen toxicity, which is now of use not only in critical care medicine but also in research for space and undersea exploration. This research not only has included exposure to different ambient concentrations of oxygen for varying periods of time but also has included exposures at subatmospheric and superatmospheric pressures. The generalized conclusions of these studies are that there are individual and species differences in susceptibility to oxygen exposure and that duration of oxygen exposure and absolute pressure of oxygen breathed are key determinants of oxygen toxicity[(149)]. In normal humans, exposure to 100% oxygen at 1 atm generates symptoms after approximately 12 hours. Dolezal (150) documented that exposure to very high levels of oxygen could last as long as 110 hours and yet be reversible.

As mentioned above, the pattern of pulmonary edema formation and of ultimate irreversible lung damage is species dependent. In rats[(151)], high oxygen exposure for 48 hours results in significant damage to the pulmonary capillary en-

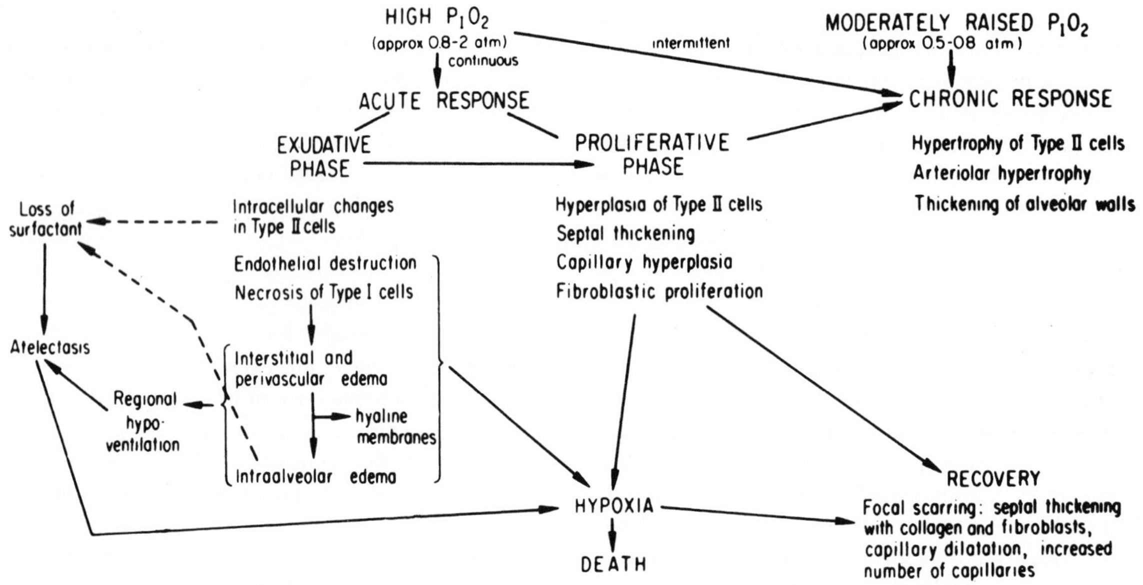

Figure 13.10. Lung response to increased oxygen exposure. Note that the response to diffuse injury is limited and not specific to the injurious agent. (From Winter PM, Miller JD. Oxygen toxicity. In: Shoemaker WC, Thompson WL, Holbrook PR, eds. Textbook of critical care medicine. Philadelphia: WB Saunders, 1984:218.)

dothelium, capillary leak as well as hemorrhage, and alveolar edema. There seems to be significant variability in individual members of species in their response, and it may be that this variability increases in higher level animals[152]. The ability of some animals to survive while others succumb to a similar insult in a matter of days is well documented. The reasons for these differences are not clear, although the general pattern of response seems similar. Early in the response to high oxygen exposure, there is an exudative phase, with capillary injury and leak resulting in pulmonary edema, which can be hemorrhagic. If there is survival of this acute phase, there is proliferation of fibroblasts and scarring. A pattern of lung response to oxygen exposure is shown in Figure 13.10, which is adopted from a review of the subject by Winter and Miller[149].

The mechanism by which oxygen produces its toxicity has been under intense investigation. Most authorities support the contention that oxygen toxicity involves oxygen radicals, which may be in the form of the superoxide anion ($O_2^{-}\cdot$), the hydroxyl radical ($OH\cdot$), or free singlet oxygen ($O_2\cdot$)[153]. It has been recognized for some time that oxygen radicals could be the cause of pulmonary damage. Two conditions have supported this hypothesis. Paraquat poisoning, whether from accident or suicidal ingestion, is known to produce lung injury, which can be exacerbated by exposure to high ambient oxygen and can be limited by exposure to low ambient oxygen concentrations. This is believed to be related to oxygen-free radical formation in the lung, where paraquat is concentrated after ingestion. A similar mechanism of oxygen-induced lung injury is thought to occur in response to ionizing radiation, which is believed to produce free radical injury. Oxygen toxicity may be mediated by cytokines released in response to hyperoxia. These agents exert direct adverse hemodynamic and hematologic effects, promote lipid peroxidation and also are potent chemotactic agents[153A]. Endothelial damage and its consequences are an early feature of oxygen toxicity. A number of investigations have tried to explain the observation that young animals are more tolerant of oxygen exposure than older animals because of their ability to scavenge free radicals[154]. Mead[155] indicated that lipid membranes, such as those found in the lung, are composed of polyunsaturated fatty acids that are particularly susceptible to hydrogen abstraction, resulting in the formation of fairly stable free radicals. In the presence of oxygen, however, there may be initiation of a radical chain, leading to autoxidation. Furthermore, the presence of substances such as superoxide dismutase, catalase, and glutathione peroxidase protect against oxidant injury. Species with neonates that have long survival time when exposed to high oxygen concentrations have high levels of antioxidant enzyme activity. Mead concluded not only that radical formation results in lipid and other membrane protein damage but also that this process may play a role in aging.

In conclusion, it is clear that among the early clinical signs of oxygen toxicity is pulmonary capillary leakage with pulmonary edema. Furthermore, it is likely that the toxicity of oxygen is related to free radical-generated lipid membrane injury. This is discussed again in the next section, Immune Responses, Hypersensitivity, and Pulmonary Edema, because there is some overlap with the pathophysiology of pulmonary edema produced by the oxidative products of arachidonic acid and other mediators of immediate hypersensitivity.

Immune Responses, Hypersensitivity, and Pulmonary Edema

Many allergic reactions involve the lung and include a series of cellular and biochemical events such as vasodilation, increased vasopermeability, and edema formation. Regardless of the initiating event, many allergic reactions can lead to pulmonary edema formation by this mechanism. A full review of immunology is not appropriate in this section, but it is clear that when immunoglobulin E (IgE) antibody and an antigen interact on the surface of a mast cell, many vasoactive substances are released. As can be seen in Figure 13.11, it is now believed that this mast cell activation results in primary mediator release and release of prostaglandin D_2 and results in the activation of other cell types. It is now believed[156] that mast cell activation results in secondary release of leukotriene and other oxidative arachidonate metabolites from pulmonary interstitial mononuclear cells.

The importance of activation of the lipoxygenase pathway production of leukotrienes in the production of pulmonary edema in response to allergic reactions can be understood on the basis of some new work on the effect of leukotriene D_4 (LTD_4) on the production of pulmonary edema. Using a rabbit model, Farrukh et al.[157] demonstrated that LTD_4 had direct effects on pulmonary vascular permeability, as demonstrated by measuring fluid conductance at four different levels of left atrial pressure. This direct effect of LTD_4 on vascular permeability was by direct stimulation of the LTD_4 pulmonary receptor, which increased membrane fluid conductance and resulted in the production of pulmonary edema. This effect could be blocked by pretreatment with a LTD_4 receptor blocker.

It is now possible to consider that at least some of the pulmonary edema produced by allergic reactions involves IgE-mediated release of substances that activate leukotriene synthesis and release LTD_4 from pulmonary interstitial

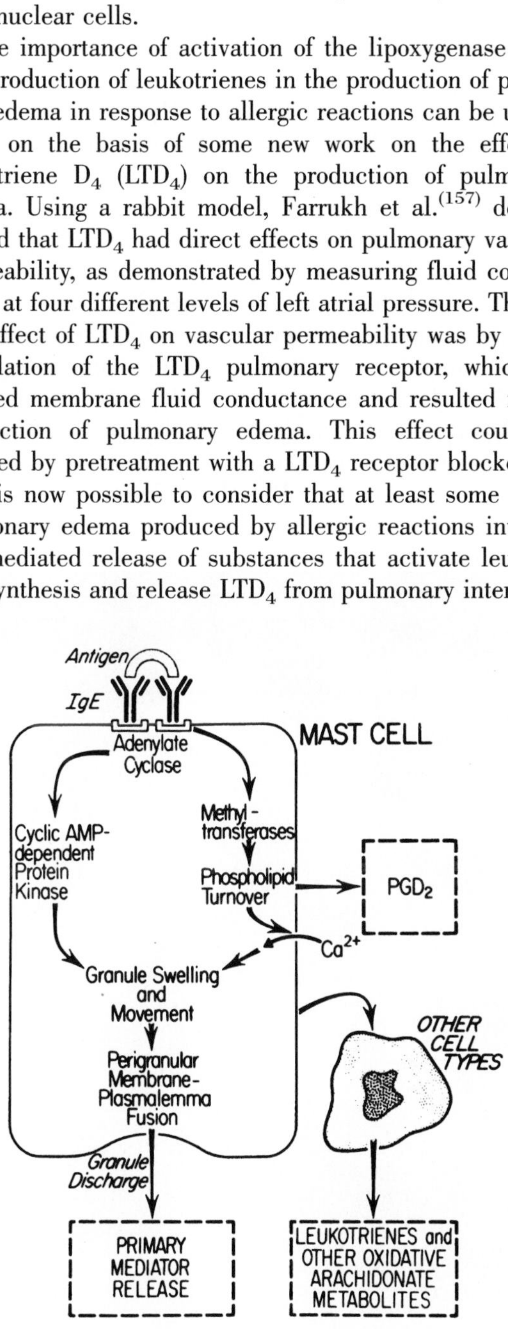

Figure 13.11. Pathway of mast cell activation-secretion to primary mediator release and arachidonic acid metabolism. Note the ultimate formation of leukotrienes. (From Lewis RA, Austen KF. Mediation of local homeostasis and inflammation by leukotrienes and other mast cell-dependent compounds. Nature 1981;293:103.)

cells. This results in increased pulmonary capillary fluid conductance and pulmonary edema. It is also possible that this may be an important mechanism in disease states such as ARDS[158]. Furthermore, arachidonic acid pathways may be activated to produce similar pathophysiologic mechanisms in pulmonary oxygen toxicity, as the results of infusion of substances such as tert-butyl hydroperoxide (t-buOOH) into pulmonary arteries have suggested[159].

Salicylate-Induced Pulmonary Edema

Scattered reports of salicylate-induced pulmonary edema have been reported for decades[160] and include reports of the syndrome in children[161]. The syndrome appears to be more common in patients over 30 years of age[162]. A review of clinical studies indicates that in adult patients with salicylate pulmonary edema, distinguishing characteristics included an acute intoxication on top of chronic administration, a history of smoking, an increased incidence of neurologic abnormalities, and proteinuria. Higher salicylate levels (greater than 40 mg/dl) were also associated with a higher incidence of pulmonary edema[160]. In a group of 36 consecutive adult patients with serum salicylate levels greater than 30 mg/dl, 8 patients developed pulmonary edema. Four of these patients had Swan-Ganz catheters placed, and none had elevated wedge pressures. In fact, mean results were a pulmonary artery pressure of 24 per 11 mm Hg, with a pulmonary capillary wedge pressure of 6.5 mm Hg, and no patient with pulmonary edema had a wedge pressure greater than 11 mm Hg. The authors of this series concluded that pulmonary edema clears in response to measures designed to lower the salicylate level.

This problem has also been examined in an experimental sheep model in which a buffered aspirin solution was infused intravenously[163]. Comparisons were made on the effects of this infusion on lung lymph flow and lymph protein concentration, with the same findings produced by mechanical elevation of pulmonary vascular pressures. As can be seen in Figure 13.12 derived from this study, salicylate infusion has actually resulted in imperceptible changes in left atrial pressure and pulmonary artery pressure but an increase in lymph protein concentration and flow. The latter result was associated with a statistically significant decrease in PaO_2. We concluded that salicylate pulmonary edema is noncardiac in origin but is a result of increased permeability to fluid and protein in the pulmonary vascular bed. Whereas general supportive measures for pulmonary edema, ranging from oxygen and diuretics to intubation and mechanical ventilation, may be needed, lowering of salicylate levels is the key ingredient in treatment.

Croup, Epiglottitis, and Pulmonary Reexpansion

In 1977, Travis et al.[133] reported two patients with pulmonary edema associated with croup and epiglottitis. The X-ray of one of the patients is shown in Figure 13.13. They postulated that there were three possible physiologic mechanisms: *(a)* a catechol-mediated shift of blood volume

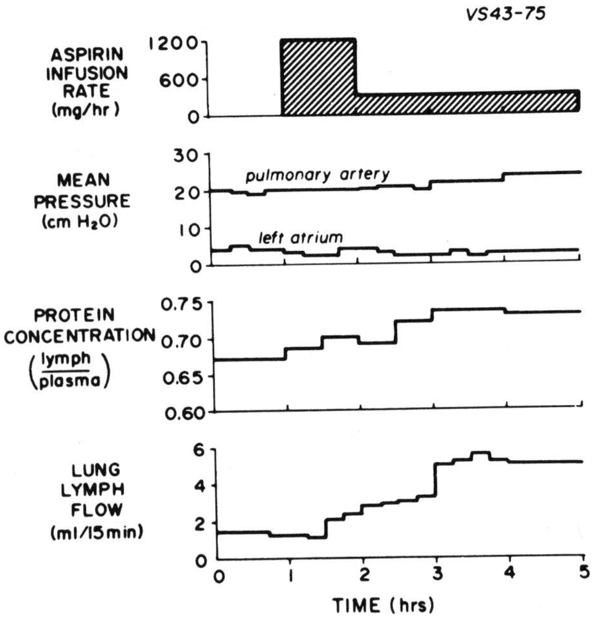

Figure 13.12. Effects of salicylate infusion on lung vascular pressures, lung lymph flow, and lymph-to-plasma protein concentration in a sheep. (From Bowers RE, Brigham KL, Owen PJ. Cardiorespiratory control. Am Rev Respir Dis 1977;115:261.)

from the systemic to the pulmonary circuit; *(b)* hypoxia-induced capillary leakage; *(c)* an increase in negative pleural pressure, resulting in an increase in the alveolar capillary transmural pressure gradient; and *(d)* negative intrathoracic pressure afterloads the left ventricle. As discussed in Chapter 11, this could result in increased flow from pulmonary capillaries into the alveoli.

Together, these changes would increase the volume of blood in the pulmonary capillaries, increase the pore size in the pulmonary capillaries, and increase the hydrostatic driving pressure of fluid into the lungs (Fig. 13.8). The authors also postulated that it was likely that the same physiology could be responsible for pulmonary edema associated with other forms of upper airway obstruction, such as chronic enlargement of the adenoids and tonsils. This same explanation has been implicated as explaining the observation that sudden reexpansion of a collapsed lung (such as in application of suction to a chest to be placed for a pneumothorax) may result in pulmonary edema[164 to 166]. Free radical damage may also contribute to the pulmonary edema associated with lung reexpansion. It has recently been reported that in rabbits, collapsed lung tissue contains decreased amounts of mitochondrial superoxide dismutase and cytochrome oxidase[167]. If this is also true in humans, oxygen radical injury would be enhanced during reoxygenation of reexpanded lung tissue.

Heroin- and Narcotic-Induced Pulmonary Edema

The need to discuss narcotic-induced pulmonary edema in a textbook on the care of children is a sad but necessary commentary on the times. It is of small consolation to note that the first report of this entity took place over a century ago in a patient who took opium by mouth[168]. When heroin was virtually the only street drug used and only a small percentage of the addicts developed pulmonary edema, it was postulated that it was not the heroin but impurities that caused the pulmonary edema. Many narcotics have now been recognized as producing the syndrome, including methadone, which is used as a heroin substitute[169].

The edema fluid in heroin overdose is virtually identical with serum proteins[170]. In fact, while heroin overdose can cause renal failure, myocardial infarction, brain infarction, and rhabdomyolysis, the lungs are the most frequent organ affected[171]. There are several mechanisms postulated for the production, but most involve the cerebral edema documented in these patients[172] and the lack of elevated wedge pressure in this syndrome. Most data suggest that the cause is not primary myocardial failure. The consensus is that narcotic-depressed respiration, caused by central nervous system hypoxia, produces a variety of neurogenic pulmonary responses. Additionally, CNS depression can cause loss of airway control and aspiration. Both of these may be implicated in the syndrome.

Patients with heroin-induced somnolence may develop pulmonary edema up to several hours after ingestion. The treatment requires intubation, ventilation, and airway control. Although narcotic reversal can be of help in arousing the patient, naloxone can cause vomiting and provoke aspiration in nonintubated comatose patients. As discussed in Chapter 39, the arousal produced by naloxone may be

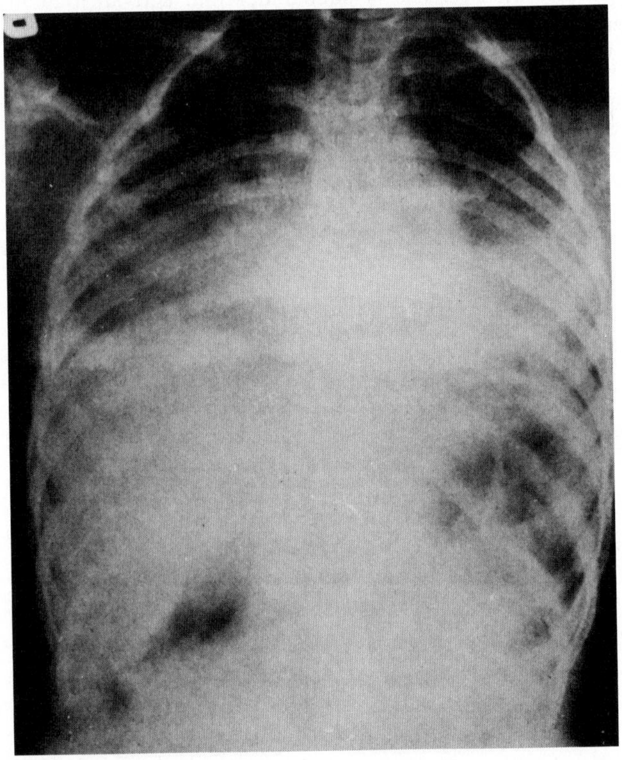

Figure 13.13. Radiograph of chest showing bilateral pulmonary edema in a patient with upper airway obstruction. (From Travis KW, Todres ID, Shannon DC. Pulmonary edema associated with croup and epiglottitis. Pediatrics 1977;59:695.)

short lived (20 minutes), and narcosis can occur again. More general approaches to narcotic overdose are also discussed in Chapter 39.

Neurogenic Pulmonary Edema

The relationship between neurologic injury and hemodynamic instability was recognized even before the description of the classic Cushing reflex, and pulmonary edema has been observed after head trauma in both adults and children[173,174].

In animals, pulmonary edema has been produced by a variety of experimental methods inducing increases in intracranial pressure. All the evidence suggests massive sympathetic discharge in the production of this neurogenic edema. Electrolytic lesions placed in the basal portion of the preoptic nucleus, or midline destruction of the periventricular system below the preoptic region of the hypothalamus, produced fulminant pulmonary edema in rats. Furthermore, animals pretreated with CNS depressants such as phenobarbital had significantly less or no pulmonary edema, compared with nontreated animals with increased intracranial pressure[175]. In addition, pulmonary edema secondary to increased intracranial pressure, like epinephrine-induced pulmonary edema, is completely blocked by pretreatment with α-adrenergic blockers[176], and cervical cord transection, which also interrupts the sympathetic pathways, is noted to abolish the phenomenon completely[177]. These experimental studies are in keeping with the clinical observations made on soldiers who died in Vietnam of head injuries but who had cervical cord transections and were not noted to have pulmonary edema.

The hemodynamic consequences of increased intracranial pressure and massive sympathetic discharge have been shown to involve marked increases in aortic, systemic arterial, pulmonary arterial, pulmonary venous, and superior vena cava pressures. When peripheral resistance increases, it causes a large shift of blood to the relatively low-resistance pulmonary circuit and an increase in pulmonary blood volume. The result is a significantly increased pulmonary vascular pressure, which may be responsible for increased pulmonary capillary permeability and exudation of a plasma-like fluid high in protein content. The hemodynamic effects have been shown to be transient in nature, lasting only 5 to 15 minutes, after which vascular pressures return to normal. Indeed, central venous and pulmonary wedge pressures measured during ongoing neurogenic pulmonary edema have been normal. A change in vascular permeability persists, however, leading to ongoing pulmonary edema in spite of these normal vascular pressures.

The mechanism of neurogenic pulmonary edema may be conceptualized as a process in which trauma, hypoxia, or increased intracranial pressure initiates a hypothalamic reflex, which results in massive sympathetic discharge. This sympathetic discharge then causes a marked but transient increase in both systemic and pulmonary vascular pressures. The result is a shift of blood from the systemic to the low-resistance pulmonary circulation. The further increase in pulmonary capillary pressure leads to capillary wall damage and increased permeability, which persists and causes ongoing pulmonary edema. As the vascular pressures return to normal values, heart failure is averted. Unfortunately, the pulmonary edema persists and can be life threatening in itself.

High-Altitude Pulmonary Edema

High-altitude pulmonary edema occurs in patients subjected to high altitude but can be reversed on return to a lower altitude or by administration of oxygen. It shares with neurogenic pulmonary edema the fact that there is normal pulmonary artery wedge pressure, suggesting lack of left ventricular failure despite documented pulmonary vascular hypertension[178,179]. There are many theories on the pathophysiology, however, and these include hypoxia-induced disruption of arteries and arterioles and hypoxia-induced increase in capillary permeability. Sympathetic nervous system discharge causing central hypervolemia is also said to be a contributing cause[180].

Treatment

With the physiologic approach to patients with pulmonary edema, it should be apparent that there may be many different approaches to the patient with pulmonary edema. For instance, chronic pulmonary edema in patients with heart disease treated with digitalis and diuretics may be compensated and may not require admission to the hospital, let alone the pediatric ICU. One of the principles of management, however, is that patients with unexplained or unusual causes of respiratory distress thought to be pulmonary edema require admission to the pediatric ICU earlier than do patients with more usual forms of cardiac failure. The reason is the rapidity with which altered permeability pulmonary edema can develop. Early observation of these patients and assessment of the rate of change in the pulmonary edema are critical to their treatment plan.

All patients admitted to the pediatric ICU require frequent assessment of vital signs. Patients should also have a chest X-ray to document baseline radiographic signs of pulmonary edema and associated cardiomegaly, if applicable. A baseline arterial blood gas should be documented. The authors emphasize that it is very useful to have samples obtained in room air, if possible, in order to evaluate the degree of intrapulmonary shunting. Samples obtained with nasal oxygen or on oxygen masks are frequently assumed to represent preset inspired oxygen concentrations, but this is very unreliable in anxious children who may have one sample with the mask on and another with the mask over the side of the face. The authors have been avoiding putting indwelling arterial lines in patients for longer periods since the advent of noninvasive oximetry, but they still believe that an indwelling arterial line for arterial blood gas monitoring is indicated if blood gases are required more frequently than every 2 or 3 hours.

In seriously ill or rapidly changing patients, particularly those who will need or already need respiratory support with positive end-expiratory pressure (PEEP) or continuous positive airway pressure (CPAP), the authors frequently employ a balloon-tipped thermodilution cardiac output catheter. The ability to measure left atrial "wedge" pressure for both diagnosis and therapy and the ability to measure intrapulmonary shunt, systemic vascular resistance, and other hemodynamic variables are often invaluable. The various catheter techniques used to measure lung water in patients with pulmonary edema have proven to be useful in the treatment of infants and children with pulmonary edema.

The primary therapy for pulmonary edema is supplemental oxygen. The use of oxygen masks that have reservoir bags (see Chapter 5) allows high levels of supplemental oxygen to be delivered. Face mask CPAP circuits may be effective. Indications for intubation include progressive hypoxemia despite supplemental oxygen, an increasing P_aCO_2, or a respiratory rate and pattern indicating the likelihood of impending respiratory fatigue. Young children out of the neonatal period who are in distress but who will not tolerate their face mask require intubation.

Intubation of patients in cardiorespiratory distress requires a knowledge of the rapid-sequence intubation techniques (Chapter 2). Once the patient is intubated, CPAP may be successful in older children who will breathe spontaneously and cooperate with medical direction. Infants and small children often require positive pressure ventilation and have a higher incidence of need for paralysis neuromuscular blockade in order to avoid inefficient ventilatory patterns. The mechanism by which PEEP works to improve hypoxemia and decrease right-to-left shunting is not by pushing fluid out of the alveoli, as originally postulated. Total lung water does not change and PEEP does not protect against increasing extracellular lung water.[180A,180B)] PEEP clearly increases functional residual capacity (FRC), expands fluid-filled alveoli, and improves compliance. The net effect is to improve arterial oxygen tension.

Specific measures beyond this clearly depend on the cause of the pulmonary edema. Cardiac failure may require digitalis, catecholamine, diuretics, and even afterload-reducing agents, depending on the specific nature of the cardiac failure. Morphine, which is used commonly in adults, is not generally used in small children as frequently because of concern about respiratory depression, although other supportive measures, such as head elevation, can be useful. The use of agents such as steroids directed at capillary permeability injury has generally not proved useful in any specific pulmonary edema syndrome and, because they may impair responses to infection, are not widely used at present. For similar reasons, the indiscriminate use of wide-spectrum antibiotics is rarely indicated because of the possibility of subsequent nosocomial infections.

Inhaled nitric oxide has recently been suggested to be useful in the treatment of ARDS[(180C,180D)]. Nitric oxide (NO), originally indentified as an endothelium derived relaxing factor (EDRF) is a naturally produced substance in the body. When administered at pharmacologic doses (5 to 40 ppm) in the inhaled gas mixture, the compound exerts a potent and selective vasodilatory effect on the pulmonary vascular bed[(180E)]. In clinical trials in neonates, NO therapy seems to result in dramatic improvement in patients with meconium aspiration and with persistent fetal circulation[(180F)]. The agent also may provide potentially significant benefit in postoperative cardiac patients that manifest elevated pulmonary vascular resistance. There are few reported adverse effects in the newborns who have received NO treatment. Because ARDS is associated with significant elevations in pulmonary vascular resistence, some investigators have used NO therapy to reduce the pulmonary resistence, improve pulmonary perfusion and thereby, to improve oxgenation and ventilation[(180G;180H)]. Clinical trials of inhaled NO treatment in pediatric acute respiratory failure outside the neonatal period are also suggest a beneficial effect of NO in this patient population[(180I)]. Children receiving NO demonstrated an acute improvement in oxygenation, lower pulmonary artery pressure and intrapulmonary shunting. Multicenter trials are under way to evaluate whether long term NO therapy will reduce morbidity and improve survival from ARDS. The possible adverse effects include systemic hypotension and methemoglobinemia which may require treatment (see below).

A point of therapy that should be emphasized is the high likelihood for pulmonary edema to develop in patients during the recovery period as the patient is weaned from PEEP or CPAP. The increased venous return, which develops as the level of PEEP or CPAP is decreased, often requires a decrease of fluid administration, diuresis, or both. Similar concerns should be expressed in critically ill patients with pulmonary edema, hypoxia, and hypercarbia who receive high levels of PEEP and CPAP. The harmful central nervous system effects of hypoxia or hypercarbia, when combined with the potential for elevated airway pressure to decrease blood pressure and increase intracranial pressure, must be considered when neurologic symptoms develop that are not explained by the degree of hypoxia or hypercarbia.

CYANOSIS

Introduction

Cyanosis is "a bluish purple discoloration of the mucous membranes and skin, because of excess amounts of reduced hemoglobin in capillaries, or less frequently to the presence of methemoglobin"[(181)]. The presence of 4 to 5 g of reduced hemoglobin per deciliter of blood is necessary to produce cyanosis. "Any state where a physiologically inadequate amount of oxygen is available to, or used by, tissue without respect to cause or degree" is referred to as hypoxia[(181)]. The presence of cyanosis is clinically significant because it implies severely decreased oxygen content of blood (hypoxemia), an important consequence of which is inadequate oxygen delivery to tissues for metabolic needs (hypoxia). A review of the physiologic causes of cyanosis is presented in **Table 13.5.** As insufficient tissue oxygen delivery is the chief concern in a cyanotic patient, it is appropriate to review the normal mechanisms of oxygen delivery first and then to consider the pathologic factors that alter the normal situation and lead to hypoxemia and cyanosis. A discussion of clinical situations associated with cyanosis and the relevant therapeutic interventions follows.

Determinants of Normal Oxygen Delivery

The supply of oxygen available to tissue beds is determined by the oxygen content of arterial blood (C_aO_2) and tissue flow ($\dot{Q}_{tiss}$. In this section, the determinants of oxygen content are addressed first, followed by a discussion on tissue flow in the normal adult.

Oxygen Content of Arterial Blood

The oxygen content of blood is dependent on several factors whose relationship can be expressed by the formula:

$$C_aO_2 = Hb \times Cap \times S_aO_2 + (0.003 \times P_aO_2) \quad \text{(Eq. 13.2)}$$

C_aO_2 is the content of oxygen in arterial blood (milliliters per deciliter). Hb is the hemoglobin concentration (grams per deciliter). Total oxygen-carrying capacity (Cap)—the amount of O_2 that can be transported by a fully saturated gram of Hb—is 1.34 ml (O_2 per gram Hb per deciliter)[182]. Experimental results suggest that this value may actually be less, ranging from 1.30 to 1.34[182,183]. The percent of Hb saturated with oxygen is represented by S_aO_2. The last value is the amount of oxygen dissolved in 100 ml of blood at body temperature (37° C) and 1 atm of pressure. This value varies directly with the partial pressure of oxygen (P_aO_2) (see below).

Table 13.5. Physiologic Causes of Cyanosis

Environmental decreased availability of oxygen
Altitude
Inhalation of nonphysiologic gas mixtures
Alveolar hypoventilation
CNS depression (e.g., trauma, drugs, infection)
Upper airway obstruction (e.g., tracheal rings, epiglottitis, etc.)
Hypotonia (e.g., CNS insults, spinal cord insults, drugs)
Restricted lung movement (e.g., diaphragmatic hernia, tension pneumothorax)
Major diffusion abnormalities
Interstitial fibrosis
Oxygen toxicity
ARDS
Pulmonary edema
Abnormalities of hemoglobin and oxygen-carrying capacity
Abnormal hemoglobin (e.g., methemoglobin, carboxyhemoglobin, sulfhemoglobin)
Alterations in oxyhemoglobin affinity (e.g., changes in 2,3-diphosphoglycerate content, pH, temperature)
Too much reduced hemoglobin (e.g., hyperviscosity)
Abnormalities of pulmonary blood flow
Congenital obstruction to heart disease with pulmonary blood flow (and/or right-to-left shunting, e.g., tetralogy of Fallot, pulmonary atresia)
Primary pulmonary hypertension
Persistent fetal circulation
Intracardiac chronic heart disease with right-to-left shunts
Hypotension
Abnormalities of $\dot{V}/\dot{Q}$ matching
Pharmacologic effects, e.g., sodium nitroprusside
Poor tissue perfusion
Shock with inadequate compensation for tissue perfusion (e.g., septic, hemorrhagic, cardiac etiology)
Impaired rheology (hyperviscosity)

Alveolar Oxygen

The process of oxygen delivery to tissues begins with inspiration. The concentration of oxygen in this air (F_IO_2) varies as it travels inward from ambient air through the upper and lower airways. The atmospheric pressure (P_{atm}) at sea level ("standard pressure") is 760 mm Hg. The fraction of this pressure that is exerted by oxygen is termed the "partial pressure of oxygen" (PO_2) and equals 160 mm Hg for inspired air (P_IO_2 = 0.21 X 760 mm Hg). As air travels through the upper airways, it is warmed to body temperature (37° C) and humidified. At 37° C, water has a vapor pressure of 47 mm Hg and comprises 6% of the air, diluting the oxygen (to 20%) and reducing the PO_2 (to 149 mm Hg). Continuing toward the alveolus, inspired air is further diluted by expired carbon dioxide in the alveolus (P_ACO_2 equals 40 mm Hg). The combined effects of this dilution result in a P_aO_2 of 104 mm Hg in the alveolus (Fig. 13.14)[182,183]. The relationships are expressed by the alveolar gas equation[184]. There are many forms of this equation, but, stated simply:

$$P_AO_2 = [F_IO_2 \times (BP - P_{H2O})] - P_ACO_2[F_IO_2 + (1 - F_IO_2)/R] \quad \text{(Eq. 13.3)}$$

where P_AO_2 is alveolar PO_2; F_IO_2 is the inspired fraction of oxygen in inspired gas, BP is the barometric pressure, and P_{H2O} is the water vapor pressure; P_ACO_2 is the alveolar PCO_2 and is approximately the same as the arterial PCO_2; R is the respiratory exchange ratio (or quotient), which has a normal value of 0.8[184].

If the atmospheric pressure changes, the partial pressure of oxygen in inspired air (P_IO_2) will also vary, while the concentration of oxygen (F_IO_2) remains unaltered. If P_{atm} decreases, P_IO_2 will decrease; conversely, when P_{atm} increases, P_IO_2 increases. The effect of changes in atmospheric pressure on P_IO_2 is shown in **Table 13.6**[183]. In addition, **Table 13.6** contains the maximum level of Hb saturation associated with various values of PO_2. It is evident from this information that significant amounts of desaturated Hb sufficient to produce cyanosis may exist in an otherwise normal individual exposed to hypobaric conditions.

The P_AO_2 is also affected by the rate of air delivery to the alveolus (ventilation). A child normally requires approximately 100 ml of air per kilogram of body weight per minute (minute ventilation or $\dot{V}$ neonates may require 150

Table 13.6. Effects on Alveolar Gas Concentrations and on Arterial Oxygen Saturation of Acute Exposure to Low Atmospheric Pressures[a]

			Breathing air			*Breathing 100% O_2*		
Altitude (ft)	*Barometric pressure (mm Hg)*	*PO_2 in air (mm Hg)*	*PCO_2 in alveoli (mm Hg)*	*PO_2 in alveoli (mm Hg)*	*Arterial oxygen saturation (%)*	*PCO_2 alveoli (mm Hg)*	*PO_2 in alveoli (mm Hg)*	*Arterial oxygen saturation (%)*
0	760	159	40	104	97	40	673	100
10,000	523	110	36	67	90	40	436	100
20,000	349	73	24	40	70	40	262	100
30,000	226	47	24	21	20	40	139	99
40,000	141	29	24	8	5	36	58	87
50,000	87	18	24	1	1	24	16	15

[a] *From Guyton AC. Textbook of medical physiology. 6th ed. Philadelphia: WB Saunders, 1981.*

to 200 ml/kg/min)[185]. An increase in ventilation will usually produce a higher P_AO_2, whereas hypoventilation can cause a reduction (Fig. 13.15). This inverse relationship is explained by the alveolar gas equation. It is obvious from the equation that the P_AO_2 rises, approaching P_IO_2, as P_ACO_2 decreases (hyperventilation). Conversely, an increased P_ACO_2 (hypoventilation) results in lower alveolar oxygen tensions (P_AO_2).

Diffusion in Alveolar-Capillary Unit

Once oxygen has been brought to the alveolus, it must diffuse into the pulmonary capillary blood before it can be transported to the tissues. The alveolar-capillary membrane across which diffusion occurs is of approximately 0.2 to 0.5 μ thickness[182]. Blood entering an alveolar capillary has a PO_2 of 40 mm Hg (P_cO_2), while the arterial PO_2 is 104 mm Hg. Oxygen diffuses along this gradient, forcing a net movement of oxygen into the capillary. Equilibrium of capillary and alveolar oxygen normally occurs within one third of the time required for blood to traverse the alveolar-capillary unit (Fig. 13.16)[182,186]. Changes in the diffusion distance (membrane thickness), gradient of arterial to capillary oxygen (P_aO_2 to P_cO_2), and/or transit time of the capillary blood can affect the transfer of O_2. This assumes that alveolar ventilation ($\dot{V}A$) and capillary blood flow ($\dot{Q}$) are closely matched; i.e., that an alveolar-capillary unit that is adequately ventilated also receives proportionately adequate perfusion ($\dot{V}_A/\dot{Q}$ matching). If capillary blood is exposed to decreased alveolar oxygen or is not exposed to O_2 at all, because of a change in the $\dot{V}_A/\dot{Q}$ relationship (intrapulmonary shunt), that blood will exit the alveolar capillary still desaturated. The contribution of each of these factors in producing cyanosis is elaborated in later sections. In general

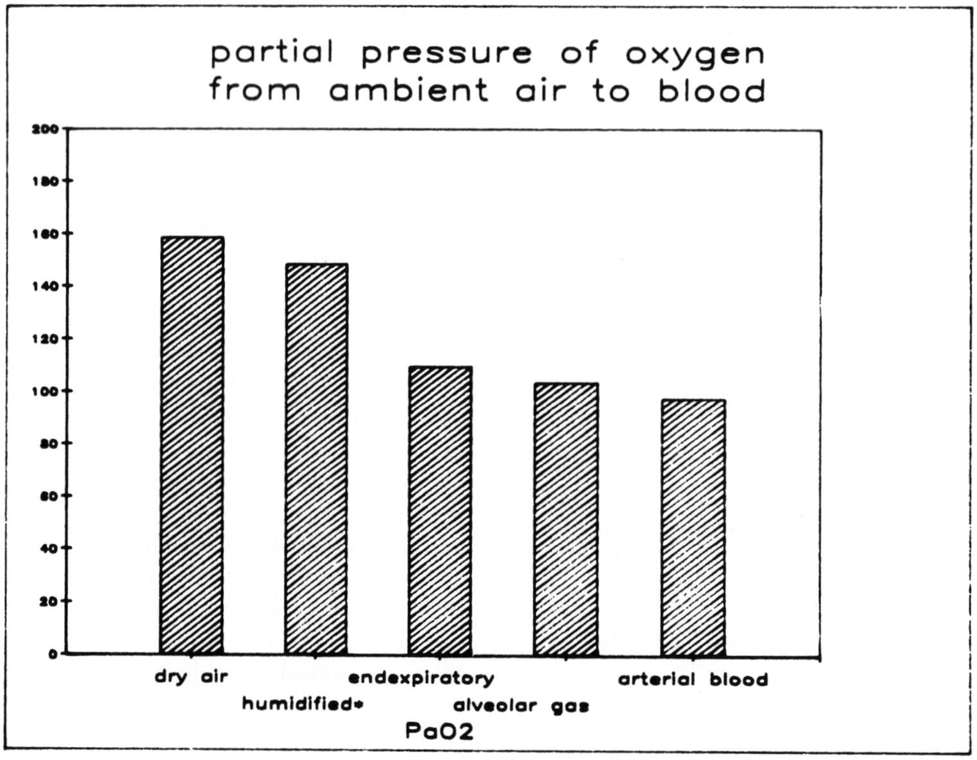

Figure 13.14. Changes in PO_2 from ambient air to blood. The slight decrease in PO_2 from alveolar gas to arterial blood is due to the effect of mixing of capillary blood with shunt blood.

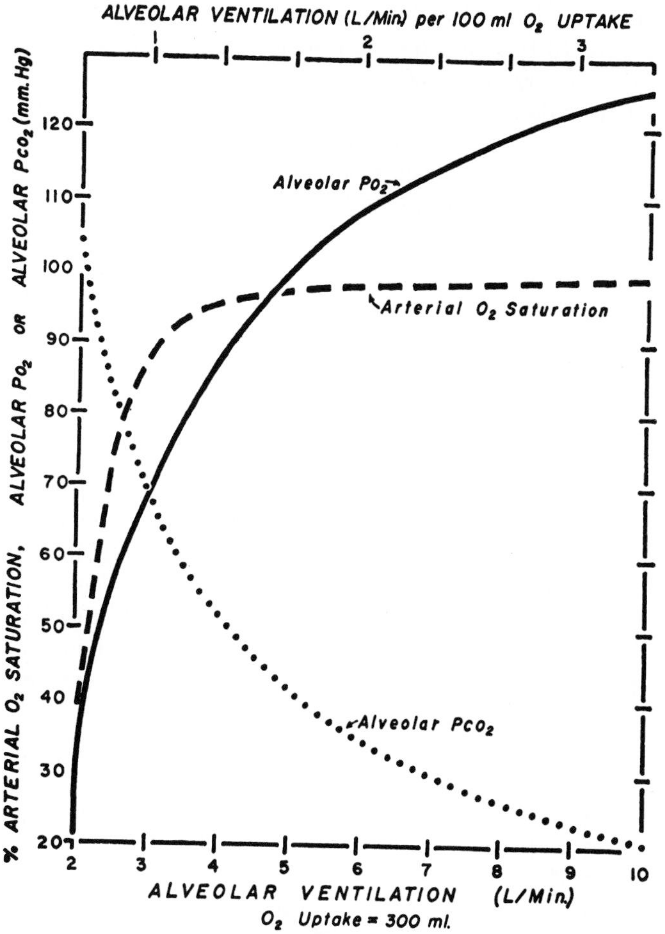

Figure 13.15. Relationship between alveolar ventilation and alveolar PO_2 and PCO_2. (From Comroe JH, Forster RE II, Dubois AB, Briscoe WA, Carlsen E. The lung, clinical physiology and pulmonary function tests. Chicago: Year Book Medical Publishers, 1955.)

hypoxemia in the PICU is a result of increased intrapulmonary shunt (low V/Q areas).

Oxygen Uptake in Blood

Once oxygen has diffused into the capillary, it must be transported in blood to the cells. This task is accomplished by binding to Hb and dissolution in blood. Binding of O_2 to Hb is determined by the PO_2 and influenced by characteristics of the Hb molecule and its biochemical environment. The classic oxygen-Hb dissociation curve defines these interrelationships (Fig. 13.17)[182,184,187]. The relationship between P_aO_2 and Hb saturation (S_aO_2) in blood is sigmoid. In the range of higher PO_2 (greater than 60 mm Hg), the curve is nearly flat. Thus, in the normal range of P_aO_2, Hb is nearly 100% saturated, and large changes in oxygen tension minimally affect O_2 saturation. Below 60 mm Hg, there is a rapid descent of the curve. Small decreases in PO_2 effect large decreases in oxygen saturation, releasing significant amounts of oxygen to the tissues, which normally have an oxygen tension of 10 to 40 mm Hg. The partial pressure of oxygen, at which half of the Hb is

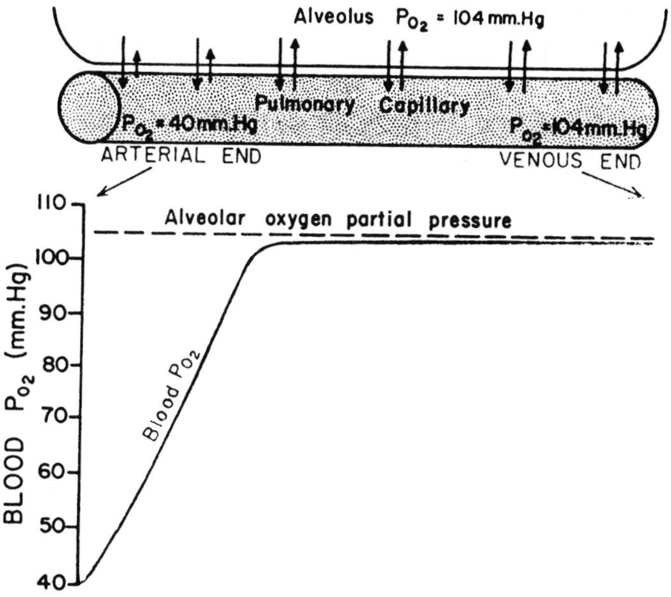

Figure 13.16. Oxygen equilibration in the alveolar-capillary unit. (From Guyton AC. Textbook of medical physiology. 6th ed. Philadelphia: WB Saunders, 1981:504.)

oxygen-bound and the other half is deoxyhemoglobin, is termed the P_{50} (26.3 mm Hg for normal adult Hb). This value is used to compare the oxygen affinities of different Hb or blood samples.

In addition to Hb-bound oxygen, blood contains dissolved oxygen (see Eq. 13.1). Normally, this dissolved O_2 contributes minimally to C_aO_2 (0.003 ml O_2 per millimeter Hg per deciliter or 0.3 ml at a PaO2 of 100 mm Hg). The amount of oxygen in solution increases as a higher P_AO_2 increases the P_aO_2. If the concentration of inspired oxygen is 100%, P_aO_2 is approximately 713 mm Hg (760 to 47 mm Hg P_{H2O}).The amount of O_2 in solution becomes 2.1 ml/dl). A subsequent elevation in ambient pressure will cause

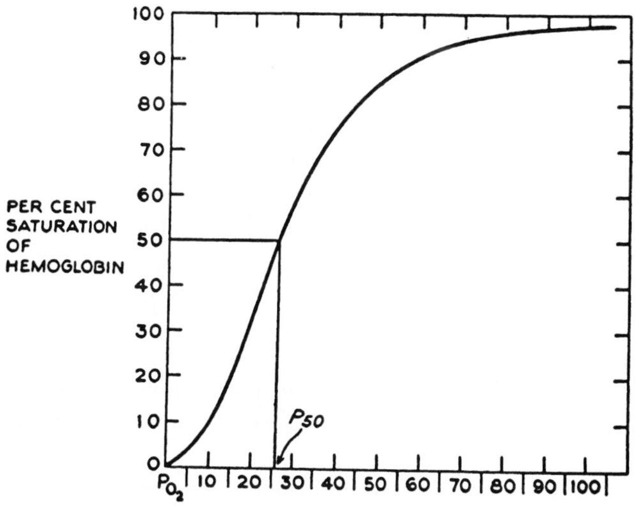

Figure 13.17. Oxygen-hemoglobin dissociation curve. (Adapted from Comroe JC. Physiology of respiration. 2nd ed. Chicago: Year Book Medical Publishers, 1974:184.)

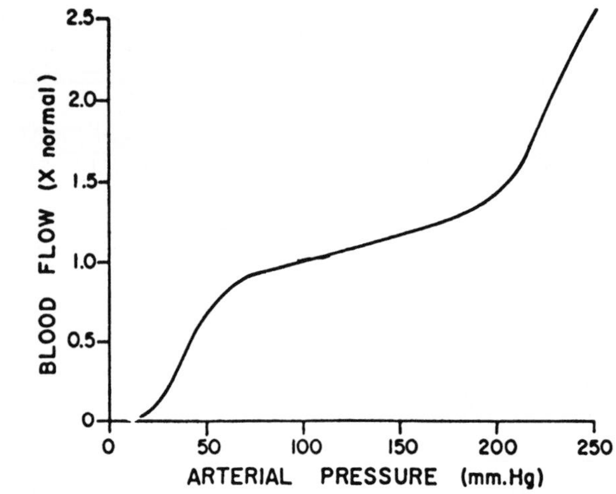

Figure 13.18. Changes in tissue blood flow ($Q\dot{Q}_{tiss}$) with changes in arterial blood pressure. (Adapted from Guyton AC. Textbook of medical physiology. 6th ed. Philadelphia: WB Saunders, 1981:236.)

more O_2 to dissolve (e.g., 4.2 ml/dl at 2 atm and 6.4 ml/dl at 3 atm).

Tissue Flow

Transport of oxygenated blood to tissue beds depends on the blood flow to the respective areas. This tissue flow ($\dot{Q}_{tiss}$) is determined by the perfusion pressure (PP_{tiss}) propelling the blood and the local vascular resistance (R_{tiss})[183,188]. The primary determinants of PP_{tiss} are inflow pressure, generally equal to mean arterial pressure (P_a), and outflow pressure, generally equal to mean central venous pressure (Pcv) which fluctuates with respiration, cardiac function, and body position:

$$PP_{tiss} = P_a - P_{cv} \qquad \text{(Eq. 13.4)}$$

These concepts are generalized for normal conditions but may vary in specific organ beds under local conditions, such as in the intracranial vault. Regardless, under normal conditions, as the mean systemic blood pressure is usually much greater than central venous pressure, one can consider PP_{tiss} directly proportional to mean blood pressure. For a given PP_{tiss}, tissue blood flow ($\dot{Q}_{tiss}$) is inversely proportional to R_{tiss}:

$$\dot{Q}_{tiss} = PP_{tiss}/R_{tiss} \qquad \text{(Eq. 13.5)}$$

Of importance is the fact that tissue blood flow is maintained well over a wide range of perfusion pressures (Fig. 13.18). This is because of the regulation of R_{tiss} by the tissue beds themselves (autoregulation). As blood pressure decreases, the resistance decreases, and changes in flow are minimized. Blood flow autoregulation in specific regions, such as in the brain, is discussed in the appropriate chapters.

Metabolic demands of individual tissue beds are a major factor in determining the local vascular resistance[183,188,189]. Changes in the requirement for oxygen, glucose, and other substances will directly alter R_{tiss} (Fig. 13.19). The primary factor is the need for oxygen. As oxygen availability decreases, tissue blood flow rises sharply. Figure 13.19 illustrates the response of tissue flow over a range of oxygen saturations of arterial blood. This autoregulation of flow results in a different amount of blood flowing to various organs, depending on the work performed by each. **Table 13.7** lists blood flow values to different organs under basal conditions. The sum of these local tissue blood flows usually determines the cardiac output. Normally, the heart plays a "permissive" role in blood flow by pumping out the venous return that it receives[183]. In fact, the venous return is merely the sum of blood entering the venous circulation from the individual tissues and is determined by their respective tissue blood flow. Thus cardiac output is linked to tissue needs.

Anatomic intrapulmonary shunts, which divert venous blood away from alveoli, normally exist in the lungs and heart[184,190]. The bronchial vessels and Thebesian veins comprise two groups of such shunts. So-called physiologic shunts are also present in the lungs. The distribution of blood flow through the lungs may be altered, affecting $\dot{V}_A/\dot{Q}$ matching. The primary determinant of $\dot{V}_A/\dot{Q}$ matching is the pulmonary vascular response to local oxygen tension.

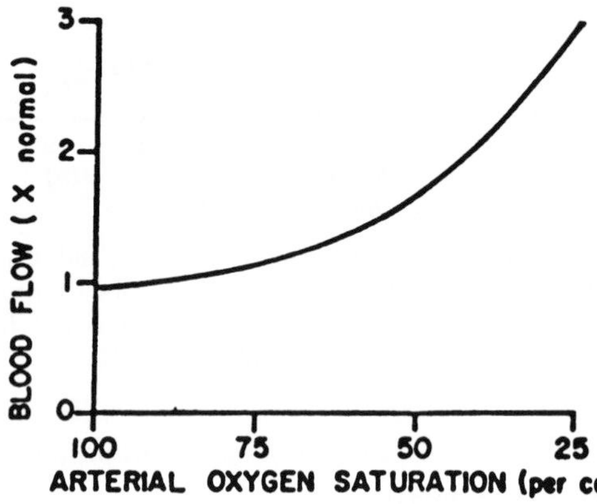

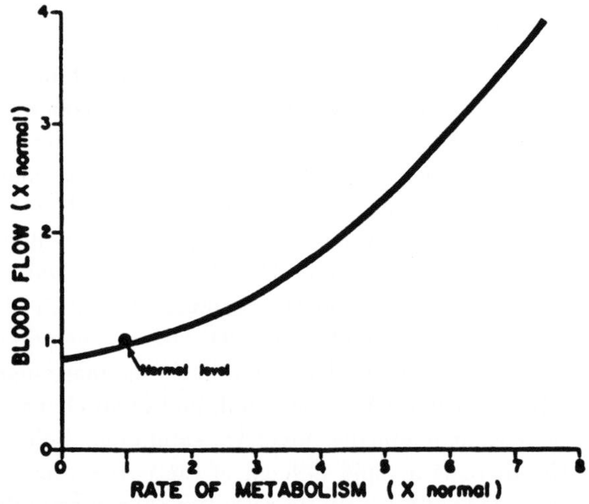

Figure 13.19. Changes in tissue blood flow with decreases in arterial oxygen saturation *(upper graph)* and with increasing metabolic rates *(lower graph)*. *Point,* normal level. (From Guyton AC. Textbook of medical physiology. 6th ed. Philadelphia: WB Saunders, 1981:234 and 233, respectively.)

In alveolar-capillary units where P_AO_2 is low (low $\dot{V}_A$), pulmonary vascular resistance increases because of hypoxic pulmonary vasoconstriction[184,191]. The blood flow is diverted away from these low $\dot{V}_A$ units to better-ventilated alveoli, resulting in improved $\dot{V}_A/\dot{Q}$.

Factors Altering Normal Oxygen Delivery

Decreased Availability of Oxygen in Inspired Air

Oxygen in adequate concentrations and partial pressures in the inspired gases is essential for adequate oxygen delivery to tissues. A decrease in the partial pressure of inspired oxygen may cause a significant decrease in arterial oxygen content. With increasing altitude, the partial pressure of oxygen decreases while its concentration (%) remains unchanged. Therefore, arterial PO_2, which depends on the PO_2 of ambient air, will decrease as the altitude at which a person breathes increases. The changes in PO_2 of ambient air for various altitudes is listed in **Table 13.6.** Similarly, inhalation of nonphysiologic gas mixtures, such as automobile exhaust, will decrease the PO_2.

Hypoventilation

Hypoventilation may cause a reduction in P_AO_2 by delivering less oxygen to the alveolus than is needed to meet metabolic demands. Clinical situations that are associated with hypoventilation[192] include:

1. Upper airway obstruction from choanal atresia, meconium aspiration, laryngeal or tracheal web, vascular rings, and tumors and masses of the neck, including adenotonsillar hypertrophy.
2. Central nervous system depression from sedative medications (such as phenobarbital), perinatal hypoxia (with or without intracranial hemorrhage), and infection (such as meningitis or cerebral abscess).
3. Hypotonia of central or neuromuscular origin.
4. Disorders that restrict normal lung movement, such as diaphragmatic hernia or eventration, pneumothorax, lobar emphysema, hypoplastic lung, and intrathoracic tumors.

If the hypoventilation caused by any one of these conditions leads to systemic desaturation, cyanosis occurs.

Table 13.7. Blood Flow to Different Organs and Tissues under Basal Conditions (in Adults)[a]

	%	ml/min
Brain	14	700
Heart	4	200
Bronchial	2	100
Kidneys	22	1100
Liver	27	1350
Portal	(21)	(1050)
Arterial	(6)	(300)
Muscle (inactive state)	15	750
Bone	5	250
Skin (cool weather)	6	300
Thyroid gland	1	50
Adrenal glands	0.5	25
Other tissues	3.5	175
Total	100.0	5000

[a] *From Guyton AC. Textbook of medical physiology. 6th ed. Philadelphia: WB Saunders, 1981.*

Major Diffusion Abnormalities

Primary abnormalities of diffusion are extremely rare in children. Interstitial fibrosis (Hamman-Rich syndrome) is usually seen in adult patients[193] and not impaired alveolar-capillary diffusion per se. Other clinical entities commonly included under this heading are really abnormalities in the $\dot{V}_A/\dot{Q}$ relationship, in that alveolar hypoventilation is associated with a decreased alveolar surface area[182,193]. Congenital lobar emphysema, hypoplasia of a lung, diaphragmatic hernia and atelectasis in hyaline membrane disease, ARDS, and aspiration pneumonia result in reduced alveolar surface area and hamper normal oxygenation of blood because of decreased $\dot{V}_A/\dot{Q}$ ratio (increased shunt). If ventilation is significantly reduced, not all the Hb traversing the pulmonary capillaries will be saturated with oxygen. When a sufficient amount of Hb remains desaturated, cyanosis results. This can be conceptualized in another way. The ventilation/perfusion ratio ($\dot{V}_A/\dot{Q}$) of the lungs is the sum of the $\dot{V}_A/\dot{Q}$ for each area, multiplied by its fraction of the total surface area. If perfusion is unaltered, the $\dot{V}_A/\dot{Q}$ ratio may be decreased because of a decrease or an absence of ventilation to the affected alveolar-capillary unit. For simplicity, all such decreases in $\dot{V}_A/\dot{Q}$ can be considered a result of perfusion of unventilated units.

Thus, a $\dot{V}_A/\dot{Q}$ ratio of 0.5, for example, may be produced by half the lungs having a $\dot{V}A/\dot{Q}$ equal to 1.0 and by the other half having a $\dot{V}_A/Q$ equal to 0.0 [(½ × 1.0) + (½ × 0 = 0.5)]. The effect of this decrease on Hb saturation can be significant. Blood from the alveolar-capillary units with $\dot{V}_A/\dot{Q}$ equal to 1.0 will be fully saturated (100%), whereas blood in the units with $\dot{V}_A/\dot{Q}$ equal to 0 will have the same saturation as the pulmonary venous blood entering the capillary (40%). The S_aO_2 for blood leaving the lungs can then be calculated to have a S_aO_2 of only 70% [(0.5 × 100%) + (0.5 × 40%)]. Even in the presence of adequate levels of inspired oxygen, altered $\dot{V}_A/\dot{Q}$ ratios may result in significant degrees of desaturation.

Hemoglobin and Oxygen-Carrying Capacity

The effect of Hb concentration on oxygen content (C_aO_2) is shown in **Table 13.8.** A consequence of this relationship is that an anemic patient may manifest inadequate C_aO_2 and tissue oxygen delivery in the presence of an adequate arterial O_2 and saturation. Tissue hypoxia will occur in the absence of cyanosis. An anemic patient is also susceptible to tissue hypoxia caused by significant Hb desaturation associated with low P_aO_2. Cyanotic discoloration will not occur because the patient does not have the necessary 4 to 5 g desaturated Hb.

Table 13.8. Oxygen Content of Blood at Various Hemoglobin Concentrations

Hb(g/dl)	*CaO_2 (ml/dl)*[a]
30	40.5
25	33.8
20	27.1
18	24.4
16	21.7
14	19.1
12	16.4
10	13.4
8	10.8
6	8.1

[a] *Assuming an oxygen-carrying capacity of 1.34 and 100% saturation.*

Conversely, polycythemia can produce cyanosis even in the absence of profound hypoxia. Polycythemia involves an increased number of circulating erythrocytes and an associated elevated blood volume[(194,195)]. In an adult, a Hct of 60% or greater strongly suggests the presence of this condition. In neonates who normally have high erythrocyte counts, a Hct of 65% or greater supports a diagnosis of polycythemia. The causes of erythrocytosis can be divided into primary and secondary. Primary polycythemia, or polycythemia vera, is a myeloproliferative disorder that commonly begins in middle life and is rare in the pediatric population. In the neonate with Down's syndrome or trisomy D, a transient marrow dysfunction may produce primary polycythemia[(195)]. Secondary polycythemia results from an increased production of erythropoietin or from transfusion of red cells[(194,195)]. The stimuli for erythropoietin formation include hypoxia and various endocrine abnormalities. Congenital heart defects with significant right-to-left shunts produce a chronic hypoxic state and polycythemia in the neonate and child[(190)]. Endocrine abnormalities such as congenital adrenal hyperplasia, neonatal thyrotoxicosis, and maternal diabetes are associated with an increased metabolic demand for oxygen and increased erythropoiesis and polycythemia[(185,195)]. Under normal conditions, the PO_2 in the venous circulation is approximately 40 to 50 mm Hg, and Hb saturation is reduced to 70 to 80%[(183,195)]. In the polycythemic patient, even this normal 30% desaturation provides the minimum 4 to 5 g total desaturated Hb per deciliter needed to produce cyanosis[(183)]. In the neonate with a normal Hct of approximately 60%, this is responsible for the commonly observed discoloration in the hands, feet, and skin (acrocyanosis or peripheral cyanosis).

Normal adult Hb (HbA_2), composed of two α and two δ chains, is represented by *curve A* in Figure 13.20. Production of HbA_2 commences by 24 weeks gestation and increases progressively[(194,195)]. However, the primary Hb in the fetus and newborn is Hb F (HbF), composed of two α and two δ chains, which comprises 70% of the total Hb in the neonate[(194)]. Over the first 6 months of life the concentration of HbF diminishes to negligible levels, while the concentration of HbA_2 increases. Blood containing HbF demonstrates an oxygen affinity that is less than that of HbA_2 (P_{50} = 26.3 mm Hg), as reflected by a leftward shift of the oxygen-Hb saturation curve (P_{50} = 19.2 mm Hg) (Fig. 13.20*A*, *curve A*)[(182,183)]. The sigmoid curve plateaus near 50 mm Hg PO_2 and signifies that fetal blood requires a lower PO_2 than adult blood to be fully saturated. Therefore, cells with HbF are well suited for oxygen uptake from the placental circulation, which has a low PO_2. However, the steep slope of the curve below 40 mm Hg implies that cells with HbF release O_2 less readily than those with HbA_2. Thus, fetal blood is less well suited for the task of oxygen delivery to tissues than is adult blood. The explanation for the dissimilar oxygen affinities of fetal and adult blood lies in the biochemical environment of the cells. Free HbA_2 and HbF, when studied in buffered solution, have been demonstrated to have identical oxygen affinities[(196,197)]. Within the erythrocyte, the influence of organic phosphates, particularly 2,3-diphosphoglycerate (2,3-DPG), alters these affinities. The interaction of 2,3-DPG with Hb produces a decrease in oxygen affinity[(198,199)]. The higher the concentration of 2,3-DPG in the erythrocyte, the greater the rightward shift of the O_2-Hb dissociation curve (lower P_{50}), indicating a greater amount of O_2 released for a unit change of PO_2. However, HbF is affected to a lesser degree by 2,3-DPG, and the resultant decrease in oxygen affinity is much less, producing the functional differences[(197)]. Elevation of 2,3-DPG levels in response to tissue hypoxia is discussed later.

Temperature and hydrogen ion concentration (pH) also greatly influence the oxygen affinity of Hb. An increased temperature will facilitate the release of oxygen and may be beneficial in cases of hyperthermia, with its accompanying increased metabolic demand for O_2. Lower temperatures have the reverse and potentially adverse effect. The P_{50} is reduced because of a greater affinity for oxygen, which reduces the amount of O_2 released for a given change in PO_2 (Fig. 13.20)[(182,183,200)].

During states of reduced oxygen consumption, such as hypothermia, dissolved O_2 may contribute more significantly to the total oxygen content. Basal oxygen consumption is approximately 3 to 4 ml/kg body weight per minute in adults[(183)]. The requirement is decreased by 50% at 31° C (approximately 2 ml/kg/min) and by an additional 25% at 20° C (to 1 ml/kg/min)[(182)]. Thus, during hypothermia, the oxygen requirements may be satisfied in large part or solely by the dissolved O_2 (assuming a cardiac output of 100 ml/kg/min)[(190)].

In their classic work, Bohr et al.[(201)] demonstrated that the binding of oxygen is affected by changes in pH ("Bohr effect"), as reflected by the CO_2 tension in the system (Fig. 13.20). An elevated pH (alkalosis) will cause a leftward shift of the curve (lower P_{50}). The oxygen affinity increases, binding O_2 more readily. The lower P_{50} is beneficial at the alveolar level, where the pH is relatively alkalotic (7.44) and promotes O_2 binding to Hb[(183)]. In the presence of systemic alkalosis, a leftward shift of the O_2-Hb dissociation curve may compromise oxygen delivery in an ill patient. Such a state may arise with alkalosis after sodium bicarbonate administration, renal dysfunction (chloride and H^+ loss from intrinsic lesions or diuretics), or gastrointestinal disorders that cause acid loss (e.g., vomiting). A low pH (acidosis and/or acidemia) will decrease O_2 binding, increasing the P_{50} and shifting the O_2-Hb dissociation curve to the right. The effect is useful at the tissue level where the pH is normally low and facilitates release of O_2 to the cells[183]. However, in systemic acidosis, this benefit is counteracted by the reduced uptake of oxygen by acidotic blood in the lungs.

A change in the redox state of the heme iron will alter O_2 delivery by affecting oxygen content. Methemoglobin (MetHb) contains oxidized iron (Fe^{3+}), which is unable to reversibly bind oxygen[202, 203]. It is constantly formed under normal circumstances but comprises less than 1 to 2% of total Hb[194,195]. The concentration is maintained at low levels by active enzymes, NADH- and NADPH-dependent methemoglobin reductase, which reduce Fe^{3+} to Fe^{2+}, a form that can transport oxygen[194,195]. If MetHb levels rise (methemoglobinemia), cyanosis occurs. The discoloration is evident with as little as 1.5 g MetHb per deciliter, compared with the 4 to 5 g desaturated normal Hb. Methemoglobinemia may be produced by a variety of causes including a congenital defect in Hb formation (M-hemoglobinopathy)[194,203], in a defect in the reducing enzyme[203], in nitrite toxicity[204], or in exposure to other toxins[202,205,206] **(Table 13.9).** Cyanide toxicity will also result in the accumulation of MetHb. Chapter 39 includes a discussion of the pathophysiology and treatment of poisoning with cyanide.

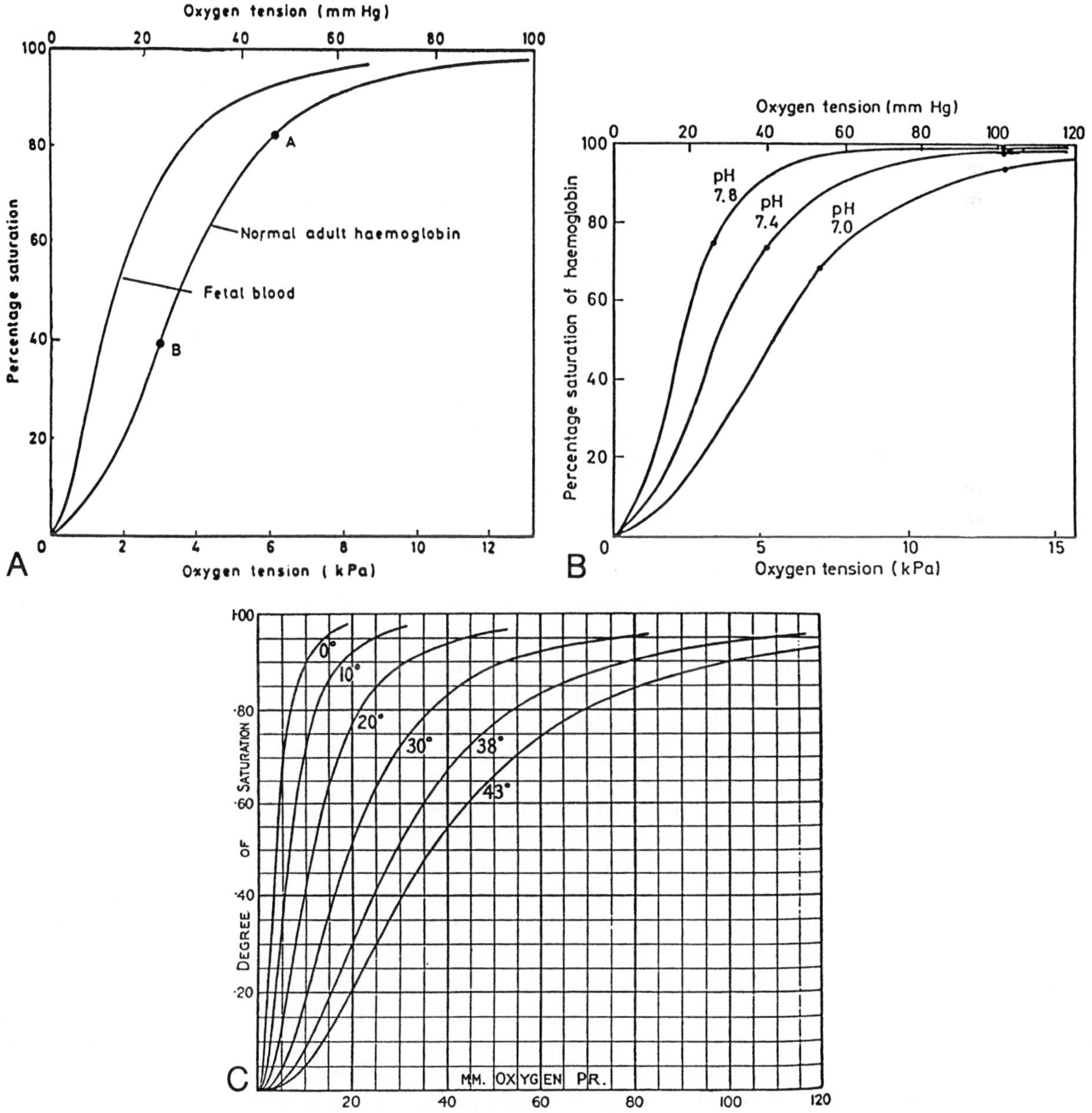

Figure 13.20. Shifts in the O_2-Hb dissociation curve as a result of fetal blood (A), hydrogen ion concentration (B), and temperature (C). (Adapted from Nunn JF. Applied respiratory physiology. 2nd ed. London: Butterworths, 1977:104; and from Barcroft J, King WOR. The effect of temperature on the dissociation curve of blood. J Physiol (Lond) 1909;39:374, 384.)

Table 13.9. Amino and Nitro Compounds Producing Methemoglobinemia[a]

Aromatic drugs	*Aliphatic and inorganic drugs*
Aniline	Sodium nitrite
Phenacetin	Hydroxylamine
Sulfanilamide	Dimethylamine
Sulfapyridine	Nitroglycerin
Sulfathiazole	Sodium nitroprusside
Phenylenediamine	Amyl nitrite
Phenylhydroxylamine	Ethyl nitrite
Nitrobenzene	Bismuth subnitrate
Dinitrobenzene	Ammonium nitrate
Trinitrotoluene	

[a] *Adapted from Finch CA. Methemoglobinemia and sulfhemoglobinemia. N Engl J Med 1972;239:470.*

Abnormalities of Pulmonary Blood Flow

A shunt that produces cyanosis is an abnormality that permits mixing of blood from the venous and systemic (arterial) circulations. Therefore, venous blood must bypass normal flow pathways to cause cyanosis. Mixing of desaturated blood with systemic blood produces variable degrees of systemic desaturation, depending on the fraction of desaturated blood. If significant portions of cardiac output are diverted through a shunt, cyanosis occurs. Shunts that produce cyanosis may be divided into those of intrapulmonary origin and those of intracardiac origin.

Intrapulmonary shunts include anatomic and physiologic pulmonary arteriovenous connections. There are normally left-to-right shunts in the lung. As an example, the bronchial circulation carries less than 1% of the cardiac output(182,183,190). However, in aortic coarctation or bronchiectasis the flow through these channels may be greatly increased(190). Potential right-to-left anatomic shunts that are normally closed are also present in the lung(182). These shunts can open and may accommodate up to 20% cardiac output during conditions of elevated pulmonary pressure and produce cyanosis(182,190). Abnormal ventilation/perfusion relationships also produce intrapulmonary shunts. Here, it is appropriate to mention flow-related phenomena that may contribute to $\dot{V}_A/\dot{Q}$ mismatching. In the alveolar-capillary unit, the relationship of alveolar ventilation to capillary perfusion ($\dot{V}_A/\dot{Q}$) is essential to any consideration of oxygen delivery (see Chapter 4). Pulmonary perfusion is matched to ventilation in an uneven manner over the surface of the lung, with an idealized summation ($\dot{V}_A/\dot{Q}$) of 1.06(182,184). The concept of matching perfusion to ventilation in this manner, as discussed in Chapter 4, is a physiologic mechanism by which different zones of the lung receive appropriate amounts of blood flow in order to ensure the maximum gas exchange across the alveolar capillary membrane. Hypoxic pulmonary vasoconstriction plays a key role in this effort by limiting blood flow to hypoxic areas of the lung, thus limiting physiologic right-to-left shunting.

Prominent factors determining appropriate pulmonary perfusion include matching of perfusion to ventilation in the alveolar-capillary unit, the transit time of blood in the pulmonary capillary, and pulmonary vascular resistance. With regard to transit time, blood traverses the alveolar-capillary unit in approximately 0.76 second, but only 0.25 second is normally required for equilibration of alveolar gas and blood. It is conceivable that an increased cardiac output and the associated decreased transit time may result in incomplete equilibration and, thus, lower P_aO_2. In the patient with normal diffusion capacity, however, the evidence is sparse for the occurrence of such an event. Normal matching of perfusion to ventilation is achieved by local hypoxic vasoconstriction. A mismatch of flow to ventilation will occur if this vasoreactivity is disturbed. Vasodilator drugs such as sodium nitroprusside, nitroglycerin, and dobutamine attenuate pulmonary vasoconstrictor response to alveolar hypoxia(207–209), leading to perfusion of poorly ventilated lung regions and hindering oxygenation of blood. If the fraction of blood thus diverted is significant, systemic desaturation and cyanosis result(207,208).

The final saturation of systemic blood depends on (a) the fraction of shunted blood, i.e., the amount of blood not exposed to ventilated lungs, (b) the oxygen content of the venous ("shunted") blood, and (c) the oxygen content of the pulmonary venous blood. If there is either low cardiac output or increased oxygen consumption, mixed venous oxygen content may be very low, and thus the impact of any given shunt will be greater. For example, a 20% intrapulmonary shunt with a venous saturation of 80% would result in 96% arterial saturation $\{[(4 \times 100) + (1 \times 80)] \div 5\}$. If venous saturation is 50%, the arterial saturation would be 90%.

Pulmonary perfusion may be compromised by inappropriate hypoxic pulmonary vasoconstriction. Hypoxic pulmonary vasoconstriction is usually localized and reversible in children and adults. In neonates and infants exposed to alveolar hypoxia, however, severe, diffuse vasoconstriction can occur in response to hypoxia(211,212). Even after the hypoxia has been corrected, pulmonary vasoconstriction and its associated reduction in total pulmonary flow may persist, producing elevated pressures in the pulmonary artery, right ventricle, and right atrium. In the neonate, if right-sided pressures become greater than those on the left, the foramen ovale and ductus arteriosus may open to produce a right-to-left shunt. This can perpetuate a pathophysiologic state termed "persistent fetal circulation (PFC)"(185,190,210). Diminished total effective pulmonary flow lowers oxygen saturation of blood and subsequently produces cyanosis.

Anatomic shunts of cardiac origin also divert blood away from the regular flow pathway. Right-to-left shunts that divert venous blood to the systemic circulation are common causes of cyanosis. These cyanotic congenital heart defects include tetralogy of Fallot, truncus arteriosus, transposition of the great arteries (TGA), tricuspid atresia, total anomalous pulmonary venous return, and single ventricle(190). In addition, admixture can also occur in the absence of pathologic intracardiac shunts when, because of obstruction to right ventricular outflow as a result of pulmonic stenosis or pulmonic atresia, increases in right ventricular and right atrial pressures cause the foramen ovale to open.

The amount of left-to-right intracardiac shunting is expressed as the ratio of the pulmonary flow ($\dot{Q}_p$) to the systemic flow ($\dot{Q}_s$). Shunt flow for a left-to-right shunt is therefore:

$$\dot{Q}_p - \dot{Q}_s = \dot{Q}_{(L \rightarrow R)} \text{ shunt}$$

When the Fick equation is applied,

$$\dot{Q}_p = \dot{V}O_2/(C_aO_2 - C_{pa}O_2)$$

where C_aO_2 and $C_{pa}O_2$ are the oxygen content of arterial and pulmonary arterial blood, respectively. Systemic flow is:

$$\dot{Q}_s = \dot{V}O_2/(C_aO_2 - C_{mv}O_2)$$

where $C_{mv}O_2$ is the mixed venous O_2 contents. When saturations are rearranged and substituted for content,

$$\dot{Q}_p/\dot{Q}_s = (S_aO_2 - S_{mv}O_2)/(S_aO_2 - S_{pa}O_2)$$

where S is now the oxyhemoglobin saturation of the respective blood samples.

For R → L, cyanotic intracardiac shunts, the Fick principle is also useful but must be modified to consider the concept of effective pulmonary blood flow ($\dot{Q}_{ep}$):

$$\dot{Q}_{ep} = \dot{V}O_2/(C_{pv}O_2 - C_{mv}O_2)$$

Pulmonary venous blood continues to be 97 to 98% saturated in the absence of an intrapulmonary shunt; thus,

$$\dot{Q}_{(R \rightarrow L)} = \dot{Q}_s - \dot{Q}_{ep}$$

and

$$\dot{Q}_{(R \rightarrow L)} = (S_{pv}O_2 - S_aO_2)/(S_{pv}O_2 - S_{mv}O_2)$$

and

$$\dot{Q}_{(L \rightarrow R)} = \dot{Q}_p - \dot{Q}_{ep}$$

or

$$(S_{pa}O_2 - S_{mv}O_2)/(S_aO_2 - S_{mv}O_2)$$

The presence and extent of admixture and cyanosis in many conditions with communications between the right and left heart may be understood by examining the ratio of pulmonary vascular resistance (PVR) to systemic vascular resistance (SVR). Normally, the SVR is several times greater than the PVR. When pulmonary resistance increases or systemic resistance decreases, blood flow may be shunted into the systemic circulation if a communication exists. These "dependent" or "dynamic" shunts can determine the level of arterial desaturation and cyanosis in conditions such as persistent fetal circulation or tetralogy of Fallot. In tetralogy of Fallot, the degree of right ventricular outlet obstruction is determined by an embryologic anomaly of the infundibulum, producing a subvalvular stenosis that can occur with pulmonic valve and/or pulmonary artery stenosis. Clinical presentation ranges from completely normal (acyanotic), because of minimal obstruction, to severe cyanosis[190,210]. Cyanosis may increase with age in patients who develop increasing obstruction as a result of pulmonary vascular changes or hypertrophy of the infundibulum. Intermittent obstruction may be caused by infundibular spasm, producing the syndrome of "paroxysmal hyperpnea." This topic, which is important in the pediatric ICU, is covered below.

Poor Tissue Perfusion Secondary to Inadequate Perfusion Pressure

In the earlier consideration of tissue blood flow, the arterial blood pressure (thus, tissue perfusion pressure) was taken as constant. As the PP_{tiss} is progressively reduced, vasodilation maintains local blood flow ($\dot{Q}_{tiss}$). Once maximum local vasodilation has been achieved, $\dot{Q}_{tiss}$ will be dependent on the perfusion pressure (Fig. 13.18). Inadequate PP_{tiss} results in insufficient flow to meet metabolic needs, a condition that occurs during congestive heart failure and in classic shock conditions. Congestive heart failure with low cardiac output, poor perfusion, and cyanosis may result from a primary myopathy, such as endocardial fibroelastosis, or numerous other causes[212]. A set of events common to the various causes may be observed. Peripheral perfusion is decreased. Increased sympathetic activity causes tachycardia and vasoconstriction of various arteriolar beds, further compromising peripheral blood flow. The net result may be a child with cool extremities, decreased blood pressure, and diminished peripheral pulses; secondary cardiomegaly may occur. If congestive heart failure is prolonged, growth delay can also ensue[190]. Because of the reduced perfusion, oxygen delivery is significantly impeded. When congestive heart failure is of moderate severity, cyanotic discoloration may be seen peripherally (acrocyanosis). More severe failure may result in systemic desaturation and "central cyanosis."

Poor Tissue Perfusion Secondary to Altered Rheology

The rheologic properties of blood normally determine the flow characteristics through the microcirculation. Blood viscosity depends on red cell deformability, the dynamics of viscoelastic fluid flow through vessels, and the influence of the individual blood components[213]. Tissue flow (and thus cardiac output) is inversely affected by viscosity. In particular, increased blood viscosity may impede flow through small vessels, which will decrease oxygen transport to the tissue[183,213]. A primary determinant of blood viscosity is the erythrocyte concentration (Hct)[214]. As shown in Figure 13.21, this relationship is nonlinear, since above a Hct of 55 to 60%, steep rises in viscosity occur with small elevations in Hct. This figure also shows the changes in O_2 delivery (reflecting cardiac output) associated with the increased viscosity. It can be inferred from the two graphs that the optimum Hct may be 40 to 45%. In the neonate,

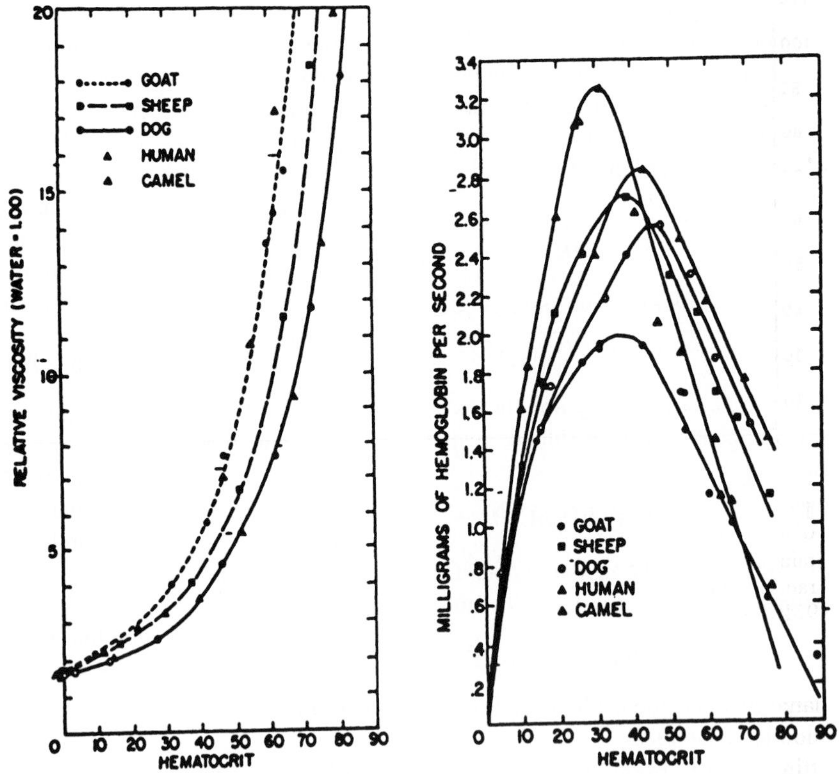

Figure 13.21. Effect of hematocrit on blood viscosity of an albumin solution *(left)* and on hemoglobin transport (oxygen delivery), which at higher hematocrits probably reflects changes in cardiac output *(right)*. (From Stone HO, Thompson HK, Schmidt-Nielsen K. Influence of erythrocytes on blood viscosity. Am J Physiol 1968;214:913.)

a significant rise in viscosity is observed above a Hct of 63%(215), and adverse effects may be observed at a Hct of 65% or greater(185,194,216).

Adaptive Changes to Hypoxia

An inadequate supply of oxygen incites multiple physiologic responses aimed at optimizing oxygen delivery. When the P_aO_2 falls below 60 mm Hg and the arterial saturation to 93%, carotid, aortic, and central chemoreceptors are activated(183,217,218). This triggers an increase in minute ventilation, which causes both the P_AO_2 and P_aO_2 to rise (Fig. 13.16)(184). Sympathetic activity is also stimulated, producing an elevated heart rate and systemic arterial blood pressure(219,220). In addition, tissue hypoxia causes a decrease in local tissue vascular resistance. Thus, tissue flow increases because of the increased tissue perfusion pressure and lower tissue vascular resistance. This results in a higher cardiac output if hypoxia is not profound and prolonged. In turn, pulmonary perfusion also increases, producing greater pulmonary capillary blood flow and increasing flow through the lungs(182,183), both of which promote oxygen uptake. In addition, distribution of systemic blood flow is affected by the sympathetic activity(183,219). Blood flow is preferentially shunted away from the muscular bed, while renal, hepatic, and cerebral flows increase.

Sustained systemic hypoxia engenders further adaptive changes geared to improve tissue oxygen availability. Minute ventilation and heart rate remain elevated and may rise further. Levels of 2,3-DPG can increase as rapidly as 24 hours after sustained hypoxia. The interaction of 2,3-DPG with Hb effects a shift of the oxygen-Hb dissociation curve to the right(198,199), which facilitates release of oxygen, making more O_2 available to the tissues for a given change in PO_2. A similar effect on oxygen dissociation is seen with a decreased pH(183,221), which is normally found in tissue capillaries. Further decreases in tissue pH may result from hypoxia-associated anaerobic metabolism and lactic acid formation, effecting a greater shift to the right.

Continued hypoxia stimulates production of erythropoietin, resulting in increased circulating Hb and red blood cell levels after 2 to 3 weeks(195,222). The elevated concentrations of Hb allow more oxygen to be transported by increasing C_aO_2 (Eq. 13.1). The polycythemia may also make the appearance of cyanosis more likely, as discussed previously. Finally, a prolonged hypoxic challenge can also induce a greater efficiency of mitochondrial oxidative systems, which optimizes cellular utilization of delivered oxygen(183,223). However, long-standing cyanosis may produce myocardial dysfunction as reflected in diminished left ventricular reserve(224).

In the adult, acute, severe hypoxia will also result in the respiratory and cardiovascular changes mentioned previously. A rapid deterioration of clinical status occurs because of depression of the myocardium and central respiratory centers, followed closely by death. In the neonate, the cardiovascular responses to acute, moderate, or severe hypoxia are different. Instead of tachycardia or increased blood pressure, *significant bradycardia and hypotension* may occur, placing the neonate at added risk(185,212).

Physiologic adaptations to hypoxia are an attempt to improve oxygen delivery and utilization. A failure of these

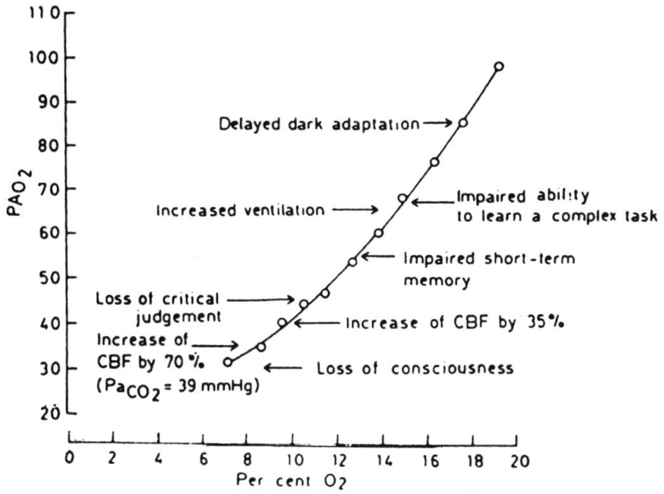

Figure 13.22. CNS responses to hypoxia. *CBF*, cerebral blood flow. (Adapted from Siesjo BK, Johannsson H, Ljunggren B, Norberg K. Brain dysfunction in cerebral hypoxia and ischemia. In: Plum F, ed. Brain dysfunction in metabolic disorders. New York: Raven Press, 1974:75.)

changes to provide sufficient oxygen for normal function is followed by malfunction of various organ systems. In this setting, bradycardia, hypoventilation, and shock result. Thus, for care of the critically ill patient it is of particular importance to understand disturbances of the central nervous system, pulmonary vasculature, kidney, and liver produced by hypoxia.

The cerebral oxygen uptake ($CMRO_2$) is approximately 3 ml O_2 per 100 grams per minute (or 45 ml O_2 per minute for an adult brain). The brain has no anaerobic metabolism and requires a continuous supply of oxygen to sustain normal function[183]. Depletion of oxygen because of any one of the previously mentioned reasons produces abnormal cerebral function. Figure 13.22 is a graphic representation of the cerebral responses to hypoxia. Impairment of short-term memory occurs at approximately P_aO_2 of 60 mm Hg. Soon thereafter (P_aO_2 of 50 mm Hg), drowsiness, lassitude, and mental fatigue are accompanied by loss of critical judgment. Euphoria, nausea, and headaches are apparent at slightly lower P_aO_2 (less than 50 mm Hg). Further decrease in arterial oxygenation (less than 40 mm Hg) produces twitching and seizures. Finally, arterial oxygen tensions less than 30 to 40 mm Hg profoundly depress the CNS to loss of consciousness (coma), which may progress to death[225] (see Chapters 20 and 21).

Renal blood flow is normally high, approximately 420 ml/kg/min **(Table 13.7).** This perfusion is required to supply oxygen for the high renal O_2 consumption necessary for tubular reabsorption. The relationship of tubular reabsorption (e.g., of Na^+) to oxygen consumption is correlated over a wide range of values (Fig. 13.23)[226]. From this figure, it can be seen that a reduced availability of oxygen reduces the reabsorptive work of the kidney. Renal oxygen deprivation from hypoxemia or ischemia significantly depresses or halts these transport mechanisms and eventually produces the pathophysiologic abnormalities of acute renal failure[183,226]. Neurohumoral responses, such as activation of the renin-angiotensin system, are also incited by ischemic hypoxia (see Chapter 37).

Liver blood supply is composed of flow from the portal vein and from the hepatic artery. The portal vein contributes blood with low PO_2[183] and comprises the larger portion (70%) of total flow. This blood perfuses first the peripheral and then the centrilobular cells, which are exposed thus to an even lower PO_2. During hypoxic conditions, hepatic arterial flow is significantly decreased[227], placing centrilobular cells at increased risk of damage and can produce centrilobular necrosis, hepatic dysfunction, and clotting abnormalities[183] (see Chapters 35 and 40).

Evaluation

The variety of clinical situations that can lead to cyanosis requires a methodical approach for efficient evaluation of the affected patient. In a sense, that is one of the purposes of the entire book. An extremely shortened conceptual approach is all that can be presented here, however.

History

A history is important not only for detection of congenital defects but also for beginning the process by which a decision is made regarding whether or not the current episode is an acute problem, a chronic problem, or both. A history of cyanotic congenital heart disease does not ensure that the current episode of cyanosis is solely a result of that heart disease and not to an episode of aspiration. Even cyanotic

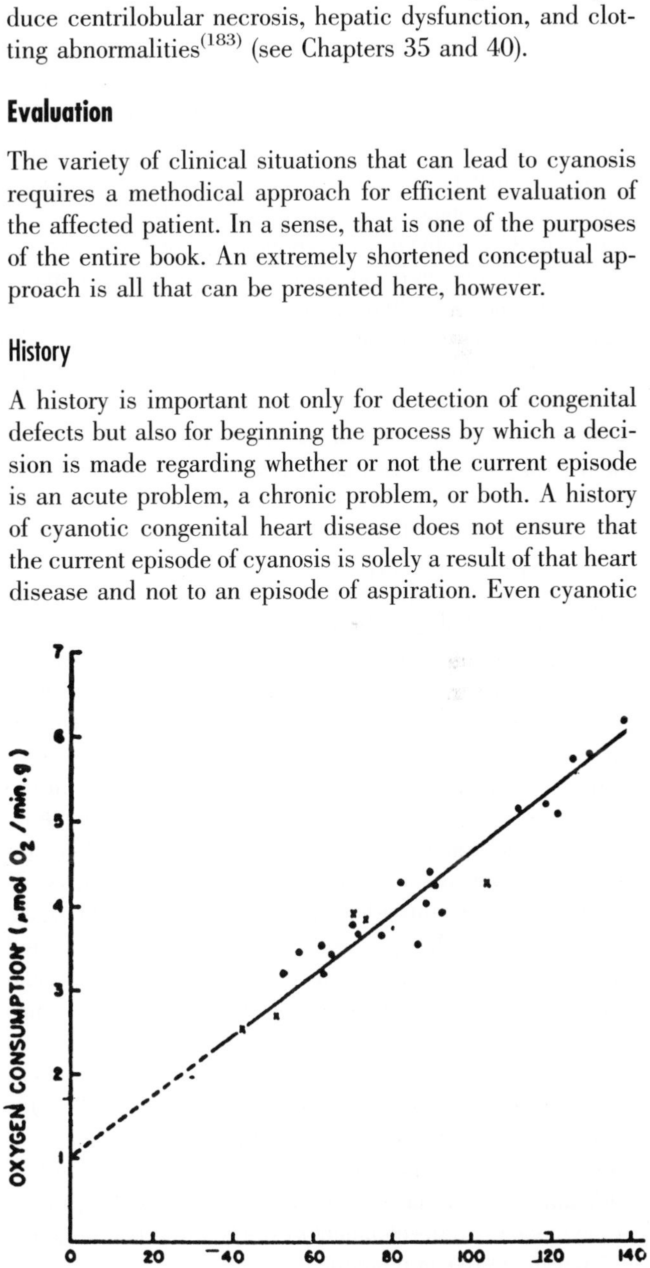

Figure 13.23. Relationship of renal oxygen consumption and tubular reabsorption of sodium. (From Thurau K. Renal Na-reabsorption and O_2-uptake in dogs during hypoxia and hydrochlorothiazide infusion. Proc Soc Exp Biol Med 1961;106:714.)

children ingest poisons, for example. The history in a patient with obvious cyanosis from pulmonary disease may seem irrelevant if the patient looks as if he or she has pneumonia, but a history may reveal an underlying immune deficiency or other additional cause of the cyanosis.

Each section of this book includes detailed chapters that explain how CNS disease, heart disease, pulmonary disease, gastrointestinal disease, and other diseases can cause cyanosis. The history is vital if the intensivist is to be effective in understanding the underlying cause of the cyanosis in addition to its symptomatic treatment.

Physical Examination

Physical examination can often clarify the reason for the cyanosis. The presence of gastric contents in the nostrils or pharynx suggests aspiration. This may be the primary cause of the cyanosis or may be secondary to it. Cyanosis with hypotonia, apnea, or bradypnea is commonly associated with CNS disorders caused by asphyxia or infection, with neuromuscular disease, or with effects of pharmacologic agents. Clubbing of the digits indicates hypoxia of several months duration. Signs of progressive hyperviscosity include plethora, lethargy, tachycardia, tachypnea, grunting, and retractions. More dramatic evidence of the polycythemia-hyperviscosity syndrome is the presence of nonspecific neurologic abnormalities as well as arterial or venous thromboses, including those in intracranial sites(215,216).

The respiratory pattern may be of help in diagnosing the cause of cyanosis. Tachypnea, use of accessory muscles, retractions, stridor, and grunting are usually manifestations of pulmonary pathology. Nasal obstruction can produce a snorting respiratory sound; laryngeal obstruction is frequently associated with inspiratory stridor; and bronchial and lower airway obstruction can produce expiratory wheezing. However, localization of the obstruction is sometimes difficult in the neonate, who may show similar signs in the presence of many causes of airway obstruction. Asymmetrical chest movements may occur because of bronchial obstruction, pneumothorax, diaphragmatic injury, or mass lesions. Inadequate muscular effort and air movement suggest a neuromuscular disorder or drug effect as the cause of the cyanosis. No monitoring equipment in the pediatric ICU can substitute for a physical examination in detecting findings of this type.

The cardiac examination may suggest the cause and extent of cyanosis(190,212). Rate, location, and characteristics of precordial impulses, intensity of pulses, and blood pressure in the upper and lower extremities should be noted. Although tachycardia is common in patients with cyanosis of any cause, the development of bradycardia is a prognostic sign suggestive of profound cyanosis. A shift of the maximal impulse may occur as a result of ventricular hypoplasia or hypertrophy related to valvular or septal abnormalities or as a result of cardiac malposition (dextrocardia). The presence of a murmur may also indicate congenital heart disease, but it is important to remember that right-to-left shunts by themselves do not produce murmurs, since the flow required would be incompatible with life. This fact is important in certain disease states, such as profound respiratory failure in the neonatal period when an enormous ductal flow producing a massive right-to-left shunt is inaudible. The specifics of cyanotic spells are covered at the end of this section.

Examination of the abdomen may be diagnostic(192). A scaphoid contour indicates that abdominal contents have possibly been displaced into the thorax because of diaphragmatic herniation. Bowel sounds heard on auscultation of the chest add further support to this diagnosis. Hepatomegaly is suggestive of congestive heart failure as the cause of the cyanosis.

Although not commonly remembered, examination of the musculoskeletal system may be vital in the evaluation of a patient with cyanosis. Fractured bones, particularly long bones, can produce fat emboli, which can clearly occur in children. Thromboembolism is generally more frequent in adults than in children, but pulmonary emboli also occur in children and have resulted in patients with cyanosis in our pediatric ICU.

Central Nervous System causes of cyanosis are well known but are not always considered. Isolated head trauma can produce both CNS-induced pulmonary edema and intrapulmonary shunting from alterations in neural control of the matching pulmonary ventilation and flow (see the chapter on CNS trauma).

Cyanotic Spells

Children with cyanotic congenital heart defects, particularly with tetralogy of Fallot, may develop an alarming complication known by various names such as "cyanotic spells," "paroxysmal hyperpnea," "tet spells," "hypoxic spells," "anoxic spells," "blue spells," or "syncopal episodes"(228,229). These episodes are characterized by paroxysmal hyperpnea and increased cyanosis. Patients often proceed to exhibit limpness, generalized stiffness, and rolling back of the eyes. Systemic acidosis accompanies these attacks(229,230). Occasionally, convulsions, cerebral vascular accidents, and/or death may also occur. In the early stages, a patient may spontaneously assume the squatting (or knee-chest) position in order to alleviate the symptoms(228,229). Patients range in age from 1 month to 12 years, with the peak incidence occurring in patients between 1 and 3 months of age. Although the paroxysms may occur at any time, the majority occur in the morning, usually on awakening(228,229). The duration of an episode ranges from minutes to several hours, with most lasting 15 to 60 minutes. Several factors precipitating the attacks have been identified. Most commonly, these are crying, defecation, and feeding(229). There seems to be no correlation between the resting arterial PO_2 and the incidence of the attacks.

Several causes have been suggested for the episodes, including spasm of the pulmonary infundibulum(231,232), acute rises of pulmonary vascular resistance (PVR)(190), and sudden decreases in systemic vascular resistance (SVR)[190,231]. Regardless, the result is an increased ratio of PVR to SVR with a decrease in pulmonary blood flow relative to systemic flow. In a normal person, hyperpnea is associated with a reduced P_aCO_2, an elevated P_aO_2, and an increased output from both the left and the right ventricle. In patients with decreased pulmonary blood flow, including those with tetralogy of Fallot, the response is altered. Although the cardiac output increases and systemic venous return also rises, the pulmonary flow can decrease. This results in a greater oxygen demand, an increase in PCO_2, a decrease in P_aO_2, and acidosis. Medical responses to cyanotic spells are covered in the section of this chapter dealing with therapy.

Laboratory Tests

Laboratory tests should complete the evaluation of cyanotic patients. Elevated Hb and/or Hct suggests the possibility of polycythemia[185,215]. In infants and children, polycythemia may be secondary to hypoxia of cardiac, pulmonary, or other cause. An elevated or depressed white cell count, with or without an increase in immature forms, implicates infections. A sample of blood drawn from a patient with suspected MetHb can be placed on filter paper and exposed to air. The blood will appear chocolate brown after a few minutes[202].

Serum or blood glucose and calcium levels should be determined. Hypoglycemia is defined as blood glucose of 40 mg/dl in infants older than 4 days[185]. However, between birth and 3 days of age, levels of less than 20 mg/dl on two determinations in premature infants and 30 mg/dl in term infants are considered to be indicative of hypoglycemia[186,233]. Calcium levels are normally in the range of 10 mg/dl; the ionized calcium is approximately 5 mg/dl. At levels less than 3 to 4 mg ionized calcium, the patient may display symptoms of hypocalcemia, including cyanosis[185,212].

Arterial blood gas determinations provide important information concerning the etiology of cyanosis. The P_aCO_2 is usually decreased in cyanosis of cardiac origin because of hypoxia-triggered tachypnea in the presence of normal gas exchange. Pulmonary disease associated with cyanosis indicates respiratory failure, which results in a normal or elevated P_aCO_2 despite the associated tachypnea. Most often, cyanosis is associated with hypoxic conditions and low P_aO_2. Commonly, in hypoxia due to hypoventilation or pulmonary disease, inspiration of 100% oxygen elevates the P_aO_2 significantly (greater than 100 to 150 mm Hg). In the case of congenital cardiac defects, the response to 100% inspired O_2 may be minimal because of the effects of right-to-left shunts[234,235]. Cyanosis may also be present in the face of a normal P_aO_2. This apparent paradox occurs *(a)* in patients with polycythemia because of the desaturated blood normally present in the venous circulation and *(b)* in patients who have suffered smoke inhalation with carboxyhemoglobin elevation (see Chapter 44). Of particular concern is the effect of carboxyhemoglobin and MetHb on the oxygen saturation of Hb (S_aO_2) determined by pulse oximetry. Pulse oximetry has become a routinely used tool for monitoring the arterial oxygen saturation and, in most circumstances, accurately correlates with the hemoglobin saturation as measured by co-oximetry. However, in the presence of carboxyhemoglobin and MetHb the S_aO_2 may be falsely and significantly elevated, thus masking the presence of hypoxemia[236].

X-rays of the chest may provide extremely valuable information. Both anteroposterior and lateral X-rays should be obtained. Symmetry of the lung fields should be noted. Classic signs of pneumothorax, pulmonary parenchymal disease, lobar emphysema, or hyaline membrane disease may be apparent[204]. A bowel gas pattern in the chest and a "gasless" abdomen point to diaphragmatic hernia. An elevated diaphragm is seen with eventration. Evaluation of pulmonary blood flow should be conducted to determine whether it is elevated or decreased. This can be extremely helpful in differentiating certain cardiac lesions. The cardiac silhouette may prove helpful in the diagnosis of congenital heart disease in a cyanotic patient. A normal-sized heart with a cocked-up apex (couer-en-sabot or boot shape) caused by right ventricular dominance is the pathognomonic sign of tetralogy of Fallot. Commonly, the mediastinal shadow is narrow, the pulmonary vascular markings are decreased, and a right aortic arch is present in 25% of cases.

An ECG should be obtained on all cyanotic patients. Most patients with cyanosis of noncardiac etiology are expected to have a normal ECG[190,192,234]. However, a child with upper airway obstruction or chronic hypoxia from other causes may develop cor pulmonale, which would manifest as right-axis deviation and right ventricular strain and hypertrophy. A prolonged Q-T interval is observed in hypocalcemia. A decrease in body temperature less than 30° C induces lengthening of all time intervals—R-R, P-R, QRS, Q-T; and "J-point deflections" may be obvious in the mid-precordial leads[190].

The use of the echocardiogram has been increasingly useful in patients with cyanosis. It has, of course, been instrumental in the diagnosis of anatomic causes of heart disease. It has also been used, with increasing sophistication, to localize and to quantitate shunts.

There are, of course, an unlimited number of tests that can be performed on cyanotic patients. In this era of concern about medical costs, we must be conscious that the history and physical examination must determine which laboratory tests are indicated.

Therapeutic Considerations

The appearance of cyanosis in the neonate or in a child of any age must be considered an emergency. While a search for the cause is being conducted, supplemental oxygen should be administered to all patients. The presence of respiratory failure, confirmed by a low P_aO_2 and elevated P_aCO_2, requires the institution of ventilatory support, usually in the form of endotracheal intubation and mechanical ventilation (see Chapter 5).

Cardiac Considerations

Successful management of congestive heart failure requires prompt identification of the underlying cause. In the interim, the patient should be resting in a semisitting position. Supplemental oxygen should be administered, and ventilatory support should be instituted as dictated by the clinical evaluation. Total fluid intake is usually restricted. Most patients with congestive heart failure also require pharmacologic treatment. Digoxin administration improves myocardial performance and yields a higher cardiac output[(211)]. Guidelines and dosage schedules are presented in **Table 13.10.** Careful and regular monitoring of the ECG, serum levels of digoxin and electrolytes, and renal function are required to prevent digoxin toxicity. In cases of severe congestive heart failure, diuretic agents may be necessary to accelerate water excretion[(211)]. However, serum levels of sodium, potassium, chloride, and bicarbonate must be monitored closely in order to prevent electrolyte disturbances caused by these agents.

Additional therapeutic measures may be necessary if initial therapy of congestive heart failure proves insufficient. Intravenous sympathomimetics, e.g., dopamine or dobutamine isoproterenol, can improve cardiac output[(207,211)]. Sedation, for example with morphine (0.05 mg/kg), fentanyl (1 to 2 micrograms/kg) or midazolam (0.05 to 0.1 mg/kg), may decrease metabolic demands[(207,211)] but must raise concerns about respiratory depression. In addition to the sedative effect, morphine produces systemic vasodilation and increases cardiac output. Afterload reduction alone or in combination with an inotrope often results in significant clinical improvement. A single agent such as amrinone may exert both an afterload reducing effect and increased inotropy, resulting in improved cardiac performance. Caution is advised however, as decreased afterload in the presence of right ventricular outflow obstruction (e.g., tetralogy of Fallot) may have adverse consequences. If the congestive failure is still inadequately controlled with medical therapy, corrective or palliative surgery of the underlying cardiac defect, which may have been scheduled for a later date, will need to be performed[(207,212)].

Cyanotic Spells

Treatment of these spells is aimed at improving arterial PO_2 and acidosis by decreasing obstruction to right ventricular outflow, improving pulmonary blood flow, and reducing the PVR/SVR ratio[(190,212)]. Supplemental oxygen is administered by face mask or oxygen hood. The patient is placed in a knee-chest position, which is physiologically similar to squatting. Squatting has been shown to increase effective pulmonary blood flow and to redistribute systemic flow to the upper body by increasing the SVR. During this maneuver, the arterial oxygen saturation remains unchanged, but the venous saturation increases, implying improved capillary and tissue oxygenation[(228)].

Intravenous fluids should be instituted. Acidosis is corrected by administration of $NaHCO_3$ after a sample for blood gas and pH has been obtained. Initially, the patient may be given 2 mEq $NaHCO_3$ per kilogram (0.5 mEq/ml)

Table 13.10. Digoxin Therapy[a]

Preparation	*Route of administration*	*Effect (onset maximum)*	*Effect (duration)*	*Total excretion*	*Oral absorption*	*Dose (digitalizing)*	*Dose (daily maintenance)*
Digoxin (lanoxin)	IV	5–30 min	24 hr	48–72 hr	40–90%	p.o. (μg/kg)	p.o. (μg/kg)
Available in	i.m.	15–60 min				Preterm: 20–30	Preterm: 20–30% of oral loading dose
Tablets: 0.125, 0.25, 0.5 mg	p.o.	1–2 hr				Full term: 25–35	Full term to adult: 25–35% of oral loading dose
		2–5 hr				1–24 months: 35–60	Maintenance dose is given q 12 hr IV (μg/kg)
Elixir: 0.05 mg/ml		2–5 hr				2–5 yr: 30–40	Preterm: 20–30% of IV loading dose
Ampules: 0.1, 0.25 mg/ml		4–8 hr				5–10 yr: 20–35	Full term to adult: 25–35% of IV loading dose
						10 yr–adult: 10–15	
						i.m. or IV (μg/kg)	
						Preterm: 15–25	
						Full term: 20–30	
						1–24 months: 30–50	
						2–5 yr: 25–35	
						5–10 yr: 15–30	
						10 yr to adult: 8–12	
						* Parenteral digitalizing doses are 80% of oral digitalizing doses; 1/2 TDD[b] is given stat, then 1/4 TDD is given q 6 to 8 hr × 2	

[a] *Adapted from Cole CH, ed. The Harriet Lane handbook. 10th ed. Chicago: Year Book Medical Publishers, 1984:132.*
[b] *TDD, total digitalizing dose.*

over 5 minutes. Subsequent doses may be administered as needed according to the following formula:

$$NaHCO_3 \text{ dose (mEq)} = 0.3 \times \text{body weight (kg)} \times \text{base deficit} \quad \text{(Eq. 13.6)}$$

Half the dose is given over 30 minutes, and the remainder over 4 hours[207,230].

Morphine administration (0.1 to 0.2 mg/kg s.c. or IV) is often effective in relieving a spell. The probable mechanism of action is a reduction of infundibular spasm and improved pulmonary blood flow[236–238]. β-Adrenergic antagonists given intravenously may also reverse a spasm. Propranolol (0.2 mg/kg IV) has been shown to terminate a spell, probably by relaxing the right ventricular outlet[187,238]. More recently, the use of esmolol, a very short-acting β-adrenergic antagonist that is administered intravenously, has offered a titratable alternative to the longer acting propranolol. Chronic oral therapy with propranolol (1 to 2 mg/kg 4 times daily) has been shown to decrease the frequency of the paroxysms[238]. However, the use of propranolol in the newborn is discouraged because it may cause severe cardiac depression[211]. Conversely, inotropic agents may exacerbate the obstruction to right ventricular outflow and cause further deterioration. Therefore, their use in the treatment of cyanotic spells is best avoided. Calcium blockers can alleviate pulmonary hypertension and are potentially useful in the treatment of cyanotic spells[239]. However, hypoxia may actually be exacerbated if cardiac performance is significantly depressed by the effects of the calcium blockers on myocardium[240]. Therefore, caution is advised until more experience has been gained with these agents in the treatment of paroxysms. Once the condition of a child with hypoxic spells has been stabilized, prompt surgical correction must be considered. Details of the operative and postoperative care are discussed in Chapter 14.

Pulmonary Considerations

Cyanosis may be a result of a pulmonary parenchymal disease such as ARDS, hyaline membrane disease, pneumonia, or aspiration. Its presence requires the administration of supplemental oxygen and may necessitate ventilatory support. Such support may take the form of CPAP or mechanical ventilation. These therapeutic measures are discussed at greater length in Chapter 5.

Surgical intervention is necessary to treat certain pulmonary causes of cyanosis. Obstruction of the airway from intrinsic lesions such as choanal atresia or congenital webs requires operative correction[193]. Surgery is also needed to treat cyanosis resulting from extrinsic lesions that restrict lung movement, which include lobar emphysema and diaphragmatic herniation[193]. A pneumothorax may be relieved by needle aspiration of the free air and/or placement of a thoracostomy tube. Pharmacologic depression of ventilation sufficient to produce cyanosis requires mechanical ventilatory support until the effects of the agent have subsided. Antagonists are available for some pharmacologic agents, such as narcotics, and may be administered to reverse respiratory depression. Morphine, meperidine (Demerol), fentanyl, and other opioids may be reversed by naloxone (Narcan), at a dose of 0.01 mg/kg i.m. or IV, and should be repeated as needed[26].

Metabolic Considerations

Metabolic abnormalities that produce cyanosis should be treated promptly while a concurrent search for cause is begun. Hypothermia can be reversed by the use of warming lights, warm coverings, and adjustment of the ambient temperature. Patients with symptomatic hypoglycemia should receive intravenous glucose. The usual dose is 1 to 2 ml/kg of 25% dextrose (50% dextrose diluted 1:1 in sterile water). We avoid direct administration of 50% glucose in order to minimize adverse effects of hyperosmolality. For infants of diabetic mothers, the dose is adjusted to deliver 150 mg/kg or 1 ml of 15% dextrose per kilogram. The initial dose is followed by an infusion of dextrose delivering 4 to 8 mg/kg/min in order to maintain a normal serum level of glucose[241,242]. The blood glucose should be determined periodically to ascertain that the patient is normoglycemic. Further therapy with hydrocortisone may be needed to maintain normal glucose levels if dextrose therapy alone is insufficient.

Hypocalcemia that is severe enough to cause cyanosis is usually associated with other symptoms, including extreme irritability and convulsions. Symptoms may be reversed by a slow intravenous push of calcium gluconate (10% in water) at a rate of 1 ml/min (to a maximum of 3 mg/kg), until a clinical response is obtained. Calcium levels may then be maintained in the normal range with an infusion of calcium. Either calcium gluceptate or calcium gluconate can be used, and the infusion adjusted, to deliver 24 to 35 mg calcium per kilogram per day[185,243,244].

Therapy for methemoglobinemia (MetHb)[202] starts with general supportive care and removal of any possible toxin. The latter may entail removal of contaminated clothes, washing of the skin, and emptying of gastric contents with induced emesis or lavage. Because normal mechanisms convert MetHb to Hb over 15 to 20 hours, no other treatment for toxin-induced methemoglobinemia is needed in the absence of hypoxic symptoms. However, if signs of hypoxia are present or the level of MetHb is greater than 30%, drug therapy should be considered. Pharmacologic treatment is aimed at converting the ferric iron (Fe^{3+}) in heme to the ferrous state. The preferred agent is methylene blue (tetramethylthionine chloride), which forms an NADPH-dependent oxidation-reduction system for heme. This is accomplished through activation of NADPH-MetHb reductase, with methylene blue as a cofactor (Fig. 13.24).

The usual dosage of methylene blue is 1 to 2 mg/kg (in a 1% solution) administered IV over 5 minutes. Most MetHb should be converted within 30 to 60 minutes[245]. If needed,

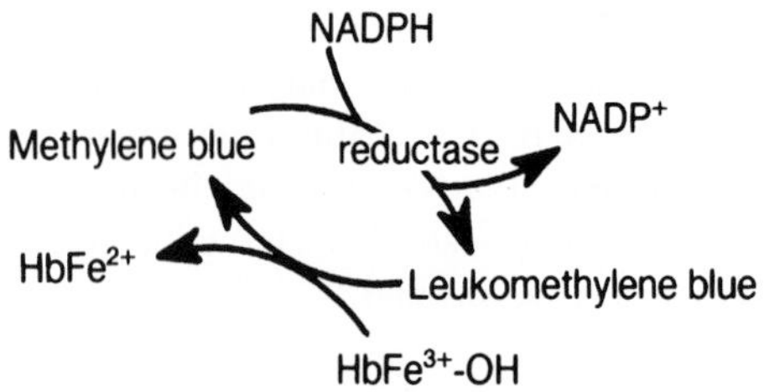

Figure 13.24. Conversion of methemoglobin ($HbFe^{3+}-OH$) to hemoglobin ($HbFe^{2+}$).

the dose may be repeated after 1 hour (maximum dose 7 mg/kg). Side effects are seen with higher doses and include precordial pain, dyspnea, restlessness, tremors, and apprehension. Dysuria and urinary frequency may also be present. High concentrations of methylene blue can occasionally cause mild hemolysis and may actually produce methemoglobinemia by reversing the reaction (Eq. 13.4). Failure of methylene blue treatment may require blood transfusion or exchange transfusion therapy. Treatment failure suggests the possibility of glucose 6-phosphate dehydrogenase deficiency or sulfhemoglobinemia[246], for which no specific therapy exists. Therapy with transfusions, exchange transfusions, or hyperbaric oxygen may alleviate the acute symptoms. This intervention can be followed by treatment with ascorbic acid, which reduces MetHb slowly. Carboxyhemoglobin is generally associated with smoke inhalation, and its evaluation and treatment are discussed in Chapter 44.

Treatment of polycythemia and/or hyperviscosity is direct at achieving an isovolemic reduction in the erythrocyte count. This is accomplished by performing a partial or "reduction" exchange transfusion. Catheters are placed for the withdrawal and infusion of blood. In the neonate, an umbilical venous or arterial catheter may be used. The total amount of blood to be exchanged is calculated as follows:

$$V = \text{weight} \times (80 \text{ ml/kg}) \times [(\text{observed Hct} - \text{desired Hct})/\text{observed Hct}] \quad \text{(Eq. 13.7)}$$

where V equals total volume to be exchanged.

The desired Hct is less than 55%. Blood is withdrawn in 5 to 10-ml aliquots and discarded; the removed blood is replaced by an equal volume of plasma solution. The process is repeated until the calculated volume has been removed and an equal amount has been reinfused. The patient's temperature should be closely monitored in order to maintain normothermia. Resuscitation drugs and equipment should be readily accessible in case severe hypotension, seizure, or cardiac arrest occur.

SUMMARY

The traditional cardiologic approaches to heart disease are a useful starting point for the intensivist caring for a child in the pediatric ICU with pulmonary edema, myocardial ischemia, or cyanosis. These approaches must be expanded upon, however, by a knowledge of the myriad of unusual entities that can cause these conditions in the pediatric ICU patient without congenital heart disease. A knowledge of these entities is absolutely necessary if the intensivist is to be helpful in responding to the care of the children with these unusual but often fascinating conditions.

References

1. Braunwald E, Sobel BE. Coronary blood flow and myocardial ischemia. In: Braunwald E, ed. Heart disease—a textbook of cardiovascular medicine. Philadelphia: WB Saunders, 1980;2:1279.
2. Klocke FJ, Braunwald E, Ross J Jr. Oxygen cost of electrical activation of the heart. Circ Res 1966;18:357.
3. Sonnenblick EH, Skelton CL. Myocardial energetics: basic principles and clinical implications. N Engl J Med 1971;285:668.
4. Evans CL, Matsuoka Y. The effect of various mechanical conditions on the gaseous metabolism and efficiency of the mammalian heart. J Physiol 1915;49:378.
5. Sonnenblick EH, Parmley WW, Urschel CW. The contractile state of the heart as expressed by force-velocity relations. Am J Cardiol 1969;23:488.
6. Ross J Jr, Sonnenblick EH, Kaiser GA, et al. Electroaugmentation of ventricular performance and oxygen consumption by repetitive application of paired electrical stimuli. Circ Res 1965;16:332.
7. Graham TP Jr, Covell JW, Sonnenblick EH, et al. Control of myocardial oxygen consumption: relative influence of contractile state and tension development. J Clin Invest 1968;47:375.
8. Sonnenblick EH, Ross J Jr, Covell JW, et al. Velocity of contraction as a determinant of myocardial oxygen consumption. Am J Physiol 1965;209:919.
9. Parmley WW, Tyberg JV. Determinants of myocardial oxygen demand. In: Yu PN, Goodwin JF, eds. Progress in cardiology. Philadelphia: Lea & Febiger, 1976:19.
10. Sarnoff SJ, Braunwald E, Welch GH Jr, et al. Hemodynamic determinants of oxygen consumption of the heart with special reference to the tension-time index. Am J Physiol 1958;192:148.
11. Boerth RC, Covell JW, Pool PE, et al. Increased myocardial oxygen consumption and contractile state associated with increased heart rate in dogs. Circ Res 1969;24:725.
12. Coleman HN, Sonnenblick EH, Braunwald E. Myocardial oxygen consumption associated with external work: the Fenn effect. Am J Physiol 1969;217:291.
13. Urschel CW, Covell JW, Graham TP, et al.. Effects of acute valvular regurgitation on the oxygen consumption of the canine heart. Circ Res 1968;23:33.
14. Powers ER, Powell WJ Jr. Effect of arterial hypoxia on myocardial oxygen consumption. Circ Res 1973;33:749.
15. Becker LC. Effect of tachycardia on regional left ventricular blood flow after coronary artery occlusion. Am J Cardiol 1975;35:122.
16. Moir TW. Subendocardial distribution of coronary blood flow and the effect of antianginal drugs. Circ Res 1972;30:621.
17. Neill WA, Oxendine J, Phelps N, et al. Subendocardial ischemia provoked by tachycardia in conscious dogs with coronary stenosis. Am J Cardiol 1975;35:30.
18. Franciosi RA, Blanc WA. Myocardial infarcts in infants and children. I. A necropsy study in congenital heart disease. J Pediatr 1968;73:309.
19. Cabal LA, Devaskar U, Siassi B, et al. Cardiogenic shock associated with perinatal asphyxia in preterm infants. J Pediatr 1980;96:705.
20. Setzer E, Ermocilla R, Tonkin I, et al. Papillary muscle necrosis in a neonatal autopsy population: incidence and associated clinical manifestations. J Pediatr 1980;96:289.
21. Stryker WA. Coronary occlusive disease in infants and in children. Am J Dis Child 1946;71:280.
22. Gault MH, Usher R. Coronary thrombosis with myocardial infarction in a newborn infant. Clinical, electrocardiographic and post-mortem findings. N Engl J Med 1960;263:379.
23. Sapire DW, Markowitz R, Valdes-Dapena M, et al. Thrombosis of the left coronary artery in a newborn infant. J Pediatr 1977;90:957.
24. James TN, Froggat P, Marshall TK. De subitaneis mortibus. II. Coronary embolism in the fetus. Circulation 1973;48:890.
25. Oppenheimer EH, Esterly JR. Some aspects of cardiac pathology in infancy and childhood. III. Coronary embolism. Johns Hopkins Med J 1967;120:317.

26. Rowe RD, Hoffman T. Transient myocardial ischemia of the newborn infant: a form of severe cardiorespiratory distress in full-term infants. J Pediatr 1972;81:243.
27. Finley JP, Howman-Giles RB, Gilday DL, et al. Transient myocardial ischemia of the newborn infant demonstrated by thallium myocardial imaging. J Pediatr 1979;94:263.
28. Bucciarelli RL, Nelson RM, Egan EA, et al. Transient tricuspid insufficiency of the newborn: a form of myocardial dysfunction in stressed newborns. Pediatrics 1977;59:330.
29. Donnelly WH, Bucciarelli RL, Nelson RM. Ischemic papillary muscle necrosis in stressed newborn infants. J Pediatr 1980;96:295.
30. Primhak RA, Jedeikin R, Ellis G, et al. Myocardial ischaemia in asphyxia neonatorum. Electrocardiographic, enzymatic and histological correlations. Acta Paediatr Scand 1985;74:595.
31. Oh KS, Bender TM, Bowen A, et al. Transient myocardial ischemia of the newborn infant. Pediatr Radiol 1985;15:29.
32. Kilbride H, Way GL, Merenstein GB, et al. Myocardial infarction in the neonate with normal heart and coronary arteries. Am J Dis Child 1980;134:759.
33. Robertson AF, Alpert BS. Transient heart disease in the newborn. South Med J 1982;75:841.
34. Esterly JR, Oppenheimer EH. Some aspects of cardiac pathology in infancy and childhood. I. Neonatal myocardial necrosis. Bull Johns Hopkins Hosp 1966;119:191.
35. Keith JD. Diseases of coronary arteries and aorta. In: Keith JD, Rowe RD, Vlad P, eds. Heart disease in infancy and childhood. 3rd ed. New York: Macmillan, 1978:1013.
35a. Lipsett J, Cohle SD, Berry PJ, et al. Anomalous coronary arteries: a multicenter pediatric autopsy study. Ped Pathol 1994;14:287–300.
36. Lure PR, Takahashi M. Abnormalities and diseases of the coronary vessels. In: Adams FH, Emmanouilides GC, eds. Moss' heart disease in infants, children and adolescents. 3rd ed. Baltimore: Williams & Wilkins, 1983:501.
37. Bharati S, Chandra N, Stephenson LW, et al. Origin of the left coronary artery from the right pulmonary artery. J Am Coll Cardiol 1984; 3:1565.
38. Tamer DF, Mallon SM, Garcia OL, et al. Anomalous origin of the left anterior descending coronary artery from the pulmonary artery. Am Heart J 1984;108:341.
39. Perry LW, Scott LP. Anomalous left coronary artery from pulmonary artery. Circulation 1970;41:1043.
40. Midgley FM, Watson DC Jr, Scott LP III, et al. Repair of anomalous origin of the left coronary artery in the infant and small child. J Am Coll Cardiol 1984;4:1231.
41. Matson JR, Loughlin GM, Strunk RC. Myocardial ischemia complicating the use of isoproterenol in asthmatic children. J Pediatr 1978;92:776.
42. Kurland G, Williams J, Lewiston NJ. Fatal myocardial toxicity during continuous infusion intravenous isoproterenol therapy of asthma. J Allergy Clin Immunol 1979;63:407.
43. Mikhail MS, Hunsinger SL, Goodwin SR, et al. Myocardial ischemia induced by isoproterenol in a young asthmatic. Pediatrics in press.
44. Furman WR, Summer WR, Kennedy TP, et al. Comparison of the effects of dobutamine, dopamine and isoproterenol on hypoxic pulmonary vasoconstriction in the pig. Crit Care Med 1982;10:371.
45. Winsor T, Mills B, Winbury MM, et al. Intramyocardial diversion of coronary blood flow: effects of isoproterenol-induced subendocardial ischemia. Microvasc Res 1975;9:261.
46. Kahn D, Rona G, Chappel C. Isoproterenol-induced cardiac necrosis. Ann N Y Acad Sci 1969;156:285.
47. Kurland G, Williams J, Lewiston NJ. Fatal myocardial toxicity during continuous infusion intravenous isoproterenol therapy of asthma. J Allergy Clin Immunol 1979;63:407.
48. Strubelt O, Hoffman A, Siegers C, et al. On the pathogenesis of cardiac necrosis induced by theophylline and caffeine. Acta Pharmacol Toxicol (Kbh) 1976;39:383.
49. Wetzel RC, Rogers MC. Unusual medical causes of pediatric heart failure. In: Shoemaker WC, Thompson WL, Holbrook PR, eds. Textbook of critical care. Philadelphia: WB Saunders, 1984:384.
50. Kawasaki T, Kosaki F, Okawa S, et al. A new infantile acute febrile mucocutaneous lymph node syndrome (MLNS) prevailing in Japan. Pediatrics 1974;54:271.
51. Yanagisawa M, Nobayahi N, Matsuya S. Myocardial infarction due to coronary thromboarteritis, following acute febrile mucocutaneous lymph node syndrome (MLNS) in an infant. Pediatrics 1974;54:277.
52. Bell DM. Kawasaki syndrome: still a mystery after 20 years. JAMA 1985;254:801.
53. Shackelford PG, Strauss AW. Kawasaki syndrome. N Engl J Med 1991;324:1664–666.
54. Melish M. Kawasaki syndrome (the mucocutaneous lymph node syndrome). Pediatr Ann 1982;11:255.
55. Scully RE, Mark EJ, McNeely WF, et al. Case records of the Massachusetts General Hospital: case 43-1990. N Engl J Med 1990;323:1189–1199.
56. Burns JC, Wiggins JW Jr, Toews WH, et al. Clinical spectrum of Kawasaki disease in infants younger than 6 months of age. J Pediatr 1986;109:759–763.
57. Price J. Kawasaki syndrome. Br Med J 1984;288:262.
58. Hallagan LF, Dawson PAJ, Eljaiek LF. Pediatric chest pain: Case report of a malignant cause. Am J Emerg Med 1992;10:43–45.
59. Hiraishi S, Yashiro K, Oguchi K, et al. Clinical course of cardiovascular involvement in the mucocutaneous lymph node syndrome. Am J Cardiol 1981;47:323.
60. Tizard EJ, Susuki A, Levin M, et al. Clinical aspects of 100 patients with Kawasaki disease. Arch Dis Child 1991;66:185–188.
61. Yanagihara R, Todd JK. Acute febrile mucocutaneous lymph node syndrome. Am J Dis Child 1980;134:603.
62. Yoshikawa J, Yanagihara K, Owaki T, et al. Cross-sectional echocardiographic diagnosis of coronary artery aneurysms in patients with the mucocutaneous lymph node syndrome. Circulation 1979;59:133.
63. Chung KJ, Brandt L, Fulton DR, et al. Cardiac and coronary arterial involvement in infants and children from New England with mucocutaneous lymph node syndrome (Kawasaki disease). Angiographic-echocardiographic correlations. Am J Cardiol 1982;50:136.
64. Rowe RD, Rose V. Kawasaki disease: Canadian update. Can Med Assoc J 1985;132:25.
65. Nakano H, Nojima K, Saito A, et al. High incidence of aortic regurgitation following Kawasaki disease. J Pediatr 1985;107:59.
66. Ohyagi A, Hirose K, Tsujimoto S, et al. Kawasaki disease complicated by acute myocardial infarction 9 years after onset. Am Heart J 1985;110:670.
67. Bierman FZ, Gersony WM. Kawasaki disease: clinical perspective. J Pediatr 1987;111:789–793.
68. Burns JC, Glode MP, Clarke SH, et al. Coagulopathy and platelet activation in Kawasaki syndrome: identification of patients at high risk for development of coronary artery aneurysms. J Pediatr 1984; 105:206.
69. Grenadier E, Allen HD, Goldberg SJ, et al. Left ventricular wall motion abnormalities in Kawasaki disease. Am Heart J 1984;107:966.
70. Novelli VM, Galbraith A, Robinson PJ, et al. Cardiovascular abnormalities in Kawasaki disease. Arch Dis Child 1984;59:405.
71. Yanagisawa M, Yano S, Shiraishi H, et al. Coronary aneurysms in Kawasaki disease: follow-up observation by two-dimensional echocardiography. Pediatr Cardiol 1985;6:11.
72. Yasuda T, Palacios IF, Dec GW, et al. Indium-111 monoclonal antimyosin antibody imaging in the diagnosis of acute myocarditis. Circulation, 1987;76:306–11.
73. Arensman FW, Sharp CG, Covitz W, et al. Diagnosing coronary artery aneurysms in patients with mucocutaneous lymph node syndrome (Kawasaki disease). J Med Assoc Ga 1984;73:491.
74. Nakanishi T, Takao A, Nakazawa M, et al. Mucocutaneous lymph node syndrome: clinical, hemodynamic and angiographic features of coronary obstructive disease. Am J Cardiol 1985;55:662.
75. Fujiwara H, Hamashima Y. Pathology of heart in Kawasaki disease. Pediatrics 1978;61:100.
76. Fujiwara H, Fujiwara T, Kao T-C, et al.. Pathology of Kawasaki disease in the healed stage. Acta Pathol Jpn 1986;36:857–867.
77. Harada K, Uesato T, Toyoda H, et al. Acute febrile mucocutaneous lymph node syndrome with multiple aneurysms: report of a case. Pediatr Cardiol 1983;4:215.
78. Koren G, Rose V, Lavi S, et al. Probable efficacy of high-dose salicylates in reducing coronary involvement in Kawasaki disease. JAMA 1985;254:767.
79. Kato H, Sigeyuki K, Yokoyama T. Kawasaki disease: effect of treatment on coronary artery involvement. Pediatrics 1979;63:175.
80. Newberger JW. The treatment of Kawasaki syndrome with intravenous gammaglobulin. N Engl J Med 1986;315:341.
80a. Steere AC, Grodziecki RL, Kornblatt AN, et al. The spirochetal etiology of Lyme Disease. NEJM 1983; 308:733–740.
81. Newberger JW, Takahashi M, Beiser AS, et al. A single intravenous in-

fusion of gamma globulin as compared with four infusions in the treatment of acute Kawasaki disease. N Engl J Med 1991;324:1633–1639.
82. Steere AC, Lyme Disease. N Engl J Med August 31, 1989; 321(9): 586–96.
83. Steere AC, Malawista SE, Snydman DR, et al. Lyme arthritis: an epidemic of oligoarticular arthritis in children and adults in three Connecticut communities. Arthritis Rheum 1977; 20:7–17.
84. Cox J, Krajden M. Cardiovascular manifestations of Lyme Disease. American Heart Journal, 1991 November; 122(5); 1449–55.
85. Ciesielski CA, Markowitz LE, Horsley R, et al. Lyme disease surveillance in the United States, 1983–1986. Rev Inf Dis 1989; 11(supp)1425–41.
86. Rowley AH, Shulman ST. Current therapy for acute Kawasaki syndrome. J Pediatr 1991;118:987–991.
87. Hersch C. Electrocardiographic changes in head injuries. Circulation 1961;23:853.
88. Fabinyi G, Hunt D, McKinley L. Myocardial creatinine kinase isoenzyme in serum after subarachnoid hemorrhage. J Neurol Neurosurg Psychiatry 1977;40:818.
89. Kaste M, Somer H, Konttinen A. Heart type creatinine kinase isoenzyme (CK MB) in acute cerebral disorders. Br Heart J 1978;40:802.
90. Wetzel RC, Rogers MC. Echocardiography in pediatric patients with head trauma. Crit Care Med 1981;9:224.
91. Greenhoot JH, Reichenbach DD. Cardiac injury and subarachnoid hemorrhage. A clinical, pathological and physiological correlation. J Neurosurg 1969;30:521.
92. Hawkins WE, Clower BR. Myocardial damage after head trauma and simulated intracranial hemorrhage in mice: the role of the autonomic nervous system. Cardiovasc Res 1971;5:524.
93. Milley JR, Nugent SK, Rogers MC. Neurogenic pulmonary edema in childhood. J Pediatr 1979;94:706.
94. Chen HI, Sun SC, Chai CY. Pulmonary edema and hemorrhage resulting from cerebral compression. Am J Physiol 1973;224:223.
95. Melville KI, Blum B, Shister HE, et al. Cardiac ischemic changes and arrhythmias induced by hypothalamic stimulation. Am J Cardiol 1963;12:781.
96. Cruickshank JM, Neil-Dwyer G, Stott AW. Possible role of catecholamines, corticosteroids, and potassium in production of electrocardiographic abnormalities associated with subarachnoid hemorrhage. Br Heart J 1974;36:697.
97. Connor RCR. Fuchsinophilic degeneration of myocardium in patients with intracranial lesions. Br Heart J 1970;32:81.
98. Harley DP, Mena I, Narahara KA, et al. Traumatic myocardial dysfunction. J Thorac Cardiovasc Surg 1984;87:386.
99. Langer JC, Winthrop AL, Wesson DE, et al. Diagnosis and incidence of cardiac injury in children with blunt thoracic trauma. J Pediatr Surg 1989;24:1091–1094.
100. Sutherland GR, Calvin JE, Driedger AA, et al. Anatomic and cardiopulmonary responses to trauma with associated blunt chest injury. J Trauma 1981;21:1.
101. Rothstein RJ. Myocardial contusion. JAMA 1983;250:2189.
102. Symbas P. Trauma to the heart and great vessels. New York: Grune & Stratton, 1978:38.
103. Rheuban KS, Tompkins DG, Nolan SP, et al. Myocardial necrosis and ventricular aneurysm following closed chest injury in a child. J Trauma 1981;21:170.
104. Silver GN, Spampinato N, Favolara R, et al. Ventricular aneurysms and blunt chest trauma. Chest 1973;63:628.
105. Bainborough AR, Watty EI. Coronary artery disease in children. Clin Invest Med 1984;7:1.
106. Carter GA, Lauer RU. Atherosclerosis. In: Adams FH, Emmanouilides GC, eds. Moss' heart disease in infants, children and adolescents. 3rd ed. Baltimore: Williams & Wilkins, 1983:646.
107. Philips JB, Ruiz-Castaneda N, Setzer ES. Coronary sinus thrombosis: a central venous catheter complication. J Pediatr Surg 1981;16:733.
108. Strong JP, McGill HC Jr. The pediatric aspects of atherosclerosis. J Atheroscler Rev 1969;9:251.
109. Haust MD. Atherosclerosis in childhood, perspectives in pediatric pathology. Chicago: Year Book Medical Publishers, 1978;4:155.
110. Stryker WA. Coronary occlusive disease in infants and children. Am J Dis Child 1946;71:280.
111. Lipshultz SE, Frassica JJ, Orav EJ. Cardiovascular abnormalities in infants prenatally exposed to cocaine. J Pediatr 1991;118:44–51.
112. Simpson RW, Edwards WD. Pathogenesis of cocaine-induced ischemic heart disease. Arch Pathol Lab Med 1986;110:479–484.
113. Koren G, Weiss AT, Hasin Y, et al. Prevention of myocardial damage in acute myocardial ischemia by early treatment with intravenous streptokinase. N Engl J Med 1985;313:1384.
114. Walther FJ, Siassi B, Ramadan NA, et al. Cardiac output in newborn infants with transient myocardial dysfunction. J Pediatr 1985; 107:781.
115. Staub NC. Pulmonary edema. Physiol Rev 1974;54:678.
116. Robin ED, Cross CE, Zelis R. Pulmonary edema. N Engl J Med 1973;288:239, 292 (2 parts).
117. Fliff LD. Extra-alveolar vessels and edema formation in the excised dog lungs. Circ Res 1971;28:524.
118. Low FN. Extracellular components of the pulmonary arterial wall. Arch Intern Med 1971;127:847.
119. Starling EH. On the absorption of fluids from the connective tissue spaces. J Physiol (Lond) 1896;19:312.
120. Boysen PG, Modell JH. Pulmonary edema. In: Shoemaker WC, Thompson WL, Holbrook PR, eds. Textbook of critical care medicine. Philadelphia: WB Saunders, 1984:238.
121. Mellins RB, Levine OR, Skalak R, et al. Interstitial pressure of the lung. Circ Res 1969;24:197.
122. Staub NC, Nagano H, Pearce ML. Pulmonary edema in dogs, especially the sequence of fluid accumulation in the lungs. J Appl Physiol 1967;22:227.
123. Staub NC. Pulmonary edema. Physiologic approaches to management. Chest 1978;74:559.
124. Stovin PGI, Micthinson MJ. Pulmonary hypertension due to obstruction of the intrapulmonary veins. Thorax 1967;20:106.
125. Brown CH, Harrison CV. Pulmonary veno-occlusive disease. Lancet 1966;2:61.
126. Heath D, Scott O, Lynch J. Pulmonary veno-occlusive disease. Lancet 1966;2:61.
127. Robin ED, Thomas ED. Some relations between pulmonary edema and pulmonary inflammation (pneumonia). Arch Intern Med 1954;93:713.
128. Petersdorf RG, Fusco JJ, Harter DH, et al. Pulmonary infections complicating Asian influenza. Arch Intern Med 1959;103:262.
129. Ketai LH, Williamson MR, Telepak RJ, et al.. Hantavirus pulmonary syndrome: radiographic findings in 16 patients. Radiology 1994 June; 191 (3): 665–8.
130. Cameron GR, Courtice FC. The production and removal of oedema fluid in the lung after exposure to carbonylchloride (phosgene). J Physiol (Lond) 1946;105:175.
131. Bils RF. Ultrastructural alterations of alveolar tissue of mice. III. Ozone. Arch Environ Health 1970;20:468.
132. Sherwin RP, Richters V. Lung capillaries permeability: nitrogen dioxide exposure and leakage in tritiated serum. Arch Intern Med 1971;128:61.
133. Snell JD Jr, Ramsey LH. Pulmonary edema as a result of endotoxemia. Am J Physiol 1969;217:170.
134. Abroug, F. Boujdaria R, Belghith M, et al. Cardiac dysfunction and pulmonary edema follwoing scorpion envenomation. Chest 1991 Oct; 199(4):1057–9.
135. Ramsey HW, Snyder GK, Taylor WJ. Pulmonary hemodynamics after infusion of *Micrurus fulvius* (coral) venom. Clin Res 1971;19:335.
136. Pietra GG, Szidon JP, Leventhal MM, et al. Histamine and interstitial pulmonary edema in the dog. Circ Res 1971;29:323.
137. Majno G, Shea SM, Leventhal M. Endothelial cell contraction induced by histamine-type mediators: an electron microscopic study. J Cell Biol 1969;42:647.
138. Wetzel RC. The intensivist's system. Crit Care Med 21:s341-s344, 1993.
139. Stephens KE, Ishizaka A, Larrick JW, et al. Tumor necrosis factor causes increased pulmonary permeability and edema. Am Rev Respir Dis 1988;137:1364–1370.
140. Rusznyak I, Foldi M, Szabo G. The lung. In: Youlten L, ed. Lymphatics and lymph circulation. 2nd Engl ed. Oxford: Pergamon Press, 1967:637.
141. Eraslan S, Turman MD, Hardy JD. Lymphatic regeneration following lung reimplantation in dogs. Surgery 1964;56:970.
142. Travis KW, Todres ID, Shannon DC. Pulmonary edema associated with croup and epiglottitis. Pediatrics 1977;59:695.
143. Lichtenstein S, Goldberg H, Mitzner W, et al. Respiratory effects on cardiac function. Fed Proc 1975;34:436.
144. Trapnell DH, Thurston JGB. Unilateral pulmonary oedema after pleural aspiration. Lancet 1970;1:1367.
145. Von Hoff DD, Rosencweig M, Piccart M. The cardiotoxicity of anticancer agents. Semin Oncol 1982;9:23.
146. Doroshow JH. Doxorubicin-induced cardiac toxicity [Editorial]. N Engl J Med 1991;324:843–845.
147. Unverferth DV, Magorien RD, Unverferth BP, et al. Human myocardial,

morphologic, and functional changes in the first 24 hours after doxorubicin administration. Cancer Treat Rep 1981;65:1093.
148. Meyers CE, McGuire WP, Liss RH, et al. Adriamycin: the role of lipid peroxidation in cardiac toxicity and tumor response. Science 1977;197:165.
149. Minow RA, Benjamin RS, Lee ET, et al. Adriamycin cardiomyopathy—risk factors. Cancer 1977;39:1397.
150. Goorin AM, Chauvenet AR, Perez-Atayde AR, et al. Initial congestive heart failure, six to ten years after doxorubicin chemotherapy for childhood cancer. J Pediatr 1990;116:144–147.
151. Lipshultz SE, Lipsitz SR, Mone AM, et al. New England Journal of Medicine. 1995 June;332(26):1738–43.
152. Olson RD, Mushlin PS. Doxorubicin cardiotoxicity: analysis of prevailing hypotheses. FASEB J 1990;4:3076–3086.
153. Lipshultz SE, Colan SD, Gelber RD, et al. Late cardiac effects of doxorubicin therapy for acute lymphoblastic leukemia in childhood. N Engl J Med 1991;324:808–815.
154. Alexander J, Dainiak N, Berger HJ, et al. Serial measurements of doxorubicin cardiotoxicity with quantitative radionuclide angiocardiography. N Engl J Med 1979;300:278.
155. Morgan GW, McIlveen BM, Freedman A, et al. Radionuclide ejection fraction in doxorubicin cardiotoxicity. Cancer Treat Rep 1981;65:629.
156. Biancaniello T, Meyer RA, Wong KY, et al. Doxorubicin cardiotoxicity in children. J Pediatr 1980;97:45.
157. Lewis AB, Crouse VL, Evans W, et al. Recovery of left ventricular function following discontinuation of anthracycline chemotherapy in children. Pediatrics 1981;68:67.
158. Smith JL. The pathological effects due to increase of oxygen tension in the air breathed. J Physiol 1899;24:19.
159. Winter PM, Miller JD. Oxygen toxicity. In: Shoemaker WC, Thompson WL, Holbrook PR, eds. Textbook of critical care medicine. Philadelphia: WB Saunders, 1984:218.
160. Dolezal V. The effect of long lasting oxygen inhalation upon respiratory parameters in men. Physiol Bohemoslov 1962;11:149.
161. Kistler GS, Caldwell PRB, Weibel ER. Development of fine structural damage to alveolar and capillary lining cells in oxygen-poisoned rat lungs. J Cell Biol 1967;21:605.
162. Kyle JD. The effects of 100% oxygen inhalation on adult and newborn rat lungs. South Med J 1965;58:1592.
163. Crapo JD, Tierney DF. Superoxide dismutase and pulmonary oxygen toxicity. Am J Physiol 1974;226:1401.
164. Frank L. Development aspects of experimental pulmonary oxygen toxicity. Free Radical Biology and Medicine 1991; 11(5):463-94.
165. Frank L, Bucher JR, Roberts RJ. Oxygen toxicity in neonatal and adult animals of various species. J Appl Physiol 1978;45:699.
166. Mead JF. Free radical mechanisms of lipid damage and consequences for cellular membranes. In: Pryor WA, ed. Free radicals in biology. Orlando, Florida: Academic Press, 1976;1:51.
167. Lewis RA, Austen KF. Mediation of local homeostasis and inflammation by leukotrienes and other mast cell-dependent compounds. Nature 1981;293:103.
168. Farrukh IS, Sciuto AM, Spannhake EW, et al. Leukotriene D_4 increases vascular permeability and pressure by different mechanisms in the rabbit. Am Rev Respir Dis 1986;134:229.
169. Matthay MA, Eschenbacher WL, Goetzel EJ. Elevated concentration of leukotriene D_4 in pulmonary edema fluid of patients with adult respiratory distress syndrome. J Clin Immunol 1984;4:479.
170. Farrukh IS, Michael JR, Summer WR, et al. Thromboxane-induced pulmonary vaso-constriction: involvement of calcium. J Appl Physiol 1985;58:34.
171. Heffner JE, Sahn SA. Salicylate-induced pulmonary edema. Ann Intern Med 1981;95:405.
172. Kahn A, Blum D. Fatal respiratory-distress syndrome and salicylate intoxication in a two-year-old. Lancet 1979;2:1131.
173. Walters JS, Woodring JH, Stelling CB, et al. Salicylate-induced pulmonary edema. Radiology 1983;146:289–293.
174. Bowers RE, Brigham KL, Owen PJ. Cardiorespiratory control. Am Rev Respir Dis 1977;115:261.
175. Hartley PH-S. Albuminous expectoration following paracentesis of the chest. St Barth Hosp Rev 1905;41:77.
176. Ziskind MM, Weil H, George RA. Acute pulmonary edema following the treatment of spontaneous pneumothorax with excessive negative intrapleural pressure. Am Rev Respir Dis 1965;92:632.
177. Trapnell DH, Thurston JGB. Unilateral pulmonary oedema after pleural aspiration. Lancet 1980;1:1367.
178. Jackson RM, Brannen AL, Veal CF, Fulmer JD. Superoxide dismutase and cytochrome oxidase in collapsed lungs: possible role in reexpansion edema. J Appl Physiol 1988;65:235–241.
179. Osler WS. Oedema in the left lung in morphia poisoning. Montg Gen Hosp Rev 1880;1:291.
180. Fraser DW. Methadone overdose: illicit use of pharmaceutically prepared parenteral narcotics. JAMA 1971;217:1387.
181. Katz S, Aberman A, Frand V, et al. Heroin pulmonary edema: evidence for increased pulmonary capillary permeability. Am Rev Respir Dis 1972;106:472.
182. Duberstein JD, Kaufman DM. A clinical study of an epidemic of heroin intoxication and heroin-induced pulmonary edema. Am J Med 1972;51:704.
183. Cerebral edema seen in many "sudden death" heroin victims [Editorial]. JAMA 1970;212:967.
184. Ducker TB. Increased intracranial pressure and pulmonary edema. Part I. Clinical study of eleven patients. J Neurosurg 1968;28:112.
185. Milley JR, Nugent SK, Rogers MC. Neurogenic pulmonary edema in childhood. J Pediatr 1979;94:706.
186. Bean JW, Beckman DL. Centrogenic pulmonary pathology in mechanical head injury. J Appl Physiol 1969;27:807.
187. Mackay EM. Experimental pulmonary edema. Proc Soc Exp Biol 1950;74:695.
188. Chen HI, Sun SC, Chai CY. Pulmonary edema and hemorrhage resulting from cerebral compression. Am J Physiol 1971;224:223.
189. Hultgren HN, Lopez CE, Lundberg E, et al. Physiologic studies of pulmonary edema at high altitude. Circulation 1964;29:393.
190. Fisher AB, Hydre RW, Reif J. Insensitivity of the alveolar septum to local hypoxia. Am J Physiol 1972;223:770.
191. Roy SB, Guleria JS, Khanna PK, et al. Immediate circulatory response to high altitude pulmonary oedema. Nature 1968;217:1177.
192. Dreyfuss D, Saumon G. American Review of Respiratory Disease. 1993;148:1194–203.
193. Wickerts CJ, Berg B, Blomqvist H. Acta Anaesthesiologica Scandinavica 1992 May; 36(4): 309–17.
194. Rossaint R. Falke KJ, Lopez F, Slama K, et al: Inhaled nitric oxide for the adult respiratory distress syndome. New England Journal of Medicine; 1993;328:399.
195. Gerlach H, Pappert D, Lewandowski K, Int Care Med 1993;19:443.
196. Wetzel RC. Aerosolized Prostacyclin. Anesthesiology 1995 June; 82(6):1315–1317.
197. Kinsella JP, Neish SR, Ivy DD, et al. Clinical responses to prolonged treatment of the newborn with low doses of inhaled nitric oxide. J Peds 1993;123:103.
198. Fierobe L, Brunet F, Dhainaut JD, et al. Effect on inhaled nitric oxide on right ventricular function in adult respiratory distress syndome. American Journal of Respiratory and Critical Care Medicine.1995 May; 151(5): 1414–9.
199. Bigatello LM, Hurford WE, Kacmarek RM, et al. Prolonged inhalation of low concentrations of nitric oxide in patients with severe adult respiratory distress syndrome. Effects and pulmonary hemodynamics and oxygenation. Anesthesiology 1994 April;80(4):761–70.
200. Abman SH, et al. J Pediatr 1994;124:881–8.
201. Blakiston's pocket medical dictionary. 4th ed. New York: McGraw-Hill, 1979.
202. Nunn JF. Applied respiratory physiology. 2nd ed. London: Butterworths, 1977.
203. Guyton AC. Textbook of medical physiology. 6th ed. Philadelphia: WB Saunders, 1981.
204. West JB. Respiratory physiology—the essentials. 2nd ed. Baltimore: Williams & Wilkins, 1979.
205. Schaffer AJ, Avery ME. Diseases of the newborn. 4th ed. Philadelphia: WB Saunders, 1977.
206. Staub NC. Alveolar-arterial oxygen tension gradient due to diffusion. J Appl Physiol 1963;18:673.
207. Lambertsen CJ, Bunce PL, Drabkin DL, Schmidt CF. Relationship of oxygen tension to hemoglobin oxygen saturation in the arterial blood of normal men. J Appl Physiol 1952;4:873.
208. Krogh A. The supply of oxygen to the tissues and the regulation of the capillary circulation. J Physiol (Lond) 1919;52:457.
209. Duling B. Oxygen metabolism, and microcirculatory regulation. In: Kaley G, Altura BM, eds. Microcirculation. Baltimore: University Park Press, 1977;II.
210. Adams FH, Emmanouilides GC, eds. Moss' heart disease in infants, children and adolescents. 3rd ed. Baltimore: Williams & Wilkins, 1983.
211. Marshall BE, Marshall C. Continuity of response to hypoxic pulmonary vasoconstriction. J Appl Physiol 1980;40:189.

212. Alexson CG. Cyanosis. In: Ziai M, ed. Bedside pediatrics diagnostic evaluation of the child. Boston: Little, Brown, 1983:307.
213. Kendig EL Jr, Chernick V. Disorders of the respiratory tract in children. Philadelphia: WB Saunders, 1983.
214. Nathan DG, Oski FA. Hematology of infancy and childhood. 2nd ed. Philadelphia: WB Saunders, 1981.
215. Williams WJ, Beutler E, Erslev AJ, Rundles RW, eds. Hematology. 2nd ed. New York: McGraw-Hill, 1977.
216. Allen DW, Wyman J Jr, Smith CA. The oxygen equilibrium of fetal and adult human hemoglobin. J Biol Chem 1953;203:81.
217. Oski FA. The unique fetal red cell and its function. Pediatrics 1973;51:494.
218. Benesch R, Benesch RE. The effect of organic phosphates from the human erythrocyte on the allosteric properties of hemoglobin. Biochem Biophys Res Commun 1967;26:162.
219. Chanutin A, Curnish RR. Effect of organic and inorganic phosphates on the oxygen equilibrium of human erythrocytes. Arch Biochem Biophys 1967;121:96.
220. Barcroft J, King WOR. The effect of temperature on the dissociation curve of blood. J Physiol (Lond) 1909;39:374–384.
221. Bohr C, Hasselbalch K, Krogh A. Ueber einen in biologischer Beziehung wichtigen Einfluss, den die Kohlensauerespannung des Blutes auf dessen Sauerstoffbinding übt. Skan Arch Physiol 1904;16:408.
222. Curry S. Methemoglobinemia. Ann Emerg Med 1982;11:214.
223. Jaffe ER, Hsieh HS. DPNH-methemoglobin reductase deficiency and hereditary methemoglobinemia. Semin Hematol 1971;8:417.
224. Martin H, Huisman THJ. Hematology-formation of ferrihaemoglobin of isolated human haemoglobin types of sodium nitrite. Nature 1963;200:898.
225. Ewing MC, Mayon-White RM. Cyanosis in infancy from nitrates in drinking water. Lancet 1957;1:931.
226. Smith RP, Olson MV. Drug-induced methemoglobinemia. Semin Hematol 1973;10:253.
227. Colley PS, Cheney PW. Sodium nitroprusside increases Q_S/Q_T in dogs with regional atelectasis. Anesthesiology 1977;47:338.
228. Wildsmith JAQ, Drummond GB, MacRae WR. Blood gas changes during induced hypotension with sodium nitroprusside. Br J Anaesth 1975;47:1205.
229. Gilman AG, Goodman LS, Gilman A. Goodman and Gilman's the pharmacological basis of therapeutics. 6th ed. New York: Macmillan, 1980.
230. Rudolph AM, Barnett HL, Einhorn AH. Pediatrics 17. New York: Appleton-Century-Crofts, 1982.
231. James S, Rowe RD. The pattern of response of pulmonary and systemic arterial pressure in newborn and older infants to short periods of hypoxia. J Pediatr 1957;51:5.
232. Sulayman RF, Thilenius OG. Complications of heart disease in children: congestive heart failure, cyanotic spells and infective endocarditis. Paediatrician 1981;10:99.
233. Chmiel H, Walitza E. On the rheology of blood and synovial fluids. New York: John Wiley, 1980.
234. Stone HO, Thompson HK, Schmidt-Nielsen K. Influence of erythrocytes on blood viscosity. Am J Physiol 1968;214:913.
235. Ramamurthy R, Brans YW. Neonatal polycythemia. 1. Criteria for diagnosis and treatment. Pediatrics 1981;68:168.
236. Brans YW, Shannon DL, Ramamurthy RS. Neonatal polycythemia. II. Plasma blood and red cell volume estimates in relation to hematocrit levels and quality of intrauterine growth. Pediatrics 1981;68:175.
237. von Euler C, Soderberg U. Medullary chemosensitive receptors. J Physiol (Lond) 1952;118:545.
238. Bouckaert JJ, Dautrebande L, Heymans C. Sinus caroticus and respiratory reflexes. Influence of CO_2, hydrogen ion concentration and anoxaemia. J Physiol (Lond) 1931;71:V.
239. Korner PI. Circulatory adaptations in hypoxia. Physiol Rev 1959;39:687.
240. Heistad DD, Abboud FM. Circulatory adjustments to hypoxia. Circulation 1980;61:463.
241. Garby L, Robert M, Zaar B. Proton- and carbamino-linked oxygen affinity of normal human blood. Acta Physiol Scand 1972;84:482.
242. Adamson JW, Finch CA. Hemoglobin function, oxygen affinity, and erythropoietin. Ann Rev Physiol 1975;37:351.
243. Robin ED, Simon LM. Oxygen transport and cellular respiration. In: Frolich ED, ed. Pathophysiology. 2nd ed. Philadelphia: JB Lippincott, 1976:167.
244. Barragry TP, Blatchford JW, Tuna IC, et al. Left ventricular dysfunction in a canine model of chronic cyanosis. Surgery 1987;102: 362–370.
245. Siesjo BK, Johannsson H, Ljunggren B, et al. Brain dysfunction in cerebral hypoxia and ischemia. In: Plum F, ed. Brain dysfunction in metabolic disorders. New York: Raven Press, 1974:75.
246. Cohen JJ, Kamm DE. Renal metabolism: relation to renal function. In: Brenner BM, Rector FC, eds. The kidney. 2nd ed. Philadelphia: WB Saunders, 1981:141.
247. Hughes RL, Mathie RT, Campbell D, et al. Systemic hypoxia and hyperoxia, and liver blood flow and oxygen consumption in the greyhound. Pflugers Arch 1979;381:151.
248. Brotmacher L. Hemodynamic effects of squatting during repose. Br Heart J 1957;19:559.
249. Morgan BC, Guntheroth WG, Bloom RS, et al. A clinical profile of paroxysmal hyperpnea in cyanotic congenital heart disease. Circulation 1965;31:66.
250. Gootman NL, Scarpelli EM, Rudolph AM. Metabolic acidosis in children with severe cyanotic congenital heart disease. Pediatrics 1963;31:251.
251. Guntheroth WG, Morgan BC, Mullins GL. Physiologic studies of paroxysmal hyperpnea in cyanotic congenital heart disease. Circulation 1965;31:70.
252. Johnson AM. Norepinephrine and cyanotic attacks in Fallot's tetralogy. Br Heart J 1961;23:197.
253. Cornblath M, Wybregt S, Baens G, et al. Symptomatic neonatal hypoglycemia. Studies of carbohydrate metabolism in the newborn infant, VIII. Pediatrics 1964;33:388.
254. Arensman FW. The cyanotic newborn: keys to early diagnosis and emergency management. J Med Assoc Ga 1984;73:627.
255. Yabek SM. Neonatal cyanosis, reappraisal of response to 100% oxygen breathing. Am J Dis Child 1984;138:880.
256. Watcha MF, Connor MT, Hing AV. Pulse oximetry in methemoglobinemia. Am J Dis Child 1989;143:845–847.
257. Wood P. Attacks of deeper cyanosis and loss of consciousness (syncope) in Fallot's tetralogy. Br Heart J 1958;20:282.
258. Braudo JL, Zion MM. The cyanotic (syncopal) attack in Fallot's tetralogy. Br Med J 1959;1:1323.
259. Ponce FE, Williams LC, Webb HM, et al. Propranolol palliation of tetralogy of Fallot: experience with long-term drug treatment in pediatric patients. Pediatrics 1973;52:100.
260. Rubin LJ, Nicod P, Hillia LD et al. Treatment of primary pulmonary hypertension with nifedipine. Ann Intern Med 1983;99:433.
261. Packer M, Medina N, Yushak M. Adverse hemodynamic and clinical effects of calcium channel blockade in pulmonary hypertension secondary to obliterative pulmonary vascular disease. J Am Coll Cardiol 1984;4:890.
262. King K, Adam P, Clemente G, et al. Infants of diabetic mothers: attenuated glucose uptake without hyperinsulinemia during continuous glucose infusion. Pediatrics 1969;44:381.
263. Haworth J, Dilling L. Relationships between maternal glucose intolerance and neonatal blood glucose. J Pediatr 1976;89:810.
264. Robertson N, Smith M. Early neonatal hypocalcemia. Arch Dis Child 1973;50:604.
265. Ramamurthy R, Harris V, Pildes R. Subcutaneous calcium deposition in the neonate associated with intravenous administration of calcium gluconate. Pediatrics 1973;55:802.
266. Finch CA. Methemoglobinemia and sulfhemoglobinemia. N Engl J Med 1972;239:470.

Postoperative Management of the Cardiac Surgical Patient 14

Gwenn E. McLaughlin
Nancy A. Setzer
Charles L. Schleien

INTRODUCTION

The immediate postoperative intensive care of the infant or child who has undergone surgery for the palliation or correction of congenital heart disease is an important part of the overall sequence of surgical management of congenital heart disease. This care requires a multidisciplinary approach with coordination of multiple services.

The general principles of care, as outlined in the first part of the chapter, apply to all patients. The preoperative condition, the intraoperative course, and the underlying cardiac defect must all be taken into account. Regardless of the specific cardiac lesion and the nature of the surgery performed, it is necessary for the pediatric intensive care physician caring for these patients to have a broad fund of knowledge in the fields of cardiology, cardiovascular surgery, cardiac anesthesia, pulmonology, neonatology, and other associated medical disciplines. For example, **Table 14–1** lists many of the medical problems which may be seen in infants with congenital heart disease. This chapter will address important issues of postsurgical care, including specific intraoperative problems, the initial assessment of the postoperative cardiac patient, aspects of multiorgan dysfunction seen in the postoperative period, and the management issues specific to the various common cardiac lesions.

Table 14.1. Preoperative Problems in Neonates

Metabolic	• ↓ glucose—poor glycogen stores • ↓ calcium—↓ parathyroid hormone activity • Acidosis • Electrolyte disturbance
Temperature	• Increased heat loss • ↓ ability to generate heat
Pulmonary	• Difficult airway • Premature—hyaline membrane disease, BPD • ↑ Pulmonary vascular resistance —(persistant fetal circulation) —reactive pulmonary vascular bed —vasoconstriction to ↑ PCO_2 and ↓ PO_2 • Pneumothorax
Liver	• ↑ bilirubin • ↓ metabolism of many drugs
Central Nervous System	• Intraventricular hemorrhage

OPEN HEART SURGERY—INTRAOPERATIVE CONCERNS

The postoperative course of the pediatric cardiac surgical patient is dictated to a large extent by intraoperative events, including not only the operation, but also the anesthetic and cardiopulmonary bypass (CPB) management. It is important for the pediatric intensive care physician to understand these events and their impact on the patient to make appropriate decisions in the postoperative period. The surgical procedure for the patient with congenital heart disease is divided into several distinct periods, which include anesthetic induction, pre-bypass surgery, the actual procedure during cardiopulmonary bypass, and the post-bypass period; information regarding each of these periods should be relayed when report is given in the ICU postoperatively.

Presurgical and Anesthetic Management

Anesthesia for congenital heart repair may be induced safely by a variety of methods, including intravenous agents such as ketamine or thiopental, intramuscular injections such as ketamine, or by inhalation agents depending on the child's disease and underlying physical condition. Anesthetic selection is based upon knowledge of the child's cardiovascular lesion and the cardiovascular effects of the various anesthetic drugs. A child with tetralogy of Fallot and good ventricular function, as an example, may tolerate anesthetic induction with inhalation halothane, intravenous fentanyl or thiopental, or intramuscular ketamine[1,2]. The common goal which can be achieved with each of these is to avoid increases in inotropy or decreased systemic vascular resistance (SVR), either of which might exaggerate right-to-left intracardiac shunting. Other anesthetic agents which decrease SVR or increase right ventricular outflow obstruction might be detrimental because they lead to an increased shunt and cyanosis.

At the other end of the clinical spectrum, the child with ventricular failure and congenital heart disease will poorly tolerate general anesthesia with any of the agents which depress myocardial contractility, such as halothane. Frequently, anesthesia is induced in these infants with agents which are more hemodynamically "neutral", such as fentanyl or sufentanil[3–5].

Table 14.2. Physiologic Factors That May be Altered By Anesthetic Agents

Respiratory	• Airway reactivity; bronchomotor tone • Chemoreceptor response to pCO_2 • Hypoxic pulmonary vasocontriction • Ciliary function
Central Nervous System	• Intracranial pressure • Cerebral blood flow • Cerebral oxygen consumption • Seizure threshold • Cognitive function
Cardiovascular	• Heart rate • Cardiac output • Systemic vascular resistance • Pulmonary vascular resistance • Baroreceptor response • Coronary blood flow • Arrhythmia threshold
Endocrine	• Catecholamine release • Growth hormone, insulin, steroid release
Immunologic	• Immune response
Miscellaneous	• Renal blood flow • Hepatic blood flow • Gastric motility

Coexisting diseases or anatomic abnormalities also influence selection of the anesthetic agent. Formulation of an anesthetic plan for any congenital heart surgery will be based on consideration of the child's cardiovascular abnormality and any other medical problems as well as the physiological effects of the individual anesthetic agents **(Table 14–2)**. As an example, anesthesia induction in the child in whom tracheal intubation is anticipated to be difficult may best be approached by a spontaneous ventilation, mask induction with halothane. Once the airway is secured, a change from this to another anesthetic technique is easily done. Similarly, in a child with severe asthma and cardiac disease, the effects of the anesthetic agents on bronchomotor tone must be considered. It should be remembered that anesthetic agents frequently have additive, and at times widely differing effects, when used in combination rather than alone.

After anesthetic induction, the child is endotracheally intubated, either via the nasal or the oral route. Nasal intubation may be preferred when it is anticipated that several days of mechanical ventilatory support will be needed in the uncooperative infant to decrease the risk of accidental extubation. One example is the infant with elevated preoperative pulmonary vascular resistance (PVR) who will likely have episodes of pulmonary hypertension necessitating controlled ventilation for several days postoperatively. There are, however, additional risks associated with nasotracheal intubation, including an increased incidence of bacteremia, sinusitis, and nasopharyngeal bleeding, which will be compounded by subsequent systemic heparinization used for bypass. These can be eliminated by administration of preoperative antibiotics and by gentle introduction of the tube into the nasopharynx.

Once the child has been successfully induced, anesthesia may be maintained with a variety of agents. Intravenous narcotics, such as fentanyl and sufentanil in anesthetic rather than analgesic doses, are the most frequently used agents in anesthetizing infants for complex, high-risk procedures because of their hemodynamic stability[5–7]. In contrast to the potent inhalational anesthetics, such as isoflurane and halothane, these drugs have been shown to have minimal effect on SVR or cardiac output and to lower an elevated PVR[8]. However, because of the long half-life of narcotics, they may delay extubation for several hours postoperatively. Adjuncts, such as midazolam given to ensure amnesia, compounds these effects on the respiratory and central nervous system (CNS) **(Table 14–3)**.

There is a wider variety of agents which can be used in children undergoing simple repairs, such as elective patent ductus arteriosus (PDA) ligation or atrial septal defect (ASD) repair. Anesthesia for children who do not have congestive heart failure may be provided with shorter-acting agents, such as the inhalation anesthetics. These allow faster awakening and tracheal extubation shortly after surgery ends.

After tracheal intubation and before surgical incision, invasive monitors, including an arterial line and central venous catheters, are placed. Currently, flow-directed pulmonary artery (PA) catheters are not used for the majority of small infants, because of obstructions, holes, and detours to the "normal" intracardiac blood flow pattern present in the majority of children with congenital heart disease. One group has successfully placed intraoperative balloon-tipped PA catheters with the use of fluoroscopy[9]; however, this adds to the preoperative time. Alternatively, pulmonary artery pressure, mixed venous saturation, and left atrial filling pressure can be measured via a transthoracic catheter placed during surgery and left in place for use postoperatively. More recently, intraoperative monitoring of cardiac function and efficacy of surgical repair by echocardiographic studies are being used. The transesophageal approach can be used in infants and children for continuous monitoring[10], although the relatively large probe size lim-

Table 14.3. Comparative Hemodynamic Effices of Induction Doses of Anesthetic Agents

	Heart Rate	*SVR*	*CO*
Halothane (1MAC)*	↓	↓←→	↓
Isoflurane (1MAC)*	↑	↓	↑
Ketamine	↑	↑	↑
Thiopental	↑	↓	↓
Fentanyl	↓	↓←→	←→
Midazolam	←→	↓←→	←→
Sufentanil	↓	↓←→	←→
Propofol	←→	↓	↓
Etomidate	←→	←→	←→

**MAC, minimum alveolar concentration, is a description of the amount of anesthetic necessary to prevent movement to a given stimulus in an unparalyzed patient. It is a method of comparing equivalent "doses" of inhalation agents when serum levels measurements cannot be done or are inappropriate. SVR, systemic vascular resistance; CO, cardiac output.*

its the use of this technology in very small infants. Epicardial imaging using a sterile-sheathed transducer can be used in these circumstances[11].

Surgery

Knowledge of the actual surgical procedure is essential in formulating a plan for care in the postoperative period. Surgery may be palliative or curative. Surgical access may be through a thoracotomy or via median sternotomy. Repair may be done with or without cardiopulmonary bypass (CPB) support.

Thoracotomy entails collapse of one lung during the operation. This approach, which is used for PDA ligation, placement of a Blalock-Taussig shunt, coarctation of the aorta repair, and pulmonary artery banding in some instances, may result in pulmonary problems due to atelectasis postoperatively. Additionally, intrathoracic structures, such as the thoracic duct or phrenic nerve, may be injured. These may manifest themselves as management problems in the ICU with chylothorax, or diaphragmatic paralysis several days postoperatively.

Procedures may be done with or without bypass support of the circulation. The same procedure under different clinical circumstances may be done either way. For those procedures in which CPB is used, knowledge of the systemic effects of bypass and the mechanism by which the myocardium is preserved intraoperatively is fundamental to understanding postoperative hemodynamics.

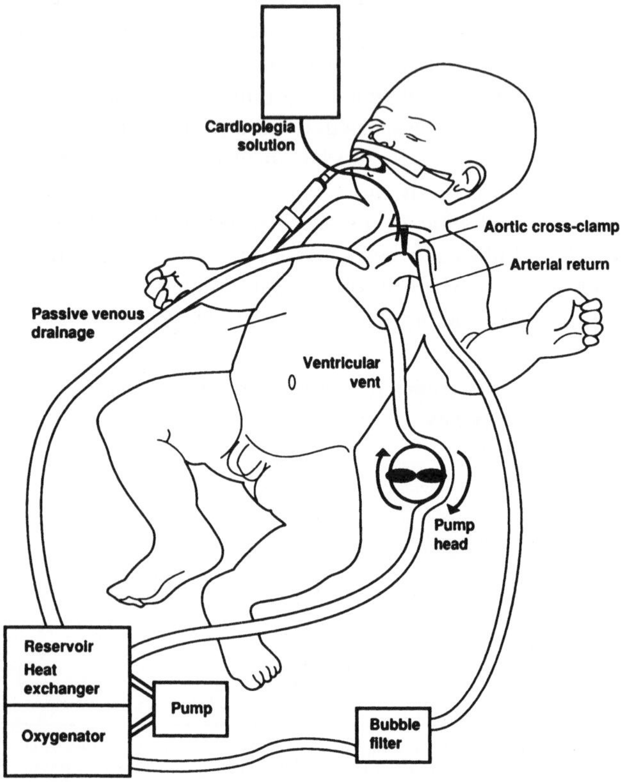

Figure 14.1. Cardiopulmonary bypass schematic. Note positions of venous and arterial cannulae, aortic cross-clamp, and cardioplegia infusion site.

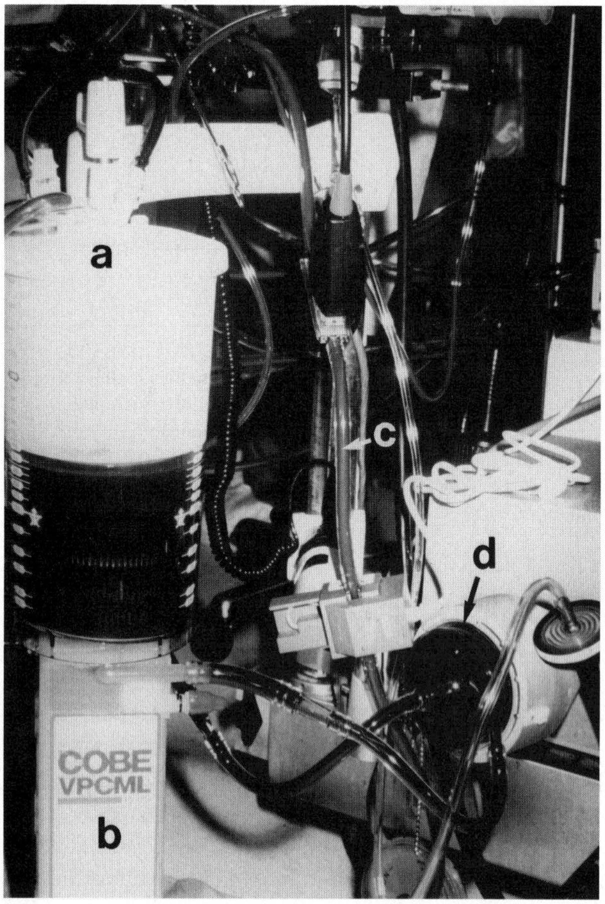

Figure 14.2. Components of cardiopulmonary bypass circuitry. Venous blood is passively drained from the patient into reservoir (a) then is pumped into the membrane oxygenator (b) where oxygen and carbon dioxide exchange occurs. From the base of the oxygenator, blood is pumped back into the child (c). In this setup, a centrifugal pump head is used (d).

Cardiopulmonary Bypass

CPB has several essential components which will be described below in detail (Figs. 14–1, 14–2, and 14–3). Conceptually, anticoagulated blood passively drains from the systemic veins or right atrium via a large cannula into a reservoir. Following "ventilation" in a mechanical oxygenator, the blood is filtered and actively pumped into the systemic circulation via an aortic cannula. During bypass, while the heart is inactive, nutrients are supplied either by continuous perfusion from bypass through the coronary arteries, or by a cardioplegia solution which relaxes the heart and decreases its metabolism. While on bypass, venous return to the heart from the periphery is diverted by cannulae placed in the inferior and superior vena cavae or a single cannula in the right atrium and allowed to drain by gravity to the venous reservoir on the circuit. Blood is not actively pumped from the body and any impediment to venous return may lead to venous engorgement. This may result in

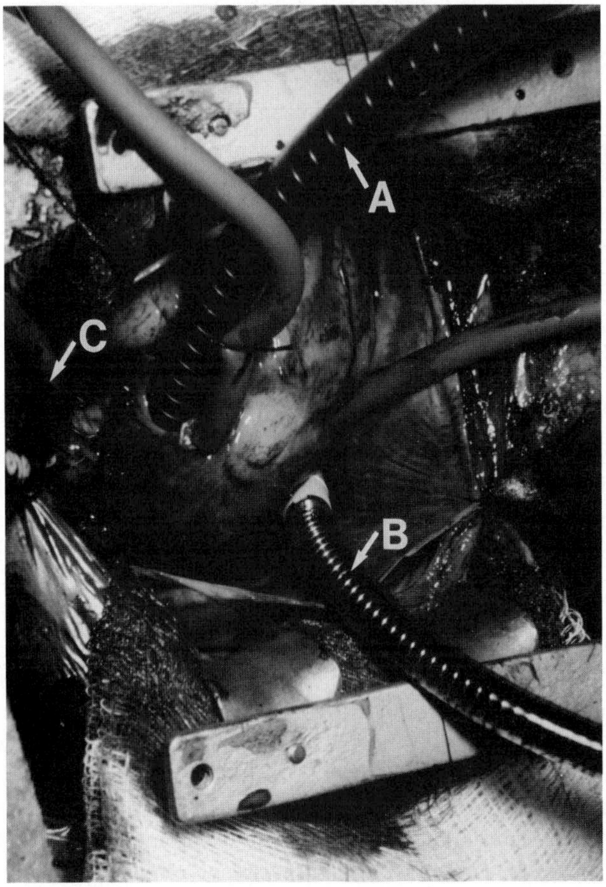

Figure 14.3. Perfusion cannulae in situ during cardiopulmonary bypass. Venous return to the pump from cannula in the SVC (a) and IVC (b) via the right atrium. Arterial return to the infant's aorta is through cannula in the aorta (c).

inadvertent cerebral venous hypertension and cerebral edema if the superior vena cava (SVC) cannula is obstructed, or passive hepatic congestion if the inferior vena cava (IVC) cannula is obstructed. In addition to the venous cannulae, blood return to the reservoir also comes from a separate (pump) suction, which scavenges blood from the operative field, and a myocardial vent, which continuously empties the heart.

All venous return from the patient is drained into a common reservoir where heating and cooling occurs. It is then pumped through an oxygenator where CO_2 removal and O_2 addition occurs. This "ventilation" may be done with either a membrane or a bubble oxygenator. These differ in the type of interface between the patient's blood and the added gas. Membrane oxygenators are currently the predominant type in clinical use for children. Gas supply and blood are separated by a thin, semipermeable membrane with no direct contact between them. Oxygenation occurs by passive diffusion across a concentration gradient. In bubble oxygenators, oxygen is bubbled directly through the blood, and residual air bubbles are filtered before blood is returned to the heart. These oxygenators are relatively inexpensive and simple, but produce significant hemolysis with prolonged bypass. Additionally, there is a theoretically greater risk of micro-air-bubble embolization, despite the use of arterial line filters. After passage through either type of oxygenator, the blood is filtered and actively pumped into the child's aorta.

Pump flow rates are generally adjusted to approximate normal cardiac output, i.e., 2.4 liters/m^2/min during normothermia. These can be safely reduced during hypothermia when metabolic requirements are decreased[12,13]. Monitoring during bypass for physiological well-being and adequacy of perfusion currently consists of on-line continuous mixed venous saturation and periodic arterial blood gas determinations[14]. Decreases in mixed venous saturation, or development of metabolic acidosis may indicate inadequate perfusion and tissue oxygen delivery. Other parameters monitored episodically include hematocrit, serum electrolytes (including potassium and ionized calcium), and glucose[15]. Ionized hypocalcemia commonly occurs during bypass, due at least in part to large volumes of crystalloid and blood to prime the pump. This may adversely affect cardiac function and alter cardiac rhythm post-bypass if uncorrected. Currently, the optimal management for serum glucose during bypass and surgery is a matter of debate. Retrospective data as well as prospective animal studies have suggested that preexisting mild hyperglycemia (serum glucose >140 mg/dl) may aggravate brain ischemia-induced neurological injury[16,17]. To confuse the issue further, fasted children may be hypoglycemic preoperatively with minimal clinical symptoms, or may develop hypoglycemia intraoperatively with symptoms masked by general anesthesia[18]. It is also recognized that children may develop hyperglycemia with serum glucose >180 mg/dl intraoperatively, even with relatively low levels of glucose infusion of 2 mg/kg/min[19]. In this context, most centers have opted to either infuse glucose at low levels intraoperatively, or withhold glucose and closely monitor glucose levels. Hemodilution to a hematocrit in the 20 to 25% range is used during hypothermia to prevent problems with viscosity and sludging in the microcirculation. Hemodilution is achieved on bypass by using either an asanguinous bypass pump prime or diluted blood to prime the pump. The final hematocrit can be calculated from the patient's blood volume and hematocrit and the pump prime volume.

Anticoagulation to prevent clotting in the bypass tubing is required for CPB. Levels of anticoagulation are monitored serially by activated coagulation time (ACT) determinations throughout bypass. Heparin at a dose of 300 μ/kg is chosen for bypass because of its easy reversibility by protamine. Adequacy of anticoagulation is assessed before bypass, and periodically during bypass by following the ACT, which is maintained above 400 seconds. Levels below this have been associated with the development of clotting, fibrin deposition on bypass tubing, and low grade disseminated intravascular coagulopathy (DIC) with secondary fibrinolysis. Rare patients exhibit resistance to the anticoagulant effects of heparin[20], usually because of antithrombin III deficiency, which is, ironically, usually acquired during chronic heparin therapy.

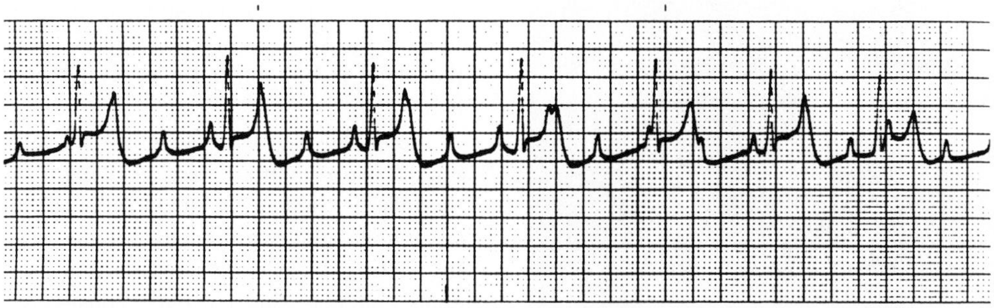

Figure 14.4. Transient third degree heart block at temperature of 26°C after aortic cross clamp removal and during rewarming on bypass after ventricular septal defect repair. This reverted to sinus rhythm at 29°C.

After separation from bypass, the heparin effect is reversed with protamine to control excessive bleeding. Although this is generally uneventful, heparin-protamine complexes form which can activate the classical complement cascade. Hemodynamic reactions to protamine, when they occur, are of three types[21]. The most common reaction is a mild drop in blood pressure, related to a decrease in contractility or SVR, presumed to be due to histamine release and requiring little or no hemodynamic support. Less frequently, catastrophic pulmonary vasoconstriction with frank right ventricular failure is seen, usually in patients with preoperative pulmonary hypertension[22]. Patients allergic to fish, or taking protamine-containing insulin preparations, appear to be at greatest risk. These hemodynamic responses occur more often with rapid central venous administration. True anaphylaxis is rare; this reaction must be treated with aggressive vasopressor support[23,24]. In some instances reheparinization and a return to bypass may be needed to rest the heart[25].

Generalized systemic hypothermia to a core temperature of 25 to 28°C is used for most procedures on bypass to aid in organ preservation. Transient arrhythmias, particularly heart block, during rewarming after the surgical repair are common (Fig. 14–4).

Myocardial Function and Protection During Bypass

The myocardium is subjected to several traumatic and metabolic insults during open heart surgery, particularly during CPB. It is important to minimize myocardial metabolism and myocardial work during this period. Myocardial metabolism is increased by mechanical and electrical activity, and minimized during asystole. During the normal cardiac cycle, coronary blood flow to the left ventricle occurs primarily during diastole. Coronary perfusion pressure is typically defined as the aortic diastolic blood pressure minus the left ventricular end-diastolic pressure (LVEDP), the downstream pressure limiting coronary flow. During CPB, as during the awake state, coronary perfusion can be maximized by minimizing LVEDP.

A still, nonbeating heart is a requirement for intracardiac repair. This can be achieved in several ways, including using hypothermia or electrically induced ventricular fibrillation, or by instilling a cardioplegia solution into the coronary arteries to arrest the heart. All of these methods decrease myocardial oxygen consumption, particularly if the heart is empty. A left ventricular vent, which ensures an empty heart, is inserted to return venous blood from the heart back into the bypass circuit.

Simple, short operations, such as an uncomplicated secundum (atrial septal defect ASD) repair can be done while the heart is fibrillating and continuously perfused by the bypass circuit. More complex procedures require an empty bloodless field with no movement. This is best provided by arresting the heart in diastole, after hypothermia is achieved. Cardioplegia is given through a cannula inserted into the aortic root which perfuses the coronary arteries. The solution does not leak into the systemic circulation because an aortic cross-clamp is placed above the cardioplegia cannula and proximal to the aortic inflow cannula from the bypass machine.

The most essential components of cardioplegia are a high concentration of potassium and a cold temperature, which cause the heart to arrest in diastole **(Table 14–4).** It has been demonstrated that in the absence of electrical activity and mechanical work, at a temperature of 5°C, myocardial metabolism is reduced to 5% of baseline; although quiescent, a low level of oxygen consumption continues. Any increase in myocardial metabolism can produce myocardial cellular ischemia, resulting in cellular swelling, breakdown of the mitochondrial apparatus, depletion of cellular ATP stores, and accumulation of the breakdown products of anaerobic metabolism with reactive oxygen species production. It is therefore important that the heart remain cold and arrested throughout the period of aortic cross-clamping, which may require several doses of cardioplegia for more complicated procedures with longer bypass times. This, combined with systemic hypothermia, will generally maintain a low myocardial temperature.

Table 14.4. Components of Cardioplegia

- Lactated ringers solution
- Glucose
- Potassium
- Lidocaine
- Mannitol
- β-blockers*
- Steroids*

Sometimes added.

Table 14.5. Systemic Effects of Cardiopulmonary Bypass

Neurologic	• Emboli (both air and debris)
	• Lower cerebral blood flow
	• Lower $CMRO_2$
	• Intact autoregulation
Cardiac	• Ischemia—coronary exclusion
	• Emboli
	• Director coronary injury
Pulmonary	• Vascular exclusion during bypass
	• Complement-induced endothelial damage
Renal	• Nonpulsate perfusion
	• Elevated ADH levels
Gastrointestinal	• Emboli
Coagulation	• Complement activation
	• Platelet consumption
	• Altered platelet aggregation
	• Coagulation factor dilution
Endocrine	• Elevated growth hormone, insulin
	• Elevated glucose

There are several other components of cardioplegia solution which may be added for myocardial protection, including lidocaine, glucose, β-adrenergic blockers, or calcium channel blockers. Additionally, blood from the patient may be mixed with the crystalloid solution in an effort to provide increased oxygen substrate as "more efficient" hemoglobin-bound oxygen rather than dissolved oxygen during the cross-clamp period. There have been no definitive studies demonstrating the absolute superiority of any of these methods, and so the composition of cardioplegia solution varies, largely reflecting individual beliefs.

Aside from the damage due to ongoing myocardial metabolism, additional myocardial injury can occur during bypass **(Table 14–5).** Coronary artery structural abnormalities, such as stenosis, may prevent adequate cardioplegia solution from perfusing the distal myocardium. Although this is primarily a problem during adult coronary surgery, it may occur in children. Microbubbles of air, or particulate emboli, may be inadvertently flushed into the coronary circulation during cardioplegia instillation, producing transient abnormalities noted during reperfusion (Fig. 14–5). Finally, the coronary arteries may be injured either directly or by kinking during the surgical procedure itself, resulting in subsequent myocardial damage (Fig. 14–6). Although these effects are generally self-limited, subtle myocardial dysfunction requiring vasopressor support after bypass may occur, particularly with longer aortic cross-clamp times **(Table 14–6).**

Pulmonary Effects During Cardiopulmonary Bypass

The lungs are uniquely susceptible to injury following CPB. The passage of blood through the bypass circuit is associated with neutrophil and complement activation with cytokine release, while diminished blood flow can lead to activation of the xanthine oxidase enzyme. When normal flow is established, the vast endothelial network of the lung is injured by neutrophil release of reactive oxygen species and elastases[26,27]. In the presence of oxygen, xanthine oxidase activity promotes the formation of superoxide anion and the hydroxyl radical. Unlike other organs, the lungs have a dual blood supply from both the pulmonary artery and bronchial arteries while receiving oxygen from both the systemic circulation and through local alveolar diffusion; this may allow more exposure to reactive oxygen species during a deleterious low flow bypass state. Children with severe cyanosis and extensive bronchial collateral circulation seem

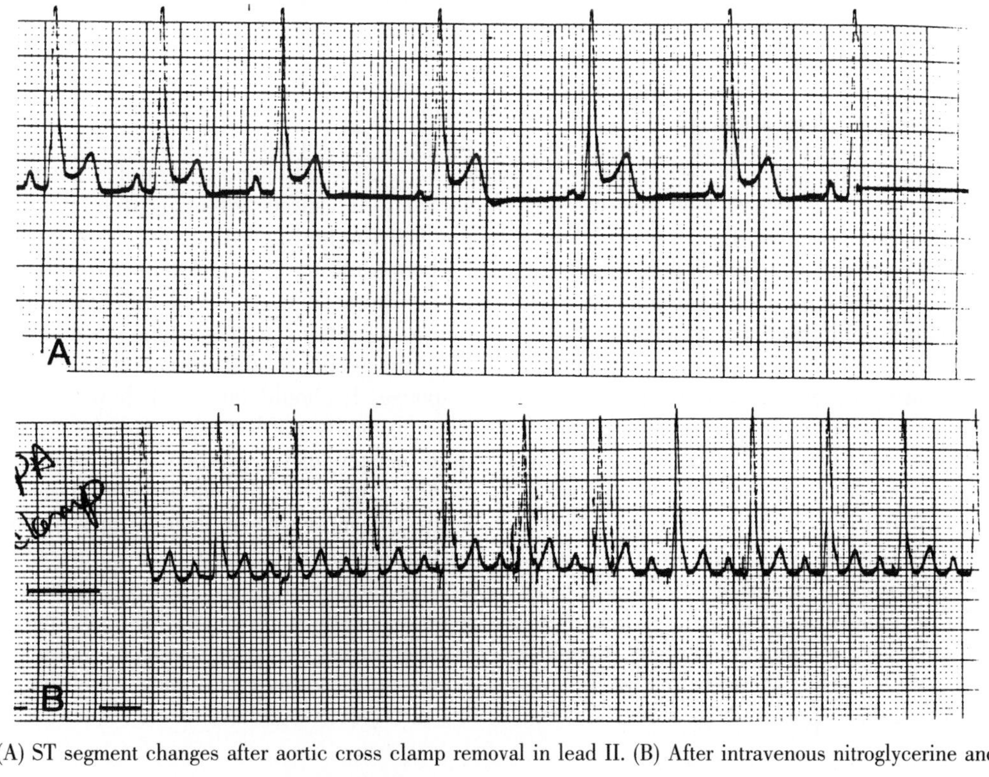

Figure 14.5. (A) ST segment changes after aortic cross clamp removal in lead II. (B) After intravenous nitroglycerine and reperfusion.

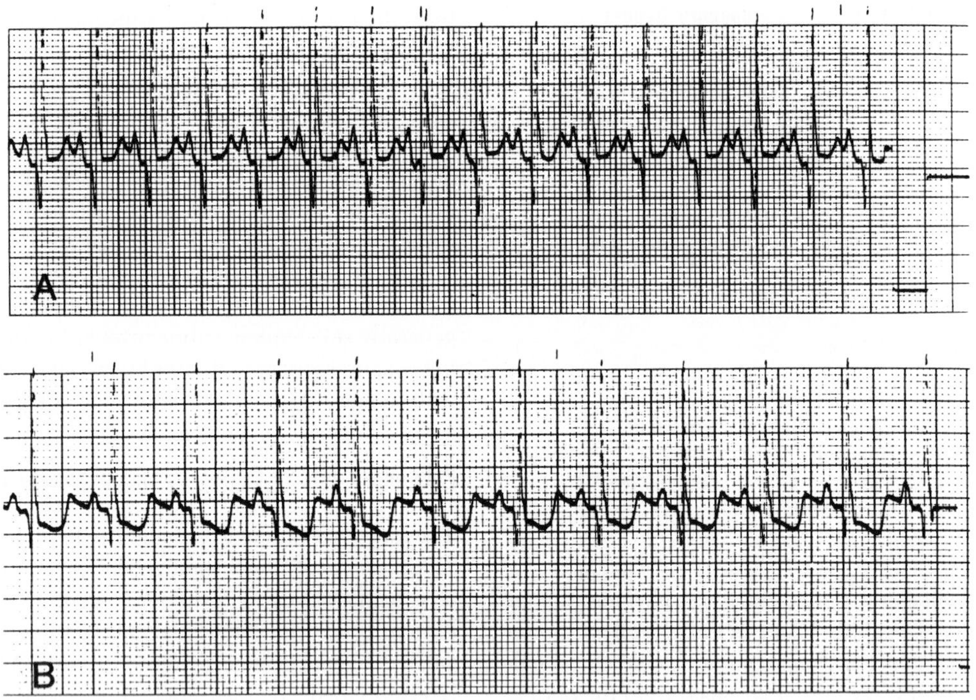

Figure 14.6. Intraoperative myocardial ischemia in child with anomalous coronary artery. (A) Baseline trace from lead II; q wave related to previous inferior wall myocardial infarction. (B) Intraoperative tracing during manipulation; note ST segment depression.

to be particularly affected. Pulmonary endothelial damage results in capillary leak or increased protein permeability, culminating in increased lung water and decreased pulmonary function and hypoxemia post-bypass. This endothelial injury is thought to primarily occur at the level of the post-capillary venule and can contribute to pulmonary hypertension. CPB is also associated with a loss of surfactant activity[28], possibly through inactivation. If left atrial pressure is high, the pulmonary capillaries may be subjected to high hydrostatic pressure, with resulting pulmonary edema and hemorrhage.

Renal Effects During Cardiopulmonary Bypass

The kidneys are affected during bypass by several physiological variables. Generally, renal perfusion pressure during CPB is lower than when awake. This is perceived by the juxtaglomerular apparatus as hypovolemia, which responds by increasing renin release. Other hormonal changes include release of antidiuretic hormone, which is normally elevated during surgery and further increased by lack of pulsatile perfusion during bypass. Natriuretic peptide levels also rise during bypass. Additional renal injury can occur after red cell hemolysis which results from shear trauma produced by bypass. The free hemoglobin is seen first as hematuria during and after bypass. Although a severe renal functional abnormality is unlikely to result from iron deposition in the renal tubules, it is important to maintain urine flow. Other causes of hemolysis, particularly a hemolytic-transfusion reaction, must be excluded. Finally, hemodynamic instability before or during weaning from bypass may result in further decreases in perfusion pressure and may contribute to decreased renal blood flow and oliguria. All of these effects are predictable; to offset oliguria, osmotic diuretics (such as mannitol) and loop diuretics (such as furosemide) are often given during bypass to maintain urine flow. Continued postoperative oliguria is currently seen almost exclusively in the setting of myocardial dysfunction and a global low cardiac output state.

Endocrine Effects During Cardiopulmonary Bypass

Recently, research has focused on the stress response of newborns and infants to anesthesia, surgery, and cardiopulmonary bypass. Anand et al. first noted that newborns undergoing PDA ligation under a "light" general anesthesia using nitrous oxide and oxygen had a generalized stress response to the surgery characterized by elevations in plasma epinephrine and norepinephrine concentrations lasting for 24 hours into the postoperative period[29]. A group of similar newborns, who received intravenous fentanyl in addition to nitrous oxide, had complete ablation of the norepinephrine response and a markedly depressed epinephrine response. It should be noted, however, that these babies were clinically stable at the time of surgery and did not require exogenous catecholamine circulatory support.

The response of the endocrine system during open heart surgery in newborns undergoing more complex procedures, including the arterial switch procedure and hypoplastic left heart repair, have been studied[30]. These infants, despite general anesthesia with halothane and morphine, had a generalized stress response to surgery distinguished by elevations in the catabolic hormones which persisted throughout the perioperative period. Overall, there was a 26% mortality in these infants, possibly due in part to inadequate perioperative control of this catabolic response. This study was followed by a randomized trial comparing this anesthetic technique with anesthesia with high-dose sufentanil in a similar group of sick neonates(31). The sufentanil group had milder elevations in stress hormones, with lower postoperative morbidity and mortality.

Central Nervous System Effects During Cardiopulmonary Bypass

Central nervous system (CNS) sequelae following open heart surgery and CPB are not uncommon(32). Currently, no exact figures exist for congenital heart surgery, although it is estimated that as many as 40% of patients undergoing open heart surgery have subtle neurological deficits as measured by neuropsychiatric testing preoperatively and postoperatively(33). Severe brain damage after bypass has been found in some adult series to be the second most common cause of death, after myocardial failure, following cardiac surgery.

Table 14.6. Frequently Used Cardiovascular Medications

Agent	*Dosage Range (μg/kg/min)*	*Effects*
Dopamine	1–3	renal vasodilator
	5–10	inotrope
	>10	$\alpha >> \beta$, ↑ PVR, ↑ SVR
Dobutamine	1–20	β_1-agonist; mild β_2-agonist inotrope, chronotrope vasodilator, ↓ PVR, ↓ SVR arrhythmogenic weak α effect
Isoproterenol	0.05–1	β-agonist (nonselective) inotrope, chronotrope vasodilator, ↓ PVR, ↓ SVR arrhythmogenic
Epinephrine	0.05–0.3	potent β-agonist, inotrope, chronotrope
	0.3–2	$\alpha > \beta$ effect, ↑ SVR
Norepinephrine	0.05–1.0	α agonist, some β effect at low doses vasoconstriction
Amrinone	5–10	loading dose- 0.75–4 mg/kg given slowly, t½ 4 hr vasodilator, ↓ PVR, ↓ SVR inotrope (not chronotrope) thrombocytopenia
Sodium Nitroprusside	0.05–10	arterial > venous vasodilator ↑ ICP, may ↑ hypoxia by blunting HPV response, cyanide toxicity, tachyphylaxis
Nitroglycerine	1–20	venous > arterial vasodilator ↓ preload, ↑ ICP
Esmolol	50–300	β_1 antagonist- short t½ 8 min, may load with 500 mcg/kg negative inotrope and chronotrope potentially useful for tachycardia, tachyarrhythmias and infundibular spasm, may cause bronchospasm
Labetalol	100–1000	$\beta > \alpha$ antagonist, vasodilator, negative inotrope, t½ 5 hr

Other consequences, including cerebral infarcts, hemorrhage, choreoathetosis, spinal cord infarcts and neuropsychiatric syndromes have been recognized for years(34–36). Very little objective data on the incidence of these complications exist, perhaps because of reticence of centers to report on them and the paucity of preoperative and postoperative comparative studies. In one prospective study, one-third of all children evaluated by computed tomography and magnetic resonance imaging scans before cardiac surgery had unsuspected central nervous system abnormalities, including cerebral infarctions, absence of corpus callosum, and ventriculomegaly(37).

There may be multiple causes for central nervous system damage during CPB. Macroemboli and microemboli, both particulate and air, may occur, despite de-airing procedures, particularly during open-chamber procedures. Intracranial hemorrhage can occur after systemic heparinization associated with CPB(38). Global CNS hypoperfusion may result from incorrect cannulae placement, preexisting cerebrovascular disease, or inadequate cerebral perfusion(39). Cerebral blood flow during bypass can be affected by impaired venous drainage from mechanical factors such as superior vena cava cannula placement, resulting in elevation of intracranial pressure. Similarly, postoperatively, the interatrial baffle placed during the Senning or Mustard procedure may inadvertently obstruct venous return, as may the elevated SVC pressures which are necessary for pulmonary perfusion after the Fontan and Glenn procedures.

Global CNS injury may also occur during cardiopulmonary bypass, when cerebral blood flow is inadequate to meet the brain's metabolic demands. Autoregulation of cerebral blood flow during hypothermia, and CPB has been an area of controversy and extensive research; however, what constitutes an adequate perfusion pressure during CPB and hypothermia in children is still unknown. Hypothermia has been demonstrated to decrease both cerebral metabolism and blood flow. Management of arterial blood gases, and in particular CO_2 during hypothermia, may have important effects on total cerebral blood flow and thus global neurological outcome after bypass(39,40). The pCO_2 level can be measured and regulated to 40 mmHg either at the temperature at which the body is functioning (α-stat, or temperature uncorrected) or at normal body temperature (pH stat, or temperature corrected). pH-stat regulation is based on the premise that pH should be maintained constant despite hypothermia during bypass. It has been widely observed in poikilothermic animals, however, that pH may fluctuate with changing body temperature, reflecting decreased CO_2 levels. Intracellular electrochemical neutrality is maintained, however, despite the change of pH because of the constant ratio between H^+ and OH^- ions intracellularly. Intracellular neutrality (albeit at a different pH) helps to maintain an optimal milieu for homeostatic cellular function, including enzyme reaction rates, concentration of metabolic intermediates, and intracellular protein structure and function. α-Stat regulation strives to maintain intracellular electrochemical neutrality as the patient cools. Alpha refers to the α-imidazole group of the protein buffer histidine, the most significant of the intracellular buffers. In terms of practical bypass management, pCO_2 and pH tend to decrease with hypothermia; in order to maintain a pH of 7.4, when the blood gas is temperature corrected to normal body temperature, extra CO_2 must be added to the gas flows to the oxygenator. This is not necessary when temperature uncorrected, or α-stat regulation of blood gases is used during bypass.

Using radioactive-xenon cerebral blood flow determinations in humans during bypass, it has been demonstrated that cerebral autoregulation with coupling of cerebral blood flow to cerebral metabolism remains intact using α-stat regulation of blood gases[(41,42)]. Regional cerebral blood flow autoregulation remains intact even during hypothermia with mean arterial pressures in the 30–40 mmHg range, when α-stat management of CO_2 during CPB is used[(42)]. pH-stat, or temperature correction of blood gases and pCO_2 regulation, requires additional CO_2 being added to the CPB. This results in vasodilation and excessive cerebral flow, with the potential for elevated intracranial pressure, or intracerebral steal phenomenon. Although these effects have been demonstrated in vitro, a prospective study in adults undergoing cardiac surgery found no differences in neuropsychiatric complications between the two methods[(43)]. Cerebral blood flow autoregulation across the normal range of perfusion pressures has been demonstrated when α-stat regulation of blood gases is used, including during deep hypothermia. In a special exception, children who undergo deep hypothermic circulatory arrest, despite α-stat regulation of blood gases, lose the ability to autoregulate cerebral blood flow upon resumption of bypass, and have pressure dependent flow[(44)].

After CPB, blood-brain barrier abnormalities were not observed in a canine model of hypothermia and bypass[(45)], although intracranial pressure is elevated during resumption of circulation[(46,47)]. Elevated intracranial pressure during a time of low cardiac output may impair cerebral perfusion.

Basal ganglia abnormalities manifested by choreoathetosis and movement disorders have been described[(48–50)] after cardiopulmonary bypass with hypothermia and appear to be more common after deep hypothermia. However, this complication is also seen after bypass without deep hypothermia and may result from a localized difference between oxygen supply and demand. One study correlated the development of choreoathetosis with hypocapnia as measured by the α-stat method during rewarming, suggesting that relative ischemia was responsible[(50)]. Similarly, choreoathetosis was associated with pulmonary collaterals arising from the neck, which may induce a steal phenomenon[(51)].

Cerebral protection during CPB is being explored with renewed enthusiasm as mortality from myocardial failure has lessened. Barbiturates were demonstrated to have "cerebral protective" effects during open chamber cardiac surgery in adults[(52)]; however, criticisms of this study include the use of normothermic bypass and the lack of filters in the bypass apparatus. Prophylactic barbiturate administration did not alter the incidence of stroke after adult coronary surgery[(53)].

Hypothermic Circulatory Arrest

Several procedures in congenital heart surgery are performed with total circulatory arrest, which facilitates repair of complex lesions in the small heart. This results in a totally bloodless field and allows removal of the venous cannulae which may obscure visualization of small intracardiac structures. The technique for cold circulatory arrest is relatively simple; the body is systemically cooled both topically and on bypass to a temperature of less than 20°C. Bypass is then stopped to allow repair of the lesion. After repair, the cannulae are replaced, circulation on bypass is resumed, and the patient is warmed[(54)].

Unique central nervous system problems related to hypothermic circulatory arrest are related to the duration of arrest and to body temperature[(55)]. At a core temperature of 18–20°C, 50 to 60 minutes of circulatory arrest is tolerated with minimal risk of gross motor or intellectual deficits; however, approximately 5–10% of these patients will have postoperative seizures[(56)]. Despite hypothermia to temperatures less than 20°C and electrocerebral silence, cerebral metabolism and oxygen consumption continue, as documented by continuously decreasing cerebral oxyhemoglobin content during circulatory arrest. The use of an even lower core temperature, to further decrease metabolism, has so far proven untenable because of microcirculatory disturbances. Other problems associated with hypothermic circulatory arrest in infants are elevated anterior fontanelle pressure and delayed normalization of visual evoked responses[(46,47)]. Other organs, including the kidneys, lungs, and liver, appear to be more tolerant of total circulatory arrest than the brain. Clinically these organs are rarely affected.

Cardiopulmonary Bypass Effects on ICU Course

Many of the physiological derangements which begin during CPB continue to manifest themselves during the initial period in the ICU **(Table 14–5).** Despite warming on bypass and subsequent passive warming measures, some degree of hypothermia is typically present upon admission of the child to the ICU. As warming progresses, the peripheral capillary bed continues to dilate, necessitating volume infusion to maintain cardiac filling pressures and volume. This can be partially offset by the earlier use of systemic vasodilators, such as nitroprusside during rewarming on bypass and while in the operating room.

Although heparin is reversed by protamine at the end of bypass, clinical bleeding may continue. Platelets are destroyed or rendered dysfunctional by CPB and are sequestered in the oxygenator. Plasma coagulation factors may be diluted in the bypass prime, or during blood loss after bypass, and may require replacement. Despite initial neutralization, residual rebound heparin effect may be seen sev-

Table 14.7. Information Required on Transfer to Pediatric Intensive Care Unit Team

Surgery	• Type of lesion • Procedure—correction, palliation, shunts, (take-downs?) • Post-repair anatomy • Cardiopulmonary bypass time • Aortic cross-clamp time
History	• Previous medical illnesses • Medications • Allergies • Previous cardiac surgery

Anesthesia	• Intraoperative problems—surgical, anesthetic, bypass
	• Respiratory parameters
	• Airway (easy?, endotracheal tube size, taped, leak?)
	• Ventilator settings
	• Anesthetic agents—reversal, dosage, last medications given
	• Cardiac rate and rhythm
	• Intravascular lines
	• Filling pressures (optimal)
	• Transport problems—bleeding
	• Any vasoactive agents
	• Most recent monitoring of vital signs—heart rate, blood pressure, temperature, urine output
	• Most recent laboratory data
	  • hematocrit
	  • K^+
	  • arterial blood gases
	  • temperature

eral minutes to hours after bypass, as measured by an elevated ACT. Additional protamine may be needed in this case. Coagulation studies should be drawn immediately on admission and replacement factors given if clinically indicated. Excessive postoperative bleeding, particularly if accompanied by hemodynamic instability, may require surgical reexploration to look for a bleeding source. (See hematology section for a full discussion of treatment of coagulopathy postoperatively.)

Many of the postoperative complications of CPB, including pulmonary edema, myocardial edema, and dilution of clotting factors and platelets, are related to or influenced by fluid overload; therefore, many centers now hemofilter the patient's blood as the patient is coming off bypass(57). In a randomized trial in 32 children undergoing tetralogy of Fallot repair, hemofiltration was associated with a higher mean arterial pressure, decreased postoperative blood loss, and a shorter time to extubation; however, these differences were not clinically significant, as no patient required transfusion, and the difference between groups in the duration of ventilation was only 4 hours(58). Of interest, despite the removal of as much 569 ± 223 ml by hemofiltration, the left atrial pressure did not differ between the two groups, suggesting that postoperative fluid management does not need to be adjusted to account for hemofiltration. This modality may be more effective in very small children undergoing prolonged bypass procedures. The improved systolic blood pressure may be secondary to improved cardiac output and a lower pulmonary vascular resistance. These hemodynamic improvements may, in turn, be related to removal of cytokines with negative hemodynamic properties(59).

INITIAL ASSESSMENT IN THE ICU

Postoperative cardiac care of children should begin before surgery by obtaining the necessary data base regarding the patient's cardiac catheterization data and other medical history. Immediately after surgery, a system to smoothly transfer the child from the surgery-anesthesia team to the critical care team should be in place. Fundamental to this transfer of care is the maintenance and continued monitoring of vital signs, including the ECG, blood pressure, ventilation, and oxygenation. During the period of transfer, any essential information pertinent to the patient's preoperative and intraoperative course is communicated, with special regard to the nature of the cardiac lesion and surgical procedure problems during surgery, most recent laboratory results (including hematocrit, electrolytes, arterial blood gases, urine output, temperature, ventilation parameters, optimal filling pressures, and cardiac rate and rhythm) **(Table 14–7).**

Particular attention should be given to bypass time, aortic cross-clamp time, and surgical and anesthetic complications. The rate of post-bypass bleeding, especially during the transport, should be noted. The anesthesiologist must relate information regarding anesthesia, monitoring, and complications. The dosage and time of administration

Table 14.8. Initial Assessment—Physical Examination

Respiratory	• Breath sounds • Endotrachial tube size, taped?, if no cuff-leak? • Chest excursion

Cardiovascular	• Heart rate
	• Blood pressure—waveform
	  • correlate with noninvasive blood pressure
	  • if coarctation—residual upper: lower extremity gradient
	• Heart sounds, murmurs, shunt flow
	• Cardiac output
	  • capillary refill
	  • temperature of distal extremities
	  • peripheral perfusion (color)
	  • precordial activity
	  • pulse volume
	  • wave form (dicrotic notch)
	• Filling pressure—RA, LA
	• Rhythm—ECG
	  • paced?
	  • pacemaker settings

Skin	• Turgor, cyanosis
Central Nervous System	• Level of wakefulness • Pupils (atropine/scopolamine given?) • Motor, sensory (postoperative palsies), deep tendon reflexes, bulbar reflexes
General Abdomen	• Vascular line position • Distended or flat • Liver, spleen size

Table 14.9. Initial Laboratory Values

CBC	• Low platelets • Hematocrit
Electrolytes	• Na ↑ ↓ • K ↓(↑) • Ca^{++} ↓ • Acidosis
Arterial Blood Gas	• pO_2, pCO_2, pH
Coagulation	• PT, PTT, platelets
Liver Function Tests	• SGOT, SGPT, bilirubin • Glucose
Chest x-ray	• Position of endotracheal tube, chest tubes, vascular lines • Heart size • Lung parenchyma, congestion, atelectasis • Pulmonary vascular markings • Pneumothorax or hemothorax • Pericardial effusion

of muscle relaxants and whether a reversal agent has been administered is noted. The dosage and timing of narcotic administration, if given, is important so that there is an appropriate expectation regarding the length of residual narcotic anesthesia. The use of other long-acting sedatives, such as benzodiazepines or droperidol, and the recent use of diuretics, including mannitol or furosemide, should be noted.

The infant or child's respiratory status should be reviewed at this time by assessing skin color, chest movement, air entry, bilateral presence of breath sounds, proper positioning of the endotracheal tube, and blood gas and pH analysis. A rapid assessment of the hemodynamic status of the child is also made, with attention to peripheral perfusion, pulse volume, precordial activity, heart rate and rhythm, blood pressure, urine output, and right and left atrial filling pressures when available. Depending on this assessment, appropriate therapy can be promptly instituted **(Table 14–8).**

A chest x-ray is obtained, noting the position of the tip of the endotracheal tube; the location of central vascular catheters; the position of mediastinal, chest, and nasogastric tubes; heart size; and the condition of the lung fields, including the presence of atelectasis, pneumothorax, or hemothorax and the status of pulmonary vascular markings. Blood studies monitored in the first 10 minutes after arrival of the patient to the ICU include hematocrit, arterial blood gases, pH, serum electrolytes, ionized calcium levels, coagulation studies (including prothrombin time [PT], partial thromboplastin time [PTT], and a platelet count) **(Table 14–9).**

POSTOPERATIVE MONITORING

Noninvasive Monitoring (Table 14–10)

Ongoing surveillance is the key to optimal care for the postoperative patient. Thorough monitoring and continuous surveillance of the acquired data is necessary to direct further therapies for the patient. Noninvasive monitoring techniques with inherently less discomfort and fewer complications are aesthetically preferable to invasive monitoring techniques but frequently do not provide adequate information on a continuous basis, which is needed for the care of the rapidly changing postoperative patient. Choosing between noninvasive and invasive monitoring techniques requires knowledge of the limitations of these techniques, the individual patient, and the nature of the cardiac lesion(60). Standard noninvasive monitoring modalities are employed on all patients. More critically ill patients will require more invasive monitoring(61).

Electrocardiogram

Continuous display and observation of a child's heart rate and rhythm is essential to postoperative management. Each child's rhythm should be immediately monitored on admission to the ICU as ventricular tachycardia, fibrillation, and asystole can occur postoperatively with alarming rapidity. Appropriate adjustment of low- and high-rate alarms should provide sufficiently early warning to allow effective diagnosis and treatment. Lead II allows assessment of amplitude, axis, and the presence or absence of P waves. A full 12-lead electrocardiogram should be obtained soon after surgery and at regular intervals thereafter to accurately analyze cardiac arrhythmias, conduction disturbances, and

Table 14.10. Postoperative Monitoring

Noninvasive	*Method*	*Information Gained*
ECG	Leads II and V5	Ischemia Arrhythmias
Temperature	Core: rectal, PA catheter, esophageal, tympanic membrane Peripheral: skin, great toe	Cardiac output Hypothermia
Blood Pressure	Manual, automated systems	Hypotension or hypertension
Oxygenation	Pulse oximeter	O_2 saturation Perfusion of limb
Urine output	Foley, diaper weighing	Renal perfusion Cardiac output
CO_2	Mainstream or sidestream end tidal CO_2 transcutaneous CO_2	pCO_2 correlate ↑ in respiratory dead space
Invasive		
Arterial Line	• Blood Pressure, blood sampling	
CVP (RA Line)	• Right atrial pressure • Fluid infusion • Monitor tracing (a, v waves)	
PA Line	• Pulmonary pressure • Cardiac output • Derived SVR, PVR • Mixed venous blood gas → O_2 consumption, O_2 extraction • Core temperature	
LA Line	• Left atrial filling pressure • LA:RA pressure difference (differentiate pulmonary hypertension)	
Chest Tubes	• Blood drainage—mediastinum, pleural space	
Pacing Wires	• Diagnosis of atrial arrhythmias • Ability to pace atria, ventricles	

ischemic and metabolic changes. Monitoring of a lateral precordial lead such as V5 (or V3R in patients with dextrocardia) will reveal septal or lateral wall ischemia with ST alteration. The atrial pacing wire can be used to assess P waves in order to differentiate between supraventricular and ventricular tachycardia.

Blood Pressure

A blood pressure cuff should be placed on every patient returning from surgery even when an arterial catheter is in place. A manual blood pressure measurement can determine the accuracy of the arterial line tracing. Arterial catheter systolic pressures may be exaggerated, especially at high heart rates, due to the particular harmonics of the system. In addition, the cuff can be used to occlude flow should the arterial catheter leak. After repair of coarctation of the aorta, measurements of blood pressure in both upper and lower extremities should be performed to estimate the residual pressure gradient across the site of repair. Blood pressure should not be measured in the extremity where an artery has been used for surgical repair (i.e., coarctation repair with subclavian flap).

Pulse Oximetry

Pulse oximetry is a safe and reliable way of continuously monitoring arterial oxygen saturation and should be used in all critically ill children[62]. In the postoperative cardiac patient, decreasing oxygen saturation may indicate decreased cardiac output, increasing intracardiac shunting, or increasing intrapulmonary shunting. Continuous pulse oximetry is particularly helpful in patients with reactive pulmonary hypertension, in whom a small decrease in oxygen saturation may be the first sign of increased pulmonary artery pressure with right-to-left shunting. This monitoring technique also provides close continuous surveillance of the efficacy of ongoing respiratory support before any complication occurs.

Urine output

In all but the simplest cardiac cases, a Foley catheter should be placed to adequately monitor urine output. Analgesics can induce urinary retention, which complicates assessment of urine output. The hourly rate of urine output should be noted as this is an excellent clinical indicator of renal perfusion; however, this indicator is often invalid in the first 2 postoperative hours after diuretic administration. Patients who have uncomplicated operative procedures with stable vital signs and good peripheral perfusion, and who are noted to void spontaneously, do not need urinary catheterization. Urine output can instead be measured directly or by weighing diapers.

Temperature

Temperature is closely monitored in the operating room, which should continue in the ICU. Continuous monitoring by rectal, skin, or esophageal temperature probes is almost universally available. If not, rectal temperature should be taken hourly. Central temperature can also be measured by the pulmonary artery thermistor catheter when available. Skin and oral temperature are frequently affected by environmental conditions, whereas central temperature is more constant.

Monitoring of peripheral as well as core temperature serves as an important objective guide to peripheral perfusion. A difference between peripheral and core temperature of greater than 2°C is associated with severely compromised cardiac output[63]. Poor peripheral perfusion diminishes the effective surface area for radiant heat loss so that any heat generated cannot be dissipated. For this reason, poor cardiac output is often accompanied by hyperthermia, which in turn increases metabolic demands. The relation of great toe temperature to ambient temperature has also been used as an indicator of cardiac output but is less reliable[64].

The pediatric intensivist must remain aware of the importance of a neutral thermal environment in the early postoperative period. After cardiac surgery, the infant or child is usually hypothermic as a result of CPB, a cold operating room, and transport. Hypothermia increases oxygen consumption and metabolic demands by causing shivering in older children. Hypothermia also activates nonshivering thermogenesis in infants and pharmacologically paralyzed older children[65,66], and induces peripheral vasoconstriction thereby increasing systemic vascular resistance. Hyperthermia, like hypothermia, increases oxygen consumption and metabolic demand. Temperature elevations may also herald an infection or malignant hyperthermia. Failure to detect and respond to alterations in body temperature leads to increased stress on an already potentially compromised circulatory system.

Invasive Monitoring (Table 14–10)

Arterial Pressure Monitoring

In patients with all but the simplest cardiac defects (i.e., PDA), intra-arterial blood pressure monitoring is usually warranted. A cuff blood pressure may be difficult to obtain in the immediate postoperative period when peripheral perfusion is poor. If vasoactive drugs are being administered, continuous blood pressure readings are mandatory for minute-to-minute medication adjustments. The presence of an arterial catheter allows frequent measurements of arterial blood gases and other tests requiring blood sampling. In addition, observation of the arterial tracing itself provides additional information from analysis of the waveform and calculation of the pulse pressure. Although embolic and ischemic complications of invasive arterial cannulation do occur, no other system provides truly continuous assessment of blood pressure.

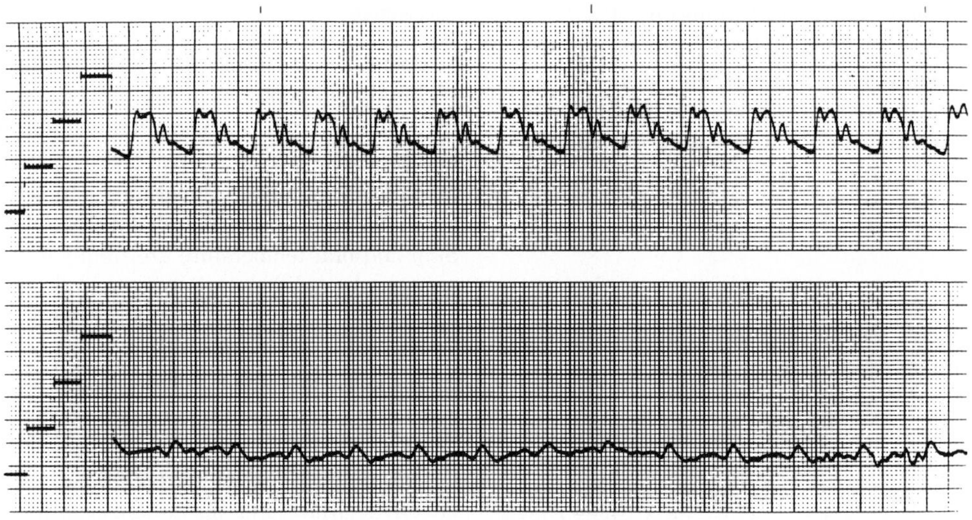

Figure 14.7. Arterial line and central venous pressure trace in child with insufficiency and acute inferior wall infarction related to an anomalous coronary artery. Note large v wave caused by tricuspid regurgitation.

Right Atrial Pressure Monitoring

Invasive monitoring of central pressures may be done via catheters placed intraoperatively or postoperatively. The selection of monitoring lines depends on the nature of the cardiac lesion, the surgical procedure performed, and the degree of myocardial dysfunction expected postoperatively.

Right atrial pressure or central venous pressure reflects right ventricular end-diastolic pressure and is related to end-diastolic volume. However, in patients with right ventricular hypertrophy or a very dilated right atrium this may not be the case. In patients with reactive pulmonary hypertension, an elevation of right atrial pressure may indicate elevated pulmonary artery pressure or poor right ventricular function rather than right ventricular volume overload. The right atrial pressure tracing is also useful to observe large or unusual waves (i.e., a large v wave associated with tricuspid regurgitation) (Fig. 14–7). Taking these limitations into account, right-sided filling pressures are helpful in postoperative management decisions. Information regarding optimal right atrial pressure can be obtained from the surgical-anesthesia team. Alternatively, by infusing volume and observing right atrial pressure along with blood pressure, heart rate, and oxygen saturation, the clinician can experimentally determine the optimal filling pressure for that patient at that time.

Measurement of right-sided pressure is warranted in most cardiac defects. Such measurements are particularly useful in patients with right-sided lesions, such as pulmonic stenosis and tetralogy of Fallot, and for those who require high right atrial pressures, such as after a Fontan procedure. Right-sided intrathoracic catheters also provide reliable vascular access for vasoactive infusions and rapid fluid boluses and therefore are used in most intrathoracic operations.

Pulmonary Artery Pressure Monitoring

PA pressure can be measured via a catheter placed through the wall of the right atrium into the pulmonary artery during cardiac surgery. The complication rate from transthoracic PA catheters is 1%; hemodynamically significant bleeding is the most common complication(67). Alternatively, a standard PA catheter may be passed intravascularly(68,69). The decision to place such a catheter postoperatively should only be made in conjunction with the surgeon who is most familiar with the anatomic status of the right ventricular outflow tract. Unpredictable hemodynamic compromise occurs in 0.5% of pediatric patients when intravascular PA catheters are placed postoperatively(68).

PA catheters have multiple applications but are most frequently used in conditions in which pulmonary hypertension is expected postoperatively, such as in repair of endocardial cushion defects. Measurements of PA pressure and/or pulmonary vascular resistance guide the medical management of pulmonary hypertension. Pulmonary capillary wedge pressure can be determined by occlusion of pulmonary artery blood flow, providing information regarding left atrial filling pressure. Simple, accurate measurement of cardiac output using the thermodilution technique is possible when a thermistor probe is present on the PA catheter(70). For adults, it has been found that clinicians are correct in their estimation of cardiac output and systemic vascular resistance less than 50% of the time(71), meaning that more direct measurement of these variables is often beneficial. PA catheters allow access to mixed venous samples, permitting direct calculation of oxygen consumption, oxygen delivery, and intrapulmonary shunt(72).

Newer PA catheters are capable of continuous oximetry, providing minute-to-minute measurement of mixed venous oxygen saturation (SvO_2). SvO_2 reflects the balance between oxygen delivery and oxygen consumption. Alterations in SvO_2 occur in many clinical conditions, such as anemia, shock, left-to-right shunting, right-to-left shunting, and cirrhosis. Changes in SvO_2 may precede detectable changes in hemodynamics by 2 to 10 minutes[73]. In 1978, De La Rocha demonstrated excellent correlation between SvO_2 and cardiac output in children undergoing cardiac surgery[74], but other investigators have not been able to confirm this correlation[75–77].

Left Atrial Pressure Monitoring

Left atrial (LA) pressure is monitored directly by a catheter inserted intraoperatively[78]. The LA pressure reflects the left ventricular end-diastolic volume in much the same way that RA pressure reflects right ventricular end-diastolic volume. Clearly, the consequences of air and particulate embolization are greater with left atrial than right atrial catheters; however, rigorous attention to the care of these catheters minimizes such risks. Blood return should be documented prior to infusion of medications or fluids through the line. The LA pressure tracing should be monitored at all times, and tubing connections should not be broken except in the case of an emergency. LA pressure monitoring can be particularly useful in patients with mitral valve dysfunction, such as after repair of endocardial cushion defects.

Management of Transthoracic Pressure Monitoring Lines

Transthoracic pressure monitoring lines, like all invasive vascular catheters, should be removed as soon as they are no longer needed. Clinically significant intrathoracic bleeding after the removal of these catheters is greater with LA than RA catheters (0.13% versus 0%)[67]. The risk of bleeding is greatest with PA catheters which are placed through the wall of the pulmonary artery rather than through the right atrium. Although the overall risk of hemorrhage is low, hypovolemia and pericardial tamponade which occur after hemorrhage can have serious consequences.

Chest tubes should generally not be removed until after the uneventful removal of all intracardiac catheters, so that bleeding may be detected and tamponade avoided. In a study of over 6,000 intracardiac monitoring lines, most catheters were removed within 72 hours[67]. This early removal of transthoracic pressure lines, theoretically before a tract has developed, does not reduce the risk of hemorrhage when compared with delayed removal; transthoracic catheters have remained in place for hyperalimentation several weeks after removal of chest tubes without bleeding complications[67].

Bleeding is suspected when fresh blood is seen in the mediastinal chest tubes, or when a previously stable patient becomes unstable after removal of a transthoracic catheter. If hemodynamic instability occurs, fluid, either as colloid or crystalloid, should be infused to maintain cardiac output while the operating room is prepared for an exploratory thoracotomy. If profound hemodynamic instability occurs, the chest should be opened in the ICU so that tamponade can be relieved and bleeding controlled. At times, removal of sternal wires can relieve the symptoms of tamponade.

Transthoracic pressure monitoring lines can produce other complications[67]. Catheter occlusion by thrombus formation is usually heralded by loss of the pressure tracing and no blood return. When this happens, the catheter should be removed rather than flushed to avoid embolization of the clot. Inability to remove a catheter necessitates a return to the operating room for thoracotomy.

Epicardial Pacing Wires

After open heart surgery, temporary epicardial pacing wires are frequently attached to the right atrium and/or right ventricle[79]. Access to cardiac pacing is particularly important after surgery in the vicinity of the cardiac conduction system, as in closure of a ventricular septal defect (VSD) or repair of transposition of the great arteries (TGA), truncus arteriosus, or endocardial cushion defects. Atrial wires may be used either for atrial pacing with an intact conduction system with an inadequate heart rate or for AV sequential pacing when the conduction system is disrupted. Ventricular wires can be used for AV sequential pacing or ventricular pacing alone. Atrial and ventricular wires can also provide atrial and ventricular electrograms for analysis of postoperative rhythms.

Pacing wires are brought out through the skin individually and generally are—from the patient's right to left—ground, atrial, and ventricular. Labeling the wires is good practice. The atrial or skin ground wire is connected to the positive pole, while the ventricular wire is connected to the negative pole of the pacemaker. In most instances when the pacemaker is functioning as a fail-safe system, the sensitivity is adjusted to ventricular demand pacing and the output to the minimum setting. The heart rate is then adjusted to 20 to 30 beats per minute more than the patient's intrinsic rate. The pacer output is then increased until the ventricle is captured and paced beats are observed on the ECG monitor. To ensure a margin of safety, the output is increased 2 mA above the capture output. The heart rate is then decreased to the minimum acceptable ventricular rate. Thus, ventricular capture is guaranteed should the patient's intrinsic rate fall below the set heart rate.

Chest Drainage Tubes

Mediastinal and pleural tubes are routinely employed for thoracic drainage after cardiac surgery. A suction pressure of 15 to 20 cm H_2O should be applied via a sealed system to facilitate drainage of blood and other fluid. These tubes should be stripped frequently to maintain patency. Chest tube drainage should be monitored closely during the immediate postoperative period. Although early chest tube drainage may actually reflect drainage of irrigation fluid used in the operating room, generally, blood loss greater than 10 ml/kg/hr warrants a return to the operating room for exploration and control of surgical bleeding. In addition, the patient should be reexplored when chest tube bleeding is bright red, its rate is increasing or not decreasing with time, after cardiac tamponade, or in the unstable patient with moderate amounts of chest tube drainage. If uncertainty exists as to the nature of the bleeding, serial comparisons of the patient's hematocrit and the hematocrit of fluid drained from the chest may indicate whether the bleeding is slowing down or persisting. Medical bleeding can be controlled with platelet transfusions, infusions of fresh frozen plasma or cryoprecipitate, protamine administration to reverse residual heparin effect, or administration of DDAVP to improve platelet function.

Excessive serous drainage from the chest tubes can arise from fluid overload and pulmonary edema. Extracardiac GORE-TEX® shunts can weep serous fluid through the interstices of the fabric, causing a pleural effusion. Excessive clear fluid can also indicate a chylothorax seen secondary to thoracic duct dysfunction before enteral feeding is instituted.

Chest tubes can be removed when drainage becomes serous and minimal, usually by the third postoperative day. Generally, drainage should be less than 3 ml/kg/day, although this is a very conservative estimate. Chest tubes should not be removed until after transthoracic intracardiac catheters, particularly LA and PA lines, are removed. Fresh blood in the chest tube at any time may be the first sign of impending tamponade or hypovolemia. An increase in the volume of chest tube drainage should prompt a thorough investigation for possible causes, including pulmonary edema, chylothorax, and increased bleeding. When possible, chest tubes should be removed prior to tracheal extubation as splinting from chest-tube-related pain may cause respiratory embarrassment.

PRINCIPLES OF POSTOPERATIVE MANAGEMENT

Hemodynamic Management

On the patient's admission to the ICU, the intensivist should anticipate hemodynamic instability, regardless of the underlying cardiac lesion, and be prepared to intervene. After the initial assessment and immediate stabilization, continued close observation remains imperative. If cardiac output is adequate, blood pressure will be in the normal range, although normal blood pressure does not preclude decreased cardiac output. Urine output should equal or exceed 0.5 ml/kg/hr. Warm peripheral extremities and brisk capillary refill are good indicators of adequate cardiac output. Sedation from analgesia or residual anesthesia impairs use of mental status as an indicator of adequate perfusion. However, disorientation or agitation may indicate hypoxia, hypercapnia, or inadequate perfusion.

Cardiac output is dependent on heart rate and stroke volume. Stroke volume is determined by preload, afterload, contractility, adequate heart rate, and an optimal rhythm. Any of these can fluctuate rapidly in the immediate postoperative period, and each must be considered and addressed in order to maintain adequate tissue perfusion.

Heart Rate and Rhythm

As mentioned above, heart rate is an important determinant of cardiac output. This is especially true in infants whose ventricles are less compliant and therefore less responsive to changes in filling pressure. Bradycardia in infants and children can severely compromise cardiac output. Tachycardia, although generally better tolerated in children than in adults, limits ventricular filling time, thereby decreasing stroke volume. Arrhythmias may disrupt appropriate coordination of atrial and ventricular contraction. Lack of atrial-ventricular synchrony decreases ventricular filling and thus cardiac output. The initial management of any arrhythmia begins with optimization of arterial blood gases, pH, and serum electrolytes. The position of intracardiac catheters should be known and their contribution to an arrhythmia ruled out. Ventricular tachycardia in the postoperative period must be treated immediately with lidocaine (1 mg/kg). If this is not successful, cardioversion should be attempted. Ventricular fibrillation should, of course, be treated with immediate cardiopulmonary resuscitation (CPR) and electrocardioversion. (See Chapter 1 for a full discussion of CPR). Specific dysrhythmias which are most commonly encountered in postoperative cardiac patients are discussed below **(Table 14–11).** Other dysrhythmias are discussed in Chapter 15.

Bradycardia

Bradycardia is common after open heart surgery. In patients undergoing hypothermic arrest, bradycardia is proportional to the degree of hypothermia. Bradycardia occurs frequently after extensive atrial surgery, the atrial switch procedure, and repair of total anomalous pulmonary venous return. Injury to the sinus node may result from incision of the node, placement of suture through the node, or interruption of the blood supply to the sinoatrial (SA) node by surgical trauma. The latter may lead to degeneration of the sinus node, which may not be apparent for months or years after surgery[80]. Clinical bradycardia may be due to sinus atrial block, sinus asystole, or AV junctional block.

If the cardiac rate is sufficiently slow to compromise cardiac output, atropine or isoproterenol may increase the conduction rate of sinus or junctional rhythms. Alternatively, the heart may be paced. Permanent pacing may be necessary. As edema around the conduction system resolves 3 to 4 days after surgery, normal sinus rhythm generally returns[81].

Tachycardia

Postoperative tachycardia may be due to pain, agitation, or hypovolemia and will respond to specific treatment. Tachycardia due to a conduction disturbance is usually junctional

Table 14.11. Common Postoperative Arrhythmias

Anatomy	*Arrhythmia*	*Lesion*
• SA node	• bradycardia	Senning or Mustard procedure (TGV)
	• sick sinus syndrome	Tetralogy of Fallot
	• sinus asystole	ASD
	• PAT	AV Canal
• Intranodal pathway	• atrial flutter	Mustard procedure (TGV)
	• SVT	TAPVR
	• junctional bradycardia	
• Junctional injury	• junctional tachycardia	Mustard procedure (TGV)
• AV node	• AV block (1°, 2°, 3°)	Endocardial cushion defect
• His' bundle		Membranous VSD
• Intraventricular conduction pathways	• RBBB	Tetralogy of Fallot
	• RBBB with LAH	AV canal
	• trifascicular block	Ostium primum ASD
		VSD
		Membranous VSD—associated with complex CHD
		Resection of pulmonary infundibulum
• Ventricle	• PVCs	Tetralogy of Fallot
	• ventricular tachycardia	Right ventriculotomy—especially with ventricular dilatation or hypertension

in origin. The ECG shows narrow QRS complexes and the absence of P waves. The junctional rate is usually 120 to 280 beats per minute. The loss of atrial contractility and the rapid ventricular response rate impair ventricular filling. If hemodynamic instability exists, cardioversion should be attempted. If atrial pacing wires are present, atrial contraction can be induced or overdrive pacing can be performed. Junctional tachycardia does not respond to vagal maneuvers. Digitalization or β-adrenergic blockade may reduce an excessive conduction rate or induce AV block, thereby slowing the ventricular rate.

Junctional ectopic tachycardia (JET) is a life-threatening arrhythmia defined as a heart rate greater than 200 and a narrow QRS complex with or without P waves. If P waves are present, there is invariably AV dissociation. This arrhythmia is thought to result from enhanced automaticity in the bundle of His and is more often seen in patients receiving inotropic support[82]. Treatment of this rhythm must be instituted early and includes conservative management, such as avoidance of vagolytic compounds, aggressive use of sedation, and avoidance of sympathomimetics[82,83]. Cooling can also slow the ventricular rate and improve cardiac output[84,85]. Recent clinical reports suggest that propafenone and amiodarone can lower heart rate in some patients[86,87]. JET has also been controlled with paired ventricular pacing and radiofrequency ablation[88,89]. JET usually subsides spontaneously 48 to 72 hours after surgery.

Cardiac Pacing

In the presence of an abnormal cardiac rhythm, cardiac pacing can be used to augment cardiac output. Atrial wires may be used for either atrial pacing when an intact conduction system is associated with a slow rate or AV sequential pacing when the conduction system is disrupted in order to augment ventricular filling. Ventricular wires can be used for AV sequential pacing or ventricular pacing alone. Should the epicardial pacing system malfunction, transesophageal pacing may be useful. A pacing catheter is passed through the esophagus to the atrial level, which is detected by the appearance of P waves[90]. Atrial capture can be accomplished easily with little discomfort[91]; however, ventricular contraction requires the presence of an intact intracardiac conduction system. Transesophageal pacing is particularly useful for application of overdrive pacing for supraventricular tachycardia[91].

Stroke Volume

Preload

Stroke volume depends on the degree of diastolic filling of the ventricle or preload. Stroke volume increases as preload increases, until the ventricle becomes overly dilated. After bypass and in the ICU, rewarming gradually occurs with a corresponding decrease in PVR. Consequently, the RA pressure decreases. This initial fall in venous return may be compensated by an increased heart rate, but as preload decreases further, peripheral perfusion will decrease. Fluid boluses in quantities of 5 to 10 ml/kg will improve venous return, right atrial pressure, and heart rate. Procedures involving ventriculotomy, prolonged cardioplegia, cardiopulmonary bypass, and those with residual outflow tract obstruction will require higher right atrial pressures. An RA pressure of 14 to 16 cm H_2O is usually adequate. Further increases in RA pressure may lead to pulmonary edema. Evidence of poor cardiac output with hypotension and poor peripheral perfusion despite adequate filling pressures warrants the use of inotropic support[92].

Contractility

Myocardial contractility is impaired after open-heart surgery due to ischemia, hypoxia, inflammation, and a ventriculotomy, when used. The selection of inotropes to improve myocardial contractility depends on the nature of the lesion and the pathophysiology present. Dopamine, for example, at low doses may be well tolerated and sufficient in some patients; however, the α-adrenergic effects of dopamine may be detrimental in other patients[93,94]. Dobutamine improves inotropy and is quite useful in the postoperative patient with poor contractility[95–97]. Complications of dobutamine that are not well tolerated include tachycardia and arrhythmias. Isoproterenol provides chronotropy, which is particularly useful after repair of total anomalous pulmonary venous return, and in the denervated heart after transplantation[98]. When diastolic blood pressure is so low that coronary perfusion is impaired, epinephrine with its α- and β-adrenergic effects may be needed[99]. Amrinone, a phosphodiesterase F-III inhibitor, a positive inotropic agent as well as a peripheral vasodilator without a chronotropic effect, is very useful in the postoperative patient[100]. Selection of the appropriate combination of inotropic agents requires full knowledge of the effects of these medications[101].

Afterload

In the presence of myocardial dysfunction, increases in afterload, which is defined as end-diastolic ventricular wall tension, are poorly tolerated. Elimination of physiologic factors that increase SVR—such as acidosis, hypoxemia, pain, and hypothermia—should be the first step in reducing afterload. Pharmacologic afterload reduction can also be instituted with smooth muscle relaxants such as nitroprusside, nitroglycerin, hydralazine, and diazoxide; β-blockers such as phentolamine, prazosin, and chlorpromazine; and the ganglionic blocking agent trimethaphan[102–105]. Vasodilators with a rapid onset and short duration of action, such as nitroprusside, are preferable in the acute postoperative period[105]. When vasodilator therapy is instituted, it is often necessary to infuse volume to maintain preload.

Aortic balloon counterpulsation, which increases coronary artery perfusion pressure and decreases afterload, has been used in older patients with a failing circulatory system[106]. Smaller catheters now permit intra-aortic balloon pumping in children, although the technique is still difficult in infants due to the distensibility of the infant's aorta and other issues related to size[107,108].

Oxygen Consumption After Cardiac Surgery

The ultimate goal of postoperative care is to maintain adequate oxygen delivery to meet the body's metabolic demands. In the immediate postoperative period, when cardiac output and oxygenation may be compromised, it is important to limit increased metabolic demand. An increase in oxygen consumption during this period may be detrimental to the infant or child at a time when oxygen delivery is already marginal. Oxygen consumption postoperatively is increased due to shivering secondary to hypothermia, endogenous and exogenous secretion of catecholamines, and muscle activity, including muscles used for respiration. To increase the oxygen supply-to-demand ratio, every effort should be made to decrease oxygen consumption while improving the level of oxygen delivery.

As previously discussed, both hypothermia and hyperthermia increase metabolic demand. Thus monitoring and control of temperature are important aspects of postoperative care.

The use of neuromuscular blocking agents to decrease oxygen consumption is controversial. D-tubocurarine did not decrease oxygen consumption in unsedated, normoxemic newborn lambs[109]. When these lambs were made hypoxemic, d-tubocurarine did decrease oxygen consumption; however, oxygen delivery was decreased to an even greater extent, creating an unfavorable balance between oxygen consumption and delivery. In anesthetized dogs, d-tubocurarine did not affect oxygen consumption, while succinylcholine actually increased oxygen consumption[110]. In a human study, d-tubocurarine decreased oxygen consumption when administered to unsedated, hypoxemic adults. A decrease in oxygen consumption was also observed after pancuronium administration in hypoxemic, nonparalyzed patients[111]. No change in oxygen consumption was seen when patients were normoxemic or had no muscle activity prior to the administration of the drug[112]. Muscle relaxants may be effective in decreasing oxygen consumption in some patients by abolishing voluntary and involuntary muscle activity. In infants, because shivering does not usually occur, muscle relaxation would not be expected to decrease oxygen consumption to as great a degree.

Sedatives or analgesics may be used to decrease oxygen consumption by decreasing endogenous catecholamine secretion. In one study of critically ill adults, morphine decreased oxygen consumption 9 to 21%[113]. In a pediatric study of children undergoing cardiac catheterization, administration of meperidine, promethazine, and chlorpromazine decreased oxygen consumption by 34%[65]. (See section on intraoperative—endocrine effects for further discussion.)

Pulmonary Hypertension

Episodic pulmonary hypertension is a life-threatening event which may occur postoperatively in those patients with cardiac lesions where there has been long-standing excessive pulmonary blood flow (e.g., a large VSD, endocardial cushion defects, and truncus arteriosus). This leads to pulmonary vascular remodeling, causing hypertrophy of the elastic lamina and narrowing of the arterial diameter. After CPB, endothelial injury of the postcapillary venules narrows the diameter of venular structures, while circulating vasoactive substances such as endothelin cause further constriction of the already narrowed arterial lumen. It is thought that venular injury persists for approximately 24 to 48 hours postoperatively and is not amenable to any intervention. In contrast, while the arterial contribution to pulmonary vascular resistance which is due to structural changes is not acutely reversible, it may be possible to acutely relax the arterial smooth muscle.

Patients susceptible to pulmonary hypertension (i.e., those with a history of excessive pulmonary blood flow) should be monitored postoperatively with a PA catheter. Acute pulmonary hypertension is detected when the PA pressure rises. This is usually followed by a sudden fall in oxygen saturation. As the PA pressure rises higher, LA pressure and mean arterial pressure will fall due to a decrease in left-sided preload. In patients without invasive monitoring, pulmonary hypertension is suspected only by a sudden drop in oxygen saturation and systemic blood pressure. An acute event may be related to agitation associated with awakening from anesthesia or suctioning or by a metabolic acidosis. Acute intervention consists of manual ventilation with 100% oxygen in order to raise both alveolar oxygen and pH through CO_2 elimination. If the patient fails to respond, pH can be increased further by sodium bicarbonate administration. Additional sedation with a narcotic such as fentanyl will also help. A variety of vasodilating agents, including sodium nitroprusside, the phosphodiesterase inhibitors, amrinone and milrinone, prazosin, and thorazine have been used to lower PA pressure; however, these agents can worsen hypoxemia by overriding the hypoxic pulmonary vasoconstriction response and cause systemic hypotension. Inhaled nitric oxide, a potent pulmonary vasodilator, has been used investigationally to reduce PA pressure postoperatively[(113,114)]. This therapy appears to be very promising in that it exerts only local effects, thereby improving ventilation-perfusion matching. Nitric oxide is rapidly inactivated intravascularly as it binds to hemoglobin and thus has no systemic hemodynamic effects, although methemoglobin concentrations need to be monitored.

Acute pulmonary hypertension is best avoided. In patients at risk, a protocol for the management of pulmonary hypertension may be put in place for 48 hours postoperatively. This includes ensuring adequate oxygenation through slow weaning of inspired oxygen to not less than 50%, mild hyperventilation to a $PaCO_2$ of 30 to 35 torr, and sedation and analgesia for those patients who are expected to have pulmonary hypertension postoperatively. Paralysis does not appear to be indicated if sedation can be maintained. In fact, muscle paralysis may mask the need for sedation, allowing the pulmonary artery pressure to rise acutely. Suctioning should be limited as it is a noxious stimulus and may coincide with hypercarbia. Additional sedation and manual ventilation prior to suctioning, and suctioning only just beyond the tip of the endotracheal tube without stimulation of the carina, may help avoid pulmonary hypertension.

Cardiac Tamponade

Cardiac tamponade in the postoperative cardiac surgical patient is a life-threatening condition that is easily reversible if it is promptly recognized and treated. Blood in the mediastinum restricts cardiac filling, reducing stroke volume and increasing afterload. Tamponade most often results from an occluded mediastinal drainage tube with ongoing postoperative bleeding. The diagnosis should always be suspected when a patient's initially benign postoperative course deteriorates, especially in the setting of diminished chest tube drainage.

Cardiac tamponade can be heralded by a narrowed pulse pressure or pulsus paradoxus present on the arterial pressure tracing. Other clinical signs include a rising RA pressure with jugular venous distension, decreased blood pressure, muffled heart sounds, tachycardia, and poor peripheral perfusion. The treatment for cardiac tamponade is prompt volume infusion to maintain cardiac output. The operating room and cardiac surgeon should be immediately notified of an impending return to the operating room for thoracotomy. If severe cardiovascular failure does not permit time for transport, the sternal wound can be opened in the ICU and a finger inserted into the pericardium to evacuate blood and clots. Needle aspiration of the pericardial cavity is dangerous, ineffective, and time-consuming when the chest can be easily opened[(115)]. Definitive exploration of the chest for a source of persistent bleeding should be undertaken.

A clinical syndrome of poor cardiac function without evidence of tamponade has been described in infants and children[(116)]. The pathophysiology of this syndrome appears to be an alteration in compliance of the left ventricle due to edema of the myocardium and surrounding structures. Hemodynamic improvement is observed when the sternum is opened. The sternum can be closed electively 24 to 72 hours later, when hemodynamics have improved. Late cardiac tamponade occurring more than 7 days postoperatively is a recognized complication and may occur as a result of postpericardiotomy syndrome[(117,118)].

Postpericardiotomy Syndrome

The postpericardiotomy syndrome (PPS) can also lead to cardiac tamponade. PPS is characterized as a febrile illness which occurs after the pericardium is opened[(119–121)]. There is pericardial and pleural reaction with effusion and occasional pulmonary parenchymal involvement. Clinically, the syndrome is heralded by fever beyond the first postoperative week. The fever is variable, with occasional spikes as high as 40°C, usually subsiding within 2 to 3 weeks. The child may be mildly irritable, with a decreased appetite, or very ill, especially in the presence of high fever and cardiac tamponade. Precordial chest pain worsens with inspiration and in the supine position and may radiate to the left shoulder.

On physical examination, a pericardial friction rub appears sometime during the course of the syndrome but is not present for as long a duration as the electrocardiographic or radiologic signs of a pericardial effusion. The rub disappears either with improvement or further accumulation of pericardial fluid. Cardiac tamponade may occur with progressive accumulation of pericardial fluid. On chest x-ray,

Table 14.12. Postpericardiotomy Syndrome

Symptoms
Persistent fever
Precordial chest pain
Irritability
Decreased appetite
Left shoulder pain
Physical examination
Pericardial friction rub
Pleural friction rub
Fever
Laboratory results
Enlarged heart
ECG changes
Elevation of ST segments
Nonspecific T-wave changes
Low amplitude (with large effusions)
Echocardiography-pericardial effusion
Anti-heart antibody present in high titer

the cardiac silhouette is enlarged due to pericardial fluid accumulation, and a left-sided pleural effusion may be seen[122]. Pulmonary parenchymal disease is seen less often than pleural reaction **(Table 14–12).**

In patients with PPS, postoperative ECG changes such as flattened or inverted T-waves may persist beyond the first week. The QRS amplitude decreases when the pericardial effusion is very large. Echocardiography should be performed to evaluate the presence and size of the pericardial effusion. The echocardiogram is also helpful in differentiating this syndrome from that of congestive heart failure with decreased cardiac contractility[123].

PPS was reported in 27% of children after intrapericardiac surgery but is unusual in patients younger than 2 years of age[124]. It is frequently associated with the development of anti-heart antibodies. A fourfold or greater rise in antibody titers against various viral agents, including adenovirus, coxsackie B virus, and cytomegalovirus, occurred in 70% of patients with the syndrome, suggesting an autoimmune response in association with a viral infection[124].

PPS is diagnosed based on the signs and symptoms described above and should be differentiated from congestive heart failure and endocarditis. The detection of anti-heart antibody in high titer is a confirmatory diagnostic test. The patient with a moderate to large pericardial effusion is best managed with strict bed rest until the fever has resolved and chest x-ray and ECG findings indicate that the condition has dissipated. For severe illness, aspirin and corticosteroids are used. Corticosteroids (2 mg/kg/day for the first week, 1 mg/kg/day for the second week, then 0.5 mg/kg/day for the last week) are associated with a more prompt clinical response and a more rapid decrease in anti-heart antibodies than aspirin alone[125].

Chylothorax and Chylopericardium

Chylothorax and chylopericardium are unusual after cardiac surgery, but important to recognize when they occur. Chylothorax, first reported by Blalock et al.[126], most frequently follows extrapericardiac procedures for correction or palliation of congenital heart disease[126–130]. These operations include repair of coarctation of the aorta, the Blalock-Taussig or Waterston shunts, Potts' anastomosis, the Glenn procedure, and ligation of a PDA. Postoperative chylothorax results from injury to the thoracic duct or its intrathoracic tributaries. It may also be due to rupture of collateral vessels which dilate secondary to postsurgical adhesions. After the Glenn procedure, chylous effusions may occur due to acute or chronic venous hypertension associated with the SVC syndrome[131].

Symptoms and signs associated with chylothorax include dyspnea, shoulder pain, pleural friction rub, pleural effusions, and fever. Effusions usually develop in the first few days postoperatively but may develop as late as 1 month after surgery. The pleural fluid appears milky and does not clot once feedings have been instituted. More commonly, the absence of chylomicrons prior to resumption of a fat-containing diet causes the fluid to appear serous or serosanguineous. Microscopic examination of the fluid for abundant lymphocytes is necessary to make the correct diagnosis in those situations.

Complications secondary to chylothorax include respiratory compromise and malnutrition. Malnutrition is caused by the loss of chyle, which is rich in proteins, lipids, and lymphocytes[132]; severe lymphocyte depletion can also occur[133].

The therapy for chylothorax ranges from conservative medical treatment to surgical ligation of the thoracic duct. Medical management of chylothorax includes strict monitoring and control of nutritional intake and drainage of pleural effusions to prevent atelectasis and ventilatory insufficiency[132]. A high-protein, high-carbohydrate, medium-chain triglyceride diet with reduced fat content decreases lymph flow[133]. This can be delivered by parenteral hyperalimentation or by an enteral medium-chain triglyceride diet. Medium-chain triglycerides are absorbed directly into the portal venous system from the gastrointestinal tract, which decreases total lymph production and attenuates fat loss via chyle[132].

If conservative management is unsuccessful, surgical ligation of the thoracic duct may be indicated. The surgical approach was first performed by Lampson in 1948[134]. Indications for surgery, according to Selle et al., include an average daily chyle loss exceeding 1500 ml in adults or 100 ml per year of age in children after a 5-day period of medical management, a flow of chyle that is not diminished after 2 weeks of medical management, or severe nutritional complications[135].

Chylopericardium, as a complication of chylothorax after cardiac surgery, was first described in 1971[136]. This complication is usually associated with intrapericardiac surgery after coronary bypass surgery, aortic or pulmonary valvular surgery, or VSD repair[137]; however, it has also been reported after palliative shunt procedures and repair of total anomalous pulmonary venous return[138,139]. Chylopericardium may occur secondary to direct trauma to the intrapericardiac lymphatics or thoracic duct obstruction due to thrombosis or intravascular catheter placement[137]. When

Table 14.13. Postoperative Respiratory Problems

Hypoventilation	• Residual anesthetics and muscle relaxants • Central nervous system disease • Upper airway (obstruction)—swelling, vocal cord paresis, plugged ETT • Diaphragmatic paralysis
Chest Wall Compliance	• Chest wall edema (fluid overload, CHF, SVC syndrome) • Splinting—(pain)
Lung Parenchyma	• Pulmonary edema (fluid overload, CHF, ARDS) • Atelectasis • Effusion (hemothorax, chylothorax)
Barotrauma	• Pneumothorax • Pneumopericardium • Pneumomediastrinum
Other Physiologic Abnormalities	• ↓ cardiac output → ↑ dead space • Anesthetics, vasodilators → ↓ HPV reflex

ETT, endotracheal tube; CHF, congestive heart failure; SVC, Superior Vena Cava; ARDS, acute respiratory distress syndrome; HPV, hyponic pulmonary vasoconstricture.

this complication is associated with extrapericardiac surgery, it may be due to inadvertent ligation of the thoracic duct or ligation of an abnormal lymphatic channel proximal to the entry of cardiac lymphatics resulting in retrograde flow of chyle into the pericardial cavity(138).

Symptoms of chylopericardium are those of cardiac tamponade or those of coincident chylothorax. Echocardiography demonstrating a pericardial effusion is helpful in making the diagnosis. Needle pericardiocentesis may be necessary to confirm the presence of chyle and for relief of cardiac tamponade. A single percutaneous pericardial aspiration may be sufficient to treat this condition. However, if the pericardial effusion recurs, surgical management consisting of partial pericardiotomy with or without ligation of the thoracic duct may be necessary(137).

Respiratory Support

Postoperative Respiratory Function

Cardiac surgery introduces many physiologic changes which affect pulmonary function **(Table 14–13).** Many of these changes are those seen after any general anesthetic, as discussed in Chapter 46, Pain, Sedation, and Postoperative Anesthetic Management in the Pediatric Intensive Care Unit. In addition, the thoracic incision and accompanying chest tubes cause postoperative pain and splinting of the chest wall in spontaneously breathing patients, with a resultant decrease in deep breathing and coughing and decreased chest wall compliance(140). Anesthetic agents and muscle relaxants depress cough reflexes, interfere with mucociliary action, and lead to diminished clearance of secretions(141). Mucous obstruction can lead to atelectasis and loss of lung volume, particularly in children with relatively small terminal airways. In addition, muscle relaxants stop periodic sighing and deep breathing, which normally work to counteract collapse and maintain functional residual capacity. Anesthetic agents dilate the pulmonary vascular bed, thereby altering hypoxic pulmonary vasoconstriction(142,143). Low cardiac output causes an increase in physiologic dead space(144).

Lung compliance may be adversely affected by an increase in LA pressure or by left ventricular failure, resulting in an increase in intravascular hydrostatic pressure(145). Moreover, an increase in RA pressure with obstruction to pulmonary lymphatic flow may also lead to increased lung water. With fluid extravasation into the alveoli, there is an increase in ventilation-perfusion mismatch due to intrapulmonary shunting and increased work of breathing due to diminished lung compliance. Postoperative persistence of a left-to-right shunt may also cause an increase in ventilation-perfusion mismatching.

The effects of CPB on postoperative lung function are varied. Prolonged CPB, especially followed by a low cardiac output, may induce pulmonary capillary endothelial damage, leading to pulmonary edema and increased lung water(146,147). This syndrome, termed *pump lung*, may be caused by trauma, neutrophil and complement activation, or foreign protein from the oxygenator(26,27,147). However, when using the double indicator-dilution technique, no correlation of extravascular lung water with the length of CPB or deep hypothermia, preoperative or postoperative left atrial pressure, postoperative serum protein, albumin, hematocrit, or cardiac index was seen(148).

Postoperative complications observed in children can involve every aspect of the respiratory system. These include upper airway complications such as stridor due to subglottic tracheal mucosal swelling, vocal cord paralysis due to damage to the recurrent laryngeal nerve, and problems associated with the endotracheal tube itself, including mucus plugging or kinking of the tube. Direct trauma to the lungs during surgery may worsen lung injury and atelectasis.

Direct trauma, edema, or stretch of the phrenic nerve can also occur, causing diaphragmatic paralysis. A decrease in diaphragmatic movement can result in significant respiratory impairment due to the infant's greater dependence on the diaphragm for respiratory work. Ventilation is less efficient in infancy due to the tendency for retraction of the elastic thoracic cage with inspiration, especially when large intrapleural pressures are generated. Limited diaphragmatic motion can also be due to abdominal distension. Diaphragmatic paralysis can be diagnosed by observation of paradoxical motion of a hemidiaphragm under fluoroscopy. Care should be taken to observe diaphragmatic motion when positive pressure is not being applied during spontaneous breathing so that the diaphragms do not appear falsely operational.

Postoperative Respiratory Care

Preoperative assessment of pulmonary function can improve postoperative respiratory care. Simple spirometry and arterial blood gases can help predict the postoperative course and avoid unexpected episodes of respiratory failure.

The respiratory management of the pediatric patient after cardiac surgery takes an understanding of both the pathophysiology of congenital heart diseases and open-heart surgery and the physiology of the respiratory system of the infant or small child. As discussed earlier in the chapter, early assessment of respiratory function is made postoperatively in the ICU, by the physical examination, chest x-ray, arterial blood gases, ventilator parameters, end-tidal CO_2, lung compliance, and bedside pulmonary function tests.

Inadequate ventilation in the immediate postoperative period occurs as a result of residual anesthesia or oversedation, residual muscle paralysis, inability to perform the work of breathing after a surgical incision and general anesthesia, airway obstruction, central nervous system depression, or alterations in chest wall mechanics, as discussed previously. Hypoventilation from any cause results in increased levels of arterial pCO_2 and, if severe, hypoxemia. Hypercapnia and the resultant respiratory acidosis may produce sympathetic stimulation and cause hypertension and tachycardia, susceptibility to cardiac arrhythmias, increased pulmonary vascular resistance, and, if very severe, a decrease in cardiac or cerebral function[149,150]. Even in the most stable postoperative patient, respiratory support is indicated until residual effects of anesthetic agents are no longer present. As a period of mechanical ventilatory support is expected in most pediatric patients who undergo cardiac surgery, narcotics and muscle relaxants are not reversed at the completion of surgery. Supplemental doses may be given for pain, agitation, and interference with effective ventilation. If agitation exists, causes such as hypoxemia, hypercapnia, and hypoperfusion should be ruled out.

Management of Mechanical Ventilation

Assessment of the endotracheal tube in terms of appropriateness of size and position should be made at the time of admission. When uncuffed endotracheal tubes are used, a leak between 10 and 30 cm H_2O is preferred. When a cuffed tube is used, the cuff is inflated until the leak just disappears. An inappropriately sized endotracheal tube can be electively changed soon after admission when the patient is still anesthetized. Extreme caution should be used in changing the tube if there is evidence of laryngeal or facial edema which may occur postpump.

Warming and humidification of inspired gases will avoid heat loss and thickened secretions. This is particularly important in small infants, in whom even small amounts of secretions may cause critical obstruction of the airway or the endotracheal tube. The temperature near the airway should be monitored to prevent overheating and thermal injury to the airway. Temperature of inhaled gases should be kept below 40°C.

During the initial assessment, all postoperative patients except those undergoing simple procedures such as an ASD repair or PDA ligation should be placed on 100% oxygen. Thereafter, by pulse oximetry and by arterial blood gas evaluation, FiO_2 should be reduced to that required to maintain a pO_2 between 75 and 125 torr and an oxygen saturation of greater than or equal to 96%. Of course, patients undergoing a palliative procedure who remain cyanotic cannot be expected to reach high oxygen saturation. Initial tidal volume and rate, or positive inspiratory pressure if using a pressure-cycled ventilator, can be set according to the respiratory parameters obtained intraoperatively and then adjusted according to clinical exam and arterial pH and pCO_2. Metabolic acidosis is common after open-heart surgery. In those patients who cannot independently correct their pH over time or are critically ill, intravenous sodium bicarbonate may be indicated. Mechanical ventilation should be used to correct respiratory acidosis and mild metabolic acidosis. For the most part, in the absence of pulmonary hypertension, maintenance of normal pH, pCO_2, and pO_2 is the goal of respiratory support. In patients with pulmonary hypertension or in those in whom it may be expected (i.e., preoperative VSD with a large left-to-right shunt), respiratory support is altered so that pO_2 is weaned in small increments and the patient is mildly hyperventilated **(Table 14–14).**

Table 14.14. Principles of Management of Increased Pulmonary Vascular Resistance

- Oxygenation
  - small increments in weaning FiO_2
  - maintain PaO_2 >100
- Hyperventilation
  - pCO_2 25—30
- Sedation and analgesia
  - fentanyl: begin 1–2 μg/kg/hour infusion
  - midazolam: begin 0.1 mg/kg/hour infusion
- Muscle relaxation
  - pancuronium 0.1 mg/kg bolus every 60–90 minutes
  - vecuronium 0.1 mg/kg/hour infusion
- Drugs
  - β-agonists with minimal α-agonist activity—dobutamine, isoproterenol, low-dose epinephrine
  - direct vasodilators nitroglycerine, nifedipine, PGE-1, tolazoline
  - phosphodiesterase inhibitors—amrinone, milrinone
- Inhaled Nitric Oxide

When severe intrapulmonary shunting or severe ventilation-perfusion mismatching exists, even 100% inspired oxygen may not be sufficient to oxygenate the patient adequately. In this situation, continuous positive airway pressure (CPAP) or positive end expiratory pressure (PEEP) may be applied to the lungs. The use of CPAP or PEEP improves oxygenation by increasing functional residual capacity and decreasing atelectasis and small airway closure[151]. Of course, by transmission of airway pressure to the pulmonary vasculature and right atrium, PEEP can decrease cardiac output[152–157]. The degree to which airway pressure is transmitted depends on the compliance of the lungs themselves[155,157]. PEEP contributes to barotrauma and the risk of subsequent complications such as pneumothorax, pneumomediastinum, and interstitial emphysema; however, benefits of PEEP in postoperative patients have been well documented[151,158–162]. As with other treatment modalities, PEEP must be used judiciously.

For patients who have had an uncomplicated closed-heart procedure without CPB or even simple bypass procedures such as repair of ASD, incomplete AV septal defect, or correction of aortic or pulmonary obstruction, the endotracheal tube can usually be removed soon after completion of the surgery[163]. The child should be sufficiently awake to maintain a patent airway and be able to oxygenate and ventilate without mechanical ventilation. In addition, the patient should be hemodynamically stable, usually off vasoactive medications, and should not be bleeding.

Patients in whom prolonged ventilation is expected are those with preexisting pulmonary disease, pulmonary edema, or pulmonary hypertension. In addition, patients who have had prolonged cardiopulmonary bypass for repair of a difficult lesion will have hemodynamic instability and should have respiratory support continued. Patients with severe systemic disease complicated by malnutrition may also need prolonged ventilatory support.

To wean the patient from mechanical support, an orderly procedure is followed. Weaning is greatly facilitated by the use of intermittent mechanical ventilation (IMV). Once the patient has recovered to begin spontaneous ventilation, the IMV rate is decreased in increments of two to five breaths per minute, with arterial blood gases evaluated at each step for hypercarbia or hypoxemia. FiO_2 is decreased as tolerated to 30% before extubation is considered. If at any step in the weaning process hypercarbia or hypoxemia occurs, respiratory support is increased to the level which previously provided adequate ventilation and oxygenation. When the patient is able to maintain normal pH, pO_2 and pCO_2 on minimal ventilatory support (physiologic CPAP with an FiO_2 of 0.30 or less), extubation is considered. Other requirements for extubation at this juncture are hemodynamic stability, normal electrolytes, paucity of secretions, and a neurologic status consistent with maintenance of a patent airway.

Simple bedside pulmonary function tests can be used to assess patient readiness for extubation. A vital capacity greater than 10 ml/kg and a maximum negative inspiratory force greater than −20 cm H_2O are usually associated with a successful tracheal extubation[164]. These tests are difficult to perform in infants and children; however, crying vital capacity greater than 15 ml/kg with a maximum negative inspiratory force greater than −45 cm H_2O allows successful extubation in infants[164].

At the time of tracheal extubation, the stomach is emptied via a nasogastric tube, and the upper airway is cleared of secretions. All the necessary equipment and medications for reintubation should be available at the bedside. After preoxygenation, the endotracheal tube is removed while applying positive pressure to the airway. The pharynx is suctioned, and the child is placed in an oxygen environment at least 10% higher than that before extubation. Oxygenation should be monitored by pulse oximetry throughout the extubation and thereafter. Arterial blood gases are determined 10 to 20 minutes after extubation to document adequate ventilation and oxygenation.

Clinically significant edema of the larynx and subglottic area of the trachea is common in infants and young children. Postextubation stridor occurs in approximately 25% of PICU patients[165], which usually responds well to racemic epinephrine by nebulization. Corticosteroids to prevent postoperative stridor are probably not indicated[166]. Pain control is particularly important after extubation to avoid splinting and atelectasis. Chest physiotherapy, while widely used, may not be particularly beneficial[167].

Supplemental oxygen is gradually withdrawn as indicated by physical examination, pulse oximetry, and arterial blood gases. A postextubation chest x-ray may be indicated in infants when looking for atelectasis and lobar collapse.

Prolonged endotracheal or nasotracheal intubation is a relatively safe alternative to tracheostomy in infants and children[168]. Good nursing care and selection of an appropriate endotracheal tube can avoid laryngeal or tracheal complications. Such complications should only occur when these structures are abnormal prior to intubation. Tracheostomy is now performed in most institutions when respiratory support is anticipated for longer than 30 days, or when a congenital or acquired airway lesion is documented[169,170].

Fluids, Electrolytes, and Renal Function

Fluids

Immediate postoperative fluid management is greatly facilitated by measurements of intracardiac pressure. Optimal intracardiac pressures are determined by clinical observation of heart rate, blood pressure, perfusion, and urine output as fluid boluses are being administered. Initially, optimal RA pressure and/or LA pressure as determined in the operating room should be communicated by the anesthesiologist when transferring the care of the patient. The optimal RA pressure is then maintained by fluid boluses of colloid or blood while maintaining the hematocrit at approximately 35%. One must remember, however, that the optimal filling pressure will vary over time and is dependent on myocardial function.

Although intraoperative hemofiltration, commonly called modified ultrafiltration (MUF), may reduce fluid overload, patients who have undergone CPB are total body fluid overloaded although intravascularly depleted. While acute volume expansion is often required, open-heart patients should have their continuous infusion rate adjusted to provide only one-half to two-thirds of normal maintenance. This is an attempt to limit the amount of fluid one must remove with diuretics when the hemodynamic status has stabilized. In contrast, patients who have not undergone CPB (i.e., after shunting procedures or repair of moderate coarctation of the aorta) can receive maintenance fluid or have their fluids adjusted according to their volume status. Those patients with large ongoing fluid losses through chest tube drainage or urine output in response to diuretics will need greater fluid volumes. Many patients have an increased volume requirement as they warm and the vascular space expands with dilatation. In addition, postoperative fever will increase insensible losses by 10% for each 1°C increase in body temperature.

Electrolytes

Because the CPB circuit is primed with normal saline or lactated Ringer's solution, patients are typically sodium as well as free water overloaded[171,172]. Most patients can maintain a normal sodium while receiving only free water for the first 24 to 48 hours postoperatively. During this time, hyponatremia reflects free water excess. Sodium may be started at 1 mEq/kg/day on the second postoperative day. More sodium may be necessary if diuresis is occurring with sodium losses. It is important to remember that infants receiving saline via intravascular catheters even at low rates may be receiving large doses of sodium.

If the patient has adequate urine output, maintenance potassium is initiated on admission to the ICU in order to avoid hypokalemia. The daily dose can then be adjusted or augmented on the basis of frequent (at least every 4 hours) serum potassium concentration determinations. A decrease in total body potassium with a negative potassium balance after cardiac or other types of surgical procedures has been observed[173–175]. Striking increases in potassium excretion or an intracellular shift of potassium during the first 2 days after major vascular procedures is common[176]. This may occur as a result of a neurohumoral factor secondary to surgery or cellular injury with potassium release and secondary excretion of potassium[172]. Of course, preoperative hypokalemia is frequently observed secondary to diuretic therapy. Other causes include hyperglycemia and hyperventilation with alkalosis. Hypokalemia should be expected after cardiac surgery and frequently leads to arrhythmias. It can be corrected by boluses of 0.2 to 0.5 mEq/kg administered over 30 minutes to 1 hour, preferably via a central line.

Hyperkalemia occurs less commonly in postoperative cardiac patients. When it occurs, it is usually a consequence of altered renal function. The treatment for severe hyperkalemia, if acute, or when life-threatening arrhythmias co-exist, consists of infusions of calcium chloride (0.2 to 0.5 ml/kg of a 10% solution over 2 to 5 minutes), and sodium bicarbonate (2 mEq/kg), along with glucose (0.5 gm/kg) and insulin (0.3 units per gram of glucose) administered over 2 hours.

Calcium homeostasis is often altered after cardiothoracic surgery by a number of factors. Ionized calcium levels and total protein are diluted by pump priming solutions[177]. Citrate added to transfused blood as an anticoagulant binds some available calcium[178]. Calcium is also excreted in urine as a response to diuretic therapy[179]. The use of albumin to expand intravascular volume decreases the proportion of ionized calcium available for cellular interaction by binding calcium. Neonates, particularly the premature, infants of diabetic mothers, and severely stressed or asphyxiated infants, are commonly hypocalcemic[180]. Hypomagnesemia, also reported after cardiac surgery, can contribute to both hypocalcemia and hypokalemia.

The treatment of hypocalcemia depends on whether or not hypocalcemic symptoms are present. Regardless of the serum level of calcium, rapid infusion of calcium generally increases contractility and cardiac output. Rapid boluses can induce bradycardia and hypotension. Measurements of ionized calcium levels should be used whenever possible to guide calcium replacement therapy. For symptomatic patients with tetany, seizures, or ECG changes, 0.1 to 0.2 ml/kg of a 10% calcium chloride solution is administered, preferably via a central catheter to avoid tissue necrosis from extravasation. Maintenance calcium requirements can be met by administration of 100 to 300 mg/kg/day of calcium gluconate parenterally or by enteral calcium containing compounds.

Hypophosphatemia has been observed in 50% of patients after surgery[181]. This may be due to a dilutional effect, intracellular shifts of phosphate which occur after glucose administration[182], or to an alteration of cellular permeability after cardiopulmonary bypass[183]. Urinary losses as well as gastrointestinal losses due to vomiting or nasogastric suctioning need to be replaced. Clinically, hypophosphatemia can lead to impaired oxygen delivery[184], myocardial depression[185], and respiratory insufficiency[186]. Phosphate can be replaced using sodium phosphate (5 to 10 mg/kg/dose over 6 hours) or by substituting potassium chloride with potassium phosphate.

Glucose

Hyperglycemia and hypoinsulinemia have been documented during cardiac surgery, associated with hypothermia[187,188]. Children may have a diminished and delayed insulin response compared with adults, resulting in severe hyperglycemia[189]. The elevation of glucose levels could also result from exogenous glucose infusion, surgical stress, or decreased peripheral glucose utilization[188]. High levels of hyperglycemia may result in an osmotic diuresis, increasing free water loss and leading to intravascular dehydration. If severe hyperglycemia results with a large amount of glucose in the urine, regular insulin should be administered by intravenous infusion. See Chapter 2, and section on preoperative concerns (this chapter) for further discussion of hyperglycemia.

Hypoglycemic coma has also been observed after cardiac surgery, possibly due to early postoperative normalization of previously inhibited pancreatic insulin release, acute liver failure, peripheral hypoperfusion with lactic acidosis secondary to low cardiac output, and partial inhibition of the adrenergic response to hypoglycemia by narcotics[190]. Monitoring of blood glucose is part of routine postoperative care.

Postoperative Renal Function

Renal Physiology

A number of preoperative conditions affecting renal function in children with congenital heart disease may play an important role in the postoperative period. Various anomalies of the genitourinary tract are associated with congenital heart disease. In the presence of congestive heart failure, decreased renal blood flow accentuates the difference between juxtamedullary and cortical blood flow normally seen in children[191]. The kidneys may be affected by chronic hypoxia, with malnutrition and growth retardation also adversely affecting renal function. Patients with cyanotic lesions may be polycythemic, resulting in the formation of renal vascular thromboses and parenchymal infarcts. Structural and functional changes demonstrated in some cardiac patients include a decrease in total glomerular mass with increased size and hyalinization or sclerosis of individual glomeruli, decreased renal plasma flow, increased filtration fraction, decreased para-aminohippurate clearance, a shift of blood flow from cortical to medullary nephrons, and a change in the ability to reabsorb sodium[192].

The use of CPB may have an adverse effect on renal function in terms of fluid balance, as discussed above, although glomerular filtration rate is generally not adversely affected by uncomplicated cardiac surgery[193]. With the possible release of antidiuretic hormone[194] and aldosterone[176] related to general anesthesia and surgery, extracellular fluid and total body water usually increase. In addition, a decrease in sodium excretion occurs along with an increase in total body sodium from uptake of sodium from the oxygenator prime[173]. Muscle cells gain sodium, chloride, and water after major vascular procedures, also pointing to cellular changes underlying the cause of water and sodium retention[195]. The glomerular filtration rate has been shown to increase as a result of cardiopulmonary bypass, which may represent a compensatory body mechanism in response to increased extracellular fluid volume[196].

Renal Failure

It is likely that postoperative renal failure occurs more frequently after cardiovascular surgery compared to other surgical procedures. The greatest risk factor for postoperative renal failure, perioperative hypotension, can occur preoperatively, during CPB, and in low perfusion conditions postoperatively. The incidence of renal failure after cardiac surgery in adults is reportedly 1 to 30%[197,198], with an incidence of 8% in one study of 248 infants and children[199]. Postoperative acute renal failure was associated with many anatomic lesions[200]. Left-sided obstructive lesions such as aortic stenosis and coarctation of the aorta with low renal perfusion may compromise an already low cortical blood flow. Cyanotic cardiac lesions may result in renal cortical hypoxia, increased blood viscosity, acidosis, and hypoglycemia[201,202]. The intraoperative use of halothane and other anesthetic agents may also affect the distribution of intrarenal blood flow away from the cortex, possibly potentiating the deleterious effects of these other factors. Other risk factors include arrhythmias, the administration of α-adrenergic agonists, exposure to nephrotoxic drugs, hypertonic dye used for cardiac catheterization, prolonged CPB, and hypothermia[203,204].

Aggressive management of renal failure in the postoperative cardiac patient should be instituted early. When low urine output or anuria exists in the patient after cardiac surgery due to impaired water and electrolyte homeostasis, the increased intravascular volume is often difficult to manage with fluid restriction, especially when multiple vasoactive and other drugs need to be administered. The increase in intravascular volume also causes a further strain on an already compromised myocardium after surgical incision. In addition, the metabolic problems associated with renal failure including metabolic acidosis and hyperkalemia are poorly tolerated in the cardiac surgical patient, leading to arrhythmias and further compromise of myocardial contractility.

Once a diagnosis of acute renal failure is established, treatment should include the elimination or careful restriction of potassium intake and limitation of fluids. Fluid administration is limited to insensible losses of 300 ml per square meter per day plus urine output, nasogastric losses, diarrhea, or other fluid losses. The patient should be weighed twice a day, if possible, to monitor fluid balance, with a loss of 1 to 2% of body weight expected on this regimen. Hyponatremia in these patients usually indicates excess body water rather than diminished body sodium levels. For this reason, fluid restriction rather than sodium, administration is indicated. If sodium is administered, it can be given as sodium bicarbonate to correct metabolic acidosis. Many children who do not develop renal failure have increased serum uric acid levels postoperatively, associated with decreases in renal excretion. The use of diuretics in the patient with acute renal failure is controversial. The administration of very high doses of furosemide (200 mg per day) in adults with acute renal failure shortens the duration of oliguria[205], although some have observed no difference between treated and untreated patients[206].

Hypertension caused by the expansion of extracellular fluid volume is common in the setting of acute renal failure. Hypersecretion of renin may also play a role, especially in patients with coarctation of the aorta after surgery. Treatment of hypertension includes the restriction of fluids and the use of diuretics and antihypertensive drugs. Nitroprusside may be the drug of choice due to its ease of use, short half-life, easy titratability, and lack of toxicity when used in doses less than 10 ug/kg/minute.

Other manifestations of acute renal failure include hypocalcemia and hyperphosphatemia, anemia, infection, and tissue catabolism, all of which are discussed in Chapter 38, "Renal Failure." Of course, all drugs that are excreted by the kidneys should have their dosing schedule reevaluated to avoid toxic levels. Plasma drug levels should be measured, whenever possible, to regulate dosing further.

Due to the sensitive physiologic state of the cardiac patient, metabolic problems associated with acute renal failure are poorly tolerated and most other therapeutic modalities of limited usefulness; therefore, dialysis is administered more aggressively and earlier in the course of renal failure than in other conditions. Dialysis is now recommended in patients with abnormal expansion of the extracellular fluid volume with hypertension and congestive heart failure, intractable hyperkalemia or acidosis, or signs of uremic encephalopathy such as disorientation, seizures, stupor, or coma. Dialysis should also be instituted in the presence of hyponatremia or hypernatremia, anemia, and malnutrition in the face of fluid overload[(207)].

The decision to use hemodialysis or peritoneal dialysis is generally determined by the patient's clinical state. Peritoneal dialysis is associated with fewer episodes of hypotension when compared with hemodialysis in this patient population. In addition, peritoneal dialysis appears to be more efficacious in the infant and young child because of the presence of a relatively large peritoneal surface area[(208)]. Complications of peritoneal dialysis include infection, hyperglycemia, hyperosmolality, hypotension, protein loss, and abdominal distension with restriction of diaphragmatic movement leading to respiratory compromise[(209)]. Continuous arteriovenous or veno-venous hemofiltration (CAVH) has been used in patients with fluid overload who do not have significant metabolic derangements. It can be used even in patients with hemodynamic instability and is effective in decreasing total body water[(210)]. This may allow increased caloric intake to maintain metabolic homeostasis.

Recovery from acute renal failure is likely with aggressive and meticulous care[(207)]. The duration of oliguria varies greatly, from 3 days to 3 weeks, with an average duration of 10 to 12 days. Polyuria may ensue, so that careful attention to fluid, electrolyte, and acid-base balance is necessary during this period until the ability of the kidneys to maintain homeostasis returns.

Hematology

Congenital heart disease and cardiac surgery produces a myriad of hematological changes. This is particularly true in the child with congenital heart disease and polycythemia, placing the patient at great risk for thrombotic complications[(211,212)]. These children have a high incidence of intraoperative and postoperative bleeding due to qualitative and quantitative platelet abnormalities. Qualitative disorders include impaired platelet adhesion[(213–214)] and abnormalities of platelet release[(215)]. Other problems in patients with cyanotic congenital heart disease are prolongation of the PT and PTT[(216)], elevated fibrin degradation products, decreased fibrinogen, decreased clotting factors 5, 7, 8, and 9, and evidence of fibrinolysis[(217,218)]. Coagulation factors that are synthesized in the liver (factors 1, 2, 5, 7, 9, and 10) may be reduced on the basis of liver parenchymal disease secondary to chronic passive congestion with right-sided heart failure[(218)]. In addition, low-grade DIC has been observed in cyanotic patients preoperatively, leading to bleeding complications in the postoperative period[(218)]. Patients with low cardiac output postoperatively, both cyanotic and acyanotic, with inadequate tissue perfusion, have the highest incidence of DIC. Postoperative problems in polycythemic children may be attenuated by preoperative phlebotomy to achieve a final hematocrit of 55 to 60%[(219)]. Children with cyanotic heart disease tend to have enlarged bronchial collateral vessels which may bleed extensively during surgery and postoperatively. Similarly, the newborn infant, because of deficiency of the vitamin K dependent coagulation factors II, VII, IX, X, protein S and protein C, can also be expected to have increased blood loss perioperatively.

Table 14.15. Coagulation Cascade Factors Inhibited by Heparin

- Factor XI
- Factor Ixa
- Thrombin
- Factor Xa
- Factor IIa

Seemingly innocuous medications, such as aspirin and other nonsteroidal anti-inflammatory agents which inhibit prostaglandin synthesis, can dramatically alter perioperative hemostasis. Platelets are irreversibly deactivated for their life, lasting 10 to 14 days. Function returns only with the generation and release of new platelets from the bone marrow.

After cardiac surgery, the hematologic complications are as diverse as the number of disorders and complications secondary to coagulopathies and generalized surgical bleeding in all patients. This section will cover the major disorders seen in the pediatric patient after cardiac surgery and CPB. For a more detailed explanation of bleeding disorders, refer to Chapter 41, Hematologic Disorders in the Pediatric Intensive Care Unit.

Hemolysis after cardiac surgery can result from severe shear stress as blood is scavenged from the operative field to the cardiotomy reservoir and suctioned from the ventricular vent (when this is used). Hemolytic transfusion or drug reactions are distinctly uncommon but need to be considered if hemolysis persists or there are other clinical suspicions. Hemolysis manifests most commonly during bypass and immediately afterward as hematuria, but is generally a benign, self-limited phenomenon. Ensuring adequate urine output by the use of loop or osmotic diuretics is generally the only therapy needed. Continuing hematuria, particularly with coexisting oliguria, may be a harbinger of a low cardiac output with renal hypoperfusion.

Several events occur simultaneously during CPB which effect coagulation postoperatively. Passage through the CPB circuit causes altered platelet structure and function, as well as frank platelet destruction[(220–224)]. This may be of little significance in patients with short bypass times and simple procedures, but more important with longer bypass times. Similarly, plasma coagulation factors are diluted on bypass. Heparin in a dose of 300 units/kg is given to prevent clotting in the bypass tubing (and patient). Heparin prevents clotting by inactivating antithrombin III[(225)] **(Table 14–15).** Protamine is administered after CPB to reverse heparin's effect, although protamine itself may have hemodynamic effects such as systemic hypotension and pulmonary hypertension[(21–25)]. Despite protamine administration there may be residual heparin effect. While protamine is a specific antidote to heparin's effect on antithrombin III, it does not alter heparin's effect on platelet aggregability. When administered alone, or in excessive amounts, protamine may have anticoagulant activity due to platelet and fibrinogen inhibition. Lastly, heparin may be initially neutralized by protamine after bypass, a phenomenon known as *heparin rebound* has been described from several minutes to hours later, characterized by an increased ACT and clinical bleeding due to heparin release from body tissue.

Bleeding problems secondary to blood transfusion are common in the postoperative period. Stored banked blood is diluted with an anticoagulant and is deficient in clotting factors 5 and 8 and platelets, all of which need to be replaced when massive transfusions are given (typically greater than a single blood volume)[171,226,227]. Also, when massive transfusions are administered, there is a large load of citrate or other preservative that binds calcium, causing a fall in ionized calcium and hemodynamic effects[228]. As hypocalcemia causes a coagulopathy, calcium gluconate or chloride should be administered if bleeding problems occur after large transfusions. Blood lost intraoperatively causes loss of plasma coagulation factors and platelets which are less likely to be replaced than red blood cells. Transfusion therapy has other complications; the 2,3-diphosphoglycerate level is depleted, which shifts the oxyhemoglobin dissociation curve to the left[229], although this does not appear to be a problem clinically. Other consequences of transfusions include microembolization with consequent hypoxemia due to particulate debris found in the pulmonary capillary bed[230], changes in red blood cell deformability[231], protein denaturation secondary to banked blood or bubble oxygenators, and a possible increase in serotonin and histamine levels or release of other mediators[232].

The patient who has had previous cardiac surgery, particularly through a sternotomy, can be expected to have increased bleeding, because of friable scar tissue and adhesions. Finally, although this may seem self- evident, those patients with extensive intracardiac and intrathoracic suture lines have greater overall blood loss than those with simple procedures.

A careful assessment of blood loss during the postoperative period due to losses through chest tubes, from surgical wounds, and secondary to blood sampling should be made. An accurate flow sheet with blood balance, especially for the infant or very small child, should be kept at the bedside and measurements recorded every 15 minutes for the first postoperative hour and on a hourly basis thereafter. A hematocrit is obtained on a regular basis until blood replacement is unnecessary. The hematocrit does not signify blood volume but aids in deciding on the type of fluid replacement. The hematocrit is maintained at 35% in children and greater than 40% in infants. Of course, cyanotic patients after a palliative procedure may remain polycythemic. In addition, after simple procedures, the hematocrit may be maintained at lower levels in order to avoid transfusion.

Coagulation studies, including platelet count, PT, and PTT should be drawn on admission to the intensive care unit; unfortunately, this will not provide any information about platelet function. The ACT should be checked after protamine administration, and additional protamine given if necessary. It should be remembered, however, that a prolonged ACT is not specific for heparin effect; deficiency of coagulation factors and nonfunctional platelets can also cause a prolonged ACT. The thromboelastogram has been studied in a number of centers as a method of evaluating clot formation after surgery, with specific patterns identified for various deficiencies. There are several drawbacks to this which have precluded its universal acceptance, including expense, length of time required to run the test, and expertise in interpreting results.

Therapy for bleeding after bypass should always be considered in the context of patient stability. Since platelet deficiency or dysfunction is the most common cause of continued oozing after surgery when major blood loss occurs in children, administration of platelets should be the first intervention[233]. Fresh frozen plasma or cryoprecipitate administration should not be deferred pending laboratory results in patients with rapid diffuse oozing and no discernable bleeding site in the operating room. Brisk bleeding, 5 ml/kg of fresh blood in the first hour and 3 to 4 ml/kg in subsequent hours, which persists after correction of the coagulopathy, necessitates surgical reexploration. Supportive transfusion therapy with both packed cells and coagulation components should be given while the patient is returned to the operating room.

Desmopressin (DDAVP), a vasopressin analogue, enhances platelet adhesiveness by increasing von Willebrand's factor, which in turn enhances platelet function and factor VIII activity. It has been shown to reduce the transfusion requirement in adults having a repeat sternotomy incision[233]. In preliminary evaluations, however, it has not been demonstrated to decrease the amount of transfusion in children with cyanotic congenital heart disease[234], or in routine adult patients. Hemodynamic side effects, including hypotension, have been reported in 35% of patients[235,236]. Epsilon-aminocaproic acid, a fibrinolysis inhibitor, may also be useful[237].

The use of fresh, whole blood, in contrast to component therapy perioperatively, has been recently evaluated in the context of neonatal open heart surgery. It was demonstrated that whole blood (less than 48 hours old) decreased the amount of overall transfusion in comparison to using component therapy[238]. Whole blood also decreases the number of donor exposures; it is, unfortunately, frequently difficult to obtain fresh whole blood.

Neurologic Complications

The neurologic system should be thoroughly evaluated when the child is sufficiently awake for a reasonable examination. In the patient who remains flaccid or weak, prolonged effects from muscle relaxants should be considered. Serial examinations can be performed to rapidly assess gross abnormalities such as hemiparesis, cranial nerve abnormalities, peripheral neuropathy, or the presence of seizures. Once the patient is even partially awake, the physical examination should include the level of consciousness with a Glasgow Coma Score, and the assessment of brainstem reflexes, including pupillary responses to light, doll's eyes, cold caloric responses if the examination is questionable, and gross motor responses. Specific note should be made of drug administration that may interfere with central nervous system function. For instance, atropine or other peripheral or ganglionic parasympatholytic drugs will cause pupillary dilatation, whereas narcotics cause pupillary constriction.

The etiology of CNS complications and the pathophysiologic principles governing CNS damage were discussed in the section on CNS effects during cardiopulmonary bypass. All intravenous lines should be meticulously cleared of air bubbles to avoid air embolism across a right-to-left intracardiac shunt. Metabolic derangements including acid-base imbalance and electrolyte disorders that cause neurologic sequelae should be avoided by closely monitoring blood gases and serum electrolytes. Glucose should also be monitored frequently, especially when acute hepatic failure occurs after cardiac surgery. Episodes of hypoxia and hypotension which affect all organ systems will have a detrimental effect on the central nervous system.

When central nervous system problems arise, supportive care is indicated. Anticonvulsant therapy for seizures and treatment of any metabolic derangement causing seizures should be administered rapidly. Airway and ventilatory support with continued intubation may be necessary due to the seizures themselves or obtundation of the patient from anticonvulsant medications. In the newborn, metabolic causes of seizures are frequent due to hypoglycemia, hypocalcemia, or hypomagnesemia. After drawing appropriate laboratory specimens, glucose (100 to 200 mg per kilogram slowly), calcium gluconate (100 mg/kg) or magnesium sulfate (1 to 2 ml per kilogram of 3% solution slowly) may be given. Management of the child in a coma with intracranial hypertension may include the usual supportive maneuvers for that problem (See Chapter 21).

Peripheral neuropathies should be sought after cardiac surgery. Diaphragmatic paralysis secondary to phrenic nerve laceration or trauma was discussed previously. Paraplegia secondary to spinal cord ischemia during coarctation repair occurs (see section on coarctation of the aorta). Vocal cord paralysis secondary to recurrent laryngeal nerve trauma has been seen after ligation of a PDA or shunting procedure. Brachial plexus injury usually involving the medial cord of the plexus is related to traction of the plexus by adverse positioning of the patient in the operating room[(239)], associated with median sternotomy[(240)]. Other peripheral neuropathies, especially an ulnar nerve palsy, may be seen after surgery.

Gastrointestinal Complications

Gastrointestinal complications are unusual after cardiac surgery, but are catastrophic when they do occur. The initial assessment should include the presence or absence of bowel sounds and measurement of abdominal girth. The liver and spleen should be percussed for position and span, specifically to assess the degree of right ventricular failure. Many factors may interfere with normal gastrointestinal function after cardiac surgery, including pain, narcotics, electrolyte imbalance (particularly hypokalemia), and drugs which alter smooth muscle function, such as nitroprusside. Acute gastric dilatation is frequently observed after chest surgery in infants and children, so a nasogastric tube should be routinely placed.

A number of special considerations involving the gastrointestinal system should be noted. The postcoarctectomy syndrome (see section on coarctation of the aorta) usually presents with abdominal pain, vomiting, and ileus, 1 to 5 days postoperatively. Prolonged restriction of oral feedings and treatment of hypertension with antihypertensive medications are the treatments of choice. A condition similar to necrotizing enterocolitis due to a local ischemic phenomenon may occur in the postoperative period in the first year of life, especially after hypothermic arrest[(241–243)]. These children present with abdominal distention, peritoneal signs, ileus, and bloody or Guaiac positive stools in the first 24 hours after surgery. Abdominal x-rays typically reveal bowel distention, pneumatosis intestinalis, and air in the hepatic portal system. This may result from either intense splanchnic vasoconstriction from marked localized sympathetic stimulation or from ischemia secondary to inadequate local perfusion[(242–245)].

Frank bowel infarction may present at any age due to poor perfusion with low cardiac output or an embolus to the mesenteric arterial system, occurring during bypass or in the postoperative period[(243)]. In one large adult series, the incidence of this complication was 0.1%. These patients presented an average of 9 days after undergoing bypass and were demonstrated to have nonocclusive vascular lesions[(244)]. As patients who underwent early surgical intervention did well, a high index of suspicion is necessary to reduce mortality.

Jaundice in the early postoperative period is seen in 2 to 9% of cases after surgery for congenital heart disease[(246,247)]. The most striking biochemical feature is an increased bilirubin level peaking between the second and the tenth postoperative day. The alkaline phosphatase level may be elevated, peaking after the seventh postoperative day, with a normal or slightly raised serum glutamic pyruvate transaminase. Jaundice may occur secondary to perioperative liver dysfunction, hemolysis, postoperative congestive heart failure, or viral hepatitis. A prospective study including 154 adult patients after open-heart surgery revealed early postoperative jaundice in 23% of the patients[(248)]. Important contributing factors to jaundice in this study were right-sided heart failure, perioperative hypotension or hypoxemia, and the amount of blood transfused perioperatively.

Acute hepatic failure in the postoperative period was described in 11 children with jaundice, increase in serum ammonia, hypoglycemia, and marked prolongation of the prothrombin time, with failure of hemostasis resulting from low levels of clotting factors 5, 7, and 9[249]. Acute hepatic failure is usually the result of poor hepatic perfusion in combination with high right-sided venous pressure[249–251]. Acute hepatic failure in the postoperative period appears to occur in children who have a decreased cardiac output for a prolonged period (greater than 24 hours), necessitating inotropic support and high right-sided vascular pressure[249]. Children at particular risk include those in whom a modified Fontan procedure was performed or those in whom elevated right atrial pressure was required to maintain pulmonary blood flow when high pulmonary vascular resistance coexisted. The presence of passive congestion predisposes patients to the development of centrilobular necrosis if an episode of shock occurs because the pressure gradient across the hepatic vascular bed is decreased[252]. The centrilobular region is most susceptible to necrosis because it is the most distant from oxygen-carrying blood vessels[253]. Patients with right-sided congestive heart failure without poor perfusion do not develop the typical pattern of centrilobular necrosis[254,255].

Regular surveillance of patients at risk for acute hepatic failure includes bilirubin, serum transaminase levels, prothrombin time, and glucose levels[249,256]. Appropriate treatment of the coagulopathy, hypoglycemia, or hyperammonemia should be started. Renal failure is a frequent concomitant of acute hepatic failure in these patients, so fluid restriction may be necessary with early institution of dialysis. Right atrial pressure should be maintained at the lowest possible level to maintain cardiac output.

A protein-losing enteropathy secondary to obstruction of the superior or inferior vena caval conduit of the intra-atrial baffle after the Mustard procedure has been described[257]. This disorder is apparently caused by increased venous pressure secondary to superior or inferior vena caval conduit obstruction, leading to obstruction of the entry of lymph into the central veins, with a resultant increase in thoracic duct pressure. It can present a year or more after surgery.

Nutrition

In the well-nourished child, adequate substrate from liver glycogen and intravenous infusions of glucose are sufficient to maintain normoglycemia. In the stressed child or newborn, hypoglycemia may occur in the postoperative period. It is important therefore to monitor blood glucose and to administer glucose if hypoglycemia is present.

Maintenance of adequate nutrition is not a problem for most children in the postoperative period. Controversy still exists regarding the timing of enteral feeds postoperatively. After simple procedures such as a PDA ligation or simple ASD or VSD closure, enteral feeds can begin as early as the first postoperative day. In some centers enteral feeds are withheld after coarctectomy for 1 to 3 days postoperatively. In more complicated operations, typically mechanical ventilation is stopped and the child is extubated before feeding is instituted. If the patient's ventilator course is more protracted with myocardial or respiratory failure, then enteral feeds can begin once the child's condition is stable. In the unstable patient or if enteral feeds cannot be started due to a primary GI problem, then parenteral feeding should be instituted (by the third postoperative day) via a central venous line. Nutritional status is usually a problem when the postoperative period is long and complicated, if the child has preexisting failure to thrive or chronic malnutrition, or if the patient is a small infant with high metabolic needs. For a discussion of the complete management and complications of hyperalimentation, see Chapter 35, Nutrition and Metabolism in the Critically Ill Child.

Infection

The child with congenital heart disease is at increased risk for infection due to chronic congestive heart failure, hypoxia, malnutrition, failure to thrive, and, most important, the number and duration of invasive vascular catheters. Structural abnormalities of the heart predispose the child to bacterial endocarditis. Surgery increases the risk due to surgical trauma, immunologic depression, and surgical entry of micro-organisms. The high risk of postoperative infection may have an immunologic basis. Open heart surgery is associated with a decrease in T- and B-lymphocyte number and function[265,266]. These decreases have not been associated with an increase in T-suppressor lymphocytes[267], although other suppressor cells such as prostaglandin-producing monocytes have been implicated with this finding[268]. Immunoglobulin levels may be decreased immediately after surgery[269,270]. Typically, children are treated prophylactically with a second-generation cephalosporin postoperatively. A loading dose is given before surgery and continued for 24 to 48 hours postoperatively.

Systemic signs of infection include fever, leukocytosis, septic shock, impaired respiratory function with adult respiratory distress syndrome, and impaired neurologic function. In the newborn, signs of infection are nonspecific and include lethargy, poor feeding, hypothermia, jaundice, hypoglycemia, and seizures. Low-grade fever in the first 48 hours postoperatively is common; fever and leukocytosis may be unreliable parameters for the diagnosis of septic complications in adults in the first postoperative week, although one study showed a high correlation between the presence of fever and infection after the third postoperative day. Therefore, fever persisting after 48 hours should be worked up with appropriate blood, urine, sputum, and wound cultures. Multiple blood cultures should be obtained to rule out bacterial endocarditis. In a patient with signs or symptoms of a central nervous system disorder, a lumbar puncture and cerebrospinal fluid cultures should be obtained. If signs and symptoms of systemic infection are present, antibiotics should be administered after obtaining cultures. Respiratory infection should be treated with antibiotics specific against organisms grown from tracheal aspirates. Urinary tract infections are usually caused by contamination from a Foley catheter. Treatment consists of the removal of the contaminated catheter and the use of an appropriate antibiotic. Low-grade fever occurring 5 to 7 days after surgery may be due to postpericardiotomy syndrome.

Sternal and costochondral infections have been reviewed extensively in adults and children[(258–262)]. In children, most mediastinitis is caused by staphylococci[(261)], but gram-negative organisms and fungi have also been implicated[(258)]. The incidence of mediastinitis after repair of congenital heart disease is 0.4 to 1%[(258)]. All sternal wounds should be examined daily for signs of erythema, superficial drainage, sternal instability, excessive incisional pain, or frank dehiscence with purulent drainage. The presence of spiking fevers, leukocytosis, positive blood cultures, or systemic sepsis should lead one to investigate the sternal wound for signs of infection while other sources of infection are being excluded. The overall incidence of sternal infections may be increased with postoperative hemorrhage or the need for thoracic reexploration. Other infectious diseases, such as hepatitis and cytomegalovirus, are common after blood transfusions and should be sought when fever presents postoperatively[(264)].

SPECIFIC SURGICAL PROCEDURES

Palliative Shunt Operations

Palliative procedures correct the physiologic defects arising from cardiac anomalies without addressing the anatomic defects **(Table 14–16).** Such procedures were originally undertaken because corrective surgery was unavailable. Today, these procedures are more commonly used to maintain a more normal physiology until the infant is large enough to undergo corrective surgery. Systemic to pulmonary artery shunts are used as palliative procedures when there is inadequate or ductal-dependent pulmonary blood flow. Critical pulmonic stenosis or pulmonary atresia and tricuspid atresia are the most common indications for shunting in the newborn period[(271)]. Advances in corrective surgery have made shunt procedures beyond the newborn period uncommon **(Table 14–17).**

Table 14.16. Types of Surgical Corrections

Total correction—no residual abnormality
VSD repair
PDA repair
Total correction—mild residual abnormality
Repair tetralogy of Fallot
Mild to moderate residual abnormality
Mustard or Senning repair for TGA
Aortic stenosis repair
Palliative procedures (final treatment) with persistent abnormalities
Fontan procedure
Palliative procedure (staged treatment)
Shunt placement
Pulmonary artery banding

Table 14.17. Types of Shunts

Blalock-Taussig
Subclavian artery to pulmonary artery
Modified Blalock-Taussig
Synthetic shunt from subclavian artery to pulmonary artery
Waterston
Ascending aorta to pulmonary artery
Potts
Descending aorta to left pulmonary artery
Glenn
Right pulmonary artery to superior vena cava

The Potts procedure, a descending aorta to pulmonary artery shunt, was first described in 1946[(272)]. Inability to control the size of the communicating orifice and its tendency to grow with time frequently lead to congestive heart failure and pulmonary hypertension. Distortion of the pulmonary artery and aneurysms of the pulmonary artery also occur[(273)].

The Waterston shunt, an ascending aorta to pulmonary artery shunt was first described in 1962[(274)]. This procedure also frequently results in distortion of the pulmonary artery. Kinking of the right pulmonary artery leads to a majority of shunt flow going into the right pulmonary artery and exaggerated ventilation-perfusion mismatch. Complications with these shunts have minimized their use.

The Blalock-Taussig shunt was first performed at the Johns Hopkins Hospital in 1945[(275)]. The original procedure involved anastomosis of a subclavian artery with the pulmonary artery. The subclavian artery provides appropriate pulmonary blood flow resulting in a low incidence of congestive heart failure and subsequent pulmonary vascular disease. Other advantages include the ease of ligation of the shunt at the time of later corrective surgery and the infrequency with which it causes distortion of the pulmonary artery.

After the classic Blalock-Taussig shunt is performed, blood pressure should not be taken in the arm on the side of the shunt. Color and warmth of that arm should be observed carefully to assess its vascular supply from collateral channels off the subclavian artery. The arm may initially be cold and pulseless; however, this gradually improves over the ensuing 48 to 72 hours[(276)], and gangrene is a rare complication[(277)]. True ischemic changes may be reversible with reconstructive arterial surgery[(278)]. Decreased muscle blood flow and impaired arm development with decreased longitudinal growth and muscle mass[(279)] can be seen in the first year after shunting, although these differences are not seen over time[(280)].

Dissatisfaction with complications of the classical Blalock-Taussig shunt led to the development of the modified Blalock-Taussig shunt, which is the most common systemic to pulmonary artery shunt used today (Fig. 14–8). This shunt is created by interposing a synthetic tube graft, usually GORE-TEX®, between the subclavian artery and the pulmonary artery. This is generally performed on the side of the aortic arch to facilitate take-down at the time of definitive repair[281]. The upper and lower lobe pulmonary branches must be identified and dissected separately to ensure that the graft is placed into a main branch pulmonary artery. Flow through the graft is primarily regulated by the size of the subclavian artery so that the size of the graft itself is not critical.

The principal disadvantage to the Blalock-Taussig shunt is a significant increase in early shunt thrombosis in neonates. This complication can be avoided with diligent postoperative care, which includes maintenance of adequate cardiac output and blood pressure in the early postoperative period, and its frequency may be related to surgical technique. Dopamine may be used to increase systolic pressure postoperatively. Early shunt occlusion occurs more frequently in cyanotic children with increased red cell mass. As viscosity increases due to an elevated hematocrit, blood flow decreases. Therefore, partial exchange transfusion or phlebotomy to lower hematocrit and avoidance of hemoconcentration by appropriate hydration perioperatively may help maintain shunt patency. Maintenance fluids or greater are administered and diuretics should be avoided in the early postoperative period, if possible. Systemic anticoagulation with heparin is used during the creation of the shunt and may be continued for 24 to 48 hours thereafter to prevent early shunt thrombosis[282]. Long-term shunt patency may be improved by the use of low dose aspirin (1 mg/kg every other day). A modified Blalock-Taussig shunt may have a lower incidence of thrombosis than the classical Blalock-Taussig shunts[283].

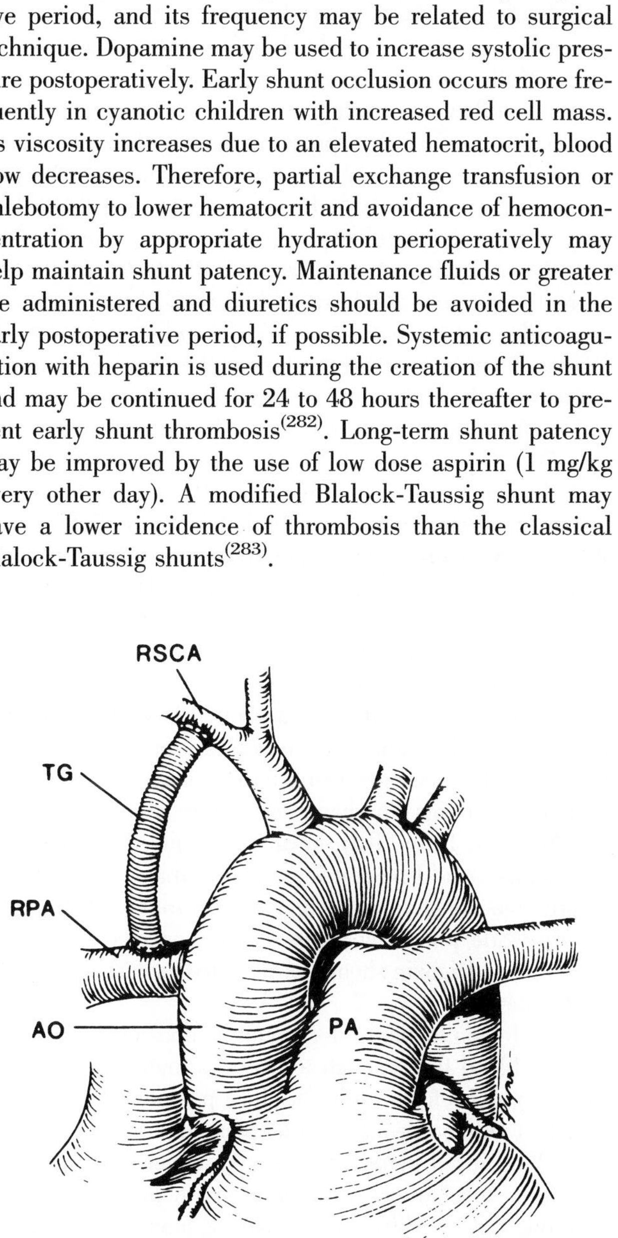

Figure 14.8. Modified Blalock-Taussig shunt. RSCA = right subclavian artery; RPA = right pulmonary artery; AO = aorta; PA = pulmonary artery; TG = tube graft. (From Ariniegas E, ed. Pediatric Cardiac Surgery. Chicago: Year Book Medical Publishers, 1985.)

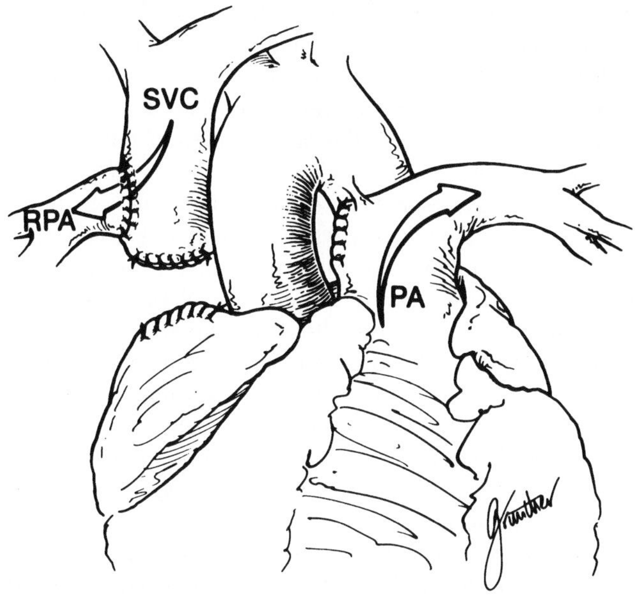

Figure 14.9. Glenn shunt, an end-to-end anastomosis of the superior vena cava to the distal end of the divided right pulmonary artery. The superior vena cava-right atrial junction and the proximal right pulmonary artery are ligated. (From Lowe DA: Abnormalities of the atrioventricular valves. (ed) Lake CL. In:Pediatric Cardiac Anesthesia, Chapter 17, Appleton and Lange, Connecticut 1988, p 305.)

Infrequent complications after Blalock-Taussig shunt procedures include chylothorax and chylopericardium. GORE-TEX® shunts may leak excessive serous fluid through the interstices of the fabric, resulting in excessive and prolonged chest tube drainage and localized seroma formation around the graft[284,285]. Management of chylothorax was previously discussed. Localized seroma can be drained by transthoracic needle aspiration. In addition, a transient unilateral increase in pulmonary blood flow and pulmonary edema can be observed on the side of the shunt. It usually clears within 48 hours.

The Glenn shunt is an anastomosis between the SVC and the right pulmonary artery to increase pulmonary blood flow in children with cyanotic congenital disease (Fig. 14–9). Unlike more traditional shunts, such as the Blalock Taussig or central aorta to pulmonary artery shunt, systemic venous pressure rather than arterial pressure is the driving force for pulmonary blood flow through the pulmonary circuit. As such, this procedure can only be performed in patients with low or normal pulmonary vascular resistance, which precludes its application in the neonate. Generally the Glenn shunt is used in older children with lesions such as tricuspid atresia and single ventricle, as part of a staged Fontan-type correction. The end result of this surgery will be separate pulmonary and systemic circulations, with pulmonary blood flow solely supplied by venous driving pressure. Preoperative problems are the same as for patients undergoing the Fontan operation (see below).

The Glenn shunt can be performed through either a right thoracotomy or a median sternotomy, depending on surgical preference, and generally is done without CPB. One exception to this is a surgical variation termed the *bidirectional* Glenn-Haller, in which the SVC is attached to both pulmonary arteries to enhance blood flow and promote "growth" of the pulmonary arteries. For this later procedure, CPB is used because of the manipulation of total pulmonary blood flow.

A right thoracotomy necessitates a period of "one lung" ventilation intraoperatively, when the right lung is collapsed and the right pulmonary artery transected from the main pulmonary artery. Usually this is well tolerated, although some deterioration in arterial oxygen saturation can be anticipated. Additional intraoperative and postoperative difficulties related to this approach, as for any thoracotomy, include pulmonary hemorrhage and plugging of the endotracheal tube. Monitoring of SVC pressure above the suture line should be done with either a jugular or subclavian central venous pressure (CVP) line. As with the Fontan procedure, care must be taken during catheter placement to not advance the CVP too distally, where it may be inadvertently sutured into the anastomosis. Elevated SVC pressure, with the potential for elevated cerebral venous pressure can be expected postoperatively. This is generally of no clinical consequence, except when cerebral perfusion pressure is compromised by low cardiac output and low mean arterial pressure. Augmenting venous return to the right pulmonary artery can be accomplished by the head-up position and manipulation of ventilatory parameters to lower mean airway pressure. Venous return is promoted by spontaneous ventilation with negative intrapleural pressure. Negative intrathoracic pressure (relative to atmospheric pressure) is transmitted to the pulmonary vascular tree, lowering pulmonary artery pressure and thus increasing the perfusion pressure. When circumstances preclude spontaneous ventilation such as residual anesthetic, narcotic, or muscle relaxants, minimizing peak inspiratory pressure and end-expiratory pressure will help to maintain forward flow. Hypercarbia and hypoxemia are potent pulmonary vasoconstrictors and should be avoided; premature tracheal extubation can be deleterious if these result.

Balloon Atrial Septostomy and Blalock-Hanlon Operation

Transposition of the great arteries (TGA) results in the presence of two noncommunicating circuits. To improve systemic oxygenation, a communication between the two circuits must be created. An intra-atrial communication can be created in the cardiac catheterization laboratory by the Rashkind procedure using a balloon septostomy catheter. This catheter is passed from the right atrium through the foramen ovale into the left atrium. After documentation of the location of the balloon by radiography or echocardiography, the catheter is rapidly withdrawn into the right atrium, tearing the atrial septum[286]. Complications of balloon septostomy are rare but include perforation of a heart chamber or AV valve and damage to the pulmonary veins or inferior vena cava[287,288]. Embolization of air or balloon fragments due to balloon rupture has also been reported. Balloon atrial septostomy is successful in 80 to 90% of children with TGA.

Should balloon septostomy fail to create an adequate communication, a Blalock-Hanlon procedure may be required. First described in 1950, an interatrial septal defect is created by excising the posterior portion of the atrial septum in a closed heart procedure[289]. Transient atrial arrhythmias usually of little clinical significance have been described after this procedure[290]. Children who do not have adequate mixing despite the creation of a large ASD require early corrective surgery.

Pulmonary Artery Banding

A palliative surgical approach to congestive heart failure due to excessive left-to-right shunting was first proposed in 1952. Muller and Dammann were able to decrease pulmonary blood flow by creating an artificial stenosis of the pulmonary artery[291]. This procedure was subsequently employed in patients with various anatomic causes of increased pulmonary blood flow[292]. Residual stenosis of the pulmonary artery after band removal and lack of growth of the branch pulmonary arteries may complicate later definitive corrective surgery. As corrective surgery is now performed on smaller infants, pulmonary artery banding is reserved for lesions deemed noncorrectable by other measures, and in neonates with single ventricle or its variant, to preserve low pulmonary vascular resistance and the feasibility of a future Fontan procedure.

Pulmonary artery banding is usually performed using a lateral thoracotomy incision. Through a pericardial incision, the main pulmonary artery is exposed and dissected free, and then constricted by siliconized tape. The band is generally constricted to reduce pulmonary artery pressure to less than half the systemic artery pressure. Frequently, oxygen saturation will also be decreased.

Because of the acute increase in right ventricular afterload induced by pulmonary artery banding, inotropes may be required. This increased afterload may not be well tolerated by patients who have preexisting tricuspid or mitral insufficiency. In the ICU, because of congestive heart failure, fluids should be restricted to two-thirds maintenance. Aggressive use of diuretics may be required to control heart failure while providing adequate fluid to meet caloric requirements. Digoxin should be resumed as early as possible postoperatively.

Initially, pulmonary artery banding does not restrict pulmonary blood flow enough to avoid pulmonary congestion. This is purposeful in order to allow potential space for the patient's pulmonary artery to increase in size as growth occurs. Weaning a patient with severe congestive heart failure from mechanical ventilation after pulmonary artery banding may be difficult but can be facilitated by avoidance of maneuvers which lower pulmonary vascular resistance. Oxygen, a potent pulmonary vasodilator, can increase pulmonary blood flow even in the banded patient. It is therefore important to remember that an arterial oxygen saturation in these patients greater than 90%, although achievable, is not desirable and may lead to excessive pulmonary blood flow. Pulmonary edema can be avoided by maintaining oxygen saturation in the mid to low 80% range. Patients who are banded too tightly are cyanotic postoperatively. Chest x-ray typically shows a paucity of pulmonary blood flow. Reoperation may be necessary in this situation.

Atrial Septal Defect (Secundum)

The ASD accounts for approximately 10% of all congenital cardiac malformations[293]. This intracardiac defect was the first to be corrected using CPB[293]. The most common type of ASD is the ostium secundum defect, in which the lesion is located in the region of the fossa ovale. Early repair of the secundum-type ASD is indicated in infants with significant left-to-right shunts (Qp/Qs greater than 1.5 : 1)[294]. Primary closure by approximation and suture of the edges of the defect is sufficient for small defects. Larger defects are repaired with a pericardial or Teflon patch.

Perioperative mortality for ASD repair approaches zero, and postoperative complications are uncommon. Postoperative arrhythmias such as atrial flutter, atrial fibrillation, sinus tachycardia, paroxysmal atrial tachycardia, and nodal rhythms can occur[295]. AV block has also been described but is rare. Most arrhythmias are transient, occurring only in the immediate postoperative period[295]. Only 2% of arrhythmias are persistent and are most likely due to surgical trauma to the sinus node or its arterial supply[296]. Persistent arrhythmias are more common in patients undergoing repair of sinus venosus defects but are still rarely clinically significant[297].

Postoperative care after repair of a simple ASD with a short cardiopulmonary bypass period is relatively routine. Most patients can be extubated in the operating room or shortly after arrival in the ICU. Extubation should be delayed, however, until rewarming is completed, the distal extremities are well perfused, and any metabolic acidosis has been corrected. As rewarming occurs along with diuresis from agents given as the patient comes off bypass, central venous pressure falls and fluid boluses are frequently required during the first few hours in the ICU. As usual, IV fluids are otherwise maintained at two-thirds of maintenance requirements until the second 24-hour period. If urine output is slow (less than 0.5 ml/kg/hour) despite adequate perfusion and filling pressures, a small dose of furosemide (0.5 mg/kg IV) can be used to induce a diuresis. A mild degree of acute tubular necrosis secondary to poor perfusion on CPB may explain diminished urine output in this situation.

A large ASD with long-standing increased pulmonary blood flow can lead to pulmonary hypertension and ventricular dysfunction preoperatively that may persist in the postoperative period[295,298]. In most young patients, however, right ventricular hypertrophy and dilatation resolve 6 months to a year after surgery[295]. In the occasional patient with cardiomegaly and more severely compromised preoperative cardiac function, poor distensibility of the left ventricle postoperatively can lead to elevated LA pressure, pulmonary edema, and hypoxemia[296,299].

Preliminary efforts at transcatheter closure of atrial septal defects using button or umbrella devices are promising[300,301]. This nonsurgical approach would avoid the inherent risks of cardiopulmonary bypass and related postoperative morbidities.

Endocardial Cushion Defect

Endocardial cushion defect describes a variety of cardiac lesions having a common embryologic abnormality. These defects include a primum ASD, isolated cleft of the mitral valve, and a complete AV canal. Successful repair of complete AV canal depends on the presence of a low pulmonary vascular resistance. Surgical repair is usually attempted at 1 year of age but has been performed earlier with low postoperative mortality and excellent long-term results[302,303].

Repair of a complete endocardial cushion defect is performed through a right atriotomy. The common leaflet of the tricuspid and mitral valves is divided. After patching of the ventricular septal defect, the cleft in the mitral valve is sutured and attached to the left side of the patch. The atrial septal defect is closed primarily, the cleft tricuspid valve is sutured, and the valve is attached to the right side of the ventricular patch[303] (Fig. 14–10).

The postoperative course is typically uncomplicated

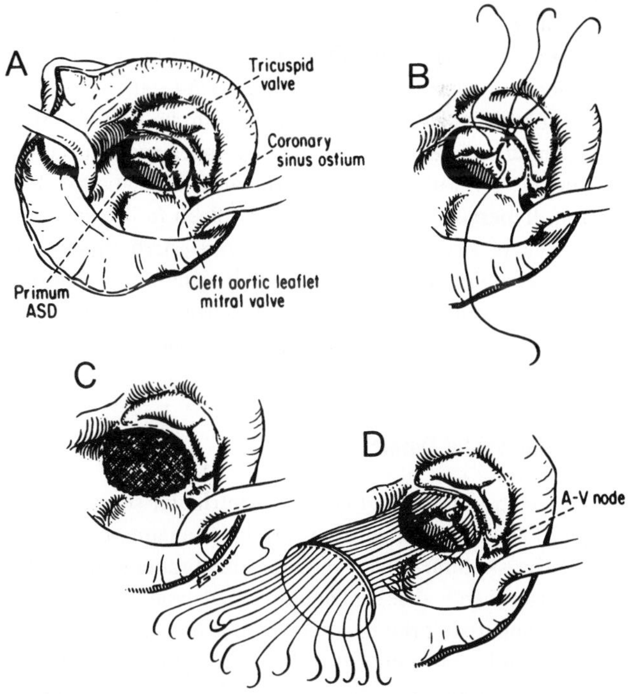

Figure 14.10. Repair of partial atrioventricular canal. (A) Surgical exposure. (B) Closure of mitral valve cleft. (C) Prosthetic patch closure of ostium primum defect. (D) Repair completed. (From Danielson GK: Endocardial cushion defects. In: Ravitch MM, Welch KJ, Benson CD, Aberdeen E, Randolph JG (eds): Pediatric Surgery, ed 3. Chicago, Year Book 1979, Vol 1, p 720.)

when repair is timed appropriately before the development of pulmonary hypertension. As no ventriculotomy is required for repair of this lesion, postoperative hemodynamic insufficiency is related to the duration of cardiopulmonary bypass and the degree of mitral insufficiency postoperatively. If inotropic support is required, dobutamine and amrinone, agents which decrease afterload and do not aggravate mitral regurgitation, are preferable to dopamine. Because of persistent mitral valve regurgitation, left atrial pressure monitoring can be particularly helpful in the management of these patients. Mitral regurgitation can be detected by inspection of the left atrial tracing for the presence of v waves. Care should be taken to use the left atrial end-diastolic pressure as the indicator of left ventricular filling pressure, as mean pressure is elevated due to the presence of v waves. Mitral regurgitation can be managed medically by minimizing afterload through the avoidance of α-adrenergic agonists and agitation while optimizing vasodilation.

When significant mitral regurgitation occurs, prolonged mechanical ventilation can be anticipated. Pulmonary edema develops due to the high left atrial pressure. To avoid pulmonary edema, the intravascular volume should be reduced as much as possible. When mitral regurgitation is expected, the rate of fluid administration should be restricted to one-half maintenance. Along with aggressive diuretic therapy and fluid restriction, continuous arteriovenous hemofiltration may be useful to permit adequate caloric intake. In time, many patients adjust to their altered physiology with decreased left-sided filling pressures. Prolonged hemodynamic instability necessitates mitral valve replacement[303]. Significant tricuspid regurgitation is rare.

Other postoperative complications of AV canal repair include pulmonary hypertension, which can be minimized by early repair before hypertension develops, and various arrhythmias[304]. Pulmonary hypertension is managed with oxygen, hyperventilation to a $PaCO_2$ of 25 to 30, sedation, avoidance of stimulation, and paralysis. Arrhythmias, including complete heart block, which necessitates cardiac pacing, are generally transient. A permanent pacemaker should be placed if heart block persists more than 3 weeks after surgery.

Ventricular Septal Defect

There are several distinct types of ventricular septal defects (VSDs), classified according to their anatomic location within the septum. These include membranous, muscular, supracristal, and atrioventricular canal-type defects, with membranous being the most common. Muscular lesions are often multiple and may be difficult to completely identify and close intraoperatively. Atrioventricular canal type defects result from incomplete genesis of the endocardial cushion, and as such are associated with insufficiency of the tricuspid and mitral valves. The supracristal VSD is located high in the ventricular septum adjacent to the aortic valve. Because of its location, this abnormality is often associated with aortic insufficiency when the septal leaflet of the aortic valve is drawn into the cavity during diastole.

Preoperatively, infants and children with VSD comprise a large, diverse group ranging from 2-month-old infants with a large defect, severe congestive heart failure, and pulmonary hypertension, to the child with an isolated "heart murmur" presenting for repair to prevent complications later in life. As such, the postoperative course can be quite variable, depending on the infant's anatomy and physiology.

Most simple VSD repairs are completed via a right atrial incision through the tricuspid valve. When exposure is not adequate, or repair is impossible with this approach, a ventricular incision is used. This, however, causes more ventricular dysfunction and need for hemodynamic support post-bypass. An attempt is made to correct coexisting valvular pathology. The postoperative course is determined by the preoperative condition, the intraoperative course, and the success of the valvular repair, if any.

In the infant with a long-standing VSD, persistent elevation of PVR is expected, with episodic pulmonary hypertensive "crises" and right ventricular failure anticipated after surgery[305]. These babies frequently have pulmonary problems, including left lower lobe collapse resulting from bronchial compression by an enlarged left atrium, pneumonia, and reactive airways. Electrolyte abnormalities secondary to chronic diuretic use result in alkalosis and hypokalemia and may persist into the postoperative period.

Ventricular function after bypass can be adversely effected by several factors; preexisting congestive heart failure, the need for ventriculotomy for repair, and poor myocardial preservation during bypass are all associated with an increased need for inotropic support postoperatively.

Pulmonary arteriolar hypertrophy and elevated pulmonary vascular resistance do not involute immediately after surgery[305,306]. The infant with pulmonary hypertension preoperatively can be expected to have episodic pulmonary hypertension, which can cause acute right ventricular failure, for several days after surgery, and may be monitored with a PA catheter placed transthoracically during surgery. Specific therapies to blunt these crises in the ICU include mild deliberate hyperventilation, ensuring adequate oxygenation, and sedation with fentanyl infusion. Muscle paralysis may also be added. If inotropic support is necessary, agents which lower PVR, such as isoproterenol, dobutamine, and amrinone may be good initial choices. Prostaglandin E_1 and nitroprusside may be useful to lower PVR[307]. Inhaled nitric oxide, a potent pulmonary vasodilator, has an advantage over these intravascular agents in that it will not cause systemic hypotension[113,114]. One exciting new development in the management of VSD is the ability to close defects in the catheterization lab using a transcatheter placement of an umbrella device which straddles the defect[308].

The older asymptomatic child usually requires little or no myocardial support postoperatively. Under these circumstances, a relatively short ICU stay can be anticipated. Weaning from mechanical ventilation and extubation may occur several hours postoperatively in the hemodynamically stable child. These patients can be managed with maintenance fluids.

Tetralogy of Fallot

Complete correction of tetralogy of Fallot was developed by Lillehei and associates in 1955[309]. This is now performed in infants with low operative mortality and excellent long-term results[310]. The repair is performed through a right ventriculotomy at the level of the outflow tact. The VSD is closed with a patch. Both ventriculotomy and patch placement must be done carefully to avoid damage to the annulus or leaflets of the overriding aorta[311]. The techniques to relieve obstruction of the right ventricular outflow tract varies according to the anatomy. In the absence of pulmonary hypertension, valvar pulmonic stenosis is repaired by incision of the pulmonary valve annulus. Infundibular stenosis is relieved by the insertion of a Dacron or pericardial patch. Complete pulmonary valve atresia is repaired by use of a conduit attached to the ventriculotomy incision and connected to the main pulmonary artery. At the time of repair of tetralogy of Fallot, previous palliative shunts (i.e., Blalock-Taussig shunt) are taken down (Fig. 14–11).

After repair of tetralogy of Fallot, diminished cardiac output results from poor right ventricular function caused by ventriculotomy, CPB, and residual right ventricular outflow obstruction. Central venous pressure may be elevated in the presence of residual outflow obstruction and yet not reflect the patient's intravascular volume. Maintenance of a high RA pressure postoperatively is important both to improve cardiac output and overcome right-sided obstruction. Under these conditions RA pressure should be increased with blood or colloid until peripheral perfusion is adequate. This

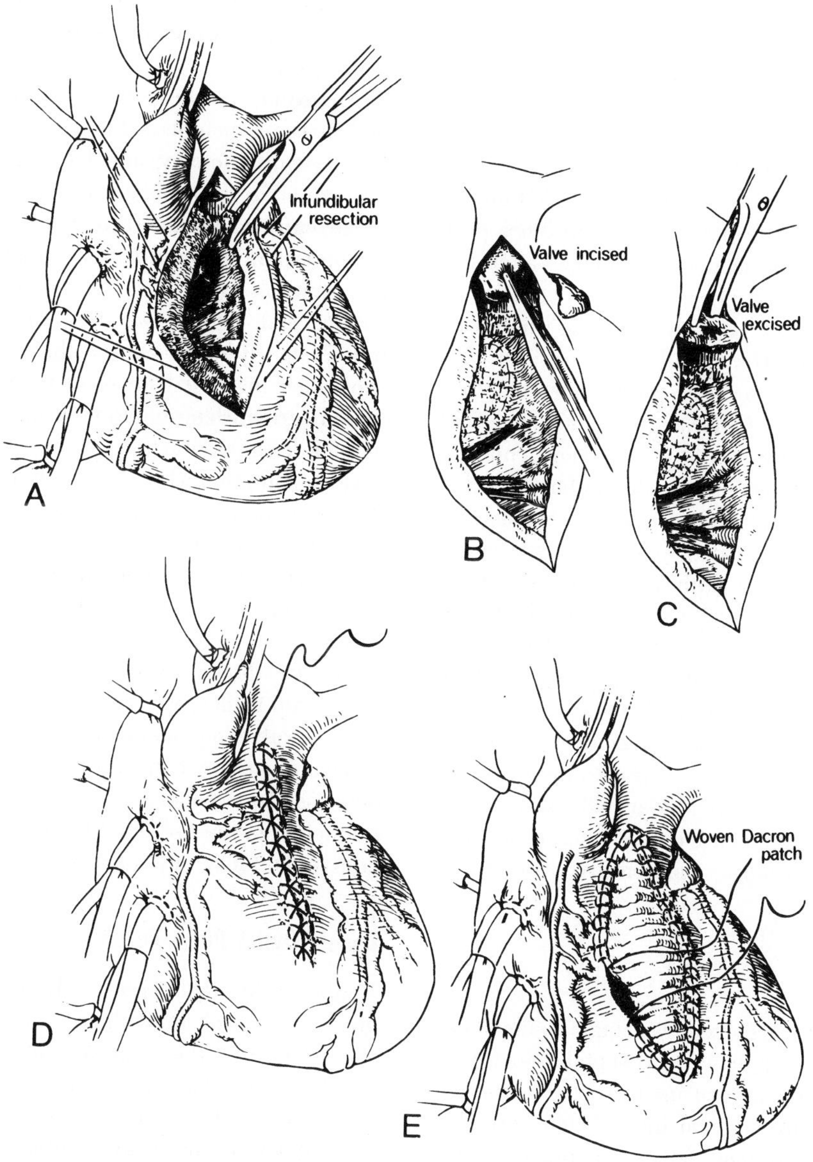

Figure 14.11. Methods of reconstructing the right ventricular outflow tract. (From Cooley DA: Total correction of tetralogy of Fallot. In: Techniques in Cardiac Surgery, Second Edition, Chapter 12. WB Saunders, Houston, Texas 1984, p 135.)

often requires a RA pressure of 16 to 18 mm Hg. Inotropic drugs should be used judiciously, and after the RA pressure is maximized. Tachycardia and an increase in the dynamic component of outflow tract obstruction can result from the use of an inotropic agent, worsening the patient's condition.

As outflow tract edema decreases and ventricular function improves, inotropes may be weaned. Mechanical ventilation is continued until the patient requires minimal hemodynamic support and is tolerating a FiO_2 of 0.35 or less. Fluids are generally restricted to two-thirds maintenance until peripheral edema has resolved. If recovery is prolonged, fluids must be liberalized to provide adequate calories with a concurrent increase in diuretic therapy. Depending on the extent of the ventriculotomy and myocardial dysfunction, digitalization may be necessary at the time of weaning from inotrope infusions.

Because electrocardiographic abnormalities are common after tetralogy of Fallot repair, temporary pacing wires are placed in all patients at the time of surgery. Right bundle branch block (RBBB) may be caused by right ventriculotomy with or without trauma to the right main bundle branch or proximal conducting system[(312)]. RBBB is often associated with left anterior hemiblock (LAH) and may be due to peripheral injury to the AV conduction system or secondary to a His' bundle lesion[(313)]. RBBB and LAH are associated with a high incidence of complete heart block postoperatively[(314)]. If complete heart block persists after 2 to 3 weeks or recurs, a permanent pacemaker should be inserted. Complete heart block is likely to persist when it results from an injury to the His' bundle.

Ventricular arrhythmias are a recognized late complication of repair of tetralogy of Fallot and are associated with a high incidence of sudden death[(315,316)]. Ventricular arrhythmias were initially thought to be due to long-standing pulmonary outflow tract obstruction; however, there is recent evidence that ventricular arrhythmias also are caused by volume overload as seen with pulmonary regurgitation[(317)]. Incision of the pulmonary valve annulus is thought to be well tolerated. Children who undergo this type of outflow tract repair may need future pulmonary valve replacement. Children who undergo repair early in life have a lower incidence of ventricular ectopy and sudden death compared to children who are repaired late[(318)]. Due to the high incidence of sudden death and ventricular arrhythmias, patients with tetralogy of Fallot should have careful long-term follow-up, including electrophysiologic and hemodynamic evaluation.

Truncus Arteriosus

Truncus arteriosus is characterized by a single common ventricular outflow tract with a ventricular septal defect. Children with truncus arteriosus and unobstructed pulmonary blood flow do not require surgical intervention until their pulmonary vascular resistance falls at approximately 3 months of age. At that time significant pulmonary congestion may develop[(319)].

The exact nature of the repair depends on the cardiac anatomy. There are four anatomic types of truncus arteriosus described by the Edwards classification. In type I, a main pulmonary artery arises from the truncus; in type II, the left and right branch pulmonary arteries arise from the posterior aspect of the truncus; type III differs from type II only in that the branch pulmonary arteries arise from the lateral aspects of the truncus. Type IV, also called pseudotruncus, is a severe form of tetralogy of Fallot in which pulmonary blood flow is provided by bronchial collaterals off the descending aorta. With the exception of type IV, the repair for each type is fundamentally the same. After aortic cannulation and cardioplegia, the pulmonary arteries are tourniqueted, excised from the truncus, and anastomosed to a conduit which is in turn attached to the right ventricular outflow tract via a vertical ventriculotomy. Conduits can be fashioned from porcine-valved Dacron conduits or aortic or pulmonary homograft. Homograft is preferable as it has greater longevity and flexibility. A VSD is easily visible through the ventriculotomy and closed with a Dacron patch.

Immediate postoperative complications of truncus arteriosus repair include a diminished cardiac output secondary to ventriculotomy, and labile pulmonary hypertension. Postoperative management of children undergoing truncus repair can be facilitated by right atrial and pulmonary artery pressure determinations. Management of pulmonary hypertension with mild hyperventilation, aggressive sedation, and muscle paralysis may be required for the first 24 to 48 hours. During the period of instability, CVP should be increased to augment cardiac output. As mentioned earlier, determination of the "best" CVP is made by clinical examination, observing peripheral perfusion and oxygen saturation while gradually infusing volume. Fluid is otherwise administered at two-thirds of maintenance requirements. Mechanical ventilation should be set to maintain pCO_2 between 30 and 35 torr and pO_2 greater than 90 torr as alkalosis and oxygen are potent pulmonary vasodilators.

Infants who do poorly after truncus repair generally have significant truncal valve regurgitation and may benefit from truncal valve replacement[(319)]. Cardiac catheterization or echocardiography can rule out a residual ventricular septal defect and pulmonary conduit obstruction. Despite the introduction of the use of aortic homografts, the early postoperative mortality rate for truncus arteriosus is 16.5%[(319)].

Double Outlet Right Ventricle

Double outlet right ventricle (DORV) occurs when all of one great artery and more than 50% of the other great artery originates from the right ventricle[(320)]. There are multiple anatomic variations. It may occur with concordance or discordance of atrial and ventricular relationships, with or without a VSD, and with or without pulmonic stenosis. Embryologically, DORV, like tetralogy of Fallot and TGA, likely results from abnormal rotation and septation of the semilunar valve region[321]. Double outlet right ventricle with a subpulmonic VSD is referred to as a Taussig-Bing malformation[322]. The first successful repair of DORV was performed in 1957[323]. Theoretically, all forms of DORV are surgically repairable, although the postoperative cardiac performance is unpredictable[324].

The most common type of DORV has concordant atrioventricular relation with d-position of the aorta[324]. The surgical repair in this lesion depends on the orientation of the VSD with respect to the semilunar and tricuspid valves. When a subaortic VSD is present, an internal baffle is placed from the VSD to the aorta through a right ventriculotomy. Other variations of DORV are corrected with modifications of Rastelli and Fontan procedures using extracardiac conduits to direct blood flow, or modifications of the Mustard procedure to redirect intracardiac blood flow. Most recently the Lecompte maneuver, whereby the posteriorly positioned pulmonary artery is brought anteriorly underneath the transected aorta, has been used to approximate normal arterial configuration with low postoperative mortality[325,326].

Early postoperative mortality after DORV repair is approximately 20%[324,327]. Early complications include a low cardiac output state due to ventriculotomy and tachyarrhythmias. As with other lesions where ventriculotomy is necessary, the CVP should be kept high postoperatively. Extracardiac conduits such as a modified Fontan procedure will require more fluid (see Fontan procedure). Inotropic support with dobutamine or amrinone may be necessary. Pulmonary hypertension occurs in DORV when there is no coexisting pulmonic stenosis[324]. Management of pulmonary hypertension with oxygen, hyperventilation, and sedation is indicated; however, the presence of pulmonary hypertension greatly increases postoperative mortality.

The incidence of sudden death after repair of DORV is 18%[327]. Sudden death generally occurs within the first postoperative year. Risk factors for sudden death include older age at time of repair, history of perioperative tachyarrhythmias, and third degree AV block[327]. Patients with DORV should therefore undergo surgical correction early. Careful electrophysiology follow-up is required postoperatively.

Hypoplastic Left Heart Syndrome

Hypoplastic left heart syndrome occurs when there is severe hypoplasia of the ascending aorta associated with a hypoplastic left ventricle and stenosis or atresia of the mitral valve. This is the fourth most common congenital heart lesion and was universally fatal prior to 1985 accounting for 25% of cardiac deaths in the first week of life[328]. Preoperatively, these infants generally present with total circulatory collapse due to closure of the ductus. They can be stabilized with prostaglandin E_1 and inotrope infusions. Cardiac transplantation was once thought to be the only possible intervention for these children; however, the severe shortage of available organs has lead to continued efforts to perfect surgical palliation.

Norwood, Kirklin, and Sanders described a palliative procedure for hypoplastic left heart syndrome in 1980[328]. Now referred to as the Stage 1 Norwood, this procedure involves the formation of a new, or neoaorta, from the ascending aorta which is augmented with the proximal pulmonary artery[329]. The distal segment of the main pulmonary artery is closed with a patch. Pulmonary flow is provided by a systemic-to-pulmonary artery shunt; adequate mixing between the left and right ventricle is ensured by an atrial septostomy. Complete circulatory arrest is required for aortic reconstruction.

Postoperatively, either limited pulmonary blood flow due to pulmonary hypertension or excessive pulmonary blood flow when pulmonary vascular resistance is low can occur. Pulmonary hypertension is managed as previously discussed with hyperventilation, sedation, and minimizing mean airway pressure. Excessive pulmonary blood flow, which may lead to systemic hypotension, is usually heralded by a paO_2 of 50 mm Hg or greater. In this situation, maneuvers to increase pulmonary vascular resistance by decreasing the FiO_2 to 0.21 and allowing the pCO_2 to rise to 50 mm Hg will restrict pulmonary blood flow and increase systemic blood pressure[329]. If the patient does not respond to these maneuvers, a hypoxic mixture of 95% air and 5% CO_2 is used to raise PVR. This is preferable to decreasing ventilation, which results in atelectasis and intrapulmonary shunting[330]. Other complications in the postoperative period are related to coronary insufficiency secondary to hypoplastic coronary arteries and ostia and/or a hypertrophied single ventricle. The mortality after stage 1 palliation is approximately 40%[330].

The second stage of the repair involves separation of the pulmonary and systemic circulations. This procedure is performed when the pulmonary vascular resistance should have reached its nadir, usually at 18 months of age. In the first description of the second stage of the repair a modified Fontan procedure was performed[329,331]. The postoperative management of these patients is similar to that for patients with tricuspid atresia undergoing a Fontan with similar postoperative problems. The immediate postoperative mortality for this second stage procedure is reported as 34%. Long-term survival (4 years) was 52%; however, patients required prolonged hospitalization (median 32 days) primarily due to significant pleural effusions. The high postoperative mortality in these children may be due to acute changes in ventricular volume load of the single ventricle. Lower mortality may be achieved when a Glenn-type hemi-Fontan procedure is performed before the Fontan is completed[332].

Interrupted Aortic Arch

Interruption of the aortic arch may occur anywhere along the transverse arch, but is seen most frequently near the origin of the left subclavian artery, as with coarctation of the aorta. Distal perfusion is provided by the ductus arteriosus; as such this lesion presents in the neonatal period with sudden onset of hypoperfusion and shock at the time of ductal closure. Preoperative stabilization is similar to that for hypoplastic left heart syndrome, including the use of prostaglandin E1 to maintain ductal patency, support of the circulation with vasopressors if necessary, and correction of metabolic abnormalities, including acidosis, if feasible, before bringing the patient to the operating room.

Surgical correction of interrupted aortic arch is generally done on bypass, with cold circulatory arrest. Distal aortic flow is maintained through the ductus arteriosus until the time of hypothermic circulatory arrest. An end-to-end anastomosis, or a dacron graft may be used for the repair[333].

Postoperative problems after repair of interrupted aortic arch are the same as those for any newborn infant undergoing surgery with CPB. These include the potential for elevated PVR, coagulopathy with the potential for extensive hemorrhage, postoperative respiratory insufficiency and fluid and electrolyte disturbances. Myocardial failure in the post-bypass period is due to several factors, including preexisting myocardial failure, and lack of complete recovery of the myocardium after cardioplegia intraoperatively. Hemodynamic support of the circulation with vasopressors such as dobutamine or epinephrine, will be similar to any other newborn with congestive heart failure. Similarly, the infant should be screened for neurological deficits after awakening from anesthesia, particularly if the aortic interruption was contiguous with the origin of any of the carotid vessels.

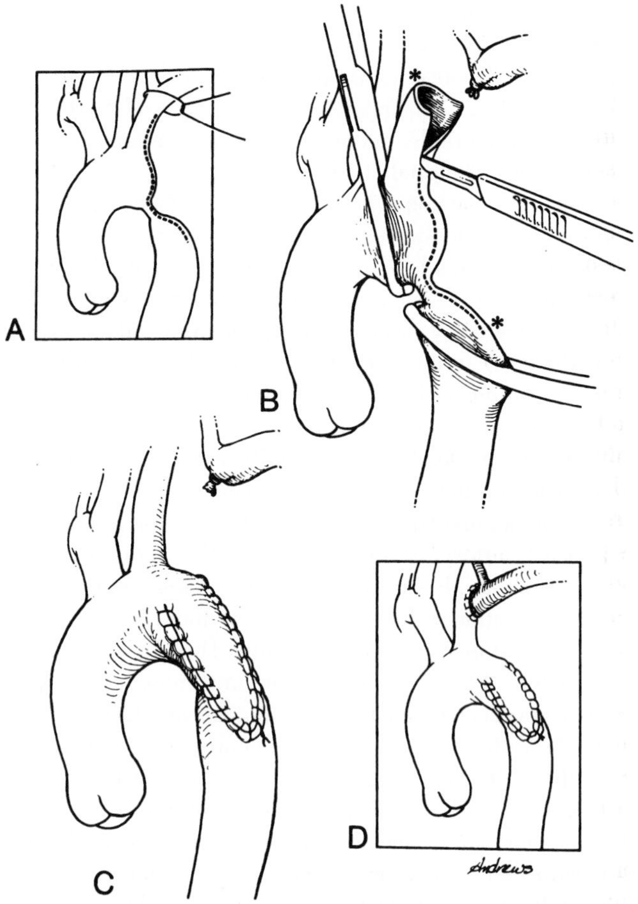

Figure 14.12. Repair technique proposed by Waldhausen. (A) and (B) The left subclavian artery is ligated distally at the level of the first branches and is then opened longitudinally. (C) The open subclavian artery is then used as a pedicle flap or patch to enlarge the stenotic isthmus. (D) A disadvantage of this method is the need to sacrifice arterial flow through a major aortic arch tributary supplying the left shoulder and vertebral artery. An end-to-side anastomosis between the divided subclavian artery and the adjacent left common carotid artery can be used to solve this problem. (From Cooley DA: Repair of coarctation of the thoracic aorta. In:Techniques in Cardiac Surgery, Second Edition, Chapter 3. WB Saunders, Houston Texas 1984, p 40.)

Coarctation of the Aorta

Aortic coarctation occurs in the descending thoracic aorta, opposite the insertion of the ductus arteriosus, and adjacent to the origin of the left subclavian artery. Symptomatology correlates with the amount of narrowing, and the presence or absence of collateral circulation to supply the distal body. Perioperative problems related to coarctation of the aorta are related to the age at presentation, type of surgical correction, and coexisting medical illness, particularly congestive heart failure.

There is a bimodal age distribution at presentation. Coarctation in the newborn usually manifests as acute onset of congestive heart failure at the time of closure of the ductus arteriosus, with decreased femoral pulses. Medically, these patients should be stabilized before coming to the operating room with an infusion of prostaglandin E1 to reopen the ductus arteriosus and reduce left ventricular afterload. Frequently, this is all that is necessary, although severe congestive failure may require endotracheal intubation with positive pressure ventilation, inotropic support with a β-adrenergic agonist, and correction of metabolic acidosis[334]. In older children with well-developed collateral circulation, coarctation is usually initially found on careful physical examination with decreased femoral pulses, and cardiac murmur; hypertension may or may not be present.

There are two types of surgical correction, the subclavian aortoplasty and end-to-end anastomosis. Choice of the procedure is related to age of the child and experience of the individual surgeon. Subclavian aortoplasty is frequently done in the newborn. This technique involves use of the proximal left subclavian artery as a patch across the narrowed segment of the aorta (Fig. 14–12). Late-onset complications from this procedure include recurrence of the coarctation in 10% of patients, due to formation of an intra-aortic shelf which may arise from retained ductal tissue[335,336]. Interestingly, although there is no subclavian flow to the left arm, perfusion to the arm remains adequate[337]. The only long-term problem referable to subclavian aortoplasty is mild growth retardation in the left arm compared to the right. End-to-end aortic anastomosis, with or without a Dacron graft, is usually used in the older infant and child. There is a 20% incidence of recoarctation requiring reoperation in these children. Postoperative aneurysm formation seen in 5 to 16% of children has been associated with the use of a Dacron patch for repair[335,338].

The most difficult intraoperative problems during coarctation repair are due to the need to cross-clamp the aorta during the repair. During the period of aortic cross-clamp, distal perfusion may be inadequate, depending on the extent of collateral circulation. Ischemia of the spinal cord, kidneys, and gastrointestinal tract may result from hypoperfusion. Measurement of distal aortic blood pressure during cross-clamp (which presumably reflects blood flow from collateral circulation) and use of a temporary shunt around the cross-clamped area has been advocated when the distal pressure is less than 40 mm Hg. Management of proximal aortic blood pressure during aortic cross-clamping can be difficult intraoperatively[339]; sudden increases in left ventricular afterload may be poorly tolerated by the patient with preexisting congestive heart failure, especially when there is poorly developed collateral circulation. Afterload reduction using direct vasodilators such as nitroprusside is potentially hazardous, if distal perfusion pressure below the cross-clamp is inadequate.

The most severe complication of aortic cross clamping is paraplegia, which has been described in 0.14% of patients postoperatively[340]. The circulation to the spinal cord is provided by the anterior spinal artery, which originates at the base of the skull as a branch of the vertebral arteries. As the anterior spinal artery descends along the length of the spinal cord, there are usually multiple areas of frank interruption or very marginal blood supply along its course. Blood supply to the spinal cord is supplemented, or even totally supplied in these marginal areas by radicular arteries which originate from the intercostal arteries; the largest of these is the artery of Adamkiewicz. The anterior spinal artery syndrome seen after coarctation repair is characterized by paralysis with preserved proprioception and temperature sensation. Intraoperatively, the duration of aortic cross-clamping, temperature, and the use of deliberate hypotension to limit left ventricular afterload increase the risk of paralysis.

Other intraoperative requirements which may create postoperative problems include the need for left lung collapse to gain access to the aorta through a left thoracotomy incision. In newborns and other children this is achieved by manual compression and packing down the lung in the operative field; adolescents can be managed with one lung ventilation through a double lumen endobronchial tube which allows independent ventilation of each lung. A large amount of intrapulmonary shunt can occur during one lung ventilation, with resultant hypoxemia. Hypoxic pulmonary vasoconstriction, which decreases blood flow to the collapsed lung and redirects blood flow to the ventilated lung, is only partially inhibited by anesthetic agents in the majority of clinical circumstances, thus maintaining an equitable matching of ventilation and perfusion. Postoperatively, although the lung is reexpanded with manual ventilation, areas of atelectasis may remain in the collapsed lung. Similarly, bleeding into the pulmonary parenchyma and bronchi can result from manipulation, which may occlude the endotracheal tube with blood clots acutely, either intraoperatively or in the ICU. A high index of suspicion for this occurrence must be maintained throughout the period of intubation. Occlusion of the endotracheal tube is associated with an increase in peak airway pressure in patients on volume controlled ventilation and a progressive decrease in end-tidal CO_2 in patients monitored by capnography. Endotracheal tube occlusion necessitates rapid reintubation before clinical deterioration occurs. Other intrathoracic complications, including phrenic nerve and recurrent laryngeal nerve injury, may create problems with weaning from mechanical ventilation and extubation after surgery. Although it is rare, thoracic duct injury with chylothorax can occur. Despite these concerns, the older child with coarctation can be extubated as soon as he or she is fully awake with adequate neuromuscular tone and minute ventilation. Prolonged episodes of gagging and coughing on the endotracheal tube may aggravate postoperative hypertension.

Persistent hypertension is seen in the majority of children after coarctation repair, both immediately postoperatively and as a long-term effect. Initially, hypertension is attributed to both elevated plasma catecholamines during the surgery and elevated plasma renin levels, with abnormal baroreceptor autoregulatory responses. Catecholamines, particularly norepinephrine, are released during the period of aortic cross-clamping[342]. Renin levels are elevated after revascularization, and continue to remain so for several months, suggesting an intrinsic abnormality in renal receptor sensitivities[342,343]. If untreated, hypertension can lead to stress on the aortic suture line which may bleed extensively postoperatively and require transfusion or surgical reexploration. Interestingly, this hypertension and the hormonal changes associated with it were not observed in patients who undergo balloon dilatation of the coarctation[344]. If untreated, uncontrolled hypertension can lead to reflex mesenteric vasoconstriction and splanchnic hypoperfusion, the so called post-coarctectomy syndrome. Intestinal ischemia, leading in some cases to frank bowel infarction, had been one of the leading causes of early postoperative morbidity and mortality in this group of patients in the past. Early aggressive management of postoperative hypertension and expectant treatment with continuous nasogastric suction and withholding feedings for two or more days has decreased the frequency of this complication.

A wide variety of medications have been used for the control of blood pressure postoperatively, including β-blockers, α-blockers, and direct vasodilators. Direct vasodilators, such as nitroprusside offer the advantage of being simple to titrate in the operating room and in the ICU, particularly during rapidly changing physiological circumstances such as emergence from anesthesia. Cyanide toxicity only occurs when nitroprusside is administered in high doses, greater than 10 μg/kg/minute, for long periods of time. β-blockers are frequently used as an adjunctive agent in treating hypertension in the child with coarctation[343]. They may be undesirable in the neonate and infant because of the infant's dependence on heart rate for cardiac output. Other agents, such as the α-adrenergic blocker phentolamine, may be given by continuous infusion, although it is not as rapidly titratable as nitroprusside.

Blood pressure monitoring perioperatively should be done in the right arm (proximal to the coarctation) and checked in the legs for presence of a residual gradient. Obviously, the left arm should not be used for blood pressure checks, intravenous access, or arterial puncture when the surgical procedure was a left subclavian aortoplasty.

Aortic Stenosis

There is a wide variability in children presenting for correction of aortic stenosis, ranging from the relatively asymptomatic child with a large gradient across the aortic valve, to the newborn infant with left ventricular failure and ductal dependent systemic blood flow on prostaglandin E_1 who requires emergency surgery. Although the older child may be relatively asymptomatic, myocardial compromise may be severe. Symptoms such as syncope and congestive heart failure are relatively late manifestations of end-stage disease in these patients[344]. Aortic stenosis as an isolated entity after rheumatic fever without coexisting mitral valve disease is rarely seen. In most instances, the etiology of isolated aortic stenosis is congenital; a bicuspid aortic valve is the most common anatomic defect.

Aortic stenosis may be surgically corrected by either aortic valvuloplasty or aortic valve replacement, depending on the clinical circumstances. Valvuloplasty is used in the infant as a means of dilating the valve orifice; a small degree of aortic regurgitation afterward is common. Aortic valve replacement is usually performed in the older child. Mechanical valves require life-long anticoagulation. Additionally, if the orifice size is insufficient as the child grows, the valve may need to be replaced by a larger valve in sequential operations. Allografts do not require anticoagulation but tend to deteriorate over time. The Ross procedure is a more complex operation. It consists of replacement of the aortic root with the native pulmonic valve and replacement of the native pulmonic valve with an allograft which is more durable in the pulmonic position[345,346]. The autograft has the potential to remain viable and grow in proportion to the growth of the child[347].

Patients with uncorrected severe aortic stenosis will have severe left ventricular hypertrophy and elevated left ventricular intracavitary pressures. Coronary perfusion pressure, the difference between diastolic blood pressure and left ventricular end-diastolic pressure, is decreased. Maintenance of coronary perfusion, therefore, relies on maintenance of the diastolic perfusion pressure and avoiding tachycardia, which decreases diastolic perfusion time. Due to limited coronary reserve, angina and myocardial ischemia can be seen in this disease, even in the absence of coronary stenosis (Fig. 14–7). Intra-aortic balloon pump, which provides aortic counterpulsation during diastole and improves coronary perfusion, may be beneficial in the adult with myocardial ischemia related to aortic stenosis, although this has been used infrequently in children due to size.

Due to myocardial hypertrophy, the ability to protect the myocardium intraoperatively with cardioplegia may be somewhat limited. This will manifest postoperatively as depressed myocardial function, despite the relief of obstruction, requiring inotropic support after bypass. Ventricular arrhythmias with ventricular tachycardia and premature ventricular contractions are common, particularly when the patient is hypokalemic. Aggressive potassium replacement may be necessary, as well as a lidocaine infusion.

Pulmonary Stenosis

Children with isolated pulmonary stenosis requiring surgery fall into two major groups: those who require urgent intervention in the neonatal period because of cyanosis and right-sided failure, and those older children with obstruction and milder clinical symptoms.

Neonates with critical pulmonary stenosis usually begin to deteriorate when the ductus arteriosus closes, generally on the second or third day of life. Preoperatively, they are generally stabilized with prostaglandin E1 infusion to maintain ductal patency and provide pulmonary blood flow, correction of electrolyte disorders, particularly systemic acidosis, and ventilatory support if needed. A common coexisting cardiac defect is right ventricular hypertrophy with a relatively small hypoplastic ventricular cavity. Surgical correction for these infants is palliative and involves dilation of the pulmonary outflow tract, which may be done with or without cardiopulmonary bypass and creation of a systemic to pulmonary shunt, such as a modified Blalock Taussig, to augment pulmonary blood flow[347]. In neonates with adequate right ventricular cavity size and isolated pulmonary stenosis, total correction of the pulmonary stenosis may be performed on bypass. In some centers, balloon dilatation of the pulmonary artery is performed as the initial intervention, with surgery reserved as a back-up modality[348].

Older children with pulmonary stenosis can have preoperative right-to-left shunting at the level of the foramen ovale, particularly when intrathoracic pressure is elevated, and will have right ventricular hypertrophy. The surgical procedure for the older child with pulmonary stenosis, or one who has undergone previous palliative surgery, entails enlarging the pulmonary outflow tract using pericardium while on cardiopulmonary bypass, and take-down of the Blalock Taussig shunt. Those patients with supravalvular pulmonary stenosis may also require augmentation of the distal pulmonary arteries. Severe right ventricular hypertrophy, particularly if it is contributing to outflow obstruction, may also be resected during bypass. Medical problems which commonly coexist are related to the degree of preexisting right-to-left shunting and include cyanosis, polycythemia, and development of an extensive bronchial collateral circulation.

The child with pulmonary stenosis and relative hypoplasia of the distal pulmonary arteries and arterioles is more difficult to manage. Frequently, these children require staged repairs with systemic to pulmonary artery shunts designed to enhance pulmonary blood flow and arteriolar growth. Single stage repair, in the face of distal pulmonary vascular hypoplasia, frequently leads to acute right-sided heart failure[349].

Major problems related to correction of isolated pulmonary stenosis which influence the ICU course are related to right ventricular dysfunction, which can occur for several reasons. Right ventricular ischemia may occur with inadequate intraoperative myocardial preservation. Pulmonary insufficiency normally occurs after pericardial outflow patch reconstruction, although this is usually of minor clinical consequence. The need for an extensive incision in the ventricle intraoperatively will also contribute to ventricular dysfunction.

The need for inotropic support after surgery and in the ICU will be dictated by the amount of right ventricular dysfunction. With relief of outflow obstruction, overall function of the right ventricle usually improves, and there is little, or no need for inotropic support. Factors which cause elevation of the pulmonary vascular resistance, such as hypercarbia or hypoxemia, may cause the ventricle to fail, and should be avoided. Otherwise, postoperative care is directed toward rewarming, volume repletion and correction of electrolyte abnormalities, as for any open heart procedure. For the uncomplicated procedure in a hemodynamically stable child, early extubation is anticipated.

Patent Ductus Arteriosus

Isolated PDA requiring surgical ligation is commonly encountered in the newborn intensive care unit as a result of prematurity[350,351]. Congestive heart failure in these babies and pulmonary plethora may aggravate neonatal respiratory distress syndrome and contribute to subsequent bronchopulmonary dysplasia. Runoff into the pulmonary artery from the aorta can compromise mesenteric perfusion and may result in necrotizing enterocolitis. Surgical ligation is indicated if indomethacin (a prostaglandin synthase inhibitor) fails to cause ductal closure[352,353]. Less frequently, older asymptomatic infants and children with a PDA undergo elective ligation to prevent complications later on in life, especially the development of pulmonary hypertension and Eisenmenger's syndrome from long-standing left-to-right shunting, and bacterial endocarditis. Ligation of the ductus arteriosus is done through a left thoracotomy. The duct may be either ligated with suture and divided or occluded with a hemoclip. Recanalization of the duct has been described in infants in whom simple suture ligation was done. Intraoperative time is generally less than 30 minutes and may be performed in the neonatal ICU[354].

Intraoperatively, problems occur while the left lung is collapsed. This maneuver alters ventilatory compliance and increases ventilation-to-perfusion mismatch. This is particularly problematic in the sick premature infant with hyaline membrane disease who already requires a high inspired concentration of oxygen. Usually, this can be overcome by increasing inspiratory pressure and end-expiratory pressure during the procedure. Other complications related to thoracotomy, including intrapulmonary hemorrhage, and occlusion of the endotracheal tube with blood clots or secretions perioperatively are sometimes seen. A devastating but extremely rare complication of this procedure is tearing of the duct, with exsanguination. This occurs more frequently in the older child, when ductal tissue has become more friable.

Postoperative problems that can be anticipated are generally related to the pulmonary system. Atelectasis occurs in almost all patients due to intraoperative collapse of the left lung, but is rarely severe. It is anticipated that the infant and child can be extubated almost immediately postoperatively, once the residual effects of anesthesia have worn off and neuromuscular blockade reversed. Other uncommon, but reported complications are injuries to the phrenic nerve resulting in diaphragmatic paralysis, thoracic duct resulting in chylothorax, and recurrent laryngeal nerve resulting in vocal cord paralysis—all of which occur more commonly in premature infants[355]. In addition, other intraoperative complications include inadvertent ligation of the pulmonary artery or distal aorta. Transcatheter closure of the PDA has recently been developed and may alter the approach in the older child[356].

Transposition of the Great Vessels

As with other cyanotic congenital heart disease, transposition of the great vessels (TGV) generally presents in the neonatal period. The degree of cyanosis differs in each infant and depends on the extent of intracardiac and extracardiac mixing of pulmonary and systemic blood flow. Infants with an absent or restrictive atrial septal defect and no other sites of intracardiac or extracardiac mixing of blood flow tend to deteriorate clinically during the early neonatal period, particularly when the ductus arteriosus closes. Prostaglandin E_1 infusion is required to maintain ductal patency until atrial septectomy, either via balloon or Blalock-Hanlon or definitive Jatene repair, can be performed.

Currently two different surgical procedures are used for correction of TGV, the arterial (Jatene) switch procedure[357] and the atrial switch (Senning or Mustard) procedure[358]. Indications for each of these procedures are based upon the individual child's anatomy, left ventricular pressure, and surgical experience and preference. Although atrial switch procedures can be performed with 80% long-term survival[359,360], the incidence of atrial arrhythmias approaches 100% after 20 years, and failure of the systemic right ventricle in patients occurs in approximately 10% of patients[361]. The discovery that the success of the arterial switch procedure was dependent on the timing of the procedure in the newborn period when the "left" ventricle is still adjusted to a relatively high pulmonary resistance led to renewed interest in this procedure[362,363]. For either switch procedure, postoperative care is affected by the type of correction done and the child's underlying physiological status.

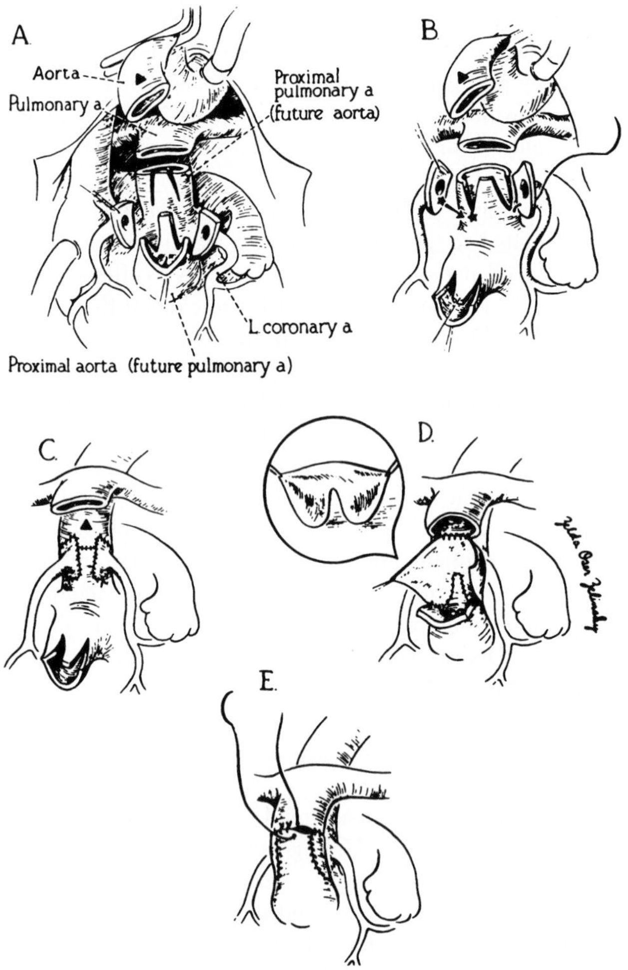

Figure 14.13. Atrial switch operative technique. Preliminary steps prior to transfer of the coronary artery-aortic cuffs include transection of the main pulmonary artery distal of valve commissures with inspection of pulmonary (neoaortic) valve and subvalvar region; and transection of the aorta about 2 mm (in neonate) distal to the coronary ostia. (A) The left and right coronary arteries are removed from their corresponding aortic sinus location with a cuff of aortic wall. (B) Incisions are made into the left and right anterior sinuses of the pulmonary artery (neoaortic) stump, and the coronary cuffs are positioned for suturing in place. (C) The distal aortic segment (solid triangle), previously anterior in A and B, is passed posterior to the bifurcation of the pulmonary artery as described by Lecompte et al.[297]. This distal aortic segment is sutured to the reconstructed (coronary ostia bearing) pulmonary artery stump of the left ventricular outflow tract. (D) A pantaloon-shaped patch of autologous pericardium is used to fill the defects in the aortic (neopulmonary) stump that were created by removal of the coronary cuffs, and the patch also forms the free edge of the stump reconstruction. (E) The distal pulmonary artery is approximated and anastomosed to the right ventricular outflow stump. (From Idriss FS, Ilbawi MN, DeLeon SY, et al.: Arterial switch in simple and complex transposition of the great arteries. J Thorac Cardiovasc Surg 1988;95:29.)

The Jatene procedure involves reimplanting both the aorta and the pulmonary artery onto their "normal" ventricle under circulatory arrest. Specifically, the pulmonary artery is transected above its origin on the left ventricle and attached to the right ventricle, while the aorta is joined to the left ventricle by suturing it to the remnant of pulmonary artery as it originates from this ventricle. The coronary arteries cannot "stretch" to accommodate this move, and as a consequence need to be removed from the aorta at their origin along with a surrounding button of aortic tissue, and reimplanted into the aorta in its new site (Fig. 14–13).

This procedure can only be done when the left ventricle is able to withstand pumping against systemic vascular resistance, rather than the lower pulmonary vascular resistance. Physiologically, this occurs under three different sets of circumstances. The first is during the weeks immediately after birth, when the pulmonary vascular resistance is sufficiently high to maintain left ventricular muscle tone. The second occurs when left ventricular pressure, and consequently muscle mass, remains high in the older child with TGV and nonrestrictive VSD. Finally, in older children with TGV without a VSD, left ventricular muscle mass can be increased acutely over several days by surgically banding temporarily the pulmonary artery, allowing the left ventricle to hypertrophy, and then performing the arterial switch[364–367]. This last maneuver has been used successfully in children with right (systemic) ventricular failure several years after Mustard or Senning type repairs[368–370].

Perioperative complications include extensive hemorrhage, elevated pulmonary vascular resistance, and myocardial ischemia related to coronary artery reimplantation[371]. Hemorrhage is related to several factors, including the relatively large priming volume used for CPB when compared to the infant's blood volume, and the decreased platelet number and function during bypass and hypothermia. The large number and extent of suture lines may also lead to excessive bleeding in the post-bypass period. These suture lines often exist in hard to control areas, such as the posterior wall of the aorta, which are difficult to access safely once bypass is terminated. It is not unusual for the infant to require more than one to two blood volumes of transfusion products, including platelets, fresh frozen plasma, and packed red cells post-bypass. The use of only fresh blood (less than 48 hours old) for surgery rather than component therapy may result in an overall decrease in total postoperative blood product requirement[238]. Elevated PVR in the neonatal period may contribute to postoperative right ventricular dysfunction. A high index of suspicion and avoiding physiological perturbations which increase PVR such as hypercarbia or hypoxemia are typically all that is needed to avoid pulmonary hypertension. Pharmacological intervention, using pulmonary vasodilators or inhaled nitric oxide, may be required when there is preexisting severe pulmonary hypertension, or during the early neonatal period, when there is persistence of the normal intrauterine elevation of pulmonary vascular resistance. A wide variety of drugs have been used to lower pulmonary vascular resistance. These include isoproterenol and dobutamine, amrinone, and direct vasodilators such as nitroglycerine, nitroprusside, and prostaglandin E_1.

Myocardial ischemia, characterized by elevations in ST segments after coronary reimplantation is seen after cross-clamp removal. Ischemia may be related to air or other microscopic debris in the coronary arteries. Significant embolization can result in overt ventricular failure. Appropriate therapy for ischemia in this setting is not known; allowing the heart to rest on cardiopulmonary bypass while the coronaries are passively reperfused may wash all the emboli distally and resolve the ischemia. Coronary artery kinking during the surgical anastomosis also causes ventricular hypoperfusion and ischemia, which requires a high index of suspicion for early diagnosis in the operating room and surgical correction. Nitroglycerine has been used as a coronary artery vasodilator perioperatively in the setting of myocardial ischemia after the Jatene operation, although control studies establishing its efficacy are lacking[(371)].

The most common long-term complication related to the arterial switch procedure thus far is aortic regurgitation (22%)[(372,373)]. Other complications include coronary artery occlusion, pulmonary hypertension, and supravalvular pulmonary stenosis[(374)]. Transient arrhythmias including supraventricular tachycardia and complete heart block have been noted in 20% of patients. Overall, the long-term survival (as late as 5 years) is 82%[(375)].

The atrial switch operation is usually not performed in the newborn period; therefore, these patients with TGV have previously undergone an atrial septectomy[(361)]. The atrial switch procedure entails constructing an intra-atrial baffle to direct systemic venous return to the left ventricle and out the pulmonary artery to the lungs, and pulmonary venous return to the right ventricle and out the aorta. The Senning and Mustard procedures are both used; they differ in the anatomy of the baffle and in the choice of material used. Pericardium or Dacron patch material is used in the Mustard procedure; native atrial tissue is used in the Senning. In one study comparing long-term outcome after these two procedures, the only difference detected was a higher incidence of sinus node dysfunction after the Mustard procedure[(359)]. Although the circulation is physiologically corrected with these procedures, the child is left with an anatomic right ventricle providing systemic perfusion for life (Fig. 14–14).

A large number of potential complications, both early and long term, have been ascribed to the atrial switch operations. Obstruction to systemic or pulmonary venous drainage into the atria can result from the intracardiac baffle within the atria. Obstruction at the right atrial to the SVC junction is suspected if there is unexplained elevation in SVC pressure. This manifests clinically as a picture of SVC syndrome, with facial plethora and jugular venous distention. Obstruction at the junction of the pulmonary veins as they enter the left atrium is more difficult to diagnose. This may clinically manifest only as pulmonary edema, often difficult to differentiate from systemic ventricular failure without the aid of diagnostic studies including echocardiography and cardiac catheterization[(376)].

Myocardial failure occurs as both an early and late complication. After these procedures, the anatomic right ventricle remains the systemic ventricle, lacking the muscular makeup and trabeculations of an anatomic left ventricle. Early postoperative ventricular failure result from the effects of CPB and surgery, and usually responds to appropriate inotropic support. Long-term follow-up studies demonstrate a 10% incidence of symptomatic ventricular failure[(361,376)]. These patients may require cardiac transplant. Alternatively, pulmonary artery banding can be done to strengthen the anatomic left ventricle, followed several weeks later by an arterial switch operation[(365)].

As extensive atrial sutures are required for atrial switch procedures, conduction system injury occurs in over 95% of children after atrial switch operations when studied with Holter monitoring. The SA node and atrial myocardium are most commonly injured[(377)]. Immediately postoperatively, AV block is common and is related to myocardial hypothermia and transient myocardial and conducting system cellular injury; with complete heart block, this may require temporary pacing in the ICU to generate adequate cardiac output. Both ventricular pacing and atrioventricular sequential pacing have been used, depending on the clinical requirements. Frequently this type of heart block will resolve over a period of several days. A more insidious form of heart block, characterized by the slow development of sick sinus syndrome with brief periods of symptomatic sinus arrest, requiring a permanent pacemaker, has been shown to develop with increased frequency. These children are at increased risk for sudden death[(378)]. Often they are admitted from the emergency room to the ICU for temporary cardiac pacing until a permanent pacemaker can be placed.

Fontan Procedure

The Fontan procedure, in essence a right heart bypass procedure, was originally employed for surgical correction in children with tricuspid atresia and normal pulmonary vascular resistance, to separate the pulmonary and systemic circulations. More recently, it has been applied in children with complex congenital heart disease and a single ventricle type of cardiac physiology and normal PVR, such as hypoplastic left or right hearts[(329,379)]. Conceptually, the procedure entails connection of all systemic venous drainage to the pulmonary arteries, either directly or through the right atrium. Pulmonary blood flow in this procedure, is not provided by "pumping" of blood, but instead relies on a pressure gradient between systemic venous pressure and pulmonary arterial pressure. For this reason, the Fontan procedure is not done in the neonatal period or first few months of life because of the normal neonatal elevation of pulmonary vascular resistance. Normal, or low PVR, less than 4 Woods units, and absence of left heart obstructive lesions such as severe mitral stenosis, are considered criti-

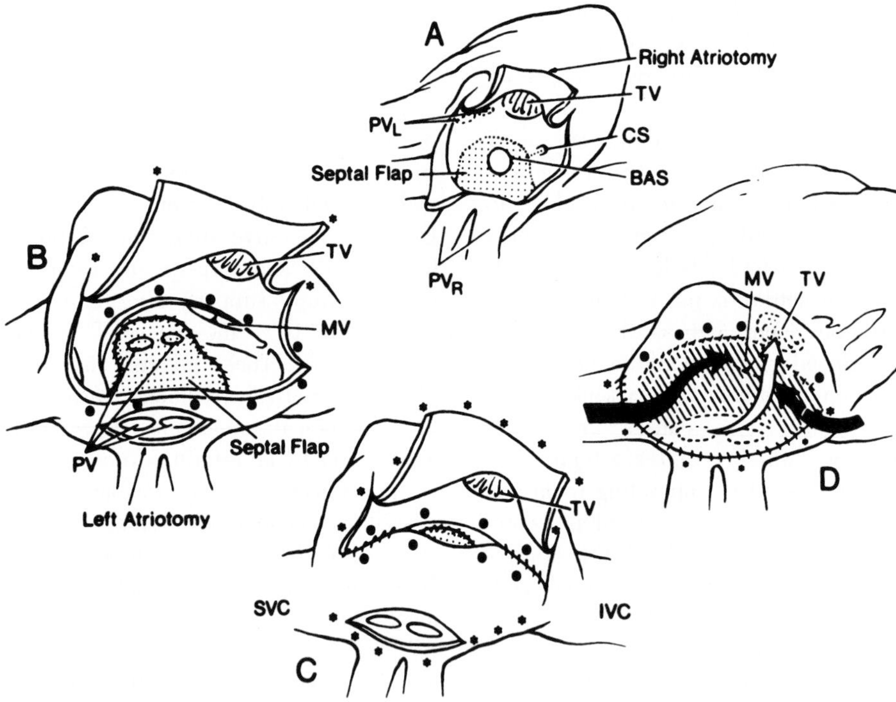

Figure 14.14. Atrial switch operation (Senning technique). Operation if performed using cardiopulmonary bypass with cold cardioplegic myocardial protection, or during profound hypothermia with total circulatory arrest. (A) A right atriotomy is made in front of and parallel to the caval veins and extended into the atrial appendage. This exposes the atrial septum with its balloon septostomy defect. The atrial septum is now incised anteriorly, superiorly, and inferiorly to form a septal flap (stippled area) as large as possible which remains fixed posteriorly between the caval entrances. The wall between the coronary sinus (CS) and left atrium may be incised so as to provide a large posterior lip for the inferior septal flap suture line (B), and direct coronary sinus return to the newly formed systemic venous chamber and conduit to the mitral valve is formed posteriorly by the repositioned septal flap, (stippled area), and the conduit is then completed anteriorly by suturing the posterior right atrial free wall flap (•••) anteriorly to the anterior septal limbus (•••) as in C. A left atriotomy is made as long as possible in the internal atrial groove (exposing the orifices of the right pulmonary veins). (C) and (D) The pulmonary venous chamber and pathway to the tricuspid valve is completed with the suturing of the anterior right free wall atrial flap (***) over the right pulmonary veins to the anterior lip of the left atriotomy (***). (D) Black arrows indicate systemic venous caval flow through the newly created atrial tissue conduit and systemic venous chamber (\\\\\\\) toward the mitral valve: the white arrow indicates pulmonary venous flow path in pulmonary venous atrium passing behind, rightward, and anterior to the systemic venous chamber toward the tricuspid valve (TV). BAS, balloon atrial septostomy; IVC and SVC, inferior and superior venae cavae; MV, mitral valve; PV, PV_L and PV_R, pulmonary veins, left and right. (From Milton H, Paul MD: Complete transposition of the great arteries and splenic syndromes. Adams FH, Emmanouilides GC, Reimenschneider TA (eds). In: Heart Diseases in Infants, Children, and Adolescents, Fourth Edition, Chapter 19. Williams and Wilkins, Baltimore, Maryland 1968, p 403.)

cal requirements for the Fontan procedure. In infants, a palliative shunt procedure is performed. It is important to size the circumference of the shunt appropriately; too much pulmonary blood flow may result in the development of reactive elevated PVR, which may preclude the Fontan operation later in life.

After the Fontan procedure, systemic venous pressure may remain high due to high PVR or an elevated end diastolic pressure in the single ventricle. Chronic elevation of systemic venous pressure leads to pericardial effusions and pleural effusions, usually right-sided, which may require drainage. Ascites and a protein-losing enteropathy have also been described in these patients. This is particularly true of the classic Fontan procedure (Fig. 14–15), in which the SVC is connected to the right pulmonary artery, and the right atrium is connected via a homograft to the main pulmonary artery[380]. When the superior vena caval and inferior vena caval connections are done as separate surgical procedures, the postoperative morbidity and mortality is reduced[331]. Alternatively, the Fontan may be performed with one or more fenestrations between the vena cava and the pulmonary venous drainage chamber. By allowing flow from the systemic venous system to the pulmonary venous system, the systemic venous pressure is reduced and cardiac output is increased[331,381,382]. Although oxygen saturation is somewhat lower (88 to 90%), and effusions still develop, they generally are less persistent[331,382]. In theory, the incidence of arrhythmias should be lower with less dilatation of the right atrium[381]. The fenestrations generally close spontaneously over time or by a transcatheter closure without hemodynamic consequences.

Children and adults presenting for the Fontan procedure usually have had long-standing cyanosis and all its attendant problems. Preoperative polycythemia can lead to inadequate perfusion and sludging at the microcirculatory capillary level, resulting in chronic metabolic acidosis. Hypoglycemia is also frequently observed, so prolonged fasting and dehydration should be avoided preoperatively.

Similarly, because of the potential impact of severe hyperglycemia on neurological sequelae, glucose levels should be monitored intraoperatively and glucose administered judiciously. Coagulation tests including prothrombin time and partial thromboplastin time are usually elevated. This has been attributed to chronic low grade diffuse intravascular coagulopathy, as well as a laboratory artifact from decreased total amount of plasma in the specimen because of increased red cell mass.

The focus of post-bypass care of the child with a Fontan procedure is on augmenting pulmonary blood flow, minimizing pulmonary vascular resistance, and optimizing myocardial function[383]. Therefore, a superior vena caval central line (CVP) is important for monitoring; this is not only a monitor for venous pressure in the SVC (and presumably the brain), but also represents the filling pressure for the pulmonary arteries. Right heart return and pulmonary blood flow are maintained through adequate intravascular volume repletion and patient positioning. SVC return of blood to the pulmonary vascular bed is aided by gravity, and so simply elevating the head of the bed or sitting the patient up is important. Drainage from the IVC can be promoted by the use of cyclically inflated MAST or leg elevation[384,385]. Compared to the preoperative status, SVC pressure and cerebral venous pressure is elevated postoperatively, with pressures of 12 to 15 mm Hg being common. Although elevated SVC pressure has the potential for decreasing cerebral perfusion, this has not generally been a problem, except when cardiac output and mean arterial pressure are decreased. In children with a right atrium, normal sinus rhythm may be necessary for adequate pulmonary blood flow[386] (Fig. 14–16).

Minimizing PVR in the post-bypass period can be accomplished by decreasing airway pressure and lowering pCO_2. Pressure is transmitted from the airways to the pulmonary vascular bed when the chest is closed. Early return of spontaneous ventilation is optimal; negative intrathoracic pressure will augment venous return. Although early extubation is preferred, it is also frequently impractical because of the residual effects of anesthetics, narcotics, muscle relaxants, and the surgery itself. Inadequate ventilation after early tracheal extubation can be deleterious, and even catastrophic rather than helpful, if hypercarbia and hypoxia increase the PVR. Mechanical ventilation, with minimal peak inspiratory pressure and PEEP, and prolonged expiratory time, are advantageous under these circumstances. Sinus rhythm is important in maintaining a low left atrial pressure which will decrease pulmonary venous pressure. Similarly, inotropic agents which dilate the pulmonary vascular bed and lower PVR, such as dobutamine, amrinone, iso-

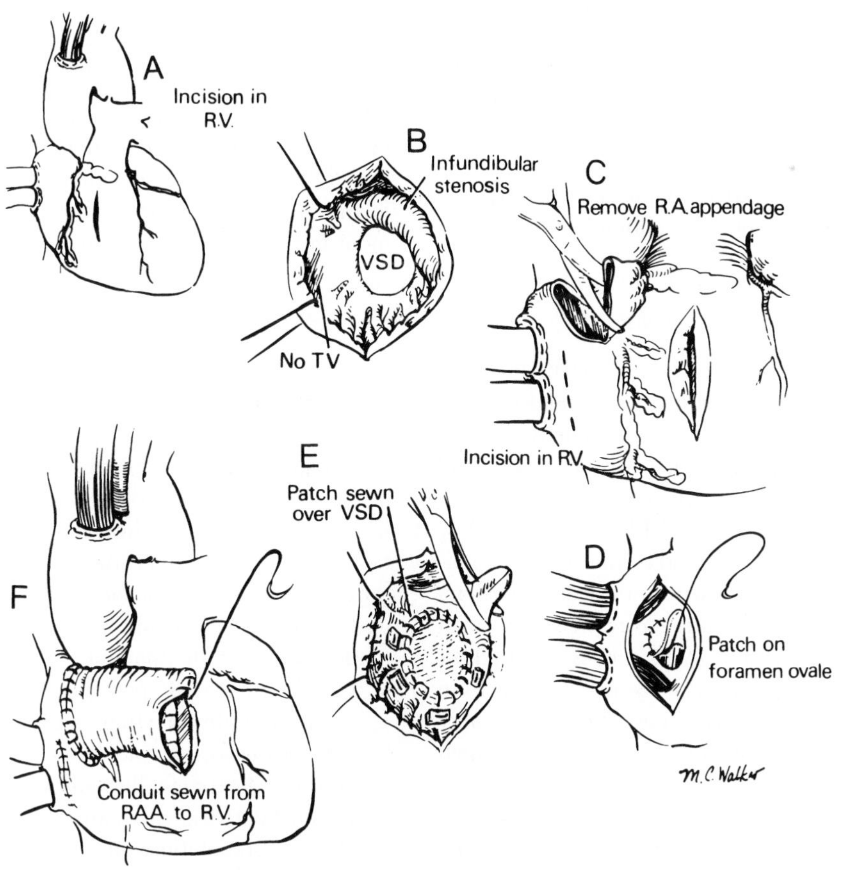

Figure 14.15. Fontan procedure for correcting congenital tricuspid atresia. In the case depicted, the patient has a ventricular septal defect, patent foramen ovale, and normal pulmonary valve, making him an ideal patient for this technique. RV, right ventricle; RA, right atrium; RAA, right atrial appendage. (From Cooley DA: Lesion of the tricuspid valve. In: Techniques in Cardiac Surgery, Second Edition, Chapter 17. WB Saunders, Houston, Texas 1984, p 218.)

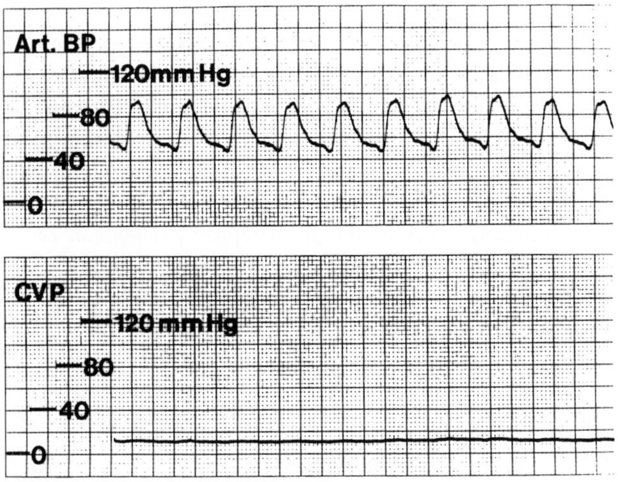

Figure 14.16. Central venous pressure (CVP) and arterial trace after Fontan procedure. Note absence of pulsatile trace in CVP as measure in the superior vena cava.

proterenol, and low dose epinephrine may be ideal. Other agents which directly lower PVR, such as nitroprusside and prostaglandin E1 may also be used, although these may also lower systemic blood pressure.

Long-term studies of patients who have undergone Fontan repair have demonstrated a relatively high incidence (24%) of both tachyarrhythmias and bradyarrhythmias requiring atrial pacing[387]. Other causes of late morbidity and mortality include sudden death (presumably due to an arrhythmia), mitral regurgitation, and poor left ventricular myocardial function[388,389]. Patients who have had previous pulmonary artery banding appear to be at unique risk for progressive subaortic obstruction postoperatively; this has been described in 85% of such patients, with a 50% mortality[390].

Total Anomalous Pulmonary Venous Return

Total anomalous pulmonary venous return (TAPVR) usually presents in the first days of life with cyanosis and respiratory symptoms. At the time of surgical correction, these neonates can be quite ill, with diminished cardiac output and metabolic acidosis requiring ventilatory support.

There are three anatomic types of TAPVR with widely different mortality. These are classified by the site of anomalous drainage of the pulmonary veins: supracardiac, cardiac, and infracardiac (Fig. 14–17). Infracardiac TAPVR, with pulmonary venous return to the liver, carries the highest mortality. In all instances, pulmonary venous drainage is to the right atrium with systemic oxygenation occurring only with atrial mixing through an obligatory patent foramen ovale or atrial septal defect[391].

The surgical correction of this lesion involves reimplanting the confluence, where the pulmonary veins join, into the posterior wall of the left atrium and closing the ASD. Important intraoperative considerations include the need for hypothermic circulatory arrest, and developmental hypoplasia of the left atrium, which may limit left ventricular filling and output. In selected instances when this is present, the ASD may be left open to accommodate the sudden increase in left atrial volume, with resultant left-to-right shunting. Pulmonary vascular resistance is usually elevated postoperatively, resulting in altered right ventricular myocardial function, which can culminate in episodic right-to-left shunting through the ASD, particularly if there is a residual pulmonary venous obstruction[392].

Postoperatively, these infants experience pulmonary hypertension, decreased myocardial function, and arrhythmias. Several factors contribute to the frequency of pulmonary hypertension, including normally elevated neonatal PVR, elevated left atrial pressure, obstruction to pulmonary venous drainage at the anastomotic site, and congenital pulmonary vascular hypoplasia. In the absence of reparable anatomic causes of pulmonary hypertension, therapy is aimed at minimizing PVR with ventilation as well as pharmacotherapy. Inotropic support is best provided by agents which are also direct pulmonary vasodilators, such as isoproterenol, dobutamine, amrinone. In infants with longstanding congestive failure, decreased density of β-receptors in the myocardium may occur. Agents which increase output by non β-receptor mediated actions, such as amrinone and calcium, may be especially beneficial under these circumstances. Arrhythmias occur as a result of atrial manipulation; junctional bradycardia is common and can be managed with an isoproterenol infusion. Other forms of heart block may require epicardial pacing.

There appear to be few long-term cardiac problems related to this repair; approximately 10% will have residual pulmonary venous obstruction necessitating reoperation[392,393]. Some may develop pulmonary hypertension due to intrapulmonary venous obstruction, which has no treatment other than lung transplantation.

HEART TRANSPLANTATION

Introduction/History

Pediatric heart transplantation has become accepted therapy for children with end-stage myocardial failure, palliated congenital heart disease, and noncorrectable congenital heart disease. As is true with other "high-tech" procedures, as the number of successful operations increases, the use of this procedure and thus ICU resources increases dramatically. These infants and children require ICU care not only in the immediate postoperative period, but also during episodes of acute rejection or when other problems related to immunosuppression occur.

In 1967, Christian Barnard performed the first human-to-human heart transplantation[394], followed the next year by 102 transplantations in multiple centers, with generally poor results[395]. The first child's heart transplantation was performed at that time by Kantrowitz, who transplanted a heart from an anencephalic infant to a 3-week-old infant with tricuspid atresia[396]. The following year, Cooley trans-

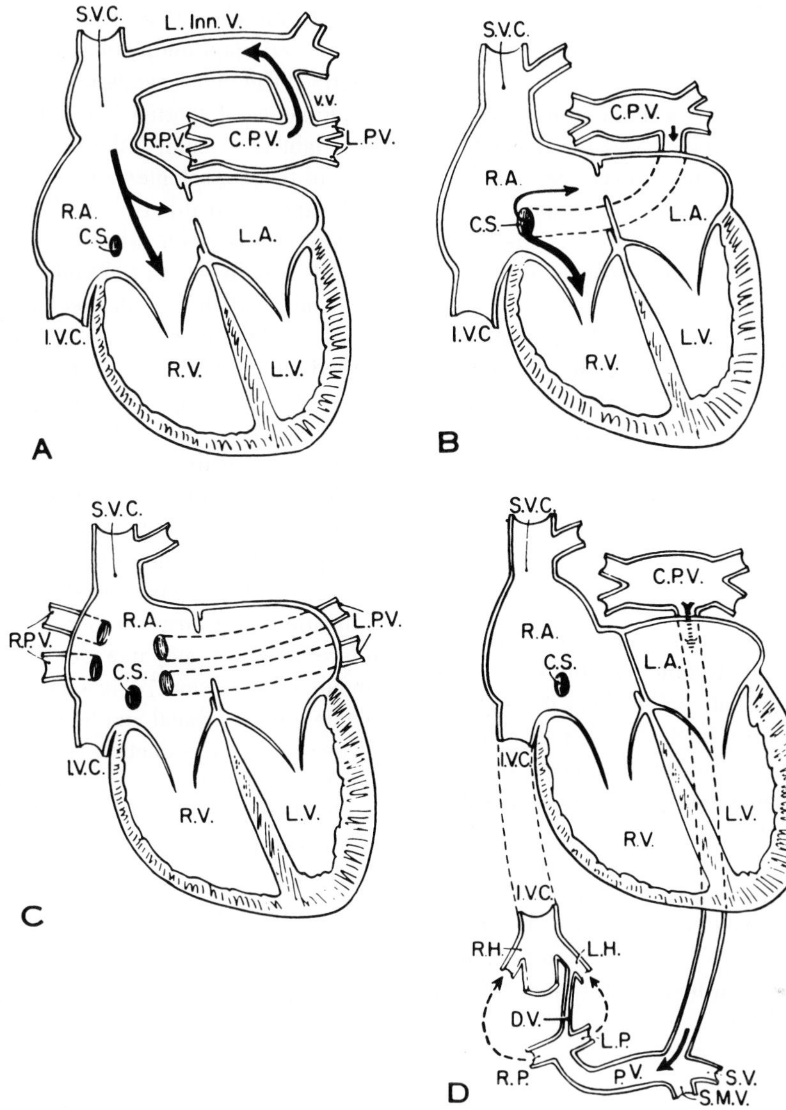

Figure 14.17. Common forms of TAPVR. (A) TAPVR to the left innominate vein (L. Inn. V.) by way of a vertical vein (V.V.). (B) TAPVR to coronary sinus (C.S.). The pulmonary veins join to form a confluence designated common pulmonary vein (C.P.V.), which connects to the coronary sinus. (C) TAPVR to right atrium. The right an left pulmonary veins (L.P.V. and R.P.V.) usually enter the right atrium separately. (D) TAPVR to the portal vein (P.V.). The pulmonary veins form a confluence, from which an anomalous channel arises. This connects to the portal vein, which communicates with the I.V.C. by way of the ductus venosus (D.V.) or the hepatic sinusoids S.V., splenic vein; S.M.V., superior mesenteric vein; R.P. and L.P., right and left portal veins; R.H. and L.H., right and left hepatic veins; S.V.C., superior vena cava; R.A. and L.A., right and left atrium; R.V. and L.V., right and left ventricle. (From Lucas RV Jr., Krabill KA: Anomalous venous connections, pulmonary and systemic. (eds) Adams FH, Emmanouilides GC, Reimenschneider TA. In: Heart Diseases in Infants, Children, and Adolescents, Fourth Edition, Chapter 27. Williams and Wilkins, Baltimore, Maryland 1968, p 588.)

planted the heart and lungs from an anencephalic infant to an infant with an endocardial cushion defect(397). Unfortunately, both of these patients died within hours of surgery. The first series of successful pediatric heart transplants was performed at Stanford University in 1981. That group reported seven successful transplantations in adolescents(398). As with other types of solid organ transplantation, the introduction of cyclosporine coincided with increased survival. As the indications for pediatric heart transplantation continue to evolve and immunosuppressive therapy becomes more fine-tuned, survival rates are expected to improve.

Selection of Patients

Donors

As the need for transplantable organs increases, recruitment and selection of available donors becomes more important. Intensivists are intimately involved with selection and preoperative care of organ donors. At the moment, all organ donors are required to meet the criteria for brain death in their particular jurisdiction (see Chapter 27 for a full discussion of brain death), although harvesting of organs after cardiac arrest is also under discussion(399). Consent for organ donation must be obtained. Cardiac function of the donor is considered adequate for transplantation if the ECG is normal without evidence of ischemia, an echocardiographic evaluation reveals a normal left ventricular shortening fraction (28 to 44%), and the donor heart is structurally normal[400]. Donors may be receiving vasoactive infusions at the time of evaluation, making decisions regarding function more difficult. The donor needs to be free of active infection, although the patient may be on antibiotics.

Loma Linda University reported that the precipitating causes of death in pediatric cardiac donors were metabolic abnormalities (48%), trauma (36%), and sudden infant death syndrome (16%). Cardiac arrest had occurred in 76% of these 25 donors, including one patient who required CPR for 30 minutes with a pH of 6.5. Thirty-six percent received inotropic support[400].

Recipients

Dilated cardiomyopathy, palliated congenital heart disease with irreversible myocardial dysfunction, life-threatening arrhythmias resistant to conventional medical therapy, and lethal neonatal heart disease, including hypoplastic left heart syndrome or variants of this complex, are current indications for heart transplantation. The majority of pediatric cardiac transplantations are performed in infants younger than 1 year, and the majority of these in infants younger than 1 month. Eighty-one percent of transplantations in infants are performed for congenital heart disease[401]. In children over 1 year of age, 64% of transplantations are performed for a cardiomyopathy and 30% for congenital heart disease[401].

With the exception of immunodeficiency and active infection, all contraindications to cardiac transplantation are relative. The major concern prior to cardiac transplantation is pulmonary hypertension which causes early postoperative right ventricular failure of the graft[402]. Sudden exposure of the transplanted right ventricle to a very high PVR will cause it to dilate or fail[403]. While no perioperative mortality was seen when the preoperative PVR index (PVRI) was less than 6 Woods units[404], the absolute upper limit of PVRI which precludes successful transplantation is unknown. Successful transplantation has been reported with PVRI between 6 and 12 Woods units[404–406]. This was especially true when the pulmonary vascular bed was responsive to vasodilators[406,407] and the ischemic time of the donor heart was kept to less than 6 hours[408]. While anatomically inadequate pulmonary arteries had previously been thought to be a relative contraindication for heart transplantation, repair of the pulmonary arteries at the time of transplantation gives good results[409,410]. Other contraindications to transplantation are also relative. Pulmonary infarction which may increase the risk of lung abscess with immunosuppression[411] has not precluded successful transplantation[412]. Renal and hepatic dysfunction, if secondary to myocardial dysfunction, may be reversible after transplantation. Decisions regarding patients with coexisting medical problems such as malignancy, diabetes mellitus, and cystic fibrosis must be individualized. Social and psychological considerations, which affect postoperative morbidity, also play a role in including or excluding a candidate for transplantation.

Donor and recipient matching is presently based on ABO compatibility and CMV status. If the recipient is serologi-

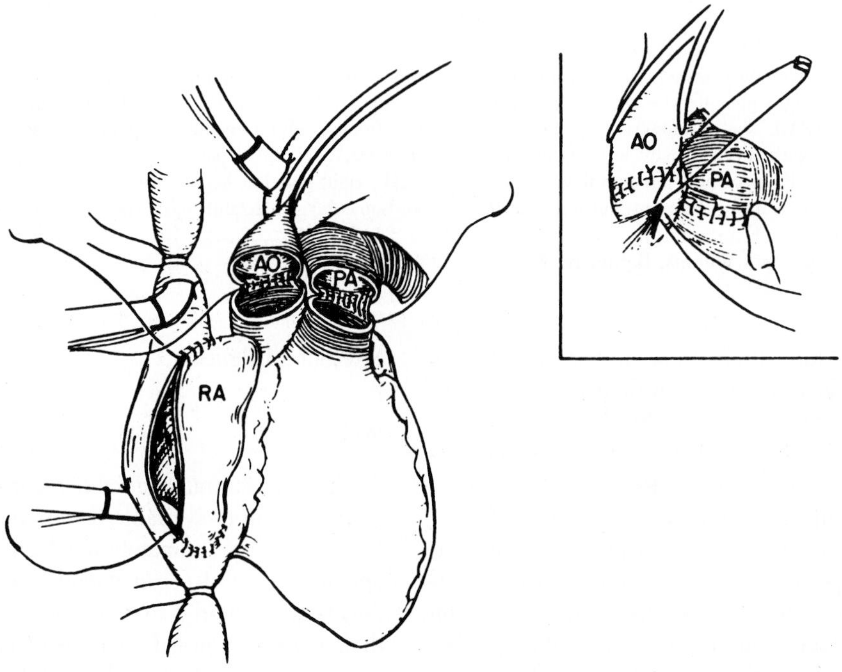

Figure 14.18. The medial aspect of the right atrial anastomosis has been completed, and the figure shows the methods of the anastomosis of the aorta and pulmonary artery. The insert demonstrates the technique of venting air from the ascending aorta as the aortic cross-clamp is released, restoring perfusion to the donor heart. (From Bolman RM III: Cardiac transplantation: The operative technique. Clinical Aspects 1990, p 140.)

cally negative for CMV, every effort is made to obtain a CMV negative heart[413]. Generally, the donor is within 80% of the body mass of that of the selected recipient. The scarcity of pediatric donors though, has necessitated considerably greater flexibility in donor-recipient size matching than is considered acceptable for adult transplantation[414], and in infants the donor to recipient body mass may vary by more than 100%[415].

Surgery

The technique of heart transplantation is based on the 1960 description by Lower and Shumway, with minor modifications[416] (Figs. 14–18 and 14–19). A midline sternotomy is performed and after appropriate dissection and securing of the pericardium, the aorta, and right atrium are mobilized. The ascending aorta is then cannulated in the routine fashion, and the cavae are cannulated, allowing preservation of a generous cuff of posterior right atrium for anastomosis to the donor heart. The patient is placed on cardiopulmonary bypass, the body temperature is lowered to 28°C, and the aorta is cross-clamped. The recipient's diseased heart is then excised, leaving posterior cuffs of left and right atrium, aorta, and pulmonary artery.

When harvesting the donor heart, the aorta and pulmonary arteries are separated; the superior vena caval orifice is overseen, and the cuffs of left and right atrium are created, matching those in the recipient, by excising the posterior wall of the left atrium and making an incision in the right atrium from the inferior vena caval orifice extending to the right atrial appendage. After placing the donor heart into the operative field the left atrial anastomosis is performed, from free wall to atrial septum. From a technical standpoint the surgeon prefers to perform the pulmonary anastomosis and right atrial anastomosis surrounding the coronary sinus prior to releasing the aortic cross-clamp. In situations in which the donor heart's ischemic time is excessive, the aortic anastomosis is performed first, followed by removal of the aortic cross-clamp to restore perfusion to the donor heart. Systemic rewarming is begun at the beginning of the aortic anastomosis, and at least 30 minutes is allowed for reperfusion of the donor heart. When hemostasis is ensured and the patient is normothermic, atrial and ventricular pacing wires are attached, isoproterenol infusion is instituted to increase heart rate above 100 beats per minute, and the patient is separated from the bypass circuit.

Postoperative Care

In patients returning to the ICU from the operating room after heart transplantation, general principles of postoperative cardiac management are adhered to, as outlined in earlier sections of the chapter. In addition, some centers adhere to a protocol of full reverse isolation. The patient typically is mechanically ventilated overnight to maintain normal oxygenation and ventilation. In patients with a reactive pulmonary vascular bed, episodes of pulmonary hypertension are avoided by hyperventilation, sedation, and limited stimulation. Intravenous catecholamines are typically used in the early postoperative period. Isoproterenol is infused at a rate that results in a slight tachycardia relative to age. Low-dose dopamine may also be administered to maintain renal blood flow. If sinus node function is not present during this period, atrial or sequential atrioventricular pacing is used. In patients who were hemodynamically very compromised in the preoperative state, weaning from mechanical ventilatory and vasopressor support may take additional days. In 25 infants who received transplants at Loma Linda University, the mean time of mechanical ventilation after transplantation was 7 ± 6 days (range 1 to 29 days)[417]. Patients are also maintained on a cephalosporin while invasive vascular lines are still in place, and on sulfamethoxazole and trimethoprim chronically to minimize the risk of *Pneumocystis carinii* infection (see below). H_2-receptor blockers are also administered as prophylaxis for stress ulcers due to the use of high dose corticosteroids.

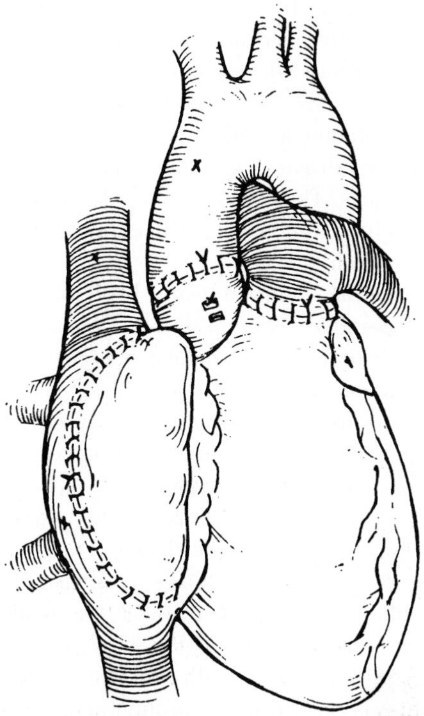

Figure 14.19. This is the completed preparation. Right atrial, aortic, and pulmonary suture lines are visible, and the cardiopulmonary bypass cannulas have been extracted. (From Bolman RM III: Cardiac transplantation: The operative technique. Clinical Aspects 1990, p 141.)

Immediately postoperatively, there are elevations in right- and left-sided filling pressures, which gradually recede[418]. The reduction in right-sided pressures may be attributable to a decrease in pulmonary artery pressure, improvement of right ventricular contractility, and a decrease in tricuspid regurgitation[418,419]. Decreasing left-sided filling pressures likely correlate with recovery of the left ventricle from its ischemic state during transport and surgery. Systemic hypertension is frequently seen as a side effect of immunosuppressive therapy and may increase the cardiac work, requiring afterload reduction. The incidence of cardiac arrhythmias is frequent in the postoperative period. While postoperative use of catecholamines stimulates arrhythmias, cardiac denervation theoretically protects against arrhythmias[420–422]. Primary malignant arrhythmias after transplantation are likely related to acute rejection, coronary artery disease, or ventricular dysfunction from some other cause. Thus, this high incidence of arrhythmias postoperatively is probably a reflection of the high incidence of rejection (see below)[423,424].

Acute rejection occurs in nearly 100% of patients in the early postoperative period despite immunosuppressive therapy[425]. In order to monitor for acute rejection, endomyocardial biopsy remains the only reliable diagnostic tool[426] and initially is usually done on a weekly basis. The presence of clinical signs of acute rejection, including fever, tachycardia, arrhythmias, hypotension, weakness, lethargy, and fluid retention, are an indication for emergency endomyocardial biopsy. In infants, for whom the risks of biopsy are higher, the need for noninvasive surveillance for rejection led to identification of recognizable patterns of alterations in echocardiography associated with rejection[427,428]. When compared prospectively with endomyocardial biopsy, changes in systolic and diastolic function missed only one out of 13 episodes of rejection in 42 infants, with 85 clinically suspected episodes of rejection. Left ventricular shortening fraction was not predictive of rejection, while evidence of diastolic dysfunction as evidenced by a decreased stroke volume, decrease in end-diastolic volume, and a reduction in peak filling rate was more suggestive[428].

Immunosuppressive therapy for cardiac transplantation continues to evolve (see Chapter 37 on liver transplantation for a full discussion of immunosuppression). Most data is reported for triple-drug therapy, including cyclosporine A, corticosteroids, and azathioprine[429], although FK506 appears superior in its ability to prevent acute graft rejection[430]. Corticosteroids are frequently not part of the prophylactic regimen in infants who have less rejection and diminished natural killer function[431–433]. Clinical or histologic rejection events are treated with high-dose intravenous solumedrol. Steroid-resistant rejection is treated with polyclonal antibodies, antithymocyte globulin, or monoclonal antibody (OKT3).

The complications of immunosuppression are well known and are discussed extensively in the liver transplant chapter and so will be discussed only briefly here. Complications include infection, hypertension, and renal dysfunction in the perioperative period. As many as 75% of pediatric patients may develop an infection during their initial hospitalization[412,434], although infection rates as low as 27% have been reported[425]. Infections include bacterial (47%); viral (41%), particularly cytomegalovirus, fungal (8%), and protozoal (4%); and *P. carinii* infection[412,434]. The single most frequent infecting organism was cytomegalovirus (26%). Pulmonary infections are the most frequent, although any of the usual sites of infection should be investigated when there are clinical signs of infection. Overall mortality per infection was 13% and was highest with fungal infections[434].

Hypertension is the most common hemodynamic abnormality following heart transplantation and is probably related to cyclosporine A. It occurs in virtually 100% of all pediatric patients and may be related to renal vasoconstriction. Therapeutic regimens include all antihypertensive medications, including diuretics, direct-acting vasodilators, angiotensin blocking agents, calcium channel blocking agents, and α- and β-blockers.

Renal dysfunction following heart transplantation is also due to drug toxicity[435], although it is also associated with cardiac dysfunction in the perioperative period. Serum creatinine level usually returns to baseline in the first month after transplantation, and then increases slowly to reach a plateau at about 1 year[409]. It may remain more elevated, though, in association with persistent hypertension[436].

Neurologic complications after heart transplantation have been described in pediatric and adult populations. In an adult autopsy series, ischemic-hypoxic damage was present in up to 50% of patients[437]. These changes, usually associated with encephalopathy, seizures, and focal neurologic deficits in the early postoperative period, are related to perioperative hypoxic-ischemic insults, focal cerebral infarction from fat and thromboembolus, metabolic disturbances, elevated levels of cyclosporine, and central nervous system infection[438,439]. The incidence of postoperative neurologic complications appears to decrease with increasing experience with children[439]. Cyclosporine A has been associated with a leukoencephalopathy in noncardiac transplant patients[440].

The most frequent neurologic complication presently seen in children after transplantation is seizures, which are observed in approximately 15% of patients after transplantation[439]. When seizures occur, benzodiazepines are the recommended choice for treatment. Barbiturates and dilantin should be avoided, if possible, to prevent induction of the hepatic enzymes responsible for metabolism of cyclosporine and corticosteroids. A second commonly seen complication is stroke which may be related to CPB, acute rejection, or catheterization[438,439].

Denervation

Denervation of the transplanted heart is, in the minds of many, the most fascinating aspect of the physiology of heart transplantation. Its effects on the patient, both short and long term, are important. The types of problems expected and the classes of drugs that are effective in the perioperative period are determined to a great extent by this "abnormal" physiology. The long-term effects of denervation and its duration play a critical role in the ultimate lifestyle and morbidity and mortality for patients undergoing heart transplantation.

Normal Anatomy

Both the sympathetic and parasympathetic components of the autonomic nervous system innervate the heart with efferent and afferent fibers. Sympathetic afferents arise from the chemoreceptor and mechanoreceptors in the pericardium and myocardium, terminating in the thalamus. Sympathetic preganglionic efferent fibers arise from the third and fourth segments of the thoracic cord and synapse in the paravertebral cervical and thoracic sympathetic ganglia. These postsynaptic fibers pass through the stellate ganglia and cardiac plexus to innervate the SA and AV nodes, atrial and ventricular myocardium, and epicardial veins and arteries[(441)]. Parasympathetic afferents with their cell bodies in the nodose ganglia, terminate in the medulla via the vagus nerve. Fibers originating in the left coronary artery system may mediate the Bezold-Jarisch reflex, resulting in hypotension and bradycardia[(442)]. Parasympathetic efferent fibers to the heart originate in the vagal nuclei in the medulla, leaving the brainstem via the vagal nerves bilaterally. They eventually synapse on the SA and AV nodes, atrial and possibly ventricular myocardium, and the ventricular coronary veins and arteries[(443)]. At the time of transplantation, afferent and efferent fibers can come only from native atrial tissue; the donor heart itself is denervated.

Physiology of the Denervated Heart

Electrical Activity

The influence of the autonomic nervous system on the heart's conduction system results from complex integration of both the sympathetic and parasympathetic afferent and efferent nervous systems. The donor's SA node, previously under the continual influence of the vagus nerve, now fires the donor's atria at a faster rate than the recipient's atria as it is no longer under the influence of tonic vagal tone[(444)]. The native atria's electrical activity does not cross the suture line, so while it continues to respond to reflex stimuli and medications, it no longer plays a role in the regulation of ventricular rate[(445)]. The rise in heart rate in response to exercise or stress is delayed, as is the time to return to baseline[(446)]. Denervation does not, however, alter conduction time through the AV node, nor does it affect ventricular conduction[(444)]. Denervation may, in fact, protect the heart from stress-induced arrhythmias[(420–422)], although arrhythmias are reported in the transplanted heart associated with tissue rejection, coronary artery disease, and ventricular dysfunction from other causes[(423,424)]. In the transplanted heart, coronary artery disease generally produces silent ischemia, since the heart is also afferently denervated and cannot sense pain. Other afferent output, such as from cardiac volume receptors, is also not detected; heart transplant recipients appear to have other mechanisms by which blood volume can be regulated by altering plasma ADH levels independent of cardiac volume receptors[(447)].

Effects of Drugs

Optimal inotropic support after transplantation is critical since there may be both primary ventricular dysfunction in the immediate postoperative period and ventricular dysfunction secondary to tissue rejection later on. Since the transplanted heart is denervated, drugs that act primarily through the autonomic nervous system will be ineffective in maintaining cardiac output. Similarly, drugs that act both directly on the heart and indirectly via the autonomic nervous system will have only their direct effects expressed. The loss of the presynaptic neuronal catecholamine uptake system[(448)] after denervation leads to a loss of norepinephrine stores beyond the early postoperative period. Indirect-acting catecholamines are therefore much less effective. In this condition, dopamine, which can no longer be converted to norepinephrine, will manifest its effects solely as a dopaminergic and α-receptor agonist. The transplanted heart appears to be supersensitive to exogenous norepinephrine and epinephrine due to a loss of presynaptic reuptake of these drugs[(449)]. In addition, upregulation of β_2-adrenergic receptors has been noted, which means that β_1-selective drugs such as norepinephrine will not occupy the entire β-receptor population at clinical doses[(450)]. Thus, nonselective agents such as epinephrine, dobutamine, and isoproterenol are more effective for inotropic support.

Other medication effects are also altered in the transplanted heart after denervation. The AV nodal blocking property of digitalis is reduced because of the interruption of preganglionic parasympathetic efferent nerves[(451)], although its inotropic effect remains intact[(452)]. As the anticholinergic properties of quinidine are virtually absent[(453)], atrial flutter can be treated with quinidine without fear of accelerating AV conduction, while digoxin is ineffective in patients with this condition. Similarly, without parasympathetic innervation, atropine cannot be used to accelerate SA or AV node conduction[(444)]. Calcium channel blockers also do not induce any major rhythm effects in the denervated heart[(454)].

Coronary Artery Dynamics

Although the coronary arteries are richly innervated by both sympathetic and parasympathetic nerves, denervation does not appear to change coronary blood flow changes associated with metabolic need[(455)]. The local influences modulating autoregulation of coronary blood flow most likely play a more important role in this setting.

Duration of Denervation

After transplantation, the heart remains denervated for years. Animal models of surgical denervation have demonstrated functional autonomic reinnervation 3 to 6 months after autotransplantation or allotransplantation[(445,456)], but recent human studies measuring myocardial catecholamines[(457,458)] and nerve density[(459)], and displaying denervation physiology and pharmacology in the transplanted heart[(444,449)], refute these findings and have been unable to show reinnervation at any point up to 5 years after surgery[(457)]. Still, there are anecdotal reports of the reestablishment of sensory innervation as evidenced by the onset of angina pectoris in patients with graft atherosclerosis[(460,461)] and evidence of late (more than 1 year) sensory reinnervation after transplantation has been shown[(461)].

Long-Term Complications

A number of long-term complications may arise in the pediatric patient after cardiac transplantation. Accelerated coronary arteriosclerosis in adults is the most common cause of mortality or allograft failure after the first year[462]. Coronary artery disease is the cause of death in 8% of infants and 16% of children over 1 year of age[401], accounting for 37% of late deaths[463]. Six of 21 children (28%) studied by angiography or autopsy 6 months to 6 years after transplantation showed evidence of arteriosclerosis[463]. Coronary angiography is generally performed at one- to two-year intervals, although the outcome after retransplantation for this complication is poor[463–466].

The histology of graft coronary artery disease is diffuse concentric intimal hyperplasia with invasion by lymphocytes and macrophages. An immune-mediated cellular or humoral injury to the coronary artery endothelium may be the primary pathogenic mechanism, with subsequent release of cytokines causing proliferation[467]. Alternatively, cytomegalovirus infection may cause smooth muscle or endothelial cell injury, inducing an inflammatory response, although little evidence for viral infection has been found in children[468]. The patients who died of this complication all had multiple episodes of clinical and histologic rejection, with ongoing evidence of histologic rejection to the graft. Ten of 49 patients with coronary artery disease had documented noncompliance with immunosuppression. Other possible risk factors to the development of coronary artery disease are hypertension, hyperglycemia, and hyperlipidemia[469], which are frequently associated with immunosuppression.

Other cardiovascular problems are observed in the long term. The incidence of hypertension caused by corticosteroids and cyclosporine A is high, necessitating chronic antihypertensive therapy[409]. Cardiac function, when not affected by acute rejection, appears adequate, with normal cardiac output and filling pressures observed 8 months to 2 years after transplantation[470]. Coarctation of the aorta or obstruction at other anastomotic sites has been reported[470].

Lymphoproliferative disease in children receiving immunosuppression has been described[471]. Armitage et al. reported that five out of 54 patients (9.2%) developed lymphoproliferative disease; three as early as 4 months after transplantation[430]. Eighty percent of these tumors were associated with Epstein-Barr infection and responded to reduction in immunotherapy. The overall mortality from lymphoproliferative disease is 60%[430]. In the majority of reported cases, patients had been treated with cyclosporine A; the incidence of lymphoproliferative disease in patients who receive FK506 is unknown but may be similar. Other neoplasias, such as leiomyosarcomas, have also been reported in immunosuppressed transplant patients[472].

Survival

The survival rate for children receiving heart transplants has improved as operative techniques, immunosuppression, and postoperative care have improved. Two centers reported no postoperative deaths for over 70 noninfant transplantations, including 28 children who had previously undergone pulmonary artery reconstruction[401]. From 1984 to 1992, 1668 pediatric heart transplantations were reported to the international registry, with a 30-day mortality of 16.6%. Actuarial 3-year survival, excluding infant transplantations, was 71%. The principle causes of death were infection (14%), acute rejection (18%), and coronary artery disease (16%). Loma Linda University has reported the largest number of infant cardiac transplantations, with an acute mortality rate of 9% and a five-year actuarial survival of 84%[473]. The international registry reported an overall survival rate of infants of 66% at 3 years, with a higher rate of early graft failure. Infants were more likely to die of infection (23%) than older children, but less likely to die of coronary artery disease (8%)[401].

Advances in operative technique and postoperative care have greatly reduced the perioperative mortality for children undergoing cardiac transplantation. As improvements in immunosuppression, surveillance for rejection, and treatments for other complications are experienced, improvements in overall survival will continue. Unfortunately, the donor supply will remain limited.

References

1. Greeley WJ, Bushman GA, Davis DP, Reves JG: Comparative effects of halothane and ketamine on systemic arterial oxygen saturation in children with cyanotic heart disease. Anesthesiology. 1986;65:666.
2. Laishley RS, Burrows FA, Lerman J, Roy WL: Effect of anesthetic induction regimens on oxygen saturation in cyanotic congenital heart disease. Anesthesiology 1986;65:673.
3. Davis PJ, Cook DR, Stiller RL, Davin-Robinson KA: Pharmacodynamics and pharmacokinetics of high-dose sufentanil in infants and children undergoing cardiac surgery. Anesth Analg 1987;66:203.
4. Moore RA, Yang SS, McNicholas KW, Gallagher JD, Clark DL: Hemodynamic and anesthetic effects of sufentanil as the sole anesthetic for pediatric cardiovascular surgery. Anesthesiology 1985;62:725.
5. Hickey PR, Hansen DD: Fentanyl-and sufenanil-oxygen-pancuronium anesthesia for cardiac surgery in infants. Anesth Analg 1984;86:823. 1987;1:137.
6. Hickey PR, Hansen DD, Wessel DL, Lang P, Jonas RA: Pulmonary and systemic hemodynamic responses to fentanyl in infants. Anesth Analg 1985;64:483.
7. Morgan P, Lynn AM, Parrot C, Morray JP: Hemodynamic and metabolic effects of two anesthetic techniques in children undergoing surgical repair of acyanotic congenital heart disease. Anesth Analg 1987;66:1028.
8. Rao C, Boyer M, Krishna G, et al.: Increased sensitivity of the isometric contraction of the neonatal isolated rat atria to halothane, isoflurane, and enflurane. Anesthesiology 1986;64:13.
9. Introna RPS, Martin DC, Pruett JK, Philpot TE, Johnston JF: Percutaneous pulmonary artery catheterization in pediatric cardiovascular anesthesia: Insertion techniques and use. Anesth Analg 1990;70:562.
10. Gentles TL, Rosenfeld HM, Sanders SP, Laussen PC, Burke RP, Van der Velde ME: Pedaitric biplane transesophageal echocardiography: preliminary experience. Am Heart J 1994;128:1225.
11. Ungerleider RM, Greeley WJ, Sheikh KH, et al.: Routine use of intraoperative, epicardial echo and doppler color flow imaging to guide and evaluate repair of congenital heart lesions: A prospective study. J Thorac Cardiovasc Surg 1990;100:287.
12. Michenfelder JD, Milde JH: The relationship among canine brain temperature, metabolism, and function during hypothermia. Anesthesiology 1991;75:130.
13. DeWall RA, Lillehei CW: Simplified total body perfusion: Reduced flows, moderate hypothermia, and hemodilution. JAMA 1962;179:430.
14. Baraka A, Baroody M, Haroun S, et al.: Continuous venous oximetry during cardiopulmonary bypass: Influence of temperature changes, perfusion flow, and hematocrit levels. J Cardiothorac Anesth 1990;4:35.
15. Nicolson SC, Jobes DR, Steven JM, Hillyer P, Handrahan JV: Evalua-

tion of a user-operated patient-side blood gas and chemistry monitor in children undergoing cardiac surgery. J Cardiothorac Anesth 1989;3:741.
16. Lanier WL: Glucose management during cardiopulmonary bypass: Cardiovascular and neurologic implications. Anesth Analg 1991;72:423.
17. Steward DJ, DaSilva CA, Flegel T: Elevated blood glucose levels may increase the danger of neurological deficit following profoundly hypothermic cardiac arrest. Anesthesiology 1988;68:653.
18. Ellis DJ, Steward DJ: Fentanyl dosage is associated with reduced blood glucose in pediatric patients after hypothermic cardiopulmonary bypass. Anesthesiology 1990;72:812.
19. Mikawa K, Maekawa N, Goto R, et al.: Effects of exogenous glucose on plasma glucose and lipid homeostasis in anesthetized children. Anesthesiology 1991;74:1017.
20. Anderson EF: Heparin resistance prior to cardiopulmonary bypass. Anesthesiology. 1986;64:504.
21. Horrow J: Protamine a necessary evil. In: Ellison N, Jobes DR (eds). Effective hemostasis in cardiac surgery: A society of cardiovascular anesthesiologists monograph. WB Saunders, Philadelphia 1988:15.
22. Lowenstein E, Zapol W: Protamine reactions, explosive mediator release, and pulmonary vasoconstriction. Anesthesiology 1990;73:373.
23. Colman RW: Humoral mediators of catastrophic reactions associated with protamine neutralization. Anesthesiology 1987;66:595.
24. Ullman DA, Bloom BS, Danker PR, Chalmers PC, Sheikh F: Protamine-induced hypotension in a two-year-old child. J Cardiothorac Anesth 1988;2:497.
25. Lock R, Hessel EA II. Probable reversal of protamine reactions by heparin administration. J Cardiothorac Anesth 1990;4:604.
26. Haga Y, Hatori N, Yoshizu H, Okuda E, Uriuda Y, Tanaka S. Granulocyte superoxide amino and elastase release during cardiopulmonary bypass. Artif Organs 1993;17:837.
27. Johnson D, Thomson D, Hurst T et al : Neutrophil-mediated acute lung injury after extracorporeal perfusion. J Thorac Cardiovasc Surg 1994; 107:1193.
28. McGowan FX, Ikegami M, del Nido PJ et al: Cardiopulmonary bypass significantly reduces surfactant activity in children.
29. Anand KJS, Sippell WG, Aynsley-Green A: Randomized trial of fentanyl anesthesia preterm neonates undergoing surgery: Effects on stress response. Lancet 1987;1:243.
30. Anand KJS, Hansen DD, Hickey PR: Hormonal-metabolic stress responses in neonates undergoing cardiac surgery. Anesthesiology 1990;73:661.
31. Anand KJS, Hickey PR. Halothane-morphine compared with high-dose sufentanil for anesthesia and postoperative analgesia in neonatal cardiac surgery. N Engl J Med 1992; 326:1.
32. Slogoff S, Girgis KZ, Keats AS: Etiologic factors in neuropsychiatric complications associated with cardiopulmonary bypass. Anesth Anal 1992;61:903.
33. Govier AV: Central nervous system complications after cardiopulmonary bypass. In: Tinker JH (ed) Cardiopulmonary bypass current concepts and controversies. A society of cardiovascular anesthesiologists monograph. WB Saunders, Philadelphia 1989:41.
34. Ferry PC: Neurologic sequelae of open-heart surgery in children. AJDC 1990;144:369.
35. Ferry PC: Neurologic sequelae of cardiac surgery in children. AJDC 1987;141:309.
36. DeLeon S, Ilbawi M, Arcilla R, et al.: Choreoathetosis after deep hypothermia without circulatory arrest. Ann Thorac Surg 1990;50:714.
37. McConnell JR, Fleming WH, Chu WK, et al.: Magnetic resonance imaging of the brain in infants and children before and after cardiac surgery. AJDC 1990;144:374.
38. Phornphutkul C, Rosenthal A, Nadas AS, et al.: Cerebrovascular accidents in infants and children with cyanotic congenital heart disease. Am J Cardiol 1973;32:329.
39. Brunberg JA, Reilly EI, Doty DB: Central nervous system consequences in infants of cardiac surgery using deep hypothermia and circulatory arrest. Circulation 1974;50[Suppl 2]:60.
40. Tinker JH, Campos JH: Blood gases should be corrected for temperature during hypothermic cardiopulmonary bypass:pH-stat mode. J Cardiothorac Anesth 1988;2:701.
41. Murkin JM, Farrar JK, Tweed WA, McKenzie FN, Guiraudon G: Cerebral autoregulation and flow/metabolism coupling during cardiopulmonary bypass: The influence of $PaCO_2$. Anesth Analg 1987;66:825.
42. Prough DS, Stump DA, Roy RC, et al.: Response of cerebral blood flow to changes in carbon dioxide tension during hypothermic cardiopulmonary bypass. Anesthesiology 1986;64:576.
43. Bashein G, Townes BD, Nessley ML, et al.: A randomized study of carbon dioxide management during hypothermic cardiopulmonary bypass. Anesthesiology 1990;72:7.
44. Greely WJ, Ungerleider RM, Smith LR, Reves JG: The effects of deep hypothermic cardiopulmonary bypass and total circulatory arrest on cerebral blood flow in infants and children. J Thorac Cardiovasc Surg 1989;97:737.
45. Gillinov M, Schleien CL, Curtis W, et al.: Hypothermic cardiopulmonary bypass does not disrupt the blood-brain barrier. Surgical Forum 1991 [Abstract].
46. Burrows FA, Hillier SC, McLeod ME, Iron KS, Taylor MJ: Anterior fontanel pressure and visual evoked potentials in neonates and infants undergoing profound hypothermic circulatory arrest. Anesthesiology 1990;73:632.
47. Friesen RH, Thieme R: Changes in anterior fontanelle pressure during cardiopulmonary bypass and hypothermic circulatory arrest in infants. Anesth Analg 1991;66:94.
48. Blackwood MJA, Haka-Ikse K, Steward DJ: Developmental outcome in children undergoing surgery with profound hypothermia. Anesthesiology 1986;65:437.
49. Brunberg JA, Doty DB, Reilly EL: Choreoathetosis in infants following cardiac surgery with deep hypothermia and circulatory arrest. J Pediatr 1974;84;232.
50. Curless RG, Fatz DA, Perryman RA, Ferrer PL, Gelblum J, Wiener WJ: Choreoathetosis after surgery for congenital heart disease. J Pediatr 1974;124:737.
51. Wong PC, Barlow CF, Hickey PR, et al .: Factors associated with choreoathetosis after cardiopulmonary bypass in children with congenital heart disease. Circulation 1992; 86:II118.
52. Nussmeier NA, Arlund C, Slogoff S: Neuropsychiatric complications after cardiopulmonary bypass: Cerebral protection by a barbiturate. Anesthesiology 1986;64:165.
53. Zaidan JR, Kochany A, Martin WM, Ziegler JS, Harless DM, Andrews RB: Effect of thiopental on neurologic outcome following coronary artery bypass grafting. Anesthesiology 1991;74:406.
54. Hickey PR, Anderson NP: Deep hyperthermic circulatory arrest: A review of pathophysiology and clinical experience as a basis for anesthetic management. J Cardiothorac Anesth 1987;66:1028.
55. Wells FC, Coghill S, Caplan HL, Lincoln C, Kirklin JW: Duration of circulatory arrest does influence the psychological development of children after cardiac operation in early life. J Thorac Cardiovasc Surg 1983;86:823.
56. Ehyai A, Fenichel GM, Bender HW, Jr: Incidence and prognosis of seizures in infants after cardiac surgery with profound hypothermia and circulatory arrest. JAMA 1984;252:3165.
57. Elliot MJ: Ultrafiltration and modified ultrafiltration in pediatric open heart operations. Ann Thorac Surg 1993;56:1518.
58. Naik SK, Knight A, Elliot M. A prospective randomized study of a modified technique of ultrafiltration during pediatric open-heart surgery. Circulation 1991;84:III422.
59. Journois D, Pouard P, Greely WJ, Mauriat P, Vouhe P, Safran D: Hemofiltration during cardiopulmonary bypass in pediatric cardiac surgery: effects on hemostasis, cytokines and complement components. Anesthesiology 1994;81:1181.
60. Piepenbrock S, Hempelman G: Intraoperative and post-operative monitoring of cardiocirculatory function in pediatric and adult cardiosurgical patients. Int Anesthesiol Clin 1976;14:49.
61. Baker RJ: Monitoring in critically ill patients. Surg Clin North Am 1977;57:1139.
62. Fait, CD, Wetzel RC, Dean JM, Schleien CL, Gioia FR: Pulse oximetry in critically ill children. J Clin Monit 1985;1:232.
63. Henning RJ, Wiener F, Valdes S, Weil MH: Measurement of toe temperature for assessing the severity of acute circulatory failure. Surg Gynecol Obstet 1979;149:1.
64. Knight RW, Opie JC: The big toe in the recovery room: peripheral warm-up patterns in children after open heart surgery. Can J Surg 1981;24:239.
65. Adamsons SK, Gandy GM, James LS: The influence of thermal factors upon oxygen consumption of the newborn human infant. J Pediatr 1965;66:495.
66. Dawkins M, Hull D: Brown adipose tissue and the response of newborn rabbits to cold. Am J Physiol 1964;172:216.
67. Gold JP, Jonas RA, Lang P, Elixson EM, Mayer JE, Castaneda AR: Transthoracic intracardiac monitoring lines in pediatric surgical patients: a ten year experience. Ann Thorac Surg. 1986;42:185.
68. Pollack MM, Reed TP, Holbrook PR, et al: Bedside pulmonary artery catheterization in pediatrics. J Pediatr 1980;96:274.

69. Callaghan ML, Weintraub WH, Coran AH: Assessment of the thermodilution cardiac output in small subjects. J Pediatr Surg 1976;11:629.
70. Freed MD, Keane JF: Cardiac output measured by thermodilution in infants and children. J Pediatr 1978;92:39.
71. Connors AF Jr., McCaffree DR, Gray BA: Evaluation of right-heart catheterization in the critically ill patient without acute myocardial infarction. N Engl J Med 1983;308:263.
72. Dean JM, Wetzel RC, Gioia FR, Rogers MC: Use of oxygen-derived variables for estimation of pulmonary shunt in critically ill children. Crit Care Med 1984;12:280.
73. Watson CB: The PA catheter as an early warning system. Anesthesiology Rev 1983;10:34.
74. De La Rocha AG, Edmonds JF, Williams WG, et al.: Importance of mixed venous oxygen saturation in the care of critically ill patients. Can J Surg 1978;21:221.
75. Jameison WRE, Turnbull KW, Laurrieu AJ, et al.: Continuous monitoring of mixed venous oxygen saturation in cardiac surgery. Can J Surg 1982;25:538.
76. Nelson LD: Continuous venous oximetry in surgical patients. Ann Surg 1986;203:99.
77. Schranz D, Schmitt S, Oerlert H, et al.: Continuous monitoring of mixed venous saturation in infants after cardiac surgery. Intensive Care Med 1989;15:228.
78. Loomis JC: Care of the pediatric patient following cardiovascular surgery. In: Ream AK, Fogdall RF (eds). Acute cardiovascular management. JB Lippincott, Philadelphia.
79. Harris PD, Malm JR, Bowman FO, Hoffman BF, Kaisar GA, Singer DH: Epicardial pacing to control arrhythmias following cardiac surgery. Circulation 1996;37(Suppl II):II178.
80. Angelini P, Feldman M, Lufschanowski R, Leachman RD: Cardiac arrhythmias during and after heart surgery: Diagnosis and management. Prog Cardiovasc Dis 1974;16:469.
81. Krongrad E: Postoperative arrhythmias in patients with congenital heart disease. Chest 1984;85:107.
82. Gillette PC: Diagnosis and management of postoperative junctional ectopic tachycardia. Am Heart J 1989;118:192.
83. Garson A, Gillette PC, Gutgesell HP, McNamara DG: Stress-induced ventricular arrhythmia after repair of tetralogy of Fallot. Am J Cardiol 1980;46:1006.
84. Bash SE, Jitendra SJ, Albers WH, Geiss DM. Hypothermia for the treatment of post-surgical greatly accelerated junctional ectopic tachycardia. J Am Coll Cardiol 1987;10:1095.
85. Balaji S, Sullicvan I, Deanfield J, James I. Moderate hypothermia in the management of resistant automatic tachycardias in children. Br Heart J 1991: 66; 221.
86. Paul T, Reimer A, Janousek J, Kallfeiz HC. Efficacy and safety of propafenone in congenital junctional ectopic tachycardia. J Am Coll Cardiol 1992; 20:911.
87. Raja P, Hwaker RE, Chaikitpinyo A, et al. Amiodarone management of junctional ectopic tachycardia after cardiac surgery in children. Br Heart J 1994:72; 261.
88. Sluysmans T, Moulin D, Jaumin P, Rubay J, Vliers A, DeJonghe D. Ventricular paired pacing to control intractable junctional ectopic tachycardia following open heart surgery in a child. Intens Care Med 1989:15;203.
89. Young ML, Mehta MB, Martinez RM, Wolff GS, Gelband. Combined α-adrenergic blockade and radiofrequency ablation to treat junctional ectopic tachycardia successfully without atrioventricular block. Am J Cardio 1993:71; 883.
90. Benson DW Jr.. Transesophageal pacing and electrocardiography in the neonate: diagnostic and therapeutic uses. Clin Perinatol 1988; 15:619.
91. Harte MT, Teo KK, Horgan JH. The diagnosis and management of supraventricular tachycardia by transesophageal cardiac stimulation and recording. Chest 1988;93:339.
92. Kouchoukos NT, Sheppard LC, Kirklin JW: Effect of alterations in arterial pressure on cardiac performance early after open intracardiac operations. J Thorac Cardiovasc Surg 1972;64:563.
93. Driscoll DJ, Gillette PC, Duff DF, et al: The hemodynamic effect of dopamine in children. J Thorac Cardiovasc Surg 1979;78:765.
94. Kleigman R, Fanaroff AA: Caution in the use of dopamine in the neonate. J Pediatr 1978;93:540.
95. Bohn DJ, Poirier CS, Edmonds JF, Barker G: Hemodynamic effects of dobutamine after cardiopulmonary bypass in children. Crit Care Med 1980;8:367.
96. Perkin RM, Levin DL, Webb R, Aquino A, Reedy J: Dobutamine: a hemodynamic evaluation in children with shock. J Pediatr 1982; 100:977.
97. Loeb HS, Bredakis J, Gunnar RM: Superiority of dobutamine over dopamine for augmentation of cardiac output in patients with chronic low output cardiac failure. Circulation 1977;55:375.
98. Kersting F, Follath F, Moulds R, et al: A comparison of cardiovascular effects of dobutamine and isoprenaline after open heart surgery. Br Heart J 1976;38:622.
99. Koehler RC, Michael JR, Guerci A, Chandra N, Schleien CL: Beneficial effect of epinephrine infusion on cerebral and myocardial blood flows during CPR. Ann Emerg Med 1985;14:744.
100. Colucci W, Wright R, Braunwald E: New positive inotropic agents in the treatment of congestive heart failure. N Engl J Med 1986; 3145:349.
101. Notterman DA: Pharmacologic support of the failing circulation an approach for infants and children. Probl Anesth 1989;3:288.
102. Applebaum A, Blackstone EH, Kouchoukos NT, Kirklin JW: Afterload reduction and cardiac output in infants early after intracardiac surgery. Am J Cardiol 1977;39:445.
103. Miller RR, Vismara LA, Williams DO, Amsterdam EA, Mason DT: Pharmacological mechanisms for left ventricular unloading in clinical congestive heart failure. Circ Res 1976;39:127.
104. Stinson EB, Holloway EL, Derby G, et al: Comparative hemodynamic responses to chlorpromazine, nitroprusside, nitroglycerin, and trimethaphan immediately after open heart operations. Circulation 1975;51(Suppl 1):I26.
105. Benzing G, Helmsworth JA, Schrieber JT, Loggie J, Kaplan S: Nitroprusside after open-heart surgery. Circulation 1976;54:467.
106. Pennington DG, Swartz M, Codd JE, et al.: Intraaortic balloon pumping in cardiac surgical patients: a nine-year experience. Ann Thorax Surg 1983;36:125.
107. Pollock JC, Charlton MC, Williams WG, et al.: Intra-aortic balloon pumping in children. Ann Thorac Surgery 1980;29:522.
108. Al Mofada S, Edmonds J, Vobecky S, Paret G, Bohn D, Barker G: Intra aortic balloon pumping in children. Crit Care Med 1990;18:230.
109. Cameron CB, Gregory GA, Rudolph AM, Heymann M: The effects of curare on oxygen consumption in hypoxic lambs. Anesthesiology 1981;55:A325 [Abstract].
110. Muldoon SM, Theye RA: The effects of succinylcholine and d-tubocurarine on oxygen consumption. Anesthesiology 1969;31:437.
111. Rosenthal MH, Smith DE, Trimble C: Cardiovascular effects and oxygen consumption with d-tubocurarine in awake man. Anesthesiology 1972:15A [Abstract] .
112. Palmisano BW, Fisher DM, Willis M, Gregory GA, Ebert PA: The effect of paralysis on oxygen consumption in normoxic children after cardiac surgery. Anesthesiology 1984;61:518.
113. Roberts JD, Lang P, Bigatello LM, Vlahakes GJ, Zapol WM: Inhaled nitric oxide in congenital heart disease. Circulation 1993;87:447.
114. Journois D, Pouard P, Mauriat P, Malhers T, Vouhe P, Safran D. Inhaled nitric oxide as a therapy for pulmonary hypertension after operations for congenital heart disease. J Thorac and Cardiovasc Surg 1994: 107; 1129.
115. Thomas T: Emergency evacuation of acute pericardial tamponade. Ann Thorac Surg 1970;10:566.
116. Shore DF, Capuani A, Lincoln C: Atypical tamponade after cardiac operation in infants and children. J Thorac Cardiovasc Surg 1982; 83:449.
117. Kron IL, Rheuban K, Nolan SP: Late cardiac tamponade in children. Ann Surg 1984;199:173.
118. Ofori-Krackne SK, Tyberg TI, Geha AS, et al.: Late cardiac tamponade after open heart surgery: incidence, role of anticoagulants in its pathogenesis and its relationship to the postpericardiotomy syndrome. Circulation 1981;63:1323.
119. Engle MA, Ito T: The postpericardiotomy syndrome. Am J Cardiol 1961;7:73.
120. Ito T, Eagle MA, Goldberg HP: Postpericardiotomy syndrome following surgery for nonrheumatic heart disease. Circulation 1958;17:549.
121. Fyfe D, Moddie DS, Gill CC: Postpericardiotomy syndrome following surgery for congenital heart disease. Cleve Clin Q 1981;48:352.
122. Ellis K, Malm JR, Bowman OB Jr., King DL: Roentgenographic findings after pericardial surgery. Radiol Clin North Am 1971;9:327.
123. Feigenbaum H, Waldhausen JA, Hyde LP: Ultrasound diagnosis of pericardial effusion. JAMA 1965;191:711.
124. Engle MA, Zabriskkie JB, Senterfit LB, Gay WA, O'Loughlin JE, Ehlers KH: Viral illness and the postpericardiotomy syndrome. Circulation 1980;62:1151.

125. Engle MA, Zabriskie JB, Senterfit LB et al. Immunologic and virologic studies in postpericardiotomy syndrome. J Pediatrics 1975:87; 1103.
126. Blalock AR, Cunningham RS, Robinson CS: Experimental production of chylothorax by occlusion of superior vena cava. Ann Surg 1936;104:359.
127. Higgins CB, Mulder DG: Chylothorax after surgery for congenital heart disease. J Thorac Cardiovasc Surg 1971;61:411.
128. Rubin JW, Moore V, Ellison RG: Chylothorax: Therapeutic alternatives. Am Surg 1977;292:297.
129. Verunelli, Giorgini V, Luisi VS, Eufrate S, Cornali, Resginato E: Chylothorax following cardiac surgery in children. J Cardiovasc Surg 1983;24:227.
130. Joyce LD, Linsday WG, Nicholoff DM: Chylothorax after median sternotomy for intrapericardiac cardiac surgery. J Cardiovasc Surg 1976;17:476.
131. Palken M, Weller LW: Chylothorax and chyloperitoneum. Report of a case occurring after embolism of the left subclavian vein with thoracic duct obstruction. JAMA 1951;147:566.
132. Kosloske AM, Martin LW, Schubert WK: Management of chylothorax in children by thoracentesis and medium-chain triglyceride feedings. J Pediatr Surg 1974;9:365.
133. Dahlgren S: Anatomy of the thoracic duct from the standpoint of surgery for chylothorax. Acta Chir Scand 1963;125:201.
134. Lampson LS: Traumatic chylothorax. A review of the literature and report of a case treated by mediastinal ligation of the thoracic duct. J Thorac Cardiovasc Surg 1948;17:778.
135. Selle JG, Snyder WH, Schreiber JT: Chylothorax: Indications of surgery. Ann Surg 1973;177:245.
136. Thomas CS Jr, McGoon DC: Isolated massive chylopericardium following cardiopulmonary bypass. J Thorac Cardiovasc Surg 1971;61:945.
137. Rose DM, Colvin SB, Danilowicz D, Isom OW: Cardiac tamponade secondary to chylopericardium following cardiac surgery: Case report and review of the literature. Ann Thorac Surg 1982;34:333.
138. Feteih W, Rao PS, Whisennand HH, Mardini MK, Lawrie GM. Brief communications. Chylopericardium: new complication of Blalock-Taussig annastamosis. J Thorac Cardiovasc Surg 1983; 85:791.
139. Pugliese P. Sanit C, Eufrate S. Isolated chyloperiacrdium after successful correction of total anomlaous pulmonary venous drainage. J Cardiovasc Surg 1983; 25:75.
140. Beecher HK: The measured effect of laparotomy on the respiration. J Clin Invest 1933;12:639.
141. Lister G: Management of the pediatric patient after cardiac surgery. Yale J Biol Med 1984;57:7.
142. Mathers J, Benumof JL, Wahrenbrock EA: General anesthetics and regional hypoxic pulmonary vasoconstriction. Anesthesiology 1977; 46:111.
143. Fordham RMM, Resnekov L: Arterial hypoxemia: A side-effect of intravenous isoprenaline used after cardiac surgery. Thorax 1968;23:19.
144. Smith G, Cheeney FW, Winter PM: The effect of change in cardiac output on intrapulmonary shunting. Br J Anaesth 1974;46:337.
145. Lees MH, Way RC, Ross BB: Ventilation and respiratory gas transfer of infants with increased pulmonary blood flow. Pediatrics 1967;40:259.
146. Ashmore PG, Wakeford J, Harterre D: Pulmonary complications of profound hypothermia with circulatory arrest in the experimental animal. Can J Surg 1964;7:93.
147. Culliford AT, Thomas S, Spencer FC: Fulminating noncardiogenic pulmonary edema: A newly recognized hazard during cardiac operations. J Thorac Cardiovasc Surg 1980;80:868.
148. Vincent RN, Lang P, Elixson M, et al.: Measurement of extravascular lung water in infants and children after cardiac surgery. Am J Cardiol 1984;54:161.
149. Cullen DJ, Eger EI: Cardiovascular effects of carbon dioxide in man. Anesthesiology 1974;41:345.
150. Rasmussen JP, Dauchot PJ, DePalma RG, et al.: Cardiac function and hypercarbia. Arch Surg 1978;113:1196.
151. Gregory GA, Edmunds LH Jr., Kitterman JA, Phibbs RH, Tooley WH: Continuous positive airway pressure and pulmonary and circulatory function after cardiac surgery in infants less than three months of age. Anesthesiology 1975;43:426.
152. Cournand A, Motley HL, Werko L, Richards DW: Physiological studies of the effects of intermittent positive pressure breathing on cardiac output in man. Am J Physiol 1948;152:162.
153. Qvist J, Pontoppidan H, Wilson RS, et al.: Hemodynamic responses to mechanical ventilation with PEEP: The effect of hypervolemia. Anesthesiology 1975;42:45.
154. Sykes MK, Adams AP, Finlay WEI, et al.: The effects of variations in end-expiratory inflation pressure on cardio-respiratory function in normo-, hypo-, and hypervolemic dogs. Br J Anaesth 1970;42:669.
155. Powers SR, Mannal R, Neclerio M, et al.: Physiologic consequences of positive end-expiratory pressure (PEEP) ventilation. Ann Surg 1973;178:265.
156. Jenkins J, Lynn A, Edmonds J, Barker G: Effects of mechanical ventilation on cardiopulmonary function in children after open-heart surgery. Crit Care Med 1985;13:77.
157. Levett JM, Culpepper WS, Lin CY, Arcilla RA, Replogle RL: Cardiovascular responses to PEEP and CPAP following repair of complicated congenital heart defects. Ann Thorac Surg 1983;36:411.
158. Downes JJ, Nicodemus HF, Pierce WS, Waldhausen JA: Acute respiratory failure in infants following cardiovascular surgery. J Thorac Cardiovasc Surg 1970;59:21.
159. Colgan FJ, Stewart S: PEEP and CPAP following open-heart surgery in infants and children. Anesthesiology 1979;40:336.
160. Stewart S, Edmunds LH Jr., Kirklin JV, Allarde RR: Spontaneous breathing with continuous positive airway pressure after open intracardiac operations in infants. J Thorac Cardiovasc Surg 1973;65:37.
161. Crew AD, Varkonyi PI, Gardner LG, Robinson QLA, Wall E, Deverall PB: Continuous positive airway pressure breathing in the postoperative management of the cardiac infant. Thorax 1974;29:437.
162. Hatch DJ, Taylor RW, Glover WJ, Cogswell JJ, Battersby EF, Kerr A: Continuous positive-airway pressure after open-heart operations in infancy. Lancet 1973;2:469.
163. Schuller JL, Bovill JG, Nijveld A, Patrick MR, Marcelletti C: Early extubation of the trachea after open heart surgery for congenital heart disease. Br J Anaesth 1984;56:1101.
164. Bendixen HH, Egbert LD, Hedley-Whyte J, Laver MB, Pontoppidan H: In: Respiratory Care: Fundamental considerations. St. Louis, CV Mosby, 1965:3.
164a. Shimada Y, Yoshiya I, Tanaka K, Yamazaki T, Kumon K: Crying vital capacity and maximal inspiratory pressure as clinical indicators of readiness for weaning of infants less than a year of age. Anesthesiology 1979;51:456.
165. Koka BV, Jeon ID, Andre JM, Mackay I, Smith RM: Postintubation croup in children. Anesth Analg 1977;56,501.
166. Tellez DW, Galvis AG, Storgion SA, Amer HN, Hoseyni M, Deakers TW: Dexamethasone in the prevention of postextubation stridor in children. J Pediatr 1991;118:289.
167. Reines D, Sade R, Bradford B, Marshall J: Chest physiotherapy fails to prevent postoperative atelectasis in children after cardiac surgery. Ann Surg 1982;195:451.
168. Allen TH, Steven IM: Prolonged nasotracheal intubation in infants and children. Br J Anaesth 1972;44:835.
169. Battersby EF, Hatch DJ, Towey RM: The effects of prolonged nasoendotracheal intubation in children. Anaesthesia 1977;32:154.
170. Aberdeen E. Downes JS: Artificial airways in children. Surg Clin North Am 1974;54:1155.
171. Breckenridge NM, Digerness SB, Kirklin JW: Increased extracellular fluid after open intracardiac operation. Surg Gynecol Obstet 1970;131:53.
172. Pacifico AD, Digerness S, Kirklin JW: Acute alterations of body composition after open intracardiac operations. Circulation 1970; 131:53.
173. Breckenridge MM, Deverall PB, Kirklin JW, Digerness SB: Potassium intake and balance after open intracardiac operations. J Thorac Cardiovasc Surg 1972;63:305.
174. Clark RE, Beasley WE, Sode J, Mills MM: Influence of hemodilutional perfusion on total body and intracellular potassium: critical prospective study. Surg Forum 1969;20:40.
175. Ebert P, Jude J, and Gaertner RA: Persistent hypokalemia following open-heart surgery. Circulation 1965;32(Suppl 1):137.
176. Cohn LH, Powell MP, Seidlitz L, Hamilton WK, Wylie EJ: Fluid requirements and shifts following reconstruction of the aorta. Am J Surg 1970;120:182.
177. Yoshioka K, Tsuchioka H, Abe T, Iyomasa Y: Changes in ionized and total calcium concentrations in serum and urine during open heart surgery. Biochem Med 1978;20:135.
178. Das JB, Eraclis AJ, Adams JG, Gross RE: Changes in serum ionic calcium during cardiopulmonary bypass with hemodilution. J Thorac Cardiovasc Surg 1971;62:449.
179. Chambers DJ, Dunham J, Braimbridge MV, Slavin B, Quiney J, Chayen J: The effect of ionized calcium, pH, and temperature on bioactive parathyroid hormone during and after open-heart operations. Ann Thorac Surg 1983;36:306.

180. Tsang RC, Donovan EF, Steichen JJ: Calcium physiology and pathology in the neonate. Pediatr Clin North Am 1976;23:611.
181. Goldstein J, Vincent JL, Leclerc J, Vanderhoeft P, Kahn RJ: Hypophosphatemia after cardiothoracic surgery. Intensive Care Med 1985;11:144.
182. Swaminathan R, Bradley P, Morgan DB, Hill GL: Hypophosphatemia in surgical patients. Surg Gynecol Obstet 1979;148:448.
183. England PC, Duari M, Tweedle DEF, Jones RA, Gowland E: Postoperative hypophosphatemia. Br J Surg 1979;66:340.
184. Knochel JP: The pathophysiology and clinical characteristics of severe hypophosphatemia. Arch Intern Med 1977;137:203.
185. O'Connor LR, Wheeler WS, Bethune JE: Effect of hypophosphatemia on myocardial performance in man. N Engl J Med 1977;297:901.
186. Newman JH, Nelf TA, Ziporin P: Acute respiratory failure associated with hypophosphatemia. N Engl J Med 1977;296:1101.
187. Shida H, Mormimoto M, Inokawa K, Ikeda Y: Inhibitory mechanisms of insulin secretion associated with hypothermic open-heart surgery. Jpn J Surg 1981;11:67.
188. Benzing G, Francis PD, Kaplan S, Helmsworth JA, Sperling MA: Glucose and insulin changes in infants and children undergoing hypothermic open-heart surgery. Am J Cardiol 1983;52:133.
189. Baum D, Dillar DH, Porte D Jr.: Inhibition of insulin release in infants undergoing deep hypothermic cardiovascular surgery. N Engl J Med 1968;279:1309.
190. Criado A, Dominguez E, Carmon J, Gomez-Arnau J, Avello F: Hypoglycemic coma after cardiac surgery. Crit Care Med 1984;12:409.
191. Spitzer A: Renal physiology. Pediatr Clin North Am 1971;18:377.
192. Gruskin AB: The kidney in congenital heart disease—An overview. Adv Pediatr 1977;24:133.
193. Bourgeois BFD, Donath A, Paunier L, et al.: Effects of cardiac surgery on renal function in children. J Thorac Cardiovasc Surg 1979;77:283.
194. Oka Y, Wakayama S, Oyama T, et al.: Cortisol and antidiuretic hormone responses to stress in cardiac surgical patients. Can Anaesth Soc J 1981;28:334.
195. Flear TG, Ackering J, McNeill IF: Observations on water and electrolyte changes in skeletal muscle during major surgery. J Surg Res 1969;9:369.
196. Cohn CH, Angell WW, Shumway E: Body fluid shifts after cardiopulmonary bypass: Effects of congestive heart failure and hemodilution. J Thorac Cardiovasc Surg 1971;63:423.
197. Abel RM, Buckley MJ, Austin CW, et al.: Etiology, incidence and prognosis of acute renal failure following cardiac operations: Results of a prospective analysis of 500 consecutive patients. J Thorac Cardiovasc Surg 1976;12:409.
198. Yeboah ED, Petrie A, Pead JL: Acute renal failure and open heart surgery. Br Med J 1972;1:415.
199. Chesney RW, Kaplan BS, Freedom RM, Haller JA, Drummond KN: Acute renal failure: An important complication of cardiac surgery in infants. J Pediatr 1975;87:381.
200. Porter GA, Kloster FE, Bristow JD, Griswold HE: Inter-relationship of hemodynamic alterations of valvular heart disease and renal function: Influences on renal sodium reabsorption. Am Hear J 1972;84:189.
201. Connolly JE, Kountz SL, Guernsey JM, Stemmer EA: Acidosis as a cause of renal shutdown during extracorporeal circulation: Its correction by the use of THAM. J Thorac Cardiovasc Surg 1963;46:680.
202. Subramanian S: Early correction of congenital cardiac defects using profound hypothermia and circulatory arrest. Ann R Coll Surg Engl 1974;54:178.
203. Mundth BD, Keller AR, Austen WG: Progressive hepatic and renal failure associated with low cardiac output following open-heart surgery. J Thorac Cardiovasc Surg 1967;53:275.
204. Yeh TJ, Brackney EL, Hall DP, Ellison RG: Renal complications of open heart surgery: Predisposing factors, prevention and management. J Thorac Cardiovasc Surg 1964;47:79.
205. Cantarovich F, Galle C, Benedetti L, et al.: High dose furosemide in established acute renal failure. Postgrad Med J 1971;47[Suppl1]:13.
206. Ganeval D, Kleinknecht D, Gonzales-Dugue LA: High dose furosemide in renal failure. Br Med J 1974;1:244.
207. John EG, Levitsky S, Hastreiter AR: Management of acute renal failure complicating cardiac surgery in infants and children. Crit Care Med 1980;8:562.
208. Esperana MJ, Collins DC: Peritoneal dialysis efficiency in relation to body weight. J Pediatr 1966;1:62.
209. Vaamonde CA, Micheal UF, Metzger RA, Carroll KE: Complications of acute peritoneal dialysis. J Chronic Dis 1975;28:637.
210. Zobel G, Stein JI, Kuttnig M, Beitzke A, Metzler H, Rigler B: Continuous extracorporeal fluid removal in children with low cardiac output after cardiac operations. J Thorac Cardiovasc Surg 1992;103(5):1021.
211. Bahnson HT, Ziegler RF: A consideration of the causes of death following operation for congenital heart disease of the cyanotic type. Surg Gynecol Obstet 1950;90:60.
212. Naeman JL: Clotting and bleeding in cyanotic congenital heart disease. J Pediatr 1970;76:333.
213. Ekert H, Schneers M: Preoperative and postoperative platelet function in cyanotic heart disease. J Thorac Cardiovasc Surg 1974;67:184.
214. Ware JA, Reaves WH, Horak JK, Sollis RT: Defective platelet aggregation in patients undergoing surgical repair of cyanotic congenital heart disease. Ann Thorac Surg 1983;36:289.
215. Ekert H, Dowling SV: Platelet release abnormality and reduced prothrombin levels in children with cyanotic congenital heart disease. Aust Paediatr J 1977;13:17.
216. Wedemeyer AL, Castaneda AR, Edson JR, Krivit W: Serial coagulation studies in patients undergoing Mustard procedure. Ann Thorac Surg 1973;15:120.
217. Pike GJ, Turner RL, Manohitharaja SM, Deverall PB: Fibrinolysis in cyanotic and acyanotic children before and after open intracardiac operations. J Thorac Cardiovasc Surg 1975;69:922.
218. Kontras SB, Sirak HD, Newton WA: Hematologic abnormalities in children with congenital heart disease. JAMA 1966;195:611.
219. Wedemeyer AL, Lewis JH: Improvement in hemostasis following phlebotomy in cyanotic patients with heart disease. J Pediatr 1973;83:46.
220. Andersen MN, Kuchiba K: Blood trauma produced by pump oxygenators: A comparative study of five different units. J Thorac Cardiovasc Surg 1969;57:238.
221. Schmidt PJ, Peden JC Jr., Brecher G, Baranovsky A: Thrombocytopenia and bleeding tendency after extracorporeal circulation. N Engl J Med 1961;265:1181.
222. Ashmore PG, Svitek V, Ambrose P: The incidence and effects of particulate aggregation and microembolism in pump oxygenator systems. J Thorac Cardiovasc Surg 1968;55:691.
223. DeLeval MR, Hill JD, Mielke CH, Macur MF, Gerbode F: Blood platelets and extracorporeal circulation. J Thorac Cardiovasc Surg 1975;69:144.
224. Harding AS, Shakoor MA, Grindon JA: Platelet support for cardiopulmonary bypass surgery. J Thorac Cardiovasc Surg 1975;70:350.
225. Hirsh J: Heparin. N Engl J Med 1991;324:1565.
226. Lim RC, Olcott C, Robinson A, Blaisdell FW. Platelet response and coagulation changes following massive blood replacemnt. J Trauma 1973;13:577.
227. Miller RD, Robbins TO, Tong MJ,. Coagulation defects associated with massive blood transfusions. Ann Surg 1971; 174:794.
228. Perkins HA, Snyder M, Thacher C, Rolfs MR: Calcium ion activity during rapid exchange transfusion with citrated blood. Transfusion 1971;11:204.
229. Valleri CR, Collins FB: Physiologic effects of 2, 3-DPG-depleted red cells with high affinity for oxygen. J Appl Physiol 1971;31:823.
230. Connell RS, Swank RL: Pulmonary microembolism after blood transfusion: An electron microscopic study. Ann Surg 1973;177:40.
231. LaCelle PL: Alteration of deformability of the erythrocyte membrane in stored blood. Transfusion 1969;9:238.
232. Strauss HW, Smith RB, Polimeni P, et al.: Plasma serotonin levels in stored human blood. Angiology 1967;18:535.
233. Czer LSC: Mediastinal bleeding after cardiac surgery: Etiologies, diagnostic considerations, and blood conservation methods. J Cardiothorac Anesth 1989;3:760.
234. Seear MD, Wadsworth LD, Rogers PC, Sheps S, Ashmore PG: The effect of desmopressin acetate (DDAVP) on postoperative blood loss after cardiac operations in children. J Thorac Cardiovasc Surg 1989; 98:217.
235. Frankville DD, Harper GB, Lake CL, Johns RA: Hemodynamic consequences of desmopressin administration after cardiopulmonary bypass. Anesthesiology 1991;74:988.
236. Israels SJ, Kobrinsky NL: Serious reaction to desmopressin in a child with cyanotic heart disease. N Engl J Med 1989;320:1563.
237. Fremes SE, Wong BI, Lee E, et al. Meta-analysis of prophylactic drug treatment in the prevention of postoperative bleeding. Ann Thorac Surg 1994;58.1580.
238. Manno CS, Hedberg KW, Kim HC, et al: Comparison of the hemostatic effects of whole blood, stored whole blood, and components after open heart surgery in children. Blood 1991;77:930.
239. Kwaan JHM, Rappaport I: Postoperative brachial plexus palsy. Arch Surg 1970;101:612.
240. Graham JG, Pye IF, McQueen INF: Brachial plexus injury after median sternotomy. J Neurol Neurosurg Psychiatry 1981;44:621.
241. Kleinman PK, Winchester P, Brill PW: Necrotizing enterocolitis after

open heart surgery employing hypothermia and cardiopulmonary bypass. AJR 1976;127:757.
242. Silane MF, Symchych PS: Necrotizing enterocolitis after cardiac surgery. A local ischemic lesion? Am J Surg 1977;133:373.
243. Ohri SK, Desai JB, Gaer JA, Roussak JB, Hashemi M, Smith PL, Taylor KM: Intraabdominal complications after cardiopulmonary bypass. Ann Thorac Surg 1991;54(4):826.
244. Allen KB, Salam AA, Lumsden AB: Acute mesentric ischemia after cardiopulmonary bypass. J Vasc Sur;16(3):391.
245. Hebra A, Brown MF, Hirschl et al. Mesenteric ischemia in hypoplastic left heart syndrome. J Pediatrics 1993;28:606.
246. Lockey E, McIntyre N, Ross DN, Brookes EWA, Sturridge MF: Early jaundice after open-heart surgery. Thorax 1967;22:165.
247. Sanderson RG, Ellison JH, Benson JA Jr., Starr A: Jaundice following open-heart surgery. Ann Surg 1967;65:217.
248. Chu CM, Chang CH, Liaw YF, Hsieh MJ: Jaundice after open heart surgery: A prospective study. Thorax 1984;39:52.
249. Jenkins JG, Lynn AM, Wood AE, Trusler GA, Barker GA: Acute hepatic failure following cardiac operation in children. J Thorac Cardiovasc Surg 1982;84:865.
250. Hill DM, Warren SE, Mitas JA, Swerdlin AHR: Hepatic coma after open heart surgery. South Med J 1980;73:906.
251. Nunes G, Blaisdell W, Margaretten W: Mechanism of hepatic dysfunction following shock and trauma. Arch Surg 1970;100:546.
252. Arcidi JM Jr., Moore GW, Hutchins GM: Hepatic morphology in cardiac dysfunction. Am J Pathol 1981;104:159.
253. Sherlock S: The liver in heart failure: Relation of anatomical functional and circulatory changes Br Heart J 1951;13:273.
254. Ellenberg M, Osserman KE: The role of shock in the production of central liver cell necrosis. Am J Med 1951;11:170.
255. Clark WTW: Centrilobular hepatic necrosis following cardiac infarction. Am J Pathol 1950;26:249.
256. Rogers EL, Rogers MC: Fulminant hepatic failure and hepatic encephalopathy. Pediatr Clin North Am 1980;27:701.
257. Moddie DS, Feldt RH, Wallace RB: Transient protein-losing enteropathy secondary to elevated caval pressures and caval obstruction after the Mustard procedure. J Thorac Cardiovasc Surg 1976;72:379.
258. Culliford AT, Cunningham JN Jr., Zeff RH, Isom WE, Tieko P, Spencer FC: Sternal and costochondral infections following open-heart surgery. J Thorac Cardiovasc Surg 1974;72:714.
259. Bryant LR, Spencer FC, Trinkle JK: Treatment of median sternotomy infection by mediastinal irrigation with an antibiotic solution. Ann Surg 1969;169:914.
260. Engelmann RM, Williams CD, Gouge TH, et al.: Mediastinitis following open heart surgery. Review of two year experience. Arch Surg 1973;107:772.
261. Barois A, Grosbuis S, Simon N, et al.: Treatment of mediastinitis in children after cardiac surgery. Intensive Care Med 1978;4:35.
262. Jimenez-Martinez M, Arguero-Sanchez R, Perez-Alvarez JJ, Mina-Castaneda P: Anterior mediastinitis as a complication of median sternotomy incisions. Diagnosis and surgical considerations. Surgery 1970;67:929.
263. Thurer RJ, Bognolo D, Vargas A, Isch JH, Kaiser GA: The management of mediastinal infection following cardiac surgery. J Thorac Cardiovasc Surg 1974;68:962.
264. Paloheimo JA, Von Essen R, Klemola E, Kaariainen L, Siltanen P: Subclinical cytomegalovirus infections and cytomeglavirus mononucleosis after open heart surgery. Am J Cardiol 1968;22:624.
265. Salo M: Effect of anaesthesia and open heart surgery on lymphocyte responses to phytohaemagglutinin and concanavalin A. Acta Anaesthesiol Scan 1978;22:471.
266. Ryhanen P, Herva E, Hollmen A, Nuutinen L, Pihlajaniemi R, Saarela E: Changes in peripheral blood leukocyte counts, lymphocyte subpopulations and in vitro transformation after heart valve replacement. Effect of oxygenator type and postoperative parenteral nutrition. J Thorac Cardiovasc Surg 1979;77:259.
267. Salo M, Soppe E, Lassila O, Ruuskanen O: Suppressor lymphocytes during open heart surgery. J Clin Lab Immunol 1981;5:159.
268. Goodwin JS, Webb DR: Regulation of the immune response by prostaglandins. Clin Immunol Immunopathol 1980;15:106.
269. Velangi SV, Taskar SP: Preoperative and postoperative changes in immunoglobulin levels in open heart surgery. Indian J Med Res 1981;73:280.
270. Parker DJ, Cantrell JW, Karp RB, Stroud RM, Digerness SB: Changes in serum complement and immunoglobulins following cardiopulmonary bypass. Surgery 1972;72:824.
271. Del Nido PJ, Williams WG, Cole JG, Trusler GA, Freedom RM: Closed heart surgery for congenital heart disease in infancy. Clin Perinatol 1988;15:681.
272. Potts WJ, Smith S, Gibson S: Anastomosis of the aorta to a pulmonary heart: certain types in congenital heart disease. JAMA 1946;132:627.
273. Ebert PA: Past, present, and future of palliative shunts. Adv Cardiol 1979;26:127.
274. Waterston DJ: Treatment of Fallot's tetralogy in children under one year of age. Rozhl Chir 1962;4:184.
275. Blalock A, Taussig HB: The surgical treatment of malformation of the heart in which there is pulmonary stenosis or pulmonary atresia. JAMA 1945;128:189.
276. Taussig HB, Croecetti A, Eshaghpour E, et al.: Long-time observations on the Blalock-Taussig operation. I. Results of first operation. Hopkins Med J 1971;129:243.
277. Webb WR, Burford TB: Gangrene of the arm following use of the subclavian artery in pulmonosystemic (Blalock) anastomosis. J Thorac Cardiovasc Surg 1952;23:199.
278. Mears AJ, Deverall PB, Kester RC: Revascularization of an arm for incipient gangrene after Blalock-Taussig anastomosis. Br J Surg 1978;65:467.
279. Currarino G, Engle MA: The effects of ligation of the subclavian artery on the bones and soft tissues of the arms. J Pediatr 1965;67:808.
280. Skrovanek J, Goetzova J, Samenek M: Changes in muscle blood flow and development of the arm following the Blalock-Taussig anastomosis. Cardiology 1975;61:131.
281. DeLeval Mr, McKay R, Jones M, et al: Modified Blalock-Taussig shunt. J Thorac Cardiovasc Surg 1981;81:112.
282. Amato JJ, Marbey ML, Bush C, Galdieri RJ, Cotroneo, Bushong J: Systemic-pulmonary polytetrafluoroethylene shunts in palliative operations for congenital heart disease. revival of the central shunt. J Thorac Cardiovasc Surg 1988;95:62.
283. Bove EL, Kohman L, Sereika S, et al.: The modified Blalock-Taussig shunt: analysis of adequacy and duration of palliation. Circulation 1987;76:III19–23.
284. LeBlanc J, Albus R, Williams WG, et al.: Serous fluid leakage: A complication following the modified Blalock-Taussig shunt. J Thorac Cardiovasc Surg 1984;88:259.
285. Damus PS: Seroma formation after implantation of GORE-TEX vascular grafts in cyanotic children. J Thorac Cardiovasc Surg 1984;88:310.
286. Lin AE, DiSessa TG, Williams RG: Balloon and blade atrial septostomy facilitated by two dimensional echocardiography. Am J Cardiol 1986;57:273.
287. Rashkind WJ: The complications of the balloon atrioseptostomy. J Pediatr 1970;76:649.
288. Ehmke DA, Durnin RE, Lauer RM: Intra-abdominal hemorrhage complicating a balloon atrial septostomy for transposition of the great arteries. Pediatrics 1970;45:289.
289. Blalock A, Hanlon CR: The surgical treatment of complete transposition of the aorta and the pulmonary artery. Surg Gynecol Obstet 1950;90:1.
290. Moene RJ, Roos JP, Eygelaar A: Cardiac arrhythmias following the creation of an atrial septal defect in patients with transposition of the great arteries. Thorax 1973;28:147.
291. Muller WH, Dammann JF: The treatment of certain congenital malformations of the heart by the creation of pulmonic stenosis to reduce pulmonary hypertension and excessive pulmonary blood flow. Surg Gynecol Obstet 1952;95:213.
292. Van Nooten G, Deuvart FE, De Paepe J, Primo G: Pulmonary artery banding: Experience with 69 patients. J Cardiovasc Surg 1989; 30:334.
293. Borow KM, Karp R: Atrial septal defect-lessons from the past, directions for the future. N Engl J Med 1990;323:1698.
294. Moss AJ, Siassi B: The small atrial septal defect-operate or procrastinate. J Pediatr 1971;79:854.
295. Sealy WC, Farmer JC, Young WG, Brown IW: Atrial dysrhythmia and atrial secundum defects. J Thorac Cardiovasc Surg 1969;57:245.
296. Young D: Later results of closure of secundum atrial septal defect in children. Am J Cardiol 1973;31:14.
297. Kyger ER, Frazier OH, Cooley DA, et al.: Sinus venous atrial septal defect: Early and late results following closure in 109 patients. Ann Thorac Surg 1978;25:44.
298. Beyer J: Atrial septal defect: Acute left heart failure after surgical closure. Ann Thorac Surg 1978;25:36.
299. Popio KA, Gorlin R, Reichholz LE, et al.: Abnormalities of left ventricular function and geometry in adults with an atrial septal defect. Am J Cardiol 1975;36:302.
300. Lloyd TR. Rao PS. Beekman RH, Mendelsohn AM, Sidiris EB. Atrial

septal defect occlusion with the buttoned device (a multi-institutional U.S. trial). Am J Cardiol 1994;73:286.
301. Rome JJ, Keane JF, Perry SB, Spevak PJ, Lock JE. Double-umbrella closure of atrial defects: initial clinical applications. Circulation 1990;82:751.
302. Fox LS: Optimal management of patients with complete atrioventricular septal defect. Clin Cardiol 1989;:12:145.
303. Urban AE: Total correction of complete atrioventricular canal: Surgical technique and analysis of long-term results. Prog Pediatr Surg 1990;25:18.
304. Midgley FM, Galioto FM, Shapiro SR, Perry LW, Scott LP: Experience with repair of complete atrioventricular canal. Ann Thorac Surg 1980;30:151.
305. Haworth SG: Pulmonary vascular disease in ventricular septal defect: Structural and functional correlations in lung biopsies from 85 patients, with outcome of intra-cardiac repair. J Path 1987;152:157.
306. Cullen M, Splittgerber F, Sweezer W, Hakimi M, Arciniegas E, Klein M: Pulmonary hypertension postventricular septal defect repair treated by extracorporeal membrane oxygenation. J Pediatr Surg 1986; 21:675.
307. Prielipp RC, Rosenthal MH, Pearl RG: Hemodynamic profiles of prostaglandin E_1, isoproterenol, prostacyclin, and nifedipine in vasoconstrictor pulmonary hypertension in sheep. Anesth Analg 1988;67:722.
308. Bridges ND, Perry SB, Keane JF, et al: Preoperative transcatheter closure of congenital muscular ventricular septal defects. N Eng J Med 1991;324:1312.
309. Lillehei CS, Cohen M, Warden HE, et al.: Direct vision intracardiac surgical correction of the tetralogy of Fallot, pentalogy of Fallot, and pulmonary atresia defects: report of first ten cases. Ann Surg 1955;142:418.
310. Pacifico AD, Bargeron LM, Kirklin JW: Primary total correction of tetralogy of Fallot in children less than four years of age. Circulation 1973;68:1085.
311. Cooley, DA: In: Techniques in cardiac surgery: Total correction of tetralogy of Fallot. second edition, WB Saunders, Philadelphia 1984:133.
312. Zimmerman HA, Martins DG, Oliveria J, Nogueira C, Mendelsohn D, Kay EB: The electrocardiogram in open heart surgery: Disturbances in right ventricular conduction. J Thorac Cardiovasc Surg 1958;36:12.
313. Gelband H, Waldo AL, Kaiser GA, Bowman FO, Malm JR, Hoffman BF: Etiology of right bundle-branch block in patients undergoing total correction of tetralogy of Fallot. Circulation 1971;64:1022.
314. Wolff GS, Rowland TW, Ellison RC: Surgically induced right bundle-branch block with left anterior hemiblock: An ominous sign in postoperative tetralogy of Fallot. Circulation 1972;51:1026.
315. James FW. Kaplan S, Chou T: Unexpected cardiac arrest in patients after surgical correction of tetralogy of Fallot: Circulation. 1975;52:691.
316. Quattlebaum TG, Varghese J, Neill CA, Donahoo JS: Sudden death among postoperative patients with tetralogy of Fallot: A follow-up study of 243 patients for an average of twelve years. Circulation 1976;54:289.
317. Zahka KG, Horneffer PJ, Rowe SA, et al: Long-term valvular function after total repair of tetralogy of fallot: relation to ventricular arrhythmias. Circulation 1988;78(Suppl III):III14.
318. Chandar JS, Wolff GS, Garson A Jr, et al: Ventricular arrhythmias in postoperative tetralogy of Fallot. Am J Cardiol 1990;65:655.
319. Jonas RA, Lang P: Open repair of cardiac defects in neonates and young infants. Clin Perinatol 1988;15:659.
320. Kirklin JK: The postperfusion syndrome: Inflammation and the damaging effects of cardiopulmonary bypass. In: Tinker JH (ed) Cardiopulmonary bypass: Current concepts and controversies. A society of cardiovascular anesthesiologists monograph. WB Saunders, Philadelphia 1989:131.
321. Bostrom MP, Hutchins GM: Arrested rotation of the outflow tract may explain double-outlet right ventricle. Circulation 1988;77:1258.
322. Taussig HB, Bing RJ: Complete transposition of the aorta and the levoposition of the pulmonary artery: clinical physiological, and pathological findings. Am Heart J 1949;37:155.
323. McGoon DC: Origin of both great vessels from the right ventricle. Surg Clin North Am 1961;41:1117.
324. Pacifico AD, Kirklin JW, Bargeron LM: Complex congenital malformations: surgical treatment of double-outlet right ventricle and double-outlet left ventricle, in Kirklin JW (ed): Advances in Cardiovascular Surgery. Grune and Stratton, London 1973;57.
325. Brawn WJ: Early results for anatomic correction of transposition of the great arteries and for double-outlet right ventricle with subpulmonary ventricular septal defect. J Thorac Cardiovasc Surg 1988;95:230.
326. Musumeci F, Shumway S, Lincoln C, Anderson RH: Surgical treatment for double-outlet right ventricle at the Brompton Hospital, 1973–1986. J Thorac Cardiovasc Surg 1988;96:278.
327. Shen WK, Holmes DR Jr, Porter CJ, McGoon DC, Ilstrup DM: Sudden death after repair of double-outlet right ventricle. Circulation 1990; 81:128–36.
328. Norwood WI, Kirklin JK, Sanders SP. Hypoplastic left heart syndrome: experience with palliative surgery. Am J Cardiol. 1980;45:87.
329. Norwood WI, Lang P, Hansen DD: Physiologic repair of hypoplastic left heart syndrome. N Engl J Med 308:23, 1983.
330. Pigott JD, Murphy JD, Barber G, Norwood WI. Palliative reconstructive surgery for hypoplastic left heart syndrome. Ann Thorac Surg 1988;45:122.
331. Farrell PE, Chang AC, Murdison KA, et al: Outcome and assessment after the modified fontan procedure for hypoplastic left heart syndrome. Circulation 1992;85:116.
332. Jacobs ML, Norwood WI. Fontan operation: influence of modifications on morbidity and mortality. Ann Thorac Surg 1994; 58:945.
333. Monro JL, Bunton RW, Sutherland GR, Keeton BR: Correction of interrupted aortic arch. J Thorac Cardiovasc Surg 1989;98:421.
334. Zimer G, Jonas RA, Perry SB, Freed MD, Castaneda AR: Surgery for coarction of the aorta in the neonate. Circulation 1986;74 (Suppl 1):I25.
335. Kron IL, Flanagan TL, Rheuban KS, et al.: Incidence and risk of reintervention after coarctation repair. Ann Thorac Surg 1990;49:920.
336. Van Son JA, Daniels O, Vincent JG, Van Lier HJ, Lacquet LF. Appraisal of resection and end-to-end anastomosis for repair of coartcatation of the aorta in infancy: preference for resection: Ann Thorac Surg 1989;48:496.
337. Shenberger JS, Prophet SA, Waldhausen JA, Davidson WR Jr., Sinoway LI: Left subclavian flap aortoplasty for coarctation of the aorta: Effects on forearm vascular function and growth. J Am Coll Cardiol 1989;14:953.
338. Del Nido PJ, Williams WG, Wilson GJ, et al.: Synthetic patch angioplasty for repair of coarctation of the aorta: Experience with aneurysm formation. Circulation 1986;74(Suppl 1):I32.
339. Wilkinson C, Clark H: Refractory hypertension during coarctectomy. Anesthesiology 1982;57:540.
340. Brewer LA, Fosburg RG, Mulder GA, Berska JJ: Spinal cord complications following surgery for coarctation of the aorta: A study of 66 cases. J Thorac Cardiovasc Surg 1972;64:368.
341. Bojar RM, Weiner B, Cleveland RJ. Intravenous labetolol for the control of hypertension following repair of coarctation of the Clin Cardiol 1988:11;639.
342. Gidding SS, Rocchini AP, Beekman R, et al.: Therapeutic effect of propranolol on paradoxical hypertension after repair of coarctation of the aorta. N Engl J Med 1985;312:1224.
343. Choy M, Rocchini AP, Beekman RH, et al : Paradoxical hypertension after repair of coarctation of the aorta in children: balloon angioplasty versus surgical repair. Circulation 1987:75;1186.
344. Liberthson RR: Aortic stenosis. In: Congenital heart disease: Diagnosis and management in children and adults. Little, Brown and Company, Boston 1989:17.
345. Ross DN. Replacement of aortic and mitral valves with a pulmonary autograft. Lancet 1967;2:956.
346. Kouchoukos NT, Davila-Roman VG, Spray TL, Murphy SF, Perrillo JB: Replacement of the aortic root with a pulmonary autograft in children and young adults with aortic-valve disease. N Engl J Med 1994;330:1.
347. Elkins RC, Knott-Craig CJ, Ward KE, Lane MM. Pulmonary autograft in children: realized growth potential. Ann Thorac Surg 1994; 57:1387.
348. Merrill WH, Shuman TA, Graham TP Jr., Hammon JW Jr., Bender HW Jr.: Surgical intervention in neonates with critical pulmonary stenosis. Ann Surg 1987;205:712.
349. Caspi J, Coles JG, Benson LN, et al.: Management of neonatal critical pulmonic stenosis in the balloon valvotomy era. Ann Thorac Surg 1990;49:273.
350. Millikan JS, Puga FJ, Danielson GK, Schaff HV, Julsrud PR, Mair DD: Staged surgical repair of pulmonary atresia, ventricular septal defect, and hypoplastic, confluent pulmonary arteries. J Thorac Cardiovasc Surg 1986;91:818.
351. Oxnard SC, McGough, Jung AL, Ruttenberg HD: Ligation of the patent ductus arteriosus in the newborn intensive care unit. Ann Thorac Surg 1977;23:564.
352. Coster DD, Gorton ME, Grooters RK, Thieman KC, Schneider RF, Soltanzadeh H: Surgical closure of the patent ductus arteriosus in the neonatal intensive care unit. Ann Thorac Surg 1989;48:386.

353. Mavroudis C, Coo LN, Fleischaker JW, et al.: Management of patent ductus arteriosus in the premature infant: Indomethacin versus ligation. Ann Thorac Surg 1983;36:561.
354. Palder SB, Schwartz MZ, Tyson KRT, Marr CC: Management of patent ductus arteriosus: A comparison of operative vs. pharmacologic treatment. J Pediatr Surg 1987;22:1171.
355. Fan LL, Campbell DN, Clarke DR, Washington RL, Fix EJ, White CW: Paralyzed left vocal cord associated with ligation of patent ductus arteriosus. J Thorac Cardiovasc Surg 1989;98:611.
356. Latson LA, Hofschire PJ, Kugler JD, Cheatham JP, Gumbiner CH, Danford DA: Transcatheter closure of patent ductus arteriosus in pediatric patients. J Pediatr 1989;115:549.
357. Bove EL, Beekman RH, Snider AR: Arterial repair for transposition of the great arteries and large ventricular septal defect in early infancy. Circulation 1988;78(Suppl III):III26.
358. Aghaji MAC, Litwin SB: Results of Mustard's repair for dextro-transposition of the great arteries. Cardiovasc Surg 1990;31:7.
359. Helbing WA, Hansen B, Ottenkamp J, Rohmer J, Chin JG, Brom AG, Quaegebeur JM: Long-term results of atrial correction for transposition of the great arteries. Comparison of mustard and senning operations. J Thorac Cardiovasc Surg 1994;108(2):363–72.
360. Myridakis DJ, Ehlers KH, Engle MA: Late follow-up after venous switch operation (mustard procedure) for simple and complex transposition of the great arteries. Am J Cardiol 1994;74(10):1030–6.
361. Williams WG, Trusler GA, Kirklin JW, et al.: Early and late results of a protocol for simple transposition leading to an atrial switch (Mustard) repair. J Thorac Cardiovasc Surg 1988;95:717.
362. Di Donato Rm, Fujii AM, Jonas RA, Casteneda AR: Age-dependent ventricular response to pressure overload. Considerations for the arterial with operation. J Thorac Cardiovasc Surg 1992;104(3):713–22.
363. Alexander JA, Knauf DG, Greene MA, van Miercop LH, O'Brien DJ: The changing strategies in operation for transposition of the great vessels. Annals Thorac Surg 1994;58(4):1278–81.
364. Jonas RA, Giglia TM, Sanders SP, et al.: Rapid, two-stage arterial switch for transposition of the great arteries and intact ventricular septum beyond the neonatal period. Circulation 1989;80:I203.
365. Davis AM, Wilkinson JL, Karl TR, Mee RB: Transposition of the great arteries with intact ventricular septum. Arterial switch repair in patients 21 days of age or older. J Thorac Cardiovasc Surg 1993;106(1): 111–5.
366. Boutin C, Jonas RA, Sanders SP, Wernovsky G, Mone SM, Colan SD: Rapid two-stage arterial switch operation. Acquisition of left ventricular mass after pulmonary artery banding in infants with transposition of the great arteries. Circulation 1994;90:1304–9.
367. Boutin C, Wernovsky G, Sanders SP, Jonas RA, Casteneda AR, Colan SD: Rapid two-stage arterial switch operation. Evaluation of left ventricular systolic mechanics late after an acute pressure overload stimulus in infancy. Circulation 1994;90:1294–303.
368. Mee RBB: Severe right ventricular failure after Mustard or Senning operation: Two-stage repair: Pulmonary artery banding and switch. J Thorac Cardiovasc Surg 1986;92:385.
369. Chang AC, Wernovsky G, Wessel DL, et al.: Surgical management of late right ventricular failure after mustard or Senning repair. Circulation 1992;86(5 Suppl): II140–9.
370. Cochrane AD, Karl TR, Mee RB: Staged conversion to arterial switch for late failure of the systemic right ventricle. Ann Thorac Surg 1993;56(4):854–61.
371. Takada K, Fujita M, Satoh M, et al.: Anesthetic management in the arterial switch "Jatene" operation for transposition of the great arteries. J Cardiothorac Anesth 1987;1:531.
372. Di Donato RM, Wernovsky G, Walsh EP, et al.: Results of the arterial switch operation for transposition of the great arteries with ventricular septal defect. Circulation 1989;80:1689.
373. Hourihan M, Colan SD, Wernovsky G, Mahaeswari U, Mayer JE, Sanders SP: Growth of the aortic anastomosis, annulus and root after the arterial switch procedure performed in infancy. Circulation 1993;88(2): 615–20.
374. Saxena A, Fong LV, Ogilvie BC, Keeton BR: Use of balloon dilatation to treat supravalvar pulmonary stenosis developing after anatomical correction for complete transposition. Br Heart J 1990;64:151.
375. Kirklin JW, Blackstone EH, Tchervenkov CI, et al. Clinical outcomes after the arterial switch operation for transposition. Patient, support, procedural and institutional factors. Circulation 1992:86;1501.
376. Uejima T, Ilbawi MN, Idriss FS: Mustard takedown and arterial switch in a patient with transposition of the great vessels. J Cardiothorac Anesth 1989;3:607.
377. Bink-Boelkens MTE, Bergstra A, Cromme-Dijkhuis AH, Eygelaar A, Landsman MJ, Mooyaart EL: The asymptomatic child a long time after the Mustard operation for transposition of the great arteries. Ann Thorac Surg 1989;47:45.
378. Deanfield J, Camm J, Maccartnet F et al. Arrhythmia and later mortality after Mustard and Senning operation for transposition of the great arteries: an eight-year prospective study. J Thorac Cardiovasc Surg 1988; 3:607.
379. Stellin G, Mazzucco A, Bortolotti U, et al. Tricuspid atresia versus other complex lesions: comparison of results with a modified Fontan procedure. J Thorac Cardiovasc Surg 1988: 96; 204.
380. Fontan F, Baudet E. Surgical repair of tricuspid atresia. Thorax 1971; 26:240.
381. Jonas RA. Indications and timing for the bidirectional Glenn shunt versus the fenestrated Fontan circulation. J Thorac Cardiovasc Surg 199:108:522.
382. Mavroudis C, Zales VR, Backer CL, Muster AJ, Latson. Fenestrated Fontan with delayed catheter closure. Effects of volume loading and baffle fenestration on cardiac index and oxygen delivery. Circulation 1992; 86(5 Suppl):II85–92.
383. Fyman PN, Good man K, Casthely PA, Griepp RB, Ergin MA, Smith P: Anesthetic management of patients undergoing Fontan Procedure. Anesth Analg 1986; 65; 51.
384. Tobias JD, Schleien CL, Reitz BA. Use of the MAST suit in the postoperative care of patients after the Fontan procedure. Crit Care Med 1990;18; 781.
385. Heck DA, Doty DB. Assisted circulation by phasic external lower body compression. Circulation 1981; 64; 118.
386. Sharratt GP, Johnson AM, Monro JL. Persistence and effects of sinus rhythm after Fontan procedure for tricuspid procedure. Br Heart J 1979; 42;74.
387. Case CL, Gillette PC, Zeigler V, Sade RM. Problems with permanent atrial pacing in the Fontan patient. PACE 1989:12; 92.
388. Graham TP, Franklin RCG, Wyse RKH, Gooch V, Deanfield JE. Left ventricular wall stress and contractile function in childhood: normal values and comparison of Fontan versus repair palliation only in tricuspid atresia. Circulation 1986; 74: I161.
389. Girod DA, Fontan F, DeVille C, Ottenkamp J, Choussat A. Long-term results after the Fontan procedure for tricuspid atresia. Circulation 1987;75;605.
390. Myers JL, Waldenhausen JA, Weber HS, et al. A reconsideration of risk factors for the Fontan operation. Ann Surg 1990;211:738.
391. Sano S, Brawn WJ, Mee RBBB. Total anomalous pulmonary venous drainage. J Thoracic Cardiovasc Surg 1989; 97:886.
392. Yee ES, Turley K, Hseih WR, Ebert PA. Infant total anomalous pulmonary venous connection: factors influencing timing of presenation and operative outcome. Circulation 1987;76:III83.
393. Jaumin P, Rubay J, Moulin D. et al. Total anomalous pulmonary venous connection. Long term results following repair under 3 months of age. J Cardiovasc Surg 1989; 30:11.
394. Barnard CN. A human cardiac transplant: an interim report of a successful operation performed at Groote Schuur Hospital, Cape Town. S Afr Med J 1967;41:1271.
395. Cooper DKC. Experimental development of cardiac transplantation. Br Med J 1968;4:174.
396. Kantrowitz A, Haller SD, Joos H, et al. Transplantation of the heart in an infant and an adult. Am J Cardiol 1968;22:782.
397. Cooley, DA, Bloodwell RD, Hallman GL, et al.: Organ transplantation for advanced cardiopulmonary disease. Ann Thorac Surg 1969;8:30.
398. Baum D, Stinson EB, Shumway NE: The place for heart transplantation in children. Pediatric Cardiology 1981;4:741.
399. Younger SJ, Arnold RM et al : Ethical, psychosocial and public policy implications of procuring organs from non-heart-beating cadaver donors. JAMA 1993; 269;2769.
400. Boucek MM, Kanakriyeh MS, Mathis CM, Trimm RF III, Bailey L: Cardiac transplantation in infancy: Donors and recipients. J Pediatr 1990;116:171.
401. Kaye MR: Pediatric Thoracic Transplantation: The World Experience. J Heart Lung Transplant 1993;12:S344.
402. Griepp RB, Stinson EB, Dong E, et al. Determination of operative risk in human heart transplantation. Am J Surg 1971;129.
403. Taquini AC, Fermoso JD, Aramendia P: Behavior of the right ventricle following acute constriction of the pulmonary artery. Circ Res 1960; 8:315.
404. Addonizio LJ, Gersony WM, Robbins RC, et al.: Elevated pulmonary vascular resistance and cardiac transplantation. Circulation 1987; 76[Suppl V]:V52.

405. Zales VR, Pahl E, Backer CL, Crawford S, Mavroudis C, Benson DW: Pharmacologic reduction of pretransplantation pulmonary vascular resistance predicts outcome after pediatric heart transplantation. J Heart Lung Transplant 1993;12:965.
406. Addonizio LJ, Gersony WM, Rose EA: Cardiac transplantation in children with high pulmonary vascular resistance. Am Heart J 1986;112:647.
407. Costard-Jackle A, Fowler MB. Influence of preoperative pulmonary artery pressure on mortality after heart transplantation: testing of potential reversibility of pulmonary hypertension with nitroprusside is useful in defining a high risk group. J Am Coll Cardiol 1992;19:48.
408. Fukushima N, Gundry SR, Razzouk AJ, Bailey LL. Risk factors for graft failure associated with pulmonary hypertension after pediatric transplantation. J Thorac Cardiovasc Surg 1994;107:985.
409. Trento A, Griffith BP, Fricker FJ, Kormos RL, Armitage J, Hardesty RL: Lessons learned in pediatric heart transplantation. Ann Thorac Surg 1989; 48:617.
410. Webber SA, Fricker J, Michaels M, Pickering RM, del Nido PJ, Griffith BP, Armitage JM: Orthotopic heart transplantation in children with congenital heart disease. Ann Thorac Surg 1994;58:1664.
411. Young JN, Yazbeck J, Espositio G, et al.: The influence of acute preoperative pulmonary infarction on the results of heart transplantation. J Heart Transplant 1986;5:20.
412. Fricker FJ, Trento A, Griffith BP. Pediatric cardiac transplantation. Cardiovasc Clin 1990;116:171.
413. Macoviak JA: The perioperative and surgical aspects of heart transplantation. Cardiology Clinics 1990;8:73.
414. Jacobs ML, Williams JF: Pediatric heart transplantation. Cardiology Clinics 1990;8:149.
415. Tweddell JS, Canter CE, Bridges ND, Moorhead S, Huddleston CB, Spray TL. Predictors of operative mortality and morbidity after infant heart transplantation. Ann Thorac Surg 1994:58;972.
416. Lower RR, Shumway NE: Studies on orthotopic transplantation of the canine heart. Surg Forum 1960;11:18.
417. Bailey LL, Assaad AN, Trimm RF, et al.: Orthotopic transplantation during early infancy as therapy for incurable congenital heart disease. Ann Surg 1988; 208:279.
418. Young JB, Leon CA, Short HD, et al.: Evolution of hemodynamics after orthotopic heart and heart-lung transplantation: Early restrictive patterns in occult fashion. J Heart Transplant 1987;6:34.
419. Bhatia SJS, Kirschenbaum J, Shemin RJ, et al.: Time course of resolution of pulmonary hypertension and right ventricular remodeling after orthotopic cardiac transplantation. Circulation 1987;76:819.
420. Ebert PA: The effects of norepinephrine infusion on the denervated heart. Cardiovasc Surg 1968;29:414.
421. Schaal SF, Wallace AG, Sealy WC. Protective influence of cardiac denervation against arrhythmias of myocardial infraction Cardiovasc Res 1969;3;241.
422. Mason JW, Stinson EB, Harrison DC. Autonomic nervous system and arrhythmias: studies in transplanted denervated human hearts. Cardiology 1967:61:75.
423. Alexopulos D, Yusuf S, Bostock J, et al.: Ventricular arrhythmias in long term survivors of orthotopic and heterotopic heart transplantation. Br Heart J 1988;59:648.
424. Uretsky BF: Physiology of the transplanted heart. Cardiovasc Cl 1990; 20:23.
425. Braunlin EA, Canter CE, Olivari MT, Ring WS, Spray TL, Bolman RM: Rejection and infection after pediatric cardiac transplantation. Ann Thorac Surg 1990;49:385.
426. Zales VR, Crawford S, Backer CL, Pahl E, Webb CL, Lynch P, Mavroudis C, Benson DW: Role of endomyocardial biopsy in rejection surveillance after heart transplantation in neonates and children. J Am Coll Cardiol 1994;23:766.
427. Boucek MM, Mathis CM, Boucek RJ, et al.: Serial echocardiographic evaluation of cardiac graft rejection after infant heart transplantation. J Heart Lung Transplant 1993;12: 824.
428. Boucek MM, Mathis CM, Boucek RJ, et al.: Prospective evaluation of echocardiography for primary rejection surveillance after infant heart transplantation: comparison with endomyocardial biopsy. J Heart Lung Transplant 1994; 13: 66–73.
429. Yacoub M, Alivizatos P, Khaghani A, Mitchell A: The use of cyclosporine, azathioprine and antithymocyte globulin with or without low dose steroids for immune suppression of cardiac transplant patients. Transplant Proc 1985;17:221.
430. Armitage JM, Fricker FJ, del Nido P et al.: A decade (1982–1992) of pediatric cardiac transplantation and the impact of FK506 immunosuppression. J Thorac Cardiovasc Surg 1993;105:464.
431. Bailey L, Kahan B, Nehlsen-Cannarella S, Sprent J, Starnes V, Yacoub M: Session V: The neonatal immune system: Window of opportunity? J Heart Lung Transplant 1991;10:II828.
432. Chiavarelli M, Gundry SR, Razzouk AJ, Bailey LL: Cardiac transplantation for infants with hypoplastic left-heart syndrome. JAMA 1993;270:2944.
433. Bailey LL, Gundry SR, Razzouk AJ et al: Bless the babies:One hundred fifteen late survivors of heart transplantation during the first year of life. J Thorac Cardiovasc Surg 1993;105:805.
434. Miller LW. Naftel, Bourge RC et al. Infection after heart transplantation: a multiinstitutional study. J Heart Lung Transplant 1994; 13:381.
435. Myers BD, Ross J, Newton L, et al.: Cyclosporine associated chronic nephropathy. N Engl J Med 1984; 311:699.
436. Farge D, Julien J, Amrein C, et al.: Effect of systemic hypertension on renal function and left ventricular hypertrophy in heart transplant recipients. J Am Coll Cardiol 1990;15:1095.
437. Montero CG, Martinez AJ: Neuropathology of heart transplantation: 23 cases. Neurology 1986;36:1149.
438. Sila CA: Spectrum of neurologic events following cardiac transplantation. Stroke 1989;20:1586.
439. Martin AB, Bricker JT, Fishman M, et al. Neurologic complications of heart transplantation in children. J Heart Lung Transplant 1992; 11:933.
440. Walker RW, Brochstein JA: Neurologic complications of immunosuppressive agents. Neurol Clin 1988;6:261.
441. Angelakos ET, King MP, Millard RW: Regional distribution of catecholamines in the hearts of various species. Ann NY Acad Sci 1969;156:219.
442. Berne RM, Rubio R: Coronary circulation. In: Berne RM (ed), Handbook of physiology, Vol 1. The Heart. Bethesda, Maryland. American Physiological Society 1979:873.
443. Firestone L: Autonomic influences on cardiac function: Lessons from the transplanted (denervated) heart. Int'l Anesth Cl 1989;27:283.
444. Cannon DS, Graham AF, Harrison DC: Electrophysiologic studies in the denervated transplanted human heart; response to atrial pacing and atropine. 1973;32:268.
445. Kontos HA, Thames MD, Lower RR: Responses to electrical and reflex autonomic stimulation in dogs with cardiac transplantation before and after reinnervation. J Thorac Cardiovasc Surg 1970;59:382.
446. Donald DE, Shepherd JT: Sustained capacity for exercise in dogs after complete cardiac denervation. Am J Cardiol 1964;14:853.
447. Convertino VA, Thompson CA, Benjamin BA, et al.: Hemodynamic and ADH responses to central blood volume shifts in cardiac-denervated humans. Cl Physiology 1990;10:55.
448. Vatner DE, Lavallee M, Amano J, Finizola A, Homcy CJ, Vatner SF: Mechanisms of supersensitivity to sympathomimetic amines in the chronically denervated heart of the conscious dog. Circ Res 1985; 57:55.
449. Gilbert EM, Eiswirth CC, Mealey PC, Larrabee P, Herrick CM, Bristow MR. β-adrenergic supersensitivity of the transplanted human heart is presynaptic in origin. Circulation 1989;79:344.
450. Port JD, Skerl L, O'Connell JB, Renlund DG, Larrabee P, Bristow MR. Increased expression of β_2-adrenergic receptors in surgically denervated, previously transplanted human ventricular myocardium. J Am Coll Cardiol 1990;15:84A [Abstract].
451. Goodman DJ, Rossen RM, Cannom DS, Rider AK, Harrison DC: Effect of digoxin on atrioventricular conduction. Circulation 1975;51:251.
452. Leachman RD, Cokkinos DV, Cabrera R, et al.: Response of the transplanted, denervated human heart to cardiovascular drugs. Am J Cardiol 1977;27:272.
453. Mason JW, Winkle RA, Rider AK, Stinson EB, Harrison DC: The electrophysiologic effects of quinidine in the transplanted human heart. J Clin Invest 1977;59:481.
454. Bexton RS, Cory-Pearce R, Spurrell RAJ, et al. Electrophysiological effects of nifedipine and verapamil in the transplanted human heart. Heart Transplant 1984;3:97.
455. Gregg DE, Khouri EM, Donald DE, et al. Coronary circulation in the conscious dog with cardiac neural ablation. Circ Res 1972;31:129.
456. Willman VL, Cooper T, Hanlon CR. Return of neural responses after autotransplantation of the heart. Am J Physiol 1964;207:187.
457. Regitz V, Bossaller C, Strasser R, Schuler S, Hetzer R, Fleck E: Myocardial catecholamine content after heart transplantation. Circulation 1990;82:620.

458. Port JD, Gilbert EM, Larrabee P, et al. Neurotransmitter depletion compromises the ability of indirect acting amines to provide inotropic support in the failing human heart. Circulation 1990;81:929.
459. Rowan RA, Billingham ME. Myocardial innervation in long-term heart transplant survivors: A quantitative ultrastructural survey. J Heart Transplant 1988;7:448.
460. Schroeder JS. Chest pain in heart-transplant recipients. New Engl J Med 1991;321:1805.
461. Stark RP, McGinn AI, Wilson RF. Chest pain in cardiac-transplant recipients: Evidence of sensory reinnervation after cardiac transplantation. New Engl J Med 1991;321:1791.
462. Uretsky BF, Murali S, Reddy PS, et al. Development of coronary artery disease in cardiac transplant patients receiving immunosuppressive therapy with cyclosporine and prednisone. Circulation 1987;76:827.
463. Pahl E, Fricker FJ, Armitage J. Coronary arteriosclerosis in pediatric heart transplant survivors: Limitation of long-term survival. J Pediatr 1990;116:177.
464. Pahl E, Zales VR, Fricker FJ, Addonzia L. Posttransplant coronary artery disease in children: a multicenter national survey. Circulation 1994;90:II56.
465. Gao SZ, Schroeder JS, Hunt S, Stinson EB. Retransplantation for severe accelerated coronary artery disease in heart transplant recipients. Am J Cardiol 1988;62:876.
466. Berry GJ, Rizeq MN, Weiss LM, Billingham ME. Graft coronary disease in pediatric heart and combined heart-lung transplant recipients: a study of fifteen cases. J Heart Lung Transplant 1993;12:S309.
467. Gao SZ, Schroeder JS, Alderman EL, et al. Clinical and laboratory correlates of accelerated coronary artery disease in the cardiac transplant patient. Circulation 1987;76[Suppl V]:V56.
468. McDonald K. Rector EB, Olivari MT. Cytomegalovirus infection in cardiac transplant recipients predicts the incidence of allograft atherosclerosis. J Am Coll Cardiol 1989;13:213A[Abstract].
469. Zimmerman J, Fainaru M, Eisenberg S. The effects of prednisone therapy on plasma lipoproteins and apolipoproteins: a prospective study. Metabolism 1984; 33:521.
470. Kanakriyeh MS, Mullins CE, Parisi F, Petry EL, Bailey LL. Late hemodynamic results after orthotopic heart transplantation in early infancy. Cath Cardiovasc Diagnosis 1989;18:232.
471. Starzl TE, Porter KA, Iwatsuki S, et al. Reversibility of lymphomas and lymphoproliferative lesions developing with cyclosporine-steroid therapy. Lancet 1986;1:583.
472. Penn I. Incidence and treatment of neoplasia after transplantation. J Heart Lung Transplant 1993;12:S328.
473. Chiaverelli M, Boucek MM, Nehlsen-Cannarella SL, Gundry SR, Razzouck AJ, Bailey LL. Neonatal Cardiac Transplantation: Intermediated-term results and incidence of rejection. Arch Surg 1992;127:1072.

Dysrhythmias and Their Management 15

Randall C. Wetzel

INTRODUCTION

In the setting of pediatric critical care medicine the rapid recognition of abnormal heart rates and rhythms is essential. In critically ill children, disorders of cardiac rate and rhythm frequently complicate noncardiac disease processes as well as primarily cause life-threatening conditions. Cardiac dysrhythmias may frequently go unrecognized until the child acutely decompensates and presents either with syncope due to central nervous system (CNS) hypoperfusion or with the signs and symptoms of cardiac failure. In addition, the fact that cardiac output tends to rely more heavily on alterations in heart rate than in stroke volume in the fetus, neonate, and young child than in the adult indicates that the pathologic consequences of alteration in heart rate and rhythm in children differ from those in adults.

Cardiac output is the product of stroke volume and heart rate. The inotropic state of the heart, the end-diastolic volume of the heart (preload), and the myocardial afterload all combine to determine stroke volume. Just as these three factors are interdependent, they are also affected by the timing and sequencing of electrical depolarization of the myocardium, and in several instances, alterations in electrical depolarization affect preload and contractility. In addition, the heart rate and rhythm may also be affected by alterations in myocardial preload and afterload. Clearly, both heart rate and heart rhythm as well as the inotropic state of the heart are simultaneously affected by alterations in autonomic and adrenergic stimulation. During the following discussion of cardiac dysrhythmias, the interrelationship of the determinants of stroke volume and heart rate should be remembered.

In children, heart rates vary over a wide range (Fig. 15.1). As can be seen, heart rate tends to decrease with age, and the range that is considered normal also decreases. Although a heart rate of 100 beats/min is considered a bradycardia in the newborn, in adolescents this heart rate is considered a tachycardia. Whereas in newborns heart rate may be normal in a range between 100 and 200 beats/min, such a wide range of normal does not exist in older children. It should be remembered that in neonates and younger children, very rapid heart rates occur physiologically and should not be confused with abnormal supraventricular tachydysrhythmias. For reasons that have been discussed earlier, it is clear that in infants and small children the cardiac output is rate dependent[1–4] (see Chapter 11, Cardiorespiratory Interactions). In summary, younger children gen-

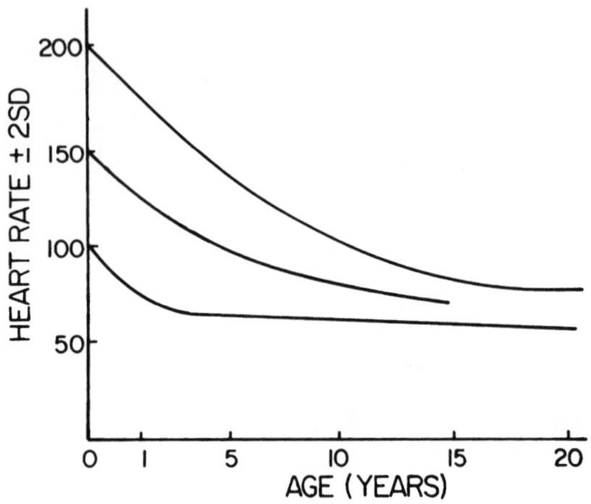

Figure 15.1. Heart rate ± 2 SD versus age. There is wide normal variation in the first year of life. (From Wetzel RC, Rogers MC. Pediatric hemodynamic monitoring. In: Shoemaker WC, Thompson WL, eds. Critical care—state of the art. Fullerton, California: Society of Critical Care Medicine, 1981;2:II[L]8.)

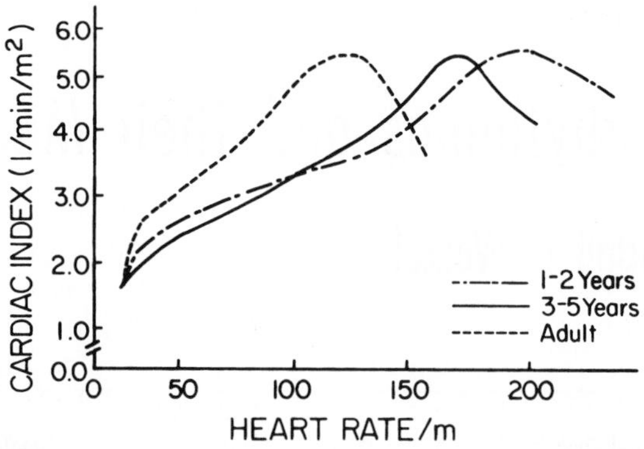

Figure 15.3. This graph demonstrates changes in cardiac index with heart rate for three different age groups. The graph is derived from normative data and illustrates the increased dependence of cardiac output on heart rate in young children. (From Wetzel RC, Rogers MC. Pediatric hemodynamic monitoring. In: Shoemaker WC, Thompson WL, eds. Critical care—state of the art. Fullerton, California: Society of Critical Care Medicine, 1981;2:II[L]9.)

erally respond to stress by increasing heart rate rather than by augmenting stroke volume.

Developmentally, stroke volume increases with age, whereas there is a concurrent decrease in heart rate (Fig. 15.2). As expected, the maximally achievable cardiac index occurs at higher heart rates in younger children than in adults (Fig. 15.3). In critically ill children, an efficacious way of providing maximal cardiac output is by maintaining near-maximal heart rates for age. Whereas the risk of ischemia under these conditions is certainly increased by rapid heart rate, this is of far less concern in children than in adults. In children, the necessary increase in oxygen consumption that follows increased heart rate is readily met by an increase in myocardial oxygen delivery; in adults, cardiovascular disease may critically limit this ability. Despite this, myocardial ischemia during rapid heart rates is occasionally noted in children, and it would be wise to consider myocardial oxygen supply-demand relationships when dealing with tachydysrhythmias in children. Either the pharmacologic or the electrical stimulation directed at increasing heart rate should be considered a means of augmenting cardiac output in low-output states in children. Conversely, from the above discussion it should be apparent that cardiac dysrhythmias would have more detrimental effects on cardiac output in younger children, with a decreased ability to enhance stroke volume, than in older children.

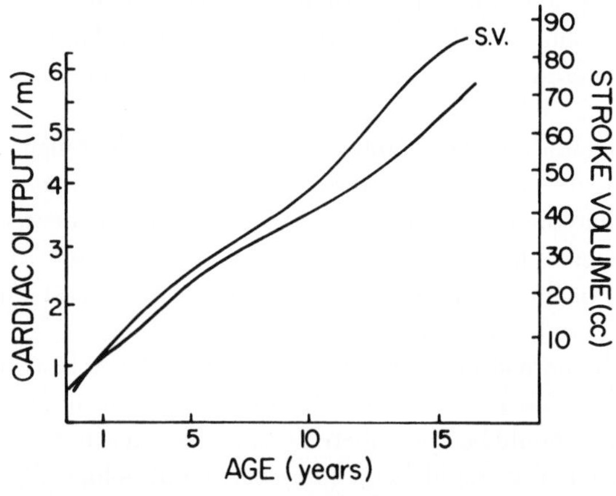

Figure 15.2. Stroke volume and cardiac output versus age derived from normative data. (From Wetzel RC, Rogers MC. Pediatric hemodynamic monitoring. In: Shoemaker WC, Thompson WL, eds. Critical care—state of the art. Fullerton, California: Society of Critical Care Medicine, 1981;2:II[L]9.)

It is the purpose of this chapter to develop the critical care physician's ability to rapidly detect, analyze, and treat the most common and seriously threatening cardiac dysrhythmias that occur in children. It is not intended to be a discussion of the complex cardiac dysrhythmias that are being increasingly reported to occur in childhood. A brief review of the physiology of myocardial depolarization and the symptomatology and diagnosis of cardiac dysrhythmias in children is followed by specific cardiac dysrhythmias and their therapy. In pediatrics, the presence of an underlying structural defect in children who present with a dysrhythmia must always be considered.

PHYSIOLOGY

A basic understanding of the physiology that underlies the generation and conduction of cardiac action potentials is necessary for understanding cardiac dysrhythmias. All myocardial tissues demonstrate characteristic action potentials. Figure 15.4 shows the characteristic action potential of non-Purkinje myocardial muscle cells and the timing with respect to the electrocardiogram (ECG). Phase 0 is the period of rapid depolarization followed by the spike potential, which reaches approximately 40 mV positive and is followed by a brief period of rapid repolarization (phase 1), a plateau (phase 2), and a rapid repolarization (phase 3). Phase 4 is, in general, a steady state of resting negative (approximately −80 mV) membrane potential preceding phase 0. In pacemaker cells the characteristic feature is spontaneous depolarization during phase 4 (automaticity). During diastole, membrane polarization constantly decays, and this automatically gives rise to an action potential (Fig. 15.4). This spontaneous depolarization occurs at different rates in various pacemaker cells throughout the myocardium, and this hierarchy of automaticity is distributed in a characteristic fashion. The sinoatrial node contains the most rapid spontaneously depolarizing cells and thus serves as the cardiac pacemaker. The rate of spontaneous depolarization decreases in order from the sinoatrial node through atrial conducting tissue toward the atrioventricular (AV) node and along the conducting pathways of bundle of His. Normally, the ventricular myocardium demonstrates the slowest spontaneously depolarizing resting membrane potential. The normally generated sinoatrial activity is conducted through the atria to the AV node along the bundle of His through the left and right bundle branches and, via the Purkinje fibers, is distributed throughout the ventricular myocardium. The most rapidly depolarizing group of cells within the myocardium suppresses other sites of spontaneous depolarization (overdrive suppression) and determines the heart rate. In general, this function is performed by the sinoatrial node. In the absence of the rapidly depolarizing sinoatrial node, successively lower areas such as the AV node or the ventricular sites may take over pacemaker function and thus generate an "escape" rhythm. Escape rhythms are defined as those rhythms in which there is sinus node depression, and one of the lower subsidiary sites performs the pacemaker function of the heart[5]. Any of these subsidiary sites

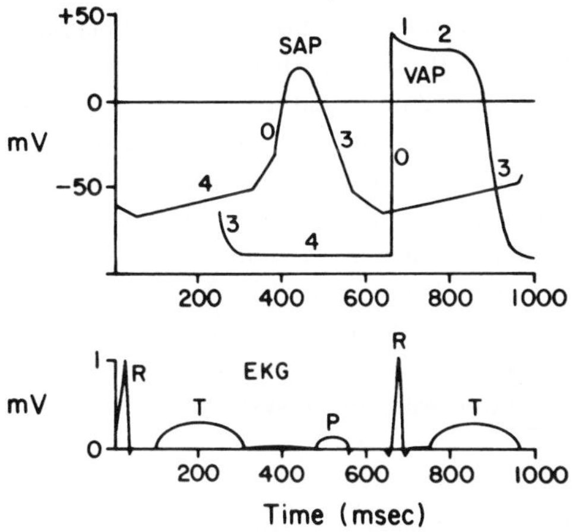

Figure 15.4. Schematic representation of a sinus node action potential *(SAP)*, ventricular myocardial cell action potential *(VAP)*, and ECG *(EKG)*. Note that the SAP undergoes spontaneous depolarization during phase 4, in contrast to the VAP. In addition, there is very little phase 2 plateau in the SAP. The timing of these events should also be noted. Sinoatrial node cells have repolarized before the ventricular myocardium depolarizes. Clearly, another SAP occurring at 625 msec after the first one would be conducted to the ventricular myocardium and would reach it during phase 3 (approximately 300 msec later) when the ventricle is refractory, thus giving the appearance of a nonconducted beat. In addition, it should be noted that sinoatrial depolarization occurs during the T-wave of the preceding QRS when the ventricle is refractory. Alterations in the timing of these events or aberrancies in conduction are a primary cause of arrhythmias.

may increase its intrinsic rate of spontaneous depolarization and lead to tachydysrhythmias, thus giving rise to sinus, nodal, and ventricular tachycardias (VTs). The lack of impulse formation, as may occur in the sick sinus syndrome[6] or blocked or delayed sinoatrial conduction, gives rise to bradydysrhythmias.

Reentry phenomena account for the majority of dysrhythmias, both ventricular and supraventricular. Pathways that conduct at different velocities and that have different repolarization characteristics set the stage for reentry. These heterogeneous pathways may occur congenitally, such as in Wolff-Parkinson-White syndrome (e.g., a bundle of Kent), or be caused by injury (e.g., ischemia, trauma, myocarditis). Theoretically, a slow (α) and a fast (β) pathway can exist. Normally, the impulse is conducted along the β pathway to depolarize the ventricle. When the slower α impulse arrives, the conducting tissue is depolarized. Repolarization is slower in the β pathway, so that a premature beat will find the β pathway blocked and be conducted down the α pathway. It may then find the β pathway able to conduct retrograde, rapidly gaining access (in the event of atrial reentry) to the atria, causing depolarization (atrial echo) and reentering the α pathway initiating the tachydysrhythmia. This is the so-called antegrade slow-retrograde fast variety of reentry. Similar reentry phenomena can occur entirely within the ventricles in the setting of unidirectional block and heterogeneous conduction rates.

Triggered activity arises from after depolarizations of the membrane potential. The low amplitude secondary depolarizations occur during either phase 3 or phase 4 of the normal action potential. Early after depolarizations (EADs) are probably caused by enhanced sodium or calcium ion entry. They occur during acidosis, hyperkalemia, and hypoxia and can be initiated by a variety of antidysrhythmic agents. Delayed after depolarizations (DADs) occur during phase 4 and are caused by excess intracellular calcium as occurs in digoxin toxicity and catechol excess. If an after depolarization achieves activation threshold, it triggers an action potential closely coupled to the first, causing a premature beat. If the after depolarization is also accompanied by a further after depolarization the process is continuous and results in a sustained dysrhythmia.

Cardiac dysrhythmias arise from (a) abnormal or delayed impulse formation at any level in the myocardium, including abnormal automaticity, (b) abnormal or blocked conduction of normal impulse formation, (c) reentry phenomena, and (d) triggered activity (after depolarization) **(Table 15.1).**

Etiology

Many congenital heart diseases are associated with a predilection toward the development of cardiac dysrhythmias. One of the best-known examples of this is the Wolff-Parkinson-White syndrome. Children with this condition are particularly prone to develop supraventricular tachydysrhythmias. Congenital complete heart block also occurs and

Table 15.1. Mechanisms of Arrhythmias

Altered automaticity
Delayed automaticity
Bradydysrhythmias
Escape rhythms
Enhanced automaticity
Atrial ectopic tachycardia
Junctional ectopic tachycardia
Accelerated junctional tachycardia
Accelerated idioventricular tachycardia
Ventricular tachycardia
Conduction block
Sinus node exit block
AV node conduction block
Bundle branch blocks
Reentry
Atrial flutter and fibrillation
Sinus node reentry tachycardia
AV* node reentry tachycardia
Junctional reentry tachycardia
AV reciprocating tachycardia (e.g., WPW)**
Ventricular tachycardia
Triggered activity
Digitalis toxicity
Torsade de pointes
Ventricular tachycardia

**AV, atrioventricular; **WPW, Wolff-Parkinson-White syndrome.*

is associated with structural abnormalities such as Epstein's anomaly, transposition of the great arteries (TGA), and mitral stenosis. Apart from structural abnormalities, congenital complete heart block may also occur in children of mothers with systemic illnesses such as lupus erythematosus; in addition, it may occur familially or idiopathically[7–9]. It is now apparent that the leading cause of congenital complete heart block is maternal connective tissue disease as demonstrated by the presence of anti-Ro (SS-A) antibody[10]. Complete heart block also occurs after surgery for congenital heart disease in children, but it is often transient[11,12]. Another intriguing group of familial cardiac abnormalities is associated with a predilection to sudden, frequently fatal, ventricular dysrhythmias. This group consists of abnormalities of ventricular repolarization as described by Jervell and Lange-Nielsen[13] and James[14] and is associated with deafness and the Romano-Ward autosomal dominant syndrome[15]. These are both characterized by a prolonged Q-T interval. Another member of this group of abnormal ventricular repolarization is manifested by prominent U-waves in association with a short P-R interval, which is also associated with sudden ventricular fibrillation[16].

Cardiac dysrhythmias may complicate a variety of systemic diseases. A most obvious systemic cause of dysrhythmias is disordered serum electrolytes, which may lead to supraventricular bradydysrhythmias or both supraventricular and ventricular tachydysrhythmias. Hyperkalemia is a frequent and, when unrecognized, a fatal cause of ventricular dysrhythmias and should consistently be considered in the intensive care unit (ICU). Because the action potential is determined by ion conductance and ion conduction depends on the environmental ionic concentration, electrolyte abnormalities alter all phases of the action potential. Altered automaticity, the repolarization duration of the plateau phase, and resting membrane potential (Nernst equation) are all altered by electrolyte abnormalities. Hypokalemia increases automaticity, thus precipitating ectopic activity, and prolongs repolarization, giving rise to U-waves and prolonged T-waves and setting the stage for reentry VT (Fig. 15.5). Hyperkalemia decreases phase 0 depolarization, leading to blocked conduction and again facilitating reentry tachydysrhythmias. Hypercalcemia increases phase 2, prolonging the Q-T-wave and leading to VT. In addition, low concentrations of magnesium and phosphorus alter ion conductances and may result in drug-resistant tachycardias. Magnesium supplementation should be considered for resistant rhythm disturbances and is particularly useful for torsade de pointes. Sodium concentration abnormalities have to be quite severe before dysrhythmias occur, and other clinical problems are generally manifested earlier.

In the critical care unit, abnormally slow cardiac rates and, therefore, compromised cardiac output may also occur in conjunction with CNS abnormalities such as elevated intracranial pressure[17]. Friedreich's ataxia and the muscular dystrophies are examples of neuromuscular disorders that are also associated with adverse effects on myocardial rate and rhythm. Other systemic diseases associated with cardiac dysrhythmias include endocrine disorders, collagen vascular diseases, and the glycogen storage diseases. A leading cause of cardiac dysrhythmias in the pediatric ICU and one that should always be considered is drug toxicity. Digitalis, sympathomimetic drugs, β-blockers, aminophylline, barbiturates, tricyclic antidepressants, and many other pharmacologic agents may lead to profound and fatal disturbances in heart rate and rhythm.

Cardiac dysrhythmias that may be associated with acute illnesses that are not of congenital origin are frequently seen in the pediatric ICU. For example, myocardial contusions, which may accompany thoracic trauma, may lead to conduction abnormalities, ventricular dysrhythmias and, most commonly, sinus tachycardia (ST). In addition, ECG abnormalities will suggest predisposition to dysrhythmias and ventricular dysrhythmia may follow acute neurologic injuries[17]. Children with severe systemic infections frequently

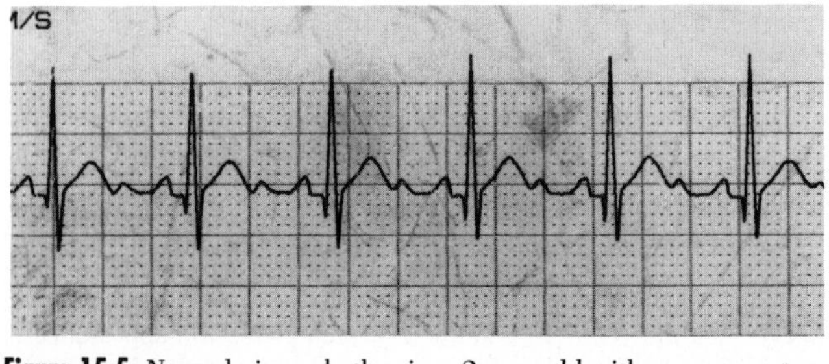

Figure 15.5. Normal sinus rhythm in a 2-year-old with a serum potassium of 2.0 mEq/ml. Note prominent U-wave after each T-wave and the potential for confusing U-waves with P-waves. U-waves resolved with potassium replacement.

have associated cardiac dysrhythmias, and again, ST is the most common. Iatrogenically induced cardiac dysrhythmias may occur in patients in the postanesthetic state or secondary to oncologic chemotherapy and as a result of therapeutic interventions in critically ill children, such as the use of sympathomimetic drugs administered as inotropic agents or the treatment of asthma with theophylline and isoproterenol.

DIAGNOSIS

Cardiac dysrhythmias in children may lead to a wide number of symptoms from the subtle to the bizarre. Children may initially be diagnosed as having seizure disorders, hysteria, or CNS pathology when, in fact, the primary cause is an underlying cardiac dysrhythmia. Symptoms that occur during cardiac dysrhythmias in children result from either acute or subacute decreases in cardiac output. A sudden decrease in cardiac output causes a sudden decrease in cerebral blood flow and can cause a host of symptoms, including abnormal and inappropriate behavior, vertigo, screaming, delirium, and syncope. Less acute changes in cardiac output caused by cardiac dysrhythmias cause symptoms that are associated with cardiac failure, such as pallor, diaphoresis, dyspnea, feeding intolerance, vomiting, and decreased peripheral perfusion, as well as failure to thrive. Although these are the most common presentations of cardiac dysrhythmias in children, it should be remembered that although the situation is rare, children may present with angina due to very fast heart rates, and in infants, this may be manifested by uncontrollable screaming and irritability. In older children, consciously sensed abnormalities in heart rhythm, such as racing hearts or skipped heart beats and angina, may be described and can be quite distressing.

The cornerstone of both evaluation and diagnosis of abnormalities in cardiac rate and rhythm is the ECG. Frequently, the first indication that a child's symptoms are due to underlying cardiac dysrhythmias is the routine electrocardiographic monitoring that is performed in the pediatric ICU. In all critically ill children, as well as those who present with abnormal mental status or sudden loss of consciousness, electrocardiographic monitoring is mandatory. The specific diagnosis of life-threatening abnormalities in cardiac rate and rhythm depends on an understanding of the normal electrocardiographic pattern in children and how it changes at various developmental stages. There are well-defined standards for the developmental alterations in heart rate, P-R interval, QRS duration, and Q-T interval in standard pediatric textbooks[18–20]. A 12-lead ECG is mandatory for all children who are suspected of manifesting disturbances in cardiac rate and rhythm, and even if this appears normal, a continuous recording for several minutes should also be obtained. Traditionally, this rhythm strip is a recording of lead II; however, all leads should be investigated to determine the morphologic characteristics of the P-wave, QRS complex, and T-wave and to delineate their relationships. Frequently, an anterior chest lead, such as V_1 or V_2, is the optimal lead to provide clear-cut morphologic relationships. Identification of all components of the ECG from the onset of the P-wave to the end of the T-wave and of their relationships to each other is the diagnostic basis of all cardiac dysrhythmias. If more prolonged monitoring is required, a Holter-type monitor should be considered. Rarely, for the diagnosis of difficult dysrhythmias, unorthodox positions such as the intracardiac or the transesophageal position for ECG recording may be necessary in the pediatric ICU. Postoperatively, pacing wires can also be used to record ECG patterns to aid in diagnosis.

SPECIFIC DYSRHYTHMIAS

Bradydysrhythmias

Asystole

Asystole is the total absence of ventricular electrical activity. Total absence of ventricular electrical activity may result from either sinoatrial node arrest or complete sinoatrial ventricular conduction blockade. During complete AV blockade, asystole occurs when a subsidiary escape rhythm from either the AV node or the ventricular site fails to occur. Because both the AV and the sinus nodes are under vagal influence, sinoatrial arrest and AV block may occur simultaneously. Fortunately, in most cases of sinoatrial generator arrest, an escape rhythm arises from the AV node or from the ventricles. This escape rhythm may or may not provide adequate hemodynamic function and generally indicates a need for therapy. Obviously, total asystole is fatal, and its therapy is the same as that outlined for cardiac arrest (Chapter 2, Emergency Management of the Upper Airway). Asystole occurs in the setting of severe myocardial damage and is the final stage after multiple severe systemic injury. Hypoxia, ischemia, direct myocardial injury, and severe electrolyte abnormalities are the major underlying causes of asystole.

Sinus Bradycardia

Sinus bradydysrhythmias may occur from either abnormally slow generator potential from the sinus node, the total absence of sinoatrial generator potential, or conduction failure of this potential. Bradydysrhythmias may occur either with or without escape rhythms from subsidiary sites. The term *bradycardia* refers to the ventricular rate, and bradydysrhythmias other than sinus bradycardia are due to failure of subsidiary sites to serve as adequate pacemakers. In these rhythms the frequency of QRS complexes is abnormally slow for either the patient's age or the clinical setting. For example, a sinus rate of 75 beats/min in an 18-month-old after cardiac surgery is abnormally slow, whereas in a sleeping child of the same age, this heart rate would be normal. A guide to the normal lower limit of heart rate in awake children is the following: 60 for children over the age of 5 years, 80 for children up to the age of 5 years, 100 for children in the first year of life, and 95 for children in the first week of life. During sleep, these limits are below 50 for children age 5 years and above and below 60 for infants. When sinus bradycardia is severe, subsidiary pacemakers may arise. These escape rhythms may be nodal, originating from the AV node, and are frequently differentiated into high, medium, or low by the morphology and timing of the P-wave with respect to the QRS complex. Frequently, these P-waves show an abnormal axis, and they are often inverted. Most commonly, a junctional escape rhythm shows P-waves positive in lead I and negative in aVF. If, in addition, the P-wave occurs before the QRS complex, it is low atrial or high nodal in origin. P-waves occurring either within or after QRS complex indicate that these are truly junctional escape rhythms in nature. Of course, idioventricular rhythms may also occur, and their QRS complexes may be morphologically identical with a premature ventricular contraction (PVC); however, they may also occur with a regular QRS pattern.

Sick Sinus Syndrome

Sick sinus syndrome may be caused by either a congenital abnormality or a direct injury to the sinus node and results in decreased sinus impulse formation or the inability of the generator potential to exit the sinus node (sinus exit block). In children, these most frequently occur after surgery, especially after the Mustard procedure for correction of TGA[21]. Sick sinus syndrome may also result from cardiomyopathies, ischemia, or myocarditis[22,23].

The electrocardiographic manifestations of sick sinus syndrome are varied and may include periods of sinus arrest and profound, unresponsive sinus bradycardia, with or without the occurrence of escape rhythms from subsidiary pacemakers. These escape rhythms may be quite varied and may be nodal or ventricular in origin, giving rise to tachydysrhythmias and, hence, the name bradycardia-tachycardia syndrome. Occasionally, atrial fibrillation occurs. Patients with sick sinus syndrome may present with either Stokes-Adams attacks or profound bradycardia and hypoperfusion. The diagnosis of sick sinus syndrome requires recognition of the characteristics and ECG abnormalities, such as sinus bradycardia and sinus arrest, or the concurrence of bradycardia and tachycardia in the same patient, in the appropriate clinical setting. Absolute diagnosis generally requires intracardiac ECG measurement of sinoatrial conduction and sinoatrial recovery times after pacing[24]. Patients with sick sinus syndrome who become symptomatic almost always require permanent intracardiac pacemaking.

Bradycardia frequently occurs in the clinical situation of increased vagal tone. In the ICU this is frequently associated with pharyngeal stimulation from, for example, nasogastric or endotracheal tube suctioning, elevated intracranial pressure, elevated blood pressure, abdominal distention, and increased intraocular pressure. In addition, metabolic derangements such as hypoglycemia, hypothermia, hypoxia, acidosis, and hypercalcemia are also causes of acute bradycardia. Drug toxicity from, for example, digitalis or propranolol may also be a contributing factor. In addition to these general conditions, direct myocardial trauma, which may occur in multiple trauma but more commonly occurs after surgery, is also a leading cause of bradycardia. Because escape rhythms frequently occur during bradycardias, it should be remembered that the clinical setting defined above is also the clinical setting in which escape rhythms are seen. The treatment of escape rhythms is directed at correcting the primary, underlying rhythm disturbance that allows the escape rhythm to develop.

Conduction Abnormalities

Bradycardias also arise from conduction abnormalities between the normally generated sinoatrial action potential and the ventricles. This AV conduction delay or block results in an inordinately slow ventricular rate and decreased cardiac output or hemodynamically unstable escape rhythms. Conduction interference occurs in a broad spectrum including first-, second- and third-degree AV block. Recognition of AV conduction delay and complete AV nodal block are important because they may herald the catastrophic deterioration of cardiac rhythm with total loss of ventricular contraction. Identification of these serves as a clue to underlying causes of syncopal episodes **(Table 15.2).** This conduction blockade may occur at any level and may be within the atrium, the AV node itself, the bundle of His, or any of the bundle branches.

First-degree AV block occurs when all sinus impulses are conducted, but with delay, as indicated by a prolonged P-R interval. The rhythm is regular with normal QRS morphology. Developmental standards for the normal duration of the P-R interval exist and need to be referred to for exact diagnosis; however, conduction times greater than 0.20 second in children should always raise suspicion. A P-R interval that is greater than 0.14 second in infants, greater than 0.16 second in children, and greater than 0.18 second in adolescents is abnormally prolonged.

Second-degree AV block is associated with failure of conduction of some, but not all, atrial beats to the ventricles and is divided into Mobitz type I and Mobitz type II block. Mobitz type I (Wenckebach phenomenon) describes a situation in which the P-R interval becomes progressively longer until eventually the atrial impulse is not conducted and a dropped beat occurs. This may occur over two, three, four, or even five beats before nonconduction happens. Mobitz type I heart block is invariably associated with conduction delay within the AV node[25,26]. Mobitz type II block is recognized by the irregular and intermittent sudden dropping of beats expected to follow P-waves (Fig. 15.6). These are not preceded by progressive P-R prolongation. The QRS morphology may alter. Mobitz type II block is the more ominous abnormality of AV conduction because it frequently progresses to complete AV block. It is generally thought to

Table 15.2. Etiology of AV Conduction Delay or Block

Congenital Heart Disease	
	ASD
	Anomalous veins
	Ebsteini's anomaly
	PDA
Increased Vagal Tone	
	Airway suctioning
	Pain
	Intubation
	Abdominal distention
Electrolytes	
	Hypo or hyperkalemia
	Hypo or hypercalcemia
	Hypoglycemia
	Hypomagnesemia
Drugs	
	β-blockade
	Digoxin
	Amiodarone
	Calcium channel blockers
Hypothermia	
Infections	
	Lyme disease
	Mumps
	Rubella
	Diptheria
	Rocky Mountain Spotted Fever
	Viral myocarditis
	Chagas' disease
	Rheumatic fever
Myopathies	
	Duchenne's muscular dystrophy
	Myotonic dystrophy
	Polio

occur via conduction blockade in the bundle of His or the bundle branches[27]. A subset of type II block is *fixed ratio AV block,* wherein QRS complexes are absent at regular intervals (i.e., 2:1, 3:1 or 4:1). This is less ominous than Mobitz II.

Complete AV block, either congenital or acquired, is the most common bradydysrhythmia in childhood. Complete AV block (third degree) means that there is total lack of conduction between the atria and the ventricles, and its diagnosis depends on the recognition of (a) an abnormally slow QRS rate for a particular age and (b) a regular atrial rhythm but an irregular P-R interval[9,28]. In children, the AV node is the most common site of conduction blockade, and for this reason, escape rhythms, when they do occur, originate from the bundle of His. One would, therefore, expect the QRS pattern to mimic that of normal sinus beats. Clearly, if there is concurrent damage to the conducting tissue of the bundle of His, which may occur during surgery, then the QRS pattern either may be consistent with bundle branch blockade or may resemble a ventricular extrasystole. The remaining criterion for complete AV blockade is complete AV dissociation. For this reason, a nonconducted P-wave should also be identifiable. As the AV node is generally refractory for 300–400 msec, P-waves that occur within 400 msec of the preceding QRS complex are not normally conducted. However, P-waves occurring 500–600 msec after the preceding QRS complex that are not conducted are clearly abnormal. As a guide, the Q-T interval is approximately 400 msec in duration; thus, P-waves occurring during the T-wave that are not conducted are not an indication of AV blockade. However, P-waves that occur after the end of the T-wave that are not conducted may be an indication of AV conduction blockade. Two final points need to be made: total nodal dissociation can occur in the presence of any atrial rhythm, and generally, the ventricular rhythm is slow and regular.

Treatment of Bradydysrhythmias

Hemodynamic compromise manifested by hypotension and hypoperfusion are the indications for therapy of the bradydysrhythmias. In addition, certain dysrhythmias, such as Mobitz type II block, are so highly associated with catastrophic deterioration that therapy may also be indicated. Treatment for all dysrhythmias initially requires correction of hypoxia, acidosis, hyperkalemia or hypokalemia, hypovolemia, hypotension, hypothermia, removal of drugs where appropriate, and treatment of elevated intracranial pressure where indicated. Therefore, oxygenation and ventilation should be ensured and intravascular volume restored. Hyperkalemia should be treated as outlined in **Table 15.3.** Vagolytic medications such as atropine frequently increase heart rate and are the first line of therapy. Thus, this treatment is useful in overriding lower escape rhythms of either junctional or ventricular origin. If atropine is unsuccessful in increasing heart rate, intravenous isoproterenol is often efficacious. Frequently, severely compromised sinus node function, such as occurs in sick sinus syndrome, is refractory to such therapy. If sinus bradycardia persists and is

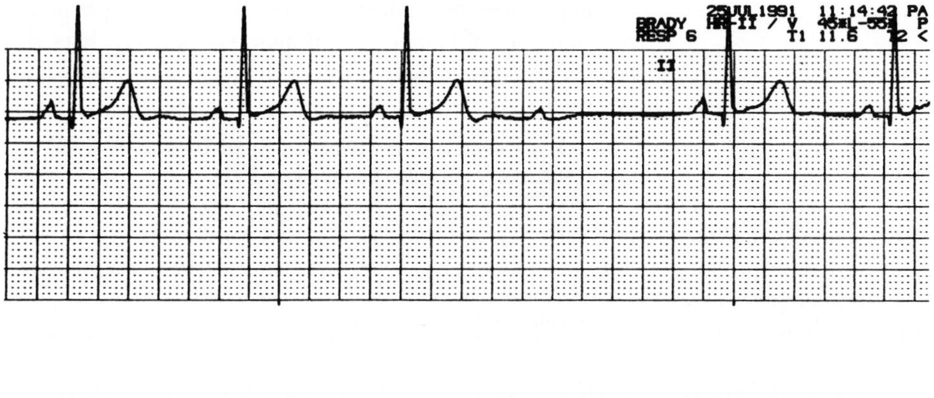

Figure 15.6. Mobitz type II second-degree heart block. Note the sinus rhythm with a regularly timed P-wave and no QRS.

Table 15.3. Treatment of Hyperkalemia

Remove all potassium from all intravenous (IV) solutions
Calcium chloride 10 mg/kg IV, or
Calcium gluconate 30 mg/kg slowly
Sodium bicarbonate 1 mEq/kg IV
clear calcium from the line first
5% dextrose 1–2 ml/kg/hr IV
Insulin 0.1 unit/kg/hr, check glucose
Kayexalate 1–2 gm/kg orally or rectally

associated with hemodynamic compromise, cardiac pacing is indicated.

The emergent treatment of bradycardias associated with conduction delay and blockade also follows the same approximate schema. Although atropine is frequently used initially, it is often unsuccessful. Isoproterenol or even epinephrine may be required for conduction delay and may provide sufficient time for either transvenous or transthoracic pacemaking to be instituted. If hemodynamic compromise is associated with conduction delay, the possibility of providing temporary or permanent electrical cardiac pacemaking should be strongly considered. Obviously, cardiac pacemaking must be at the ventricular level in AV conduction defects. Ventricular pacemaking can be provided through a number of techniques. Whenever the threat of AV conduction delay occurs or sinoatrial node dysfunction can be expected, such as after surgery on the atrium or ventricular septum, ventricular pacing wires should be placed on the ventricle for several days after surgery. In the absence of ventricular pacing wires, transvenous balloon-tipped, flow-directed pacing catheters may be passed with electrocardiographic and pressure monitoring in the absence of fluoroscopic guidance and can provide ventricular pacemaking. Transcutaneous pacing may be effective when available. Transthoracic pacing can also be performed during acute circulatory failure and cardiac arrest from complete AV block[29]. A newer approach to ventricular pacing is transesophageal pacing; however, this approach is inappropriate in the presence of AV conduction delay[30]. The duration of pacemaking after the acute onset of AV conduction delay is a matter of concern. Frequently, normal conduction may be expected to return in 1–2 weeks. After 2 weeks, however, if AV conduction has not returned to normal, permanent cardiac pacemaking will probably be required[29,31]. Pacemaker use is described below.

Tachydysrhythmias

Atrial Extrasystoles and Tachydysrhythmias

Atrial extrasystoles frequently occur in healthy individuals and children admitted to the pediatric ICU. Atrial extrasystole is readily recognized by the early, premature occurrence of a P-wave followed by a QRS complex **(Table 15.4)**. The premature QRS complex may have the morphology identical with that of the preceding QRS complexes, or it may be aberrantly conducted and thus be dissimilar from preceding QRS complexes. Because of the extremely rapid rate of repolarization of the conducting tissue in the infant's myocardium, aberrant conduction rarely occurs in children under 18 months of age. Although simple premature atrial beats are frequently considered benign, they should still be sought, as they have the ability to initiate serious cardiac dysrhythmias. Theoretically, the most serious atrial dysrhythmias always occur in response to an atrial (or nodal) extrasystole initiating multiple reentry pathways leading to supraventricular tachydysrhythmias or atrial fibrillation. Differentiation of atrial extrasystoles from ventricular extrasystoles may be difficult, especially in children **(Table 15.5)**. The knowledge that aberrancy does not occur in children younger than 18 months of age should be borne in mind. In addition, the right bundle branch block (RBBB) pattern occurs more frequently in aberrantly conducted premature atrial contractions (PACs), and therefore the recognition of the rsr′ pattern in V_1 makes the extrasystole more likely an aberrantly conducted PAC than a PVC (Fig. 15.7). Another useful differentiating point is the occurrence of a compensatory pause, suggesting that the premature beat is a ventricular ectopic beat. Finally, PVCs generally demonstrate a different initial vector from the preceding sinus beats, whereas PACs do not. Despite these differences, it may not be possible to differentiate a given PAC with aberrancy from a PVC.

Table 15.4. ECG Forms of Premature Atrial Contractions

Early P-wave, normal QRS
Early P-wave blocked in AV node
Early P-wave, blocked in bundle branches, wide QRS with high likelihood of right bundle branch block (RBBB)

Sinus Tachycardia

ST, although defined in adults as heart rates greater than 100 beats/min, cannot be so readily defined in children, and recognition of the appropriate heart rate range for age is necessary to determine if a sinus rhythm is pathologic. ST is identified by recognizing one-to-one AV conduction, regular R-R intervals, regular QRS morphology, and an abnormally fast rate. ST frequently occurs in response to stress and is often not associated with any hemodynamic impairment. Indeed, treatment of ST, which is a normal physiologic compensation for a pathologic state, not only is not indicated but can be disastrous. ST occurs in children after exercise and surgery, with fever, with certain drug ingestions, in the postanesthetic state, during anemia, during hypothyroidism, and, of course, during pain and anxiety. It is also the correct physiologic response to such states as volume

Table 15.5. Comparison of Premature Atrial Contraction (PAC) and Premature Ventricular Contraction (PVC)

PAC—resets sinus node, no compensatory pause
PVC—does not reset sinus node, compensatory pause
PAC—most have normal QRS; some have no QRS (blocked); some have RBBB pattern
PVC—wide and bizarre in any shape

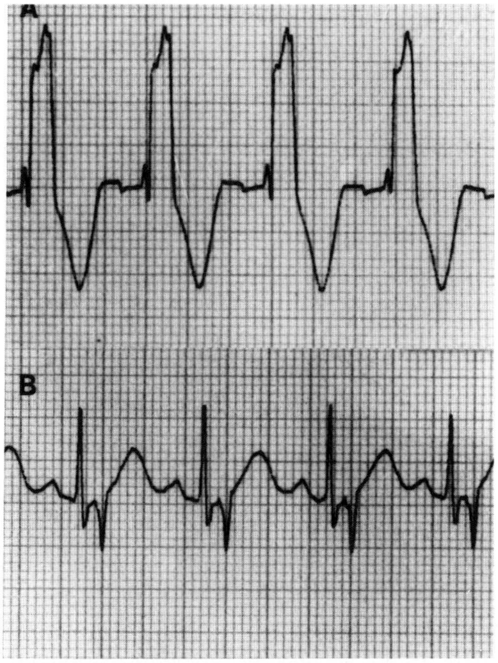

Figure 15.7. Tachycardia in a child following an AV canal repair with right bundle branch block. In **A,** lead V_1, note the rsr′ pattern, as would be seen in an aberrantly conducted PAC. In **B,** lead 2, the P-QRS relationship is obvious.

contraction after hemorrhagic, septic, or anaphylactic shock; hypoxemia; and hypercarbia, and it usually accompanies heart failure of any cause. Treatment should be directed at the underlying cause.

Supraventricular Tachydysrhythmia

The most frequently observed pathologic dysrhythmia in pediatric practice is paroxysmal supraventricular tachycardia (SVT), which includes paroxysmal atrial tachycardia (PAT). This is defined as a rapid heart rate originating from an abnormal mechanism proximal to the bifurcation of the bundle of His that, additionally, is morphologically dissimilar to atrial flutter[32,33]. Morphologically, the ECG demonstrates regular R-R intervals and narrow QRS complexes (Fig. 15.8A). However, abnormal P-wave morphology and a deranged P-R relationship with prolonged P-R intervals and absent or difficult-to-define P-waves usually occur (Fig. 15.8B). In infants and neonates SVT may be at rates of 200–300 beats/min, whereas in older children heart rates of 150–250 beats/min are more common. Characteristically, the onset of SVT is paroxysmal with a rapid sudden onset and offset. The majority of children with SVT demonstrate a normal P-R interval and a normal QRS complex. One exception to this is in the Lown-Ganong-Levine syndrome with a short P-R interval and a normal QRS complex. In children between the ages of 3 and 16 years, the P-R interval is greater than 100 msec, and in adults it is greater than 120 msec, whereas in children under 3 years it is greater than 80 msec. In the majority of patients with SVT, both atria and ventricles are beating abnormally rapidly.

SVT with aberrant AV conduction is extremely uncommon in children. For this reason, QRS morphology is generally normal, and virtually invariably so in children under 18 months of age. When the QRS is abnormally wide, it is

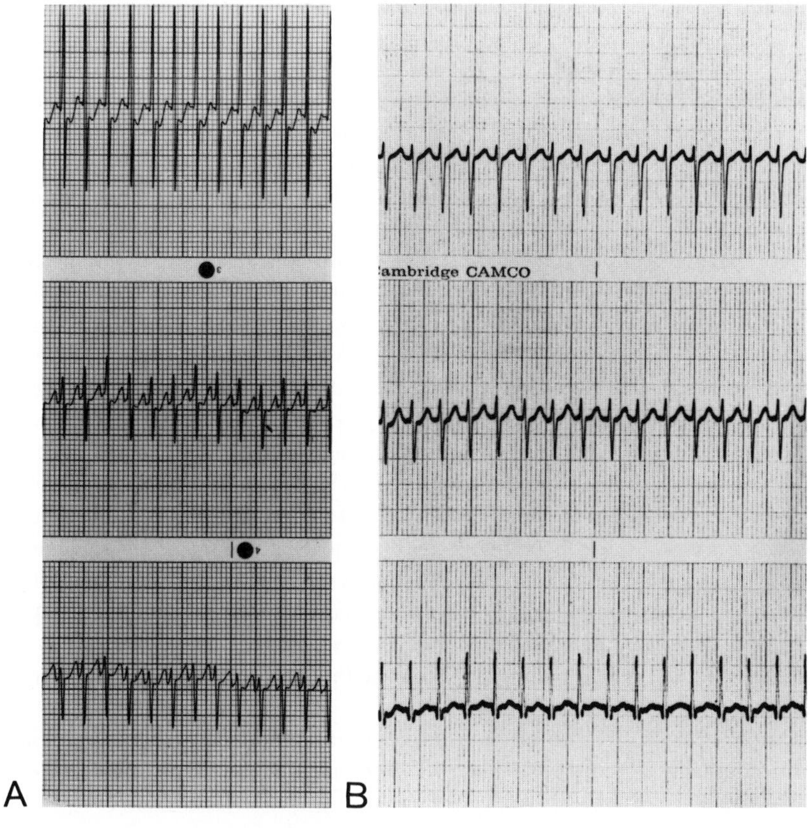

Figure 15.8. Two examples of neonatal SVT. Note narrow, regular QRS complexes, regular P-R intervals, and a heart rate of 300 beats/ min. The regular P-waves that are evident in **A** are not as clearly defined in **B.**

usually of a similar morphology to that seen during normal sinus rhythm. When aberrancy does occur, it may be extremely difficult to differentiate SVT from VT; however, a RBBB pattern is more commonly seen with SVT, and a left bundle branch block pattern is more frequently seen with VT.

SVT is caused by the *reentry* phenomenon. This occurs when the atria are excited through the aberrant, retrograde entry of an electrical impulse along a conducting pathway back into the atria, causing a circular movement of depolarization. This can occur through the AV node (AV nodal reentry tachycardia, AVNRT) or, commonly, through accessory conducting tissue pathways such as the bundle of Kent or James' bundle (AV reciprocating tachycardia, AVRT)[34,35]. The ability of atrial tissue to rapidly repolarize, especially in children, is the underlying reason why this aberrant circular movement can be effective. The Wolff-Parkinson-White syndrome was the first pattern of reentry phenomena described in which the bundle of Kent leads to recurrent paroxysmal SVT. Patients characteristically have widened QRS complexes with a short P-R interval and a slurred upstroke (δ-wave), indicating the aberrant pathway of early depolarization through the anomalously conducting bundle of Kent. Reentry is usually triggered by an atrial premature beat that produces unidirectional block in one of the reentry pathways. Dual AV nodal pathways are common in children[36]. Any premature beat, junctional or ventricular, may initiate the reentry phenomenon and thus initiate SVT. Another mechanism that may initiate reentry is that of sinus slowing with an atrial, junctional, or ventricular escape beat initiating the SVT[37].

Sinus node reentrant tachycardia resembles sinus tachycardia with regular P waves but is truly a reentrant tachycardia caused by reentry at the sinus node. It is characterized by a sudden onset and offset. This rhythm, with the consequences of tachycardia, may persist after therapeutic measures directed at alleviating a sinus tachycardia (volume, analgesia, antipyrexials, etc.) and may require therapy directed at interrupting reentry pathways. Superventricular tachycardia also arises from true deranged automaticity, such as in atrial ectopic tachycardia. This may be resistant to conventional therapy[35,38,39]. Although this is uncommon postoperatively, it may give rise to a resistant atrial tachycardia postoperatively.

In general, children with SVT present with congestive cardiac failure. SVT may occur in utero and lead to the birth of a hydropic newborn infant. The diagnosis of fetal SVT in utero can be made by ultrasound or by fetal electrocardiographic studies[40]. The identification of fetal dysrhythmias may indicate underlying congenital heart disease or impending fetal distress. In utero therapy is possible[41]. Frequently, in older children who present with failure, SVT may be confused with any of several other causes of low output, including cardiac failure, fever, sepsis, septic shock, and volume contraction. Chest pain may also be the presenting symptom in children with SVT, and screaming and irritability may be the only symptoms in infants. In older age groups, the onset of rapid heart rate may lead to the diagnosis of SVT. Most commonly, the onset of SVT occurs in children before they reach 6 months of age and is slightly more common in males than in females. Although it may reflect underlying Wolff-Parkinson-White syndrome, frequently there are no predisposing factors. Two additional forms of SVT occur and result from non-reentry atrial tachycardia and junctional tachycardias[42,43]. Both of these are due to rapid depolarization of an ectopic focus in either nodal or atrial tissue. In contrast to other forms of SVT, they are nonparoxysmal and are, unfortunately, quite resistant to therapy. They are almost always associated with severe underlying organic heart disease, such as ischemia or myocarditis, or with symptoms of digitalis toxicity[42,43].

Treatment of Supraventricular Tachycardia

After adequate oxygenation has been assured, the first priority is to abort the SVT. Frequently, children with SVT are well compensated; however, this hemodynamic compensation may be at the expense of important peripheral vascular beds. Acute decompensation may follow further physiologic challenges or prolonged SVT, in which case time is of the essence. In addition, chronic SVT may cause an underlying cardiomyopathy. Finally, diagnosis of the underlying disorder cannot adequately proceed without the reestablishment of sinus rhythm. This is of more than diagnostic importance, as the therapy for the Wolff-Parkinson-White syndrome and other causes of SVT may be different from the treatment of the idiopathic varieties of SVT.

It is appropriate to consider treating all children who present with SVT with maneuvers that increase vagal tone. This increased vagal tone may interrupt electrical depolarization caused by the irregular circus movement and is frequently rapidly successful in converting SVT to sinus rhythm. In older children and in adults, these maneuvers include carotid sinus massage and Valsalva's maneuver. In younger children, this can be done by merely applying firm abdominal pressure, which often leads to a bearing-down response in children. Although ocular pressure is occasionally successful, this technique carries with it a high risk of retinal detachment and is therefore no longer recommended.

Another modality of treating SVT is eliciting the diving reflex[44–46]. This complex neurologic reflex is elicited by providing an iced water (0°C) stimulus to the head and/or face of the child. This gives rise to both an increase in vagal tone and a withdrawal of sympathetic tone and, frequently, rapidly aborts SVT. This technique is particularly efficacious in infants and small children; however, it has also been successfully applied to older children. One important caveat is essential in performing all of these physiologic maneuvers; i.e., one should be prepared to rapidly treat profound bradycardias and even asystole, which may result from vagotonic methods of aborting supraventricular dysrhythmias.

Two other techniques for increasing neurally mediated suppression of SVT deserve mention. *Edrophonium chloride*

(Tensilon) can be given intravenously (0.1 mg/kg). This short-acting cholinesterase inhibitor increases concentrations of endogenous acetylcholine and thus vagal tone. Another means of suppressing SVT is the use of α-adrenergic sympathomimetic agents that lead to an elevation in systemic vascular resistance and reflex vagal stimulation of the myocardium. Both methoxamine and phenylephrine (5–10 mg/kg) have been reported to be useful for this purpose. It may be necessary to increase the blood pressure to twice the baseline before conversion is achieved. In children who have already maximally compensated for decreased cardiac output secondary to SVT, a further increase in peripheral vascular resistance may lead to catastrophic myocardial decompensation. For this reason, this technique must be applied with caution, especially in older children.

In the past, *digitalization* was the standard first-line therapy for conversion of SVT in infants and older children. Rapid digitalization intravenously, if necessary over 4–6 hours, frequently converts supraventricular tachydysrhythmias. Continuation of digitalis in children who have been converted from SVT to sinus rhythm seems to be warranted; although the incidence of attacks may not be decreased, the rapidity of conversion of future attacks seems to be enhanced. Recent concerns about the use of digoxin in patients with Wolff-Parkinson-White syndrome have cast doubt on the wisdom of using digoxin as the first line of therapy in undiagnosed patients presenting with SVT. As digoxin may enhance AV conduction, it could cause early conduction of atrial beats to a nonrefractory ventricle, which could result in VT or ventricular fibrillation[(47)]. For this reason, the use of digoxin for initially converting SVT, atrial fibrillation, and atrial flutter in children may be contraindicated, and it is no longer the first line of therapy.

Adenosine has become the drug of first choice for the treatment of reentry SVT in adults[(48,49)]. Multiple reports document its usefulness in children. Because most SVT in children is initiated by reentry mechanisms, adenosine is particularly useful. Because of its short half-life, few side effects, and ability to be used with other drugs, it is rapidly becoming the drug of first choice for SVT in children (see below)[(50)]. *Propranolol* and other β-blocking agents, such as esmolol, have proven useful in converting supraventricular tachydysrhythmias. β-Blockade prolongs AV conduction time by increasing the refractory period of the conducting pathways and thus blocks reentry. It is therefore useful for converting as well as preventing future episodes of SVT. Propranolol can be given intravenously when indicated and repeated hourly as long as the blood pressure and heart rate tolerate it. Propranolol is particularly effective in treating SVT resulting from Wolff-Parkinson-White syndrome. In severe cases of refractory SVT, other agents that block intraventricular conduction, such as quinidine and procainamide, may be useful in converting the tachydysrhythmia. *Verapamil*, a calcium channel blocker, has been reported to be useful therapy for converting SVT in infants and children. It is a useful alternative to propranolol as a first-line treatment in Wolff-Parkinson-White syndrome[(51)]. Because of the myocardial depressant and peripheral vasodilator actions of verapamil, hypotension may be a complication[(52)]. These two effects explain why it must be used with great care in combination with β-blockade.

In the child who presents with hypoperfusion or becomes acutely hypoperfused, hypotensive, or acidotic or in whom pharmacologic therapy has been ineffective, further therapy is urgently required. Such is generally the situation in neonates with SVT and congestive heart failure. Synchronized direct-current *cardioversion* with a dose of 0.5–2 J/kg is usually effective. Repeated attempts are indicated, and the dose may be increased to 5 J/kg. Anesthesia and sedation may be considered before cardioversion is undertaken if the child is otherwise stable with appropriate airway management. Previous digitalization is not a contraindication to cardioversion in the face of life-threatening SVT with hemodynamic collapse. If cardioversion is successful, maintenance therapy should be initiated as indicated by the underlying defect.

It should be remembered that cardioversion can result in asystole or severe bradycardia. If all of the above methods have failed, intra-atrial cardiac pacing may be required. The atrial rate is increased above that of the supraventricular rate and then suddenly withdrawn. Frequently, cardioversion to a sinus rhythm follows this maneuver; however, it may need to be repeated frequently. This is relatively simple if atrial pacemaking wires are in place, such as after cardiac surgery, but insertion of atrial pacing electrodes in an emergency situation can be difficult. For this reason, the recent report of esophageal overdrive pacing for SVT provides promise[(53)].

All of the above techniques may be only temporary, as they only transiently inhibit the underlying pathophysiologic mechanism that causes the circus movement initiating the SVT. For this reason, after conversion of the SVT, other agents may be required to maintain sinus rhythm. After sinus rhythm has been restored, further therapy will be guided by the patient's clinical condition and the definitive diagnosis. If conversion has been achieved, diagnosis will guide the required maintenance therapy. If conversion has not occurred, further pharmacologic therapy is indicated if time and the patient's condition allow. After conversion, those children without Wolff-Parkinson-White syndrome are best treated by digitalization. Those with Wolff-Parkinson-White syndrome are best maintained on propranolol, preferably administered orally.

Atrial Fibrillation and Flutter Treatment

Tachydysrhythmias that are initiated in the atria include atrial fibrillation and atrial flutter. These often occur in the pediatric ICU setting and need to be differentiated from more serious supraventricular tachydysrhythmias. Atrial fibrillation results from rapid chaotic depolarization of multiple atrial foci; results in disorganized, irregular, ineffective, atrial contraction; and is accompanied by a variable response from the ventricles. Recent evidence suggests that local microreentry phenomena are the cause of the chaotic depolarization. Electrocardiographically, one sees a rapid, irregular, ventricular response with irregular R-R intervals and absent P-waves (Fig. 15.9). The atrial rate may vary between 350 to 600 times/min with prominent (coarse), small (fine), or inapparent P-waves. Occasionally, distorted complexes indicating aberrant conduction are present. Atrial fibrillation may occur in rheumatic heart disease, mitral valve disease, hyperthyroidism, pulmonary embolus, pericarditis, atrial septal defects, Epstein's anomaly, and cardiomyopathies. The loss of atrial filling during atrial fibrillation is usually better tolerated in children than in adults.

Atrial flutter appears less frequently in children and is characterized by a rapid, regular, uniform, sawtooth flutter wave that occurs between 250 to 500 times/min. Flutter waves are atrial depolarizations that last for up to 180 msec (Fig. 15.10A) and are caused by a reentry mechanism. It should be noted that the flutter waves may not be present in all electrocardiographic leads. Leads II, III, aVF, and V_1 are the leads that most frequently show flutter waves. AV conduction is almost always blocked to some degree, resulting in an irregular ventricular response (Fig. 15.10B). QRS morphology is the same as that for normal sinus beats, though aberrant conduction may also occur. In a large survey of patients it was found that 75% of these patients with atrial flutter had an operation to correct a congenital heart defect[54,55]. This was most commonly a Mustard or Senning procedure, atrial septal defect repair, Blalock-Hanlon

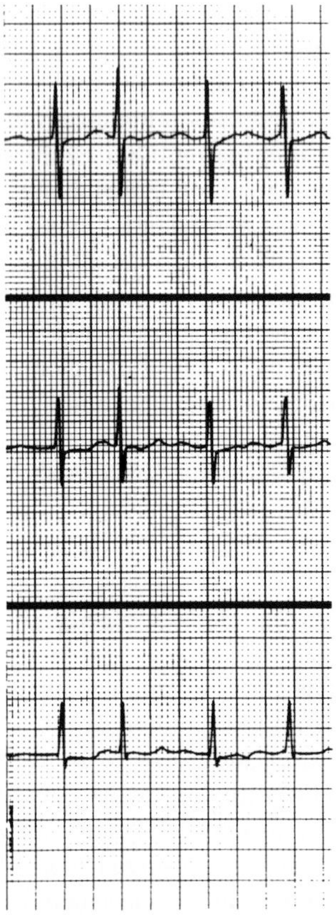

Figure 15.9. Atrial fibrillation. Note the absence of P-waves and the irregular P-R interval with normal QRS morphology ($V_4 = V_6$).

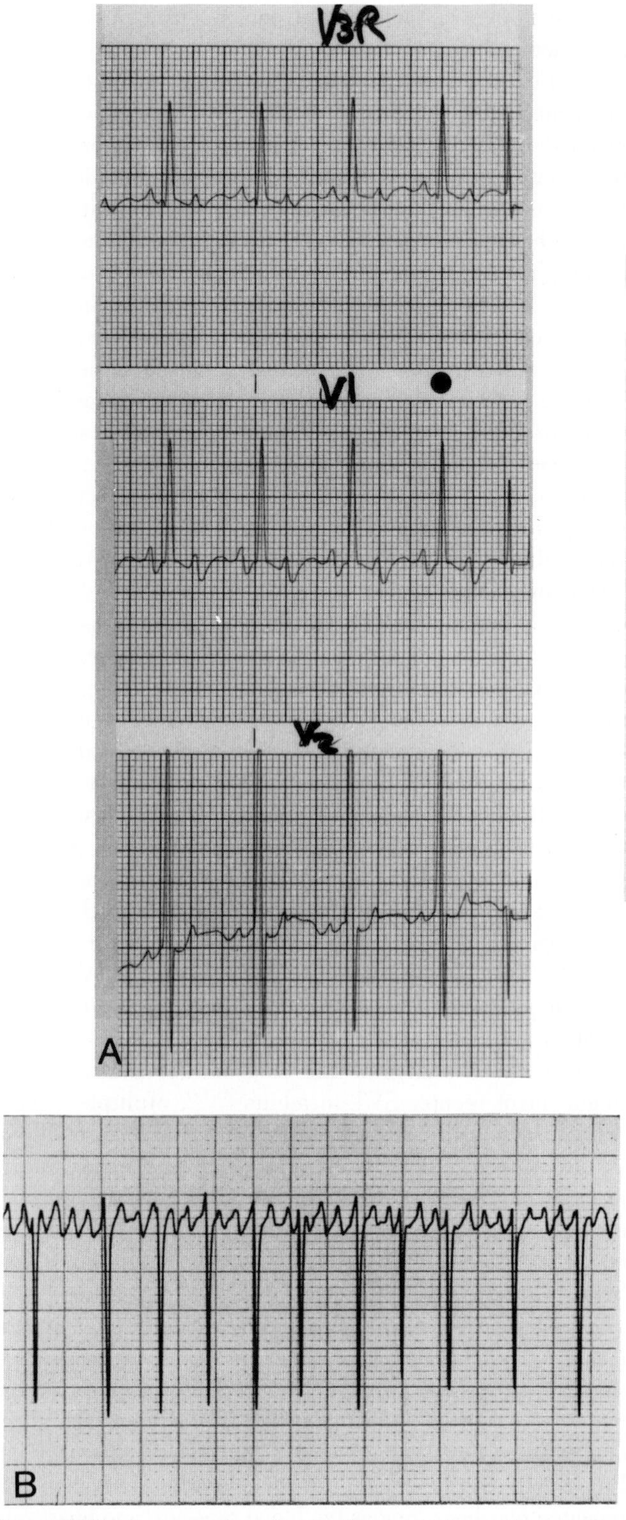

Figure 15.10. Two examples of atrial flutter. **A** shows flutter with a regular 2:1 AV conduction block and regular P-R intervals with a rate of 104 (leads I–III). This example of flutter is more subtle than that for another patient **(B)** (lead V_1), showing the characteristic sawtooth pattern with variable R-R intervals.

septectomy, or a Fontan procedure. Other causes of atrial flutter were various types of congenital heart disease, cardiomyopathies, rheumatic disease, mitral valve prolapse, and pericarditis; occasionally, atrial flutter occurs in an anatomically normal heart. When atrial flutter occurs in a child younger than 1 year of age, it is likely to be associated with the Wolff-Parkinson-White syndrome.

Treatment. As in other dysrhythmias, the underlying hemodynamic status and diagnosis dictate the therapy. In patients who are hemodynamically stable, atrial flutter and fibrillation may best be treated with intravenous digitalization. However, if the underlying diagnosis includes the Wolff-Parkinson-White syndrome, digitalization is best avoided, and intravenous propranolol or a short-acting β-blocker may be useful in slowing the ventricular response. Disopyramide and verapamil have been used to treat flutter and fibrillation. Procainamide and quinidine have also been useful in treating refractory flutter and fibrillation.

In the acutely ill child or one in whom the above pharmacologic maneuvers have been unsuccessful, the safest method of converting atrial flutter is overdrive atrial pacing. This can be performed with an indwelling intracardiac catheter or via an esophageal pacing electrode. Atrial pacing should be at a rate approximately 20–30 beats greater than the intrinsic atrial rhythm and should be continued for at least 60 seconds. The pacing voltage should be 3 or 4 times greater than the atrial capture threshold. It should then be rapidly terminated. The underlying cause for atrial flutter and fibrillation could be sinus node disease, in which case rapid conversion could lead to an inordinately slow bradycardia and potentially to asystole. For this reason, means of atrial pacing and increasing atrial rate should be available. The most efficacious way of converting atrial fibrillation and flutter is by synchronized direct-current cardioversion. Again, standby pacing should be available, and appropriate anesthesia should be provided. If cardioversion is followed by rapid relapse, intravenous digitalization may be indicated, as well as the addition of procainamide. An alternative to this tactic is the use of propranolol, which, through slowing AV conduction, may maintain the conversion to sinus rhythm.

Multifocal atrial tachycardia has been reported to occur in children as young as 1 week of age[(56)]. The ECG shows a rate over 100 atrial beats/min, discrete nonsinus P-waves with at least three morphologies. The P-P, P-R, and R-R intervals are irregular with an isoelectric baseline. Altered automaticity may underlie this rhythm, although the cause is not certain. The rhythm occurs postoperatively in myocarditis and mitral valve disease. Fifty percent of these patients may have no underlying disease. Treatment requires correction of the underlying abnormalities. β-Blockers (metoprolol, esmolol) and calcium channel blockers are the major therapeutic choices. Magnesium and amiodarone have worked[(57)]. Electrical cardioversion and digoxin are not recommended[(43)].

Junctional Ectopic Tachycardia

Junctional ectopic tachycardia (JET) is the most severe form of SVT that can occur in children[(42,58)]. In JET, the QRS rate is abnormal for age, with the rate usually between 120 and 220 beats/min and occasionally as high as 350 beats/min. The R-R interval is regular, and QRS morphology is similar to that of normal sinus beats. Although occasionally P-waves cannot be seen, retrograde conducted P-waves follow each QRS. The dysrhythmia is incessant, narrow, and complex and often results in hemodynamic compromise. This arrhythmia may be a manifestation of AV block and is most commonly seen in the postoperative period (ventricular septal defect, Mustard, and tetralogy of Fallot) but can occur with myocarditis. It also occurs in infants younger than 6 months of age.

Therapy of this dysrhythmia is generally unsatisfactory but should initially include correction of hypovolemia, hyperthermia, inadequate analgesia, electrolyte abnormalities, hypoxia, and hypercarbia. If possible, catecholamine inotropes should be decreased or stopped. The underlying cause may be surgical or other injury (trauma) at or near the bundle of His. Metabolic abnormalities may exacerbate the dysrhythmia. Although the administration of digitalis and β-blockers may lower the rate, it is often unsuccessful in converting this dysrhythmia to sinus rhythm. Surface cooling to 33° to 35°C has been somewhat successful. Overdrive pacing may be tried but is usually not effective. A newer technique described by Waldo and colleagues and known as paired ventricular pacing has been described[(59)]. Ventricular pacing is adjusted to such a rapid rate that although every beat causes an electrical QRS complex, effective ventricular contraction only occurs with every other beat. Unfortunately, this technique may not increase cardiac output, and therefore close monitoring of cardiac output and perfusion is necessary. If pacing is unsuccessful, intravenous propranolol may be effective. Severe bradydysrhythmias may follow and may require ventricular pacing. In addition, myocardial depression, especially in the postoperative heart, may not be tolerated. Amiodarone has yielded some success in the treatment of this arrhythmia in adults and children[(60,61)], but it must be given orally. In severe cases, especially postoperatively, ablation of the ectopic site by surgical manipulation may be necessary and should be considered before the patient is moribund[(62)]. Propafenone has been successfully used to convert this dysrhythmia[(63)]. Intravenous magnesium may also be beneficial. In treating JET, the ability to pace the heart should be readily available.

Ventricular Dysrhythmias

Ventricular tachydysrhythmias can present dramatically and pose a serious threat to life. For this reason, the rapid recognition of predisposing factors and effective therapy is vitally important. A PVC is characterized by a wide, abnormal, slurred QRS complex, usually followed by a T-wave with an inverted axis without a preceding P-wave (Fig. 15.11). A PVC is defined by a QRS complex not preceded by a premature P-wave. Differentiation from aberrantly conducted PAC may be difficult. The best way to differentiate these two phenomena is to note the presence of a P-wave or a compensatory pause between QRS complexes (twice the normal R-R interval), which

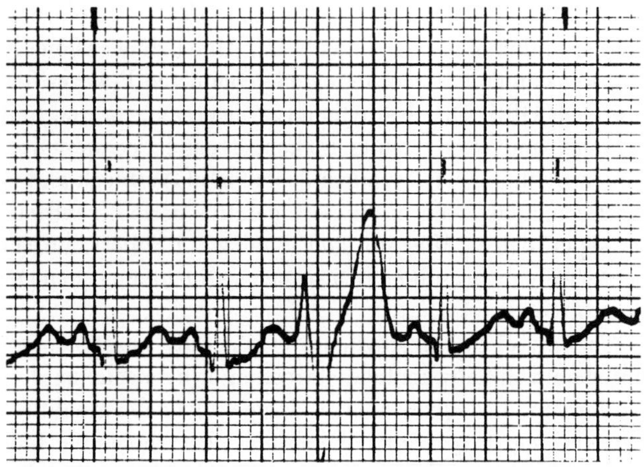

Figure 15.11. A single ventricular extrasystole. Note wide QRS with opposite vector from sinus QRS, abnormal T-morphology, and fully compensatory pause.

indicates a ventricular ectopic beat. In addition, PVCs generally demonstrate a different initial vector from the preceding sinus beats, whereas PACs do not, and the QRS vector is different from that of the preceding normal QRS complexes **(Table 15.4)**.

PVCs can be described morphologically as uniform or multiform (old terms: unifocal or multifocal). The term multiform merely refers to the morphology of the QRS being different. It does not necessarily indicate multiple ectopic ventricular foci. Fusion beats also occur. Their ECG appearance results from the fusion of an ectopic ventricular beat with a supraventricular beat, and thus their morphology lies between that of a sinus beat and a PVC (Fig. 15.12). Because a fusion beat requires ventricular ectopic focus, the significance of a fusion beat is the same as that of any other PVC. The significance of individual PVCs or couplets and triplets (VT) of PVCs is that they indicate damaged areas of myocardium resulting from ischemia, drugs, or direct trauma that alone gives rise to an area of myocardial irritability. These damaged foci constantly pose the risk of deterioration to a sustained VT or ventricular fibrillation with hemodynamic collapse (Figs. 15.13 and 15.14).

VT can arise from an electrolyte or metabolic imbalance, cardiac tumor, cardiac damage after surgery, myocarditis,

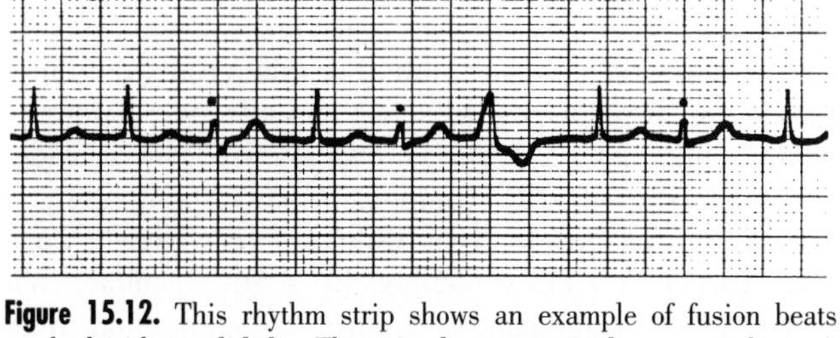

Figure 15.12. This rhythm strip shows an example of fusion beats marked with a *solid dot.* There is also a ventricular ectopic beat. A fusion beat represents a combination of a ventricular ectopic beat with a supraventricular beat and is intermediate in form between the two. Their significance is the same as for ventricular ectopic beats.

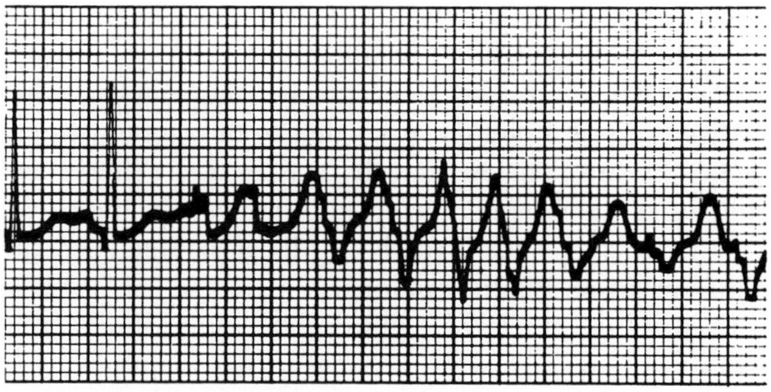

Figure 15.13. Sinus rhythm degenerating into VT tachycardia.

or a cardiomyopathy, or it may be idiopathic[64]. It can also occur in the prolonged Q-T syndromes (Jervell, Lange-Nielsen, or Romano-Ward)[65]. Frequently in prolonged Q-T syndromes, torsade de pointes is seen (Fig. 15.15)[66]. Hemodynamic compromise follows VT and leads to syncope or sudden death. VT may be very regular and even occur with narrow QRS complexes. Ventricular fibrillation is manifest by chaotic, irregular ventricular depolarization and is characterized by the absence of regular recognizable QRS complexes. The therapy for ventricular fibrillation is the same as that for cardiac arrest.

It is frequently difficult to differentiate SVT from VT. Rates greater than 150 beats/min, wide QRS complexes, and inadequate circulation may occur in both. Preexisting AV dissociation, however, suggests VT, as does the presence of preexisting fusion beats. An rsr pattern in V_1 suggests SVT, as does the presence of a preexcitation phenomenon. Frequently, a trial of therapy is required to differentiate SVT and VT. Vagomimetic maneuvers rarely affect VT and frequently slow or abort SVTs. Adenosine may be of particular help in diagnosing the tachycardia.

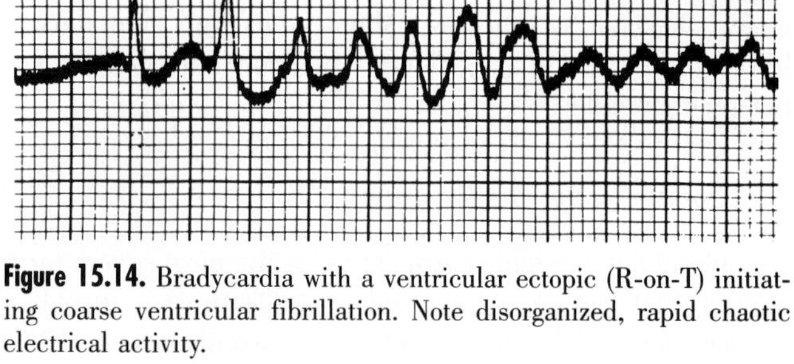

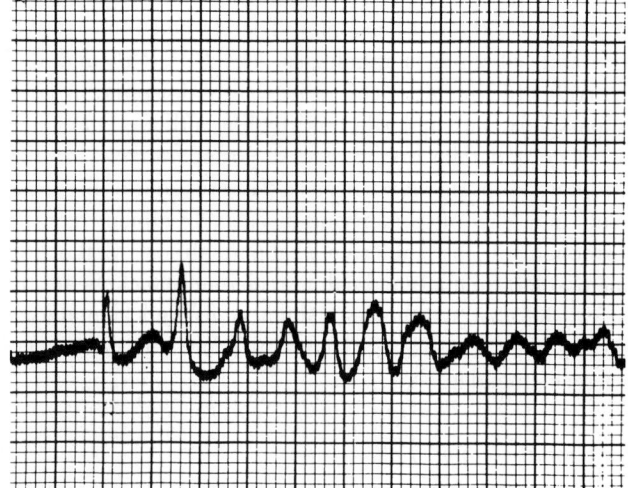

Figure 15.14. Bradycardia with a ventricular ectopic (R-on-T) initiating coarse ventricular fibrillation. Note disorganized, rapid chaotic electrical activity.

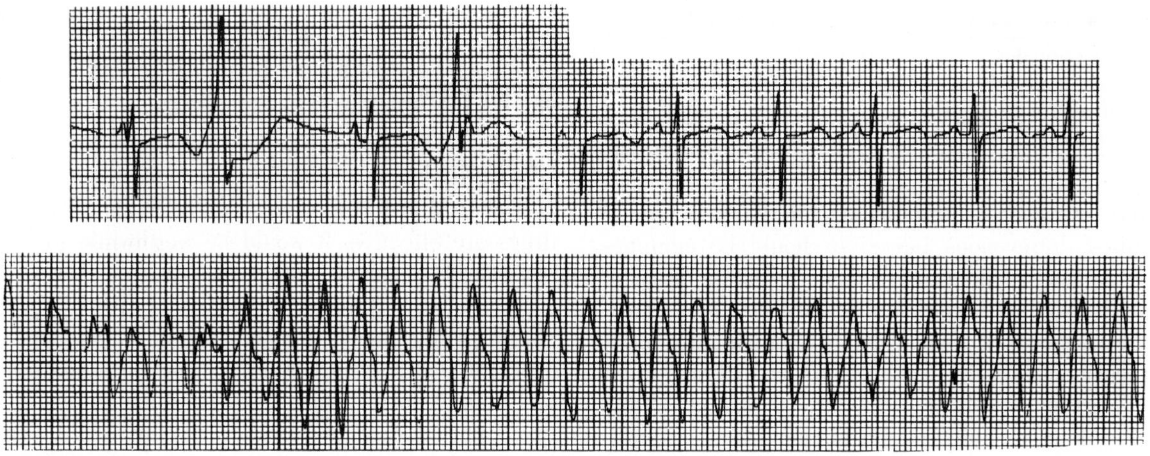

Figure 15.15. A 6-year-old who presented with syncope and an ECG suggesting bigeminy. The sinus Q-T_c is 0.52 seconds. Moments later torsade de pointes developed. This was successfully treated by intravenous magnesium, suggesting acquired Q-T syndrome. The child was receiving amiodarone.

Therapy

Treatment of rhythms that predispose to VT and ventricular fibrillation is indicated when there is either hemodynamic compromise or a rhythm that may rapidly deteriorate. The rhythms that may deteriorate are those with PVCs in couplets or triplets, multiform ventricular premature beats, PVCs occurring on or near the T-wave (Fig. 15.13), and more than 6 PVCs/min. Although ventricular bigeminy is a stable dysrhythmia, the presence of hemodynamic compromise caused by the inadequate ventricular contractions during the ectopic beat may require therapy directed at preventing the PVCs **(Table 15.6).**

After metabolic stabilization and correction of hypoxia and hypercarbia, the acute therapy for PVCs is intravenous lidocaine. If this is unsuccessful in altering the pattern of PVCs, it may be repeated and a continuous intravenous lidocaine infusion with serum levels to guide therapy is indicated. Intravenous procainamide is the next therapeutic step and may be continued either orally or intravenously. Disopyramide, a quinidine-like drug, is an oral agent that prevents and suppresses PVCs and may eventually be available for intravenous use in the United States[67]. Oral quinidine is also effective in the long-term suppression of PVCs.

The treatment of VT is again guided by the hemodynamic status of the patient. If cardiac output is maintained, the first drug of choice is intravenous lidocaine repeated twice and followed by a continuous infusion. If VT persists, intravenous procainamide or phenytoin is frequently successful. Recently, bretylium tosylate, an adrenergic nerve-blocking drug given intravenously, has proven very effective in terminating ventricular fibrillation and VT in children and should be considered in children with resistant VT[68]. Although it works within several minutes in ventricular fibrillation, it may take up to 2 hours to be effective in VT. Intravenous amiodarone has also occasionally been used to treat resistant VT in children. A short-acting blocker such as esmolol may be useful in suppressing recurrent VT.

If pharmacologic treatment has been unsuccessful and hemodynamic compromise is present, electrocardioversion is the therapy of choice. VT with hypotension requires cardioversion (Fig. 15.16). Again, anesthetic and airway management aspects of the child should be ensured prior to defibrillation. Doses of 1–4 J/kg are necessary and may be repeated until sinus rhythm occurs. For ventricular fibrillation or VT refractory to defibrillation, overdrive ventricular pacing may suppress an ectopic focus, and paired ventricular pacing may also be efficacious therapy.

The therapy for ventricular fibrillation is the same as that for cardiac arrest. Correction of underlying acidosis, airway maintenance, intubation, and ventilation with 100% F_IO_2

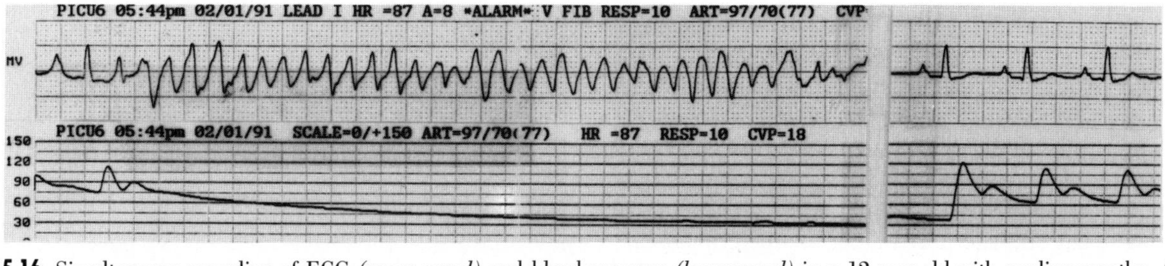

Figure 15.16. Simultaneous recording of ECG *(upper panel)* and blood pressure *(lower panel)* in a 12-year-old with cardiomyopathy. A fusion beat initiated VT. Blood pressure fell rapidly; cardioversion successfully restored sinus rhythm and pressure.

Table 15.6. When to Treat a Premature Ventricular Contraction

High frequency (>6/min)
Three or more in a row (VT)
Multifocal (different QRS forms)
Vulnerable period (PVC on T-wave)

is essential, as well as correction of underlying metabolic abnormalities. Intravenous lidocaine should be administered and repeated if there is evidence of deterioration of the underlying rhythm toward ventricular fibrillation. However, in all instances of ventricular fibrillation, cardiopulmonary resuscitation and treatment of the arrhythmia by direct cardioversion is indicated. A starting dose of 2 J/kg, followed by doubling until cardioversion occurs, is indicated. As mentioned above, intravenous bretylium tosylate may be efficacious. A note concerning coarse and fine ventricular fibrillation is worthwhile. Fine ventricular fibrillation may mimic an isoelectric ECG and is generally thought to be more difficult to convert. The addition of a potent catecholamine such as isoproterenol or epinephrine and even the use of intravenous calcium may convert a fine ventricular fibrillation or apparent asystole into coarse ventricular fibrillation or VT, which is more amenable to electrical cardioversion. This therapy may be useful in the desperate situation of apparent asystole or fine ventricular fibrillation.

Torsade de pointes is a variant of polymorphic VT frequently difficult to treat. It is characterized by variation in the QRS height, so that the complexes (points) appear to twist (torsade) around the baseline[(65,66)]. The mechanism is poorly understood, but the presence of prominent U-waves and T-U-wave abnormalities suggests delayed ventricular repolarization and a reentry mechanism. On the other hand, afterdepolarizations may be occurring. This rhythm occurs in antidysrhythmic drug toxicity, especially from type I (quinidine) and II drugs, tricyclic overdose, hypovolemia, and prolonged Q-T syndromes. Ventricular tachydysrhythmias that occur in prolonged Q-T syndromes may be either pause dependent (usually acquired or drug induced) or adrenergic dependent (usually congenital or familial). The former respond to magnesium, pacing, isoproterenol, and even atropine[(65,66)]. The latter respond to β-blockade. In the acute ICU setting, torsade de pointes has been treated with propranolol, lidocaine, and phenytoin, but with little success. Recently, intravenous magnesium sulfate (10 mg/kg) has been reported to be very efficacious, especially in acquired prolonged Q-T syndromes[(69)].

Understanding and recognition of abnormalities in cardiac rate and rhythm are the cornerstones of providing rapid therapeutic interventions aimed at restoring circulation. Once recognition occurs, therapy is fairly straightforward. It must be guided by the underlying basics of resuscitation, the patient's hemodynamic status, and the underlying diagnosis. The provision of routine critical care and specific antidysrhythmic therapy is usually rewarded with a successful outcome in treating cardiac dysrhythmias in children.

THERAPEUTICS

Specific Pharmacotherapy

Introduction

To understand the mechanisms by which antidysrhythmic drugs are effective, it would be worthwhile to review the physiology of cardiac depolarization. As shown in Figure 15.4, the action potential consists of five distinct phases starting with phase 0, during which rapid depolarization occurs, through phases 1 and 2 to phase 3 (or repolarization) and finally phase 4 (or the period of maintained or spontaneously decaying membrane depolarization). There are characteristic ion movements during each of these phases, and certain antidysrhythmic agents appear to alter these ion fluxes. During phase 0, the voltage-dependent sodium channel allows rapid, intense entry of sodium ions for a brief period, leading to depolarization. Phase 1 is a period of partial repolarization due to several factors but including potassium ion egress and chloride ion ingress. During phase 2, the slow channels open, allowing calcium and sodium ion entry in a fashion analogous to phase 0 sodium ion entry. During phase 3 repolarization, there is a constant, rapid, outward potassium ion movement that leads to a progressively more negative membrane potential. Also, during phase 3 the sodium channels are reactivated, and until this occurs, the cell is refractory to further depolarization. The timing of these ion movements accounts for the characteristics of cardiac action potentials. During phase 4, most myocardial cells remain constantly depolarized and will remain so indefinitely unless depolarized by an outside, propagated action potential. This resting diastolic membrane potential is maintained by a sodium potassium exchange pump. However, in the Purkinje system a decreased outward potassium current and an inward, probably sodium ion current leads to spontaneous depolarization. These ion currents are altered by the action of several antidysrhythmic drugs, and alterations in action potential duration, refractory period, conduction times, and responsiveness are primarily due to underlying alterations in the ion currents.

Antidysrhythmics have been classified into four classes **(Table 15.7).** Class I drugs depress the fast inward sodium ion channels and thus increase the refractory period and delay the return of excitability. Resting membrane potential is generally unchanged in phase 4 and may, in fact, be depressed. Class I drugs can be further divided into those agents that shorten total action potential duration (e.g., lidocaine) and those that lengthen it (e.g., quinidine). Their major effect is to slow repolarization and depress spontaneous depolarization. This class of drugs has wide clinical usage. Class II drugs act by inhibiting the catecholamine-dependent spontaneous depolarization of phase 4. Thus automaticity is slowed. Class III drugs act as potassium channel blockers and thus prolong phase 3 repolarization and thus prolong the effective refractory period. These drugs are very useful for treating and suppressing ventricular tachydysrhythmias. Class IV drugs block the calcium channels, and the effect of this is to prolong conduction and increase nodal and bundle of His tissue refractory time. They are, therefore, quite effective in treating reentry-type dysrhythmias.

This brief summary of how antidysrhythmics appear to function aids in the understanding of why certain agents are more useful for certain dysrhythmias; however, it should be remembered that there is considerable overlap between classes. Several drugs alter many phases of the action potential—for example, verapamil (a calcium channel blocker) has the ability to alter phases 1 and 2 and depress phase 4. The overall antidysrhythmic attributes of all of the antidysrhythmic drugs depend on many factors, only a few of which are clearly understood. In addition, developmental aspects of the cardiac conducting system suggest that the action of agents in adults cannot necessarily be extrapolated directly to children **(Table 15.7).**

Quinidine (Class IA)

Quinidine is one of the oldest antidysrhythmic agents known, and its use for atrial flutter was first described in 1749. More recently, Wenckebach's description of its effects in atrial fibrillation in the early 1900s led to its widespread clinical usage. The electrophysiologic effects of quinidine include a slight decrease in total action potential duration and a major increase in duration of the effective refractory period, thus making it suitable for treating SVT. In addition, phase 4 is stabilized and thus spontaneous depolarization is retarded. Also, by slow-channel inactivation, the activation threshold is increased and the rapidity of depolarization (phase 0) is decreased. These factors cause decreased automaticity and decreased conduction in atrial nodal and ventricular tissue. In atrial flutter, prolongation of refractoriness is cited as the major cause of its success, but quinidine also depresses conduction velocity and this would tend to oppose the prior effect. Quinidine usually slows the heart rate and prolongs the P-R, QRS, and Q-T intervals **(Table 15.8).**

Table 15.7. Classification of Antidysrhythmics

Class I—sodium channel blockers
A. Quinidine
 Procainamide
 Disopyramide
B. Lidocaine
 Phenytoin
 Mixetelene
 Tocainide
C. Propafenone
 Flecainide
 Encainide
Class II—β-blockers
Propranolol
Timolol
Class III—prolonged repolarization
Bretylium
Amiodarone
Sotalol
Class IV—calcium channel blockers
Verapamil
Nifedipine
Diltiazem
Class V
Adenosine
Digoxin

Quinidine has a broad spectrum of action as an antidysrhythmic. The major limiting factors to its use are the necessity of oral administration and its many untoward side effects. Quinidine is useful for reliably treating and providing prophylaxis for SVT, atrial flutter, and atrial fibrillation. In the Wolff-Parkinson-White syndrome, it is quite effective in preventing SVT. Although quinidine is an effective therapy for PVCs, its use in treating ventricular tachydysrhythmias has been abandoned. It prolongs the Q-T interval and may predispose to VT, especially torsade de pointes. Newer agents and countershock are safer.

The dose of quinidine is titrated against the ECG and rhythm changes. Effective serum levels are 2–5 μg/ml. Usual doses started at 5–10 mg/kg orally every 6 hours and are titrated to effect. The side effects of quinidine are legion and include cinchonism, diarrhea, hypotension, VT, and hypersensitivity reactions. Quinidine tends to increase serum levels of concurrently administered digoxin, and this poses a serious potential risk[70]. Another potentially serious response during therapy for atrial fibrillation is slowing of the atrial rate, which allows an increase in the ventricular rate that is due to increased conduction (decreased block) of atrial contractions. This may seriously compromise cardiac function.

The role of quinidine in the ICU is limited. Frequently, patients may already be receiving it when they arrive. It may occasionally be useful to treat PACs and fibrillation and/or flutter in addition to digoxin when these dysrhythmias are refractory to digoxin alone. In addition, as it prolongs the QT_c interval, it may predispose patients to torsade de pointes in the ICU. The high incidence of side effects during intravenous administration decreases its utility. When a quinidine-like class IA drug is indicated emergently, procainamide is the wise choice. In addition, procainamide is a more potent agent for treating ventricular dysrhythmias.

Lidocaine (Class IB)

Lidocaine is clearly the most widely used drug for acute treatment of ventricular dysrhythmias and PVCs. It has been in general use for over 30 years. The main electrophysiologic effect of lidocaine is to increase ventricular refractoriness and the threshold for ventricular fibrillation[71]. It has very little effect on atrial or nodal tissue and is thus a selective ventricular antidysrhythmic. Lidocaine depresses conductivity and intraventricular muscle and does not alter conductivity in normal myocardial tissue[72]. It also blocks ventricular reentry currents.

The major adverse effect of lidocaine is CNS toxicity with excitability and seizures. In addition, lidocaine has been accused of being a myocardial depressant; however, this effect is not clear. Bolus doses of lidocaine of 1 mg/kg are used to treat acute dysrhythmias. For suppression and prophylaxis, a continuous infusion after a loading bolus is use-

Table 15.8. Drug Therapy for Dysrhythmias

Drug	*Dose*	*Route*	*Drug Level*	*Side Effects*
Therapy for SVT				
Adenosine	50–250 μg/kg	IV bolus, every 1 minute	—	Hypotension, bradycardia, sinus arrest
Digoxin	See digitalizing schedule	Orally, intramuscularly, IV	1–3 ng/ml	Dysrhythmias, conduction delay, diarrhea, nausea, vomiting
Edrophonium	0.04 mg/kg × 3	IV	—	Profound bradydysrhythmias
Methoxamine	5–15 μg/kg/min, titrate to blood pressure	IV infusion	—	Hypertension
Phenylephrine	0.5–5 μg/kg/min, titrate to blood pressure	IV infusion	—	Hypertension
Verapamil	0.05–0.15 mg/kg, over 15 minutes × 2 − 3	IV bolus, p.o.	100–300 ng/ml	Hypotension
Therapy for ventricular dysrhythmias				
Bretylium	5 mg/kg bolus	IV bolus	—	Hypotension
Lidocaine	1–3 mg/kg, repeat if necessary 30–50 μg/kg/hr	IV bolus, infusion	1–7 μg/ml	Convulsions, tremor
Magnesium sulfate	15–30 mg/kg	IV bolus	—	Hypotension
Phenytoin	1–2 mg/kg	IV bolus, p.o.	15–20 μg/ml	Heart block
Therapy effective for SVT and ventricular dysrhythmias				
Disopyramide	2–5 mg/kg	orally	2–5 μg/ml	—
Esmolol	100–1000 μg/kg/min, increase every 2 minutes	IV infusion	0.15–0.2 μg/ml	Hypotension
Propranolol	0.01–0.1 mg/kg slowly	IV bolus	20–150 ng/ml	Hypotension, asystole, bronchospasm
Procainamide				
Infants	5–7 mg/kg	Slow IV bolus, infusion, p.o.	3–10 μg/ml	Nausea, vomiting, sudden death
Children	7–15 mg/kg	—	—	Hypotension
Quinidine	15–60 mg/kg/day	Orally	2–8 μg/ml	PVCs, AV block, hypotension
Therapy for bradydysrhythmias				
Atropine	0.01 mg/kg not < 0.1 mg	Intramuscularly, IV bolus	—	Flushing, tachycardia, fever, pupillary dilatation
Isoproterenol	0.1–1.0 μg/kg/min, titrated	IV infusion	—	PVCs, tachycardia

ful[73]. Because of CNS toxicity, dosage should be restricted to less than 5–7 mg/kg over 6 hours.

Encainide, Flecainide, Propafenone (Class IC)

Encainide, flecainide, and propafenone, all administered orally, block sodium channels[74]. There they decrease the phase 0 slope and slow conduction velocity. Their effects include prolonged atrial and ventricular conduction slowing and increased atrial and ventricular refractory periods. Accessory and retrograde conduction are also retarded. Propafenone has additional β-blocking and calcium channel-blocking characteristics that may make it a safer drug to use in ventricular dysrhythmias. These drugs are effective in blocking reentry dysrhythmias at both the atrial and the ventricular levels. Their major clinical indication is for treating sustained resistant VT. Encainide and flecainide have been used with moderate success in treating refractory reentry SVT, Wolff-Parkinson-White syndrome, AV nodal reentry tachydysrhythmias, and atrial flutter. Propafenone may be useful in JET[63]. All of these agents are proarrhythmic; VT and SVT can be triggered or worsened. Careful monitoring is essential during their use.

Propranolol (Class II)

Propranolol was the first nonselective β-antagonist to achieve general clinical use. Its antidysrhythmic properties are largely explained by direct β-antagonism. In addition to this β-blocking effect, propranolol also acts to stabilize the membrane and impede depolarization in a fashion similar to that of quinidine. This is a dual effect mediated by suppression of both the outward potassium current and the inward sodium current[75]. As a β-blocker, propranolol increases the refractory period of the AV node, and this phenomenon is the basis of its major indication as an antidysrhythmic agent. In the face of SVT, atrial flutter, or atrial fibrillation, propranolol effectively reduces ventricular response, which is the goal of therapy. In addition, AV nodal reentrant arrhythmias, such as many SVTs, are beneficially treated with propranolol for this reason. There is sufficient evidence that propranolol also slows intramyocardial conduction and decreases threshold potentials and excitability[76]. In addition, ventricular action potentials are prolonged. Propranolol also decreases the phase 4 slope, thus slowing automaticity and decreasing heart rates. This effect is moderated by β-blockade and by a membrane-stabilizing quinidine-like effect on outward potassium current. As is expected from the above information, electrocardiographic propranolol changes are multiple. The P-R interval is generally prolonged and the $Q\text{-}T_c$ decreased. The QRS duration is usually unchanged.

The major clinical use of propranolol is in treating supraventricular tachydysrhythmias such as SVT, atrial fibrillation, and atrial flutter. In general, the ventricular response is reliably decreased, with consequent improved function. In SVT, reentrant pathways may be blocked, thus terminating the dysrhythmias. Propranolol is also useful in preventing recurrent SVTs, especially in the Wolff-Parkinson-White syndrome. Propranolol is also efficacious in treating digitalis-induced ventricular dysrhythmias; however, both phenytoin and lidocaine therapy have fewer side effects. Propranolol is also an effective prophylaxis against PVCs and therapy of ventricular dysrhythmias in prolonged Q-T syndromes.

The side effects of propranolol treatment include hypotension and bronchospasm. Severe bradycardia may also occur. β-Blockade in patients with impaired hemodynamic function should only be undertaken with caution and consideration of its potentially negative inotropic effects. Newer blockers are more cardioselective. Acebutolol is useful for VT. Esmolol is a very short-acting ($t_{1/2}$ = 9 min) β_1-antagonist useful for atrial SVT and possibly VT. Its short duration makes it ideal as a trial of β-blockade. If bradycardia and hypotension develop, the effect is short-lived. Atenolol is an orally active, long-acting blocker used to treat SVT and suppress VT, especially in long Q-T syndromes.

Bretylium Tosylate (Class III)

The original use of bretylium as an acute, antihypertensive agent was superseded by guanethidine in the 1950s. It was not until 1978 that it became a clinically significant antidysrhythmic agent. Since Leveque's initial report[(77)], it has been shown that bretylium elevates the ventricular fibrillation induction threshold in normal and ischemic myocardium[(78,79)]. In acute myocardial infarction it suppresses recurrent ventricular dysrhythmias[(80)]. The effects of bretylium on the myocardium may be related to two factors. Clearly, its adrenergic blocking properties are important. Bretylium first leads to norepinephrine release and then to subsequent inhibition of catecholamine release. This may account for the initial increase in automaticity occasionally seen, but this effect is transient. The second effect is to prolong Purkinje and ventricular action potentials and thus to increase ventricular refractoriness. This occurs in the absence of atrial effects. Bretylium does not interfere with myocardial conduction or contractility. In summary, bretylium, like amiodarone and sotalol, increases refractoriness and does not affect conduction. The ECG effects include increased P-R and Q-T intervals, but QRS duration is unchanged. These characteristics indicate that it is most useful for the management of ventricular tachydysrhythmias.

The major indication for bretylium is in the treatment of ventricular dysrhythmias that do not respond to lidocaine and procainamide, and it may even be useful in cases in which countershock has proven unsuccessful[(81)]. Bretylium is given intravenously (5 mg/kg) slowly. Ventricular fibrillation may rapidly convert, whereas frequent PVCs and VT may take somewhat longer. The major side effect is hypotension, and thus it should only be administered in a critical care setting. The major role for bretylium in the pediatric ICU is in the acute management of resistant ventricular tachydysrhythmias.

Amiodarone (Class III)

Although amiodarone is not available for intravenous administration and is not generally useful for the immediate conversion of ventricular dysrhythmias, its use in refractory dysrhythmias should be familiar to the critical care pediatrician. Due to its current use in treating refractory ventricular and supraventricular dysrhythmias, children admitted to the pediatric critical care unit may already be receiving it. Amiodarone prolongs the action potential, decreases automaticity, and markedly prolongs the refractory period. In addition, it has α- and β-blocking as well as calcium channel-blocking activity. It seems to alter the way in which thyroxine affects the heart[(82)]. The exact relationship between these properties and its antidysrhythmic effects is not clear. However, the ability of amiodarone to increase the threshold of ventricular fibrillation, increase conduction time, and suppress VT is well documented[(83)].

As mentioned above, amiodarone is used for chronic control of life-threatening ventricular tachydysrhythmias. Large oral loading doses have been used in the acute situation to treat both SVT and VT[(84,61)]. There may even be a place for acute intravenous therapy, but this is undocumented in children. Amiodarone is also used to treat SVT especially associated with the Wolff-Parkinson-White syndrome. The side effects include hypotension and negative inotropism, skin discoloration, and corneal microdeposits as well as deranged thyroid function.

Verapamil (Class IV)

Calcium slow-channel blockade has effects that are widespread in muscle and other excitable tissues. With respect to cardiac dysrhythmias, the slow inward calcium current is responsible for phase 2 of the action potential. Phase 0 slope is decreased, as is resting membrane potential. Other effects include decreased contractility and coronary systemic and pulmonary vasodilation. Verapamil appears to be the most effective antidysrhythmic calcium ion channel blocker, whereas nifedipine and diltiazem are predominantly smooth-muscle relaxants.

The electrophysiologic effects of verapamil are of interest. In isolated tissue, automaticity is depressed, and thus sinus rate is reduced. In vitro, however, the vasodilating action of verapamil leads to a reflex stimulation of sinus rate, and thus the depression of automaticity is less marked. Verapamil also decreases the rate of phase 4 depolarization. The most useful effect of verapamil is in decreasing conduction velocity specifically in the AV node[(85)]. Thus it increases the refractory period. This effect is not prevented by atropine and propranolol and thus cannot be treated by the former and may be adversely potentiated by the latter. Clearly, verapamil should be expected, therefore, to slow the ventricular response rate to SVTs and to block reentry phenomena and convert SVT. Nodal suppression may also be useful in treating junctional tachydysrhythmias. The sole electrocardiographic effect of verapamil is the prolongation of the P-R interval in patients in sinus rhythm. Ventricular response is decreased in atrial flutter and fibrillation.

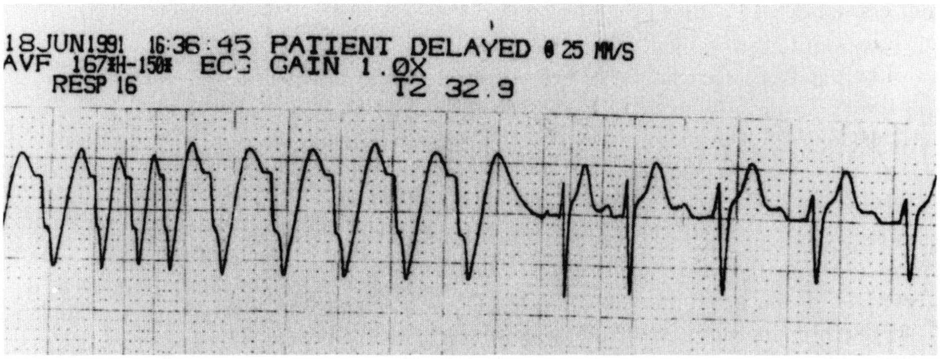

Figure 15.17. Wide complex tachycardia. SVT converted to sinus rhythm 12 seconds after an intravenous adenosine bolus, indicating its supraventricular origin.

Verapamil is a first-choice drug in adults to convert SVT due to reentry phenomena and the Wolff-Parkinson-White syndrome[86]. It has been seriously considered as such in children. Its use in narrow complex tachycardia to differentiate SVT and VT is limited to children who have not had surgery and are not in failure. In wide complex tachycardia its use is risky, as ventricular fibrillation has been reported. It is also extremely successful in immediately decreasing ventricular response in atrial flutter and fibrillation. Probably the major reason that this drug is less widely used in children than in adults is the still continued preference for digoxin in treating atrial tachydysrhythmias. In addition, reports of serious hypotension, bradycardia, and arrests in infants have limited its use. Digoxin also decreases AV conduction, and the concurrent use of digoxin and verapamil may lead to total heart block and is, therefore, best avoided.

Verapamil is given as an intravenous bolus of 50–70/kg. Its main side effect is hypotension. There is always the potential for heart block. Myocardial depression is rare. In addition to the above-mentioned digoxin interaction, concurrent use of β-blockade and verapamil is dangerous for similar reasons. One further note: verapamil also tends to increase digoxin levels in a fashion analogous to that of quinidine. Verapamil is the most useful calcium channel blocker in the pediatric ICU; however, its use for acute control of SVT has not become common, and adenosine will probably supplement it.

Adenosine (Class V)

Adenosine plays a central biochemical role in energy production and transmission[87]. In view of this, it is perhaps not surprising that intravenous administration of adenosine has an immediate impact on cardiac rhythm, but it is surprising that its effects are limited and specific. Its short half-life and ubiquitous presence tend to limit its effects. Adenosine is both a negative chronotrope and a negative dromotrope (delays spread of excitation) agent[74]. It stimulates extracellular adenosine A_1 receptors, depressing calcium slow channels and enhancing potassium conduction. It slows sinus rhythm and develops AV conduction. As such, it is superbly suited to block nodal reentry phenomena, the most frequent cause of SVT in children. Multifocal atrial tachycardia, flutter, or fibrillation is almost always resistant[35]. Multiple studies now testify to its efficacy in terminating SVT (both AVNRT and AVRT), more so than verapamil and digoxin, with fewer side effects[50,74,88]. It is rapid acting (seconds), has no negative inotropy, and has no proarrhythmic effects (Fig. 15.17)[74]. Although it is a vasodilator, hypotension is uncommon and readily reverses about 20 seconds after a bolus or discontinuation of a drip. It does cause bradycardia and has caused transient sinus arrest. Its short half-life has made this drug very popular for the acute treatment of SVT. In adults it has supplanted verapamil[48]. Because verapamil has not caught on for children, adenosine has become the first line of therapy for conversion of reentrant SVT in pediatrics[49].

Digoxin (Class V)

Although the diuretic and salutary cardiac effects of digitalis glycosides have been known since before the time of Withering, it is not clear when the potent antidysrhythmic effects became known. Digoxin is the most commonly used digitalis preparation, and the discussion is confined to its properties and use in treating dysrhythmias. Digoxin has both direct and indirect electrophysiologic effects on myocardial cells. With regard to ion currents, digoxin in low doses does not alter sodium conductance, and thus phases 4 and 0 are not altered. In higher doses, phase 4 slope is increased, resting membrane potential decreased, and sodium channels inhibited. Thus phase 4 is shorter, and the slope of phase 0 is decreased. In addition, phase 2 is altered, possibly due to alterations in calcium ion conductance. The effect of digoxin in therapeutic doses on Purkinje tissue is thus to decrease the threshold, shorten the action potential, prolong phase 0, and decrease conduction velocity. In AV nodal tissue, digoxin in large doses retards AV conduction, increases the refractory period, and can totally block AV conduction. Action potentials in ventricular muscle are shortened, and threshold potential is decreased, providing an explanation for digoxin-induced ventricular dysrhythmias. Although these direct effects are important, especially in high doses, the indirect autonomically mediated electrophysiologic effects of digoxin are clinically more significant in controlling dysrhythmias. The glycosidic moiety of digoxin enhances carotid sinus baroreceptor activity and leads to increased vagal and decreased sympathetic tone. In addition, there seems to be direct central parasympathetic stimulation. The summation of the opposing direct and indirect action leads to the important clinical role of digoxin and helps to explain its toxicity. Digoxin classically alters the ECG. First, normal sinus rhythm is slowed, the P-R interval is prolonged due to prolongation of AV conduction, and alteration occurs in the ST segment to a classic down-sloping pattern (digitalis effect). The QRS is not affected, even by toxic doses. T-waves may be flattened or inverted, and the Q-T interval is shortened due to hastened ventricular repolarization.

The major antidysrhythmic indication for digoxin is in the treatment of SVT, atrial fibrillation, and atrial flutter. The major purpose is to slow AV conduction and to decrease the ventricular response to these atrial dysrhythmias. Digoxin reliably decreases ventricular rate for atrial flutter and fibrillation, but the abnormal rhythm is rarely converted to sinus rhythm. In SVT, digoxin enhances vagal activity and may suppress or convert SVT to sinus rhythm. There are two important caveats in treating SVT. First, digoxin may shorten accessory pathway refractoriness and increase ventricular response and should be used, if at all, with caution in accessory pathway dysrhythmias such as the Wolff-Parkinson-White syndrome. Second, SVT with partial AV block may result from digoxin toxicity, and further digoxin could prove disastrous.

Digoxin has a wide spectrum of toxicity. Apart from the classic effects of digitalis intoxication, i.e., visual disturbances, nausea, diarrhea, and vomiting, it also causes PVCs, ventricular tachydysrhythmias, and AV blockade. It has been said that virtually any dysrhythmia may arise during digoxin treatment. The dysrhythmias are due to digoxin alterations in ventricular repolarization and an increase in the likelihood of reentry excitation phenomena. The impact of digoxin on sodium, potassium, and calcium ion conductance are, to some extent, due to ion concentrations, especially potassium. Therefore, hypokalemia greatly accentuates the risk of digoxin-induced ventricular dysrhythmias. Therapy for digoxin-induced ventricular dysrhythmias includes withholding digoxin, diuretics, and administration of potassium. Diphenylhydantoin and lidocaine are the most useful agents for treating digoxin dysrhythmias. Digoxin-induced bradycardia, however, will not respond to these drugs, and pacing may be required.

The wide variability in serum levels from digoxin therapy and the low therapeutic index indicate a need to monitor digoxin levels. This is mandatory in the acute care setting. Children tolerate higher levels of digoxin than adults, and the therapeutic serum range is from 1 to 3 ng/ml[89]. Alterations in renal function affect levels, as digoxin is entirely dependent on renal excretion. Digoxin interacts with several drugs. Quinidine coadministration increases digoxin levels. Thus conduction abnormalities are due to not only summation of their effects but also the high digoxin levels. Verapamil, amiodarone, and propafenone act similarly. Serum digoxin levels must be monitored with concurrent administration of these agents. The effects of β-blockade on nodal conduction may be additive and may lead to AV block if digoxin is administered concurrently. Drugs that alter potassium ion concentrations may also enhance digoxin toxicity. Not surprisingly, the use of succinylcholine, which may acutely alter potassium ion flux, can precipitate digoxin-induced dysrhythmias. The use of digoxin in the ICU is reserved for controlling heart rate and decreasing ventricular response to rapid atrial dysrhythmias, especially atrial fibrillation and flutter. It may be useful in converting SVT, but care must be exercised; digoxin is not the drug of first choice for SVT unless the precise diagnosis is known.

Magnesium

Magnesium is the first line of therapy for dysrhythmia in the presence of hypomagnesemia. In addition, there is anecdotal evidence of its efficacy in torsade de pointes and prolonged QT-associated VT. It may cause hypotonia (with respiratory consequences) and hypotension. It should be considered in refractory VT.

Electrical Cardioversion

Delivery of a direct-current electric shock across the thoracic wall to cause conversion of dysrhythmias is slightly more than 25 years old[90]. Since then, it has become a mainstay of emergent and elective rhythm control, both with and without other pharmacologic antidysrhythmic agents. Direct-current countershock (DCC) is most useful in treating dysrhythmias arising from reentrant phenomena, including atrial flutter, atrial fibrillation, SVT, VT, and ventricular fibrillation. It is thought to act by interrupting the abnormal reentry depolarization currents and allowing resumption of an orderly conducted sinus pacemaker rhythm. The major indication for DCC is life-threatening tachydysrhythmias with hemodynamic instability that have not responded to medical therapy and for which medical therapy may not act rapidly enough. The individual clinical situation must be evaluated, but a fast rhythm with no blood pressure requires urgent therapy. In the absence of cardiac output, parenterally administered drugs may be expected to fail. DCC may also be used to convert less threatening dysrhythmias such as atrial flutter and fibrillation, and its use in these cases is considered elective.

DCC for life-threatening ventricular dysrhythmias should be performed with the greatest possible speed. The electrodes are placed over the fifth intercostal space in the midaxillary line and in the second intercostal space just right of the sternum. Electrode impedance should be reduced by the liberal use of conducting electrode jelly; however, the conducting jelly areas should not be contiguous to avoid "shorting" the circuit. When possible, anterior-posterior electrode placement is used, because smaller currents are then required. A dose of 1–4 J/kg is recommended for VT and SVT.

For electrical cardioversion of conscious patients, cooperation between clinician and anesthesiologist is recommended. Adequate sedation is mandatory, and in children, a short-acting general anesthetic is probably indicated. In elective DCC, the shock is synchronized with the patient's ECG to avoid the T-wave and potential deterioration into life-threatening ventricular dysrhythmias. The rest of the procedure is the same as stated previously. Usually, lower doses are effective for SVT (0.5–2 J/kg).

In general, DCC has excellent results, with sinus rhythm being restored in 85% of patients with atrial fibrillation[91] and 95% of patients with atrial flutter, SVT, and ventricular tachydysrhythmias[92]. Its efficacy in cardiac arrest situations depends on the underlying viability of the heart; however, conversion of VT and coarse ventricular fibrillation can usually be relied on early in an arrest situation. The complications of DCC are rare but not insignificant. Superficial burns are the most common. Bradycardias due to enhanced vagal tone with heart block and sinus exit block can occur and frequently require atropine[93]. Occasionally, total sinus arrest may occur, and acute cardiac pacing may be emergently required.

PACEMAKERS

Advances in pacemaker technology and greater knowledge about dysrhythmias are responsible for more extensive use of pacemakers in the pediatric population. The earliest reported use of a voltage applied to a child's heart was in 1929, when Mark C. Lidwill applied 16 V to the ventricles of a stillborn infant via a transthoracic needle and successfully resuscitated the baby[94]. Since that time, developments in the design of the power source, electrodes, and implantation techniques have made pacemakers an effective and reliable means for treating cardiac dysrhythmias in children. In pediatric ICU patients, temporary pacemakers after cardiac surgery, permanently implanted pacemakers, or emergency pacing capabilities for the urgent management of cardiac dysrhythmias may be found.

Design

A current passed through the myocardium will cause cardiac contraction if it is of sufficient strength to reach threshold potential and to propagate depolarization. Pacemakers are simply controlled pulse generators in which output current (in milliamperes), pulse interval (in milliseconds), and the ability to be inhibited are incorporated (Fig. 15.18). These factors make it possible to vary the rate and output and to override the pacemaker output when indicated in response to the child's intrinsic heart rate. In addition, AV sequential pacemakers can deliver paired pulses at fixed intervals to provide physiologic synchronization of atrial and ventricular contractions when necessary. Permanently implanted pacemakers are externally programmable, and the timing and output circuits can be varied according to the child's needs and, indeed, even altered transtelephonically[95]. In addition, pacemakers can have the synchronizing mode blocked if indicated. Manufacturers have

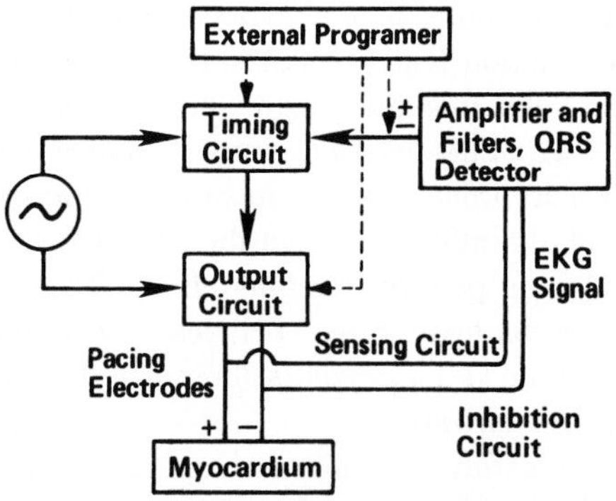

Figure 15.18. Pacemaker schematic. The timing and output circuits are programmable, and the sensing loop provides inhibition to the timing circuit. It can be disabled and rendered asynchronous if desired. For implantable pacemakers, the functions can be externally altered. *EKG*, ECG.

developed smaller-sized implantable models and improved circuits that have helped eliminate many of the problems and failures of the past.

Electrodes may be either unipolar or bipolar and may be attached to the heart in various fashions. Clearly, both an anode (positive electrode that causes hyperpolarization) and a cathode (negative electrode that causes reduction in membrane potential) are necessary to cause a cardiac contraction. In so-called unipolar pacemakers, the anode is not in direct contact with the heart. In temporary pacemakers, the anode is usually a skin wire or electrode patch, and in permanent pacemakers, it is most usually the generator case itself. Bipolar pacemakers have both an anode and a cathode in contact with the myocardium. Transvenous pacemakers are of this type. Briefly, bipolar electrodes sense better, and the pacemaker artifact is less noticeable. In addition, as anodal stimulation is more likely to lead to a ventricular dysrhythmia than is cathodal stimulation, bipolar pacers are more frequently implicated as a cause of ventricular dysrhythmias. Generally, in children, permanent pacemaking is done with epicardial electrodes, and temporary pacing is done with removable epicardial wires—systems that are virtually the same. Epicardial screw-in leads have made new implant techniques possible. However, reports comparing the screw-in (sutureless) electrode and the sutured-in electrode show a greater incidence of pacemaker exit block with screw-in type leads[96]. Epicardial electrodes remain the method of choice for permanent pacemaking in children. The transvenous implantation of pacing electrodes is technically difficult and impractical for permanent pacemaking because the transvenous wires lose ventricular contact as the child grows[97]. Nevertheless, transvenous pacemaker implantation in the pediatric population, even in infants[98,99], despite occasional reports of fatal complications from infections[100,101], is becoming more frequently used[102]. Transvenous pacing is also used when emergency temporary pacing is required.

Permanent pacemakers comprise a pulse generator and one or two electrodes. The pacing impulse is triggered by the cathode (negative terminal). The implantable pacemakers now in use have lithium iodide batteries with a life span of 4–10 years or more, depending on the type of battery, pacing rate, amount of output needed, and lead resistance[102,103]. Generators have been implanted in the anterior abdominal wall, beneath the rectus abdominis, and in the axilla, perirenal space, and even pleural cavity, and—as mentioned above—they can be externally programmed **(Table 15.9)**[102,104,105].

Indications

Symptomatic bradydysrhythmias or anticipation thereof are the major indications for pacemakers in children. These include both sinus node dysfunction and AV block. The single most common indication for cardiac pacing in children is now postoperative heart block[105–109], whereas previously the most common indication was nonsurgical sinus node dysfunction[110]. The types of surgery that commonly result in the need for pacing include repair of TGA[111], AV canal[112], tricuspid atresia[113], tetralogy of Fallot[114], and complex congenital heart disease with Wolff-Parkinson-White syndrome[115]. The other major cause of bradyarrhythmias is nonsurgical complete heart block[116], which may be congenital[117–119] and associated with various disease states, such as endocardial fibroelastosis[120], prolonged Q-T interval[121], myotonic dystrophy[122], and mesothelioma[123]. Pacemakers have also been reported as effective therapy for recurrent, severe vasovagal syncope[124], atrial arrhythmias associated with Emery-Dreifuss muscular dystrophy[125], recurrent VT[126], and SVT[127]. Tachydysrhythmias that may be readily fatal are also an indication. Guidelines for permanent pacemaker implantation are shown in **Table 15.9** [102,128–131].

Table 15.9. Indications for Cardiac Pacing

Congenital AV block
1. Ventricular rate <55 beats/min in a neonate or <50 beats/min in an older child
2. Atrial rate >140 beats/min
3. Association with other congenital heart defects
4. Congestive heart failure from low heart rate not responsive to medical therapy
5. Syncope, history of Stokes-Adams attacks
6. Decreasing exercise tolerance
7. Block located at or below bundle of His in the asymptomatic patient
8. Dizziness associated with arrhythmia or combined with Q-T prolongation
9. Ventricular ectopy refractory to drug treatment

Surgical heart block
1. Complete or second-degree AV block present 2 weeks after surgery and located at or below the bundle of His
2. Symptoms of syncope, low cardiac output, and congestive heart failure no matter what the site of block is

Acquired nonsurgical heart block

If symptomatic or if block is at or below bundle of His

Sinus bradycardia
1. Symptoms of dizziness
2. Sleeping heart rate <35 beats/min

Sick sinus syndrome

SVT refractory to medical treatment
1. Inability to be treated with surgical ablation and medication causes severe bradycardia
2. Demonstration that slow atrial pacing controls SVT in the catheterization laboratory
3. Surgical destruction of the normal AV conduction system necessary and pacemaker needed to ensure adequate ventricular response
4. Primary treatment for SVT

Temporary Pacing

Temporary pacing is indicated for patients in the ICU for similar disorders until a permanent pacemaker can be implanted. It is also used to support patients through life-threatening but reversible situations. These situations include profound bradycardias; conduction blockade; SVT; VT (rarely); escape rhythms; drug toxicity from digitalis, propranolol, or verapamil; and electrolyte imbalances such as hypokalemia or hyperkalemia. Temporary pacing is also used immediately after cardiac surgery to provide backup and support for the transiently depressed myocardium that may have a rate-dependent output. Temporary pacing is also increasingly used to aid in the diagnosis of several arrhythmias.

Transvenous insertion of a pacing catheter can be performed in the cardiac catheterization laboratory, the operating room, or the ICU. The pacemaker may be placed through the jugular, subclavian, brachial, or femoral veins. The techniques for cannulation of these vessels have been described elsewhere. ECG guidance is recommended, and pacemaker operation in the VOO mode will demonstrate capture. Atrial or ventricular pacing is possible.

Temporary pacemakers either routinely attached to postoperative cardiac patients by surgically implanted wires or used in conjunction with transvenous or transthoracic emergent pacing consist of the essential elements outlined above. Transthoracic pacing is readily established by placing a pacing wire into the right or left ventricle via a spinal needle inserted either subxiphoid or through the left fifth intercostal space. These pacemakers provide the most rapid means of pacing the arrested heart and are indicated if time does not allow transvenous insertion.

Two alternatives for emergency pacing exist that are less invasive. The first, transesophageal cardiac pacing, has been widely used[30,95,132]. The esophagus is intimately related to the left atrium, and thus electrode placement can be established without surgery or transvenous pacing. This mode of pacing is especially useful for overdrive suppression pacing of SVT and terminating reentrant phenomenon-dependent dysrhythmias[132,133]. In addition, it has proved successful for atrial flutter and fibrillation conversion[95,102]. Clearly, it is of less use for treating ventricular dysrhythmias and not useful at all for managing heart block, since only atrial pacing is achieved. Its use requires a stronger pulse generator because cardiac tissue is further from the electrode (0–40 mA at a pulse width of 0–10 msec). A standard bipolar intracardiac pacing catheter can be positioned in the esophagus with ECG guidance. This technique provides a useful approach to atrial dysrhythmias in pediatric ICU patients. Transcutaneous pacing is also possible. Large pacing electrodes are placed on the chest and back. Special equipment is required. Current is increased until ventricular capture is produced. Figure 15.19 shows a typical pacemaker and the controls available on its front panel.

Use

The pacemaker rate is set according to the patient's need, and in pediatric patients, this varies widely with age (Fig. 15.1). In critically ill children, the higher range of normal is appropriate. For treatment of bradydysrhythmias, the rate should be set within the normal range for the age group. Once an ECG QRS complex is produced (capture), the blood pressure should be assessed. If it is not improved, then increasing pacemaker output will not help. An increased rate may help, however. If there is capture without pressure generation, electromechanical dissociation exists and requires appropriate therapy, not more pacing. Tachydysrhythmias are treated either by slow *underdrive* atrial pacing, which may interrupt SVT, or by overdriving the abnormal rhythm with a very fast rate and acutely discontinuing pacing. For this reason, the pacemaker must be capable of high rates (200–600/min).

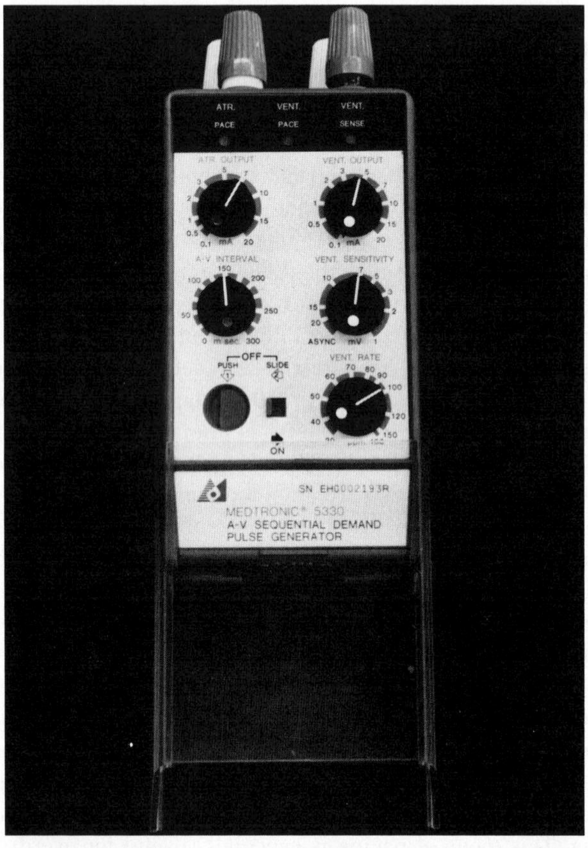

Figure 15.19. Meditronics AV sequential external pacemaker. Notice four electrode terminals. At the top are indicator lights showing when atrial and ventricular pacing occur and sensing of ventricular activity. Both atrial and ventricular outputs can be adjusted from 0.1–20 mA. Ventricular sensing sensitivity from asynchronous to 1 mV can be set. The AV interval can range from 0 to 300 msec, and the ventricular rate can be adjusted from 30 to 180 beats/min. The "on" switch requires the use of one hand, whereas the "off" switch requires the use of two hands. A clear plastic shield protects against inadvertent alterations.

The output current to achieve the threshold potential that is generally required by a temporary pacemaker is usually below 1 mA, often 0.5 mA or less. The maintenance current should be set 2–5 times above this threshold to ensure constant capture. The threshold current required should be routinely checked and the output control adjusted. In an emergency situation when the electrode position is questionable, the pacer can be set to maximum output (20 mA) to capture, and the current can then be slowly decreased as proper positioning is obtained.

Pacemaker function is described by a multiletter code. The first letter A(trial), V(entricular), D(ual), or S(ingle) indicates the paced cardiac chamber. The second letter indicates the sensed chamber: A, V, D, or 0 for no sensing. The third letter indicates the pacemaker's response to sensed beats: I(nhibited), T(riggered), D(ual), or 0 for no response. A fourth letter is used to note special features, such as R for rate responsive. Thus, V00 is a nonsensing ventricular pacemaker. VVI indicates a ventricular pacemaker which is inhibited by sensed ventricular beats.

Temporary pacing in the critical care setting is usually provided in the synchronous-demand pacemaking mode. This is provided by using a sensing circuit to inhibit ventricular pacing in the critical period after an intrinsic cardiac contraction. Thus, in the synchronized mode, the heart is ventricularly paced and sensed, and the pacemaker is inhibited (VVI mode). Competition with the patient's own intrinsic rhythm is prevented, and there is less chance that ventricular tachydysrhythmias will occur. Also in this VVI mode, a backup rate can be set below the patient's intrinsic rate as a safety feature should a sudden bradydysrhythmia occur. In this mode, the sensing dial should be set with sensitivity to greater than 6 mV consistently, and it should be noted that the sensing indicator is being triggered. In the emergency situation when there is not intrinsic rhythm, the asynchronous mode is used. In this mode the heart is ventricularly paced, not sensed, and there is no response to the patient's intrinsic rate (V00 mode). This mode is not indicated if the patient has an intrinsic rate.

Recently there has been wider use of the physiologic AV sequential pacemaker (Fig 15.19), especially in children with hemodynamic compromise. These pacemakers, now routinely used in our ICU, have the ability to pace independently both atrially and ventricularly and thus have four terminals (anode and cathode for each chamber). The operator can set both atrial and ventricular output and set the ventricular rate. In addition, the duration between the atrial impulse and the ventricular impulse (P-R interval) can be varied. These pacemakers are thus double-chamber pacing (atrial and ventricular) and double-chamber sensing and can have double-mode response (atrial inhibited, ventricular paced) and can be programmed to the universal mode (DDD). This system most closely mimics the normal cardiac electrical sequence and can provide dramatic improvement in hemodynamic function compared with the VVI or V00 mode.

The complications of cardiac pacing are multiple but clinically uncommon. The pacing wires inserted temporarily are occasionally associated with pericardial bleeding and tamponade, especially when removed. All electrodes and implantable generators carry some risk of infection, which must be constantly watched for. During permanent pacing, lead fracture, desensitization, and generator malfunction have all been reported but hopefully are becoming less frequent with improved technology. Complications subsequent to pacing include ventricular dysrhythmias and the potential for decreased cardiac output as the result of poorly timed pacing at an inadequate rate. The most common ICU complication in the emergent situation is failure to capture, due to either myocardial damage or improper electrode replacement.

In summary, electrical cardiac pacing can be used not only to cause an asystolic heart to beat but also to convert certain dysrhythmias and to optimize cardiac output in the critically ill child. Pacemaking can be permanent or, more commonly, temporary, as used in the ICU(134). Familiarity with the simple basic techniques of pacing and the principles underlying it can be lifesaving in the pediatric ICU and deserves the attention of all physicians caring for critically ill children.

RADIOFREQUENCY CATHETER ABLATION AND SURGICAL TREATMENT OF DYSRHYTHMIAS

The ablation of the necessary conduction pathways in Wolff-Parkinson-White syndrome(135) introduced the concept of surgical treatment for dysrhythmias. Surgical ablative techniques have since been used to treat a wide variety of refractory pediatric dysrhythmias(136). Surgical techniques have progressed from ablation of the AV mode(137), with resultant third-degree heart block and pacemaker placement, to specific interruption of reentry pathways(138). The exciting development of percutaneous nonoperative catheter ablative techniques(139,140), using either direct-current ablation(141) or, more recently, radiofrequency ablation(142,140), has further increased the potential for nonpharmacologic treatment of cardiac dysrhythmias. Nevertheless, for refractory arrhythmias in children, the surgical approach remains attractive especially for AVNRT and VT(143). Although the major application is for treatment of chronic or relapsing tachydysrhythmias, therapy for refractory life-threatening situations is also possible(136,144). Not only may reentry dysrhythmias be treated, but foci of ectopic activity can be ablated(136,145). SVT, VT, atrial tachycardia, flutter and fibrillation, JET, and AV nodal reentry phenomena have all been treated by this approach(58,62,145,146). Precise electrophysiologic mapping is essential no matter which technique is used. Specialized, interventional cardiology techniques and

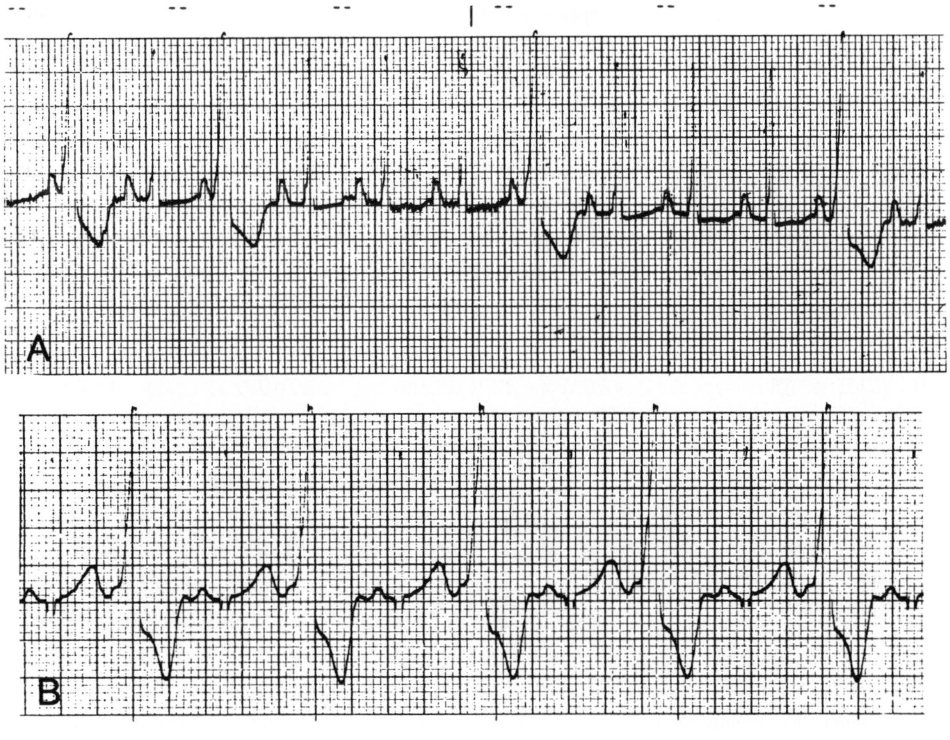

Figure 15.20. Two different examples of wide QRS complexes. Timing is crucial. Is **A** an example of ventricular extrasystoles, fusion beats, or preexcitation with aberrant conduction? The P-P interval is regular (sinus node not reset). The abnormal QRS complexes are premature. The P-R intervals in the first three abnormal complexes are shorter than the last, while QRS morphology is constant. Thus, these are most likely ventricular ectopics occurring before AV nodal conduction has occurred. In **B**, the P-waves are regular, but every other one is variably lost in the QRS. These have a compensatory pause. In effect, these are more obviously ectopic PVCs than those in **A.**

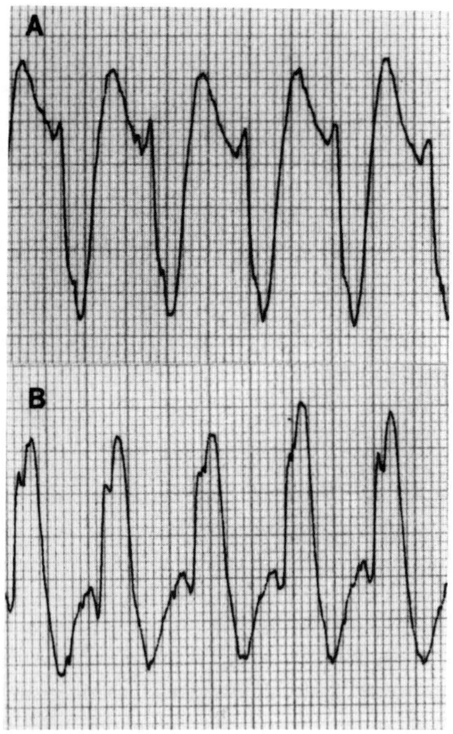

Figure 15.21. Wide complex tachycardia (145 beats/min, regular). In **A,** obvious P-waves are absent in lead V_1. By observing lead II **(B),** clear P-waves and a P-QRS 1 : 1 relationship are seen, identifying this as SVT.

expertise are required. In the life-threatening situation, this approach may present a useful option for the refractory tachydysrhythmia.

THE PROBLEM TACHYCARDIA

Treating specific dysrhythmias follows reasonably clear guidelines once the rhythm disturbance is correctly diagnosed. This may not be so simple. Many dysrhythmias encountered in the ICU defy ready diagnosis. In the absence of an ECG before the dysrhythmia in a sick child with a fast heart, what do you do? Recently, the terms *narrow complex tachycardia* and *wide complex tachycardia* have become fashionable. This reflects the occasional difficulty of differentiating between SVT and VT, which would guide therapy in the emergent situation. In addition, it has been recognized that the urgency with which these need to be differentiated is perhaps more dependent on the clinical situation than on precise diagnosis, since similar therapeutic approaches are frequently appropriate for both. Thus, using the terms narrow or wide complex tachycardia has some practical application and honestly reflects the occasional impossibility of knowing the source of a particular dysrhythmia.

Narrow complex tachycardias can be atrial, junctional, or even ventricular in origin, especially in children. Wide complex tachycardias are due to either VT or aberrantly conducted SVT[69]. The urgency to treat these tachycardias is dictated by the presence of hemodynamic instability or a concern for injury that may arise from the imbalance of oxygen supply-and-demand relationships, leading to ischemic injury. Clearly, if the child has hypotension, blunted level of consciousness, or other evidence of hypoperfusion, therapy is more urgent than precise diagnosis (see below). If the child is hemodynamically stable and in no distress, meticulous diagnosis will be possible. Diagnosis depends on whether or not there is a P-wave, and its timing, morphology, and relationship to the QRS complexes. In SVT, clear P-waves should have a constant relationship to the QRS complex. If AV dissociation is present, the tachycardia has a lower origin (JET or VT). QRS morphology is of little help in differentiating narrow complex tachycardias. Comparison to the normal rhythm complexes may be of some help. If the frontal plan axis alters, then atrial origin is unlikely. In wide complex tachycardias, previous QRS morphology is important. The presence of aberrantly conducted PACs before the onset of the tachycardia with similar morphology to the tachycardia complex suggests SVT, but this is not always easy to determine (Fig. 15.20). Frontal axis is also important; a shift from regular sinus beats suggests VT. Detailed 12-lead ECG analysis may reveal the underlying source of the tachycardia (Fig. 15.21).

The presence of fusion beats is also critical (Figs. 15.12 and 15.22). Premature beats with a combination of atrial

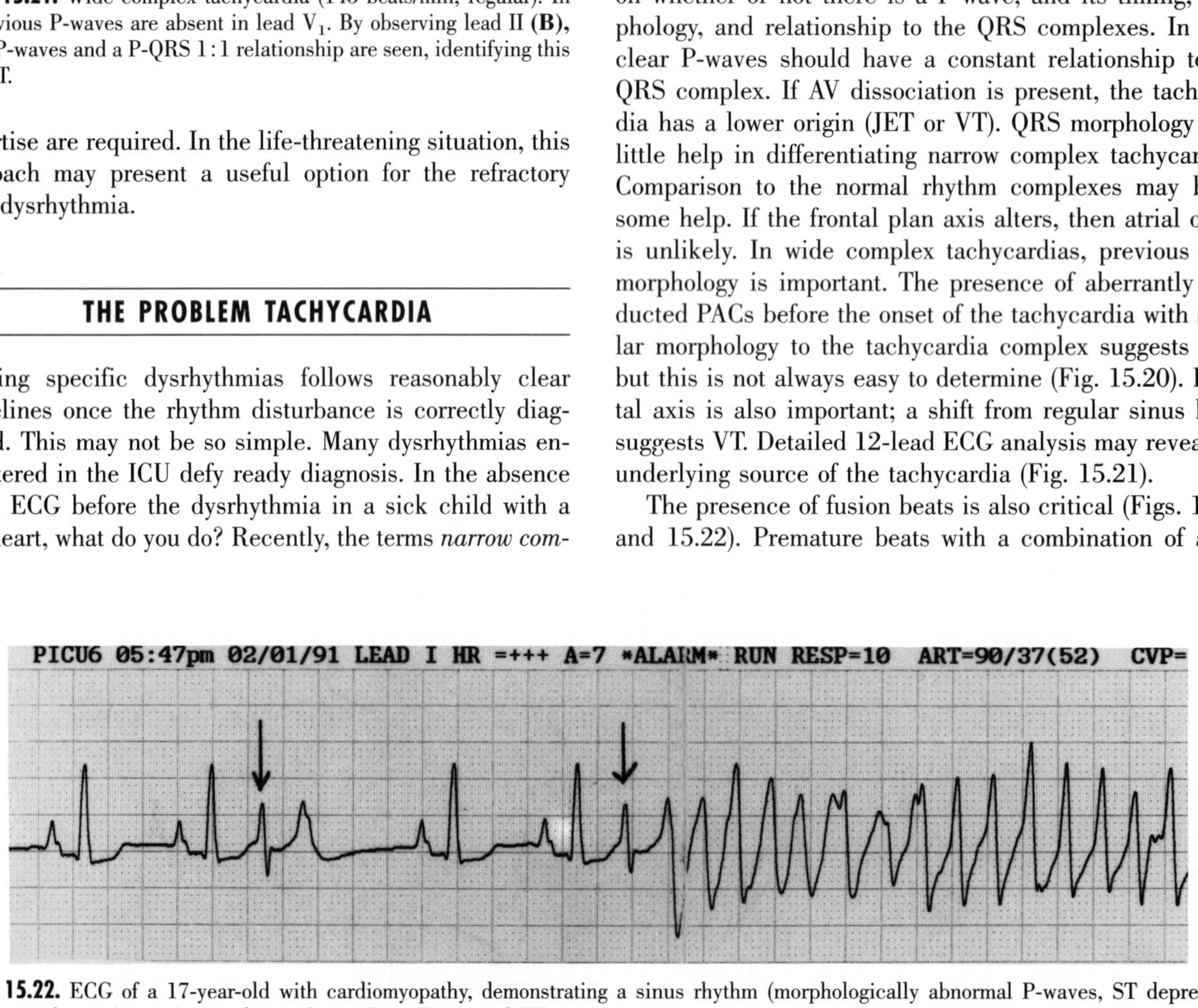

Figure 15.22. ECG of a 17-year-old with cardiomyopathy, demonstrating a sinus rhythm (morphologically abnormal P-waves, ST depression) with fusion beats *(arrows)* preceding a fusion R-on-T-initiated VT.

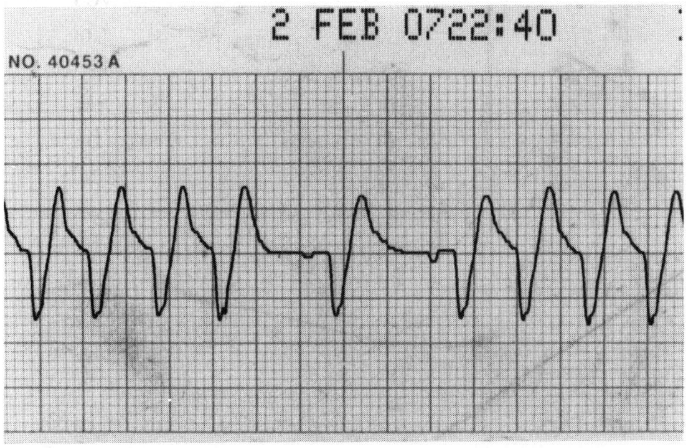

Figure 15.23. Wide complex tachycardia that was slowed, with emergence of P-waves, by carotid sinus massage. This suggests that the underlying rhythm is SVT.

and ventricular characteristics occur when an atrial beat occurs near simultaneously with an ectopic ventricular beat(69). They may have a wide spectrum of forms, depending on the timing and site of the ectopic ventricular beat. QRS width is also variable. Fusion beats can be narrow, especially if atrial, aberrantly conducted beats are also present. Fusion beats indicate that there is a ventricular ectopic focus and suggest that the tachycardia is ventricular in origin.

In addition to a full ECG, nonconventional recordings can be made to determine the presence of atrial activity and its relationship to the QRS complexes. Recordings may be taken from epicardial wires or esophageal leads. Recording these leads on a V_1 or a bipolar limb lead may show the P-QRS relationship. Simultaneously recording three or more leads may help to identify this relationship. AV dissociation indicates VT. Unfortunately, a 1:1 relationship does not always indicate SVT. Retrograde atrial depolarization may occur in VT and even JET. The total absence of atrial activity is diagnostic(148).

Frequently, vagal maneuvers may slow or convert SVT (Fig. 15.23). Responses to carotid massage, Valsalva's maneuver, or ice to the face (diving reflex) may demonstrate the atrial origin of the tachycardia and guide further therapy(147). Slowing or even brief interruption of the rhythm may indicate the atrial origin, but total absence of effect does not help differentiate VT from SVT. If sinus rhythm is restored at any time by physiologic, pharmacologic, or electrical means, a full ECG should immediately be obtained. Even a few sinus beats may provide the key to diagnosing underlying rhythm disturbance. The occurrence of PACs, aberrancy, preexcitation, PVCs, or fusion beats will guide further therapy.

So what should be done if, in consultation with a cardiologist and after several diagnostic ECGs, the rhythm remains undiagnosed and the patient's clinical condition warrants therapy? Every effort should be made to diagnose the rhythm, but if this is not possible, how does one proceed? If the child is hypotensive and in need of urgent therapy, direct-current countershock starting at 1 J/kg and increasing to 4 J/kg will convert both SVT and VT 85–95% of the time. QRS synchronization is preferred but may be difficult in wide complex tachycardia. Digoxin-induced tachycardias should not be cardioverted as more unstable VT or ventricular fibrillation may result. Electrolyte abnormalities should be corrected, volume resuscitation ensured, and oxygen given. Pacing, if readily available, may also terminate the tachycardia, especially if it is an escape rhythm-initiated dysrhythmia. Overdrive pacing should be tried if leads are in situ in the unstable patient.

If the patient is relatively stable and the rhythm still uncertain, a trial of therapy is indicated. The choice is between drugs and pacing and depends on the clinical situation and availability of equipment. Pharmacologic therapy is often more readily available. At this stage a hunch must be played. In wide complex tachycardia, if VT is more likely, lidocaine should be given as many as three times. In narrow complex tachycardia, a bolus of adenosine has few side effects and will rapidly convert SVT (and possibly JET). If there is any conversion, future therapy should take the rhythm, the drug, and the response into account. The short duration of action of adenosine also suggests its use (Fig. 15.17)(150). An alternative might be esmolol(147). This short-acting cardioselection β_1-agent may convert SVT and VT in children(151). Obviously, myocardial depression is a concern; however, the short duration (3–5 minutes) of esmolol makes this a low risk. In addition, interactions between β-blockers and calcium channel blockers or digoxin can also be avoided(74,152). Procainamide is a second-line drug for VT and may be used to treat SVT, although it is

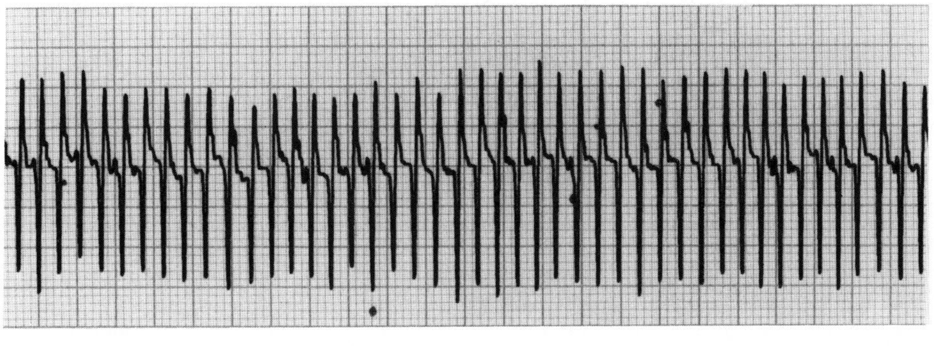

Figure 15.24. An ECG with apparent narrow complex tachycardia at a rate of nearly 600 beats/min. The patient is a 6-year-old child during a prolonged myoclonic seizure. It did not respond to adenosine. Valium resolved the rhythm disturbance. Despite the alarming ECG appearance, 1:1 conduction at a rate of 600, or a ventricular rate of 600, is extremely unlikely, if not impossible. This is a neurologic, not cardiac, problem.

not a preferred choice. Magnesium may be of help and has few side effects. Surface cooling may be tried if JET is considered.

If the rhythm persists, unresponsive to the above therapy, and no clues have been gained, pacing and cardioversion should be considered. Other drugs (bretylium, digoxin) have significant risks and are best avoided in an uncertain situation, especially after the above agents have been tried. Generally, these refractory undiagnosable rhythms are rare. Intracardiac electrophysiologic studies are indicated if the rhythm persists and remains unresponsive. Constant review of the ECG responses to therapy and the child's condition, with vigilance, are necessary in this setting. Finally, understanding the child's entire condition and interpreting this with the cardiac status may occasionally resolve the most difficult ECG dysrhythmia problem (Fig. 15.24).

References

1. Downing SE, Talner NS, Gardner TH. Ventricular function in the newborn lamb. Am J Physiol 1965;208:931.
2. Heymann MA, Rudolph AM. Effect of increasing preload on right ventricular output in fetal lambs in utero. Circulation 1973;48(Suppl 4):37.
3. Rudolph AM, Heymann MA. Cardiac output in the fetal lamb: the effects of spontaneous and induced changes in heart rate and left ventricular output. Am J Obstet Gynecol 1976;124:183.
4. Friedman WF. Intrinsic properties of the developing heart. Prog Cardiovasc Dis 1972;15:87.
5. Garson A. The electrocardiogram in infants and children: a systematic approach. Philadelphia: Lea & Febiger, 1983:195.
6. Kugler JD. Sinoatrial node dysfunction. In: Gillette PC, Garson A, eds. Pediatric cardiac dysrhythmias. New York: Grune & Stratton, 1981:265.
7. Vetter VL, Rashkind WJ. Congenital complete heart block and connective-tissue disease. N Engl J Med 1983; 309:236.
8. Husson GS, Blackman MS, Rogers MC, Bhavati S, Lev M. Familial congenital bundle branch system disease. Am J Cardiol 1973;32:365.
9. Pinsky WW. Diagnosis and management of congenital complete atrioventricular block. In: Gillette PC, Garson A, eds. Pediatric cardiac dysrhythmias. New York: Grune & Stratton, 1981:383.
10. Scott JS, Maddison PJ, Taylor PV, Esscher E, Scott O, Skinner RP. Connective-tissue disease, antibodies to ribonucleoprotein, and congenital heart block. N Engl J Med 1983;309:209.
11. Anderson PAW, Rogers MC, Canent RB, Spach MS. Reversible complete heart block following surgery: analysis with His bundle electrocardiograms. Circulation 1972;46:514.
12. Garson A, Nihill MR, McNamara DG, et al. Status of the adult and adolescent after repair of tetralogy of Fallot. Circulation 1979;59:1232.
13. Jervell A, Lange-Nielsen F. Congenital deaf-mutism, functional heart disease with prolongation of the Q-T interval and sudden death. Am Heart J 1957;54:59.
14. James TN. Congenital deafness and cardiac arrhythmias. Am J Cardiol 1967;19:627.
15. Ward OC. A new familial cardiac syndrome in children. Ir Med J 1964;54:103.
16. McRae JR, Wagner GS, Rogers MC, Canent RV. Paroxysmal familial ventricular fibrillation. J Pediatr 1974; 84:515.
17. Rogers MC, Zahka KG, Nugent SK, Gioia FR, Epple L. Electrocardiographic abnormalities in infants and children with neurological injury. Crit Care Med 1980;8:213.
18. Gillette PC, Garson A, Porter CJ, McNamara DG. Arrhythmias. In: Adams FH, Emmanouilides GC, eds. Heart disease in infants, children and adolescents. Baltimore: Williams & Wilkins, 1983:725.
19. Guntheroth WG. Pediatric electrocardiograms. Philadelphia: WB Saunders, 1965.
20. Garson A, Gillette PC, McNamara DG. A guide to cardiac dysrhythmias in children. New York: Grune & Stratton, 1980.
21. Kaplan BM, Langendorf R, Lev M, Pick A. Tachycardia-bradycardia syndrome (so-called "sick sinus syndrome"). Am J Cardiol 1973;31:497.
22. Alpert MA, Flaker GC. Arrhythmias associated with sinus node dysfunction. JAMA 1983;250:2160.
23. Kugler JD, Gillette PC, Mullins CE, McNamara DG. Sinoatrial conduction in children: an index of sinoatrial node function. Circulation 1979;59:1266.
24. Schiller MS, Levin AR, Haft JI, Engle MA, Ehlers KH, Klein AA. Electrophysiologic studies in sick sinus syndrome following surgery for d-transposition of the great arteries. J Pediatr 1977;91:891.
25. Helfant RH. Bellet's essentials of cardiac arrhythmias. 2nd ed. Philadelphia: WB Saunders, 1979.
26. Chung EK. Principles of cardiac arrhythmias. 2nd ed. Baltimore: Williams & Wilkins, 1977.
27. Zipes DP. Second-degree atrioventricular block. Circulation 1979;60:465.
28. Michaelsson A, Engle MA. Congenital complete heart block: an international study of the natural history. In: Brest AN, Engle M, eds. Cardiovascular clinics. Philadelphia: FA Davis, 1972:85.
29. Driscoll DJ. Surgical complete atrioventricular block. In: Gillette PC, Garson A, eds. Pediatric cardiac dysrhythmias. New York: Grune & Stratton, 1981:397.
30. Backofen JE, Schauble JF, Rogers MC. Transesophageal pacing for bradycardia. Anesthesiology 1984;61:777.
31. Morriss JH, Gillette PC, Barrett FF. Atrioventricular block complicating meningitis; treatment with emergency cardiac pacing. Pediatrics 1976;58:866.
32. Garson A, Gillette PC, McNamara DG. Supraventricular tachycardia in children: clinical features, response to treatment and long-term follow-up in 217 patients. J Pediatr 1981;98:875.
33. Fisher DJ, Gross DM, Garson A. Rapid sinus tachycardia—differentiation from supraventricular tachycardia. Am J Dis Child 1983;37:164.
34. Gallagher JJ, Pritchett ELC, Sealy WC, et al. The preexcitation syndromes. Prog Cardiovasc Dis 1978;20:285.
35. Ganz LI, Friedman PL. Supraventricular tachycardia. N Engl J Med 1995; 332:162-173.
36. Casta A, Wolff GS, Mehta AV, Tamer D, Garcia OL, Pickoff AS, Ferrer PL, Sung RJ, Gelband H. Dual atrioventricular nodal pathways: a benign finding in arrhythmia-free children with heart disease. Am J Cardiol 1980;48:1013.
37. Levy AM, Bonazinga BJ. Sudden sinus slowing with junctional escape: a common mode of initiation of juvenile supraventricular tachycardia. Circulation 1983;67: 84–87.
38. Bauersfeld U, Gow RM, Hamilton RM, Izukawa T. Treatment of atrial ectopic tachycardia in infants < 6 months old. Am Heart J 1995; 129:1145-1148.
39. Dhala AA, Case CL, Gillette PC. Evolving treatment strategies for managing atrial ectopic tachycardia in children. Am J Cardiol 1994; 74:283–286.
40. Lingman G, Lundstrom N-R, Marsal K, Ohrlander S. Fetal cardiac arrhythmia: clinical outcome in 113 cases. Acta Obstet Gynecol Scand 1986;65:263–267.
41. Lingman G, Ohrlander S, Ohlin P. Intrauterine digoxin treatment of fetal paroxysmal tachycardia. Br J Obstet Gynaecol 1980;87:340–342.
42. Garson A, Gillette PC. Junctional ectopic tachycardia in children: electrocardiography, electrophysiology and pharmacology response. Am J Cardiol 1979;44:298.
43. Kastor JA. Multifocal atrial tachycardia. N Engl J Med 1990;322:1713.
44. Hamilton J, Moodie D, Levy J. The use of the diving reflex to terminate supraventricular tachycardia in a 6 week old infant. Am Heart J 1979;97:371.
45. Grahame IFM, Hann IM. Use of the diving reflex to treat supraventricular tachycardia in an infant. Arch Dis Child 1978;53:515.
46. Bissett GS, Gaum W, Kaplan S. The ice bag: a new technique for interruption of supraventricular tachycardia. J Pediatr 1980;97:593.
47. Dreifus LS, Haiat R, Watanabe Y, et al. Ventricular fibrillation: a possible mechanism of sudden death in patients with WPW syndrome. Circulation 1971;43:520.
48. Drugs for cardiac arrhythmias. Med Lett 1991;33:55–60.
49. DeWolf D, Rondia G, Verhaaren H, Matthys D. Adenosine triphosphate treatment for supraventricular tachycardia in infants. Eur J Pediatr 1994; 153:668-671.
50. Till J, Shinebourne EA, Rigby ML, Clarke B, Ward DE, Rowland E. Efficacy and safety of adenosine in the treatment of supraventricular tachycardia in infants and children. Br Heart J 1989;62:204–211.
51. Porter CJ, Gillette PC, Garson A, Hesslein PS, Karpawich PP, McNamara DG. The effects of verapamil on supraventricular tachycardia in children. Am J Cardiol 1981;48:487.

52. Gibson R, Driscoll DJ, Hartley CJ, Gillette PC. The comparative electrophysiologic and hemodynamic effects of verapamil in puppies and adult dogs. Dev Pharmacol Ther 1981;2:104.
53. Benson DW, Dunnigan A, Benditt DG, Pritzker MR, Thompson TR. Transesophageal study of infant supraventricular tachycardia: electrophysiologic characteristics. Am J Cardiol 1984;53:63.
54. Garson A. Atrial flutter in the young: a collaborative study of 380 cases. J Am Coll Cardiol 1985;6:871.
55. Ashraf MH, Cotroneo J, DiMarco D, Subramanian S. Fate of long-term survivors of mustard procedure (inflow repair) for simple and complex transposition of the great arteries. Ann Thorac Surg 1986;42:385–389.
56. Yeager SB, Hougen TJ, Levy AM. Sudden death in infants with chronic atrial rhythm. Am J Dis Child 1984; 138:689–692.
57. Zeevi B, Berant M, Sclarovsky S, Blieden LC. Treatment of multifocal atrial tachycardia with amiodarone in a child with congenital heart disease. Am J Cardiol 1986; 57:344–345.
58. Gillette PC, Garson A Jr, Hesslein PS, Karpawich PP, Tierney RC, Cooley DA, McNamara DG. Successful surgical treatment of atrial, junctional, and ventricular tachycardia unassociated with accessory connections in infants and children. Am Heart J 1981;102:984.
59. Waldo AL, Krongrad E, Kupersmith J, et al. Ventricular paired pacing to control rapid ventricular heart rate following open heart surgery. Circulation 1976;53:176.
60. Garson A, Hesslein PS, McVey P, Porter CJ, Gillette PC. Amiodarone in the young: treatment of choice for atrial flutter [Abstract 682]. Circulation 1982;66(Suppl II):II.
61. Paul T, Guccione P. New antiarrhythmic drugs in pediatric use: amiodarone. Pediatr Cardiol 1994; 15:132–138.
62. Gillette PC, Garson A, McVey P, Porter CJ. Junctional ectopic tachycardia: new proposed treatment by transcatheter His bundle ablation. Am Heart J 1983;106:619.
63. Garson A, Smith RT, Moke JP. Control of postoperative junctional ectopic tachycardia with propafenone. J Am Coll Cardiol 1985;5:428.
64. Yabek SM. Ventricular arrhythmias in children with an apparently normal heart. J Pediatr 1991;119:1–11.
65. Jackman WM, Friday KJ, Anderson JL, et al. The long QT syndromes: a critical review, new clinical observations and a unifying hypothesis. Prog Cardiovasc Dis 1988; 31:115–172.
66. Tzivoni D, Banai S, Schuger C, et al. Treatment of torsades de pointes with magnesium sulfate. Circulation 1988;77:392–397.
67. Koch-Weser J. Disopyramide. N Engl J Med 1979; 300:957.
68. Koch-Weser J. Bretylium. N Engl J Med 1979;300:473.
69. Rinkenberger RL, Naccarelli GV. Evaluation and acute treatment of wide complex tachycardias. Crit Care Clin 1989;5:599.
70. Hager WD, Fenster P, Mayersohn M, Perrier D, Graves P, Marcus FI, Goldman S. Digoxin-quinidine interaction. Pharmacokinetic evaluation. N Engl J Med 1979; 300:1238.
71. Gerstenblith G, Spear JF, Moore EN. Quantitative study of the effect of lidocaine on the threshold for ventricular fibrillation in the dog. Am J Cardiol 1972;30:242.
72. Kupersmith J, Shiang H, Litwak RS, Herman MV. Electrophysiological and antiarrhythmic effects of propranolol in canine acute myocardial ischemia. Circ Res 1976;38:302.
73. Greenblatt DJ, Bolognini V, Koch-Weser J, Harmatz JS. Pharmacokinetic approach to the clinical use of lidocaine intravenously. JAMA 1976;236:273.
74. Case CL, Trippel DL, Gillette PC. New antiarrhythmic agents in pediatrics. Pediatr Clin North Am 1989; 36:1293.
75. Stagg AL, Wallace AG. The effect of propranolol on membrane conductance in canine cardiac Purkinje fibers. Circulation 1974;50(Suppl 3):145.
76. Davis LD, Temte JV. Effects of propranolol on the transmembrane potentials of ventricular muscle and Purkinje fibers of the dog. Circ Res 1968;22:661.
77. Leveque PE. Antiarrhythmic action of bretylium. Nature 1965;207:203.
78. Kniffen FJ, Lomas T, Counsell RE, Lucchesi BR. The antiarrhythmic and antifibrillatory actions of bretylium and its *o*-iodobenzyltrimethylammonium analog, UM-360. J Pharmacol Exp Ther 1975;192:120.
79. Anderson JL, Patterson E, Conlon M, Pasyk S, Pitt B, Lucchesi BR. Kinetics of antifibrillatory effects of bretylium: correlation with myocardial drug concentrations. Am J Cardiol 1980;46:583.
80. Bernstein JG, Koch-Weser J. Effectiveness of bretylium tosylate against refractory ventricular arrhythmias. Circulation 1972;45:1024.
81. Roberts WC, ed. Symposium on the management of ventricular arrhythmias. Am J Cardiol 1984;54:1.
82. Singh BN. Amiodarone. Am Heart J 1983;106:788.
83. Saksena S, Rothbart ST, Shah Y, Cappello G. Clinical efficacy and electropharmacology of continuous intravenous amiodarone infusion and chronic oral amiodarone in refractory ventricular tachycardia. Am J Cardiol 1984; 54:347.
84. Rakita L, Sobol SM. Amiodarone in the treatment of refractory ventricular arrhythmias. Importance and safety of initial high-dose therapy. JAMA 1983;250:1293.
85. Wit AL, Cranefield PF. Effect of verapamil on the sinoatrial and atrioventricular nodes of the rabbit and the mechanism by which it arrests re-entrant atrioventricular tachycardia. Circ Res 1974;35:413.
86. Nademanee K, Singh BN. Advances in antiarrhythmic therapy. The role of newer antiarrhythmic drugs. JAMA 1982;247:217.
87. Pantely GA, Bristow JD. Adenosine: renewed interest in an old drug. Circulation 1990;82:1854–1856.
88. Clarke B, Till J, Rowland E, et al. Rapid and safe termination of supraventricular tachycardia in children by adenosine. Lancet 1987;1:299–301.
89. Roger MC, Willerson JT, Goldblatt A, Smith TW. Serum digoxin concentrations in the human fetus, neonate and infant. N Engl J Med 1972;287:1010.
90. Lown B, Amarasingham R, Newman J. New method for terminating cardiac arrhythmias. Use of synchronized capacitor discharge. JAMA 1962;182:548.
91. Resnekov L, McDonald L. Appraisal of electrocardioversion in treatment of cardiac dysrhythmias. Br Heart J 1968;30:786.
92. Razavi M, Duarte EP, Tahmooressi P. Cardioversion: ten year Cleveland Clinic experience. Cleve Clin Q 1976; 43:175.
93. Lown B, Kleiger R, Wolff G. The technique of cardioversion. Am Heart J 1964;67:282.
94. Gold RD. Cardiac pacing—from then to now. Med Instrum 1984;18:15.
95. Dick M, Campbell RM. Advances in the management of cardiac arrhythmias in children. Pediatr Clin North Am 1984;31:1175.
96. DeLeon SY, Ilbawi MN, Koster N, Idriss FS. Comparison of the sutureless and suture-type epicardial electrodes in pediatric cardiac pacing. Ann Thorac Surg 1982;33:273.
97. DeLeon SY, Ilbawi MN, Idriss FS. Pacemaker implantation in infants and children: a simplified approach. Ann Thorac Surg 1980;30:599.
98. Fraedrick G, Mulch J, Netz H, Scheld HH. Actively adhering endocardial leads for pacing in children. Thorac Cardiovasc Surg 1981;29:242.
99. Holmes DR, Maloney JD, Feldt RH. The use of percutaneous subclavian techniques for permanent cardiac pacing in childhood. Mayo Clin Proc 1980;55:579.
100. Brunswick RA, Moynihan PC, Webb WR. Treatment of pacemaker infection in the neonate. J Thorac Cardiovasc Surg 1980;80:123.
101. DeLeon SY, Bojar R, Kosta NK, Ilbawi MN, Munez H, Idriss FS. Recurrent sepsis from retained endocardial electrode in children: successful removal with cardiopulmonary bypass. PACE 1984;7:166.
102. Kugler JD, Danford DA. Pacemakers in children: an update. Am Heart J 1989;117:665–679.
103. Gillette PC. Recent advances in mechanisms, evaluation and pacemaker treatment of chronic bradydysrhythmias in children. Am Heart J 1981;102:920.
104. Hafez A, Conso JF, Belhaj M, Planche C, Binet JP. Perirenal space implantation of permanent cardiac pacemakers in infants and small children. Thorac Cardiovasc Surg 1983;31:101.
105. Young D. Permanent pacemaker implantation in children: current status and future considerations. PACE 1981;4:61.
106. Driscoll DJ, Gillette PC, Hallman GL, Cooley DA, McNamara DG. Management of surgical complete atrioventricular block in children. Am J Cardiol 1979;43:1175.
107. McCue CM, Robertson LW, Goldstein S. Grand rounds: pacemakers in children. Va Med 1981;108:460.
108. Waelkens JJJ. Cardiac pacemakers in infants and children. Pediatr Cardiol 1982;3:337.
109. Ward DE, Signig M, Oldershaw P, Jones S, Shinebourne EA. Cardiac pacing in children. Arch Dis Child 1982;57:514.
110. Fleming WH, Sarafain LB, Kugler JD, Hofschire PJ, Clarke EB. Changing indications for pacemakers in children. Ann Thorac Surg 1981;31:329.

111. Mahoney L, Turley K, Ebert P, Heymann MA. Long term results after atrial repair of transposition of the great arteries in early infancy. Circulation 1982;66:253.
112. Bender HW, Hammon JW, Hubbard SG, Muirhead J, Graham TP. Repair of atrioventricular canal malformation in the first year of life. J Thorac Cardiovasc Surg 1982;84:512.
113. Gale AW, Danielson GK, McGoon DC, Wallace RB, Mair DD. Fontan procedure for tricuspid atresia. Circulation 1980;62:91.
114. Bolens M, Friedle B. Progressive atrioventricular block after total correction of Fallot's tetralogy, documented by repeat electrophysiological studies. Cardiology 1982; 69:185.
115. Benson DW, Gallagher JJ, Oldham HN, Sealy WC, Sterba R, Spach MS. Corrected transposition with severe intracardiac deformities with Wolff-Parkinson-White syndrome in a child. Circulation 1980; 61:1256.
116. Vanetti A, Donzeau-George GP, Frank R, Fourate M, Evans J, Ismail MB, Daumet P. Surgical treatment for a complicated congenital aortic stenosis. J Thorac Cardiovasc Surg 1979;77:230.
117. Esscher EB. Congenital complete heart block in adolescence and adult life. A follow-up study. Eur Heart J 1981;2:281.
118. Koga Y, Toita M, Shibata K, Onitsuka T. Pacemaker implantation in a neonate with congenital complete heart block. Jpn J Surg 1982;12:30.
119. Reid JM, Coleman EN, Doig W. Complete congenital heart block. Br Heart J 1982;48:236.
120. Rios B, Duff J, Simpson JW. Endocardial fibroelastosis with congenital complete heart block in identical twins. Am Heart J 1984;107:1290.
121. Nicholic G, Arnold J, Coles DM. Torsade de pointes and asystole in a child with complete heart block and prolonged QT interval. Aust Paediatr J 1983;19:187.
122. Komayder M, Frank R, Verdel S, Fontaine G, Petitot J, Grosgogeat Y. Intracardiac conduction defects in dystrophia myotonica. Br Heart J 1980;43:315.
123. Hellmans IM, Van Hemel NM, Kooyman CA. Atrioventricular block in childhood causes by mesothelioma. PACE 1983;4:216.
124. Sapire DW, Casta A, Safely W, O'Riordan AC, Balsara RK. Vasovagal syncope in children requiring pacemaker implantation. Am Heart J 1983;106:1406.
125. Dickey RP, Ziter FA, Smith RA. Emery-Dreifuss muscular dystrophy. J Pediatr 1984;104:555.
126. DiSegni E, David D, Katzenstein M, Kleins HO, Kaplinsky E, Levy MJ. Permanent overdrive pacing for the suppression of recurrent ventricular tachycardia in a newborn with long QT syndrome. J Electrocardiol 1980;13:189.
127. Gillette PC. Advances in the diagnosis and treatment of tachydysrhythmias in children. Am Heart J 1981; 102:111.
128. Esscher E. Congenital complete heart block. Acta Pediatr Scand 1981;70:131.
129. Gillette PC, Garson A. Pediatric cardiac dysrhythmias. New York: Grune & Stratton, 1981.
130. Karpawich PP, Gillette PC, Garson A, Hesslein PS, Porter C, McNamara DG. Congenital complete atrioventricular block: clinical and electrophysiologic predictors of need for pacemaker insertion. Am J Cardiol 1981;48:1098.
131. Pinsky WW, Gillette PC, Garson A, McNamara DG. Diagnosis, management and long-term results of patients with congenital complete atrioventricular block. Pediatrics 1982;69:729.
132. Benson DW, Gallagher JJ. Electrophysiologic evaluation and surgical correction of Wolff-Parkinson-White syndrome in children. Clin Pediatr 1980;19:575.
133. Gallagher JJ, Smith WM, Kerr CR, et al. Esophageal pacing: a diagnostic and therapeutic tool. Circulation 1982;65:336.
134. Wood M, Ellenbogen KA. Bradyarrhythmias, emergency pacing, and implantable defibrillation devices. Crit Care Clin 1989;5:551.
135. Rinkenberger RL, Naccarelli GV. Evaluation and treatment of narrow complex tachycardias. Crit Care Clin 1989;5:569.
136. Akhtar M, Shenasa M, Jazayeri M, Caceres J, Tchou PJ. Wide QRS complex tachycardia: reappraisal of a common clinical problem. Ann Intern Med 1988;109:905–912.
137. Greco R, Musto B, Arienzo V, et al. Treatment of paroxysmal supraventricular tachycardia in infancy with digitalis, ATP, and verapamil: a comparative study. Circulation 1982;66:504–508.
138. DiMarco JP, Sellers TD, Lerman BB, Greenberg ML, Berne RM, Belardinelli L. Diagnostic and therapeutic use of adenosine in patients with supraventricular tachyarrhythmias. J Am Coll Cardiol 1985;6:417–425.
139. Trippel DL, Wiest DB, Gillette PC. Cardiovascular and antiarrhythmic effects of esmolol in children. J Pediatr 1991;119:142–147.
140. DiMarco JP, Sellers TD, Lerman BB, et al. Diagnostic and therapeutic use of adenosine in patients with supraventricular tachycardia. J Am Coll Cardiol 1985;6:417–425.
141. Benson DW Jr, Gallagher JJ. Electrophysiologic evaluation and surgical correction of Wolff-Parkinson-White syndrome in children. Clin Pediatr 1980;19:575–583.
142. Case CL, Crawford FA, Gillette PC. Surgical treatment of dysrhythmias in infants and children. Pediatr Clin North Am 1990;37:79.
143. Ott DA, Garson A, Cooley DA, et al. Definitive operation for refractory cardiac tachyarrhythmias in children. J Thorac Cardiovasc Surg 1985;90:681–689.
144. Pritchett ELC, Anderson RW, Kasell JH, et al. Reentry within the atrioventricular node: surgical cure with preservation of atrioventricular conduction. Circulation 1979;60:440–446.
145. Ruskin JN. Catheter ablation for supraventricular tachycardia. N Engl J Med 1991;324:1660–1662.
146. VanHare GF. Radiofrequency catheter ablation of cardiac arrhythmias in pediatric patients. Adv Pediatr 1994; 41:83–109.
147. Gallagher JJ, Svenson RH, Kasell JH, et al. Catheter technique for closed chest ablation of the atrioventricular conduction system: a therapeutic alternative for the treatment of refractory supraventricular tachycardia. N Engl J Med 1991;306:194–200.
148. Jackman WM, Wang X, Friday KJ, Roman CA, Moulton KP, Beckman KJ, McClelland JH, Twidale N, Hazlitt HA, Prior MI, Margolis PD, Calame JD, Overholt ED, Lazzara R. Catheter ablation of accessory atrioventricular pathways (Wolff-Parkinson-White syndrome) by radiofrequency current. N Engl J Med 1991;324:1605–1611.
149. Crawford Jr FA, Gillette PC. Surgical treatment of cardiac dysrhythmias in infants and children. Ann Thorac Surg 1994; 58:1262–1268.
150. Campbell RM, Hamman JW Jr, Echt DS, Graham TP Jr. Surgical treatment of pediatric cardiac arrhythmia. J Pediatr 1987;110:501–508.
151. Scheinman MM, Laks MM, DiMarco J, Plumb V. Current role of catheter ablative procedures in patients with cardiac arrhythmias: a report for health professionals from the subcommittee on electrocardiography and electrophysiology, American Heart Association. Circulation 1991;83:2146–2153.
152. Kennedy EE, Westerman GR, Moss MM, Dungan WT, Bissett JK. Cardiac arrhythmia surgery. J Arkansas Med Soc 1987;84:201–204.

Shock and Multi-Organ System Failure 16

Joseph R. Tobin
Randall C. Wetzel

INTRODUCTION

Shock is a clinical syndrome of acute disruption of both microcirculatory and macrocirculatory function, leading to a general insufficiency of tissue perfusion, oxygen utilization and cellular energy production that ultimately results in deranged homeostatic mechanisms and irreversible cellular damage. Despite this academic definition, shock remains a clinical diagnosis. In general, all shock states eventually involve decreased delivery or impaired utilization of essential cellular substrates. This, in turn, causes disruption and eventual loss of normal cellular metabolism and function. Because circulatory function depends on blood volume, vascular tone, and cardiac function, shock states result from abnormalities in one or more of these factors or from cellular metabolic dysfunction from inability to utilize substrates delivered via the circulatory system. It must be emphasized that hypotension is not the sine qua non of shock. Indeed, children in shock may frequently have a normal blood pressure and a normal or even increased cardiac output. Conversely, hypotension frequently occurs in the absence of shock. Shock occurs in a wide variety of clinical settings in children just as it does in adults. Shock states in children, unlike those in adults, often occur in the absence of other chronic or debilitating diseases, and the predisposing factors to shock may not be obvious. As shock frequently occurs in previously healthy children, the diagnosis may be delayed. Nevertheless, the outcome of shock may be better in children than in adults.

The rapid onset of gastroenteritis and the limited intravascular volume reserve in children explain why hypovolemic shock is the number one worldwide cause of death during childhood, often affecting otherwise healthy children. Among the most common causes of shock in children in developed countries is hypovolemia, resulting from severe hemorrhage after accidental injury that usually occurs in the absence of any predisposing illness. Septic shock also arises de novo in otherwise apparently healthy children and can be caused by organisms that are unusual causes of shock in adults, such as β-hemolytic streptococci, *Haemophilus influenzae* and *Neisseria meningitidis*. Although, as in adults, septic shock may occur after surgery or arise as an intercurrent illness during hospitalization for other diseases (especially oncologic conditions), there are frequently no predisposing factors in children.

Although shock occurs in children of all ages, the distribution of the various types of shock may vary with age. For example, neonates are more likely to develop septic shock and are less likely to suffer accidental injury than are older children. Some children are particularly at risk for developing shock. For example, children with oncologic and urologic problems are at risk for septic shock. On the other hand, hyperactive and economically deprived children are at greater risk for accidental injury and hemorrhagic shock because of difficulties in supervision. Obviously, children with congenital heart disease may develop insidious or acute cardiogenic shock.

This chapter reviews the basic pathophysiology of shock, including the newer insights into the neurohumoral, endothelial, and mediator basis of shock syndromes, and their sequela, multiple-organ system failure (MOSF). It also presents those features of both diagnosis and therapy unique to infants and children that will guide the care of children in the pediatric intensive care unit (PICU).

PHYSIOLOGY

Defending the Blood Pressure

The body has a host of regulatory systems designed to maintain adequate perfusion pressures to vital vascular beds. These can be broadly divided into neural reflexes and humoral reflexes **(Table 16.1).** The complex interplay of these reflexes in defending the blood pressure plays a key role in the survival of the patient when threatened with a wide variety of hypotensive stimuli, including endotoxemia, hemorrhage, and anaphylaxis. Despite this key survival role, it must also be remembered that prolonged tonic neurohumoral reflex activity to maintain perfusion pressure at the expense of regional blood flow can have deleterious effects on several vital vascular beds and thus impair long-term survival. To emphasize some of these complex interactions, physiologic review of the systemic response to hypotension is in order.

Patients who have suffered significant hemorrhage demonstrate several cardiovascular findings. Arterial systolic, diastolic, and pulse pressures are all diminished, and the peripheral pulses are rapid and weak. In addition, peripheral perfusion is decreased with decreased capillary filling, empty veins, pallor, and slightly cyanotic or ashen skin color. The patient is frequently dyspneic. The study of the physiologic responses to blood shedding in animals has revealed several interesting findings. After hemorrhage to a mean arterial pressure of 50% of normal, all animals demonstrate an initial return toward baseline pressures over the next 30 to 60 minutes. In some animals, baseline blood pressure is restored after several hours. In other animals, however, blood pressure falls after an initial elevation, until the animal dies (Fig. 16.1). Another way of examining hemorrhage in animals is by a constant pressure reservoir method to allow the animal to exsanguinate to a blood pressure of between 30 and 40% of control. Observation using this method reveals that as the blood pressure is maintained, the animal first continues to lose blood volume for an hour or two, indicating vasoconstriction. After a couple of hours, blood returns to the animal from the reservoir, indicating vasodilatation. If this low pressure is maintained for several hours despite a transient improvement after return of the shed blood to the animal, there is an accelerating decline in arterial pressure and death ensues, even with additional massive transfusion of donor blood (Fig. 16–1 B). This progressive deterioration in hemodynamic function represents irreversible shock. These two simple experi-

Table 16.1. Major Factors That Defend the Blood Pressure

Neural sympathetic via vasomotor center
Baroreceptors
Carotid body
Aortic arch
Volume receptors
Right atrium
Pulmonary vascular
Chemoreceptors
Aortic and carotid
Medullary
Cerebral ischemic response
Humoral
Adrenal medulla—catecholamines
Hypothalamopituitary response
Adrenocorticotropic hormone and vasopressin
Renin-angiotensin-aldosterone system

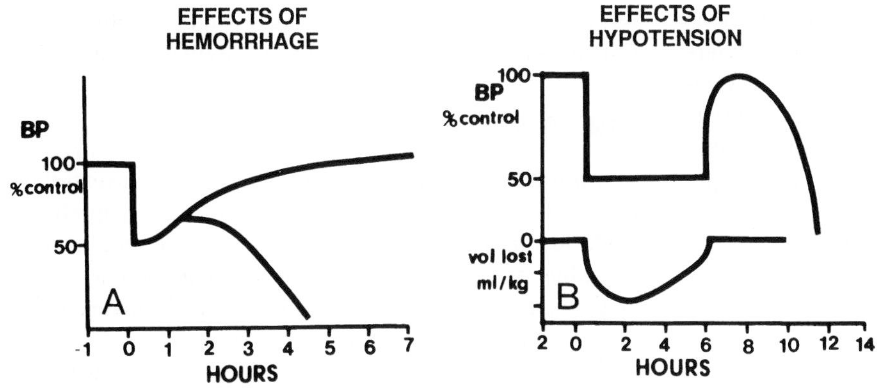

Figure 16.1. **A.** Effects of hemorrhage. The results of acute blood shedding severe enough to reduce the mean arterial blood pressure (*BP*) by 50% are shown. Initially, all animals demonstrate a rise in blood pressure, and several survive. Others, however, after initial improvement, perish. **B.** Effects of 6 hours of controlled hypotension. See the text for explanation.

ments indicate that there are compensatory reflex mechanisms that help maintain arterial blood pressure after hemorrhage. Clearly, this regulatory mechanism is beneficial after hemorrhage, at least transiently. Additionally, if hypotension is prolonged, volume resuscitation is inadequate to assure survival. The major elements of this response include (a) baroreceptor reflexes, (b) chemoreceptor reflexes, (c) cerebral ischemic responses, (d) release of humoral vasoactive substances, (e) renal, salt, and water retention, (f) altered endothelial metabolic function and (g) alteration in the Starling forces leading to resorption of fluid (autotransfusion).

Baroreceptors

A reduction in mean arterial or pulse pressure results in decreased stimulation of carotid sinus and aortic arch baroreceptors. Baroreceptors are also located in both right and left atrial walls, at the junction of the superior and inferior venae cavae and pulmonary veins with the atria, in the left ventricle, and in the pulmonary circulation. Baroreceptor firing increases with stretch and is decreased with hypotension. Baroreceptor central input affects both the vasomotor center and the cardioinhibitory center. Impulses generated by baroreceptors excite the cardioinhibitory center, and produce vasodilatation, hypotension, bradycardia, and decreased cardiac output. They also inhibit the tonic discharge of vasoconstrictor tone from the vasomotor center. Thus hypotension leads to decreased baroreceptor firing, which releases inhibition of the vasomotor center, resulting in vasoconstriction. In addition, the decrease in excitation of the cardioinhibitory center also results in vasoconstriction. This alteration in baroreceptor tone leads to multiple cardiovascular responses aimed at returning arterial pressure toward normal. A combined reduction in vagal tone and an enhancement in sympathetic activity leads to a positive inotropic effect and an increase in heart rate. Increased sympathetic vasomotor tone leads to both arterial and venous constriction.

Clearly, this acute activity results in increased cardiac preload, cardiac contractility, and cardiac afterload, all of which act to return blood pressure toward normal. In several species, increases in venomotor tone and mobilization of reservoir blood (i.e., from the spleen) may lead to considerable preload augmentation (autotransfusion). In humans, this function is served by the hepatic, pulmonary, and cutaneous venous systems. The contribution of various baroreceptor reflexes can be seen in a series of experiments performed by Edis[1]. An 8% blood loss in control animals led to a 12% decrease in blood pressure. With both vagi cut and carotid sinus baroreceptors intact, this degree of hemorrhage led to a 14% decrease in blood pressure not significantly different from that of the control. When aortic baroreceptors were intact and carotid sinuses were denervated, the same blood volume reduction caused a 38% decline in blood pressure. With both groups of baroreceptors denervated, the decline was 48%. As can be seen from this series of experiments, although both sets of baroreceptors are important, carotid sinus baroreceptors make the major contribution to the increase of sympathetic tone in hemorrhage.

The vasoconstrictor response to hemorrhage is, however, not uniform throughout all vascular beds. Vasoconstriction is most severe in skeletal, splanchnic, and cutaneous vascular beds, however, regional flow is preserved in the cerebral, coronary, and retinal circulations (autoregulation) until the systems are overwhelmed. Vascular resistance decreases in the adrenal medulla and neuro-hypophysis during hemorrhagic shock. These increases (up to 300%) occur despite falling perfusion pressures[2]. Clearly, this mechanism is important in facilitating the catecholamine and vasopressin response in shock. During hemorrhage, the perfusion decreases in the renal vascular bed only when hemorrhage is severe, because of a result of renovascular autoregulation. With severe hemorrhage, intense renal vasoconstriction occurs, and blood flow is diverted from cortical to medullary tissues in the kidney. If the hemorrhage is very severe, renal cortical and papillary necrosis occur, and the characteristic vasomotor nephropathy (acute tubular necrosis) is seen.

Chemoreceptors

The baroreceptor response reaches a maximum at around 60 mm Hg, and reductions in blood pressure below this do not further enhance sympathetic tone. When pressure continues to fall, chemoreceptor reflexes occur because of local tissue hypoxia and acidosis because of inadequate local perfusion. These reflexes enhance vasoconstrictor tone and are similar to baroreceptor responses. In addition, there is marked respiratory stimulation. This enhanced respiratory pattern may provide an auxiliary cardiac pumping mechanism during hypotension by alterations in intrathoracic pressure that enhance venous return and increase peripheral blood flow (Chapter 11). A separate discussion of blood volume restitution in trauma, including the shift of fluid from the extravascular to the intravascular spaces, is included in Chapter 44.

Cerebral Ischemic Receptors

When cerebral perfusion pressure falls below 40 mm Hg, below the range where cerebral autoregulation occurs, cerebral blood flow begins to decrease, and massive sympathetic discharge occurs. This response is many times greater than that which is achieved by peripheral baroreceptor activity. When this response is very severe, however, vagal activity also increases, which may lead to profound bradycardia and may aggravate the hypotensive situation.

In addition to these central nervous system (CNS) responses, several authors have raised the possibility that CNS damage resulting from the early stages of shock may antecede other peripheral tissue damage[3]. This early CNS damage may lead to neurogenic circulatory influences that precipitate irreversible shock. Certainly, early CNS endothelial vascular damage occurs in hemorrhagic shock and is associated with impaired cortical perfusion and a perivascular distribution of lesions[4]. An intriguing question remains: Is irreversible shock the cause or the result of CNS hypoperfusion and injury?

Humoral Responses to Hypovolemia

Several humoral systems are activated in hemorrhagic shock when mean arterial pressure is lowered to 40 mm Hg in experimental animals. Circulating epinephrine and norepinephrine increase by 50-fold and 10-fold, respectively. Abundant evidence confirms this massive increase in catecholamine levels in several species, including humans. The catecholamine increase is in response to the same stimuli that cause increased sympathetic tone. Whereas epinephrine is released from the adrenal medulla, norepinephrine is released from both the adrenal medulla and systemic adrenergic nerve endings. The effect of norepinephrine is vasoconstriction in all vascular beds, whereas epinephrine tends to lead to dilatation in skeletal muscle and the hepatic circulation, and vasoconstriction elsewhere. Both agents increase myocardial contractility. The overall effect is to enhance the sympathetic stress response during hemorrhage.

A blood volume reduction of 20% in experimental animals leads to a 40-fold increase in the rate of vasopressin secretion from the neurohypophysis. This response is mediated through carotid and aortic baroreceptors as well as atrial volume receptors. Vasopressin, in addition to being a peripheral vasoconstrictor, also leads to enhanced free water absorption from the renal tubules and collecting ducts, thus maintaining or expanding intravascular volume.

Renal, Salt, and Water Retention

The third humoral mechanism, and perhaps the most potent, is the renin-angiotensin system. Renal hypoperfusion leads to renin secretion from the juxtaglomerular apparatus, which is a proteolytic enzyme acting on the α_2-globulin angiotensinogen to release angiotensin I. Angiotensin I is converted to the potent vasoconstrictor angiotensin II by endothelial angiotensin- converting enzyme. Angiotensin II, in addition to being an extremely potent vasoconstrictor, stimulates the release of aldosterone from the adrenal cortical glomerulosa cells, leading to renal tubular sodium resorption. Interestingly, there is evidence that angiotensin II also enhances vasopressin secretion by direct hypothalamic stimulation. It has been suggested that vasopressin can, in turn, reduce renin secretion by the juxtaglomerular apparatus and thus form a potential negative feedback loop on angiotensin formation. Angiotensin II contributes to the increased resistance of multiple peripheral vascular beds during hypovolemic shock. Initially, angiotensin release leads to increased peripheral vascular resistance and maintains blood pressure; if this release is prolonged, however, these effects are deleterious. Ischemic renal tubular necrosis appears after prolonged angiotensin exposure and peripheral hypoperfusion, and profound alterations in vascular tone can lead to irreversible circulatory decompensation, which may contribute to the state of irreversible shock[5]. For this reason, angiotensin-converting enzyme inhibitors such as captopril have been suggested as potentially beneficial in shock. The summation of these renal responses leads to increased sodium and water retention. However, these physiologic adaptive responses will result in pathophysiologic alterations in the perfusion of multiple organs if circulatory volume is not restored.

Whereas the above neurohumoral systems seem to decrease renal blood flow and glomerular filtration rate and to increase renal vascular resistance, these are not the only responses that occur during shock. The role of endothelially derived vasoactive substances in the renal circulation is increasingly appreciated. Failure of endothelially derived relaxing factors could lead to decreased renal perfusion and acute vasomotor nephropathy[6]. Renal vasodilator prostaglandins are locally released during both hemorrhage and endotoxemia[7]. Cyclo-oxygenase inhibition during these stressed states leads to renal vasoconstriction. In addition, endogenous prostaglandins also appear to regulate sodium excretion. Conversely, uncontrolled local release of constricting factors could critically alter renal perfusion. Thus the net effect of shock on renal blood flow is a combination of systemic neurohumoral regulatory mechanisms in defense of intravascular volume and blood pressure and local vasodilator mechanisms in defense of renal perfusion. Understanding the complex interplay between the components that regulate the renal circulation in shock may provide insight into overall cardiovascular regulation in the various shock states.

Autotransfusion

The net fluid flux across the basement membrane, $\dot{Q}$, is defined as

$$\dot{Q} = K_f [(P_{mv} - P_{pmv}) - \sigma(\pi_{mv} = \pi_{pmv})]$$

where K_f is the filtration coefficient; P_{mv} and P_{pmv} are hydrostatic pressures within the microvasculature ($_{mv}$) and in the perimicrovascular space ($_{pmv}$), respectively; π is oncotic pressure; and σ is the reflectance coefficient. It can be seen that if P_{mv} falls (decreased blood pressure) and intravascular oncotic pressure increases, there will be a net force to increase intravascular volume. Both K_f and σ are related to the physical characteristics of the basement membrane, such as pore size, and can be altered in various shock states, leading to altered transcapillary fluid flux.

In arterial hypotension with arteriolar constriction and reduced venous pressures, capillary hydrostatic pressure is low. This leads to resorption of interstitial fluid into the vascular compartment. Considerable quantities of fluid may be added to the intravascular circulation in this way. Approximately 15 ml/kg/hr or 1 liter/hr in the average adult can be autotransfused after acute intravascular volume depletion. Clearly, this is a dynamic process. The fall in hematocrit and colloid oncotic pressure tends to counteract this autotransfusion. In addition to the extracellular- to-intravascular fluid transfusion, intracellular-to-extracellular fluid translocation also occurs, albeit at a much slower rate. This appears to be enhanced by cortisol. This augments fluid restitution over the ensuing 24 to 48 hours.

As outlined in Chapter 12, there are significant differences between newborns and adults in myocardial autonomic innervation and function. The immature autonomic system may also be accompanied by underdeveloped or incompletely regulated humoral responses to shock; however, this has not been clearly demonstrated. In review, several of the factors that may cause the response in the neonates to differ from that seen in adults[8–11] are (a) the incomplete development of the sympathetic nervous system as reported by Friedman and colleagues, (b) decreased myocardial contractility, (c) decreased enzyme levels, and (d) decreased muscle fiber density. In addition, the extracellular fluid volume is proportionately greater in neonates than adults, and this has a significant impact on the response to hypovolemic shock. In one of the few studies of hemorrhagic shock in newborn animals, Horton and Cohen[9] demonstrated that neonatal dogs showed less of a blood pressure fall after hemorrhage than did adult dogs and this was accompanied by a smaller fall in the extracellular fluid volume in younger (-27%) than in older (-42%) animals for a given blood loss. In these same experiments, however, neonatal dogs demonstrated an inadequate sympathoadrenal response manifested by persistent bradycardia and an inadequate increase in systemic vascular resistance. In addition, a sustained decrease in myocardial blood flow greater than in adult animals and a generalized failure of reflex compensatory mechanisms to maintain myocardial function and coronary flow occurred in neonates. Not surprisingly, impaired contractility during shock and after resuscitation was more apparent in the newborn group. The significance of this complex interplay of poorly integrated sympathoadrenal responses along with apparently maintained extracellular fluid volume in younger animals is not clear with regard to survival.

MEDIATORS OF TISSUE DAMAGE IN SHOCK

Altered Oxygen Metabolism

The critical role oxygen plays places oxygen metabolism in the foremost position when shock states are considered. Disruption in the delivery and utilization of oxygen and the increased oxygen demand indicate the basic importance of understanding oxygen metabolism in shock. In addition, the recent recognition of the reperfusion syndrome and its role in shock and MOSF highlights the fact not only that too little oxygen is bad but also that too much oxygen at the wrong time is not good.

Hypoxic-Ischemic Injury in Shock

Hypoxic (oxygen deficit) and ischemic (oxygen plus substrate deficit) injury occurs at some time during all types of shock. In hypovolemic shock, hypoxic-ischemic injury occurs early and is the primary cause of circulatory disruption; in septic shock, on the other hand, hypoxic-ischemic injury occurs as a result of mediator-induced circulatory and cellular metabolic abnormalities. The tissue insult caused by hypoxia and ischemia, although similar, are not identical and are worth considering separately. In addition, reperfusion injury that occurs after ischemia plays a critical role in tissue damage that is almost certainly as significant as the hypoxic insult itself. Furthermore, this injury affects multiple organ systems and leads to the release of locally and distally acting metabolites that amplify tissue injury in shock.

Cellular hypoxia results from several causes. Hypoxic hypoxia occurs either when atmospheric pO_2 is low or when the lungs are abnormal, causing marked ventilation/perfusion ($\dot{V}/\dot{Q}$) mismatch. Both conditions lead to arterial blood not being fully saturated. Stagnant hypoxia occurs when there is deficient or absent blood flow to the cells. Anemic hypoxia results from an inability of circulating blood to transport sufficient oxygen because of either deficient or abnormal hemoglobin. Any of these types of hypoxia can occur during any type of shock and at various stages during shock. For example, during septic shock when arteriovenous shunting occurs, part of the peripheral vascular bed is underperfused and stagnant hypoxia can occur. In addition, if adult respiratory distress syndrome (ARDS) occurs, hypoxic hypoxia may complicate the shock

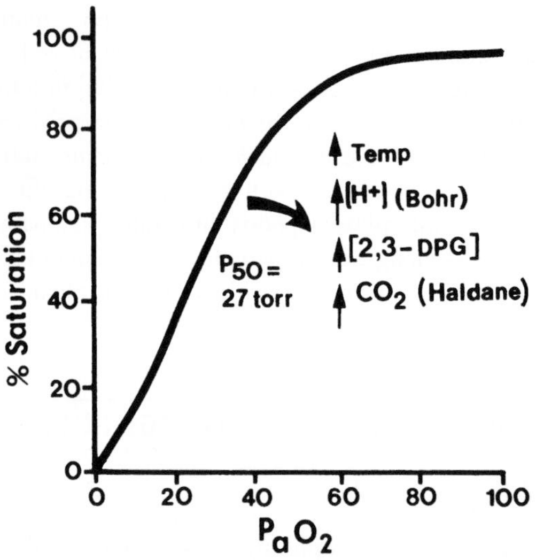

Figure 16.2. Oxyhemoglobin dissociation curve: hemoglobin saturation *(% Saturation)* versus partial pressure of oxygen (P_aO_2). Increases in temperature, hydrogen ion concentration (acidosis), carbon dioxide, and 2,3-diphosphoglyceraldehyde *(2,3-DPG)* all shift the curve to the right and decrease hemoglobin oxygen affinity, thus releasing more oxygen to the tissues.

picture. Anemic hypoxia, which can clearly occur during hemorrhage, can also complicate septic shock after, for example, disseminated intravascular coagulation (DIC) with intravascular hemolysis and hemorrhage. A significant cause of anemic hypoxia is a significant metabolic disturbance that shifts the oxyhemoglobin dissociation curve (Fig. 16.2). For example, a leftward shift of the curve (decreased P_{50}) occurs with alkalosis, hypocarbia, or deficient 2,3-diphosphoglyceraldehyde (all of which occur during shock) and leads to less oxygen delivery to the tissues, which may contribute to peripheral tissue hypoxia.

The effects of acute tissue hypoxia are legion[12,13]. Although an exhaustive discussion of the metabolic alterations of hypoxia is not appropriate here, a summary of the effects is useful. Approximately 90% of the cellular oxygen supply of the body is consumed by the mitochondrial electron transport chain, which under normal conditions provides over 95% of the total energy needs of the body. Clearly, both adequate mitochondrial function and oxygen delivery are necessary to ensure energy supply. The electron transport mechanism, which passes electrons via the various cytochromes and which finally results in the reduction of atmospheric oxygen, is the final sequence in cellular oxidative metabolism. This begins with glucose and, via the Embden-Meyerhof (glycolytic) pathway and Krebs (tricarboxylic acid) cycles, generates 36 high-energy adenosine 5'-triphosphate (ATP) molecules per glucose molecule. In contrast, anaerobic glycolysis leads to the production of a mere 2 ATP molecules per glucose molecule.

During hypoxia, mitochondrial function rapidly becomes depressed[14]. One of the earliest findings is inhibition of mitochondrial calcium transport, leading to nearly complete inhibition of mitochondrial calcium uptake[15]. Thus cytosolic calcium levels rise, and the calcium-scavenging ability of the mitochondria is lost. In addition, both adenosine triphosphatase (ATPase) activity and adenine nucleotide translocase activity are severely depressed and lead to an excess of adenosine 5'-diphosphate (ADP) compared with ATP and a depression of the normal ADP-facilitated respiratory activity[16]. Interestingly, because of the exceedingly high affinity of the cytochrome system for oxygen, the electron transport reaction along the respiratory chain is generally not depressed[17]. Although cellular energy needs are not met during hypoxia, it appears that as long as tissue oxygen tension is above the critical level necessary to provide electron transport (1 torr), the mitochondrial membrane system remains intact[18].

At low oxygen levels (30 to 40 torr), mitochondria actually adapt to hypoxia as long as electron transport is intact[19]. Low oxygen tensions induce enhanced respiratory activity and the ability to perform energy-generating reactions as measured by increased activity when the mitochondria return to normal substrate and normoxic conditions. Indeed, mitochondrial respiratory activity appears to double after 30 minutes of in vivo hypoxia. An interesting developmental change occurs in this system after birth and is, in a sense, the opposite of that which occurs in adults after hypoxia[20]. The fetal cellular metabolism is adapted to extremely low levels of tissue oxygen (approximately 10 torr pO_2) and yet maintains a level of respiratory capability above that of adults. This may, in part, explain the resistance of the fetus and newborn to hypoxia and may indicate an active resistance of neonatal mitochondria to damage in shock states[20,21]. Postnatally, the respiratory capability decreases rapidly toward adult levels as tissue oxygen tension rises. It is apparent that although cellular energy metabolism breaks down during hypoxia, mitochondrial function is maintained. However, it is known that tissue ischemia and sepsis lead to irreversible mitochondrial damage. Thus it appears that mitochondrial damage is probably a result of factors other than hypoxia. These factors are dependent on the delivery of substrates, the removal of toxic wastes, or elaboration of direct mitochondrial toxins[19]. Although in shock, the mitochondria may remain viable, the profound disturbance of energy metabolism usually affects cytosolic and plasma membrane function. ATP shortage causes an early breakdown in the cell membrane ionic pumps and leads to an influx of sodium and efflux of potassium. Abnormal cytosolic calcium levels lead to inhibition of high-energy systems, including phosphodiesterases, and insoluble ATP complexing with further, irreversible loss of cellular energy substrate.

Histologically, the cell shows distinct changes that accompany this biochemical alteration. As the sodium-potassium transmembrane ion pumps break down, intracellular edema occurs with swelling of the cell. Eventually, intracellular organelles swell, and mitochondrial swelling occurs late. As the membrane structures break down, membrane permeability increases and cellular enzyme patterns and distribution are disrupted. In addition, lysosomal enzymes enter the cytosol, leading to further structural disruption. Ultimately, as this irreversible step occurs, intranuclear chromatin is destroyed. Dystrophic calcification occurs throughout the now indistinct cell contents, reflecting cell death. All of these stages reflect the absence of essential energy needs and are characteristic of substrate depletion as well as hypoxia. Clearly, hypoxia and ischemia lead to significant cellular damage per se. This summary, however, does not take into account other toxic substances such as superoxides, lysosomal products, interleukins (IL-1, IL-2, etc.), tumor necrosis factor (TNF), and other toxic substances released by cells in response to hypoxia and ischemia. These are discussed later. In addition, in shock a wide variety of other mediators, such as endotoxin in septic shock, may lead to greater and earlier disruption of essential cellular metabolism than does the hypoxic-ischemic insult.

The derangement in energy metabolism may not only acutely alter cell function but may also be responsible for triggering the hypermetabolic state that follows hemodynamic catastrophe and is seen in septic shock[(22)]. The contribution in carbohydrate, fat, and protein metabolism to MOSF and death is becoming increasingly appreciated. Therapy specifically designed to have a clinically significant impact on this metabolic catastrophe is gaining increasing attention (see below).

Reperfusion

The role of reperfusion injury in the pathophysiology of human disease has been elucidated in the coronary and cerebral circulations. Total ischemia after embolic or thrombotic phenomena or cardiac arrest sets the stage for a wide spectrum of responses when oxygen and substrate are reintroduced to the ischemic tissues[(23)]. This phenomenon has been invoked to explain occurrences that follow hypoperfusion in various shock states, when areas of the body may be ischemic, or traumatized with impaired circulation. Certainly, clinical syndromes that follow tissue trauma in the absence of clear bacterial infection suggest the possibility of reperfusion injury occurring[(24,25)]. During reperfusion, activation of several of the systems (neutrophils, complement activation, fibrin, and products of factor XII) occurs. These systems provide amplification of the initial insult and lead to widespread tissue damage, which may in fact be the basis of MOSF.

During cell ischemia, xanthine dehydrogenase is converted to xanthine oxidase, and ATP is converted to xanthine and hypoxanthine. When the cells are reperfused, xanthine oxidase converts available oxygen to superoxide anion[(26)]. Superoxide anion, hydrogen peroxide, peroxynitrite, and hydroxyl radicals are capable of initiating a cascade of events. Cyclo-oxygenase and eicosanoid products are generated, chemoattractants with leukotaxis are stimulated, the complement cascade is triggered. Direct endothelial injury occurs. Failure of numerous local regulatory mechanisms follows. The widespread access of these mediators to the systemic circulation may form the basis of MOSF. Ischemia and reperfusion in any vascular bed leads to both local and distal injury. An example of local significance of this occurs in the splanchnic circulation. The splanchnic circulation undergoes ischemia fairly readily during shock. On resuscitation, reperfusion initiates reperfusion injury, superoxide generation, and local damage to the endothelium and gut epithelium. This breakdown of gut barrier function leads to bacterial translocation with seeding of bacteria to the peritoneum, mesenteric lymph nodes, and hepatic portal circulation. These multiple septic foci activate a host of other biologic cascade systems that amplify the initial hypoperfusion injury into full-blown MOSF[(27)].

Hypermetabolism

The work of Cerra and his associates has highlighted the impact of hypermetabolism in the MOSF syndrome[(22)]. Patients who have had surgery, trauma, and sepsis after shock demonstrate increased oxygen consumption, CO_2 production, and catabolism, peaking around the third day after injury and abating by the seventh day. In some patients after this initial response, however, there is prolonged hypermetabolism that proceeds toward death. There are multiple initiators of this hypermetabolism syndrome. There is much evidence to support the idea that appropriate nutritional therapy may be effective in maintaining protein nitrogen balance, altering immunologic responses, limiting gut bacterial translocation, and limiting the contribution of hypermetabolism to MOSF[(28)]. Although our understanding of this area is in its infancy, pediatricians should be aware of the significant impact of appropriate nutrition on a wide host of critical illnesses. Appropriate nutritional support, supplementation with arginine, zinc, iron, vitamins C, A, D, and E, limiting 6ω fatty acids, and increasing the amount of 3ω fatty acids have a positive impact on this syndrome[(29)]. Specifically tailoring nutritional support and considering tailored replacement therapy as critical as antibacterial therapy may ultimately have an impact on the outcome of shock.

Oxygen Balance

Dantzker and colleagues[(30)] first described an apparent relationship between oxygen delivery and consumption in ARDS. This same phenomenon has been described in nearly all critical illnesses[(31)]. In general, oxygen consumption is independent of oxygen delivery above a certain critical point. Below this point, oxygen consumption becomes limited by the amount of oxygen delivery because delivery falls below basal oxygen consumption. Above this point, there is a plateau phase in which oxygen consumption does not increase with increased oxygen delivery. In ARDS, septic shock, hemorrhagic shock, and burns, it has been demonstrated that this relationship breaks down[(30–32)]. As long as oxygen delivery is increased, oxygen consumption increases, frequently to 2 to 3 times normal oxygen consumption. This observation has been interpreted in various ways. It should be mentioned that not the least of these is the fact that it may be artifactual[(33)]. The Fick equation and thermodilution cardiac output are used to compute both consumption and delivery, and thus both parameters have a common factor. Others have said that this relationship demonstrates a significant oxygen lack in shock states. Recognition of the hypermetabolism syndrome suggests that the increased use of oxygen that occurs may indeed be delivery limited in hypoperfusion states.

Although the occurrence of this observation is without doubt, its implications are less clear. Shoemaker and others[34] have championed the concept that oxygen delivery should be driven until consumption plateaus. They have demonstrated some improvement in outcome if this strategy of optimizing oxygen delivery is achieved. Conversely, driving hypermetabolism by delivering increased oxygen, stoking the hypoperfusion/reperfusion mechanism, and demanding cardiac output and oxygen delivery in an injured system has potentially deleterious benefits. In a clinical study, Bihari et al.[35] demonstrated that when oxygen consumption increased in patients who went on to die, oxygen delivery was increased by prostacyclin infusion[35]. Those patients in whom extraction fell (increased delivery, steady consumption) survived. In complicated shock states, the value of determining oxygen delivery and consumption must be weighed against the risks of obtaining this information and the lack of certainty concerning whether driving oxygen delivery is indeed beneficial in the long term, or merely an indicator of subgroups of patients with severe pathology.

The Endothelium

The pivotal role of the endothelium as both a target and a source of mediators of tissue injury has become increasingly apparent. Knowledge of this dual role is important for understanding how many mediators of shock-induced injury interact. The central role of the endothelium in maintaining vascular integrity and tone, its strategic location, and its role in the metabolism of numerous vasoactive substances has gained increasing appreciation in recent years[36]. A few years ago, this apparently insignificant vascular lining was thought to contribute to maintaining blood viscosity, coagulation, and performing a mundane barrier function. Over the past few years, this relatively limited view of the endothelium has been exploded[37]. Obviously, to enter the parenchyma of any organ a substance must cross and therefore interact with the endothelium. All invading organisms, all pharmacologic substances, and everything absorbed from the gastrointestinal tract must interact with the endothelium in order to access any other organ system. The endothelium has tight junctions, as well as the ability for a substance to move across the endothelium without entering cells. Endothelial cells are actively pinocytotic and endocytotic and can ingest bacteria, circulating small particles, and circulating substrate[38]. In addition to this, a large number of vasoactive substances primarily interact with the endothelium to alter vascular tone[39]. All of the circulating blood is exposed to the systemic as well as the pulmonary endothelial organs. This vast endothelial surface area is ideally situated to modulate a wide variety of pharmacologically active substances and to interact with every circulating cell and macromolecular system. Of critical interest in shock states are the interactions with circulating leukocytes and platelets.

Although the barrier function of the endothelium has long been recognized, recent appreciation of the importance of endothelial injury, which disrupts this physical barrier and thus underlies the capillary leak seen particularly in ARDS, has been more clearly appreciated. Furthermore, the biologic impairment that results from shock-induced "endotheliopathy" further augments and amplifies the insult. A total breakdown in the endothelial cell barrier, synthetic and metabolic function may well be a common lesion in every organ system affected by shock. As such it may be the basis for widespread MOSF. It has clearly been demonstrated that the endothelium is a premier target of all the activated mediator systems in ARDS[40]. This "endotheliopathy" may also be a final common pathway of pathophysiology in the coronary, renal, and cerebral circulations in shock[36,41].

Although it is well known that the endothelium is the source of eicosanoid metabolites, notably the potent vasodilator prostacyclin, the work of Furchgott and Zawadzki[42] awakened interest in the role of the endothelium in vasoregulation. The conundrum of "why acetylcholine acted as a vasodilator in vivo, but a vasoconstrictor in vitro" was resolved by their clear demonstration of the key role of the endothelium[42]. Their realization that an intact endothelium was necessary for acetylcholine to cause an endothelial-dependent relaxation in the underlying vascular smooth muscle opened the way to the description of endothelium-derived relaxing factors (EDRFs)[43]. A wide variety of biologically vasoactive substances assert their vasoregulatory effects through EDRF[44]. At least one EDRF has been characterized and identified as nitric oxide (NO)[45].

Nitric oxide is formed from arginine by nitric oxide synthases (NOS) and has a half-life of 7 to 14 seconds. Multiple isoforms of the enzymes have been delineated[46]. The endothelium contains one isoform (endothelial constitutive nitric oxide synthase-eNOS) and other isoforms are found in neurons, glia and macrophages. Endothelial NOS activity is present in most vascular beds and is at least one component of the flow-dependent vasodilation response. Nitric oxide may act on other endothelial intracellular systems, but the prominent activity is via diffusion to adjacent vascular smooth muscle where it activates guanylate cyclase increasing cyclic GMP production. This cGMP stimulates calcium sequestration and relaxes actin-myosin tension generation thereby resulting in smooth muscle relaxation.

Along with this tonic or constitutive NOS activity, cytokines and endotoxin induce an isoform of NOS (iNOS) in macrophages, endothelial cells and vascular smooth muscle[46]. When transcribed, this second isoform increases NO production dramatically in a short time (4 to 16 hours). This increase in NO likely is a critical mechanism of host defense bacteriocidal activity of macrophages. Nitric oxide also causes profound vasodilation and anti-platelet aggregation. It is unknown if these are adaptive physiologic responses to increase local microcirculatory flow or if these responses are pathophysiology of the host initiated by microorganism invasion. Although other stimuli mediate increases in endothelial NOS activity, the greatest current interest is in understanding this response in sepsis.

The endothelium has been recognized for its multiple critical roles and the disruption of these functions in sepsis[47]. Increased endothelial NO production contributes to the systemic vasodilation and endothelial permeability alterations seen in sepsis. Understanding in altered endothelial metabolism, clinicians have hoped to control this response using NOS antagonists. Although these may improve systemic blood pressure in shock, survival has not yet improved. Early reports of use of NOS antagonists demonstrate profound increases in systemic vascular resistance[48] similar to early studies and use of norepinephrine. We are awaiting newer studies with more isoform specific antagonists and dose response studies[49]. Impairment of local EDRF/NO function or production in maintaining decreased smooth muscle tone may play a central role in pulmonary hypertension, and myocardial hypoperfusion and ischemia. The early and intermediate stages of septic shock are associated with increased EDRF/NO release and vasomotor paresis. Late stages of septic shock with severe endothelial lesions may lead to loss of EDRF and widespread vasoconstriction. It is interesting that intensivists have used pharmacologic EDRF substitutes (nitroglycerin and sodium nitroprusside) for years.

The discovery of a role of EDRF led Yanagisawa and others[50] to search for an endothelial-derived constricting factor (EDCF). Indeed, polypeptide EDCF was identified in 1987, and it is now realized that this EDCF is the most potent vasoconstrictor known to humans[50]. EDCF has a suggested role in essential hypertension and hypertensive crisis, and deranged EDCF secretion may lead to local vasoconstriction and ischemia in shock states[51]. Understanding the interplay between the multiple endothelially derived vasoactive substances provides a crucial insight into local vasoregulation and autoregulation.

There is a plethora of metabolic functions of the endothelium[52]. In addition to the presence of angiotensin-converting enzyme in the endothelium, bradykinin, kallikrein, histamine, catecholamines, and multiple other compounds are also metabolized by the endothelium. The key role that the endothelium plays in eicosanoid metabolism must also be noted[53]. The widespread activation of endothelial eicosanoid release may well account for a host of changes in underlying vascular tone. The central role that eicosanoids play on activation of other key cell functions also suggests the important consequences of shock-related endotheliopathies.

The potential for the metabolism of circulating vasoregulatory substrate by the endothelium is great. Derangement in this function, which accompanies shock, could be critical. The impact of endothelial injury on the coagulation cascade, blood clotting, and physical properties of blood flow cannot be underestimated. Loss of this important property can lead to sludging in the microcirculation and further tissue ischemia. In addition, DIC may be triggered by endothelial dysfunction[54]. Endothelial injury likely occurs in reperfusion injury, with a generation of locally active superoxide radicals during reperfusion leading to widespread endothelial insult and EDRF failure[55]. A second common cause of injury occurs when the endothelium becomes a target for activated neutrophils[56]. There is widespread recognition that the CD_{11}/CD_{18} glycoprotein complex on leukocytes plays a key role in binding to endothelial cells[57]. In these protected microenvironments between the endothelial cells and the white cells, the elaboration of a host of proteolytic enzyme systems as well as superoxides can cause widespread endothelial disruption. It has been demonstrated that inhibition of this disruption alters the pathology of shock states, can prevent the development of the MOSF that accompanies septic shock in experimental animals, and improve survival[58]. The interplay of the vascular endothelium with the coagulation cascade and platelets also provides another source of endothelial derangement. The interaction between endothelial cells, TNF, and interleukins demonstrates the complexity and central role of the endothelium in a wide variety of shock states, especially septic shock[59,60].

That endothelial injury and derangement of endothelial function (endotheliopathy) occurs prior to multiple-organ system impairment and failure. This suggests a central role for the endothelial organ system in a wide variety of critical illnesses, especially shock states[36,41]. The endothelium, if considered as an organ in its own right, forms the largest organ system in the body. Fifty percent of this intravascular organ is located in the lungs. In this critical location, it is exposed to all circulating blood with which it can interact. This supports the potential for a central role for endothelium in all shock states. In the future, therapies designed to ameliorate endothelial injury and alter the endothelial response in multiple pathophysiologic states may provide a wide variety of therapeutic modalities specifically designed with the realization of the central role of the endothelium in critical illness[36].

Endotoxin

Tissue damage to the endothelium of multiple organs precedes parenchymal failure. There are numerous factors involved in the widespread tissue damage that occurs in all shock states. Although much of the following discussion is centered around the impact of bacterial sepsis, it must be emphasized that other shock stimuli, in many instances, trigger many of the same tissue-disrupting mechanisms. In addition, growing appreciation of the potential occurrence of bacterial translocation in all forms of shock suggests the importance of understanding the mechanisms that underlie septic shock[27].

In 1892, Pfieffer first recognized endotoxins as being bacterial products that were different from the previously described exotoxins[61]. Exotoxins are synthesized and secreted by live bacteria, mainly Gram-positive organisms but also a few Gram-negative organisms. In contradistinction to exotoxins, endotoxins appear to be unique to Gram-negative organisms and form an essential component of their cell walls. These toxins, when released from the cell wall either during active cell wall growth or by the death of the organism, have a vast potential for interacting with mammalian cells. It is a basic precept of endotoxin shock research that the consequences of these interactions are responsible for the myriad responses seen during Gram-negative septic shock. Thorough research into the structure, active site, and potential receptor interaction of endotoxin as well as the interlinking reactions between endotoxin and the clinical syndrome of septic shock has provided many useful insights on which to base our therapy and continues to be necessary to delineate potential future therapies. All Gram-negative bacteria (GNB) so far studied produce a macromolecular glycolipid referred to as lipopolysaccharide (LPS)[62]. Although LPS is synthesized in the cytosol, it is located on the cell membrane and, together with various proteins and phospholipids, forms the external membrane of GNB. This exposed portion of the cell membrane forms the site at which the GNB react with their environment[63]. Indeed, the antigenic site of GNB located within this LPS is synonymous with the term "O-specific antigen," which is often used interchangeably with LPS.

There is great diversity in the chemical structure of the various endotoxins produced by different bacteria. Indeed, a pure bacterial culture will elaborate several chemically distinct endotoxins. Whether this wide variety of individual endotoxins has distinct effects or whether all endotoxins trigger similar responses is not known. It is clear, however, that the greater the heterogeneity of the endotoxins produced, the greater the toxicity. Study of the nature of LPS derived from many sources has disclosed a basic common structure. Chemically, these macromolecules are made up of three distinct components: a lipid-rich area, a hydrophilic component, and a central acidic core[64]. The hydrophilic chain that forms the O-specific antigen and the linking core form a heteropolysaccharide chain that is covalently linked to the lipid moiety called lipid A. This chemically defined LPS molecule thus contains both the somatic antigens and the endotoxic activity of GNB (Fig. 16.3).

The O-specific polysaccharide chain is a large unit containing repeating oligosaccharide subunits. The different oligosaccharide content of this unit, the structure of the repeating sugars, and their glycosidic linkages determine the

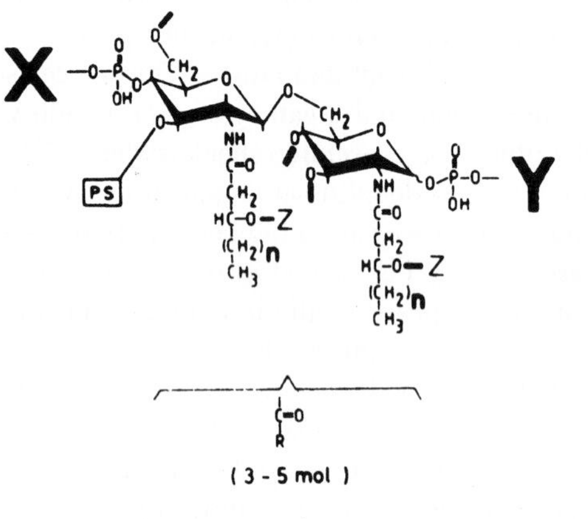

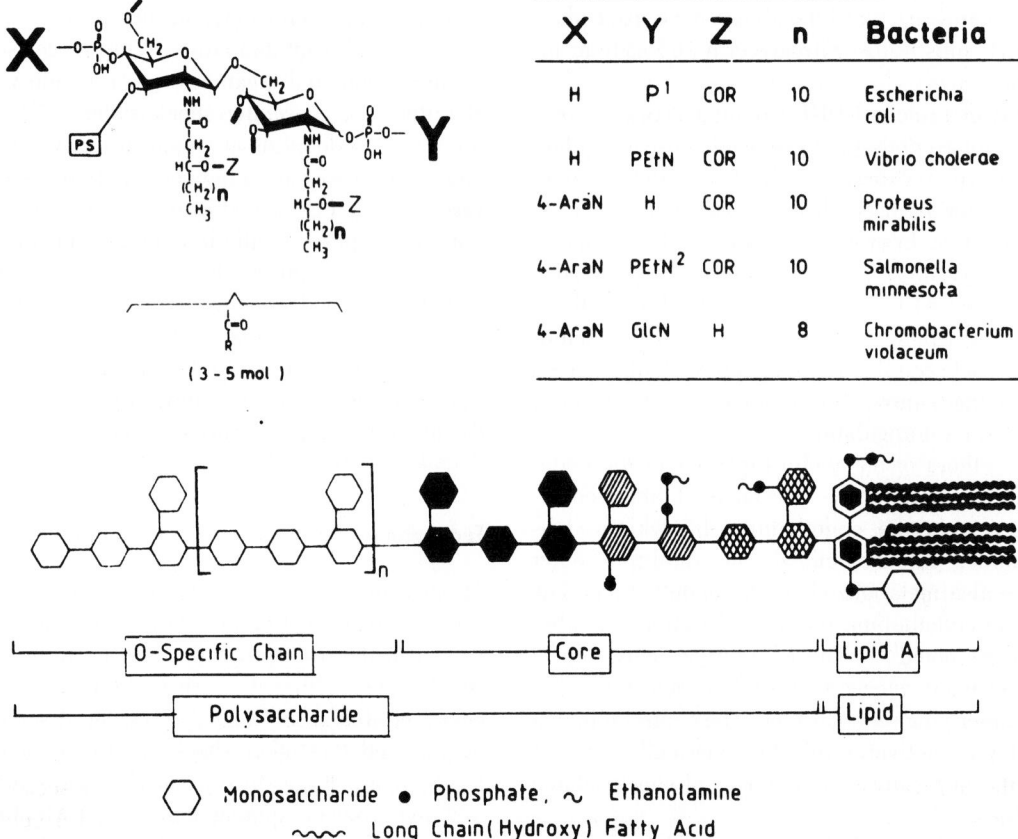

X	Y	Z	n	Bacteria
H	P[1]	COR	10	Escherichia coli
H	PEtN	COR	10	Vibrio cholerae
4-AraN	H	COR	10	Proteus mirabilis
4-AraN	PEtN[2]	COR	10	Salmonella minnesota
4-AraN	GlcN	H	8	Chromobacterium violaceum

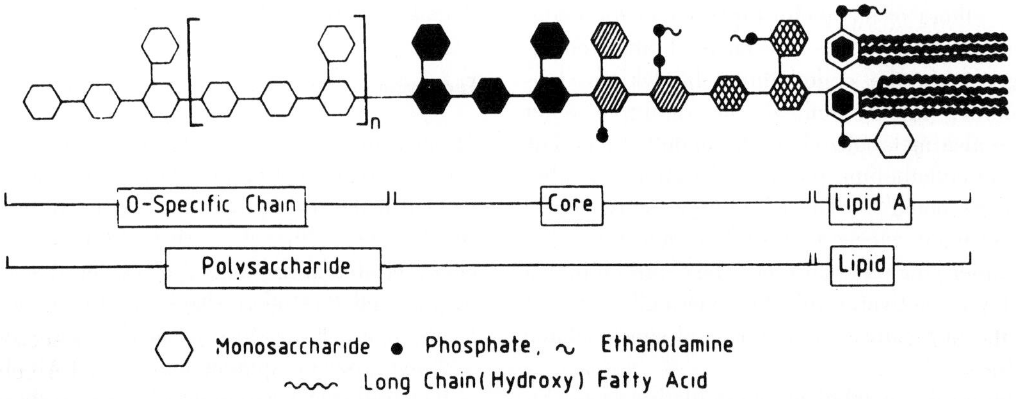

Figure 16.3. *Upper panel:* Generalized structure of lipid A. The central element is a phosphorylated β-1,6-linked *d*-glucosamine disaccharide with the *d*-3-hydroxy fatty acids amide-linked as indicated. *Lower panel:* Schematic representation of the *Salmonella* LPS molecule. (Reprinted from The Almqvist and Wiksell Periodical Company, Stockholm, Sweden, and from Rietschel ET, Schade U, Jensen M, Wollenweber HW, Luderritz O, Greisman SG. Bacterial endotoxins: chemical structure, biological activity and role in septicaemia. Scand J Infect Dis Suppl 1982;31:10 and 12.)

serologic properties of the individual GNB[65]. The complexity of these polysaccharides is immensely variable, with some consisting of repeating units of identical polysaccharides and others consisting of heteropoly- saccharides with complex side chain linkages. The analysis of the actual sugars that make up these chains has revealed many new sugars and even new classes of monosaccharides apparently unique to GNB[65]. This complexity accounts for the wide variety of distinct antigenic characteristics of closely related GNB.

The O-specific unit is linked to a core acidic oligosaccharide unit of less structural heterogeneity that contains glucose, galactose, and several phosphoethanolamine side residues. In addition, the core contains two unusual sugars, heptose and ketodeoxyoctonic acid, through which it is linked to lipid A. It has been known for a long time that GNB in agar culture undergo transformation characterized by morphologic colony mutation from smooth to rough forms (SR activation) with loss of their O-specific antigen. Thus the LPS of R mutants consists only of this core or R-specific unit and lipid A. There are only a few distinct R-specific antigens shared by GNB and directed by a genetic locus distinct from the O-specific antigens. These findings may have important implications concerning immunologic aspects of therapy for septic shock[65].

Lipid A is the structurally distinct lipid portion of LPS and has a strongly conserved structure with very little variability between widely different groups of GNB[62,66]. Isolated lipid A is an extremely potent bacterial toxin that interacts with and perturbs mammalian cell membranes and evokes a wide variety of distinct biochemical and clinical responses. The toxic activity of isolated lipid A is similar to that of intact LPS isolated from various sources[67]. It would appear that lipid A is probably the active, toxic moiety of LPS and the portion of the molecule responsible for the wide variety of effects seen in endotoxic shock. The unique structure of lipid A is characterized by a phosphorylated, central β-1,6-linked *d*-glucosamine disaccharide that is linked to *d*-3-hydroxy fatty acids by an amide group (Fig. 16 to 3). Various polar groups are bound to phosphate residues in the 1,4 positions and include phosphoethanolamine, *d*-glucosamine, and aminodeoxyarabinose. The lipid molecule is thus both hydrophilic and hydrophobic and contains both acidic and basic residues (amphoteric). These unique structural attributes make lipid A a vital constituent of GNB cell walls, which plays both a structural and a functional role. This physicochemical heterogeneity partially explains the ability of lipid A to interact with other cellular membranes[62,65].

In summary, the endotoxic properties reside in the LPS constituent of the cell walls of GNB. This consists of a polysaccharide unit made up of an O somatic antigen moiety and an R core-specific subunit that contribute to the antigenic properties of GNB. In addition, the polysaccharide portion serves to solubilize the toxic lipid A and may contribute to the distribution of LPS within the animal as well as the site specificity of LPS in its interaction with cell membranes. Lipid A seems to be responsible for the toxic biologic effects of GNB endotoxins, and a focus on the cellular interactions of lipid A has provided interesting insights into many aspects of septic shock.

Interaction with Cell Membranes

In the endotoxin-exposed animal, every organ system is either primarily or secondarily affected. The clinical characteristics of endotoxin shock are extremely well known. Studies over the past several decades have disclosed that LPS, particularly lipid A, seems to affect virtually every mammalian cell and seems to be responsible for the characteristics of endotoxin shock. What is not so well understood, however, is how one reasonably well defined chemical entity triggers such a diverse spectrum of biologic reactions. Several lines of evidence indicate that the net effect of lipid A is to stimulate individual cell types to perform their usual function[63,66]. This may be proliferation and division as for B-cells or secretion of humoral substances. An example of the latter is a variety of interleukins released from macrophages incubated with LPS, leading to the multifaceted pyrexial response seen during endotoxemia[68]. The wide varieties of cell types stimulated would lead to a host of biologic responses including release of various humoral mediators, which in turn are responsible for the clinical aspects of endotoxin shock. These mediators include histamine, bradykinin, eicosanoids, endorphins, colony- stimulating activity, platelet-activating factor, monocytes, macrophage cytokines (interleukins, TNF), glucocorticoid- antagonizing factor, collagenases, nitric oxide and others, depending on with which cell LPS interacts. Also endotoxin exposure initiates the production of new gene products such as inducible (Type II) nitric oxide synthase. These products may directly alter cellular metabolism or initiate secretion of materials which secondarily affect other organ systems. It is unclear if gene products transcribed secondary to endotoxin exposure represent host adaptive physiology or pathophysiologic response induced by the invading microorganism. Several of these are discussed in detail below.

LPS initiation of specific, individual cellular responses has several implications. Clearly, LPS must interact at a specific site with a given cell membrane. This site could be a nonspecific interaction of the hydrophobic lipid A with membrane phospholipid[69] or a highly specific interaction actually involving LPS and cell membrane receptors[64,70]. After cell membrane binding, membrane reaction must lead to transmembrane signaling that stimulates the cell to perform its preprogrammed response. This signaling could occur directly via translocation of LPS into the cytosol (endocytosis) or indirectly by mobilization of second messengers. Alterations of cell membranes by lipid A could lead to hypersensitivity of other membrane receptors or mimic bona fide transmembrane triggering of normal intracellular biochemical responses and cellular activation[66]. Whether some or all of these mechanisms are important in determining the effects of LPS on mammalian cells and to what extent is as yet not clear. Whatever may be the exact sequence of events, the ability of LPS to stimulate widespread humoral responses from host cells is clearly great. Inhibition or alteration of this process of transmembrane signaling may provide future therapeutic strategies.

Interactions with Subcellular Components

Endotoxin, apart from transmembrane signaling, which initiates the release of humoral mediators, may also enter the cell (phagocytosis) and interact with subcellular components. Although interactions have been reported with most subcellular components, of particular interest are those with lysosomes and mitochondria. Phagocytosis, leading to the formation of a phagosome (endosome), has been known to occur since Metchnikoff. Classically, this phagosome interacts with lysosomes and forms phagolysosomes. This, in turn, leads to the release of lysosomal enzymes and bacteriocidal activity. Clearly, in terms of this process being bacteriocidal, it is beneficial. LPS plays a crucial role in activating lysosomes by destabilizing their membranes; consequently, this may unfortunately lead to the exposure of other cellular components to potent lysosomic enzymes. LPS enhances the release of the hydrolases, cathepsin, and β-glucuronidase, a reaction that can be prevented by the membrane-stabilizing effects of hydrocortisone pretreatment[(71)]. In human cells, LPS evokes β-glucuronidase and acid phosphatase lysosomal enzyme activity[(72)]. Triggering of massive lysosomal enzyme release by LPS may contribute to the cellular toxicity in endotoxemia.

Mitochondria contain key respiratory and metabolic enzymes (i.e., cytochrome reductases and oxidases, β-hydroxybutyrate dehydrogenase, and adenylate kinase) that are fundamental to cellular integrity. There is ample evidence that mitochondrial function is globally depressed by endotoxin. For example, mitochondrial succinate dehydrogenase, a key tricarboxylic acid cycle enzyme, is depressed in LPS-exposed animals[(73)]. For years it has been known that mitochondria from endotoxin-treated animals have depressed oxidative phosphorylation and energy production, neither of which is seen in hemorrhagic shock[(74)]. Investigators have advanced the concept that endotoxin depresses mitochondrial electron transport[(70)]. In addition, mitochondria exposed to endotoxin show abnormal potassium, calcium, and water transport. Morphologic changes are also seen including mitochondrial swelling and cristae disruption. Although mitochondrial preparations treated with large concentrations of LPS demonstrate these findings, there is also strong evidence that the majority of mitochondrial dysfunction in vivo arises as a secondary phenomenon in endotoxemia[(64,70)]. Whether mitochondrial dysfunction is a primary or a secondary phenomenon does not alter the fact that the profound disruption of fundamental cellular energy metabolism seen during endotoxemia is a major determinant of cell death and MOSF.

Endotoxin affects a wide array of cellular metabolism, not the least of which is basic carbohydrate metabolism. Endotoxin rapidly depletes carbohydrate stores[(75)]. The usual response to endotoxin is an initial rise in serum glucose over 1 to 2 hours, followed by a decline and subsequent hypoglycemia. In addition, succinate dehydrogenase activity, serum pyruvate, and liver glycogen are all depleted[(64,73)]. There is evidence that endotoxin interferes with both glycolysis and gluconeogenesis, thus doubly interfering with glucose metabolism. The activity of the key enzyme, pyruvate kinase, which is responsible for the conversion of phospho*enol*pyruvate (PEP) to pyruvate is enhanced during endotoxemia. This enhancement is because of lipid A and is blocked by cortisone[(70)]. Pyruvate kinase is responsible for increasing glucose entry into the tricarboxylic acid (TCA) cycle and reducing PEP levels, thus inhibiting gluconeogenesis. In addition, phospho*enol*pyruvate carboxykinase (PEPCK) activity is greatly decreased by endotoxemia, further blocking gluconeogenesis. It appears that this effect is because of the elaboration of a hormone, glucocorticoid-antagonizing factor, by macrophages in the liver (Kupffer cells), which inhibits the cortisol-induced increased activity of PEPCK during sepsis[(76)]. This basic metabolic disruption clearly has the potential for severe cellular derangement. Similarly, amino acid and protein metabolisms are severely disrupted during endotoxemia[(70)].

The critical interaction of endotoxin with the immunologic system provides a key link in the understanding of septic shock. As early as 1955, evidence that endotoxin activated the complement system was demonstrated. In the past 30 years the activation of complement has been realized to play an important role in mediating endotoxin-induced biologic responses[(77)]. Further investigation demonstrated an alternate pathway of complement activation (non-antigen-antibody complex induced) or the properdin system[(70,78)]. It now appears that LPS can activate complement by both the classic and the alternate pathways. The consequences of complement activation are legion. Classically, opsonization and enhanced phagocytosis occur as well as widespread chemotaxis and participate in the presentation of the systemic inflammatory response syndrome (SIRS). In addition, C3a and C5a (anaphylotoxins) are capable of causing leukocyte degranulation and massive histamine release with marked systemic consequences. Chemotaxis, leukoaggregation, and embolization triggered by C5a have been implicated as causes of the widespread tissue damage that occurs during shock[(79)].

Effects of Endotoxin on the Microvasculature

Septic shock is invariably accompanied by hypoproteinemia, increased fluid requirements, and edema. Endotoxin-induced increases in microvascular permeability are at least partially responsible for this triad[(80)]. Damage to the endothelium directly caused by endotoxin, complement activation, or leukocyte activation is commonly regarded as a universal accompaniment of septic shock. The timing of this endothelial injury is, however, debatable. The ability of endotoxin to cause endothelial damage in early shock has been questioned[81]. Nevertheless, endothelial changes are noted as early as four hours after exposure to endotoxin. Microvascular injury with increased permeability and decreased perfusion certainly contributes to the physiologic derangement in the later stages of shock.

Endotoxemia has other important effects on the microvasculature. Peripheral vessels are less responsive to catecholamines in endotoxin-shocked animals. This may underlie the failure of normal adrenergic compensatory mechanisms in shock[82]. Several authors have suggested that prostaglandins play a part in blocking this response[83]. Others have suggested a direct blocking of neurotransmitter release[84]. Another possible mechanism for this peripheral vasodilatation is endotoxin interference with smooth muscle calcium metabolism and membrane ATPase activity[85]. Recently, the key role of the endothelium in the regulation of vasomotor tone has been appreciated, including the preeminent role of nitric oxide[36,39,42,46,47,49,50]. In this light, it is not surprising that endotoxin-induced endothelial damage has multiple consequences. By multiple mechanisms endotoxin leads to peripheral vasodilatation and decreased peripheral resistance as an integral and early part of septic shock.

Endotoxin interferes with normal cellular function in multiple cell types, the function of subcellular components, and primary energy metabolism. It triggers a host of humoral responses that ultimately cause widespread hemodynamic alterations and tissue destruction. Endotoxins, specifically the lipid A moiety of LPS, have profound perturbing effects on many aspects of cellular function, which ultimately leads to multiple organ failure and, if severe enough, death. Gram positive bacterial exotoxins as well as products of rickettsia, fungi and viruses also induce profound physiologic disturbances by both parallel and other novel mechanisms. Recently, the contribution of bacterial infection to other forms of shock has been realized (bacterial translocation), and thus aspects of septic shock may play a role in all forms of shock and other critical illness.

Gut Translocation of Bacteria

Hypoperfusion of the splanchnic circulation occurs in virtually every form of shock[86]. Among the compensatory mechanisms outlined above is shunting flow away from the splanchnic circulation toward more critically important areas. This sets the stage for widespread splanchnic insult that may result in a breakdown in barrier function. The body becomes exposed to the threat of a large load of bacterial flora, which are normally contained within the gut. It is clear that this can trigger a number of tissue disruptive systems activated in shock. Endotoxin itself play a critical role in inducing bacterial translocation from the gut[27,86,87]. In addition to this, although other systems such as complement activation, leukoaggregation, and endothelial injury that aggravates mucosal injury in the gut are involved, it is clear that reperfusion injury plays a crucial role[23–25]. Reperfusion injury leads to the breakdown of the mucosal barrier in the gallbladder, stomach, and large intestines and to increased gut permeability that underlies translocation of bacteria. This effect can be ameliorated by the use of allopurinol, a xanthine oxidase inhibitor, which ameliorates reperfusion injury[88]; however clinical utility is not yet accepted.

The central importance of bacterial translocation in shock and in critically ill patients as a crucial etiologic factor in MOSF is increasingly recognized[27,87]. Bacterial translocation initiates an ongoing nidus of infection in mesenteric lymph tissue and in the portal system, which in turn activates a host of mediator systems. This leads to other organ system failure, with the lungs bearing the early brunt (ARDS), followed by sequential organ system failure. In addition to this, bacterial translocation is implicated as a cause of nosocomial pneumonia. Even as a greater cause of nosocomial pneumonias in critically ill patients than recurrent silent aspiration[89]. Furthermore, recent evidence suggests that the degree of splanchnic ischemia (sigmoid ischemia) that accompanies large abdominal aortic operations is directly correlated to the risk of postoperative infections and ongoing critical illness[90]. Recognition of the significant role that gut-associated bacteria play in the ongoing pathogenesis of MOSF highlights a potential role for gut decontamination early in the treatment of shock[91]. Stress ulceration from gastric ischemia, cholecystitis, and peritonitis may all form part of a spectrum of critical illness-associated splanchnic ischemia syndrome[92]. Although the exact significance of bacterial translocation, which has been demonstrated in multiple experimental animals and supported by evidence that it occurs in humans, has not been conclusively demonstrated in critical illnesses, further attention to the development of these concepts will no doubt yield significant insights into MOSF in intensive care.

Coagulation

No discussion of the pathogenesis of shock would be complete without a review of the coagulation system. Perturbations in coagulation are most striking during septic shock but occur in all other forms of shock, especially in the terminal phases. The most striking clinical manifestations include thrombocytopenia, purpura fulminans, peripheral gangrene, and, of course, DIC. Some derangement of clotting function occurs in all cases of endotoxemia, with thrombocytopenia being the most frequent. It is now abundantly clear that endotoxin directly activates the coagulation cascade[93], most probably by activating factor XII (Stuart-Hageman factor)[94]. Activation of factor XII is intimately interlinked with the generation of bradykinin and other kinins, plasminogen conversion, and even complement activation[95]. This is in addition to its initiation of the coagulation cascade. Thus, factor XII plays a pivotal role in the pathogenesis of endotoxin shock.

Platelet activation and consumption readily occur in shock states. Widespread tissue damage releases thromboplastins, and intravascular endothelial damage exposes subendothelial platelet activators, procoagulants, and phospholipase A_2 (PLA_2) activity releases platelet-activating factor (PAF)[96]. Acidosis and widespread tissue damage seen in the later stages of shock potentiates platelet aggregation. In septic shock, endotoxin is a potent platelet activator not only directly but also via complement activation and endothelial damage. This massive platelet activation makes a significant contribution to the coagulopathies seen in shock and plays an important role in inducing DIC[97].

In DIC the coagulation process becomes self-perpetuating. Massive amounts of thrombin are released into the circulation, leading to consumption of fibrinogen, platelets, and decreased factors II, V, VII, VIII, IX, and XI. In turn, the fibrinolytic system is activated, and large amounts of fibrin degradation products are formed. These lead to defective fibrin formation, inhibited coagulation, impaired platelet activity, pulmonary vasoconstriction, hypoperfusion, and hypotension. In the end, essential clotting factors are consumed and coagulation is actively inhibited. In an already-impaired microcirculation, which may be hypoperfused and have significant endothelial damage, thrombosis and necrosis are inevitable and potentiate the situation. Purpura fulminans and distal gangrene are dramatic manifestations of these coagulopathies seen in shock states.

Complement

The role of complement in the immune response to pathogenic invasion has been exhaustively described since the 19th century. Complement forms a major component of humoral immunity and plays a central linking role in host defense. Complement is a mediator of widespread tissue damage, most notably in ARDS. This mechanism may underlie the widespread injury seen in various types of shock. For these reasons, a brief review of the complement system, its activation, and the consequences of that activation is in order.

The complement system is composed of the group of serum proteins that were first described as heat-labile, nonspecific agents that cause cell lysis on reacting with the heat-stable serum components (antibodies). Originally, a complement cascade that was specifically antibody dependent was described and characterized as the classic complement pathway. In the 1950s, it became apparent that yeasts (zymosan) and bacterial pathogens activated the complement cascade by an alternate, nonclassical, or properdin pathway. Components of both pathways have been isolated and characterized **(Table 16.2).** Classical complement activation is triggered by adherence of antibody molecules to the globular C1 circulating complex. Specifically, C1q binds to the Fc fragment of the antibody and the cascade is initiated. Only G (IgG)- and M (IgM)-class immunoglobulins are capable of classic complement activation. The next sequence of activity is mediated via the protease, esterase, and convertase activity of the various complement components (Fig. 16.4). As each component of the system can cleave several other components, there is marked amplification inherent in this cascade. The early stages of the cascade (C1–C5) are facilitated by being cell bound, as large protein-protein interactions are required; however, with the formation of C5 convertase (C423b), C5a is released into solution, and C5b can bind to cell sites distant from the convertases. The effect of this is that the cytolytic sequence can continue in the absence of its initial activator and involve innocent bystander cells. This mechanism accounts for the widespread tissue damage that may occur during shock. The C5b moiety serves as a focus for C6–C9 binding, and the C5–C9 attack complex is responsible for cel-

Table 16.2. Complement Proteins

Pathway	*Serum (μg/mg)*	*Molecular Weight* $\times 10^7$
Classical pathway		
C9	160	79
C8	80	163
C7	55	120
C6	60	95
C5	75	206
C3	1400	190
C2	30	117
C4	430	209
C1 (q.r.s.)	80	110
	100	188
	190	390
Alternate pathway		
B (C3 proactivator)	200	100
D (C3 proactivator)	1–5	25
D (properdin)	25	223
Modulating proteins		
CT inhibitor	180	105
C36 inactivator	50	100
C4-binding protein		1570

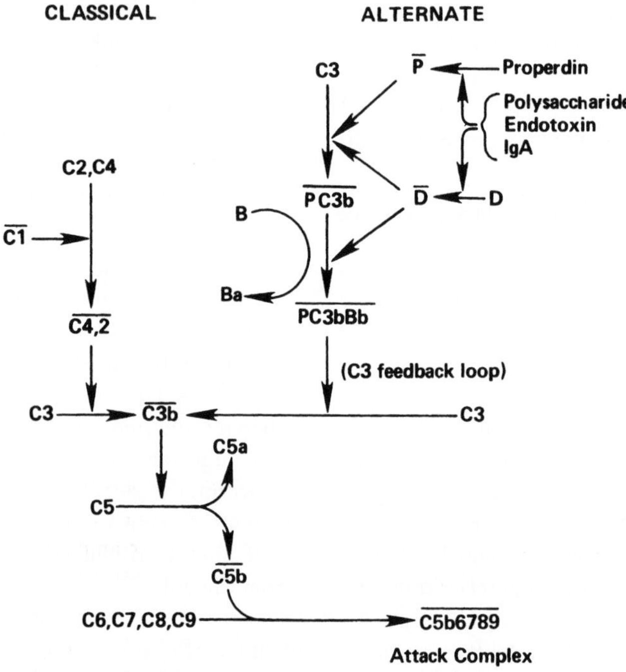

Figure 16.4. Complement cascade showing both classical and alternate pathways. Note the central role of C3 activation and the C3 feedback loop, which serves to potentiate the alternate pathway response.

lular disruption, either by intercalation into the lipid bilayer or by membrane pore formation ("punching holes"). The formation of a hole in the cell membrane leads to osmotic cell lysis. A single complement hole is sufficient to cause cell destruction (the "one-hit phenomenon").

Alternate activation in the absence of specific antibodies, a phylogenetically more primitive pathway, also occurs through the formation of convertases and cascade amplification. Endotoxin, lipid A, polysaccharides, yeast, immunoglobulin A (IgA), immunoglobulin E (IgE), and multiple other surface activators are potent alternative pathway activators. In this pathway, factors B and D function as C3, C4, and C2 and ultimately feed into the classic pathway by forming a C5-convertase complex (C3bBb), thus leading to C5a and C5b formation with the same effects as in the classic pathway. Both systems are potent amplifiers of the initial response, leading to the formation of large amounts of C5a and C5b, the widespread consequences of which have recently been delineated[(98)]. Clearly, intrinsic control mechanisms must be available to damp down this autoamplification, and there are several serum inhibitors of complement activation. In addition, the individual complexes require high density to act on other components and are also short lived, a factor that further limits the effects of their activation.

The role bacterial pathogens play in complement activation is central to understanding septic shock. From a host-defense point of view, complement activation with adherence to bacterial cell membranes and consequent lysis is beneficial. The teleologic raison d'etre for the alternate and antibody-mediated classic complement cascades is bacterial destruction. In general, acute bacterial infections are associated with normal or even elevated complement levels[(99)]. However, in shock, particularly those associated with GNB, the complement system goes beyond this beneficial, defensive role. In patients with septic shock and especially in those who die from their Gram-negative infections, serum C3 is reduced because of massive activation of the alternate complement pathway[(99)]. Other components of the complement system, i.e., C5, C6, and C9, are also decreased, thus indicating completion of complement activation in these patients. Although the widespread activation of attack complexes, release of C5a and C5b, and cell lysis are fatal to GNB, other systemic effects of complement activation and lysis of innocent bystander cells (i.e., endothelium, erythrocytes) is deleterious and potentially fatal. A host protective adaptive physiologic response has become pathophysiologic.

The biologic consequences of complement activation are multiple. The C3 and C5 convertase reactions release fragments that attract phagocytic cells and further amplify the inflammatory response. Larger fragments serve as opsonins and activate the reticuloendothelial system. Both C3a and C5a, also cell anaphylatoxins, cause histamine release from mast cells and stimulate neutrophils and macrophages that lead to degranulation with release of potent vasoactive and tissue toxic substances, as well as increased production of free oxygen radicals. Platelet clumping and the release of other vasoactive prostanoids is also enhanced by complement. These smaller complement peptides also cause smooth muscle contraction, i.e., tracheal, uterine, and ileal smooth muscle. Thus complement activation can mimic the reactions of classic anaphylaxis with hypotension, endothelial damage, and increased vascular permeability. Clearly, complement activation in shock states may serve as a potentiating cause of the observed physiologic derangement or may further aggravate the homeostatic defects.

In addition to the above, C5a is a potent chemotactic agent that leads to leukoactivation and leukoaggregation and sets the stage for disseminated leukoembolization to multiple peripheral vascular beds and, most dramatically, to the lungs. The work of Jacob and coworkers has delineated this mechanism as a key pathogenic mechanism in ARDS, Purtscher's retinopathy, myocardial infarction, and hemodialysis-associated pulmonary dysfunction[(98)]. In early ARDS, plugging of the pulmonary circulation with granulocytes has been noted, a phenomenon that can be mimicked with C5a infusion. Generation of toxic oxygen radicals, thrombosis, and endothelial damage lead to deranged vasoregulation, autocoid release, and permeability edema. In patients with ARDS, increased C5a activity has been described, and increased C5a appeared before the development of ARDS in patients with shock[(98,100)]. Complement activation, specifically C5a activation, occurs in endotoxemia, traumatic shock, burns, and pancreatitis and underlies, at least in part, the pulmonary injury (ARDS) and endothelial injury in other organ systems, i.e., myocardial and renal vascular beds, seen in multiple shock states[(98,100)].

Leukoactivation

Neutrophilic polymorphonuclear leukocytes are extremely well designed killer cells. There are two main processes associated with leukoactivation. The first, degranulation, occurs after phagocytosis and discharge of lysosomal contents into the phagolysosomes. The second, the respiratory burst, is associated with increased oxygen uptake by the polymorphonuclear leukocyte and formation of toxic oxygen radicals. Both of these processes summate to cause bacterial killing. Unfortunately, both of these processes also are indiscriminate and cause host cellular dysfunction. Although it was formerly believed that these toxic substances were wholly contained within the cell, it has recently become abundantly clear that they also have considerable extracellular activity that may have both local and remote effects[(56)].

Leukoactivation can occur through various mechanisms. As described above, complement, especially C5a, is responsible for chemotaxis and leukoaggregation and can begin the leukoactivation process. Obviously, bacteria covered with antibodies, particularly the Fc portion of the immunoglobulins, can cause leukoactivation. Many other substances can lead to activation, such as latex spherules, zymosan, certain calcium ionophores, and concanavalin A. In critically ill children, the role of interleukins and TNF appears central. All of these are capable of activating both degranulation and the respiratory burst. Degranulation is a calcium ion-dependent process of increased membrane fluidity and transiently increased sodium-potassium permeability[56,101]. Although the lysosomal products are generally maintained in a safe, intravacuolar environment, not infrequently, especially during massive pathogen challenge, the vacuoles may open and allow host tissue attack. The enzymes responsible for the tissue damage are cathepsin G, oxygen radicals, collagenases, elastases, and proteases[56].

After leukoactivation, cellular metabolism shifts from anaerobic to aerobic. There are four key factors to this respiratory burst: (a) increased oxygen uptake, (b) oxygen radical production, (c) hydrogen peroxide production, and (d) increased hexose monophosphate shunt activity and thus increased glucose metabolism. The increased oxygen uptake fuels superoxide anion and other oxygen radical production. Although the exact mechanism is not entirely understood, it is clear that the generation of superoxide anion, singlet oxygen, hydroxyl radical, hydrogen peroxide, nitric oxide and peroxynitrite and halous acids occurs by a series of simple reactions dependent on a single enzyme system **(Table 16.3).** Although superoxide anion is probably not in itself responsible for bacterial killing, it is essential for the formation of other oxygen radicals. For example, the reaction with hydrogen ion catalyzed by superoxide dismutase is responsible for the formation of hydrogen peroxide. In the presence of halide ion and myeloperoxidase, extremely efficient bacterial killing occurs. The central electron donor for this system appears to be nicotinamide adenine dinucleotide phosphate (NADPH), and a membrane-bound flavoprotein NADPH oxidoreductase (OR) catalyzes the initial superoxide-forming reaction.

$$NADPH + 2O_2 \rightarrow 2\ O_2^- + NADP^+ + H^+$$

In addition, quinone, a *b*-type cytochrome, and an oxidase are essential membrane-associated components of this enzyme system. The formation of these very reactive compounds leads rapidly to bacterial killing. They are, however, also released into the environment, and these free oxygen radicals mediate serious host tissue damage, such as the endothelial capillary damage seen in ARDS. This mechanism is especially active during reperfusion.

Considering the fact that leukoactivation leads to generation of such severely toxic compounds, it is perhaps surprising that host demise does not instantly follow bacterial invasion. Fortunately, there are also host defense mechanisms provided against the extracellular escape of these products of leukoactivation. For example, α_1-antitrypsin and α_2-macroglobin are both enzyme systems designed to scavenge extracellular elastase, protease, and other lysosomal contents. With regard to superoxide generation, several systems exist to scavenge these free radicals, including ceruloplasmin, superoxide dismutase, and catalase[56,101]. Another mechanism is the downregulation of NADPH-OR by negative feedback mediated by toxic oxygen metabolites themselves, as was suggested by the work of Zimmerman et al. on critically ill children[102]. This limits the autodigestive process initiated by the amplification of host defense mechanisms in critically ill children. Only when these resources are overwhelmed does host tissue damage occur.

Another aspect of leukoactivation is the formation of arachidonic acid metabolites from the lipid layer of the polymorphonuclear cell membrane that may make a significant impact on the host responses during sepsis and other forms of shock that lead to leukoactivation. Initially, this may also be viewed as a defense mechanism because it serves a role in scavenging toxic oxygen metabolites. These reactions lead to endoperoxide, thromboxane A_2, formation of preleukotriene compounds, and eventually stable prostaglandins such as prostacyclin and leukotrienes C_4 and D_4. The formation of these eicosanoid derivatives, when viewed as free radical scavengers, can be thought of as anti-inflammatory. On the other hand, the wide variety of biologic activity demonstrated by the eicosanoids indicates a far wider role in shock states.

Table 16.3. Oxygen Radicals

H_2O_2 formation: superoxide dismutase
$2O_2^- + 2H^+ \rightarrow H_2O_2 + O_2$
Hypohalite ions: myeloperoxidase
$X^- + H_2O_2 \rightarrow XO^- + H_2O$
$X^- = Cl^-, Br^-, I^-$
Hydroxyl radical: Haber-Weiss reaction
$O_2^- + H_2O_2 \rightarrow OH\cdot + OH^- + O_2$
$O_2^- + R - OOH \rightarrow OH\cdot + OR^- + O_2$
Singlet O_2
$OCl^- + H_2O_2 \rightarrow O2\cdot + Cl^- + H_2O$
$O_2^- + H_2O_2 \rightarrow O2\cdot + OH\cdot + OH^-$
$2O^2_- + 2H^+ \rightarrow O2\cdot + H_2O_2$

Eicosanoids

Aspirin blocks several typical effects of endotoxin, including fever, hypotension, pulmonary hypertension, shock, and abortion, as does the nonsteroidal cyclo-oxygenase inhibitor, indomethacin[103,104]. That potent inhibitors of arachidonic acid metabolism block some of the effects of endotoxin suggests that prostaglandins may be involved in the septic shock response. Serum levels of both thromboxane A_2 and prostacyclin, among others, rise in response to endotoxin challenge, and their levels parallel the hemodynamic sequelae[105,106]. Thromboxane is a potent vasoconstrictor and platelet aggregator-activator that can mimic several sequelae of shock. Prostacyclin is a potent vasodilator, alters platelet function, and can lead to profound hypotension. These earlier observations have been extended to explain other aspects of endotoxin shock. For example, thromboxane synthesis inhibition has been shown to increase survival[103], stabilize lysosomes, enhance splanchnic blood flow, and block the hypoglycemia associated with endotoxemia[104]. In addition to the cyclo-oxygenase metabolites, the lipoxygenase products, leukotrienes, have also received much attention. It has been shown that endotoxins stimulate leukotriene release[107]. In addition to promoting cyclo-oxygenase activity, leukotrienes mediate anaphylactic and inflammatory responses and can mimic symptoms of endotoxin shock[106,108]. Decreased cardiac output, vasoconstriction, and increased vascular permeability are known leukotriene effects[109]. Additional evidence provided by inhibitor studies supports a key role for leukotrienes in endotoxin shock[110]. Clearly, both prostaglandins and leukotrienes play a key role in endotoxin shock. This evidence is outlined in **Table 16.4.**

The effects of endotoxin, TNF, and interleukins are, at least in part, mediated by local eicosanoid release. These autocoids (locally synthesized immediately before release, locally acting, short-acting substance) are produced by many cell types. There is ample evidence that a source of eicosanoids is the LPS-stimulated macrophage for both the prostaglandins[111] and leukotrienes[107]. Platelets are also a rich source of thromboxanes. The vascular endothelium is probably the most important source of prostaglandins. Although all mammalian cells have the capability of eicosanoid production, the specific cellular source, i.e., endothelium or macrophage, may be related to the manifestations of particular shock states. All eicosanoids are formed from membrane-bound fatty acids. Phospholipases cleave the precursors from these phospholipid membrane components. PLA_2 is the best understood of these systems. Its activity yields not only arachidonate as the primary eicosanoid precursor, via lipoxygenase and cyclo-oxygenase pathways, but also PAF. Regulation of eicosanoid metabolism is complexly interrelated. Substrate availability seems critical. For example, PLA_2 inhibition (i.e., steroids) depletes both pathways. Cyclo-oxygenase inhibition "shunts" arachidonate toward lipoxygenase metabolites. These interactions probably account for the variability in effectiveness of various synthesis inhibitors. A potentially more successful therapeutic strategy may be specific receptor antagonism. These autocoids are an example of an LPS-cell-mediated response that is central to the understanding of the effects of endotoxin. It is obvious that this central role of prostaglandins and leukotrienes may have profound implications for future pharmacologic interventions in the therapy of septic and, potentially, other shock states.

Arachidonic acid is released from the phospholipid ester linkages in cellular plasma membranes by PLA_2[112]. Arachidonic acid (Fig. 16.5) then serves as a substrate for

Table 16.4. Support for Role of Eicosanoids

Administration of arachidonate, leukotrienes, and prostaglandins produces shock-like states.
In shock models and humans, hemorrhagic, anaphylactic, ischemic, burn, and septic shock are associated with increased levels of prostaglandins, thromboxanes, and leukotrienes.
Inhibitors of lipoxygenase, cyclo-oxygenase, and thromboxane synthetase, as well as receptor antagonists, inhibit or ameliorate many shock state responses.
Animals deficient in arachidonate substrate and with deficits in prostaglandin synthesis are resistant to endotoxic shock.

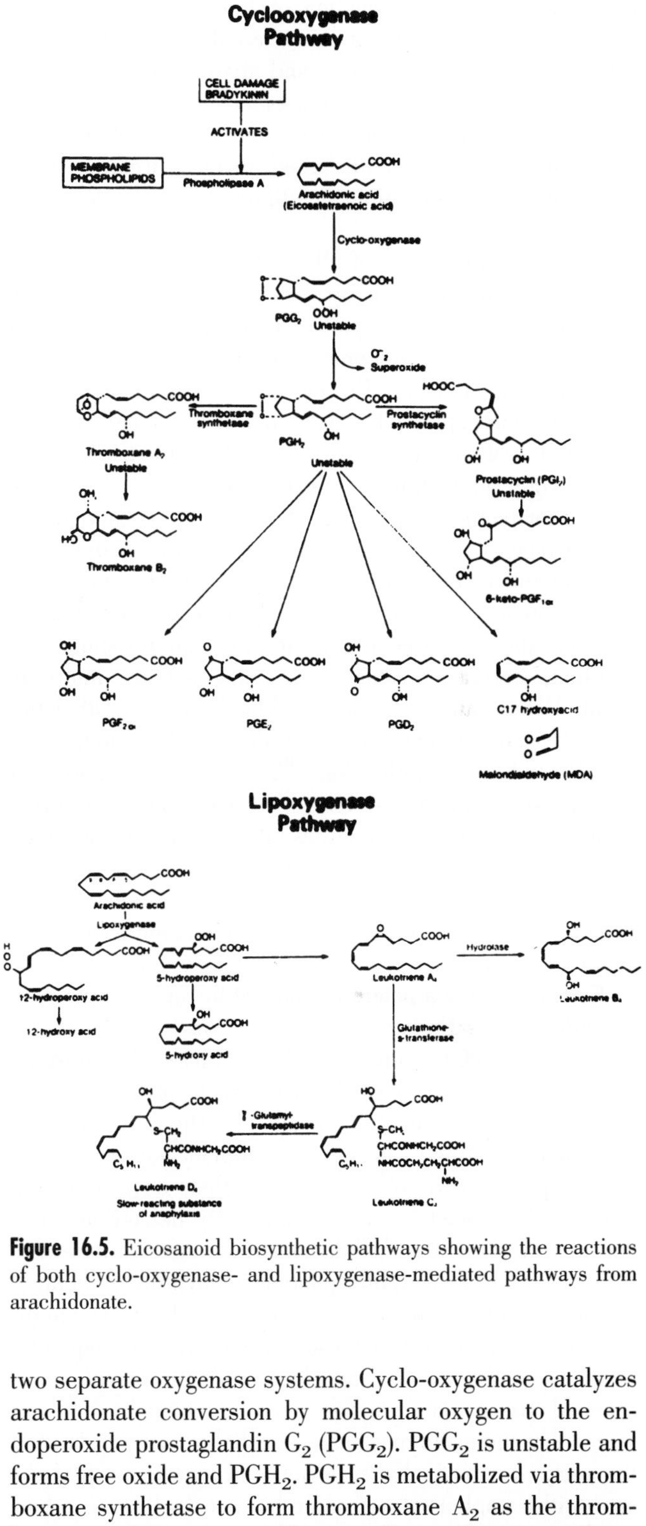

Figure 16.5. Eicosanoid biosynthetic pathways showing the reactions of both cyclo-oxygenase- and lipoxygenase-mediated pathways from arachidonate.

two separate oxygenase systems. Cyclo-oxygenase catalyzes arachidonate conversion by molecular oxygen to the endoperoxide prostaglandin G_2 (PGG_2). PGG_2 is unstable and forms free oxide and PGH_2. PGH_2 is metabolized via thromboxane synthetase to form thromboxane A_2 as the thromboxane series precursor. Prostacyclin synthetase catalyzes the conversion of PGH_2 to prostacyclin (PGI_2). PGH_2 is also spontaneously unstable and gives rise to a host of prostanoids, such as PGF_2, PGE_2, and PGD_2. The other oxygenase pathway is the lipoxygenase pathway. Lipoxygenase catalyzes the formation of hydroxyeicosotetranoic acid (HETE), the precursor of the leukotriene series of eicosanoids. Both the lipoxygenase and cyclo-oxygenase pathways are intimately interrelated. For example, blockade of cyclo-oxygenase enhances formation of lipoxygenase products, blockade of thromboxane synthetase enhances prostacyclin synthetase product formation, and anything that increases free arachidonic acid formation, especially in the presence of free oxygen radicals, enhances the formation of all of the eicosanoids. As already discussed, in the setting of septic shock and leukoactivation, conditions are ideal for eicosanoid formation.

Although the actions of all of the arachidonic acid derivatives are as yet undefined, several have been closely studied in various shock states. Thromboxane A_2 is a potent pulmonary and systemic vasoconstrictor as well as a platelet aggregator[(113)]. Prostacyclin, on the other hand, seems to inhibit platelet activation and is a potent pulmonary and systemic vasodilator[(114)]. The leukotrienes also have several interesting actions. Leukotriene B_4[(115)] is a potent chemotactic agent and is capable of leukoactivation. Leukotrienes C_4 and D_4 are the constituents of the slow-reacting substance of anaphylaxis and are, therefore, pulmonary smooth muscle constrictors, causing bronchoconstriction and increased pulmonary vascular resistance. In addition, several prostaglandins also act as inotropic agents[(116)] and increase coronary blood flow[(117)]. Other potentially salutary activities include vasodilatation, lysosomal membrane stabilization[(118)], and even modulation of the autonomic nervous system[(119)]. Clearly, these multiple, frequently antagonistic activities of the various eicosanoids make delineation of their precise physiologic role in shock states difficult to define; however, there is a great deal of evidence suggesting that they play a significant role during shock.

Endotoxemia is a potent initiator of the arachidonic acid cascade[(120,121)]. Endotoxin rapidly causes an increase in thromboxane, PGF_2, and PGI_2. Furthermore, thromboxane synthetase inhibitors have been shown to protect animals from the lethal effects of endotoxin[(104)]. The role of PGI_2 is less clearly defined, and several authors suggest that it plays a protective role[(104)], whereas others have indicated that it may indeed be hemodynamically deleterious. Recently, Halushka et al.[(122)] demonstrated massive increases in 6-keto-PGF_1 (the stable spontaneous hydrolysis metabolite of prostacyclin) in patients with septic shock. The highest levels were found in those patients who subsequently died. Recently, a role for eicosanoids in complement-induced tissue damage has been elucidated[(123,124)]. It seems that the cyclo-oxygenase metabolites are involved in the early pulmonary hypertension and hypoxemia that are seen with complement activation but not implicated in leukoaggregation or in the microvascular injury. The formation of lipoxygenase products is stimulated by complement activation. It seems that C5a may directly modulate lipoxygenase activity and, in part, act to regulate the proportion of arachidonate that is directed via the different oxygenase pathways[(124)]. The evidence that eicosanoids play a role in shock states continues to accumulate. Because of their wide variety of frequently opposing activities, it is not yet clear whether they are simply epiphenomena (concentrations correlated with clinical outcome) or whether they play a central causative role in the hemodynamic and metabolic consequences of shock.

Cyclo-oxygenase, lipoxygenase, combined cyclo-oxygenase and lipoxygenase inhibition, and eicosanoid receptor antagonism have been demonstrated to improve outcomes in multiple experimental models of septic shock in many species. In addition to this, several studies have demonstrated that the infusion of prostacyclin and PGE1, in both experimental animals and humans, demonstrate short-term improvements in multiple physiologic indices in septic shock[(35,125)]. Holcroft et al.[(126)] demonstrated that PGE_1 in ARDS improved oxygenation and hemodynamic parameters. PGI_2 has also been shown to improve short-term cardiorespiratory function, albeit not affect outcome[(35)]. This contrasts with results of a recent study that demonstrated that intravenous indomethacin improved studied parameters and outcome[(127)]. What are we to make of the fact that both inhibitors of, and infusions of eicosanoids improve outcomes? These results highlight the complex nature of the eicosanoid response in shock syndromes. Perhaps future therapeutic strategies will lie in the inhibition of phospholipases or of total cyclo-oxygenase and lipoxygenase with replacement of a beneficial eicosanoid compound, such as PGI_2 and PGE_1[(128–130)], in controlled concentrations.

Platelet-Activating Factor

Several of the pathophysiologic events that occur during endotoxemia and sepsis are mediated by PAF[(131,132)]. Acetyldiacyl ether phosphorylcholine (PAF) is released from numerous cells, including endothelial cells, leukocytes, monocytes, and platelets, after PLA2 activation by a host of stimuli[(133,134)]. The major biologic effects of PAF include increased pulmonary and systemic vascular permeability, superoxide release, platelet aggregation, leukoaggregation and leukoactivation, release of cyclo-oxygenase and lipoxygenase products, and pulmonary and systemic vasoconstriction and dilatation, depending on the report and the circumstances[(133,134)]. PAF antagonists block the cardiovascular changes that accompany endotoxic shock[(134,135)]. Development of PAF antagonists may be useful in ameliorating the cardiovascular and permeability defects associated with shock syndromes.

Vasoactive Neuropeptides

Endogenous Opioids

In 1973, the characterization of specific opiate receptors was rapidly followed by the discovery of endogenous opiate polypeptides. Collectively, these endogenous opiates function to modulate the nervous systems by acting as hormones and neurotransmitters[(136)]. The similarity of morphine overdose and shock, i.e., hypotension, suggested to Holaday and Faden[(137)] that endogenous opioids may play a role in shock states. In 1978, report of their simple but dramatic experiment greatly stimulated research into the role of opiates in physiologic regulation and shock states[137]. Further work by these and other investigators demonstrated the role of endogenous opiates in several types of experimental shock: hemorrhagic, spinal, anaphylactic, and endotoxin in numerous species[136–139]. However, both animal and human studies have failed to demonstrate that long-term survival increased. As endotoxin and other shock states are complex entities, it is possible that other pathophysiologic effects of shock obscure the effect of opiate-induced hemodynamic depression on overall survival. What is without doubt is that opiate antagonism readily restores the blood pressure in a wide variety of shock states. The endogenous opiate system consists of several distinct polypeptides and their widespread receptors. The actions of this family of peptides are found in the CNS, peripheral nervous system, and many other systems[140].

Most endorphins and enkephalins share the amino acid sequence Try-Gly-Gly-Phe at their N terminus. Several fragments and larger precursors have also been identified. There appear to be at least three distinct genetic loci for these opiate hormone systems[141]: (a) proenkephalin A, which gives rise to the enkephalins; (b) prodynorphin, which gives rise to dynorphin and related polypeptides; and (c) pro-opiomelanocortin, from which β-endorphin, adrenocorticotropic hormone (ACTH), melanocyte-stimulating hormone, and β-lipotropic hormone are derived[140]. The presence of these common precursors suggests physiologically related secretion of both ACTH and β-endorphin[142]. Dynorphin is secreted from the posterior pituitary in a manner analogous to vasopressin[140]. The origin of circulating enkephalins is the sympathetic nerve terminals and the adrenal medulla, where their secretion is closely tied to catecholamines[143]. Even though catecholamines and enkephalins are related, (coexpression in some cells) different control mechanisms exist for their release, and this suggests the potential for new therapeutic strategies[144]. Endogenous and exogenous opioid compounds act as inhibitors of catecholamine secretion during stress. These endogenous opiates are also associated with specific neuron groups throughout the CNS and periphery[140,142,143].

At least three receptors have been identified for the endorphins: δ, μ, and κ; additionally, σ, ϵ, and λ opiate-binding sites have been suggested[141]. Evidence is emerging that various endorphins have different affinities for these binding sites and that stimulation of specific receptors leads to distinct physiologic effects[138,140]. For example, morphine-μ-receptor interaction leads to bradycardia, and hypotension seems to rely on morphine-δ interaction. Development of specific agonists and antagonists for the individual opiate receptors may provide useful therapeutic modalities in the future. In low doses, naloxone binds preferentially to the μ-receptors and is thus a good antagonist of morphine effects. However, in larger doses, such as those used to treat shock, naloxone blocks δ-, κ-, and μ-receptors and therefore provides little receptor-specific information. The use of other antagonists such as ICM M154,129, which selectively inhibits δ-receptors and blocks the hypotensive effects of endotoxin while not antagonizing morphine analgesia, indicates that the δ-receptor is involved in the shock response[145].

Although the role of endogenous opiates in shock is well founded, their exact site of action and source in shock are not firmly established. Antagonist/agonist investigations, experiments on hypophysectomized and adrenalectomized animals, and serum assays of β-endorphin-like activity (as well as the profoundly hypertensive endorphin, dynorphin) have given rise to conflicting results[140,141]. Nevertheless, the evidence seems to indicate that in shock, both central and peripheral endorphin effects are mediated via the sympathoadrenal medullary system. Stimulation of central endorphin receptors plays an important role in the modulation of these sympathoadrenal responses to all forms of shock. Peripheral effects may involve direct vascular and myocardial depression, prostaglandin-mediated calcium ion transport, inhibition of catecholamine release, inhibition of the release of myocardial depressants, or even modulation of macrophage responses to shock[141,146]. With these variable potential mechanisms, it is not surprising that the site and the mode of action of naloxone in shock remain controversial. Holaday and Faden[147] favor a central site of activity but agree that there is ample evidence to support peripheral myocardial, vascular, and adrenal effects. The interaction of naloxone and corticosteroids is also confusing. It would seem that as feedback suppression of pro-opiomelanocortin occurs with steroid treatment, β-endorphin levels would be suppressed, and thus the effect of naloxone would be diminished. However, naloxone and corticosteroids may actually be synergistic in ameliorating shock[148]. An endorphin role seems evident in shock, unfortunately, naloxone administration has no proven clinical efficacy[149,150].

Thyrotropin-Releasing Hormone

In addition to opiate neuropeptides, other CNS-associated neuropeptides may play a role in shock. These include vasoactive intestinal polypeptides and thyrotropin-releasing hormone (TRH). Although their interactions are less well delineated than opioids, they have a potentially important role in shock states. TRH (a tripeptide), apart from its well-known endocrine effects, has a host of pharmacologic effects, such as arousal, tachypnea, tachycardia, hypertension, enhancement of peristalsis, increased body temperature, and mydriasis. These effects suggested that the use of TRH as a therapeutic opiate antagonist would be feasible, and TRH inhibited or attenuated several opiate effects with the important exception of analgesia[141]. These findings prompted a trial of TRH in shock, and as was expected, TRH improved physiologic parameters and even survival in various shock states[151,152]. In addition, it is worth noting that TRH is effective in experiments involving leukotriene, anaphylactic, lipoxygenase, and PAF-induced shock that have not been shown to involve opioids. TRH does not appear to be a specific antagonist but rather appears to be a centrally acting nonspecific factor in reversing shock. Its effect is mediated via central autonomic pathways and is not observed in a pithed animal. Another hypothesis is that TRH increases free T_3 (triiodothyronine) which is depressed in critical illness, however this does not appear so. In addition, the effects of naloxone and TRH are additive[153].

After the initial reports of TRH induced improvement in physiologic variables in shock, further studies found no effect of TRH on mortality[154,155]. In large doses (a bolus of 2 mg/kg and infusions of 2 mg/kg/hr) in cats and rats, a significant pressor response was seen; however, this was transient. Also, TRH did not attenuate measured biochemical indices of the severity of shock (myocardial depressant factor, plasma amino-nitrogen concentrations, or cathepsin D). Compared with controls, survival time and regional blood flows were not improved[154]. Difficulty in interpretation of interspecies responses to TRH has also diminished the early enthusiasm for TRH as a treatment in different shock states[152,155].

Vasoactive Intestinal Polypeptide

Another neuropeptide, vasoactive intestinal polypeptide (VIP), a potent vasodilator, may contribute to the hypotension in shock. VIP is a 28-residue polypeptide that was isolated from pig intestines and subsequently identified as an important central and peripheral neurotransmitter[156]. VIP-containing neurons occur in exocrine organs, gut, autonomic nerve fibers, and in close relationship with blood vessels. Several reports implicate VIP as a mediator in septic and hemorrhagic shock[156,157]. Its activity does not rely on the cholinergic, adrenergic, or eicosanoid systems. It is more potent than either secretin or glucagon. Although VIP is present in the CNS, this is not the major source. It has been shown that total removal of the gastrointestinal tract blocks the increase in plasma VIP levels that accompany hypotension seen with endotoxin[157]. An association of endotoxin and circulatory VIP has been reported in patients with meningococcal sepsis. After institution of antibiotic and fluid therapy, VIP levels rapidly declined. Recent information points to VIP as a physiologic mediator of endotoxin-induced vasodilatation[158]. Although VIP is not significantly elevated in hemorrhagic hypotension, it is increased during reperfusion in mesenteric artery occlusion. With these interesting findings, VIP merits further investigation.

Corticotropin-Releasing Factor

Corticotropin-releasing factor (CRF) is a 41-amino acid peptide that is the primary regulator of the hypophyseal-pituitary- adrenal axis. Its role as a neurotransmitter has recently been established. CRF stimulates the sympathetic autonomic nervous system and the adrenal medulla when administered into the cerebrospinal fluid or brain. CNS administration of CRF causes increased blood pressure and systemic catecholamine levels, and CRF-receptor antagonist administration prevents stress-induced increases in catecholamines. This suggests an adaptive physiologic role for CRF neurotransmission in stress. In comparison, peripheral CRF administration produces vasodilatation and hypotension. This interesting paradox is currently under investigation as CRF has now been identified in the adrenal cortex.

The intricacy and the complexity of interactions between CRF- and dynorphin-related peptides are slowly being unveiled, which promises to advance our knowledge of adaptive and pathophysiologic responses to stress and shock[159]. Current understanding is too limited to substantiate CRF neurotransmission abnormalities in shock, but this area will be of great interest in the future.

Histamine and Kallikrein-Bradykinin

Histamine release occurs under a wide variety of circumstances that lead to or occur during shock. Mast cell degranulation is triggered by a host of stimuli, including anaphylaxis, sepsis, and widespread tissue injury. Locally formed histamine is also important in the regulation of the microcirculation. Histamine causes peripheral vasodilatation, profound hypotension, pulmonary hypertension, and microvascular injury, probably caused by postcapillary venular spasm. Histamine leads to portal and splanchnic venous pooling and decreased venous return. Not surprisingly, decreased venous return and increased right ventricular afterload lead to impaired cardiac output. This coupled with peripheral vasodilatation, explains the hypotension with histamine release. Histamine release occurs as an integral part of anaphylactic shock[160], and the hemodynamic consequences of anaphylaxis can be blocked by antihistamines. Antagonists of both H_1- and H_2-receptor subtypes are required. Endotoxin is also a potent histamine releaser[161], and there is a similarity between early sepsis and anaphylaxis, possibly as a result of histamine release[162]. Antihistamines ameliorate septic shock[163]. Histamine release clearly occurs in various shock states and probably contributes to the hemodynamic picture. The exact role requires further elucidation.

Bradykinin is a potent vasoactive nonapeptide released by the action of trypsin and kallikrein (proteases) on its circulating precursor α2-globulin, bradykininogen. Kallikrein is released as part of the stress response whenever sympathetic activity is increased and acute phase reactants appear. Bradykinin is a potent vasodilator of small vessels whose actions are most marked on the coronary, skin, capillary, and skeletal circulations. Bradykinin increases capillary permeability and along with other vasoactive agents, may be responsible for the capillary leak seen in shock. Bradykinin is an extremely short-lived compound, and its activity is probably local, where it is formed and is unlikely to act as a circulating vasodilator.

Cardioinhibitory Factors in Shock

Since the observations of Blalock nearly 50 years ago[164], it has been known that toxic substances circulate in the blood of animals who have been subjected to shock. It was not until 1966 that Brand and Lefer[165] and Baxter et al.[166] concurrently described myocardial depressant factor (MDF) in the blood of dogs in shock after both burns and hemorrhage. In the past 20 years, substances that depress myocardial function have been described in hemorrhagic, cardiogenic, endotoxin, burn, and splanchnic ischemic shock and in acute pancreatitis in numerous species[167]. The suggestion of Siegel et al.[168] that myocardial decompensation significantly contributed to mortality in shock led to renewed interest in myocardial function in the later stages of shock. In the 1970s, there were numerous reports of myocardial dysfunction during shock, especially endotoxin shock, but the presence of humoral cardioinhibitory factors and their role were specifically questioned; other etiologies of cardioinhibition, such as myocardial hypoperfusion and direct myocardial depression by endotoxin, were raised[169–171]. In humans, although a fall in cardiac output occurs in hemorrhagic and cardiogenic shock, in endotoxin shock, increased cardiac output rather than cardiac depression is almost always seen in the early stages.

Confusion concerning myocardial depression almost certainly arises from the myriad technicalities of experimental preparations, the definitions of cardiac contractility, and the difficulty of separating peripheral vascular effects of shock from effects on myocardial function[171]. In addition, the failure to recognize and stratify different types of shock and to realize that the hemodynamic picture varies at different stages of shock has also led to confusion. Myocardial depression may accompany shock associated with blood loss, trauma (myocardial contusion), and global ischemia, and MDFs have been reported to occur in all of these. Recently, much attention has been focused on myocardial depression in endotoxin shock, and Parrillo et al.[172] have demonstrated myocardial depressant activity in serum from patients with septic shock. Although the remainder of this discussion is focused on endotoxin shock, several of the general principles also apply to other forms of shock.

Myocardial Depression in Endotoxin Shock

It has been conclusively demonstrated in several species that myocardial functional impairment occurs during septic shock and as a response to endotoxin. Furthermore, myocardial dysfunction appears to occur not only preterminally but also in the intermediate and even early stages of endotoxin shock[173,174]. Although peripheral vascular paralysis may be the major cause of hypotension in early septic shock, demonstrable decreased contractility does occur, and as the shock state progresses, this negative inotropism becomes progressively more severe and eventually is a major determinant of survival[173].

In humans, it is unusual to see a hypodynamic picture with a low cardiac index in septic shock, although it is occasionally noted. Even so, this does not preclude abnormal myocardial function, and recent investigations of cardiac performance that used more sensitive parameters have demonstrated decreased contractility during human septic shock. Parker et al.[174] clearly demonstrated myocardial depression in humans with septic shock. They demonstrated early abnormalities in the ejection fraction (less than 40%) and increased end-systolic and end-diastolic volumes. In survivors over the next 10 days, these abnormalities resolved. Other investigators have demonstrated depressed cardiac function curves and abnormal responses to volume loading and correlated survival with cardiac index[175]. Although cardiac index may be within the normal range, this alone may be inadequate in shock states, and in fact, cardiac performance may be impaired sufficiently for the patient to be unable to respond adequately to the stress of septic shock.

Several possible mechanisms underlying myocardial decompensation include (a) global metabolic defects of the myocardium resulting from shock, (b) decreased response to the sympathoadrenal support, (c) circulating cardiotoxic substances, (d) myocardial ischemia resulting from increased workload and decreased supply, or (e) coronary vascular endothelial injury, (f) endocardial/myocardial nitric oxide production, and (g) endocardial endothelial injury. The occurrence of widespread metabolic derangements is well documented. Protein, carbohydrate, and fat metabolisms are adversely altered in septic shock. Altered pH, increased lactate levels, decreased oxygenation, altered insulin metabolism, and amino acid profiles are apparent. Siegel et al.[176] have suggested that a feedback mechanism involving basic metabolic functions eventually leads to myocardial failure. Other evidence indicates that myocardial metabolism is deranged and that abnormal calcium metabolism is the cause of myocardial failure[173]. Altered catecholamine response has been suggested, and although the levels of endogenous catechols are high, impaired end-organ response has been reported[176,177].

Circulating cardioinhibitory substances have received a great deal of attention. Among these are histamine, endorphins, complement, TNF, IL-1 and IL-2, and prostaglandins[174,178–180]. Specific MDFs such as those championed by Lefer and colleagues have received a great deal of enthusiastic support. There have been multiple demonstrations that serum, plasma, or blood from shocked animals depresses the function of isolated myocardium. Indeed, polypeptides have been isolated and even analyzed that have cardioinhibitory properties such as IL-2. It has been claimed that MDF is dialyzable and can be removed from the circulation with salutary consequences[167]. The source of most of these factors appears to be the region supplied by the splanchnic circulation, particularly the pancreas. It would appear that factors that depress myocardial function are elaborated during shock and that the pancreas is a major source. The existence of circulating cardioinhibitory factors in human shock states has been established[172,180–182]. What is less clear is whether these factors have a significant role to play in shock. The role of other metabolic derangements and the elaboration of cardiotoxic substances may indeed be additive in their deleterious myocardial effects. Clearly, in shock, myocardial performance is impaired. The cause of this dysfunction is almost certainly multivariant[178,182]. Most likely, metabolic derangements, circulating cardiodepressant factors, and altered myocardial metabolism in addition to impaired myocardial oxygen and substrate supply-to-demand ratios aggravated by endothelial injury are all responsible for the profound myocardial depression seen in the end stages of all forms of shock. Recent investigations challenge the hypothesis of insufficient oxygen delivery to the myocardium until very late stages of shock or during diastolic hypotension, and limited myocardial O_2 delivery is probably not a significant contributor to cardiac dysfunction. Interesting new work demonstrated local increases in endocardial nitric oxide production after endotoxin exposure and that this increased NO mediates a negative inotropic activity or myocardium[183,184].

The widespread derangement of endothelial function in shock may cause myocardial depression. Coronary vascular endotheliopathy with ischemia could certainly depress myocardial function. It is also now clear that the endocardial endothelium significantly alters myocardial contractility[185,186]. Local release of mediators of myocardial myocyte function, including the positive inotrope, endothelin[186], regulate the heart's perfusion and inotropic state.

We have also shown that the endocardial endothelium also releases unique, potent, depressors of myocardial function[187]. Perhaps the widespread endotheliopathy seen in shock states accounts for the depressed myocardial function as well.

Cytokines

Although endotoxin has many direct effects on endothelial cell and various tissue/organ functions, much interest has been displayed in other mediators of sepsis, e.g., host response proteins that may be released and induce further physiologic perturbations. Activated complement and coagulation cascade factors are examples previously mentioned. Cytokines, which are polypeptides released by activated monocytes and macrophages, have been shown to induce the shock state in experimental animals similar to human septic shock[188–193]. These cytokines are numerous and include TNF-α, interleukins (IL-1, IL-2, and IL-6), and interferons (INF-α and INF-γ). Each of these cytokines are released by monocytes or lymphocytes activated in the immune response by endotoxin and other antigens. Once released, these cytokines demonstrate autocrine, paracrine, and endocrine activity[194]. Endothelial cells are target sites of action for many of these substances. Despite intense effort and success in isolating mechanisms of action of these substances in vitro, prediction of in vivo activity has been less precise. For example, different endothelial cells (renal versus pulmonary versus umbilical vein) behave differently in response to exposure to various cytokines[194].

In vivo studies of cytokines in shock states were initially descriptive. In patients with meningococcemia, TNF-α, IL-1, and IFN-γ were found to correlate with severity of disease[195,196]. Hack et al.[188] found increases in IL-6 with the septic state. In another study, Damas and colleagues[197] measured TNF-α and IL-1β in patients developing sepsis. Of the 27 patients studied, 10 survived. Nonsurvivors had a statistically significant greater lactatemia and TNF-α level. IL-1 levels were not different in the survivors versus nonsurvivors. Further analysis revealed a greater mortality with a TNF-α level greater than 200 pg/ml (12 of 13 died) than those with TNF-α levels less than 200 pg/ml (5 of 14 died). Calandra and coworkers[198] found a correlation between TNF and IL-1β levels but not IFN-α or IFN-γ with mortality in septic shock[198]. Infusions of TNF and IL-1 each induce a shock state in animals[189–193]. Neilson et al.[199] found that in rats, shock was not induced by large infusions of TNF alone, whereas individually sublethal doses of TNF and endotoxin caused 100% mortality when given together. Administration of small doses of endotoxin to human volunteers resulted in increased TNF[187]. IL-6 acts as an endogenous pyrogen and is increased in patients with burns, solid organ transplant rejection, and meningococcemia. As new host mediators are identified, further insight into the timing, course, and effects of mediator release is being gained to provide a more complete understanding of the shock syndrome. Investigations utilizing neutralizing antibodies to cytokines continues to undergo evaluation for prophylaxis and treatment of sepsis and is discussed further under "Immunotherapy."

Heat Shock Proteins and Others

Ischemia with reperfusion has been shown to induce expression of the early intermediate genes c-*fos*, c-*jun*, and heat shock protein 70 (hsp70—70,000 molecular weight)[200–202]. Exposure to endotoxin has been demonstrated to initiate expression of "inducible" nitric oxide synthase (NOS Type II) in macrophages and multiple NOS isoforms in other tissues[46]. These genes and gene products are recognized as important in cell growth and differentiation, and cellular metabolism and bacteriocidal properties. These gene products are known mediators of transcription of other proteins. As cells are stressed by acidosis, hyperthermia, or hypoxia, increased transcription of hsp70 occurs to the exclusion of other proteins[203]. It is highly likely that our understanding of the mechanisms of cellular injury and responses to the shock state will be enhanced as we elucidate the expression and function of these types of genes, which may be critical as adaptive physiologic responses to stress or pathophysiologic in some situations initiating secondary injury.

Classification of Shock States

Shock has been classified in many ways. The lack of a single universally accepted system indicates the complexity of the underlying pathologic processes and their tremendous variability. Furthermore, for any given shock state, the pathophysiologic characteristics vary widely over time. Therefore, in addition to delineating the underlying abnormalities for a given shock state, it is necessary to know the

Table 16.5. Classification of Shock

Hypovolemic
Dehydration
Gastroenteritis
Deprivation
Heat stroke
Burns
Hemorrhage
Distributive
Anaphylaxis
Neurogenic
Drug toxicity
Septic
Cardiogenic
Congenital heart disease
Ischemic heart disease
Anoxia
Kawasaki disease
Traumatic
Infectious cardiomyopathies
Drug toxicity
Tamponade
Obstructive
Pulmonary embolism (air, blood, fat)
Cardiovascular Obstructive Lesions
Dissecting aortic injury or aneurysm
Asymmetric septal hypertrophy/idiopathic hypertrophic subaortic stenosis
Aortic stenosis
Critical pulmonic stenosis
Mitral stenosis
Critical coarctation of the aorta
Interrupted aortic arch
Septic shock
Miscellaneous
Heat stroke
Adrenal insufficiency (congenital adrenal hyperplasia, HIV, autoimmune, steroid use, idiopathic)
Pancreatitis
Drug overdose
Barbiturates
β-Antagonists
Ca^{++} channel antagonists

time course of each particular syndrome. Any classification of shock must allow for various overlaps. A classic example of distributive shock is septic shock; however, septic shock also has characteristics of both hypovolemic and cardiogenic shock. Any given patient in shock may have pathophysiologic characteristics of several classifications of shock. For example, the child suffering from a motor vehicle accident may initially suffer from hypovolemic shock caused by hemorrhage and neurogenic shock secondary to head injury. She may eventually suffer from septic shock after aspiration pneumonia. With these reservations, shock can be etiologically classified into (a) hypovolemic (lack of blood volume), (b) distributive (altered vascular tone, either primary or secondary to neurologic or neurohormonal alterations), (c) cardiogenic (cardiac pump failure), and (d) septic shock, which has characteristics of all of the previous types of shock and is important enough and has enough unique characteristics to require separate classification **(Table 16.5).** Because the diversity of shock states makes classification difficult, several types cannot be neatly classified. Some of these are shown in the miscellaneous section of Table 16.5.

In addition to the above classification, it is of help to consider three stages in shock: compensated, uncompensated, and irreversible. In the early compensated stage, homeostatic mechanisms are functioning to maintain essential organ perfusion. Blood pressure, urine output, and cardiac function may all seem to be normal, however early cellular metabolic alterations are underway. In the decompensated stage, this circulatory compensation fails because of ischemia, endothelial injury, the elaboration of host inducible gene products and toxic materials from host and microorganisms, and often the deleterious impact of physiologic compensatory mechanisms. Eventually, cellular function deteriorates and widespread abnormalities occur in all organ systems. When this process has caused such significant, irreparable functional loss in essential organs that death is inevitable despite temporary support, the terminal or irreversible stage of shock is reached. Many investigators are in search of a specific metabolic marker or physiologic parameter as an assessment of the threshold of no return from "irreversible shock." No currently measured parameter is sufficiently sensitive and specific to act as a gold standard indicator of irreversible shock. By this stage, no matter what the initial classification of a given shock state may have been, there are gross abnormalities in volume status, vascular tone, cardiac function, and cellular energetics and multiorgan failure.

Hypovolemic Shock

Hypovolemic shock results from decreased intravascular volume and, therefore, decreased venous return and myocardial preload. This intravascular fluid depletion may be a result of hemorrhage, water and electrolyte losses, or plasma losses **(Table 16.6),** all of which may be either external or internal (third space losses). The major cause of infant mortality in the world is shock resulting from dehy-

Table 16.6. Hypovolemic Shock

Water and electrolyte loss
Diarrhea
Vomiting
Diabetes insipidus
Renal losses
Heat stroke
Intestinal obstruction
Burns
Hemorrhage
Trauma
Surgery
Gastrointestinal bleeding
Plasma losses
Burns
Nephrotic syndrome
Sepsis
Intestinal obstruction
Peritonitis

dration resulting from the diarrhea and vomiting that accompany infectious gastroenteritis. It is estimated that between 7 and 20 million children die annually throughout the world from this condition. Although gastroenteritis affects many children in this country, it can be effectively treated by volume resuscitation and electrolyte replacement. In the United States, trauma is the leading cause of death in children over 1 year of age and hypovolemic shock is a major contributor to the mortality caused by trauma[204].

Hemorrhagic shock resulting from trauma may occur because of external or internal blood loss. A ruptured viscus, usually the spleen, mesentery, or the liver, can lead to profound hypovolemic shock in a very short time and mandates immediate surgery. Soft tissue trauma and long bone fractures can also lead to massive blood loss and edema formation, thus causing shock that may be less obvious than frank external hemorrhage. Among the most obvious sites of external blood loss are vascular lacerations (or penetrating trauma) and scalp lacerations that may bleed profusely and rapidly compromise the circulation[205].

Gastrointestinal hemorrhage, another leading cause of hemorrhagic shock in children, can occur as part of a systemic illness or gastrointestinal infection, or it can result directly from a gastrointestinal tract primary lesion. Gastrointestinal hemorrhage occurs in patients with generalized coagulopathies such as those that occur in leukemias, in idiopathic thrombocytopenic purpura, after chemotherapy, or with DIC from many causes, including septic shock. Severe gastrointestinal hemorrhage can accompany salmonellosis and shigellosis, further complicating the volume depletion that occurs in these diseases. Specific gastrointestinal lesions that may lead to hemorrhagic shock are different for different age groups **(Table 16.7).** In infancy, the most likely diagnosable cause of hemorrhagic shock from the gastrointestinal tract is associated with coagulopathies, notably hemorrhagic disease of the newborn. However, it is worth noting that nearly 50% of the cases of gastrointestinal hemorrhage in the newborn remain undiagnosed. Gastric wall irritation, ulceration, or perforation may occur from nasogastric tube placement or persistent suction applied for gastrointestinal decompression in any child (preterm newborn through adolescence). In children older than 1 year of age, upper gastrointestinal bleeding from ulceration, esophageal varices, or the Mallory-Weiss syndrome can lead to rapid, life-threatening exsanguination and requires emergent attention. Infrequently but still notable etiologies are gastrointestinal hemorrhage from corticosteroid therapy or critical illness such as severe closed head injury. Lower gastrointestinal bleeding can occur suddenly and profusely in children with intestinal polyposis (i.e., Peutz-Jeghers syndrome), colitis, intussusception, and rarely but dramatically a Meckel's diverticulum.

Table 16.7. Causes of Gastrointestinal Hemorrhage

Neonates
Hemorrhage diseases of the newborn
Anorectal trauma
Infectious diarrhea
Colitis (milk and soy)
Necrotizing enterocolitis
Volvulus
Gastric ulcer/perforation
Idiopathic
Infants
Intussusception
Gastritis
Esophagitis and varices
Duodenal ulcers
Gangrenous bowel
Gastric ulcers
Children
Colonic polyps
Esophagitis and varices
Gastric and duodenal ulcers
Ulcerative colitis and Crohn's disease
Mallory-Weiss syndrome
Meckel's diverticulum
Intussusception
Henoch-Schönlein purpura

Loss of fluid and electrolytes from vomiting and diarrhea is the major cause of world infant mortality, and although it is less common in this country, children still present with profound dehydration and shock after gastroenteritis. A child can lose 10 to 20% of his or her circulating volume in 1 to 2 hours with fulminant gastroenteritis, and because of the frequent inability of voluntarily restoring this volume loss by oral rehydration or because of accompanying vomiting, shock rapidly ensues. In this country, viral gastroenteritis (rotavirus, enterovirus, and adenovirus) is the most common cause. Bacterial gastroenteritis caused by *Salmonella, Shigella, Yersinia enterocolitica,* and *Campylobacter* can also lead to profound dehydration. Cholera, although rare in the United States, affects children of all ages. In the newborn, enteropathogenic *E. coli* and staphylococcus also present a profound threat.

Dehydration from other sources can occasionally lead to shock. Rarely, renal diseases such as nephrotic syndrome and acute tubular necrosis, especially during the diuretic phase, can result in massive volume loss. Infants with congenital adrenal hyperplasia (adrenogenital syndrome) frequently present with shock resulting from intravascular volume depletion (see Chapter 38). Diabetes insipidus, especially in infants, can readily lead to fatal volume depletion. Nephrogenic diabetes insipidus from cystic kidney disease also allows excessive fluid loss if not countered by increased intake. Excessive cutaneous water losses can occur in early heat stroke, fever, and overbundling, especially in small infants. Additionally, intentional water deprivation, which may occur as part of the spectrum of child abuse, may lead to hypovolemic shock in unfortunate children.

Patients who suffer burns may rapidly die from hypovolemic shock. Initially, soft tissue damage leads to massive fluid sequestration (third spacing) in the wounded areas, and this is often worse in second-degree burns than in third-degree burns. Tissue robbed of its epidermal covering has massive evaporation losses; in addition, exposure of and damage to blood vessels can lead to significant blood loss both internally and externally. In the 24 hours after burns, major loss becomes exudative, and large amounts of plasma are lost. Thus burn patients suffer volume contraction from water, electrolyte, blood, and plasma loss and sequestration immediately and for several days after a burn. Children with more than 20% full-thickness burns can rapidly become volume depleted. Although thermal injury burns are the most common in children, burns from other sources, such as caustic chemicals and electricity, may lead just as readily to volume depletion and therefore require exacting observation and aggressive fluid management.

The patient with early compensated hypovolemic shock presents with cool extremities, decreased peripheral perfusion, tachycardia, and decreased urine output as described earlier. Hemodynamically, they have normal to reduced filling pressures, increased systemic vascular resistance, and decreased cardiac output but generally normal blood pressure. Flow is diverted away from the skin and splanchnic circulation to preserve CNS, myocardial, adrenal medulla, and central perfusion. Release of antidiuretic hormone (vasopressin) and stimulation of the renin-angiotensin-aldosterone system tend to restore and preserve intravascular volume. In addition, alterations in the forces that control fluid flux across the capillary endothelium (Starling forces) lead to "autotransfusion" in the microcirculation from the uninjured peripheral tissues. However, with ongoing uncorrected volume loss, uncompensated shock leads to tissue damage, inadequate central circulation, unresponsiveness of microcirculation, fatigue of compensatory systems, and the release of products of tissue hypoxia and ischemia that may further aggravate the already-serious situation (vide supra). Hypotension, mental dysfunction, anuria, and respiratory and cardiac failure occur. Eventually, tissue hypoperfusion is so profound and so widespread that permanent myocardial damage and widespread cell death occur and recovery is impossible.

Distributive Shock

Abnormalities in vasomotor tone can cause maldistribution of a normal circulatory volume, which, if severe enough, may lead to shock. Consequent peripheral pooling and vascular shunting lead to a state of "relative hypovolemia." In addition, loss of arterial tone leads to marked hypotension. Although distributive shock may clinically resemble hypovolemic shock, it generally arises from different causes. Distributive shock occurs classically but not exclusively during anaphylaxis, drug toxicity, neurologic injury, or sympathectomy and septic shock **(Table 16.8).**

Shock is one facet of anaphylaxis[206]. The immune response is generated in a previously sensitized host when an antigen reacts with fixed IgE antibody. This triggers a complex series of reactions within circulating mast cells, eosinophils, and perivascular connective tissue mast cells and leads directly to complement activation, causing a massive release of a wide variety of vasoactive mediators. Among these are histamine, leukotrienes C_4 and D_4 (slow-reacting substances of anaphylaxis), eosinophilic chemotactic factor, bradykinin, and various vasoactive prostanoid compounds. Hemodynamically, the initial responses are widespread vasodilatation, intravascular pooling, and decreased venous return, followed by microvascular endothelial injury and intravascular volume depletion via this capillary leak. Cardiac output is diminished as a result of decreased venous return and potentially from the action of myocardial depressant factors. Clearly, profound hypotension can be the most dramatic manifestation of anaphylaxis; however, upper airway obstruction, obstructive bronchoconstrictive airway disease, pulmonary edema, cutaneous manifestations, and gastrointestinal disturbances also occur and can be life-threatening. In patients with anaphylactic shock, volume restitution, and restoration of vasomotor tone are essential in preventing the development of uncompensated shock.

Neurogenic shock is most familiar after high spinal cord transection but may occur in severe brainstem and isolated intracranial injuries. Hypotension accompanying CNS injuries can obviously have grave consequences with regard to the adequacy of CNS perfusion. Spinal shock occurs with cord transections above T1 which cause total loss of sympathetic cardiovascular tone. This leads to profound hypotension with systolic pressures of less than 40 mm Hg and may be accompanied by bradycardia as a result of interrupted conduction of the integrated output of the cardiac accelerator center. Not surprisingly, mentation is affected and urine output is very low. In the setting of trauma, the concurrence of hemorrhagic shock can be disastrous. Hypotension and bradycardia should alert one to the possibility of spinal cord transection in children after trauma. Clinical experience dictates that isolated head injury is rarely the etiology of hypotension in trauma. The rare circumstance of posterior fossa hemorrhage (spontaneous or traumatic) inducing isolated brainstem etiology of hypotension should be considered only after initial attempts at volume resuscitation for potential occult hemorrhage elsewhere.

Table 16.8. Distributive Shock

Anaphylaxis
Antibiotics
Vaccines
Blood
Local anesthetics
Iodine contrast media
Insects
Foods
Latex
Neurologic injury
Head injury (brainstem)
Spinal shock
Septic shock
Early phase
Drugs
Barbiturates
Phenothiazines
Tranquilizers
Antihypertensives

Drug intoxication, which may be accidental in young children and self-inflicted in older children, can lead to profound peripheral vasodilatation and distributive shock. This topic is further discussed in Chapter 39. The major tranquilizers, barbiturates, and antihypertensive drugs (beta-blockers, clonidine and calcium channel blockers) are frequent offenders. In young children who present with shock with no apparent injury or septic focus, drug or toxin ingestion should be considered.

Cardiogenic Shock

Cardiogenic shock does not occur frequently in children, but it does account for a large number of admissions to pediatric ICUs. Cardiogenic shock can result from congenital heart disease, a wide spectrum of infectious and noninfectious acquired cardiomyopathies, trauma, ischemia, or surgical intervention. Hypoplastic left heart syndrome is a major cause of neonatal death and is a common cause of cardiogenic shock in the first few weeks of life[207]. Recent advances in the surgical treatment of this condition make early recognition and effective therapeutic support more important than they were in the past[208]. In the pediatric ICU, the major cause of cardiogenic shock is surgical repair of congenital heart disease. Myocardial impairment after inflammatory processes (myocarditis), ischemic infarction (as can occur in infants with anomalous left coronary artery, isoproterenol-treated asthmatics, or children with Kawasaki disease), primary cardiomyopathy (either obstructive, metabolic, or degenerative), secondary cardiomyopathy (infectious, toxic, and radiation), and high-output cardiac failure (shunt related, catecholamine-induced) also contribute to the number of children seen with cardiogenic shock in the pediatric ICU. Other causes of myocardial impairment in children that may lead to shock include hypoglycemia, metabolic abnormalities, hypothermia, asphyxial episodes, various drug intoxications, and sepsis[209–212]. In addition to direct myocardial impairment, cardiogenic shock may result from cardiac dysrhythmias such as supraventricular tachycardia typically seen in neonates, junctional escape tachycardia (JET) after surgical repair of congenital heart disease, and ventricular arrhythmias. Obstructive cardiac lesions are sometimes classified as causes of cardiogenic shock, however we have chosen to list these separately along with other causes and classified as causes of "obstructive shock".

Septic Shock

Shock that occurs during sepsis may result from deficient intravascular volume, maldistribution of intravascular volume, and impaired myocardial function, and tissue cellular metabolic derangements which make tissues unable to utilize whatever substrates are delivered by the compromised cardiovascular system. All of these abnormalities occur at different times during the course of septic shock. Thus septic shock has distinct similarities to the previously described types of shock at various times during its course.

Table 16.9. Common Pathogens Causing Septic Shock

Neonates
Group B β-hemolytic streptococci
Enterobacteriaceae
Listeria monocytogenes
Staphylococcus aureus
Herpes simplex
Infants
Haemophilus influenzae
Streptococcus pneumoniae
Staphylococcus aureus
Children
Streptococcus pneumoniae
Neisseria meningitidis
Staphylococcus aureus
Enterobacteriaceae
Haemophilus influenzae
Immunocompromised
Enterobacteriaceae
Staphylococcus aureus
Pseudomonadaceae
Candida albicans

In addition, although in other forms of shock circulatory insufficiency precedes derangement of cellular metabolism, septic shock is remarkable for the early occurrence of impaired cellular metabolism. The invasive organism triggers myriad patient response mechanisms that, along with beneficial effects, may ultimately lead to widely impaired endothelial and parenchymal cellular function resulting in metabolic dysfunction and circulatory collapse. The diversity of the pathophysiologic deficits and the marked early metabolic derangement justify a separate classification for septic shock.

The exact incidence of septic shock in children is difficult to document. Estimates of the mortality in the United States (adults and children) from Gram-negative septic shock approach 100,000 deaths annually. In addition, viral, fungal, rickettsial, and Gram-positive septic shock have significant mortalities. Clearly, septic shock is a serious and common disease. Septic shock arises in a variety of clinical settings. Most familiarly, in pediatrics it occurs in immunocompromised children such as neonates and those with leukemia and congenital immunodeficiencies; it also occurs after chemotherapy. Children with congenital urinary tract abnormalities and congenital heart disease are also at increased risk. Children with extensive burns or multiple traumas and critically ill children in ICUs frequently develop septic shock. In addition, reticuloendothelial depression follows hemorrhagic shock and can predispose children to developing septic shock. Translocation of bacteria from the gut can complicate virtually any critical illness and lead to septic shock[27,213]. Septic shock also occurs de novo in otherwise-healthy children and can be rapidly fatal. Meningococcemia, pneumococcemia, and infection with *H. influenzae* are frequently complicated by septic shock, and these organisms have a particular predilection for children.

The pathogens responsible for initiating septic shock in children vary with age **(Table 16.9).** Although septic shock is generally caused by bacterial pathogens, it should be remembered that viral (dengue, herpes, varicella, adenovirus, influenza), rickettsial (Rocky Mountain spotted fever and typhus), chlamydial, protozoal (malaria), and fungal *(Candida)* pathogen infections may be accompanied by septic shock. Although in the past it was believed that the type of pathogen determined the pattern of hemodynamic response, this now seems less likely[214]. A wide variety of pathogens appear to be able to trigger the host mechanisms responsible for the clinical syndrome of septic shock and to initiate common metabolic and hemodynamic sequelae. Although the pattern of response does not rely on the exact pathogen, much previous work has made Gram-negative shock and endotoxin shock synonymous with septic shock. Vast numbers of animal studies with endotoxin have contributed to our understanding of septic shock. Although all of the responses to pathogenic invasion are not the result of the elaboration of endotoxins, these have been best categorized.

Invasion by pathogenic organisms leads to a wide variety of responses. The immunologic system is activated, and this initially limits pathogenic invasion. Ongoing stimulation of the immune system leads to widespread release of many mediators, which in turn may lead to circulatory derangement. Among these are histamine, complement, VIP, interleukins, TNF, activated coagulation cascade factors and fibrinolysins, bradykinin, nitric oxide and eicosanoids. Tissue damage may result as a direct effect of the pathogen, a response to endotoxin, or an evoked response of the immune system, such as the generation of superoxide free radicals (superoxide, nitric oxide and peroxynitrite) or leukoaggregation and leukoembolization leading to microvascular obstruction and ischemia. Pathogenic endotoxins may alter the response to normal homeostatic mechanisms. For example, endotoxin antagonizes the effect of epinephrine and norepinephrine on blood vessel tone[215,216].

Septic shock, regardless of the organisms involved, undergoes distinct physiologic stages. Although the exact nature of the underlying hemodynamic derangements in septic shock has been the topic of much discussion, it is now becoming clear that a characteristic common hemodynamic picture can be delineated. The early compensated stage of septic shock in humans is characterized by decreased vascular resistance (distributive shock), increased cardiac output, tachycardia, warm extremities, and adequate urine output. At this stage, coexisting hypovolemia may lead to a decreased output, but overt myocardial depression is not characteristic of the early, hyperdynamic shock secondary to sepsis. Later, the uncompensated phase occurs, with intravascular volume depletion and myocardial depression becoming more apparent. The child is now cold, listless, anuric, and in respiratory distress and has a high vascular resistance and decreasing cardiac output. This clinical picture progresses with the addition of ischemic injury to that caused by endotoxins, and irreversible shock is reached when multiorgan and myocardial damage is profound. This final pattern is not dissimilar to that seen in other forms of shock. The distinct characteristics of septic shock are the early appearance of metabolic breakdown including impaired oxygen utilization[217], acidosis, and depression of myocardial function that occurs earlier in septic shock than in other forms of shock.

Sepsis Syndrome

The septic process may result from any infectious process, either as a primary cause of septic shock or secondary to other shock processes, most significantly by translocation of gut bacteria and secondary sepsis. Infection and bacteremia can occur with little consequence in a wide variety of clinical settings; however, when these trigger a wide spectrum of host responses, sepsis or the sepsis syndrome occurs. This pattern of response to sepsis has been more generally characterized as a response in many illnesses as a generalized inflammation and has been termed the Systemic Inflammatory Response Syndrome (SIRS). Bone and colleagues[25], have recently defined the sepsis syndrome **(Table 16.10).**

The syndrome definition relies on clinical criteria, with the most significant being the actual presence or a high suspicion of infection. Other accompaniments of the septic syndrome include leukocytosis, proteinuria, eosinopenia, hypoferrinemia, liver function abnormalities, hyperglycemia, further manifestations of CNS injury, coagulation abnormalities with thrombocytopenia, and DIC. Even in the absence of profound DIC, prolongation of prothrombin time (PT) and partial thromboplastin time (PTT) frequently occurs. Clearly, there is a high incidence of cardiovascular collapse, as well as MOSF in patients with septic syndrome, and recognition of this syndrome is common to critical care clinicians. Although cardiovascular instability may not be present at the time of presentation of sepsis syndrome, management and expectant therapy for the development of septic shock is wise. Positive identification and isolation of an organism is not necessary for definition of the septic syndrome. This broadened definition of sepsis is useful for prospectively identifying patients at risk for the development of shock and MOSF. In a large, multicenter study, this definition was used to guide methylprednisolone therapy[218]. In the 382 patients identified with sepsis syndrome, there was nearly 30% mortality. Only 45% of the patients had positive blood cultures, although nearly two-thirds either had shock on entry or developed shock during the study.

Table 16.10. Findings of Sepsis Syndrome

Tachypnea/hyperpnea
Tachycardia
Fever or hypothermia with some clinical evidence of infection
Hyperdynamic circulation followed by hypoperfusion
Altered CNS function
Oliguria
Lactic acidemia
Impaired organ system function
Hypoxemia
Renal failure

Twenty-five percent of this population developed ARDS. Despite the absence of positive blood cultures in half the patients, the significant morbidity and mortality suggests the importance of recognizing this syndrome.

Obstructive Causes of Shock

Pulmonary Embolism

In adults, pulmonary embolism is a frequent cause of death in the United States[219]. Although traditionally pulmonary embolism is said to be extremely uncommon in children, with more invasive, aggressive care it has been increasingly recognized[220,221]. The most commonly fatal pulmonary emboli consist of thrombus, fat, or air. Although venous thromboembolism is the most common, fat and air emboli can occur after trauma and surgery, and air embolism can occur as an iatrogenic complication in the care of critically ill children. The pathophysiologic characteristics of these various types of pulmonary emboli share many common features, and the hemodynamic responses to acute, nonfatal emboli are similar. Acute massive pulmonary thromboembolism can occur in children after the following: surgery, especially pelvic surgery; instrumentation of the heart vessels; cardiac catheterization; hemodialysis; hyperalimentation; ventriculojugular catheterization; pulmonary artery catheterization; trauma, especially to the pelvis; and hypercoagulopathies such as polycythemia, severe thrombocytosis, and, antithrombin III, protein C, or protein S deficiency. It may also occur secondary to other illnesses such as dehydration and heat stroke, and although it is not embolic, sickle cell disease can lead to massive pulmonary artery thrombosis, which has characteristics in common with massive pulmonary embolism.

Acute pulmonary embolism leads to circulatory failure via several mechanisms. First, total blockage of the pulmonary artery prevents venous return to the left heart, mimics acute hypovolemic shock, and is rapidly fatal. Second, acute right ventricular afterloading with right ventricular failure also leads to ventricular septal shift and to decreased left-heart end-diastolic length/volume and performance, preload, and shock. Right ventricular failure is due both to mechanical blockage of the pulmonary arteries and to reflex pulmonary vasoconstriction. Hypoxemia leads to multiple-organ as well as myocardial failure. The massive release of vasoactive mediators from the pulmonary circulation, which in turn can lead to circulatory failure, also occurs *pari passu* with these. This appears to occur particularly with fat and air embolization. In addition, stasis and activation of leukocytes and platelets that may occur with embolism lead to pulmonary capillary endothelial damage that may result in hemorrhagic pulmonary edema and initiate further systemic vascular abnormalities. This is frequently seen in fat embolism and may lead to intravascular volume depletion.

Fat embolism occurs in a wide variety of clinical settings that give rise to bone trauma[222]. Although traumatic fracture is the most common of these, it may also follow orthopedic surgery and even occur in sickle cell disease[223]. Although fat embolism after long bone fracture is said to be rare in children, it still requires consideration. The picture of acute massive fat embolism is that of shock secondary to low output as a result of sudden right ventricular failure. As in pulmonary thromboembolism, fat globules in the pulmonary arteries lead to pulmonary vasoconstriction and pulmonary capillary endothelial damage with resulting shock. Mediators of vascular permeability will again be released and systemic resistance may fall or be maintained only as a result of intense baroreceptor activity, which will eventually fail.

Entry of air into central vessels may be rapidly fatal or may give rise to a shock state. Air emboli can occur when large vessels are lacerated after trauma, during spinal surgery or neurosurgery, and iatrogenically by accidental air entry during intravenous therapy. "Air block" of the right ventricular outflow tract, main pulmonary artery, or distal alveolar arterioles leads to decreased right and left ventricular output and decreased systemic perfusion. There is also reflex pulmonary vasoconstriction that increases right ventricular afterload. In addition, paradoxic systemic emboli may occur, giving rise to CNS signs and myocardial ischemia. Profound hypotension and cyanosis with hyperpnea indicate a grave shock state.

Diagnosis of pulmonary embolization relies on a high index of suspicion and recognition of early clinical signs. All pulmonary emboli are associated with low output states, hypoxia, and hypercarbia. Aspiration of pulmonary arterial blood if a catheter is in situ may reveal air or fat globules. Microscopic urinalysis may reveal fat globules if a fat embolus has occurred, but this is not completely sensitive, and the appearance may be delayed many hours. The final diagnosis of thromboembolism is best performed by a pulmonary ventilation/perfusion scan and less frequently requires pulmonary angiography. Therapy consists of hemodynamic support, oxygen, prevention of further embolization, and removal of emboli. Thromboembolus may be dissolved by the use of heparin or by thrombolytic therapy such as streptokinase, urokinase, or tissue plasminogen activator (tPA)[224]. Air should be aspirated from the pulmonary artery or right ventricular outflow tract when possible. There are no effective methods of removing fat emboli. Although unusual, pulmonary emboli may lead to shock on their own or may complicate the course of children with shock from other causes.

Obstructive Cardiac and Great Vessel Lesions

Just as acute pulmonary thromboembolism may cause shock, many congenital or acquired structural heart and great vessel lesions are responsible for shock. Newborns and young infants may present in shock from poor cardiac output secondary to a valvular stenosis. Critical aortic stenosis, atrioventricular valve stenosis, and pulmonic valve stenosis are tolerated in utero but may present catastrophically in the young infant. The myocardial contractility may be normal, but the stenotic lesions prevent forward ventricular output and inadequate oxygen delivery to the tissues. Critical pulmonic stenosis presents with cyanosis and shock unresponsive to airway intervention and assisted ventilation. Mitral stenosis prevents pulmonary venous return to the left ventricle, and left-sided output is impaired. Elevated pulmonary venous pressures result in pulmonary congestion and edema and increased right ventricle afterload, reducing its performance.

Critical aortic stenosis, subaortic stenosis (as a result of a subaortic membrane or idiopathic hypertrophic subaortic stenosis), impairs left ventricular output, and the tissues suffer from ischemia. This is also seen in an infant with critical coarctation of the aorta or interrupted aortic arch. The use of PGE_1 (alprostadil) has gained widespread acceptance for use in the shocked neonate, since it may save the infant's life by improving pulmonary or systemic circulation by opening the ductus arteriosus when an obstructive lesion impedes forward flow. Trauma to the aorta may also cause a dissection that results in an obstruction to left ventricular output and shock. These lesions along with pulmonary embolism can be collectively considered etiologies of "obstructive" shock.

Miscellaneous Causes of Shock

Heat Stroke

Cardiovascular collapse secondary to excessive body temperature can result from increased heat production or decreased heat dissipation. Both of these types of heat stroke occur in children. The former usually occurs in older children after a pyrexial illness or exercise, and the latter occurs in younger infants and neonates who may be kept excessively warmed and covered. Cardiovascular failure as a result of excessive body heat may accompany a febrile illness in children and should be considered in hot, shocked children. Elevated body temperature may aggravate shock from other causes. Fever increases oxygen consumption, carbon dioxide formation, and the demand for augmented cardiopulmonary performance that the child may not be capable of generating. Fever may be an appropriate host response to infection, however it is undesirable physiologically in the presentation of heat stroke and should be aggressively managed.

Heat is lost from the body by convection, radiation, conduction, and evaporation. Clearly, all of these depend on a body-to-environment temperature gradient. Evaporation is unique to biologic systems. Clothing and blankets generally decrease conduction and convection, leaving radiation and evaporation as the major sources of heat dissipation. As ambient temperature approaches body temperature, heat loss becomes limited to evaporative losses only. Increased humidity impairs heat dissipation even further. As body temperature increases, evaporative loss increases (up to 20 to 40 ml/kg/hr), and peripheral vasodilatation increases radiation losses. The removal of clothing and contact with surfaces below body temperature increase convective and conductive losses. Thus with increased body temperature, there is increased water and salt loss, decreased peripheral vascular resistance, and increased cardiac output. In excess, these can lead to a hypovolemic and distributive type of shock picture in the extreme.

As core temperature rises (above 42°C), direct tissue damage occurs, oxygen consumption is vastly increased, leukoactivation occurs, and several vasoactive mediators and heat shock proteins are released, all of which may lead to further cardiovascular impairment. Tissue damage arises from protein and enzyme denaturation, protease release, phospholipid structural alterations with cellular and intracellular membrane breakdown, uncoupling of oxidative phosphorylation, and mitochondrial death. Anaerobic metabolism, systemic acidosis, and vascular endothelial breakdown occur and lead to intravascular volume loss and edema. Anhidrosis is a symptom of cellular sweat gland damage resulting from hyperthermia and cardiovascular collapse rather than a cause of heat stroke. The stages of heat stroke shock are similar to those of the other forms, with decreased intravascular volume, loss of vascular tone, cardiac impairment, and irreparable organ failure.

Children who develop high fevers, are overbundled, or who may have a congenital failure of the heat-dissipating mechanism (Riley-Day syndrome among others) are clearly at risk. In addition, heat stroke is obviously more common in hot weather. Limitation of liberal water intake, as may occur in infants, or intentional deprivation is also an aggravating feature. In children who present with acidosis, hemodynamic dysfunction, and fever of higher than 42°C, heat stroke is a major, life-threatening consideration.

A clinical syndrome of hemorrhagic shock, hyperpyrexia, and encephalopathy has been described in infants and children[(225–227)]. Levin et al.[(225)] described "hemorrhagic shock and encephalopathy syndrome" as a clinical presentation in infants and young children with a mild prodromal illness progressing to encephalopathy, shock, DIC, and negative bacterial cultures. These children had fevers ranging from 38°C to 41.5°C. Later reports by other authors described children with similar clinical courses where hyperpyrexia was more severe (higher than 41.5°C)[(226,227)]. Postmortem examination and microbiologic analysis could not demonstrate either viral or bacterial pathogens. The etiology of the syndrome is unclear, but moderate or severe hyperthermia appears to be a consistent finding. Whether resulting from dysfunction of endogenous thermoregulatory mechanisms or accelerated heat production initiated by unknown mechanisms, hyperpyrexia appears to contribute to the endotheliopathy seen and the catastrophic presentation of shock and rapidly fatal MOSF.

Acute Pancreatitis

Acute pancreatitis represents another cause of shock that has been increasingly recognized in children. Acute hemorrhagic pancreatitis can readily give rise to hypotension, hemoconcentration, anuria, hypocalcemia, fever, and acidosis, which may require therapy aimed at correcting the shock state. Although cholelithiasis and alcoholism are the leading causes of this condition in adults, in children it is most commonly associated with drug therapy (thiazides, prednisone, azathioprine), congenital biliary disease, mumps or occurs idiopathically[(228)]. Pancreatitis is classically divided into interstitial and hemorrhagic forms. Shock is most common in the hemorrhagic form and occurs in 16% of children with pancreatitis[(228)].

In pancreatic shock, severe pancreatic damage occurs with widespread liquefaction, thrombosis, and massive peripancreatic edema and is occasionally complicated by massive gastrointestinal bleeding. Metabolic disturbances include hyperglycemia and hypocalcemia. Volume loss and the release of vasoactive substances including bradykinin, histamine, platelets, myocardial depressant factor and TNF, and leukocyte thrombi lead to circulatory dysfunction and systemic shock. ARDS is an invariable accompaniment of profound pancreatic shock, probably as a result of C5a activation. Septic shock may either precipitate or complicate acute pancreatitis. The diagnosis relies on recognizing the clinical constellation and measuring serum amylase and lipase and amylase clearance[(229)]. Therapy is directed at reversing shock, correcting metabolic abnormalities, and providing respiratory support. Surgery carries an immense risk and should be avoided if at all possible.

Drug Overdose and Poisonings

A shock-like picture is frequently seen after inadvertent and intentional drug overdoses. The characteristics of this shock-like state may be those of both distributive and hypovolemic shock, and, indeed, there are several drugs that have myocardial depressant characteristics. Thus shock states after drug overdoses may have complex underlying pathophysiology and require an understanding of the physiologic abnormalities in these types of shock. Several groups of drugs produce a shock-like picture, including the narcotics, barbiturates, tricyclic antidepressants, and β-blockers (see Chapter 39).

Barbiturate intoxication provides an example of shock seen after drug overdose. Patients in this state initially demonstrate decreased intravascular volume with low central filling pressures and significantly decreased cardiac outputs. Frequently, peripheral vascular resistance is elevated. However, in much more massive overdoses, peripheral vascular resistance may be low. Respiratory compromise subsequent to barbiturate intoxication leads to diffuse, hypoxic insult that aggravates the situation. Intravascular fluid depletion is a result of third-space losses from a capillary endothelial defect. In addition, barbiturates are well recognized as direct myocardial depressants, and this certainly plays a role in shock states seen after overdoses. Shock also occurs after morphine and heroin abuse, and this, again, is multifactorial in origin. Histamine release may lead to hypotension, and respiratory depression may cause diffuse hypoxic insult. In addition, pulmonary edema is frequently associated with narcotic abuse, and this may be severe enough to lead to marked intravascular volume depletion and the signs of hypovolemic shock. Antidepressants cause severe cardiac dysrhythmias which may induce shock (ventricular tachycardia and fibrillation).

The management of patients who are suspected of having shock secondary to drug intoxication involves the removal and detoxification of the suspected offending agent. This may include such maneuvers as gastric lavage, charcoal administration, or induction of emesis, hemodialysis, peritoneal dialysis, and therapy with specific antidotes (see Chapter 39). In addition, respiratory support is indicated, especially in those patients who manifest hemodynamic instability. The general therapy of shock states as outlined later is, of course, also concurrently undertaken to ensure adequate vital organ perfusion while the patient is being detoxified. Discussion of other specific overdoses and poisonings including cyanide toxicity is located in Chapter 41.

Adrenal Shock

Although infrequent in childhood, adrenal shock should be considered when the etiology of shock is not obvious. Appreciation of adrenal function in shock has recently been addressed, and a multifactorial cause for failure is suspected[(230,231)]. A more thorough discussion of hypocortisolism and adrenal shock is found in Chapter 38. Any newborn less than 30 days of age should be considered at risk for adrenal insufficiency or congenital heart disease as occult etiologies of shock and empiric stress glucocorticoid and PGE_1 should be administered until definitive diagnosis is achieved. In older infants and children, adrenal insufficiency is also an infrequent cause of shock, which must be considered and treated until the diagnosis is confirmed or excluded.

Summary

These are only a few examples of the miscellaneous causes of shock that demonstrate characteristics of several different classifications of shock. Under all circumstances, when faced with a shock situation, it is important to remember that the cardiovascular picture may have characteristics that resemble hypovolemic, distributive, and cardiogenic shock and that none of these forms are mutually exclusive. In addition, the hemodynamic picture characteristic of these types of shock may vary over time.

DIAGNOSIS OF SHOCK

Shock is a clinical diagnosis. The recognition of a child who is lethargic, ashen gray, tachypneic, cold, with diminished peripheral pulses and a blood pressure of 60/30 mm Hg as being in shock presents no difficulties. Unfortunately, by this stage the likelihood of successful intervention is limited. To apply aggressive, lifesaving therapeutic interventions, early recognition of shock or impending shock is crucial. Previously well children with intact homeostatic mechanisms can compensate extremely well during hypoperfusion states. For this reason, the early stages of all types of shock are difficult to differentiate from the patient's normal status. Of course, the child who has lost 70% of her blood volume after a traffic accident and is cold and acidotic presents no early phase, and therapy is clearly and immediately indicated. On the other hand, the burned child compensates for volume contraction well and ideally will never develop tissue hypoperfusion. However, he or she still needs to be managed as if in shock since it will ensue if adequate anticipation of fluid needs is not addressed. Consistent vigilance is required to identify the early stage of shock and facilitate therapy. Because of the rapidity of change and the possibility of catastrophic deterioration, early transfer to a pediatric ICU when there is even the suspicion of shock is warranted to allow compulsive monitoring while diagnostic evaluation is continuing.

The early diagnosis of shock requires a high index of suspicion and a knowledge of which conditions predispose children to shock. Clearly, the age of the child will provide some diagnostic clues, and previous medical conditions such as congenital heart disease, immunodeficiencies, suspected ingestions, and a history of trauma will raise the suspicion that the child may be suffering from a shock state. In children, shock can also occur after surgery, especially cardiac surgery. Clearly, children who are febrile, have an identifiable source of an infection, or are hypovolemic from any cause are at great risk of developing shock. It may be very difficult to determine that children have crossed from being dehydrated and febrile to developing shock. The diagnostic problem hinges on the dilemma concerning the diagnosis of shock. For example, when does the child with pyelonephritis, tachycardia, fever, and tachypnea cross from sepsis to septic shock? Clearly, identifying patients who are susceptible to shock states before they are hypotensive, comatose, acidotic, and anuric is preferable. Therefore, the recognition of states in which shock is likely to develop is more important than the recognition and definition of shock states. Expectant treatment to prevent circulatory collapse is preferable. Therapeutic interventions, as if one were treating shock, are indicated in these patients before they actually develop shock. Although the diagnostic definition of shock may be vague, the recognition of tissue hypoperfusion demands management as if shock were present.

What differentiates the child with fever and urinary tract infection from the child with fever, urinary tract infection, and septic shock? When does the transition from dehydration caused by diarrhea to hypovolemic shock occur? The answer to these questions is when tissue hypoperfusion or exposure to endotoxin leads to breakdown of cellular function and tissue damage. This may be identified by the recognition of lactic acidosis and is often accompanied by alterations in platelets, coagulation factors, complement, altered mental status, and stress response with the hypercatecholaminergic state. The historical and physical findings that accompany these occurrences can clearly be identified and form the basis for the diagnosis of hypoperfusion and shock states.

The early diagnosis of shock requires knowledge of which children are predisposed to shock. Interrogation of the child's parents or the physicians, nurses, and emergency transfer personnel caring for the child may provide valuable clues. The child's age may suggest possible etiologies for the shock state. In the case of neonates, a clear maternal history with respect to peripartum fevers, premature rupture of membranes, intrapartum blood loss, fetal distress, lethargy or irritability, and possibly even bacterial cultures is necessary. In the case of trauma, witnesses, emergency personnel, and parents may provide an indication of severity, amount of blood loss, and status before arrival, and all of this information should be sought. A history of underlying immunodeficiency state such as exists in children who have received chemotherapy may arouse suspicion of sepsis. Assessment of activity with regard to the development of lethargy, decreased oral intake, apathy, and general responsiveness may be valuable in indicating the severity and duration of the abnormality. Clearly, information concerning the amount of excessive fluid loss from diarrhea or vomiting is necessary in dehydration, and a history of decreased urine output is an essential guide to assessing the adequacy of intravascular volume and its replacement. Details of environmental exposure, potential drug ingestion, previous medical problems, and allergies are also worthwhile not only to aid in diagnosis but also to guide therapeutic endeavors. In the case of children with previous medical problems, the examination of past records for details of chemotherapy, surveillance cultures, cardiac diagnosis, and other potential problems is, of course, necessary. Frequently, the essential details of the patient's history can be obtained in a matter of minutes and contribute to the patient's entire management.

With regard to the physical examination, it is possible to identify signs reflecting the underlying physiologic process[232]. Decreased tissue perfusion can be identified by changes in body surface temperature, capillary refill, and impaired function of several organ systems. Body surface temperature is a time-honored, simple, and effective method of assessing adequate tissue perfusion. Cold extremities or increased peripheral-core temperature gradients (greater than 2°C) indicate intact homeostatic mechanisms that have decreased nonessential cutaneous perfusion in the face of contracted intravascular volume[233]. This system is very efficient and therefore serves as an early indicator of decreased intravascular volume. Decreased capillary refill is also a sensitive indicator of tissue perfusion. The exact technique for determining capillary refill must be determined by each physician, because there are no universally recognized standards. The rate of refill after firm compression of soft tissues and nail beds for 5 seconds is related to the site of determination, because of the intricacy of the capillary bed, the temperature, and the amount of circulation through the microvasculature. In general, refill over the face is faster than that over the chest, which is faster than that over the hands and feet. Normally, a blanched area disappears extremely rapidly, in less than 3 seconds[234]. Capillary refill that takes longer than 5 seconds is clearly abnormal. Although this is a very nonspecific indicator of tissue hypoperfusion, it is also a very sensitive one. In addition, stasis as a result of peripheral vasoconstriction may lead to peripheral cyanosis. Although peripheral hypoperfusion is the physiologic response to intravascular volume contraction, it does not in itself indicate shock; however, it clearly heralds it. In addition, the physical findings of dehydration may also be present and can indicate the severity of hypovolemia **(Table 16.11).** Vital organ hypoperfusion can be assumed to occur if oliguria from renal hypoperfusion exists or if altered mentation occurs, indicating CNS hypoperfusion.

The physical findings of acidosis are primarily respiratory. Decreased CNS pH is a potent stimulus to the chemoreceptors located in the area postrema of the medulla. Chemoreceptor stimulation causes increased minute ventilation by increasing both tidal volume and respiratory rate. Therefore, tachypnea, hyperpnea, and hyperventilation are frequently seen as early findings in shock states. Respiratory alkalosis is frequently an early accompaniment of all stages of all types of shock.

By far, the most significant physical findings in shock result from autonomic responses to stress. Clearly, peripheral vasoconstriction is an early phase of this response. In children, tachycardia also occurs early. The younger the child, the more dependent the cardiac output is on heart rate in comparison with increases in stroke volume. Extremely rapid heart rates occur before notable alterations in mean arterial pressure in infants and small children, however close attention to pulse pressure and pulse intensity by clinical exam reveals early alterations. As heart rate varies considerably with age, reference to age-related standards is necessary (see Chapter 12).

Alteration in mean arterial pressure is a late manifestation of hypovolemia in children. Blood pressure is well defended, and only when hemodynamic compromise is severe does mean arterial pressure begin to fall. Initially, pulse pressure is decreased, often because of a minor decrease in systolic pressure and an increase in diastolic pressure. As stroke volume deteriorates because of decreases in venous return, systolic pressure slowly falls, but the increased tone of the arterial circulation maintains diastolic and mean arterial pressures. Eventually, systolic and diastolic pressures fall. This stage indicates major hemodynamic compromise. Apart from blood pressure, pulse characteristics should also be noted. Clearly, absent pulses are more significant than weak pulses. Unequal pulses may indicate underlying cardiac disease such as coarctation or interrupted aortic arch. Bounding full pulses occur in sepsis, and in the neonate they may indicate a patent ductus arteriosus. Pulsus paradoxus occurs with decreased lung compliance but may also indicate decreased myocardial contractility or myocardial tamponade. Examination of the pulses and the electrocardiogram (ECG) for abnormalities in rhythm, axis, and voltage is equally important in patients with all types of hemodynamic compromise.

The physical findings vary according to the type of shock and, perhaps more importantly, to the stage. Perhaps early septic shock is most anomalous. Physical examination during the early stage usually reveals increased peripheral pulses, warm, overperfused extremities, widened pulse pressure, and a hyperdynamic precordium. Although the patient is hyperdynamic, the presence of acidosis supports the diagnosis of early shock. Clearly, this is a very different clinical picture from that seen in the child with the early stages of hypovolemic shock. With time, as myocardial contractility fails, intravascular volume becomes depleted, and multiple organ systems begin to fail, the patient with septic shock becomes cold, with decreased pulses, low blood pressure, and all the findings of late shock common to other types of shock. Hemorrhagic shock can be divided into four classes according to the amount of blood loss and the severity of symptoms. **Table 16–12** shows these classes as defined by the Advanced Trauma Life Support Standards of the American College of Surgeons. This classification can be used to guide therapy, assess severity, and standardize various shock states as well as to provide a useful basis for information transfer between caretakers of children in shock.

Further assessment of the severity and cause of shock states is greatly assisted by several laboratory investigations. Routine laboratory tests such as serum electrolytes, blood cell counts, platelet counts, and hematocrits (for the reasons discussed earlier) are obviously necessary to delineate the extent of metabolic disturbance. Serum calcium

Table 16.11. Clinical Signs of Dehydration in Children

Clinical signs[a]	*Mild*	*Moderate*	*Severe*
Activity	Normal	Lethargic	Lethargic to coma
Color	Pale	Gray	Mottled
Urine output	Decreased (<2–3 ml/kg/hr)	Oliguric (<1 ml/kg/hr)	Anuria
Fontanel	Flat	Depressed	Sunken (retreated)
Mucous membranes	Dry	Very dry	Cracked
Skin turgor	Slight decrease	Marked decrease	Tenting
Pulse	Normal to increased	Increased	Grossly tachycardic
Blood pressure	Normal	Normal	Decreased
Weight loss	5%	10%	15%

[a] Hypernatremic dehydration may occur with only moderate changes in clinical signs.

Table 16.12. Advanced Trauma Life Support Classification of Shock

Class I
15% or less acute blood volume loss
Blood pressure normal
Pulse increased 10–20%
No change in capillary refill
Class II
20–25% loss of blood volume
Tachycardia >150 beats/min
Tachypnea 35–40 breaths/min
Capillary refill prolonged
Systolic blood pressure decreased
Pulse pressure decreased
Orthostatic hypotension >10–15 torr
Urine output >1 ml/kg/hr
Class III
30–35% blood volume loss
All of the above signs
Urine output <1 ml/kg/hr
Lethargic, clammy, and vomiting
Class IV
40–50% blood volume loss
Nonpalpable pulses
Obtunded

should be determined in all shock states because hypocalcemia occurs frequently and can further compromise respiratory muscle, myocardial, and metabolic function. Although ionized hypocalcemia may be a homeostatic protective mechanism of unclear significance, replacement is indicated if cardiovascular performance is unacceptable. Measurements of serum protein, albumin, and colloid oncotic pressure serve as guides to volume replacement and the severity of the capillary endothelial defect.

Probably the most frequently performed and most valuable laboratory investigation is the arterial blood gas analysis. Clearly, arterial oxygen content and carbon dioxide tension aid in the evaluation of the adequacy of ventilatory function that is frequently impaired in shock. In addition, pH and base deficit determination serves as one of the most readily available methods of quantifying tissue hypoperfusion. The degree of metabolic acidosis correlates with the severity of tissue hypoperfusion and readily guides the adequacy of therapy. Persistent acidosis indicates inadequate or ineffective therapy and the need for further intervention and investigation. Restoration of normal pulse and blood pressure but with persistence of acidosis mandates further action, cautious monitoring, and therapeutic support. In addition to arterial blood gas analysis, the assessment of mixed venous oxygen tension, saturation and content can add further information about the adequacy of tissue perfusion, cardiovascular compensation and performance, and guide optimization of oxygen consumption and delivery. Since a major therapeutic intervention in shock is respiratory support, the arterial blood gas and venous blood gas may be very discordant indicating adequate respiratory support but severe cellular injury, poor cardiac performance, and persistent venous acidosis[235].

MONITORING OF SHOCK

The purpose of monitoring children who are potentially shocked is for rapid detection of alterations in physiologic status and for assessment of the outcomes of therapeutic interventions[232]. The exact type and extent of monitoring of these children will depend on the severity and complexity of the child's underlying illness and shock state. There are certain essential minimum requirements for baseline monitoring that should be applied to all children who are at risk for shock. All monitoring for children with shock is best facilitated by admission to a pediatric ICU.

It cannot be emphasized too strongly that the most effective and sensitive physiologic monitoring available is the repeated and careful examination of the child's physical status by a competent and experienced clinician. Observations for alteration in peripheral perfusion, color, presence of cyanosis, characteristics of the pulse, blood pressure, respiratory pattern, and level of consciousness are absolutely essential in the continuous, ongoing monitoring of children with shock. Careful nursing observation of vital signs and activity of the child and clear, concise display of these data form the central core of information from which the child's therapy is determined. In addition, the minimum monitoring of a child with shock or at risk for shock includes continuous ECG monitoring, pulse oximetry, and temperature and blood pressure measurements. In younger infants, blood glucose should frequently be determined (Dextrostix). In all but the most mild cases, blood pressure determination will probably necessitate invasive intra-arterial cannulation. In addition, these indwelling arterial cannulae can be used for continuous monitoring of blood gases that, as mentioned earlier, provide the key laboratory measurements in monitoring patients with shock. Relying on sphygmomanometry in children with shock has many pitfalls and is remarkably unreliable. The unstable and potentially catastrophic compromise in circulation requires beat-to-beat continuous blood pressure measurement and display. In addition to ECG and blood pressure monitoring, close attention to intake and output and urine production is essential. Urine output in children is normally 2 to 3 ml/kg/hr, and urine outputs of less than 1 ml/kg/hr are indicative of renal hypoperfusion and activation of homeostatic water and sodium conservation mechanisms in shock states. It is usual for oliguria to occur early in shock states and injury before the alterations in mean arterial pressure or the development of the significant tachycardia. Alterations in urine-specific gravity should be noted. (Naturally, intake should be carefully recorded, and the patient's weight should also be monitored.)

In patients with severe shock and certainly in children with myocardial compromise, consideration must be given to invasive venous and pulmonary arterial pressure monitoring. In the past decade, there has been increasing use of this form of monitoring in critically ill children[232]. It now has an historically established role to play in providing quick, accurate assessment of not only cardiac performance as determined by cardiac output but also both right and left ventricular filling pressures and alterations in pulmonary vascular resistance. Frequently, the determination of central filling pressures is considered to reflect intravascular volume accurately. This concept can be dangerously misleading. Although total circulating blood volume is one contributing factor to both right and left atrial filling pressures, it is not the most important. This can readily be appreciated by considering the child after pure hemorrhagic shock. Central venous filling pressure in this state is low (0 to 1 mm Hg) and may remain so despite adequate intravascular filling. The normal central venous pressure, although usually described as less than 10 mm Hg, is in actuality only 1 to 3 mm Hg, and intravascular volume expansion by as much as 30% does not alter right atrial pressure significantly. The major determinants of cardiac filling pressure are, in fact, ventricular function and compliance[(236,237)]. With a constant intravascular volume, changes in right ventricular contractility, afterload (pulmonary vascular resistance), and compliance will significantly affect central venous pressure. A similar argument pertains to left atrial and pulmonary artery occlusion pressures (pulmonary capillary wedge pressures). This concept must be borne soundly in mind when monitoring includes measurements of central venous filling pressures. In pure hypovolemic shock without myocardial compromise, it is unlikely that central venous pressure measurement adds anything to careful, repeated determinations of peripheral perfusion and observation of blood pressure, respiratory pattern, acid-base balance, and, of course, urine output. Indeed, attempts to elevate filling pressures (5 to 10 cm H_2O) are unnecessary and almost certainly deleterious, as they will lead to volume overload and increased tissue edema. On the other hand, when myocardial function is compromised or renal impairment has occurred and urine output cannot be followed, central venous pressure monitoring may be necessary to avoid excessive fluid administration.

The use of a balloon-tipped, flow-directed multilumen pulmonary artery catheter (Swan-Ganz catheter)[(238,239)] has increased our understanding of shock states. Measurement and monitoring of changes in pulmonary artery occlusion pressure in addition to central venous pressure with these catheters adds an extra dimension of information about left ventricular function. In addition, combining pressure measurements with the determination of cardiac output, either by the dye dilution technique or by the addition of a thermistor as in the thermodilution technique, has allowed us to accurately quantitate cardiac performance. In children with a complex disease such as septic shock who have myocardial impairment in the face of hypotension or hypoperfusion, this monitoring can be very helpful to tailor therapy accurately. The relationship of filling pressures in cardiac output allows theoretic construction of cardiac function curves relating changes in filling pressure to changes in cardiac index. For example, when monitoring reveals a fall in cardiac index of an elevated filling pressure, it is clear that myocardial contractility has been impaired.

The placement of a pulmonary artery catheter allows measurement of mixed venous oxygen tension and hemoglobin saturation. Calculation of oxygen delivery, extraction, and utilization are then possible, and newer evidence demonstrates the potential importance of this information[(240,241)]. Resuscitation of the shocked child does not end at obtaining a normal blood pressure, and this newer evidence suggests that obtaining "physiologic" cardiac output and cardiopulmonary indices may not be sufficient. There may be some value in attaining supraphysiologic values for many parameters. If this work receives further confirmation and acceptance, then invasive monitoring may have more widespread use.

Measurements of continuous mixed venous oxygen saturation allows minute-to-minute assessment of interventions in cardiorespiratory support[(242)] and resuscitation[(235)]. An oximetric catheter assists in titration of positive end-expiratory pressure (PEEP), in minimizing barotrauma, and in assessing changes in mode of ventilatory support. Minute-to-minute changes in cardiac output are indirectly assessed as vasoactive agents are varied. Further advances in technology offer promise for monitoring the shocked child. With continuously improving microminiaturization, intravascular continuous blood gas analysis will soon be available. Currently used in critically ill adults and patients on cardiopulmonary bypass, continuous intravascular blood gas monitoring minimizes blood sampling and allows extremely rapid titration in support of the patient.

TREATMENT OF SHOCK

The treatment of shock states in children is aimed at optimizing perfusion of critical vascular beds, i.e., coronary, cerebral, and renal vascular beds, and preventing or correcting metabolic abnormalities arising from cellular hypoperfusion. The ultimate goals are to prevent or reverse the defects in cellular substrate delivery and metabolism as well as to support the entire patient until homeostasis is restored and adequate nutritional support can be instituted to allow healing to commence. Attaining normal hemodynamic values, adequate urine output, and normal blood gases, although a good start, may not be sufficient. Hemodynamic and oxygen transport profiles of patients with shock who ultimately survive are generally "supranormal"[(243,244)]. Although little information exists on children concerning optimal hemodynamic values, obtaining "normal" values is merely a start in overall patient management.

General Principles

For all forms of shock, treating the underlying cause is mandatory. Hemorrhage, either external or internal, should be stopped and replaced, and surgery may be required. If sepsis is the underlying cause, identification and eradication of the offending organism are essential. Administration of broad-spectrum antibiotics aimed at the most likely organisms in neonates and children and the location and draining of sites of infection, where possible, are crucial. Although infection may be eradicated, toxic products may remain, and therapy directed at the metabolic consequences of these products is offering new excitement among shock researchers. In the case of volume loss as a result of diarrhea, treatment of the specific cause, i.e., *Salmonella* or *Shigella,* is required to remove gastrointestinal irritants and to prevent the increased gut osmotic load. In neurogenic shock, neuroresuscitative measurements must be undertaken concurrently with other therapy to substitute for the compromised autonomic nervous system components including assisted ventilation, cardiac and vascular contractile support (see Chapter 20).

In attempting to restore homeostasis, metabolic abnormalities require correction. Always start with the ABCs of basic life support. Hypoxemia is the essential abnormality to correct and to avoid. Increasing arterial oxygen content by ensuring 95 to 100% saturation and adequate hemoglobin content for oxygen delivery is the goal. The first pharmacologic therapy in shock is oxygen. All children with compromised circulation should receive supplemental oxygen because the risks are minimal. In preterm neonates, the risk of retrolental fibroplasia requires caution and close monitoring, but if a neonate is critically ill, hypoxia should not be tolerated.

The correction of acid-base disturbances allows better cellular function and myocardial performance, allows decreased systemic and pulmonary vascular resistance, and decreases the need for the respiratory compensation of metabolic acidosis. Base deficits greater than 10 mEq/liter in septic or cardiogenic shock are generally associated with a poor outcome; profound metabolic acidosis as a result of hypovolemia and renal bicarbonate loss, however, is generally better tolerated. A base deficit greater than 6 mEq/liter in acute shock states should probably be corrected. Renal compensation and correction may be of help in correcting the acidosis over time, but acidosis in an acute life-threatening situation requires bicarbonate and volume supplementation. Hepatic metabolic conversion of lactate or acetate to correct acidosis in most shock states is impaired and will be inadequate.

Bicarbonate supplementation can be given by repeated slow boluses of sodium bicarbonate of 1 to 2 mEq/kg; in neonates, a solution of 0.5 mEq/ml is used to avoid acute change in osmolarity, which may lead to intraventricular hemorrhage[245]. Frequently, 10 to 20 mEq/kg may be required to correct profound acidosis. The formula required to half-correct acidosis [0.3 (body weight in kg) $\times$ (base deficit) = mEq $NaHCO_3$] may serve as a rough guide. If bolus therapy is not effective or the metabolic acidosis persists or grows more severe, a continuous intravenous sodium bicarbonate infusion may be required. The major limitation in bicarbonate replacement therapy is sodium overload and hyperosmolarity. Close monitoring of serum sodium is required if massive bicarbonate replacement (more than 10 mEq/kg) is undertaken. If serum sodium increases over 150 mEq/liter, another method of correcting acidosis may be required. Tromethamine (or THAM) has been recommended; however, serious problems are associated with its use, and in general it is best to avoid this unfamiliar agent. Carbicarb has also been recommended but has not yet received widespread acceptance.

If sodium bicarbonate supplementation is ineffective, peritoneal dialysis may be necessary to remove excess acid, lactate, phosphate, and hydrogen ion, as well as to correct hypernatremia and to allow further bicarbonate administration. In severe metabolic acidosis with hemodynamic collapse, which may occur in aspirin overdose and with inborn errors of metabolism or sepsis, peritoneal dialysis may be lifesaving not only by removing excess acid but also by alleviating the underlying cause of shock. Adequate peritoneal perfusion is necessary for effective peritoneal dialysis, so initial blood pressure and intravascular volume resuscitation is mandatory.

It is important to remember that when correcting acidosis with bicarbonate replacement, other electrolyte abnormalities may be expected. A fall in serum ionized calcium occurs as the pH returns toward normal, and this, in addition to possible renal calcium loss or parathyroid ischemia, may result in profound hypocalcemia. Decreased serum ionized calcium can lead to alterations in level of consciousness, tremors, seizures, tetany, hypotension, tachycardia, myocardial depression, and acidosis[246]. As serum ionized calcium bears little relationship to total serum calcium, ionized calcium must be measured (see Chapter 38). Levels of ionized calcium below 0.90 mm should probably be treated. Either calcium gluconate (100 mg/kg i.v. slow bolus) or calcium chloride (20 mg/kg) will rapidly restore serum ionized calcium. As pH returns toward normal, serum potassium levels fall as potassium reenters the cells, and hypokalemia may occur. Again, serial serum potassium measurements and urine output monitoring with slow continuous correction and/or replacement are essential. However, the danger of rapid potassium therapy can not be overemphasized. Potassium therapy should be given prudent consideration and slow administration (0.1 to 0.3 mEq/kg/hour).

Hyperglycemia frequently accompanies severe stress and shock states in children. It may provide an excessive osmotic load and act as an osmotic diuretic. Generally, correction of the underlying stress leads to homeostatic control of glucose levels before insulin supplementation is required. Hypoglycemia may occur in infants in shock as glycogen reserves are exhausted and homeostatic mechanisms in support of blood sugar fatigue (cortisol, growth hormone, catecholamines, glucagon, and somatostatin). Frequent monitoring is important.

Cardiovascular Support

Rate and Rhythm

Assuring adequate cardiac rate and rhythm is basic to life support. Heart rates are acceptable within a wide range of normal for age, and monitoring the heart rate is essential in guiding therapy. Treatment of arrhythmias includes correction of hypoxia, acidosis, hypocalcemia, hypomagnesemia, and hypokalemia or hyperkalemia and the use of cardioactive drugs such as atropine, isoproterenol, or epinephrine for bradydysrhythmias; adenosine, β-blockers, digoxin or potentially verapamil for supraventricular tachydysrhythmias, and lidocaine for ventricular ectopy. Temporary pacing and cardioversion may be needed in certain situations and are discussed in Chapter 15.

Stroke Volume

Preload Augmentation

Rapid intravascular volume expansion guided by the clinical examination and urine output is frequently adequate to restore blood pressure and peripheral perfusion in children with shock. In the case of otherwise-normal cardiorespiratory function, volume overload resulting in pulmonary edema is rare. Volume replacement of 10 to 20 ml/kg over 10 minutes can generally be safely given and repeated if necessary. Replacement of losses as a result of excess urine output, stool output, or hemorrhage can be guided by body weight changes, careful monitoring of intake and output, and repeated physical examinations. When volume resuscitation greater than 50 to 100 ml/kg in the first 1 to 2 hr is required, more invasive monitoring and diagnostic investigations should be considered. Severe third-space losses because of capillary leak can occur, but occult hemorrhage must not go undiagnosed.

Another method of increasing venous return and augmenting preload is by application of military antishock trousers, which are manufactured in pediatric sizes. Application of these in the field or hospital for children suffering from severe hypotension may prove lifesaving and provide a means of maintaining blood pressure until more definitive therapy is provided. Unfortunately, despite widespread use, only recently have data become available to assess the efficacy of pneumatic antishock garments (PASG). In the field, no difference was found in survival or morbidity for patients treated with PASG compared with those not treated with PASG[(247)]. Further confirmation or follow-up of these results may change the priority of recommendation to use the antishock garment.

The use of colloid versus crystalloid replacement for shock is an ongoing debate in pediatrics[(248–250)]. For simple dehydration, the estimated fluid and electrolyte deficits should be replaced[(251)]. For sepsis and trauma, the underlying arguments of vascular leak, intravascular oncotic pressure maintenance, pulmonary edema (ARDS), and cost versus risks are ongoing. At present, a judicious mixture of crystalloid, blood products to maintain hemoglobin and clotting factors, and colloid (albumin and hetastarch) to maintain colloid oncotic pressure seems appropriate and most reasonable. Recent evidence suggests that hypertonic fluid replacement may have a role to play[(239,252–254)], but caution is advised, since detrimental results have also been noted in the laboratory[(255)]. **Table 16.13** provides guidelines for fluid therapy in dehydration.

Preload augmentation in patients with septic shock, myocardial impairment, or pulmonary disease may require central pressure monitoring. A central venous pressure line may be useful to protect against volume overload. If the central venous pressure remains low, volume overload is unlikely. However, a central venous pressure that is rising or greater than 7 to 10 mm Hg indicates either myocardial dysfunction, increased right ventricular afterload, or volume overload. In these cases, further fluid management may require more invasive hemodynamic monitoring[(256,257)].

The absolute limitation of preload augmentation in children is a persistent elevation in ventricular filling pressures without an increase in cardiac output. Further preload augmentation does not improve peripheral perfusion and may, by increasing venous pressure, decrease perfusion pressure in several critical vascular beds. Increased venous pressures may increase vascular leak, leading to increased tissue edema, most notably pulmonary edema. In patients with ARDS, central filling pressure should be maintained on the low side (less than 10 mm Hg) if possible to optimize hy-

Table 16.13. Fluid Therapy Guidelines

	H_2O (ml/kg)	*Na*	*K (mEq/kg)*	*Cl*	*HCO_3*
To Correct 10% Dehydration					
Isotonic	150	7–10	7–10	4–8	8–15
Hypotonic (Na <130 mEq/liter)	75	10–15	10–15	5–10	10–20
Hypertonic (Na >150 mEq/liter)	125	2–5	2–5	2–4	4–10
Maintenance					
Calories					
900/m^2/day or by weight:	1–10 kg	—	—	—	—
100 cal/kg	11–20 kg	—	—	—	—
1000 + 50 cal/kg	>20 kg	—	—	—	—
1000 + 20 cal/kg	—	—	—	—	—
Water	100 ml/100cal/day	Na = 3–5 mEq/kg/day	—	—	—
Electrolytes[a]	K = 2–3 mEq/kg/day	Ca^+ = 2–5 mEq/kg/day	—	—	

[a] Balance anion as chloride, bicarbonate, or phosphate guided by laboratory tests.

drostatic fluid gradients and to minimize or reduce interstitial edema. Neurologically injured patients with elevated intracranial pressure also require cautious fluid management. Any increase in intracranial volume can rapidly lead to disastrous increases in intracranial pressure, with a consequent risk of decreased cerebral perfusion pressure and cerebral herniation[258]. In the patient with elevated intracranial pressure, inotropic support may be warranted before preload is fully augmented. As our monitoring capabilities and understanding of intracranial pathophysiology improve, this question may be definitively answered.

Cardiac Contractility

The use of pressor agents to increase myocardial function in children is well described. Although for years digitalis glycosides have been advocated, their use in children with potential electrolyte abnormalities, myocardial impairment, irritable myocardium, acid-base disturbances, and questionable renal function carries a high risk. For this reason, more specific inotropic agents with a rapid onset of action, ability to be titrated, and short half-lives are preferable. The use of dopamine, dobutamine, isoproterenol, epinephrine and other catecholamine pressor agents is well described in both infants and older children **(Table 16.14)**[259–262]. Although there is some question on the value of dopamine in neonates because of their functionally immature autonomic nervous system, it is frequently of value in increasing hemodynamic performance. All of these agents augment myocardial contractility[263–266]. In children with septic cardiomyopathy or myocarditis or in children after cardiac surgery, an imbalance in the myocardial oxygen supply-to-demand ratio may become important, and catecholamine-induced cardiomyopathies may occur. Children who are unstable enough to require more than minimal support also require and deserve comprehensive invasive monitoring.

Specific Catecholamines

The complexity of the cardiovascular derangement in shock states makes it difficult to predict the response to individual hemodynamically active therapeutic agents. This has two implications. First, the response to any agent may not be the textbook response. For example, dobutamine in a volume-depleted patient may cause significant vasodilatation (systemic and pulmonary) and increased intrapulmonary shunting and therefore actually decrease cardiac output and oxygen delivery despite enhancing contractility.

Table 16.14. Specific Agents

Agent	*Site of action*	*Dose (μg/kg/min)*	*Effect*[a]
Dopamine	Dopaminergic	0.5–4	Renal vasodilator
	β	4–10	Inotrope
	α > β	11–20	Peripheral vasoconstriction Increased PVR Dysrhythmias
Dobutamine	β_1 and β_2	1–20	Inotrope Vasodilatation (β2) Lowers PVR Weak α-activity Tachycardia and extrasystoles
Isoproterenol	β_1 and β_2	0.05–2.0	Inotrope Vasodilatation Lowers PVR $M\dot{V}O_2$ Dysrhythmias
Epinephrine	β > α	0.05–2.0	Inotrope Tachycardia Decreased renal flow $M\dot{V}O_2$ Dysrhythmias
Norepinephrine	α > β	0.05–2.0	Profound constrictor Inotrope $M\dot{V}O_2$, SVR
Sodium nitroprusside	Vasodilator: arterial greater than venous	0.5–10	Rapid onset, short duration Increases ICP $\dot{V}/\dot{Q}$ mismatch Cyanide toxicity
Nitroglycerin	Vasodilator: venous greater than arterial	1–20	Decreased PVR Increases ICP
PGE_1	Complex	0.05–0.2	Vasodilatation Open ductus arteriosus
Amrinone	PDE_3 inhibitor	1–20	Inotrope Chronotrope Vasodilatation

[a] PVR, pulmonary vascular resistance; SVR, systemic vascular resistance; ICP, intracranial pressure; and PDE3, phosphodiesterase inhibitor.

Second, as the responses may vary, invasive hemodynamic arterial monitoring and measurement of cardiac output is indicated in children ill enough to require advanced hemodynamic support. This needs to be remembered during the coming discussion of the cardiovascular support drugs. Table 16.14 summarizes key points concerning these agents.

Although pediatricians have traditionally been unconcerned about the effects of therapeutic agents on myocardial oxygen supply-demand relationships, this approach is no longer warranted. Our increasing sophistication has allowed us to support increasingly ill children, frequently with significant myocardial disease and occasionally even with ischemic heart disease. The occurrence of myocardial ischemia in Kawasaki disease, during isoproterenol therapy for asthma, and in congenital heart disease[267,268] indicates that myocardial ischemia occurs in children. Thus, consideration of myocardial oxygen supply-demand relationships is important even in children (see Chapter 13). A basic understanding of how individual catecholaminergic agents alter both myocardial oxygen consumption ($M\dot{V}O_2$) and oxygen delivery is necessary in dealing with children whose myocardia have been hypoperfused and exposed to numerous myocardial depressant factors and have an increased demand placed on them. All of these occur in shock.

Isoproterenol was the first synthetic catecholamine and has found extensive application in a wide host of clinical settings. Isoproterenol is almost a pure β-agonist and is thus a positive inotropic and chronotropic agent. In addition, both peripheral vasodilatation, as manifested by a fall in diastolic blood pressure, and pulmonary vasodilatation occur. Also, renal, splanchnic, muscle, and cutaneous flows are increased. The latter may unfortunately lead to perfusion of nonessential vascular beds and a relative "steal" phenomenon. The fall in diastolic pressure may have adverse effects on myocardial perfusion. This, in combination with significantly increased $M\dot{V}O_2$ because of its positive inotropic and chronotropic effects, may lead to aggravated myocardial ischemia[269,270]. Isoproterenol is also a potent pulmonary vasodilator. As such, it is a very useful agent in children with right heart failure and elevated pulmonary vascular resistance. Isoproterenol blunts hypoxic pulmonary vasoconstrictor activity and may thus increase intrapulmonary shunting. Hypoxia may be exacerbated secondary to increased $\dot{V}/\dot{Q}$ mismatch. For this reason, oxygen delivery should be monitored in the critical situation with significant lung disease when isoproterenol is administered. Finally, isoproterenol has β-adrenergic metabolic effects causing hyperglycemia, albeit less than that seen with epinephrine (with its α and β actions), and increased release of free fatty acids. Apart from the tendency to aggravate myocardial ischemia, it is additionally dysrhythmogenic. The clinical use of isoproterenol is best reserved for those situations in which potent inotropic stimulation is required, especially in conjunction with pulmonary vascular dilatation.

Dobutamine was synthesized in 1973[271] and approved for clinical use in the United States in 1978. The goal was to find a catecholaminergic agent specifically designed to provide an inotropic effect without the untoward effects of isoproterenol. In animals, dobutamine causes a predominantly inotropic rather than chronotropic effect, compared to isoproterenol[272]. Like isoproterenol, peripheral vasodilatation, pulmonary vasodilatation, attenuated pulmonary vascular hypoxic vasoconstriction, and, occasionally, unwanted tachycardia can occur. Dobutamine is less likely to give rise to ventricular dysrhythmias than either epinephrine or isoproterenol. Dobutamine has been shown to enhance myocardial performance under certain circumstances[273], but if falling blood pressure and increased $M\dot{V}O_2$ occur concurrently, myocardial ischemia is still a serious threat. Dobutamine has very little metabolic effect and only 1/45th the α effect of norepinephrine and 1/180th the β_2 effect of isoproterenol. It does not selectively enhance renal perfusion. In summary, dobutamine is the intravenous drug that is at present closest to being a pure inotropic agent[274,275].

Dopamine remains the most commonly used therapeutic agent in shock states[259–263,276]. This is true in spite of or perhaps because of its less than pure effects. Dopamine stimulates α-, β-, and dopaminergic sympathetic receptors and thus has a variety of effects. In low doses (0.5 to 4 μg/kg/min), it acts primarily by causing renal and splanchnic vasodilatation, thus serving as a diuretic and protecting renal perfusion[277]. In medium doses (4 to 10 μg/kg/min), increasing inotropic effect is seen, with increased stroke volume and cardiac output. In larger doses (more than 10 μg/kg/min), increasing α- vasoconstrictor activity is seen, and decreased peripheral and renal perfusion and increased myocardial afterload may occur. The exact degree to which these mixed effects occur in an individual varies, and careful monitoring to assess the response to dopamine in each patient is required. Tachycardia and extrasystoles may occur but are less of a problem with dopamine than with the previously mentioned agents. Pulmonary vascular resistance may be increased, and this should be remembered in treating newborns and patients at risk for pulmonary hypertension. In addition, because of the arguments given earlier concerning the neonatal myocardium, there is some debate concerning its efficacy in neonates.

Epinephrine stimulates both α- and $\beta_{1,2}$-receptors. The response to it mimics that of generalized autonomic stimulation. In general, increased cardiac output, blood pressure, and heart rate, a hypermetabolic state, CNS stimulation, and increased $M\dot{V}O_2$ occur. Both pulmonary and systemic vascular resistances are elevated, and renal ischemia is a potential complication. Ventricular tachydysrhythmias are serious threats. Epinephrine can certainly be expected to enhance myocardial contractility and to lead a still heart to beating, but its myriad untoward activities cause its use to be reserved only for dire cases.

Norepinephrine has a long, if somewhat unglorified, clinical position. Although it is both an α- and β_1-agonist, its potent peripheral vasoconstrictor effects overshadow the positive inotropic effects. Severe systemic, pulmonary, peripheral, renal, and splanchnic vasoconstriction occur with its use, and these acutely elevate the blood pressure. Although cardiac contractility is enhanced in the setting of increased myocardial afterload, cardiac output may not be increased, and the significantly enhanced $M\dot{V}O_2$ may cause myocardial ischemia. For these reasons, its use had largely been abandoned. Recently, however, clinicians have again begun to consider it as a potentially valuable therapeutic agent[278,279]. Better monitoring and understanding of the hemodynamic abnormalities underlying shock states have made it possible to apply this potent vasoconstrictor with salutary effects. Clearly, when myocardial perfusion pressures must be acutely maintained, norepinephrine can assuredly elevate perfusion pressures and enhance perfusion. In addition, when peripheral vascular resistance is low, such as during anaphylaxis, in neurogenic shock, and, most remarkably, in septic shock, enhancing peripheral vasomotor tone with norepinephrine may be the most beneficial single therapy. The combination of enhanced contractility and a return to normal peripheral vascular resistance should rapidly restore blood pressure and perfusion to multiple vascular beds. The use of norepinephrine in these circumstances may be beneficial but requires exact hemodynamic diagnosis and careful hemodynamic monitoring. Providing generalized exogenous delivery of the potent hormone (and neurotransmitter) should not be regarded as replacement for the intricate control of the sympathetic nervous system.

A newer agent available for inotropic and chronotropic support is amrinone. This bipyridine derivative differs from catecholamines in structure and in mechanism of action. Amrinone is a phosphodiesterase type III inhibitor that by its action slows the myocardial intracellular cyclic adenosine monophosphate (cAMP) degradation[280,281]. This augments myocardial contractility and has been demonstrated to increase cardiac output and decrease left ventricular end-diastolic and pulmonary capillary wedge pressures. Amrinone also induces relaxation of vascular smooth muscle, thereby reducing systemic vascular resistance. Since its mechanism of action differs from catecholamines, amrinone may be used in combination with catecholamines to achieve further increases in cardiac output and a decrease in afterload. This agent has been most efficacious in the postoperative period in patients with impaired myocardial performance after cardiotomy. Amrinone is administered intravenously (given in a bolus of 750 μg/kg over 1 to 3 minutes, followed by continuous infusion as listed in Table 16.14).

Afterload Reduction

Afterload reduction plays a role in improving myocardial performance in children with cardiogenic shock after surgery, myocarditis, or ischemic heart disease or in the later stages of septic shock with myocardial failure. In the late stage of septic shock, high systemic vascular resistance, poor peripheral perfusion, and decreased cardiac output may respond to afterload reduction. Afterload-reducing agents may also benefit children who require epinephrine or norepinephrine as an inotropic agent to decrease the α-adrenergic effects of increased systemic vascular resistance[282]. This combination of afterload reduction with inotropic support may provide the optimal benefit for a profoundly impaired myocardium. Both nitroprusside and nitroglycerin lower systemic vascular resistance in children and are useful afterload-reducing agents (nitroprusside > nitroglycerin)[283,284]. These agents act via generation of nitric oxide (NO). It has been suggested that nitroglycerin is a more potent venodilator and pulmonary vasodilator than is nitroprusside, whereas nitroprusside has more potent peripheral arterial vasodilating effects. The physiologic profile differences in these drug actions is not yet adequately explained, however, some speculation of a nitroglycerin receptor in discrete locations has been reported.

The pulmonary circulation plays an important role in children with hemodynamic compromise who have increased pulmonary vascular resistance secondary to congenital heart disease, ARDS, or sepsis. Children tend to have a more dramatic pulmonary vascular response than adults. Reduction of pulmonary vascular resistance and right ventricular afterload may be required to decrease intracardiac shunting and to prevent right ventricular failure. Correction of hypoxia, optimization of respiratory support, and correction of metabolic abnormalities are essential in reducing pulmonary vascular resistance. Unfortunately, no truly specific pulmonary vasodilator is available at the present time. The α-adrenoreceptor-blocking agent, tolazoline, has traditionally been used, but it is also a potent peripheral vasodilator[285]. PGI_2 (prostacyclin) has been reported to be efficacious, with less (but still present) systemic vasodilatation, but widespread clinical experience is lacking[286]. The predominantly β effects of isoproterenol also serve as a useful pulmonary vasodilator, but again, systemic hypotension and intrapulmonary shunting are problematic. In older children, isoproterenol is the drug of choice, but the use of nitroprusside or nitroglycerin may also be advantageous. Close monitoring and volume augmentation are frequently required when vasodilators are used to decrease pulmonary vascular resistance. Calcium channel-blocking agents such as nifedipine have the potential for decreasing pulmonary vascular resistance, but there is little experience in children at the present time. Other experimental therapies (ATP, ATP-MgCl, adenosine, and nitric oxide) continue to be developed, but further characterization of their effects and experience are required prior to recommendations for widespread use. Currently, inhaled nitric oxide has been used for many causes of respiratory failure (sepsis, pulmonary hypertension, meconium aspiration and others) with some promising results.

Steroids

The use of glucocorticoids in shock was reported as efficacious in early trials[287–291]. In many laboratory and human trials, however, high-dose steroid use has been associated with increased morbidity and no improvement in mortality and no longer should be recommended[218,292]. Nonetheless, children and all patients with human immunodeficiency virus (HIV) infection may have a predilection to adrenal failure during sepsis. Adrenal cortical failure is associated with cardiovascular hyporesponsiveness to endogenous mediators and exogenous therapies. Glucocorticoid replacement or stress doses should be considered. Physiologic doses (12.5 mg/m^2/day) or stress doses (50 to 100 mg/m^2/day) of hydrocortisone have not been shown to be detrimental and may be lifesaving in adrenal failure. When adrenal function may be impaired, such as in the Waterhouse-Friderichsen syndrome after meningococcal or *H. influenzae* infection, or in congenital adrenal hyperplasia, glucocorticoid replacement is essential, and mineralocorticoid replacement should be considered. A more detailed discussion can be found in Chapter 38.

Naloxone

Naloxone has been shown to reverse hypotension and improve short-term survival in many experimental studies. Naloxone has also been reported anecdotally to lead to hemodynamic recovery in children[(293)] and neonates[(294)]. Since these encouraging findings were reported between 1978 and 1984, there has been much enthusiasm for the potential of opiate antagonists. Unfortunately, the promise remains unfulfilled[(150)].

Immunotherapy

As was noted earlier in the section on endotoxin, Gram-negative LPSs consist of the toxic, lipid A moiety, an R core antigen, and an O-specific somatic antigen. Immunization with the O-specific somatic antigen provides no cross-protectivity to other Gram-negative organisms involved with bacteremia and septic shock. On the other hand, immunization with the R core antigen stimulates cross-reactive antigens, because the central core of the LPS is a primitive, well-conserved antigenic structure common to many GNB. These facts have suggested that vaccination with rough mutants would provide protection against heterologous GNB, and this has, in fact, been demonstrated[(295,296)].

One of the most exciting developments in treating septic shock has been the realization that patients can passively be immunized against the effects of LPS. Ziegler et al.[(297)] demonstrated that treating patients suffering from Gram-negative bacteremia with antiserum from volunteers exposed to the J5 rough mutant of *E. coli* 0111:B4 significantly reduced mortality. They reported that 42 of 109 control patients died in comparison with 23 of 103 patients treated with the J5 antisera (*P* of 0.011). In patients with septic shock, 30 of 39 controls died compared with 18 of 41 treated patients. These data demonstrated that human antisera to LPS core antigen substantially reduce the mortality resulting from Gram-negative bacteremia. Recently, this work has been extended. Baumgartner et al.[(298)] have used this approach in prophylactically treating patients at high risk for Gram-negative bacteremia with J5 antibody. They reported that 15 of 136 control patients acquired Gram-negative infections and 9 died. In the treated patients, only 6 of 126 patients acquired Gram-negative infections and only 2 died. Again, human antiserum to *E. coli* J5 was used. To eliminate the reliance on human antiserum volunteer donors, Teng et al.[(299)] and Braude[(300)] have developed a technique for harvesting human monoclonal IgM antibodies to the J5 mutant in laboratory hybridomas[(299,300)]. This monoclonal antibody is directed toward the covalently bound lipid A, which is the least variable structural component of LPS. For this reason, it can be expected that monoclonal antibodies will have a broad spectrum of anti-GNB activity[(299)].

Continuing their earlier work, Ziegler and colleagues[(301)] have reported recent results with HA-1A human monoclonal antibody. They conducted a double-blind, randomized trial in patients with sepsis and presumed sepsis. Of the 200 patients with Gram-negative bacteremia in the study, placebo-treated patients had a 49% mortality rate, with only a 30% mortality rate noted in the HA-1A-treated group (*P* of 0.014). Of the patients classified as in shock at entry to the study, 57% of placebo-treated patients and 33% of the HA-1A-treated patients died (*P* of 0.017). Treatment with HA-1A did not adversely affect septic patients who did not have Gram-negative sepsis. They concluded that treatment was safe and efficacious. Fisher et al.[(302)] also studied the effects of HA-1A antibody administration and found the treatment was well tolerated. No patient developed antibodies to HA-1A, and capillary leak syndrome did not alter the predicted pharmacokinetic model of HA-1A distribution. Subsequent data has been less supportive[(303)]. Recently a large multicenter trial of E5 monoclonal endotoxin antibody failed to show reduced mortality in Gram-negative sepsis without shock. Some improvement in the incidence of respiratory distress was suggested.

Other immunotherapeutic investigations are currently in progress. Besides antibody to endotoxin moieties, antibodies to proposed endogenous mediators of endotoxin action are being studied. One such mediator is TNF. Anti-TNF monoclonal antibody has been administered to anesthetized baboons after lethal doses of *E. coli*. Control group baboons lived an average of 19 hours. Antibody-treated animals survived more than 7 days and demonstrated a high quality of life and activity until killed[(304)]. Postmortem examination on the two groups of animals demonstrated marked differences in many organs, most notably the lungs, adrenal gland, kidneys, and liver. Histopathologic changes were severe in the control group, and the treated animals were protected from edema, fibrin deposition, necrosis, vascular congestion, and neutrophil accumulation. Another immunologic approach is to specifically design antibodies that interfere with leukocyte endothelial interaction. Antibodies to the leukocyte CD_{11}/CD_{18}-binding site have been demonstrated to decrease mortality in rabbits in septic shock. This therapy may prevent or ameliorate the endotheliopathy of septic shock[(57,58)].

The use of immunotherapy represents the application of years of mechanistic research to the care of critically ill patients. Unfortunately, the extensive research has not yet significantly improved our outcomes. So far anticytokine therapy has not fulfilled the promise[305,306]. Thus our understanding of the complex immunologic responses in septic shock is still insufficient. Additionally, better definition of sub-populations that may benefit from this therapeutic approach is necessary[305].

Supportive Therapy

The management of the multisystem deterioration with shock states is as important as treating the underlying condition. Renal, gastrointestinal, CNS, and hematologic abnormalities in shock need to be diligently searched for, identified, and treated. Coagulation abnormalities probably occur to some extent in all forms of septic shock and may complicate hypoperfusion states of any etiology[307–308]. Monitoring of PT, PTT, platelet count, evidence of fibrinolysis, and observation for excessive bleeding are essential. Replacement therapy specifically designed to replace absent clotting factors seems to provide the most advantageous therapy currently available. Use of vitamin K, fresh frozen plasma, and platelet transfusions should correct most coagulopathies. If replacement therapy is ineffective and peripheral gangrene from thrombosis occurs, heparinization may be of value[309]. Other therapies that have been reported in few patients include the use of regional anesthetic blocks[310] and fibrinolytic therapy. More experience is necessary before these can be widely applied.

Gastrointestinal disturbances after hypoperfusion and stress include bleeding, ileus, brush border cell and enzyme loss, and bacterial translocation. Ileus may result from electrolyte abnormalities and may lead to abdominal distention with respiratory compromise. Endothelial damage with diffuse gut edema and ischemia may underlie a host of other problems. Gastrointestinal blood loss from either acute gastritis or peptic ulceration should be prevented by using antacids and/or an H_2-receptor blocker such as cimetidine or gastric mucosal coating with sucralfate. Intensive investigations into metabolic changes in the gastrointestinal tract may reveal important new therapies. The gastrointestinal tract may not be a functional route for nutrition for some time, and parenteral nutrition will be necessary. However, trophic enteral feedings may play an important role in decreasing gastrointestinal pathology. Bacterial translocation is discussed in a previous section.

Renal support is essential to avoid prolonged renal shutdown in hypoperfusion states. Volume augmentation and the use of diuretics such as mannitol, furosemide, and ethacrynic acid have been advocated for early use to encourage renal blood flow and to maintain tubular function. Low-dose dopamine (0.5 to 4 g/kg/min) also improves renal blood flow and may be beneficial in preventing acute renal failure in shock states[311]. Acute renal failure leading to anuria may require treatment with either peritoneal dialysis or hemodialysis. High-output renal failure may occur in shock states without any previous episodes of oliguria. This may falsely indicate adequate renal perfusion and adequate prerenal augmentation at a time when the patient's intravascular volume is, in fact, being depleted. Therefore renal function should be assessed by response to current circulatory status and serial measurements of serum creatinine.

Respiratory Support of the Child in Shock

One of the major goals in shock therapy is to ensure optimal oxygen delivery. The child with acute circulatory failure may have ineffective oxygen delivery not only on a hemodynamic basis but also on a decreased respiratory muscle function basis, causing hypoventilation and hypoxemia[312]. This may be because of decreased respiratory muscle perfusion, acidosis, hypoxia, and electrolyte abnormalities. Under these circumstances, children may rapidly fatigue. They will compensate until complete, and sometimes alarmingly rapid deterioration occurs. A second cause of respiratory failure in shock is the development of intrapulmonary shunting as a result of noncardiac pulmonary edema (ARDS), which may further aggravate ventilation/perfusion abnormalities[313,314]. For these reasons, increased inspired oxygen is essential in all children with shock. Furthermore, to ensure the airway provides optimal relief from respiratory muscle fatigue and facilitates provision of positive airway pressure, early intubation of the trachea should be considered in all children with shock[312,315].

In children with cardiogenic shock and pulmonary edema, intubation and mechanical ventilation may rapidly improve myocardial function by relieving deleterious cardiorespiratory interactions. Increased negative pleural pressure leads to increased left ventricular transmural pressure that may have the same deleterious effect on the myocardium as increased afterload[316]. Children can develop negative intrathoracic pressures (-60 cm of H_2O can occur in neonates), and this can contribute to myocardial afterload. If left ventricular transmural pressure is considered an index of left ventricular afterload, in a patient with a mean arterial pressure of 50 mm Hg, an intrathoracic pressure of -40 mm Hg can increase left ventricular transmural pressure by 60%. This significantly increases myocardial afterload. Intubation and synchronization of ventilation may improve myocardial function by decreasing this afterload effect. Furthermore, expansion of functional residual capacity, improvement in pulmonary compliance, and a decreased intrapulmonary shunting greatly improve oxygen delivery and decrease pulmonary vascular resistance, improving right ventricular performance.

Mechanical ventilation in children may be provided in both intermittent mandatory ventilation (IMV) mode (volume cycled) or by pressure-controlled ventilation. Close observation of chest movement, ventilator pressures and flows, and arterial blood gases is essential to ensure adequate oxygenation and ventilation. Changes in compliance or obstruction of the endotracheal tube can lead to inadequate alveolar ventilation and oxygenation, and vigilance must be maintained.

The management of the ARDS in children is achieved

with an increase in PEEP, leading to an increase in end expiratory lung volume, a decrease in intrapulmonary shunt, and improvement in oxygenation[313]. Increasing intrathoracic pressure can impair venous return and may lead to decreased cardiac output and oxygen delivery if cardiac preload is not maintained. For this reason, children in shock with severe ARDS requiring PEEP greater than 15 cm H2O should have cardiac output, central pressure, and oxygen transport data monitored.

Extracorporeal Circulatory Support

Despite the maximal cardiopulmonary support used, the shocked child still is at high risk of death and developing prolonged MOSF. Newer extracorporeal technology has been applied in select circumstances to rescue nonresponders to conventional support. Extracorporeal membrane oxygenation (ECMO) has been in use for neonates for more than 15 years for neonatal respiratory distress. Neonates and certain older children in shock develop early respiratory distress or ARDS, pulmonary hypertension, and/or heart failure and may be unresponsive to conventional maximal therapies. ECMO has been used successfully to treat infants in septic shock[317]. In this study, 10 infants in septic shock with predicted 80% mortality were placed on ECMO. The survival rate of these infants was a striking 100%. However, along with encouraging survival statistics comes an increased morbidity. In comparison with other (nonseptic) infants placed on ECMO, the septic infants had a higher incidence of chronic lung disease and intracranial hemorrhage. These authors also cite the National ECMO Registry reporting of 68% survival in septic infants. These results are encouraging, compared with earlier data without such survival utilizing ECMO[318]. ECMO has also been used as therapy for cardiogenic shock. Rogers et al.[319] reported their experience in neonates and young children (less than 5 years) with use of ECMO after cardiotomy where severe postoperative right or biventricular failure was refractory to maximal support. Seven of ten patients survived. Other reports of ECMO use for cardiac support have varied from 40 to 80% survival in children with predicted mortality of greater than 80%[320,321]. ECMO has been used in older patients with refractory cardiogenic shock from varied etiologies[322]. Nine of 38 patients (24%) were discharged as long-term survivors, and from their experience, the authors suggest criteria for selective use of ECMO.

Extracorporeal technology (extracorporeal CO2 exchange, intravascular oxygenators (IVOX), and hemoperfusion) has been used in critically ill adults. Many of these devices have not yet been miniaturized for use in infants and small children. The intra-aortic balloon pump has been used in children, and many children have received benefit from continuous arteriovenous hemofiltration for volume overload and renal failure. Recently, DeCarlo et al.[323] reported that arteriovenous hemofiltration and/or dialysis could improve gas exchange in critically ill children. Charcoal hemoperfusion has also been used to remove circulatory infectious agents and host mediators in septic shock, but further experience is necessary before this is recommended for widespread use.

Multiorgan System Failure

After severe injury, hypotension or sepsis, each organ is at risk for dysfunction. With initial resuscitation from hemorrhage, hypotension or sepsis, the restitution of normal perfusion pressure is only an early goal. Extremely short lived insult with adequate resuscitation may result in no serious organ dysfunction. However, acute organ ischemia (or hypoxia) may initiate moderate or severe impairment in isolated or multiple organ function. The greater the severity or duration of the insult the more organs at risk.

After acute battlefield trauma and resuscitation, renal failure was a common secondary injury. With more aggressive fluid resuscitation the kidneys were more frequently spared, but acute lung injury became more problematic. With our increased sophistication in postoperative support, technical monitoring and intensive care, we are now able to successfully support children through single organ failure. However, multiple organ failure is more commonly seen than ever before as a result of aggressive therapy for children who would not have survived previously.

Causes of multiorgan failure include the causes of shock previously listed in this chapter. Organ failure occurs from the initial event and the associated host responses. It is clear that hypoxia-ischemia will deplete cells of energy production and if oxygen and substrates are not urgently restored, then cellular organelles are damaged. A large percentage of energy production is used to maintain electrochemical balance, synthetic function and cellular repair. In sepsis and certain poisonings, cellular function is disrupted directly by endotoxin or the toxic agent despite adequate delivery of oxygen and substrates. In hypermetabolic crises (i.e. malignant hyperthermia, thyrotoxicosis) complex cellular dysfunction occurs in an excessive energy productive state.

The lengthy list of host response mediators discussed earlier includes many molecules which can initiate or maintain organ failure. The host response may be not just adaptive physiologic protection but secondarily pathophysiologic in the progression of multiorgan system failure. Some of the compounds include interleukins, prostaglandins, oxygen free radicals, neuropeptides, eicosanoids and complement. These multiple substances mediate not only end organ metabolic dysfunction, but alter cardiovascular and endothelial function as well.

Endothelial dysfunction allows microvascular platelet aggregation, vasoparesis, interstitial fluid accumulation (which may increase extravascular pressure sufficiently to impair venocapillary channels and impairs transport of nutrients and waste products. Endotheliopathy is probably a major component of multiorgan dysfunction.

Cellular processes affected in multiorgan failure and shock continue to be unraveled. Carbohydrate metabolism is affected in the glycolytic pathway, tricarboxylic acid cycle and in mitochondrial oxidation. Endotoxin increases hexose monophosphate cycle activity. The many catabolic "stress" hormones released in shock mediate lipolysis. Proteolysis is also increased, probably to provide glucogenic amino acids. Since maintaining the integrity and function of the cell membrane demands a high percentage of cellular energy production, these processes including electrochemical balance and transmembrane signaling are at risk early during energy failure. When cell membrane function is lost, organ failure will occur along with release of intracellular contents into the circulation which may extend the injury to other organs.

The clinical pattern of multiorgan failure is variable. After apparent early successful resuscitation from shock, one organ, then another, show dysfunction which slowly worsens rather than improving. This can occur over many hours or many days. In the acute onset pattern, shock likely produced the multiorgan failure by nutrient and oxygen deficiency. The multiorgan failure presents with circulatory, respiratory, renal, hepatic, CNS and coagulation cascade failure. This overwhelming insult is fatal. The second pattern of subacute development of multiorgan failure occurs after initial successful resuscitation, but over the next few days slowly rising creatinine, hepatic transaminase levels and hyperbilirubinemia appear, and progressive respiratory or circulatory dysfunction evolve. During this pattern, the host response factors, bacterial translocation or other source of secondary infection, and products of mesenteric ischemia are contributing to the development of multiorgan failure.

Supportive Care

Each component organ involved in multiorgan failure may require technologic support in addition to meticulous overall clinical care. Respiratory support for isolated respiratory failure as a result of any cause is also required in multiorgan failure. Airway control as well as mechanical ventilation is usually essential to maintain oxygenation and ventilation during the dynamic processes in multiorgan failure. Newer ventilation strategies to diminish barotrauma and volutrauma by allowing hypercapnia and accepting lower oxygenation parameters have not been studied in a randomized fashion to demonstrate superior or inferior results. Specifics of mechanical ventilation support are given in Chapter 6. Ongoing trials with high frequency ventilation and surfactant replacement may offer new progress in this area.

Circulatory support with volume replacement and inotropic agents sometimes assisted with pulmonary artery catheter placement is necessary. Although studies in adults conclude that achieving "supranormal oxygen delivery" is correlated with improved survival after trauma, data in children are lacking. Currently cardiovascular support is provided to achieve satisfactory circulatory profile as assessed clinically.

Renal support includes optimization of circulatory status, monitoring of acid/base status and azotemia and providing extracorporeal assistance as needed. This may be in the form of hemodialysis, ultrafiltration or peritoneal dialysis. These techniques are more fully explained in Chapter 39.

Support for hepatic dysfunction is multifactorial including glucose support, coagulation factor replacement, extraction of ammonia from the body, nutrition (enteral or parenteral) and recognition of the inadequate liver function in prescribing the multitude of pharmacologic agents in intensive care. Dialysis to remove "middle molecules" resulting from liver dysfunction may improve hepatic encephalopathy.

Immune modulation and nutritional support promise to be areas of potential improvement in outcome for patients with multiorgan failure, but first we must develop a more complete comprehension of the cellular and organ processes which result in organ failure and improve our abilities to support or enhance the healing processes.

Summary

An aggressive multimodal approach to shock consists of consideration of all of these therapies, often simultaneously. Ensuring a patent airway and adequate oxygenation is, as always, the first step. Preload augmentation with intravascular fluid therapy should rapidly follow and is the most important therapy in nearly every instance. It should be considered at every stage of shock therapy and for every type of shock. Therapy directed at the underlying cause, whether it be instituting antibiotics, converting a cardiac dysrhythmia, or stopping hemorrhage, should occur concurrently. Frequently, oxygenation, ventilation, and fluid therapy are all that is required and, even in severe circumstances, will often delay further deterioration requiring more aggressive therapy. The administration of pharmacologic agents to correct metabolic abnormalities and restoring cardiovascular function is the final step in completing the multimodality therapy of shock states. Figure 16.6 provides an abbreviated algorithm for shock therapy.

ASSESSING OUTCOMES

Aggressive management of children in shock can be intensely rewarding as the restoration of a child to full potential is frequently the outcome, especially if therapy is started early. It is, however, not entirely clear what our therapeutic goals should be and how we determine the severity of shock. Perhaps most importantly, the question of which of the recent therapeutic advances alleged to have shown the ability to increase at least short-term survival in animal models will be truly advantageous in children. Considering these studies, it should be remembered that "increased survival time" or "increased survival" in a short-term study may not indicate whether there is, in fact, improved survival, which is, after all, our ultimate goal[324].

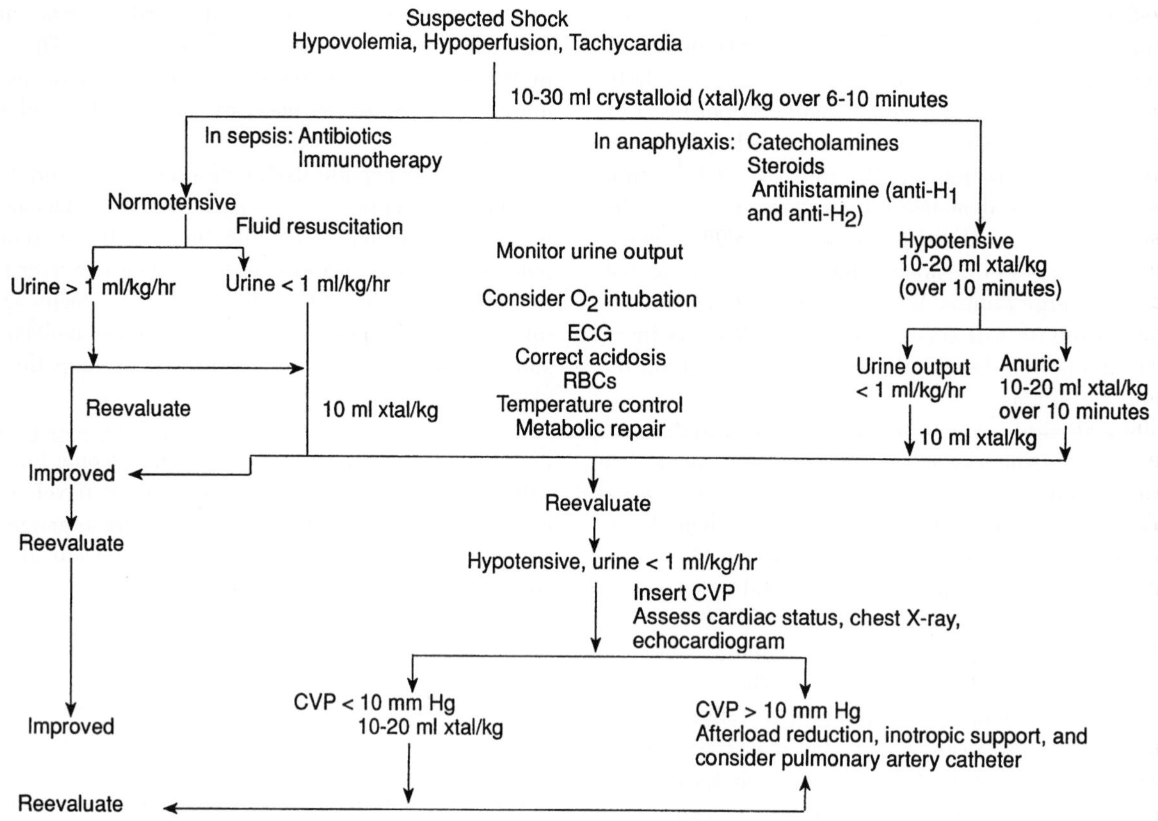

Figure 16.6. Abbreviated algorithm for shock therapy.

With regard to therapeutic goals, these are only just beginning to be defined. The work in adults of Siegel et al.[(178)], vanLanschot[(325)], and Shoemaker and others[(240,326–328)] has indicated that merely attaining "normal" physiologic parameters during the therapy of shock states is not adequate. It is more likely that "supraphysiologic" responses are required to meet the hypermetabolic needs of shock states. A general approach to determining goals in shock therapy has been to measure the mean of multiple parameters in patients who survived shock states[(329)]. In adults, it has been demonstrated that therapy aimed at achieving these goals improves survival[(240,330)]. In children who survive septic shock, Pollack and associates[(331)] have determined the median levels of multiple physiologic parameters and assessed which of these levels best correlate with outcome. Based on this, they have gone a step further and tentatively suggested therapeutic goals in children suffering from septic shock[(332)] **(Table 16.15).** Although there is as yet no confirmation of the notion that attaining these goals improves survival in children, they at least offer a starting point for further investigation. As has been noted, outcome is improved in patients with increased cardiac output, elevated oxygen consumption, and elevated oxygen extraction and without significant pulmonary disease. On the other hand, low body temperature (less than 37°C, no survivors), pulmonary disease, low cardiac index (less than 3.3 liters/min/m^2), and decreased oxygen utilization are all poor prognostic indicators in shock. It would seem logical that therapeutic endeavors aimed at preventing or correcting abnormalities in these areas would be useful. Caution is necessary; these variables are descriptive indicators of mortality. Achieving supraphysiologic parameters with therapeutic interventions may be valuable for only a select group, and these responders might have been the survivors at the start.

Table 16.15. Prognostic Indicators[a]

Variable	*% Survival in range*	*Range*
Oxygen consumption	75	>200 ml/min/m^2
Arteriovenous O_2 gradient	71	>5.5 ml/dl
pH	69	>7.4 units
$\dot{Q}_S/\dot{Q}_T$	69	<12%
WEDGE[b]	69	<11.3 torr
Cardiac index	67	3.3–6.0 liter/min/m^2
Oxygen extraction	59	>28%
Core temperature	58	>37°C

[a] From Pollack MM, Fields AI, Ruttiman VE. Distribution of cardiopulmonary variables in pediatric survivors and nonsurvivors of septic shock. Crit Care Med 1985;13:454.
[b] WEDGE, pulmonary artery occlusion pressure.

Although the past several years have seen the interesting introduction of exciting modalities of therapy, and in these years we have advanced our knowledge regarding components of the pathophysiology of shock, the fact that septic shock still has a greater than 50% mortality rate in children[332] indicates that we still are less than halfway to our goal. Further information on the earliest defects in shock states, factors controlling the distribution of blood flow, endothelial cell and microcirculatory function, utilization of central substrates, alterations in gene expression, and rapid identification of children in the early stages of shock are still required. Means of preventing the late sequelae of shock, such as myocardial, renal, and pulmonary failure, or at the very least of reversing the damage to these vital organs are still a long way off. A major effort toward prophylaxis still remains essential. Protection of children from burns and trauma by accident safety programs deserves every physician's support. The exciting developments in endotoxin and host mediator immunology suggest methods of preventing endotoxin shock and will possibly become more prominent in the future. Finally, awareness of the serious threat that shock poses to the child and constant vigilance aimed at providing early aggressive therapy for children at risk for shock states will improve the efficacy of all of our therapeutic endeavors.

References

1. Edis AJ. Aortic baroreflex function in the dog. Am J Physiol 1971;221:1352.
2. Breslow MJ, Mennen A, Koehler RC, Traystman RJ. Adrenal medullary and cortical blood flow during hemorrhage. Am J Physiol 1986;250:954.
3. Kovach AGB, Sandor P. Cerebral blood flow and brain function during hypotension and shock. Annu Rev Physiol 1976;38:571.
4. Badonnel MC, DeGirolami U, Joris I, Majno G. The intracerebral microcirculation of the rat in hemorrhagic shock. J Neuropathol Exp Neurol 1983;42:561.
5. Fettman MJ, Hand MS, Chandrasina LG, Cleek JL, Mason RA, Brooks PA, Phillips RW. Effects of captopril on hemodynamic and metabolic parameters in awake endotoxemic Yucatań minipigs. Circ Shock 1984;12:25.
6. Kon V, Harris RC, Ichikawa I. A regulatory role for large vessels in organ circulation: endothelial cells of the main renal artery modulate intrarenal hemodynamics in the rat. J Clin Invest 1990;85:1728.
7. Fink MP, MacVittie T, Casey E. Effects of non-steroid inflammatory drugs on renal function in septic dogs. J Surg Res 1984;36:516.
8. O'Brien WF, Golden SM, Davis SE, Bibro MC. Endotoxemia in the neonatal lamb. Am J Obstet Gynecol 1985;151:671.
9. Horton JW, Cohen D. Cardiovascular function and fluid compartments in newborn canine hemorrhagic shock. Am J Physiol 1985; 248:R724.
10. McCartney FA. Heart and circulation. In: Godfrey S, Bower JD, eds. Clinical pediatric physiology. Oxford: Blackwell Scientific Publications, 1979:284.
11. Friedman WF. The intrinsic physiologic properties of the developing heart. Prog Cardiovasc Dis 1972;15:87.
12. Friedman WF, Kirkpatrick SE. Fetal cardiovascular adaptation to asphyxia. In: Gluck L, ed. Intrauterine asphyxia and the developing fetal brain. Chicago: Year Book Medical Publishers, 1977:149.
13. Guyton AC. Circulatory shock and physiology of its treatment. In: Guyton AC, ed. Textbook of medical physiology. Philadelphia: WB Saunders, 1976:357.
14. Kariman K, Hempel FG, Jobsis FF, Burns SR, Saltzman HA. In vivo comparison of cerebral tissue PO_2 and cytochrome aa_3 reduction-oxidation state in cats during hemorrhagic shock. J Clin Invest 1981;68:21.
15. Mela L, Bacalzo LV, Miller LD. Defective oxidative metabolism of rat liver mitochondria in hemorrhagic and endotoxin shock. Am J Physiol 1971;220:571.
16. Mela L. Mitochondrial metabolic alterations in experimental circulatory shock. In: Urbaschek B, Urbaschek R, Neter E, eds. Gram-negative bacterial infections and mode of endotoxin actions. New York: Springer-Verlag, 1975:288.
17. Mela L. Mechanism and physiological significance of calcium transport across mammalian mitochondrial membranes. Curr Top Membr Transp 1977;9:103.
18. Chance B, O'Shino N, Sugano T, Mayersky A. Basic principles of tissue oxygen determination from mitochondrial signals. In: Bicher HI, Bruley DF, eds. Oxygen transport to tissue. New York: Plenum, 1983:277.
19. Mela L, Miller LD, Bacalzo LV, Olofsson K, White RR. Role of intracellular variations of lysosomal enzyme activity and oxygen tension in mitochondrial impairment in endotoxemia and hemorrhage in the rat. Ann Surg 1973;178:727.
20. Mela L, Goodwin CW, Miller LD. In vivo adaptation of O_2 utilization to O_2 availability: comparison of adult and newborn mitochondria. In: Jobsis FF, ed. Oxygen and physiological function. Dallas: Professional Information Library, 1977:285.
21. Thurston JH, McDougal DB. Effect of ischemia on metabolism of the brain of the newborn mouse. Am J Physiol 1969;216:348.
22. Cerra FB. Metabolic manifestations of multiple systems organ failure. Crit Care Clin 1989;5:119.
23. Kirsch JR, Helfaer MA, Koehler RC, Traystman RJ. Brain ischemia and reperfusion injury. Update. In: Bihari D, Holaday JW, eds. Intensive care and emergency medicine. Vol 9: brain failure. Berlin: Springer-Verlag, 1989.
24. Deitch EA, Bridges W, Baker J, et al. Hemorrhagic shock-induced bacterial translocation is reduced by xanthine oxidase inhibition or inactivation. Surgery 1988; 104:191.
25. Balk RA, Bone RC. The septic syndrome: definition and clinical implications. Crit Care Clin 1989;5:1.
26. Parks D, Granger D. Xanthine oxidase: biochemistry, distribution and physiology. Acta Physiol Scand 1986;598:87.
27. Deitch EA, Taylor M, Grisham M, et al. Endotoxin induces bacterial translocation and increases xanthine oxidase activity. J Trauma 1989;29:1679.
28. Alexander JW, Gottschlich MM. Nutritional immunomodulation in burn patients. Crit Care Med 1990;18:S149.
29. Alexander JW, Peck MD. Future prospects for adjunctive therapy: pharmacologic and nutritional approaches to immune system modulation. Crit Care Med 1990; 18:S159.
30. Danek SJ, Lynch JP, Weg JG, Dantzker DR. The dependence of oxygen uptake on oxygen delivery in the adult respiratory distress syndrome. Am Rev Respir Dis 1980;122:387.
31. Dantzker DR, Foresman B, Gutierrez G. Oxygen supply and utilization relationships: a reevaluation. Am Rev Respir Dis 1991;143:675.
32. Lucking SE, Williams TM, Chaten FC, Metz RI, Mickell JJ. Dependence of oxygen consumption on oxygen delivery in children with hyperdynamic septic shock and low oxygen extraction. Crit Care Med 1990;18:1316.
33. Vermeij CG, Feenstra BWA, Bruining HA. Oxygen delivery and oxygen uptake in postoperative and septic patients. Chest 1990;98:415.
34. Shoemaker WC, Appel PL, Kram HB. Tissue oxygen debt as a determinant of lethal and nonlethal postoperative organ failure. Crit Care Med 1988;16:1117.
35. Bihari D, Smithies M, Gimson A, Tinker J. The effects of vasodilation with prostacyclin on oxygen delivery and uptake in critically ill patients. N Engl J Med 1987;317:397.
36. Wetzel RC. The endothelium: the intensivists system. Crit Care Med 1993;21:S341.
37. Vane JR, Anggard EE, Botting RM. Regulatory functions of the vascular endothelium. N Engl J Med 1990; 323:27.
38. Ryan US. Phagocytic properties of endothelial cells. In: Ryan US, ed. Endothelial cells. Boca Raton, Florida: CRC Press, chap 30, 1988;III:33.
39. Furchgott RF. The role of endothelium in the responses of vascular smooth muscle to drugs. Am Rev Pharmacol Toxicol 1984;24:175.
40. Bersten A, Sibbald WJ. Acute lung injury in septic shock. Crit Care Clin 1989;5:49.
41. Maeda K, Abello PA, Abraham MR, Wetzel RC, Robothan JL, Buchman TG. Endotoxin induces organ-specific endothelial cell injury. Shock 1995;3(1):46.
42. Furchgott RF, Zawadzki JV. The obligatory role of endothelial cells in the relaxation of arterial smooth muscle by acetylcholine. Nature 1980;288:373.

43. Angus JA, Cocks TM. Vasodilatation and the discovery of endothelium-derived relaxing factor. Med J Aust 1987;146:250.
44. Peach MJ, Loeb AL, Singer HA, Saye J. Endothelium-derived vascular relaxing factor. Hypertension 1985;7 (Suppl 1):I94.
45. Palmer RMJ, Ferrige AG, Moncada S. Nitric oxide release accounts for the biological activity of endothelium-derived relaxing factor. Nature 1987;327:524.
46. Szabó C. Alterations in nitric oxide production in various forms of circulatory shock. New Horizons 1995;3(1):2.
47. Daniel TO, Ives HE. Endothelial control of vascular function. News Physiol Sci 1989;4:139.
48. Petros A, Bennett D, Vallance P. Effect of nitric oxide synthase inhibitors on hypotension in patients with septic shock. Lancet 1991;338:1557.
49. Booke M, Meyer J, Lingnau W, Hinder F, Traber LD, Traber DL. Use of nitric oxide synthase inhibitors in animal models of sepsis. New Horizons 1995;3(1):123.
50. Yanagisawa M, Kurihara H, Kimura S, Tomobe Y, Kobayashi M, Mitsui Y, Yazaki Y, Goto K, Masaki T. A novel potent vasoconstrictor peptide produced by vascular endothelial cells. Nature 1988;332:411.
51. Luscher TF. Endothelin: key to coronary vasospasm? Circulation 1991;83:701.
52. Mautone AJ. Metabolic activity of vascular endothelium. In: Scarpelli EM, ed. Pulmonary physiology: fetus, newborn, child, and adolescent. Philadelphia: Lea & Febiger, chap 7, 1990:173.
53. MacIntyre DE, Pearson JD, Gordon JL. Localization and stimulation of prostacyclin production in vascular cells. Nature 1978;271:549.
54. Harker LA. Endothelium and hemostasis. In: Ryan US, ed. Endothelial cells. Boca Raton, Florida: CRC Press, chap 11, 1988;I:168.
55. Rubanyi GM, Vanhoutte PM. Oxygen-derived free radicals, endothelium, and responsiveness of vascular smooth muscle. Am J Physiol 1986;250:H815.
56. Weiss SJ. Tissue destruction by neutrophils. N Engl J Med 1989;320:365.
57. Vedder NB, Winn RK, Rice CL, Harlan JM. Neutrophil-mediated vascular injury in shock and multiple organ failure. Perspectives in shock research: metabolism, immunology, mediators, and models. New York: Alan R Liss, 1989:181.
58. Vedder NB, Winn RK, Rice CL, Chi EY, Artors KE, Harlan JM. A monoclonal antibody to the adherence-promoting leukocyte glycoprotein, CD_{18}, reduces organ injury and improves survival from hemorrhagic shock and resuscitation in rabbits. J Clin Invest 1988;81:939.
59. Warren JS, Ward PA. Review: oxidative injury to the vascular endothelium. Am J Med Sci 1986;292:97.
60. Aoki N, Siegfried M, Lefer AM. Anti-EDRF effect of tumor necrosis factor in isolated, perfused cat carotid arteries. Am J Physiol 1989;256:H1509.
61. Westphal O, Westphal U, Sommer T. The history of pyrogen research. Microbiology 1977:229.
62. Rietschel ET, Schade U, Jensen M, Wollenweber HW, Luderitz O, Greisman SG. Bacterial endotoxins: chemical structure, biologic activity and role in septicemia. Scand J Infect Dis Suppl 1982;31:8.
63. Nikaido HG, Nakae T. The outer membrane of Gram negative bacteria. Adv Microb Physiol 1979;8:163.
64. Bradley SG. Cellular and molecular mechanism of action of bacterial endotoxins. Annu Rev Microbiol 1979;33:67.
65. Westphal O, Jann K, Himmelspach K. Chemistry and immunochemistry of bacterial lipopolysaccharides as cell wall antigens and endotoxins. Prog Allergy 1983;33:9.
66. Morris RC, Rudbach JH. Endotoxin cell-membrane interactions leading to transmembrane signalling. Contemp Top Mol Immunol 1981:187.
67. Galanos C, Luderitz O, Rietschel ET, Westphal O. Newer aspects of the chemistry and biology of bacterial polysaccharides, with special reference to their lipid A component. Int Rev Biochem 1977;14:239.
68. Rafter GW. Stimulation of pyrogen production by lipopolysaccharide-leukocyte interactions. Microbiology 1980:154.
69. Morrison DC, Ryan JL. Bacterial endotoxins and host immune responses. Adv Immunol 1979;28:293.
70. Berry LJ. Bacterial toxins. CRC Crit Rev Toxicol 1977;5:239.
71. Weissman G, Thomas L. Studies on lysosomes. 1. The effects of endotoxin, endotoxin tolerance and cortisone on the release of acid hydrolases from a granular fraction of rabbit liver. J Exp Med 1962;116:433.
72. McGivney AL, Bradley SG. Effects of bacterial endotoxin on malic dehydrogenase activities in primary cultures of a mouse liver. Va J Sci 1978;29:107.
73. Kun E, Miller CP. Effect of bacterial endotoxins on carbohydrate metabolism of rabbits. Proc Soc Exp Biol Med 1948;67:221.
74. DePalma RG, Harevno Y, Robinson AV, Holden WD. Structure and function of hepatic mitochondria in hemorrhage and endotoxemia. Surg Forum 1970;21:3.
75. Shands JW, Miller V, Marlin H, Senterfitt V. Hypoglycemic activity of endotoxin. 2. Mechanism of the phenomenon in BCG-infected mice. J Bacteriol 1969;98:494.
76. McCallum RE. Mediated inhibition of hepatic gluconeogenesis by endotoxin. Microbiology 1980:87.
77. Gerwisz H, Snyderman R, Mergenhagen SE, Shin SH. Effects of endotoxic lipopolysaccharides on the complement system. In: Kadis D, Weinbaum G, Ajl SJ, eds. Microbial systems: a comprehensive treatise. New York: Academic Press, 1971;5:127.
78. Gotze P, Miller-Eberhard HJ. The alternative pathway of complement activation. Adv Immunol 1976;24:1.
79. Jacob HS. Complement mediated leucoembolization: a mechanism of tissue damage during extracorporeal perfusions, myocardial infarction and in shock. A review. Q J Med 1983;207:289.
80. Brigham K, Bower R, Haynes J. Increased sheep lung vascular permeability caused by *E. coli* endotoxin. Circ Res 1979;45:292.
81. Demling RH, Wong C, Wenger H. Effect of endotoxin on the integrity of the peripheral microcirculation. Circ Shock 1984;12:191.
82. Bond RF. Peripheral vascular adrenergic depression during hypotension. Adv Shock Res 1983;9:157.
83. Bond RF, Bond CH, Peissner LC, Manning ES. Prostaglandin modulation of adrenergic vascular control during hemorrhagic shock. Am J Physiol 1981;241:H85.
84. Pearson RJ. Actions of endotoxin excitation secretion coupling at the neural membrane. Prog Clin Biochem Res 1981:65.
85. Soulsby M, Bennett C, Hess M. Canine arterial calcium transport during endotoxin shock. Circ Shock 1980;7:139.
86. Fiddian-Green RG. Studies in splanchnic ischemia and multiple organ failure. In: Marston A, Bulkley GB, Fiddian-Green RG, Haglund UH, eds. Splanchnic ischemia and multiple organ failure. St Louis: CV Mosby, chap 32, 1989:349.
87. Berg RD, Garlington AW. Translocation of certain indigenous bacteria from the gastrointestinal tract to the mesenteric lymph nodes and other organs in a gnotobiotic mouse model. Infect Immun 1979;23:403.
88. Deitch EA, Specian RD, Berg RD. Endotoxin-induced bacterial translocation and mucosal permeability: role of xanthine oxidase, complement activation, and macrophage products. Crit Care Med 1991;19:785.
89. Fiddian-Green RG, Baker S. Nosocomial pneumonia in the critically ill: product of aspiration or translocation? Crit Care Med 1991;19:763.
90. Fiddian-Green RG, Gantz NM. Transient episodes of sigmoid ischemia and their relation to infection from intestinal organisms after abdominal aortic operations. Crit Care Med 1987;15:835.
91. Kever AJH, Rommes JH, Meuessen-Verhage EAE, et al. Prevention and colonization of infection in critically ill patients: a prospective randomized study. Crit Care Med 1988;16:1087.
92. Meakins JL, Marshall JC. The gut as the motor of multiple system organ failure. In: Marston A, Bulkley GB, Fiddian-Green RG, Haglund UH eds. Splanchnic ischemia and multiple organ failure. St Louis: CV Mosby, chap 31, 1989:339.
93. Beller FK. Sepsis and coagulation. Clin Obstet Gynecol 1985;28:46.
94. Morrison DC, Cochrane C. Direct evidence by Hageman factor activation by bacterial lipopolysaccharides. J Exp Med 1974;140:797.
95. Schreiber AD, Austin KF. Inter-relationships of the fibrinolytic, coagulation kinin generating and complement system. Semin Hematol 1973;6:593.
96. Semerano N, Lattazio A. Interaction of platelets with bacterial endotoxins. Agents Actions 1983;13:461.
97. McCabe WR, Treadwell TL, DeMaria A. Pathophysiology of bacteremia. Am J Med 1983;75:7.
98. Jacob HS, Craddock PR, Hammerschmidt DS, Moulow CF. Complement-induced granulocyte aggregation. An unsuspected mechanism of disease. N Engl J Med 1980;302:789.
99. Fearon DT, Ruddy S, Schur PH, McCabe WR. Activation of the properdin pathway of complement in patients with Gram-negative bacteremia. N Engl J Med 1975;292:937.
100. Zimmerman GA, Renzetti AD, Hill HR. Functional and metabolic activity of granulocytes from patients with adult respiratory distress syndrome. Am Rev Respir Dis 1983;127:290.
101. Babior BM. Oxygen dependent microbial killing by phagocytes. N Engl J Med 1978;298:659.
102. Zimmerman JJ, Shelhamer JH, Parrillo JE. Quantitative analysis of polymorphonuclear leukocyte superoxide anion generation in critically ill children. Crit Care Med 1985;13:143.

103. Wise WC, Cook JA, Knapp DR, Holushka PV. Protective effects of thromboxane synthetase inhibitors in endotoxic shock. Circ Res 1980;46:854.
104. Holushka PV, Cook JA, Wise WC. Beneficial effects of UK 37248, a thromboxane synthetase inhibitor, in experimental endotoxic shock in the rat. Br J Clin Pharmacol 1983;15:133.
105. Boston GD, Johnson MA, Roesel OF. Endotoxin-induced hemodynamic changes in dogs: role of thromboxane and prostaglandin I2. Am J Vet Res 1983;44:1497.
106. Fletcher JR, Ramwell PW. Prostaglandins in shock. Adv Shock Res 1978;24:154.
107. Leideritz TH, Rietschel ET, Schade U. Release of leukotrienes from macrophages stimulated by lipopolysaccharide. Immunobiology 1983; 165:312.
108. Hagman W, Denzlinger C, Keppler D. Role of peptide leukotrienes and their hepatobiliary elimination in endotoxin shock. Circ Shock 1984;14:223.
109. Lewis RA, Austin KE. The biologically active leukotrienes. J Clin Invest 1984;73:889.
110. Hagman W, Keppler D. Leukotriene antagonists prevent endotoxin lethality. Naturwissenschaften 1982;69:594.
111. Rietschel ET, Schade U, Luderitz O, Fischer H, Peskar B. Prostaglandins in endotoxicosis. Microbiology 1980:66.
112. Flynn JT, Lefer AM. Prostaglandin metabolism during circulatory shock. Biochim Biophys Acta 1977;497:775.
113. Moncada S, Vane JR. Pharmacology and endogenous roles of prostaglandin endoperoxides, thromboxane A_2, and prostacyclin. Pharmacol Rev 1979;30:293.
114. Malik AB, Perlman MB, Cooper JA, Noonan T, Bizios R. Pulmonary microvascular effects of arachidonic acid metabolites and their role in lung vascular injury. Fed Proc 1985;44:36.
115. Samuelsson B. Leukotrienes: mediators of immediate hypersensitivity reactions and inflammation. Science 1983;220:568.
116. Katori M, Takeda K, Imai S. Effect of prostaglandin E_1 and F_1 on the heart lung preparation of the dog. Tohoku J Exp Med 1970;101:67.
117. Hollenberg M, Walder PS, McCormick D. Cardiovascular responses to intracoronary infusion of PGE_1, F_1 and F_2. Arch Int Pharmacodyn Ther 1968;174:66.
118. Raflo GT, Wangenstein SL, Glenn TM, Lefer AM. Mechanisms of protective effects of prostaglandins E_1 and F_2 in canine endotoxin shock. Eur J Pharmacol 1973;24:86.
119. Hedgvist P. Studies on the effects of PGE_1 and E_2 on the sympathetic neuromuscular transmission in some animal tissues. Acta Physiol Scand 1970;79(Suppl 345):1.
120. Wise WC, Cook JA, Halushka PV, Knapp DR. Protective effects of thromboxane synthetase inhibitors in rats in endotoxic shock. Circ Res 1980;46:854.
121. Emau P, Giri SN, Bruss ML. Role of prostaglandins, histamine and serotonin in the pathophysiology induced by *Pasteurella hemolytica* endotoxin in sheep. Circ Shock 1984;12:47.
122. Halushka PV, Reines HD, Barrow SE, Blair IA, Dollery CT, Rambo W, Cook JA, Wise WC. Elevated plasma 6-keto-prostaglandin F_1 in patients with septic shock. Crit Care Med 1985;13:451.
123. Clancy RM, Dahinden CA, Hugli TE. Complement-mediated arachidonate metabolism. Prog Biochem Pharmacol 1985;20:120.
124. Gee MH, Perkowski SZ, Tahamont MV, Flynn JT. Arachidonate cyclooxygenase metabolites as mediators of complement-initiated lung injury. Fed Proc 1985;44:46.
125. Lefer AM. Leukotrienes as mediators of ischemia and shock. Biochem Pharmacol 1986;35:123.
126. Holcroft JW, Vassary MJ, Weber CJ. Prostaglandin E_1 and survival in patients with the adult respiratory distress syndrome: a prospective trial. Ann Surg 1986; 203:371.
127. Steinberg SM, Rodriguez JL, Bitzer LG, Rhee JW, Kelley KA, Flint LM. Indomethacin treatment of human adult respiratory distress syndrome. Circ Shock 1990;30:375.
128. Young JS, Passmore JC. Hemodynamic and renal advantages of dual cyclooxygenase and leukotriene blockade during canine endotoxic shock. Circ Shock 1990; 32:243.
129. Turner CR, Quinian MF, Schwartz LW, Wheeldon EB. Therapeutic intervention in a rat model of ARDS: 1. Dual inhibition of arachidonic acid metabolism. Circ Shock 1990;32:231.
130. Bihari DJ, Tinker J. The therapeutic value of vasodilator prostaglandins in multiple organ failure associated with sepsis. Intensive Care Med 1988;15:2.
131. Salari H, Demos M, Wong A. Comparative hemodynamics and cardiovascular effects of endotoxin and platelet-activating factor in rat. Circ Shock 1990;32:189.
132. Qi M, Jones SB. Contribution of platelet activating factor to hemodynamic and sympathetic responses to bacterial endotoxin in conscious rats. Circ Shock 1990; 32:153.
133. Lefer A. Significance of lipid mediators in shock states. Circ Shock 1989;27:3.
134. Feuerstein G, Siren A. Platelet-activating factor and shock. Prog Biochem Pharmacol 1988;22:181.
135. Fink A, Geva D, Zung A, Konichezky S, Eliraz A, Bentwich Z. Adult respiratory distress syndrome: roles of leukotriene C_4 and platelet activating factor. Crit Care Med 1990;18:905.
136. Faden Al, Holaday JW. Experimental endotoxin shock. The pathophysiologic function of endorphins and treatment with opiate antagonists. J Infect Dis 1980;142:229.
137. Holaday JW, Faden AI. Naloxone reversal of endotoxin hypotension suggests role of endorphins in shock. Nature 1978;275:450.
138. Holaday JW. Cardiovascular effects of endogenous opiate systems. Annu Rev Pharmacol Toxicol 1983;23:541.
139. Murray MJ, Offord KP, Yarsh TL. Physiologic and plasma hormone correlates of survival in endotoxic dogs: effects of opiate antagonists. Crit Care Med 1989;17:39.
140. Bernton SW, Long JB, Holaday JW. Opioids and neuropeptides. Mechanisms in circulatory shock. Fed Proc 1985;44:290.
141. Faden AI. Opiate antagonists and thyrotropin releasing hormone. JAMA 1984;252:1177.
142. Bloom FE. The endorphins. Annu Rev Pharmacol Toxicol 1983;23:151.
143. North RA, Egan TM. Actions and distribution of opiate peptides in peripheral tissues. Br Med Bull 1983;39:71.
144. LaGamma EF, Adler JE, Black IB. Impulse activity differentially regulates (Leu) enkephalin and catecholamine characters in the adrenal medulla. Science 1984; 224:1102.
145. Cox BM. Endogenous opioid peptides. A guide to structure and terminology. Life Sci 1982;31:1654.
146. Faden AI, Holaday JW. Opiate antagonists: a role in treatment of hypovolemic shock. Science 1979;205:317.
147. Holaday JW, Faden AI. Naloxone acts at central opiate receptors to reverse hypotension, hypothermia and hypoventilation in spinal shock. Brain Res 1980;194:608.
148. Weinglas IS, Hinchey EJ, Chier RC. Naloxone and methylprednisone in the treatment of experimental septic shock. J Surg Res 1982;33:131.
149. Hackshaw KV, Parker GA, Roberts JW. Naloxone in septic shock. Crit Care Med 1990;18:47.
150. Rock P, Silverman H, Plump D, Kecala Z, Smith P, Michael JR, Summer W. Efficacy and safety of naloxone in septic shock. Crit Care Med 1985;13:28.
151. Reynold DC, Gwill NJ, Holaday JW, Ganes E. Thyrotrophin releasing hormone in primate endotoxin shock. Physiologist 1982;25:309.
152. Gurll NJ, Holaday JW, Reynolds DG, Ganes E. Thyrotropin releasing hormone: effects in monkeys and dogs subjected to experimental circulatory shock. Crit Care Med 1987;15:574.
153. Holaday JW, Faden AI. Naloxone and TRH have additive effects in reversing endotoxin shock. In: Takagi H, Simon EJ, eds. Advances in endogenous and exogenous opioids. Oxford: Pergamon Press, 1981:367.
154. Hock CE, Lefer AM. Lack of effect of thyrotropin releasing hormone (TRH) in circulatory shock. Peptides 1985;6:547.
155. McIntosh TK, Faden AI. Thyrotropin-releasing hormone (TRH) and circulatory shock. Circ Shock 1986;18:241.
156. Said SI. Vasoactive peptides. Hypertension 1983;5:17.
157. Revhaug A, Hygren I, Lindgren TI, Anderson OK, Burhol PG, Gierck-sky KE. Increased plasma levels of VIP in pigs during endotoxemia. Eur Surg Res 1985;17:75.
158. Brandtzaeg P, Oktedalen O, Kierulf P, Opstad PK. Elevated VIP and endotoxin plasma levels in human Gram-negative septic shock. Regul Pept 1989;24:37.
159. Fisher LA. Corticotropin-releasing factor: endocrine and autonomic integration of responses to stress. Trends Pharmacol Sci 1989;10:189.
160. Bochner BS, Lichtenstein LM. Anaphylaxis. N Engl J Med 1991;324:1785.
161. Hinshaw LB, Jordan MM, Vick JA. Histamine release and endotoxin shock in the primate. J Clin Med 1961;40:1631.
162. Vick JA, Mehlman B, Heiffer MH. Early histamine release and death due to endotoxin. Proc Soc Exp Biol Med 1971;137:902.
163. Kraus SM, Hess ML. Diphenhydramine protection of the failing myocardium during Gram-negative endotoxemia. Circ Shock 1979;6:75.
164. Blalock A. A study of thoracic duct lymph in experimental crush in-

jury and injury produced by gross trauma. Bull Johns Hopkins Hosp 1943;72:54.
165. Brand ED, Lefer AM. Myocardial depressant factor in plasma from cats in irreversible post-oligemic shock. Proc Soc Exp Biol Med 1966;122:200.
166. Baxter CR, Cook WA, Shires GT. Serum myocardial depressant factor of burn shock. Surg Forum 1966;17:1.
167. Lefer A. Properties of cardioinhibitory factors produced in shock. Fed Proc 1978;37:2734.
168. Siegel JH, Greenspan M, Del Guekicio LR. Abnormal vascular tone, defective oxygen transport and myocardial failure in human septic shock. Ann Surg 1967;165:504.
169. Hinshaw LB, Archer LT, Spitzer JJ, Black MR, Peyton MD, Greenfield LJ. Effects of coronary hypotension and endotoxin on myocardial performance. Am J Physiol 1974;227:1051.
170. Hinshaw LB. Myocardial function in endotoxin shock. Circ Shock 1979;1(Suppl):43.
171. Goldfarb RD. Cardiac dynamics following shock. Role of circulating cardiodepressant substances. Circ Shock 1982;9:317.
172. Parrillo JE, Burch C, Shelhamer JH, Parker MM, Natanson C, Schuette W. A circulating myocardial depressant substance in humans with septic shock: septic shock patients with a reduced ejection fraction have a circulating factor that depresses in vitro myocardial cell performance. J Clin Invest 1985;76:1539.
173. Parker JL, Adam R. Development of myocardial dysfunction in endotoxin shock. Am J Physiol 1985;248:H818.
174. Parker MM, Shelhamer JH, Bacharach SL, Green MV, Natanson C, Frederick TM, Damske BA, Parrillo JE. Profound but reversible myocardial depression in patients with septic shock. Ann Intern Med 1984;100:483.
175. Weil MH, Nishijima H. Cardiac output in bacterial shock. Am J Med 1978;64:920.
176. Siegel JH, Cerra F, Coleman B, Giovannini I, Shetye M, Border JR, McMenamy RH. Physiologic and metabolic correlations in human sepsis. Surgery 1979;86:163.
177. Archer LT, Black MR, Hinshaw LB. Myocardial failure with altered response to adrenaline in endotoxin shock. Br J Pharmacol 1975; 54:145.
178. Cunnion RE, Parrillo JE. Myocardial dysfunction in sepsis: recent insights. Chest 1989;95:941.
179. Ognibene FP, Rosenberg SA, Lotze M, Skibber J, Parker MM, Shelhamer JH, Parrillo JE. Interleukin-2 administration causes reversible hemodynamic changes and left ventricular dysfunction similar to those seen in septic shock. Chest 1988;94:750.
180. Hollenberg SM, Cunnion RE, Lawrence M, Kelley JL, Parrillo JE. Tumor necrosis factor depresses myocardial cell function: results using an in vitro assay of myocyte performance. Clin Res 1989;37:528A.
181. Reilly JM, Cunnion RE, Burch-Whitman C, Parker MM, Shelhamer JH, Parrillo JE. A circulating myocardial depressant substance is associated with cardiac dysfunction and peripheral hypoperfusion (lactic acidemia) in patients with septic shock. Chest 1989;95:1072.
182. Parrillo JE, Parker MM, Natanson C, Suffredini AF, Danner RL, Cunnion RE, Ognibene FP. Septic shock in humans: advances in the understanding of pathogenesis, cardiovascular dysfunction, and therapy (NIH Conference). Ann Intern Med 1990;113:227.
183. Finkel MS, Oddis CV, Jacob TD, Watkins SC, Hattler BG, Simmons RL. Negative inotropic effects of cytokines on the heart mediated by nitric oxide. Science 1992;257:387.
184. Brady AJB, Poole-Wilson PA, Harding SE, Warren JB. Nitric oxide production within cardiac myocytes reduces their contractility in endotoxemia. Am J Physiol 1992;263:H1963.
185. Brutsaert DL, Meulemans AL, Sipido KR, Sys SU. Effects of damaging the endocardial surface on the mechanical performance of isolated heart muscle. Circ Res 1988;62:358.
186. Mebazaa A, Mayoux E, Maeda K, Martin L, Lakatta EG, Robotham JL, Shah AM. Paracrine effects of endocardial endothelial cells on myocyte contraction mediated via endothelin. Am J Physiol 1993; 265:H1841.
187. Shah AM, Mebazaa A, Wetzel RC, Lakatta EG. Novel cardiac myofilament desensitizing factor released by endocardial and vascular endothelial cells. Circulation 1994;89:2492.
188. Hack CE, DeGroot ER, Felt-Bersma RJF, Nuijens JH, Strack VanSchijndel RJM, Eerenberg-Belmer AJM, Thijs LG, Aarden LA. Increased plasma levels of interleukin-6 in sepsis. Blood 1989;74:1704.
189. Cerami A, Beutler B. The role of cachectin/TNF in endotoxin shock and cachexia. Immunol Today 1988;9:28.
190. Okusawa S, Gelfand JA, Ikejima T, Conolly RJ, Dinarello CA. Interleukin-1 induces a shock-like state in rabbits. Synergism with tumor necrosis factor and the effect of cyclooxygenase inhibition. J Clin Invest 1988;81:1162.
191. Waage A, Espevik T. Interleukin 1 potentiates the lethal effect of tumor necrosis factor α/cachectin in mice. J Exp Med 1988;167:1987.
192. Remick D, Kunkel RG, Larrick JW, Kunkel SL. Acute in vivo effects of human recombinant tumor necrosis factor. Lab Invest 1987; 56:583.
193. Stephens KE, Ishizaka A, Larrick JW, Raffin TA. Tumor necrosis factor causes increased pulmonary permeability and edema. Comparison to septic acute lung injury. Am Rev Respir Dis 1988;137:1364.
194. Pober JS, Cotran RS. Cytokines and endothelial cell biology. Physiol Rev 1990;70:427.
195. Waage A, Halstensen A, Espevik T. Association between tumour necrosis factor in serum and fatal outcome in patients with meningococcal disease. Lancet 1987;1:355.
196. Girardin E, Grau GE, Dayer JM, Roux-Lambard P, J5 Study Group, Lambert P-H. Tumor necrosis factor and interleukin-1 in the serum of children with severe infectious purpura. N Engl J Med 1988; 319:397.
197. Damas P, Reuter A, Gysen P, Demonty J, Lamy M, Franchimont P. Tumor necrosis factor and interleukin-1 serum levels during severe sepsis in humans. Crit Care Med 1989;17:975.
198. Calandra T, Baumgartner J-D, Grau GE, Wu M-M, Lambert P-H, Schellekens J, Verhoef J, Glauser MP, Swiss-Dutch J5 Immunoglobulin Study Group. Prognostic values of tumor necrosis factor/cachectin, interleukin-1, interferon-α, and interferon-γ in the serum of patients with septic shock. J Infect Dis 1990;161:982.
199. Neilson IR, Neilson KA, Yunis EJ, Rowe MI. Failure of tumor necrosis factor to produce hypotensive shock in the absence of endotoxin. Surgery 1989;106:439.
200. Verrier B, Muller D, Bravo R, Muller R. Wounding of fibroblast monolayer results in the rapid induction of the *c-fos* protooncogene. EMBO J 1986;5:913.
201. Bukh A, Martinez-Valdez H, Freedman SJ, Freedman MH, Cohen A. The expression of *c-fos*, *c-jun*, and *c-myc* genes is regulated by heat shock in human lymphoid cells. J Immunol 1990;144:4835.
202. Deguchi Y, Negoro S, Kishimoto S. *c-fos* expression in human skin fibroblasts by reperfusion after oxygen deficiency: a recovery change of human skin fibroblasts after oxygen deficiency stress. Biochem Biophys Res Commun 1987;149:1093.
203. Craig EA, Gross CA. Is hsp 70 the cellular thermometer? Trends Biochem Sci 1991;April:135.
204. National Safety Council. Accident facts. National Safety Council Annual Report. Chicago: National Safety Council, 1981.
205. Jaffe D, Wesson D. Emergency management of blunt trauma in children. N Engl J Med 1991;324:1477.
206. Haupt MT. Anaphylaxis and anaphylactic shock. In: Parrillo JE, ed. Current therapy in critical care medicine. 2nd ed. Philadelphia: BC Decker, 1991:58.
207. Fyler DC. Report of the New England Regional Infant Cardiac Program. Pediatrics 1980;65:37.
208. Norwood W, Lang P, Hansen DD. Physiologic repair of aortic atresia hypoplastic left heart syndrome. N Engl J Med 1983;308:23.
209. Levin D. Congestive heart failure. In: Levin DL, Morris FC, Moore GC, eds. A practical guide to pediatric intensive care. St Louis: CV Mosby, 1979:55.
210. Benzing G, Schubert W, Hug G, Kaplan S. Simultaneous hypoglycemia and acute congestive heart failure. Circulation 1969;40:209.
211. Cabal LA, Devaskar U, Siassi B, Hodgman J, Emmanouilides G. Cardiogenic shock associated with perinatal asphyxia in preterm infants. J Pediatr 1980;96:705.
212. Weisel RD, Vito L, Dennia RC. Myocardial depression during sepsis. Am J Surg 1977;133:512.
213. Deitch EA, Bridges W, Ma L, Berg R, Specian RD, Granger DN. Hemorrhagic shock-induced bacterial translocation: the role of neutrophils and hydroxyl radicals. J Trauma 1990;30:942.
214. Wiles JB, Cerra FB, Siegel JH, Border JR. The systemic septic response: does the organism matter? Crit Care Med 1980;8:55.
215. Baker CH, Sutton ET, Zhou Z, Reynolds DG. Reduced microvascular adrenergic receptor activity due to opioids in endotoxin shock. Circ Shock 1990;32:101.
216. Goto M, Griffin AJ, Chiemmongkoltip P, Ohya N. β-Adrenergic drug therapy in newborn canine endotoxic shock. Circ Shock 1990; 32:123.

217. Astiz M, Rackow EC, Weil MH, Schumer W. Early impairment of oxidative metabolism and energy production in severe sepsis. Circ Shock 1988;26:311.
218. Bone RC, Fisher CJ, Clemmer TP, Slotman GJ, Metz CA, Balk RA, Methylprednisolone Severe Sepsis Study Group. A controlled clinical trial of high-dose methylprednisolone in the treatment of severe sepsis and septic shock. N Engl J Med 1987;317:653.
219. Wolfe WG, Sabiston DC. Pathogenesis, incidence and clinical significance of pulmonary embolism. Major Probl Clin Surg 1980;25:9.
220. Buck JR, Connors RH, Coon WW, Weintraub WH, Wesley JR, Coran AG. Pulmonary embolism in children. J Pediatr Surg 1981;16:385.
221. Jones RH, Sabiston DC. Pulmonary embolism in childhood. Monogr Surg Sci 1966;3:35.
222. Peltier LF. Fat embolism. An appraisal of the problem. Clin Orthop 1984;187:3.
223. Shapiro MP, Hayes JA. Fat embolism in sickle cell disease. Report of a case with brief review of the literature. Arch Intern Med 1984;144:181.
224. Sharma GVRK, Cella G, Parisi AF, Sasahara AA. Thrombolytic therapy. N Engl J Med 1982;306:1263.
225. Levin M, Kay JDS, Gould JD, et al. Hemorrhagic shock and encephalopathy: a new syndrome with a high mortality in young children. Lancet 1983;2:64.
226. Chaves-Carballo E, Montes JE, Nelson WB, Chrenka BA. Hemorrhagic shock and encephalopathy: clinical definition of a catastrophic syndrome in infants. Am J Dis Child 1990;144:1079.
227. Caspe WB, Nucci AT, Cho S. Extreme hyperpyrexia in childhood: presentation similar to hemorrhagic shock and encephalopathy. Clin Pediatr 1989;28:76.
228. Jordan SC, Ament ME. Pancreatitis in children and adolescents. J Pediatr 1977;91:211.
229. Warshaw AL, Fuller AF Jr. Specificity of increased renal clearance of amylase in diagnosis of acute pancreatitis. N Engl J Med 1975; 292:325.
230. Garcia R, Abarca S, Municio AM. Adrenal gland function in reversible endotoxic shock. Circ Shock 1990;30:365.
231. Togari H, Sugiyama S, Ogino T, Suzuki S, Ito T, Ichiki T, Kamiya K, Watanabe I, Ogawa Y, Wada Y, Takaoka T. Interactions of endotoxin with cortisol and acute phase proteins in septic shock neonates. Acta Paediatr Scand 1986;75:69.
232. Wetzel RC, Rogers MC. Pediatric monitoring. In: Shoemaker WC, Ayres S, Grenvik A, Holbrook PR, Thompson WL, eds. Textbook of critical care. Philadelphia: WB Saunders, chap 22, 1989:215.
233. Aynsley-Green A, Pickering D. Use of central and peripheral temperature measurements in care of critically ill children. Arch Dis Child 1974;49:477.
234. Saavedra JM, Harris GD, Li S, Finberg L. Capillary refilling (skin turgor) in the assessment of dehydration. Am J Dis Child 1991; 145:296.
235. Bergman KS, Harris BH. Arteriovenous pH difference—a new index of perfusion. J Pediatr Surg 1988;23:1190.
236. Sibbald WJ, Calvin J, Driedger AA. Right and left ventricular preload and diastolic ventricular compliance: implications for therapy in critically ill patients. In: Shoemaker WC, Thompson WL, eds. Critical care—state of the art. Fullerton, California: Society of Critical Care Medicine, 1982;III:III(F)1.
237. Guyton AC. The pumping ability of the heart as expressed by cardiac function curves. In: Guyton AC, Jones CE, Coleman TG, eds. Circulatory physiology: cardiac output and its regulation. Philadelphia: WB Saunders, 1973:147.
238. Todres ID, Crone RK, Rogers MC, Shannon DC. Swan-Ganz catheterization in the critically ill newborn. Crit Care Med 1979;7:330.
239. Stanger P, Heymann MA, Hoffman JI, Rudolph AM. Use of the Swan-Ganz catheter in cardiac catheterization of infants and children. Am Heart J 1972;83:749.
240. Shoemaker WC, Appel PL, Kram HB, Waxman K, Lee T-S. Prospective trial of supranormal values of survivors as therapeutic goals in high-risk surgical patients. Chest 1988;94:1176.
241. Villar J, Slutsky AS, Hew E, Aberman A. Oxygen transport and oxygen consumption in critically ill patients. Chest 1990;98:687.
242. Rah KH, Dunwiddie WC, Lower RR. A method for continuous post-operative measurement of mixed venous oxygen saturation in infants and children after open heart procedures. Anesth Analg 1984; 63:873.
243. Shoemaker WC. Shock states: pathophysiology, monitoring, outcome prediction, and therapy. In: Shoemaker WC, Ayres S, Grenvik A, Holbrook PR, Thompson WL, eds. Textbook of critical care. Philadelphia: WB Saunders, chap 109, 1989:977.
244. Mercier J-C, Beaufils F, Hartmann J-F, Azema D. Hemodynamic patterns of meningococcal shock in children. Crit Care Med 1988;16:27.
245. Simmon MA, Adcock EW, Bard H, Battaglia FC. Hypernatremia and intracranial hemorrhage in infants. N Engl J Med 1974;291:5.
246. Sorell M, Rosen JF. Ionized calcium: serum levels during symptomatic hypocalcemia. J Pediatr 1975;87:67.
247. Mattox KL, Bickell W, Pepe PE, Burch J, Feliciano D. Prospective MAST study in 911 patients. J Trauma 1989;29:1104.
248. Baxter CR. Problems and complications of burn shock resuscitation. Surg Clin North Am 1978;58:1313.
249. DeFelippi J, Timoner J, Velasco IT, Lopes OU, Silva MR. Treatment of refractory hypovolemic shock by 7.5% sodium chloride injections. Lancet 1980;2:1002.
250. Novak I, Konigova R, Dornak F. Fluid supply to burned children during the period of shock. Acta Chir Plast 1981;23:189.
251. Dell RB. Pathophysiology of dehydration. In: Winters RW, ed. The body fluids in pediatrics. Boston: Little, Brown, 1973:134.
252. Jelenko C, Williams JB, Wheeler ML, Callaway BD, Fackler UK, Albers CA, Barger AA. Studies in shock and resuscitation. 1. Use of a hypertonic, albumin-containing, fluid demand regimen (HALFD) in resuscitation. Crit Care Med 1979;7:157.
253. Landau EH, Gross D, Assalia A, Krausz MM. Treatment of uncontrolled hemorrhagic shock by hypertonic saline and external counterpressure. Ann Emerg Med 1989;18:1039.
254. Bitterman H, Triolo J, Lefer AM. Use of hypertonic saline in the treatment of hemorrhagic shock. Circ Shock 1987;21:271.
255. Gross D, Landau EH, Klin B, Krausz MM. Treatment of uncontrolled hemorrhagic shock with hypertonic saline solution. Surg Gynecol Obstet 1990;170:106.
256. Demling RH. Correlation of changes in body weights and pulmonary vascular pressures with lung water accumulation during fluid overload. Crit Care Med 1979;7:153.
257. Packman M, Rachow E. Optimum left heart filling pressure during fluid resuscitation of patients with hypovolemic and septic shock. Crit Care Med 1983;11:165.
258. Raphaely RC, Swedlow DB, Downes JJ, Bruce OA. Management of severe pediatric head trauma. Pediatr Clin North Am 1980;27:715.
259. Driscol AS, Gillette PC, McNamara DC. The use of dopamine in children. J Pediatr 1978;92:309.
260. Lang P, William RG, Norwood W, Castenena R. The hemodynamic effects of dopamine in infants with corrective cardiac surgery. J Pediatr 1980;96:630.
261. Perkin RM, Levin DC, Webb R, Aquino A, Reedy J. Dobutamine: a hemodynamic evaluation in children with shock. J Pediatr 1982; 10:977.
262. Seri I. Cardiovascular, renal and endocrine actions of dopamine in neonates and children. J Pediatr 1995;126(3):333.
263. MacConnell KL, McNay JL, Meyer MB, Goldberg LI. Dopamine in the treatment of hypotension and shock. N Engl J Med 1966;275:1399.
264. Ruiz CE, Weil MH, Carlson RW. Treatment of circulatory shock with dopamine. JAMA 1979;242:165.
265. Talley RC, Goldberg LI, Johnson CE, McNay JL. A hemodynamic comparison of dopamine and isoproterenol in shock. Circulation 1969;39:361.
266. Weil MH, Shubin H, Carlson R. Treatment of circulatory shock. JAMA 1975;231:1280.
267. Finley JP, Howman-Giles RG, Gilday DL, Rowe RD. Transient myocardial ischemia of the newborn infant demonstrated by thallium myocardial imaging. J Pediatr 1979;94:263.
268. Kurland G, Williams J, Lewiston NJ. Fatal myocardial toxicity during continuous infusion intravenous isoproterenol therapy of asthma. J Allergy Clin Immunol 1979;63:407.
269. Parmley WW, Tyberg JV. Determination of myocardial oxygen demand. Prog Cardiol 1976;5:9.
270. Sakamato T, Yamada T. Hemodynamic effects of dobutamine on patients following open heart surgery. Circulation 1977;55:525.
271. Tuttle R, Mills J. Dobutamine. Circ Res 1975;36:185.
272. Sonnenblock EH, Frishman WH, LeJemtel TH. Dobutamine. N Engl J Med 1979;300:17.
273. Stephens J, Ead H, Sourrell R. Hemodynamic effects of dobutamine with special reference to myocardial blood flow. Br Heart J 1979;42:43.
274. Loeb HS, Bredakis J, Gunnar RM. Superiority of dobutamine over dopamine for augmentation of cardiac output in patients with chronic low output cardiac failure. Circulation 1977;55:375.

275. Jewitt D, Birkhead J, Mitchell A, Dollery C. Clinical cardiovascular pharmacology of dobutamine. A selective inotropic catecholamine. Lancet 1974;2:363.
276. Ruiz CE, Weil MH, Carlson RW. Treatment of circulatory shock with dopamine. Studies on survival. JAMA 1979;242:165.
277. MacDonald RH, Goldberg LI, McNay JL, Tuttle EP. Effects of dopamine in man. J Clin Invest 1964;43:1116.
278. Schaer GL, Mitchell PF, Parrillo JE. Norepinephrine alone versus norepinephrine plus low dose dopamine. Enhanced renal blood flow with combination pressor therapy. Crit Care Med 1985;13:492.
279. Abboud FM. Shock. In: Wyngaarden JB, Smith LH, eds. Cecil textbook of medicine. Philadelphia: WB Saunders, 1982:155.
280. Alousi AA, Farah AE, Lesher GY, Opalka CJ Jr. Cardiotonic activity of amrinone—Win 40680 [5-amino-3,4′-bipyridin-6(1H)-one]. Circ Res 1979;45:666.
281. Braunwald E. A symposium: amrinone. Introduction. Am J Cardiol 1985;56:1B.
282. Benzing G, Helmsworth JA, Schreiber JT, Kaplan S. Nitroprusside and epinephrine for treatment of cardiac output in children after open heart surgery. Ann Thorac Surg 1979;27:523.
283. Applebaum A, Blackstone EH, Kouchoukos NT, Kirklin JW. Afterload reduction and cardiac output in infants early after intracardiac surgery. Am J Cardiol 1977;39:445.
284. Benson LN, Bohn D, Edmonds JF, Fortune RL, Price SA, Williams WG, Rowe RD. Nitroglycerin therapy in children with low cardiac index after heart surgery. Cardiovasc Med 1979;4:207.
285. Drummond WH, Gregory GA, Heymann MA, Phibbs RA. The independent effects of hyperventilation, tolazoline and dopamine on infants with persistent pulmonary hypertension. J Pediatr 1981;98:603.
286. Lock JE, Olley PM, Coceani F, Swyer PR, Rowe RD. Use of prostacyclin in persistent fetal circulation. Lancet 1979;2:1343.
287. Machiedo GW, Rush BF. Comparison of corticosteroids and prostaglandins in treatment of hemorrhagic shock. Ann Surg 1979;190:753.
288. Brigham KL, Borvers RE, McKeen CR. Methylprednisolone prevention of increased lung vascular permeability following endotoxemia in sheep. J Clin Invest 1981;67:1103.
289. Schumer W. Steroids in the treatment of clinical septic shock. Ann Surg 1976;184:333.
290. Smith JAR, Norman JN. Use of glucocorticoids in refractory shock. Surg Gynecol Obstet 1979;149:369.
291. Weitzman S, Berger S. Clinical trial design in studies of corticosteroids for bacterial infections. Ann Intern Med 1974;81:36.
292. Veterans Administration Systemic Sepsis Cooperative Study Group. Effect of high-dose glucocorticoid therapy on mortality in patients with clinical signs of systemic sepsis. N Engl J Med 1987;317:659.
293. Tiengo M. Naloxone in irreversible shock. Lancet 1980;2:690.
294. Furman WL, Menke JA, Barson WJ, Miller RR. Continuous naloxone infusion in two neonates with septic shock. J Pediatr 1984;105:649.
295. Ziegler EJ, Douglas H, Sherman JE, Davis CE, Braude AI. Treatment of *E. coli* and *Klebsiella* bacteremia in agranulocytic animals with antiserum to a UDP-Gal epimerase-deficient mutant. J Immunol 1973;111:433.
296. McCabe QR. Immunization with R mutants of *S. minnesota*. 1. Protection against challenge with heterologous Gram-negative bacilli. J Immunol 1972;108:601.
297. Ziegler EJ, McCutchan JA, Fierer J, Glauser MP, Sadoff JC, Douglas H, Braude AI. Treatment of Gram-negative bacteremia and shock with human antiserum to a mutant *Escherichia coli*. N Engl J Med 1982;307:1225.
298. Baumgartner JD, McCutchan JA, Van Melle G, Vogt M, Luethy R, Glauser MP, Ziegler EJ, Klauber EJ, Klauber MR, Muehlen E, Chiolero R, Geroulanos S. Prevention of Gram-negative shock and death in surgical patients by antibody to endotoxin core glycolipid. Lancet 1985;2:59.
299. Teng NNH, Kaplan HS, Herbert JM, Moore C, Douglas H, Wunderlich A, Braude AI. protection against Gram-negative bacteremia and endotoxemia with human monoclonal IgM antibodies. Proc Natl Acad Sci U S A 1985;82:1790.
300. Braude AI. Endotoxic immunity. Adv Intern Med 1980;26:427.
301. Ziegler EJ, Fisher Jr CJ, Sprung CL, Straube RC, Sadoff JC, Foulke GE, Wortel CH, Fink MP, Dellinger RP, Teng NNH, Allen IE, Berger HJ, Knatterud GL, LoBuglio AF, Smith CR, HA-1A Sepsis Study Group. Treatment of Gram-negative bacteremia and septic shock with HA-1A human monoclonal antibody against endotoxin: a randomized, double-blind, placebo-controlled trial. N Engl J Med 1991; 324:429.
302. Fisher Jr CJ, Zimmerman J, Khazaeli MB, Albertson TE, Dellinger RP, Panacek EA, Foulke GE, Dating C, Smith CR, LoBuglio AF. Initial evaluation of human monoclonal anti-lipid A antibody (HA-1A) in patients with sepsis syndrome. Crit Care Med 1990;18:1311.
303. Greenman RL, Schein RMH, Martin MA, et al: A controlled clinical trial of E5® murine monoclonal IgM antibody to endotoxin in the treatment of Gram-negative sepsis. JAMA 1991; 266:1097–1102.
304. Hinshaw LB, Tekamp-Olson P, Chang ACK, Lee PA, Taylor Jr FB, Murray CK, Peer GT, Emerson Jr TE, Passey RB, Kuo GC. Survival of primates in LD100 septic shock following therapy with antibody to tumor necrosis factor (TNFα). Circ Shock 1990;30:279.
305. Bone RC, Balk RA, Fein AM, Perl TM, Wenzel RP, Reines HD, Quenzer RW, Iberti TJ, Macintyre N, Schein RMH, The E5 Sepsis Study Group. A second large controlled clinical study of E5, a monoclonal antibody to endotoxin: Results of a prospective, multicenter, randomized, controlled trial. Crit Care Med 1995; 23:994–1006.
306. Wherry J, Wenzel R, Wunderink R, et al: Monoclonal antibody to tumor necrosis factor (TNF MAb): Multicenter efficacy and safety study in patients with sepsis syndrome. Abstract 696. Presented at the 33rd International Conference on Antimicrobial Agents and Chemotherapy, New Orleans, LA, October 17–20, 1993, p 246.
307. Wolff SM. The treatment of Gram-negative bacteremia and shock. N Engl J Med 1982;307:1267.
308. Colman RW, Robboy SJ, Minna JD. Disseminated intravascular coagulation: a reappraisal. Annu Rev Med 1979;30:359.
309. Sloder BE, Buchanan GR. The bleeding neonate. Pediatrics 1976;58:548.
310. Tobias JD, Haun SE, Helfaer M, Nichols DG. Use of continuous caudal block to relieve lower-extremity ischemia caused by vasculitis in a child with meningococcemia. J Pediatr 1989;115:1019.
311. Parker S, Carlon GC, Issacs M, Howland WS, Kahn RC. Dopamine administration in oliguria and oliguric renal failure. Crit Care Med 1981;9:630.
312. Ward ME, Roussos C. The respiratory muscles in shock: service or disservice? Intensive Crit Care Dig 1985;4:3.
313. Lyrene RK, Truog WE. Adult respiratory distress syndrome in a pediatric intensive care unit: predisposing conditions, clinical course and outcome. Pediatrics 1981;67:790.
314. Nussbaum E. Adult-type respiratory distress syndrome in children: experience with seven cases. Clin Pediatr (Phila) 1983;22:401.
315. Newth CJL. Recognition and management of respiratory failure. Pediatr Clin North Am 1979;26:617.
316. Buda AJ, Pinsky MR, Ingels NB, Daughters ST, Stinson EB, Alderman EL. Effects of intrathoracic pressure in left ventricular performance. N Engl J Med 1979;301:453.
317. McCune S, Short BL, Miller MK, Lotze A, Anderson KD. Extracorporeal membrane oxygenation therapy in neonates with septic shock. J Pediatr Surg 1990;25:479.
318. Kornhausen MS, Gilbert PL, Desai HJ, et al. The efficacy of extracorporeal membrane oxygenation (ECMO) in meconium aspiration syndrome and group B streptococcal pneumonia. Pediatr Res 1988; 23:414A.
319. Rogers AJ, Trento A, Siewers RD, Griffith BP, Hardesty RL, Pahl E, Beerman LB, Fricker FJ, Fischer DR. Extracorporeal membrane oxygenation for postcardiotomy cardiogenic shock in children. Ann Thorac Surg 1989;47:903.
320. Kanter KR, Pennington DG, Weber TR, Zambie MA, Braun P, Martychenko V. Extracorporeal membrane oxygenation for postoperative cardiac support in children. J Thorac Cardiovasc Surg 1987; 93:27.
321. Redmond CR, Graves ED, Falterman KW, Ochsner JL, Arensman RM. Extracorporeal membrane oxygenation for respiratory and cardiac failure in infants and children. J Thorac Cardiovasc Surg 1987; 93:199.
322. Reedy JE, Swartz MT, Raithel SC, Szukalski EA, Pennington DG. Mechanical cardiopulmonary support for refractory cardiogenic shock. Heart Lung 1990;19:514.
323. DiCarlo JV, Dudley TE, Sherbotie JR, Kaplan BS, Costarino AT. Continuous arteriovenous hemofiltration/dialysis improves pulmonary gas exchange in children with multiple organ system failure. Crit Care Med 1990;18:822.
324. Beller BK, Archer LT, Lane MM, Murray CK, Parker DE, Hinshaw LB. Invited commentary. Preventing versus delaying death in shock therapy studies: evaluating "survival". Circ Shock 1983;11:351.
325. vanLanschot JJB, Feenstra BWA, Vermeij CG, Bruining HA. Outcome prediction in critically ill patients by means of oxygen consumption in-

dex and simplified acute physiology score. Intensive Care Med 1988;14:44.
326. Bland B, Shoemaker WC, Shabot MM. Physiologic monitoring goals for the critically ill patient. Surg Gynecol Obstet 1978;147:833.
327. Shoemaker WC, Elwyn DH, Levin H, Rosen AL. Use of nonparametric analysis of cardiorespiratory variables as early predictors of death and survival in postoperative patients. J Surg Res 1974;17:301.
328. Shoemaker WC, Appel PL, Bland R, Hopkins JA, Chang P. Clinical trial of an algorithm for outcome prediction in acute circulatory failure. Crit Care Med 1982;10:390.
329. Shoemaker WC, Pierchala C, Chang P, State D. Prediction of outcome and severity of illness by analysis of the frequency distributions by cardiorespiratory variables. Crit Care Med 1977;5:82.
330. Shoemaker WC, Appel PL, Waxman K, Schwartz S, Chang P. Clinical trial of survivors' cardiorespiratory patterns as therapeutic goals in critically ill postoperative patients. Crit Care Med 1982;10:398.
331. Pollack MM, Fields AI, Ruttimann UE. Sequential cardiopulmonary variables of infants and children in septic shock. Crit Care Med 1984;12:554.
332. Pollack MM, Fields AI, Ruttimann UE. Distributions of cardiopulmonary variables in pediatric survivors and nonsurvivors of septic shock. Crit Care Med 1985;13:454.

Hemodynamic Monitoring Considerations in Pediatric Critical Care

17

Eugenie S. Heitmiller and Randall C. Wetzel

INTRODUCTION

Hemodynamic monitoring provides information concerning perfusion of the patient's vital organs, and is used to direct therapy and assess the results of interventions. Basic monitoring for all patients in the Pediatric Intensive Care Unit (PICU) includes electrocardiogram (ECG), respiratory rate, noninvasive blood pressure measurement, pulse oximetry, and temperature. Capnography should be used for all intubated patients. The use of invasive monitoring depends on the patient's clinical status and includes arterial blood pressure, central venous pressure (CVP), pulmonary artery pressure, and urinary output (bladder catheter). Left atrial catheters placed intraoperatively by the surgeon during cardiac surgery are used to monitor filling pressures in the PICU postoperatively. More extensive monitoring is becoming available as technology progresses with echocardiography, continuous mixed venous saturation, and continuous cardiac output monitoring.

The purpose and goals of hemodynamic monitoring are as follows:

1. Diagnostic: Continual monitoring of physiologic data is necessary for assessing the severity of and diagnosing the underlying condition that causes physiologic impairment.
2. Therapeutic: Hemodynamic monitoring is necessary to indicate the need for therapeutic intervention and to quantitate the response to that therapeutic intervention.
3. Prognostic: Trends in hemodynamic parameters can indicate the likelihood of survival and may be useful for prediction of outcomes.

4. Warning: The provision of alarm systems by alarms, tones, and visible signals is one of the most obvious uses of continuous, on-line hemodynamic monitoring.

Several considerations determine the type and amount of monitoring that a child requires. Clearly, when the appropriateness of monitoring technologies in the PICU is being assessed, it is helpful to determine the following factors:

1. Monitoring systems should have minimal risk for the patient.
2. Whenever possible, monitoring should be noninvasive and painless.
3. Monitoring should track the rapid changes in the parameters that are monitored.
4. Monitoring should provide continuous visual and/or auditory display of information for ready assessment of the child's condition.
5. The data provided should be specific, reproducible, and readily understood by the child's caretakers; it should also be relevant to the child's underlying condition.
6. A means of continuously recording the information graphically or storing it on a computer database, as well as keeping a bedside record, should be available. Trends contain much more information than individual data points.
7. Monitoring systems should require low maintenance.

Incredible advances in microcircuit computer technology and data retrieval have created an avalanche of monitoring systems available for the PICU. Computer applications are constantly being developed[1]. Newer monitors can measure multiple parameters, record them, produce graphic charts, and store the data. Frequently, they can manipulate the data and do all of this in color. The sophisticated technology and style of these monitoring systems should not detract critical care physicians from evaluating their patients with the goals outlined in this chapter. To make critical decisions involving the child's hemodynamic status, the clinician must have an understanding of the underlying physiology of the child and combine this with the knowledge of reliability and accuracy of information that can be obtained from the multiple monitoring modalities. Intensivists, through their understanding of critical illness and the ability to evaluate critically ill children, should control, rather than be controlled by, these monitoring technologies.

The intensivist who does not understand the basics behind advanced hemodynamic monitoring is doomed to be enslaved by it or to be merely a technician who manipulates numbers rather than a clinician who treats children. In critical situations, the clinician's ability to derive information by physical examination is quicker, more efficient, and more reliable and certainly should receive priority over more advanced monitoring modalities. Although advanced hemodynamic monitoring provides a necessary dimension to pediatric critical care, it should serve as an adjunct to, and not a replacement for, superb clinical skills.

PHYSICAL EXAMINATION

Repeated observation of critically ill children is the cornerstone of hemodynamic monitoring. Observation of the state of consciousness, the state of hydration, and the activity level of the child will provide valuable clues. Observation of rate and rhythm of respirations may indicate whether the child is acidotic or has underlying lung disease. Frequently, the first indication of hemodynamic compromise is rapid, shallow tachypnea. For example, respiratory alkalosis is frequently an initial finding in sepsis. Respiratory compensation from metabolic acidosis may first be apparent on physical examination, and in the hemodynamically compromised patient, air hunger may indicate profound acidosis.

Examining a child's microcirculation by examining his or her peripheral perfusion is critical. Firm pressure over a bony prominence such as the forehead, anterior tibia, or sternum for 5 seconds should be followed by loss of blanching and hyperemia within 3 to 5 seconds. More than 5 seconds is clearly prolonged. In patients whose capillary refill takes longer than 7 to 10 seconds, marked hemodynamic compromise is present. Changes in peripheral perfusion occur very rapidly with volume resuscitation.

Another means of examining the microcirculation or the adequacy of peripheral perfusion is by noting the core-peripheral temperature gradient[2,3]. A core-peripheral temperature gradient of more than 5° C indicates marked hypoperfusion. After cardiopulmonary bypass in children, the core temperature may be 37° C, but the periphery will not rewarm until perfusion is restored[4]. Great toe temperature after cardiac surgery correlates with peripheral perfusion[5]. During rewarming, as peripheral perfusion increases, the expected rise in toe temperature should be observed. If this ceases, or if the toe temperature falls while the core temperature remains the same, perfusion is inadequate. Routine monitoring of peripheral temperature and observations of the change in the core-peripheral temperature gradient provide an objective measure of perfusion and can be a more sensitive indicator of the adequacy of the peripheral circulation than blood pressure or heart rate. The exceptions to this are septic shock or the use of vasodilatory agents that cause peripheral vasodilation. These need to be considered in the setting of hemodynamic compromise. A well-perfused child with palpable pulses and warm extremities usually has an adequate cardiac output. Because the child's homeostatic mechanisms are able to sacrifice peripheral perfusion in preference to core perfusion in most settings, a warm periphery is assurance of adequate central perfusion in the absence of septic shock.

The presence and characteristics of the pulse should also be examined. Obviously, if peripheral pulses are not palpable, peripheral perfusion is inadequate and resuscitation is required. Pulse characteristics, apart from rate, should also be noticed. A low-volume rapid pulse is clearly a sign

Table 17.1. Age-Specific Heart Rates (Beats per Minute)

Age	*2%*	*Mean*	*98%*
<1 day	93	123	154
1–2 day	91	123	159
3–6 day	91	129	166
1–3 wk	107	148	182
1–2 mo	121	149	179
3–5 mo	106	141	186
6–11 mo	109	134	169
1–2 yr	89	119	151
3–4 yr	73	108	137
5–7 yr	65	100	133
8–11 yr	62	91	130
12–15 yr	60	85	119

Adapted from Davignon A, Rautaharju P, Boiselle E, et al. Normal ECG standards for infants and children. Pediatr Cardiol 1979;1:123–152.

of inadequate perfusion. The presence of pulsus paradoxus in the spontaneously breathing patient may indicate either severe obstructive lung disease or myocardial decompensation.

Changes in pulse volume in the mechanically ventilated patient are also important to assess. An increase in pulse volume with mechanical ventilation may indicate impaired contractility, while a decrease in pulse volume with a mechanical breath may indicate decreased preload (see Chapter 11). If these findings are severe enough to be palpable, they indicate an underlying compromised circulation. These findings may also be obvious on an arterial pressure waveform tracing.

Renal perfusion is a commonly assessed parameter of vital organ perfusion. Urine output less than 0.5 ml/kg/hr in a child with normal renal function indicates intravascular volume depletion or excessive antidiuretic hormone secretion. Normal urine output of 1 to 3 mg/kg/hr may be a better indicator of adequate intravascular volume than cardiac filling pressures.

Assessment of heart rate requires knowledge of the child's intrinsic basic heart rate and normal standards for age **(Table 17.1)**. Continuous display of heart rate and ECG and watching for changes in heart rate with therapeutic intervention are basic routine intensive care monitoring. The child is more dependent than the adult on heart rate for cardiac output. Due to the relatively small stroke volumes and the nature of the neonatal myocardium, changes in an infant's heart rate may have significant impact on cardiac output (Fig. 17.1). Examination of the intensity of the heart sounds, the presence of murmurs by auscultation, and the placement of the apical beat may indicate underlying cardiac disease and form a crucial part of hemodynamic monitoring.

ARTERIAL BLOOD PRESSURE

Pressure is defined as the force exerted per unit cross-sectional area of a surface. The systemic pressure is an indirect measurement of perfusion, as dictated by the equation:

$$\dot{Q} = \Delta P/R$$

where $\dot{Q}$ represents blood flow, Δ P is the arteriovenous pressure gradient, and R is the resistance to flow through the vascular structures. As seen in the discussion of pulmonary artery catheterization that follows, R does not necessarily remain constant; hence, a constant blood pressure does not always indicate constant blood flow. For example, hypovolemia can result in an R that may be dramatically increased, resulting in low tissue perfusion in spite of a "normal" blood pressure value.

The arterial pressure may be measured either indirectly, with a blood pressure cuff placed around an arm or leg, or directly, with a catheter in an artery that is connected to a pressure transducer. The noninvasive measurement of arterial blood pressure has the considerable advantage of being repeatable over a long period of time with minimal risk or discomfort to the patient. Normal arterial blood pressure varies with a child's age (Fig. 17.2).

Noninvasive Methods of Measurement

When the blood pressure is measured indirectly with a blood pressure cuff on the arm, pressure in the cuff is raised higher than the arterial pressure and is then lowered slowly until the return pulsation can be detected by palpation, a Doppler probe, or listening over the brachial artery to the Korotkoff's sounds (Fig. 17.3). When the first pulsation is palpated or the first sound is heard, the corresponding pressure on the manometer is the systolic pressure. The dia-

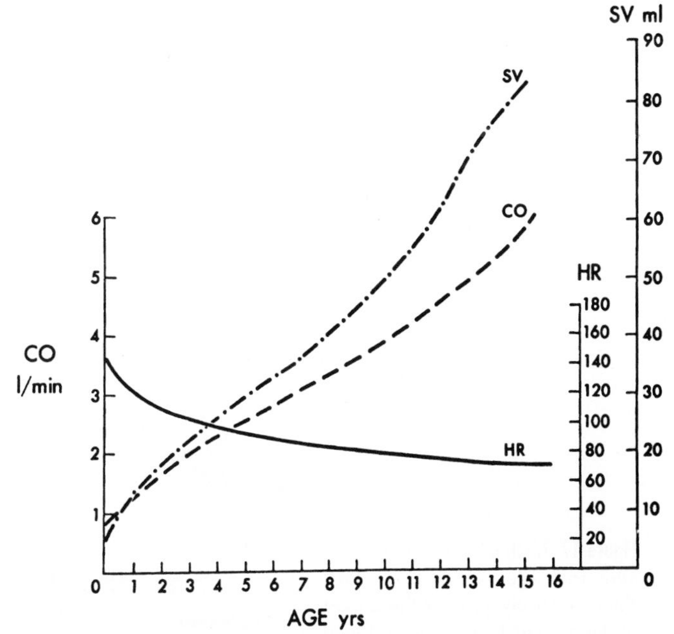

Figure 17.1. Changes in cardiac output *(CO)*, stroke volume *(SV)*, and heart rate *(HR)*, with age. (From Rudolph AM. Congenital diseases of the heart. Chicago: Year Book Medical Publishers. 1974:27.)

stolic pressure may be obtained with the auscultatory method and seems to correspond best to the fourth Korotkoff phase (when compared with direct measurements), where there is a muffling of a sound, although it is often taken at the fifth Korotkoff phase when the sound disappears. The sound may not disappear in states with low diastolic pressure, such as aortic insufficiency, and exercise is also reported to produce a low disappearance point[6].

Cuff size is particularly important in measuring blood pressure. If the cuff is too wide, it may produce readings that underestimate the blood pressure; if it is too narrow, the pressure may be overestimated because too short a length of artery is occluded (Fig. 17.4). The cuff should be about 20% wider than the diameter of the limb or, as the American Heart Association recommends, 40% the circumference of the midpoint of the limb[7]. Careful technique will permit measurement of systolic and diastolic pressure, with less than 15% error when this technique is compared with invasive techniques[8].

Cuff placement is also very important. An incorrectly placed cuff may give inaccurate information or may directly compress a nerve, resulting in a neuropathy (see Complications of Noninvasive Monitoring, below). In infants, a thigh cuff may be used if the upper arm cuff interferes with peripheral venous catheter flow or if descending aortic pressure is to be monitored, as in children having undergone an aortic coarctation repair. Systolic pressures in the thigh are normally higher than in the arm, but diastolic pressures are usually about the same[9].

The method of noninvasive blood pressure measurement using the detection of Korotkoff 's sounds with a stethoscope requires the cuff to be inflated above the systolic pressure and then deflated slowly (2 to 3 mm Hg per second). As the cuff pressure falls below the systolic pressure, the arterial wall is partially opened, allowing turbulent flow to pass. This turbulent flow is audible through the stethoscope. As the cuff pressure falls below diastolic pressure, the Korotkoff sounds disappear because the obstruction to flow by the cuff is eliminated. In some patients the sounds never totally disappear, and in these the diastolic pressure is taken as the point of fading or dampening of the sounds rather than their disappearance.

If a stethoscope is not available, or if the sounds are difficult to hear, as is often the case in infants, the systolic pressure may be determined using palpation, ultrasonic flow probes, or the pulse oximeter. Riva-Rocci described the palpation method in 1896, which involved placing a cuff around the arm, filling it with air until the radial pulse disappeared, and then slowly deflating the cuff until the pulse reappeared. The two readings were averaged, and the result was taken as the systolic pressure. Diastolic pressure cannot be determined by this method.

Ultrasonic blood flow detectors, also called Doppler flow probes, are very accurate in detecting the systolic pressure. The detector is placed over the artery distal to the blood pressure cuff, which is slowly deflated. The pressure at which the characteristic swishing sound of arterial blood flow is first heard is the systolic blood pressure. The pulse oximeter can be used to monitor systolic blood pressure in a similar fashion. As the cuff is slowly deflated, a sudden

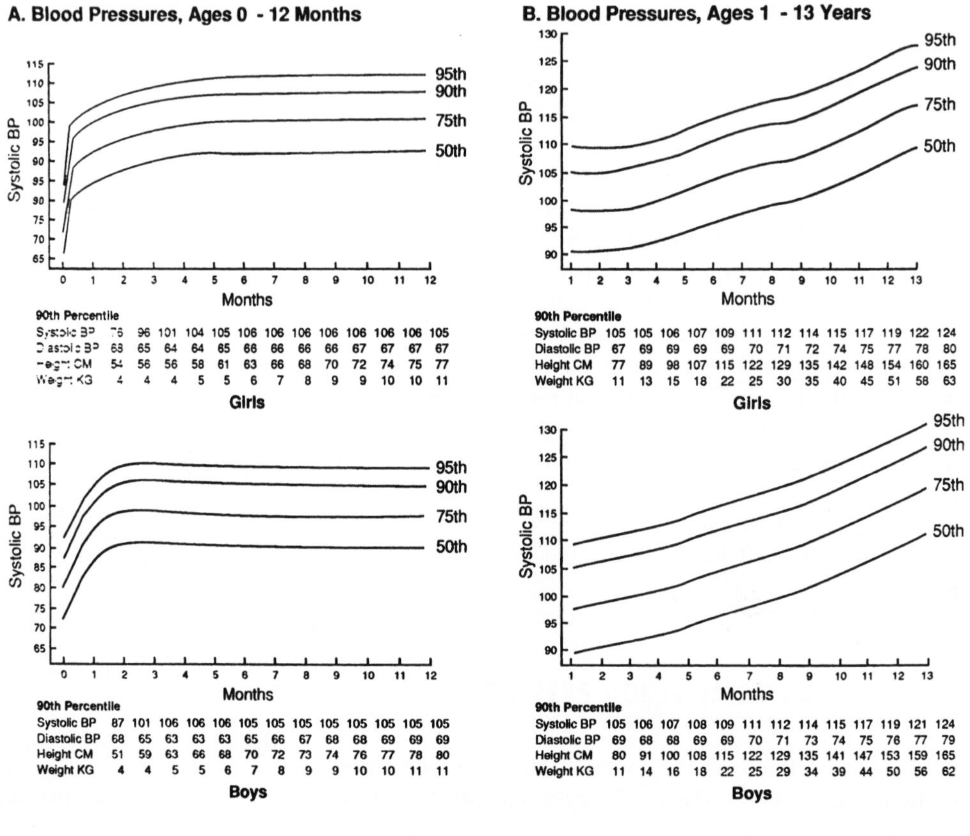

A. Girls, 90th Percentile (Months 0–12)

Systolic BP	76	96	101	104	105	106	106	106	106	106	106	106	105
Diastolic BP	68	65	64	64	65	66	66	66	66	67	67	67	67
Height CM	54	56	56	58	61	63	66	68	70	72	74	75	77
Weight KG	4	4	4	5	5	6	7	8	9	9	10	10	11

B. Girls, 90th Percentile (1–13)

Systolic BP	105	105	106	107	109	111	112	114	115	117	119	122	124
Diastolic BP	67	69	69	69	69	70	71	72	74	75	77	78	80
Height CM	77	89	98	107	115	122	129	135	142	148	154	160	165
Weight KG	11	13	15	18	22	25	30	35	40	45	51	58	63

A. Boys, 90th Percentile (Months 0–12)

Systolic BP	87	101	106	106	106	105	105	105	105	105	105	105	105
Diastolic BP	68	65	63	63	63	65	66	67	68	68	69	69	69
Height CM	51	59	63	66	68	70	72	73	74	76	77	78	80
Weight KG	4	4	5	5	6	7	8	9	9	10	10	11	11

B. Boys, 90th Percentile (1–13)

Systolic BP	105	106	107	108	109	111	112	114	115	117	119	121	124
Diastolic BP	69	68	68	69	69	70	71	73	74	75	76	77	79
Height CM	80	91	100	108	115	122	129	135	141	147	153	159	165
Weight KG	11	14	16	18	22	25	29	34	39	44	50	56	62

Figure 17.2. Changes in blood pressure with age. (From Horan MJ, Sinaiko AR: Synopsis of the Report of the Second Task Force on Blood Pressure Control in children, *Hypertension* 10:115–121, 1987; with permission.)

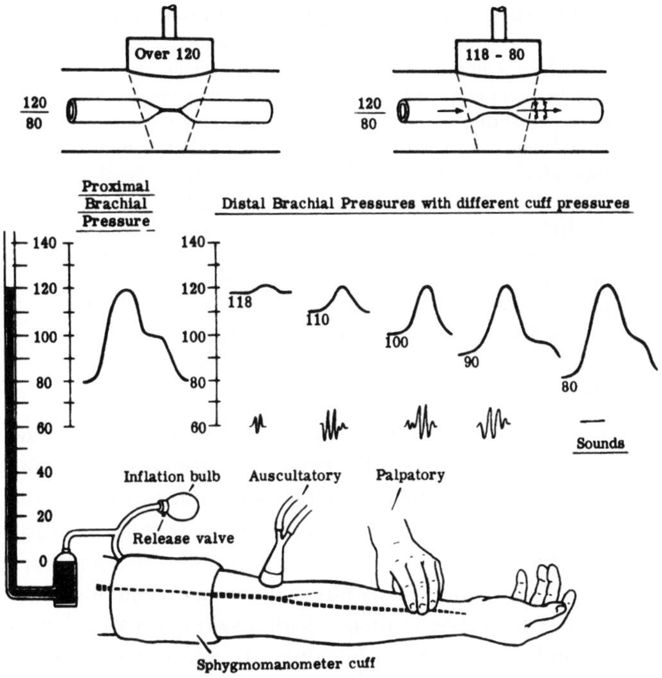

Figure 17.3. Method of obtaining blood pressure with a blood pressure cuff and Korotkoff sounds. (From Abel FL, McCutcheon EP. Cardiovascular function principles and applications. Boston: Little Brown, 1979:231.)

oscillation in the output of the blood flow detector of the pulse oximeter correlates with the systolic pressure. This method was found to correlate with Doppler ultrasonography ($r = 0.996$) and arterial cannulation ($r = 0.88$)[10]. However, movement of the detector or constriction of blood vessels beneath the detector can result in erroneous measurements.

How well do noninvasive methods correlate with invasive (direct) methods of blood pressure measurement? Many studies have been carried out to examine this question. It seems that the best correlation results when the systolic pressure, determined noninvasively by the Riva-Rocci palpation method, is compared with the pressure measured by the return-to-flow method with an arterial catheter. This is performed by placing a blood pressure cuff on the same arm as the radial artery catheter and inflating it until the pulsatile trace disappears. The air is then slowly released, and the pressure at which the first pulsatile trace reappears on the arterial tracing is the systolic blood pressure[11].

Automated Methods

The development of automated sphygmomanometers have largely replaced the use of the stethoscope and cuff in the operating room and PICU. The Dinamap was the first automated oscillometric device. The name stands for *d*evice for *i*ndirect *n*oninvasive *a*utomated *m*ean *a*rterial *p*ressure. This device, as well as models of other manufacturers, now measures heart rate and systolic, diastolic, and mean arterial blood pressure. Studies assessing the accuracy of the Dinamap have shown it to produce reliable trend information for infants and children during anesthesia[12,13]. Compared with direct intra-arterial pressure in patients, the Dinamap was found to have correlation coefficients of 0.95, 0.85, and 0.87 for systolic, diastolic, and mean arterial pressures (MAPs), respectively[13]. The diastolic pressure was consistently higher than intra-arterial values. It should be remembered that initially the cuff is automatically inflated to a pressure of 160 mm Hg for the adult cuff and 130 mm Hg for the pediatric cuff, with subsequent inflations to 35 mm Hg above the previous systolic pressure. If there are large changes in blood pressure over a short time, the readings may not be accurate, and the blood pressure in patients with severe arrhythmias may not be accurately measured.

Measurement of blood pressure using finger cuffs has become popular in recent years. One method is to use a neonatal oscillometric cuff placed around the finger of older children and young adults (aged 7 to 20 years). When com-

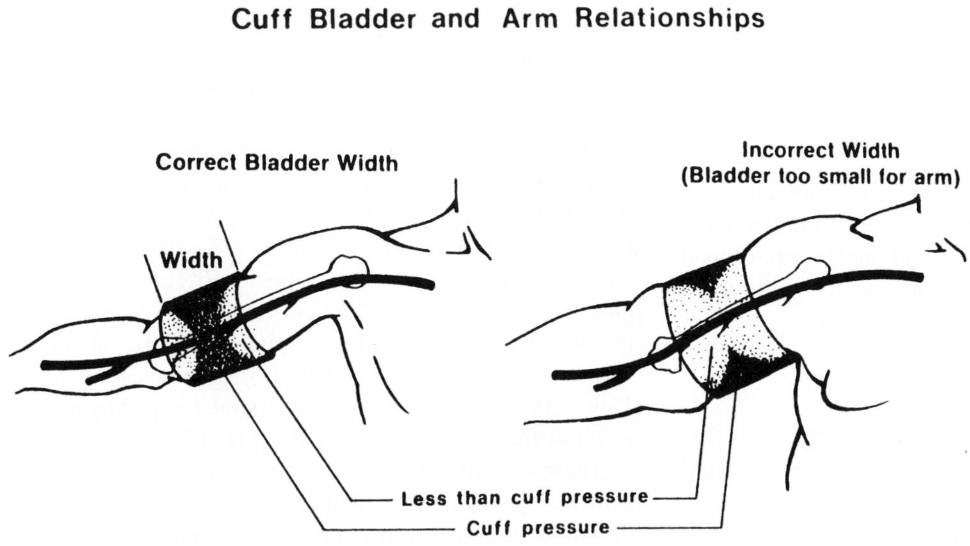

Figure 17.4. Bladder and cuff. (From Kirkendall W, Feinleib M, Freis E, et al. Recommendations for human blood pressure determination by sphygmomanometers. Subcommitee of the AHA Postgraduate Education Committee. Circulation 1980; 62:1147A)

pared with arm cuffs, the oscillometric forefinger cuffs correlated well with systolic blood pressure ($r = 0.85$), but not so well with the mean or diastolic pressure[14].

A second method using noninvasive, nonocclusive blood pressure measurement was described by Peñaz, whereby arterial pressure can be measured continuously by unloading the arterial wall of the finger and generating an arterial waveform[15]. The first commercially marketed device to use this method is Finapres (Ohmeda, Englewood, Colorado); it consists of a finger pressure cuff and infrared photoplethysmograph. The Finapres device correlates with arterial pressure measured by the auscultatory method and direct intra-arterial pressure measurement[16]. Although the finger cuff is continuously inflated at MAP, it has been used for prolonged periods without adverse sequelae[17]. Another device, developed by Wong and coworkers in Canada[18], is a pulse monitor, which operates on the principle of a finger plethysmograph. It was found to be as accurate as the Doppler ultrasound technique in estimating systolic blood pressure, and it has the advantage of less critical sensor positioning and not being subject to electric interference.

The use of arterial tonometry as an indirect method of beat-to-beat blood pressure measurement has been studied by several investigators over the past 5 years. The sensors initially did not perform as well in children as in adults[19]. A new sensor has been developed to improve performance and has been found to provide accurate, continuous, noninvasive measurement of arterial blood pressure in children aged 1 to 6 years. However, measurements could not be made in approximately 30% of the patients studied because of insufficient pulse contour[20].

Complications of Noninvasive Monitoring

Automated methods of noninvasive blood pressure monitoring have become standard practice in the operating room and PICU because they are relatively safe, generally reliable, and easy to use. However, if the cuff is inflated too frequently or for a prolonged time, skin avulsion and venostasis can result[21–23]. In addition, ulnar neuropathies have been reported to result from a poorly positioned cuff[24,25].

Invasive Methods of Blood Pressure Measurement

Arterial cannulation for direct blood pressure measurement is used to continuously monitor arterial pressure, provide access for arterial blood sampling, and enable rapid blood withdrawal in cases in which cardiac output will be measured by the indocyanine green dye technique.

Catheter-Manometer Systems

Sir William Harvey (1578—1657) pioneered the work that initiated cardiovascular physiology. In 1733, the Reverend Stephen Hales (1677—1761) became the first person to measure animal blood pressure directly[26]:

> In December I caused a mare to be tied down alive on her back, she was fourteen hands high, and about 14 years of age, had a fistula on her withers, was neither very lean, nor yet lusty. Having laid open the left crural artery about 3 inches from her belly, I inserted into it a brass pipe whose bore was one sixth of an inch in diameter; and to that, by means of another brass pipe which was fitly adapted to it, I fixed a glass tube of nearly the same diameter, which was 9 feet in length. Then untying the ligature on the artery, the blood rose in the tube 8 feet 3 inches perpendicular above the left of the left ventricle of the heart. But it did not attain to its full height at once; it rushed up about half way an instant, and afterwards gradually at each use, twelve, eight, six, four, two and sometimes one inch. When it was at its full height, it would rise and fall at and after each pulse, 2, 3, or 4 inches.

The theory of manometer design for recording pulsatile pressure has changed little since its introduction by Otto Frank in 1903[27], who used large-bore catheters connected to rubber membrane manometers. The advent of the early electronics revolution in the 1940s allowed the miniaturization of pressure manometers and an improvement in their frequency response. Catheters with smaller bores were then used, and their safety in humans was established. For accurate measurement of blood pressure, the catheter-manometer system must precisely reproduce the arterial pressure waveform. Therefore, the system must have a flat frequency response over the range of frequencies contained in the waveform. How does one determine the bandwidth needs of the system? The Fourier series is applicable to the analysis of complex periodic biologic waveforms with a period T by representing them as a sum of simple sinusoids (sine and cosine waves) of the form[28]:

$$f(x) = Ao + An[\cos(2nx/T)] + Bn[\sin(2nx/T)]$$

where Ao, An, and Bn are the Fourier coefficients, which can be determined by the Euler formulae (Fig. 17.5):

$$Ao = 1/T[f(x)dx]$$

$$An = 2/T[f(x)\cos(2n/T)xdx]$$

$$Bn = 3/T[f(x)\sin(2n/T)xdx]$$

Nichols et al.[27] and Patel et al.[30] have demonstrated that the magnitude of the harmonic components of the pressure tracing rapidly decreases with the harmonic number. The first 10 harmonics contain 99.5% of the information needed to reproduce the arterial curve, and little additional information is supplied by extending the frequency response (Fig. 17.6). That is, for heart rates up to 240 beats/min (4 Hz), an accurate waveform is achieved with a system that has a flat frequency response up to 40 Hz with minimal phase lag. Gersh et al.[31], however, demonstrated that to measure reliably the first-order time derivative of the left ventricular pressure curve (dP/dT), harmonics up to the 15th to the 20th were significant, thereby requiring a bandwidth of from 0 to at least 90 Hz (Fig. 17.7).

These requirements are easily met by the modern catheter-tip manometers that have resonant frequencies in the kilohertz range with unmeasurable phase lag[29]. There

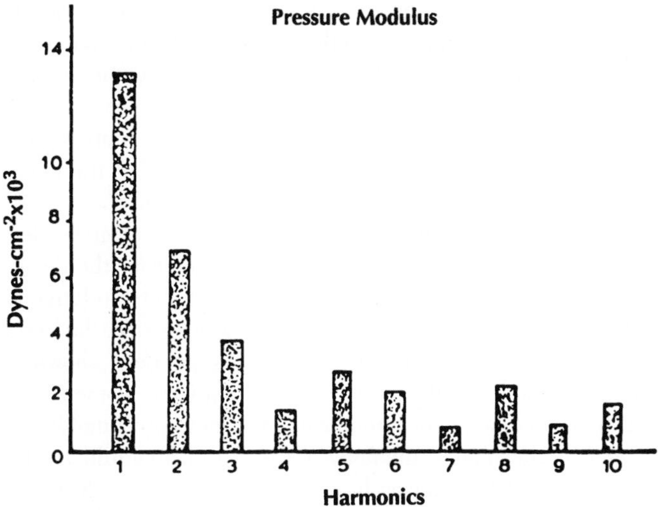

Figure 17.5. Fourier or harmonic components (N = 10) of a high-fidelity recording of an ascending aortic pressure wave in a dog. (From Katona Z, Bolvary G. Automatic sphygmomanometer. Adv Cardiovasc Phys 1983;5:148.)

are basically four types of catheter-tip manometers: electrolytic, inductance, optical, and strain gauge. Their descriptions can be found elsewhere[27]. In contrast to the catheter-tip manometers, the fluid-filled catheter-manometer systems are more commonly used in clinical practice because of their greater flexibility, durability, and ease of handling under sterile conditions. However, their bandwidth is more severely restricted (20 to 40 Hz), which increases the probability of waveform distortion. Inaccuracies can also be introduced by the presence of entrapped air bubbles, catheter bores, and tubing length. (Small air bubbles cause an overestimation of blood pressure values, while large bubbles lead to underestimation. Small bores may produce an underestimation, and excessive lengths dampen the arterial waveforms, causing an underestimation.) These problems can be minimized by continuous flushing of the system and placement of the manometer as close to the patient as possible. One hundred cm 5-, 6-, and 7-French catheters can produce frequency responses of up to 75 Hz with a 5% flat frequency response up to 25 Hz[27]. These provide adequate response for physiologic pressure monitoring (Fig. 17.7).

Part of the increased performance is achieved by the equalization of the catheter-manometer system by use of a second-order electrical circuit[32]. Basically, the frequency spectrum is divided into several bands by means of bank filters. The circuit automatically determines the resonance frequency of the system (which gives a false elevation of the signal amplitude at the area of the spectrum) by determining the highest output voltage in the parallel series of filters. A compensation network is then tuned to this filter set and applies a negative feedback to the operational amplifier, thus providing a flat response in the region of the resonance frequency.

When direct and indirect methods of measuring blood pressure are compared, direct measurements usually average 5 to 20 mm Hg higher than indirect measurements. Several explanations attribute these discrepancies to changes in the pulse waveform as it travels toward the periphery[33]. There are different rates of transmission of the various parts of the wave. The standing wave phenomenon within vessels

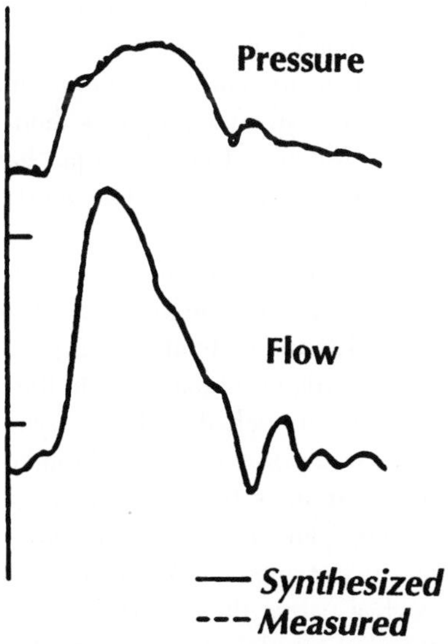

Figure 17.6. Resynthesis of the pressure and flow curves by 10 harmonic components recorded in the dog descending aorta. Sampling rate was 100/sec. (From Katona G, Bolvary G. Automatic sphygmomanometer. Adv Cardiovasc Phys 1983;5:147.)

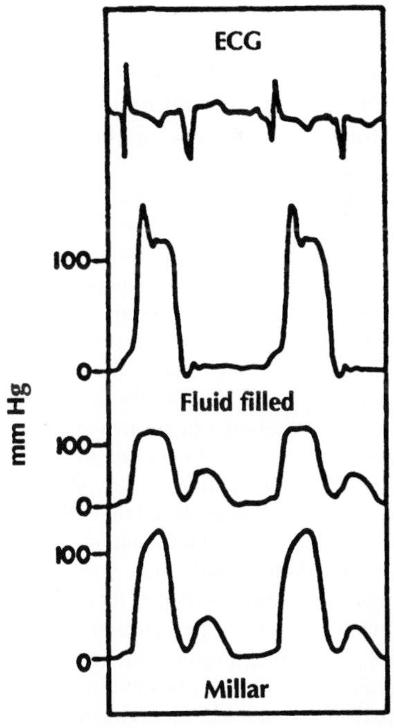

Figure 17.7. Simultaneous left ventricular pressures recorded in a dog with two fluid-filled catheter-manometer systems and a Millar catheter-tip transducer during premature ventricular contractions (PVCs). The response of the system used to record the *upper pressure tracing* was too slow (resonance frequency 8 Hz) to detect the PVC values. This pressure tracing also shows a large overshoot in early systole. The PVC values, however, were detected with the system with a higher resonance frequency (42 Hz; *middle tracing*) and the Millar-tip transducer *(lower tracing)*. (From Katona Z, Bolvary G. Automatic sphygmomanometer. Adv Cardiovasc Phys 1983;5:156.)

can result in reinforcement and cancellation of wave components. Changes in the elasticity of the vessel walls occur. The vessels may distort the various wave components. Part of the kinetic energy of the pulse wave may be converted to hydrostatic pressure. Last but not least, there may be changes within the catheter-manometer system itself.

Other factors leading to inconsistencies between direct and indirect measurements of blood pressure include the use of an oversized cuff, which would give lower blood pressure values by sphygmomanometry, and improper calibration of the transducer. If indirect measurements are higher than direct pressures, the discrepancies are almost always due to calibration or other technical problems. Variations of 20 to 30 mm Hg usually occur in the patient with shock or hypothermia, where the indirect measurements will falsely read lower. Other considerations include (a) peripheral vascular disease, in which direct pressures recorded distally may be significantly lower than proximal readings with the cuff, and (b) the electronic monitors, whereby the highest pressure is read every 3 to 7 seconds, whereas with use of the cuff method the pressure is read beat to beat[33]. Disparities of greater than 30 mm Hg are almost always due to systolic overshoot by the catheter-manometer system. This can occur when the resonance frequency of the system is low (within the bandwidth of the pressure wave), the heart rate is high (thereby causing the harmonic components of the pressure wave to approach the resonance frequency of the system), and the rate of rise of dP/dT is excessively steep. To minimize these problems, the shortest possible length of the stiffest plastic tubing available should be used with care in preventing the entrapment of air bubbles and the possible formation of clots in the line. The following guidelines are recommended[33]:

> Allow the transducer and monitor to warm up at least 10 minutes before calibration and testing. The effects of heating within equipment on the various electronic components can cause initial fluctuations in measured pressure values. Mechanically zero the transducer by positioning it at the same level as the heart and opening the distal end of the connector tubing to the atmosphere. Purge all air from the system. Use the shortest length of very stiff tubing extension, and minimize the number of stopcock connectors. Check all fittings for tightness. Electrically zero and then calibrate the system with a mercury manometer. Avoid withdrawing blood the full length of the system to minimize the risk of clot formation. This consideration is especially important in neonates, since the volume withdrawn is a more significant portion of their total blood volume. Use a continuous infusion of heparinized (0.25 units heparin/ml) saline solution to help prevent clot formation. Place extension tubing near the patient to prevent a pulsating line. Whenever the patient is moved, recheck the mechanical and electrical zero of the system and recalibrate if necessary. Avoid making changes to the amplifier except at the time of calibration. The electrical and mechanical zeroes should be frequent, once in an 8-hour shift and should be recalibrated if necessary.

Catheters

The most commonly used technique for peripheral artery catheterization is the catheter-over-needle, first describe by Barr in 1961[34]. Catheters are manufactured from a variety of materials, including Teflon, polypropylene, polyvinyl chloride, and polyethylene. Polypropylene catheters are stiffer and are more prone to thrombus formation in radial arteries than Teflon catheters[35–38]. Heparin impregnation of catheters may be good for short-term use, but the heparin is lost from the catheter in 24 to 48 hours[39].

The size of the catheter is important for optimal monitoring and patient safety. An important factor for the development of thrombosis is the size of the catheter relative to the size of the vessel; the smaller the catheter size, the lower is the incidence of thrombosis[40]. This has been shown in adults, whereby with the same-sized catheter, women have a higher incidence of thrombosis than men, presumably because of the smaller diameter of the vessel. In adults a 30% incidence of thrombosis has been reported when 20-gauge catheters are left in for 7 to 10 days[41,42]. In newborns the incidence of radial artery occlusion has been reported to be as high as 72% when 22-gauge catheters are in place for 10 days[43]. A 24-gauge catheter can be used in small infants to monitor blood pressure but may not be reliable for withdrawing blood samples.

The small-sized catheters used in children also tend to kink more easily than the larger catheters used in adults. A study in adults showed that 20% of 20-gauge catheters kink within 24 hours of insertion[40]. Methods of unkinking a catheter include rotating it through a 180-degree arc or applying distal traction and withdrawing it slightly[44]. The often-used method of hyperextending the wrist may be associated with median nerve injury[44].

Arterial Cannulation

The major uses for arterial cannulation are to monitor arterial pressure continuously, to sample arterial blood with minimal pain and discomfort to the patient without disturbing the steady-state measurements, and to provide access for rapid blood withdrawal. In certain settings, it is also used to measure cardiac output and shunts via the indocyanine green dye technique, although the use of the hemodilution cardiac output technique has limited the use of arterial cannulation for cardiac output determination.

The requirements for use of any artery for direct pressure measurements are that the vessel be large enough to reflect accurately the true systemic blood pressure and that there be sufficient collateral blood flow to the distal tissues perfused by the vessel such that these tissues remain viable if the cannulated vessel becomes thrombosed. Another important consideration is the effect of the anatomic site on the measured oxygen values of blood sampling. This becomes critical in patients with right-to-left extracardiac shunting through a patent ductus arteriosus. In this situation, the right radial arterial blood represents blood oxygen saturation to the brain, since the right subclavian, right common, and left common carotid arteries originate from the aorta, proximal to the ductus arteriosus. The left subclavian artery and the descending aorta represent postductal blood oxygen saturation, which will be lower than that going to the brain. Hence, reliance on the oxygen values from the left arm and both lower extremities will result in unnecessarily vigorous medical treatment to raise the PO_2, the patient's brain oxygen delivery is adequate. Finally, when an upper extremity is used, the nondominant side is preferable, in the unlikely event that there is a complication.

Radial Artery Cannulation

The radial artery is the most frequently used site for arterial cannulation because it is easy to access and there is a very low complication rate at this site when the catheter is properly inserted and maintained. The decision to place the radial artery catheter on the right or left depends on whether the blood flow to the arm is expected to be interrupted. For example, the arterial catheter is placed in the right arm if the left subclavian artery is to be used as a flap for aortic coarctation repair. The arterial catheter is placed in the left arm if the right subclavian artery is to be used for an arterial-to-pulmonary shunt. As stated above, in patients with right-to-left shunting through a patent ductus arteriosus, the right radial artery represents the blood oxygen saturation and pressure to the brain, since the right subclavian and common carotid arteries arise from the aorta proximal to the ductus arteriosus. In this case, a right artery catheter would be indicated.

Collateral blood flow to the hand may be assessed by Allen's test before inserting a catheter(45). This is performed in older children by applying pressure over the area of the radial and ulnar arteries at the wrist and having the patient squeeze the hand several times until the blood is exsanguinated. The pressure is then released from the ulnar artery, and the time until the nail bed capillaries refill is measured. Collateral flow is considered normal if the refill time is 5 seconds(40,46). In young children and infants, this test requires two persons, one to compress the arteries and one to compress the patient's hand approximately 10 times. When the ulnar compression is released, normal color should appear in the hand within 5 seconds. When performing the test, the patient's hand should be warm; if it is not, it should be immersed in warm water. A 6 to 15 second delay suggests slowed filling, while greater than a 15-second delay indicates no ulnar collateral blood flow. To test radial arterial blood flow, repeat the above test, but release pressure over the radial artery. Despite its widespread use, the predictive value of Allen's test is questionable. Marshall and associates(47) reported a large series of children who underwent arterial catheterization without a preliminary Allen's test and had no complications. On the other hand, Mangano and Hickey(48) reported a case of hand ischemia requiring amputation in a patient with normal Allen's test results. In addition to Allen's test, collateral blood flow to the hand can be assessed by Doppler ultrasonography (probe placed over the lateral aspect of the superficial palmar arch) and pulse oximetry (probe placed on the thumb)(49,50).

The radial artery of the nondominant arm is located at the wrist within the groove bounded laterally by the distal radius and medially by the tendon of the flexor carpi radialis. The equipment needed includes the following: First, one must have 20-, 22-, or 24-gauge Teflon-coated catheter-over-needles 1 to 2 inches in length; the catheter gauge is determined by the age and size of the patient, with recommended sizes being 22 to 24 gauge for neonates and small infants, 22 gauge for larger infants and children and 20 gauge for children over 40 kg or 12 years of age. A syringe with heparinized solution (125 units of heparin in 500 ml of 0.9% saline or 5% dextrose-water) is connected to a stopcock with a short extension tube. The remaining items are a short arm board, gauze pads, adhesive tape, iodine and alcohol solutions, a 16-gauge straight needle, a 0.5% lidocaine solution, and sterile gloves. A Doppler flow detector may be used to locate arteries that are difficult to palpate(51).

The distal forearm and hand should be secured onto the arm board in a semidorsiflexed position, with gauze pads placed under the wrist for support(52). Palpate the artery and visualize its position. Wash the skin surface with an iodine solution (assuming no allergy to topical iodine), allow to dry, and wipe clean with alcohol. Drape the field with sterile towels. Infiltrate the skin over and to the sides of the artery with 0.5% lidocaine for local anesthesia, using a 25-gauge needle and small syringe. Make a skin puncture with the 16-gauge needle at the planned site of catheter insertion, taking care to do so superficially so as not to puncture the artery accidentally. This will facilitate catheter entry and minimize skin drag.

Cannulation can then be performed in one of two ways (Fig. 17.8). The transfixation method is accomplished by inserting the catheter-over-needle through the skin puncture site at a 45-degree angle with respect to the skin, aiming centrally. Continue insertion until blood is seen in the hub (the needle is now within the vessel lumen), and insert a short distance further until blood return stops, indicating posterior vessel wall puncture. Sometimes, blood return is not seen because smaller catheters were used, i.e., 22 to 24 gauge, or because the patient's artery is very small, especially in neonates and young children. It is better to continue with the following instructions than to pull the needle and the catheter out for another try because of the possibility of already having punctured the artery. Carefully, remove the catheter at a 30-degree angle with respect to the skin until blood return is seen. At that point, the catheter tip is now within the lumen. Advance the catheter slowly up to the hub, recheck for blood flow, and attach the extension tubing, checking for tightness of fittings, and withdraw blood to confirm successful cannulation. Always try to avoid intra-arterial injection of air bubbles. If no blood return is seen, remove the catheter and reinsert the needle. Follow the above instructions again.

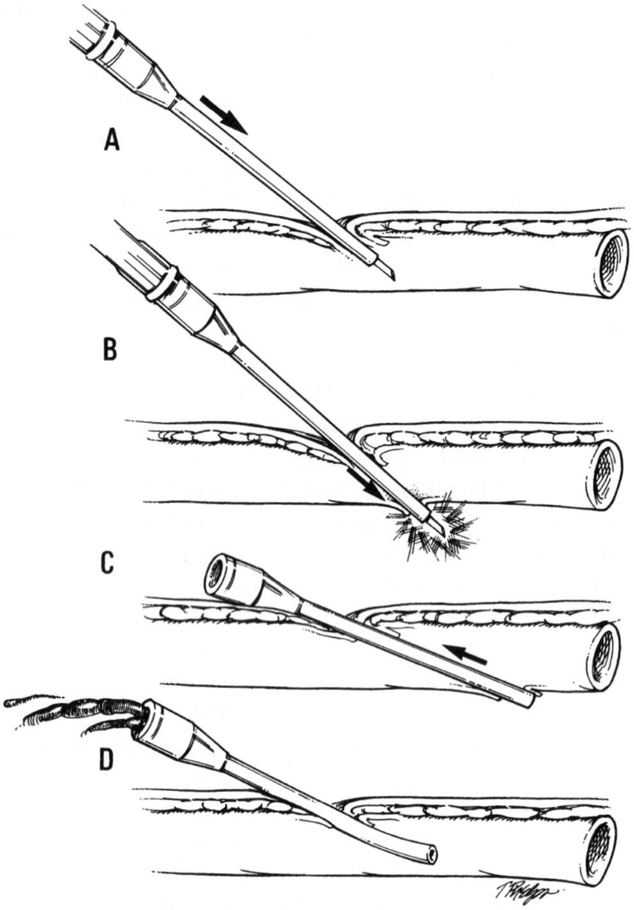

Figure 17.8. Radial artery cannulation. the catheter-over-needle unit is inserted into the artery **(A).** When arterial blood flow is seen in the needle hub, the catheter may be advanced over the needle into the artery. Another technique is to further advance the catheter and needle until blood flow ceases, thereby transfixing the artery **(B),** and then remove the needle **(C)** and withdraw the catheter until blood flow is seen. The catheter is then advanced into the artery **(D).**

The direct-threading technique involves the insertion of the catheter-over-needle through the skin at a 30-degree angle. As soon as blood is seen in the hub, the catheter is inserted into the lumen over the needle, with care taken not to move the needle. The catheter is then secured with skin sutures, a clear occlusive dressing such as Uniflex® or Op-Site® (Smith & Nephew United, Inc., Largo, Florida), or well-applied strips of adhesive tape.

Surgical cut-down may be required in patients who have undergone repeated arterial catheterizations or multiple failures of the percutaneous technique. The anatomic landmarks used for this technique are shown in Figure 17.9.

Alternative Sites for Arterial Catheterization

Other sites for arterial cannulation include the ulnar, femoral, axillary, dorsalis pedis, and posterior tibial arteries. The ulnar artery may be used if the radial artery cannot be cannulated and collateral flow is still present. The femoral artery is a frequently used cannulation site in children and provides reliable blood pressure measurements. Its use may be limited in patients who have had multiple cardiac catheterizations via the femoral vessels. Catheterization of both the femoral artery and vein in the same extremity may lead to limb ischemia in patients likely to experience low flow states; infants appear to be at greatest risk in this regard. The axillary artery also provides a centrally located catheter, but because of its position close to the aortic arch, there is an increased risk of cerebral embolus from air or debris when the catheter is flushed[53]; however, embolus can occur with arterial cannulation at any site. The femoral and axillary arteries are both most reliably cannulated with the Seldinger technique.

DORSALIS PEDIS AND POSTERIOR TIBIAL ARTERIES. The dorsalis pedis and posterior tibial arteries are the second choice for arterial cannulation in the PICU. They are the extensions of the anterior and posterior tibial arteries. The dorsalis pedis courses superficially along the dorsum of the foot, lateral to the extensor hallucis longus. The posterior tibial is located medially behind the malleolus[54]. Collateral blood flow to the foot is supplied by both the anterior and posterior tibial arteries. Collateral circulation can be tested in a manner analogous to the modified Allen test[55]. Make sure that the foot is warm—if it is not, immerse it in warm water. Occlude the dorsalis pedis artery. Blanch the great toenail by pressing hard on it for several seconds. Release the pressure and note the color change of the nail. Rapid filling indicates good collateral circulation. The incidence of thrombosis noted with use of this technique is about 7%[56]. The risk factors for infection are the same as those for radial artery cannulation.

AXILLARY ARTERY. The axillary artery is a large branch from the subclavian artery at the base of the neck, near the lateral aspects of the first thoracic rib; it enters the arm as the brachial artery. It has a rich collateral circulation via the thyrocervical trunk of the subclavian artery and the subscapular artery, which arises from the axillary artery distally. Therefore, axillary artery occlusion

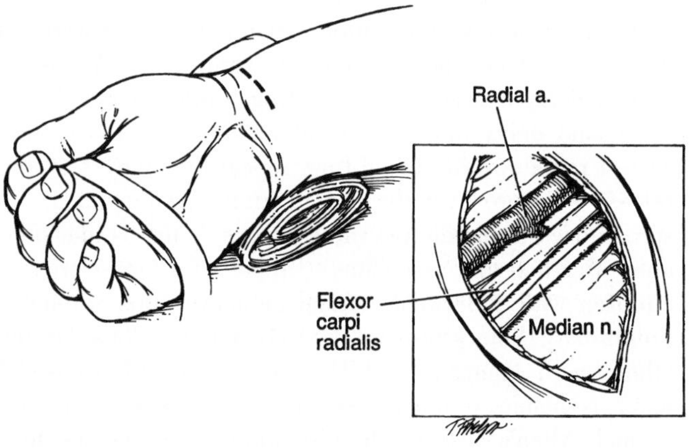

Figure 17.9. Surgical cut-down for radial artery cannulation.

does not usually lead to impaired circulation of the arm[57]. Although it has frequently not been used because of potential complications such as embolism and because of theoretical concerns of brachial plexus injury, it is used in the pediatric population[58]. Cantwell et al.[59] showed no permanent complications occurred from axillary artery cannulation, with catheters in place from 24 hours to 24 days. Equipment needed to insert an axillary artery catheter depends on whether the Seldinger technique or the catheter-over-needle method is used. For the former, a long, 20-gauge Teflon catheter (16 cm for adults) with flexible guide wire and a 3-inch, 20-gauge needle are required. For the latter, a 20-gauge, 3-inch catheter-over-needle is needed. Other equipment is the same as that used for radial artery cannulation.

The technique is as follows: Immobilize the hyperabducted and supinated arm. Identify the axillary artery by palpation. Shave the skin and clean the axilla with iodine and alcohol solutions. Infiltrate the skin with lidocaine for local anesthesia. Insert a long needle into the axilla as proximal as possible. If you are using the Seldinger technique, as soon as blood flow is freely obtained, insert a guide wire into the arterial lumen and remove the needle. If the catheter-over-needle method is used, insert it until free blood return occurs, and then advance it a little further until it stops, indicating posterior wall puncture. Remove the needle and slowly withdraw the catheter until blood flows back freely (indicating the tip is within the lumen), then advance the catheter into the artery. If you are unsuccessful after three attempts, try another site. Secure the catheter with skin sutures and apply a sterile dressing. Observe closely for the development of hematoma.

Thrombosis is seldom seen from axillary cannulation because of the excellent collateral blood flow. However, embolism is of greater concern because of the artery's proximity to the circulation of the aortic arch, and compulsive care must be given so as not to vigorously flush the system. This may have more bearing on the right axillary artery, which branches off the brachiocephalic artery. The brachiocephalic artery also gives rise to the right internal and external carotids. Theoretically, neurologic injury in the distal arm may occur as the result of direct injury from attempted punctures or compression injury by hematoma formation to the brachial plexus that courses with the axillary artery and vein to form a neurovascular bundle.

FEMORAL ARTERY. The femoral artery arises from the external iliac artery below the inguinal ligament. It forms the midpoint of a line drawn from the symphysis pubis to the anterior iliac spine. Medial to it is the femoral vein, and the femoral nerve lies lateral to it. Historically, the cannulation of this vessel was avoided because earlier catheters and catheterization techniques produced vascular problems and ischemia of the leg. In addition, there was concern about fecal and urinary contamination. It should be avoided in the presence of occlusive vascular disease of the leg and perhaps in neonates and young infants because of the greater risk of thrombosis[60]. In addition, the femoral vein and artery in the same leg should not be cannulated if at all possible.

Equipment needed for femoral artery cannulation is the same as that used for axillary artery cannulation. Identify the femoral artery by palpation, and choose a site below the inguinal ligament. Shave the skin and cleanse with iodine and alcohol solutions. Wear cap, mask, and sterile gloves. Drape the site with sterile towels. Place the middle three fingers over the femoral artery to identify its location and course. The insertion site is between the index and middle fingers. Infiltrate the skin with lidocaine for local anesthesia. If you are using the Seldinger technique, insert the needle cephalad at a 45-degree angle with respect to the skin. As soon as free blood flow is achieved, insert a flexible guide wire gently into the arterial lumen. It should pass with minimal resistance. The use of force can result in arterial wall dissection. If the artery is not punctured, withdraw the needle completely and repeat the above steps. If the artery is entered but the wire cannot be advanced, remove the needle and wire. Compress the artery and obtain hemostasis before the next attempt. If the wire passes easily, slip the catheter over the wire and advance it into the artery. Remove the wire and attach the catheter to the manometer system. Secure the catheter with skin sutures and adhesive tape. Apply iodine ointment and sterile dressings. If the catheter-over-needle technique is used, insert it in the same manner as described for insertion in the Axillary Artery section, and when free blood return is seen, slide the catheter into the artery while keeping the needle in place. Remove the needle.

Thrombosis may occur in 1 to 4% of femoral artery cannulations[60,61]. Risk factors for thrombosis include larger catheter sizes, prolonged cannulation, presence of peripheral vascular disease, and excessive pressure for hemostasis after catheter removal. Pressure for hemostasis should be applied for 10 minutes and should not occlude the femoral pulse. Embolic phenomena may result in gangrene to the distal foot. Doppler flowmeters should be used for periodically checking the integrity of circulation in the popliteal, posterior tibial, and dorsalis pedis arteries. Hematoma formation commonly occurs after catheter removal. Care must be taken not to puncture the artery above the inguinal ligament because of the risk of occult retroperitoneal hemorrhage[62]. Infection is most commonly associated with the insertion site's close proximity to the genitourinary and anal tracts. Therefore, constant ongoing care should be provided to keep the dressings free of urine and fecal contamination. The use of occlusive dressings can help to protect the insertion site but cannot guarantee freedom from infection.

BRACHIAL ARTERY. The brachial artery should never be used for continuous intra-arterial monitoring. This vessel is a continuation of the axillary artery and courses through the upper arm below the medial border of the biceps tendon. In the antecubital fossa it is palpable lateral to the median nerve and medial to the biceps tendon. In the forearm, it branches into the radial and ulnar arteries. Around the elbow are a few branches of the inferior ulnar collateral artery that anastomose with branches of the ulnar artery. Thus the paucity of collateral circulation makes the brachial artery the least desirable vessel for cannulation. Brachial artery occlusion can lead to loss of the entire distal arm. In one adult study(63), 14 to 25 patients who underwent brachial artery cannulation had absent peripheral pulses and vascular abnormalities noted on angiography after catheter removal. Four of the 11 patients seen at 6-month follow-up still had evidence of vascular abnormalities seen on angiography, with narrowing at the site of brachial puncture. For these reasons, the brachial artery should always be avoided.

TEMPORAL ARTERY. The temporal artery is part of the external carotid circulation and passes anteriorly to the auditory meatus on both sides of the head. It has been used clinically for intermittent arterial blood sampling. In several case reports of its use in neonates and young infants, it has resulted in brain infarction on follow-up computed tomography scans of the head, presumably secondary to retrograde passage of air and clot emboli through the external carotid artery into the common and internal carotid arteries with catheter flushing(64). For this reason, its use is absolutely contraindicated.

Complications of Invasive Arterial Blood Pressure Monitoring

Many of the complications of invasive arterial catheters have been discussed above. In general, monitoring blood pressure via an arterial catheter in a child is a safe procedure in most cases. However, serious complications that have been associated with arterial catheters include bleeding, infection, vascular compromise, nerve damage, and accidental injection(53,65–67). Development of arteriovenous fistula and carpal tunnel syndrome have been reported as late sequelae(68).

Bleeding due to line placement is usually not a problem in the absence of coagulopathy(67), but a hematoma may result after the catheter is removed or after several unsuccessful attempts. Hematoma formation at the site of radial artery cannulation has been reported to be associated with a greater incidence of vascular occlusion(42). Significant hemorrhage may occur if the catheter and tubing become disconnected. Pediatric intravenous "T" connectors are prone to disconnect and should be used with caution, if at all, when the cannula site is not visible. The use of Luer-Lok tubing prevents such disconnection.

The risk of infection due to arterial catheters has been reported as low. In children, the risk of bacteremia from an arterial catheter becomes significant when the catheter has been in place for more than 1 week(67), although in one prospective study in adults, catheter-related septicemia was observed in 4% of patients, and localized infection at the insertion site was noted in 18%(69). Associated risk factors included cannulation for more than 4 days, insertion by surgical cut-down, and inflammation at the entry site. Infection can also develop within the manometer system but can be reduced by the use of disposable transducer domes and continuous flushing just distal to the transducer(70) with non-dextrose-containing solutions(69).

The incidence of thrombosis and diminished blood flow has been found to be high, but studies have shown this not to be clinically significant in most cases(65,66). The risk of thrombosis increases with prolonged cannulation, particularly beyond the first 24 to 36 hours(71). Thirty percent of 333 radial artery cannulations in adults resulted in thrombosed vessels at the time of removal; this incidence decreased to 24% after the first week. The injection of hyperosmolar solutions can lead to vessel wall spasm and/or endothelial damage, thereby increasing the risk of thrombosis.

As discussed above, catheter size is a risk factor. The larger the bore, the greater the likelihood of thrombosis. There is greater intima damage associated with a catheter that occupies a larger percentage of the vessel lumen. A lower incidence of thrombosis was noted with the use of 20-gauge rather than 18-gauge catheters in adults(40); conversely, patients with smaller arteries (e.g., women and children) ran a higher risk of thrombosis(72). Multiple puncture attempts before successful insertion also increased thrombosis risk(39). Teflon-coated(40,41), nontapered(37,39) catheters had the lowest incidence of thrombosis in adult studies. However, in one pediatric study(47) in which Medicut (tapered polypropylene) catheters were used, no clinical signs of vascular insufficiency in 70 radial arterial cannulations on 62 patients occurred, and in 64 of 67 patients, radial pulses were equal in both wrists one year later. Children seem to do better than adults.

Clinically significant ischemia is extremely rare. In one study of 12,000 arterial cannulations in adults (radial, femoral, and brachial), only 15 developed digital necrosis(73). Risk factors for distal ischemia include peripheral occlusive and/or spastic vascular disease, systemic hypotension, and the use of vasopressor drugs. Some cases of impaired circulation may be due to spasm, although one study found all cases to be due to thrombosis(74). Hence, one should check distal perfusion at least once every 8 hours, observing capillary filling, skin temperature, and color. If poor perfusion is detected, blood withdrawal is difficult, or if the arterial tracing remains constantly damped, the catheter should be removed. The loss of extremities from peripheral arterial catheters has been reported(75). Vasospasm may be seen after the catheter is removed, but this is usually transient.

Retrograde flow has been shown to occur during routine flushing of both peripheral and umbilical artery catheters(53). This can result in flushing of air bubbles and debris into major vascular systems, including the carotid and superior mesenteric arteries. Butt and associates[53] showed that this can be prevented in infants by flushing 0.5 ml of fluid over a 5-second period.

Arterial Waveform Interpretation

Fundamental to the interpretation of the data obtained from direct arterial blood pressure is an understanding of the effect of Bernoulli's principle on the observed pressure. The Bernoulli equation for the total energy stored in blood includes terms for the pressure (P), the gravitational potential energy ($\rho \times g \times h$), and the kinetic energy ($\frac{1}{2}\rho v^2$), where ρ is the density, g is the force of gravity, h is the height of the column of blood, and v is the velocity of blood. Further knowledge of the physical properties of the measurement system is useful to recognize errors or artifacts in these data.

The most common application of Bernoulli's principle is in the changes in pressure with posture. The gravitational term ($\rho \times g \times h$) predicts the change in pressure of one part of the circulation relative to another or relative to an external pressure-measuring device. In the supine position, the relative pressure difference between the head and feet in both arterial and venous circulations is slight. However, in the standing position, the gravitational forces are no longer equally distributed from head to foot. The arterial pressure in the foot relative to the midchest level is greater due to the force of a column of blood equal to that distance. In a child, if this distance is 60 cm, then the difference in pressure will be

$$1.05\ g/\text{ml} \times 980\ \text{cm/sec}^2 \times 60\ \text{cm} = 61{,}740\ \text{dyne/cm}^2 \text{ or } 46\ \text{torr}$$

Similarly, if the distance between the midchest and the head is 30 cm, the arterial pressure difference will be 23 torr, and the total pressure difference between the head and feet will be 69 torr. The pressure differences in the venous circulation would be exactly the same, although the absolute values would be different.

These concepts must be applied when a circulatory pressure is compared with an outside reference such as a pressure transducer or manometer. Zero reference or atmospheric pressure must be set, with the transducer at exactly the same level as the chamber or vessel being measured. In general, for patients in the supine position, this is at the level of the heart or approximately midchest level. As explained previously, in the supine position, the error introduced by the difference in height of a monitoring line in the head or foot rather than in the heart is minor. Consider a child sitting up in bed with a catheter in the dorsalis pedis artery. If zero is defined as atmospheric pressure at the midchest level, then the arterial pressure measured in the foot will be artifactually decreased in proportion to the distance between the transducer and the measuring site in the foot. Alternatively, if central venous pressure is being measured by a catheter in the superior vena cava, with the child supine and with reference to a transducer at the midchest position, then sitting the child up without changing the position of the transducer will increase the measured pressure. Thus, to ensure accurate and reproducible pressure measurements, all recordings should be made with the child in the supine position and the transducer at midchest level.

The kinetic energy term of the Bernoulli equation ($\frac{1}{2}\rho v^2$) must be considered in at least a qualitative manner when pressures in an area with high velocity are measured. As illustrated in Figure 17.10, if a fluid is traveling at low velocity in a large-bore tube, most the energy is stored as pressure. If the tubing narrows, the velocity of the flow must increase in proportion to the decrease in cross-sectional area of the tube. The increase in velocity results in an increase in the kinetic energy of the fluid; thus, because total energy must be constant, the increase in kinetic energy must be offset by a decrease in potential energy or pressure. If the tube is level, the gravitational portion of the energy is constant, and the energy transferred to the kinetic term must come from the pressure portion of energy. Thus, the pressure measured in the high-velocity area will be lower than that measured in the low-velocity area. If the fluid then enters a tube with a cross-sectional area identical with the initial portion, the pressure will be increased because the kinetic energy is converted back to potential energy. The clinical correlation of this phenomenon is found in children with valvar stenosis. If an end-hole catheter is placed in the main pulmonary artery in a child with severe pulmonic valve stenosis, the kinetic energy of the high-velocity jet will tend to decrease the measured pulmonary arterial pressure.

In most clinical settings, vascular pressure is measured with a fluid-filled catheter connected to a strain gauge pressure transducer. The signal from the transducer is amplified, displayed on an oscilloscope, or recorded on a strip chart. Systolic, mean, or diastolic pressure is often electronically determined and displayed on a digital readout. Each step in the measurement process may introduce error, which will degrade the quality of the signal and introduce artifacts into the pressure measurement.

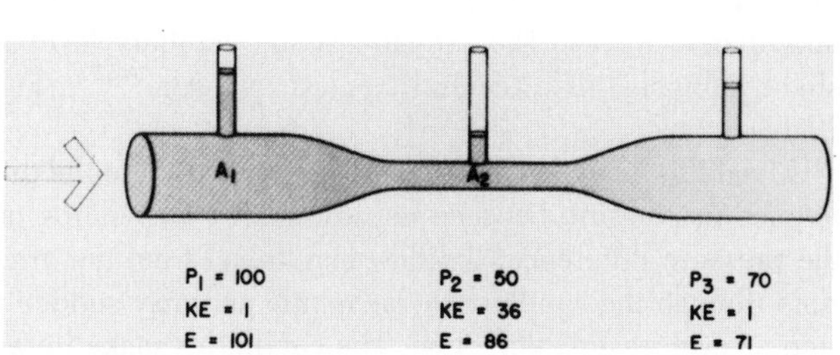

Figure 17.10. Principle of continuity and Bernoulli equation. *P*, pressure; *KE*, kinetic energy; and *E*, total energy. As the tube narrows, lateral pressure decreases and kinetic energy increases. As the tube widens, lateral pressure increases and the kinetic energy decreases. (From Abel FL, McCutcheon EP. Cardiovascular function principles and applications. Boston: Little, Brown, 1979:7.)

The most critical of these errors is overdamping due to long, narrow, compliant catheters, air bubbles, or blood in the system. This may be recognized in the arterial circulation by a slow upstroke, a poorly defined dicrotic notch, and a narrow pulse pressure. The measured systolic pressure in an overdamped system may be substantially less than the actual vascular pressure and may result in unwarranted changes in clinical management based on faulty data. Careful flushing of the catheter and pressure tubing to remove blood and even small air bubbles, as well as the choice of the shortest, stiffest, and largest catheter safe for the measurement, will minimize these errors.

In contrast, an underdamped system will result in overshoot of the actual arterial pressure. This may be identified by a notch in the tracing immediately after the peak systolic pressure. This usually is remedied by electronically damping the signal at high frequencies by a filter switch found on many amplifiers. Motion of the catheter (fling) will result in oscillation of the pressure tracing, which may also be seen in some tracings from pulmonary artery catheters. Many of these catheter-induced artifacts may be eliminated by the use of catheter-tipped manometers in which the pressure transducer itself is mounted on the end of a catheter. These catheters have several disadvantages, which have limited their routine clinical use, including poor durability, expense, and the inability to draw blood samples, since they frequently do not have lumens. Errors introduced by properly maintained transducers, amplifiers, and recorders, such as drift and nonlinear response, are infrequent and may be minimized by occasional recalibration with a mercury manometer.

Blood is directed away from the heart via large arteries, which branch into small arteries. The small arteries then branch into arterioles, which are about 50 to 100 μm in diameter, and subsequently branch into terminal arterioles, which are 30 to 50 μm in diameter[76]. The arterioles are considered to be the beginning of microcirculation. Blood arrives at the arteriole with a mean arterial pressure (MAP) approximately the same as that of the aorta. The pressure begins to decrease rapidly at the terminal arteriole. The terminal arterioles then branch into capillaries, which are the smallest blood vessels, and range from 4 to 15 μm in diameter. These endothelial tubes have no muscular elements. The pressure at the capillary level is slightly higher than central venous pressure[6,77] (Fig. 17.11).

Blood flows through the capillary in proportion to the difference in pressure between its two ends[6]. Depending on the pressure difference, the flow may travel from the arteriole through the capillary to the venule and may suddenly stop or even reverse direction. The capillaries make up an extensive network in the body, with a large number of alternate pathways to help protect any particular region from ischemia[6].

Substances travel from the capillary to the tissue in a number of ways. Capillary walls have pores through which substances may passively diffuse, travel by bulk flow, or

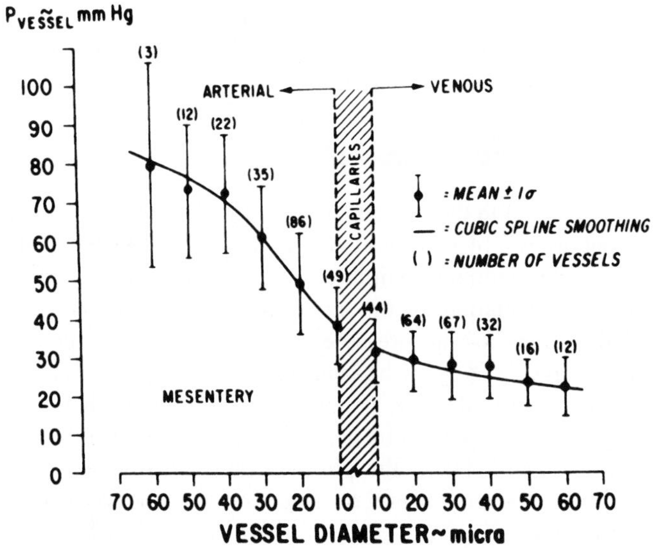

Figure 17.11. Distribution of blood pressure along the microcirculation. The arterial pressure decreases slightly from 70- to 40-μm vessels. There is less than a 10-mm Hg fall along the length of the capillary. (From Abel Fl, McCutcheon EP. Cardiovascular function principles and applications. Boston: Little, Brown, 1979:240.)

flow by osmosis. However, the supply of nutrients and the removal of metabolic wastes at the capillary level are ultimately dependent on the blood flow to the area.

If the pressure is measured in the ascending aorta and then withdrawn and measured at 10-cm intervals, waveforms are obtained (Fig. 17.12). The waveform consists of an ascending or anacrotic limb to a peak, which is the systolic pressure; an incisura corresponding to the closure of the semilunar valves; and a slower descending catacrotic limb (Fig. 17.13). The lowest pressure is the diastolic pressure, and the difference between the systolic and diastolic pressure is the pulse pressure.

The MAP can be calculated from a pulse pressure tracing by calculating the area of the waveform and dividing it by the length of the base; the height of the rectangle formed is the MAP[6,78] (Fig. 17.14). The MAP may also be calculated from the systolic pressure (SP) and diastolic pressure (DP) as follows:

$$MAP = DP + [(SP - DP)/3]$$

Vascular Impedance

The position of the dicrotic notch is associated with changes in vascular resistance. To fully understand these changes, a knowledge of vascular impedance is necessary. Although frequently used synonymously with vascular resistance to imply the opposition to blood flow, vascular impedance is more precisely the quantitative characterization of the physical properties of the vascular bed. Vascular resistance is a function of the diameter, length, and number of small arterioles in the distal circulation. Impedance is determined by the distensibility, diameter and length of the large arteries, and reflected waves off branch points in the circulation, as well as the arterial resistance. Resistance is a phenomenon of steady-state nonpulsatile blood flow and is the

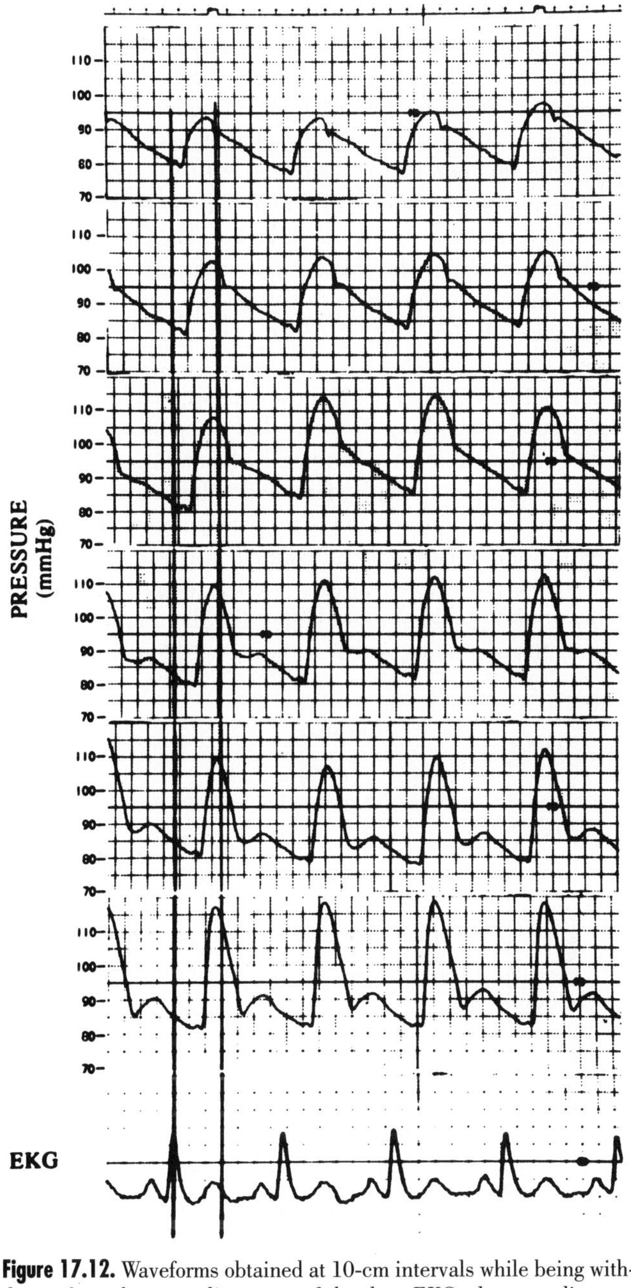

Figure 17.12. Waveforms obtained at 10-cm intervals while being withdrawn from the ascending aorta of the dog. *EKG*, electrocardiogram. (From Able FL, McCutcheon EP. Cardiovascular function principles and applications. Boston: Little, Brown, 1979:33.)

ratio of the mean pressure drop and mean blood flow across the arterial bed. Impedance can be determined only by analyzing the pulsatile properties of the blood flow on an instantaneous rather than a steady-state basis. By considering both components of blood flow, vascular impedance also permits quantification of the total energy expended by the heart to move blood through the vascular tree. These concepts have led to the use of impedance to describe the total afterload of the ventricle[79,80].

The calculation of arterial impedance requires the simultaneous recording of high-fidelity pressure and flow velocity signals in a large artery. In clinical practice, this is done with a catheter-tip manometer and flow probe, in either the aorta or the main pulmonary artery. The individual signals are subjected to mathematical analysis to break the complex waveforms into a series of sinusoidal components called harmonics. These waves have a frequency that is a multiple of the heart rate, a modulus or amplitude, and a phase angle that describes the timing of the waves. The impedance spectrum has two components: the impedance modulus and the phase angle, both of which are plotted as a function of frequency. The impedance modulus is the ratio of the pressure and flow moduli and of each frequency or harmonic. Typically, the impedance modulus is greatest at zero frequency. It falls rapidly to a minimum value at a frequency twice the heart rate and then oscillates around a mean value at higher frequencies. The impedance modulus at zero frequency is equivalent to the arterial resistance. The mean value of the impedance modulus at higher frequencies is the characteristic impedance. The phase angle of the impedance spectrum is the degree to which the pressure wave precedes or follows the flow wave at any given frequency (Fig. 17.15).

In general, an increase in the impedance modulus at all frequencies implies a stiffening of the large arteries or a decrease in their diameter. A shift in the initial minimum of the impedance modulus indicates an increase in the wave velocity or a change in the reflections sites. Dampening of the oscillations around the characteristic impedance suggests decreased reflection of the pulse wave from the distal sites. These reflections may be dampened by distal vasodilatation, increased distensibility, or recruitment of new vascular beds[79].

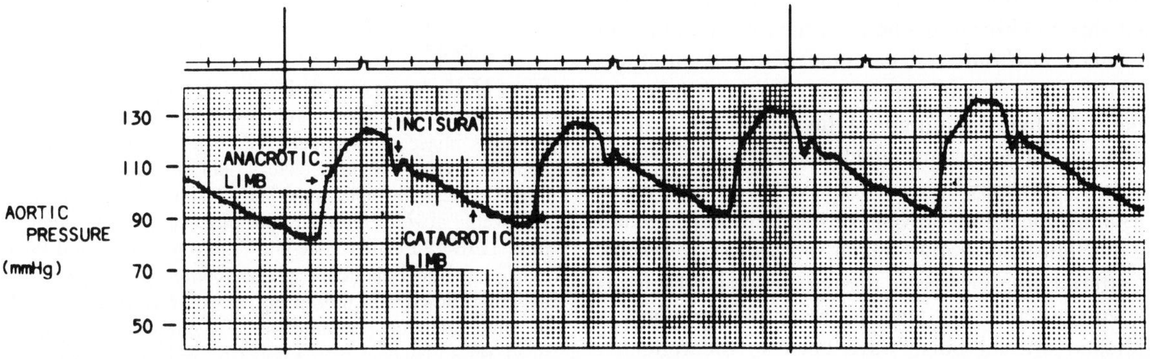

Figure 17.13. Central aortic pressure tracing in the human. (From Abel FL, McCutcheon EP. Cardiovascular function principles and applications. Boston: Little, Brown, 1979:230.)

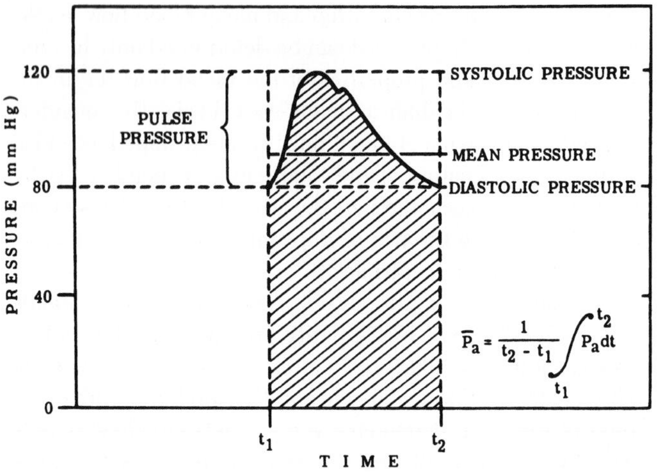

Figure 17.14. Calculation of the mean arterial pressure from a pressure pulse tracing. (From Abel FL, McCutcheon EP. Cardiovascular function principles and applications. Boston: Little, Brown, 1979:230.)

The calculation of the hydraulic energy associated with pulsatile blood flow has shown that more energy is required to move blood in a pulsatile fashion than in a steady-state manner. The pulsatile components of both potential and kinetic energy ordinarily make up approximately 10% of the total energy in the systemic circulation and 30% of the total energy in the pulmonary circulation. Thus, the properties of the large arteries, including distensibility, diameter, and reflected waves make a relatively greater contribution to the afterload of the right ventricle than to the afterload of the left ventricle. Alternatively, proportionately less energy is needed to move the blood in a pulsatile fashion by the left ventricle; thus, it is more efficient[79].

Systemic vasoconstriction or vasodilation has effects on the aortic impedance in both experimental and clinical studies. O'Rourke and Taylor[81], studying the femoral artery impedance in dogs, showed that vasodilation not only lowers the peripheral arterial resistance but also flattens the impedance curve, with a loss of the minimum value and a decrease in the phase difference between pressure and flow. Vasoconstriction affected the systemic resistance primarily with little change in the remainder of the spectrum. This and other experiments suggest that with vasodilation, there is a decrease in the pulse wave velocity and in the reflected waves from the arteriolar bed. These changes may be recognized as a shift to lower frequencies of the first minimum of the impedance modulus and damping of the oscillations around the characteristic impedance. Because reflected waves contribute to the amplitude of the arterial pressure after the dicrotic notch, loss of reflections and the decreased pulse wave velocity may be recognized on the arterial pulse tracing as a low-amplitude wave after the dicrotic notch and as a low diastolic and dicrotic notch pressure. In contrast, lowered arterial pressure with normal arteriolar tone, as might be encountered with low cardiac output, produces a normal-shaped arterial pulse wave because the reflected waves are maintained[82].

Vasoconstriction tends to accentuate reflections, and as the arterial pressure rises, the aortic wall becomes less distensible, increasing the pulse wave velocity. This shifts the impedance spectrum toward higher frequencies, accentuates the oscillations around the characteristic impedance, and tends to increase the characteristic impedance. The change in characteristic impedance may be blunted by the associated increase in arterial diameter. The changes in the reflected waves may be manifested on the arterial pressure waveform as a notch on the upstroke in early systole because the reflected wave is superimposed on the incoming wave[83].

These findings may also be used to help explain the dramatic pulse wave amplification that is commonly seen in children when the ascending and descending aortic pressures are compared. With aging and stiffening of the aortic wall, the pulse pressure tends to increase, and the systolic pressure amplification is attenuated. The stiffer aorta increases the pulse wave velocity so that the reflected waves return to the proximal aorta before the dicrotic notch, thus making the ascending and descending aortic pressures more

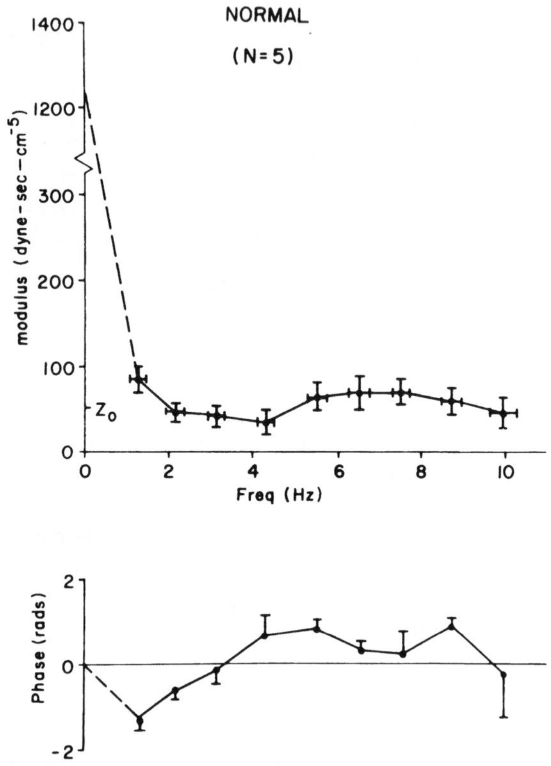

Figure 17.15. Average aortic input impedance of five normal adult subjects. *Vertical* and *horizontal bars* represent the mean ± SE of the modulus, phase, and frequency. Z_0 is the estimated characteristic impedance (53 ± 4 dyne·sec·cm^{-5}) obtained by averaging the moduli above 2 Hz. The input impedance modulus *(top panel)* falls from a high value at zero frequency (mean aortic pressure divided by mean flow, 1218 ± 147 dyne·sec·cm^{-5}) to a minimum and then rises to a maximum. the impedance phase *(bottom panel),* which is initially negative (flow leads pressure), crosses zero in the neighborhood of the first modulus minimum and becomes positive (pressure leads flow). (From Nichols WW, Conti CR, Walker WE, Milnor WR. Input impedance of the systemic circulation in man. Circ Res 1977;40:451.)

similar. In children, because the reflections return more slowly, the reflected waves in the proximal aorta are added to the pressure after the dicrotic notch, while in the distal aorta they are superimposed on the pressure prior to aortic valve closure.

There has been considerable interest in the use of arterial impedance as a measure of ventricular afterload, one of the important determinants of myocardial function. In classic isolated-muscle experiments, afterload is the force per unit area or stress that the muscle is forced to generate. Unfortunately, attempts to extend this approach to the intact ventricle have been hampered by the difficulty in measuring wall stress directly and by the multiple assumptions required to estimate wall stress. Furthermore, if afterload is considered the total opposition to forward flow, then wall stress may not be an appropriate measure of afterload. During ventricular ejection, wall stress is continually changing, yet the physical properties of the vascular bed are relatively constant. Furthermore, some of the energy produced by the ventricle must distend the aorta rather than generate pressure, and this would not be included in the wall stress calculations. Similarly, because arterial impedance more completely describes the characteristics of the arterial bed, it is superior to limiting the concept of afterload to the peripheral resistance.

The concept of arterial impedance can provide the most complete understanding of the physical properties of the arterial bed. Changes in the *impedance spectrum* reflect alterations in the large arteries, including diameter, distensibility, and reflected waves in addition to peripheral vascular resistance. Thus, the two terms should never be used interchangeably. Although complex, studies of aortic or pulmonary impedance in the PICU could provide valuable insight into the pathophysiology of a number of disease states, including shock and cor pulmonale.

Central Venous Pressure

CVP monitoring is indicated for children undergoing cardiovascular surgery or surgical procedures that can involve large blood loss or fluid shifts. Central venous catheters are often used for children requiring vasoactive drugs, parenteral hyperalimentation, or venous access (in the face of inadequate peripheral venous access).

Venous Circulation

The capillaries combine to form venules, which subsequently join to form small veins. These join to form large veins, which drain into the vena cava. The venous system is a reservoir that contains 65 to 75% of the total blood volume at any given time[6]. Veins have a system of valves that break up the vessel into segments so that dependent areas such as the upper and lower extremities do not receive the entire hydrostatic pressure generated by the venous circulation. In the healthy person, when standing upright, most of the venous volume is below the level of the heart. Deep veins in the leg are surrounded by muscles, which increase venous return when contracted. CVP is measured with a needle or catheter in a central vein, which is connected either to a pressure transducer or to a calibrated tube filled with sterile saline. The level in the tube corresponds to the venous pressure in centimeters of H_2O. Venous pressure, as all vascular pressures, must be measured with a reference pint known at the level of the right atrium. If the manometer is too high, the pressure will be falsely low, and if placed below the reference level, the pressure reading will be falsely high. Because the venous pressures are normally low and a few points difference either way may change a patient's treatment, accurate measurement is important.

Several factors influence venous return. First is the difference between the peripheral venous pressure and right atrial pressure. The mean venous capillary pressure is the arterial pressure that remains after blood has passed through the capillaries into the venous system and is about 15 mm Hg; the right atrial pressure is about 5 mm Hg[6]. The pressure difference of 10 mm Hg is what drives the blood back to the heart. Gravity affects the venous circulation, so that when a patient is standing, blood pools in the lower extremities and the jugular veins collapse, causing increased resistance to flow and decreased venous return. Placing the patient's head down (the Trendelenburg position) is used to increase venous return through gravity, although in the spontaneously ventilating patient this may decrease vital capacity, and elevating the legs with the head and trunk flat may be just as effective.[6,84].

As stated before, contraction of muscles surrounding the veins together with one-way valves in the veins will increase venous return to the heart. During spontaneous breathing, inspiration will increase venous return by increasing thoracic pressure, causing a favorable pressure gradient for flow of blood into the thorax (Fig. 17.16). During positive pressure ventilation, the pressure in the thorax will be increased and the effect reversed, so that inspiration will now decrease venous return, while expiration will increase venous return[6] (Fig. 17.17).

Insertion Sites and Techniques

CVP catheters can be placed via the external or internal jugular, subclavian, basilic, or femoral vein. CVP catheters are usually placed in children intraoperatively after the induction of anesthesia and tracheal intubation, or in the PICU with sedation and local anesthesia. Before placement of a CVP catheter, the ECG must be monitored, because arrhythmias may be induced with the wires or catheters as they enter the heart. Patients are placed in the Trendelenburg position if they can tolerate this; alternatively, the legs may be raised with the patient flat or in a slight head-up position. This positioning distends the internal jugular veins

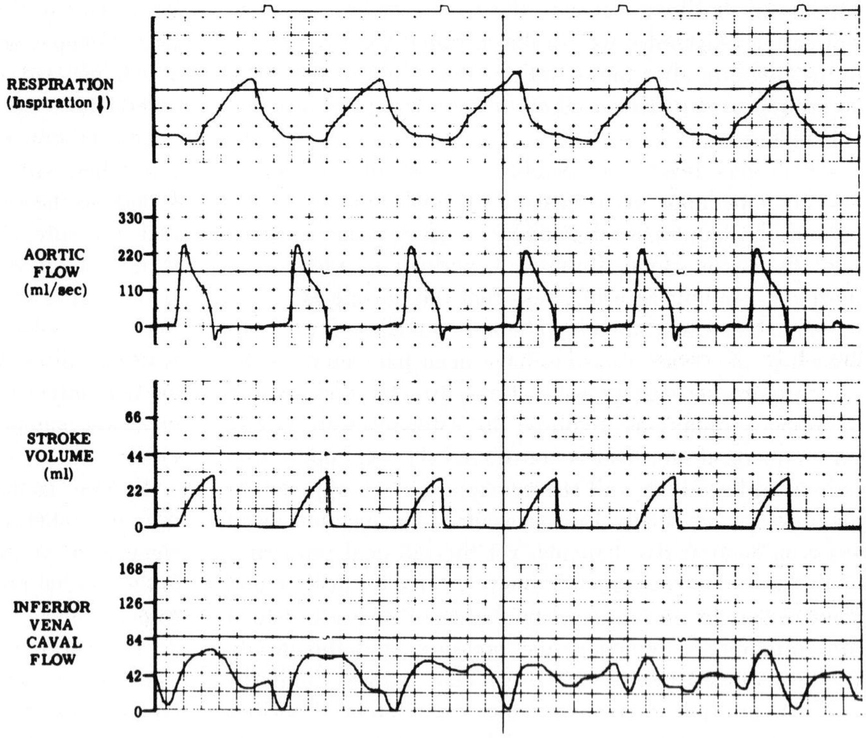

Figure 17.16. Effect of quiet respiration on stroke volume and aortic and venous flow in the sheep. (From Abel FL, McCutcheon EP. Cardiovascular function principles and applications. Boston: Little Brown, 1979:276.)

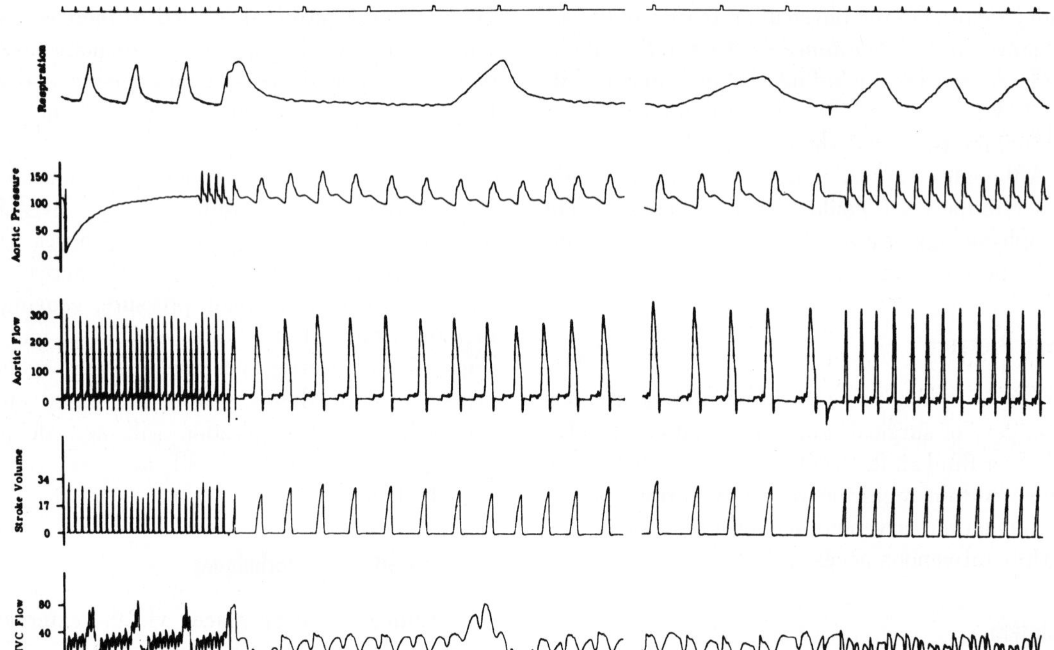

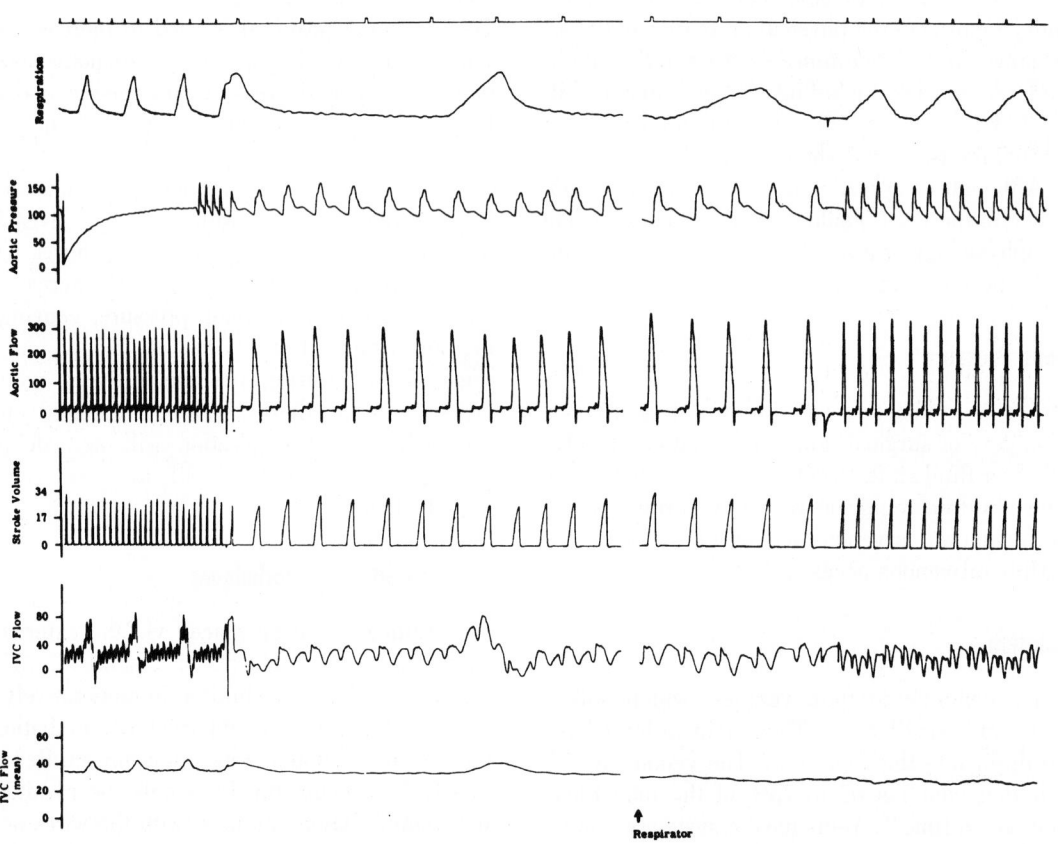

Figure 17.17. Effect of normal respiration versus positive pressure ventilation on venous and aortic flow. The animal was placed on positive pressure ventilation at the *arrow. IVC,* inferior vena cava. (From Abel FL, McCutcheon EP. Cardiovascular function principles and applications. Boston: Little, Brown, 1979:275.)

and decreases the risk of embolism. The area is prepared with an iodine-containing solution (assuming there is no allergy to iodine; otherwise, alcohol is used) and draped with sterile towels. If the patient is not anesthetized, 0.5 to 1% lidocaine is used for local anesthesia. A small needle (25 or 22 gauge) is often used to locate the vein, then the larger needle is inserted after the same line (Fig. 17.18). When venous blood is freely aspirated, a wire is placed through the needle, and the needle is removed leaving the wire in place.

The size of catheter to be used is related to the size of the child. A rough rule of thumb is to use a 3-French catheter in infants weighing less than 3 kg, 4-French in children under 10 kg, 5-French in those 10 to 20 kg, and 6-French in those over 20 kg. If two catheters are to be placed, the second needle insertion is performed before inserting the catheter over the wire, because catheter shearing and embolization can occur if the needle inadvertently cuts into the first catheter. After the catheter is placed over the wire, placement in the vein is confirmed by the lack of pulsatile flow and by measuring the pressure waveforms.

Waveform Interpretation

The normal CVP trace has three positive waves: *a*, *c*, and *v*, and two negative waves: *x* and *y* (Fig. 17.19). Normal and abnormal characteristics of the CVP trace are summarized in **Table 17.2.** The *a* wave is caused by atrial contraction, the *a* wave by ventricular contraction against a closed tricuspid valve, and the *a* wave by atrial filling. The *v* wave is normally lower in amplitude than the *a* wave, but in the presence of an atrial septal defect the higher left atrial pressure may be transmitted to the right atrium during atrial filing, causing the *a* and *v* waves to be equal in amplitude.

Right atrial and wedge pressures, in the presence of normal tricuspid and mitral valve function, reflect their respective ventricular end-diastolic pressures. Ventricular end-diastolic pressure is determined by ventricular compliance (the relationship between volume and pressure), afterload, and function. High filling pressures primarily reflect poor function, not intravascular volume. For example, in children who have undergone cardiac surgery, aortic cross-clamping may have impaired ventricular function so that filling pressures for given intravascular volume and output must be higher. Changing filling pressures reflect changes in cardiac function. Increasing left atrial pressures in the postoperative period may indicate deteriorating left ventricular function, while falling pressures with adequate perfusion are generally more encouraging. Finally, the temptation to equate filling pressures with volume must be assiduously resisted. Although fluid overload may cause high filling pressures, these usually indicate the need for adequate preload (intravascular volume). As with all monitored parameters, their interpretation requires a thorough understanding of the child's clinical condition.

Normal values for CVP in infants are difficult to define. Healthy babies generally have CVP values from −2 to +4 mm Hg. In infants with congenital heart disease, the values are in the range of 4 to 8 mm Hg. Infants ventilated for respiratory disease have values of 2 to 6 mm Hg and often do not tolerate lower values from 0 to 3 mm Hg. CVP measurements above 8 mm Hg are often associated with myocardial dysfunction or high intrathoracic pressure, such as with pneumothorax[85]. Pressures measured at end expiration from femoral catheters positioned in the inferior vena cava give accurate CVP values[86].

Table 17.2. Characteristics of Abnormal Central Venous Pressure Trace

Wave	*Physiology*	*Associated Disease*
"Cannon" a	Right atrium contracts against obstructed tricuspid valve	Complete heart block Tricuspid stenosis Right atrial myxoma
	Resistance to right ventricular filling	Pulmonary hypertension Pulmonary stenosis
Absent a	No effective atrial contraction	Atrial fibrillation
"Giant" v	Right ventricular pressure transmitted to right atrium	Tricuspid regurgitation

Artifacts and Errors in Measurement

The transducer position, which is particularly important for accurate measurement of CVP, is conventionally at the level of the right atrium. If the patient's position changes, measurements that are erroneously high (if the transducer is too low) or low (if the transducer is too high) will result. Because changes in the CVP of just a few millimeters of mercury can be a significant finding, one must be vigilant to keep the transducer level in the correct position and accurately zeroed. It is also necessary to check the pressure waveform, because the catheter may be long enough to pass through the tricuspid valve into the right ventricle in some patients, or the waveform may be overdamped if the catheter is against the chamber wall or if blood or air bubbles are in the tubing.

Complications

One study found the rate of successful cannulation of the internal jugular vein to be significantly decreased in children under 3 months of age and weighing less than 4.0 kg[87], but other studies found no relation to these factors[88,89]. The most common complication of internal jugular vein catheterization is inadvertent carotid artery puncture. Other complications of insertion include local hematoma, air embolism, catheter malposition (resulting in infiltration or extravasation of drugs and fluid into neck tissue, mediastinum, or pericardial or pleural cavities), pneumothorax, hemothorax, trauma to the brachial plexus, and subclavian artery puncture. Some patients may have a higher risk of insertion complications because of preexisting clinical conditions, such as contralateral diaphragmatic dysfunction; congenital abnormalities, including short or webbed necks; or previous internal jugular catheterizations. Complications related to indwelling catheters include infection, thrombophlebitis, superior vena cava thrombosis, and intracardiac thrombus formation.

The risk of infection related to internal jugular vein catheterization has been reported to be 11% in children[90], and the risk of catheter-related septicemia 0.5% to 1.0%[90,91]. The incidence of having positive catheter-tip cultures without complications related to culture positivity is 5%[92]. Catheter in situ time and open heart surgery in infants under 1 year of age have proven to be the most significant independent risk factors for a positive tip culture. The safe in situ time has been reported to be 3 days for infants and 6 days for older children[92].

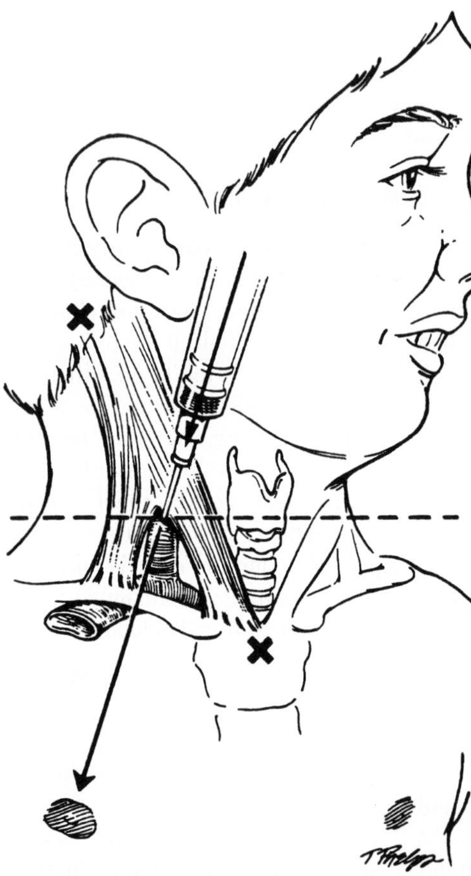

Figure 17.18. Internal jugular cannulation. Head turned to the opposite side. Needle puncture at the apex of the triangle formed by the heads of the sternocleidomastoid muscle (midway between the sternal notch and the mastoid process). Needle aimed at the ipsilateral nipple. (From Schleien CL: *Cardiopulmonary resuscitation.* In: Nicholes DG, Yaster M, Lappe DG, Buck JR, editors. *Golden Hour–the handbook of advanced pediatric life support,* St. Louis, 1991, Mosby–Year Book, p. 124; with permission.)

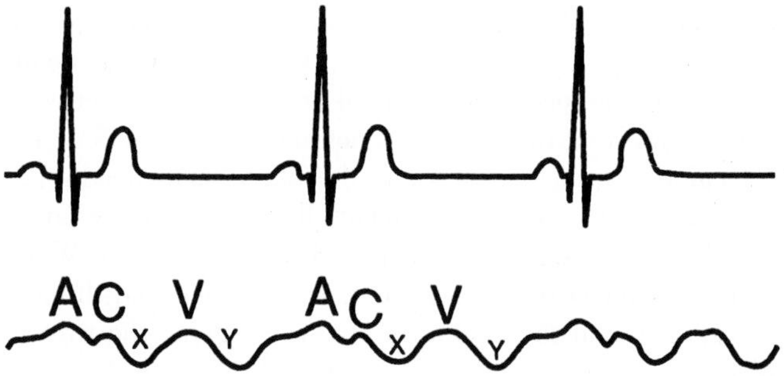

Figure 17.19. Central venous pressure trace with corresponding electrocardiogram (ECG). The a wave is produced by atrial contraction, occurring after the P wave on the ECG. The c wave is produced by bulging of the tricuspid valve upward into the right atrium after valve closure. The x descent is caused by the tricuspid valve being pulled away from the right atrium by the contracting ventricle during systole. The v wave occurs prior to the opening of the tricuspid valve and is the result of a rapid late systolic filing of the atrium. The y descent occurs as the tricuspid valve opens and blood enters the ventricle. (From O'Rourke RA: *The measurement of systemic blood pressure: normal and abnormal pulsations of the arteries and veins.* In Hurst JW, editor: *the heart,* New York, 1990, McGraw-Hill, p 159; with permission.)

PULMONARY ARTERY PRESSURE

Swan et al.[93] first described in 1970 the use of a balloon-tipped catheter inserted into the pulmonary artery for the measurement of the pulmonary artery occlusion pressure (PAOP), also known as the wedge pressure, in critically ill patients. Two years later, Forrester et al.[94] used a triple-lumen catheter with a thermistor tip that allowed measurement of cardiac output by the thermodilution technique. Today, pulmonary artery catheterization is an indispensable tool in the PICU and is increasingly used in children[95]. A more precise description of the circulatory state of a given patient is now possible, allowing the appropriate selection and titration of medical therapy to optimize cardiovascular performance.

A primary role of pulmonary artery pressure monitoring is to provide the functional characteristics of the left and right ventricles by measuring the filling pressures of each ventricle (PAOP and right atrial pressures) and cardiac output[96]. Measurement of cardiac output by the thermodilution technique is reliable in animals, adults, and children over a wide range of flow values (2 to 14% for flows between 200 and 500 ml/min)[97–100]. Maintaining an adequate cardiac output helps to ensure the ability to meet organ tissue metabolic demands, and maintaining normal values of PAOP prevents exudation of fluid into the pulmonary interstitial space.

The second function of monitoring is to estimate values of those parameters that affect left and right ventricular outputs as well as right atrial pressure and PAOP[96]. For example, systemic pressure and vascular resistance affect the impedance to left ventricular outflow, while pulmonary artery pressure and pulmonary vascular resistance (PVR) are related to the impedance to right ventricular outflow. Additional calculations of left and right ventricular volume indices and stroke work indices give additional description to the functional characteristics of the cardiovascular system.

Access to mixed venous blood permits the measurements of arterial minus mixed venous O_2 content difference, O_2 consumption, and intrapulmonary shunt fraction. These parameters aid in the management of both cardiovascular and/or respiratory diseases.

Catheter Description

Pulmonary artery catheters (Fig. 17.20) come in several sizes. In general, the 5-French catheter is used for children weighing 10 to 18 kg, and the 7-French is used for patients 18 kg and over. The 7-French catheter is usually placed via the femoral vein in children weighing 18 to 40 kg. The 5-French catheter may be placed through internal jugular or subclavian vein insertion in children over 25 kg. For small patients, 2- and 3-French double-lumen catheters consisting of a distal port and thermistor are available. They can be used in children under 10 kg of weight for the measurement of cardiac output, with the separate insertion of a right atrial catheter for the injection of cold saline. The pulmonary artery catheter is placed through an introducer sheath which is one-half to one size larger than the catheter itself, depending on the manufacturer's design.

The 5- and 7-French catheters both have proximal (right atrial) and distal (pulmonary artery) ports and an inflatable balloon. A fourth lumen supports wiring to the thermistor located near the tip. The thermistor is used for thermodilution cardiac output measurement. Black marks are spaced every 10 cm of catheter length. The two sizes differ in four ways[95] **(Table 17.3)**. The smaller catheter does not allow rapid infusion of fluids, which would falsely elevate pressure readings. Its use in small infants with the neck as the insertion site may be made difficult by the distance between the proximal and distal ports. While the tip may be properly wedged in the pulmonary artery, the proximal port may be outside of the right atrium or even outside of the catheter introducer sheath, hence, the injectate may be infused outside of the body.

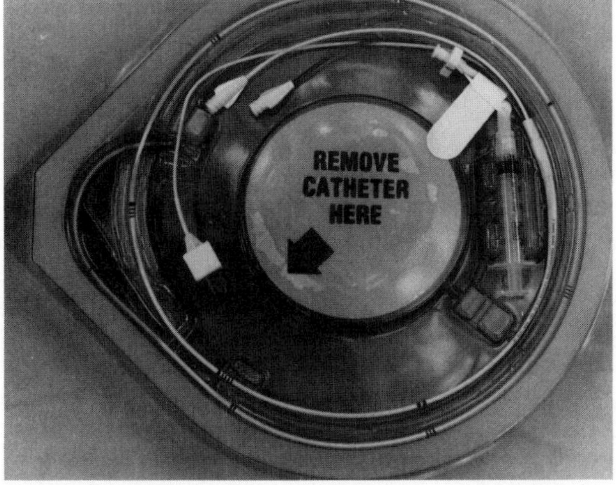

Figure 17.20. Quadruple-lumen pulmonary artery catheter (Swan-Ganz catheter).

Table 17.3. Differences in Quadruple-Lumen Pulmonary Artery Catheters

Description	*5 French*	*7 French*
Thermistor distance from tip (cm)	2.5 ± 0.5	3.5 ± 0.5
Balloon capacity/diameter	0.75 ml/8 mm	1.5 ml/12 mm
Usable length (cm)	70	110
Introducer size (French)	5.6	7.8

From Katz RW, Pollack M, Welbley R. Pulmonary artery catheterization in pediatric intensive care. Adv Pediatr 1984; 30:169.

Insertion Technique

Equipment for this technique should include the following: pulmonary artery catheter; pressure transducers to hook to proximal and distal ports via three-way stopcocks; small syringe for balloon inflation; equipment for the percutaneous or cut-down insertion of the catheter introducer sheath; and sterile drapes, gowns, gloves, masks, and alcohol and iodine solutions.

The insertion of a pulmonary artery catheter may induce arrhythmias by direct irritation to the atrial and ventricular walls. Therefore, the patient must be continuously monitored by ECG, and intravenous access must be established, with lidocaine, atropine, and a defibrillator immediately available. The pressure manometer systems should be flushed with heparinized 0.9% saline solution, checked for leaks, electrically zeroed, and mechanically calibrated with a mercury manometer. The insertion site should then be cleaned vigorously with iodine solution. Strict aseptic technique should be observed to minimize risk of infection, especially when the catheter will remain in the patient for several days.

The catheter is inserted through an introducer sheath which is placed in the same manner as a CVP catheter. Common insertion sites include the internal and external jugular veins, the subclavian vein, the median basilic vein within the antecubital fossa, and the femoral vein. The major problem with the antecubital fossa approach is that the catheter may get caught within the shoulder area and not pass into the right atrium or that the catheter is more likely to dislodge if the arm is moved, requiring immobilization. The femoral route, due to its length, may make catheter passage more difficult. Entry may be by percutaneous or cut-down route, depending on the experience of the operator. The operator should be gowned, gloved, and masked, and the entry site should be draped with sterile towels.

After the catheter sheath is inserted, the pulmonary artery catheter is removed from the container by using sterile technique. The syringe is attached to test the integrity of the balloon. Air is normally used for this purpose, but in patients with intracardiac shunts, the risk of air embolism may be reduced by the use of carbon dioxide. The distal and proximal ports are connected to the pressure manometer system and flushed with heparinized saline solution. The thermistor is connected to the cardiac output computer, and the patient's blood temperature should be displayed. Depending on the type of equipment, the thermistor will register as functioning.

There are several important considerations during catheter insertion. Never use more than the recommended volume of air for balloon inflation to avoid rupture. Never use force during insertion, as this may damage the catheter lumens. Whenever withdrawing the catheter, always deflate the balloon to avoid valvular and/or vessel rupture. This is best done by disconnecting the syringe and opening the valve to atmospheric pressure, rather than by actively removing air with the syringe, which may lead to balloon damage.

The catheter length necessary to reach the right atrium can initially be measured by noting the length from the insertion site to the manubriosternal notch. In the adult, the right atrium is entered from the internal and external jugular veins, with 15 to 20 cm of catheter inserted. Entry at the right arm requires about 40 cm of length, while for the left arm it is 50 cm. Femoral venous insertion requires about 50 cm.

After the catheter is introduced through the sheath, it is advanced into the right atrium. Measured pressures (accentuated by the patient coughing or performing a Valsalva's maneuver) vary with patient and condition, but venous waves are present. While the distal port pressures and waveform tracings are being continuously monitored, the balloon is inflated and the catheter is advanced through the tricuspid valve to the right ventricle. Entry into the ventricle is characterized by a sudden rise in systolic pressure and a rapid fall to zero in diastole (Fig. 17.21). Further advancement places the catheter in the pulmonary artery, where the diastolic pressure rises. When the catheter is advanced to the wedged position, the tracing becomes damped, mean pressure decreases, and the appearance of *a* and *c* venous waves becomes more pronounced. The mean wedge or pulmonary artery occlusion pressure should be equal to or less than pulmonary artery diastolic pressure. When the balloon is deflated, the tracing should immediately revert to that of the pulmonary artery (Fig. 17.21).

It is important not to use an excessive length of pulmonary artery catheter during insertion. It may curl within the right atrium or ventricle, knotting on itself, possibly making removal of the catheter difficult or impossible. In the adult, the 7-French catheter reaches the pulmonary artery by 50 cm of catheter length from the neck veins and 70 cm from the arms and femoral veins. If insertion is not successful on the first approach, deflate the balloon and carefully pull the catheter back to the 10 to 20 cm distance and repeat the above procedure. In children, the 5-French catheter is used and reaches the pulmonary artery with less catheter length, depending on the size of the child.

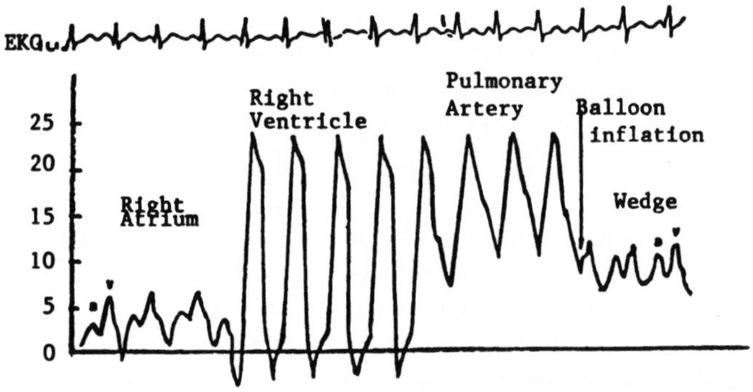

Figure 17.21. Pressure wave tracing during a Swan-Ganz catheter insertion, passing from the right atrium into the pulmonary artery. The pulmonary artery wedge pressure is lower than the pulmonary artery diastolic pressure. Mechanical obstruction of the catheter (air bubbles, catheter placement in West zone 1 and 2, overinflation of the balloon) may lead to excessive dampening of the wedge tracing or higher wedge pressure than pulmonary artery diastolic pressure. *EKG,* electrocardiagram. (From Wiedermann H, Matthay M, Matthay R. Cardiovascular-pulmonary monitoring in the intensive care unit. Chest 1984;85:540.)

Catheter placement may be difficult in patients with tricuspid regurgitation, pulmonary hypertension, and low cardiac output. Having the child make deep inspiratory efforts may facilitate catheter passage. Also, having the child positioned slightly head up and right-side down may help pass the catheter into the pulmonary artery. Otherwise, fluoroscopy will be needed to assist catheter passage. Cold saline may be injected into the catheter to help stiffen it, since prolonged exposure to the heat of the vascular compartment softens it, making passage harder. More difficulty occurs in the smaller patient. Repeated passages may be required. Attention should be paid to the preformed curve of the catheter tip and to orienting the curve in such a way as to facilitate advancement through the atrium and ventricle.

Cardiac dysrhythmias (premature atrial and ventricular contractions and transient right bundle branch block) may occur during catheter insertion, but they most commonly occur when the catheter is entering the right ventricle. Removal of the catheter from the affected chamber is usually sufficient to correct the dysrhythmia. If it is not sufficient, drug therapy and/or countershock therapy may be indicated. Pulmonary artery catheters with ventricular pacing capacity (e.g., Paceport, Baxter Healthcare Corp., Irvine, California) are available for patients with left bundle branch block because of the high risk of third-degree heart block developing if right bundle branch block ensues during catheter placement. These catheters capable of pacing the heart are usually 7.5-French because of the extra pacing wire lumen.

After the catheter has been placed into the pulmonary artery, confirm catheter position with a chest x-ray, which will also exclude such complications as pneumothorax. Maintain a length of sterile catheter in a protective sheath to allow for catheter manipulation should it migrate out of or further into the pulmonary vasculature.

Complications of Pulmonary Artery Catheters

The complications of passing the pulmonary artery catheter include arrhythmias, the development of right bundle branch or complete heart block, pulmonary artery rupture, pulmonary infarction, air embolus, catheter knotting or kinking, and valvular damage. Arrhythmias can be precipitated by the catheter touching the atrium or ventricle. This is more likely to happen if the balloon is not inflated or if the catheter coils in the right ventricle. Administration of lidocaine (1 mg/kg) may help decrease ventricular arrhythmias. The development of a right bundle branch or complete heart block has been reported during the passage of the pulmonary artery catheter through the right ventricle. As discussed above, if a patient has a preexisting left bundle branch block, a pulmonary artery catheter with pacing capability can be used in older children so that the heart can be paced if complete heart block develops.

Knotting or kinking of the catheter can occur if an excessive amount of catheter is passed into the heart in an attempt to enter the pulmonary artery or to wedge the catheter[(67)]. The catheter can curl and develop a knot. This is more likely in patients with large atrial and/or ventricular cavities as well as in low-flow states. Damage to tricuspid or pulmonary valves can occur if the catheter is pulled back through a closed valve while the balloon is inflated. For this reason, it is important to be vigilant about allowing the balloon to deflate before withdrawing the catheter.

Even with successful, uncomplicated insertion, complications can develop with an indwelling pulmonary artery catheter. Intracardiac thrombus formation can occur if a thrombus forms from the tip of the catheter. The thrombus can then embolize to the pulmonary artery or lead to thrombocytopenia. Pulmonary infarction can occur if the catheter is allowed to remain in the wedge position for an extended period[(101–103)]. Careful continuous monitoring of the pulmonary artery waveform is essential to prevent this complication.

Pulmonary artery rupture can occur if the balloon is inflated in a small or diseased pulmonary arterial branch, causing the vessel to tear; patients with pulmonary hypertension are at greater risk for this complication. Patients will immediately develop hemoptysis or blood via the endotracheal tube[(104,105)]. Depending on the severity of the bleeding, therapy ranges from conservative support to the use of a double-lumen endotracheal tube to protect the normal lung, which is possible only in larger children. In some cases, surgery may be required for massive hemorrhage[(106)].

Air embolus can be introduced by attempts to inflate a ruptured balloon or by inadvertent introduction of air through one of the catheter ports. This is particularly important to watch for in patients with low right atrial pressure or who generate large negative inspiratory pressures. If these patients are in the sitting position and the introducer or a catheter port is open to air, entrainment of air can occur during inspiration. The amount of air introduced into the circulation can have dire consequences for patients with intracardiac shunts. In this group, it may be advisable to use CO_2 because this is more rapidly absorbed and excreted by the lungs.

Prolonged catheterization increases the risk of infection. This risk can be minimized if (a) the patient is aseptic at the time of insertion, (b) less than three repositionings of the catheter were performed, and (c) the catheter is removed after 3 days[(107,108)]. Valvular damage[(102)] and thromboembolic phenomena[(102,103,109)] may also occur. Constant line flushing with heparinized solution should minimize the latter risk.

Interpretation of Measured Pressures and Waveforms

Interest in the measurement of CVP stemmed from the initial hypothesis that it accurately reflected intravascular volume and therefore was an indicator of myocardial preload[(110)]. Toussaint and associates[(111)] measured CVP and PAOP in 27 postoperative hypoxemic patients. In 14 patients with no history of cardiac disease, the correlation coefficient between the two parameters was only 0.68. In the remaining patients with pulmonary hypertension or cardiac disease, the correlation was worse. Other studies[(112)] have shown the lack of correlation between CVP and PAOP in a variety of disease states, emphasizing the disparity between left and right ventricular function and the danger in relying on CVP as an indicator of left ventricular function. Clearly, PAOP accurately reflects left atrial pressure (LAP) only when there is a continuum between the wedged pulmonary artery catheter and the left atrium[(113)].

Accurate interpretation of pulmonary artery catheter data often depends on the location of the catheter tip and the patient's pulmonary status. To obtain accurate pulmonary catheter measurements, the catheter tip must be in an area where the pulmonary artery blood pressure is greater than the pulmonary venous blood pressure or the pulmonary alveolar pressure. West and colleagues[(114)] described three zones of the lung, illustrated in Figure 17.22. If the catheter tip is in zone 1, the alveolar pressure will be greater than the pulmonary artery or pulmonary venous pressure, so airway pressure will be transmitted to the catheter, and the resulting waveform will be significantly affected by changes in ventilation.

A chest X-ray may be used to confirm the position of the catheter tip, and if it is above the left atrium, it should be repositioned below the left atrium. The correlation between PAOP and LAP has been very good in a variety of studies[(115–118)]. But the correlation of LAP with PAOP is affected by mechanical ventilation and positive end-expiratory pressure (PEEP). PEEP can be transmitted to the pulmonary vasculature and interrupt the continuum between the pulmonary artery catheter tip and left atrium.

Nevertheless, Tooker and associates[119] demonstrated that with pulmonary artery catheters located below the left atrium, LAP was accurately measured by PAOP at all levels of PEEP up to 30 cm H_2O. Berryhill and Benumof[120] noted that LAP correlated well with PAOP up to levels of PEEP of 20 cm H_2O, especially during spontaneous breathing with PEEP (continuous positive airway pressure [CPAP]), even if the catheter tip was above the left atrium[120]. Nonetheless, PAOP, also referred to as pulmonary capillary wedge pressure (PCWP), should be measured during the spontaneous phase of intermittent mandatory ventilation during CPAP. If a patient is spontaneously breathing but the breathing is labored or obstructed, a large negative intrapleural pressure can be generated during inspiration, which can then be transmitted to the pulmonary circulation and cause negative filling pressures. If the patient is receiving positive pressure ventilation (PPV), the positive pressure can be transmitted, resulting in falsely high pulmonary artery pressure measurements.

PAOP, LAP, and left ventricular end-diastolic pressure (LVEDP) are virtually interchangeable in patients with normal cardiovascular systems who are breathing spontaneously. This relationship fails in the presence of left ventricular dysfunction, mechanical ventilation, pulmonary hypertension, and mitral valve disease. Jardin et al.[121] demonstrated that PAOP was higher than LVEDP in adult patients with adult respiratory distress syndrome who were mechanically assisted with PEEP greater than 10 cm H_2O.

In the presence of atrial contractions making significant contributions to ventricular filling, PAOP tends to underestimate LVEDP, in that PAOP measures mean LAP, not the atrial contraction portion of the waveform[122]. Therefore, measurement of the *a* wave pressure may be more accurate in assessing LVEDP[123]. However, the *a* wave is less distinct in children because of the smaller catheter sizes. The presence of a large *v* wave can indicate mitral regurgitation or a decrease in ventricular compliance (Fig. 17.23). Large or "cannon" *a* waves occur with nodal rhythm and complete heart block.

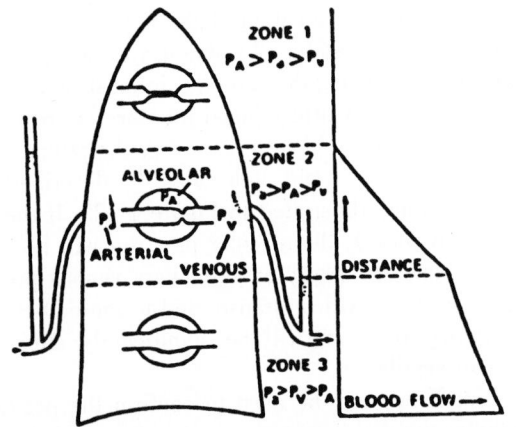

Figure 17.22. Wedge pressure reflects left atrial pressure only if there is a continuous column of blood. This relationship is influenced by three factors: P_A (pulmonary alveolar pressure), P_a (pulmonary artery pressure), and P_v (pulmonary venous pressure). It is in zone 3 that both P_a and P_v exceed P_A. This relationship may change under varying conditions (increased P_A with positive pressure ventilation; decreased P_a and P_v with intravascular volume depletion) and change zone 3 into zone 1 or 2 functionally. (From Wiedermann H, Matthay M, Matthay R. Cardiovascular-pulmonary monitoring in the intensive care unit. Chest 1984;85:542.)

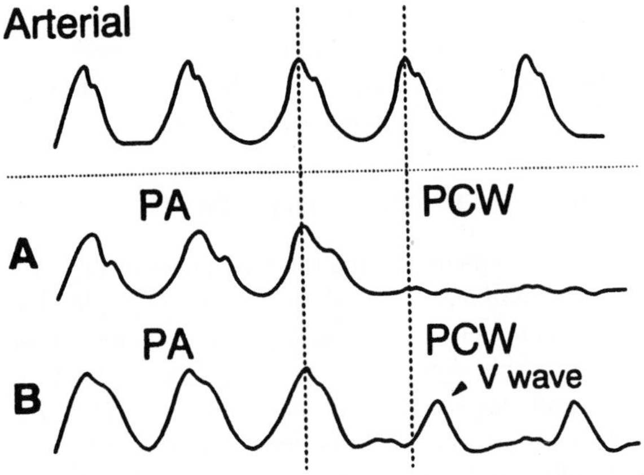

Figure 17.23. The relationship of a systemic arterial waveform, a pulmonary artery *(PA)* waveform, and a pulmonary capillary wedge *(PCW)* waveform in the normal patient **(A)** and in the presence of a v wave **(B).** From Reich DL, Kaplan JA: *Hemodynamic monitoring.* In Kaplan JA, editor: *Cardiac anesthesia,* Philadelphia, 1993, WB Saunders, p 276; with permission.)

PARAMETERS MEASURED BY PULMONARY ARTERY CATHETERS

Intracardiac Measurements

Pulmonary artery catheters directly measure right atrial pressure (proximal port), pulmonary artery pressure (distal port), PAOP (from the distal port when the balloon is inflated), cardiac output, and blood temperature (using the wiring to the thermistor). By drawing blood samples from the two ports, oxygen saturations can be directly measured. Normal intracardiac pressures and oxygen saturations are shown schematically in Figure 17.24. From these parameters, indices of both hemodynamic function **(Table 17.4)** and respiratory function **(Table 17.5)** can be derived. With this information, volume status, ventricular function, and the presence of pulmonary hypertension can be assessed. Interpretation of abnormal values is shown in **Table 17.6.**

Pulmonary artery catheters directly measure cardiac output using the thermodilution technique. This and other methods of cardiac output measurements are discussed in the next section of this chapter.

Oxygen Saturations

One might think that in the absence of intracardiac shunts, the oxygen saturation in the superior vena cava (SVC), the right atrium (RA) and the pulmonary artery (PA) would be equal. However, due to variations in the patient's status (both cardiac and respiratory) and sampling/measurement errors, this may not always be so. Despite this, measurement of oxygen saturation from the right side of the heart

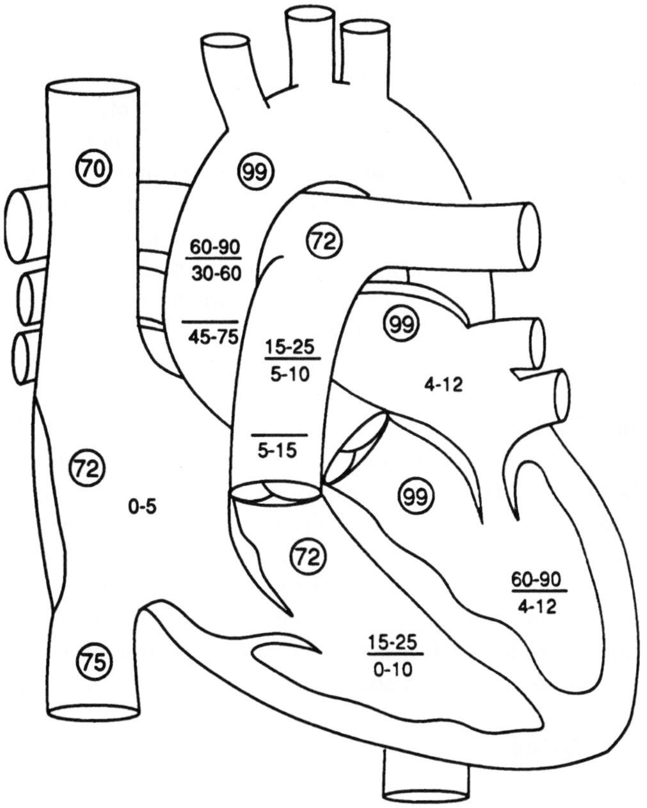

Figure 17.24. Normal cardiac catheterization values in an infant. Oxygen saturation numbers are circled. Systolic, diastolic, and mean pressures are expressed as ranges.

can be very helpful in understanding the patient's clinical status (Fig. 17.24).

Oxygen saturation of the SVC should be sampled in the midportion above the entrance of the azygous vein. A high saturation may be indicative of a high output state, an anomalous pulmonary venous connection to the SVC, or an arteriovenous fistula. A low saturation may be due to pulmonary venous desaturation, a right-to-left shunt, or a low cardiac output state. The right atrial sample from the proximal port of the PA catheter should be about the same as the SVC saturation. A step-up of more than 9% in the oxygen saturation is suggestive of a left-to-right shunt at the atrial level[98]. A right ventricular sample can be obtained from pulmonary artery catheters with pacing capability, which have a right ventricular port through which to pass a pacing wire if necessary. The right ventricular saturation should be approximately equal to the RA. A step-up of 6% suggests a left-to-right shunt[98]. Similarly, the pulmonary artery sample from the distal port on the PA catheter should approximate the RA and RV samples. A greater than 6% step-up in oxygen saturation at the level of PA suggests a left-to-right shunt[98].

A true mixed venous oxygen saturation is measured by drawing a blood sample from the pulmonary artery (distal) port of the pulmonary artery catheter. It is important that the balloon be deflated and the catheter not be in a wedged position when the sample is drawn, otherwise an arterialized pulmonary venous sample will be obtained rather than a mixed venous pulmonary artery sample. The mixed venous oxygen saturation (Svo_2) may reflect the adequacy of perfusion. Under normal circumstances, Svo_2 is 75% (Ppo_2 = 40 mm Hg) compared with an arterial oxygen saturation (Sao_2) of 95 to 100%. Svo_2 varies directly with hemoglobin, cardiac output, and arterial O_2 saturation, and indirectly with metabolic rate. Therefore, when Svo_2 falls, it indicates that hemoglobin, cardiac output, and arterial oxygen saturation should be directly measured. If these indices are stable, it suggests that the metabolic rate may have significantly increased. This can occur, for example, in the postoperative period when a hypothermic patient begins shivering as the muscle paralysis wears off. Svo_2 is more difficult to interpret under conditions of intracardiac shunts, peripheral shunts, sepsis, cirrhosis, and cyanide poisoning.

LEFT ATRIAL PRESSURE

Direct measurement of left atrial pressure is indicated when pulmonary artery catheter monitoring is technically difficult or if the patient's anatomy or clinical condition makes the use of a pulmonary artery catheter impossible. Such conditions exist with tricuspid stenosis or atresia, pulmonary stenosis or atresia, severe pulmonary hypertension, and right heart failure.

The left atrial pressure waveform has *a*, *c*, and *v* waves similar to the waveform from the right atrium and pulmonary capillary wedge tracing. Left atrial pressure measured

Table 17.4. Derived Physiologic Values

Value	*Formula*	*Physiologic Range*	*Units*
Cardiac index (CI)	CI=CO/BSA	3.5–5.5	liters/min/m^2
Stroke volume (SV)	SV=CO/HR	50–80	ml
Stroke index (SI)	SI=CI/HR	30–60	ml/m^2
Systemic vascular resistance index (SVRI)	SVR index=79.9(MAP-CVP)/CI	800–1600	dyn-sec/cm^5/m^2
Pulmonary vascular resistance (PVR) index	PVR index=79.9 (MPAP-PCWP)/CI	80–240	dyn-sec/cm^5/m^2
Arterial-mixed venous O_2 content difference ($avDO_2$)	$avDO_2=C_aO_2-C_vO_2$	3.0–5.5	ml/dl
Left ventricular stroke work index (LVSWI)	LVSWI=SI×MAP×0.0136	56±6	g-m/m^2
Left cardiac work index (LCWI)	LCWI=CI×MAP×0.0136	4.0±0.4	kg-m/m^2
Right ventricular stroke work index (RVSWI)	RVSWI=SI×MPAP×0.0136	6.0±0.9	g-m/m^2
Right cardiac work index (RCWI)	RCWI=CI×MPAP×0.0136	0.5±0.06	kg-m/m^2

Abbreviations: CO, cardiac output (liters/min); HR, heart rate (beats/min); BSA, body surface area (m^2); MAP, mean arterial pressure (mm Hg); CVP, central venous pressure (mm Hg); MPAP, pulmonary arterial pressure (mm Hg); C_aO_2, arterial O_2 content (ml/dl); and C_vO_2, venous O_2 content (ml/dl).

Table 17.5. Derived Indices of Gas Transport

$$Qs/Qt = \frac{Cco_2\ Cao_2}{Cco_2\ Cvo_2}\ (normal < 5\%)$$

A-aO_2 = $P_AO_2 - PaO_2$ (normal <9 mm Hg if $FiO_2 = 0.21$; <34 mm Hg if $FiO_2 = 1.0$)

$\dot{V}O_2$ = CI (a-vO_2) × 10 (normal = 140–160 ml · min · m^{-2})

DO_2 = CI(CaO_2) × 10 (normal = 400–600 ml · min · m^{-2})

$avDO_2$ = $CaO_2 - CvO_2$ (normal = 4 to 6 ml/dl)

where:

Qs/Qt = intrapulmonary shunt

CcO_2 = capillary O_2 content (Hgb × 1.39[a]) + [FiO_2 × 713 − ($PaCO_2$)] × 0.0031

CaO_2 = arterial O_2 content (Hgb × 1.39 × SaO_2) + (PaO_2 × 0.0031)

CvO_2 = mixed venous O_2 content (Hgb × 1.39 × SVO_2) + (PVO_2 × 0.0031)

A–aO_2 = alveolar-arterial O_2 gradient

P_AO_2 = alveolar O_2 tension (PB[b] − 47) (FiO_2) − ($PACO_2$/R)

PaO_2 = arterial O_2 tension

$\dot{V}O_2$ = O_2 consumption (l/min)

$\dot{C}O$ = cardiac output

$\dot{D}O_2$ = tissue oxygen delivery

$avDO_2$ = arteriovenous O_2 content difference

PvO_2 = mixed venous oxygen tension

SvO_2 = mixed venous oxygen saturation

SaO_2 = arterial oxygen saturation

[a] *Assumes FiO_2 <0.35 (SaO_2 = 100%).*
[b] *Assumes barometric pressure (P_B) = 760 mm Hg and respiratory quotient (R) = 1.*

directly is more accurate than PCWP because it is not affected by the lungs. It is important to note that the left atrial catheter must be placed surgically and has the serious disadvantage of being a possible site for air entry into the left side of the heart. The consequences of thrombosis and air or clot embolism on the left (systemic) circulation may be profound, with neurologic or coronary vascular occlusion and possibly devastating consequences.

CARDIAC OUTPUT

Cardiac output is defined as the amount of blood ejected by the left ventricle in one minute; it is equal to the heart rate multiplied by the stroke volume. In neonates, cardiac output is normally 400 to 500 ml/kg/min because of residual left-to-right shunts (patent foramen ovale, patent ductus arteriosus). In normal infants, these shunts close after the first week of life, and the cardiac output falls to 150 to 200 ml/kg/min. As cardiac output falls, an increase in peripheral vasoconstriction occurs to produce the gradual rise in blood pressure with age. Premature infants have a relatively higher cardiac output than full-term babies with a cardiac index of 5.5 L/min/m^2[124].

It is self-evident that the ability to measure cardiac output is important for the clinical management of critically ill patients. The most commonly used methods to measure cardiac output are the indicator-dilution technique and the Doppler-flow probes. The indicator-dilution technique uses either oxygen, cold injectate (thermodilution), or green dye as the indicator. The thermodilution, green dye, and Fick methods for measuring cardiac output are, for the most part, equally accurate when carried out properly[125].

The presence of either a left-to-right or a right-to-left shunt will result in erroneous cardiac output measurements. In a left-to-right shunt, the area under the curve is falsely elevated because of recirculation, so the cardiac output will be erroneously low. In a right-to-left shunt, some of the cold injectate will be shunted to the left side without affecting the blood reaching the thermistor, resulting in a falsely high cardiac output. In addition to these problems, the pulmonary artery catheter measures only right heart cardiac output and reflects left heart output only if the two are equal, i.e., in the absence of shunts.

Fick Method

The Fick method can be used to measure either pulmonary or systemic blood flow. According to the Fick principle, cardiac output is equal to the oxygen consumption divided by the arteriovenous oxygen difference. Oxygen consumption is approximately 140 to 160 ml/min/m^2. Thus, for pulmonary blood flow, the oxygen uptake by the lungs is divided by the difference between the pulmonary venous and pulmonary arterial oxygen content. For systemic blood flow, the oxygen consumption is divided by the difference between the arterial and mixed venous oxygen content. This knowledge of systemic and pulmonary blood flows makes it possible to calculate the amount of intracardiac shunt, Qp/Qs:

$$Qp/Qs = \frac{S_{O_2}(Ao) S_{O_2}(RA)}{S_{O_2}(PV) S_{O_2}(PA)}$$

where

So_2 = oxygen saturation
Ao = aorta
RA = right atrium
PV = pulmonary vein
PA = pulmonary artery

Table 17.6. Interpretation of Abnormal Hemodynamic Values

	CVP	*PCWP*	*SVR*	*CI*	*Comment*
Hypovolemia	↓	↓	↑	↓	Confirm diagnosis with fluid challenge
Cardiogenic shock	↑	↑	↑	↓	PCWP is low in isolated right heart failure
Septic shock	↓	↓	↓ or ↑	variable	EF is decreased; SV and CO are maintained by LV dilation and increased HR; mixed venous O_2 saturation may be high
Tamponade	↑	↑	↑	↓	Equalization of diastolic pressures

Abbreviations: CVP, central venous pressure; PCWP, pulmonary capillary wedge pressure; SVR, systemic vascular resistance; CI, cardiac index; EF, ejection fraction; SV, stroke volume; CO, cardiac output; LV, left ventricular; HR, heart rate.

The arterial (C_{aO_2}) minus mixed venous oxygen content ($C_{mv}O_2$), i.e., the arterial venous oxygen difference ($avDO_2 = C_aO_2 - C_{mv}O_2$), is related to cardiac output (CO) using the Fick principle:

$$CO = \text{oxygen consumption}/avDO_2$$

If O_2 consumption remains stable, then CO is inversely related to $avDO_2$. Oxygen consumption does change in the critically ill patient, and $avDO_2$ therefore represents only the adequacy of CO in meeting the body's metabolic needs. Mixed venous oxygen saturation can be of help in following cardiac output, provided O_2 consumption and hemoglobin concentration remain constant. Normal mixed venous oxygen saturation values are 75 to 80% with a mixed venous PO_2 of 36 to 42 torr. Higher values are seen in patients with lower $avDO_2$ values (septic shock, elevated CO, left-to-right shunting). Lower values occur in patients with decreased CO and anemia. Mixed venous PO_2 values below 27 mm Hg (50% saturation) correlated with increased concentrations of lactate and are therefore thought to be indicative of insufficient O_2 supply to the body[110,126]. Because streaming and inadequate mixing occur in the right atrium, only blood samples from the pulmonary artery should be used to measure mixed venous PO_2.

Oxygen transport can be assessed in various ways:

Value	*Formula*	*Normal Units*
O_2 availability	$\dot{D}O_2 = C_aO_2 \times CI \times 10$	620 ± 50 ml/min/m^2
O_2 consumption	$\dot{V}O_2 = CI \times avDO_2 \times 10$	120 to 200 ml/min/m^2
O_2 extraction	$O_2\ ext = avDO_2/C_{aO2} \times 100$	28 to 33%

$\dot{D}O_2$ represents the amount of oxygen generally available to the tissues. $\dot{V}O_2$ is the oxygen-required-tissue metabolic oxygen needs. CI is the cardiac index measured in liters per minute per square meter, and C_aO_2 (arterial oxygen content) and $avDO_2$ are measured in milliliters per deciliter. Extraction refers to the rate of oxygen consumption divided by availability, and it therefore reflects the adequacy of oxygen delivery to meet tissue needs.

These data may also be used to calculate the intrapulmonary shunt fraction that represents the fraction of blood passing through unventilated lungs:

$$\dot{Q}s/\dot{Q}t = (C_{pv}O_2 - C_aO_2/(C_{pv} - C_vO_2)$$

where $C_{pv}O_2$ equals:

$$C_{pv}O_2 = P_AO_2\ (bp - wp) - (P_aCO_2/0.8)$$
(alveolar gas equation)

where $C_{pv}O_2$, C_aO_2, and C_vO_2 are the O_2 contents in pulmonary venous, arterial, and venous blood, respectively; P_AO_2 and P_aO_2 are the partial pressures of alveolar and arterial O_2; bp and wp are the barometric and water vapor pressures, respectively; and a respiratory quotient of 0.8 is assumed. Normal values are 3 to 7%. Values of 50% are not uncommon with adult respiratory distress syndrome or pulmonary edema.

Dye Dilution

The dye dilution technique uses indocyanine green (also known as Cardio-Green or green dye) because it is nontoxic, is rapidly removed from the circulation by the liver, and has a half-life in circulation of about 10 minutes. It has a peak absorption wavelength at 805 nm, which is near the point at which the absorption of light by oxygenated and reduced hemoglobin is identical, so changes in blood oxygen concentrations will not affect the cardiac output determination.

The technique requires a central vein and an arterial catheter. The dye solution is injected rapidly into the CVP catheter, and continuous sampling of arterial blood from the arterial catheter (withdrawn at a constant rate by a syringe in a calibrated pump) is begun. The blood passes through a densitometer, and the change in indicator concentration is measured over time, generating a dye concentration-versus-time curve. The area under the curve is calculated, and the cardiac output is computed by the Stewart-Hamilton equation[127], whereby cardiac output is equal to the amount of injected indicator divided by the area under the curve:

$$\text{Indicator dye cardiac output} = \frac{60xi}{AxCF}\ \frac{60 \times i}{Cxt}$$

where

i = amount of dye injected (mg)

A = area of first pass of green dye curve measured in millimeters deflection multiplied by duration of first pass in seconds and

CF = calibration factor of standard measured in milligrams green dye per L/per mm deflection

$\overline{C}$ = mean concentration of dye under the curve (mg/L)

t = duration of curve (sec)

In the presence of a shunt, the normal cardiac output curve is distorted (Fig. 17.25). Right-to-left shunting results in an early-appearing hump on the build-up slope due to dye that has bypassed the pulmonary vasculature. Left-to-right shunting results in a decreased peak concentration of dye, a prolonged disappearance time, and a slow return to baseline with a loss of the recirculation peak.

Thermodilution

The measurement of cardiac output cardiac output by the thermodilution technique uses a known volume (usually 5 or 10 ml) of 5% dextrose in water or 0.9% normal saline solution either iced or at room temperature. After a stable baseline blood temperature is measured, the solution is injected into the proximal (right atrial) port of the pulmonary artery catheter, and the temperature change is monitored by the distal thermistor in the pulmonary artery. The temperature change integrated over time yields the cardiac output[99,127,128].

$$\dot{Q} = \frac{V(T_B - T_I)K_1K_2}{\int_0^{\infty} T_B(t)dt}$$

where

$\dot{Q}$ = cardiac output

V = volume injected

T_B = blood temperature

T_I = injectate temperature

K_1 = empiric factor used to correct for injectate warming, which is specific for catheter size (e.g., for 7-French catheters, $K_1 = 0.825$), and adjusts units to L/min

$\int_0^{\infty} K_2$ = computational constants for the specific gravity and specific heat of the blood and the injectate (D_5W), the product of which equals approximately 1.08

$T_B(t)\,dt$ = the change in blood temperature as a function of time (the area under the curve)

Thus, the change in blood temperature over time is inversely proportional to the cardiac output.

The accuracy of this method relies on very rapid injection rates, accurate measurement of the injectate temperature, thorough mixing, no loss of injectate, and having the appropriate constant entered into the cardiac output computer. Falsely elevated cardiac output will occur with injection rates that are too slow and injectate volumes that are too small. Falsely depressed cardiac output values occur with the use of solutions cooler than or injectate volumes greater than the values programmed on the cardiac output computer. In addition, simultaneous infusions of IV fluids through a peripheral or central vein may cause artifacts in cardiac output measurements[129]. When cardiac output has been calculated, it is possible to construct a ventricular function curve with cardiac output on the y-axis as a function of CVP (right ventricle) and/or PAOP (left ventricle) on the x-axis. Other determinants of left and right ventricular function can then be estimated.

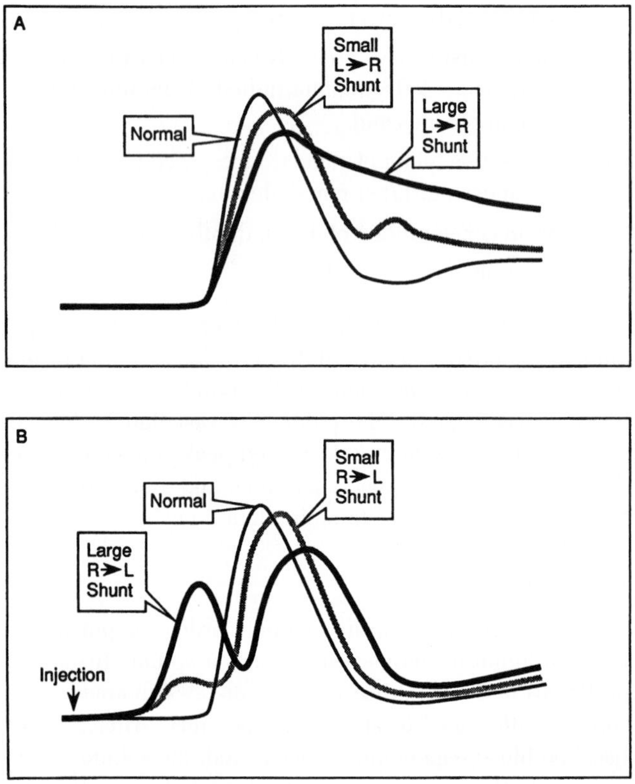

Figure 17.25. Examples of cardiac output curves obtained by the dye dilution method in normal, left-to-right (**A**), and right-to-left (**B**) shunt. In **A** the normal recirculation curve can be seen. The effect of a small left-to-right shunt is decreased peak height and apparent "early" recirculation. A large left-to-right shunt shows slurring of the dye peak with no second peak. In **B**, a small right-to-left shunt has an early peak as contrast material rapidly enters the systemic circulation. This pattern is more pronounced with a large right-to-left shunt.

Doppler (Flow Probe) Techniques

The Doppler principle was first enunciated by Christian Doppler in 1842[130]. The Doppler effect is the occurrence of a change in frequency of sound, light, or other electromagnetic radiation, caused by motion of either the source or the observer. If an ultrasound beam is reflected from a moving target, a frequency shift in proportion to the velocity of the moving target will occur. This is described by the Doppler equation:

$$V = (C \times \Delta f)/2\ f_o \cos\Theta$$

where V is the velocity of the target, C is the speed of sound in the tissue, f_o is the baseline frequency, Δf is the change in frequency, and Θ is the angle of incidence. It can be seen that since the cosine of 90 degrees is 0, the smaller the angle of incidence, the less important this angle becomes. Ideally, the ultrasound beam should be aimed directly incident on the direction of flow, i.e., parallel with the direction of flow (Fig. 17.26). This allows determination of the movement of the target, which is red blood cells, and direct measurement of the average velocity. Obviously, the Doppler waveform will vary with ejection. It also assumes that the red cells are moving in a laminar flow pattern without turbulent flow.

The Doppler technique can be used to measure ascending aortic blood flow velocity[131,132]. Cardiac output is equal to the product of the blood flow velocity and the cross-sectional area of the vessel. Because the cross-sectional area of the aorta can be measured, the product of the mean velocity and the cross-sectional area gives a flow rate. The aortic root dimension and thus the diameter of the cross-sectional area can be determined by either M-mode or two-dimensional echocardiography. The assumptions inherent in the Doppler technique for determining cardiac output are that the aortic root dimension can be accurately determined and that the cosine of the angle of incidence, Θ, is close to 1.

The ultrasound waves can be emitted and detected via transthoracic transducers[131,133,134], esophageal transducers[135], transducers mounted on the tip of an endotracheal tube[136], or miniaturized flow probes implanted directly onto the ascending aorta[137,138]. The cardiac output calculated is a left heart output without coronary blood flow, since the measurement is made above the take-off of the coro-

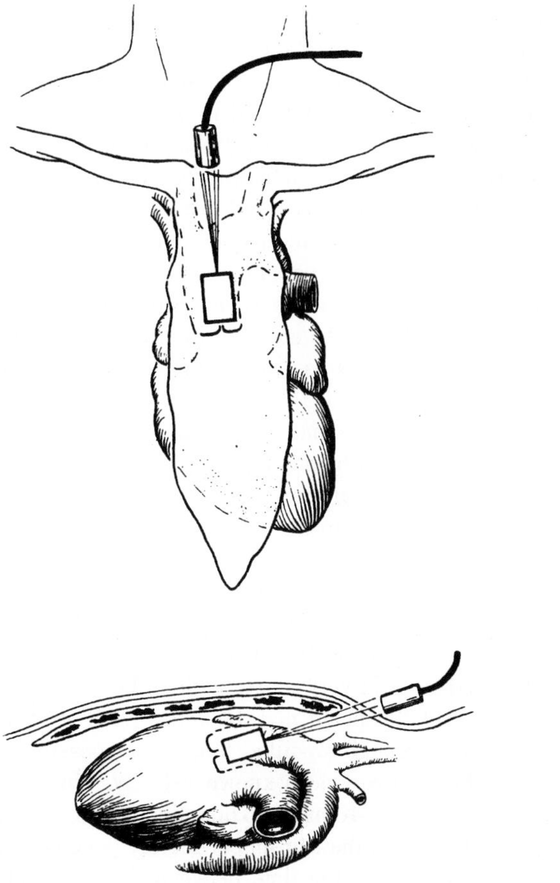

Figure 17.26. Doppler ultrasound transducer position to determine flow velocities in the aortic root. The ultrasound beam should be directly incident (parallel to) the blood flow for the optimal Doppler velocity determinations. (From Alverson DC, et al. Noninvasive pulsed Doppler determination of cardiac output in neonates and children. J Pediatr 1982;101:47.)

nary arteries. It will therefore be less than the cardiac output measured by the indicator dilution technique.

The Doppler method of determining cardiac output is subject to measurement inaccuracies at several points: incorrect determination of vessel diameter, incorrect determination of the mean velocity by measuring only one point within the vessel, or a beam angle greater than 20 degrees to the axis of blood flow.

A transthoracic ultrasound transducer placed in the suprasternal notch and directed toward the ascending aorta is a noninvasive method of measuring aortic blood flow velocity[132,134]. The pulsed Doppler technique has been shown to have a good correlation with the Fick method for calculating cardiac output in children[132,139], and the dual-beam Doppler technique had acceptable agreement with thermodilution-measured cardiac output in critically ill infants[134,140].

Transesophageal echocardiography probes with continuous-wave Doppler capability are now commercially available in sizes suitable for use in infants and small children. There are a limited number of early studies of transesophageal pulse wave Doppler echocardiography in adults, with variable results[135,141]. Data in children will undoubtedly be available in the near future. Transtracheal Doppler cardiac output measurements do not correlate well with thermodilution cardiac output in adults[136]. Our experience with children has been complicated by the fact that we were unable to position the endotracheal tube to maintain an adequate signal.

A more invasive method of measuring cardiac output entails intraoperatively attaching a miniature ultrasound probe to the adventitia of the ascending aorta. This probe is connected to monitoring equipment by wires that exit the chest wall through a small stab wound[137]. It allows continuous monitoring of cardiac output in the postoperative period. The aortic diameter measurements are made intraoperatively, and the probe is removed by gentle traction.

Bioimpedance Cardiac Output

Kubicek and coworkers[142,143] pioneered a method, called impedance cardiography, for determining cardiac output. Here the change in electrical impedance of the thoracic cavity is related to the change in content of blood within the thoracic cavity, which is the stroke volume (SV) (Fig. 17.27). Kubicek's original formula was

$$SV = (\rho \times L^2)/(Z_o^2 \times VET \times dZ/dt)$$

where ρ is the specific resistivity of blood, L is the length of thoracic segment, Z_o is the basic thoracic impedance, VET is the ventricular ejection time, and dZ/dt is the first

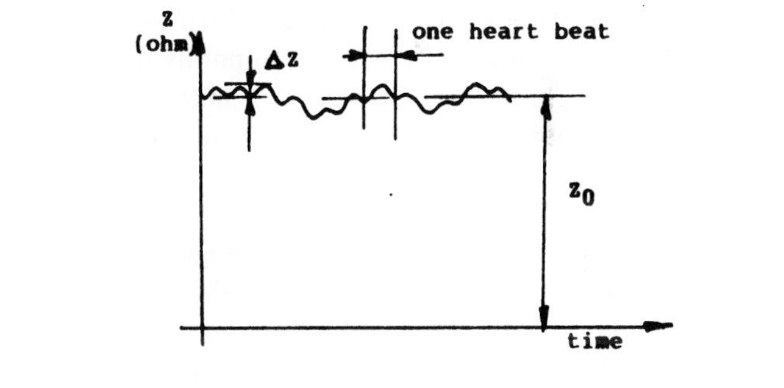

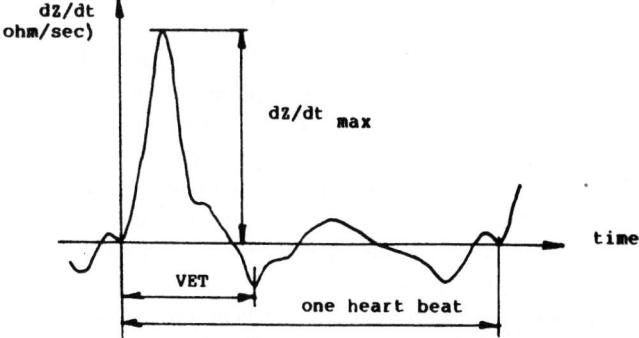

Figure 17.27. Bioimpedance waveform. *Upper panel:* Mean thoracic bioimpedance (Z_0) versus time. *Lower panel:* First differential of this waveform. *VET,* ventricular ejection time. This signal is the basis for stroke volume determination (see text). (From Spinale FG, et al. Relationship of bioimpedance to thermodilution and echocardiographic measurements of cardiac function. Crit Care Med 1990;18:415.)

derivative of electrical impedance. This formula gives stroke volume. In a well-controlled experimental setting, this technique or variations on the algorithms used to manipulate dZ/dt have given close correlation with cardiac output determined by multiple techniques(83,144–146).

The technique of bioimpedance cardiac output uses an alternating current of low amplitude and high frequency which is introduced and simultaneously sensed by two sets of electrodes placed around the neck and lower thorax. Changes in thoracic impedance are induced by ventilation and pulsatile blood flow, and only the cardiac-induced pulsatile component is analyzed when measuring cardiac output. Approximately 70 to 80% of the pulsatile component originates from the thoracic aorta(147). The correlation between thoracic impedance and thermodilution cardiac output is reported to be good by some(146,148) but not all(149,150) reports. In children less than 125 cm in length, the measured thoracic length did not result in accurate bioimpedance cardiac output measurements(151). In addition, intracardiac shunts interfere with measurements(46).

ECHOCARDIOGRAPHIC ASSESSMENT OF HEMODYNAMIC FUNCTION

Two-Dimensional Echocardiography

Rapid, instantaneous, noninvasive study of dynamic cardiac function has become increasingly possible with ultrasound technology(152–154). Not only is it possible to study direct cardiac motion on a real-time basis, but it is also possible now to determine flows, shunts, and cardiac output by using ultrasound and Doppler techniques. A rudimentary understanding of ultrasound technology is useful because of the widespread application of this technology in the PICU. Noninvasive types of monitoring are particularly suitable for small children because of their small size and the fact that there is frequent technical difficulty with more invasive forms. In addition, the anatomic relationships and the close distance of the heart to the chest suggest that the quality of imaging would be somewhat better in children than in adults.

In the early 1950s, Edler and Hertz pioneered ultrasonography to study the heart(155); Feigenbaum in the mid-1960s was crucial in introducing equipment and techniques into the United States(156). Since the early amplitude mode (A-mode) echocardiograph, echocardiographic machines now display real-time, two-dimensional pictures with video display, stop-action flow, and derived variables, all available within one machine. These are all based on the same underlying principles.

Ultrasound is sound energy that is at a higher frequency than detectable by the human ear. This frequency is 20,000 Hz (cycles per second). In medical practice, the usual range is actually in megahertz (MHz) (or 10^6 Hz) frequencies. This ultrasound is generated by a piezoelectric crystal. A piezoelectric crystal vibrates when subjected to an electrical current and thus generates a high-frequency sound beam. The piezoelectric crystal also works in the reverse, i.e., sound energy will stimulate an electric signal from it. Thus, the piezoelectric crystal is the heart of ultrasonography because it both generates the signal and senses its return. The piezoelectric crystal is enclosed in a transducer that can focus, aim, and direct the sound beam emitted by the piezoelectric crystal. In practice, piezoelectric crystals emit bursts of sound or pulses and are silent while sensing for the return of the reflected (echo) sound. It is the returning echoes from the various soft-tissue structures in the body that generate the images seen. Sound is reflected from acoustic interfaces. An acoustic interface is a boundary region between two areas of different acoustic impedance. Acoustic impedance is the product of tissue density and the velocity of sound in that tissue. This varies for various tissues (i.e., between blood and myocardium or between pericardium and myocardium). In most cases, most of the ultrasound beam is transmitted through the tissues, and only a small part is reflected back to the transducer for sensing; however, this allows detection of multiple acoustic interfaces that are used to build up an image of the soft tissues underlying the beam. When the gradient between acoustical impedances is very great, such as between air and tissue, most of the beam may be reflected. For this reason, penetration through air-filled lung is not possible. The reflected beam travels at a known velocity, which in human tissue averages 1540 m/sec. Thus, the distance of an acoustic interface from the transducer merely becomes the product of velocity and the time between the sound pulse and return of the echo generated from any acoustic interface:

$$\text{Distance} = \text{Velocity} \times \text{Time}$$

Obviously, for an echo to be detected it must be reflected back to the transducer; thus, if the ultrasound beam is deflected at 90 degrees from the structure being interrogated, there will be no reflected sound, and this structure will not be seen. If it is reflected 180 degrees perpendicular to the incidence of the sound beam, the structure will appear quite dense. If, as is common in human tissues, the acoustic interface is curvilinear, only part of the ultrasound beam will return.

Synchronization with an ECG allows understanding of how cardiac structures moved in relation to the cardiac cycle. In a two-dimensional echocardiogram, the piezoelectric crystal itself swings in an arc, generally around 45 to 60 degrees, thus building up a two-dimensional sector of the myocardium. By experience and understanding of placement of the echocardiographic beam and recognition of the dynamic heart structures, it is possible to measure cardiac dimensions. Left ventricular and end-diastolic and end-systolic diameters, great vessel dimensions such as those of the aorta and pulmonary artery, the opening and closing of the valvular structures, and, with the addition of Doppler technology, the flow velocity, both antegrade and retrograde across valve structures, can be objectively measured (Fig. 17.28). All of this information can be synthesized into an understanding of volume changes within the heart and of measures of contractility, such as stroke volume, shortening fraction, and ejection fraction. Measurement of the ratios of the systolic time intervals—preejection and the ejection times—of the right and left ventricles also gives an indication of myocardial contractility, as well as PVR[157–159]. In addition, abnormal structures can be readily seen, such as a thrombus prolapsing through the mitral valve[160,161], and the presence of bacterial endocarditis have also been assessed echocardiographically[160–162].

Transesophageal Echocardiography

The development of transesophageal echocardiography (TEE) has provided the possibility of continuous, detailed, real-time observation of the heart during surgery and, potentially, in the PICU. Transesophageal echocardiography is a well-accepted procedure for diagnosis and monitoring in adults[163], and it is becoming increasingly used in children[164–171]. The use of this technology in children has been limited for several reasons. First, transthoracic echocardiography provides high-quality images of the heart in the majority of children, thus the need for this procedure is restricted to certain clinical conditions. Second, the standard probes used in adults are too large for use in infants and small children (less than 12 kg), necessitating a smaller and equally expensive probe for their evaluation. Third, TEE is performed in children under heavy sedation or general anesthesia. For this reason, the majority of studies are in children who are undergoing general anesthesia for surgery or cardiac catheterization or who are in the intensive care unit.

Although high-quality images of the heart can be obtained using transthoracic echocardiography, there are some patients in whom clarity of images obtained by transesophageal echocardiography may redirect the clinical management. Indications for TEE include evaluation for the presence of valvular vegetations, subaortic membranes, and left atrial thrombus[163,172] (Fig. 17.28). Transesophageal echocardiography is also used in children who are "poor imagers" due to chest wall abnormalities, cardiac malpositions, and chronic lung disease. Patients who are in the PICU after cardiac surgery are usually very difficult to image because of air between the sternum and heart. Transesophageal echocardiography can be used to evaluate ventricular function in these patients when hemodynamic management issues arise[173,174].

Children undergo TEE using sedation or general anesthesia. The use of ECG, blood pressure, and pulse oximetry to monitor the child during the procedure is the standard of care for these patients. Indeed, the importance of carefully monitoring these patients cannot be stressed too strongly, especially in light of a case report of bronchial obstruction by a transesophageal echocardiography probe in a 5-year-old, 15-kg child who had an endotracheal tube in place[175]. At our institution, children who weigh more than 20 kg and are over the age of 9 years usually tolerate this procedure without endotracheal intubation, while younger children who weigh less than 20 kg undergo endotracheal intubation to prevent upper airway obstruction. This is consistent with studies describing the technique of upper gastrointestinal endoscopy in children[176–178]. The adult TEE probe which measures 11 mm in diameter at the tip is usually too large to be safely used in children under 12 kg or under the age of 3 years. The esophagus in the full-term infant measures 4 to 6 mm in diameter and is able to accommodate a 7.6-mm pediatric gastrointestinal endoscope[178], which is about the size of the new pediatric probes that have become commercially available.

Transesophageal echocardiography can be used in the PICU for both diagnostic and monitoring purposes[179]. Parker et al. stated that one-third to one-half of all mechanically ventilated patients cannot be studied transthoracically as a result of poor image quality; those requiring more than 10 cm PEEP have uniformly unsatisfactory transthoracic

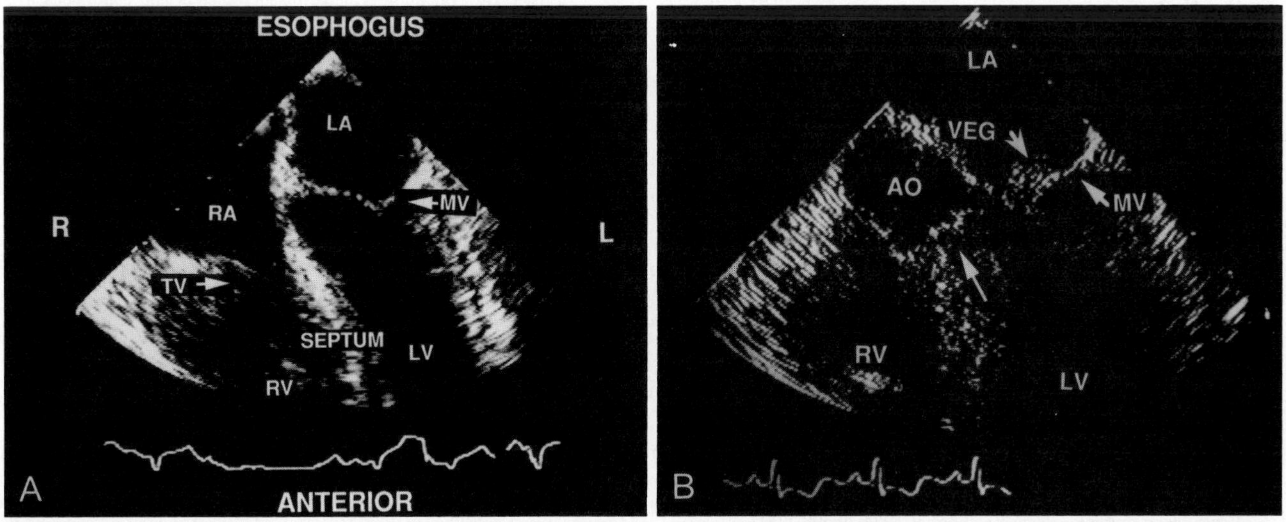

Figure 17.28. Two-dimensional transesophageal echocardiograms. **A.** Four-chamber view showing left atrium *(LA)*, right atrium *(RA)*, right ventricle *(RV)*, left ventricle *(LV)* with the septum and atrioventricular *(AV)* valves in the normal position. **B.** Four-chamber view showing the aortic outflow *(AO)*, *LA*, *RV*, and *LV*. In the center of the mitral valve *(MV)* is a highly echogenic vegetation *(VEG)*. There is also a subaortic membrane *(arrow)*.

studies. Transesophageal echocardiography allows continuous cardiac evaluation in patients treated with up to 15 cm PEEP[180]. Koenig et al.[181] were able to diagnose one case each of ventricular septal and papillary muscle rupture by TEE after acute myocardial infarction. The sudden onset of cardiogenic shock requiring tracheal intubation and mechanical ventilation had made transthoracic images suboptimal. Postoperative cardiac surgery patients or those with significant thoracic trauma may have bandages that interfere with transthoracic probes[182]. Cardiac tamponade, a common complication of either trauma or cardiac surgery, often can be diagnosed echocardiographically[183,184].

Transesophageal echocardiography is a field which has evolved through the collaborative efforts of several disciplines, including pediatric and adult cardiology, anesthesiology, cardiac surgery, and radiology. Several authors have raised the question regarding the possibilities and expectations of the various disciplines with regard to this procedure[185–187]. In essence, each discipline provides unique expertise in the performance and interpretation of transesophageal echocardiography studies.

References

1. Sittig DF, Gardner RM. Summary of the 10th Annual International Symposium on Computers in Critical Care, Pulmonary Medicine and Anesthesia. Int J Clin Monitoring Computing 1990;7(1):33–39.
2. Joly H, Weil M. Temperature of the great toe as an indicator of the severity of shock. Circulation 1969;39:131–138.
3. Henning R, Wiener F, Valdes S, Weil M. Measure of toe temperature for assessing the severity of acute circulatory failure. Surg Gynecol Obstet 1979;149:1–7.
4. Ryan C, Soder C. Relationship between core/peripheral temperature gradient and central hemodynamics in children after open heart surgery. Crit Care Med 1989;17:638–640.
5. Knight R, Opie J. The big toe in the recovery room: Peripheral warm-up patterns in children after open-heart surgery. Can J Surg 1981;24: 239–242.
6. Abel F, McCutcheon E. Cardiovascular function: Principles and application. Boston: Little, Brown, 1979.
7. Kirkendall W, Feinleib M, Freis E, Mark A. Recommendations for human blood pressure determination by sphygmomanometers. Subcommittee of the AHA Postgraduate Education Committee. Circulation 1980;62:1146A–1155A.
8. Raferty E, Ward A. The indirect method of recording blood pressure. Cardiovasc Res 1968;2:210.
9. Pascarelli E, Bertrand C. Comparisons of blood pressures in the arms and legs. N Engl J Med 1964;270:693.
10. Talke P, Nichols RJ, Traber D. Does measurement of systolic blood pressure with a pulse oximeter correlate with conventional methods? J Clin Monit 1990;6:5–9.
11. Bruner J, Krenis L, Kunsman J, Sherman A. Comparison of direct and indirect methods of measuring arterial blood pressure, part III. Med Instrum 1981;15:182–188.
12. Friesen R, Lichtor J. Indirect measurement of blood pressure in neonates and infants utilizing an automatic noninvasive oscillometric monitor. Anesth Analg 1981;60:742–745.
13. Hutton P, Dye J, Prys-Roberts C. An assessment of the Dinamap 845. Anaesthesia 1984;39:261–267.
14. Lyew M, Jamieson J. Blood pressure measurement using oscillometric finger cuffs in children and young adults. Anaesthesia 1994;49: 895–899.
15. Peñaz J. Current photoelectric recording of blood flow through the finger. Ceskoslovenska Fysiologie 1975;24(4):349–352.
16. Molhoek G, Wesseing K, Settels J, et al. Evaluation of the Peñaz servoplethysmo-manometer for the continuous, non-invasive measurement of finger blood pressure. Basic Res Cardiol 1984;79:598–609.
17. Gravenstein J, Paulus D, Feldman J, McLaughlin G. Tissue hypoxia distal to a Peñaz finger blood pressure cuff. J Clin Monit 1985;1: 120–125.
18. Wong D, Volgyesi G, Bissonnette B. Systolic arterial pressure determination by a new pulse monitor technqiue. Can J Anaesth 1992;39: 596–599.
19. Kemmotsu O, Otsuka H, Vedo M, Yamamura T, Eckerle J, Winter D. Arterial tonometry for blood pressure monitoring in pediatric anesthesia. Anesth Analg 1991;72:S135.
20. Kemmotsu O, Ohno M, Takita K, et al. Noninvasive, continuous blood pressure measurement by arterial tonometry during anesthesia in children. Anesthesiol 1994;81:1161–1168.
21. Bause G, Weintraub A, Tanner G. Skin avulsion during oscillometry. J Clin Monit 1986;2:262–263.
22. Sanford T, Jones B, Smith N. Noninvasive blood pressure measurement. Anes Clin North Am 1988;6:721–741.
23. Showman A, Betts E. Hazard of automatic noninvasive blood pressure monitoring. Anesthesiol 1981;55:717–718.
24. Miller R, Camp P. Postoperative ulnar neuropathy. JAMA 1979; 242:1636–1639.
25. Sy W. Ulnar nerve palsy possibly related to use of automatically cycled blood pressure cuff. Anesth Analg 1981;60:687–688.
26. Hales S. Statistical Essays. New York: New York Academy of Medicine, 1964 The History of Medicine Series; Vol. 22.
27. Nichols W, et al. Catheter tip manometer system: Pressure and velocity measurement. Adv Cardiovasc Phys 1983;5:144.
28. Petersen R, Myers G. Waveform analysis in medicine. Springfield, IL: Charles C Thomas, 1976:119.
29. Nichols W, et al. Percutaneous left ventricular catheterization with an ultraminiature catheter tip pressure transducer. Cardiovasc Res 1978; 12:566.
30. Patel D, et al. Harmonic analysis of pressure pulses obtained from the heart and great vessels of man. Am Heart J 1965;69:785.
31. Gersh B, et al. Physical criteria for measurement of left ventricular pressure and its first derivative. Cardiovasc Res 1971;5:32.
32. Falsetti H, et al. Analysis and correction of pressure wave distortion in fluid-filled catheter systems. Circulation 1974;49:165.
33. Kaye W. Invasive monitoring techniques: Arterial cannulation, bedside pulmonary artery catheterization, and arterial puncture. Heart Lung 1983;12:395.
34. Barr P. Percutaneous puncture of the radial artery with a multipurpose Teflon catheter for indwelling use. Acta Physiol Scand 1961; 51:343.
35. Bedford R, Major M. Percutaneous radial-artery cannulation—increased safety using Teflon catheters. Anesthesiology 1977b;42:219–222.
36. Davis F. Radial artery cannulation: Influence of catheter size and material on arterial occlusion. Anaesth Intensive Care 1978;6:49.
37. Downs J, Rackstein A, Klein EJ, Hawkins IJ. Hazards of radial-artery catheterization. Anesthesiology 1973;38:283–286.
38. Kim J, Arakawa K, Bliss J. Arterial cannulation: Factors in the development of occlusion. Anesth Analg 1975;54:836–841.
39. Downs J, Chapman RJ, Hawkins IJ. Prolonged radial-artery catheterization. An evaluation of heparinized catheters and continuous irrigation. Arch Surg 1974;108:671–673.
40. Bedford R. Radial arterial function following percutaneous cannuluation with 18- and 20-gauge catheters. Anesthesiology 1977a;47:37–39.
41. Bedford R. Long-term radial artery cannulation: Effects on subsequent vessel function. Crit Care Med 1978a;6:64–67.
42. Cederholm I, Sorensen J, Carlsson C. Thrombosis following percutaneous radial artery cannuluation. Acta Anaesthesiol Scand 1986;30: 227–230.
43. Barr P, Sumners J, Wirtschafter D, Porter R, Cassady G. Percutaneous peripheral arterial cannulation in the neonate. Pediatrics 1977;59 suppl:1058–1062.
44. Bedford R, Shah N. Blood pressure monitoring: Invasive and Noninvasive. In: Blitt C, Hines R, ed. Monitoring in anesthesia and critical care medicine. New York: Churchill Livingstone, 1995: 108.
45. Allen E. Thromboangitis obliterans: Methods of diagnosis of chronic occlusive arterial lesions distal to the wrist with illustrated cases. Am J Med Sci 1929;178:237.
46. Reich D, Kaplan J. Hemodynamic monitoring. In: Kaplan J, ed. Cardiac anesthesia. Philadelphia: WB Saunders, 1993: 261–298.
47. Marshall A, Erwin D, Wyse R, Watch D. Percutaneous arterial cannulation in children. Concurrent and subsequent adequacy of blood flow at the wrist. Anaesthesia 1984;39:27–31.
48. Mangano D, Hickey R. Ischemic injury following uncomplicated radial artery catheterization. Anesth Analg 1979;58:55–57.

49. Pillow K, Herrick I. Pulse oximetry compared with Doppler ultrasound for assessment of collateral blood flow to the hand. Anaesthesia 1991;46:388–390.
50. Raju R. The pulse oximeter and the collateral circulation. Anesthesiol 1986;41:783–784.
51. Chinyanga H, Smith J. A modified Doppler flow detector probe—an aid to percutaneous radial arterial cannulation in infants and small children. Anesthesiology 1979;50:256–258.
52. Cole F, Todres I, Shannon D. Technique for percutaneous cannulation of the radial artery in the newborn infant. J Pediatr 1978;92:105–107.
53. Butt W, Gow R, Whyte H, Smallhorn J, Koren G. Complications resulting from use of arterial catheters: Retrograde flow and rapid elevation in blood pressure. Pediatrics 1985;76:250–254.
54. Spahr R, MacDonald H, Holzman I. Catheterization of the posterior tibial artery in the neonate. Am J Dis Child 1979;133:945–946.
55. Johnstone R, Greenhow D. Catheterization of the dorsalis pedis artery. Anesthesiol 1973;39:654.
56. Youngberg J, Miller E. Evaluation of percutaneous cannulations of the dorsalis pedis artery. Anesthesiol 1976;44:80.
57. De Angelis J. Axillary arterial monitoring. Crit Care Med 1976;4:205.
58. Lawless S, Orr R. Axillary arterial monitoring of pediatric patients. Pediatr 1989;84:273.
59. Cantwell G, Holzman B, Caceres M. Percutaneous catheterization of the axillary artery in the pediatric patient. Crit Care Med 1990;18:880.
60. Graves P, Davis A, Maggi J, Nussbaum E. Femoral artery cannulation for monitoring in critically ill children: Prospective study. Crit Care Med 1990;18:1363.
61. Shah A, et al. Complications of selective coronary arteriography by the Judkins technique and their prevention. Am Heart J 1975;90:353.
62. Morris T, Bouhoutsos J. The dangers of femoral artery puncture and catheterization. Am Heart J 1975;89:260.
63. Bjork L, Enghoff E, et al. Local circulatory changes following brachial artery catheterization. Vasc Dis 2:283.
64. Prian G, Wright G, Rumach C, O'Meara O. Apparent cerebral embolization after temporal artery catheterization. J Pediatr 1978;93:115–118.
65. Miyasaka K, Edmonds J, Conn A. Complications of radial artery lines in the paediatric patient. Can Anaesth Soc J 1976;23:9–14.
66. Slogoff S, Keats A, Arlund C. On the safety of radial artery cannulation. Anesthesiol 1983;59:42–47.
67. Smith-Wright D, Green T, Lock J, Egar M, Fuhrman B. Complications of vascular catheterization in critically ill children. Crit Care Med 1984;12:1015–1017.
68. Steven J, Nicolson S. Monitoring the pediatric patient. In: Blitt C, Hines R, ed. Monitoring in anesthesia and critical care medicine. New York: Churchill Livingstone, 1995: 687.
69. Band J, Maki D. Infections caused by arterial catheters used for hemodynamic monitoring. Am J Med 1979;67:735–741.
70. Shinozaki T, et al. Bacterial contamination of arterial lines: A prospective study. JAMA 1983;249(223).
71. Bedford R, et al. Complications of percutaneous radial-artery cannulation: An objective prospective study in man. Anesthesiol 1973; 38:228.
72. Bedford R. Wrist circumference predicts the risk of radial arterial occlusion after cannulation. Anesthesiol 1978b;48:377.
73. Shapiro B. Monitoring gas exchange in acute respiratory failure. Respir Care 1983;28:605.
74. Crossland S, Neviaser R. Complications of radial artery catheterization. Hand 1977;9:287.
75. Tyson J, deSa D, Moore S. Thromboatheromatous complications of umbilical arterial catheterization in the newborn period. Arch Dis Child 1976;51:744–754.
76. Hislop A, Reid L. Intrapulmonary arterial development during fetal life—branching pattern and structures. J Anat 1972;113:35.
77. Zweifach B. Quantitative studies on microcirculatory structure and function. I. Analysis of pressure distribution in the terminal vascular bed in cat mesentery. Circ Res 1974;34:843.
78. Selkurt E. Physiology. Boston: Little, Brown, 1976.
79. Milnor W. Pulsatile blood flow. N Engl J Med 1972;287:27.
80. O'Rourke M. Vascular impedance studies of arterial and cardiac function. Physiol Rev 1982;62:570.
81. O'Rourke M, Taylor M. Input impedance of the systemic circulation. Circ Res 1967;20:365.
82. Hamilton W. The patterns of the arterial pressure pulse. Am J Physiol 1944;141:235.
83. Miles D, Gotshall R, Golden J, Tuuri D, Beekman RI, Dillon T. Accuracy of electrical impedance cardiography for measuring cardiac output in children with congenital heart defects. Am J Cardiol 1988;61:612–616.
84. Case E, Stiles J. The effect of various surgical positions on vital capacity. Anesthesiol 1946;7:29.
85. Skinner J, Milligan D, Hunter S, Hey E. Central venous pressure in the ventilated neonate. Arch Dis Child 1992;67:374–377.
86. Lloyd T, Donnerstein R, Berg R. Accuracy of central venous pressure measurement from the abdominal inferior vena cava. Pediatrics 1992;89(3):506–508.
87. Hayashi Y, Uchida O, Takaki O, et al. Internal jugular vein catheterization in infants undergoing cardiovascular surgery: An analysis of the factors influencing successful catheterization. Anesth Analg 1992;74:688–693.
88. Cote C, Jobes D, Schwartz A, Ellison N. Two approaches to cannuluation of a child's internal jugular vein. Anesthesiology 1979;50:371–373.
89. Prince S, Sullivan R, Hackel A. Percutaneous catheterization of the internal jugular vein in infants and children. Anesthesiol 1976;44: 170–174.
90. Krausz M, Berlatzky Y, Ayalon A, Freund H, Schiller M. Percutaneous cannulation of the internal jugular vein in infants and children. Surg Gynecol Obstet 1979;148:591–594.
91. Hall D, Geefhuysen J. Percutaneous catheterization of the internal jugular vein in infants and children. J Pediatr Surg 1977;12:719–722.
92. Damen J. Positive bacterial cultures and related risk factors associated with percutaneous internal jugular vein catheterization in pediatric cardiac patients. Anesthesiology 1987;66:558–562.
93. Swan H, Ganz W, et al. Catheterization of the heart in man with use of a flow-directed balloon-tipped catheter. N Engl J Med 1970;283:447.
94. Forrester J, Ganz W, et al. Thermodilution cardiac output determination with a single flow-directed catheter. Am Heart J 1972;83:306.
95. Katz R, Pollack M, Weibley R. Pulmonary artery catheterization in pediatric intensive care. Adv Pediatr 1984;30:169.
96. Swan H, Ganz W. Measurement of right atrial and pulmonary arterial pressures and cardiac output: Clinical application of hemodynamic monitoring. Adv Pediatr 1982;27:453.
97. Sorensen M, Bille-Brahe N, Engell H. Cardiac output measurement by thermal dilution: Reproducibility and comparison with dye-dilution technique. Ann Surg 1978;65:67.
98. Freed M. Invasive diagnostic and therapeutic techniques. Part I. In: Adams F, al. e, ed. Moss' Heart Disease in Infants and Children, and Adolescents. Baltimore: Williams & Wilkins, 1989: 130–147.
99. Wyse S, Pfitzner J, et al. Measurement of cardiac output by thermodilution in infants and children. Thorax 1975;30:262.
100. Moodie D, Feldt R, Kaye M, et al. Measurement of cardiac output by thermodilution: Development of accurate measurements at flow applicable to the pediatric patient. J Surg Res 1978;25:305.
101. Katz J, Cronau L, et al. Pulmonary artery flow-guided catheters in the perioperative period: Indications and complications. JAMA 1977b; 237:2832.
102. Elliott C, Zimmerman G, et al. Complications of pulmonary artery catheterization in the care of critically ill patients: A prospective study. Chest 1979;76:647.
103. Foote G, Schabel S, Hodges M. Pulmonary complications of the flow-directed balloon-tipped catheter. N Engl J Med 1974;290:927.
104. Golden M, Pinder T, et al. Fatal pulmonary hemorrhage complicating use of a flow-directed balloon-tipped catheter in a patient receiving anticoagulant therapy. Am J Cardiol 1973;32:865.
105. Pape L, Haffajee C, et al. Fatal pulmonary hemorrhage after use of the flow-directed balloon-tipped catheter. Ann Intern Med 1979;90:344.
106. Urschel J, Myerowitz P. Catheter-induced pulmonary artery rupture in the setting of cardiopulmonary bypass. Ann Thorac Surg 1993;56: 585–589.
107. Michel L, McMirchan J, Marsh H. Pulmonary artery catheter colonization and related sepsis. Crit Care Med 1979;7:131.
108. Appelfeld J, Caruthers T, et al. Assessment of the sterility of long-term cardiac catheterization using the thermodilution Swan-Ganz catheter. Chest 1978;74:377.
109. Pace N, Horton W. Indwelling pulmonary artery catheters: Their relationship to aseptic thrombotic endocardial vegetations. JAMA 1975;233:893.
110. Simmons D, Alpas A, et al. Hyperlactatemia due to arterial hypoxemia or reduced cardiac output or both. J Appl Physiol 1978;45:195.
111. Toussaint G, Burgess J, et al. Central venous pressure and pulmonary wedge pressure in critical surgical illness. Arch Surg 1974;109:265.
112. Civetta J, Gabel J, Laver M. Disparate ventricular function in surgical patients. Surg Forum 1971;22:131.

113. Geer R. Interpretation of pulmonary-artery wedge pressure when PEEP is used. Anesthesiol 1977;46:383.
114. West J, Dollery C, Naimark A. Distribution of blood flow in isolated lung: Relation to vascular and alveolar pressures. J Appl Physiol 1964;19:713.
115. Fitzpatrick G, Hampson L, et al. Bedside determination of left atrial pressure. Can Med Assoc J 1972;106:1293.
116. Humphrey C, Oury J, et al. An analysis of direct and indirect measurements of left atrial filling pressure. J Thorac Cardiovasc Surg 1976;71:643.
117. Lappas D, Lell W, et al. Indirect measurement of left atrial pressure in surgical patients: Pulmonary-capillary wedge and pulmonary-artery diastolic pressures compared with left-atrial pressure. Anesthesiol 1973;38:394.
118. Walston A, Kendall M. Comparison of pulmonary wedge and left atrial pressure in man. Am Heart J 1973;86:159.
119. Tooker J, Huseby J, Butler J. The effect of Swan-Ganz catheter height on the wedge pressure-left atrial pressure relationship in edema during positive-pressure ventilation. Am Rev Respir Dis 1978;117:721.
120. Berryhill R, Benumof J. PEEP-induced discrepancy between pulmonary arterial wedge pressure and left atrial pressure. Anesthesiol 1979;51:303.
121. Jardin F, Farcot J, et al. Influence of positive end-expiratory pressure on left ventricular performance. N Engl J Med 1981;304:387.
122. Fisher M, DeFelice C, Parigi A. Assessing left ventricular pressure with flow-directed (Swan-Ganz) catheters: Detection of sudden changes in patients with left ventricular dysfunction. Chest 1975b;68:542.
123. Rahimtoola S. Left ventricular end-diastolic and filling pressures in assessment of ventricular function. Chest 1973;63:858.
124. Hatch D, Sumner E. Neonatal anesthesia.Chicago: Mosby-Year Book, 1981:75–85.
125. Stetz C, Miller R, Kelly G, Raffin T. Reliability of the thermodilution method in the determination of cardiac output in clinical practice. Am Rev Respir Dis 1982;126:1001–1004.
126. Scheinman M, Evans G, et al. Relationship between pulmonary artery end-diastolic pressure and left ventricular filling pressure in patients in shock. Circulation 1973;47:317.
127. Hamilton W, Riley R, Ahyah A, et al. Comparison of the Fick and dye injection methods of measuring the cardiac output in man. Am J Physiol 1948;153:309.
128. Freed M, Keane J. Cardiac output measured by thermodilution in infants and children. J Pediatr 1978;92:39–42.
129. Wetzel R, Latson T. Major errors in thermodilution cardiac output measurement during rapid volume infusion. Anesthesiol 1985;62:684-687.
130. Doppler C. Uber das fabirge der doppelsterne. Abhandlungen der konglich bomchen gessellschaft ab wisenschaften. 4 to Prog 1842;II:465.
131. Zhang Y, Nitter-Hauge S, Ihlen H, Myhre E. Doppler echocardiographic measurement of cardiac output using the mitral orifice method. Br Heart J 1985;53:130–136.
132. Alverson D, Eldridge M, Dillon T, Yabek S, Berman WJ. Noninvasive pulsed Doppler determination of cardiac output in neonates and children. J Pediatr 1982;101:46–50.
133. Seear M, D'Orsogna L, Sandor G, de Souza E, Popov R. Doppler-derived mean aortic flow velocity in children: An alternative to cardiac index. Pediatr Cardiol 1991;12:197–200.
134. Wipperman C, Schranz D, Huth R, Zepp F, Oelert H, Jungst B. Determination of cardiac output by an angle and diameter independent dual beam Doppler technique in critically ill infants. Br Heart J 1992;67:180–184.
135. Muhiudeen I, Kuecherer H, Lee E, Cahalan M, Schiller N. Intraoperative estimation of cardiac output by transesophageal pulsed Doppler echocardiography. Anesthesiol 1991;74:9–14.
136. Siegel L, Fitzgerald D, Engstrom R. Simultaneous intraoperative measurement of cardiac output by thermodilution and transtracheal Doppler. Anesthesiol 1991;74:664–669.
137. Keagy B, Wilcox B, Lucas C, et al. Constant postoperative monitoring of cardiac output after correction of congenital heart defects. J Thorac Cardiovasc Surg 1987;93:658–664.
138. Van Orden D, Farley D, Fastenow C, Brody M. A technique for monitoring blood flow changes with miniaturized Doppler flow probes. Am J Physiol 1984;247:H1005–H1009.
139. Goldberg S, Sahn D, Allen H, Valdes-Cruz L, Hoenecke H, Carnahan Y. Evaluation of pulmonary and systemic blood flow by two-dimensional Doppler echocardiography using fast Fourier transform spectral analysis. Am J Cardiol 1982;50:1394–1400.
140. Kapusta L, Hopman J, Daniels O. The agreement between pulmonary and systemic blood flow measurements in babies by dual beam Doppler echocardiography. Eur Heart J 1991;12:112–116.
141. Perrino AJ, Fleming J, LaMantia K. Transesophageal Doppler ultrasonography evidence for improved cardiac output monitoring. Anesth Analg 1990;71:651–657.
142. Kubicek W, Karnegis J, Patterson R, Witsoe D, Mattson R. Development and evaluation of an impedance cardiac output system. Aerosp Med 1966;37:1208–1212.
143. Lababidi Z, Ehmke D, Durnin R, Leaverton P, Lauer R. Evaluation of impedance cardiac output in children. Pediatr 1971;47:870–879.
144. Gotshall R, Miles D. Noninvasive assessment of cardiac output by impedance cardiography in the newborn canine. Crit Care Med 1989;17:63–65.
145. Tibballs J. A comparative study of cardiac output in neonates supported by mechanical ventilation: Measurement with thoracic electrical bioimpedance and pulsed Doppler ultrasound. Pediatr 1989;114:632–635.
146. Spinale F, Smith A, Crawford F. Relationship of bioimpedance to thermodilution and echocardiographic measurements of cardiac function. Crit Care Med 1990;18:414–418.
147. Thys D. Cardiac output. Anes Clin North Am 1988;6:803–824.
148. Castor G, Molter G, Helms J, Niedermark I, Altmayer P. Determination of cardiac output during positive end-expiratory pressure—noninvasive electrical bioimpedance compared with standard thermodilution. Crit Care Med 1990;18:544–546.
149. Siegel L, Shafer S, Martinez G, et al. Simultaneous measurements of cardiac output by thermodilution, esophageal Doppler, and electrical impedance in anesthetized patients. J Cardiothorac Anesth 1988;2:590.
150. Smith S, Russell A, West M, Chalmers J. Automated non-invasive measurement of cardiac output: Comparison of electrical bioimpedance and carbon dioxide rebreathing techniques. Br Heart J 1988;59:292–298.
151. Introna R, Pruett J, Crumrine R, Cuadrado A. Use of transthoracic bioimpedance to determine cardiac output in pediatric patients. Crit Care Med 1988;16:1101–1105.
152. Bennett E, Barclay S, Davis A, Mannering D, Mehta N. Ascending aortic blood velocity and acceleration using Doppler ultrasound in the assessment of left ventricular function. Cardiovasc Res 1984;18: 632–638.
153. Nicolosi G, Pungercic E, Cervesato E, Modena L, Zanuttini D. Analysis of interobserver and intraobserver variation of interpretation of the echocardiographic and Doppler flow determination of cardiac output by the mitral orifice method. Br Heart J 1986;55:446–448.
154. Robson S, Dunlop W, Moore M, Hunter S. Combined Doppler and echocardiographic measurement of cardiac output: Theory and application in pregnancy. Br J Obstet Gynaecol 1987;93:1014–1027.
155. Edler I, Hertz C. Use of ultrasonic reflectoscope for continuous recording of movements of heart walls. Kung Fysiograf Sallsk Lund Fordhandl 1954;24:40.
156. Feigenbaum H, Zaky A. Use of diagnostic ultrasound in clinical cardiology. J Indiana State Med Assoc 1966;59(140).
157. Riggs T, Hirschfeld S, Fanaroff A, et al. Persistence of fetal circulation syndrome: An echocardiographic study. J Pediatr 1977;91:626–631.
158. Hirschfeld S, Meyer R, Schwartz D, Korfhagen J, Kaplan S. Measurement of right and left systolic time intervals by echocardiography. Circulation 1975a;51:304–309.
159. Hirschfeld S, RA M, Schwartz D, Korfhagen J, Kaplan S. The echocardiographic assessment of pulmonary artery pressure and pulmonary vascular resistance. Circulation 1975b;52:642–650.
160. Reeves W, Chitwood WJ. Assessment of left atrial myxoma using transesophageal two-dimensional echocardiography and color flow Doppler. Echocardiography 1989;6:547.
161. Horowitz M, Rossen R, Harrison D. Echocardiographic diagnosis of pericardial disease. Am Heart J 1979;97:420–427.
162. Wann L, Dillon J, Weyman A, Feigenbaum H. Echocardiography in bacterial endocarditis. N Engl J Med 1976;295:135–139.
163. Seward J, Khndheria B, Oh J, et al. Transesophageal echocardiography: Technique, anatomic correlations, implementation, and clinical applications. Mayo Clinic Proceedings 1988;63:649–680.
164. Kyo S, Omoto R, Matsumura M, Shah P, Ito H. Intraoperative transesophageal echocardiography in pediatric patients. J Thorac Cardiovasc Surg 1990;99:373–375.
165. Ritter S. Transesophageal real-time echocardiography in infants and children with congenital heart disease. JACC 1991;18(2):569–580.
166. Stumper O, Elzenga N, Hess J, Sutherland G. Transesophageal echocardiography in children with congenital heart disease: An initial experience. J Amer Coll Cardiol 1990;16:443–441.

167. Sreeram N, Stumper O, Kaulitz R, Hess J, Roelandt J, Sutherland G. Comparative value of transthoracic and transesophageal echocardiography in the assessment of congenital abnormalities of the atrioventricular junction. J Amer Coll Cardiol 1990;16:1205–1214.
168. Cyran S, Kimball T, Meyer R, et al. Efficacy of intraoperative transesophageal echocardiography in children with congenital heart disease. Amer J Cardiol 1989;63:594–596.
169. Dan M, Bonato R, Mazzucco A, et al. Value of transesophageal echocardiography during repair of congenital heart defects. Ann Thorac Surg 1990;50:637–643.
170. Lam J, Neirotti R, Nijveld A, Schuller J, Blom-Muilwijk C, Visser C. Transesophageal echocardiography in pediatric patients: Preliminary results. J Amer Soc Echocardiogr 1991;4:43–50.
171. Stumper O, Witsenburg M, Sutherland G, Cromme-Kijkhuis A, Godman M, Hess J. Transesophageal echocardiographic monitoring of interventional cardiac catheterization in children. JACC 1991a; 18(6): 1506–1514.
172. Matsuzaki M, Toma Y, Kusukawa R. Clinical applications of transesophageal echocardiography. Circulation 1992;82:709–722.
173. Stumper O, Sutherland G, Geuskens R, Roelandt J, Bos E, Hess J. Transesophageal echocardiography in evaluation and management after a Fontan procedure. JACC 1991b;17(5):1152–1160.
174. Fyfe D, Kline C, Sade R, Greene C, Gillette P. The utility of transesophagreal echocardiography during and after Fontan operations in small children. Am Heart J 1991;122:1403–1415.
175. Gilbert T, Panico F, McGill W, Martin G, Halley D, Sell J. Bronchial obstruction by transesophageal echocardiography probe in a pediatric cardiac patient. Anesth Analg 1992;74:156–158.
176. Ament M, Christie D. Upper gastrointestinal fiberoptic endoscopy in pediatric patients. Gastroenterology 1977;72:1244–1248.
177. Cadranel S, Rodesch P, Peeters J, Cremer M. Fiberendoscopy of the gastrointestinal tract in children. Am J Dis Child 1977;131:41–45.
178. Caulfield M, Wyllie R, Sivak M, Michener W, Steffen R. Upper gastrointestinal tract endoscopy in the pediatric patient. J Pediatr 1989;115:339–345.
179. Parker M, Cunnion R, Parrillo J. Echocardiography and nuclear cardiac imaging in the critical care unit. JAMA 1985;254:2935.
180. Terai C, Uenishi M, Sugimoto H, et al. Transesophageal echocardiographic dimensional analysis of four cardiac chambers during positive end-expiratory pressure. Anesthesiol 1985;63:640.
181. Koenig K, Kasper W, Hofmann T, et al. Transesophageal echocardiography for diagnosis of rupture of the ventricular septum or left ventricular papillary muscle during acute myocardial infarction. Am J Cardiol 1987;59:362.
182. Kyo S, Takamoto S, Matsumura M, et al. Immediate and early postoperative evaluation of results of cardiac surgery by transesophageal two-dimensional Doppler echocardiography. Circulation 1987;76(Suppl V):V–113.
183. D'Cruz I, Kensey K, Campbell C, et al. Two-dimensional echocardiography in cardiac tamponade occurring after cardiac surgery. J Am Coll Cardiol 1985;5:1250.
184. Singh S, Wann L, Schuchard G, et al. Right ventricular and right atrial collapse in patients with cardiac tamponade—a combined echocardiographic and hemodynamic study. Circulation 1984;70:966.
185. Hickey P. Transesophageal echocardiography in pediatric cardiac surgery. Anesthesiol 1992;77:610.
186. Muhiudeen I, Silverman N. Transesophageal echocardiography in pediatric cardiac surgery. Anesthesiol 1992;77:610–611.
187. Sahn D, Weintraub R. Transesophageal echocardiography in pediatric cardiac surgery. Anesthesiol 1992;77:611.

Neurologic Intensive Care

Section Four

Section Editor

J. Michael Dean

Pathophysiology and Management of the Intracranial Vault

18

W. Bradley Poss
Douglas L. Brockmeyer*
Bonnie Clay
J. Michael Dean

INTRODUCTION

The pathophysiology and management of the intracranial vault is an extraordinarily complex and challenging subject. Major strides have been made in the last 10 years in understanding the regulation of intracranial pressure, largely because of an increased knowledge of the regulation of cerebral blood flow as well as advancements in our ability to measure both cerebral blood flow and intracranial pressure.

The goal of this chapter is to present a unified approach to understanding the physiologic mechanisms involved in maintaining normal cerebral homeostasis as well as the pathophysiology of intracranial hypertension. We will also present techniques for monitoring intracranial pressure and

*University of Utah School of Medicine Department of Pediatrics and Department of Neurosurgery
Address for Correspondence: J. Michael Dean, M.D.
Acting Chairman, Department of Pediatrics
Director, Division of Pediatric Critical Care
University of Utah School of Medicine
Primary Children's Medical Center
100 North Medical Drive
Salt Lake City, Utah 84113

a rational approach to the prevention and treatment of intracranial hypertension.

PATHOPHYSIOLOGY OF INTRACRANIAL PRESSURE

General Concepts

Intracranial pressure (ICP) is normally thought of as the pressure within the intracranial vault that results from the interaction of the brain, the cerebral blood volume (CBV), and the cerebrospinal fluid (CSF). These components may undergo alterations in their individual volumes but the total volume of the intracranial contents must remain fixed. Thus, alterations in the volume of one compartment must be compensated for by opposite changes in another compartment in order for the ICP to remain the same. This concept is known as the modified Monro-Kellie doctrine[60,85] and is familiar to most clinicians. This concept is demonstrated in Figure 18.1, where arterial and venous blood, brain, and CSF are shown in the first chamber at equilibrium along the pressure-volume curve thus producing a normal resting ICP. If an intracranial mass such as a hematoma is introduced into this equilibrium, compensatory mechanisms must occur for the ICP to remain within the normal range. These compensatory mechanisms normally consist of displacement of CSF and blood from the intracranial vault as the brain is relatively incompressible. A further increase in the mass in Figure 18.1 has shifted the system farther to the right on the pressure-volume curve but the ICP remains constant. Eventually, these compensatory mechanisms will be exhausted (the blood and CSF maximally displaced) and a further increase in the size of the mass will produce a sharp rise in the ICP. It is important to

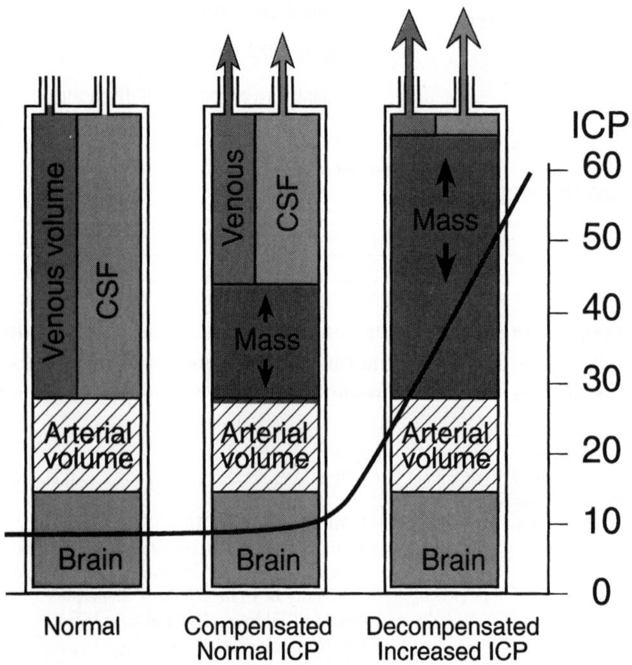

Figure 18.1. Intracranial compensation for an expanding mass lesion.

remember that once decompensation has occurred, small increases in any compartment will lead to large increases in ICP. It is also important to realize that measuring a normal ICP gives you no information on where the patient lies on the pressure-volume curve and how much of her compensatory mechanisms are intact.

The concept of brain elastance was developed to help assess the compensatory reserve of the intracranial system[82]. This involves the rapid (1 second) addition or removal of CSF to determine the effect on ICP. This is then quantified as the volume-pressure response (VPR) with normal being 0 to 2 mm Hg/ml and levels of greater than 5 mm Hg/ml representing abnormal compliance. This concept was further expanded with the creation of the pressure-volume index (PVI) which is defined as the volume of fluid that needs to be injected to increase the ICP by a factor of 10[74]. The PVI is calculated from the formula:

$$\text{PVI} = \text{V}/\log(\text{P1}/\text{P2})$$

where V is equal to the amount injected, P_1 is the baseline ICP, and P_2 is the ICP value after the injection. In the normal adult, the PVI is 25 ml while a PVI of less than 13 ml is considered consistent with significantly altered compliance[59]. A recent study using brain compression in a dog model indicated that PVI appears to be more of a measure of cerebral vascular compressibility than total intracranial compliance[110]. PVI's and VPR's are rarely used in the management of children with elevated ICP but the concepts are important in understanding altered intracranial compliance and the various treatment modalities.

It is clear that the concepts presented in the previous section and the simple pressure-volume curve are somewhat simplistic and may sometimes be misleading. As discussed earlier, the addition of volume to the intracranial vault must be associated with an extracranial translocation of CSF or blood (or even ultimately of the brain itself). However, some patients herniate with relatively small subdural hematomas, while other patients present with very large brain tumors and only a mild headache.

There are other problems with this simple model. For instance, it is assumed that differences in the type and location of volume added to the intracranial vault do not affect the ultimate pressure change within the vault. In fact, this is not correct because pressure increases produced by equal amounts of CSF and epidural balloon inflation do not result in the same increases in ICP as shown in Figure 18.2[122]. There may be a variety of explanations for this phenomenon, such as varying rates of CSF removal or the balloon inflation producing mass effect and resulting in CSF obstruction. Regardless of the underlying reasons, it should be apparent that simple assumptions regarding ICP dynamics are often incorrect, and the concept of the ICP pressure-volume curve fails to entirely explain laboratory and clinical observations.

From the preceding section, an appreciation can be gained that the concept of ICP is much more involved and

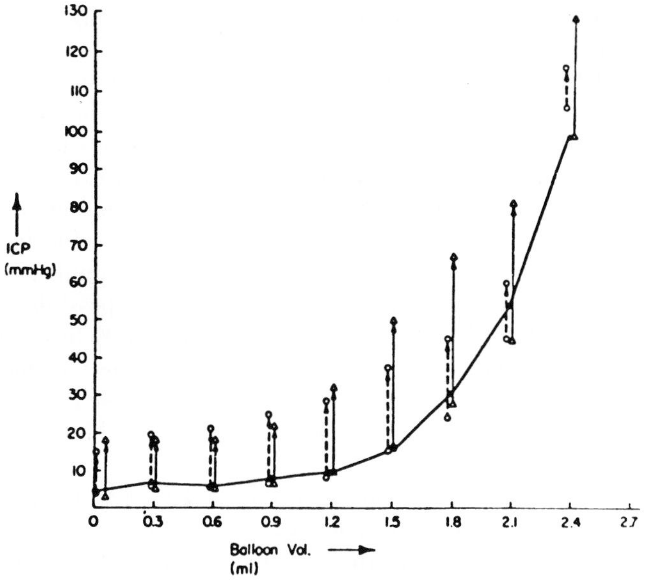

Figure 18.2. ICP pressure changes in an animal after bolus loading of an epidural balloon (triangles) or an equivalent ventricular volume of CSF (open circles). Note that as the pressure-volume curve enters the steep portion of the curve, a volume of CSF infusion produces less of a rise in ICP than an equal volume of epidural balloon inflation. (From Sullivan HG, Miller JD, Griffith RL, et al. CSF pressure transients in response to epidural and ventricular volume loading. Am J Physiol 1978;234(5):R169.)

complex than the simplistic manner in which it is sometimes presented. A more complete understanding of the many factors involved in the determination and regulation of ICP can be best obtained by taking a close look at each of the components of the intracranial vault and the multitude of factors involved in their regulation under normal and abnormal situations.

Components of the Intracranial Space

Brain

The brain normally comprises about 90% of the intracranial vault. 75 to 80% of the brain contents consist of water, which is further divided into intracellular and extracellular compartments. The intracellular compartment consists of gray and white matter which possess important structural differences[36]. The gray matter consists of tightly woven neural cells with limited compliance. The white matter is a much looser network of tissue and can accommodate increases in water content of 10% or more[36]. The extracellular compartment consists of a thin layer of fluid similar to CSF that makes up 15 to 20% of the brain volume[8].

The brain has generally been thought of as incompressible and therefore to be of a constant volume[84]. This implies that as intracranial volume increases because of blood, tumor, or edema, the compensatory mechanisms involving displacement of CSF or blood will eventually be exceeded. The end result will be brain tissue loss or herniation from the fixed and rigid skull. However, there is evidence that the brain is capable of volume regulation which may help to explain the difference in time at which various pathophysiological conditions may present. This concept has been well presented in an excellent review article[23] and is summarized briefly in the following paragraph.

Under normal circumstances, the blood-brain barrier allows only minimal change in brain volume. The blood-brain barrier consists of tight endothelial junctions that result in relative impermeability to both protein and solutes. The relatively dilute fluid that is filtered across the capillary membranes into the interstitial space is quickly reabsorbed because of the osmotic gradient that exists between the plasma and interstitium[35]. However, in certain pathophysiological states such as hypertonic dehydration, the brain does not behave in an idealized manner. Active uptake and release by the brain of osmotically active particles such as Na^+, Cl^-, and K^+ allows the brain to slowly shrink. Thus, water loss is only about one third of the predicted loss[19,64]. Other experimental evidence has demonstrated that therapeutic osmotic agents have no effect on brain cell volume. Instead, their effect actually results from a reduction of brain extracellular water[19]. There is also increasing experimental evidence that the brain is able to further regulate its fluid balance using a variety of hormones such as vasopressin, atriopeptin, and angiotensin[23]. There are currently several investigators looking at novel ways of influencing the neuro-endocrine control of the CNS in an effort to reduce cerebral edema formation[27,91]. The regulation of the blood-brain barrier is also much more complex than previously thought and a variety of messengers involved in transport regulation have been identified[57].

The volume of brain can obviously be altered by the presence of blood, tumor, or cerebral edema. Cerebral edema occurs in infections, tumors, head injury, Reye syndrome, asphyxia, and a wide variety of other diseases encountered in pediatric intensive care. There are three types of cerebral edema (vasogenic, cytotoxic, and interstitial) as defined by Fishman in 1975[37]. First, vasogenic edema is characterized by increased permeability of brain capillary endothelial cells. This type of edema is encountered around tumors, abscesses, intracerebral hematomas, etc. It is also present in inflammatory conditions, such as encephalitis and meningitis, as well as in experimental models of brain edema, such as freezing lesions. It is important to understand the basis of vasogenic edema. In vasogenic edema, the neurons are not primarily injured, and the edema does not reflect neuronal injury. Reduction of vasogenic edema can help maintain perfusion and prevent ischemia to normal neurons.

The second type, cytotoxic edema, is a result of cellular swelling secondary to cell injury. Cytotoxic edema reflects failure of ATPase-dependent sodium exchange and may involve all cells within the brain, including neurons, astrocytes, and oligodendroglia. Although reversible cytotoxic edema might be seen (e.g., with water intoxication), the pediatric intensivist most often encounters states of irreversible cytotoxic edema as seen in diffuse axonal injury. In such instances, of course, therapy does not dramatically alter the outcome because the edema and swelling are more an epiphenomenon of cell death than they are contributors to further damage. The situation is more complex because cytotoxic edema and swelling in one area of the brain may cause compression of the arterial supply of another region.

Interstitial edema, the third type of brain edema, is a result of increased CSF hydrostatic pressure. This is most often encountered in hydrocephalic states but may be seen in other situations as well. For instance, if CSF absorption is decreased at the arachnoid villi level, hydrocephalus and interstitial edema may develop. Treatment of this type of edema is usually directed at managing the direct cause of hydrocephalus and timely therapy is almost universally successful.

Cerebrospinal Fluid

CSF makes up about 10% of the total intracranial volume, and the amount of fluid present reflects the balance between the rate of production and the rate of absorption. 70% of the CSF is normally produced in the choroid plexus with the remainder produced at various sites within the brain and spinal cord. The average CSF volume is 90 ml in children from ages 4 to 13 and 150 ml in adults with the average rate of CSF production being 0.35 ml/min or 500 ml/day[34]. The rate of CSF production is generally constant but has been shown to decrease as CSF pressure increases. This has been felt to likely be a result of decreased perfusion of the choroid plexus[100]. Drugs such as furosemide and acetazolamide have also been shown to decrease CSF production by their effect on chloride transport and carbonic anhydrase, respectively[131].

CSF absorption is primarily through the arachnoid villi but also takes place at various sites throughout the brain and spinal cord. CSF absorption rates are much more sensitive to changes in pressure and can increase to three times the rate of production as ICP rises. Resistance to flow has also been shown to decrease with elevated CSF pressures thus compensating for increased ICP by both increased CSF flow and absorption[131].

Severe head injuries may have a multitude of effects on CSF fluid balance besides the already mentioned effects of elevated ICP on CSF production and absorption. Brain edema has been shown to be partially cleared via the ventricular system which would further elevate ICP[106]. The presence of intraventricular blood or compression of normal CSF pathways may also impede CSF flow. The CSF volume can be altered by several means, but the usual method involves placing a shunt or drain to allow removal of CSF from the intracranial vault.

Blood

Blood comprises about 10% of the total intracranial volume. It is important to distinguish CBV from cerebral blood flow (CBF) because there are different therapeutic implications of each. CBV is an important contributor to intracranial volume and pressure; while CBF does not primarily affect ICP[5].

CBF is the amount of blood in transit through the brain; in physical terms, it is the flux of blood across the intracranial compartment. CBF is influenced by numerous factors such as the mean arterial blood pressure, the ICP, the viscosity of the blood, and the diameter of the arteries and arterioles[7]. CBV is the volume of the blood contained within the intracranial vasculature and is primarily determined by the diameter of the arterioles and venules. It is possible to increase the CBV, and ICP, and to decrease CBF. In more physical terms, when the CBV is increased, the pressure gradient across the compartment is altered because it is enclosed by the skull and, therefore, flow through the system is decreased.

Recently, new techniques have been developed to measure CBV in acutely ill patients, although this work must be considered still experimental. In a study of 15 head injured patients, Bouma and Muizelaar found no correlation between CBV and CBF[7]. The PVI's in 10 of these patients were also measured. PVI correlated well with CBV, thus supporting the evidence that CBV, rather than CBF, is a primary determinant of brain tightness and ICP. The same investigators also found that patients with increased CBV were at greater risk for ICP fluctuations.

REGULATION OF CEREBRAL BLOOD FLOW

To maintain homeostasis, the brain depends on a constant supply of blood to provide oxygen and metabolic substrates. Its minimal ability to store energy dictates that aerobic metabolism be maintained at all times. Anaerobic metabolism may produce deleterious and toxic end-products such as free radicals and excitatory amino acids[7]. The normal adult CBF is estimated to be 50 ml/100 g/min, however, the CBF is generally higher in children. The minimum flow that is required to prevent ischemia is unknown but may depend on several factors such as patient age, cerebral metabolic rate, and associated injuries. The regulation of CBF is accomplished through a variety of mechanisms, many of which are now just being elucidated. The mechanisms involved can generally be divided into four categories; chemical (metabolic products and arterial blood gases), myogenic, neurogenic, and endothelium-dependent factors. Each of these will be discussed in greater detail below.

Autoregulation of Cerebral Blood Flow

Autoregulation refers to the brain's ability to maintain CBF despite fluctuations in the systemic blood pressure. This is accomplished by changes in cerebral resistance in response to the alterations in systemic mean arterial pressure (MAP). Normally, CBF is well maintained with MAP's of 60 to 150 mm Hg (Fig. 18.3). When the MAP reaches either end of this range, alterations in CBF will occur. The cerebral vasculature is maximally dilated at 60 mm Hg and further re-

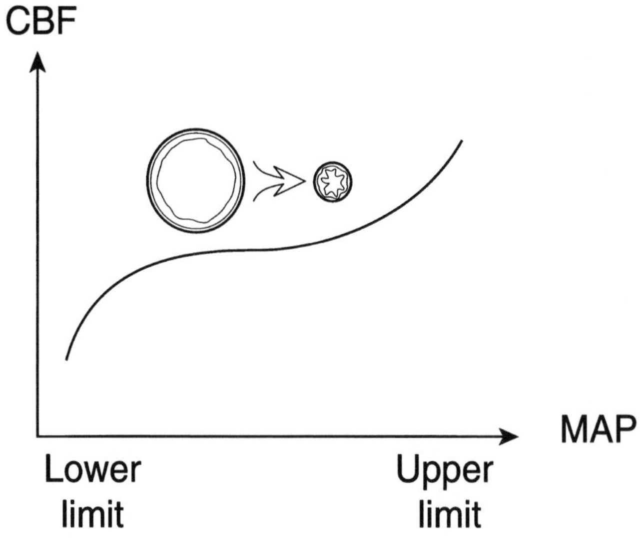

Figure 18.3. The relationship of mean arterial pressure (MAP) and cerebral blood flow (CBF). In addition, cerebral vessel diameter at each limit of the normal autoregulatory range is shown.

ductions in MAP will be accompanied by reductions in CBF and possible ischemia (Fig. 18.4). Hypertension, on the other hand, may disrupt the vasoconstrictive response with resultant increases in CBF and disruption of the blood-brain barrier.

Brain perfusion is dependent on the same factors that determine fluid flow through any system. The driving force for blood flow through the brain is the systemic arterial blood pressure. Venous pressure (or ICP in the case of intracranial hypertension) represents the downstream pressure. This introduces the concept of cerebral perfusion pressure (CPP) which is normally defined as: CPP = MAP − ICP. It is important to define cerebral perfusion pressure in a more rigorous manner than simply the arterial blood pressure minus the intracranial pressure. For instance, a child with Reye syndrome undergoing ICP monitoring may have an ICP of 35 mm Hg, an arterial pressure of 65 mm Hg and a central venous pressure of 5 mm Hg. In this child, the cerebral perfusion pressure is 30 mm Hg, and the central venous pressure is not a determinant of cerebral perfusion pressure. In contrast, an infant with severe cardiac failure who has an open and soft anterior fontanelle, a blood pressure of 50 mm Hg, and a central venous pressure of 25 mm Hg, does not have a normal cerebral perfusion pressure (assuming that a soft fontanelle means low ICP). In this case the cerebral perfusion pressure is only 25 mm Hg because the higher central venous pressure is the back pressure to CBF. This circumstance may arise in children or adults who undergo cardiac bypass; after a period with fairly low arterial and high venous pressures, such patients are at risk for post-ischemic complications.

Mechanisms of Cerebral Blood Flow Regulation

Metabolic

CBF is normally tightly coupled to cerebral metabolism as seen in Figure 18.5. The cerebral metabolic rate of oxygen ($CMRO_2$) is calculated from the equation: $CMRO_2 = CBF \times AVDO_2$ where $AVDO_2$ is the cerebral arteriovenous difference in oxygen content. CBF is measured by techniques

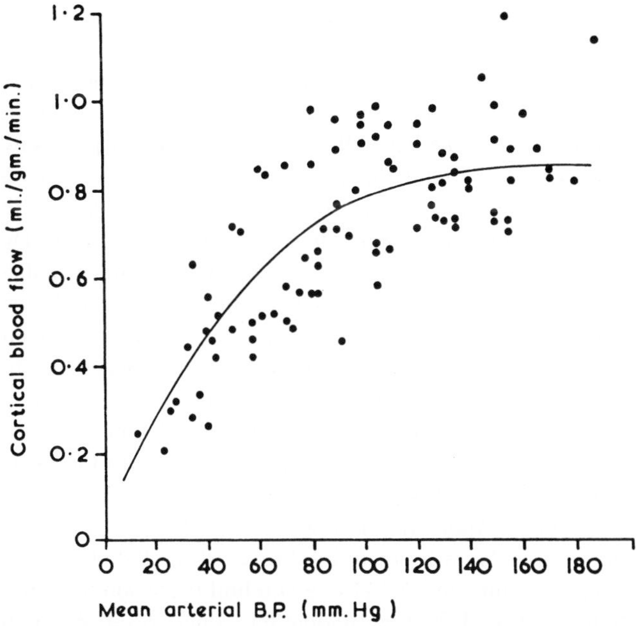

Figure 18.4. Effect of lowering mean arterial blood pressure on cortical blood flow in a series of normocapneic dogs. Flow is expressed as a percentage of the control value and the line is the best polynomial fit. (From Harper AM. Autoregulation of cerebral blood flow; influence of the arterial blood pressure on the blood flow through the cerebral cortex. J Neurol Neurosurg Psychiatry. 1966;29:400.)

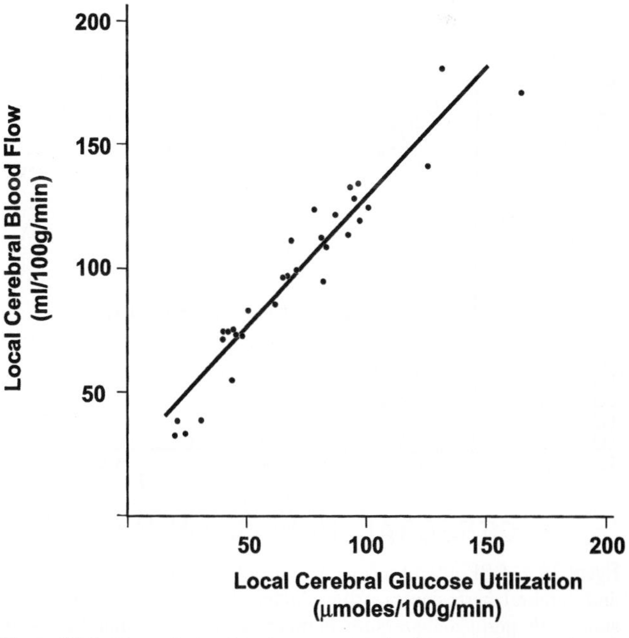

Figure 18.5. The relationship between cerebral metabolism and cerebral blood flow in a rat model. Each point represents the data from one cerebral region. (From Kuschinsky W. Coupling of blood flow and metabolism in the brain. Journal of Basic & Clinical Physiology & Pharmacology. 1990;1(1-4):195.)

discussed elsewhere in this book and the $AVDO_2$ is calculated from measuring the oxygen content in arterial and jugular venous blood. Jugular venous bulb catheterization has been accomplished in infants and children[40]. The normal $AVDO_2$ during normocapnia has been calculated at 6 vol% and the normal $CMRO_2$ is 3.2 ml/100g/min[62,63].

Clinical situations with increased cerebral metabolic activity (such as seizures or fever) will be accompanied by an increase in CBF. Many of the treatment modalities discussed later in this chapter involve the reduction or control of cerebral metabolism (sedation, antipyretics, and antiepileptics) in order to preserve the balance between CBF and metabolic requirements. This is one basis for the use of barbiturate coma in the treatment of head injury.

The mechanism coupling CBF to cerebral metabolism remains elusive but most authors believe it involves vasodilators released from neurons. Adenosine appears to be the most likely agent and has been shown to be a potent cerebral vasodilator. Other authors have proposed factors such as changes in extracellular ions, changes in capillary density and activity, and cyclo-oxygenase products in addition to adenosine[52,65].

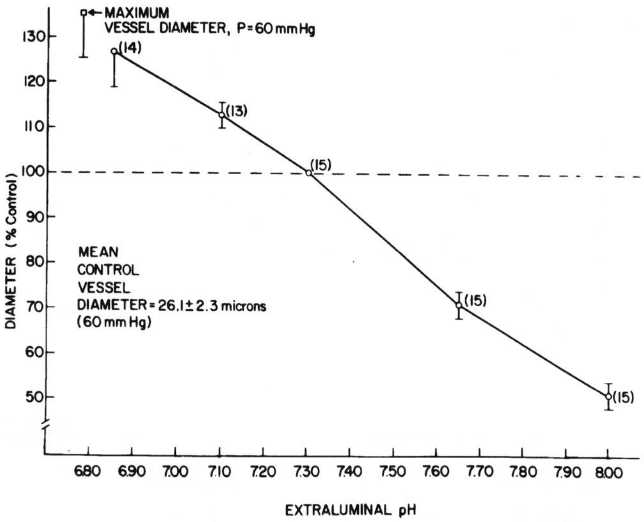

Figure 18.7. Effect of perivascular pH on the mean vessel diameter (± SEM) of the rat intracerebral arteriole. Numbers in parentheses indicate number of vessels studied at that pH. (From Dacey RG and Duling BR. A study of rat intracerebral arterioles: methods, morphology, and reactivity. Am J. Physiol. 1982;243 Heart Circ. Physiol. 12):H598).

Oxygen and Carbon Dioxide

The effect of arterial blood gases on CBF is important in the management of patients with elevated intracranial hypertension and therefore will be covered in detail (Fig. 18.6). Although oxygen and carbon dioxide are really metabolic components, it is advantageous to discuss their proposed mechanisms separately as they are easy to manipulate in the Pediatric Intensive Care Unit (PICU) setting. Changes in oxygen pressure have been shown to produce significant effects on vascular smooth muscle. Hypoxia has been shown to greatly increase CBF by vasodilatation. Rises in oxygen content have also been shown to produce vasoconstriction but to a lesser degree. It is unclear if oxygen's effect on vascular smooth muscle is by a direct mechanism or by the production of the metabolic substrates discussed in the previous section. No matter the mechanism, it is clear that maintenance of an adequate PaO_2 is essential in the management of intracranial hypertension.

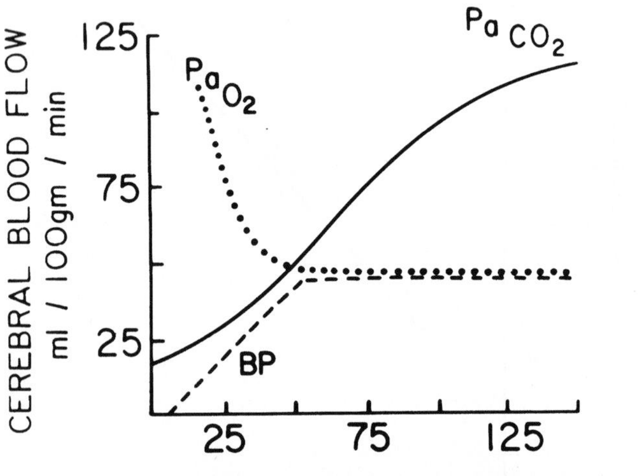

Figure 18.6. CBF alterations as a result of changes in $PaCO_2$, PaO_2, and cerebral perfusion pressure. Notice that CBF is relatively constant with perfusion pressure between 50 and 150 mm Hg, is increased as PaO_2 drops below approximately 50 mm Hg and is related linearly to $PaCO_2$ in the normal range of $PaCO_2$ encountered (20-70 mm Hg). (From Rogers MC, Traystman RJ. An overview of the intracranial vault: physiology and philosophy. Crit Care Clin 1985;1:199.)

$PaCO_2$ has also been shown to have a significant effect on CBF with hypercapnia increasing flow up to 350% of normal and hypocapnia producing smaller reductions in flow[125]. Again, these changes appear to be accomplished via an indirect method; alterations in tissue pH producing changes in arteriolar diameter (Fig. 18.7). Carbon dioxide has been shown to readily cross the blood-brain barrier and lower CSF pH via its reaction with carbonic anhydrase. The changes in pH occur rapidly as does the resultant change in vessel diameter. These mechanisms are preserved even when normal autoregulation has been lost. Therefore changes in $PaCO_2$ are often used by the clinician to alter ICP. It is important to realize that the response to sustained hyperventilation appears to be lost after 24 hours because of accumulation of lactic acid and alterations in the bicarbonate buffer system.

Initially, hyperventilation was thought to be beneficial to the injured brain by restoring brain pH, restoring cerebral autoregulation, and increasing cerebral perfusion by reductions in ICP. Hyperventilation has since been shown to produce cerebral ischemia, hypoxia, and local inverse steal[21,61,81]. Several recent studies have shown prolonged hyperventilation to have an adverse effect on outcome in head-injured patients[13,87]. The liberal use of hyperventilation in children with increased ICP must be approached with caution because of the concerns mentioned in this section. It is our policy to maintain $PaCO_2$ between 30-35 mm Hg in head-injured patients as will be discussed later in this chapter.

Myogenic

A myogenic mechanism for cerebral autoregulation was first proposed in 1902[(6)]. Numerous investigators have since expanded on the notion that the vascular smooth muscle has an intrinsic capacity to respond to changes in the arterial pressure. This was originally thought to be the primary mechanism for cerebral autoregulation because the rapid response of the actin-myosin complex would account for the rapid responses of the cerebral vasculature in maintaining CBF. However, it has been recently suggested that critical review of many of the earlier studies led to the conclusion that the myogenic mechanism plays a secondary role to the other mechanisms discussed here and is mainly involved in dampening arterial pulsations[(125)].

Neurogenic

The nervous system has been proposed to have a significant effect on cerebrovascular regulation for many years. Most of the experimental work has been hampered by the enormous complexity and fragility of the system[(125)]. The sympathetic nervous system has been shown to shift autoregulation towards higher pressures and sympathetic blockade or denervation to shift it downwards[(7)]. The sympathetic nervous system has also been shown to have an effect on the regulation of CBV and CSF formation[(111)].

Endothelium-Dependent Mechanisms

Recently, there has been much speculation on the role of nitric oxide (NO) in the regulation of cerebral blood flow under a variety of normal and pathological conditions[(30,31)]. NO has been shown to be produced by a variety of cells under static conditions as well as when stimulated by a variety of factors such as cytokines. NO has been shown to produce relaxation of both cerebral arteries and arterioles (Figure 18.8) and appears to be important in maintaining basal tone. NO has been implicated in a variety of pathological conditions such as ischemia, hypoxia, stroke, and subarachnoid hemorrhage; as well as playing a role in both the coupling of cerebral metabolism and CBF and the effects of hyperventilation[(31)]. This promises to be an area of extensive research over the next several years.

Loss of Autoregulation

The ability to regulate CBF over a broad range of perfusion pressures has been shown to be impaired by a variety of pathophysiological insults such as head trauma. Most investigators have demonstrated metabolic uncoupling and hyperemia after head injury[(69,88,93)] as well as impairment of the vasomotor response to $PaCO_2$. The etiology of these findings remains elusive as does their significance. To date,

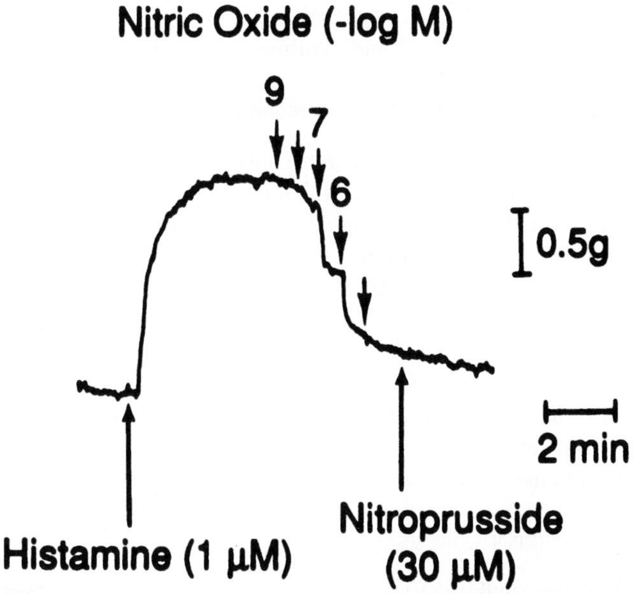

Figure 18.8. Effect of various concentrations of nitric oxide (NO) on a ring of the rabbit middle cerebral artery. The artery was precontracted with histamine and concentrations of NO are shown above the tracing. (From Faraci FM and Brian JE. Nitric oxide and the cerebral circulation. Stroke. 1994;25:693.)

no studies have demonstrated a correlation of outcome or clinical status with the loss of autoregulation[(7)]. It is anticipated that this relationship will continue to be examined as techniques to measure CBF are further refined.

INTRACRANIAL PRESSURE MONITORING

ICP monitoring is frequently used in the management of patients with intracranial hypertension. As previously discussed in this chapter, maintaining an adequate cerebral perfusion pressure is an important factor in the survival of patients with neurological injuries. Invasive monitoring is the only available way to accurately measure ICP. This technology can be used, along with frequent clinical assessment, to manage the patient at risk for complications secondary to intracranial hypertension.

Historical Perspective

The effects of increased ICP on cerebral function were first examined in 1824 using animal models[(14)]. However, it was not until 1951 that ICP monitoring in humans became accepted and widespread[(70)]. In 1965 Lundberg published a report stating, "continuous recording of the ventricular fluid pressure in cases of severe traumatic injury of the head facilitates the evaluation of intracranial dynamics and offers a more rational basis for treatment than do conventional measures."[(71)]. The earliest ICP monitors consisted of a catheter placed directly into the ventricle and this continues to be the most accurate method of determining ICP. Ventricular catheterization, however, is not without risk and subsequently less invasive catheters and monitoring devices have been developed and continue to be refined.

Types of Intracranial Pressure Monitors

ICP monitors may exist in one of several locations: intraventricular, intraparenchymal, subarachnoid, or epidural. They can be further classified into fiberoptic, strain gauge, or fluid coupled, depending on the method of operation of the individual system (Fig. 18.9). Fluid coupling implies that a fluid chamber communicates with a transducer by a fluid pathway. Since fluid is relatively incompressible, if there are pressure fluctuations in the fluid cavity it will be transmitted to the transducer[124]. The ideal ICP monitor would be accurate, consistent, sensitive, specific, reproducible, cost effective, easy to use, and expose the patient to minimal risk[67].

Intraventricular Catheters

Intraventricular catheters are commonly used, and are considered to be the standard by which other ICP monitoring devices are compared. An intraventricular catheter may be placed in the operating room, emergency department, or the PICU. To place the catheter, a patch of hair is shaved on the appropriate coronal suture in the mid-pupillary line. The area is prepped with an anti-microbial solution and local injection of lidocaine with epinephrine is performed. Systemic analgesia and sedation should be considered if the cardiovascular status is adequate. Once the ventricle is entered and fluid returns through the drain, an opening ICP can be obtained and the system connected to a standard pressure transducer system.

There are several advantages of the intraventricular catheter. The CSF pressure measurement within the ventricle is dampened the least compared to other monitoring techniques, and therefore is logically the most accurate. Pressure tracings should be clear and sufficiently accurate for diagnostic purposes. Re-zeroing or re-calibration of the monitor can be accomplished as needed, as the transducer lies outside of the head.

Undoubtedly the most important advantage of the intraventricular catheter is the ability to withdraw CSF to emergently or continuously lower ICP, as well as to perform cultures on CSF fluid. Injection of preservative-free normal saline into the ventricle can also be performed to determine the volume-pressure response. Another advantage of the intraventricular catheter is that it may be used with standard pressure transducer systems, such as those that monitor blood pressure, and rarely requires additional capital expenditure.

Although intraventricular catheters are frequently used for ICP monitoring, their placement carries several risks. As with all invasive procedures there is the risk of infection. There is little recent evidence concerning the rate of infection for indwelling intraventricular catheters. The overall infection rate of all ICP monitors is generally reported as low, less than 10%[76]. However in a study performed in 1986, an infection rate of 21% was described while using an intraventricular catheter[3]. More recently in 1993, the infection rate for an intraventricular catheter was described as 7.1%[133].

In our experience, there have been few cases of infection secondary to intraventricular catheters. Our approach to the use and ongoing care of these catheters includes strict aseptic technique upon insertion and maintenance of this sterility whenever the system is violated. The nursing staff draws daily CSF cultures and the results are followed for increasing white blood cell count and the presence of organisms. Only if a catheter becomes infected will it be replaced with a new one. This practice supports the findings of a study in 1993 that suggested the infection rate of intraventricular catheters did not increase after 5 days[133] as had previously been reported in the literature[76]. Systemic antibiotic coverage is provided for the duration of the cath-

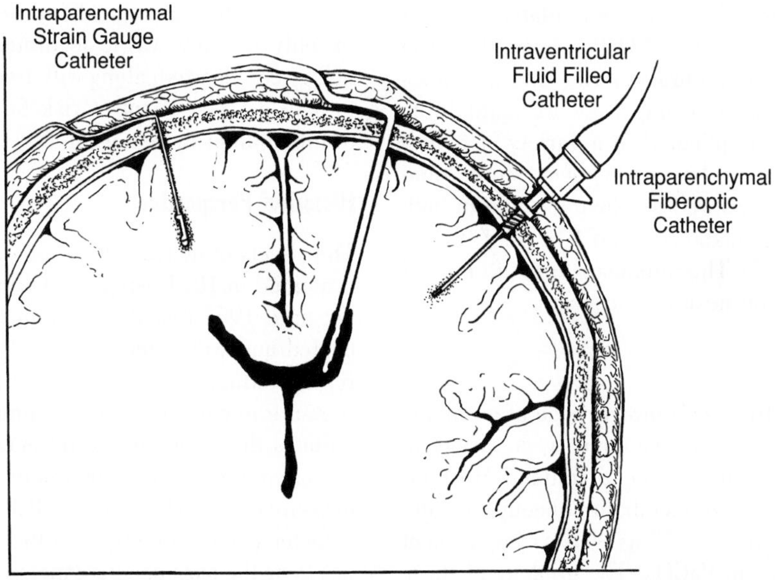

Figure 18.9. Location of various intracranial monitors as described in the text.

eter's placement. This topic warrants further investigation and research. Several papers have supported the use of prophylactic antibiotic coverage(133,134) while others suggest there is no significant difference in the infection rates of patients receiving prophylactic nafcillin and those patients on no antibiotic coverage(76). Other techniques to minimize infection are the changing of dressings saturated with CSF or blood, and the removal of the catheter as soon as ICP monitoring is no longer indicated.

Hemorrhage secondary to the insertion or removal of an intraventricular catheter is a second potential risk. Although the literature is scant concerning the frequency with which these bleeds occur, in our personal experience it is low. One study in 1982 suggests the rate of hemorrhage to be approximately 1 to 2%(92). Coagulation studies should be performed prior to the insertion or removal of any invasive ICP monitoring system.

Placement of the intraventricular catheter in ventricles that are small or slit-like, or in those patients with a significant midline shift may be very difficult and therefore is suggested as another potential disadvantage of this type of catheter. Once the catheter is in place, it is important to establish an appropriate drainage height in order to avoid excessive CSF withdrawal and ventricular collapse. The usual height of the drain is 15 cm H_2O above ear level. With external systems, such as the Becker system, ICP can be measured continuously or intermittently as prescribed (Fig. 18.10).

Although not adequately documented in the literature, the risk of seizures is also present with ICP catheter placement. We believe the risk is minimal and do not recommend routine anti-epileptic medications. Finally, blockage of the drain may occur, resulting in dampening of the wave form and erroneously transduced pressures. This may occur secondary to blood or tissue blocking the tip of the catheter. Flushing of the catheter will usually relieve the obstruction. When indicated, flushing of the system should be performed by experienced personnel using strict aseptic technique. In our institution, back flushing of the drainage system itself is done by experienced nursing staff, while flushing of the catheter into the ventricle is performed by neurosurgical personnel or the intensivist.

In summary, the intraventricular catheter is an excellent means of accurately monitoring ICP and can usually be placed without significant complications. However, because of the risks and disadvantages reviewed above, intraventricular catheters should be reserved for those patients with, or at significant risk for, increased ICP.

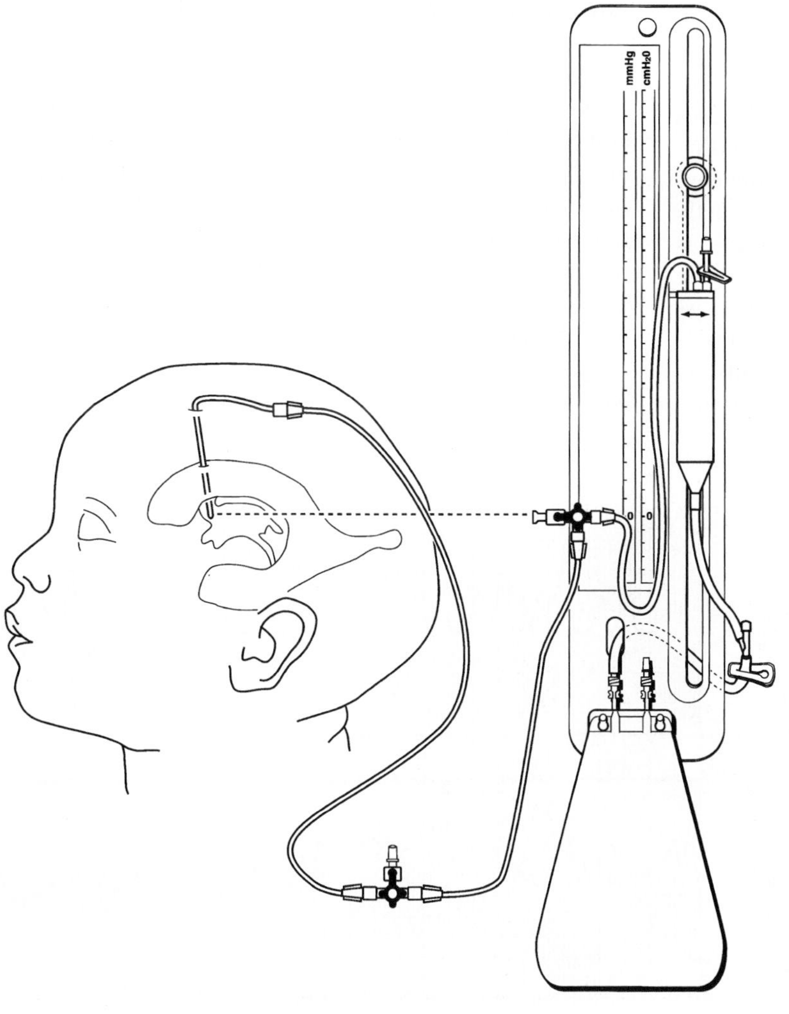

Figure 18.10. Intraventricular intracranial pressure monitor with attached drainage system.

Intraparenchymal Monitors

In recent years there have been advances made in the use of fiberoptic tipped catheters to measure ICP. The major component in these devices is a monitor that can sense variations in the amount of light reflected from a pressure-sensitive diaphragm that is located at the tip of the catheter[24]. These monitors are placed directly into the brain parenchyma, approximately 1 cm below the subarachnoid space, via a bolt device and offer several advantages over the intraventricular catheter[41].

The first advantage of the fiberoptic catheter is the relative ease of insertion into the brain parenchyma that can be accomplished despite increased ICP, mid-line shift, or slit-like ventricles. As previously discussed, appropriate sedation and analgesia should be used prior to placement of the catheter.

In 1990, Crutchfield et al. looked at intercompartmental pressure relationships utilizing an animal model. Despite various manipulations of the ICP, the pressure within the subdural, intraventricular and intraparenchymal compartments responded simultaneously and to the same degree[17]. A recent adult human study demonstrated minimal differences between intraventricular pressures, measured with a standard intraventricular catheter, and intraparenchymal pressures in the contralateral hemisphere utilizing a fiberoptic catheter. The intraventricular pressure was consistently 2 mm Hg higher than the intraparenchymal pressure. ICP wave forms were similar[38]. In a more recent pediatric study, groups of patients with similar Glasgow Coma Scores and days of ICP monitoring were compared utilizing either an intraventricular catheter or an intraparenchymal catheter. The difference in pressure was consistently 3 ± 2 mm Hg lower in the intraparenchymal space as compared to the intraventricular space. The authors of the study suggest that the difference is greatest with increasing severity of cerebral trauma[39]. In summary, a major advantage of the fiberoptic catheter is the ability to accurately measure subdural, intraventricular, and intraparenchymal pressures by placing a catheter in the intraparenchymal space only.

Despite the advantages of the intraparenchymal catheter listed above, disadvantages do exist. First is the inability to withdraw CSF. This is not a consideration if monitoring is the only goal of measuring the ICP. However, in patients where removal of CSF is an integral part of ICP management, then a second catheter needs to be placed in the ventricle. Another disadvantage of the fiberoptic catheter is the inability to re-calibrate once the catheter has been placed, because the transducer lies inside the head. This is a potential problem as the drift of the fiberoptic catheter has been stated to be up to 6 mm Hg over a 5 day period[67]. The positive side of an implantable transducer, however, is that leveling of equipment is not necessary with patient position changes, as is necessary with external transducers. Another problem with a fiberoptic catheter is the potential for breakage or dislodgment. These are problems that can be managed with experienced bedside nurses. Finally, any fiberoptic system requires dedicated hardware and can significantly add to capital expenditure.

The most recent intraparenchymal catheter system consists of a miniature transducer mounted on a pressure-sensing diaphragm. The pressure sensor is composed of two semiconductor strain gauges mounted on an extremely thin diaphragm which bends in proportion to applied pressure. Wires from the gauge run in a flexible nylon cable to a resistor network to complete the bridge circuit[44]. Like the fiberoptic catheters, this catheter requires dedicated hardware, cannot be recalibrated once inserted and cannot be used for CSF withdrawal at this time. Advantages of this system include the flexibility of the catheter which can be kinked without breaking or disturbing the pressure signal, and a suggested drift of only 1 mm Hg at nine days. Early animal studies also support the accuracy of the strain gauge catheter when compared to the intraventricular catheter[44].

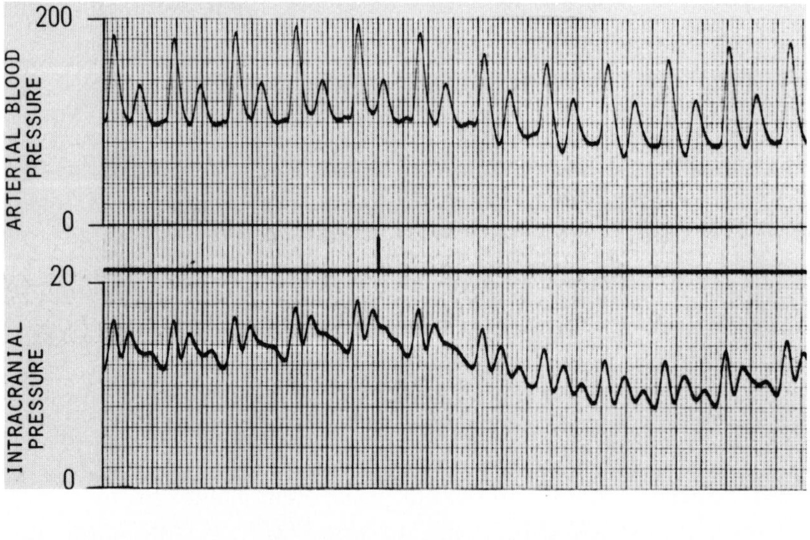

Figure 18.11. Intracranial pressure waveforms closely resemble arterial waves; differences between arterial and intracranial pressure waveforms are a result of brain vascular capacitance and resistance, the presence or absence of cerebral edema, and the compliance of the intracranial vault.

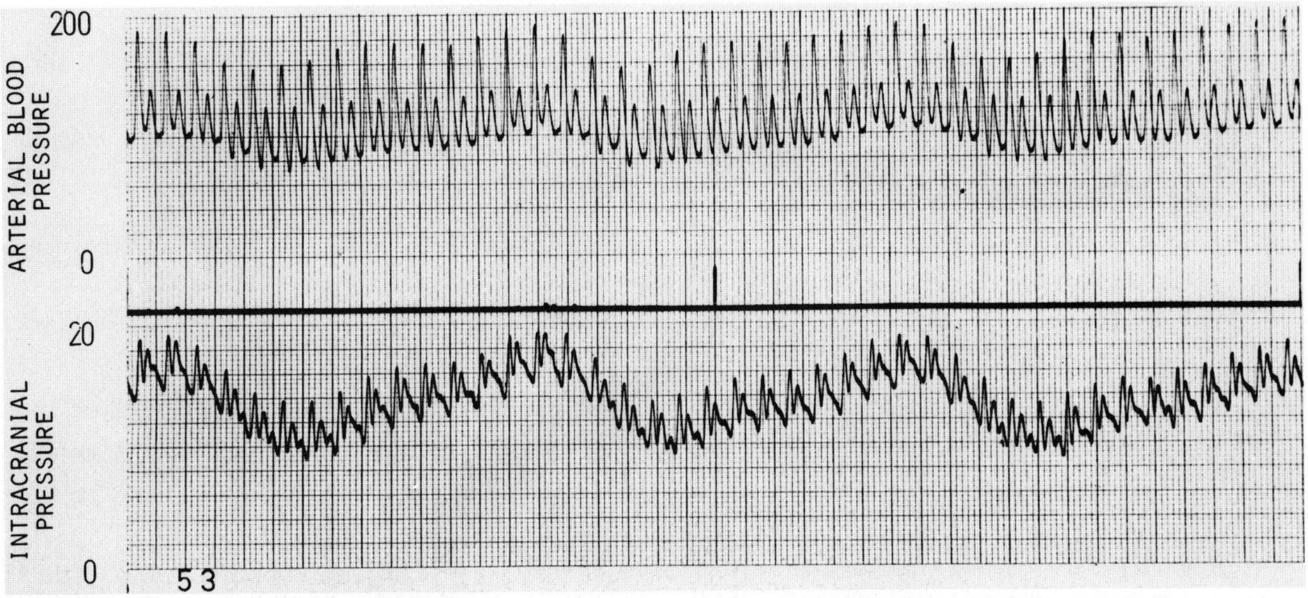

Figure 18.12. Effect of respiratory excursions on intracranial pressure. This effect is mediated both by transmission of intrapleural pressure to the intracranial vault and by effects on cardiac output. This patient was on a mechanical ventilator.

In summary, intraparenchymal monitoring is a safe alternative to intraventricular monitoring in those patients who do not require CSF drainage as part of their management plan. Further research is needed on these newer catheters in regards to their accuracy, their potential for drift and their degree of potential infectious complications, which are rarely mentioned.

Subarachnoid/Epidural Monitors

Subarachnoid and epidural monitors have been extensively used with moderate success in previous years to measure ICP when an intraventricular catheter could not be used. Their present role in management of ICP, however, has been limited secondary to the development of fiberoptic and catheter tip strain gauge transducers. Their placement, function, advantages and disadvantages will not be discussed as their use has become limited.

Types of Intracranial Pressure Waveforms

There are several types of waveforms and fluctuations that are seen when monitoring intracranial pressure. The intracranial pressure waveform resembles an arterial waveform (Fig. 18.11), although the amplitudes of the different frequency components of the waveform are different. There may be obvious respiratory excursions consistent with transmission of intrapleural pressure to the intracranial vault (Fig. 18.12), although these waves have been attributed to reflexes[71]. Finally, B-waves (Fig 18.13) and plateau waves

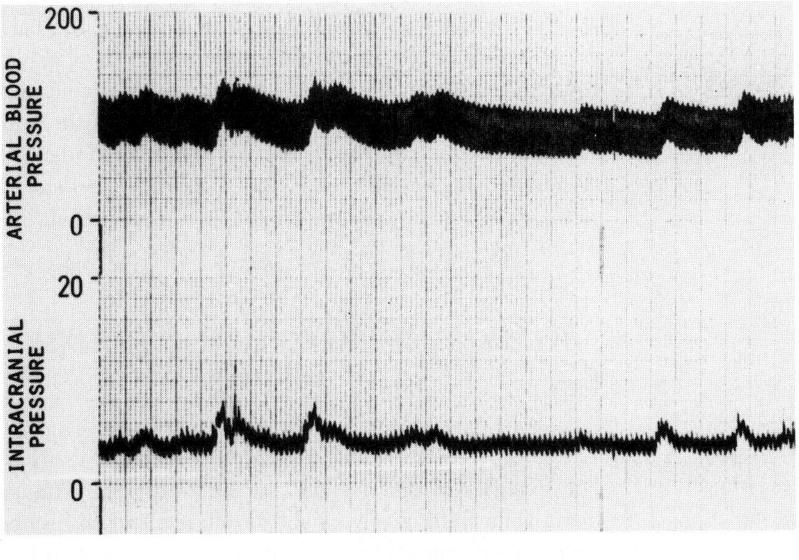

Figure 18.13. B-waves in a child after removal of a subdural hematoma. Although such waves may be innocuous, they may presage the occurrence of plateau waves.

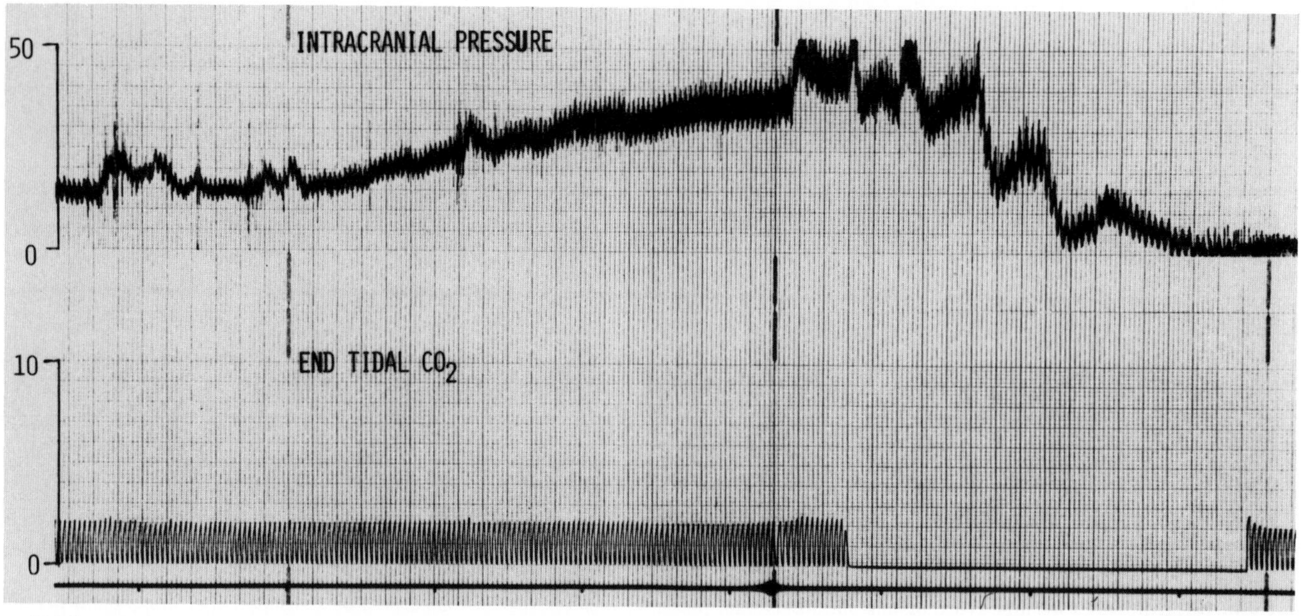

Figure 18.14. Plateau waves in a 12-year old boy with severe cerebral edema after closed head trauma. Notice the B-waves, which occurred prior to the plateau wave. The elevated ICP was effectively treated by hyperventilation, as shown by the disconnection of the end-tidal $PaCO_2$ monitor.

(Fig. 18.14) may be encountered. The etiology of either wave is uncertain, but both are probably related to cerebral vasodilatation and an increase in CBV. The more dangerous wave is the plateau wave; the prolonged elevated intracranial pressure may result in global ischemia, brainstem compression, or herniation.

Summary

Although there are limitations to any method of measuring ICP, these authors support the use of ICP monitoring as part of an overall management plan in treating patients with intracranial hypertension. The clinician is offered several options with which to measure ICP. Before utilizing any of the above systems it is imperative that the physician and nursing staff alike be familiar with their use. For example, an improperly zeroed fiberoptic or strain gauge catheter, already in place in the brain parenchyma will be of no value to the clinician caring for the patient, and may in fact lead to inappropriate medical intervention. Consistent zeroing of the external transducers also ensures greater accuracy from day to day. We recommend that the external transducer be zeroed 3 cm above and 3 cm anterior to the auricle of the ear (Fig. 18.15). This position more accurately reflects the placement of the third ventricle and therefore the site of desired measurement.

The decision to invasively monitor ICP should be made jointly by the pediatric intensivist and neurosurgeon. This form of monitoring should be reserved for those patients in whom it is truly indicated. All participants in the care of the patient must be aware of the inherent risks of this procedure, as previously discussed. ICP monitoring can be an important adjunct to the care and treatment of the patient with intracranial hypertension. The complications of this procedure can be minimized by experienced bedside personnel, as well as an organized, rational approach to the use of invasive monitoring.

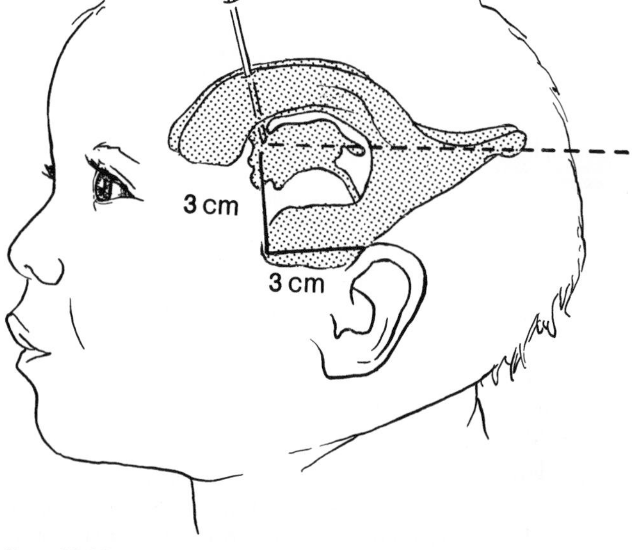

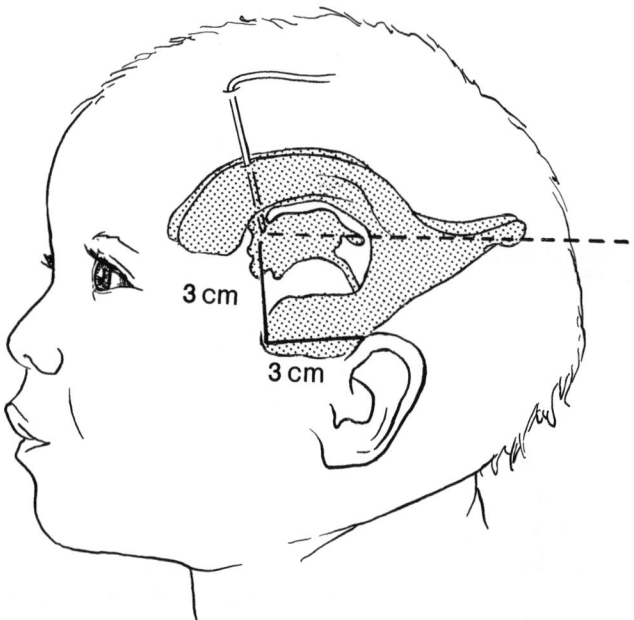

Figure 18.15. Properly zero-referenced intraventricular monitor system as described in the text.

TREATMENT OF INTRACRANIAL HYPERTENSION IN CHILDREN

Introduction

The experience documented by the Children's Traumatic Coma Data Bank gives insight into the nature and scope of the problems encountered when managing increased ICP in children[2,68]. If one considers solely traumatic brain injuries, there is a strong association with poor outcome when bilateral parenchymal swelling (with or without midline shift) and mass lesions are seen on the initial CT scan. These finding underscore the critical role increased ICP management plays in the ultimate outcome of children with traumatic brain injuries. The outcome is poorest in the 0 to 4 year-old age group, with distinctive features consisting of subdural hematomas in 20%, hypotension in 32% and a 62% overall one year mortality. The most favorable outcome is in the 5 to 10 year-old age group, with two thirds of these patients having a good Glasgow outcome score at one year. The most important prognostic indicators in the Data Bank study were the lowest post-resuscitation Glasgow Coma Score and pupillary reactivity. It is clear that much can be done to improve these statistics, and rational management strategies directed toward the prevention and treatment of increased ICP must be the cornerstone of that effort.

In this subsection, we will first address basic concepts and controversial issues involving management of mass lesions within the intracranial vault. Next, we will discuss the basic science fundamentals upon which therapeutic decisions concerning ICP are made. Finally, we describe our current approach to the management of elevated ICP in children.

Surgical Evacuation of Mass Lesions

Although a comprehensive review dealing with the management of mass lesions within the intracranial vault is beyond the scope of this chapter, it is appropriate to discuss this issue first because often a patient's survival depends on the timely evacuation of a life-threatening mass. The management of the patient's ICP before, during and after surgical intervention must be the primary concern of the pediatric team. In fact, preservation of neurological function depends upon it. Certain concepts discussed earlier in this chapter must be stressed here. First, all mass lesions are not alike. They differ by their rapidity of onset, location, size and underlying pathophysiologic mechanism. Thus, a lesion such as a moderate-sized temporal epidural hematoma is treated as a neurosurgical emergency while a large posterior fossa tumor may be treated with steroids and operated at the next elective opportunity. The point is that hematomas, tumors, cysts, abscesses and the like are all very different, and the goal is to use sound judgment and knowledge of the lesion's natural history in order to preserve and restore neurological function. A second point to consider is that certain intracranial lesions are more ominous than others. A large epidural hematoma may be evacuated with minimal or no neurological sequelae, while a thin holohemispheric subdural hematoma is often associated with significant underlying parenchymal injury and increased ICP[129]. Understanding these differences is important when evaluating and treating children with mass lesions in the ICU setting.

There are several controversial issues concerning the management of traumatic mass lesions of the intracranial vault. For instance, it is felt by several authors that not all epidural hematomas need to be evacuated. These authors have managed anywhere from 9% to 24% of medium to large epidural hematomas in a conservative fashion[10,96,101]. However, there are still neurosurgeons who feel all epidural hematomas should be surgically evacuated no matter what the size or location. Another controversy concerns the management of thin, holohemispheric, "rim" subdural hematomas overlying a swollen and contused hemisphere. Some neurosurgeons would perform a craniotomy, evacuate the subdural hematoma and leave the dura open and the bone flap out. Others would perform a small twist drill craniotomy for placement of an ICP device, let the subdural hematoma express itself through the hole, and then place the monitoring device for medical management of the increased ICP. Still others would manage the problem only medically, without the aid of an ICP monitoring device[121]. Obviously, there are many ways to manage a given problem, and the overall poor outcomes associated with severe head injuries are testimony to the fact that no one "right" way has been developed over the years to combat the challenge of increased ICP.

Physiologic Basis for Medical ICP Control

General Measures

Temperature Control

The increased metabolic demand that results from fevers can increase CBF, CBV and ICP. Increased CBV and pressure may lead to worsening of cerebral edema, reduced CBF and deterioration of the brain's oxygen supply and demand ratio. Therefore, it is imperative that hyperthermia be aggressively treated when increased ICP is present.

Temperature control may be accomplished with cooling mattresses and the administration of rectal acetaminophen. Shivering, which can increase ICP by increasing intrathoracic pressure, can be prevented by muscle paralysis. Overcooling to the point of hypothermia is to be avoided; rather, the goal is normothermia. Rectal, esophageal, or pulmonary arterial (via a Swan-Ganz catheter) temperature probes should be used to provide continuous temperature monitoring.

Head Position

Keeping the head of the patient's bed flat or raising the head to a 30 degree angle may have different theoretical effects on optimizing CPP. Specifically, remembering that CPP = MAP − ICP, the mean arterial pressure to the brain is highest in the supine position, while the ICP is lowest when the head is elevated. The question is, which position has the predominant effect on influencing CPP? To address this issue, Feldman et al.[33] studied 22 head injured patients and concluded that keeping the head of the bed elevated to 30 degrees provided the optimal benefit for ICP control. In an earlier study, Durward et al.[26] concluded that moderate head elevation to 15 to 30° optimized cerebral perfusion pressure. At head elevation levels above 30° the arterial pressure measured at head level failed to maintain cerebral perfusion, which was significantly reduced[94]. Similar effects have been noted in newborn infants[28], supporting the concept of moderate head elevation in infants with asphyxial injuries or intraventricular hemorrhage.

Another important issue concerning head position is preventing inadvertent neck constriction secondary to cervical collars or endotrachial tube tape. These maneuvers maximize jugular venous outflow and improve ICP control. Once the cervical spine has been cleared radiographically (usually by fluoroscopic flexion-extension views), the patient may be log rolled side to side at one to two hour intervals to prevent pressure sores on the body or back of the head.

Seizure Control and Prophylaxis

During seizure activity, the brain's metabolic rate, blood flow and oxygen consumption increase significantly[66,117], thus diminishing its capacity for maintaining a normal ICP. If the brain is injured and has loss of autoregulatory activity, seizures can result in dangerous ICP elevations, and need to be treated aggressively. Ongoing seizures may be treated with lorazepam 0.1 to 0.2 mg/kg IV repeated twice every five minutes or until the seizures cease. At the same time, the patient should be loaded with either phenytoin 10 mg/kg IV and repeated in 30 minutes (if the patient is over 2 years of age) or phenobarbital 10 mg/kg IV and also repeated in 30 minutes (if the patient is under 2 years of age).

Prophylactic administration of antiepileptic drugs is an important part of preventing unwanted ICP elevations. However, this is a complex topic, and no study has been able to define clear-cut risk groups for which prophylactic anticonvulsant therapy is indicated. Hahn et al.[49] found that the more severe the brain injury, either by Glasgow Coma Scale criteria or by the CT findings of acute subdural hematoma or cerebral swelling, the higher the incidence of seizures. Jennett et al.[56] studied the incidence of post-traumatic epilepsy in patients with depressed skull fractures. If dural laceration, early epilepsy (one or more seizures in the first week) or post-traumatic amnesia longer than 24 hours were present, there was up to 20% risk of seizures. A 45% risk of seizures is seen once the patient has experienced a "late" post-traumatic epileptic event[51]. Other high risk groups seem to include patients with parenchymal abnormalities such as contusions, lacerations, or surgical evacuation sites. Our approach has been to prophylactically treat patients with anticonvulsants if there is a late post-traumatic seizure or if a parenchymal abnormality is seen on the CT scan. Similarly, if a patient is being treated for increased ICP and still has sustained, unexplained ICP elevations, subclinical seizures must be considered as a cause and EEG evaluation is warranted.

Fluid Management

Traditional views of head injury management have advocated restricting fluid and sodium administration in hopes of preventing cerebral edema in areas of injured brain and subsequently, increased ICP[79,114]. However, in a recent study, Schmoker et al.[112] indicated that patients kept normovolemic during their period of increased ICP management fare just as well as those kept deliberately hypovolemic. In the first study of its kind they retrospectively reviewed the fluid and sodium intake of 57 adults with severe head injury. They found that maintenance of normovolemia does not predispose head injured patients to uncontrolled ICP. This is in contrast to the old concept of "drying out" a head injury patient by restricting fluids and giving large amounts of osmotic diuretics. Current practice based on this new concept has so far met with encouraging results in several centers, including ours.

The type of intravenous maintenance and replacement fluid to use is subject to debate, although we prefer using an isotonic fluid such as Ringer's lactate or 0.9% saline with 20 mEq/L of KCl. Relatively hypotonic fluids such as 0.45% saline are often used in pediatric patients, but one must be vigilant that hyponatremia does not occur. D_5W is never indicated except in the circumstance of fluid replacement for significant hypernatremia as a result of neurogenic diabetes insipidus.

Sedation and Neuromuscular Blockade

Perhaps no issue in this discussion is more controversial than the management of sedative and paralytic drugs in the ICU setting, especially in patients being treated for increased ICP. The typical scenario involves a child with a severe head injury, and an ICP monitoring device in place, who is receiving continuous IV infusions of a sedative/hypnotic agent, a narcotic, and a non-depolarizing paralytic agent. While many times such management is appropriate, the amount, timing and duration of such therapy remains to be elucidated. A known complication of indiscriminate usage of non-depolarizing paralytic agents involves prolonged weakness and continued need for ventilatory support beyond the expected, appropriate amount of time[29,53]. The cause of this problem is unclear, but is probably multifactorial. The use of nerve stimulators should be standard during neuromuscular blockade and will minimize the risk of prolonged neuromuscular weakness.

A reasonable approach to sedation and paralyzation for children with increased ICP involves the step-wise institution of first a sedative/hyponotic (such as midazolam) with or without a narcotic (such as fentanyl), followed by a non-depolarizing neuromuscular blocker if ICP control is still a problem. Once ICP control has been achieved, the sequence can be reversed at the appropriate time. Another approach involves the use of the IV general anesthetic propofol as the sole agent for sedation[46,97,104,108,119,126,127]. This agent has the benefit of rapid onset and emergence from sedation, thus making timely neurological assessment easier. However, propofol has also been implicated as the source of a fatal metabolic acidosis in the intensive care unit[120], and its use should be monitored closely.

CSF Removal

External Ventricular Drains

As mentioned earlier, the gold standard for ICP measurement is ventricular catheterization. However, an external ventricular drain (EVD) also has therapeutic potential by allowing CSF removal once the ICP has reached a dangerous level. Removing CSF in this fashion is a physiologic way to reduce ICP and avoid unwanted side effects from medications. Obviously, the ventricle needs to be large enough to cannulate, but in experienced hands, this problem is usually surmounted. The benefits of EVD insertion for ICP control seem to far outweigh the potential risks (such as intracranial hematomas or infection), although no controlled study has addressed this issue.

Lumbar Drains

Once medical therapy for ICP control has been exhausted and barbiturate coma therapy is being considered, further CSF removal via a lumbar drain may produce dramatic and long-lasting changes in ICP. This has been documented by Baldwin and Rekate(4). Caveats to remember are that a supratentorial EVD must first be in place, and the basilar cisterns must be open (documented by CT scan) in order to prevent tonsillar herniation and brainstem compression. Although this practice seems counter-intuitive to traditional teachings, it has met with considerable success in our hands and many times eliminated the need for barbiturate coma in patients with severe, refractory increased ICP.

Osmotic Agents and Diuretic Therapy

A great deal has been learned recently about osmotic agents such as mannitol and diuretic therapy for increased ICP. The following discussion will review what is currently known about these treatment modalities and their interactions between each other. Urea and glycerol are now rarely used for ICP control, and will not be discussed further(43,48,55,72,90,98,102,128).

Mannitol is the most commonly used agent for control of increased ICP and produces an intracranial chain of events that has recently been clarified. Upon intravenous administration, mannitol decreases blood viscosity (maximum effect at 10 minutes, with a duration of 75 minutes)(4,89,103) and transiently increases CBV, CBF and ICP(4,89,103). Cerebral oxygen transport then improves(18,86) and adenosine levels decrease(89). If autoregulation is intact, cerebral vasoconstriction occurs in response to the decreased adenosine levels, and CBF is kept constant(86,89). ICP is then decreased as a result of a lower CBV. If autoregulation is impaired, as in the case of diffuse axonal injury, less of an effect is seen(86). If the CPP is greater than 70, mannitol may not work as well as when the CPP is less than 70 because cerebral vasoconstriction may already be near maximal(109).

It is important to remember to give no more mannitol than is absolutely necessary. Negative long-term effects on ICP control may occur if previous excessive amounts have been given(77). In fact, there is no proof that 1 gm/kg of mannitol works any better than 0.25 gm/kg, so therefore it is probably prudent to give the smaller amount. Also, there is no proof that osmotic agents lower ICP by decreasing brain water content(50,89). Mannitol's effects probably have more to do with altering CBF and CBV, as outlined above. Rapid administration of mannitol seems to be more effective in lowering ICP(107), although clinical experience has also indicated that mannitol drips may bring about a favorable responses in ICP control.

The loop diuretic furosemide is also helpful when managing increased ICP. Two proposed mechanisms of action are responsible for furosemide's effect on ICP. They include 1) interference with CSF formation and sodium and water movement across the blood-brain barrier and 2) preferential excretion of water over solute in the distal renal tubule(99). It has been documented that furosemide and mannitol work better together than either one used alone(99,132). It has also been shown that giving mannitol 15 minutes before furosemide has the largest effect on ICP control(107).

Although the carbonic anhydrase inhibitor acetazolamide is often discussed in ICP management, it is most often used as a temporizing measure for control of CSF production in hydrocephalic patients. It is almost never used in the ICU setting except for premature infants with post-hemorrhagic hydrocephalus from an intraventricular/germinal matrix hemorrhage.

Hyperventilation and Ventilator Management

Hyperventilation produces hypocapnea and cerebral vasoconstriction, which results in decreased CBV and ICP. In fact, the change in CBV resulting from carbon dioxide control and variation is 0.05 ml/100 gm/torr $PaCO_2$ in normal volunteers. For example, when the $PaCO_2$ falls from 40 mm Hg to 25 mm Hg, the CBV will decrease by 0.75 ml/100 gm(45), thus making hyperventilation a useful tool in the management of acute increases in ICP. This reduction in CBV persists for approximately 15 minutes after the $PaCO_2$ returns to its original value(45). The magnitude of the acute drop in ICP after hyperventilation is similar to that produced by the ventricular drainage of a few milliliters of CSF. However, the effects of routine, long-term hyperventilation for ICP control are now being called into question, and new management strategies are emerging.

Besides the obvious advantage of cerebral vasocontriction for ICP control, hyperventilation also has the theoretical advantage of reversing brain and CSF acidosis. The disadvantages of hyperventilation are possible cerebral ischemia because of regional or global over-vasoconstriction and a short-lived effect on CSF pH from loss of the bicarbonate buffer system. Recent evidence indicates that mild hyperventilation in head injured patients, with $PaCO_2$ levels 30 to 35 mm Hg, is tolerated over long periods of time and may produce better overall outcomes(13).

In a randomized, controlled trial involving patients with

severe head injuries, Muizelaar et al.[87] studied three groups of patients. The first group had $PaCO_2$ levels held at 35 mm Hg, the second group had $PaCO_2$ level held at 25 mm Hg, and the third group had $PaCO_2$ levels held at 25 mm Hg and THAM (tromethamine, an alkaline CSF buffer) was given. The first and third group's outcome were better at a statistically significant level. They concluded that chronic hyperventilation to a $PaCO_2$ level of 25 mm Hg is deleterious. Also, Cold et al.[13], in a study measuring CBF in head injured patients, found a correlation between hyperventilation ($PaCO_2$ 25 to 30 mm Hg) and poor outcome. They hypothesized that chronic, aggressive hyperventilation produces areas of oligemia in marginally perfused brain tissue. How long does the effect of hyperventilation last, and what happens when it is discontinued too quickly? Albrecht et al.[1], using a goat model, found that the effects of hyperventilation lasted only up to about 6 hours, and sudden discontinuation of hypocapnea caused a rebound increase in ICP. These findings have important implications in the clinical management of children with increased ICP.

Therefore, while aggressive hyperventilation ($PaCO_2$ 25 to 30 mm Hg) is a useful tool in the management of increased ICP in the acute setting (i.e. during trauma transport, in the emergency room, or during a sudden ICP spike), chronic hyperventilation to such levels is potentially harmful. PaC02 levels in the chronic hyperventilatory state probably should be kept in the 30 to 35 mm Hg range.

Other ventilator parameters, such as PEEP, may also have a negative influence on ICP. However, Cooper et al.[15] found that PEEP up to 10 cm H_20 had minimal effects on ICP. Beyond that level, increased intrathoracic pressure may impede jugular venous outflow and raise ICP. If high frequency jet ventilation is needed for management of severe pulmonary disease, Hurst et al.[54] found that ICP is minimally influenced, or even improved, without significant hemodynamic or oxygen transport compromise.

Several authors have discussed the use of jugular venous saturation monitors in the treatment of increased ICP. Using the Fick principle, the difference in arterial-venous oxygen saturation measured from an arterial site and the jugular vein gives a rough estimate of the brain's oxygen extraction fraction and it's current aerobic/anaerobic status[111]. Cruz et al.[18] found that continuous monitoring of cerebral oxygenation using fiberoptic catheter oximetry was valuable in identifying decreased brain oxygenation even when CPP was adequate. Gayle et al.[40] documented the use of jugular venous bulb catheters in 26 infants and children, and found them useful during increased ICP management. However, the potential benefit and added information given by jugular venous saturation monitors must be weighed against their potential risks, which include infection, venous thrombosis and inadvertent carotid puncture during insertion[40].

Near-infrared (near-IR) spectroscopy may be used to non-invasively monitor brain vascular hemoglobin saturation in a non-invasive fashion[118]. This technique supposedly allows continuous monitoring of brain capillary oxygenation and may be sensitive enough to alert the clinician to situations where blood flow and oxygenation are inadequate. Used in conjunction with an ICP monitor and arterial blood gasses, one may gain sophisticated insight into a patient's ongoing cerebral oxygenation status and manage cardiorespiratory support in a more intelligent fashion. Although there are no reports of clinical experience with near-IR spectroscopy in the pediatric head injured population, it holds some promise for future development and use.

Barbiturate Coma

Much has been written in the past regarding the use of barbiturate coma in the management of increased ICP refractory to other medical means. The proposed mechanism of action for ICP control involves both the reduction of $CMR0_2$, thereby reducing oxygen need and blood flow, as well as a direct reduction in CBF and CBV. Cerebral vasoconstriction probably plays a role in the barbiturate effect, but whether this results from reduction in $CMR0_2$ or is a direct vascular effect is unknown. Messeter et al.[80] have shown that preservation of cerebral $C0_2$ reactivity can predict the response of ICP in barbiturate coma. When $C0_2$ responsivity was normal, barbiturates reduced CBF and normalized ICP in 75% of patients. When this response was reduced or absent, CBF was unchanged or increased, and ICP was reduced in only 20%.

However, several studies document that barbiturate use provides no better outcome than routine management in emperic therapy for coma[83,130]. Specifically, Schwartz et al.[113] found no significant difference between using standard mannitol therapy and barbiturates. In another large, randomized controlled trial (53 patients) by Ward et al.[130], barbiturates showed no statistical benefit in outcome when administered in a prophylactic fashion. Complicating Ward et al.'s study, as well as other studies, is the fact that significant side effects, such as hypotension, may occur in the barbiturate group[123,130]. Our current use of barbiturates in managing increased ICP is restricted to patients with pressures refractory to maximal medical and surgical therapy (including a lumbar drain), and as prophylaxis in vascular neurosurgical cases.

If barbiturates must be used in the treatment of increased ICP, we administer them as a continuous drip. The loading dose is 5 to 10 mg/kg of pentobarbital, but we emphasize that more drug is often required. This is followed by continuous infusions of 1 to 5 mg/kg/hr of pentobarbital. One seeks a target effect of reducing ICP or until burst suppression is achieved on continuous EEG monitoring, and this type of therapy is true brinksmanship. One uses as much barbiturate as needed to control intracranial hypertension, supporting the cardiovascular system against its toxicities. It is a difficult tightrope, for which reason we recommend invasive and extensive hemodynamic monitoring during such therapy.

Steroid Therapy

Steroids, with their antiinflammatory and cell membrane stabilization effects, have long been used in the management of increased ICP. Their effect is most commonly seen in the reduction of vasogenic edema surrounding tumors, abscesses or hematomas. In this setting, steroids are useful, and in some instances, life saving. However, as with barbiturate therapy, there is no evidence that steroids, even in high doses, improve ICP control or outcome in severe head injuries. In a prospective, double-blind controlled trial, Dearden et al.[22] found no difference between high-dose dexamethasone therapy versus placebo in the Glasgow Outcome Score of severely head injured patients with increased ICP. Giannnotta et al.[42] documented that although high dose methylprednisolone resulted in lower mortality (6%) than low-dose or placebo groups (43%) in patients under 40 years old, there was an increase in the poor outcome categories for the high-dose group.

Steroids also have significant side effects, including gastrointestinal bleeding, glucose intolerance, and increased risk of infection[16,20,47,75]. It is unclear to what degree steroids increase the risk of GI hemorrhage over and above the risk associated with head injury alone[20,75].

Needless to say, in the absence of steroid's clear benefit in the use of ICP control in severe head injury, their use should be limited to control of vasogenic edema surrounding certain mass lesions such as tumors or abscesses.

Infants

Very little has been written in the past regarding the management of infants with increased ICP. Needless to say, this is an important patient subgroup and there is much to be learned regarding the pathophysiological mechanisms that influence the immature, developing brain. Several factors contribute to our incomplete understanding of the effect of increased ICP on the infant brain. These include the presence of open sutures and fontanelles (turning the intracranial cavity into a non-rigid container), the fact that the normal tolerance range for ICP in infants is unknown, and the high degree of cerebral deformability because of the brain's high water content at that age. The lack of guidelines concerning the management of this patient subgroup contributes to the poor outcomes referred to earlier in the Children's Traumatic Coma Data Bank.

Kaiser and Whitelaw studied the hypertensive response to raised ICP in infants[58]. They concluded that aggressive blood pressure support (including the use of inotropes) to maintain CPP is often needed because the reflex rise in MAP in response to increased ICP may be insufficient. For practical purposes, aiming for a CPP of at least 50 mm Hg is reasonable, although there is no hard evidence to substantiate that recommendation. Other practical matters concern the use of ICP monitors in infants. Our own bias is to place an external ventricular drain if the ventricles are of sufficient size to cannulate. If this is not possible, a fiberoptic intraparenchymal catheter may be placed in an infant over approximately 4 months of age. Before that age, the skull is too thin to hold the threads of the monitoring device's housing unit. The new "strain gauge" intraparenchymal monitors do not need to be tightly mounted into the skull, and therefore offer an advantage over other types of monitors in this situation.

Lidocaine and Etomidate

Lidocaine has been used with success to blunt the intracranial pressure rise seen with intubation[78,102]. Lidocaine is probably safer than thiopental in patients with hemodynamic instability and is effective for rapid reduction of intracranial pressure. The dose is 1.5 mg/kg as an intravenous bolus.

Etomidate has been used in the past to control intracranial pressure in patients with head injuries. The drug is not currently on the market because of concern over its safety[78]. Currently, there is no place for its use in pediatric intensive care.

Surgical Decompression

Surgical decompression has been used in various settings, without substantial information concerning its efficacy. It is tempting to consider this therapy in extreme cases of increased ICP, but unfortunately, too much damage is usually done before the decision is made. The authors continue to withhold final judgment on this mode of therapy, which may be indicated in very specific and rare circumstances.

Experimental and Future Therapies

Several new therapeutic strategies are being investigated for the use of ICP control. Many of these are byproducts of greater understanding of brain injury at the cellular and molecular level, and hold potentially promising results. While not much can be done to prevent effects caused by a primary brain injury (such as a laceration), there is increasing evidence that much can be done to prevent effects caused by delayed primary or secondary injury[9,25,78,116,117]. Delayed primary injury is defined as cells in which deleterious, and perhaps ultimately fatal, biochemical events are initiated at the time of trauma and proceed, over time, to completion. Secondary injury refers to otherwise healthy brain cells which are permanently injured as a result of the influence of other local or systemic effects. The cascade of biochemical pathways responsible for delayed primary and secondary injury are currently being studied, and agents to interrupt those pathways are being developed. These agents include free radical scavengers, lipid peroxidase antagonists, cyclooxygenase inhibitors, opioid antagonists, calcium channel blockers, and neurotransmitter modulators[9,25,78,116,117].

The use of hypothermia in the treatment of increased ICP

has recently undergone a resurgence around the world. Hypothermia has been used since the 1940's as a specific treatment measure for increased ICP(32), although the degree of cooling used (30 °C) caused significant side effects such as cardiac dysrhythmias, coagulopathies, and fluid-electrolyte/acid-base disturbances. Recently, Shiozazi et al.(115) reported favorable outcomes when moderate hypothermia (to 34 °C) was used to treat patients with severe head injuries. However, Marion et al.(73) offered a more restrained opinion of the beneficial effects of moderate hypothermia, citing a trend in better outcome using hypothermia, but no statistically significant benefit. Further clinical experience with hypothermia has been reported(12,95,105), including a phase II clinical trial(11), but there is obviously a need for a better understanding of this type of treatment. Randomized, controlled trials involving moderate hypothermia for head injury management are currently underway.

Tromethamine (THAM), mentioned earlier, is a buffer that maintains the level of CSF alkalization in chronically hyperventilated patients. By decreasing CSF acidosis with THAM, Muizelaar et al(87), found improved stabilization of ICP courses in head-injured patients. Further work with this agent will reveal whether it will become part of the standard therapy for increased ICP.

Potentially Contraindicated Therapeutic Agents

No discussion regarding the treatment of increased ICP in children would be complete without considering therapeutic actions and agents that may be harmful. Using the previous discussions of the intracranial compartments as an outline (i.e. blood, brain and CSF), one may construct a list of potentially harmful agents in the setting of severe head injury. First, any agent that increases CBV might have direct detrimental effects on ICP. Nitroglycerin and nitroprusside have direct cerebral vasodilatory effects and are considered unsafe in the setting of severe head injury, even when indicated for cardiovascular purposes. Ketamine also causes a marked increase in CBV, and is contraindicated when increased ICP is suspected. Second, any agent that might increase brain swelling is also relatively contraindicated. This most commonly concerns the use of D_5W as an

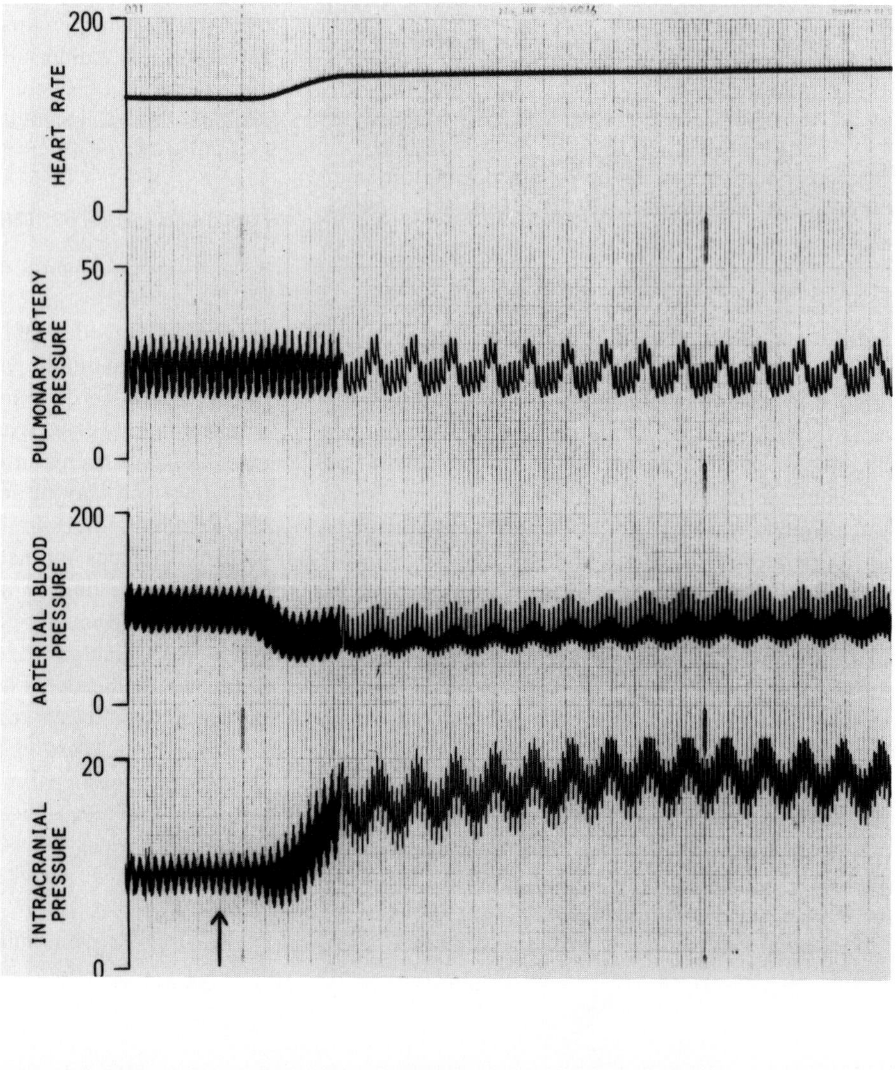

Figure 18.16. Administration of isoproterenol to a child with severe cerebral edema. The arrow indicates the start of the drug (0.05mg/kg/min). The drug was discontinued within 30 seconds, but the intracranial pressure remained elevated for 5 minutes.

intravenous replacement fluid. Neuronal swelling, increased ICP and possibly cell death may result from the cellular edema caused by administering free water. Since there is no medication that directly increases CSF formation or decreases CSF absorption, this third element of the intracranial compartment is less of a concern.

An often overlooked element in the equation regarding potentially contraindicated therapeutic agents is the role of the blood-brain barrier. Epinephrine, dopamine, and isoproterenol do not cross the blood-brain barrier of normal subjects; hence, these drugs are often used without consideration of CNS effects. However, after neurologic injury, the blood-brain barrier may be disrupted. Figure 18.16 is an example, showing the effect of a low-dose infusion of isoproterenol in a child with Reye syndrome. Isoproterenol, in this patient, presumably crossed the BBB, caused cerebral vasodilatation, and resulted in increased ICP at a time when the arterial blood pressure actually dropped. This example serves to show that even drugs that ordinarily are not active in the cerebral vasculature may have dramatic effects in the setting of neurologic injury.

SUMMARY

Intracranial hypertension is the end product of a variety of neurological insults. Prompt recognition and treatment requires both an understanding of the pathophysiology of intracranial hypertension as well as meticulous attention to general intensive care. The cornerstone of neurological intensive care remains the same as other intensive care: basic airway protection and provision of oxygenation and ventilation. Intracranial pressure monitoring has become an integral part of pediatric intensive care and should be provided to any child at risk for increased ICP. In addition, recent experimental evidence has revealed new insights into both the treatment of ICP as well as the prospect of innovative techniques to measure cerebral metabolic activity. It is hoped that proper application of this knowledge will lead to improved neurological recovery in pediatric patients with intracranial hypertension.

References

1. Albrecht RF, Miletich DJ, Ruttle M. Cerebral effects of extended hyperventilation in unanesthetized goats. Stroke 1987;18(3):649-655.
2. Aldrich EF, Eisenberg HM, Saydjari C, et al. Diffuse brain swelling in severely head-injured children. A report from the NIH Traumatic Coma Data Bank. J Neurosurg 1992;76:450-454.
3. Aucoin PJ, Kotilainen HR, Gantz NM, Davidson R, Kellogg P, Stone B. Intracranial pressure monitors: Epidemiologic study of risk factors and infections. Am J of Medicine 1986;80:369-376.
4. Baldwin HZ, Rekate HL. Preliminary experience with controlled external lumbar drainage in diffuse pediatric head injury. Pediatr Neurosurg 1991;17(3):115-120.
5. Barie PS, Ghajar JB, Firlik AD, Chang VA, Hariri RJ. Contribution of increased cerebral blood volume to posttraumatic intracranial hypertension. J Trauma 1993;35(1):88-95.
6. Bayliss WM. On the local regulation of the arterial wall to changes of internal pressure. J Physiol London 1902;28:220.
7. Bouma GJ, Muizelaar JP. Cerebral blood flow, cerebral blood volume, and cerebrovascular reactivity after severe head injury. Journal of Neurotrauma 1992;9(Supplement 1):S333-S448.
8. Bradbury MWB. The concept of a blood-brain barrier. New York: Wiley, 1979.
9. Bullock R, Fujisawa H. The role of glutamate antagonists for the treatment of CNS injury. J Neurotrauma 1992;9:443-473.
10. Chen T, Wong C, Chang C, et al. The expectant treatment of asymptomatic supratentorial epidural hematomas. Neurosurgery 1993;32:176-179.
11. Clifton GL, Allen S, Barrodale P, et al. A phase II study of moderate hypothermia in severe brain injury. J Neurotrauma 1993;10(3):263-271.
12. Clifton GL, Allen S, Berry J, Koch SM. Systemic hypothermia in treatment of brain injury. J Neurotrauma 1992;9:487-495.
13. Cold GE. Does acute hyperventilation provoke cerebral oligaemia in comatose patients after acute head injury? Acta Neurochirurgica 1989;96(3-4):100-106.
14. Cooper A. Lectures on the Principles and Practices of Surgery with Additional Notes and Cases by Frederick Tyrell. London: T&G Underwood, 1824: 282.
15. Cooper KR, Boswell PA, Choi SC. Safe use of PEEP in patients with severe head injury. J Neurosurg 1985;63:552-555.
16. Cooper PR, Moody S, Clark WK, et al. Dexamethasone and severe head injury. A prospective double-blind study. J Neurosurg 1979;51:307.
17. Crutchfield JS, Narayan RK, Robertson CS, Michael LH. Evaluation of a fiberoptic intracranial pressure monitor. J Neurosurg 1990;72(3):482-487.
18. Cruz J, Miner ME, Allen SJ, Alves WM, Gennarelli TA. Continuous monitoring of cerebral oxygenation in acute brain injury: injection of mannitol during hyperventilation. J Neurosurg 1990;73(5):725-730.
19. Cserr HF, Patlak CS. Regulation of brain volume under isosmotic and anisosmotic conditons. In: Gilles R, ed. Advances in comparative and enviromental physiology. Berlin, Heidelberg, New York, Tokyo: Springer, 1991:62-80.
20. Cushing H. Peptic ulcers and the interbrain. Surg Gynecol Obstet 1932;55:1.
21. Darby JM, Yonas H, Marion DW, Latchaw RE. Local "inverse steal" induced by hyperventilation in head injury. Neurosurgery 1988;23:84-88.
22. Dearden NM, Gibson JS, McDowall DG, Gibson RM, Caomeron NM. Effect of high-dose dexamethasone on outcome from severe head injury. J Neurosurg 1986;64:81-88.
23. Doczi T. Volume regulation of the brain tissue-a survey. Acta Neurochir 1993;121:1-8.
24. Doyle DJ, Mark PW. Analysis of intracranial pressure. J Clin Monit 1992;8:81-90.
25. Duhaime A. Exciting your neurons to death: Can we prevent cell loss after brain injury? Pediatr Neurosurg 1994;21:117-123.
26. Durward QJ, Amacher AL, Del MR, Sibbald WJ. Cerebral and cardiovascular responses to changes in head elevation in patients with intracranial hypertension. J Neurosurg 1983;59:938.
27. Dytko G, Kinter LB. Prevention of hyponatremia in experimental Schwartz-Bartter syndrome with the vasopressin antagonist SK & F 101926. In: Cserr HF, ed. The neuronal microenviroment: Ann NY Acad Sci, 1986:369-371. (vol 481).
28. Emery JR, Peabody JL. Head position affects intracranial pressure in newborn infants. J Pediatr 1983;103:950.
29. Fahy BG, Matjasko MJ. Disadvantages of prolonged neuromuscular blockade in patients with head injury. J Neurosurg Anesth 1994;6:136-138.
30. Faraci FM. Regulation of the cerebral circulation by endothelium. Pharmacology & Therapeutics 1992;56(1):1-22.
31. Faraci FM, Brian JE Jr. Nitric oxide and the cerebral circulation. Stroke 1994;25(3):692-703.
32. Fay T. Observations on generalized refrigeration in cases of severe cerebral trauma. Trauma of the Central Nervous System. Proceedings of the Assocation 1945:611-619.
33. Feldman Z, Kanter MJ, Robertson CS, et al. Effect of head elevation on intracranial pressure, cerebral perfusion pressure, and cerebral blood flow in head-injured patients. J Neurosurg 1992;76:207-211.
34. Fenichel GM. Clinical Pediatric Neurology. Philadelphia: W. B. Saunders, 1988: 89-90.
35. Fenstermacher JD. Volume regulation of the central nervous system. In: Staub NC, Taylor AE, ed. Oedema. New York: Raven, 1984:383-404.
36. Fenstermacher JD, Rapoport SI. Blood brain barrier. In: Renkin EM, Michel CC, ed. Handbook of Physiology. Sect. 2: The cardiovascular system. Bethesda: AM Phys Soc, 1984:969-1000.

37. Fishman RA. Brain edema. N Engl J Med 1975;293:706-711.
38. Gambardella G, D'Aveela D, Staropoli C, Toscano S, Tomasello F. Bilateral interparenchymal pressure in patients with unilateral supratentorial mass lesions. In VIII International Symposium on Intracranial Pressure. Rotterdam, 1991:A39.
39. Gambardella G, Zaccone C, Cardia E, Tomasello F. Intracranial pressure monitoring in children: comparison of external ventricular device with the fiberoptic system. Childs Nervous System 1993;9(8):470-473.
40. Gayle MO, Frewen TC, Armstrong RF, et al. Jugular venous bulb catheterization in infants and children. Crit Care Med 1989;17(5):385-388.
41. Germon K. Intracranial pressure monitoring in the 1990's. Critical Care Nursing Quarterly 1994;17(1):21-32.
42. Giannotta SL, Weiss MH, Apuzzo ML, Martin E. High dose glucocorticoids in the management of severe head injury. Neurosurgery 1984;15(4):497-501.
43. Gilsanz V, Reballar RL, Buencuerpo J, Chantres MT. Controlled trial of glycerol versus dexamethasone in the treatment of cerebral edema in acute cerebral infarction. Lancet 1975;1:1049.
44. Gopinath SP, Cherian L, Robertson CS, Narayan RK, Grossman RG. Evaluation of a microsensor intracranial pressure transducer. Journal of Neuroscience Methods 1993;49(1-2):11-15.
45. Greenberg JH, Alavi A, Reivish M, et al. Local cerebral blood volume response to carbon dioxide in man. Circ Res 1978;43:324-331.
46. Grounds RM, Lalor JM, Lumley J, Royston D, Morgan M. Propofol infusion for sedation in the intensive care unit: preliminary report. British Med Journal 1987;294:397-400.
47. Gudeman SK, Miller JD, Becker DP. Failure of high-dose steroid therapy to influence intracranial pressure in patients with severe head injury. J Neurosurg 1979;51:301.
48. Hagnevik K, Gordon E, Lins LE, Wilhelmsson S, Forster D. Glycerol induced haemolysis with haemoglobinuria and acute renal failure. Lancet 1974;1:75.
49. Hahn YS, Fuchs S, Flannery AM, Barthel MJ, McLone DG. Factors influencing posttraumatic seizures in children. Neurosurgery 1988;22(5):864-867.
50. Hartwell RC, Sutton LN. Mannitol, intracranial pressure, and vasogenic edema. Neurosurgery 1993;32(3):444-450.
51. Hauser WA. Post-traumatic epilepsy in children. In: K S, ed. Pediatric Head Trauma. New York: Futura Publishing Co., 1983:271-287.
52. Hougaard K, Nillson B, Wieloch T. Fatty acid cyclo-oxygenase inhibitors and the regulation of cerebral blood flow. Acta Physiol Scand. 1983;117:585-587.
53. Hsiang JK, Chesnut RM, Crisp CB, Klauber MR, Blunt BA, Marshall LF. Early, routine paralysis for intracranial pressure control in severe head injury: Is it necessary? Crit Care Med 1994;22:1471-1476.
54. Hurst JM, Saul TG, De Haven CB, Branson R. Use of high frequency jet ventilation during mechanical hyperventilation to reduce intracranial pressure in patients with multiple organ system injury. Neurosurgery 1984;15(4):530-534.
55. Javid M. Urea-New use of an old agent. Reduction of intracranial and intraocular pressure. Surg Clin North Am 1958;38:907.
56. Jennett B, Miller JD, Braakman R. Epilepsy after non missile depressed skull fracture. J Neurosurg 1974;41:208-216.
57. Joo F. Minireview: regulation by second messengers of permeability in the cerebral microvessels. Neurobiology 1993;1(1):3-10.
58. Kaiser AM, Whitelaw AG. Hypertensive response to raised intracranial pressure in infancy. Arch Dis Child 1988;63(12):1461-1465.
59. Kanter MJ, Narayan RK. Intracranial Pressure Monitoring. Neurosurgery Clinics of North America 1991;2(2):257-265.
60. Kellie G. An account of the appearances observed in the dissection of two of three individuals presumed to have perished in the storm of 3rd, and whose bodies were discovered in the vicinity of Leith on the morning of the 4th November 1821 with some reflections on the pathology of the brain. Trans. Med. Chir. Sci. Edinb. 1824;1:84-169.
61. Kennealy JA, McLennan JE, Loudon RG, McLaurin RL. Hyperventilation induced cerebral hypoxia. Am Rev Respir Dis 1980;122(3):407-412.
62. Kennedy C, Sokoloff L. An adaptation of the nitrous oxide method to the study of the cerebral circulation in children; normal values for cerebral blood flow and cerebral metabolic rate in childhood. J Clin Invest. 1957;36:1130-1137.
63. Ketty SS, Schmidt CF. The nitrous oxide method for the quantitative determination of cerebral blood flow in man: Theory, procedure, and normal values. J Clin Invest. 1948;27:476-483.
64. Kuncz A, Doczi T, Bodosi M. The effect of skull and dura on brain volume regulation after hypo- and hyperosmolar fluid treatment. Neurosurgery 1990;27:509-515.
65. Kuschinsky W. Coupling of blood flow and metabolism in the brain. Journal of Basic & Clinical Physiology & Pharmacology 1990;1(1-4):191-201.
66. Lassen NA. Control of cerebral circulation in health and disease. Circ. Res. 1974;34:749-760.
67. Lehman LB. Intracranial pressure monitoring and treatment: a contemporary view. Ann Emerg Med 1990;19(3):295-303.
68. Levin HS, Aldrich EF, Saydjari C, et al. Severe head injury in children: experience of traumatic coma data bank. Neurosurgery 1992;31(3):435-44.
69. Lewelt W, Jenkins LW, Miller JD. Autoregulation of cerebral blood flow after experimental fluid percussion injury of the brain. J. Neurosurg. 1980;53:500-511.
70. Lundberg N. Continuous recording and control of ventricular fluid pressure in neurosurgical patients. Acta Psychiatr Scand 1960;149(Suppl 36):1.
71. Lundberg N, Troupp H, Lorin H. Continuous recording of the ventricular fluid pressure in patients with severe acute traumatic brain injury. J Neurosurg 1965;22:581.
72. MacDonald JT, Uden DL. Intravenous glycerol and mannitol therapy in children with intracranial hypertension. Neurology 1982;32:437.
73. Marion DW, Obrist WD, Carlier PM, Penrod LE, Darby JM. The use of moderate therapeutic hypothermia for patients with severe head injuries: a preliminary report. J Neurosurg 1993;79(3):354-362.
74. Marmarou A, Shulman K, Lamorgese J. Compartmental analysis of compliance and outflow resistance of the cerebral spinal fluid system. J Neurosurg 1976;43:523-534.
75. Marshall LF, King J, Langfitt TW. The complications of high-dose corticosteroid therapy in neurosurgical patients: A prospective study. Ann Neurol 1977;1:201.
76. Mayhall CG, Archer NH, Lamb VA, et al. Ventriculostomy related infections: A prospective epidemiologic study. N Engl J Med 1984;310:553.
77. McGraw CP, Howard G. Effect of mannitol on increased intracranial pressure. Neurosurgery 1983;13:269.
78. McIntosh TK. Pharmacologic strategies in the treatment of experimental brain injuries. J Neurotrauma 1992;9:201-209.
79. McLaurin RL, King LR, Elam EB. Metabolic response to craniocerebral trauma. Surg Gynecol Obstet 1960;110:282-286.
80. Messeter K, Nordstrom CH, Sundbarg G. Cerebral hemedynamics in patients with acute severe head trauma. J Neurosurg 1986;64:231.
81. Michenfelder JD, Sundt TM. The effect of $PaCO_2$ on the metabolism of ischaemic brain in squirrel monkeys. Anesthesiology 1973;38:445-453.
82. Miller JD. Volume and pressure in the craniospinal axis. Clin Neurosurg 1975;22:76-105.
83. Miller JD, Becker DP, Ward JD, Sullivan HG, Adams WE, Rosner MJ. Significance of intracranial hypertension in severe head injury. J Neurosurg 1977;47:503.
84. Miller JD, Stanek AE, Langfitt TW. Cerebral blood flow regulation during experimental brain compression. J Neurosurg 1973;39:186-196.
85. Monro A. Observations on the structure and function of the nervous system. Edinburgh: Creech and Johnson, 1783.
86. Muizelaar JP, Lutz HA, Becker DP. Effect of mannitol on ICP and CBF and correlation with pressure autoregulation in severely head-injured patients. J Neurosurg 1984;61(4):700-706.
87. Muizelaar JP, Marmarou A, Ward JD, et al. Adverse effects of prolonged hyperventilation in patients with severe head injury: a randomized clinical trial. J Neurosurg 1991;75:731-739.
88. Muizelaar JP, Ward JD, Marmarou A, Newlon PG, Wachi A. Cerebral blood flow and metabolism in severely head-injured children. Part 2: Autoregulation. Journal of Neurosurgery 1989;71(1):72-76.
89. Muizelaar JP, Wei EP, Kontos HA, Becker DP. Mannitol causes compensatory cerebral vasoconstriction and vasodilation in response to blood viscosity changes. J Neurosurg 1983;59:822.
90. Nahata MC, Kerzner B, McClung HT, Sherard ES, Hilty MD. Variations in the glycerol kinetics in Reye's syndrome. Clin Pharmacol Ther 1981;29:782.
91. Nakao N, Itakura T, Yokote H, Nakai K, Komai N. Effect of atrial naturetic peptide on ischaemic oedema. Changes in brain water and electrolytes. Neurosurgery 1990;27:39-44.
92. Narayan RK, Kishore PRS, Becker DP, et al. Intracranial pressure: To monitor or not to monitor? J Neurosurg 1982;56:650-659.
93. Obrist WD, Langfitt TW, Jaggi JL, Cruz J, Gennarelli TA. Cerebral blood flow and metabolism in comatose patients with acute head injury. J. Neurosurg. 1984;61:241-253.

94. Palafox BA, Johnson MN, McEwen DK, Gazzaniga AB. ICP changes following application of the MAST suit. J Trauma 1981;21:55.
95. Palmer AM, Marion DW, Botscheller ML, Redd EE. Therapeutic hypothermia is cytoprotective without attenuating the traumatic brain injury-induced elevations in interstitial concentrations of aspartate and glutamate. J Neurotrauma 1993;10(4):363-72.
96. Pang D, Horton JA, Herron JM, Wilberger JE, Vries JK. Nonsurgical management of extradural hematomas in children. J Neurosurg 1983;59:958-971.
97. Pinaud M, Lelausque JN, Chetanneau A, Fauchoux N, Menegalli D, Souron R. Effects of propofol on cerebral hemodynamics and metabolism in patients with brain trauma. Anesthesiology 1990;73(3):404-409.
98. Pitlick WH, Pirikitakuhlr P, Painter MJ, Wessel HB. Effects of glycerol and hyperosmolarity on intracranial pressure. Clin Pharmacol Ther 1982;31:466.
99. Pollay M, Fullenwider C, Roberts PA, Stevens FA. Effect of mannitol and furosemide on blood-brain osmotic gradient and intracranial pressure. J Neurosurg 1983;59:945.
100. Pollay M, Stevens FA, Robets PA. Alteration in choroid plexus blood flow and cerebrospinal fluid formation by increased ventricular pressure. In: Wood JH, ed. Neurobiology of Cerebrospinal Fluid 2. New York: Plenum Press, 1983:687-695.
101. Pozzati E, Tognetti F. Spontaneous healing of acute extradural hematomas: Study of twenty-two cases. Neurosurgery 1986;18:696-700.
102. Quandt CM, de lRR. Pharmacologic management of acute intracranial hypertension. Drug Intell Clin Pharm 1984;18:105.
103. Ravussin P, Archer DP, Tyler JL. Effects of rapid mannitol infusion on cerebral blood volume. J Neurosurg 1986;64:104-113.
104. Ravussin P, Guinard JP, Ralley F, Thorin D. Effect of propofol on cerebrospinal fluid pressure and cerebral perfusion pressure in patients undergoing craniotomy. Anaesthesia 1988;43(suppl):37-41.
105. Resnick DK, Marion DW, Darby JM. The effect of hypothermia on the incidence of delayed traumatic intracerebral hemorrhage. Neurosurgery 1994;3(2):252-255.
106. Reulen HJ, Tsuyumu M, Prioleau GR. Further results concerning the resolution of vasogenic brain edema. Brain Edema: Pathology, Diagnosis, and Therapy. Advances in Neurology. New York: Raven Press, 1980:375-381.
107. Roberts PA, Pollay M, Engles C, Pendleton B, Reynolds E, Stevens FA. Effect on intracranial pressure of furosemide combined with varying doses and administration rates of mannitol. J Neurosurg 1987;66:440-446.
108. Ronan KP, Gallagher TJ, George B, Hamby B. Comparison of propofol and midazolam for sedation in intensive care unit patients. Crit Care Med 1995;23:286-293.
109. Rosner MJ, Coley I. Cerebral perfusion pressure: a hemodynamic mechanism of mannitol and the postmannitol hemogram. Neurosurgery 1987;21(2):147-156.
110. Schettini A, Walsh EK. Contribution of brain distortion and displacement to CSF dynamics in experimental brain compression. Am J Physiol 1991;260(1 Pt 2):R172-R178.
111. Schmidt JF. Changes in human cerebral blood flow estimated by the (A-V)O_2 difference method. Danish Medical Bulletin 1992;39(4):335-342.
112. Schmoker JD, Shackford SR, Wald SL, Pietropaoli JA. An analysis of the relationship between fluid and sodium administration and intracranial pressure after head injury. Journal of Trauma 1992;33:476-481.
113. Schwartz ML, Tator CH, Rowed DW, Reid SR, Meguro K, Andrews DF. The University of Toronto head injury treatment study: a prospective, randomized comparison of pentobarbital and mannitol. Can J Neurol Sci 1984;11(4):434-440.
114. Shenkin HA, Bezier HS, Bouzarth WF. Restricted fluid intake: Rational management of the neurosurgical patient. J Neurosurg 1976;45:432-437.
115. Shiozaki T, Sugimoto H, Taneda M, et al. Effect of mild hypothermia on uncontrollable intracranial hypertension after severe head injury. J Neurosurg 1993;79(3):363-368.
116. Siesjo BK. Pathophysiology and treatment of focal cerebral ischemia. I. Pathophysiology. J Neurosurg 1992;77:169-184.
117. Siesjo BK, Carlsson C, Hagerdal M. Brain metabolism in the critically ill. Crit. Care Med. 1976;4:283-294.
118. Smith DS. Noninvasive measurement of brain vascular hemoglobin saturation. In: Sperry RJ ST, ed. Anesthesia and the Central Nervous System. The Netherlands: Kluwer Academic Publishers, 1993: 93-102.
119. Stephan H, Sonntag H, Schenk HD, Kohlhausen S. Effect of Disoprivan (propofol) on the circulation and oxygen consumption of the brain and CO_2 reactivity of brain vessels in the human [Ger]. Anaesthesist 1987;36(2):60-65.
120. Strickland RA, Murray MJ. Fatal metabolic acidosis in a pediatric patient receiving an infusion of propofol in the intensive care unit: Is there a relationship? Crit Care Med 1995;23:405-409.
121. Stuart GG, Merry GS, Smith JA, Yelland JD. Severe head injury managed without intracranial pressure monitoring. J Neurosurg 1983; 59(4):601-605.
122. Sullivan HG, Miller JD, Griffith RL, Becker DP. CSF pressure transients in response to epidural and ventricular volume loading. Am J Physiol 1978;234(5):R167-R171.
123. Traeger SM, Henning RJ, Dobkin W, Giannotta S, Weil MH, Weiss M. Hemodynamic effects of pentobarbital therapy for intracranial hypertension. Crit Care Med 1983;11:697.
124. Unwin DH, Giller CA, Kopitnik TA. Central system monitoring. What helps, what does not. Surgical Clinics of North America 1991;71(4):733-747.
125. Ursino M. A mathematical study of human intracranial hydrodynamics. Part 2-Simulation of clinical tests. Annals of Biomedical Engineering 1988;16(4):403-416.
126. Van HJ, Fitch W, Mattheussen M, Van AH, Plets C, Lauwers T. Effect of propofol on cerebral circulation and autoregulation in the baboon. Anesth Analg 1990;71(1):49-54.
127. Van HJ, Van AH, Plets C, Goffin J, Vermaut G. The effects of propofol on intracranial pressure and cerebral perfusion pressure in patients with brain tumors. Acta Anaesthesiologica Belgica 1989;40(2): 95-100.
128. Wald SL, McLauren RL. Oral glycerol for the treatment of traumatic intracranial hypertension. J Neurosurg 1982;56:323.
129. Walker ML, Storrs BB, Mayer TA. Head injuries. In: TA M, ed. Emergency management of pediatric trauma. Philadelphia: WB Saunders, 1985:272-286.
130. Ward JD, Becker DP, Miller JD, et al. Failure of prophylactic barbiturate coma in the treatment of severe head injury. J Neurosurg 1985;62(3):383-388.
131. Ward JD, Moulton RJ, Muizelaar JP, Marmarou A. Cerebral Homeostasis and Protection. In: Wirth FP, Ratcheson RA, ed. Neurosurgical Critical Care. Baltimore: Williams and Wilkins, 1987:187-213.
132. Wilkinson HA, Rosenfeld SR. Furosemide and mannitol in the treatment of acute experimental intracranial hypertension. Neurosurgery 1983;12(4):405-410.
133. Winfield JA, Rosenthal P, Kanter RK, Casella G. Duration of intracranial pressure monitoring does not predict daily risk of infectious complications. Neurosurgery 1993;33(3):424-430.
134. Wyler AR, Keeley WA. Use of antibiotics with external ventriculostomies. J Neurosurg 1972;37:185-187.

Monitoring the Central Nervous System

19

Francis Filloux,
J. Michael Dean
Jeffrey R. Kirsch

INTRODUCTION

The ultimate goal of intensive care for children with severe central nervous system (CNS) dysfunction is that of survival with the minimum degree of neurologic morbidity. To this end, the intensivist and pediatrician attempt to continuously assess the function and state of the nervous system using a variety of clinical and technological means in order to(1) make appropriate therapeutic interventions designed to improve outcome and(2) accurately determine prognosis so as to best guide the intensity and duration of medical care.

Presumably it is the localized tissue metabolic status that is the crucial variable to be maintained in an optimal range. Ideally, this is the parameter that would be (continuously) monitored. However, such is not practically feasible. Consequently, a number of other related variables are measured as frequently as possible in neurologically critically ill children. These include cerebral metabolic rate (of oxygen or glucose), cerebral blood flow, other neurochemical parameters (e.g., lactate and pyruvate), intracranial pressure, and spontaneous or evoked cerebral electrical activity. In general, since these various methods for monitoring the nervous system all have their specific advantages and disadvantages, they are typically used in combination. A thorough understanding of the information they provide along with their limitations is essential to ideal monitoring of the CNS in the critically ill child. The reader is referred to a number of updated reviews for additional information[1–4].

ANATOMY

The predominant flow of arterial blood to the brain is via paired carotid arteries anteriorly and the paired vertebral arteries posteriorly (Fig. 19.1). The carotid arteries provide blood flow to the brain via the internal carotid arteries, as well as to the extracranial circulation via the external carotid arteries. This explains why the carotid arterial pulsations may yet be palpable in a brain-dead child with no cerebral blood flow (CBF) (i.e., persistent flow to external but not internal carotid arteries). The internal carotid arteries branch to give rise to the anterior cerebral arteries (connected by the anterior communicating artery) and the middle cerebral arteries. The proximal middle cerebral arteries are joined to the posterior cerebral arteries via the posterior communicating arteries (Fig. 19.1). The posterior cerebral arteries are derived from the basilar artery, which arises at the level of the brainstem as the fusion of the vertebral arteries. This network of connections between the anterior, middle, and posterior cerebral arteries is called the *circle of Willis.* It should be noted that a complete circle of Willis (one in which all major cerebral arteries are joined symmetrically) is the exception rather than the rule in humans. Variations, in which one or more anastomoses (such

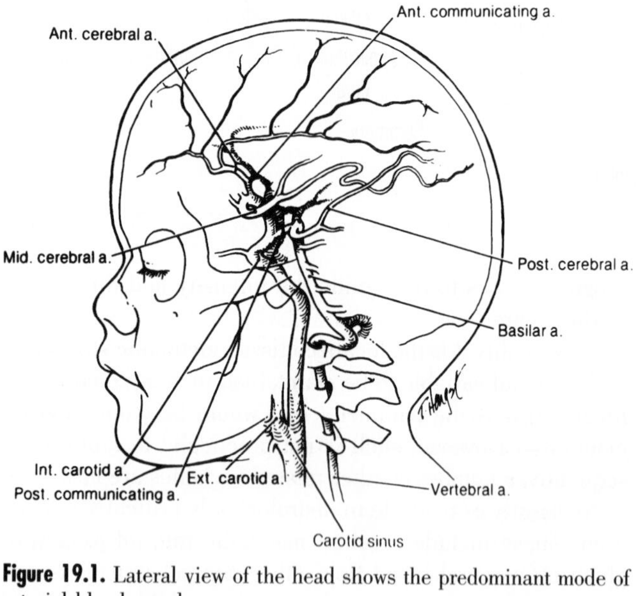

Figure 19.1. Lateral view of the head shows the predominant mode of arterial blood supply.

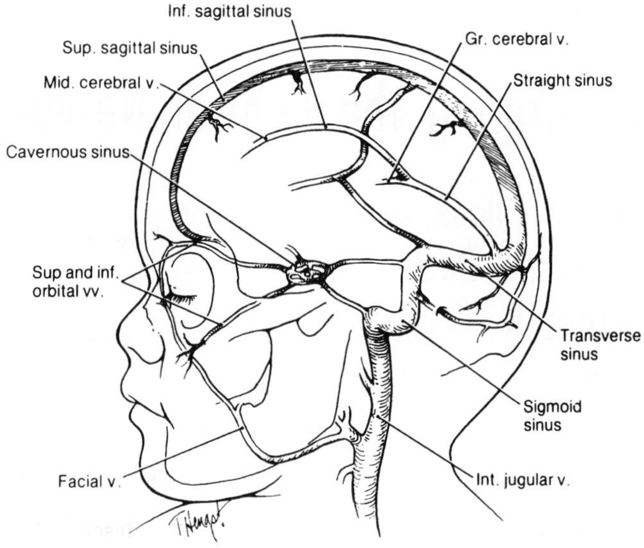

Figure 19.2. Lateral view of the head shows the predominant mode of venous drainage.

as one or both posterior communicating arteries) are missing are common.

The brain has two systems of venous drainage: the first consists of venous branches similar to the arterial circulation; the second drains blood from the cortex directly into the overlying venous sinuses (Fig. 19.2). The predominant drainage from the deep system is via the great cerebral vein (of Galen), which eventually joins the sinus system by connecting with the inferior sagittal sinus to form the straight sinus. The straight sinus continues posteriorly to connect with the superior sagittal sinus, which then bifurcates (transverse sinuses) to continue anteroinferiorly as the sigmoid sinuses. The latter exit the cranium to join the petrosal sinuses (facial drainage) at the level of the internal jugular bulb. Hence, the internal jugular veins do not carry blood purely from the cerebral circulation.

As alluded to above, anatomic variations[5,6] complicate this simple presentation of CBF. External carotid artery branches such as the trigeminal, auditory, and hypoglossal arteries may, on occasion, communicate with the cerebral circulation. It must be noted also that the internal jugular veins do not carry all the cerebral venous blood. A portion is drained via the vertebral veins. It should be emphasized that, as stated above, a large amount of extracranial blood may drain into the internal jugular veins (e.g., from the maxillary, facial, and ophthalmic veins), thereby introducing error into any technique that relies on catheterization of the internal jugular bulb.

CEREBRAL BLOOD FLOW MEASUREMENT TECHNIQUES

Over the past several decades, it has become clear that alterations in CBF reflect and may greatly influence the potential for recovery and survival in the critically ill child suffering from a variety of medical and surgical conditions. Of particular interest to pediatricians and intensivists is the role of alterations in CBF in the pathophysiology of such diverse disease states as head trauma, Reye's syndrome, intraventricular hemorrhage, meningitis and near-drowning.

If attempts are to be made to alter CBF when caring for patients with these conditions, one must be able to measure CBF accurately, reliably, and repeatedly. Unfortunately, the most accurate techniques currently available are invasive, while the others are fraught with difficulties in interpretation. Therefore, it is important that the physician maintain a healthy respect and skepticism concerning the application of CBF measurements to critically ill pediatric patients.

This section focuses on the basic techniques used in human CBF studies. It summarizes the physiologic principles, advantages, and limitations of the techniques described.

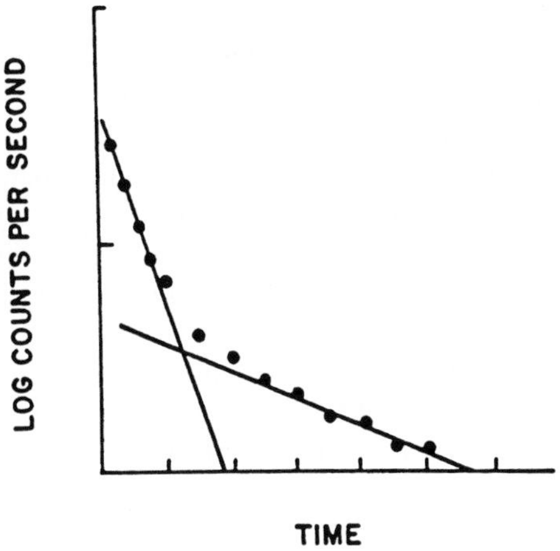

Figure 19.3. Logarithmic transformation of a typical ^{133}Xe clearance curve.

Radioactive Isotopes

Radioactive isotopes can be used in both qualitative and quantitative methods.

Qualitative

Radionucleotide angiography is a qualitative technique that is useful in identifying regions of the brain with increased or decreased blood flow. The radionucleotide is injected into a peripheral vein, and brain activity is measured by an externally placed collimated scintillation detector. Resolution by this technique is 2 to 3 cm at best. The percent contribution of extracranial circulation cannot be determined.

Static scintigraphy is associated with the same disadvantages as those of radionucleotide angiography. Furthermore, in using this technique it may be difficult to distinguish ischemic from hemorrhagic areas, and it may be days before an area of infarction can be identified.

Quantitative

^{133}Xe Clearance

One quantitative method uses ^{133}Xe as a tracer isotope (half-life of 5.2 days). A small amount is administered via the intravenous, intracarotid, or inhalational route. The activity of the isotope is measured externally by scintillation detectors placed around the head. The resulting washout curve shows two exponential components: the first hypothetically represents blood flow to the gray matter, and the second, flow to white matter of the brain (Fig. 19.3).

Studies have been performed using ^{133}Xe isotope in the measurement of CBF in children. Lou et al.[7] injected small amounts of ^{133}Xe into an umbilical arterial catheter with its tip at the innominate artery, at the left carotid artery, or within the aortic arch at the entrance to the above arteries. Younkin et al.[8] modified the technique by injecting their isotope intravenously.

Ment et al.[9] used the inhalation technique on infants weighing less than 1200 g. The CBF values in the study by Ment et al.[9] correlated well with those measured by Lou et al.[7] for newborns with respiratory distress and with those measured by Younkin et al.[8] for neurologically normal infants.

Huttenlocher et al.[10] used the ^{133}Xe inhalation method to measure CBF in older children (3 to 16 years) with sickle cell disease. Their results correlated well with those of Kennedy and Sokoloff[11], who used a different method of measuring CBF for same-aged children.

The calculation of CBF by use of ^{133}Xe assumes that the isotope is not metabolized by the brain, that it is physiologically inert with respect to the brain and is freely diffusible through tissue, and that the blood-brain partition coefficient remains constant. The first assumption is true. ^{133}Xe, however, does have biochemical effects in the brain; i.e., in high concentrations, xenon has general anesthetic effects and has been shown to elevate CBF significantly[12,13].

Furthermore, there have been observations that suggest diffusion is not homogenous under a variety of conditions and that variations in blood-brain partition coefficients occur under pathologic states[14]; partition coefficient differences between children and adults may also exist[15]. Hence, comparison of CBF values between different groups, or even in the same child at different times, may be invalid. There is also controversy regarding the validity of the different mathematical methods used to calculate CBF values. However, values obtained using different paradigms have corresponded remarkably well[7,16].

Contamination from extracerebral sources may also invalidate the measurements of CBF via these methods. It may be secondary to the intermixing of cerebral and extracerebral circulations, as outlined above, or to the inability to discriminate between radiation originating from cerebral versus extracerebral sources when scintillation detectors are placed over the intact cranium. Another disadvantage to the ^{133}Xe clearance technique is that the patient is exposed to radiation, the long-term effects of which remain unknown. Lassen[17] estimated the following amounts of absorbed radiation: for the brain, 0.001 rad; for the gonads, 0.001 rad;

and for the lungs, 0.017 rad (equivalent to approximately 10 chest roentgenograms). Patlak et al.(18) have critically discussed the errors made in measuring CBF via the ^{133}Xe washout technique.

In summary, the ^{133}Xe clearance technique may be used to measure CBF. However, its validity and accuracy in children are open to question. Contamination from the extracerebral circulation or failure to correct for isotope recirculation may result in erroneous measurements, and the blood-brain partition coefficient is probably not constant with age and across differing disease states. Established normative data do not exist, since most clinical measurements reported to date have been from abnormal infants. The risks of radiation exposure further limit the frequency with which the technique may be applied to a given child. In short, its use in routine monitoring is unlikely to become widespread.

Positron Emission Tomography

Another technique for measurement of CBF uses isotopes that emit positrons. Volpe et al.(19) have modified the technology of positron emission tomography (PET) for use in neonates. The principle of PET is based on the emission of a low-energy particle, called a positron, from an administered isotope. The particle collides with an electron in the tissue, causing emission of γ-rays, which are measured by external detectors. In the study by Volpe et al. the infants were all premature, and all had major intraventricular hemorrhage. To estimate CBF, each neonate was given the positron-emitting isotope ^{15}O as $H_2[^{15}O_2]$ intravenously by bolus injection. An emission scan was then obtained with an in-plane resolution of 11.7 mm. The tomograph was calibrated to obtain the actual regional isotope concentration in each part of the brain. Finally, blood flow was calculated based on several factors, including(1) the local radiotracer concentration over the time period of the scan,(2) the concentration of the radiotracer measured in arterial blood over the time of the scan, and(3) the blood-brain partition coefficient for the tracer. An attempt to test the validity of this technique in adult baboons has shown that measurement of CBF with PET probably slightly underestimates actual CBF.

There are several drawbacks to the use of this approach, not the least of which are the extremely high cost and technical sophistication required. The measurements, of course, cannot be made at the bedside. Furthermore, although the half-life of each of these isotopes is very short (e.g., $t_{1/2}$ ^{15}O equals 123 seconds), performance of a scan still exposes the child to the radiation of the scan in addition to the radiation of the lateral skull roentgenogram that is used for positioning. In a 1-kg child, the total absorbed radiation is approximately 63 mrem, whereas the absorbed dose to the brain is approximately 100 mrem. The proponents of this technology argue that this is still smaller than the radiation from conventional computed tomography (CT). Obtaining accurate values for CBF depends on the ability to obtain adequate quantities of arterial blood to follow the level of the radioisotope during the time period of the scan. This may be very difficult in small neonates. In addition, accurate CBF values also depend on having an appropriate value for the blood-brain partition coefficient. Therefore, as with the ^{133}Xe technique, comparisons of CBF values between individuals or over time in the same individual may not be valid. Finally, although the resolution of the scans is currently considerably greater than it was at the time of the study by Volpe et al.(19), the equipment and technical expertise required are extensive and markedly expensive. This, and the requirement for a nearby cyclotron to generate the isotopes, limits the technology to a few major centers.

In summary, PET is a valuable experimental technology that may be useful in measuring cerebral hemodynamics in addition to cerebral metabolism in the child. It is hoped that the potential problems with the technology do not discourage future research on its clinical applicability to children. On the other hand, its practical applicability to critical care medicine is likely to be limited, particularly in view of new developments in magnetic resonance imaging (MRI) which now permit at least qualitative assessment of local cerebral perfusion (see below).

Single Photon Emission Computed Tomography

With positron emission tomography providing the impetus, radionucleotide scintigraphy has recently been adapted to allow for the generation of three-dimensional images reflecting CBF or metabolism in brain. The resulting technique, known as single photon emission computed tomography (SPECT), has been referred to as the poor man's PET. Its distinct advantages derive from its greater affordability (less than one-tenth the cost of PET) and accessibility (the isotopes and scanning equipment are available in most nuclear medicine facilities)(20,21).

Currently employed SPECT systems typically depend on a standard nuclear medicine camera (a γ-camera) that is adapted to rotate 360 degrees around the head. Alternatively, circular arrays of sensors have been employed. In either case, the data acquired are digitized, computer processed, and corrected for tissue absorption, and tomographic images of the brain in a particular plane are generated.

Initially, the SPECT technique used ^{133}Xe as the photon source. Subsequently, other radionucleotides providing greater photon flux were developed, and several are now routinely employed(22). Thus, ^{123}I-iodoamphetamine, ^{99m}Tc-hexamethyl propyleneamine, and ^{99m}Tc-ethyl cysteinate dimer(23) have allowed for greater image quality and resolution. By using any of these agents, quantitative measurements of CBF or cerebral metabolic rate are possible but, as with PET, are not particularly practical in critically ill patients, as they cannot be performed at the bedside(20). More fruitful are qualitative measurements of CBF with these agents. Such studies can be very useful in the evaluation of patients with cerebral ischemia, stroke, subarachnoid hemorrhage, seizures, and movement disorders[20,21,24]. In such children, the functional imaging provided by SPECT scanning can uncover abnormalities not apparent with use of structural imaging techniques such as CT or standard MRI[24]. Finally, modifications in SPECT technology promise to improve the resolution affordable with this methodology to near that achievable with PET (i.e., less than 1 cm in the axial and transaxial directions)[20,22].

Magnetic Resonance Imaging of Cerebral Perfusion

The techniques described above all allow for qualitative or quantitative assessment of cerebral blood flow or perfusion, but all rely on radioisotopes. Thus, all have the disadvantage of radiation exposure, which limits the number of times the measurements may be carried out in a single patient. Furthermore, most of the techniques rely on expensive equipment which may not be readily available or applicable to the critically ill child. In contrast, probably all facilities in the United States with pediatric intensive care units have available a dedicated magnet and associated hardware/software for MRI. Newly developed techniques allow for at least qualitative evaluation of cerebral blood flow using this technology, thereby without exposing the patient to radiation.

A basic description of magnetic resonance theory and techniques is beyond the scope of this chapter. However, the reader should be aware of certain imaging paradigms which permit assessment of cerebral perfusion[25,26]. Echo planar imaging and other "ultrafast" MRI techniques have paved the way for sophisticated approaches to MRI of cerebral perfusion[25,26]. Such imaging can be accomplished either with or without the injection of contrast agents. The former is perhaps easiest to understand. In these instances, a paramagnetic contrast agent (such as gadolinium) is injected. This agent rapidly courses through normally perfused brain regions, producing a powerful magnetic field gradient in the capillary vasculature and adjacent tissue. This produces a decrease in signal intensity in normally perfused areas, while ischemic (unperfused) regions do not manifest a signal change[25]. Although these techniques currently provide primarily anatomic, qualitative assessments of cerebral perfusion, it is anticipated that quantitative estimates of CBF and blood volume will become feasible in the future[25,26]. Thus, these and similar techniques hold promise for clinical application.

Kety-Schmidt Technique

In the 1940s, Kety and Schmidt[27] applied the Fick principle to the brain's uptake of nitrous oxide (N_2O) to calculate CBF. The Fick principle states that the quantity of a substance taken up by an organ is equal to the total amount of substance delivered to the organ minus the amount taken away in a given time period; i.e.,

$$\text{Brain uptake} = (\text{arterial content} - \text{venous content}) \times \text{CBF}$$

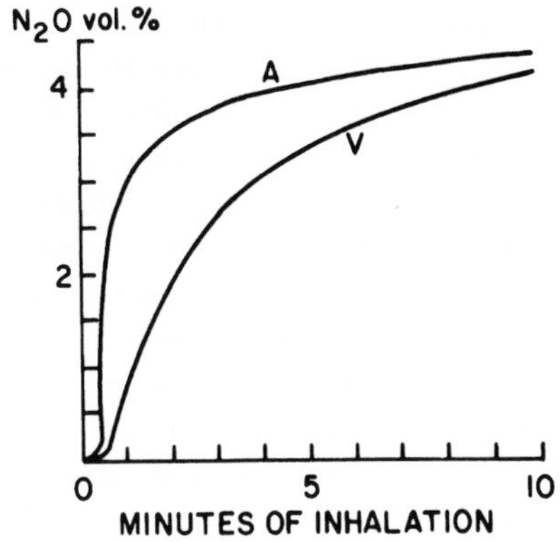

Figure 19.4. Response time for the elevation of arterial and venous N_2O concentration with inhalation of 15% N_2O as originally described by Kety and Schmidt.

Since N_2O is not metabolized by the brain, the rate of uptake is determined by the substance's blood-brain partition coefficient and by the CBF. The blood-brain partition coefficient is assumed to remain constant; thus, the brain becomes saturated with N_2O with time. Therefore, the venous content approaches the arterial content as extraction declines (Fig. 19.4). CBF is determined by measuring the rate at which venous content approaches arterial content.

$$\text{CBF} = (100 \times V_t \times S) / \int_0^\infty (A - V)dt \text{ (ml/100g/min)}$$

where V_t is the cerebral venous content of N_2O at equilibrium, S is the blood-brain partition coefficient, and $\int_0^\infty (A - V)dt$ is the integral of the arteriovenous difference of N_2O from the beginning of inhalation to the time of equilibrium.

While the arterial sample may be obtained from any artery, the venous sample should not be contaminated with extracerebral blood if the result is to be accurate. The cerebral venous blood is usually obtained from the internal jugular bulb. Catheterization of the internal jugular bulb may be difficult in a neonate. Once inserted, the catheter position should be confirmed with a lateral skull roentgenogram in an attempt to avoid as much extracerebral contamination as possible. Kety and Schmidt[28] estimated that under their ideal experimental conditions, 6.5% of blood in the internal jugular bulb represented flow from the external cerebral circulation. This can be increased by withdrawing blood too quickly from the bulb, resulting in retrograde flow from structures of the neck and face. Kety and Schmidt[28] have also shown that up to 20% of a substance injected into the internal carotid artery could be retrieved in the external jugular veins. As a whole, this information suggests that the 6.5% contamination figure that has been proposed may be an underestimate under certain circumstances. To complicate matters further, Batson[29] demonstrated that the sagittal sinus may drain predominantly into just one jugular vein. Thus, if measurement is made via the contralateral nondominant vein, the measurement may be even less valid.

Nevertheless, the N_2O technique has been shown to be safe for use in children[30] and has been modified to use smaller blood samples[31]. Continuous monitoring of A-V oxygen extraction has also been recently described[32–34]. The major disadvantage of this technique is that it requires catheterization of the jugular bulb for cerebral venous blood sampling. In awake children, anxiety interferes with success of the procedure. Obviously, in the intensive care setting most children subjected to this intervention will be either paralyzed and sedated or will be comatose, so issues of cooperation are minimized. Swedlow et al.[35], using the N_2O technique, measured CBF in children with head trauma and Reye's syndrome and described the technical problems associated with this method.

Other limitations with this technique include (1) the inability to calculate regional blood flow, (2) evidence that N_2O is an anesthetic and may itself cause alterations in CBF, (3) evidence that the N_2O blood-brain partition coefficient may not be constant under pathologic conditions[14] and as the patient ages[15], and (4) evidence that the uptake of N_2O by the brain not only is dependent on CBF but also is dependent on uptake by the cerebral spinal fluid (CSF). Therefore, uptake may not be constant across different brain regions because of variations in diffusion which depend in part on degrees of tissue involvement by disease processes. For these reasons, comparison of CBF values between and within groups of patients with different disease states may be invalid. Finally, in the one instance where serial measurements of CBF were formally obtained in children using the Kety-Schmidt approach[36], no evidence of clinical benefit was provided. Thus, the value of this challenging technique may be limited[37].

Other Means for Measuring Cerebral Metabolic Rate for Glucose

Recently, several groups of investigators have used a modification of ^{133}Xe measurements of CBF combined with jugular venous and arterial blood sampling to calculate the cerebral metabolic rate for glucose ($CMRO_2$)[38–40]. This approach also relies on the Fick principle:

$$CMRO_2 = CBF \times C_{(a-v)}O_2,$$

where $C_{(a-v)}O_2$ represents a value for the difference in O_2 content between arterial and jugular venous blood ($avDO_2$). Typically, a radiopaque catheter is inserted transcutaneously into a jugular vein and is then advanced into the jugular bulb[38]. Simultaneous samples of jugular venous and arterial blood are obtained at the same time as CBF measurements are made by means of ^{133}Xe inhalation technique. Estimates of O_2 content are derived from the measured blood gas values.

Unfortunately, recent application of this technique to evaluation of traumatic coma has been somewhat disappointing[35–37]. CBF measurements have failed to correlate well with outcome (except in the extreme)[39–41]. The $CMRO_2$ measurement is more predictive of outcome, with a positive correlation existing between $CMRO_2$ and the Glasgow coma scale on one hand[39] and on clinical outcome on the other[39,40]. However, the range of variation is so great as to make application of $CMRO_2$ measurements to the prediction of outcome impossible in the individual case[40]. The only exception is in the extreme when decrease in $CMRO_2$ to less than 1 ml/100 g/min invariably indicates eventual brain death[39,42]. Thus, this invasive, time-consuming, and labor-intensive technique is unlikely to be of great practical value to intensivists in the foreseeable future.

Alternative Means of Estimating Cerebral Blood Flow

Doppler Flow Velocity

The Doppler technique has found wide application in the detection and characterization of blood flow. It is used for intrapartum fetal monitoring, blood pressure measurement, and assessment of peripheral vascular disease. The principle is easily understood. Sound waves are directed toward the blood vessels, reflected by moving cells, and returned to the transducer. A frequency shift occurs when the cells are in motion, i.e., red blood cells (RBCs), and the shift is proportional to their velocity. If the blood vessel diameter is known, total flow may be calculated from the RBC velocity. Unfortunately, in the clinical setting, vessel caliber is usually unknown.

A Doppler probe may be positioned on the head of children with an open anterior fontanel and directed toward the anterior cerebral artery. Alternatively, transcranial Doppler measurements are feasible, typically through a transtemporal direction, whereby proximal major cerebral vessels can be imaged using pulsed Doppler equipment[43,44]. The signal is displayed with an oscilloscope as a series of peaks and troughs that correspond to the systolic and diastolic amplitude (Fig. 19.5). Measurements are standardized by calculating a value known as the pulsatile index (PI), which was designed to negate the variations in frequency shifts secondary to such factors as probe position, or by computing the Pourcelot resistance index (RI)[45]. Other investigators have elected to express their values in velocity units (centimeters per second) by calibrating their output with an in vitro system.

Both the PI and the RI can serve as indices of distal resistance to blood flow: high values indicate high resistance, and low values indicate low resistance[45,46]. Greisen et al.[47] have suggested that the PI may be determined by the blood pressure curve and amplitude, blood velocity, and heart rate. The values appear to be the same whether measured on the left or right anterior cerebral artery. A fluctu-

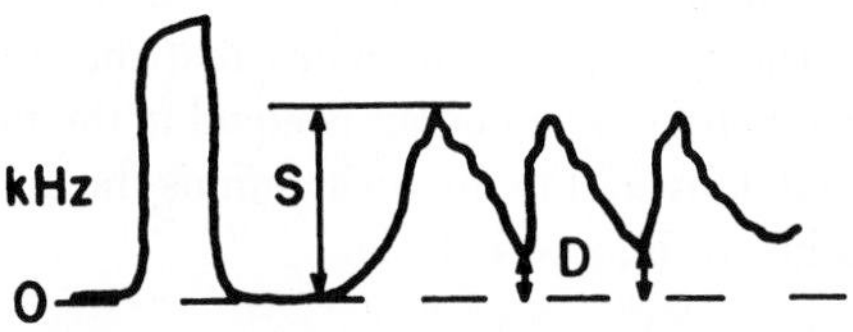

Figure 19.5. Electrical signal from a Doppler probe, corresponding to the systolic *(S)* and diastolic *(D)* pressure amplitudes.

ating or low PI is said to predispose infants with respiratory distress to intraventricular hemorrhage(46,48). Mortality rates are greater for infants with high PI values than for those with lower PI values(49). The RI, on the other hand, is calculated as the peak systolic velocity minus the end diastolic velocity divided by the former of these two values(45). In a study applying this technique to the monitoring of CBF velocity in pyogenic meningitis, a linear correlation between the mean arterial pressure and the RI was encountered in the one neonate who eventually died. The authors took this to be an indication of a pressure passive CBF velocity response (i.e., loss of cerebral autoregulation), which they propose could be a useful prognostic sign(45). Hence, noninvasive transcranial Doppler may allow for the identification of alterations in CBF velocity which portend a deterioration in cerebral hemodynamics.

The major advantage of Doppler flow velocity measurements is the noninvasive nature of the technique. Furthermore, the equipment required is modest in cost and portable, and therefore can be applied in the intensive care unit (ICU) without disturbing the patient. Valuable information concerning CBF can be obtained as described above(50,51). However, specific disadvantages also exist(52): first, CBF cannot be directly quantitated as such; and second, an increase in blood velocity does not necessarily mean an increase in blood flow, since the vessel diameter may not remain constant under all physiologic conditions. For example, vasoconstriction could produce increased blood velocity with either no change or even a decrease in net blood flow. Furthermore, measured values obtained from the anterior cerebral vessels alone do not necessarily reflect total brain blood flow. Greisen et al.(47) compared the values of PI obtained via the Doppler technique with CBF measurements obtained via the ^{133}Xe washout technique. CBF increased as PI decreased but with a linear correlation coefficient of −0.56, suggesting poor overall reliability of the Doppler technique.

More recently, technical developments in optical laser equipment has permitted the elaboration of thin, flexible optical probes which can be placed on the cortical surface or can be directly implanted into the brain parenchyma with relatively minor trauma. This allows for a technique known as laser Doppler flowmetry, whereby blood flow velocity measurements can be obtained from the microcirculation of specific brain regions(53). Such probes permit light emitted by a helium-neon laser tube to be directed to a localized region of brain by the flexible light conductor. The backscattered light is transmitted by the same flexible tube to photodetectors which measure the Doppler shift. Obviously, this invasive technique is subject to the same limitations discussed above with reference to transcranial Doppler flow measurements. Furthermore, laser Doppler flowmetry provides information referable only to a very limited volume of brain tissue. Theoretically, this would allow for more precise correlation of intracranial pressure with regional CBF in zones of particular interest to the neurosurgeon(53), but the technique has yet to demonstrate any clinical benefit.

Vascular Occlusion Plethysmography

Application of vascular occlusion plethysmography is limited to infants. Use of this technique requires that the investigator be able to measure the cranial dimensions of an infant accurately. Cross et al.(54,55) used a mercury stain gauge plethysmograph around the occipital-frontal circumference (OFC) of their patients. This device produces an electrical signal proportional to the amount it is stretched. The jugular veins are occluded for a preset time, and the CBF is calculated from the rate of the subsequent increase and reduction of the skull volume. This technique works because of the pliability of the newborn skull, whose plates are not yet fused. This feature allows the skull to expand in the presence of increased blood volume during venous outflow occlusion (Fig. 19.6). Skull volume in these studies is estimated from the OFC. Postmortem experimentation(56) has revealed that the brain volume is equal to the OFC raised to the fourth exponential power, multiplied by a constant that was experimentally derived. Leahy et al.(57) demonstrated that an accurate constant must be obtained and that it changed between different age groups of infants.

The accuracy of vascular occlusion plethysmography has never been validated, since no direct comparisons have been made with other accepted techniques. It probably underestimates CBF for several reasons. In any case, the technique is clearly of limited value and is not likely to be widely applied even in neonatal ICU.

Rheoencephalography

Rheoencephalography is a noninvasive method of measuring CBF in humans. First described by Jenkner(58), it measures the electrical impedance of the head. Namon et al. (59) demonstrated that the resulting signal was pulsatile, hypothesizing that it varied linearly with CBF. While the brain blood volume does contribute to the impedance changes, the signal appeared to follow stroke volume and not flow velocity or pressure. In human subjects, the signal de-

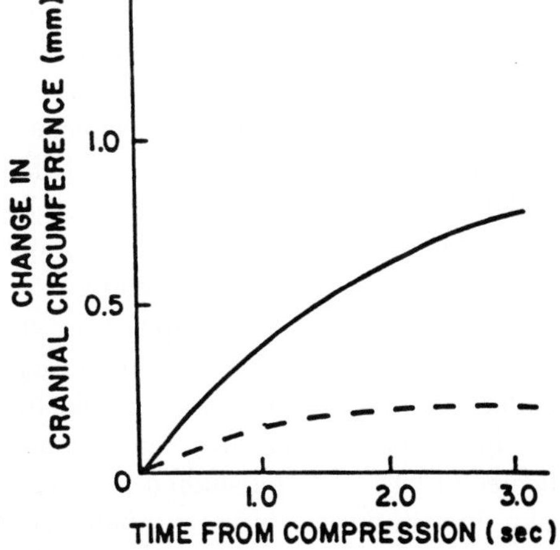

Figure 19.6. Typical response of the cranial circumference to bilateral jugular vein compression *(solid line)* and unilateral jugular vein compression *(dotted line).*

creased in amplitude in response to hyperventilation and increased in amplitude during inhalation of 5% CO_2. However, Namon et al.[59] showed that inhaling 100% O_2 decreased the electrical impedance, while exposure to high CO_2 concentrations raised it. They concluded that it was ". . . not possible to state what the various impedance amplitudes and wave shapes obtained from the head signify in terms of the cerebral circulation." Jelsma and McQueen[60] found no correlation between electrical head impedance and CBF. Costeloe et al.[49] modified the technique for use in children and compared rheoencephalography to vascular occlusion plethysmography. The former was found to lack reproducibility, most likely because of noise in part due to body and respiratory movements. Another limitation is that as much as 20% of the total impedance may be accounted for by the extracerebral circulation[61]. Thus, not only is this method unable to give quantitative values of CBF, but it may at worst have no correlation with CBF[59].

Infrared Technique

Brazy et al.[62] described a method of continuously measuring cerebral oxygenation in preterm infants at the bedside. The instrument, which they refer to as a near-infrared oxygen sufficiency scope (NIROS-SCOPE), delivers light with wavelengths between 760 and 904 nm to an infant's head. Based on the changes in the light absorbance collected on the other side of the patient's head, the relative oxidation-reduction state of cytochrome aa_3, the amounts of oxygenated and deoxygenated hemoglobin, and the hemoglobin volume in the light field can be estimated. Light in the near-infrared spectrum is used based on the relative transparency of the infant's skin and skull to light in this range.

Proctor et al.[63] have shown that relative CBF could be determined by a different modification of infrared technology. In this case, indocyanine green (with an absorption peak of 800 nm) was injected into a central venous catheter in a cat model, and CBF was determined by integrating under the curve generated by its transit through the illuminated field. Others have described instrumentation and algorithms necessary for the measurement of cerebral oxygen saturation (cerebral oximetry) and intracranial hemodynamics using infrared spectroscopy in humans[64,65]. The apparatus described by McCormick and colleagues[65] does not require transmission from one surface of the skull to the other. Light in the near infrared spectrum (650 to 1100 nm) is delivered to the subject's scalp by a fiberoptic cable. Light entering the skull and brain is scattered within tissue, and some passes back to the scalp surface at the same entry point. There, a second set of fiberoptic light cables receive, collect, and return this scattered light back to detectors. Cerebral hemodynamics (cerebral transit time, and even estimates of CBF) can be studied by monitoring the transmission through the cerebrum of a bolus of the infrared tracer, indocyanine green. This is compared with transit through an arterial vessel generating time activity curves for passage through the head or through the peripheral arterial vessel, respectively. A mathematical algorithm[65] allows for cerebral transit time to be calculated from these time activity curves. Alternatively, a mathematical algorithm[65] is provided for calculation of an estimate of the regional hemoglobin saturation based on infrared spectroscopy without the need for the tracer dye.

The infrared technology is appealing because it is noninvasive, portable, and useful for continuous monitoring. Its use, however, should not be considered to be without potential risks. The lasers that were used in the Brazy et al.[62] study deliver a significant amount of energy to the infant's head. The lasers used were class IIIB and, although not considered to be hazardous to the skin, may be hazardous to the infant's eyes if the lasers are viewed directly. For this reason, shielding of the eyes is required. At this time, the infrared technique has unfortunately not developed to the point where data other than those documenting qualitative trends can be obtained. The technique is promising, but much work remains before clinical applicability to cerebral pathophysiology becomes routine.

Summary

In the past several years, interest in the pathophysiology of the cerebral circulation as it applies to neurologic intensive care has grown tremendously. A variety of methods designed to measure or estimate CBF in various pathologic states have been developed. Before any conclusions can be made regarding their utility, the physician must have a basic understanding of the principles involved, their limitations, and the potential for misinterpretation. Ultimately this should allow the patient to receive medical care of greatest benefit at minimal risk.

INTRACEREBRAL MICRODIALYSIS

Intracerebral microdialysis is a technique that has undergone widespread recent application in experimental neurochemistry and neuropharmacology. The principle relies on a double-bore hollow probe, the tip of which is covered by a semipermeable membrane. This microdialysis probe is implanted within brain tissue and is continuously perfused with sterile artificial CSF or some similar balanced salt solution at a constant rate (usually 2 μL/min). At regular intervals the fluid so introduced into the brain which has reentered the collecting chamber through the semipermeable membrane (the dialysate) is collected, and aliquots can then be subjected to analysis (usually by high-pressure liquid chromatography [HPLC]) for various metabolites or amino acids such as lactate, pyruvate, hypoxanthine, and glutamate. This then provides estimates of the extracellular fluid (ECF) concentrations of these various neurochemicals or metabolites. The technique has provided extremely valuable in vivo neurochemical data in animal models of stroke, in neuropharmacological studies, and so forth.

Persson and Hillered have described application of this

technique to human patients in the intensive care setting[66]. Four patients underwent implantation of such a microdialysis probe in parallel with placement of an intraventricular catheter (no additional burr hole required). Patients were monitored for up to eight days with no complications recognized as secondary to this additional piece of hardware. Numerous chemical analyses from serial ECF samples were taken generating estimates of ECF concentrations of lactate, pyruvate, hypoxanthine, and several amino acids. The lactate-to-pyruvate ratio was also calculated. Fluctuations in the ECF levels or ratios so measured could be found in many instances to correspond to specific clinical or pathophysiological events (e.g., increased lactate to pyruvate ratio with seizures). The authors conclude[66] that the technique is applicable to humans, is safe, and may provide valuable information regarding pathophysiological processes affecting the CNS. Increased sophistication, such as on-line detection of pH[67], may eventually allow for true continuous monitoring of ECF in the clinical setting. The actual benefit of such approaches in the ICU remains to be clarified.

INTRACRANIAL PRESSURE MONITORING

In contrast to serial measurements of CBF that truly have little application to the routine care of critically ill children, the monitoring of intracranial pressure (ICP) is commonly employed in the pediatric ICU. A clear understanding of the methodology is vital to the management of patients with head trauma as well as those various illnesses accompanied by elevated ICP. The methodologic aspects of this subject are discussed here. Clinical applications of the technique are covered in detail elsewhere and thus are not repeated in this chapter.

Historical Perspective

As far back as 1866, Leyden[68] described a method by which ICP variations were recorded through burr holes in the skull. The technique of lumbar puncture was introduced by Quincke in 1891[69], and since that time, single and repeated measurements of spinal fluid pressure were used to assess ICP. It was not until 1951 that Guillaume and Janny[70] continuously recorded ICPs and noted that clinical neurologic signs were unreliable as indicators of increased ICP. However, it is the work of Lundberg[71,72] and others which firmly established the usefulness of continuous ICP monitoring.

Principles

The principles of ICP monitoring are reviewed in great detail in the discussion of the pathophysiology of the intracranial vault in Chapter 18. In brief, the Monro-Kellie hypothesis maintains that intracranial volume (consisting of brain tissue, blood, and CSF) must remain constant since it lies within a rigid structure—the skull. Infants are an exception, given unfused sutures and open fontanels that allow for considerable expansion of intracranial volume. Through a compensation process, any increase in one component must result in a reduction of at least one other component. However, in the presence of brain disease, such changes may be poorly tolerated.

Brain damage due to a CNS insult, whether it be the result of trauma, metabolic alterations, or hypoxic-ischemic encephalopathy, involves three processes of tissue injury: primary brain injury, secondary injury resulting from brain-tissue responses to the original insult, and additional subsequent CNS damage occurring as a consequence of systemic responses to the CNS disturbance. Primary injury induces tissue necrosis and, in the presence of trauma, vascular disruption, hemorrhage, and axonal shearing or stretching. Secondary brain injury evolves over a longer period of time. It involves complex pathophysiologic and biochemical mechanisms, commonly including loss of CBF autoregulation, development of cerebral edema, breakdown of the blood-brain barrier, and release of potentially toxic endogenous substances such as glutamate. These lead to a marked increase in brain volume that can produce functional impairment directly or, more seriously, may engender ischemia and/or herniation. Further CNS injury may result from disturbances of the cardiopulmonary system, such as hypertension or hypotension, hypercapnia, hypoxia, and decreased cardiac output. A major consideration in such a situation is the cerebral perfusion pressure (CPP), defined as[73,74].

$$\text{CPP} = (\text{MAP} - \text{ICP}) \text{ or } (\text{MAP} - \text{CVP})$$

whichever is lower, where MAP is mean arterial blood pressure. In general, CPP must be kept above 50 mm Hg to maintain adequate CBF. Once neurologic damage has occurred, increased ICP is associated with poor outcome[75–77]. Since clinical assessment cannot provide reliable information regarding ICP, aside from neurologic signs that indicate impending or progressing transtentorial herniation, ICP monitoring is crucial to allow the clinician to take appropriate measures toward reduction of ICP and maintenance of adequate CPP before irreversible catastrophic consequences supervene.

Criteria for Monitoring

Criteria for ICP monitoring is discussed extensively in Chapters 18 and 24. Briefly, there are no absolute criteria for the use of intracranial monitoring. Mayer and Walker[78] used a Glasgow coma scale[79] score of 7 or less or head injury with loss of consciousness and inability to utter words or follow commands. In their series of 56 patients, which included trauma, Reye's syndrome, and near-drowning, 80% had ICP elevations that required treatment. Their complication rate was less than 5%, which the authors believed was an acceptable risk-benefit ratio. In other series reporting on traumatic brain injury, between 50 and 70% of monitored patients developed ICP elevations requiring treatment[75,80,81]. On the other hand, whether or not ICP monitoring (presumably accompanied by appropriate therapeutic interventions) actually improves outcome in nontraumatic encephalopathies such as near-drowning and other forms of hypoxic-ischemic CNS insult is uncertain[82].

Intracranial Monitoring Devices

A number of different methods have been employed over the years for ICP monitoring[83]. The ventricular catheter has been described as the gold-standard and has the advantages of allowing for regular checking of zero drift and permitting removal of CSF from the ventricular space as one management option. On the other hand, it is often difficult, if not impossible, to place ventricular catheters when ICP is associated with collapsed or slit ventricles, a circumstance often present in nontraumatic coma[84]. For this and other reasons, an entire array of alternative devices have been designed to allow for measurement of ICP from the ventricular cavity to the subarachnoid space[83,84]. Each has distinct advantages and disadvantages with which the intensivist should be familiar (the reader is referred to two recent reviews for further detail,[82,83]).

Epidural Devices

Epidural devices consist of a balloon radiotransmitter or a fiberoptic transducer placed within the epidural space, or the signal is transmitted to an extracranial sensor via an extradural screw. They afford easy placement and a low incidence of infection. Major disadvantages include sensor plate-dura interrelationships, signal dampening, a tendency to overread compared with ventricular pressure, and inability to measure brain compliance and withdraw excess CSF[85].

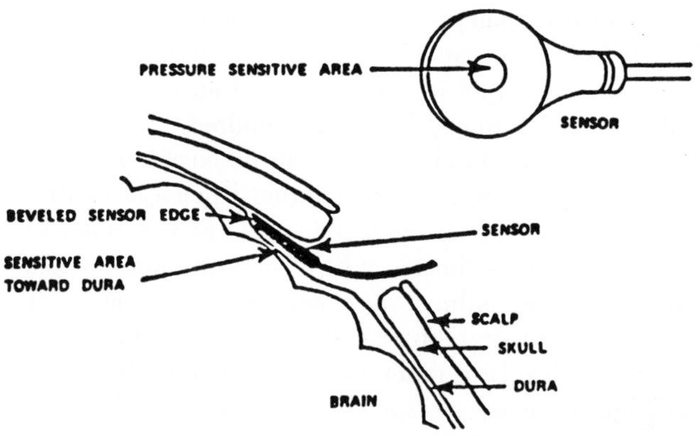

Figure 19.8. Cross-sectional diagram showing the placement of the fiberoptic pressure transducer (Ladd's device) within the skull. (From Ivan LP, Choo SH, Ventureyra ECG. Intracranial pressure monitoring with the fiberoptic transducer in children. Childs Brain 1980;7:306.)

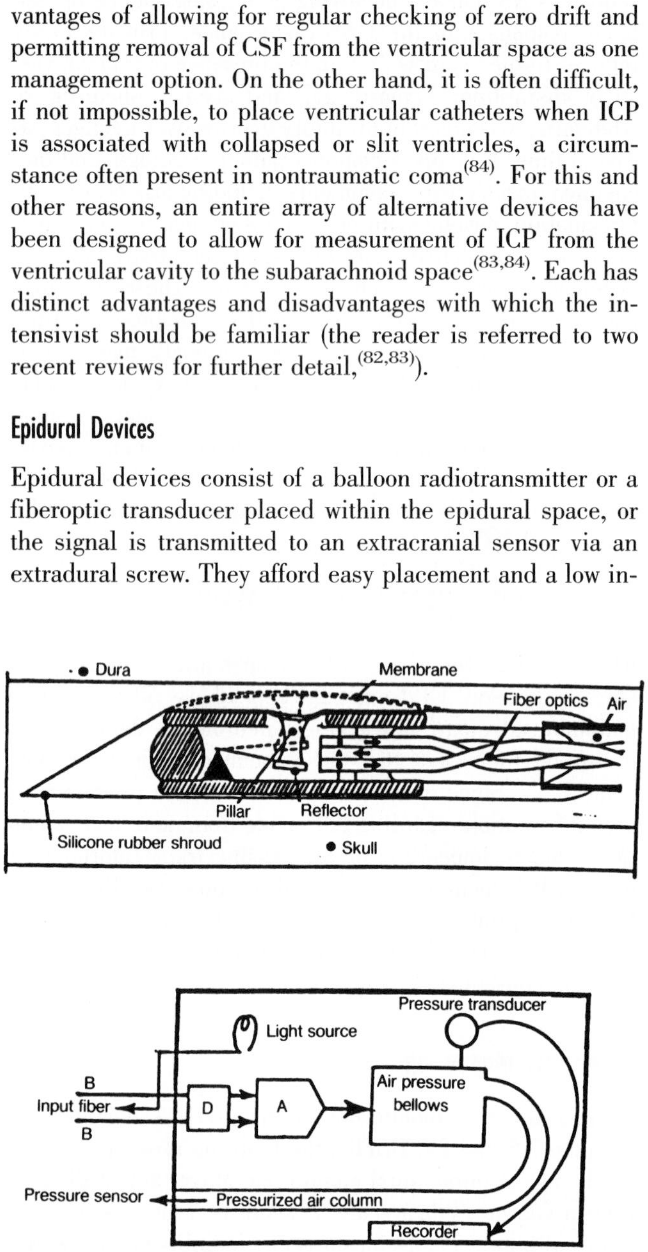

Figure 19.7. *Top:* Cross-section of the epidural pressure transducer (Ladd intracranial monitor) based on the principle of the Numoto pressure switch. *A,* input fibers; *B,* output fibers; and *arrows* which indicate direction of light. *Bottom:* Schematic of the monitor control unit. *A,* amplifier; *B,* output fiber; and *D,* photocell light detectors. (From Ivan L, Choo SH, Ventureyra ECG. Intracranial pressure monitoring with the fiberoptic transducer in children. Childs Brain 1980;7:305.)

The fiberoptic sensor (Fig. 19.7) marketed as the Ladd ICP monitor by Roche measures from −37 to +185 mm Hg. The sensor, encased in silicone, contains three fiberoptic columns, a pneumatic tube, and a pressure-sensitive membrane. A mirror is placed on the membrane and deflects a beam of incoming light in the center fiberoptic column toward two outgoing optic fibers. Pressure of the dura against the membrane moves the mirror, casting uneven light on the two outgoing fibers. The monitor contains photoelectric sensors that detect the light difference; it applies an external pneumatic pressure to balance the mirror so that the light output is again equal. The pressure readout is the pressure of the system required to balance the mirror. Equalization of the dural pressure occurs at frequent intervals to give a continuous reading.

The sensor is placed through a burr hole in the right or left frontal area (Fig. 19.8). Its accuracy and reliability still need confirmation through prospective studies. Ivan et al.[85] showed excellent outcome in 52 patients who received epidural devices for the measurement of ICP. No direct comparison was made with intraventricular or subarachnoid devices; hence, one cannot be sure of the accuracy of the readings obtained.

Subarachnoid Devices

Subarachnoid devices consist of a subarachnoid catheter or extradural screw placed in the subdural or subarachnoid space, connected to a fluid-filled manometer system. They provide ease of insertion, avoidance of brain puncture, and ability to obtain some information of brain compliance and withdrawal of CSF (Fig. 19.9). Disadvantages include the possible obstruction or leakage of CSF and the risk of infection. Mendelow et al.[86] observed that Richmond and Leeds screws underread in the subdural space at ICP val-

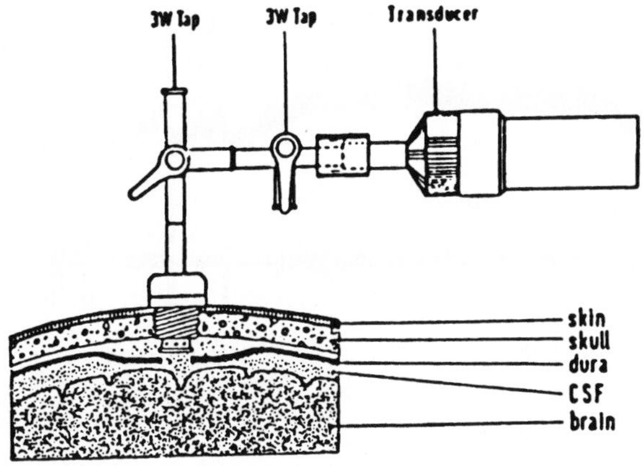

Figure 19.9. Diagram showing the cross-section of the cranium and the position of the Leed's device for measuring subarachnoid pressure. (From Dearden NM, McDowall DG, Gibson RM. Assessment of Leeds device for monitoring intracranial pressure. J Neurosurg 1984;60:124.)

ues greater than 20 mm Hg. This was confirmed by Dearden et al.[87]. Weaver et al.[88] reported that subarachnoid pressures may vary by site in patients with unilateral brain pathology.

The subarachnoid bolt was first used in 1972 by Vries et al.[89]. A burr hole is made in the skull with a small incision placed in the dura. The bolt is then screwed into the cranium, where the sensor tip is then positioned in the subarachnoid space. It is used in children older than 1 year (because it does not sit well within the table of the infant's skull) and when the ventricles are small.

Intraventricular Devices

The intraventricular catheter is inserted through a burr hole into the nondominant or nonaffected hemisphere[83,84]. The tip is then positioned within the frontal or occipital horn of the lateral ventricle. Various catheters may be used, which are then connected to a fluid-filled manometer system, with the transducer positioned at the level of the lateral ventricle or external auditory meatus.

The major advantages of this device are direct measurement of CSF pressure, testing for brain compliance by the injection of air or contrast media, and withdrawal of CSF to decrease pressure and/or for sampling purposes[90,91]; regular adjustment of zero drift is also possible. Disadvantages include leakage of CSF, infection (1%), intracerebral bleeding, and difficulty of insertion in patients with small ventricles.

Intraparenchymal Devices

Recent progress in the technology of fiberoptics has led to the development of fiberoptic pressure transducers which measure changes in light reflected off a pressure-sensitive membrane located at the tip of the fiberoptic device[84,92]. Such catheters can be designed to be inserted into any of the intracranial compartments (subdural, intraparenchymal, or intraventricular). In particular, the use of these devices for implantation directly into cerebral tissue (intraparenchymal placement) has gained support. Proponents of these catheters[84,92] claim they are (1) as accurate as the gold standard (intraventricular catheter); (2) easy to implant on a single pass (reducing trauma); (3) safe and rarely associated with infection; (4) particularly advantageous because the reference pressure point is at the tip of the catheter, thereby obviating a need for calibration adjustments with changes in head position, etc.; and (5) subject to minimum drift (cumulative drift of ≤6 mm Hg per 5-day period, although this could be clinically significant). Their main disadvantage is that the fiberoptic catheter itself cannot be used for CSF drainage. The relative risk of such devices is yet to be elucidated[93,94].

At our institutions (University of Utah Medical Center and Primary Children's Medical Center), the preferred device is the Camino system[84,92] fitted in a ventricular catheter or, if the ventricles are too compressed, inserted directly into the brain parenchyma.

Waveforms

The normal ICP ranges from 0 to 15 mm Hg or 0 to 200 cm H_2O[96,97]. However, even in the normal patient pressure may transiently rise 30 to 50 mm Hg during a Valsalva's maneuver or coughing without a deleterious effect. However, sustained elevations can be harmful by decreasing cerebral perfusion pressure, resulting in parenchymal ischemia.

The tracing should show definite waveforms, fluctuating with the patient's respirations. Three distinct waveforms have been described[61–63]: A, B, and C (Fig. 19.10).

A-waves, also known as plateau waves, have a large amplitude with a steep rise. They may be sustained for 5 to 20 minutes, resulting in marked rises of ICP from 50 to 110 mm Hg. They represent loss of cerebral autoregulation and can result in severe cerebral hypoperfusion. Clinically, the patient may complain of severe headaches with decreasing level of consciousness. Decerebrate or decorticate posturing usually indicates progressive brainstem compression from either central or uncal herniation. These findings, of course, constitute a medical or neurosurgical emergency.

B-waves are of lower amplitude (0 to 50 mm Hg) and occur more frequently, and their significance is more controversial, with some experts stating that they have no clinical significance and others believing that they may be associated with decreased mental status and/or Cheyne-Stokes breathing.

C-waves have the smallest amplitudes (0 to 20 mm Hg) and appear to be the result of fluctuations of systemic blood pressure and of brainstem dysfunction.

Analysis and Interpretation of ICP Monitoring

Aside from the identification of waveforms and calculation of the CPP as described above, a number of other methods of ICP analysis have been employed[95–97]. These include (1) generation of ICP histograms, (2) continuous statistical

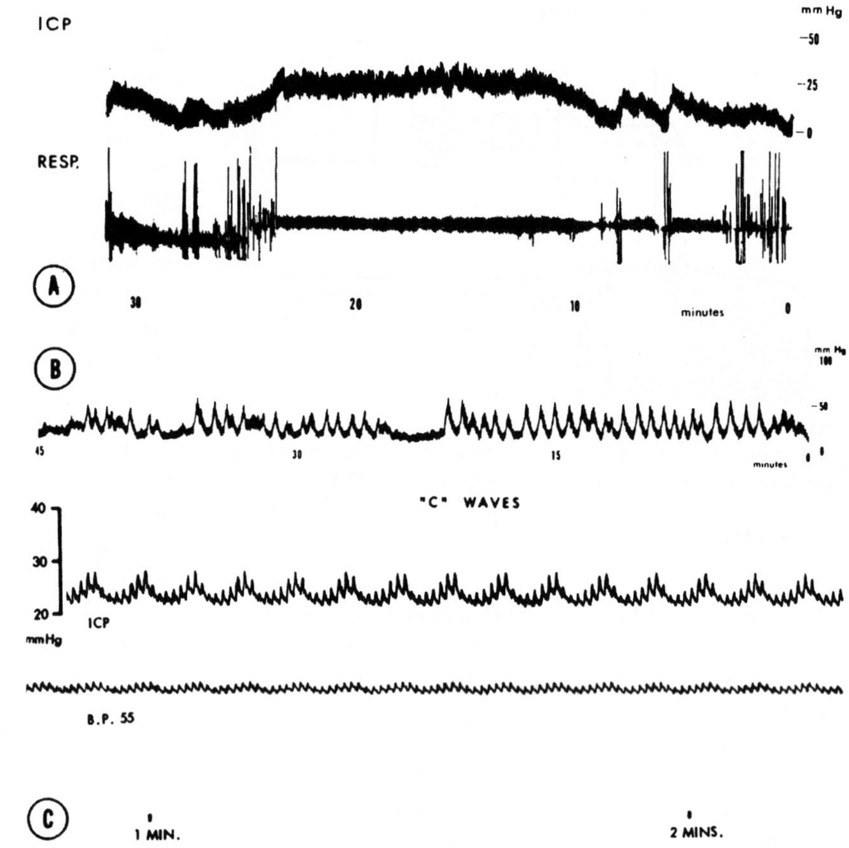

Figure 19.10. Depiction of three distinct ICP waves (according to Lundberg). **A.** A typical plateau or A wave is shown. Note the sustained rise in pressure lasting 11 to 12 minutes. B and C waves are shown in **B** and **C,** respectively. Both are of much shorter duration than the plateau waves, with the C-wave fluctuations being paralleled by systemic blood pressure *(B.P.)* oscillations. (From Hanlon K. Description and uses of intracranial pressure monitoring. Heart Lung 1976;5:277.)

analysis of ICP trends, (3) estimation of intracranial compliance, (4) systems analysis of intracranial pressure, and (5) other computerized methods.

The generation of ICP histograms simply provides a profile of ICP ranges over a specified period (e.g., one day). Its clinical benefit thus far appears dubitable. Continuous statistical analysis of ICP providing ongoing values for mean ICP and ICP variance has been performed in an effort to predict sudden rises in intracranial pressure. In some cases, abrupt rises in ICP can be anticipated by the prior appearance of significant increases in ICP variance[95]. Alternatively, efforts to estimate intracranial compliance have been made in accordance with the presumption that decreasing compliance may indicate need for specific therapeutic interventions and/or may be of prognostic significance. Mathematical estimates of intracranial compliance have been based both on analysis of ICP changes in response to an infusion into or withdrawal of fluid from the intracranial space as well as on more sophisticated analyses of ICP waveforms. No consensus on these approaches exists at present[95]. Finally, other computerized analytic methods including systems analysis are currently being developed, but these remain primarily investigational tools with an uncertain clinical future.

Interventions

The treatment of elevated ICP is discussed elsewhere in this book. The reader is also referred to several excellent recent papers on the subject[83,90,91,98–100]. In summary, management involves the prevention of hypoxemia, hypotension, hypercapnia, and ICP elevations. Elevating the head by 30 to 45° facilitates venous drainage from the cranium. Increased arterial blood oxygen content helps to decrease secondary brain injury[101,102]. Hyperventilation (i.e., keeping PCO_2 at 25 to 29 mm Hg) prevents cerebral vasodilatation and thereby decreases ICP[90,91,98,102]. Maintaining normal systemic blood pressure, i.e., systolic blood pressure greater than 80 plus 2 times the age in years but less than 140 mm Hg, allows for adequate CPP and better clinical outcome[78,90,91,100,103].

Elevations of ICP may be further managed with diuretic therapy: mannitol 0.25 to 1 g/kg every 4 hours (maintain high serum osmolarity of less than 320 mOsm) and/or furosemide 0.5 to 1 mg/kg lowers ICP by reducing the brain water content. Their use requires bladder catheterization for accurate recording of fluid output. Hypothermia decreases brain metabolism and cerebral blood volume. Temperature should be maintained above 30 to 31°C because of cardiac arrhythmias associated with lower values[102].

When the above modalities fail, barbiturate coma may lower ICP through as-yet unknown mechanisms (thiopental sodium: 2 to 4 mg/kg initially, 2 mg/kg/hr maintenance with serum levels between 25 and 35 μg/mm) and with induction of a burst-suppression pattern on electroencephalogram (EEG). However, since barbiturates lower cardiac output, careful monitoring of ICP and cardiovascular function is required[75].

Summary

ICP monitoring and consequent therapeutic interventions are aimed at treatment of marked elevations of ICP and have been shown (at least in traumatic encephalopathies) to produce better patient outcome[100]. The key to their use is the understanding of ICP physiology and its ultimate effects on CBF and metabolism. There are more precise methods of measuring the latter two parameters (nuclear magnetic resonance spectroscopy and PET CBF measurement techniques), but they are unfortunately available only in selected institutions because of their high cost and complicated technology. Hence, if physicians are to continue using ICP monitoring, they must be aware of the advantages, disadvantages, and pitfalls in the interpretation of the data.

ELECTRICAL MONITORING OF THE CENTRAL NERVOUS SYSTEM

Strictly speaking, standard multichannel electroencephalography is not practically applicable to continuous monitoring or even to frequent intermittent monitoring of the CNS in the ICU setting. However, until recently, serial EEG recordings have represented the primary means of evaluating brain electrical activity in critically ill patients. Furthermore, routine electroencephalography continues to be necessary as a complement to actual electrical monitoring systems (cerebral function monitor [CFM] and compressed spectral array [CSA]) currently available for ICU use. Finally, understanding the electronic and technical principles of routine electroencephalography is a prerequisite to the comprehension of these newer methods of electroencephalographic averaging and to the theory and use of evoked potentials (EPs). Thus, an initial introduction to standard electroencephalography technology is followed by discussion of newer means of compressing EEG readings and then by an overview of EPs.

Electrical monitoring of the CNS is of crucial value to the proper evaluation of the intensive care child with neurologic disease[104]. In fact, reliance on electrical monitoring is growing as technologic advances in critical care medicine increasingly require interventions that impair the clinician's ability to evaluate the patient on the basis of physical and neurologic examinations (e.g., use of sedative and anticonvulsant drugs, induction of pentobarbital coma, skeletal muscle paralysis)[104,105]. In many such patients on life support systems, measurement of electroencephalographic activity may provide the only information available to the clinician as to the functional status of the brain. In addition, the EEG or EPs may provide valuable diagnostic or prognostic information in the management of patients with intractable seizures and of those with obtundation or coma due to various causes. Thus, the importance of electroencephalographic techniques to modern critical care management of pediatric patients cannot be overstated. On the other hand, the interpretation of these methods of CNS monitoring is challenging, is easily contaminated by artifact, and typically requires the close availability of a clinical neurophysiologist trained in the interpretation of such studies, particularly as they pertain to encephalopathic patients.

ROUTINE ELECTROENCEPHALOGRAPHY

Resting electrical activity was first definitively demonstrated in the brains of animals by the Englishman Richard Caton in the late 19th century[106]. In a paper presented in 1876 to the British Medical Association, he described the presence of spontaneous electrical variation recorded from the cortical surface of animals, and he noted this activity to be sensitive to anoxia and anesthesia. He also described cerebral EPs, a technique that was promptly exploited for the determination of sensory receptive areas in the CNS. It was, however, the reclusive Hans Berger, a German psychiatrist, who first recorded human cerebral electrical activity. He is responsible for coining the term *Electroenkephalogramm,* using it in the title of his publication on the subject in 1929[106]. Since that seminal manuscript, the sophistication of electroencephalographic measurement has grown, but the principles remain essentially unchanged.

Principles and Technique of Electroencephalography

Routine electroencephalography consists of the recording of scalp electrical activity for a finite (limited) period of time (usually less than or equal to 30 minutes). Metal cup electrodes are applied to selected sites on the scalp and ears, based on specific positions relative to the inion, the nasion, and right and left preauricular sites defined by the international 10 to 20 electrode convention (Fig. 19.11). These are, in turn, connected in pairs to differential amplifiers (an amplifier that compares the relative voltage at its two inputs, G_1 and G_2). By convention, if the voltage present at the electrode connected to input 1 (G_1) is negative with respect to the voltage present at the electrode connected to input 2 (G_2), a positive signal (upward pen deflection) is generated (Fig. 19.12).

Most currently employed electroencephalography machines consist of 18 channels (i.e., 18 differential amplifiers, each of which drives one pen). The hardware of the machine allows for different pairs of scalp electrodes to be connected to different amplifiers resulting in a predefined set of montages. In other words, a montage refers to the pattern in which scalp electrodes are compared with one another in order to generate a set of 18 tracings, 16 of which typically represent the voltages from various scalp regions and the other two of which are often used to depict noncerebral activity, such as the ECG, the electromyogram (EMG), or the electro-oculogram (EOG) (eye movements). Two general types of electrode connections (montages) can be used. *Referential* montages refer each scalp electrode to the same (reference) electrode, such as the ipsilateral ear. In contrast, in *bipolar* montages, an electrode is referred to

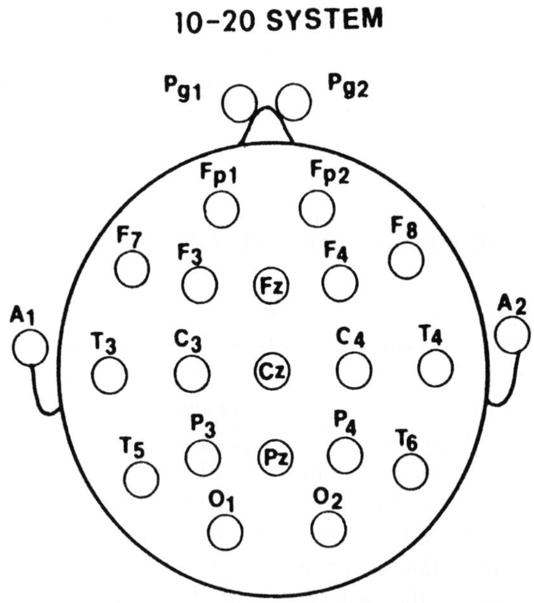

Figure 19.11. Electrode placement according to the 10 to 20 electrode convention. *Circles* represent electrode locations on this schematic depiction of the scalp. All electrodes from the left side of the head bear an *odd number subscript;* those from the right, an *even number subscript.* A_1 and A_2 represent electrodes typically attached to the ear lobes.

a neighboring electrode, and that electrode is, in turn, compared with a subsequent neighboring electrode to generate the output of the next channel, and so forth. Examples of such montages and their output are shown in Figure 19.13. Modern data storage systems also allow for the more condensed collection of longer recordings of conventional EEG. Analog recordings are now often stored on electromagnetic tape. Alternatively, machines are now routinely available for collection of digitized, real-time EEG, in which optical disks allow for the storage of well over 24 hours of EEG on a single disk. Furthermore, with digital processing of the EEG, montages can be changed subsequent to the recording, as can the filtering and time dependence. This allows for greater flexibility and more efficient data management.

In routine electroencephalography, the brain's electrical activity is recorded from a supine, resting patient in awake and sleep states, if possible. Allowances must, of course, be made for the immature child, the combative child, a seizing patient, etc. The (uncontaminated) output of the EEG recording consists of 18 horizontal tracings of the potential differences measured on a continuous basis by the 18 differential amplifiers. In general, this output ranges from a few microvolts to several hundred microvolts in amplitude and by convention is divided into four frequency bands (Fig. 19.14). From lower (slower) frequency to higher (faster) frequency waves, these consist of the following frequency

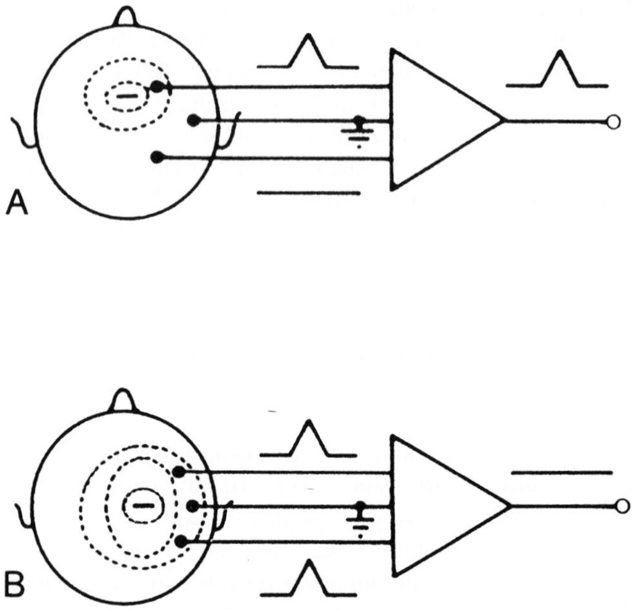

Figure 19.12. Schematic depiction of differential amplification of the EEG. In each diagram, a negative voltage source is emanating from the scalp as shown. *Triangle* represents the differential amplifier. The *top line* to the scalp is input 1, whereas the *bottom line* is input 2. The voltage is always measured with reference to ground, which in this case is defined as the middle lead. In **A,** input 1 is negative *relative to* input 2, so an upgoing deflection (shown to the *right*) is drawn by the pen. In **B,** inputs 1 and 2 sense the same potential relative to ground; thus there is no *difference* in potential between the two inputs, and no pen deflection results. (Adapted from Spehlmann R. EEG primer. New York: Elsevier, 1981.)

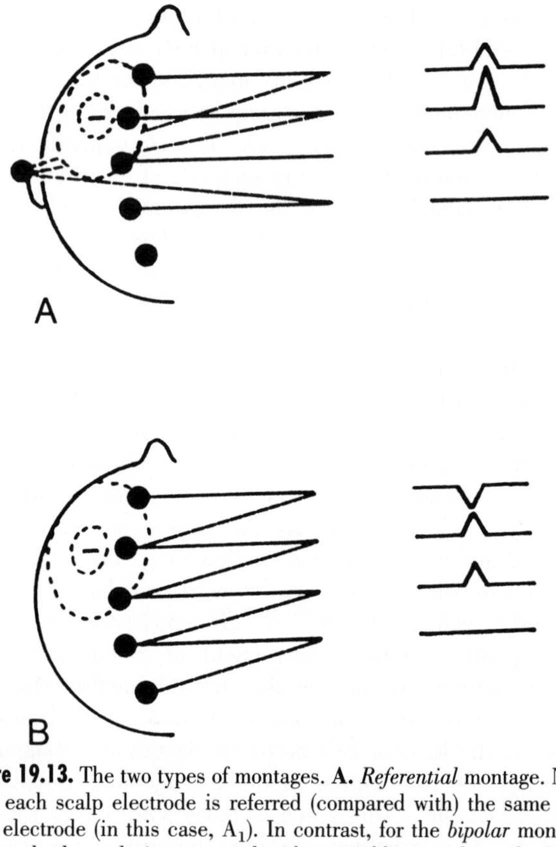

Figure 19.13. The two types of montages. **A.** *Referential* montage. Note how each scalp electrode is referred (compared with) the same distant electrode (in this case, A_1). In contrast, for the *bipolar* montage **(B)** each electrode is compared with a neighboring electrode. Even though the signal at the scalp is the same, different tracings result. (Adapted from Spehlmann R. EEG primer. New York: Elsevier, 1981.)

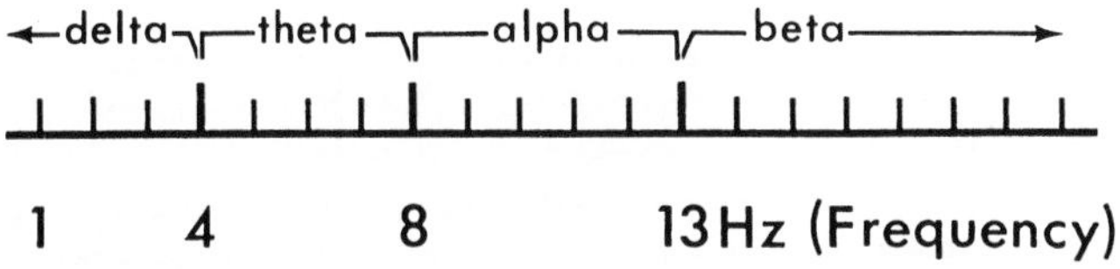

Figure 19.14. Frequency bands of the EEG. By convention, EEG waves are divided into four frequency bands: delta (δ), theta (θ), alpha (α), and beta (β), as shown. (Adapted from Spehlmann R. EEG primer. New York: Elsevier, 1981.)

bands: δ (less than 4 Hz), θ (4 to 7 Hz), α (8 to 13 Hz), and β (more than 13 Hz). In the typical EEG of a resting, wakeful older child or adult, an occipital (posterior) α-rhythm predominates, whereas anterior β-rhythms of lower amplitude are seen over frontal head regions. Younger children have slower rhythms in general (Fig. 19.15)[95]. Each stage of sleep also has its typical EEG features, but full discussion of normal and abnormal EEG patterns is beyond the scope of this chapter. The reader is referred to several excellent reviews or texts[107–110].

Actual cerebral activity is of relatively low amplitude, compared with signals generated by various artifacts intrinsic or extrinsic to the patient (e.g., eye movements, eye blinks, temporal muscle contraction, jaw movements, intravenous pumps, and other electrical equipment). Such artifacts can severely contaminate a record and make discernment of underlying cerebral activity (normal or abnormal) extremely difficult. In general, portable recordings in the ICU are far more susceptible to contamination by artifact, and often Herculean efforts must be made by staff and technicians to curtail such contamination or to identify it repeatedly on the record when it cannot be eliminated. Elec-

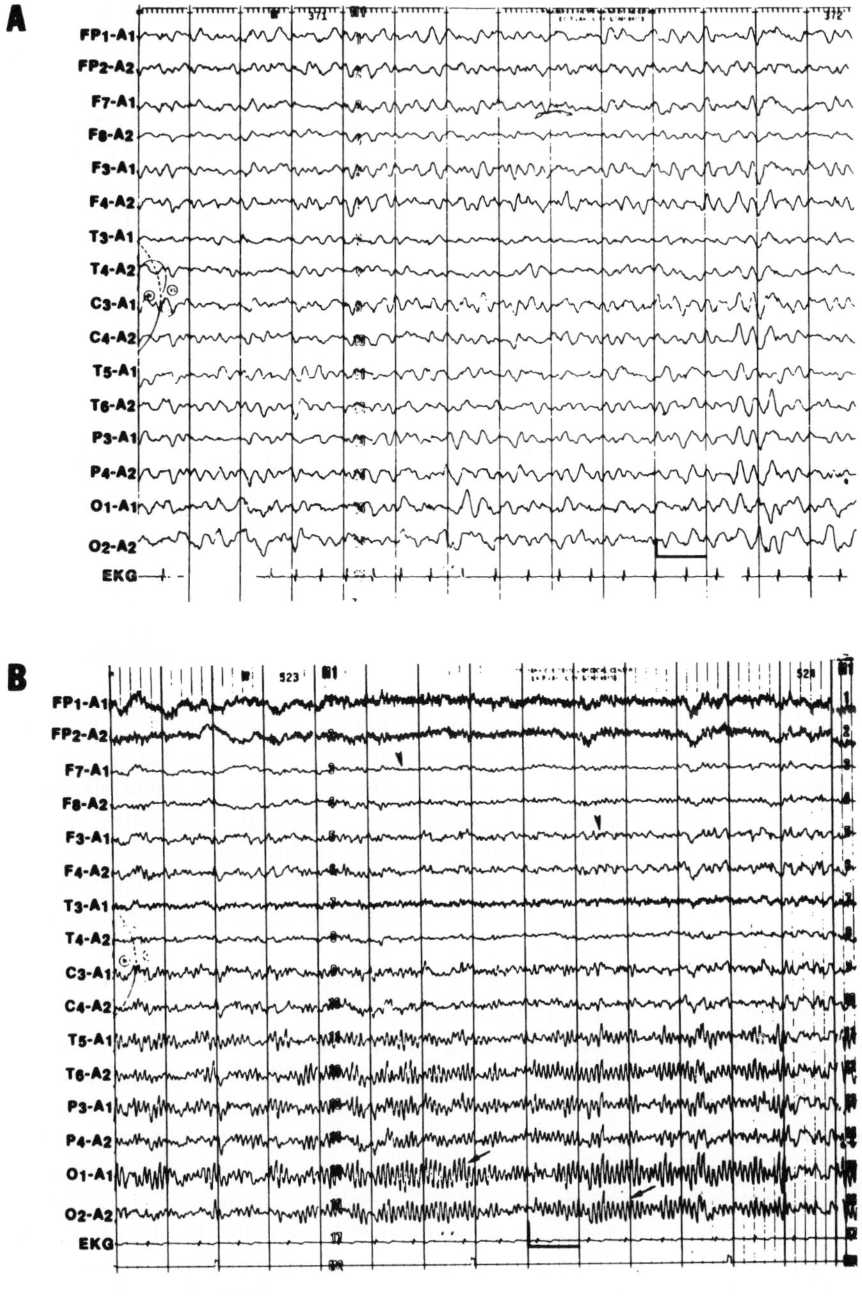

Figure 19.15. Normal EEG patterns. Note how the EEG of a 6-month-old boy **(A)** displays slower frequencies than those of a 15-year-old boy **(B)**, whose activity is that of an adult. The dominant frequency for the infant is in the θ-range (4 to 5 Hz), whereas the older boy's EEG demonstrates a well-formed, regular, sinusoidal, occipital α-rhythm *(arrows)*. Lower-amplitude β-frequency activity can be appreciated anteriorly *(arrowheads)*. *Horizontal bar,* 1 second; *vertical bar,* 100 μV.

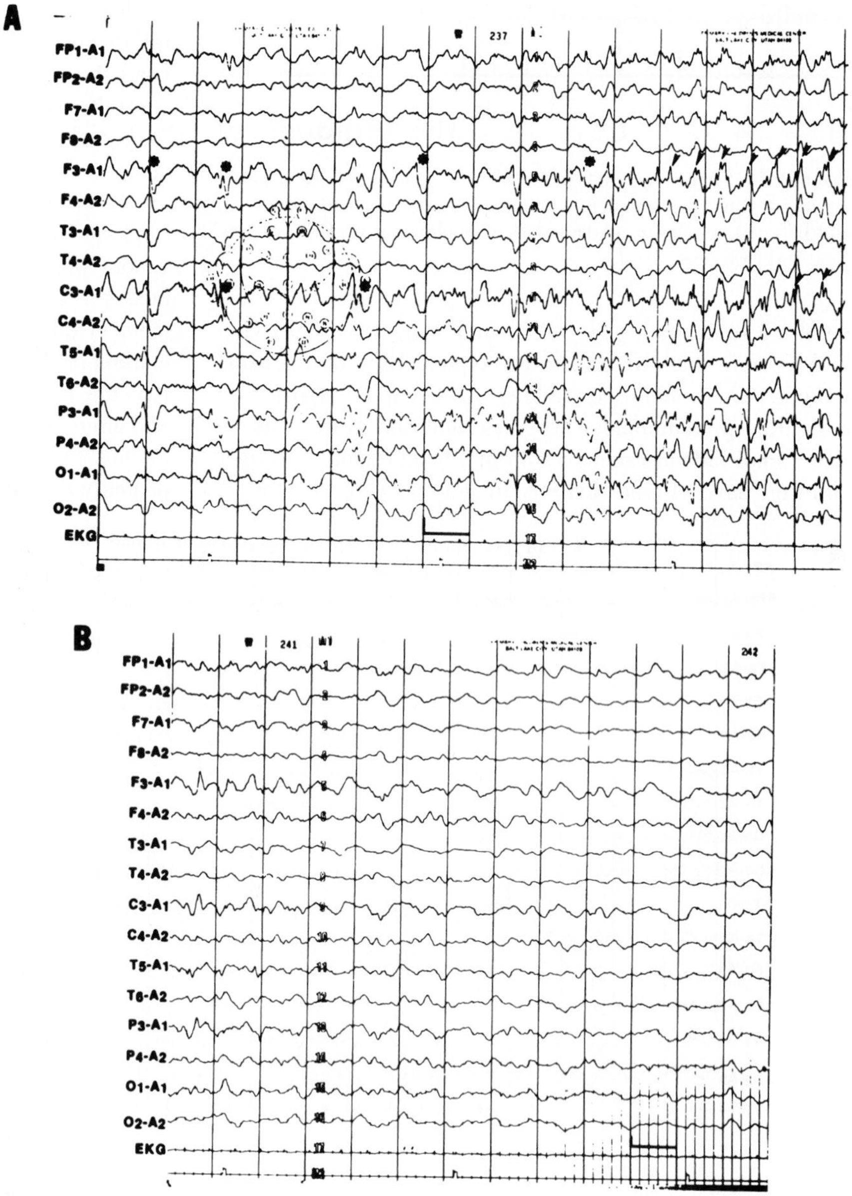

Figure 19.16. This 3 1/2-year-old girl with Burkitt's lymphoma was admitted to the ICU with encephalopathy. The routine EEG demonstrated an electrographic seizure unaccompanied by recognized clinical signs. **A.** depicts buildup of left hemisphere epileptiform discharges *(asterisks)*, resulting finally in the repetitive discharges of the seizure *(arrowheads)*, which lasted another 10 seconds. **B.** The EEG was slower and attenuated 20 to 30 seconds later. Such seizure activity was believed to be contributing to the child's encephalopathy. *Horizontal bar,* 1 second; *vertical bar,* 100 μV.

troencephalographers are trained to identify such artifacts, but sufficient contamination may make a record uninterpretable. Unfortunately, the issue of artifact identification and contamination becomes far more problematic in electroencephalography monitoring systems (described below).

Use of the Routine Electroencephalogram in Intensive Care

The EEG has long been used in the evaluation and follow-up (intermittent monitoring) of the critically ill child[111,112]. Its greatest value, lies in the assessment of the obtunded, comatose, or seizing individual, wherein it may provide both valuable diagnostic as well as prognostic information[113]. It may also be used to measure cerebral activity in therapeutically paralyzed or anesthetized patients and may help to ascertain the effects of various therapeutic interventions (such as therapy for intracranial hypertension or anticonvulsant administration). The method, as is clarified below, is most limited by the sheer volume and breadth of the information it generates. The amount of paper alone makes continuous or even frequent electroencephalography monitoring a practical impossibility (as well as an ecologic extravagance). In addition, the continued requirement for technician time and labor-intensive interpretation further limits its applicability for ongoing CNS monitoring.

The routine EEG is the most accurate means of identifying the electrical footprints of seizure activity[112]. In critical care medicine, it frequently becomes necessary to identify the presence of ongoing cerebral seizure activity that does not result in clinical manifestations, e.g., silent seizures, subclinical seizures, or nonconvulsive status (Fig. 19.16)[113–115]. Such epileptic disorders may represent the primary cause of an encephalopathy or may accompany a variety of CNS insults, thereby complicating their treatment and the interpretation of the patient's level of consciousness. In some series as many as 50 to 70% of comatose patients in the ICU setting were found to exhibit periods of nonconvulsive status. Unfortunately, available methods for compressing (averaging) EEG recordings may make the identification of repeated or ongoing subclinical seizures difficult; therefore, ICUs equipped with such monitoring systems must nevertheless rely on the periodic routine EEG also(116,117).

Electrographic seizure activity can thus be identified in encephalopathic patients with idiopathic epilepsy, as in absence status (Fig. 19.17) or focal epilepsy, e.g., psychomotor status (Fig. 19.18). The routine EEG is very useful in locating regions of excessive cortical irritability or in identifying seizure foci, such as in encephalitic illnesses (Fig. 19.19). In fact, the identification of temporal lobe epileptiform discharges is often crucial to the accurate diagnosis of herpes encephalitis. The recognition of continued electrographic seizures in obtunded patients is critical to proper anticonvulsant management and also helps determine duration of general anesthesia or pentobarbital coma in cases of intractable status epilepticus(114,115).

Use of the EEG as an aid in the diagnosis of stupor and coma has been curtailed to some extent with the advent of improved neuroimaging. Nevertheless, it remains invaluable in the serial evaluation of coma and in prognostication with regard to both traumatic and nontraumatic encephalopathies. In general, the EEG in coma (aside from effects of ongoing seizure activity, if present) is characterized by generalized slowing of EEG activity with or without accompanying amplitude attenuation. The degree of slowing, the severity of amplitude suppression, and the relative presence or absence of fluctuation in EEG frequencies over time represent the major variables that relate to eventual outcome(104,111,112). In general, the slower the frequencies, the greater the amplitude suppression, and the more in varying the EEG frequency spectrum, the poorer the prognosis(104,111,112), although predictive power is weak except for extremes of abnormality or normalcy, respectively. For example, Pampiglione and Harden(111) reported on 120 children with hypoxic-ischemic encephalopathy from cardiac arrest. Four general EEG patterns were described: pattern A, in which EEG features were relatively "well-preserved"; pattern B, which is characterized by generalized δ-frequency slowing; pattern C, which consists of periods of marked EEG attenuation interrupted by brief bursts of high-amplitude slow waves with or without intermixed waves of other frequencies (burst-suppression EEG); and pattern D, which is described as an equipotential (isoelectric) EEG (Fig. 19.20). In this group of patients(111), pat-

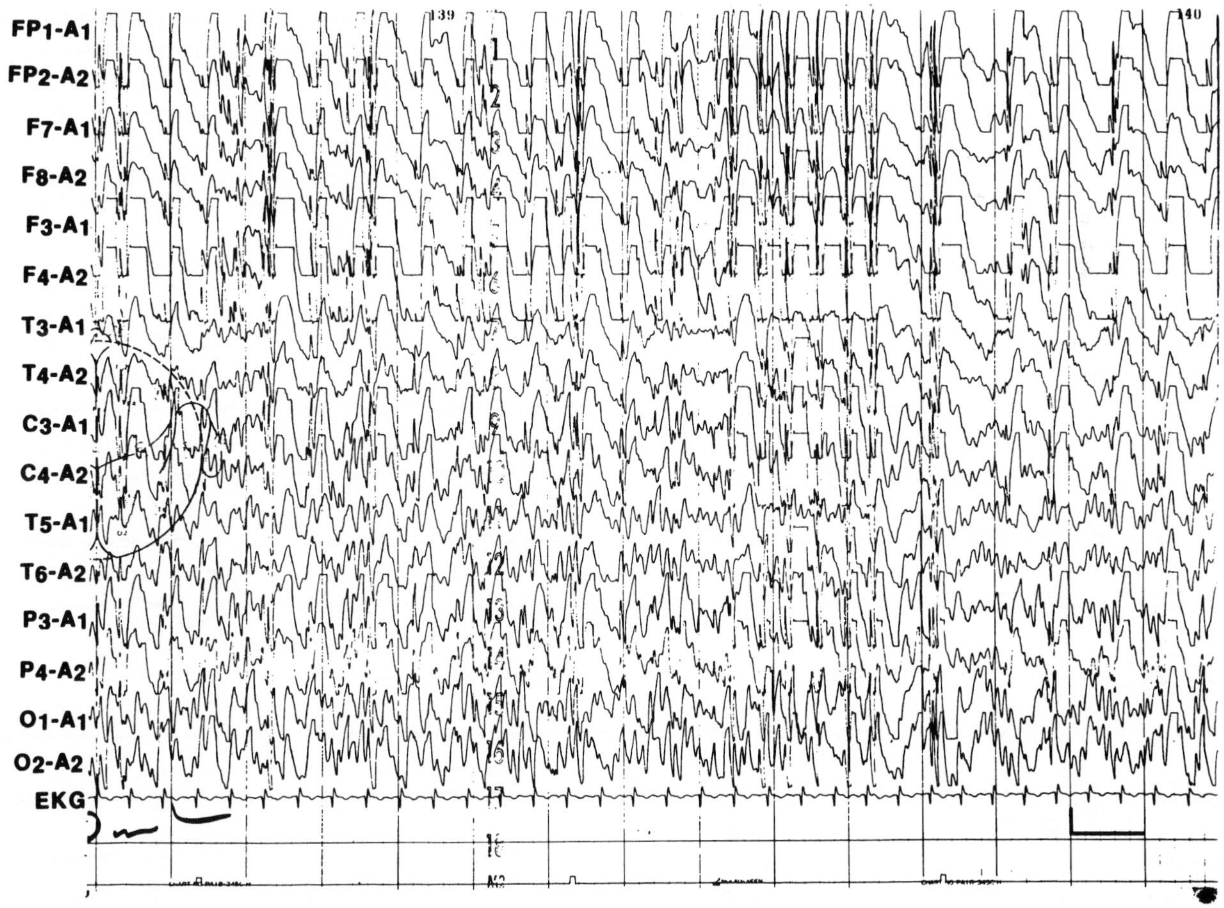

Figure 19.17. Absence status in an encephalopathic patient. This 9-year-old boy was being treated with phenytoin for idiopathic epilepsy. He presented in a dazed state, able to ambulate and converse but appearing distant and confused. His EEG depicts continuous generalized spike-wave activity. Treatment with intravenous lorazepam and discontinuation of phenytoin terminated the episode. *Horizontal bar,* 1 second; *vertical bar,* 100 μV.

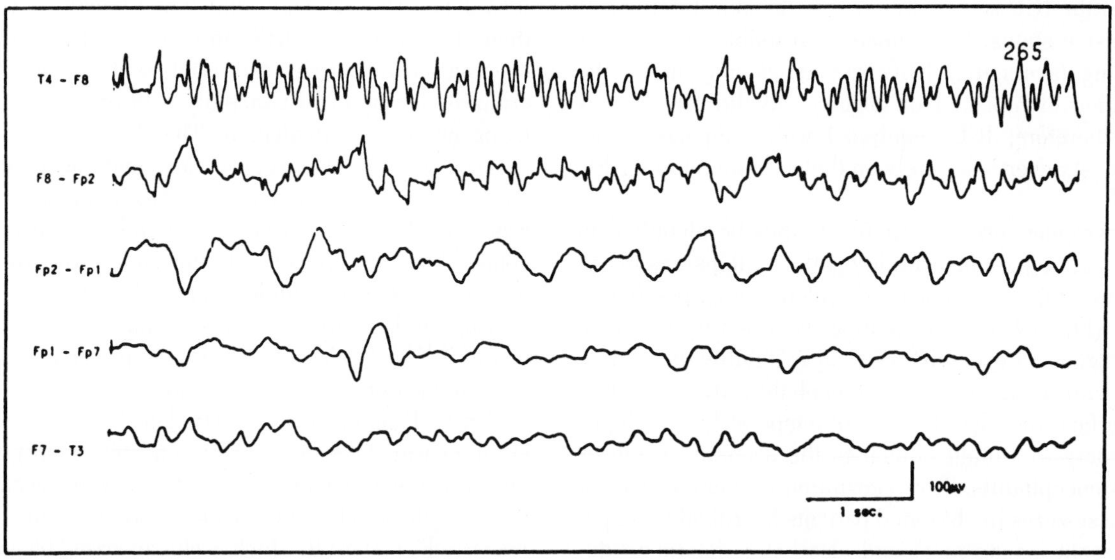

Figure 19.18. Partial-complex (psychomotor) status. This 5-year-old girl developed unexplained stupor and alteration of consciousness after surgery for craniopharyngioma. She appeared awake but made no visual contact. She could not follow simple commands and mumbled nonsensically. No definite convulsive movements were observed. Her EEG shows continuous spike and spike-wave discharges in the midtemporal region on the right (i.e., *upper trace* labeled *T4–F8*). (From Mayeux R, Lueders H. Complex partial status epilepticus. Case report and proposal for diagnostic criteria. Neurology 1978;28:957.)

terns B, C, and D, evident within 2 to 12 hours of the CNS insult, invariably predicted a poor outcome (death or severe neurologic dysfunction). Those children with pattern A all recovered promptly (although some had subsequent cardiorespiratory arrests). On the other hand, other reports of anoxic encephalopathy have not provided as clear-cut a set of prognostic criteria. For instance, in reports of freshwater near-drownings, Kruus and colleagues[118] described patients with at least early EEG features compatible with Pampiglione and Harden's pattern A who developed severe neurologic sequelae and others with pattern B who had a "favorable" recovery. Nevertheless, most studies document that burst-suppression patterns (Pampiglione and Harden's pattern C) and isoelectric EEGs invariably indicate fatal or severely compromised functional outcomes.

EEG criteria are frequently used in the diagnosis of brain

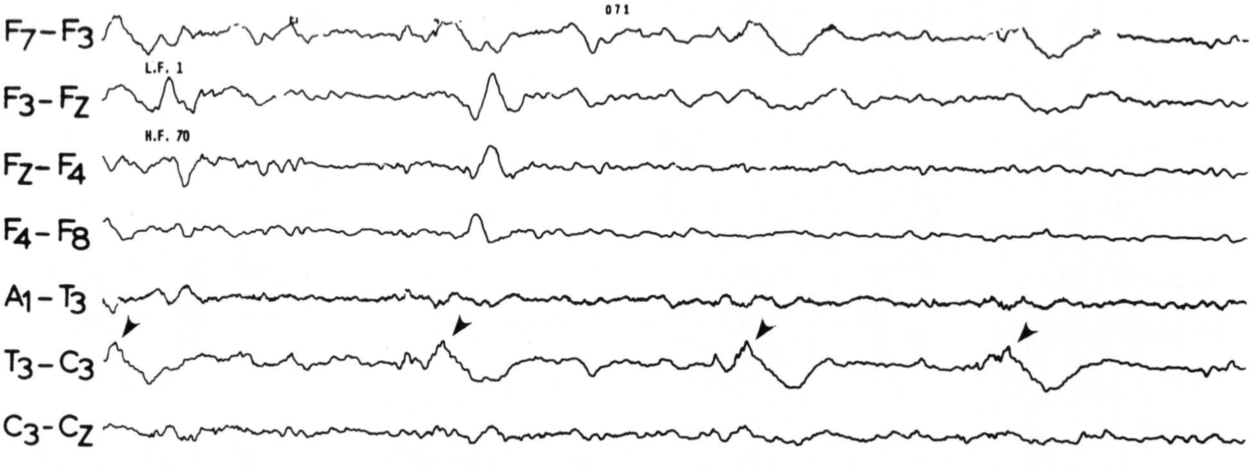

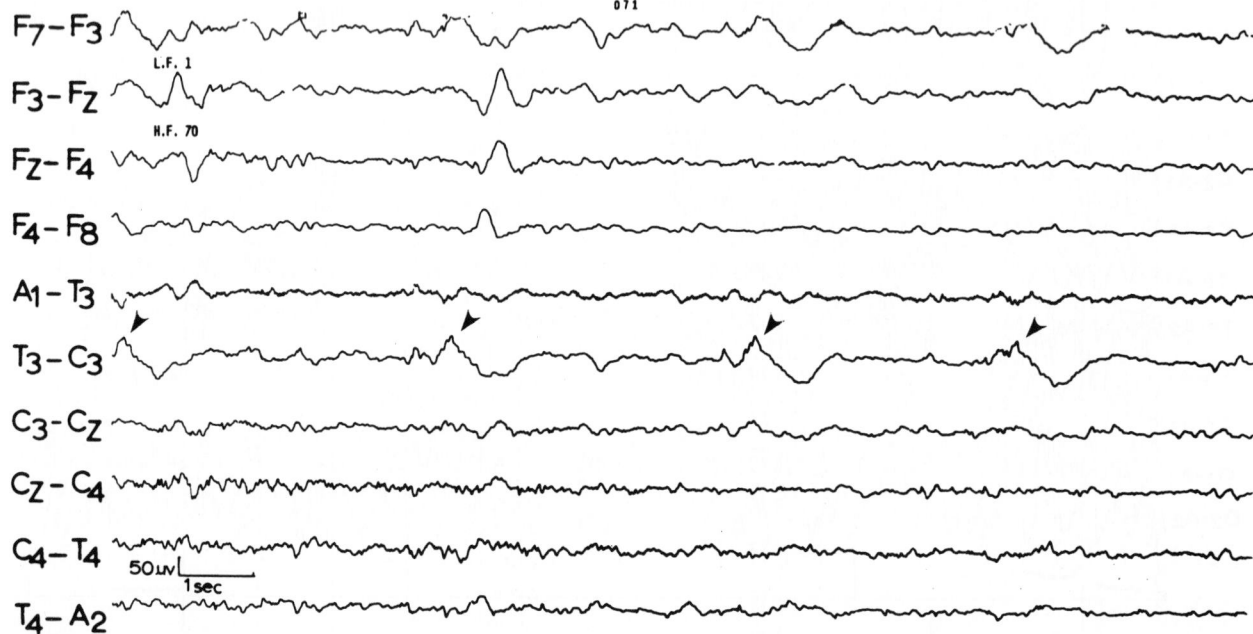

Figure 19.19. Focal epileptiform discharges in a patient with herpes simplex encephalitis. Severe headache and photophobia developed in this previously healthy individual, followed by fever and the onset of seizures. The EEG demonstrates left temporal periodic sharp transients *(arrows)*. A diagnosis of herpes simplex encephalitis was made on clinical grounds. (Figure and history are provided courtesy of Dr. F. Matsuo, Department of Neurology, University of Utah School of Medicine.)

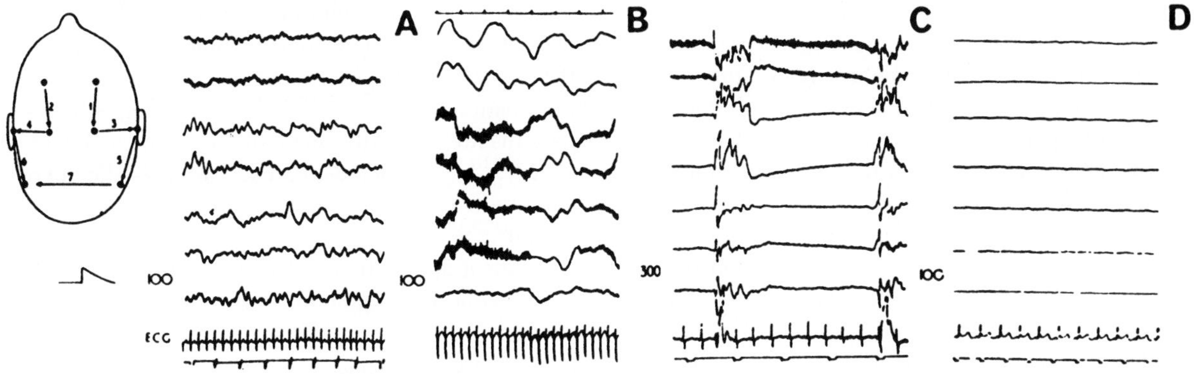

Figure 19.20. Four EEG patterns of coma (according to Pampiglione). **A.** EEG shows some excess slow rhythms but is only mildly abnormal. **B.** Diffuse δ-wave activity without faster frequencies. This is the most common pattern seen in encephalopathies of diverse causes. **C.** So-called burst-suppression pattern, in which prolonged periods of marked EEG attenuation are interrupted by briefer bursts of irregular waves of intermixed frequencies. **D.** Isoelectric (equipotential) EEG. The latter two patterns are only rarely compatible with survival. (From Pampiglione G, Harden A. Resuscitation after cardio-circulatory arrest. Lancet 1968;1:1261.)

death, (see Chapter 27 for details). It must be stressed that these criteria may be different for children than for adults. In fact, the younger the infant, the less reliable the EEG for determination of CNS viability. Extreme caution is required in defining cerebral death in the setting of the profoundly comatose child under the age of 2 months. On the other hand, clinical judgment of outcome in the severely ill, comatose neonate is rarely faulty if the cause of the encephalopathy is properly identified. Although references to unexpected survival in infants with extremely abnormal EEGs abound in the medical literature, such survivors are virtually invariably severely handicapped. Finally, there are reports in children (primarily infants) in whom apparent cessation of CBF was accompanied by persistent low-amplitude EEG activity[(119)]. Fortunately, such unusual cases are rare, but they, too, emphasize the need to use the EEG as one in a series of different means of determining CNS function and viability.

In traumatic coma, the EEG is perhaps less predictive, although again the extremes of abnormality (burst-suppression pattern or isoelectric tracings) strongly indicate unfavorable results. Finally, in the ICU setting, the confounding effect of CNS depressant medication on EEG activity should always be taken into account[(104,110)]. Thus, high levels of barbiturates, benzodiazepines, or tricyclic antidepressants (among others) may themselves induce generalized δ-frequency slowing or even burst-suppression and isoelectric tracings. Indeed, the endpoint of pentobarbital coma for the treatment of intractable status epilepticus is the induction of a burst-suppression EEG. It is primarily for this reason that prognostication based on EEG findings is critically dependent on an accurate determination of the cause of the encephalopathy.

Techniques of Electroencephalographic Monitoring

As mentioned earlier, the main drawback to the use of the EEG in continuous monitoring of the critically ill patient is the tremendous volume of detailed information it entails. Collecting and interpreting this wealth of material quickly becomes a practical impossibility. For this reason, in part, various means of consolidating, averaging, or compressing EEG data have been developed[(120,121)]. These have become increasingly available and sophisticated due to progress in computer hardware and software. Numerous different methods for condensing the EEG have been described[(120)], including channel integration, filtering, subtraction, and more standardized digital methods known as the cerebral function monitor (CFM)[(122)] and the compressed spectral array (CSA)[(123)]. Only the latter two, which are the more readily available and best applicable to intensive care monitoring, are described in detail here. Both have been used for CNS monitoring of children in the ICU setting. The reader interested in other systems is referred to several excellent sources[(115,121,124)].

Cerebral Function Monitor

The CFM was developed in the late 1960s by Maynard[(122)]. The original model and related systems are currently commercially available. The details of their functioning and use have been described extensively by Prior and Maynard[(122)].

The various forms of this monitoring system are relatively inexpensive and are easily admitted into the ICU setting. They share the following characteristics: The monitor displays as an on-line paper trace the condensed data obtained from a single EEG channel (i.e., single pair of electrodes). The EEG data are processed in several ways to produce a tracing that depicts the variation in and range of summated EEG amplitude over time. Amplitude is plotted in the vertical direction on a partially logarithmic scale, with the range of amplitude (peak to peak) at any one time depicted by a vertical line whose upper and lower endpoints indicate the maximum and minimum EEG amplitudes, respectively, over that particular period of time (Fig. 19.21). The device automatically assigns different weights to different frequencies to compensate for the fact that slower waves (e.g., δ-frequency activity) are in general of greater amplitude than are waves of faster frequencies (e.g., α- and β-frequency activity). Finally, the mechanism includes several means of artifact rejection. Thus, the final tracing consists of a continuous band, the upper edge of which indicates the maximum EEG amplitude at any one time, while the lower edge represents minimum EEG amplitude (Fig. 19.21). Typically, paper speed is set such that 1 to 2 minutes of EEG activity is condensed into a 1-cm distance on the tracing.

As can be determined from the above description, the simplest form of the CFM provides no information regarding the frequency distribution of the original EEG activity. This is a serious drawback to the system[116,117]. Subsequent models have addressed this problem by providing simultaneous crude estimates of the percentage contribution of various frequencies (δ, θ, α, and β) to the net EEG amplitude. One such model (the cerebral function analyzing monitor (CFAM))[122] will provide an estimate of percent suppression. Finally, the CFAM also presents a continuous readout of muscle artifact and electrode impedance, both representing measures that may aid in artifact identification (Fig. 19.22).

It should be immediately obvious that both the CFM and the CFAM markedly condense the EEG. The routine EEG requires at least three pages to depict the amount of time condensed into 1 cm of CFM output. On the other hand, a tremendous amount of detail is, of necessity, lost. Nevertheless, the resultant tracings can be very useful in the continuous monitoring of critically ill, comatose, or encephalopathic patients. Occasional routine EEG recordings, however, are necessary to complement the CFM and to aid in its proper interpretation[116,117].

Interpretation, and training in interpretation, of the CFM tracing is claimed to be relatively simple and to be accessible to ICU staff with modest training[122]. By and large, interpretation rests on the recognition of trends (e.g., progressively declining amplitude over time (Fig. 19.23) in the case of increasing CNS dysfunction from increased ICP or the sequelae of hypoxic-ischemic brain damage) or of distinct patterns[116,117,122,125–128]. For example, classic comb patterns are seen with burst-suppression EEG activity (Fig. 19.24)[116,117], whereas periodic or episodic increases in amplitude can accompany cerebral seizure activity (Fig. 19.25)[129,130].

Clinical applications of the CFM are summarized in the next section in conjunction with CSA.

Compressed Spectral Array

Of the currently available methods of EEG monitoring, the so-called compressed spectral display, often referred to in the literature as the compressed spectral array (CSA), probably represents the most widely used method[120,123]. It may also retain and depict a greater amount of detail than the aforementioned CFM.

The CSA produces a pseudo-three-dimensional image of the temporal evolution of EEG frequency distribution and relative amplitude over time. The system, originally described by Bickford and colleagues[123], relies on computerized Fourier analysis of the underlying EEG. This computational process allows for extraction of relative contributions of various frequencies to the overall EEG trace and thereby generates a frequency spectrum.

In this approach, the EEG derived over a certain predefined interval of time (epoch) is analyzed (Fig. 19.26). The frequency spectrum of a given epoch is plotted as a horizontal tracing in which upward deflections represent the presence of EEG activity at a given frequency. By convention, low to high frequencies are depicted from left to right, and the intensity (power or amplitude squared) of a given

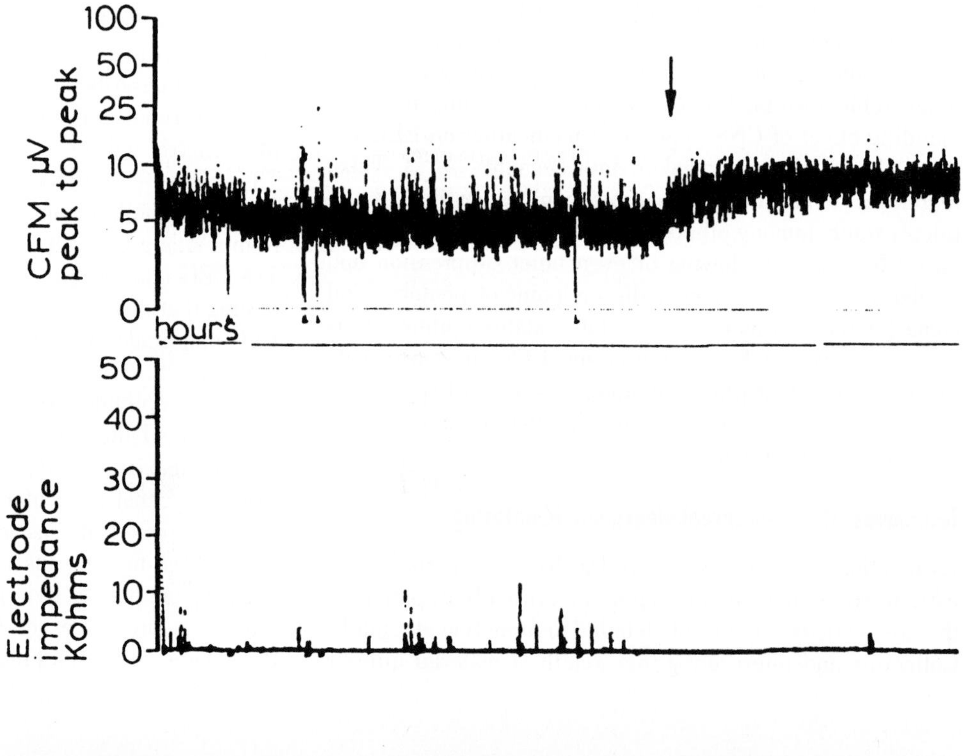

Figure 19.21. Typical cerebral function monitor (CFM) tracing. Summated EEG amplitude is depicted in the thick band in the upper portion of the printout. Thus, at the beginning of this tracing, maximum amplitude is around 7 to 8 μV, and minimum amplitude averages 5 μV or less. At the *arrow*, the patient fell asleep, with a resultant change in amplitude distribution. The *bottom scale* registers electrode impedance. Upward deflections on this scale usually indicate movement or other causes of poor electrode contact. Note that the tracing provides no information about frequency distribution of EEG activity. The entire length of this recording is less than 2 hours. Another normal CFM tracing can be seen in Figure 19.25*A*. (From Prior PF, Maynard DE. Monitoring cerebral function. New York: Elsevier, 1986.)

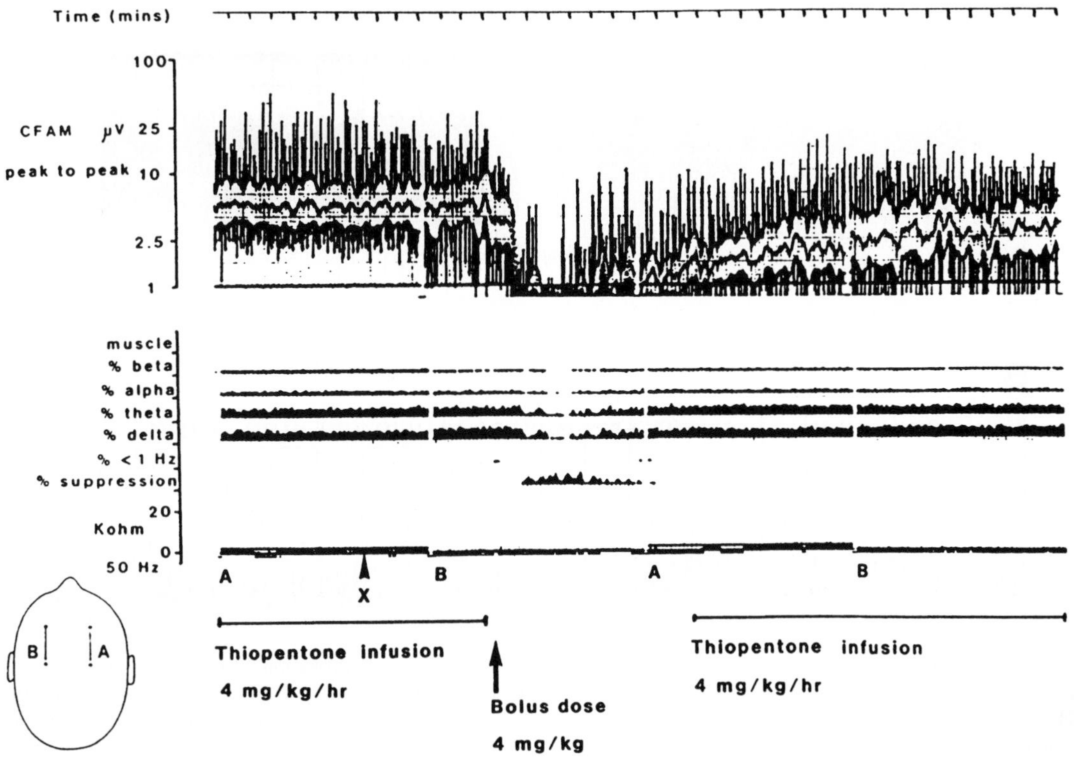

Figure 19.22. Typical cerebral function analyzing monitor (CFAM) tracing. The *upper trace* is similar to the output of the CFM (Fig. 19.21), except that an amplitude envelope is depicted (upper and lower extremes of amplitude), with the *central line* in the *clear region* indicating the median summated amplitude at any one time. Below the amplitude tracing are individual outputs that give an estimate of percent contribution of the various frequency ranges (delta, theta, etc.) to the overall EEG. An estimate of *% suppression* is also provided. In this case, note how the large intravenous bolus of thiopentone induces marked EEG attenuation (i.e., amplitude declines drastically, and *% suppression* increases in the interval immediately after the *arrow* indicating bolus dose). Note also that activity from any given electrode pair must be recorded separately (two pairs are recorded alternately in this case). (From Tasker RC, et al. The cerebral function analyzing monitor in paediatric medical intensive care: applications and limitations. Intensive Care Med 1990;16:60.)

frequency is proportional to the height of the resultant deflection (or peak). The CSA then plots the spectra of subsequent epochs above the previous epoch's tracing. Finally, the computer subtracts out (or suppresses) portions of the tracing that would otherwise appear behind (actually above) a previous epoch (Fig. 19.27). This hidden line suppression creates the illusion of a three-dimensional figure in which the x-axis represents frequency, the y-axis represents time, and the (imagined) z-axis represents intensity (amplitude squared).

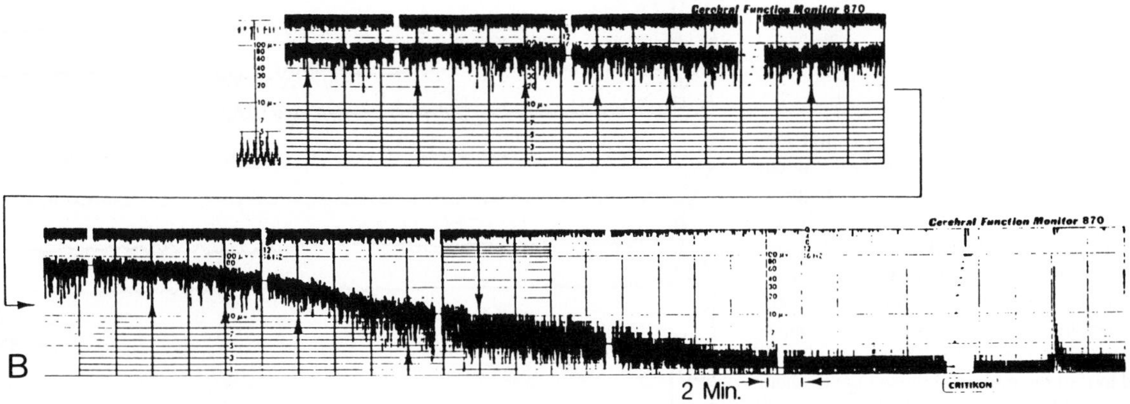

Figure 19.23. Gradual decline in amplitude of CFM tracing. Progressive decrease in EEG activity is clearly shown by the CFM. In this case, the decline in amplitude is secondary to repeated doses of an anticonvulsant, but a similar pattern could accompany progressive cerebral edema, increasing intracranial pressure, worsening metabolic status, etc. Recognition of patterns such as this could perhaps prompt appropriate therapeutic intervention. (From Talwar D, Torres F. Continuous electrophysiologic monitoring of cerebral function in the pediatric intensive care unit. Pediatr Neurol 1988;4:137.)

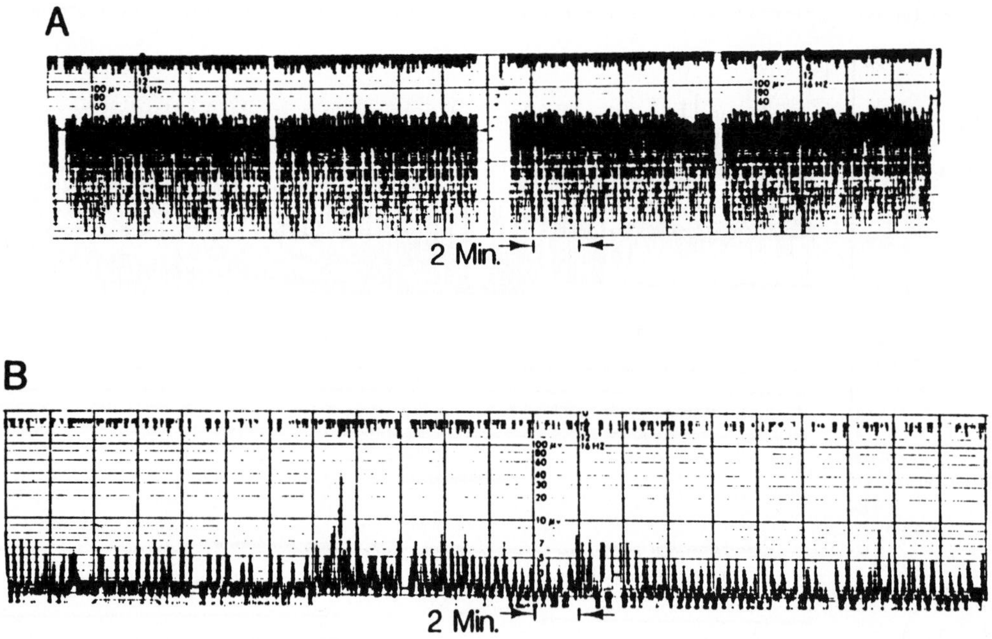

Figure 19.24. Comb patterns on the CFM. Comb patterns such as these indicate a burst-suppression EEG. In **A,** the periods of relative EEG activity are interrupted by briefer bursts of attenuation, resulting in a downward comb pattern. In **B,** the opposite holds, with relatively greater attenuation resulting in an upward comb pattern. (From Talwar D, Torres F. Continuous electrophysiologic monitoring of cerebral function in the pediatric intensive care unit. Pediatr Neurol 1988;4:137.)

Typically, unlike the CFM, CSA data are usually generated from multichannel montages[120]. Frequencies from 0.5 to 20 Hz are generally included. Epochs are most often 4 to 10 seconds in duration, and the longer the epoch, the greater the averaging and the greater the loss of detail. In most cases, CSA monitors produce two parallel records, with each representing the compressed spectral output from one hemisphere (Fig. 19.28). It is also possible to produce a fi-

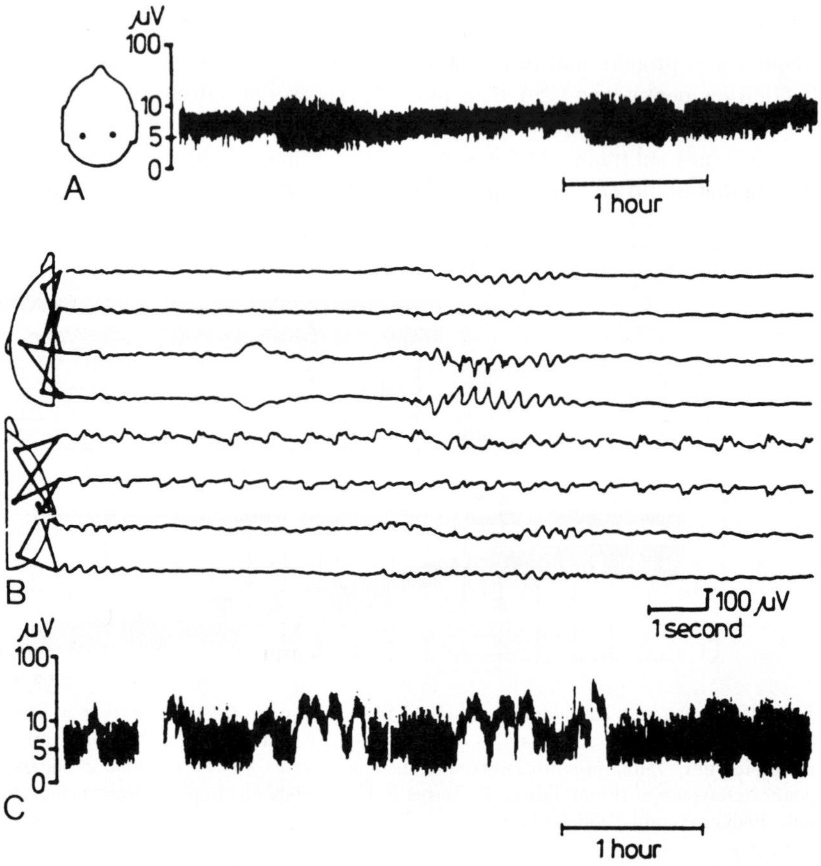

Figure 19.25. Sawtooth seizure pattern on CFM. Compared with a normal tracing **(A),** the CFM will record episodic electrographic seizure activity as sudden increases in amplitude punctuated by erratic returns toward baseline **(C).** This will result in a sawtooth pattern, as seen in **C.** The routine EEG tracing **(B)** from the same patient (not simultaneous, however) illustrates how such an amplitude increase is generated. The electrographic seizure noted toward the middle of the left hemisphere tracing **(B)** would contribute markedly to increasing the amplitude of the CFM tracing. The more such activity, the higher (and longer) the period of increased amplitude recorded by the CFM would be. (From Bjerre I, Hellstrom-Westas L, et al. Monitoring of cerebral functions after severe asphyxia in infancy. Arch Dis Child 1983;58:997.)

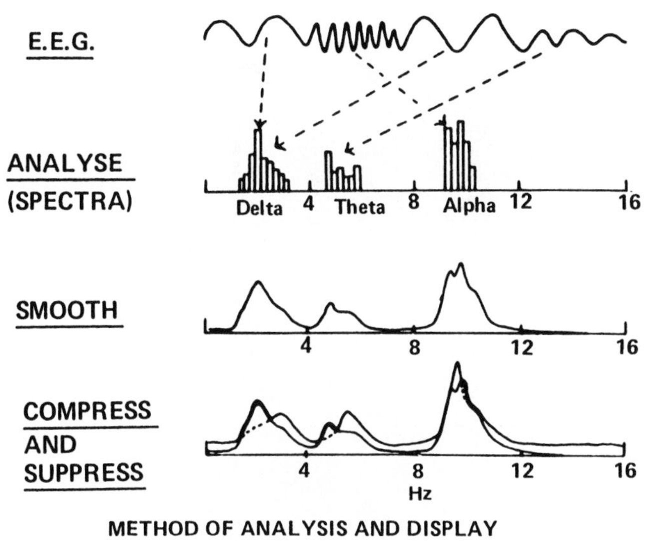

Figure 19.26. Schematic diagram illustrating means of creating compressed spectral EEG tracing. An "epoch" of EEG activity is shown at the *top*. Fourier analysis breaks this epoch down into constituent frequency contributions. The crude frequency spectrum is then smoothed. In the *lowest frame,* a second epoch has been analyzed and is depicted behind (actually above) the first. Elimination of that portion of the second spectrum appearing behind the first is depicted with *dotted lines.* (From Bickford RG. Newer methods of recording and analyzing EEGs. In: Klass DW, Daly DD, eds. Current practice of clinical electroencephalography. New York: Raven Press, 1979:451.)

nal display including spectral data from several different brain regions arranged topographically[(120)], but this becomes unwieldy and less applicable to critical care monitoring.

It should be noted that the CSA and the CFM share certain advantages. Both are able to compress data and thereby make continuous or frequent intermittent EEG monitoring manageable. Both theoretically allow for EEG monitors at the bedside in the ICU without requiring continuous technician support and at a lower cost (than could be achieved with conventional EEG equipment). In practice, however, proper interpretation of the CFM (and most assuredly of the CSA) requires that occasional (serial) standard EEGs be obtained so as to validate the conclusions drawn from the monitor tracing and to identify potential artifact or EEG signals (e.g., epileptiform discharges) not always readily discernible with CFM or CSA[(116,117,124)]. Other potential advantages include easy comprehensibility and consequent ease of interpretation.

The CFM (or CFAM) or the CSA may be useful in the monitoring of nontraumatic and traumatic patients in coma, in the monitoring of the neurologically endangered patient in whom clinical examination is substantially curtailed, in the evaluation of treatment effectiveness in status epilepticus, in the management of increased ICP, in the monitoring of neurologically ill patients at risk from cardiovascular instability, and in the recognition of patient care procedures that may have deleterious effects (e.g., endotracheal suctioning in the patient with increased ICP). In addition, response to treatment in metabolic encephalopathies can also be followed over time.

In contrasting the two methods, it should be noted that the CFM is limited by single-channel output, thus the findings are highly dependent on appropriate selection of recording electrode placement[(130)]. Furthermore, information regarding frequency distribution is less detailed with the CFM[(117)], making recognition of fluctuating patterns in coma (see below) more challenging. On the other hand, the identification of epileptic phenomena may be more difficult with CSA[(117)], although this is variable. To date, no study has compared these two tools with regard to diagnostic or prognostic accuracy or in terms of cost or ease of interpretation[(117)].

The CSA may be useful in most of the situations described previously in reference to the CFM. Perhaps its greatest alleged utility has been in the prediction of outcome from coma[(104,128)]. In this regard, most studies have demonstrated that a fluctuating frequency spectral pattern carries a better prognosis than a continuous, unrelenting (invariable) slow-wave spectrum (Fig. 19.28)[(131–134)]. In the former (the fluctuating pattern), the CSA readily demonstrates that in addition to the high-amplitude, persistent δ-peak typical of most encephalopathies, an intermittent, often irregular θ- or α-peak (of lower amplitude) occasionally appears over a prolonged (8 to 24 hour) period. The appearance of this second peak tends to confer a more positive outlook for neurologic recovery. In contrast, shifting the CSA spectrum from the fluctuating to the invariable type portends a more negative ultimate outcome. A shift in the opposite direction (invariable to fluctuating) may be more favorable. The discernment of such subtle EEG frequency

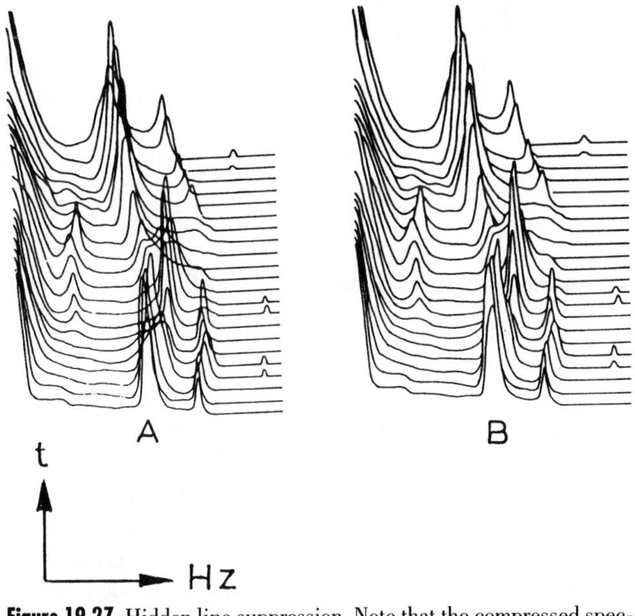

Figure 19.27. Hidden line suppression. Note that the compressed spectral display in **B** is identical with that originally produced (in **A**), except that portions of subsequent lines, which are overlapped by a previous line, are removed (suppressed). This creates the illusion of three dimensions and improves the visual clarity of the resultant display. (Adapted from Prior PF, Maynard DE. Monitoring cerebral function. New York: Elseiver, 1986.)

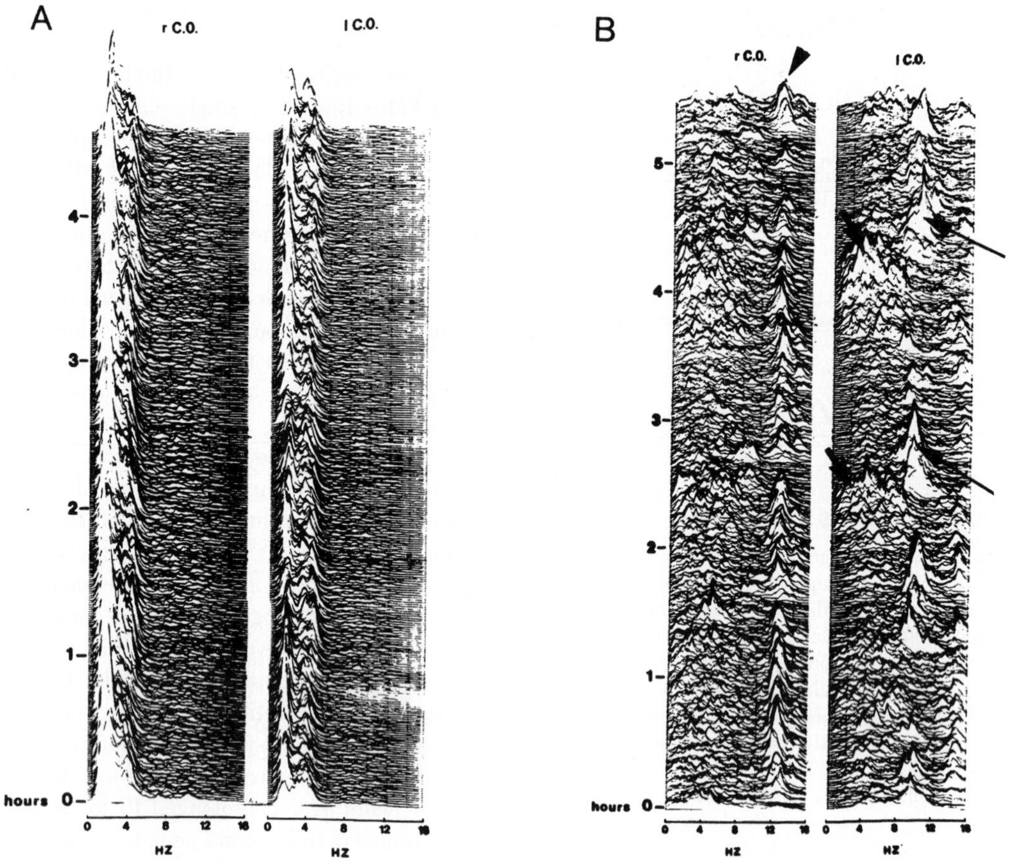

Figure 19.28. Invariable versus fluctuating compressed spectral array (CSA) tracings. Note that in **A,** the frequency spectrum is limited to monotonous activity in the δ-wave range throughout this prolonged recording. In contrast, in **B,** the left hemisphere *(l C.O.)* shows periods of predominant slow activity *(short arrows),* but frequent peaks in the α-wave range are also seen *(long arrows).* (The right hemisphere *[r C.O.]* shows a sleep-like pattern with β-wave peaks *[arrowhead].*) The monotonous (or invariable) pattern similar to that seen in **A** predicts a poorer prognosis than the fluctuating pattern (**B,** *l C.O.*). (Adapted from Bricolo A, et al. Electrophysiological monitoring in the intensive care unit. Electroencephalogr Clin Neurophysiol 1987;39(Suppl):255.)

fluctuations may be difficult or impossible with either serial standard EEGs or the CFM[104,131–134]. In the case of the former, EEG frequency fluctuations either may not be adequately sampled or may simply be sufficiently subtle to escape detection by even the trained encephalographer. The CFM usually does not provide adequate detail regarding frequency spectra to discern these shifts.

Electroencephalographic Monitoring Precautions

Several disadvantages of electroencephalographic monitoring systems have been alluded to. First, although some artifact rejection or identification is built into the equipment, contamination and misinterpretation remain significant problems. Although on the surface interpretation is much simpler (than with conventional electroencephalography), all staff members (from physicians to nursing personnel) caring for patients should have a basic understanding of the tracing and be able to recognize significant patterns or changes if the full value of the technique is to be realized. Perhaps of greatest importance is that undue reliance on these technologic marvels not produce unwarranted complacency in the evaluation of neurologically impaired or comatose children and not lead to careless application of the physical and neurologic examination. The physician caring for critically ill patients must remember that, to date, routine electroencephalography monitoring has never been demonstrated to result in improved outcome.

EVOKED POTENTIALS

EPs consist of a heterogeneous group of neurophysiologic phenomena in which a particular stimulus results in a predictable, characteristic change in the EEG. The resultant EEG change or wave, the EP, represents the ". . . electrical manifestation of the brain's reception of and response to a given external stimulus"[135]. Different generic types of EPs can be defined[121,135]. Short-latency EPs refer to EEG events occurring immediately after a stimulus (within intervals of several msec to 100 msec), whereas long-latency EPs appear in the EEG after a longer delay. Short-latency EPs have a greater predictability, demonstrate less interpersonal variability, and appear at very consistent time intervals (latencies) following the stimulus. They are not particularly influenced by level of cognitive awareness, nor are they suppressed by high levels of sedative drugs. Long-latency EPs, which include event-related or endogenous potentials such as the P300 EP, are less reproducible and are subject to greater influence by psychologic factors, particularly by selective attention. All EP measurements applicable to clinical intensive care medicine are of short latency, whereas event-related potentials are primarily used in psychophysiologic research.

In any case, the recording of EPs has become a routine adjunct to the clinical evaluation of many neurologic conditions, including circumstances requiring critical care[135]. Strictly speaking, EP measurements cannot be used for continuous or even frequent intermittent monitoring of patients in the ICU setting. However, they may have a place in the serial evaluation of certain neurologic conditions, particularly encephalopathies. In this regard, three different short-latency EPs are used on the basis of the three different sensory modalities that can be readily activated: visual, auditory, and somatosensory.

General Methodology of Evoked Potentials

In general, the methodologic principles underlying the different stimulus-elicited EPs are very similar. They are first described in generic terms, and then specifics are detailed for each EP type.

EPs are of very low amplitude (less than 20 μV) relative to spontaneous background EEG activity. Thus, a single stimulus results in an EP that cannot be readily discerned from this continuous background. The ability to summate intervals of EEG activity accurately following and time-locked to serial identical stimuli allows for the magnification of the EP signal relative to the background noise[120,121,135]. This step, which depends on a signal averager, is the crucial technologic advance that has allowed EP measurements to become clinically applicable. In effect, the summation of sequential epochs of EEG that follow serial identical stimuli allows for magnification of any electrical event that follows the stimulus by a specific, reproducible, identical time interval (latency) (Fig. 19.29). In contrast, EEG activity that is random in relation to the stimulus tends to be canceled out. Thus, there is a resultant (and progressive) increase in the signal-to-noise ratio as greater numbers of stimulus repetitions are summated (Fig. 19.29).

The end product of this process consists of one or more tracings of amplitude versus time. Each tracing represents the summed output of a given electrode pair connected to a differential amplifier (as in the routine EEG). The tracing will have a stimulus artifact at its inception (marking the time of stimulus delivery) and subsequent (hopefully) recognizable waves will be present. The most useful data to be derived from these tracings consist of time intervals between waves (interpeak latencies) and the actual presence or absence of recognizable waves. Amplitude values (either absolute or in the form of wave-amplitude ratios) are less reliable and are infrequently used for routine clinical purposes.

Successful obtaining of EPs is dependent, therefore, on reproducible serial production of an identical stimulus (although the patient need not be cognitively aware of the stimulus delivery). The signal averager must be able to mark the precise time of stimulus delivery in order to sum sequential responses accurately. Sufficient vertical (amplitude) and horizontal (temporal) resolution is essential, as well as adequate memory capacity to store information that is then averaged. Artifact is a common obstacle to the quality of the test, and considerable sophistication is required on the part of both the technician and the interpreter.

The clinician attempting to gain an understanding of EPs for the first time is frequently frustrated by the fact that few conventions have been established regarding nomenclature in this rapidly developing field. Specifically, the naming of particular EP waveforms varies tremendously, as does the description of polarity of peaks (positive or negative). Furthermore, norms for various measured parameters (e.g., interpeak latencies, absolute latencies) must be established for each machine and each laboratory[135]. This not only complicates clinical application of these laboratory tests but often makes comparison of findings in different laboratories difficult. Attempts at understanding results published in the literature can literally become a nightmarish experience. In the descriptions that follow, an effort is made to

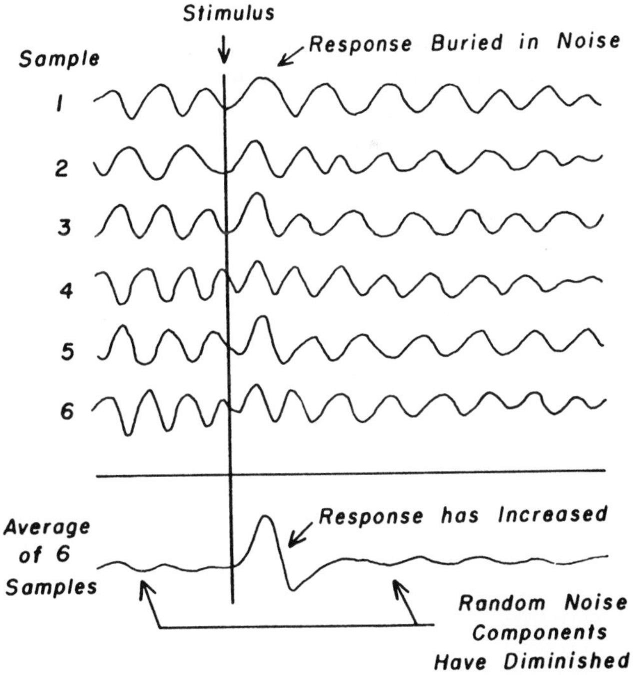

Figure 19.29. Principle of signal averaging. Six samples of EEG activity after a similar stimulus are shown. Note that the response that is poorly distinguished from background occurs at approximately the same time interval after the stimulus. Other waves are random relative to the stimulus. If the samples are summed, the tracing shown below is generated, in which the response has been amplified and the background decreased. (From Bickford RG. Newer methods of recording and analyzing EEGs. In: Klass DW, Daly DD, eds. Current practice of clinical electroencephalography. New York: Raven Press, 1979;451–480.)

use only commonly encountered nomenclature, but the reader must remain aware of this problem in terminology.

Visual Evoked Potentials: Methodology

Of the three commonly performed EPs, the visual evoked potential (VEP) is by far the simplest and easiest to understand(135,136).

Stimulus

In the awake patient, the most commonly used stimulus is the so-called pattern-shift visual target, in which a checkerboard pattern on a video monitor shifts from light to dark repeatedly. In the ICU setting, a repetitive flash stimulus is more likely to be used (specifically with comatose or obtunded children)(137).

Electrode Placement and Channels

The active electrode is typically placed over the occipital lobes, usually in the midline. The reference electrode is distant, over the mastoid, earlobe, or frontal head region. A single channel comparing these two electrodes is usually sufficient.

Resulting Waveforms

The typical VEP consists of a large biphasic or triphasic wave whose most prominent (positive) peak occurs (in adults) approximately 100 msec after the stimulus (Fig. 19.30). The main parameter used in the evaluation of the VEP is the absolute latency of this P100 wave (i.e., time from stimulus to P100 peak). Since this temporal interval reflects transmission time from retina to occipital cortex, different latencies may be elicited with monocular stimulation of either eye. (This occurs, for example, when demyelination of one optic nerve slows conduction relative to the other.) Thus, the comparison of P100 latencies elicited by monocular stimulation may also represent a useful measure (although less commonly so in the ICU setting).

Brainstem Auditory Evoked Potentials: Methodology

Brainstem auditory evoked potentials (BAEP) occur at differing time intervals after an auditory stimulus. For all intents and purposes, only those occurring within the first 10 msec are sufficiently reproducible to be of clinical value. These short-latency EPs are generated within brainstem structures and the cochlear nerve, thus their integrity and latencies reflect brainstem function(135,138,139). Although the electrical signals are generated in the brainstem, they are volume conducted through CNS substance and are recorded from the scalp. Therefore, they are referred to as far-field potentials.

Stimulus

A click stimulus is delivered manually to one ear while the other is masked with white noise. Typically, the click represents an electrical square wave lasting 100 to 200 msec, deflecting the device toward (condensation) or away from (rarefaction) the tympanic membrane. Stimulus repetition

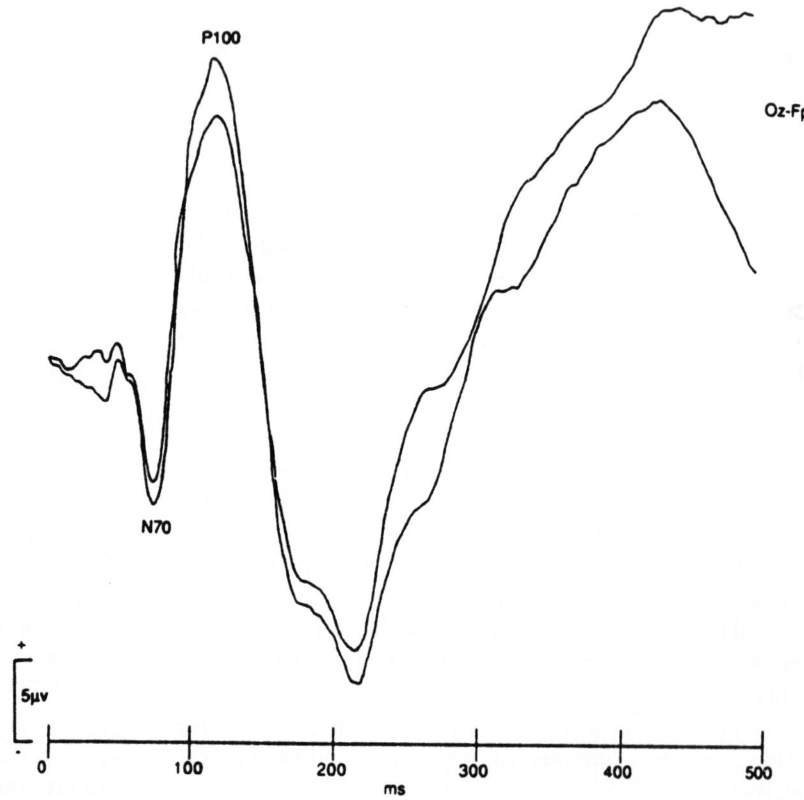

Figure 19.30. Typical visual evoked potential (VEP). The typical (normal) VEP consists of a negative deflection followed by a larger positive peak occurring approximately 100 msec after the stimulus. (Adapted from Taylor MJ, Farrell EJ. Comparison of the prognostic utility of VEPs and SEPs in comatose children. Pediatr Neurol 1989;5:145–150.)

rate is usually 10/sec, and over 1000 repetitions are necessary. Rarefaction clicks are preferable because wave I (see below) is better elicited. Interpretation of the BAEP is not possible without wave I (135, 140), hence the importance of this choice. Stimulus intensity significantly affects results, thus an intensity of at least 60 dB over threshold is usually employed.

Electrode Placement and Channels

Interpretation of the BAEP is facilitated by recordings from at least four channels[118]. Typically, a scalp electrode at the vertex (C_z) is referred to each ear ($A_i - C_z$, $A_c - C_z$, where A_i and A_c designate the ipsilateral and contralateral ears, respectively), a channel is used to compare the signal at one ear with the signal at the other ($A_i - A_c$), and an additional channel may compare vertex activity with that at the inion (C − inion). Wave I, which is believed to represent reception of stimulus by and activation of the cochlear nerve, is best delineated on the interconnected ear channel, whereas waves II to V are better seen from channels including scalp electrodes[135].

Resulting Waveforms

The resulting normal tracing typically consists of five waves with vertex positivity (named waves I to V), whereas later waves occurring at 7 to 10 msec (waves VI, VII) are less reliably elicited (Fig. 19.31). Proper identification of wave I is crucial, since its appearance guarantees that the stimulus has entered the nervous system (i.e., has activated the cochlear nerve). If wave I is not seen, the study must be considered uninterpretable, since no alternative means of proving stimulus effectiveness is available[135,140]. Successive waves are believed to represent activation of various points along the brainstem auditory pathways, with wave V probably representing neuronal activity at the level of the inferior colliculus (mesencephalic level)[138,139].

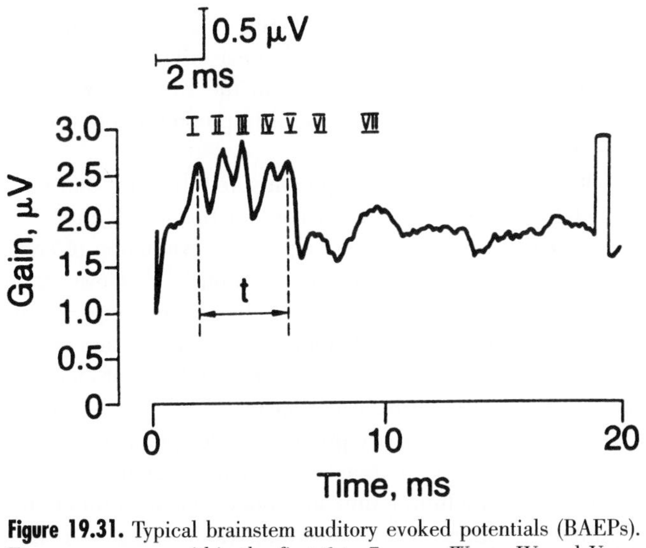

Figure 19.31. Typical brainstem auditory evoked potentials (BAEPs). Five waves occur within the first 6 to 7 msec. Waves IV and V are often part of a common peak. (Adapted from Lutschg J, et al. Brainstem auditory evoked potentials and early somatosensory evoked potentials in neurointensively treated comatose children. Am J Dis Child 1983;137:421, copyright 1983, American Medical Association.)

The most useful parameters obtained from the BAEP include calculation of interpeak latencies, particularly the I to V interpeak latency. In the ICU setting, loss of waves subsequent to wave I represents a critical finding (see below).

Somatosensory Evoked Potentials: Methodology

Of the clinically relevant EPs, somatosensory evoked potentials (SEPs) are perhaps the most fraught with difficulty, in terms of consistency in both methodology and interpretation. In general, SEPs can be obtained from stimulation of either the upper or the lower extremity. The latter is by far more challenging[141] and, although commonly used for intraoperative monitoring of spinal surgery, is perhaps less critical to the intensive care of children. Thus, only the upper extremity SEPs are described here. The reader is referred to Chiappa's authoritative text[135] and to other reviews[142,143] for further details.

Stimulus

The median nerve is stimulated at the wrist with an electrical square wave stimulus of 100 to 200 msec in duration and of 10 to 15 mA. The intensity is typically adjusted to achieve perceptible movement of the thumb in response to each stimulus. A total of fewer than five stimulations per second is desirable, and care must be taken, particularly in obtunded patients, to avoid tissue damage from high-repetition frequency or long pulse durations. As in BAEPs, over 1000 repetitions are generally required.

Electrode Placement and Channels

Median nerve stimulation elicits a series of EPs that appear to emanate from several sequential sites along somatosensory pathways[135,142]. The volley of activity passing through the brachial plexus elicits a wave (referred to as Erb's point potential or, unfortunately, EP). Subsequently, activation of the dorsal root entry zone through the medial lemniscus contributes to a second wave complex occurring approximately 13 msec after the stimulus and consisting of negative and positive components (the order of these depends on polarity conventions). This is the N/P13 wave, best recorded from the scalp. Finally, thalamic and thalamocortical contributions generate the N19/P22 biphasic wave. Electrodes are thus placed at or around Erb's point in the supraclavicular fossa, at a site overlying the spinous process of the second cervical vertebra (C2) and over the scalp in the midline and over the somatosensory cortex bilaterally. At least four channels are desirable to allow for proper identification of all waves. As with the BAEPs, failure to record the 1st wave (Erb's point potential) makes interpretation impossible, since proof of

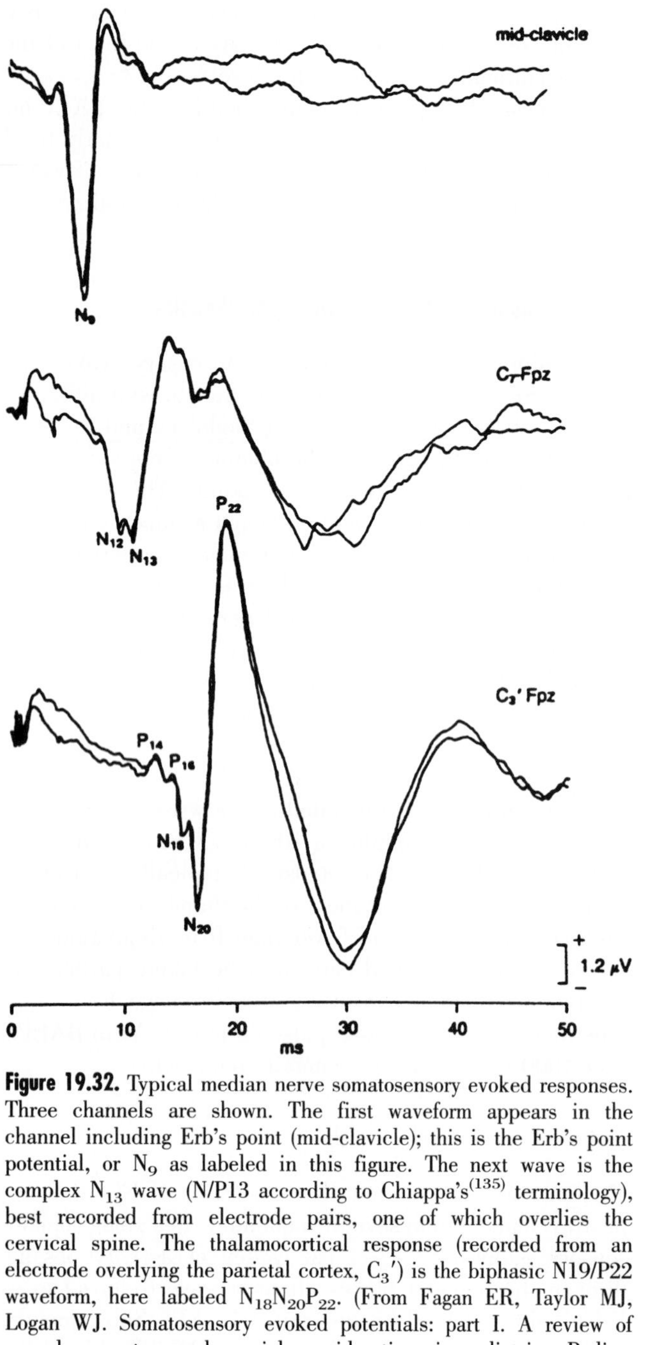

Figure 19.32. Typical median nerve somatosensory evoked responses. Three channels are shown. The first waveform appears in the channel including Erb's point (mid-clavicle); this is the Erb's point potential, or N_9 as labeled in this figure. The next wave is the complex N_{13} wave (N/P13 according to Chiappa's[135] terminology), best recorded from electrode pairs, one of which overlies the cervical spine. The thalamocortical response (recorded from an electrode overlying the parietal cortex, C_3') is the biphasic N19/P22 waveform, here labeled $N_{18}N_{20}P_{22}$. (From Fagan ER, Taylor MJ, Logan WJ. Somatosensory evoked potentials: part I. A review of neural generators and special considerations in pediatrics. Pediatr Neurol 1987;3:189.)

activation of the proximal peripheral nervous system is lacking in such instances[135].

Resulting Waveforms

The median nerve SEP produces three identifiable waveforms, as described above (Fig. 19.32): (1) the Erb's point potential (EP) best recorded from the Erb's point electrode; (2) the N/P13 wave, well seen in channels obtained from electrode pairs including the C2 electrode; and (3) the N19/P22 waveform best recorded from the contralateral somatosensory scalp electrode. As with the other EPs, the most useful parameters (assuming an Erb's point potential is recorded) include presence or absence or subsequent waves and interpeak latencies.

Application of Evoked Potentials to Critical Care

With rare exceptions, there is only a single common application of EP determinations to the critical care of children, and that is in the evaluation and/or prognostication of the encephalopathic child[135,137,144–147]. A particular advantage of EPs over routine or averaged EEG in this regard derives from the fact that EPs are generally unaffected by even high levels of pharmacologic agents that typically markedly affect spontaneous EEG activity[135,144,145,147]. Thus, confounding effects of high anticonvulsant levels or of other sedative agents are not a serious factor in the interpretation of EPs in coma. In addition, some anatomic specificity is afforded by particular EPs. This is at once an advantage and a disadvantage. For example, although BAEPs may provide alternative information specifically about brainstem pathways[144], they are less useful prognostically, since abnormal BAEPs may be associated with intact cognitive function (as in the locked-in syndrome), while normal BAEPs do not preclude the development of a persistent vegetative state[139,144,149]. Although VEPs and SEPs provide some specific information regarding visual and somatosensory pathways, respectively, the latter are clearly the most useful in the prognostic evaluation of coma[137,140,145,146].

In this regard, it has now been repeatedly shown[135,137,140,144,147,150,151] that in children, as in adults, bilateral absence of cortical SEPs in the setting of coma portends poor outcome (brain death or persistent vegetative state) (Fig. 19.33). As alluded to above, such is not necessarily the case with regard to absence or impairment of BAEPs[146,149]. Furthermore, persistent unilateral absence of or latency delay in the cortical SEP is strongly indicative of subsequent contralateral hemiparesis after recovery from coma (Fig. 19.34)[137,144]. Thus, of the EPs, the SEP appears to be the single most useful in prediction of outcome in comatose children.

Other investigators have promulgated the view that multimodality EP studies (i.e., a combination of all three EP types) may be of even more help in the evaluation of coma than any single EP determination alone[152]. However, it should be emphasized that few studies have compared the prognostic accuracy of EP studies with other means of predicting outcome. In rare instances where different modes of prognostication have been contrasted[139,153,154], electrical studies do not necessarily provide greater precision than is afforded by other basic items of information (such as historical variables, including time to spontaneous respiration and pupillary findings in near-drowning victims; e.g., see Ref. 155). Therefore, caution must be exercised in espousing these sophisticated techniques as the best means of gaining prognostic information regarding comatose children[148].

Finally, EP studies may be useful in some other condi-

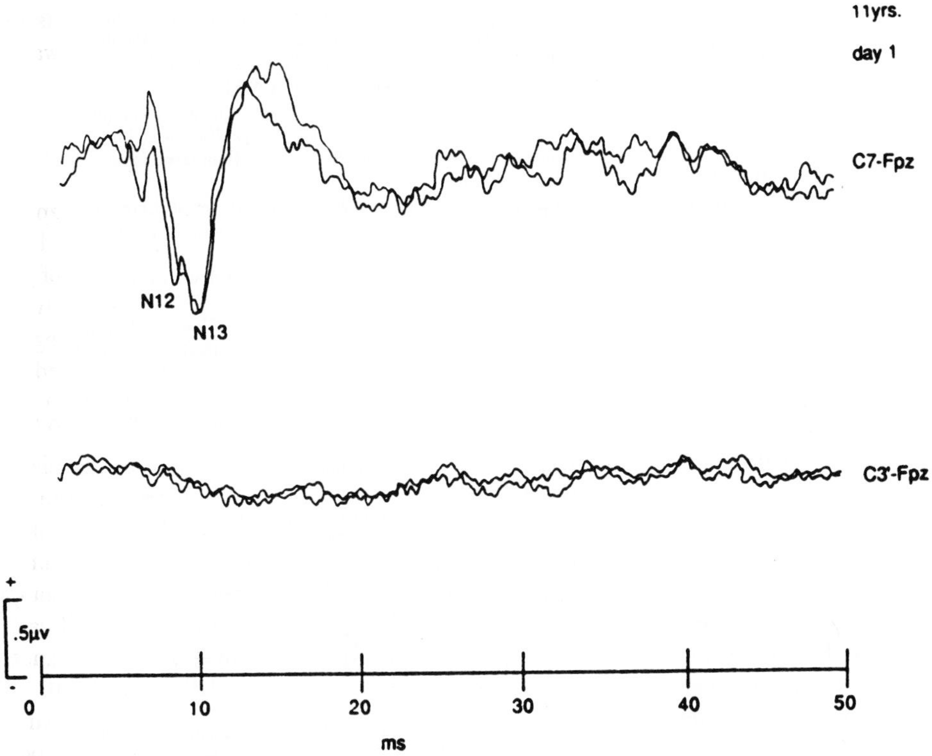

Figure 19.33. Absence of cortical somatosensory evoked potentials (SEPs) in coma. In this comatose child, although the cervical component (N13) of the SEP is present *(upper trace)*, indicating successful activation of the central nervous system by the stimulus, no thalamocortical component is recorded from this hemisphere *(lower trace)*. Similarly, no cortical response was present on the opposite side. The child did not survive. (From Taylor MJ, Farrell EJ. Comparison of the prognostic utility of VEPs and SEPs in comatose children. Pediatr Neurol 1989; 5:145–150.)

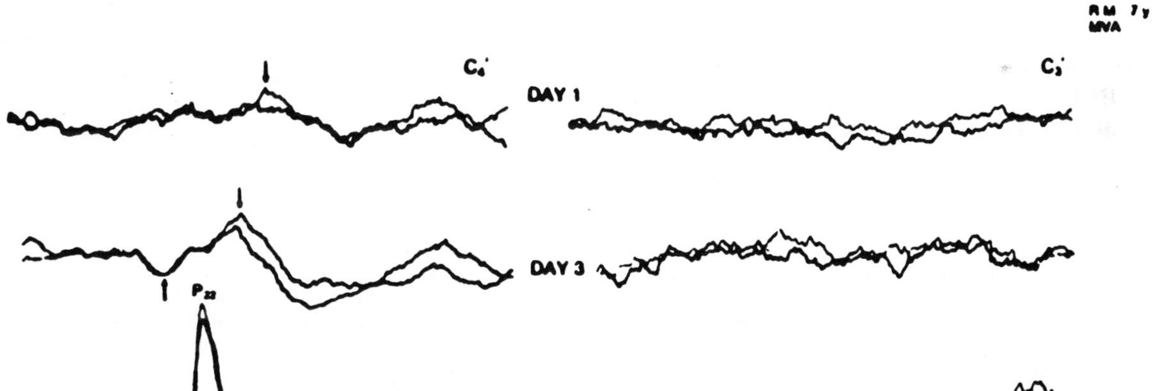

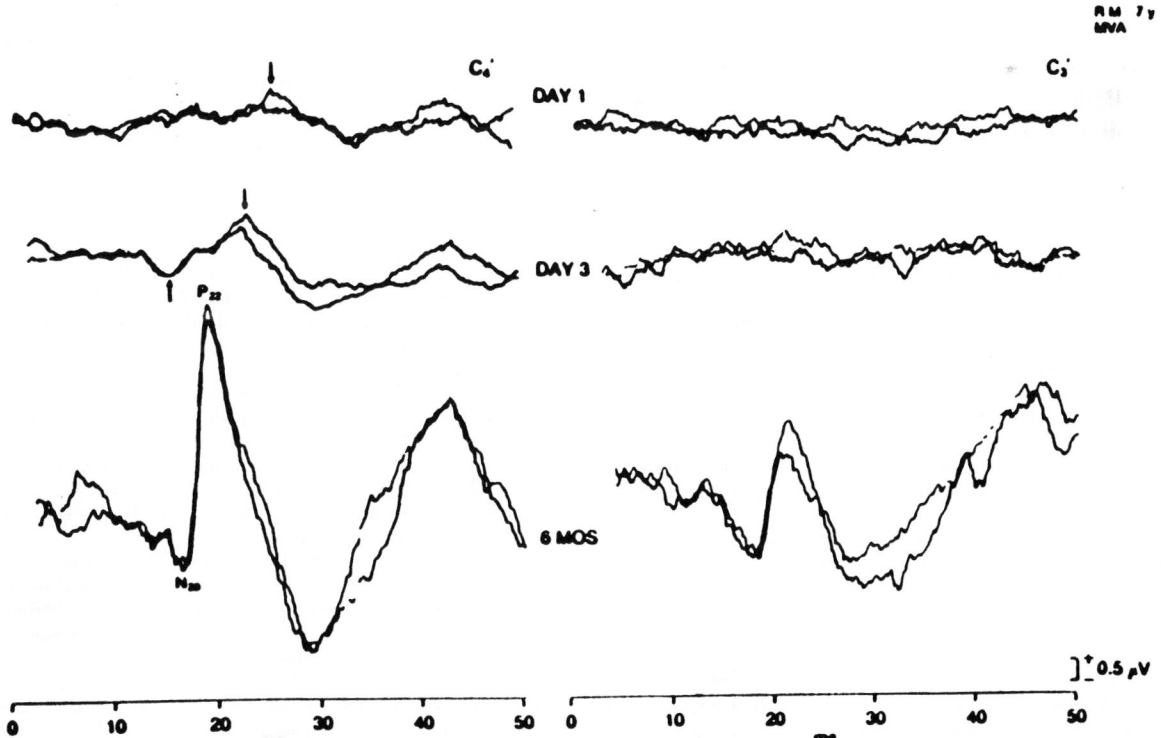

Figure 19.34. Asymmetry of cortical SEPs. Responses were recorded from the right (C_4') and left (C_3') parietal areas on three different occasions. On day 1, a small response was obtained from the right hemisphere *(top trace, left side)*, whereas no response was recorded from the left. This asymmetry persists. The patient recovered with a right hemiparesis. (From DeMeirleir LJ, Taylor MJ. Prognostic utility of SEPs in comatose children. Pediatr Neurol 1987;3:78.)

tions encountered in the critical care setting. For example, lower extremity SEPs could be used to monitor response to treatment (chemotherapy, radiation, or corticosteroids) of an inoperable malignant tumor compressing the spinal cord. Recovery from transverse myelitis could also be quantitated in this manner. Again, it is perhaps appropriate to question whether such electrical studies are actually preferable to other more standard clinical means of evaluating and monitoring these neurologic conditions.

SUMMARY

The importance of electrical monitoring of the CNS in critically ill children cannot be overemphasized. For this purpose, routine serial EEGs can be very valuable but are limited by the unwieldy amount of information produced, as well as by the requirements for the technical and interpretive sophistication they entail. Computerized methods for averaging the EEG (the CFM and CSA, in particular) may alleviate some of these problems, but they do not entirely obviate the need for the routine EEG. In addition, the use of these methods of electroencephalographic compression may introduce additional difficulties of their own, such as artifact recognition and the masking of irregular brief CNS events such as electrographic seizures. Finally, although EPs provide yet another means of assessing the CNS with some anatomical specificity, their interpretation requires considerable skill and experience, and their presumed advantages over other means of CNS evaluation remain largely unproven. These caveats are not meant to dissuade the clinician caring for critically ill children from employing these methods. Rather, they are intended to encourage thorough understanding of the methodologies to be applied so as to allow for their wise and efficient use, to the patient's greatest benefit.

References

1. Harrington GR, Hnatiuk, MW. Noninvasive Monitoring. The American Journal of Medicine 1993;95:221.
2. Pfenninger J. Neurological intensive care in children. Intensive Care Med 1993;19:243.
3. Richards P. Monitoring of cerebral function. British J of Hosp Med 1992;48:390.
4. Ropper AH, ed. Neurological and neurosurgical intensive care, 3d ed New York: Raven Press, 1993.
5. Altmann F. Anomalies of the internal carotid artery and its branches: their embryological and comparative anatomical significance. Laryngoscope 1947;57:313.
6. Gros CL, Minvielle J, Viahovitch B. Anastomoses arterielles intracraniennes, etude arteriographic et clinique. Neurochirurgie 1956;2:281.
7. Lou HC, Lassen NA, Friis-Hansen B. Impaired autoregulation of cerebral blood flow in the distressed newborn infant. J Pediatr 1979;94:118.
8. Younkin DP, Reivich M, Jaggi J, et al. Noninvasive method of estimating human newborn regional cerebral blood flow. J Cereb Blood Flow Metab 1982;2:415.
9. Ment LR, Ehrenkranz RA, Lange RC, et al. Alterations in cerebral blood flow in preterm infants with intraventricular hemorrhage. Pediatrics 1981;68:763.
10. Huttenlocher PR, Moohr JW, Johns L, et al. Cerebral blood flow in sickle cell cerebrovascular disease. Pediatrics 1984;73:615.
11. Kennedy C, Sokoloff L. An adaptation of the nitrous oxide method to the study of the cerebral circulation in children: normal values for cerebral blood flow and cerebral metabolic rate in childhood. J Clin Invest 1957;36:1130.
12. Junck L, Dhawan V, et al. Effects of xenon and krypton on regional cerebral blood flow in the rat. J Cereb Blood Flow Metab 1985;5:126.
13. Giller CA, Purdy P, Lindstrom WW. Effects of inhaled stable xenon on cerebral blood flow velocity. AJNR 1990;11:177.
14. Kelcz F, Hilal SK, Hartwell P, et al. Computed tomographic measurement of the xenon brain/blood partition coefficient and implications for regional cerebral blood flow: a preliminary report. Radiology 1978;127:385.
15. Hernandez MJ, Brennan RW, Vannuci RC, et al. Cerebral blood flow and oxygen consumption in the newborn dog. Am J Physiol 1972;24:R209.
16. Zierler KL. Equations for measuring blood flow by external monitoring of radioisotopes. Circ Res 1965;16:309.
17. Lassen NA. Assessment of tissue radiation dose in clinical use of radioactive inert gases with examples of absorbed doses from He^3, Kr^{85}, and Xe^{133}. Minerva Nucl 1964;8:211.
18. Patlak CS, Blasberg RG, Fenstermacher JD. An evaluation of errors in the determination of blood flow by the indicator fractionation and tissue equilibration (Kety) methods. J Cereb Blood Flow Metab 1984;4:47.
19. Volpe JJ, Herscovitch P, Perlman JM, et al. Positron emission tomography in the newborn: extensive impairment of regional cerebral blood flow with intraventricular hemorrhage and hemorrhagic intracerebral involvement. Pediatrics 1983;72:589.
20. Ell PJ, Jarritt PH, Costa DC, Cullum ID, Lui D. Functional imaging of the brain. Semin Nucl Med 1987;17:214–229.
21. Maurer AH. Nuclear medicine: SPECT comparisons to PET. Radiol Clin North Am 1988;26:1059–1074.
22. Walovitch RC, Williams SJ, Lafrance ND. Radiolabeled agents for SPECT imaging of brain perfusion. Int J Rad Appl Instrum [B] 1990;17:77.
23. Grünwald F, Menzel C, Pavics L, et al. Ictal and interictal brain SPECT imaging in epilepsy using technetium-99m-ECD. J Nuclear Med 1994;35:1896.
24. Vles JSH, Demandt E, Ceulemans B, deRoo M, Casaer PJM. Single photon emission computed tomography (SPECT) in seizure disorders in childhood. Brain Dev 1990;12:385–389.
25. Fisher M, Sotak C, Minematsu K, et al. New magnetic resonance techniques for evaluating cerebrovascular disease. Ann Neurol 1992;32:115.
26. Pickens D. Perfusion/Diffusion Quantitation with Magnetic Resonance Imaging. Investig Radiol 27(suppl.2) 1992;S12.
27. Kety SS, Schmidt CF. The determination of cerebral blood flow in man by the use of nitrous oxide in low concentrations. Am J Physiol 1945;143:53.
28. Kety SS, Schmidt CF. The nitrous oxide method for the quantitative determination of cerebral blood flow in man: theory, procedure and normal values. J Clin Invest 1948;27:476.
29. Batson OV. Anatomical problems concerned in the study of cerebral blood flow. Fed Proc 1944;3:139.
30. Goetting MG, Preston G. Jugular bulb catheterization does not increase intracranial pressure. Intensive Care Med 1991;17:195.
31. Baird HW, Garfunkel JM. A method for the measurement of cerebral blood flow in infants and children. J Pediatr 1953;42:570.
32. Cruz J, Raps EC, Hoffstad OJ, et al. Cerebral oxygenation monitoring. Crit Care Med 1993;21:1242.
33. Cruz J. Combined continuous monitoring of systemic and cerebral oxygenation in acute brain injury: preliminary observations. Crit Care Med 1993;21:1225.
34. Cruz J. Cerebral oxygenation. Monitoring and management. Acta Neurochir Suppl Wien 1993;59:86.
35. Swedlow DB, Kettrick RG, Raphaely RC. Jugular venous bulb catheterization in children. Crit Care Med 1981;9:287.
36. Sharples PM, Stuart AG, Aynsley-Green A, et al. A practical method of serial bedside measurement of cerebral blood flow and metabolism during neurointensive care. Arch Disease in Childhood 1991;66:1326.
37. Hantson PH, Mahieu P. Usefulness of cerebral venous monitoring through jugular bulb catheterization for the diagnosis of brain death. Intensive Care Med 1992;18:59.
38. Obrist WD, Langfitt TW, Jaggi JL, et al. Cerebral blood flow and metabolism in comatose patients with acute head injury. J Neurosurg 1984;61:241.
39. Jaggi JL, Obrist WD, Gennarelli TA, Langfitt TW. Relationship of early cerebral blood flow and metabolism to outcome in acute head injury. J Neurosurg 1990;72:176–182.
40. Robertson CS, Contant CF, Gokaslan ZL, et al. Cerebral blood flow, arteriovenous oxygen difference, and outcome in head injured patients. J Neurol Neurosurg Psychiatry 1992;55:594.

41. Muizelaar JP, Marmarou A, DeSalles AAF, Ward JD, Zimmerman S, Li Z, Choi SC, Young HF. Cerebral blood flow and metabolism in severely head-injured children. J Neurosurg 1989;71:63–76.
42. Shalit W, Beller AJ, Feinsod M. Clinical equivalents of cerebral oxygen consumption in coma. Neurology 1972;22:115.
43. Aaslid R, Markwalder T-M, Nornes H. Non-invasive transcranial Doppler ultrasound recording of flow velocity in basal cerebral arteries. J. Neurosurgery 1982;57:769.
44. Newell DW, Aaslid R, Transcranial doppler. New York: Raven Press, 1992.
45. Goh D, Minns RA. Cerebral blood flow velocity monitoring in pyogenic meningitis. Archives of Disease in Childhood 1993;68:111.
46. Bada HS, Hajjar W, Chua C, et al. Noninvasive diagnosis of neonatal asphyxia and intraventricular hemorrhage by Doppler ultrasound. J Pediatr 1979;95:755.
47. Greisen G, Johansen K, Ellison PH, et al. Cerebral blood flow in the newborn infant: comparison of Doppler ultrasound and 133-xenon clearance. J Pediatr 1984;104:411.
48. Perlman JM, McMenamin JB, Volpe JJ. Fluctuating cerebral blood-flow in respiratory-distress syndrome. Relation to the development of intraventricular hemorrhage. N Engl J Med 1983;309:204.
49. Costeloe K, Smyth DP, Murdoch N, et al. A comparison between electrical impedance and strain gauge plethysmography for the study of cerebral blood flow in the newborn. Pediatr Res 1984;18:290.
50. deBray JM, Granry JC, Monrigal JP, et al. Effects of thiopental on middle cerebral artery blood velocities: a transcranial doppler study in children. Child's Nerv Syst 1993;9:220.
51. Newell DW, Aaslid R, Stooss R, Reulen HJ. The relationship of blood flow velocity fluctuations to intracranial pressure B waves. J Neurosurgery 1992;76:415.
52. Sanker P, Richard KE, Weigl HC, et. al. Transcranial doppler sonography and intracranial pressure monitoring in children and juveniles with acute brain injuries or hydrocephalus. Childs Nerv Syst 1991;7:391.
53. Meyerson BA, Gunasekera L, Linderoth B, et al. Bedside monitoring of regional cortical blood flow in comatose patients using laser Doppler flowmetry. Neurosurgery 1991;29:750.
54. Cross KW, Dear PRF, Warner RM, et al. An attempt to measure cerebral blood flow in the newborn infant. J Physiol 1976;260:42.
55. Cross KW, Dear PRF, Hathorn MKS, et al. An estimate of intracranial blood flow in the new-born infant. J Physiol 1979;289:329.
56. Leahy FAN, Cates D, MacCallum M, et al. Effects of CO_2 and 100% O_2 on cerebral blood flow in preterm infants. J Appl Physiol 1980;48:468.
57. Leahy FAN, Sankaran K, Cates D, et al. Quantitative noninvasive methods to measure cerebral blood flow in newborn infants. Pediatrics 1979;64:277.
58. Jenkner FL. Rheoencephalography: a method for the continuous registration of cerebrovascular changes. Springfield, Illinois: Charles C Thomas, 1962.
59. Namon R, Gollan F, Shimojyo S, et al. Basic studies in rheoencephalography. Neurology 1967;17:239.
60. Jelsma LF, McQueen JD. Changes in impedance pulsations and carotid blood flow during intracranial hypertension. In: Bain WH, Harper AM, eds. Blood flow through organs and tissues. Edinburgh: Churchill Livingstone, 1968:328.
61. Weindling AM, Murdoch N, Rolfe P. The effect of electrode size in the contributions of intracranial and extracranial blood flow to the cerebral electrical impedance plethysmogram. Med Biol Eng Comput 1982;20:545.
62. Brazy JE, Lewis DV, et al. Noninvasive monitoring of cerebral oxygenation in preterm infants: preliminary observations. Pediatrics 1985;75:217.
63. Proctor HJ, Cairns C, Fillipo D, et al. Brain metabolism during increased intracranial pressure as assessed by niroscopy. Surgery 1984;96:273.
64. Wyatt JS, Cope M, Delpy DT, Wray S, Reynolds EOR. Quantification of cerebral oxygenation and haemodynamics in sick newborn infants by near infrared spectroscopy. Lancet 1986;2:1063.
65. McCormick P, Stewart M, Goetting M, et al. Noninvasive cerebral optical spectroscopy for monitoring cerebral oxygen delivery and hemodynamics. Crit Care Med 1991;19:89.
66. Persson L, Hillered L. Chemical monitoring of neurosurgical intensive care patients using intracerebral microdialysis. J Neurosurg 1992;76:72.
67. Landolt H, Langemann H, Gratzl O. On-line monitoring of cerebral pH by microdialysis. Neurosurgery 1993;32:1000.
68. Leyden D. Beitrage und Untersuchungen zur Physiologie und Pathologie des Gehirns. Über Hirndruck und Hirnbewegungen. Virchows Arch 1866;37:519.
69. Quincke H. Über hydrocephalus. Verh Dtsch Ges Inn Med 1891;10:321.
70. Guillaume J, Janny P. Manometrie intracranienne continue. Rev Neurol (Paris) 1951;84:131.
71. Lundberg N. Continuous recording and control of ventricular fluid pressure in neurosurgical practice. Acta Psychiatr Neurol Scand 1960;36(Suppl 149):7.
72. Lundberg N. Monitoring of intracranial pressure. Proc R Soc Med 1972;65:19.
73. Miller JD, Stanek A, Langfitt TW. Concepts of cerebral perfusion pressure and vascular compression during intracranial hypertension. Prog Brain Res 1971;35:411.
74. Jennet WB, Harper AM, Miller JD, et al. Relation between cerebral blood flow and cerebral perfusion pressure. Br J Surg 1970;57:390.
75. Marshall LF, Smith RW, Shapiro HM. The outcome with aggressive treatment in severe head injuries. 1. The significance of intracranial pressure monitoring. J Neurosurg 1979;50:20.
76. Bruce DA, Schut L, et al. Outcome following severe head injuries in children. J Neurosurg 1970;48:679.
77. Miller JD, Becker DP, et al. Significance of intracranial hypertension in severe head injury. J Neurosurg 1977;24:233.
78. Mayer T, Walker ML. Emergency intracranial pressure monitoring in pediatrics. Clin Pediatr 1982;21:391.
79. Jennett B, Bond M. Assessment of outcome after severe brain damage. A practical scale. Lancet 1975;1:480.
80. Miller JD, Butterworth JF, et al. Further experience in the management of severe head injury. J Neurosurg 1981;54:298.
81. Miller JD, Sweet RC, et al. Early insults to the injured brain. JAMA 1978;240:439.
82. Le Roux PD, Jardine DS, Kanev PM, et al. Pediatric intracranial pressure monitoring in hypoxic and nonhypoxic brain injury. Child's Nerv Syst 1991;7:34.
83. Pickard JD, Czosnyka M. Management of raised intracranial pressure. J of Neurology, Neurosurgery, and Psychiatry 1993;56:845.
84. Gambardella G, Zaccone C, Cardia E, et al. Intracranial pressure monitoring in children: comparison of external ventricular device with the fiberoptic system. Child's Nerv Syst 1993;9:470.
85. Ivan L, Choo SH, Ventureyra ECG. Intracranial pressure monitoring with the fiberoptic transducer in children. Childs Brain 1980;7:303.
86. Mendelow AD, Rowan JO, et al. A clinical comparison of subdural screw pressure measurements with ventricular pressure. J Neurosurg 1983;58:45.
87. Dearden NM, et al. Assessment of Leeds device for monitoring intracranial pressure. J Neurosurg 1984;60:123.
88. Weaver DD, Winn HR, Jane JA. Differential intracranial pressure in patients with unilateral mass lesions. J Neurosurg 1982;56:660.
89. Vries JK, Becker DP, Young HF. A subarachnoid screw for monitoring intracranial pressure. J Neurosurg 1973;39:416.
90. Borel C, Hanley D, Diringer MN, Rogers MC. Intensive management of severe head injury. Chest 1990;98:180–189.
91. Lehman LB. Intracranial pressure monitoring and treatment: a contemporary view. Ann Emerg Med 1990;19:295–303.
92. Tasker RD, Matthew DJ. Cerebral intraparenchymal pressure monitoring in non-traumatic coma: clinical evaluation of a new fiberoptic device. Neuropediatrics 1991;22:47.
93. Piek J, Bock WJ. Continuous monitoring of cerebral tissue pressure in neurosurgical practice—experiences with 100 patients. Intensive Care Med 1990;16:184.
94. Clark WC, Muhlbauer MS, Lowrey R, Hartman M, Ray MW, Watridge CB. Complications of intracranial pressure monitoring in trauma patients. Neurosurgery 1989;25:20–24.
95. Doyle DJ, Mark PWS. Analysis of intracranial pressure. J Clin Monit 1992;8:81.
96. Czosnyka M, Price DJ, Williamson M. Monitoring of cerebrospinal dynamics using continuous analysis of intracranial pressure and cerebral perfusion pressure in head injury. Acta Neurochir Wien 1994;126:113.
97. Taylor FA, Schutz H. Symptoms caused by intracranial pressure waves. J Neurosurg Nurs 1977;9:144.
98. Mendelow AD. The early management of head injury. Curr Opinion Neurol Neurosurg 1991;4:5–11.
99. Tasker RC, Matthew DJ, Helms P, Dinwiddie R, Boyd S. Monitoring in non-traumatic coma. Part I: invasive intracranial measurements. Arch Dis Child 1988; 63:888–894.
100. Barnes MP. Outcome of head injury. Curr Opinion Neurol Neurosurg 1991;4:12–16.

101. Venes J. Intracranial pressure monitoring in perspective. Childs Brain 1981;7:236.
102. Bruce DA, Berman WA, Schut L. Cerebrospinal fluid pressure monitoring in children: physiology, pathology and clinical usefulness. Adv Pediatr 1977;24:233.
103. Shankaran S, Woldt E, Bedard MP, et al. Feasibility of invasive monitoring of intracranial pressure in term neonates. Brain Dev 1994; 16:121.
104. Chiappa KH. Electrophysiologic monitoring. In: Ropper AH, ed. Neurological and neurosurgical intensive care. 3rd ed. New York, Raven Press 1993;147–184.
105. Price HL, Matthew DJ. Evaluation of pediatric intensive care scoring systems. Intensive Care Med 1989;15:79–83.
106. Brazier MAB. The emergence of electrophysiology as an aid to neurology. In: Aminoff MJ, ed. Electrodiagnosis in clinical neurology. 3rd ed. New York: Churchill Livingstone, 1992:1–16.
107. Hahn JS, Tharp BP. Neonatal and pediatric electro-encephalography. In: Aminoff MJ, ed. Electrodiagnosis in clinical neurology. 3rd ed. New York: Churchill Livingstone, 1992:93–141.
108. Aminoff MJ. Electroencephalography: general principles and clinical applications. In: Aminoff MJ, ed. Electrodiagnosis in clinical neurology. 3rd ed. New York: Churchill Livingstone, 1992:41–91.
109. Epstein CM, Andriola MR. Introduction to EEG and evoked potentials. Philadelphia: JB Lippincott, 1983.
110. Fisch BJ. Spehlmann's. EEG primer. New York: Elsevier, 1991.
111. Pampiglione G, Harden A. Resuscitation after cardiocirculatory arrest. Lancet 1968;1:1261–1264.
112. Tasker RC, Boyd S, Harden A, Matthew DJ. Monitoring in non-traumatic coma. Part II: electroencephalography. Arch Dis Child 1988;63:895–899.
113. Lowenstein DH, Aminoff MJ. Clinical and EEG features of status epilepticus in comatose patients. Neurology 1992;42:100.
114. Grand'Maison F, Reiher J, Leduc CP. Retrospective inventory of EEG abnormalities in partial status epilepticus. Electroencephalogr Clin Neurophysiol 1991;79:264.
115. Jordan KG. Continuous EEG and evoked potential monitoring in the neuroscience intensive care unit. J Clin Neurophysiology 1993;10:445.
116. Tasker RC, Boyd SG, Harden A, Matthew DJ. The cerebral function analysing monitor in paediatric medical intensive care: applications and limitations. Intensive Care Med 1990;16:60–68.
117. Talwar D, Torres F. Continuous electrophysiologic monitoring of cerebral function in the pediatric intensive care unit. Pediatr Neurol 1988;4:137–147.
118. Kruus S, Bergstrom L, Suutarinen T, Hyvonen R. The prognosis of near-drowned children. Acta Paediatr Scand 1979;68:315–322.
119. Ashwal S, Schneider S. Failure of electroencephalography to diagnose brain death in comatose children. Ann Neurol 1979;6:512–517.
120. Bickford RG. Newer methods of recording and analyzing EEGs. In: Klass DW, Daly DD, eds. Current practice of clinical electroencephalography. New York: Raven Press, 1979:451–480.
121. Gevins AS. Quantitative aspects of EEG and evoked potentials. In: Aminoff MJ, ed. Electrodiagnosis in clinical neurology. 2nd ed. New York: Churchill Livingstone, 1986:149–203.
122. Prior PF, Maynard DE. Monitoring cerebral function: long-term monitoring of EEG and evoked potentials. New York: Elsevier, 1986.
123. Bickford RG, Billinger TW, Fleming N, Stewart L. The compressed spectral array (CSA). A pictorial EEG. Proc San Diego Biomed Symp 1972;11:365–370.
124. Hellstrom-Westas I. Comparison between tape-recorded and amplitude-integrated EEG monitoring in sick newborn infants. Acta Paediatr 1992;81:812.
125. Verma UL, Archbald F, Tejani NA, Handwerker SM. Cerebral function monitor in the neonate. I: normal patterns. Dev Med Child Neurol 1984;26:154–161.
126. Archbald F, Verma UL, Tejani ND, Handwerker SM. Cerebral function monitor in the neonate. II: birth asphyxia. Dev Med Child Neurol 1984;26:162–168.
127. Bjerre I, Hellstrom-Westas L, Rosen I, Svenningsen NW. Monitoring of cerebral functions after severe asphyxia in infancy. Arch Dis Child 1983;58:997–1002.
128. Thornberg E, Ekström-Jodal B. Cerebral function monitoring: a method of predicting outcome in term neonates after severe perinatal asphyxia. Acta Paediatr 1994;83:596.
129. Hellstrom-Westas L, Rosen I, Svenningsen NW. Silent seizures in sick infants in early life: diagnosis by continuous cerebral function monitoring. Acta Paediatr Scand 1985;74:741–748.
130. Tasker RC, Boyd SG, Harden A, Matthew DJ. EEG monitoring of prolonged thiopentone administration for intractable seizures and status epilepticus in infants and young children. Neuropediatrics 1989;20:147–153.
131. Bricolo A, Turazzi S, Faccioli F, Odorizzi F, Sciaretta G, Erculiani P. Clinical application of compressed spectral array in long-term EEG monitoring of comatose patients. Electroencephalogr Clin Neurophysiol 1978;45:211–225.
132. Bricolo A, Faccioli F, Grosslercher JC, Pasut ML, Dinna GP, Turazzi S. Electrophysiological monitoring in the intensive care unit. Electroencephalogr Clin Neurophysiol Suppl 1987;39:255–263.
133. Cant BR, Shaw NA. Monitoring by compressed spectral array in prolonged coma. Neurology 1984;34:35–39.
134. Karnaze DS, Marshall LF, Bickford RG. EEG monitoring of clinical coma: the compressed spectral array. Neurology 1982;32:289–292.
135. Chiappa KH. Evoked potentials in clinical medicine. New York: Raven Press, 1990.
136. Sokol S. Visual evoked potentials. In: Aminoff MJ, ed. Electrodiagnosis in clinical neurology. 3rd ed. New York: Churchill Livingstone, 1992:491–502.
137. Taylor MJ, Farrell EJ. Comparison of the prognostic utility of VEPs and SEPs in comatose children. Pediatr Neurol 1989;5:145.
138. Picton TW, Taylor MJ, Durieux-Smith A, Edwards CG. Brainstem auditory evoked potentials in pediatrics. In: Aminoff MJ, ed. Electrodiagnosis in clinical neurology. 3rd ed. New York: Churchill Livingstone, 1992:537–569.
139. Krieger D, Adams HP, Schwartz S, et al. Prognostic and clinical relevance of pupillary responses, intracranial pressure monitoring, and brainstem auditory evoked potentials in comatose patients with acute supratentorial mass lesions. Crit Care Med 1993;21:1944.
140. Goldie WD, Chiappa KH, Young RR, Brooks EB. Brainstem auditory and short-latency somatosensory evoked response in brain death. Neurology 1981;31:248–256.
141. White CP, Cooke RWI, Somatosensory evoked potentials following posterior tibial nerve stimulation predict later motor outcome. Developmental Med and Child Neuro 1994;36:34.
142. Fagan ER, Taylor MJ, Logan WJ. Somatosensory evoked potentials. Part I. A review of neural generators and special considerations in pediatrics. Pediatr Neurol 1987;3:189–196.
143. Fagan ER, Taylor MJ, Logan WJ. Somatosensory evoked potentials. Part II. A review of the clinical applications in pediatric neurology. Pediatr Neurol 1987;3:249–255.
144. DeMeirleir LJ, Taylor MJ. Evoked potentials in comatose children: auditory brainstem responses. Pediatr Neurol 1986;2:31–34.
145. DeMeirleir LJ, Taylor MJ. Prognostic utility of SEP's in comatose children. Pediatr Neurol 1987;3:78–82.
146. Goitein KJ, Amit Y, Fainmesser P, Sohmer H. Diagnostic and prognostic value of auditory nerve brainstem evoked responses in comatose children. Crit Care Med 1983;11:91–94.
147. Lutschg J, Pfenninger J, Ludin HP, Vasella F. Brainstem auditory evoked potentials and early somatosensory evoked potentials in neurointensively treated comatose children. Am J Dis Child 1983;137:421–426.
148. Goodwin SR, Friedman WA, Bellefleur M. Is it time to use evoked potentials to predict outcome in children and adults? Crit Care Med 1991;19:1518.
149. Frank LM, Furgiuele TL, Etheridge JE Jr. Prediction of chronic vegetative state in children using evoked potentials. Neurology 1985;35:931–934.
150. Judson JA, Cant BR, Shaw NA. Early prediction of outcome from cerebral trauma by somatosensory evoked potentials. Crit Care Medicine 1990;18:363.
151. Moulton RJ, Shedden PM, Tucker WS, et al. Somatosensory evoked potential monitoring following severe closed head injury. Clin Investr Med 1994;17:187.
152. Barelli A, Valente MR, Clemente A, et al. Serial multimodality-evoked potentials in severely head-injured patients: Diagnostic and prognostic implications. Crit Care Med 1991;19:1374.
153. Lindsay KW, Carlin J, Kennedy I, Fry J, McInnes A, Teasdale GM. Evoked potentials in severe head-injury-analysis and relation to outcome. J Neurol Neurosurg Psychiatry 1981;44:796–802.
154. Lindsay K, Pasoghi A, Hirst D, Allardyce G, Kennedy I, Teasdale G. Somatosensory and auditory brain stem conduction after head injury: a comparison with clinical features in prediction of outcome. Neurosurgery 1990;26:278–285.
155. Frates RC. Analysis of predictive factors in the assessment of warm-water near-drowning in children. Am J Dis Child 1981;135:1006–1008.

Theories of Brain Resuscitation

20

Steven E. Haun
Jeffrey R. Kirsch
J. Michael Dean

"Anoxaemia not only stops the machine but wrecks the machinery."
J.S. Haldane

INTRODUCTION

One of the most disheartening aspects of the practice of pediatric critical care medicine is to care for a brain dead child following a "successful" cardiopulmonary resuscitation. Management of children with severe hypoxic-ischemic brain injury is usually a discouraging prospect, and it is natural that clinicians seek means to ameliorate brain damage in such patients. The term *brain resuscitation* has been coined to include a large variety of interventions that attempt to limit the consequences of hypoxic-ischemic brain injury. However, the term brain resuscitation has proven to be a oxymoron.

The past two decades has witnessed an explosion of research on hypoxic-ischemic brain injury and brain resuscitation. Initially, there were many attempts to use existing pharmacological agents, e.g., barbiturates and calcium channel blockers, to ameliorate hypoxic-ischemic brain injury. After initial excitement, none of these therapies proved efficacious. It is unlikely that there will be a "quick fix," and effective therapy can only be developed with a more complete understanding of the pathophysiology of hypoxic-ischemic brain injury. More recently, research emphasis has shifted away from trials of the "magic bullet du jour" to studies dealing with mechanisms of injury. Ongoing research in this area may ultimately provide the background knowledge on which new therapies can be based, permitting us to salvage sublethally injured brain tissue.

The remainder of this chapter is divided into three parts. The first part reviews the pathophysiology of hypoxic-ischemic brain injury, the second part discusses potential therapies, and the final part outlines a pragmatic approach to the child with hypoxic-ischemic brain injury.

PATHOPHYSIOLOGY OF HYPOXIC-ISCHEMIC BRAIN INJURY

The processes leading to neuronal death after a hypoxic-ischemic insult are exceedingly complex, and our understanding of the pathophysiology of hypoxic-ischemic injury is far from complete. In this section we will review current knowledge of the pathophysiology of hypoxic-ischemic brain injury. After a brief review of terminology, we first consider the changes in cerebral blood flow (CBF) that occur after global cerebral ischemia. Next we discuss the histologic changes that have been described after global cerebral ischemia. Subsequently, we briefly review biochemical mechanisms of hypoxic-ischemic brain injury, including cellular energy depletion, acidosis, excitatory amino acids, calcium metabolism, phospholipid hydrolysis, eicosanoid metabolism, oxygen radicals, nitric oxide, protein phosphorylation, protein synthesis, gene expression, and inflammation. We conclude with a brief discussion of developmental differences in tolerance to hypoxic-ischemic insults.

Definitions

Hypoxic-ischemic brain injury results from inadequate oxygen delivery to the brain. Barcroft[1] eloquently describes three mechanisms leading to inadequate oxygen delivery in his oft-cited treatise: (1) hypoxic hypoxia or hypoxia resulting from a low partial pressure of oxygen in the arterial blood, (2) anemic hypoxia or hypoxia resulting from inadequate hemoglobin concentration in the arterial blood, and (3) ischemic hypoxia or hypoxia resulting from inadequate blood flow. Hypoxic brain injury results from inadequate delivery of oxygen to the brain despite normal or increased CBF. This can result via several different mechanisms: (1) inadequate partial pressure of oxygen in arterial blood, (2) inadequate hemoglobin concentration in arterial blood, or (3) impaired binding of oxygen to hemoglobin, e.g., carbon monoxide poisoning or methemoglobinemia. Ischemic brain injury results from inadequate blood flow to the brain. Ischemic insults may be further classified into focal and global categories. Global ischemia results from inadequate flow to the entire brain, e.g., during cardiac arrest. Focal ischemia results from inadequate flow to a particular region of the brain, usually representing the area supplied by a particular vasculature. Focal ischemia may result from localized disruption of the blood supply during trauma (see Chapter 24, Head and Spinal Cord Injury) or stroke (see Chapter 25, Cerebrovascular Disease and Vascular Anomalies). Focal ischemia can be further classified by whether the occlusion of the vascular supply is transient or permanent. We limit the discussion in this chapter to global ischemia because focal ischemia is relatively uncommon in children. For the interested reader, focal ischemia has recently been reviewed[2,3]. Finally, ischemia and hypoxia are relative parameters, and the effects of each depend on the relative severity of the perturbation. Hypoxia can be quantified by a variety of means, e.g., PaO_2, CaO_2. Ischemia can also be quantified by the level of CBF that remains during the ischemic event. Global ischemia is often categorized as complete or incomplete. For example, severe hypotension may produce partial or incomplete ischemia, whereas unresuscitated cardiac arrest would cause complete ischemia.

Cardiorespiratory arrest and resultant global ischemia in children is usually the result of asphyxia, i.e., respiratory arrest leading to cardiac arrest, as opposed to the primary cardiac arrest usually seen in adults. In asphyxial cardiorespiratory arrest, global cerebral ischemia is preceded by severe hypoxia and hypercarbia, whereas in cardiorespiratory arrest secondary to dysrhythmia, the global ischemic insult is sudden and usually not preceded by hypoxia and hypercarbia. Thus, in children, the injury is usually a combination of hypoxia and ischemia or hypoxic-ischemic brain injury. In summary, the variety of terms and definitions emphasizes the complexity of the situation, and the reader should recognize that each type of injury may have vastly different consequences.

Cerebral Blood Flow

CBF during and after cerebral ischemia has been studied extensively. In this section, we discuss the ischemic threshold and the patterns of CBF observed during the early reperfusion period. The ischemic threshold, i.e., level of CBF at which the brain begins to exhibit energy failure, is fairly well defined. Reduction of CBF below 15 ml/min/100 g results in failure of electrical activity[4], and a reduction to less than 10 ml/min/100 g results in ionic pump failure[5]. Cellular energy failure appears to be the inciting event for nearly all the deleterious biochemical processes occurring during ischemia (see below). It is important to note that the severity of the hypoxic-ischemic insult is a function of both the duration and the degree of CBF reduction. For example, a reduction of CBF to zero for several seconds may produce no permanent injury, whereas a small amount of CBF for many minutes may produce severe injury.

A characteristic pattern of CBF after global cerebral ischemia (Fig. 20.1) has been demonstrated in different species[6–9], different models in the same species[6,10], and at different stages of development in the same species[9]. When blood flow is restored, there is an initial hyperemia that generally lasts less than 30 minutes. This hyperemic phase is followed by a phase of relative hypoperfusion (delayed hypoperfusion) that may persist for hours. Of historical note is the concept of *no reflow*, which is well known to most neurologists, neurosurgeons, and intensivists, having been proposed by Ames and colleagues[11] in the 1960s. Simply stated, these investigators noted that after a period of global cerebral ischemia, reflow could not be reestablished. What is less often remembered, however, is that the original studies were decapitation studies conducted in rabbits. What was actually found was that carbonized spheres could not successfully be perfused into decapitated rabbit heads after prolonged periods of ischemia. Although the

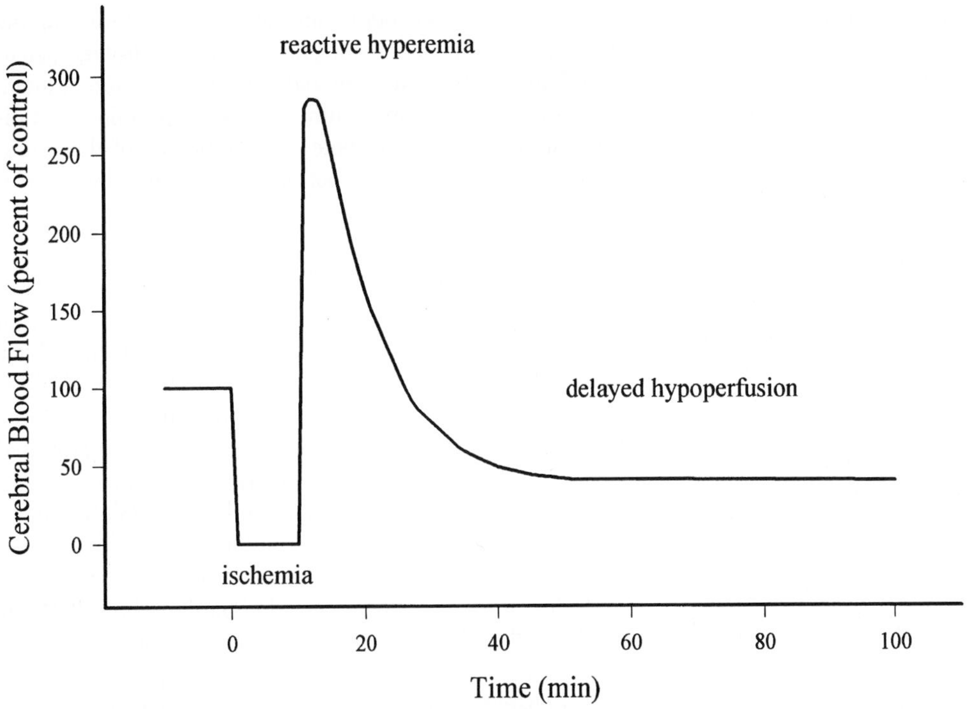

Figure 20.1. Characteristic pattern of cerebral blood flow after global ischemia.

concept may be valid, extrapolation to the clinical situation is unwarranted.

Early attempts at brain resuscitation were based on the concept that preventing no reflow would improve neurologic outcome. Examples of such early therapeutic attempts include induced hypertension, hemodilution, and carotid artery flushing. However, the relationship between delayed hypoperfusion and brain injury is unclear. Is delayed hypoperfusion a cause of ongoing ischemic brain injury, or is it merely the result of decreased metabolism in the injured brain? Michenfelder and Milde[(12)] studied the effect of the duration (for 3, 9, 12, or 18 minutes) of global ischemia on CBF and cerebral metabolic rate for oxygen during the early reperfusion period in a canine model. At 90 minutes of reperfusion, the magnitude of the reduction of CBF and cerebral metabolic rate for oxygen correlated with the duration of ischemia. However, the duration of ischemia had no effect on the ratio of CBF to cerebral metabolic rate for oxygen or the oxygen content of sagittal sinus blood. The authors concluded that postischemic CBF appears to be determined by the metabolic needs of the brain and that delayed hypoperfusion is probably not a significant cause of neuronal injury. Thus, delayed hypoperfusion is probably the result of brain injury rather than the cause.

Histologic Changes

Several histologic changes have been described after total cessation of brain blood flow. Brown and Brierley[(13)] and Brierley and coworkers[(14,15)] demonstrated mitochondrial, endoplasmic reticulum, perineuronal, and astrocytic swelling. With prolonged ischemia, the cell develops eosinophilia, and intracellular organelles become disrupted. Eventually, the cells shrink and become karyorrhectic. It is often assumed that early stages indicated by cellular swelling are reversible but that when intracellular organelles are disrupted, the injury is irreversible. The disruption of organelles is evidenced by the loss of Nissl substance, the formation of ribosomal rosettes, and swelling of the smooth endoplasmic reticulum.

Brief periods of global ischemia typically do not lead to infarction but rather to selective neuronal necrosis, i.e., glia and endothelium are spared. Pannecrotic lesions (involving neurons, glia, and endothelium) occur after ischemia of longer duration[(16,17)] and after brief periods of ischemia in animals who are hyperthermic[(18,19)] or hyperglycemic[(20)] (see below). Neuronal populations from different regions of the brain are not affected in the same manner during global ischemia. The most sensitive, i.e., selectively vulnerable, neurons are located in the CA1 sector of the hippocampus, layers 3, 5, and 6 of the cerebral cortex, and portions of the caudate and cerebellum[(14,21–23)]. These areas are similar to the most vulnerable areas during status epilepticus (see Chapter 22, Status Epilepticus), suggesting neurochemical events common to both processes[(24)]. The mechanisms responsible for this selective vulnerability remain controversial[(25)]. Glutamate toxicity mediated by the N-methyl-D-aspartate (NMDA) receptor (see below) has been proposed to explain selective vulnerability[(26)]. However, this hypothesis is problematic. As recently reviewed by Pulsinelli and colleagues[(27)], there is minimal correlation between NMDA receptor density and sensitivity to ischemia. For example, the ischemia-resistant granule cells of the dentate gyrus have a concentration of NMDA receptors equal to that of the ischemia-sensitive pyramidal cells of the CA1 sector, and cerebellar Purkinje cells, highly vulnerable to ischemia, are nearly devoid of NMDA receptors.

Neuronal injury appears to continue after the ischemic event. Maturation of the ischemic injury may take up to one week to be completed[28–30]. Mechanisms leading to "delayed neuronal death" are unclear. Delayed neuronal death is probably the result of biochemical processes that are initiated during global ischemia but that require time to result in neuronal death[31]. Oxygen radical-induced injury, changes in protein phosphorylation, and alterations in gene expression and protein synthesis are possible candidates. Cells appear to die via one of two mechanisms: necrosis or apoptosis[32]. Necrosis results from severe alterations of the extracellular environment, e.g., ischemia, that lead to cell swelling and, ultimately, increased permeability of the cell membrane. Apoptosis is gene-directed cellular self-destruction which can be triggered by either the cell's internal "clock" or external stimuli such as viral infections, toxic exposures, and cytokines. Apoptosis requires protein synthesis and usually involves endonucleolytic cleavage of cellular DNA[32]. DNA fragmentation characteristic of apoptotic cell death has been demonstrated after both focal[33–36] and global[37,38] cerebral ischemia. After a global ischemic insult, DNA fragmentation is most pronounced in neurons of the CA1 region of the hippocampus[37,38], suggesting that apoptosis may play a role in both selective neuronal necrosis and delayed neuronal death. The concept of delayed neuronal death is important for two reasons. First and foremost, the concept of delayed neuronal death implies that there is a window of opportunity for treatment after global ischemia, i.e., injurious processes initiated during ischemia may be interrupted with pharmacotherapy during the early reperfusion period. Second, delayed neuronal death is important to consider when evaluating animal models that use histology as an outcome measure. Results from models that do not allow for "maturation" of the ischemic injury must be interpreted with caution.

Finally, clinical correlation with histopathology is unclear. For example, Steen and colleagues[39] have shown that the calcium antagonist nimodipine improved postischemic neurologic outcome in pigtailed monkeys, but failed to improve histopathologic outcome. In fact, there were striking discrepancies in several animals between the neurologic outcome and the histopathology observed on autopsy. Conversely, in a study on the effect of hypothermia on outcome after global ischemia in the dog, postischemic hypothermia initiated after 15 minutes of reperfusion resulted in improved histologic but not neurologic outcome[40]. Obviously, from a clinician's (and patient's) standpoint, neurologic outcome is by far the most important endpoint.

Biochemical Changes

Innumerable biochemical events occur during and after ischemia in the brain. It is not our purpose here to review the subject exhaustively; rather, we provide a brief overview, with an emphasis on recent advances. We discuss adenosine 5′-triphosphate depletion, acidosis, excitatory amino acids, calcium metabolism, phospholipid hydrolysis, eicosanoid metabolism, oxygen radicals, nitric oxide, protein phosphorylation, protein synthesis, gene expression, and inflammation. It is vital to note the complexity of these processes and, even more importantly, how they are interrelated.

Adenosine 5′-Triphosphate Depletion

Cellular energy depletion is postulated to be the triggering event that initiates the plural cascades of injury during ischemia[41,42]. Adenosine 5′-triphosphate (ATP) is the energy source that drives, directly or indirectly, all cellular physiologic processes. One of the most vital processes performed at the expense of ATP is preservation of membrane ionic gradients. In fact, under normal conditions, ionic pumping accounts for approximately 50% of total cellular energy expenditure[43]. Seconds after the onset of ischemia, oxygen is depleted and oxidative phosphorylation stops. Cellular work can then be performed only at the expense of phosphocreatine stores, and ATP produced via glycolytic pathways. Phosphocreatine stores are rapidly exhausted, and the brain's minimal glucose and glycogen stores are rapidly depleted because of the relatively inefficient production of energy characteristic of the glycolytic pathway (2 mol ATP produced per mol glucose versus 36 mol ATP per mol glucose in oxidative phosphorylation). Numerous studies[44–47] have demonstrated nearly total depletion of ATP after less than 5 minutes of complete ischemia. ATP depletion leads to membrane depolarization and massive transmembrane ionic fluxes. Lack of sodium/potassium adenosine triphosphatase (ATPase) activity leads to net influx of sodium, chloride, and calcium and net efflux of potassium[48] (Fig. 20.2).

Although energy depletion occurs very rapidly, phosphocreatine levels and adenylate energy charge can be restored to near normal levels during reperfusion after periods of ischemia as long as 10 minutes[49] and even 15 minutes[45]. Furthermore, there appears to be rapid recovery of mitochondrial function during reperfusion[50,51], although more recent studies[52–54] have demonstrated abnormal mitochondrial respiration after ischemia. To summarize, energy depletion, the event that initiates hypoxic-ischemic injury, occurs very early in the course of an ischemic insult and appears to be reversible if the ischemic insult is of limited duration.

Acidosis

During complete global ischemia, substrate delivery to the brain is interrupted. The oxygen supply is depleted almost immediately, but glucose is available to the brain for a short time during the ischemic period via the breakdown of brain glycogen. Since glycogen stores in brain are small and the anaerobic degradation of glucose is relatively inefficient, the energy obtained by this mechanism is not sufficient for normal brain metabolism. As glycolysis proceeds, so does

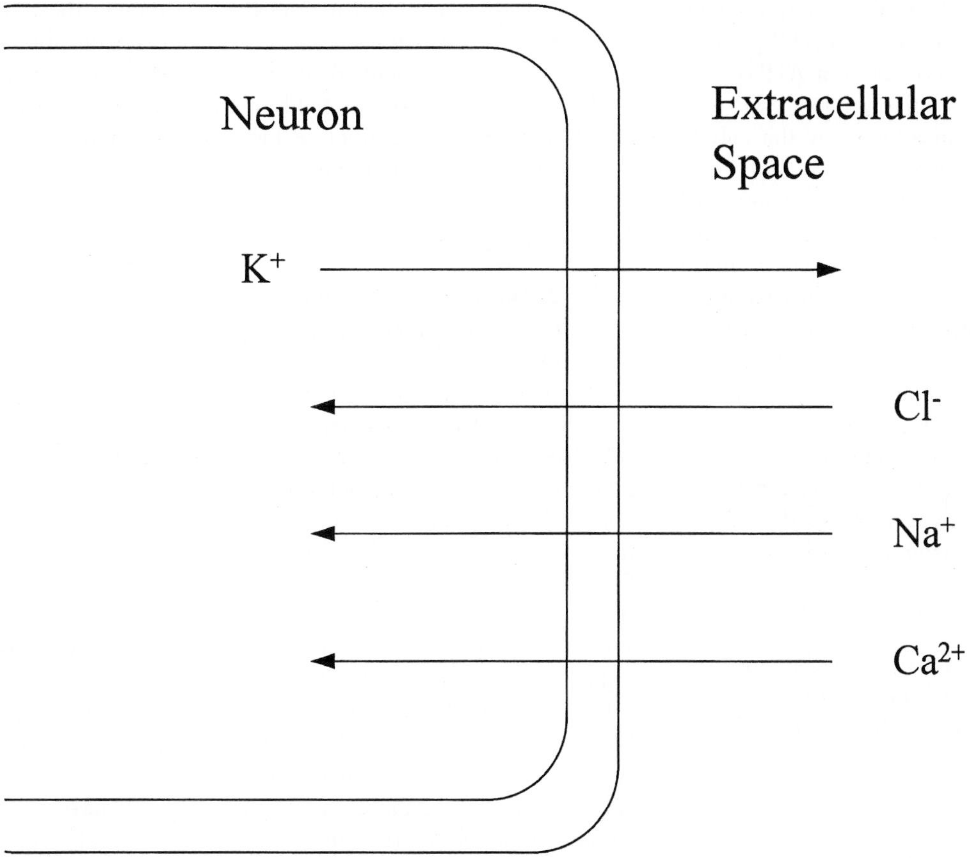

Figure 20.2. Ionic fluxes during ischemia. (Modified from Siesjo BK, Bengtsson F, Grampp W, Theander S. Calcium, excitotoxins, and neuronal death in the brain. Ann NY Acad Sci 1989;568:238.)

the buildup of lactate and hydrogen ion, and the latter is proposed to be a mediator of actual tissue damage(55).

In 1974, Ljunggren and colleagues(56) demonstrated that lactate production during ischemia is directly related to preischemic stores of glucose and glycogen. In other words, hyperglycemic rats had much higher brain lactate levels during ischemia than normoglycemic or hypoglycemic rats. However, the brain energy charge of the animals was not different, and during reperfusion, identical degrees of restitution of energy charge were noted in both normoglycemic and hyperglycemic animals. In a subsequent study(57), the same laboratory noted that hyperglycemic animals in which lactate accumulation occurred had impaired restitution of energy charge as well as nonrecovery of evoked responses. Preischemic hyperglycemia has been shown to result in a more pronounced fall in both intracellular and extracellular brain pH during ischemia(58,59). More importantly, researchers from several laboratories(20,60–63) have demonstrated that when subjected to the same ischemic insult, hyperglycemic animals have a more pronounced histopathologic injury than normoglycemic animals. Thus, preischemic hyperglycemia leads to accelerated production of lactate and hydrogen ion and appears to be detrimental during global ischemia.

Based on these results, it has also been suggested that in the face of impaired oxygen delivery, ongoing delivery of glucose may be detrimental. This may occur, for instance, in states of incomplete ischemia during which glucose delivery would continue at a rate exceeding the oxygen delivery required for aerobic metabolism. This could result in ongoing anaerobic metabolism and tremendous accumulation of lactate and hydrogen ion(64). However, there are alternative mechanisms by which incomplete ischemia may be worse than total ischemia, including the possibility that a trickle of oxygen permits ongoing release of oxygen radicals(55). The premise that incomplete ischemia is worse than total ischemia is controversial, as there are data to suggest that incomplete ischemia is less(65–73) or more(50,52,57,74) damaging than total ischemia. It is plausible that in normoglycemic animals a small amount of CBF may improve recovery. In the absence of acidosis, a low level of CBF may provide enough oxygen to support some energy production and thus confer relative protection. In other words, unless conditions favor production of large amounts of lactate and hydrogen ion, e.g., hyperglycemia, incomplete ischemia probably causes less injury than complete ischemia.

The mechanisms by which acidosis may augment cellular injury during ischemia remain unclear. Direct cytotoxicity, cellular swelling, oxygen radical-mediated damage, and alterations in intracellular calcium homeostasis have been proposed as mechanisms of acidosis-induced injury(55). In vitro studies have demonstrated that direct cytotoxicity of acidosis is a function of both pH and duration of exposure(75–77). For example, astroglial cultures required exposure to pH 6.0 for 60 minutes to cause significant cell death(76), and if exposure is limited to 10 minutes, the critical pH appears to be near 5.0[75]. Acidosis may promote cellular swelling by inhibiting mitochondrial ATP production[78] and thereby reduce sodium/potassium ATPase activity. In addition, in cells with relatively intact ATP production, swelling may occur in an attempt by the cell to regulate intracellular pH at the expense of intracellular volume via activation of sodium/hydrogen ion antiporters. Potentiation of oxygen radical-mediated processes may occur via one of several mechanisms. First, acidosis may decrease binding of iron to iron-binding proteins and thus facilitate iron-catalyzed oxygen radical production[79] (see below). Second, acidosis has been demonstrated to potentiate lipid peroxidation reactions in vitro[80] (see below). Third, acidosis may convert superoxide radical ($O_2{\cdot}^-$) to its protonated, more lipid-soluble form ($HO_2{\cdot}$). Last, acidosis may promote nitric oxide (NO) coupled production of hydroxyl radicals. In the presence of superoxide radical, nitric oxide and superoxide radical react to form peroxynitrite.

$$NO\cdot + O_2{\cdot}^- \rightarrow ONOO^- + H^+ \rightarrow ONOOH$$

Obviously, the formation of peroxynitrite would be promoted by an increased concentration of H^+. Peroxynitrite then decomposes to yield nitrogen dioxide and the highly toxic hydroxyl radical.

$$ONOOH \rightarrow OH\cdot + NO_2$$

The proposed roles of oxygen radicals and nitric oxide in the pathophysiology of hypoxic-ischemic brain injury are discussed below. Acidosis may lead to an increase in the intracellular concentration of unbound calcium, leading to many deleterious processes (see below). This speculation was recently supported by Araki and colleagues[81], who demonstrated that intracellular concentration of calcium returned to normal after transient ischemia more slowly in hyperglycemic animals than in normoglycemic animals. This rise in intracellular calcium concentration may result from one of several mechanisms. First, hydrogen ion competes directly with calcium for intracellular binding sites, and an increased intracellular concentration of hydrogen ion would displace calcium from these binding sites, leading to an increase in unbound or "free" intracellular calcium. Next, acidosis leads to increased activity of the sodium/hydrogen ion antiporters (see above), which creates conditions that favor reversal of sodium/calcium exchange, i.e. influx of calcium.

Recently, it has been suggested that acidosis is not as harmful as previously thought and that mild acidosis may, in fact, be neuroprotective via its modulating effect on the excitotoxic component of ischemic injury[82] (see below). Tombaugh and Sapolsky[83] demonstrated that several hours of oxygen and glucose deprivation damaged cultures of hippocampal neurons at pH 7.4, but this same perturbation failed to cause injury when the extracellular pH was reduced to 6.5. Similar results were found in cortical cultures exposed to glucose and oxygen deprivation at pH 6.6[84]. Acidosis appears to block NMDA gated cell currents[84] and therefore NMDA receptor-mediated calcium accumulation[85]. Thus, it is plausible that mild acidosis decreases NMDA receptor-mediated neurotoxicity. Although the role of acidosis in the pathogenesis of hypoxic-ischemic brain injury is still being defined, it appears that acidosis does contribute to injury and probably produces its detrimental effects by augmenting other pathways of destruction, i.e., oxygen radicals, calcium, etc.

Excitatory Amino Acids

In 1959, Van Harreveld[86] suggested that glutamate might be involved in the pathophysiology of hypoxic-ischemic brain injury. There is now considerable evidence supporting the role of glutamate, an excitatory neurotransmitter, as a mediator of hypoxic-ischemic brain injury, especially in selectively vulnerable brain regions[26]. First, extracellular glutamate levels in brain increase dramatically during ischemia[87–89] and, after 30 minutes of ischemia, exceed by sixfold the concentration required to kill neurons after a 5-minute exposure in vitro[90]. Second, intrahippocampal injection of the competitive glutamate antagonist 2-amino-7-phosphonoheptanoate decreased the loss of CA1 neurons induced by transient cerebral ischemia in the rat[91]. Third, selective ablation of glutamatergic inputs into the hippocampus resulted in significantly less hippocampal injury when the animal was later subjected to an ischemic insult[92,93]. Fourth, glutamate receptor antagonists have been shown to ameliorate injury in animal models of focal[94] and global[95] ischemia. Finally, glutamate receptor antagonists attenuate injury of cultured neurons when the neurons are exposed to oxygen deprivation[96,97] or glucose and oxygen deprivation[98]. Thus, evidence is accumulating in support of a role for glutamate in hypoxic-ischemic brain injury. In this section we discuss the different types of excitatory amino acid receptors, the relationship between receptors and ionic channels, and the proposed mechanisms of injury induced by excitatory amino acids.

Application of molecular biology to the study of glutamate receptors has led to an explosion of information in this area which is well beyond the scope of this chapter[99–101]. The following summary is obviously a simplification but in adequate detail for an understanding of glutamate receptors and their role in the pathophysiology of ischemia. Glutamate receptors can be broadly classified into two major categories, ionotropic and metabotropic, based on pharmacological, electrophysiological, and biochemical studies. Ionotropic glutamate receptors gate cation channels that allow movement of cations through the cell membrane, whereas metabotropic glutamate receptors are coupled to adenylate cyclase or phospholipase C via G proteins[99] **(Table 20.1).** G proteins are membrane proteins that facilitate transmembrane signalling. The ionotropic glutamate receptors are further subdivided into the NMDA and the α-amino-3-hydroxy-5-methyl-4-isoxazole-4-propionic acid (AMPA)-kainate receptor based on their selective agonist. The AMPA-kainate receptor is also referred to as the non-NMDA receptor.

The NMDA receptor is the most widely studied glutamate receptor. The channel gated by this receptor allows

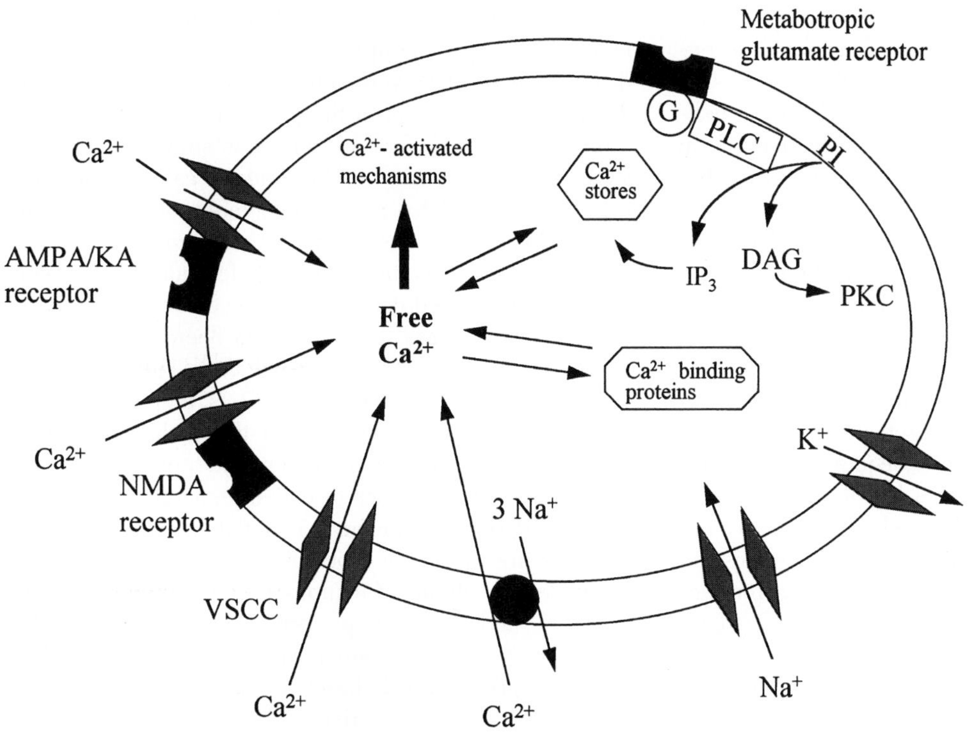

Figure 20.3. Events leading to accumulation of intracellular calcium during ischemia. Extracellular calcium may enter the neuron via NMDA and AMPA/KA gated calcium channels, voltage-sensitive calcium channels, and via reversal of the sodium/calcium exchanger. Sequestered calcium may be mobilized by IP_3 produced after stimulation of the metabotropic glutamate receptor and bound calcium may be displaced by hydrogen ions produced during ischemia. AMPA, α-amino-3-hydroxy-5-methyl-4-isoxazole-4-propionic acid; DAG, diacylglycerol; G, G protein; IP_3, inositol 1,4,5-trisphosphate; KA, kainate; NMDA, N-methyl-D-aspartate; PI, phosphoinositides; PKC, protein kinase C; PLC, phospholipase C; and VSCC, voltage-sensitive calcium channel. (Modified from Morley P, Hogan MJ, Hakim AM. Calcium-mediated mechanisms of ischemic injury and protection. Brain Pathol 1994; 4:39.)

entry of sodium, potassium, and calcium[(99)] (Fig. 20.3), and calcium accumulation via this channel[(102–104)] is felt to be responsible for the neurotoxicity of glutamate[(105–107)]. The NMDA receptor-ion channel complex is unique in that calcium entry is modulated by several factors including glycine, polyamines, magnesium, and zinc[(99)] (Table 20.1).

The non-NMDA receptor has been shown to exhibit significant functional and structural heterogeneity[(99,100)]. Until recently, this receptor-ion channel complex was felt to be permeable to only monovalent cations (sodium and potassium) and relatively impermeable to calcium. However, it has been shown that the ion channel gated by the non-NMDA receptor allows direct influx of calcium[(108)] and that ischemia may induce changes in receptor subunits that change the non-NMDA receptor-ion channel from calcium-impermeable to calcium permeable[(109)] (Fig. 20.3). Consistent with this work, non-NMDA receptor antagonists have

Table 20.1. Glutamate Receptors

Receptor	*Effector*
Ionotropic	
NMDA	cation channels (Na^+, K^+, and Ca^{2+})
AMPA/kainate (non-NMDA)	cation channels (Na^+, K^+, and Ca^{2+})
Metabotropic	
mGluR1	stimulate phospholipase C
mGluR2	inhibit adenylate cyclase
mGluR3	inhibit adenylate cyclase
mGluR4	inhibit adenylate cyclase
mGluR5	stimulate phospholipase C
mGluR6	inhibit adenylate cyclase
mGluR7	inhibit adenylate cyclase

NMDA, N-methyl-D-aspartate; AMPA, α-amino-3-hydroxy-5-methyl-4-isoxazole-4-propionic acid.

been shown to reduce neuronal injury after focal and global ischemia[(110)].

The metabotropic glutamate receptors are coupled to second messenger pathways via G proteins[(99,101)] (Table 20.1). Metabotropic receptors can be distinguished from ionotropic receptors by the use of (1S,3R)-1-aminocyclopentane-1,3-dicarboxylic acid (1S,3R-ACPD), a selective agonist for metabotropic glutamate receptors[(111)]. Metabotropic receptors are coupled to phospholipase C[(112,113)] or adenylate cyclase[(114)]. Thus, stimulation of the metabotropic receptor leads to increased production of diacylglycerol and inositol 1,4,5-trisphosphate (Fig. 20.3) or decreased production of cyclic adenosine monophosphate. Seven subtypes of the metabotropic glutamate receptor have been identified[(99,115)]; subtypes 1 and 5 are coupled phospholipase C, whereas subtypes 2, 3, 4, 6, and 7 are coupled to adenylate cyclase.

Evidence supporting the role of glutamate neurotoxicity in hypoxic-ischemic brain injury was outlined above. How does glutamate exposure induce neuronal death? Current thinking[(105–107)] suggests that calcium (see below) plays a pivotal role in glutamate neurotoxicity. Choi and Hartley[(106)] proposed that glutamate-induced neuronal death is a three-stage process, as follows: (1) induction, (2) amplification, and (3) expression. During induction, glutamate activates neuronal receptors. Activation of NMDA receptors leads to an influx of calcium, whereas activation of non-NMDA receptors leads to influx of sodium and an obligatory influx of chloride and water. As described above, non-NMDA receptor stimulation may also lead to influx of calcium. Stimulation of the metabotropic receptor leads to increased production of inositol 1,4,5-trisphosphate and diacylglycerol. The cellular injury cascades initiated during the induction stage can be divided into two components: acute cellular swelling (sodium dependent) and delayed neuronal degeneration (calcium dependent)[(116)]. Both of these processes can be interrupted in cell culture models of glutamate neurotoxicity by removing sodium or calcium, respectively, from the extracellular space[(117)]. Amplification results from the damaging cascades initiated by increased concentrations of calcium, inositol 1,4,5-trisphosphate, and diacylglycerol. Altered calcium homeostasis leads to activation of many deleterious processes (see below), including activation of phospholipases, proteases, endonucleases, protein kinases, and calmodulin-regulated enzymes, e.g., nitric oxide synthase. There is preliminary evidence that nitric oxide is an important mediator of glutamate neurotoxicity[(118)]. Inositol 1,4,5-trisphosphate causes release of sequestered intracellular calcium[(119)], resulting in further increases in intracellular calcium concentrations, and diacylglycerol causes activation of protein kinase C[(120)] (Fig. 20.3). The expression stage consists of actual cell destruction resulting from activation of catabolic enzyme systems and oxygen radical production.

However, our understanding of glutamate neurotoxicity is incomplete. For example, what is the role of the metabotropic receptor? Koh and colleagues[(121)] demonstrated that 1S,3R-ACPD, a selective metabotropic receptor agonist, failed to produce cellular injury in neuronal cultures. The role of the metabotropic receptor may depend on the predominant receptor subtype that is expressed on the cell being studied, e.g., subtype 1 may potentiate injury (increases inositol 1,4,5-trisphosphate and diacylglycerol), whereas subtype 2 (decreases cyclic adenosine monophosphate) may be protective. Further work in this area will continue to yield valuable information to our understanding of the pathophysiology of hypoxic-ischemic brain injury. In summary, there is increasing evidence that glutamate plays a significant role in hypoxic-ischemic brain injury, and the mechanism of glutamate-induced injury appears to be initiated by alterations in calcium homeostasis, leading to the activation of many deleterious processes (see below).

Calcium Metabolism

Calcium plays a strategic role in the regulation of many cellular metabolic processes, and therefore the concentration of cytosolic free calcium is tightly controlled. Hypoxic-ischemic injury is postulated to interrupt intracellular calcium homeostasis, resulting in massive increases in the intracellular concentration of calcium[(105,122–124)]. This calcium accumulation is felt to promote irreversible cellular injury by activating phospholipases, proteases, and endonucleases and uncoupling oxidative phosphorylation[(125)]. Recent work suggests that calcium plays a key role in triggering nitric oxide synthase, protein kinases, oxygen radical production, and alterations in gene expression[(31)] (see below). What is the evidence supporting the speculation that altered calcium homeostasis contributes to ischemic cell death? It has been conclusively demonstrated that calcium accumulation occurs during and after ischemia[(126–128)]. The role of calcium in ischemia-induced cell death is less definitively substantiated. Indirect evidence for the role of calcium in the pathophysiology of ischemic injury exists in the form of numerous studies that demonstrate that pharmacological blockade of calcium entry during and/or after global ischemia confers protection, i.e., improves outcome (see below). Several in vitro studies provide more direct evidence favoring a role for calcium accumulation in ischemic cell death. Removing calcium from the extracellular space has been shown to decrease cellular injury in neuronal[(129,130)] and astroglial[(131)] cultures exposed to oxygen and glucose deprivation. Thus, it appears that calcium may play a pivotal role in the pathophysiology of hypoxic-ischemic injury. In the remainder of this section we review the different types of calcium channels and potential mechanisms of calcium accumulation.

There are two major types of calcium channels located in the cell membrane of neurons: voltage-sensitive calcium channels and receptor-operated calcium channels (see above). Four voltage-sensitive calcium channels have been identified **(Table 20.2)** based on electrophysiological and pharmacological characteristics[(132)]; they are designated L (long lasting), T (transient), N (neuronal, neither L nor T), and P (Purkinje cells). The L-type channel has properties of high voltage activation, high conductance, and slow inactivation and therefore may make a larger direct contribution to calcium influx during ischemia than the other subtypes. Of note, the L-type channel is the only subtype to be blocked by calcium channel blockers of the dihydropyridine class, e.g., nimodipine. The N-type channel, with properties of high voltage activation and moderate inactivation, appears to be linked to neurotransmitter release and is blocked by conotoxins. The P-type channel also requires high voltage activation but has very slow inactivation. The P-type channel appears to be linked to neurotransmitter release, and its distribution in the central nervous system (CNS) is much greater than initially thought[(133)]. T-type channels have properties of low voltage activation and rapid inactivation and are involved in pacemaker activity, e.g., conducting system of the heart. Thus, during ischemia, the L-type channel could allow direct postsynaptic entry of calcium, whereas presynaptic calcium entry via the P- or N-type channel could lead to glutamate release and resultant calcium entry via glutamate-gated calcium channels (see above). Early theories regarding calcium-related neuronal injury[(134)] speculated that calcium entered cells

Table 20.2. Voltage-Sensitive Calcium Channels[a]

Channel	*Activation*	*Inactivation*	*Function*
L	high voltage	slow	dihydropyridine sensitive
N	high voltage	moderate	neurotransmitter release
P	medium voltage	very slow	neurotransmitter release
T	Low voltage	rapid	pacemaker activity

[a] *Modified from Spedding M, Paoletti R. Classification of calcium channels and the sites of drugs modifying channel function. Pharmacol Rev 1992;44:368.*

primarily via these voltage-sensitive calcium channels. However, it has become apparent that calcium entry also occurs via receptor-operated calcium channels gated by NMDA[102–104] and non-NMDA[108] receptors (see above).

Intracellular free calcium may increase during ischemia either by influx of extracellular calcium or by release of bound or sequestered intracellular calcium (Fig. 20.3). Cerebral ischemia is accompanied by a significant decrease in extracellular calcium concentration[135,136], which is consistent with an intracellular shift of calcium. Energy failure during ischemia results in membrane depolarization, which allows calcium influx via voltage-sensitive calcium channels[103,137] and causes glutamate release[87–89]. Glutamate can promote calcium influx by three different mechanisms. The first and most obvious mechanism is via opening the NMDA receptor-gated calcium channel[102–104]. Second, stimulation of non-NMDA receptors opens sodium channels (see above) and results in massive influx of sodium and subsequent membrane depolarization. Membrane depolarization would then allow calcium entry via voltage-sensitive calcium channels. Third, the ion channel gated by non-NMDA receptors allows direct influx of calcium[108,109]. Two additional possibilities exist for calcium entry during ischemia: (1) reversal of sodium/calcium exchanger and (2) nonspecific membrane leak. As described above, massive influx of sodium during ischemia creates conditions that inhibit or even reverse sodium/calcium exchange, leading to further calcium influx. It is also possible that calcium enters through areas of the cell membrane that have been damaged by the ischemic insult. Release of bound or sequestered calcium probably occurs via two different mechanisms. First, as described above, hydrogen ion which accumulates during ischemia can directly displace bound calcium. Second, sequestered intracellular calcium may be mobilized by inositol 1,4,5-trisphosphate[119], which is produced by glutamate-stimulated hydrolysis of polyphosphoinositides mediated by the metabotropic receptor[112,113] (see above).

How much does each mechanism contribute to the rise in intracellular calcium seen during and after ischemia? This remains unclear. It is also unclear whether influx of calcium or release from intracellular stores is predominant. While most work has centered on the role of calcium influx, recent work points to the importance of release of sequestered calcium. Mitani and colleagues[138] demonstrated that two-thirds of the increase in intracellular concentration of calcium seen in cultures of hippocampal neurons subjected to glucose and oxygen deprivation is due to release of sequestered calcium, and one-third is due to influx of extracellular calcium. Research from the same laboratory[139] showed that dantrolene, which blocks the release of sequestered calcium, produced significant protection against delayed neuronal death in a gerbil model of transient forebrain ischemia. Thus, the relative contribution of influx and release from internal stores is still not clear, but there is evidence accumulating that release from internal stores does indeed play a role. To summarize, intracellular calcium accumulation is assumed to play a significant role in ischemic brain injury, and its accumulation appears to be initiated by energy failure and glutamate-mediated events.

Phospholipid Hydrolysis

Metabolism of membrane phospholipids is postulated to play a key role in the pathophysiology of ischemic brain injury[140,141]. Early in the course of ischemia, fatty acids are released from membrane phospholipids by enzymatic hydrolysis[142,143]. Fatty acids appear to be released via two pathways (Fig. 20.4): (1) membrane phospholipid degradation by the action of phospholipase A_1 and phospholipase A_2[144,145] and (2) degradation of phosphoinositides by the action of phospholipase C, leading to the production of diacylglycerol which is then hydrolyzed by diacylglycerol and monoacylglycerol lipases[146–149]. Release of free fatty acids and diacylglycerol may simply be an epiphenomenon of ischemic brain injury or, as discussed below, may directly contribute to brain damage.

The mechanisms leading to the activation of phospholipid hydrolysis during ischemia are unclear. Phospholipid turnover normally is a balance between synthesis and degradation[150]. Energy depletion leading to a greater rate of deacylation relative to reacylation (energy dependent) is one potential mechanism leading to free fatty acid production during ischemia. Also plausible is receptor-stimulated phospholipid hydrolysis. Stimulation of NMDA receptors leads to activation of phospholipase A_2[151–155]; this activation appears to be calcium-mediated. Farooqui and colleagues[156] have shown that NMDA receptor stimulation also leads to activation of monoacylglycerol and diacylglycerol lipases. As described above, stimulation of certain metabotropic receptor subtypes leads to activation of phospholipase C[111–113]. Thus, in neurons, both enzymic pathways leading to liberation of arachidonic acid are modulated, at least in part, by glutamate receptors.

Free fatty acids and diacylglycerols produced during ischemia appear to have directly injurious effects. As alluded to above, diacylglycerol is a substrate for further free fatty acid release. Furthermore, diacylglycerol and inositol 1,4,5-trisphosphate, produced by the action of phospholipase C on polyphosphoinositides, have been implicated as second messengers in intracellular signal transduction. Inositol 1,4,5-trisphosphate mobilizes intracellular calcium[103], which is postulated to initiate many destructive processes during ischemia (see above), and diacylglycerols activate protein kinase C[120] and inhibit sodium/potassium ATPase[157]. Free fatty acids inhibit sodium/potassium ATPase[158,159], promote brain edema[160], uncouple oxidative phosphorylation[161–163], promote release of neurotransmitters[164], inhibit uptake of neurotransmitters[159,165–167], and activate protein kinase C[168]. In addition, release of free fatty acids at the onset of ischemia provides the substrate (arachidonic acid) for production of eicosanoids[169] and oxygen radicals[170] during reperfusion. In summary,

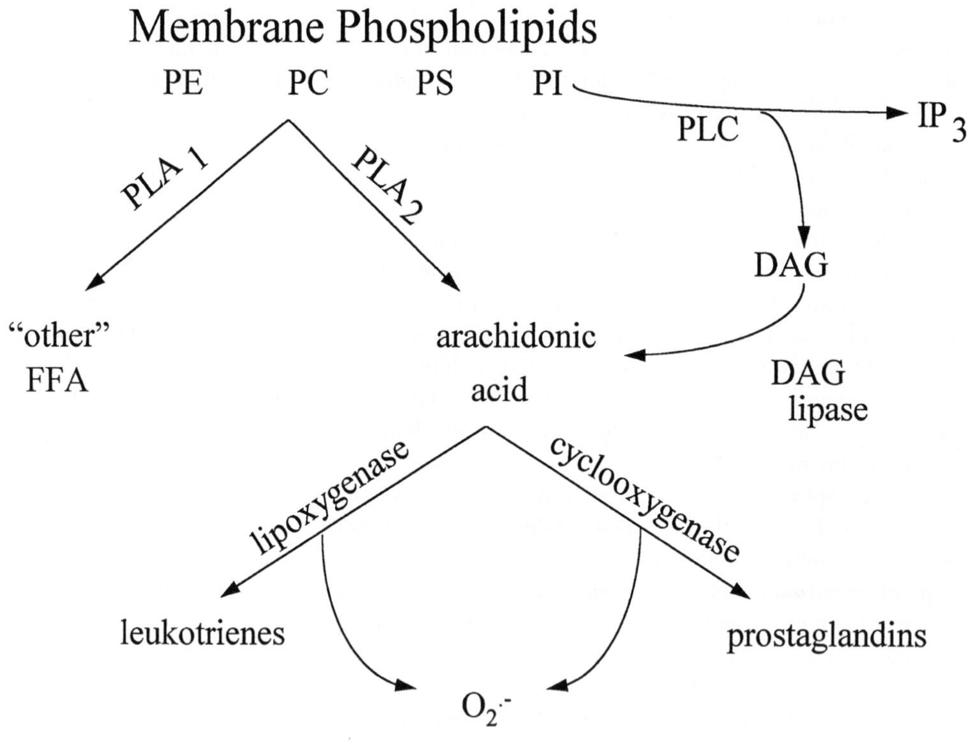

Figure 20.4. Phospholipid metabolism during ischemia. Membrane phospholipids are hydrolyzed by two pathways: PLA_1/PLA_2 pathway and PLC/DAG lipase pathway. Arachidonic acid produced by phospholipid hydrolysis is the substrate for eicosanoid synthesis and oxygen radical production. DAG, diacylglycerol; FFA, free fatty acids; IP_3, inositol 1,4,5-trisphosphate; PC, phosphatidylcholine; PE, phosphatidylethanolamine; PI, phosphatidylinositol; PS, phosphatidylserine; PLA_1, phospholipase A_1; PLA_2, phospholipase A_2; PLC, and phospholipase C.

free fatty acids and diacylglycerols are released during ischemia; this release appears to be at least partially induced by receptor-mediated events, and free fatty acids and diacylglycerols seem to be directly involved in cellular injury.

Eicosanoid Metabolism

Arachidonate released at the onset of ischemia becomes the substrate for eicosanoid production during reperfusion (see Figure 20.4). Products of the cyclooxygenase pathway[(169,171–174)], i.e., thromboxane and prostaglandins, and the lipoxygenase pathway[(169,175)], i.e., leukotrienes, are formed during reperfusion after ischemia. The role of eicosanoids in ischemic brain injury is unclear, but they appear to affect primarily the cerebral circulation. Thromboxane causes vasoconstriction and platelet aggregation and thus may play a role in delayed hypoperfusion. Likewise, leukotrienes have been shown to cause vasoconstriction of cerebral vessels[(176,177)] and may also be one of the mediators of delayed hypoperfusion. In addition, the cyclooxygenase and lipoxygenase pathways produce superoxide radical[(170)], and these pathways may be a significant source of oxygen radicals during reperfusion (see below).

Oxygen Radicals

Oxygen radicals have been implicated in numerous disease processes, including pulmonary oxygen toxicity[(178)], carcinogenesis[(179)], and reperfusion injury after ischemia[(180)]. Relevant to this discussion, oxygen radicals have long been implicated as mediators of reperfusion injury after cerebral ischemia[(181)]; however, until recently, direct evidence for production of oxygen radicals during reperfusion has been lacking[(182,183)]. Validation has been difficult because oxygen radicals are extremely volatile compounds with extraordinarily short half-lives (see below), which makes their measurement problematic. Indirect evidence in support of oxygen radical-mediated injury after cerebral ischemia includes decreases in tissue antioxidant levels during ischemia and reperfusion[(181,184,185)], increased production of lipid peroxides during reperfusion[(186–190)], improved outcome after global[(191–193)] and focal[(194–197)] ischemia in animals treated with antioxidants, and reduction in infarct volume after focal ischemia in transgenic mice that overexpress superoxide dismutase[(198,199)]. Direct evidence documenting the role of oxygen radicals in the pathophysiology of hypoxic-ischemic brain injury has begun to accumulate largely due to the development of methods that allow measurement of oxygen radicals in vivo. Nitroblue tetrazolium reduction[(200,201)], electron spin resonance spectroscopy[(202,203)], and salicylate trapping[(204,205)] have been used to document oxygen radical production during and/or after cerebral ischemia. In this section, we review the different oxygen radical species allegedly involved in reperfusion injury, their mechanisms of production, and the mechanisms by which they may produce cellular injury.

It is appropriate first to define an oxygen radical. Radicals are molecules that contain at least one unpaired electron in the outer (valence) electron orbital. Some of the more common oxygen radicals include superoxide radical ($O_2^{\cdot -}$), hydroxyl radical ($OH^{\cdot}$), and hydrogen peroxide (H_2O_2)[(206–208)]. These molecules are very reactive and, as a result, very short lived. These properties make the study

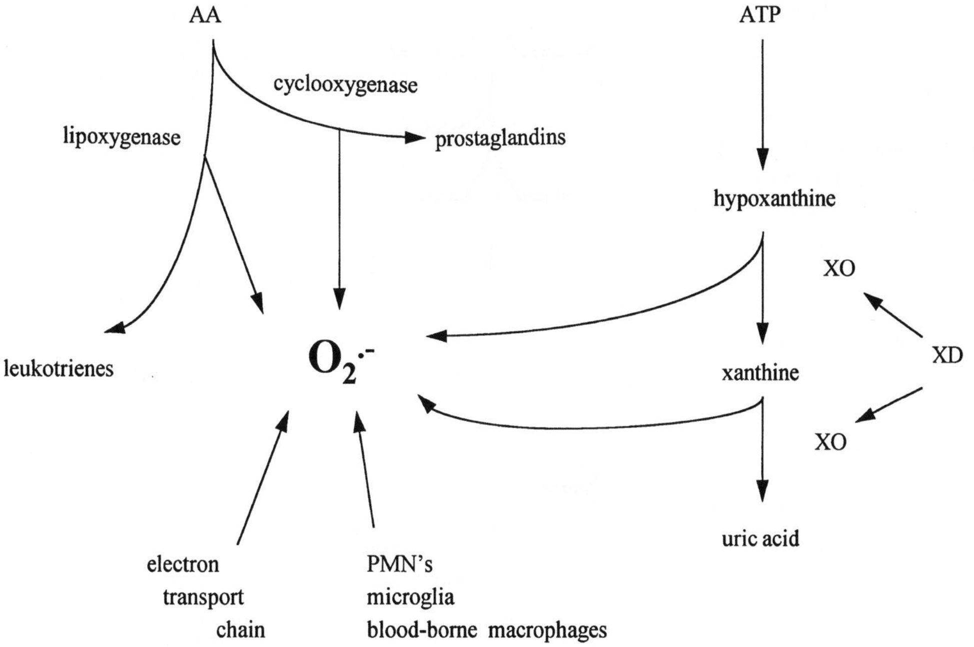

Figure 20.5. Potential mechanisms of superoxide radical production during ischemia and reperfusion. Important pathways leading to production of superoxide radical include the cyclooxygenase and lipoxygenase pathways and the purine degradation pathway. Other potential sites of superoxide radical production include the electron transport chain and inflammatory cells. AA, arachidonic acid; ATP, adenosine triphosphate; PMN, polymorphonuclear leukocyte; XD, xanthine dehydrogenase; and XO, xanthine oxidase.

of oxygen radical-mediated processes extremely difficult, hence the paucity of data either confirming or refuting their role in reperfusion injury.

Superoxide radical is formed after the addition of a single electron to diatomic oxygen (O_2)[207,209]. The multiple pathways of superoxide radical production are diagrammed in Figure 20.5. It is formed when the electron transport chain operates in the presence of oxygen. Regardless of the tightness of the control of the electron transport chain, there is always "electron leak," which allows oxygen to accept single electrons, and superoxide radical formation occurs. During ischemia, highly reduced conditions may lead to enhanced production of superoxide radical via this mechanism. Potential mechanisms of oxygen radical production during reperfusion include oxidation of hypoxanthine by xanthine oxidase[210] and arachidonate metabolism via the cyclooxygenase and lipoxygenase pathways[170]. The relative contribution of each of these two mechanisms to oxygen radical production during reperfusion is unclear. Shortly after the onset of global ischemia, adenine nucleotides are metabolized through a series of intermediates to hypoxanthine, the substrate for xanthine oxidase. Adenosine[211] and hypoxanthine[212] concentrations in brain increase dramatically within seconds after the onset of ischemia. Thus, there appears to be an abundance of substrate, but whether there is adequate enzyme present for this pathway to contribute significantly to oxygen radical production during reperfusion remains speculative. Xanthine oxidase activity is very low in brain[213] but is substantial in cerebral vascular endothelium[214]. More importantly, ischemia has been shown to induce the conversion of xanthine dehydrogenase to xanthine oxidase, leading to significant levels of xanthine oxidase in brain[215]. This conversion appears to be a calcium dependent process. Recent work by Phillis and Sen[203] provides direct evidence that the xanthine oxidase pathway contributes to oxygen radical production during reperfusion. They demonstrated that oxypurinol, a xanthine oxidase inhibitor, significantly decreased production of hydroxyl radical after cerebral ischemia in rats. The contribution of arachidonate metabolism to oxygen radical production after cerebral ischemia appears to be supported by preliminary evidence. Kontos et al.[216] demonstrated that when arachidonate is directly applied to the cortex of cats, providing a substrate for the cyclooxygenase and lipoxygenase pathways, superoxide radical is generated. More significantly, Armstead et al.[200] demonstrated superoxide radical production during reperfusion after global cerebral ischemia in piglets. This superoxide radical production was reduced nearly to control levels by pretreatment with indomethacin. Thus, results of these preliminary studies suggest that superoxide radical may be produced through pathways of arachidonate metabolism. Additional mechanisms for production of oxygen radicals include polymorphonuclear leukocytes, microglia, and blood-borne macrophages[182,183]. These are discussed below.

The superoxide radical is an extremely reactive compound and undergoes a dismutation reaction that produces hydrogen peroxide:

$$2O_2{\cdot}^- + 2H^+ \; H_2O_2 + O_2$$

This reaction is spontaneous but is greatly enhanced by the presence of superoxide dismutase[217]. Under normal conditions, hydrogen peroxide is not produced in quantities that will overwhelm the cells' antioxidant defenses. Hydrogen peroxide is degraded by two enzymes. One reaction is catalyzed by catalase:

$$2H_2O_2 \rightarrow O_2 + 2H_2O$$

A more important mechanism may be the reaction catalyzed by glutathione peroxidase:

$$2GSH + H_2O_2 \rightarrow GSSH + 2H_2O$$

The oxidized glutathione (GSSH) produced in this reaction can be quickly reduced by glutathione reductase to provide an ongoing supply of reduced glutathione (GSH). Under certain conditions, e.g., reperfusion after ischemia, hydrogen peroxide is produced in quantities that overwhelm intracellular scavenging mechanisms, and hydrogen peroxide is converted into the highly reactive hydroxyl radical. In the presence of Fe^{2+}, hydrogen peroxide can cause a Fenton-type reaction forming hydroxyl radicals:

$$Fe^{2+} + H_2O_2 \rightarrow Fe^{3+} + OH\cdot + OH^-$$

Iron in brain exists in the oxidized state (Fe^{3+}) and is tightly bound to proteins such as ferritin or transferrin. Superoxide radical can reduce and mobilize bound iron, resulting in unbound ferrous ion[218]:

$$O_2\cdot^- + \text{ferritin-}Fe^{3+} \rightarrow O_2 + \text{ferritin} + Fe^{2+}$$

If the above reaction is coupled to the Fenton-type reaction, the sum of the two reactions is the Haber-Weiss reaction:

$$O_2\cdot^- + H_2O_2 \rightarrow O_2 + OH\cdot + OH^-$$

In other words, hydrogen peroxide is converted to hydroxyl radical via a superoxide-dependent, iron-catalyzed reaction. Hydroxyl radical is also produced by decomposition of peroxynitrite formed by superoxide radical and nitric oxide (see above).

Hydroxyl radical is extremely reactive and combines with most molecules at rates that are limited by diffusion. The radical cannot cross membranes, largely because it reacts with them immediately, wreaking havoc and causing lipid peroxidation. This ion is probably responsible for most of the damage caused by oxygen radicals. It is much more reactive than either superoxide or hydrogen peroxide, there are no intrinsic scavenging mechanisms for this radical, and it has a propensity to react with lipid membranes.

There are at least four mechanisms by which these oxygen radicals may produce cellular injury during reperfusion. First, oxygen radicals may potentiate injury produced by excitatory amino acids. Oxygen radicals have been shown to promote release of excitatory amino acids[219] and inhibit their uptake[220]. Second, Oliver and coworkers[221] demonstrated a significant increase in protein oxidation and a decrease in glutamine synthetase activity during reperfusion after global ischemia in gerbils. Other important enzymes may lose their activity after oxidative injury, thus contributing to neuronal injury and death. In addition, loss of glutamine synthetase activity should lead to increased levels of glutamate and may contribute to neuronal injury via glutamate-mediated mechanisms (see above). Third, oxygen radicals have been demonstrated to cause strand scission of nucleic acids[222], and this may also contribute to delayed neuronal death. Finally, oxygen radicals (more specifically, hydroxyl radicals) cause peroxidation of membrane phospholipids[186–190]. Lipid peroxidation is probably the most important of these four mechanisms of injury and thus is discussed here in greater detail.

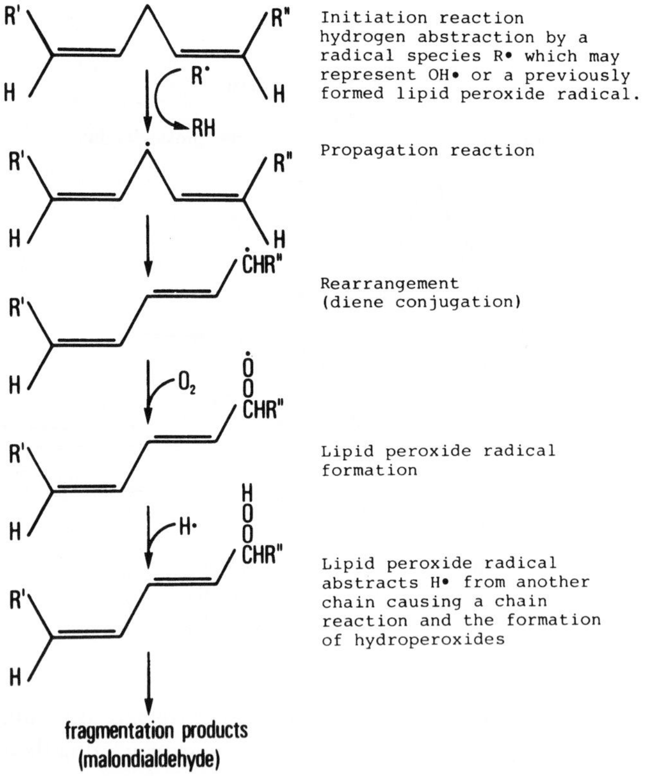

Figure 20.6. Schematic representation of polyunsaturated fatty acid peroxidation. (From Del Maestro R. An approach to oxygen radicals in medicine and biology. Acta Physiol Scand [Suppl] 1980;492:161.)

Lipid peroxidation is an iron-dependent process in which oxygen radicals oxidatively rearrange the structure of double bonds of unsaturated fatty acids of membrane phospholipids[207]. A hydrogen atom is removed from polyunsaturated fatty acids; this can only be done by the hydroxyl radical (not by superoxide or hydrogen peroxide). This creates a carbon radical, which is quickly rearranged to form a conjugated diene. This combines with molecular oxygen to form the peroxy radical, which then reacts with other fatty acids and causes a chain reaction. The process is diagrammed in Figure 20.6. The hydroperoxides that are formed in this process are stable unless they come into contact with transition metals such as iron or copper. The presence of heme proteins such as the cytochromes and hemoglobin ensures the availability of such transition metals, and the lipid hydroperoxides are decomposed, thus perpetuating the chain reaction. In addition, these lipid peroxidation reactions are intensified in the presence of calcium[223] and acidosis[80].

Lipid peroxidation may contribute to cellular injury and death via several different mechanisms. Most importantly, changes in fatty acid configuration may lead to alterations of membrane fluidity and permeability[224], resulting in dis-

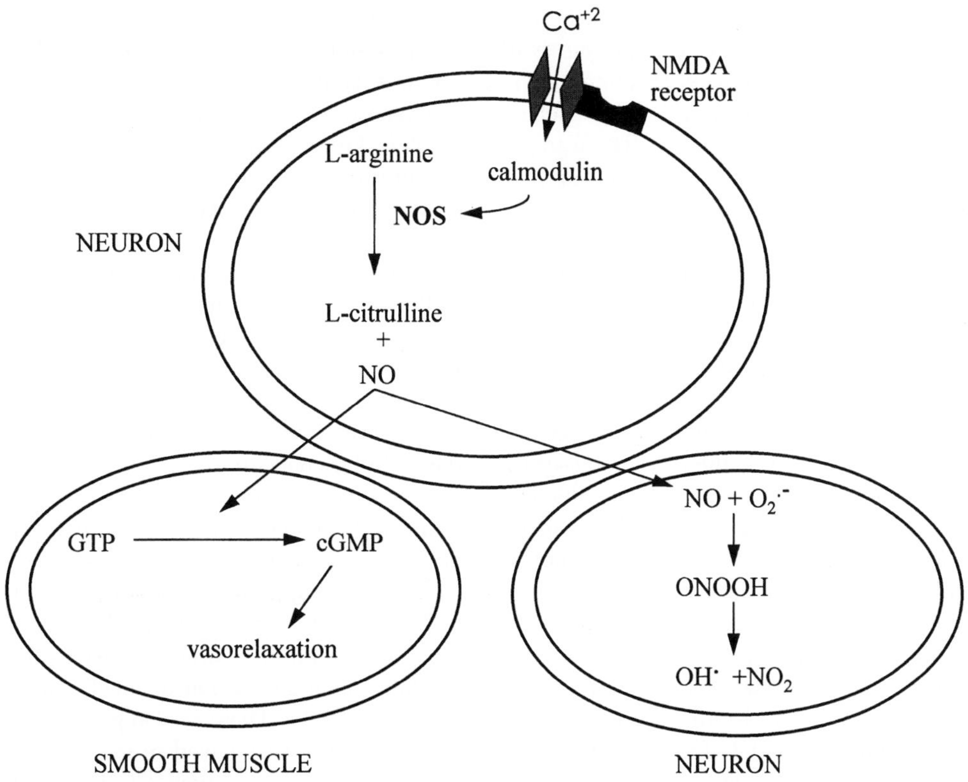

Figure 20.7. Nitric oxide metabolism during ischemia and reperfusion. Nitric oxide is formed by the reaction catalyzed by nitric oxide synthase, which converts L-arginine to L-citrulline and nitric oxide. Nitric oxide diffuses to target cells, where it stimulates guanylate cyclase leading to vasorelaxation, or it can react with superoxide radical leading to the production of hydroxyl radical. cGMP, cyclic guanosine monophosphate; GTP, guanosine triphosphate; NMDA, N-methyl-D-aspartate; NO, nitric oxide; NOS, nitric oxide synthase; OH·, hydroxyl radical; $O_2{}^{\cdot-}$, superoxide radical; and ONOOH, peroxynitrite.

ruption of organelles and even the cell as a whole. In addition, lipid peroxidation products activate phospholipase A_2[(225)] and protein kinase C[(226)] and inhibit sodium/potassium ATPase[(227)]. Thus, lipid peroxidation may significantly contribute to cellular injury during reperfusion.

It is important to reemphasize the interrelatedness of the numerous pathways of cellular destruction during ischemia and reperfusion. Acidosis appears to exacerbate oxygen-radical mediated injury (see above). Alterations in calcium homeostasis lead to activation of phospholipase A_2, conversion of xanthine dehydrogenase to xanthine oxidase, and activation of nitric oxide synthase. All three of these processes may lead to oxygen radical formation (see above). In turn, oxygen radicals inhibit glutamate uptake and lipid peroxides increase phospholipase A_2 activity (see above).

In summary, oxygen radicals may play a significant role in reperfusion injury after cerebral ischemia. The extremely reactive and short-lived nature of these molecules makes documentation of their role in hypoxic-ischemic brain injury very difficult. Nonetheless, data continue to accumulate that support a very significant role for these processes in cellular injury after ischemia.

Nitric Oxide

Over the past 9 years, nitric oxide has become established as an important molecular messenger in mammals[(228–233)]. It is an uncharged molecule and thus readily diffuses across cell membranes. It has an unpaired electron and therefore reacts rapidly with oxygen in aqueous solutions to form nitrite and nitrate[(230)]. As a result, it has an extremely short half-life. It has been implicated in processes as diverse as immune cell-mediated cytotoxicity, inhibition of platelet aggregation, smooth muscle relaxation, and neuronal signalling[(228)]. Nitric oxide is produced in a reaction catalyzed by nitric oxide synthase in which oxygen and L-arginine are converted into citrulline and nitric oxide (Fig. 20.7). Nitric oxide synthase requires several cofactors including flavin adenine dinucleotide, flavin mononucleotide, nicotinamide adenine dinucleotide phosphate, tetrahydrobiopterin, and heme[(232)]. Three isoforms of nitric oxide synthase have been described. There are two constitutive isoforms: neuronal and endothelial. An inducible isoform has also been described and has been demonstrated in macrophages, microglia, and astrocytes[(233)]. The constitutive enzymes are calcium-calmodulin dependent enzymes, whereas the inducible isoform is calcium independent. Neuronal nitric oxide synthase is present in highest concentration in the cerebellum and lowest in the medulla[(234)], and there are neurons that express nitric oxide synthase in all brain regions. The function of nitric oxide in the CNS is far from elucidated. It appears to be involved in regulation of CBF[(229,233)] and in cell-cell signalling[(230–232)]. In some neurons, nitric oxide synthase activity is regulated by the NMDA receptor (Fig. 20.7). NMDA receptor stimulation results in calcium influx and activation of nitric oxide synthase. Nitric oxide is produced and then diffuses to target cells and stimulates guanylate cyclase, leading to the production of cyclic guanosine monophosphate (GMP) (Fig. 20.7). Cyclic GMP then produces the physiological effect, e.g., vasorelaxation, cell signalling, etc. Inducible nitric oxide synthase is expressed by several cell types (including macrophages, microglia, and astrocytes) in response to stimulation by cytokines. Nitric oxide produced by this enzyme is involved in cell-mediated cytotoxicity[228,232]. The mechanism of this cytotoxicity is not yet fully understood but may involve inhibition of key enzymes necessary for DNA replication and mitochondrial energy production[232].

Nitric oxide appears to be a mediator of glutamate neurotoxicity[118]. It is postulated that NMDA receptor overstimulation leads to massive calcium influx and activation of nitric oxide synthase. Nitric oxide produced via this mechanism contributes to the cytotoxity of glutamate, presumably via hydroxyl radical production (Fig. 20.7). Nitric oxide contributes to hydroxyl radical production through its reaction with superoxide radical. Nitric oxide and superoxide radical react to form peroxynitrite. Peroxynitrite then decomposes to yield nitrogen dioxide and the highly toxic hydroxyl radical (see above). Obviously, hydroxyl radical formation is dependent on the presence of superoxide radical. Recent work by Lipton and colleagues suggests that nitric oxide produced by NMDA receptor stimulation may be neurotoxic or neuroprotective based on the redox state of nitric oxide[235]. Neurotoxicity results if the redox state favors peroxynitrite formation and subsequent hydroxyl radical production. Neuroprotection results if the redox state favors formation of nitrosonium ion, which may protect by nitrosylating NMDA receptors, resulting in their downregulation. The role of nitric oxide in cerebral ischemia remains unclear. Nitric oxide is produced during both focal[236] and global[237] ischemia. However, one can easily envision that nitric oxide could be both beneficial and detrimental to the brain during ischemia and reperfusion. Possible beneficial effects include vasodilation, inhibition of platelet aggregation, and downregulation of NMDA receptors, whereas possible detrimental effects include production of hydroxyl radicals and inhibition of key enzymes necessary for DNA replication and mitochondrial energy production[238]. Accordingly, animal studies using nitric oxide synthase inhibitors for treatment of both global and focal ischemia have yielded mixed results[229,233,238] (see below). Thus, nitric oxide, a novel molecular messenger, appears to play a significant role in the pathophysiology of cerebral ischemia. However, our understanding of this role is still in its infancy.

Protein Phosphorylation

Many cellular processes are regulated by protein phosphorylation. Protein phosphorylation leads to either activation or inhibition of the function of the phosphorylated protein. The phosphorylation state depends on the relative activities of two opposing types of enzymes: kinases and phosphatases. As their names imply, kinases add phosphate groups to proteins, whereas phosphatases remove phosphate groups. Protein kinases are activated by second messengers such as calcium, diacylglycerol, arachidonic acid, and cyclic adenosine monophosphate; the regulation of phosphatases is not well understood. Protein kinases regulate important neuronal functions, including ion channel activity, transmitter release, receptor function, gene expression, and protein synthesis. It has therefore been proposed that alterations in protein kinase activity during and/or after cerebral ischemia may contribute to neuronal death[31,239]. Three important protein kinases have been shown to have changes in activity after cerebral ischemia: protein kinase C, calcium-calmodulin dependent kinase II, and casein kinase II.

Activation of protein kinase C requires translocation from cytosol to cell membrane; this translocation is promoted by a rise in the intracellular concentration of calcium. After association with membrane phospholipids, protein kinase C becomes fully activated in the presence of diacylglycerol[240]. As described above, ischemia leads to increases in the intracellular concentrations of both calcium and diacylglycerol, creating conditions conducive to activation of protein kinase C. Indeed, protein kinase C has been shown to translocate from cytosol to plasma membrane during ischemia[241–243]; however, during reperfusion, its activity is inhibited[241,244]. This postischemic inhibition of protein kinase C may contribute to neuronal injury as this enzyme is an important modulator of ion channel activity and neurotransmitter release[245]. There is also preliminary evidence that protein kinase C is involved in the intracellular response to growth factor stimulation[246]; thus, inhibition of protein kinase C may lead to impairment of important reparative processes after ischemia.

Similar to protein kinase C, calcium-calmodulin dependent kinase II activity is decreased after ischemia[244,247–249]. This impairment has been proposed to contribute to depressed neurotransmitter release after ischemia[239] because calcium-calmodulin dependent kinase II phosphorylates synapsin I, a protein involved in mobilization of synaptic vesicles. Postischemic inhibition of protein kinase C [244] and calcium-calmodulin dependent kinase II[244,247] occurs in resistant as well as vulnerable brain regions, suggesting that inhibition of these enzymes may not play a significant role in selective neuronal necrosis. In contrast to both protein kinase C and calcium-calmodulin dependent kinase II, casein kinase II activity is decreased in selectively vulnerable regions but increased in resistant brain regions[250]. Casein kinase II phosphorylates proteins involved in regulation of gene expression, and protein synthesis and inhibition of this kinase may explain postischemic inhibition of protein synthesis in selectively vulnerable regions of the brain[239] (see below). In summary, our knowledge of the role of protein phosphorylation in the pathophysiology of hypoxic-ischemic brain injury is limited. However, in light of the importance of protein kinases and phosphatases in normal cellular functions, it is likely that altered protein phosphorylation will prove to play an important role in ischemic injury.

Protein Synthesis

Protein synthesis is essential for cell survival. Proteins are involved in nearly every process in the cell, e.g., enzymatic reactions, transport, storage, intracellular signalling, intercellular signalling, and cytoskeletal support. Obviously, intact protein synthesis is important for cellular recovery after hypoxic-ischemic injury. Over two decades ago, Kleihues and Hossmann[251,252] first demonstrated that total protein synthesis is impaired after cerebral ischemia. This work was rapidly confirmed and expanded on by other investigators. Of interest, in vitro protein synthesis in brain homogenates from animals exposed to ischemia without reperfusion is normal, whereas ischemia and reperfusion produces profound inhibition of protein synthesis[253,254]. This suggests that events during reperfusion lead to the impairment in protein synthesis. Inhibition of protein synthesis is slow to recover, requiring hours to days to return to normal levels[251,254–256]. The inhibition of protein synthesis is not regionally homogeneous; inhibition is more severe and prolonged in the cortex, hippocampus, and caudate[255–259]. Failure of protein synthesis to recover after ischemia is the biochemical correlate of cell death[239,260]. Protein synthesis in neurons of the vulnerable CA1 region of the hippocampus fails to recover after even short periods of ischemia[256–259]. Inhibition of protein synthesis after cerebral ischemia and eventual recovery in cells that are destined to survive is a well established phenomenon, but mechanisms leading to the inhibition of protein synthesis after ischemia remain elusive.

Protein synthesis requires (1) energy (i.e., ATP and guanosine triphosphate), (2) intact DNA, (3) functional transcription mechanisms, (4) processing and transport of messenger RNA from the site of transcription to the site of translation, and (5) functional translation mechanisms[261]. The concentration of high-energy phosphates rapidly decreases during ischemia (see above), and this is adequate to explain inhibition of protein synthesis during ischemia. However, the energy state of the brain is restored long before the recovery of protein synthesis[254]; consequently, inadequate energy does not explain inhibition of protein synthesis after cerebral ischemia. Brain DNA does not sustain significant damage after 20 minutes of ischemia followed by 8 hours of reperfusion[262]. Total RNA synthesis does not appear to be impaired during reperfusion[263], implying that transcription is intact. Several studies suggest that during reperfusion, newly synthesized messenger RNA accumulates in the nucleus[263,264], suggesting that there is a block in the process beyond transcription, i.e., at the processing/transport level or the translational level[260,261]. To summarize: (1) total protein synthesis is inhibited after cerebral ischemia, (2) recovery of protein synthesis correlates with cell survival, and (3) the mechanisms leading to the inhibition of protein synthesis remain to be elucidated. Understanding the mechanisms leading to irreversible inhibition of protein synthesis may yield yet another way to intervene during the postischemic period.

Gene Expression

While total protein synthesis is decreased after cerebral ischemia, the synthesis of some proteins is actually increased. It is enticing to postulate that these proteins may play an important role in reparative processes after cerebral ischemia; however, it is equally plausible that the selective expression of some genes may contribute to delayed neuronal death, possibly via apoptotic mechanisms (see above). Ischemia appears to cause dramatic changes in gene expression[265–268]. Genes that have received the most attention in models of cerebral ischemia include the immediate early genes (*c-fos* and *c-jun*), heat shock genes, and trophic factor genes. Immediate early genes code for proteins (fos, jun, and others) that function as transcription factors that control the expression of many genes in the CNS[268]. Increased expression of *c-fos* [268–270] and *c-jun*[268,270] has been demonstrated after global cerebral ischemia. However, the functional significance of this increased expression remains unclear.

Heat shock genes are a large family of genes that are induced during periods of stress[265]. Heat shock proteins probably play an important role in cellular defense against environmental stresses, possibly by handling denatured proteins and restoring ribosomal function[266,267]. The *hsp70* gene is the heat shock gene that has been best characterized after cerebral ischemia. Numerous studies have demonstrated increased transcription of *hsp70* messenger RNA[268,271] and increased synthesis of HSP70 protein[272,273] after global cerebral ischemia. This gene appears to be expressed in proportion to the duration of ischemia. Increasing durations of ischemia lead to *hsp70* expression first in neurons from selectively vulnerable regions, e.g., CA1 region of the hippocampus, then relatively resistant neurons, then glia, and, finally, endothelial cells[265]. Ongoing work in this area will hopefully delineate the role of heat shock proteins in the modulation of neuronal death after cerebral ischemia.

Trophic factors appear to be produced in the CNS after ischemic brain injury and may contribute to the repair of damaged cells[266]. Fibroblast growth factor and nerve growth factor are two growth factors elaborated in the CNS that appear to be important for the survival and development of neurons. Takami et al.[274] demonstrated increased production of fibroblast growth factor messenger RNA and fibroblast growth factor after global ischemia in the rat. Nerve growth factor levels have also been shown to increase after cerebral ischemia[275]. Both fibroblast growth factor[276] and nerve growth factor[277], administered via injection into the lateral ventricle, have been shown to decrease neuronal injury after cerebral ischemia in gerbils. Thus, increased expression of growth factors after ischemia appears to be an attempt by the injured brain to prevent further injury and promote repair. In summary, our understanding of gene expression after cerebral ischemia is far from complete, but it is an exciting start in the application of the techniques of molecular biology to the study of cerebral ischemia.

Inflammation

The role of inflammation in the pathophysiology of hypoxic-ischemic brain injury is unclear. In this section we briefly review current knowledge of the role of polymorphonuclear leukocytes, macrophages, and interleukin-1 in the pathogenesis of global hypoxic-ischemic brain injury. It is plausible that polymorphonuclear leukocytes may contribute to hypoxic-ischemic brain injury by causing delayed hypoperfusion and/or producing oxygen radicals[(278)]. However, the evidence supporting this notion is lacking. First, in a canine model of global ischemia, Anderson and colleagues[(279)] failed to demonstrate significant infiltration of polymorphonuclear leukocytes at 3 hours of reperfusion after 40 minutes of ischemia. In contrast, Dietrich et al.[(280)] were able to demonstrate polymorphonuclear leukocyte infiltration in a rat model of global ischemia (1 hour of reperfusion after 20 minutes of ischemia). Preischemic administration of antipolymorphonuclear leukocyte antibody prevented delayed hypoperfusion in a rat model of global ischemia[(281)], whereas postischemic administration failed to prevent delayed hypoperfusion after global ischemia in the rat[(281)] or gerbil[(282)]. Furthermore, postischemic administration of antipolymorphonuclear leukocyte antibody failed to improve neurological outcome in a canine cardiac arrest model of global ischemia[(283)]. There is no compelling evidence supporting the role of the polymorphonuclear leukocytes in global hypoxic-ischemic brain injury.

Infiltration of blood-borne macrophages and microglia can be detected as early as 20 minutes after global ischemia. However, infiltration becomes pronounced at 24 hours of reperfusion and maximal at 4 to 6 days of reperfusion[(284)]. Blood-borne macrophages and microglia could contribute to delayed neuronal death by producing tumor necrosis factor, nitric oxide, hydrogen peroxide, superoxide radical, and interleukin-1[(285)]. Interleukin-1 is a cytokine that acts as a mediator of host defense responses to injury and is also a mediator of fever[(286)]. Interleukin-1 is synthesized in the brain, primarily by microglia. Interleukin-1 production increases dramatically after global ischemia[(287)], and an interleukin-1 receptor antagonist has been shown to cause a 50% reduction in infarct volume in a rat model of focal ischemia[(288)]. Interleukin-1 receptor antagonists have not been studied in global ischemia. In light of these preliminary data, further work in the area of cytokines and ischemic injury is clearly warranted. In summary, the role of inflammation in the pathophysiology of hypoxic-ischemic brain injury remains to be defined. Further understanding of the contribution of microglia and cytokines to the process of delayed neuronal death may provide another target for pharmacological intervention during the reperfusion period.

Developmental Differences

Traditionally, it has been held that children and infants seem to be more tolerant of hypoxic-ischemic insults than adults[(289)]. However, there are little clinical or laboratory data to support this concept. In the 1930s, Kabat[(290)] subjected dogs of different ages to global ischemia (cervical tourniquet) and found that younger animals were able to endure longer periods of ischemia with complete neurologic recovery. Twenty years later, Brockman and Jude[(291)] examined neurologic outcome in a canine model of global cerebral ischemia (aortic cross-clamp) and demonstrated that puppies after 14 minutes of ischemia recovered without neurologic deficits, whereas adult dogs exposed to more than 12 minutes of ischemia either died or had permanent neurologic deficits. These early studies were plagued by small numbers of subjects in each group and lack of control of important physiologic variables, e.g., blood pressure, temperature, and arterial blood gases, during the reperfusion period. More recent work by Kirsch and coworkers[(9)] studied CBF, cerebral oxygen consumption, and electrophysiologic parameters after 10 minutes of global cerebral ischemia (aortic cross-clamp) in immature (1 to 2 weeks of age) and mature swine. Immature pigs were found to have a more rapid recovery of CBF, cerebral oxygen consumption, and somatosensory evoked potentials than mature pigs. Using a different model of global ischemia (increased intracranial pressure), Ichord and colleagues[(73)] found that immature swine also had more rapid recovery of CBF, cerebral oxygen consumption, and somatosensory evoked potentials after complete ischemia when compared to mature swine. However, it is unclear exactly how these parameters relate to neurologic outcome, and these animals were not studied (i.e., neurologic examination or neuropathology) beyond 2 hours of reperfusion. In summary, it remains unclear whether younger animals are more resistant than adult animals to a comparable hypoxic-ischemic insult.

Summary

The processes leading to neuronal death after an hypoxic-ischemic insult are extremely complex and interrelated. Data acquired over the last two decades have produced more questions than definitive answers. As we gain greater understanding of the pathophysiology, only then will we begin to design therapies that will impact the outcome of this tragic injury.

POTENTIAL THERAPIES

In this section we review both animal and human studies of therapeutic measures directed at hypoxic-ischemic brain injury, i.e., brain resuscitation. As pointed out earlier, we confine the discussion, for the most part, to studies of global cerebral ischemia. We also limit our discussion in this section to studies with either histologic or neurologic outcome measures and to therapies that have potential clinical implications; e.g., we do not discuss drugs that can only be administered via intracerebral injection. We review barbiturates, oxygen radical scavengers, calcium antagonists, glutamate receptor antagonists, nitric oxide synthase inhibitors, and hypothermia.

Barbiturates

Barbiturates may be considered the prototype drugs of brain resuscitation, and their use continues in many intensive care units today. Although barbiturates can be used for treating seizures (see Chapter 22) and lowering intracranial pressure (see Chapter 18), this discussion is limited to the use of barbiturates in the treatment of hypoxic-ischemic brain injury. The primary purpose of this section is to review the history of the use of these drugs for brain resuscitation and to suggest that there is no role for these agents in the treatment of hypoxic-ischemic brain injury. The history itself is instructive because it points out many major problems with research in this field and should reinforce for the clinician the need to be very cautious when extrapolating animal research results to human patients.

Barbiturates were first shown to be effective in global brain ischemia (as a pretreatment) by Goldstein and colleagues(292), though others could not reproduce the results a decade later. Early studies were plagued by the difficulty of achieving a reproducible global ischemic insult. The first large animal model (rhesus monkeys) in which barbiturates were tested was described by Nemoto et al.(293) and made use of a high-pressure neck tourniquet (1500 mm Hg) combined with systemic hypotension. The ischemia time was 16 minutes. In 1978, Bleyaert and colleagues(294) reported that thiopental ameliorated brain damage in this model even when it was administered as late as 60 minutes after the 16-minute ischemic period. Briefly, the authors reported that at 90 mg/kg, thiopental significantly ameliorated neurologic damage if given 5 or 15 minutes after ischemia (Fig. 20.8) and, at 120 mg/kg, ameliorated damage if given 60 minutes after ischemia (Fig. 20.9). Of interest, the authors found an ameliorative effect when thiopental at 120 mg/kg was administered after 60 minutes of reperfusion, but they found no effect when the drug was given at 30 minutes (Fig. 20.9). These exciting results were the first suggestion that clinical neuroprotection could be achieved after a prolonged period of global cerebral ischemia when pharmacological agents were administered after the insult. However, there are several methodological problems with this study that are worthy of detailed consideration. First, the number of animals (N equals 5 in experimental groups) in each group was too small to provide reliable information. Second, the earlier publication regarding the control animals(293) suggests that the control and experimental groups were not run concurrently, further confounding the conclusions. Last, there was a natural selection process occurring in these experiments. In the paper by Bleyaert and colleagues(294), it was pointed out that 9 of 19 control animals(293) had to be excluded because of premature death or failure to keep the animals on the protocol; 16 of 43 animals treated with thiopental were excluded for similar reasons. The higher exclusion rate for the control animals, which was published earlier, suggests that the investigators improved their ability to keep animals on the protocol. Exclusion of experimental subjects on the basis of predefined criteria is certainly valid, but the absence of concurrent controls is unacceptable from a methodological standpoint. In spite of its limitations, this study directly led to a multicenter clinical trial of thiopental loading after cardiac arrest (the study is described below).

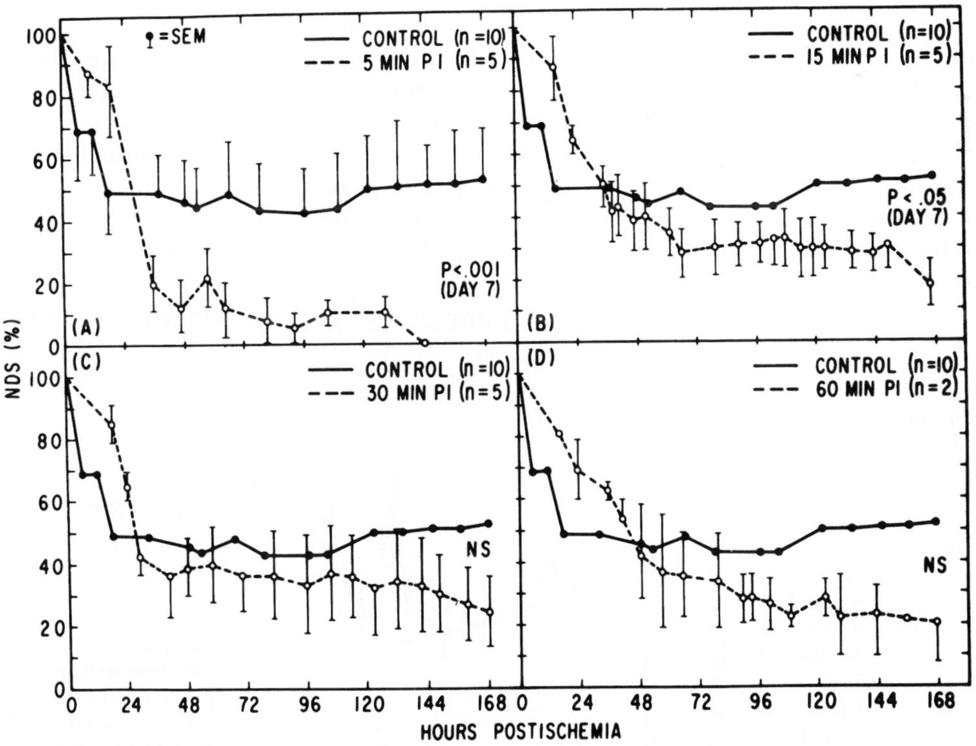

Figure 20.8. Neurologic deficit scores *(NDS)* in rhesus monkeys for 7 days, after 16 minutes of global ischemia of the brain produced by a high-pressure neck tourniquet and trimethaphan-induced hypotension. Ten untreated monkeys served as controls for four treatment groups *(A-D)*. Treated monkeys received thiopental, 90 mg/kg, infused intravenously beginning 5, 15, 30, and 60 minutes postischemia, respectively, with one-third of the original dose infused in the first 5 minutes and two-thirds over the subsequent 55 minutes. (From Bleyaert AL, Nemoto EM, Safar P, Stezoski SW, Mickell JJ, Moossy J, Rao GR. Thiopental amelioration of brain damage after global ischemia in monkeys. Anesthesiology 1978;49:392.)

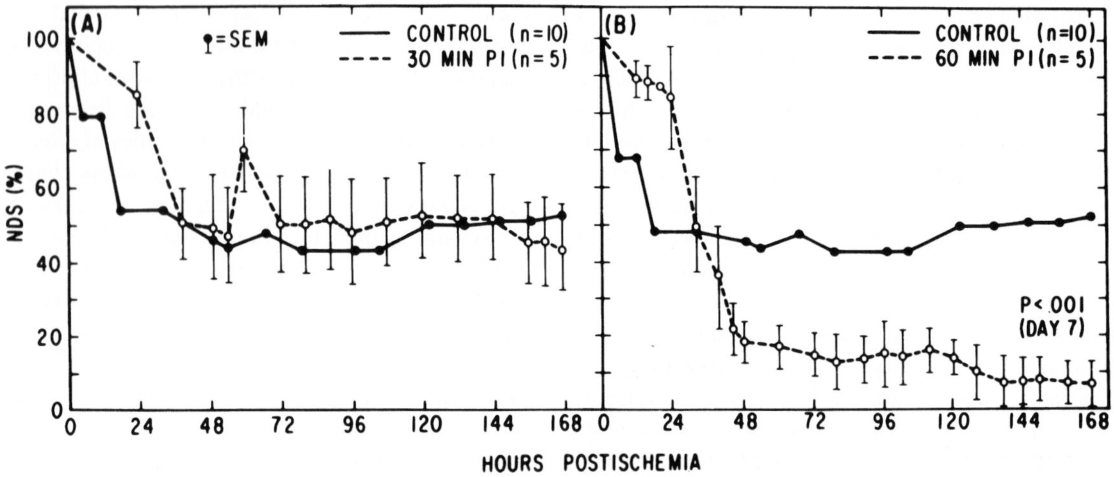

Figure 20.9. Neurologic deficit scores (NDS) in rhesus monkeys for 7 days, after 16 minutes of global ischemia of the brain produced by a high-pressure neck tourniquet and trimethaphan-induced hypotension. Ten untreated monkeys served as controls for two treatment groups (**A** and **B**). Treated monkeys received thiopental, 120 mg/kg, infused intravenously beginning 30 and 60 minutes postischemia, respectively, with one-third of the total dose infused in the first 5 minutes and two-thirds over the subsequent 55 minutes. (From Bleyaert AL, Nemoto EM, Safar P, Stezoski SW, Mickell JJ, Moossy J, Rao GR. Thiopental amelioration of brain damage after global ischemia in monkeys. Anesthesiology 1978;49:393.)

Unfortunately, the ameliorative effects of thiopental on total cerebral ischemia could not be reproduced by other investigators[295,296], and, even worse, it could not be confirmed later by researchers in the same laboratory[297]. In this latter study, the blood pressure was tightly controlled between the different animal groups (Fig. 20.10); this had not been achieved in the earlier study, in which the nonconcurrent controls had been hypotensive slightly longer after ischemia than the treated animals. Finally, the neurologic deficit scores in this study were essentially identical between the groups of animals (Fig. 20.11). Notably, at least 10 animals were used in each group in this study. In spite of their inability to reproduce their own results, Gisvold and colleagues[297] concluded, "There is clearly insufficient support at the present time for recommending clinical use of large doses of barbiturate after GBI [global brain ischemia], as in cardiac arrest. The ongoing clinical trial of thiopental loading after cardiac arrest hopefully will provide more conclusive information." In our opinion, this is a reversal of sound investigative medical progress: firm laboratory evidence should exist for a therapy before an ongoing clinical trial is instituted.

On the basis of the study by Bleyaert and colleagues[294], the use of thiopental after cardiac arrest in humans was proposed by Breivik and colleagues[298]. In this anecdotal list of patients, a possible ameliorative effect was noted, and a multi-institutional trial was instituted. In 1986, the results of this multi-institutional study were published, and no beneficial effect could be demonstrated in the barbiturate-treated group[299], thus confirming the results obtained in the laboratory.

To summarize, barbiturates have been proposed for use

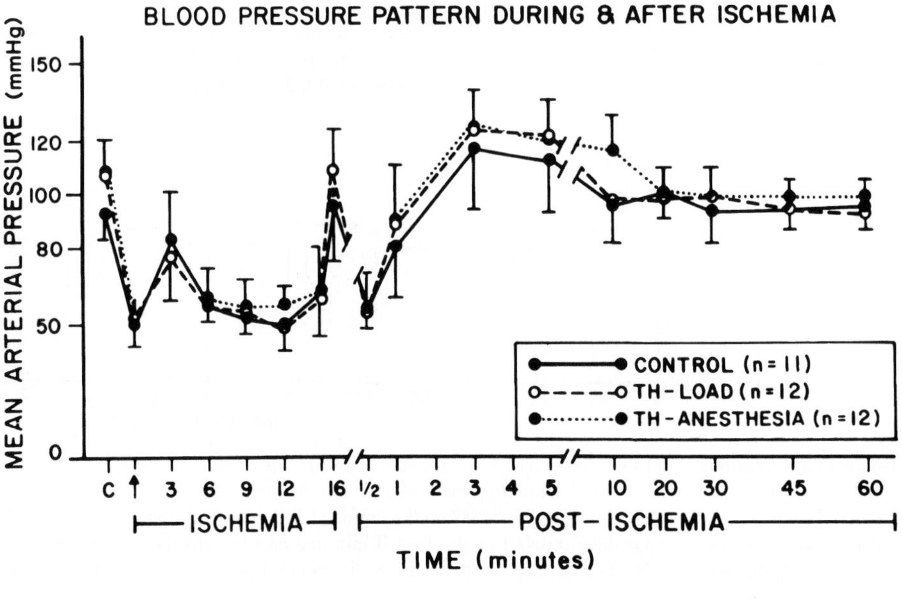

Figure 20.10. Mean arterial pressure (MAP) pattern during and after ischemia in three groups of monkeys subjected to 16 minutes of total cerebral ischemia. *TH-LOAD* equals 90 mg of thiopental per kilogram, with one-third of the dose infused in the first 5 minutes and two-thirds infused over the subsequent 55 minutes. *TH-ANESTHESIA* equals 90 mg of thiopental per kilogram, infused over 12 hours. As always with this model, there is a tendency for MAP to rise during the first 3 minutes of ischemia. At no point was there a significant difference in MAP between the three groups. (From Gisvold SE, Safar P, Hendrickx HHL, Rao G, Moossy J, Alexander H. Thiopental treatment after global brain ischemia in pigtailed monkeys. Anesthesiology 1984;60:91.)

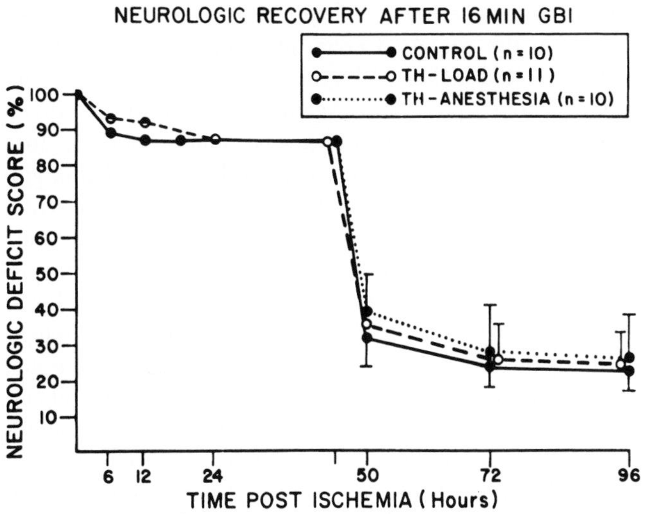

Figure 20.11. Neurologic deficit scores (NDS) in the three groups of monkeys described in the legend to Figure 20.10. Only the animals surviving 96 hours are included; the final score thus expresses quality of survival in the respective groups. In the strict sense, NDS are not evaluable until after 48 hours postischemia, when muscle relaxation is reversed and nitrous oxide is discontinued. The final NDS at 96 hours postischemia were almost identical in the three groups. (From Gisvold SE, Safar P, Hendrickx HHL, Rao G, Moossy J, Alexander H. Thiopental treatment after global brain ischemia in pigtailed monkeys. Anesthesiology 1984;60:93.)

after global cerebral ischemia. Their use in this setting is not supported by data obtained in animals or humans, and the drugs should not be employed for this purpose. Although there are legitimate uses for barbiturates in neurologic intensive care, e.g., status epilepticus and intracranial hypertension, such uses should be tempered by recognition of the risk-to-benefit ratio of these drugs.

Oxygen Radical Scavengers

As discussed above, oxygen radicals are postulated to be mediators of injury during the reperfusion period. In this section we review the use of oxygen radical scavengers in animal models of hypoxic-ischemic brain injury. We confine our discussion to superoxide dismutase and 21-aminosteroids.

Superoxide Dismutase

Before proceeding to some of the models that have been used to explore the role of oxygen radicals in cerebral ischemia, we should spend a few moments discussing superoxide dismutase[(300–302)]. Superoxide dismutases are very efficient catalysts, providing a 2000-fold increase in the dismutation reaction of the superoxide radical (see above). There are two distinct types of superoxide dismutases in mammalian cells: copper-zinc superoxide dismutase and manganese superoxide dismutase. Copper-zinc superoxide dismutase is located in the cytosol, whereas manganese superoxide dismutase is located in the mitochondria. Superoxide dismutases are widely distributed throughout the body[(303)], but the plasma level is very low[(304)] as a result of efficient renal clearance.

Copper-zinc superoxide dismutase has been proposed as a therapeutic agent for reperfusion injury because of its ability to scavenge oxygen radicals. Superoxide dismutase has two drawbacks as a therapeutic agent. First, it is rapidly cleared by the kidney and has a circulatory half-life of approximately 8 minutes[(305)]. Second and more importantly, copper-zinc superoxide dismutase is a large, water-soluble molecule (molecular mass of 32 kDa)[(217)] and therefore cannot readily penetrate cell membranes[(306,307)] or cross the blood-brain barrier in significant quantities after intravenous administration[(308)]. Thus, if access to intracellular compartments is required for therapeutic efficacy, it appears unlikely that copper-zinc superoxide dismutase would provide a protective effect. A 1987 study demonstrated that treatment with a combination of copper-zinc superoxide dismutase and deferoxamine in an apnea-induced cardiac arrest model of global ischemia in the dog resulted in improved recovery of CBF and somatosensory evoked potentials during the early reperfusion period[(309)]. It is unclear from this study whether superoxide dismutase contributed to this enhanced recovery. Indeed, pretreatment with copper-zinc superoxide dismutase and catalase failed to improve neurologic outcome after global ischemia in dogs[(310)], and pretreatment with copper-zinc superoxide dismutase alone failed to prevent delayed hypoperfusion after global ischemia in rats[(311)]. To add further confusion, more recent work with recombinant human superoxide dismutase[(312,313)] suggests that pretreatment with this form of the enzyme can reduce injury to vulnerable hippocampal neurons after global ischemia in gerbils.

Investigators have tried two different modifications in the delivery of superoxide dismutase in an effort to increase the circulatory half-life and intracellular access of the intravenously administered enzyme: liposome-entrapped superoxide dismutase and polyethylene glycol-conjugated superoxide dismutase. Superoxide dismutase delivered in positively charged liposomes has a circulatory half-life of approximately 4 hours[(305)] and has dramatically increased access into cultured endothelial cells[(306)]. Administration of liposome-entrapped superoxide dismutase has been shown to both increase brain superoxide dismutase activity[(195,314)] and reduce infarct volume in a rat model of focal cerebral ischemia[(195)]. Liposome-entrapped superoxide dismutase has not been studied in a model of global ischemia. Conjugation of polyethylene glycol monomers to superoxide dismutase increases its circulatory half-life to approximately 37 hours[(315)] and increases its uptake into cultured endothelial cells[(307)]. However, polyethylene glycol-conjugated superoxide dismutase does not appear to increase brain superoxide dismutase activity[(316)]. Nonetheless, pretreatment with polyethylene glycol-conjugated superoxide dismutase and polyethylene glycol-conjugated catalase has been shown to reduce infarct volume in a rat model of focal cerebral ischemia[(194)], and polyethylene glycol-conjugated superoxide dismutase alone has been shown to decrease in-

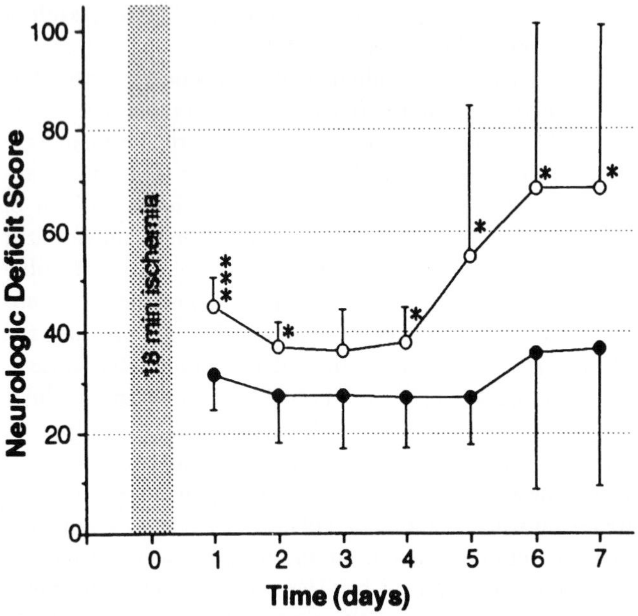

Figure 20.12. Neurologic deficit scores (0 = normal; 100 = coma or death) after 18 minutes of global ischemia produced by aortic cross-clamp in control (open circles) and SM-SOD treated (filled circles) dogs. (From Takeda Y, Hashimoto H, Kosaka F, Hirakawa M, Inoue M. Albumin-binding superoxide dismutase with a prolonged half-life reduces reperfusion brain injury. Am J Physiol 1993;264:H1713.)

farct volume in cat(196) and rat(197) models of focal ischemia. Although polyethylene glycol-conjugated superoxide dismutase has not been shown to be neuroprotective in a model of global ischemia, pretreatment with polyethylene glycol-conjugated superoxide dismutase and polyethylene glycol-conjugated catalase has been shown to prevent delayed hypoperfusion after asphyxia in newborn lambs(317). Furthermore, Kirsch and colleagues(318) demonstrated that treatment with polyethylene glycol-conjugated superoxide dismutase improved the response of CBF to hypercapnia after global ischemia in piglets. However, there was no improvement in cerebral metabolic rate for oxygen or somatosensory evoked potentials in the treated animals. Recently, a novel superoxide dismutase derivative, poly-(styrene-co-maleic acid)butyl ester covalently linked to superoxide dismutase, has been shown to ameliorate delayed hypoperfusion and improve neurological outcome after global ischemia in dogs (Fig. 20.12)(319).

21-Aminosteroids

The 21-aminosteroids are potent inhibitors of lipid peroxidation but lack classic steroidal activities(320). The most extensively studied 21-aminosteroid, U74006F or tirilazad mesylate, appears to possess multiple antioxidant properties, including the ability to scavenge lipid peroxyl and hydroxyl radicals and stabilize membranes(321). However, preliminary studies using this agent in global cerebral ischemia have yielded mixed results. Hall and Yonkers(322) studied the effect of postischemic administration of U74006F on CBF and recovery of somatosensory evoked potentials after 5 minutes of severe incomplete global ischemia (neck tourniquet) in the cat. At 3 hours of reperfusion, treated animals exhibited higher CBF and greater recovery of somatosensory evoked potentials. Again, the relationship between these parameters and neurologic outcome is unclear. In a canine cardiac arrest (ventricular fibrillation) model of global ischemia, animals treated with U74006F after circulation was restored had a significantly higher survival rate and improved neurologic outcome at 24 hours after the arrest (192). In a canine model of global ischemia, Perkins et al(193) demonstrated significant improvements in neurological outcome in animals treated with U74006F before and after 12 minutes of ischemia. Interestingly, Helfaer and colleagues(323) failed to note any improvement in early neurophysiologic (somatosensory evoked responses) and metabolic (ATP, phosphocreatine, and pH) parameters after 10 minutes of complete global ischemia in dogs treated with U74006F. However, researchers in the same laboratory noted striking improvements in similar parameters in U74006F-treated dogs subjected to 30 minutes of incomplete global ischemia and hyperglycemia. The effect of U74006F on histologic outcome after global ischemia is unclear. In rat models of global ischemia, investigators in two laboratories(324,325) failed to show any improvement with U74006F, and two groups(326,327) showed protection in the cortex but no effect in the hippocampus or striatum. Thus, while there have been encouraging results with U74006F, further studies of this drug and related compounds(328) will be necessary.

To summarize, it is obvious that there is no current role for oxygen radical scavenger therapy in children with brain injury. Animal studies of oxygen radical scavengers suggest that oxygen radicals play a significant role in hypoxic-ischemic brain injury. Nonetheless, at present there is only preliminary evidence supporting the efficacy of these agents after a global ischemic insult.

Calcium Antagonists

It has been pointed out that cerebral ischemia results in alterations of cellular calcium homeostasis that lead to intracellular calcium accumulation, and this calcium accumulation is postulated to cause neuronal injury. Based on this mechanism, investigators have explored the role of calcium channel blockers in ameliorating hypoxic-ischemic neuronal injury. As mentioned above, these calcium antagonists act by blocking the influx of calcium via voltage-sensitive calcium channels. In addition, they are potent relaxers of vascular smooth muscle and may minimize delayed hypoperfusion because of their ability to inhibit cerebral vasoconstriction. However, as discussed above, the relationship between delayed hypoperfusion and ongoing brain injury is unclear. In this section, the use of calcium channel blockers after global cerebral ischemia is considered; we discuss several agents that have been studied, specifically flunarizine, lidoflazine, and nimodipine.

Flunarizine

Flunarizine is a diphenylalkylamine calcium channel antagonist that is nonselective, i.e., it does not block a specific voltage-sensitive calcium channel[132]. Unfortunately, studies regarding the protective effect of this agent have yielded conflicting results. White and coworkers[329] administered flunarizine to dogs after 20 minutes of total cerebral ischemia induced by placing the animals on cardiac bypass and then turning off the machine. At the end of ischemia, the bypass machine was turned on again, and reperfusion was initiated. The authors reported that postischemic administration of flunarizine prevented the delayed hypoperfusion described earlier in this chapter. Deshpande and Wieloch[330] demonstrated that rats treated with flunarizine either before or after 9 minutes of global ischemia had improved histologic outcome, but there was no improvement in postischemic hypoperfusion or recovery of high-energy phosphates. Moreover, flunarizine was found to improve recovery of the EEG after global ischemia in dogs[331]. However, in an important study that evaluated neurological outcome, Newberg and coworkers[332] showed that flunarizine had no effect on CBF, cerebral metabolism, or outcome in dogs after 10 minutes of total cerebral ischemia.

Lidoflazine

Lidoflazine is a nonselective voltage-sensitive calcium channel antagonist that in early animal studies appeared to ameliorate hypoxic-ischemic brain injury. However, later studies, including a large clinical trial, failed to substantiate the early experiments. Winegar and colleagues[333] demonstrated improvement in early (12 hours) neurological outcome after global ischemia (cardiac arrest model) in dogs treated with lidoflazine. A subsequent study was published suggesting that lidoflazine improves neurologic outcome after total cerebral ischemia (Fig. 20.13)[334]. The authors also hypothesized that a mechanism different from flow preservation might underlie this effect because preliminary studies in their laboratory failed to demonstrate an effect of lidoflazine on CBF. Unfortunately, these results were not confirmed by other investigators. Dean and colleagues[335] failed to demonstrate any effect of pretreatment with lidoflazine on CBF after 12 minutes of global cerebral ischemia in dogs; cerebrovascular resistance was similarly unaffected. They proposed that if the drug had any ameliorative effect, i.e., effect on neurologic outcome, it must be by some mechanism other than flow preservation. In a canine model of global ischemia (cardiac arrest), treatment with lidoflazine and deferoxamine failed to alter histologic outcome after 15 minutes of ischemia[336]. Furthermore, work from Fleischer and colleagues failed to demonstrate any improvement in neurological outcome after global ischemia in dogs[337] or monkeys[338] treated with lidoflazine. In spite of these equivocal data, a large multicenter clinical trial of treatment with lidoflazine after cardiac arrest was initiated, and, unfortunately, lidoflazine

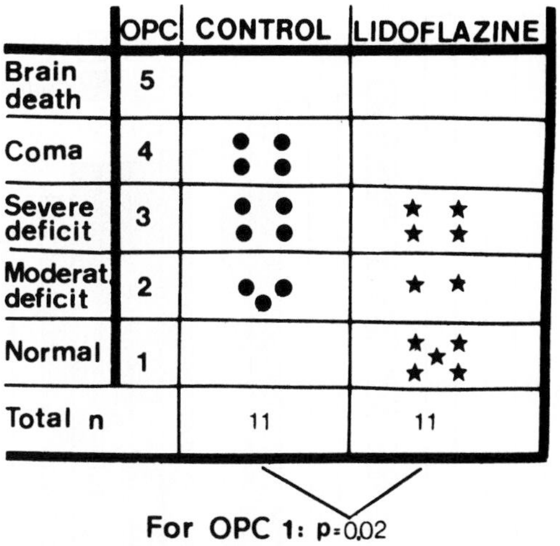

Figure 20.13. Best overall performance category (OPC) scores during the 96-hour period of observation after 10 minutes of ventricular fibrillation and cardiopulmonary resuscitation in control and lidoflazine-treated dogs. (From Vaagenes P, Cantadore R, Safar P, Moossy J, Rao G, Diven W, Alexander H, Stezoski W. Amelioration of brain damage by lidoflazine after prolonged ventricular fibrillation cardiac arrests in dogs. Crit Care Med 1984;12:852.)

treatment failed to alter neurological outcome in these patients[339].

Nimodipine

Nimodipine, a dihydropyridine compound that selectively blocks the L-type calcium channel, has been studied in animal models of global cerebral ischemia and in human survivors of cardiac arrest. Using a canine model, Steen and colleagues demonstrated that preischemic treatment with nimodipine resulted in increased CBF and improved neurological outcome after 10 minutes of global ischemia[340]. However, when the drug was administered after ischemia, the results were intermediate; i.e., CBF was improved, but outcome was unchanged[341]. These results are particularly notable because this same group of investigators failed to find a beneficial effect from barbiturates or flunarizine in this model, results that we already discussed. Furthermore, this same group[39] demonstrated improved neurologic outcome (Fig. 20.14) in pigtailed monkeys treated with nimodipine after 17 minutes of total cerebral ischemia induced with a neck tourniquet similar to that employed for barbiturate studies by Nemoto and coworkers[293]. Subsequently, Milde and colleagues[342] studied the effect of postischemic treatment with nimodipine on CBF in the early reperfusion period. Nimodipine-treated dogs had significantly higher CBF, but interestingly, nimodipine treatment had no effect on cerebral metabolism. Again, this raises the question of whether improving blood flow in the early reperfusion period has any effect on neurologic outcome. These results culminated in a clinical trial of nimodipine treatment in survivors of cardiac arrest (ventricular fibrillation)[343]. There was no difference in neurological outcome or survival at 3 or 12 months post-arrest. However, post hoc analysis sug-

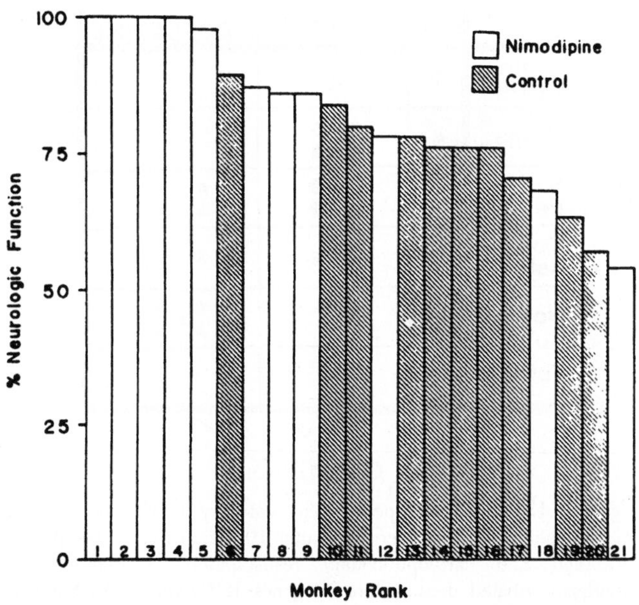

Figure 20.14. Neurologic function (0 = brain death; 100 = normal) in pigtailed monkeys 96 hours after 17 minutes of global ischemia of the brain produced by a high-pressure neck tourniquet and trimethaphan-induced hypotension. Nimodipine-treated monkeys had significantly better neurologic outcome. (From Steen P, Gisvold SE, Milde JH, Newberg LA, Scheithauer BW, Lanier WL, Michenfelder JD. Nimodipine improves outcome when given after complete cerebral ischemia in primates. Anesthesiology 1985;62:410.)

gested that in patients with long delays in initiation of advanced life support measures, nimodipine treatment resulted in improved survival at 12 months post-arrest.

To summarize, calcium channel blockers have been studied in a variety of animal models of global ischemia and have been subjected to clinical trials. Despite some encouraging results in animal models, the clinical trials have failed to yield positive results. New calcium channel antagonists are currently being evaluated and may prove to be more effective than those discussed above. For example, recent work by Buchan and coworkers[344] showed that treatment with SN-111, a selective N-type calcium channel blocker, resulted in significant histological improvement even when treatment was delayed up to 24 hours after global ischemic injury in rats. Thus, ongoing work with these agents may ultimately lead to the development of a neuroprotective agent.

Glutamate Antagonists

As previously discussed, excitotoxic mechanisms appear to play a significant role in hypoxic-ischemic brain injury, and NMDA and non-NMDA receptor antagonists have been studied extensively in numerous animal models of cerebral ischemia. Although numerous antagonists have been studied, we will limit our discussion to dizocilpine maleate (MK-801) and 2,3-dihydroxy-6-nitro-7-sulfamoylbenzoquinoxaline (NBQX) as these are the most widely studied NMDA and non-NMDA receptor antagonists, respectively.

MK-801

MK-801 is a noncompetitive NMDA antagonist; i.e., it does not compete with glutamate for binding to the NMDA receptor but rather blocks influx of extracellular calcium by binding to a site within the NMDA receptor-gated calcium channel. Results of numerous studies strongly suggest that this agent is neuroprotective in the setting of focal ischemia[27,345–347]; however, results of MK-801 treatment in the setting of global ischemia are, for the most part, discouraging. As usual, initial studies demonstrated protective effects. A 1988 study[348] demonstrated that preischemic treatment with MK-801 resulted in decreased neuronal damage in the CA1 region of the hippocampus of rats subjected to 10 minutes of forebrain ischemia. In a model of forebrain ischemia in gerbils, Gill and associates demonstrated that treatment with MK-801 either before[349] or after[350] ischemia resulted in significantly less neuronal damage in the CA1 region of the hippocampus. In another study demonstrating a protective effect[8], pretreatment with MK-801 resulted in improved EEG recovery, higher CBF, preserved cerebrovascular reactivity to changes in arterial CO_2, and less blood-brain barrier disruption in cats subjected to 15 minutes of global ischemia.

Subsequently, other investigators have not been able to demonstrate a protective effect of MK-801 in large animal models of global ischemia. Fleischer and coworkers[351] were unable to demonstrate any improvement in neurologic or histologic outcome after cardiac arrest in cats treated with MK-801. Michenfelder and colleagues[352] studied the effect of MK-801 on histologic and neurologic outcome in a canine model of global ischemia (aortic cross-clamp) and were also unable to demonstrate any improvement in neurologic or histologic outcome in dogs treated with MK-801 after 11 minutes of ischemia. Researchers in the same laboratory[353] also failed to demonstrate any improvement in neurologic or histologic outcome in pigtailed monkeys treated with MK-801 after 17 minutes of total cerebral ischemia induced with a neck tourniquet similar to that employed for the barbiturate studies by Nemoto and coworkers[293].

Follow-up studies in rodents have been predominantly negative[354,355]. Buchan and Pulsinelli[356] studied the effect of MK-801 in the gerbil model in which Gill and coworkers (see above) had previously demonstrated a protective effect of MK-801[349,350] and demonstrated that the protective effect of MK-801 was largely mediated by prolonged postischemic hypothermia. They demonstrated that when body temperature was carefully controlled, MK-801-treated animals fared no better than control animals with regard to histologic outcome (Fig. 20.15). Furthermore, untreated animals subjected to the same degree of postischemic hypothermia as that induced by MK-801 were afforded an identical degree of protection, compared with MK-801-treated animals in whom temperature was not controlled. Even moderate hypothermia is neuroprotective[357,358] (see below), and the importance of meticulously controlling temperature during an experimental protocol cannot be overemphasized. In summary, MK-801 appears to have neuroprotective properties in the setting of focal ischemia but does not appear to be neuroprotective after global ischemia. Of interest, MK-801 will not be subjected to clinical trials in focal ischemia because of concerns regarding its psychomimetic effects and potential toxicity. Because it acts at the same site within the NMDA-gated calcium channel, it has psychomimetic effects similar to those of phencyclidine and ketamine(359). With regard to toxicity, MK-801 has been shown to cause cytoplasmic vacuoles(360) and induce heat shock proteins(361) in neurons of the posterior cingulate and retrosplenial cortices of rats.

NBQX

NBQX is a non-NMDA receptor antagonist that appears to have neuroprotective properties in the setting of both focal and global ischemia(27,110,362). Studies have primarily used

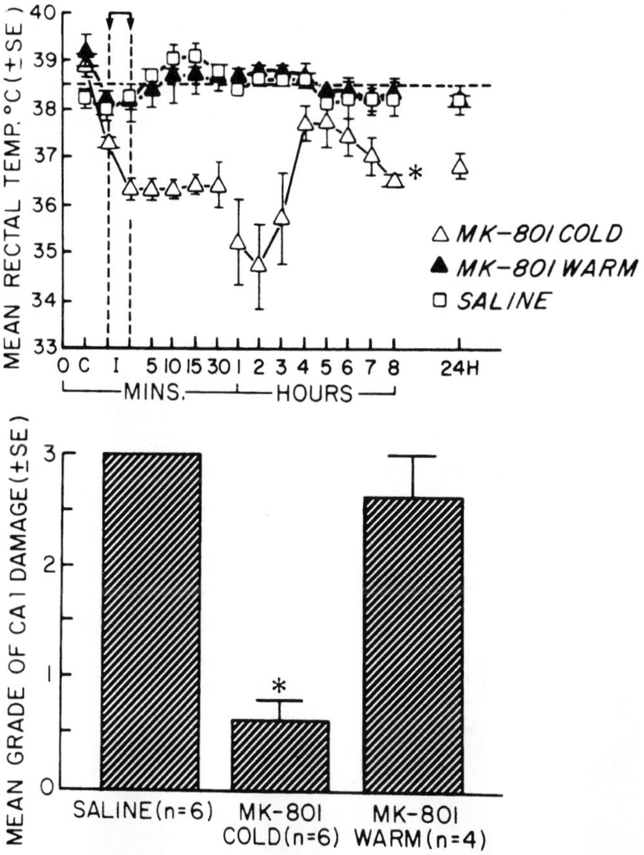

Figure 20.15. Mean rectal temperatures and CA1 damage in gerbils subjected to 5 minutes of forebrain ischemia. The saline-treated and MK-801 WARM groups were maintained normothermic during the first 8 hours after ischemia, whereas the MK-801 COLD group was allowed to become hypothermic. The MK-801 COLD group had significantly better histologic outcome than the saline-treated and MK-801 WARM groups. There was no difference in histologic outcome between the saline-treated and MK-801 WARM groups. (From Buchan AM, Pulsinelli WA. Hypothermia but not the N-methyl-D-aspartate antagonist, MK-801, attenuates neuronal damage in gerbils subjected to transient global ischemia. J Neurosci 1990;10:314.)

histology as the outcome measure. Sheardown and colleagues(363) demonstrated protection of the CA1 region of the hippocampus after global ischemia in gerbils treated with NBQX. Several investigators(95,364–366) have shown that NBQX confers histologic protection in the cortex and/or hippocampus in rat models of global ischemia. Of interest, delayed treatment with NBQX appears to be effective. Treatment 12 hours after global ischemia in the rat(367) and 24 hours after global ischemia in the gerbil(368) resulted in significantly decreased delayed neuronal death in the CA1 region of the hippocampus.

The effect of NBQX on neurologic outcome after global ischemia has not been extensively studied. In a gerbil model of global ischemia, Judge and colleagues(369) demonstrated that postischemic NBQX administration resulted in histologic protection of the hippocampus and diminished locomotor hyperactivity after global ischemia in gerbils. In a more clinically relevant model, Redmond and coworkers(370) studied the effect of NBQX treatment (2 hours after ischemia) on neurologic and histologic outcome after 2 hours of global ischemia in a canine model of hypothermic (18°C) circulatory arrest. NBQX-treated dogs had dramatically improved neurologic and histologic outcome (Fig. 20.16). Although further work is required, these early data suggest that NBQX is neuroprotective after global ischemia, and that a significant window of opportunity exists for administration of the drug after global ischemia.

To summarize, despite a large body of research supporting the excitotoxic hypothesis of neuronal injury during ischemia, NMDA receptor antagonists do not appear to be protective after global ischemia. However, recent data suggest that non-NMDA receptor antagonists may be neuroprotective in both focal and global ischemia. Further experiments with NBQX in other animal models, especially those using neurological outcome as an endpoint, are warranted.

Nitric Oxide Synthase Inhibitors

As described above, nitric oxide could be both beneficial and detrimental to the brain during ischemia and reperfusion. Possible beneficial effects include vasodilation, inhibition of platelet aggregation, and down-regulation of NMDA receptors, whereas possible detrimental effects include production of hydroxyl radicals and inhibition of key enzymes necessary for DNA replication and mitochondrial energy production(238). It is not surprising then, that animal studies using nitric oxide synthase inhibitors for treatment of cerebral ischemia have yielded both positive and negative results(229,233). Nitric oxide synthase inhibitors are analogues of L-arginine, the substrate for nitric oxide synthase. These analogues competitively inhibit the conversion of L-arginine to L-citrulline and nitric oxide. In the setting of focal ischemia, studies with nitric oxide synthase inhibitors have shown both dramatic increases and dramatic decreases in infarct volume(229,233). Currently available data in models of global ischemia are similarly unclear. Two studies have shown that inhibition of nitric oxide synthase causes even further decrements in CBF during the period of delayed hypoperfusion (Fig. 20.1) after global ischemia[371,372]. Thus it is plausible that inhibition of nitric oxide synthase during reperfusion could lead to impaired oxygen delivery to the brain and thus worsen outcome. However, in the study by Clavier and coworkers[372], the decrement in CBF was not accompanied by a decrement in cerebral oxygen consumption, suggesting that cerebral oxygen consumption was not limited by CBF. There have been few studies examining the effect of nitric oxide synthase on histologic outcome after cerebral ischemia. In a gerbil model of global ischemia, Weissman et al.[373] found that preischemic treatment with N-omega-nitro-L-arginine (50 mg/kg) led to increased neuronal death in the hippocampus and other brain regions. This same group of investigators (Shapira et al.)[374] later performed a dose-response curve with N-omega-nitro-L-arginine and found that 5 mg/kg prevented injury to the CA1 region of the hippocampus, whereas higher doses resulted in potentiation of injury. In another gerbil study, Caldwell and colleagues[375] found that postischemic administration of N-omega-nitro-L-arginine resulted in significantly greater neuronal survival in the CA1 region of the hippocampus compared to untreated animals. Finally, in a well-characterized model of global ischemia in the rat, Buchan and coworkers[376] showed that N-omega-nitro-L-arginine failed to reduce injury to the CA1 region and in higher doses resulted in increased mortality. Thus, while the effect of nitric oxide synthase inhibitors on outcome after global ischemia remains to be clarified, available evidence suggests that this therapy is unlikely to be significantly neuroprotective.

Hypothermia

The concept of deep hypothermia conferring protection to the brain during ischemia is not new; hypothermia has been successfully applied during cerebrovascular and cardiovascular surgery for several decades[377,378]. However, recent work suggests that even mild hypothermia (30 to 34°C) applied either during or immediately after global ischemia can cause significant neuroprotection[357,358]. Potential mechanisms for the protective effect of hypothermia include inhibition of glutamate release[379–383], inhibition of adenine nucleotide depletion[384–387], prevention of brain acidosis[387–390], and preservation of protein kinase activity[391,392]. Interest in this area of research was rekindled by Busto and coworkers[393], who performed a controlled study looking at the effect of brain temperature on histologic outcome after global ischemia in the rat. These investigators showed that variations in intraischemic brain temperature as little as 2°C could lead to dramatic differences in histologic outcomes. This study was important for two reasons. First, it demonstrated that even mild intraischemic hypothermia is neuroprotective. Second, it pointed out the critical importance of monitoring brain temperature in models of ischemia (see above).

Subsequent to the work by Busto and colleagues, numerous investigators studied the effect of mild and moderate hypothermia on outcome in animal models of both focal and global ischemia. To briefly summarize the work in focal ischemia, intraischemic hypothermia appears to decrease infarct volume[394–399]; however, the effect appears to be more consistent in models of transient focal ischemia as opposed to permanent focal ischemia[400,401]. We will review the effect of hypothermia in global ischemia in more detail. First, we will briefly examine the effect of intraischemic hypothermia on outcome after global cerebral ischemia. Numerous investigators[18,402–404] have shown that mild (32 to 35°C) hypothermia confers significant protection in terms of histologic outcome after global ischemia in the rat. Intraischemic hypothermia has been shown to improve neurologic outcome after global ischemia in rats[405,406] and dogs[407,408]. Postischemic hypothermia, if efficacious, would have clinical implications for resuscitation after glo-

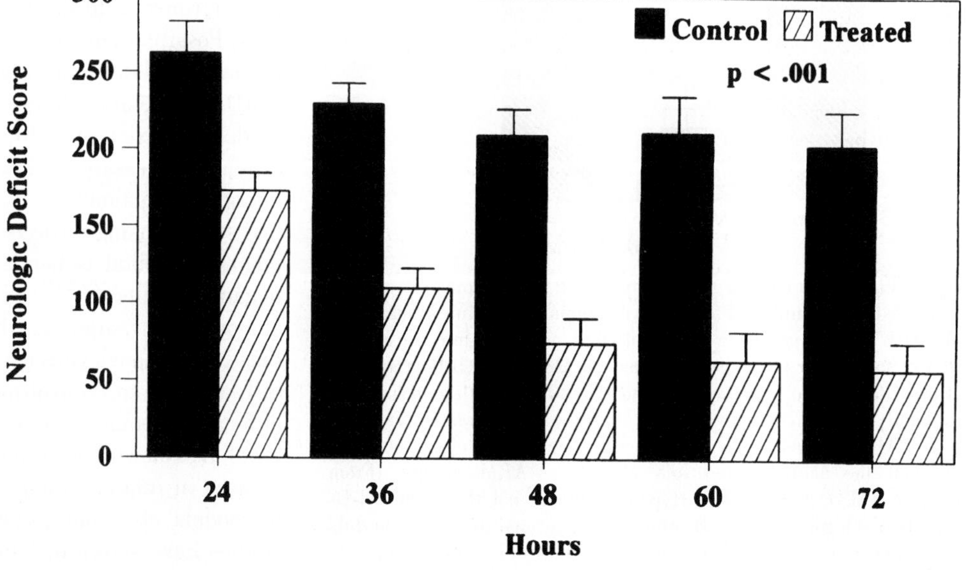

Figure 20.16. Neurologic deficit scores (0 = normal; 500 = brain death) in control and NBQX-treated dogs after 2 hours of hypothermic (18°C) circulatory arrest. NBQX-treated dogs had significantly better outcome at all time points. (From Redmond JM, Zehr KJ, Blue ME, Lange MS, Gillinov AM, Troncoso JC, Cameron DE, Johnston MV, Baumgartner WA. AMPA glutamate receptor antagonism reduces neurologic injury after hypothermic circulatory arrest. Ann Thorac Surg 1995;59:581.)

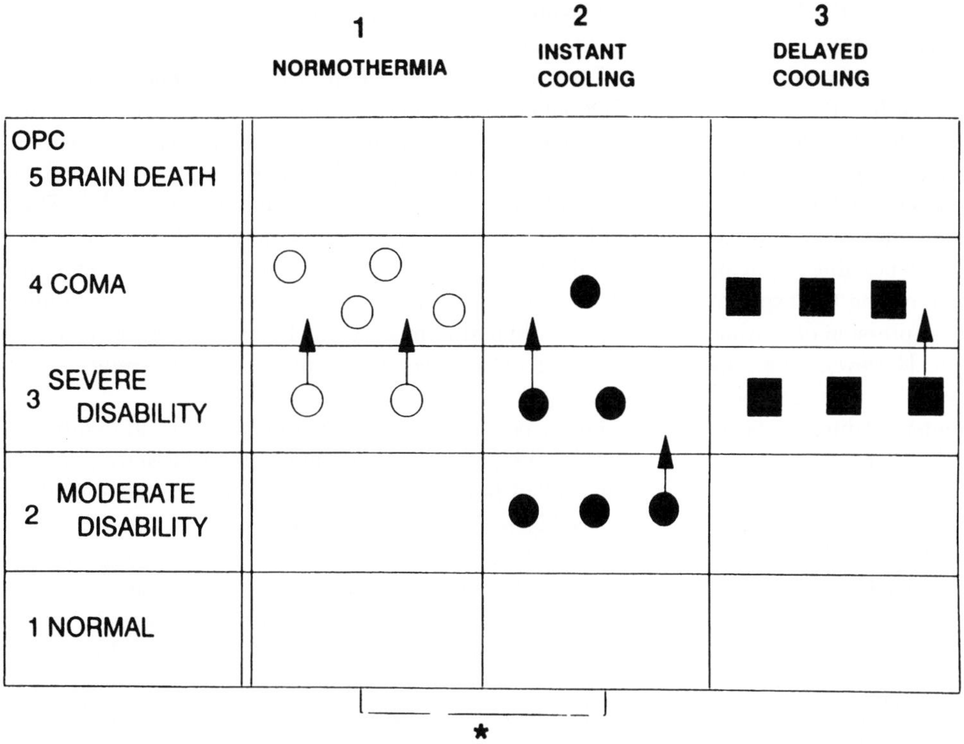

Figure 20.17. Best overall performance categories (OPC) between 24 and 96 hours of resuscitation after 12.5 minutes of ventricular fibrillation. Arrows indicate deterioration from best to final OPC. Animals cooled immediately after ischemia (instant cooling group) had significantly better OPC than normothermic animals, whereas delayed cooling (15 minutes after ischemia) failed to provide neuroprotection. (From Kuboyama K, Safar P, Radovsky A, Tisherman SA, Stezoski SW, Alexander H. Delay in cooling negates the beneficial effect of mild resuscitative cerebral hypothermia after cardiac arrest in dogs: A prospective, randomized study. Crit Care Med 1993;21:1354.)

bal ischemia. Postischemic hypothermia has been shown to confer significant neuroprotection after global ischemia in rats[409–411], gerbils[356,412], cats[413], and dogs[40,414,415]. However, the degree of neuroprotection resulting from postischemic hypothermia appears to depend on the time elapsed from the onset of recirculation to the onset of cooling. Busto and colleagues[409] demonstrated that 3 hours of postischemic hypothermia (30°C) initiated 5 minutes after global ischemia in the rat resulted in histologic protection, whereas postischemic hypothermia initiated 30 minutes after ischemia was not protective. However, in a similar model, 5 hours of postischemic hypothermia initiated 2 hours after 10 minutes of global ischemia resulted in significant histologic protection[410]. In a gerbil model of global ischemia, Carroll and Beek[412] showed that 6 hours of postischemic hypothermia (28 to 32°C) was effective if initiated within 1 hour of reperfusion but not if initiated at 3 hours of reperfusion. Similar work has been done in a canine cardiac arrest model[40,414]. Postischemic hypothermia (34°C for 1 hour) initiated at the onset of reperfusion resulted in significant improvements in neurologic and histologic outcome[40,414], whereas a delay of 15 minutes resulted in improved histologic but not neurologic outcome (Fig. 20.17)[40]. Thus, the therapeutic window of efficacy appears to be limited for postischemic hypothermia, which has curtailed enthusiasm for this treatment modality. Furthermore, deeper levels of hypothermia are not practical in the postischemic period because of cardiovascular complications[415].

One of the most important points learned from the study of the effect of temperature on outcome from global ischemia is that hyperthermia, both intraischemic and postischemic, can dramatically worsen outcome after ischemia[416]. Three studies published in 1990 demonstrated the detrimental effects of hyperthermia both during and after ischemia. Both Minamisawa et al.[18] and Dietrich et al.[19] demonstrated dramatically worse histologic outcome after global ischemia in rats exposed to intraischemic hyperthermia (39°C). Both groups showed that ischemia under hyperthermic conditions led to overt pannecrosis or infarction. In a gerbil model of global ischemia, Kuroiwa and coworkers[417] demonstrated that postischemic hyperthermia resulted in significantly worse histologic outcome than in animals that were maintained normothermic during the immediate postischemic period.

To summarize, intraischemic hypothermia is protective in both focal and global cerebral ischemia. Postischemic hypothermia is protective after global ischemia provided that it is initiated very soon after the onset of reperfusion. This narrow window of opportunity will limit the application of hypothermia in the clinical setting. Hyperthermia is deleterious during and immediately after the ischemic insult, and this has obvious implications in the treatment of patients after cardiorespiratory arrest.

Summary

In this section we reviewed both animal and human studies of therapeutic measures directed at hypoxic-ischemic brain injury, i.e., brain resuscitation. As was demonstrated with several of the agents reviewed above, initial studies often suggested a neuroprotective effect only to be disproven with well-controlled, well-designed experiments. Our search for a neuroprotective drug for use in the setting of global ischemia has been comparable to the search for the Holy Grail. As our understanding of the pathophysiology of hypoxic-ischemic brain injury grows, therapies based on this understanding will be developed, and hopefully, these interventions will prove effective. For example, it is tempting to predict that in the future we will apply "gene therapy" after cerebral ischemia. Altering gene expression after cerebral ischemia may allow us to intervene in the processes that lead to delayed neuronal death. A possible application of gene therapy might consist of increasing the expression of growth factors or decreasing the expression of detrimental proteins after cerebral ischemia. However, it is important to reiterate that the development of such therapies is dependent on a more complete understanding of the processes leading to neuronal death after cerebral ischemia.

APPROACH TO THE PATIENT WITH GLOBAL HYPOXIC-ISCHEMIC BRAIN INJURY

The underlying foundation of neurointensive care is excellent supportive care (see Chapter 18, Pathophysiology and Clinical Management of the Intracranial Vault). Until a neuroprotective agent is developed, state-of-the-art care for a patient who has suffered an hypoxic-ischemic injury consists of maintenance of adequate blood pressure, oxygenation, ventilation, and electrolyte homeostasis and prevention of hyperglycemia, hyperthermia, and seizures. There are, however, several features of postischemic intensive care that warrant further discussion. These include hyperventilation, corticosteroids, glucose homeostasis, temperature regulation, and anticonvulsant therapy.

Hyperventilation has been advocated after cerebral injury as a means to decrease intracranial pressure. However, the use of hyperventilation, even after traumatic brain injury, is being reevaluated[(418)]. There is no evidence of beneficial effect of hyperventilation after hypoxic-ischemic brain injury, and its use should be avoided. Although CBF response to lowering $PaCO_2$ is impaired immediately after cerebral ischemia[(419)], hyperventilation may lead to cerebral hypoperfusion and worsening of the ischemic injury.

Steroid compounds appear to inhibit lipid peroxidation[(420)] and for many years were routinely administered to patients after cardiac arrest in an attempt to ameliorate hypoxic-ischemic brain injury. However, postischemic administration of corticosteroids results in significantly increased neuronal injury after global ischemia in the rat[(421)]. Furthermore, two large retrospective clinical studies[(422,423)] have failed to demonstrate any improvement in neurological outcome after cardiac arrest; thus there is no role for steroids after hypoxic-ischemic brain injury.

As described above, hyperglycemia is deleterious during and after cerebral ischemia. Furthermore, due to high levels of endogenous catecholamines and other counter-regulatory hormones, it is not uncommon to see high blood glucose levels after hypoxic-ischemic injury. Care should be taken to maintain normoglycemia during the postischemic phase. Blood glucose levels should be monitored frequently and insulin administered as needed to lower the serum glucose to normal levels.

Temperature regulation after hypoxic-ischemic injury is of paramount importance. As described in detail above, hypothermia initiated immediately after ischemia appears to be neuroprotective[(40,356,409–415)], whereas hyperthermia is extremely detrimental to the ischemic brain[(18,19,417)]. Thus, until clinical trials have been performed that prove a beneficial effect of postischemic hypothermia, normothermia (36 to 37°C) is recommended after hypoxic-ischemic injury. However, hyperthermia should be avoided; aggressive, active treatment with cooling blankets and antipyretics is warranted.

Postischemic seizures are not uncommon and require aggressive therapy because prolonged seizure activity per se can lead to brain damage[(24)]. Clinical seizures should be treated aggressively with benzodiazepines and phenytoin (see Chapter 22). If these agents are unsuccessful, barbiturates may be added. The downside to barbiturates in this setting is that they will further depress the sensorium and make prognostication difficult. Treatment of subclinical seizures, i.e., manifest only on the EEG, is controversial; there are little data regarding the effect of treating subclinical seizure activity on outcome after global ischemia.

To summarize, the most important treatment of hypoxic-ischemic brain injury is to provide excellent supportive care. Aggressively treating hyperglycemia, hyperthermia, and seizure activity will allow the best possible outcome. Unfortunately, the most difficult decisions to be made during postischemic management involve ethical decisions regarding withdrawal of support.

CONCLUSION

In this chapter we reviewed the pathophysiology of hypoxic-ischemic brain injuries and described some of the laboratory and clinical investigations of brain resuscitation. These include studies of barbiturates, calcium antagonists, glutamate antagonists, oxygen radical scavengers, nitric oxide synthase inhibitors, and hypothermia. It seems likely that there will never be a simple answer, and ultimately, successful therapies will be based on years of investigation of the mechanisms leading to neuronal death. Neurointensive care and resuscitation are areas of complex physiology and biochemistry that are not susceptible to simplistic analysis. Too often we are reminded of the words of H. L. Mencken, i.e., that ". . . for every complex problem, there is a solution that is simple, direct, and wrong." After the initial excitement about brain resuscitation, the progress is likely to continue to be slow and difficult. Progress is always difficult if you ask the right questions.

Acknowledgments

The authors thank Ms. Anita Smith for transforming illegible scribbles on pieces of paper into Figures 20.2 to 20.5 and 20.7.

References

1. Barcroft J. On anoxemia. Lancet 1920;2:485–489.
2. Siesjo BK. Pathophysiology and treatment of focal cerebral ischemia. Part II: Mechanisms of damage and treatment. J Neurosurg 1992;77:337–354.
3. Siesjo BK. Pathophysiology and treatment of focal cerebral ischemia. Part I: Pathophysiology. J Neurosurg 1992;77:169–184.
4. Branston NM, Symon L, Crockard HA, Pasztor E. Relationship between the cortical evoked potential and local cortical blood flow following acute middle cerebral artery occlusion in the baboon. Exp Neurol 1974;45:195–208.
5. Astrup J, Symon L, Branston NM, Lassen NA. Cortical evoked potential and extracellular K^+ and H^+ at critical levels of brain ischemia. Stroke 1977;8:51–57.
6. Snyder JV, Nemoto EM, Carroll RG, Safar P. Global ischemia in dogs: Intracranial pressures, brain blood flow and metabolism. Stroke 1975;6:21–27.
7. Kagstrom E, Smith ML, Siesjo BK. Local cerebral blood flow in the recovery period following complete cerebral ischemia in the rat. J Cereb Blood Flow Metab 1983;3:170–182.
8. Stevens MK, Yaksh TL. Systematic studies on the effects of the NMDA receptor antagonist MK-801 on cerebral blood flow and responsivity, EEG, and blood-brain barrier following complete reversible cerebral ischemia. J Cereb Blood Flow Metab 1990;10:77–88.
9. Kirsch JR, Helfaer MA, Blizzard K, Toung TJ, Traystman RJ. Age-related cerebrovascular response to global ischemia in pigs. Am J Physiol 1990;259:H1551–H1558.
10. Miller C, Lampard D, Alexander K, Brown W. Local cerebral blood flow following transient cerebral ischemia. I. Onset of impaired perfusion within the first hour following global ischemia. Stroke 1980;11:534–541.
11. Ames A I, Wright RL, Kowada M, Thurston JM, Majno G. Cerebral ischemia II. The no-reflow phenomenon. Am J Pathol 1968;52:437–452.
12. Michenfelder JD, Milde JH. Postischemic canine cerebral blood flow appears to be determined by cerebral metabolic needs. J Cereb Blood Flow Metab 1990;10:71–76.
13. Brown AW, Brierley JB. The earliest alterations in rat neurones and astrocytes after anoxia-ischemia. Acta Neuropathol (Berl) 1973;23:9–22.
14. Brierley JB, Meldrum BS, Brown AW. The threshold and neuropathology of cerebral "anoxia-ischemic" cell change. Arch Neurol 1973;29:367–374.
15. Brierley JB. The no-reflow phenomenon. In: Langfitt TW, McHenry LCJ, Reivich M, Wollman H, eds. Cerebral Circulation and Metabolism. New York: Springer-Verlag, 1975:
16. Pulsinelli WA, Brierley JB. A new model of bilateral hemispheric ischemia in the unanesthetized rat. Stroke 1979;10:267–272.
17. Smith ML, Auer RN, Siesjo BK. The density and distribution of ischemic brain injury in the rat following 2–10 min of forebrain ischemia. Acta Neuropathol (Berl) 1984;64:319–332.
18. Minamisawa H, Smith ML, Siesjo BK. The effect of mild hyperthermia and hypothermia on brain damage following 5, 10, and 15 minutes of forebrain ischemia. Ann Neurol 1990;28:26–33.
19. Dietrich WD, Busto R, Valdes I, Loor Y. Effects of normothermic versus mild hyperthermic forebrain ischemia in rats. Stroke 1990;21:1318–1325.
20. Pulsinelli WA, Waldman S, Rawlinson D, Plum F. Moderate hyperglycemia augments ischemic brain damage: A neuropathological study in the rat. Neurology 1982;32:1239–1246.
21. Brierley JB, Graham DI. Hypoxia and vascular disorders of the central nervous system. In: Adams JH, Corsellis JAN, Duchen LW, eds. Greenfield's Neuropathology. New York: Wiley Medical, 1984:125–56.
22. Schmidt-Kastner R, Freund TF. Selective vulnerability of the hippocampus in brain ischemia. Neuroscience 1991;40:599–636.
23. Kuroiwa T, Okeda R. Neuropathology of cerebral ischemia and hypoxia: recent advances in experimental studies on its pathogenesis. Pathol Int 1994;44:171–181.
24. Siesjo BK, Wieloch T. Epileptic brain damage: pathophysiology and neurochemical pathology. Adv Neurol 1986;44:813–847.
25. Paschen W. Molecular mechanisms of selective vulnerability of the brain to ischemia. Circ Metab Cerveau 1989;6:115–139.
26. Choi DW, Rothman SM. The role of glutamate neurotoxicity in hypoxic-ischemic neuronal death. Annu Rev Neurosci 1990;13:171–182.
27. Pulsinelli W, Sarokin A, Buchan A. Antagonism of the NMDA and non-NMDA receptors in global versus focal brain ischemia. Prog Brain Res 1993;96:125–135.
28. Pulsinelli WA, Brierley JB, Plum F. Temporal profile of neuronal damage in a model of transient forebrain ischemia. Ann Neurol 1982;11:491–498.
29. Kirino T. Delayed neuronal death in the gerbil hippocampus following ischemia. Brain Res 1982;239:57–69.
30. Petito CK, Feldmann E, Pulsinelli WA, Plum F. Delayed hippocampal damage in humans following cardiorespiratory arrest. Neurology 1987;37:1281–1286.
31. Siesjo BK. A new perspective on ischemic brain damage. Prog Brain Res 1993;96:1–9.
32. Hockenbery D. Defining apoptosis. Am J Pathol 1995;146:16–19.
33. Li Y, Sharov VG, Jiang N, Zaloga C, Sabbah HN, Chopp M. Ultrastructural and light microscopic evidence of apoptosis after middle cerebral artery occlusion in the rat. Am J Pathol 1995;146:1045–1051.
34. Li Y, Chopp M, Jiang N, Zaloga C. In situ detection of DNA fragmentation after focal cerebral ischemia in mice. Brain Res Mol Brain Res 1995;28:164–168.
35. Li Y, Chopp M, Jiang N, Yao F, Zaloga C. Temporal profile of in situ DNA fragmentation after transient middle cerebral artery occlusion in the rat. J Cereb Blood Flow Metab 1995;15:389–397.
36. Linnik MD, Zobrist RH, Hatfield MD. Evidence supporting a role for programmed cell death in focal cerebral ischemia in rats. Stroke 1993;24:2002–8; discussion 2008–9.
37. MacManus JP, Buchan AM, Hill IE, Rasquinha I, Preston E. Global ischemia can cause DNA fragmentation indicative of apoptosis in rat brain. Neurosci Lett 1993;164:89–92.
38. Sei Y, Von Lubitz KJ, Basile AS, et al. Internucleosomal DNA fragmentation in gerbil hippocampus following forebrain ischemia. Neurosci Lett 1994;171:179–182.
39. Steen PA, Gisvold SE, Milde JH, et al. Nimodipine improves outcome when given after complete cerebral ischemia in primates. Anesthesiology 1985;62:406–414.
40. Kuboyama K, Safar P, Radovsky A, Tisherman SA, Stezoski SW, Alexander H. Delay in cooling negates the beneficial effect of mild resuscitative cerebral hypotherma after cardiac arrest in dogs: A prospective, randomized study. Crit Care Med 1993;21:1348–1358.
41. Siesjo BK. Mechanisms of ischemic brain damage. Crit Care Med 1988;16:954–963.
42. Krause GS, White BC, Aust SD, Nayini NR, Kumar K. Brain cell death following ischemia and reperfusion: a proposed biochemical sequence. Crit Care Med 1988;16:714–726.
43. Erecinska M, Silver IA. ATP and brain function. J Cereb Blood Flow Metab 1989;9:2–19.
44. Lowry OH, Passonneau JV, Hasselberger FX, et al. Effect of ischemia on known substrates and cofactors of the glycolytic pathway in brain. J Biol Chem 1964;239:18–30.
45. Ljunggren B, Ratcheson RA, Siesjo BK. Cerebral metabolic state following complete compression ischemia. Brain Res 1974;73:291–307.
46. Nilsson B, Norberg K, Nordstrom CH, et al. Rate of energy utilization in the cerebral cortex of rats. Acta Physiol Scand 1975;93:569–571.
47. Nordstrom CH, Siesjo BK. Effects of phenobarbital in cerebral ischemia. Part I:Cerebral energy metabolism during pronounced incomplete ischemia. Stroke 1978;9:327–335.
48. Hansen AJ, Nedergaard M. Brain ion homeostasis in cerebral ischemia. Neurochem Pathol 1988;9:195–209.
49. Onodera H, Iijima K, Kogure K. Mononucleotide metabolism in the rat brain after transient ischemia. J Neurochem 1986;46:1704–1710.
50. Schutz H, Silverstein PR, Vapalahti M, Bruce DA, Mela L, Langfitt TW. Brain mitochondrial function after ischemia and hypoxia. I. Ischemia induced by increased intracranial pressure. Arch Neurol 1973;29:408–416.
51. Ginsberg MD, Mela L, Wrobel-Kuhl K, Reivich M. Mitochondrial metabolism following bilateral cerebral ischemia in the gerbil. Ann Neurol 1977;1:519–527.
52. Rehncrona S, Mela L, Siesjo BK. Recovery of brain mitochondrial function in the rat after complete and incomplete cerebral ischemia. Stroke 1979;10:437–446.
53. Linn F, Paschen W, Ophoff BG, Hossmann KA. Mitochondrial respiration during recirculation after prolonged ischemia in cat brain. Exp Neurol 1987;96:321–333.
54. Sims NR, Pulsinelli WA. Altered mitochondrial respiration in selectively vulnerable brain subregions following transient forebrain ischemia in the rat. J Neurochem 1987;49:1367–1374.
55. Siesjo BK, Katsura K, Mellergard P, Ekholm A, Lundgren J, Smith ML. Acidosis-related brain damage. Prog Brain Res 1993;96:23–48.
56. Ljunggren B, Norberg K, Siesjo BK. Influence of tissue acidosis upon restitution of brain energy metabolism following total ischemia. Brain Res 1974;77:173–186.
57. Rehncrona S, Rosen I, Siesjo BK. Brain lactic acidosis and ischemic

cell damage. I. Biochemistry and neurophysiology. J Cereb Blood Flow Metab 1981;1:297–311.
58. Smith ML, von Hanwehr R, Siesjo BK. Changes in extra- and intracellular pH in the brain during and following ischemia in hyperglycemic and in moderately hypoglycemic rats. J Cereb Blood Flow Metab 1986;6:574–583.
59. Chopp M, Welch KM, Tidwell CD, Helpern JA. Global cerebral ischemia and intracellular pH during hyperglycemia and hypoglycemia in cats. Stroke 1988;19:1383–1387.
60. Kalimo H, Rehncrona S, Soderfeldt B, Olsson Y, Siesjo BK. Brain lactic acidosis and ischemic cell damage: 2. Histopathology. J Cereb Blood Flow Metab 1981;1:313–327.
61. Myers RE, Yamaguchi M. Effects of serum glucose concentration on brain response to circulatory arrest. J Neuropathol Exp Neurol 1976;35:301.
62. Lanier WL, Stangland KJ, Scheithauer BW, Milde JH, Michenfelder JD. The effects of dextrose infusion and head position on neurologic outcome after complete cerebral ischemia in primates: examination of a model. Anesthesiology 1987;66:39–48.
63. Natale JE, Stante SM, D'Alecy LG. Elevated brain lactate accumulation and increased neurologic deficit are associated with modest hyperglycemia in global brain ischemia. Resuscitation 1990;19:271–289.
64. Siesjo BK. Acidosis and ischemic brain damage. Neurochem Pathol 1988;9:31–88.
65. Marshall LF, Durity F, Lounsbury R, Graham DJ, Welsh F, Langfitt TW. Experimental cerebral oligemia and ischemia produced by intracranial hypertension. I. Pathophysiology, electroencephalography, cerebral blood flow, blood-brain barrier and neurological function. J Neurosurg 1975;43:308–317.
66. Marshall LF, Graham DJ, Durity F, Lounsbury R, Welsh F, Langfitt TW. Experimental cerebral oligemia and ischemia produced by intracranial hypertension. 2. Brain morphology. J Neurosurg 1975;43:318–322.
67. Marshall LF, Welsh F, Durity F, Lounsbury R, Graham DI. Experimental cerebral oligemia and ischemia produced by intracranial hypertension. Part 3: brain energy metabolism. J Neurosurg 1975;43:323–328.
68. Steen PA, Michenfelder JD, Milde JH. Incomplete versus complete cerebral ischemia. Improved outcome with a minimal blood flow. Ann Neurol 1979;6:389–398.
69. Shibuya M, Suzuki Y, Takayasu M, et al. The effects of an intracellular calcium antagonist HA 1077 on delayed cerebral vasospasm in dogs. Acta Neurochir (Wien) 1988;90:53–59.
70. Dietrich WD, Busto R, Yoshida S, Ginsberg MD. Histopathological and hemodynamic consequences of complete versus incomplete ischemia in the rat. J Cereb Blood Flow Metab 1987;7:300–308.
71. Yoshida S, Busto R, Martinez E, Scheinberg P, Ginsberg MD. Regional brain energy metabolism after complete versus incomplete ischemia in the rat in the absence of severe lactic acidosis. J Cereb Blood Flow Metab 1985;5:490–501.
72. Rehncrona S, Rosen I, Smith ML. Effect of different degrees of brain ischemia and tissue lactic acidosis on the short-term recovery of neurophysiologic and metabolic variables. Exp Neurol 1985;87:458–473.
73. Ichord RN, Kirsch JR, Helfaer MA, Haun S, Traystman RJ. Age-related differences in recovery of blood flow and metabolism after cerebral ischemia in swine. Stroke 1991;22:626–634.
74. Hossmann KA, Zimmerman V. Resuscitation of the monkey brain after one hour's complete ischemia. I. Physiological and morphological observations. Brain Res 1974;81:59–74.
75. Goldman SA, Pulsinelli WA, Clarke WY, Kraig RP, Plum F. The effects of extracellular acidosis on neurons and glia in vitro. J Cereb Blood Flow Metab 1989;9:471–477.
76. Norenberg MD, Mozes LW, Gregorios JB, Norenberg LO. Effects of lactic acid on astrocytes in primary culture. J Neuropathol Exp Neurol 1987;46:154–166.
77. Staub F, Baethmann A, Peters J, Kempski O. Effects of lactacidosis on volume and viability of glial cells. Acta Neurochir Suppl 1990;51:3–6.
78. Hillered L, Ernster L, Siesjo BK. Influence of in vitro lactic acidosis and hypercapnia on respiratory activity of isolated rat brain miochondria. J Cereb Blood Flow Metab 1984;4:430–437.
79. Rehncrona S, Hauge HN, Siesjo BK. Enhancement of iron-catalyzed free radical formation by acidosis in brain homogenates: difference in effect by lactic acid and CO_2. J Cereb Blood Flow Metab 1989;9:65–70.
80. Siesjo BK, Bendek G, Koide T, Westerberg E, Wieloch T. Influence of acidosis on lipid peroxidation in brain tissues in vitro. J Cereb Blood Flow Metab 1985;5:253–258.
81. Araki N, Greenberg JH, Sladky JT, Uematsu D, Karp A, Reivich M. The effect of hyperglycemia on intracellular calcium in stroke. J Cereb Blood Flow Metab 1992;12:469–476.
82. Tombaugh GC, Sapolsky RM. Evolving concepts about the role of acidosis in ischemic neuropathology. J Neurochem 1993;61:793–803.
83. Tombaugh GC, Sapolsky RM. Mild acidosis protects hippocampal neurons from injury induced by oxygen and glucose deprivation. Brain Res 1990;343–345.
84. Giffard RG, Monyer H, Christine CW, Choi DW. Acidosis reduces NMDA receptor activation, glutamate neurotoxicity, and oxygen-glucose deprivation neuronal injury in cortical cultures. Brain Res 1990;506:339–342.
85. Takadera T, Shimada Y, Mohri T. Extracellular pH modulates N-methyl-D-aspartate mediated neurotoxicity and calcium accumulation in rat cortical cultures. Brain Res 1992;572:126–131.
86. Van Harreveld A. Compounds in brain extracts causing spreading depression of cerebral cortical activity and contraction of crustacean muscle. J Neurochem 1959;3:300–315.
87. Benveniste H, Drejer J, Schousboe A, Diemer NH. Elevation of the extracellular concentrations of glutamate and aspartate in rat hippocampus during transient cerebral ischemia monitored by intracerebral microdialysis. J Neurochem 1984;43:1369–1374.
88. Hagberg H, Lehmann A, Sandberg M, Nystrom B, Jacobson I, Hamberger A. Ischemia-induced shift of inhibitory and excitatory amino acids from intra- to extracellular compartments. J Cereb Blood Flow Metab 1985;5:413–419.
89. Drejer J, Benveniste H, Diemer NH, Schousboe A. Cellular origin of ischemia-induced glutamate release from brain tissue in vivo and in vitro. J Neurochem 1985;45:145–151.
90. Choi DW, Maulucci-Gedde M, Kriegstein AR. Glutamate neurotoxicity in cortical cell culture. J Neurosci 1987;7:357–368.
91. Simon RP, Swan JH, Griffiths T, Meldrum BS. Blockade of N-methyl-D-aspartate receptors may protect against ischemic damage in the brain. Science 1984;226:850–852.
92. Johansen FF, Jrgensen MB, Diemer NH. Ischemic CA-1 pyramidal cell loss is prevented by preischemic colchicine destruction of dentate gyrus granule cells. Brain Res 1986;377:344–347.
93. Onodera H, Sato G, Kogure K. Lesions to Schaffer collaterals prevent ischemic death of CA1 pyramidal cells. Neurosci Lett 1986;68:169–174.
94. Buchan AM, Slivka A, Xue D. The effect of the NMDA receptor antagonist MK-801 on cerebral blood flow and infarct volume in experimental focal stroke. Brain Res 1992;574:171–177.
95. Buchan AM, Li H, Cho S, Pulsinelli WA. Blockade of the AMPA receptor prevents CA1 hippocampal injury following severe but transient forebrain ischemia in adult rats. Neurosci Lett 1991;132:255–258.
96. Goldberg MP, Weiss JH, Pham PC, Choi DW. N-methyl-D-aspartate receptors mediate hypoxic neuronal injury in cortical culture. J Pharmacol Exp Ther 1987;243:784–791.
97. Rothman SM, Thurston JH, Hauhart RE, Clark GD, Solomon JS. Ketamine protects hippocampal neurons from anoxia in vitro. Neuroscience 1987;21:673–678.
98. Kaku DA, Goldberg MP, Choi DW. Antagonism of non-NMDA receptors augments the neuroprotective effect of NMDA receptor blockade in cortical cultures exposed to prolonged deprivation of oxygen and glucose. Brain Res 1991;554:344–347.
99. Nakanishi S. Molecular diversity of glutamate receptors and implications for brain function. Science 1992;258:597–603.
100. Wisden W, Seeburg PH. Mammalian ionotropic glutamate receptors. Curr Opin Neurobiol 1993;3:291–298.
101. Schoepp DD, Conn PJ. Metabotropic glutamate receptors in brain function and pathology. Trends Pharmacol Sci 1993;14:13–20.
102. MacDermott AB, Mayer ML, Westbrook GL, Smith SJ, Barker JL. NMDA-receptor activation increases cytoplasmic calcium concentration in cultured spinal cord neurones. Nature 1986;321:519–522.
103. Mayer ML, MacDermott AB, Westbrook GL, Smith SJ, Barker JL. Agonist- and voltage-gated calcium entry in cultured mouse spinal cord neurons under voltage clamp measured using arsenazo III. J Neurosci 1987;7:3230–3244.
104. Murphy SN, Thayer SA, Miller RJ. The effects of excitatory amino acids on intracellular calcium in single mouse striatal neurons *in vitro.* J Neurosci 1987;7:4145–4158.
105. Choi DW. Calcium: still center-stage in hypoxic-ischemic neuronal death. Trends Neurosci 1995;18:58–60.
106. Choi DW, Hartley DM. Calcium and glutamate-induced cortical neuronal death. In: Waxman SG, ed. Molecular and Cellular Approaches to

the Treatment of Neurological Diseases. New York: Raven Press,Ltd. 1993:23–34.
107. Westbrook GL. Glutamate Receptors and Excitotoxicity. In: Waxman SG, ed. Molecular and Cellular Approaches to the Treatment of Neurological Disease. New York: Raven Press, Ltd. 1993:35–50.
108. Iino M, Ozawa S, Tsuzuki K. Permeation of calcium through excitatory amino acid receptor channels in cultured rat hippocampal neurons. J Physiol 1990;424:151–165.
109. Pellegrini-Giampietro DE, Zukin RS, Bennett MV, Cho S, Pulsinelli WA. Switch in glutamate receptor subunit gene expression in CA1 subfield of hippocampus following global ischemia in rats. Proc Natl Acad Sci U S A 1992;89:10499–10503.
110. Buchan AM, Lesiuk H, Barnes KA, et al. AMPA antagonists: do they hold more promise for clinical stroke trials than NMDA antagonists?. Stroke 1993;24(suppl I):I–148–I–152.
111. Desai MA, Conn PJ. Selective activation of phosphoinositide hydrolysis by a rigid analogue of glutamate. Neurosci Lett 1990;109:157–162.
112. Sladeczek F, Pin JP, Recasens M, Bockaert J, Weiss S. Glutamate stimulates inositol phosphate formation in striatal neurones. Nature 1985;317:717–719.
113. Sugiyama H, Ito I, Hirono C. A new type of glutamate receptor linked to inositol phospholipid metabolism. Nature 1987;325:531–533.
114. Schoepp DD, Johnson BG, Monn JA. Inhibition of cyclic AMP formation by a selective metabotrophic glutamate receptor agonist. J Neurochem 1992;58:1184–1186.
115. Okamoto N, Hori S, Akazawa C, et al. Molecular characterization of a new metabotropic glutamate receptor mGluR7 coupled to inhibitory cyclic AMP signal transduction. J Biol Chem 1994;269:1231–1236.
116. Rothman SM, Olney JW. Glutamate and the pathophysiology of hypoxic—ischemic brain damage. Ann Neurol 1986;19:105–111.
117. Choi DW. Ionic dependence of glutamate neurotoxicity. J Neurosci 1987;7:369–379.
118. Dawson VL, Dawson TM, London ED, Bredt DS, Snyder SH. Nitric oxide mediates glutamate neurotoxicity in primary cortical cultures. Proc Natl Acad Sci U S A 1991;88:6368–6371.
119. Berridge MJ, Irvine RF. Inositol trisphosphate, a novel second messenger in cellular signal transduction. Nature 1984;312:315–321.
120. Kishimoto A, Takai Y, Mori T, Kikkawa U, Nishizuka Y. Activation of calcium and phospholipid-dependent protein kinase by diacylglycerol, its possible relation to phosphatidylinositol turnover. J Biol Chem 1980;255:2273–2276.
121. Koh J, Palmer E, Lin A, Cotman C. A metabotropic glutamate receptor agonist does not mediate neuronal degeneration in cortical culture. Brain Res 1991;561:338–343.
122. Siesjo BK, Bengtsson F. Calcium fluxes, calcium antagonists, and calcium-related pathology in brain ischemia, hypoglycemia, and spreading depression: a unifying hypothesis. J Cereb Blood Flow Metab 1989;9:127–140.
123. Choi DW. Calcium-mediated neurotoxicity: relationship to specific channel types and role in ischemic damage. Trends Neurosci 1988;11:465–469.
124. Morley P, Hogan MJ, Hakim AM. Calcium-mediated mechanisms of ischemic injury and protection. Brain Pathol 1994;4:37–47.
125. Cheung JY, Bonventre JV, Malis CD, Leaf A. Calcium and ischemic injury. N Engl J Med 1986;314:1670–1676.
126. Deshpande JK, Siesjo BK, Wieloch T. Calcium accumulation and neuronal damage in the rat hippocampus following cerebral ischemia. J Cereb Blood Flow Metab 1987;7:89–95.
127. DeLeo J, Toth L, Schubert P, Rudolphi K, Kreutzberg GW. Ischemia-induced neuronal cell death, calcium accumulation, and glial response in the hippocampus of the Mongolian gerbil and protection by propentofylline (HWA 285). J Cereb Blood Flow Metab 1987;7:745–751.
128. Silver IA, Erecinska M. Intracellular and extracellular changes of [Ca2+] in hypoxia and ischemia in rat brain in vivo. J Gen Physiol 1990;95:837–866.
129. Goldberg WJ, Kadingo RM, Barrett JN. Effects of ischemia-like conditions on cultured neurons: protection by low Na+, low Ca2+ solutions. J Neurosci 1986;6:3144–3151.
130. Goldberg MP, Choi DW. Combined oxygen and glucose deprivation in cortical cell culture: calcium-dependent and calcium-independent mechanisms of neuronal injury. J Neurosci 1993;13:3510–3524.
131. Haun SE, Murphy EJ, Bates CM, Horrocks LA. Extracellular calcium is a mediator of astroglial injury during combined glucose-oxygen deprivation. Brain Res 1992;593:45–50.
132. Spedding M, Paoletti R. Classification of calcium channels and the sites of action of drugs modifying channel function. Pharmacol Rev 1992;44:363–376.
133. Hillman D, Chen S, Aung TT, Cherksey B, Sugimori M, Llinas RR. Localisation of P-type calcium channels in the central nervous system. Proc Natl Acad Sci U S A 1991;88:7076–7080.
134. Siesjo BK. Cell damage in the brain: A speculative synthesis. J Cereb Blood Flow Metab 1981;1:155–185.
135. Nicholson C, Bruggencate GT, Steinberg R, Stockle H. Calcium modulation in brain extracellular microenvironment demonstrated with ion-selective micropipette. Proc Natl Acad Sci USA 1977;74:1287–1290.
136. Hansen AJ, Zeuthen T. Extracelluar ion concentrations during spreading depression and ischemia in the rat brain cortex. Acta Physiol Scand 1981;113:437–445.
137. Thayer SA, Murphy SN, Miller RJ. Widespread distribution of dihydropyridine-sensitive calcium channels in the central nervous system. Mol Pharmacol 1986;30:505–509.
138. Mitani A, Yanase H, Sakai K, Wake Y, Kataoka K. Origin of intracellular Ca2+ elevation induced by in vitro ischemia-like condition in hippocampal slices. Brain Res 1993;601:103–110.
139. Zhang L, Andou Y, Masuda S, Mitani A, Kataoka K. Dantrolene protects against ischemic, delayed neuronal death in gerbil brain. Neurosci Lett 1993;158:105–108.
140. Siesjo BK, Katsura K. Ischemic brain damage: focus on lipids and lipid mediators. Adv Exp Med Biol 1992;318:41–56.
141. Farooqui AA, Horrocks LA. Excitatory amino acid receptors, neural membrane phospholipid metabolism and neurological disorders. Brain Res Rev 1991;16:171–191.
142. Bazan NG. Effects of ischemia and electroconvulsive shock on free fatty acid pool in the brain. Biochim Biophys Acta 1970;218:1–10.
143. Bazan NG, DeBazan HEP, Kennedy WG, Joel CD. Regional distribution and rate of production of free fatty acids in rat brain. J Neurochem 1971;18:1387–1393.
144. Edgar AD, Strosznajder J, Horrocks LA. Activation of ethanolamine phospholipase A2 in brain during ischemia. J Neurochem 1982;39:1111–1116.
145. Hirashima Y, Moto A, Endo S, Takaku A. Activities of enzymes metabolizing phospholipids in rat cerebral ischemia. Mol Chem Neuropathol 1989;10:87–100.
146. Yoshida S, Ikeda M, Busto R, Santiso M, Martinez E, Ginsberg MD. Cerebral phosphoinositide, triacylglycerol, and energy metabolism in reversible ischemia: origin and fate of free fatty acids. J Neurochem 1986;47:744–757.
147. Ikeda M, Yoshida S, Busto R, Santiso M, Ginsberg MD. Polyphosphoinositides as a probable source of brain free fatty acids accumulated at the onset of ischemia. J Neurochem 1986;47:123–132.
148. Abe K, Kogure K, Yamamoto H, Imazawa M, Miyamoto K. Mechanism of arachidonic acid liberation during ischemia in gerbil cerebral cortex. J Neurochem 1987;48:503–509.
149. Sun GY, Lu FL, Lin SE, Ko MR. Decapitation ischemia-induced release of free fatty acids in mouse brain. Relationship with diacylglycerols and lysophospholipids. Mol Chem Neuropathol 1992;17:39–50.
150. Sun GY, Su KL, Der OM, Tang W. Enzymic regulation of arachidonate metabolism in brain membrane phosphoglycerides. Lipids 1978; 14:229–235.
151. Dumuis A, Sebben M, Haynes L, Pin JP, Bockaert J. NMDA receptors activate the arachidonic acid cascade system in striatal neurons. Nature 1988;336:68–70.
152. Lazarewicz JW, Wroblewski JT, Palmer ME, Costa E. Activation of N-methyl-D-aspartate-sensitive glutamate receptors stimulates arachidonic acid release in primary cultures of cerebellar granule cells. Neuropharmacology 1988;27:765–769.
153. Dumuis A, Pin JP, Oomagari K, Sebben M, Bockaert J. Arachidonic acid released from striatal neurons by joint stimulation of ionotropic and metabotropic quisqualate receptors. Nature 1990;347:182–184.
154. Lazarewicz JW, Wroblewski JT, Costa E. N-methyl-D-aspartate-sensitive glutamate receptors induce calcium-mediated arachidonic acid release in primary cultures of cerebellar granule cells. J Neurochem 1990;55:1875–1881.
155. Sanfeliu C, Hunt A, Patel AJ. Exposure to N-methyl-D-aspartate increases release of arachidonic acid in primary cultures of rat hippocampal neurons and not in astrocytes. Brain Res 1990;526:241–248.
156. Farooqui AA, Anderson DK, Horrocks LA. Effect of glutamate and its analogs on diacylglycerol and monoacylglycerol lipase activities of neuron-enriched cultures. Brain Res 1993;604:180–184.
157. Goldberg WJ, Dorman RV, Dabrowiecki Z, Horrocks LA. The effects of

ischemia and CDPamines on Na+, K+-ATPase and acetylcholinesterase activities in rat brain. Neurochem Pathol 1985;3:237–248.
158. Ahmed K, Thomas BS. The effects of long chain fatty acids on sodium plus potassium ion-stimulated adenosine triphosphatase of rat brain. J Biol Chem 1971;246:103–109.
159. Chan PH, Kerlan R, Fishman RA. Reductions of gamma-aminobutyric acid and glutamate uptake and (Na^+ + K^+)-ATPase activity in brain slices and synaptosomes by arachidonic acid. J Neurochem 1983;40:309–316.
160. Chan PH, Fishman RA. Brain edema: Induction in cortical slices by polyunsaturated fatty acids. Science 1978;201:358–360.
161. Kuwashima J, Fujitani B, Nakamura K, Kadokawa T, Yoshida K, Shimizu M. Biochemical changes in unilateral brain injury in the rat: A possible role of free fatty acid accumulation. Brain Res 1976;110:547–557.
162. Hillered L, Chan PH. Role of arachidonic acid and other free fatty acids in mitochondrial dysfunction in brain ischemia. J Neurosci Res 1988;20:451–456.
163. Hillered L, Chan PH. Effects of arachidonic acid on respiratory activities in isolated brain mitochondria. J Neurosci Res 1988;19:94–100.
164. Rhoads DE, Osburn LD, Peterson NA, Raghupathy E. Release of neurotransmitter amino acids from synaptosomes: Enhancement of calcium-independent efflux by oleic and arachidonic acids. J Neurochem 1983;41:531–537.
165. Rhoads DE, Kaplan MA, Peterson NA, Raghupathy E. Effects of free fatty acids on synaptosomal amino acid uptake systems. J Neurochem 1982;38:1255–1260.
166. Yu ACH, Chan PH, Fishman RA. Effects of arachidonic acid on glutamate and gamma-aminobutyric acid uptake in primary cultures of rat cerebral cortical astrocytes and neurons. J Neurochem 1986;47:1181–1189.
167. Volterra A, Trotti D, Cassutti P, et al. High sensitivity of glutamate uptake to extracellular free arachidonic acid levels in rat cortical synaptosomes and astrocytes. J Neurochem 1992;59:600–606.
168. Sumida C, Graber R, Nunez E. Role of fatty acids in signal transduction: modulators and messengers. Prostaglandins Leukot Essent Fatty Acids 1993;48:117–122.
169. Dempsey RJ, Roy MW, Meyer K, Cowen DE, Tai HH. Development of cyclooxygenase and lipoxygenase metabolites of arachidonic acid after transient cerebral ischemia. J Neurosurg 1986;64:118–124.
170. Kukreja RC, Kontos HA, Hess ML, Ellis EF. PGH synthase and lipoxygenase generate superoxide in the presence of NADH or NADPH. Circ Res 1986;59:612–619.
171. Gaudet RJ, Alam I, Levine L. Accumulation of cyclooxygenase products of arachidonic acid metabolism in gerbil brain during reperfusion after biolateral common carotid artery occlusion. J Neurochem 1980;35:653–658.
172. Gaudet RJ, Levine L. Transient cerebral ischemia and brain prostaglandins. Biochem Biophys Res Commun 1979;86:893–901.
173. Crockard HA, Bhakoo KK, Lascelles PT. Regional prostaglandin levels in cerebral ischaemia. J Neurochem 1982;38:1311–1314.
174. Kempski O, Shohami E, von Lubitz D, Hallenbeck JM, Feuerstein G. Postischemic production of eicosanoids in gerbil brain. Stroke 1987;18:111–119.
175. Moskowitz MA, Kiwak KJ, Hekimian K, Levine L. Synthesis of compounds with properties of leukotrienes C4 and D4 in gerbil brains after ischemia and reperfusion. Science 1984;224:886–889.
176. Busija DW, Leffler CW, Beasley DG. Effects of leukotrienes C4, D4, and E4 on cerebral arteries of newborn pigs. Pediatr Res 1986;20:973–976.
177. Tagari P, Du Boulay GH, Aitken V, Boullin DJ. Leukotriene D4 and the cerebral vasculature in vivo and in vitro. Prostaglandin Leukotriene Med 1983;11:281–297.
178. Deneke SM, Fanburg BL. Normobaric oxygen toxicity of the lung. N Engl J Med 1980;303:76–86.
179. Floyd RA. Role of oxygen free radicals in carcinogenesis and brain ischemia. FASEB J 1990;4:2587–2597.
180. McCord JM. Oxygen-derived free radicals in postischemic tissue injury. N Engl J Med 1985;312:159–163.
181. Flamm ES, Demopoulos HB, Seligman ML, Poser RG, Ransohoff J. Free radicals in cerebral ischemia. Stroke 1978;9:445–447.
182. Traystman RJ, Kirsch JR, Koehler RC. Oxygen radical mechanisms of brain injury following ischemia and reperfusion. J Appl Physiol 1991;71:1185–1195.
183. Phillis JW. A "radical" view of cerebral ischemic injury. Prog Neurobiol 1994;42:441–448.
184. Yoshida S, Abe K, Busto R, Watson BD, Kogure K, Ginsberg MD. Influence of transient ischemia on lipid-soluble antioxidants, free fatty acids and energy metabolites in rat brain. Brain Res 1982;245:307–316.
185. Cooper AJ, Pulsinelli WA, Duffy TE. Glutathione and ascorbate during ischemia and postischemic reperfusion in rat brain. J Neurochem 1980;35:1242–1245.
186. Yoshida S, Inoh S, Asano T, et al. Effect of transient ischemia on free fatty acids and phospholipids in the gerbil brain. Lipid peroxidation as a possible cause of postischemic injury. J Neurosurg 1980;53:323–331.
187. Watson BD, Busto R, Goldberg WJ, Santiso M, Yoshida S, Ginsberg MD. Lipid peroxidation in vivo induced by reversible global ischemia in rat brain. J Neurochem 1984;42:268–274.
188. Krause GS, Nayini NR, White BC, et al. Natural course of iron delocalization and lipid peroxidation during the first eight hours following a 15-minute cardiac arrest in dogs. Ann Emerg Med 1987;16:1200–1205.
189. Bromont C, Marie C, Bralet J. Increased lipid peroxidation in vulnerable brain regions after transient forebrain ischemia in rats. Stroke 1989;20:918–924.
190. Sakamoto A, Ohnishi ST, Ohnishi T, Ogawa R. Relationship between free radical production and lipid peroxidation during ischemia-reperfusion injury in the rat brain. Brain Res 1991;554:186–192.
191. Yamamoto M, Shima T, Uozumi T, Sogabe T, Yamada K, Kawasaki T. A possible role of lipid peroxidation in cellular damages caused by cerebral ischemia and the protective effect of alpha-tocopherol administration. Stroke 1983;14:977–982.
192. Natale JE, Schott RJ, Hall ED, Braughler JM, DAlecy LG. Effect of the aminosteroid U74006F after cardiopulmonary arrest in dogs. Stroke 1988;19:1371–1378.
193. Perkins WJ, Milde LN, Milde JH, Michenfelder JD. Pretreatment with U74006F improves neurologic outcome following complete cerebral ischemia in dogs. Stroke 1991;22:902–909.
194. Liu TH, Beckman JS, Freeman BA, Hogan EL, Hsu CY. Polyethylene glycol-conjugated superoxide dismutase and catalase reduce ischemic brain injury. Am J Physiol 1989;256:H589–H593.
195. Imaizumi S, Woolworth V, Fishman RA, Chan PH. Liposome-entrapped superoxide dismutase reduces cerebral infarction in cerebral ischemia in rats. Stroke 1990;21:1312–1317.
196. Matsumiya N, Koehler RC, Kirsch JR, Traystman RJ. Conjugated superoxide dismutase reduces extent of caudate injury after transient focal ischemia in cats. Stroke 1991;22:1193–1200.
197. He YY, Hsu CY, Ezrin AM, Miller MS. Polyethylene glycol-conjugated superoxide dismutase in focal cerebral ischemia-reperfusion. Am J Physiol 1993;265:H252–6.
198. Kinouchi H, Epstein CJ, Mizui T, Carlson E, Chen SF, Chan PH. Attenuation of focal cerebral ischemic injury in transgenic mice overexpressing CuZn superoxide dismutase. Proc Natl Acad Sci U S A 1991;88:11158–11162.
199. Yang G, Chan PH, Chen J, et al. Human copper-zinc superoxide dismutase transgenic mice are highly resistant to reperfusion injury after focal cerebral ischemia. Stroke 1994;25:165–170.
200. Armstead WM, Mirro R, Busija DW, Leffler CW. Postischemic generation of superoxide anion by newborn pig brain. Am J Physiol 1988;255:H401–H403.
201. Nelson CW, Wei EP, Povlishock JT, Kontos HA, Moskowitz MA. Oxygen radicals in cerebral ischemia. Am J Physiol 1992;263:H1356–H1362.
202. Zini I, Tomasi A, Grimaldi R, Vannini V, Agnati LF. Detection of free radicals during brain ischemia and reperfusion by spin trapping and microdialysis. Neurosci Lett 1992;138:279–282.
203. Phillis JW, Sen S. Oxypurinol attenuates hydroxyl radical production during ischemia/reperfusion injury of the rat cerebral cortex: an ESR study. Brain Res 1993;628:309–312.
204. Cao W, Carney JM, Duchon A, Floyd RA, Chevion M. Oxygen free radical involvement in ischemia and reperfusion injury to brain. Neurosci Lett 1988;88:233–238.
205. Hall ED, Andrus PK, Althaus JS, VonVoigtlander PF. Hydroxyl radical production and lipid peroxidation parallels selective post-ischemic vulnerability in gerbil brain. J Neurosci Res 1993;34:107–112.
206. Del Maestro R. An approach to free radicals in medicine and biology. Acta Physiol Scand [Suppl] 1980;492:153–169.
207. Halliwell B, Gutteridge JM. Oxygen toxicity, oxygen radicals, transition metals and disease. Biochem J 1984;219:1–14.
208. Schmidley JW. Free radicals in central nervous system ischemia. Stroke 1990;21:1086–1090.
209. Holmberg P. The physics and chemistry of free radicals. Med Biol 1984;62:68.

210. McCord JM, Fridovich I. The reduction of cytochrome c by milk xanthine oxidase. J Biol Chem 1968;243:5753–5760.
211. Van Wylen DG, Park TS, Rubio R, Berne RM. Increases in cerebral interstitial fluid adenosine concentration during hypoxia, local potassium infusion, and ischemia. J Cereb Blood Flow Metab 1986;6:522–528.
212. Nihei H, Kanemitsu H, Tamura A, Oka H, Sano K. Cerebral uric acid, xanthine, and hypoxanthine after ischemia: the effect of allopurinol. Neurosurgery 1989;25:613–617.
213. Al-Kyalidi UAS, Chaglassian TH. The species distribution of xanthine oxidase. Biochem J 1965;97:318–320.
214. Betz AL. Identification of hypoxanthine transport and xanthine oxidase activity in brain capillaries. J Neurochem 1985;44:574–579.
215. Kinuta Y, Kimura M, Itokawa Y, Ishikawa M, Kikuchi H. Changes in xanthine oxidase in ischemic rat brain. J Neurosurg 1989;71:417–420.
216. Kontos HA, Wei EP, Ellis EF, et al. Appearance of superoxide anion radical in cerebral extracellular space during increased prostaglandin synthesis in cats.. Circ Res 1985;57:142–151.
217. McCord JM, Fridovich I. Superoxide dismutase. An enzymic function for erythrocuprein (hemocuprein). J Biol Chem 1969;244:6049–6055.
218. Thomas CE, Morehouse LA, Aust SD. Ferritin and superoxide dependent lipid peroxidation. J Biol Chem 1985;260:3275–3280.
219. Pellegrini-Giampietro DE, Cherici G, Alesiani M, Carla V, Moroni F. Excitatory amino acid release from rat hippocampal slices as a consequence of free-radical formation. J Neurochem 1988;51:1960–1963.
220. Volterra A, Trotti D, Tromba C, Floridi S, Racagni G. Glutamate uptake inhibition by oxygen free radicals in rat cortical astrocytes. J Neurosci 1994;14:2924–2932.
221. Oliver CN, Starke Reed PE, Stadtman ER, Liu GJ, Carney JM, Floyd RA. Oxidative damage to brain proteins, loss of glutamine synthetase activity, and production of free radicals during ischemia/reperfusion-induced injury to gerbil brain. Proc Natl Acad Sci U S A 1990;87:5144–5147.
222. Brawn K, Fridovich I. DNA strand scission by enzymically generated oxygen radicals. Arch Biochem Biophys 1981;206:414–419.
223. Braughler JM, Duncan LA, Goodman T. Calcium enhances in vitro free radical-induced damage to brain synaptosomes, mitochondria, and cultured spinal cord neurons. J Neurochem 1985;45:1288–1293.
224. Farber JL. Biology of Disease. Membrane injury and calcium homeostasis in the pathogenesis of coagulative necrosis. Lab Invest 1982;47:114–123.
225. Sevanian A, Kim E. Phospholipase A2 dependent release of fatty acids from peroxidized membranes. J Free Radic Biol Med 1985;1:263–271.
226. O'Brian CA, Ward NE, Weinstein IB, Bull AW, Marnett LJ. Activation of rat brain protein kinase C by lipid oxidation products. Biochem Biophys Res Commun 1988;155:1374–1380.
227. Demopoulos HB, Flamm ES, Pietronigro DD, Seligman ML. The free radical pathology and the microcirculation in the major central nervous system disorders. Acta Physiol Scand 1980;492:91–119.
228. Moncada S. The 1991 Ulf von Euler Lecture. The L-arginine:nitric oxide pathway. Acta Physiol Scand 1992;145:201–227.
229. Iadecola C, Pelligrino DA, Moskowitz MA, Lassen NA. Nitric oxide synthase inhibition and cerebrovascular regulation. J Cereb Blood Flow Metab 1994;14:175–192.
230. Vincent SR. Nitric oxide: A radical neurotransmitter in the central nervous system. Prog Neurobiol 1993;42:129–160.
231. Bruhwyler J, Chleide E, Liegeois JF, Carreer F. Nitric oxide: A new messenger in the brain. Neurosci Biobehav Rev 1993;17:373–384.
232. Lowenstein CJ, Dinerman JL, Snyder SH. Nitric oxide: A physiologic messenger. Ann Intern Med 1994;120:227–237.
233. Faraci FM, Brian JE, Jr. Nitric oxide and the cerebral circulation. Stroke 1994;25:692–703.
234. Forstermann U, Gorsky LD, Pollock JS, Schmidt HHHW, Heller M, Murad F. Regional distribution of EDRF/NO-synthesizing enzyme(s) in rat brain. Biochem Biophys Res Commun 1990;168:727–732.
235. Lipton SA, Choi Y, Pan Z, et al. A redox-based mechanism for the neuroprotective and neurodestructive effects of nitric oxide and related nitroso-compounds. Nature 1993;364:626–632.
236. Malinski T, Bailey F, Zhang ZG, Chopp M. Nitric oxide measured by a porphyrinic microsensor in rat brain after transient middle cerebral artery occlusion. J Cereb Blood Flow Metab 1993;13:355–358.
237. Sato S, Tominaga T, Ohnishi T, Ohnishi ST. EPR spin-trapping study of nitric oxide formation during bilateral carotid occlusion in the rat. Biochim Biophys Acta 1993;1181:195–197.
238. Choi DW. Nitric oxide: foe or friend to the injured brain? Proc Natl Acad Sci U S A 1993;90:9741–9743.
239. Wieloch T, Bergstedt K, Hu BR. Protein phosphorylation and the regulation of mRNA translation following cerebral ischemia. Prog Brain Res 1993;96:179–191.
240. Huang KP, Huang FL. How is protein kinase C activated in CNS. Neurochem Int 1993;22:417–433.
241. Wieloch T, Cardell M, Bingren H, Zivin J, Saitoh T. Changes in the activity of protein kinase C and the differential subcellular redistribution of its isozymes in the rat striatum during and following transient forebrain ischemia. J Neurochem 1991;56:1227–1235.
242. Domanska-Janik K, Zalewska T. Effect of brain ischemia on protein kinase C. J Neurochem 1992;58:1432–1439.
243. Cardell M, Wieloch T. Time course of the translocation and inhibition of protein kinase C during complete cerebral ischemia in the rat. J Neurochem 1993;61:1308–1314.
244. Aronowski J, Grotta JC, Waxham MN. Ischemia-induced translocation of Ca^{2+}/calmodulin-dependent protein kinase II: Potential role in neuronal damage. J Neurochem 1992;58:1743–1753.
245. Nishizuka Y. The family of protein kinase C for signal transduction. JAMA 1995;262:1826–1833.
246. Hama T, Huang K, Guroff G. Protein kinase C as a component of nerve growth factor sensitive phosphorylation system in PC 12 cells. Proc Natl Acad Sci U S A 1986;83:2353–2357.
247. Yamamoto H, Fukunaga K, Lee K, Soderling TR. Ischemia-induced loss of brain calcium/calmodulin-dependent protein kinase II. J Neurochem 1992;58:1110–1117.
248. Morioka M, Fukunaga K, Yasugawa S, Nagahiro S, Ushio Y, Miyamoto E. Regional and temporal alterations in Ca2+/calmodulin-dependent protein kinase II and calcineurin in the hippocampus of rat brain after transient forebrain ischemia. J Neurochem 1992;58:1798–1809.
249. Churn SB, Taft WC, Billingsley MS, Sankaran B, DeLorenzo RJ. Global forebrain ischemia induces a posttranslational modification of multifunctional calcium- and calmodulin-dependent kinase II. J Neurochem 1992;59:1221–1232.
250. Hu BR, Wieloch T. Casein kinase II activity in the postischemic rat brain increases in brain regions resistant to ischemia and decreases in vulnerable areas. J Neurochem 1993;60:1722–1728.
251. Kleihues P, Hossmann KA. Protein synthesis in the cat brain after prolonged cerebral ischemia. Brain Res 1971;35:409–418.
252. Kleihues P, Hossmann KA. Regional incorporation of L-[^{3}H]tyrosine into cat brain proteins after one hour of complete ischemia. Acta Neuropathol (Berl) 1973;25:313–324.
253. Cooper HK, Zalewska T, Kawakami S, Hossmann KA. The effect of ischemia and recirculation on protein synthesis in the rat brain. J Neurochem 1977;28:929–934.
254. Nowak TS, Fried RL, Lust WD, Passonneau JV. Changes in brain energy metabolism and protein synthesis following transient bilateral ischemia in the gerbil. J Neurochem 1985;44:487–494.
255. Bodsch W, Barbier A, Oehmichen M, Grosse Ophoff B, Hossmann KA. Recovery of monkey brain after prolonged ischemia. II. Protein synthesis and morphological alterations. J Cereb Blood Flow Metab 1986; 6:22–33.
256. Dienel GA, Pulsinelli WA, Duffy TE. Regional protein synthesis in rat brain following acute hemispheric ischemia. J Neurochem 1980; 35:1216–1226.
257. Thilmann R, Xie Y, Kleihues P, Kiessling M. Persistent inhibition of protein synthesis precedes delayed neuronal death in postischemic gerbil hippocampus. Acta Neuropathol (Berl) 1986;71:88–93.
258. Araki T, Kato H, Inoue T, Kogure K. Regional impairment of protein synthesis following brief cerebral ischemia in the gerbil. Acta Neuropathol (Berl) 1990;79:501–505.
259. Widmann R, Kuroiwa T, Bonnekoh P, Hossmann KA. [14C]leucine incorporation into brain proteins in gerbils after transient ischemia: relationship to selective vulnerability of hippocampus. J Neurochem 1991;56:789–796.
260. Hossmann KA. Disturbances of cerebral protein synthesis and ischemic cell death. Prog Brain Res 1993;96:161–177.
261. Krause GS, Tiffany BR. Suppression of protein synthesis in the reperfused brain. Stroke 1993;24:747–755.
262. White BC, Tribhuwan RC, Vander Laan DJ, DeGracia DJ, Krause GS, Grossman LI. Brain mitochondrial DNA is not damaged by prolonged cardiac arrest or reperfusion. J Neurochem 1992;58:1716–1722.
263. Matsumoto K, Yamada K, Hayakawa T, Sakaguchi T, Mogami H. RNA synthesis and processing in the gerbil brain after transient hindbrain ischaemia. Neurol Res 1990;12:45–48.
264. Maruno M, Yanagihara T. Progressive loss of messenger RNA and delayed neuronal death following transient cerebral ischemia in gerbils. Neuroscience Letters 1990;115:155–160.

265. Sharp FR, Kinouchi H, Koistinaho J, Chan PH, Sagar SM. HSP70 heat shock gene regulation during ischemia. Stroke 1993;24:I72–5.
266. Kogure K, Kato H. Altered gene expression in cerebral ischemia. Stroke 1993;24:2121–2127.
267. Abe K, Kogure K. Selective gene expression after brain ischemia. Prog Brain Res 1993;96:221–236.
268. Nowak TS, Jr., Osborne OC, Suga S. Stress protein and proto-oncogene expression as indicators of neuronal pathophysiology after ischemia. Prog Brain Res 1993;96:195–208.
269. Onodera H, Kogure K, Ono Y, Igarashi K, Kiyota Y, Nagaoka A. Proto-oncogene c-fos is transiently induced in the rat cerebral cortex after forebrain ischemia. Neurosci Lett 1989;98:101–104.
270. Wessel TC, Joh TH, Volpe BT. In situ hybridization analysis of c-fos and c-jun expression in the rat brain following transient forebrain ischemia. Brain Res 1991;567:231–240.
271. Abe K, Tanzi RE, Kogure K. Induction of HSP70 mRNA after transient ischemia in gerbil brain. Neurosci Lett 1991;125:166–168.
272. Vass K, Welch WJ, Nowak TS. Localization of 70-kDa stress protein induction in gerbil brain after ischemia. Acta Neuropathol (Berl) 1988;77:128–135.
273. Gonzalez MF, Lowenstein D, Fernyak S, Hisanaga K, Simon R, Sharp FR. Induction of heat shock protein 72-like immunoreactivity in the hippocampal formation following transient global ischemia. Brain Res Bull 1991;26:241–250.
274. Takami K, Iwane M, Kiyota Y, Miyamoto M, Tsukuda R, Shiosaka S. Increase of basic fibroblast growth factor immunoreactivity and its mRNA level in rat brain following transient forebrain ischemia. Exp Brain Res 1992;90:1–10.
275. Shozuhara H, Onodera H, Katoh Semba R, Kato K, Yamasaki Y, Kogure K. Temporal profiles of nerve growth factor beta-subunit level in rat brain regions after transient ischemia. J Neurochem 1992;59:175–180.
276. Wen, TC, Matsuda S, Yoshimura H, Aburaya J, et al. Protective effect of basic fibroblast growth factor-heparin and neurotoxic effect of platelet factor 4 on ischemic neuronal loss and learning disability in gerbils. Neuroscience 1995; 65:513–521.
277. Shigeno T, Mima T, Takakura K, et al. Amelioration of delayed neuronal death in the hippocampus by nerve growth factor. J Neurosci 1991;11:2914–2919.
278. Kochanek PM, Hallenbeck JM. Polymorphonuclear leukocytes and monocytes/macrophages in the pathogenesis of cerebral ischemia and stroke. Stroke 1992;23:1367–1379.
279. Anderson ML, Smith DS, Nioka S, et al. Experimental brain ischaemia: assessment of injury by magnetic resonance spectroscopy and histology. Neurol Res 1990;12:195–204.
280. Dietrich WD, Halley M, Valdes I, Busto R. Interrelationships between increased vascular permeability and acute neuronal damage following temperature-controlled brain ischemia in rats. Acta Neuropathol Berl 1991;81:615–625.
281. Grogaard B, Schurer L, Gerdin B, Arfors KE. Delayed hypoperfusion after incomplete forebrain ischemia in the rat: The role of polymorphonuclear leukocytes. J Cereb Blood Flow Metab 1989;9:500–505.
282. Aspey BS, Jessimer C, Pereira S, Harrison MJ. Do leukocytes have a role in the cerebral no-reflow phenomenon. J Neurol Neurosurg Psychiatry 1989;52:526–528.
283. Schott RJ, Natale JE, Ressler SW, Burney RE, D'Alecy LG. Neutrophil depletion fails to improve neurologic outcome after cardiac arrest in dogs. Ann Emerg Med 1989;18:517–522.
284. Morioka T, Kalehua AN, Streit WJ. The microglial reaction in the rat dorsal hippocampus following transient forebrain ischemia. J Cereb Blood Flow Metab 1991;11:966–973.
285. Lees GJ. The possible contribution of microglia and macrophages to delayed neuronal death after ischemia. J Neurol Sci 1993;114:119–122.
286. Rothwell NJ, Relton JK. Involvement of interleukin-1 and lipocortin-1 in ischaemic brain damage. Cerebrovasc Brain Metab Rev 1993;5:178–198.
287. Minami M, Kuraishi Y, Yabuuchi K, Yamazaki A, Satoh M. Induction of interleukin-1 beta mRNA in rat brain after transient forebrain ischemia. J Neurochem 1992;58:390–392.
288. Relton JK, Rothwell NJ. Interleukin-1 receptor antagonist inhibits ischemic and excitotoxic neuronal damage in the rat. Brain Res Bull 1992;29:243–246.
289. Garcia JH. Morphology of global cerebral ischemia. Crit Care Med 1988;16:979–987.
290. Kabat H. The greater tolerance of very young animals to arrest of the brain circulation. Am J Physiol 1940;130:588–599.
291. Brockman SK, Jude JR. The tolerance of the dog brain to total arrest of circulation. Bull Johns Hopkins Hosp 1960;106:74–80.
292. Goldstein A, Jr., Wells BA, Keats AS. Increased tolerance to cerebral anoxia by pentobarbital. Arch Int Pharmacodyn Ther 1966;161:138–143.
293. Nemoto EM, Bleyaert AL, Stezoski SW, Moossy J, Rao GR, Safar P. Global brain ischemia: A reproducible monkey model. Stroke 1977;8:558–564.
294. Bleyaert AL, Nemoto EM, Safar P, et al. Thiopental amelioration of brain damage after global ischemia in monkeys. Anesthesiology 1978;49:390–398.
295. Steen PA, Milde JH, Michenfelder JD. No barbiturate protection in a dog model of complete cerebral ischemia. Ann Neurol 1979;5:343–349.
296. Todd MM, Chadwick HS, Shapiro HM, Dunlop BJ, Marshall LF, Dueck R. The neurologic effects of thiopental therapy following experimental cardiac arrest in cats. Anesthesiology 1982;57:76–86.
297. Gisvold SE, Safar P, Hendrickx HH, Rao G, Moossy J, Alexander H. Thiopental treatment after global brain ischemia in pigtailed monkeys. Anesthesiology 1984;60:88–96.
298. Breivik H, Safar P, Sands P, et al. Clinical feasibility trials of barbiturate therapy after cardiac arrest. Crit Care Med 1978;6:228–244.
299. Brain Resuscitation Clinical Trial I Study Group. Randomized clinical study of thiopental loading in comatose survivors of cardiac arrest. N Engl J Med 1986;314:397–403.
300. Dunbar J, Johansen J. Structural and functional properties of Cu, Zn superoxide dismutases. Bull Eur Physiopathol Respir 1981;17:51
301. Pain R. Dressing the SOD. Nature 1983;306:228
302. Tainer J, Getzoff ED, Richardson JS, Richardson DC. Structure and mechanism of copper, zinc superoxide dismutase. Nature 1983; 306:284–287.
303. Marklund SL. Extracellular superoxide dismutase in human tissues and human cell lines. J Clin Invest 1984;74:1398–1403.
304. Marklund S, Holme E, Hellner L. Superoxide dismutase in extracellular fluids. Clin Chim Acta 1982;126:41–51.
305. Turrens JF, Crapo JD, Freeman BA. Protection against oxygen toxicity by intravenous injection of liposome-entrapped catalase and superoxide dismutase. J Clin Invest 1984;73:87–95.
306. Freeman BA, Young SL, Crapo JD. Liposome-mediated augmentation of superoxide dismutase in endothelial cells prevents oxygen injury. J Biol Chem 1983;258:12534–12542.
307. Beckman JS, Minor RL, White CW, Repine JE, Rosen GM, Freeman BA. Superoxide dismutase and catalase conjugated to polyethylene glycol increases endothelial enzyme activity and oxidant resistance. J Biol Chem 1988;263:6884–6892.
308. Petkau A, Chelack WS, Kelly K, Barefoot C, Monasterski L. Tissue distribution of bovine 125I-superoxide dismutase in mice. Res Comm Chem Pathol Pharmacol 1976;15:641–654.
309. Cerchiari EL, Hoel TM, Safar P, Sclabassi RJ. Protective effects of combined superoxide dismutase and deferoxamine on recovery of cerebral blood flow and function after cardiac arrest. Stroke 1987;18:869–878.
310. Forsman M, Fleischer JE, Milde JH, Steen PA, Michenfelder JD. Superoxide dismutase and catalase failed to improve neurologic outcome after complete cerebral ischemia in the dog. Acta Anaesthesiol Scand 1988;32:152–155.
311. Schurer L, Grogaard B, Gerdin B, Arfors KE. Superoxide dismutase does not prevent delayed hypoperfusion after incomplete cerebral ischemia in the rat. Acta Neurochir (Wien) 1990;103:163–170.
312. Uyama O, Matsuyama T, Michishita H, Nakamura H, Sugita M. Protective effects of human recombinant superoxide dismutase on transient ischemic injury of CA1 neurons in gerbils. Stroke 1992;23:75–81.
313. Tagaya M, Matsumoto M, Kitagawa K, et al. Recombinant human superoxide dismutase can attenuate ischemic neuronal damage in gerbils. Life Sci 1992;51:253–259.
314. Yusa T, Crapo JD, Freeman BA. Liposome mediated augmentation of brain SOD and catalase inhibits CNS O2 toxicity. J Appl Physiol 1984;1674–1681.
315. White CW, Jackson JH, Abuchowski A, et al. Polyethylene glycol-attached antioxidant enzymes decrease pulmonary oxygen toxicity in rats. J Appl Physiol 1989;66:584–590.
316. Haun SE, Kirsch JR, Helfaer MA, Kubos KL, Traystman RJ. Polyethylene glycol-conjugated superoxide dismutase fails to augment brain superoxide dismutase activity in piglets. Stroke 1991;22:655–659.
317. Rosenberg AA, Murdaugh E, White CW. The role of oxygen free radicals in postasphyxia cerebral hypoperfusion in newborn lambs. Pediatr Res 1989;26:215–219.
318. Kirsch JR, Helfaer MA, Haun SE, Koehler RC, Traystman RJ. Polyethylene glycol-conjugated superoxide dismutase improves recovery of postischemic hypercapnic cerebral blood flow in piglets. Pediatr Res 1993;34:530–537.

319. Takeda Y, Hashimoto H, Kosaka F, Hirakawa M, Inoue M. Albumin-binding superoxide dismutase with a prolonged half-life reduces reperfusion brain injury. Am J Physiol 1993;264:H1708–15.
320. Braughler JM, Pregenzer JF, Chase RL, Duncan LA, Jacobsen EJ, McCall JM. Novel 21-aminosteroids as potent inhibitors of iron-dependent lipid peroxidation. J Biol Chem 1987;262:10438–10440.
321. Hall ED. Cerebral ischaemia, free radicals and antioxidant protection. Biochem Soc Trans 1993;21:334–339.
322. Hall ED, Yonkers PA. Attenuation of postischemic cerebral hypoperfusion by the 21-aminosteroid U74006F. Stroke 1988;19:340–344.
323. Helfaer MA, Kirsch JR, Hurn PD, Blizzard KK, Koehler RC, Traystman RJ. Tirilazad mesylate does not improve early cerebral metabolic recovery following compression ischemia in dogs. Stroke 1992;23:1479–1485.
324. Beck T, Bielenberg GW. Failure of the lipid peroxidation inhibitor U74006F to improve neurological outcome after transient forebrain ischemia in the rat. Brain Res 1990;532:336–338.
325. Buchan AM, Bruederlin B, Heinicke E, Li H. Failure of the lipid peroxidation inhibitor, U74006F, to prevent postischemic selective neuronal injury. J Cereb Blood Flow Metab 1992;12:250–256.
326. Lesiuk H, Sutherland G, Peeling J, Butler K, Saunders J. Effect of U74006F on forebrain ischemia in rats. Stroke 1991;22:896–901.
327. Sutherland G, Haas N, Peeling J. Ischemic neocortical protection with U74006F—a dose-response curve. Neurosci Lett 1993;149:123–125.
328. Hall ED, Pazara KE, Braughler JM, Linseman KL, Jacobsen EJ. Nonsteroidal lazaroid U78517F in models of focal and global ischemia. Stroke 1990;21:III83–7.
329. White BC, Gadzinski DS, Hoehner PJ, et al. Effect of flunarizine on canine cerebralcortical blood flow and vascular resistance post cardiac arrest. Ann Emerg Med 1982;11:119–126.
330. Deshpande JK, Wieloch T. Flunarizine, a calcium entry blocker, ameliorates ischemic brain damage in the rat. Anesthesiology 1986;64:215–224.
331. Abiko H, Mizoi K, Suzuki J, Oba M, Yoshimoto T. Cerebral protective effect of flunarizine in a canine model of cerebral ischaemia. Neurol Res 1988;10:145–150.
332. Newberg LA, Steen PA, Milde JH, Michenfelder JD. Failure of flunarizine to improve cerebral blood flow or neurologic recovery in a canine model of complete cerebral ischemia. Stroke 1984;15:666–671.
333. Winegar CP, Henderson O, White BC, et al. Early amelioration of neurologic deficit by lidoflazine after fifteen minutes of cardiopulmonary arrest in dogs. Ann Emerg Med 1983;12:471–477.
334. Vaagenes P, Cantadore R, Safar P, et al. Amelioration of brain damage by lidoflazine after prolonged ventricular fibrillation cardiac arrest in dogs. Crit Care Med 1984;12:846–855.
335. Dean JM, Hoehner PJ, Rogers MC, Traystman RJ. Effect of lidoflazine on cerebral blood flow following twelve minutes total cerebral ischemia. Stroke 1984;15:531–535.
336. Kumar K, White BC, Krause GS, et al. A quantitative morphological assessment of the effect of lidoflazine and deferoxamine therapy on global brain ischaemia. Neurol Res 1988;10:136–140.
337. Fleischer JE, Lanier WL, Milde JH, Michenfelder JD. Effect of lidoflazine on cerebral blood flow and neurologic outcome when administered after complete cerebral ischemia in dogs. Anesthesiology 1987;66:304–311.
338. Fleischer JE, Lanier WL, Milde JH, Michenfelder JD. Lidoflazine does not improve neurologic outcome when administered after complete cerebral ischemia in primates. J Cereb Blood Flow Metab 1987;7:366–371.
339. Brain Resuscitation Clinical Trial II Study Group. A randomized clinical study of a calcium-entry blocker (lidoflazine) in the treatment of comatose survivors of cardiac arrest. N Engl J Med 1991;324:1225–1231.
340. Steen PA, Newberg LA, Milde JH, Michenfelder JD. Nimodipine improves cerebral blood flow and neurologic recovery after complete cerebral ischemia in the dog. J Cereb Blood Flow Metab 1983;3:38–43.
341. Steen PA, Newberg LA, Milde JH, Michenfelder JD. Cerebral blood flow and neurologic outcome when nimodipine is given after complete cerebral ischemia in the dog. J Cereb Blood Flow Metab 1984;4:82–87.
342. Milde LN, Milde JH, Michenfelder JD. Delayed treatment with nimodipine improves cerebral blood flow after complete cerebral ischemia in the dog. J Cereb Blood Flow Metab 1986;6:332–337.
343. Roine RO, Kaste M, Kinnunen A, Nikki P, Sarna S, Kajaste S. Nimodipine after resuscitation from out-of-hospital ventricular fibrillation. A placebo-controlled, double-blind, randomized trial. JAMA 1990;264:3171–3177.
344. Buchan AM, Gertler SZ, Li H, et al. A selective N-type Ca(2+)-channel blocker prevents CA1 injury 24 h following severe forebrain ischemia and reduces infarction following focal ischemia. J Cereb Blood Flow Metab 1994;14:903–910.
345. Albers GW. Potential therapeutic uses of N-methyl-D-aspartate antagonists in cerebral ischemia. Clin Neuropharmacol 1990;13:177–197.
346. Buchan AM. Do NMDA antagonists protect against cerebral ischemia: Are clinical trials warranted? Cerebrovasc Brain Metab Rev 1990;2:1–26.
347. McCulloch J. Excitatory amino acid antagonists and their potential for the treatment of ischaemic brain damage in man. Br J Clin Pharmacol 1992;34:106–114.
348. Church J, Zeman S, Lodge D. The neuroprotective action of ketamine and MK-801 after transient cerebral ischemia in rats. Anesthesiology 1988;69:702–709.
349. Gill R, Foster AC, Woodruff GN. Systemic administration of MK-801 protects against ischemia-induced hippocampal neurodegeneration in the gerbil. J Neurosci 1987;7:3343–3349.
350. Gill R, Foster AC, Woodruff GN. MK-801 is neuroprotective in gerbils when administered during the post-ischaemic period. Neuroscience 1988;25:847–855.
351. Fleischer JE, Tateishi A, Drummond JC, et al. MK-801, an excitatory amino acid antagonist, does not improve neurologic outcome following cardiac arrest in cats. J Cereb Blood Flow Metab 1989;9:795–804.
352. Michenfelder JD, Lanier WL, Scheithauer BW, Perkins WJ, Shearman GT, Milde JH. Evaluation of the glutamate antagonist dizocilipine maleate (MK-801) on neurologic outcome in a canine model of complete cerebral ischemia: correlation with hippocampal histopathology. Brain Res 1989;481:228–234.
353. Lanier WL, Perkins WJ, Karlsson BR, et al. The effects of dizocilpine maleate (MK-801), an antagonist of the N-methyl-D-aspartate receptor, on neurologic recovery and histopathology following complete cerebral ischemia in primates. J Cereb Blood Flow Metab 1990;10:252–261.
354. Buchan AM, Li H, Pulsinelli WA. The N-methyl-D-aspartate antagonist, MK-801, fails to protect against neuronal damage caused by transient, severe forebrain ischemia in adult rats. J Neurosci 1991;11:1049–1056.
355. Nellgard B, Gustafson I, Wieloch T. Lack of protection by the N-methyl-D-aspartate receptor blocker dizocilpine (MK-801) after transient severe cerebral ischemia in the rat. Anesthesiology 1991;75:279–287.
356. Buchan AM, Pulsinelli WA. Hypothermia but not the N-methyl-D-aspartate antagonist, MK-801, attenuates neuronal damage in gerbils subjected to transient global ischemia. J Neurosci 1990;10:311–316.
357. Ginsberg MD, Sternau LL, Globus MY, Dietrich WD, Busto R. Therapeutic modulation of brain temperature: relevance to ischemic brain injury. Cerebrovasc Brain Metab Rev 1992;4:189–225.
358. Maher J, Hachinski V. Hypothermia as a potential treatment for cerebral ischemia. Cerebrovasc Brain Metab Rev 1993;5:277–300.
359. Koek W, Woods JH, Winger GD. MK-801, a proposed noncompetitive antagonist of excitatory amino acid neurotransmission, produces phencyclidine-like behavioral effects in pigeons, rats, and rhesus monkeys. J Pharmacol Exp Ther 1988;245:969–974.
360. Olney JW, Labruyere J, Price MT. Pathological changes induced in cerebrocortical neurons by phencyclidine and related drugs. Science 1995;244:1360–1362.
361. Sharp FR, Jasper P, Hall J, Noble L, Sagar SM. MK-801 and ketamine induce heat shock protein HSP72 in injured neurons in posterior cingulate and retrosplenial cortex. Ann Neurol 1991;30:801–809.
362. Diemer NH, Valente E, Bruhn T, Berg M, Jorgensen MB, Johansen FF. Glutamate receptor transmission and ischemic nerve cell damage: evidence for involvement of excitotoxic mechanisms. Prog Brain Res 1993;96:105–123.
363. Sheardown MJ, Nielsen EO, Hansen AJ, Jacobsen P, Honore T. 2,3-Dihydroxy-6-nitro-7-sulfamoyl-benzo(F)quinoxaline: a neuroprotectant for cerebral ischemia. Science 1990;247:571–574.
364. Diemer NH, Jorgensen MB, Johansen FF, Sheardown M, Honore T. Protection against ischemic hippocampal CA1 damage in the rat with a new non-NMDA antagonist, NBQX. Acta Neurol Scand 1992;86:45–49.
365. Le Peillet E, Arvin B, Moncada C, Meldrum BS. The non-NMDA antagonists, NBQX and GYKI 52466, protect against cortical and striatal cell loss following transient global ischaemia in the rat. Brain Res 1992;571:115–120.
366. Nellgard B, Wieloch T. Postischemic blockade of AMPA but not NMDA receptors mitigates neuronal damage in the rat brain following transient severe cerebral ischemia. J Cereb Blood Flow Metab 1992;12:2–11.
367. Li H, Buchan AM. Treatment with an AMPA antagonist 12 hours fol-

lowing severe normothermic forebrain ischemia prevents CA1 neuronal injury. J Cereb Blood Flow Metab 1993;13:933–939.
368. Sheardown MJ, Suzdak PD, Nordholm L. AMPA, but not NMDA receptor antagonism is neuroprotective in gerbil global ischemia, even when delayed 24 h. Eur J Pharmacol 1993;236:347–353.
369. Judge ME, Sheardown MJ, Jacobsen P, Honore T. Protection against post-ischemic behavioral pathology by the alpha-amino-3-hydroxy-5-methyl-4-isoxazolepropionic acid (AMPA) antagonist 2,3-dihydroxy-6-nitro-7-sulfamoyl-benzo(f)quinoxaline (NBQX) in the gerbil. Neurosci Lett 1991;133:291–294.
370. Redmond JM, Zehr KJ, Blue ME, et al. AMPA glutamate receptor antagonism reduces neurologic injury after hypothermic circulatory arrest. Ann Thorac Surg 1995;59:579–584.
371. Prado R, Watson BD, Wester P. Effects of nitric oxide synthase inhibition on cerebral blood flow following bilateral carotid artery occlusion and recirculation in the rat. J Cereb Blood Flow Metab 1993;13:720–723.
372. Clavier N, Kirsch JR, Hurn PD, Traystman RJ. Cerebral blood flow is reduced by N omega-nitro-L-arginine methyl ester during delayed hypoperfusion in cats. Am J Physiol 1994;267:H174–81.
373. Weissman BA, Kadar T, Brandeis R, Shapira S. NG-nitro-L-arginine enhances neuronal death following transient forebrain ischemia in gerbils. Neurosci Lett 1992;146:139–142.
374. Shapira S, Kadar T, Weissman BA. Dose-dependent effect of nitric oxide synthase inhibition following transient forebrain ischemia in gerbils. Brain Res 1994;668:80–84.
375. Caldwell M, O'Neill M, Earley B, Leonard B. NG-Nitro-L-arginine protects against ischemia-induced increases in nitric oxide and hippocampal neuro-degeneration in the gerbil. Eur J Pharmacol 1994;260:191–200.
376. Buchan AM, Gertler SZ, Huang ZG, Li H, Chaundy KE, Xue D. Failure to prevent selective CA1 neuronal death and reduce cortical infarction following cerebral ischemia with inhibition of nitric oxide synthase. Neuroscience 1994;61:1–11.
377. Botterell EH, Lougheed WM, Scott JW, Vandewater SL. Hypothermia and interruption of carotid or carotid and vertebral circulation, in the management of intracranial aneurysms. J Neurosurg 1956;13:1–42.
378. Lewis FJ, Taufic M. Closure of atrial septal defects with aid of hypothermia: experimental accomplishments and the report of one successful case. Surgery 1953;33:52–59.
379. Mitani A, Kataoka K. Critical levels of extracellular glutamate mediating gerbil hippocampal delayed neuronal death during hypothermia: brain microdialysis study. Neuroscience 1991;42:661–670.
380. Simpson RE, Walter GA, Phillis JW. The effects of hypothermia on amino acid neurotransmitter release from the cerebral cortex. Neurosci Lett 1991;124:83–86.
381. Baker AJ, Zornow MH, Grafe MR, et al. Hypothermia prevents ischemia-induced increases in hippocampal glycine concentrations in rabbits. Stroke 1991;22:666–673.
382. Busto R, Globus MY, Dietrich WD, Martinez E, Valdes I, Ginsberg MD. Effect of mild hypothermia on ischemia-induced release of neurotransmitters and free fatty acids in rat brain. Stroke 1989;20:904–910.
383. Duhaime AC, Ross DT. Degeneration of hippocampal CA1 neurons following transient ischemia due to raised intracranial pressure: evidence for a temperature-dependent excitotoxic process. Brain Res 1990;512:169–174.
384. Welsh FA, Sims RE, Harris VA. Mild hypothermia prevents ischemic injury in gerbil hippocampus. J Cereb Blood Flow Metab 1990;10:557–563.
385. Stocker F, Herschkowitz N, Bossi E, et al. Cerebral metabolic studies in situ by 31P-nuclear magnetic resonance after hypothermic circulatory arrest. Pediatr Res 1986;20:867–871.
386. Michenfelder JD, Theye RA. The effects of anesthesia and hypothermia on canine cerebral ATP and lactate during anoxia produced by decapitation. Anesthesiology 1970;33:430–439.
387. Sutton LN, Clark BJ, Norwood CR, Woodford EJ, Welsh FA. Global cerebral ischemia in piglets under conditions of mild and deep hypothermia. Stroke 1991;22:1567–1573.
388. Norwood WI, Norwood CR. Influence of hypothermia on intracellular pH during anoxia. Am J Physiol 1982;243:C62–C65.
389. Chopp M, Knight R, Tidwell CD, Helpern JA, Brown E, Welch KM. The metabolic effects of mild hypothermia on global cerebral ischemia and recirculation in the cat: comparison to normothermia and hyperthermia. J Cereb Blood Flow Metab 1989;9:141–148.
390. Chen H, Chopp M, Vande Linde AM, Dereski MO, Garcia JH, Welch KM. The effects of post-ischemic hypothermia on the neuronal injury and brain metabolism after forebrain ischemia in the rat. J Neurol Sci 1992;107:191–198.
391. Cardell M, Boris-Moller F, Wieloch T. Hypothermia prevents the ischemia-induced translocation and inhibition of protein kinase C in the rat striatum. J Neurochem 1991;57:1814–1817.
392. Churn SB, Taft WC, Billingsley MS, Blair RE, DeLorenzo RJ. Temperature modulation of ischemic neuronal death and inhibition of calcium/calmodulin-dependent protein kinase II in gerbils. Stroke 1990;21:1715–1721.
393. Busto R, Dietrich WD, Globus MY, Valdes I, Scheinberg P, Ginsberg MD. Small differences in intraischemic brain temperature critically determine the extent of ischemic neuronal injury. J Cereb Blood Flow Metab 1987;7:729–738.
394. Xue D, Huang ZG, Smith KE, Buchan AM. Immediate or delayed mild hypothermia prevents focal cerebral infarction. Brain Res 1992;587:66–72.
395. Chen H, Chopp M, Zhang ZG, Garcia JH. The effect of hypothermia on transient middle cerebral artery occlusion in the rat. J Cereb Blood Flow Metab 1992;12:621–628.
396. Baker CJ, Onesti ST, Solomon RA. Reduction by delayed hypothermia of cerebral infarction following middle cerebral artery occlusion in the rat: a time-course study. J Neurosurg 1992;77:438–444.
397. Baker CJ, Onesti ST, Barth KN, Prestigiacomo CJ, Solomon RA. Hypothermic protection following middle cerebral artery occlusion in the rat. Surg Neurol 1991;36:175–180.
398. Onesti ST, Baker CJ, Sun PP, Solomon RA. Transient hypothermia reduces focal ischemic brain injury in the rat. Neurosurgery 1991;29:369–373.
399. Kader A, Brisman MH, Maraire N, Huh JT, Solomon RA. The effect of mild hypothermia on permanent focal ischemia in the rat. Neurosurgery 1992;31:1056–1060.
400. Ridenour TR, Warner DS, Todd MM, McAllister AC. Mild hypothermia reduces infarct size resulting from temporary but not permanent focal ischemia in rats. Stroke 1992;23:733–738.
401. Morikawa E, Ginsberg MD, Dietrich WD, et al. The significance of brain temperature in focal cerebral ischemia: histopathological consequences of middle cerebral artery occlusion in the rat. J Cereb Blood Flow Metab 1992;12:380–389.
402. Sano T, Drummond JC, Patel PM, Grafe MR, Watson JC, Cole DJ. A comparison of the cerebral protective effects of isoflurane and mild hypothermia in a model of incomplete forebrain ischemia in the rat. Anesthesiology 1992;76:221–228.
403. Lundgren J, Smith ML, Siesjo BK. Influence of moderate hypothermia on ischemic brain damage incurred under hyperglycemic conditions. Exp Brain Res 1991;84:91–101.
404. Minamisawa H, Nordstrom CH, Smith ML, Siesjo BK. The influence of mild body and brain hypothermia on ischemic brain damage. J Cereb Blood Flow Metab 1990;10:365–374.
405. Green EJ, Dietrich WD, van Dijk F, et al. Protective effects of brain hypothermia on behavior and histopathology following global cerebral ischemia in rats. Brain Res 1992;580:197–204.
406. Kuluz JW, Gregory GA, Yu AC, Chang Y. Selective brain cooling during and after prolonged global ischemia reduces cortical damage in rats. Stroke 1992;23:1792–1796.
407. Natale JA, D'Alecy LG. Protection from cerebral ischemia by brain cooling without reduced lactate accumulation in dogs. Stroke 1989;20:770–777.
408. Leonov Y, Sterz F, Safar P, et al. Mild cerebral hypothermia during and after cardiac arrest improves neurological outcome in dogs. J Cereb Blood Flow Metab 1990;10:57–70.
409. Busto R, Dietrich WD, Globus MY, Ginsberg MD. Postischemic moderate hypothermia inhibits CA1 hippocampal ischemic neuronal injury. Neurosci Lett 1989;101:299–304.
410. Coimbra C, Wieloch T. Hypothermia ameliorates neuronal survival when induced 2 hours after ischaemia in the rat. Acta Physiol Scand 1992;146:543–544.
411. Chopp M, Chen H, Dereski MO, Garcia JH. Mild hypothermic intervention after graded ischemic stress in rats. Stroke 1991;22:37–43.
412. Carroll M, Beek O. Protection against hippocampal CA1 cell loss by post-ischemic hypothermia is dependent on delay of initiation and duration. Metab Brain Dis 1992;7:45–50.
413. Horn M, Schlote W, Henrich HA. Global cerebral ischemia and subsequent selective hypothermia. A neuropathological and morphometrical study on ischemic neuronal damage in cat. Acta Neuropathol (Berl) 1991;81:443–449.
414. Sterz F, Safar P, Tisherman S, Radovsky A, Kuboyama K, Oku K. Mild

hypothermic cardiopulmonary resuscitation improves outcome after prolonged cardiac arrest in dogs. Crit Care Med 1995;19:379–389.
415. Weinrauch V, Safar P, Tisherman S, Kuboyama K, Radovsky A. Beneficial effect of mild hypothermia and detrimental effect of deep hypothermia after cardiac arrest in dogs. Stroke 1992;23:1454–1462.
416. Ginsberg MD, Globus MY, Dietrich WD, Busto R. Temperature modulation of ischemic brain injury—a synthesis of recent advances. Prog Brain Res 1993;96:13–22.
417. Kuroiwa T, Bonnekoh P, Hossmann KA. Prevention of postischemic hyperthermia prevents ischemic injury of CA1 neurons in gerbils. J Cereb Blood Flow Metab 1990;10:550–556.
418. Muizelaar JP, Marmarou A, Ward JD, et al. Adverse effects of prolonged hyperventilation in patients with severe head injury: a randomized clinical trial. J Neurosurg 1991;75:731–739.
419. Helfaer MA, Kirsch JR, Haun SE, Koehler RC, Traystman RJ. Age-related cerebrovascular reactivity to CO2 after cerebral ischemia in swine. Am J Physiol 1991;260:H1482–H1488.
420. Hall ED. The neuroprotective pharmacology of methylprednisolone: A review. J Neurosurg 1992;76:13–22.
421. Sapolsky RM, Pulsinelli WA. Glucocorticoids potentiate ischemic injury to neurons: therapeutic implications. Science 1985;229: 1397–1400.
422. Jastremski M, Sutton Tyrrell K, Vaagenes P, Abramson N, Heiselman D, Safar P. Glucocorticoid treatment does not improve neurological recovery following cardiac arrest. Brain Resuscitation Clinical Trial I Study Group. JAMA 1989;262:3427–3430.
423. Grafton ST, Longstreth WT. Steroids after cardiac arrest: a retrospective study with concurrent nonrandomized controls. Neurology 1988;38:1315–1316.

Evaluation of the Comatose Child

21

Gitte Y. Larsen
Donald D. Vernon
J. Michael Dean

INTRODUCTION

Perhaps one of the most striking aspects of central nervous system (CNS) disorders is the enormous variety of causes that result in impairment of neurologic function. "Consciousness" is a state of awareness of self and environment. The comatose state necessitates absence of function in both cerebral hemispheres and/or the dysfunction of the reticular activating system within the brainstem[1,2]. The comatose condition represents a medical emergency and may herald imminent death. The critical care approach to the comatose child involves a different exam from the traditional neurologic evaluation because of the limited cooperation from the patient and the limited history typically available during the initial evaluation[6]. Results of a specific coma exam facilitates location of the lesion and direction of therapy, diagnosis, and possibly prognosis. Thus, in this chapter, discussion of the subject is divided into three sections: (a) the emergent management and stabilization of the comatose child, (b) the physical examination of such children, and (c) the differential diagnosis of coma using a pragmatic, therapeutically oriented approach.

Address correspondence to:
Gitte Y. Larsen
Pediatric Critical Care Fellow
Division of Pediatric Critical Care
University of Utah Department of Pediatrics
Primary Children's Medical Center
100 North Medical Drive
Salt Lake City, UT 84113

STABILIZATION AND EMERGENCY MANAGEMENT

It is extremely important to manage comatose patients as if they were in imminent danger of death. An emergent, compulsive approach to such patients will prevent further contribution to the primary neurologic injury.

Although the most striking aspect of a comatose patient may be the comatose state itself, the clinician must adhere to the emergent principles of airway, breathing, and circulation. The initial approach should first focus on vital signs and the provision of supplemental oxygen. Attention should be paid to stabilizing the airway, breathing and circulation. The degree of neurologic injury, regardless of the etiology, can then be addressed to facilitate planning of further evaluations, such as a computed tomography (CT) scan or neurosurgical intervention. Finally, there must be vigilance for further neurologic deterioration and a preparedness to deal with possible cerebral edema and[2,4,7,8].

Airway

As with any medical emergency, the first priority is assurance of a patent airway. In assessing and maintaining the airway, it is crucial to remember that cervical spine injuries may be present in cases of traumatic injury and, therefore, manipulation of the neck should be kept to a minimum. To clear the airway, the jaw should be thrust forward in the usual "jaw thrust" with no significant movement of the cervical spine. Extension of the neck should be avoided until X-rays have been obtained and the clinician is certain that no cervical fracture or dislocation is present.

Breathing

It is important to remember that comatose patients often have a high incidence of hypercapnia and hypoxia, both of which may exacerbate the original neurologic injury. Supplemental oxygen should be provided during the initial evaluation. One of the cornerstones of neurologic intensive care is the goal of preventing secondary injury. Thus, children with coma often require endotracheal intubation and assisted ventilation in the triage area[(9)]. When there is impairment of airway protection, intubation is preferable, no matter what the level of consciousness. In the immediate management of the comatose child, it is routine to intubate and control ventilation. It is especially important to consider intubation prior to the interhospital transport of children by skilled personnel[(10–13)].

At this juncture, it is worthwhile to comment on the issue of nasotracheal intubation, particularly in the setting of cervical injury. First, blind nasotracheal intubation is facilitated by spontaneous ventilation of the patient; the severely comatose child may be apneic. Second, nasal cannulation with any tubes (nasotracheal or nasogastric) is contraindicated in the presence of a basilar skull fracture, often impossible to rule out in the acute setting. Third, the child with hypoxia and hypercapnia who is being intubated in the emergency situation should be intubated in the most facile manner possible. In the case of significant facial or oropharyngeal injuries, intubation over a fiberoptic flexible bronchoscope, placing an emergent tracheostomy, or instrumentation of the cricothyroid membrane may be required[(14)].

If the child is struggling, appropriate sedation and muscle relaxation are in order. Muscle relaxants must be used cautiously in patients with CNS injury. Use of nondepolarizing muscle relaxants will make intubation easier for the clinician and may partially ameliorate the increases in intracranial pressure that occur during intubation. It is obvious that the clinician who uses these drugs must be certain that he or she can ventilate the patient. Depolarizing muscle relaxants (e.g. succinylcholine) may increase intracranial pressure, and depolarizing agents are contraindicated when spinal cord, crush injuries, burn injuries, or neuromuscular disease are present. An increased sensitivity to acetylcholine in these injuries can lead to sustained muscular fasciculation, increased intracranial pressure, and life threatening hyperkalemia when depolarizing muscle relaxants are used[(15–17)]. Pretreatment with lidocaine when using depolarizing muscle relaxants may help diminish the increase in ICP occasionally associated with their use[(16,17)]. In addition, lidocaine may ameliorate the increase in ICP associated with airway manipulation. A long-acting agent such as pancuronium bromide precludes the possibility of a complete neurologic examination for a prolonged period of time. The following sequence is one option for rapid-sequence intubation in the head-injured patient: preoxygenation with 100% oxygen, pretreatment with low dose vecuronium (0.01 mg/kg), lidocaine (1.5 mg/kg), and fentanyl (3 to 5 mcg/kg) followed by neuromuscular blockade and sedation with thiopental (50% of usual dose if hypotensive) and succinylcholine (1.5 mg/kg)[(17)].

Circulation

There are no neurologic problems that take priority over stabilization of the patient's hemodynamic status and maintenance of adequate blood pressure. Blood pressure must be high enough to maintain appropriate cerebral perfusion pressure and also high enough to maintain renal function, coronary perfusion, and splanchnic organ flow. In the patient with a severe brain injury, the superimposition of renal failure or necrotic bowel complicates management, making it difficult to treat intracranial hypertension. Fluid administration in the emergent period must be tailored to hemodynamic stabilization and therefore, fluid restriction is not indicated. In addition, the clinician must select fluids that are least likely to cause harm to the CNS. Appropriate normotonic or hypertonic fluids include Ringer's lactate, 0.9% saline, and 0.45% saline with 5% dextrose (as a maintenance fluid only). Blood and colloid are also appropriate in many circumstances. Hypotonic solutions such as 5% dextrose in water can increase cerebral edema and are inappropriate fluids for resuscitation of hypovolemia.

The already injured brain is absolutely intolerant to further insults such as unappreciated hypoxia occurring after the injury, hypercapnia in the hours after resuscitation, and low blood pressure because of inadequate fluid resuscitation[(18,19)]. The safest way to manage respiratory support is to titrate therapy by frequent monitoring of arterial blood gases, end-tidal pCO2 or continuous pulse oximetry. One of the keys to improved outcome in children with neurologic injury is excellent supportive care. Indeed, it is often suggested that improved results in patients receiving intracranial pressure monitoring actually accrue from the increased attention paid to the patients by nurses and physicians rather than from the monitoring itself.

Initial Neurologic Assessment

Rapid neurologic assessment should be performed as soon as cardiopulmonary stabilization is assured. It is important at the outset to have some idea of the severity of neurologic injury. This can help the clinician gauge the prognosis and appropriate level of intervention. Emergency stabilization is often conducted by physicians who do not eventually care for the patient. For example, the child might well be resuscitated initially at some distance from the ICU to which he or she will be transferred. Early neurologic assessment greatly assists the intensivist by providing important prognostic and triage information. Therefore, the physician can

Table 21.1. Glasgow Coma Scale

	Score
Eye opening	
Spontaneous	4
To speech	3
To pain	2
None	1
Best verbal response	
Oriented	5
Confused	4
Inappropriate words	3
Incomprehensible sounds	2
None	1
Best motor response	
Obeys	6
Localizes	5
Withdraws	4
Abnormal flexion	3
Extensor response	2
None	1

develop a trend by comparing the child's current status (in the ICU) with the child's previous status in the community hospital. Some of the therapies used in the emergency room, such as anticonvulsants and muscle relaxants, may compromise future neurologic examinations, at least temporarily, making the baseline assessment critical. Anticonvulsants have sedative effects and may impair the oculomotor exam at higher doses. Muscle relaxants, often necessary for intubation, obliterate the neurologic examination until their effects are extinguished.

The Glasgow coma scale is useful in the emergent setting as the information required for this score is quickly available and places no reliance on history. The components of the score are shown in **Table 21.1**. The scale was developed to provide care providers with objective criteria to assess the level of consciousness and to direct treatment[20]. The Glasgow coma scale has some advantages over a more thorough neurologic examination: simplicity, validity, and practicality[21]. Its simplicity permits frequent reexamination and recording of the scores, and thus is a useful tool for communication. A variety of pediatric modifications have been suggested, including a best score based on age-appropriate skills[22–26]. The ability of the Glasgow coma scale to predict outcome in a variety of disease states has been assessed[27–30]. However there are limitations to the ability of the Glasgow coma scale to predict outcome[29,31,32]. In addition, the Glasgow coma scale is limited by the exclusion of brainstem function in measurement parameters.

In addition to assessment of the depth of coma of the child, further assessment of the child's neurologic status must obviously be accomplished in the emergency period. Patients can be divided into three categories: (a) traumatic injuries involving the head and other systems, (b) traumatic injuries believed to be restricted to the head, and (c) brain injury not associated with trauma. The priorities of assessment are slightly different.

Traumatic Injuries Involving the Head and Other Organ Systems

Children with mixed systemic and CNS traumatic injuries are evaluated by a trauma team that includes a trauma surgeon, an emergency physician, and a pediatric intensivist. The essential question to answer is whether an abdominal or thoracic injury offers an acute threat to the patient's life. Hypotension in such patients is a result of systemic trauma, not head injury, and efforts must be made to control shock. If the child has a life-threatening major abdominal or thoracic injury requiring operative intervention, this intervention has priority over most head injuries. However, during such therapy, the clinician must anticipate and be prepared to treat the possibility of cerebral edema and herniation. If the child is hemodynamically stable enough to have a neurosurgical assessment prior to going to the operating room, this should be accomplished. However, neurosurgical treatment may initially be less important than care of general surgical emergencies. If the pupils are unequal or there are focal or localizing signs, a subdural or epidural hematoma may be strongly suspected, and neurosurgical evaluation may proceed in the operating room while the abdominal or thoracic emergency is being treated.

Traumatic Injuries Restricted to the Head

The child with an "isolated head injury" should be considered a child with mixed injuries in whom the systemic injury is so mild as to be of less concern in the emergency treatment phase. In this category of patients, neurosurgical intervention takes priority. Generally, systemic trauma is not going to preempt neurosurgical intervention or evaluation in such patients, but careful evaluation and attention to hemodynamic stability must be maintained throughout the evaluation. Figure 21.1 shows an example of a patient with traumatic brain injury.

Coma Without a History of Trauma

Finally, comatose children with no documented history of trauma also require expeditious evaluation of their CNS, including evaluation with a head CT scan. Figures 21.2 and 21.3 show examples of brain lesions resulting in coma. The absence of a trauma history does not rule out either trauma or the necessity of neurosurgical intervention. For example, spontaneous intracerebral hemorrhage, brain tumors with resultant hydrocephalus, or shaken baby syndrome may present with sudden coma. **(Table 21.2)** The most important tool for the clinician is the physical examination.

PHYSICAL EXAMINATION OF THE COMATOSE CHILD

The directed coma examination has the purpose of localizing the anatomy of the coma (i.e. bilateral hemispheres or brainstem) and thus its cause. The major features of the specialized exam addresses consciousness, cranial nerve func-

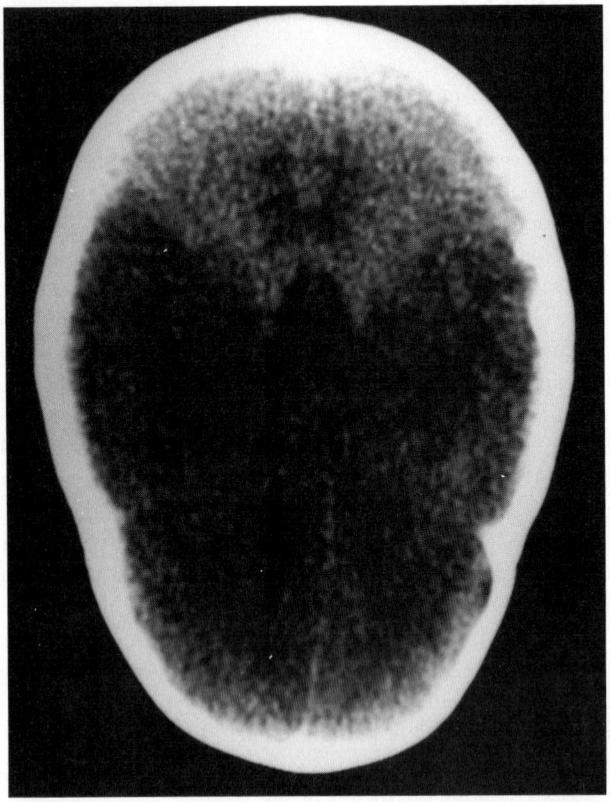

Figure 21.1. CT scan (without contrast) of a patient with traumatic brain injury reveals diffuse attenuation of the hemiparesis with loss of the gray-white interface. The left hemisphere is swollen with a shift of the falx toward the right. The basilar cisterns are compressed by the diffuse cerebral edema.

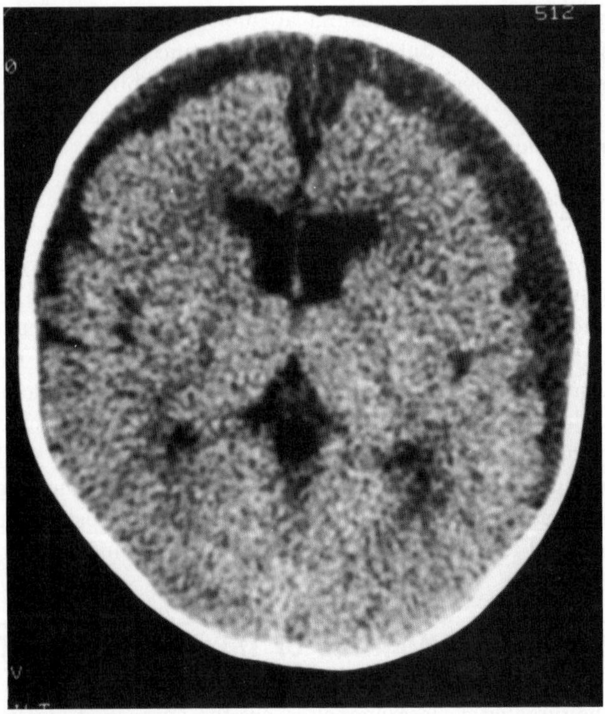

Figure 21.2. Unenhanced CT scan of a child with nonaccidental trauma reveals large extra-axial fluid collections. Especially over the right frontal lobe, areas of variable attenuation suggest chronic subdurals of varying ages.

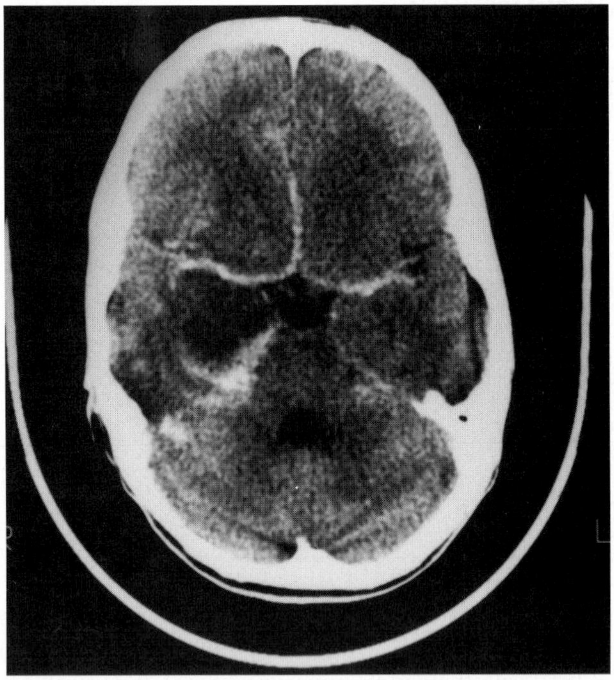

Figure 21.3. Enhanced CT scan of a boy with herpes encephalitis reveals an area of decreased attenuation in the right temporal lobe (adjacent to an area of increased attenuation along the petrous ridge).

tion, and motor function[2,18]. Figures 21.4, 21.5, and 21.6 depict the signs of central transtentorial herniation, uncal herniation, and late herniation.

Level of Consciousness

The initial neurologic examination must be directed to assessing the level of consciousness. Sequential stimulation with loud voice, touch, and finally pain should be used. Adjectives to describe the patient's level of consciousness, such as lethargic or stuporous, are fraught with variable definitions and generally should be avoided in favor of direct descriptions of the patient's response to stimuli.

There are several noxious stimuli acceptably used to assess the mental status of the comatose patient. Ungual pressure with a blunt object, sustained pressure to the superior

Table 21.2. Traumatic and Physical Causes of Coma[a]

Acute subdural hematoma
Brain tumor
Chronic subdural hematoma
Concussion
Contusion
Decompression sickness (caisson disease)
Electrocution
Epidural hematoma—middle cerebral artery laceration
Extreme hypothermia
Hanging[51]
Heatstroke
Non-accidental trauma or child abuse (incl. shaken baby syndrome)
Sunstroke

[a]*Adapted from Lockman LA. Coma. In: Swaiman K & Manning S, eds. Pediatric neurology: Principles and Practice, St Louis: Mosby Year Book Inc., 1994.*

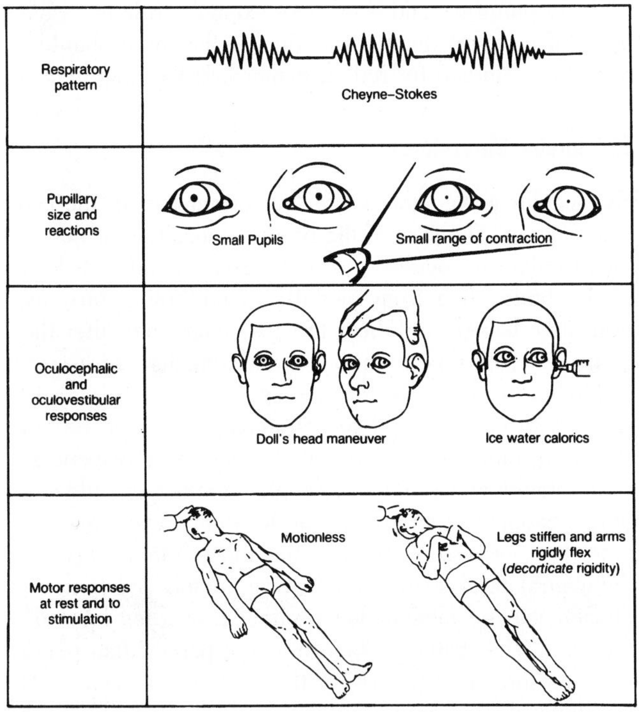

Figure 21.4. Signs of central transtentorial herniation. (From Plum F, Posner JB. The diagnosis of stupor and coma. 3rd ed. Philadelphia: FA Davis, 1982:104.)

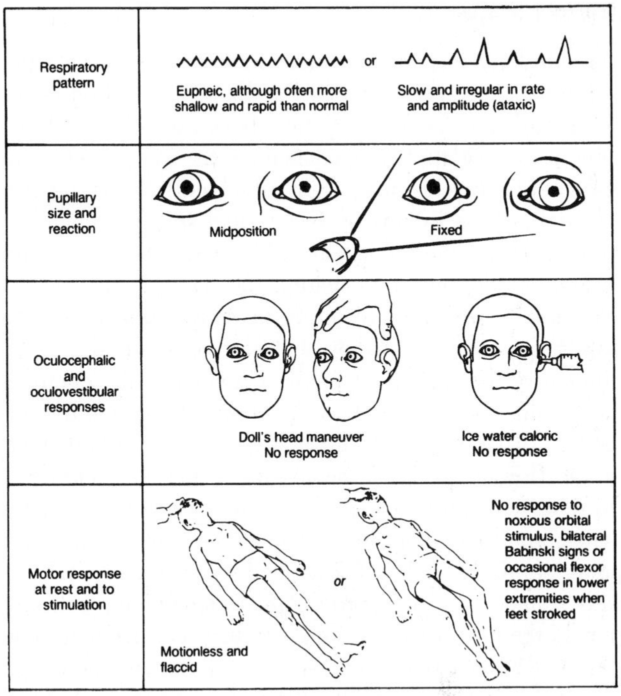

Figure 21.6. Signs of late herniation, with lower pons upper medulla involvement. Either central or uncal herniation may progress to this stage. (From Plum F, Posner JB. The diagnosis of stupor and coma. 3rd ed. Philadelphia: FA Davis. 1982:108.)

medial orbit or pinna, and rubbing of the sternum are examples of stimuli used to produce motor responses that correlate with different behavioral and pathologic states. With avoidance behavior demonstrated for each limb and the head, the examiner can infer that the patient, under conditions of noxious stimulation, can access hemispheric cognitive centers. Weak, poorly sustained, or stereotyped (decorticate or decerebrate pattern) responses for one limb or one side of the body are suggestive of a supratentorial mass lesion[2,33].

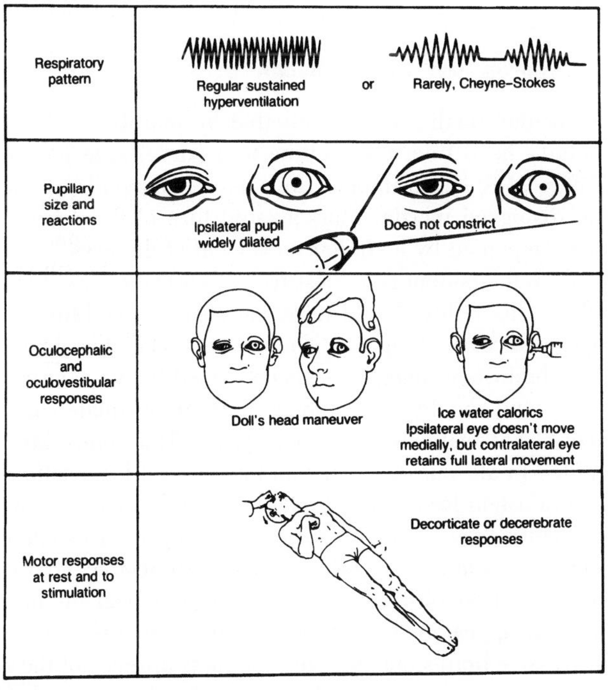

Figure 21.5. Signs of uncal herniation, demonstrating third nerve involvement. (From Plum F, Posner JB. The diagnosis of stupor and coma. 3rd ed. Philadelphia: FA Davis, 1982:110.)

Respiratory Pattern

Comatose patients will typically have an altered pattern of respiration. Patients with bilateral cerebral hemisphere dysfunction may have a normal pattern of breathing or they may demonstrate a Cheyne-Stokes pattern, characterized by an increasing depth and rate of breathing in an accelerating-decelerating pattern followed by a brief apneic period. Patients with a midbrain lesion will often hyperventilate as a central neurogenic process, not in response to hypercarbia or hypoxemia. This pattern of respiration is also associated with metabolic acidosis, with salicylate overdose, or with a primary pulmonary process. The patient with a pontine lesion may demonstrate an apneustic pattern of breathing characterized by a prolonged inspiratory phase, followed by a short expiratory phase. Finally, lesions in the medulla may have an associated ataxic respiratory pattern that is disorganized and ineffective, characterized by hyperventilation, apnea, or apneustic breathing. In addition, an assessment of the ability to generate a cough and gag with pharyngeal stimulation suggests the risk to airway protection. Intubation at this point is recommended to insure adequate ventilation, oxgenation, and protection of the patient's airway[2,14,33].

Pupillary Response

The pupillary response to bright light is an important part of the comatose examination. Pupillary constriction is mediated by the parasympathetic fibers travelling with the third nerve. Dilation is mediated by the sympathetic system, which travels from the hypothalamus to the superior cervical ganglia by way of the cervical spinal column. Lesions involving the brainstem will interrupt these pathways. Lesions in the midbrain disrupt the parasympathetic and sympathetic pathways resulting in midposition unreactive pupils. In uncal herniation, the most sensitive sign is the dilation of the ipsilateral pupil attributed to the compression of the third cranial nerve as it passes through the tentorium, leaving sympathetic influence on the pupil unopposed. However, even in the absence of herniation or direct third nerve involvement, pupils are often dilated in the presence of midbrain damage. Lesions in the pons result in pinpoint pupils because of disrupted sympathetic pathways with intact and unopposed parasympathetic pathways though the mechanism for this pupillary constriction is not well understood. Medullary lesions result in nonreactive pupils of a normal size.[2,33] Pupillary changes associated with the area of anatomic involvement are shown in Figure 21.7.

The pupillary response to light is usually unaffected in metabolic processes and can be a guide to the underlying etiology. Medications given in the emergency room and ICU can cause pupillary changes, but generally the pupils will remain reactive. Atropine and scopolamine cause full dilation and nonreactivity of the pupils. Glutethimide usually causes mydriasis and may cause them to be nonreactive to light. Muscle relaxants will affect extraocular movements, but pupillary responses should be normal. Narcotics generally cause pinpoint but reactive pupils. Examination of pupils should be done with a bright and abrupt exposure to light. Any reactivity, whether sluggish or not, is indicative of intact pathways and would, for example, rule out a diagnosis of cerebral death. And finally, the fundi should always be examined for retinal hemorrhages or papilledema.

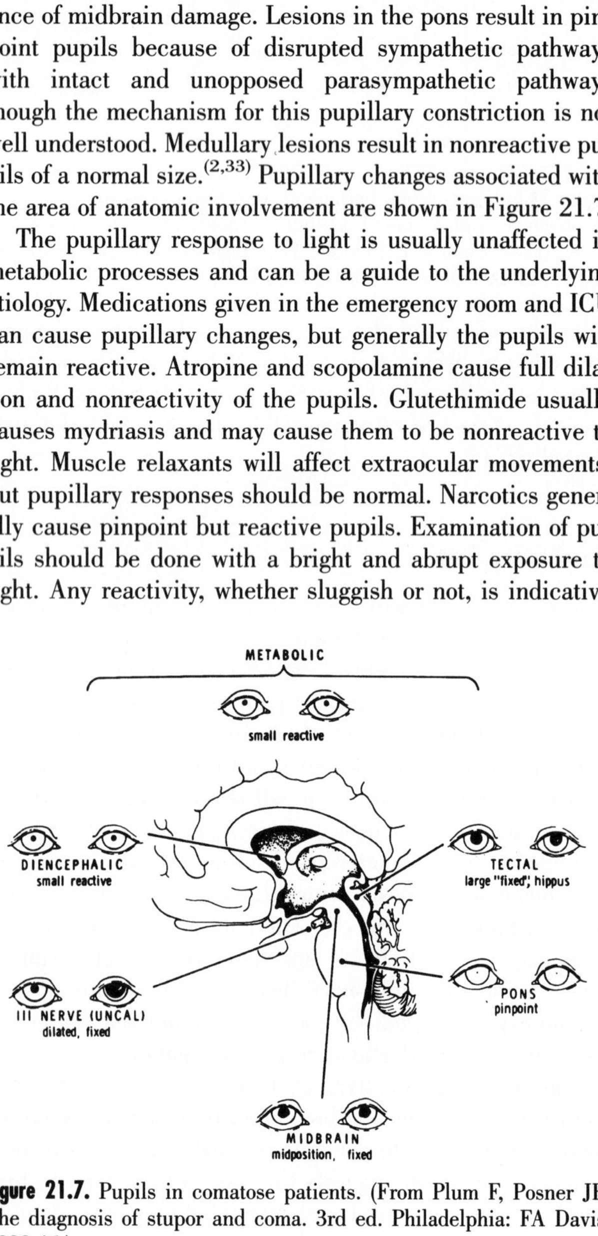

Figure 21.7. Pupils in comatose patients. (From Plum F, Posner JB. The diagnosis of stupor and coma. 3rd ed. Philadelphia: FA Davis, 1982:46.)

Extraocular Movements

Extraocular movements are an important part of the coma examination. The area of the brain responsible for the oculovestibular and oculocephalic reflexes extends the length of the brain stem from medulla to midbrain; thus, most brainstem lesions sufficient to cause coma may alter these pathways. Analysis of these eye movements can assist in localizing the anatomic lesion responsible for the comatose state. With continuing, long-term compression of the brain stem, eye movements cease, including reflex responses to head rotation and to ice water applied to the tympanic membrane. Symmetric and conjugate horizontal eye movements requires coordination beween the third cranial nerve and the contralateral sixth cranial nerve nuclei. This is accomplished via the median longitudinal fasciculus located in the pons. The system is known as the paramedian pontine reticular formation (PPRF) or the pontine gaze center. The vestibular nuclei, cranial nerve eight, is responsible for reacting to movements of the head and body and coordinates this with horizontal gaze. The interaction among these systems account for the immediate reflexive realignment of the eyes to the orientation of the head and body. This is a tonically active system, with a balance between right and left sides, and is the basis of the oculovestibular reflex. The PPRF is also a part of the reticular activating system responsible for maintaining consciousness and thus changes in its activity indicate structural abnormalities in the brainstem[2,33].

Oculocephalic (Doll's Head) Reflex

The oculocephalic reflex is elicited by sharply turning the patient's head from the midline to a lateral gaze position. (Figure 21.8) Old-fashioned dolls often had mobile eyeballs that displayed inertia. Thus a rapid turn of the head was unaccompanied by a similar movement of the eyes. Such a result in the patient is a "positive" or normal oculocephalic reflex. This reflex should never be tested in children with suspected cervical injuries. The information that is obtained about brainstem function is also obtained by the caloric response and should be postponed until an adequate assessment of cervical spine integrity occurs. This reflex can be elicited in all four directions and may assist localization of the brainstem lesion. For example, midbrain tectal lesions may cause selective loss of reflex upward gaze. This change often occurs in young children with early rostrocaudal deterioration from obstructed ventricular peritoneal shunts. In short, disappearance or absence of the response indicates progressive brainstem damage. Complete absence of the response is a component of the criteria for diagnosing brain death.

Oculovestibular Reflex

The oculovestibular reflex (or cold caloric response) tests the same pathways as the oculocephalic but can be accomplished even in patients with cervical injuries. The tympanic membrane must be intact prior to initiating the test. To test lateral eye movements, the head is elevated 30° by elevating the bed and up to 120 mL of ice water is gently introduced via a catheter over several minutes into the canal. (Figure 21.8) The absence of the reflex should not be diagnosed until the maximum volume has been used; lesser volumes can be used if the response is apparent. Testing of the opposite ear should not be attempted for at least 5 minutes to allow the vestibulo-ocular system to stabilize. In awake patients with an intact brainstem, nystagmus is produced by these maneuvers, with the slow eye deviation towards the cold stimulus and a rapid nystagmus in the opposite direction. As cerebral hemisphere disease develops, including metabolic depression of cortical function, the fast component disappears with tonic deviation of the eyes towards the cold stimulus. Such deviation may persist for several minutes. As metabolic depression continues to severe levels (such as barbiturate coma) or in the presence of brainstem damage, the caloric reflex is abolished. The oculovestibular (cold caloric) reflex is more persistent than the oculocephalic reflex and thus may be present despite absence of the oculocephalic reflex.

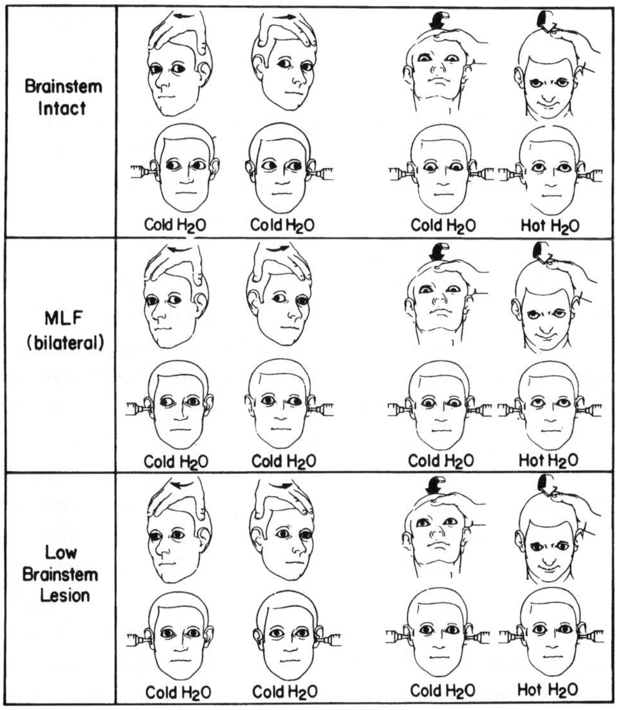

Figure 21.8. Vestibulo-ocular response in unconscious patients. In patients with intact brainstem function (*upper panel*), a positive doll's eye response is elicited, and cold water stimulus causes tonic deviation toward the cold side. *Middle panel* illustrates the findings with involvement of the medial longitudinal fasciculus (*MLF*). Severe brainstem disease leads to abolition to the vestibulo-ocular reflex (*lower panel*). (Adapted from Plum F, Posner JB. The diagnosis of stupor and coma. 3rd ed. Philadelphia: FA Davis, 1982:55.)

Corneal Response

The corneal response assesses the sensory component of the fifth cranial nerve and the motor component of the seventh cranial nerve. Afferent stimuli are generated by touching the cornea with a cotton wisp and observing the stimulated eye for constriction of the orbicularis oculi (a blink response). The contralateral eye should have a consensual blink. If the consensual response is the only response that occurs, then sensation is intact on the stimulated side, and there is an ipsilateral facial nerve palsy. For some obtunded patients, light touch will not produce a response, but gentle scleral pressure with a cotton swab elicits orbicularis oculi constriction.

A weak motor response can be noted by closely following the lower eyelid's medial lashes: they deviate toward the midline and then relax. This corneal reflex is a good test for mid- and low-pontine dysfunction. To test other branches of the seventh nerve, a cotton swab can be used to irritate the nasal mucosa. This stimulus produces widespread facial muscular contraction with a grimace response.

Motor Response

Motor response is one of the three components of the Glasgow coma scale. A patient's motor performance gives a form of cognitive testing in the unconscious patient. Purposeful motor behavior requires intact motor pathways and an awareness of self and surroundings.

The speed, strength, and symmetry of motor responses are functions that can be quantified in detail when the patient is awake. For the unresponsive patient, these functions are best described qualitatively and typically require a noxious stimulus to elicit a response. Eye opening or any form of speech, including poorly defined grunts and groans, suggests some degree of reticular activating system function. Speech and/or purposeful withdrawal from painful stimuli is a sign of cortical function and hence cortical preservation. If asymmetry is noted in the motor response, the limb in question should be stimulated several times to validate the finding. Decorticate postures are associated with cortical or hemispheric dysfunction. Decerebrate postures (arm and leg extension) correlate with high pontine and midbrain lesions below the level of the red nucleus. This is attributed to the compromised function of the rubrospinal and corticospinal systems, which normally exert a net facilitatory effect on flexor muscles, and the consequent release of the vestibulospinal system, which facilitates extensor muscle groups[2,33]. The motor response to noxious stimulation in comatose patients is depicted in Figure 21.9.

The muscle tone of an extremity and the deep tendon reflexes should be evaluated to confirm the finding of an asymmetric response to pain. Hypotonia occurs acutely with

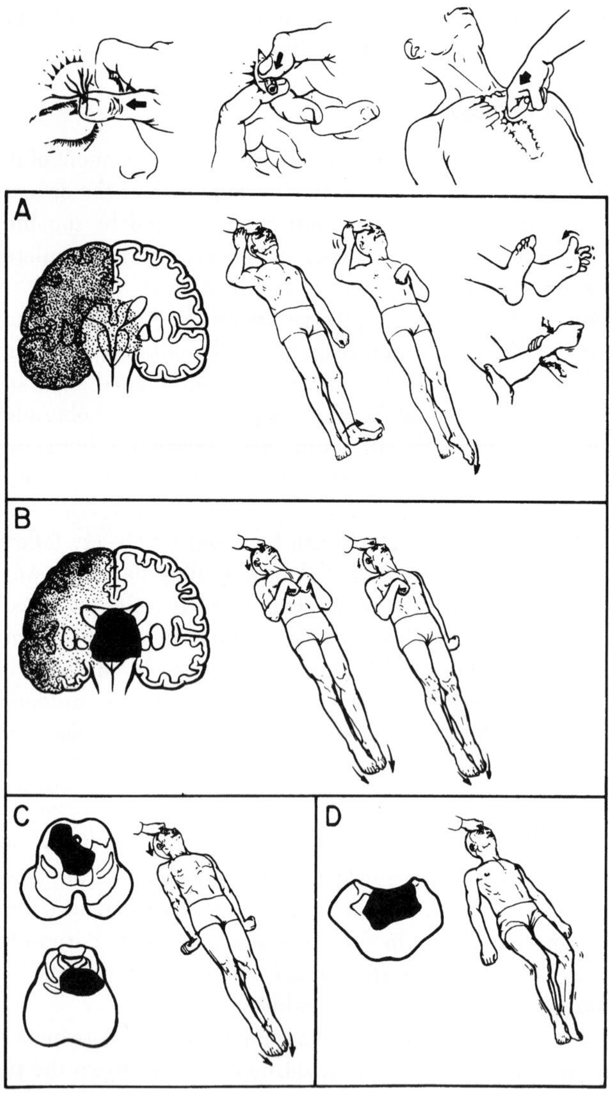

Figure 21.9. Motor responses to noxious stimulation in comatose patients. **A** demonstrates localization of pain as the patient reaches for the inciting stimulus; **B** shows decorticase rigidity; **C** demonstrates decerebrate rigidity; **D** shows a flaccid patient with no response to pain. (From Plum F, Posner JB. The diagnosis of stupor and coma. 3rd ed. Philadelphia: FA Davis, 1982:66.)

hemispheric, medullary, and spinal cord lesions. Hypertonia is usually a late sign or a sign of preexistent corticospinal tract injury. The major exception is acute injury to the midbrain or pons. When this occurs, the vestibulospinal motor system continues to exert a tonic influence on the spinal cord, but the more rostral corticospinal system is disrupted. Hypertonia, hyperreflexia, clonus, and the Babinski sign can be elicited acutely in this situation. Decerebrate rigidity can be thought of as an extreme manifestation of these unopposed vestibulospinal reflexes. Flaccidity and the absence of any motor response are indicative of severe low (pontomedullary junction and caudal) brainstem dysfunction. Flaccidity strongly suggests spinal shock and should be associated immediately with cervical spine and medullary lesions; both are life threatening[2,33].

CAUSES OF COMA

Causes of coma may be classified in numerous ways, but from a diagnostic standpoint, the Plum and Posner method is difficult to improve[2]. As previously discussed, unconsciousness is a product of abnormal function of the brainstem reticular activating system and/or both cerebral hemispheres. By careful consideration of the history and the physical examination, it is possible to classify comatose patients into one of four pathophysiologic categories:

1. Supratentorial mass lesions
2. Subtentorial mass lesions or destructive lesions
3. Metabolic disorders
4. Psychogenic coma

For the critical care physician initially evaluating the comatose patient, an alternative classification may be more useful:

1. Metabolic coma that is immediately treatable
2. Rapidly progressive supratentorial or subtentorial masses or destructive lesions
3. Nonprogressive (stable) coma

The purpose of this system is not the complete evaluation of the differential diagnosis of the comatose child. The primary goal of the system is to ensure that the clinician prevents early death or permanent sequelae to the patient during the diagnostic process.

Immediately Treatable Metabolic Coma

A metabolic cause for the comatose state should be suspected if the neurologic examination (including physical findings, electrophysiologic studies, and CT scans) cannot be reconciled. **(Table 21.3)** For example, any structural lesion that completely eliminates respiration would do so by compression or destruction of medullary structures, and supramedullary structures would precede in such destruction. Thus, fixed and dilated pupils would be expected.

Hypoglycemia is one etiology of metabolic coma that is easily treated and may cause irreversible CNS damage when not treated. Naloxone or other narcotic antagonist administration is appropriate if the patient shows severe effects of narcotics, such as hypoventilation, hypotension, miosis, or pulmonary edema[64]. The same is true of benzodiazepine overdose, characterized by tachycardia, hypotension, somnolence, miosis, and hypoventilation. Flumazenil, a benzodiazepine antagonist, is an appropriate agent to use in the case of severe intoxication[65,66]. However, its use is contraindicated in the case of coingestion with tricyclic antidepressants or cocaine. In these cases, benzodiazepines are felt to provide a protective antiepileptic effect[65–70].

If the child has fever, meningismus, or a suggestive history, and meningitis is a possibility, then a lumbar puncture should be performed when the child is stabilized. Antibiotics should be instituted promptly, prior to the lumbar

Table 21.3. Metabolic Causes of Coma[a]

Acidosis
Alkalosis
Hemolytic-Uremic Syndrome[42]
Henoch-Schonlein Purpura
Hepatic failure, portosystemic shunts
Hyperammonemia
Ornithine transcarbamylase deficiency[47]
Reyes Syndrome[48]
Hypercalcemia and hypocalcemia
Hypercapnia (Pickwickian syndrome)
Hypermagnesemia, hypomagnesemia
Hypoglycemia
Hypoxia
Hyperosmolar states
Hypertonic dehydration
Infection (see Table 21.4)
Juvenile rheumatoid arthritis[43]
Kearns-Sayre syndrome[44,45]
Poisonings
Anticholinergic eye drops[34]
Isoniazid toxicity[35]
Methotrexate/Ara-C therapy[36,37]
Organophosphate/carbamate poisoning[38]
Phenothiazine/Butyrphenone poisoning[39]
Sertraline overdose[40]
Tricyclic overdose[41]
Porphyria
Status epilepticus[46]
Thyrotoxicosis[49]
Uremia
Vitamin deficiency or dependency states
Carnitine deficiency[50]
Nicotinic acid
Pantothenic acid
Pyridoxine
Thiamine (Leigh's disease)
Vitamin B_{12}

[a]Adapted from Lockman LA. Coma. In: Swaiman K & Manning S, eds. Pediatric neurology: Principles and Practice, St Louis: Mosby Year Book Inc., 1994.

puncture if the child is too unstable. Other infectious etiologies for coma are outlined in **Table 21.4**.

Other causes of metabolic comas are myriad and include diffuse brain anoxia or ischemia, accidental poisoning (including ethanol, opiates, barbiturates, heavy metals, and aspirin), acid-base derangements, hyper- or hypocalcemia, pulmonary disease (carbon dioxide narcosis, carbon monoxide poisoning), uremia, liver failure, hypo- or hyperthermia, and meningitis. Simple bedside maneuvers may assist the clinician in diagnosing these disorders. For instance, calculation of the anion gap may alert the clinician to an exogenous anion causing a metabolic acidosis. It is also possible to calculate an osmolal gap, which is the difference between the measured and calculated osmolality. Finally, the finding of any strongly abnormal value should alert the clinician to a metabolic cause[2,7,8].

Rapidly Progressive Intracranial Lesions

Supratentorial lesions cause coma by depressing function of large parts of the cerebral cortex, and thus, relatively small focal supratentorial lesions are unlikely to cause

Table 21.4. Infectious Causes of Coma[a]

Brain abscess with ventricular rupture
Empyema, epidural or subdural
Encephalitis[60], bacterial
Myocoplasma[46]
Encephalomyelitis, post-infectious
Encephalitis[60], viral
Herpes
Sleeping Sickness[61]
Typhoid fever
Varicella zoster
Hemorrhagic shock and leukoencephalopathy[62,63]
Meningitis, bacterial
Meningitis, fungal
Cryptogenic[52]
Meningitis, tuberculous
Protozoan infections—amebic, malarial, cysticercosis
Malaria[53–59]
Severe systemic infection, sepsis

[a]Adapted from Lockman LA. Coma. In: Swaiman K & Manning S, eds. Pediatric neurology: Principles and Practice, St Louis: Mosby Year Book Inc., 1994.

coma. Subtentorial lesions may depress consciousness by exerting pressure on or causing dysfunction or destruction of the brainstem, including the reticular activating system. Unlike supratentorial lesions, a small lesion in the brainstem is capable of depressing consciousness. In either case, onset of coma from an intracranial lesion is nearly always rapidly progressive and must be approached in an emergent manner. The differential diagnoses of supratentorial lesions and subtentorial lesions differ, but the ramifications for the emergent management and approach are the same[2,7,8].

Focal findings support the possibility of intracranial pathology; their absence should not lull the physician into believing that the coma is based on metabolic causes.

Any patient in whom brainstem abnormalities can be demonstrated should be considered to have a mass lesion until the clinician can rule out such a possibility. Examples include abnormal cranial nerve function, or abnormal oculovestibular or oculocephalic reflexes. Whether such abnormalities arise from a supratentorial or a subtentorial source may be suggested by the changes in the neurologic exam over time. Clear rostral-to-caudal deterioration, though uncommon, is highly suggestive of a supratentorial mass. Patients with abnormalities of brainstem function should be presumed to have serious intracranial pathology with a potential for further deterioration. The most expedient way to evaluate patients for intracranial mass lesions is the CT scan.

Nonprogressive (Stable) Coma

This category refers to all causes of coma for which there is no immediately reversible condition. Patients with coma from this etiology will suffer mortality and morbidity in the absence of compulsive intensive care. By the time the clinician arrives to this point, all emergent therapies have been started and most treatable causes of coma have been identified. In this context, elective intubation and ventilation, early CT scanning, and admission to the ICU provide a safe basis on which to begin more sophisticated consideration of the differential diagnosis of coma. Thereafter, the physician can more carefully consider the history and plan his or her work-up of the patient. The approach to comatose children should be aggressive and pragmatic.

SUMMARY

This chapter presents a pragmatic approach to the comatose patient. This approach includes appropriate management of the airway, breathing, and circulatory systems. Supplemental oxygen is provided, hypoglycemia is treated preemptively, antibiotics are begun if meningitis is probable, and the timing of neuroimaging studies is considered. Thereafter, the myriad causes of coma should be carefully considered once life-threatening causes of coma have been treated. In this manner, the intensive care physician can combine emergent management with an intelligent diagnostic approach and be ready to organize or define further neurologic care.

References

1. Kelly D. Disorders of Sleep and Consciousness. In: Kandel ER SJ, ed. Principles of Neural Science, 2nd Edition. New York: Elsevier Science Publishing, 1985:659–670.
2. Plum F, Posner J. The Diagnosis of Stupor and Coma. (3 ed.) Philadelphia: F.A. Davis Company, 1982:377. Contemporary Neurology Series; vol 19.
3. Goldstein B, Powers KS. Head trauma in children. Pediatr Rev 1994;15(6):213–9; quiz 219.
4. James HE. Neurologic evaluation and support in the child with an acute brain insult. Pediatr Ann 1986;15(1):16–22.
5. Kaufman BA, Dacey RG, Jr. Acute care management of closed head injury in childhood. Pediatr Ann 1994;23(1):18–20, 25–8.
6. Michaud LJ, Duhaime AC, Batshaw ML. Traumatic brain injury in children. Pediatr Clin North Am 1993;40(3):553–65.
7. Lockman L. Impairment of Consciousness. In: Swaiman K, Manning S, ed. Pediatric Neurology: Principles and Practice. 2 ed. St. Louis, MO: Mosby-Year Book Inc., 1994:183–195. vol 1.
8. Pfenninger J. Neurological intensive care in children. Intensive Care Med 1993;19(5):243–50.
9. Redan JA, Livingston DH, Tortella BJ, Rush BF, Jr. The value of intubating and paralyzing patients with suspected head injury in the emergency department. J Trauma 1991;31(3):371–5.
10. Sarnaik AP, Lieh-Lai MW. Transporting the neurologically compromised child. Pediatr Clin North Am 1993;40(2):337–54.
11. Andrews PJ, Piper IR, Dearden NM, Miller JD. Secondary insults during intrahospital transport of head-injured patients. Lancet 1990;335(8685):327–30.
12. Macnab AJ. Optimal escort for interhospital transport of pediatric emergencies. J Trauma 1991;31(2):205–9.
13. Gentleman D, Jennett B. Audit of transfer of unconscious head-injured patients to a neurosurgical unit [published erratum appears in Lancet 1990 Mar 3; 335(8688):554.] Lancet 1990;335(8685):330–4.
14. Noah Z, Hahn Y, Rubenstein J, Aronyk K. Management of the child with severe brain injury. Critical Care Clinics 1992;3(1):59–77.
15. Gronert G, Theye R. Pathophysiology of hyperkalemia induced by succinylcholine. Anesthesiology 1975;43(1):89–99.
16. O'Connor M, Roizen M. Use of muscle relaxants in the intensive care unit. Journal of Intensive Care Medicine 1993;8:34–46.
17. Walls R. Rapid-sequence intubation in head trauma. Ann Emerg Med 1993;22(6):1008–1013.
18. Chesnut RM, Marshall LF, Klauber MR, et al. The role of secondary brain injury in determining outcome from severe head injury. J Trauma 1993;34(2):216–22.
19. Pigula FA, Wald SL, Shackford SR, Vane DW. The effect of hypotension and hypoxia on children with severe head injuries. J Pediatr Surg 1993;28(3):310–4; discussion 315–6.
20. Teasdale G, Jennett B. Assessment of coma and impaired consciousness: a practical scale. Lancet 1974;2:81–84.
21. Sagy M. Scoring systems in emergency pediatrics: "one cannot see the forest for the trees" [see comments]. Pediatr Emerg Care 1989;5(2): 142–4.
22. Morray JP, Tyler DC, Jones TK, Stuntz JT, Lemire RJ. Coma scale for use in brain-injured children. Crit Care Med 1984;12(12):1018–20.
23. Simpson D, Reilly P. Pediatric coma scale [letter]. Lancet 1982; 2(8295):450.
24. Simpson DA, Cockington RA, Hanieh A, Raftos J, Reilly PL. Head injuries in infants and young children: the value of the Paediatric Coma Scale. Review of literature and report on a study. Childs Nerv Syst 1991;7(4):183–90.
25. Yager JY, Johnston B, Seshia SS. Coma scales in pediatric practice. Am J Dis Child 1990;144(10):1088–91.
26. Raimondi AJ, Hirschauer J. Head injury in the infant and toddler. Coma scoring and outcome scale. Childs Brain 1984;11(1):12–35.
27. Kalff R, Kocks W, Pospiech J, Grote W. Clinical outcome after head injury in children. Childs Nerv Syst 1989;5(3):156–9.
28. Kennedy F, Gonzalez P, Dang C, Fleming A, Sterling-Scott R. The Glasgow Coma Scale and prognosis in gunshot wounds to the brain. J Trauma 1993;35(1):75–7.
29. Groleau GA, Tso EL, Olshaker JS, Barish RA, Lyston DJ. Baseball bat assault injuries. J Trauma 1993;34(3):366–72.
30. Chan B, Gaudry P, Grattan-Smith TM, McNeil R. The use of Glasgow Coma Scale in poisoning. J Emerg Med 1993;11(5):579–82.
31. Humphreys RP, Hendrick EB, Hoffman HJ. The head-injured child who "talks and dies". A report of 4 cases. Childs Nerv Syst 1990;6(3): 139–42.
32. Lieh-Lai MW, Theodorou AA, Sarnaik AP, Meert KL, Moylan PM, Canady AI. Limitations of the Glasgow Coma Scale in predicting outcome in children with traumatic brain injury. J Pediatr 1992;120(2 Pt 1):195–9.
33. Rolak L. Critical care evaluation of coma. In: Taylor R, Shoemaker W, eds. The Society of Critical Care Medicine. Society of Critical Care Medicine, 1991: 81–90.
34. Nadal J, De la Fuente V, Abadias M, Torrent J, Jane F. Toxic coma induced by anticholinergic eye drops [letter]. Br Med J (Clin Res Ed) 1987;295(6609):1352.
35. Orlowski JP, Paganini EP, Pippenger CE. Treatment of a potentially lethal dose isoniazid ingestion. Ann Emerg Med 1988;17(1):73–6.
36. von der Weid NX, de Crousaz H, Beck D, Deonna T, Miklossy J, Janzer RC. Acute fatal myeloencephalopathy after combined intrathecal chemotherapy in a child with acute lymphoblastic leukemia. Med Pediatr Oncol 1991;19(3):192–8.
37. Gerrard MP, Eden OB, Lilleyman JS. Acute encephalopathy during induction therapy for acute lymphoblastic leukemia. Pediatr Hematol Oncol 1986;3(1):49–58.
38. Sofer S, Tal A, Shahak E. Carbamate and organophosphate poisoning in early childhood. Pediatr Emerg Care 1989;5(4):222–5.
39. Knight ME, Roberts RJ. Phenothiazine and butyrophenone intoxication in children [published erratum appears in Pediatr Clin North Am 1988 Aug; 35(4):following vii]. Pediatr Clin North Am 1986;33(2):299–309.
40. Kaminski CA, Robbins MS, Weibley RE. Sertraline intoxication in a child. Ann Emerg Med 1994;23(6):1371–4.
41. Wedin GP, Oderda GM, Klein-Schwartz W, Gorman RL. Relative toxicity of cyclic antidepressants. Ann Emerg Med 1986;15(7):797–804.
42. Kelles A, Van Dyck M, Proesmans W. Childhood haemolytic uraemic syndrome: long-term outcome and prognostic features. Eur J Pediatr 1994;153(1):38–42.
43. Hadchouel M, Prieur AM, Griscelli C. Acute hemorrhagic, hepatic, and neurologic manifestations in juvenile rheumatoid arthritis: possible relationship to drugs or infection. J Pediatr 1985;106(4):561–6.
44. Welch E, Gelband H. Hyperglycemic acidosis with mortality in Kearns-Sayre syndrome [letter]. Am J Dis Child 1989;143(10):1135–6.
45. Curless RG, Flynn J, Bachynski B, Gregorios JB, Benke P, Cullen R. Fatal metabolic acidosis, hyperglycemia, and coma after steroid therapy for Kearns-Sayre syndrome. Neurology 1986;36(6):872–3.
46. Hulihan JF, Bebin EM, Westmoreland BF. Bilateral periodic lateralized epileptiform discharges in Mycoplasma encephalitis. Pediatr Neurol 1992;8(4):292–4.
47. Coskun T, Ozalp I, Monch S, Kneer J. Lethal hyperammonaemic coma due to ornithine transcarbamylase deficiency presenting as brain stem

encephalitis in a previously asymptomatic ten-year-old boy. J Inherit Metab Dis 1987;10(3):271.
48. Dezateux CA, Dinwiddie R, Helms P, Matthew DJ. Recognition and early management of Reye's syndrome. Arch Dis Child 1986;61(7): 647–51.
49. Radetti G, Dordi B, Mengarda G, Biscaldi I, Larizza D, Severi F. Thyrotoxicosis presenting with seizures and coma in two children [letter]. Am J Dis Child 1993;147(9):925–7.
50. Stanley CA, De Leeuw S, Coates PM, et al. Chronic cardiomyopathy and weakness or acute coma in children with a defect in carnitine uptake. Ann Neurol 1991;30(5):709–16.
51. Vander Krol L, Wolfe R. The emergency department management of near-hanging victims. J Emerg Med 1994;12(3):285–92.
52. David TJ. Cryptogenic meningitis and unexplained episodes of coma in a young child [letter]. Lancet 1989;2(8661):513–4.
53. Kawo NG, Msengi AE, Swai AB, Chuwa LM, Alberti KG, McLarty DG. Specificity of hypoglycaemia for cerebral malaria in children. Lancet 1990;336(8713):454–7.
54. Kawo NG, Msengi AE, Swai AB, et al. Hypoglycaemia and cerebral malaria [letter]. Lancet 1990;336(8723):1128–9.
55. Molyneux ME, Taylor TE, Thomas CG, Mansor S, Wirima JJ. Efficacy of quinine for falciparum malaria according to previous chloroquine exposure. Lancet 1991;337(8754):1379–80.
56. Wright PW, Avery WG, Ardill WD, McLarty JW. Initial clinical assessment of the comatose patient: cerebral malaria vs. meningitis. Pediatr Infect Dis J 1993;12(1):37–41.
57. Carlson J, Helmby H, Hill AV, Brewster D, Greenwood BM, Wahlgren M. Human cerebral malaria: association with erythrocyte rosetting and lack of anti-rosetting antibodies. Lancet 1990;336(8729):1457–60.
58. Brewster DR, Kwiatkowski D, White NJ. Neurological sequelae of cerebral malaria in children. Lancet 1990;336(8722):1039–43.
59. Hypoglycaemia and cerebral malaria [letter; comment]. Lancet 1990; 336(8720):950–2.
60. Koskiniemi M, Rautonen J, Lehtokoski-Lehtiniemi E, Vaheri A. Epidemiology of encephalitis in children—A 20 year survey. Ann Neurol 1991;29:492–497.
61. Pepin J, Milord F, Guern C, Mpia B, Ethier L, Mansinsa D. Trial of prednisolone for prevention of melarsoprol-induced encephalopathy in gambiense sleeping sickness. Lancet 1989;1(8649):1246–50.
62. Chesney PJ, Chesney RW. Hemorrhagic shock and encephalopathy: reflections about a new devastating disorder that affects normal children. J Pediatr 1989;114(2):254–6.
63. Levin M, Pincott JR, Hjelm M, et al. Hemorrhagic shock and encephalopathy: clinical, pathologic, and biochemical features. J Pediatr 1989;114(2):194–203.
64. Hoffman JR, Schriger DL, Luo JS. The empiric use of naloxone in patients with altered mental status: a reappraisal. Ann Emerg Med 1991;20(3):246–52.
65. Sprenger H, Sharpe MD, McLachlan RS. Flumazenil as a diagnostic tool in the differential diagnosis of coma in a critically ill patient. Can J Anaesth 1994;41(1):52–5.
66. Chern TL, Hu SC, Lee CH, Deng JF. Diagnostic and therapeutic utility of flumazenil in comatose patients with drug overdose. Am J Emerg Med 1993;11(2):122–4.
67. Lheureux P, Vranckx M, Leduc D, Askenasi R. Flumazenil in mixed benzodiazepine/tricyclic antidepressant overdose: A placebo-controlled study in the dog. Am J Emerg Med 1992;10:184–188.
68. Mordel A, Winkler E, Almog S, Tirosh M, Ezra D. Seizures after flumazenil administration in a case of combined benzodiazepine and tricyclic antidepressant overdose. Crit Care Med 1992;20(12):1733–1734.
69. Sugarman JM, Paul RI. Flumazenil: A review. Ped Emerg Care 1994;10(1):37–43.
70. Derlet RW, Albertson TE. Flumazenil induces seizures and death in mixed cocaine-diazepam intoxications. Ann Emerg Med 1994;23(3): 494–498.

Status Epilepticus 22

Robert C. Tasker
J. Michael Dean

INTRODUCTION

Status epilepticus is a condition in which epileptic activity persists for 30 minutes or longer, causing a wide spectrum of clinical symptoms, and with a highly varied pathophysiologic, anatomic and etiologic basis[1]. From the perspective of pediatric critical illness, it is a medical emergency that requires prompt recognition and immediate vigorous treatment. If patients are left untreated or poorly treated, or if there is delay in effective treatment, permanent neurologic sequelae or even death may ensue[2].

At the present time, with the majority of children receiving appropriate management for life-threatening status epilepticus, secondary complications are fortunately rare[3]. However, this should not lead to a complacency in our present practice or understanding of the condition because some infants and children are at special risk. These patients include those referred for intensive care because of the continued need for frequent intravenous anticonvulsants, refractory status epilepticus[4–6], or difficult management involving more than one organ system[6–9], of which frequent seizures or status epilepticus is a "symptom" or complication of some underlying pathophysiologic process.

Since status epilepticus is a common neurologic emergency, with sometimes complex clinical management problems, the pediatric intensivist should be familiar with the range of clinical manifestations in infants and children, potential systemic and central nervous system (CNS) complications, causal pathophysiology, required clinical evaluation, and therapy.

CLINICAL PRESENTATION

Clinical Appearance

Seizures associated with status epilepticus in infants and children include a number of forms or types seen only at particular ages **(Table 22.1)**[10]. Therefore the pediatric

Table 22.1. Forms of Status Epilepticus in Relation to Age at Presentation

Age	*Type of Status Epilepticus*	*Features*
Neonate	Neonatal status epilepticus	—subtle, tonic, clonic, myoclonic, apneic, fragmentary
	Neonatal epilepsy syndromes	
	• early infantile epileptic encephalopathy	—tonic
	• neonatal myoclonic encephalopathy	—erratic, myoclonic
	• benign familial neonatal seizures	—clonic
Infant and Child	Febrile status epilepticus	—convulsive or hemiconvulsive (tonic-clonic)
	Infantile spasms (West syndromes)	—salaam attacks
	Status in childhood myoclonic syndromes)	—myoclonic ± absence
	Status in benign partial epilepsy	—complex partial seizures
Child and Adult	Tonic-clonic status epilepticus	—tonic-clonic,subtle
	Absence status epilepticus	—absence
	Epilepsia partialis continua	—simple partial
	Myoclonic status epilepticus in coma	—myoclonic
	Myoclonic status in epilepsy syndromes	—myoclonic
	Complex partial status epilepticus	—complex partial
	Status epilepticus in mental retardation	—atypical absence, tonic, minor motor

Adapted from classification by Shorvon SD, In: Shorvon SD, ed. Status epilepticus: its clinical features and treatment in children and adults. New York: Cambridge University Press, 1994.

specialist should not place all clinical emphasis on generalized tonic-clonic episodes, although this is the most common form in both children and adults.

At the neonatal end of our clinical spectrum, seizure episodes or "status epilepticus" have a poorly organized and polymorphic appearance[11], sometimes resembling isolated fragments of seizures seen in older patients. Subtle or minimal seizures are seen in both premature and term infants. These episodes take the form of jerks, spasms, and automatisms and may continue for hours to days. Tonic seizures in neonates are commonly seen in the premature infants. The motor form, which may be stimulus sensitive, is manifested by the rapid extension of all four limbs (or flexion of the upper and extension of the lower limbs), sometimes apnea, deviation of the eyes, and tremor of the extended limbs. Clonic seizures are rarely seen in premature babies. They may be either focal or multifocal, with random or organized jerks of the limbs that may spread or fluctuate.

In the infant and child, clonic or tonic-clonic episodes are most commonly seen and may be unilateral or focal—a characteristic feature not usually observed in older children[2]. Classically, the motor concomitants of these episodes have the same tonic and clonic features as isolated seizures, with an average duration of 90 seconds, shortening as the status progesses to less than 1 minute[12]. Other forms of status epilepticus in children, of critical care relevance, include epilepsia partialis continua, myoclonic status epilepticus in coma, and tonic status epilepticus seen in patients with mental retardation.

Epilepsia partialis continua is defined as spontaneous regular or irregular clonic twitching of cerebral cortical origin, sometimes aggravated by action or sensory stimuli, confined to one part of the body, and continuing for hours, days, or weeks[13]. This jerking can occur in clusters, and the distribution may vary over time with involvement of facial, palatal, and pharyngeal muscles.

A variety of seizures can occur in comatose patients, e.g., tonic-clonic, tonic, simple, and complex partial episodes. However, continuous myoclonia is the most typical and has been named myoclonic status epilepticus in coma, differentiating it from the myoclonic status seen in mental retardation, primary generalized epilepsy, and progressive myoclonic epilepsies. In this context the patients are usually comatose with seizure episodes involving irregular, asynchronous, small amplitude, repetitive myoclonic jerking of the facial muscles, and less consistently of the limbs[14–16].

Finally, in mentally retarded patients one frequent type of status which occurs comprises severe and repeated tonic seizures. The features are similar to isolated tonic attacks but may become transformed as the status progresses with lessening motor phenomena and marked autonomic features[12].

Etiology

In pediatric practice, status epilepticus may occur either in those known to have epilepsy or in those who have never had a seizure. Among epileptic children the incidence of status epilepticus may approach Lennox and Lennox's figure of 8%[17], and in 50 to 86% of such children it may be the presenting seizure[2,3,17–21]. However, considering the broader spectrum of status epilepticus in infants and children, various studies[2,3,17–25] indicate that causes differ widely **(Table 22.2)**, probably reflecting factors such as age distribution of the group studied and the referral base of the institution performing the analysis. Certain causes special to infants and children may be indicated by the age at presentation **(Table 22.3)**, e.g., neonatal or infancy, or the form of status epilepticus **(Table 22.4)**, e.g., infantile spasms, epilepsia partialis continua, and myoclonic status epilepticus in coma, and should be sought for appropriately. Also, fever may be the sole precipitating event for recurrent seizures and status epilepticus in children[2,3] and indeed accounts for approximately 25% of all such episodes.

A comparison of underlying causes among a number of recent studies indicates that the largest group with status

Table 22.2. Causes of Status Epilepticus

	Percentage of Cases by Selected Series					
Cause	*Janz[25] 1961*	*Aicardi and Chevrie[2] 1970*	*Rowan and Scott[22] 1970*	*Yager et al.[20] 1988*	*Phillips and Shanahan[21] 1989*	*Maytal et al.[3] 1989*
Symptomatic	—	14	4	15	14	6
Tumor	25	—	5	4	1	1
Trauma	24	1	26	0	5	4
Cerebrovascular	4	—	7	2	1	2
Infection	3	12	5	19	14	8
Congenital/asphyxia	3	27	16	23	14	23
Miscellaneous	7	—	2	4	6	9
Unknown	34	52 (28 febrile)	26 (5 febrile)	33 (21 febrile)	45 (29 febrile)	48 (24 febrile)
Total patients	95	239	43	52	218	193
Mortality	7%	11%	21%	6%	6%	4%

epilepticus consists of patients with known epilepsy who are suffering from an acute exacerbation of seizures. A second large group is nonepileptic patients with acute CNS lesions precipitating status epilepticus. In these patients, a variety of cerebrovascular diseases, CNS infections, head trauma, neoplasms, anoxic metabolic disorders, and toxins may precipitate status epilepticus (Figures 22.1 to 22.3).

Aicardi and Chevrie[2] found that in their group of 239 children, approximately half of the status epilepticus episodes were idiopathic, and half were caused by definable precipitants. In the latter patients, slightly more than half of the episodes were due to acute injury (e.g., meningitis, encephalitis, and dehydration) and slightly less than half were seen in children with prior cerebral damage. Of the 126 children with no discernable cause for their status epilepticus, more than half of the episodes were associated with fever. The highest incidence of fever-associated episodes occurred in children between the ages of 6 months and 3 years. In such a context as this, with significant likelihood of finding underlying disease, Janz[25] has stated that an episode of status epilepticus is presumably always the expression of organic brain damage, and he has suggested that patients exhibiting status epilepticus should have a thorough diagnostic work-up to identify underlying brain disease. **Table 22.2** supports this approach, and it seems reasonable that an episode necessitating admission to an intensive care unit warrants complete investigation for specific causes (see later section).

PROGNOSIS

Mortality

Before 1960, mortality rates as high as 50% were reported after convulsive status epilepticus. Current mortality of tonic-clonic status epilepticus in children is in the range of 4 to 6% (**Table 22.2**) [26]. In cases with documented underlying causes (trauma, tumor, infections, etc.), it cannot be determined whether mortality is related to the underly-

Table 22.3. Potential "Nonidiopathic" Causes of Status Epilepticus According to Age at Presentation

	Newborn	*First 1–2 Months*	*Later Infancy and Childhood*
Acute insult	Hypoxic-ischemic	CNS infection	CNS infection
	CNS infection	Subdural hematoma	Intracranial hemorrhage
	Intracranial hemorrhage	—	Anoxia
Genetic and Metabolic	Hypoglycemia	Hypoglycemia	Hypoglycemia
	Hypernatremia	Hypernatremia	Hypernatremia
	Hyponatremia	Hyponatremia	Hyponatremia
	Hypocalcemia	Hypocalcemia	Hypocalcemia
	Hypomagnesemia	—	—
	Hyperbilirubinemia	—	—
	Organic acidemia	Organic acidemia	Lysosomal defects
	Urea cycle defects	Urea cycle defects	Uremia
	Nonketotic hyperglycinemia	Phenylketonuria	Liver failure
	Congenital lactic acidosis	Riley-Day syndrome	—
	Pyridoxine dependency	—	—
Malformation	Neuronal migration defect	Sturge-Weber syndrome	—
	Chromosome anomaly	Neurofibromatosis	—
		Tuberous sclerosis	—
Other	Toxins	Cocaine toxicity	Febrile convulsion
	Drugs	—	—
	Narcotic withdrawal	—	—
	Epilptic encephalopathies	—	—

Table 22.4. Causes of Specific Forms of Status Epilepticus

Infantile Spasms	*Epilepsia Partialis Continua*	*Myoclonic Status in Coma*
Cerebral malformation	*Brain tumors*	*Hypoxic-ischemic encephalopathy*
—neuronal migration defect	—astrocytoma	—cardiopulmonary bypass
—neurocutaneous syndrome	—oligodendroglioma	—post resuscitation syndrome
		—carbon monoxide poisoning
Genetic metabolic disease	*CNS infection*	—CO_2 narcosis
—phenylketonuria	—brain abscess	—subarachnoid hemorrhage
—nonketotic hyperglycinemia	—tuberculosis	
—pyridoxine dependency	—viral encephalitis	*Toxic-metabolic encephalopathy*
—histidinemia	—cysticercosis	—hepatic failure
—hyperornithinemia-hyperammonemia		—uremia and dialysis syndrome
—homocitrullinemia	*Vascular*	—hyponatremia
—maple syrup urine diseae	—cortical vein thrombosis	—heavy metal poisoning
—leucine-sensitive hypoglycemia	—malformation	—drug toxicity with tricyclic antidepressants, anticonvulsants, penicillin, and opiates
Degenerative disease	*Trauma*	—nonketotic hyperglycinemia
—*Leigh's encephalopathy*	—posttraumatic cyst	
—*leucodystrophies*	—chronic subdural	*Injury*
—*Alpers' disease (neuronal degeneration)*	—focal gliosis	—posttraumatic
—*Sandhoff's disease*		—heat stroke
—*Tay-Sachs disease*		—lightning
Perinatal or acute insult		*Inflammatory*
—hypoxia-ischemia		—viral encephalitis
—hemorrhage		—subacute sclerosing panencephalitis
—infection		—postinfectious encephalomyelitis
—trauma		—opportunistic CNS infection
		—progressive leukoencephalopathy

CNS, central nervous system.

ing process, the episode of status epilepticus and its secondary systemic consequences, therapy, or even lack of therapy. In the 1970 pediatric series of Aicardi and Chevrie[2], half of the 11% mortality was attributed to a cerebral lesion. A better prognosis was indicated by a later follow-up study in 1984 of 482 children with seizures starting between 1 and 12 months of age: 66 had status, of whom only 3% died in the follow-up period[27]. In 1989 Maytal et al.[3] described 193 children of whom only 7 died, all of whom had acute or progressive cerebral insults. While it may be suggested that "status was now not as dangerous as once taught"[28] because of current prompt and appropriate treatment dramatically reducing mortality, Aicardi and Chevrie have warned against any complacency in dealing with what remains a medical emergency[29].

In 1989 Phillips and Shanahan also reported a study of childhood status epilepticus[21], which had been designed to update Aicardi and Chevrie's data from 1970[2]. Of 218

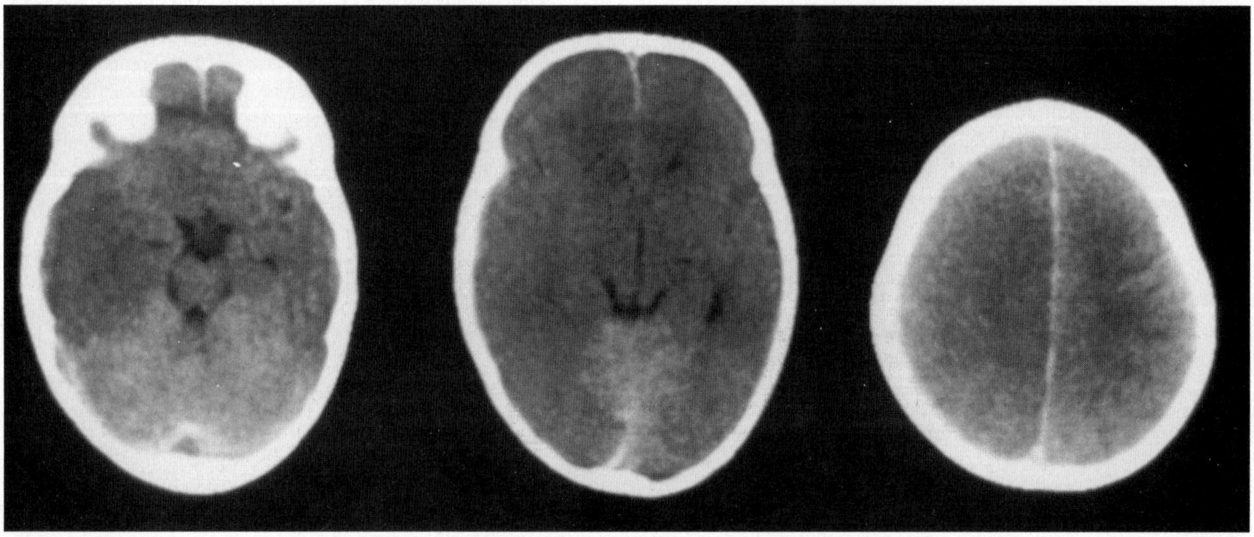

Figure 22.1. Cranial computed tomography (CT) scan of a 5-month-old infant with an encephalitic illness who presented with status epilepticus of at least 60 minutes in duration. The scan shows diffuse supratentorial edema.

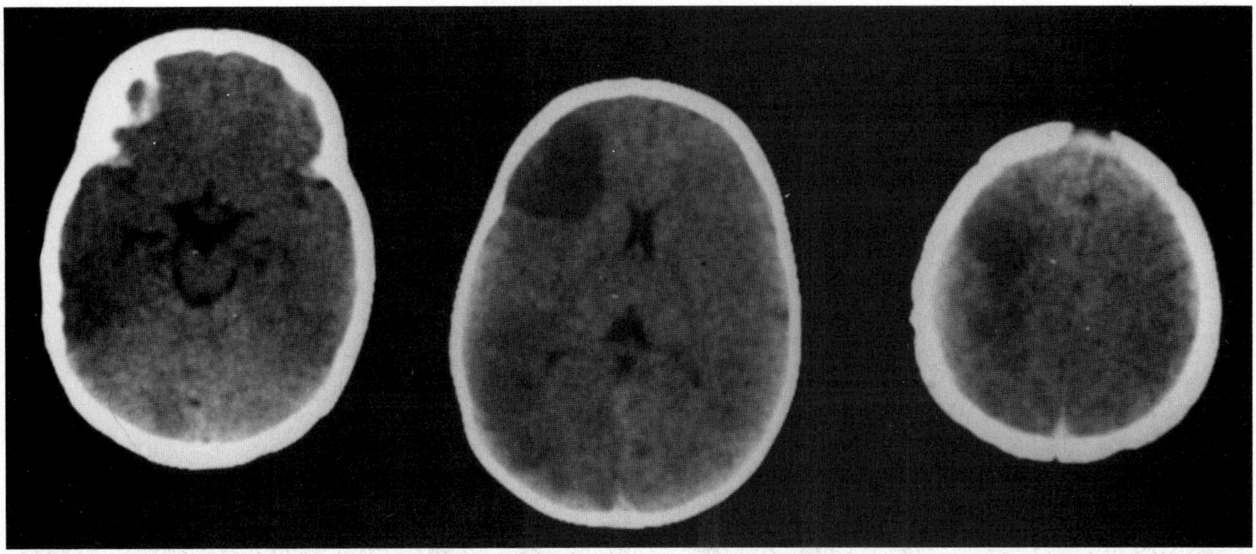

Figure 22.2. Cranial CT scan of a 4-month-old infant with viral encephalitis complicated by shock, hypoxia, and status epilepticus. The scan shows bilateral supratentorial low density most marked in the right middle cerebral artery distribution.

episodes of status seen on a pediatric intensive care unit, 13 ended fatally. Three children died within 24 hours of presentation and the other 10 in the subsequent days or weeks. In 11 children there was an underlying causal cerebral insult, and one child died with an unidentified cerebral encephalopathy. Importantly, there was only one death among the 99 episodes of idiopathic status epilepticus.

Neurologic Sequelae

In 1970 Rowan and Scott[22] found that 26% of their patients had neurologic sequelae seemingly related to status epilepticus, and more recently (1988) Yager et al.[20] reported a figure of 28%. However, an estimation of neurologic morbidity directly attributable to an episode of status epilepticus is fraught with difficulties. We often observe a multifactorial process; therefore, trying to separate factors or apportion morbidity to the type and duration of status, independent of underlying cause and disease time course, consequent physiologic derangements, and prescribed therapy is almost impossible[6,9]. For instance, Oxbury and Whitty[30] found deterioration in 5 of 86 patients, 3 of whom had encephalitis that presumably contributed substantially to their outcome.

Aicardi and Chevrie[2] found that in children who had seizures prior to their episode of status epilepticus, there were changes in type of seizure activity after status epilepticus that were "associated with organic damage," which is in keeping with electroclinical observations in adults[31], infants[9], and children[6]. Of previously normal children in their series, 20% showed permanent neurologic deficits (e.g., hemiplegia), and 33% had mental retardation after status epilepticus. The disability was greatest in patients under the age of 40 months, and 78% of infants under 6

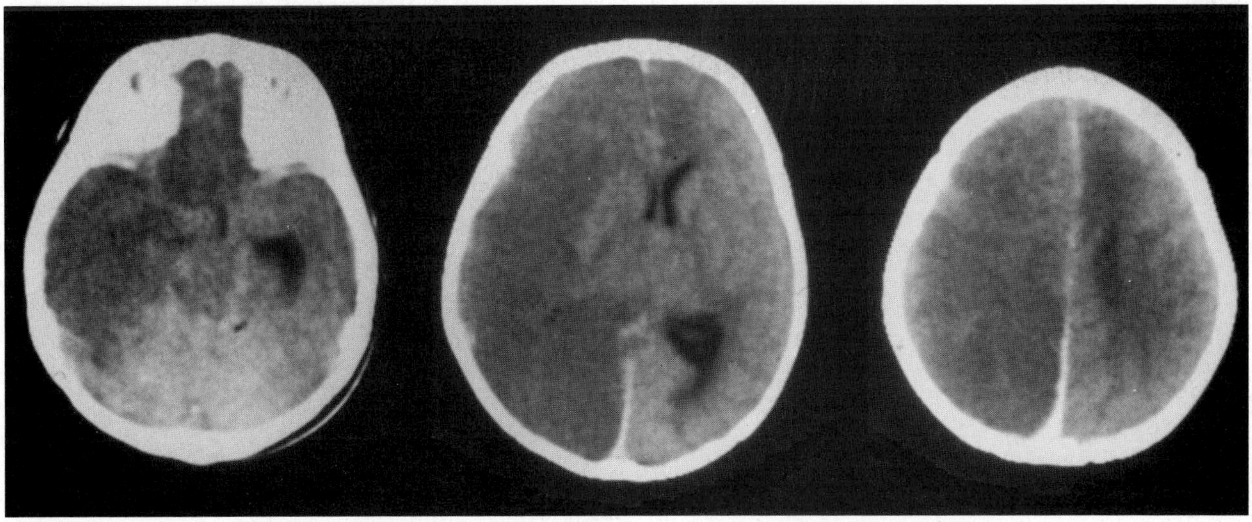

Figure 22.3. A 6-month-old child after acute onset of coma and focal status epilepticus. The CT scan shows diffuse low density of the right hemisphere with midline shift and dilatation of the left lateral ventricle.

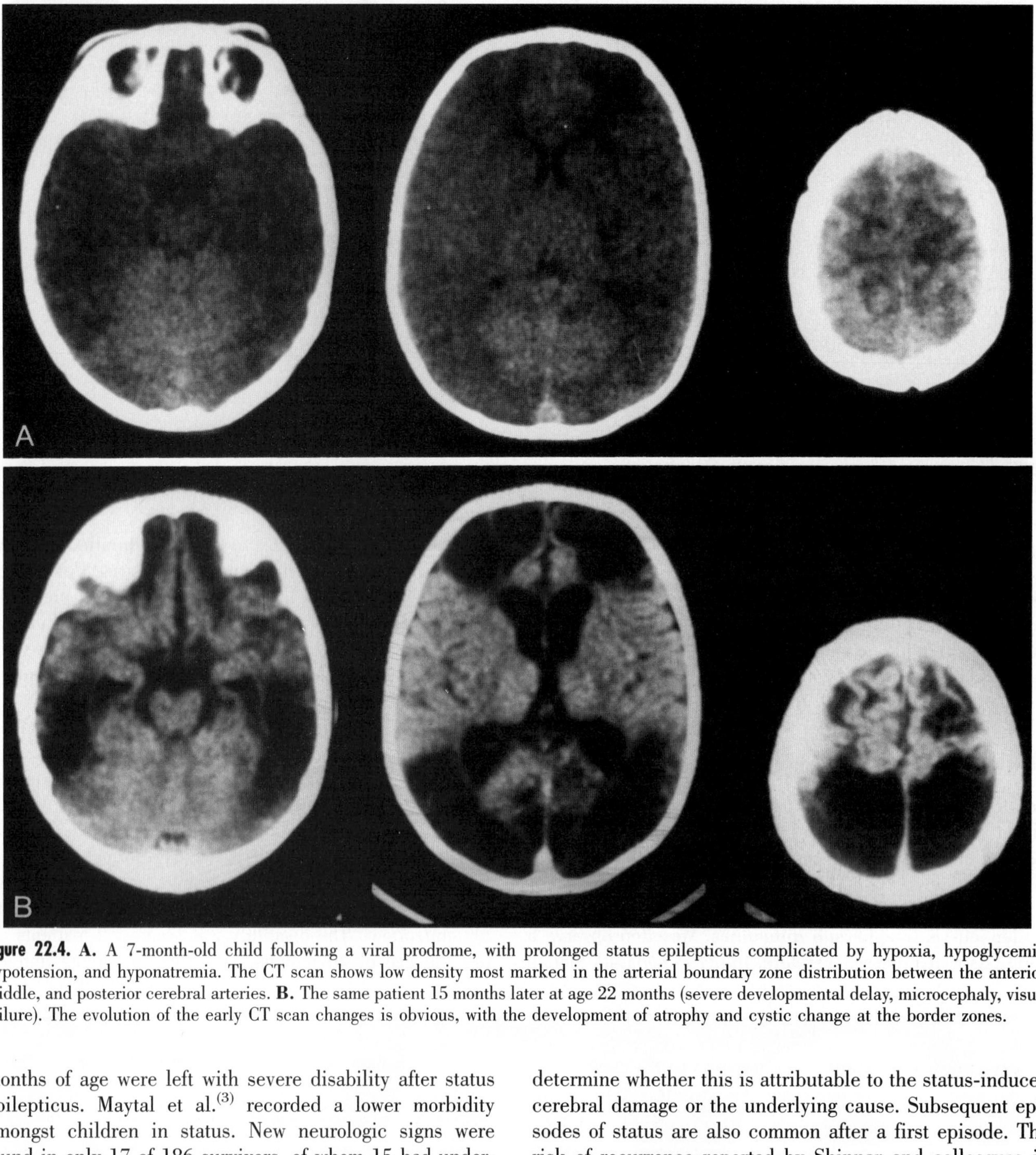

Figure 22.4. **A.** A 7-month-old child following a viral prodrome, with prolonged status epilepticus complicated by hypoxia, hypoglycemia, hypotension, and hyponatremia. The CT scan shows low density most marked in the arterial boundary zone distribution between the anterior, middle, and posterior cerebral arteries. **B.** The same patient 15 months later at age 22 months (severe developmental delay, microcephaly, visual failure). The evolution of the early CT scan changes is obvious, with the development of atrophy and cystic change at the border zones.

months of age were left with severe disability after status epilepticus. Maytal et al.[3] recorded a lower morbidity amongst children in status. New neurologic signs were found in only 17 of 186 survivors, of whom 15 had underlying disease that could have contributed to the new deficits. Although there are insufficient data to determine whether these historical differences in morbidity are due to study selection bias or better treatment, it is the authors' impression that with current vigorous management, most episodes of status epilepticus in "normal" children can be controlled and that neither mortality nor morbidity is a necessary consequence of status epilepticus. However, it should be remembered that the underlying or "triggering" encephalopathy or specific developmental vulnerability[32,33] may be of particular relevance (Fig. 22.4).

Epilepsy is a common sequel to initial status epilepticus and may be as high as 77%[2], although it is impossible to determine whether this is attributable to the status-induced cerebral damage or the underlying cause. Subsequent episodes of status are also common after a first episode. The risk of recurrence reported by Shinnar and colleagues in 1992[34] was 16 (17%) of a cohort of 95 children for a second episode, and 5 (5%) for further attacks. In relation to premorbid state, the recurrence risk was about 50% in those with prior neurologic abnormalites and about 3% in the neurologically normal at the time of the first episode.

Motor problems following an episode of status epilepticus include hemiplegia, diplegia, and extrapyramidal and cerebellar disturbance[2]. The status-induced hemiconvulsion-hemiplegia (HH) and hemiconvulsion-hemiplegia-epilepsy (HHE) syndromes seen in children, typically between 6 months and 2 years of age, rarely occurs when status is of short duration. Most of these patients (80 to 100%) go on to develop a permanent epileptic condition.

Table 22.5. Medical Complications of Status Epilepticus

Interictal coma
Cumulative anoxia
cerebral and systemic
Cardiovascular complications
tachycardia, bradycardia
cardiac arrest
hypertension
cardiac failure, hypotension, cardiogenic shock
Respiratory system failure
apnea
Cheyne-Stokes breathing
tachypnea
neurogenic pulmonary edema
aspiration, pneumonia
pulmonary embolism
respiratory acidosis
cyanosis
Renal failure
oliguria, uremia
acute tubular necrosis
rhabdomyolysis
lower nephron necrosis
Autonomic system disturbance
hyperpyrexia
excessive sweating, vomiting
hypersecretion (salivary, tracheobronchial)
airway obstruction
Metabolic and biochemical abnormalities
acidosis (metabolic, lactate)
anoxemia
hypernatremia, hyponatremia
hyperkalemia
hypoglycemia
hepatic failure
dehydration
acute pancreatitis
Infections
pulmonary
bladder
skin
Other
disseminated intravascular coagulation
multiple organ system dysfunction
fractures
thrombophlebitis

Systemic Complications

Systemic changes and complications of status epilepticus are protean with the involvement of all organ systems **(Table 22.5)** (35–37). Of additional importance in relation to etiology and specific therapy is the observation that leukocytosis is a frequent finding, occurring in approximately 67% of episodes(24,38), even in the absence of infection(36), potentially resulting in some diagnostic confusion. Also, there may be minimal elevation in cerebrospinal fluid (CSF) white blood cell (WBC) count attributable to status epilepticus alone. Woody et al.(38) found more than 5 WBCs/mm^3 in 5 of 20 CSF specimens obtained from children with status epilepticus who had no evidence of CNS infection; Dunn(24) found CSF WBCs between 8 and 25 cells/mm^3 in 6 of 64 similar children.

The systemic derangements listed in **Table 22.5** undoubtedly contribute to the ultimate mortality seen in patients with status epilepticus. Avoiding these is imperative. Early recognition may be aided by considering findings from adult human studies of generalized tonic-clonic status epilepticus, which have reported a distinct natural history with predictable effects(31,35,36,39). As the duration of status epilepticus progresses, there is systemic alteration, with worsening of general clinical state associated with an evolution of motor phenomena, and a specific sequence of electroencephalographic (EEG) findings. The final stages are characterized by respiratory compromise, hypotension, hyperthermia, and ongoing epileptiform paroxysms without motor accompaniments. During this evolving picture, neurologic morbidity and mortality are seemingly related to the combination and interaction of the following processes:

1. Damage to the CNS caused by the acute insult precipitating status epilepticus
2. Systemic stress from repeated generalized tonic-clonic convulsions
3. Injury from repetitive epileptic discharges within the CNS

Further comprehensive description with a more detailed understanding of the phenomenology of status epilepticus has been gleaned from animal studies and is discussed in the following section on pathophysiology (see below).

PATHOPHYSIOLOGY AND EXPERIMENTAL STATUS EPILEPTICUS

In the experimental setting, when studying phenomena and pathology akin to clinical status epilepticus, models have been achieved by using intact animals. However, it should be remembered that in an effort to reduce and simplify the experimental system, certain pathologic, temporal, and developmental factors that contribute to the familiar clinical "syndromes" seen in our practice (see above) may not necessarily be inherent to the models used **(Table 22.6)**(40–42).

In the experimental models, the pathophysiology of status epilepticus involves a complex interaction of multiple

Table 22.6. Experimental Animal Models of Status Epilepticus

Model	*Precipitant*	*Proposed Mechanism*
Chemical		
Enhances excitatory	Pentylenetetrazol	Antagonizes GABA-mediated inhibition
	Kainate	Stimulates excitatory receptor
Block inhibitory	Picrotoxin, penicillin, bicuculline	Block effect of GABA at receptor
	Allylglycine	Block GABA synthesis
Block electrolyte transport	Ouabain	Inhibit Na/K-ATPase[a]
Electrical	Electroconvulsive stimulation	
Genetic	Light or auditory stimulus	

[a] ATPase, adenosine 5′-triphosphatase.

systemic stress changes as well as intrinsic brain effects due to the status epilepticus itself, with the latter being manifested by inadequate cortical oxygen metabolism and parenchymal neurotoxic effects. An overview of the systemic alterations, physiology, and cerebral metabolic and neuropathologic events associated with experimental status epilepticus is schematically summarized in Figure 22.5[43]. In several models there are distinct stages and phenomena, many of which bear resemblance to observations in adult and pediatric clinical studies.

Motor and Electroencephalographic Events

In some models of convulsive status epilepticus, there is an evolution of motor activity[44], starting with generalized convulsions, followed by myoclonic jerking and ending with "electromechanical dissociation"[35,45] characterized by abnormal EEG discharges without any motor correlates. On the EEG (Fig. 22.6), the occurrence of discrete electrographic seizures with spiking ceasing simultaneously in all channels marks the beginning of status epilepticus. This is followed by a brief period of postictal low-voltage slow activity. After several minutes the distinct seizure offset is no longer seen. Instead, irregular 1 to 3 Hz spike and wave activity follows rapid spiking, with spike amplitude increasing rapidly over time. Spiking eventually becomes relatively constant at a high amplitude and rate of occurrence, sometimes interspersed with brief flat periods. When status epilepticus is induced by lithium and pilocarpine, continuous spiking persists for 1 to 2

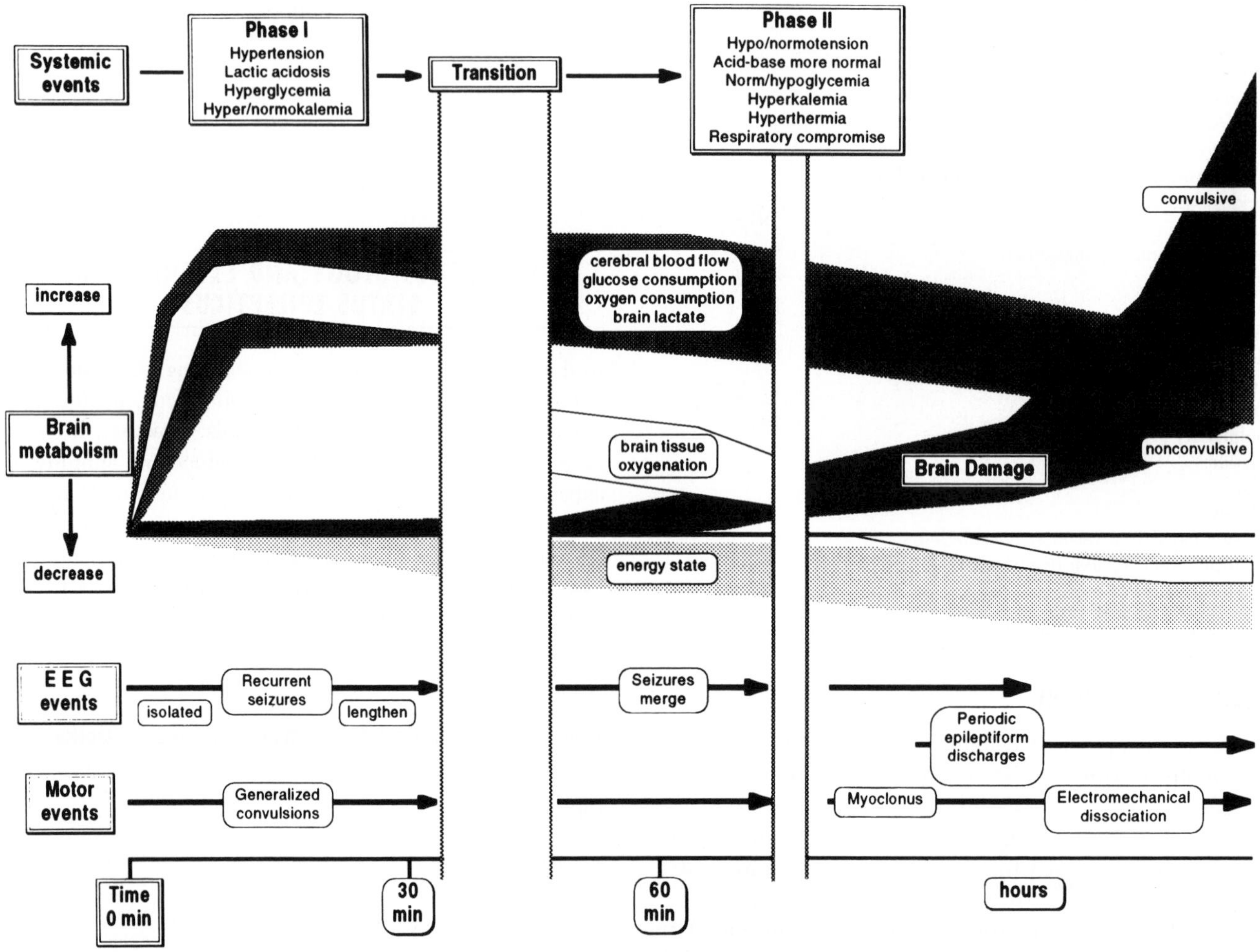

Figure 22.5. Schematic overview of systemic alterations, neurophysiology, and cerebral metabolic and neuropathologic events associated with experimental status epilepticus (see text). After the initiation of status epilepticus, systemic changes *(upper portion)* pass through an initial phase (phase I less than 30 minutes, see Table 22.2), followed by a period of transition culminating in phase II, characterized by severe systemic distress. Over this period, motor and EEG events *(lower portion)* demonstrate a sequence from generalized convulsions associated with recurrent EEG seizures progressing to a merging of EEG discharges and then a "dissociated" period with lack of motor activity associated with repetitive or periodic epiliptiform discharges (see Fig. 22.4). The *middle portion* crudely summarizes the studies of brain metabolism. In the initial period, there is an increase in cerebral blood flow, glucose consumption, oxygen consumption, and brain tissue oxygenation with increased brain lactate production. There is no deficit in brain energy state until later when parenchymal oxygenation falls (see Figs. 22.5–22.10). Associated with this time course is the development of brain damage. (Modified from Lothman E: The biochemical basis and pathophysiology of status epilepticus, Neurology 1990;40(S2):13.)

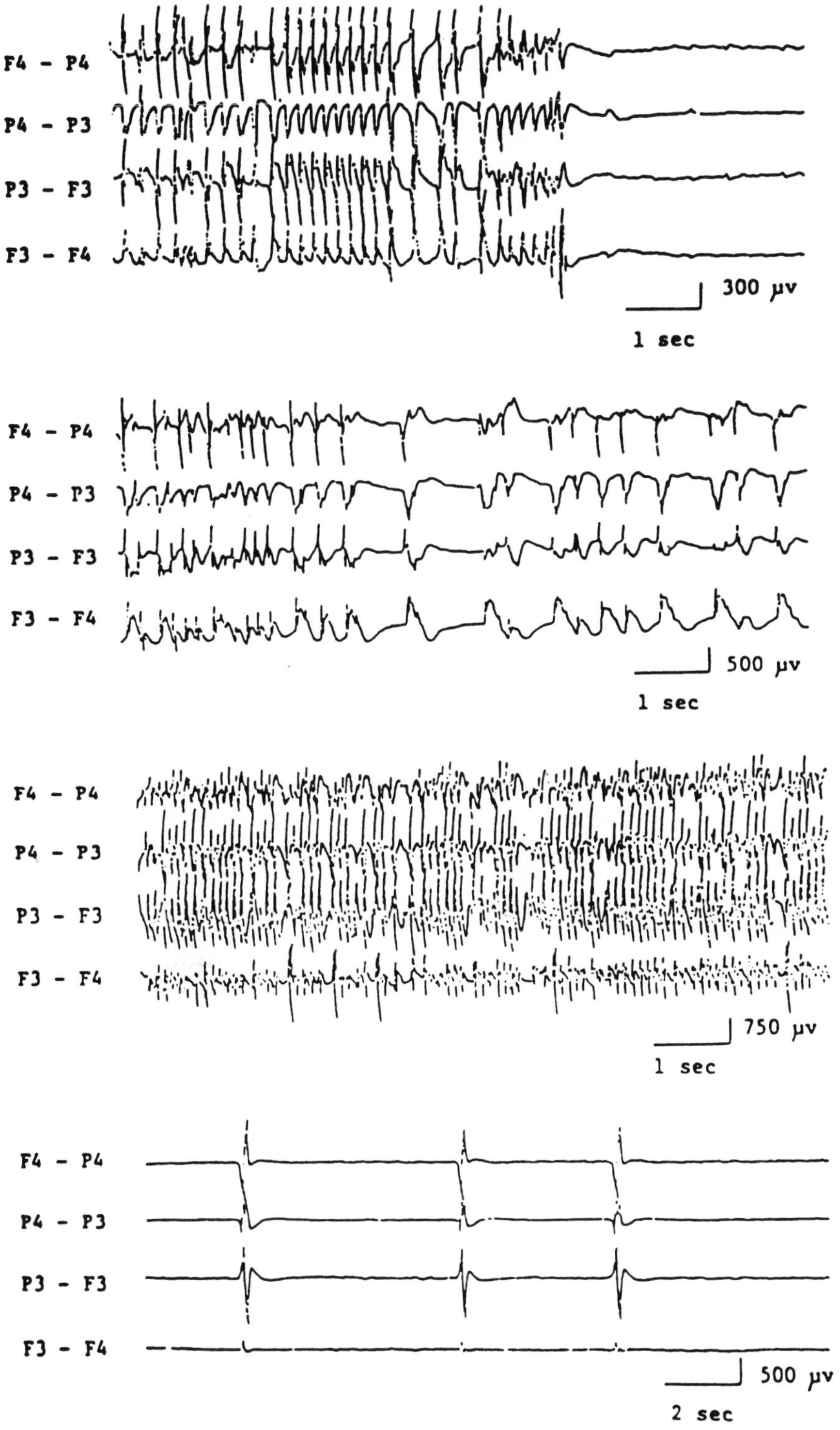

Figure 22.6. Progressive changes in EEG pattern during status epilepticus induced by lithium and pilocarpine. *Upper trace:* EEG showing discrete electrographic seizures, recorded 1 minute after onset of status epilepticus. *Second trace:* EEG showing waxing and waning epiliptiform activity, recorded 10 minutes after onset of status epilepticus. *Third trace:* continuous high-amplitude, rapid-spiking EEG recorded 34 minutes after onset of status epilepticus. *Lower trace:* EEG showing periodic epileptiform discharges on a relatively flat background, recorded 6 hours 6 minutes after onset of status epilepticus. (From Walton NY, Trieman DM. Response of status epilepticus induced by lithium and pilocarpine to treatment with diazepam. Exp Neurol 1988;101:267.)

hours. After this, periodic epileptic discharges separated by periods of lower amplitude activity begin to appear in runs lasting several seconds. These discharges gradually increase in frequency and duration of occurrence until the animal dies.

Systemic and Organ-System Effects

In patients, autonomic changes can be prominent. They include cardiac tachyarrythmias, hypertension, apnea, pupillary dilatation, hypersecretion, and sweating. In addition, respiration may be compromised by excessive salivation and tracheobronchial secretions. A more detailed analysis of the status-associated physiologic changes was first undertaken by Meldrum et al.[46–49]. In their baboon model of convulsive status epilepticus using systemic bicuculline as the inducing agent, two phases of systemic alteration were identified and characterized by (a) changes in hemodynamic state, (b) biochemistry, and (c) temperature control (**Table 22.7,** Figure 22.7).

Table 22.7. Time-Related Systemic Complications of Status Epilepticus

Parameter	*Phase I Early (<30 Min)*	*Phase II Late (>30 Min)*	*Complications Observed*
Blood pressure	increase	decrease	hypotension
Arterial oxygen	decrease	decrease	hypoxia
Arterial CO_2	increase	variable	increased ICP
Serum pH	decrease	decrease	acidosis
Temperature	increase by 1°C	increase by 2°C	fever
Autonomic activity	increase	increase	arrhythmias
Lung fluids	increase	increase	atelectasis
Serum potassium	increase or normal	increase	arrhythmias
Serum CPK	normal	increase	renal failure
Cerebral blood flow	increase 900%	increase 200%	cerebral bleed
$CMRO_2$	increase 300%	increase 300%	ischemia

CO_2—carbon dioxide, ICP—intracranial pressure, CPK—creatine phosphokinase, $CMRO_2$—cerebral metabolic rate for oxygen

Arterial and Cerebral Venous Blood Pressures

At the onset of seizure activity and during the first 25 minutes (phase I), both arterial and central venous pressures rose dramatically with each convulsion, with arterial systolic pressures often over 200 mm Hg. Within an hour the

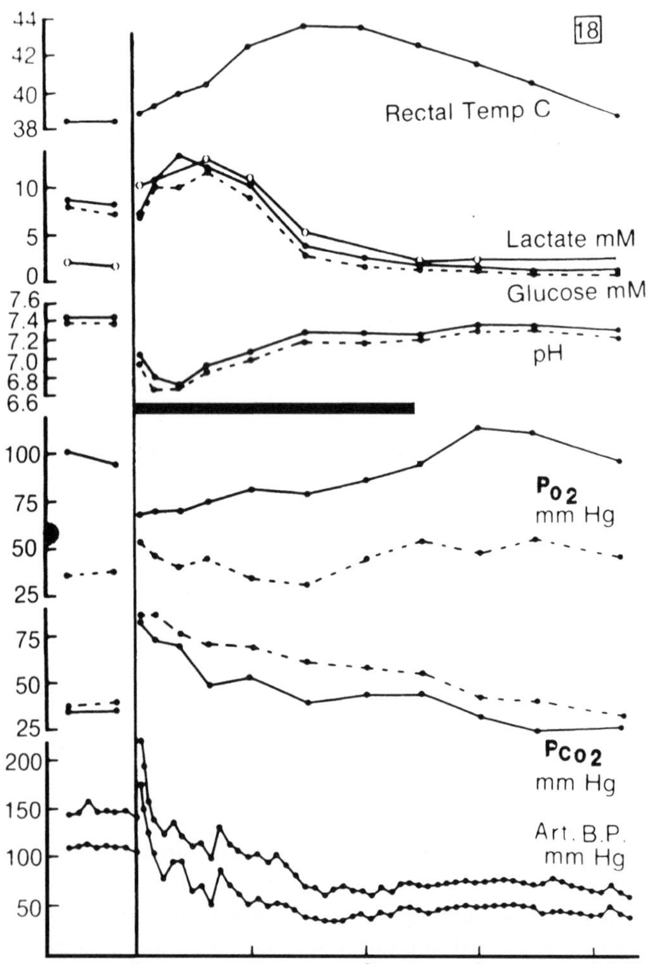

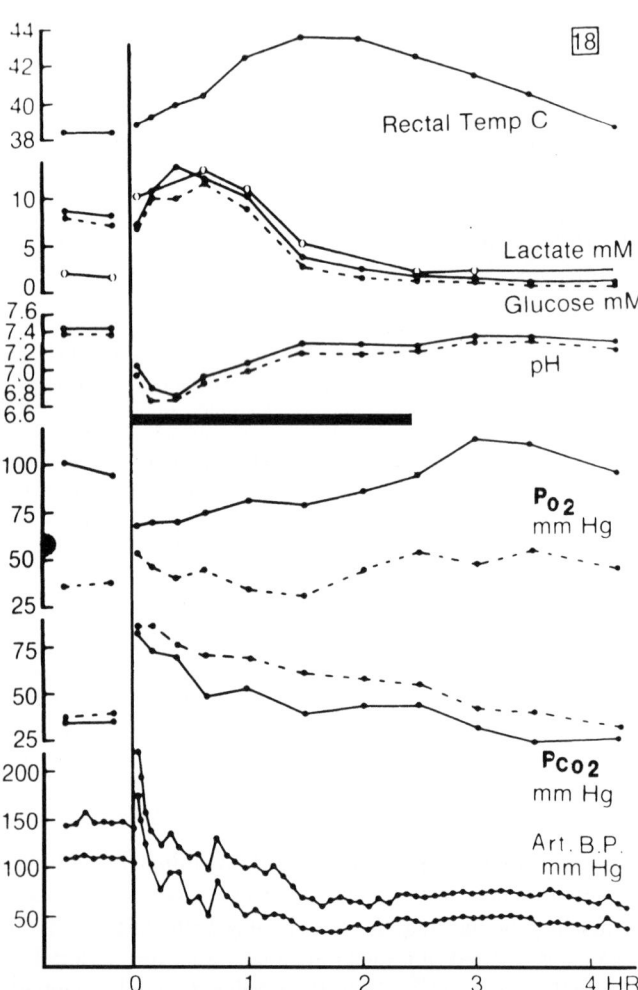

Figure 22.7. Physiologic changes during status epilepticus in baboons. *Vertical line,* injection of bicuculline (0.5 mg/kg) at time zero; *open circles,* lactate; *dashed lines,* venous values; *horizontal bar,* generalized seizure activity lasting 148 minutes. (From Meldrum BS, Horton RW. Physiology of status epilepticus in primates. Arch Neurol 1973;28:8, copyright 1973, American Medical Association.)

blood pressure returned to normal or subnormal levels, but the mean arterial pressure did not drop below the level considered adequate for cerebral perfusion (i.e., 60 mm Hg). Since the initial rise in blood pressure can be blocked by phentolamine hydrochloride, it is presumably due to massive sympathetic discharge. Such findings have been further examined by Simon et al.[50,51] and Benowitz et al.[52] in a sheep bicuculline model. Status epilepticus was found to cause a rise in circulating norepinephrine and epinephrine concentrations, indicating, respectively, adrenergic stimulation and adrenomedullary activation. However, the later decline of blood pressure (during phase II) despite sympathetic activation has yet to be explained. Likely mechanisms include desensitization of vascular adrenergic receptors[53] and/or hypovolemia, produced by intense vasoconstriction with movement of vascular fluid into extracellular spaces[54].

In the baboon model, cerebral venous pressure also increased dramatically (Fig. 22.8) due to cerebral vasodilatation, increases in intrathoracic and right atrial pressure due to myoclonus, and increases in cerebral blood flow. The increase in cerebral venous pressure has been shown to be lessened by general anesthesia, which reduces the contribution of myoclonus and "back pressure" from the thorax. Measured intracranial pressure may exceed cerebral venous pressure[55], suggesting the occurrence of sudden cerebral vasodilatation. In dogs subjected to electroshock seizures the combination of these events have led to punctate hemorrhages[55].

Late in status epilepticus, while arterial blood and cerebral venous pressures return to normal or even hypotensive levels, cerebral blood flow continues to be higher than normal. (In animals, cerebral blood flow as high as 900% of normal has been measured during status epilepticus[56,57]). However, there may be differences between models. For instance, the magnitude of the increase in cerebral blood flow is progressively smaller, as seizures continue in models using sustained seizures[56–60]. Although the increase in cerebral blood flow is presumably compensatory for the increased metabolic rate of the brain, the precise mechanism that contributes to the increased flow rates remains to be determined[61]. The involvement of metabolic factors such as prostaglandins, local acidosis, ionic flux (both calcium and potassium), and adenosine has been suggested[62,63]. In

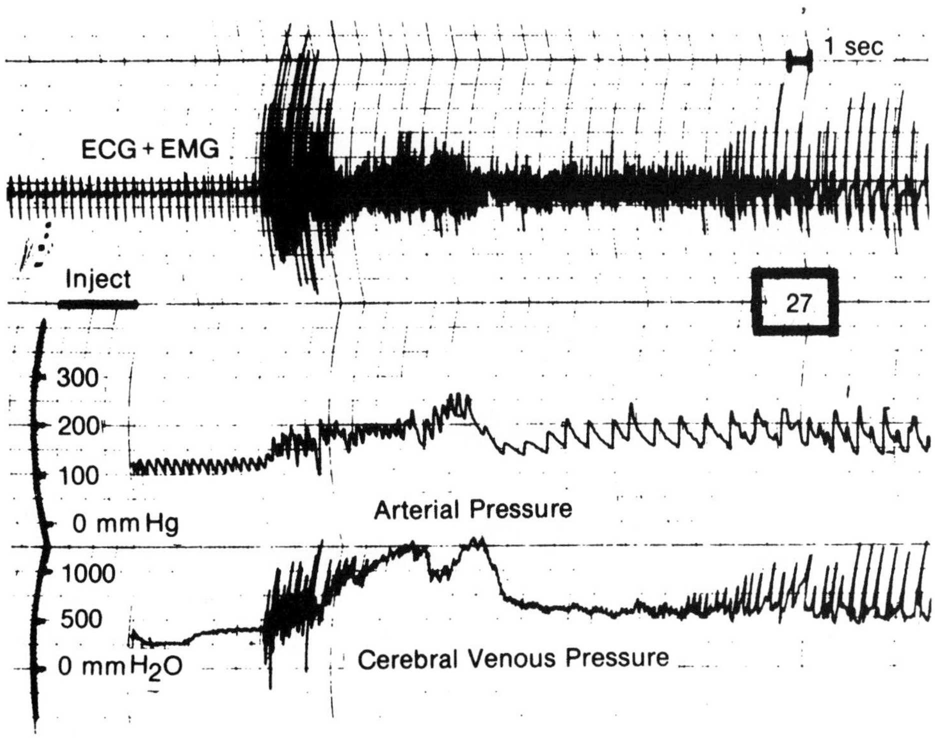

Figure 22.8. Polygraph records showing rise in arterial and cerebral venous pressure at onset of seizure in a baboon. Electrocardiogram plus electromyogram *(ECG + EMG)* is recorded between electrodes in the left arm and chest wall. *Horizontal bar (inject)*, intravenous injection of bicuculline (0.4 mg/kg). After 3 seconds of irregular generalized jerks, tonic flexor spasm developed. Highest mean arterial and cerebral venous pressures occurred during the first 6 seconds of this spasm. Subsequently, bradycardia developed, associated with widening of pulse pressure. (From Meldrum BS, Horton RW. Physiology of status epilepticus in primates. Arch Neurol 1973;28:7, copyright 1973, American Medical Association.)

addition, activation of vasodilator nervous pathways either extrinsic to the brain, as proposed by Meldrum et al.[57], or intrinsic[64,65] could be responsible for the seizure-induced hyperemia. Of developmental interest is the observation that in some neonatal models, immature cortical vessels appear unable to respond with an increased cerebral blood flow commensurate with the increased metabolic rate[66]. In human infants the situation may be more complex, given their propensity to develop germinal matrix rupture and intraventricular hemorrhage, which in itself may be exacerbated by any cerebral hyperemia[67].

Blood Gases

During the early phase of status epilepticus, changes occurred in arterial blood gas values (Fig. 22.7). Within 15 to 20 minutes the blood pH dropped dramatically to an average low of 6.61 on the arterial side. Serum bicarbonate was reduced to an average low of 5.4 mEq/liter. The arterial PCO_2 was increased, exacerbating the acidosis, and cerebral venous PCO_2 was increased to an average value of 68 mm Hg. Finally, arterial oxygen tension dropped to approximately 70 to 80 mm Hg, and cerebral venous increased PO_2 slightly. Despite this, the arterial oxygen was never low enough to be expected to cause hypoxic damage and over time gradually improved.

Such blood gas changes could exacerbate other physiologic events. Studies dealing with cortical oxygen metabolism (discussed later in the text) are highly suggestive of inadequate oxygen delivery. The drop in pH (as low as 6.51 in cerebral venous blood) would shift the oxyhemoglobin dissociation curve, reducing the actual oxygen content. The cerebral venous oxygen content, which was often less than 1 ml/dl[46], indicates that maximum oxygen extraction was occurring in these animals. The increase in carbon dioxide may contribute to cerebral vasodilatation, and this, in combination with increased metabolic activity due to seizures, probably leads to a maximally dilated, nonautoregulated cerebral vascular bed. This would be expected to cause significant cerebral edema, prolonged intracranial hypertension, and ultimately, if brain edema is severe, regional cerebral ischemia. Indeed, cerebral herniation has been observed in this animal model[47].

Finally, in some animals, pulmonary edema and hypoxia presumably of neurogenic origin have been shown to develop[50]. These changes, along with pulmonary vascular changes[68], occur relatively late in status epilepticus, at a time when arterial hypotension occurs. This may be an additional mechanism for inadequate cortical oxygen delivery late in status epilepticus.

Glucose, Lactate, and Electrolyte Levels

In the baboon bicuculline model, serum glucose increased initially and later dropped to normal or hypoglycemic levels. Meldrum and Horten[46] and Blennow et al.[69] even observed that seizure activity was sometimes increased or resumed when the hypoglycemia was treated, suggesting that hypoglycemia could eventually limit seizure activity. Early hypoglycemia was not seen in baboons with status epilepticus incited by allylglycine[70], but late in status epilepticus severe hypoglycemia predominated.

Arterial lactate rises immediately when status epilepticus is induced, reaching levels as high as 11.6 mEq/liter within minutes; this eventually returns to normal (Fig. 22.7). Measurement of arterial and cerebral venous blood suggests net uptake of lactate by the brain, which supports the notion that lactate production results from tonic-clonic mani-

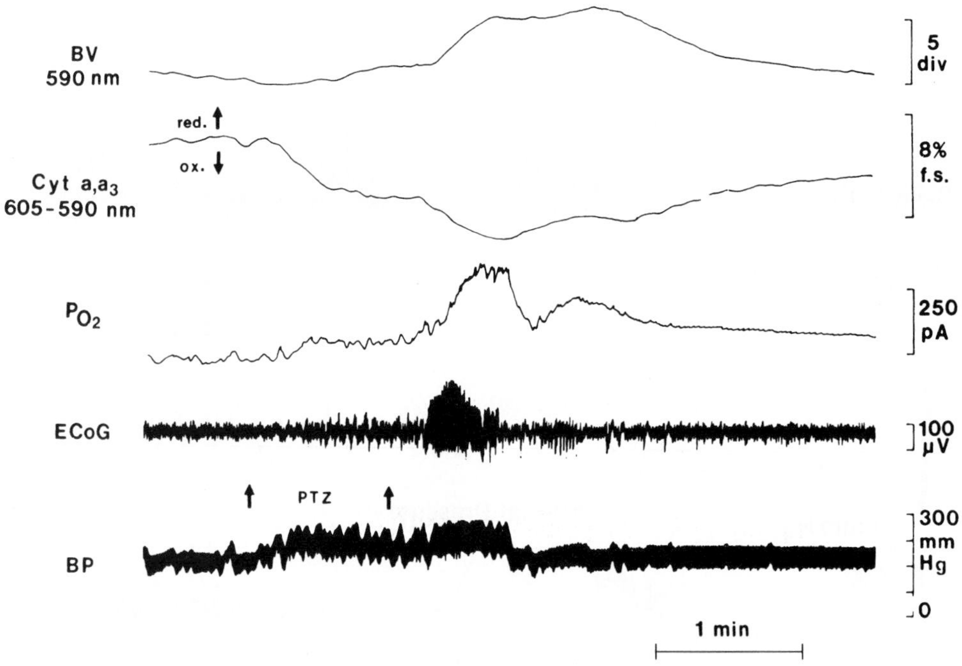

Figure 22.9. Changes in cerebral blood volume *(BV)*, cytochrome *(Cyt* a,a_3*)* redox level, PO_2, and blood pressure *(BP)* accompanying an initial seizure of a series showing onset of responses during electrocorticogram *(ECoG)* activation prior to the ECoG burst. *PTZ*, pentylenetetrazol. (From Kreisman NR, LaManna JC, Rosenthal M, Sick TJ. Oxidative metabolic responses with recurrent seizures in rat cerebral cortex: role of systemic factors. Brain Res 1981;218:179.)

festations of status epilepticus. (Neuromuscular blockade and mechanical ventilation are associated with negligible systemic acidosis[48], although serum lactate was not measured in the study). Direct measurement of brain lactate during status epilepticus in paralyzed rats has suggested intracerebral lactate production and accumulation[49]. A possible explanation for this difference is that measurement of arteriovenous lactate difference may not be accurate at the very high cerebral blood flow rates seen during status epilepticus.

These lactate metabolic changes could also be explained by the following. During early status epilepticus, cerebral glucose consumption has been noted to greatly exceed cerebral oxygen consumption (stoichiometrically)[71,72], and by 1 hour it gradually decreases to equal oxygen consumption. Anaerobic glycolysis is required and lactate is produced. When the glucose consumption rate drops to match oxygen consumption, lactate production decreases, a fact consistent with the finding that cerebral lactate levels stop increasing after the first hour of status epilepticus[49]. In the nonparalyzed animal, muscle lactate production greatly exceeds cerebral production and hence obscures lactic acid alterations stemming from CNS metabolism.

Changes in sodium, potassium, and urea nitrogen were also noted by Meldrum and Horten[46]. In the baboons, the most significant change during seizure activity was hyperkalemia, with levels near 9 mEq/liter. This was believed to be the cause of death in at least one experiment. Presumably during the tonic-clonic activity, potassium is released from muscle, and this is further exacerbated by the systemic acidosis.

Severe Hyperpyrexia

In Meldrum and Horten's baboons, severe hyperpyrexia developed during prolonged seizures induced by bicuculline[46]; a similar, although less dramatic, response followed allylglycine-induced seizures[70]. The temperature can reach as high as 43°C. After seizure activity ceases, the temperature drifts downward, eventually becoming subnormal. The increase in temperature during status epilepticus is blunted but not abolished by paralysis[48]. Hyperpyrexia may reflect hypothalamic dysfunction as well as increased total oxygen consumption in the body.

Brain Metabolism

Although cerebral blood flow, glucose consumption, and oxygen consumption increase greatly during status epilepticus[57,71–74], it remains to be determined whether or not the observed increase in cerebral blood flow is always able to supply adequate substrate and oxygen to meet the brain's demands.

Blennow et al.[69] and Meldrum[75] "clamped" key systemic factors such as blood pressure, oxygenation, and pH at normal physiologic levels in ventilated paralyzed rats and measured brain metabolism after status epilepticus had been induced by bicuculline. Although they found a sustained increase in glucose and oxygen metabolism, they did not observe a "mismatch" with decreased cerebral blood flow.

In a rodent pentylenetetrazol model that permitted separate seizures to be induced as often as desired, Kreisman and colleagues[76–78] measured the electrocorticogram, cerebral tissue oxygen tension, reduction/oxidation state of cytochrome aa_3, and cerebral blood volume (Fig. 22.9). With onset of seizure activity, cortical oxygen actually rose, the cytochrome system was oxidized, and cerebral blood volume increased. This suggests that cerebral oxygen delivery was adequate to meet metabolic demand during acute seizures. However, when seizures were reinstituted and com-

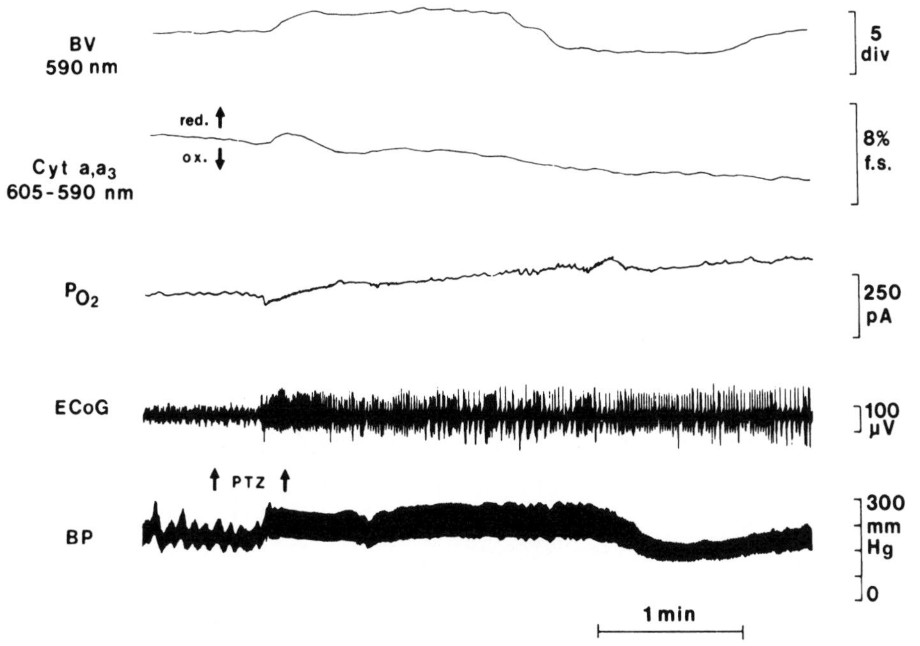

Figure 22.10. Transitional responses of cerebral blood volume *(BV)*, cytochrome (*Cyt.* a,a_3) redox level, PO_2, and blood pressure *(BP)* in association with later seizures in a series. Note the prolonged increase in blood pressure. (From Kreisman NR, LaManna JC, Rosenthal M. Sick TJ. Oxidative metabolic responses with recurrent seizures in rat cerebral cortex: role of system factors. Brain Res 1981;218:180.)

parable electrical activity was induced, several differences were noted. In contrast to the initial seizure, later seizures were not accompanied by an increase in oxygen delivery, and PaO_2 initially fell slightly (Fig. 22.10). Cerebral blood volume rose but not as much as with previous seizures. The arterial blood pressure rose and remained elevated well beyond the ictal period. In subsequent seizures, PaO_2 dropped and there was no increment of arterial blood pressure or cerebral blood volume. Although these investigators attributed the decreased cortical oxygenation to insufficient blood flow, no quantitative measurements of cerebral blood flow were made in conjunction with measurements of cerebral tissue oxygen levels.

Kreisman et al.[77] further questioned whether the difference in response to an initial versus subsequent seizure was related to the durations of previous seizures; perhaps it might be expected that seizures of long duration lead to more problems than those of short duration. Interestingly, the investigators found opposite results. Repetitive short-duration seizures were less adequately compensated (cortical oxygen delivery was impaired, cerebral vascular response was lost, oxidation was not demonstrable) than were long seizures (Fig. 22.11). Kreisman et al. suggested that seizures of a long duration are better able to induce compensatory changes in the cerebral vasculature than are short repetitive seizures.

More recently, by measuring focal cortical cerebral blood flow in addition to relative changes in the oxidation/reduction level of cytochrome aa_3, Kriesman et al.[80] reported that during early seizures, cortical cerebral blood flow increased to 350% of control and cortical oxygenation also rose markedly. During later seizures, the increases in both cerebral blood flow and cortical oxygenation were attenuated progressively. This was also accompanied by attenuation of the associated increases in blood pressure. Cortical oxygenation decreased during a seizure if the increase in cerebral blood flow failed to exceed 150 to 200% of control, which was defined as the critical value of cerebral blood flow. Ventilating the rats on 97% oxygen resulted in restoration of the seizure-associated decreases in cortical oxygenation in 50% of the animals. The elevation of inspired oxygen was effective only if cerebral blood flow increasd once again above 150 to 200% of control levels (Fig. 22.12). Hence, during repetitve seizures, cerebral blood flow must rise to greater than 200% of control levels to provide sufficient oxygen to meet the enhanced metabolic requirements of repetitive seizures.

Extrapolation of these investigations suggests that with respect to oxygen delivery, prolonged continuous status epilepticus might even be better tolerated than inadequately controlled repetitive seizures, because shorter seizures are less well compensated. Furthermore, with repeated seizures, the associated rise in cerebral blood flow progressively attenuates to a threshold or critical value, below which there is insufficient oxygen delivery to meet enhanced metabolic demands, a deficit that cannot be improved by ventilation alone. The probable role of a cerebrovascular compensation is additionally supported by recent observations of nitric oxide synthase inhibition in kainic acid and pilocarpine models of status epilepticus[81]. The authors found that treatment for 4 days with Nw-nitro-L-arginine (an endothelial and neuronal nitric oxide synthase inhibitor) greatly potentiates seizures induced by convulsants, suggesting that at least nitric oxide mediated vasodilation is an important compensatory mechanism.

The above discussion has concentrated on laboratory findings in mature animal models. Of developmental interest is a recent study of pentylenetetrazol-induced status epilepticus in the immature rat[82]. The results showed that changes in local cerebral blood flow with seizures are age

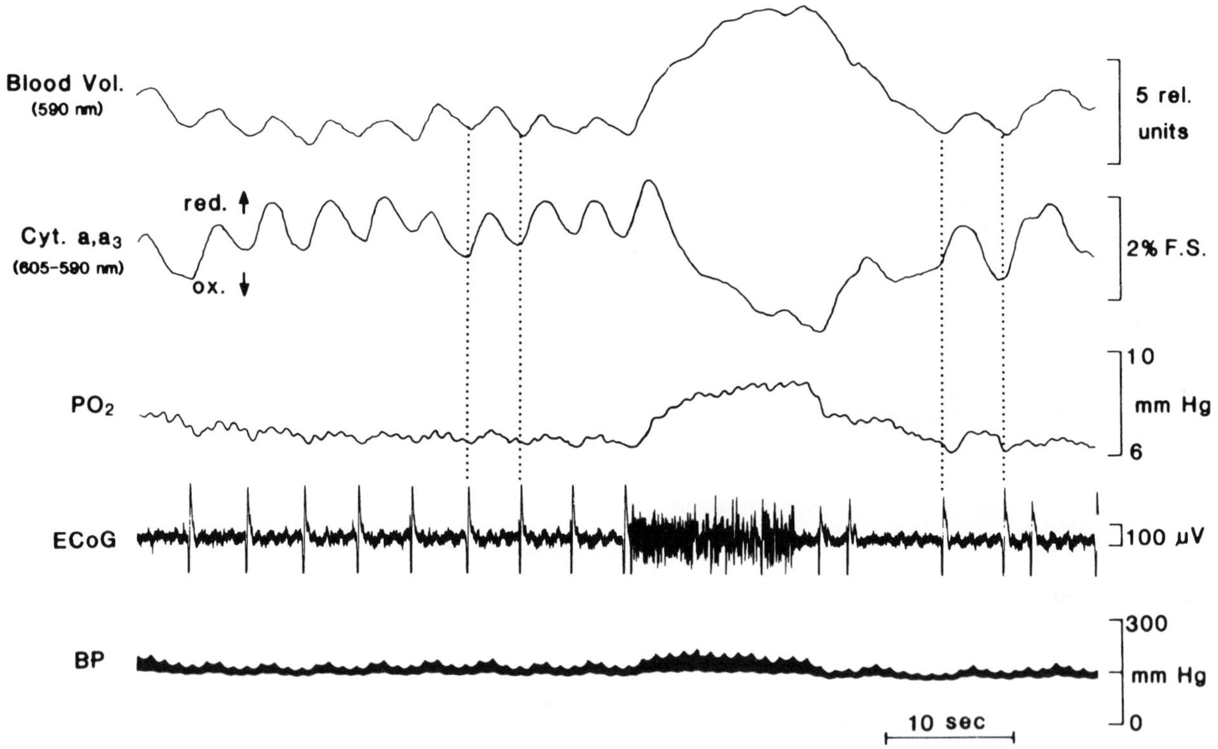

Figure 22.11. Segment of chart record taken 28 minutes after initiation of PTZ-induced status epilepticus in a rat anesthetized with 70% nitrous oxide. Compare changes in local cortical blood volume, cytochrome *(Cyt.* a,a_3*)* redox levels, cortical tissue PO_2, and systemic blood pressure in association with interictal spikes rather than ictal bursts. *Dotted lines* show synchrony between traces. (From Kreisman NR, Sick TJ, Rosenthal M. Importance of vascular responses in determining cortical oxygenation during recurrent paroxysmal events of varying duration and frequency of repetition. J Cereb Blood Flow Metab 1983;3:333.)

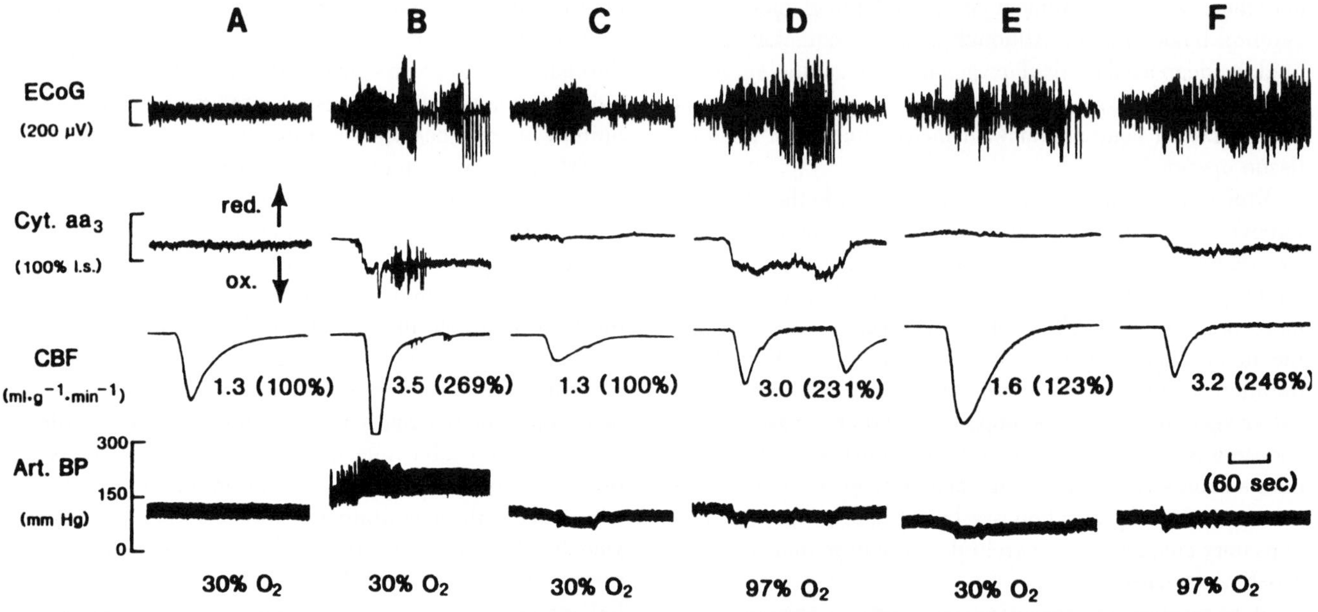

Figure 22.12. Sample records from an experiment showing changes in cortical oxygenation and cerebral blood flow *(CBF)* during serial pentylenetetrazol-induced seizures in a rat anesthetized with pentobarbital. A downward deflection of the cytochrome aa_3 *(Cyt.* aa_3*)* trace signals a decrease in the fraction of reduced/oxidized cytochrome aa_3 (i.e., an increase in cortical tissue oxygenation). An upward deflection of the trace indicates an increase in the fraction of reduced/oxidized cytochrome aa_3 (i.e., a decrease in tissue oxygenation). Absolute values of cerebral blood flow in ml/g/min and as a percentage of the preseizure values (in *parentheses*) are shown next to each of the H_2 traces (which are inverted). **A.** Preseizure control period. **B.** Third seizure. **C.** Fifth seizure (*CBF* and *Cyt.* aa_3 oxidation both fail to increase). **D.** Sixth seizure (increase in *CBF* and phasic oxidation of *Cyt.* aa_3 are both restored by breathing 97% oxygen). **E.** Eighth seizure (returning to 30% oxygen reinstates cerebral hypoxia). **F.** Ninth seizure (breathing 97% oxygen once again restores the increase in both *CBF* and *Cyt.* aa_3 oxidation). *ECoG,* electrocorticogram, and *Art. BP,* arterial blood pressure. (From Kreisman NR, Magee JC, Brizzee BL. Relative hypoperfusion in rat cerebral cortex during recurrent seizures. J Cereb Blood Flow Metab 1991;11:77.)

dependent. At the most immature ages, (postnatal rats aged 10 to 14 days), both local cerebral blood flow and local cerebral metabolic rate for glucose were largely increased by long-lasting seizures. In 17- to 21-day-old rats, the blood flow response to status epilepticus becomes more heterogeneous, with specific decreases in the hippocampus and cortex in the 21-day-old animals. In this model the authors also observed an absence of mismatch between blood flow and metabolism at all ages and suggested that their findings may explain, at least in part, why the immature brain is more resistant to seizure-induced damage than the adult brain.

NEUROPATHOLOGY

The neuropathologic features associated with status epilepticus have been recognized for over 100 years[(83)]. Changes including hippocampal necrosis, widespread cerebellar necrosis, and degeneration of Purkinje cells as well as neuronal necrosis and loss in the cortex have been described[(84–86)]. However, in many instances the cerebral findings are strikingly normal. Grossly, there may be only minimal brain swelling with no evidence of compartment herniation. The hippocampus may be swollen but with most of the gray and white matter grossly normal. In children with a history of long-standing epilepsy, the hippocampus may be shrunken into a scar—the so-called mesial temporal sclerosis[(87)]. In addition, atrophy of the cerebellum, thalamus, and cerebral cortex may be seen.

Evaluating the significance of these changes in terms of cause or effect of status is confounded by the variety of accompanying illnesses seen with severe episodes, metabolic complications, and sometimes underlying chronic epileptic disorders. In an attempt to elucidate possible causes of any acquired neuropathology, animal models have been used to study the effects of altered systemic physiology hypotension; complicating tissue hypoxia, hyperpyrexia, and acidosis; and intrinsic CNS mechanisms related to electrical activity.

Animal Models

In the baboon bicuculline model, Meldrum and Brierley[(47)] reported cerebral herniation in 4 of 10 animals. In half of the animals, microscopic changes were seen in the cerebral cortex, hippocampus, thalamus, and cerebellum. However, the histology in the other five animals was completely normal, and there were no gross abnormalities in the six animals without herniation. Although the interpretation of these findings is made the more complicated by any concomitant deranged systemic physiology[(46)], Meldrum and Brierley found that seizure-induced hyperpyrexia was the only variable other than duration of status epilepticus that was correlated with residual CNS damage[(47)]. Specifically, none of the five animals with normal histology had incurred hyperpyrexia greater than 40°C. Furthermore, in baboons who were paralyzed, ventilated, and well oxygenated and did not have hypotension, severe acidosis, or hyperpyrexia (greater than 40°C), the cerebellum was completely spared, but histologic changes were observed in the cortical areas, hippocampus, and thalamus[(48)]. Using allylglycine-induced status epilepticus in baboons, Meldrum et al.[(70)] observed much less severe hyperpyrexia and less severe hypoxia and acidosis with relatively stable blood pressure. As would be expected, the neuropathologic findings in these animals spared the cerebellum and were similar to the changes seen in paralyzed ventilated baboons subjected to bicuculline-induced status epilepticus. Based on these observations, Meldrum et al. suggested that a mismatch between metabolism and blood flow was not critical for brain damage and speculated that electrical seizure activity caused the histologic changes in the cortex, hippocampus, and thalamus by the release of an intrinsic "toxic" chemical[(75)]. This cellular injury could be further exacerbated by hyperpyrexia (from muscle rigidity).

In other models, in which the metabolic consequences of status epilepticus in the brain have been examined, a mismatch between brain metabolism and substrate delivery has been proposed as the major explanation for the functional and structural disturbances of neurons in vulnerable areas. This could be due to some abnormality in cerebrovascular responsiveness[(80)] that develops during prolonged episodes of recurrent seizures and may explain the mechanism for ischemic histologic changes documented in some neuropathologic studies[(46–49,88,89)]. However, while the mismatch between substrate delivery and metabolism certainly may complicate neuronal injury[(75)], others have shown that neuronal damage in status epilepticus does not primarily involve tissue hypoxia. Pinard et al.[(90)] reported that the hippocampus can sustain seizure-induced damage in the absence of accompanying tissue hypoxia. Despite these findings, the role of hypoxia and ischemia in neuronal damage after status epilepticus remains controversial.

CNS Mechanisms

In support of a primary CNS mechanism responsible for neuronal injury, Sloviter[(91)] demonstrated, in vivo, that electrical stimulation of a single excitatory afferent to the rat hippocampus appeared to reproduce the "epileptic" pattern of hippocampal damage without causing motor convulsions. It was suggested that seizure-associated brain damage could be caused by excessive presynaptic release of an excitatory transmitter, which then induces intracellular postsynaptic changes that lead to dendritic swelling and cell death[(91,92)]. Further support for an excitatory mechanism is the finding that selective neuronal necrosis observed in experimental status epilepticus develops with a characteristic sequence[(93,94)]; i.e., first the dendrites swell, and later the neuronal cell bodies are affected. Because such lesions develop only in regions where receptors for excitatory amino acids exist[(95)], the excitatory amino acids have been implicated in the development of this selective neuronal necrosis[(94,96,97)]. It has been suggested that either these amino

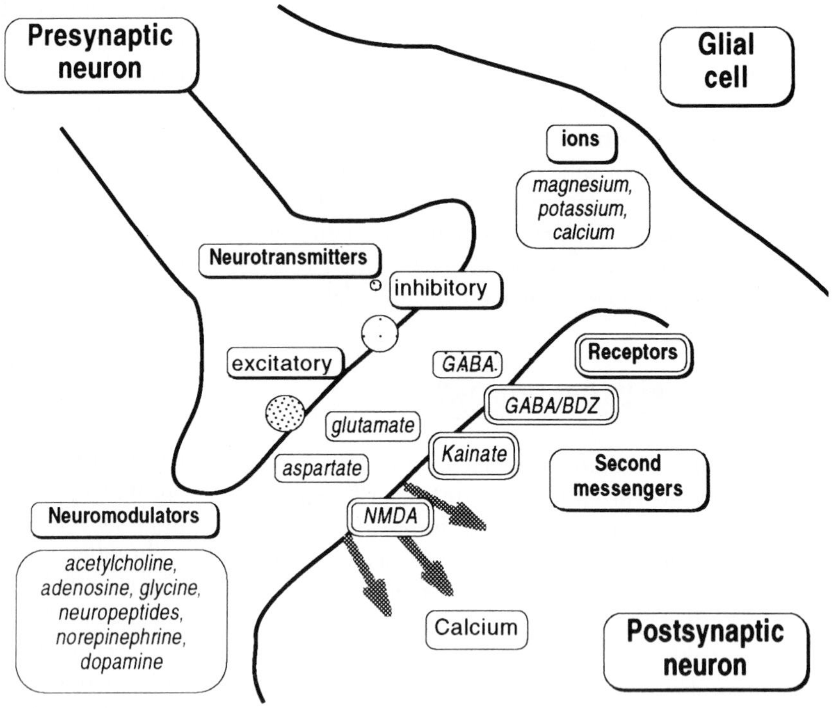

Figure 22.13. Schematic diagram of the neuronal synapse, illustrating the complex interrelationship that may be responsible for seizure activity. *G.A.B.A.*, γ-aminobutyric acid; *GABA/BDZ*, γ-aminobutyric acid/benzodiazepine; and *NMDA*, *N*-methyl-D-aspartate.

acids are released excessively or the ability of the tissues to deactivate them is impaired or overridden[93].

An alternative CNS mechanism would be to implicate an inhibitory-excitatory interaction. In an in vivo "continuous hippocampal stimulation" model of limbic seizures, it was found that there is a diminution of γ-aminobutyric acid (GABA) mediated inhibition, which further deteriorates after stimulation stops[98,99]. This not only provides a molecular substrate for chronic spontaneous seizures but also suggests why status epilepticus might be more difficult to control the longer it persists. Concurrent with the changes in GABA-ergic inhibition is the implication that there is an unmasking of excitatory glutamate (N-methyl-D-aspartate [NMDA] subtype) receptor channel-mediated events. Despite these findings, central to an excitatory and/or inhibitory hypothesis would be the notion that excitatory amino acids with neurotoxic effects increase in the extracellular fluid during prolonged periods of seizures[100]. Studies with brain microdialysis do not consistently support this notion, which is in contrast to hypoglycemia and ischemia[101–104]. For instance, after 2 hours of status induced by folate injection into the amygdala in a rabbit, a 50 to 75% increase in extracellular glutamate concentrations was measurable in the hippocampus[104]. In contrast, in the kainic acid-, bicuculline-, and pilocarpine-induced seizure models, investigators failed to detect any increase in extracellular glutamate levels[105,106]. However, there may be confounding factors such as glutamate reuptake systems and signal-to-noise difficulties (i.e., transmitter signal compared with metabolic pools).

Finally, although there has been much emphasis on an excitatory neurotoxic mechanism in status epilepticus supported by encouraging neuroprotective effects of NMDA receptor antagonists[107,108], other mechanisms of equal or even greater importance should not be overlooked (Figures 22.13 and 22.14). For instance, Mikati et al.[109] demonstrated that brain injury attributable to kainic acid -induced seizures in the developing rat could be prevented by phenobarbital, a medication working through an inhibitory mechanism. Also, Tecott et al.[110] showed that mice lacking 5-HT2C serotonin receptors have a lowered seizure threshold, and some develop fatal spontaneous seizures, suggesting that 5-HT2C receptor-mediated tonic inhibition of neuronal network excitability is important in maintaining the normal state.

Status-Induced Chronic Epilepsy

A question of great importance is whether status-epilepticus-induced brain damage results in chronic epilepsy. In adults with temporal lobe epilepsy the most common pathologic lesion seen is mesial temporal sclerosis, which consists of selective neuronal loss and reactive gliosis in the hippocampus and other mesial temporal structures[87]. Experimental studies indicate that prolonged seizures constitute only an initial factor that causes mesial temporal sclerosis[111]. It has been suggested that prolonged seizures induce neuronal loss which, in turn, leads to formation of new synaptic connections that can express abnormal hyperexcitability and result in a propensity to develop seizures. A vicious cycle of neuronal injury and synaptic reorganization can then emerge which may under-

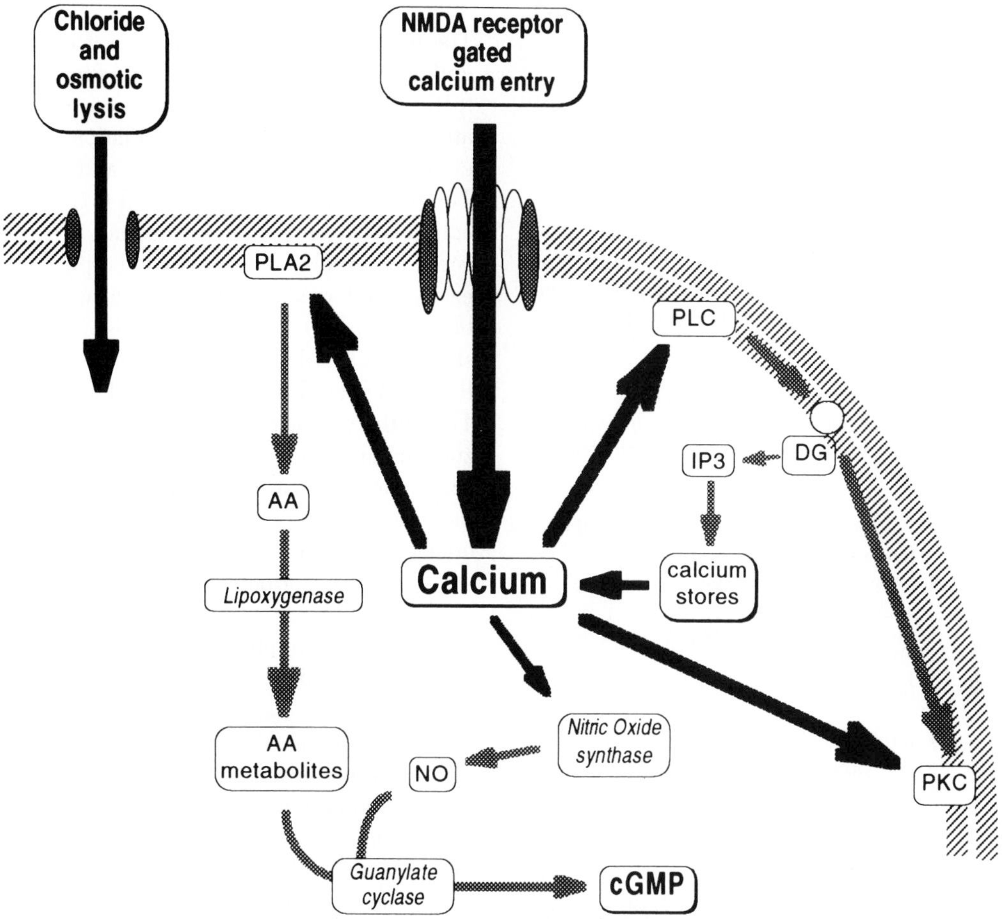

Figure 22.14. Schematic representation of *N*-methyl-D-aspartate (NMDA) receptor-linked signal transduction, which when abnormally activated leads to neuronal injury, cell lysis, and death. *PLA2,* phospholipase A_2; *AA,* arachidonic acid; *PLC,* phospholipase C: *DG,* 1,2-diacylglycerol; *PKC,* protein kinase C; *NO,* nitric oxide; and *IP3,* inositol 1,4,5-triphosphate.

lie an uncontrollable progression to a state of refractory or recurrent seizures. Illustrative of this is the long-term effect of kainic acid-induced status which results in recurrent seizures in primates, cats, and rodents[(112)]. Also, age may be an important factor, as shown by Holmes and Thompson[(113)], who found that an enhanced hippocampal kindling response was found in adult rats in which status had been induced during the fourth week of life, even though no cerebral damage could be observed on pathologic examination. Even so, the immature brain is not specifically sensitive to the effects of status, since epilepsy can be induced by status in the mature rat.

Clinical support for the influence of status epilepticus in the pathogenesis of mesial temporal sclerosis and epilepsy has been suggested by a variety of reports. Corsellis and Bruton examined the brain tissue of 20 patients who died during or shortly after status[(86)]. The most vulnerable part of the brain was the hippocampus. Wasterlain et al. reported that in three patients who died 11 to 27 days after the onset of nonconvulsive status epilepticus lasting from 2.5 hours to 3 days, status caused neuronal loss in the hippocampus, amygdala, piriform cortex, dorsomedial thalamic nucleus, cerebellum, and cerebral cortex[(114)]. Corsellis and Bruton found that of 25 patients who had sustained one or more recorded episodes of status epilepticus before lobectomy for refractory seizures, 16 had a sclerotic hippocampus[(86)]. Finally, in a review of brain magnetic resonance images from 53 children with medically refractory temporal lobe epilepsy, Grattan-Smith et al.[(115)] found that hippocampal sclerosis was present in 30 children (57%). Mesial temporal sclerosis was frequently associated with a history of neurologic insults, primarily febrile seizures.

CLINICAL MANAGEMENT

The clinical approach to management and therapy for status epilepticus in children must include the provision of an appropriate level of care, intervention, supervision, support for vital functions, and anticonvulsant treatment. In addition, there must be directed consideration for possible underlying causes that may necessitate and benefit from specific therapies.

Table 22.8. Summary of Standard Emergency Management of Status Epilepticus from Emergency Department to Intensive Care[a]

Immediate	
Airway	• Protect—use 100% oxygen and endotracheal tube if necessary
Breathing	• Support and use muscle relaxants if necessary
Circulation	• Verify good blood pressure—support if necessary
	• Establish secure intravenous line
Draw	• Laboratory samples for glucose, blood urea nitrogen, electrolytes, calcium, phosphate, complete blood count, toxicology
Administer	• 2–4 ml of 25% dextrose in water per kg (500 mg/kg)
Anticonvulsants	• See **Tables 22.9 and 22.10**
First-line	• Diazepam (0.2–0.4 mg/kg) or lorazepam (0.1–0.2 mg/kg) given over 2 minutes, maximum of 10 mg
	OR
	• Phenytoin (15–20 mg/kg) up to 1000 mg (no faster than 25 mg/min)
Second-line	• Phenytoin if not already give (dose as above)
	• Phenobarbital (10 mg/kg) no more than 30 mg/kg × 2
	Intubate if Respiratory Depression Occurs
Critical care	
CNS protection	• Intubate and mechanically ventilate
	• See **Tables 22.11 and 22.12**
Drugs	• Phenytoin—rebolus and give according to levels
	• Paraldehyde (0.15 ml of 4% solution per kg per hr) by continuous intravenous line
	• Anesthesia with short-acting barbiturates

[a]Based on the history, progression to critical care may be appropriate within minutes of presentation.

Management Priorities

The longer generalized convulsive status epilepticus persists, the harder it is to control, and the worse the likely morbidity and risk of mortality become[16]. It is therefore imperative that the sequence of escalating treatment be planned. An approach such as the one outlined in **Table 22.8** should be known to everyone involved in administering and supervising emergency care. In this context, the underlying goals are as follows:

1. To stabilize the patient:
   a. By ensuring adequate cardiorespiratory function and oxygenation
   b. By correcting and preventing metabolic imbalance of hydration, electrolytes, glucose, and lactate
2. To treat the treatable
   a. By stopping clinical and electrical seizure activity as soon as possible, preferably within 30 minutes
   b. By preventing the recurrence of seizures
   c. By preventing or correcting any systemic complications
   d. By evaluating for and treating specific causes of status epilepticus

Stabilizing the Patient

The top priority in the management of patients with status epilepticus is preservation of vital function, i.e., airway protection, maintenance of ventilation, assurance of oxygenation, and support of the circulation. Patients with status epilepticus often have hypoxia and impaired ventilation. The patient should be positioned to avoid aspiration, suffocation, or physical injury. Adequate aeration should be ensured, and a plastic airway may be placed if it can be done easily. The forced use of such an airway or the use of tongue blades or metal objects may cause severe oral injury and should be avoided. In the presence of poor air exchange, the child should be intubated and mechanically ventilated. The authors also recommend that a patient in whom seizure activity does not cease after appropriate anticonvulsants are administered should be intubated and ventilated proactively. It is wrong to wait long enough for the development of florid systemic complications such as cyanosis, severe acidosis, or hemodynamic instability before proceeding to intubation.

To accomplish intubation, neuromuscular blockade is often necessary. Moreover, because it should be assumed that all such patients have a full stomach and are at significant risk of aspiration, the rapid sequence technique with cricoid pressure is mandatory. (For further information concerning intubation, see Chapter 2.) Of course, once having used a muscle relaxant, anticonvulsant therapy can no longer be titrated against a clinical endpoint, if indeed this were one's sole aim. If clinical parameters for treatment evaluation are used, a short-acting agent is preferable. However, in some patients with complex multisystem pathology, a long-acting agent may be more preferable for optimal treatment of their other problems, and alternative monitoring should be used (discussed later).

After intubation is accomplished, or if it is deemed unnecessary, the child should be placed in 100% oxygen to avoid the development of hypoxia. Subsequent oxygen therapy should be guided by arterial blood gases and other appropriate oxygen monitoring, with the caveat that a seizure-associated decline in cortical oxygenation may respond to such treatment (see above).

Patient Monitoring

As with any patient receiving neurologic intensive care, clinical surveillance should include regular observations of motor, sensory, and pupillary function; blood pressure, pulse, and electrocardiographic state; and oximetry and temperature. In the more severely affected patients, more complete and invasive monitoring should be undertaken, e.g., capnography, central venous pressure, and Swan-Ganz pulmonary artery pressure monitoring. Given that metabolic abnormalities may cause or result from status epilepticus, it is also important to review serum biochemistry, blood glucose, blood gases, pH, clotting and hematologic parameters.

Nursing care is also vitally important. Tracheobronchial secretions may be excessive, and bronchial or endotracheal tube obstruction is a significant hazard. Scrupulous attention should therefore be given to airway care. In addition, if the patient is comatose, all of the measures applied to standard care (e.g., early tube feeding for nutrition, regular turning to avoid pressure sores, and eye care) should be applied.

In the acute setting, intravenous lines should be used for fluid and drug administration. The lines should be placed in large veins, as many anticonvulsants can cause severe phlebitis and thrombosis at the infusion site. When more than one anticonvulsant is used, more than one line or lumen is necessary, mainly because of incompatibilities in mixing or precipitation if added to glucose infusions (discussed later). Arterial lines are commonly used for monitoring, and in emergencies some drugs have been given via this route. However, anticonvulsants should not be administered in this way because severe arterial spasm and necrosis may develop. If there is a lack of access for administering anticonvulsants, the intraosseous or intramuscular route can be used (discussed later).

Emergency Investigations

Blood gases, pH, blood sugar level, renal and liver function, calcium and magnesium levels, haematologic parameters (including platelet count), and anticonvulsant levels should be measured. In addition, blood and urine should be kept for toxicologic or metabolic screening at a later time, if this is subsequently deemed necessary.

Further investigations depend on the clinical circumstances, whether or not there is a history of epilepsy, and age of presentation **(Tables 22.3 and 22.4).** When the episode of status is unexplained, focal, or coexistent with an acute illness, cranial computed tomography scanning is warranted. The CSF should be examined only when there is no risk to the patient.

Circulatory Support

When seizures have continued for a significant period, cerebral autoregulation is impaired and cerebral blood flow becomes perfusion pressure dependent; i.e., systemic arterial pressure is a major determinant. Maintaining blood pressure within normal levels is therefore of utmost importance. During the first 60 minutes of continuing seizures the blood pressure is usually normal, but in untreated status, hypotension can become more of a problem. Hypotension may be further exacerbated by respiratory failure and intravenous anticonvulsants, with a cardiodepressant effect. Hence, abatement of hypotension should include attention to general respiratory status, anticonvulsant infusions and levels, and administration of inotropic agents. If necessary, dopamine is usually adequate, and the dose (5 to 20 μg/kg/min) can be titrated against the desired hemodynamic and renal response. Persistent hypotension which is unresponsive to supportive therapy represents a severe state in protracted seizures and may portend a poor outcome. Hypertension as a consequence of seizures may also occur.

Other Physiologic Changes and Management

Status epilepticus may produce a variety of acute metabolic, autonomic, and cardiovascular derangements which require active intervention. Frequently observed problems include the following:

Acidosis Lactic acidosis is common and can contribute to a compromised hemodynamic state. If the patient is in shock, appropriate fluid and pressor therapy should be administered. Rarely, intravenous bicarbonate is necessary, but it can be given to half correct an acidosis when the pH is less than 7.2. In most instances correction of respiratory abnormalities and cessation of convulsive movements will adequately contain an acquired metabolic problem.

Hypoglycemia Hypoglycemia may cause or be a consequence of status epilepticus. This abnormality should be considered early and, when present, treated with intravenous dextrose, 500 mg/kg stat dose. Appropriate blood and urine investigation is also necessary, since profound hypoglycemia may be a "symptom" of inherited metabolic disease (see Chapter 23).

Hypercarbia, Pulmonary Artery Hypertension, and Pulmonary Edema There may be a variety of factors accounting for these abnormalities, which may be fatal. Treatment should be aimed primarily at optimizing mechanical ventilation. Thereafter, diuretics and vasoactive agents may be needed.

Hyperthermia In the patient with uncontrolled seizures, hyperpyrexia may develop. Generally this can be limited by neuromuscular blockade, adequate fluid resuscitation, and the use of body-temperature cooling aids, e.g., temperature-controlled water mattresses.

Disseminated Intravascular Coagulation This may develop rapidly and requires appropriate treatment. More importantly, deranged clotting may herald the onset of complicating liver failure or drug toxicity.

Renal failure Hypotension, severe metabolic acidosis, or rhabdomyolysis may compromise renal function. Oliguria is an important sign and protective attempts to avoid renal failure should be initiated; ensure adequate cardiac output, hydration, and urine flow.

Electrolyte and Fluid Balance The fluid requirements of a patient with status epilepticus will vary. Initially, if the patient is hyperthermic and shocked, active fluid resuscitation to achieve a good blood pressure and urine output must be initiated. Thereafter, a balance is achieved, providing enough to avoid renal failure, yet not so much as to compromise pulmonary alveolar-capillary leak and any cerebral edema. Electrolytic abnormalities in potassium and sodium are treated when present.

Cerebral Edema Persistent seizures may result in the development of cerebral edema and raised intracranial pressure. On occasion, seizures may continue unabated, despite

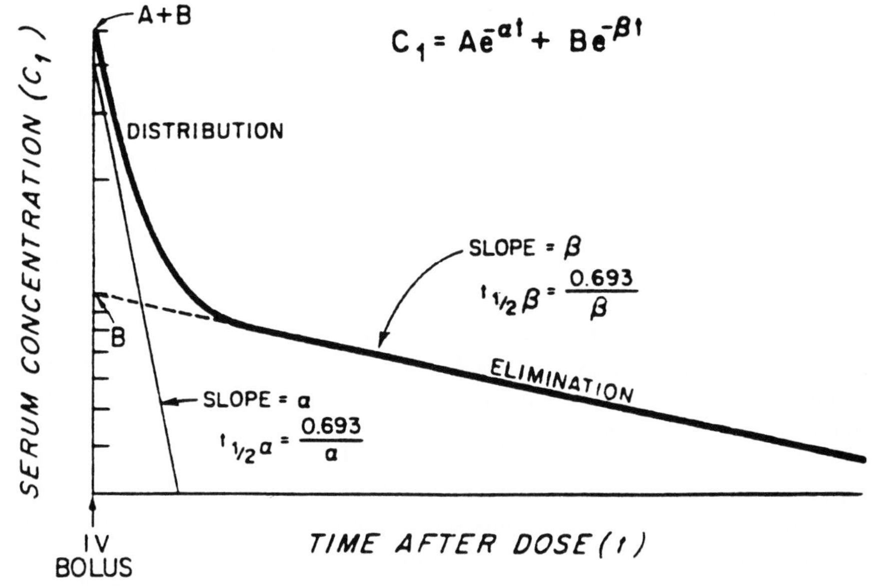

Figure 22.15. Schematic graph of serum concentration (C_1) plotted on a logarithmic scale, versus time *(t)* after a single intravenous *(IV)* bolus of a drug as predicted by the two-compartment open model. (From Greenblatt DJ, Koch-Weser J. Drug Therapy, clinical pharmacokinetics. N Engl J Med 1975;293:702, reprinted by permission of *The New England Journal of Medicine.*)

seemingly adequate anticonvulsant therapy, until specific cerebral edema therapy is given (mannitol 0.25 gm/kg stat dose). In patients in whom status is a symptom of underlying brain insult, regular mannitol or even neurosurgery may be necessary.

Implementing Drug Therapy

To control status epilepticus quickly and to prevent recurrence, a therapeutic serum concentration of a long-acting anticonvulsant medication must be achieved. However, when treating status epilepticus, the therapeutic endpoint is not the production of a particular drug concentration but rather a clinical and/or electrical endpoint. Clinical experience suggests that virtually any antiepileptic drug, sedative, hypnotic, or general anesthetic agent works, but dangerously high concentrations of hypnotics are often needed. It is not the particular choice of drug but rather the timing, route, and vigor of therapy that are major determinants of the duration of status epilepticus and subsequent morbidity. Furthermore, early therapy is far more effective than later therapy, suggesting that vigorous intravenous therapy early in a seizure may abort status epilepticus.

Once the acute episode of status epilepticus has been controlled, the therapeutic priorities change. Drug concentrations become an important consideration in preventing seizure recurrence. To help minimize confusion and provide a rational basis for what to do next if treatment becomes complex, an understanding of pharmacokinetic principles and alternative therapeutic strategies is essential.

Pharmacokinetics

None of the current drug classes used to treat seizures and status epilepticus is ideal. The drugs cannot leave intact the level of consciousness and respiratory function while entering the brain rapidly, having a long therapeutic half-life, and treating associated somatic manifestations and cerebral electrical events[117]. They are all lipid-soluble agents, and the pertinent pharmacokinetic properties outlined below describe their ability to enter and be maintained in the brain.

First, the volume of distribution of a lipid-soluble drug increases in proportion to the degree of its solubility[118]. Second, two pharmacokinetic phases are seen after such a drug is administered: an initial distribution phase, in which the drug is distributed from the plasma to the various tissues, and a later elimination phase, in which the drug is metabolized and/or excreted directly (Fig. 22.15)[119]. With highly lipid-soluble drugs, free brain concentration corresponds to the free serum concentration[120]. Third, a loading dose equal to twice the dose per elimination half-life will immediately attain a therapeutic serum concentration[121] and will be sustained indefinitely if maintenance therapy is begun at this time. Without a loading dose, a time equivalent to 5 or more elimination half-lives is required to attain a steady-state serum concentration. Fourth, in determining toxicity, the rate of administration of a drug may be more important than the total amount administered slowly. Such a "bolus" effect[117] is the probable cause of cardiac depression associated with rapid intravenous infusion of phenytoin; i.e., a relatively high concentration is presented to the heart and then delivered to the brainstem.

Standard Anticonvulsant Therapy

The three most commonly used classes of anticonvulsant drugs included in the acute treatment of status epilepticus are benzodiazepines, phenytoin, and barbiturates. An outline of these drugs and their dosages is shown in **Table 22.9.**

Diazepam and Lorazepam

Diazepam is the most lipid-soluble drug used to treat status epilepticus, and it has the largest volume of distribu-

Table 22.9. First-Line Anticonvulsants for Status Epilepticus

Drug	Loading Dose	Route	Blood Level	Side Effects	Idiosyncratic Effects[a]
Diazepam					
Neonatal	0.2–0.4 mg/kg	i.v.		Sedation, hypotension, respiratory depression, laryngospasm, arrest	Absence status may convert to tonic status, leukopenia (neutropenia, granulocytopenia), agranulocytosis, aplastic anemia, hemolytic anemia, transient decrease in renal function, increased AST (SGOT), ALT (SGPT), LDH, alkaline phosphatase, and total and direct bilirubin
Infant/child	0.2–0.4 mg/kg	i.v.			
	0.5 mg/kg	p.r.			
Adult	10 mg	i.v.			
Lorazepam					
Infant/child	0.1–0.2 mg/kg	i.v.		As above	As above
Adult	4–8 mg	i.v.			
Phenytoin			10–20 μg/ml		
Neonatal	20 mg/kg	i.v.		Hypotension, cardiac conduction defects, less sedation	Blood dyscrasia, lupus-like syndrome, reduced IgA, rash, peripheral neuropathy, hepatotoxicity, lymphoma
Infant/child	20 mg/kg	i.v.			
Adult	15–20 mg/kg	i.v.			
Phenobarbital			10–40 μg/ml		
Neonatal	20 mg/kg	i.v.		Same as diazepam, may act synergistically	Maculopapular rash, hepatotoxicity, toxic epidermal necrolysis, exfoliation
Infant/child	20 mg/kg	i.v.			

[a] *AST, aspartate transaminase; SGOT, serum glutamic oxaloacetic transaminase; ALT, alanine transaminase; SGPT, serum glutamic pyruvic transaminase; LDH, lactic dehydrogenase; IgA, immunoglobulin A.*

tion. It gained popularity because of its rapid distribution in the brain (within 10 seconds) and its relatively low toxicity[(120)]. In addition, it is effective in virtually all types of status epilepticus, including grand mal, focal motor, absence, myoclonic, and secondarily generalized grand mal status epilepticus[(122)]. It is, however, associated with an extensive drop in serum concentration during the distribution phase, with limitation of anticonvulsant activity to approximately 20 minutes and a greater than 70% fall in serum concentration within the first 2 hours after administration. This fall may be associated with seizure recurrence.

The lipid solubility, volume of distribution, and distribution half-life of lorazepam are approximately half those of diazepam. Like diazepam, lorazepam rapidly enters the brain; the onset of lorazepam and diazepam action in status epilepticus is similar 3 and 2 minutes, respectively[(123)]. However, unlike diazepam, redistribution is minimal, and effective levels persist in the brain several hours after a single intravenous dose[(124)], extending the anticonvulsant effect, though with a somewhat rapid development of tolerance. Finally, since lorazepam does not have any significant metabolites, side effects including respiratory depression and apnea are less severe with lorazepam than with diazepam.

Phenytoin

Phenytoin is extremely effective in controlling tonic-clonic status epilepticus in adults and children[(125,126)] and in neonates and young infants[(127)]. Compared with other drugs used to treat status epilepticus, phenytoin has relatively low lipid solubility and therefore enters and equilibrates in the brain slowly. The elimination kinetics are nonlinear, and approximately 30% of children have a degree of saturated metabolism that makes it difficult to adjust phenytoin concentration within the therapeutic range[(128)]; this also means that there is a nonlinear relationship between clinically relevant doses and concentrations achieved. Hence, whenever phenytoin doses are increased, the serum concentration increases disproportionately. In practice, this phenomenon is compounded by another consequence of the nonlinear elimination kinetics: the apparent half-life for phenytoin progressively increases as the serum concentration increases.

With a loading dose of 18 to 20 mg/kg, peak brain drug levels may not be reached for 10 to 30 minutes, though the level should have equilibrated by 1 hour and a subsequent therapeutic level maintained for 24 hours. Such kinetics form the rationale for the present practice of using phenytoin as a second-line drug in status epilepticus and waiting at least 30 minutes after a dose before drug failure is concluded. As already discussed, the rate of intravenous administration should be limited to 25 mg/min in older children or 0.5 to 1.0 mg/kg/min in younger children.

Phenobarbital

Phenobarbital is highly effective in the therapy of status epilepticus and has been the initial agent of choice for many years. Phenobarbital is the least lipid-soluble drug commonly used to treat status epilepticus and, therefore, has the slowest onset of action. The distribution phase lasts 1 hour or longer, and there is a long elimination half-life. During status epilepticus, the entrance of phenobarbital into the brain is enhanced, largely due to changes in blood pH and blood pressure changes[(129)].

Compared with shorter-acting barbiturates, such as pentobarbital and thiopental (discussed later), phenobarbital is many times more potent an anticonvulsant when related to equal CNS depressant effects[(130–132)]. However, the short and medium half-life barbiturates can be used with more rapid effect, though at the expense of inducing anesthesia.

Therapeutic Strategies

Treatment in Relation to Age

In newborns the relationship between drug dose and concentration is highly unpredictable and changing. In comparison with older patients, there are lower concentrations of serum proteins, which means a lesser degree of drug protein binding and increased free levels[(133,134)]. Furthermore, there is an evolving ability and capacity to eliminate drugs, which results in an enormous range of required doses, with often-quoted average doses being of value only as initial treatment. Both phenobarbital and phenytoin are effective for status epilepticus; at high levels, however, phenobarbital produces an increasing anesthetic effect, with progressive anticonvulsant effect. This is avoided with phenytoin, though at extremely high levels this drug may exacerbate seizures. Therefore, while phenytoin has been effective as an initial drug[(135)], dosage should not exceed 20 to 30 mg/kg before blood levels are monitored (particularly because of the nonlinear elimination kinetics with a half-life ranging 7 to 140 hours). For safer longer-term administration, phenobarbital is preferable to phenytoin. At all ages, benzodiazepines including both diazepam and lorazepam are effective in stopping status epilepticus, but high dosages are required. The major drawback of diazepam is the short duration of anticonvulsant action after bolus dosing and the uncertainty of the actual dose administered when delivered by infusion. With lorazepam there is rapid development of tolerance despite the relatively long duration of action. If status epilepticus recurs within 48 hours and lorazepam is used repeatedly, it becomes progressively less effective.

Infants have the highest relative capacity to eliminate anticonvulsant drugs. The half-life of phenobarbital diminishes from 114 to 45 hours. Phenytoin is rapidly eliminated, and its nonlinear kinetics mean that when phenytoin concentrations are low, the apparent half-life is usually very short, sometimes necessitating the use of maintenance doses as high as 20 mg/kg/day to produce consistent therapeutic levels[(136)].

After infancy, relative drug clearance progressively declines until adult values are achieved at age 10 to 15 years. Benzodiazepines are extremely effective in stopping status epilepticus. Since diazepam has a short duration of anticonvulsant action, a longer-acting drug should be coadministered to prevent seizures from recurring. Lorazepam has been put forward as a better alternative[(137)] since it has proved effective (between 80% and 100%) in a number of studies[(138–141)]; thus, the need for early institution of a second anticonvulsant is avoided. However, in most patients treated with lorazepam, a second anticonvulsant must be started in the first 12 to 24 hours after status epilepticus, which in practice would confer little advantage over the coadministration of diazepam with another anticonvulsant. Finally, it should be remembered that the benzodiazepines have not been demonstrated to be superior to phenobarbital[(142)].

Treatment According to Duration of Seizure

Of the variety of anticonvulsants which can be used to treat a seizure, some are more appropriate than others as the duration of an individual episode increases **(Table 22.10).** For practical purposes an unrelenting seizure can be divided into four phases[(143)]. The first is a prodromal stage which is predictable in patients with established epilepsy and presages status. Emergency treatment with diazepam or midazolam usually halts evolution to true status. The second phase comprises the initial 30 minutes of a seizure; lorazepam and diazepam with phenytoin are potential first-line choices. The third phase is established status epilepticus of 30 to 60 minutes duration, when the therapeutic objective of merely trying to control the seizure changes to one of cerebral protection and limiting morbidity and mortality. If the patient is seen for the first time at this stage, possible treatments are diazepam, lorazepam, or phenytoin, and

Table 22.10. Anticonvulsant Treatment According to Duration of Seizure

Prodromal Stage	*Initial 30 Minutes*	*Status 30–60 Minutes*
First line		
Diazepam	Lorazepam	Diazepam
or midazolam	*or* diazepam	*or* lorazepam
(0.15–0.3 mg/kg i.m.)		*or* phenytoin
Second line	Phenytoin	Phenytoin
	Clonazepam (neonate 0.25 mg i.v. bolus) (child 0.5 mg i.v. bolus)	Phenobarbital
	Midazolam (0.05–0.4 mg/kg/hr i.v. after bolus)	
	Paraldehyde (0.15 ml of 4% solution/kg/hr/i.v.)	
Other		Chlormethiazole (0.08 mg/kg/min, increasing to hourly)
		Clonazepam (repeat bolus 0.01 mg/kg up to 4 times)
		Midazolam
		Paraldehyde

Doses of diazepam, lorazepam, phenytoin, and phenobarbital are quoted in Table 22.9.

Table 22.11. Alternative Anticonvulsants for Refractory Status Epilepticus

Drug	*Initial i.v. Dose*	*Rate of Infusion*	*Notes*	*Side Effects*
Paraldehyde	0.15 ml/kg (4% solution)	Divide over 1 hour	Give under EEG control and titrate dose against effect. More than 1 ml is rarely needed (use <5–10 ml)	Drowsiness and coma, pulmonary embolus, pulmonary hemorrhage, hepatic toxicity, renal toxicity
		Repeat dose in 1-4 hours	Use fresh solution: half-life 6-9 hours	
Lidocaine	1–2 mg/kg	2–4 mg/kg/hr (neonates 2–6 mg/kg/hr)	ECG monitoring for changes such as prolonged PR interval and in QRS complex	Hypotension, heart block, arrhythmia, and CNS toxicity
Clonazepam	0.25-mg neonate 0.5-mg child	Repeat bolus 0.01 mg/kg (10–40 μg/kg/min)	More potent than diazepam in sedation. Long half-life (20 ± 50 hr) so infusion not usually used	Hypotension—can paradoxically worsen tonic status
Chlormethiazole	0.08 mg/kg/min or 0.1 ml/kg/min (0.8% solution)	Increase dose every 2 hours until seizures abolished	Accumulates—metabolism is affected by changes in hepatic blood flow	Risk of hypotension, heart block, tachycardia, fluid overload, and electrolyte disturbance

phenobarbital. In those patients who do not respond to or cannot be controlled despite standard doses of these drugs, higher doses of phenobarbital should be tried before additional drugs are used (discussed below). The other agents which can be coadministered with the above drugs are chlormethiazole, clonazepam, diazepam, midazolam, and paraldehyde. The use of high-dose diazepam is limited by acute tolerance to anticonvulsant effect and progressive resistance to additional doses. Lorazepam should not be used as short-acting monotherapy. High-dose phenytoin with rapid loading in the emergent situation has potential cardiotoxic side effects[117,144–146]. In the fourth phase, in which resistant status epilepticus lasts longer than 60 minutes, the primary aim is cerebral protection by suppression of CNS activity and metabolism with the use of anesthetic agents (discussed below).

Refractory Status Epilepticus and Treatment Failure

As the episode of status epilepticus increases in duration, a variety of alternative anticonvulsant agents may prove beneficial **(Table 22.11).** However, once convulsive status epilepticus has continued for 60 minutes despite treatment, the episode should be deemed refractory, and emergency therapy with anesthetic agents must be employed. Initiation of such treatment before 60 minutes has elapsed is often guided by personal experience. In addition, one must weigh the advantages of rapid suppression of CNS metabolism with induction of anesthesia by short or medium half-life barbiturates or inhalational agents **(Table 22.12)**[6,147–151] against the risks of hemodynamic instability during therapy and difficulties in seizure control during weaning.

Suppression of CNS metabolism with short-acting barbiturates such as thiopentone and pentobarbitone can be achieved rapidly with acute control of seizures and status epilepticus (Fig. 22.16). A protocol such as the one outlined in **Table 22.13** has proved effective, without hemodynamic compromise, in a variety of critically ill infants and children with intractable seizures and status epilepticus[6]. Few guidelines exist regarding depth or duration of anesthesia, and although acute seizure control can be achieved, difficulties in control may arise on weaning. Other nonbarbiturate anesthetic agents (e.g., propofol and isoflurane) have been used in this context, but experience with them is very limited, and, paradoxically, they bear little intrinsic anticonvulsant activity and may even be proconvulsant.

As an alternative to adopting the above protocol of anesthesia to control status epilepticus and limit morbidity and mortality, Crawford et al.[5] have suggested that more treatment with phenobarbital at an earlier stage should be used. In the controlled environment of the intensive care unit, there does not appear to be a maximum dose of phenobarbital. In a large series of children with refractory status epilepticus, the authors found that seizures were eventually controlled by repeated bolus doses of 5 to 20 mg/kg, spaced by an adequate time to allow for penetration of the drug into the CNS (approximately 30 to 60 minutes). Maximum doses administered in 24 hours ranged from 30 to 120 mg/kg (median 60 mg/kg), and the maximum blood levels achieved were 70 to 344 μg/ml (median 114 μg/ml). Despite such a regimen of very high dose administration and continuing high serum levels of phenobarbital, many patients were weaned from respiratory support, and there did not appear to be any acute drug-related complications. The authors concluded that such an approach would in most cases obviate the need for intubation, mechanical ventilation, and EEG monitoring. However, while these data support the use of higher doses of phenobarbital, further prospective evaluation for such treatment is needed, particularly to address the question of duration in clinical and electrical status epilepticus. In an emergency such as refractory status epilepticus, it is the authors' experience that rapid control of the clinical state is essential. This can

Table 22.12. Anesthesia for Control of Status Epilepticus

Drug	*Dose*	*Notes*	*Side Effects*
Thiopental sodium	See Table 22.13	Saturable kinetics, active metabolite	Hypotension, hypersensitivity—laryngeal edema, bronchospasm, and erythema 1/30,000. Pancreatitis and hepatic dysfunction.
Pentobarbitone sodium	5–20 mg/kg loading 0.5–3 mg/kg/hr infusion (5–20 mg/kg bolus for breakthrough seizures)	Advantage over thiopental: nonsaturable kinetics, no active metabolites, longer duration of action, and GABA-ergic action	Hypotension and cardiac dysfunction Decerebrate posturing and flaccid paralysis during anesthesia, and weakness may persist for weeks.
Isoflurane	End-tidal concentration 0.8–2%—dose titrated to maintain burst suppression	Pupils are rendered small. Isoflurane can be used in liver and renal disease.	Muscle relaxant effect. After prolonged use a transient movement disorder may become evident.
Etomidate	0.3 mg/kg 20 μg/kg/min infusion	Corticosteroid coadministration is required	Hypotension, drug-induced myoclonus, and muscular twitching. Interferes with adrenocorticoid function.
Propofol	2 mg/kg bolus 5–10 mg/kg/hr initially then reduced to 1–3 mg/kg/hr		Proconvulsant Prolonged infusion results in lipemia and accumulation of inactive gluconuride metabolites with metabolic acidosis—especially in children.

be achieved with induction of anesthesia, and there appears to be little advantage in a more delayed approach given the facility of modern intensive care. However, phenobarbital is a better anticonvulsant than pentobarbitone or thiopentone, and it may be effective as long-term maintenance therapy.

Finally, as with any emergency situation, when the clinical course does not follow an expected pattern of response to therapy and improvement, it is always valuable to reassess all the correctable factors systematically. This will occur either during the initial hours of treatment or during the weaning stage of anesthesia. The following questions need to be asked:

- Has inadequate drug therapy been used? In response to this question, check the individual drugs administered and their doses.
- Has appropriate maintenance antiepileptic therapy been initiated?. Check to verify that long-term maintenance treatment has been started.
- Have all systemic and metabolic derangements been excluded and appropriately controlled? See **Table 22.5.**
- Has a treatable underlying structural, metabolic, or infective cause been missed? See **Tables 22.3 and 22.4.**

Table 22.13. Thiopental Infusion Therapy for Status Epilepticus

Aim of therapy	
To control the physical effects of seizures	
To suppress electrical correlates of seizure activity	
To induce either burst suppression or electrocerebral silence	
To avoid toxic drug levels and complications	
Basics of critical care	
Mechanically ventilate	
(Muscle relaxation)	Muscle rest (see text)
Maintain physiologic parameters	Normoxia and normocarbia Normotension Normoglycemia Normothermia
Monitor	Blood pressure, ECG, capnography, oximetry, EEG Drug levels
Therapy	
Loading dose	2–8 mg/kg thiopental in increments of 2 mg/kg under EEG
Infusion	1–10 mg/kg via central intravenous line (giving the minimum necessary to achieve the above aims)

Treatment for Non-tonic-clonic Forms of Status Epilepticus

So far, the treatment strategies outlined have concentrated on the approach to neonatal status epilepticus and the tonic-clonic form of status, in which it is imperative to control seizure activity and avoid the systemic and central pathologic consequences. In non-tonic-clonic forms of status epilepticus, systemic derangements are generally less evident, and in practice such changes usually result from the unwanted effects of anticonvulsants used. The presence or absence of generalized motor concomitants of status epilepticus should not be the sole determinant of aggressive and prompt treatment, since even nonconvulsive status epilepticus results in a rise in serum neuron-specific enolase, indicating at least a transient neuronal injury[152]. However, in non-tonic-clonic forms of status epilepticus, treatment escalation invariably occurs at a different pace, and by the

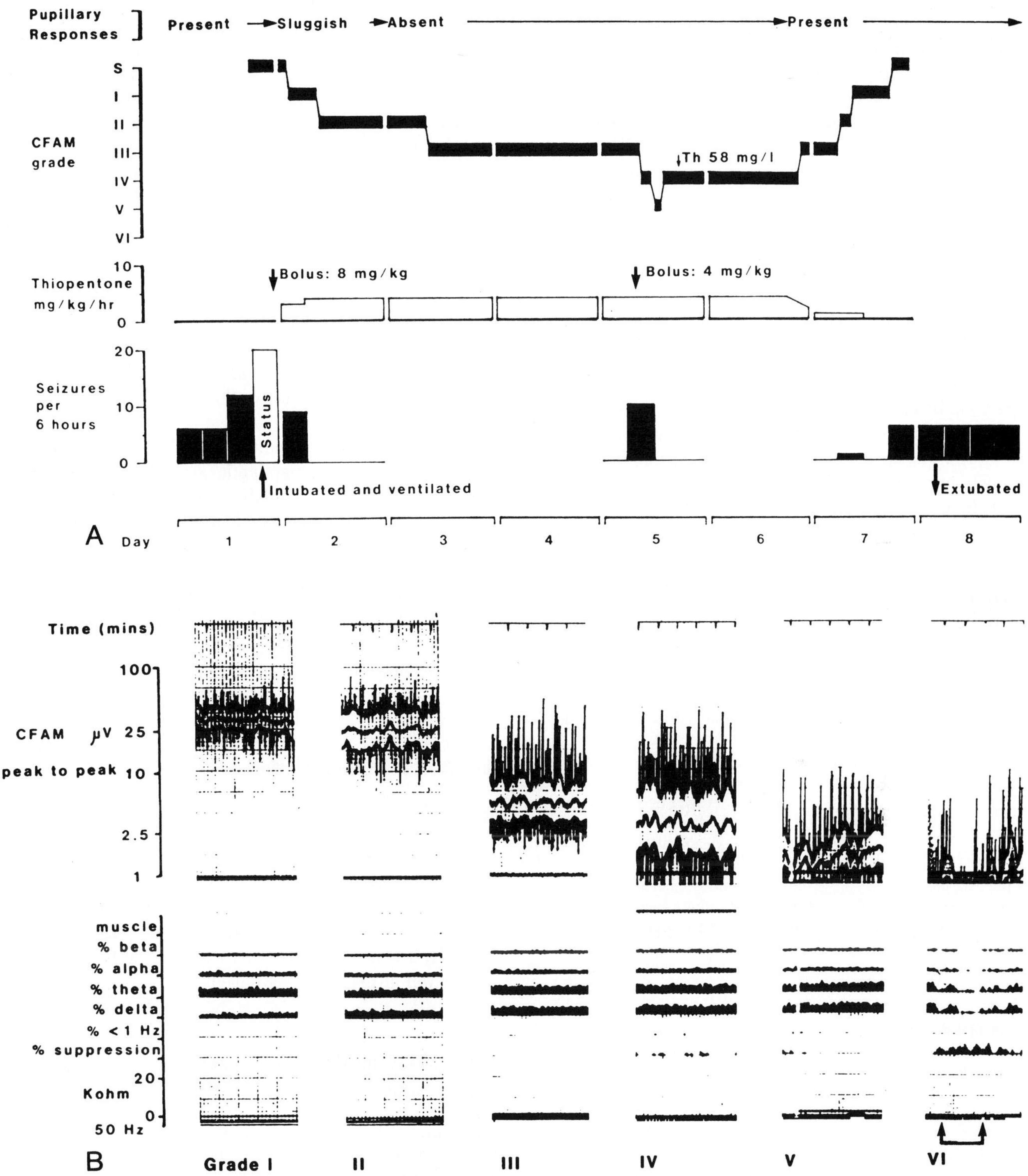

Figure 22.16. A. A 5-year-old child with intractable seizures who exhibited acute exacerbation of seizure control. Seizure frequency, EEG monitoring (see **B**), and pupillary responses are recorded during prolonged intravenous thiopental therapy. Status epilepticus was controlled and cortical electrical activity was depressed to a burst-suppression pattern by titrating drug administration against EEG effect *(CFAM grades IV–VI).* On stopping, thiopental cortical activity and baseline seizure frequency returned. *Th,* plasma thiopental concentration; *CFAM,* cerebral function analyzing monitor. **B.** Continuous processed EEG using the CFAM. The grading scale illustrates increasing cortical depression (i.e., decreasing amplitude plotted as the range, mean, 10th percentile, and 90th percentile of cerebral activity on the *upper part* of the *trace* and decreasing frequency plotted as percent cerebral activity within standard EEG frequency bands, including <1 Hz and burst-suppression) with the administration of thiopental, a short-acting barbiturate. *Grades IV–VI* represent burst suppression to electrocerebral silence. (From Tasker RC, Boyd SG, Harden A, Matthew DJ. EEG monitoring of prolonged thiopentone administration for intractable seizures and status epilepticus in infants and young children. Neuropediatrics 1989;20:147).

time such patients are admitted to the intensive care unit, they are receiving a complex anticonvulsant cocktail which may be difficult to rationalize. Management of these patients is complex. Simply adding or discontinuing an anticonvulsant may result in converting one type of seizure into another, more resistant form. In the authors' experience, optimal treatment of these patients can be successfully achieved only with full support from clinical neurophysiologic and neurologic services. For the common forms of status epilepticus outlined in the section on clinical presentation, the range of preferred treatments are listed in **Table 22.14.**

Investigational Antiepileptic Drugs

Several new antiepileptic drugs are in various stages of clinical testing. Some of these compounds show potential for treatment of the catastrophic childhood epilepsies which are complicated by episodes of status epilepticus and are notoriously unresponsive to currently available antiepileptic drugs. The agents that appear to be of value include felbamate, vigabatrin, clobazam, and lamotrigine(153).

Felbamate is structurally similar to meprobamate and has been approved by the U.S. Food and Drug Administration. It has been evaluated in a multicenter double-blind, placebo-controlled, add-on trial in 73 patients with Lennox-Gastaut syndrome, with encouraging results(154). Felbamate significantly decreased the frequency of atonic and tonic-clonic seizures. Vigabatrin is an analogue of GABA that irreversibly binds to the enzyme GABA-transaminase, thus inhibiting GABA degradation; resulting in a prolonged increase in brain GABA levels(155). It may play an important role in the treatment of infantile spasms. Chiron et al.(156) reported that 32 of 34 children with infantile spasms had at least a 50% decrease in seizure frequency; 11 were completely controlled. Clobazam is a benzodiazepine not fundamentally different from diazepam, nitrazepam, or clonazepam, although it may be less sedating(155). In a double-blind crossover study of children with medically refractory seizures, clobazam reduced the seizure frequency by more than 50% in half of the patients(157).

Lamotrigine (3,5-diamino-6[2,3-dichlorophenyl]-1,2,4-triazine) is a novel antiepileptic drug that is structurally unrelated to currently available drugs. It has weak antifolate activity which is independent of its anticonvulsant activity(155). It acts by limiting presynaptic glutamate release. Dulac et al.(158) reported in 1991 preliminary findings on 36 of 193 children who participated in an open add-on trial. Of the 36, 15 (41%) had a decrease in seizure frequency of at least 50%. The seizure types that responded best included myoclonic, myoclonic absence, tonic, and atonic. A single case report suggests that it might be effective in status epilepticus(159).

Table 22.14. Preferred Anticonvulsants for Non-tonic-clonic Forms of Status Epilepticus

Infantile spasms (West's syndrome)	Treat any underlying cause, e.g., hypoglycemia, metabolic disorders, endocrine abnormalities, infection. • ACTH 150 IU/day in 2 divided doses for 1 week —then 75 IU/day in 2 divided doses for 1 week —then lower over 5–8 weeks • Other drugs: benzodiazepines, valproate, vigabatrin, pyridoxine phosphate, gamma globulin
Epilepsia partialis continua	This may remit spontaneously. • First choice anticonvulsants: phenytoin, carbamazepine, phenobarbitone • Other treatment: corticosteroids or gamma globulin, nimodipine, surgery
Status epilepticus in mental retardation	Sedation may worsen all types of seizures. Tonic status is usually resistant to treatment, and occasionally benzodiazepines may worsen the episode. • First choice anticonvulsants: valproate, clonazepam, clobazam, lamotrigine • In emergencies, high-dose ACTH 80 IU/day or corticosteroids 0.3–1 mg/kg/day • Surgery
Status epilepticus in myoclonic syndromes	This is highly resistant to therapy. Urgently treat any fever or infection. • ACTH (as above) • Valproate and ethosuximide • Other drugs: acetazolamide, nitrazepam, corticosteroids
Myoclonic status epilepticus in coma	• Phenytoin or phenobarbitone • Corticosteroids can be tried.

Drug Toxicities in Status Epilepticus

Knowledge of the potential drug toxicities occurring during the treatment of status epilepticus is essential, not least because they are almost always iatrogenic **(Tables 22.9, 22.11, and 22.12).** An important distinction to make is between an anticonvulsant-related toxicity and that produced by a drug which has also induced seizures **(Table 22.15).** Treatment in the latter case will be helped by the withdrawal of the implicated agent.

Table 22.15. Drugs That Cause Seizures

Antimicrobials
Isoniazid
Penicillins
Nalidixic acid
Metronidazole
Anesthetics, narcotics, analgesics
Halothane, enflurane
Cocaine, fentanyl, meperidine
Ketamine
Psychopharmaceuticals
Antihistamines
Antidepressants
Antipsychotics
Phencyclidine
Tricyclic antidepressants

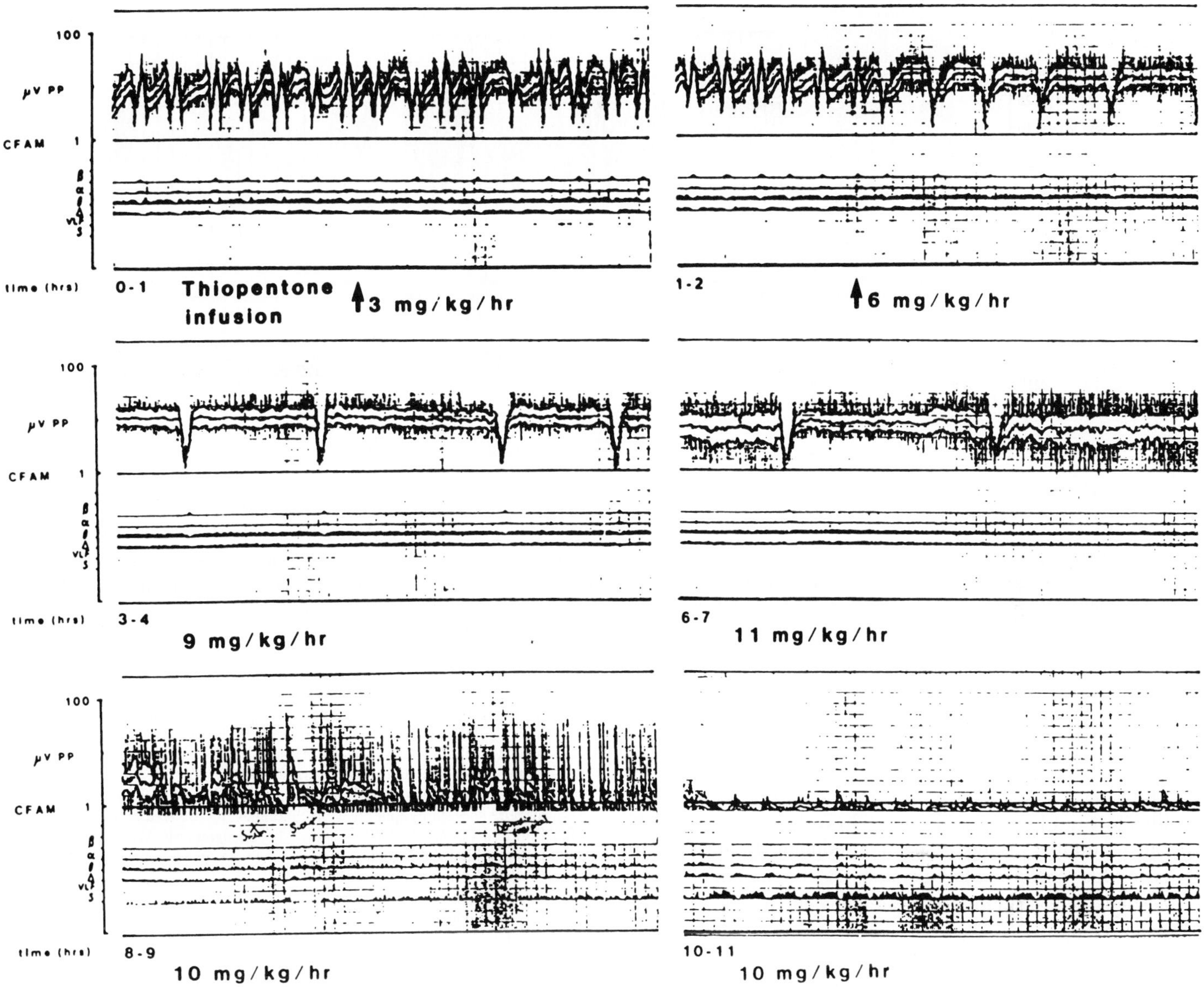

Figure 22.17. A sequence of 1-hour continuous processed EEG traces using the CFAM during the monitoring of an infant receiving prolonged intravenous thiopental for status epilepticus. Note the amplitude and frequency fluctuations related to seizures, which gradually diminish with increasing drug administration until burst-suppression and/or electrocerebral silence is induced. (From Tasker RC, Boyd SG, Harden A, Matthew DJ. The cerebral function analysing monitor in paediatric medical intensive care: application and limitation. Intensive Care Med 1990;16:60.)

Electroencephalography

Electroencephalography has an important place in the management of patients with seizures. Occasionally it provides information of diagnostic importance, but mainly its value is in providing an observable endpoint for anticonvulsant treatment when this is not clinically discernable. In status epilepticus multichannel electroencephalograms (EEGs) have the advantage that global findings and changes are well represented. However, when used over many days, they have obvious disadvantages, particularly with large volumes of data and continuous bedside interpretation.

The single- or two-channel signal processed EEG, such as that illustrated in Figure 22.16, presents data in an easily interpretable form. This can be used as a monitor of electrical seizures in the patient receiving neuromuscular blockers or as a monitor of general anesthesia therapy (Fig. 22.17). When considering the monitoring of seizures, it is important to first perform a multichannel EEG and select an appropriate channel for continuous monitoring. In previous studies[6,9,160,161] we have shown that many critically ill infants and young children have multifocal or variable focal rather than generalized discharges. Therefore, "blind" use of a standard single channel will inevitably lead to the possibility of missing certain events. Furthermore, the varied appearance and pattern of discharges may produce differing features on signal processing (Fig. 22.18). Unless these are specifically identified, bedside monitoring may be uninterpretable.

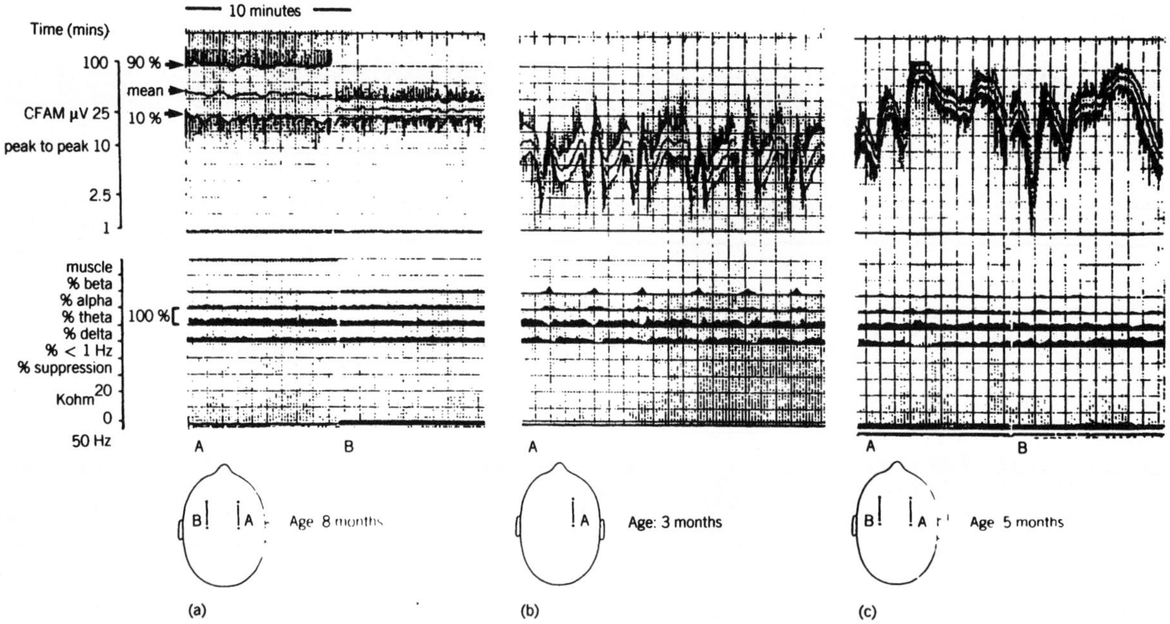

Figure 22.18. Paroxysmal changes observed using continuous signal processed EEG from the CFAM. **A.** Unchanging high-amplitude trace due to continuous repetitive discharges of fixed morphology—note that the left and right hemisphere discharges have a different amplitude. **B.** Consistently repetitive stereotyped fluctuations in amplitude and frequency due to episodic repetitive discharges. **C.** Irregular and chaotic fluctuations in amplitude and frequency due to discharges changing in rate, amplitude, and morphology.

When using signal processed EEG monitoring for assessing a pharmacologic endpoint such as burst-suppression with thiopentone, one would expect a generalized effect which should not be missed by a standardized channel. As illustrated in Figures 22.16 and 22.17, drug administration can be titrated against a specific endpoint. In our experience this enables administration of the minimum dose needed, thereby limiting or avoiding potential toxicities with unnecessary overdosing.

SUMMARY

Status epilepticus causes significant mortality and morbidity and must be regarded as a medical emergency. Delayed treatment disregards an enormous amount of pathologic evidence that status epilepticus per se is harmful to the brain. The longer seizures are permitted to continue, the more difficult they become to control, and the worse the prognosis. Immediate, rational, and potentially aggressive therapy is essential to reduce the mortality and long-term morbidity of status epilepticus. With the present level of expertise and sophistication of pediatric intensive care, it is doubtful that recent assessments of mortality can be improved on. What is hoped for in the future are newer and safe pharmacologic strategies aimed at suppressing activity resulting in neuronal injury, with applicability to some of our most difficult patients—those with non-tonic-clonic forms of status epilepticus.

References

1. Delgado-Escueta AV, Wasterlain CG, Trieman DM, Porter RJ, eds. Status epilepticus: summary. Adv Neurol 1983;34:537.
2. Aicardi J, Chevrie JJ. Convulsive status epilepticus in infants and children: a study of 239 cases. Epilepsia 1970;11:187.
3. Maytal J, Shinnar S, Moshe SL, Alvarez LA. Low morbidity and mortality of status epilepticus. Pediatrics 1989;83:323.
4. Orlowski JP, Erenberg G, Hans L. Hypothermia and barbiturate coma for refractory status epilepticus in children. Crit Care Med 1984;12:367.
5. Crawford TO, Mitchell WG, Fishman LS, Snodgrass SR. Very-high-dose phenobarbital for refractory status epilepticus in children. Neurology 1988;38:1035.
6. Tasker RC, Boyd SG, Harden A, Matthew DJ. EEG monitoring of prolonged thiopentone administration for intractable seizures and status epilepticus in infants and young children. Neuropediatrics 1989; 20:147.
7. Aubourg PO, Dulac P, Plouin C, Diebler. Infantile status epilepticus as a complication of 'near-miss' sudden infant death. Develop Med Child Neurol 1985;27:40.
8. Constantinou JEC, Gillis J, Ouvrier RA, Rahilly PM. Hypoxic-ischaemic encephalopathy after near miss sudden infant death syndrome. Arch Dis Child 1989;64:703.
9. Tasker RC, Boyd SG, Harden A, Kendall B, Harding BN, Matthew DJ. The clinical significance of seizures in critically ill young infants requiring intensive care. Neuropediatrics 1991;22:129.
10. Gastaut H. Classification of status epilepticus. Adv Neurol 1983;34:15.
11. Dreyfus-Brisac C, Monod N. Neonatal status epilepticus. In: Remond A, ed. Handbook of electroencephalography and clinical neurophysiology. Amsterdam: Elsevier, 1977;38.
12. Roger J, Lob H, Tassinari CA. Status epilepticus. In: Magnus O, Lorentz de Haas OM, eds. Handbook of clinical neurology. Amsterdam: North Holland Publishing Company, 1974;145.
13. Obeso JA, Rothwell JC, Marsden CD. The spectrum of cortical myoclonus. Brain 1985;108:193.
14. Celesia GG, Grigg MM, Ross E. Generalized status myoclonicus in acute anoxia and toxic-metabolic encephalopathies. Arch Neurol 1988;45:781.
15. Jumao-as A, Brenner RP. Myoclonic status epilepticus: a clinical and electroencephalographic study. Neurology 1990;40:1199.
16. Lowenstein DH, Aminoff MJ. Clinical and EEG features of status epilepticus in comatose patients. Neurology 1992;42:104.
17. Lennox WG, Lennox MH. Epilepsy and related disorders. Boston: Little, Brown 1960:1.
18. Fujiwara T, Ishida S, Miyakoshi M et al. Status epilepticus in childhood. A retrospective study of initial convulsive status and subsequent epilepsies. Folia Psychiatr Neurol Jpn 1979;33:337.

19. Vigevano F, DiCapua M, Fusco L, et al. Status epilepticus in infancy and childhood. J Pediatr Neurosci 1985;1:101.
20. Yager JY, Cheang M, Seshia SS. Status epilepticus in children. Can J Neurol Sci 1988;14:402.
21. Phillips SA, Shanahan RJ. Etiology and mortality of status epilepticus in children: a recent update. Arch Neurol 1989;46:74.
22. Rowan AJ, Scott DF. Major status epilepticus: A series of 42 patients. Arch Neurol Scand 1970;46:573.
23. Zhang Z, Feng Y. A clinical study of 100 status epilepticus cases. Chin Med J [Engl] 1982;95:113.
24. Dunn DW. Status epilepticus in children. Etiology, clinical features and outcome. J Child Neurol 1988;3:167.
25. Janz D. Etiology of convulsive status epilepticus. Adv Neurol 1983;34:47.
26. Dunn DW. Status epilepticus in infancy and childhood. Neurol Clin 1990;8:647.
27. Cavazzuti GB, Ferrari P, Lalla M. Follow-up study of 482 cases with convulsive disorders in the first year of life. Dev Med Child Neurol 1984;26:425.
28. Freeman JM. Status epilepticus: it's not what we've thought or taught. Pediatrics 1989;83:444.
29. Aicardi J, Chevrie JJ. Status epilepticus. Pediatrics 1989;84:939.
30. Oxbury JM, Whitty CWM. Causes and consequences of status epilepticus in adults—a study of 86 cases. Brain 1971;94:733.
31. Trieman DM, Walton NY, Wickholdt C, DeGiorgio C. Predictable sequence of EEG changes during generalized convulsive status epilepticus in man and three experimental models of status epilepticus in the rat. Neurology 1987;34:244.
32. McDonald JW, Johnston MV. Physiological and pathophysiological roles of excitatory amino acids during central nervous system development. Brain Res Rev 1990;15:41.
33. McDonald JW, Johnston MV, Young AB. Differential ontogenic development of three receptors comprising the NMDA receptor/channel complex in the rat hippocampus. Exp Neurol 1990;110:237.
34. Shinnar S, Maytal J, Krasnoff L, Moshé SL. Recurrent status epilepticus in children. Ann Neurol 1992;31:598.
35. Aminoff MJ, Simon RP. Status epilepticus: causes, clinical features and consequences in 98 patients. Am J Med 1980;657.
36. Simon RP. Physiologic consequences of status epilepticus. Epilepsia 1985;26(suppl 1):58.
37. Glaser GH. Medical complications of status epilepticus. Adv Neurol 1983;34:395.
38. Woody RC, Yamauchi T, Bolyard K. Cerebrospinal fluid cell counts in childhood idiopathic status epilepticus. Pediatr Infect Dis J 1988;7:298.
39. Treiman DM, Walton NY, Kendrick CW. A progressive sequence of electroencephalographic changes during generalized convulsive status epilepticus. Epilepsy Res 1990;5:49.
40. Woodbury DM. Experimental models of status epilepticus and mechanisms of drug action. Adv Neurol 1983;34:149.
41. Fisher RS. Animal models of the epilepsies. Brain Res Rev 1989;14:245.
42. Lombroso CT, Burchfiel JL. Etiologic and preventive aspects of epilepsy in the child bridging the gap between laboratory and clinic. Epilepsia 1987;28(suppl 1):25.
43. Lothman E. The biochemical basis and pathophysiology of status epilepticus. Neurology 1990;40(suppl 2):13.
44. Walton NY, Treiman DM. Experimental secondarily generalized convulsive status epilepticus induced by D.L. homocysteine thiolactone. Epilepsy Res 1988;2:79.
45. Walton NY, Treiman DM. Response of status epilepticus induced by lithium and pilocarpine to treatment with diazepam. Exp Neurol 1988;101:267.
46. Meldrum BS, Horten RW. Physiology of status epilepticus in primates. Adv Neurol 1973;28:1.
47. Meldrum BS, Brierley JB. Prolonged epileptic seizures in primates: ischemic cell damage and its relation to ictal physiological events. Arch Neurol 1973;28:10.
48. Meldrum BS, Vigouroux RA, Brierley JB. Systemic factors and epileptic brain damage: prolonged seizures in paralyzed, artificially ventilated baboons. Arch Neurol 1973;29:82.
49. Meldrum BS. Physiological changes during prolonged seizures and epileptic brain damage. Neuropediatrie 1978;9:203.
50. Simon RP, Bayne LL, Tranbaugh RF et al. Elevated pulmonary lymph flow and protein content during status epilepticus in sheep. J Appl Physiol 1982;52:91.
51. Simon RP, Aminoff MJ, Benowitz NL. Changes in plasma catecholamines after tonic-clonic seizures. Neurology 1984;34:255.
52. Benowitz NL, Simon RP, Copeland JR. Status epilepticus: divergence of sympathetic activity and cardiovascular response. Ann Neurol 1986;19:197.
53. Davies JB, Mathias CJ, Sudera D, et al. Agonist regulation of adrenergic receptor response in man. J Cardiovasc Pharmacol 1982;4:139.
54. Finnerty FA, Buckholz H, Guillaudeu RI. The blood volumes and plasma protein during levarterenol-induced hypertension. J Clin Invest 1958;37:425.
55. Hendley CD, Spudis EV, de la Torre E. Intracranial pressure during electroshock convulsions in the dog. Neurology 1965;15:351.
56. Penfield W, Saitha K, Cipriani I. Cerebral blood flow during induced epileptiform seizures in animals and man. J Neurophysiol 1939;2:258.
57. Meldrum BS, Nilsson B. Cerebral blood flow and metabolic rate early and late in prolonged epileptic seizures induced in rats by bicuculline. Brain 1976;99:523.
58. Horten RW, Meldrum BS, Pedley TA, McWilliam JR. Regional cerebral blood flow in the rat during prolonged seizure activity. Brain Res 1980;192:399.
59. Ingvar M, Siesjo BK. Local cerebral blood flow and glucose consumption in the rat during sustained bicuculline induced seizure. Acta Neurol Scand 1983;25:191.
60. Ingvar M, Soderfeldt B, Folbergrova J, Kalimo H, Olsson Y, Siesjo BK. Metabolic, circulatory and structural alteration in the rat brain induced by sustained pentylenetetrazole seizure. Epilepsia 1984;25:191.
61. Baldy-Moulinier M, Ingvar DH, Meldrum BS. Current problems in epilepsy: cerebral blood flow, metabolism and epilepsy. London: John Libbey, 1983.
62. Kuschinsky W, Wahl M. Perivascular pH and pial arterial diameter during bicuculline induced seizure in cats. Pflugers Arch Ges Physiol 1979;382:81.
63. Winn HR,, Welch J, Rubio R, Berne RM. Changes in brain adenosine during bicuculline-induced seizures in rat. Effects of hypoxia and altered systemic blood pressure. Circ Res 1980;47:481.
64. Marovitch S, Pinard E, Seylaz F. Two neural mechanisms in rat fastigial nucleus regulating systemic and cerebral circulation. Am J Physiol 1986;251:H153.
65. Nakai M, Iadecola C, Ruggiero D, Tucker L, Rens DJ. Electrical stimulation of the cerebral fastigial nucleus increases cerebral cortical blood flow without change in focal metabolism: evidence for an intrinsic system in brain for primary vasodilation. Brain Res 1983;260:35.
66. Fujikawa DG, Dwyer BE, Lake RR, Wasterlain CG. Cerebral blood flow and metabolism during neonatal seizures. In: Vert P, Wasterlain CG, eds. Neonatal seizures. New York: Raven Press,1990.
67. Perlman JM, Volpe JT. Seizures in the preterm infant: effect on cerebral blood flow velocity, intracranial pressure and arterial blood pressure. J Pediatr 1983;102:288.
68. Bayne LL, Simon RP. Systemic and pulmonary vascular pressures during generalized seizures in sheep. Annals of Neurology 1981;10:566.
69. Blennow G, Brierley JB, Meldrum BS, Siesjo BK. Epileptic brain damage: the role of systemic factors that modify cerebral metabolism. Brain 1978;101:687.
70. Meldrum BS, Horten RW, Brierley JB. Epileptic brain damage in adolescent baboons following seizures induced by allylglycine. Brain 1974;97:407.
71. Miller AL. Brain intermediary metabolism in vivo: changes with carbon dioxide, development and seizures. Int Rev Neurobiol 1981; 22:47.
72. Plum F, Poosner JB, Troy B. Cerebral metabolic and circulatory response to induced convulsions in animals. Arch Neurol 1968;18:1.
73. Borgstrom L, Chapman AG, Siiesjo BK. Glucose consumption in the cerebral cortex of rats during bicuculline induced status epilepticus. J Neurochem 1976;27:971.
74. Chapman AG. Cerebral energy metabolism and seizures. In: Pedley TA, Meldrum BS, eds. Recent advances in epilepsy 2. London: Churchill Livingstone, 1985:19.
75. Meldrum BS. Metabolic factors during prolonged seizures and their relation to nerve cell death. Adv Neurol 1983;34:261.
76. Kreisman NR, La Manna JC, Rosenthal M, Sick TJ. Oxidative metabolic responses with recurrent seizures in rat cerebral cortex: role of systemic factors. Brain Res 1981;218:175.
77. Kreisman NR, Sick TJ, Rosenthal M. Importance of vascular responses in determining cortical oxygenation during recurrent paroxysmal events of varying duration and frequency of repetition. J Cereb Blood Flow Metab 1983;3:330.
78. Kreisman NR, Rosenthal M, La Manna JC, Sick TJ. Cerebral oxygenation during recurrent seizures. Adv Neurol 1983;34:231.
79. Jobsis FF, Keizer J, La Manna JC, Rosenthal M. Reflectance spectro-

photometry of the intact cerebral cortex. I. Dual wavelength technique. J Appl Physiol 1977;43:858.
80. Kreisman NR, Magee JC, Brizzee BL. Relative hypoperfusion in rat cerebral cortex during recurrent seizures. J Cereb Blood Flow Metab 1991;11:77.
81. Maggio R, Fumagalli F, Donati E, Barbier P, Raragni G, Corsini GV, Riva M. Inhibition of nitric oxide synthase dramatically potentiates seizures induced by kainic acid and pilocarpine in rats. Brain Res 1995;679:184.
82. Pereira de Vasconcelos A, Boyet S, Koziel V, Nehlig A. Effects of pentylenetetrazol-induced status epilepticus on local cerebral blood flow in the developing brain. J Cerebral Blood Flow and Metabolism 1995; 15:270.
83. Sommer W. Erkrankung des ammonshorns als ätiologisches moment der epilepsie. Archiv für Psychiatrie Nervenkrankheiten 1880;10:631.
84. Meldrum BS, Corsellis JAN. Epilepsy. In: Adams JH, Corsellis JAN, Duchen LW, eds. Greenfield's neuropathology. London: Edward Arnold, 1984:921.
85. Norman RM. The neuropathology of status epilepticus. Med Sci Law 1964;4:46.
86. Corsellis JAN, Bruton CJ. Neuropathology of status epilepticus in adults. Adv Neurol 1983;34:129.
87. Babb T, Brown W. Pathological findings in epilepsy. In: Engel J, ed. Surgical treatment in epilepsy. New York: Raven Press, 1987; 511.
88. Soderfeldt B, Kalimo H, Olsson Y, Siesjo BK. Bicuculline induced epileptic brain injury. Acta Neuropathol 1983;62:87.
89. Nevander G, Ingvat M, Auer R, Siesjo BK. Status epilepticus in well oxygenated rats causes neuronal necrosis. Ann Neurol 1985;18:281.
90. Pinard E, Rigaud AS, Riche D, Naquet R, Seylaz J. Continuous determination of the cerebrovascular changes induced by bicuculline and kainic acid unanaesthetized spontaneously breathing rats. Neuroscience 1987;23:943.
91. Sloviter RS. Epileptic brain damage in rats induced by sustained electrical stimulation of the perforant path. I. Acute electrophysiological and light microscopic studies. Brain Res Bull 1983;10:675.
92. Olney JW, DeGubareff T, Sloviter RS. Epileptic brain damage in rats induced by sustained electrical stimulation of the perforant path. II. Ultrastructural analysis of acute hippocampal pathology. Brain Res Bull 1983;10:699.
93. Collins R, Olney J. Focal cortical seizures cause distant thalamic lesions. Science 1982;218:177.
94. Ingvar M, Morgan PF, Auer RW. The nature and timing of excitotoxic neuronal necrosis in the cerebral cortex, hippocampus and thalamus due to flurothyl-induced status epilepticus. Acta Neuropathol 1988;75:362.
95. Monaghan D, Holets V, Toy D, Cotman C. Anatomical distribution of four pharmacologically distinct ^{3}H-L - glutamate binding sites. Nature 1983;306:176.
96. Olney JW. Excitatory transmitters and epilepsy-related brain damage. Int Rev Neurobiol 1985;27:337.
97. Ingvar M. Seizure-induced damage in the substantia nigra pars reticulata: lesion in the frontal cortex prior to the seizure period mitigate the damage. Exp Brain Res 1989;75:369.
98. Woodbury DM. Experimental models of status epilepticus and mechanisms of drug action. Adv Neurol 1983;34:149.
99. Kapur J, Lothman EW. loss of inhibition precedes delayed spontaneous seizures in the hippocampus after tetanic electrical stimulation. J Neurophysiol 1989;61:426.
100. Lehman A, Hamberger A. Extracellular levels of amino acids in epilepsy: methods and findings. In: Fisher RS, Coyle JT, eds. Neurotransmitters and epilepsy: frontiers of clinical neuroscience. New York: Alan R Liss, 1991.
101. Benveniste H, Drejer J, Schousboe A, Diemer NH. Elevation of the extracellular concentrations of glutamate and aspartate in rat hippocampus during transient cerebral ischemia monitored by intracerebral microdialysis. J Neurochem 1984;43:1369.
102. Hagberg H, Lehmann A, Sandberg M, Nystrom B, Jacobson I, Hamberger A. Ischemia-induced shift of inhibitory and excitatory amino acids from intra- to extracellular compartment. J Cereb Blood Flow Metab 1985;5:413.
103. Sandberg M, Butcher SP, Hagberg H. Extracellular overflow of neuroactive amino acids during severe insulin-induced hypoglycemia: in vivo dialysis of the rat hippocampus. J Neurochem 1986;47:178.
104. Lehmann A. Alterations in hippocampal extracellular amino acids and puring metabolites during limbic seizures induced by folate injections into the rabbit amygdala. Neuroscience 1987;22:573.
105. Lehmann A, Hagberg H, Jacobson I, Hamberger A. Effects of status epilepticus on extracellular amino acids in the hippocampus. Brain Res 1985;359:147.
106. Fujikawa DG, Cheung MC. Extracellular glutamate and aspartate concentrations in the amygdala are unchanged by pilocarpine seizures and microinjection of AP7. J Cereb Blood Flow Metab 1989;11(suppl 2):107.
107. Ormandy GC, Jope RS, Snead OC. Anticonvulsant actions of MK-801 on the lithium-pilocarpine model of status epilepticus in rats. Exp Neurol 1989;106:172.
108. Sparenborg S, Brennecke LH, Juax NK, Braitman DJ. Dizocilpine (MK-801) arrests status epilepticus and prevents brain damage induced by soman. Neuropharmacology 1992;331:357.
109. Mikati MA, Holmes GL, Chronopoulos A et al. Phenobarbital modifies seizure-related brain injury in the developing brain. Ann Neurol 1994;36:425.
110. Tecott LH, Sun LM, Akana SF, Strack AM, Lowenstein DH, Dallman MF, Julius D. Eating disorder and epilepsy in mice lacking 5-HT2C serotonin receptors. Nature 1995;374:542.
111. Liu Z, Mikati M, Holmes GL. Mesial temporal sclerosis: pathogenesis and significance. Pediatr Neurol 1995;12:5.
112. Lothman EW, Bertram EH. Epileptogenic effects of status epilepticus. Epilepsia 1993;34(suppl 1):559.
113. Holmes GL, Thompson JL. Effects of kainic acid on seizure susceptibility in the developing brain. Dev Brain Res 1988;39:51.
114. Wasterlain CG, Fujikawa DG, Penix L, Sankar R. Pathophysiological mechanisms of brain damage from status epilepticus. Epilepsia 1993;34(suppl 1):37.
115. Grattan-Smith JD, Harvey AS, Desmond PM, Chow CW. Hippocampal sclerosis in children with intractable temporal lobe epilepsy: detection with MR imaging. AJR 1993;161:1045.
116. Simon PR. Management of status epilepticus. In: Pedley TA, Meldrum BS, eds. Recent advances in epilepsy 2. Edinburgh: Churchill Livingstone, 1985:137.
117. Browne TR. The pharmacokinetics of agents used to treat status epilepticus. Neurology 1990;40(suppl 2):28.
118. Arendt RM, Greenblatt DJ, DeJong RH. In vivo correlates of benzodiazepine cerebrospinal fluid uptake, pharmacodynamic action and peripheral uptake. J Pharmacol Exp Ther 1983;227:98.
119. Greenblatt DJ, Koch-Wesser J. Clinical pharmacokinetics. N Engl J Med 1975;293:702.
120. Ramsay RE, Hammond EJ, Perchalski RJ, et al. Brain uptake of phenytoin, phenobarbital and diazepam. Arch Neurol 1979;36:355.
121. Browne TR. Clinical pharmacology of antiepileptic drugs. Drug Ther Rev 1979;2:469.
122. Tassinari CA, Daniele O, Michelucci R, Bureau M, Dravet C, Roger J. Benzodiazepines: efficacy in status epilepticus. Adv Neurol 1983; 34:465.
123. Leppik IE, Derivan AT, Homan RW, Walker JE, Ramsay RE, Patrick B. Double-blind study of lorazepam and diazepam in status epilepticus. JAMA 1983;249:1452.
124. Kyriakopoulos AA, Greenblatt DJ, Shader RI. Clinical pharmacokinetics of lorazepam: a review. J Clin Psychiatry 1978;39:16.
125. McWilliam PKA, Leeds MB. IV phenytoin sodium in continuous convulsions in children. Lancet 1958;2:1147.
126. Wallis W, Kott M, McDowell F. Intravenous diphenylhydantoin in treatment of acute repetitive seizures. Neurology 1968;18:513.
127. Albani M. Phenytoin in infancy and childhood. Adv Neurol 1983;34:457.
128. Dodson WE. Nonlinear kinetics of phenytoin in children. Neurology 1982;32:42.
129. Simon RP, Copeland JR, Benowitz NL, Jacob P, Bronstein J. Brain phenobarbital uptake during prolonged status epilepticus. J Cereb Blood Flow Metab 1987;7:783.
130. Aston R, Domino EF. Differential effects of phenobarbital, pentobarbital and diphenylhydantoin on motor cortical and reticular thresholds in the rhesus monkey. Psychopharmacologia 1961;2:304.
131. Macdonald RL, Barker JL. Different actions of anticonvulsant and anesthetic barbiturates revealed by use of cultured mammalian neurons. Science 1978;200:775.
132. Raines A, Blake GJ, Richardson B, Gilbert MB. Differential selectivity of several barbiturates on experimental seizures and neurotoxicity in the mouse. Epilepsia 1979;20:105.
133. Kurz H, Mauser-Ganshorn A, stickel HH. Differences in the binding of drugs to plasma protein from newborn and adult man. Eur J clin Pharmacol 1977;11:436.

134. Ehrnebo M, Agurell S, Jalling B, Boreur LO. Age differences in drug binding by plasma proteins in studies on human foetuses, neonates and adults. Eur J Clin Pharmacol 1971;3:189.
135. Cloyd JC, Gumnit RJ, McLain LW Jr. Status epilepticus. The role of intravenous phenytoin. JAMA 1980;244:1475.
136. Dodson WE. Special pharmacokinetic consideration in children. Epilepsia 1987;28(suppl 1):56.
137. Mitchell WG, Crawford TO. Lorazepam is the treatment of choice for status epilepticus. T Epilepsy 1990;3:7.
138. Lacey DJ, Singer WD, Horwitz SJ, Gilmore H. Lorazepam therapy of status epilepticus in children and adolescents. J Pediatr 1986;108:771.
139. Deshmukh A, Wittert W, Schnitzler E, Mangurten HH. Lorazepam in the treatment of refractory neonatal seizures. Am J Dis Child 1986;140:1042.
140. Crawford TO, Mitchell WG, Snodgrass SR. Lorazepam in childhood status epilepticus and serial seizures: effectiveness and tachyphylaxis. Neurology 1987;37:190.
141. Celesia GG, Grigg MM, Ross E. Generalized status myoclonus in acute anoxic and toxic-metabolic encephalopathies. Arch Neurol 1988; 45:781.
142. Gabor AJ. Lorazepam versus phenobarbital: candidates for drug of choice for treatment of status epilepticus. J Epilepsy 1990;3:3.
143. Shorvon SD. Tonic-clonic status epilepticus. J Neurology Neurosurgery Psychiatry 1993;56:1 25.
144. Cranford RE, Leppik IE, Patrick B, et al. Intravenous phenytoin in acute seizure disorders. Neurology 1978;28:874.
145. Louis S, Kutt H, McDowell F. The cardiocirculatory changes caused by dilantin and its solvent. Am Heart J 1967;74:523.
146. Cranford RE, Leppik IE, Patrick B, Anderson CB, Kostick B. Intravenous phenytoin: clinical and pharmacokinetic aspects. Neurology 1978;28:874.
147. Delgado-Escueta AV, Wasterlain C, Treiman DM, Porter RJ. Management of status epilepticus. N Engl J Med 1982;306:1337.
148. Opitz A, Marshall M, Degan R, Koch D. General anesthesia in patients with epilepsy. Adv Neurol 1983;34:531.
149. Orlowski JP, Erenberg G, Hans L. Hypothermia and barbiturate coma for refractory status epilepticus. Crit Care Med 1984;12:367.
150. Rawal K, D'Souzo BJ. Status epilepticus. Crit Care Clin 1985;1:339.
151. Kofke WA, Snider MT, Young RSK, Ramer JC. Prolonged low-flow isoflurane anesthesia for status epilepticus. Anesthesiology 1985;62:653.
152. Rabinowicz AL, Correale JD, Bracht KA, Smith TD, DeGiorgio CM. Neuron-specific enolase is increased after nonconvulsive status epilepticus. Epilepsia 1995;36:475.
153. Shields WD. Investigational drugs for the treatment of childhood seizure disorders: a review of efficacy and safety. Epilepsia 1994;35(Suppl 2):24.
154. Ritter FJ, Leppik IE, Dreifuss FE, et al. Felbamate: a double-blind controlled trial in Lennox-Gastaut syndrome. N Eng J Med 1993;328: 29.
155. Rogawski MA, Porter RJ. Antiepileptic drugs: pharmacological mechanisms and clinical efficacy with consideration of promising developmental stage compounds. Pharmacol Rev 1990;42:223.
156. Chiron C, Mondragon S, Dulac O, Beaumont D, Palacios L, Luna D. Clinical trial of vigabatrin in infantile spasms. Epilepsia 1989;30:661.
157. Keene DL, Whiting S, Humphreys P. Clobazam as an add-on drug in the treatment of refractory epilepsy of childhood. Can J Neurol Sci 1990;17:317.
158. Dulac O, Withers RM, Yuen AWC. Add-on lamotrigine in pediatric patients with treatment resistant epilepsy. Epilepsia 1991;32(suppl 1):95.
159. Pisani F, Gallitto G, Di Perri R. Could Lamotrigine be useful in status epilepticus? A case report. J Neurology Neurosurgery Psychiatry 1991;54:845.
160. Tasker RC, Boyd SG, Harden A, Matthew DJ. The cerebral function analysing monitor in paediatric medical intensive care: application and limitations. Intensive Care Med 1990;16:60.
161. Tasker RC, Boyd S, Harden A, Matthew DJ. Monitoring in non-traumatic coma. Part II: electroencephalography. Arch Dis Child 1988;63:895.

Reye Syndrome and Metabolic Encephalopathies 23

Robert C. Tasker
W. Bradley Poss
J. Michael Dean

INTRODUCTION

Many metabolic disturbances may produce a fluctuation in level of consciousness or coma. During the course of an acute illness—whether at presentation or developing as a secondary complicating factor—these changes may result in or be symptomatic of significant morbidity and even lead to death. For the pediatric intensivist, no condition has more exemplified the acute encephalopathic progression than *acute toxic encephalopathy*[(1,2)], of which Reye syndrome[(3–5)], characterized by nonicteric hepatic dysfunction, has been the most common in recent years. Although for the present Reye syndrome is infrequently seen[(6,7)], in the wider context of clinical management during toxic-metabolic derangement and nontraumatic coma it should be considered prototypic. Historically, the development of a refined critical care approach to children with Reye syndrome has generally shaped our present practice of pediatric intensive care[(8)]. Indeed, many of the techniques used for its treatment have found beneficial application in some cases of overwhelming liver disease, renal disease, hyperammonemia, and inborn errors of metabolism.

Extensive review of the symptoms, natural history, biochemistry, and management of individual toxic-metabolic disorders can be found in standard pediatric, metabolic, and toxicologic texts[(9–11)]. Although many of the genetic and toxic-metabolic disorders are rare, particular clinical scenarios not unusual for intensive care should alert the physician to an appropriate differential diagnosis, especially if the working diagnosis is unsubstantiated or the clinical course is atypical.

The scope of this chapter is a discussion of the following:

1. The extent to which metabolic derangements contribute to the differential diagnosis of familiar intensive-care scenarios

2. The pathophysiology and neurotoxicity of common metabolic encephalopathies
3. Specific therapies that may be required at the time of acute presentation to reduce morbidity and optimize outcome

ETIOLOGY AND DIFFERENTIAL DIAGNOSIS

There are a variety of toxic-metabolic disorders that may produce an acute depression in level of consciousness **(Table 23.1),** with some being more common at particular ages (see below). In some patients, etiology may be complex, with more than one known factor being implicated as the cause for coma. For practical application in the context of critical care, patient presentation can be in one of two ways:

1. A characteristic history and findings, not infrequently seen and suggestive of certain disorders, the so-called classic syndromes of critical illness:
   a. Reye syndrome and Reye-like illness
   b. Raised intracranial pressure
   c. Hepatic encephalopathy
   d. Fulminant infantile encephalopathy
2. An identified profound biochemical derangement requiring further management, e.g., acidosis, hyperammonemia, hypoglycemia, electrolyte imbalance

Table 23.1. Causes of Acute Toxic-Metabolic Encephalopathy in Childhood

Acid-base disturbance
Acidosis—diabetic ketoacidosis, organic acidemia, renal tubular acidosis
Alkalosis
Fluid and electrolyte derangement
Dehydration
Adrenal crisis
Water intoxication—inappropriate ADH[a] secretion, psychogenic polydipsia
Hypercalcemia/hypocalcemia
Hypernatremia/hyponatremia
Hypomagnesemia/hypermagnesemia
Deprivation of oxygen, substrate, or metabolic cofactor
Hypoxia/ischemia
Hypoglycemia
(Seizure postictally)
Vitamin/cofactor deficiency—thiamine, niacin, pyridoxine
Diseases of organs other than brain
Liver failure/hyperammonemia—infection, urea-cycle, Reye-like
Renal failure—uremia
Lung—carbon dioxide narcosis
Endocrine—thyroid, parathyroid, adrenal, diabetes
Endogenous (inherited metabolic disorders)
Aminoaciduria
Organic acidemia
Galactosemia
Porphyria

[a] ADH, antidiuretic hormone.

Classic Syndromes of Critical Illness

Reye Syndrome and Reye-like Illness

Reye syndrome is a disorder of unknown etiology and historically of high mortality[(3–5)]. It is exemplified by the child who, while recovering from a viral prodrome, unexpectedly develops pernicious vomiting and, subsequently, a deteriorating level of consciousness. Abnormalities related to hepatic failure may occur, including enzyme elevations, coagulation disorders, and alterations of carbohydrate, amino acid, and lipid metabolism. Other accompaniments of multisystem failure may occur, including myocardial failure[(12)], dehydration and shock, acute renal failure[(13)], peptic ulcers[(14)], pancreatitis[(15,16)], and sepsis. Patients who die have severe cerebral edema and fatty infiltration of the viscera, including the heart (Fig. 23.1) and kidneys (Fig. 23.2). Although the usual cause of death is brain tissue herniation secondary to intracranial hypertension, it may also result from myocardial failure, gastrointestinal bleeding, status epilepticus, renal failure, respiratory failure, or cardiovascular collapse.

Etiology

The cause of Reye syndrome has remained elusive. Since the original description in 1963[(3–5)], it has been seen in large clusters as well as more sporadically during the 1970s. Over this time the debate about etiology has encompassed ideas concerning associated trigger factors and specific genetic-metabolic defects or some combined interaction. For example, several studies have documented a controversial association between the use of aspirin in children with viral illnesses and the subsequent development of Reye syndrome[(17–21)]. In support of this, a national campaign during the 1980s, aimed at reducing the use of aspirin in children,

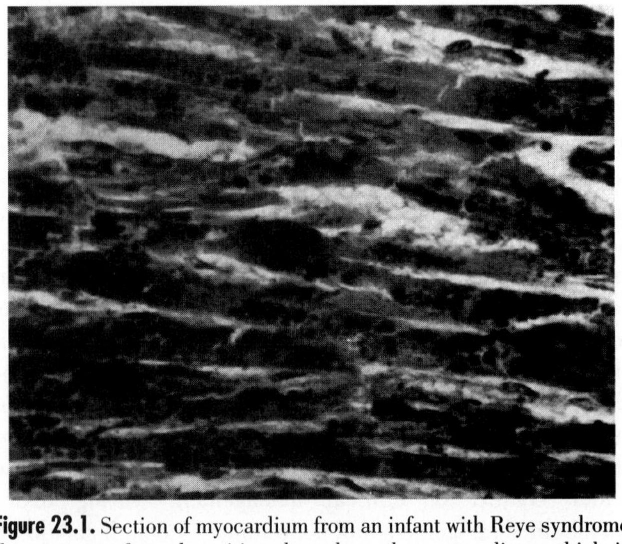

Figure 23.1. Section of myocardium from an infant with Reye syndrome demonstrates fatty deposition throughout the myocardium, which is microvesicular (×200). Osmium stain. (Courtesy of Grover Hutchins, M.D., Department of Pathology, The Johns Hopkins University School of Medicine.)

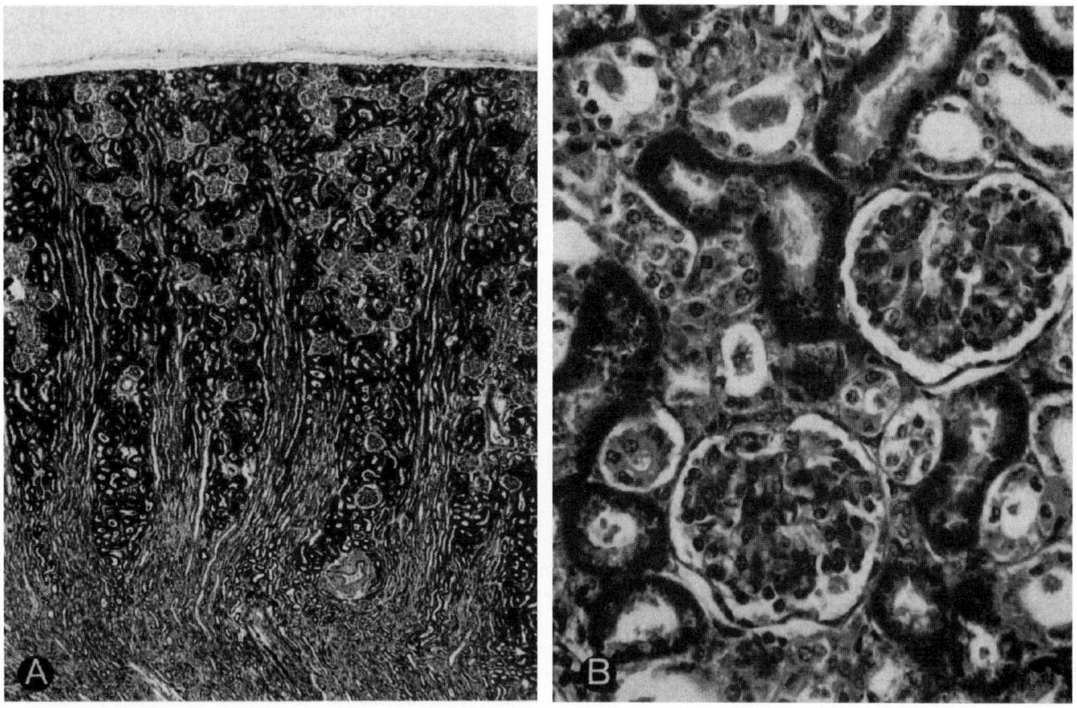

Figure 23.2. Sections of kidney from a child with Reye syndrome. **A.** Diffuse involvement of the proximal tubuli with fatty deposition and relative sparing of the glomeruli and distal tubuli (×40). **B.** Subnuclear distribution of the microvesicular fatty deposits (×400). Osmium stain. (Courtesy of Grover Hutchins, M.D., Department of Pathology, The Johns Hopkins University School of Medicine.)

was linked with a subsequent decline in Reye syndrome reporting[22]. This decline was seen at the same time as knowledge of metabolic diseases was rapidly expanding, and an alternative explanation may be that fewer patients with an underlying genetic-metabolic disease were being incorrectly labeled as Reye syndrome[23–25]. Despite this, Reye syndrome has not disappeared[26,27], although the 25 cases reported in the United States in 1989 was the lowest since the institution of national surveillance in 1979[28].

The likely candidate for a metabolic defect is a hepatic mitochondrial β-oxidation disorder[29]. Possible triggering factors include antecedent viral infection, particularly influenza B, and to a lesser extent influenza A and varicella[30,31], though others have been reported, e.g., adenovirus, Coxsackie A and B, cytomegalovirus, dengue, echoviruses, Epstein-Barr virus, herpes viruses, mumps, parainfluenza, and respiratory syncytial virus[32–34]. The exact mechanisms involved in the viral pathogen's disruption of mitochondrial oxidation remains unproven, although most experimental evidence has speculated on co-triggers salicylate ingestion, endotoxins, cytokines, or tumor necrosis factor[29]. Other authors have demonstrated mitochondrial changes in mice secondary to changes in mitochondrial lipid peroxidation[35], increased hepatic mitochondrial cholesterol[36], increases in dicarboxylic acids[37], and free radicals[38].

Differential Diagnosis

Of recent interest and importance has been the recognition and description of a variety of conditions presenting with what has been termed Reye-like illness or secondary Reye syndrome[39]. Patients with these conditions meet the standard clinical diagnostic criteria of Reye syndrome as defined by the Centers for Disease Control **(Table 23.2)**[40]. The differential diagnoses include the spectrum of inflammatory encephalopathies, toxic ingestions, and primary infections of the liver (i.e., hepatitis). Multiple types of genetic metabolic disorders may look like Reye syndrome **(Table 23.3)**, including ornithine transcarbamylase deficiency[41], carnitine deficiency[42], arginosuccinic acid synthetase deficiency[43], pyruvate dehydrogenase and pyruvate carboxylase deficiencies[44], fatty acid oxidative abnormalities[45], and urea cycle abnormalities[46]. Of these, the most metabolic disorders which mimic Reye's syndrome are urea cycle disorders, organic acidemias, and disorders of fat oxidation.

Table 23.2. Centers for Disease Control (1980) Case Definition of Reye Syndrome[a]

Acute noninflammatory encephalopathy
- Microvesicular fatty metamorphosis of the liver confirmed by biopsy or autopsy
- Serum glutamic oxaloacetic transaminase (SGOT), or Serum glutamic pyruvic transaminase (SGPT), or Serum ammonia greater than 3 times normal

Cerebrospinal fluid
If obtained, there must be less than 9 leukocytes/m^2

Exclusion of other diagnoses
There should be no other more reasonable explanation for the neurologic presentation of the hepatic abnormality

[a] From Centers for Disease Control. Follow-up on Reye's syndrome—United States. MMWR CDC Surveill Summ 1980;29:321.

Table 23.3. Conditions Producing a Reye-like Illness

Infective conditions
Acute liver failure (viral hepatitis, antituberculous drugs, monoamine oxidase inhibitors, acetaminophen, ischemia)
Severe infection (endotoxic shock)
Inherited disorders of urea cycle
Carbamoyl-phosphate synthase deficiency
Ornithine carbamoyltransferase deficiency
Citrullinemia
Arginosuccinic aciduria
Arginase deficiency (rare)
Organic acidemias
Proprionic and methylmalonic acidemia
Other inherited metabolic disease
Triple H syndrome (hyperammonemia, hyperornithinemia, homocitrullinuria)
Hyperlysinemia
Fat oxidation defects (medium- and long-chain and multiple acetyl-CoA[a] dehydrogenase deficiency)
Toxins and medications
Drugs (salicylates, valproate, warfarin)
Toxins (aflatoxin, hypoglycine, ackee, pteridine, calcium hopantenate, isopropyl alcohol methobromide, lead, margosa oil, diallylacetate)

[a] acyl-CoA, acylocoenzyme A.

Urea Cycle Disorders Metabolic acidosis and hypoglycemia are not usually found, but hyperammonemia is present and often severe. The plasma and urine amino acid profiles are abnormal, and urinary orotic acid is elevated in most of these disorders. In the most serious cases, patients are affected in the neonatal period, but there is a wide spectrum of severity, and patients may be affected at any age in childhood. The female carrier of the X-linked disorder ornithine carbamylase deficiency, as well as the homozygous male with partial enzyme deficiency, may present with mild episodic symptoms.

Organic Acidemias The main distinguishing feature in the organic acidemias is usually an overriding metabolic acidosis. Hyperammonemia, at times as dramatic as that associated with urea cycle disorders, is commonly seen in critically ill neonates, whereas it is less consistently observed in older children. These conditions arise from a defect in amino acid breakdown, and the most common are propionic acidemia, methylmalonic acidemia, and maple syrup urine disease. The plasma amino acid profile is diagnostic in the latter, but to establish the diagnosis in the majority of these disorders gas chromatography of plasma and urine organic acids is required.

Disorders of Fat Oxidation Medium- and long-chain acyl CoA dehydrogenase deficiency may resemble Reye syndrome. Typically these patients have nonketotic hypoglycemia and hyperammonemia, but the metabolic acidosis is not striking. Episodes of encephalopathy are often associated with hepatomegaly (due to fatty infiltrates) and tend to become less frequent with time. Serum carnitine is low, which probably results from urinary losses of acyl carnitine. Some children may have primary systemic carnitine deficiency present with a Reye-like illness(47). The cause of this primary carnitine deficiency is unclear but is possibly due to a combination of impaired gastrointestinal absorption and renal tubular resorption.

Pathology

The most significant histologic abnormalities in patients with Reye syndrome are found in the liver. A diffuse, panlobular, microvesicular steatosis with central nuclei and glycogen depletion are seen at autopsy or on liver biopsy specimens(48). Electron microscopy studies reveal deformed hepatic mitochondria with decreased matrix density and cristae in affected patients. Interestingly, Tonsgard(37) reproduced identical morphologic changes in murine hepatic cells using serum from patients with Reye syndrome.

The other key pathologic findings in patients with Reye syndrome is fatty infiltration of the heart and kidney and cerebral edema. The brain pathology has been variable but classically consists of cytotoxic cerebral edema with swelling of astrocytic foot processes(49). Ischemic changes from increased intracranial pressure are often noted, as cerebral herniation is the usual cause of death. Autopsy studies have not demonstrated a primary cerebral mitochondrial defect(49), and hyperammonemia has usually been implicated as the cause of the encephalopathy(50).

Historical Treatment and Outcome

Historically, the treatment of Reye syndrome has been instrumental in developing a rational approach to the current treatment of patients with acute encephalopathy complicated by hypoglycemia, raised intracranial pressure, and hyperammonemia.

The treatment of Reye syndrome consisted of basic intensive care with attention to airway management, preservation of perfusion and oxygenation, prevention of hypoglycemia, and treatment of intracranial hypertension. Therapy was essentially supportive, with prompt recognition and correction of problems. Hypoglycemia was corrected by the initiation of appropriate glucose-containing intravenous solutions. Intracranial pressure was monitored with invasive catheters and limited by a protocol of hyperventilation, fluid restriction, and osmotic diuresis(51–53). Hyperammonemia was treated by a variety of ammonia-reducing approaches, including peritoneal dialysis(54,55), exchange transfusions(51), charcoal hemoperfusion(56), and even total body washout with the use of cardiopulmonary bypass(57,58). Apart from individual case reports, none of these treatments has had a major impact on outcome.

During the 1970s mortality rates between 12 and 40% were seen. Long-term sequelae in survivors included learning disabilities, behavioral difficulties, and speech disorders in as much as 50%(59,60). A more recent report from Great Britain comparing Reye syndrome survivors with matched siblings was more optimistic(61). Most (82%) of the survivors were performing well in school and differed only in their performance on basic math skills when compared

Table 23.4. Toxic-Metabolic Encephalopathies in Which Significant Cerebral Edema Has Been Reported[a]

Inherited metabolic
Aminoacidopathies
Organic acidemias
Hyperammonemia
Porphyria
Nonketotic hyperglycinemia
Organ failure
Uremia
Hepatic failure
Electrolytes, minerals, and vitamins
Hypercalcemia
Hypernatremia
Water intoxication
Lead poisoning
Vitamin A toxicity
Other
Hypoglycemia
Hypoxia/ischemia

[a] This list, rather than being exhaustive, reflects the diversity of disease categories associated with cerebral edema.

to siblings. Other complications of Reye syndrome have included Ondine's curse[62] and vocal cord paralysis[63].

Raised Intracranial Pressure

In the absence of an intracranial space-occupying lesion or hydrocephalus, raised intracranial pressure can result from increased venous pressure (as in dural sinus thrombosis), increased resistance of arachnoid villi to resorption of cerebrospinal fluid, hypersecretion of cerebrospinal fluid (as seen in certain endocrine abnormalities), and cerebral edema. The toxic-metabolic causes are listed in **Table 23.4.** Early symptoms and signs of raised intracranial pressure are nonspecific **(Table 23.5),** and the late identification of this problem is often indicated by signs of brain-tissue herniation **(Table 23.6).**

Pathologic Types of Cerebral Edema

Cerebral edema is defined as an increase in brain volume due to an increase in its water content. When generalized, it will cause raised intracranial pressure. Localized edema however, may result merely in an alteration in cerebral function with no change in fluid dynamics. Cranial imaging will aid the diagnosis of cerebral edema: computed tomography (CT) scanning may show diffuse or localized low attenuation as a result of high water content; T2-weighted magnetic resonance imaging (MRI) will show an intense signal. Cerebral edema can result from a variety of brain insults, with specific types of edema being associated with certain pathologic processes, although in many instances more than one of the processes may be implicated.

Vasogenic Edema An increase in cerebral capillary endothelial permeability will result in the exudation of proteinaceous fluid into surrounding cerebral white matter. Whether there is focal or global cerebral edema will be determined by the underlying cause of the change in cerebral vascular permeability (e.g., infection, trauma, toxins, focal seizures, and hypertension).

Table 23.5. Nonspecific Symptoms and Signs of Raised Intracranial Pressure

	Infant	*Child*
General state	Poor feeding, vomiting Irritability-coma Seizures	Anorexia, nausea, vomiting Lethargy-coma Seizures
Head/eyes	Full fontanele Scalp vein distention False localizing signs	False localizing signs *(see Table 23.13)*
Other	Altered vital signs Hypertension Pulmonary edema	Altered vital signs Hypertension Pulmonary edema

Cytotoxic Edema All cells within the brain can undergo rapid swelling as a result of membrane ionic pump failure secondary to intracellular energy failure. This may be due to hypoxic-ischemic insult, severe infection, toxins, status epilepticus, and low cerebral blood flow.

Hypo-osmotic Edema Osmotic dysequilibrium between a low osmolality plasma compartment and higher osmotic pressure within glial cells will result in astrocytic water accumulation and brain tissue edema. This may occur with hyponatremia, excessive fluid resuscitation for diabetic ketoacidosis, and dialysis dysequilibrium syndrome.

Interstitial Edema In patients with raised intracranial pressure and hydrocephalus, periventricular interstitial edema may occur, caused by transependymal resorption of cerebrospinal fluid into the extracellular space.

Hydrostatic Edema When an increased intravascular pressure is transmitted to the capillary bed, there is a net efflux of water into the extracellular space. Such hydrostatic edema may be seen in states of deranged autoregulation, as occurs in systemic hypertension and hypercapnia.

Benign Intracranial Hypertension

The syndrome of benign intracranial hypertension is characterized by raised intracranial pressure in the absence of focal neurologic dysfunction, intracerebral mass lesion, obstructive hydrocephalus, chronic meningitis, hypertension, and pulmonary encephalopathy. In most cases the cause and pathogenesis are poorly understood **(Table 23.7).** What distinguishes this clinical condition of raised intracranial pressure from that of cerebral edema is the apparent well-being of these patients. On the intensive care unit this may pose a problem when interpreting the clinical significance of elevated intracranial pressure in some patients who have multiple reasons for coma. In the conscious patient, headache is the most common complaint, with signs including nerve VI palsy, visual acuity loss, papilledema, vertical strabismus or other oculomotor abnormalities, pupillary abnormalities, facial palsy, and ataxia[64].

Table 23.6. Clinical Signs of Brain Downward Herniation

	Tentorial	Foramen Magnum
Mechanism	1. Diencephalon and hypothalamus move downward and caudally • Optic chiasm stretched and twisted • Infundibulum displaced • Brainstem torsion • Vertebral arteries displaced 2. Compression of • Cerebral peduncle • Nerve VI • Posterior cerebral artery 3. Secondary hemorrhage in brain stem	1. Tentorial downward shift continues to the posterior fossa 2. Cerebellar tonsils herniate at the side of the cord (may be down to C5)
Signs		
Consciousness	Decreased, tonic seizures	Comatose
Motor	Decerebrate responses	Hypotonia/spinal flexion Brisk flexor withdrawal Tongue fasciculation, bulbar palsy Erb's palsy
Eyes	Nerve palsy III and VI "Sunsetting" Cortical blindness	Absent calorics or doll's eyes response Absent ciliospinal reflex
Respiration	Central neurogenic hyperventilation Cheyne-Stokes respiration	Bradypnea, apnea Laryngeal stridor
Other	Loss of temperature control Cardiac irregularity	Hypotension

Hepatic Encephalopathy

Hepatic encephalopathy complicates both acute and chronic liver failure. This complex syndrome may be caused by potentially reversible metabolic abnormalities and in its extreme form can lead to coma and death. The differential diagnosis of the variety of possible causes is discussed in Chapter 36.

Table 23.7. Causes and Differential Diagnosis of Benign Intracranial Hypertension

1. Intracranial venous sinus thrombosis
   Ear infection—related to lateral sinus thrombosis
   After head trauma
   Idiopathic
   Secondary to vena cava and other venous thrombosis and obstruction
2. Endocrine and metabolic disorders
   Corticosteroid withdrawal
   Chronic hypocalcemia (hypoparathyroidism)
   Pseudohypoparathyroidism
   Vitamin D deficient rickets
   Chronic carbon dioxide retention
   Addison's disease
   Obesity
3. Drugs and toxins
   Excess dose of vitamin A
   Nalidixic acid
   Tetracycline and minocycline
   Amiodarone
4. Hematologic disorders
   Iron-deficiency anemia
   Infectious mononucleosis
   Wiskott-Aldrich syndrome

Fulminant Neonatal Encephalopathy

In the first postnatal month and early infantile period, the clinical presentation of metabolic disease may include a varied combination of biochemical derangement (e.g., glucose, acid base, liver function), and hepatic failure **(Table 23.8)**. The most common causes associated with various constellations of metabolic derangement are shown in **Table 23.9**. Of particular note with respect to neurologic distress are the *neonatal sepsis syndrome* and *infantile seizure-myoclonic syndromes.*

Neonatal Sepsis Syndrome

Nonspecific clinical signs and symptoms indistinguishable from the presentation of sepsis may be seen in the neonate presenting with one of a number of diseases of carbohydrate, fat, or protein metabolism **(Table 23.8)**. In some infants, a history of apparent normality in the early neonatal period is deceptive, but it merely indicates that either the metabolic disturbances have taken time to accumulate to toxic levels or the toxic process has taken time to evolve. Although in general there are few pathognomonic findings during the neonatal period, many of the disorders appearing at this age are associated with an anion-gap acidosis and some with hyperchloremic acidosis[65].

Infantile Seizure—Myoclonic Syndromes

A variety of names have been given to the occurrence of repeated and intractable seizures, spasms, or subtle episodes starting in the neonatal period (see Chapter 22). These syndromes are important in that seizure control is

Table 23.8. Infantile Encephalopathic Presentation of Metabolic Disease[a]

	Seizures	*Acidosis*	*Renal Dysfunction*	*Liver Dysfunction*	*Hypoglycemia*	*Other*
Organic acidemia						
MSUD[b]	+	+	−	−	+	Bone marrow depression,
Propionic acidemia	+	+	−	−	+	increased lactate,
Isovaleric acidemia	+	+	−	−	+	hyperammonemia (applies to
Methylmalonic acidemia	+	+	−	−	+	*all* organic acidemias)
HMG CoA lyase deficiency	+	+	−	−	+	
Urea cycle defects						
CPS deficiency	+	±	−	+	−	
OTC deficiency	+	±	−	+	−	Orotic acid crystals
Citrullinemia	+	+	−	+	−	
Carbohydrate disorders						
Galactosemia	−	+	+	+	+	Jaundice
Hereditary fructose intolerance	+	+	+	+	+	Decreased serum phosphate
Aminoacidopathies						
Hereditary tyrosinemia	−	+	+	+	−	Coagulopathy
Homocystinuria	+	−	−	−	−	
Nonketotic hyperglycine	+	−	−	−	−	Hypsarrhythmia
Endocrinopathies						
Congenital adrenal hyperplasia	+	±	−	−	±	Virilization, hyperkalemia
Congenital diabetes	−	+	−	−	−	Hyperglycemia, ketonemia

[a] Adapted from Nyhan WL. An approach to the diagnosis of overwhelming metabolic disease in early infancy. Curr Prob Pediatr 1977; 7:1.
[b] MSUD, maple syrup urine disease; HMG, 3-hydroxy-3-methylglutarate; CPS, carbamyl-phosphate synthase; and OTC, ornithine transcarbamylase.

poor and outcome is usually dismal. In some, there is the possibility that an inborn error of metabolism (e.g., pyridoxine-dependent seizures and nonketotic hyperglycinemia) may be responsible—particularly in the infant with no documented history of acute central nervous system insult **(Table 23.9).** Two epileptic syndromes that fall into this category are the early myoclonic encephalopathy and the early infantile epileptic encephalopathy syndromes.

Early Myoclonic Encephalopathy[66,67] is characterized clinically by the occurrence of erratic fragmentary myoclonus of early onset, usually in association with other types of seizures, and from electroencephalography (EEG) by the intermittent or suppression-burst pattern (Fig. 23.3). This clinical picture may be seen in infants affected by various neurologic disorders[68]. However, it has been suggested by some that specific metabolic disorders should be sought, e.g., glycine abnormalities[69–71].

Early Infantile Epileptic Encephalopathy[72] may be a variant of West's syndrome with onset in early infancy, typified by mainly intractable tonic spasms, invariant intermittent activity on EEG, severe neurodevelopmental deficits, and multiple causes, especially brain malformations.

Profound Biochemical Derangement

A variety of biochemical disturbances, such as hypoglycemia, acidosis, electrolyte abnormalities, and endogenous toxins in either isolation or combination, may account for an altered level of consciousness as well as specific clinical signs or features.

Hypoglycemia

Hypoglycemia may result from a variety of causes which can be categorized as deficient substrate provision; deranged endocrine balance; inborn errors of carbohydrate, lipid, or amino acid metabolism; drug-induced hypoglycemia; hepatic failure; and **(Table 23.10),** as follows:

Deficient Substrate Provision in patients dependent on intravenous fluids with glucose is always a risk at times of fasting or when access has been lost.

Deranged Endocrine Balance resulting from hyperinsulinism, hypopituitarism, growth hormone deficiency, adrenal insufficiency, hypothyroidism, and glucagon deficiency may all account for hypoglycemia.

Table 23.9. Most Common Metabolic Causes of Infantile Coma and Seizures Associated with Various Constellations of Metabolic Derangement[a]

Acidosis	−	+	+	−	−
Ketosis	+	+	+	−	−
Hyperammonemia	−	+	−	+	−
Hyperlactacidemia	−	−	+	−	−
		Acidemias			
Most frequent diagnoses	1. Maple syrup urine disease	1. Methylmalonic 2. Propionic 3. Isovaleric	1. Congenital lactic acidosis	1. Urea cycle defects	1. Hyperglycinemia 2. Peroxisomal 3. Sulfite oxidase deficiency 4. Respiratory chain diseases

[a] Adapted from Saudubray JM, et al. Clinical approach to inherited metabolic disease in the neonatal period: a 20 year survey. J Inherited Metab Dis 1989;12(S1):25.

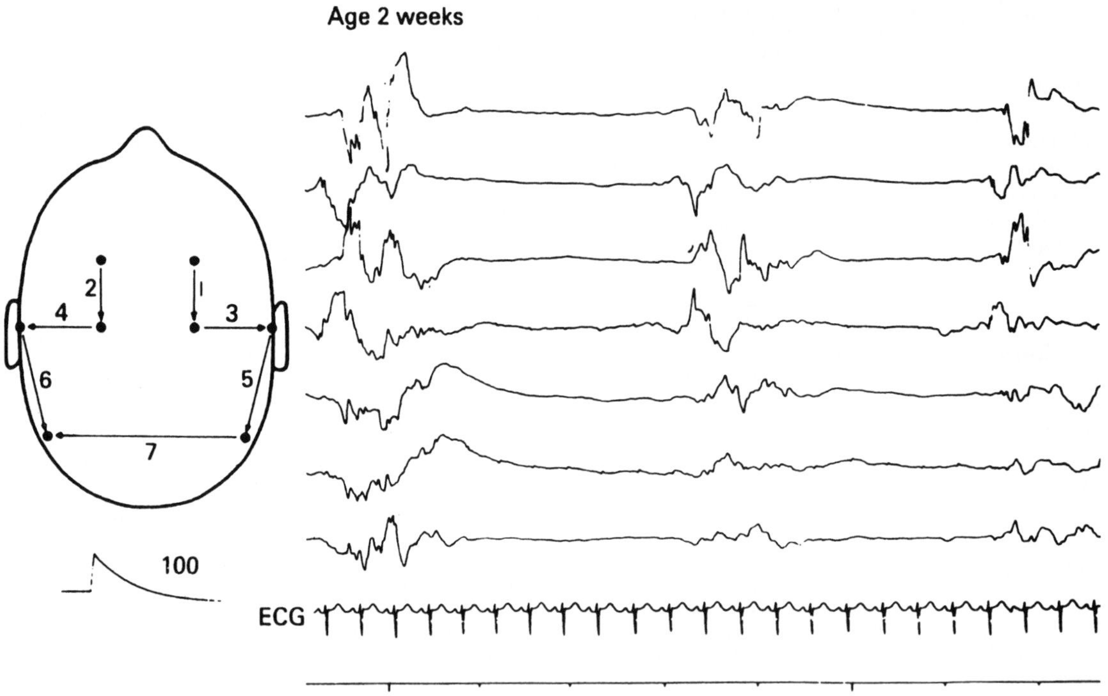

Figure 23.3. A 2-week-old infant with nonketotic hyperglycinemia who had seizures from birth. The EEG shows a grossly abnormal pattern with intermittent bursts of activity typically, but not exclusively, seen in this condition. (From Leonard JV. Inherited metabolic disease: urea cycle disorders, organic acidemias and non-ketotic hyperglycinemia. In: Brett EM, ed. Paediatric neurology. New York: Churchill Livingstone, 1991:220.)

Table 23.10. Causes of Hypoglycemia

Deficient substrate provision
Ketotic hypoglycemia
Inadequate infused glucose during total intravenous therapy
Deranged endocrine balance
Hyperinsulinism: nesidioblastosis, leucine-induced, islet cell adenoma
Adrenal insufficiency
Hypothyroidism
Glucagon deficiency
Inborn errors of carbohydrate metabolism
Glycogen storage disease types I, III, IV
Galactosemia
Fructose intolerance
Pyruvate carboxylase deficiency
Phosphoenolpyruvate deficiency
Inborn errors of lipid metabolism
Medium- and long-chain acetyl CoA dehydrogenase deficiency
Inborn errors of amino acid metabolism
Maple syrup urine disease
Methylmalonic aciduria
Propionic acidemia
Isovaleric acidemia
Drug-induced hypoglycemia
Insulin
Sulfonylureas
Salicylates
Acetaminophen
Propranolol
Hepatic failure

Inborn Errors of Carbohydrate Metabolism which prevent the release of glucose from glycogen cause hypoglycemia, e.g., glycogen storage disease types I, III, IV; galactosemia; fructose intolerance; pyruvate carboxylase deficiency; and phosphoenolpyruvate deficiency.

Inborn Errors of Lipid Metabolism producing the Reye-like syndrome have hypoglycemia as a major feature (see above and **Table 23.3**,)

Inborn Errors of Amino Acid Metabolism such as maple syrup urine disease, methylmalonic aciduria, propionic acidemia, and isovaleric acidemia, are associated with hypoglycemia.

Drug-Induced Hypoglycemia is seen with insulin, sulfonylureas, salicylates, acetaminophen, and propranolol.

Hepatic Failure caused by drugs, hepatitis, and Reye syndrome will cause hypoglycemia.

Hyperammonemia

Hyperammonemia refers to an accumulation of ammonia in blood and brain in sufficient concentrations to cause neurologic symptoms. In both neonates and older children, the acute presentation can be a catastrophic illness. The hyperammonemia can result from acquired diseases such as toxic or infectious hepatic failure(73) or Reye syndrome(74) and from a number of inborn errors of metabolism that affect nitrogen metabolism(75). Untreated, these latter diseases lead to permanent brain damage or death. Less acute presentations of hyperammonemic disorders are more var-

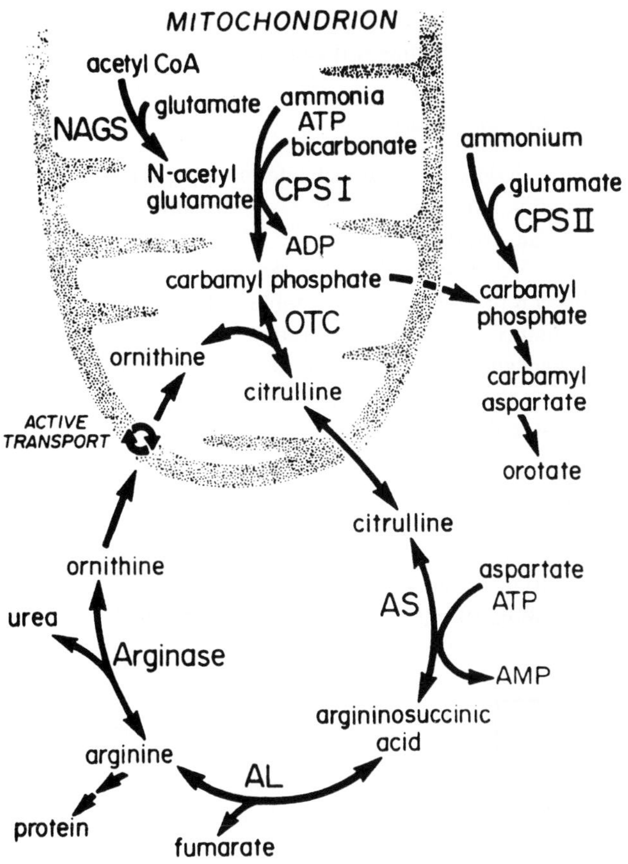

Figure 23.4. Urea cycle. Enzymes are divided between the mitochondrial and cytosolic compartments with ornithine and citrulline crossing the mitochondrial membrane. *NAGS*, *N*-acetylglutamate; *ATP*, adenosine triphosphate; *CPS*, carbamyl-phosphate synthetase; *ADP*, adenosine diphosphate; *OTC*, ornithine transcarbamylase; *AS*, arginosuccinate synthetase; *AMP*, adenosine monophosphate; and *AL*, arginosuccinate lyase. (From Batshaw ML. Hyperammonemia. In: Lockhart JD, et al, eds. Current problems in pediatrics. Chicago: Year Book Medical Publishers, 1984.)

ied, and coma may ensue only after significant stress, such as intercurrent illness, pregnancy, or augmented protein intake. Algorithms for the differential diagnosis of neonatal and childhood onset hyperammonemia are shown in Figures 23.4–23.6.

Electrolyte Disturbance

Any central neurologic disturbance in patients hydrated by the intravenous or nasogastric tube route should prompt the search for an abnormal electrolyte concentration, e.g., sodium, calcium, and magnesium.

Hypernatremia may produce varying degrees of impaired consciousness, fever, spasticity, and subdural hemorrhage. It can be due to severe dehydration, body water loss, diabetes insipidus, salt poisoning, or sodium retention seen in hyperaldosteronism or Cushing's disease.

Hyponatremia may produce an altered level of consciousness and seizures. Its causes include injudicious solute-poor intravenous fluid administration, water retention in cardiac or liver failure, the syndrome of inappropriate secretion of antidiuretic hormone, and drugs such as vincristine and carbamazepine.

Calcium and Magnesium metabolism are closely linked. When profoundly low, focal or multifocal seizures may be observed. Hypermagnesemia can induce weakness, hypotonia, stupor, and respiratory failure.

Encephalopathy Seen in Systemic Disturbance or Disease

A variety of disease states are known to induce encephalopathic features. Those that could be attributed to a metabolic or toxic process are discussed below.

Vitamin Deficiency

Thiamine (vitamin B_1), pyridoxine (vitamin B_6), and vitamin A deficiencies may result in an alteration in level of consciousness, sometimes rather precipitously.

Thiamine plays an important role in the decarboxylation of pyruvate and of α-ketoglutarate (two steps of the Krebs cycle), and the conversion of 5-carbon to 6-carbon sugars by means of the enzyme transketolase. Thiamine deficiency will therefore decrease energy available to the brain and increase the concentration of the two keto acids. In patients receiving total parenteral nutrition[76], chronic dialysis[77], or high-carbohydrate diet during debilitating illness[78,79], Wernicke's encephalopathy may be observed. In these settings, the features are highly variable and may be manifested by sudden collapse and death or seizures, or by the classic ataxia, confusion, and ocular abnormalities.

Pyridoxine in the form of pyridoxal-5-phosphate is essential for normal brain function. It is particularly necessary for the decarboxylation of glutamic acid to γ-amino butyric acid (GABA), an essential inhibitory neurotransmitter. In deficiency states such as that seen in patients who are receiving isoniazid or penicillamine, seizures may be observed.

Vitamin A deficiency can result in a rise in intracranial pressure[80], which may be reversed by replacement (see above) benign intracranial hypertension).

Diabetes Mellitus

Encephalopathy may complicate various abnormal biochemical states associated with diabetes mellitus.

Diabetic Ketoacidosis may result in a marked impairment in cerebral blood flow and oxygen uptake by the brain, cerebral edema, and focal neurologic deficit[81–83].

Nonketotic Hyperosmolar Coma occurs in children and results in generalized or focal seizures, ophthalmoplegia, and hemiparesis[84].

Hypoglycemia may result in a spectrum of clinical findings ranging from transient focal neurologic signs to coma and focal or generalized seizures[85].

Renal Disease

The encephalopathies associated with underlying renal disease are invariably multifactorial and may be attributable to electrolyte disturbance, hypertension, or specific disease toxins. Those that require specific mention are listed below.

Uremic Encephalopathy is characterized by obtundation, hypotonia, seizures, athetoid movements, nystagmus, and ataxia(86–87), and it is the main neurologic complication of renal insufficiency. Focal cerebral symptoms, hemiparesis, and cortical blindness are more usually due to hypertensive encephalopathy.

Dialysis Dysequilibrium Syndrome is caused by a failure of urea to rapidly establish equilibrium between brain and blood during dialysis, thus resulting in a net shift of extracellular water into the brain.

Rejection Encephalopathy that is not due to electrolyte disturbance, hypertension, steroids, or fever occurs in some renal transplant patients(88). More recently cyclosporin toxicity has been implicated. This produces a syndrome of coma, cortical blindness, quadriplegia, and seizures(89).

Septic Encephalopathy

An encephalopathy seen in bacteremic patients, not due to meningitis, abscess, cerebritis, or emboli, has been described in critically ill adults(90). Mortality and morbidity is high. The causes of this state may include microabscesses in the cerebral cortex (appreciable only at autopsy), metabolic disturbance such as the ratio of branched-chain to unbranched and aromatic amino acids(91), cerebral microcirculatory dysfunction, cerebral edema(92), and drugs administered.

Poisons and Drugs

Drug intoxication is an important cause of encephalopathy in children. **Table 23.11** summarizes the findings in the more commonly seen episodes.

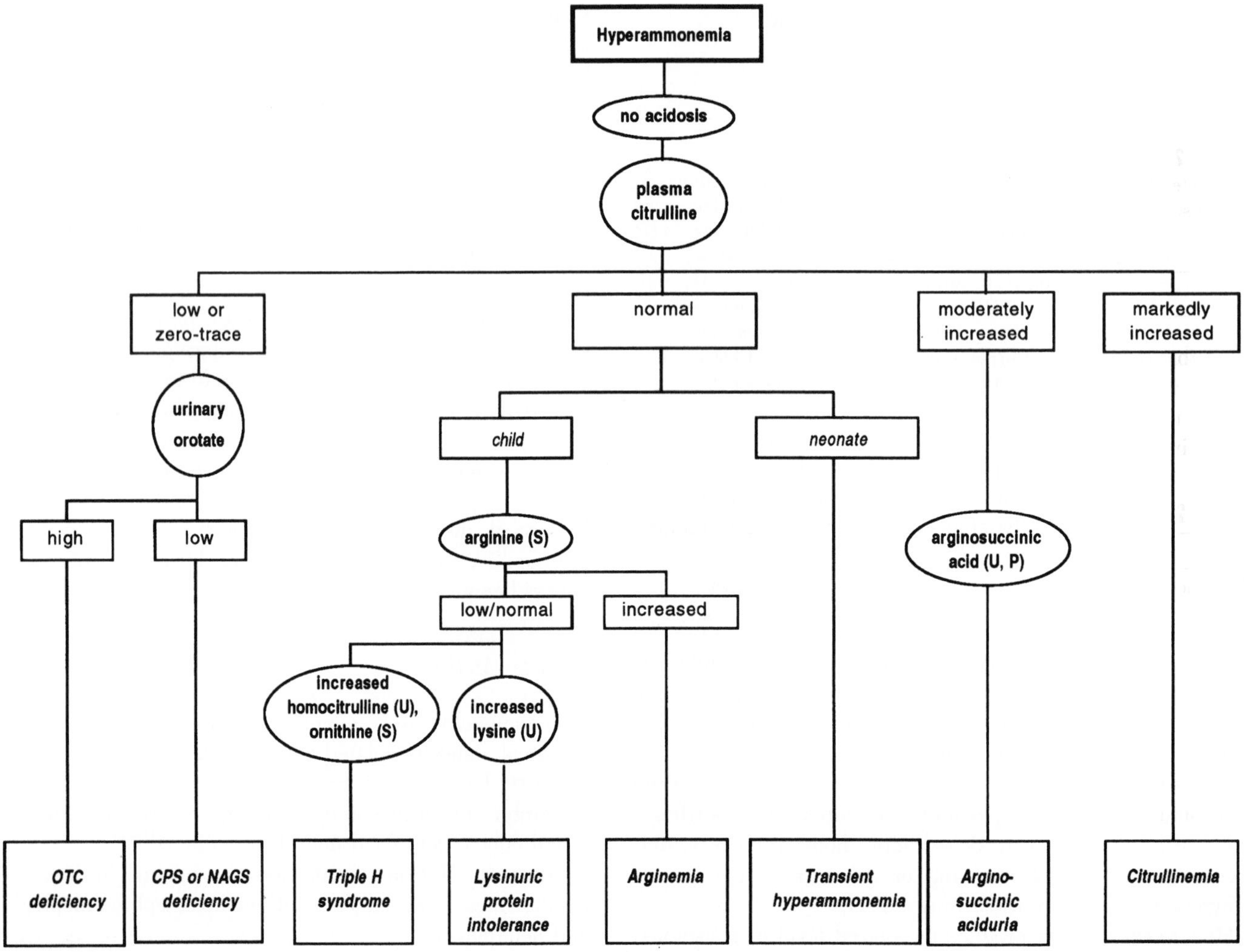

Figure 23.5. Algorithm for the differential diagnosis of hyperammonemia in the absence of acidosis. *U*, urine; *S*, serum; *OTC*, ornithine transcarbamylase; *CPS*, carbamyl-phosphate synthetase; and *NAGS*, *N*-acetylglytamate. (Adapted from Batshaw ML. Hyperammonemia. In: Lockhart JD, et al, eds. Current problems in pediatrics. Chicago: Year Book Medical Publishers, 1984.)

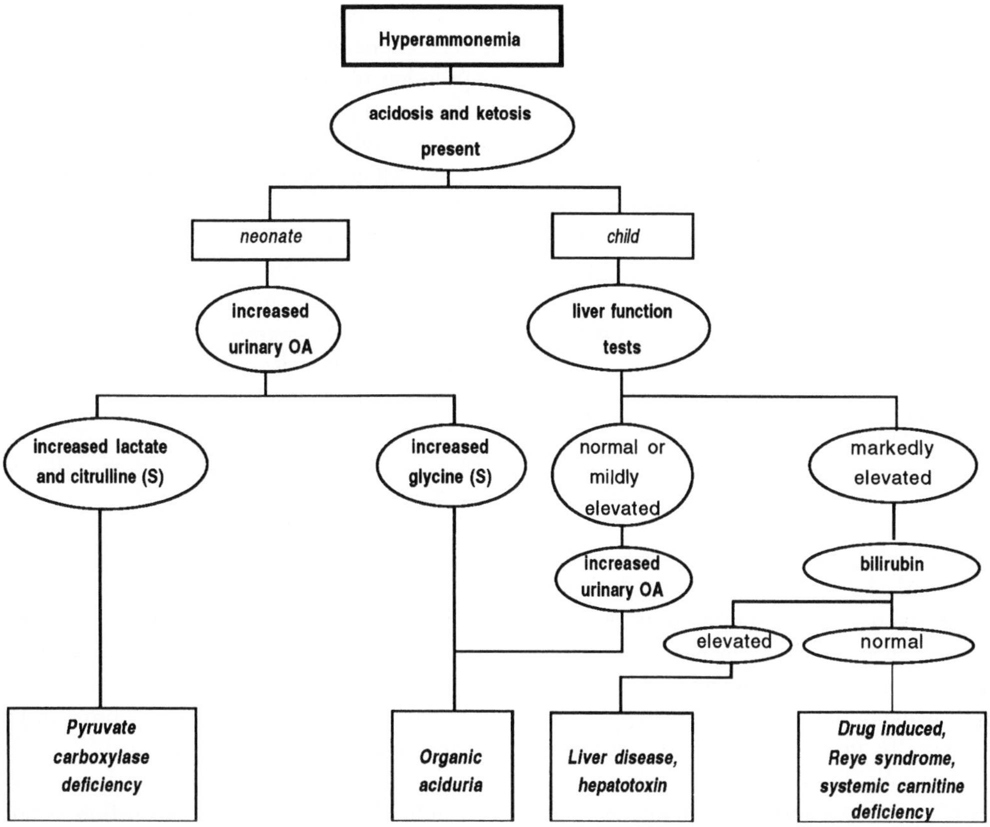

Figure 23.6. Algorithm for the differential diagnosis of hyperammonemia with associated acidosis and ketosis. *OA*, organic acids; and *S*, serum. (Adapted from Batshaw ML. Hyperammonemia. In: Lockhart JD, et al, eds. Current problems in pediatrics. Chicago: Year Book Medical Publishers, 1984.)

PATHOPHYSIOLOGY

Metabolic encephalopathy may result from a variety of insults, not unusually multifactorial. While many of these insults may result in the nonspecific development of brain swelling with resultant effects on blood flow, cerebral metabolism, and neuronal survival, it is also likely that specific or selective neurotoxicity may result from the release of endogenous toxins and neuromodulators or the accumulation of a toxic metabolite. A discussion of intracranial vault pathophysiology with cytotoxic cerebral edema can be found in Chapter 18. Concerning neurotoxicity, the most

Table 23.11. Drug Intoxication and Encephalopathy

Drug	*Neurology*	*Eyes*	*Cardiac*	*Other Organ Systems*
Amphetamines	Depressed consciousness Delirium Agitation Chorea Hyperreflexia	Mydriasis	Cardiac arrhythmia Tachycardia Hypertension	Hyperpyrexia Sweating
Tricyclic antidepressants	Agitation Muscle rigidity Seizures Coma	Mydriasis	Tachycardia	Sweating Vomiting
Antihistamines	Depressed consciousness Hallucinations Tremor Seizures	Mydriasis	Hypotension	Dry mouth Urinary retention
Barbiturates	Ataxia Coma Arreflexia	Miosis	Hypotension	Hypothermia Respiratory depression
Methadone	Depressed consciousness	Miosis	Hypotension	Urinary retention Respiratory depression

studied and characterized metabolic insult other than ischemia has been the neurologic injury produced by hypoglycemia, hyperammonemia, and hepatic failure. A basic understanding of these insults is invaluable, since they encompass theories related to endogenous neurotoxin production, neuronal energy failure, and neuronal excitatory and inhibitory mechanisms.

Neurotoxic processes seen with other common causes of metabolic encephalopathy in patients coming to intensive care are summarized in **Table 23.12;** a more detailed analysis of many of these conditions can be found in Chapters 35–38.

Neurochemistry and Toxicity

Hypoglycemia

A variety of experimental approaches have been used to explain how hypoglycemia kills neurons[93]. Of relevance to an understanding of hypoglycemic neurotoxicity in pediatrics is the difference observed between neonatal hypoglycemia and adult experimental hypoglycemia, which may be a reflection of development and maturity of metabolic neurotransmitter systems. In the mature brain, hypoglycemia less than 20 mg/dl usually gives rise to an isoelectric EEG and brain damage[94]. In the neonatal brain, glucose levels in this range, if the neonate is asymptomatic, rarely give rise to permanent neurologic deficit[95]. Unfortunately, even though the pathology has been characterized for over 20 years[96–98], the developmental neurobiology of hypoglycemia remains poorly understood. The emphasis of this discussion relates primarily to adult experimental studies that also have relevance to children, since there is a paucity of neonatal and infant data.

In the adult, neuronal necrosis as a result of hypoglycemia is absent unless the EEG becomes isoelectric, regardless of the blood sugar level at which the EEG goes flat[94]. Furthermore, the duration of electrocerebral silence roughly determines the degree of resultant brain damage. Results of studies in humans[99] as well as in animals[100] on the relationship between cerebral blood flow and brain metabolism lend support to the concept that simple energy failure (i.e., inadequate substrate delivery and low levels of high-energy phosphates) does not account for the encephalopathy observed. Indeed, cerebral blood flow does not fall significantly during hypoglycemia.

Experimental studies have shown that a number of ionic and metabolic changes occur in the brain abruptly at the onset of cerebral EEG isoelectricity[101–105]. Whole-brain neurochemical analyses reveal that with profound hypoglycemia, cellular redox systems are oxidized and brain pH is increased, which is in contrast to the changes induced by ischemia (see Chapter 20)[100,106,107]. The formation of ammonia from deamination of amino acids, the consumption of metabolic acids, and the absence of lactic acid formation account for the alkalosis. Considering the normal dependence of the brain on both oxygen and glucose, which are consumed in a stoichiometric relationship[108], the observed energy failure is less than would be expected. Depression of cerebral oxygen consumption is also less than that expected in proportion to depression of glucose utilization, indicating that the brain is versatile in oxidizing fuels other than glucose to maintain a stable energy state[100,109–112]. (It should be remembered that although production of lactic acid during hypoglycemia is not possible because of glucose deficiency, it can be burned as fuel, thereby reversing hypoglycemic stupor. However, this functions only in immature animals because of failure of blood lactate to enter the central nervous system in mature animals.)

The oxidation of endogenous substrates such as proteins and fats for fuel also explains why during hypoglycemia, adenosine 5-triphosphate (ATP) levels remain over one-third of normal values[101,104,105,111,112], even when the hypoglycemia is profound enough to cause an isoelectric EEG (i.e., cessation of cerebral electrical activity). This is in contrast to experimental ischemia, in which neuronal ATP levels quickly drop to less than 5% of the normal[108,113]. It is also of interest that additional cerebral insult during hypoglycemia (e.g., lowering of blood pressure) results in no further increase in neuronal necrosis[114,115], despite the increased cellular release of potassium and enhanced energy failure. This suggests that blood flow is not the critical determinant of hypoglycemia-induced neuronal injury.

As well as the above ionic and chemical changes occurring at the onset of a hypoglycemia-induced isoelectric EEG, significant changes occur in cerebral amino acids. It has been suggested that the 300–400% increase in brain tissue aspartate and the fall in glutamate[101,116–119] may be involved in the endogenous neurotoxicity of hypoglycemia and are related to any or all of the following:

1. Protein breakdown
2. Lack of protein synthesis
3. Pooling of amino acids
4. A shift in the aspartate-glutamate transaminase reaction toward aspartate

By using cerebral intraparenchymal dialysis techniques, increased extracellular levels of aspartate and, to a lesser extent, glutamate, have been found in models of hypoglycemic coma[119,120]. It has been proposed that the excess aspartate originates from the neuronal metabolic pool[121,122] and results in toxic glutamate (*N*-methyl-D-aspartate) receptor activation. Indeed, attention and protection of hypoglycemic neurotoxicity both in vitro[123,124] and in vivo[125] have been achieved by inhibition of these receptors.

Hyperammonemia

In children, severe hyperammonemia is accompanied by cytotoxic changes, cerebral edema, and increased intracranial pressure. The toxicity associated with hyperammonemia has been attributed to a number of mechanisms, including the

Table 23.12. Summary of Pathogenic Mechanisms and Pertinent Clinical Features of Not Uncommon Encephalitic Conditions Seen in Patients Presenting for Intensive Care[a]

	Pathogenesis	*Clinical Notes*
Renal disease		
Uremia	Chronic progressively worsening uremia produces a spectrum of CNS[b] signs. A. ***Implicated*** • Imbalance of neurotransmitters (GABA, dopamine, and serotonin) due to plasma amino acid levels • Increased CSF and brain guanidino compounds that inhibit inhibitory GABA and glycine systems • Increased brain tissue osmolality • Increased gray matter calcium B. ***Contributory factors in renal failure*** • Hypercalcemia, hypertension, hemorrhage, drug toxicity C. ***Noncontributory*** • Energy state (normal levels of cerebral ATP and phosphocreatine, secondary reduction of glycolysis)	***Examination*** • Sensorium: headache, nausea, vomiting • Motor: tremor, myoclonus, asterixis • Neurology: focal signs often seen • Seizures: focal and generalized
Dialysis dysequilibrium	Occurs during or immediately after hemodialysis or peritoneal dialysis. A. ***Implicated*** • Brain edema (increased brain tissue water content due to blood-brain osmotic gradient, idiogenic osmoles) • CNS acidosis	***Examination*** • Sensorium: headache, confusion, and heightening of preexisting obtundation and coma • Motor: muscle twitching • Seizures: focal and generalized
Hypercalcemia	Cerebral infarction due to arterial spasm has been reported. A. ***Implicated*** • ? Brain parathormone levels • ? CSF citrate and lactate buffering B. ***Contributory*** • Azotemia, dehydration C. ***Noncontributory*** • Normal CSF content of calcium and phosphate	***Examination*** • Neurology: focal findings • Seizures: generalized and focal
Acute electrolyte disturbance		
Hyponatremia	Acute presentation with seizures and obtundation. A. ***Implicated*** • Cytotoxic cerebral edema with increased brain water	***Examination*** • Motor: rare asterixis and multifocal myoclonus Neurology: occasional focal signs, hemiparesis, monoparesis, unilateral corticospinal tract signs • Seizures: frequent (Na <115, acute) ***Treatment*** • Slow/rapid/overcorrection (*cf.* central pontine myelinosis) • Hypertonic saline (to correct Na 120–125), water restriction
Hypernatremia	Factors responsible for the obtundation are unclear but: A. ***Implicated*** • Increased brain tissue osmolality • Increased osmotically active particles (Na, K, Cl, and "idiogenic osmoles," e.g., urea and amino acids	***Examination*** • Motor: tremor, hyperreflexia • Neurology: focal signs related to hemorrhage (subdural-bridging veins or multiple intraparenchymal) • Seizures: frequent, often progress to coma
Hypocalcemia	Hypocalcemic states often present with neurologic manifestations. A. ***Implicated*** • ? Acute lowering or absolute level of serum calcium • ? Alteration in neurotransmitter synthesis as well as uptake and release of catecholamines • ? Brain parathormone levels	***Examination*** • Sensorium: confusion-coma • Motor: tetany, movement disorder • Seizures: generalized and partial complex

[a] The range of conditions illustrates the diversity of implicated mechanisms.
[b] CNS, central nervous system; GABA, γ-aminobutyric acid; CSF, cerebrospinal fluid; ATP, adenosine triphosphate; RBC, red blood cell(s); and 2,3-DPG, 2,3-diphosphoglyceric acid.

Continued.

Table 23.12. Summary of Pathogenic Mechanisms and Pertinent Clinical Features of Not Uncommon Encephalitic Conditions Seen in Patients Presenting for Intensive Care[a] (continued)

	Pathogenesis	Clinical Notes
Hypomagnesemia	Usually associated with other abnormalities, including alkalosis, hypocalcemia, and hypophophatemia. A. ***Implicated*** • ? Brain parathormone levels	***Examination*** • Sensorium: delirium, vertigo • Motor: choreoathetosis • Seizures: generalized and focal
Hypophosphatemia	A. ***Implicated*** • ? Related to change in RBC metabolism and affinity for oxygen (decreased RBC ATP and 2,3-DPG heightens affinity for oxygen and decreases availability for tissues) B. ***Noncontributory*** • CSF phosphorus remains constant	***Examination*** • Sensorium: stupor-coma • Motor: tremor, ballismus • Seizures: generalized
Glucose		
Hyperglycemia	Hyperosmolality rather than hyperglycemia appears to be associated with depression of sensorium. A. ***Implicated*** • Rapid water loss by the brain • Increased brain tissue concentration of ions and metabolites B. ***Contributory factor*** • Focal circulatory impairment	***Examination*** • Hyperosmotic hyperglycemic nonketotic • Sensorium: obtunded • Neurology: focal signs • Seizures: focal, (epilepsia partialis continua) Ketotic hyperglycemia is seldom associated with seizures or focal signs.
Miscellaneous		
Thyrotoxicosis	A. ***Implicated*** • Acute neuronal accumulation of thyroid hormone • ? Altered catecholamine sensitivity B. ***Noncontributory*** • Cerebral oxygen consumption not increased • Brain mitochondria do not undergo changes that occur in other tissues	***Examination*** • Motor: tremor-chorea/athetosis • Neurology: acute reversible bulbar dysfunction, progressive myelopathy with paraplegia • Seizures: generalized
Intussusception encephalopathy	Intestinal intussusception with the most prominent presenting feature of depressed level of consciousness and reported apparent responses to naloxone. A. ***Implicated*** • ? Gastrointestinal release of neurotoxins, vasoactive peptides, and neuroactive gut hormones • ? Age-related pain release of endorphins B. ***Contributory*** • Blood loss, dehydration, electrolyte imbalance, and sepsis	***Examination*** • Sensorium: coma • Motor: hypotonia, hyporeflexia • Neurology: miosis

direct effects of ammonia on cerebral blood flow, blood-brain barrier integrity and function, cerebral metabolism, and toxin or neurotransmitter balance. The development of raised intracranial pressure and consequent altered cerebral blood flow accompanying a predominantly cytotoxic cerebral edema may further compound the underlying toxic process. However, it is of note that changes in cerebral blood flow are variable, with only some animal models exhibiting an increase in flow(126), altered cerebral blood flow regulation, and elevated intracranial pressure(127–130). This does not exclude the probability that the end-stage common pathophysiologic pathway for the variety of metabolic derangements resulting in hyperammonemia may still be due to changes in intracranial fluid and tissue dynamics.

At an early stage, the observation that the neuropathology of hyperammonemia involves astrocytic swelling without opening of endothelial tight junctions or other structural alterations(131) suggests that at an early stage, severe damage is not inevitable; indeed, the toxicity may be reversible.

Ammonia is normally detoxified in astrocytes by glutamate dehydrogenase and glutamine synthetase, which occupy an important position in the brain because there is no functional urea cycle for clearing ammonia in the central nervous system(132,133). These reactions form glutamic acid and glutamine with the consumption of ATP, reduced nicotinamide adenine dinucleotide (NADH), and α-ketoglutarate(134). In hyperammonemia, brain ammonia concentration increases in proportion to blood level, since it crosses the blood-brain barrier by diffusion. In addition, altered physical properties or permeability of the blood-brain barrier, e.g., selective damage of brain amino acid transport systems(135), increases brain aromatic acid concentrations, which can further disturb and compound neuronal energy metabolism or alter neurochemical or neurotransmitter balance(136). During hyperammonemia, glutamine synthesis is insufficient to clear ammonia and maintain intracerebral ammonia at normal levels. From whatever mechanism, the abnormally high ammonia levels may then directly interfere with glial and neuronal function. Increased intraneuronal ammonia (which is enhanced by increased pH) can produce subtle influences in membrane potential and ionic shifts[137], which then causes alterations in neuronal transmission. Alternatively, the changes in neuronal function and astrocyte swelling may be the consequence of energy depletion. However, there have been conflicting results from studies in different animal models directly measuring high-energy phosphates[136]. Of more significance may be regional energy failure involving certain cerebral centers, e.g., ATP depletion in the brainstem reticular formation but not in the colliculi[138], suggesting a specific effect of ammonia in the cerebral locus known to be important for maintaining consciousness.

Hepatic Failure

The neurobiology of hepatic encephalopathy remains an area of much speculation[136]. The basic premise is that altered liver function produces a disturbance of metabolism, which in turn causes cerebral dysfunction. Over the past several decades, research has focused on the role of several agents as potential toxins, including ammonia, short-chain fatty acids, mercaptans, phenols, false neurotransmitters (octopamine), and, more recently, GABA. For the present, not one of these seems likely to be completely responsible for the disease.

A review of the various hypotheses concerning hepatic encephalopathy has been succinctly summarized by Lockwood[136] and Jones et al.[139]. The accepted hypotheses include the following:

1. The synergistic neurotoxins hypothesis suggests that coma results from the ". . . synergistic effects of accumulating toxins with coma-producing potential and augmenting endogenous metabolic abnormalities"[140]. Ammonia was considered to play a central role in pathogenesis. Other implicated toxins are mercaptans, fatty acids, and phenol[141].
2. The false neurotransmitter hypothesis[142–144] suggests that a plasma amino acid imbalance with elevated brain serotonin and false neurotransmitters such as octopamine cause encephalopathy and coma.
3. The neural inhibitory hypothesis implicates the GABA neurotransmitter system in the pathogenesis of hepatic encephalopathy[139].

Historically, the first two of these hypotheses arose from measurement of the concentrations of neuroactive substances of pathogenic importance or their metabolites in plasma, cerebrospinal fluid (CSF), and brain. In contrast, the third hypothesis arose from an alternative approach, which was to consider which of the established mechanisms that mediate changes in neuronal activity in the brain could conceivably contribute to the pathogenic basis of the neural inhibition seen in hepatic encephalopathy[145].

There has been much interest in the possibility that GABA causes hepatic encephalopathy. Experimental findings have shown that when the liver fails, GABA, which is produced by the enteric bacterial flora, crosses an abnormally permeable blood-brain barrier and binds to neuronal postsynaptic GABA receptors[146–149]. It has been suggested that this exogenous GABA contributes to the neural inhibition of hepatic coma. However, conflicting data indicate that brain GABA levels are very resistant to change by mechanisms operating outside the brain[150]. An adjunct to the neural inhibitory hypothesis of hepatic encephalopathy is the possible role for an endogenous benzodiazepine-like ligand[151].

It is noteworthy that experimental findings have shown a markedly elevated concentration of benzodiazepine-binding inhibitors in the CSF of patients with hepatic encephalopathy[152]. This suggests that an endogenous substance with benzodiazepine-like characteristics contributes to the encephalopathy, presumably via an effect on GABAergic neurotransmission. In fact, the elevation in inhibitors correlated with encephalopathy and was not seen in those patients with liver disease and normal cognitive function. Furthermore, reports such as the observation that rapid improvement of hepatic encephalopathy can be achieved with administration of flumazenil[153,154], a benzodiazepine antagonist, lend support to an endogenous benzodiazepine-GABA hypothesis.

Neuropathology

The main neuropathologic findings associated with metabolic encephalopathy include both specific regional toxic effects as well as nonspecific global effects, with the latter often being attributable to acute brain swelling.

Specific or selective damage of particular groups of brain cells or regions of the brain is seen with a variety of disorders. Of note are the disorders that have a predilection for either basal ganglia or cerebellar or cortical disease. Although these are often identified macroscopically postmortem, they can now be appreciated grossly with modern imaging techniques **(Table 23.13).**

Microscopically, hypoglycemia produces selective neuronal necrosis of the superficial cortical layers, sparing nonneuronal elements unless hypoglycemia is severe and prolonged[96,97]. Infarction is usually absent, even after a severe hypoglycemic insult[93]. Neuronal degenerative changes can also be seen throughout the putamen, caudate nucleus, and cerebellar granular layer. In contrast, in Reye syndrome the histopathology is nonspecific for a primary cytotoxic cerebral edema[155], with swelling of astrocytic foot processes. The cortical neurons are either swollen or shrunken and deeply staining. Astrocytes and oligodendroglia are swollen without microglial proliferation. The hallmark of hepatic coma is the enlargement and proliferation of the protoplasmic astrocyte, the so-called Alzheimer type II astrocyte. Long-standing or recurrent hepatic encephalopathy may lead to the development of degenerative changes in the brain involving layers 5 and 6 of the cortex, underlying white matter, basal ganglia, and cerebellum[156].

Table 23.13. Predominant Region of Involvement Inferred from Computed Tomography Scanning or Magnetic Resonance Imaging of the Head

Primary destructive or calcification abnormality of basal ganglia and brainstem (examples)	
Leigh disease	Barbiturate intoxication
Mitochondrial cytopathies	Heavy metals
Hypoglycemia	Carbon monoxide
Hypocalcemia	Cyanide poisoning
Central pontine myelinosis	Methylmalonic acidemia
Sulfite oxidase deficiency	
Primary diffuse myelin (white matter) involvement (examples)	
Defects of protein metabolism	
• Maple syrup urine disease	
• Phenylketonuria	
Nonspecific predilection: diffuse changes with or without demyelination, ischemic change, calcification, and hemorrhage (examples)	
Hypoglycemia	Nonketotic hyperglycinemia
Organic acidemias	Hartnup disease
Congenital lactic acidosis	Mitochondrial cytopathies

CLINICAL MANAGEMENT

The rapid assessment and management of the infant or child with an altered level of consciousness is a pediatric emergency. A review of an appropriate clinical approach including resuscitation, investigation, and institution of initial therapy of the comatose child is discussed in Chapter 21. In the context of a child referred with a presumed or identified metabolic encephalopathy, the priority is not only supportive therapy but also the identification and treatment of treatable problems, which should reduce morbidity and optimize outcome **(Tables 23.14 and 23.15).**

In practice, at an early stage the likelihood of neuronal injury may be limited by prompt therapy and correction of biochemical derangement. However, it is possible that even with the most aggressive management and correction of metabolic upset, central neurotoxic processes continue because of either a secondary complication (e.g., cytotoxic cerebral edema and raised intracranial pressure) or a persistent brain neurochemical or transmitter imbalance.

The rest of this chapter provides a framework for clinically evaluating and monitoring the patient with a metabolic encephalopathy, as well as a discussion of specific and supportive therapies.

Table 23.14. Hierarchical Approach to the Encephalopathic Child

	Assessment	*Action*
Vital signs	Respiratory	Maintain oxygenation
	Cardiovascular	Maintain circulation
	? Seizures	Treat and check blood gas, electrolytes, glucose, blood count, toxicology (see Table 23.15)
	? Hypoglycemia	
	? Coagulopathy	
Level of coma	Neurologic	Treat and monitor trends
	? Deteriorating	(see Tables 23.17–23.19)
	? Raised ICP[a]	(see Fig. 23.15)
	? Seizures	(see Chapter 22)
Diagnosis	Full history/ examination	Specific or supportive therapy (see Table 23.20)
	? CT scan	
	? Neurophysiology	

[a] ICP, intracranial pressure; CT, computed tomography.

Clinical Presentation and Findings

An infant or child with metabolic derangement and encephalopathy may be seen during an apparent prodromal phase of illness, when it is often difficult to differentiate a solely infectious cause of irritability, mild pyrexia, and upper re-

Table 23.15. Investigations and Screening in Infants and Children with Suspected Metabolic Cause of Encephalopathy

Primary investigations that will facilitate initial therapy

Blood
- Acid-base balance (arterial)
- Glucose
- Urea, electrolytes, and creatinine
- Osmolality
- Full blood count, coagulation screen
- Toxicology screen

Urine
- Sedative and toxic drug screen

Bedside urinary screening tests

Odor
- Maple syrup/burned sugar (MSUD)[a]
- Cheesy/sweaty feet (isovaleric acidemia)
- Cat's urine (multiple carboxylase deficiency, HMG CoA lyase deficiency)

Ferric chloride test: place 2 drops of 10% ferric chloride in 1 ml of fresh urine; mix and observe color immediately on standing (negative test does not exclude disease)
- Green (PKU, tyrosinemia, direct hyperbilirubinemia)
- Blue-green (histidinemia)
- Gray-green (MSUD)
- Purple (ketones, salicylates)

Reducing substances
- Galactose (galactosemia, severe liver disease)
- Fructose (hereditary fructose intolerance)
- Glucose
- *p*-Hydroxyphenylpyruvic acid (tyrosinemia)

Secondary investigations that might provide specific diagnosis

Blood
- Liver function tests
- Ammonia
- Amino acids
- Organic acids
- Ketones
- Pyruvate/lactate, octanoic acid, carnitine, fructose, porphyrins

Urine
- Organic acids
- Amino acids
- Ketones
- Orotic acid
- Carnitine

Further definitive diagnostic tests

Deep-freeze urine and plasma.

Initiate fibroblast culture for specific enzyme assay.

Obtain liver biopsy for histology and enzyme assay.

[a] MSUD, maple syrup urine disease; PKU, phenylketonuria.

spiratory tract symptoms from metabolic disease precipitated or exacerbated by infection. Alternatively, patients may be seen after a seizure, in coma, or occasionally with multiorgan disease particularly marked by severe cardiorespiratory impairment[1,2].

Evaluation of the patient in general, with assessment of all organ systems, is essential, since some of the therapies that are used to manage severely affected children are aggressive, invasive, and dangerous. Such an approach is covered in other sections of this book. Concerning the specific central nervous system features of an encephalopathy found on examination, most causes produce a relatively stereotyped array of symptoms and signs[157,158]. It is the authors' practice to evaluate these in the context of a methodical and meticulous clinical examination (see Chapter 21). Of course, in the infant and child, interpretation will be influenced by the stage of development and expected normal responses. Generally, the neurologic findings fall into one of the following categories:

1. A generalized depression of predominantly cerebral hemisphere function: consciousness is depressed, motor tone becomes diminished, pupils are small but reactive, and reflex eye movements are disinhibited. Asterixis, one of the hallmarks of metabolic encephalopathy, may relate to intermittent depression of motor function.
2. A heightened excitability of neural tissue resulting from a direct lowering of the threshold for neuronal excitability or because of a selective depression of inhibitory influences on neuronal function: Cheyne-Stokes respiration may result from bilateral hemispheric inhibition, and certain types of seizures from neuronal excitability.
3. Selective vulnerability or focal involvement of a specific brain region to a systemic metabolic insult. This may be due to regional differences in tissue metabolic requirements for oxygen, glucose, or amino acids or, alternatively, regional differences in neurotransmitters and receptors. It is not uncommon for focal findings to remain unexplained (e.g., those occurring during hypoglycemia, hyperglycemia, uremia, and hypercalcemia) or possibly be representative of an anamnestic response to a previous (perhaps occult) neurologic injury.
4. Progressive deterioration with features and signs indicative of raised intracranial pressure and brain-tissue shifts, which may represent a cytotoxic cerebral edema **(Tables 23.4–23.6).**

Laboratory Investigation

Once clinical suspicion of metabolic disease is aroused, general supportive measures and laboratory investigation must be undertaken immediately. The initial approach for investigation is set out in **Table 23.15.** Laboratory sample handling is important, since inappropriate handling may lead to unnecessary effort and further investigation because of spurious results. Of particular importance is the determination of the plasma ammonia concentration. Blood should be collected in ammonia-free heparinized tubes, placed on ice at the bedside, and transferred by hand to the laboratory, where the plasma is separated immediately. The analysis should be undertaken without delay, but if storage of samples is unavoidable, they should be frozen at −70°C, since breakdown of some nitrogenous compounds occurs at −20°C. Measurement of the arterial ammonia level may be very helpful because venous levels may be artificially high, especially after the application of a tourniquet, which tends to cause the release of ammonia from ischemic muscle. Likewise, measurement of pyruvate, 3-hydroxybutyrate, and acetoacetate should be carried out on plasma deproteinized within minutes of collection. Urine for amino and organic acid assays should be fresh. If this is not feasible, the samples should be centrifuged and frozen.

In general, if there is sufficient suspicion of metabolic disease, it is important to store adequate quantities of plasma, urine, and if collected, cerebrospinal fluid samples, at the time of presentation: they reflect the time of maximal metabolic stress, when the likelihood of defining the metabolic abnormality is optimal. It should also be obvious that the use of these precious samples needs to be carefully planned with the advice from specialists in metabolic medicine. In the event of such a child dying, adequate diagno-

Table 23.16. Perimortem Genetic-Metabolic Diagnostic Protocol for Infants and Children with Encephalopathy of Unknown Cause[a,b]

	Samples	*Storage and Usage*
Body fluids		
Blood	Heparinized Unheparinized	Serum and plasma are separated prior to freezing at −20°C
	Incubated with phytohemagglutinin	For metaphase chromosome analysis
	Whole blood in ethylenediamine tetraacetic acid	Store at 4°C for up to 5 days, used to extract DNA from leukocytes
Urine	Centrifuge to remove blood and debris	Stores at −20°C
Fibroblast culture		
Skin	Punch biopsy sample fully immersed in tissue culture media or patient's serum	Store at 4°C
Tissue enzyme activity		
Liver	Needle or open biopsy	Snap-freezing: immerse immediately in liquid nitrogen or isopentane chilled on dry ice
Muscle	Needle or open biopsy	Store at −70°C
Histology		
Liver	Needle or open biopsy	Tissue fixed in formalin for light microscopy
Muscle	Needle or open biopsy	Tissue fixed in glutaraldehyde for electron microscopy

[a] From Kronick JB, Seriver CR, Goodyear PR, Kaplan PB. A perimortem protocol for suspected genetic disease. Pediatrics 1983;71:960.
[b] Prior to invasive investigation, appropriate informed consent, according to institutional requirements, should be gained.

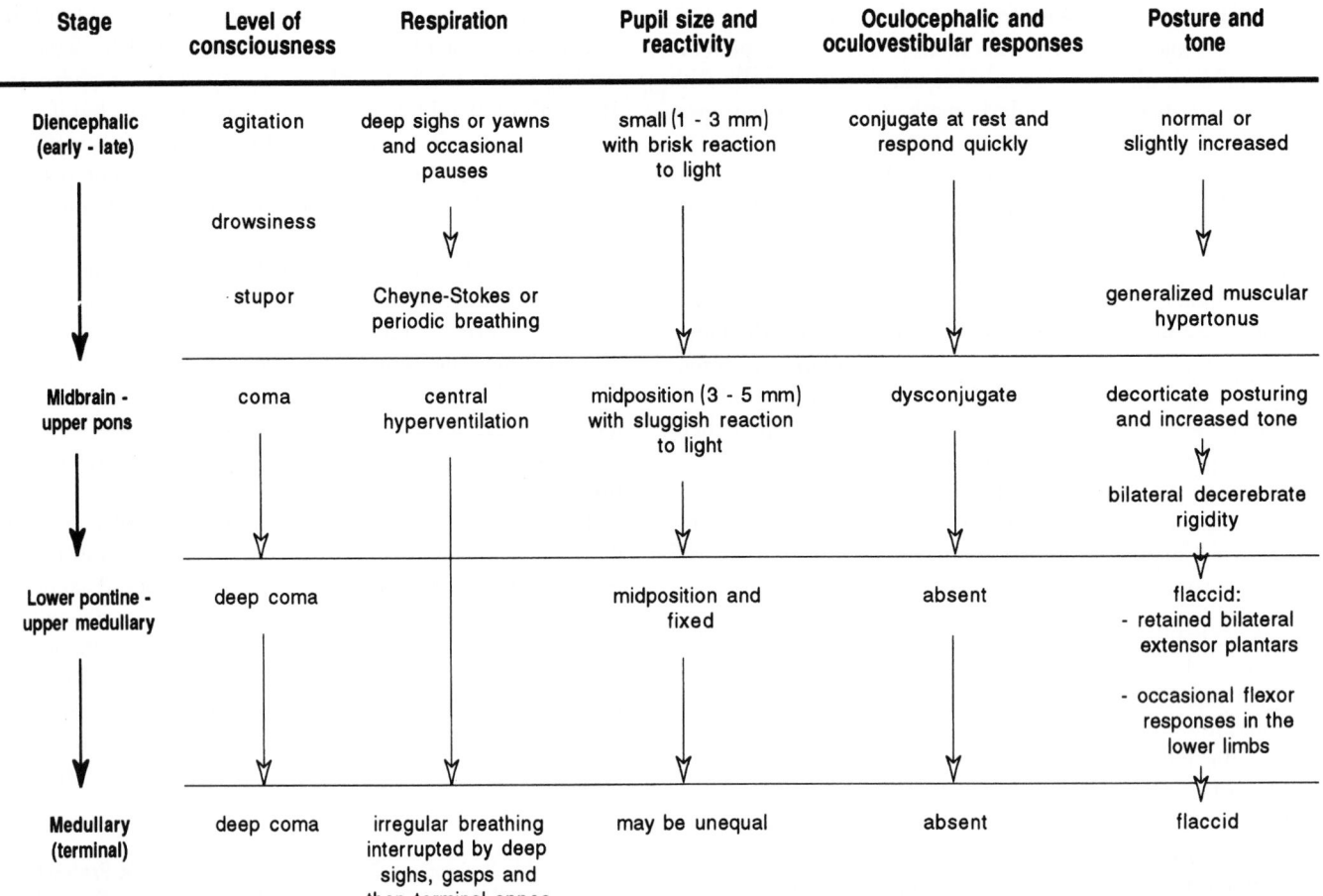

Stage	Level of consciousness	Respiration	Pupil size and reactivity	Oculocephalic and oculovestibular responses	Posture and tone
Diencephalic (early - late)	agitation ↓ drowsiness ↓ stupor	deep sighs or yawns and occasional pauses ↓ Cheyne-Stokes or periodic breathing	small (1 - 3 mm) with brisk reaction to light	conjugate at rest and respond quickly	normal or slightly increased ↓ generalized muscular hypertonus
Midbrain - upper pons	coma	central hyperventilation	midposition (3 - 5 mm) with sluggish reaction to light	dysconjugate	decorticate posturing and increased tone ↓ bilateral decerebrate rigidity
Lower pontine - upper medullary	deep coma		midposition and fixed	absent	flaccid: - retained bilateral extensor plantars - occasional flexor responses in the lower limbs
Medullary (terminal)	deep coma	irregular breathing interrupted by deep sighs, gasps and then terminal apnea	may be unequal	absent	flaccid

Figure 23.7. Clinical features of central syndrome or rostrocaudal deterioration. (Adapted from Plum F, Posner JB. Diagnosis of stupor and coma. Philadelphia: FA Davis, 1966.)

sis is important for family genetic counseling. An autopsy protocol similar to the one outlined in **Table 23.16** should be developed so that items such as biopsy needles (e.g., liver, kidney, and skin), dry ice, and culture media can be made readily available and samples can be appropriately stored at any time.

Neurologic Severity Staging and Monitoring

Clinical

For patients needing frequent neurologic review to monitor for significant change or evaluate the need for specific cerebral protective therapy, there are obvious advantages to using a screening assessment that can be carried out quickly and reliably by different bedside attendants. With these considerations, a number of clinical neurologic scoring/severity systems have been applied to infants and young children in nontraumatic coma[159–162]. All of these have similarities with the description of progressive rostrocaudal neurologic deterioration or central syndrome highlighted by Plum and Posner[158] (Fig. 23.7).

For the pediatrician, the most well-known assessment of metabolic encephalopathy was developed for staging Reye syndrome and was described by Lovejoy et al.[163]. The clinical stages divide the progress of disease into five relatively arbitrary levels of severity and their associated metabolic and EEG features. To simplify this, a Reye syndrome consensus statement in 1981[164] resulted in the following purely clinical staging system—the similarities with Plum and Posner's description of central syndrome[158] can be easily identified:

1. Stage I: lethargy, follows verbal commands, normal posture, purposeful response to pain, brisk pupillary light reflex, and normal oculocephalic reflex
2. Stage II: combative or stuporous, inappropriate verbalizing, normal posture, purposeful or nonpurposeful response to pain, sluggish pupillary reflexes, and conjugate deviation on doll's eyes maneuver
3. Stage III: comatose, decorticate posture, decorticate response to pain, sluggish pupillary reaction, conjugate deviation on doll's eyes maneuver
4. Stage IV: Comatose, decerebrate posture and decerebrate response to pain, sluggish pupillary reflexes, and inconsistent or absent oculocephalic reflex
5. Stage V: Comatose, flaccid, no response to pain, no pupillary response, no oculocephalic reflex

The Glasgow coma scale (GCS) **(Table 23.17)** is a modification of the central syndrome that assigns scores for

Table 23.17. Glasgow Coma Scale[a]

			Score
Eyes	Open	Spontaneous	4
		To verbal command	3
		To pain	2
		No response	1
Best motor response	To verbal command	Obeys	6
	To painful stimulus	Localizes pain	5
		Flexion withdrawal	4
		Flexion abnormal	3
		Extension	2
		No response	1
Best verbal response	Adult	Oriented and converses	5
		Disoriented and converses	4
		Inappropriate words	3
		Incomprehensible sounds	2
		No response	1
	Child	Oriented	5
		Words	4
		Vocal sounds	3
		Cries	2
		None	1
Total	Eyes (1–4) + motor (1–6) + verbal (1–5)		3–15

[a] Compiled from Teasdale G, Jennett B. Assessment of coma and impaired consciousness. A practical scale. Lancet 1974;2:81; and from Reilly PL, Simpson DA, Sprod R, Thomas L. Assessing the conscious level in infants and young children: a paediatric version of the Glasgow coma scale. Childs Nerv Syst 1988;4:30.

clinical developments that follow head injury[159]. In the wider context of nontraumatic coma and encephalopathy in infants and children, it should be remembered that there has been little in the way of prospective validation[162]. Although many authors would advocate the use of a pediatric scale to facilitate rapid screening review and assessment[165–167], in practice multiobserver interpretation of vocal sounds, cries, and arousal behavior is very difficult and for the most part probably inadequate. It remains to be seen whether or not in the spectrum of conditions producing metabolic encephalopathy as well as in expected or potential complications (e.g., raised intracranial pressure), the total score or change in score is of any early diagnostic value. In Reye syndrome, deterioration in GCS appeared to be more sensitive than the change in Lovejoy staging for clinical deterioration due to raised intracranial pressure[165]. A more basic approach would be to consider that a deviation from assumed or expected normal scores indicates that more formal review is needed to explain any observed change. An alternative scoring assessment, which can also be used effectively in intubated patients, has been described by Morray et al.[161] **(Table 23.18).** In contrast to the pediatric GCS, inclusion of brainstem reflexes allows reference to the neurologic features of central syndrome.

Neurophysiology

Appropriately chosen clinical neurophysiologic techniques have been used in combination with clinical assessment in a variety of encephalopathic disorders in both adults and children[168]. They are particularly useful in patients in whom clinical evaluation is unreliable because of administration of sedatives, hypnotics, or muscle relaxants. Although there may be difficulty in obtaining this type of testing at the time of admission, there is considerable information to be gained. During the acute phase of illness, EEG may provide information about the severity and distribution of altered cerebral function of the cortex, presence of discharges (seizure activity), and even on occasion a clue to the possible cause. Boyd and Harden[169] reviewed the role of clinical neurophysiologic investigation (e.g., combined use of evoked potentials and EEG) in the comatose infant or child.

Regardless of etiology, EEG during an acute encephalopathic process usually shows varying degrees of slow activity. This was used by Aoki and Lombroso[170] when they described the relationship between increasing severity of encephalopathy and worsening EEG changes in children with Reye syndrome (Fig. 23.8). The system they used, which was subsequently incorporated in clinical staging of Reye syndrome by Lovejoy et al.[163], graded for degree of EEG abnormality between normal for age and electrocerebral silence (i.e., absence of all cerebral activity). The predominant abnormal background activity was classified as follows:

1. Normal for age
2. Borderline normal for age
3. Abnormal for age: graded 1–5 according to frequency and amplitude of slow activity (as patients deteriorated, predominant EEG activity became slower—4–6 cycles/sec to 0.5–2 cycles/sec—and of lower amplitude—less than 50 μV—then intermittent)
4. Electrocerebral silence

A similar version of this EEG staging has been used in the wider context of nontraumatic coma[171], in which evaluation of severity was successfully carried out in a variety of

Table 23.18. Clinical Assessment of Cortical and Brainstem Function[a]

Best Response	*Score*
Cortical function: scores 0–6	
Purposeful, spontaneous movement	6
Purposeful movement to command	5
Localizing pain	4
Nonpurposeful movement, withdrawal response	3
Decorticate posturing	2
Decerebrate posturing	1
Flaccidity	0
Brainstem function: scores 0–3	
Pupillary light reflex, corneal reflex, oculovestibular and oculocephalic	
All normal	3
Some absent or diminished	2
All absent, but breathing	1
All absent and apneic (normal carbon dioxide)	0
Total score: cortical (0–6) + brainstem (0–3)	0–9

[a] From Morray JP, et al. Coma scale for use in brain-injured children. Crit Care Med 1984;12:1018.

metabolic encephalopathies complicated by raised intracranial pressure (Fig. 23.9).

Neuroimaging

Cranial CT in the comatose child is invaluable for assessing potential underlying cerebral disease and need for surgical intervention. In the context of metabolic encephalopathy, the CT scan is particularly useful in the evaluation of cerebral edema and raised intracranial pressure[172,173]. The likelihood of the latter can be determined by reviewing the presence or absence of CSF spaces both above and below the tentorium. Loss of spaces below the tentorium (i.e., the basal cisterns) is indicative of severe swelling. A grading system for the worsening generalized loss of CSF spaces **(Table 23.19)** has been used in this context, and worsening loss of CSF spaces was associated with more increased levels of intracranial pressure (Figs. 23.10–23.13).

In comparison with cranial CT, MRI of the brain will not provide more information of therapeutic relevance. However, proton magnetic resonance spectroscopy (^{1}H-MRS) can provide information on the biochemical state of the brain. Metabolites measured with measured ^{1}H-MRS include *N*-acetylaspartate, a neuronal marker; creatine, composed of phosphocreatine and its precursor, which are bioenergetic metabolites; choline-containing compounds, including free choline, phosphoryl, and glycerophosphoryl choline, which are released during membrane disruption; lactate, which accumulates in response to tissue damage; glutamate; and immediately formed glutamine and *myo*-inositol. Abnormal ^{1}H-MRS spectra have been observed in patients with hepatic encephalopathy, diabetic ketoacidosis, stroke, ornithine transcarbamylase deficiency, aminoacidopathies, mitochondrial encephalopathies, and peroxisomal disorders. Recently Auld and colleagues[174] used ^{1}H-MRS in 30 infants and children with acute central ner-

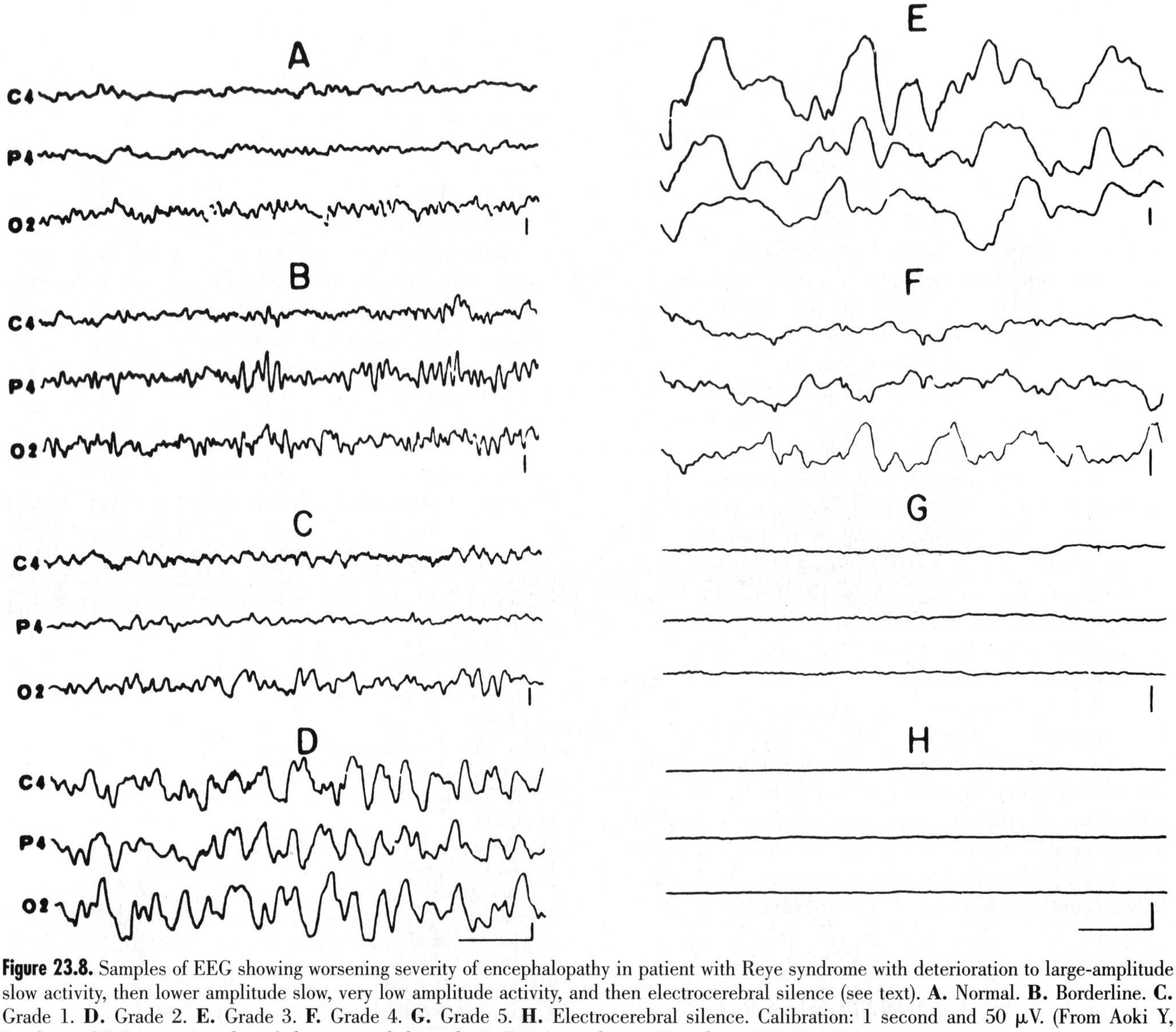

Figure 23.8. Samples of EEG showing worsening severity of encephalopathy in patient with Reye syndrome with deterioration to large-amplitude slow activity, then lower amplitude slow, very low amplitude activity, and then electrocerebral silence (see text). **A.** Normal. **B.** Borderline. **C.** Grade 1. **D.** Grade 2. **E.** Grade 3. **F.** Grade 4. **G.** Grade 5. **H.** Electrocerebral silence. Calibration: 1 second and 50 μV. (From Aoki Y, Lombroso CT. Prognostic value of electroencephalography in Reye's syndrome. Neurology 1973;23:333.)

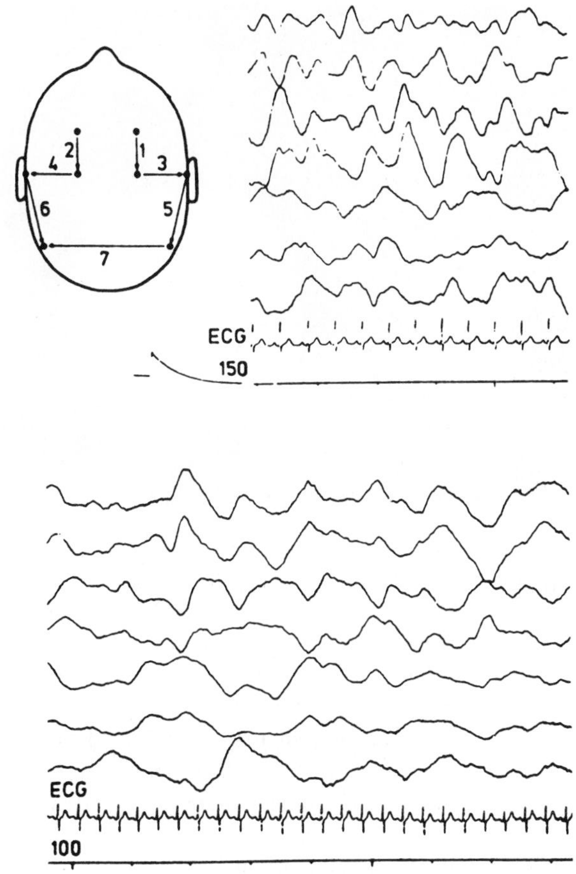

Figure 23.9. An infant aged 18 months with a metabolic encephalopathy had generalized large-amplitude slow activities on initial EEG *(upper trace)*. Nine days later *(lower trace)*, slow activity is even more prominent. (From Tasker RC, Boyd S, Harden A, Matthew DJ. Monitoring in non-traumatic coma: electroencephalography. Arch Dis Child 1988;63:895.)

Table 23.19. Worsening Severity of Generalized Loss of Cerebrospinal Fluid Spaces on Cranial Computed Tomography (CT) Scan[a]

Grade	*CT Scan Features*
N	Normal CT scan
I	Loss of sulci cerebri and/or interhemispheric fissure and/or sylvian fissure and/or occlusion of body lateral ventricle
II	Complete loss of sulci and fissures and/or chiasmatic cistern and/or quadrigeminal cistern and/or interpeduncular cistern
III	Complete loss of sulci, fissures, and all (perimesencephalic) cisterns

[a] From Tasker RC, Matthew DJ, Kendall B. Computed tomography in the assessment of raised intracranial pressure in nontraumatic coma. Neuropediatrics 1990;21:91.

vous system injuries to determine the value of cerebral biochemical indices in predicting outcome. Use of spectroscopy variables (ratios of *N*-acetylaspartate : creatine, *N*-acetylaspartate : choline, choline : creatine, and presence of lactate) alone correctly classified 81% of patients. The combination of clinical and ^{1}H-MRS variables correctly classified all patients, suggesting that spectroscopy may be a useful adjunct in patient assessment.

Specific Clinical Treatment

The management of children with metabolic encephalopathy ranges from the relatively simple provision or correction of electrolytes or metabolic substrate to the extremely complex neurointensive care for children with more severe complications, such as renal failure, fulminant hepatic failure, or raised intracranial pressure. In general, care rests on the firm foundation of strict attention to fluid and electrolyte balance, adequate oxygenation and perfusion, tem-

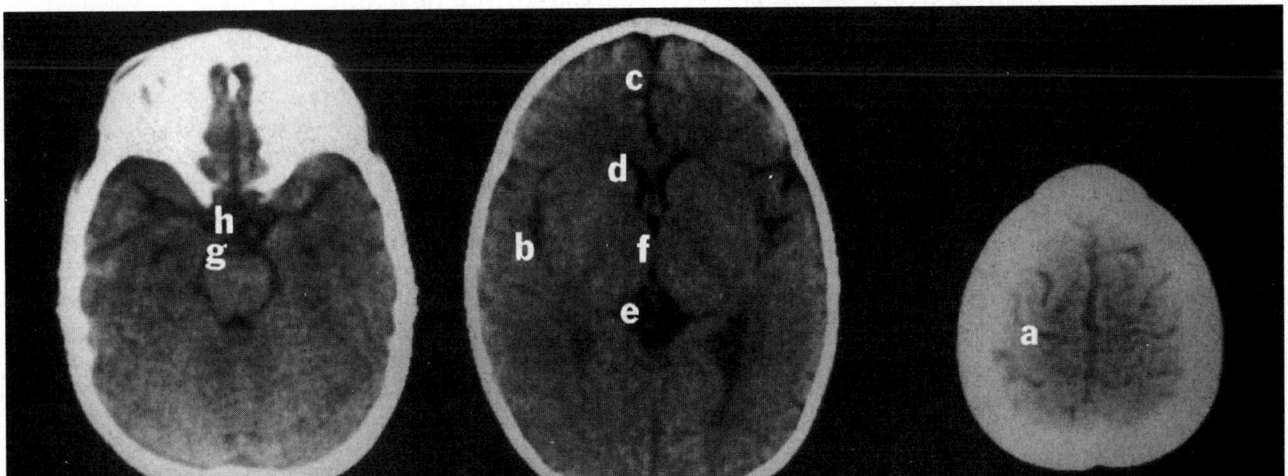

Figure 23.10. Normal head CT scan in a 7-year-old with an encephalopathic illness. *a*, sulci cerebri; *b*, Sylvian fissure; *c*, interhemispheric fissure; *d*, body of lateral ventricle; *e*, quadrigeminal cistern; *f*, third ventricle; *g*, interpeduncular cistern; and *h*, chiasmatic cistern.

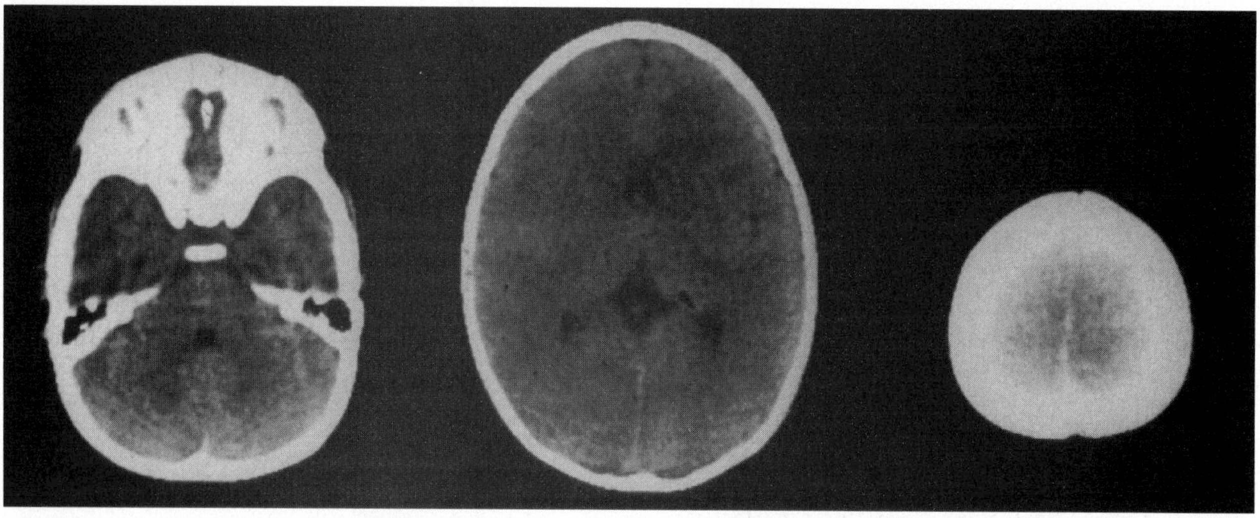

Figure 23.11. A 3-year-old who presented postoperatively with repeated episodes of profound hypoglycemia. Note the loss of CSF spaces above and below the tentorium, as well as gray-white differentiation indicative of marked cerebral edema.

perature control, prevention of infection, and seizure control. More specific therapy for individual organ system failure as well as the total care of patients with multisystem disease is described in other chapters of this book.

Many of the specific metabolic therapies oriented toward the underlying process and etiology of encephalopathy, outlined in earlier sections of this chapter, are covered elsewhere in the book. This discussion is mainly restricted to the therapeutic considerations for reducing ammonia levels.

Ammonia Reduction Therapy

Several types of therapy have been designed to lower ammonia levels in infants and children with a hyperammonemic disorder. Immediate therapy includes elimination of protein intake and caloric supplementation with hypertonic glucose to decrease catabolism. This can be achieved by infusing concentrated solutions of glucose at 75–100 g/m^2/day (2.5–3.5 g/kg/day) plus insulin if hyperglycemia becomes a problem. Acidosis should be corrected with sodium bicarbonate, and if this is ineffective or hypernatremia develops, bicarbonate peritoneal dialysis should be instituted.

In some patients, removal of ammonia by dialysis is the only effective treatment. This can be undertaken in one of three ways: continuous peritoneal dialysis, episodic hemodialysis, or continuous arteriovenous/venovenous hemofiltration with dialysis[(175–178)]. More aggressive extracorporeal techniques, including exchange transfusion[(179–182)], charcoal hemoperfusion[(183,184)], and heart-lung bypass total-body washout[(185–187)], previously used in hepatic coma and Reye syndrome, are now fortunately solely of historical interest, since they were ineffective and labor intensive.

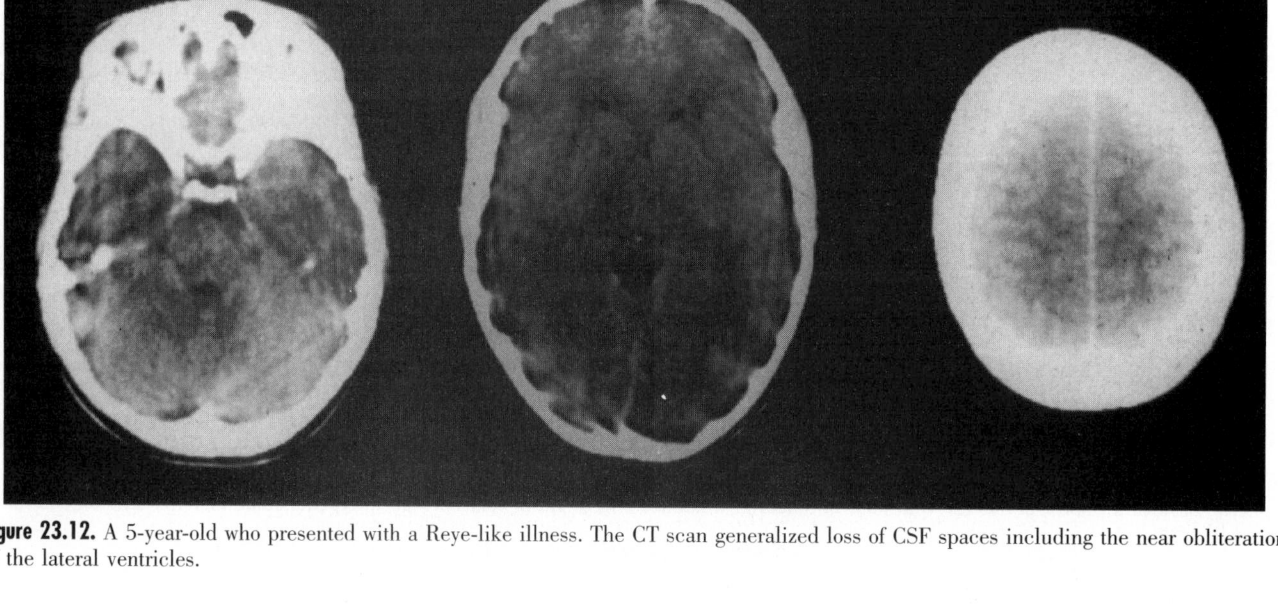

Figure 23.12. A 5-year-old who presented with a Reye-like illness. The CT scan generalized loss of CSF spaces including the near obliteration of the lateral ventricles.

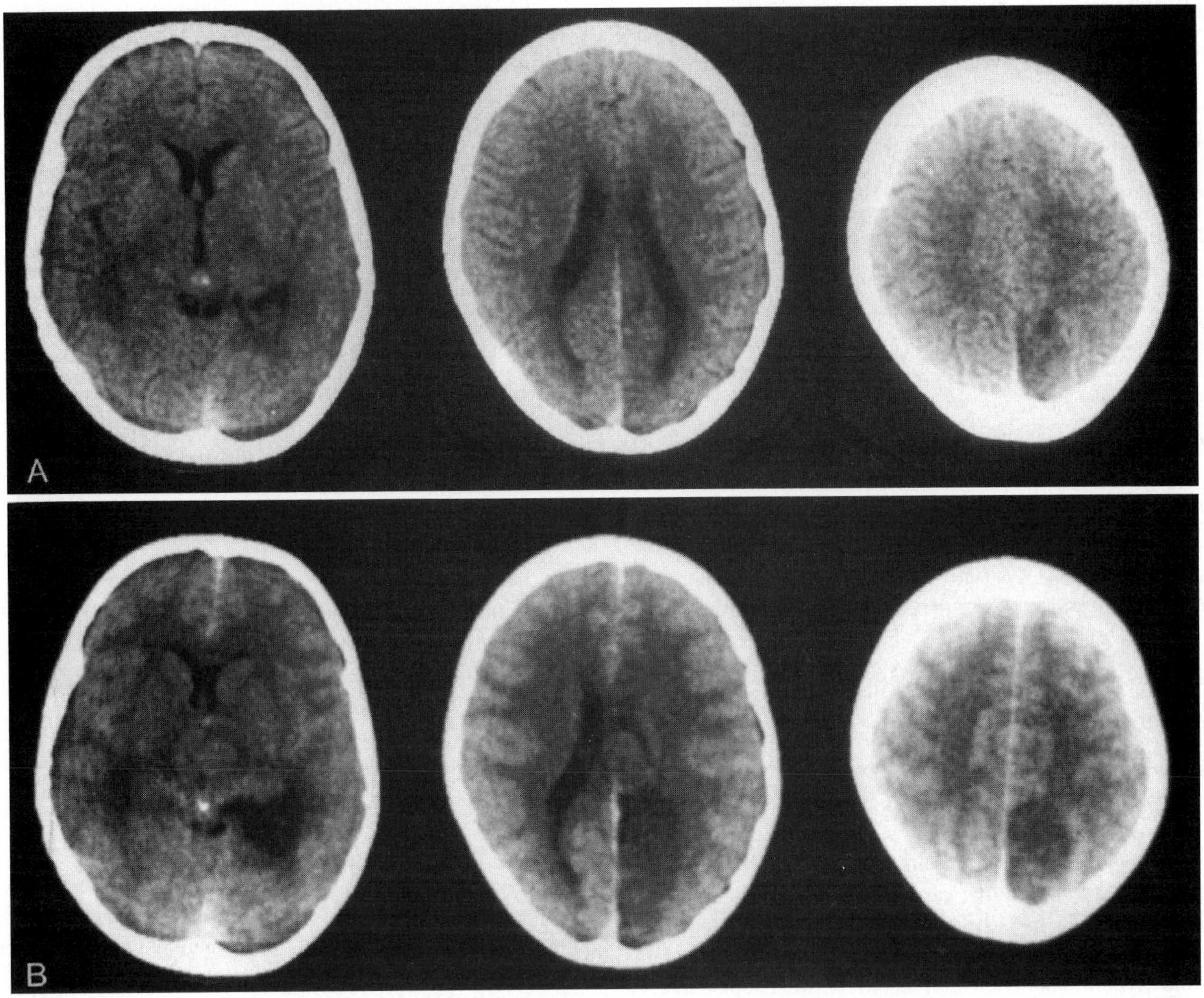

Figure 23.13. A. A 9-year-old girl who presented 12 hours into fluid resuscitation therapy for diabetic ketoacidosis. Her level of consciousness was depressed. The CT scan shows prominent lateral ventricles and an area of low density in the occipital region on the right. **B.** The same patient 2 weeks later with a CT scan showing evolution of the occipital low density indicative of posterior cerebral artery infarction secondary to tentorial herniation.

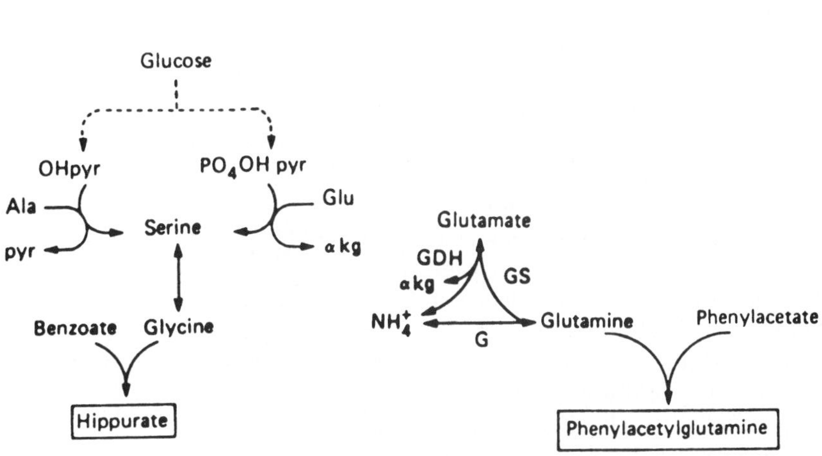

Figure 23.14. Pathways of waste nitrogen synthesis in patients with deficiencies of carbamyl-phosphate synthetase and ornithine transcarbamylase, treated with sodium benzoate and phenylacetate. Hippurate and phenylacetylglutamine serve as the waste nitrogen products. *GDH*, glutamate dehydrogenase; *GS*, glutamine synthetase; *G*, glutaminase; and α*kg*, α-ketoglutarate. (From Brusilow SW. Inborn errors of urea synthesis. Butterworths Int Med Rev 1985;5:140.)

Table 23.20. Metabolic Therapies

Agents Activating Alternative or Normal Pathways of Nitrogen Balance

Medication	*Metabolic Mechanism of Action*	*Product and Excretion Rate*	*Atoms of Waste Nitrogen/Molecule*
Sodium benzoate load: 0.25 g/kg i.v. then: continuous i.v. 0.25–0.5 g/kg/day	Conjugates with glycine to form hippuric acid	Hippurate 5 times glomerular filtration rate	1
Arginine hydrochloride load: 0.8 g/kg i.v. then: continuous i.v. 0.2–0.8 g/kg/day	Provides substrate for intact part of urea cycle—ensures ornithine deficiency does not limit detoxification	Citrulline 25% glomerular filtration rate	1
Phenylacetate load: 0.25 g/kg then: continuous i.v. 0.25–0.5 g/kg/day	Conjugates with glutamine to form phenylacetylglutamine	Phenylacetylglutamine Glomerular filtration rate	2
Phenylbutyrate	Oxidized in vivo to its active metabolite phenylacetate		

Vitamins and Cofactors

Enzyme Deficiency	*Medication*	*Daily Dosage*	*Other Therapy*
Multiple carboxylase deficiency	Biotin	10–20 mg	
Methylmalonic acidemia	B_{12}	1–2 mg or less	L-carnitine 100 mg/kg i.v. in 6 hr, then 100 mg/kg/day
Maple syrup urine disease	Thiamine	5–20 mg/kg	
Multiple acyl-CoA dehydrogenase deficiency	Riboflavin	300 mg	L-carnitine 100 mg/kg i.v. in 6 hr, then 100 mg/kg/day

Peritoneal dialysis has the advantage of not requiring large intravascular access. This method will remove ammonium (albeit slowly, 5–8 ml/min/m^2, see below), as well as other nitrogen-containing waste molecules (glutamine, glutamate, and alanine). Episodic hemodialysis, in contrast, enables a clearance of ammonium 10 times higher, but rebound hyperammonemia may occur between episodes. To avoid such problems continuous hemofiltration with dialysis has been used, with similarly more rapid clearance rates.

Metabolic therapies designed to accelerate the detoxification of ammonia or to decrease its rate of production rely in part on the cause of the hyperammonemia **(Table 23.20** and Fig. 23.14). For example, in the neonate, the intramuscular administration of biotin and hydroxycobalamin (vitamin B_{12}) for suspected organic acidemia[188] and the intravenous administration of arginine and sodium benzoate to facilitate alternative pathway excretion of ammonia in suspected urea cycle defects[189–191] are appropriate. Propionic acidemia in some instances responds to biotin therapy, and methylmalonic acidemia may be responsive to hydroxycobalamin. In urea cycle disorders such as citrullinemia and arginosuccinic aciduria, arginine supplementation promotes function of the urea cycle up to the point of the deficient enzyme[192]. Both citrulline and arginosuccinic acid are then excreted in the urine, providing an alternative route for nitrogen excretion. In the older child with a urea cycle defect, therapy with sodium benzoate, phenylacetic acid, arginine, or *N*-carbamyl glutamate can be used to gain the most efficient excretion of nitrogen atoms. Likewise, vitamin cofactors, bicarbonate, or carnitine therapy may be used for organic acidemias. In addition, carnitine supplementation may be beneficial in several of the organic acidemias to remedy secondary carnitine deficiency.

Hepatic Encephalopathy

Encephalopathy due to acute or chronic hepatic disease requires a variety of measures to affect ammonia production **(Table 23.21).** It is also important to recognize and treat precipitating factors that may have led to increased ammonia production or poor clearance, e.g., gastrointestinal bleeding, infection, and an increase in dietary protein **(Table 23.22).**

Raised Intracranial Pressure

Any child with a metabolic encephalopathy who is seriously ill, with an impaired level of consciousness, should be considered to have raised intracranial pressure. In these patients, careful thought should be given to monitoring their

Table 23.21. Factors That Affect Ammonia Production and Levels

Source	*Action to Limit Ammonia*
Gastrointestinal	
Dietary nitrogen	Restrict
Bacterial production	Increase gut motility with cathartics Reduce bowel flora with antibiotics
Renal production	Correct metabolic alkalosis
Brain accumulation	
Ammonia diffusion	Correct metabolic alkalosis Accelerate ammonia detoxification by providing substrate for brain transamination of α-keto amino acids

Table 23.22. Precipitants of Hepatic Encephalopathy

Drugs	Sedatives
	Tranquilizers
	Narcotics
	Diuretics
Electrolyte imbalance	Hyponatremia
	Hypokalemic alkalosis
Excessive nitrogen load	Gastrointestinal hemorrhage
	Excess dietary protein
	Azotemia
	Constipation
Other	Infection
	Hypoxia
	Hypovolemia

intracranial pressure and instituting standard management (Fig. 23.15). However, although this form of therapy has been used in Reye syndrome, hepatic encephalopathy, and many other types of metabolic derangement, it is unlikely that this form of treatment controls or reverses a cytotoxic edema.

Hypoglycemia

The treatment of hypoglycemia is discussed elsewhere in this book. **Table 23.23** summarizes the initial management approach.

Table 23.23. Treatment of Hypoglycemia

Newborns and infants
- 0.25 g glucose 0.25 g/kg i.v. followed by increase in maintenance

Repeat if persistent
- Hydrocortisone 5 mg/kg/day

If adrenal insufficiency or hypopituitarism suspected, 20–60 mg/m^2/day
- Glucagon 0.03 mg/kg/day i.v. or i.m. up to 1 mg if hyperinsulinemia suspected
- Diazoxide 10–25 mg/kg/day oral or i.v. in hyperinsulinism

Children
- 0.25 g glucose/kg i.v. followed by increase in maintenance

Repeat if persistent
- Hydrocortisone 5 mg/kg/day up to 100 mg
- Glucagon 0.03 mg/kg/day i.v. or i.m. up to 1 mg
- Diazoxide 10–25 mg/kg/day oral or i.v.

CONCLUSION

In the infant or child with an acute encephalopathic process, a variety of metabolic causes may account for the acute brain dysfunction. Given the highly selected population referred for intensive care, the intensivist should be aware of the more common differential diagnoses, necessary investigation, and therapeutic priorities if neurologic morbidity is to be minimized.

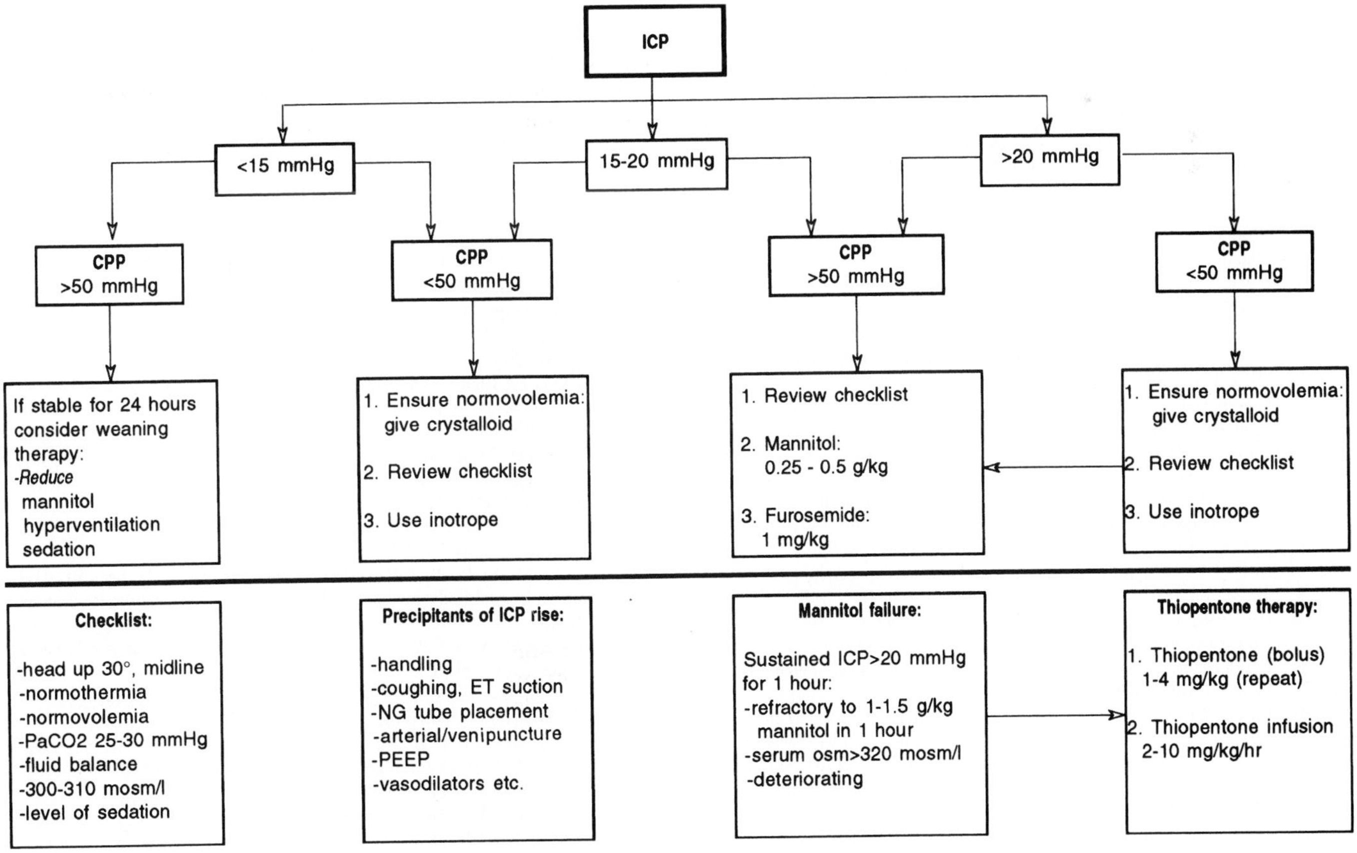

Figure 23.15. Guidelines for the treatment of raised intracranial pressure in the monitored and mechanically ventilated patient. *ICP*, intracranial pressure; *CPP*, cerebral perfusion pressure; *ET*, endotracheal; *NG*, nasogastric; and *PEEP*, positive end-expiratory pressure.

References

1. Brown JK, Habel AH. Toxic encephalopathy and acute brain-swelling in children. Dev Med Child Neurol 1975;17:659.
2. Seshia SS, Seshia MMK, Sachdeva RK. Coma in childhood. Dev Med Child Neurol 1977;19:614.
3. Reye RDK, Morgan G, Baral J. Encephalopathy and fatty degeneration of the viscera: a disease entity in childhood. Lancet 1963;2:749.
4. Anderson RMD. Encephalitis in childhood: pathological aspects. Med J Aust 1963;1:573.
5. Johnson GM, Scurletis TD, Carroll NB. A study of sixteen fatal cases of encephalitis-like disease in North Carolina children. N C Med J 1963;24:464.
6. Hurwitz ES, Barrett MJ, Bregman D. Public Health Service study of Reye's syndrome and medication. JAMA 1987;257:1905.
7. De Vivo DC. Reye's syndrome. In: Johnson RT, ed. Current therapy in neurologic disease. Philadelphia: BC Decker, 1990;3:346.
8. Roger MC. Introduction: the development of pediatric intensive care. In: Rogers MC, ed. Textbook of pediatric intensive care, First edition. Baltimore: Williams & Wilkins, 1987:1.
9. Swaiman KF, ed. Pediatric neurology. Principles and practice. St Louis: CV Mosby, 1989.
10. Behrman RE, Vaughan VC, eds. Nelson's textbook of pediatrics. Philadelphia: WB Saunders, 1987.
11. Stanbury JB, Wyngaarden JB, Frederickson DS, Goldstein JL, Brown MS, eds. The metabolic basis of inherited disease. New York: McGraw-Hill, 1983.
12. Morales AR, Bourgeois CH, Chulacharit E. Pathology of the heart in Reye's syndrome (encephalopathy and fatty degeneration of the viscera). Am J Cardiol 1971;27:314.
13. Baliga R, Fleischmann LE, Chang CH, et al. Acute renal failure in Reye's syndrome. Am J Dis Child 1979;133:1009.
14. Manning R, Kearney PJ. Peptic ulcer in Reye's syndrome. Br Med J 1983;287:1105.
15. Ellis GH, Mirkin LD, Mills MC. Pancreatitis and Reye's syndrome. Am J Dis Child 1979;133:1014.
16. Chaves-Carballo E, Menezes AH, Bell WE, Hernriquez EM. Acute pancreatitis is Reye's syndrome: a fatal complication during intensive supportive care. South Med J 1980;73:152.
17. Forsyth BW, Horwitz RI, Acampora D, et al. New epidemiologic evidence confirming that bias does not explain the aspirin/Reye's syndrome association. JAMA 1989;261:2517.
18. Starko KM, Ray CG, Dominquez LB, Stromberg WL, Woodstall DF. Reye's syndrome and salicylate use. Pediatric 1980;66:864.
19. Waldman RJ, Ng HW, McGee H, Van Amburg G. Aspirin as a risk factor in Reye's syndrome. JAMA 1982;247:3089.
20. Orlowski JP, Campbell P, Goldstein S. Reye's syndrome: a case control study of medication use and associated viruses in Australia. Cleve Clin J Med 1990;57:323.
21. Orlowski JP, Gillis J, Kilham HA. A catch in the Reye. Pediatrics 1987;5:638.
22. Arrowsmith JB, Kennedy DL, Kuritsky JN, Faich GA. National patterns of aspirin use and Reye syndrome reporting, United States, 1980 to 1985. Pediatrics 1987;79:858.
23. Gauthier M, Guay J, Lacroix J, Lortie A. Reye's syndrome: a reappraisal of diagnosis in 49 presumptive cases. AJDC 1989;143:1181.
24. Green A, Hall SM. Investigation of metabolic disorders resembling Reye's syndrome. Arch Dis Child 1992;67:1313.
25. Greene CL, Blitzer MG, Shapira E. Inborn errors of metabolism and Reye syndrome: differential diagnosis. J Pediatr 1988;113:156.
26. Hukin J, Junker AK, Thomas EE, Farrell K. Reye syndrome associated with subclinical varicella zoster virus and influenza A infection. Pediatr Neurol 1993;9:134.
27. Poss WB, Vernon DD, Dean JM. A reemergence of Reye's syndrome. Arch Pediatr Adolesc Med 1994;148:879.
28. Centers for Disease Control. Reye syndrome surveillance—United States, 1989. MMWR 1991;40:88.
29. Corkey BE, Geschwind J, Deeney JT, Hale DE, Douglas SD, Kipatrick L. Ca2+ responses to interleukin 1 and tumor necrosis facot in cultured human skin fibroblasts. J Clin Invest 1991;87:778.
30. Sullivan-Bolyai JZ, Corey L. Epidemiology of Reye syndrome. Epidemiol Rev 1981;3:1.
31. Jenkins R, Dvorak A, Patrick J. Encephalopathy and fatty degeneration of the viscera associated with chickenpox. Pediatrics 1967;39:769.
32. Joske RA, et al. Hepatitis-encephalitis in humans with reovirus infection. Arch Intern Med 1964;113:811.
33. Powell HC, et al. Reye's syndrome: isolation of parainfluenza virus. Arch Neurol 1973;29:135.
34. Morens DM, Halsey NA, Schonberger LB, et al. Reye syndrome associated with vaccination with live virus vaccines. Clin Pediatr (Phila) 1979;18:42.
35. Brown RE, Koh SJ, BhuVaneswaran C, Brewster MA. Lipid peroxidation and hepatocellular degeneration in Reye syndrome. Ann Clin Lab Sci 1982;12:327.
36. Schwarz KB, Larroya S, Vogler C, et al. Role of influenza B virus in hepatic steosis and mitochondrial abnormalities in a mouse model of Reye syndrome. Hepatology 1991;13:96.
37. Tonsgard JH. Effect of Reye's syndrome serum on the ultrastructure of isolated liver mitochondria. Lab Invest 1989;60:568.
38. Saibara T, Himeno H, Ueda H, et al. Acute hepatic failure with swollen mitochondria and microvesicular fatty degeneration of hepatocytes triggered by free radical inhibitor. Lab Invest 1994;70:517.
39. Robinson RO. Differential diagnosis of Reye's syndrome. Dev Med Child Neurol 1987;29:110.
40. Centers for Disease Control. Follow-up on Reye's syndrome—United States. MMWR CDC Surveill Summ 1980;29:321.
41. LaBreque DR, Latham PS, Reily CA, et al. Heritable urea cycle enzyme deficiency—liver disease in 16 patients. J Pediatr 1979; 94:580.
42. Glasgow AM, Eng G, Engel AC. Systemic carnitine deficiency simulating recurrent Reye syndrome. J Pediatr 1980;96:889.
43. Brown T, Hug G, Lansky L, et al. Transiently reduced activity of carbamyl-phosphate synthetase and ornithine transcarbamylase in liver of children with Reye's syndrome. N Engl J Med 1976;294:861.
44. Robinson BH, Gall DG, Cutz E. Deficient activity of hepatic pyruvate dehydrogenase and pyruvate carboxylase in Reye's syndrome. Pediatr Res 1977;11:279.
45. Truscott RJW, Hick L, Pullin C, et al. Dicarboxylic aciduria: the response to fasting. Clin Chim Acta 1979;94:31.
46. Snodgrass PJ, DeLong GR. Urea-cycle enzyme deficiencies and an increased nitrogen load producing hyperammonemia in Reye's syndrome. N Engl J Med 1976;294:855.
47. Engel AG, Rebouche CJ. Carnitine metabolism and inborn errors. J Inherited Metab Dis 1984;7(suppl 1):38.
48. Kimura S, Kobayashi T, Tanaka Y, Sasaki Y. Liver histopathology in clinical Reye syndrome. Brain Dev 1991;13:95.
49. Blisard KS, Davis LE. Neuropathologic findings in Reye syndrome. J Child Neurol 1991;6:41.
50. Delong GR, Glick TH. Encephalopathy of Reye's syndrome: a review of pathogenic hypotheses. Pediatrics 1982;69:53.
51. Berman W, Pizzi F, Schut L, et al. The effects of exchange transfusion on intracranial pressure in patients with Reye syndrome. J Pediatr 1975;87:887.
52. Kindt GW, Waldman J, Kohl S, et al. Intracranial pressure in Reye's syndrome. JAMA 1975;231:822.
53. Lovejoy FH, Bresnan MJ, Lombroso CT, Smith AL. Anticerebral oedema therapy in Reye's syndrome. Arch Dis Child 1975;50:933.
54. Nadler H. Therapeutic delirium in Reye's syndrome. Pediatrics 1974;54:265.
55. Samaha FJ, Blau E. The role of peritoneal dialysis in Reye's syndrome. In: Pollack JD, ed. Reye's syndrome. New York: Grune & Stratton 1975:295.
56. Engle WD, Jacobs JF, Swartz RD, et al. Severe coagulopathy complicating charcoal hemoperfusion in children with Reye's syndrome. J Pediatr 1978;93:972.
57. Talmage EA, Thomas JM, Weeks JH. Total blood washout for Reye's syndrome. Anesth Anal 1973;42:563.
58. Lansky LL, Fixley M, Romig DA, Ketges PW, Boggan M, Reis RL. Hypothermic total body-washout with survival in Reye' syndrome. Lancet 1974;2:1019.
59. Shaywitz SE, Cohen PM. Long-term consequences of Reye syndrome. J Pediatr 1982;100:41.
60. Reitman MA, Kasper J, Koplin J. Motor disorders of voice and speech in Reye syndrome survivors. AJDC 1984;138:1129.
61. Duffy J, Glasgow JFT, Patterson CC, Clarke MJ, Turner IF. A sibling controlled study of intelligence and academic performance following Reye syndrome. Dev Med 1991;33:811.
62. Leibhaber MM, Robin E, Lynne-Davis P, Sinatra F. Reye syndrome complicated by Ondine's curse. West J Med 1977;126:118.
63. Thompson JW, Rosenthal P, Camilon FS. Vocal cord paralysis and superior laryngeal nerve dysfunction in Reye's syndrome. Arch Otolaryngol Head Neck Surg 1990;116:46.

64. Fishman RA. Cerebrospinal fluid in diseases of the nervous system. Philadelphia: WB Saunders, 1980.
65. Collins J. A practical approach to the diagnosis of metabolic disease in the neonate. Dev Med Child Neurol 1990;32:79.
66. Aicardi J, Goutieres F. Encephalopathie myoclonique neonatale. Rev Electroencephalogr Neurophysiol Clin 1978;8:99.
67. Dalla Bernardina B, Dulac O, Fejerman N, Dravet C, Capovilla G, Roger J. Early myoclonic epileptic encephalopathy (EMEE). Eur J Pediatr 1983;140:248.
68. Aicardi J. Early myoclonic encephalopathy. In: Roger J, Dravet C, Bureau M, Dreifuss FE, Wolf P, eds. Epileptic syndromes in infancy, childhood and adolescence. London: John Libbey Eurotex, 1985:12.
69. Dalla Bernardina B, Colamaria V, Capovilla G, Bondavalli S. Nosological classification of epilepsies in the first three years of life. In: Nistico G, Di Perri R, Meinardi H, eds. An update on research and therapy. New York: Alan R Liss, 1983:165.
70. Aicardi J. Epilepsy in children. New York: Raven Press, 1986:165.
71. Lombroso CT. Early myoclonic encephalopathy, early infantile epileptic encephalopathy, and benign and severe infantile myoclonic epilepsies: a critical review and personal contribution. J Clin Neurophysiol 1990;7:380.
72. Ohtahara S, Ishida T, Oka E. On the specific age dependent epileptic syndrome. The early infantile epileptic encephalopathy with suppression-burst. No To Hattatsu 1976;8:270.
73. Flannery DB, Hsia YE, Wolf B. Current status of hyperammonemic syndromes. Hepatology 1982;2:495.
74. Delong GR. Reye's syndrome. In: Dickerman JD, Lucey JF, eds. Smith's the critically ill child: diagnosis and medical management. Philadelphia: WB Saunders, 1985:173.
75. Batshaw ML. Hyperammonemia. Curr Probl Pediatr 1984;14:1.
76. Meyers CC, Schochet SS, McCormick WF. Wernicke's encephalopathy in infancy: development during parenteral nutrition. Acta Neuropathologica 1978;43:267.
77. Jagadha V, Deck JHN, Halliday WC, Smyth HS. Wernicke's encephalopathy in patients on peritoneal dialysis or hemodialysis. Ann Neurol 1987;21:78.
78. Seear MD, Norman MG. Two cases of Wernicke's encephalopathy in children: an undiagnosed complication of poor nutrition. Annals of Neurology 1988;24:85.
79. Pihko H, Saarinen U, Paetau A. Wernicke encephalopathy: a preventable cause of death. Report of 2 children with malignant disease. Pediatr Neurol 1989;5:237.
80. Keating JP, Feigin RD. Increased intracranial pressure associated with probable vitamin A deficiency in cystic fibrosis. Pediatrics 1970; 46:41.
81. Rosenbloom AL, Riley WJ, Weber FT, Malone JI, Donelly WH. Cerebral edema complicating diabetic ketoacidosis in childhood. J Pediatr 1980;96:357.
82. Krane EJ, Rockoff MA, Wallman JK, Wolfsdorf JI. Subclinical brain swelling in children during treatment of diabetic ketoacidosis. N Engl J Med 1985;312:1147.
83. Greene SA, Jefferson IG, Baum JD. Cerebral oedema complicating diabetic ketoacidosis. Dev Med Child Neurol 1990;32:633.
84. Vernon DD, Postellon DC. Nonketotic hyperosmolar diabetic coma in a child: management with low dose insulin infusion and intracranial pressure monitoring. Pediatrics 1986;77:770.
85. Koh THHG, Aynsley-Green A, Tarbit M, Eyre JA. Neural dysfunction during hypoglycaemia. Arch Dis Child 1988;63:1353.
86. Foley CM, Polinsky MS, Gruskin AB, Baluarte HJ, Grover WD. Encephalopathy in infants and children with chronic renal disease. Arch Neurol 1981;38:656.
87. Rotundo A, Nevins TE, Lipton M, Lockman LA, Mauer SM, Michael AF. Progressive encephalopathy in children with chronic renal failure. Kidney Int 1982;21:486.
88. Gross MLP, Sweny P, Pearson RM, Kennedy J, Fernando ON, Moorhead JF. Rejection encephalopathy: an acute neurological syndrome complicating renal transplantation. J Neurol Sci 1982;56:23.
89. Berden JHM, Hoitsma AJ, Merx JL, Keyser A. Severe central nervous system toxicity associated with cyclosporin. Lancet 1985;1:219.
90. Young GB, Bolton CF, Austin TW, et al. The electroencephalogram in sepsis-associated encephalopathy. J Clin Neurophysiol 1992;9:145.
91. Freund H, Atamian S, Holroyde J, et al. Plasma amino acids as predictors of the severity and outcome of sepsis. Ann Surg 1979;190:571.
92. Jeppson B, Freund HR, Gimmon Z, et al. Blood-brain barrier dysfunction in sepsis: cause of septic encephalopathy? Am J Surg 1981;141:136.
93. Auer RN. Progress review: hypoglycemic brain damage. Stroke 1986;17:699.
94. Auer RN, Olsson Y, Siesjo BK. Hypoglycemic brain injury in the rat. Correlation of density of braindamage with EEG isoelectric time: a quantitative study. Diabetes 1984;33:1090.
95. Haworth JC, McRae KN. The neurological and developmental effects of neonatal hypoglycemia: a follow-up of 22 cases. Can Med Assoc J 1965;92:861.
96. Banker BQ. The neuropathological effects of anoxia and hypoglycemia in the newborn. Dev Med Child Neurol 1967;9:544.
97. Anderson JM, Milner RDG, Strich JJ. Effects of neonatal hypoglycemia on the nervous system: a pathological study. JNNP 1967;30:295.
98. Jones EL, Smith WT. Hypoglycemic brain damage in the neonatal rat. In: Brierley JB, Meldrum BS, eds. Brain hypoxia. London: William Heinemann Medical Books, 1971:231.
99. Eisenberg S, Seltzer HS. The cerebral metabolic effects of acutely induced hypoglycemia in human subjects. Metabolism 1962;11:1162.
100. Sieber FE, Derrer SA, Saudek CD, Traystmann RJ. Effect of hypoglycemia on cerebral metabolism and carbon dioxide responsivity. Am J Physiol 1989;256:H697.
101. Tews JK, Carter SH, Stone WE. Chemical changes in the brain during insulin hypoglycemia and recovery. J Neurochem 1965;12:679.
102. Lewis LD, Ljunggren B, Norberg K, Siesjo BK. Changes in carbohydrate substrates, amino acids and ammonia in the brain during insulin-induced hypoglycemia. J Neurochem 1974;23:659.
103. Norberg K, Siesjo BK. Oxidative metabolism of the cerebral cortex of the rat in severe insulin induced hypoglycemia. J Neurochem 1976;26:345.
104. Agardh C-D, Folbergrova J, Siesjo BK. Cerebral metabolic changes in profound insulin-induced hypoglycemia, and in the recovery period following glucose administration. J Neurochem 1978;31:1135.
105. Wieloch T, Harris RJ, Symon L, Siesjo BK. Influence of severe hypoglycemia on brain extracellular calcium and potassium activities, energy and phospholipid metabolism. J Neurochem 1984;43:160.
106. Pelligrino D, Siesjo BK. Regulation of extra- and intracellular pH in the brain in severe hypoglycemia. J Cereb Blood Flow Metab 1981;1:85.
107. Pelligrino D, Almquist L-O, Siesjo BK. Effects of insulin-induced hypoglycemia on intracellular pH and impedance in the cerebral cortex of the rat. Brain Res 1981;221:129.
108. Siesjo BK. Cell damage in the brain: a speculative synthesis. J Cereb Blood Flow Metab 1981;1:155.
109. Kety SS, Woodford RB, Harmel MH, Freyhan FA, Appel KE, Schmidt CF. Cerebral blood flow and metabolism in schizophrenia. The effect of barbiturate semi-narcosis, insulin coma and electroshock. Am J Psychiatry 1948;104:765.
110. Pappenheimer JR, Setchell BP. Cerebral glucose transport and oxygen consumption in sheep and rabbits. J Physiol 1973;233:529.
111. Agardh C-D, Chapman AG, Nilsson B, Siesjo BK. Endogenous substrates utilized by the rat brain in severe insulin-induced hypoglycemia. J Neurochem 1981;36:490.
112. Ghajar JBG, Plum F, Duffy TE. Cerebral oxidative metabolism and blood flow during acute hypoglycemia and recovery in unanesthetised rats. J Neurochem 1982;38:397.
113. Ljunggren B, Schutz H, Siesjo BK. Changes in energy state and acid-base parameters of the rat brain during complete compression ischemia. Brain Res 1974;73:277.
114. Pelligrino D, Yokoyama H, Ingvar M, Siesjo BK. Moderate arterial hypotension reduces cerebral cortical blood flow and enhances cellular release of potassium in severe hypoglycemia. Acta Physiol Scand 1982;115:511.
115. Auer RN, Hall P, Ingvar M, Siesjo BK. Hypotension as a complication of hypoglycemia leads to enhanced energy failure but no increase in neuronal necrosis. Stroke 1986;17:442.
116. Gorell JM, Dolkhart PH, Ferrendelli JA. Regional levels of glucose, amino acids, high energy phosphates, and cyclic nucleotides in the central nervous system during hypoglycemic stupor and behavioural recovery. J Neurochem 1976;27:1043.
117. Agardh C-D, Kalimo H, Olsson Y, Siesjo BK. Hyoglycemic brain injury. I. Metabolic and light microscopic findings in rat cerebral cortex during profound insulin-induced hypoglycemia and in the recovery period following glucose administration. Acta Neuropathol (Berl) 1980;50:31.
118. Behar KI, den Hollander JA, Petroff OAC, Hetherington HP, Prichard JW, Shulman RG. Effect of hypoglycemic encephalopathy upon amino acids, high energy phosphates, and pH_i in the rat brain in vivo. Detection by sequential ^{1}H and ^{31}P NMR spectroscopy. J Neurochem 1985;44:1045.

119. Sandberg M, Nystrom B, Hamberger A. Metabolically derived aspartate-elevated extracellular levels in vivo in iodoacetate poisoning. J Neurosci Res 1985;13:489.
120. Sandberg M, Butcher SP, Hagberg H. Extracellular overflow of neuroactive aminoacids during severe insulin-induced hypoglycemia: in vivo dialysis of the rat hippocampus. J Neurochem 1986;47:178.
121. Engelsen B, Fonnum F. Effects of hypoglycemia on the transmitter pool and the metabolic pool of glutamate in rat brain. Neurosci Lett 1983;42:317.
122. Engelsen B, Westerberg E, Fonnum F, Wieloch T. Effect of insulin-induced hypoglycemia on the concentrations of glutamate and related aminoacids and energy metabolism in the intact and decorticated rat neostriatum. J Neurochem 1986;47:1634.
123. Monyer H, Goldberg MP, Choi DW. Glucose deprivation neuronal injury in cortical culture. Brain Res 1989;483:347.
124. Tasker RC, Coyle JT, Vornov JJ. The regional vulnerability to hypoglycemia-induced neurotoxicity in organotypic hippocampal culture: protection by early TTX or delayed MK-801. J Neurosci 1992;12:4298.
125. Wieloch T. Hypoglycemia-induced neuronal damage prevented by *N*-methyl-D-aspartate antagonist. Science 1985;230:681.
126. Voorhies TM, Ehrlich ME, Duffy TE, Petito CK, Plum F. Acute hyperammonemia in the young primate: physiologic and neuropathologic correlates. Pediatr Res 1983;17:970.
127. Barzilay Z, Britten AG, Koehler RC, Dean JM, Rogers MC, Traystman RJ. Cerebral metabolic and vascular response to changes in P_aCO_2 with acute hyperammonemia. Crit Care Med 1984;12:217.
128. Barzilay Z, Britten AG, Koehler RC, Dean JM, Rogers MC, Traystman RJ. Cerebral hemodynamic and metabolic responses to changes in P_aCO_2 with continuous sodium acetate infusion. Crit Care Med 1984;12:226.
129. Barzilay Z, Britten AG, Koehler RC, Dean JM, Rogers MC, Traystman RJ. Cerebral hemodynamic and metabolic effects of acute hyperammonemia in dogs. Crit Care Med 1984;12:254.
130. Barzilay Z, Britten AG, Koehler RC, Dean JM, Traystman RJ. Interaction of CO_2 and ammonia on cerebral blood flow and O_2 consumption in dogs. Am J Physiol 1985;248:H500.
131. Zimmermann A, Bachmann C, Colombo JP. Ultrastructural pathology in congenital defect of the urea cycle: ornithine transcarbamylase and carbamyl-phosphate synthetase deficiency. Virchows Arch [A] 1981;393:321.
132. Benjamin AM. Ammonia. In: Lajtha A, ed. Handbook of neurochemistry. 2nd ed. Vol 1: Chemical and cellular architecture. New York: Plenum, 1982:117.
133. Wicklas WJ. Amino acid metabolism in the central nervous system: role of glutamate dehydrogenase. Adv Neurol 1984;41:245.
134. Batshaw ML, Brusilow S, Waber L, et al. Treatment of inborn errors of urea synthesis. Activation of alternative pathways of waste nitrogen systems and excretion. N Engl J Med 1982;306:1387.
135. Mans A, Biebuyk J, Hawkins R. Brain tryptophan abnormalities in hyperammonemia and liver disease. In: Bieder DA, Joseph MH, Kochen W, Steinhart H, eds. Progress in tryptophan and serotonin research. Berlin: Walter de Guyter, 1987:207.
136. Lockwood AH. Hepatic encephalopathy: experimental approaches to human metabolic encephalopathy. CRC Crit Rev Neurobiol 1987;3:105.
137. Raabe ME, Gumnit JJ. Disinhibition in cat motor cortex by ammonia. J Neurophysiol 1975;38:347.
138. McCandless DW, Schenker S. Effects of Acute ammonia intoxication on energy stores in the reticular activating system. Exp Brain Res 1981;44:325.
139. Jones EA, Schafer DF, Ferenci P, Pappas SC. The neurobiology of hepatic encephalopathy. Hepatology 1984;4:1235.
140. Zieve L. The mechanism of hepatic coma. Hepatology 1981;1:360.
141. Windus-Podehl G, Lyftogt C, Zieve L, et al. Encephalopathic effect of phenol in rats. J Lab Clin Med 1983;101:586.
142. Fischer JE, Baldessarini RJ. False neurotransmitters and hepatic failure. Lancet 1971;2:75.
143. Fischer JE, Baldessarini RJ. Pathogenesis and therapy of hepatic coma. Prog Liver Dis 1976;V:363.
144. James JH, Ziparo V, Jeppsson B, et al. Hyperammonemia, plasma aminoacid imbalance and blood-brain aminoacid transport: a unified theory of portal-systemic encephalopathy. Lancet 1979;2:772.
145. Roberts E. The γ-aminobutyric acid (GABA) system and hepatic encephalopathy. Hepatology 1984;4:342.
146. Ferenci P, Pappas SC, Munson PJ, et al. Changes in the status of neurotransmitter receptors in a rabbit model of hepatic encephalopathy. Hepatology 1984;4:186.
147. Schafer DE, Fowler JM, Munson PJ, et al. γ-Aminobutyric acid and benzodiazepine receptors in animal model of fulminant hepatic failure. J Lab Clin Med 1983;102:870.
148. Ferenci P, Pappas SC, Munson PJ, et al. Changes in glutamate receptors on systemic membranes associated with hepatic encephalopathy or hyperammonemia in the rabbit. Hepatology 1984;4:25.
149. Schafer DE, Jones EA. Hepatic encephalopathy and the γ-aminobutyric acid neurotransmitter system. Lancet 1982;1:18.
150. Butterworth RF, Giguere J-F, Fournier H, Bergeron M. Aminoacid neurotransmitter function in portal-systemic encephalopathy. J Cereb Blood Flow Metab 1987;7:S385.
151. Butterworth RF, Layrargues GP, eds. Hepatic encephalopathy, pathophysiology and treatment. Clifton, New Jersey: Humana Press, 1989.
152. Rothstein JP, McKhann G, Guarneri P, et al. Cerebrospinal fluid content of diazepam binding inhibitor in chronic hepatic encephalopathy. Ann Neurol 1989;26:57.
153. Mullen KD, Szauter KM, Kaminsky-Russ K. "Endogenous" benzodiazepine activity in body fluids of patients with hepatic encephalopathy. Lancet 1990;336:81.
154. Vander Ritt CCD, Schalm SW, Meulstee J, Stijren TH. Flumazenil therapy for hepatic encephalopathy: a double blind cross-over study. Hepatology 1989;10:590.
155. Blisard KS, Davis LE. Neuropathologic findings in Reye syndrome. J Child Neurol 1991;6:41.
156. Adams RD, Foley JM. The neurologic disorder associated with liver disease. Assoc Res Nerv Ment Dis Proc 1953;32:198.
157. Reeves AG, Posner JB. The ciliospinal response in man. Neurology 1969;19:1145.
158. Plum F, Posner JB. The diagnosis of stupor and coma. 3rd ed. Philadelphia: FA Davis, 1980.
159. Teasdale G, Jennett B. Assessment of coma and impaired consciousness. A practical scale. Lancet 1974;2:81.
160. Simpson DA, Reilly PL. Pediatric coma scale [letter]. Lancet 1982;2:450.
161. Morray JP, Tyler DC, Jones TK, Stuntz JT, Lemire RJ. Coma scale for use in brain-injured children. Crit Care Med 1984;12:1018.
162. Reilly PL, Simpson DA, Sprod R, Thomas L. Assessing the conscious level in infants and young children: a paediatric version of the Glasgow coma scale. Childs Nerv Syst 1988;4:30.
163. Lovejoy FH, Smith AL, Bresnan MJ, et al. Clinical staging in Reye syndrome. Am J Dis Child 1974;128:36.
164. National Institutes of Health Consensus Conference on Reye's syndrome. Diagnosis and treatment of Reye's syndrome. JAMA 1981;246:2441.
165. Duncan CC, Ment LR, Shaywitz BA. Evaluation of level of consciousness by the Glasgow coma scale in children with Reye's syndrome. Neurosurgery 1983;13:650.
166. Gordon NS, Fois A, Jacobi G, Minns RA, Seshia SS. The management of the comatose child. Neuropediatrics 1983;14:3.
167. Sinclair JF, Skeoch CH, Hallworth D. Prognosis of meningococcal septicaemia [letter]. Lancet 1987;2:862.
168. Markand ON. Electroencephalography in diffuse encephalopathies. J Clin Neurophysiol 1984;1:357.
169. Boyd SG, Harden A. Clinical neurophysiology of the central nervous system. In: Brett EM, ed. Paediatric neurology. 2nd ed. New York: Churchill Livingstone, 1991:717.
170. Aoki Y, Lombroso CT. Prognostic value of electroencephalography in Reye's syndrome. Neurology 1973;23:333.
171. Tasker RC, Boyd S, Harden A, Matthew DJ. Monitoring in non-traumatic coma II: electroencephalography. Arch Dis Child 1988;63:895.
172. Kendall B, Wilson J. Neuroradiology. In: Gordon I, ed. Diagnostic imaging in paediatrics. London: Chapman & Hill, 1987:259.
173. Tasker RC, Matthew DJ, Kendall B. Computed tomography in the assessment of raised intracranial pressure in non-traumatic coma. Neuropediatrics 1990;21:91.
174. Auld KL, Ashwal S, Holshouser BA, et al. Proton magnetic resonance spectroscopy in children with acute central nervous system injury. Pediatr Neurol 1995;12:323.
175. Donn SM, Swartz RD, Thoene JG. A comparison of exchange transfusion, peritoneal dialysis and hemodialysis for the treatment of hyperammonemia in the anuric newborn infant. J Pediatr 1979;95:67.
176. Wiegand C, Thompson T, Bock GH, Mathis RK, Kjellstrand CM, Mauer SM. The management of life-threatening hyperammonemia: a comparison of several therapeutic modalities. J Pediatr 1980;96:142.

177. Thompson GN, Butt WW, Shann FA, et al. Continuous venovenous hemofiltration in the management of acute decompensation in inborn errors of metabolism. J Pediatr 1991;118:879.
178. Reeves JH, Butt WB, Sathe AS. A review of venovenous haemofiltration in seriously ill infants. J Pediatr Child Health 1994;30:50.
179. Berman W, Pizzi F, Schut L, et al. The effects of exchange transfusion on intracranial pressure in patients with Reye's syndrome. J Pediatr 1975;87:887.
180. Huttenlocher PR. Reye's syndrome: relation of outcome to therapy. J Pediatr 1972;80:845.
181. Schubert WK, Partin JC, Bobo R, Partin JS. Exchange transfusion in Reye's syndrome. In: Pollock JD, ed. Reye's syndrome. New York: Grune & Stratton, 1975:301.
182. Bobo RC, Schubert WK, Partin JC, Partin JS. Reye syndrome: treatment by exchange transfusion with special reference to the 1974 epidemic in Cincinnati, Ohio. J Pediatr 1975;87:881.
183. Gazzard BG, Weston MJ, Murray-Lyon IM, et al. Charcoal hemoperfusion in the treatment of fulminant hepatic failure. Lancet 1974;1:1301.
184. Engle WD, Jacobs JF, Swartz RD, et al. Severe coagulopathy complicating charcoal hemoperfusion in children with Reye syndrome. J Pediatr 1978;93:972.
185. Talmage EA, Thomas JM, Weeks JH. Total body washout for Reye's syndrome. Anesth Analg 1973;52:563.
186. Lansky LL, Fixley M, Romig DA, et al. Hypothermic total-body washout with survival in Reye's syndrome. Lancet 1974;2:1019.
187. Klebanoff G, Hollander D, Cosmi AB, et al. Asanguinous hypothermia total body perfusion (TBW) in the treatment of stage IV hepatic coma. J Surg Res 1972;12:1.
188. Mahoney MJ. Organic acidemias. Clin Perinatol 1976;3(Suppl 1):61.
189. Batshaw ML, Brusilow S, Waber, et al. Treatment of inborn errors of urea synthesis: activation of alternative pathways of waste nitrogen synthesis and excretion. N Engl J Med 1982;306:1387.
190. Brusilow SW. Arginine, an indispensible amino acid for patients with inborn errors of urea synthesis. J Clin Invest 1984;74:2144.
191. Brusilow SW. Urea cycle enzymes. In: Scriver CR, Beaudet AL, Sly WS, Valle D, eds. The metabolic basis of inherited disease 6th ed. New York: McGraw-Hill, 1989;629.
192. Msall M, Batshaw ML, Suss R, et al. Neurologic outcome in children with inborn errors of urea synthesis: outcome of urea-cycle enzymopathies. N Engl J Med 1984;310:1500.

Head and Spinal Cord Injury 24

Elizabeth M. Allen
Richard Boyer
W. Bruce Cherny
Douglas Brockmeyer
Vera Fan Tait

INTRODUCTION

Head injury is one of the major causes of morbidity and mortality in children today. Trauma is the leading cause of death in children older than 1 year of age in the United States. Most of these trauma deaths are from head injury[1–4]. Injuries lead to more days of hospital care than any disease, cause the highest proportion of discharges to long-term care facilities, and result in the highest proportion of children requiring home health care after being discharged from the hospital[5]. It is obvious that the emotional, psychological, and economic cost of childhood head injury is staggering.

Approximately 5% of pediatric deaths from head injury occur at the site of the accident, underscoring the importance of safety issues and accident prevention[6]. To decrease the mortality and the morbidity of the remaining 95% of head-injured children, intense research has focused on the pathophysiologic features and therapeutic modalities in these children. Few areas in medicine have undergone such a radical change in the past several years. The focus of head injury management has shifted from maintaining a normal intracranial pressure (ICP) to optimizing cerebral perfusion and matching it with cerebral metabolic needs. Recognition of potential regional differences in oxygen delivery and utilization in the injured brain is increasing. Newer technology to measure these parameters more closely in a noninvasive, clinically feasible fashion are being investigated. Therapeutic modalities that have been conventionally considered to be standard of care are being reconsidered, and new modalities are being evaluated. Differences between the adult and pediatric populations are being refined. The impact of all these changes on the eventual outcome of this large population of critically ill children remains to be seen.

EPIDEMIOLOGY

Incidence

Each year an estimated 600,000 children are hospitalized because of injuries, and almost 16 million more are treated in emergency departments[1]. The overall incidence of head injury in the pediatric population is estimated to be approximately 200 per 100,000; this includes all head injury resulting in hospitalization or death or both[6]. In more than half of children, head injuries are classified as mild using the Glasgow Coma Scale; 8% are moderate, and 6% are severe[6]. Because pediatric intensive care units are unlikely to care for children with minor head injuries, they participate in the care of only a small proportion of the total number of head-injured children.

Approximately 7000 children (ages 0 to 19 years) died of head injury in 1985[6]. Based on death certificate information, the National Center for Health Statistics estimates that approximately 29% of pediatric trauma deaths are caused by head trauma[6,7]. However, this may be an underestimation of the problem. Case series from multiple trauma centers show that 75 to 97% of trauma deaths in children result from head injury, making it the leading cause of trauma death[2–4].

Gender, Age, and Seasonal Distribution

Boys are approximately twice as likely to become victims of head injury as are girls[2,6]. The rate of head injury is relatively stable throughout childhood, then increases at approximately 15 years of age for both genders[6]. The rate of increase during adolescence is more dramatic in boys than in girls (Fig. 24.1)[6]. This seems to coincide with their involvement in developmentally appropriate activities such as sports activities and driving. Unfortunately, a large increase

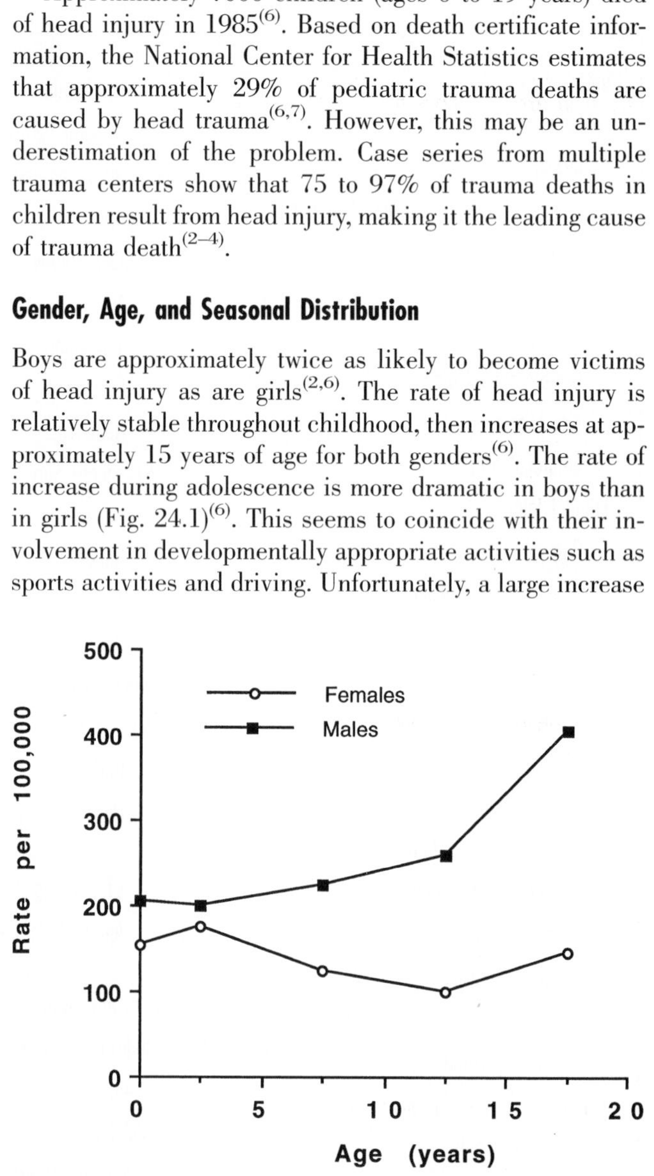

Figure 24.1. Age-specific brain injury rates per 100,000 by gender, San Diego County, California, 1981. Reprinted with permission from Kraus J, Rock A, Hemyari D. Brain injuries among infants, children, adolescents, and young adults. Am J Dis Child 1990;144:686. Copyright 1990, American Medical Association.

Table 24.1. Brain Injuries by Major Causes and Percentage Seriously Injured* According to Age Groups

		External Cause											
		Motor Vehicles		Falls		Assault		Recreation		Others		Total	
Age Group (yrs)	No. of Cases	No.	Serious (%)	No.	Serious (%)	No.	Serious (%)	No.	Serious (%)	No.	Serious (%)	No.	Serious (%)
<1	54	4	50	37	8	9	56	1	100	3	67	54	24
1–4	185	41	23	94	6	9	90	30	3	11	45	185	16
5–9	229	71	31	71	4	2	0	73	7	11	18	229	14
10–14	241	58	22	43	9	12	25	104	7	24	4	241	12
15–19	525	289	31	47	10	89	28	53	4	53	19	525	25

**Percentage seriously injured includes those patients with moderate, severe, or fatal brain injuries*
(Modified from Kraus J, Rock A, Hemyari P. Brain injuries among infants, children, adolescents, and young adults. Am J Dis Child 1990;144:687. Copyright 1990, American Medical Association.)

has occurred in the incidence of head injury from gunshot wounds in teenagers, especially in boys[8,9]. Some series have found another peak in the incidence of head injury in children younger than 1 year of age that is related to falls and nonaccidental abuse[10]. Most series show an increase in head injury during the spring and summer months, when children are outdoors more often[6,10].

Etiology

The major causes of head injury in children include motor vehicle crashes, falls, recreational activities, and assaults **(Table 24.1)**[6,10]. The percentage of injuries caused by each type of accident varies somewhat between studies and depends on the inclusion criteria. The cause of head injury also varies, depending on the age and gender of the child[6,10].

Motor vehicle crashes account for 27 to 37% of all pediatric head injuries **(Table 24.1)**[6,10]. The severity of brain injury is greater after motor vehicle crashes than after falls or recreational activities. In the most comprehensive pediatric study to date, 29% of all pediatric brain injury caused by motor vehicle crashes was classified as moderate, severe, or fatal[6]. In another multiinstitutional study, 70% of children with head and extracranial injuries who died were injured in a motor vehicle crash, whereas a motor vehicle crash was the cause of injury in 25% of patients with an isolated fatal head injury[2]. In most cases involving children younger than 15 years of age, the child is a pedestrian or a bicyclist and is not an occupant of the motor vehicle[7]. Pedestrian accidents are the second leading cause of death in children 5 to 9 years of age, surpassed only by cancer in this age group[1,7]. In teenagers, the victim is usually an occupant of the vehicle, and alcohol often is involved[7]. Properly used passenger restraints often are effective in preventing injury in children and adolescents, and it is hoped that airbags will further reduce the incidence of injury[7,10].

Falls account for 24% of all brain injuries requiring hospitalization **(Table 24.1)**[6,10]. Most falls result in mild brain injury[6]. However, in a multiinstitutional study that examined pediatric trauma deaths, falls are the cause of injury in 60% of the patients with fatal isolated head injury, and in 20% of children who had both head and extracranial injuries and died[2]. The highest incidence is found in children 4 years of age or younger[6]. Most of the falls that result in head injury, especially those involving small children, are from an elevation[6,11].

Recreational activities account for 21% of pediatric brain injuries **(Table 24.1)**[6]. Half of these injuries occur during a bicycle accident that does not include a motor vehicle[7].

The incidence of assault on children is difficult to ascertain, because the diagnosis of child abuse may be missed unless a high degree of suspicion and investigative vigilance are maintained. It has been estimated that assault is the cause of 10% of all childhood head injury **(Table 24.1)**[6]. Additionally, the severity of head injury caused by assault is greater than that from any other cause[6,12]. Child abuse is an important subcategory of assault that is more commonly seen in younger children[12,13]. In a recent series of 100 head-injured children younger than 2 years of age who were admitted to the hospital, abuse was diagnosed in 24% and suspected in another 32%[14].

Pediatric deaths caused by firearms, another assault-related subcategory, are increasing at an alarming rate[8,9]. Adolescent boys, especially blacks, account for most firearm fatalities among the pediatric population[1,9]. Gang involvement is related to this trend in some parts of the country[15]. The most common organ system injury leading to death in adolescents suffering from gunshot wounds is the central nervous system[8].

ANATOMY

The anatomy of the cranial vault renders the brain uniquely susceptible to injury. The brain itself is a semisolid structure without means of internal support. It is bathed and supported by a fluid medium, the cerebrospinal fluid (CSF). It is invested in a delicate membrane, the pia-arachnoid, and further enveloped by a tough membranous covering, the dura mater. The brain is enclosed in a rigid cranium that has irregular bony buttresses at the frontal poles in the anterior fossa and at the temporal poles in the middle fossa (Fig. 24.2). It is further compartmentalized into left and right hemispheres by the falx cerebri and into supratentorial and infratentorial compartments by the tentorium (Fig. 24.3). Each of these is a tough membranous structure with unyielding edges. The brainstem (the major conduit of the

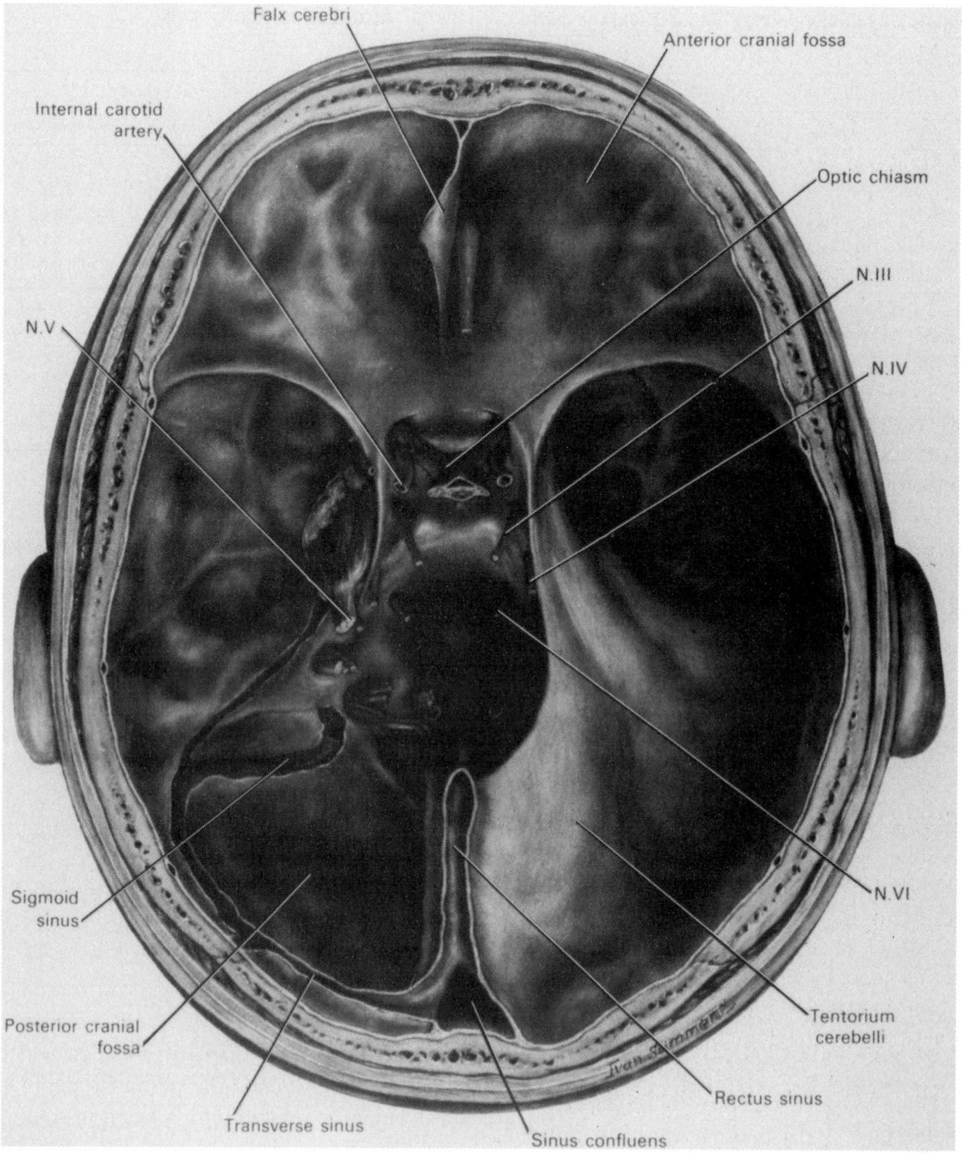

Figure 24.2. View of the base of the skull with dura mater. The falx cerebri and tentorium cerebeli have been removed to visualize the posterior cranial fossa. (Reprinted with permission from Mettler FA. Neuroanatomy. St Louis: CV Mosby, 1948:51.)

central nervous system) and the spinal cord traverse the only opening of the calvarium of significant size, the foramen magnum. At the moment of injury, the brain can be thrown against any of these bony irregularities and membranous slings, or it can be compressed against these surfaces because of intracranial volume shifts after the injury.

Blood is delivered to the brain by four vessels. The paired internal carotid arteries supply most of the supratentorial brain. The paired vertebral arteries supply most of the infratentorial brain. Branches of these vessels travel along the cerebral surface in the subarachnoid space until they enter the brain parenchyma, where they undergo significant arborization. Each branch supplies a specific portion of the brain without significant overlap from other vessels. This territorial arrangement of blood supply results in "watershed" regions of the brain, which occur at the interface of two or more vascular territories. The metabolic needs of the brain in these areas are met tenuously by the end vessels of two or more major vascular divisions. During periods of relative global hypoperfusion, these areas are most susceptible to ischemic injury.

Fine veins in the brain parenchyma drain blood into cerebral veins that pass through the subarachnoid space to empty into endothelial-lined sinuses of the dura mater. These venous sinuses eventually return blood to the internal jugular vein, which in turn empties into the right atrium through the superior vena cava.

PHYSIOLOGY

Cerebrospinal Fluid

The CSF plays an important role in maintaining brain homeostasis. CSF has multiple functions, including suspending and cushioning the intracranial contents and maintaining the internal milieu for the brain parenchyma. Normally, CSF flows from the primary site of formation, the choroid plexus of the lateral and fourth ventricles, through the foramina of Magendie and Luschka into the subarachnoid space. Once in the subarachnoid space, CSF circulates around the spinal cord and over the convexities of the brain. Further details of the production and absorption of CSF are provided in Chapter 18.

Blood-Brain Barrier

Under normal circumstances, a unique functional barrier exists between the intracerebral blood vessels and the brain parenchyma, so many substances cannot pass freely from the blood vessels into the parenchyma. This blood-brain barrier is formed by the tight junctions between capillary endothelial cells in the brain. Solute characteristics such as size, lipid solubility, and polarity affect the ability of substances to penetrate this blood-brain barrier. Active transport mechanisms exist that allow some substances to cross this barrier. Injury to the brain often damages the blood-brain barrier, and substances that are normally excluded from the brain parenchyma may enter.

Autoregulation

Because the brain has minimal ability to store energy, it depends on a constant supply of glucose and oxygen to meet its metabolic needs. Neurons are quickly damaged when this supply is interrupted. *Autoregulation* refers to the intrinsic mechanisms that match cerebral blood supply with brain metabolism. A detailed discussion of cerebral autoregulation is provided in Chapter 18. Pressure autoregulation refers to the ability of the brain to maintain a constant cerebral blood flow across a wide range of mean arterial pressures, so cerebral blood flow is typically independent of mean arterial pressure from approximately 50 to 150 mm Hg[16]. Beyond these blood pressure limits, autoregulation is lost, and cerebral blood flow becomes directly related to arterial pressure. Global and local injury also can disrupt pressure autoregulation, thus cerebral blood flow passively follows arterial pressure.

Various regional mediators exert control over local blood supply by modulating arteriolar tone and thereby resistance[17,18]. These vessels are also exceptionally responsive to changes in $PaCO_2$ and PaO_2. A change in $PaCO_2$ by 1 mm Hg leads to a 3 to 4% change in cerebral blood flow[19,20]. The cerebral vasculature is less sensitive to changes in PaO_2 until a PaO_2 of 50 mm Hg is reached; cerebral blood flow increases dramatically with increasing hypoxia below this level[21]. This autoregulatory system is less sensitive to disruption from injury compared with pressure autoregulation.

PRIMARY INJURY

Pathophysiology

In general, there are two phases of a head injury which ultimately impact on the outcome of the pediatric trauma victim. The primary injury is the damage sustained at the time

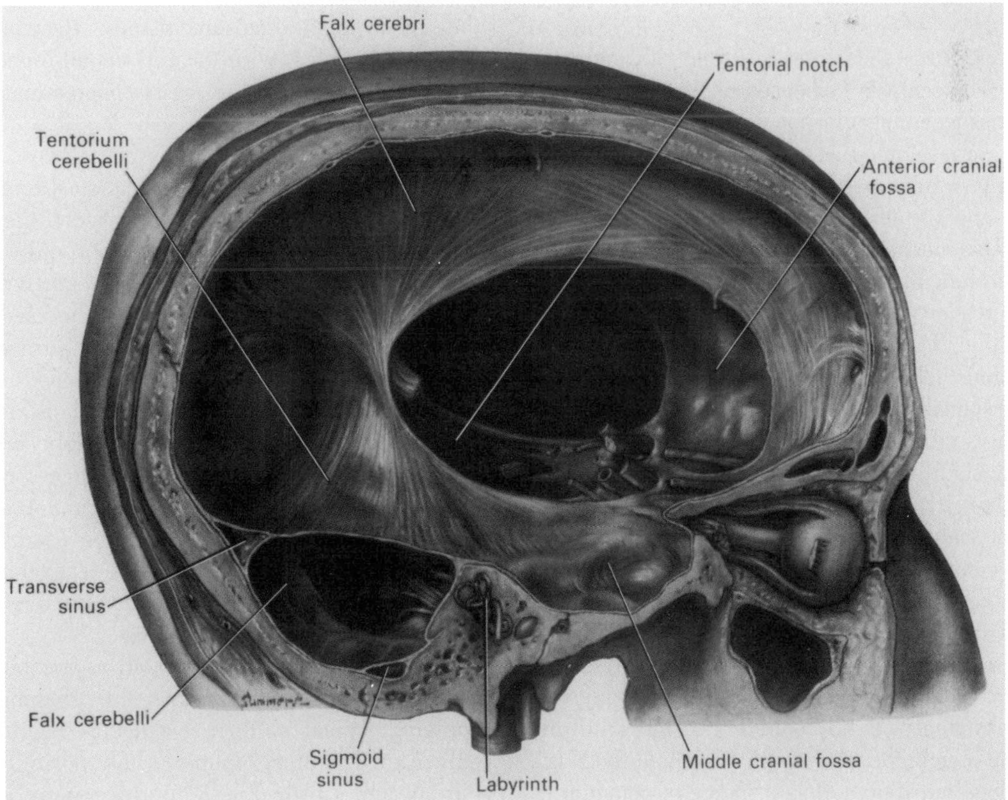

Figure 24.3. Parasagittal section of the head showing the falx cerebri, falx cerebelli, and tentorium cerebelli. (Reprinted with permission from Mettler FA. Neuroanatomy. St. Louis: CV Mosby, 1948:52.)

of impact. It is proportional to the magnitude and duration of the applied force, as well as the direction of the impact[22]. Two mechanisms are primarily involved. Direct injury of brain parenchyma occurs as it impacts on bony protuberances of the skull or dural surfaces, or from penetration of the brain parenchyma by bony fragments. Because of the compliant nature of a young child's skull, the mechanism of injury is usually direct impact of the deformed skull on the underlying brain, resulting in a coup lesion. In adults, the direct impact often causes the semiliquid brain to be compressed against the bony buttresses opposite the point of impact, resulting in a contrecoup lesion. Injury to vascular structures results in tearing of the vessels and intracranial hemorrhage.

The second mechanism of primary injury involves injury to the long white-matter tracts from stretching during an acceleration force. This shearing can lead to axonal disruption and eventual cell death. Animal studies show that the degree of this type of injury depends on the magnitude, direction, and duration of acceleration applied[22]. Axonal injury is correlated with an increased duration of the acceleration pulse[22].

Depending on the degree and type of impact, patients may experience a single type or a combination of primary injuries. Because this phase of injury occurs at the time of the accident, it is generally not amenable to medical intervention.

Specific Types of Primary Injury

Scalp Injuries

Scalp injuries often are seen in association with traumatic brain injuries. The scalp is composed of five layers: skin, subcutaneous tissue, a musculoaponeurotic layer, an areolar layer, and the periosteum. Each layer plays a role in the pathophysiologic characteristics of scalp injury and in considerations for appropriate treatment. The skin is the hair-bearing layer. This must be kept in mind when issues of cosmesis arise. The subcutaneous layer consists mainly of fat in the superficial portion and large blood vessels and nerves in the deeper portion. The musculoaponeurotic layer contains the galea, a fibrous helmet that covers the cranial vault. The galea is also responsible for most of the tensile strength of the scalp; being a very noncompliant structure, it stretches little. Thus any significant scalp closure must include this layer, but this layer may be the limiting factor when considering closure of scalp defects. The areolar layer is a potential space that contains the emissary veins. This layer gives rise to scalping injuries, in which large portions of the skull are denuded. This layer also gives rise to possible planes of infectious spread through the emissary veins as well as the accumulation of other materials, such as blood and serous fluid. The periosteum is tightly adherent to the skull and forms a limiting membrane between the skin and the skull. It is vital for bone nutrition and as a source of potential fibroblasts for secondary coverage of the denuding injury.

The scalp carries a rich blood supply that is interconnected by an extensive network of anastomoses. Blood loss from a laceration can be rapid and extensive enough to result in hypotension, shock, and even death, especially in infants and small children. Direct digital tamponade at the wound edges provides the best control for bleeding. This should not be performed if a laceration overlies a depressed skull fracture. In this case, pressure should be applied at the edge of the palpably intact cranial bone. Surgical clamps, such as hemostats, should not be placed on the skin except under extreme circumstances, because tissue damage and possible necrosis may occur. Most bleeding subsides with adequate pressure and sufficient time. A pressure dressing with a firm head wrap minimizes further blood loss until primary repair can be performed. Especially brisk bleeding can be controlled with a full-thickness figure-of-eight suture around the skin edge at the bleeding vessel or with surgical scalp clips. These methods are temporary until definitive debridement and repair can be performed.

When underlying skull and intracranial pathologic lesions have been ruled out, the treatment of scalp injuries is usually straightforward. Uncomplicated subgaleal hematomas and cephalohematomas are treated conservatively. Antibiotics rarely are needed. Simple lacerations are treated by using the usual general surgical techniques and principles. Adequate anesthesia is mandatory. Close inspection and digital probing are needed before the wound is closed, looking for evidence of foreign body or bony disruption indicating a fracture. A simple one-layer closure is most often used, but care must be taken to include the galea in the closure planes. Because of the rich vascular supply of the scalp, wound infection is rarely encountered. Even so, a grossly contaminated wound may warrant delayed closure.

Avulsion lacerations with tissue loss pose a slightly more difficult surgical problem. Defects smaller than 3 to 4 cm often can be closed primarily because of the compliance of the scalp. However, larger defects require some form of grafting. When the vascular periosteum has been left intact, a split-thickness skin graft can be used. Hair grafting can be undertaken later for cosmetic purposes. If the vascular periosteum is not intact or the blood supply is otherwise uncertain, various forms of skin flaps and pedicle flaps must be used. The same principles apply in cases of total scalp avulsion. Except in rare instances of microvascular reimplantation, the avulsed scalp cannot be replaced. If suitable, however, the scalp may be used as a donor for split-thickness skin grafting or tissue coverage. If the scalp is unsuitable and the periosteum remains normal, grafts from other donor sites may be used.

Burns of the scalp are treated as are burns elsewhere. First-degree burns may be treated by shaving the scalp and applying topical antibiotics such as bacitracin zinc and polymyxin B sulfate ointment (Polysporin) or sulfadiazine. Partial- and full-thickness injuries require grafting. Again, hair grafting may be undertaken later for cosmetic purposes.

Skull Fractures

Many children presenting for evaluation of head trauma have skull fractures[23,24]. The types of skull fractures include linear, comminuted, depressed, and diastatic. Ninety percent of the fractures found in these children are linear. The importance of the presence of a linear fracture is twofold. First, the force required to fracture a child's skull is significant. Therefore, the potential for underlying brain damage is more likely with fracture[25]. The other important feature of a skull fracture is related to its location. A fracture crossing the path of a known major vascular structure, such as the middle meningeal artery or large dural sinus, holds potential for significant intracranial bleeding and subsequent complications. Childhood fractures tend to be more diastatic than their adult counterparts. Thus their radiographic appearance may be more impressive. However, most are uncomplicated. Most children tend to be symptomatic, but observation is the treatment of a closed simple linear fracture that does not involve a major vascular structure. Children who are completely asymptomatic may be discharged to the home environment with a safe, reliable caregiver[24]. However, if significant neurologic signs or symptoms are found or if there are worrisome or significant radiographic findings, the patient should be admitted to the hospital for observation. This includes patients with protracted bouts of nausea and vomiting, a common occurrence after occipital or posterior fossa fractures. Most of these children recover without sequelae. One potential complication of skull fractures unique to the pediatric population is the so-called growing fracture or leptomeningeal cyst. Growing skull fractures consist of resorbing bone edges overlying a dural defect. Interposed between the bone and dural defect are leptomeninges or a porencephalic cyst lined with gliotic brain[26]. Leptomeningeal cysts occur more often in fractures involving the suture line. CSF pulsations and the active growth and resorption of the bone result in a persistently enlarging defect. Growing skull fractures sometimes resolve with age. However, surgical intervention may be necessary, and patients with such potential must be followed closely for at least 1 to 2 years.

If the linear fracture is associated with an overlying laceration, it is by definition an open fracture. Although this fracture is open with respect to the underlying bone, in addition, a potential opening to the central nervous system exists. Therefore, neurosurgical evaluation is mandatory to decide whether operative repair should be undertaken. CSF leaking from the wound or collecting under the scalp is obvious evidence of a dural laceration, and operative exploration is indicated. When managing these wounds, routine aseptic principles must be adhered to strictly. If surgical closure is not indicated, the wound should be copiously irrigated and meticulously debrided. The child should be admitted not only for a period of observation but also for antibiotic coverage, especially in the case of gross contamination of the wound. In these instances, the rate of infection is low, and the posttraumatic complications are few.

A depressed skull fracture is present when the inner table of the skull is displaced by more than one thickness of the entire bone. This type of fracture usually requires a greater amount of force and thus represents a more severe injury. The location of depressed skull fractures, in descending order of relative frequency, is the frontal, parietal, temporal, and occipital bones. Although plain skull radiographs are helpful, computed tomography (CT) scanning with appropriate bone windows is the best method of evaluating depressed skull fractures and clearly shows the location and degree of depression of the fracture. It also shows underlying cerebral trauma, giving clues to potential dural laceration or cortical laceration (Fig 24.4). Of all depressed fractures, one-third are simple, one-third are associated with dural laceration, and one-fourth are associated with cortical lacerations[27].

When the diagnosis of depressed skull fracture has been made and the lesion evaluated radiographically, no further probing or exploration of the wound nor any attempt at removal of bony fragments or foreign objects is justified in the emergency department. In such attempts, there is a great risk of removing a fragment that may be tamponading a torn or lacerated blood vessel. Also, further probing may push fracture fragments further into the brain.

Indications for surgical elevation of a depressed skull fracture are: 1) cerebral spinal fluid leak, 2) probable dural compromise, 3) the presence of focal neurologic deficits, 4) a depression in a cosmetically important area, or 5) a segment of depression greater than or equal to the thickness or table width of the skull in that region. Left unrepaired, depressed fractures with significant compression of the cerebral cortex are believed to be associated with an increased incidence of focal neurologic deficits or seizure development.

Open depressed skull fractures are still considered relative surgical emergencies primarily because of the risk of bacterial spread into the central nervous system. However, because of the vascular nature of the pediatric skull and scalp, even moderate contamination of bony fragments does not result in a prohibitive rate of infection. In most instances, the infection rate is lower than 5%. With modern broad-spectrum antibiotic therapy and prompt surgical care, chronic infections and osteomyelitis of the skull are rarely seen. The optimal choice of antibiotics and the length of antibiotic therapy for open depressed skull fractures is not concrete and is influenced by the extent of the wound contamination and the length of time from injury to surgical repair. In general, broad-spectrum antibiotic coverage should be used for at least 72 hours, but under special circumstances, it may be warranted for 10 to 14 days.

Definitive treatment of depressed skull fractures in the operating room consists of meticulous debridement of devitalized scalp, hair, or any contaminants, and copious irrigation. Wide surgical exposure is necessary, and the skin flap should completely expose the entire fracture area. A circumferential craniectomy is made at the edge of the fracture site, and all depressed fragments are elevated and re-

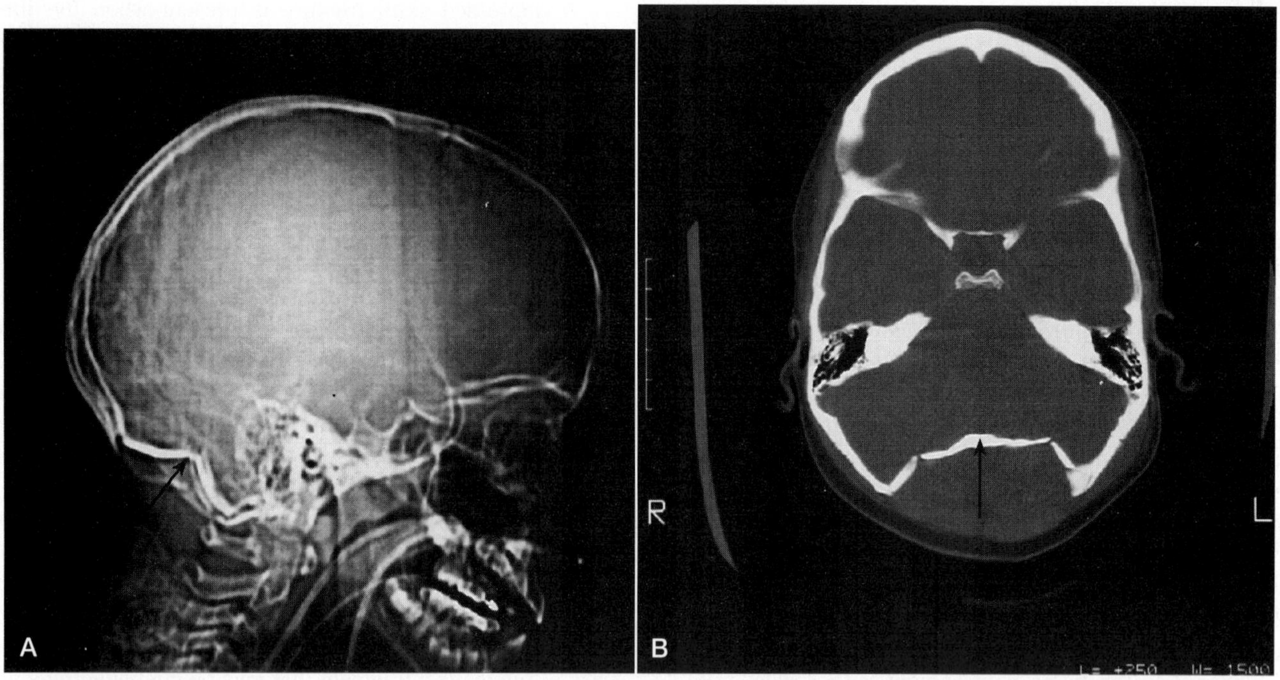

Figure 24.4. Depressed skull fracture. Lateral digital radiograph, or scanogram (A), and axial CT scan (B) through the posterior fossa in a child with a direct blow to the occiput show a markedly depressed occipital skull fracture (arrows). Brain-window images (not shown) showed intraventricular hemorrhage and acute hydrocephalus.

moved. The underlying dura is closely inspected for evidence of dural laceration or underlying subdural hematoma. Subdural hematoma or free fracture fragments driven into the brain warrant further exploration. In these cases, the dura is incised or the dural laceration is extended, yielding an adequate view of the underlying cortex. Any bleeding points are controlled, and any grossly devitalized cortical tissue is carefully debrided. Deeper penetration of the brain tissue with or without a foreign body may require further exploration. This occurs at the discretion of the surgeon, and the primary indication is for control of hemorrhage. In many instances, deep-seated foreign objects are not removed because of the risk of creating hemorrhage and the risk of further damage to the brain.

The dura is closed in a water-tight fashion, often with the aid of grafting or dural patches. Previously removed bone fragments should be cleansed and replaced. Neurologic outcome of depressed skull fractures relates directly to the extent of cortical injury.

Basilar Skull Fracture

Fractures of the base of the skull are common injuries in childhood. They are seen in 6 to 14% of children who sustain head injuries[28,29]. A tremendous force is required to fracture the base of the skull; thus a basilar skull fracture is not a trivial injury. However, in most instances, an uncomplicated basilar skull fracture has an excellent prognosis for recovery.

The diagnosis of basilar skull fracture is made from a combination of clinical and radiographic findings. A history of a blow sustained to the back of the head raises the suspicion of the possibility of the diagnosis. There may or may not be an associated loss of consciousness, seizures, or other manifestations of neurologic injury. On physical examination, certain findings are pathognomonic of basilar skull fracture. Battle's sign, which is retroauricular or mastoid ecchymosis without history or evidence of direct trauma to the area, is one such finding. Battle's sign represents a dissection of blood from the disrupted skull cortex in the occipital and mastoid regions. A laceration of the external auditory canal without history or evidence of trauma to the ear or canal indicates a fractured petrous bone. This may be further complicated by concomitant laceration or disruption of the facial and auditory nerves. Blood behind the tympanic membrane, imparting a bluish discoloration and often resulting in a bulging membrane, likewise indicates a deeper fracture of the petrous temporal bone and also may be associated with disruption of facial and auditory nerves. Periorbital ecchymosis without other evidence of trauma to the region, the so-called "raccoon eyes," also indicates basilar skull fracture. This results from the forward dissection of blood from the disrupted skull cortex into the soft areolar spaces of the periorbital regions. In most instances, one or a combination of these clinical findings leads to the diagnosis of basilar skull fracture.

Leaking of CSF from the ears or nose, CSF otorrhea or rhinorrhea, occurs secondary to disruption of the leptomeninges by a basilar skull fracture. Therefore, the presence of CSF otorrhea or rhinorrhea is another useful clinical indication that this type of fracture has occurred. CSF rhinorrhea develops within 48 hours of the injury in 60 to 70% of patients[30,31]. The differentiation between CSF rhinorrhea and the usual nasal discharge is classically made by testing the specimen on glucose oxidase test tapes. However, caution must be exercised, because these tapes are sometimes sensitive to the mucopolysaccharides in ordinary nasal discharge. Because the sinuses are not well pneumatized in the first decade, CSF rhinorrhea is rare during this time[32,33]. Similarly, CSF otorrhea is unusual before 5 years of age because of underdeveloped mastoid air cells.

Although the diagnosis of basilar skull fracture is often based on the aforementioned clinical signs, radiographic studies can be useful in evaluating these patients. Skull radiographs rarely identify a fracture, even in cases of clinically evident basilar skull fractures. However, a CT scan localizes the area of fracture, but perhaps more important, identifies associated brain injury (Fig. 24.5).

Patients with a basilar skull fracture are more prone to prolonged symptoms of nausea, vomiting, and general malaise than with other types of fractures, especially without other evidence for underlying brain injury. This may be partially because of the close proximity of the fracture to the emesis centers and vestibular centers of the brainstem. In general, the management of these patients involves close observation, intravenous hydration, pain control, and antiemetic agents. Because of the disruption of the cribiform plate, nasotracheal intubation and placement of nasogastric tubes are to be avoided in these patients; orotracheal and orogastric tubes should be placed instead. The course usually is uncomplicated, and an excellent recovery can be expected.

The most significant complication of basilar skull fractures is CSF leak. In 80% of patients, CSF rhinorrhea heals spontaneously within 1 week, and only a few of the remaining unresolved cases require surgical intervention[34,35]. As with CSF rhinorrhea, most CSF otorrhea resolves spontaneously[36]. Rarely, the CSF leak persists without resolution and requires surgical intervention. Keeping the head elevated with or without serial lumbar puncture may be sufficient to lower the CSF pressure and allow spontaneous resolution. In some instances, surgical repair is necessary. Before the surgical repair is undertaken, the area of leakage must be precisely identified. This has been done in the past by use of radionuclide cysternography. More recently, this technique has been coupled with high-resolution CT scanning.

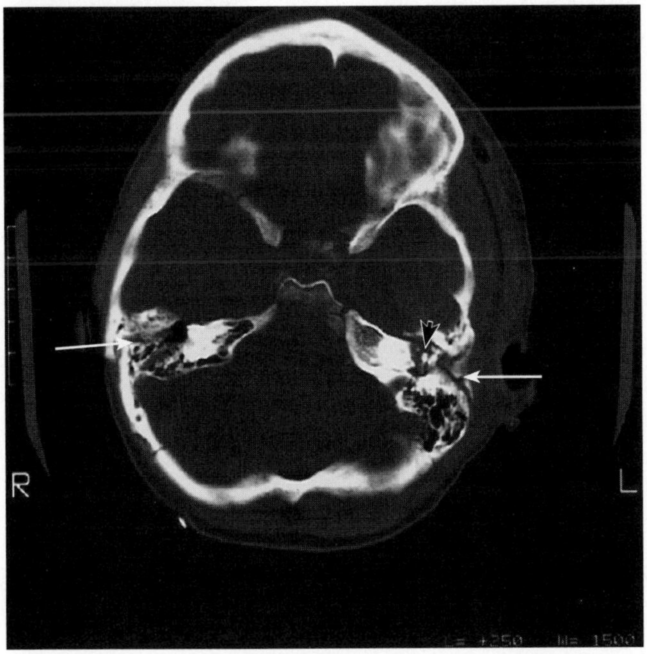

Figure 24.5. Basilar skull fracture. Head CT scan through the petrous temporal bones and skull base displayed in bone window in a child with severe closed head trauma shows a complex basilar skull fracture (arrows) extending in a coronal plane across the petrous portion of both temporal bones. Note that there is fluid opacification (blood or CSF) in the left middle ear cavity with dislocation of the ossicles (arrowhead).

Other major complications of basilar skull fracture are meningitis and cranial nerve injury. Meningitis occurs in 3 to 25% of patients with CSF rhinorrhea and in approximately 4.5% of patients with CSF otorrhea[30,36,37]. Prophylactic antibiotics are no longer believed to be indicated[35,37–39]. The injudicious use of prophylactic antibiotics may lead to a nosocomial infection with an agent resistant to antibiotics and thus much more difficult to treat[40]. Therefore, the trend has been to avoid antibiotics except in actual cases of meningitis or in special situations in which clinical judgment deems it necessary. Cranial nerve injury ensuing from the fractured bone also is a significant problem. Three to ten percent of patients are anosmic at the time of discharge, and this deficit tends to be permanent[41]. Ocular nerve palsy develops in 1 to 10% of patients. The order of decreasing frequency is sixth, third, and fourth cranial nerves[42]. Oculomotor nerve palsies rarely are complete, and 75% of patients make a full recovery[28,29,43]. Facial nerve palsies appear in 1 to 12% of patients with basilar skull fractures, and 90% can be expected to make a spontaneous recovery. Dizziness, tinnitus, and sensory hearing loss from eighth nerve injury may also occur. Complete sensorineural hearing loss occurs in approximately 1.5% of cases[41].

Concussion

Concussion is defined as "a transient loss of consciousness which occurs as the consequence of head trauma"[44]. The term *concussion* is descriptive and does not denote any specific anatomical or physiologic abnormalities.

Because the concussive injury is transient, patients often have a normal neurologic examination when examined by a physician. Therefore, the diagnosis of mild concussion is made primarily on a historical basis. The history differs in patients of varying age groups. In infants and very young children, the incidence of benign posttraumatic seizures is higher, but unconsciousness is uncommon. In this group, the history often uncovers a syndrome of delayed somnolence and vomiting[45]. This becomes less common as the child gets older. In older children more able to cooperate with a medical historian, posttraumatic amnesia is an important finding. In general, the length of posttraumatic amnesia is proportional to the severity of the injury[46]. Also in the older child, more waxing and waning of the level of consciousness occurs without attendant physical damage.

Obtaining a head CT scan is recommended in patients with loss of consciousness and concussion. In most cases of mild concussion, the studies are negative, although one study reported that 31% of patients with a score of 12 or more on the Glasgow Coma Scale had an abnormal CT scan(47). Even in the case of traumatic subarachnoid hemorrhage, one can expect an excellent recovery. The patient's neurologic function usually normalizes in approximately 1 week. However, for periods of months to even a year, the child may continue to have slight behavioral difficulties and some slowness in the acquisition of new knowledge(48,49). This may be associated with mild headaches. This is the postconcussive syndrome and can be expected to resolve completely without significant impact on outcome.

Contusion

A brain contusion is defined as an area of intraaxial posttraumatic bruising or microscopic hemorrhage. In the pediatric population, contusions are usually caused by direct injury to the head, with the focal energy being transferred to the underlying brain. Contusions also may occur when the brain strikes skull-base bony protuberances during rapid acceleration or deceleration. Brain contusion is often associated with other forms of brain injury. Normally, it is other concomitant injury that dictates the aggressiveness with which the patient is treated. However, the contusion itself has its own clinical consequences.

The clinical course typically seen is one of gradual neurologic deterioration caused by progressive local edema, infarction, or late-developing hematomas. Medical management to control increased ICP, as described later in this chapter, should be instituted if necessary. In some instances, the hemorrhage may extend, leading to a late-developing intracerebral hematoma. Surgical intervention may be indicated to relieve significant mass effect. Unless the course is complicated by other neurologic injury, the outcome can be expected to be favorable(50).

Epidural Hematoma

An epidural hematoma is a collection of blood occurring between the skull and the dura. Classically, it has been presumed that these lesions occur with a low frequency in childhood(51). The reason is that the dura is adherent to the inner table of a child's skull, especially at the suture lines. Yet in one series, 25% of all posttraumatic intracranial hematomas occurring in the 0- to 20-year-old age group were epidural(52).

The sequence of events leading to an epidural hematoma begins with a head injury of sufficient force to cause separation of dura from the underlying bone(53). As the epidural blood accumulates, the hematoma usually encounters a limiting border at a suture line, which it rarely crosses unless a concomitant skull fracture is present that disrupts the dural adherence at the suture. A high percentage of patients with epidural hematomas have overlying skull fractures(24). Depending on the location and vascular structures involved, the hemorrhage may be of arterial or venous origin. The arterial pressure may be of sufficient magnitude to allow further separation of the dura from the bone, resulting in an enlarging mass.

By history, the initial injury may seem minor, and the associated loss of consciousness may be brief or absent altogether(51). The classic "lucid interval" between initial loss of consciousness and subsequent rapid neurologic deterioration occurs in 50 to 60% of adult patients with epidural hematomas, but is much less common in pediatric patients. In 85% of infants, no altered mental status at the time of injury was noted(54).

If an epidural hematoma is not recognized promptly and properly treated, rapid deterioration may ensue. Initially, only focal pressure effects are seen. However, as the hematoma enlarges and as the compensatory mechanisms of the brain are exhausted, significant mass effect causes temporal lobe herniation and brainstem compression. These events are reflected in the sequential neurologic examination. The patient may be awake initially and complaining of headache associated with vomiting and nuchal rigidity. Contralateral hemiparesis may progress to unconsciousness with posturing and ipsilateral pupillary dilatation. Seizures are uncommon. Emergent CT scanning is mandatory. The epidural hematoma has a characteristic CT scan appearance as a localized, lenticular, high-density lesion with obvious mass effect (Fig. 24.6).

Although most epidural hematomas are treated with emergent craniotomy and clot evacuation, up to 20% of

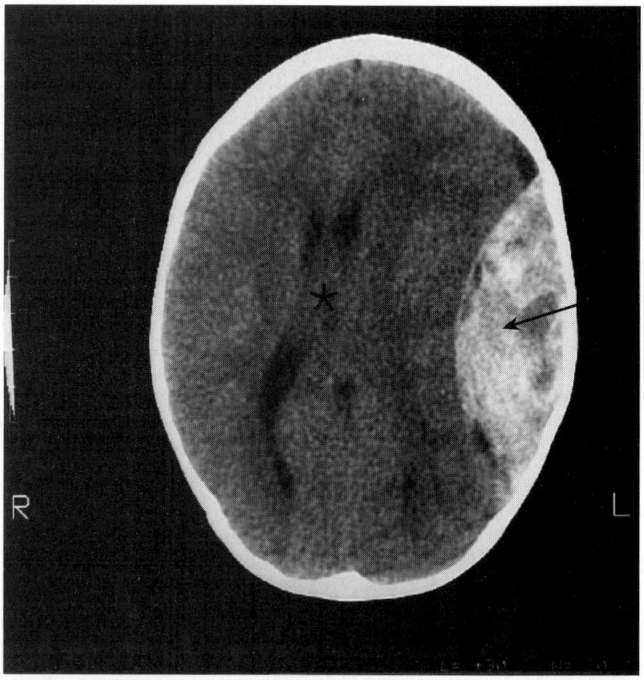

Figure 24.6. Epidural hematoma with subfalcine herniation. Head CT scan of a young child after head injury shows a large epidural hematoma (arrow) compressing the left cerebral hemisphere and shifting the midline to the right (asterisk). In this setting, the anterior cerebral artery on the side of the hematoma is compressed against the free margin of the falx, possibly leading to herniation.

them can be treated by conservative measures alone. Aggressive medical management of intracranial hypertension, using measures discussed later in this chapter, is important to stabilize the patient's rapidly deteriorating neurologic status while awaiting surgery. Burr-hole evacuation of clotted blood is technically difficult and usually unsuccessful, and should not be attempted in the emergency department. However, under extreme circumstances, burr holes may be of help as a diagnostic procedure in the absence of adequate radiologic evaluation[55].

Patients who are managed conservatively should be closely monitored, both clinically and radiographically. Surgical evacuation should be performed immediately if the patient becomes symptomatic or if the hematoma seems to be enlarging on CT scan. In general, epidural hematomas of arterial origin reach their peak size by 6 to 8 hours after the injury; those of venous origin may continue to grow for the first 24 hours and possibly longer. Epidural hematomas in the posterior fossa may grow silently and become symptomatic just before the patient's rapid deterioration and herniation. For this reason, there is generally a low threshold for surgical removal of these hematomas when they are diagnosed.

The results of the surgical evacuation and overall clinical outcome are directly related to the promptness of adequate medical care. The usual mortality is approximately 17%, although of these, approximately 66% are in a coma from associated brain injury[54,56]. With prompt intervention, mortality rates as low as 5% have been obtained, with 89% good recovery[57].

Subdural Hematoma

A subdural hematoma is a collection of blood located on the surface of the cortex beneath the dura. In most instances, there is associated cortical damage from lacerated vessels or direct cortical contusion[58]. This results in a much less favorable prognosis than that seen with epidural hematomas[59]. Subdural hematomas are usually classified as acute and chronic subdural hematomas.

Acute subdural hematomas are almost always traumatic. A great amount of force is required to cause this injury, and often the underlying cortical disruption is severe. Occasionally, subdural hematomas occur secondary to birth trauma. In this instance, changes are seen within 12 hours of life. The child is often listless and dyspneic, with a full fontanelle, anisocoria, and subhyaloid hemorrhages. Emergent CT scanning is mandatory in these patients.

Subdural hematomas arise from bleeding points on the surface of the brain. This may be from laceration or tearing of a bridging vein or cortical arteries, or from direct trauma imparted by the deformed skull. Subdural hematomas usually occur over the convexities of the brain, but can be found anywhere. Unlike epidural hematomas, hematomas in the subdural space are not limited by suture lines and may become holohemispheric.

The clinical presentation is that of an acutely head-injured child. The lucid intervals seen in patients with epidural hematoma are rarely seen in patients with subdural hematomas because they usually are associated with severe parenchymal injury. Rather, the child often presents with profound and progressive neurologic deterioration. The physical examination depends on the severity of the injury, the size of the hematoma, and the time since injury. Radiologic evaluation of a head-injured patient with subdural hematoma is performed by emergent CT scanning. The typical CT appearance of a subdural hematoma consists of a hyperdense crescentic mass located along the cerebral convexities (Fig. 24.7). Often, there is considerable mass effect from the hematoma, underlying contusion, and associated brain edema. In many cases, a significant amount of hemispheric edema already may be present.

The initial approach to the patient with a subdural hematoma is medical management of intracranial hypertension, using measures to be outlined later in this chapter and in Chapter 18. Large subdural hematomas should be surgically evacuated without delay. The hematoma is evacuated through an appropriately placed craniotomy, with control of hemorrhage, and possible resection of badly damaged brain. In some instances, the brain may be so swollen and tense that closure of the dura or replacement of the craniotomy defect is difficult or impossible. The outcome of children with subdural hematomas is less favorable than of those with epidural hematomas. This is primarily because of the frequent association of underlying brain injury. The eventual outcome seems to be strongly related to the initial presentation of the child.

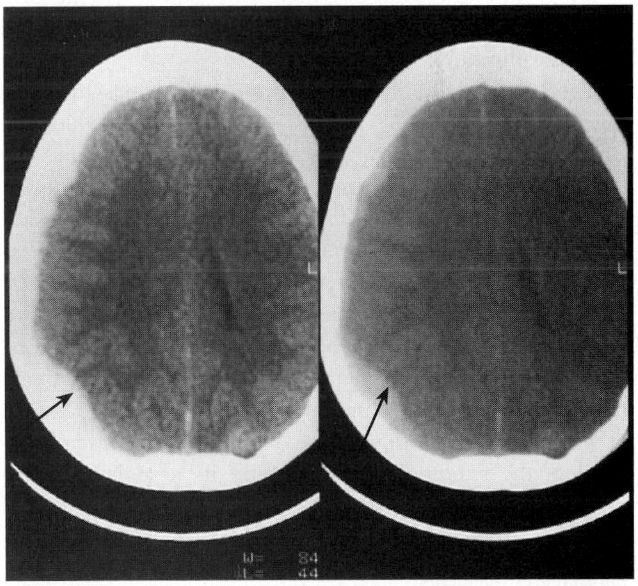

Figure 24.7. Subdural hematoma. Head CT scan at the level of the top of the lateral ventricles in a child with head injury shows a moderately large acute subdural hematoma (arrows) with mass effect on the adjacent hemisphere and effacement of the right lateral ventricle. Note that the blood is better seen in the right image, which is photographed at intermediate windows, because it can be distinguished from the adjacent calvarium. In the left image, photographed at brain windows, the blood blends with the high attenuation of the overlying calvarium and is more difficult to detect.

Chronic subdural hematomas occur from various sources. In many cases, the term "hematoma" is a misnomer, in that the fluid represents serous exudate and accumulation of blood breakdown products. Chronic subdural hematomas are rare in children older than 2 years of age, except in instances of intracranial shunt complications. The usual cause is trauma, although in many instances no history of trauma can be elicited. It is believed that the compliant nature of the infant's skull, with an open fontanelle and pliable sutures, allows the slow accommodation of the subdural fluid. Additionally, many subdural hematomas in this age group arise from long-standing cases of child abuse, and the patient may present a long time after the initial insult[60].

The clinical features of chronic subdural hematomas are characterized by seizures caused by cortical irritation from the fluid, and intracranial hypertension Thus the clinician sees a poorly thriving, irritable child with evidence of intracranial hypertension. Focal neurologic deficits are unusual. The occipital frontal circumference is enlarged, and the fontanelle is often tense. Retinal hemorrhages are seen in approximately 10% of the cases. A significant amount of force is required to produce retinal hemorrhages, and its association with subdural hematoma is almost pathognomonic for child abuse[61]. Very young infants may have associated anemia. However, this is usually on a nutritional basis. Evaluation may be by ultrasound or CT scanning. The typical CT findings are that of a hypodense collection located over the cerebral convexities in a crescentic shape. Mass effect and midline shift are unusual, but occasionally occur. In fact, the sulci are often widened, as are the CSF spaces. A subdural tap may be performed to determine the nature of the fluid.

The treatment of chronic subdural hematomas in childhood is controversial[62,63]. Considerations must include the liquid portion of the chronic subdural hematoma and the subdural membrane. Failure to remove the membrane results in reaccumulation of the subdural fluid. Bilateral subdural tapping alone is usually reserved for relief of intracranial hypertension. However, in many cases, subdural taps alone, singly or in series, result in permanent resolution of the subdural hematoma. In instances in which the taps alone fail, the placement of a subdural shunt effectively treats the subdural accumulation. Craniotomy for removal of membrane is not often required but is the definitive treatment of the subdural hematoma and its associated membrane.

Intracerebral Hematoma

An intracerebral hematoma is a solid clot of blood in the brain parenchyma. Intracerebral hematomas in children are an infrequent complication of head injury. Most arise as an extension or late development from cortical contusion. The prognosis of children with intracranial hematoma, especially those in deep locations, is poor because of the association of this problem with injury to the surrounding brain parenchyma. However, in some cases, isolated hematomas in polar locations do not cause significant neurologic deterioration. Indications for surgical evacuation of the hematoma include 1) easy accessibility, polar location, 2) progressive neurologic deterioration, and 3) intracranial hypertension intractable to medical therapy.

Penetrating Injury

Penetrating injuries occur from various sources. These injuries should be considered neurosurgical emergencies. The penetrating body or bodies should be left in place in the field or the emergency department, because its removal could result in further neurologic injury or uncontrollable hemorrhage. CT scanning and other studies such as angiography or magnetic resonance imaging (MRI), when appropriate, should be obtained as quickly as possible to guide the surgical approach. Such injuries require prophylactic antibiotics and possibly anticonvulsants if the cerebral cortex is involved.

Definitive treatment is surgical removal of all accessible foreign bodies and debridement of necrotic and grossly contaminated brain. Missile injuries from gunshot wounds, unfortunately a frequent occurrence in many parts of the country, are often especially severe. Patients presenting with a Glasgow Coma Score of 5 or lower after initial resuscitation, with an interhemispheric trajectory of the bullet, have an especially poor prognosis. Injuries to the dominant hemisphere also indicate a poor potential for recovery.

Intraventricular Hemorrhage

Most intraventricular hemorrhage from trauma is minor and resolves spontaneously. However, obstructive hydrocephalus may occur with larger hemorrhages, especially those located at the foramen of Monroe or the aqueduct of Sylvius. In these cases, the hydrocephalus may require external ventricular drainage. Large bilateral intraventricular hemorrhage may require a drain to be placed on each side. Posthemorrhagic hydrocephalus may occur secondary to a diminished capacity for normal CSF absorption. The mechanism is a proteinaceous obstruction of the arachnoid villi. Significant, symptomatic hydrocephalus requires shunting. Although the number is not precisely known, it is believed that only a small percentage of patients with intraventricular hemorrhage require a shunting procedure.

Subarachnoid Hemorrhage

Subarachnoid hemorrhage is the most common type of posttraumatic intracranial hemorrhage. Small blood vessels on the cerebral cortex are disrupted; this bleeding tends to occur on the outer cortical surface or along the falx cerebri or tentorium. Subarachnoid hemorrhage usually does not require specific treatment, but blood in the subarachnoid space is chemically irritating to the meninges, and patients may complain of headaches, nuchal rigidity, fever, restlessness, and nausea or vomiting. Supportive care with acetaminophen is often sufficient to alleviate minor symptoms. However, severe cases may require treatment with oral or intravenous corticosteroids. Subarachnoid hemorrhage, in and of itself, usually is not associated with significant neurologic sequelae and rarely causes posttraumatic hydrocephalus.

Diffuse Axonal Injury

Diffuse axonal injury is a disruption of small axonal pathways as a result of rapid cranial acceleration and deceleration. This injury often involves the deep hemispheric nuclei, the thalamus and basal ganglia, and the crossing white-matter tracts (corpus callosum), because their weight and angle of momentum are different from the rest of the cerebral cortex. Thus, shear forces tend to preferentially affect these structures.

Often the patient's initial CT scan shows no significant intracranial pathology despite a severely compromised neurologic state. Occasionally, numerous small petechial hemorrhages may be seen. Evidence of parenchymal swelling also may be present. When an ICP monitor is placed, the initial ICP is often normal, but may become elevated later in the patient's hospital course.

As noted above, despite the frequent lack of intracranial pathologic lesions seen on CT scanning, these patients invariably present in various states of coma, and they often remain in long-term vegetative states. MRI scanning of these patients is a valuable tool to understand their underlying anatomical abnormality. Typical findings include high-signal intensity lesions, best seen on T_2 or proton density images, involving the aforementioned areas. The prognosis for full recovery is often poor. Many medical, surgical, and rehabilitative resources are required to care for these patients.

SECONDARY INJURY

Pathophysiology

Neurons that are damaged, but not irreversibly destroyed, at the time of impact need optimal delivery of oxygen and nutrients for their recovery. Injured neurons are especially susceptible to further damage during this critical time because of impaired or absent normal reparative reflexes. Secondary insults that occur during this recovery phase inhibit the ability of injured cells to survive. These secondary insults include systemic events such as hypotension or hypoxia, or intracranial events that occur in response to the primary injury. Such insults may lead to a widening area of microcirculatory disruption and neuronal damage. This phase of injury evolves across time, beginning immediately after the primary injury and peaking in a matter of several days. The outcome of the patient depends on the extent of the primary and secondary injuries. Most of the medical therapies used in head-injured patients are aimed at reducing or eliminating secondary insults.

Systemic Events

The two most significant systemic insults leading to secondary neuronal damage are hypotension and hypoxia. Hypotension lowers cerebral perfusion pressure (CPP), leading to cerebral ischemia, especially in the face of impaired autoregulation. The Traumatic Coma Data Bank reported that 35% of seriously injured adult patients presented with both hypotension and head trauma[(64,65)]. Hypovolemia caused by blood loss or vasodilation caused by spinal cord injury are two of the most common causes of hypotension in head-injured victims. Cardiac contusions or arrhythmias may lead to low cardiac output and hypotension. The Traumatic Coma Data Bank found that the mortality of head-injured patients who are hypotensive was 50% compared with 27% in head-injured patients without hypotension[(64,65)].

Many unconscious victims develop hypoxia secondary to airway obstruction from positioning, vomitus, or blood. Additional causes of hypoxemia include hypoventilation caused by direct brainstem injury, high arterial-alveolar gradient secondary to pulmonary contusion or tension pneumothorax. Previously, the presence of hypoxia (PaO_2 less than 60 mm Hg) in head-injured patients was associated with an increased mortality[(66)]. However, recent data did not find this association of early hypoxia with increased mortality[(64,65)]. It is hypothesized that modern methods of emergency management and transport of head-injured patients may have some impact on minimizing hypoxia and thereby secondary hypoxic damage. Prompt attention to securing an airway, administration of supplemental oxygen and resolution of hypotension have a significant impact on limiting secondary cerebral damage in severely head-injured patients.

Intracranial Events

Inflammatory Events

A myriad of biochemical perturbations occur in the brain parenchyma in response to injury. These perturbations activate many inflammatory cascades that result in microcirculatory disruption and neuronal death extending beyond the limits of the original damage. One of the biomolecular responses to neuronal injury that has been directly measured is an increase in oxygen free radicals in the brain[(67,68)]. These free radicals are generated from arachidonic acid, mitochondria, and eventually from neutrophils[(67,69)]. An increase in brain neutrophils has been measured in rats at 2 hours postinjury secondary to an increase in cerebral blood volume. By 4 to 8 hours postinjury, there is an accumulation of polymorphonuclear cells independent of blood volume[(70)]. Free iron that is released from extravasated red blood cells or from storage molecules such as ferritin helps to catalyze oxygen radical formation[(67,68,71)]. In postischemic reperfusion injury, free radicals are responsible for membrane lipid peroxidation in neurons, glial cells, and blood vessels[67,71,72]. Membrane peroxidation subsequently continues as a chain reaction unless halted by a specific event[64,69]. Membrane oxidation leads to ionic fluxes into and out of the cells, enzyme impairment, and eventual cell disruption.

Several avenues of indirect evidence support the presumption that oxygen radicals cause membrane peroxidation after traumatic injury as well. In an animal model, generation of oxygen radicals by topical application of arachidonate causes an increase in the blood-brain barrier permeability that was blocked by the antioxidant superoxide dismutase[67,73]. A 21-aminosteroid compound, U-74006F, is an example of a new class of drug called lazaroids that act as antioxidants by terminating radical chain reactions. In a rat model of percussive head injury, U-74006F restores the blood-brain barrier and improves neurologic function[74]. In a later animal study of percussive injury, administration of U-74006F reduced brain water content in the hemisphere contralateral to the injured side[75]. Thus oxygen radicals are strongly implicated in microvascular dysfunction and generation of vasogenic edema after brain injury.

Another group of chemical mediators thought to be responsible for brain injury are excitatory neurotransmitters such as glutamate and aspartate[76]. When directly applied to neurons in experimental conditions, these molecules cause cell swelling, vacuolization, and cell death[77]. Excitatory neurotransmitters may bind to any of four classes of neurotransmitter receptors, leading to ionic fluxes across neuronal membranes[78]. Activation of these receptors causes an influx of sodium and an efflux of potassium, resulting in a change of membrane polarity that eventually may allow a massive influx of calcium into the cells[78]. Excess calcium entry leads to an inhibition of phosphorylation, activation of proteases and phospholipases, and membrane hydrolysis[78]. It has been hypothesized that glutamate-induced neurotoxicity is mediated by two processes, an early sodium-dependent acute neuronal swelling, and a later calcium-dependent neuronal disintegration.

Cerebral Edema and Intracranial Pressure

Cerebral edema is a principal result of the primary and secondary injuries that occur after traumatic brain injury. The three types of cerebral edema are discussed in detail in Chapter 18. Cytotoxic edema develops in the injured area because of neuronal death. Vasogenic edema caused by disruption of the blood brain barrier develops secondary to primary vascular injury and the aforementioned secondary inflammatory responses. Hydrocephalus, or extra CSF accumulation in the ventricular system of the brain, can occur after certain types of trauma when hemorrhage into the fourth ventricle or basal cisterns causes meningeal inflammation, scarring, and obstruction of the egress of CSF.

According to the Monro-Kellie Doctrine discussed in Chapter 18, the total volume of the three intracranial components, brain, blood, and CSF, must remain fixed within the bony cranium. In addition to cerebral edema, increased cerebral blood volume secondary to altered autoregulatory mechanisms is seen after head trauma. Extravasated extraparenchymal blood is another source of increased cerebral blood volume. Some compensatory mechanisms exist that allow volume shifts out of the cranium when brain or blood volumes increase after traumatic injury. These include extrusion of CSF through the foramen magnum into the spinal subarachnoid space, thus decompressing the ventricular system. Cerebral venous blood volume may be relieved through the jugular veins, thus lowering cerebral blood volume. When these compensatory mechanisms are exhausted, further increases in the volume of any of the constituents lead to increasing ICP.

The ICP represents the outflow pressure of the cerebral perfusion equation (see Chapter 18). ICP often is elevated after traumatic brain injury[21,79–81]. Increased ICP may impede cerebral perfusion, leading to ischemic damage to the already injured brain. The elevated pressure may eventually lead to various herniation syndromes (Fig. 24.8). Significant transtentorial herniation causes brainstem distortion and failure, leading to respiratory and circulatory collapse.

Hyperemia

As discussed previously, an increase in cerebral blood volume can lead to elevated ICP. A common finding in children after a significant head injury is diffuse bilateral cor-

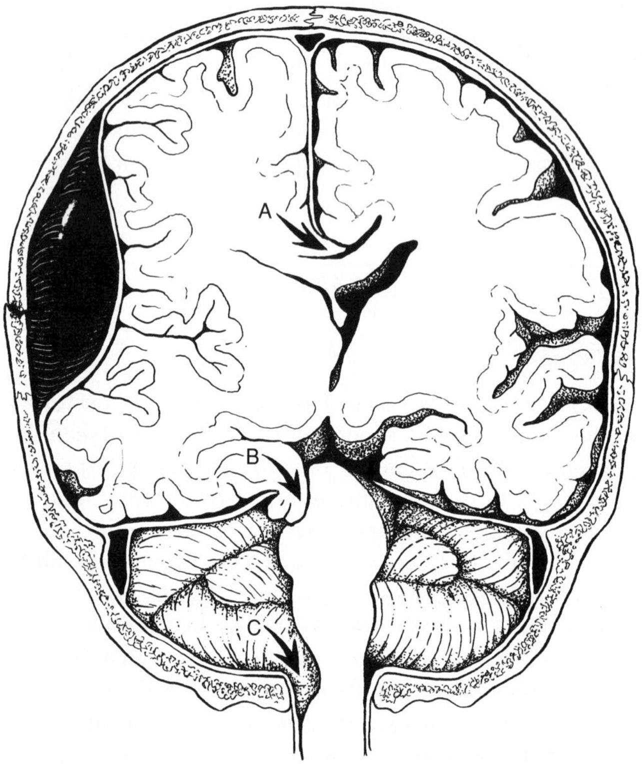

Figure 24.8. Subfalcine herniation occurs when one cerebral hemisphere is displaced under the falx cerebri across the midline (A). Uncal herniation refers to displacement of supratentorial structures inferiorly under the tentorium cerebelli, causing distortion and compression of the blood supply to infratentorial structures (B). Downward herniation of the cerebellum causes compression of the brainstem (C).

tical swelling on CT[79,82–84]. Bruce et al[82] identified hyperemia, or increased cerebral blood volume, instead of cerebral edema as the cause of "malignant" cerebral swelling in children. Using direct measurement of cerebral blood flow, other investigators have found a high percentage of patients with increased global cerebral blood flow[20,21,85,86]. Although posttraumatic cerebral hyperemia is seen in the adult population, children seem more prone to its development[20,21]. In a recent study of percussive injury in a rat model, immature animals had less cerebral hypoperfusion than did mature animals[87]. The cause of this age-related difference is unclear.

The cause of posttraumatic cerebral hyperemia has been thought to be loss of autoregulatory mechanisms. However, little evidence for this concept can be found. Cerebral vasculature almost always is initially sensitive to changes in $PaCO_2$ except in the most severely damaged patients[20,88]. The loss of pressure autoregulation has been shown in fewer than 50% of adult patients[18,89]. Therefore, the concept of "vasomotor paralysis" after trauma does not seem to be valid. Hyperemia often occurs in patients with decreased cerebral metabolic needs, suggesting that a metabolic uncoupling occurs after traumatic injury[18,21].

Increased cerebral blood flow has been correlated with increases in ICP in some studies[20]. However, not all studies have found a relationship between cerebral blood flow and ICP. One pediatric study that measured global cerebral blood flow using ^{133}Xe found no correlation between cerebral blood flow and ICP or score on the Glasgow Coma Scale[21]. However, cerebral blood volume correlated strongly with the pressure-volume index, which reflects cerebral compliance[21]. This suggests that cerebral blood volume, not flow, may play a role in cerebral compliance and ICP. In a study of 15 adult head-injured patients, no correlation between cerebral blood flow and blood volume was apparent[18]. While cerebral vessel diameter determines blood volume, cerebral blood flow depends on blood pressure, ICP, and blood viscosity, as well as vessel diameter. Therefore, cerebral vasodilatation always results in an increase in cerebral blood volume and possibly an increase in ICP if compensatory mechanisms are exhausted. At the same time, cerebral blood flow may be diminished, normal, or increased, depending on the interplay of the other variables.

Potential regional differences of blood volume or flow or both in the injured brain add to the confusion about the role of hyperemia in cerebral swelling and increased ICP. Technology to evaluate regional cerebral blood flow is available only on an experimental basis. Various therapeutic modalities such as hyperventilation that are designed to decrease cerebral vascular diameter and cerebral blood volume may improve regions of injured brain with hyperemia, but at the same time cause other areas with previously normal cerebral blood flow to become ischemic[18].

Cerebral Perfusion Pressure and Ischemia

As discussed above, the presence of cerebral edema or hyperemia or both after head injury may lead to an elevated ICP and lowered cerebral perfusion. Ongoing low cerebral blood flow may potentially exacerbate ischemic damage to the injured brain. Current medical therapy of head-injured patients focuses on preserving CPP in an attempt to minimize secondary damage caused by ischemia. A detailed discussion of the calculation of CPP is provided in Chapter 18. Briefly, CPP can be lowered by systemic hypotension or an increase in ICP. Therefore, prevention of systemic hypotension is paramount in preventing secondary ischemic damage. As discussed previously, an increase in ICP occurs when intracranial compensatory mechanisms are exceeded by an increase in the volume of the brain, cerebral blood, or CSF. Therefore, drainage of CSF, minimizing cerebral edema, and lowering cerebral blood volume while maintaining cerebral blood flow theoretically lowers ICP and optimizes perfusion pressure.

Evidence for the occurrence of posttraumatic ischemia was first identified more than 20 years ago. Postmortem studies performed in the 1970s showed lesions suggestive of global or regional ischemic damage in 50% of patients dying of severe head injury[90]. Watershed areas in the frontoparietal area were most often involved, suggesting a selective vulnerability to ischemia in these areas[90]. Up to 40% of adults have been found to have cerebral vasospasm after head injury[91]. More recent studies measuring cerebral blood flow in hemodynamically stable adult trauma victims using ^{133}Xe scans showed regions of low cerebral blood flow in some severely injured patients[20,85,92]. Although less common in the pediatric population, regions of low flow have been identified in children after head trauma[21]. All of these patients were being managed with measures to decrease ICP, which may have caused some modulation of the cerebral blood flow.

More emphasis is now being placed on identifying the link between cerebral blood flow and cerebral metabolic needs. Neurons sustaining a significant primary injury may not recover, regardless of oxygen delivery, so a low cerebral blood flow in these areas may not matter. Obrist et al[20] showed a linear correlation between cerebral oxygen consumption and Glasgow coma score in adult trauma patients; however, 15 patients with a "low flow" state also had low oxygen extraction ratios, suggesting that flow was not rate-limiting and still exceeded metabolism. Additionally, there may be regional differences in oxygen demand and supply that our current bedside technology is unable to measure.

INITIAL CLINICAL ASSESSMENT

History

Knowing a trauma victim's mechanism of injury is helpful in anticipating problems and establishing priorities. Therefore, obtaining an accurate description of the accident is an important and fundamental part of trauma management. If possible, a detailed description of the type of accident and estimated degree of force should be obtained from available witnesses and emergency personnel as soon as possible. The position of the victim when found and the state of consciousness should be ascertained. Any subsequent deterioration in the level of consciousness indicates decreasing cerebral perfusion and should be acted on promptly. This decrease could be caused by an intracranial process such as an extending hematoma, or could be caused by a systemic effect such as hypotension caused by hemorrhage.

Primary Survey

Many victims of severe head injury also have sustained traumatic injury to other organs. Recognition and treatment of life-threatening respiratory or circulatory injuries always takes precedence in the resuscitation of trauma victims. Besides being potentially life-saving, prompt resolution of hypoxia, hypercapnia, and hypotension is crucial in minimizing secondary cerebral injury.

The primary survey consists of a rapid, focused physical examination designed to quickly identify and treat life-threatening injuries. A more detailed description of these injuries is given in Chapter 43; the subsequent sections focus on how the primary survey relates specifically to head-injured patients.

Airway

Establishing a secure airway should be the initial maneuver in the resuscitation of any trauma victim. This is especially crucial in head-injured patients to prevent hypoxia or hypercarbia, which may lead to secondary brain injury. The threshold for endotracheal intubation should be low in any child who sustains a head injury. Indications for intubation are listed in **Table 24.2.** Any child who is unable to open his or her eyes or verbalize should be considered a candidate for intubation because of concerns about absent or impaired airway protective reflexes. Intracranial hypertension with impending herniation may be inferred from the presence of dilated, unresponsive pupils or Cushing's triad, a symptom complex consisting of hypertension, bradycardia, and an abnormal respiratory pattern. Intubation also may be performed as a prophylactic measure before transportation. Oral intubation occasionally may be impossible in patients with severe maxillofacial trauma. In these cases, establishing an airway by performing a cricothyroidotomy or tracheotomy should be considered. Nasal intubation and even nasogastric tubes should be avoided in the initial resuscitation of head-injured patients until the absence of an anterior basilar skull fracture has been confirmed.

The intubation technique should be modified to protect the cervical spine and minimize the rise in ICP associated with intubation. The patient's neck should be maintained in a neutral position, with axial traction applied by a person whose sole responsibility is to maintain the position of the neck. A rapid-sequence induction as outlined in Chapter 2 should be performed, because it must be assumed that the patient has eaten recently. Sufficient sedation to minimize the ICP response to intubation should be administered. All sedatives that lower ICP also have the potential to cause hypotension, especially in hemodynamically unstable trauma victims. Because hypotension leads to impaired cerebral perfusion, meticulous attention should be given to maintaining the blood pressure within a normal range during sedation. Additionally, lidocaine (1 mg/kg) may be given intravenously before muscle relaxants to blunt the rise in ICP during intubation[93]. Although succinylcholine often is used in rapid sequence intubations because of its rapid action, short duration, and reliable muscle relaxation properties, there are concerns about its use in head-trauma patients because it may raise ICP[94]. This response may be attenuated by defasciculating doses of a nondepolarizing muscle relaxant[95].

Table 24.2. Indications for Airway Management in the Pediatric Trauma Victim

Upper Airway Obstruction
Loss of pharyngeal muscle activity and tone
Inability to clear secretions
Foreign body
Direct trauma
Seizures
Loss of Protective Airway Reflexes
Abnormalities of Respiratory Rate and Rhythm
Chest Wall Dysfunction
Respiratory Muscle Dysfunction
Fatigue
Shock states
Secondary to nerve dysfunction
Pulmonary Disease
Failure of oxygenation
Failure of ventilation
Pulmonary hypertension
Intracranial Hypertension
Prophylactic

Ventilation

Hypoventilation caused by several pulmonary or neurologic causes is common in head-injured patients. Hypercarbia is a potent cerebral vasodilator, and should be strenuously avoided in these patients. Although the value of long-term hyperventilation in controlling intracranial hypertension has been questioned, the short-term use of moderate hyperventilation in the immediate resuscitation of any seriously head-injured patient is recommended. Patients with physical findings suggestive of brainstem compression from herniation such as Cushing's triad or dilated and unreactive pupils should be hyperventilated as soon as possible to acutely lower ICP.

Supplemental oxygen should be provided for all patients with moderate to severe head trauma to prevent hypoxia that may cause secondary brain injury. The patient's oxygen saturation should be monitored with a pulse oximeter and should be maintained 90% or higher.

Circulation

When the adequacy of the airway and ventilation have been established, the next therapeutic goal should be the assessment and optimization of perfusion. Shock, or an inadequate delivery of oxygen and nutrients to meet the metabolic de-

Table 24.3. Glasgow Coma Score

Activity	*Best Response*	*Score*
Eye opening	Spontaneous	4
	To verbal stimuli	3
	To pain	2
	None	1
Verbal	Oriented	5
	Confused	4
	Inappropriate words	3
	Nonspecific sounds	2
	None	1
Motor	Follows commands	6
	Localizes pain	5
	Withdraws in response to pain	4
	Flexion in response to pain	3
	Extension in response to pain	2
	None	1

mands of the tissue, can result from multiple causes. The injured brain is one of the most susceptible organs to inadequate perfusion, and unless prompt resolution of shock occurs, secondary injury results. Hypovolemic shock from blood loss is commonly seen in trauma victims. Except in small infants, it is impossible to lose enough blood in the cranium to cause hypotension. Therefore, other sources of blood loss besides head injury should be sought in these patients. The primary goal should be the restoration of adequate perfusion, and adequate fluid resuscitation should not be withheld because of concerns about cerebral edema. However, isotonic fluid should be used to minimize free water administration.

Other causes of hypotension besides hypovolemia can occur and should be diagnosed quickly. Cardiac contusions may lead to cardiogenic shock and arrhythmias; inotropic and antiarrhythmic medications are beneficial in these cases. Spinal cord injury may lead to the loss of sympathetic tone, vasodilatation, and hypotension. Although adequate fluid administration is required in these cases, alpha adrenergic agonists to increase systemic vascular resistance often are necessary.

Neurologic

The neurologic examination during the primary survey should be succinct, and aimed primarily at diagnosing and treating life-threatening intracranial hypertension with incipient herniation. Evaluation of pupillary response to light can be performed quickly, and can be helpful in diagnosing herniation. The pupillary light reflex consists of an afferent pathway through the optic nerve and an efferent pathway consisting of sympathetic and parasympathetic fibers. Transtentorial herniation causes compression of the parasympathetic fibers along the third cranial nerve and results in ipsilateral pupillary dilation with no response to direct or consensual stimulation. Bilaterally dilated pupils that are unresponsive are an ominous sign, whether caused by bilaterally compressed third nerves or severe cerebral anoxia and ischemia. Their presence is an indication for rapid therapeutic maneuvers to decrease ICP. Hyperventilation and other maneuvers to acutely lower ICP should be instituted immediately if a unilateral or bilateral dilated, unresponsive pupil is found.

If possible, the level of consciousness should be rapidly assessed at this stage. This examination will have to be delayed in patients who have received muscle relaxants or sedatives or both during intubation or transport. In describing the level of consciousness, terms such as *obtunded, comatose ,or awake* should be avoided because of differences in interpretation. The level of consciousness should be evaluated using the Glasgow Coma Scale. This descriptive scoring system evaluates performance in three areas: eye opening, which relates to the level of arousal; verbalization, which relates to content and mentation; and motor ability **(Table 24.3).** The score has been modified to apply to preverbal infants **(Table 24.4).** To assess motor ability, the extremities are observed for the presence and symmetry of spontaneous movement. Diminished spontaneous movement may be attributed to local or spinal cord injury. Mildly painful stimuli can be applied to the extremities by asserting pressure on the nailbed, or between the fingers or toes, to elicit a motor response. Central painful stimuli such as sternal rubbing or supraorbital pressure may elicit purposeful movement, decorticate posturing, decerebrate posturing, or no response.

This scoring system is consistent between observers and predicts outcome[96]. It is a useful tool for ongoing evaluation of the patient; changes across time help diagnose improving or deteriorating neurologic function.

Secondary Survey

The secondary survey involves a thorough physical examination of the patient. The aim of the secondary survey is to identify all traumatic injuries and to begin to prioritize treatment. A more detailed explanation of this survey is provided in Chapter 43. Specific areas of the secondary survey are especially important in head-trauma patients.

Head

Careful inspection of the head for depressions, swellings, lacerations, or ecchymoses that would indicate underlying injury should be performed. Exploration of all lacerations

Table 24.4. Modified Glasgow Coma Score for Infants

Activity	*Best Response*	*Score*
Eye opening	Spontaneous	4
	To speech	3
	To pain	2
	None	1
Verbal	Coos and babbles	5
	Irritable cries	4
	Cries to pain	3
	Moans to pain	2
	None	1
Motor	Normal spontaneous movements	6
	Withdraws to touch	5
	Withdraws to pain	4
	Abnormal flexion	3
	Abnormal extension	2
	None	1

with a gloved finger should be performed to diagnose underlying open or depressed skull fractures or foreign material that warrants surgical attention.

Discoloration of the eyelids and retromastoid areas, or the raccoon eyes and Battle's sign, respectively, are signs of basilar skull fractures. The facial area should be palpated for signs of instability or swelling suggestive of underlying fractures. Facial fractures may be associated with fracture of the cribiform plate. Leakage of CSF from the nose or ears, or the presence of hemotympanum, also indicate a basilar skull fracture. Any of the aforementioned signs are absolute contraindications to the placement of a nasogastric tube because of concerns that disruption of the basilar skull allows entry into the intracranial vault.

The anterior fontanelle should be palpated in infants, because its tone (bulging, soft, sunken) is a general indication of ICP.

Neck

Injury to the cervical spine should be assumed in any head-injured patient until it has been definitively ruled out by methods discussed later in this chapter. The neck should remain immobilized in an appropriately sized collar, and manipulation should be kept to a minimum. If the collar is removed for any reason, the neck should be held in a midline position and gentle axial traction applied by a person whose sole responsibility is supporting the cervical spine. Obvious deformity, swelling, or ecchymosis of the neck should be visible on inspection. Palpation of the neck may show a malalignment, stepoff, or splaying of the spinous processes suggesting a ligamentous and unstable injury.

Thorax

The chest wall should be observed for the pattern and adequacy of ventilation. Specific patterns of breathing are seen with head injury and may have important localizing value (Fig. 24.9). Posthyperventilation apnea indicates forebrain damage. Cheyne-Stokes respiration or alternating phases of hyperpnea is caused by dysfunction deep within the cerebral hemispheres or diencephalon. Hyperventilation or persistent rapid respiration is caused by damage in the rostral brainstem or tegmentum. Apneustic respiration, or prolonged sustained end-inspiratory pauses, is caused by damage at the midpontine or caudal pontine level. Ataxic respiration, or completely random and irregular breathing, indicates medullary damage. Complete apnea or paralysis of the diaphragm occurs with high cervical cord damage.

Neurologic

A rapid evaluation of the eyes is included in the primary survey, but should be expanded on during the secondary survey. The presence of eye opening, as indicative of mental responsiveness, is evaluated as part of the Glasgow Coma

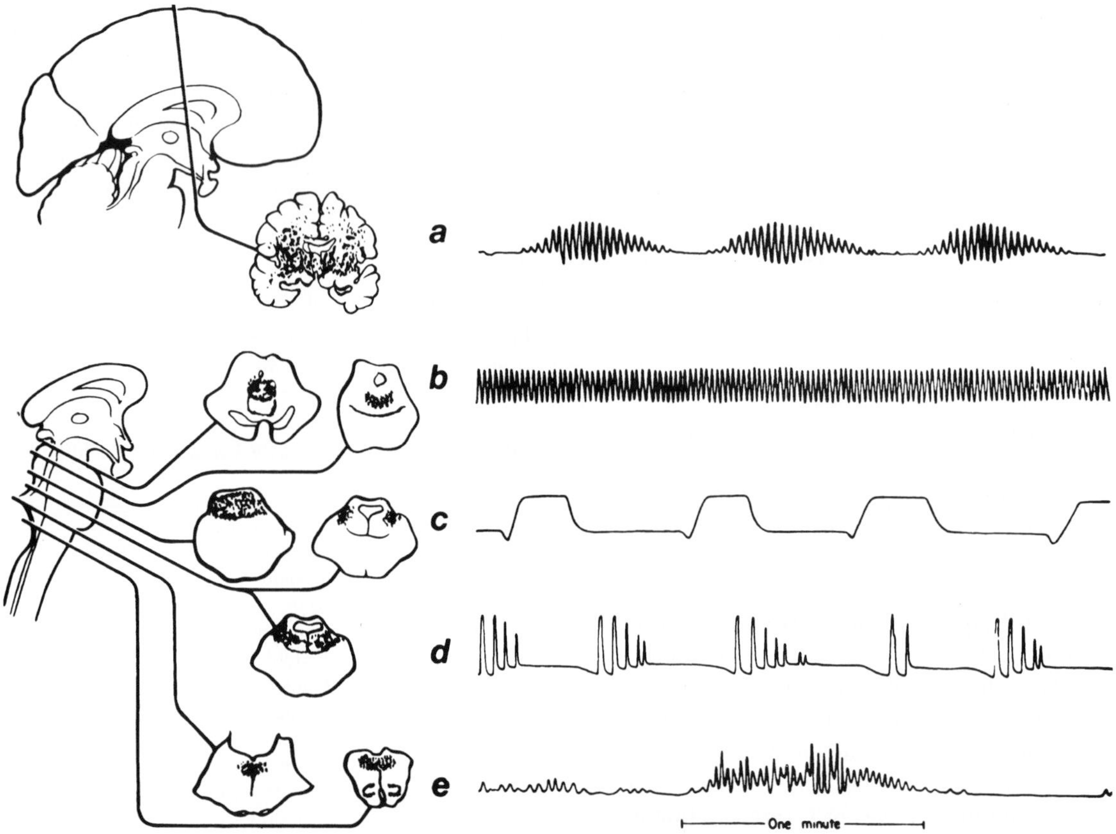

Figure 24.9. Injury to different portions of the brain leads to distinctive abnormal breathing patterns that may help localize the area of injury. A prolonged abnormal respiratory pattern may interfere with oxygenation and ventilation. (Reprinted with permission from Mettler FA. Neuroanatomy. St Louis: CV Mosby, 1948:816.)

Scale. As discussed in the primary survey, assessment of pupillary response to light to detect brainstem compression should be performed early in the patient assessment. However, this reflex should be monitored across time, because changes in pupillary response signify important intracranial changes.

It is possible for head-injured patients to suffer afferent disruption of the light reflex. It is important to examine the consensual response to light because this differentiates a nonreactive pupil caused by disruption of efferent versus afferent pathways. Unilateral pupil dilation unreactive to direct stimulation but consensually reactive is caused by absent light perception in that eye or a deafferented pupil. Alternately shining the light into each eye reveals the paradoxical dilation on the affected side with direct stimulation. This is the Marcus Gunn pupil and represents dilation of the affected pupil after consensually stimulated constriction. When the light is shone into the deafferented eye, both eyes perceive darkness, and both pupils dilate accordingly.

Damage to the hypothalamic region can interrupt sympathetic pathways and cause ipsilateral pupillary constriction associated with ptosis and anhidrosis. This is Horner's syndrome and may be an early sign of transtentorial herniation.

Pupillary size may be helpful in delineating the level of injury. Injury to the midbrain tectum may result in pupils that are midposition and fixed to light but retain hippus, the ciliospinal reflex, and response to accommodation. Pinpoint pupils are associated with pontine lesions. Medications used during the resuscitation of these patients, such as atropine or narcotics, may alter pupillary size and obscure this part of the physical examination.

The eyes should be observed for conjugate gaze or abnormal movement. Conjugate gaze is evaluated in the awake and cooperative patient by use of a flashlight. The light, when looked at by the patient, should reflect from the same spot on each pupil. Voluntary movement is evaluated in all primary directions. The inability to move the eyes in a given direction can indicate orbital entrapment or cranial nerve paresis. Nystagmus may be noted and is often secondary to cerebellar or vestibular injury. In the unconscious patient, gaze paresis is more difficult to show. When observed at rest, the eyes may show roving movements of a conjugate or dysconjugate nature. This implies intact oculomotor centers. Tonic deviation of one or both eyes can be caused by ipsilateral cortical lesions, cranial nerve dysfunction, or seizure activity.

A fundoscopic examination should be performed, especially when physical abuse is suspected. The presence of retinal hemorrhages signifies a significant degree of injury, and almost always represents nonaccidental trauma.

In a comatose patient, testing of brainstem reflexes is helpful in evaluating the degree of injury and the prognosis. Examination of the pupillary response to light has been discussed. The corneal reflex may be tested using a wisp of cotton. The oculovestibular reflex (cold-water calorics), gag reflex, and respiratory effort should be assessed. The evaluation of the oculocephalic reflex (doll's eyes reflex) requires manipulation of the neck, and should be postponed until the cervical spine has been cleared of any injury.

The extremities should be tested individually for sensory functions to assess spinal cord injury function. Although it is optimal to test multiple sensory modalities such as pain, temperature, light touch, and two-point discrimination, most of these tests require patient cooperation. In cooperative patients, pain may be assessed using a sterile needle. The patient is lightly and repeatedly stimulated from the periphery toward the center. Any change in sensation is noted and the level demarcated. The sacral and perineal area should also be examined. In younger infants or patients with decreased mentation, these modalities cannot be performed. Although not as accurate, mildly painful peripheral and central stimuli as described during the Glasgow coma score, may be used to assess sensory function in these patients.

The deep tendon reflexes should be elicited in each extremity and compared from right to left. Asymmetric reflexes may be helpful in lateralizing the injury. Bilateral hyperactive reflexes may be associated with head or spinal cord injuries, but should be symmetric and not associated with pathologic reflexes. Rapid sustained dorsiflexion of each ankle to test for clonus should be performed. Stroking the sole of the foot with a firm object should cause a flexion of the great toe; a positive Babinski reflex occurs when the patient dorsiflexes his or her toe. Many infants retain a dorsiflexion response to this maneuver, and the presence of a Babinski reflex has little localized value.

Laboratory Evaluation

Several laboratory studies are important in the overall management of head-injured patients and should be obtained after the initial physical evaluation of the patient has been completed. A CBC, platelet count, electrolytes, type and cross, amylase, and a coagulopathy panel (PT, PTT, fibrinogen level) should be obtained as soon as possible. A pulse oximeter should be placed on the patient as soon as possible, but an arterial blood gas should be obtained to verify oxygenation and to assess ventilation.

Neuroradiologic Evaluation

Background

CT is the modality of choice for urgent neuroimaging of patients with apparently serious head injuries. The ability to rapidly define posttraumatic intracranial abnormalities has reduced the morbidity and mortality of head-injured patients[97–99]. Posttraumatic lesions that are amenable to surgical intervention are uncommon in children[80,99]. However, the ability to rapidly visualize these abnormalities often has allowed specific decompressive surgery to be performed in a timely fashion, before the patient has advanced clinical symptoms[100]. Although MRI has some advantages (discussed later) in imaging the brain, the limitations of a strong magnetic field and increased scan times make it less useful in the acute setting[101–103]. CT is readily available and is not limited by the constraints of a strong magnetic field. Because of its frequent use for patients in the critical care unit, the critical care physician must be capable of evaluating the head CT scan. Therefore, this section will concentrate on an approach to the evaluation of the head CT scan in the setting of the critical care unit, with brief comments about the use of other modalities.

Understanding the CT Image

To understand the CT image, it is essential to remember that the cross-sectional CT image, as displayed on a monitor or on film, represents a display of numerical data portrayed in a gray-scale image on a spatial matrix. To generate an image in current generation CT scanners, a narrowly collimated beam of x-ray photons is passed through the affected part of the patient. Some of the photons are absorbed by the body, depending on the atomic properties of the elements contained within the volume of tissue that is scanned. The nonabsorbed photons are recorded by multiple detectors and converted to electrical signals. The computer then uses sophisticated reconstruction algorithms to quantitate the electrical signals and assign a numerical value to the correct spatial location in the image. Photon absorption is measured in Hounsfield units (HU) (named for Sir Godfrey Hounsfield, who received the Nobel Prize for discovery of this technology). An HU is assigned to each voxel in the matrix and displayed on a computer monitor.

Understanding the gray scale of the CT image is critical. Two operator-selective variables determine the appearance of the image as displayed on the monitor. These variables are similar to the contrast and brightness controls on a television screen. One variable, the window width, determines the breadth of the HUs that will be displayed by the gray scale. This is similar to the contrast control on a television monitor. With a wide window width (i.e., more than 1000 HU), there is a broad separation of the gray scale, producing a low-contrast image that allows distinction between bone, air, and soft tissue. This window width typically would be used to create a "bone-window" image (Fig. 24.10,A). Alternatively, a narrow window width produces a high contrast image that discriminates between subtle differences in attenuation of photons such as might be necessary in distinguishing gray from white matter structures in the brain. A typical window width for "brain windows" would be 80 to 100 HU (Fig 24.10,B).

A second variable, the window center, determines what HU attenuation number will be placed at the numerical center of the gray-scale display. This is similar to the brightness control on a television monitor. Tissues beyond the margins of the window width are seen as white or black. Only those within the window are seen as variations of gray. The window center is properly set at approximately the attenuation number of the tissue being examined. For instance, in typical "brain windows," the window level is set at approximately 40 HU, corresponding to the attenuation coefficient of brain parenchyma. Alternatively, with "bone-window" images, the window center is at approximately 250 HU, closer to the attenuation of bone.

The term "density" is incorrectly applied to description of findings in the CT image. The correct term for description of differences in photon absorption is *attenuation*. Therefore, in the standard gray-scale image, a structure that is brighter on the screen represents greater photon absorp-

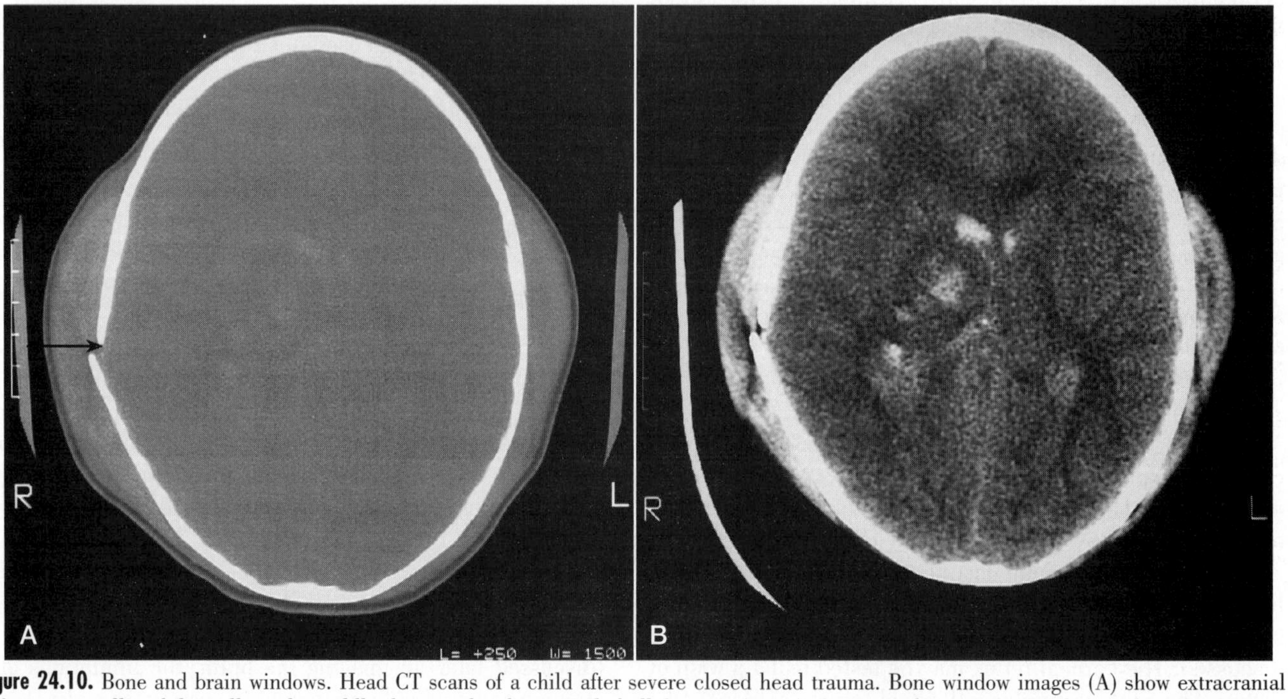

Figure 24.10. Bone and brain windows. Head CT scans of a child after severe closed head trauma. Bone window images (A) show extracranial soft tissue swelling bilaterally and a mildly depressed right parietal skull fracture (arrow). Brain window images (B) do not show the fracture and swelling as well, but show the structures of the brain at the same level and multiple foci of parenchymal hemorrhage.

tion (attenuation) than a structure that looks darker on the screen. The lowest attenuation seen on a head CT scan is that of air, which absorbs essentially no x-ray photons. Progressively greater attenuation (brighter intensity) is seen by fat, water, soft tissues, contrast material, bone, and metal. Blood has variable attenuation depending on its age, clotting, and dilution (Fig. 24.11). The differences in attenuation of these structures allow discrimination of the various intracranial structures and abnormalities.

CT Imaging Protocols

The standard CT brain scan is performed with 5- to 10-mm thick contiguous scans from the foramen magnum to the vertex in the axial (transverse) plane. Scans are displayed with a narrow window width, or brain windows, for discrimination of the soft-tissue structures of the brain. Wide window images, or bone windows, are also displayed if there has been trauma, surgery, or concern about a calvarial lesion. Thin-section scans of the skull base, facial region, and orbits are helpful for resolution of subtle fractures. Intravenous iodinated contrast is given and the scan series repeated if there is concern for inflammatory, neoplastic, or vascular disease. If the patient has compromised renal function, non-ionic contrast is indicated. Direct coronal scanning is preferable to computer reconstruction of axial images in the coronal plane for better visualization of facial and temporal bone structures and the vertex of the skull.

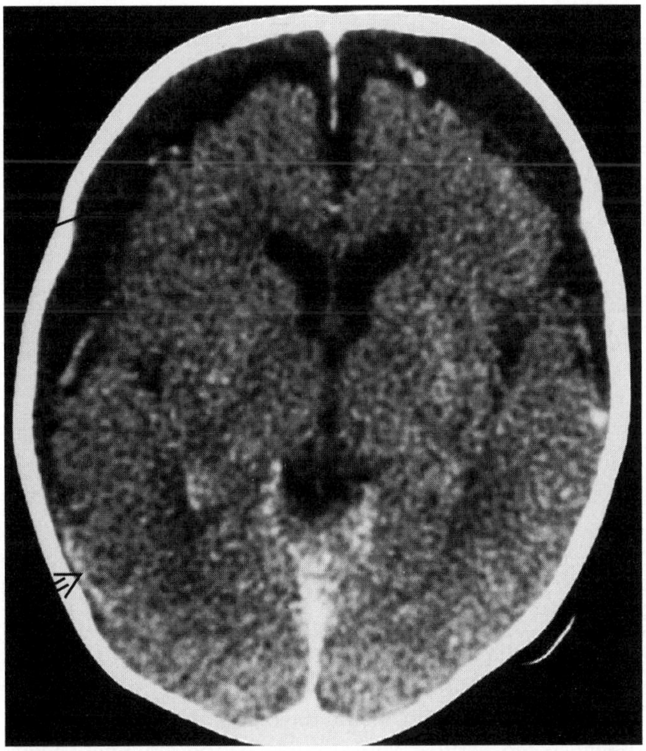

Figure 24.11. Varying attenuation of blood. Head CT scan of an abused child shows both acute (bright) blood (open arrow) and chronic (dark) blood (closed arrow) in the subdural space, indicating multiple episodes of intracranial hemorrhage secondary to nonaccidental head trauma.

However, coronal positioning may not be possible in the setting of cervical spine injury or may require sedation in the uncooperative patient. In addition, patients who are agitated or combative may require sedation for a satisfactory study. Otherwise, sedation is not generally used for routine head CT scanning of critical care patients. Additional techniques that may be used in brain CT scanning include three-dimensional reconstructions, CT angiography and xenon brain scanning (with special equipment). Interpretation of these studies is not expected of the critical care physician.

Approach to the Head CT Scan

An orderly approach in evaluating a head CT study is helpful. The bone-window images (if available) are reviewed first, looking for soft-tissue swelling (indicating acute injury), fractures, spread sutures, bulging fontanels, foreign bodies, and surgical changes. Careful attention to the skull base, temporal bones, sinuses, mastoids, and maxillofacial-orbital structures is important. Linear skull fractures that approximate the angle of the scan plane may not be visible on the axial scan images. Coronal scanning may be helpful in this setting. Plain skull radiographs may be necessary to accurately visualize the entire course of a fracture. Reference to the digital radiograph, or scanogram, obtained at the beginning of the CT study may be helpful in visualizing a fracture not seen on the axial images. Diastasis, depression, and fragmentation of fractures are important observations (Fig. 24.4).

The brain-window images are then evaluated. Structures to be assessed may be approached by a caudal to rostral review of the images. Attention should be directed specifically to the appearance of the normal structure and the appearance of the brainstem, cerebellum, basal ganglia, cerebral hemispheres, ventricles, basilar cisterns, and convexity extraaxial fluid spaces. After reviewing the normal structures, look for abnormalities such as hemorrhage (acute or chronic, parenchymal, intraventricular, or extra-axial); areas of increased attenuation (calcification, foreign body, or tumor); or decreased attenuation (edema, infarction, contusion, cerebritis, abscess, cyst, or tumor). Evaluation of the gray-white interface is crucial. In current-generation scanners, the interface between gray (brighter) and white (darker) matter is well seen in both the cerebral and cerebellar hemispheres. Loss of distinction of the gray-white interface may be an early sign of edema, even before mass effect or shift occurs (Fig. 24.12).

It is important to evaluate mass effect and shift, if present. Infarction, contusion, hemorrhage, tumor, and abscess cause local mass effect and may lead to shift of the intracranial contents. Cerebral edema, focal or diffuse, also leads to shift. If the mass effect is unilateral in the cerebrum, the shift is from side to side. The midline falx is a relatively rigid structure. There may be injury to the brain or blood vessels as the brain shifts from side to side (subfalcine herniation). The distal anterior cerebral artery on the side of the mass effect is especially prone to injury or com-

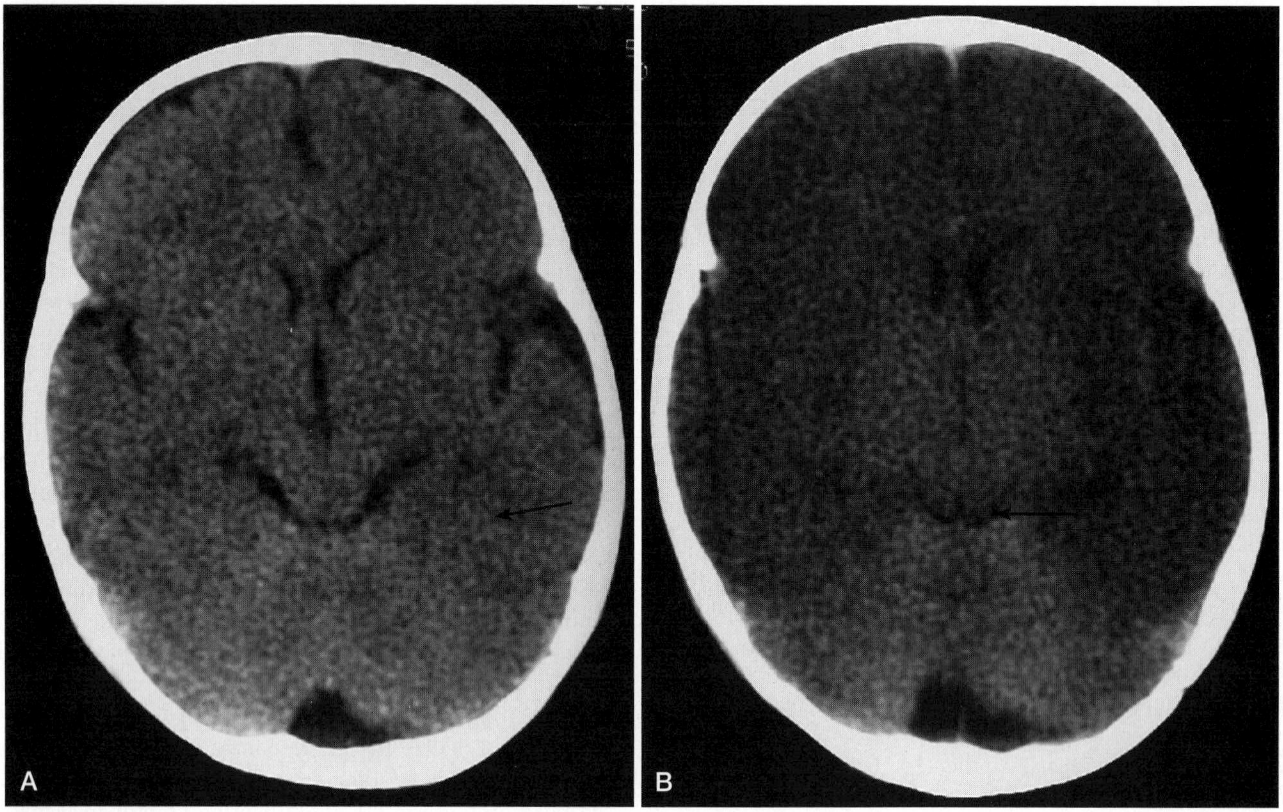

Figure 24.12. Signs of cerebral edema. Head CT scans of a 6-month-old infant with near sudden infant death syndrome event. Initial scan (A) on the day of admission shows only subtle decrease in the normal contrast between gray and white matter structure, best seen in the posterior temporal lobes (arrow). Follow-up scan (B) performed 3 days later shows diffuse low attenuation of the brain indicative of severe cerebral edema. Note effacement of the lateral ventricles and quadrigeminal plate cistern (arrow).

pression in this setting as it impinges on the falx (Fig. 24.6). When the mass effect is generalized in the cerebral hemispheres, the shift is downward through the incisural opening of the tentorium (descending transtentorial herniation) (Fig. 24.13). Clinically this is often heralded by pupillary dilatation, indicating compression of cranial nerve III. A much less common form of herniation through the incisura occurs when the mass effect is in the posterior fossa and the herniation is upward (ascending transtentorial herniation.) (Fig. 24.14). The relatively rigid margins of the tentorium at the incisura compress vessels adjacent to them when herniation occurs. With descending herniation, the posterior cerebral arteries are compressed against the tentorium, leading to bilateral occipital lobe infarction; in ascending herniation, bilateral cerebellar infarction may occur with compression of the superior cerebellar arteries against the under surface of the tentorium. Downward herniation through the foramen magnum may be difficult to detect on CT studies. A "tight" appearance to the posterior fossa, absence of fluid in the cisterna magna, or posterior displacement of the fourth ventricle may be helpful signs.

The appearance of the ventricles may be helpful in detecting mass effect and shift. A lateral ventricle may be compressed by a mass in the cerebral hemisphere adjacent to it. The third ventricle may be compressed or displaced by mass effect deep in the cerebrum, i.e., in the basal ganglia and thalamus. The fourth ventricle is displaced or distorted by mass effect in the cerebellum. Generalized enlargement of the ventricular system may indicate developing hydrocephalus secondary to intraventricular hemorrhage, inflammation, or blockage by mass effect. Not all large ventricles indicate hydrocephalus. The ventricles may enlarge passively secondary to loss of brain tissue ("ex vacuo dilatation"), especially after the acute phase of a global brain injury resolves. Serial measurements of head size may be helpful in making this distinction, especially in younger children with more mobile cranial sutures.

Extraaxial fluid may be difficult to evaluate. There is normally some CSF in the subarachnoid space over the convexities of the cerebral hemispheres. This fluid should have identical attenuation to that of normal intraventricular CSF. If the attenuation of an extraaxial collection is greater than that of intraventricular CSF, the fluid contains increased protein or cellular content, most likely secondary to previous hemorrhage or inflammation. It is normal to have an increased volume of the subarachnoid space in infants and toddlers, but the fluid should have normal CSF attenuation. Because the cortical veins course in the arachnoid membrane, when the subarachnoid space enlarges, the veins are displaced off the surface of the brain (the "cortical vein sign") (Fig. 24.15). Careful inspection of the location of the cortical veins can be helpful in correctly assigning the space

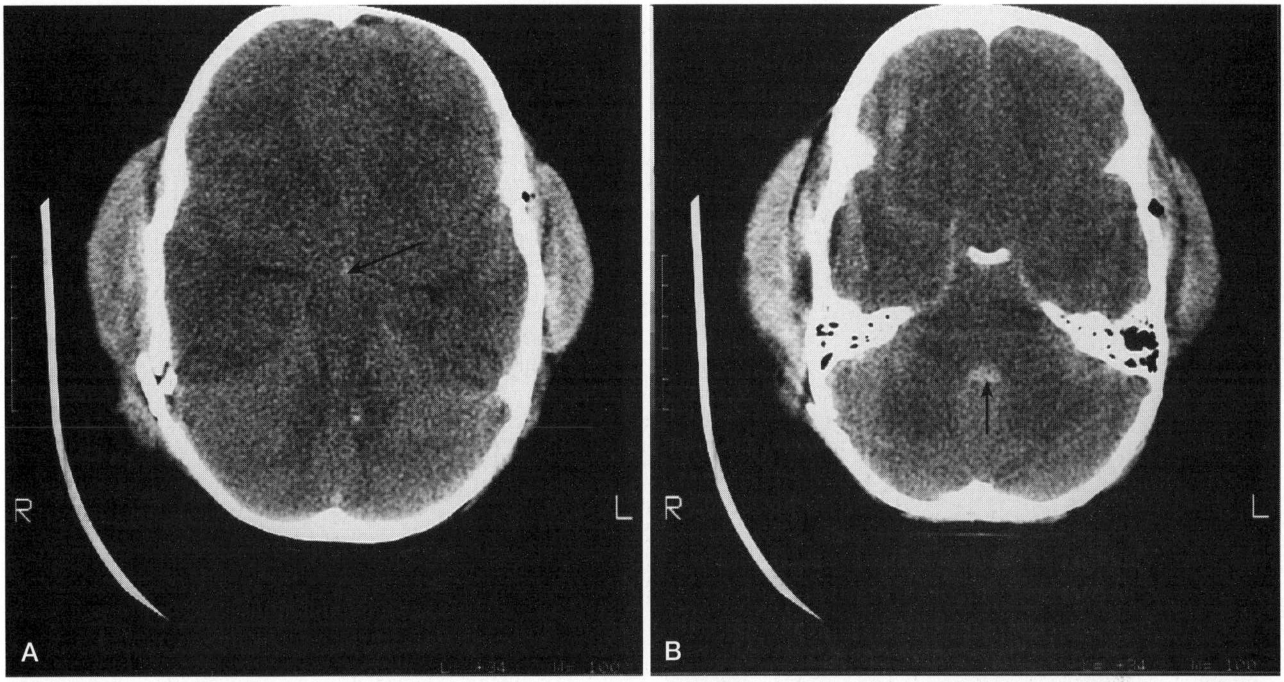

Figure 24.13. Descending transtentorial herniation. Head CT scans of a child with severe closed head injury (same patient as in Figure 24.10) at the level of the tentorial incisura (A) and the fourth ventricle (B) show effacement of the cisterns at the skull base and in the posterior fossa and compression of the brainstem at the incisura. There are also signs of tonsillar herniation. Note the blood in the third (arrow in A) and fourth (arrow in B) ventricles.

of low-attenuation extraaxial fluid. Alternatively, if the veins are closely applied to the surface of the brain with the fluid peripheral to them, especially if the fluid has greater attenuation than normal CSF, the collection is most like a chronic subdural hematoma or hygroma.

It is also important to evaluate the basilar extracerebral spaces. Basilar cisterns containing CSF normally exist at all ages. If not present, the possibility of brain swelling should be considered. These are best seen in the suprasellar region and around the midbrain above the level of the incisura. One of the early signs of cerebral edema is effacement of the normal basilar cisterns. Nonvisualization of the basilar cisterns may be caused by the presence of a lumbar CSF drain or shunt.

Appearance of blood in the extracerebral spaces is discussed in a previous section of this chapter. Blood in the subdural compartment may be "isodense" to brain as it evolves from the phase of increased attenuation (acute) to decreased attenuation (chronic) relative to the brain. Careful attention to the displacement of the gray-white junction medially or the "hematocrit effect" caused by layering of cellular and serum elements of blood may be helpful in detecting subtle subdural hemorrhage.

Hemorrhage in the parenchyma of the brain may be subtle and diffuse, as in hemorrhagic infarction or contusion; focal and discrete, as in an hematoma; linear in the cortex, as in laminar cortical necrosis; or punctate at the gray-white interface, as in diffuse axonal injury. Intraventricular hemorrhage usually is caused by trauma, shunt placement, or rupture of an arteriovenous malformation.

A frequently seen pattern of hemorrhage and extracerebral fluid accumulation is seen in the shaking-impact form of child abuse. In this setting, acute hemorrhage often occurs in the extracerebral compartment (usually subdural) frequently adjacent to the falx or tentorium or the tips of the occipital or temporal lobes. This acute hemorrhage is adjacent to more chronic-looking hemorrhage in the subdural space over one or both convexities. In addition, there may be diffuse brain swelling, indicating cerebral edema caused by diffuse axonal injury or suffocation. The constellation of these findings is highly suggestive of nonaccidental injury to the infant or young child (Figs. 24.11 and 24.15).

If intravenous contrast has been given, it is important to evaluate the enhancing pattern of the brain, blood vessels, brain coverings, and any abnormal structures. Areas of increased parenchymal enhancement may indicate inflammation, tumor, infarction, "luxury perfusion," or other cause of loss of the normal blood-brain barrier. Decreased enhancement may indicate infarction, cerebral edema, or nonenhancing tumor. Attention to the caliber of the vessels at the skull base may detect decreased size indicating spasm, inflammation, vasculitis, or encasement. If the vessels are large, there may be loss of autoregulation, a vascular malformation, or a high flow tumor. Enhancement of the leptomeninges covering the brain may indicate inflammatory change as in meningitis, with development of subdural effusion or empyema, postoperative inflammation, or spread of tumor to the subarachnoid space or membrane adjacent to a subacute or chronic subdural hematoma.

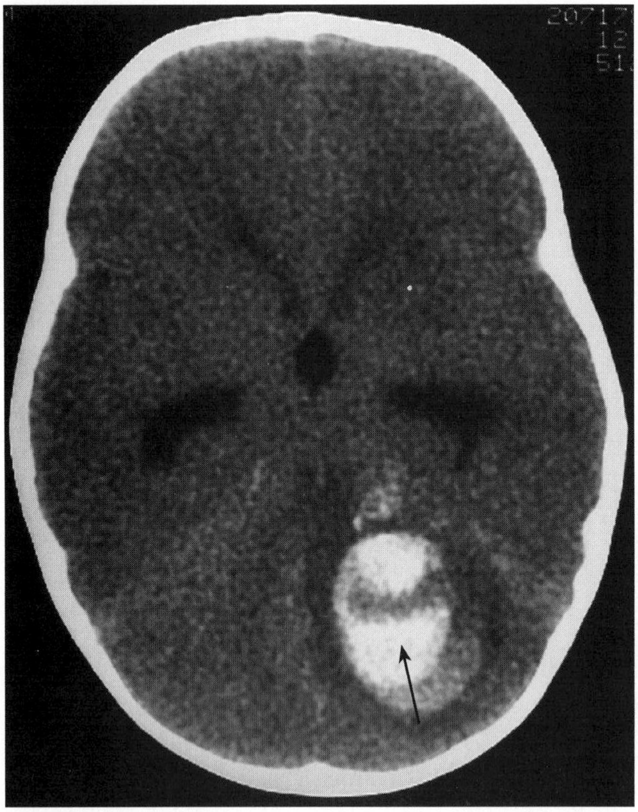

Figure 24.14. Ascending transtentorial herniation. Head CT scan of an infant with hemorrhage (arrow) of a cerebellar vascular malformation shows effacement of the posterior fossa and basilar cisterns and acute hydrocephalus secondary to obstruction of CSF flow at the level of the aqueduct.

Other Modalities

Other modalities for neuroimaging of the child in the critical care unit will be discussed briefly. As mentioned, CT is the modality of choice and is sufficient for most neuroimaging indications.

MRI is a powerful modality for brain imaging, with the ability to display the brain in exquisite detail in multiple planes, distinguish soft tissues much better than CT, detect various stages of hemoglobin degradation, assess maturity of myelination, and evaluate hemorrhage in or around the brain. However, it is limited by the environment of a strong magnetic field, precluding the use of intravenous pumps, most respirators and other life-support equipment. It also requires the patient to be still for several minutes at a time. MRI usually is used to clarify findings initially seen on CT or to reveal abnormalities that may escape detection by CT. A robust application of MRI is the ability to create vascular images (MRI angiography without the need for contrast or vascular catheterization). Future applications of MRI to the critical care patient may include metabolic assessment of brain function with functional MRI and MRI spectroscopy.

Nuclear medicine studies are of limited application to the head injured patient. The most frequently performed study is to assess cerebral perfusion in the determination of brain death (see Chapter 27). Using newer isotope formulations, it is possible to obtain both flow and static images of the brain to establish the presence or absence of cerebral perfusion.

Xenon CT is available in few centers. Xenon gas is inhaled until a steady state is attained, and a CT scan is performed. The attenuation of the brain reflects the perfusion of the brain and may be useful in the critical care patient to assess the effect on brain perfusion of interventional measures such as hyperventilation, volume expansion, and pharmacologic intervention. Special equipment for ventilation of the gas and modifications to the CT scanner are necessary for this technique.

Indications for Acute Surgical Intervention/Intracranial Monitoring

Indications for placement of an ICP monitor in head-injured patients include a Glasgow coma score lower than 8, rapid deterioration in the patient's neurologic examination, or loss of the ability to follow the patient's neurologic examination during surgery or while he or she is receiving muscle relaxants or sedatives. Occasionally patients with diffuse cerebral edema visualized on a CT scan have an ICP monitor placed in anticipation of intracranial hypertension developing, even though their initial Glasgow coma score is higher than 8. Additionally, intraventricular hemorrhage with secondary hydrocephalus should be drained with a ventricular drain-monitor. The various types of intracranial monitors and the technical aspects of their placement are described in Chapter 18.

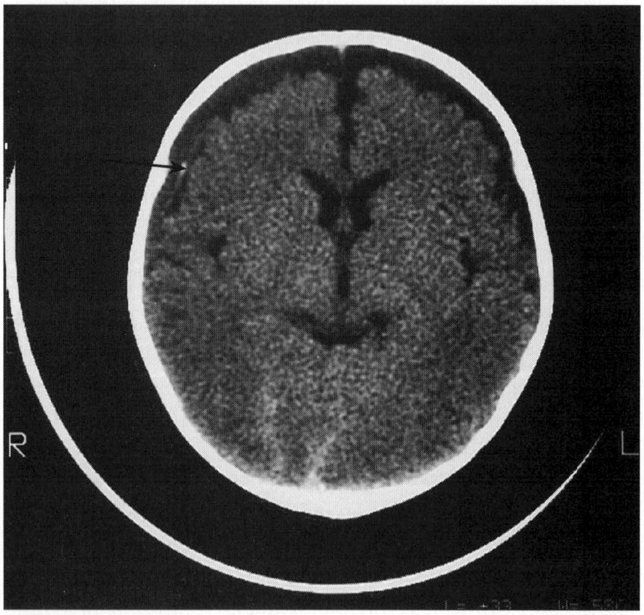

Figure 24.15. Cortical vein sign. Head CT scan of an abused child shows bilateral chronic subdural hematomas. A cortical vein (arrow) can be seen at the interface of the subdural hematoma (peripheral to the vein, which runs in the arachnoid membrane) and the underlying CSF in the subarachnoid space (between the brain and the cortical vein).

A selected group of posttraumatic lesions in children benefits from surgical treatment[80,99]. Rapidly expanding mass lesions such as subdural or epidural hematomas that cause focal compression of the underlying brain, and rapidly increasing ICP, should be surgically decompressed as soon as possible. Prompt surgical resolution of these injuries in patients sustaining no other underlying brain injury has a major impact on morbidity and mortality[100]. Patients who have suffered more diffuse brain injury in addition to hematomas still may have a dismal outcome despite surgical decompression. Smaller focal lesions that seem to be symptomatic also are considered likely to benefit from surgical evacuation. Exceptions include deep contusions or hematomas that require dissection of large areas of the brain to access them, or lesions in eloquent areas of the brain such as the speech or motor cortex.

CLINICAL MANAGEMENT

Pulmonary Management

Pulmonary complications are common after serious head injury. Neurogenic pulmonary edema (NPE) is the most dramatic of these pulmonary complications. Medical attention was first focused on this entity in Vietnam, where NPE was diagnosed in more than 85% of casualties suffering from isolated head injures[104]. The high incidence of pulmonary edema after severe head injury also was found in an adult autopsy series; in this series most of the patients experiencing NPE died within an hour of their injury[105]. A much lower incidence of NPE was found in less severely injured adult patients who eventually recovered[106]. Therefore, NPE seems to occur predominantly in massive, often fatal, injuries.

Classically, NPE develops within 2 to 12 hours of the injury, but can be delayed up to several days[107]. Patients present with hypoxia, hyperventilation, and hypocarbia. Radiographic examination reveals diffuse "fluffy" infiltrates. Measurement of wedge pressure by a Swan-Ganz catheter are generally low, suggesting that the origin of the edema is noncardiac and caused by increased pulmonary permeability[108]. Other causes of noncardiogenic pulmonary edema, such as direct chest trauma with contusion or aspiration, should be considered in the diagnosis. The diagnosis of NPE is made by exclusion of these other causes of pulmonary edema in a patient with a compatible history.

Animal models suggest that medullary ischemia is responsible for initiating the cascade of events that ultimately leads to NPE[107–109]. Medullary injury causes a massive transient neural discharge, which leads to a sudden increase in sympathetic activity. This increased sympathetic tone causes a sudden increase in pulmonary vascular pressure, as well as a shift in blood distribution from the systemic to the pulmonary vessels[107,108,110]. This transient response leads to pulmonary endothelial "stress" damage and impaired permeability that allows the transudation of protein-rich fluid into the alveoli[107,108,110]. In addition, sympathetically induced constriction of the pulmonary lymphatics, microemboli caused by disseminated intravascular coagulopathy, and lung ischemia caused by severe pulmonary vasoconstriction have been proposed to play a role in the development of NPE[107]. Medullary ischemia may be caused by the primary cerebral injury or to secondary ischemia. Clinical studies have failed to correlate increased ICP with the development or degree of NPE[108,111,112]. However, cerebral perfusion pressure has been correlated with NPE, suggesting that cerebral ischemia is necessary in the development of NPE[108]. Animals treated with beta blockers or cervical cord transection fail to develop NPE after head injury, verifying the central role of sympathetic discharge in this process[113,114].

Generally, NPE resolves if the patient survives. Few, if any, of these patients die of respiratory failure; most succumb from their neurologic injury. However, if not aggressively treated, NPE may lead to prolonged hypoxia and increase the secondary hypoxic damage in the injured brain. Additionally, NPE may complicate the management of these patients. High levels of positive end-expiratory pressure (PEEP) often are necessary to treat hypoxia in these patients; this amount of PEEP may impair venous return from the head, thereby increasing ICP.

NPE seems to be most severe in the spectrum of pulmonary complications after head injury. Other, less severe, forms of hypoxic respiratory failure are more common. In adult series, 50 to 85% of head-injured patients had an increase in the alveolar-arterial gradient and hypoxia[112,115]. Pulmonary edema is not recognized on physical examination or radiographically in most of these patients. Although the cause of this hypoxia is unclear, many factors have been implicated. These include neurally induced ventilation-perfusion mismatch, sympathetically induced depletion of surfactant, microemboli secondary to disseminated intravascular coagulopathy, and abnormal breathing patterns leading to atelectasis[107,108,116,117]. Abnormal breathing patterns after head injury are common[117] (Fig. 24.9).

Pulmonary infections are the most common infectious complication in head-injured patients[107,108]. Prolonged intubation and impaired airway protective reflexes are common causes. The organisms responsible for pneumonia in head-injured patients are the same as in any critically ill patient[118]. Pneumonia tends to develop early in these patients compared with other trauma victims[118]. Poor airway protection and aspiration immediately after the injury have been implicated, but no substantiating data exist.

Pulmonary management of head-injured patients is primarily supportive. Indications for intubation and positive pressure ventilation are delineated earlier in the chapter. Supplemental oxygen often does not resolve the hypoxia that develops in these patients. The judicious use of PEEP to recruit alveoli, lessen ventilation-perfusion mismatching, and improve pulmonary compliance is recommended. It should be recognized that high levels of PEEP impair cerebral venous return, thereby potentially increasing cerebral blood volume and ICP if brain compliance is low. The goal of therapy should be to maintain oxygen saturation at 90% or higher if possible to optimize cerebral oxygen delivery.

Other aspects of pulmonary care should be maximized in these patients. Overhydration should be avoided to minimize pulmonary and cerebral edema. Aggressive pulmonary toilet minimizes atelectasis. Airway manipulation is a potent stimulus for elevated ICP. Lidocaine (1 mg/kg) intravenously before suctioning may be helpful in minimizing this central response[93]. Intubation may increase the amount of agitation in these patients, potentially increasing ICP. Appropriate sedation techniques and neuromuscular blockade may be necessary to prevent patient-induced injury, allow hyperventilation, and decrease ICP. This issue will be discussed subsequently in this chapter.

Cardiovascular Management

A hyperdynamic cardiovascular response occurs after head injury, and is directly related to sympathetically mediated elevations of plasma epinephrine and norepinephrine[107,119]. As with NPE, injury to the medulla and hypothalamus are implicated as the cause of the sympathetic outpouring[107]. This hyperdynamic state can be blocked by beta antagonists[120]. Primary or secondary injury to the brainstem also may cause an increase in vagal tone.

The blood pressure of all patients with moderate to severe head injuries should be monitored closely. Patients with ongoing hemorrhage or third-space fluid losses may become hypotensive secondary to hypovolemia. The massive vasodilatation secondary to spinal trauma that will be discussed in the following section also may lead to hypotension. Conversely, hypertension is common in adults after head injury; no data exist on the incidence in the pediatric population[107]. There are two patterns of hypertension: associated with transient increases in blood pressure during posturing, and sustained hypertension[119]. The ominous association of hypertension with bradycardia and an abnormal respiratory pattern, or Cushing's triad should be recognized as signifying brainstem compression and impending herniation. However, in 25% of adult patients, hypertension is not related to increases in ICP[119]. In patients with impaired pressure autoregulation, hypertension may lead to increased vasogenic cerebral edema. However, the rapid and unmonitored lowering of blood pressure may lead to localized ischemia in some portions of the injured brain in patients with impaired autoregulation[119]. Therefore, treatment of hypertension should be done cautiously, and with close monitoring of cerebral perfusion pressure. The use of calcium channel blockers or beta blockers should be considered instead of direct vasodilators if treatment of hypertension is deemed necessary.

All patients admitted to the pediatric intensive care unit after head injury should have continuous electrocardiographic monitoring. The incidence of arrhythmias after head injury is unknown, but may be more common than previously appreciated in children[112]. Fifteen of 20 children without heart disease who were admitted to the pediatric intensive care unit after a neurologic insult had rhythm disturbances, including ST-T wave abnormalities and ventricular arrythmias[121]. Areas on the right and left ventricles receive sympathetic innervation from only the right or left stellate ganglion, respectively[122]. Additionally, some degree of lateralization of sympathetic tone exists in the hypothalamus in relation to the right and left ventricles[123]. It has been proposed that brain injuries may produce differentially right- or left-sided alterations in sympathetic tone that produce repolarization differences and allow reentry arrhythmias to occur[121]. In patients with multiple injuries, myocardial contusions also may cause arrhythmias, and evidence of myocardial damage such as the presence of new murmurs or elevated myocardial isoenzymes should be sought in these patients. If these findings are absent, neurogenic arrythmias should be considered. Standard therapy for tachycardic or bradycardic arrythmias should be instituted if they are associated with hemodynamic instability.

Hematologic Support

In a recent study, approximately one third of pediatric patients had disseminated intravascular coagulopathy (DIC) after head injury[124]. Another one third of the patients had one or more abnormal clotting test[124]. Brain tissue is a potent stimulator of DIC. The severity of the hematologic abnormalities correlated with the severity of the head injury[125]. Because of concerns about excessive bleeding, the presence of DIC complicates potential surgical procedures, including the placement of intracranial monitoring devices. Additionally, DIC has been associated with delayed and recurrent intracerebral hematomas[107,124,125]. For those reasons, it is recommended to treat DIC aggressively with replacement factors.

Nutritional Support

A hypermetabolic response occurs shortly after any traumatic injury, including head injury, and can last for several weeks[107]. An increase in sympathetic tone leads to a sudden increase in plasma catecholamine concentrations, which causes an increase in oxygen consumption[107]. Abnormalities in temperature regulation may lead to fever or hypothermia with shivering, which also increases metabolic demands. Excessive muscle activity such as seizures or posturing can increase oxygen consumption. Therapeutic modalities such as sedation or neuromuscular blockade or both may alter these changes. All of these factors make estimating the nutritional needs of these patients extremely difficult[126].

The massive catecholamine release also leads to a mobilization of carbohydrate and fat stores as well as enhanced hepatic gluconeogenesis, so hyperglycemia often occurs[107]. Hyperglycemia has been associated with a poor outcome in animal models of global ischemia[127,128]. However, its effect on localized ischemia is controversial[129].

Since the brain generally can use only glucose for energy metabolism, hypoglycemia should be avoided to prevent worsening secondary brain injury[128].

Several studies show an improved outcome in head-injured patients who receive early nutritional support[129]. The goals of nutritional support should be to provide adequate calories to support cellular metabolism, prevent catabolism, and promote healing. A positive nitrogen balance is optimal, but often difficult to achieve in these patients. Sufficient glucose should be provided to prevent protein-wasting; maintaining a normal serum glucose concentration is recommended. Either the enteral or parenteral route may be considered, depending on the patient's overall condition. Appropriate monitoring of nutritional support using standard methods is recommended.

Seizure Control

Posttraumatic seizures occur in 6.5 to 10% of children[130-132]. Posttraumatic seizures are classified as impact or early seizures (within 1 week of injury) and late seizures (occurring more than 1 week after an injury). Children are more prone than adults to develop early seizures, given the same degree of injury[133,134]. Early convulsions occur in 5% of children with minor head injury and 35% of children with severe head injuries[130,131]. Predisposing factors include a depressed skull fracture, dural or cortical laceration, hematomas, and posttraumatic amnesia longer than 24 hours[135]. Children are less prone to late-onset seizures than adults[133,134]. The risk of late epilepsy in children sustaining early or impact seizures is 15%[132].

Seizure activity has multiple adverse effects on the injured brain. Convulsions may interfere with effective oxygenation and ventilation, thereby potentially worsening secondary hypoxic brain injury and causing cerebral vasodilatation with a concurrent increase in ICP. Even if oxygenation and ventilation are maintained, seizure activity increases the metabolic demands of the injured brain. For these reasons, convulsions should be aggressively treated with standard anticonvulsants. Lorazepam (0.1 to 0.3 mg/kg) usually is effective in stopping seizure activity; its half-life is short, however, and long-acting agents such as phenytoin or phenobarbital should be administered. Phenytoin has some advantage over phenobarbital because of its nonsedating qualities.

CEREBRAL PERFUSION PRESSURE MANAGEMENT

Introduction

As opposed to global hypoxic-ischemic injury, aggressive treatment to maintain an adequate cerebral perfusion pressure has been shown to improve the morbidity and mortality in children with head injuries[81,136]. The specific treatment modalities commonly used are mentioned briefly below, but are extensively reviewed in Chapter 18.

Positioning

Traditional practice has been to maintain the head at a 30° angle and in a midline position to improve cerebral venous drainage. This lowers cerebral blood volume, thereby lowering ICP, especially when cerebral compliance is low[137,138]. Some investigators have questioned the effect of head elevation on cerebral perfusion pressure and blood flow[139]. However, a recent study showed a significant decline in ICP but no reduction in cerebral blood flow or perfusion pressure when patients' heads were elevated from 0° to 30°[140].

Sedation/Paralysis

Agitation and muscular activity increases ICP; presumably, increased respiratory tone interferes with cerebral venous return[141]. Patients with an altered mental status and agitation after a head injury may injure themselves or medical staff. Therefore, muscle relaxants or sedatives or both are commonly used in head-injured patients. Potential adverse effects of these medications are becoming more apparent[142]. Additionally, these agents alter patients' neurologic examination, making it difficult to assess changes over time that may reflect changes in ICP. Careful patient selection and frequent monitoring using a nerve stimulator minimizes side effects of these medications. Direct monitoring of ICP is recommended in patients who require sedation or neuromuscular blockade after head injury.

Fluid and Osmolality Therapy

Traditionally, head-injured patients were maintained in a negative fluid balance to minimize cerebral edema, but current management is aimed at maintaining euvolemia[143,144]. In an animal model, rats given large volumes of isotonic fluid did not develop more brain edema or have a worse neurologic outcome compared with fluid-restricted animals[145]. Maintaining adequate filling pressures helps ensure a normal cardiac output, thereby optimizing systemic blood pressure and cerebral perfusion. Overaggressive administration of fluid, especially hypotonic solutions, should be avoided. A central venous or pulmonary arterial catheter may be indicated in some patients to guide fluid administration.

Loop and osmotic diuretics are frequently used in head-injured patients. One goal of diuretic therapy is to maintain euvolemia. However, both types of diuretics have actions on the injured brain independent of their ability to remove excess fluid via the kidney. The loop diuretic, furosemide, has been shown to decrease CSF production, which may be beneficial when cerebral compliance is low[146]. Mannitol lowers blood viscosity and thereby improves cerebral blood flow[147]. Its effects on reducing cerebral edema remain unproved[148].

CSF Drainage

CSF is one of the three normal components of intracranial volume. The volume of CSF may be small when compared with brain and cerebral blood volume, especially in patients with hyperemia and cerebral edema after head trauma. However, patients with low intracranial compliance may experience a large change in ICP even with small changes in intracranial volume. Removal of CSF often improves intracranial hypertension in these patients. Further discussion about this issue is provided in Chapter 18.

Hyperventilation

Long the mainstay therapy in head-injured patients, recent evidence suggests that prolonged hyperventilation may be deleterious to these patients(149–153). Most patients initially retain their cerebrovascular responsiveness to changes in $PaCO_2$ after head injury, making it possible to reduce cerebral blood volume by lowering $PaCO_2$(18,86). However, evidence from animal models suggests that the cerebrovascular response to $PaCO_2$ diminishes after 24 hours of hyperventilation(154). Additionally, by lowering bicarbonate concentration and thereby altering the buffer capacity, prolonged hyperventilation seems to change the baseline cerebral vascular tone in an animal model, and renders the vessels more susceptible to changes in $PaCO_2$(154). Even short-term hyperventilation produces local cerebral ischemia and inverse steal in some patients(18,150–153). Several studies show that prolonged hyperventilation has an adverse effect on the outcome of head-injured patients(149). Therefore, hyperventilation as a therapeutic modality should be viewed with caution in head-injured patients. Ideally, intracranial hypertension should be treated using the other modalities enumerated herein, with hyperventilation being reserved to treat acute, severe rises in ICP that impair cerebral perfusion.

Corticosteroids and Barbiturates

Multiple studies have showed that corticosteroids are ineffective in reducing intracranial hypertension in head-injured patients(155–157). More specific, potent antioxidant therapies are being investigated(71,74,75,158).

The use of barbiturates in treating intracranial hypertension is controversial(159–162). The cardiodepressant effect of barbiturates makes their use in head-injured patients especially challenging because of concerns about lowering blood pressure and thereby cerebral perfusion pressure(162). At most, barbiturate therapy should be reserved for patients with intractable intracranial hypertension(160).

Experimental Therapies

Animal models of brain injury suggest that moderate hypothermia may protect the central nervous system(163). Presumed mechanisms by which hypothermia may reduce secondary brain injury include reducing cerebral metabolism, stabilizing cellular membranes, or suppressing excitatory amino acid release(164). Several prospective, randomized human studies in severely brain-injured adults cooled to 32 to 33° for 24 to 48 hours postinjury show hypothermia reduces ICP, decreases cerebral blood flow, and may improve neurologic outcome(164–166). No significant increase in side effects has been noted in the hypothermic patients(164–166). Further studies about the use of hypothermia in brain-injured patients seem warranted.

Other experimental modalities being examined for use in head-injured patients focus on minimizing the inflammatory reaction that leads to secondary brain damage. Antagonists of N-methyl-D-aspartate receptors are one example of these newer forms of treatment. These agents block excitatory amino acid receptor binding, potentially inhibiting the inflammatory cascade that results in secondary brain injury. Potent antioxidants such as the 21-aminosteroid U-74006F, have been studied in animal models of head injury. The administration of exogenous gangliosides has been shown to improve behavioral outcome in animal models of ischemic and traumatic brain injury. The data about the use of these experimental modalities has been extensively reviewed(71).

OUTCOME

Multiple studies have shown that the outcome of head-injured children is better than adults with a comparable degree of injury(4,167–171). However, these data do not seem to be true for children younger than 7 years of age; this may be partially because of the high incidence of abuse-related injuries in this age group(102,169,171,172). In general, the length of coma correlates with the degree of long-term functional impairment(102). Children with multiple trauma that includes head injury fare worse than children with isolated head injuries(2,3,4). Although the Glasgow coma score can be used as an early predictor of outcome in the pediatric population, it cannot be accurately applied to individual patients(173-175). The long-term rehabilitative process in these children will be discussed later in this chapter.

SPINAL CORD INJURY

Anatomy

The structure of the spine allows for a significant amount of unrestricted movement in the axial skeleton, while providing protection for delicate neural structures. The basic elements of the spine include the spinal cord, vascular structures, bony vertebrae, and encasing ligaments and musculature.

The spinal column is composed of 7 cervical, 12 thoracic, 5 lumbar vertebrae, and the sacrum and coccyx. Except for the first two cervical vertebrae, all of the vertebrae

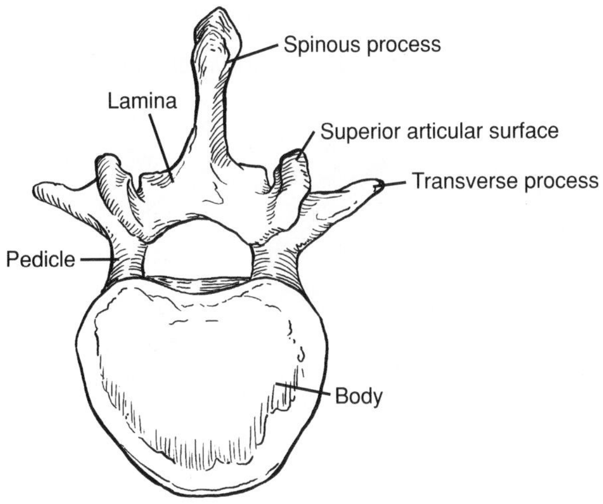

Figure 24.16. A transverse section view of a normal thoracic vertebra, which is composed of the vertebral body, paired pedicles with superior and inferior articular surfaces, paired laminae with transverse processes, and a posterior spinal process.

have a similar anatomic appearance (Fig. 24.16). The individual vertebrae interarticulate at the segmental level by virtue of the intervertebral disks and the superior and inferior facets (Fig. 24.17). The intervertebral disks are located between the vertebral bodies and are composed of a gelatinous center, the nucleus pulposus, and a tough fibrous covering. These disks provide a flexible and mobile articulation surface and also act as shock absorbers. The superior and inferior articulating facets are the lateral articulations of the vertebrae. The paired pedicles and laminae form a bony canal surrounding the dural tube that consists of the spinal cord, CSF, and vessels. Lateral openings, or foramina, allow the nerve roots to exit the canal. A complex system of tough ligaments provides strength and stability for the spine. The anterior and posterior aspects of the vertebral bodies are invested by ligaments. The ligamentum flavum covers each interlaminar space in the spinal canal in an interrupted fashion. The interspinous ligaments connect the spinous processes. Intracapsular ligaments are located at the facet joints. This osseoligamentous complex is essential for spinal column stability.

The spinal cord courses through the bony spinal column, traveling dorsal to the vertebral bodies (Fig. 24.18). Similar to the brain, it is enveloped in a dura mater and pia-arachnoid membranes. It is surrounded by CSF in the subarachnoid space. In general, the motor functions are concentrated ventrally, and sensory functions are located dorsally. Segmental nerve roots emerge from the dorsal and ventral aspects of the cord to merge as spinal nerves that exit through the neural foramina.

The blood supply to the spine is provided by the paired posterior spinal arteries, a single anterior spinal artery, and multiple radicular arteries (Fig. 24.19). The posterior and anterior spinal arteries are derived from the vertebral arteries and course down the spinal cord (Fig. 24.20). At times they become so small as to seem discontinuous. The radicular arteries are derived from segmental arteries (ascending cervical, intercostal, and lumbar) and course along the ventral surface of the dorsal roots. They are the principal blood supply for the thoracic, lumbar, and sacral spinal regions. Although the radiculating arteries anastamose with the posterior and anterior spinal arteries, these anastamoses may not provide sufficient blood supply to watershed areas in the thoracic spine during periods of hypotension.

The first two cervical vertebrae are designed to allow maximum rotational movement. The first cervical vertebrae, the atlas, is ring-shaped and articulates with the base of the skull. The axis, or second cervical vertebrae, has an anteriorly placed peg of bone named the dens, or odontoid process, that protrudes through the ring of the atlas. The dens is secured to the inner surface of the atlas by the transverse ligament; the integrity of the transverse ligament is crucial to the stability of the atlantoaxial complex.

Epidemiology

It is estimated that 1,200 new cases of traumatic spinal cord injury occur yearly; 1065 of these involve children(176). Spinal cord injury is more likely to occur in the 16- to 30-year-old age group than in all other age groups combined(177). Many adolescent patients are cared for in pediatric intensive care units. The leading causes of spinal cord injury in the adolescent and adult population are motor vehicle crashes, industrial accidents, gunshot wounds, and recreational activities(176,177).

Although uncommon, spinal cord injuries occur in younger children. Figure 24.21 shows the age distribution of spinal injuries in the pediatric population(178). Similar to older patients, boys are much more likely than girls to sustain spinal cord injury(178). **Table 24.5** shows the age-related differences in causes of spinal cord injury(178). Mo-

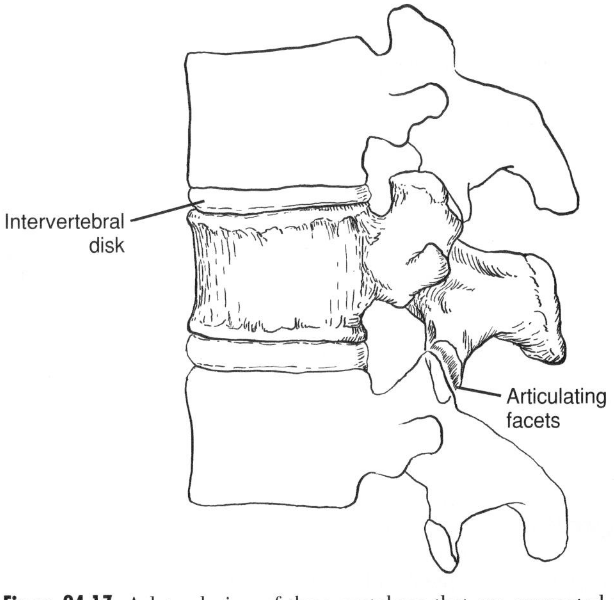

Figure 24.17. A lateral view of three vertebrae that are connected to each other via the intervertebral disks and superior/inferior articulating facets.

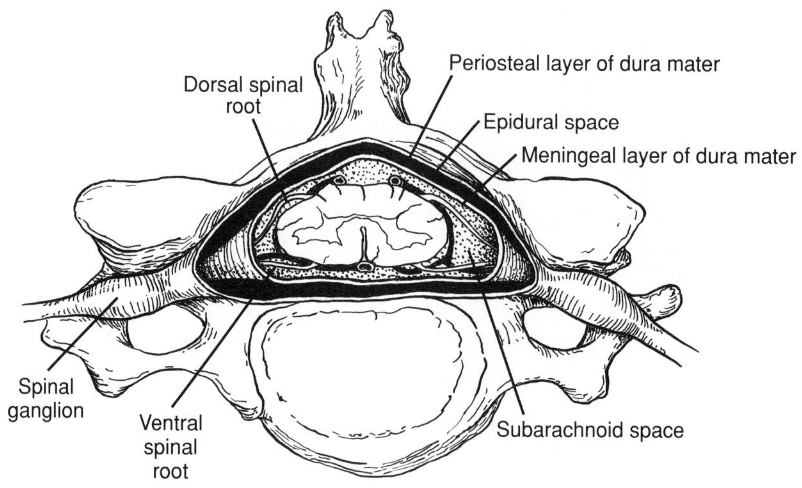

Figure 24.18. A transverse section view of the spinal cord with its associated membranes within the bony vertebrae. Segmental nerve roots and blood vessels pass through the neural foramina.

tor vehicle crashes are the leading cause of spinal cord injuries in all age groups[178–180]. Younger children are more likely to sustain a spinal cord injury secondary to a fall and are much less likely to suffer this type of injury during athletic activities. The location and type of primary injury differ in younger children compared with adolescents and adults; this will be discussed further in the next section.

Spinal cord injuries in children are often associated with traumatic injury to other organs. Head injury is the most common injury associated with spinal cord injury[178]. These patients often have decreased consciousness, making it difficult to diagnose a spinal injury on physical examination. Therefore, a high index of suspicion for these injuries should be maintained in all head-injured patients.

Primary Injury

Introduction

Injury to the spinal column occurs when traumatic force exceeds the structural tensile strength of the spinal column[181]. The location, type, and severity of the primary injury is proportional to the direction and magnitude of the traumatic force. It is possible for bony or ligamentous injuries or both to occur without injury to the spinal cord. Alternatively, spinal cord injury without radiographic evidence of bony or ligamentous injury can occur, especially in the pediatric population[178,182]. Identified by the acronym SCIWORA, or Spinal Cord Injury Without Radiographic Abnormality, this type of injury occurs when the excessive flexibility and elasticity of the pediatric osseoligamentous complex allows transient segmental subluxation followed by spontaneous reduction.

Bony Injury

Fractures in the bony elements of the spinal column are classified as stable or unstable. Stable fractures involve nonarticulating surfaces or bony elements anterior to the spinal cord, such as the vertebral bodies. They also include fractures of the transverse and spinal processes. Stable fractures are fractures that do not result in abnormal movement of spinous elements. Although the stability of the spine is not jeopardized, the possibility of bony fragments or disk material being forced into the spinal canal still exists. Un-

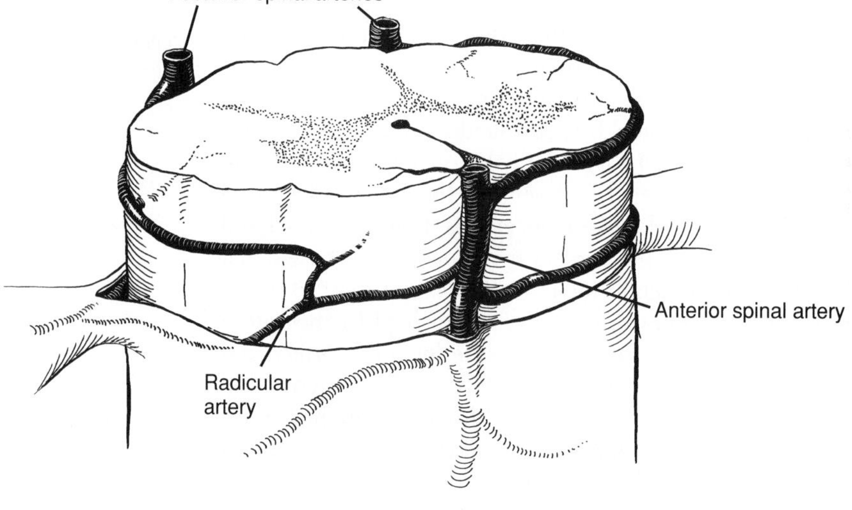

Figure 24.19. The posterior and anterior spinal arteries anastamose with the segmental radicular arteries to provide the blood supply to the spine. Disruption or compression of this blood supply secondary to injury may result in ischemic damage to the spinal cord.

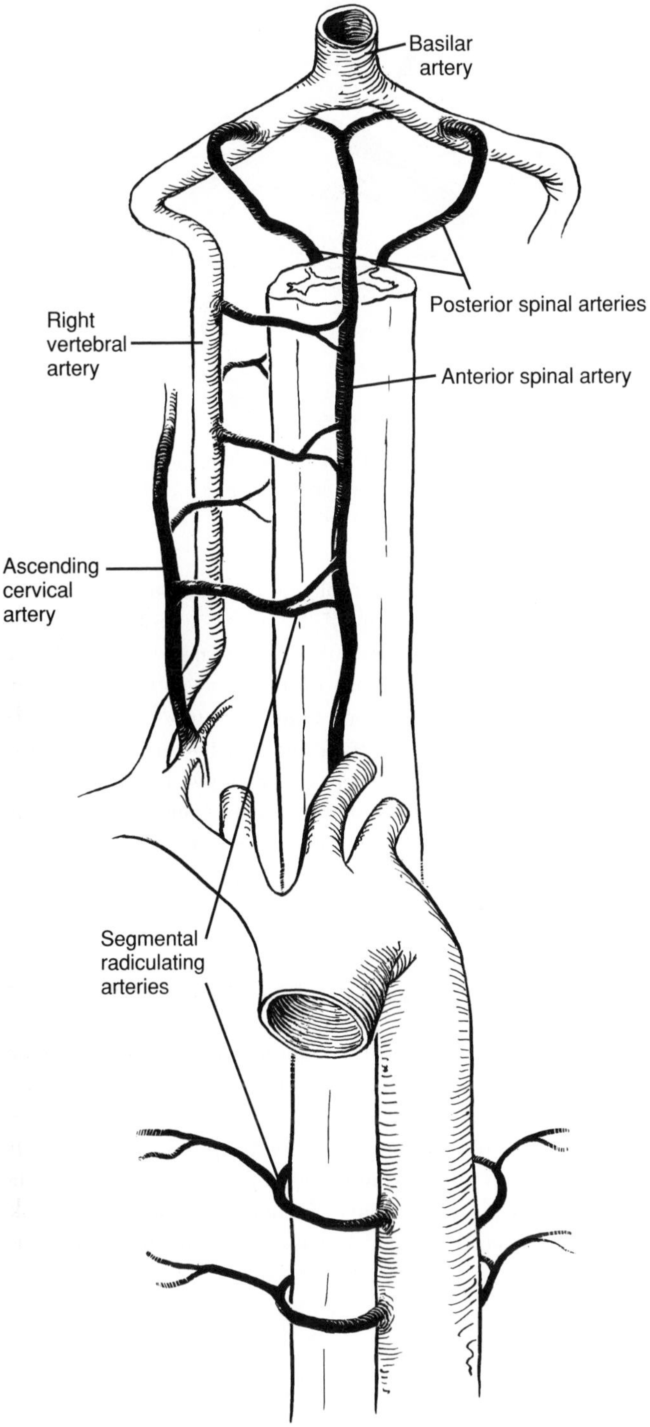

Figure 24.20. The paired posterior spinal arteries and anterior spinal artery are derived from the vertebral arteries. Radicular spinal arteries arise from segmental arteries such as the cervical, intercostal, and lumbar arteries.

stable fractures result in the potential for abnormal movement of the spinal column, with resultant spinal cord trauma. Because the posterior osseoligamentous complex is crucial in the stability of the spinal column, fractures involving the posterior articulating elements, the pedicles or facets, often are unstable.

Supporting Structure Injury

The accessory supporting or shock-absorbing structures of the spinal column also can be injured. Pure ligamentous injury can occur and lead to spinal instability. Similarly, traumatic disk herniation in the absence of a bony fracture can occur and lead to neural compression syndromes. Disk herniation in an anterior or posterior position occurs because of excessive flexion or extension. These injuries often are initially recognized by neurologic examination because the initial plain radiographs may be normal.

Spinal Cord Injury

Primary spinal cord injury is defined as the neuronal damage occurring to the spinal cord at the time of impact. Primary injuries may be classified according to location, type, and severity. Location refers to the specific vertebral level(s) involved. Neurologic deficits that are present are dictated by the level of cord that is injured.

Several types of primary spinal cord injury occur. The spinal cord may be compressed by displaced bony elements or herniated disks (Fig. 24.22). An impact injury refers to direct spinal cord injury from the cord striking bony elements at the time of injury (Fig. 24.23). A missile or laceration injury occurs when a projectile, such as bony fragments, a bullet, or a knife enters the spinal cord (Fig. 24.24). Finally, a distraction injury refers to stretching of the spinal cord (Fig. 24.25). Rarely is the cord transected at the time of injury; most primary injuries to the cord involve compression[(183)].

Spinal cord injuries can also be classified as complete or partial according to the resulting neurologic deficit, as determined on the initial examination. Determination of complete and partial injuries is discussed in more detail in subsequent sections. Although many factors may eventually influence the patient's outcome, this initial classification has some prognosticating value. In a recent pediatric series, approximately half of the children showed a complete spinal cord injury, and half had a partial deficit[(178)].

Table 24.5. Cause of Spinal Injury According to Age Groups

Cause	*Group I (0–8 yrs)*	*Group II (9–16 yrs)*	*Total*
Vehicular crashes	28 (45%)	72 (61%)	100 (56%)
Passenger	22	67	89
Pedestrian	6	5	11
Falls	15 (24%)	15 (13%)	30 (17%)
Athletics	1 (2%)	23 (20%)	24 (13%)
Birth trauma	10 (16%)	—	10 (5%)
Penetrating injuries	3 (5%)	5 (4%)	8 (4%)
Miscellaneous	5 (8%)	2 (2%)	7 (4%)
Total	62 (100%)	117 (100%)	179 (100%)

From Osenbach R, Menezes A. Pediatric spinal cord and vertebral column injury. Neurosurgery 1992;30:386.

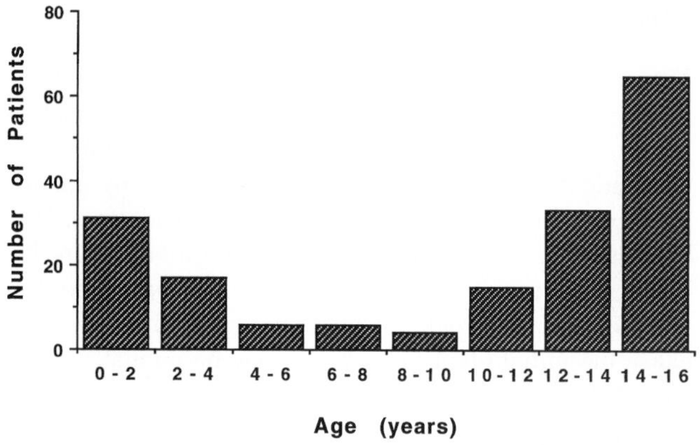

Figure 24.21. The age distribution of children with spinal cord injury. Printed with permission and modified from Osenbach R, Menezes A. Pediatric spinal cord and vertebral column injury. Neurosurgery 1992;30:386).

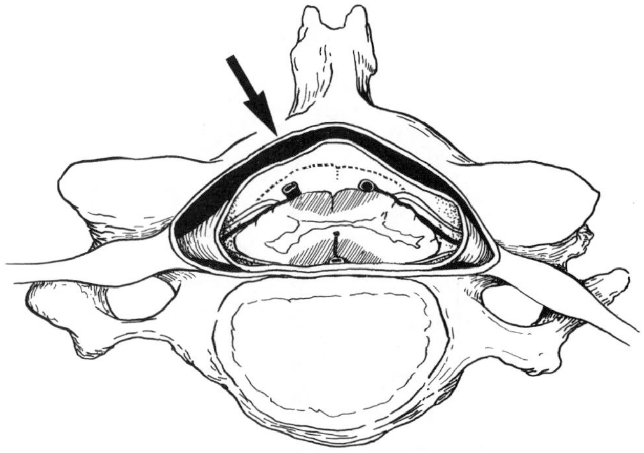

Figure 24.23. A transverse section view depicting impact of the spinal cord on the bony edges of the vertebral column and distraction as two mechanisms of primary spinal cord injury.

Pediatric Considerations

The vertebral levels involved in spinal cord injury differ in younger children compared with adolescents and adults. Children are more likely to sustain a cervical cord injury, and thoracic and lumbar spinal injuries are more common in adolescents[178,184]. Additionally, of all children sustaining cervical cord injuries, younger children are more prone to have high cervical injuries, and older children are more likely to have lower cervical spine injuries[178,184,185]. This may be related to the relatively larger head in younger children (causing a more rostral fulcrum in the cervical spine), incompletely ossified wedge-shaped vertebrae, and more horizontally positioned facet joints (allowing excessive translational motion in an anterioposterior motion). Minor trauma may lead to cervical cord injury in children with abnormalities of the bony structures such as juvenile rheumatoid arthritis or achondroplasia, or ligamentous complex such as Down's syndrome[186–188].

Nondisplaced bony fractures occur more commonly in adolescents and adults, but children seem to have more subluxation injuries without bony fractures[178,182,184,185]. The pediatric spine is hypermobile because of factors mentioned above. Increased ligamentous laxity and immature paraspinal musculature also contribute to the hypermobility. While ligamentous laxity protects the bony spine from fractures, it also allows for a high chance of ligamentous injury in children. Transient subluxation can lead to the SCIWORA syndrome in children.

Pathophysiology of Secondary Injury

In the past, most of the clinical management of patients with spinal injuries was focused on rehabilitation, which improved their functional outcome but did not alter their physiologic outcome. Similar to head-injured patients, little can be done to alter the neuronal damage in the spine that occurs at the time of impact. Secondary damage in the injured spinal cord occurs, and seems to add to the neuro-

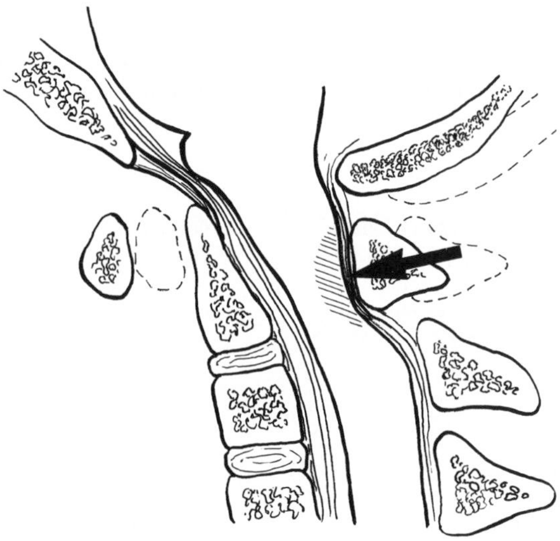

Figure 24.22. A lateral view depicting compression from displaced bony elements causing spinal injury. This is a common mechanism of primary spinal cord injury in children because of their hypermobile vertebral column.

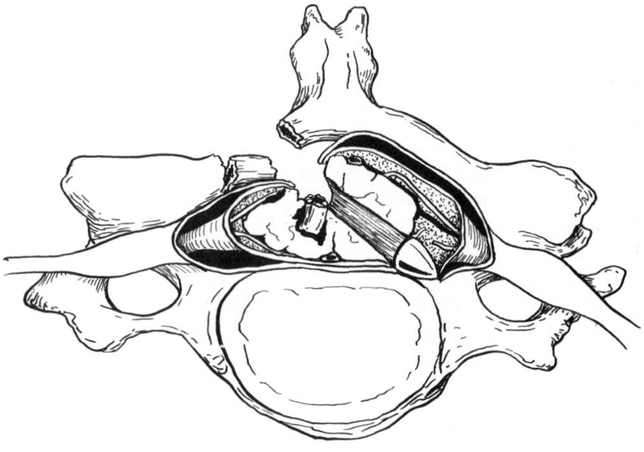

Figure 24.24. A transverse section view depicting laceration by a foreign body as a mechanism of primary spinal cord injury.

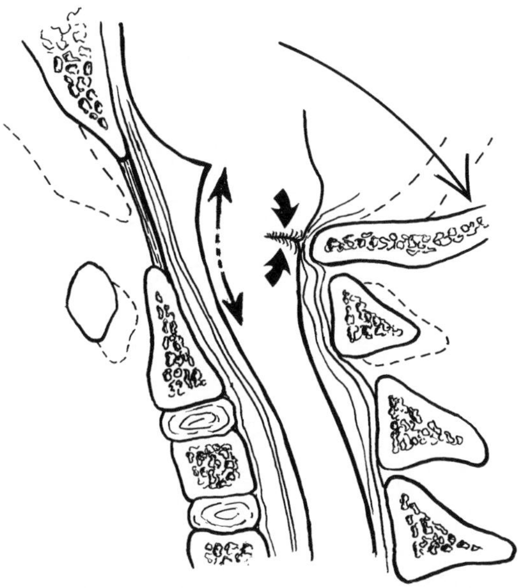

Figure 24.25. A lateral view depicting a hyperextension injury, which causes distraction on one side of the spinal cord and compression on the other side. Additionally, subluxation caused by ligamentous or bony injuries or both can cause further spinal cord compressive injury.

logic deficits ultimately experienced by the patient. Recent advances are beginning to improve our understanding of the pathophysiologic processes involved in this type of injury, and clinical management is beginning to focus on this issue.

Secondary damage to the spine can occur when respiratory compromise leads to hypoxia, or hemodynamic instability occurs. Patients with an injury above the fourth cervical vertebrae have paralysis of the respiratory muscles. Hypoxia from respiratory failure quickly ensues unless an airway is provided and positive pressure ventilation is performed. Patients with multiple injuries may be hypovolemic from blood loss, leading to hypotension and impaired perfusion to the spinal cord. Additionally, patients with disruption of sympathetic outflow secondary to spinal injury lose vascular tone and become hypotensive from decreased vascular resistance. This also leads to hypoperfusion to the spinal cord. Mechanical compression of the spinal or radiculating arteries from dislocated bony elements or hematomas also may lead to ischemic damage of the spinal cord.

However, secondary damage to the spine also may occur even in patients without obvious respiratory or hemodynamic instability. Similar to cerebral injury, activation of membrane phospholipases, release of excitatory amino acid neurotransmitters, initiation of lipid peroxidation, and the production of free radicals all have been implicated as the initiating events that ultimately result in cellular death after spinal injury[189–193]. These factors seem to lead to the production of eicosanoids, which produce vasoconstriction, enhance vascular permeability, produce edema, promote platelet aggregation, and cause neutrophil infiltration[189,194–196]. The result is that membrane permeability is disrupted, intracellular calcium accumulates, and cellular degradation occurs[197].

Injury to the spinal cord also is accompanied by mechanical damage to the microvasculature, which may contribute to secondary changes in oxygen and metabolite delivery. This phenomenon has been studied in animal models. Within seconds of injury to the spinal cord, petechial hemorrhages occur in the gray matter of the injured area. By 10 minutes of the injury, these hemorrhages are visualized in the white matter[198]. A reduction in spinal cord blood flow can be measured, which worsens over time[183,199,200]. By 24 to 48 hours after the injury, the injury site is necrotic. These pathologic changes seem to occur at the arteriolar level, while the major spinal cord vessels generally remain patent[183,199].

Initial Clinical Assessment

Primary Survey

Because the consequences of a cervical spinal injury are so devastating, any injured patient should be assumed to have sustained such an injury, and appropriate precautions to prevent further spinal injury should be taken by emergency personnel at the scene. These precautions include meticulous attention to immobilization of the cervical spine during extrication, mobilization, and transportation. If injury to the thoracic or lumbar spine is suspected, the patient should be immobilized on a backboard.

Similar to head-injured victims, the initial assessment and management of patients with a suspected spinal cord injury should focus on restoring and maintaining respiratory and hemodynamic stability. The primary survey should focus on airway, breathing, and circulation. Indications for establishing an airway and positive pressure ventilation are discussed in the previous section. Protection of the cervical spine during intubation in any injured patient should always occur. Spinal injury above the level of the fourth cervical vertebrae results in paralysis of all the muscles involved in respiration. These patients have poor to absent spontaneous respiratory effort. Injuries to the lower cervical spinal cord spare the diaphragm but abolish some of the accessory muscle strength, resulting in decreased vital capacity and retention of secretions. Although these patients have adequate respirations initially, they may develop respiratory failure over time as the diaphragm fatigues.

Interruption of the sympathetic outflow in patients with spinal injury above the level of the fourth thoracic vertebrae can result in neurogenic shock, with vasodilatation, decreased systemic vascular resistance, and hypotension. This form of shock may be difficult to differentiate from hypovolemia in patients with multiple injuries. The presence of a relative bradycardia considering the patient's age and hypotensive state can help to diagnose neurogenic shock; most hypovolemic patients have a compensatory tachycardia. Restoration of blood volume alone may not improve patients with injury-induced vasodilatation, and alpha-adrenergic

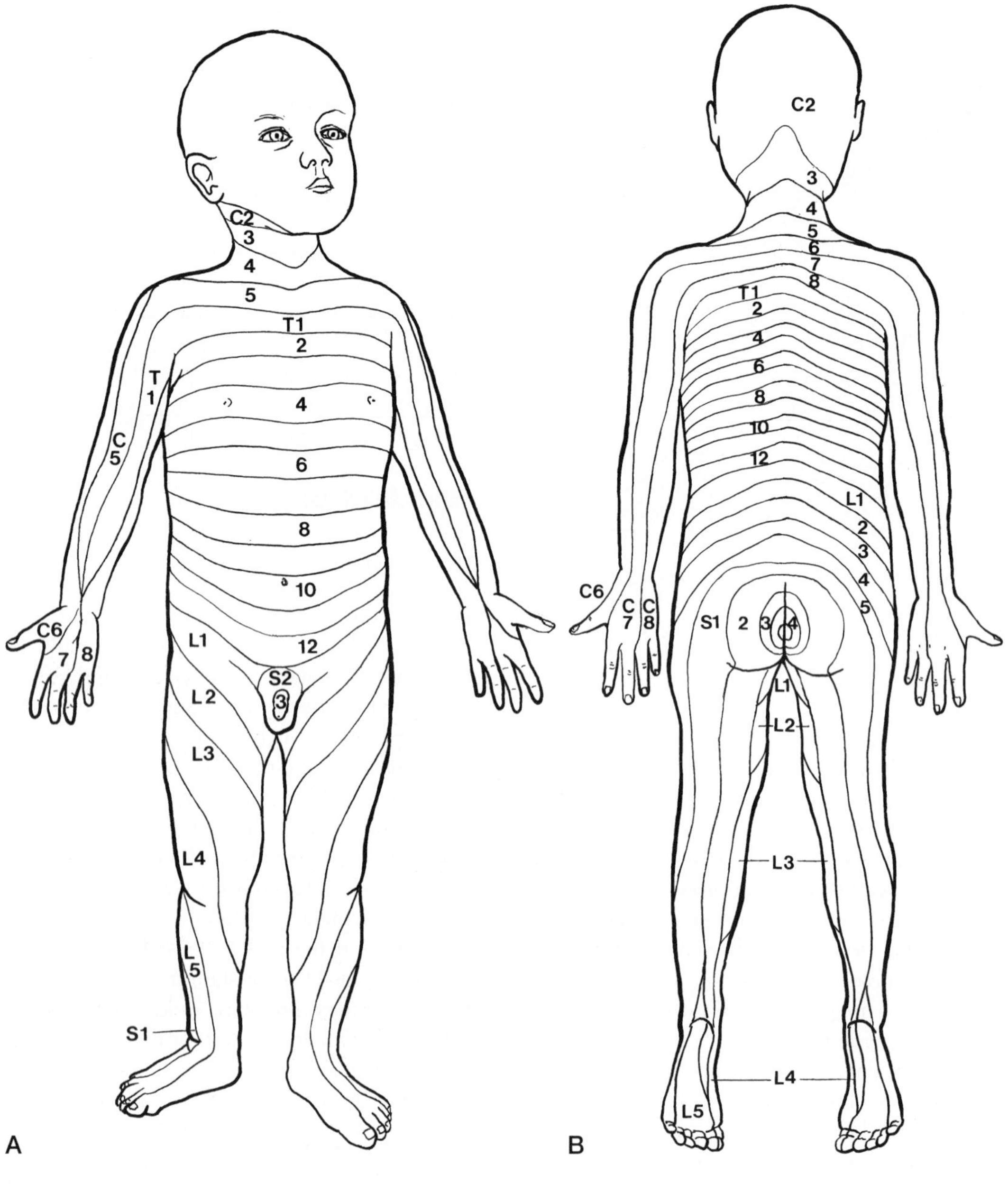

Figure 24.26. Segmental dermatomes are reproducible and helpful in identifying the level of spinal cord injury.

agents such as dopamine or epinephrine, as well as military antishock trousers, may be needed to raise systemic vascular resistance and blood pressure.

Secondary Survey

Other injuries should be identified and treated during a secondary survey. Although some of these injuries may be life-threatening, and therefore will take precedence over identification of a spinal injury, precautions to immobilize the spine to prevent further damage should occur during this time.

When feasible, the entire spine should be examined carefully. The patient should be logrolled to perform this examination. Ecchymoses indicate trauma in the region, and should be noted. The spinal column should be palpated, and widening of the spaces between adjacent spinous processes, malalignment of the spine, or stepoff of the spinous processes may indicate underlying distraction or dislocation.

The functional integrity of the spinal cord is evaluated by a thorough neurologic examination. The sensory and motor examinations have been described in the previous section. The sensory level is described according to the lowest dermatome in which sensation is normal (Fig. 24.26)[179,201]. The motor level is defined as the lowest segment in which muscle strength is assessed as able to move and hold in an antigravity position[179,201]. Key muscles for determination of motor level are shown in **Table 24.6.** Superficial reflexes such as the abdominal, cremasteric, and anal reflexes are helpful in localizing the level of injury in patients with spinal injury. Absent or diminished superficial reflexes suggest corticospinal lesions above the seg-

Table 24.6. Key Muscle Groups and Reflexes

Nerve Root	*Muscles and Function*	*Reflexes*
C-4	Diaphragm: inspiration	
C-5	Deltoid: shoulder flexion and abduction	Biceps (C-5, C-6)
	Biceps: elbow flexion	
C-6	Extensor carpi radialis: wrist extension	
C-7	Triceps: elbow extension	Triceps (C-7, C-8)
C-8	Flexor digitorum superficialis: finger flexion	
T-1	Interossei: finger abduction and adduction	
T-2–T-7	Intercostals: expiration, forced expiration	
T-8–T-12	Abdominals: expiration, trunk flexion	Superficial abdominals
L-2	Iliopsoas: hip flexion	Cremasteric (L-1,L-2)
L-3	Quadriceps: knee extension	Knee (L-3,L-4)
L-4	Tibialis anterior: foot dorsiflexion	
L-5	Extensor hallucis longus: great toe extension	Hamstring (L-5,S-1)
S-1	Gastrocnemius: foot plantar flexion	Ankle (S-1,S-2)
S-2–S-4	Anal sphincter: fecal continence	Anal wink, bulbocavernosus

From Massagli T. Jaffe K. Pediatric spinal cord injury: treatment and outcome. Pediatrician 1990;17:246, published by S. Karger, AG, Basel.

mental innervation of this reflex. Complete loss of sensation, segmental reflexes, and motor function below a given level indicates a complete lesion. Retention of any function below the level of injury indicates an incomplete lesion. The function classically retained is that of the sacral nerves. Thus it is imperative that perianal sensation and reflexes be tested and documented. A rectal examination should be performed to evaluate anal sphincter tone. An incomplete lesion has the potential for improvement.

Several patterns of incomplete lesions are recognized. The Brown-Sequard syndrome consists of ipsilateral motor weakness, decreased position, and vibratory sensation, and contralateral diminution of pain sensation below the level of injury. This results from lateral damage to the spinal cord, especially in penetrating injuries. The anterior cord syndrome consists of absent motor function and pain sensation with preservation of position and vibratory sensation. This results from injury to the anterior spinal artery that supplies motor tracts, the central gray matter, and the spinothalamic tracts. This may be seen in fractures involving displacement of intervertebral disk into the spinal cord. The central cord syndrome consists of bilateral arm weakness with relative sparing of lower-extremity function and perianal functions. This is caused by injury to the central portions of the cord from compression.

The presence of a spinal cord injury above the seventh thoracic vertebrae may mask the tenderness normally associated with an intraabdominal injury. A high index of suspicion is needed in these patients to diagnose intraabdominal bleeding. Ongoing physical examinations to evaluate increasing abdominal distention and rapid radiologic examination of the abdomen are helpful in diagnosis.

Neuroradiologic Evaluation

Contrary to neuroimaging of the head, in which CT is the modality of choice, plain film radiographs are the preferred imaging modality for imaging the cervical spine. Interpretation of these radiographs is often difficult, especially in children. The simple mnemonic ABC'S is useful in approaching a radiograph of the cervical spine. The letters of the mnemonic stand for: A, alignment; B, bones; C, cartilage (disks); and S, soft tissues.

Alignment is evaluated first. The lateral radiograph is most important for this purpose, and should be obtained as soon as it is clinically feasible. The radiograph must show the entire cervical spine from skull base to upper thoracic spine. Fortunately, this is much easier in children than in adults. Three curved lines can be followed easily with the examining eye. They are the anterior body line, the posterior body line, and the laminar junction line, which is

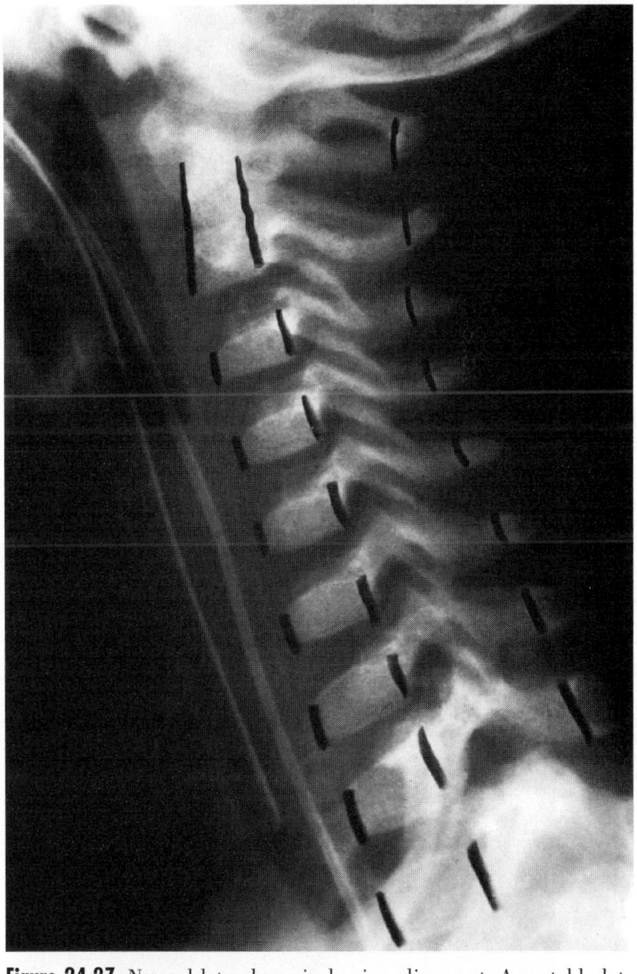

Figure 24.27. Normal lateral cervical spine alignment. A portable lateral cervical spine radiograph obtained in the emergency department on an injured child must show all seven cervical vertebra and the cervicothoracic junction. Three curvilinear lines are followed in assessing alignment. These are, from anterior to posterior, the anterior body line, the posterior body line, and the laminar junction line (each marked on the radiograph with a wax pencil).

formed by the union of the lamina in the posterior arch of each cervical vertebra (Fig. 24.27). With the spine in neutral position, these lines form a gentle curve reflecting the normal lordosis of the cervical spine. This curve may be straightened by the presence of a cervical collar or by muscle spasm from trauma or inflammation. In the younger child, physiologic subluxation, or pseudosubluxation, because of ligamentous laxity is normal. This is most apparent at the level of the C2-3 interspace, especially with the neck in any degree of forward flexion (Fig. 24.28)[181]. Alignment at the cranial cervical junction also should be evaluated. Without using all the formulas proposed in the literature, a normal relationship of the tip of the clivus to the top of the odontoid usually can be determined (Fig. 24.29). Flexion and extension lateral films of the cervical spine may be used to supplement the neutral position films. These films require the supervision of a qualified member of the neurosurgical or critical care team in a patient with impaired level of consciousness. Ligamentous instability and subluxation that is not present on the neutral views may be apparent on these films[178,181].

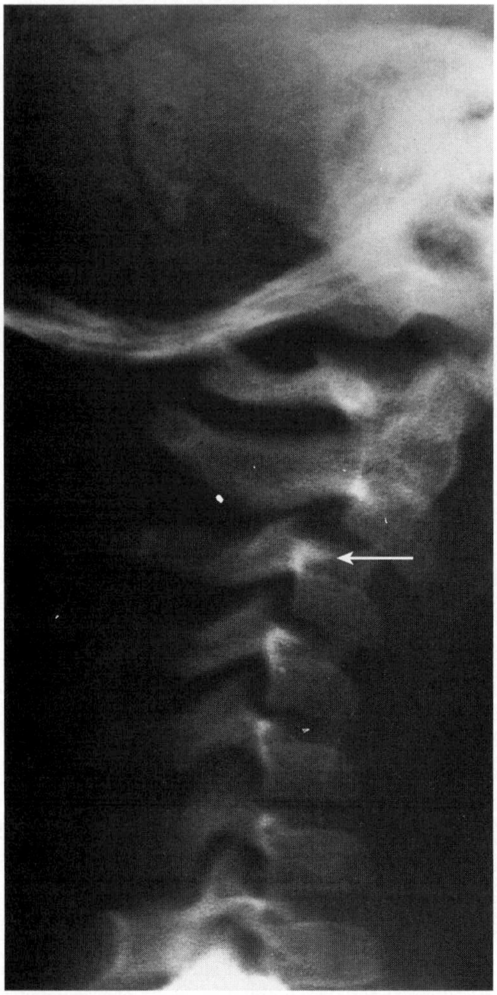

Figure 24.28. Pseudosubluxation of the upper cervical spine. Lateral cervical radiograph in a young child shows physiologic forward subluxation of the vertebrae of the upper cervical spine (pseudosubluxation), most prominent at the C2 to 3 level (arrow).

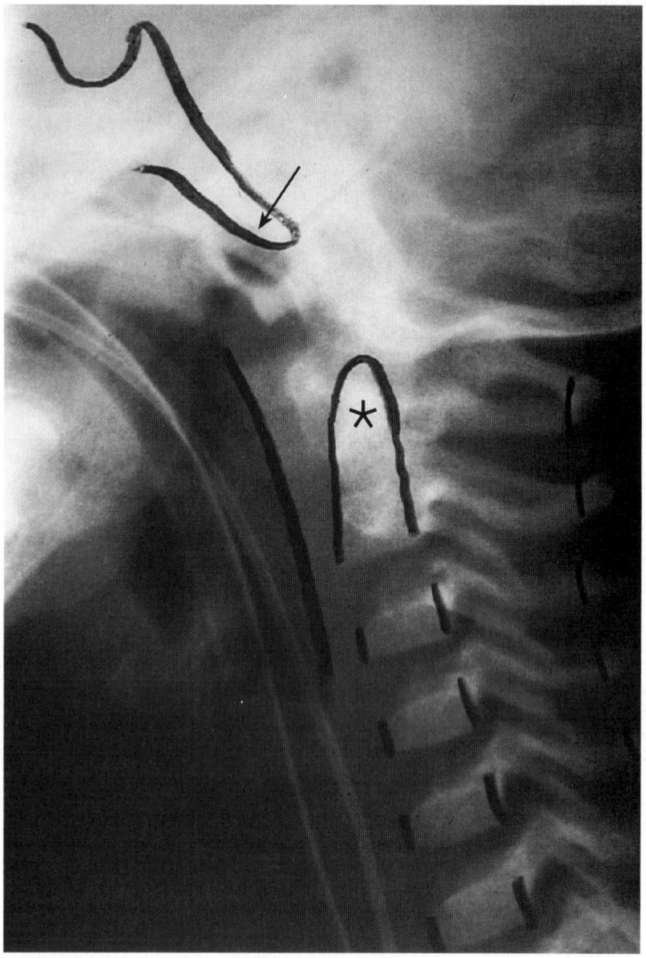

Figure 24.29. Normal craniocervical relationship. Normal lateral radiograph of the upper cervical spine and skull base in a child shows normal relationships of the tip of the clivus (arrow) to the odontoid (asterisk). Note also the cephalad portions of the three lines of normal alignment and the prevertebral soft-tissue line (all outlined on the radiograph in wax pencil).

Alignment seen in the frontal radiograph of the cervical spine is seldom abnormal, except in cases of vertebral fracture. However, the open-mouth view of the C1-2 relationship is important. This film is difficult to obtain at best, and almost impossible in children younger than age 3 years. The odontoid should be symmetrically positioned with regard to the lateral masses of C-1 (Fig. 24.30). Mild asymmetry usually relates to some rotation of the patient on the film. Significant asymmetry suggests rotatory subluxation. Odontoid fractures and os odontoideum are best evaluated by this technique. A pitfall in evaluation of this film is called "pseudospread of the atlas." In children between approximately 3 and 8 years of age, the atlas (C-1) grows faster than the axis (C-2), so that there is normal overlap of the lateral margins of C-1 on C-2 by 1 to 3 mm on each side. This simulates a ring fracture (Jefferson's fracture) of C-1, but is physiologic at this age. If necessary, CT of C-1 is confirmatory.

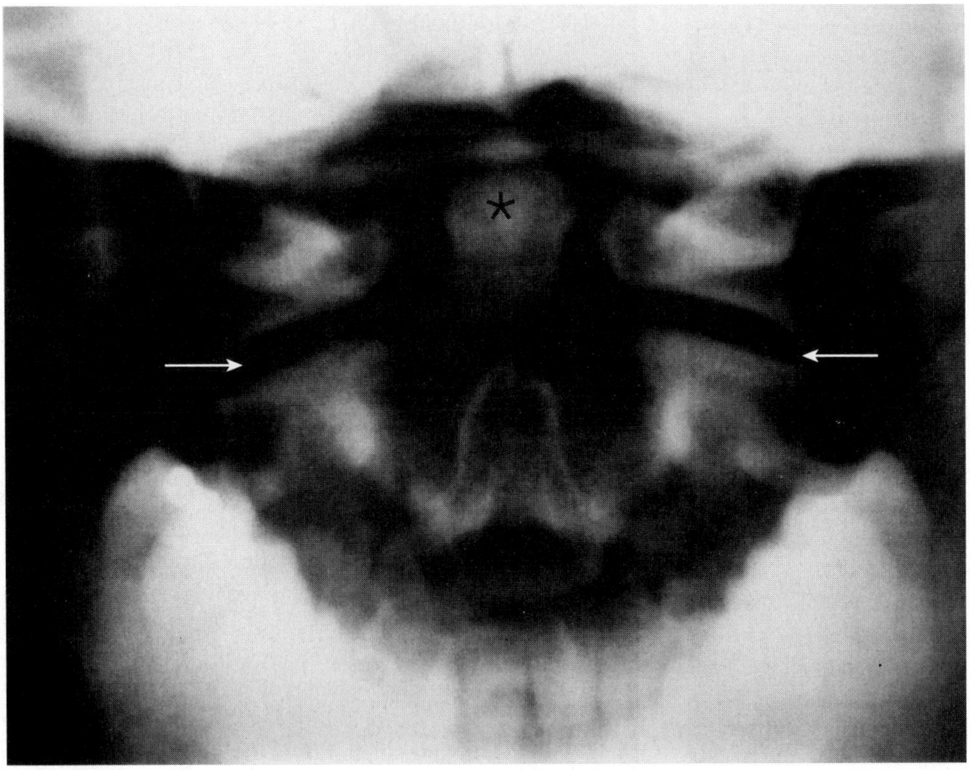

Figure 24.30. Normal open-mouth view. Anteroposterior radiograph of the upper cervical spine through an open mouth shows the normal relationship of C-1 and C-2 with the odontoid (asterisk) in the midline and symmetrical alignment between the lateral masses of C-1 and C-2 on each side (arrows). Minor asymmetry in children is usually caused by rotation or muscle spasm secondary to pain rather than to significant bone or soft-tissue injury.

The bones are evaluated for fracture (trauma), destructive change (histiocytosis, tumor, and infection), and congenital malformation (achondroplasia, dysplasias, segmentation, and fusion anomalies). It is important to evaluate the cartilage (disk) spaces for their normal height. Loss of the normal disk space may reflect a congenital malformation, disk herniation, or inflammatory change.

The soft tissues are evaluated for swelling in the prevertebral space of the upper cervical spine, which may be caused by trauma (ligamentous injury, fracture, penetrating injury), inflammation (retropharyngeal abscess, osteomyelitis, or diskitis), or tumor. Assessment of airway compromise from inflammatory or neoplastic mass may be possible.

Other modalities are occasionally useful in evaluation of the cervical spine. CT is used to evaluate fractures, especially at the craniocervical junction, or ring fractures of the vertebral bodies and posterior elements. Sagittal and coronal reconstructions of thin, overlapping scans obtained in the axial plane may have sufficient spatial resolution for diagnostic purposes when cervical spine injury precludes positioning for directly obtaining these projections.

MRI is the modality of choice for assessment of the cervical spinal cord in the setting of trauma (contusion, laceration, hematoma, penetrating injury, or infarction), inflammation (myelitis, abscess), demyelination (multiple sclerosis, postviral encephalomyelopathy) and congenital abnormality (syringohydromyelia, split cord syndromes, Chiari's malformations). MRI is also best for detecting hemorrhage or inflammation in the extraaxial (usually epidural) space of the cervical canal and is excellent for demonstration of vertebral body and disk abnormalities secondary to inflammatory or neoplastic disease (Figs. 24.31 and 24.32).

Nuclear medicine bone scans may be helpful in detecting traumatic, inflammatory, or neoplastic disease. Single photon emission CT nuclear scintigraphy is especially helpful in detecting subtle skeletal abnormalities of the cervical spine. MRI spectroscopy requires a motionless patient for approximately 30 minutes, often requiring sedation in the critical care setting.

Angiography of the carotid and vertebral arteries is indicated when the clinical findings and other imaging studies suggest injury or other abnormality of one or more of these vessels. This may occur in the setting of penetrating injury, skull base or cervical fracture, dissection, stroke, tumor, or retropharyngeal abscess.

Clinical Management

Spinal Cord

The first step in preventing further spinal cord damage from compression or laceration is immobilization. Next, if a subluxation is present, the bony vertebrae must be realigned and the spinal cord decompressed. This is often accomplished with cervical traction by gentle manipulation under fluoroscopic control, or Gardner-Wells tongs with weights. Acute surgical indications include a penetrating wound with an associated cerebrospinal leak or hematoma, failure of closed reduction, nerve root impingement, spinal cord compression from bony fragments, and initial fixation of some unstable fractures. Patients with a partial spinal cord injury and progressive neurologic deficit also should be considered operative candidates for decompression procedures. There is no evidence that surgery results in an improved neurologic outcome in patients with a stable neurologic exam. Halo braces and various external fixation devices also are used to maintain long-term immobilization while allowing vertebral column fractures to heal. In some patients, bone grafting and rigid internal fixation may be necessary to maintain stability of the vertebral column and to facilitate rapid remobilization.

Recent evidence shows that patients who receive intravenous corticosteroids shortly after spinal cord injury have an improved long-term physiologic outcome[202]. This is true for patients with a partial or complete spinal cord injury. Methylprednisolone 30 mg/kg followed by a 23-hour infusion of 5.4 mg/kg/hour should be administered to any patient with suspected spinal cord injury as soon as possible. The proposed mechanisms of action involve more than glucocorticoid receptor activation, and include facilitation of spinal cord impulse generation, enhancement of spinal cord blood flow, and decreased spinal cord lipid peroxidation[203].

Pulmonary Management

Pulmonary complications are the leading cause of death in hospitalized patients with spinal cord injuries, primarily secondary to pneumonia[204]. Patients with injuries above the fourth cervical vertebrae have an impaired respiratory effort secondary to muscle weakness, and initially often require intubation and positive pressure ventilation. Unless lung disease coexists with muscle weakness, these patients usually are easily oxygenated and ventilated using moderate conventional ventilator settings. Adequate pulmonary toilet to minimize atelectasis is essential. Patients with a loss of sympathetic tone may develop profound bradycardia during suctioning because of the unopposed parasympathetic tone; atropine should be administered to these patients before suctioning. The use of kinetic beds to improve pulmonary toilet has been suggested; however, no well-controlled studies showing a benefit are available. The use of theophylline to increase diaphragmatic function is controversial.

Independence from mechanical ventilation is a major determinant of functional outcome, as well as mortality, in patients with cervical spinal injuries. A recent adult study showed a significantly higher 5-year mortality in adults with

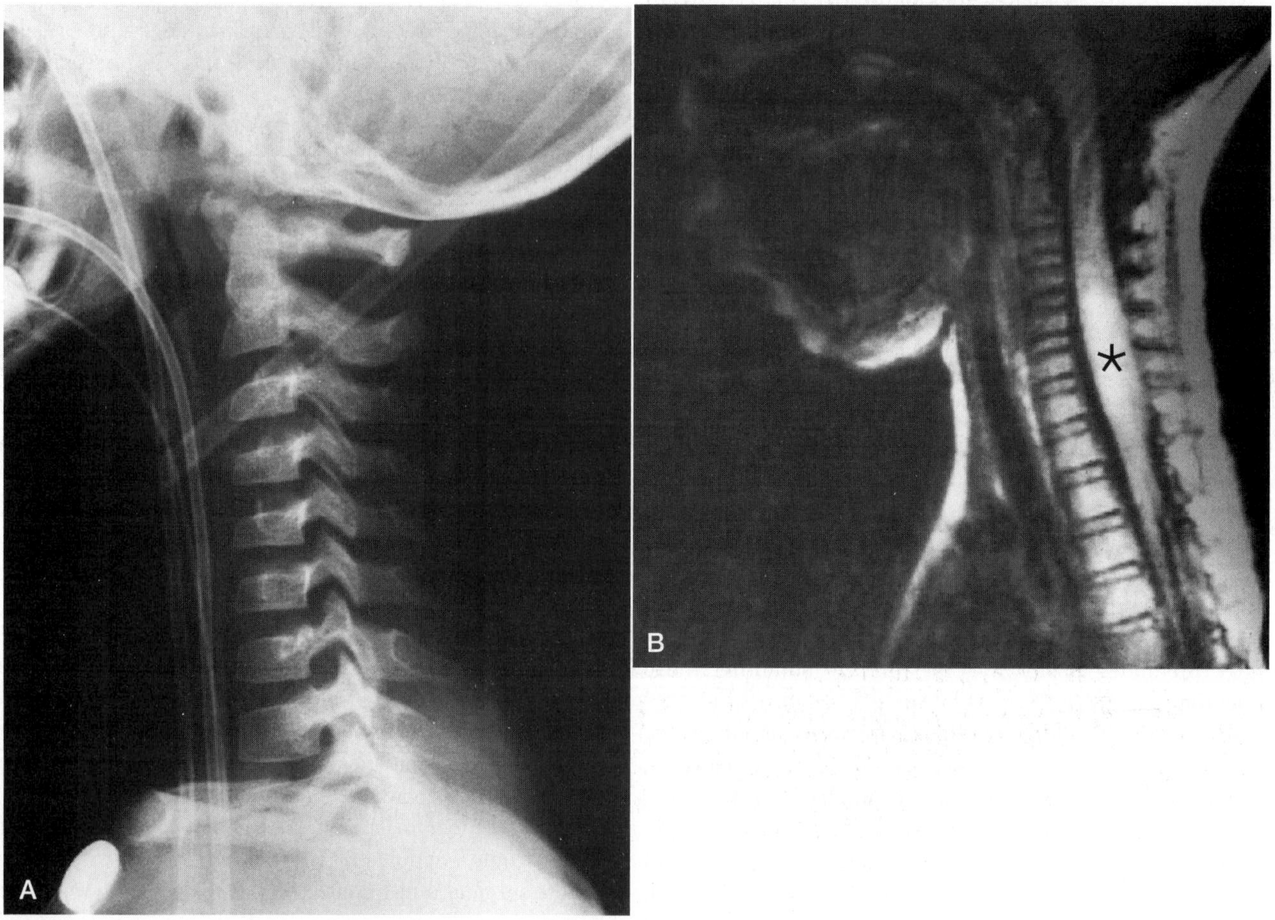

Figure 24.31. Cervical cord contusion. Lateral cervical spine radiograph of a child with upper spine trauma (A) is normal, except for loss of the normal cervical lordosis. However, sagittal T_1-weighted MRI scan (B) of the cervical spine shows fusiform swelling and increased signal in the mid-cervical spine cord (asterisk), indicating cord contusion or infarction.

quadriplegia who were ventilator-dependent versus those who were ventilator-independent[205]. Almost all patients with a C-4 or lower spinal lesion can be weaned from mechanical ventilation. No data are available in pediatric patients, but a study of adults with quadriplegia showed that more than half of patients with C2-4 lesions were eventually weaned from mechanical ventilation[205]. Because pulmonary function tends to improve during the first 4 months after spinal injury, weaning from mechanical ventilation can be a slow process. Data comparing the various modes of weaning patients with cervical spine injuries from mechanical ventilation do not exist. Various strategies, such as pressure support, designed to slowly increase the work of breathing may be helpful in these patients. Some patients may become ventilator-independent during the day, but require long-term nighttime ventilation. Newer techniques to improve the patient's chances for independent ventilation include diaphragmatic pacing. However, these patients need an intact phrenic nerve-diaphragm axis and chest wall stability.

Cardiovascular Management

Neurogenic shock with sympathetic interruption is associated with hypotension, hypothermia, and bradycardia. These patients may not mount a tachycardic response to hypovolemia, so aggressive monitoring of the intravascular space is required. For this reason, appropriate fluid resuscitation may require the placement of a central venous catheter. Vasopressor support also may be required. Bradycardia is generally responsive to atropine, but prolonged infusions of epinephrine or isoproterenol may be necessary. A transvenous pacemaker may also be considered. Although neurogenic shock eventually resolves, the patient may experience prolonged dysautonomia, with postural hypotension. Close attention should be paid to blood pressure changes associated with position changes in these patients.

Supportive Care

The long-term management of the spine-injured patient centers on meticulous nursing care and eventual rehabilitation. Frequent turning and careful skin care prevent decubitus ulcers. Foley catheterization with later intermittent catheterization prevents unnecessary bladder distention. Passive range-of-motion exercise several times a day keeps joints supple and prevents contractures. Early mobilization, subcutaneous minidose heparin, and intermittent pneumatic compression minimize the risk of deep vein thrombosis. Adequate nutritional support prevents muscle wasting. As discussed in the next section, early participation in the patient's care by a coordinated rehabilitation team is optimal.

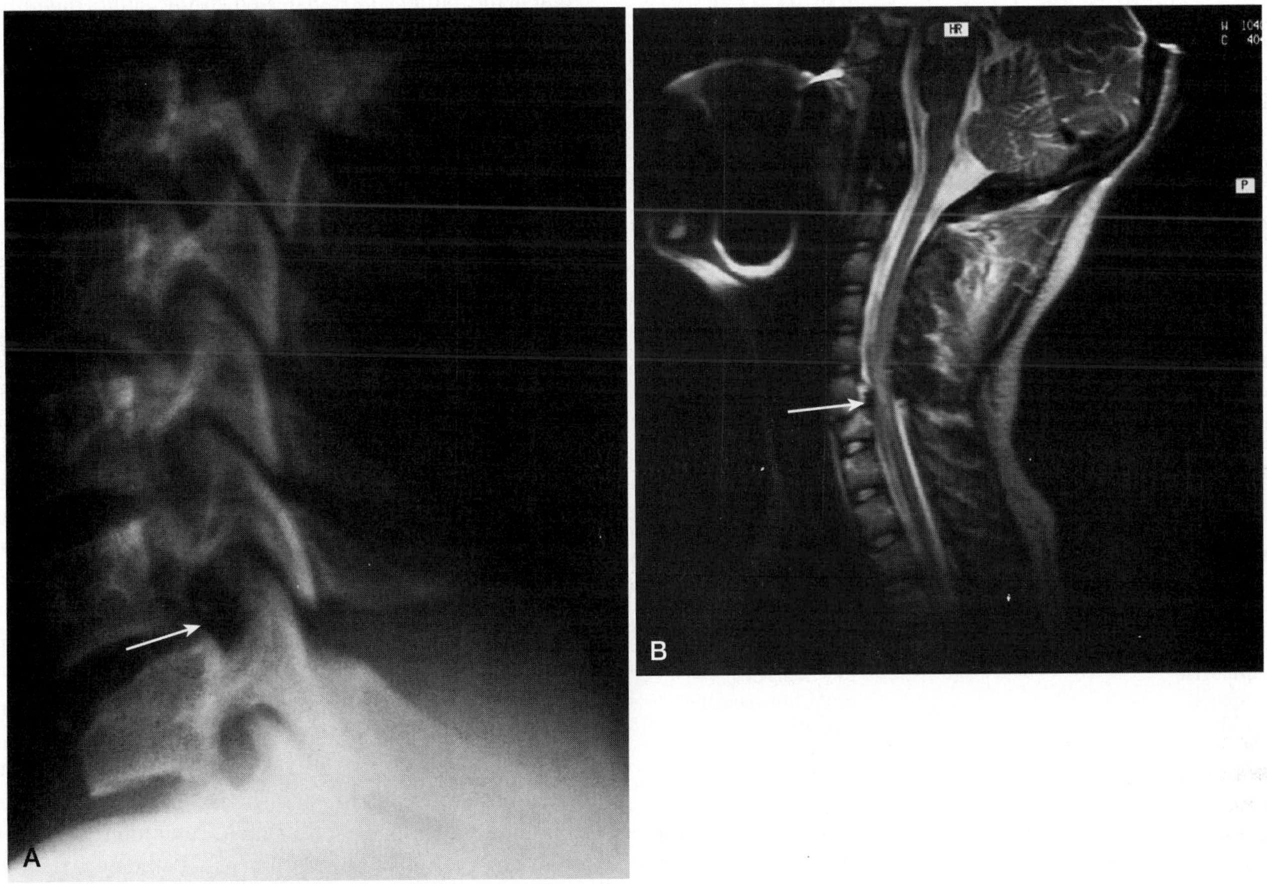

Figure 24.32. Cervical spine fracture with disk herniation. Lateral cervical radiograph (A) of a young teenager shows angular deformity of alignment at C6 to 7 (arrow) with anterior wedging of C-7, indicating a hyper-flexion injury. Sagittal T_2-weighted spine MRI (B) shows the bone abnormalities with hemorrhage and disk herniation at C6 to 7 impinging on the adjacent spinal cord (arrow).

TRAUMATIC BRAIN INJURY REHABILITATION

Introduction

As emphasized in the previous section of this chapter, head injury is a significant cause of morbidity in children today. During the past decade there has been an enormous increase in knowledge about the rehabilitation necessary after traumatic brain injury. The old adages "go home and learn to live with it" or "nothing more can be done" should no longer apply[(206)]. An increasing number of traumatic brain injury rehabilitation programs are available to help with the problem[(207)]. In addition, the US government, in its Education of the Handicapped Act Amendments of 1990, has added traumatic brain injury as a new category of disability, thus increasing funded research and services.

Definition

Interdisciplinary and interagency task forces throughout the United States have met to develop recommendations for providing services (within the education system, rehabilitation facilities, and public agencies) to persons with traumatic brain injury. One such task force defined traumatic brain injury as "an insult to the brain, not of a degenerative or congenital nature, but caused by a physical event, that may produce a diminished or altered state of consciousness." The injury may result in impairment of cognitive function, physical abilities, communication, or social behavior. These impairments may be temporary or permanent and may cause partial or total functional disability, as well as psychosocial maladjustments[(208)].

Rehabilitation of traumatic brain injury consists of an transdisciplinary team of professionals who coordinate the treatment and recovery of the patient with his or her family **(Table 24.7).** British colleagues have described the overall aim of rehabilitation as "the re-establishment of the maximum physical, intellectual, and emotional independence and dignity that is possible for that person in their particular environment"[(209)]. The World Health Organization defines *impairment* as any loss or abnormality of psychological, physiologic, or anatomical structure or function. A *disability* is a restriction or lack of ability (caused by an impairment) to perform an activity in the manner or within the range considered normal at a certain age. A *handicap* is a disadvantage (because of impairment or disability) that limits or prevents the fulfillment of a role that is normal for the individual[(210)]. Rehabilitation, through the interdisciplinary process, improves the impairment and thereby decreases the disability and the handicap. A transdisciplinary team often includes many people, as listed in **Table 24.7.**

Table 24.7. Rehabilitation Transdisciplinary Team

Patient	Social worker
Family	Nutritionist
Primary care physician	Audiologist
Neurologist	Psychologist
Physiatrist	Child life specialist
Consultants	Financial assistant
Nurses	Neuropsychologist
Occupational therapist	Teacher
Physical therapist	School personnel
Speech language pathologist	Educational specialist
Recreational therapist	Orthotist
Adaptive equipment specialist	Discharge planner
Case manager	Respiratory therapist

Obviously, even with "perfect" collaboration and cooperation, the number of people involved in the child's care can be overwhelming, especially in a crisis. Involvement of patient and parents with the team, improvement of communication, and coordination of services are critical to optimize care.

Medical Management

Rehabilitation can begin early in a child's hospitalization. Preventive and therapeutic intervention should begin in the intensive care unit during the acute stages of the recovery process. For example, active and passive range-of-motion exercise, proper positioning, splinting, and casting can help increase tone and thereby prevent contractures. Appropriate skin care and position changes helps avoid decubiti. A speech/language pathologist can assess comprehension, establish a functional communicative response, and evaluate bulbar function. Early family education about traumatic brain injury helps to decrease stress[(211)].

When the patient is transferred to the acute rehabilitation inpatient unit, continued careful management of medical problems is paramount to prevent complications and maximize rehabilitation[(212,213)]. Respiratory status must be carefully monitored, because aspiration is a danger after a head injury. Specifically, patients may have oral motor problems resulting in chewing and swallowing difficulties. If there is any concern about bulbar function, a videofluoroscopy swallowing study is obtained in conjunction with a complete feeding and swallowing evaluation by a speech/language pathologist. Adequate and safe nutrition, whether by the oral, nasogastric tube, gastrostomy, or parenteral route, is achieved by consultation with the dietitian, speech/language pathologist, occupational therapist, and physician.

Rehabilitation nursing is crucial in all stages of recovery. Decubiti are decreased by careful observation of the patient, with frequent turning and appropriate skin care. Special skin precautions are necessary when splints, casts, or braces are used[(214)]. Bowel and bladder problems must be anticipated and treated. Urinary tract infections are common, because many of the children are catheterized when in the intensive care unit. Occasionally a more complete urologic evaluation, including a cystometrogram, is necessary for appropriate bladder treatment and "retraining."

Orthopedic problems are common, because many children sustaining head injury also have skeletal fractures, usually of the long bones or clavicle. Nonunion of fractures can prolong the rehabilitation process. Pathologic fractures can occasionally occur secondary to osteoporosis. Periarticular heterotopic ossification can occur 1 to 6 months after head injury and is characterized by pain and swelling of the joint with decreased joint motion, especially at the hip, shoulder, elbow, and knee. This heterotopic ossification may be diagnosed by bone scan 2 to 3 weeks before radiographic changes are seen. Medical treatment of heterotopic ossification is controversial, but prophylaxis is not currently a routine practice in pediatrics[215].

Neurologic sequelae must be carefully evaluated, diagnosed, and treated. Obviously, the goal of treatment of posttraumatic seizures is control, it is hoped without the undesirable side effects of medications. Duration of treatment with anticonvulsants is controversial, but recent studies suggest carefully weighing the benefits of treatment against the possibility of additional neurobehavioral problems from the drugs themselves[216–219]. Decisions about long-term prophylaxis must therefore be individualized and should be made in conjunction with neurosurgeon, neurologist, and physiatrist. Before discharge, seizure precautions with regards to bathing, swimming, climbing, and hiking must be discussed with the parents and the patient.

Cranial nerve dysfunction after traumatic brain injury is common, often interfering with both acute rehabilitation and, ultimately, with schooling. Fractures of the anterior fossa may produce anosmia, at times associated with rhinorrhea. Visual impairment may be caused by direct trauma to the optic nerve, optic atrophy, extraocular movement palsies (resulting in diplopia), cortical visual field deficits, or complex disturbances of gaze and tracking. Although surgical correction is often delayed to observe spontaneous recovery, an early ophthalmologic evaluation is advised. Eighth nerve dysfunction is frequent in children with fractures of the temporal bone. A complete audiologic evaluation is necessary to diagnose this sensorineural hearing loss. Dysphagia and dysphonia are usually secondary to end-organ injury (or supranuclear injury) rather than cranial nerve dysfunction[212].

Posttraumatic hydrocephalus must be considered if clinical deterioration occurs in the patient. Symptoms of hydrocephalus (or shunt malfunction) often include decreasing responsiveness or increased agitation, headache, vomiting, or increasing spasticity. A comparative CT scan usually is diagnostic. However, often the radiographic changes are subtle, so neurosurgical consultation is critical.

Spasticity may be difficult to manage, even with intense therapy and medications. Other movement disorders requiring treatment may include dystonic posturing, ataxia, choreoathetosis, or tremor[220]. Specific treatment modalities are discussed in the next section.

Motor Dysfunction: Mobility

Independence in mobility (and the activities of daily living) is a primary goal, achieved by individual programs established by the transdisciplinary team. Through therapy, it is hoped that the child will regain developmental milestones and learn new skills for circumventing deficits. The transdisciplinary approach may be exemplified by the following example: occupational therapy may focus on the fine motor control and activities of daily living. However, the fine motor control is very closely related to proximal trunk control, one of the more classic physical therapy goals. Physical, occupational, and speech/language therapy integrate sensory discrimination abilities, visual motor abilities, perceptual-motor abilities, and general cognition[221,222].

Various physical and occupational therapy techniques are used to improve motor function while preventing contractures or deformities. In addition to the traditional exercises for strengthening and range of motion, management of spastic contractures may include splints, progressive inhibitive serial casting, motor point or nerve blocks used in conjunction with this casting, and, ultimately, tendon releases or transfers. Correct positioning and seating not only provides comfort but also helps decrease abnormal tone, thereby preventing scoliosis and contractures[212].

When physical modalities are not controlling spasticity, pharmacologic treatment must be considered, although side effects of these medications are common among head-injured patients. Dantrolene, diazepam, and baclofen are three of the most commonly used medications[223]. The benzodiazepines (diazepam and clorazepate) may cause sedation, enhance truncal hypotonia, and worsen bulbar function. Baclofen also may cause lethargy. Dantrolene may be less sedating but has increased potential for hepatotoxicity[215,223–225]. Recently, intramuscular injections of botulinum toxin in combination with increased stretching and splinting have proved to be effective in decreasing spasticity and contractures and increasing function[226-229].

Disorders of Language and Communication

Oral motor and bulbar function are initially assessed in relation to swallowing and feeding. The bedside examination performed by the speech/language pathologist or occupational therapist is an important screening procedure before any oral feeding. This initial evaluation includes a detailed history searching for factors that could cause bulbar dysfunction (e.g., neck injuries, prolonged intubation, brainstem trauma) and a history of problems with swallowing.

Behavioral and cognitive assessments evaluate alertness, combativeness and impulsiveness. The orosensory examination includes reaction to taste, temperature, and texture. The cranial nerve and swallow evaluation assess voluntary and reflexive control. Obviously, the gag reflex and protective cough reflex must be intact for safe feedings. Identification and treatment of abnormal reflexes are also critical. All patient care providers should be aware of signs and symptoms of oral and pharyngeal swallowing problems. These may include coughing during meals, difficulty chewing or manipulating food orally, increase in secretions during or after a meal, "gurgly" voice quality, spiking a temperature within 2 hours of a meal, and recurrent pneumonia. The importance of family counseling cannot be overemphasized, because parents often feel that if a child can eat, discharge is imminent[230–233].

If there is any concern about pharyngeal dysfunction that could result in aspiration, a videofluoroscopy swallow study must be performed. The purpose of this study is to provide the therapist with diagnostic information, including the efficiency of the oral, pharyngeal, laryngeal, and esophageal structures during swallowing; the adequacy of the patient's airway protection; the ways in which position, food consistency, and amount and method of presentation affect swallowing[234,235].

The specific cause of difficulties in speech production may be difficult to diagnose because often there are problems with dysarthria, dysphasias, and dyspraxias. Formal and informal assessment must include evaluation of the patient's receptive, expressive, and integrative language, and verbal memory. As with cognitive deficits, the identification of language disorders or comprehension deficits depends on the sensitivity of the assessment tools that are used. For example, the verbal proportion of the Wechsler Intelligence Scale for Children-R is inadequate to predict language disorders after traumatic brain injury because it relies heavily on the retrieval of information acquired before the injury, instead of requiring rapid, efficient processing of verbal information within a time limit, as is required in normal conversation or at school. Treatment of the communication problems obviously depends on the type and severity of the problem. Hearing must be adequately assessed in evaluating an auditory input deficit. Testing of central auditory processing also may be useful. Initially communication aids such as a picture board may be helpful. In the more severely involved children, augmentative communication may be necessary. At every stage of treatment, cognitive problems must be carefully evaluated for their impact on communication[212,236].

Cognitive Deficits

Cognitive deficits are often the most important sequelae of head injury, sometimes persisting long after the resolution of physical injuries. During the past decade there has been a significant increase in the therapeutic intervention of these deficits. Comprehensive cognitive assessment is critical to identify deficits (as well as assets), plan treatments, and establish appropriate programs at home and in the educational system.

Cognition consists of a myriad of interwoven cerebral activities by which we perceive our environment, store and retrieve information, make judgments, and respond through language or motor activities. Problems with cognition after traumatic brain injury may involve attention, perception, memory, organizing processes, reasoning, knowledge base, "executive" function, and functional-integrative performance[237,238]. Knowledge-base deficits involve the organized system of general information, without which new information is difficult to interpret, organize, and remember. Loss of this base also may imply a loss of social rules that apply to conversational exchange. The executive system relates to functions necessary to formulate goals and execute these plans effectively. Areas of executive system problems include self-awareness and goal-setting, volition, planning, self directing/initiating, self-inhibiting, self-monitoring, self-evaluating, and flexible problem-solving[239–242]. Problems with functional-integrative performance involve cognitive components that break down under the stress of time pressure, a demanding context, or interpersonal encounters.

Debate exists about the efficacy of cognitive rehabilitation but not about the impact of these problems on the patient and family[243–246]. Three basic treatment strategies have been suggested. The first involves *specific cognitive retraining,* in which the therapist helps the patient try to relearn or redevelop lost cognitive skills. The second approach, *functional remediation,* places the patient in a therapeutic setting in which cognitive skills must be exercised to achieve a specific goal. The third approach teaches *compensatory techniques* to cope with persistent cognitive deficits[247,248].

Behavioral and Psychological Sequelae

Various long-term behavioral problems are seen after traumatic brain injury. These problems often are a result of the injury itself, the child's frustration at his loss of ability, and misinterpretation of the child's behavior as intentionally inappropriate[249]. Because these problems are considered "organic," often it is believed that they are not amenable to change and that attempts to do so would be futile. These factors may combine to create a downward spiral of failure and further behavioral deterioration[250].

During the initial recovery from head injury, agitation is common, often making nursing care difficult. The patient may respond to internal, external, and environmental stimuli otherwise not normally perceived. All possible sources of discomfort must be removed, with care given in a structured, secure environment. Safety is an obvious concern. Consistent one-to-one supervision by family and nursing staff often is necessary. Transdisciplinary behavioral intervention often is ineffective at this stage, and physical restraints may exacerbate the behavioral problem. Medications are used sparingly, because they may sedate and further cloud the sensorium[251].

Various behavioral problems may present in the later stages of recovery from traumatic brain injury. Increased irritability and frustration, disinhibition, emotional lability, aggression, and socially inappropriate behavior may alter the way a child is viewed by family and friends. In addition, as patient insight occurs, depression and anxiety may complicate these behavioral problems[252,253].

A multifaceted approach to treatment is often most effective. Education (of patient, parents, and peers) about causes of the behavioral changes is critical to prevent escalation of the problems. Specifically, the abnormal behavior may be a combination of the direct result of the injury, the decrease in child or family coping ability after the injury, and the exacerbation of preinjury problems. More traditional behavioral modification techniques may be effective if they are modified to address the unique impairments of the head-injury population. Cooperation and consistency in behavior management helps eliminate undesirable behaviors and reinforces appropriate skills. Group interventions may provide support, feedback, and modeling, thus decreasing isolation and facilitating acceptance and reintegration. Often, counseling by various health care professionals is necessary to help head injury patients accept the trauma and adjust to the resultant changes and challenges[250,254–257].

Predictors of neurobehavioral outcome are varied and include the age of child, localization and severity of lesion, premorbid personality, previous injuries, and parental involvement. Pharmacologic treatment may be used in extreme conditions that are unresponsive to other methods. Medications are most commonly used in treatment of severe agitation and aggression. Varying success has been achieved with different agents, including neuroleptics, antidepressants, stimulants, lithium, anticonvulsants, benzodiazepines, and beta blockers. Any medication must be used with caution because it may lower the seizure threshold, adversely affect cognition, or produce a paradoxical reaction[258–270].

Educational Needs

When patients have left the inpatient rehabilitation setting, the public education system becomes a primary provider of services and a facilitator of ongoing recovery. The Education for All Handicapped Children Act (Public Law 94-142, Section 504 of the Rehabilitation Act), passed in 1975 and amended in 1986, required intervention for children with the following conditions: deaf, blind, hard of hearing, mentally retarded, multihandicapped, orthopedically impaired, other health-impaired, seriously emotionally disturbed, learning-disabled, speech-impaired, and visually handicapped. Unfortunately, children with traumatic brain injury often were not appropriate for these categories, and therefore did not receive the needed services. However, the 1990 amendments (Individuals with Disabilities Education Act, P.L. 101-476) added two new categories of disability: autism and traumatic brain injury.

Obviously, individual education programs are necessary for children with traumatic brain injury. They often perform "differently" from other students, even learning-disabled students. For example, because of confusion and lack of internal control, students with traumatic brain injury may be more impulsive, distractible, or verbally intrusive. In addition to inconsistent patterns of performance, discrepancies in ability levels may be more extreme. There may be more problems with generalization, organization, and integration of skills or information. There may be severe problems with organization of thoughts, cause-effect relationships and problem-solving[271–275]. Rate of recovery is often unpredictable, so programs must be flexible, with frequent reviews of the appropriateness of the school programs.

A smooth transition from the rehabilitation setting to the school setting requires early communication and an understanding of the demands and limitations of the systems. It is essential that a solid groundwork of communication and planning be established between health care professionals, rehabilitation professionals, educators, and families. Shortly after admission to rehabilitation, the school should be notified and previous baseline school records obtained. With appropriate patients, neuropsychological cognitive testing continues throughout the admission to plan (with the school), the appropriate goals, placement, and educational program[276]. Modification in the school program often is necessary to design optimal education programs for children with traumatic brain injury. Some characteristics of quality educational systems for traumatic brain injury pupils are listed in **Table 24.8**[277,278].

Family Issues

Traumatic brain injury can have a devastating impact on the family. The initial shock and fear about survival soon give way to concerns about the uncertain future. Stresses on the family unit are severe and often long-term. Bereavement is the normal response of parents who mourn their child's loss of certain abilities and characteristics. Emotional reactions are varied, but often include denial, anxiety, guilt, anger, frustration, depression, and despair. Understanding that these emotions are the "usual" responses to the crisis of traumatic brain injury helps the family, as well as the professionals who deal with the family.

Stress also may be reduced if parents are actively involved in the assessment and treatment process. Hopes, expectations, and fears must be discussed so that staff and parents are working toward the same goals. Family-oriented professionals can aid the coping process by being sensitive to the individual family needs and by being prepared for the stormy emotions that invariably surface[279–283].

Siblings are often the most overlooked of family members, but may be affected directly and indirectly in many ways. They may feel neglected and resent the time required to care for the patient. They may be angry about new or additional responsibilities or feel guilty about surviving and being normal. Adequate explanations concerning the injured child's injuries and limitations may help decrease

Table 24.8. Characteristics of Quality Educational Systems for Children with Traumatic Brain Injury

Flexibility
Low pupil-teacher ratio
Identification of appropriate environments
Cuing, shadowing experiences
Progressive functional and process-oriented instruction
Behavioral programming
Greatest possible degree of independence
Readjustment counseling
Simulation experiences
Reduced demands
Staff knowledge of traumatic brain injury
Ongoing evaluation and determination of services
Preparation for transitions

awkwardness in interactions within the family. Specific treatment and counseling depend on the age of the siblings and the situation surrounding the trauma. Support groups may be helpful in preadolescent and adolescent siblings[(284)].

Discharge Planning

The important process of coordinating and implementing an appropriate discharge should begin at admission to the acute rehabilitation unit. The successful critical transition from the inpatient unit to the home with outpatient services requires intensive planning by all of the professionals involved. A "seamless" continuum of care is the goal, often facilitated by day treatment programs. The case manager must consider current and future funding and community resources. The correct timing of home, school, and community reintegration must be carefully considered. The amount and type of continued therapeutic modalities is based on patient and family needs.

As has been previously discussed, successful school reentry is critical to avoid failure. Parents and professionals must communicate to prevent service gaps and to ensure continuity in programming. Communication between health care professionals, rehabilitation professionals, educators, and families must be established *before* discharge.

Compensation for functional disabilities may require many forms of equipment. Wheelchairs and accessories and orthopedic equipment may be required for variable periods of time. The home must be evaluated as soon as possible for necessary furnishing or architectural renovations. Often vehicular accessories and modifications are necessary.

Careful follow-up after discharge is critical. Accessibility of inpatient and outpatient health care professionals can help decrease the fear and stress surrounding discharge and thereby ensure successful transitions[(285,286)].

Outcome

Traumatic brain injury is a devastating event in the life of a patient and his or her family and friends. Early and effective integration of rehabilitation services into the system of trauma care is believed to decrease impairments and disabilities, thereby improving ultimate function and independence. However, with the changes in health care financing, demands for cost containment and outcome accountability are increasing daily[(287)]. Clearly defined goals with continuing reviews of the patient's progress are critical. In addition, every rehabilitation program must monitor and document its performance with standardized data collection and long-term follow-up. Results of rehabilitation to date suggest positive results, but appropriate documentation, standardized evaluation, and controlled studies are necessary to improve therapeutic intervention[(288–291)].

Possibly the most important aspect of traumatic brain injury is prevention. Injuries must be recognized as a major public health problem, with support being given for injury prevention research and for professional training. Organizations must be developed to help establish a broad-based education campaign. Causes of intentional injury must be addressed as part of the problem. Finally, safer environments for children may be established through legislation and regulation[(5,292)].

References

1. Division of Injury Control, Center for Environmental Health and Injury Control, Centers for Disease Control. Childhood injuries in the United States. Am J Dis Child 1990;144:627–646.
2. Lescohier I, DiScala C. Blunt trauma in children: causes and outcomes of head versus extracranial injury. Pediatrics 1993;91:721–725.
3. Walker M, Storrs B, Mayer T. Factors affecting outcome in the pediatric patient with multiple trauma: further experience with the modified injury severity scale. Childs Brain 1984;11:387–397.
4. Tepas JJ, DiScala C, Ramenofsky ML, Barlow B. Mortality and head injury: the pediatric perspective. J Pediatr Surg 1990;25:92–96.
5. Rosenberg M, Rodriguez J, Chorba T. Childhood injuries: where we are. Pediatrics 1990(suppl);86:1084–1091.
6. Kraus J, Rock A, Hemyari P. Brain injuries among infants, children, adolescents, and young adults. Am J Dis Child 1990;144:684–691.
7. Rivera F. Epidemiology and prevention of pediatric traumatic brain injury. Pediatr Ann 1994;23:12–17.
8. Beaver B, Moore V, Peclet M, Haller JA, Smialek J, Hill JL. Characteristics of pediatric firearm fatalities. J Pediatr Surg 1990;25:97–100.
9. Christoffel KK. Pediatric firearm injuries: time to target a growing population. Pediatr Ann 1992;21:430–436.
10. Callahan Henry P, Pickett Hauber R, Rice M. Factors associated with closed head injury in a pediatric population. J Neurosci Nurs 1992;24:311–316.
11. Kraus J, Fife D, Cox P, Ramstein K, Conroy C. Incidence, severity, and external causes of pediatric brain injury. Am J Dis Child 1986;140: 687–693.
12. Goldstein B, Kelly M, Bruton D, Cox C. Inflicted versus accidental head injury in critically injured children. Crit Care Med 1993;21:1328–1332.
13. Willging J, Bower C, Cotton R. Physical abuse of children: a retrospective review and an otolaryngology perspective. Arch Otolaryngol Head Neck Surg 1992;118:584–590.
14. Duhaime AC, Alario AJ, Lewander WJ, et al. Head injury in very young children: mechanisms, injury types, and opthalmologic findings in 100 hospitalized patients younger than 2 years of age. Pediatrics 1992;90:179–185.
15. Levy M, Masri L, Levy K, et al. Penetrating craniocerebral injury resultant from gunshot wounds: gang-related injury in children and adolescents. Neurosurgery 1993;33:1018–1025.
16. Reivich M. Regulation of the cerebral circulation. Clin Neurosurg 1969;16:378–418.
17. Siesjo B. Cerebral circulation and metabolism. J Neurosurg 1984;60:883–908.
18. Bouma G, Muizelaar JP. Cerebral blood flow, cerebral blood volume, and cerebrovascular reactivity after severe head injury. J Neurotrauma 1992;9;S333–348.
19. Cold G, Jensen FT, Malmros R. The effects of $PaCO_2$ reduction on regional cerebral blood flow in the acute phase of brain injury. Acta Anaesthesiol Scand 1977;21:359–367.
20. Obrist W, Langfitt T, Jaggi J, Cruz J, Gennarelli TA. Cerebral blood flow and metabolism in comatose patients with acute head injury. J Neurosurg 1984;61:241–253.
21. Muizelaar JP, Marmarou A, DeSalles A, et al. Cerebral blood flow and metabolism in severely head-injured children, 1: relationship with GCS score, outcome, ICP and PVI. J Neurosurg 1989;71:63–71.
22. Gennarelli TA, Thibault LE, Adams JH, Graham DI, Thompson C, Marcincin R. Diffuse axonal injury and traumatic coma in the primate. Ann Neurol 1982;12:564–574.
23. Levi L, Guilburd JN, Linn S, Feinsod M. The association between skull fracture, intracranial pathology and outcome in pediatric head injury. Br J Neurosurg 1991;5:617–625.
24. Rosenthal BW, Bergman I. Intracranial injury after moderate head trauma in children. J Pediatr 1989;115:346–350.
25. Bonadio WA, Smith DS, Hillman S. Clinical indicators of intracranial lesion on computed tomographic scan in children with parietal skull fracture. Am J Dis Child 1989;143:194–196.
26. Lende RA, Erickson RC. Growing skull fractures of childhood. J Neurosurg 1961;19:479.
27. Jamieson KG, Yelland JD. Depressed skull fractures in Australia. J Neurosurg 1972;37:150–155.

28. Henrick EB, Harwood-Nash DC, Hudson AR. Head injuries in children: a survey of 4465 consecutive cases at the Hospital for Sick Children, Toronto, Canada. Clin Neurosurg 1964;11:46.
29. Mealey J Jr. Pediatric head injuries. Springfield, IL, Charles C Thomas, 1968.
30. Lewin W. Cerebrospinal fluid rhinorrhea in non-missile head injuries. Clin Neurosurg 1964;12:23–52.
31. Robinson RG. Cerebrospinal fluid rhinorrhea, meningitis and pneumocephalus due to non-missile injuries. Aust N Z J Surg 1970;39: 328–334.
32. Jamieson KG, Yelland JDN. Surgical repair of the anterior fossa because of rhinorrhea, aerocele, or meningitis. J Neurosurg 1973;39: 328–331.
33. Jefferson A, Reilly G. Fractures of the floor of the anterior cranial fossa: the selection of patients for dural repair. Br J Surg 1972;59:585–592.
34. Rasf J. Post-traumatic cerebrospinal fluid leaks. Arch Surg 1967;95:648–651.
35. Mincy JE. Post-traumatic cerebrospinal fluid fistula of the frontal fossa. J Trauma 1966;6:618–622.
36. Leech PH, Paterson A. Conservative and operative management for cerebrospinal fluid leakage after closed head injury. Lancet 1973;1:1013–1016.
37. MacGee EE, Cauthen JR, Brackett CE. Meningitis following acute traumatic cerebrospinal fluid fistula. J Neurosurg 1970;33:312–316.
38. Klastersky J, Sadeghi M, Brihaye J. Antimicrobial prophylaxis in patients with rhinorrhea or otorrhea: a double-blind study. Surg Neurol 1976;6:111–114.
39. Shulman K. Late complications of head injuries in children. Clin Neurosurg 1972;19:371–380.
40. Einhorn A, Mizrah EM. Basilar skull fractures in children. Am J Dis Child 1978;11:1121–1124.
41. Hughes BJ. The results of injury to special parts of the brain and skull. In: Rowbotham GF, ed. Acute injuries of the head, their diagnosis, treatment, complications and sequels. Baltimore: Williams & Wilkins, 1964:408.
42. Rucker CW. The causes of paralysis of the third, fourth and sixth nerves. Am J Opthalmol 1966;61:1293–1298.
43. Bruce D, Schut L. Concussion and contusion following pediatric head trauma. In: McLaurin R, Schut L, Venes J, Epstein F, eds. Pediatric Neurosurgery: Surgery of the Developing Nervous System. Philadelphia: WB Saunders, 1989:271.
44. Ommaya AK, Gennarelli TA. Cerebral concussion and traumatic unconsciousness: correlations of experimental and clinical observations on blunt head injuries. Brain 1974;97:633–654.
45. Pickles W. Acute general edema of the brain in children with head injuries. N Engl J Med 1950;242:607.
46. Russell WR, Smith A. Post-traumatic amnesia in closed head injury. Arch Neurol 1961;5:4.
47. Rivara F, Tanaguchi D, Parish RA, Stimac GK, Mueller B. Poor prediction of positive computed tomographic scans by clinical criteria in symptomatic pediatric head trauma. Pediatrics 1987;80:579–584.
48. Levin HS, Eisenberg HM. Neuropsychological outcome of closed head injury in children and adolescents. Childs Brain 1979;5:281–292.
49. Rutherford WH. Sequelae of concussion caused by minor head injuries. Lancet 1977;1:1–4.
50. Niroshi T, Shozo N. Specific types of head injury in children, report of 5 cases. Childs Brain 1980;7:124.
51. Singounas EG, Volikas ZG. Epidural haematoma in a paediatric population. Childs Brain 1984;11:250–254.
52. Jamieson KG, Yelland JDN. Extradural hematoma: report of 167 cases. J Neurosurg 1968;29:13–23.
53. Ford LE, McLaurin RL. Mechanisms of extradural hematomas. J Neurosurg 1963;20:760.
54. Galbraith S, Teasdale G. Predicting the need for operation in the patient with an occult traumatic intracranial hematoma. J Neurosurg 1981;55:75.
55. Andrews BT, Ross AM, Pitts LH. Surgical exploration before computed tomography scanning in children with traumatic tentorial herniation. Surg Neurol 1989;32:434–438.
56. Tomei G, Gaini SM, Giovarnelli M, Paging CA, Villani R. Traumatic brain lacerations in children: surgical results and follow-up. Childs Brain 1981;8:434–443.
57. Bricolo AP, Pasut LM. Extradural hematoma: toward zero mortality. Neurosurgery 1984;14:8–12.
58. Shenkin HA. Acute subdural hematoma: review of 39 consecutive cases with high incidence of cortical artery rupture. J Neurosurg 1982;57: 254–257.
59. Britt RH, Hamilton RD. Large decompressive craniotomy in the treatment of acute subdural hematoma. Neurosurgery 1978;2:195–200.
60. Sinal SH, Ball MR. Head trauma due to child abuse: serial computerized tomography in diagnosis and management. South Med J 1987;80:1505–1512.
61. Johnson DL, Braun D, Friendly D. Accidental head trauma and retinal hemorrhage. Neurosurgery 1993;33:231–235.
62. McLaurin RL, Isaacs E, Lewis HP. Results of nonoperative treatment in 15 cases of infantile subdural hematoma. J Neurosurg 1971;34: 753–759.
63. Ransohoff J. Chronic subdural hematoma treated by subdural-pleural shunt. Pediatrics 1957;20:561.
64. Doberstein C, Hovda D, Becker D. Clinical considerations in the reduction of secondary brain injury. Ann Emerg Med 1993;22:993–997.
65. Chestnut RM, Marshall LF, Klauber M et al. The role of secondary brain injury in determining outcome from severe head injury. J Neurosurg 1993;34:216–222.
66. Miller JD, Becker DB. Secondary insults to the injured brain. J R Coll Surg Edinb 1982;27:292–298.
67. White B, Krause G. Brain injury and repair mechanisms: the potential for pharmacologic therapy in closed-head trauma. Ann Emerg Med 1993;22:970–979.
68. Kontos HA, Povlishock JT. Oxygen radicals in brain injury. Centr Nerv Syst Trauma 1986;3:257–263.
69. Hall E. Lipid antioxidants in acute central nervous system injury. Ann Emerg Med 1993;22:1022–1027.
70. Schoettle R, Kochanek P, Magargee MJ, Uhl M, Nemoto E. Early polymorphonuclear leukocyte accumulation correlates with the development of posttraumatic cerebral edema in rats. J Neurotrauma 1990;7: 207–217.
71. McIntosh T. Novel pharmacologic therapies in the treatment of experimental traumatic brain injury: a review. J Neurotrauma 1993;10: 215–261.
72. Siesjo B. Basic mechanisms of traumatic brain damage. Ann Emerg Med 1993;22:959–969.
73. Wei EP, Ellison MD, Kontos HA, Povlishock J. O_2 radicals in arachidonate-induced increased blood-brain barrier permeability to proteins. Am J Physiol 1986;25:H693–699.
74. Hall ED, Yonkers PA, McCall JM, Braughler JM. Effects of the 21-aminosteroid U74006F on experimental head injury in mice. J Neurosurg 1988;68:456–461.
75. McIntosh TK, Thomas M, Smith DF, Banbury M. The novel 21-aminosteroid U74006F attenuates cerebral edema and improves survival after brain injury in the rat. J Neurotrauma 1992;9:33–46.
76. Faden AI, Demediuk P, Panter SS, Vink R. The role of excitatory amino acids and NMDA receptors in traumatic brain injury. Science 1989;244:798–800.
77. Olney JW. Inciting excitotoxic cytocide among central neurons. Adv Exp Mol Biol 1986;203:631–645.
78. Gentile N, McIntosh T. Antagonists of excitatory amino acids and endogenous opioid peptides in the treatment of experimental central nervous system injury. Ann Emerg Med 1993;22:1028–1034.
79. Aldrich EF, Eisenberg HM, Saydjari C, et al. Diffuse brain swelling in severely head-injured children: a report from the NIH Traumatic Coma Data Bank. J Neurosurg 1992;76:450–454.
80. Bruce D, Raphaely R, Goldberg A, et al. Pathophysiology, treatment and outcome following severe head injury in children. Childs Brain 1979;5:174–191.
81. Saul T, Ducker T. Effect of intracranial pressure monitoring and aggressive treatment on mortality in severe head injury. J Neurosurg 1982;56:498–503.
82. Bruce D, Alavi A, Bilaniu, L, Dolinskas C, Obrist W, Uzzell B. Diffuse cerebral swelling following head injuries in children: the syndrome of "malignant brain edema." J Neurosurg 1981;54:170–178.
83. Zimmerman R, Bilaniuk L, Bruce D, Dolinskas C, Obrist W, Kuhl D. Computed tomography of pediatric head trauma: acute general cerebral swelling. Radiology 1978;126:403–408.
84. Lang D, Teasdale G, MacPherson P, Lawrence A. Diffuse brain swelling after head injury: more often malignant in adults than children? J Neurosurg 1994;80:675–680.
85. Overgaard J, Mosdal C, Tweed W. Cerebral circulation after head injury, 3: does reduced regional cerebral blood flow determine recovery of brain function after blunt head injury? J Neurosurg 1981; 55:63–74.
86. Jaggi J, Obrist W, Gennarelli T, Langfitt T. Relationship of early cerebral blood flow and metabolism to outcome in acute head injury. J Neurosurg 1990;72:176–182.

87. Grundl P, Biagas K, Kochanek P, Schiding J, Barmada M, Nemoto E. Early cerebrovascular response to head injury in immature and mature rats. J Neurotrauma 1994;11:135–148.
88. Enevoldsen E, Jensen F. Autoregulation and CO_2 responses of cerebral blood flow in patients with acute severe head injury. J Neurosurg 1978;48:689–703.
89. Bouma FG, Muizelaar JP. The relationship between cardiac output and cerebral blood flow in patients with intact and with impaired autoregulation. J Neurosurg 1990;73:368–374.
90. Graham DI, Adams JH. Ischaemic brain damage in fatal head injuries. Lancet 1971;1:265–266.
91. Weber M, Grolimund P, Seiler RW. Evaluation of postraumatic cerebral blood flow velocities by transcranial doppler ultrasonography. Neurosurgery 1990;27:106–112.
92. Bouma G, Muizelaar JP, Stringer W, Choi S, Fatouros P, Young H. Ultra-early evaluation of regional cerebral blood flow in severely head-injured patients using xenon-enhanced computerized tomography. J Neurosurg 1992;77:360-368.
93. Hamill JF, Bedford RF, Weaver DC, Colohan AR. Lidocaine before endotracheal intubation: intravenous or laryngeotracheal? Anesthesiology 1981;55;578–581.
94. Minton MD, Grosslight K, Stirt JA, Bedford RF. Increases in intracranial pressure from succinylcholine: prevention by prior nondepolarizing blockade. Anesthesiology 1986;65:165–169.
95. Stirt JA, Grosslight KR, Bedford RF, Vollmer D. "Desfasciculation" with metocurine prevents succinylcholine-induced increases in intracranial pressure. Anesthesiology 1987;67:50–53.
96. Teasdale G, Knill-Jones R, Van der Sande J. Observer variability in assessing impared consciousness and coma. J Neurol Neurosurg Psychiatry 1978;41:603–610.
97. Zimmerman RA, Bilaniuk LT, Gennarelli T. Computerized tomography of shearing injuries of the cerebral white matter. Radiology 1978;127:393–396.
98. Johnson M, Lee SH. Computed tomography of acute cerebral trauma. Radiol Clin North Am 1992;30:325–352.
99. Pascucci RC. Head trauma in the child. Intensive Care Med 1988;14:185–195.
100. Khellemmes P, Lejeune JP, Christiaens JL, Combelles G. Traumatic extradural hematomas in infancy and childhood. J Neurosurg 1985;62:861–864.
101. Sklar E, Quencer R, Bowen B, Altman N, Villanueva P. Magnetic resonance applications in cerebral injury. Radiol Clin North Am 1992; 30:353–366.
102. Gomori J, Grossman R, Goldberg H, Zimmerman R, Bilaniuk L. Intracranial hematomas: imaging by high-field MR. Radiology 1985;157: 87–93.
103. Goldstein B, Powers K. Head trauma in children. Pediatr Rev 1994;15:213–219.
104. Simmon R, Martin A, Heisterkamp C, Ducker TB. Respiratory insufficiency in combat casualties, II: pulmonary edema following head injury. Ann Surg 1969;17:39–62.
105. Weisman S. Edema and congestion of the lungs resulting from intracranial hemorrhage. Surgery 1939;6:722–729.
106. Singbartl G, Cunitz G, Hamrouni H. Disturbed pulmonary gas exchange in patients with cerebral edema. Anesthetist 1982;31:228–233.
107. Kaufman H, Timberlake G, Voelker J, Pait TG. Medical complications of head injury. Med Clin North Am 1993;1:43–60.
108. Demling R, Riessen R. Pulmonary dysfunction after cerebral injury. Crit Care Med 1990;18:768–774.
109. Chen H, Liao J, Kuo L, Ho S. Centrogenic pulmonary hemorrhagic edema induced by cerebral compression in rats. Circ Res 1980;47:366–373.
110. Theodore J, Robin E. Speculations on neurogenic pulmonary edema. Am Rev Respir Dis 1976;113:405–411.
111. Mackersie R, Christensen J, Pitts L, Lewis F. Pulmonary extravascular fluid accumulation following intracranial injury. J Trauma 1983;23: 968–975.
112. Baigelman W, O'Brien J. Pulmonary effects of head trauma. Neurosurgery 1981;9:729–740.
113. Malik A. Mechanisms of neurogenic pulmonary edema. Circ Res 1985;57:1–18.
114. Ducker TB, Simmons RL. Increased intracranial pressure and pulmonary edema, 2: the hemodynamic response of dogs and monkeys to increased intracranial pressure. J Neurosurg 1968;28:118–123.
115. Katsurada K, Yamada R, Sugimoto T. Respiratory insufficiency in patients with severe head injury. Surgery 1973;73:191–199.
116. Beckman D, Bean J, Baslock P. Neurogenic influence on pulmonary compliance. J Trauma 1974;14:111–115.
117. North JB, Jennett S. Abnormal breathing patterns associated with acute brain damage. Arch Neurol 1974;31:338–344.
118. Helling T, Evans L, Fowler D, Hays L, Kennedy F. Infectious complications in patients with severe head injury. J Trauma 1988;28:1575–1577.
119. Clifton G, Robertson C, Kyper K, Taylor A, Dhekne RD, Grossman R. Cardiovascular response to severe head injury. J Neurosurg 1983;59:447–454.
120. Talman WT. Cardiovascular regulation and lesions of the central nervous system. Ann Neurol 1985;18:1–12.
121. Rogers M, Zakha K, Nugent S, Gioia F, Epple L. Electrocardiographic abnormalities in infants and children with neurologic injury. Crit Care Med 1980;8:213–214.
122. Yanowitz F, Preston JB, Abildskov JA. Functional distribution of right and left stellate innervation to the ventricles. Circ Res 1966;18: 416–428.
123. Rogers MC, Abildskov JA, Preston JB. Neurogenic ECG changes in critically ill patients: an experimental model. Crit Care Med 1973;1:192–196.
124. Miner M, Kaufman H, Graham S, Haar F, Gildenberg P. Disseminated intravascular coagulation fibrinolytic syndrome following head injury in children: frequency and prognostic implications. J Pediatr 1982; 100:687–691.
125. Stein S, Young G, Talucci R, Greenbaum B, Ross S. Delayed brain injury after head trauma: significance of coagulopathy. Neurosurgery 1992;30:160–165.
126. Phillips R, Ott L, Young B, Walsh J. Nutritional support and measured energy expenditure of the child and adolescent with head injury. J Neurosurg 1987;67:846–851.
127. Siemkowicz E, Hansen AJ. Clinical restitution following cerebral ischemia in hypo-, normo- and hyperglycemic rats. Acta Neurol Scand 1978;58:1–8.
128. Sieber F, Traystman R. Special issues: glucose and the brain. Crit Care Med 1992;20:104–114.
129. Rapp RP, Young B, Twyman D, et al. Favorable effect of early parenteral feeding on survival in head-injured patients. J Neurosurg 1983;58:906–912.
130. Humphreys R. Complications of pediatric head injury. Pediatr Neurosurg 1991-92;17:274–278.
131. Hahn YS, Fuchs S, Flannery AM, Barthel MJ, McLone DG. Factors influencing posttraumatic seizures in children. Neurosurgery 1988;22:864–867.
132. Hendrick EB, Harris L. Post-traumatic epilepsy in children. J Trauma 1968;8:547–556.
133. Annergers JF, Grabow JD, Broover RV, Laws ER, Elveback LR, Kurland LT. Seizures after head trauma: a population study. Neurology 1980;30:683–689.
134. Yablon S. Posttraumatic seizures. Arch Phys Med Rehabil 1993; 74:983–1001.
135. Weiss GH, Caveness WF. Prognostic factors in the persistence of posttraumatic epilepsy. J Neurosurg 1972;37:164–169.
136. Marshall LW, Smith RW, Shapiro HM. The outcome with aggressive treatment in severe head injuries, 1: the significance of intracranial pressure monitoring. J Neurosurg 1979;50:20–25.
137. Kenning JA, Toutant SM, Saunders RL. Upright patient positioning in the magagement of intracranial hypertension. Surg Neurol 1981; 15:148–152.
138. Durward QJ, Amacher AL, Del Maestro RF, et al. Cerebral and cardiovascular responses to changes in head elevation in patients with intracranial hypertension. J Neurosurg 1983;59:938–944.
139. Rosner M, Coley I. Cerebral perfusion pressure, intracranial pressure, and head elevation. J Neurosurg 1986;65:636–641.
140. Feldman Z, Kanter M, Robertson C, et al. Effect of head elevation on intracranial pressure, cerebral perfusion pressure, and cerebral blood flow in head-injured patients. J Neurosurg 1992;76:207–211.
141. Shapiro HM. Intracranial hypertension: therapeutic and anesthetic considerations. Anesthesiology 1975;43:445–471.
142. Hsiang J, Chestnut R, Crisp C, Klauber M, Blunt B, Marshall L. Early, routine paralysis for intracranial pressure control in severe head injury: is it necessary? Crit Care Med 1994;22:1471–1476.
143. Davis RJ, Tait VF, Dean JM, Goldberg A, Rogers M. Head and spinal cord injury. In: Rogers M, ed. Textbook of Pediatric Intensive Care. 2nd ed. Baltimore: Williams & Wilkins, 1992:805–857.
144. Rosner M, Daughton S. Cerebral perfusion pressure management in head injury. J Trauma 1990;30:933–941.
145. Shapira Y, Artru A, Cotev S, Muggia-Sulam M, Freund H. Brain edema and neurologic status following head trauma in the rat. Anesthesiology 1992;77:79–85.

146. Buhrley L, Reed DJ. The effect of furosemide on sodium-22 uptake into cerebrospinal fluid and brain. Exp Brain Res 1972;14:503–510.
147. Cruz J, Miner M, Allen S, Alves W, Gennarelli T. Continuous monitoring of cerebral oxygenation in acute brain injury: injection of mannitol during hyperventilation. J Neurosurg 1990;73:725–730.
148. Hartwell RC. Mannitol, intracranial pressure and vasogenic edema. Neurosurgery 1993;32:444–450.
149. Muizelaar JP, Marmarou A, Ward J, et al. Adverse effects of prolonged hyperventilation in patients with severe head injury: a randomized clinical trial. J Neurosurg 1991;75:731–739.
150. Kennealy JA, McLennasn JE, Loudon RG, McLaurin RL. Hyperventilation induced cerebral hypoxia. Am Rev Respir Dis 1980;122: 407–412.
151. Darby JM, Yonas H, Marion DW, Latchaw RE. Local "inverse steal" induced by hyperventilation in head injury. Neurosurgery 1988;23: 84–88.
152. Sheinberg M, Kanter M, Robertson C, Contant C, Narayan R, Grossman R. Continuous monitoring of jugular venous oxygen saturation in head-injured patients. J Neurosurg 1992;76:212–217.
153. Cruz J, Miner M, Allen S, Alves W, Gennarelli T. Continuous monitoring of cerebral oxygenation in acute brain injury: assessment of cerebral hemodynamic reserve. Neurosurgery 1991;29:743–749.
154. Muizelaar JP, Van der Poel H, Li Z, Kontos H, Levasseur J. Pial arteriolar vessel diameter and CO_2 reactivity during prolonged hyperventilation in the rabbit. J Neurosurg 1988;69:923–927.
155. Gudeman S, Miller JD, Becker D. Failure of high-dose steroid therapy to influence intracranial pressure in patients with severe head injury. J Neurosurg 1979;51:301–306.
156. Dearden NM, Gibson J, McDowall DG, Gibson RM, Cameron M. Effect of high-dose dexamethasone on outcome from severe head injury. J Neurosurg 1986;64:81–88.
157. Cooper P, Moody S, Clark WK, et al. Dexamethasone and severe head injury: a prospective double-blind study. J Neurosurg 1979;51: 307–316.
158. Hall E. The neuroprotective pharmacology of methylprednisolone. J Neurosurg 1992;76:13–22.
159. Pittman T, Bucholz R, Williams D. Efficacy of barbiturates in the treatment of resistant intracranial hypertension in severely head-injured children. Pediatr Neurosci 1989;15:13–17.
160. Eisenberg H, Frankowski R, Contant C, Marshall L, Walker M, Comprehensive central nervous system trauma centers: high-dose barbiturate control of elevated intracranial pressure in patients with severe head injury. J Neurosurg 1988;69:15–23.
161. Marshall L, Smith R, Shapiro H. The outcome with aggressive treatment in severe head injuries, II: acute and chronic barbiturate administration in the management of head injury. J Neurosurg 1979,50: 26–30.
162. Ward J, Becker D, Miller D, et al. Failure of prophylactic barbiturate coma in the treatment of severe head injury. J Neurosurg 1985;62: 383–388.
163. Clifton GL, Jiang JY, Lyeth BG, Jenkins LW, Hamm RJ, Hayes RL. Marked protection by moderate hypothermia after experimental traumatic brain injury. J Cereb Blood Flow Metab 1991;11:114–121.
164. Marion D, Obrist W, Carlier P, Penrod L, Darby J. The use of moderate therapeutic hypothermia for patients with severe head injuries: a preliminary report. J Neurosurg 1993;79:354–362.
165. Shiozaki T, Sugimoto H, Taneda M, et al. Effect of mild hypothermia on uncontrollable intracranial hypertension after severe head injury. J Neurosurg 1993;79:363–368.
166. Clifton G, Allen S, Barrodale P, et al. A phase II study of moderate hypothermia in severe brain injury. J Neurotrauma 1993;10: 263–271.
167. Levin H, Aldrich F, Saydjari C, et al. Severe head injury in children: experience of the traumatic coma data bank. Neurosurgery 1992;31:435–444.
168. Miner ME, Ewing-Cobbs L, Kopaniky DR, Cabrera J, Kaufmann P. Experimental and clinical studies: the results of treatment of gunshot wounds to the brain in children. Neurosurgery 1990;26:20–25.
169. Johnston M, Gerring J. Head trauma and its sequelae. Pediatr Ann 1992;21:362–368.
170. Luerssen T, Klauber M, Marshall L. Outcome from head injury related to patient's age: a longitudinal prospective study of adult and pediatric head injury. J Neurosurg 1988;68:409–416.
171. Mahoney WJ, D'Souza BJ, Haller JA, et al. Long-term outcome of children with severe head trauma and prolonged coma. Pediatrics 1983;71:756–762.
172. Kriel RL, Krach LE, Panser LA. Closed head injury: comparison of children younger and older than 6 years of age. Pediatr Neurol 1989;5: 296–300.
173. Grewal M, Sutcliffe AJ. Early prediction of outcome following head injury in children: an assessment of the value of Glasgow Coma Scale Score trend and abnormal plantar and pupillary light relfexes. J Pediatr Surg 1991;26:1161–1163.
174. Choi S, Ward J, Becker D. Chart for outcome prediction in severe head injury. J Neurosurg 1983;59:294–297.
175. Marshall L, Gautille T, Klauber M, et al. The outcome of severe closed head injury. J Neurosurg 1991;75:S28–S36.
176. Parsons K, Lammertse K. Rehabilitation in spinal cord disorders, 1: epidemiology, prevention, and system of care of spinal cord disorders. Arch Phys Med Rehabil 1991;72:S293–294.
177. Carter RE. Etiology of traumatic spinal cord injury: statistics of more than 1,100 cases. Tex Med 1977;73:61–65.
178. Osenbach R, Menezes A. Pediatric spinal cord and vertebral column injury. Neurosurgery 1992;30:385–390.
179. Massagli T, Jaffe K. Pediatric spinal cord injury: treatment and outcome. Pediatrician 1990;17:244–254.
180. Kewalramani LS, Orth MS, Kraus JF, Sterling HM. Acute spinal-cord lesions in a pediatric population: epidemiological and clinical features. Paraplegia 1980;18:206–219.
181. Connolly JF, ed. DePalma's the management of fractures and dislocations, an atlas. 3rd ed. Philadelphia: WB Saunders, 1981.
182. Pang D, Wilberger JE. Spinal cord injury without radiographic abnormalities in children. J Neurosurg 1982;57:114–129.
183. Tator CH, Fehlings MG. Review of the secondary injury theory of acute spinal cord trauma with emphasis on vascular mechanisms. J Neurosurg 1991;75:15–26.
184. Hadley MN, Zabramski J, Browner CM, Rekate H, Sonntag V. Pediatric spinal trauma: review of 122 cases of spinal cord and vertebral column injuries. J Neurosurg 1988;68:18–24.
185. Hill S, Miller C, Kosnik E, Hunt W. Pediatric neck injuries: a clinical study. J Neurosurg 1984;60:700–706.
186. Pueschel SM, Herndon JA, Gelch MM, Senft K, Scola F, Goldberg M. Symptomatic atlantoaxial subluxation in persons with Down Syndrome. J Pediatr Orthop 1984;4:682–688.
187. Nathan FF, Bickel WH. Spontaneous axial subluxation in a child as the first sign of juvenile rheumatoid arthritis. J Bone Joint Surg Am 1968;50:1675–1678.
188. Yang SS, Corbett DP, Brough AJ, Heidelberger KP, Bernstein J. Upper cervical myelopathy in achondroplasia. Am J Clin Pathol 1977;68: 68–72.
189. Anderson DK, Hall ED. Pathophysiology of spinal cord trauma. Ann Emerg Med 1993;22:987–992.
190. Demediuk P, Saunders RD, Anderson DK, Means E, Horrocks L. Membrane lipid changes in laminectomized and traumatized cat spinal cord. Proc Natl Acad Sci U S A 1985;82:7071–7075.
191. Faden AI, Chan PH, Longar S. Alterations in lipid metabolism, Na,+K+-ATPase activity, and tissue water content of spinal cord following experimental traumatic injury. J Neurochem 1987;48: 1809–1816.
192. Demediuk P, Saunders RD, Clendenon NR, Means E, Anderston DK, Horrocks L. Changes in lipid metabolism in traumatized spinal cord. Prog Brain Res 1985;63:211–226.
193. Panter SS, Yum SW, Faden AI. Alteration in extracellular amino acids after traumatic spinal cord injury. Ann Neurol 1990;27:96–99.
194. Hsu CY, Halushka PV, Hogan EL, Banik NL, Lee WA, Perot PL. Alteration of thromboxane and prostacyclin levels in experimental spinal cord injury. Neurology 1985;35:1003–1009.
195. Griffiths IR. Vasogenic edema following acute and chronic spinal cord compression in the dog. J Neurosurg 1975;42:155–165.
196. Means ED, Anderson DK. Neuronophagia by leukocytes in experimental spinal cord injury. J Neuropath Exp Neurol 1983;42:707–719.
197. Balentine JD, Spector MN. Calcification of axons in experimental spinal cord trauma. Ann Neurol 1977;2:520–523.
198. Dohrmann GJ, Wagner FC Jr, Bucy PC. The microvasculature in transitory traumatic paraplegia: an electron microscopic study in the monkey. J Neurosurg 1971;35:263–271.
199. Wallace MC, Tator CH, Frazee P. Relationship between posttraumatic ischemia and hemorrhage in the injured rat spinal cord as shown by colloidal carbon angiography. Neurosurgery 1986;18: 433–439.
200. Fried LC, Goodkin R. Microangiographic observations of the experimentally traumatized spinal cord. J Neurosurg 1971;35:709–714.
201. American Spinal Injury Association. Standards for neurological classification of spinal injury patients. Chicago: ASIA, 1989.

202. Bracken M, Shepard MJ, Collins W, et al. A randomized, controlled trial of methylprednisolone or naloxone in the treatment of acute spinal-cord injury: results of the second national acute spinal cord injury study. N Engl J Med 1990;332:1405–1411.
203. Hilton G, Frei J. High-dose methylprednisolone in the treatment of spinal cord injuries. Heart Lung 1991;20:675–680.
204. Mansel JK, Norman JR. Respiratory complications and management of spinal cord injuries. Chest 1990;97:1446–1452.
205. Wicks AB, Menter RR. Long-term outlook in quadriplegic patients with initial ventilator dependency. Chest 1986;90:406–410.
206. Shahani B, Scheinberg L. Neurologic rehabilitation. In: Scheinberg L, Shahani BT, eds. Neurologic clinics. Philadelphia: W.B. Saunders Company, 1987:519–522.
207. Burke WH, Wesolowski MD, Guth ML. Comprehensive head injury rehabilitation: an outcome evaluation. Brain Inj 1988;2:313–22.
208. Bean SW, Kukic S, Hostetter C. Guidelines for serving students with traumatic brain injuries. Salt Lake City: Utah State Office of Education, 1993.
209. Hall DMB, Johnson SLJ, Middleton J. Rehabilitation of head injured children. Arch Dis Child 1990;65:553–556.
210. World Health Organization. International classification of impairments, disabilities and handicaps: a manual of classification relating to the consequences of disease. Geneva: World Health Organization, 1980.
211. Cowley RS, Swanson B, Chapman P, Kitik BA, Mackay LE. The role of rehabilitation in the intensive care unit. J Head Trauma Rehabil 1994;9:32–43.
212. Perrin JCS. Head injury. In: Molnar GE, ed. Pediatric rehabilitation. Baltimore: Williams & Wilkins, 1985:207–232.
213. Chamovitz I, Chorazy AJL, Hanchett JM, Mandella PA. Rehabilitative medical management. In: Ylvisaker M, ed. Head injury rehabilitation: children and adolescents. San Diego: College-Hill Press, 1985:119–139.
214. Woolsey RM, McGarry JD. The cause, prevention, and treatment of pressure sores. Neurol Clin 1991;9:797–808.
215. Bontke CF, Brockman N, Cilo MP, Robert V, Worthington L. Acute care and rehabilitation. In: Deutsch PM, Fralish KB, eds. Innovations in head injury rrehabilitation. New York: Matthew Bender & Co, 1991;4: 1–23.
216. Temkin NR, Dikmen SS, Wilensky AJ, Keihm J, Chabal S, Winn R. A randomized, double-blind study of phenytoin for the prevention of post-traumatic seizures. N Engl J Med 1990;323:497–502.
217. Dikmen SS, Temkin NR, Miller B, Machamer J, Win HR. Neurobehavioral effects of phenytoin prophylaxis of postttraumatic seizures. JAMA 1991;265:1271–1277.
218. Willmore JL. Post-traumatic seizures. Neurol Clin 1994;11:823–835.
219. Yablon SA. Post traumatic seizures. Arch Phys Med Rehabil 1993;74:983–1001.
220. Bachman DL. The diagnosis and management of common neurologic sequelae of closed head injury. J Head Trauma Rehabil 1992;7:50–59.
221. Jaffe MB, Mastrilli JP, Molitor CB, Valko AS. Intervention for motor disorders. In: Ylvisaker M, ed. Head injury rehabilitation: children and adolescents. San Diego: College-Hill Press, 1985:167–194.
222. Haley SM, Cioffi MI, Lewin JE, et al. Motor dysfunction in children and adolescents after traumatic brain injury. J Head Trauma Rehabil 1990;5:77–90.
223. Young RR, Delwaide PJ. Drug therapy: spasticity (pt 1 of 2). N Engl J Med 1981;304:28–33.
224. Young RR, Delwaide PJ. Drug therapy: spasticity (pt 2 of 2). N Engl J Med 1981;304:96–99.
225. Young RR. Physiologic and pharmacologic approaches to spasticity. In: Scheinberg L, Shahani BT, eds. Neurologic clinics. Philadelphia: W.B. Saunders Company, 1987:529–539.
226. Cosgrove AP, Cory IS, Graham HK. Botulinum toxin the management of lower limb in cerebral palsy. Dev Med Child Neurol 1994;36: 386–396.
227. Das TK, Park DM. Botulinum toxin in treating spasticity. Br J Clin Pharmacol 1989;43:401–403.
228. Koman CA, Modney JF, Smith B, Goodman A, Mulvaney T. Management of cerebral palsy with botulinum A toxin: preliminary investigation. J Pediatr Orthop 1993;13:489–495.
229. Snow BJ, Tsui JD, Bhatt MH. Treatment of spasticity with botulinum toxin: a double blind study. Ann Neurol 1990;28:512–515.
230. Lazarus C, Logemann JA. Swallowing disorders in closed head trauma patients. Arch Phys Med Rehabil 1987;68:79–87.
231. Logeman JA. Evaluation and treatment planning for the head-injured patient with oral intake disorders. J Head Trauma Rehabil 1989;4: 24–33.
232. Lazarus CL. Swallowing disorders after traumatic brain injury. J Head Trauma Rehabil 1989;4:34–41.
233. Logeman JA, Pepe J, Mackay LE. Disorders of nutrition and swallowing: intervention strategies in the trauma center. J Head Trauma Rehabil 1994;9:43–56.
234. Ylvisaker M, Logemann J. Therapy for feeding and swallowing disorders following head injury. In: Ylvisaker M, ed. Head injury rehabilitation: children and adolescents. San Diego: College-Hill Press, 1985:195–218.
235. Splaingard ML, Hutchins B, Sulton LD, et al. Aspiration in rehabilitation patients: videofluoroscopy vs bedside clinical assessment. Arch Phys Med and Rehabil 1988;69:637–40.
236. Ylvisaker M. Language and communication disorders following pediatric head injury. J Head Trauma Rehabil 1986;4:48–56.
237. Baxter R, Cohen SB, Ylvisaker M. Comprehensive cognitive assessment. In: Ylvisaker M, ed. Head injury rehabilitation: children and adolescents. San Diego: College-Hill Press, 1985:247–274.
238. Bleiberg J, Cope DN, Spector J. Cognitive assessment and therapy in traumatic brain injury. Physical medicine and rehabilitation: state of the art reviews, vol 3. Philadelphia: Hanley and Belfus, Inc, 1989;3:123–142.
239. Ylvisaker M, Szekers SF. Metacognitive and executive impairments in head-injured children and adults. Top Lang Disorders 1989;9:34–49.
240. Crosson B, Barco PP, Velozo CA, et al. Awareness and compensation in postacute head injury rehabilitation. J Head Trauma Rehabil 1989;4:46–54.
241. Lezak M. Newer contributions to the neuropsychological assessment of executive functions. J Head Trauma Rehabil 1993;8:24–31.
242. Varney NR, Menefee L. Psychosocial and executive deficits following closed head injury: implication for orbital frontal cortex. J Head Trauma Rehabil 1993;8:32–44.
243. Berrol S. Issues in cognitive rehabilitation. Arch Neurol 1990;47: 219–220.
244. Volpe BT, MacDowell FH. The efficacy of cognitive rehabilitation in patients with traumatic brain injury. Arch Neurol 1990;47:220–222.
245. Levin HS. Cognitive rehabilitation: unproved but promising. Arch Neurol 1990;47:223–224.
246. Levin HS. Memory deficit after closed-head injury. J Clin Exp Neuropsychol 1989;12:129–153.
247. Namerow NS. Cognitive and behavioral aspects of brain-injury rehabilitation. In: Scheinberg L, Shahani BT, eds. Neurologic clinics. Philadelphia: W.B. Saunders Company, 1987:569–583.
248. Sohlberg MM, Mateer CA, Stuss DT. Contemporary approaches to the management of executive control dysfunction. J Head Trauma Rehabil 1993;8:45–58.
249. Ylvisaker M. Cognitive and psychosocial outcome following head injury in children. Children 1989;16:203–216.
250. Deaton A. Behavioral change strategies for children and adolescents with severe brain injury. J Learn Dis 1987;20:581–589.
251. Jaffe KM, Hay RM. Pediatric head injury: rehabilitative medical management. J Head Trauma Rehabil 1986;1:30–40.
252. Silver JM, Yudofsky SC, Hales RE. Depression in traumatic brain injury. Neuropsychiatry, Neuropsychol, and Behav Neurol 1991; 1:12–23.
253. McGuire TL, Rothenberg MB. Behavioral and psychosocial sequelae of pediatric head injury. J Head Trauma Rehabil 1986;1:1–6.
254. Divack JA, Herrle J, Scott MB. Behavior management. In: Ylvisaker M, ed. Head injury rehabilitation: children and adolescents. San Diego: College-Hill Press, 1985:347–360.
255. Barin JJ, Hanchett JM, Jacob WL, Scott M. Counseling the head injured patient. In: Ylvisaker M, ed. Head injury rehabilitation: children and adolescents. San Diego: College-Hill Press, 1985:361–379.
256. Cole JR. Psychosocial rehabilitation. In: Deutsch PM, Fralish KB, eds. Innovations in head injury rehabilitation. New York: Matthew Bender & Co, 1991;10:1–32.
257. Rao N, Jellinek HM, Woolston DC. Agitation in closed head injury: haloperidol effects on rehabilitation outcome. Arch Phys Med Rehabil 1985;66:30–34.
258. Elliott FA. Propranolol for the control of behavior following acute brain damage. Ann Neurol 1977;1:489–491.
259. Yudofsky S, Williams D, Gorman J. Propranolol in the treatment of rage and violent behavior in patients with chronic brain syndromes. Am J Psychiatry 1981;138:218–220.
260. Mansheim P. Treatment with propranolol of the behavioral sequelae of brain damage. J Clin Psychiatry 1981;42:132.
261. Hale MS, Donaldson JO. Lithium carbonate in the treatment of organic brain syndrome. J Nerv Ment Dis 1982;170:362–365.

262. Jackson RD, Corrigan JD, Arnett JA. Amitriptyline for agitation in head injury. Arch Phys Med Rehabil 1985;66:180–181.
263. Evans RW, Gualtieri CT. Carbamazepine: a neuropsychological and psychiatric profile. Clin Neuropharmacol 1985;1:221–241.
264. Hall RCW, Disook S. Paradoxical reations to benzodiazepines. Br J Clin Pharmacol 1981;11:995–1045.
265. Parmalee DX, O'Shanick GJ. Neuropsychiatric interventions with head injured children and adolescents. Brain Inj 1987;1:41–47.
266. Evans RW, Gualtiere CT. Psychostimulant pharmacology in traumatic brain injury. J Head Trauma Rehabil 1987;2:29–33.
267. Mysiw WJ, Jackson RD. Tricyclic antidepressant therapy after traumatic brain injury. J Head Trauma Rehabil 1987;2:34–42.
268. O'Shanick GJ. Psychotropic management of behavioral disorders after a head trauma. Psychiatr Med 1988;6:67–82.
269. Blieberg J, Gaumoe W, Cedarquist J, Reeves D, Lux W. Effects of dexadrine on performance consistancy following brain injury. Neuropsychiatry Neuropsychol Behav Neurol 1993;6:245–248.
270. Sutton RL, Weaver MS, Feeney DM. Drug-induced modifications of behavioral recovery following cortical trauma. J Head Trauma Rehabil 1987;2:50–58.
271. Cohen SB, Joyce CM, Rhoades KW, Welks DM. Educational programming for head injured students. In: Ylvisaker M, ed. Head injury rehabilitation: children and adolescents. San Diego: College-Hill Press, 1985:247–274.
272. Savage RC. Identification, classification, and placement issues for students with traumatic brain injuries. J Head Trauma Rehabil 1991;6:1–9.
273. Carney J, Gerring J. Return to school following severe closed head injury: a critical phase in pediatric rehabilitation. Pediatrician 1990;17:222–229.
274. Pollock E, Fue LD, Goldstein S. A teachers guide: managing children with brain injury in the classroom. Salt Lake City: The Neurology, Learning and Behavior Center, 1993:1–16.
275. Savage R, Wolcott G. Educational dimensions of acquired brain injury. Austin: Pro-Ed, 1994.
276. Ylvisaker M, Hartwick P, Stevens M. School reentry following head injury: managing the transition from hospital to school. J Head Trauma Rehabil 1991;6:10–22.
277. Telzrow CF. Management of academic and educational problems in head injury. J Learn Dis 1987;20:536–545.
278. Cohen S. Adapting educational programs for students with head injuries. J Head Trauma Rehabil 1991;6:56–63.
279. Barin JJ, Leger D, Bachman KM. Working with the family. In: Ylvisaker M, ed. Head injury rehabilitation: children and adolescents. San Diego: College-Hill Press, 1985:93–115.
280. Lash M. Getting help and coping when your child is seriously injured. Boston: Tufts University/New England Medical Center, 1990:20–24.
281. Florian V, Katz S, Lahav V. Impact of traumatic brain damage on family dynamics and functioning: a review. Brain Inj 1989;3:219–233.
282. Simons R. After the tears: parents talk about raising a child with a disability. Denver: The Children's Museum of Denver, 1985:11–13.
283. DeBoskey DS, Hecht JS, Calub CJ. Educating families of the head injured: a guide to medical, cognitive and social issues. Aspen: Gaithersberg, 1991:155–169.
284. Orsillo SM, McCaffrey RJ, Fisher JM. Siblings of head-injured individuals: a population at risk. J Head Trauma Rehabil 1993;8: 102–115.
285. Deutsch PM. Discharge planning: studying the home environment. In: Deutsch PM, Fralish KB, eds. Innovations in head injury in rehabilitation. New York: Matthew Bender & Co, 1991;16:1–41.
286. Cohen SB, Titonis J. Head injury rehabilitation: management issues. In: Ylvisaker M, ed. Head injury rehabilitation: children and adolescents. San Diego: College-Hill Press, 1985:429–443.
287. Hall KM, Cope DN. The benefit of rehabilitation in traumatic brain injury: a literature review. J Head Trauma Rehabil 1995;10:1–13.
288. Gans BM. Rehabilitation of severely injured children. West J Med 1991;154:566–568.
289. Namerow NS. Cognitive and behavioral aspects of brain-injury rehabilitation. Neurol Clin 1987;5:569–583.
290. Cope, DN. Traumatic closed head injury: status of rehabilitation treatment. Semin Neurol 1985;5:212–220.
291. Keith RA. The comprehensive treatment team in rehabilitation. Arch Phys Med Rehabil 1991;72:269–274.
292. Bergman AB, Rivera FP. Sweden's experience in reducing childhood injuries. Pediatrics 1991;88:69–74.

Cerebrovascular Disease and Vascular Anomalies 25

A. Marc Harrison
Madolin Witte
J. Michael Dean

INTRODUCTION—DEFINITIONS AND EPIDEMIOLOGY

Although strokes are much less common in neonates and children than in adults, acute central nervous system pathology secondary to cerebrovascular disease represents a clinical challenge to the pediatric intensivist. The term *stroke* denotes an ischemic or hemorrhagic injury to the brain, producing neurologic symptoms that last at least 24 hours. Neurologic deficits which resolve within 24 hours are termed *transient ischemic attacks,* and as they are associated primarily with atherosclerotic disease, are uncommon in children. Strokes in children are generally caused by one of two etiologic final common pathways: vascular occlusion (e.g., thrombus, embolus, or spasm) and intracerebral hemorrhage (e.g., breach in vascular integrity or a hypocoagulable state). A 1978 study in Rochester, Minnesota, estimated annual stroke incidence in children age 0 to 14 years at 2.52 cases per 100,000[1]. This study was limited by a relatively small number of resident children. In Cincinnati, Ohio, between 1988 and 1989, a much larger study of 295,577 resident children younger than 15 years old described an incidence rate of 3.1 per 100,000 for African-American children and 2.6 per 100,000 for white children[2]. The Minnesota and Ohio data concur with an Italian study which found that the causes of strokes in children are roughly equally divided between ischemic and hemorrhagic causes. This is in contrast to cerebrovascular disease in adults, in whom the vast majority of strokes are ischemic and caused by atherosclerotic disease[3]. Strokes in infants and children are more commonly caused by a wide range of disease processes, often congenital or genetic **(Table 25.1)**.

Studying the epidemiology of a rare disease, such as stroke in children, presents significant practical and methodological stumbling blocks. In adults, stroke incidence varies widely in the literature based upon the ethnicity and nationality of the population studied[4]. These data are most accurate when collected longitudinally from a large, heterogeneous, stable population.

ANATOMY OF THE CEREBRAL VASCULATURE

The cerebrum receives its arterial blood via anterior and posterior circulations. Anteriorly, the internal carotid arteries branch into the anterior and middle cerebral arteries (Fig. 25.1). Clinically, occlusion of these arteries or their tributaries leads to syndromes with varied symptoms ranging from motor aphasia (posterior frontal branch of middle cerebral arteries MCAs) to lower extremity paralysis (pericallosal branch of ACA).

Posteriorly, paired vertebral arteries merge into the basi-

Table 25.1. Causes of Cerebrovascular Disease

Intracranial Hemorrhage	**Ischemic Stroke**
Cardioembolic	Cardioembolic
Arterial dissection	Arterial dissection
trauma	trauma
spontaneous	spontaneous
Disordered clotting	Disordered clotting
sickle cell disease	sickle cell disease
hemophilia	Antithrombin-III
DIC	Protein-S, protein-C
hypofibrinoginemia	hyperfibrinoginemia
ITP	dehydration
Tumor	antiphospholipid syndrome
Hypertension	Malignancy
Moyamoya	Moyamoya
Venous thrombosis	Venous thrombosis
Vascular malformations	metabolic disease
aneurysm	Vasculitis
arteriovenous malformation	autoimmune
angioma	CNS infection
Trauma	drug abuse
Idiopathic	Idiopathic

DIC, disseminated intravascular coagulation; ITP, idiopathic thrombocytopenic purpura; CNS, central nervous system.

lar artery (Fig. 25.2). The basilar artery branches into the anterior, posterior, and superior cerebellar arteries, as well as the posterior cerebral arteries. Symptoms caused by disturbance of the posterior circulation secondary to occlusion or hemorrhage are very diverse and may be subtle. They may include cranial neuropathies, difficulty with balance and coordination, tremor, and even decreased wakefulness.

There is anatomic variability in the vascular supply of the circle of Willis (Fig. 25.3). The anterior circulation is dominant in some patients, with the posterior cerebral artery arising from the internal carotid artery instead of the basilar artery. Significant collateral flow exists, primarily via the posterior communicating artery. Adequacy of collateral flow is evidenced by the degree to which ligation of the internal carotid artery is tolerated during traditional ECMO, without vascular reconstruction.

Cerebral venous anatomy consists of a deep system penetrating the intracranial vault and a system of superficial dural sinuses (Fig. 25.4). There is extensive anastamotic connection between the two systems. Thrombotic cerebrovascular disease often involves both systems simultaneously. The sagittal sinus, cavernous sinus, and great vein of Galen are commonly involved in pathology seen in the pediatric intensive care unit (PICU).

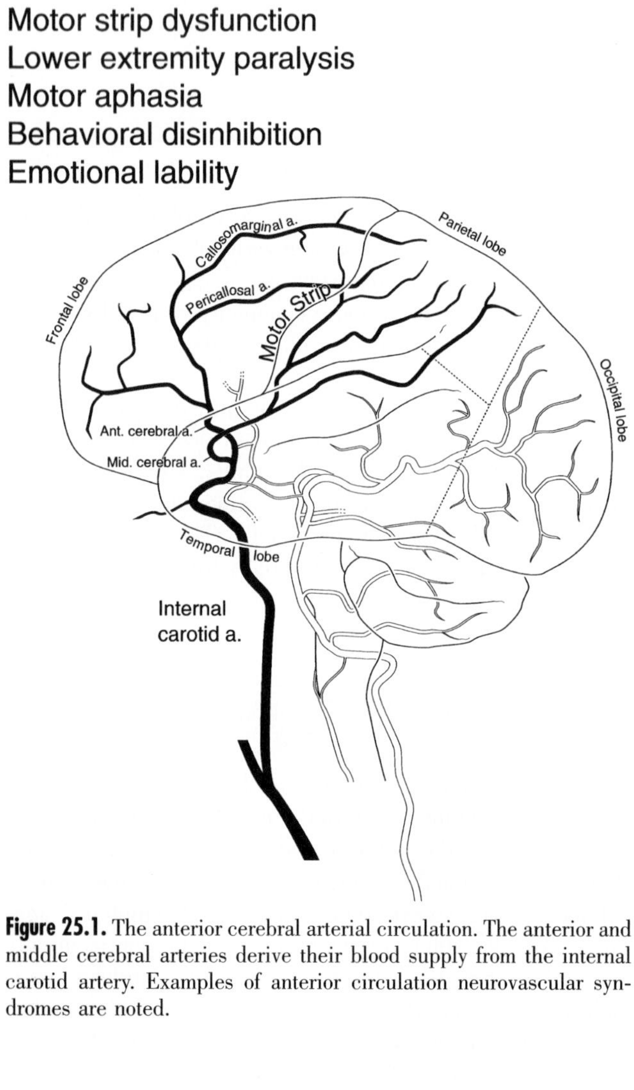

Figure 25.1. The anterior cerebral arterial circulation. The anterior and middle cerebral arteries derive their blood supply from the internal carotid artery. Examples of anterior circulation neurovascular syndromes are noted.

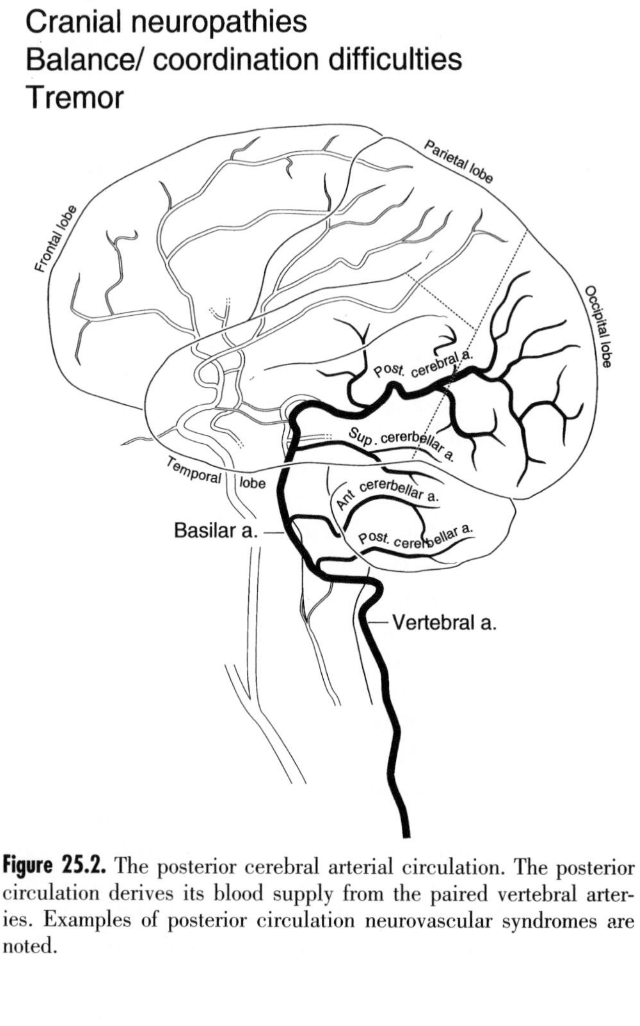

Figure 25.2. The posterior cerebral arterial circulation. The posterior circulation derives its blood supply from the paired vertebral arteries. Examples of posterior circulation neurovascular syndromes are noted.

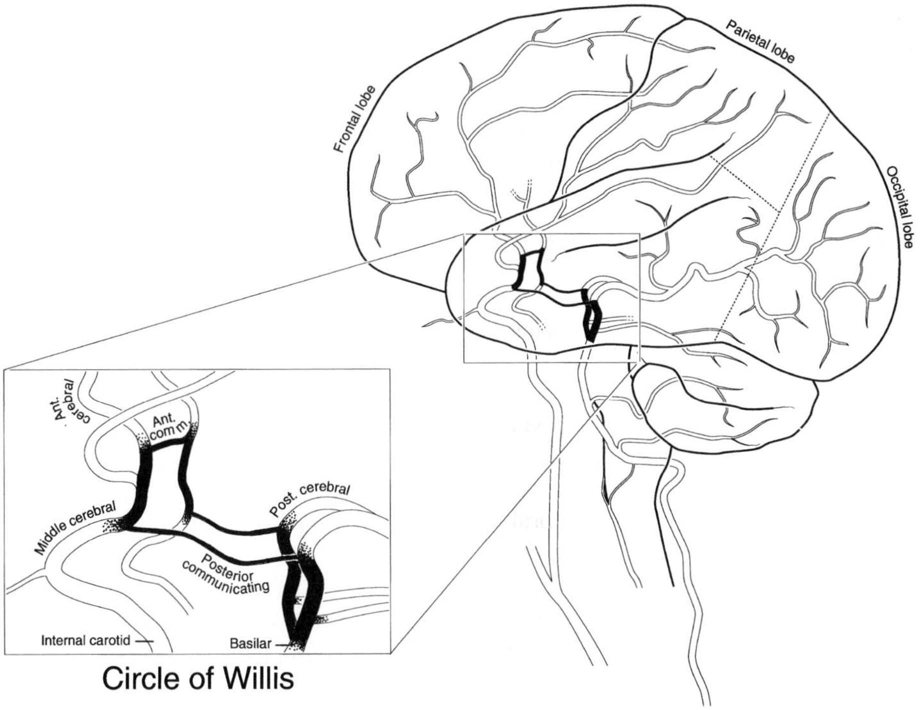

Figure 25.3. The circle of Willis, which is formed by the internal carotid artery, the anterior and posterior cerebral arteries, and the anterior and posterior communicating arteries.

CAUSES OF CEREBROVASCULAR DISEASE

Intracranial Hemorrhage

As previously noted, hemorrhagic stroke and subarachnoid hemorrhage (SAH) account for up to 60% of acute, nontraumatic cerebrovascular disease in children[2]. These two entities are forms of intracranial hemorrhage (ICH). Unlike ICH in the elderly, which is almost uniformly caused by atherosclerosis, childhood ICH can be caused by coagulopathy, recreational drugs, brain tumors, arterial hypertension, and structural vascular disease.

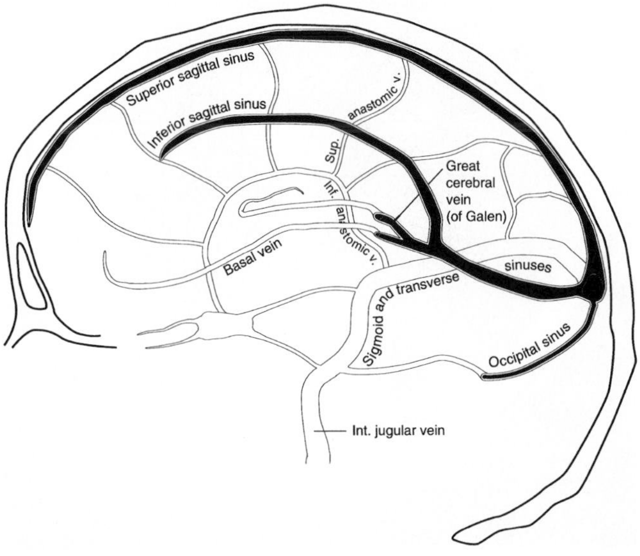

Figure 25.4. Venous system of the brain. The dural sinuses collect blood from the skull, meninges, and brain. They drain anteriorly and inferiorly toward the face and pharynx, respectively. Deep penetrating veins primarily drain the brain parenchyma.

Hemorrhagic disease of the newborn (HDN) is a cause of spontaneous intracranial hemorrhage that merits brief discussion. This entity occurs in infants who are exclusively or predominantly breast-fed and do not receive vitamin K at birth. Classic, early-onset HDN usually results in mild and self-limited bleeding (most commonly gastrointestinal) during the first 2 weeks of life. However, Chaou et al. describe intracranial hemorrhage in 32 infants, aged 2 weeks to 6 months, who were breast-fed and did not receive vitamin K[5]. Prothrombin time and partial thromboplastin time were prolonged in all infants in whom these studies were performed. Subarachnoid hemorrhage was seen in most patients, sometimes in combination with subdural, parenchymal, and intraventicular hemorrhage. Evaluation 2 to 18 months after hemorrhage revealed a high incidence of microcephaly and developmental delay.

Coagulopathy

Disseminated intravascular coagulation (DIC) is one of the most common causes of coagulopathy in the PICU. Poorly regulated coagulation may cause both inappropriate bleeding and clotting. DIC may be precipitated by triggers as diverse as sepsis, malignant hyperthermia, and envenomation. ICH is most commonly seen in the cerebral cortex and is caused by depletion of clotting factors and platelets[6].

Heparin and warfarin are anticoagulants used therapeutically and prophylactically in the PICU, especially in patients with structural heart disease or known venous thrombosis. ICH may be a complication of these drugs[7]. In adults, long-term warfarin therapy has been associated with an eightfold increased risk of ICH. This is increased with excessive anticoagulation[8]. No studies specifically address these risks in children.

ICH is the most feared complication of thrombocytopenia. Bleeding is rare unless the platelet count is less than 10,000. A variety of disease states may cause thrombocytopenia, with idiopathic thrombocytopenic purpura as the most common in the school-age child. Fewer than 2% of children with ITP will develop CNS bleeding[9,10].

The full spectrum of clotting factor deficiencies have been implicated in childhood ICH. Five percent of children with hemophilia (factor VIII or IX deficiency) develop parenchymal, subdural, or subarachnoid bleeds[11].

Deficiency of vitamin K dependent clotting factors (II, VII, IX, X) may cause significant coagulopathy and is found in congenital deficiency, hemorrhagic disease of the newborn, liver disease, starvation, and intestinal malabsorption[12]. Von Willebrand's disease, afibrinogenemia, and hypothrombinogenemia may also contribute to ICH.

Arterial Hypertension

Arterial hypertension is a cause of ICH in young adults. A prospective study at the University of Mississippi found that 78% of patients who suffered ICH had a history of arterial hypertension[13]. While most adults have primary hypertension, children are more likely to have a definable disorder such as renal vascular or parenchymal disease, coarctation of the aorta, or pheochromocytoma.

Illicit drugs, particularly those with sympathomimetic effects (e.g., hypertension), have been associated with ICH. Amphetamines and cocaine are the most commonly implicated substances[14–16] (Fig. 25.5). Recreational abuse of phenylpropanolamine may also cause ICH[17]. A case-controlled study at Stanford described a 6.5 relative risk of hemorrhagic stroke for drug-abusers compared with controls. In patients younger than 35 years old, drug abuse was the single most commonly identified risk-factor for stroke[18].

Cocaine may also cause vasospasm and ischemic stroke. This is especially true of crack cocaine (alkaloidal cocaine). Up to 80% of crack-associated strokes are ischemic compared with less than 50% caused by cocaine hydrochloride[19]. In vitro experiments suggest that cerebral vascular spasm may be precipitated by cocaine-induced loss of intracellular free Mg^{++} ions[20]. Cocaine predisposes individuals to ICH by blocking norepinephrine uptake and increasing sensitivity to catecholamines[21]. Preexisting arteriovenous malformations (AVMs) and aneurysms are the source of bleeding in some who have ICH associated with drug abuse[21,22]. Thus angiographic evaluation remains important in drug abusers with ICH.

Tumors

Intracranial tumors can cause ICH. Malignant histology is more commonly associated with hemorrhage. The tumor may be either metastatic or primary. Primary tumors may be of either neuronal (e.g., medulloblastoma) or supporting (e.g., glioblastoma) cellular origin[23,24].

Vascular Malformations

The central nervous system vascular malformations encompass a variety of diagnoses, including AVMs, capillary telangiectasias, cavernous angiomas, and venous malformations. Four percent of the United States population has one of these lesions[25].

A capillary telangiectasia represents an abnormally dense collection of capillaries within normal brain tissue. The vessels are composed of a single layer of endothelial cells and are extremely fragile. They are generally identified at autopsy as an incidental finding. In rare instances, they may bleed. Persons with Rendu-Osler-Weber disease have multiple telangiectasias throughout the body, including the brain[26].

Histologically, cavernous malformations are composed of clustered dilated blood vessels. There is little neural tissue interspersed between the vessels. They may be located in normal parenchyma, periventricularly, or subarachnoid[26].

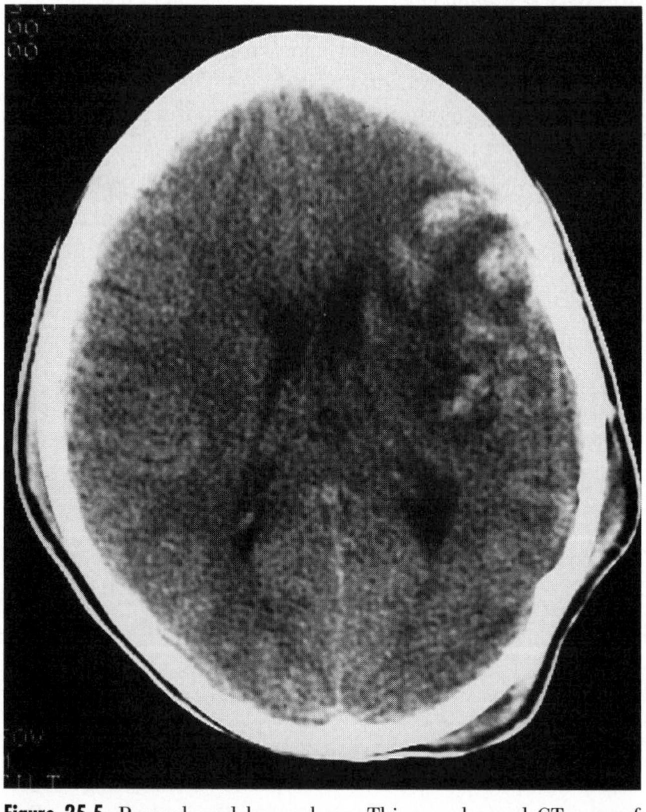

Figure 25.5. Parenchymal hemorrhage. This unenhanced CT scan of the brain demonstrates fresh parenchymal hemorrhage in the left middle cerebral artery distribution of a 15-year-old male who smoked methamphetamine.

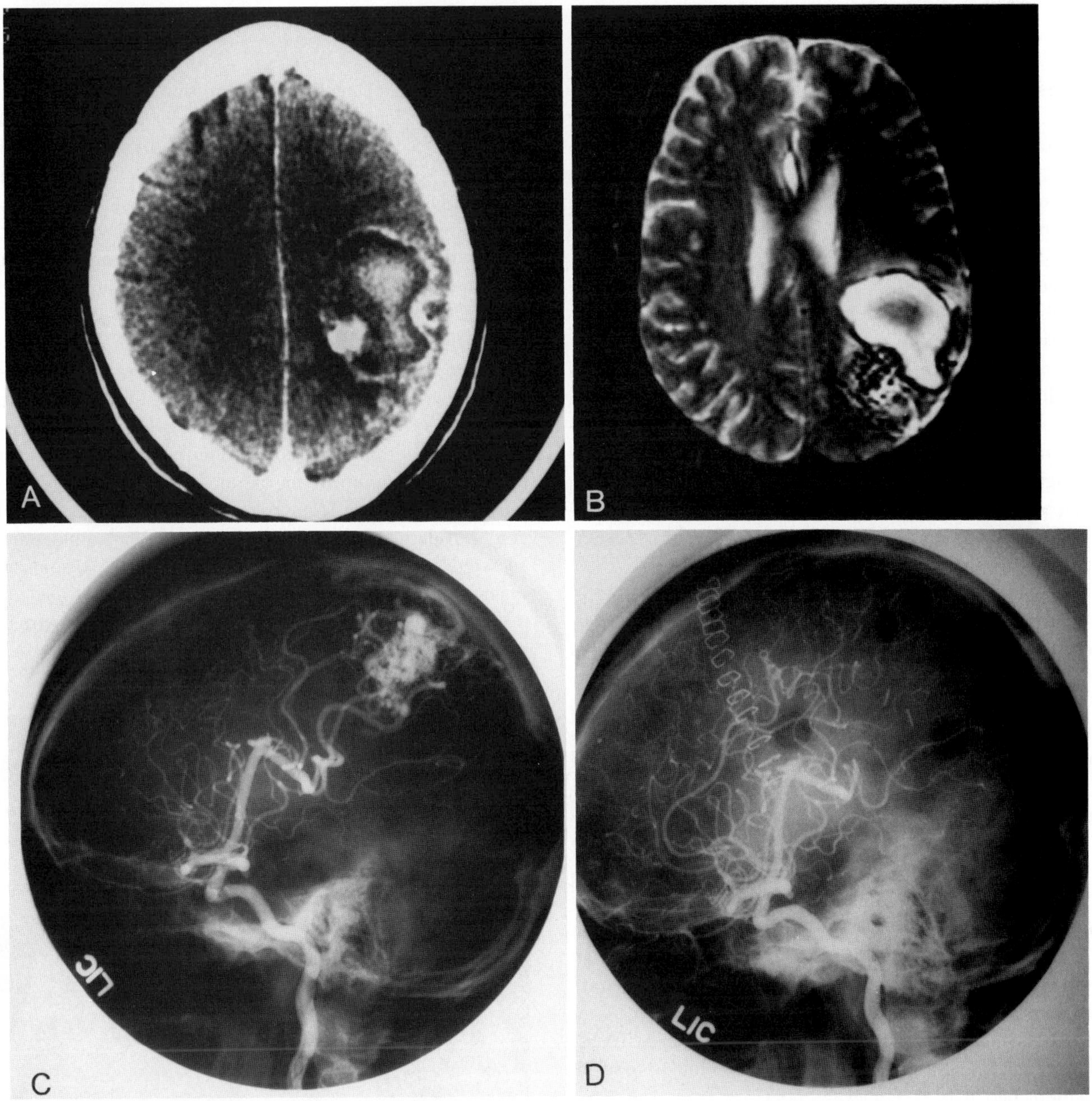

Figure 25.6. A. Enhanced CT scan in a patient who presented with sudden onset headache, right hemiparesis, and dysphasia. This scan shows an area of subacute hemorrhage in the left parietal region with an unusual nodule of enhancement posteriorly. This is suggestive of an arteriovenous malformation. **B.** T-2-weighted MRI scan of the same patient. In this study, the high-intensity signal in the left parietal region represents the subacute hematoma. The punctate "salt and pepper" appearance of vessels posterior to this hematoma is the arteriovenous malformation. **C** and **D.** Lateral internal carotid angiograms demonstrating the serpiginous arteriovenous malformation of the left parietal region **(C).**

These lesions may affect 0.5 to 0.7% of the United States population. Cavernous malformations may occur sporadically or be inherited in an autosomal dominant fashion. The familial form accounts for over half of the cases and is characterized by multiple lesions[(27)]. In adults, the hemorrhage rate per lesion per year is between 0.1 and 1.1%[(27,28)]. Given the low rate of spontaneous hemorrhage, surgery is reserved for symptomatic (e.g., seizures or headache) lesions.

An AVM is a mixture of abnormal arteries and veins. These lesions are generally in the subarachnoid space, although some have an intraparenchymal component. They are most commonly located near the Sylvian fissure[(26)] (Fig. 25.6). 40% are found in the posterior fossa[(29)]. AVMs may account for 30 to 50% of ICH in children. In a series of 166 adults, re-bleeding occurred at a rate of 4% per year, with a mortality rate of 1% per year[(30)].

AVMs represent a low-resistance portion of the vascular circuit, with a correspondingly high blood flow. The feeding vessels for AVMs are functionally abnormal. They lack vasoreactivity to CO_2. Hyperventilation induces more hemodynamic changes in normal vessels than in vessels that feed an AVM[(31)].

Treatment strategies for AVMs vary according to region, medical center, and neurosurgical preference. Modalities may be used solo and in combination. These include embolization, microneurosurgery, and radiosurgery. Choice of treatment depends on size, location, and operability of the lesion.

At our institution, the majority of AVMs are approached

in stages. Preoperative anatomy is defined angiographically. Feeding vessels are embolized endovascularly to reduce risk of intraoperative bleeding. At microneurosurgery, feeding vessels are clipped and the lesion is excised. Follow-up angiography confirms complete eradication of the AVM. Additional embolization and surgery is occasionally necessary.

Successful treatment of an AVM may be assessed during embolization and surgery. Some advocate continuous monitoring of jugular bulb oxygen saturations during embolization to determine adequacy of embolization[32]. Doppler ultrasound provides another option for assessing postembolization flow[33]. Improved surgical success for difficult to visualize AVMs may be achieved with intraoperative angiography[34].

Series of surgically treated AVMs describe normal neurologic outcome in 67 to 85% of cases. Morbidity associated with embolization and surgery ranged from 2 to 15%, with periprocedural mortality of less than 2%[35–38].

Radiosurgery refers to the destruction of intracranial targets, such as AVMs and tumors, with single, large doses of stereotactically guided ionizing radiation generated in a linear accelerator. Appropriate use of this technology, also known as the gamma knife, for treatment of AVMs remains controversial. Critical evaluation of this therapy is limited by absence of a controlled, randomized study in the literature.

This therapy has been used effectively in lesions of varying size, grade, and location[39]. No studies report early morbidity associated with radiosurgery. The most comprehensive study reports obliteration of 100% of AVMs less than 1 cm in diameter, decreasing to 58% in lesions larger than 4 cm[40]. Another study reports an 81% thrombosis rate without correlation between AVM size and success[41]. A report from Boston describes complete obliteration of AVMs in five of eight children. In the 12-month follow-up period, no patient had ICH[42].

A single study compares microneurosurgery to radiosurgery for hard-to-reach AVMs smaller than 3 cm in diameter. The radiosurgery data were compiled from five centers using this modality. Success was comparable. These authors suggest that radiosurgery should be reserved for AVMs that are truly inoperable with standard techniques[43].

The vein of Galen aneurysm predisposes children to ICH. As with other dural AVMs, arterial supply comes from both the tentorial artery (internal carotid system) and the meningeal artery (external carotid system)[44]. Clinical presentation of this large, low-resistance lesion varies with the age of the patient. At the Hospital for Sick Children in Toronto, 88% of affected neonates presented with high-output heart failure[45]. Hydrocephalus and bleeding predominate later in infancy and childhood (Fig. 25.7). Bleeding may originate from the fragile feeding vessels as well as from the dural malformation itself.

Saccular, or berry, aneurysms are diagnosed less commonly in children than in adults. In two large studies, 0.5 and 0.6% of all aneurysms were found in patients younger than 19 years of age[46]. Most intracranial saccular aneurysms are located in the anterior circulation (Fig. 25.8)[47,48]. Debate exists in the literature regarding whether pediatric and adult aneurysms are distributed differently throughout the brain. The most common locations are the bifurcation of the internal carotid artery (26%), the anterior cerebral-anterior communicating artery complex (20%), and the vertebral-basilar artery complex (20%)[45].

Multiple aneurysms are present in 5% of children as opposed to 10 to 20% of adults[49]. Intracranial aneurysms have been shown to be familial in some rare circumstances[50]. Saccular aneurysms may be associated with Marfan's syndrome, autosomal dominant polycystic kidney disease, coarctation of the aorta, fibromuscular dysplasia, Moyamoya, pituitary tumors, and defects in type III collagen. Ten percent of patients with an AVM also have an associated aneurysm[51]. The combination of AVM and aneurysm increases the risk of ICH[52].

Treatment is largely surgical. Vascular reconstruction may be necessary in some instances.

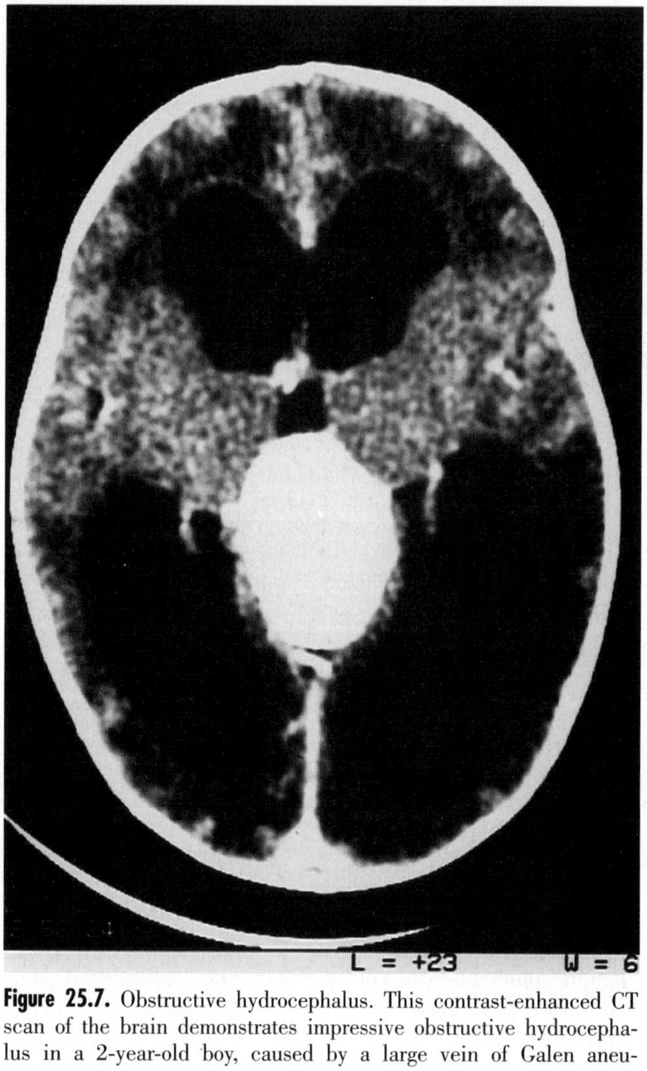

Figure 25.7. Obstructive hydrocephalus. This contrast-enhanced CT scan of the brain demonstrates impressive obstructive hydrocephalus in a 2-year-old boy, caused by a large vein of Galen aneurysm.

Cardioembolic Stroke

Cardioembolic events cause approximately 25% of strokes in infants and children[1]. These strokes may be bland or hemorrhagic, and are rarely preceded by TIAs. Typically, the patient's symptoms are maximal at the time of the event. Cardiac origin of the stroke may be inferred by the presence of structural heart disease, contractile dysfunction, or cardiac rhythm disturbance. Precise questioning may identify a history of palpitations, lightheadedness, or syncope. Physical examination may reveal stigmata of systemic embolism.

If cardioembolic disease is entertained as a possible cause for a stroke, evaluation should include a chest radiograph, 12-lead EKG, and transthoracic echocardiography. Some patients will need additional investigation of their heart rhythm or search for intracardiac thrombus. Complementary studies include Holter monitor, cardiac MRI, high-speed cardiac CT, and transesophageal echocardiography (TEE). In the setting of a convincing history, negative studies for thrombus must be viewed with skepticism.

Many clinicians, including those at our institution, feel that TEE is the most sensitive examination for cardiac thrombus. Unfortunately, even this technology is imperfect. Black et al. reported cerebral embolism in adult patients with atrial fibrillation after TEE showed no evidence of intracardiac thrombus[53].

Atrial fibrillation and sick-sinus syndrome are the arrhythmias most commonly associated with embolic CNS disease. De novo atrial fibrillation is extremely rare in children. It is usually seen in patients with Wolff-Parkinson-White syndrome or hyperthyroidism. The sick-sinus syndrome often manifests itself as a "tachy-brady" rhythm[54]. Both arrhythmias predispose individuals to atrial thrombus formation and thromboembolism.

Hemodynamic stasis in dilated cardiomyopathy predisposes individuals to intracardiac thrombus and embolism. Adult studies describe left ventricular mural thrombus in up to two-thirds of patients with dilated cardiomyopathy[55,56]. Clinically significant embolization occurs at a rate of approximately 4% per year[49].

Most significant structural heart disease is diagnosed early in childhood. Children with atrial or ventricular septal defects are at particular risk for cerebral emboli. Emboli from the great veins may pass from the right to the left circulations across a septal defect. Thus, a small embolus has the potential to cause a significant stroke instead of a relatively innocuous pulmonary embolism. This process is referred to as *paradoxical embolization.* Patent foramen ovales are generally clinically silent, are present in 10% of

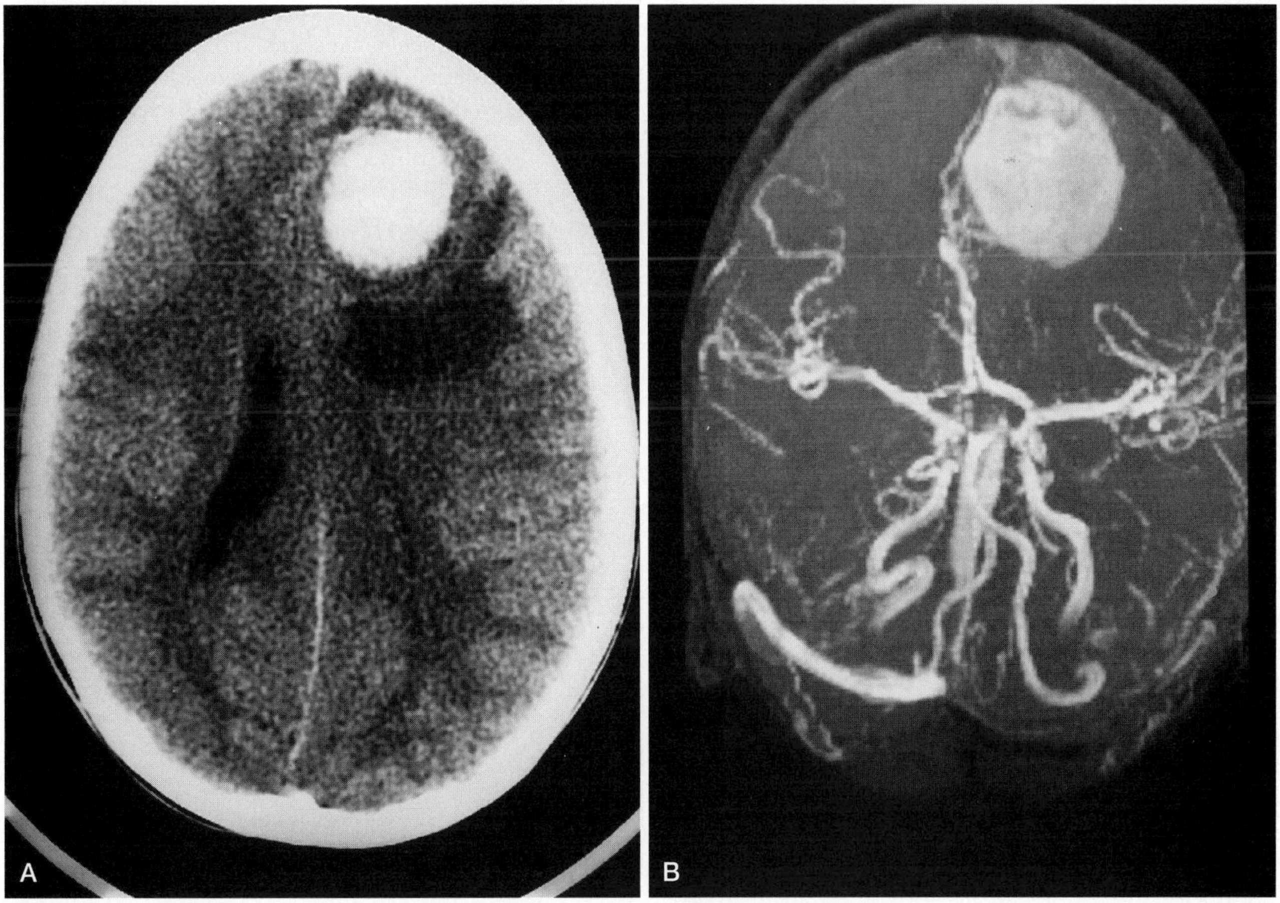

Figure 25.8. Aneurysmal vascular malformation. **A.** A contrast-enhanced CT scan of a 14-year-old boy's brain; the boy complained of frontal headaches. **B.** Angiography delineates a large aneurysm of the left anterior cerebral artery.

the population, and may be a source of paradoxical emboli. Two studies report up to 40% incidence of patent foramen ovale in otherwise unexplained, apparently embolic stroke[(57,58)].

Valvular heart disease may cause cerebral embolism. Rheumatic heart disease may lead to mitral stenosis, left atrial enlargement, and occasionally to atrial fibrillation. These factors predispose patients to atrial thrombus formation and thromboemboli. Mitral valve prolapse has been linked to otherwise unexplained cerebral ischemia[(59)]. Septic thrombi may embolize systemically in the setting of infectious endocarditis[(60)].

Central Nervous System Vasculitis

CNS vasculitis is histologically characterized by obliterative, necrotizing arteritis. Large and small vessels of the meninges and brain may be affected. This disease process must be suspected in any patient with central nervous system infection, drug abuse, evidence of systemic autoimmune disease, or with multiple and/or recurrent strokes. The strokes may be either ischemic or hemorrhagic **(Table 25.2)**.

Bacterial meningitis may cause significant intracranial arteritis. Any of the common pathogens (group B streptococcus, *Haemophilus influenzae*, pneumococcus, or meningococcus) may cause vascular inflammation. Unfortunately, stroke is a common complication of meningitis, especially in the very young patient (Fig. 25.9)[(61)]. Early sterilization of the spinal fluid does not necessarily protect against stroke, suggesting that the bacteria is not the sole inflammatory culprit.

Table 25.2. Evaluation of Central Nervous System Vasculitis

Drug screen
Antinuclear antibodies
Rheumatoid factor
C3, C4, CH50
Neutrophilic cytoplasmic antibody (antineutrophil cytoplasm antibody)
Coomb's test
Cerebrospinal fluid studies
Tissue biopsy
Visceral angiography
Erythrocyte sedimentation rate

A comparison of 17 children with *H. influenzae* meningitis with age-matched controls showed sixfold increases in platelet-activating factor (PAF) in the CSF of the children with meningitis[(62)]. PAF is a potent inflammatory mediator and vasoconstrictor, and causes vascular injury in experimental models of necrotizing enterocolitis. PAF or other proinflammatory substances may contribute to strokes in bacterial meningitis.

Other CNS infections can also cause vasculitis and stroke. These include tuberculosis, fungus, syphilis, mycoplasma, HIV, and cat-scratch disease[(63–69)].

Amphetamines may precipitate ICH secondary to sympathomimetic effect. These drugs may also cause cerebral vasculitis and stroke. Two articles describe angiographic and pathologic findings of vasculitis in several young adult users of dextroamphetamine and methamphetamine[(70,71)]. The mechanism may be immune-complex mediated.

A variety of systemic inflammatory diseases have been

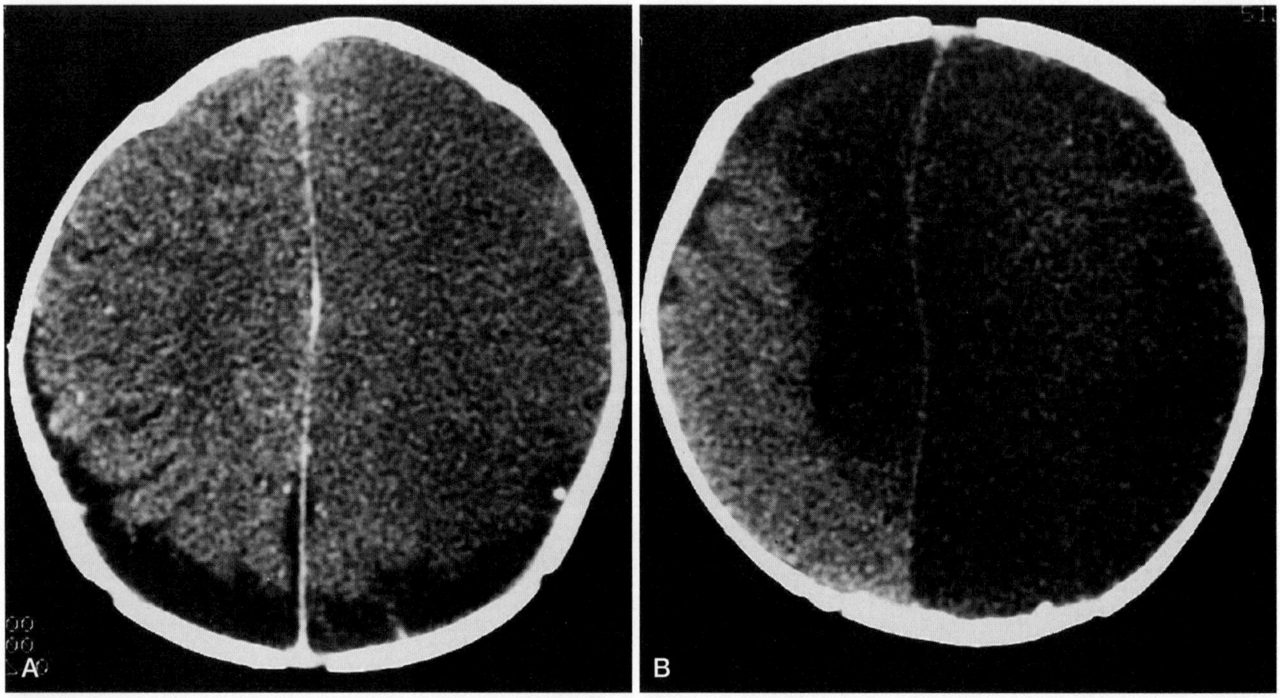

Figure 25.9. Bland cerebral infarction and bacterial meningitis. These unenhanced brain CT scans demonstrate evolution of bland cerebral infarction in a previously healthy 5-month-old girl with pneumococcal meningitis. CT scan **A** was obtained on hospital day 2 and **B** was obtained on hospital day 6. The stroke involves the entire left hemisphere and the anterior cerebral artery distribution on the right side. Support was withdrawn on hospital day 6.

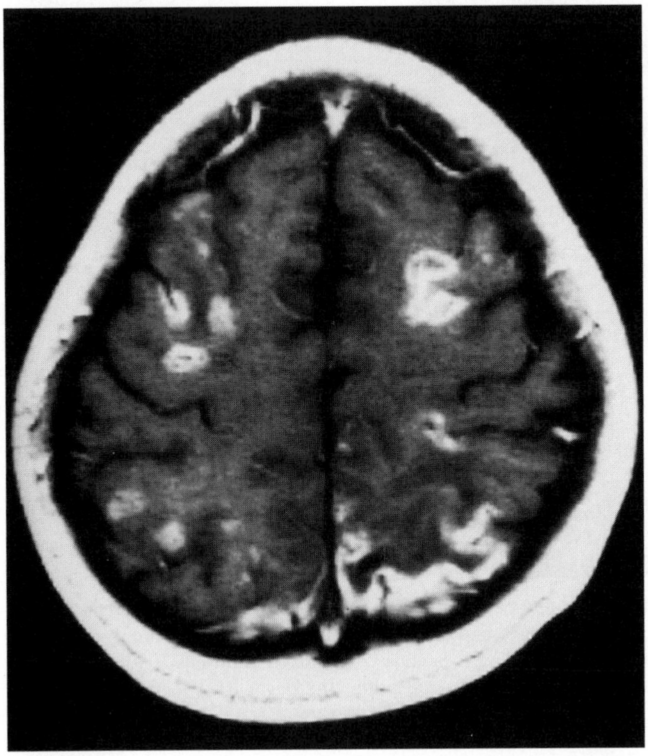

Figure 25.10. Noninfectious cerebral vasculitis. This T-2 weighted brain MRI scan shows multiple sites of abnormal enhancement representing stroke. The patient is an 11-year-old girl with idiopathic vasculitis affecting her kidneys, lungs, and brain.

associated with stroke. The mechanism of stroke in these diseases is not well understood but are believed to be secondary to vasculitis. They include polyarteritis nodosa, systemic lupus erythematosis, ulcerative colitis (another PAF-associated disease), Takayasu's arteritis, Henoch-Schonlein purpura, and mixed-connective tissue disease[72–76]. General laboratory findings are indicative of nonspecific inflammation (e.g., elevated erythrocyte sedimentation rate).

Primary idiopathic cerebral vasculitis is a rare and confusing disease. Presentation varies dramatically from case to case. Lesions may be multiple or single (Fig. 25.10). Patients may have a spectrum of neurological symptoms from focal to generalized encephalopathy. Strokes may be hemorrhagic or ischemic. Brain biopsy is the diagnostic gold standard. Given the spotty, unpredictable nature of this disease, a negative biopsy does not rule out cerebral vasculitis. Angiography may show evidence of vasculitis but is highly variable. CSF and serologic studies may be normal or show nonspecific signs of inflammation[77,78]. Making this difficult diagnosis is important, as treatment with high-dose steroids and cyclophosphamide may be clinically helpful[79].

Thrombotic Stroke

Thrombotic, or bland, stroke may occur secondary to deranged hemostasis, vascular disease, or genetic disorders or in association with migraine.

Table 25.3. Evaluation of Coagulation in Cerebrovascular Disease

Complete blood count
Prothrombin time, partial thromboplastin time
Fibrin degradation products
D-dimer
Plasma fibrinogen
Plasminogen levels
Factor V, VII, IX, X, XI, XIII assay
Plasma antithrombin-III activity
Protein C and S levels
Plasma fibrinogen
Bleeding time
Antiphospholipid antibodies
Anticardiolipin antibodies

Hemostatic Disorders

Two to seven percent of ischemic strokes in children and young adults are caused by thrombotic disorders[80]. These hypercoagulable states may be either primary or secondary **(Table 25.3)**.

A primary hypercoagulable state should be suspected in a child if there is a personal or family history of deep venous thrombosis, pulmonary embolus, or previous ischemic stroke. Antithrombin III, protein S, and protein C deficiencies are the most common inherited causes of hypercoagulability[81]. Resistance to activated protein C has recently been implicated in thromboembolism[82]. These entities are inherited independently in an autosomal dominant fashion. Homozygous disease may be early and fulminant (e.g., protein S—purpura fulminans neonatalis). Heterozygosity predisposes the patient to thrombosis (especially venous) and thromboembolism. All of these disorders may lead to stroke. The event may be spontaneous or related to damage to the cerebral vasculature, as in minor head trauma[83].

Antiphospholipid antibodies are a well-recognized cause of hypercoagulability in adults, causing deep vein thrombosis, stroke, and fetal loss. The two most common antiphospholipid antibodies are the lupus anticoagulant and anticardiolipin antibodies. These antibodies may be found in otherwise healthy people as well as those with lupus erythematosis, other autoimmune diseases, cancer, and chronic infections (e.g., HIV). A subgroup with arterial and venous thromboses have been termed as having the *antiphospholipid syndrome*[84–86].

Decreased production of anti-thrombin III, inhibition of protein C activation, and platelet dysfunction have been invoked as possible mechanisms of antiphospholipid syndrome hypercoagulability. At this time, no explanation is definitive[87]. Recently, several groups have identified antiphospholipid antibodies in children with otherwise unexplained ischemic stroke[88,89].

Hyperviscocity secondary to polycythemia (e.g., cyanotic heart disease) and sickle cell disease leads to microvascular sludging and predisposes to thrombotic stroke. Risk for stroke in sickle cell disease increases with fever, dehydration, and low oxygen tension[90,91]. Patients with sickle cell disease most commonly suffer cerebral infarction or dural sinus thrombosis (Fig. 25.11). They are also at risk for ICH.

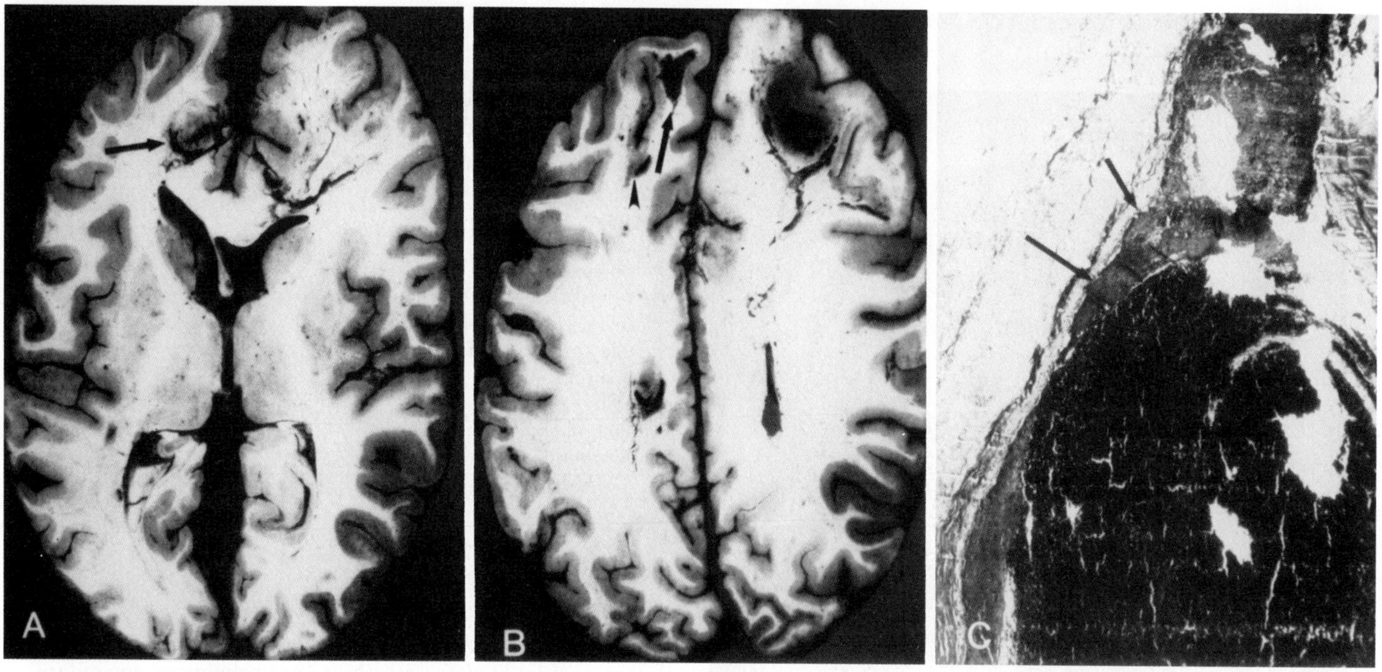

Figure 25.11. Thrombosis of the superior sagittal sinus in a 7-year-old child with sickle cell anemia; the child survived 5 days after the stroke. **A** and **B** demonstrate subarachnoid hemorrhage, subcortical brain hemorrhages *(arrows)*, and marked softening of the right frontal white matter. **C.** Cross-section of superior sagittal sinus showing incomplete occlusion by organizing thrombus. Hematoxylin and eosin. (Original magnification ×250.) (From Garcia JH, Anderson ML. Circulatory disorders and their effects on the brain. In: Davis RL, Robertson DM, eds. Textbook of neuropathology. 2nd ed. Baltimore: Williams & Wilkins, 1991:674.)

Stroke occurs in 6 to 9% of patients with sickle cell disease[92]. Cerebrovascular events may be decreased with exchange transfusions to keep hemoglobin S less than 30%[93]. Sickle cell patients with acute stroke are aggressively transfused to achieve hemoglobin S less than 20% of total.

Thrombosis of the dural sinuses may lead to ICH; however, ischemic stroke is more common. The bleeding may be subarachnoid or intraparenchymal. The most common causes are severe dehydration, trauma, and infection[94]. Hypercoagulable states and childhood cancer, especially acute lymphoblastic leukemia, have been implicated[95].

As with other venous thromboses, cavernous sinus thrombosis is also caused by dehydration and trauma, but is most strongly associated with bacterial infections of the face, bony sinuses, and orbits. The internal carotid artery, and cranial nerves III, IV, and VI pass through this unique venous sinus. Thrombosis may present with headache, ophthalmoplegia, or cranial nerve palsy. This entity is especially well imaged with magnetic resonance angiography.

Genetic/Metabolic Disease

Several rare genetic disorders may predispose a child to stroke. Homocystinuria is caused by a deficiency of cystathionine synthase. It is inherited in an autosomal recessive fashion. Affected individuals may have platelet dysfunction, leading to thrombotic events, including pulmonary embolism and stroke. Accumulation of homocysteine may also damage vascular endothelium, leading to occlusion[96]. These patients are treated with vitamin B_6 and antiplatelet drugs[97,98].

Recently, urea cycle defects have been added to the list of genetic causes for stroke. Ornithine transcarbamalase deficiency has been associated with repeated strokes[99].

Rarely, bland stroke may be caused by mitochondrial myopathy, encephalopathy, lactic acidosis, and stroke-like episodes (MELAS). Abnormal mitochondria are found in the blood vessels, muscle, and brain of these patients. Intermittent vasospasm and focal metabolic failure have been invoked as possible mechanisms for stroke[100].

Other inherited diseases uncommonly associated with stroke include Leigh's disease, methylmalonic acidemia, propionic acidemia, isovaleric acidemia, and Fabry's disease.

Vascular Disease

Vascular malformation, injury, and disease may cause ischemic stroke. Moyamoya is a noninflammatory vasculopathy. Moyamoya means "puff of smoke" in Japanese and is descriptive of this disorder's angiographic findings in the basal ganglia (Fig. 25.12). Histologically, affected vessels are tortuous with endothelial thickening and fibrosis. This thickening starts at the terminal internal carotid artery, extends to the proximal anterior and middle cerebral arteries, and causes progressive narrowing. The vertebral circulation is generally spared.

While Moyamoya can cause both hemorrhagic and bland strokes, ischemic manifestations predominate in children[101]. Repeated ischemic strokes are often seen. Infarctions are generally found in watershed areas of the brain. Surgical therapy may be fraught with difficulty, given the diffuse nature of this vasculopathy.

Cervicocephalic arterial dissection causes up to 22% of ischemic strokes in patients under 30 years of age[102]. It is the most common nonatherosclerotic vasculopathy leading to cerebral infarction in all age groups[103]. Dissection occurs when blood works its way between the intima and

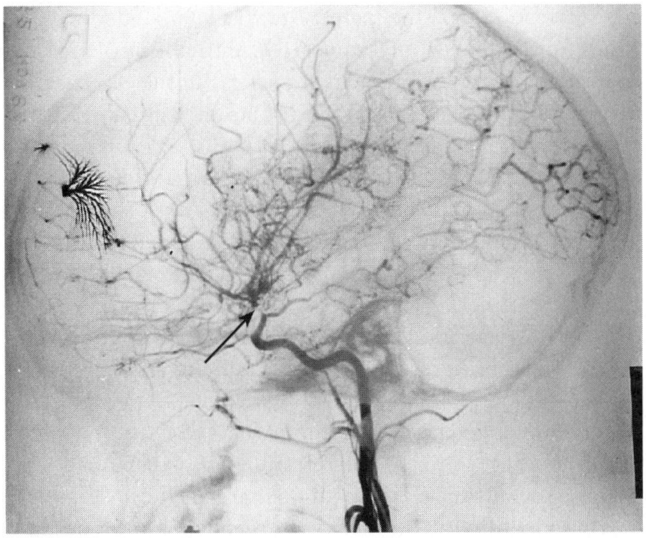

Figure 25.12. Moyamoya. This lateral cerebral angiogram demonstrates truncation of the right internal carotid artery (arrow) and associated disorganized vasculature characteristic of Moyamoya.

media. The dissection propagates distally and causes narrowing or occlusion of the vessel. Dissections start in the cervical internal carotid or vertebral arteries. The origin of the lesion is rarely intracranial.

Dissections may occur spontaneously, secondary to trauma, or in association with Marfan's syndrome, cystic medial degeneration, fibromuscular dysplasia, luetic arteritis, Moyamoya, and tonsillitis[(49)]. Injury to the high cervical spine is associated with vertebral artery dissection. Falls with a sharp object (e.g., a pencil) in the mouth are associated with internal carotid artery dissection[(104)].

Arterial dissection must be considered in any child with unexplained cerebral infarction. Angiographic resolution of spontaneous internal carotid artery dissection occurs within 3 months in 85% of cases[(49)]. Prognosis for neurologic recovery is good in stroke secondary to arterial dissection[(105)]. Surgery rarely plays a role in the therapy of cervicocephalic arterial dissection.

Migraine

Migraine headaches affect 10% of the United States population[(106)]. A subset of patients have neurologic symptoms such as aphasia, paralysis, and sensory changes associated with the headache. For over a century, physicians have recognized that during the course of a migraine these symptoms can become permanent[(107)]. A variety of pathophysiologic mechanisms linking migraine to cerebral infarction have been postulated. These include arterial dissection, platelet dysfunction, and vasospasm[(108–110)].

No proposed mechanism has proven to be definitive, and the cause of stroke in these patients may be multifactorial. For example, antiphospholipid antibodies may coexist in a patient with migraine. There is evidence that some patients with migraine have abnormal brain energy metabolism. In a recent study, 9 of 12 patients with a history of migraine had high adenosine diphosphate concentration and low phosphorylation potential in their brains as measured by ^{31}P magnetic resonance spectroscopy[(111)]. The authors suggest that these patients have relatively little cerebral metabolic reserve and that deficiencies of cerebral energy production may be important to migrainous symptoms. As with MELAS, these patients may be at risk for focal metabolic failure and stroke.

Documented cerebral infarction occurs in less than 1% of children with migraine. Although a causal relationship has not been shown in any pediatric cases, a history of migraines may be a contributory risk factor for childhood stroke[(112)].

Flunarizine is an oral, nonspecific calcium antagonist used as prophylaxis against hemiplegic migraines[(113)]. An intravenous formulation has been proposed as therapy for evolving stroke in patients with migraine.

DIAGNOSTIC APPROACH

Presentation and Initial Diagnosis

The clinical presentation of cerebrovascular diseases in children are as diverse as the neurologic repertoire of the affected brain and will depend on the type, extent, and distribution of the vascular event. Cerebral thrombotic disease classically evolves over several hours, and embolic events are typically sudden and complete at onset, although this distinction in presentation tends to be much more subtle in infants and children than in older patients. Symptoms may include decreased sensorium, frank coma, generalized or focal seizures, headache, or discrete functional deficits (Fig. 25.13). In general, the more anterior an ischemic lesion is, the more likely it is to result in impairment of motor and speech function, whereas posterior lesions are associated with sensory and visual field impairment. The distribution of the middle cerebral artery is most often involved in embolic and thrombotic ischemic injury, and lesions in this area may produce the symptom complex of hemiplegia and hemianesthesia, apraxias, agnosias, and homonymous hemianopsia. Seizures at the onset of stroke are more common in infants and children younger than age 4 years.

Fever or other evidence of infection is common in pediatric patients with stroke, with over half of children presenting with ischemic infarcts having evidence of infection. Meningitis and infections of the ears, mastoids, paranasal sinuses, and soft tissues of the face are the commonest infections associated with ischemic cerebral injury. Close attention to concurrent medical problems such as structural heart disease or acute drug intoxication may be helpful in guiding a work-up.

A patient who presents with acute, unexplained neurologic changes should receive an imaging study of the brain (see subsequent sections), chemistry profile, complete blood count, and coagulation studies. Further work-up should be dictated by physical examination, history, and radiologic findings. In many instances, initial treatment of symptoms (e.g., status epilepticus) will take precedence over definitive diagnosis.

Emergent evaluation must focus on airway protection, cardiovascular stabilization, and exclusion of a surgically remediable cause for the symptoms.

Computed Tomography

The CT scan remains the initial radiological examination of choice in nearly all pediatric patients with an acute change in neurologic status. For the unstable patient, a CT scan of the brain is fast (less than 15 minutes), rarely requires sedation, does not prevent rapid access to the patient in an emergency, and is easily interpretable. It also remains the most sensitive test for fresh bleeding, which appears hyperdense (very white). As such, it is very useful in determining the need for immediate surgical intervention.

An acute brain infarction may be difficult to detect if the CT scan is obtained when the lesion is less than 24 hours old. A study in adult patients demonstrated 54% sensitivity at detecting cerebral infarcts in the first 24 hours[(114)]. The lesions become more clearly demarcated over the next several days, as the affected brain becomes hypodense. A contrast-enhanced study will demonstrate luxury perfusion around a stroke between 1 and 3 weeks postinfarct.

CT is not the optimal study for pathology suspected in the brain stem, basal ganglia, and posterior fossa. While superior at imaging bone and fresh blood, it does not offer the anatomic detail of magnetic resonance imaging (MRI).

Magnetic Resonance Imaging

MRI is a valuable tool in the routine evaluation of the child with suspected cerebrovascular disease who is stable from a cardiorespiratory standpoint. Drawbacks include length of study (up to 1 hour for brain MRI); difficulty in assessing the patient and lack of emergent access to the patient during the study; and magnetic constraints on ventilators, monitors, and intravenous pumps.

MRI is excellent for diagnosis of small lesions and disease in the anatomic areas in which CT is weak (brain stem, basal ganglia, and posterior fossa). MRI is especially sensitive (84%) in the diagnosis of ischemic stroke in the first 24 hours[(114)].

An MRI scan can provide useful information about the cerebral vasculature. Blood moving through vessels is interpreted by MRI as very low density and represented as black. This phenomenon is referred to as *flow void.* Absence of flow void in the anatomic distribution of a major vessel suggests occlusion or markedly decreased flow[(115)]. AVMs may be identified by flow void in an unusual location. Specifically, Moyamoya is noted to have MRI characteristics of MCA flow void, basal ganglia hypodensities, and strokes in the carotid distribution[(116,117)].

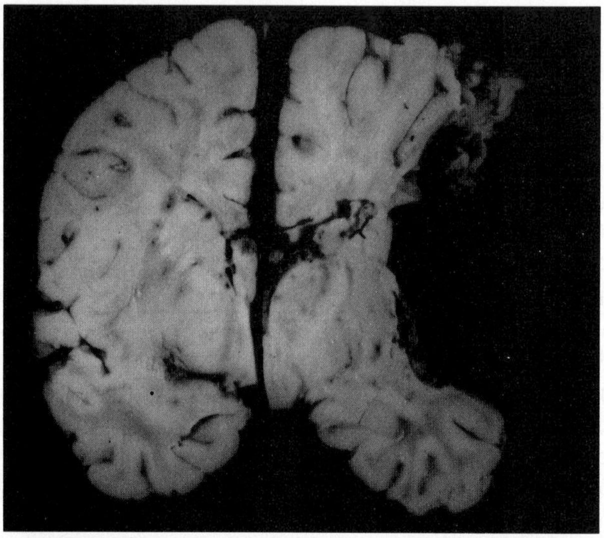

Figure 25.13. Brain section from a 3-month-old infant with biliary atresia and severe coagulopathy who suffered an abrupt episode with one high-pitched cry followed by a coma, intracranial hypertension, and absence of cerebral blood flow on angiogram. Section demonstrates the large area occupied by the clot, which had ruptured from its intracerebral origin into the subdural space. (Courtesy of Grover Hutchins, M.D., Department of Pathology, The Johns Hopkins Medical Institutions.)

Angiography

Cerebral angiography remains the gold standard for evaluating cerebrovascular disease and is the most valuable study for determining pathogenesis of a stroke. Any intracranial hemorrhage without a traumatic history and with normal coagulation studies and platelet count necessitates thorough evaluation of the cerebral vasculature. The clinician must aggressively search for a surgically correctable lesion such as AVM, aneurysm, or vasculopathy.

In preparation for surgery, angiographic evaluation of nontraumatic hemorrhage should proceed once the child is stable from a hemodynamic and respiratory standpoint. Given the 3% yearly risk of bleeding from an AVM and the 40% combined morbidity and mortality from each bleed, there is good evidence to support rapid radiological evaluation and prompt surgical excision of accessible vascular lesions[(118,119)].

While some debate exists in the literature regarding the need for formal angiography versus noninvasive magnetic angiography (MRA)[(120)], the pediatric neurosurgeons at our institution will rarely operate without the angiogram. At this time, no large, controlled study of MRA or transcranial ultrasound versus traditional angiography has been performed in children. Anecdotally, our pediatric neuroradiologists feel that MRA misses some important pathologic findings, especially the inflammatory vasculopathies.

The role of angiography in ischemic stroke is less clear. Generally, if the cause is known (e.g., protein S deficiency), angiography will add little to patient care. However, angiography remains important in the evaluation of a cerebral infarction of unknown cause and may have therapeutic implications (e.g., steroids and cyclophosphamide for inflammatory vasculopathies).

Cerebral angiography has some drawbacks and relative contraindications. Young patients need sedation for the procedure, occasionally necessitating prophylactic intubation.

Caution should be used regarding intravenous contrast in patients with diminished renal function. Theoretic concerns exist regarding angiography precipitating reembolization of intraarterial thrombus. Extrapolating from the adult literature, transient neurologic symptoms occur after 2.7% of angiograms, and 0.4% of studies are associated with permanent neurologic impairment[121]. In comprehensive studies, these sequelae are not reported in patients under 30 years of age.

Magnetic Resonance Angiography

MRA represents a promising and evolving technology with regard to cerebrovascular disease. This study adds approximately 15 minutes to a standard brain MRI scan, requires no additional sedation, and is noninvasive. Some authors suggest that MRA may offer sufficient preoperative imaging for certain pediatric AVMs[120–123]. This may be so for low-grade AVMs in less functionally dense areas of the brain. MRA represents an effective technology for following defined vascular lesions after conventional or radiosurgery[25]. It also offers an alternative to angiography to patients with poor renal function or known intraarterial thrombus.

Transcranial Doppler Ultrasound

Transcranial Doppler ultrasound fills much of the same noninvasive niche as MRA. It is highly dependent on operator skill. Furthermore, there is considerable intersubject variability[124].

Some institutions use Doppler studies to determine the efficacy of preoperative AVM embolization[33]. This technology is also used to screen for cerebrovascular disease in children with sickle cell disease[125]. The utility of this study in the work-up of the acutely ill PICU patient remains unproved.

TREATMENT

Supportive Therapy

PICU care of the stroke patient revolves around meticulous attention to basic management, supporting critical organ system function. Patients with a Glascow coma score of less than 8, increased intracranial pressure (ICP), or poor airway protective reflexes should be intubated. Intracranial pressure monitoring, with an external ventricular drain (EVD), should be considered in patients with focal CNS lesions and evidence of ICP.

Increased ICP is treated with mild hyperventilation, pCO_2 30 to 35. The head of the patient's bed is elevated to 30 degrees. Osmotic diuretics may be helpful. Sedatives, analgesics, and pharmacological paralysis are useful adjuncts in controlling ICP (see Chapter 18, Pathophysiology and Clinical Management of the Intracranial Vault).

Blood pressure control is paramount in the acute management of stroke. Although chronic hypertension is a less commonly associated medical condition in pediatric stroke patients, it may be present in children with a systemic vasculitis underlying their cerebral ischemia. As cerebral autoregulation is maintained at a higher level than in normotensive patients, significant diminution in cerebral blood flow may occur with any decrease in blood pressure. Since autoregulation of cerebral blood flow may also be impaired following stroke, overzealous correction of hypertension may extend areas of ischemia even in previously normotensive patients. In the event of malignant hypertension, calcium channel blockers and nitroprusside are effective and well tolerated. Beta-blockers should be avoided, given concerns regarding unopposed alpha effect and excessive cerebral vasoconstriction.

Careful attention is paid to a patient's coagulation status. Coagulopathy should be treated aggressively with FFP, vitamin K, cryoprecipitate, protamine, and specific clotting factors, as the clinical situations demands. Hemophiliacs should have factor levels corrected to at least 50% of normal activity.

Surgical Therapy

In very rare instances of uncontrollable ICP secondary to a large ischemic stroke, surgical intervention may be warranted. A small study in adults with massive cerebral artery infarction documents good neurologic outcome in patients who underwent strokectomy for declining level of consciousness[126].

Anticoagulant and Thrombolytic Therapy

Cardioembolic strokes, especially large embolic infarcts, have a propensity to undergo hemorrhagic transformation, with resulting increase in neurologic impairment, thus the decision to administer anticoagulation must be based on the relative risks of recurrent embolization versus bleeding complications. Despite a risk of bleeding into an ischemic stroke, heparinization and warfarinization are indicated for patients with intracardiac thrombus. Patients with primary hypercoagulable states (e.g., protein C deficiency) should be heparinized (PTT 1.5 times normal) then maintained on warfarin (PT 1.5 times normal). Patients with AT III deficiency should receive replacement with plasma as well as heparin. Anticoagulation of children with idiopathic thrombotic stroke is not well studied.

The potential role of exogenous thrombolytics (urokinase, streptokinase, and recombinant tissue plasminogen activator) has received considerable attention in the literature on adult ischemic stroke. Several studies have shown that early arterial recanalization with superselective catheterization and infusion of thrombolytics is associated with improved clinical outcome. Intravenous administration may also result in arterial recanalization. Late thrombolytic therapy (more than 6 hours after onset of symptoms) has been associated with hemorrhagic transformation. This body of literature is limited by a lack of randomized, controlled studies[127].

In the future, interventional thrombolysis may result in improved neurologic outcome in selected pediatric stroke patients who are rapidly diagnosed and have no radiologic evidence of intracranial hemorrhage.

Neuroprotective Therapy

Brain that is completely deprived of blood flow loses viability within a matter of minutes. Newly completed ischemic stroke is surrounded by an area of marginally perfused and potentially viable brain, the penumbra. The goal of neuroprotective therapy, including hemodilution, pentoxifylline, and calcium channel blockers, is to maximize salvage of the penumbra.

Of these modalities, hemodilution has been most extensively studied. Several randomized, controlled trials of isovolemic or hypervolemic hemodilution using varying degrees of phlebotomy and colloid replacement have been performed in adults with ischemic stroke. Improved short-term and long-term neurologic outcomes have been reported in patients randomized to isovolemic or hypervolemic hemodilution compared with control patients, whose stroke therapy was the same except for the exclusion of hemodilution[128,129]. One study noted the significant prevalence of dehydration in the setting of acute ischemic stroke and observed improvement in neurologic outcome in patients with initial hematocrits greater than 45% who received crystalloid without phlebotomy[130].

There have been no studies of hemodilution for therapy of acute stroke in infants and children. Prophylactic phlebotomy may prevent cerebrovascular accidents in patients with polycythemic states. At this time, it is appropriate to correct hemoconcentration associated with dehydration and volume depletion. Further study of active hemodilution via phlebotomy and colloid administration is needed before this treatment is used in pediatric stroke victims.

Pentoxifylline decreases blood viscosity by improving the deformability of the formed elements of blood and by decreasing fibrinogen levels. Given intravenously, it improves early neurologic symptoms in adults with acute ischemic stroke. It does not affect mortality or late neurologic outcome[131].

Calcium channel blockers relax vascular smooth muscle. In doses that maintain normal blood pressure, these drugs do not significantly reduce calcium influx into neurons[131a]. Several adult studies have shown that early (less than 12 hours after initial symptoms occurred), daily treatment with 60 or 120 mg of nimodipine resulted in improved neurologic outcome[132–134].

Relaxation of cerebral vasospasm secondary to aneurysmal subarachnoid hemorrhage is the best defined role for calcium channel blockers in the PICU[135].

OUTCOME

The outcome following stroke is dependent on the type and location of the event, the age of the patient, and the underlying disease process. Children with hemorrhagic stroke fare worse from a functional standpoint than do those with ischemic stroke. In the Cincinnati study, ischemic stroke carried a 14%, 30-day mortality rate, as opposed to 22% for hemorrhagic stroke[2]. In surviving patients, the prevalence of neurologic disability is similar with either type of stroke and is approximately 75%. Despite this high incidence of residual deficit, most young stroke victims have normal or near normal functional motor development and global cognitive function.

SUMMARY

Childhood strokes fall into two categories: ischemic and hemorrhagic. Causes are diverse. Most imaging strategies should include a study of the cerebral vasculature. Patient care revolves around management of increased intracranial pressure, appropriate blood pressure manipulations, and attention to the child's coagulation status.

References

1. Schoenberg B, Mellinger J, Schoenberg D. Cerebrovascular disease in infants and children: a study of incidence, clinical features, and survival. Neurology 1978;28:763–768.
2. Broderick J, Talbot G, Prenger E, Leach A, Brott T. Stroke in children within a major metropolitan area: the surprising importance of intracerebral hemorrhage. Journal of Child Neurology 1993;8(3):250–255.
3. Daniels S, Bates S, Lukin R, et al. Cerebrovascular arteriopathy and ischemic childhood stroke. Stroke 1982;13:360–365.
4. Modan B, Wagener D. Some epidemiological aspects of stroke: mortality/morbidity trends, age, sex, race, socioeconomic status. Stroke 1992;23:1230–1236.
5. Chaou W, Chou M, Eitzman D. Intracranial hemorrhage and vitamin K deficiency in early infancy. Journal of Pediatrics 1984;105:880–884.
6. Schwartzman R, Hill S. Neurologic complications of disseminated intravascular coagulation. Neurology 1982;32:791–797.
7. Silverstein A. Neurologic complications of anticoagulation therapy: a neurologist's review. Archives of Internal Medicine 1979;139:217–220.
8. Forfar J. Prediction of hemorrhage in patients for long-term coumarin anticoagulation by excessive prothrombin ratio. American Heart Journal 1982;102:445–446.
9. Woerner S, Abildgaard C, French B. Intracranial hemorrhage in children with idiopathic thrombocytopenic purpura. Pediatrics 1981; 67:570–571.
10. Krivit W, Tate D, White J, Robison L. Idiopathic thrombocytopenic purpura and intracranial hemorrhage. Pediatrics 1981;67:570–571.
11. Martinowitz U, Heim M, Tadmor R, et al. Intracranial hemorrhage in patients with hemophilia. Neurosurgery 1986;18:538–541.
12. Matthay K, Koerper M, Ablin A. Intracranial hemorrhage in congenital factor VII deficiency. Journal of Pediatrics 1979;94:413–415.
13. Haerer A, Smith R. Cerebrovascular disease of young adults in a Mississippi teaching hospital. Stroke 1970;1:466–476.
14. Delaney P, Estes M. Intracranial hemorrhage with amphetamine abuse. Neurology 1980;30:1125–1128.
15. Klonoff D, Andrews B, Obana W. Stroke associated with cocaine use. Archives of Neurology 1989;46:989–993.
16. Green R, Kelly K, Gabrielsen T, et al. Multiple intracerebral hemorrhages after smoking "crack" cocaine. Stroke 1990;21:951–962.
17. Bernstein E, Diskont B. Phenylpropanolamine: a potentially hazardous drug. Annals of Emergency Medicine 1982;11:311–315.
18. Kaku, Lowenstein D. Emergence of recreational drug abuse as a major risk factor for stroke in young adults. Annals of Internal Medicine 1990;113(11):821–827.
19. Levine S, Brust J, Futrell N. A comparative study of the cerebrovascular complications of cocaine: alkaloidal versus hydrochloride—a review. Neurology 1991;41(8):1173–1177.
20. Altura B, Zhang A, Cheng T. Cocaine induces rapid loss of intracellular free Mg2+ in cerebral vascular smooth muscle cells. European Journal of Pharmacology 1993;246(3):299–301.

21. Oyesiku N, Colohan A, Barcow D, et al. Cocaine induced aneurysmal rupture: an emergent negative factor in the natural history of intracranial aneurysms. Neurosurgery 1993;32(4):518–526.
22. Lukes S. Intracranial hemorrhage from an arteriovenous malformation after amphetamine injection. Archives of Neurology 1983;40:60–61.
23. Little J, Dial B, Bellenger G, Carpenter S. Brain hemorrhage from intracranial tumor. Stroke 1979;10:283–288.
24. Wakai S, Yamakawa K, Manaka S, Takakura K. Spontaneous intracranial hemorrhage caused by brain tumor. Its incidence and clinical significance. Neurosurgery 1982;10:437–444.
25. Zabramski J, Wascher T, Spetzler R, et al. The natural history of familial cavernous malformations: results of an ongoing study. Journal of Neurosurgery 1994;80(3):422–432.
26. Edwards M, Hoffman H, eds. Cerebral Vascular Disease in Children and Adoloscents. Baltimore: Williams & Wilkins, 1989:101–102.
27. Rigamonti D, Hadley M, Drayer B, et al. Cerebral cavernous malformations. Incidence and familial occurrence. New England Journal of Medicine. 1988;319:343–347.
28. Curling OJ, Kelly DJ, Elster A, et al. An analysis of the natural history of cavernous angiomas. Journal of Neurosurgery 1991;75:702–708.
29. Humphreys B, Hendrick E, Hoffman H. Vascular malformations of the brainstem in childhood. Concepts in Pediatric Neurosurgery 1980;1:36–48.
30. Ondra S, Treup P, George E, Schwab K. The natural history of symptomatic arteriovenous malformations of the brain: a 24-year follow-up assessment. Journal of Neurosurgery 1991;73(3):387–391.
31. DeSalles A, Manchola I. CO_2 reactivity in arteriovenous malformations of the brain: a transcranial Doppler ultrasound study. Journal of Neurosurgery 1994;80(4):624–630.
32. Katayama Y, Tsubokawa T, Hirayama T, et al. Continuous monitoring of jugular bulb oxygen saturation as a measure of the shunt flow of cerebral arteriovenous malformations. Journal of Neurosurgery 1994; 80(5):826–833.
33. Westra S, Curran J, Duckwiler G, et al. Pediatric intracranial vascular malformations: evaluation of treatment results with Doppler US. Work in progress. Radiology 1993;186(3):775–783.
34. Anegawa S, Hayashi T, Torigoe R, et al. Intraoperative angiography in the resection of arteriovenous malformations. Journal of Neurosurgery 1994;80(1):73–78.
35. Morgan M, Johnston I, Hallihan J, et al. Complications of surgery for arteriovenous malformations of the brain. Journal of Neurosurgery. 1993;78(2):176–182.
36. Piepgras D, Sundt TJ, Ragoowansi A, et al. Seizure outcomes in patients with surgically treated cerebral arteriovenous malformations. Journal of Neurosurgery 1993;78(1):5–11.
37. Vinuela F, Dion J, Duckwiler G, et al. Combined endovascular embolization and surgery in the management of cerebral arteriovenous malformations: experience with 101 cases. Journal of Neurosurgery 1991;75(6):856–864.
38. Fox A, Pelz D, Lee D. Arteriovenous malformations of the brain: recent results of endovascular therapy. Radiology 1990;177(1):51–57.
39. Lunsford L, Flickinger J, Coffey R. Stereotactic gamma knife radiosurgery. Initial North American experience in 207 patients. Archives of Neurology 1990;47(2):169–175.
40. Lunsford L, Kondziolka D, Flickinger J, et al. Stereotactic radiosurgery for arteriovenous malformations of the brain. Journal of Neurosurgery 1991;75(4):512–524.
41. Friedman W, Boua F. Linear accelerator radiosurgery for arteriovenous malformations. Journal of Neurosurgery 1992;77(6):832–841.
42. Loeffler J, Rossitch E, Siddon R, et al. Role of stereotactic radiosurgery with a linear accelerator in treatment of intracranial arteriovenous malformations and tumors in children. Pediatrics 1990;85(5):774–782.
43. Sisti M, Kader A, Stein B. Microsurgery for 67 intracranial arteriovenous malformations less than 3 cm in diameter. Journal of Neurosurgery 1993;79(5):653–660.
44. Vidyasager C. Persistent embryonic veins in the arteriovenous malformations of the dura. Acta Neurochir 1979;48:199–216.
45. Hoffman H, Chuang S, Hendrick E, et al. Aneurysms of the vein of Galen: Experience at the Hospital for Sick Children, Toronto. Journal of Neurosurgery 1982;57:316–322.
46. Locksley H. Report on the Cooperative Study of Intracranial Aneurysms and Subarachnoid Hemorrhage, Section V, Part I: Natural history of subarachnoid hemorrhage, intracranial aneurysms and arteriovenous malformations. Based on 6,368 cases in the Cooperative Study. Journal of Neurosurgery 1966;25:219–239.
47. Ostergaard J, Voldby B. Intracranial arterial aneurysms in children and adolescents. Journal of Neurosurgery 1983;58:832–837.
48. Hourihan M, Gates P, McAllister V. Subarachnoid hemorrhage in childhood and adolescence. Journal of Neurosurgery 1984;60:1163–1166.
49. Biller J, Mathews K, Love B, eds. Strokes in Children and Young Adults. Boston: Butterworth-Heineman, 1994:210.
50. Brisman R, Abbassion K, Brissman R. Familial intracranial aneurysms. Journal of Neurosurgery 1971;34:678–682.
51. Cunha e Sa M, Stein B, Solomon R, McCormick P. The treatment of associated intracranial aneurysms and arteriovenous malformations. Journal of Neurosurgery 1992;77(6):853–859.
52. Brown RJ, Weibers D, Forbes G. Unruptured intracranial aneurysms and arteriovenous malformations: frequency of intracranial hemorrhage and relationship of lesions. Journal of Neurosurgery 1990;73(6):859–863.
53. Black I, Fatkin D, Sagar K, et al. Exclusion of atrial thrombus by transesophageal echocardiography does not preclude embolism after cardioversion of atrial fibrillation. A multicenter study. Circulation 1993;89(6):2509–2513.
54. Ferrer M. Sick sinus syndrome. Journal of Cardiovascular Medicine 1981;6:743–748.
55. Johnson R, Palacios I. Dilated cardiomyopathies of the adult. (First of two parts). New England Journal of Medicine 1982;307:1051–1058.
56. Johnson R, Palacios I. Dilated cardiomyopathies of the adult (Second of two parts). New England Journal of Medicine 1982;307:1119–1126.
57. Webster M, Chancellor A, Smith H, et al. Patent foramen ovale in young stroke patients. Lancet 1988;2:11–12.
58. Lechat P, Mas J, Lascault G, et al. Prevalence of patent foramen ovale in patients with stroke. New England Journal of Medicine 1988;318:1148–1152.
59. Barnett H, Boughner D, Taylor D, et al. Further evidence relating mitral-valve disease to cerebral ischemic events. New England Journal of Medicine 1980;302:139–144.
60. Greenlee J, Mandell G. Neurologic manifestations of infective endocarditis. Stroke 1973;4:958–962.
61. Igarashi M, Gilmartin R, Gerald B, et al. Cerebral arteritis and bacterial meningitis. Archives of Neurology 1984;41:531–535.
62. Arditi M, Mongue K, Caplan M. Cerebrospinal fluid cachectin/tumor necrosis factor- alpha and platelet-activating factor concentrations and severity of bacterial meningitis in children. The Journal of Infectious Diseases 1990;162(1):139–147.
63. Hsieh F, Chia L, Shen W. Location of cerebral infarctions in tuberculous meningitis. Neuroradiology 1992;34:197–199.
64. Beal M, O'Carroll C, Kleinman G, et al. Aspergillosis of the central nervous system. Neurology 1982;32:473–479.
65. Salaki J, Louria D, Chmel H. Fungal and yeast infections of the central nervous system. A clinical review. Medicine 1984;63:108–132.
66. Simon R. Neurosyphilis. Archives of Neurology 1985;42:606–613.
67. Parker P, Puck S, Fernandez P. Cerebral infarction association with *Mycoplasma pneumoniae.* Pediatrics 1981;67:373–375.
68. Selby G, Walker G. Cerebral arteritis in cat scratch disease. Neurology 1979;29:1413–1418.
69. Park Y, Belman A, Kim T. Stroke in pediatric acquired immune deficiency syndrome. Annals of Neurology. 1990;28:303–311.
70. Citron B, Halpern M, McCarron M, et al. Necrotizing angiitis associated with drug abuse. New England Journal of Medicine 1970; 283:1003–1011.
71. Rumbaugh C, Bergeron F, Fang H, et al. Cerebral angiographic changes in the drug abuse patient. Radiology 1971;101:335–344.
72. Sams W. Necrotizing vasculitis. Journal of the American Academy of Dermatology 1980;2:1–13.
73. Mayeux R, Fahn S. Strokes and ulcerative colitis. Neurology 1978;28:571–574.
74. Kohrman M, Huttenlocher R. Takayasu arteritis: a treatable cause of stroke in infancy. Pediatric Neurology 1986;12:154–158.
75. Belman A, Lerchner C, Moshe S, et al. Neurologic manifestations of Schonlein-Henoch Purpura: report of three cases and review of the literature. Pediatrics 1985;75:687–692.
76. Graf W, Milstein J, Sherry D. Stroke and mixed connective tissue disease. Journal of Child Neurology 1993;8(3):256–259.
77. Kennodle G, Bullard D, Caldwell D. Isolated angiitis of the central nervous system. Neurosurgery 1986;7:1–6.
78. Cupps T, Moore P, Fauci A. Isolated angiitis of the central nervous system. American Journal of Medicine 1983;74:97–105.
79. Koo E, Massey E. Therapy for granulomatous angiitis. Clinical Neuropharmacology 1986;9:132–137.
80. Hart R, Kanter M. Hematologic disorders and ischemic stroke. Stroke 1990;21:1111–1121.

81. Nathan D, Oski F, eds. Hematology of Infancy and Childhood. 4th ed. Philadelphia: W.B. Saunders Co., 1993:
82. Dahlback B. Physiologic anticoagulation. Resistance to activated protein C and venous thromboembolism. Journal of Clinical Investigation 1994;94:923.
83. Rich C, Gill J, Wernick S, et al. An unusual cause of cerebral thrombosis in a four-year-old child. Stroke 1993;24(4):603–605.
84. Levine S, Welch K. Antiphospholipid antibodies. Annals of Neurology 1989;26:386–389.
85. Briley D, Coull B, Goodnight SJ. Neurologic disease associated with antiphospholipid antibodies. Annals of Neurology 1989;25:221–227.
86. Eisenberg G. Antiphospholipid syndrome. Hospital Practice 1992;:119–131.
87. Coull B, Goodnight S. Antiphospholipid antibodies, pre-thrombotic states and stroke. Current Concepts Cerebrovascular Disease Stroke 1990;25:13–18.
88. Olson J, Konkol R, Gill J, et al. Childhood stroke and lupus anticoagulant. Pediatric Neurology 1994;10(1):54–57.
89. Schoning M, Klein R, Krageloh-Mann I, et al. Antiphospholipid antibodies in cerebrovascular ischemia and stroke in childhood. Neuropediatrics 1994;25(1):8–14.
90. Greenberg J, Massey E. Cerebral infarction in sickle cell trait. Annals of Neurology 1985;18:354–355.
91. Ohene-Frempong K. Stroke in sickle cell disease: demographic, clinical and therapeutic considerations. Seminars in Hematology 1991; 28(3):213–219.
92. Powars D, Wilson B, Imbus C. The natural history of stroke in sickle cell disease. American Journal of Medicine 1978;65:461–471.
93. Wang W, Kovnar E, Tonkin I, et al. High risk of recurrent stroke after discontinuance of five to twelve years of transfusion therapy in patients with sickle cell disease. Journal of Pediatrics 1991;118:377–382.
94. Yang D, Sohn D, Anand H. Thrombosis of superior longitudinal sinus during infancy. Journal of Pediatrics 1969;74:570.
95. Lockman L, Mastri A, Priest J, et al. Dural venous thrombosis in acute lymphoblastic leukemia. Pediatrics 1980;66:943–947.
96. Boers G, Smals A, Trijbels F, et al. Heterozygosity for homocystinuria in premature peripheral and cerebral occlusive arterial disease. New England Journal of Medicine 1985;313:709–715.
97. Mudd S. Vascular disease and homocystein metabolism. New England Journal of Medicine 1985;313:751–753.
98. Harker L, Slichter S, Scott C, et al. Homocystinemia, vascular injury and arterial thrombosis. New England Journal of Medicine 1974; 291:537–543.
99. Christodoulo J, Qureshi I, Clarke J. Ornithine transcarbamalase deficiency presenting with stroke like episodes. Journal of Pediatrics 1993;122(3):423–425.
100. Roach E. Cerebrovascular disorders and trauma in children. Current Opinions in Pediatrics 1993;5(6):660–668.
101. Gordon N, Isler W. Childhood moyamoya disease. Developmental Medicine and Child Neurology 1989;31:98–107.
102. Bogousslavsky J, Regli F. Ischemic stroke in adults younger than 30 years of age. Archives of Neurology 1987;44:479–482.
103. Adams HJ, Butler M, Biller J, et al. Nonhemorrhagic cerebral infarction in young adults. Archives of Neurology 1986;43:793–796.
104. Graham C, Schwartz J, Stacy T. Stroke following oral trauma in children. Annals of Emergency Medicine 1991;20(9):1029–1031.
105. Gary B, Otleinger C, Smith R, et al. Strokes in children due to vertebral artery trauma. Neurology 1993;43(12):2555–2558.
106. Kurtzke J. The current neurologic burden of illness and injury in the United States. Neurology 1982;32:362–367.
107. Welch K, Levine S. Migraine-related stroke in the context of the International Headache Society classification of head pain. Archives of Neurology 1990;47(4):458–462.
108. D'Angelan-Chatillon J, Ribeiro V, Mas J. Migraine—a risk factor for dissection of cervical arteries. Headache 1989;29:560–561.
109. Joseph R, Welch K. The platelet and migraine: a non-specific association. Headache 1987;27:375–380.
110. Spierings E. Angiographic changes suggestive of vasospasm in migraine complicated by stroke. Headache 1990;30:727–728.
111. Barbiroli B, Montagna P, Cortelli P, et al. Abnormal brain and muscle energy metabolism shown by ^{31}P magnetic resonance spectroscopy in patients affected by migraine with aura. Neurology 1992;42:1209–1214.
112. Rossi L, Penzien J, Deonna T, et al. Does migraine-related stroke occur in childhood? Developmental Medicine and Child Neurology 1990;32(11):1016–1021.
113. Isler H. Flunarizine in migraine attack. Journal of Cardiovascular Pharmacology 1991;18(Supp8):515–516.
114. Bryan R, Levy L, Whitlow W, et al. Diagnosis of acute cerebral infarction: comparison of CT and MRI imaging. American Journal of Neuroradiology 1991;12:611–620.
115. Yuh W, Crain M, Loes D, et al. MR imaging of cerebral ischemia: findings in the first 24 hours. American Journal of Neuroradiology 1991;12:621–629.
116. Welch W, McBride M, Kido D, Nelson C. Moyamoya disease in an infant with autonomic dysfunction: angiographic and MRI findings. Journal of Child Neurology 1988;3:110–113.
117. Bruno A, Yuh W, Biller J, et al. Magnetic resonance imaging in young adults with cerebral infarction due to Moya-moya. Archives of Neurology 1988;45:303–306.
118. King W, Martin N. Intracerebral hemorrhage due to arteriovenous malformations and fistulae. In: Batjer H, ed. Spontaneous Intracerebral Hemorrhage. Philadelphia: W.B. Saunders Co., 1992: 577–590. Neurosurgery Clinics of North America; vol. 3).
119. Heros R, Yong-Kwang T. Is surgical therapy needed for unruptured arteriovenous malformations? Neurology 1987;37:279–286.
120. Zimmerman R, Bogdan A, Gusnard D. Pediatric magnetic resonance angiography: assessment of stroke. Cardiovascular and Interventional Radiology 1992;15(1):60–64.
121. Dion J, Gates P, Fox A, et al. Clinical events following neuroangiography: a prospective study. Stroke 1987;18:997–1004.
122. Ross J, Masaryk T, Modie M, et al. Magnetic resonance angiography of the extra-cranial carotid arteries and intracranial vessels: a review. Neurology 1989;39:1369–1376.
123. Vogl T, Balzer J, Stemmler J, Bergman C, Egger E, Lissner J. MR angiography in children with cerebral neurovascular diseases: findings in 31 cases. American Journal of Roentgenology 1992;159(4):817–823.
124. Raju T. Cerebral doppler studies in the fetus and newborn. Journal of Pediatrics 1991;119:165–174.
125. Seibert J, Miller S, Kirby R, et al. Cerebrovascular disease in symptomatic and asymptomatic patients with sickle cell anemia: screening with duplex transcranial Doppler US—correlation with MR imaging and MR angiography. Radiology 1993;189(2):457–466.
126. Kalia K, Yonas H. An aggressive approach to middle cerebral artery infarction. Archives of Neurology 1993;50(12):1293–1297.
127. Boysen G, Overgaard K. Thrombolysis in ischaemic stroke—how far from a clinical breakthrough? Journal of Internal Medicine 1995; 237:95–103.
128. Strand T, Asplund K, Eriksson S, et al. A randomized, controlled trial of hemodilution therapy in acute ischemic stroke. Stroke 1984; 15:980–9.
129. Strand T. Evaluation of long-term outcome and safety after hemodilution therapy in acute ischemic stroke. Stroke 1992;23(5):657–662.
130. Goslinga H, V E, JHA H, et al. Custom-tailored hemodilution with albumin and crystalloids in acute ischemic stroke. Stroke 1992;23:181–8.
131. Hsu C, Norris J, Hogan E, et al. Pentoxifylline in acute nonhemorrhagic stroke. A randomized, placebo-controlled double-blind trial. Stroke 1988;19:716–22.
131a. Grotta JC, Pettigrew LC, Rosenbaum D., et al. Efficacy and mechanism of action of a calcium channel blocker after global cerebral ischemia in rats. Stroke 1988; 19: 447–54.
132. Grotta J. Why do all drugs work in animals but none in stroke patients? 2 Neuroprotective therapy. Journal of Internal Medicine 1995;237:89–94.
133. The International Nimodipine Study Group. Meta-analysis of nimodipine trials in acute ischemic stroke. Stroke 1992;23:148.
134. Bridgers S, Koch G, Munera C. Intravenous nimodipine in acute stroke: interim analysis of randomized trials. Stroke 1991;22:29.
135. Grotta J. Clinical aspects of the use of calcium antagonists in cerebrovascular disease. Clinical Neuropharmacology 1991;14:373–390.

Pediatric Drowning and Near-Drowning 26

Mark E. Rowin
David Christensen
Elizabeth M. Allen

INTRODUCTION

Submersion events include both drowning and near-drowning episodes. Drowning is death from asphyxia, caused by submersion in water[1,2]. Death is usually at the time of the submersion event or within a 24-hour period. Near-drowning is defined as an immersion event of sufficient severity to require medical treatment in which the patient survives for at least 24 hours, regardless of eventual outcome[1–4].

Submersion injuries remain one of the most frequent causes of morbidity and mortality in children[3–7], and victims of drowning and near-drowning events are frequently seen among the pediatric intensive care population. Although these children suffer hypoxic damage to many of their organs, it is hypoxic damage to the central nervous system (CNS) which is usually the limiting factor in their recovery. While new therapeutic modalities are being sought, currently available medical interventions have not been shown to significantly alter the pathophysiology of hypoxic encephalopathy resulting from drowning. Some dramatic recoveries have been reported, but many children are left with severe neurologic debilitation. However, the true tragedy of drowning is not only that in a matter of minutes a previously healthy child dies or is left with a permanent neurologic deficit, but rather that these episodes are often preventable. Increased emphasis by the medical community should be placed upon safety issues in an attempt to prevent this childhood tragedy.

INCIDENCE AND EPIDEMIOLOGY

Drowning is the third most common cause of death by unintentional injury among persons of all ages in the United States, and the second leading cause of injury death in children younger than 15 years of age[5,8–10]. An average of 6500 people drown each year in the United States[2,11]. For all children (infants through age 19 years), 1 in every 1098 boys and 1 in every 3333 girls will die from drowning[12]. Near-drowning statistics are equally impressive in that 1 out of every 301 boys and 1 out of every 913 girls will be hospitalized after a nonfatal immersion event[12]. For every child admitted through the emergency department after a near-drowning event, it is estimated that four were treated and sent home[13].

In the United States, the drowning rate for all children younger than 19 years of age is approximately 2.9 per 100,000[14]. There is a racial difference in the incidence of pediatric drowning in the United States, with whites having the lowest incidence and Native Americans having the highest[5].

Regional differences in the incidence of pediatric drownings exist within the United States (Fig. 26.1). The west-

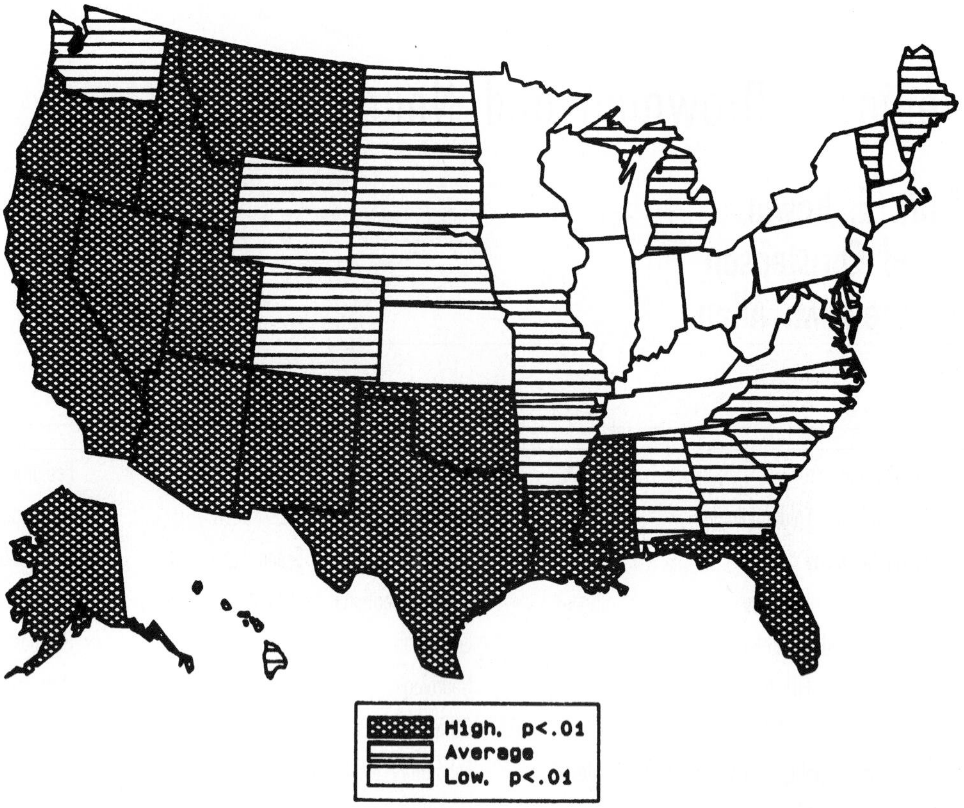

Figure 26.1. Drowning deaths by state, children ages 0 to 14 years, in the United States, 1980 to 1985. (From Waller AE, Baker SP, Szocka A. Childhood injury deaths: national analysis and geographic variations. Am J Public Health 79:310–315, 1989, with permission.)

ern states, Alaska, and the Gulf Coast region have the highest incidence of pediatric drownings, while the northeast has the lowest[11–13]. This may be due to an increased number of in-ground swimming pools throughout the southern and western United States[15]. In a nation-wide analysis from 1980-1985, 10 states (Alaska, Arizona, California, Florida, Hawaii, Montana, Nevada, Oregon, Utah, and Washington) demonstrated drowning as the leading cause of death from injury in children ages 0 to 14 years[5]. Surprisingly, even in states that border the oceans or other large bodies of salt water, most pediatric drownings occur in fresh water[3,6,12,16]. Seasonal variations occur as well. Approximately 50% of drownings occur from June through August[7,11,17]. While submersion accidents occur more frequently in warm-weather months, they can occur at any time of the year (Fig. 26.2).

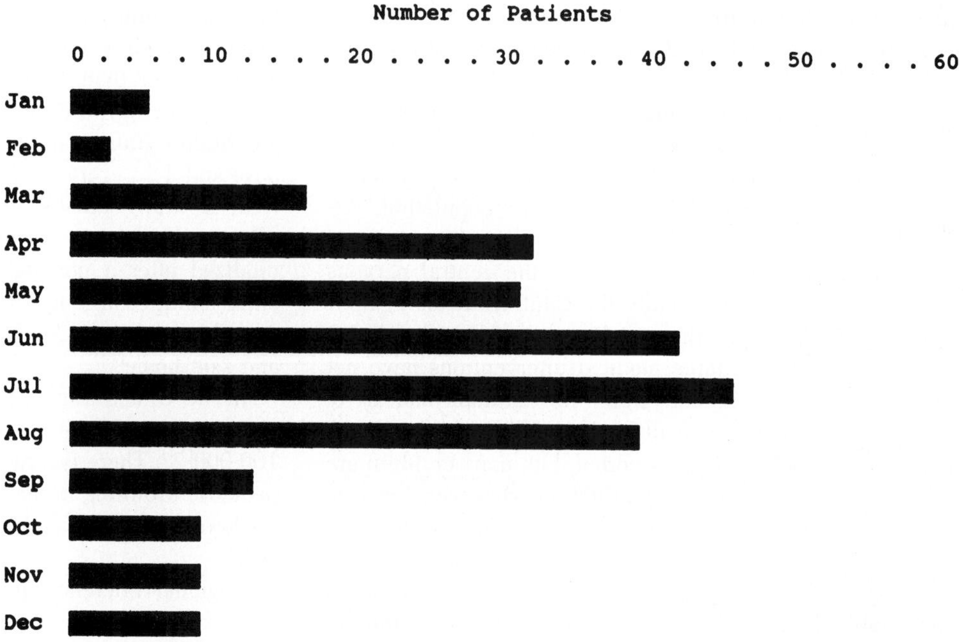

Figure 26.2. Months of near-drowning accidents, Children's Medical Center, Dallas, Texas (1975 to 1991). (From Levin DL, Morriss FC, Toro LO, Brink LW, and Turner GR. Drowning and near-drowning. Pediatr Clin North Am 40:321–336, 1993, with permission.)

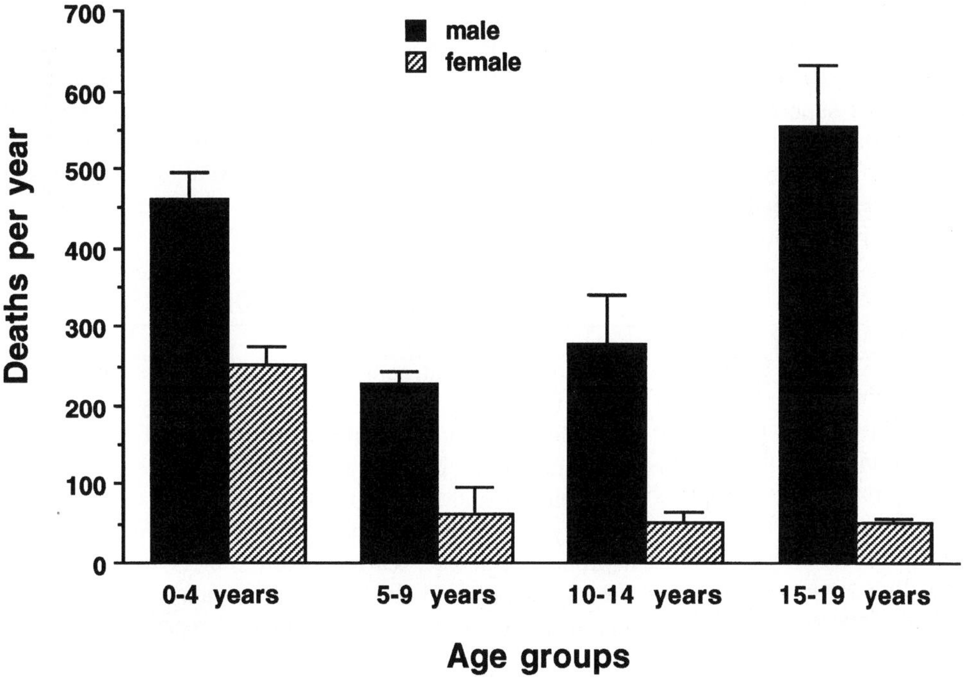

Figure 26.3. Age related drowning rates in the United States, 1971 to 1988, for males and females. (data from Waller AE, Baker SP, Szocka A. Childhood injury deaths: national analysis and geographic variations. Am J Public Health 79:310–315, 1989 and Wintemute GJ. Childhood drowning and near-drowning in the United States. AJDC 144:663–669, 1990 and Brenner RA, Smith GS, Overpeck MD. Divergent trends in childhood drowning rates, 1971–1988. JAMA 271:1606–1608, 1994.)

Males outnumber females as drowning victims. Males account for 78% of all deaths from drowning. When children older than 5 years of age are evaluated, males account for 86% of all drowning deaths[12]. In males, mortality from drowning shows a bimodal age distribution, with a peak among boys younger than 5 years of age, and again in adolescents 15 to 19 years of age (Fig. 26.3). The second peak is most likely related to water sports, boating, recklessness from bravado, swimming in undesignated or unprotected areas, voluntary hyperventilation, illegal drug use, and, most importantly, alcohol[4,7,14,16,18]. Alcohol is involved in approximately 50% of adolescent drownings[11,12,18]. Drowning deaths in female pediatric patients show a peak in children younger than 5 years of age, but no adolescent peak (Fig. 26.3).

The location associated with pediatric drownings tends to vary with the age of the victim **(Table 26.1).** Approximately 40% of infant drownings occur in bathtubs[9]. A classic description of a bathtub drowning victim is an infant younger than 1 year of age, often the youngest or second youngest member of the family, who is left in the care of an older sibling or is momentarily left unsupervised by a parent[19,20]. Bathtub drownings are an increasingly recognized form of child abuse among infants and toddlers[21]. Fourteen percent of 44 cases in a 2-year study examining infants drowning in a bathtub were judged to be intentional homicide. Also, there were features highly suggestive of child abuse in an additional 9%[19]. A 6-year retrospective study in Seattle showed that 8.5% of infant drowning cases were referred to Children's Protective Services for suspicion of abuse or neglect[22]. Other sites in which infants tend to drown include buckets, toilets, and residential swimming pools. However, these incidents occur less often than bathtub drownings[6,9,23,24].

Preschool-aged children are most likely to drown in residential swimming pools[6,15,25,26]. Children in the 0 to 4 age group accounted for approximately 50 to 90% of all pool drownings[7,12,14,15,25,27]. In a 5-month prospective study involving residential swimming pools, 142 immersion events were recorded in children younger than 5 years of age[27]. Two-thirds of these children were being supervised by one

Table 26.1. Submersion Injury Epidemiology

Age Group	*Common Sites*	*Comments*
Infant	Bathtub	Consider intentional injury Commonly associated with inadequate adult supervision
Toddler	Swimming pool/spa Bucket Toilet Bathtub Canal	Key features include inadequate supervision, curiosity, no fear of water, and inability to swim White > black (except with bucket near-drownings) Male ≥ female Limited success of prevention programs
Preschool and school-age	Swimming pool/spa Bathtub	Male > female Black > white
Adolescent	Natural bodies of water	Key features include risk-taking behavior, difficulty of rapid rescue, illegal drug use, and alcohol Medical illnesses are occasional factors Male > Female Highest case fatality rate Associated injuries are common

or both parents at the time of the accident. However, most parents reported brief lapses in supervision while they were occupied with household chores. Similarly, a 10-year study in King County, Washington, showed adult supervision in 84% of cases, but only 18% witnessed the actual immersion event[26]. Most immersion times in residential pool near-drownings were less than 5 minutes. The high incidence of toddlers drowning in a private or residential pool may not apply to the most northern areas of the country, where in-ground pools are less common[15].

Other important drowning sites in this age group include bathtubs, hot tubs, spas, and buckets[6,9,23,28]. In a recent 4-year study, 24% of all toddler drownings were caused by the toddler falling into 5-gallon industrial buckets[29]. One hundred sixty bucket-related drownings occurred in children younger than 2 years of age from 1984 through 1989[23]. A toddler's center of gravity is high and coordination poor, making it feasible that a child may fall head-first into a bucket and not have the strength to escape. In a recent survey from California, 6% of all drownings in children under 2 years of age occurred in hot tubs, whirlpools, and spas [28]. This number is dramatically increasing, as only 15 drownings in spas occurred between 1960 through 1979, but 59 cases were reported between 1980 to 1985.

Adolescents tend to drown in natural bodies of water, such as rivers, lakes, canals, and beaches; swimming pool drownings are much less frequent in this group[9,12,26]. Although preschool children have the highest incidence of total drownings and near-drownings, adolescents have the highest fatality rate[26]. In fact, in male adolescents, drowning is the second leading cause of nonintentional injury death after motor vehicle crashes[7]. Rapid rescue is likely affected by the deep water and poor water clarity associated with natural bodies of water. This problem is probably compounded by lack of supervision, increased time to initiate a rescue, and the physiologic effects of alcohol.

Certain medical illnesses have been associated with an increased risk of drowning, including seizure disorders and cardiac dysrhythmias such as prolonged QTC syndrome[30,31]. Children with seizure disorders have four to 10 times the risk of drowning or having a near-drowning incident[32–34]. In a 2-year retrospective study from England, 4% of submersion incidents followed an epileptic seizure[32]. Data from a 16-year analysis on risk factors related to epilepsy and drowning show that these children tend to be older than 5 years of age, show an even sex distribution, and were more likely to drown in a bathtub[33]. Like children without seizure activity, a majority of these children's submersion incidents (88%) were not witnessed.

The impact of childhood drowning is immense, not only in terms of psychosocial and emotional stress, but also in terms of direct medical costs to the family and economic costs to society. It has been estimated from 1982 data that drowning was responsible for $4.4 million per year in direct costs to the American health care system[35]. Drowning was also responsible for an estimated 100,000 years of productive life lost in children aged 0 to 19 years in 1985 alone[35]. Near-drowning has an estimated indirect societal economic cost of $350–$650 million per year[35,36]. This makes it the third most costly childhood injury, after motor vehicle and pedestrian injuries, to the United States health care system. The annual cost of care for a neurologically impaired survivor of a near-drowning event in a chronic care facility is approximately $100,000[37].

PATHOPHYSIOLOGY

The most important consequence of near-drowning is decreased oxygen delivery to tissues, specifically the CNS. To some degree, hypoxemia affects all organ systems. It is the magnitude of the hypoxic insult, as well as the body's ability to endure and recover from oxygen deprivation, that ultimately affects the patient's chances for survival and good neurologic outcome. Early reinstitution of tissue oxygenation is the current hallmark of therapy and is the best regimen available to improve neurologic outcome.

Sequence of Events

A specific sequence of events during a drowning episode has been well documented in animal models[38]. A similar description has also been documented in humans[39,40]. The sequence of events classically described begins with an initial period of panic and voluntary breath-holding. During this time, there is violent struggling as well as automatic swimming movements. Breath-holding continues until a breaking point is reached. The break point is determined by both hypercarbic and hypoxic drives[40]. Evaluation of voluntary apnea has shown a mean duration in normal subjects of 87 seconds with a $PACO_2$ of 51 torr and a PAO_2 of 73 torr[41]. With hyperventilation followed by vigorous exercise, breath-holding could be maintained for 85 seconds. During this time, the $PACO_2$ increased to 49 torr, while the PAO_2 fell to 43 torr[41]. As the victim's PCO_2 rises, the diaphragm begins to have episodic contractions, reducing intrathoracic pressure. Inspiration is prevented only by voluntary closure of the glottis. Eventually, an involuntary gasp occurs. Water may be aspirated into the lungs at this time. In 10 to 20% of drowning cases, inadequate ventilation is not caused by fluid within the respiratory tree, but rather by severe laryngeal spasm[40]. This prevents water from entering the lungs and is often referred to as dry drowning (Figs 26.4 and 26.5). It appears that a small amount of water, upon entering the larynx or trachea, triggers a parasympathetic response which produces a severe laryngeal spasm. This is followed quickly by secretion of a thick mucus which, in some cases, forms a physical mucous plug[40]. Within seconds of the first submerged breath, a stage of secondary apnea occurs. This is followed by involuntary gasping which may continue for several minutes before final respiratory arrest occurs. Water may be aspirated into the lungs at this time, or the laryngeal spasm may persist. The victims often swallow a large volume of water, which may

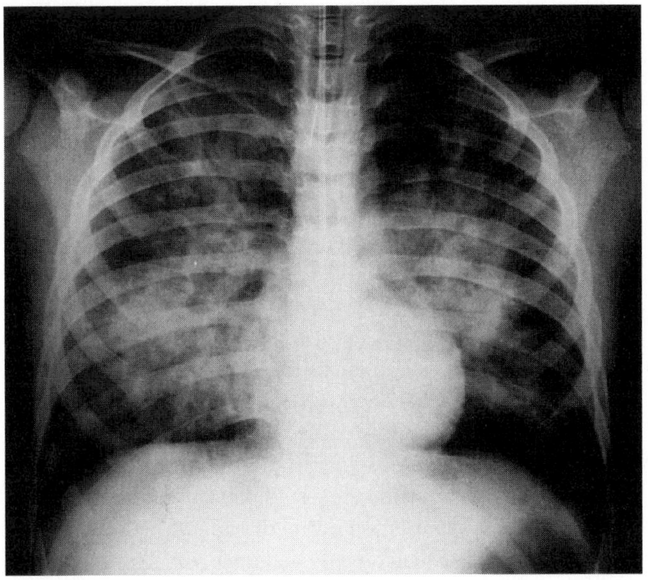

Figure 26.4. Chest x-ray of a 9-year-old victim of a pool near-drowning, demonstrating fluid aspiration and a wet drowning appearance to the radiograph. (Courtesy of the resident teaching files, Department of Radiology, University of Utah School of Medicine, Salt Lake City.)

induce emesis and subsequent aspiration. Consciousness is usually lost within 3 minutes due to cerebral hypoxia. As the hypoxemia worsens, the laryngeal spasm may relax, and water can then passively enter the lungs. Cardiac arrhythmias may develop. Convulsions and spasmodic efforts then precede death[38].

Fluids and Electrolytes

For many years, there has been controversy regarding different pathophysiologic mechanisms in freshwater versus saltwater drownings. Initial animal studies showed that the tonicity of the water appeared to cause biochemical differences[38,42,43]. It was commonly thought that large volumes of fluid were aspirated by human victims, followed by large fluid shifts across the alveoli. Experimental models reflected this hypothesis and used direct intratracheal installation of large volumes of fluid. These studies demonstrated alterations in electrolytes, blood volume, and hemoglobin that were highly dependent on the salinity of the drowning medium. Ventricular fibrillation commonly occurred as a terminal event, believed to be due to dramatic electrolyte shifts. It was concluded from these experiments that freshwater drowning caused hemodilution and hemolysis that produced hyperkalemia, hyponatremia, hemoglobinemia, and an elevated circulating blood volume[42,43]. In contrast, seawater drowning (approximately 3.5% NaCl) produced hypernatremia, hemoconcentration, and contraction of circulating blood volume[42,43].

Despite evidence from these studies in animal models, clinical correlation in humans has not been found[44]. Clinically important electrolyte abnormalities, fluid shifts, and changes in hematocrit are unusual in near-drowning patients, regardless of the tonicity of the water[1]. Electrolytes are usually within a normal physiologic range, whether the patient's near-drowning experience occurred in fresh or salt water[45–47]. Ventricular fibrillation is also uncommon in human victims who have not suffered concomitant hypothermia, supporting the notion that electrolytic shifts are usually not life threatening. The difference between the animal models and human correlates appears to be the amount of fluid aspirated during the drowning event. The majority of human drowning victims appear to aspirate less than 22 ml/kg of fluid, the fluid volume used in the animal models. Therefore, generally the therapeutic approach to both freshwater and saltwater near-drownings is similar[1,2,11,45,46].

Drowning victims can exhibit either hypervolemia or hypovolemia. Systemic fluid overload may be secondary to fluid absorbed through both the pulmonary and gastric circulations. The exact volume of fluid in the pulmonary tree varies from victim to victim but is generally less than 5 ml/kg[48]. However, 80 to 90% of near-drowning victims will swallow large volumes of water into their stomach. Not only will this potentially cause systemic fluid overload, but it very often causes gastric distention and increases the risk of vomiting and aspiration during resuscitation. Additionally, overzealous administration of intravenous fluids during the early phases of resuscitation may contribute to fluid overload[45]. More often, near-drowning victims exhibit hypovolemic shock. The hypovolemia is most likely due to excessive capillary permeability secondary to endothelial damage from hypoxia and resultant loss of protein-rich fluid into the third space. Glucose metabolism appears to be altered in near-drowning victims[49]. Hyperglycemia has been noted after the stress of a near-drowning episode and is believed to be secondary to excessive endogenous catecholamines. Hyperglycemia may potentiate neurologic damage in an ischemic brain. In children with a severe neurologic insult, blood glucose levels of greater than 250 mg/dl

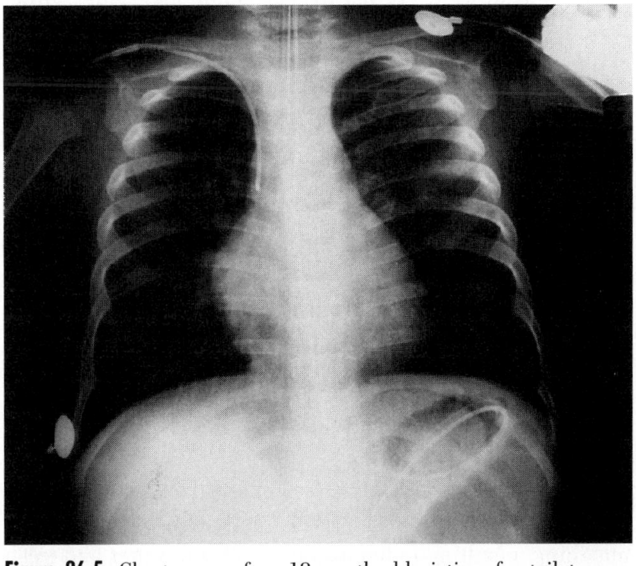

Figure 26.5. Chest x-ray of an 18-month-old victim of a toilet near-drowning, demonstrating a dry drowning appearance to the radiograph. (Courtesy of Richard Boyer, M.D., Department of Radiology, University of Utah School of Medicine, Salt Lake City.)

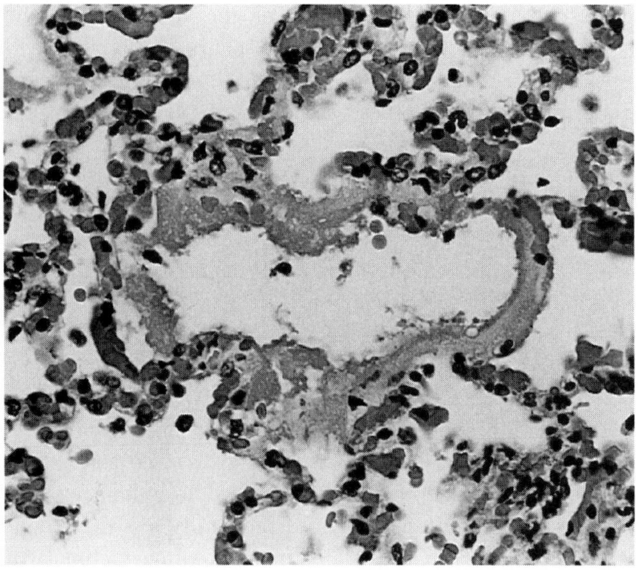

Figure 26.6. Lung section from a 2-year-old drowning victim demonstrating breakdown of the alveolar membrane, resulting in fluid and fibrin deposition within the alveolus. (Slides, courtesy of Dr. Edward Leis, State of Utah Medical Examiner's Office; photomicrographs, courtesy of Dr. Edward C. Klatt, Department of Pathology, University of Utah School of Medicine, Salt Lake City.)

have been associated with an increased likelihood of death or poor neurologic outcome when compared to children with similar injuries who were normoglycemic[49]. Similarly, rats treated with insulin after a hypoxic-ischemic event to maintain normoglycemia demonstrated an improved neurologic outcome when compared to hyperglycemic controls[50]. However, hypoglycemia produced by the overzealous use of insulin may have neurologic effects as well. Hypoglycemia has been shown to increase cerebral blood flow as much as 300%[49]. This can dramatically increase intracranial pressure (ICP) in a patient with cerebral edema from hypoxia. There is also evidence that hypoglycemia may cause direct neuronal injury[50]. The exact blood glucose levels at which neuronal injuries occur is unknown.

Pulmonary Effects

During the breath-holding portion of the near-drowning event, the functional residual capacity of the lung is the only source of gas exchange for the pulmonary capillaries. As oxygen uptake and carbon dioxide elimination are compromised, hypoxia and hypercarbia rapidly develop. A mixed metabolic and respiratory acidosis subsequently develops. If the victim is rescued prior to fluid aspiration, this hypoxia and acidosis tend to resolve rapidly as lung damage and pathophysiologic changes are minimal.

Aspiration of fluid into the airway triggers a cascade of pathophysiologic events. The primary effect of water aspiration on the lung is to increase ventilation-perfusion mismatching, resulting in hypoxemia. Both salt water and fresh water affect pulmonary surfactant, but by different mechanisms. Fresh water causes surfactant to denature and become nonfunctional. Sea water either dilutes surfactant concentrations or washes the surfactant out of the alveolus entirely[11,40]. This change in surfactant alters the surface tension properties of the alveoli and results in atelectasis, decreased lung compliance, and increased intrapulmonary shunting[7,40]. This increased intrapulmonary shunting may take days to return to normal, even in children who are no longer hypoxemic and otherwise appear clinically well[40].

Secondary pulmonary edema may develop in response to water aspiration during drowning. Inhaled water may disrupt the alveolar membrane, moving across the alveolar epithelium and into the basement membrane. Here, it is eventually removed by lymphatic and capillary drainage. An intense inflammatory reaction may occur, resulting in the destruction of alveolar pneumocytes. The alveolar capillary membrane is disrupted, leading to an outpouring of a plasma-rich exudate into the alveolus[45,51].

Postmortem examination of the drowned lung reveals diffuse edema with occasional focal hemorrhages. Histologic examination shows foreign material as well as proteinaceous fluid and fibrin deposition within the alveolus. Both type 1 and type 2 pneumocytes are damaged. Pulmonary vascular endothelial changes show microvesicle formation, mitochondrial swelling, detachment from the basement membrane, and disruption of the cells[45,52] (Figs. 26.6 and 26.7).

In addition to its effects on alveoli, aspiration of water into the lung can cause changes in the airways and pulmonary vasculature. Small amounts of aspirated fresh water (1 ml/kg) have been shown to cause pulmonary vasoconstriction, with the immediate development of pulmonary hypertension[40]. Aspirated water also causes a distal airway bron-

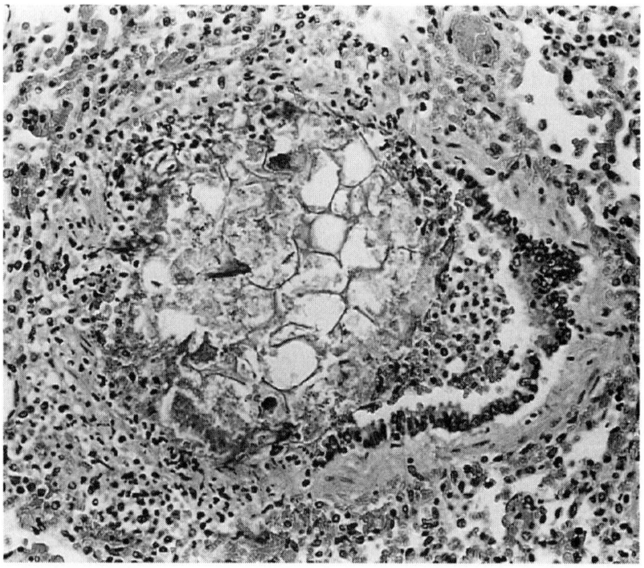

Figure 26.7. Lung section from a 2-year-old drowning victim found in an irrigation canal. The patient died 18 hours after rescue. The section shows a distal bronchiole occluded with organic material and an intense inflammatory reaction to the foreign material. (Slides, courtesy of Dr. Edward Leis, State of Utah Medical Examiner's Office; photomicrographs, courtesy of Dr. Edward C. Klatt, Department of Pathology, University of Utah School of Medicine, Salt Lake City.)

chiolar constriction which is believed to be a vagally mediated reflex[53].

All of these pathophysiologic changes within the lung interfere with gas exchange and result in systemic hypoxemia, hypercapnea, and acidosis[45,54]. With proper medical management, gas exchange is rapidly reestablished, and the hypercarbia and acidosis tend to resolve rapidly in a near-drowning victim. However, hypoxemia can persist for days.

There is a subset of patients who initially respond well to pulmonary management but later demonstrate significant respiratory deterioration. In many of these patients, surfactant loss can continue even after a rescue[51]. This loss of surfactant may be secondary to a persistent chemical degradation (i.e., chlorine, detergents) or osmotic and inflammatory damage to the pneumocytes themselves[51]. Ultimately, this leads to significant alveolar collapse. This form of severe pulmonary dysfunction seen after a victim has been resuscitated is known as secondary drowning and probably occurs in less than 5% of survivors[51]. It is defined as the occurrence of respiratory deterioration after "successful" resuscitation due to primary alveolar membrane dysfunction. Secondary drowning can occur from 3 to 72 hours after rescue[55]. Other causes of postrescue pulmonary deterioration include bacterial pneumonia, barotrauma, an inflammatory response to a foreign body aspiration (sand, mud, debris), hypoventilation from neurologic deterioration, and oxygen toxicity.

Cardiovascular Effects

The pediatric heart is remarkably tolerant of a hypoxic-ischemic insult, and electrical activity can often be generated after a prolonged period of oxygen deprivation. Electrocardiographic changes usually mimic those seen in primary respiratory arrest, showing bradycardia which progresses to asystole[17,45,56]. However, in one pediatric series, supraventricular tachycardia was noted in 16% of near-drowning victims[57]. Ventricular fibrillation does occur but is a relatively uncommon dysrhythmia in the pediatric victim[57,58]. It was initially thought to be due to hyperkalemia and hypocalcemia that were believed to be a common occurrence in freshwater drowning[39]. However, it is most likely the result of hypothermia and hypoxia rather than electrolyte abnormalities[58,59].

Although it is often possible to obtain cardiac electrical activity after aggressive resuscitation, cardiogenic shock after near-drowning is common. Poor contractility after a hypoxic insult is common[2,60]. Additionally, an increased capillary permeability due to anoxia may lead to transudation of fluid into the interstitial space and intravascular hypovolemia, which may worsen the clinical picture of shock. The systemic vascular resistance is typically elevated[46,60]. These hemodynamic effects are similar in all near-drowning victims, regardless of the tonicity of the water[46]. Inadequate tissue perfusion due to ongoing cardiogenic and hypovolemic shock may continue the ischemic damage to the heart and other organs, especially the CNS.

Histologically, hearts from animals drowned in either fresh or salt water demonstrate similar results. Diffusely distributed focal lesions are noted where the normal striation patterns are disrupted, resembling necrosis or myofibrillar degeneration[61]. The myocytes are hypereosinophilic and hypercontracted into contraction bands, and they show evidence of disruption of the intercalated discs[59]. In these areas, the mitochondria are swollen and demonstrate increased lucency, while the nuclei show marginal crenation and chromatin clumping. While these histologic changes occur in hypoxic-ischemic hearts, similar lesions have also been noted to be produced by excess exogenous catecholamines[59]. Elevated cytosolic calcium and oxygen-derived free radical production have also been suggested to participate in myocardial injury after reperfusion of a hypoxic-ischemic heart[62].

Renal, Hepatic, and Gastrointestinal Effects

Various organ systems can be affected by the hypoxic-ischemic insult commonly seen in the near-drowning victim. Renal dysfunction is common. Albuminuria, hemoglobinuria, hematuria, oliguria, and anuria can occur. Renal dysfunction was initially thought to occur as a result of the hemolysis and hemoglobinemia that were presumed to accompany freshwater near-drownings. The cause is now believed to be anoxic injury to the kidney itself, resulting in acute tubular necrosis[7,45,63].

The liver is also susceptible to anoxic injury, which can be manifested by elevation of bilirubin levels, elevated transaminase levels, and impaired production of procoagulant factors. Liver dysfunction undoubtedly plays a role in the disseminated intravascular coagulation that can be seen after near-drowning.

Gastrointestinal injury from hypoxia and ischemia is well described. The intestinal mucosa is sensitive to anoxic injury and will often slough after a hypoxic-ischemic event. The patient passes large quantities of foul-smelling, bloody, mucus-filled stools. These patients are at risk for bacterial translocation, or, in severe cases, perforation of the gastrointestinal tract. In general, while these complications can be severe, with supportive care they rarely pose a threat to overall survival in an otherwise salvageable patient.

Neurologic Effects

Submersion injuries involve a variable combination of ischemia and hypoxia to all organs. However, brain-tissue energy stores are small, and the brain has limited ability to use anaerobic metabolism, making it exquisitely dependent upon an uninterrupted oxygen delivery for aerobic metabolism. Acidosis and hypercarbia are undoubtedly also important in cerebral injury, but it is irreversible hypoxic-ischemic damage to the brain that ultimately determines the outcome in the majority of near-drowning patients.

Not all neurons are equally vulnerable to the effects of hypoxia. Those that participate in visual-motor coordination are particularly sensitive[64], as are the pyramidal cells of the hippocampus and neocortex, and neurons in the caudate, putamen, and thalamic nuclei[65]. However, all neurons are damaged by hypoxia after a long enough duration.

The primary injury to the brain is a result of hypoxia and ischemia during the drowning event itself. On a biochemical level, this primary insult is due to adenosine triphosphate (ATP) depletion, which occurs after approximately 2 minutes of ischemia. Without ATP, cell membrane gradients are lost, intracellular communication stops, and intracellular macromolecules are broken down. The result is cytotoxic edema and ultimately neuronal death.

There are a number of biochemical responses within the brain which result from the primary hypoxic injury and may cause further CNS damage, referred to as secondary injury[65,66]. One example involves the excitatory amino acids, L-glutamate and L-aspartate. The extracellular concentrations of these amino acids rise during hypoxic-ischemic events, probably because release is enhanced and re-uptake is inhibited[65,67]. These neurotransmitters act on specific postsynaptic receptors that increase transmembrane conductance for sodium and calcium[65,68]. As the ATP-dependent Na^+-K^+ pump fails due to the effects of hypoxia, intracellular concentrations of sodium increase. Chloride and water then passively enter the cell and cellular edema occurs. Loss of ATP prevents sequestering of calcium in the mitochondria and endoplasmic reticulum, allowing increased cytosolic calcium concentrations. Increased intracellular calcium is believed to be responsible for neuronal dysfunction and death. The consequences of increased intracellular calcium include calcium-activated phospholipid hydrolysis followed by lipid peroxidation and release of fatty acid metabolites (i.e., arachidonic acid), oxygen free radical formation, and increases in calcium-activated proteases[67,68].

Membrane phospholipid breakdown by elevated intracellular calcium causes the release of arachidonic acid. This triggers a series of biochemical reactions that result in increased production of prostacyclin and thromboxanes[69]. During hypoxia, synthesis of prostaglandins generates an increased production of oxygen free radicals. Overproduction of thromboxane A2 causes vasoconstriction and platelet aggregation, thereby worsening ischemia[67].

Oxygen free radicals are another important biochemical response to cerebral hypoxia and are implicated as important pathologic mediators in CNS injury. Free radicals are highly reactive molecules that are normally neutralized by an array of endogenous antioxidants. Overproduction of oxygen free radicals (such as superoxide, hydroxyl, hydroperoxyl, alkoxy, and peroxy radicals) occurs both during hypoxia and during the reperfusion phase of oxygen-deprived neuronal tissue[66,67]. These substances are very reactive and interact with lipid membranes and DNA to produce additional cellular damage.

Additionally, secondary cerebral injury may result from systemic factors. Cardiogenic shock and hypovolemia may cause hypotension, which may worsen cerebral ischemic damage. As previously discussed, fluid aspiration and subsequent pulmonary dysfunction may result in hypoxia, which may worsen cerebral damage.

As a result of both the primary and secondary injuries discussed above, cerebral edema usually develops within 24 to 72 hours of a severe near-drowning event. The three types of cerebral edema are discussed in detail in Chapter 18. Due to loss of neuronal membrane integrity, cytotoxic cerebral edema often develops after near-drowning. This is an indirect measure of cell death and occurs as a consequence of the primary neuronal insult (hypoxia) and the subsequent cascade of secondary biochemical events. Hypoxia and the secondary free radical formation also lead to vasogenic edema. The tight junctions of the cerebral endothelial cells appear to become dysfunctional during hypoxia, leading to a breakdown in the blood-brain barrier which allows passage of intravascular fluid into the parenchyma[70,71].

As the cranial vault has a fixed volume, increases in intraparenchymal fluid can quickly elevate ICP. Increased ICP alone is not generally responsible for neuronal death[72]. However, increased ICP may impair cerebral perfusion, potentially worsening CNS injury. Cerebral perfusion pressure (CPP) is defined as the difference between mean arterial pressure (MAP) and ICP. Thus, as the ICP increases, cerebral perfusion will decrease unless the MAP also increases. This relationship is discussed in greater detail in Chapter 18.

Loss of the normal autoregulatory mechanisms after an anoxic injury may compound cerebral damage. Restoration of cerebral circulation after a severe hypoxic-ischemic insult causes a transient vasodilatation, followed by a marked decrease in cerebral blood flow[66,73]. Thus, neuronal injury due to ischemia may continue even after restoration of adequate systemic circulation and oxygenation. Calcium entry into the vascular smooth muscles of the cerebral arteriolar system may play a role in producing spasm, thereby worsening postresuscitation cerebral ischemia[66,74]. There is strong evidence that free-radical production may be a crucial mechanism for CNS vascular injury after reperfusion[65,75,76]. Reperfusion delivers oxygen to previously oxygen-deprived tissues, which is used as a substrate for superoxide and hydrogen peroxide production[77]. CNS acidosis from ischemia may promote iron (in the Fe^{2+} form)-mediated catalysis of hydrogen peroxide to form hydroxyl radicals[65]. These radicals are very unstable and rapidly initiate lipid peroxidation[66,75] and widespread cellular injury.

Hypothermia and the Diving Reflex

There have been several reported cases of children surviving prolonged submersions with good neurologic outcome[78–80]. Often, these children fell into very cold water and arrived at the hospital profoundly hypothermic. Two theories have been proposed to explain this phenomenon: hypothermia and the diving response. Hypothermia has been shown to develop rapidly after submersion in cold water[45]. Heat loss presumably occurs both through the skin and due to cold-water ingestion and aspiration. Ethanol may potentiate heat loss due to its vasodilatory properties. Children have larger surface areas and decreased insulation from fat than adults and can lose heat much more rapidly[81].

The brain in these cases is rapidly cooled, and cerebral metabolism is depressed. Cerebral oxygen consumption is 50% of normal at 28°C, and 25% of normal at 20°C[82]. Cerebral blood flow decreases 6 to 7% per 1°C temperature drop[2]. If cerebral oxygen consumption decreases at an equal or greater rate than oxygen delivery, the brain will be able to withstand longer periods of hypoxia. This may explain the beneficial effect of hypothermia on cerebral salvage.

A number of pathophysiologic effects are associated with hypothermia. As the internal temperature drops to 32°C, the victim becomes increasingly disoriented and uncoordinated and eventually loses consciousness. Pupils dilate at temperatures below 30°C and are minimally reactive[83]. At 28°C cardiac dysrhythmias are common, especially ventricular fibrillation[83]. Blood viscosity is increased from hemoconcentration, and the oxygen-hemoglobin dissociation curve shifts to the left. Hypothermia may also decrease white cell functions, allowing an increased risk of infection[84]. Lastly, hypothermia decreases insulin production and impairs tissue glucose utilization, with resultant hyperglycemia[83].

The diving reflex, noted in many marine mammals, acts as an oxygen-conserving adaptation in response to submersion. It appears to be triggered by breath-holding and cold stimulation. Several cardiovascular changes occur which conserve oxygen for those tissues that are most sensitive to hypoxia. Cardiac output is markedly reduced, mostly because of bradycardia. Peripheral and mesenteric vasoconstriction shifts blood away from the skeletal muscles, skin, gut, and kidneys. Coronary blood flow reduces to about 10% of the pre-dive level. Systemic oxygen consumption and metabolic rates decrease, but cerebral blood flow and oxygen delivery are maintained[82].

There is controversy as to whether humans retain a diving reflex. Some authors believe this primitive reflex in children is weak and does not afford much protection[83,85]. They point out the decreased ability of children to hold their breath in cold water. Others claim that while seen to a lesser extent in humans, in icy water about 15% of volunteers exhibited a profound diving response[82].

INITIAL ASSESSMENT AND RESUSCITATION

The goal of initial assessment and management is to improve tissue oxygen delivery as rapidly as possible in order to minimize cerebral hypoxic-ischemic damage. Improving oxygen delivery optimally begins at the scene and continues during transport to a medical facility. Unfortunately, the lack of cardiopulmonary resuscitation (CPR) training among rescuers often results in the near-drowning victim waiting for the arrival of a paramedic team before CPR is started. In a study from California, 42% of children who died after a submersion event did not receive resuscitative efforts until emergency medical technicians arrived[18]. Another study demonstrated that providing CPR at the scene of a near-drowning event significantly increased the chances of a good outcome[86].

Management at the Scene

At the scene of the near-drowning accident, mouth-to-mouth resuscitation should be started as soon as possible, beginning when the victim reaches the surface of the body of water. During attempted ventilation, air can easily enter the stomach. This causes gastric distention and an increased risk of regurgitation and aspiration. There is some question as to whether the Heimlich maneuver should be performed prior to the initiation of rescue breathing. It was initially believed that fluid in the airways was obstructive and may prevent attempted ventilation[87]. However, in a majority of patients, the amount of fluid aspirated is small, usually less than 5 ml/kg[48]. It is likely that this fluid is rapidly absorbed and does not physically obstruct the airways[88,89]. Also, the Heimlich maneuver may increase the risk of aspiration of regurgitated stomach contents[90,91]. Since the most devastating aspect of drowning is hypoxemia, time should not be wasted attempting to clear the airway of water.

The hemodynamic status should be evaluated soon after the victim is removed from the water. If the patient is pulseless, closed-chest compressions should be started. Chest compressions are ineffective in water, therefore they should be initiated after the patient reaches solid ground and is determined to be pulseless[11].

Activation of emergency medical services and transport to a medical facility should be arranged as soon as possible.

Airway/Breathing

If the patient has adequate respiratory effort, then supplemental oxygen is all that is indicated. The presence of a weak respiratory effort does not mean that adequate oxygenation and ventilation are occurring. The threshold for endotracheal intubation should be very low in these patients. Indications for endotracheal intubation include (1) loss of airway protective reflexes due to a depressed level of consciousness, (2) a deteriorating neurologic examination, (3) severe respiratory distress or severe hypoxia despite administration of supplemental oxygen, (4) cardiorespiratory arrest, and (5) severe hypothermia (core temperature less than 30°C).

Once the patient arrives at the hospital, initial resuscitation should continue to focus on stabilization of the respiratory system. The initial respiratory examination should evaluate the presence of equal and adequate air entry. Oxygen saturations should be monitored using pulse oximetry, and oxygen administration should be adjusted to keep saturations greater than 90%. However, if severe pulmonary injury has occurred, supplemental oxygen alone may not be sufficient to treat the hypoxemia. As discussed previously, aspirated water can cause significant intrapulmonary shunting due to distal airway obstruction and alveolar collapse which may not respond to increasing the FiO2. Positive end-expiratory pressure (PEEP) may be necessary. PEEP improves oxygenation and ventilation by alveolar recruitment and increasing functional residual capacity of the lungs, thus decreasing ventilation-perfusion mismatching[90]. The goal of airway management should be maintaining sufficient arterial oxygen saturation in order to maximize oxygen delivery to tissue beds, especially the CNS.

Circulation

Once the airway is established and adequate ventilation is obtained, the circulatory status should be assessed. The goal of initial cardiovascular stabilization is return of end-organ perfusion. Arrhythmias can occur in the drowning patient, especially if the patient is hypothermic. Common rhythms include bradycardia and asystole in warm-water drownings, while atrial and ventricular fibrillation are seen in cold-water drownings[56,83]. Continuous electrocardiographic monitoring should begin soon after arrival of emergency medical personnel.

Perfusion should be assessed quickly. Indications of poor perfusion include prolonged capillary refill, mottled appearance of the skin, poor pulses, cool extremities, small urine output, and altered sensorium. Frequently, the near-drowning patient exhibits hypovolemia and marked vasoconstriction secondary to fluid transudation. This may make detection of distal pulses extremely difficult. Judicious intravenous fluid administration should proceed. Administration of large volumes of hypotonic fluid is contraindicated because of the lack of effective volume expansion. Additionally, the free water in hypotonic fluids may worsen cerebral edema and cause hyponatremia, thereby lowering the seizure threshold. A central venous or pulmonary artery catheter may be needed to monitor fluid administration. Intravenous fluids should not be withheld secondary to concerns regarding cerebral edema, since optimizing cerebral perfusion is one of the most important goals of cardiovascular management. If poor perfusion continues once the intravascular volume has been adequately expanded, the use of inotropic agents to improve cardiac contractility should be considered.

Neurologic

The initial support of the CNS is best accomplished by ensuring adequate oxygenation combined with circulatory stability. After reestablishing respiratory and circulatory stability, a brief but thorough neurologic examination should be performed. Serial neurologic examinations can distinguish intact survivors from those with a poor neurologic outcome as early as 24 hours after the accident[92].

The level of consciousness should be assessed using the Glasgow Coma Scale (GCS). The GCS is well known to most emergency and critical care physicians. This scoring system is based on three areas of evaluation: eye opening, verbalization, and motor response. Eye opening relates to level of arousal, verbalization relates to mentation, and motor ability relates to response to external stimuli. The GCS minimizes interobserver variability and provides a framework in which to evaluate the patient over time. It has also shown prognostic value in drowning patients[129].

The evaluation of brainstem reflexes may aid in determining the extent of cerebral damage and has been shown to have some prognostic value. In a 1994 study, patients who demonstrated spontaneous, purposeful movements and had a normal brainstem examination at 24 hours progressed to full recovery[92]. Children without these findings by 24 hours suffered severe neurologic deficits or death.

The pupillary response to light can be evaluated relatively quickly. Unilateral pupillary dilation and unresponsiveness generally indicates an increased ICP with transtentorial herniation causing compression of the blood supply to the brainstem. Bilaterally unresponsive pupils are an ominous sign, indicating severe cerebral dysfunction from the hypoxic-ischemic injury or bilateral uncal herniation. When these findings are noted on examination, hyperventilation and other modalities to lower ICP should be initiated immediately. Other brainstem reflexes to be assessed include the corneal, gag, oculovestibular, and oculocephalic reflexes and spontaneous respiratory effort.

Other associated injuries may occur and need to be considered. Closed-head injuries can occur in diving into shallow water. These may cause intracranial accumulations of blood which rapidly raise ICP. Injury to the cervical vertebrae and spinal cord may also occur. This type of injury is especially prevalent among adolescents involved in diving or boating accidents[93,94]. In a recent study spanning 11 years, 9.0% of adolescent diving injuries involved documented neck fractures[95]. In all patients in whom a cervical spine injury is suspected, midline traction and cervical immobilization should be employed.

Other Systems

Intra-abdominal trauma should be considered if abdominal bruising is present and the story of the injury is consistent (i.e., diving accident or possible child abuse). When the suspicion of child abuse is high, possible fractures or evidence of previous injury should be evaluated.

Laboratory Evaluation

Initial laboratory assessment should include an assessment of arterial blood gas to evaluate the degree of acidosis and hypoxia and the effectiveness of ventilation. Serum electrolyte levels should be obtained. Initial blood glucose levels may be predictive of eventual outcome after near-drowning in children. A 1990 study showed that glucose levels obtained on admission had a predictive value of 68%[96]. An elevated initial glucose level (465 to 511 mg%) was seen in children who died or remained in a persistent vegetative state when compared to children with a good outcome (238 mg%). However, the study group was small (16 children), and confounding variables such as glucose-containing intravenous fluids are not mentioned. Other tests to be considered include renal and hepatic function tests, especially if the degree of hypoxia is severe. Adolescent near-drownings are often associated with illegal drug and alcohol use. When appropriate, toxicologic tests should be evaluated. A chest radiograph is needed for all intubated patients to check the location of the endotracheal tube, assess the degree of pulmonary edema, and evaluate possible barotrauma.

Hypothermia

Hypothermia from cold-water near-drownings presents a unique clinical challenge. Efforts at rewarming should begin as soon as possible. Wet clothing should be removed to prevent continued conductive heat loss(83). Active external (surface) rewarming should be instituted in patients with core temperatures greater than 30°C(97). These methods include electric warming devices, hot water bottles, warm bedding, and radiant heat sources. For near-drowning victims with core temperatures less than 30°C, active internal rewarming is needed(97). Rewarming the peripheral circulation first increases the risk of cardiac collapse. It creates a vasodilated, metabolically active tissue bed whose needs cannot be met by a cold, poorly contractile heart(56,83). Additionally, by-products of anaerobic metabolism are circulated back to the heart and may contribute to worsening cardiac function. External rewarming of a markedly hypothermic patient also increases the risk of severe localized burns at the sites of rewarming. Poor peripheral circulation from vasoconstriction or a cardiogenic source does not adequately dissipate the heat emitted from localized sources. Core rewarming can be accomplished by warmed intravenous fluids, warmed humidified oxygen, gastric or rectal lavage with warmed fluids, and peritoneal lavage(56,83,97). Cardiopulmonary bypass has also been successfully used to rewarm near-drowning patients(78,80).

Hypothermia often confounds the initial physical examination of the near-drowning patient. The patient may appear clinically dead due to decreased cardiac and neurologic activity from the hypothermia itself. As the patient becomes normothermic during resuscitation, hypoxic injury to organ systems becomes more readily apparent. Often, the injury is too severe and the organs will not recover function. However, many clinicians report remarkable recoveries after prolonged submersions(78–80,98). Unless a drowning victim is clearly dead, with no hope of responding to appropriate resuscitative efforts, it seems reasonable that a patient should not be declared legally dead until the core temperature is 32°C or greater(11).

A hypothermic heart is extremely irritable and prone to ventricular fibrillation(97). Additionally, the hypothermic heart is resistant to the effects of defibrillation and cardiotonic agents. Attempts at electrical defibrillation are not likely to be successful if core temperature is less than 30°C(97). Three attempts at defibrillation should be attempted. If ventricular fibrillation persists, then CPR should be continued as before. The patient should be aggressively rewarmed and repeat defibrillation attempted as the temperature increases(97,99). Cardiotonic mediations should be used with caution in hypothermic patients. Hypothermia slows renal and hepatic excretion of drugs(83) so that routine doses may result in extremely high plasma concentrations. Epinephrine, lidocaine, and procainamide may accumulate to toxic levels if used repeatedly(97). For these reasons, it is recommended that a single dose of lidocaine or bretylium be given to a hypothermic patient in ventricular fibrillation(99), but that subsequent doses be held until the patient's core temperature is greater than 30°C(97).

PEDIATRIC INTENSIVE CARE UNIT MANAGEMENT

The near-drowning event is a global hypoxic-ischemic insult that results in multi-organ dysfunction. The degree of organ dysfunction tends to correlate with the severity and length of hypoxia and ischemia. While all organ systems may be damaged, the cornerstone of modern therapy is directed toward cerebral resuscitation and protection. Intensive care unit management attempts to minimize secondary neurologic damage from hypoxia, ischemia, acidosis, seizure activity, and fluid/electrolyte abnormalities.

All near-drowning patients admitted to the pediatric intensive care unit (PICU) require continuous electrocardiograms and pulse oximetry. For the unstable near-drowning patient, arterial and central venous pressure monitoring is almost always required. The placement of a flow-directed pulmonary artery catheter may also provide useful information in the patient showing severe cardiac and/or pulmonary dysfunction. Urine output should be monitored as a measure of end-organ perfusion.

Respiratory Management

Patients admitted to the PICU must have their respiratory system monitored closely. Spontaneously breathing patients must be watched closely for the development of tachypnea, retractions, decreased breath sounds, a change in level of consciousness, or other signs of respiratory distress. Serial examinations are also important in intubated mechanically ventilated patients to ensure the adequacy of the ventilatory assistance being provided. Deterioration of the respiratory system is possible up to 24 to 72 hours after a near-drowning episode from secondary drowning, adult respiratory distress syndrome, chemical pneumonitis, or pneumonia.

Hypoxia should be treated as quickly as possible; the aggressiveness of the therapy should be dictated by the severity of the patient's condition. The administration of supplemental oxygen is the first line in therapeutic intervention. A PaO2 of less than 60 mm Hg while on 50% oxygen, oxygen saturation less than 90%, or worsening hypercapnea may indicate the need for ventilatory support. However, severe pulmonary dysfunction after a near-drowning episode is often unresponsive to supplemental oxygen and is best treated with PEEP[1,2,4,7,11,56,100]. This reduces intrapulmonary shunting, increases functional residual capacity, increases lung compliance, and is extremely effective in reversing hypoxemia. PEEP should be gradually increased to the point where oxygen saturations are greater than 90% while on FiO2 of 0.5 or less. In general, patients tolerate PEEP well, but it can impair cardiac output, especially in the hypovolemic patient[100]. Maintenance of normal intravascular volume should be ensured in patients receiving high levels of PEEP. Barotrauma, including pneumothoraces and subcutaneous emphysema, is another complication of high PEEP. The pulmonary dysfunction associated with drowning is usually limited. Regeneration of surfactant and a decrease in pulmonary capillary leak typically occur in 3 to 4 days, after which time the pulmonary manifestations of near-drowning tend to resolve, and PEEP can be rapidly weaned[56] (Fig. 26.8a and b).

A moderate degree of hyperventilation may be helpful in patients who show evidence of cerebral edema. A PaCO2 in the 30 to 35 mm Hg range is adequate. Some authors advocate hyperventilation to PaCO2 level of 20 to 25 mm Hg to treat suspected cerebral edema[101], but excessive hyperventilation may induce vasoconstriction to a degree that cerebral perfusion is impaired. Additionally, the efficacy of prolonged hyperventilation is questionable.

On rare occasions, conventional ventilatory methods are ineffective in resolving hypoxia. Case reports have described the successful use of high-frequency jet ventilation after near-drowning[80,102]. In the most severe cases of pulmonary insufficiency, extracorporeal membrane oxygenation (ECMO) has been attempted[7,103,104]. To date, controlled studies comparing ECMO to conventional ventilation after near-drowning have not been reported in the literature[7].

Prophylactic use of corticosteroids for treatment of pulmonary complications after near-drowning has been shown to be of no benefit, and its use is uniformly discouraged[4,7,54]. A retrospective review of 91 near-drowning victims showed an increased mortality in those who received steroids[54]. The prophylactic use of antibiotics is somewhat more controversial. In general, the use of prophylactic antibiotics has not been shown to improve survival, and there are concerns that its use will select out antibiotic-resistant organisms[54]. In one published study, 64% of mechanically ventilated patients developed pneumonia despite the prophylactic use of antibiotics, and a majority of the organisms were resistant to the antibiotics being used to treat the patients[105]. Secondary bacterial infections due to aspiration or as a consequence of ventilation are seen in chil-

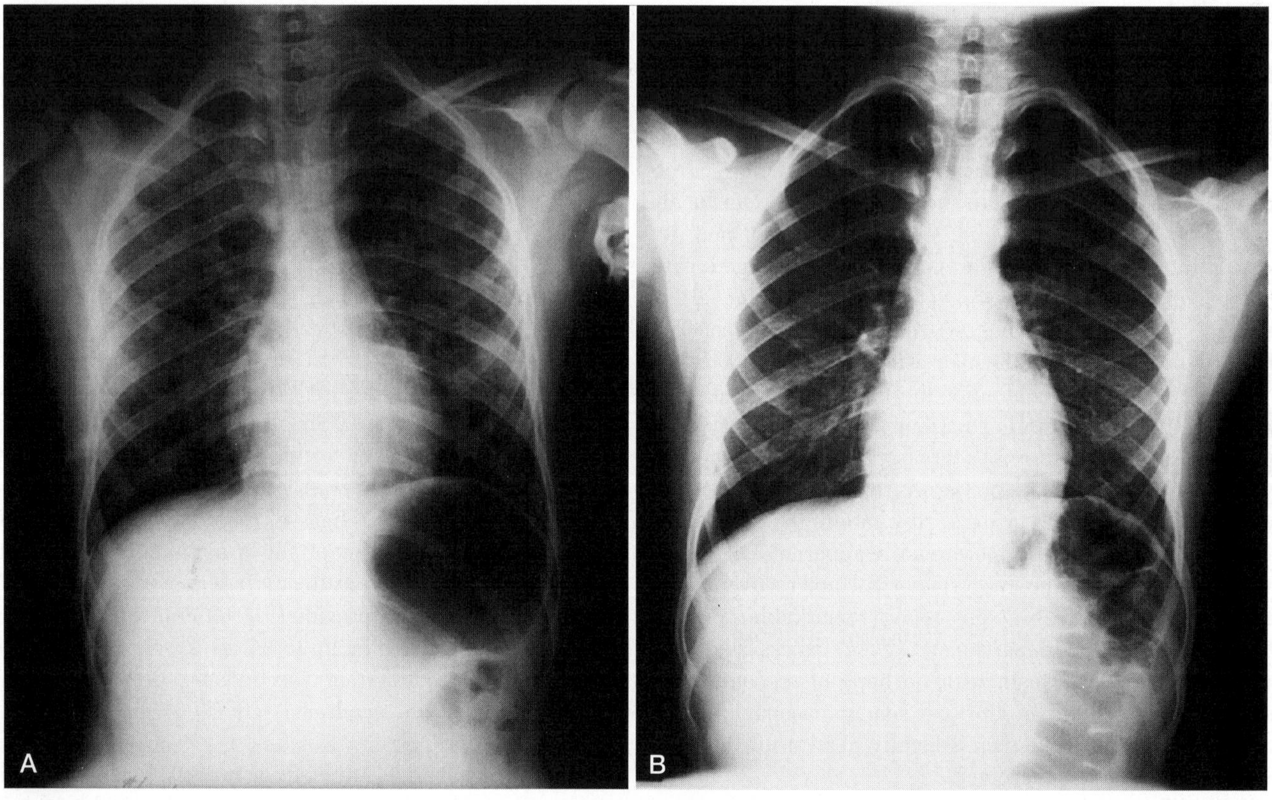

Figure 26.8. Chest x-ray of a 6-year-old near-drowning victim who was found floating unconscious in a pool. Radiographs A and B both demonstrate clearing of pulmonary infiltrates with 48 hours. (Courtesy of Richard Boyer, M.D., Department of Radiology, University of Utah School of Medicine, Salt Lake City.)

dren[106,142] (Fig. 26.9). The exact incidence of early infections after aspiration is not known. In a 1992 study involving risk analysis for bacterial infections after aspiration events, 39% of pediatric near-drowning victims developed clinical signs of infection as well as bacteremia[106]. No diagnostic features in the first 2 days of hospitalization reliably separated those who developed infections from those who did not. The authors recommended beginning intravenous antibiotics in all children after aspiration events. It seems rational to consider use of prophylactic antibiotic coverage in patients who aspirate grossly contaminated water, or water from untreated hot tubs and spas (a likely reservoir of Pseudomonas). Close observation of the patient's clinical examination, laboratory data, and chest x-rays,[8] with early consideration of diagnostic procedures (protected specimen brushes and bronchoalveolar lavage), should be used as a guide for starting antibiotic therapy.

Recently, a number of new therapies directed toward increasing pulmonary function after near-drowning have been published. Artificial surfactant has been used in humans to replace the inactivated surfactant seen in fresh water aspirations[107]. Vaporized n-butyl alcohol has been used in an animal model to improve oxygenation after saltwater near-drowning[47]. It is believed to work by a "defoaming" action on the fine foam bubbles produced in the alveoli after near-drowning that may cause small airway obstruction. It also acts as a perhydroxyl radical scavenger agent. Significant improvement in PaO2 was noted in 15 minutes in those animals receiving the n-butyl alcohol vapor plus oxygen compared to oxygen alone. These studies are inconclusive at present,[9] and further clinical trials are warranted before their use can be recommended.

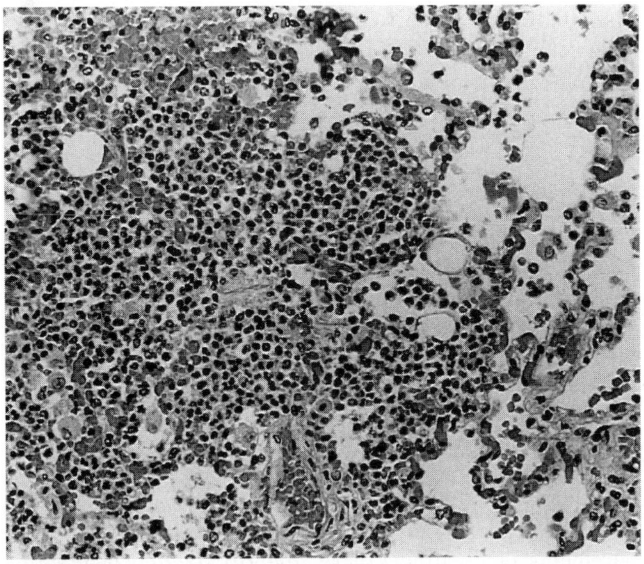

Figure 26.9. Lung section shows diffuse pneumonia in a 2-year-old male who was found in a river and died 48 hours after rescue. Cultures grew Streptococcus pneumoniae. (Slides, courtesy of Dr. Edward Leis, State of Utah Medical Examiner's Office; photomicrographs, courtesy of Dr. Edward C. Klatt, Department of Pathology, University of Utah School of Medicine, Salt Lake City.)

Cardiovascular Management

The goal of cardiovascular management is to maintain adequate cardiac output and organ perfusion. Anoxic and ischemic injury to the heart after a near-drowning episode can occur. The electrocardiogram may show nonspecific ST- and T-wave changes[56]. Cardiac isoenzymes may be elevated. Persistent cardiac dysfunction is often due to hypoxic cardiomyopathy. Ensuring adequate intravascular volume will help cardiac function and ensure improved end-organ perfusion. Excessive administration of intravascular fluids may increase symptoms of left-sided heart failure and worsen cerebral edema. Poor cardiac function may need to be augmented by inotropic support. In patients with significant hypoxic organ injury, a flow-directed pulmonary artery catheter may be useful in assessing cardiac function and oxygen delivery.

Neurologic Management

The concept of cerebral resuscitation has changed dramatically in the past two decades. In the late 1970s, Conn et al. reported improved recovery of near-drowning victims using aggressive brain-preservation techniques aimed primarily at controlling cerebral edema, treating elevated ICPs, and decreasing cerebral metabolic requirements[108,109]. This form of therapy initially caused a great deal of enthusiasm, but subsequent studies have shown no benefit from therapies geared toward decreasing ICP in order to prevent secondary CNS damage after hypoxia-ischemia[84,110–114].

There is increasing evidence that monitoring ICPs in hypoxic-ischemic cerebral injury does not affect outcome[16,79,114–117]. It appears that cerebral edema and resultant intracranial hypertension is a direct result of the original hypoxic cerebral injury and not a manifestation of a reversible process. Classically, high ICPs and low CPPs allow separation of nonsurvivors from survivors in near-drowned deeply comatose children. However, they have been unable to separate neurologically intact survivors from those in a persistent vegetative state, as an increased ICP does not always occur in children who have a poor neurologic outcome. It is questionable whether aggressive treatment of increased ICPs improves survival[118]. Additionally, aggressive treatment of intracranial hypertension has not decreased the incidence of poor neurologic outcome[113]. A series of studies noted no significant differences in neurologic outcomes when children treated with ICP monitoring were compared with near-drowning children in which no ICP monitoring occurred[79,117]. As therapies attempting to control cytotoxic cerebral edema and subsequent intracranial hypertension appear futile, the use of ICP monitoring after hypoxic-ischemic cerebral injury is becoming much less frequent in the PICU.

Current neurologic intensive care is directed at conservative management, and attempts to decrease possible secondary injury to the brain. Cerebral resuscitation therapy consists of rapid restoration and stabilization of oxygenation and cerebral circulation. Correction of acid-base and electrolyte abnormalities is important. Maintenance of normoglycemia and normothermia is optimal. Hyperthermia should be avoided since it can increase cerebral metabolic demands and lower seizure thresholds. Control of seizure activity is important as seizure activity increases cerebral oxygen consumption and cerebral blood flow. Control of suspected intracranial hypertension should not increase potential risk factors. Recommended therapies include mild hyperventilation, sedation, elevating the head of the bed, avoiding fluid overload, and limiting potential noxious stimuli. The use of neuromuscular blocking agents decreases the amount of useful information available through neurologic examination, but may be necessary to improve ventilation status in severe pulmonary dysfunction.

A number of experimental therapies have been considered in order to limit the neuronal damage associated with hypoxia. These therapies have their basis in the cellular pathophysiology that is believed to occur with hypoxia-ischemia. They include calcium channel blockers, free radical scavengers, excitatory neurotransmitter (L-glutamate and L-aspartate) blockade, and lazaroids (lipid peroxidation inhibitors)[66,67,119,120]. It was hoped that these therapies would limit the damage hypoxia-ischemia produces in its penumbra, and they initially produced much excitement in critical care neurologic research, but clinical results over the last decade have been frankly disappointing.

The best predictor of outcome currently remains the neurologic examination over time[11,92,112]. However, because of pulmonary disease, some patients require neuromuscular blockade and/or sedation, thus preventing an accurate examination. Additionally, an ability to predict outcome early in the patient's hospital course would facilitate decision making by the family and physicians. For these reasons, a number of radiologic techniques, neurophysiologic tests, and laboratory studies have been evaluated as adjuncts in determining the extent of neurologic damage and eventual outcome. Studies have found that a normal head computed tomography (CT) scan after anoxic cerebral injury is poorly predictive of outcome[121,122]. However, an abnormal CT scan in the initial 36 hours after the near-drowning event is nearly always associated with a dismal prognosis. A commonly noted abnormal CT finding in hypoxic cerebral injury is the reversal sign, which consists of a diffusely decreased density in the cerebral cortical gray and white matter, with a loss of the gray/white interface and relative increased density of the thalami, brainstem, and cerebellum (Fig. 26.10). Neurophysiologic testing has included the use of brainstem auditory-evoked responses (BAERs) and electroencephalographic monitoring[114,123]. Relevant EEG findings associated with a poor prognosis are low amplitude activity, isoelectric tracings, burst-suppression patterns, uninterrupted seizure activity, or alpha activity in the presence of clinical coma (termed alpha-coma). However, EEG tracings must be interpreted with caution as they can be influenced by hypothermia, illegal drug use, and barbiturate therapy. BAERs have been demonstrated to be useful in differentiating survivors from nonsurvivors after near-drownings, often within 6 hours of admission. They are less useful in differentiating survivors with neurologic deficits. Patients in persistent vegetative states normalize some aspects of their BAERs, but cannot be completely differentiated from neurologically intact survivors until day 3 of hospitalization[123].

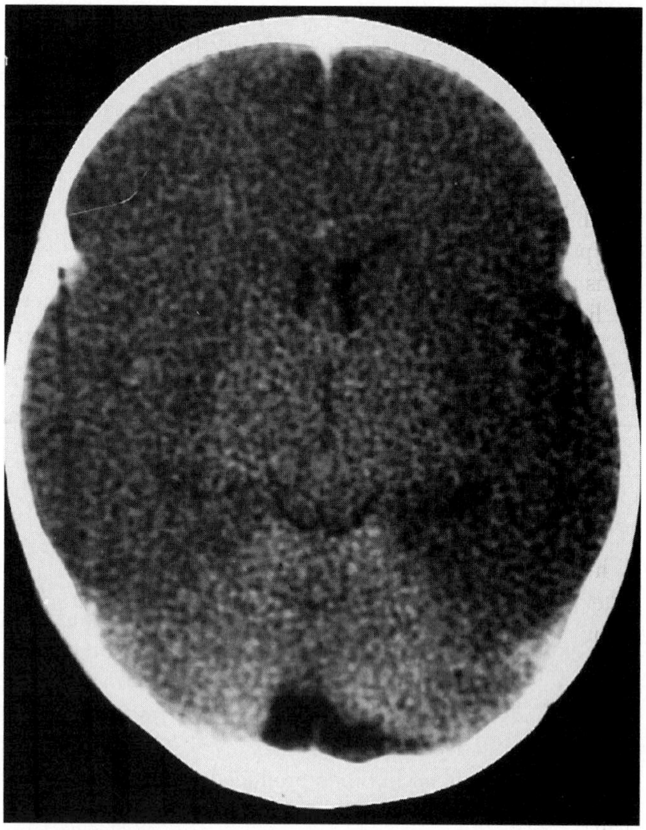

Figure 26.10. Cranial computed tomography scan of a 4-year-old near-drowning victim shows findings consistent with the reversal sign, including diffusely decreased density in the cortical gray and white matter, with loss of the gray/white interface and relative increased density of the thalamic nuclei, brainstem, and cerebellum. (Courtesy of Richard Boyer, M.D., Department of Radiology, University of Utah School of Medicine, Salt Lake City.)

Cerebral blood flow and oxygen utilization studies have also been used to predict recovery[96,118]. These studies demonstrate that global cerebral blood flow does not relate prognostically to functional neurologic outcome. However, children with a normal neurologic examination who survive demonstrate a significantly higher cross-brain oxygen content difference at 24 hours and have a higher oxygen metabolic rate at 48 hours[118].

Recently, cerebrospinal fluid analysis has been used to evaluate the extent of neuronal injury in adults[124]. Measurements of creatine kinase, the BB fraction of creatine kinase, and lactate dehydrogenase (isoenzymes 1–3) were all found to peak 76 hours after a hypoxic-ischemic cerebral insult in all patients who either died or were neurologically disabled. Patients who recovered normally had no change in their cerebrospinal fluid analysis. A difference could be seen between these groups as early as 28 hours after resuscitation.

PROGNOSTIC EVALUATION

An ability to accurately prognosticate the eventual outcome of a patient early in the hospital course would allow physicians to more appropriately counsel parents. A number of studies have attempted to predict what variables affect a near-drowning victim's outcome. However, no prognostic scoring system to date has been found to be entirely accurate[(11)].

Submersion time has been considered an important factor in eventual outcome; unfortunately, it is often difficult to ascertain an accurate submersion time[(125)]. Death or severe neurologic impairment predictably occur in victims with submersion times longer than 10 minutes in non-icy water, and resuscitation (CPR) durations greater than 25 minutes[(17,89)]. Good outcomes are more likely in children with a 5-minute or less submersion time, and less than a 10-minute duration of CPR[(17)]. Good outcomes could also be predicted when the child was found to have sinus rhythm, reactive pupils, and neurologic responsiveness at the scene. Many studies have shown that the need for ongoing CPR in the emergency department is predictive of a dismal prognosis. In these studies, most children who arrived at an emergency department with no heart rate (i.e., requiring ongoing CPR) either died or remained in a persistent vegetative state[(79,86,115,126)]. Similarly, the use of cardiotonic medications was associated with death in 70% of patients and severe neurologic impairment in the remaining 30%[(115)]. However, there have recently been a number of reports documenting full neurologic recovery in normothermic pediatric near-drowning patients who arrived at the emergency department without vital signs, required prolonged CPR, and received cardiotonic medications[(112,127)].

Features of the near-drowning patient's physical examination and initial laboratory data have also been used to predict prognosis. One of the earliest of these prognostic systems was devised by Fandel and Bancalari[(128)]. They showed that all children with a pH less than 7.0, coma, the need for CPR, and the need for ventilatory support had a dismal prognosis. Orlowski constructed a prognostic scoring system using five criteria: age younger than 3 years, immersion time longer than 5 minutes, no resuscitation for 10 minutes, coma at initial presentation, and arterial pH less than 7.1[(125)]. A point was given for each item present. With this scoring system, he was able to define whether a child had a 90% chance of normal recovery (scores of 0–1) or less than 5% chance of recovery (scores of ≥3). This system is somewhat flawed in that lack of information is not handled well, the historical information regarding submersion and resuscitation time is often unreliable, and laboratory measurements may not be predictive because they are subject to many factors, including previous treatment and timing of blood samples. Conn et al. used a scoring system based on depth of coma and postural tone[(109)]. Patients are placed in categories A, B, and C based on depth of coma, and in subclasses 1 to 4 based on postural tone (decorticate, decerebrate, and flaccid) at time of assignment. His findings showed deep coma with flaccid tone (category C3) to be associated with a 14% chance of recovery.

The GSC has also been used extensively to predict outcomes of pediatric near-drownings[(92,112,129,130)]. Multiple studies have demonstrated that an initial GCS less than 5 was highly predictive of death or severe neurologic sequelae[(92,129,130)]. Additionally, no improvement in the GCS over 24 hours was also highly predictive of a dismal outcome[(92,112)]. Since the GCS is easily, rapidly, and reproducibly assessed from physical findings alone, it is suggested as an initial tool in assessing the extent of cerebral damage, particularly in the prehospital setting.

There is a great deal of controversy regarding when to limit resuscitation of a near-drowning victim[(131)]. Some argue that there is no practical medical index or score that will predict with 100% certainty which patients will and will not survive a near-drowning accident neurologically intact. Therefore, all children should initially receive aggressive resuscitation. Others argue that aggressive therapy increases the number of neurologically devastated survivors. This creates emotional and financial hardships for the patient's family and drains limited national resources available for medical care. There is no easy answer to this question. Our approach is to provide aggressive initial resuscitative attempts, then consider withdrawing life support within a few days if neurologic improvement is not seen[(135)].

OUTCOME

Pulmonary dysfunction was once the leading cause of mortality after near-drowning episodes. With improvements in cardiovascular and pulmonary intensive care, pulmonary insufficiency is no longer a significant cause of death in the hospitalized near-drowning patient. After the near-drowning patient is successfully stabilized, the main determinant of morbidity and mortality is the degree of posthypoxic encephalopathy. However, determining the degree of a hypoxic-ischemic cerebral insult may be difficult initially. As it is difficult to predict the outcome for any patient using prehospital prognostic criteria or scoring systems, aggressive resuscitation should be continued until the physician believes that further resuscitative efforts are hopeless. In those patients that survive to reach the PICU, intact neurologic survival ranges from 50 to 80%[(11)]. Mortality rates are 25 to 35%, and approximately 10% of patients survive with neurologic impairment **(Table 26.2.)**

Long-term outcomes of near-drowning victims with neurologic impairment have been studied. In patients who suffer anoxic encephalopathy, musculoskeletal changes are common. The posturing and spasticity in children with anoxic encephalopathy secondary to near-drowning has been

Table 26.2. Outcomes of Pediatric Near-Drownings in a Tertiary Care Setting

Authors	*Total Number of Near-Drownings*	*Intact Survival*	*Died*	*Profound Neurologic Damage*
Biggart et al.[79]	55	32 (58%)	18 (33%)	5 (9%)
Nichter et al.[115]	93	67 (72%)	19 (20%)	7 (8%)
Abrams and Mubarak[132]	290	220 (76%)	38 (13%)	32 (11%)
Levin et al.[7]	248	134 (54%)	86 (35%)	28 (11%)
Jensen et al.[6]	119	84 (71%)	29 (24%)	6 (5%)
Lavelle and Shaw[112]	44	25 (56%)	14 (32%)	5 (12%)

shown to progress rapidly and be more severe than that associated with either head trauma or cerebral palsy[(132)]. The most common musculoskeletal problems were contractures, especially equinus (82%), hip adductor (53%), hamstring (33%), and quadriceps (26%). Hip dislocation or subluxation occurred in 34% of patients, while scoliosis developed in 18%. Of children who suffered severe anoxic encephalopathy after near-drowning, 69% were nonambulatory[(132)].

In addition to musculoskeletal problems, anoxic encephalopathy after near-drowning can cause a multitude of other neurologic sequelae. As a group, neurologically injured near-drowning patients had longer durations of unconsciousness, decreased verbal skills after recovery, poorer cognitive outcomes, and a higher incidence of dystonic rigidity[(12,133)]. In one study of 20 neurologically injured near-drowning victims, 13 remained in persistent vegetative states. The remaining seven made good recoveries but showed mild coordination or gross motor deficiencies. All of these children were conscious within 2 weeks of injury[(133)]. A second study showed that 73% of near-drowning victims unconscious for at least 24 hours after the injury remained in persistent vegetative states. The remaining 27% were conscious but profoundly neurologically impaired[(134)].

The cessation of life support for severely impaired near-drowning patients is a problem faced by many intensive care physicians[(3,135)]. Consideration of limitation and withdrawal of therapy for these patients, in whom quality of life is questionable, has become increasingly acceptable in the critical care community. Decisions regarding life-sustaining therapy should be made with the input of the family.

CONCLUSION

Drowning and near-drowning episodes produce global hypoxia, with the CNS being particularly sensitive to the effects of decreased tissue oxygenation. Therapies directed toward decreasing the extent and amount of neuronal damage have met with limited success. Until more effective neuronal salvage techniques are available, prevention of the submersion event itself is the most powerful tool available[(37,136–140)].

There is cause for hope and cause for concern. In a recent survey evaluating childhood trends in drowning over a 15-year period, a decreased incidence was noted in older children (<5.8% per year for children ages 10 to 14, and <5.4% per year for adolescents[(9)]. However, only a slight decline was noted in toddlers, while the incidence of drownings among infants actually increased. This is unusual, as most prevention programs are aimed at infants and toddlers. As such, the U.S. Public Health Service objectives for the year 2000 call for a reduction in drowning rates among all children but emphasize targeting children ages 4 and younger[(141)]. Unfortunately, this may be difficult to implement. A recent survey showed that the proportion of pool owners endorsing risk reduction behaviors (voluntary CPR training, pool barrier requirements) is much larger than the proportion actually adopting them[(140,143)]. This suggests that public education may have less effect than originally hoped. Regardless of this finding, the role of the clinician in preventive education remains paramount.

References

1. Witte M, Near-drowning, in A Practical Guide to Pediatric Intensive Care, J. Blumer, Editor. 1990, Mosby-Year Book: St. Louis.
2. Sarnaik A, Lieh-Lai M, Near-Drowning, in Pediatric Critical Care, B. Fuhrman and J. Zimmerman, Editor. 1992, Mosby Year Book: St. Louis.
3. Kallas HJ, O'Rourke PP: Drowning and immersion injuries in children. Curr Opin Pediatr 5:295–302, 1993.
4. Fields AI: Near-drowning in the pediatric population. Crit Care Clin 8:113–129, 1992.
5. Waller AE, Baker SP, Szocka A: Childhood injury deaths: national analysis and geographic variations. Am J Public Health 79:310–315, 1989.
6. Jensen LR, Williams SD, Thurman DJ, Keller PA: Submersion injuries in children younger than 5 years in urban Utah. West J Med 157:641–644, 1992.
7. Levin D, Morriss F, Toro L, Brink L, Turner G: Drowning and near-drowning. Pediatr Clin North Am 40:321–336, 1993.
8. Baker S, O'Neill B, Ginsburg M, Guohua L, The Injury Fact Book. 1992, New York: Oxford University Press.
9. Brenner RA, Smith GS, Overpeck MD: Divergent trends in childhood drowning rates, 1971 through 1988. JAMA 271:1606–8 Issn:12 0098–7484, 1994.
10. Baker S, Waller A, Childhood Injury State by State Mortality Facts. 1989, Baltimore: The Johns Hopkins Injury Prevention Center.
11. Shaw KN, Briede CA: Submersion injuries: drowning and near-drowning. Emerg Med Clin North Am 7:355–370, 1989.
12. Wintemute GJ: Childhood drowning and near-drowning in the United States. Am J Dis Child 144:663–669, 1990.
13. Spyker D: Submersion injury: epidemiology, prevention, and management. Pediatr Clin North Am 32:113–125, 1985.
14. Fatal injuries to children—United States, 1986. MMWR Morb Mortal Wkly Rep 39:442–445, 451, 1990.
15. Wintemute G: Drowning in early childhood. Pediatr Ann 21:417–421, 1992.
16. Orlowski J: Drowning, near-drowning, and ice-water submersions. Pediatr Clin North Am 34:75–92, 1987.
17. Quan L, Kinder D: Pediatric submersions: prehospital predictors of outcome. Pediatrics 90:909–913, 1992.
18. Wintemute G, Kraus J, Teret S, Wright M: Drowning in childhood and adolescence: a population-based study. Am J Public Health 77:830–832, 1987.
19. Kemp AM, Mott AM, Sibert JR: Accidents and child abuse in bathtub submersions. Arch Dis Child 70:435–438, 1994.
20. Pearn J, Nixon J: Bathtub immersion accidents involving children. Med J Aust 1:211–213, 1977.
21. Griest KJ, Zumwalt RE: Child abuse by drowning. Pediatrics 83:41–46, 1989.
22. Feldman K, Monastersky C, Feldman G: When is childhood drowning neglect? Child Abuse & Neglect 17:329–336, 1993.
23. Mann NC, Weller SC, Rauchschwalbe R: Bucket-related drownings in the United States, 1984 through 1990. Pediatrics 89:1068–1071, 1992.

24. Budnick L, Ross D: Bathtub-related drownings in the United States. Am J Public Health 75:630–633, 1985.
25. Wintemute GJ, Drake C, Wright M: Immersion events in residential swimming pools. Evidence for an experience effect. Am J Dis Child 145:1200–1203, 1991.
26. Quan L, Gore EJ, Wentz K, Allen J, Novack AH: Ten-year study of pediatric drownings and near-drownings in King County, Washington: lessons in injury prevention. Pediatrics 83:1035–1040, 1989.
27. Present P. Child drowning study: a report on the epidemiology of drownings in residential pools to children under age five. in US Consumer Product Safety Commission. 1987. Washington, D.C.
28. Shinaberger CS, Anderson CL, Kraus JF: Young children who drown in hot tubs, spas, and whirlpools in California: a 26-year survey. Am J Public Health 80:613–614, 1990.
29. Jumbelic M, Chambliss M: Accidental toddler drowning in a 5-gallon bucket. JAMA 263:1952–1953, 1990.
30. Weintraub RG, Gow RM, Wilkinson JL: The congenital long QT syndromes in childhood. J Am Coll Cardiol 16:674–680, 1990.
31. Harris E, Knapp J, Sharma V: The Romano-Ward syndrome: a case presenting as near-drowning with a clinical review. Pediatr Emerg Care 8:272–275, 1992.
32. Kemp AM, Sibert JR: Epilepsy in children and the risk of drowning. Arch Dis Child 68:684–685, 1993.
33. Diekema DS, Quan L, Holt VL: Epilepsy as a risk factor for submersion injury in children. Pediatrics 91:612–616, 1993.
34. Pearn J: Epilepsy and drowning in childhood. Br Med J 1:1510–1511, 1977.
35. Guyer B, Ellers B: Childhood injuries in the United States. AJDC 144:649–652, 1990.
36. Rodgers GB: Factors contributing to child drownings and near-drownings in residential swimming pools. Hum Factors 31:123–132, 1989.
37. American Academy of Pediatrics Committee on Injury and Poison Prevention: Drowning in infants, children, and adolescents. Pediatrics 92:292–294, 1993.
38. Karpovich P: Water in the lungs of drowned animals. Arch Path 15:828–833, 1933.
39. Noble C, Sharpe N: Drowning: its mechanism and treatment. Canad Med Assoc J 89:402–405, 1963.
40. Pearn J: Pathophysiology of drowning. Med J Aust 142:586–588, 1985.
41. Craig A: Causes of loss of consciousness during underwater swimming. J Appl Physiol 16:583–586, 1961.
42. Redding J, Cozine R, Voight G: Resuscitation from drowning. JAMA 178:1136–1139, 1961.
43. Swann H, Spafford N: Body salt and water changes during fresh and sea water drowning. Tex Rep Biol Med 9:356–382, 1951.
44. Modell J, Davis J: Electrolyte changes in human drowning victims. Anesthesiology 30:414–420, 1969.
45. Beyda DH: Pathophysiology of near-drowning and treatment of the child with a submersion incident. Crit Care Nurs Clin North Am 3:273–280, 1991.
46. Orlowski J, Abulleil M, Phillips J: The hemodynamic and cardiovascular effects of near-drowning in hypotonic, isotonic, and hypertonic solutions. Ann Emerg Med 18:1044–1049, 1989.
47. Waugh W: Potential use of warm butyl alcohol vapors as adjunct agent in the emergency treatment of sea water near-drowning. Am J Emerg Med 11:20–27, 1993.
48. Modell J, Moya F: Effects of volume of aspirated fluid during chlorinated fresh water drowning. Anesthesiology 27:262–272, 1966.
49. Michaud L, Rivara F, Longstreth W, Grady M: Initial blood glucose levels and poor outcome following severe brain injuries in children. J Trauma 31:1356–1362, 1991.
50. Sieber F, Traystman R: Glucose and the brain. Crit Care Med 20:104–114, 1992.
51. Pearn J: Secondary drowning in children. Br Med J 281:1103–1105, 1980.
52. Nopanitanya W, Gambill T, Brankhous K: Fresh water drowning: pulmonary ultrastructure and systemic fibrinolysis. Arch Pathol 98:361–366, 1974.
53. Colebatch H, Halmagyi D: Effect of vagotomy and vagal stimulation on lung mechanics and circulation. J Appl Physiol 18:881–887, 1963.
54. Modell J, Graves S, Ketover A: Clinical course of 91 consecutive near-drowning victims. Chest 70:231–238, 1976.
55. Clarke E, Niggemann E: Near-drowning. Heart Lung 4:946–955, 1975.
56. Fiser D: Near-drowning. Pediatrics in Review 14:148–151, 1993.
57. Peterson B: Morbidity of childhood near-drowning. Pediatrics 59:364–370, 1977.
58. Harries M: Drowning in man. Crit Care Med 9:409–410, 1981.
59. Karch S: Pathology of the heart in drowning. Arch Pathol Lab Med 109:176–178, 1985.
60. Hildebrand C, Andreas G, Edgardo L, Gomez R, Bing R: Cardiac performance in pediatric near-drowning. Crit Care Med 16:331–335, 1988.
61. Oehmichen M, Pedal I, Hohmann P: Diagnostic significance of myofibrillar degeneration of cardiocytes in forensic pathology. Forensic Sci Int 48:163–173, 1990.
62. Opie L: Reperfusion injury and its pharmacologic modification. Circulation 80:1049–1062, 1989.
63. Walsh EA, Ioli JG: Childhood near-drowning: nursing care and primary prevention. Pediatr Nurs 20:265–269, 1994.
64. Pearn J: Survivors of childhood freshwater immersion accidents: neurologic and psychometric studies. Lancet 1:7–9, 1977.
65. Siesjo B: Mechanisms of ischemic brain injury. Crit Care Med 16:954–963, 1988.
66. Rogers M, Kirsch J: Current concepts in brain resuscitation. JAMA 261:3143–3147, 1989.
67. Giacoia G: Asphyxial brain damage in the newborn: new insights into pathophysiology and possible pharmacologic interventions. South Med J 86:676–681, 1993.
68. Johnston M: Cellular alterations associated with perinatal asphyxia. Clin Invest Med 16:122–132, 1993.
69. Wolfe L: Eicosanoids: prostaglandins, thromboxanes, leukotrienes, and other deviations of carbon 20 unsaturated fatty acids. J Neurochem 38:1–14, 1982.
70. Itoh U, Omno K, Nakamura R: Brain edema during ischemia and after restoration of blood flow: measurement of water, sodium, potassium content and plasma protein permeability. Stroke 10:542–547, 1979.
71. Lataste X: The blood brain barrier in hypoxia. Int J Sports Med 13:45–47, 1992.
72. Kogura K, Busto R, Scheinberg P: The role of hydrostatic pressure in ischemic brain edema. Ann Neurol 9:273–282, 1981.
73. Ames A, Wright L, Masayoshi K, Thurston J, Majno G: Cerebral ischemia: the no-reflow phenomenon. Am J Pathol 52:437–447 1968.
74. White B, Gadzinski D, Hoehner P, Krome C, Hoehner T, White J, Trombley J: Effects of flunarizine on canine cerebral cortical blood flow and vascular resistance post cardiac arrest. Ann Emerg Med 11:119–126, 1982.
75. Sano K, Asano T, Tanishima T: Lipid peroxidation as a cause of cerebral vasospasm. Neurol Res 2:253–257, 1980.
76. Wei E, Kontos H, Dietrich W: Inhibition by free radical scavengers and by cyclooxygenase inhibitors of plial arteriolar abnormalities from concussive brain injury in cats. Circ Res 48:95–99, 1981.
77. McCord J: Oxygen derived free radicals in postischemic tissue injury. N Engl J Med 312:159, 1985.
78. Bolte R, Black P, Bowers R, Thorne J, Corneli H: The use of extracorporeal rewarming in a child submerged for 66 minutes. JAMA 260:377–379, 1988.
79. Biggart MJ, Bohn DJ: Effect of hypothermia and cardiac arrest on outcome of near-drowning accidents in children. J Pediatr 117:179–183, 1990.
80. Norberg W, Agnew R, Brunsvold R, Sivanna P, Browdie D, Fisher D: Succesful resuscitation of a cold water submersion victim with use of cardiopulmonary bypass. Crit Care Med 20:1355–1357, 1992.
81. Corneli H: Accidental hypothermia. J Pediatr 120:671–679, 1992.
82. Gooden B: Why some people do not drown: hypothermia versus the diving response. Med J Aust 157:629–632, 1992.
83. Elixson EM: Hypothermia. Cold-water drowning. Crit Care Nurs Clin North Am 3:287–292, 1991.
84. Bohn D, Biggar W, Smith C, Conn A, Barker G: Infuence of hypothermia, barbiturate therapy, and intracranial pressure monitoring on morbidity and mortality after near-drowning. Crit Care Med 14:529–534, 1986.
85. Hayward J, Hay C, Matthews B: Temperature effects on human dive response in relation to cold water near-drowning. J Appl Physiol 56:202–208, 1984.
86. Kyriacou DN, Arcinue EL, Peek C, Kraus JF: Effect of immediate resuscitation on children with submersion injury. Pediatrics 94:137–142, 1994.
87. Heimlich H: Subdiaphragmatic pressure to expel water from lungs of drowning persons. Ann Emerg Med 10:476–480, 1981.
88. Quan L: Drowning issues in resuscitation. Ann Emerg Med 22:366–369, 1993.
89. Quan L, Wentz K, Gore E, Copass M: Outcome and predictors of outcome in pediatric submersion victims receiving prehospital care in King County, Washington. Pediatrics 86:586–593, 1990.

90. Beyda DH: Prehospital care of the child with a submersion incident. Crit Care Nurs Clin North Am 3:281–285, 1991.
91. Orlowski J: Vomiting as a complication of the Heimlich maneuver. JAMA 258:512–513, 1987.
92. Bratton SL, Jardine DS, Morray JP: Serial neurologic examinations after near drowning and outcome. Arch Pediatr Adolesc Med 148:167–170, 1994.
93. Ornato J: The resuscitation of the near-drowning victim. JAMA 256:75–77, 1986.
94. Osenbach R, Menezes A: Pediatric spinal cord and vertebral column injury. Neurosurgery 30:385–390, 1992.
95. Bailes J, Herman J, Quigley M, Cerullo L, Meyer PJ: Diving injuries of the cervical spine. Surg Neurol 34:155–158, 1990.
96. Ashwal S, Schneider S, Tomasi L, Thompson J: Prognostic implications of hyperglycemia and reduced cerebral blood flow in childhood near-drowning. Neurology 40:820–823, 1990.
97. Emergency Cardiac Care Committee and Subcommittees AHA: Guidelines for cardiopulmonary resuscitation and emergency cardiac care-special resuscitation situations. JAMA 268:2244–2246, 1992.
98. Sekar T, MacDonnel K, Namsirikul P: Survival after prolonged submersion in cold water without neurologic sequelae. Arch Intern Med 140:775–779, 1980.
99. The Medical Letter: treatment of hypothermia. The Medical Letter 25:9–11, 1983.
100. Luttrell P: Care of the pediatric near-drowning victim. Crit Care Nurs Clin North Am 3:293–306, 1991.
101. Nussbaum E, Pediatric Intensive Care. Second edition ed. Changing trends in cerebral and cardiopulmonary resuscitation in nearly drowned children, ed. E. Nussbaum. 1989, Mount Kisco, NY: Futura Publishing.
102. Smith DW, Frankel LR, Derish MT, Moody RR, Black LE, Chipps BE, Mathers LH: High-frequency jet ventilation in children with the adult respiratory distress syndrome complicated by pulmonary barotrauma. Pediatr Pulmonol 15:279–286, 1993.
103. Bonis S, Heaton J, Fajardo E. Extracorporeal membrane oxygenation in pediatric patients. in Fourth Annual Children's Hospital National Medical Center ECMO Symposium. 1988.
104. Steiner RB, Adolph VR, Heaton JF, Bonis SL, Falterman KW, Arensman RM: Pediatric extracorporeal membrane oxygenation in posttraumatic respiratory failure. J Pediatr Surg 26:1011–1014, 1991.
105. Oakes D, Sherck J, Maloney J: Prognosis and management of victims of near-drowning. J Trauma 22:544–549, 1982.
106. Kennedy GA, Kanter RK, Weiner LB, Tompkins JM: Can early bacterial complications of aspiration with respiratory failure be predicted? Pediatr Emerg Care 8:123–125, 1992.
107. McBrien M, Katumba J, Mukhtar A: Artificial surfactant in the treatment of near-drowning. Lancet 342:1485–1486, 1993.
108. Conn A, Edmonds J, Barker G: Cerebral resuscitation in near-drowning. Pediatr Clin North Am 26:691–701, 1979.
109. Conn A, Montes J, Barker G: Cerebral salvage in near-drowning following neurologic classification by triage. Can Anaesth Soc J 27:201–209, 1980.
110. Modell J: Drowning. NEJM 328:253–256, 1993.
111. Modell J, Graves S, Kuck E: Near-drowning: correlation of level of consciousness and survival. Can Anaesth Soc J 27:211–215, 1980.
112. Lavelle J, Shaw K: Near drowning: is emergency department cardiopulmonary resuscitation or intensive care unit resuscitation indicated? Crit Care Med 21:369–373, 1993.
113. Nussbaum E, Maggi J: Pentobarbital therapy does not improve neurologic outcome in nearly drowned, flaccid-comatose children. Pediatrics 81:630–634, 1988.
114. Pfenninger J: Neurological intensive care in children. Intensive Care Med 19:243–250, 1993.
115. Nichter M, Everett P: Childhood near-drowning: is cardiopulmonary resuscitation always indicated? Crit Care Med 17:993–995, 1989.
116. Dean J, McComb J: Intracranial pressure montoring in severe pediatric near-drowning. Neurosurgery 9:627–630, 1981.
117. Sarnaik A, Preston G, Lieh-Lai M, Eisenbrey A: Intracranial pressure and cerebral perfusion pressure in near-drowning. Crit Care Med 13:224–227, 1985.
118. Connors R, Frewen TC, Kissoon N, Kronick J, Sommerauer J, Lee R, Singh N, Tiffin N, Brown T: Relationship of cross-brain oxygen content difference, cerebral blood flow, and metabolic rate to neurologic outcome after near-drowning. J Pediatr 121:839–844, 1992.
119. Prehn J, Welsch M, Backhaub C, Nuglisch J, Ausmeier F, Karkoutly C, Krieglstein J: Effects of serotonergic drugs in experimental brain ischemia: evidence for a protective role of serotonin in cerebral ischemia. Brain Res 630:10–20, 1993.
120. Gunn A, Williams C, Mallard E, Tan W, Gluckman P: Flunarizine, a calcium channel antagonist, is partially prophylactically neuroprotective in hypoxic-ischemic encephalopathy in the fetal sheep. Pediatr Res 35:657–663, 1994.
121. Han BK, Towbin RB, De Courten Myers G, McLaurin RL, Ball WS Jr.: Reversal sign on CT: effect of anoxic/ischemic cerebral injury in children. Am J Roentgenol 154:361–368, 1990.
122. Romano C, Brown T, Frewen TC: Assessment of pediatric near-drowning victims: is there a role for cranial CT? Pediatr Radiol 23:261–263, 1993.
123. Fisher B, Peterson B, Hicks G: Use of brainstem auditory-evoked response testing to assess neurologic outcome following near drowning in children. Crit Care Med 20:578–585, 1992.
124. Karkela J, Pasanen M, Kaukinen S, Morsky P, Harmoinen A: Evaluation of hypoxic brain injury with spinal fluid enzymes, lactate, and pyruvate. Crit Care Med 20:378–386, 1992.
125. Orlowski J: Prognostic factors in pediatric cases of drowning and near-drowning. Ann Emerg Med 8:176–179, 1979.
126. Weinberg H: Prognostic variables in nearly drowned, comatose children [letter]. Am J Dis Child 140:329, 1986.
127. Christesen D, Jansen P, Perkin R: Characteristics of children with unpredictable good outcome after severe warm water near-drowning. Crit Care Med 23:199, 1995.
128. Fandel I, Bancalari E: Near-drowning in children: clinical aspects. Pediatrics 58:573–579, 1976.
129. Dean J, Kaufman N: Prognostic indicators in pediatric near-drowning: the Glasgow coma scale. Crit Care Med 9:536-539, 1981.
130. Beyda D, Tellez D, Liu P: Casuality of pediatric submersion injuries. Crit Care Med 18:S2377, 1990.
131. Modell J: Drowning: to treat or not to treat—an unanswerable question? Crit Care Med 21:313–315, 1993.
132. Abrams RA, Mubarak S: Musculoskeletal consequences of near-drowning in children. J Pediatr Orthop 11:168–175, 1991.
133. Kriel RL, Krach LE, Luxenberg MG, Jones Saete C, Sanchez J: Outcome of severe anoxic/ischemic brain injury in children. Pediatr Neurol 10:207–212, 1994.
134. Bell T, Ellenberg L, McComb J: Neuropsychological outcome after severe pediatric near-drowning. Neurosurgery 17:604–608, 1985.
135. Vernon DD, Dean JM, Timmons OD, Banner W Jr., Allen Webb EM: Modes of death in the pediatric intensive care unit: withdrawal and limitation of supportive care. Crit Care Med 21:1798–1802, 1993.
136. Hazinski M, Francescutti L, Lapidus G, Micik S, Rivara F: Pediatric injury prevention. Ann Emerg Med 22:456–467, 1993.
137. Kemp A, Sibert JR: Drowning and near drowning in children in the United Kingdom: lessons for prevention. BMJ 304:1143–1146, 1992.
138. Coffman SP: Parent education for drowning prevention. J Pediatr Health Care 5:141–146, 1991.
139. Press E: The health hazards of saunas and spas and how to minimize them. Am J Public Health 81:1034–1037, 1991.
140. Wintemute GJ, Wright MA: Swimming pool owners' opinions of strategies for prevention of drowning. Pediatrics 85:63–69, 1990.
141. Service UPH, Healthy People 2000: National Health Promotion and Disease Prevention Objectives. 1991, US Dept of Health and Human Services, US Public Health Service.
142. Vernon DD, Banner W, Cantwell GP, Holzman BH, Bolte RG, Dean JM: Streptococcus pneumoniae bacteremia associated with near-drowning. Crit Care Med 18:1174–1176, 1990.
143. Wintemute GJ, Wright MA: The attitude-practice gap revisited: risk reduction beliefs and behaviors among owners of residential swimming pools. Pediatrics 88:1168–1171, 1991.

Brain Death, Organ Donation, and Withdrawal of Life Support

27

Donald D. Vernon
Mary Jo Grant
Nancy A. Setzer

INTRODUCTION

Historically, death was identified with the cessation of pulse and respiratory effort, since these findings invariably heralded ultimate dissolution of the individual. With the advent of intensive care units (ICUs) and artificial ventilation in the 1950s and 1960s, a group of patients appeared who exhibited persistent pulse and circulation in the absence of detectable neurologic function. It soon became obvious that absence of neurologic function on serial examinations dictated a hopeless prognosis; there was no recovery from this situation, and indeed, such patients universally progressed to cardiac asystole despite maximal cardiopulmonary supportive care[1–3]. Care of these patients consumed large amounts of intensive care resources and was distasteful for both medical staff and family, who wondered whether such a person was actually alive[4]. Concomitantly, broad advances in transplant technology were making life possible for patients with previously fatal end-stage diseases, and with refinements in immunologic management, transplantation of organs from unrelated cadaver donors became a reality. Although brain dead patients offered a potential source of organs for these transplant programs, early transplants from seemingly "brain dead" patients occasionally created highly publicized legal difficulties for the transplant teams, with allegations of homicide rendered against transplant surgeons, both in the United States and in Japan[5,6]. Obviously, a medical and legal definition of brain death was needed before routine "harvesting" of organs from these patients would be possible. Thus, beginning in the 1960s, attempts were made to formulate a workable definition of brain death which would be legally equated with the death of the person. The issue was not, however, that of redefining death; death is a unitary phenomenon signifying the end of human existence. Rather, the issue was that of expansion of the way in which death is identified, i.e., to add a neurologic formulation of death to the cardiopulmonary formulation that had traditionally been used. (Pallis[3] argued that neurologic criteria are actually the most fundamental, because "cardiopulmonary death," or cardiac asystole, could be equated with the death of a person only if it persisted long enough to result in neurologic death or brain death.) Over the past three decades, the concept of brain death has achieved broad acceptance, so that at least in the United States, most of Europe, Australia, the Middle East, Mexico, and Russia brain death is equated legally and medically with the death of the person.

DEVELOPMENT OF BRAIN DEATH CRITERIA

Brain death certification was first proposed by the Ad Hoc Committee of the Harvard Medical School, which introduced the first set of brain death criteria to the medical community in 1968 **(Table 27.1)**[7]. A number of other, mostly similar criteria were proposed in following years. Nearly all proposed sets of brain death criteria, despite variations in their specific requirements, attempt to identify complete lack of function of both the cerebral hemispheres and the brain stem; this is known as the "whole-brain" formulation for brain death[8]. The demonstration of brain death further requires that the cause of brain dysfunc-

Table 27.1. Harvard Brain Death Criteria (1968)

1. Unresponsiveness, temperature greater than 32.2°C
2. Absence of depressant drugs
3. No spontaneous movements
4. Apnea off respirator for 3 minutes at room air
5. No reflexes, including:
Decerebrate or decorticate posturing
Pupils fixed and dilated
Swallowing, vocalization
Corneal and pharyngeal reflexes
Stretch and deep tendon reflexes
6. Isoelectric EEG
7. All of the above should be repeated after 24 hours

From: A definition of irreversible coma: report of the Ad Hoc Committee of the Harvard Medical School to Examine the Definition of Brain Death. JAMA 1968;205:337.

tion be known; that irreversibility be demonstrated (by showing that the brain death state persists over a period of time); and that confounding factors such as hypothermia, circulatory shock, and drug intoxication be excluded.

The functional whole-brain formulation for brain death is generally accepted, but other approaches to brain death have also been proposed. A *higher-brain* formulation (also termed *neocortical death*) would hold that the death of human beings should be equated with irreversible loss of those brain functions that are uniquely human, including emotion, self-awareness, and cognitive reasoning[8–10]. Under this formulation, death could be diagnosed in patients in a persistent vegetative state or perhaps those with severe senile dementia a prospect likely unacceptable to society at large[9]. In addition, such a formulation would be inadequate for evaluating young children, particularly infants, in whom assessment of cognitive function is difficult. Conversely, others have argued that mere loss of brain function is inadequate proof and that demonstration of anatomic destruction of the brain is necessary to define death[11]. There are practical difficulties, however, inherent in an anatomic definition of brain death, in particular with the "premortem" demonstration of brain necrosis. Finally, functional standards for brain death are consistent with the traditional cardiopulmonary criteria for brain death, which are also functional in nature; they do not require that the heart be necrotic, only that it has irreversibly ceased to beat[8].

An important step in validation of the concept of brain death was taken by the multicenter National Collaborative Study for the Determination of Cerebral Death, established by the National Institute for the Neurological Disorders and Stroke in the United States in 1971; its purpose was to examine prospectively the clinical characteristics of severely comatose patients over a 3-month period[12]. The study presumed at its inception that brain death criteria would, when satisfied, predict nonsurvival over a 3-month observation period despite maximum supportive care. Here, it was assumed that the most important validation of the brain death concept was the observation that patients in this condition inevitably and invariably progress to cardiac asystole (cardiovascular death), usually within a few days[1]. A total of 503 patients met the study entry criteria of cerebral unresponsiveness and apnea (defined as failure to override mechanical ventilation); 462 died within the 3-month period. These criteria alone thus did not adequately diagnose brain death, since 12.9% of the patients identified survived the period of observation. The Collaborative Study then examined the Harvard criteria (cerebral unresponsiveness, apnea, absent brain stem reflexes, and two isoelectric electroencephalograms (EEGs) obtained 24 hours apart), which were strictly satisfied by only 19 of these patients, all of whom died.One hundred two patients satisfied the Harvard criteria on one occasion (clinical brain death plus one isoelectric EEG), and all of these patients died also. Therefore, although the Harvard criteria could be used reliably to predict death, they failed to identify many patients with hopeless prognoses. The Collaborative Study then proposed the criteria of apnea, cerebral unresponsiveness, and electrocerebral silence, which proved more sensitive than the Harvard criteria; 187 patients met these criteria, and 185 died within the 3-month period (the remainder appear to have been cases of drug intoxication). Major differences between the National Collaborative Study criteria and the Harvard criteria included the period of observation (24 versus 6 hours), the presence of spinal stretch reflexes, and the need for a single corroborative EEG **(Table 27.2).**

Since this pioneering study, a number of others have been conducted to examine the natural history of patients identified as brain dead. Powner et al.[13] in 1977 reported 489 patients diagnosed with brain death for whom supportive care was continued until there was cardiac asystole, which occurred for most within 24 hours, and within 9 days for all. Jennett et al.[14] examined criteria devised by the Conference of Royal Colleges and Faculties of the United Kingdom in 609 brain dead patients, 326 of whom continued to receive supportive care and all of whom progressed to cardiac arrest. He also reviewed the records of 1003 survivors of severe head trauma, none of whom even briefly met the Royal College criteria for brain death, reinforcing

Table 27.2. National Collaborative Study Brain Death Criteria (1976)

1. Unresponsive coma—absent decorticate or decerebrate posturing
2. Apnea no effort to override mechanical ventilation
3. Dilated, fixed pupils
4. Absent cephalic reflexes
Corneal
Oculocephalic
Oculovestibular
Oculoauditory
Ciliospinal
Snout
Cough
Pharyngeal
Swallow
5. Isoelectric EEG

Prerequisites: Diagnosis established for coma and deemed irreversible. Criteria should be present over a 30-minute observation period, at least 6 hours after the onset of coma. From: An appraisal of the criteria of cerebral death: a summary statement. A collaborative study. JAMA 1976;237:982.

Table 27.3. Royal College Brain Death Criteria (1976)

1. Absent brain stem reflexes:
   Pupillary
   Corneal
   Absent cranial motor response
   Oculovestibular
   Gag and cough
2. Apnea—with ventilator disconnection
3. Spinal reflexes may be present
4. Testing should be repeated after observation
5. EEG and cerebral blood flow studies are not needed
6. Certifying physician should be consultant in charge of case or his or her deputy and one other doctor

Prerequisites: deep coma and need for intracranial ventilation, temperature greater than 35°C. Diagnosis established with coma due to irremediable structural brain damage, not due to metabolic disorder.
From: Conference of Royal Colleges and Faculties of the United Kingdom: Diagnosis of brain death. Lancet 1976;2:1069.

the concept that these criteria would not falsely identify patients with coma as being brain dead. In addition, Pallis[15] reviewed 16 studies, representing a total of 1036 brain dead patients who were maintained on mechanical ventilation; all of these progressed to cardiac asystole.

Other sets of brain death criteria **(Tables 27.3–27.5)** have been proposed, including those from the Royal Colleges[16] and the Report of the Medical Consultants on the Diagnosis of Death to the President's Commission for the Study of Ethical Problems in Medicine and Biomedical and Behavioral Research[8]. Overall, these various criteria are similar in their fundamental premise; i.e., that brain death can only be declared in a normothermic, nonintoxicated patient with no evidence of central nervous system (CNS) function after a defined period of observation. There are, however, several differences among these sets of criteria, involving the presence of spinal reflexes, pupillary changes, the need for corroborative testing, and the period of observation necessary prior to declaring brain death.

The Harvard criteria, when initially presented in 1968, considered the presence of spinal deep tendon stretch reflexes to be inconsistent with the diagnosis of brain death[7]. However, in a prospective study of 63 patients with absent intracranial circulation on four-vessel angiography, Jörgensen[17] noted that in 50% of the patients, spinal deep tendon stretch reflexes were preserved. He observed that

Table 27.4. Minnesota Brain Death Criteria (1971)

1. No spontaneous movement
2. Apnea—disconnect from ventilator for 4 minutes
3. Absent brain stem reflexes
   Fixed, dilated pupils
   Corneal
   Ciliospinal
   Tonic neck
   Gag
   Oculocephalic
   Oculovestibular
4. 12-hour observation period

Prerequisite: Diagnosis of irreparable cerebral lesion
From: Mohandas A, Chou SN. Brain death: a clinical and pathological study. J Neurosurg 1971;35:211.

Table 27.5. Medical Consultants to the President's Commission—Brain Death Criteria (1982)

1. Absence of hypothermia, shock, and drug intoxication
2. Cerebral unresponsiveness
3. Apnea with PCO_2 over 60 mm Hg and O_2 insufflation
4. Absent brain stem reflexes
   Pupillary
   Corneal
   Oculovestibular
   Oculocephalic
   Oropharyngeal
5. Observation for 6 hours if corroborative testing is used
6. Observation for 12 hours if corroborative testing is not used
7. Corroborative tests: EEG, cerebral angiography, radionuclide flow study

Prerequisite: Diagnosis is established with no possibility of recovery.
From: Report of the Medical Consultants on the Diagnosis of Death to the President's Commission for the Study of Ethical Problems in Medicine and Biomedical and Behavioral Research. Guidelines for the determination of death. Crit Care Med 1982;10:62.

spinal reflexes were generally absent during periods of cardiovascular instability and during the first 24 hours after the CNS insult but frequently returned after restitution of a stable systemic circulation. Other prospective studies of comatose patients, including the National Collaborative Study[12], have found spinal reflexes frequently preserved in many brain dead patients, and contemporary criteria for brain death certification generally recognize this fact.

The pupillary findings characteristic of brain dead patients have been debated. Fixed, dilated pupils most frequently accompany brain death, but many contend that fixed midposition pupils are also consistent with the diagnosis if sedative drug intoxication is not present. Although drug intoxication can generally be excluded through a careful history and drug toxicology screen, dilated as well as fixed pupils are required by most major brain death criteria.

CORROBORATIVE TESTING

Perhaps the most controversial and variable aspect of brain death determination is the use of various corroborative studies to obtain "objective" verification of brain death. These studies fall into two groups: those that evaluate brain electrical activity and those that evaluate brain blood flow. Corroborative testing is most heavily employed when there is diagnostic uncertainty or the presence of confounding factors such as hypothermia or barbiturate administration[14,15,18,19]. Absent such considerations, there appears to be a recent trend toward greater reliance on clinical determination of brain death and less use of these corroborative tests.

Electroencephalography (EEG) was required by the Harvard criteria and subsequently recommended by the National Collaborative Study. An isoelectric EEG predicts nonsurvival in comatose patients with clinically absent brain stem function, as demonstrated in a multicenter study by Silverman et al.[20]. While EEG possesses the advantages of being a portable procedure easily and safely performed at the bedside, it has several limitations. EEG is susceptible to electrical artifact at the high sensitivity settings necessary to confirm electrocerebral silence, especially in the electrically hostile environment of a busy ICU; EEG brain activity has been seen shortly before death in patients who were found to have total brain autolysis on autopsy[21,22]. Another major shortcoming of the EEG is that it only reflects cortical (not brain stem) activity, and will be suppressed in many clinical settings besides brain death, such as circulatory shock, hypothermia, and particularly drug intoxication. It has been argued that small amounts of isolated electrical cortical activity in a patient with clinical brain stem death are meaningless[23]; indeed, Pallis[15] noted that none of the patients with brain stem death in his series, despite small amounts of electrical activity on EEG, showed clinical evidence of CNS function, and all had cardiac asystole within days despite maximal supportive care. Ashwal and Schneider[21] reported similar results in children. In addition, the EEG may not be reliable in very young and particularly premature infants, since there are reports of return of neuronal function and EEG activity after the demonstration of electrocerebral silence[23–26]. Despite these shortcomings, however, an isoelectric EEG in the absence of sedative drugs still represents hard evidence of absent cortical function (Fig. 27.1)[23,24,27,28]. It remains a useful confirmatory test for brain death[19,29].

Demonstration of absent intracranial circulation has been thought by many to be the best confirmation of brain death[30,31], since absent cerebral blood flow is incompatible with neuronal survival because of inadequate cellular substrate provision. Two different mechanisms have been hypothesized to be responsible for this absence of perfusion in the setting of brain death. Massive cerebral edema, with a concomitant rise in intracranial pressure to levels greater than mean arterial pressure, prevents arterial flow. Alternatively, it has been speculated that progressive cerebral vascular endothelial swelling occurs with cerebral death, resulting in an absence of flow. Angiographically, one of two different patterns may be seen: total absence of intracranial circulation or the cessation of circulation at the level of the circle of Willis. Currently, cerebral angiography is not widely used to confirm brain death because of its inconvenience (requiring transport to the radiology suite) and the invasive nature of the examination. Radionuclide flow studies with intravenous 99Tc have been used during the past decade to assess intracranial blood flow (Figs. 27.2 and 27.3). This scanning technique offers advantages over four-vessel angiography in that it is relatively noninvasive and technically easier and can often be done in the ICU using a portable scanner. Several studies have correlated absent flow on these scans with brain death as diagnosed by clinical examination and EEG in both adults and children[21,32–34]. Additionally, Schwartz et al.[35,36] correlated absent flow on these brain scans with absent cerebral flow on four-vessel cerebral angiography. Two distinct imaging patterns have been recognized in brain dead patients. Most patients show no evidence of cerebral blood flow; others demonstrate late filling of the sagittal sinus only, which is thought to represent venous drainage of extradural perforating arteries. Radionuclide flow studies appear to have limitations, at least in infants; however, Ashwal[26] and Ashwal et al.[37] reported a number of babies clinically brain dead who had persistent cerebral blood flow identified, and Toffol et al.[38] reported persistent cerebral perfusion on radionuclide scan in a 3-year-old child who was clinically

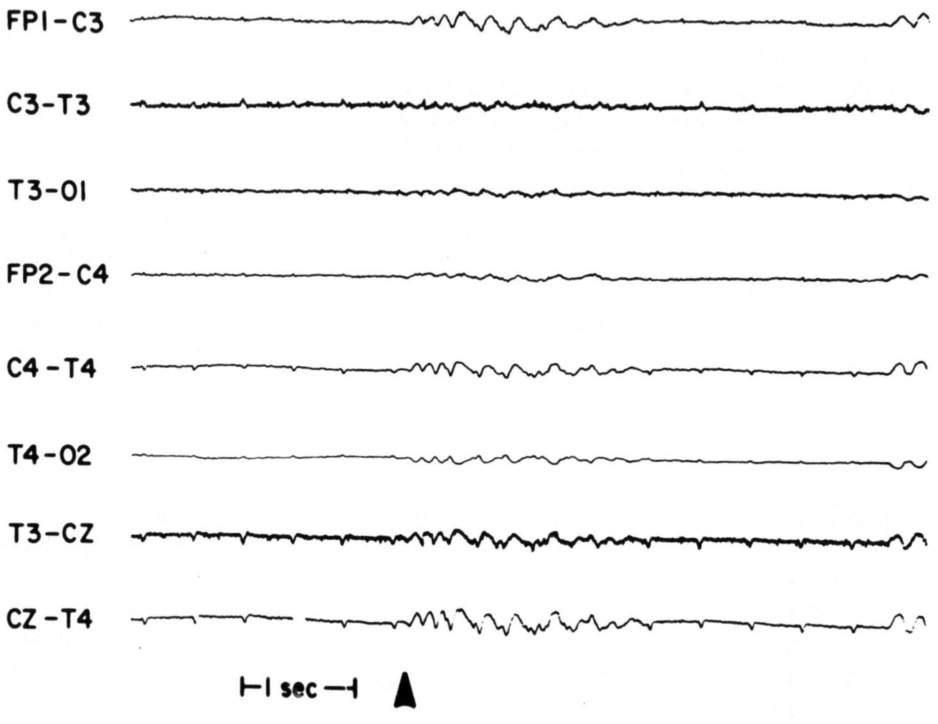

Figure 27.1. Isoelectric EEG obtained from 9-year-old girl who was brain dead. Solid arrowhead indicates artifact produced by mechanical ventilator. (From Setzer N. Brain death: physiologic definitions. Crit Care Clin 1985;1:375.)

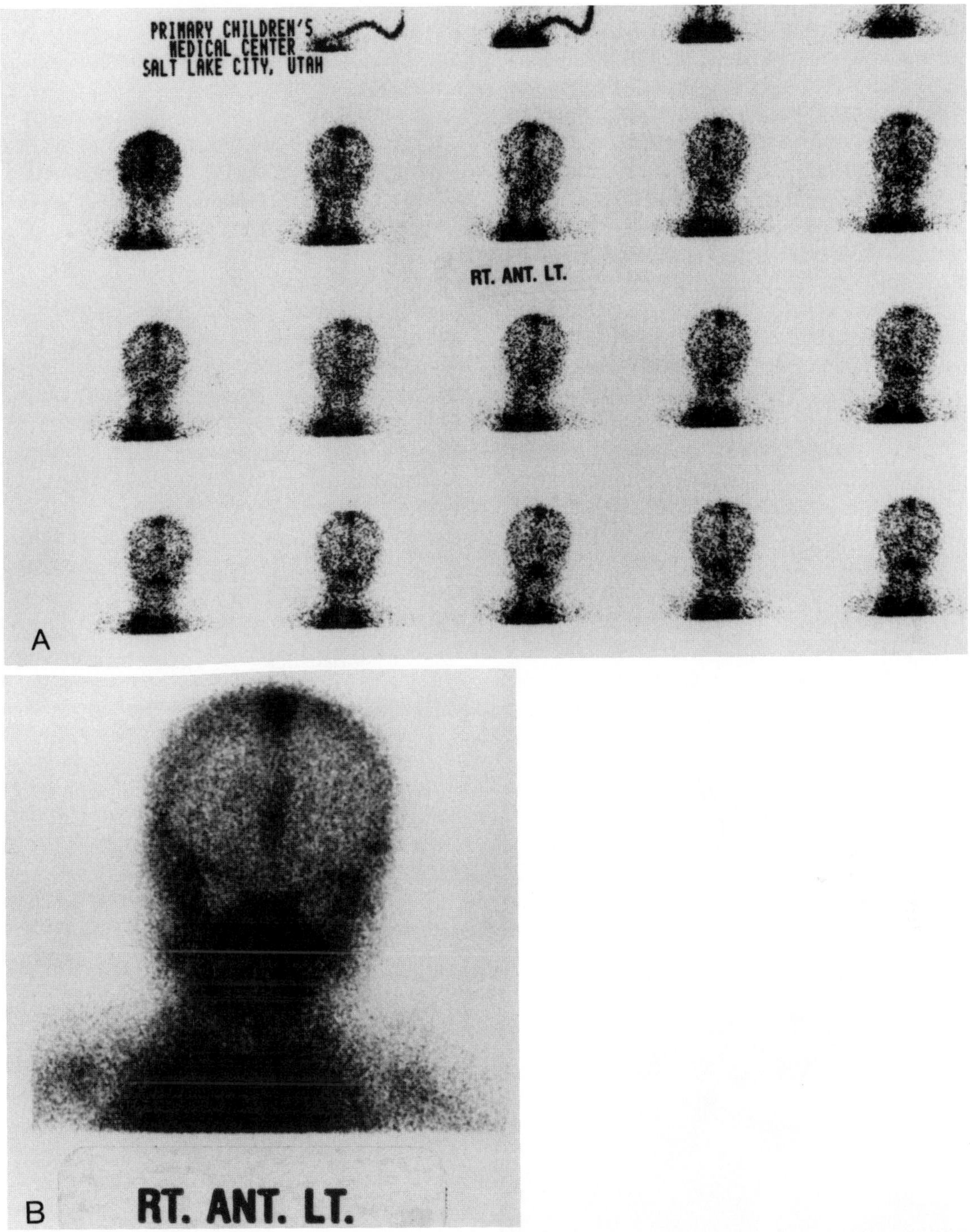

Figure 27.2. A. Dynamic 99Tc scan showing normal cerebral blood flow. Dynamic images were taken at 2-second intervals immediately after radionuclide injection. B. Static 99Tc scan showing normal cerebral blood flow. Image was taken 5 minutes after radionuclide injection.

brain dead and had repeated isoelectric EEG tracings. Conversely, it has been suggested that values of cerebral blood flow too low to be detected by radionuclide flow studies are possibly consistent with neuronal survival in young infants[39].

In addition to EEG, cerebral angiography, and radionuclide flow studies, a number of other corroborative studies for brain death have been described, although none has achieved widespread use. Examination of carotid blood flow by transcranial Doppler studies is a simple measurement which has been used to evaluate cerebral flow at the bedside in the ICU; in brain death, there is no detectable flow in the middle cerebral artery[40,41]. Cerebral blood flow assessment by contrast computerized axial tomography or xenon computed tomography have also been advocated[37,42,43], although these methods offer little practical advantage over radionuclide imaging, because patient transport from the ICU to the radiology suite is still required. Echoencephalography detects anterior and middle cerebral artery pulsations in infants with open fontanels,

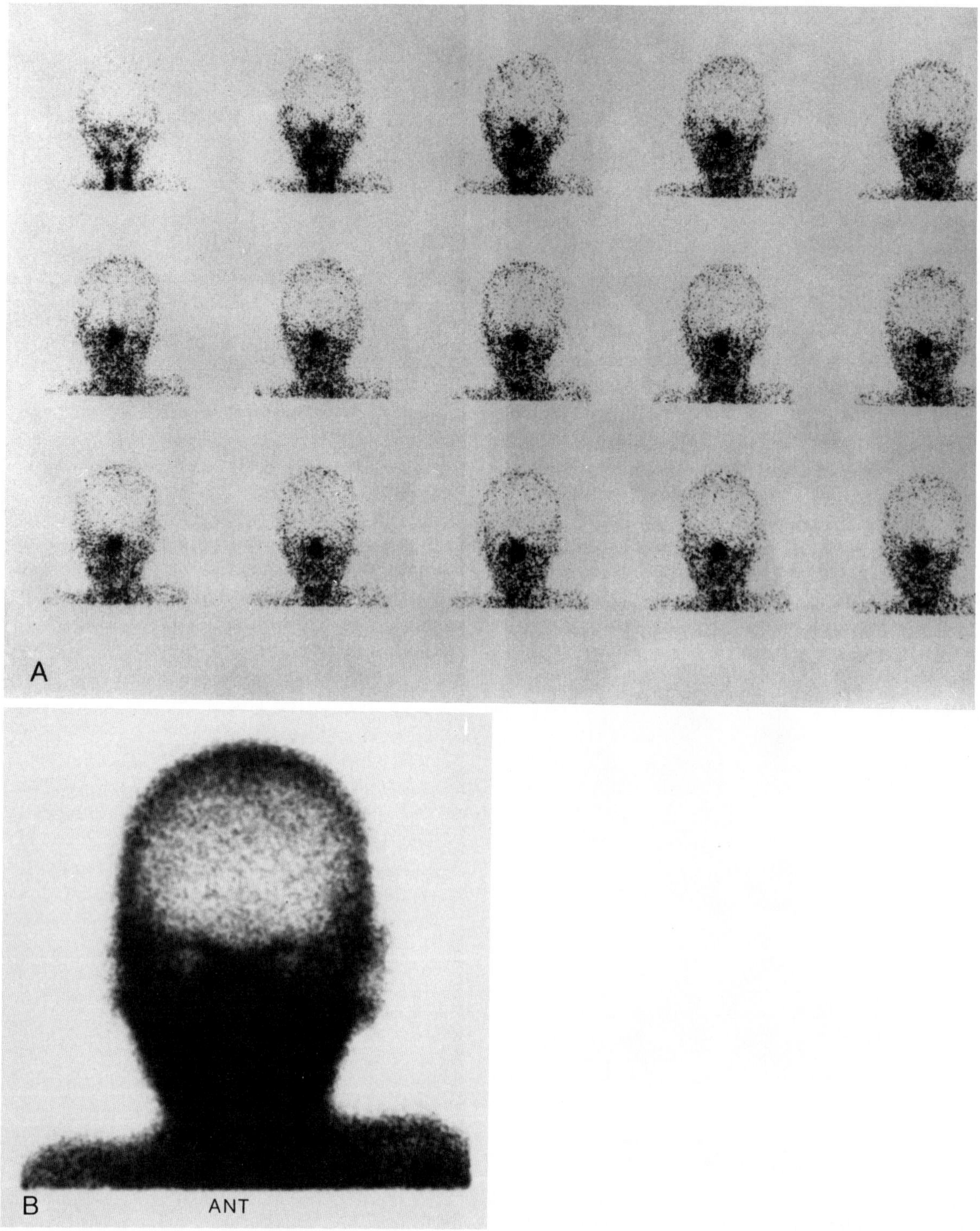

Figure 27.3. A. Dynamic 99Tc scan showing complete absence of cerebral blood flow. Dynamic images were taken at 2-second intervals immediately after radionuclide injection. B. Static 99Tc scan showing complete absence of cerebral blood flow. Image was taken 5 minutes after radionuclide injection.

evaluating cortical (but not brain stem) blood flow in a limited fashion[44]. In the study of Furgiuele et al.[45], describing over 800 children, 11 of 12 with absent pulsations met conventional brain death criteria. Similarly, absence of anterior cerebral artery flow on serial Doppler ultrasonography studies through the anterior fontanel has also been described in brain dead infants, but as with radionuclide flow studies, occasionally persistent flow has been seen in infants who are clinically brain dead[46,47].

Magnetic resonance imaging after gadopentetate dimeglumine contrast injection has also been used to evaluate intracranial anatomical and flow derangements in the setting of brain death. Characteristic findings include carotid artery enhancement, indicative of cerebral infarction, and enhanced uptake in the nose and scalp (the so-called "hot nose sign"), reflecting enhanced flow to these areas(48). It has been stated that intracranial pressure greater than mean arterial pressure (cerebral perfusion pressure less than zero) is presumptive evidence of absent cerebral perfusion(3). However, periods of intracranial pressure greater than arterial pressure as long as 1 hour have been reported in patients who went on to survive, apparently in at least one case with only minor neurologic deficits(49), although this finding may largely reflect technical difficulties with the measurement of intracranial pressure.

Experimentally, multimodality evoked potential studies have been evaluated in several clinical studies in both adults and children as a possible corroborative test to confirm brain death(50–53). Evoked potentials measure cerebral electrical responses to a given clinical stimulus, such as an auditory click, an electrical shock, or a visual pattern. These electrical responses differ from ordinary EEG activity in that the evoked potential waves are of extremely small microvoltage, ordinarily hidden among normal cerebral electrical activity, and are only detected by repetitive stimulation and measurements which are computer recorded, summed, and averaged to produce the final wave pattern. Unlike routine EEG analysis, evoked potentials are not suppressed by sedative anesthetic drugs, including barbiturates, but can only measure activity along specific anatomical pathways and do not represent global cortical or brain stem activity. The three different types of clinically utilized sensory evoked responses (brain stem auditory (BAERs), somatosensory, and visual) measure function across different pathways; all of these evoked potentials have been evaluated in the clinical setting of brain death. BAERs obtained by using a click stimulus show only a wave I (indicating auditory nerve activity) or no waves at all in brain dead individuals (Fig. 27.4A)(54,55). Caution must be applied in interpreting these, however, because a totally flat response may also be seen in a patient with auditory nerve failure (as occurs with certain types of deafness and middle ear trauma or fluid). In addition, brain stem responses have (rarely) been detected with BAER testing in patients who are clinically brain dead, suggesting that either the test is flawed or that some brain stem function may persist, at least for a time, in patients who lack clinical signs of brain stem function(56). Conversely, a loss of auditory evoked potentials has been reported in a man who continued to breathe, indicating the presence of clinical brain stem function(57) in areas of the brain stem remote from the pathway measured by the BAER. BAER testing is, therefore, merely confirmatory of absent brain stem function and not, by itself, diagnostic of brain death.

Somatosensory evoked potentials show no cortical waves (after peripheral nerve electrical stimulus) in patients who are brain dead. The majority of those studied, however, have a single negative deflection detectable over the upper cervical brain with a mean latency of 14–15 msec. The origin of this wave has been widely debated; currently, it is thought to arise from the lower medulla or cervical cord near the cervicomedullary junction (Fig. 27.4B). Also, absent corti-

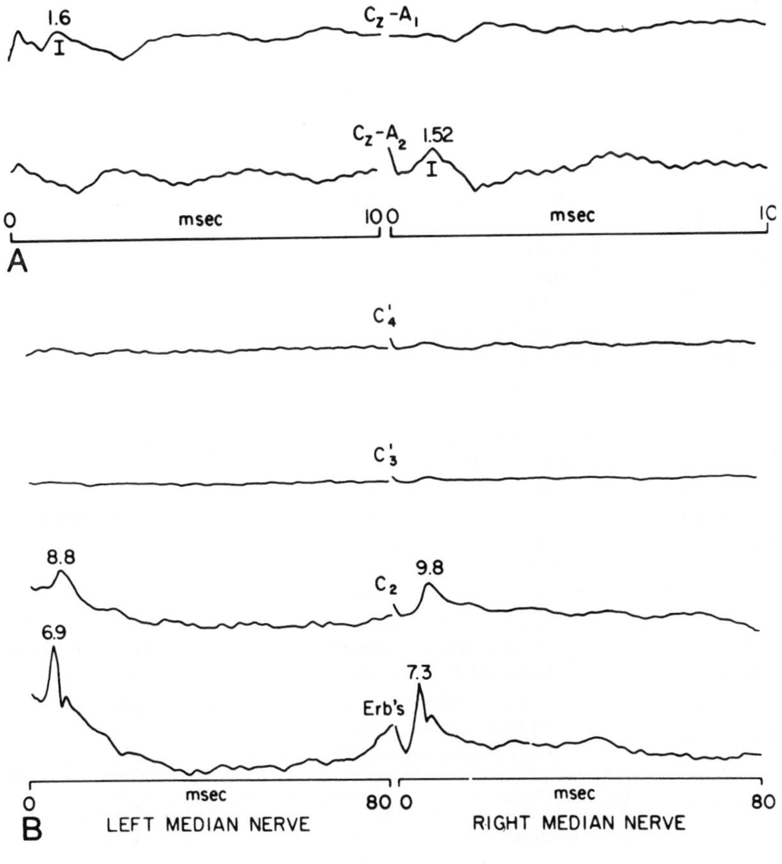

Figure 27.4. A. Brain stem auditory evoked potential tracing obtained in a 2-year-old boy who was brain dead. Note the preservation of wave I only, indicating peripheral auditory nerve activity. B. Short-latency somatosensory evoked potential after median nerve stimulation in a 2-year-old child with brain death diagnosed. Electrical activity is recorded over Erb's point (brachial plexus and C2 (cervicomedullary junction). This latter wave has been identified in the majority of brain-dead adults; here the latency is shorter because of the shorter nerve length in children. There is no cortical activity recorded (C3', C4'). (From Setzer N. Brain death: physiologic definitions. Crit Care Clin 1985;1:375.)

cal waves may be seen after severe cerebral trauma and are not specific indicators of brain death. Visual evoked potentials measure cortical responses to flashing light stimuli; they are uniformly flat in brain dead patients. Flat responses are not specific for brain death, however, in that interruption anywhere from the retina, the optic nerve, or the optic radiation pathways may produce a similar pattern. Currently, evoked potentials are infrequently used as corroborative evidence of brain death, although they are useful in detection of CNS failure during therapeutic drug coma.

From the discussion, it should be clear that no corroborative test is foolproof and that both false-positives and false-negatives may occur. Indeed, Fackler and Rogers[(58)] described a clinically brain dead child who had small amounts of both EEG activity and cerebral blood flow by angiography (although not on radionuclide scan). Rigid insistence that certain corroborative tests be performed to "prove" brain death in every case will inevitably lead to confusion and anguish, especially for the families of patients.

PATHOLOGIC CORRELATES

The diagnosis of brain death, from its conceptual inception by the Ad Hoc Committee of the Harvard Medical School until today, has been functionally rather than anatomically or pathologically defined. Some investigators have attempted to derive a pathologic definition of brain death based on the correlation of clinical examination with autopsy findings, albeit without notable success. Overall, no specific pathologic characterization has been found except at the extreme of brain liquefaction necrosis, the so-called respirator brain. This brain autolysis was present on autopsy in only 40% of comatose apneic patients who died; the rest exhibited a wide constellation of pathologic findings. The characteristic changes seen in patients with respirator brain were detailed after a multicenter survey of neuropathologists by Walker et al. in 1975[(59)]. These changes included cortical congestion with swelling, softening, cerebellar fragmentation, and pituitary infarction. Microscopically, vascular congestion was noted with a generalized lack of inflammatory response. Here, it was noted that these gross structural and microscopic changes were seen predominantly in those brain dead patients who had received ventilator support for more than 12 hours. Ironically, in a few patients with complete liquefaction necrosis, EEG activity has been recorded just a few hours before cardiac arrest, casting further doubt on the validity of the EEG in diagnosing brain death. Also, areas of architecturally normal cells are sometimes seen in the brain on microscopic examination of brain dead patients. Autopsy studies done on brain dead patients supported for more than 4 days after the onset of coma have shown evidence of an intracranial meningoencephalitic reaction, possibly indicating partial resumption of brain perfusion after resolution of intracranial hypertension[(60)].

BRAIN DEATH CRITERIA FOR CHILDREN

Initial brain death criteria did not specifically address determination of brain death for infants and children. With some exceptions[(61)], most suggested a cautious approach to the diagnosis of brain death in children, reflecting a belief that brain death in children was "different" or more difficult to diagnose, or the (poorly supported) hypothesis that the brains of infants and children are more resistant to hypoxic damage than are those of adults[(39)]. The Report of the President's Commission reflected this attitude, stating that "physicians should be particularly cautious in applying neurologic criteria to determine death in children younger than 5 years"[(8)], and Masland et al.[(62)] stated that studies of brain dead individuals "cannot be applied to infants and young children." In an attempt to clarify the issue, the Task Force on Brain Death in Children was organized and in 1987 proffered its *Guidelines for the Determination of Brain Death in Children,* published simultaneously in four major medical journals[(63,64)] **(Table 27.6).** These guidelines differ from criteria used for adults in several important areas. First, they specify that, at least for perinatal insults, 7 days must pass before neurologic assessment is valid, meaning that brain death cannot be di-

Table 27.6. Guidelines for the Determination of Brain Death in Children—Report of the Task Force for the Determination of Brain Death in Children

1. Coma and apnea must coexist
2. Absence of brain stem function:
   - Pupils unreactive to light (midposition or dilated)
   - Absence of eye movement spontaneously and in response to oculocephalic and oculovestibular (caloric) testing
   - Absence of corneal, gag, cough, sucking, and rooting reflexes, as well as of spontaneous movement of bulbar musculature
   - Absence of spontaneous respiratory effort
3. Normal blood pressure and temperature
4. Flaccid muscle tone, absence of spontaneous movements (spinal reflexes acceptable)
5. Examination consistent with brain death throughout the period of testing and observation; observation periods and testing are specific for age groups
6. Observation and testing according to age:
   - Age 7 days to 2 months:
     - Two examinations and EEGs separated by 48 hours
   - Age 2 months to 1 year:
     - Two examinations and EEGs separated by 24 hours, except that repeat examination and EEG are not necessary if radionuclide brain blood flow study demonstrates absence of cerebral perfusion
   - Older than 1 year:
     - Corroborative testing not required if an irreversible cause is identified. An observation period of 12 hours is recommended, except that when assessment of extent and irreversibility of brain damage is difficult, specifically after hypoxic-ischemic insults, an observation period of at least 24 hours is recommended (may be shortened by use of EEG or radionuclide flow study).

From: Report of special task force. Guidelines for the determination of brain death in children. American Academy of Pediatrics Task Force on Brain Death in Children. Pediatrics 1987;80:298.

agnosed in infants younger than 7 days. Second, different criteria are specified for children of different ages. Third, at least for infants, a longer period of observation (48 hours) is specified than in other criteria. Fourth, a specific test (the EEG) is specified as a requirement for the declaration of brain death, at least in the younger age groups. Interestingly, these criteria completely avoid the issue of the declaration of brain death in premature infants. They also have been criticized for making little use of tests for brain blood flow, which are "optional"[(65)], and it has been questioned whether the prolonged periods of observation suggested for the youngest infants are appropriate[(66)]. Although the intent of the task force was presumably to clarify the issue of brain death for children, they do not appear to have achieved this goal[(67)]; the American Academy of Pediatrics, one of the sponsoring bodies of the task force, specifically stated that their official position is not represented by these guidelines[(68)]. However, these criteria are associated with several respected academic bodies and, as such, may well become accepted as standard guidelines despite the lack of evidence or consensus that they are superior to other brain death criteria. Interestingly, at least two other proposed brain death criteria sets for children appeared in the literature at roughly the same time as these guidelines[(43,69)], differing from them in several respects, such as specifying shorter observation periods, placing less reliance on the EEG, and making less of age-related differences.

The need for special pediatric brain death criteria has been questioned; Alvarez et al.[(24)] retrospectively reviewed 52 brain dead children younger than 5 years of age and noted that criteria similar to those used for adults (clinical brain death persistent for 24 hours and one flat EEG) would have adequately identified those older than 3 months. However, newborn and, especially, premature infants do appear to present special problems. Ashwal[(26)] and Ashwal and Schneider[(43)] proposed that clinical determination of brain death, i.e., as determined by the clinical history and the physical examination, can reasonably diagnose brain death in the newborn, with the proviso that observation periods of at least 2 days (for term infants) and 3 days (for preterm infants) are necessary.

Several studies have examined the validity and applicability of brain death criteria in children; a few children have been included along with adults in most of the large prospective studies of brain death criteria. Rowland et al.[(70)] retrospectively evaluated children who had absent cortical and brain stem function and an isoelectric EEG, finding that all eventually developed cardiovascular collapse despite aggressive support. Unfortunately, validation of brain death for children may not be as clear-cut as it appears to be for adults. For instance, Kohrman and Spivack[(25)] reported a 3-month-old girl who appeared clinically brain dead and had two isoelectric EEGs but who subsequently regained some cortical and brain stem function and survived on the ventilator for more than a month before dying. Additionally, case reports of prolonged somatic "survival" of brain dead children, in one case for 6 months[(70,71)], have called into question the premise of rapid inevitable, unsupportable cardiovascular collapse in brain dead patients.

DECLARATION OF BRAIN DEATH

Brain death can be established only after continuous observation of a comatose patient in a stable environment. Brain death is not properly diagnosed in the emergency department, where the patient may receive care from several physicians and undergo initial stabilization and a variety of diagnostic studies. The possibility of brain death in an unconscious child should be considered only after admission to the ICU, where evaluation can proceed in an orderly fashion. As prerequisites, the cause of coma should be known, and the lesion should be deemed irreversible[(39)]. This may easily be established in some situations, such as after catastrophic CNS trauma, but is less obvious under others, as, for example, in the patient with hypoxic or metabolic encephalopathy, or after procedures such as extracorporeal membrane oxygenation or open heart surgery with cardiopulmonary bypass[(72,73)]. Additionally, the patient's medical history should be known, and the presence of coexisting disease that might complicate neurologic evaluation should be recognized. Labyrinthine disease, for example, may cause inaccurate findings on oculovestibular testing, and clinical features mimicking those of brain death have been described both in Guillain Barré syndrome[(74)] and Miller Fisher syndrome (brain stem encephalitis)[(75)]. If unresolved questions exist regarding the circumstances under which the injury occurred, the possibility of child abuse should be considered and reported to the appropriate authorities at the time of admission.

The child should be hemodynamically stable throughout the period of observation. In adults, Jörgensen and Moller[(76)] found that CNS function ceases during cardiac arrest; they noted, however, that some return of neurologic function occurred within 15 minutes of restoration of stable blood pressure. Respiratory effort was generally the first manifestation of activity, followed by the return of other brain stem functions, over a period of hours. Neurologic testing and physical examination are performed when the patient is normothermic (core temperature at least 35°C) and hemodynamically stable in the absence of neuromuscular blockade or sedation. If the child has received muscle relaxants, residual blockade can be assessed using a peripheral nerve stimulator. Nondepolarizing agents may be reversible by cholinesterase inhibitors such as edrophonium or neostigmine; these agents should be administered with a vagolytic agent such as atropine or glycopyrrolate to prevent severe bradycardia. Note that occasionally neuromuscular blockade may persist for days in patients who have received nondepolarizing agents for a prolonged period. Prolonged, irreversible neuromuscular blockade occurs after succinylcholine administration in patients with pseudocholinesterase deficiency, possibly creating a clinical state mimicking brain death[(77)]; again, the correct diagnosis can be made with the demonstration of peripheral nerve blockade.

On physical examination, the brain dead child should have no spontaneous movements; there should be no purposeful or posturing response to noxious stimuli. Cranial nerve and brain stem function are evaluated by appropriate cephalic reflex testing: (a) Pupils should be fixed and dilated, with no response to light. Pupillary constriction, as part of a ciliospinal reflex, should be absent. (b) Cerebral reflexes, including decorticate and decerebrate posturing, should be absent, and there should be no eye movement with oculocephalic (doll's eyes) or oculovestibular (cold caloric) testing. (c) There should be no pharyngeal reflexes or gag present and no cough response to tracheal suctioning.

Apnea testing is carried out after preoxygenation with 100% oxygen. Then, mechanical ventilation is discontinued, and oxygen is passively insufflated through the endotracheal tube[(78)]. The patient is then observed for any respiratory activity for at least 5 minutes. During apnea, $PaCO_2$ rises by approximately 3–4 torr/min (may be slightly less in a brain dead patient because cerebral metabolism has ceased). If one ensures that the initial $PaCO_2$ is at least 40 torr[(78,79)], then 5 minutes of apnea should yield a $PaCO_2$ of roughly 60 torr, which should elicit at least some ventilatory effort in any patient who is not brain dead, including those with chronic obstructive pulmonary disease and abnormal chemoreceptor function[(17)]. Passive oxygen insufflation is necessary during testing to prevent hypoxemia, and ongoing monitoring of oxygenation should be done. Previously described methods for determining apnea, including the insufflation of 5% carbon dioxide or administration of hypoxic gas mixtures, are no longer recommended[(80,81)]. Hemodynamic changes frequently occur during apnea testing. Jeret and Benjamin noted hypotension in 39% of 61 comatose individuals during testing, despite normoxia[(82)].

As previously mentioned, Jörgensen noted that spinal stretch and deep tendon reflexes are found on physical examination in at least 50% of brain dead patients[(17)]. He also described two specific spinal reflexes that are seemingly present only in brain dead patients. The first, an ipsilateral flexion withdrawal after noxious stimulation in the L3–L4 dermatome, was elicited in 79% of brain dead patients. Additionally, 33% exhibited an ipsilateral extension-pronation response after arm or upper chest stimulation[(76)]. This latter response superficially resembles decerebrate posturing; however, movement occurs only ipsilaterally. Occasionally, stereotyped movements of the extremities and extensor posturing can be seen in patients who are clearly brain dead; these have been termed the *Lazarus sign*[(80)].

Once it is demonstrated that the clinical examination is consistent with brain death, then irreversibility must be demonstrated by the persistence of these findings over a period of observation. Unfortunately, there is no consensus on how long such a period must be, with intervals of 6–48 hours being suggested. Finally, many centers in the United States require some sort of corroborative test of brain death, most commonly by EEG or radionuclide cerebral blood flow study, although the reliance on such testing may be diminishing somewhat.

Several other findings are characteristic of brain death, although they are not part of the usual diagnostic criteria. Diabetes insipidus is common although not universal[(83)], and all patients require passive warming to maintain body temperature[(17,66)]. A slowing of metabolism manifested by low CO_2 production and low glucose requirement has also been described[(84)]. Although intracranial blood flow is usually absent in brain dead patients, carotid pulses are present because of the preservation of blood flow through the external carotid system. Hemodynamically, there should be no cardiac accelerator response to atropine in brain dead patients and no bradycardia with vagal maneuvers. Recently, computerized analysis of EEG tracings in brain dead children have shown diminished beat-to-beat heart rate variability compared with the rate variability in normal children[(85)]. A hypertensive response to incision in brain dead organ donors in the absence of pressor or volume administration has been described, associated with an outpouring of both epinephrine and norepinephrine after incision and increase in systemic vascular resistance (Fig. 27.5)[(86–88)]. This response is believed to be mediated at the spinal cord level and has been demonstrated in decapitated animals. Conversely, the cold pressor response to dipping the hand in ice water, which is a central brain stem cardiovascular response, is absent in brain dead children but not in children with coma[(89)].

Therapeutic barbiturate coma (pentobarbital is most commonly used) is often employed for control of intractable intracranial hypertension. Pentobarbital blood concentrations greater than 20–30 g/dl, however, will suppress neurologic function and negate the clinical examination. Barbiturate-induced suppression of electrical activity (electrical silence on EEG is possible and has been described as the therapeutic goal) eliminates the ability of the EEG to evaluate cortical activity. Although brain stem evoked potentials are little affected by barbiturates, it must be remembered that flat responses are not diagnostic of brain death. Currently, brain death can be diagnosed during barbiturate

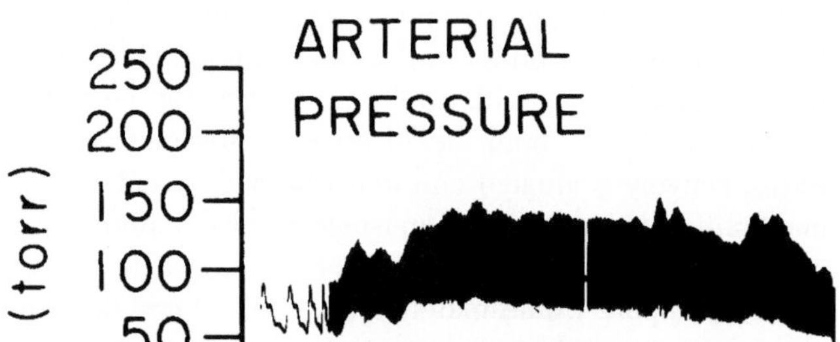

Figure 27.5. Hemodynamic tracing obtained in 30-year-old brain-dead organ donor after incision. Small open triangles indicate time in minutes. (From Wetzel RC, Setzer N, Stiff JL, Rogers MC. Hemodynamic responses on brain dead organ donor patients. Anesth Analg 1985; 64:125.)

coma only with the demonstration of absent intracranial circulation[90].

There are many potential areas of controversy regarding the concept of brain death as currently defined. As previously stated, brain death is not necessarily characterized by destruction of all intracranial neurons, and certain neurologic functions that are not routinely tested may be present in patients considered brain dead by contemporary standards. For example, human growth hormone (hGH), thyroid stimulating hormone (TSH) and ACTH are measurable in brain dead patients, including some with absent flow on cerebral angiography, indicating at least some preservation of neuroendocrine function[91,92]. Additionally, Fiser et al.[83] noted that only 38% of brain dead children exhibit diabetes insipidus. These observations correlate with autopsy studies in which islands of architecturally normal, potentially viable cells are seen microscopically in many patients with brain death. Similarly, cortical evoked potential studies have demonstrated the presence of a single central wave with a mean latency of 14–15 msec recorded over the upper cervical vertebrae in the majority of brain dead patients. The electrophysiologic origin of this wave remains uncertain, but it is most likely in the lower medulla in the dorsal column nuclei[51].

BRAIN DEATH AND THE LAW

Brain death is an accepted legal concept in the United States, and beginning with Kansas in 1970, most states have passed laws dealing with this issue[3,90]. The general message of these statutes is the same: brain death is synonymous with death of the person. Furthermore, these laws identify brain death in functional terms (irreversible cessation of function of the entire brain) and do not require that anatomic destruction of the brain be demonstrated[61]. These laws have not, by and large, defined the medical criteria by which brain death is determined, nor have they required that specific tests be performed, allowing for changing medical practice as medical expertise within this area grows. Instead, brain death laws generally specify that brain death has occurred when a physician or physicians have determined that irreversible cessation of function of the entire brain has occurred. Indeed, the variation between brain death laws among states, or even the lack of such laws in a few states, appears to have had little impact on the approach to the diagnosis of brain death across the United States. The selection of criteria by which brain death is declared has thus been left to the individual governing boards of the hospitals within the state. An example of these rules and regulations are the criteria used at Johns Hopkins Hospital **(Table 27.7).**

Table 27.7. The Johns Hopkins Hospital Criteria for Brain Death (1984)

1. Absence of hypothermia or cardiovascular shock
2. Observation for 6 hours by an attending or chief resident in neurology or neurosurgery plus the primary attending physician
3. Clinical criteria:
   Fixed, dilated pupils
   Absent oculovestibular response to 100 ml of instilled ice water
   Absent corneal reflex
   Apnea—with $PaCO_2$ greater than 60 mm Hg
   No behavioral or reflex response to stimuli that imply function above the level of the foramen magnum
   Isoelectric EEG
4. Special considerations:
   Absent cerebral blood flow as measured by bilateral carotid and arch arteriography precludes functioning of the brain and will be required in the presence of therapeutic drug intoxication.

Prerequisite: Known and untreatable structural damage to the brain or irreversible systemic metabolic derangement.
From: Medical staff policies and procedures. Baltimore: The Johns Hopkins Hospital, 1984:41.

INTERNATIONAL AND RELIGIOUS VIEWS OF BRAIN DEATH

Although the United States and most of Europe have adopted and employed the brain death concept over the last three decades, other countries, most notably Japan, have been more reluctant to accept brain death as being equivalent to death of the individual[4,93,94]. In Japan, this has been attributed to several factors, including perhaps a public mistrust of the medical profession[5], ambivalence as to when the spirit vacates the body during death, and respect by the family for the corporal remains of an individual after death. In 1985, the Japanese Ministry of Health and Welfare issued criteria for the determination of brain death[95,96] similar to those of other countries, and some transplant surgery has been undertaken. Kawashima et al.[97] reported that while a majority of Japanese considered brain death synonymous with death of the individual after experiencing brain death in a family member, only one-third had held this opinion previously. Several families in this study consented to organ donation after being approached by the physician. A major issue for those refusing transplantation was the possibility of injury to the deceased person during the procedure[97]. In the Middle East, there was a previous misconception that brain death and organ donation were not permitted under Islamic law[98]. During the past decade, Saudi Arabia, Tunisia, and Turkey have enacted laws recognizing brain death and allowing heart-beating organ donation[99–101].

BRAIN DEATH AND ORGAN DONATION: MAINTENANCE OF ORGAN DONORS

The supply of pediatric donor organs remains critically short despite an apparent societal acceptance of this concept, and in the United States there are approximately 23,000 people awaiting major organ transplantation[102]. At the same time, there are an estimated 7000–10,000 brain dead individuals, of which only 4000 become organ donors[103], indicating a need to increase efficiency in obtaining consent to donate. Several countries have taken steps to surmount this difficulty. Austria has enacted legislation providing that consent for donation is presumed unless individuals have signed cards to the contrary ("opting out")[104]. This has tripled the size of the donor pool from 10 to 32 per million persons, thus decreasing waiting time for transplant. The United States has, by way of contrast, 17 donors per million inhabitants. In Turkey, surgeons are even allowed to removed organs from brain dead individuals in whom next of kin cannot be located[100]. In Paris, a unit dedicated to the care of brain dead organ donor cadavers has been established, which provides medical care of the donor, verifies brain death, completes legal proceedings, and accomplishes organ harvesting in preparation for transplantation[105].

Consent for organ donation may be more readily obtained for the pediatric age group than for adults. Morris et al., in a series of 18 brain dead children, found that consent for organ donation was obtained from all families, and they attributed this high rate to the empathy that families of brain dead children may have with other families who are awaiting organs for their chronically ill children[106]. Organ donation has also been cited as a factor that helps parents and families with the grieving process[107].

Physicians intending to support pediatric organ donors should be prepared to treat the characteristic physiologic problems, including coexisting metabolic derangements, hemodynamic disturbances, and endocrine abnormalities, for the several hours required to mobilize the surgical team and locate potential transplant recipients[108]. An evaluation of 114 adult solid-organ donors found that 18% of the organs were obtained within 3 hours of brain death; 53% were procured within 3–7 hours, and 21% were procured 7–11 hours after determination of brain death[109]. The mean donor maintenance time for pediatric patients is 10.5 ± 6.7 hours[108]. Organ donation should be considered even when high levels of support are necessary for adequate blood pressure and perfusion, since it appears that such care can maintain donor organs in good condition for transplantation[110].

Intensive nursing care is required for the maintenance period, and facilities should have the personnel needed to provide a 1:1 or 2:1 bedside nurse-patient ratio[108]. During this time general care such as turning to avoid decubitus ulcers and maintenance of sterility for invasive procedures is necessary to decrease the risk of infection. The eyes should be protected with lubrication, airway frequently suctioned, and nasogastric tube placed on intermittent suction to prevent aspiration of gastric contents. A Foley catheter should be placed to accurately measure urine output. A temperature probe is necessary as temperature instability is a frequent finding in the brain dead patient. Serum electrolytes, glucose level, hematocrit, and arterial blood gases are monitored.

Hemodynamic instability is the most common physiologic derangement noted in pediatric organ donors, due to loss of central neurohumoral regulatory control of vasomotor tone, as well as intravascular volume abnormalities (perhaps related to diabetes insipidus) and myocardial dysfunction related to the original insult. Since the most important determinant of organ viability is the maintenance of an adequate systemic perfusion pressure, constant attention to hemodynamic status is essential to preserve donor organ function. Kidneys are especially sensitive to low perfusion, and adult studies have demonstrated an increased incidence of acute tubular necrosis and allograft failure when the donor systolic blood pressure is less than 80–90 mm Hg[111]. Because of the high likelihood of hemodynamic instability, invasive monitoring using central venous and arterial catheters is necessary for ongoing assessment, and Swan-Ganz catheters may sometimes be helpful[112]. Suggested therapeutic goals include systolic blood pressure of 70–80 mm Hg for patients younger than 6 years, with adolescent parameters similar to those of adult normals.

Volume status may be difficult to assess because of ongoing volume depletion and loss of vascular tone. It is not uncommon to find a donor on more than 10 μg of dopamine per kilogram per minute only to discover, after sternotomy, that the right atrium and ventricle are collapsed and the intravascular volume is low[113]. Initial management should include intravascular volume repletion with isotonic crystalloid or colloid solutions[114,115] and monitoring of central venous pressure.

Myocardial dysfunction is not rare in the pediatric organ donor and may result from the initial insult; for instance, anoxic cardiomyopathy may be present in a patient whose brain injury results from drowning or other asphyxial injury. Pathophysiologically, the cardiac deterioration which follows brain death has been partially verified in a pig model, in which it was demonstrated that β-adrenergic receptor density decreases and contractility deteriorates within 6 hours of brain death[114,116]. Interestingly, this decreased β-adrenergic receptor density was not demonstrated in infant piglets.

Catecholamine administration is occasionally necessary to maintain organ perfusion in the organ donor, although adequate intravascular volume must be assured first[113]. The β- and α-adrenergic effects and the potential for maintaining renal and mesenteric blood flow make dopamine a reasonable first choice. Early cardiac allograft survival does not seem affected by dopamine infusions of 10 μg/kg/min[113]. However, doses greater than this may reduce renal allograft survival by increasing the risk of acute tubular necrosis[117]. Vasoconstriction may compromise organ perfusion, so a vasopressor with significant α-adrenergic effects, such as epinephrine and norepinephrine, should be used with caution[117–119]. If additional inotropic treatment is necessary, dobutamine is preferred to isoproterenol because of isoproterenol's potential to increased myocardial oxygen demand[120].

The incidence of bradycardia and asystole is higher in the pediatric than adult population[108]. Significant dysrhythmia affecting blood pressure requires treatment. Transient bradyarrhythmias may be seen in the early phase of brain herniation, but atropine sulfate has no chronotropic effect on the brain dead patient[120]. If donation for heart transplantation is considered, an electrocardiogram, an echocardiogram, and cardiac isoenzymes may be evaluated to assess function. Hemodynamic support with catecholamines does not limit the viability of the organ for transplantation.

In the early phase of brain herniation, centrally mediated hypertension may be apparent, which is occasionally associated with histologic evidence of microinfarcts in the heart[120]. Adrenergic blocking agents are effective in controlling centrally mediated hypertension and tachycardia. Esmolol hydrochloride or labetalol hydrochloride may be used; both are short acting and can be administered by an easily titrated continuous infusion[115].

Pulmonary insufficiency may occur because of lung trauma, aspiration, or neurogenic pulmonary edema. Minute ventilation needs may be minimal in the brain dead patient because carbon dioxide production is low secondary to lowered brain metabolism, hypothermia, and decreased muscle tone; glucose metabolism and oxygen consumption are also reduced[84]. The goal of pulmonary support is maintenance of normocarbia and end-organ oxygen supply, achieved in the standard fashion with positive-end expiratory pressure and supplemental oxygen. Hemoglobin oxygen saturation should be maintained above 95% if possible. If high positive-end expiratory pressure is used to maintain oxygenation, careful attention must be given to evaluation of cardiac output to ensure organ perfusion. An alveolar-arterial oxygen difference greater than 400 mm Hg may exclude the lung from donation[115].

The maintenance fluid should contain dextrose, though as noted earlier, cerebral metabolism of glucose is nil in the brain dead patient. Potassium and sodium regulation are frequently impaired secondary to free water loss from both diabetes insipidus and diuretics. Ninety percent of brain dead patients develop hypokalemia; however, 39% of these patients also became hyperkalemic in one study[121].

Hypothermia results from lack of hypothalamic control of body temperature. Children generally are more susceptible to temperature instability due to their relatively large body surface area. Kissoon et al. found 53% of pediatric donors to have hypothermia[108]. It is necessary for the patient to be normothermic (rectal temperature 35°C) at the time of neurologic testing and physical examination. Temperature should be managed with warming blankets, radiant warmers, warmed inspired gases, and intravenous fluids. Extreme hypothermia shifts the oxygen dissociation curve to the left, thus decreasing tissue oxygen delivery, and predisposes the patient to sepsis by affecting neutrophil function and release[122].

Loss of the hypothalamic-pituitary axis, resulting in central diabetes insipidus, is noted in 38–87% of patients with brain death from trauma or global brain ischemia[83,123]. Uncontrolled, this will lead to massive fluid and electrolyte losses. Treatment for diabetes insipidus can reasonably be instituted when the patient becomes polyuric and serum sodium concentration rises above 150 mEq/L. In the intensive care setting, diabetes insipidus is easily treated using a continuous intravenous infusion of aqueous vasopressin. A reasonable starting rate is 0.5 mU/kg/hour; if no effect is noted, the rate is doubled every 30 minutes and titrated to achieve the desired urine output, generally 2–4 mU/kg/hour. Aqueous vasopressin is convenient because the effect is rapid in both onset and termination, allowing for easy dosage adjustments. Vasopressin possesses vasopressor activity, and increased vascular tone and hypertension are potential adverse effects, although this seems to be only an occasional clinical management problem in the brain dead organ donor. Alternative approaches to diabetes insipidus include hormone replacement with desmopressin, which can be given intravenously or intranasally. This agent has the advantage of being practically devoid of vasopressor activity, but the long duration of action (12 hours) makes it difficult to titrate therapy in the intensive care patient. Some clinicians advocate management of diabetes insipidus without hormone replacement, using intravenous replacement of fluids lost in the urine as the sole treatment. However, truly large volumes of fluid may be required, and in practical terms this may be difficult and may place the patient at risk of electrolyte abnormalities and significant overhydration or underhydration.

Blood concentrations of triiodothyronine (T_3) are low in most brain dead patients, thought to be consistent with the sick euthyroid syndrome; Keogh et al. found subnormal T_3 levels in 81% of brain dead patients despite normal TSH and thyroxine (T_4) levels[124]. However, hemodynamic status and transplanted organ function do not correlate with thyroid hormone levels, and there is little evidence that empirical T_3 replacement therapy improves hemodynamic function[125–127]. T_3 and T_4 are not routinely administered to brain dead organ donors, although there is a report of their successful use in treating refractory hypotension in adult donors[124]. Other anterior pituitary hormones including ACTH, prolactin, growth hormone, and gonadotropin are not markedly depleted in brain dead patients[128]. Powner et al. demonstrated that pituitary function remains relatively normal in most patients after brain death[129]. One evaluation of pediatric brain dead patients indicated that nearly half required insulin for treatment of significant hyperglycemia[108].

Antimicrobial therapy previously initiated is generally continued after the patient becomes an organ donor candidate; if such therapy is not ongoing, a single dose of a first- or second-generation cephalosporin is often administered. The use of nephrotoxic antibiotics should be avoided. A positive blood culture is not a contraindication for organ procurement. Active hepatitis B and infection with the human immunodeficiency virus are the only absolute infectious contraindications for organ procurement.

Blood products should be administered judiciously to allow pretransplantation serologies to be obtained prior to transfusions. The donor hematocrit is maintained at 25 to 35%[130]. Disseminated intravascular coagulopathy is present in up to 88% of patients with lethal head injuries[131]. Severe coagulopathy should be corrected before organ procurement.

The management of the pediatric organ donor in the operating room requires an understanding of pathophysiologic changes that accompany brain death. Simply transferring the patient to the operating room may cause hemodynamic instability. The anesthesia team should anticipate an initial increase in blood pressure and heart rate, as well as a possible reaction of spinal reflexes, after the surgical incision for procurement. The source of this response may be humoral, such as adrenal medullary stimulation by a reflex spinal arc[86]. Hypertension is frequently followed by a significant decrease in systemic vascular resistance[87]. The large incision needed for multiple organ procurement leads to a rapid decline in core temperature in a cold operating room. Thus, the temperature in the operating room should be regulated with this in mind.

BRAIN DEATH DECLARATION: APPROACH TO THE FAMILY

Brain death is usually the result of a sudden accident that leads to either catastrophic cerebral trauma or global ischemia. After the medical evaluation and stabilization of the child with coma after an intracranial catastrophe, attention should be turned toward the emotional well-being of the family. The first meeting with the family usually occurs shortly after admission and includes those one or two family members who accompanied the child to the hospital. Although this initial meeting is generally for purposes of acquiring information about the circumstances of the accident or the patient's previous medical problems, it also should be used to provide information to the family and to begin to support them. As much as possible, this and all subsequent meetings should be conducted in an unhurried manner in a quiet room away from the patient's bedside. Communication is not a matter that should be relegated as an afterthought to the junior house staff rotating through the ICU but should involve attending staff throughout the process, and involvement of the social worker is highly desirable. Although there is a clear medical and legal distinction between patients who are brain dead and those who are permanently vegetative, the general public often tends to confuse the two; it must be clearly and explicitly stated and understood by the parents and other family "spokespersons" that brain death represents the cessation of all CNS function and not just cortical areas governing consciousness, thinking, feeling, and the other functions that make up human behavior. Once brain death is determined according to hospital protocol and criteria, death is pronounced, the family informed, and a death certificate filed. The family should be approached about organ donation for transplantation only after death has been determined; frequently, they have been discussing this among themselves and may have already reached some decision. In those cases involving accidental death, the medical examiner's or the coroner's office may need to give permission for organ donation. Once a death certificate[11] has been filed, the body should be removed from the ventilator or brought to the operating room if organ donation is planned.

One may encounter families (and occasionally physicians and other medical personnel) who do not accept the brain death concept and recognize only the cessation of cardiac function as death[11]. The majority of such families will eventually understand and accept brain death when it is explained in an unhurried, compassionate manner. When parents refuse to accept the concept of brain death, they may merely be reflecting ambivalent, uninformed feelings expressed by other, respected family members, such as grandparents; then, large family and ICU staff conferences that include not only the parents but also other family spokespersons may be helpful. Should the parents adamantly insist on continued care for their brain dead child, the situation becomes very difficult for both medical and nursing staff members. Although there is no medical reason to continue supportive care, physicians have usually been very reluctant to remove supportive care over parental objections, even though there is probably very little legal liability for doing so. In one seemingly bizarre case reported in the *New York Times,* a brain dead child was evidently sent home on the ventilator (at hospital expense) when the family refused to allow withdrawal of care, despite the ruling of a court that no legal risk would have resulted from removal of supportive care[132]. Under such circumstances, many physicians have opted to continue basic ventilatory care with no escalation in supportive care when hemodynamic instability or an infectious process supervenes, although this appears no more logical than continuing mechanical ventilation for a patient with irreversible cardiac asystole.

Special family circumstances also exist when brain death is the result of child abuse or homicide. This has already been examined by the court system on several occasions, including one celebrated case in which a transplant surgeon was sued unsuccessfully for causing the "death" of a brain dead patient. Although usual hospital brain death criteria are applied, early involvement of the hospital or community social services staff may help with family difficulties and in facilitating police, family, and medical communication.

CESSATION OF SUPPORT

It should be recognized that declaration of brain death is not a necessary prerequisite to the discontinuation of supportive care[65,67]. The major reason for the "ceremony" of formal brain death declaration is the issue of organ transplantation, but the majority of patients dying in a pediatric ICU will not be organ donors. In these cases, then, there is little reason to subject the parent and the child to the process of brain death determination or to a possibly prolonged period of waiting for brain death to manifest itself.

Just as they are able to address the innumerable medical problems presented by critically ill children, physicians and nurses working in intensive care must be capable of coping with patients who are destined to die. There is some perception within both the medical profession and the general public that intensive care specialists often "do too much" by continuing to provide high-technology, invasive, and expensive care to patients for whom the prognosis is hopeless and who thus cannot benefit. Several authors have lamented that the ICU, rather than relieving suffering, may become the cause of it, and have decried the transformation of death into a "mechanized spectacle"[133,134]. Not surprisingly, the issue of determining the proper limits of medical care for hopelessly ill patients has gained the attention of the general public and the legal profession.

Over the past years the attention of the public has been drawn to a number of highly publicized legal cases dealing with issues of terminal care. The most famous of these was that of Karen Ann Quinlan, a young woman vegetative after head trauma, wherein the patient's family petitioned the court to allow withdrawal of mechanical ventilation when physicians involved were unwilling to do so. There are some similar pediatric examples as well, such as the case of a child left vegetative and ventilator-dependent after airway obstruction caused by foreign body aspiration. In this case, the parents wished to withdraw support, but the physicians refused to do so on legal grounds, since the hospital attorney had opined that this act would constitute murder under state law. Eventually, the child's father held medical personnel at gunpoint while he disconnected the ventilator and allowed his son to die[135–137]. There are a fair number of such legal cases, and although there are differences among them, as a group they present a remarkably repetitive scenario: a terminally ill patient whose family members desire to withdraw life support but find themselves in opposition with physicians or a hospital unwilling to do so. With few exceptions, courts in these cases have affirmed the right of individuals or families to make decisions to stop intensive care[138]. Clearly, most people are sympathetic of the "right to die" of hopelessly ill patients, with this right to be exercised by the patient or family[139]. Unfortunately, if the general public's knowledge of these issues is shaped solely by these few widely publicized cases, they may indeed reasonably fear the inappropriate application of invasive and painful critical care to themselves or family members at the end of their lives[140]. Interestingly, these landmark legal cases may suggest that the legal profession, and possibly the public at large, perceive that limitation and withdrawal decisions are infrequent, and that most have resulted in litigation[139]. In reality, of course, such decisions are made on countless occasions each year, in adult and pediatric hospitals throughout the United States, without court intervention.

What factors might induce physicians in intensive care to "do too much" and continue to provide care past the point of possible patient benefit? One factor is known as the "technological imperative"[141], a term which describes the tendency for a technology to be applied simply because it is available. For instance, since mechanical ventilation is commonly available in ICUs, some physicians might feel compelled to use it for every patient with respiratory difficulty, no matter the ultimate prognosis. A possibly more powerful factor is fear of litigation; physicians may be reluctant to stop providing critical care for fear of criminal or civil legal sanctions if they do less than everything within their ability, even in the face of a hopeless prognosis. The motivation in the case of the vegetative child noted above was purely fear of criminal prosecution, as no one involved had any ethical objection to the withdrawal of life support[133]. Another possible reason may be diffusion of responsibility among the several specialists often involved with each patient in the ICU, although the intensive care specialist is the logical person to assume the lead in this area[141,142]. Finally, there may be a simple reticence to accept futility and inform the family there is no more to be done, and to accept the responsibility for making such a weighty decision as the removal of life-support technology with the specific intent of allowing a person to die.

Confusion about the legal status of decisions to limit or withdraw life-support care for pediatric patients may result in part from a conflict between federal statutes and state case law. Federal law operant in this area is known as the Federal Child Abuse Amendments, which represent to some extent an iteration of the original Baby Doe laws. These laws were specifically written to mandate medical care for even severely handicapped infants, the goal being to prevent discrimination against such children[143,144]. Although they were designed to ensure that handicapped children are not denied care, these laws, if strictly interpreted, may prohibit withdrawal of supportive care from hopelessly ill children, or else the physicians and others involved might be liable to charges of child abuse[144]. For instance, the Civil Rights Commission interpreted these laws to mandate care in almost all cases, even if it is inhumane, unless the physician is sure it is virtually futile[143]. The U.S. Department of Health and Human Services, in evaluating these regulations, flatly rejected quality of life as a consideration in withdrawal of support[143]. Thus, according to the Federal Child Abuse Amendments, decisions concerning withdrawal of support should be largely made by physicians on the basis of perceived prognosis without much influence from the patient's family and other considerations such as quality of life.

The Federal Child Abuse Amendments appear to be in conflict with state case law. In a recent review article, Clark[143] reviewed six court actions involving withdrawal of life support from children. In none of these cases was the federal standard invoked, but rather, state law appears to be evolving its own distinct standard. For example, in the case of a 10-year-old girl in a persistent vegetative state after head trauma, the parents wished to withdraw support but were reported to the authorities by intensive care nursing staff members. Here, the court held that there was a right to withhold or withdraw care, to be exercised by the parents, and that the proper place for such decisions was at the bedside, with the courts serving only as a last resort to resolve conflicts. Courts held similarly in the other cases, and in no case were the Federal Child Abuse Amendments invoked. Thus, there appear to be two conflicting legal standards in this country concerning withdrawal of support from children. The first, the federal standard as stated in the Federal Child Abuse Amendments, is objective, physician-driven, and appears to make withdrawal a difficult process, possibly requiring judicial review; currently, this standard appears to be largely ignored by state courts. In contrast to this is the standard evolving from state case law, which is subjective, and largely driven by parental wishes, with decisions made at the bedside, and appears to reflect the reality of clinical, bedside decision making. The existence of legal standards apparently in conflict with one another potentially creates problems for physicians attempting to find the proper course of action[(143)].

Given this situation, then, what is the legal reality for physicians surrounding issues of withdrawal and limitation of life support? Certain cases might give one pause; in California, two physicians involved were indicted for murder after withdrawing support (with consent of the patient's family) from a man in a vegetative state[(139,141,145)]. In truth, however, the legal risk is exceedingly small (the above-noted case never came to trial). No record exists of any criminal conviction of any physician involved in a withdrawal-of-support decision, including several cases wherein decision making might appear questionable[(146)]. Generally, the courts have held that the criminal law does not exist to regulate the conduct of physicians attempting to make reasonable decisions[(145,147,148)]. For example, a Massachusetts court (1980) held that ". . . the doctor will be protected if he acts on a good faith judgment that is not grievously unreasonable by medical standards"[(145)]. As noted by Glantz[(145)], this is a powerfully pro-physician statement. Thus, although many futile therapies have been undertaken in hopes of avoiding litigation[(136)], one must conclude that criminal prosecution is not a realistic risk when making withdrawal of life support decisions. It has been noted that, considering that the majority of legal cases have originated when a physician has resisted a withdrawal-of-support decision, one is more likely to land in court by refusing to do so[(139)]. Therefore, despite the Federal Child Abuse Amendments, there appears to be no legal impediment to withdrawal-of-support decisions made at the bedside by consensus between care providers and family members.

Published surveys of physician attitudes suggest that a sizable minority of the medical profession is not comfortable with withdrawal-of-support issues[(149–151)]. A survey of attendees at a 1988 conference of critical care professionals revealed that 56% were not disturbed by withholding or withdrawing treatment, implying that 44% were disturbed; however, a majority of respondents had withheld or withdrawn treatment from hopelessly ill patients[(152)]. Caralis and Hammond[(153)] surveyed 360 medical students, house officers, and faculty physicians and found that 76% equated withdrawal and withholding of support with passive euthanasia, while a clear majority (73%) felt that withdrawal of support was different from and more disturbing than withholding; one-third of house staff and students saw no difference between withdrawal of life-support treatments and deliberate action to terminate the life of a patient[(153)]. Even when the physician claims to be comfortable with withdrawal of support, there is sometimes reluctance to stop mechanical ventilation and extubate patients who are hopelessly ill. Note that current thinking holds there is no ethical or legal difference between withholding and withdrawing care[(141,149,151,152,154)].

Several recent papers have described approaches to limitation and withdrawal of supportive care in critically ill children. Jefferson et al.[(155)] describe an interesting procedure in which parents sign a directive, similar to a living will, prior to withdrawal of supportive care; it is not clear whether the directive was required for all patients who underwent withdrawal of support. Mink and Pollack[(156)] reported that therapy was withdrawn (defined as removal of mechanical ventilation or of inotrope therapy) or limited (including do-not-resuscitate status) in 32% of 60 children dying in a pediatric ICU, while death followed a failed attempt at cardiopulmonary resuscitation in 38%. Vernon et al. reported that withdrawal of support, defined as cessation of mechanical ventilation, was the most common mode of death in 300 children dying from all causes in a pediatric ICU, occurring in 32% of cases, with support limited for 26%, and failed cardiopulmonary resuscitation being the least common mode of death (19%)[(157)]; Ryan et al. reported similar results from a Canadian pediatric ICU[(158)]. The willingness to withdraw supportive care from hopelessly ill children reflected in these studies may not be universal, however; Lantos et al. noted that mechanical ventilation was withdrawn from only one patient dying in a pediatric ICU during a 1-year study[(159)].

Compared with pediatric ICUs, withdrawal and limitation of supportive care may be more commonly done in adult units, although comparisons are clouded because of differing definitions of withdrawal of support[(160)]. Smedira et al.[(161)] reported that nearly half (89 of 198) of all deaths in two San Francisco ICUs were associated with withdrawal or withholding of therapy, although withdrawal of support was defined to include removal of catecholamine infusions for patients kept on the ventilator. Faber-Langendoen and Bartels[(162)] reported that a majority (52 of 70) of patients, including some children, dying at a university hospital had forgone some treatment modalities, primarily endotracheal intubation. It appears, however, that a majority of dying patients who received mechanical ventilation died on the ventilator, although some were undergoing stepwise decreases in the level of support ("terminal weaning"), including one brain dead child; three of the six patients who were electively extubated were brain dead[(162)]. Stern and Orlowski demonstrated that physician behavior in terminal care may be malleable over time; over a 5-year period after the adoption of a specific do-not-resuscitate policy, the percentage of dying patients given terminal resuscitative efforts decreased from 52 to 3%, with a concomitant increase in the proportion of dying patients with do-not-resuscitate orders in place increasing from 46 to 98% and an increase in the proportion of patients undergoing withdrawal of support from 23 to 73%[163].

How does one go about communicating with families of patients when discontinuation of support is to be considered? First, the physician must reach the conclusion that further care is futile. Unfortunately, absolute guarantees of futility are hard to come by as with absolute guarantees in other areas of medicine so that one must be satisfied with there being no reasonable or realistic prospect of recovery rather than absolute certainty. Families should be told, with compassion, that their loved one cannot possibly recover and that further aggressive supportive care can be of no benefit to him or her. A decision to discontinue supportive care or to possibly institute do-not-resuscitate status can be made at that time. Decisions are best made in a cooperative fashion between the physician and the family, as well as others involved in the child's care, and current standards call for such a decision to be largely made by the patient's family. However, the physician cannot simply describe the facts to the family and then ask for their decision, but must have major input into what is fundamentally a medical decision[142,148,164,165], while at the same time avoiding paternalism[166].

Once having made the decision that further care is futile, what is the proper next step? All such decisions are necessarily situational. Institution of do-not-resuscitate status is one possible course, perhaps as a temporary step while the family considers more active withdrawal of life support or whether they are reluctant to take that course. Indeed, cardiopulmonary resuscitation has been characterized as a "desperate end stage gesture"[167], and it has very limited utility in the pediatric ICU[142,168]. When a decision is made to withdraw life support, what specific kinds of support should be withdrawn? There appears to be wide variation in therapies actually withdrawn. In the study by Vernon et al., withdrawal was defined as endotracheal extubation[157], but others have used such practices as "terminal weaning", discontinuation or reduction in dose of catecholamine infusions, or "do not escalate therapy" orders[156,160,161]. Mechanical ventilation is the most important and invasive life-support technology, but some families (and physicians) may find its abrupt discontinuation too dramatic and rapid a step.

Although discussions of limitation or withdrawal of supportive care are often initiated by physicians, occasionally families may initiate them. In such cases, physicians are probably bound to carry out a family's plan as long as it meets the test of reasonableness; it does not have to be originated by the physician or even necessarily be the course with which he or she is most comfortable, it only must be a reasonable course. In some cases, families may refuse to allow or even consider the withdrawal or limitation of care, even when it is abundantly clear that the prognosis is hopeless. Generally, physicians are not bound to provide futile care, and there is some sentiment that it is unethical to provide care at the family's request when it is clearly of no benefit. In practice, however, most physicians find it difficult to refuse treatment in such cases, given that absolute proof of futility is difficult to provide[148,167]. In one case, this has reportedly even led to the discharge of a brain dead child to the home[132].

Many hospitals have ethics committees which may be involved in withdrawal-of-support decisions; however, a withdrawal-of-support decision by itself does not represent an ethical dilemma. When the case is clear-cut, as is the usual case, there is little to be gained by involvement of a committee, essentially a group of strangers with no special knowledge of the case at hand. Ethics committees should be convened to assist with resolution of conflicts or differences of opinion, but there is little need for ethics committee involvement with every decision to limit or withdraw care.

References

1. Black P. Brain death. N Engl J Med 1978;299:338.
2. Mollaret P, Goulon M. Le coma depasse. Rev Neurol (Paris) 1959;101:3.
3. Pallis C. Brain stem death the evolution of a concept. Med Leg J 1987;55 (part 2):84.
4. Bai K. The definition of death: the Japanese attitude and experience. Transplant Proc 1990;22:991.
5. Feldman EA. Culture, conflict, and cost. Perspectives on brain death in Japan. International Journal of Technology Assessment in Health Care 1994;10:447.
6. Veith F, Fein J, Tendler M, Veatch R, Klelman M, Kalkines G. Brain Death. JAMA 1977;238:1744.
7. A definition of irreversible coma: Report of the Ad Hoc Committee of the Harvard Medical School to Examine the Definition of Brain Death. JAMA 1968;205:337.
8. President's Commission for the Study of Ethical Problems in Medicine and Biomedical and Behavioral Research. Defining death. Washington, DC: Government Printing Office, 1981.
9. Devettere R. Neocortical death and human death. Law Med Health Care 1990;18:96.
10. Youngner S, Barlett E. Human death and high technology: the failure of the whole-brain formulation. Ann Intern Med 1983;99:252.
11. Byrne P, O'Reilly S, Quay P. Brain death an opposing view point. JAMA 1979;242:1985.
12. An appraisal of the criteria of cerebral death: a summary statement. A collaborative study. JAMA 1977;237:982.
13. Powner D, Snyder J, Grenvik A. Brain death certification: a review. Crit Care Med 1977;5:230.
14. Jennett B, Gleave J, Wilson P. Brain death in three neurosurgical units. Br Med J 1981;282:533.
15. Pallis C. The arguments about the EEG. Br Med J 1983;286:284.
16. Conference of Royal Colleges and Faculties of the United Kingdom. Diagnosis of brain death. Lancet 1976;2:1069.
17. Jörgensen E. Spinal man after brain death. Acta Neurochir (Wien) 1973;28:259.
18. Jennett B. Brain death. Intensive Care Med 1982;8:1.
19. Sweet W. Brain death. N Engl J Med 1978;299:410.
20. Silverman D, Masland R, Saunders M, Schwab R. Irreversible coma associated with electrocerebral silence. Neurology 1970;20:525.
21. Ashwal S, Schneider S. Failure of electroencephalography to diagnose brain death in comatose children. Ann Neurol 1979;6:512.
22. Mohandas A, Chou S. Brain death: a clinical and pathological study. J Neurosurg 1971;35:211.
23. Moshe S. Usefulness of EEG in the evaluation of brain death in children: the pros. Electroencephalogr Clin Neurophysiol 1989;73:272.

24. Alvarez LA, Moshe SL, Belman AL, Maytal J, Resnick TJ, Keilson M. EEG and brain death determination in children. Neurology 1988;38:227.
25. Kohrman MH, Spivack BS. Brain death in infants: sensitivity and specificity of current criteria. Pediatr Neurol 1990;6:47.
26. Ashwal S. Brain death in the newborn. Clin Perinatol 1989;16:501.
27. Moshe S, Alvarez L. Diagnosis of brain death in children. J Clin Neurophysiol 1986;3:239.
28. Buchner H, Schuchardt V. Reliability of electroencephalogram in the diagnosis of brain death. Eur Neurol 1990;30:138.
29. Setzer N. Brain death: physiologic definitions. Crit Care Clin 1985;1:375.
30. Ingvar D, Widen L. Brain death: Summary of a symposium. Lakartidningen 1972;69:3804.
31. Rosenklint A, Jörgensen P. Evaluation of angiographic methods in the diagnosis of brain death. Correlation with local and systemic arterial pressure and intracranial pressure. Neuroradiology 1974;7:215.
32. Holzman B, Curless R, Sfakianakis G, Ajmone-Mardan, Montes J. Radionuclide cerebral perfusion scintigraphy in determination of brain death in children. Neurology 1983;33:1027.
33. Goodman J, Hedk L, Moore B. Confirmation of brain death with portable isotope angiography: a review of 204 consecutive cases. Neurosurgery 1985;16:492.
34. Galaske R, Schober O, Heyer R. Determination of brain death in children with 123I-IMP and Tc-99m HMPAO. Psychiatry Res 1989;29:343.
35. Schwartz J, Baxter J, Brill D. Diagnosis of brain death in children by radionuclide cerebral imaging. Pediatrics 1984;73:14.
36. Schwartz J, Baxter J, Brill D, Burns J. Radionuclide cerebral imaging confirming brain death. JAMA 1983;249:246.
37. Ashwal S, Schneider S, Thompson J. Xenon computed tomography measuring cerebral blood flow in the determination of brain death in children. Ann Neurol 1989;25:539.
38. Toffol G, Lansky L, Hughes J, et al. Pitfalls in diagnosing brain death in infancy. J Child Neurol 1987;2134.
39. Volpe J. Brain death determination in the newborn. Pediatrics 1987;80293.
40. Feri M, Ralli L, Felici M, Vanni D, Capria V. Transcranial Doppler and brain death diagnosis. Critical Care Medicine 1994;22:1120.
41. Sanker P, Roth B, Frowein RA, Firsching R. Cerebral reperfusion in brain death of a newborn. Case report. Neurosurgical Review 1992;15:315.
42. Handa J, Matsuda M, Matsuda I, Nakasu S. Dynamic computed tomography in brain death. Surg Neurol 1982;17:417.
43. Ashwal S, Schneider S. Brain death in children: part II. Pediatr Neurol 1987;3:69.
44. Petty GW, Mohr JP, Pedley TA, et al. The role of transcranial Doppler in confirming brain death: sensitivity, specificity, and suggestions for performance and interpretation. Neurology 1990;40:300.
45. Furgiuele T, Frank M, Riegle C. Prediction of cerebral death by cranial sector scan. Crit Care Med 1984;12:1.
46. Glasier C, Seibert J, Chadduck W, Williamson S, Leithiser R. Brain death in infants: evaluation with Doppler US. Radiology 1989;172:377.
47. McMenamin J, Volpe J. Doppler ultrasonography in the determination of neonatal brain death. Ann Neurol 1983;14:302.
48. Orrison W, Champlin A, Kesterson O, Harshorne M, King J. MR 'hot nose sign' and 'intravascular enhancement sign' in brain death. American Society of Neuroradiology 1994;15:913.
49. Richard K, Nanassis K, Froweing R. Intracranial pressure: a reliable criterion of brain death? Neurosurg Rev 1989;1:287.
50. Goldie W, Chiappa K, Young R, Brooks E. Brain stem auditory and short-latency somatosensory evoked responses in brain death. Neurology 1981;31:248.
51. Trojaborg W, Jörgensen E. Evoked cortical potentials in patients with "isoelectric" EEG's. Electroencephalogr Clin Neurophysiol 1973; 35:301.
52. Setzer N, McPherson R, Johnson R, Gioia F. Evoked potential determinations in children with brain death. Anesthesiology 1983;59:A130.
53. Ganes T, Lundar T. EEG and evoked potentials in comatose patients with severe brain damage. Electroencephalogr Clin Neurophysiol 1988;69:6.
54. Facco E, Casartelli L, Munari M, Toffoletto F, Baratto F, Giron G. Short latency evoked potentials: new criteria for brain death? J Neurol Neurosurg Psychiatry 1990;53:351.
55. Machado C, Valdes P, Garcia-Tigera J, et al. Brain stem auditory evoked potentials and brain death. Electroencephalography and clinical Neurophysiology 1991;80:392.
56. Barelli A, Della Corte F, Calimici R, Sandroni C, Proietti R, Magalini SI. Do brain stem auditory evoked potentials detect the actual cessation of cerebral functions in brain dead patients? Crit Care Med 1990;18:322.
57. Biniek R, Ferbert A, Buchner H, H. Loss of brain stem acoustic evoked potentials with spontaneous breathing in a patient with supratentorial lesion. Eur Neurol 1990;30:38.
58. Fackler J, Rogers M. Is brain death really cessation of all intracranial function? J Pediatr 1987;110:84.
59. Walker A, Diamond E, Mostly J. The neuropathological findings in irreversible coma. J Neuropathol Exp Neurol 1975;34:295.
60. Schröauder R. Later changes in brain death. Signs of partial recirculation. Acta Neuropathol 1983;62:15.
61. Vernon D, Holzman B. Brain death: considerations for pediatrics. J Clin Neurophysiol 1986;3:251.
62. Masland R, Walker A, Mokinari G. Criteria of cerebral death. Trans Am Neurol Assoc 1975;100:29.
63. Report of special task force. Guidelines for the determination of brain death in children. American Academy of Pediatrics Task Force on Brain Death in Children. Pediatrics 1987;80:298.
64. Ad Hoc committee on Brain Death, The Children's Hospital, Boston. Determination of brain death. J Pediatrics 1987;110:15.
65. Shewmon D. Commentary on guidelines for the determination of brain death in children. Ann Neurol 1988;24:789.
66. Fackler JC, Troncoso JC, Gioia FR. Age-specific characteristics of brain death in children. Am J Dis Child 1988;142:999.
67. Freeman J, Ferry P. New brain death guidelines in children: further confusion. Pediatrics 1988;81:301.
68. Narkewicz RM. Guidelines for the determination of brain death in children. Pediatrics 1989;83:629.
69. Ashwal S, Schneider S. Brain death in children: part I. Pediatr Neurol 1987;3:5.
70. Rowland T, Donnelly J, Jackson A, Jamroz S. Brain death in the pediatric intensive care unit. Am J Dis Child 1983;137:547.
71. Parisi J, Kim R, Collins G, Hilfinger M. Brain death with prolonged somatic survival. N Engl J Med 1982;306:14.
72. DeLeon S, Ilbawi M, Egel R, et al. Perioperative spinal canal narrowing in patients with Down's syndrome. The Society of Thoracic Surgeons 1991;52:1325.
73. Price M, Galantowicz M, Stolar C. Congenital diaphragmatic hernia, extracorporeal membrane oxygenation, and death: a spectrum of etiologies. Journal of Pediatric Surgery 1991;26:1023.
74. Marti-Masso J, Suarez J, Lopez de Munain A, Carrera N. Clinical signs of brain death simulated by Guillain-Barre syndrome. Annula of the Neurological Sciences 1993;120:115.
75. Ragosta K. Miller Fisher syndrome, a brain stem encephalitis, mimics brain death. Clinical Pediatrics 1993;32:685.
76. Jörgensen E, Moller A. Cerebral prognostic signs during cardiopulmonary resuscitation. Resuscitation 1978;6:217.
77. Tyson R. Simulation of cerebral death by succinylcholine sensitivity. Arch Neurol 1974;30:409.
78. Marks S, Zisfein J. Apneic oxygenation in apnea tests for brain death. A controlled trial. Arch Neurol 1990;47:1066.
79. Rowland T, Donnelly J, Jackson A. Apnea documentation in the determination of brain death in children. Pediatrics 1984;74:505.
80. Heytens L, Verlooy J, Gheuens J, Bossaert L. Lazarus sign and extensor posturing in a brain-dead patient. Case report. J Neurosurg 1989;71:449.
81. Outwater K, Rockoff M. Apnea testing to confirm brain death in children. Crit Care Med 1984;12:357.
82. Jeret JS, Benjamin JL. Risk of hypotension during apnea testing. Archives of Neurology 1994;51:595.
83. Fiser DH, Jimenez JF, Wrape V, Woody R. Diabetes insipidus in children with brain death. Critical Care Medicine 1987;15:551.
84. Staworn D, Lewison L, Marks J, Turner G, Levin D. Brain death in pediatric intensive care unit patients: incidence, primary diagnosis, and the clinical occurrence of Turner's triad. Critical Care Medicine 1994;22:1301.
85. Kero P, Antila K, Ylitalo V, Valimaki L. Decreased heart rate variation in decerebration syndrome: quantitative clinical criterion of brain death. Pediatrics 1978;62:307.
86. Wetzel RC, Setzer N, Stiff JL, et al. Hemodynamic responses in brain dead organ donor patients. Anesth Analg 1985;64:125.
87. Pennefather SH, Dark JH, Bullock RE. Haemodynamic responses to surgery in brain-dead organ donors. Anaesthesia 1993;48:1034.
88. Gramm H, Zimmermann J, Meinhold H, Dennhardt R, Voigt K. Hemodynamic responses to noxious stimuli in brain-dead organ donors. Intensive Care Med 1992;18:493.

89. Goldstein B, DeKing D, DeLong DJ, et al. Autonomic cardiovascular state after severe brain injury and brain death in children. Critical Care Medicine 1993;21:228.
90. Ventura M, Masser P. Defining death: developments in recent law. Crit Car Clin 1985;1:397.
91. Gramm H, Meinhold H, Bickel U, et al. Acute endocrine failure after brain death. Transplantation 1992;54:851.
92. Schrader H, Krogness K, Aakvaag A, Sortland O, Purvis K. Changes of pituitary hormones in brain death. Acta Neurochir (Wien) 1980; 52:239.
93. Anderson A. Japan grapples with definition of death by brain death. Nature 1989;337:592.
94. Rix B. Danish ethics council rejects brain death as the criterion of death. J Med Ethics 1990;16:5.
95. Handa H. Diversification in the concept of "birth and death": the controversy about "brain death and organ transplantation" in Japan. Surg Neurol 1993;39:437.
96. Ebafa T, Watanabe Y, Amaha K, Hosaka Y, Takagi S. Haemodynamic changes during the apnoea test for diagnosis of brain death. Can J Anaesth 1991;38:436.
97. Kawashima T, Hasegawa T, Fuse K, et al. Organ transplantation from brain-dead individuals in Japan: results of a questionnaire in families of brain-dead patients. Transplantation Proceedings 1994;26:977.
98. Sellami MM. Islamic position on organ donation and transplantation. Transplantation Proceedings 1993;25:2307.
99. Shaheen F, Nezamuddin N, Adiku W, et al. Outcome of brain-dead patients in Jeddah kidney center. Transplantation Proceedings 1992;24:2067.
100. Haberal M, Altaca G, Tokyay R, Bilgin N. Ethics in organ procurement in Turkey. Transplantation Proceedings 1992;24:2100.
101. El Matri A, Abdallah T, Maiz H, et al. Organ transplantation in Tunisia. Transplantation Proceedings 1993;25:2350.
102. Walker J, McGrath P, MacDonald N, Wells G, Petrusic W, Nolan B. Parental attitudes toward pediatric organ donation: a survey. Can Med Assoc J 1990;142:1383.
103. Evans RW, Orians CE, Ascher NL. The potential supply of organ donors. An assessment of the efficacy of organ procurement efforts in the United States. JAMA 1992;267:239.
104. Gnant M, Goetzinger W, Sautner T, Steininger R, Muehlbacher F. The impact of the presumed consent law and a decentralized organ procurement system on organ donation: quadruplication in the number of organ donors. Transplantation Proceedings 1991;23:2685.
105. Romano J, Margenet-Baudry A, Guerrinl P, Reynaud P, Gallared, M. Organization of a brain death unit in a Paris suburb hospital. Transplantation Proceedings 1991;23:2468.
106. Morris JA, Jr., Wilcox TR, Frist WH. Pediatric organ donation: the paradox of organ shortage despite the remarkable willingness of families to donate. Pediatrics 1992;89:411.
107. Pelletier M. The organ donor family members' perception of stressful situations during the organ donation experience. Journal of Advanced Nursing 1992;17:90.
108. Kissoon N, Frewen TC, Bloch M, Gayle M, Stilre C. Pediatric organ donor maintenance: Pathophysiologic derangements and nursing requirements. Pediatrics 1989;84:688.
109. Nygaard CE, Townsend RN, Diamond DL. Organ donor management and organ outcome: a 6-year review from a Level I trauma center. J Trauma 1990;30:728.
110. Kinoshita Y, Okamoto K, Yahata K, et al. Clinical and pathological changes of the heart in brain death maintained with vasopressin and epinephrine. Pathol Res Pract 1990;186:173.
111. Lucas BA, Vaughn WK, Spees EK, Sanfilippo F. Identification of donor factors predisposing to high discard rates of cadaver kidneys and increased graft loss within one year posttransplantation. Transplantation 1987;43:253.
112. Gosh S, Bethune DW, Hardy I, Kneeshaw J, Latimer RD, Oduro A. Management of donors for heart and heart-lung transplantation. Anaesthesia 1990;45:672.
113. Kormos RL, Donato W, Hardesty RL, Griffith BP, Kiernan J, Trent BA. The influence of donor organ stability and ischemia time on subsequent cardiac recipient survival. Transplant Proceedings 1988;20:980.
114. Mertes PM, el Abassi K, Jaboin Y, et al. Changes in hemodynamic and metabolic parameters following induced brain death in the pig. Transplantation 1994;58:414.
115. Brink LW, Ballew A. Care of the pediatric organ donor. American Journal of Diseases of Children 1992;146:1045.
116. Peterseim D, Chesnut L, Meyers C, D'Amico T, Van Trigt P, Schwinn D. Stability of the β-adrenergic receptor/adenylyl cyclase pathway of pediatric myocardium after brain death. J Heart Lung Transplant 1994;13:635.
117. Whelchel JD, Diethelm AG, Phillips MG, Ryder WR, Shein LG. The effect of high-dose dopamine in cadaver donor management on delayed graft function and graft survival following renal transplantation. Transplant Proceedings 1986;20:523.
118. Yoshioka T, Sugimoto H, Masaaki U. Prolonged hemodynamic maintenance by the combined administration of vasopressin and epinephrine in brain death: a clinical study. Neurosurgery 1986;18:565.
119. Schneider A, Toledo-Pereyra LH, Aeichner WD, Allaben R, Whitten J. Effect of dopamine and pitressin on kidneys procured and harvested for transplantation. Transplantation 1983;36:110.
120. Darby JM, Stein K, Grenvik A, Stuart SA. Approach to management of the heartbeating 'brain dead' organ donor. Jama 1989;261:2222.
121. Jordan CA, Snyder JV. Intensive care and intraoperative management of the brain-dead organ donor. Transplant Proceedings 1987;19:21.
122. Briggar WE, Bohn DJ, Kent G. Neutrophil circulation and release for bone marrow during hypothermia. Infectious Immunology 1983;40:708.
123. Outwater KM, Rockoff MA. Diabetes insipidus accompanying brain death in children. Neurology 1984;34:1243.
124. Keogh AM, Howlett TA, Perry L, et al. Pituitary function in brain stem dead organ donors: A prospective study. Transplant Proceedings 1988;20:729.
125. Garcia-Fages L, Cabrer C, Valero R, Manyalich M. Hemodynamic and metabolic effects of substitutive triiodothyronine therapy in organ donors. Transplantation Proceedings 1993;25:3038.
126. Randell T, Hockerstedt K. Trilodothyronine treatment is not indicated in brain-dead multiorgan donors: a controlled study. Transplantation Proceedings 1993;25:1552.
127. Gifford RM, Weaver AS, Burg JE, et al. Thyroid hormone levels in heart and kidney cadaver donors. Journal of Heart Transplantation 1986;5:249.
128. Howlett TA, Keogh AM, L. P, et al. Anterior and posterior pituitary function in brain stem dead donors. Transplantation 1989;47:828.
129. Powner DJ, Hendrich A, Lagler RG, Ng RH, Madden RL. Hormonal changes in brain dead patients. Crit Care Med 1990;18:702.
130. Hardesty RL, Griffith BP. Multiple cadaveric organ procurement for transplantation with emphasis on the heart. Surgical Clinics of North America 1986;66:451.
131. Kaufman HH, Hui KS, Mattson JC, et al. Clinicopathologic correlations of disseminated intravascular coagulation in patients with severe head injury. Neurosurgery 1984;15:34.
132. Brain-dead Florida girl will be sent home on life support. New York Times, February 18, 1994.
133. Kjellstrand CM. Who should decide about your death? JAMA 1992;267:103.
134. Schuster DP. Everything that should be done not everything that can be done [editorial]. American Review of Respiratory Disease 1992;145:508.
135. Lantos JD, Miles SH, Cassel CK. The Linares affair. Law, Medicine & Health Care 1989;17:308.
136. Nelson LJ, Cranford RE. Legal advice, moral paralysis and the death of Samuel Linares. Law, Medicine & Health Care 1989;17:316.
137. Truog RD. Allowing to die [editorial]. Critical Care Medicine 1990;18:790.
138. Jonsen AR. What is extraordinary life support? The Western Journal of Medicine 1984;141:358.
139. Meisel A. Refusing treatment, refusing to talk, and refusing to let go: On whose terms will death occur? Law, Medicine & Health Care 1989;17:221.
140. Iserson KV. The "no code' tattoo—An ethical dilemma. The Western Journal of Medicine 1992;156:309.
141. Luce J, Raffin T. Withholding and withdrawal of life support from critically ill patients. Chest 1988;94:621.
142. Ruark JE, Raffin TA. Initiating and withdrawing life support. The New England Journal of Medicine 1988;318:25.
143. Clark FI. Intensive care treatment decisions: the roots of our confusion. Pediatrics 1994;94:98.
144. Clark F. Child abuse law. Pediatrics 1995;95:455.
145. Glantz LH. Withholding and withdrawing treatment: The role of the criminal law. Law, Medicine & Health Care 1987/88;15:231.
146. Fost N. Do the right thing: Smauel Linares and defensive law. Law, Medicine & Health Care 1989;17:330.
147. Gilfix M, Raffin TA. Withholding or withdrawing extraordinary life support. Critical Issues in Medicine 1984;141:387.
148. Nelson LJ, Nelson RM. Ethics and the provision of futile, harmful, or burdensome treatment to children. Critical Care Medicine 1992;20:427.

149. NIH Workshop Summary: Withholding and withdrawing mechanical ventilation. Am Rev Resp Dis 1986;134:1327.
150. Brennan T. Incompetent patients with limited care in the absence of family consent. Ann Intern Med 1988;109:819.
151. Reines H. Attitudes of critical care medicine professionals concerning foregoing life-sustaining treatment. Crit Care Med 1992;20:316.
152. Attitudes of critical care medicine professionals concerning foregoing life-sustaining treatments. The Society of Critical Care Medicine Ethics Committee. Crit Care Med 1992;20:320.
153. Caralis PV, Hammond JS. Attitudes of medical students, housestaff, and faculty physicians toward euthanasia and termination of life-sustaining treatment. Critical Care Medicine 1992;20:683.
154. Task Force on Ethics of the Society of Critical Care Medicine: Consensus report on the ethics of foregoing life-sustaining treatments in the critically ill. Crit Care Med 1990;18:1435.
155. Jefferson L, White B, Louis P, et al. Use of the Natural Death Act in pediatric patients. Crit Care Med 1991;19:901.
156. Mink RB, Pollack MM. Resuscitation and withdrawal of therapy in pediatric intensive care. Pediatrics 1992;89:961.
157. Vernon D, Dean J, Timmons O, Banner W, Allen-Webb E. Modes of death in the pediatric intensive care unit: Withdrawal and limitation of supportive care. Crit Care Med 1993;21:1798.
158. Ryan CA, Byrne P, Kuhn S, Tyebkhan J. No resuscitation and withdrawal of therapy in a neonatal and a pediatric intensive care unit in Canada. Journal of Pediatrics 1993;123:534.
159. Lantos JD, Berger AC, Zucker AR. Do-not-resuscitate orders in a children's hospital. Critical Care Medicine 1993;21:52.
160. Faber-Langendoen K. The clinical management of dying patients receiving mechanical ventilation. A survey of physician practice. Chest 1994;106:880.
161. Smedira NG, Evans BH, Grais LS, et al. Withholding and withdrawal of life support from the critically ill. N Engl J Med 1990;322:309.
162. Faber-Langendoen K, Bartels DM. Process of forgoing life-sustaining treatment in a university hospital: an empirical study. Crit Care Med 1992;20:570.
163. Stern SG, Orlowski JP. DNR or CPR the choice is ours. Critical Care Medicine 1992;20:1263.
164. Anonymous. American Academy of Pediatrics Committee on Bioethics: Guidelines on foregoing life-sustaining medical treatment. Pediatrics 1994;93:532.
165. Safar P, Winter P. Helping to die. Critical Care Medicine 1990; 18:788.
166. Brennan TA. Silent decisions: Limits of consent and the terminally ill patient. Law, Medicine & Health Care 1988;16:204.
167. Paris JJ, Schreiber MD, Statter M, Arensman R, Siegler M. Beyond autonomy—physicians' refusal to use life-prolonging extracorporeal membrane oxygenation. The New England Journal of Medicine 1993; 329:354.
168. Parker JM, Landry FJ, Phillips YY. Use of do-not-resuscitate orders in an intensive care setting. Chest 1993;104:1592.

Immunologic and Infectious Disease Considerations

Section Five

Section Editor

Alice D. Ackerman

Primary and Secondary Immunodeficiencies 28

Karen J. Miller
Alice D. Ackerman

INTRODUCTION

Charged with the care of critically ill children, many of whom have infectious diseases, the pediatric intensive care provider must be aware of the ways that particular microorganisms may affect the host and may potentially complicate the child's therapy. The pediatric intensive care specialist must also be aware of and avoid those conditions that make infections more likely. This chapter discusses conditions of the host that have an adverse effect on immune system function and make it more likely that the child will develop an infection. Such conditions include the congenital immunodeficiency disorders as well as acquired states, such as malnutrition, extremely young age or prematurity, bacterial and viral infections, immunosuppressive drug therapy, surgery, anesthesia, and trauma, all of which lead to inhibition of immune function.

Specific aspects of immunity are discussed as they relate to the particular diseases or states, but no attempt has been made to describe the functions of the immune system as a whole. Such discussions can be found in general immunology textbooks. This chapter is intended to serve as a reference and to provide guidelines for the practitioner faced with specific disease entities. It is hoped the reader will acquire an appreciation for the complexity of immunity as it pertains to pediatric practice in the intensive care unit (ICU), and also of the need to consider how one disease process, such as trauma, or one of its complications, such as malnutrition, may make secondary infections much more likely. Such knowledge will naturally lead to increased levels of attention to simple prophylactic measures, as well as the ability to predict likelihood of infection and therapeutically to intercede in a rapid fashion.

The chapter begins with a discussion of nonspecific and acquired alterations of immune function, which is followed by a brief overview of the inherited immunodeficiency diseases, and concludes with recommendations regarding when to suspect an underlying immune defect.

NONSPECIFIC AND ACQUIRED ALTERATIONS OF IMMUNE FUNCTION

Age

Neonates, especially when preterm, are immunologically immature. Extremely young age is associated with poor outcome with regard to critical illness. The development of the immunocompetent state requires the interaction of many genetically determined variables, which code for the expression of both specific and nonspecific host defenses. Specific immune defenses involve antibody production and cellular immunity (B-cell and T-cell function, respectively) which are specific for the offending antigen and require previous exposure to the antigen as well as the presence of an immunologic memory for full expression. Because of the neonate's relative lack of experience and exposure, he or she will have some impairment of B-cell and T-cell response on this basis alone. A description of how these responses develop in the fetus and neonate follows.

Very early B cells or pre-B cells have been documented in the fetal liver by five to eight weeks of gestation(1). By the middle of the second trimester, the absolute number of B cells has reached nearly adult levels, and differentiation has proceeded to the point where the various clones committed to synthesis of each immunoglobulin class are present in similar proportions to those in adults(2,3). Despite this apparent adequacy of B-cell numbers, the fetus has a limited ability to synthesize specific immunoglobulins. Serum concentration of IgG in the full-term baby may be as great as or may exceed that of the mother, primarily because of active and passive transplacental crossing of IgG in the final trimester(4). IgG transfer across the placenta occurs as early as 8 weeks gestation age(5). The level of IgG in premature babies is low and directly proportional to gestational age(6–11). Fetal IgG levels at less then 17 weeks gestational ages are very low and at 28 weeks are still less than 50% term levels(5). In both the premature and the full-term baby, IgG levels fall during the first four months of extrauterine life. The half-life of IgG is 25 days. Very early premature infants, therefore, may be exceedingly hypogammaglobulinemic for the first half of their first year of life, leading to higher rates of infection and rehospitalization(12). Adult levels of IgG are reached by four to six years of age(1).

The presence of maternal IgG provides some degree of passive immunity for the baby and may help defend against invading organisms. However, as suggested by the failure of term infants in the first few weeks of life to mount an antibody response to certain antigens (notably diphtheria toxoid and polio virus), the presence of placentally acquired IgG may inhibit the infant's intrinsic antibody response(13,14). Another possible cause for this failure to produce antibody is an imbalance of T-helper and suppressor interaction with B cells(15–17).

By 10 weeks of gestation, the fetus is capable of producing IgM and may make large quantities in the presence of a congenital infection(1). The noninfected newborn has an IgM concentration that is approximately 10% the normal adult value and that reaches mature levels at one to two years(18). The initial humoral response of the newborn to most antigens is an elevation of IgM that is relatively persistent but may not provide effective protection against all organisms.

IgA is not measurable until late in gestational life and is very limited in the infant, failing to reach adult values until puberty(1–3,19). Secretory IgA appears later than serum IgA, and this discrepancy accounts for, to some extent, the easy sensitization of the infant to ingested allergens in the first year of life(18). The development of B-cell-related immunity is summarized in **Table 28.1**(1).

Lymphocytes destined for the various T-cell subsets are first found at about 40 days of gestation, initially in the liver(20). The neonate does not develop a typical hypersensitivity reaction to intradermal antigen injection. In addition to this noted anergy, the neonate's T cells lack the ability to produce certain cytokines, such as interferon and monocyte migration inhibitory factor(21). The major problem with T-cellular immunity in this age group is the immature nature of the interaction between T cells and B cells; namely, there is greater reactivity of T-suppressor cells relative to T-helper cells, compared with those of the normal adult(17).

In summary, both limbs of specific immunity are impaired in the newborn, causing the newborn to be susceptible to a number of microorganisms. Immaturity of the B-cell system results in inadequate levels of specific IgG to protect against gram-negative organisms or to provide opsonization of the group B streptococcus. The immature T-cell system in the neonate causes preferential induction of suppressor Tcells in response to certain organisms, further diminishing the production of specific antibody.

Nonspecific mechanisms of host defense include all of the responses and the functions of phagocytic cells, the complement system, and specific chemical mediators of the immune response, such as opsonization and chemotaxis. Phagocytes of the newborn exhibit diminished motility, adherence, and chemotaxis(22–26), and these findings may contribute to the neonate's difficulty in localizing infections. However, phagocytosis appears normal in nonstressed full-term newborns(27,28). In the presence of illness or prematurity, phagocytosis is diminished(29–31). Bacterial killing by polymorphonuclear leukocytes, which depends on the generation of oxygen-derived free radicals, is intact in healthy term and most premature newborns(28,32–34), but quickly becomes insufficient in the stressed neonate(35–37) or in the presence of many organisms(38).

Table 28.1. B-Cell Ontogeny[a]

Type of B-cell	*Characteristics*	*Fetal Age First Noted (wk)*	*Effects of Possible Arrest at this Stage*
Pre-B-cell	Cytoplasmic IgM, no surface immunoglobulin: may show Ia antigens	5–8	Thymoma with hypogammaglobulinemia
Early B-cell, surface IgM positive	Surface IgM: show Ia antigen on surface	8–9	Congenital agammaglobulinemia (X-linked, sporadic)
Virgin B-cells; surface IgM positive (Bμ): surface IgA positive (Bα): surface IgD positive[b] (Bδ): surface IgE positive (Bє)	Surface immunoglobulin of all classes present: cytoplasmic immunoglobulin not present; complement receptor positive; Ia positive	9.5–11	Common variable immunodeficiency, selective IgA deficiency
Actively secreting B-cells (become plasma cells terminally)	Responds to pokeweed mitogen, antigens, and T-regulatory cells and factors	17	Multiple myeloma

[a] *From Cooper MD, Buckley RH. Developmental immunity and the immunodeficiency diseases. JAMA 1982;248:2658. Copyright 1982, American Medical Association.*
[b] *IgD may be another receptor present on early B-cells, resulting in double immunoglobulin-bearing early B-lymphocytes (e.g., IgM positive and IgD positive).*

Opsonization is deficient in many neonates for some organisms, specifically *Escherichia coli* and *Serratia marcescens*(36) as well as other gram-negative organisms. Failure to opsonize several types of group B streptococci increases the likelihood of infection with this organism and has helped establish the important role for this bacterium in postnatal infectious mortality, even among many otherwise healthy full-term babies(39–44).

Premature and full-term infants are deficient in all measurable products of complement activation(45,46). Placental passage of complement is minimal. Synthesis of complement by fetal tissue begins around eight weeks gestation. Levels increase dramatically during the third trimester(47–50) and are at 50% of maternal levels by term. Adult levels are reached by three to six months of life(51). The biologic activities of complement are listed in **Table 28.2.**

Specific considerations for therapy of the infected newborn and premature infant are discussed in Chapter 32. The discussion, however, should clarify the underlying reasons for the neonate's increased susceptibility to gram-negative infections, group B streptococci, and certain other organisms, such as *Listeria.* Organisms that require production of specific subclasses of immunoglobulins to induce immunity may be encountered repeatedly by the infant and young child until the ability to produce specific immunoglobulin has been developed. This is particularly true for the encapsulated bacterial organisms, the most important of which is *Haemophilus influenzae* type b, which was the most frequent cause of bacterial meningitis in childhood before the development of effective immunization(52). Specific immunity to this organism requires synthesis of IgG2, the capacity for which is limited until after 2 years of age(53). Studies of the antibody response to immunization with the purified polysaccharide vaccine as well as following natural infection have documented frequent failure of an immune response to this antigen in the child less than 24 months of age(54,55). Such findings provided the rationale for development of the *Haemophilus influenzae* type b conjugate vaccines, in which the capsule-derived polysaccharide is attached to a harmless protein antigen, allowing infants to develop an antibody response to the polysaccharide moiety(56).

Many viral infections produce less stress on the neonate because of the relatively intact T-cell function. Diseases whose defense depends primarily upon secretory IgA, such as some of the viral respiratory agents (e.g., respiratory syncytial virus) and infectious diarrheas, remain prevalent throughout infancy.

Anesthesia, Surgery, and Accidental Trauma

A significant percentage of patients admitted to most pediatric ICUs enter subsequent to surgical and anesthetic interventions or require intensive care following major accidental trauma or severe thermal injury. Therefore, it is of

Table 28.2. Biologic Activities of Complement[a]

Component	*Activities*
C4b	Viral neutralization Immune adherence
C3b	Immune adherence Opsonization Enhances antibody-dependent cellular cytotoxicity Amplifies alternative pathway via feedback loop
C3a	Stimulates B-cell lymphokine production Anaphylatoxin (induces smooth muscle contraction, histamine release from basophils and mast cells, and increased vascular permeability)
C3e	Induces granulocytosis
C5a	Chemoattractant for polymorphonuclear cells and monocytes Anaphylatoxin Induces granulocyte aggregation
C5b–C9	Membrane attack complex that leads to cell lysis
C1–C6	Endotoxin inactivation in vitro Animal protection against endotoxin in vivo
Factor B fragment	Macrophage activation

[a] *Modified from Cates KL, Rowe JC, Ballow M: The premature infant as a compromised host. In: Current problems in pediatrics. Chicago: Year Book Medical Publishers, 1983:1.*

paramount importance that the pediatric intensive care specialist recognize the potential effects that such manipulations or accidents may have on his or her patients. With regard to surgical trauma, it is difficult to separate the effects of associated anesthesia on the immune system from those of the operation itself. Underlying host disease and overall severity of illness will interact with any documented effects of both surgery and anesthesia.

Anesthesia

Table 28.3 summarizes some of the known specific effects of various anesthetic agents on the immune system. The overall consequences of general or local anesthesia on host defense mechanisms must also be considered. Issues involved with breech of normal barriers to infection associated with endotracheal intubation, mechanical ventilation, and insertion of intravenous, urinary, and epidural catheters are discussed in depth in Chapter 31. Interference with the respiratory mucosa and ciliary functions are important in the development of nosocomial infections following intubation for any reason. Such interventions make clearance of foreign materials from the airways difficult. This problem is worsened by administration of sedatives and analgesics that further diminish the host's protective airway reflexes.

One of the most commonly used inhalational anesthetics, nitrous oxide (N_2O), has long been known as a bone marrow depressant[57]. Some patients who were treated for severe tetanus in the 1950s with long-term N_2O (50%) and curarization developed aplastic anemia and sepsis[58,59]. N_2O suppresses both T-cell and B-cell function and has also been used clinically to induce (brief) remission in adults with myelogenous leukemia[60]. The agent's specific effects on complement levels and activity are not known. Halothane also has effects on the phagocytic system. In addition to suppressing bone marrow function, resulting in diminished numbers of circulating leukocytes[61], halothane also alters the cytoplasmic-to-nuclear ratio of granulocytes via a presumed effect on membrane metabolism[62]. It decreases phagocytosis, bacterial killing, and chemotaxis and has a depressant effect on reticuloendothelial phagocytic activity[63]. T-cell numbers and function are also impaired, as is specific antibody synthesis[64].

Administration of thiopental and other "short-acting" barbiturate agents at anesthetic levels for as little as 30 minutes has produced granulocytopenia[65]. Longer exposures to pentobarbital have resulted in an 80% decrement in the circulating granulocyte count[66].

The major adverse effect on immunity produced by narcotics, such as morphine sulfate, is depression of leukocyte chemotaxis[67]. The muscle relaxants pancuronium and curare impair chemotaxis, whereas succinylcholine augments the chemotactic response[57]. Local anesthetics diminish the adherence of leukocytes to damaged vascular endothelial surfaces[68].

Surgery and Trauma

Surgical and accidental trauma induce acquired immune defects in patients, the nature and extent of which vary con-

Table 28.3. Anesthetic Agents and Immune Function[a]

	Immune System Component			
Agent	*Phagocytes*	*T-cells*	*B-cells*	*Other*
Inhalational	↓ Number	↓ Number	↓ Proliferation response to antigens	
Cyclopropane	↓ Activity of reticuloendothelial and pulmonary macrophages	↓ Response to mitogen		
Enflurane	↓ Chemotaxis and same effects as cyclopropane	Same as cyclopropane	Same as cyclopropane	
Ether	↓ Peripheral phagocytosis ↓ Reticuloendothelial activity	Same as cyclopropane	Same as cyclopropane	↓ C3, C4
Halothane	Same as enflurane and alters cytoplasm to nucleus ratio ↓ Peripheral phagocytosis ↓ Bacterial killing	Same and ↓ cytotoxicity	↓ Antibody synthesis	
Methoxyflurane	↓ Pulmonary macrophage activity	Unknown	↓ Overall activity	
N_2O	Bone marrow depression or failure/aplastic anemia ↓ Phagocytosis ↓ Bacterial killing	↓ Response to mitogen	↓ Proliferation and activity	
Barbiturates	Overt granulocytopenia ↓ Phagocytosis ↓ Bacterial killing	↓ Response to mitogen ↓ cytotoxicity	↓ Antibody synthesis	
Narcotics	↓ Chemotaxis ↓ Phagocytosis and killing			
Local Anesthetics	↓ Adherence of leukocytes to damaged vascular endothelium			

[a] *See References 57–68.*

siderably according to age, presence of chronic illness, and importantly, the length and complexity of surgery or degree of trauma[69].

The immune system performs a two-fold purpose during the intraoperative and postoperative periods[70]. Production of antibodies secondary to tissue injury would potentially result in a form of autoimmunity, which must be suppressed to avoid damage to the host. However, wound healing is optimized under conditions where functional immunity is geared up, thereby promoting hemostasis and preventing wound infections and sepsis.

A surgical wound dramatically increases the circulating neutrophil count[71]. This is related to certain humoral effects of trauma, most notably, to a strong, acute catecholamine release that is part of a multifactorial, endocrinologically mediated nonspecific response to stress[72–74]. The phagocytic response is the first and most important host reaction to surgery. The presence of these inflammatory cells evokes both cell-mediated and antibody-antigen responses and helps initiate release of complement fractions by the alternate pathway. Complement components act as chemotactic factors to attract more leukocytes to the wound site. The phagocytes also ingest and kill bacteria contaminating the area.

Blood levels of B lymphocytes and T lymphocytes decrease in response to surgical stress, but large accumulations of T cells are found postoperatively in the spleen and, to a lesser extent, in the liver[75].

Cutaneous anergy may develop following surgery. It correlates predictably with a higher incidence of wound infection and sepsis[76–79]. T cells are involved in the regulation of wound healing[80]. Evaluation of wound lymphocyte populations has indicated an increased ratio of T-suppressor to T-helper cells relative to that in the peripheral blood. In addition, T cells produce a variety of lymphokines that participate in the modulation of fibroblast activity, and contribute to down-regulation of T-cell function, potentially slowing the proliferative phase of wound healing.

A number of immune function alterations have been documented following major trauma[69,81–86]. Many of these have also been implicated in the posttrauma sepsis syndrome. The commonly noted effects of trauma on immune function are listed in **Table 28.4.**

Reviews of nosocomial infections following surgery and trauma have described the most likely offending organisms in postsurgical patients at various sites[87–91] **(Table 28.5).** Aerobic Gram-negative organisms *(E. coli, Proteus, Pseudomonas, Klebsiella, Enterobacter,* and *Acinetobacter)* play the largest role in surgical infections, followed by gram-positive organisms *(Staphylococcus aureus* and *Staphylococcus epidermidis)* and the anaerobes (especially *Bacteroides*). Appropriate host defense against gram-negative species requires many aspects of immunity to be intact, because these organisms produce disease by release of both exotoxin and endotoxin. These are the organisms most implicated in postsurgical bacterial sepsis and against which antibiotic therapy alone may be of limited value. Effective protection against these microorganisms requires specific opsonization by IgG in concert with complement. IgM is produced in response to infection by these bacteria, but its effectiveness is not clear. When invasion by any of these organisms proceeds in the host who has no specific immunity to quell bacterial reproduction, endotoxin may be produced, which has widespread multisystem effects on physiologic functions. Endotoxin activates many of the interacting protein cascade systems in an indiscriminate manner and leads eventually to loss of capillary endothelial integrity, direct depression of the cardiovascular system, stimulation of clotting and fibrinolytic systems, and generation of kinins and prostaglandins[92]. The pathophysiology of the shock syndromes is discussed in Chapter 16. Infections in children undergoing cardiovascular surgical procedures have been evaluated[93]. Overall, patients who are sickest upon returning to the PICU (as measured by the PRISM score) have a greater risk of developing an infection. The site at which infection develops in this patient population most commonly is at the wound, then at the chest tube site; bacteremia related to presence of a central venous catheter also occurs. When all infections at all sites are considered, there is a predominance of gram-positive organisms (52.3%), followed by *Pseudomonas* (21%) and *Candida* species (15%). Specific issues related to catheter-induced infections are considered in Chapter 31.

As is the case in postoperative patients, the majority of infections in the trauma victim are nosocomial[94]. This is an important observation, since the second most common cause of death in the pediatric trauma victim who survives the initial postinjury period is infection[95]. The risk of nosocomial infection increases with the severity of injury[96], despite advances in care that have permitted survival of critically injured persons.

Because the risk of infection is so great, many health care centers advocate the use of prophylactic antibiotics[97], although much controversy exists[95]. Prophylactic antibiotics are most beneficial in injuries involving the large and

Table 28.4. Effect of Trauma on Immune Function

Immune System Component	*Effect*
Neutrophils	
Number	Increased
Chemotaxis	Decreased
Phagocytosis	Decreased
Lymphocytes	
T-cells (number)	Decreased
CD4 + (number)	Decreased
Response to stimulation	Decreased
Monocytes (number)	Increased
Cytokines (mediators)	
PGE_2	Increased
IL-1	Decreased
IL-2	Decreased
IL-6	Increased
TNF-α	Increased
TGF-β	Increased
Immunoglobulins	
Nonspecific IgG	Increased
Primary response to immunization	Decreased
Response to recall antigens	Unchanged

Table 28.5. Infections in the Surgical Patient: Relative Likelihood of Organisms Causing Infection at a Particular Organ Site[a]

	Gram-negative	Staphylococcus	*Anaerobes*	Enterococcus
Pneumonia	++++	++	0	0
Fecal peritonitis[b]	++++	0	++++	+
Biliary tract infection	++++	0	0	+
Wound infection	+++	+++	(+)[c]	+
Primary bacteremia and line sepsis	+++	+++	0	+
Urinary tract infection	++++	0	0	+

[a] *From Blackburn GL, Menkes E. Surgical immunology. In: Chandra RK, ed. Primary and secondary immunodeficiency disorders. New York: Churchill Livingstone, 1983:263.*
[b] *These organisms when causing peritonitis, are almost always present in combination.*
[c] *In wounds after surgery on the large bowel.*

the small bowel, and in soft tissue crush and extremity avulsion injuries[98]. The need for large-scale prospective studies of this issue remains.

Major abdominal trauma may be either blunt or penetrating. The risks of bowel perforation are greater with penetrating injuries such as stabbings and gunshot wounds. With the exception of the urban adolescent population, blunt abdominal injuries predominate throughout most of childhood. Bowel perforation from blunt trauma occurs in approximately 15% of patients who have this type of injury[99]. The risk of perforation increases with greater force, focal trauma, or the presence of associated injuries, such as pelvic fractures, splenic disruption, or damage to retroperitoneal organs with associated hematoma. Antibiotics are generally administered and are usually effective in preventing wound infections or sepsis caused by a rupture. Septic complications are more likely when perforation occurs in the presence of pelvic fracture[97,100], localized hematoma, or hemorrhage[101].

Anaerobic and polymicrobial contamination must be considered when colonic contents have spilled into the abdominal cavity, which poses the greatest risk of subsequent abscess development. When colonic contamination is possible, recommended antibiotics are an aminoglycoside plus clindamycin to ensure coverage of mixed aerobic and anaerobic organisms. Alternatively, the combination of a third-generation cephalosporin plus clindamycin may also be used in this situation. Metronidazole also provides excellent anaerobic coverage, as do the newer, extended-spectrum penicillins, such as imipenem and ticarcillin-clavulinic acid[102]. Ampicillin provides effective coverage of enterococci and should be added when this organism is suspected.

An area of special interest to the pediatric intensive care specialist is the association of closed-head trauma with infection. Severe head injury may cause suppression of cell-mediated immunity, which may contribute to the 50 to 75% of patients with severe head injury who develop infectious complications, especially pneumonia[103]. Luckily, CNS infectious complications are rare in children[104]. Closed-head injuries with the potential for serious neurologic infection are those that result in disruption of the dura, leading to communication between the subarachnoid space and the ear, nose, or sinuses. Such a communication is known as a dural fistula and may be suspected by the finding of rhinorrhea or otorrhea following closed-head trauma[105–108]. In adults, posttraumatic meningitis has been reported in up to 25% of those with basilar skull fractures[109–111]. Organisms most frequently implicated are *S. pneumoniae* (50 to 90%), *H. influenzae* type b (9%), and other streptococcal species (10%), with other organisms such as *N. meningitidis* (5%), *S. aureus* (5%), *S. epidermidis* (2%), and enteric Gram-negative organisms (4%) accounting for only a very small percentage[112–117] (see **Table 28.6**).

Some adults have developed multiple or recurrent bouts of pneumococcal meningitis. There is a 10% mortality from posttraumatic meningitis. Eighty percent of dural fistulas in adults close spontaneously in the first seven days after injury[118]. Although some retrospective studies have demonstrated a lower incidence of meningitis in patients who received prophylactic antibiotics (approximately 5%)[110,119], this practice is not currently recommended[118,120,121]. When basilar skull fracture is accompanied by severe head injury that entails the use of invasive intracranial pressure monitoring, the scope of infections differs and is considered in Chapter 30.

Burns

The effects of severe thermal injury on immunity and infection are well described. Burns suppress all aspects of specific and nonspecific immune function[122]. Chemotaxis[123–128], opsonization, phagocytosis, and bacterial killing are all inhibited[129]. The complement cascade is activated, resulting in an increased concentration of degradation products, many of which are immunosuppressive[130]. Immunoglobulin levels are decreased[108,131,132], and blastogenesis and recruitment of lymphocytes are inhibited. There is inversion of the usual T-4 to T-8 subset ratio, resulting in an absolute deficiency of the T-helper

Table 28.6. Bacteriology of Posttraumatic Meningitis[a]

Organism	*% of Cases*
S. pneumoniae	65
Other streptococci	10
H. influenzae	9
N. meningitidis	5
S. aureus	5
Enteric gram-negatives	4
S. epidermidis	2

[a] *Adapted with permission from Hirschman JV. Bacterial meningitis following closed cranial trauma. In: Sande M, ed. Bacterial meningitis. New York: Churchill Livingstone, 1985:5. Data are from References 105, 113–117, 119.*

lymphocytes and relative prevalence of the T-suppressor line[122], which inhibits the production of specific antibody.

Massive release of prostaglandin E_2 (PGE_2) occurs in a sustained fashion following thermal injury, leading to activation of the arachidonic acid pathway and inhibition of lymphocyte proliferation. High concentrations of dietary lipids, especially of the Omega-6 series, may contribute to the development of postburn sepsis, by augmenting the plasma concentration of PGE_2 and prostacyclin[130].

Other nutritional factors may be important in determining a patient's likelihood to develop infection. Feeding by the enteral route is preferable to parenteral nutrition, because food in the gut can decrease the rate of organism and toxin translocation across the gastrointestinal tract. Arginine, as a nutritional factor, has been shown to influence postburn recovery through a variety of mechanisms[133]. It stimulates wound healing, potentially through its roles in the formation of nitric oxide (endothelium-derived relaxing factor) and by enhancing growth hormone secretion from the pituitary gland. Arginine has also been shown to be a direct immune modulator[133]. Large dietary supplements of arginine (500 mg/kg/day) are nontoxic[133]. It has been suggested that the enteral diet administered to burned children should contain 2% arginine[130]. Other proteins may have similar beneficial effects, and the diet should be relatively rich in protein as a source of calories[130].

Superimposed on the induced immunoincompetence following thermal injury is the excellent bacteriologic growth medium provided by the coagulated tissue and protein exudate in the burn wound. Colonization in the first five to seven days after injury is predominantly with gram-positive bacteria, followed thereafter by gram-negative hospital-acquired organisms[134]. Complete prevention of colonization is not possible; however, prevention of significant infection is of utmost importance, since the major cause of death among burn victims who survive initial fluid resuscitation is sepsis[135]. The cornerstone of prevention of burn wound sepsis is excellent wound care, with careful attention given to debridement of devitalized tissue and administration of local antimicrobials, such as silver sulfadiazine. Surveillance is important, with routine culturing of the burn wound in many health care centers performed by skin biopsy and reported quantitatively. In this situation, a bacterial count of greater than 105 organisms per gram of tissue is considered significant and worthy of parenteral antimicrobial therapy[136,137].

Because of the severity of infections caused by β-hemolytic streptococci in the early postburn period, standard practice in many burn centers had been prophylaxis with penicillin G for the first few days of hospitalization. However, several studies have failed to support such use of prophylactic antibiotics and have pointed out the risks that can accompany the practice. Therefore, the currently recommended course of action is to provide local antimicrobial coverage but to save the use of systemic antibiotics for documented or strongly suspected invasion[138–140]. For more specific recommendations regarding burn wound management, refer to Chapter 46.

As mentioned previously, the most frequently identified organisms in the early postburn period are gram-positive. These are predominantly *S. aureus,* with streptococci making up a slightly lower percentage. The β-hemolytic streptococci make up about 10 to 15% of all wound isolates in the first several days[134]. Of the gram-negative organisms that later colonize the wound, *Pseudomonas aeruginosa* and *E. coli* are the most prevalent. *Pseudomonas* infection can be particularly dangerous, because it has a propensity to further devitalize intact tissue and may convert a partial-thickness burn to a full thickness one. *Klebsiella, Enterobacter,* and other gram-negative organisms make up the remainder of the bacterial organisms implicated in infection of the burn wound. More recently recognized are fungal wound infections and sepsis, most commonly caused by *Candida albicans* or other *Candida* species. A list of burn wound pathogens is provided in **Table 28.7.** Control of nosocomial infection in the burn unit requires meticulous attention to and elimination of possible environmental sources, such as fresh vegetables, fruits and flowers, organisms carried on the hands or clothing of personnel or visitors, and moisture-laden patient care equipment. The mechanisms in place for prevention of infection in this situation are an extension of the general measures for nosocomial disease control in critical care settings, as discussed in Chapter 31. After identification of burn wound sepsis has been made by quantitative wound cultures, by recovery of the organism in the bloodstream, or from signs and symptoms of septicemia **(Table 28.8),** appropriate antibiotic therapy must be instituted and the other aspects of burn care continued. Some authors also recommend surgical excision of an infected burn wound[141].

Malnutrition

Malnutrition is a tremendous problem worldwide. It is most pronounced in the developing countries, but seriously undernourished children may be found in industrialized nations, including the United States. Malnutrition is a complication of many chronic diseases, such as cystic fibrosis and cancer. Serious secondary problems may

Table 28.7. Burn Wound Pathogens[a]

Organism	*% Patients from Whom Organism Recovered*
S. aureus	65–85
β-Hemolytic streptococcus	3–13
Other streptococci	38–65
P. aeruginosa	21–65
Klebsiella-Enterobacter	8–70
E. coli	30–60
Other gram-negatives	20–50
Candida sp.	12–75
C. albicans	18–55

[a] *Data are from Reference 134. Percentages are for the years 1970–1978 in 821 acutely burned patients at the Cincinnati Unit of the Shriner's Burns Institute.*

Table 28.8. Common Findings in Patients with Burn Wound Sepsis[a]

	S. aureus (Gram +)	*P. aeruginosa* (Gram −)	*C. albicans*
Wounds	Dissolution of granulation	Patchy black necrosis	Dry, flat, yellow-orange, granular
Course	Insidious, 2–6 days	Rapid, 12–36 hr	Chronic
Disorientation	Severe	Mild or absent	None
Temperature	Hypothermic	Hypothermic	Normal to low
White blood cell count	Usually increased	Usually depressed	Normal to increased
Ileus	Severe	Severe	Severe
Hypotension	Insidious, followed by oliguria	Sudden, with oliguria	None
Mortality (%)	0–5	20–30	30–40

[a] *From MacMillan BG. Infections following burn injury. Surg Clin North Am 1980;60:185.*

occur related to the nutritional deficiencies in malnourished children.

Studies aimed at elucidating the specific effects of malnutrition on the immune system have been confounded by a number of issues, including the presence of concurrent infections in the study populations as well as a failure to use precise definitions of types and degrees of malnutrition. Animal studies have also yielded conflicting results. In some cases, differences were related to the species; the rapidity with which malnutrition was induced; or whether protein, calories, or other nutrients were restricted or specific dietary components were withheld. Additionally, different microorganisms may have varying responses in the face of nutritional deficits and may actually cause more harm in a well-nourished host (especially malaria, see the following text).

The relatively extreme types of protein-calorie malnutrition (PCM), namely, marasmus (lack of protein *and* calories) and kwashiorkor (protein deficiency), primarily affect cell-mediated immunity[(142–148)]. Qualitatively, this is expressed by increased incidence of infections with the viral (especially measles and disseminated herpes virus[(149,150)]), fungal *(Candida)*, opportunistic organisms (*Pneumocystis carinii* [(151–153)]) and bacteria listed in **Table 28.9.** Children with kwashiorkor have very small thymus glands[(144,154)], with relative atrophy of lymph nodes and spleen[(155)], when compared with healthy controls from the same population. They have diminished tonsil size[(155)], and often they have an absolute lymphopenia. Nearly all such children show diminished percentage and absolute deficiency of T-lymphocytes. Evaluation with monoclonal antibodies has revealed this deficiency to rest mostly in the T-4 helper cell pool, which often is less then 40% of normal with a decreased helper/suppressor ratio[(156,157)]. Malnourished subjects exhibit diminished delayed cutaneous hypersensitivity reactions[(146,158)] and, in some cases, are totally anergic. The lymphocyte proliferation response has been reported to be diminished by some groups[(146,147,159)] and to be intact by others[(160,161)].

Table 28.9. Principal Infections in PCM[a]

Mycobacterium tuberculosis
Herpes simplex
P. carinii
Measles
Malaria
Diarrheal disease caused by strains of *E. coli, Shigella,* and rotaviruses
Schistosoma and other parasites
Staphylococcal pneumonia
Gram-negative urinary tract infection and bacteremia
Hepatitis B antigenemia

[a] *Modified with permission from Cunningham-Rundles S. Nutritional factors in immune response. In: Malnutrition: determinants and consequences. New York: Alan R. Liss, 1984:233.*

Appropriate nutritional support can convert a patient with abnormal delayed cutaneous hypersensitivity response from negative to positive status over a period of several weeks[(162)]. Animals with pure protein malnutrition lose the ability to generate a positive skin test to purified protein derivative (PPD), even though they have been sensitized to it by prior injection of complete Freund's adjuvant. When placed back on a regular diet, all regain sensitivity to PPD within two weeks. However, refeeding amino acids alone in the setting of protein malnutrition is not adequate, because studies have documented the need for refeeding with both protein and calories[(162)] to regain competence of the cellular immune system.

The phagocytic system is also adversely affected by PCM. Clinically this is represented by the high incidence of pyogenic and fungal infections of the skin, often in the absence of pus[(148)]. Chemotaxis is delayed[(163,164)], but a normal number of granulocytes will eventually migrate to the site of infection if given enough time. Bactericidal and fungicidal activity are also diminished, but opsonization appears to be intact[(165–167)].

The B-cell system is relatively spared in children with moderate PCM, in that the concentration of total immunoglobulins is often normal or elevated. When looked at in the absence of concurrent infection, however, levels of most immunoglobulins are lower than normal, although the levels of serum IgA are generally elevated[(168)]. Levels of secretory IgA mostly remain low, though, and this may help explain the finding of frequent respiratory and diarrheal disease, as well as the high incidence of antibodies to food antigens in these populations[(169–172)]. Seroconversion in malnourished children in response to immunization with diphtheria and tetanus toxoids is normal, as is response to pneumococcal polysaccharide and polio vaccines[(173–175)]. Chandra and colleagues[(175)] have found a reduced affinity of antibody for tetanus toxoid antigen following immunization and persistence of immune complexes in the malnourished host and postulate that these findings may be related to the clinically apparent increased susceptibility to disease. Response to some of the viral vaccines, such as yellow fever, measles, and influenzae A, is impaired, as is response to Bacille Calmette-Guerin (BCG)[176,177]. Serum levels of IgE are consistently elevated, presumably related to dysfunctional regulation by T-cell subsets, although this finding is frequently complicated by concurrent intestinal parasitism[148].

The study of malaria in malnourished subjects and in experimental animals has yielded some interesting findings. No unusual susceptibility to malaria has been noted among malnourished groups[178,179]. In fact, a higher percentage of the often fatal cerebral form of malaria has been reported among relatively well-nourished subjects[179,180]. Experimental mice who are protein deficient on both an acute and a chronic basis are more resistant to malarial infection and exhibit shorter episodes of parasitemia than their well-nourished counterparts[151,181]. Chronically malnourished animals who are then repleted and exposed to the parasite are relatively protected, and fewer animals die from the infection, compared with those who had never been nutritionally depleted. The mechanism of their protection may lie in the inability of the host's red blood cells to resist oxidant stress caused by the parasite[182–184]. The malnourished host undergoes more rapid lysis of red blood cells during infection, which also causes death of the microorganism. The duration of parasitemia is shortened, thereby providing relative protection for the host. Humans with glucose-6-phosphate dehydrogenase deficiency are also resistant to malarial infection because of a similar mechanism. Another potential mechanism of resistance to malaria among malnourished patients is from the anemia that accompanies PCM and deprives the parasite of required amounts of iron within the erythrocyte, a mechanism similar to the resistance seen among those with thalassemia. Repletion of the iron-deficient state worsens or precipitates malarial attacks[185–188].

In PICUs in the United States, the pediatric intensive care specialist is not as likely to see children with endogenous PCM but is certainly likely to see patients with acute malnutrition, usually caused by inadequate protein-calorie and nutrient intake over a period of days to weeks following surgery, trauma, or acute illness[189–191]. More chronically depleted children are those suffering from ongoing diseases such as malignancies, where both the underlying process and its therapy combine to impair nutritional reserves[192]. In most of these subjects, it is also difficult to separate the effects of the nutritional deprivation on the immune system from those of the cancer chemotherapy or other concurrent confounding variables. As regimens for parenteral nutrition become more firmly established in pediatric units, it is hoped that health care providers will see fewer iatrogenically starved children, and immune deficiency on this basis will become less frequent. A discussion of nutritional approaches in the critically ill child is found in Chapter 36. A summary of the effects of malnutrition on the various components of the immune system is provided in **Table 28.10**[193].

Treatment with Immunosuppressive Drugs

Children with a wide variety of underlying problems are treated with drugs that suppress numerous aspects of the immune system. The major categories of patients include children who have had organ transplants[194–196], those undergoing cancer chemotherapy or irradiation[197,198], and youngsters receiving systemic steroid preparations[199–201]. Although suppression of host immunity is essential for optimal outcome of organ transplantation, it obviously puts the patient at increased risk of infection[194]. Additionally, length of stay in the ICU or hospital environment, as well as the need for invasive monitoring devices and central venous catheters for parenteral nutrition, increases the risk of nosocomial infection. The concurrent findings of azotemia, chronic malnutrition, and performance of surgical procedures further increase these risks. Infected implants (especially cadaver kidneys) or blood products may lead to rejection caused by infection with cytomegalovirus (CMV) or other viral contaminants[195]. Humoral, cellular, and phagocytic systems are all impaired, and these patients are at risk to develop infections because of normally pathogenic bacteria as well as the classic opportunistic organisms[194,196]. Older patients may experience reactivation of tuberculosis infection. Latent herpes simplex viral infection often becomes symptomatic. The total body irradiation performed before bone marrow transplant further reduces the immunologic capacity of lymph nodes, thymus, and spleen. Many of the procedures also render these patients granulocytopenic, so that the nonspecific first line of defense against invading microorganisms is ablated.

Steroids

Administration of glucocorticoids is a ubiquitous practice for therapy of inflammatory, atopic, and autoimmune diseases. Steroids have widespread and mostly nonspecific effects on the immune system. Although they do not diminish serum antibody concentrations, they decrease the circulating pool of T lymphocytes by sequestering these cells in extravascular sites[199]. Steroids impair function of monocytes and adversely affect maturation of macrophages. This results in diminished antigen processing and presentation to lymphocytes for antibody production. Steroids reduce production of IL-1 and IL-2[202]. Monocytic killing of bacteria and fungi is inhibited, but not that of the granulocytes. Glucocorticoids primarily affect cell-mediated immunity resulting in relative anergy to cutaneous stimulation in patients receiving these preparations. Chemotaxis of polymorphonuclear leukocytes is inhibited, as is adherence of granulocytes to vascular endothelial surfaces. Many of the studies of glucocorticoid effects on immunity in humans have been contradictory, and studies in animals have been species specific and not representative of the human experience, since humans are apparently much more resistant to the effects of these agents than are most other animals[203]. Regardless of mechanism, patients receiving

Table 28.10. Immunodeficiency in PCM[a]

Parameter	*Humans*	*Animals*
Size of lymphoid organs	Thymus most affected, other lymphoid organs also reduced in size	Early deficiency leads to thymic atrophy and depressed spleen size
Morphology of thymus	In fatal kwashiorkor and marasmus, either acute involution or chronic atrophy, depletion of thymocytes	Decrease of cell density in both T- and B-cell areas, greatest loss in thymic-dependent areas
Morphology of spleen	Reduced germinal center activity: kwashiorkor and marasmus; depletion of paracortical, periarteriolar (thymus-dependent) areas in kwashiorkor	↓ In intracellular cAMP, spleen was most rapidly reconstituted following repletion
Morphology of lymph nodes	Depletion of paracortical areas in under-nourished children	Germinal center forming capacity of lymph node maintained; stem cells and nonmigratory T-cells most affected; regrowth delayed, but possible
Morphology of gut-associated lymphoid tissue (Peyer's patches), tonsillar	Size reduction: depletion of paracortical areas and germinal centers	Mesenteric lymph node less affected than thymus, attributed to antigenic stimulation from bacteria in gut
Humoral immune response: B-cell function	Serum immunoglobulin levels normal or increased; occasionally, IgE decreased	Absolute reduction in antibody-forming cells and antibody titers; intrinsic B-cell function relatively intact; increased response to T-dependent antigens has been reported
Humoral immune response: T-cell helper lymphocytes	Reduced as described in studies; reduced T-cell help may account for poor viral immunization	Marked depression of antigen-binding cells; diminished T-cell help leading to primary and secondary responses
Secretory antibody	Poor secretory IgA function after immunization; serum IgA normal; secretory IgA in tears and saliva reduced, IgG increased	Not studied
T-cell number	Depressed	Depressed
Delayed cutaneous hypersensitivity	Depressed secondary response; weaker response may be elicited with stronger dose; impaired primary response	Depressed primary and secondary responses
In vitro response to lymphocyte mitogens	Slight to severe depression reversible with nutritional repletion; some cases normal response	No effect; protein deprivation alone causes enhancement
Lymphokine production	Few studies, interferon production reduced in vitro	Interferon production decreased; protein alone increased; migration inhibitory factor production; depressed in PCM
Phagocytic cell function	Defective mononuclear cell chemotaxis, normal neutrophil chemotaxis in some studies, impaired killing demonstrated in some cases	Reduction of marrow neutrophil pool, reduced neutrophil mobility

[a] *From Cunningham-Rundles S. Effects of nutritional status on immunologic function. Am J Clin Nutr 1982;35:1202.*

glucocorticoids or ACTH are more susceptible to bacterial, viral, fungal, and parasitic diseases and have a diminished ability to localize infection. Because these agents are antipyretic, they may also help mask a febrile response in an infected patient, putting the child at risk for unrecognized progressive infection and possibly worsened morbidity. Evaluation of abdominal processes is also more difficult, because steroids may partially mask the development of peritonitis.

Other Immunosuppressive Agents

A number of other agents are used clinically in inducing or maintaining immunosuppression of organ transplant recipients and in treating episodes of rejection. The major effects and complications of these agents, other than those of infection, are listed in **Table 28.11.** For more detailed descriptions of actions, mechanisms, doses, and complications, the reader is referred to various reviews[202–206]. The appropriate use of any of these agents requires meticulous attention to all components of the patients' care. The intensive care specialist and immunologist must work in close collabo-

Table 28.11. Effects and Complications of Immunosuppressive Agents[a]

Agent	*Major Effects*	*Major Complications*
Cyclosporine	↓ IL-2 production ↓ γ-Interferon	Renal failure Systemic hypertension
Azathioprine	↓ Purine synthesis	Nausea, vomiting, diarrhea
	↓ RNA and DNA synthesis	↓ WBC, platelets
Antilymphocytic agents	Bind to T-cells or specific cell-surface antigens	Fever, chills, serum sickness, nausea, vomiting

[a] *Data from References 202, 204, 205.*

ration to optimize the desired immunosuppression that limits or treats rejection of the transplanted organ, but does not put the patient in jeopardy from overwhelming infection. The risks of acquiring or reactivating certain viral infections are high, and efforts must be made not to introduce new viral organisms. Blood products should be tested and should be negative for CMV. In addition to the agents listed in **Table 28.11**, a number of new agents have been evaluated in animals and humans and may provide additional, specific immunosuppression in the not-too-distant future.

Effects of Antimicrobial Agents on Immune Function

Antimicrobial agents are widely used in clinical medicine in general and used in ICU youngsters in particular. Information on the adverse effects of various agents on host immune function has been largely ignored. Reviews of this important and interesting topic may be found elsewhere[207,208]. **Table 28.12** presents some antibiotics and their primary effects on various components of the immune system. This information is presented for the sake of completeness, because it is not clear how significant such effects are on the actual ability of the host to resist clinical infection.

Effects of Viral, Bacterial, and Parasitic Infections on the Immune Response

A list of infectious agents and the presumed mechanisms by which they impair immune response is presented in **Table 28.13.** Interaction of infectious agents with various host factors is very complex, and in many cases, it is not at all clear how the infecting organism exerts its

Table 28.12. Effects of Antimicrobial Agents on Immune Function[a]

	Immune System Component		
Agent	*Phagocytes*	*T-cells*	*B-cells*
Antibacterials			
Aminoglycosides	? ↓ Chemotaxis, ? ↓ killing	No effect	Probably no effect
Cephalosporines	No effect on chemotaxis or killing at usual doses	No effect	Some may ↓ antibody production
Chloramphenicol	Variable effects on chemotaxis, ↓ respiratory burst	Variable, probably no effect	↓ Antibody production
Clindamycin	No effect on chemotaxis, variable effects on killing	↓ Lymphocyte transformation and proliferation at high doses	
Erythromycin	↓ Chemotaxis and migration, no effect on killing	↓ Lymphocyte transformation and proliferation at high doses	
Metronidazole		↓ Cell-mediated immunity	
Penicillins	No effect on chemotaxis or killing	No adverse effects	No adverse effects
Quinolones (Ciprofloxacin)	Probably no effect on chemotaxis	↓ Lymphocyte transformation (↓ IL-1 production)	
Rifampin	↓ Chemotaxis, variable effects on killing	↓ Lymphocyte transformation, delayed type hypersensitivity, and graft rejection	Variable effects on antibody production
Tetracyclines	↓ Chemotaxis, variable effects on phagocytosis	Most preparations ↓ lymphocyte transformation	↓ Antibody production
TMP-SMX	No effect on chemotaxis, ↓ respiratory burst	↓ Lymphocyte transformation, number and graft rejection	↓ Antibody production
Antifungals			
Amphotericin B	↓ Chemotaxis, respiratory burst, and phagocytosis	↓ Lymphocyte transformation, ? ↑ delayed type hypersensitivity	↓ Antibody production
Clotrimazole		↓ Lymphocyte transformation	
5-Fluorocytosine	No effect		
Griseofulvin	No effect		
Ketoconazole			
Miconazole	May ↓ chemotaxis	↓ Lymphocyte transformation	
Nystatin	No effect		
Antivirals			
Adenosine arabinoside			
Cytosine arabinoside		↓ Cell-mediated immunity	
Inosiplex		↑ Lymphocyte transformation	↑Antibody production
5-iodo-2′ deoxyuridine		↓ Cell-mediated immunity	
Ribavirin		↓ Skin graft rejection	↓ Antibody formation
Antiparasitics			
Chloroquine		↓ Lymphocyte transformation	
Primaquine		↓ Lymphocyte transformation	
Pyrimethamine		↑ Lymphocyte transformation	↑ Antibody production
Quinine		↓ Lymphocyte transformation	

[a] *Data from References 207 and 208. TMP-SMX = trimethoprim-sulfamethoxazole. Blank spaces indicate inadequate information available to determine effect of particular agent.*

Table 28.13. Effect of Various Microorganisms on Immune Function

Organism	*Effect on Immune System*
Bacteria[a]	
Pyogenic organisms	Dysfunctional granulocyte random locomotion, chemotaxis, bactericidal activity
Tuberculosis	T-cell dysfunction
Leprosy	T-cell dysfunction, abnormal T-cell macrophage interaction
Cholera	T-cell dysfunction due to elevated cAMP levels
Viruses[b]	
Acute Infection	
Measles	T-cell dysfunction, increased tuberculosis mortality, bacterial and herpes infections
Epstein-Barr virus	Hypergammaglobulinemia, T-cell depression, abnormal T- and B-cell interaction
Rubella	T-cell dysfunction
Mumps	Unclear
Congenital Infections[b]	
Rubella	Dysgammaglobulinemia, specific antibody responses, T-cell dysfunction
CMV	↑ IgM, persistent viral excretion
Hepatitis B	Unclear
Parasites[c]	
Malaria	Altered antibody responses, variable effects on cell-mediated immunity
Trypanosomes	Impaired antibody responses T-cell dysfunction
Toxoplasmosis	T- and B-cell dysfunction
Shistosomiasis	T- and B-cell dysfunction

[a] *See Reference 22.*
[b] *See Reference 209.*
[c] *See Reference 210.*

detrimental effect on host defenses. The reader is referred to various sources for specific information[209–211]. The effects of HIV infection are considered separately in detail in Chapter 29.

Asplenia

Absence of the spleen, whether anatomic or functional, predisposes the young child to potentially fatal sepsis from encapsulated bacterial species[212–217]. The most prevalent offender is the pneumococcus in 50% of cases. *H. influenzae* type b, meningococcus, and group A Streptococci account for 25%. *S. aureus, Pseudomonas,* and other gram-negatives have also been implicated. Infants with congenital asplenia usually have associated complex cardiac defects, and the presence of Howell-Jolly bodies on the blood smear is generally detected early in their evaluation. Some babies have isolated absence of the spleen, and these infants may present within the first few months of life with overwhelming sepsis resulting from *S. pneumoniae* or *H. influenzae*[218].

The largest group of children with defective splenic function are homozygotes for sickle cell disease. In these patients, the spleen generally becomes dysfunctional during early childhood. The earlier this phenomenon occurs, the more severe the resulting immune defect and the greater the risk for bacterial sepsis. Children less than 3 years of age with absent or dysfunctional spleens are at greatest risk to develop overwhelming infections, although the increased risk of sepsis is lifelong[219].

Studies aimed at evaluating risk factors secondary to asplenia have been performed in otherwise healthy surgically splenectomized children to avoid the confounding problems with coincident immune dysfunction. In this population, the incidence of postsplenectomy fatal sepsis is approximately 2%, compared with a rate of 0.7% in children with intact spleens[214]. The long-term outcome is more favorable for patients undergoing splenectomy for trauma rather than hematologic (thrombocytopenia, hereditary spherocytosis) or malignant (lymphoma) reasons. Of trauma patients, 22 to 68% are found to have splenosis, small nodules of spleen on the omentum or serosa of the bowel that grow from viable spleen cells that dissociate from the spleen during trauma[217,220]. Although the actual incidence of septic episodes in splenectomized patients is not known, it is fatal to an estimated 50 to 70% of children in this population once sepsis occurs[216,217]. Symptoms of postplenectomy sepsis are rapid in onset and include a brief, influenzalike prodrome with fever, malaise, myalgia, headache, and vomiting. Massive bacteremia with septic shock and DIC quickly ensues with death usually occurring in 24 to 48 hours. Bacteremia is so overwhelming that bacteria may be visualized in the buffy coat.

The therapeutic approach to splenectomized patients is multifactorial. There is general agreement that immunization of asplenic patients with pneumococcal vaccine should be performed. Timing is crucial, however, and when possible, this should be accomplished at least two weeks before surgical splenectomy. Of course, this is impossible with congenital asplenia and sickle-cell disease. Additionally, as noted previously, children who are less than 2 years of age have a poor response to pure polysaccharide vaccines, so immunization at a young age is not feasible. When immunization is performed, there is an uneven response to each of the components of the pneumococcal vaccine, leading to immunity of some strains and not to others in any individual subject[213]. There are 23 pneumococcal types represented in the current vaccine, which cover approximately 90% of the strains responsible for infection in adults. The types most often responsible for childhood disease are 14, 6, 18, 19, 23, 4, 9, 7, 1, and 3[221]. Of these, types 6, 18, and 7 are *not* covered by the vaccine. However, the vaccine does cover those strains most likely to cause severe disease, such as sepsis and meningitis.

The issue of prophylactic antibiotics has not been totally resolved because of the diversity of patient groups in which splenic dysfunction occurs and because of the difficulty in performing randomized prospective studies in this area. Splenectomized mice treated with penicillin prior to challenge with pneumococci have a better outcome than those who do not receive the antimicrobial agent[222]. Subjectively, children given continuous penicillin therapy also seem to do better, although postsplenectomy deaths because of organisms resistant to the antibiotic have been reported in prophylactically treated subjects[223]. Although penicillin prophylaxis has become routine among a number of groups[224], others have suggested that prompt administration of antibiotics with any febrile illness will more reliably reduce the percentage of fatal episodes[213]. The recommended prophylaxis regimen is 250 mg/day of oral penicillin G or V. In children under the age of five years, this amount is given in two divided doses[221]. Although some health care centers choose to discontinue prophylaxis in patients with sickle-cell disease at about age 6, others continue therapy into adulthood. Whether prophylaxis is used, patients with asplenia or hyposplenia should be informed to seek medical attention immediately for any signs of infection. With early intervention, mortality from sepsis may be decreased to 10%[217].

Regardless of ambulatory practice, the sick, febrile, asplenic child who is admitted to the PICU will require coverage for the encapsulated bacteria *(S. pneumoniae, N. meningitidis,* and *H. influenzae)* as well as the pyogenic pathogens most likely to cause infection *(Staphylococcus* and *Streptococcus).* Because patients with sickle-cell anemia also have an opsonization defect, they may benefit from transfusion, exchange transfusions, or administration of fresh frozen plasma in addition to antimicrobial therapy[213]. Recent surgical studies, which have revealed a good prognosis of blunt abdominal trauma with associated splenic injury when the spleen is left in situ, have helped reduce the number of children who are at risk for postsplenectomy sepsis by encouraging pediatric surgeons to leave the spleen intact whenever possible[211].

PRIMARY OR CONGENITAL IMMUNODEFICIENCY DISORDERS

The following is a brief discussion of the primary immunodeficiency diseases, so called because of their congenital or hereditary nature. Although there are a great number of these diseases, they do not occupy much space in this chapter. Thorough descriptions and reviews are provided in the standard immunology textbooks. They are included here for the sake of completeness and to emphasize their importance in the intensive-care setting. These problems are seen predominantly in children because most tend to impair longevity. They affect all aspects of the immune system. Classification and relative frequency of the primary immunodeficiency diseases are presented in **Table 28.14,** and the characteristic clinical features common to the majority of such illnesses, regardless of classification, are presented in **Table 28.15.** A summary of the diseases discussed in this chapter can be found by consulting **Table 28.16.**

In the text, emphasis has been placed on those disorders of greatest importance to the pediatric intensive care specialist.

Table 28.14. Classification and Frequency of the Primary Immunodeficiencies[a]

	Approximate % of Total
Antibody (B-cell) immunodeficiencies	50
Secretory IgA immunodeficiency	<1
Cellular (T-cell) immunodeficiencies	40
With antibody immunodeficiencies	30
Isolated cellular immunodeficiency	10
Phagocytic immunodeficiencies	6
Mononuclear phagocytic immunodeficiency	<1
Complement immunodeficiencies	4

[a] *From Stiehm ER: Immunodeficiency disorders—General considerations. In: Stiehm ER. Fulginiti VA, eds. Immunologic Disorders in Infants and Children. Philadelphia: WB Saunders, 1980:183.*

Table 28.15. Clinical Features in Primary Immunodeficiencies[a]

Usually present
1. Recurrent upper respiratory infections
2. Repeated severe bacterial infections (e.g., pneumonia, meningitis, and sepsis)
3. Failure to thrive

Frequently present
1. Chronic diarrhea
2. Pallor and irritability
3. Sinusitis
4. Draining ears, mastoiditis
5. Skin lesions (e.g., rash, pyoderma, alopecia, eczema, and telangiectasia)
6. Thrush
7. *P. carinii* infection
8. Malabsorption
9. Chronic pneumonitis or bronchiectasis
10. Paucity of lymph nodes and tonsils

Occasionally present
1. Chronic conjunctivitis
2. Lymphadenopathy
3. Hepatosplenomegaly
4. Severe viral disease
5. Arthritis
6. Hematologic abnormalities (e.g., leukocytosis, leukopenia, thrombocytopenia, and hemolytic anemia)

[a] *Modified from Stiehm ER: Immunodeficiency disorders—General considerations. In: Stiehm ER. Fulginiti VA, eds. Immunologic Disorders in Infants and Children. Philadelphia: WB Saunders, 1980:183.*

Immunodeficiency Disorders Primarily Affecting Immunoglobulins

X-Linked Agammaglobulinemia

X-linked agammaglobulinemia (XLA) was originally known as Bruton's agammaglobulinemia, and in 1952, was the first immunodeficiency disease to be described[225]. The gene for XLA was recently identified and mapped to the long arm of the X chromosome at Xq22. The gene codes for a protein, Bruton's tyrosine kinase (Btk), necessary for maturation of pre-B cells[226,227]. Deletions and point mutations of this gene have been detected in patients with XLA[228]. Trans-

Table 28.16. Summary of Primary Immune Deficiency Disorders

Category	*Name*	*Type of Deficiency*	*Prenatal Dx Available?*	*Predominant Organisms*	*Usual Sites*	*Treatment*	*Complications and Associated Findings*
Humoral	1. X-linked agammaglobulinemia	Absent or low immunoglobulins	Yes	Enteroviruses, pyogenic bacteria	Respiratory, GI, meninges	IVIG, specific antibiotics for infections, ? gene replacement therapy	Respiratory failure, CEMA, overwhelming sepsis, diarrhea
	2. Common variable agammaglobulinemia	Low but variable immunoglobulins		Enteroviruses, pyogenic bacteria	Respiratory, GI	IVIG and specific antibiotics for infections	T-cell abnormalities in 50%, malabsorption
	3. Transient hypogammaglobulinemia	Low levels of immunoglobulins until age 4 yr	No specific suseptibilities		Respiratory	None	None
	4. Selective IgA deficiency	Secretory and serum IgA		Encapsulated bacteria, viruses	Respiratory tract, mucous membranes	Antibiotics for documented infection	Autoimmune disease common
	5. Selective IgM deficiency	Serum IgM		Gram-negative bacteria	Respiratory, meninges	Antibiotics for documented infection	Allergies, splenomegaly, malignancies
	6. Selective IgG deficiency	Specific subclasses of IgG (IgG 2 most common)		Encapsulated bacteria	Respiratory, meninges	Antibiotics for documented infection, IVIG, ? prophylactic antibiotics	Overwhelming infection possible
	7. Hyper IgM	IgA and IgG, IgM, cyclic neutropenia	Yes	Pyogenic bacteria, *P. carinii*	Respiratory	Antibiotics for specific infection, IVIG	Oral ulcers, autoimmune diseases
Cellular	1. DiGeorge syndrome	Thymic hypoplasia, absence of mature T-cells	Yes	Viruses, fungi, *P. carinii*	Respiratory, GI, skin	TMP-SMX, fetal thymic transplantation, ? BMT	Hypoparathyroidism, congenital heart disease
	2. Chronic mucocutaneous candidiasis	Defect in cell-mediated response to candidal antigen		*Candida*	Skin, scalp, nails, mucous membranes	Antifungal therapy	Endocrinopathy, liver failure, adrenal insufficiency
Combined disorders	1. Severe combined immunodeficiency disease (SCID)	Dysplastic thymus, lymphopenia, cutaneous anergy, low or absent immunoglobulins	Yes	*P. carinii*, CMV, *Candida*, all bacteria	Respiratory, mucous membranes, liver, GI, systemic sepsis	BMT, ? enzyme replacement	Often fatal by age 2 yr, adenosine deaminase deficiency
	2. Wiskott-Aldrich	Eczema, thrombocytopenia, IgA and IgE, IgM, B-cells, T-cells and macrophages	Yes	Encapsulated bacteria, viruses, fungi	Respiratory and systemic	Antibiotics for documented infection, IVIG, ? BMT	Petechiae, bleeding, hepatosplenomegaly, arthritis, malignancies
	3. Ataxia telangiectasia	IgA and IgG 2, cutaneous anergy		Viruses, fungi, various bacteria	Respiratory, sinuses	Antibiotics for documented infection, IVIG for IgG 2	Malignancies, muscle weakness
	4. Reticular dysgenesis	Absent T-cells, B-cells, and granulocytes		All bacteria, fungi, and viruses	Systemic sepsis, respiratory, GI	?BMT, ? granulocyte transfusions	Rapidly fatal
	5. Short-limbed dwarfism	Combined but variable, T-cell defect predominant	Yes	Viral, esp. varicella	Skin	VZIG for varicella, IVIG	Variable
	6. Cartilage-hair hypoplasia	Combined but variable, T-cell defect predominant		Viral, esp. varicella	Respiratory, systemic	?	?
Phagocyte	1. Chronic granulomatous disease (CGD)	Oxidative burst and bactericidal activity	Yes	Catalase-positive bacteria, fungi	Respiratory, mucous membranes, bone	Prophylactic TMP-SMX, γ-interferon, antimicrobial therapy	Death in second or third decade
	2. Chediak-Higashi syndrome	Abnormal degranulation		Pyogenic bacteria	Respiratory, skin	Ascorbic acid, folate	Lymphoma-like syndrome, thrombocytopenia, bleeding, albinism
	3. Glucose-6-phosphate dehydrogenase (G6PD) deficiency	Abnormal bactericidal function	Yes	Catalase-positive bacteria, fungi	Respiratory, mucous membranes, bone	Antibiotics for documented infection	Usually not very severe
	4. Myeloperoxidase deficiency	Abnormal bactericidal function		*Candida*, bacteria *(Staphylococcus)*	Respiratory, skin	Antibiotics for documented infection	Usually mild
	5. Hyperimmunoglobulin E syndrome	chemotaxis, IgE, T-cell and B-cell dysfunction		*Staphylococcus*, *Streptococcus*	Skin	Antibiotics for documented infection, ? chronic antistaphylococcal therapy	Job syndrome (chronic dermatitis)
	6. Cyclic neutropenia	Bone marrow production of PMNs and RBCs		Pyogenic bacteria	Skin, mucous membranes, lymphadenopathy, periodontal	ACTH, steroids	Usually nonfatal
	7. Severe congenital neutropenia	Maturation defect		Pyogenic bacteria	Sepsis, respiratory, skin	BMT	Almost always fatal
Complement	1. Hereditary angioedema	C1-esterase deficiency		*No* increased susceptibility to infection	NA	NA	Airway obstruction
	2. C1, 4, 2, C3	Opsonization and phagocytosis		Encapsulated and pyogenic bacteria	Sepsis, skin, meninges	Antibiotics for specifc infections	Autoimmune diseases
	3. C5–9	Membrane attack complex		*Neisseria* species and other gram-negatives	Sepsis, meninges	Antibiotics for specific infections	Autoimmune diseases
Asplenia	1. Congenital asplenia	Splenic absence		Encapsulated bacteria, pyogenic bacteria	Sepsis, bones, respiratory	Immunization, prophylactic antibiotics, specific antimicrobial therapy	Fewer problems in adulthood

mitted as an X-linked recessive with full penetrance[227,228], XLA occurs with an estimated incidence of 1 in 50,000 to 1 in 150,000[229,230]. The clinical course is variable, depending on the specific mutation[229]. Boys affected with XLA have profoundly decreased serum immunoglobulins, less than 10% of normal, and no antigen specific antibody to any antigen[226]. Plasma cells, germinal centers, and follicle formation are all absent from lymphoid tissue. The tonsils are usually absent or hypoplastic[231]. The underlying immunologic defect is an arrest of B-lymphocyte differentiation, resulting in less than one percent of normally 5 to 15% circulating lymphocytes in the form of B cells[226]. Circulating T lymphocytes appear functionally normal, although isolated instances of abnormal cell-mediated immunity have been described[232,233]. Clinical presentation of disease, represented by recurrent infections with extracellular pyogenic organisms such as pneumococci, streptococci, meningococci, *H. influenzae*, and *P. aeruginosa*, does not usually occur until the nadir of maternally acquired immunoglobulins is reached, at approximately 6 to 9 months of extrauterine life. Common infections include pneumonia, bronchitis, sinusitis, otitis media, pyoderma, osteomyelitis and sepsis[234,235]. *Pneumocystis carinii* pneumonia has been noted to occur occasionally[235]. If environmental exposures are limited, infections may not become a problem until 2 years of age or later. Although onset of symptoms peaks at 7 months, 40% of boys are asymptomatic at 1 year and 21% present at 3 to 5[236]. Identification of the immunodeficiency is typically made in the third of fourth year of life[237]. Because T-cell function is usually intact, most fungi and viruses are handled normally[238]. However, an increased susceptibility to recurrent enteroviral infections (polio, echo virus) has been noted[239,240], suggesting that the response to these viruses requires the presence of specific neutralizing antibody.

The syndrome of chronic enteroviral meningoencephalitis of agammaglobulinemia (CEMA) has been well described[232]. Since routine treatment of XLA with intravenous immunoglobulin (IVIG) in the early 1980s, the incidence of CEMA has been greatly reduced but not eradicated[241]. Patients with CEMA typically present with a neurologic syndrome slowly progressive in nature. Although some patients have an onset characterized by fever, headache, and seizures, most present in a subacute fashion with lethargy, ataxia, and loss of cognitive skills. Many patients have an associated dermatomyositislike syndrome (DLS), probably related to viral dissemination, and typified by edema and erythematous rashes of the extremities, muscle weakness, and contractures. Some children may also have signs and symptoms of other organ involvement, especially the liver. Although a few patients have been successfully treated (see next section), the majority of individuals with CEMA have an intermittent but chronic course, in many cases leading to severe neurologic impairment or death.

The diagnosis should be considered in a child with XLA who presents with neurologic symptoms and no other obvious etiology. In some cases, the onset of CEMA has preceded the recognition of the immune defect, so a child with persistent meningoencephalitis should be evaluated for possible hypogammaglobulinemia. Mild CSF pleocytosis is nearly always present, with the usual CSF WBC under 1000 cells/mm^3, although much higher values have been reported[232]. Differential evaluation of the WBCs generally reveals a lymphocyte predominance. Protein levels are usually elevated, and glucose concentrations are diminished.

Treatment has not been universally successful, but consists of IVIG administration aimed at maintaining a higher level of IgG (troughs of 900 to 1000 mg/dl) than is typical for the general care of these children (trough values of 400 mg/dl are generally sufficient). Because the most common strains of echovirus implicated in CEMA are also the most prevalent in the population at large (serotypes 9, 11, and 30), most preparations of IVIG will contain sufficient neutralizing antibody. If the viral isolate is an unusual strain, it is valuable to test the preparation for neutralizing capability against the patient's virus. Because very little of the systemically administered immunoglobulin crosses the blood-brain barrier, a number of these children has been treated with adjunctive intraventricular immunoglobulin, with cure reported in a few cases. Even if the virus is not totally eradicated, the combined systemic and intraventricular administration of antibody seems to aid the abatement of symptoms and limits the episodes of dissemination.

Poliovirus is also an enterovirus and likewise may cause devastating effects in children with XLA. Live polio vaccine, therefore, should not be administered. Unfortunately, since most cases of XLA are not identified in infancy, the majority of sporadic cases will have received their primary immunizations prior to diagnosis. Since the poliovirus is excreted in the stool, the live vaccine should also be withheld from other members of the family.

Chronic respiratory infections and failure to thrive occur in many affected children. Increased longevity and better growth have been achieved by treating these children with IVIG, which has been documented to be superior to intramuscular γ-globulin[242]. Peak serum levels of immunoglobulin correlate with the dose administered, but clearance appears to be related to the preparation, concentration, and individual patient variation. Prophylactic regimens consisting of monthly injections of anywhere between 100 mg/kg and 600 mg/kg have been recommended[242]. High dose IVIG (350 to 600 mg/kg every 3 weeks) has been shown to decrease number of hospital days and decrease severe pulmonary infections. An additional dose may be administered with signs of acute serious infection. Commonly available preparations of IVIG contain primarily IgG. For raising the level of IgA or IgM in these patients, infusions of fresh frozen plasma may be of help[243]. It is given at a dose of 15 to 20 ml/kg intravenously every 3 weeks. Some patients continue to have problems with respiratory infections, since secretory IgA remains deficient despite therapy with IVIG and plasma, and chronic pulmonary disease and respiratory failure often result from the bronchiectasis caused by recurrent pneumonia and sinusitis. Antibiotic usage should be reserved for instances where infections arise, despite prophylactic passive immunotherapy. Without treatment, patients typically die before 5 years of age[228]. With current treatment, most patients die of pulmonary failure in the third decade[227].

Carriers of XLA have normal immunoglobulin levels and normal numbers of B cells. They can be detected because of nonrandom X chromosome inactivation leading to selective growth of B cells possessing the normal X chromosome[244,245]. Prenatal diagnosis is possible by linkage analysis using restriction fragment length polymorphisms or, more recently, polymerase chain reaction[226].

Common Variable Agammaglobulinemia

Common Variable Immunodeficiency (CVID) is an acquired hypogammaglobulinemia mostly sporadic in nature although familial cases have been observed[246]. Some pedigrees have been observed to include members affected with either CVID or IgA deficiency, suggesting a common genetic basis[235]. The incidence of CVID is approximately 1 per 100,000 and although clinically similar to XLA, it is usually not clinically apparent until the second or third decade, and males and females are equally affected[246]. The immunologic findings in CVID include hypogammaglobulinemia with normal numbers of B cells that do not differentiate into plasma cells, resulting in impaired antibody responses. Also, defective T-cell immunity is found in 50% of patients[247]. Patients with CVID are susceptible to the same array of organisms and infections as patients with XLA and, as in XLA, bronchiectasis is a frequent complication of untreated disease[247]. CVID is complicated by autoimmune disorders in 20% of patients (hemolytic anemia, thrombocytopenia, pernicious anemia, thyroid disease), gastrointestinal disorders including diarrhea often from *Giardia lamblia* infection, ulcerative colitis, Crohn's disease, malabsorption and a 50-fold increased risk of gastric carcinoma, and a 30 to 200 fold increased risk for non-Hodgkin's lymphoma[234]. Therapy of this disease is similar to that of XLA, namely, immunoglobulin replacement.

Transient Hypogammaglobulinemia of Infancy

Some infants exhibit an exaggerated hypogammaglobulinemia when maternal antibodies wane, and their intrinsic production is delayed[238,248]. Unlike patients with XLA, they have intact ability to produce specific antibody. Most children with transient hypogammaglobulinemia of infancy (THI) recover normal immunoglobulin levels by 4 years of age although in some cases, resolution of hypogammaglobulinemia has been replaced by selective IgA deficiency[249,250]. It has been suggested that this disorder be renamed hypogammaglobulinemia of early childhood with either recovery or with development of other dysgammaglobulinemia[250]. Patients with this entity usually have a benign clinical course with recurrent upper respiratory infections. IVIG is usually not indicated unless severe infections occur and may delay spontaneous recovery of immunoglobulin production[250]. THI may be associated with atopic disease and food intolerances[251].

Selective IgA Deficiency

Selective IgA deficiency is the most common primary immunodeficiency with a frequency of 1 in 400 to 1 in 2000[252]. Although most cases are sporadic, there may be a familial association[253]. Although one-half to two-thirds of patients are asymptomatic[247,234] the remainder have mild recurrent infections of the respiratory, gastrointestinal, and genitourinary tract with encapsulated bacteria. This disorder is associated with an increased incidence of autoimmune, atopic, and malignant disorders. It has been associated with the use of phenytoin, sulfasalazine, penicillamine, and gold[254] and has also occasionally been linked to abnormalities of chromosome 18 in mentally retarded individuals[252,253]. IgA levels are usually <50 mg/dl although severe cases may be <5 mg/dl, and IgG levels are usually elevated because of recurrent infections[253]. IVIG is not used for treatment. IVIG contains only small amounts of IgA, which is not conferred to mucosal surfaces. In addition, 30 to 40% of these patients have antibodies to IgA that may result in anaphylaxis when administered blood products containing IgA[247]. When red blood cell or other component therapy is required, the blood should be frozen and washed or ideally should be obtained from an IgA-deficient donor.

Selective IgM Deficiency

Selective IgM deficiency is much less common. Patients with this disorder have IgM levels less than 20 mg/100 ml and usually have no other immune abnormalities. Affected children are susceptible to recurrent bacterial infections, mostly with gram-negative organisms, including *N. meningitidis*[255,256]. They may present with repetitive episodes of meningitis. Splenomegaly, allergic disorders, and malignancies of the reticuloendothelial system have been reported[257]. IgM deficiency has been associated with Bloom syndrome resulting from a failure of surface IgM positive B cells to mature into IgM secreting cells[258].

Selective IgG Deficiency

Isolated deficiency of IgG and IgG subclasses have been described. Low levels of total serum IgG are usually associated with hypercatabolism of IgG in patients with myotonic dystrophy[259]. There are four IgG subclasses. IgG1 (70%) and IgG3 (6%) are antibodies to protein antigens such as tetanus and diphtheria toxoids. IgG2 (20%) and IgG4 (4%) are antibodies to polysaccharide antigens such as pneumococcus and the A and B blood group antigens or isoglutinins[260]. Children with suspected immunodeficiency should have IgG subclasses quantitated, even if their total IgG level is normal or increased[261]. IgG2 deficiency is the most well-defined subclass deficiency. It is associated with recurrent upper and lower respiratory tract disease, otitis media, sinusitis, chronic lung symptoms, impaired lung function, and invasive disease with *S. pneumoniae* and *H. influenzae*[262]. Patients with chronic asthma, especially if steroid dependent or accompanied by recurrent sinopulmonary infections or bronchiectasis, deserve evaluation for IgG subclass deficiency. IgG subclass deficiency, especially IgG2, may be combined with IgA deficiency in which the risk of lung damage may be increased[263]. It is important to note that IgG2 and IgG4 levels mature late and may be low in children less than 2 years old[260]. Healthy individuals exist with decreased IgG2 who are able to produce antibody response to carbohydrate antigen[247]. Patients for whom treatment for IgG subclass deficiency is being considered should demonstrate not only low levels of that subclass but also an inability to respond to appropriate antigen. For IgG1 and IgG3 deficiencies, response to tetanus and diphtheria vaccine should be evaluated. For IgG2 and IgG4 deficiencies, response to pneumococcal vaccine in patients over 2 years and blood agglutinin titers in patients less than 2 years (except, of course, patients who are of AB blood group) should be evaluated. Treatment consists of IVIG in patients with severe infections, IgG subclass deficiency, and inability to respond to appropriate antigens[260]. Patients with IgG2 deficiency should receive conjugate vaccines and may need multiple doses to document an adequate response.

Immunoglobulin Deficiency with Increased IgM Levels

Elevated levels of IgM associated with IgA and IgG deficiency is a rare syndrome that is usually X-linked but may be autosomal dominant or autosomal recessive in inheritance[264]. In the X-linked form, a mutation occurs in the gene that codes for the membrane protein CD40 ligand on T cells. This protein is responsible for sequential switch of B-cell immunoglobulin production[265,266]. Patients usually become symptomatic at 1 to 2 years with recurrent pyogenic infections. It is associated with autoimmune phenomena (hemolytic anemia, thrombocytopenia, and neutropenia) and lymphoproliferative diseases, especially lymphoma of the gastrointestinal tract. Fifty percent of patients have hepatosplenomegaly. When treated with IVIG, IgM levels decrease and lymphoid hyperplasia resolves[247]. Patients are susceptible to opportunistic infections such as PCP, cryptococcus, and CMV. PCP often occurs in the first year of life[264,267]; therefore, all patients should be on PCP prophylaxis.

Immunodeficiencies Primarily Affecting T-Cell Function

DiGeorge Syndrome

The most widely recognized disease characterized by deficiency of cell-mediated immunity in infancy is the DiGeorge syndrome (DGS). This syndrome was described by DiGeorge in 1965[268], although the association of absent thymus, seizures, and abnormalities of the third and fourth pharyngeal pouches has been described by Harrington in 1829[269]. The complete syndrome includes thymic aplasia, parathyroid aplasia with hypocalcemia possibly leading to seizures, and a conotruncal cardiac defect[270]. Patients with partial DGS have less severe disease manifestations. Some patients undergo spontaneous restoration of T-cell function[271,272]. Facial features associated with DGS include hypertelorism, micrognathia, low-set ears, and a fish shaped mouth[234,273]. DGS has been associated with maternal diabetes, alcoholism, isotretinoin usage, and most recently, deletion or unbalanced translocation of a portion of chromosome 22, 22q11[247,273]. Using cytogenetic analysis with high-resolution banding, 25% of patients with DGS have visible lesions at chromosome 22q11[274]. With molecular analysis using DNA probes that flank the DGS gene, monosomy is found in 95% of DGS patients[275]. Velo-cardio-facial syndrome (VCFS) clinically overlaps DGS, suggesting the gene for VCFS may overlap or occur within the DGS gene region[276]. Cytogenetic and molecular studies of VCFS patients have revealed that 76% have deletions at chromosome 22q11[274]. Using molecular studies on patients with isolated conotruncal cardiac defects, 29% have been found to have deletions at 22q11[277]. Since this confers a 50% risk to offspring, molecular analysis of patients with these defects is crucial to provide genetic counseling. The most common cardiac anomalies in DGS in order of prevalence are interrupted aortic arch type B (IAA type B), persistent truncus arteriosis (PTA), tetralogy of Fallot (TOF), right aortic arch, ventricular septal defect, and patent ductus arteriosis. Of all patients with IAA type B, 68% have DGS. Of all patients with PTA and TOF, 33% and 2% respectively have DGS[278]. The congenital heart disease and hypoparathyroidism in DGS are often more clinically significant than the immunodeficiency. Those patients who manifest the immunodeficiency are most susceptible to viral and fungal infections and have chronic rhinorrhea, pneumonia, skin lesions, and diarrhea. They are also prone to develop infections with *P. carinii.* Prophylaxis against the later pathogen with TMP-SMX is recommended. The common childhood viral infections, such as varicella and measles, may prove rapidly fatal and usually noninvasive gut bacteria may cause disease requiring critical care. Therapy of the immune dysfunction with implanted (intramuscular or intraperitoneal) thymus of a 10-week-old to 14-week-old fetus is recommended[279,280]. Beyond age 14 weeks, the fetal thymus is capable of graft-versus-host disease, and therefore, the younger glands are preferable. Once reconstitution is achieved (6 hours to 4 days later), it appears to be permanent, and cellular immunity usually remains intact. Implantations of fetal thymic epithelium[281] and fetal thymus encased in a Millipore filter[282] have also been reportedly successful. More recently, use of thymic factors[272] and bone marrow transplant (BMT)[283,284] have been presented as viable options in DGS.

The pediatric intensive care specialist may first consider the diagnosis of DGS when confronted with a baby with a conotruncal cardiac defect who develops hypocalcemia with tetany and seizures. In patients with suggestive cardiac lesions or DGS type facies, serum calcium should be checked to avoid complications of untreated hypocalcemia. Use of irradiated blood products is imperative any time DGS is suspected to avoid graft-versus-host disease[270].

Immunodeficiency Disorders Involving Both B- and T-Cell Function

Severe Combined Immunodeficiency Disease

Several types of severe combined immunodeficiency (SCID) have been described. These include (1) reticular dysgenesis in which lymphoid, myeloid as well as erythroid precursor differentiation is impaired (autosomal recessive); (2) absence of T-lymphocyte and B-lymphocyte differentiation or alymphocytosis (autosomal recessive, designated T-B−); (3) the most frequent type of SCID, absence of T-cell differentiation (X-linked or autosomal recessive, designated T-B+); (4) adenosine deaminase (ADA) deficiency, found in 50% of those with autosomal recessive SCID; and (5) Omenn syndrome with oligoclonal T cells and eosinophilia[285]. ADA is an enzyme used in the purine salvage pathway. When deficient, metabolites accumulate which are toxic to T lymphocytes[286]. Fifty percent of patients with ADA SCID have osseous abnormalities, including cupping and flaring of the anterior costochondral junction (rachitic rosary) and pelvic dysplasia[287]. Purine nucleoside phosphorylase (PNP) is the next enzyme in the purine salvage pathway, and deficiency leads to similar immune manifestations[287].

The incidence of SCID is 1 in 100,000 to 1 in 150,000[285]. The first symptoms develop on average by 5 weeks of age with first hospitalization by 4 months[288]. Because of maternal T-cell engraftment, up to 50% of newborns will have mild GVHD with erythema, diarrhea, hepatitis, and eosinophilia. Clinically, patients with SCID present a significant challenge in terms of preventing and treating life-threatening infections. The course is one of chronic and sometimes progressive pulmonary disease, often with *P. carinii* or CMV pneumonia. Resistant oral candidiasis, sometimes associated with esophagitis and skin involvement, is most frequently encountered. The chronic diarrhea often becomes life-threatening, because it responds poorly to alterations in diet. This leads to profound failure to thrive[289] and malnutrition, which further limits the nonspecific aspects of the immune response. Parenteral nutrition is often required, placing the patient at risk of serious nosocomial disease. The liver enzymes are often elevated, sometimes in response to chronic viral hepatitis. Numerous skin and collagen defects have been noted in some patients with this disease[1]. Major causes of death include infection with CMV and EBV as well as parainfluenza type 3, adenovirus, enterovirus, and herpes[290]. Death without definitive treatment usually occurs in the first year of life[285]. Despite symptoms beginning at an early age, over 50% of children are undiagnosed at 6 months. It has been suggested that the majority of children with SCID would be diagnosed by 6 months if low lymphocyte counts (mean 1700, all less than 2800) obtained on CBCs were investigated[288]. Early diagnosis is imperative since survival following bone marrow transplant is more favorable if the procedure is performed at a younger age.

Therapy of infections is symptomatic and organism oriented. Prophylaxis with TMP-SMX is helpful with regard to *Pneumocystis*. Therapy with varicella zoster immunoglobulin should be given within 72 hours of any exposure to varicella. On the whole, however, the only real hope for a good outcome in these patients is with bone marrow transplantation[291]. Since the first successful transplant was accomplished in 1968[292], many new techniques have contributed to increased success of the procedure. Survival from an HLA-matched sibling is currently 80% and HLA haploidentical relative 56%[285]. Liver transplant has a survival of only 10%[285]. For ADA SCID, transfusion of irradiated RBCs, which contain ADA, every 2 to 4 weeks is no longer used because of risks such as iron overload. In 1986, polyethylene glycol (PEG) bound ADA given as IM injections one to two times a week was introduced. Since approval in 1990, it has been used in more than 40 patients with few complications[286,293]. In 1990, gene therapy using a retroviral vector was first used for ADA SCID with promising results[294]. The treatment of choice for ADA SCID remains HLA identical bone marrow transplant[286].

In providing care for these patients in the PICU, very close attention must be paid to prevention of nosocomial infections. In addition, when blood or blood products are used, they must be appropriately irradiated prior to infusion to prevent graft-versus-host disease. Transfusion-induced GVHD leads to epidermal necrolysis, bloody diarrhea, severe hepatitis, and often death[285].

The gene for X-linked SCID has been isolated on the long arm of the X chromosome, and linkage analysis has made carrier detection and prenatal diagnosis possible.

Wiskott-Aldrich Syndrome

Wiskott-Aldrich syndrome (WAS) is an X-linked, recessive disease characterized by eczema, thrombocytopenia, and recurrent infections[295]. This disorder, first described by Wiskott in 1937[296], was noted to be of X-linked inheritance in 1954 by Aldrich and colleagues[297]. Thrombocytopenia, as well as small and poorly functioning platelets, are present at birth[298]. Small platelets are found almost exclusively in WAS[234]. Boys with WAS present in the first few months of life with bleeding problems. Problems may begin with circumcision or present with petechia, epistaxis, bloody diarrhea, or intracranial bleeding[299]. Eczema occurs early in life and resembles atopic eczema[299]. Immunoglobulins have an abnormal pattern with IgM deficiency and elevated IgA and IgE. IgG may be normal or decreased[247]. Patients with WAS are unable to produce antibodies to polysaccharide antigens and therefore present with infections with *S. pneumoniae, H. influenzae,* and *N. meningitidis* at around 6 months of age when maternal antibody levels decline[298].

T-cell number and function decrease with age with profound lymphopenia by school age(247,300). Associated findings include arthritis, glomerulonephritis, and secondary malignancies, especially CNS and GI lymphomas and systemic reticuloendothelioses(301,302).

Without treatment, most patients with WAS die in early childhood from severe hemorrhage, overwhelming sepsis, or malignancy(298). Therapy is aimed at prevention of overwhelming infection and control of acute bleeding episodes. Splenectomy has been advocated to reduce platelet destruction(300,303), but this procedure worsens the risk of bacterial sepsis. With splenectomy, platelet counts consistently return to normal with serious bleeding decreased seven fold and median survival increased to 25 years(304). Prophylactic antibiotics are especially useful in splenectomized patients. Bone marrow transplant was first attempted in the late 1960s, and currently satisfactory results are obtained with HLA identical but not haploidentical transplants(304,305). HLA-matched transplant is currently the treatment of choice for WAS with splenectomy performed in cases where there is no matched donor. The gene responsible for WAS has been mapped to the short arm of the X chromosome(306), and DNA markers currently allow for carrier detection and prenatal diagnosis(302).

Ataxia Telangiectasia

Ataxia telangiectasia is a disease with much variability in clinical manifestations, as well as a spectrum of immune deficit with which it is associated. The pathogenesis of the syndrome is not clearly understood. It was first described in 1926(307) but was not defined as a specific syndrome until 1957. Sedgwick and Boder first applied the name ataxia telangiectasia and pointed out the recurrent infections that accompany the disorder(308). It is an autosomal recessive disorder with an incidence of 1 in 300,000 that has been localized to chromosome 11 at 11q22-23(309,310). The product of the gene is believed to be involved in DNA recombination. There is increased sensitivity to radiation, even in heterozygotes, with frequent chromosomal breaks(247), and lymphocytes are found to have a high frequency of translocations of chromosome 7 and 14(309). Breakpoints involve genes that encode T-cell receptors and immunoglobulin heavy chains leading to B-cell and T-cell abnormalities(235).

Clinically, ataxia is noted early, usually by the end of the second year. Other neurologic abnormalities include abnormal eye movements and dysarthria. Telangiectasias first appear on the bulbar conjunctiva and later the pinnae and flexor surfaces of the arms and are noted between 2 and 8 years of age. Cognitive function appears to be normal(311). The recurrent infections are often of the sinuses or respiratory tract. There is IgA deficiency, cutaneous anergy, and diminished responsiveness of T cells to in vitro stimulation. Early deaths generally result from associated malignancies; lymphosarcoma is the most common. Overall prognosis is difficult to specify, since the clinical manifestations are so variable. Those who live longest, however, exhibit progressive deterioration of their cerebellar function with worsening muscle weakness. There is no known cure, and various therapies have been attempted, none with spectacular results. Prophylactic antibiotics are not indicated, so therapy consists of general supportive measures and appropriate therapy of acute infections. Heterozygote detection and prenatal diagnosis on amniotic fluid or chorionic villus cells is available by measurement of chromosomal radiosensitivity(309,310).

Other Combined Disorders

A combined but variable immunodeficiency may accompany some forms of short-limbed dwarfism(312) and the cartilage-hair hypoplasia syndrome(313). Susceptibility to bacterial infection is not marked in the majority of individuals because a T-cell deficiency predominates, and the most significant, potentially life-threatening infection in these patients is varicella. A smaller subset of patients has a more severe combined immunodeficiency state and may suffer from a similar set of infectious complications as patients with SCID (as described previously).

Abnormalities of the Phagocytic System

The phagocytic system involves both leukocytes and monocytes. Polymorphonuclear leukocytes are primarily responsible for engulfment and killing of bacteria. The role of monocytes and macrophages in host defenses has only recently been delineated. Because of the difficulty enunciating the function of monocytes and macrophages, this chapter does not discuss the disorders of that system in detail. Suffice it to say that the monocyte plays many roles in host defense, and the abnormalities that affect its maturation, movement, number, and cytotoxic activity have protean effects on the host in relation to bacterial, viral, and fungal infections.

Aberrations of neutrophil function, number, and mobility have been well described. The best known of the granulocyte disorders, chronic granulomatous disease (CGD), is described in the next section. The other disorders that affect phagocytic function and have an adverse effect on killing of microorganisms are addressed only briefly because of their rarity.

Chronic Granulomatous Disease of Childhood

Probably the best known of the neutrophil disorders is CGD of childhood. This entity is caused by a defect in any one of four components of the enzyme NADPH oxidase, which generates antimicrobial oxidants such as superoxide and hydrogen peroxide essential for bacterial killing(314,315). There are many subtypes of CGD caused by a diverse number of mutations and multiple affected genes. Sixty-five percent of cases are X-linked, and the remainder are autosomal recessive in inheritance(314). The overall incidence is approximately 1 in 500,000(314–316). In these disorders, the initial leukocyte response to bacterial infection (phagocytosis) is normal, but for some organisms, killing is impaired, resulting in increased susceptibility to infections caused by these species. The secondary host response involves formation of granulomatous lesions that represent leukocytes, monocytes, and macrophages,which contain ingested but still viable bacteria or fungi. CGD phagocytes are able to use exogenously supplied hydrogen peroxide[317], so organisms such as β-hemolytic streptococci, pneumococci, and meningococci, which produce their own hydrogen peroxide, are effectively killed by these granulocytes. Therefore, they pose no additional threat to the CGD patient. Organisms capable of producing chronic infection are those that are "catalase-positive" and prevent CGD phagocytes from using microbial generated hydrogen peroxide. The most common organism causing disease in CGD include *S. aureus* and *aspergillus*. Other organisms include the gram-negative, mostly enteric, bacteria *Serratia, Pseudomonas, Salmonella, E. coli, Proteus,* and *Aerobacter*[315] and the fungi *Candida* and *Torulopsis*[314]. The majority of patients develop symptoms in the first year of life and are diagnosed by 2 years of age[316]. Infections typically involve the epithelial surfaces in contact with the environment, mainly skin, mucous membranes, the gastrointestinal tract and lungs, and the lymph nodes that drain them[316]. Granulomatous involvement of the gastrointestinal tract may be indistinguishable from Crohn's disease and can lead to obstruction. Chronic inflammation leads to lymphadenopathy, hepatosplenomegaly, anemia of chronic disease, and failure to thrive[314]. Patients may also develop osteomyelitis, visceral abscesses, and sepsis[316]. Fungal infections localized to bone or soft tissue have generally responded well to therapy[318], including systemic antifungal administration and/or surgical excision and/or granulocyte transfusion. The patient with CGD who develops a pulmonary or disseminated infection has a 20% chance of succumbing to the infection, despite therapy. Because definitive diagnosis of fungal disease in the setting of CGD often requires tissue or open-lung biopsy, some patients will die of severe pneumonitis or disseminated fungemia before the diagnosis has been made and therapy begun. For this reason, when a child with CGD is admitted to the ICU with fulminant infection of undetermined etiology, systemic antifungal therapy should probably be added to the other antimicrobial agents. *P. carinii* pneumonitis has also been described[319] and should be considered in a child with CGD who develops interstitial pneumonitis. Because cellular and humoral immunity is usually intact, these patients do not have extraordinary trouble with other microorganisms. Immunoglobulin levels are usually elevated appropriately to the severity of recurrent infections[320].

Untreated, the classic severe X-linked form of CGD generally leads to death in early adulthood. Some males have been described with a more benign course and do not manifest evidence of immunodeficiency until the late teens or early twenties[319,321,322]. Females with the autosomal recessive type of CGD also tend to have a less rapidly fatal disease[323]. Some have a normal oxidative burst in their monocytes and macrophages, although their leukocytes continue to exhibit the defects described previously.

Therapy for CGD is aimed at prevention and reducing exposure to offending organisms. Continuous administration of prophylactic antibiotics is recommended. The combination of trimethoprim (TMP) and sulfamethoxazole (SMX) is active against most of the organisms to which these patients are prone. A study[323] of continuous therapy with TMP-SMX showed a significant drop in the number of infectious episodes, the number of infecting organisms, the number of surgical procedures required for drainage of abscesses, and the number of days of hospitalization for most patients during the treatment period. Itraconazole as prophylaxis for fungal infections is currently being studied[324].

Treatment of patients with γ-interferon has been shown to partially correct the functional defect in CGD patients[325,326] and decreases serious infections by 70% and hospitalizations by two-thirds[320]. Bone marrow transplant has been successful in only a small number of patients resulting from the high degree of immunosuppression required and generally, risks are felt to outweigh benefits. The ability to detect the gene defect in the many types of CGD has made prenatal diagnosis by molecular biologic techniques on fetal DNA obtained by CVS or amniocentesis possible[315]. Genetic correction using gene therapy with retrovirus vectors is currently being studied[327].

Chediak-Higashi Syndrome

Chediak-Higashi is a rare, autosomal recessive syndrome characterized by recurrent pyogenic infections, partial oculocutaneous albinism, photophobia, and nystagmus[328,329]. Patients have pyoderma, subcutaneous abscesses, otitis, sinusitis, bronchitis, and pneumonia mostly because of *S. aureus* and β-hemolytic streptococcus[247]. Eighty-five percent of patients develop accelerated disease that presents as a lymphomalike picture with infiltration of organs by atypical lymphocytes leading to hepatosplenomegaly, lymphadenopathy, leukopenia, neurologic changes, and a bleeding tendency[247,328]. The mean age of survival is less than 6 years with most patients succumbing by 10 years[328]. In this disorder, abnormal giant granules formed by the fusion of lysosomes are seen in the cytoplasm of all cells containing lysosomes[330], including leukocytes and skin and hair bulb melanocytes. The immunodeficiency includes defective phagocytosis, chemotaxis, and lack of natural killer (NK) activity[328–330]. The leukocyte abnormalities are thought to be related to elevated levels of cAMP[331,332] and an abnormality of the cGMP system[331,333]. The administration of ascorbic acid, which reduces the concentration of the cAMP, has been shown to be of some benefit[334]. The accelerated phase is treated with chemotherapy, and recently splenectomy has been used with success when chemotherapy fails[328]. Some success with bone marrow transplantation has been demonstrated[335]. Prenatal diagnosis by light microscopy of fetal-hair[330] and fetal-blood sampling, amniocentesis and chorionic villus sampling to measure size of lysosomes[329] has been successful.

Glucose-6-Phosphate Dehydrogenase Deficiency

Patients with the usual phenotypes of glucose-6-phosphate dehydrogenase deficiency do not have evidence of increased risk of infections. However, leukocyte dysfunction ensues[336,337] when levels of the enzyme are less than 5% of normal, resulting in inability to activate the hexose monophosphate shunt to actuate bacterial killing. The defect mimics but is not as severe as CGD, and the clinical course, although similar from the standpoint of likely infecting organisms, is milder, with later onset of infectious complications.

Myeloperoxidase Deficiency

This disorder is characterized by absence of peroxidase-positive granules from leukocytes and monocytes, with normal eosinophils[338,339]. It appears to be autosomal recessive and may lead to increased frequency of candidal and bacterial infections. Bactericidal activity is diminished, but the oxidative burst increases[340,341]. In most patients, the defect is actually fairly mild, resulting in no adverse effect on longevity. There is also an acquired form of the disease, which may accompany severe bacterial or viral infections and various leukemias[342–344].

Abnormalities of Chemotaxis

Hyperimmunoglobulin E, Recurrent Infection Syndrome

Hyperimmunoglobulin E syndrome (Job syndrome) consists of recurrent serious infections, chronic eczematoid dermatitis and elevated levels of IgE[234,247]. Transmitted as an autosomal dominant disorder with incomplete penetrance, it is often associated with coarse facial features, fair skin, and light hair[345]. It is associated with skin and sinopulmonary infections, most commonly with *S. aureus* and *candida.* Chronic mucocutaneous candidiasis occurs in 50% of patients[247,346]. Although commonly classified as a disorder of chemotaxis, not all patients have defective chemotaxis and it appears only intermittently in others. T-cell and antibody responses have been found to be defective, and this syndrome may best be classified as a combined B-cell and T-cell immunodeficiency[253]. Patients may benefit from TMP-SMX prophylaxis[347] and possibly γ-interferon treatment[345].

Other Disorders With Abnormalities of Chemotaxis

A number of other hereditary and acquired disorders lead to problems with chemotaxis. These include complement deficiencies, other immunodeficiencies, certain malignancies, some clotting factor abnormalities, certain patients with severe burns, and some chronic infections that are associated with cutaneous anergy. A list of disorders affecting chemotaxis is presented in **Table 28.17.**

Table 28.17. Conditions Associated with Defects of Chemotaxis

Acrodermatitis enteropathica
Actin dysfunction
Burns
Cancer
Chediak-Higashi syndrome
Chemotactic factor inhibitors
Complement deficiencies
Corticosteroid or immunosuppressive therapy
Diabetes mellitus
Down syndrome
Elevated IgA
Elevated IgE
Ethanol intoxication
Hypophosphatemia
Infections
Lazy leukocyte syndrome
Malnutrition
Mannosidosis
Membrane glycoprotein deficiency
Rheumatoid arthritis
Uremia

Diminished Number of Phagocytes

The secondary forms of neutropenia, which develop during the course of certain malignancies or subsequent to cancer chemotherapy, and a discussion of the approach to the febrile neutropenic patient are included in Chapter 40, which deals with oncologic problems in the PICU. Some of the congenital disorders that lead to abnormalities of neutrophil number or function are described in the following section.

Cyclic Neutropenia

This is an autosomally dominant inherited disorder[348] in which bone marrow production of neutrophilic, erythrocytic, and platelet precursors waxes and wanes in a cyclic fashion[349,350]. Because red blood cells and platelets have a longer peripheral half-life, short drops in their production are of minor clinical consequence. Of clinical significance is the severe neutropenia (<200 cells/mcl) that occurs at approximately three-week intervals and lasts for 3 to 6 days. During this time, malaise, anorexia, fever, aphthous stomatitis, gingivitis, and cervical adenopathy develop[351,352]. Severe infections are unusual although rare cases of colonic ulceration, peritonitis, and bacteremia with *Clostridium* species have been described[351]. For the most part, the life span of patients with this problem tends to be normal. Treatment with granulocyte-colony-stimulating factor (G-CSF) causes cycles to occur more frequently (14 days) with larger oscillations and nadir lasting less than one day[352]. On treatment, energy level and appetite increase, and infections are reduced significantly[351]. Granulocyte-macrophage-colony-stimulating factor (GM-CSF) causes only a modest increase in neutrophils, but it dampens oscillations in neutrophil count and has been shown to improve clinical symptoms[353].

Severe Congenital Neutropenia

Also known as Kostmann syndrome[354], severe congenital neutropenia disease is characterized by a neutrophil count that remains chronically less than 200/mm^3. The problem stems from bone marrow granulocyte maturation arrest[352,355]. Affected infants have recurrent, often fatal, pyogenic infections[352]. Bone marrow transplantation has been successful[335]. Treatment with G-CSF has been shown to resolve neutropenia as well as symptoms[352].

Schwachman-Diamond Syndrome

This disorder entails a deficiency in the exocrine function of the pancreas combined with neutropenia secondary to bone marrow failure[355,357]. One-quarter of these patients have an associated pancytopenia; 10% have neutropenia accompanied by anemia. In the remainder, only the granulocytes are affected[358–360]. They chronically have granulocyte counts of less than 1000/mm^3, which, in some cases, wax and wane in cyclic fashion. Dwarfism and metaphyseal chondrodysplasia usually accompany the syndrome, compounded by chronic diarrhea and growth failure secondary to the malabsorption of pancreatic insufficiency. Pancreatic disease can be treated with replacement enzymes, but the neutropenia has been recalcitrant to most forms of attempted therapy. Patients die of infection or from secondary malignant disorders, mostly leukemias[360,361].

Disorders of the Complement System

Genetic defects of the majority of complement components have been discovered. Deficiency of components of the classical pathway, C1, C2, and C4 leads to a high incidence of systemic lupus erythematosis (SLE)[362]. Twenty percent experience systemic infections. C3 is found at the convergence of the classical and alternative pathways, and deficiency leads to an 80% risk of severe infections with encapsulated bacteria, mainly pneumococcus and meningococcus[363]. Deficiency of terminal complement components (C5, C6, C7, C8, C9) leads to susceptibility to neisserial infections, especially meningococcus. Patients with those deficiencies have a 60% incidence of meningococcal disease, typical in their teenage years, with a lower case mortality than noncomplement deficient patients but a 50% recurrence risk[364].

Hereditary Angioedema

Patients with C1 esterase deficiency, an autosomal dominant disorder, deserve special mention. Although this deficiency does not lead to immunodeficiency, patients have a one-third incidence of death before the end of their third decade because of upper airway obstruction. Most patients with this deficiency develop episodes of angioedema at sites of minor trauma or during periods of stress or temperature extremes beginning early in childhood. The episodes last 24 to 48 hours, the edema is nonpitting and causes a sensation of pressure rather than pain[364]. In addition to episodes of upper airway swelling, patients experience varying intestinal symptoms from angioedema of the bowel, which may mimic an acute abdomen. Anabolic steroids have been used in adults to prevent attacks and in children for short courses prior to surgical procedures. Purified C1 inhibitor has immediate benefit for airway obstruction and may soon be available in the United States[364].

WHEN TO SUSPECT AN IMMUNODEFICIENCY

Children in PICUs often present diagnostic dilemmas. Many of them have infections as the primary reason for admission or as a complicating or confounding factor. Not all children with infections have a primary immunodeficiency, but some children will end up in the PICU with their infection *because* of their underlying immunodeficiency. If the immune defect has been previously diagnosed, the intensive care specialist will be looking for unusual organisms or unusual manifestations of disease. In the previously undiagnosed patient, certain clues as to the possibility of an immune defect may be present. The following are a few such clues:

1. The patient has had recurrent serious bacterial infections.
2. The patient has a systemic fungal infection or is infected with a normally benign bacterial organism.
3. The patient is infected with a common microbial pathogen, but the presentation was unusual.
4. The patient with a significant infection is neutropenic.
5. The patient has had recurrent skin infections or mouth ulcers.
6. The patient gives a history of recurrent fevers with no identified source.
7. The patient has had chronic diarrhea with failure to thrive.
8. The patient has recurrent or persistent evidence of meningoencephalitis with no bacterial source identified.
9. The patient has congenital heart disease associated with hypocalcemia.
10. The family has a positive history of immunologic or autoimmune disease.

Although the presence of any one of the previously mentioned clues may not be conclusive for immunodeficiency, the intensive care specialist should use this information to broaden the scope of the differential diagnosis and probably the considerations of possible infecting organisms as well.

SUMMARY

This chapter has reviewed the major immunodeficiency disorders as they pertain to the care of the infant and child in the PICU. The "secondary" and, therefore, potentially preventable disorders have been addressed in some detail. The primary immunodeficiencies have been reviewed with much more brevity. It is hoped this discussion proves useful as a point from which the intensive care specialist can proceed when consideration of any of these disorders occurs in the context of his or her practice. Obviously missing from this chapter is a guide to the work-up of patients with potential immune defects. This omission has been intentional. First, such a description is beyond the scope of this chapter's purpose. Second, and perhaps most important, is that because most ICU patients are severely ill, secondary temporary immune defects can be fairly common, and the majority of the work-up of a potential congenital immune defect should be accomplished after the child has regained his or her usual state of health. In some situations, this may not be feasible, and under those circumstances, consultation with an immunologist or hematologist/oncologist is indicated, depending on the nature of the presumed defect.

References

1. Cooper MD, Buckley RH. Developmental immunity and the immunodeficiency diseases. JAMA 1982;248:2658.
2. Lawton AR, Cooper MD. Ontogeny of immunity. In: Stiehm ER, Fulginiti VA, eds. Immunologic disorders in infants and children. Philadelphia: WB Saunders, 1980:36.
3. Roper M, Cooper MD. Development of immunocompetent cells in humans. In: Chandra RK, ed. Primary and secondary immunodeficiency disorders. New York: Churchill Livingstone, 1983:12.
4. Kohler PF, Farr RS. Elevation of cord over maternal IgG immunoglobulin: evidence for an active placental IgG transport. Nature 1966;210:1070.
5. Whitelaw A, Parkin J. Development of immunity. BMJ 1988;44:1037–1051.
6. Hyvarinen M, Zelter P, Oh W, et al. Influence of gestational age on serum levels of alpha-1-fetoprotein, IgG globulin and albumin in newborn infants. J Pediatr 1973;82:430.
7. Berg T. Immunoglobulin levels in infants with low birth weights. Acta Paediatr Scand 1973;57:369.
8. Evans EH, Akpata SO, Glass L. Serum immunoglobulin levels in premature and full-term infants. Am J Clin Pathol 1971;56:416.
9. Yeung CY, Hobbs JR. Serum-gamma G-globulin levels in normal, premature, post-mature and "small-for-dates" newborn babies. Lancet 1968;1:1167.
10. Hobbs JR, Davis JA. Serum G-globulin levels and gestational age in premature babies. Lancet 1967;1:757.
11. Gitlin D, Biasucci A. Development of gamma G, gamma M, beta IC/beta 1A C'1 esterase inhibitor, ceruloplasmin, transferrin, hemopexin, haptoglobin, fibrinogen, plasminogen, antitrypsin, orosomucoid, B lipoproteins, B2-macroglobulin and prealbumin in the human conceptus. J Clin Invest 1969;48:1433.
12. Ballow M, Cates KL, Rowe JC, Goetz C, Desbonnet C. Development of the immune system in very low birth weight (less than 1500g) premature infants: concentrations of plasma immunoglobulins and patterns of infections. Pediatr Res 1986;20:899–904.
13. Barrett CD Jr, McClean IW Jr, Molver JG, et al. Multiple antigen immunization of infants against poliomyelitis, diphtheria, pertussis, and tetanus. Pediatrics 1962;30:720.
14. Brown GC, Volk VK, Gottshall RY, et al. Responses of infants to DTP vaccine used in nine injection schedules. Public Health Rep 1964;79:585.
15. Oldstone MBA, Tishon A, Moretta L. Active thymus derived suppressor lymphocytes in human cord blood. Nature 1977;269:333.
16. Hayward AR, Lawton PM. Suppression of B lymphocyte differentiation by newborn T lymphocytes with an Fc receptor for IgM. Clin Exp Immunol 1978;34:374.
17. Durandy A, Fischer A, Griscelli C. Active suppression of B lymphocyte maturation by two different newborn T lymphocyte subsets. J Immunol 1979;123:2644.
18. Cates KL, Rowe JC, Ballow M. The premature infant as a compromised host. In: Current problems in pediatrics. Chicago: Year Book Medical Publishers, 1983:1.
19. Allansmith M, McClennan BH, Butterworth M, Maloney JR. The development of immunoglobulin levels in man. J Pediatr 1968;72:276.
20. Berkel AI. Developmental aspects of delayed hypersensitivity. Boll Ist Sieroter Milan 1974;(Suppl 1):147.
21. Winter HS, Bryson YJ, Gard SE, et al. Deficiency of monocyte migration inhibition factor and immune interferon production in lymphocytes of normal newborns. Pediatr Res 1978;12:488.
22. Krause PJ, Maderazo EG, Scroggs M. Abnormalities of neutrophil adherence in newborns. Pediatrics 1982;69:184.
23. Cates KL. Defects in neutrophil chemotaxis. Clin Immunol Allergy 1981;1:603.
24. Miller ME. Chemotactic function in the human neonate: humoral and cellular aspects. Pediatr Res 1971;5:487.
25. Klein RB, Fischer TJ, Gard SE, et al. Decreased mononuclear and polymorphonuclear chemotaxis in newborn infants and young children. Pediatrics 1977;60:467.
26. Laurenti F, Ferro R, Marzetti G, et al. Neutrophil chemotaxis in preterm infants with infections. J Pediatr 1980;96:468.
27. Gluck L, Silverman WA. Phagocytosis in premature infants. Pediatrics 1957;20:951.
28. Conly ME, Speert DP. Human neonatal monocyte-derived macrophages and neutrophils exhibit normal nonopsonic and opsonic receptor-mediated phagocytosis and superoxide anion production. Biol Neonate 1991;60:361–366.
29. Wright WC Jr, Ank BJ, Herbert J, et al. Decreased bactericidal activity of leukocytes of stressed newborn infants. Pediatrics 1975;56:579.
30. Forman ML, Stiehm ER. Impaired opsonic activity but normal phagocytosis in low-birth-weight infants. N Engl J Med 1969;281:926.
31. Bektas S, Goetze B, Speer CP. Decreased adherence, chemotaxis and phagocytic activities of neutrophils from preterm neonates. Acta Paediatr Scand 1990;79:1031–1038.
32. Shigeoka AO, Santos JI, Hill HR. Functional analysis of neutrophil granulocytes from healthy, infected, and stressed neonates. J Pediatr 1979;95:454.
33. Park BH, Holmes B, Good RA. Metabolic activities in leukocytes of newborn infants. J Pediatr 1970;76:237.
34. Corberand J, Grozdea I, Rolland M. Leukocyte cytochemical reactions in preterm and small for date babies. Biomedicine 1976;25:334.
35. Anderson DC, Pickering LK, Feigin RD. Leukocyte function in normal and infected neonates. J Pediatr 1974;85:420.
36. Dossett JH, Williams RC Jr, Quie PG. Studies on interaction of bacteria serum factors and polymorphonuclear leukocytes in mothers and newborns. Pediatrics 1969;44:49.
37. McCracken GH Jr, Eichenwald HF. Leukocyte function and the development of opsonic and complement activity in the neonate. Am J Dis Child 1971;121:120.
38. Gabig TG, Babior BM. The killing of pathogens by phagocytes. Ann Rev Med 1981;32:313.
39. Hill HR, Shigeoka AO, Hall RT, et al. Neonatal cellular and humoral immunity to group B streptococci. Pediatrics 1979;64:S787.
40. Baker CJ. Group B streptococcal infections in neonates. Pediatr Rev 1979;1:5.
41. Baker CJ, Edwards MS, Kasper DL. Role of antibody to native type III polysaccharide of group B streptococcus in infant infection. Pediatrics 1981;68:544.
42. Christensen KK, Christensen P, Dahlander K, et al. Quantitation of serum antibodies to surface antigens of group B streptococci types Ia, Ib and III: low antibody levels in mothers of neonatally infected infants. Scand J Infect Dis 1980;12:105.
43. Edwards MS, Baker CJ, Kasper DL. Opsonic specificity of human antibody to the type III polysaccharide of group B Streptococcus. J Infect Dis 1979;140:1004.
44. Baker CJ, Edwards MS, Webb BJ, et al. Antibody independent classical pathway-mediated opsonophagocytosis of type Ia, group B streptococcus. J Clin Invest 1982;69:394.
45. Sawyer MK, Forman ML, Kuplic LS, et al. Developmental aspects of the human complement system. Biol Neonate 1971;19:148.
46. Traub B. The complement activity of the serum of healthy persons, mothers, and newborn infants. J Pathol Bacteriol 1943;55:447.
47. Colten HR, Goldberger G. Ontogeny of serum complement proteins. Pediatrics 1979;64:S775.
48. Adinolfi M. Human complement: onset and site of synthesis during fetal life. Am J Dis Child 1977;131:1015.

49. Strunk RC, Fenton LJ, Gaines JA. Alternative pathway of complement activation in full term and premature infants. Pediatr Res 1979;13:641.
50. Drew JH, Arroyave CM. The complement system of the newborn infant. Biol Neonate 1980;37:209.
51. Quie PG. Antimicrobial defenses in the neonate. Semin Perinatol 1990;14:2–9.
52. Peter G, Smith DH. *Haemophilus influenzae* meningitis at the Children's Hospital Medical Center in Boston, 1958 to 1973. Pediatrics 1975; 55:523.
53. Daum RS, Granoff DM. A vaccine against *Haemophilus influenzae* type b. Pediatr Infect Dis 1985;4:355.
54. Robbins JB, Parke JC Jr, Schneerson R, Whisnant JK. Quantitative measurement of "natural" and immunization induced *Haemophilus influenzae* type b capsular polysaccharide antibodies. Pediatr Res 1973;7:103.
55. Petola H, Kayhty H, Sivonen A, Makela H. *Haemophilus influenzae* type b capsular polysaccharide vaccine in children: a double blind field study of 100,000 vaccinees 3 months to 5 years of age in Finland. Pediatrics 1977;60:730.
56. Eskola J, Kayhty H, Takala AK, et al. A randomized, prospective field trial of conjugate vaccine in the protection of infants and young children against invasive *Haemophilus influenzae* type b disease. N Engl J Med 1990;323:1415.
57. Tsuda T, Kahan BD. The effects of anesthesia on the immune response. In: Chandra RK, ed. Primary and secondary immunodeficiency disorders. New York: Churchill Livingstone, 1983:253.
58. Lassen HC, Hendriksen E, Neukrich F, Kristensen HS. Treatment of tetanus: severe bone-marrow depression after prolonged nitrous oxide inhalation. Lancet 1956;1:527.
59. Eastwood DW, Green CD, Lambdin MA, Gardner R. Effect of nitrous oxide on the white-cell count in leukemia. N Engl J Med 1963;268:297.
60. Lassen HC, Kristensen HS. Remission in chronic myeloid leukaemia following prolonged nitrous oxide inhalation. Dan Med Bull 1959;6:252.
61. Bruce DL, Koepke JA. Changes in granulopoiesis in the rat associated with prolonged halothane anesthesia. Anesthesiology 1966;27:811.
62. Bruce DL. Effect of halothane anesthesia on experimental *Salmonella* peritonitis in mice. J Surg Res 1967;7:180.
63. Lofstrom B, Shildt B. Reticuloendothelial function under general anesthesia. Acta Anaesthesiol Scand 1974;18:34.
64. Cullen BF, Duncan PG, Ray-Kiel L. Inhibition of cell-mediated cytotoxicity by halothane and nitrous oxide. Anesthesiology 1976;44:386.
65. Usenik EA, Cronkite EP. Effect of barbiturate anesthesia on leucocyte in normal and splenectomized dogs. Anesth Analg 1965;44:167.
66. Graca JG, Garst EL. Early blood changes in dogs following intravenous pentobarbital anesthesia. Anesthesiology 1957;18:461.
67. Stanley TH, Hill GE, Portas MR, et al. Neutrophil chemotaxis during and after general anesthesia and operation. Anesth Anald 1976;55:668.
68. Giddon DB, Lindhe J. In vivo quantitation of local anesthetic suppression of leucocyte adherence. Am J Pathol 1972;68:327.
69. Lennard TWJ, Browell DA. The immunological effects of trauma. Proc Nutr Soc 1993;52:85–90.
70. Blackburn GL, Menkes E. Surgical immunology. In: Chandra RK, ed. Primary and secondary immunodeficiency disorders. New York: Churchill Livingstone, 1983:263.
71. Monjan AA, Collector MI. Stress-induced modulation of the immune response. Science 1977;196:307.
72. Moore FD. Energy and the maintenance of body cell mass. JPEN 1980;4:228.
73. Wilmore DW, Long JM, Mason AD, et al. Catecholamines: mediator of the hypermetabolic response to thermal injury. Ann Surg 1974;180:653.
74. Eskay RL, Grino M, Chen HT. Interleukins, signal transduction, and the immune system-mediated stress response. In: Porter JC, Jezova D, eds. Circulating regulatory factors and neuroendocrine function. New York: Plenum Press, 1990.
75. Howard RJ, Simmons RL. Acquired immunologic deficiencies after trauma and surgical procedures. Surg Gynecol Obstet 1974;139:771.
76. Pietsch JB, Meakin JL, MacLean LD. The delayed hypersensitivity response: application in clinical surgery. Surgery 1977;82:349.
77. McLoughlin GA, Wu AV, Saporoschetz I, Nimberg R, Mannick JA. Correlation between anergy and a circulating immunosuppressive factor following major surgical trauma. Ann Surg 1979;190:297.
78. Wilson NW, Gooding A, Peterson B, Bastian JF. Anergy in pediatric head trauma patients. Am J Dis Child 1991;145:326.
79. Balbo G, Farina EC. Secondary immunodeficiencies in surgical patients. Pharmacol Res 1992;26:86–87.
80. Barbul A, Regan MC. The regulatory role of T lymphocytes in wound healing. J Trauma 1990:30:S97.
81. Miller-Graziano CL, Szabo G, Kodys D, Griffey K. Aberrations in post-trauma monocyte (MO) subpopulation: role in septic shock syndrome. J Trauma 1990;30:S86–S97.
82. Wilson NW, Ochs HD, Peterson B, Hamvurger RN, Bastian JF. Abnormal primary antibody responses in pediatric trauma patients. J Pediatr 1989;115:424–427.
83. McRitchie DI, Girotti MJ, Rotstein OD, Teodorczyk-Injeyan JA. Impaired antibody production in blunt trauma. Possible role for T cell dysfunction. Arch Surg 1990;125:91–96.
84. Schneider RP, Christou NV, Meakins JL, Nohr C. Humoral immunity in surgical patients with and without trauma. Arch Surg 1991;126:143–148.
85. Ertel W, Faist E, Nestle C, Hueltner L, Storck M, Schildberg FW. Kinetics of interleukin-2 and interleukin-6 synthesis following major mechanical trauma. J Surg Res 1990;48:622–628.
86. Faist E, Ertel W, Cohnert T, Huber P, Inthorn D, Heberer G. Immunoprotective effects of cyclooxygenase inhibition in patients with major surgical trauma. J Trauma 1990;30:8–18.
87. Brackman P, Dan B, Haley R. Nosocomial surgical infection. Surg Clin North Am 1980;60:17.
88. Haley RW, Hooton TM, Culver DH, et al. Nosocomial infections in US Hospitals, 1975–76. Am J Med 1981;70:947.
89. McGuckin MB, Kelsen SG. Surveillance in a surgical intensive care unit: patient and environment. Infect Control 1981;2:21.
90. Ortona L, Federico G, Fantoni M, Pallavicini F, Ricci F, Antinori A. A study on the incidence of postoperative infections and surgical sepsis in a university hospital. Infect Control 1987;8:320–324.
91. Craven DE, Kunches LM, Lichtenberg DA, Kollisch NR, Barry MA, Heeren TC, McCabe WR. Nosocomial infection and fatality in medical and surgical intensive care unit patients. Arch Intern Med 1988; 148:1161–1168.
92. Schlesinger D. Microbiology. Washington DC: American Society of Microbiology, 1975:328.
93. Pollock EMM, Ford-Jones EL, Rebeyka I, Mindorff CM, Bohn DJ, Edmonds JF, Lightfoot NE, Coles J, Williams WG, Trusler GA, Barker GA. Early nosocomial infections in pediatric cardiovascular surgery patients. Crit Care Med 1990;18:378–384.
94. Caplan ES, Hoyt N. Infection surveillance and control in the severely traumatized patient. Am J Med 1981;70:638.
95. Allgower M, Durig M, Wolff G. Infection and trauma. Surg Clin North Am 1980;60:133.
96. Cheadle WG, Wilson M, Hershman MJ, Bergamini D, Richardson JD, Polk HC. Comparison of trauma assessment scores and their use in prediction of infection and death. Ann Surg 1989;209:541–546.
97. Thadepalli H. Principles and practice of antibiotic therapy for post-traumatic abdominal injuries. Surg Gynecol Obstet 1979;148:937.
98. Trunkey DD. The treatment of sepsis and other complications in the trauma patient. Clin Ther 1990;12:21(Suppl B).
99. Shick JM, Lowe RJ. Intestinal disruption due to blunt abdominal trauma. Am J Surg 1978;136:668.
100. Oosterlee J. McGeehan DF, Robbs JV. Prevention of septic complications in massive pelvic-perineal injuries. S Afr Med J 1984;66:147.
101. Reichard SA, Helikson MA, Shorter N, et al. Pelvic fractures in children—review of 120 patients with a new look at general management. J Pediatr Surg 1980;15:727.
102. Ollier DW. Infection in victims of trauma. Probl Crit Care 1990;4: 3–20.
103. Quattrocchi KB, Frank EH, Miller CH, Dull ST, Howard RR, Wagner FC. Severe head injury: effects on cellular immune function. Neurol Res 1991;13:13–20.
104. Einhorn A. Mizrahi EM. Basilar skull fractures in children: the incidence of CNS infection and the use of antibiotics. Am J Dis Child 1978;132:1121.
105. Lewin W. Cerebrospinal fluid rhinorrhea in closed injuries. Br J Surg 1954;42:1.
106. Morley TP, Hetherington RF. Traumatic cerebrospinal fluid rhinorrhea and otorrhea, pneumocephalus and meningitis. Surg Gynecol Obstet 1957;104:88.
107. Lewin W. Cerebrospinal fluid rhinorrhea in non-missile head injuries. Clin Neurosurg 1964;12:237.
108. Leech P. Cerebrospinal fluid leakage, dural fistulae and meningitis after basal skull fractures. Injury 1974;6:141.
109. Raaf J. Post-traumatic cerebrospinal fluid leaks. Arch Surg 1967;95:648.
110. MacGee E, Canthen JC, Brackett CE. Meningitis following acute traumatic cerebrospinal fluid fistula. J Neurosurg 1970;33:312.

111. Ignelzi RJ, Van der Ark GD. Analysis of the treatment of basilar skull fractures with and without antibiotics. J Neurosurg 1975;43:75.
112. Hirschman JV. Bacterial meningitis following closed head trauma. In: Sande M, ed. Bacterial meningitis. New York: Churchill Livingstone, 1985:95.
113. Jones HM. The problem of recurrent meningitis. Proc R Soc Med 1974;67:1141.
114. Applebaum E. Meningitis following trauma to the head and face. JAMA 1960;173:116.
115. Hand WL, Sanford JP. Posttraumatic bacterial meningitis. Ann Intern Med 1970;72:869.
116. Jones SR, Luby JP, Sanford JP. Bacterial meningitis complicating cranial-spinal trauma. J Trauma 1973;13:895.
117. Jefferson A, Reilly G. Fractures of the floor of the anterior cranial fossa. The selection of patients for dural repair. Br J Surg 1972;59:585.
118. Picker S. The initial assessment and management of severe head injury. Probl Crit Care 1991;5:220–239.
119. Leech PJ, Patterson R. Conservative and operative management for cerebrospinal leakage after closed head injury. Lancet 1973;1:1013.
120. Helling TS, Evans LL, Fowler DL, et al. Infectious complications in patients with severe head injury. J Trauma 1988;28:1575.
121. Wilson GL. The pathophysiology and resuscitation of infectious brain injury. Probl Crit Care 1991;5:279–291.
122. Shires GT, Dineen P. Sepsis following burns, trauma and intraabdominal infections. Arch Intern Med 1982;142:2012.
123. Warden JD, Mason AD Jr, Pruitt BA Jr. Evaluation of leukocyte chemotaxis in vitro in thermally injured patients. J Clin Invest 1974;54:1001.
124. Grogan JB. Suppressed in vitro chemotaxis of burn neutrophils. J Trauma 1976;16:985.
125. Fikrig SM, Karl SC, Suntharalingam L. Neutrophil chemotaxis in patients with burns. Ann Surg 1977;186:746.
126. Davis JM, Dineen P, Gallin JI. Neutrophil degranulation and abnormal chemotaxis after thermal injury. J Immunol 1980;127:1467.
127. Altman LC, Furukawa CT, Klebanoff SJ. Depressed mononuclear chemotaxis in thermally injured patients. J Immunol 1977;119:199.
128. Warden GC, Mason AD, Pruitt BA Jr. Suppression of leukocyte chemotaxis in vitro by chemotherapeutic agents used in the management of thermal injuries. Ann Surg 1975;181:363.
129. Alexander JW. Serum and leucocyte lysosomal enzymes. Arch Surg 1967;95:482.
130. Alexander JW. Mechanism of immunologic suppression in burn injury. J Trauma 1990;30:S70–S75.
131. Munster AM, Hoagland HC, Pruitt BA. The effect of thermal injury on serum immunoglobulins. Ann Surg 1970;172:965.
132. Daniels JC, Larson DL, Abston S, et al. Serum protein profiles in thermal burns. I. Serum electrophoretic patterns, immunoglobulins and transport proteins. J Trauma 1974;14:137.
133. Kirk SJ, Barbul A. Role of arginine in trauma, sepsis, and immunity. JPEN 1990;14:226S–229S.
134. MacMillan BG. Infections following burn injury. Surg Clin North Am 1980;60:185.
135. Sevitt S. A review of the complications of burns, their origin and importance for illness and death. J Trauma 1979;19:358.
136. Loebl EC, Jancet MA, Hock EL, et al. The method of quantitative burn wound biopsy culture and its routine use in the care of the burned patient. Am J Clin Pathol 1974;61:128.
137. Bharadwaj R, Phadke SA, Joshi BN. Bacteriology of burn wound using the quantitative full thickness biopsy technique. Indian J Med Res 1983;78:337.
138. Monafo WW, Ayvazian VH. Topical therapy. Surg Clin North Am 1978;58:1157.
139. Larkin JM, Moylan JA. The role of prophylactic antibiotics in burn care. Am Surg 1976;42:247.
140. Harvey JS, Watkins GM, Sherman RT. Emergent burn care. South Med J 1984;77:204.
141. Parks DH, Linares HA, Thomson PD. Surgical management of burn wound sepsis. Surg Gynecol Obstet 1981;153:374.
142. Edelman R. Cell-mediated immunity in protein-calorie malnutrition. New York: Academic Press, 1975.
143. Schlesinger L, Stekel A: Impaired cellular immunity in marasmic infants. Am J Clin Nutr 1974;27:615.
144. Purtila DT, Connor DH. Fatal infections in protein-calorie malnourished children with thymolymphatic atrophy. Arch Dis Child 1975;50:149.
145. Mugerwa JW. The lymphoreticular system in kwashiorkor. J Pathol 1971;105:105.
146. Smythe PM, Brereton-Stiles GG, Grace HJ, et al. Thymolymphatic deficiency and depression of cell-mediated immunity in protein calorie malnutrition. Lancet 1971;2:939.
147. McMurray DN, Loomis SA, Casazza LJ, et al. Development of impaired cell-mediated immunity in mild and moderate malnutrition. Am J Clin Nutr 1981;34:68.
148. Shearer WT, Anderson DC. The secondary immunodeficiencies. In: Stiehm ER, ed. Immunologic disorders in infants and children. Philadelphia: WB Saunders, 1989;400–438.
149. Whittle HC, Mee J, Webinska J, et al. Immunity to measles in malnourished children. Clin Exp Immunol 1981;42:144.
150. Becker W, Nande W, Du T, et al. Virus studies in disseminated herpes simplex infections: association with malnutrition in children. S Afr Med J 1963;37:74.
151. Schrimshaw NS, Taylor LE, Gordon JE. Interactions of nutrition and infection. WHO Monogr Ser 1968;57:3.
152. Suskind R, Sirisinha S, Vithayasai V, et al. Immunoglobulin and antibody response in children with protein-calorie malnutrition. Am J Clin Nutr 1976;29:835.
153. Mata LF. Malnutrition-infection interactions in the tropics. Am J Trop Med Hyg 1975;24:564.
154. Trowell HC, Davies JNP, Dean RFA. Kwashiorkor. London: Edward Arnold, 1954.
155. Chandra RK. Immunocompetence in undernutrition. J Pediatr 1972;81:1194.
156. Chandra RK. Nutrition immunity and infection: present knowledge and future direction. Lancet 1983;1:688.
157. Chandra RK, Kumari S. Nutrition and immunity: an overview. J Nutr 1994;124:1433S–1435S.
158. Moldauer LL, Nauss K, Bristrian RR, Blackburn CL. Cellular immunity in protein malnutrition: differences in vivo and in vitro responses. Surg Forum 1979;30:138.
159. Bishian RR, Blackburn GL, Scrimshaw NS. Cellular immunity in semistarved states in hospitalized patients. Am J Clin Nutr 1978;28:1148.
160. Schlesinger L, Stekel A. Impaired cellular immunity in marasmic infants. Am J Clin Nutr 1974;27:615.
161. Bristrian BR, Sherman M, Blackburn CC. Cellular immunity in adult marasmus. Arch Intern Med 1977;137:1408.
162. Daly JM, Reynolds J, Sigal RK, Shou J, Liberman MD. Effect of dietary protein and amino acids on immune function. Crit Care Med 1990;18:S86–S93.
163. Coovadia HM, Soothill JF. The effect of protein restricted diets on the clearance of 125I-labeled polyvinyl pyrrolidone in mice. Clin Exp Immunol 1976;23:373.
164. Freyre EA, Chabes A, Peornape O. Abnormal Rebvek skin-window response in kwashiorkor. J Pediatr 1973;82:523.
165. Seth V, Chandra RK. Opsonic activity, phagocytosis, and bactericidal capacity of polymorphs in undernutrition. Arch Dis Child 1972;47:282.
166. Selvoraj RJ, Bhat KS. Metabolic and bacterial activities of leukocytes in protein-calorie malnutrition. Am J Clin Nutr 1972;25:166.
167. Wunder JA, Stinnet JD, Alexander JW. The effects of malnutrition on variables of host defense in the guinea pig. Surgery 1978;84:542.
168. Cunningham-Rundles S. Nutritional factors in immune response. In: Malnutrition: determinants and consequences. New York: Alan R Liss, 1984:233.
169. Chandra RK. Reduced secretory antibody response to live attenuated measles and poliovirus vaccines in malnourished children. BMJ 1975;2:583.
170. Sirisinha S, Suskind R, Edelman R, et al. Secretory and serum IgA in children with protein-calorie malnutrition. Pediatrics 1975;55:166.
171. Chandra RK, Newberne PM. Nutrition, immunity and infection: mechanisms of interactions. New York: Plenum Press, 1977.
172. Lim TS, Messika N, Watson RR. Immune components of the intestinal mucosa of aging and protein-deficient mice. Immunology 1981;43:401.
173. Neumann CG, Lawlor GJ, Stiehm ER, et al. Immunologic responses in malnourished children. Am J Clin Nutr 1975;28:89.
174. Chandra RK, Chakraburty S, Chandra S. Malnutrition humoral immunity and infection. Indian J Pediatr 1976;43:159.
175. Chandra RK, Chandra S, Gupta S. Antibody affinity and immune complexes after immunization with tetanus toxoid in protein-energy malnutrition. Am J Clin Nutr 1984;40:131.
176. Satyanarayana K, Bhaskaran P, Seshu VC, Reddy V. Influence of nutrition on post-vaccinial tuberculin sensitivity. Am J Clin Nutr 1980;33:2334.
177. Harland PSEG. Tuberculin reactions in malnourished children. Lancet 1965;2:719.

178. Brown RE, Opio EA. Associated factors in kwashiorkor in Uganda. Trop Geogr Med 1966;18:119.
179. Edington GM. Pathology of malaria in West Africa. BMJ 1967;1:715.
180. Hendrickse RG, Hasan AH, Olumide LO, Akiunkunmi A. Malaria in early childhood. Ann Trop Med Parasitol 1971;65:1.
181. Fargett GAT. Malnutrition and immunity to protozoan parasites. In: Isliker H, Schurch B, eds. The impact of malnutrition on immune defense in parasitic infestation. Bern, Switzerland: Nestle Foundation Publication Series 2, Hans Huber, 1981:158.
182. Etkin NL, Eaton JW. Malaria-induced erythrocyte oxidant sensitivity. In Brewer GJ, ed. Erythrocyte structure and function. New York: Alan R. Liss, 1975:219.
183. Eckman JR, Eaton JW, Berger E, Jacob HS. Role of vitamin E in regulating malaria expression. Trans Assoc Am Physicians 1976;89:105.
184. Friedman MJ. Oxidant damage mediates variant red cell resistance to malaria. Nature 1979;280:245.
185. Byles AB, D'Sa A. Reduction of reaction due to iron dextran infusion using chloroquine. BMJ 1970;3:625.
186. Masawe AEJ, Muindi JM, Swai GBR. Infections in iron deficiency and other types of anemia in the tropics. Lancet 1974;2:314.
187. Murray MJ, Murray AB, Murray BM, Murray CJ. The adverse effect of iron repletion on the course of certain infections. BMJ 1978;2:1113.
188. McGregor IA. Malaria: nutritional implication. Rev Infect Dis 1982;4:798.
189. Mattar JA, Nunes RB: Nutritional status in the critically ill. Crit Care Med 1981;9:281.
190. Mickell JJ. Urea nitrogen excretion in critically ill children. Pediatrics 1982;70:949.
191. Bole JM, Garre MA, Youinou PY, et al. Nutritional status in intensive care patients: evaluation in 84 unselected patients. Crit Care Med 1983;11:87.
192. Donaldson SS, Wesley MN, DeWeys WD, et al. A study of the nutritional status of pediatric cancer patients. Am J Dis Child 1981; 135:1107.
193. Cunningham-Rundles S. Effects of nutritional status on immunologic function. Am J Clin Nutr 1982;35:1202.
194. Rubin RH, Wolfson JS, Cosimi AB, Tolkoff-Rubin NE. Infection in the renal transplant recipient. Am J Med 1981;70:405–411.
195. Spees EK, Light JA, Oakes DD, Reinmuth B. Experiences with cadaver renal allograft contamination before transplantation. Br J Surg 1982;69:482–485.
196. Ramos E, Karmi S, Alongi SV, et al. Infectious complications in renal transplant recipients. South Med J 1980;73:751–754.
197. Hughes WT, Townsend TR. Nosocomial infections in immunocompromised children. Am J Med 1981;70:412.
198. Young LS. Nosocomial infections in the immunocompromised adult. Am J Med 1981;70:398.
199. Parillo JE, Fauci AS. Mechanisms of glucocorticoid action on immune processes. Annu Rev Pharmacol Toxicol 1979;19:179.
200. Fauci AS. Mechanisms of the immunosuppressive and anti-inflammatory effect of glucocorticosteroids. J Immunopharmacol 1978;1:1.
201. Fauci AS, Dale DC, Balow JE. Glucocorticosteroid therapy: mechanisms of action and clinical considerations. Ann Intern Med 1976;84:304.
202. Bollinger RR, Kirk AD, Fabian MA, Pruitt SK. Immunosuppressive pharmacology. In Taylor RW, Shoemaker WC, eds. Critical care state of the art. 1991;12:541–568.
203. Stevenson HC, Fauci AS. Immunosuppression secondary to pharmacologic agents. In: Chandra RJ, ed. Primary and secondary immunodeficiency disorders. New York: Churchill Livingstone, 1983:232.
204. Makinodan T, Santos GW, Quinn RP. Immunosuppressive drugs. Pharmacol Rev 1970;22:189.
205. Kaplan SR, Calabresi P. Immunosuppressive agents. N Engl J Med 1973;289:952, 1234.
206. Reid MM. Splenectomy, sepsis, immunisation, and guidelines. Lancet 1994;344:970–971.
207. Thong YH. Immunomodulation by antimicrobial drugs. Med Hypotheses 1982;8:361–370.
208. Korzeniowski OM. Effects of antibiotics on the mammalian immune system. Infect Dis Clin North Am 1989;3:469–478.
209. Lamelin JP, Lenoir GM. Immunodeficiency secondary to viral infection. In Chandra RJ, ed. Primary and secondary immunodeficiency disorders. New York: Churchill Livingstone, 1983:204.
210. Terry RJ, Hudson KM. Secondary immunodeficiencies on protozoan and helminth infections. In Chandra RJ, ed. Primary and secondary immunodeficiency disorders. New York: Churchill Livingstone, 1983:219.
211. McCall CE, Bass DA, Dechatelet LR, et al. In vitro response of human neutrophils to N-formyl-methionyllencyl-phenylalanine: correlation with effects of acute bacterial infection. J Infect Dis 1979;140:270.
212. Lobel JS, Bove KE. Clinicopathologic characteristics of septicemia in sickle cell disease. Am J Dis Child 1982;136:543.
213. Overtury G, Powars D. Multi-institutional study group of pneumococcal vaccine in sickle cell disease: infections in sickle cell anemia: pathogenesis and control. Texas Rep Biol Med 1980;40:283–981.
214. McCool RE, Catalona WJ. Current management of iatrogenic splenic injuries in children. J Urol 1981;125:549.
215. Robinson RG, Adler R, Swanson VL, et al. Congenital hypoplastic anemia (CHA) associated with congenital absence of the spleen. Am J Pediatr Hematol Oncol 1982;4:341.
216. Embry JH. Fatal *Streptococcus pneumonia* infection due to hyposplenism. Ala Med 1994;64:20–22.
217. Brigden ML. Overwhelming postsplenectomy infection still a problem. West J Med 1992;157:440–443.
218. Waldman JD, Rosenthal A, Smith AL, et al. Sepsis and congenital asplenia. J Pediatr 1977;90:555.
219. Deodhar HA, Marshall RJ, Barnes JN. Increased risk of sepsis after splenectomy. BMJ 1993;307:1408–1409.
220. Hathaway JM, Harley RA, Self S, Schiffman G, Virella G. Immunological function in post-traumatic splenosis. Clin Immunol Immunopathol 1995;74:143–150.
221. Committee on Infectious Diseases, American Academy of Pediatrics. Report of the committee on infectious diseases. Elk Grove Village, American Academy of Pediatrics, 1991:373–378.
222. Dickerman JD, Bolton E, Coil JA, et al. Protective effect of prophylactic penicillin on splenectomized mice exposed to an aerosolized suspension of type III *Streptococcus pneumoniae* blood. Blood 1979; 53:498.
223. Ertel IJ, Boles ET Jr, Newton WA Jr. Infection after splenectomy. N Engl J Med 1977;296:1174.
224. Ahonkai VI, Landesman SH, Fikrig SM, et al. Failure of pneumococcal vaccine in children with sickle cell disease. N Engl J Med 1979;300:26.
225. Bruton OD. Agammaglobulinemia. Pediatrics 1952;9:722.
226. Conley ME, Parolini O, Rohrer J, Campana D. X-linked agammaglobulinemia: new approaches to old questions based on the identification of the defective gene. Immunol Rev 1994;138:5–21.
227. Timmers E, De Weers M, Alt FW, Hendriks RW, Schuurman RKB. X-linked agammaglobulinemia. Clin Immunol Immunopathol 1991; 61:S83–S93.
228. Etzioni A, Pollack S. Primary antibody deficiency disorders—insight into the pathogenesis. Isr J Med Sci 1994;30:717–720.
229. Ohta Y, Haire RN, Litman RT, et al. Genomic organization and structure of Bruton agammaglobulinemia tyrosine kinase: localization of mutations associated with varied clinical presentations and course in X chromosome-linked agammaglobulinemia. Proc Natl Acad Sci 1994; 91:9062–9066.
230. Smith CIE, Islam KB, Vorechovsky I, et al. X-linked agammaglobulinemia and other immunoglobulin deficiencies. Immunol Rev 1994; 138:159–183.
231. Conley ME, Puck JM. Carrier detection in typical and typical X-linked agammaglobulinemia. J Pediatr 1988;112:688–694.
232. McKinney RE Jr, Katz SL, Wilfert CM. Chronic enteroviral meningoencephalitis in agammaglobulinemic patients. Rev Infect Dis 1987; 9:334–356.
233. Wagner DK, Marti GE, Jaffe ES, Straus SE, Nelson DL, Fleisher TA. Lymphocyte analysis in a patient with X-linked agammaglobulinemia and isolated growth hormone deficiency after development of echovirus dermatomyositis and meningoencephalitis. Int Arch Allergy Appl Immunol 1989;89:143–148.
234. Iseki M, Heiner DC. Immunodeficiency disorders. Pediatr Rev 1993;14:226–236.
235. Buckley RH. Immunodeficiency diseases. JAMA 1992;268:2797–2806.
236. Hermaszewski RA, Webster ADB. Primary hypogammaglobulinaemia: a survey of clinical manifestations and complications. QJM 1993;86: 31–42.
237. Lederman HM, Winkelstein JA. X-linked agammaglobulinemia: an analysis of 96 patients. Medicine 1985;64:145–156.
238. Rosen FS, Janeway CA. The gammaglobulins. III. The antibody deficiency syndromes. N Engl J Med 1966;275:709.
239. Wilfert CM, Buckley RM, Mohanakumar T, et al. Persistent and fatal CNS ECHO virus infection in patients with agammaglobulinemia. N Engl J Med 1977;296:1485.
240. Wright PF, Hatch MH, Kasselberg AG, et al. Vaccine associated polio-

myelitis in a child with sex-linked agammaglobulinemia. J Pediatr 1977;91:408.
241. Misbah SA, Spickett GP, Ryba PCJ, et al. Chronic enteroviral meningoencephalitis in agammaglobulinemia: case report and literature review. J Clin Immunol 1992;12:266–270.
242. Berkman SA, Lee ML, Gale RP. Clinical uses of intravenous immunoglobulins. Semin Hematol 1988;25:140–158.
243. Buckley RH. Plasma therapy in immunodeficiency diseases. Birth Defects 1975;11:347.
244. Alterman LA, de Alwis M, Genet S, et al. Carrier determination for X-linked agammaglobulinemia using X inactivation analysis of purified B cells. J Immunol Methods 1993;166:111–116.
245. Allen RC, Nachtman RG, Rosenblatt HM, Belmont JW. Application of carrier testing to genetic counseling for X-linked agammaglobulinemia. Am J Hum Genet 1994;54:25–35.
246. Eisenstein EM, Sneller, MC. Common variable immunodeficiency: diagnosis and management. Ann Allergy 1994;73:285–292.
247. Shyur SD, Hill HR. Immunodeficiency in the 1990s. Pediatr Infect Dis J 1991;10:595–611.
248. Good RA, Kelly WD, Rotstein J, Varco RL. Immunological deficiency diseases. Prog Allergy 1962;6:187.
249. Dressler F, Peter HH, Muller W, Rieger CHL. Transient hypogammaglobulinemia of infancy. Acta Paediatr Scand 1989;78:767–774.
250. McGeady SJ. Transient hypogammaglobulinemia of infancy: need to reconsider name and definition. J Pediatr 1987;110:47–50.
251. Walker AM, Kemp AS, Hill DJ, Shelton MJ. Features of transient hypogammaglobulinaemia in infants screened for immunological abnormalities. Arch Dis Child 1994;70:183–186.
252. Cunningham-Rundles C, Fotino M, Rosina O, Peter JB. Selective IgA deficiency, IgG subclass deficiency, and the major histocompatibility complex. Clin Immunol Immunopathol 1991;61:S61–S69.
253. De Laat PCJ, Weemaes CMR, Gonera R, Van Munster PJJ, Bakkeren JAJM, Stoelinga GBA. Clinical manifestations in selective IgA deficiency in childhood. Acta Paediatr Scand 1991;80:798–804.
254. Hong R. Update on the immunodeficiency diseases. Am J Dis Child 1990;144:983–992.
255. Hobbs JR, Milner RDG, Watt PJ. Gamma-M deficiency predisposing to meningococcal septicaemia. BMJ 1967;4:583.
256. Faulk WP, Kiyasu WS, Cooper MD, Fudenberg HH. Deficiency of IgM. Pediatrics 1971;47:399.
257. Hobbs JR. IgM deficiency. Birth Defects 1975;11:112.
258. Kondo N, Ozawa T, Kato Y, et al. Reduced secreted μ mRNA synthesis in selected IgM deficiency of Bloom's syndrome. Clin Exp Immunol 1992;88:35–40.
259. Wochner RD. Hypercatabolism of normal IgG: an unexplained immunoglobulin abnormality in the connective tissue diseases. J Clin Invest 1970;49:454.
260. Shackelford PG. IgG subclasses: importance in pediatric practice. Pediatr Rev 1993;14:291–296.
261. Shield JPH, Strobel S, Levinsky RJ, Morgan G. Immunodeficiency presenting as hypergammaglobulinaemia with IgG2 subclass deficiency. Lancet 340;448–450.
262. Smith TF. IgG Subclasses. Adv Pediat 1992;39:101–126.
263. Hanson LA, Soderstrom R, Nilssen DE, et al. IgG subclass deficiency with or without IgA deficiency. Clin Immunol Immunopathol 1991; 61:S70–S77.
264. Banatvala N, Davies J, Kanariou M, Strobel S, Levinsky R, Morgan G. Hypogammaglobulinaemia associated with normal or increased IgM (the hyper IGM syndrome): a case series review. Arch Dis Child 1994; 71:150–152.
265. Fuleihan R, Ramesh N, Rosen F, Geha RS. Localization of the genetic defect in X-linked immunoglobulin deficiency with normal or elevated IgM (HIGMX-1) to the CD40 ligand gene. Trans Assoc Am Physicians 1993;107:91–95.
266. Callard RE, Smith SH, Herbert J, et al. CD40 Ligand (CD40L) expression and B cell function in agammaglobulinemia with normal or elevated levels of IgM (HIM). J Immunol 1994;153:3295–3306.
267. Ochs HD, Wedgwood RJ. Disorders of the B-cell system. In: Stiehm ER, ed. Immunologic disorders of infants and children. Philadelphia: WB Saunders, 1989:226–256.
268. DiGeorge AM. Congenital absence of the thymus and its immunologic consequences: concurrence with congenital hypothyroidism. Birth Defects 1968;4:116.
269. Harrington H. Absence of the thymus gland. Lond Med Gaz 1829;3:314.
270. Greenberg F. What defines DiGeorge Anomaly. J Pediatr 1989;115:412–413.
271. Bastian J, Law S, Vogler L, Lawton A, Herrod H, Anderson S, Horowitz S, Hong R. Prediction of persistent immunodeficiency in the DiGeorge anomaly. J Pediatr 1989;115:391–396.
272. Cunningham-Rundles S, Harbison M, Guirguis S, Valacer D, Chretien PB. New perspectives on use of thymic factors in immune deficiency. Ann NY Acad Sci 1994;730:71–83.
273. Greenberg F. DiGeorge syndrome: an historical review of clinical and cytogenetic features. J Med Genet 1993;30:803–806.
274. Driscoll DA, Salvin J, Sellinger B, et al. Prevalence of 22q11 microdeletion in DiGeorge and velocardiofacial syndromes: implications for genetic counselling and prenatal diagnosis. J Med Genet 1993;30:813–817.
275. Scambler PJ, Kelly D, Lindsay E, et al. Velo-cardio-facial syndrome associated with chromosome 22 deletions encompassing the DiGeorge locus. Lancet 1992;339:1138–1139.
276. Driscoll DA, Spinner NB, Budarf ML, et al. Deletions and microdeletions of 22q11.2 in velo-cardio-facial syndrome. Am J Med Genet 1992;44:261–268.
277. Goldmuntz E, Driscoll D, Budarf ML, et al. Microdeletions of chromosomal region 22q11 in patients with congenital conotruncal cardiac defects. J Med Genet 1993;30:807–812.
278. Van Mierop LHS, Kutsche LM. Cardiovascular anomalies in DiGeorge syndrome and importance of neural crest as a possible pathogenetic factor. Am J Cardiol 1986;58:133–137.
279. August CS, Levay RH, Berkel AI, et al. Establishment of immunological competence in a child with congenital thymic aplasia by a graft of fetal thymus. Lancet 1970;1:1080.
280. Cleveland WW, Fogel BJ, Brown WT, Kay HEM. Foetal thymic transplant in a case of DiGeorge's syndrome. Lancet 1968;2:1211.
281. Thong YH, Robertson EF, Rischbreth HG, et al. Successful restoration of immunity in the DiGeorge syndrome with fetal thymic epithelial transplant. Arch Dis Child 1978;53:580.
282. Steele RW, Limas C, Thurman GB, et al. Familial thymic aplasia: attempted reconstruction with fetal thymus in a Millipore diffusion chamber. N Engl J Med 1972;287:787.
283. Goldsobel AB, Haas A, Stiehm ER. Bone marrow transplantation in DiGeorge syndrome. J Pediatr 1987;111:40–44.
284. Borzy MS, Ridgway D, Noya FJ, Shearer WT. Successful bone marrow transplantation with split lymphoid chimerism in DiGeorge syndrome. J Clin Immunol 1989;9:386–392.
285. Stephan JL, Vlekova V, Le Deist F, et al. Severe combined immunodeficiency: A retrospective single-center study of clinical presentation and outcome in 117 patients. J Pediatr 1993;123:564–572.
286. Hilman BC, Sorensen RU. Management options: SCIDS with adenosine deaminase deficiency. Ann Allergy 1994;72:395–403.
287. Hirschhorn R. Overview of biochemical abnormalities and molecular genetics of adenosine deaminase deficiency. Pediatr Res 1993;33:S35–S41.
288. Hague RA, Rassam S, Morgan G, Cant AJ. Early diagnosis of severe combined immunodeficiency syndrome. Arch Dis Child 1994;70:260–263.
289. Rosen FS, Cooper MD, Wedgwood RJP. The primary immunodeficiencies. N Engl J Med 1984;311:235.
290. Buckley RH, Schiff SE, Schiff RI, et al. Haploidentical bone marrow stem cell transplantation in human severe combined immunodeficiency. Semin Hematol 1993;30:92–104.
291. Simmons K. SCID takes many forms; infection common. JAMA 1984;251:1935.
292. Gatti RA, Meuwissin HJ, Allen HD, et al. Immunological reconstitution of sex-linked lymphopenic immunological deficiency. Lancet 1968;2:1366.
293. Hershfield MS, Chaffee S, Sorensen RU. Enzyme replacement therapy with polyethylene glycol-adenosine deaminase in adenosine deaminase deficiency: overview and case reports of three patients, including two now receiving gene therapy. Pediatr Res 1993;33:S42–S47.
294. Blaese RM. Development of gene therapy for immunodeficiency: adenosine deaminase deficiency. Pediatr Res 1993;33:S49–S53.
295. Lenarsky C, Weinberg K, Kohn DB, Parkman R. Unrelated donor BMT for Wiskott-Aldrich syndrome. Bone Marrow Transplant 1993;12:145–147.
296. Wiskott A. Fimiliarer, angeborener Morbus Werihoff? Wschr Kinderheilk 1937;68:212.
297. Aldrich RA, Steinberg AG, Campbell DC. Pedigree demonstrating a sex-linked recessive condition characterized by draining ears, eczematoid dermatitis and bloody diarrhea. Pediatrics 1954;13:133.
298. Beard LJ, Toogood IRG, Pearson CC, Ferrante A. Early bone marrow

transplantation in an infant with Wiskott-Aldrich syndrome. Am J Pediatr Hematol Oncol 1991;13:310–314.
299. Peacocke M, Siminovitch KA. Wiskott-Aldrich syndrome: new molecular and biochemical insights. J Am Acad Dermatol 1992;27:507–519.
300. Ochs HD, Slichter SJ, Harker LA, et al. The Wiskott-Aldrich syndrome: studies of lymphocytes, granulocytes and platelets. Blood 1980;55:243.
301. Perry GS III, Spector BD, Schuman LM, et al. The Wiskott-Aldrich syndrome in the United States and Canada (1892–1979) J Pediatr 1980;97:72.
302. Standen GR. Wiskott-Aldrich syndrome: a multidisciplinary disease. J Clin Pathol 1991;44:979–982.
303. Lum LG, Tubergen DG, Corash L, Blaese RM. Splenectomy in the management of the thrombocytopenia of the Wiskott-Aldrich syndrome. N Engl J Med 1980;302:892.
304. Mullen CA, Anderson KD, Blaese RM. Splenectomy and/or bone marrow transplantation in the management of the Wiskott-Aldrich syndrome: long-term follow-up of 62 cases. Blood 1993;82:2961-2966.
305. Brochstein JA, Gillio AP, Ruggiero M, et al. Marrow transplantation from human leukocyte antigen-identical or haploidentical donors for correction of Wiskott-Aldrich syndrome. J Pediatr 1991;119:907–912.
306. Greer WL, Peacocke M, Siminovitch KA. The Wiskott-Aldrich syndrome: refinement of the localization on Xp and identification of another closely linked marker locus, OATL1. Hum Genet 1992;88:453–456.
307. Syllaba L, Henner K. Contribution a l'independance de'athetose double idiopathique et congenitale: atteinte familiale, syndrome dystrophique, signe du reseau vasculaire conjonctival, integrite psychique. Rev Neurol 1926;1:541.
308. Boder E, Sedgwick RP. Ataxia telangiectasia: a review of 101 cases. In: Wash G, ed. Cerebellum, posture and cerebral palsy. London: The National Spastics Society and Heinemann Medical Books, 1963:110.
309. Taylor AMR, Byrd PJ, McConville CM, Thacker S. Genetic and cellular features of ataxia telangiectasia. Int J Radiat Biol 1994;65:65–70.
310. Taylor AMR, Jaspers NGJ, Gatti RA. Fifth international workshop on ataxia-telangiectasia. Cancer Res 1993;53:438–441.
311. Wong V, Yu YL, Chan-Lui WY, Woo E, Yeung CY: Ataxia telangiectasia in Chinese children. Clin Neurol Neurosurg 1987;89:137–144.
312. MacDermot KD, Winter RM, Wigglesworth JS, Strobel S. Short stature/short limb skeletal dysplasia with severe combined immunodeficiency and bowing of the femora: report of two patients and review. J Med Genet 1991;28:10–17.
313. Polmar SH, Pierce GF. Cartilage hair hypoplasia: immunological aspects and their clinical implications. Clin Immunol Immunopathol 1986; 40:87–93.
314. Curnutte JT. Chronic granulomatous disease: the solving of a clinical riddle at the molecular level. Clin Immunol Immunopathol 1993;67:S2–S15.
315. Roos D. The genetic basis of chronic granulomatous disease. Immunol Rev 1994;138:121–157.
316. Thrasher AJ, Keep NH, Wientjes F, Segal AW. Chronic granulomatous disease. Biochim Biophys Acta 1994;1227:1–24.
317. Ambruso DR, Johnston RB Jr. Defects of phagocyte function. In: Chandra RK, ed. Primary and secondary immunodeficiency disorders. New York: Churchill Livingstone, 1983:133.
318. Pedersen FK, Johansen S, Rosenkrist J, et al. Refractory *Pneumocystis carinii* infection in chronic granulomatous disease: successful treatment with granulocytes. Pediatrics 1979;64:935.
319. Mark LK. Chronic granulomatous disease in the adult. J Fam Pract 1978;7:445.
320. Quie P. Chronic granulomatous disease of childhood: a saga of discovery and understanding. Pediatr Infect Dis J 1993;12:395–8.
321. Donowitz GR, Mandell GL. Monocyte function in patients with chronic granulomatous disease of childhood. Am J Med 1982;73:1151.
322. Balfour HH Jr, Shehan JJ, Speecher CE, et al. Chronic granulomatous disease of childhood in a 23-year-old man. JAMA 1971;217:7.
323. Weening RS, Kabel P, Pijman P, Roos D. Continuous therapy with sulfamethoxazole-trimethoprim in patients with chronic granulomatous disease. J Pediatr 1983;103:127.
324. Fischer A, Segal AW, Seger R, Weening RS. The management of chronic granulomatous disease. Ear J Pediatr 1993;152:896–899.
325. Gallin JI, Sechler JMG, Malech HL. Reconstitution of defective phagocytic function in chronic granulomatous disease of childhood with recombinant human interferon-γ. Trans Assoc Am Physicians 1988; 101:12–17.
326. Rex JH, Bennett JE, Gallin JI, Malech HL, DeCarlo ES, Melnick DA. In vivo interferon-γ therapy augments the in vitro ability of chronic granulomatous disease neutrophils to damage *Aspergillus hyphae*. J Infect Dis 1991;163:849–852.
327. Kume A, Dinaeur MC. Retrovirus-mediated reconstitution of respiratory burst activity in X-linked chronic granulomatous disease cells. Blood 1994;84:3311–3316.
328. Harfi HA, Malik SA. Chediak-Higashi syndrome: clinical, hematologic, and immunologic improvement after splenectomy. Ann Allergy 1992;69:147–150.
329. Diukman R, Tanigawara S, Cowen MJ, Golbus MS. Prenatal diagnosis of Chediak-Higashi Syndrome. Prenat Diagn 1992;12:877–885.
330. Durandy A, Breton-Gorius J, Guy-Grand D, Dumez C, Griscelli C. Prenatal diagnosis of syndromes associating albinism and immune deficiencies (Chediak-Higashi syndrome and variant). Prenat Diagn 1993; 13:13–20.
331. Boxer LA, Watanabe AM, Rister M, et al. Correction of leukocyte function in Chediak-Higashi syndrome by ascorbate. N Engl J Med 1976; 295:1041.
332. Malawista SE, Oliver JM, Rudolph SA. Microtubules and cyclic AMP in human leukocytes: on the order of things. J Cell Biol 1978;77:881.
333. Oliver JM, Zurier RB. Correction of characteristic abnormalities of microtubule function and granule morphology in Chediak-Higashi syndrome with cholinergic agonists: Studies in vitro in man and in vivo in the beige mouse. J Clin Invest 1976;57:1239.
334. Boxer LA, Albertini DF, Baehner RL, Oliber JM. Impaired microtubule assembly and polymorphonuclear leukocyte function in the Chediak-Higashi syndrome correctable by ascorbic acid. BMJ 1979;43:207.
335. Good, RA. Bone marrow transplantation symposium: bone marrow transplantation for immunodeficiency diseases. Am J Med Sci 1987;294: 68–74.
336. Cooper MR, DeChatelet LR, McCall CE, et al. Complete deficiency of leukocyte glucose-6-phosphate dehydrogenase with defective bactericidal activity. J Clin Invest 1972;51:769.
337. Gray GR, Stamatoyannopoulos G, Naiman SC, et al. Neutrophil dysfunction, chronic granulomatous disease, and non-spherocytic haemolytic anaemia caused by complete deficiency of glucose-6-phosphate dehydrogenase. Lancet 1973;2:530.
338. Lehrer RI, Cline MJ. Leukocyte myeloperoxidase deficiency in disseminated candidiasis: the role of myeloperoxidase in resistance to candida infections. J Clin Invest 1969;48:478.
339. Lech P, Papathanassiou, Boreux G, et al. Hereditary myeloperoxidase deficiency. Blood 1979;53:403.
340. Klebanoff SJ, Pincus SH. Hydrogen peroxide utilization in myeloperoxidase-deficient leukocytes: a possible microbial control mechanism. J Clin Invest 1971;50:2226.
341. Rosen H, Klebanoff SJ. Chemiluminescence and superoxide production by myeloperoxidase-deficient leukocytes. J Clin Invest 1976;58:50.
342. Davis AT, Brunning RD, Quie PG. Polymorphonuclear leukocyte myeloperoxidase in a patient with myelomonocytic leukemia. N Engl J Med 1971;285:789.
343. Repine JE, Clawson CC, Brunning RD. Abnormal pattern of bactericidal activity of neutrophils deficient in granules, myeloperoxidase, and alkaline phosphatase. J Lab Clin Med 1976;88:788.
344. El-Maalem H, Fletcher J. Impaired neutrophil function and myeloperoxidase deficiency in myeloid metaplasia. Br J Haematol 1976;33:144.
345. Jeppson JD, Jaffe HS, Hill HR. Use of recombinant human interferon gamma to enhance neutrophil chemotactic responses in Job syndrome of hyperimmunoglobulinemia E and recurrent infections. J Pediatr 1991;118:383–387.
346. Brown CC, Gallin JI. Chemotactic disorders. Hematol Oncol Clin North Am 1988;2:61–79.
347. Hattori K, Hasui M, Masuda K, Masua M, Ogino H, Kobayashi Y. Successful trimethoprim-sulfamethoxazole therapy in a patient with hyperimmunoglobulin E syndrome. Acta Paediatr 1993;82:324–326.
348. Reimann HA. Haemocytic periodicity and periodic disorders: periodic neutropenia, thrombocytopenia, lymphocytosis and anemia. Postgrad Med J 1971;47:504.
349. Leale M. Recurrent furunculosis in an infant showing an unusual blood picture. JAMA 1910;54:1854.
350. Guerry D, Dale DC, et al. Periodic hematopoiesis in human cyclic neutropenia. J Clin Invest 1973;53:3220.
351. Dale DC, Bolyard AA, Hammond WP. Cyclic neutropenia: natural history and effects of long-term treatment with recombinant human granulocyte colony-stimulating factor. Cancer Invest 1993;11:219–223.
352. Dunkel IJ, Bussel JB. New developments in the treatment of neutropenia. Am J Dis Child 1993;147:994–1000.
353. Wright DG, Kenney RF, Oette DH, LaRussa VF, Boxer LA, Malech HL.

Contrasting effects of recombinant human granulocyte-macrophage colony-stimulating factor (CSF) and granulocyte CSF treatment on the cycling of blood elements in childhood-onset cyclic neutropenia. Blood 1994;84:1257–1267.

354. Kostmann R. Infantile genetic agranulocytosis: a review with presentation of ten new cases. Acta Paediatr Scand 1975;64:362.

355. Hestdal K, Welte K, Lie SO, Keller JR, Ruscetti FW, Abrahamsen TG. Severe congenital neutropenia: abnormal growth and differentiation of myeloid progenitors to granulocyte colony-stimulating factor (G-CSF) but normal response to G-CSF plus stem cell factor. Blood 1993;82:2991–2997.

356. Shwachman H, Diamond LK, Oski FA, Khaw K. The syndrome of pancreatic insufficiency and bone marrow dysfunction. J Pediatr 1964;65:645.

357. Burke V, Colebatch JH, et al. Association of pancreatic insufficiency and chronic neutropenia in childhood. Arch Dis Child 1967;42:147.

358. Shwachman H, Holsclaw D. Some clinical observations on the Shwachman syndrome (pancreatic insufficiency and bone marrow hypoplasia). Birth Defects 1972;3:46.

359. Huijgens PC, van der Veen EA, et al. Syndrome of Shwachman and leukaemia. Scand J Haematol 1977;18:20.

360. Stevens MJ, Lilleyman JS, et al. Shwachman's syndrome and acute lymphoblastic leukaemia. BMJ 1978;2:18.

361. Alper CA, Colten HR, Rosen FS, et al. Homozygous deficiency of the third component of complement (C3) in a patient with repeated infections. Lancet 1972;2:1179.

362. Walport MJ. Complement deficiency and disease. Br J Rheumatol 1993;32:269–273.

363. Densen P. Complement deficiencies and meningococcal disease. Clin Exp Immunol 1991;86:57–62.

364. Rosen FS. Genetic defects of the complement system. Clin Immunol Immunopath 1991;61:S78–S82.

The Critically Ill Child with Human Immunodeficiency Virus Infection

29

John J. Farley
Robert Englander
Randall L. Tressler
Peter E. Vink

INTRODUCTION

The first cases of acquired immune deficiency syndrome (AIDS) in children were described in 1982. Since then, AIDS has become one of the leading causes of death in children. As of the end of 1994, over 6000 cases of AIDS in children less than 13 years of age had been reported in the United States[1]. Based on masked serosurveys, it is estimated that there are 10,000 to 15,000 children in the United States infected with human immunodeficiency virus type 1 (HIV), which causes AIDS[2]. Worldwide, it is estimated there are more than 500,000 HIV infected infants and children[3]. Many of these children will come under the care of a pediatric intensive care specialist who must provide medical and supportive care for both the critically ill child, as well as for family members who themselves may also be suffering from this devastating illness.

EPIDEMIOLOGY

Perinatal transmission from infected mother to infant is the most common means by which children acquire HIV infection, accounting for 86% of AIDS cases in children under 5 reported through 1994[1]. Transmission of infection by contaminated blood, blood products, and coagulation factors is responsible for most of the remaining cases. Childhood sexual abuse and undetermined risk factors account for less than 1% of cases[1,4]. Among mothers of perinatally infected children with AIDS, injection drug use as a risk factor is becoming less frequent, reported by 15% in 1994[1]. Approximately 60% of perinatally acquired AIDS cases in the United States are among African-American children and 24% among Hispanic children.

Although approximately 2000 cases of AIDS among adolescents 13 to 19 years old have been reported, more than 16,000 cases have been reported in young adults 20 to 24 years old, most of whom were presumably infected with HIV during adolescence[5]. Among AIDS cases in adolescents reported through 1994, more than 34% were related to blood product or tissue receipt, followed by male-to-male sexual contact (21%), heterosexual contact (19%), and injection drug use (10%)[1].

Perinatal Transmission

Perinatal HIV transmission can occur before, during, or after delivery. HIV has been isolated from both first and second trimester aborted fetuses[6–9]. About 30 to 50% of infants ultimately found to be HIV infected are polymerase chain reaction (PCR) or virus culture positive at birth, consistent with virus acquisition in utero. Conversely, 50 to 70% of infants do not demonstrate detectable virus until late in infancy, suggestive of acquisition during the intrapartum period[10]. In a study of twins with discordant infection outcome born to HIV infected women, the presenting twin had a three-fold greater risk of infection than the second born twin[11], presumably resulting from intrapartum transmission. HIV can be transmitted postpartum through breast feeding as well, particularly among mothers with primary HIV infection postpartum[12]. In the developed world, breast feeding by HIV infected mothers is strongly discouraged[13].

In Europe and North America, overall perinatal transmission rates have ranged from 10 to 39%, with somewhat higher rates reported in Africa. Many studies have demonstrated an association between advanced HIV disease in the mother (represented by increased viral burden, low CD4+ T lymphocyte count, or clinical AIDS) and increased risk of HIV transmission to the infant[14]. A recent study has suggested an increased risk of HIV transmission among women with recently acquired HIV infection[15].

Until recently, no interventions to prevent HIV transmission had been proven efficacious. In 1994, results of a clinical trial were announced that demonstrated the efficacy of a perinatal Zidovudine (ZDV) regimen in reducing the rate of HIV transmission. The trial was placebo controlled and consisted of a three-part regimen: mothers were treated prenatally with oral ZDV, mothers received intravenous ZDV during labor, and infants received ZDV orally for the first six weeks of life. The proportions of infants infected with HIV were 8.3% in the treatment group and 25.5% in the placebo group[16]. Although study participation was limited to women with CD4+ T lymphocyte counts $\geq$ 200 cells/ml^3, another report suggests that the beneficial effects of ZDV in reducing perinatal transmission may extend to women with lower CD4$^+$ T lymphocyte counts as well[17].

In spite of evidence that 50 to 70% of perinatal HIV transmission occurs during the intrapartum period, there have been conflicting results regarding the influence of cesarian section delivery on transmission rates[18]. A clinical trial was recently begun in Europe. A clinical trial incorporating the perinatal ZDV regimen and using HIV hyperimmune globulin was recently begun in the United States.

Transmission by Contaminated Blood Products

HIV transmission by contaminated blood is the most efficient mode of infection transmission. In a study of 694 patients who received contaminated blood, 80% became infected[19]. Among hemophiliacs, infection by infusions of clotting factor concentrates prepared from plasma pools obtained from thousands of donors was extremely common prior to universal virus inactivation procedures and antibody screening. In a survey of 7000 persons with hemophilia followed at United States treatment centers from 1985 to 1989, 70% of persons with severe factor VIII deficiency and nearly 50% of persons with severe factor IX deficiency were reported to be HIV seropositive[20].

In 1983, a donor self-exclusion program was initiated to allow high risk donors to remove their donated blood confidentially from the transfusion pool. This step was followed in 1985 by HIV antibody screening of all donated blood products. In spite of these steps, which have minimized transmission from infected units, a finite risk of transmission of HIV by blood products still remains. Blood units donated by individuals who have recently become infected but have not yet developed detectable circulating antibodies ("the window period") remain infectious[21,22].

HIV PATHOGENESIS

Clinical Perspective

In the adult, several discrete stages of HIV-1 disease progression can be observed. After the initial infection with HIV-1, some patients undergo an acute influenzalike illness. This acute infection is accompanied by a rapid but transient fall in CD4 T lymphocytes and increasing viral p24 antigenemia. The first systemic cells to be infected are activated and differentiated cells capable of supporting viral replication. Since few activated CD4 T lymphocytes circulate and peripheral blood monocytes are not susceptible to infection, the prime targets are differentiated macrophages in the spleen and activated CD4 T lymphocytes in lymphoid tissues. Within days of infection, high levels of viral replication occur in these tissues as measured by p24 antigenemia and high viremia titers. Before an antiviral response occurs, large numbers of cells within lymphoid tissues become infected. The CD8 T lymphocytes increase similar to other viral infections[23]. Within weeks, viremia is markedly reduced in response to immune reaction against HIV-1. Cellular immune responses are thought to be the first effective antiviral activity with the early production of CD8 T lymphocytes before seroconversion[24,25]. Plasma viral levels decrease before neutralizing antibodies can be detected[26,27].

As the transient acute illness passes, the patient enters a clinically asymptomatic protracted stage. This asymptomatic phase is characterized by nearly normal circulating CD4 T lymphocyte numbers, detectable circulating HIV-1 antibodies, and normal health[28]. During this phase, CD4 T lymphocytes decline at a steady rate estimated at 25 to 60 cells/μl per year[29]. During this period, the CD8 T lymphocyte population remains elevated. Several longitudinal studies reveal a slow, inexorable increase in overall viral burden (free- and cell-associated virus) over months to years.

The asymptomatic phase is eventually replaced by asymptomatic HIV infection characterized by progressive immunosuppression, further declining of CD4 T lymphocyte numbers, decreasing CD8 T lymphocyte numbers, increasing viral p24 antigenemia, and finally the appearance of opportunistic infections. In January 1995, Wei et al. and Ho et al. demonstrated that treatment of patients with multidrug regimens produces a rapid reduction in plasma viremia. In addition, concomitant increases in the number of circulating CD4 T lymphocytes occurs[30,31]. This data suggests a dynamic interplay between a responsive immune system and viral replication. Wei and Ho treated symptomatic patients and extrapolated from viremic measures that between 10^8 and 10^9 virions were being cleared every day or approximately 30% of the total viral load. Further calculations, assuming comparable daily rates of viral destruction and production, show HIV production to be around 10^8 to 10^9 virions per day. The CD4 T lymphocyte recovery on the multidrug regimen was also modeled by both Wei and Ho. Assuming that peripheral CD4 T lymphocyte elevations were also occurring in lymphoid tissues, they established that an average of 2×10^9 CD4 T lymphocytes (0.1 to 7×10^9) was produced daily. Since an overall decline in CD4 T lymphocytes occurs over months to years, the extent of daily CD4 T lymphocyte destruction exceeding the average daily production can be estimated.

This loss of CD4 T lymphocytes can no longer be explained by intrinsic HIV cytopathic effects. Coupling both the dynamic CD4 T lymphocyte production and loss with the efficient viral clearance, the immune system itself becomes the prime candidate for the immune system destruction. Cytotoxic T lymphocytes (CTL) or "killer cells" efficiently clear many viral infections. As infected cells express viral proteins, the infected cells are recognized by the CTL as foreign and are destroyed. HIV-specific CTL can infiltrate lymphoid tissues where most infected CD4 T lymphocytes reside and eliminate them[32]. In HIV-infected cells, the successful clearance of virus by CTL would account for the depletion of infected CD4 T lymphocytes. Billions of infected CD4 T lymphocytes and virions can be efficiently destroyed every day.

Concomitant with the dynamic viral replication within the lymph nodes is an associated destruction of CD4 T lymphocytes in the lymph node and lymph node architecture[33,34]. In some patients, the circulating CD4 T lymphocyte number may dramatically fall (below 200 cells/μl) over months with a return to high level circulating viral levels similar to the initial acute phase viremia[35,36,37]. In addition, a fall in circulating CD8 T lymphocytes is observed in late-stage AIDS possibly associated with a HIV-specific CTL loss. Without supportive, prophylactic, and antiretroviral therapies, the symptomatic HIV phase progresses to AIDS. Death generally results from overwhelming opportunistic infections or malignancy in these severely immunosuppressed individuals.

In children with vertically acquired HIV-1 infection, similar phases of disease progression are observed but the time scale is foreshortened. Few children have been recognized to undergo the acute influenzalike illness and primary viremia of HIV-1. This may be secondary to the timing of infection (in utero versus perinatal), the amount of viral inoculum, the route of viral inoculum (transplacental versus ingested blood), the virulence of the viral strain, or the immaturity of the infant immune system attempting to mount an acute influenzalike response.

Many children go through a protracted asymptomatic phase similar to adults. It is clear, however, this asymptomatic phase is abbreviated as compared to the adults in whom it is estimated to average 10 years. The etiology of this contracted time course in children is unclear. One hypothesis is a difference in interaction of the virus with the mature immune systems of adults versus the developing immune systems of infants and children. The stages of symptomatic HIV-1 infection and progression to AIDS are very similar to the adult. Like adults, the children generally die of overwhelming opportunistic infections or malignancy in association with their severe immunosuppression.

Cellular Perspective

HIV-1 is a member of the lenti virus group, so named because of the protracted nature of the diseases caused by members of this viral genus. The structure of the virus is complex. Viral RNA strands are covered by proteins (p9 and p7) that, with reverse transcriptase and a core-covering protein, p24/25, make up a disc-shaped core particle. The core is surrounded by shell of protein components, p17, and a host cell-derived lipid bilayer, the viral envelope. This viral envelope contains glycoproteins (gp), gp41 and gp120, which allow the virus to attach to a specific receptor for HIV, the CD4 receptor on the host cell.

The life cycle of the virus can be conceptualized as afferent and efferent components. The afferent component comprises the infection of the host cell by a virion. The efferent component comprises the production of progeny virions.

The afferent component of the viral life cycle is initiated after attachment to the host cell CD4 receptor. The viral envelope then fuses with the host cell membrane. Viral core material, the nucleoscapsid, is injected into the host cytoplasm. Reverse transcriptase translates viral RNA into double-stranded DNA or provirus that enters the host cell nucleus. Once the provirus is incorporated or integrated into the host genome, the host cell is permanently infected[38,39].

Retroviral integration can rapidly lead to progeny virion synthesis in preactivated lymphoid and macrophage cells. However, in in vitro experiments, proviral-containing cells can be dormant and remains so until a variety of stimuli result in the conversion from dormant to active virion production[40–44]. The efferent component of the viral life cycle includes the successful transcription, translation, and assembly of progeny virions. The completed virions bud from the surface of the infected cell and are capable of infecting other cells.

Clearly many children and adults experience a prolonged course of HIV infection. It has been hypothesized that these clinically slow progressors are dependent predominantly on a specific cell mediated CD4 T lymphocyte immune response known as T-helper type one (TH1) immune response[45]. TH1 cell-mediated immune responses are supported and maintained by various cytokines, particularly interleukin 2 (IL-2) and interferon beta (IFNB). IL-2, produced by CD4 T lymphocytes, autoregulates CD4 T lymphocyte resulting in increased activation and proliferation of CD4 cells. IL-2 also enhances CD8 T lymphocyte function, in particular antiviral responses. It is believed that there is sustained production of the TH1 cytokines, IL-2, and IFNB in these slow progressors that maintain CD8 T lymphocyte HIV-specific antiviral activity.

This is contrasted by rapid progressors whose CD4 T lymphocytes have switched from TH1 cell-mediated immune response to B lymphocyte "help" resulting in humoral-mediated immune response. This CD4 B lymphocyte "help" is known as T-helper type 2 (TH2) immune response. TH2 humoral-mediated immune responses are supported and maintained by various cytokines, including IL-4 and IL-10. These TH2 cytokines suppress CD8 T lymphocyte antiviral functions allowing HIV-1 disease progression. The shift at the cellular level from TH1 to TH2 immune response and cytokine production is believed to precede clinical progression of HIV-1 disease. Further, TH2 cytokines feed back to the CD4 T lymphocytes and turn off TH1 cytokine production. This effectively stops further CD8 cell-mediated antiviral activity and CD4 T lymphocyte proliferation.

When enough CD4 T lymphocytes are lost (through direct and/or indirect mechanisms such as apotosis, syntitia, complement and neutralizing antibody lysis, HIV-specific CTL), CD4 production of IL-2 is reduced sufficiently to no longer maintain CD8 T lymphocyte proliferation and function. This loss of CD8 antiviral activity results in measurable increases in viremia.

In the prolonged asymptomatic stage, thousands of viral types are being produced, perhaps secondary to the extensive immune pressure. This asymptomatic period is characterized by the heterogeneity of these viral types. With progression to symptomatic HIV and AIDS, the emergence of a single (occasionally, several) dominant HIV type occurs. This dominant homogeneous viral production is considered a virulent strain. The clinical virulence of the strain is seen in the emergence of syntitial producing, neurotropic, and/or other tissue specific strains with subsequent cellular and tissue damage and associated HIV clinical morbidity. Further disease progression may occur secondary to enhanced cellular entry. HIV-specific antibodies are generally thought to neutralize free HIV virions. However, in vitro experiments have shown that in some dominant virulent strains HIV-specific antibodies can enhance viral entry into target cells.

Further testing of the TH1 versus TH2 immune response hypothesis is needed. If correct, this pathogenic mechanism suggests new therapies and interventions for HIV-1. Clearly, the goal would be maintenance of TH1 cellular immune responses and enhancing TH1 cytokine production. This might be accomplished by regular infusions of IL-2 or other TH1 cytokines such as IFN*B*. Strategies to regulate TH2 cytokine production and prevent TH2 feedback on TH1 cytokine production could be designed. One approach may be the administration of neutralizing antibodies directed against the TH2 cytokines, IL-4 and IL-10. Enhancing CD8 T lymphocyte production and survival would help maintain HIV-specific antiviral functions. Clinical trials infusing massive volumes and numbers of ex vivo-produced autologous CD8 T lymphocytes have been initiated.

DIAGNOSIS OF HIV INFECTION

General Considerations

Although tests for antibody to HIV are the mainstay for laboratory diagnosis in adults and older children, antibody tests are inadequate for diagnosing infection in infants born to HIV-infected women. In infants younger than 18 months of age, serum tests for immunoglobulin G (IgG) antibody to HIV do not differentiate between infant and passively acquired maternal antibody. A positive HIV antibody test in an infant only indicates exposure and possible infection, prompting the need for further testing. In addition, serologic testing may lack sensitivity, since some HIV-infected infants will become hypogammaglobulinemic and will not produce antibody including antibody to HIV[46].

A number of nonserologic early diagnostic tests have been developed with high sensitivity and specificity (see the following section). In the pediatric intensive care unit, the polymerase chain reaction test (PCR) offers the highest sensitivity with the most rapid result. Criteria for definitive diagnosis of HIV infection in children have recently been revised by the Centers for Disease Control and Prevention **(Table 29.1)**[47]. Two positive nonserologic HIV detection tests are required to make the diagnosis in a child less than 18 months of age. Note that an infant less than 18 months of age born to an HIV-infected mother with an AIDS-defining condition **(Table 29.2B)** meets the criteria without further laboratory testing.

Laboratory Testing

Serologic Testing

If HIV infection is clinically suspected, the diagnosis in adults and older children is made by detecting the presence of circulating HIV antibodies[48–52]. These antibodies to HIV can usually be detected within 6 to 12 weeks of the primary infection, although an occasional patient may only become seropositive after many months. The immunosorbent assay (ELISA) detects the presence of antibody to HIV or to a semipurified extract of HIV grown in tissue culture. ELISA is the primary screening test for HIV infection because of its very high degree of sensitivity, reproducibility, and low cost. It is necessary to evaluate a positive test further since the cut-off positive value has been selected to ensure a high degree of sensitivity for blood-bank screening, but with less specificity. The positive predictive value of the ELISA test is, therefore, relatively low in regions with a low HIV endemic rate. For this reason, a positive ELISA test should be repeated and, if the results remain positive, the sample should be subject to one of several confirmatory tests.

Western blot analysis is the most widely used confirmatory test[48–52]. In this test, viral protein antigens—including envelope, core, enzyme, and regulatory proteins—are separated by electrophoresis, blotted on nitrocellulose strips, and incubated with patient's serum. Specific antibodies to viral protein components are determined by the binding of an enzyme-labeled indicator, e.g., immunoperoxidase. A colored antigen band appears at the site of antibody binding, identifying a specific antibody response to the particular viral protein. Standard criteria for interpretation of western blot tests have been published by several groups[53,54]. When bands are present but do not meet the criteria for a positive test, those results are considered indeterminate and should be repeated or another test used.

ELISA and confirmatory western blot testing is both time consuming and expensive. To date, two rapid serologic tests have been licensed in the United States. One uses a latex direct agglutination assay, and the second uses a microfil-

Table 29.1. Diagnosis of Human Immunodeficiency Virus (HIV) Infection in Children[a]

DIAGNOSIS: HIV INFECTED

a) A child <18 months of age who is known to be HIV seropositive or born to an HIV-infected mother **and:**
- has positive results on two separate determinations (excluding cord blood) from one or more of the following HIV detection tests:
  —HIV culture,
  —HIV polymerase chain reaction,
  —HIV antigen (p24),

or

- meets criteria for acquired immunodeficiency syndrome (AIDS) diagnosis based on the 1987 AIDS surveillance case definition.

b) A child ≥18 months of age born to an HIV-infected mother or any child infected by blood, blood products, or other known modes of transmission (e.g., sexual contact) who:
- is HIV-antibody positive by repeatedly reactive enzyme immunoassay (EIA) and confirmatory test (e.g., Western blot or immunofluorescence assay [IFA]);

or

- meets any of the criteria in a) above.

DIAGNOSIS: PERINATALLY EXPOSED (PREFIX E)

A child who does not meet the criteria above who:
- is HIV seropositive by EIA and confirmatory test (e.g., Western blot or IFA) and is <18 months of age at the time of test;

or

- has unknown antibody status, but was born to a mother known to be infected with HIV.

DIAGNOSIS: SEROREVERTER (SR)

A child who is born to an HIV-infected mother and who:
- has been documented as HIV-antibody negative (i.e., two or more negative EIA tests performed at 6–18 months of age or one negative EIA test after 18 months of age);

and

- has had no other laboratory evidence of infection (has not had two positive viral detection tests, if performed);

and

- has not had an AIDS-defining condition.

[a]*From Centers for Disease Control. 1994 Revised Classification System for Human Immunodeficiency Virus Infection in Children Less than 13 Years of Age. MMWR 1994; 43:RR–12.*

tration enzyme immunoassay procedure. Recent technology for testing dried blood samples collected on filter paper has been developed[55].

Viral Culture

Viral culture is one of the most sensitive and specific techniques for detecting HIV infection in infants and is used extensively in research settings. The sensitivity in children is less than 50% in the first week of life, but rises to greater than 90% by age 3 months and nearly 100% by age 6 months[56–58]. The technique involves coculturing patient peripheral blood mononuclear cells (PBMC) separated from whole blood with phytohemagglutinin-stimulated PBMC feeder cells from healthy uninfected donors. Cocultures are stimulated with interleukin-2, supplemented periodically with feeder cells and monitored for the presence of virus by antigen or reverse transcriptase production[59,60]. Viral cultures require experienced laboratory personnel, special facilities because of biosafety precautions, and take 7 to 28 days or more to complete. A serial dilution method can be used to monitor the level of HIV in blood[61].

Polymerase Chain Reaction (PCR)

The sensitivity and specificity of PCR for detection of HIV infection in infants is comparable to that of viral culture[62,63]. The procedure detects HIV proviral DNA in PBMC through a three-step repetitive amplification process: cellular double-stranded DNA is denatured into single strands, specific complementary DNA primers anneal to the target sequences, and extension of annealed primers occurs. Following amplification, a number of techniques can be used to detect the HIV DNA sequences. PCR requires a minimal amount of blood and can be performed in 1 to 2 days. A PCR system has been developed as a simplified diagnostic kit[64]. Methodology has been developed to detect HIV in specific cells or tissues, to quantitate viral load, or to measure active viral replication by detecting viral RNA in plasma[63,65,66].

p24 Antigen Detection

Enzyme immunoassays for detecting viral antigen components such as p24 core antigen are commercially available. The standard p24 antigen assay does not detect p24 that is complexed with antibody; therefore, the test may not be positive unless there are sufficient levels of circulating free p24 antigen. Although useful as a prognostic marker and for monitoring antiviral therapy, sensitivity is inadequate for early diagnosis of infants[67–69]. Modification of the standard p24 antigen assay by acidification of the sample to dissociate immune complexes increases sensitivity considerably. The modified assay can be used to diagnose HIV infection in infants[47]. However, because data is lacking regarding sensitivity in early infancy, use of this assay alone is not currently recommended to exclude HIV infection[70].

Other Tests

HIV-specific immunoglobulin A assays have been developed that can detect HIV infection in infants by age 6 months, but are generally negative in infected infants under age 3 months[71,72]. Saliva can be used as well as serum and plasma[73]. In vitro antibody production assay and the rapid alternative ELISPOT detect the presence of HIV-specific antibody producing B lymphocytes in the infant. False-positive tests in uninfected infants in the first 2 months of life have been reported, and false-negative tests have been observed in persons with advanced immunodeficiency[74].

In 1986, a second virus called HIV-2 was isolated from some patients with AIDS. Most patients infected with HIV-2 reside in West Africa, and fewer than 50 cases have been reported in the United States[75]. Serologic testing is available. In 1992, routine screening of the United States blood supply for HIV-2 was initiated.

CLINICAL MANIFESTATIONS

Disease Progression

Among perinatally infected children, the earliest clinical manifestations include lymphadenopathy, hepatosplenomegaly, hypergammaglobulinemia, and skin disease including candidal dermatitis and/or seborrhea[67,76–79]. Although these manifestations lack specificity, they should arouse clinical suspicion and recommendation for testing. At least two distinct patterns of disease progression have emerged. A group of children develop severe symptomatology in the first year of life including *Pneumocystis carinii* pneumonia, symptomatic cytomegalovirus infection, wasting syndrome, and encephalopathy. Another group of children have a more indolent course. Clinical problems noted initially include lymphoid interstitial pneumonitis, lymphadenopathy, hepatosplenomegaly, and parotid gland enlargement[80–86]. Therefore, delayed recognition of HIV infection among older children is not uncommon[87]. A recent large prospective study reported that 23% of infected children developed AIDS before the age of 1 year and nearly 40% by age 4 years. Ten percent died before age 1, and 28% before age 5[88].

Disease progression among children infected by blood transfusion is slower than among those perinatally infected[86,89,90]. In a recent report comparing children with perinatally acquired infection to those with infection acquired from neonatal transfusion, median symptom-free survival time from birth to symptomatic infection was 6.4 months and 17.8 months respectively[91]. Survival after development of symptoms did not differ by transmission mode. Among hemophiliacs with known time of HIV seroconversion, progression to AIDS is slower among children than adults. Goedert and colleagues reported a 13.3% ± 5.3%

8 year cumulative rate of AIDS among those between ages 1 and 17[92].

Adolescents are more similar to adults than children in clinical symptomatology. Common infectious AIDS defining conditions include *Pneumocystis carinii* pneumonia (32.9%), candida esophagitis (11.8%), cryptococcosis (8.8%), and chronic herpes simplex infection (7.6%). The leading noninfectious AIDS-defining condition is wasting syndrome (18.4%)[93]. Little information is known concerning the natural history of disease among nonhemophiliac adolescents.

Classification System

The classification system for HIV infection in children less than 13 years of age was revised in 1994[47]. Once defined as infected, children are classified into one of four mutually exclusive clinical categories based on signs, symptoms, or diagnoses related to HIV infection **(Tables 29.2A and 29.2B).** Conditions in Category C as well as lymphoid interstitial pneumonitis from Category B meet the AIDS surveillance case definition[94]. Children are also classified into one of three immunologic categories based on age-specific CD4+ T lymphocyte count or CD4+ percent of total lymphocytes **(Table 29.3).** A grid combining immunologic with clinical categories is then used for the classification **(Table 29.4).** Children are not reclassified to a less severe category regardless of subsequent CD4+ determinations or resolution of clinical symptomatology. Children born to HIV-infected mothers whose HIV infection status is not yet determined are classified by using the grid with a letter "E" (for perinatally exposed) placed before the appropriate classification code.

Adolescents with HIV infection are classified using the 1993 Revised Classification System for HIV Infection and Expanded Surveillance Case Definition for AIDS Among Adolescents and Adults[95]. A similar grid combining immunologic with clinical categories is used **(Table 29.5).** With publication of this system, the surveillance case definition for AIDS was broadened to include *Mycobacterium tuberculosis* infection (any site), recurrent pneumonia, invasive cervical cancer, and a CD4+ T lymphocyte count less than 200 cells/ml^3 or CD4+ percent less than 14.

MEDICAL COMPLICATIONS OF HIV INFECTION

Pulmonary Complications

Pulmonary disease occurs in almost 70% of HIV-infected children and is often the cause of death. Such patients frequently require intensive care for respiratory failure. A wide variety of diseases, both infectious and noninfectious, affect these children and are outlined in **Table 29.6**[96–100]. Some of the infections are truly opportunistic, whereas others also affect normal children. Although some patients with lung disease may have chronic complaints, others may develop rapid respiratory decompensation and require intensive care and mechanical ventilation for fulminant respiratory failure. The most important of the lung diseases in HIV-infected patients is *Pneumocystis carinii* pneumonia (PCP).

Pneumocystis carinii Pneumonia (PCP)

PCP is the most common opportunistic infection in AIDS patients in the U.S. and has affected approximately 50% of pediatric AIDS patients[101]. It has been the initial HIV-

Table 29.2A. Clinical Categories for Children with Human Immunodeficiency Virus Infection[a]

CATEGORY N: NOT SYMPTOMATIC

Children who have no signs or symptoms considered to be the result of HIV infection or who have only one of the conditions listed in Category A.

CATEGORY A: MILDLY SYMPTOMATIC

Children with two or more of the conditions listed below but none of the conditions listed in Categories B and C.

- Lymphadenopathy (≥0.5 cm at more than two sites; bilateral = one site)
- Hepatomegaly
- Splenomegaly
- Dermatitis
- Parotitis
- Recurrent or persistent upper respiratory infection, sinusitis, or otitis media

CATEGORY B: MODERATELY SYMPTOMATIC

Children who have symptomatic conditions other than those listed for Category A or C that are attributed to HIV infection. Examples of conditions in clinical Category B include but are not limited to:

- Anemia (<8 gm/dL), neutropenia (<1,000/mm^3), or thrombocytopenia (<100,000/mm^3) persisting ≥30 days
- Bacterial meningitis, pneumonia, or sepsis (single episode)
- Candidiasis, oropharyngeal (thrush), persisting (>2 months) in children >6 months of age
- Cardiomyopathy
- Cytomegalovirus infection, with onset before 1 month of age
- Diarrhea, recurrent or chronic
- Hepatitis
- Herpes simplex virus (HSV) stomatitis, recurrent (more than two episodes within 1 year)
- HSV bronchitis, pneumonitis, or esophagitis with onset before 1 month of age
- Herpes zoster (shingles) involving at least two distinct episodes or more than one dermatome
- Leiomyosarcoma
- Lymphoid interstitial pneumonia (LIP) or pulmonary lymphoid hyperplasia complex
- Nephropathy
- Nocardiosis
- Persistent fever (lasting >1 month)
- Toxoplasmosis, onset before 1 month of age
- Varicella, disseminated (complicated chickenpox)

CATEGORY C: SEVERELY SYMPTOMATIC

Children who have any condition listed in the 1987 surveillance case definition for acquired immunodeficiency syndrome, with the exception of LIP (Box 3).

[a]*From Centers for Disease Control. 1994 Revised Classification System for Human Immunodeficiency Virus Infection in Children Less than 13 Years of Age. MMWR 1994; 43:RR-12.*

Table 29.2B. Conditions Included in Clinical Category C for Children Infected with Human Immunodeficiency Virus (HIV)[a]

CATEGORY C: SEVERELY SYMPTOMATIC

- Serious bacterial infections, multiple or recurrent (i.e., any combination of at least two culture-confirmed infections within a 2-year period), of the following types: septicemia, pneumonia, meningitis, bone or joint infection, or abscess of an internal organ or body cavity (excluding otitis media, superficial skin or mucosal abscesses, and indwelling catheter-related infections)
- Candidiasis, esophageal or pulmonary (bronchi, trachea, lungs)
- Coccidioidomycosis, disseminated (at site other than or in addition to lungs or cervical or hilar lymph nodes)
- Cryptococcosis, extrapulmonary
- Cryptosporidiosis or isosporiasis with diarrhea persisting >1 month
- Cytomegalovirus disease with onset of symptoms at age 1 month (at a site other than liver, spleen, or lymph nodes)
- Encephalopathy (at least one of the following progressive findings present for at least 2 months in the absence of a concurrent illness other than HIV infection that could explain the findings): a) failure to attain or loss of developmental milestones or loss of intellectual ability, verified by standard developmental scale or neuropsychological tests; b) impaired brain growth or acquired microcephaly demonstrated by head circumference measurements or brain atrophy demonstrated by computerized tomography or magnetic resonance imaging (serial imaging is required for children <2 years of age); c) acquired symmetric motor deficit manifested by two or more of the following: paresis, pathologic reflexes, ataxia, or gait disturbance
- Herpes simplex virus infection causing a mucocutaneous ulcer that persists for >1 month; or bronchitis, pneumonitis, or esophagitis for any duration affecting a child >1 month of age
- Histoplasmosis, disseminated (at a site other than or in addition to lungs or cervical or hilar lymph nodes)
- Kaposi's sarcoma
- Lymphoma, primary, in brain
- Lymphoma, small, noncleaved cell (Burkitt's), or immunoblastic or large cell lymphoma of B-cell or unknown immunologic phenotype
- *Mycobacterium tuberculosis,* disseminated or extrapulmonary
- *Mycobacterium,* other species or unidentified species, disseminated (at a site other than or in addition to lungs, skin, or cervical or hilar lymph nodes)
- *Mycobacterium avium* complex or *Mycobacterium kansasii,* disseminated (at site other than or in addition to lungs, skin, or cervical or hilar lymph nodes)
- *Pneumocystis carinii* pneumonia
- Progressive multifocal leukoencephalopathy
- Salmonella (nontyphoid) septicemia, recurrent
- Toxoplasmosis of the brain with onset at >1 month of age
- Wasting syndrome in the absence of a concurrent illness other than HIV infection that could explain the following findings: a) persistent weight loss >10% of baseline OR b) downward crossing of at least two of the following percentile lines on the weight-for-age chart (e.g., 95th, 75th, 50th, 25th, 5th) in a child ≥1 year of age OR c) <5th percentile on weight-for-height chart on two consecutive measurements, ≥30 days apart *PLUS* a) chronic diarrhea (i.e., at least two loose stools per day for ≥30 days) OR b) documented fever (for ≥30 days, intermittent or constant)

[a]*From Centers for Disease Control. 1994 Revised Classification System for Human Immunodeficiency Virus Infection in Children Less than 13 Years of Age. MMWR 1994;43:RR–12.*

related illness in 72% of children progressing to AIDS in the first year of life[(102)]. Of particular importance is the fact that PCP may be the first manifestation of HIV-related disease in infants not previously known to be infected with this virus. It may be a lethal first manifestation, with mortality approximating 100% if untreated.

CD4+ T lymphocyte counts can be used in HIV-infected children more than 1 year of age to identify those at highest risk for PCP. In a CDC survey, 16 (84%) of 19 children 1 to 5 years of age had CD4+ T lymphocyte counts less than or equal to 500 cells/ml^3 at the time of PCP diagnosis, and all 7 children more than age 6 who developed PCP had CD4+ T lymphocyte counts less than 200 cells/ml^3. However, recent data demonstrates that CD4+ T lymphocyte counts are of limited value in identifying children at risk for PCP who are less than 1 year of age[(103)].

Etiology and Pathogenesis

Pneumocystis carinii is a unicellular organism, the taxonomic category of which is unclear. It has been considered either a protozoan parasite or a fungus and, as such, exists

Table 29.3. Immunologic Categories for Children ≥13 Years Based on Age-specific CD4+ T-lymphocyte Counts and Percent of Total Lymphocytes[a]

	Age of child					
	<12 mos		*1–5 yrs*		*6–12 yrs*	
Immunologic category	μL	(%)	μL	(%)	μL	(%)
1. No evidence of suppression	≥1,500	(≥25)	≥1,000	(≥25)	≥500	(≥25)
2. Evidence of moderate suppression	750–1,499	(15–24)	500–999	(15–24)	200–499	(15–24)
3. Severe suppression	<750	(<15)	<500	(<15)	<200	(<15)

[a]*From Centers for Disease Control. 1994 Revised Classification System for Human Immunodeficiency Virus Infection in Children Less than 13 Years of Age. MMWR 1994;43:RR–12.*

Table 29.4. Pediatric Human Immunodeficiency Virus (HIV) Classification[a]

	Clinical categories			
Immunologic categories	*N: No signs/ symptoms*	*A: Mild signs/ symptoms*	*B:† Moderate signs/ symptoms*	*C:† Severe signs/ symptoms*
1. No evidence of suppression	N1	A1	B1	C1
2. Evidence of moderate suppression	N2	A2	B2	C2
3. Severe suppression	N3	A3	B3	C3

**Children whose HIV infection status is not confirmed are classified by using the above grid with a letter E (for perinatally exposed) placed before the appropriate classification code (e.g., EN2).*
†Both Category C and lymphoid interstitial pneumonitis in Category B are reportable to state and local health departments as acquired immunodeficiency syndrome.
[a]From Centers for Disease Control. 1994 Revised Classification System for Human Immunodeficiency Virus Infection in Children Less than 13 Years of Age. MMWR 1994;43:RR–12.

as a cyst (the form usually recognized diagnostically) that contains eight intracystic bodies. These bodies are released from the cyst and form new cysts(104). The organism becomes attached to the type 1 alveolar cells of the lung. This results in an alveolitis characterized by the presence of large amounts of foamy material containing organisms within the alveolar space and interstitial edema with an interstitial mononuclear cell infiltrate. The resulting physiologic disturbance is characterized by ventilation-perfusion mismatch, decreased pulmonary compliance, and alveolar capillary block, with hypoxia and elevated alveolar-arterial oxygen gradient. Most normal children older than age 4 years have serologic infection of latent infection with *Pneumocystis carinii*(105). Therefore, this infection in older children and adults is presumably the result of reactivation of the organism. In infants, PCP may result from a primary infection, possibly accounting for the rapid progression of the disease in this age group.

Clinical Manifestations

Patients with PCP usually have the tetrad of nonproductive cough, fever, dyspnea, and tachypnea. It is often insidious in onset but may develop acutely especially in infants. Commonly observed physical findings include respiratory distress with tachypnea, retractions, and cyanosis(106–8). Hypoxemia is almost an essential element of PCP, frequently appearing more severe than would be suggested by the associated radiologic changes. Patients will not necessarily have a fever. Percussion and auscultation of the lungs are often normal, but rales, rhonchi, or wheezes may be present. Although most HIV patients infected with *Pneumocystis carinii* have pneumonia alone, disseminated disease with involvement of spleen, liver, bone marrow, heart, kidneys, adrenal glands, and retinae can occur(109).

Table 29.5. Classification System for HIV Infection and Expanded AIDS Surveillance Case Definition for Adolescents and Adults[a]

	Clinical categories*		
CD4+ T-cell categories	*(A) Asymptomatic, acute (primary) HIV or PGL†*	*(B) Symptomatic, not (A) or (C) conditions*	*(C) AIDS-indicator conditions*
1. ≥500/μL	A1	B1	C1
2. 200–499/μL	A2	B2	C2
3. <200/μL AIDS-indicator T-cell count	A3	B3	C3

**Persons with AIDS-indicator conditions (Category C) as well as those with CD4+ T-lymphocyte counts <200/μL (Categories A3 or B3) are reportable as AIDS cases in the United States and Territories, effective January 1, 1993.*
†PGL = persistent generalized lymphadenopathy. Clinical Category A includes acute (primary) HIV infection.
[a]From Centers for Disease Control. 1993 Revised Classification System for HIV Infection and Expanded Surveillance Case Definition for AIDS Among Adolescents and Adults. MMWR 1992;41:RR–17.

Diagnosis

Although a presumptive diagnosis of PCP can be made on the basis of tachypnea, hypoxia, and diffuse alveolar infiltrates, definitive diagnosis still depends on the demonstration of organisms in pulmonary tissue, respiratory secretions, or lung fluid. Definitive diagnosis is important for several of the following reasons:

1. PCP can be successfully treated but is uniformly fatal if untreated.

Table 29.6. Pulmonary Diseases in Children with AIDS

Infectious
1. Parasitic
   Pneumocystis carinii, Toxoplasma gondii, Strongyloides stercoralis
2. Viral
   Respiratory viruses: respiratory syncytial virus, influenza virus, parainfluenza virus, adenovirus
   Measles
   Opportunists: cytomegalovirus, herpes simplex, varicella zoster virus
3. Bacterial
   Streptococcus pneumoniae, Haemophilus influenzae, Staphyloccus aureus
   Nosocomial: enteric bacilli, *Pseudomonas aeruginosa*
   Actinomycetes: *Nocardia* species
   Mycobacterial: *M. tuberculosis, M. avium-intracellulare*
4. Fungal
   Cryptococcus neoformans, Histoplasma capsulatum, Coccidioides immitis, Candida sp., *Asperidillus* sp.

Noninfectious
1. Lymphoid diseases
   Pulmonary lymphoid hyperplasia
   Lymphocytic interstitial pneumonia
   Polyclonal polymorphic B-cell lymphoproliferative disorder
2. Bronchiectasis
3. Kaposi's sarcoma

2. Assuming that the pulmonary infiltrate is caused by *Pneumocystis carinii* infection, failure to treat other infections may result without laboratory confirmation. Other causes of diffuse alveolar infiltrate in HIV-infected children include cytomegalovirus, *Mycobacterium avium* intracellularae, Epstein-Barr virus, parainfluenza virus, and lymphoid interstitial pneumonitis.
3. Posttreatment prophylaxis against this infection is indicated.
4. The development of PCP in an otherwise asymptomatic HIV-infected child is an AIDS-defining condition.

The following methods may be used to obtain appropriate specimens of pulmonary fluid:

1. Induced sputum technique is the least invasive technique to obtain pulmonary secretion specimens. This method requires patient cooperation and cannot be used in infants, the largest group of affected children. The recommended procedure is as follows[(110)]:
   a. Food is withheld for 4 hours before the procedure.
   b. Rinse the mouth with 3% saline (up to 50 ml. to remove oral contaminants.
   c. Have the patient inhale a nebulized mist of 3% saline delivered from an ultrasonic nebulizer.
   d. Some patients require 20 to 30 minutes for saline inhalation.
   e. Expectorated sputum is collected in specimen cups and diluted 1:1 with sterile water.
   f. Specimens are then digested with dithiothreitol and processed for culture and cytology.
2. Deep tracheal suction or tracheobronchial lavage through an endotracheal tube is another technique used to obtain sputum. Both of the above methods are relatively insensitive but are useful if they result in positive identification of the organism.
3. Bronchoalveolar lavage is the most widely used method for obtaining lung fluid to diagnose PCP. The recommended procedure is as follows[(111)]:
   a. Premedicate with atropine 0.01 mg/kg injected intramuscularly before the procedure. When the procedure begins, give meperidine 3.0 mg/kg intravenously. Administer supplemental oxygen, and apply topical anesthesia with 1% lidocaine to nose, pharynx, vocal cords, and tracheobronchial tree.
   b. Insert flexible bronchoscope transnasally or, if intubated, through the endotracheal tube.
   c. Examine airway, and wedge bronchoscope into a subsegment of the right middle or right lower lobe.
   d. Begin lavage by instilling 2.0 ml/kg sterile normal saline (without preservative) not to exceed a total of 10 ml.
   e. After a few seconds, aspirate saline with a syringe attached to suction port. This procedure may be repeated five to seven times, depending on the amount of fluid aspirated and patient tolerance.
   f. Process specimen for cytology and cultures.

   Although the precise sensitivity of this test in children with PCP is unknown, high yields with low incidence of complications have been reported[(111,112)]. Possible complications of the procedure include transient tachypnea, fever developing 4 to 6 hours later, and a transient increase in the opacification of the lavaged area of the lung. Deterioration in pulmonary function may occur after the procedure[(108)].
4. Open-lung biopsy or transbronchial biopsy provides lung tissue for examination and expands the information that can be obtained. A biopsy is necessary for the diagnosis of lymphoid interstitial pneumonitis. Open-lung biopsy requires a thoracotomy and is used only if a diagnosis is not forthcoming with less invasive procedures.

A suggested algorithm for establishing the diagnosis of diffuse bilateral pneumonitis in immunosuppressed children is shown in Figure 29.1.

When diagnostic procedures are to be performed for PCP or other opportunistic infections, it is important that the pathologist is consulted to ensure that the specimen is appropriately handled and processed. Special stains are required. In addition, appropriate microbiology tests should be arranged. Recommended studies for specimens obtained by induced sputum, tracheobronchial lavage, or bronchoalveolar lavage are listed in **Table 29.7.**

Treatment

The treatment of PCP consists of supportive modalities, antimicrobial therapy, and steroids. Oxygen therapy, continuous positive airway pressure, and mechanical ventilation are discussed in detail in Chapter 9.

Trimethoprim-sulfamethoxazole (TMP-SMX) is recommended for the initial treatment of PCP (Fig. 29.2). TMP-SMX is administered either orally or intravenously (TMP 20 mg/kg/day and SMX 100 mg/kg/day in three to four equal doses). Initial administration should be intravenous, but the drug may be given orally once clinical improvement has occurred. Therapy should be continued for a total of 21 days, since studies in infected adults demonstrated that *Pneumocystis carinii* cysts and trophozoites may still be observed in bronchoalveolar lavage fluid after 14 days of therapy. At the completion of therapy, the drugs are reduced to prophylactic doses and continued indefinitely. AIDS patients commonly experience adverse effects, which include cutaneous eruptions, bone marrow suppression, fever, and hepatic transaminase elevation[(113)]. Patient drug intolerance may result in cutaneous rashes, but unless these are characteristic of a type 1 hypersensitivity reaction or of toxic epidermal necrolysis or Stevens-Johnson syndrome, therapy should not be discontinued.

Patients who cannot tolerate TMP-SMX or fail to respond to this therapy should be treated with pentamidine isethionate. Although as efficacious as TMP-SMX in the therapy of PCP, the drug has a wide variety of side effects when used systemically. These include pancreatitis, hypoglycemia, hyperglycemia, neutropenia, thrombocytopenia, and azotemia. Intramuscular injection frequently causes sterile abscesses. The therapeutic regimen is 4 mg/kg/day given intravenously in a single dose for 21 days.

In view of the high frequency of adverse effects of both TMP-SMX and pentamidine in AIDS patients, several alternative forms of antimicrobial chemotherapy have been evaluated and shown promise for treating PCP in adults, but are not approved for general pediatric use. In a recent double-masked study of 322 adults with PCP and AIDS, atovaquone compared favorably with TMP-SMX(114). Preliminary pharmacokinetic studies in infants and children suggest a dose of 40 mg/kg/day by mouth would be appropriate, but no efficacy studies in children have been performed(108). Aerosolized pentamidine, 8 mg/kg/day or 600 mg/day in adults, has been shown to be a less effective regimen than intravenous pentamidine for PCP(115). Trimetrexate (45 mg/m^2/day), with leucovorin rescue (80 mg/m^2/day) is an effective regimen but relapses occur(116). Dapsone alone is not adequate treatment for PCP(117).

Corticosteroids in anti-inflammatory dosages have been used as an adjunct to antimicrobial therapy in patients with PCP. Their use has been associated with improved clinical outcome in adults with moderate or severe PCP(118–120). A retrospective study of 11 HIV infected children with PCP and respiratory failure demonstrated improved short-term survival with use of methylprednisolone 1 mg/kg every 6 hours for 7 days followed by a 1 week taper(121). Doses as high as 4 mg/kg as initial therapy are in common usage.

Table 29.7. Recommended Studies for Induced Sputum, Tracheobronchial Lavage, Bronchoalveolar Lavage Specimens

Cytology
Methenamine silver nitrate stain
Toluidine blue O stain
Giemsa stain
Pneumocystis carinii indirect immunoflourescent monoclonal antibody (if available)
Microbiology
Gram stain and bacterial culture
Acid fast bacilli stain and culture
Fungal culture
Viral culture and rapid tests
Mycoplasma culture (consider)
Legionella stain and culture (consider)

Prophylaxis

PCP can be prevented by using antimicrobial chemoprophylaxis. This was first demonstrated in leukemic children who were prophylaxed with TMP-SMX(122). Among older children, PCP is clearly associated with lower CD4+ T lymphocyte counts(103). Guidelines for CD4+ T lymphocyte count monitoring and thresholds for primary prophylaxis have been established **(Table 29.8).** Recent data indicates

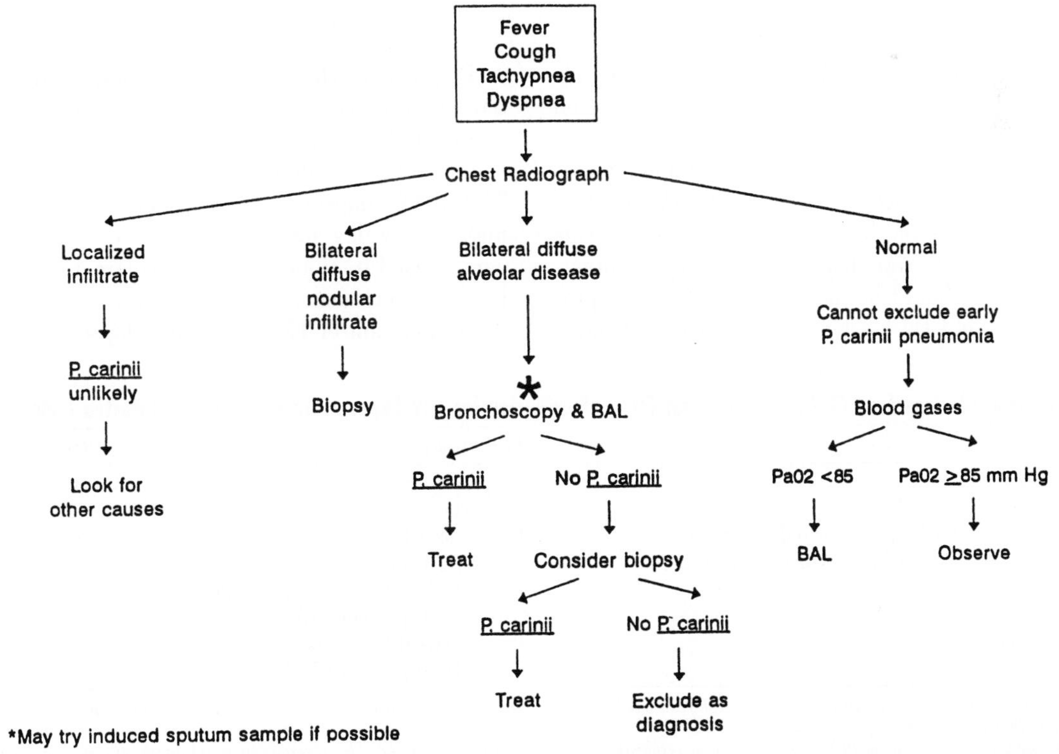

Figure 29.1. Algorithm for establishing the diagnosis of diffuse bilateral pneumonitis in immunosuppressed children. (From Hughes WT. *Pneumocystis carinii* pneumonia. In: Pizzo PA, Wilfert CM, eds. Pediatric AIDS. The challenge of HIV infection in infants, children and adolescents. 2nd Ed. Baltimore: Williams & Wilkins, 1994).

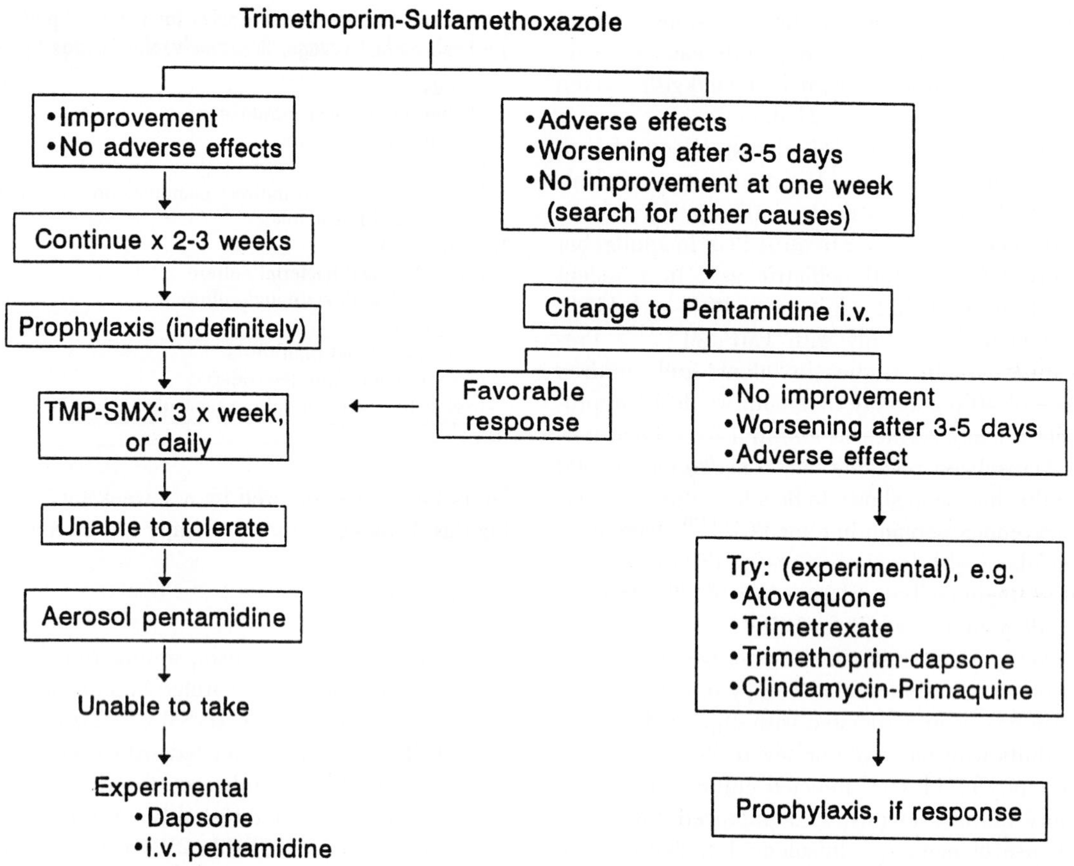

Figure 29.2. Algorithm for the treatment of Pneumocystis pneumonia. (From Hughes WT. *Pneumocystis carinii* pneumonia. In: Pizzo PA, Wilfert CM, eds. Pediatric AIDS. The challenge of HIV infection in infants, children and adolescents. 2nd Ed. Baltimore: Williams & Wilkins, 1994.)

that CD4+ T lymphocyte counts lack sensitivity among infants less than 12 months of age[103]. Therefore, revised guidelines call for administering prophylaxis to all infants less than 12 months of age born to HIV-infected mothers regardless of CD4+ T lymphocyte counts until HIV infection can be reasonably excluded based on viral diagnostic tests such as culture or PCR. Note that all children with a previous episode of PCP should be maintained on lifelong prophylaxis regardless of CD4+ T lymphocyte measurement.

Prophylaxis should consist of oral therapy with TMP-SMX in a dosage of 150 mg TMP/750 mg SMX per m^2/day, in two daily doses, given 3 days per week on either consecutive days or alternate days. For children intolerant of TMP-SMX, dapsone, 2 mg/kg/dose (maximum dose 200 mg), once a day should be used. Aerosolized pentamidine can be used in older children. Pentamidine may be administered intravenously every 2 to 4 weeks in younger children intolerant of TMP-SMX and dapsone.

Table 29.8. Recommendations for PCP Prophylaxis and CD4+ Monitoring for HIV-Exposed Infants and HIV-Infected Children

Age		*PCP Prophylaxis*	*CD4+ Monitoring*
Birth to 4–6 weeks		No prophylaxis	1,3,6,9,12 months of age
4–6 weeks to 4 months		Prophylaxis for all	
4–12 months	HIV-infected or indeterminate	Prophylaxis for all	
	HIV infection reasonably excluded[b]	No prophylaxis	None
1–5 years, HIV-infected		Prophylaxis if CD4+ count <500 or CD4+ percent <15%[c,d]	Every 3–4 months[e]
6–12 years, HIV-infected		Prophylaxis if CD4+ count <200 or CD4+ percent <15%[d]	

[a]*From Centers for Disease Control. 1995 revised guidelines for prophylaxis against* pneumocystis carinii *pneumonia for children infected with or perinatally exposed to human immunodeficiency virus. MMWR 1995;44:RR–4.)*

[b]*≥2 negative HIV diagnostic tests (culture or PCR), both of which are performed at ≥1 month of age and one of which is performed at ≥4 months of age, or ≥2 negative HIV IgG antibody tests performed at >6 months of age in a child who has no clinical evidence for HIV disease.*

[c]*Children 1–2 years of age who were on PCP prophylaxis and had a CD4+ count 50 or percent <15% in the first year of life should continue on prophylaxis.*

[d]*Prophylaxis should be considered on a case-by-case basis for children who may otherwise be at risk for PCP, such as children with rapidly declining CD4+ counts or percents or with Category C conditions.*

[e]*More frequent monitoring (e.g., monthly) is recommended for children whose CD4+ counts or percents are approaching the threshold for prophylaxis.*

Viral Pneumonia

Etiology and Pathogenesis

Viral pneumonia frequently occurs in children with HIV infection and is caused by the common pediatric respiratory pathogens—including respiratory syncytial virus (RSV), influenza virus, parainfluenza virus, rhinoviruses, caronaviruses, and adenovirus—or as a manifestation of disseminated infection with measles, herpes simplex viruses types 1 and 2 (HSV-1, HSV-2), cytomegalovirus (CMV), or varicella zoster virus (VZV)[(123)]. Viral pneumonia may be superimposed on a respiratory system already compromised by lymphocytic interstitial pneumonitis. In addition, children may be co-infected with viruses and *Pneumocystis carinii* or bacteria.

The mechanisms of immunologic protection against respiratory virus infection are frequently not the same as the mechanisms of recovery from infection, thus both serum antibody and cellular immunity are important[(123)]. Cell-mediated immunity is particularly critical in recovery from measles. Unlike the common viral pediatric respiratory pathogens, measles is always accompanied by viremia, reflected in the longer incubation time and the presence of systemic signs and symptoms. Infection with HSV-1 or HSV-2 may be asymptomatic or present as gingivostomatitis or genitalis, after which the virus becomes latent and may reactivate. Reactivation is enhanced by immunosuppression and is clinically more severe in immunocompromised patients. CMV is a ubiquitous organism that can be transmitted either vertically (mother to baby), or horizontally (person to person). As one of the herpes viruses, it remains latent in the body after the initial infection. In immunodeficient individuals, CMV may cause visceral infection following either primary infection or reactivation of latent infection[(124)]. Varicella (chicken pox) is usually a benign illness characterized by a diffuse vesicular rash caused by primary infection with VZV. The frequency of complications and severity of disease increases in immunocompromised children. Zoster (shingles), caused by reactivation of latent VZV, is seen with increased frequency among immunodeficient patients, particularly those with deficiencies in cell-mediated immunity. Among children with AIDS, the interval between chicken pox and shingles may be reduced to months instead of decades[(125,126)].

Clinical Manifestations

In normal infants, the most important cause of lower respiratory tract infections, including pneumonia, is respiratory syncytial virus (RSV). In HIV-infected children, RSV infections are more likely to cause pneumonia than bronchiolitis, and prolonged excretion of the virus is common[(123,127)]. A striking feature of case reports of RSV pneumonia among HIV-infected children is the rarity of wheezing as a physical finding[(127,111,128)]. It is important to note that the demonstration of RSV infection in a patient does not exclude the possibility of co-infection with other pathogens.

A few cases of severe influenza virus pneumonia among HIV- infected children have been described, and prolonged shedding of parainfluenza virus (both types 2 and 3), sometimes associated with wheezing, has been noted in a number of case reports[(123)]. Pneumonia accompanying fulminant hepatic failure in disseminated adenovirus infection among HIV-infected children has been described[(129)].

Measles may have devastating effects on the lung[(130)] and is highly contagious. Measles itself may be associated with pneumonia, and the lung may be secondarily infected by other viruses, in particular, herpes simplex virus and adenovirus[(131)] and by bacteria, in particular, *Staphyloccus aureus* and gram-negative bacilli. Pneumonia was documented in 5 of the 11 cases of measles among HIV-infected individuals in the United States described in the literature[(129,132,133)]. Although a rash is typical of measles, it may be absent in immunodeficient individuals.

Herpes simplex virus pneumonia in the immunocompromised host usually occurs as a part of severe disseminated disease. Patients may also exhibit hepatitis, shock, hemorrhage, disseminated intravascular coagulation, seizures, and renal failure. In AIDS patients, CMV mainly causes disease of the retina and of the gastrointestinal tract. Pneumonia attributed to CMV usually results in a diffuse interstitial process. When CMV is cultured from or demonstrated histologically in the lung of such individuals, it is usually present with other pathogens. Therefore, its significance in the pathogenesis of pneumonia is often unclear[(134)]. Generally, in AIDS patients, CMV should be considered the cause of pneumonia only when other pathogens cannot be demonstrated, or when adequate therapy directed at other associated pathogens fails to improve the health of the patient[(135)]. Complications of varicella zoster virus (VZV) infection, including pneumonia and life-threatening bacterial infections, may be more common among HIV-infected children[(125)]. Varicella pneumonia is more likely during chicken pox, but may occur in an immunocompromised patient with shingles because of virus dissemination. Respiratory symptoms may range from mild to severe hypoxemia and respiratory failure. HIV-infected children may be at increased risk for nervous system disease because of VZV and may develop acute encephalitis.

Diagnosis

The mainstay of diagnosis of the common pediatric respiratory viruses as well as measles is detection of the virus in a sample of respiratory secretion, rather than measurement of antibody in serum. Viral culture, although slow, is sensitive and reliable. Immunofluorescence is as sensitive as culture for RSV, more sensitive for measles, and acceptably sensitive for the parainfluenza viruses. An ELISA is commercially available for RSV with good sensitivity and specificity.

Scraping remains the definitive method for diagnosis of

HSV or isolation of virus from bodily fluids or skin vesicle. Cytologic examination of cells from involved sites for intranuclear inclusions and multinucleated giant cells is helpful if facilities for diagnostic virology are not available. Immunofluorescence or immunoprecipitation for the detection of HSV antigens can be performed.

Diagnosis of CMV disease, particularly in the lung, is problematic. Because CMV is common even in normal children, infection must be distinguished from disease. Diagnosis should be based on histopathologic or other evidence of disease at the organ site involved along with isolation of the virus. Cell culture is used for viral isolation. The shell vial technique is a modification of conventional technique using monoclonal antibodies to directly detect CMV antigen in cell culture or immunofluorescence. Although CMV can be detected within 12 to 24 hours of inoculation, the procedure lacks sensitivity in specimens with low quantities of virus[(124)].

VZV can be isolated from vesicular fluid obtained within the first 3 to 4 days of rash. Rapid diagnosis by immunofluorescence or immunoprecipitation can be used. Tzank smears indicate a herpes virus infection but are not specific for VZV.

Treatment

Licensed therapeutic agents for treatment of respiratory viral infections are aerosolized ribavirin for RSV[(136)] and amantadine for influenza A[(137)]. Ribavirin aerosol has also been demonstrated to be efficacious in the treatment of influenza in adults[(138)]. Invitro studies show activity against parainfluenza viruses and measles[(139,140)]. Case reports have described clearance of parainfluenza type 3 or RSV from the respiratory tract of severe combined immunodeficiency syndrome patients during ribavirin treatment[(141,142)]. The usual ribavirin aerosol administration regimen is 20 mg/ml in reservoir for 16 to 20 of each 24 hours for at least 5 days or longer if virus and symptoms persist. High-dose intravenous immunoglobulin has been used to treat RSV infection in normal infants with therapeutic results comparable to ribavirin[(143)]. Experience with use of immunoglobulin to treat severe viral respiratory infection in children with HIV infection is quite limited.

Although studies have demonstrated the efficacy of the anti-CMV drug ganciclovir in treating CMV retinitis in adults, the efficacy of the treatment of CMV pneumonia is unclear. Manifestations of disease frequently recur when drug therapy is discontinued. Ganciclovir is a toxic drug with a narrow therapeutic-toxic window. Major adverse effects include myelosuppression with neutropenia, thrombocytopenia, anemia, as well as fever, rash, liver enzyme elevation, confusion, hallucinations, psychosis, and seizures[(144)]. The myelosuppressive side effects are aggravated by concomitant use of ZDV[(145)]. Ganciclovir is usually administered intravenously in a dose of 7.5 to 15 mg/kg/day, divided into two or three doses for 10 to 21 days. This induction dose is then followed by maintenance therapy of 5 to 10 mg/kg/day. Foscarnet (phosphonoformate), an alternative therapeutic to ganciclovir, has mainly nephrotoxic side effects and is not associated with myelosuppression. The drug should be administered intravenously at 120 to 230 mg/kg/day in three doses. Considering the unclear significance of CMV in the lungs of patients with AIDS, and the significant adverse effects of anti-CMV drugs, their use to treat pulmonary disease alone is questionable.

Acyclovir is the drug of choice for disseminated varicella zoster and herpes simplex infections. The recommended dosage for varicella zoster is 1500 mg/m^2/day administered intravenously divided three times a day for 7 days. A lower dose is often used for localized HSV infection. Children with ocular involvement from HSV should receive a topical ophthalmic antiviral drug.

Bacterial Pneumonia

Bacterial pneumonia is a frequently diagnosed infection in HIV-infected children and may progress to respiratory failure[(146)]. Although the diagnosis of bacterial pneumonia is usually considered when lobar consolidation is observed, diffuse and patchy infiltrates may also have a bacterial origin. The microbial etiology of pneumonia in young children usually remains unknown, unless blood cultures or rapid diagnostic tests for bacterial antigens are positive, or diagnostic procedures such as bronchoalveolar lavage or lung biopsy are performed. The most common bacterial causes of pneumonia in children with AIDS are *Streptococcus pneumoniae, Haemophilus influenzae,* and *Pseudomonas aeruginosa.*

Children whose clinical or radiologic features suggest bacterial pneumonia should be treated presumptively. Diffuse interstitial pulmonary infiltrates, although not excluding the possibility of bacterial infection, suggest another diagnosis such as PCP. The specific approach to antimicrobial therapy in HIV-infected children with suspected bacterial pneumonia is discussed in a subsequent section on severe bacterial infection.

Mycobacterial Pneumonia

Etiology and Pathogenesis

The most important mycobacterial infections in HIV-infected children are those caused by *Mycobacterium tuberculosis* and the *Mycobacterium avium-intracellulare* complex (MAC). Tuberculosis in young children is the result of a primary infection as opposed to reactivation of disease, which often occurs in adults. The primary focus of infection is almost always in the lung. In the United States, a progressive decline in the incidence of tuberculosis reversed in 1986. The alarming increase in the number of cases of tuberculosis continues and appears closely associated with the HIV epidemic. Disseminated MAC infection has been found in 11 to 14% of HIV-infected children. A CD4 count of less than 100 cells/mm^3 was identified as the primary risk factor for this opportunistic infection.

Clinical Manifestations

The clinical features of tuberculosis are nonspecific and include fever, weight loss, and cough. Characteristic roentgenographic features include localized pulmonary infiltrate and hilar lymphadenopathy. Diffuse patchy infiltrates and lobar consolidation may also occur. Cavitation, a common finding in adults, is unusual in children. In adults with AIDS, disseminated (miliary) and focal extrapulmonary infection are common[147–149]. Although pulmonary disease will be evident in most pediatric cases, rapid hematogenous dissemination may result in severe disease, including meningitis, without obvious pulmonary findings[150]. Symptoms associated with disseminated MAC infection include fever, night sweats, malaise, and weight loss, often with anemia and neutropenia. Pneumonia because of MAC infection alone is rare.

Diagnosis

Establishing the diagnosis of tuberculosis remains very important for the following reasons: (a) the infection can be readily treated with oral drugs; (b) contacts, especially the source of infection, should be traced; and (c) respiratory isolation procedures for hospitalized patients should be instituted. The diagnosis is based on the history of exposure, the radiologic appearance of the lungs, a positive skin test (Mantoux with purified protein derivative [PPD]), and demonstration of the causative organism. Skin testing family contacts may offer supportive diagnostic evidence of tuberculosis. In children in general, and in HIV-infected children in particular, making the diagnosis may be difficult for several reasons: (a) the radiologic appearance of the lungs is not specific; (b) the skin test may be negative as a result of anergy. Although a negative test does not exclude infection with *Mycobacterium tuberculosis,* a positive test indicates infection, but not necessarily disease; and (c) since cavitary disease is rare in children, the organism is not present in large numbers in the sputum.

Tuberculin skin testing along with appropriate controls consisting of two additional antigens (*Candida,* mumps, or tetanus toxoid) should be administered by the Mantoux method in HIV-infected children who have suspected tuberculosis[151]. Acid-fast stain and mycobacterial culture are important elements in the evaluation. Obtaining appropriate culture material is essential not only to document infection but also to determine sensitivities to available antituberculous agents. Morning gastric aspirates are the most readily available samples from children. In addition, broncho-alveolar lavage should be strongly considered early in the diagnostic evaluation[152]. Since pneumonia is a relatively uncommon manifestation of MAC infection, the presence of acid-fast organisms on smears of pulmonary samples should be considered to be tuberculosis until proven otherwise.

Persistent bacteremia is common in disseminated MAC infection. Cell lysis blood culture techniques are quite sensitive. Evidence suggests that obtaining two blood cultures for mycobacteria at different times is sufficient to detect almost all MAC bacteremic episodes. Isolation of MAC from nonsterile sites such as stool and respiratory secretions must be assessed together with symptoms since colonization may precede invasive infection by months.

Treatment

The treatment of tuberculosis in AIDS patients is generally the same as in immunologically normal patients. However, therapy for pulmonary infection should be given for at least 9 months (as opposed to 6 months), or for 6 months after sputum cultures are negative. Therapy should consist of isoniazid, rifampin, and pyrazinamide daily for the first 2 months, after which it is continued with only isoniazid and rifampin daily. Because of the increased frequency of multidrug resistant tuberculosis, planned revised guidelines will recommend a four drug regimen (isoniazid, rifampin, pyrazinamide, and streptomycin or ethambutol) as initial therapy for new cases of tuberculosis until sensitivity is known.

Resistance is particularly problematic in treatment of disseminated MAC infection. Although multiple drug regimens may increase intolerance and toxicity, most experts recommend that treatment of MAC bacteremia should include at least two antimycobacterial agents, one of which should be a macrolide. Although evaluation of therapeutic agents in children is limited, a pediatric trial of clarithromycin demonstrated clinical improvement and only mild adverse reactions. Prophylaxis with oral rifabutin has proven efficacious in adults with CD4 counts <200 cells/mm^3.

Fungal Pneumonia

Although uncommon, pulmonary manifestations of fungal infections occur among HIV infected children. Although meningitis is by far the most common presentation of cryptococcosis in this population, pulmonary infiltrates have been noted. Patients with disseminated histoplasmosis have fever, pulmonary infiltrates, cutaneous lesions, and septic shock. The chest radiograph in histoplasmosis in HIV-infected patients may demonstrate various patterns, including reticulonodular, miliary, and lobar infiltrates. Patients with HIV infection in endemic areas appear to be at particularly high risk for development of disseminated coccidiomycosis. Symptoms reported in adults include fever, chills, weight loss, cough, chest pain, headache, altered sensorium, and skin rashes. Lastly, pulmonary aspergillosis can cause particularly severe disease among HIV-infected patients with granulocytopenia and thrombocytopenia. Other HIV infected patients tend to have a more chronic bronchopneumonia.

Diagnosis can usually be established by direct examination and culture of respiratory secretions or biopsy of suspicious pulmonary lesions. In the case of histoplasmosis, culture and examination of bone marrow is one of the most reliable methods to establish the diagnosis. The treatment of choice for each of these pathogens is Amphotericin B at 0.5 to 1.5 mg/kg every 24 hours. Chronic administration of Amphotericin B can be complicated by azotemia, hypokalemia, anemia, and weight loss.

Lymphoid Diseases of the Lung

Etiology and Pathogenesis

The lungs of approximately 25 to 40% of children who acquire HIV perinatally are affected by lymphocytic infiltrations that form overlapping clinical and pathologic disorders, namely, pulmonary lymphoid hyperplasia (PLH) and lymphocytic interstitial pneumonia (LIP)[(153,154)]. Pathologically, PLH is characterized mainly by peribronchial lymphoid nodules with germinal centers, while LIP is characterized mainly by diffuse interstitial infiltration of the alveolar septa with lymphocytes and plasma cells[(155)]. The interstitial process results primarily in restrictive lung disease with hypoxia and hypocapnia, whereas peribronchial disease may result in obstructive lung disease. The cause of this group of disorders is unclear, but the findings of both Epstein-Barr virus genome and HIV antigen in lung tissue suggests that these viruses play a pathogenic role[(156)].

Clinical Manifestations

Most children with lymphoid disease of the lung acquired their HIV infection perinatally. After the first year of life, these children usually have the insidious onset of cough, tachypnea, and wheezing. Other clinical manifestations include digital clubbing and evidence of lymphoid or reticuloendothelial hyperplasia, such as generalized lymphadenopathy, hepatosplenomegaly, and parotid enlargement. The previously mentioned findings, particularly if associated with high immunoglobulin levels, suggest the diagnosis of lymphoid disease of the lung rather than opportunistic pulmonary infection[(153,154)]. PCP is likely if the onset of disease is more acute with fever, cough, hypoxia, and rales.

The disease process waxes and wanes, but may result in persistent chronic hypoxia, bronchiectasis, and possibly, pulmonary B-cell neoplasia. Deterioration in pulmonary function is often caused by superimposed bacterial infection. PCP and other pulmonary infections may develop in children with lymphoid disease of the lung as well.

Diagnosis

The previously described clinical features certainly suggest the diagnosis of this group of disorders, particularly when supported by radiologic findings of a diffuse reticulonodular pattern, with nodules of 1 to 5 mm in diameter with frequently associated mediastinal lymphadenopathy, that persists for several months without evidence of other opportunistic infections[(153,154)]. If clinical deterioration occurs, further diagnostic studies should be performed including oxygen saturation monitoring, radiographic imaging, and obtaining respiratory secretions to rule out infection. Since bronchoalveolar lavage, which is useful for diagnosing PCP, is not of value in diagnosing lymphoid disease of the lung, lung biopsy may become necessary.

Treatment

The treatment of lymphoid diseases of the lung is largely supportive since there is no known specific therapy. General supportive measures include attention to nutrition and anemia, immunization against respiratory pathogens, aggressive management of respiratory infections, and appropriate monitoring of pulmonary function. Bronchodilators and oxygen may be necessary. Patients with PLH/LIP have symptomatic HIV infection and should receive antiretroviral therapy. The use of systemic corticosteroids such as prednisone, 2 mg/kg/day for 4 to 12 weeks with subsequent gradual reduction of the dose has been found to be of value, but controlled trials have not been performed[(157)]. Many patients are then maintained on a low dose daily or every other day regimen. Patients who develop an acute exacerbation of disease often respond to a 5 to 7 day steroid burst followed by a taper to their regular dose[(153)].

Cardiac Complications

Etiology and Pathogenesis

Although prospective studies are lacking, it is clear that cardiovascular problems are very common among HIV-infected children. Among those referred for cardiac testing, abnormalities have been demonstrated in as many as 90%[(158)]. Children with HIV may be admitted to a pediatric intensive care unit with severe life-threatening congestive heart failure or arrhythmias[(159)]. Cardiac involvement in children includes dilated cardiomyopathy, myocarditis, pericarditis, endocarditis, arrhythmias, conduction disturbances, and vascular disease. Although not completely elucidated, stage of HIV disease does appear to correlate with occurrence of cardiovascular disease among HIV-infected children[(160–162)]. Heart disease can develop in children with either perinatally acquired congenital infection or in older children with HIV infection acquired after contaminated blood or blood product exposure.

The etiology of HIV-associated cardiac disease is unclear but is probably multifactorial involving HIV virus, other viral infectious agents (CMV, EBV, or coxsackie virus), fungal, bacterial, or protozoan infections, an abnormal host response, and drug toxicity[(158)]. HIV could contribute to myocardial damage by the "innocent bystander" mechanism whereby myocyte damage is produced by the release of proteolytic mediators from infected monocytes and macrophages. Although myocytes do not exhibit CD4 receptors, the fact that segments of HIV genome have been detected within myocytes suggests that HIV virus could damage myocytes directly[(163)]. The host immune system may play a role in heart damage by the production of autoantibodies in a similar fashion to the pathogenesis of other forms of viral myocarditis[(164)].

Since acute and chronic lung disease so frequently complicates the course of HIV infection in infants, cor pulmonale may contribute to the etiology of heart disease as well. Malnutrition with selenium deficiency has been implicated in the etiology of HIV cardiac disease and conflicting reports exist with respect to the efficacy of replacement therapy[158]. Carnitine deficiency is another potentially reversible cause of ventricular dysfunction and has been reported among some HIV-infected malnourished adults with cardiac symptoms. Finally, other therapies may be implicated. TMP-SMX, intravenous pentamidine, and ganciclovir have each been associated with rapid onset cardiac problems[158].

Clinical Presentation

Dilated cardiomyopathy is the most frequent form of heart disease in the HIV-infected child. Early on, such affected children may be clinically asymptomatic with only echocardiographic evidence of dysfunction. More severe involvement is characterized by cardiomegaly with ventricular hypertrophy and dilation and poor contractility and signs of overt congestive heart failure[165]. The electrocardiogram may demonstrate left ventricular hypertrophy and ST-T wave changes. Frequently, intercurrent infections with fever, anemia, and sepsis precipitate clinical decompensation. In addition, the symptoms of cardiac failure may be mistaken for pulmonary or liver disease or even sepsis. Left ventricular involvement is predominant but, with advancing disease, right ventricular function is compromised. In addition, Lipshultz et al. have demonstrated a subgroup of patients with enhanced left ventricular contractility, increased left ventricular mass, and obstructive left ventricular hypertrophy. These patients are more likely to develop high-grade arrhythmias and sudden death[166].

The incidence of endocardial abnormalities is less than that of myocardial or pericardial findings among HIV-infected children. Pericardial effusions are frequently observed on echocardiographic examination of children with AIDS. Although adult effusions are usually secondary to Kaposi's sarcoma and opportunistic infectious myocarditis, those in children are not associated with such complications, are usually small, and tamponade is rare.

Some children with HIV heart disease will develop rate and rhythm disturbances. Although isolated atrial ectopic beats and wandering atrial pacemaker are the more common arrhythmias observed, potentially life-threatening arrhythmias such as supraventricular tachycardia and ventricular tachycardia have been observed in 10% of children with HIV heart involvement[166]. Patients with enhanced left ventricular function, decreased afterload, and an element of left ventricular outflow obstruction appear at increased risk for developing these arrhythmias. Prolongation of the QT interval is occasionally observed and has been attributed to sympathetic tract neuritis[166,167].

Diagnosis

Since cardiovascular abnormalities can be difficult to recognize clinically and on chest radiograph[166,167,168], the echocardiogram remains the single most useful diagnostic test to assess ventricular function and structure, pericardial disease, and cardiac vascular disease. The electrocardiograph and Holter monitor are used to assess rhythm disturbances.

Treatment

Congestive heart failure should be treated conventionally with inotropic agents such as digoxin and dopamine, with diuretics, and with afterload reducing agents, e.g., captopril[169]. Class IA antiarrhythmics (quinidine, procainamide) should be avoided in children with prolonged QTc interval. The therapeutic roles of immunoglobulin treatment, steroids, or micronutrient replacement remain to be clarified.

Renal and Electrolyte Complications

Etiology and Pathogenesis

Up to 30 to 55% of HIV-infected children will develop definitive evidence of renal disease at some point in their illness[170–173]. Renal disease in HIV-infected persons falls into three categories[173–175]: (a) acute renal failure secondary to acute tubular necrosis, either because of ischemia from volume depletion and septic shock or nephrotoxicity complicating therapeutic use of aminoglycosides, acyclovir, pentamidine, or amphotericin B; (b) a group of glomerular disorders referred to as HIV-associated nephropathy; and (c) a third group of miscellaneous parenchymal lesions that includes drug-related interstitial nephritis and an uncommon form of HIV-associated hemolytic uremic syndrome. In addition, electrolyte abnormalities may occur. Hyponatremia is the most common electrolyte disorder noted in AIDS patients. Although usually related to fluid losses from diarrhea, syndrome of inappropriate antidiuretic hormone has been reported as a complication of PCP[173]. As most of these renal disorders are discussed in Chapter 38, this section will focus on the group of glomerular disorders referred to as HIV-associated nephropathy.

This glomerulopathy is noted to occur in up to 15% of HIV-infected children[170,171,176]. Focal segmental glomerulosclerosis is the most common histologic finding in children[171] and adults[173] with HIV-associated nephropathy. Diffuse mesangial hyperplasia is common in children as well. Since focal segmental glomerulosclerosis is only a pathologic expression of disease or injury, HIV infection per se, secondary immune complex injury, hemodynamic instability, opportunistic infection, and drug toxicity may all contribute to the etiology of HIV-associated nephropathy.

Clinical Presentation

Children with HIV nephropathy may be asymptomatic or may demonstrate advanced HIV disease. Renal abnormalities may occasionally represent the first clinical manifestation of HIV disease. Presenting symptoms of HIV-associated nephropathy with focal segmental glomerulosclerosis include nephrotic range proteinuria, edema, hypoalbuminemia, and azotemia. Patients are usually normotensive and remain so despite progressive loss of renal function[177,178]. Children tend not to follow the course of rapid loss of renal function and death reported in adults[171]. Children with biopsy-confirmed mesangial hyperplasia experience a more benign course with no development of frank renal insufficiency, but they have persistent abnormalities in urinary sediment[170,171].

Diagnosis

Routine screening of HIV-infected children with urinalysis, creatinine, and blood urea nitrogen facilitates early identification and may result in reduced morbidity from renal disease. A urinalysis that is positive for blood and/or protein suggests glomerulonephropathy and warrants further investigation. Proteinuria may occur intermittently, thus routine screening is important[179]. Evaluation of the child with suspected glomerulonephropathy should include a renal ultrasound to assess renal anatomy. Renal biopsy may be indicated to differentiate nephrotoxicity from nephropathy and diagnose severity of renal involvement.

Treatment

General aspects of treatment of nephrotic syndrome, nephritis, hypertension, electrolyte abnormalities, and renal failure are outlined in Chapter 38. For patients with HIV-associated nephropathy who develop tubular dysfunction and acidosis, alkali replacement is indicated. Replacement of magnesium, calcium, and phosphorus may be required and may necessitate intravenous administration prior to oral maintenance. Children with biopsy-proven minimal change lesions or focal glomerulosclerosis have been treated with prednisone or low dosage of cyclosporin. No clear responsiveness has been demonstrated[172]. It is appropriate to initiate dialysis for the management of acute renal failure in HIV patients when potentially reversible causes such as ischemia or nephrotoxic drugs are suspect. The decision to dialyze patients with irreversible kidney disease should be made only after consideration of the extent of other organ involvement and the overall state of health[180]. Generally, peritoneal dialysis is used because it is accessible and adaptable for prolonged use.

Hematologic Complications

Hematopoietic abnormalities are a common complication of HIV infection or treatment and include anemia, neutropenia, thrombocytopenia, and coagulopathy[181]. Possible causes include (a) disruption of stem-cell function by HIV virus and other opportunistic infectious agents, (b) production of autoantibodies to stem cells[182], and (c) inhibition of colony formation of erythroid and granulocyte-macrophage progenitor cells with dideoxynucleoside treatment[183].

Anemia

Anemia is the most common hematologic disorder observed in HIV infected children. This is mostly because of HIV-induced bone marrow suppression, but other contributing factors include iron deficiency from enteric blood loss and poor nutrition, reduced endogenous erythropoietin, and a Coombs-positive autoimmune hemolysis[184]. Anemia is common among children receiving ZDV, reported in 18 to 67% of cases[181]. Perhaps related to a concurrent iron deficiency, anemia among HIV-infected children is often microcytic and hypochromic[185]. Conversely, macrocytosis is associated with ZDV therapy. In addition to iron replacement therapy when indicated, treatment of chronic anemia may include erythropoietin (150 units/kg given subcutaneously 3 days per week). Studies of erythropoietin treatment of HIV-infected adults have shown a decrease in transfusion requirement and an increase in mean hematocrit levels when the patients baseline endogenous erythropoietin level was less than 500 IU/liter[186].

Neutropenia

Neutropenia, defined as an absolute neutrophil count (ANC) less than 1500 cells/mm^3, has been reported in 43% of previously untreated children with HIV infection[187]. Associations with disease progression[185] as well as antineutrophil antibodies[188] have been described. The currently recommended ZDV dose for children of 180 mg/m^2/dose every 6 hours orally has been associated with ANC less than 750 cells/mm^3 among 48% of treated children[189]. Myelosuppression is infrequent with dideoxyinosine (ddI) treatment. Other drugs commonly prescribed for HIV-infected children, including TMP-SMX, acyclovir, and ganciclovir can have a myelosuppressive effect.

Although the increased risk for infectious complications noted in cancer patients with ANC less than 500 cells/mm^3 has not been clearly defined in HIV-infected children, an increased incidence of bacterial infections has been reported in neutropenic HIV-infected adults[190]. When fever occurs in a neutropenic HIV-infected child, prompt initiation of empiric broad spectrum antibiotics is prudent. Cytokines can be used to treat neutropenia in HIV-infected patients. Granulocyte-macrophage colony stimulating factor (GMCSF) is effective in raising the neutrophil count, but there is concern that it may enhance HIV viral replication[181]. Granulocyte colony stimulating factor (GCSF) at a dose of 1 to 2 ug/kg/day subcutaneously has been demonstrated to increase both median white blood cell count and ANC with negligible side effects when administered to neutropenic HIV-infected children receiving ZDV[191].

Thrombocytopenia

Thrombocytopenia may occasionally be so severe as to produce a bleeding diathesis. Megakaryocyte infection with HIV[192] as well as platelet-associated HIV specific IgG leading to increased platelet destruction[193] are likely etiologies. IVIG, 1 g/kg/dose over 2 to 5 days, is indicated for immune thrombocytopenia when platelet counts fall below 20,000/mm^3, although response may be transient[194]. Corticosteroids have a 40 to 60% initial response rate in HIV-infected individuals, but relapses are common after tapering[195]. No deleterious side effects have been demonstrated when a short course of steroid therapy is administered to HIV-infected children[196]. Improvement in HIV-associated thrombocytopenia has been reported with ZDV or ddI treatment[197,198].

Coagulopathy

Disorders of coagulation factors secondary to severe liver disease caused either by HIV or opportunistic pathogens are occasionally observed in critically ill children. In addition, lupuslike anticoagulants[199,200] as well as acquired antibodies with antifactor X, XI, and XII activity—although usually not of clinical significance—may contribute to bleeding. Although the HIV-infected child with hemophilia does not seem to be at increased risk for bleeding in the absence of thrombocytopenia, intracranial hemorrhages are more frequent in thrombocytopenic hemophiliac patients[201]. Bleeding tendency and platelet function can be markedly abnormal in hemophiliacs who are treated with ZDV and ibuprofen simultaneously[202]. Therapy of coagulopathy as well as platelet transfusions may be required before performing surgery or other invasive procedures.

Neurologic Complications

HIV Encephalopathy

Pediatric neuro-AIDS, the clinical manifestations of CNS involvement in HIV-1 infected children, follows a different time course from that observed in adults infected with HIV-1. In children, CNS manifestations of HIV-1 infection are more prevalent, are infrequently resulting from opportunistic infections, may be the initial presenting sign of HIV-1 infection, can be an important determinant of therapeutic efficacy, and may cause significant impairments in the child's overall functioning and quality of life[203]. In children, HIV-1 infection is associated with central (and less commonly peripheral) nervous system abnormalities caused directly or indirectly by HIV-1 infection of the CNS. In series that include asymptomatic, mildly symptomatic, and children with advanced disease, a 19.6% prevalence rate is reported[203,83,204]. Belman et al.[205] followed a group of children referred for HIV symptomatology and identified the time course for several pediatric neurodevelopmental syndromes. These syndromes include an insidious neurologic deterioration beginning subacutely showing a relentless progressive course of encephalopathy; a progressive neurologic deterioration as the initial and only manifestation of HIV infection; and an apparently static course manifested by nonprogressive cognitive and neurologic deficits that remain stable over time.

Cryptococcal Meningitis

In AIDS patients the most important systemic fungal infection is caused by the yeast *Cryptococcus neoformans*. The organism enters the body through the lungs and spreads hematogenously to cause disseminated or focal infections. The most common of these is meningitis, which may develop very insidiously. The diagnosis is confirmed by the cerebrospinal fluid features of chronic meningitis, the observation of organisms with an Indian ink stain, the presence of cryptococcal antigen, and a positive culture. The patient should be treated initially with amphotericin B, 0.5 to 1.0 mg/kg/day for 6 to 8 weeks, with or without flucytosine 50 to 150 mg/kg/day in four divided doses. Amphotericin B must be given intravenously, diluted in only 5% dextrose water. After a test dose of 0.1 given over about 4 hours, the dosage may be increased over 2 to 4 days to 0.5-1 mg/kg given daily over 6 to 8 hours. The medication has several severe adverse effects, and the most important of which is high fever, chills, and renal dysfunction with renal potassium wasting. Because the infection frequently relapses, long-term suppressive therapy with weekly amphotericin B or daily fluconazole should be used.

Toxoplasmosis

Toxoplasma gondii is an obligate intracellular protozoan parasite that has a diverse range of hosts, including mammals, birds, and some reptiles. Unlike the adult experience where most cases occur secondary to reactivation of previously acquired infection, a major mode of acquisition in children is congenital. Toxoplasmosis resulting from reactivation of previously acquired infection most commonly presents as an encephalitis with focal neurologic abnormalities[206]. The disease is the most common cause of intracerebral mass lesions in adult AIDS patients[207,208]. Computerized axial tomography performed with contrast typically reveals one or more intraparenchymal ring-enhancing lesions in various regions of the brain. Most cases of congenital toxoplasmosis that occur in infants born to mothers infected with both *Toxoplasma* and HIV are not evident at birth[209]. Symptoms developing in the first few months of life include chorioretinitis, cerebritis with intraparenchymal calcifications, pneumonitis, myocarditis, lymphadenopathy, and hepatosplenomegaly[210]. Diagnosis based on detection of *Toxoplasma*-specific antibodies is problematic because it is difficult to distinguish reliably active from chronic infection among AIDS patients using serology alone and to use IgM antibodies to diagnose congenital infection. The technically difficult Sabin-Feldman dye test has been considered the reference standard against which most other assays are compared. Generally, diagnosis is based on symptomatology with supportive serologic testing[209]. The standard regimen for treatment is pyrimethamine 15 mg/m^2/day (double dose first 2 days), sulfadiazine 85 mg/kg/day two to four times a day, and folinic acid 5 mg every 3 days. Because of the high frequency of relapse, these patients should continue to be treated with the regimen above indefinitely.

Other Neurologic Complications

Although rare, primary central nervous system lymphomas are the most common intracranial mass lesions that develop in HIV-infected children[211]. Signs and symptoms are usually rapidly progressive with new onset of seizures and neurologic deficits and progression of mental status changes.

Strokes in HIV-infected children comprise both ischemic infarction and cerebral hemorrhage[212,213]. Ischemic infarction may be the sequela of primary HIV arteriopathy of central nervous system vasculature. Hemorrhagic strokes, although rare, usually occur in association with autoimmune thrombocytopenia[214].

Gastrointestinal Complications

Malnutrition

Nearly 95% of all HIV-infected children will develop malnutrition before death. One prospective study reports infected children have comparable height and weight percentiles from birth to 3 months of age, but by 3 to 6 months of life, they are significantly smaller in height and weight percentiles than their uninfected counterparts[215]. Linear growth is most affected, resulting in patients for whom the weight for height may appear average, whereas weight and height for age are significantly decreased[215,216]. Anthropometric data indicate that the arm circumferences of HIV-infected children are smaller, but that their skinfold thickness measures, reflecting fat stores, are normal. This suggests that there is a preferential wasting of muscle mass to fat[216,217]. Growth failure in HIV-infected children often precedes a fall in CD4+ cell counts and may be an important sign of progression to symptomatic disease[215]. In its simplest form, the malnutrition associated with pediatric HIV/AIDS is the result of inadequate caloric intake, maldigestion, malabsorption, and/or increased nutrient requirements. Diarrhea may be present and is often the result of malabsorption. Standard pathogens should be ruled out. *Cryptosporidium* should be considered as well in cases of large volume secretory diarrhea that is associated with malabsorption, anorexia, and weight loss. *Mycobacterium avium-intracellulare* should be considered in cases of diarrhea, weight loss, and recurrent fevers.

Malnutrition and resultant growth failure is often a complex interaction of many factors. The Task Force on Nutritional Support in AIDS has set forth specific guidelines for nutrition in individuals with AIDS[215]. Although the daily caloric requirements for pediatric AIDS have not been established, Winter and Chang[218] recommend that the children receive 150% of the recommended daily allowance (RDA). Bentler and Spanish[219] suggest a system for establishing a minimum and maximum goal for daily caloric intake. The minimum goal is established by multiplying RDA times the weight at the 50th percentile for the child's actual height, whereas the maximum is established by multiplying the RDA times the weight at the 50th percentile for the child's age. Protein intake should be a minimum of 150% RDA for age[218], but may need to be doubled to compensate for ongoing losses[219].

Management of malnutrition is age and situation dependent and is discussed in more detail in Chapter 35. For infants, increased caloric density of feeds (24 or 27 Kcal/oz) will often suffice. For older children and adolescents, commercially available high-calorie supplements should be offered as soon as growth-curve deviation is noted. Nutritional supplements should be high protein, contain vitamins and minerals, avoid lactose and other disaccharides unless breath hydrogen challenges are normal, and avoid long-chain fatty acids if diarrhea is present. Addition of glucose polymers or medium chain triglycerides may help meet the caloric requirements. Supplemental enteral tube feedings have been shown to increase weight, body-cell mass, body fat mass, total lymphocyte count, and serum albumin[220–222]. For long-term enteral feeds, a gastrostomy tube is recommended. Peripheral parenteral nutrition is recommend only for as a short-term replacement for or supplement to enteral feeds[223]. Central parenteral nutrition should be reserved for patients with a nonfunctional GI tract, acute pancreatitis, or as a supplement to enteral feeds in patients with extraordinary caloric requirements[224].

Esophagitis

A significant and troublesome infection among HIV-infected children is candidal esophagitis. This may be suspected clinically based on the features of dysphagia, odynophagia, and chest pain. Confirmation requires esophagoscopy and biopsy and is particularly useful to rule out esophagitis resulting from other infections such as Herpes simplex virus or peptic ulcer disease. Esophageal candidiasis is a diagnostic indicator disease for AIDS. Dissemination of disease is rare. Treatment options include ketoconazole 5 to 10 mg/kg/day orally in one or two doses, fluconazole 3 to 6 mg/kg/day orally, or amphotericin B intravenously.

Pancreatitis and Abnormal Liver Function Tests

Symptoms consistent with pancreatitis accompanied by elevation of amylase and lipase are a frequent occurrence among HIV-infected children, as high as 17% in one study[225]. Pancreatitis may be caused by medications such as dideoxyinosine (ddI) and may develop as long as 8 months after starting therapy[226]. Pentamidine can cause fatal acute pancreatitis[227], and trimethoprim-sulfamethoxazole and Dapsone may cause pancreatitis as well[228]. Infectious agents including cytomegalovirus and mycobacteria have also been associated with pancreatitis. Although recovery from an acute episode of pancreatitis is possible, most HIV-infected children with pancreatitis have a chronic relapsing course. The mean survival of children with pancreatitis has been reported as 8 months after onset of disease[225]. Management of acute pancreatitis is discussed in more detail in Chapter 36.

Although hepatic dysfunction is not a common manifestation of HIV disease, many therapeutic agents used to treat children with HIV can cause hepatocellular injury or cholestasis. Sulfonamides may cause a mixed hepatocellular-cholestatic reaction, whereas zidovudine produces more of a cholestatic profile. Other medications including amphotericin B, Ketoconazole, ddI, and ketoconazole cause a mild hepatitis. Infectious agents that can result in hepatobiliary abnormalities include hepatitis A, B, and C; *Mycobacterium avium-intracellulare;* cytomegalovirus; *Cryptosporidium; Pneumocystis carinii;* toxoplasmosis; and histoplasmosis. Hepatic failure is discussed in detail in Chapter 36.

Severe Bacterial Infections

Etiology and Pathogenesis

Bacterial infections are a significant cause of morbidity among HIV-infected children. Because the T cell is the main target of HIV, infection with this virus results in severe dysfunction of the cell-mediated immune response. However, other arms of the immune system are also affected, including B cells and macrophages[229]. B-lymphocyte dysregulation results from altered T-lymphocyte help as well as direct B-lymphocyte effects and manifests as polyclonal hypergammaglobulinemia, hypogammaglobulinemia, IgG subclass deficiency, and impaired antibody responses to T-lymphocyte dependent and independent antigens[230]. CD4 bearing mononuclear phagocytes are infected by HIV, resulting in impaired function[231]. Decreased levels of complement components have been demonstrated[232]. In addition, neutropenia may occur as a result of HIV-induced bone marrow depression or autoimmunity, mycobacterial or viral infection, or as a result of drugs such as ZDV, TMP/SMX, and ganciclovir[181,233].

Clinical Manifestations

In two studies of infections in children with AIDS, bacteremia occurred in 24% and 46%, respectively[234,235]. The most common causes of bacteremia were *Streptococcus pneumoniae, Haemophilus influenzae, Staphylococcus aureus,* and *Salmonella* species. A recent prospective study demonstrated an incidence rate of pneumococcal bacteremia and other invasive disease of 11.7/100 child years among HIV-infected children less than 36 months of age, higher than the rate reported in patients with sickle-cell disease[236]. When other Gram-negative bacilli , e.g., *Pseudomonas, Escherichia coli, Enterobacter* species, and *Klebsiella* caused bacteremia, the infection was usually nosocomial and often related to a central venous catheter. *Pseudomonas aeruginosa* bacteremia must be treated vigorously and early and occurs in both neutropenic and non-neutropenic HIV-infected children[237]. Although initial reports describing bacterial infection in HIV-infected children reported an 11% incidence of bacterial meningitis in children with AIDS or AIDS-related complex, subsequent larger studies did not find a disproportionate incidence of meningitis among HIV-infected children[234,236].

Diagnosis

In normal young children with a high fever and no obvious focus of infection, bacteremia is a frequent diagnostic consideration. In HIV-infected children with high fever, this diagnosis should be even more strongly considered. In children with AIDS, a focus of infection leading to bacteremia is seldom detected. However, when such a focus is found, it is usually in the lung. Less frequently, meningitis and infections of the skin, urinary tract, and indwelling vascular catheters are responsible. *Salmonella* bacteremia is frequently associated with gastrointestinal disease[238]. Although recent data suggests fever intensity and white blood count greater than 15,000/mm^3 are significantly associated with bacteremia among febrile HIV-infected children[239], blood culture should always be strongly considered in the evaluation of febrile illnesses among this group. Cultures of urine or cerebrospinal fluid should be obtained if clinically indicated, and chest radiograph may prove useful.

Treatment

Once appropriate cultures have been obtained from a patient with suspected bacteremia, meningitis, or bacterial pneumonia, antimicrobial therapy should be instituted. In the absence of a focus of infection or material for Gram's stain, antimicrobial therapy should be directed at *Streptococcus pneumoniae, Haemophilus influenzae,* and *Salmonella* species. Although ampicillin was previously used against these organisms, the high prevalence of ampicillin-resistant *Haemophilus influenzae* precludes the empiric use of this antibiotic in this circumstance. The most suitable agents are third-generation cephalosporins such as cefotaxime or ceftriaxone. If an organism has been cultured and its antimicrobial susceptibilities have been determined, narrower spectrum antimicrobial therapy should be used to reduce the likelihood of the child developing a superinfection, particularly with *Candida* species.

Systemic salmonellosis poses a difficult therapeutic challenge in AIDS patients. The organisms remain intracellularly within macrophages and effective cell-mediated immunity is necessary for their elimination. In these patients, relapses of infection are common, and long-term suppressive antimicrobial therapy should be used[240]. Depending on the antibiotic susceptibilities of the organism, this may be accomplished with amoxicillin, TMP/SMX, or a fluoroquinolone such as ciprofloxacin. Fluoroquinolones are generally not recommended for use in children, because of the damage they cause to articular cartilage in experimental animals when used in high dosage. However, this potential adverse effect should be balanced against the possible benefits of these agents.

Nosocomial bacterial infections are often caused by multiple-resistant bacteria, especially gram-negative bacilli and staphylococci. Empiric therapy of such infections should take into account the prevalent microorganisms in the particular hospital unit and their susceptibility patterns. Therapeutic regimens may include vancomycin, directed at methicillin-resistant staphylococci and at enterococci, and amikacin, directed at gentamicin-resistant *Pseudomonas aeruginosa.*

As in any patient with bacterial infection, attention must be paid to supportive care and surgical drainage of pus. Household contacts of patients with infections caused by *Haemophilus influenzae* type b and *Neisseria meningitidis,* should be warned of their risks of infection and given chemoprophylaxis with rifampin.

Prophylaxis

The benefit of IVIG administration in asymptomatic and mildly symptomatic children has been demonstrated in a multicentered collaborative placebo-controlled study sponsored by the National Institute of Child Health and Human Development[(241)]. This study demonstrated a significant decrease in documented bacterial infections, suspected bacterial infections, and days in hospital in IVIG-treated children with CD4 count of over 200/mm^3 compared to placebo-treated children. A second multicenter placebo-controlled trial demonstrated that intravenous immune globulin decreases the risk of serious bacterial infections among children with advanced HIV disease who are receiving zidovudine[(242)]. The treatment effect was seen primarily among the children who were not receiving trimethoprim-sulfamethoxazole prophylaxis at entry. The therapeutic rather than prophylactic role of IVIG in the management of HIV-infected children with suspected bacterial infection remains controversial. Chemoprophylaxis with penicillin or other agents may reduce the incidence of infections with encapsulated bacteria; however, this has not been adequately tested in HIV-infected children. Uncontrolled data using prior pneumococcal infection in the same patients suggests penicillin may be useful in preventing invasive pneumococcal disease in this group[(243)]. Active immunization of HIV-infected children against pneumococcus and *Hemophilus influenza* type B has generally resulted in a poorer serologic response than uninfected children of the same age.

ANTIRETROVIRAL THERAPY

Although much work remains, considerable progress has been made in developing antiviral treatment strategies that improve the quality and duration of life of children infected with HIV. Currently, antiretroviral therapy is recommended for HIV-infected children who either have evidence of significant immunodeficiency or defined HIV-associated symptoms[(244)]. In the PICU setting, management of acute processes must take priority. If antiretroviral therapy is likely to complicate acute management, it should be postponed until the patient is recovering. Therapeutic options for antiretroviral therapy may also be limited by the route of administration, because only zidovudine (ZDV) is readily available in a form for intravenous administration.

The mainstay of antiretroviral therapy to date has been directed against the afferent or cell infection by the virus. Several candidate therapies against the efferent or cell production of progeny HIV are under investigation. Of afferent therapies, the reverse transcriptase inhibitor nucleoside analogues are the only currently licensed products for children.

Zidovudine (ZDV) was approved for use in children in 1990 and has clear benefits. Dramatic improvements in neurocognitive functioning have been demonstrated, as well as improvements in activity, weight gain, linear growth velocity, CD4+ lymphocyte counts, serum p24 antigen and survival[(187,189,245,246)]. Although generally well tolerated, the major side effects include anemia, neutropenia, nausea, headache, hepatic transaminase elevations, and myositis[(247–249)]. The complications of anemia and neutropenia are particularly problematic when patients are receiving a second myelosuppressive drug, such as high-dose trimethoprim/sulfamethoxasole for acute *Pneumocystis carinii* pneumonia. Initiation of ZDV therapy is generally postponed in this clinical situation. ZDV is commercially available as a syrup. Dosing every 6 hours is recommended **(Table 29.9).** The development of resistant virus through mutations in the reverse transcriptase gene is an increasing problem and has been associated with poor clinical outcome[(250)].

Therapy with 2′,3′-Dideoxyinosine (ddI) can result in improved CD4+ T lymphocyte counts and decreased levels of p24 antigen in serum[(198)]. Improvement in cognitive function has been documented as well[(198,251)]. The drug was approved for use in children in 1991. Possible toxicities include pancreatitis, peripheral neuropathy, and retinal depigmentation[(198,252,253)]. In contrast to ZDV, ddI is rarely associated with myelosuppression. ddI is acid labile and must be taken with antacids. Dosing every 12 hours is recommended **(Table 29.9).** As with ZDV, the emergence of viral resistance is problematic, particularly with prolonged therapy[(254)].

Because of the in vitro observations that ZDV and ddI have synergistic antiviral activity and a lack of viral cross-resistance[(255)], simultaneous administration of both these

Table 29.9. Currently Approved Antiretroviral Agents

	Dose	*Side Effects*
ZDV	180 mg/m^2/dose every six hrs.	anemia, neutropenia, nausea, headache, liver function elevation, myositis
ddI		
BSA m^2		
1.1–1.4	100 mg. every 12 hrs.	pancreatitis, peripheral
0.8–1.0	75 mg. every 12 hrs.	neuropathy, retinal
0.5–0.7	50 mg. every 12 hrs.	depigmentation
≤0.4	25 mg. every 12 hrs.	

agents has been studied. In children, the combination is well-tolerated at doses as high as those used as single agent therapy, and potent invivo antiviral activity is observed[256]. This observation was underscored with the 1995 announcement of the interim results of a clinical trial comparing three treatments for children with symptomatic HIV infection or AIDS (ZDV alone, ddI alone, or the combination of ZDV and ddI). ZDV alone was the least effective as the initial therapy to prevent disease progression. The children receiving ZDV as a single agent also had higher rates of side effects.

Clinical trial experience with a number of other nucleoside analogues is promising. 2′,3′-dideoxycytidine (ddC) is the most potent of these agents in vitro, and a pilot study suggests clinical efficacy[257]. ddC is approved for use in adults in combination with ZDV. However, mouth sores and peripheral neuropathy were common toxicities in the initial pediatric trial. A larger trial comparing two doses of ddC as a salvage regimen has recently been completed. Lamivudine or 3TC is an analog of ddC that is well-tolerated in children. This drug has caused interest for pediatric therapy since in adults, the combination of ZDV with 3TC has shown more pronounced and longer-lasting effects on CD4+ T lymphocyte counts and viral load than any combination therapy studied to date. Stavudine or D4T appears to have good bioavailability and CNS penetration. The major toxicity is peripheral neuropathy. A pediatric clinical trial will conclude shortly.

Other antiretroviral agents available for treatment of children enrolled in clinical trials include nonnucleoside reverse transcriptase inhibitors. These agents have a high degree of antiviral activity and minimal toxicity in common. However, the rapid emergence of viral resistance generally occurs early in the course of monotherapy. Several clinical trials are assessing the benefits of combining one of these agents with both ZDV and ddI.

The most promising area for intervention is a class of agents that block the virus-encoded protease critical in the assembly of the virus protein coat. Several of these agents are under study in adults, and a pediatric trial of this efferent therapy has begun. The greatest benefit of these agents is likely to be realized when used in combination with other agents that work at other points in the viral life cycle.

It must be pointed out that to date, supportive and antiretroviral therapies have had only modest effects on AIDS disease progression. New antiretroviral targets must be identified and new therapies developed to reach full therapeutic potential[258]. Once symptomatic HIV infection has been reached, a steady progression toward lethal immunosuppression occurs. It is thought that the immune damage at this point is so extensive that clinical therapies cannot reverse or prevent the progression to AIDS. Logically, the protracted clinically asymptomatic period following acute HIV-1 infection offers the greatest therapeutic potential. During this period of generally good health for the infected individual, the balance of active HIV-1 viral replication and active immune responsiveness is maximal. The progression of HIV-1 disease is evidenced by the slow CD4 T lymphocytes' decline. Novel strategies and therapies are being developed and applied to alter the progression from this clinically asymptomatic stage to AIDS.

TRANSMISSION PRECAUTIONS FOR HIV IN THE INTENSIVE CARE UNIT

Health care providers are understandably concerned about the risk of acquiring HIV from infected patients. A rational approach to this problem must be based on an understanding of the possible modes of transmission of HIV infection in the hospital setting.

Although HIV has been detected in many body fluids, such as blood; semen; vaginal secretions; urine; tears; cerebrospinal, pleural, pericardial, and synovial fluids; and breast milk, epidemiologic evidence suggests that blood is the single most infectious medium for HIV in the medical setting. In 1987, the CDC published guidelines based on the premise that all patients should be treated as potentially contagious for blood-borne pathogens. These guidelines proposed that blood and body fluid precautions be adopted for all patients regardless of HIV antibody status. These precautions are known as "Universal Blood and Body Fluid Precautions" or "Universal Precautions"[259,260]. The CDC guidelines are presented in **Table 29.10.**

The most likely potential sources of HIV infection for the intensive care specialist are either direct parenteral inoculation of blood by accidental needle stick exposure or exposure to mucous membranes and secretions contaminated with blood. Approximately 80% of occupationally acquired HIV infection results from contaminated needle stick injuries rather than from exposure to infected secretions[259]. Several studies involving more than 1000 cases of health care workers who sustained needle stick exposure to HIV-infected blood have been reported over the past several years. The cumulative results of these studies suggest that the risk of acquiring HIV infection under these circumstances is approximately 0.5%. The risk is approximately ten times lower than after similar exposure to hepatitis B-contaminated blood[261,262].

Gloves should be worn during venipuncture or when per-

Table 29.10. Universal Precautions[a]

1. Use appropriate barrier precautions to prevent skin and mucous membrane exposure to blood and body fluid:
   Use gloves for venipuncture or any vascular procedure.
   Use gowns, masks, and protective eyewear for procedures that may produce droplets of blood or secretions (i.e. endotracheal suctioning, transfer of blood from syringes to vacuum tubes).
2. Strict handwashing should be employed after gloves are removed or after inadvertent exposure to body fluids.
3. Do not recap, bend, or manipulate needles in any way after use. All disposable sharp items should be discarded in a conveniently located, puncture-proof container.

[a]*From Centers for Disease Control. Recommendations for prevention of HIV transmission in health care settings. MMWR 1988;361(Suppl 2):229.*

forming vascular access procedures, intubation, extubation, passage of nasogastric tubes, and oral and nasopharyngeal suctioning. They should be removed after the procedure before handling other noncontaminated articles and equipment. Further, the intensive care specialist must use appropriate barrier precautions to prevent skin and mucous membrane contamination by patients' blood and body fluids. Masks and protective eye wear—glasses or face shields—should be worn during procedures that generate droplets of blood or body fluids, for example, during major vessel cannulations and fiberoptic bronchoscopy or intubation. Hands should be washed after gloves have been removed[(260)].

Because parenteral exposure to infected blood by accidental needle stick injury is the overwhelming cause of occupationally acquired HIV infection in health care workers, extraordinary care must be taken to prevent injury to hands from needles, scalpels, and other sharp instruments. If stop-cocks are placed in intravenous lines, the use of needles for injections will be minimized. After use, needles and scalpel blades must be placed in puncture-resistant containers for disposal. To reduce the hazards of injury, needles must not be recapped, bent, or removed from disposable syringes before being discarded[(260)].

Proper application of universal precautions should decrease the incidence of HIV transmission from patients to their health care providers; however, until HIV is eliminated as a disease, health care institutions should provide anonymous HIV testing as well as counseling for health care workers who are occupationally exposed to HIV infection.

OUTCOMES FOR PEDIATRIC AIDS PATIENTS TREATED IN THE PEDIATRIC INTENSIVE CARE UNIT

Given the grim long-term prognosis for patients infected with HIV, intensive care specialists have begun to examine the efficacy of intensive care interventions. Most studies to date have looked specifically at the morbidity and mortality associated with the need for mechanical ventilation of HIV infected adults.

Studies in the mid-1980s of adult patients with acute respiratory failure (ARF) secondary to opportunistic infections demonstrated mortality rates of 86 to 100%, whereas those from the late 1980s and early 1990s showed mortality rates of 45 to 62%, demonstrating significant improvement in the short-term survival of AIDS patients with respiratory failure[(263,264)]. Potential explanations for the improved survival of adult AIDS patients with respiratory failure include (a) prehospital prophylactic treatment for PCP; (b) earlier diagnosis and treatment of the opportunistic infection causing respiratory failure; (c) antiretroviral treatment; (d) the use of corticosteroids in the treatment of PCP-related respiratory failure; and (e) improved conventional ventilator strategies with increasing knowledge of the pathophysiology of the various opportunistic infections.

Far fewer studies of outcomes in critically ill pediatric patients with HIV infection have been undertaken. The results of those studies demonstrate an encouraging improvement in outcome over the past several years. Vernon et al. reviewed their experience over a 46-month period from 1983 to 1986 and found an 84% mortality in 31 children mechanically ventilated for AIDS-related opportunistic infection and respiratory failure[(265)]. Bernstein et al. reviewed their patients with PCP and found a mortality of 39% in their 18 cases; however, the mortality was 50% for those who required mechanical ventilation for their PCP[(266)]. In a study of patients with AIDS who required assisted ventilation for acute respiratory failure (ARF), Notterman et al. found a mortality of 81%. This was compared to a mortality of only 9% in those HIV-infected children requiring mechanical ventilation for reasons other than ARF[(267)]. Most recently, Abadco et al. found a mortality of 50% for their HIV-infected patients with ARF[(268)].

We recently reviewed all admissions of HIV-infected patients to the pediatric intensive care unit (PICU) at the University of Maryland Hospital between March 1990 and September 1992. This investigation showed that 28 patients had a total of 53 admissions to the PICU during this time period. The acute mortality for the first admission was 0%. Of the 27 patient charts available for review of the first admission, six required mechanical ventilation, four of whom had ARF. All patients survived to hospital discharge.

During this interval, 12 patients had a second admission to the PICU. Of the 11 records available for review, eight patients survived to hospital discharge and one patient was discharged from the PICU but required readmission before hospital discharge. The overall mortality for the second PICU admission for this population was 18%. In this group, five patients required mechanical ventilation, all for ARF. Three of these five patients were successfully extubated and survived to hospital discharge, resulting in a mortality of 40% for those patients in their second PICU admission with ARF.

Six of the twenty-eight patients required three or more admissions to the PICU. Two of these patients died during their third PICU admission because of ARF, resulting in a 33% mortality for the third PICU admission for complications of AIDS. Three patients were admitted a fourth time, with one death (mortality = 33%). One patient survived a fifth admission and was discharged to home, and one patient had a total of seven admissions during the study period and survived all admissions to hospital discharge.

Our findings and those of other recent epidemiologic investigations discussed previously clearly support the general premise of intensive care treatment of the HIV-infected pediatric patient. They do not diminish, however, the long-term morbidity and mortality of this chronic disease. Therefore, the primary health care providers and the PICU team must maintain open, honest, and realistic communication with the patients' surrogates to evaluate the potential risks and benefits of intensive care treatment on a case-by-case basis.

References

1. Centers for Disease Control. HIV/AIDS Surveillance Report 1994;6:No.2.
2. Gwinn M, Wasser S, Fleming P, Karon J, Peterson L. Increasing prevalence of HIV infection among childbearing women, United States, 1989–1991 (Abstract PoC16–2990). Ninth International Conference on AIDS, Berlin, Jun 1993.
3. Chin J. Current and future dimensions of the HIV epidemic. Lancet 1990;336:221–224.
4. Gutman LT, St. Claire KK, Weedy C, et al. Human immunodeficiency virus transmission by child sexual abuse. Am J Dis Child 1991; 145:137–141.
5. D'Angelo L. HIV infections and AIDS in Adolescents. In: Pizzo PA, Wilfert CM, eds. Pediatric AIDS. The challenge of HIV infection in infants, children and adolescents. 2nd Ed. Baltimore: Williams & Wilkins, 1994:71–82.
6. Jovaisas E, Koch MA, Schafer A, Stauber M, Lowenthal D. LAV/HTLV-III in a 20 week fetus (Letter). Lancet 1985;2:1129.
7. Sprecher S, Soumenkoff G, Puissant F, Deguildre M. Vertical transmission of HIV in a 15 week fetus. Lancet 1986;2:288–289.
8. Courgnaus V, Laure F, Brossard A, et al. Frequent and early in-utero HIV-1 infection. AIDS Res Hum Retroviruses 1991;7:337–341.
9. Soiero R, Rubenstein A, Rasbaum WK, Lyman WD. Maternal-fetal transmission of AIDS: Frequency of human immunodeficiency virus type 1 nucleic acid sequences in human fetal DNA. J Infect Dis 1992;166:699–703.
10. Mofenson L, Wolinsky SM. Vertical transmission of HIV: Current insights regarding vertical transmission. In: Pizzo PA, Wilfert CM, eds. Pediatric AIDS. The challenge of HIV infection in infants, children and adolescents. 2nd Ed. Baltimore: Williams & Wilkins, 1994:179–206.
11. Goedert JJ, Duliege AM, Amos CI, et al. High risk of HIV-1 infection for first born twins. Lancet 1991;338:1471–1475.
12. Ziegler JV, Cooper DA, Johnson RO, et al. Postnatal transmission of AIDS-associated retrovirus from mother to infant. Lancet 1985;1: 896–897.
13. American Academy of Pediatrics Task Force on Pediatric AIDS. Perinatal Human Immunodeficiency Virus Infection. Pediatrics 1988; 82:941–944.
14. Oxtoby MJ. Vertically acquired HIV infection in the United States. In: Pizzo PA, Wilfert CM, eds. Pediatric AIDS. The challenge of HIV infection in infants, children and adolescents. 2nd Ed. Baltimore: Williams & Wilkins, 1994:3–20.
15. St. Louis ME, Kamenga M, Brown C, et al. Risk factor for perinatal transmission of human immunodeficiency virus type 1: Independent effects of high maternal CD8+ lymphocytes, low CD4+ lymphocytes and placental inflammation. JAMA 1993;269:2853–2859.
16. Connor EM, Sperling RS, Gelber R, et al. Reduction of maternal-infant transmission of human immunodeficiency virus type 1 with zidovudine treatment. N Engl J Med 1994;331:1173–1180.
17. Boyer PJ, Dillon M, Navaie M, et al. Factors predictive of maternal-fetal transmission of HIV-1: Preliminary analysis of zidovudine given during pregnancy and/or delivery. JAMA 1994;271:1925–1930.
18. Dunn DT, Newell ML, Mayaux C, et al. Mode of delivery and vertical transmission of HIV-1: A review of prospective studies. J Acquir Immune Defic Syndr 1993;6:298–302.
19. Ward JW, Bush TJ, Perkins HA, et al. The natural history of transfusion-associated infection with human immunodeficiency virus: factors influencing the rate of progression to disease. N Engl J Med 1988;318: 473–478.
20. National Hemophilia Foundation Information Exchange Medical Bulletin 137, July 1991.
21. Caldwell MB, Rogers MF. Epidemiology of pediatric HIV infection. Pediatr Clin North Am 1991;38:1–16.
22. Eyster ME. Transfusion and coagulation factor acquired disease. In: Pizzo PA, Wilfert CM, eds. Pediatric AIDS. The challenge of HIV infection in infants, children and adolescents. 1st Ed. Baltimore: Williams & Wilkins, 1991:22–37.
23. Blomberg RS, Schooley RT. Lymphocyte markers in infectious diseases. Semin Hematol 1985;22:81–114.
24. Clerici M, Giorgi JV, Chou CC, Gudeman VK, Zack JA, Gupta P, Ho HN, Nishanian PG, Berzofsky JA, Shearer GM. Cell-mediated immune response to human immunodeficiency virus (HIV) type 1 in seronegative homosexual men with recent sexual exposure to HIV-1. J Infect Dis 1992;165:1012–1019.
25. Mackewicz C, Levy JA. CD8+ cell anti-HIV activity: Non-lytic suppression of virus replication. AIDS Res Hum Retroviruses 1992; 8:1039–1050.
26. Daar ES, Chernyavskiy T, Moudgil T. The role of humoral immunity in primary HIV-1 infection, [Abstract MoA0017]. VIIIth International Conference on AIDS:Abstracts, Amsterdam, 1992.
27. Mackewicz CJ, Wu J, Levy JA. Exposure to HIV can be detected prior to seroconversion by CD8+ cell anti-HIV responsiveness, [Abstract 2:A33]. VIIIth International Conference on AIDS:Abstracts, Amsterdam, 1992.
28. Ranki A, Valle SL, Krohn M, Antonen J, Allain JP, Leuther M, Franchini G, Krohn K. Long latency preceded overt seroconversion is sexually transmitted human-immunodeficiency-virus infection. Lancet 1987; ii:589–593.
29. Lang W, Perkins H, Anderson RE, Royce R, Jewell N, Winkelstein W, Jr. Patterns of T lymphocyte changes with human immunodeficiency virus infection: From seroconversion to the development of AIDS. J Acquired Immune Defic Syndr 1989;2:63–69.
30. Wei X, Shosh SK, Taylor ME, Johnson VA, Emini EA, Deutsch P, Lifson JD, Bonhoeffer S, Nowak MA, Hahn BH, Saag MS, Shaw GM. Viral dynamics in human immunodeficiency virus type 1 infection. Nature 1995;373:117–122.
31. Ho DD, Neumann AU, Perelson AS, Chen W, Leonard JM, Markowitz M. Rapid turnover of plasma virions and CD4 lymphocytes in HIV-1 infection. Nature 1995;373:123–126.
32. Zindernagel RM, Hengartner H. T-cell-mediated immunopathology versus direct cytolysis by virus: Implications for HIV and AIDS. Immun Today 1994;15:262–268.
33. Fauci AS. Multifactorial nature of human immunodeficiency virus disease: Implications for therapy. Science 1993;262:1011–1018.
34. Pantaleo G, Graziosi C, Fauci AS. Mechanisms of disease: The immunopathogenesis of human immunodeficiency virus infection. N Engl J Med 1993;328:327–336.
35. Eyster ME, Gail MH, Ballard JO, Al-Mondhiry H, Goedert JJ. Natural history of human immunodeficiency virus infections in hemophiliacs: Effects of T-cell subsets, platelet counts, and age. Ann Inter Med 1987;107:1–6.
36. Levy JA. The mysteries of HIV: Challenges for therapy and prevention. Nature 1988;333:519–522.
37. Schellekens PR, Tersmette M, Roos MTT, Koot RO, De Wolf F, Coutinborand RA, Miedema F. Biphasic rate of CD4+ cell count decline during progression to AIDS correlates with HIV-1 phenotype. AIDS 1992;6:665–670.
38. Rosenberg ZF, Fauci AS. Immunopathogenesis of HIV infection. FASEB J 1991;5:2382–2390.
39. Bednarik DP, Folks TM. Mechanisms of HIV-1 latency. AIDS 1992;6: 3–16.
40. Clouse KA, Powell D, Washington I, Poli G, Strebel K, Farrar W, Barstad P, Kovacs J, Fauci AS, Folks TM. Monokine regulation of human immunodeficiency virus-1 expression in a chronically infected human T-cell clone. J Immunol 1989;142:431–438.
41. Butera ST, Perez VL, Wu BY, Nabel GJ, Folks TM. Oscillation of the human immunodeficiency virus surface receptor is regulated by the stat of viral activation in a CD4+ cell model of chronic infection. J Virol 1991;65:4645–4653.
42. Folks TM, Justement J, Kinter A, Schnittman S, Orienting J, Poli G, Fauci AS. Characterization of a promonocyte clone chronically infected with HIV and inducible by 13-phorbol-12-myristate acetate. J Immunol 1988;140:1117–1120.
43. Folks TM, Justement J, Kinter A, Dinarello CA, Fauci AS. Cytokine-induced expression of HIV-1 in a chronically infected promonocytic cell line. Science 1987;238:800–802.
44. Perez VL, Rowe T, Justement JS, Butera ST, June CH, Folks TM. An HIV-1 infected T-cell clone defective in IL-2 production and Ca2+ mobilization after CD3 stimulation. J Immunol 1991;147:3145–3148.
45. Mitsuya H, Yarchoan R, Kageyama S, Broder S. Targeted therapy of human immunodeficiency virus-related disease. FASEB J 1991;5:2368–2381.
46. Parks WP, Scott GB. An overview of pediatric AIDS: Approaches to diagnosis and outcome assessment. In: Broder S, ed. AIDS-modern concepts and therapeutic challenges. New York: Marcel Decker, 1987: 245–262.
47. Centers for Disease Control. 1994 Revised classification system for human immunodeficiency virus infection in children less than 13 years of age. MMWR 1994.43:RR–12.
48. Rogers JF, Ou CY, Kobourne B, Schochetman G. Advances and prob-

lems in the diagnosis of HIV infection in infants. In: Pizzo PA, Wilfert CM, eds. Pediatric AIDS. The challenge of HIV infection in infants, children and adolescents. Baltimore: Williams & Wilkins, 1991: 159–174.
49. Kraskinski K, Borkowsky W. Laboratory diagnosis of HIV infection. Pediatr Clin North Am 1991;38:17–36.
50. Arpadi S, Caspe WB. HIV testing. J Pediatr 1991;119:S8–S13.
51. Centers for Disease Control. Recommendations for assisting in the prevention of perinatal transmission of human T-lymphotropic virus type III/lymphadenopathy-associated virus and acquired immunodeficiency syndrome. MMWR 1985;34:721–732.
52. Jackson JB, Balfour Jr HH. Practical diagnostic testing for human immunodeficiency virus. Clin Microbiol Rev 1988;1:124–138.
53. Centers for Disease Control. Interpretation and use of the Western blot assay for serodiagnosis of human immunodeficiency virus type 1 infections. MMWR 1989;38:S1–S7.
54. Centers for Disease Control. Interpretive criteria used to report Western blot results for HIV-1 antibody testing—United States. MMWR 1991;40:692–695.
55. Hoff R, Berardi VP, Weiblen BJ, Mahoney-Trout L, Mitchell ML, Grady GF. Seroprevalence of human immunodeficiency virus among childbearing women. N Engl J Med 1988;318:525–530.
56. Report of a consensus workshop, Siena, Italy, January 17–18, 1992. Early diagnosis of HIV infection in infants. J Acquir Immune Defic Syndr 1992;5:1169–78.
57. McIntosh K, Pitt J, Brambilla D, et al. Blood culture in the first 6 months of life for the diagnosis of vertically transmitted human immunodeficiency virus infection. J Infect Dis 1994;170:996–1000.
58. Burgard M, Mayaux MJ, Blanche S, et al. The use of viral culture and p24 antigen testing to diagnose human immunodeficiency virus infection in neonates. N Engl J Med 1992;327:1192–1197.
59. Rayfield MA. Human immunodeficiency virus culture. In: Schochetman G, George JR, eds. AIDS testing: Methodology and management issues. New York:Springer-Verlag, 1992:111–122.
60. Hollinger FB, ed. ACTG virology manual for HIV laboratories. Bethesda: National Institutes of Health, 1993.
61. Ho DD, Moudgil T, Alam M. Quantitation of human immunodeficiency virus type 1 in the blood of infected persons. N Engl J Med 1989; 321:1621–1625.
62. Rogers MF, Ou CY, Rayfield M, et al. Use of the polymerase chain reaction for early detection of the proviral sequences of human immunodeficiency virus in infants born to seropositive mothers. N Engl J Med 1989;320:1649–1654.
63. Krivine A, Firtion G, Cao L, Francoual C, Henrion R, Lebon P. HIV replication during the first weeks of life. Lancet 1992;339:1187–1189.
64. Butcher A, Spadoro J. Using PCR for detection of HIV-1 infection. Clin Immunol Newslett 1992;12:73–76.
65. Bagasra O, Hauptman SP, Lischner HW, Sachs M, Pomerantz RJ. Detection of human immunodeficiency virus type 1 provirus in mononuclear cells by in situ polymerase chain reaction. N Engl J Med 1992;326:1385–1391.
66. Schochetman G, Sninsky JJ. Direct detection of human immunodeficiency virus infection using the polymerase chain reaction. In: Schochetman G, George JR, eds. AIDS testing: Methodology and management issues. New York:Springer-Verlag, 1992:90–110.
67. Johnson JP, Nair P, O'Neil KM, Alger L, Hines SE, Seiden SW, Revie DR, Hebel R. HIV infection in infants: natural history and serologic diagnosis of children. Am J Dis Child 1989;143:1147–1153.
68. Fahey JL, Taylor JMG, Detels R, et al. The prognostic value of cellular and serologic markers in infection with human immunodeficiency virus type 1. N Engl J Med 1990;322:166–172.
69. Chaisson RE, Allain J, Volberding PA. Significant changes in HIV antigen level in the serum of patients treated with azidothymidine. N Engl J Med 1986;315:1610–1611.
70. Centers for Disease Control. 1995 revised guidelines for prophylaxis against Pneumocystis carinii pneumonia for children infected with or exposed to human immunodeficiency virus. MMRW 1995;44:RR-4.
71. Quinn TC, Kline RL, Halsey N, et al. Early diagnosis of perinatal HIV infection by detection of viral-specific IgA antibodies. JAMA 1991;266:3439–3442.
72. Landesman S, Weiblen B, Mendez H, et al. Clinical utility of HIV-IgA immunoblot assay in the early diagnosis of perinatal HIV infection. JAMA 1991;266:3443–3446.
73. Archibald DW, Johnson JP, Nair P, et al. Detection of salivary immunoglobulin A antibodies to HIV-1 in infants and children. AIDS 1990;4:417–420.
74. Rogers MF, Schochetman G, Hoff R. Advances in diagnosis of HIV infection in infants. In: Pizzo PA, Wilfert CM, eds. Pediatric AIDS. The challenge of HIV infection in infants, children and adolescents. 2nd Ed. Baltimore: Williams & Wilkins, 1994:219–238.
75. O'Brien TR, George JR, Holmberg SD. Human immunodeficiency virus type 2 infection in the United States. JAMA 1992;267:2775–2779.
76. Oleske J, Minnefor A, Cooper Jr R, Thomas K, Dela Cruz A, Ahdiehl H, Guerrero I, Joshi V, Desposito F. Immune deficiency syndrome in children. JAMA 1983;249:2345–2349.
77. Rubinstein A, Sicklick M, Gupta A, et al. Acquired immunodeficiency with reversed T4/T8 ratios in infants born to promiscuous and drug addicted mothers. JAMA 1983;249:2350–2359.
78. Pawha S, Kaplan M, Fikrig S, et al. Spectrum of human T cell lymphotropic virus type III infection in children. JAMA 1986;225:2299–2305.
79. Rogers MF. AIDS in children: a review of the clinical, epidemiologic and public health aspects. Pediatr Infect Dis 1985;4:220–236.
80. Blanche S, Rouzioux C, Guihard Moscato ML, Veber F, Mayaus MJ, Jacomet C. A prospective study of infants born to women seropositive for human immunodeficiency virus type 1. N Engl J Med 1989; 320:1643–1648.
81. Tovo PA, DeMartino M, Gabiano C, et al. Prognostic factors and survival in children with perinatal HIV-1 infection. Lancet 1992; 339:1249–1253.
82. European Collaborative Study. Children born to women with HIV-1 infection: natural history and risk of transmission. Lancet 1991;337:253–260.
83. Blanche S, Tardieu M, Duliege A, et al. Longitudinal study of 94 symptomatic infants with perinatally acquired human immunodeficiency virus infection. Am J Dis Child 1990;144:1210–1215.
84. Turner BJ, Denison M, Eppes SC, Houchens R, Fanning T, Markson LE. Survival experience of 789 children with the acquired immunodeficiency syndrome. Pediatr Infect Dis J 1993;12:310–320.
85. MaWhinney S, Pagano M, Thomas P. Age at AIDS diagnosis for children with perinatally acquired HIV. J Acquir Immune Defic Syndr 1993;6:1139–1144.
86. Auger I, Thomas P, DeGruttola V, et al. Incubation periods for paediatric AIDS patients. Nature 1988;336:575–577.
87. Persaud D, Chandwani S, Rigaud M, et al. Delayed recognition of human immunodeficiency virus in preadolescent children. Pediatrics 1992;90:688–691.
88. European Collaborative Study. Natural history of vertically acquired human immunodeficiency virus-1 infection. Pediatrics 1994;94:815–819.
89. Jones DS, Byers RH, Bush TJ, Oxtoby MJ, Rogers MF. Epidemiology of transfusion-associated acquired immunodeficiency syndrome in children in the United States, 1981–1989. Pediatrics 1992;89:123–127.
90. Krasinski K, Borkowsky W, Holzman RS. Prognosis of human immunodeficiency virus infection in children and adolescents. Pediatr Infect Dis J 1989;8:216–220.
91. Frederick T, Mascola L, Eller A, et al. Progression of human immunodeficiency virus disease among infants and children infected perinatally with human immunodeficiency virus or through neonatal blood transfusion. Pediatr Infect Dis J 1994;13:1091–1097.
92. Goedert JJ, Kessler CM, Aledort LM, et al. A prospective study of human immunodeficiency virus type 1 infection and the development of AIDS in subjects with hemophilia. N Engl J Med 1989;321:1141–1148.
93. D'Angelo LJ. HIV infection and AIDS in adolescents. In: Pizzo PA, Wilfert CM, eds. Pediatric AIDS. The challenge of HIV infection in infants, children and adolescents. 2nd Ed. Baltimore: Williams & Wilkins, 1994:71–81.
94. Centers for Disease Control. Revision of the CDC surveillance case definition for acquired immunodeficiency syndrome. MMWR 1987; 36(suppl):1–15s.
95. Centers for Disease Control. 1993 revised classification system for HIV infection and expanded surveillance case definition for AIDS among adolescents and adults. MMWR 1992;41:RR17.
96. Falloon J, Eddy J, Wiener L, Pizzo PA. Human immunodeficiency virus infection in children. J Pediatr 1989;114:1–30.
97. Burroughs MH, Edelson PJ. Medical care of the HIV infected child. Pediatr Clin North Am 1991;38:45–68.
98. Hauger SB. Approach to the pediatric patient, with HIV infection and pulmonary symptoms. J Pediatr 1991;119:S25–S33.
99. Murray JF, Mills J. Pulmonary infectious complications of human immunodeficiency virus infection. Part 1. Am Rev Respir Dis 1990; 141:1356–1372.
100. Murray JF, Mills J. Pulmonary infectious complications of human immunodeficiency virus infection. Part 2. Am Rev Respir Dis 1990; 141:1582–1598.

101. Rogers MF, Thomas PA, Starcher ET, Noa MC, Bush TJ, Jaffee HW. Acquired immunodeficiency syndrome in children: Report of the Centers for Disease Control National Surveillance, 1982 to 1985. Pediatrics 1987;79:1008–1014.
102. Rogers MA. AIDS in children: A review of the clinical, epidemiologic, and public health aspects. Pediatr Infect Dis J 1985;4:230–236.
103. Simonds RJ, Lindegren ML, Thomas P, et al. Prophylaxis against *Pneumocystis carinii* pneumonia among children with perinatally acquired HIV infection in the United States. N Engl J Med 1995;332:786–790.
104. Matsumoto Y, Yoshida Y. Advances in *Pneumocystis* biology. Parasitology Today 1986;2:137–142.
105. Pifer LL, Hughes WT, Stagno S, Woods D. *Pneumocystis carinii* infection: Evidence of high prevalence in normal and immunosuppressed children. Pediatrics 1978;61:35–40.
106. Sanders-Laufer D, DeBruin W, Edelson PJ: *Pneumocystis carinii* infections in HIV infected children. Pediatr Clin North Am 1991;38:69–88.
107. Bye MR, Bernstein LJ, Glaser J, Kleid D: *Pneumocystis carinii* pneumonia in young children with AIDS. Pediatr Pulmonol 1990;9:251–253.
108. Hughes WT. *Pneumocystis carinii* pneumonia. In: Pizzo PA, Wilfert CM, eds. Pediatric AIDS. The challenge of HIV infection in infants, children and adolescents. 2nd Ed. Baltimore: Williams & Wilkins, 1994:405–418.
109. Kwok SO, Donnell JJ, Wood IS. Retinal cotton-wool spots in a patient with *Pneumocystis carinii* infection. N Engl J Med 1982;307:184.
110. Ognibene FP, Gill VJ, Pizzo PA, et al. Induced sputum to diagnose *Pneumocystis carinii* pneumonia in immunosuppressed patients. J Pediatr 1989;115:430–433.
111. Bye MR, Bernstein L, Shah K, Ellawie M, Rubinstein A. Diagnositic bronchoalveolar lavage in children with AIDS. Pediatr Pulmonol 1987;3:425–428.
112. de Blic J, Blanche S, Danel C, Le Bourgeois M, Caniglia M, Scheinmann P. Bronchoalveolar lavage in HIV-infected patients with interstitial pneumonitis. Arch Dis Child 1989;64:1246–1250.
113. Gordin FM, Simon GL, Wofsy CB, Mills J. Adverse reactions to trimethoprim-sulfamethoxazole in patients with the acquired immunodeficiency syndrome. Ann Intern Med 1984;100:495–499.
114. Hughes WT, Leoung G, Kramer F, Bozzette S, Framer P. Comparison of Atovaquon 566C80 and trimethoprim-sulfamethoxazole to treat *P. carinii* pneumonitis in patients with AIDS. N Engl J Med 1993;328:1521–1527.
115. Conte JE, Chernoff P, Feigal DW, Joseph P. McDonald C, Golden JA. Intravenous or inhaled pentamidine for treating *Pneumocystis carinii* pneumonia in AIDS. A randomized trial. Ann Intern Med 1990; 113:203–209.
116. Sattler FR, Allegra CJ Verdegem TD, et al. Trimetrexate-leucovorin dosage evaluation study for treatment of *Pneumocystis carinii* pneumonia. J Infect Dis 1990; 161:91–96.
117. Mills J, Leoung G, Medina I, Hopewell PC, Hughes WT, Wofsy C. Dapsone treatment of *Pneumocystis carinii* pneumonia in the acquired immunodeficiency syndrome. Antimicrob Agents Chemother 1988; 32:1057–1060.
118. Gagnon S, Boota AM, Fischl MA, Baier H, Kirksey OW, La Voie L. Corticosteroid as adjunctive therapy for severe *Pneumocystis carinii* pneumonia in the acquired immunodeficiency syndrome A double-blind, placebo controlled trial. N Engl J Med 1990;2323:1444–1450.
119. Bozzette Sa, Sattler FR, Chiu J, et al. A controlled trial of early adjunctive treatment with corticosteroid for *Pneumocystis carinii* pneumonia in the acquired immunodeficiency syndrome. N Engl J Med 1990;323:1451–1457.
120. The National Institutes of Health, University of California Expert Panel for Corticosteroids as Adjunctive Therapy for *Pneumocystis* pneumonia. Consensus statement on the use of cortocosteroid adjunctive therapy for *Pneumocystis* pneumonia in the acquired immunodeficiency syndrome. N Engl J Med 1990;323:1300–1304.
121. Sleasman JW, Hemenway C, Klein AS, Barrett DJ. Corticosteroids improve survival of children with AIDS and *Pneumocystis carinii* pneumonia. AJDC 1993;147:30–34.
122. Sanders-Laufer D, DeBruin W, Edelson PJ: *Pneumocystis carinii* infections in HIV infected children. Pediatr Clin North Am 1991;38:69–88.
123. McIntosh K. Respiratory virus infections. In: Pizzo PA, Wilfert CM, eds. Pediatric AIDS. The challenge of HIV infection in infants, children and adolescents 2nd Ed. Baltimore: Williams & Wilkins, 1994:365–376.
124. Jue S, Whitley B. Herpesvirus infections children with human immunodeficiency virus. In: Pizzo PA, Wilfert CM, eds. Pediatric AIDS. The challenge of HIV infection in infants, children and adolescents. Baltimore: Williams & Wilkins, 1994:345–364.
125. Jura E, Chadwick EG, Josephs SH et al. Varicella-zoster virus infections in children infected with the human immunodeficiency virus. Pediatr Infect Dis J 1989;8:586–590.
126. Patterson LE, Butler KM, Edwards MS. Clinical herpes zoster shortly following primary varicella in two HIV infected children. Clin Pediatr 1989;28:354.
127. Chandwani S, Borkowsky W, Krasinski K, Lawrence R, Welliver R. Respiratory syncytial virus infection in human immunodeficiency virus infected children. J Pediatr 1990;117:251–254.
128. Murphy D, Rose RC. Respiratory syncytial virus pneumonia in a human immunodeficiency virus infected man (Letter). JAMA 1989; 26:1147.
129. Krilov LR, Rubin LG, Frogel M et al. Disseminated adenovirus infection with hepatic necrosis in patients with human immunodeficiency virus infection and other immunodeficiency states. Rev Infect Dis 1990;12:303–307.
130. Kaschula ROC, Druker J, Kipps A. Late morphologic consequences of measles: a lethal and debilitating lung disease among the poor. Rev Infect Dis 1983;5:395–404.
131. Kipps A, Kaschula ROC. Virus pneumonia following measles. A virological and histological study of autopsy material. S Afr Med J 1976;50:1083–1088.
132. Centers for Disease Control. Measles in HIV infected children, United States. MMWR 1988;37:183–186.
133. Kaplan LJ, Daum RS, Smaron M, McCarthy CA. Severe measles in immunocompromised patients. JAMA 1992;267:1237–1241.
134. Vernon D, Holzman, B, Lewis P, et al. Respiratory failure in children with acquired immunodeficiency syndrome and acquired immunodeficiency syndrome-related complex. Pediatrics 1988;82:223.
135. Drew WL, Jacobson MA, Erlich KS. Cytomegalovirus: clinical presentations. In: Cohen PT, Sande MA, Volberding PA, eds. The AIDS knowledge base. Waltham, MA: The Medical Publishing Group, 1990; 6.4.6.:1–3.
136. Hall CB, McBride JT, Walsh EE et al. Aerosolized ribavirin treatment of infants with respiratory syncytial virus infection. N Engl J Med 1983;308:1443–1447.
137. Wingfield WL, Pollack D, Grunert RR. Therapeutic efficacy of amantadine HCl and rimantadine HCl in naturally occurring influenza A2 respiratory illness in man. N Engl J Med 1969;281:579–584.
138. Gilbert BE, Wilson SZ Knight V et al. Ribavirin small-particle aerosol treatment of infections caused by influenza virus strains A/Victoria/7/83 (H1N1) and B/Texas/1/84. Antimicrob Agents Chemother 1985;27: 309–313.
139. Sigwell RW, Huffman JH, Khare GP. Broad-spectrum anti-viral activity of virazole 1-beta-1-ribofuranosyl-1,2,4-triazole-3-carboximide. Science 1972;177:705–706.
140. Banks SG, Fernandez H. Clinical use of ribavirin in measles. A summarized review. In: Smith RA, Knight V, Smith JAD eds. Clinical applications of ribavirin. Orlando:Academic,1984:203–209.
141. McIntosh K, Kurachek S, Cairns LM, Burns JC, Godspeed B. Treatment of respiratory viral infection in an immunodeficient infant with ribavirin aerosol. Am J Dis Child 1984;138:305–308.
142. Gelfand EW, McCurdy D, Rao CP, Middleton PJ. Ribavirin treatment of viral pneumonitis is severe combined immunodeficiency disease. Lancet 1983; 2:732–733.
143. Hemming VG, Rodriguez W, Kim HW et al. Intravenous immunoglobulin treatment of respiratory syncitial virus infections in infants and young children. Antimicrob Agent Chemother 1987;31:1882–1886
144. Pau AK, Pitrak DL. Management of cytomegalovirus infection in patients with acquired immunodeficiency syndrome. Clin Pharm 1990;9:613–631.
145. Hochster H, Dieterich D, Bozette S, et al. Toxicity of combined ganciclovir and zidovudine for cytomegalovirus disease associated with AIDS. An AIDS clinical trials group study. Ann Intern Med 1990;113: 111–117.
146. Principi N, Marchisio P, Tornaghi R, et al. Occurrence of infections in children infected with human immunodeficiency virus. Pediatr Infect Dis J 1991;10:190–193.
147. Advisory Committee for the elimination of tuberculosis. Tuberculosis and Human Immunodeficiency Virus Infection: recommendations of the Advisory Committee for the Elimination of Tuberculosis (ACET). MMWR 1989;38:236–238,243–250.
148. Chaisson RE, Schecter GF, Theuer CP, Rutherford EW, Echenberg PF, Hopewell PC. Tuberculosis in patients with the acquired immunodeficiency syndrome. Clinical features, response to therapy, and survival. Am Rev Respir Dis 1987;136:570–574.

149. Snider DE, Hopewell PC, Mills J, Reichman LB. Mycobacterioses and the acquired immunodeficiency syndrome. Am Rev Respir Dis 1987;136:472–496.
150. Berenguer J, Moreno S, Laguan F et al. Tuberculosis meningitis in patients infected with the human immunodeficiency virus. N Engl J Med 1992; 326:668–672.
151. Centers for Disease Control. Purified protein derivative (PPD)-tuberculin anergy and HIV infection: Guidelines for anergy testing and management of anergic persons at risk for tuberculosis. MMWR 1991;40:27–32.
152. Husson RN. Mycobacterial Infections: Tuberculosis. In: Pizzo PA, Wilfert CM, eds. Pediatric AIDS. The challenge of HIV infection in infants, children and adolescents 2nd Ed. Baltimore: Williams & Wilkins, 1994:289–307.
153. Connor EM, Andiman WA. Lymphoid Interstitial Pneumonitis. In: Pizzo PA, Wilfert CM, eds. Pediatric AIDS. The challenge of HIV infection in infants, children and adolescents 2nd Ed. Baltimore: Williams & Wilkins, 1994:467–481.
154. Pitt J. Lymphocyte interstitial pneumonia. Pediatr Clin North Am 1991;38:89–96.
155. Joshi V. Pathology of children with AIDS. Pediatr Clin North Am 1991;38:97–120.
156. Andiman WA, Eastman R, Marten K, et al. Opportunistic lymphoproliferative disease associated with Epstein-Barr viral DNA in infants and children with AIDS. Lancet 1985; 2:1390–1393.
157. Lania-Howarth M, Graffino D, Oleske J, Connor E. Blood viscosity measurement in children with HIV infection. J Allergy Clin Immunol 1990;85:148.
158. Lipshultz SE. Cardiovascular Problems. In: Pizzo PA, Wilfert CM, eds. Pediatric AIDS. The challenge of HIV infection in infants, children and adolescents 2nd Ed. Baltimore: Williams & Wilkins, 1994:483–511.
159. Kavanaugh-McHugh A, Ruff AJ, Rowes A, Herskowitz A, Modlin JF. In: Pizzo PA, Wilfert CM, eds. Pediatric AIDS. The challenge of HIV infection in infants, children and adolescents. Baltimore: Williams & Wilkins, 1991:355–372.
160. Lipshultz SE, Liginbuhl LM, Saul JP, McIntosh K. Dysrhythmias, unexpected arrest and sudden death in pediatric HIV infection (Abstract). Circulation 1991;84:11–660.
161. Liginbuhl LM, Orav EJ, McIntosh K, Lipshultz SE. Cardiac morbidity and mortality in children with human immunodeficiency virus-1 infection. JAMA 1993;269:2869–2875.
162. Lipshultz SE, Liginbuhl LM, McINtosh K, Orav EJ. Cardiac morbidity and mortality in children with symptomatic HIV infection (Abstract). Circulation 1992;86:1–362.
163. Dittrich H, Chowl, Denaro F, Spector S. Human immunodeficiency virus infection, coxsackie virus and cardiomyopathy. Ann Intern Med 1988;108:308–309.
164. Herskowitz A, Ansari AA, Neumann DA, et al. Cardiomyopathy in acquired immunodeficiency syndrome: evidence for autoimmunity. Circulation 1989;80 (Suppl II):322.
165. Steinherz LJ, Brochstein JA, Robin J. Cardiac involvement in congenital acquired immunodeficiency syndrome. Am J Dis Child 1988; 140:1241–1244.
166. Lipshultz SE, Chanock S, Sanders SP, Colan SD, Perez-Atayde A, McIntosh K. Cardiovascular manifestations of human immunodeficiency virus in infants and children. Am J Cardiol 1989;63:1489–1497.
167. Stewart JM, Kaul A, Gromisch DS, Reyes E, Woolf PK, Gowitz MH. Symptomatic cardiac dysfunction in children with human immunodeficiency virus infection. Am Heart J 1988;117:140–144.
168. Mast HL, Haller JO, Schiller MS, Anderson VM. Pericardial effusion and its relationship to cardiac disease in children with acquired immunodeficiency syndrome. Pediatr Radiol 1992;22:548–551.
169. Bierman FZ. Guidelines for diagnosis and management of cardiac disease in children with HIV infection. J Pediatr 1991;119:553–556.
170. Pardo V, Meneses R, Ossa L et al. AIDS-related glomerulopathy: Occurrence in specific risk groups. Kidney Int 1987;31:1167–1173.
171. Strauss J, Abitbol C, Zilleruelo G et al. Renal disease in children with the acquired immunodeficiency syndrome. N Engl J Med 1989; 321:625–630.
172. Connor E, Gupta S, Joshi V et al. Acquired immunodeficiency syndrome-associated renal disease in children. J Pediatr 1988;113:39–44.
173. Tarshish P. Approach to the diagnosis and management of HIV associated nephropathy. J Pediatr 1991;119:550–552.
174. Wigfall DR. Renal Problems. In: Pizzo PA, Wilfert CM, eds. Pediatric AIDS. The challenge of HIV infection in infants, children and adolescents 2nd Ed. Baltimore: Williams & Wilkins, 1994.547–557.
175. Glassock RJ. HIV infection and the kidney. Ann Intern Med 1990;112:35–49.
176. Ingulli E, Tejani A, Fikrig S, Nicastri A, Chen CK, Pomrantz A. Nephrotic syndrome associated with acquired immunodeficiency syndrome in children. J Pediatr 1991;119:710–716.
177. Rao TKS. Human immunodeficiency virus (HIV) associated nephropathy. Annu Rev Med 1991;42:391–401.
178. Rao TKS, Friedman EA. AIDS (HIV)-associated nephropathy; does it exist? Am J Nephrol 1989;9:441–453.
179. Santos F, Orejas G, Foreman JW, Chan JCM. Diagnostic workup of renal disorders. Curr Probl Pediatr 1991;20:48–74.
180. Schoenfeld P, Feduska NJ. AIDS and renal disease: report of the National Kidney Foundation-National Institutes of Health Task Force on AIDS and Kidney Diseases. Am J Kidney Dis 1990;16:14–25.
181. Mueller BU. Hematological Problems and their Management in children with HIV infection. In: Pizzo PA, Wilfert CM, eds. Pediatric AIDS. The challenge of HIV infection in infants, children and adolescents 2nd Ed. Baltimore: Williams & Wilkins, 1994.591–601.
182. Hilgarten M. Hematologic manifestation in HIV-infected children. J Pediatr 1991;119:S47–S49.
183. Ganser A, Greher J, Volkers B, Staszewski S, Hoelzer D. Inhibitory effect of azidothymidine, 2'-3'-dideoxycitidine on in-vitro growth of hematopoietic progenitor cells from normal persons and from patients with AIDS. Exp Hematol 1989;17:321–325.
184. Zon LI, Groopman JE. Hematologic manifestations of the human immunodeficiency virus. Semin Hematol 1988;25:208–218.
185. Ellaurie M, Burns ER, Rubinstein A. Hematologic manifestations in pediatric HIV infection: Severe anemia as a prognostic factor. Am J Pediatr Hematol Oncol 1990;12:449–453.
186. Fischl MA, Galpin JE, Levine JD et al. Recombinant human erythropoietin for patients with AIDS treated with zidovudine. N Engl J Med 1990;322:1488–1493.
187. Pizzo PA, Eddy J, Falloon J et al. Effect of continuous intravenous infusion of zidovudine (AZT) in children with symptomatic HIV infection. N Engl J Med 1988;319:889–896.
188. McCance-Katz EF, Hoecker JL, Vitale NB. Severe neutropenia associated with anti-neutrophil antibody in a patient with acquired immunodeficiency syndrome-related complex. Pediatr Infect Dis J 1987;6: 417–418.
189. McKinney RE, Maha MA, Connor EM et al. A multicenter trial of oral zidovudine in children with advanced human immunodeficiency virus disease. N Engl J Med 1991;324:1018–1025.
190. Shaunak S, Bartlett JA. Zidovudine-induced neutropenia: Are we too cautious? Lancet 1989;2:91–92.
191. Mueller BU, Jacobsen F, Butler KM, Husson RN, Lewis LL, Pizzo PA. Combination treatment with azidothymidine and granulocyte colony-stimulating factor in children with human immunodeficiency virus infection. J Pediatr 1992;121:797–802.
192. Zucker-Franklin D, Cao YZ. Megakaryocytes of human immunodeficiency virus-infected individuals express viral RNA. Proc Natl Acad Sci 1989;86:5595–5599.
193. Karpatkin S. Autoimmune thrombocytopenia and AIDS-related thrombocytopenia. Curr Opin Immunol 1990;2:625–632.
194. Ellaurie M, Burns ER, Bernstein LJ, et al. Thrombocytopenia and human immunodeficiency virus in children. Pediatrics 1988;82:905–908.
195. Oksenhendler E, Bierling P, Farcet JP, Rabian C, Seligmann M, Clauvel JP. Response to therapy in 37 patients with HIV-related thrombocytopenic purpura. Br J Haematol 1987;66:491–495.
196. Saulsbury FT, Bringelsen KA, Normansell DE. Effects of prednisone on human immunodeficiency virus infection. South Med J 1991;84: 431–435.
197. Oksenhendler E, Bierling P, Ferchal F, Chauvel JP, Seligmann M. Zidovudine for thrombocytopenic purpura related to human immunodeficiency virus (HIV) infection. Ann Intern Med 1989;110:365–368.
198. Butler KM, Husson RN, Balis FM et al. Dideoxyinosine in children with symptomatic human immunodeficiency virus infection. N Engl J Med 1991;324:137–144.
199. Burns ER, Krieger B, Bernstien L, Rubinstein A. Acquired circulating anticoagulants in children with the acquired immunodeficiency syndrome. Pediatrics 1988;82:763–765.
200. Cohen AJ, Phillips TM, Kessler ZCM. Circulating coagulation inhibition in the acquired immunodeficiency syndrome. Ann Intern Med 1986;104:175–180.
201. Ragni MV, Bontempo FA, Myers DJ, Kiss JE, Oral A. Hemorrhagic sequelae of immune thrombocytopenic purpura in human immunodeficiency virus-infected hemophiliacs. Blood 1990;75:1267–1272.

202. Ragni MV, Miller BJ, Whalen R, Ptachcinski R. Bleeding tendency, platelet function, and pharmacokinetics of ibuprofen and zidovudine in HIV+ hemophiliac men. Am J Hematol 1992;450:176–182.
203. Scott G, Hutto C, Makuch RW, et al. Survival in children with perinatally acquired human immunodeficiency virus type 1 infection. N Engl J Med 1989;321:1791–1796.
204. Cogo P, Laverda AM, Ades AE. European Collaborative Study: Neurologic signs in young children with human immunodeficiency virus infection. Pediatr Infect Dis J 1990;9:402–406.
205. Belman AL, Ultmann MH, Horoupian D, et al. Neurological complications in infants and children with acquired immune deficiency syndrome. Annals of Neurology 1985;18:560–566.
206. Porter SB, Sande MA. Toxoplasmosis of the central nervous system in the acquired immunodeficiency syndrome. N Engl J Med 1992; 327:1643–1648.
207. Isrealski DM, Remington JS. Toxoplasmic encephalitis in patients with AIDS. Infect Dis Clin North Am 1988;2:429–445.
208. Luft JB, Remington JS. Toxoplasmic encephalitis. J Infect Dis 1988; 157:1–6.
209. Mitchell CD. Toxoplasmosis.In: Pizzo PA, Wilfert CM, eds. Pediatric AIDS. The challenge of HIV infection in infants, children and adolescents 2nd Ed. Baltimore: Williams & Wilkins, 1994.419–455.
210. Mitchell CD, Erlich S, Mastrucci M, Hutto SC, Parks WP, Scott G. Congenital toxoplasmosis occurring in infants perinatally infected with human immunodeficiency virus 1. Pediatr Infect Dis J 1990;9:512–518.
211. Epstein LG, Dicarlo F, Joshi V, et al. Primary lymphomas of the central nervous system in children with acquired immunodeficiency syndrome. Pediatrics 1998;82: 355–363.
212. Brouwers P, Belman AL, Epstein LG. Central nervous system involvement: manifestations and evaluation. In: Pizzo PA, Wilfert CM, eds. Pediatric AIDS. The challenge of HIV infection in infants, children and adolescents. Baltimore: Williams & Wilkins, 1991:318–335.
213. Park Y, Belman AL, Dickson D, et al. Stroke in pediatric AIDS. Ann Neurol 1988;24:359.
214. Belman AL, Diamond G, Dickson D, et al. Pediatric acquired immunodeficiency syndrome: neurologic syndromes. Am J Dis Child 1988;149:29–35.
215. McKinney RE. The effect of human immunodeficiency virus (HIV) infection on the growth of children less than 24 months old. Pediatr Res 1992;31:170A.
216. McKinney RE, Robertson JW. Effect of human immunodeficiency virus infection on the growth of young children. J Pediatr 1993;123:579–582.
217. Rosh J, Peters V, Mugrditchian L, et al. Expression of malnutrition in pediatric AIDS. Pediatr Res 1993;33:108A.
218. Winter HS, Chang TL. Nutrition in children with HIV infection. Pediatric Forum 1993;1:1–5.
219. Bentler M, Stanish M. Nutrition support of the pediatric patient with AIDS. J Am Diet Assoc 1987;87:480–491.
220. Hommes M, Romijn JA, Godfried MH, et al. Increased resting energy expenditure in human immunodeficiency virus infected men. Metabolism 1990;39:1186–1190.
221. Kotler DP, Tierney AR, Brenner SK, Coulture S, Wang J, Poerson RN. Preservation of short term energy valance in clinically stable patients with AIDS. Am J Clin Nutr 1990;51:7–13.
222. Hommes MJ, Romijn JA, Endert E, Sauerwein HP. Resting energy expenditure and substrate oxidation in HIV infected asymptomatic men: HIV affects host metabolism in the early asymptomatic stage. Am J Clin Nutr 1991;54:311–315.
223. Nicholas SW, Leung J, Fennoy I. Guidelines for nutritional support of HIV infected children. J Pediatr 1991;119:s59–s62.
224. Task Force on Nutrition Support in AIDS: Guidelines for nutrition support in AIDS. Nutrition 1989;5:39–46.
225. Miller TL, Winter HS, Luginbuhl LM, Orav EJ, McIntosh K. Pancreatitis in pediatric human immunodeficiency virus infection. J Pediatr 1992;120:223–227.
226. Yarchoan R, Pluda JM, Thomas RV, et al. Long-term toxicity activity profile of 2′,3′-dideoxyinosine in AIDS or AIDS-related complex. Lancet 1990;336:526–529.
227. Zuger A, Wolf BZ, El-Sadr, Simberkoff MS, Rahal JJ. Pentamidine-associated fatal acute pancreatitis. JAMA 1986;256:2282–2385.
228. Mallory A, Kern F. Drug-induced pancreatitis: a critical review. Gastroenterology 1980;78:813–820.
229. Noel GJ. Host defense abnormalities associated with HIV infection. Pediatr Clin North Am 1991;38:37–43.
230. Krasinski K. Bacterial Infections. In: Pizzo PA, Wilfert CM, eds. Pediatric AIDS. The challenge of HIV infection in infants, children and adolescents 2nd Ed. Baltimore: Williams & Wilkins, 1994;241–253.
231. Smith PD, Ohura K, Masur H et al. Monocyte function in the acquired immune deficiency syndrome. J Clin Invest 1984;74:2121–2128.
232. Lin Ry, Wildfever O, Franklin MM et al. Hypocomplementemia and human immunodeficiency virus infection: Clinical correlation and relationships to circulating immune complex and immunoglobulin G levels. Int Arch Allergy Appl Immunol 1988;87:40–46.
233. Perkocha LA, Rodgers GM. Hematologic aspects of human immunodeficiency virus infection: laboratory and clinical considerations. Am J Hematol 1988;29:94–105.
234. Bernstien LJ, Krieger BZ, Novick B, Sicklick MJ, Rubinstein A. Bacterial infection in the acquired immunodeficiency syndrome of children. Pediatr Infect Dis J 1985;4:472–475.
235. Krasinski K, Borkowsky W, Bonk S, Lawrence R, Chandwani S. Bacterial infections in human immunodeficiency virus infected children. Pediatr Infect Dis J 1988;7:323–328.
236. Farley JJ, King JC, Nair P, Hines SE, Tressler RL, Vink PE. Invasive pneumococcal disease among infected and uninfected children of mothers with human immunodeficiency virus infection. J Pediatr 1994; 124:853–858.
237. Rolides E, Butler, Husson RN, et al. Pseudomonas infections in children with human immunodeficiency virus infection. Pediatr Infect Dis J 1992;11:547–553.
238. Pelton SI, Klein JO. Bacterial diseases in infants and children with infection due to HIV. In: Pizzo PA, Wilfert CM, eds. Pediatric AIDS. The challenge of HIV infection in infants, children and adolescents. Baltimore: Williams & Wilkins, 1991:199–208.
239. King JC, Lichenstein R, Farley JJ, Vink PE. Factors associated with pneumococcal bacteremia in outpatient febrile HIV-infected children. presented 1995 Interscience Conference on Antimicrobial Agents and Chemotherapy.
240. Sperber SJ, Schleupner CJ. Salmonellosis during infection with human immunodefiency virus. Rev Infect Dis 1987;9:925–934.
241. The National Institute of Child Health and Human Development Intravenous Immunoglobulin Study Group. Intravenous immune globulin for the prevention of bacterial infections in children with symptomatic human immunodeficiency virus infection. N Engl J med 1991;325:73–80.
242. Spector SA, Gelber RD, McGrath N et al. A controlled trial of intravenous immune globulin for the prevention of serious bacterial infections in children receiving zidovudine for advanced human immunodeficiency virus infection. N Engl J Med 1994;331:1181–1187.
243. Peters V, Diamant E, Hodes D. Efficacy of penicillin prophylaxis against invasive pneumococcal infections in HIV-infected children (Abstract 909). 32nd Interscience Conference on Antimicrobial Agents and Chemotherapy, Anaheim, Oct 1992.
244. Pizzo PA, Wilfert C. Antiretroviral Treatment for Children with HIV Infection. In: Pizzo PA, Wilfert CM, eds. Pediatric AIDS. The challenge of HIV infection in infants, children and adolescents 2nd Ed. Baltimore: Williams & Wilkins, 1994;651–687.
245. Brouwers P, Moss H, Wolters P, et al. Effect of continuous infusion zidovudine therapy on neuropsychologic functioning in children with symptomatic human immunodeficiency virus infection. J Pediatr 1990;117:980–985.
246. Italian Multicenter Trial. Long term follow-up of HIV infected children treated with zidovudine (AZT): Italian multicenter trial. International Conference on AIDS 1993. Abstract PO-B26-2057.
247. Dalakas MC, Illa I, Pezeshkpour GH, Laukaitis JP, Cohen B, Griffin JL. Mitochondrial myopathy caused by long-term zidovudine therapy. N Engl J Med 1990;322:1098–1105.
248. McKinney RE, Pizzo PA, Scott GB, et al. Safety and tolerance of intermittent intravenous and oral zidovudine therapy in human immunodeficiency virus infected pediatric patients. J Pediatr 1990;116:640–647.
249. Till M, MacDonell KB. Myopathy with human immunodeficiency virus type 1 infection: HIV-1 or zidovudine? Ann Intern Med 1990;113: 492–493.
250. Tudor-Williams G, StClair MH, McKinney RE, et al. HIV-1 sensitivity to zidovudine and clinical outcome in children. Lancet 1992;339: 15–19.
251. Wolters P, Brouwers P, Moss H, et al. The effect of dideoxyinosine on the cognitive functioning of children with HIV infection after 6 and 12 months of treatment. International Conference on AIDS 1991. Abstract W.B.2051.
252. Balis FM, Pizzo PA, Butler KM, et al. Clinical pharmacology of 2′,3′-dideoxyinosine in human immunodeficiency virus infected children. Jnl of Inf Dis 1992;165:99–104.

253. Butler KM, Venzon D, Henry N, et al. Pancreatitis in human immunodeficiency virus infected children receiving dideoxyinosine. Pediatrics 1993;91:747–751.
254. Dimitrov DH, Hollinger FB, Baker CJ, et al. Study of human immunodeficiency virus resistance to 2′,3′-dideoxyinosine and zidovudine in sequential isolates from pediatric patients on long term therapy. Jnl Infect Dis 1993;167:818–823.
255. St. Clair MH, Martin JL, Tudor-Williams G, et al. Resistance to ddI and sensitivity to AZT induced by a mutation in HIV-1 reverse transcriptase. Science 1991;253:1557–1559.
256. Husson, RN, Mueller BU, Farley M, et al. Zidovudine and didanosine combination therapy in children with human immunodeficiency virus infection. Pediatrics 1994;93:316–322.
257. Pizzo PA, Butler K, Balis F, et al. Dideoxycytidine alone and in an alternating schedule with zidovudine in children with symptomatic human immunodeficiency virus infection. J Pediatr 1990;117:799–808.
258. Levy JA. HIV pathogenesis and long-term survival. AIDS 1993;7:1401–1410.
259. Centers for Disease Control. Recommendations for prevention of HIV transmission in healthcare settings. MMWR 1988;361(Suppl 2):229.
260. Centers for Disease Control. Update universal precautions for prevention of transmission of human immunodeficiency virus hepatitis B virus and other blood borne pathogens in health care settings. JAMA 1988;260:462–465.
261. Kuhls TL. Occupational risks of HIV, HBV AND HSV-2 infections in health care personnel caring for AIDS patients. Am J Public Health 1987;77:1306–1310.
262. McCray E. Cooperative Needle Stick group. Occupational risk of the acquired immunodeficiency syndrome among health care workers. N Engl J Med 1986;314:1127.
263. Wachter RM, Luce JM, Hopewell PC. Critical care of patients with AIDS. JAMA 1992; 267:541–547.
264. Rosen MT, DePalo VA. Outcome of intensive care for patients with AIDS. Crit Care Clin of N America 1993;9:107–113.
265. Vernon D, Holzman, B, Lewis P, et al. Respiratory failure in children with acquired immunodeficiency syndrome and acquired immunodeficiency syndrome-related complex. Pediatrics 1988;82:223.
266. Bernstein LJ, Bye MR, Rubinstein A. Prognostic factors and life expectancy in children with acquired immunodeficiency and syndrome and *Pneumocystis carinii* pneumonia. Am J Dis Child 1989;143:775–778.
267. Notterman DA, Greenwald BM, DiMaio-Hunter A, et al. Outcome after assisted ventilation in children with acquired immunodeficiency syndrome. Crit Care Med 1990;18:18–20.
268. Abadco DL, Rao M, Kravath RE, et al. The role of assisted ventilation in survival after respiratory failure in children with AIDS. AJDC 1992;146:1052–1055.

Nosocomial Infections in the Pediatric Intensive Care Unit

30

William T. Merritt
Michael Green

INTRODUCTION

Nosocomial, or hospital-acquired, infections remain a significant problem in the delivery of pediatric intensive care. Virtually any infection acquired in the community can be transmitted within a pediatric intensive care unit (PICU). Because approximately half of all nosocomial infections are related to invasive procedures and devices, however, this chapter will focus on infections related to those procedures and devices used in the life support of seriously ill children[1,2].

Much work in this area has been performed in adult patients, and this information is worth reviewing. An increasing body of pediatric and PICU nosocomial infection data is developing as well. It is hoped that this chapter will help those caring for sick children approach nosocomial PICU infections from an intensive care specialist's point of view. Chapters 28, 29, 31 to 34 deal with other aspects of infectious diseases important to the pediatric intensive care specialist.

DEFINITIONS OF INFECTION

Variations in study design and definitions frustrate comparison of much nosocomial work. Because of this, it is useful to review some of the definitions currently used by the Centers for Disease Control (CDC) and the National Nosocomial Infection Study (NNIS)[2–6]. A more detailed description of the criteria for various categories of nosocomial infection is found in Appendix 1[6].

Colonization implies the presence of an organism on a mucosal surface, skin, or in tissue or body fluids without clinical evidence of adverse effects. **Inflammation** is a manifestation of injury to tissue or of unusual irritation from physical, chemical, or biologically active agents. The clinical characteristics of warmth, erythema, swelling, and some degree of pain as well as pathologic findings of accumulation of leukocytes, hyperemia, fibrin deposition, and exudation of tissue fluid serve to signify an inflammatory reaction. However, they do not allow a visual distinction between inflammation and infection.

Infection requires an organism's presence in a body fluid or tissue with local or systemic adverse effect. Microbiologic or clinical confirmation is necessary to diagnose infection. Serologic or biochemical evidence of infection is a useful indirect indicator of infection but generally is not sufficient by itself to confirm infection. Unless there is reason to suspect specimen contamination, organisms cultured from normally sterile areas (e.g., blood, cerebrospinal fluid, peritoneal cavity, etc.) should be considered as pathogens. In body areas with normal flora, and/or in areas developing a colonizing flora, such organisms should not generally be considered as pathogens on their "home ground," unless evidence of infection exists.

Epidemiologic investigation of infections in hospitals requires also that infections be categorized as **community-acquired** or **hospital-acquired** (nosocomial). **Nosocomial** infections are all infections that occur during a patient's hospitalization and not present or incubating on admission. In addition, any infection that is judged to have been acquired in the hospital but does not manifest until after discharge should be judged nosocomial. Nosocomial infections may be caused by organisms that originate from endogenous sources,such as one's own normal flora, or from exogenous sources, which are animate or inanimate objects in the hospital. Since a patient's flora is often altered in association with illness and hospitalization, this distinction is often not clear. **Surgically related** infections are those involving an operative wound or deep organs, tissues, or cavities exposed during an operative procedure. Infections arising in postoperative patients but not in tissues exposed or manipulated during surgery, for example, urinary tract infection (UTI) in a tracheostomy patient, are not considered surgically related, but are nosocomial.

Intensive care involves numerous invasive medical and surgical procedures, such as vascular access by percutaneous stick or cutdown, urinary catheterization, dialysis, lumbar puncture, or ventricular drainage. Infections occurring at the site of the procedure or associated with the procedure, for example, endocarditis following pulmonary artery catheterization or cardiac catheterization, should be recognized as such and reported.

The frequency of any specific problem must also be examined to appreciate the burden of any nosocomial infection. **Sporadic** infections occur infrequently and irregularly with no discernable pattern. **Endemic** infections occur with a measurable and fairly steady ongoing frequency, whereas **hyperendemic** refers to a gradual increase in the occurrence of disease. An **epidemic** or outbreak identifies a definite increase in the infection in question. A full review of hospital epidemiology is beyond the scope of this chapter; but, as mentioned previously, some of the definitions used by the CDC and the NNIS have been paraphrased directly in Appendix 1. Appendix 2 is a brief review of important bacteria classified by Gram's stain characteristics.

OVERVIEW OF NOSOCOMIAL INFECTIONS

In a point prevalence study in 1973, 15% of patients had an active nosocomial infection at a screening bedside examination[7]. Other researchers have noted that one or more nosocomial infections will develop in approximately 5% of adult medical and surgical patients[8]. As many as 1.2% of hospital-acquired infections will cause death, and another 3.5% will contribute to death[9]. Other early studies in adult medical and surgical ICUs noted bloodstream infection rates as high as 33 per 100 admissions, and pneumonia rates were 25 per 100 admissions[10,11]. Such high rates of infection compared to hospitalized patients in general have been explained by the clustering of patients who are at high risk of infection by virtue of the seriousness of their underlying diseases and the need for highly invasive procedures[12].

The NNIS began in 1970 to standardize the approach to hospital-acquired infections. An extensive manual of nosocomial infection definitions was formulated to assist ongoing surveillance by infection control personnel[3]. A representative NNIS report[13] deals with both large and small hospitals, as well as teaching and nonteaching hospitals. Infection rates, which are the number of hospital-acquired infections per 1000 patients discharged, have generally been highest in teaching hospitals. Surgical services have the highest rate, followed by medical, gynecologic, and obstetric services. Newborn and pediatric services generally have the lowest infections. The relative ranking of service rates is similar in nonteaching hospitals as well **(Table 30.1).** In adult patients, the urinary tract is the most frequent site of infection, followed by surgical wound infection, and lower respiratory tract infections[13]. However, in pediatric and newborn services, nosocomial lower respiratory infections are the most common, with bacteremia, UTI, cutaneous, and surgical wound infection in order of frequency[13]. *Staphylococcus aureus*, coagulase-negative staphylococci, *Escherichia coli*, *Pseudomonas aeruginosa*, *Klebsiella*, entero-

Table 30.1. Infection Rates (Cases per 1000 Discharges) by Hospital Category and Service for 1983[a,b]

Hospital Category	*SURG*	*MED*	*GYN*	*OB*	*NEW*	*PED*
Nonteaching	32.1	27.8	13.5	10.3	8.9	2.2
Small teaching	42.6	35.0	35.6	15.6	11.0	11.0
Large teaching	57.5	47.5	31.4	16.9	18.4	16.8
Total	44.3	37.1	27.4	14.7	13.4	11.1

[a]Adapted from Centers for Disease Control Nosocomial infection surveillance, 1983. In: Centers for Disease Control Surveillance Summaries, 1984;33(No. 2SS):9SS–21SS.
[b]Abbreviations: SURG = surgical; MED = medical; GYN = gynecologic; OB = obstetric; NEW = newborn; PED = pediatric.

Table 30.2. Five Most Common Pathogens Isolated and Percentage of Total Within Each Site and Service, 1983[a,b]

	Site							
	UTI		*SWI*		*LRI*		*BACT*	
Service	*Pathogen*	*%*	*Pathogen*	*%*	*Pathogen*	*%*	*Pathogen*	*%*
Medicine	*E. coli*	32.7	*S. aureus*	15.7	*P. aeruginosa*	14.7	*S. aureus*	14.7
	Enterococci	14.2	Enterococci	13.4	*S. aureus*	14.1	Coag-neg *Staph.*	13.9
	P. aeruginosa	11.1	*E. coli*	11.1	*Klebsiella* spp.	13.3	*E. coli*	10.7
	Klebsiella spp.	8.2	*P. aeruginosa*	10.8	*Enterobacter* spp.	9.2	*Klebsiella* spp.	10.6
	Proteus spp.	8.0	*Enterobacter* spp.	8.0	*E. coli*	7.5	*P. aeruginosa*	7.5
Surgery	*E. coli*	28.6	*S. aureus*	19.6	*P. aeruginosa*	15.6	Coag-neg *Staph.*	13.1
	P. aeruginosa	16.2	Enterococci	11.3	*Klebsiella* spp.	12.4	*S. aureus*	12.0
	Enterococci	14.4	*E. coli*	10.9	*Enterobacter* spp.	11.4	*Enterobacter* spp.	10.3
	Klebsiella spp.	7.3	*P. aeruginosa*	9.0	*S. aureus*	11.1	Enterococci	9.6
	Proteus spp.	7.1	Coag-neg *Staph.*	8.4	*E. coli*	6.9	*E. coli*	8.8
Pediatrics	*E. coli*	38.6	*S. aureus*	28.8	*Klebsiella* spp.	16.7	Coag-neg *Staph.*	18.0
	Candida spp.	16.9	Coag-neg *Staph.*	16.4	*P. aeruginosa*	13.0	*S. aureus*	12.4
	P. aeruginosa	10.8	*E. coli*	8.2	*S. aureus*	13.0	*Klebsiella* spp.	10.1
	Enterococci	8.4	*P. aeruginosa*	6.8	*Candida* spp.	7.4	*E. coli*	9.0
	Klebsiella spp.	8.4	Enterococci	6.8	*E. coli*	3.7	*Candida* spp.	6.7
			Klebsiella spp.	6.8				
Newborn	*E. coli*	25.5	*S. aureus*	30.4	*S. aureus*	21.1	Coag-neg *Staph.*	22.0
	Klebsiella spp.	15.7	Coag-neg *Staph.*	26.2	*P. aeruginosa*	16.7	Group B *Strep.*	19.6
	Enterococci	9.8	Enterococci	13.0	Coag-neg *Staph.*	12.3	Enterococci	8.9
	S. aureus	7.8	*Klebsiella* spp.	13.0	*Klebsiella* spp.	11.4	*S. aureus*	7.1
	Enterobacter spp.	5.9	*P. aeruginosa*	8.7	*E. coli*	7.0	*E. coli*	6.0

[a]Adapted from Centers for Disease Control. Nosocomial infection surveillance, 1983. In: Centers for Disease Control Surveillance Summaries. 1984;33(No. 2SS):9SS–21SS.
[b]Abbreviations: UTI = urinary tract infection; SWI = surgical wound infection; LRI = lower respiratory infection; BACT = bacteremia; Coag-neg *Staph.* = coagulase-negative *Staphylococcus;* Group B *Strep.* = Group B *Streptococcus.*

cocci, and *Candida* species vie as significant pathogens on pediatric and medical services and in the various sites examined **(Table 30.2)**[(13)]. Infections with secondary bacteremia are most common on pediatric, medical, newborn, and surgical services in teaching hospitals **(Tables 30.3 and 30.4)**. The NNIS also follows trends in antimicrobial resistance[(9,13)].

Although the risk of nosocomial infection is almost certainly a direct consequence of severity of illness and/or surgery, the level of invasive monitoring, the indiscriminate use of antibiotics, and the nature of diagnostic procedures[(9,14,15)] this has not been adequately studied[(16–18)]. It is generally acknowledged that infections in intensive care areas, including neonatal units, may be more widespread than those on general hospital wards[(15–24)].

The 1985 study by Brown and colleagues addressed PICU infections within the context of comparing different ICUs, such as medical/surgical, coronary, PICU, newborn, and cardiac surgery, in the same hospital. It also looked at community-acquired infection as part of the burden of infection in the ICU. In general, infection rates were highest in pediatric and medical/surgical ICUs. In keeping with the age-related acquisition of community-acquired infections, the PICU had nearly twice the medical/surgical unit's rate of community-acquired infection, but the medical/surgical unit had nearly double the pediatric unit's rate of ICU-acquired infections. The PICU had high rates of respiratory, genitourinary, and cerebrospinal fluid (CSF) infections, ranging from approximately 21 to 25% of ICU infections. Unfortunately, this PICU data does not examine the relative role of nosocomial infection within the categories of infection reported and is not medical device- or procedure-specific[(21)].

Since late 1986, the NNIS has monitored intensive care nosocomial infections in coronary care, medical, medical/surgical, surgical, and pediatric units. Two important points have arisen from these data. The first recognizes that the duration of care in an ICU is important in nosocomial infection, necessitating length-of-stay as one of the denominators in nosocomial infection rate calculations. The other is the importance of invasive devices, e.g., intravascular lines, endotracheal tubes, and urinary catheters, in the de-

Table 30.3. Percentage of Infections with Secondary Bacteremia (Excluding Primary Bacteremia), by Hospital Category and Service, 1983[a,b]

	SURG	*MED*	*GYN*	*OB*	*NEW*	*PED*	*All services*
Nonteaching	3.8	5.1	1.2	3.7	1.1	0.0	4.2
Small teaching	4.4	6.3	0.6	2.6	3.0	6.7	4.7
Large teaching	6.5	7.5	2.6	3.6	9.9	12.1	6.8
All hospitals	5.2	6.5	1.6	3.2	6.0	9.6	5.5

[a]Adapted from Centers for Disease Control. Nosocomial infection surveillance, 1983. In: Centers for Disease Control Surveillance Summaries 1984;33(No. 2SS):9SS–21SS.
[b]Abbreviations: SURG = surgical; MED = medical; GYN = gynecological; NEW = newborn; PED = pediatric.

Table 30.4. Ten Pathogens with the Highest Percentage of Associated Secondary Bacteremia, by Hospital Category, 1983[a]

	Nonteaching		*Small Teaching*		*Large Teaching*		*All Hospitals*	
Pathogen	*No. of Infections*	*Percentage with Secondary Bacteremia*	*No. of Infections*	*Percentage with Secondary Bacteremia*	*No. of Infections*	*Percentage with Secondary Bacteremia*	*No. of Infections*	*Percentage with Secondary Bacteremia*
Bacteroides spp.	24	16.7	65	13.8	53	17.0	142	15.5
Serratia spp.	123	9.8	115	10.4	241	13.7	479	11.9
S. aureus	648	7.7	828	8.6	1,274	16.0	2,750	11.8
Acinetobacter	26	0.0	27	0.0	94	18.1	147	11.6
Group B *Streptococcus*	57	7.0	87	8.0	100	16.0	244	11.1
Providencia spp.	14	7.1	13	7.7	19	15.8	46	10.9
Coagulase-negative *Staphylococcus*	212	4.2	356	6.5	550	9.5	1,118	7.5
Enterobacter spp.	285	5.3	321	4.2	601	9.7	1,207	7.4
Klebsiella spp.	366	4.4	404	4.2	718	9.7	1,488	6.9
P. aeruginosa	773	5.0	644	7.6	1,209	5.7	2,626	6.0

[a]Adapted from Centers for Disease Control. Nosocomial infection surveillance, 1983. In: Centers for Disease Control Surveillance Summaries 1984;33(No. 2SS):9SS–21SS.

velopment of nosocomial infection. In addition, rates of device usage affect comparison of device-related infection[25]. For example, the presence of central lines is strongly associated with the development of bloodstream infections (BSI), regardless of the type of ICU **(Table 30.5).** Endotracheal intubation with mechanical ventilation as well as urinary catheterization are associated with the development of ventilator-associated pneumonia and nosocomial UTI **(Table 30.6).** Significant differences exist among units regarding the incidence of these complications. Pediatric units have significantly higher rates of central line-associated BSIs and significantly lower rates of ventilator-associated pneumonia (VAP) and catheter-associated UTI **(Table 30.7).** Other researchers have noted that very young age and length of PICU stay more than one week are predictive of patients with increased risk of nosocomial infection[26].

The relative importance of different etiologic factors of nosocomial infections in PICUs has been studied. Although data organization and statistical methods vary in this group, it is clear that primary and catheter-associated bacteremia, lower respiratory tract, wound, urine, skin, and eye infections are extremely important[11,27,28].

Normal flora disappears rapidly once patients are hospitalized, especially for those in ICUs. A recent study in a pediatric respiratory intensive care unit found the mean number of days after admission to abnormal colonization as follows: gastric aspirate, 2 days; stool, 4 days; tracheal aspirate, 5 days; and urine, 10 days. The acquired organisms were often antibiotic resistant and were almost exclusively gram-negative bacilli and *Staphylococcus aureus*[29].

Table 30.5. Central Line Associated Bloodstream Infections[a]

ICU Type	*CL*	*NCL*
RESP	2.1[b]	1.1
NS	4.5	0.5
M/S	5.1	0
TRAUMA	5.8	2.0
SICU	5.8	0.5
MICU	6.9	0
CCU	7.0	0
PED	11.4	0.4
BURN	30.2	1.2

[a]Adapted from Jarvis WR, Edwards JR, Culver DH, et al. Nosocomial infection rates in adult and pediatric intensive care units in the United States. Am J Med 1991;91:185S–191S.
[b]Median number of BSIs/1000 central line days or noncentral line days; CL = central line; NCL = no central line; NS = neurosurgical; M/S = medical-surgical.

INTRAVASCULAR LINES AND NOSOCOMIAL INFECTION IN PICU PRACTICE

Intensive medical and surgical care includes the ubiquitous use of vascular access devices, such as intravenous scalp vein steel needles and polyethylene catheters, arterial pressure monitoring catheters, percutaneous central venous lines, and external dialysis shunts. Of all hospitalized patients, 30 to 50% receive such intervention, and virtually all ICU patients have at least one such line[66]. Central venous and arterial catheters cause more than 90% of all intravascular device-related septicemias[67]. A common denominator of all these items is passage through the skin, either directly, or through a cutdown incision.

Implanted medical devices become covered with biofilms that can harbor discrete bacterial microcolonies surrounded by dense secretions of their own exopolysaccharide slime. Within this barrier, these bacteria are potentially 500 times more resistent to antibiotics than bacteria in general body

Table 30.6. NI Rate Differences by Unit Type[a]

Unit Type	*CL-BSI*	*VAP*	*CA-UTI*
CCU/MICU	6.9[b]	12.8[c]	10.7[d]
M/S-SURG	5.3	17.6	7.6
PED	11.4	4.7	5.8

[a]Adapted from Jarvis WR, Edwards JR, Culver DH, et al. Nosocomial infection rates in adult and pediatric intensive care units in the United States. Am J Med 1991;91:185S–191S.
[b]Median number of BSIs/1000 CL days.
[c]Medial number of ventilator associated pneumonias (VAP) per 1000 ventilator days.
[d]Median number of catheter associated UTIs (CA-UTI) per 1000 catheter.

Table 30.7. PICU Nosocomial Infection Rates[a]

	Study Number				
Data Method	*1*	*2*	*3*	*4**	*5*
# NI/100 adm	13.7			25.2	14.6
BSI/100 adm	1.1	1.7			1.8
LRI/100 adm	2.9	1.0			1.5
UTI/100 atm	2.0	0.8			
VASC cath/100 adm		0.2			3.6
CNS/100 adm		0.2			
Wound/100 adm	1.4				2.2
Eye/100 adm					0.7
Chest tube/100 adm					0.7
% Primary bacteremia			38	8	
% LRI			15	9	
% Skin			8	5	
% Eye			8	6	
% UTI			7	6	
% Wound			7	28	
% Chest tube				15	
% VASC cath				19	

All data is for admissions longer than 72 hr. NI = nosocomial infection; BSI = blood stream infection; LRI = lower respiratory infections; UTI = urinary tract infections; VASC = central and arterial catheters; CNS = central nervous system, e.g., drain, bolts, etc.; % = percent of nosocomial infections reported.
1 = Donowitz I. Crit Care Med 1986;14:26–28.
2 = Merritt W. NI in the PICU. Chap 25. In: Rogers, MC, ed: Textbook of pediatric intensive care. Baltimore: Williams & Wilkins, 1987;755–785.
3 = Milliken J, et al. Crit Care Med 1988;16:233–237.
4 = Pollack E, et al. (cardiovascular surgery only) Crit Care Med 1990;18:378–384.*
5 = Pollack E, et al. Crit Care Med 1991;19:160–165.

fluids. Detection and eradication of such infection can be extremely difficult[(68)].

Ecology of the Skin

The skin has long been recognized as an ecosystem of its own with areas rich in warmth and moisture and capable of sustaining the growth of an array of microorganisms. Resident bacteria may inhabit the hair follicle-sebaceous gland complexes, sweat glands, and the upper layers of the stratum corneum. The densest growth of bacteria is in the groin and thigh areas, the umbilicus, the axilla, and the head and scalp[(69)]. Although not all investigators have been convinced that the deep structures of the skin harbor bacteria[(70)], most have demonstrated anaerobes and some aerobes on normal skin[(71)], with changing and more pathogenic flora in hospitalized patients, presumably secondary to proximity of other colonized patients, the use of antibiotics, and the high prevalence of suboptimal nutrition in seriously ill patients. Any transcutaneous line site can become locally colonized with these organisms and may demonstrate evidence of inflammation and, presumably, of infection. A fibrin sheath readily forms along the external walls of intravascular lines[(68,72)]. It is thought that this substance facilitates growth and migration of bacteria down the catheter and toward the bloodstream, providing a ready source of bacterial dissemination and the development of clinical infection. Intravascular devices may also become colonized or contaminated by the infusate being delivered to the patient[(73)] and by bacteria from other infected sites within the body, e.g., urine, lung, and surgical wound infections, even when no demonstrable bacteremia has taken place. Also, certain drugs and solutions given intravenously may produce inflammation indistinguishable from bacterial infection. Such agents include penicillin, nafcillin[(74)], cephalothin, tetracyclines, benzodiazepines, barbiturates, etomidate, and potassium chloride[(75)]. The remainder of this section discusses vascular access devices grouped as much as possible by type and site and by the problems encountered with infection.

Peripheral Venous Access

Scalp Vein Needles, Heparin Locks, and Pliable Catheters

Among the studies concerning intravenous and intra-arterial access devices are multiple study designs and culture protocols as well as definitions of contaminant, pathogen, nonpathogen, local infection, and catheter-related sepsis. Most of the early studies in this area dealt with both ward and ICU adult patients. More recently, similar studies have produced data for the pediatric patient.

Polyethylene catheters were introduced in the mid-1940s for intravenous infusions. Then, increasing evidence arose that suggested such devices were associated with infection. Early reports documented cases of severe catheter-associated sepsis and septic thrombophlebitis and warned against prolonged catheter placement and against use of the lower extremity[(76–80)]. In 1963, Druskin and Siegel[(81)], using polyethylene catheters inserted by both cutdown and percutaneously, showed a 30% incidence of phlebitis and a 41% incidence of contamination with nonpathogens. Moran et al.[(82)] studied venous cutdowns in adults whose wounds were applied with Neosporin ointment on insertion and daily until removal, in a double-blind manner. Unlike subsequent studies, however, the researchers found a significantly lower incidence of bacteriologically positive cultures of catheter sites and catheter tips in those insertion sites treated topically with Neosporin; infected cutdowns increased after 48 hours in both treated and untreated groups. A poor correlation was found between the presence of phlebitis and positive cultures, especially in patients without phlebitis but with positive cultures[(82)]. Smits and Freedman[(83)] found that approximately 9% of positive blood cultures could be traced to patients in whom no other source of infection than an intravenous catheter could be found. They were unable to associate any positive blood cultures with scalp vein needles[(83)]. In 1986, Collins et al.[(74)] performed a study in which the insertion, maintenance, and removal of catheters was not controlled. They found also that phlebitis was a poor indicator of actual infection, in which less than half of cultures from phlebitic patients were positive. One-third of all catheters were positive, with the risk of local infection with pathogenic organisms increasing with time. Two percent of the positive catheters were associated with sepsis and were a major contribution to death in one-half of these patients. They also noted an association of phlebitis with the infusion of penicillin and especially nafcillin[(74)]. In another study using Neosporin or placebo ointment for percutaneous catheters at insertion and every other day until removal, Zinner et al.[84] found a two-fold decrease in numbers of pathogens cultured from the antibiotic-treated catheters, but no significant difference in the overall rate of colonization. Notably, there was a suggestion that the antibiotic ointment-treated group favored colonization with *Candida* species. Increasing duration of insertion was associated with increasing positive cultures in both groups[84].

Norden[85] likewise found that phlebitis is a poor predictor of positive catheter tip cultures, because the double-blind application of Neosporin ointment did not significantly alter the recovery of pathogens from catheter tips, but rather lowered the recovery of nonpathogen contaminants. Likewise, the data also suggested the antibiotic ointment may favor the growth of *C. albicans*[83].

A prospective study in 1972 looked at the difference between pediatric infections with scalp vein needles and polyethylene catheters, in which all of the polyethylene catheters were placed by cutdown. The needles and the catheter tips were cultured at the time of discontinuation of the infusion. Eight percent of the patients with catheters developed catheter-associated bacteremia (positive catheter tip and subsequent peripheral blood culture). None of the patients with scalp vein needles was found to have bacteremia. The incidence of local infection was also higher in the catheter group, 24% versus 9%, with the catheter group having 10 times more pathogens. Their incidence of positive cultures of both contaminants and pathogens increased with time for both needles and catheters and suggested that catheters should be removed at 48 hours. They also showed that the number of positive needle tip cultures after 5 days in situ was similar to that for catheters of similar duration, suggesting that long-term steel needles are of potential for inducing septicemia[86].

Steel needles are relatively safe in terms of association with septicemia, but not without reports of severe thrombophlebitis and sepsis, especially in patients with some form of malignancy[87–90]. Until 1973, the rate of associated bacteremia was judged to be about 0.2% for steel needles and up to 9% for polyethylene catheters[83,89,90], a difference possibly related to the difficulty of maintaining steel needle intravenous lines for long periods[86], especially in children.

None of the previous studies really attempted to quantitate the various bacteria isolated from catheters and sites, forcing qualitative and subjective judgments to be made about the relative pathogenicity of organisms as contaminants or noncontaminants. A few studies served to turn the direction of infusion-related sepsis toward more quantitative inquiry. The first[91] study was published in 1973 and examined cultures, including skin prior to antiseptic, skin culture prior to catheter removal, and culture of needle tip or catheter on a blood agar plate before placement in a broth solution. Gentamicin or placebo cream was applied to each site on a daily basis until the device was removed. A small portion of the study included a standardized preparation of the skin, including the use of sterile gloves. The researchers deduced that a needle or catheter was the probable source of infection if both the blood agar and the broth cultures were positive with the same organism, and as the possible source of infection, or simply colonization of the intravenous line, if one but not both cultures was positive. They found that approximately 50% of the patients with probable infection also had phlebitis, but only 10% of possibly infected devices had phlebitis. They also found no overall statistically significant difference between placebo or gentamicin-treated groups relative to developing probable sources of infection, but it is interesting to note that in the sterile-technique group, no probable infections resulted in either the placebo or gentamicin ointment groups. The researchers found no probable infections associated with steel needles used in their study[91].

The study published by Maki et al. in 1977[92] placed quantitation of catheter-associated septicemia on much stronger grounds. They studied nonburned adult patients whose lines had been placed in a noncontrolled fashion and sought catheters in place for prolonged periods. Because of concern over the potential for contamination at the time of catheter removal, a technique was standardized. The site was wiped clean with an alcohol pledget, and sterile forceps were used to withdraw the catheter. Then the wound was milked for pus. For short catheters, the entire length, beginning several millimeters inside the former skin-surface-catheter interface, was sterilely removed and cultured. For longer lines, the 5- to 7-cm intercutaneous segment, as well as the distal 5 to 7 cm were both cultured. Cultured segments were first rolled on solid medium and then incubated in broth. Because local inflammation was more common in catheters whose solid medium cultures grew 15 or more colonies, this cutoff was chosen as a positive semiquantitative culture, signifying infection. The researchers found that 70% of the catheters yielded no growth at all. Another 20% showed growth only in broth or less than seven colonies on solid medium. None of these catheters was associated with septicemia, and only 18% had local inflammation at the time of removal. Of the remaining 10% with greater than 15 colonies on solid medium and matching broth cultures, 16% produced septicemia (all with semiquantitative culture counts of greater than 1000). Of this group with positive and semiquantitative cultures, 64% also had signs of local inflammation. The placement of catheters for more than 48 hours was strongly associated with signs of local inflammation. None of the patients in this study who had bacteremia from a focus distant from the intravenous device had positive semiquantitative solid medium cultures, and only four had positive broth cultures for the same organisms; however, the researchers cautioned that with time, the risk of these lines becoming heavily infected with the distant-focus organism is presumably considerable. They concluded that positive semiquantitative cultures denote local infection that will be associated with sepsis in approximately 15% of cases, and that those lines locally infected with traditionally more invasive *S. aureus*, *Candida*, and Gram-negative organisms have a much higher risk of septicemia of approximately 57%(89).

Since 1977, several more studies have furthered an understanding of catheter-associated infections. In patients with severely limited sites for catheter insertion, Wing et al.(93) suggested that quantitative blood cultures drawn through the catheter compared with peripherally drawn cultures may help implicate the catheter as the source of positive blood culture, reassuring those who must make the decision to remove that catheter(93). Cleri et al.(94) quantitatively cultured intravenous catheters in both adults and children. Although they did not standardize catheter insertion and did not include all catheters, removal of the catheter was standardized and 90% of the patients had simultaneous peripheral blood cultures from another site. They placed both the intradermal and intravascular segments in broth and then serially diluted the broth and plated the cultures on solid media, in addition to culturing the undiluted broth. The researchers defined intravascular insert-associated bacteremia as an isolated organism of the same species and sensitivity pattern from both the intravascular segment and simultaneous blood culture, and an infected intravascular insert as having 10^3 colony-forming units (CFU). This latter definition resulted from their finding that all inserts with an associated bacteremia grew 10^3 CFU. Using a scoring system for inflammation, they found that 77% of the patients with insert-associated bacteremia had little or no inflammation; however, among those patients with marked inflammation, 30% had insert-associated bacteremia. Approximately one-third of all the patients had positive nonquantitative catheter tip broth cultures, but of this group, one-half had intravascular inserts that grew 10^3 CFU, and 54% of this group developed bacteremias. The researchers also found that 75% of the intradermal segments were colonized with the same organism found in the intravascular segment, suggesting, but not proving, that the skin insertion site was the portal of entry of the organisms(94). Others believe that migration of bacteria from the hub of the catheter or stop-cock into the lumen of the catheter is the primary source for subsequent catheter sepsis(95). It has been shown that Gram's stain examination of catheter tips is a readily performed test and very sensitive and specific for catheter-associated infection(96). Arm boards, used to restrain arms for proper positioning of intravenous and arterial lines, have also been implicated in nosocomial infections. Several published reports of cutaneous *Aspergillus* infection of the hand and arm in immunocompromised patients have found an association with *Aspergillus* colonization of the nonsterile gauze used to wrap arm boards(97–99).

A study of small-gauge (85% smaller than 22 g) Teflon catheters in non-PICU pediatric patients (no antibiotic ointment and no heparin locks), demonstrated a modest rate of colonization (10.4%), with no suppurative phlebitis, cannula-related sepsis, or suspected sepsis(100). In sick neonates, catheter tips from peripheral venous catheters are nearly three times more likely to be colonized when left in place for more than 3 days compared with those in place for less than 3 days. However, the study did not mention antibiotic ointment used, transparent dressing employed, and how the skin site was prepared at time of catheter removal. The relative risk for catheter colonization was significantly greater in the lower extremities than in the scalp(101).

Arterial Catheterization

Intra-arterial monitoring of blood pressure is a mainstay of intensive care, providing instantaneous hemodynamic information as well as providing a pain-free portal for obtaining blood for various laboratory tests. It is an easily performed procedure in all age groups, but it is not without complications(102), chiefly occlusive/thrombotic(103–114), embolic(115–117), and infectious(118,119).

Early reports of infections complicating arterial lines included that of an Osler's node proximal to a radial arterial line(120). Blood cultures and catheter tip were positive for *Proteus mirabilis*. After removal and without antibiotics, the blood became sterile. No endocarditis was found(120). Gardner et al.(108) cultured arterial catheter tips at the time of removal and found 8 of 200 (4%) to have positive cultures. Two of these were with organisms also cultured elsewhere, but all were considered insignificant colonizations. However, 38 patients in the study who died did not have catheters cultured(108). Todres et al.(110) reported that 0 of 60 transcutaneous arterial lines in neonates became infected, and that 2 of 16 developed a localized infection at the insertion site when a cutdown became necessary for insertion, but that neither of these infections proved serious. Band and Maki(121) studied 130 arterial catheters in 95 patients ranging in age from 16 to 85 years. Fourteen percent of the catheters were placed by surgical cutdown. Most of the catheters were in the radial artery, but 10% were in a brachial artery, 12% in a femoral artery, and 6% were in a dorsalis pedis artery. Duration was from 1 to 14 days (mean = 4.4). Although 11% of all catheters developed local inflammation, 18% of the catheters had local infection (see their definitions), and 28% of this group became bacteremic. In decreasing order of frequency, the organisms most responsible were *C. albicans*, *Enterococcus*, *S. epidermidis*, *S. aureus*, and *K. pneumoniae*. Catheters placed by surgical cutdown had twice the incidence of local infection and a nine-fold increase in septicemia. Local inflammation was associated with a two-fold increase in risk of local infection and a 12-fold increase in incidence of septicemia. The researchers found that catheters in place for more than 4 days were significantly (2.5%) more likely to develop local infection. Overall, 4% of all their arterial catheters caused septicemia, and 12% of all bacteremias in the study patients originated from arterial lines. However, a more recent prospective study of arterial catheters in children placed without topical antibiotic ointments suggests that local inflammation is not predictive of catheter tip colonization and correlates poorly with the duration of catheterization[119].

Femoral arterial catheter placement is often unavoidable because of the lack of other available sites or the urgency and ease of placement in such a large vessel. Ersoz et al.[122] reported in 1970 on 63 femoral arterial lines. Mean duration was 3 days (range = 1 hour to 10 days). Ersoz et al. described no local inflammation, but of the catheters that were cultured on removal, both *Candida* and *Pseudomonas* species were isolated; these were presumably not associated with clinically important bacteremias. The Maryland Institute for Emergency Medical Services, a regional adult trauma center, reported no difference in the incidence of infectious complications between radial and femoral arterial lines[123]. Other reports in adults have also found no difference in infectious complications between radial and femoral arterial lines[124–126].

A recent study of 70 arterial lines in PICU patients suggests that infectious complications are fairly low. Catheters were placed with an iodine prep, without topical antibiotic, and covered with a sterile adhesive taping. The setup included a disposable transducer and a low-flow heparinized saline infusion (3 ml/hr). Sixty of the catheters were in the upper extremity and ten were in the foot; the mean duration of catheterization was only 59.1 + 5.8 hours. Eight catheter sites became inflamed and there were no positive catheter cultures or catheter-related septicemias. In this study with relatively short period of catheterization, neither duration of use nor inflammation at the site appeared to be related to significant infectious complications[127]. Femoral and axillary arterial cannulation are also important in PICU monitoring, especially when access must be obtained quickly. Infection risk appears to be relatively low (5%)[128–132].

Long intra-arterial catheters have been placed in the brachial artery for regional delivery of chemotherapeutic agents. One report noted nine cases of *S. aureus* septic endarteritis over a 3 1/2-year period associated with discontinuation of hexachlorophene for extremity scrubbing before cannulation. Their series suggests a distinct syndrome that facilitates implicating the catheter as a source of fever in the patient receiving intra-arterial chemotherapy: early local pain and hemorrhage, distal Osler's nodes, subsequent local inflammation, purulence, and signs of systemic sepsis[133].

Arterial lines have been incriminated in the development of bacteremias in other ways as well. Colonization of an ICU ice machine and subsequent contamination of arterial line stop-cocks by iced syringes was judged responsible for an outbreak of *Flavobacterium* bacteremias[134]. *Serratia* colonized a solution used to prime arterial pressure manometers, which were thought to be isolated from direct blood contact, and caused bacteremias[135]. Transducer chamber-dome fluid has been found to become contaminated and strongly associated with subsequent bacteremia[136–139]. Entirely disposable transducer-dome combinations have recently become available. With considerations of cost and reliability set aside[140], extended use to decrease expense should be of concern regarding infection. Luskin et al.[141] recently reported on the results of a prospective randomized study in which the disposable transducers on arterial lines and pulmonary artery (PA) catheters were changed at 2, 4, and 8 days. They found that the cumulative prevalence of contamination at day 8 was significantly higher than that at day 2. The only definite transducer-related bacteremia occurred in the 8-day group. The 4-day group was found not to differ significantly from the 2-day group, and these authors thought that single-patient disposable transducers could be used for up to 4 days safely[141].

Long-term, arterial/venous mechanical circulatory assist devices in adults are highly associated with infection. Rates from 24 to 70% have been reported. Because of this, as many as 20% of patients awaiting heart transplantation will be excluded because of infection[142–146].

Central Venous Access

Internal and External Jugular, Subclavian, Antecubital, Femoral; Pulmonary Artery (PA) Catheters

Central venous access is a necessary condition for monitoring of central venous pressure, central administration of various drugs and fluids, delivery of central alimentation, and the passage of a PA catheter. Lines are placed percutaneously or by surgical cutdown, and the sites of placement include the internal and external jugular veins, the subclavian (SC) veins, antecubital veins, and femoral veins. Complications of placement include injury to adjacent structures and organs, bleeding, migration of catheter tip to an unplanned site, embolization of thrombi or pieces of catheter, and infection[72,147–150]. Although there is overlap with studies of infections in peripheral intravenous devices, a small number of reports have specifically looked at infections related to central lines. Most of this work has concerned adult patient populations. As in the studies with peripheral lines, definitions of infection, pathogen, and methods vary widely.

Bernard et al.[151] in 1971 reported on the infectious complications of 98 SC catheterizations. In this prospective study, when SC lines were placed by inexperienced persons, the subsequent infection rate was greater than twice that of experienced personnel[151]. Mogensen et al.[152] reported on cultures of blood, skin around catheter site, catheter fluid, and catheter tip taken at the time of SC catheter removal. One group of patients had the catheter placed during an episode of known sepsis or focus of infection, and a second group was not known to be infected. Their data demonstrate that catheters inserted during an active infection may well become colonized with the same organism(s), in the absence of clinical or bacteriologic evidence of bacteremia, and may subsequently provide a source for continual seeding. No description is given of catheter insertion sites at the time of removal, but approximately the same percentage of catheter tips in both groups were colonized with organisms also present in the skin site culture, suggesting migration of organisms from skin to the catheter tip, or contamination upon removal. Duration of insertion was correlated with positive cultures(152).

Michel et al.(153) reported in 1979 on 390 SC catheter tips cultured on removal in 327 patients. In those patients with a remote site of infection, 19% developed positive cultures versus only 4% with no such focus. However, in the absence of proven bacteremia, the isolation of pathogens from a catheter tip was not statistically related to the presence of a remote-infected focus but was related to the presence of a tracheostomy. They noted a 45% incidence of catheter contamination in the presence of bacteremia, and a 34% incidence of contamination when a tracheostomy was present. This rose to 81% when both were present. Positive catheter cultures increased with the duration of catheter placement. Nine percent of their bacteremias were thought to be directly caused by an infected SC catheter. They proposed that the proximity of a tracheostomy might be a relative contraindication for a SC venous line(153).

Getzen and Pollak(154) in 1979 reported retrospectively on complications of central access in critically wounded combat victims during the Vietnam War from 1967 to 1970. The manner of their skin preparation is not given nor the criteria for diagnosing infection, but 1.1% of 1021 SC, 1.4% of 759 femoral venous lines, and 3.3% of 680 antecubital lines developed local infection during catheterization of less than 72 hours. The researchers stated that no catheter-related sepsis occurred in any patient in whom the catheter was removed within 72 hours(154).

SC vein catheterization in children is a reasonable alternative to surgical cutdown and has been used in a number of centers. Infectious complications are probably less than 5% and comparable to other central venous access sites(155–157), as are femoral venous lines(158).

Burn victims are at risk of developing numerous complications related to massive fluid losses and the loss of normal cutaneous and mucosal protective barriers to infection. Pruitt et al.(159) have reviewed the experience at the Brook Army Burn Unit with infectious complications of peripheral and central lines in burn patients. Between 1969 and 1978, 32% of catheterized jugular and other central veins developed suppurative thrombophlebitis, as did 42% of leg veins and 26% of upper limb veins. Manipulation of burns during therapy causes transient bacteremia(160), which may result in colonization of intravascular catheters. Bacteria may also migrate proximally from the wound surface to colonize catheters. Diagnosis is difficult. Infection may not manifest itself until several days after removal of the intravenous device, inflammation may be absent in 68%, and fever may be absent in 30%, but clinical evidence of sepsis and bacteremia is present in greater than 80%.

Suppurative thrombophlebitis is an extremely serious condition. Effective treatment is difficult and usually requires surgical excision of any infected vein and involved tributaries. A broad range of organisms, usually found to be flora in individual patients and cyclically in individual burn units, include *Enterobacteriaceae*, staphylococci, *Candida*, enterococci, and *Pseudomonas*(159,161). Suppurative thrombophlebitis has been reported in nonburn patients as well(162).

With the introduction of PA catheters during the mid-1970s, the acquisition of accurate bedside information regarding hemodynamic function was greatly facilitated, but not without added risks, including those of vascular access and bleeding, pneumothorax, emboli, pulmonary infarction, arrhythmia, thrombocytopenia, and infection(163–165). Predictably, infectious complications have become a major concern because of the frequent need for breaks in the line to measure function or to administer drugs, and the intracardiac/transvalvular position of placement. Applefeld et al.(166) reported on a group of adult surgical ICU patients in whom PA catheters were placed. Among the variables monitored were duration of insertion, number of repositionings, approximate number of pressure readings, and the number of daily cardiac outputs. Each patient had a daily blood culture drawn through the PA port of the catheter as well as from a peripheral vein. Among the subset of patients with an easily identifiable source of actual or potential infection (perforated viscus, multiple intra-abdominal abscesses, or infection of the urinary tract), 46% had positive blood culture drawn through the PA port at some point; 25% had positive PA cultures during the first 72 hours, but all catheters remaining longer than 72 hours had positive PA blood cultures. Within the group not having an easily identifiable source of infection, 9% developed positive PA blood cultures overall, with none of the catheter blood cultures positive if the catheter was removed in less than 72 hours, and 25% were positive if the catheter was left in place for more than 72 hours. In both groups, positive PA blood cultures were associated with longer duration of catheterization, increased number of repositionings, and more frequent insertions. Although associated peripheral blood cultures were negative, all PA catheter-cultured organisms were associated in both groups with organisms grown elsewhere, e.g., endotracheal tube, wound, urine, abscess, and surgical site. Although the PA catheter itself was not implicated as a source of bacteremia in this study, the incidence of colonization was extremely high and suggests a high potential as a nidus for subsequent infection or reinfection. Catheter tips and aspiration ports were not cultured(166).

In a report of complications of PA catheters in 81 patients(167), 92 PA catheter tips were cultured. No signs of local infection were noted. Of 32 (35%) positive catheter tip cultures, 24 (75%) were thought to be related to other sites of infection, 5 were colonized, and 3 were thought to represent probable catheter septicemia. As in most studies, no mention is made of cultures of other concurrent indwelling lines.

After using full surgical scrubbing, gowning, and draping for placement of all PA catheters by percutaneous means, Michel et al.(168) then cultured catheter tips at removal. Other cultures were performed only as indicated. Of 153 consecutive catheter tip cultures, 29 (19%) were positive. For those patients with a known infected focus before catheter insertion, there was a fourfold increase in incidence of positive tip cultures (35 versus 9%). However, no positive catheter cultures were thought to be the source of a bacteremic infection, and all were attributed to either colonization with organisms recognized elsewhere or to contamination.

Miller et al.[165] studied central lines placed with full surgical antisepsis through the SC route in adults. Triple-lumen catheters (TLCs), PA catheters, and central venous pressure lines were included[165]. TLC and central venous pressure lines were used for drugs and fluids or parenteral nutrition. At the time of removal, cultures were taken at the skin puncture site, from the contents of each lumen, and from the catheter tip, and paired with a peripheral blood culture. Catheter sepsis was defined as a clinical episode of systemic infection with isolation of an organism from both the peripheral blood culture and the culture from the catheter. Catheters were considered contaminated if the peripheral blood culture was negative or did not agree with the catheter culture, and there was no clinical or laboratory evidence of sepsis. Of all catheters, 7 to 10% were thought to have caused sepsis, but no deaths occurred from this complication. Thirty-three percent of the TLCs, 20% of the PA catheters, and 10% of the central venous pressure lines were found to be contaminated. There was no significant difference between contamination of the different ports of the TLCs, a strong correlation occurred between organisms cultured from the insertion site and those found to be contaminating catheters. Triple-lumen central venous catheters have been reported to have an associated bacteremia rate of 3.1%[169]. Another recent study looked for a relatively noninvasive method to implicate venous catheters as the site of colonization. Their study suggests that a negative skin culture (3×3 cm around catheter insertion point) can rule out catheter colonization[170]. If this data stands up prospective scrutiny, such simplified culturing would decrease costs in responding to fever in those patients with central catheterization who are not otherwise experiencing clinical evidence of sepsis.

In pediatric cardiac surgery patients, 11% have positive PA catheter tip cultures at the time of removal, whereas peripheral venous, central venous, and arterial catheter tip cultures were positive 0.9, 5.9, and 3.9%. This extensive study found that time in place, young age, and inotropic support were significant independent predictors of positive catheter tip colonization. There was no catheter-related septicemia or endocarditis in this study[171].

Any intravenous device that traverses the cardiac valves and chambers may damage the endocardium with the potential for the development of endocarditis. This is not surprising, since one of the animal models of the study of endocarditis involved damaging heart valves with a polyethylene intravenous catheter before the infusion of live staphylococci[172]. Autopsy reports of patients with recent PA catheters have described both septic and nonseptic endocardial vegetations[173–177]. A high incidence is found in burn patients[178]. In consecutive autopsies at the Yale-New Haven Hospital[179], 39% of the hearts had recent PA catheters inserted. Fifty-three percent of these hearts had one or more right-sided lesions and 7% had infective endocarditis. Only 3% of the noncatheterized hearts had any lesions, and none had infective endocarditis. This has been seen, as well, in neonates with umbilical catheters extending into the right atrium[180].

A study of the microbiologic risk of almost 2300 invasive hemodynamic monitoring devices demonstrated relatively low rates of positive catheter tip cultures—intravenous catheters, 1.1%; central venous catheters, 3.9%; arterial catheters, 1.5%; and PA catheters, 2.1%. None of these patients developed catheter-related septicemia or endocarditis. PA catheters, however, did have a significantly higher incidence of positive catheter tip cultures after 72 hr in place[181].

Long-term Central and Peripheral Venous Access

Uncuffed and Cuffed Lines for Central Alimentation, Chemotherapy and Antibiotics; Implantable Venous Access Devices

In a variety of serious medical and surgical illnesses, the general condition of the patient precludes sufficient oral nutrition for metabolic demands. Increasingly, early and aggressive peripheral and central intravenous alimentation is used to circumvent this problem.

In the late 1960s, total parenteral nutrition (TPN) became widely used, but within a few years it also became painfully obvious that infectious complications were frequent, ranging from 14 to 93%. With scrupulous attention to antiseptic catheter insertion methods as well as strict adherence to a protocol that prohibits piggyback infusions and stop-cocks in TPN lines, avoidance of blood drawing through TPN catheters, and limitation of catheter care and manipulation to a team member specifically employed for TPN catheter care, TPN-related infection (and also costs) could be dramatically reduced to well below 10%, with some centers reporting a maximum rate of septicemia of 1 to 2%[182–186].

More than 50% of TPN-associated infections are caused by Gram-positive organisms, with *S. epidermidis* and *S. aureus* most frequently isolated. Approximately 30% of TPN infections are caused by fungi, with *C. albicans, Candida* species, and *Torulopsis* primarily responsible. Gram-negatives are important as well and represent about 20% of TPN-associated infections. Anaerobes are seen in about 2%.

Growth of representative organisms has been studied in parenteral nutrition fluids, and this information demonstrates ready growth of *Candida* species in amino acid-dextrose solutions, casein and fibrin hydrolysates, and lipid emulsions. *S. aureus* and many Gram-negative organisms grow well in casein hydrolysate-dextrose and lipid emulsions but proliferate less well in amino acid-dextrose solutions. *P. aeruginosa* grows poorly in casein hydrolysate-dextrose and amino acid-dextrose solutions but grows well in 5% dextrose solutions. *Enterobacter cloacae* grows well in 5% dextrose, but does poorly in fibrin hydrolysate and some crystalline amino acid solutions, and it is eventually killed by casein hydrolysates and by 50% dextrose[(66,182)]. Gram-negative bacteremias and polymicrobial bacteremias in both neonates and older pediatric patients have been associated with lipid emulsions extrinsically colonized by improper handling of multiple-dose containers, both in the ICU setting and in the pharmacy[(187,188)]. Candidemia is also associated with parenteral nutrition[(189–192)], and two reports indicated a 10 to 22% incidence of *Candida* endophthalmitis in patients so infected[(193–193a)]. *S. epidermidis,* as well, has become increasingly important as a pathogen associated with parenteral nutrition[(194,195)].

Because of the considerable literature concerning the potential for central lines to become contaminated during the course of bacteremias and, thus, to serve as a nidus for sustained seeding, conventional wisdom has dictated that all lines should be removed in the setting of documented positive blood cultures. However, catheters changed over a wire (Seldinger technique) may carry no greater risk of sustained infection than those replaced at a new site[(196)]. More recently, 65 to 78% of patients with central vein catheters with documented catheter-related sepsis, which were not removed, were cured by a regimen of antibiotics delivered through the catheter[(197,198)]. Fibrin sleeve formation around central catheters has long been thought to be important in bacterial attachment and nutrition and subsequent established infection[(199)]. It has been suggested that heparin might alter the bonding of this sleeve to the catheter and decrease the incidence of infection. Several studies have shown decreased phlebitis and improved patency of catheters through which heparin was given, as well as fewer positive catheter tip cultures[(200–202)].

The Broviac catheter introduced in 1973[(203)] and the slightly larger bore Hickman catheter introduced in 1979[(204)] are made of silicone rubber and are designed for subcutaneous tunneling before vein entry. The Broviac catheter has one Dacron cuff for the tunnel, and the Hickman catheter has two similar cuffs; one is near the venous entrance site and one near the skin exit site. In theory, these cuffs serve as anchors to prevent displacement and as barriers to infection. Patients with gastrointestinal illnesses that prevent adequate oral intake as well as oncology patients needing prolonged therapy and nutrition have been the principal recipients. In spite of placement by major cutdown procedures, infection rates are low, especially in the nononcology group. Older reviews of bacteremias in neutropenic patients with peripheral venous catheters found a high incidence of Gram-negative infections, as well as Gram-positive and fungal sepsis[(205–207)]. A more recent review of infections associated with Broviac catheters suggests that Gram-positive organisms may be more common than Gram-negative infections or fungemias in patients with similar catheters[(208)]. Shapiro et al.[(209)] addressed the problem of whether Broviac catheters need always be removed from febrile pediatric oncology patients in whom line sites are scarce and placement may require general anesthesia. Although all of the blood cultures drawn through the catheter were positive, they were able to cure 91% of their infections by administering appropriate antibiotics through the catheter without removing it[(209)]. Johnson et al.[(210)] have reviewed their experience with 70 Broviac catheters in 64 pediatric oncology patients. They noted a crude infection rate of 2.8 infections (sepsis, exit site infection, or both) per 1000 catheter-days and a catheter-related sepsis rate of 1.9/1000 catheter-days. The youngest group, less than 4 years old, had the highest infection rate. Overall, 70% of infections were cured without removal of the catheter, including 83% of those with catheter-related sepsis. Infection-free periods after cure were found to be shorter by one-half when catheters were left in place than when new catheters were inserted. As in other studies, coagulase-negative staphylococci were the most common cause of catheter-related sepsis, and Gram-positive cocci accounted for nearly 50% of all infections. Thirty percent of infections were polymicrobial[(210)]. Trooskin et al.[(211)] recently showed experimentally that central catheters pretreated with tridodecylmethylammonium chloride and an anionic antibiotic (penicillin or cephalosporin) had significantly less colonization at removal than did controls[(211)], but the significance of this sort of information remains to be determined.

Predictors of line-associated sepsis have been difficult to determine[(209)] probably because of differences in the care and maintenance of central sites from the time of insertion to the time of removal, differing culture protocols, and variations in the background use of intravenous and topical antibiotics. A more recent study of uncuffed catheters used for hyperalimentation suggests several points. Skin site erythema ≤4 mm, fever, and positive skin site culture (semiquantitative; greater than 50 colonies) were predictors of line associated infection. However, more than 50 colonies of an organism other than coagulase-negative staphylococci were better predictors than similar counts of coagulase-negative staphylococci. Quantitative cultures drawn through the line compared with simultaneous peripheral venous cultures were not generally considered helpful because of pulmonary filtering of bacteria. However, a ratio of *more than* 10 : 1 catheter to peripheral quantitative growth may be useful.[(212)].

Totally implanted vascular access (central venous) devices have been used to treat a number of conditions. The subcutaneous reservoir provides a simple site for repeated administrations of antibiotics and chemotherapeutic agents, with infection rates similar to Hickman and Broviac catheters; more than half of these infections can be treated with antibiotics through the reservoir[(213–216)]. Others are using long-term peripheral venous access systems. Resevoirs are implanted in the arm, with catheters placed radiographically into the superior vena cava. Costs appear to be greatly reduced over more formal surgical implantation, with a low infection rate[(217,218)].

Whether a central line becomes colonized through contamination at the hub (i.e., contamination proximal to the catheter), through migration of skin organisms along the outside of the catheter, or via seeding from distant sites of infection, decisions regarding removal/replacement can be extremely difficult. Pieces of a catheter can only be cultured or examined microscopically after the catheter has been removed; therefore, other criteria must be used when it is desirable to leave the catheter in place, e.g., long-term use in patients with poor venous access. Many catheter-related bacteremias can be cured with antibiotics delivered through the offending catheter. Fungemias, however, often require catheter removal for cure[(219)]. Clinical indicators (e.g., fever, erythema at catheter site) and microbiologic criteria (e.g., ratio of colony counts through the catheter relative to peripheral cultures) are evolving and should continue to improve[(198,212,220,221)].

Infections Associated with Indwelling Percutaneous Access for Hemodialysis and Extracorporeal Membrane Oxygenation

In any PICU, a small number of children will require short-term hemodialysis while awaiting resolution of acute renal failure, if that is going to occur. Some patients will have intermittent cannulation of the appropriate vessels. Others will have an externalized shunt device surgically implanted for intermittent hemodialysis[(222–224)]. Some will have a single-lumen catheter placed for intermittent dialysis[(225)]. Only those patients requiring long-term dialysis will have native arteriovenous (A-V) fistulas or prosthetic A-V fistulas created for that purpose.

Infectious complications of hemodialysis are well described. Bacteremia from contamination of the dialysis coil[(226,227)], dialysate fluid[(228–231)], and dialyzer gaskets[(232)] have been reported. Endotoxin, present in either sterile[(233)] or nonsterile dialysis fluid (when the bacterial count of dialysis fluid is less than 10^4, the patient is usually unaffected)[(234–236)] has also been noted. However, localized infections of the shunt itself are the most common sources of bacterial infection and may lead to bacteremia, septic emboli from dislodged clots, and bacterial endocarditis. Asymptomatic *Pseudomonas* bacteremia has been noted as well in patients on dialysis[(237)]. Bacteremia from distant foci may also seed an A-V shunt, with subsequent infection of the shunt and infectious complications as already mentioned. However, at least 50% of bacteremias in patients with a vascular dialysis access device may be secondary to that device[(238)]. Since percutaneous dialysis shunts are usually placed in acutely ill patients, it is useful to review briefly the associated infectious complications. Most of the published reports deal with adult populations.

Current terminology of vascular access for hemodialysis favors external shunt to mean any prosthetic shunt that is externalized, internal shunt to mean any prosthetic A-V communication that is not external to the skin, and internal fistula to mean any direct connection of the arterial to venous system, without any prosthetic graft[(222)]. Any review of infections associated with such devices is hampered somewhat by older terminology, leading to uncertainty as to the type of A-V connection in many of the earlier reports. Often, these reports are anecdotal as well.

A five-hospital review in 1972 of external shunt infections found that one-third to two-thirds of such shunts became infected with an average attack rate of 3.5 infected shunts per 100 patient months[(239)]. Similar rates have been reported in children[(240)]. Others have reported much higher rates of shunt infection[(239,241)].

Numerous investigators have noted external shunt infections to be caused by *S. aureus* 50 to 90% of the time, with *Pseudomonas, Enterobacteriaceae,* and other Gram-positive organisms (such as enterococci and *S. epidermidis*) responsible for most of the remaining infections[(222,223,239–250)]. *Listeria monocytogenes* (a Gram-positive rod) infections have also been reported[(251)]. Bacteremias associated with these infections have a high mortality of approximately 20%[(222)] and are associated with metastatic infection, including endocarditis, persistent bacteremia, empyema, meningitis, and septic pulmonary emboli[(252–258)]. Most patients are infected with their own endogenous colonizing bacteria. It is well known that patients receiving long-term hemodialysis (as well as the dialysis staff) have a high rate of *S. aureus* carriage, which contributes to the high incidence of staphylococcal infection[(241,253,255,256)]. The Hemasite needleless vascular access device has a titanium exit port for dialysis hookup. As might be expected, this device also has a high rate of infection. As was noted in a recent study by Reed et al.[(257)], 60% of these grafts required removal for infection.

Localizing signs are common with infected external shunts and include tenderness or pain, purulent drainage, or signs of skin breakdown. Such infections at the vascular access site suggest poor graft survival. Since the entire graft is often involved, early removal is important. When bacteremia is noted in a patient with no localizing signs of external shunt infection, aggressive antibiotic therapy adjusted for the degree of renal function may allow resolution of the infection without graft removal. Internal fistulas become infected much less frequently, but the organisms involved are generally the same. However, localizing signs are much less common[(240)]. Appropriate therapy will ultimately be guided by results of blood and purulent drainage cultures. A Gram's stain of any drainage may demonstrate the class of organism, whether Gram-positive or Gram-negative cocci or bacilli, and narrow the spectrum of coverage[(258)]. Initial coverage for *Staphylococcus* and possibly Gram-negative rods, including *Pseudomonas,* is warranted.

Extracorporeal circulation—for example, extracorporeal membrane oxygenation-ECMO; total extracorporeal lung assist-ECLA—either to assist ventilation in the setting of pulmonary insufficiency or to assist a failing ventricle, has become increasingly common in specialized PICU settings. Indications have included congenital diaphragmatic hernia, meconium aspiration syndrome, persistent pulmonary hypertension, adult respiratory distress syndrome, and severe pulmonary infections. In spite of the inherently invasive nature of this technology, few reports of infectious complications have arisen. A recent review states that 5% of 3876 patients had an infectious complication, but does not elaborate[(259)]. This may be related to the scrupulously fastidious protocols for line care, percutaneous sites, and breaks for drawing blood. Nevertheless, as experience is gained and problematic neurologic and thrombotic complications decrease, infectious complications may become more obvious; presumably they will resemble those infections associated with both central venous and arterial catheterization[(260–263)].

NOSOCOMIAL ILLNESS ASSOCIATED WITH THE RESPIRATORY TRACT

Colonizing Flora

From the time of birth, the infant acquires a set of indigenous bacteria in the upper respiratory system, skin, and gastrointestinal tract. In the first few months of life, aerobic species tend to dominate the normal upper respiratory flora[(30,31)], with increasing numbers of anaerobic and facultative anaerobes over the first year of life, especially after the eruption of the first teeth. By 12 months of age, the normal infant's mouth may be host to various streptococci, staphylococci, *Neisseria* and *Candida* species, as well as anaerobic streptococci, *Actinomyces, Fusobacteria,* and *Bacteroides* species[(32)]. The dorsal surface of the tongue, the gingival sulcus, and dental plaque are the main areas of growth for these organisms. Within these areas, the bacteria count may range from 10^7 to 10^8 organisms/cm^3[(30–33)].

The maintenance of normal upper respiratory flora is a dynamic process[(34,35)]. At various times, the healthy person will harbor different organisms and/or relative percentages of organisms. The pathogenicity of these colonizing organisms can also vary, with the majority of healthy people harboring relatively harmless bacteria. It is also known that some members of the normal upper respiratory flora may inhibit the growth of more pathogenic bacteria. As many as 18% of normal adults seem to harbor small numbers of Gram-negative bacillary organisms from time to time[(36–40)]. Such colonization and subsequent illness has been shown in newborns[(41,42)] and in infants[(43)], as well as in adults[(44,45)]. Asymptomatic carrier states for organisms such as staphylococci, pathogenic streptococci, and *Haemophilus influenzae* are well described.

Illness, hospitalization, and the use of antibiotics also have profound influence on indigenous flora, and extensive literature documents attendant changes in general flora, as well as upper respiratory colonization[(42–44,46–53)]. These studies and others document marked swings in microflora that can occur with initiation, changes, and discontinuation of antibiotics. It is generally accepted that the broader the spectrum of antibiotics used, the greater will be the concurrent perturbation of flora, with a tendency toward colonization by more pathogenic and antibiotic-resistant organisms.

In addition to the previously mentioned influences on upper respiratory flora, other important factors may alter flora and provide for nosocomial respiratory infection. The bacterial colonization of the patient environment, which includes room, sinks, air, infant bath sponges, phlebotomy tourniquets, spirometer tubing and mouthpieces, food, and operating room, has been extensively reviewed[(54)], but unfortunately, except for a few clear examples[(55–63)], most concerns about the hospital environment are conjectural. The hands of hospital personnel[(41,60)], other nearby patients, and patient equipment may also serve as cross-colonizing reservoirs for the patient. If organisms of sufficient pathogenicity are acquired, a nosocomial infection may result. Unfortunately, strict handwashing among hospital personnel are not universally practiced[(64)].

A recent opportunity to examine flora of inanimate objects in an old hospital and in a new hospital before and after the transfer of patients suggests little overall effect of a different physical plant on the resultant nosocomial infections[(65)].

Infections Complicating Endotracheal and Gastrointestinal Instrumentation

Bacteremia

Bacteremia has been reported in association with nasotracheal intubation[(264,265)], dental manipulation[(266)], nasal suctioning[(267)], and fiberoptic bronchoscopy[(268)]. This should be kept in mind when evaluating patients who develop fever or signs of infection shortly after such procedures or who require prophylaxis for endocarditis. The bacteremia reflects the organisms colonizing the airway, which may include Gram-negative bacteria as well as normal upper respiratory flora in hospitalized patients.

Sinusitis, Mastoiditis, Otitis Media, and Ocular Infections

The infant is not born with a complete set of paranasal sinuses. Although the maxillary and ethmoid sinuses are recognizable during midgestation and demonstrable radiographically in infancy, the frontal sinuses are recognized histologically during the latter half of the first year of life and radiographically between the third and sixth year of life. The sphenoid sinuses do not appear until approximately the third year of life and are radiographically evident by approximately the ninth year of life.

Endotracheal tubes, if passed through the nares, and nasogastric tubes come in contact with the turbinates and may alter the normal drainage of the maxillary and ethmoid sinuses by either direct trauma or by causing irritation and edema of these tissues. In addition, the presence of a nasal tube may delay pneumatization of the sinuses and the mastoid air cells during infancy. This can facilitate the development of otitis media, sinusitis, and mastoiditis, even in infancy. Diagnosis may be difficult because of poor representation on X-ray examination; obtaining purulent material by aspiration or surgical drainage is necessary. Eustachian tube dysfunction probably precedes the otitis media and mastoiditis. It is not surprising that several reports have noted maxillary and/or ethmoid sinusitis, otitis media, and mastoiditis to be a problem after nasal instrumentation in adults[269–272] as well as infants and children[273,274].

Acute sinusitis in otherwise normal adults is primarily a disease caused by *Streptococcus pneumoniae, H. influenzae,* and anaerobes[275,276]. In children less than 10 years of age, *Streptococcus* and *Branhamella catarrhalis* have been the primary cause of acute maxillary sinusitis[277]. However, hospitalized patients with nasal endotracheal tubes or nasogastric tubes are at risk of developing a maxillary or ethmoid sinusitis, which is caused chiefly by a variety of Gram-negative organisms originating in their upper respiratory tract. These include *P. aeruginosa, Klebsiella, Proteus, E. coli, Enterobacter,* and *Serratia.* Multiple organisms are not uncommon[268–272].

Although sinusitis following nasotracheal intubation may affect 2% of adult patients, it often does not produce symptoms for 1 to 2 weeks. The diagnosis of these infections is often hampered by an unconscious or sedated patient who is unable to communicate well because of the endotracheal tube. Fewer than one-third of the patients may have a purulent nasal discharge[272]. Fever, without an obvious source in a patient with a current or recent nasal tube, should raise the question of sinusitis. Occasionally, erythema or facial pain over the involved sinus may also be noted. Because the bacteriologic etiology is so varied, antimicrobial therapy should be based first on the Gram's stain and, subsequently, on culture results from material aspirated directly from the involved sinus prior to therapy. It has been clearly shown in acute sinusitis that culture of the nose or throat will often not yield organisms responsible for the sinusitis[275,277], and this is also true for nosocomial sinusitis[272]. Removal of the nasal tube and replacement with a tracheostomy or gastrostomy may accelerate the resolution of the infection[274] or be sufficient to resolve the infection in some cases[272].

Severe ocular infections, often caused by *P. aeruginosa,* have occurred in patients receiving respiratory support. These usually begin as a corneal ulcer, but may progress to hypopyon, corneal destruction, and perforation within 48 hours. This condition may be secondary to bacteremic seeding of the eye, but is more likely the result of respiratory secretions dripping into the eyes during suctioning or other procedures[278].

Nosocomial Illness Transmitted by the Respiratory Route

When a patient is admitted to the ward or to the ICU with a respiratory illness or with an infection transmitted by respiratory shedding, there is ample evidence for nosocomial spread of the organisms[279–290]. Patients with measles[284], chickenpox[286,287], influenza[288–292], respiratory syncytial virus[288,292–296], parainfluenza virus[288,292,297], rhinovirus[288,292,298], meningococcal pneumonia[299], pulmonary tuberculosis[300], pertussis[301], diphtheria[302], *Pneumocystis carinii*;[303–307], and others are capable of disseminating their organisms either by aerosol droplet or by hand-carried secretions to others, including patients and staff[288,297,298]. For example, as many as 40% of hospital-contact infants may acquire respiratory syncytial virus infection during a community outbreak[288,296]. Infants with congenital heart disease, especially those with an element of pulmonary hypertension, have a much greater likelihood of developing severe illness with a high mortality[298]. Pertussis in symptomatic children may be acquired by partially immune or nonimmune hospital staff and passed on to other infants[285]. Nosocomial *P. carinii* pneumonia outbreaks in immunoincompetent patients may be associated with respiratory spread from other infected patients or from patients not known to be immunoincompetent but who are asymptomatic carriers[303–306]. Several outbreaks of nosocomial legionellosis have occurred in sick patients. The source may be from inhalation of organisms from environmental contamination rather than from other patients[306,307]. It should also be remembered that patients with severe viral respiratory disease are predisposed to severe staphylococcal pneumonia, especially infants less than 12 months of age[308]. Such infections, if acquired on the ward or in the ICU, will predictably complicate the course of the ICU patient.

Pneumonia

Pulmonary infections consistently rank high on lists of nosocomial infection **(see Table 30–7).** It is approximately the third most common site of hospital acquired infection, roughly 15% of all nosocomial infections arise in the lungs.

Pneumonia in the nonintubated ICU patient may reflect the primary disease process or one that has been acquired in the hospital setting. Sick, obtunded patients handle oral secretions poorly because gag and cough reflexes are not optimal. This may lead to aspiration of oral secretions (and, if present, gastric/intestinal secretions as well) and to subsequent pneumonia. The organisms are usually hospital-acquired, Gram-negative, and often drug-resistant. In more debilitated or hospitalized patients, alterations in secretory immunoglobulins and bacterial adherence to epithelial cells seem to favor such colonization[38–40,44]. Also, for children the predominate cause of nosocomial pneumonia is gram negative bacilli. Fecal/oral spread probably accounts for Enterobacteriaciae getting into the airway, but environmental or caregiver contamination accounts for other organisms, such as Pseudomonas, which is not a normal GI colonizer. Nosocomial pneumonia is a serious complication, with mortality of 20 to 50%, accounting for 15% of deaths in all hospitalized patients[309].

The bacterial cause of nosocomial pneumonia is often difficult to determine, especially in small children. But the process is aided by blood cultures, and cultures and Gram's stains of secretions obtained by tracheal suctioning (high contamination), bronchoscopy, and catheters passed through endotracheal tubes[310,311].

Tracheal intubation, however, alters airway clearance mechanisms in several ways. Endotracheal tubes are passed through the nares[311–314] or oropharynx[315–317], with the potential for carrying infectious secretions into the trachea. Because they prevent glottic closure, there is also the potential for seepage of oral secretions into the trachea, even around cuffed endotracheal tubes. Indeed, it has been shown that organisms often appear in the stomach[318] or in the hypopharynx[319] just before colonizing the trachea. Some have even advocated that patients on mechanical ventilation undergo topical oropharyngeal decontamination to prevent this progression of colonization[320]. The tracheal tube cuff itself may damage the tracheal mucosa, predisposing it to infection. When cuffed tubes are used, infection is more common with high-volume, low-pressure cuffs[321–324]. Because the tube prevents expectoration, bronchial secretions may accumulate and inspissate, and the patient becomes dependent on exogenous suctioning of secretions for their removal.

Contaminated suctioning equipment has been shown to lead to respiratory infection[325,326]. In addition, since intubated patients are usually receiving respiratory support as well, they are at risk from contamination in the respiratory equipment. Awareness of the potential for equipment contamination should be an ongoing concern in all ICUs, and institution guidelines should be thoughtfully established and rigorously followed. Respiratory illness and/or colonization has been described in association with contaminated resuscitation bags[327], oxygen analyzers[328], spirometer mouthpieces and tubing[63], nebulizers[329–334], the placement of contaminated medications into nebulizers[332–336], and the readily changeable parts of ventilators[337,338]. Gas exhaust from ventilators[339] or from intermittent positive pressure breathing machines[340] used on infected patients may be contaminated with the organisms from those patients. Small Venturi medication nebulizers seem to have little risk of contaminating patients as long as the medication is sterile. Also, ventilators with humidifying cascades rather than nebulizers seem to have little role in contaminating patients if tubing changes occur every 48 hours[59,341], since these cascades generate no aerosol. however, the tubing does become colonized with the patient's own organisms. Indeed, a recent study suggests that ventilator tubing changes as infrequent as every 7 days not only result in significant cost savings but also result in no significant increase in ventilator associated pneumonia[342]. Nebulizers may also become contaminated with a patient's own organisms and subsequently lead to bacterial aerosols and pneumonia. Frequent (i.e., every treatment) cleaning decreases this risk[341]. Awareness of the potential for equipment contamination should be an ongoing concern in all ICUs.

Patients are at risk of contamination from pathogens colonizing hospital personnel as well. In one survey, more than 20% of hospital personnel had antibiotic-resistant *E. coli* and *Klebsiella* on their hands[343]. In an intensive care nursery, approximately 50% of hands were positive for aerobic Gram-negative bacilli after povidone-iodine hand washing, and more than 80% were positive after hexachlorophene washing. This study also showed that organisms may actively multiply on the hands of personnel[344]. In a surgical ICU, hexachlorophene hand washing did not prevent colonization of approximately 70% of nurses' hands with Gram-negative bacilli[345]. In another report, 17% of the staff of an ICU had strains of *Klebsiella* contaminating their hands. Minimal contact with the patient's skin was shown to be capable of transmitting this organism. Chlorhexidine hand washing can greatly reduce the problem[346,347]. Even hand cream used by nursing personnel has been implicated in an outbreak of sepsis caused by *K. pneumoniae*[348]. Persons with dermatitis are at a special risk of harboring and transmitting pathogenic organisms[349–351]. All things considered, intensive care personnel, especially physicians, have poor hand washing practices, both in the teaching hospital and private hospital setting[64,352].

Thus, many factors interplay in the acquisition of colonizing microflora. In intubated patients, as many as 70% of the *Enterobacteriaceae* and other Gram-negative organisms (e.g., *Pseudomonas*) colonizing the trachea were actually first isolated from the trachea[319], suggesting direct external contamination. Experimentally, it has been shown that *Pseudomonas* adheres especially well to tracheal cells injured by endotracheal intubation[353]. In pediatric patients who are often intubated with uncuffed endotracheal tubes, aspiration of oropharyngeal secretions may be high, for example, 80% in intubated premature infants[354]. Aspiration is seven-fold higher with noncuffed tubes in younger children[355]. Patients treated with antacids or cimetidine are at increased risk of Gram-negative bacillary colonization of their gastric secretions and subsequent colonization of the oropharynx or, if intubated, the trachea as well[356–358].

Altered states of consciousness, acidosis, hypotension/decreased perfusion, antibiotics, nasogastric/tracheal intubation, GE reflux, immunosuppression—malnutrition, chemotherapy, prematurity, AIDS—have a significant role in hospital-acquired lower respiratory infection.

Tracheostomy

Tracheostomy has been employed intermittently and with varied success for approximately 3500 years. Both the Rig Veda (sacred book of Hindu medicine) and Eber's Papyrus describe such a procedure. However, it was not until the 19th century that tracheostomy received widespread attention and acceptance. It was advocated for obstruction of the upper airway by foreign bodies, croup, diphtheria, and trauma, as well as for administration of anesthesia. However, with the introduction of the oral endotracheal tube in 1880 and its increasing acceptance by the early 1900s, the tracheostomy with its rather high rate of complications became reserved for special situations. But with the modern availability of sophisticated, long-term ventilatory support came the realization that oral and nasal endotracheal tubes had their own complications, and that converting to a tracheostomy for ventilation and pulmonary toilet was often justified[359].

Not only does a tracheostomy tube pass through a skin incision, but it also comes in direct contact with open tissues—subcutaneous, fat, thyroid, vascular, cartilage—between the skin and the trachea. Either the tracheal rings are spread apart or a section of tracheal wall is removed or displaced for the tube to pass into the lumen. As this wound heals by primary intention, ample opportunity exists for local infection, which can be quite serious[360], as well as colonization and infection of the tracheobronchial tree itself. In addition, warming and filtration of inspired gases is absent, secretions are handled poorly, and effective cough is impaired because of the tracheal opening. When discussing pulmonary infections associated with tracheostomies, it is necessary to distinguish colonization of the trachea from tracheobronchitis—increase in volume, white blood cells, and change in color of secretions—and pneumonia, for example, new or increased fever, peripheral leukocytosis, change in chest physical examination, and chest radiograph. Not all reviews of tracheostomy and infectious complications make this distinction clear, however. In addition, differences in duration of the tracheostomy at the time of study, attention to standardization of care given to the tracheostomy site, suctioning procedures, and variations in respiratory equipment handling procedures are seldom mentioned.

The patient who has a tracheostomy usually has had a lengthy endotracheal intubation, and the tracheostomy is an extension of that respiratory support. It is not surprising then that patients with tracheostomies have a higher percentage of overall respiratory infections than patients who do not require such therapy[361].

Reviews of tracheostomy-related infections are quite variable. One review of 212 tracheostomies in all age groups noted that 9% of patients had severe pneumonia or endotracheitis, and 2.4% had severe local infection[362]. Another report found a 6% incidence of tracheitis, but no wound infections or pneumonia[363]. Some reports in adults, however, have demonstrated high infection rates (25 to 78%), which may reflect differences in definition of infection or care of the site. A high incidence of *P. aeruginosa, K. pneumonia, Proteus* species, *E. coli,* and *Candida* is found in these patients[361,364,365].

Although reviews of a total of 511 tracheostomies in children found no associated local or pulmonary infectious complications[365–370], others have not had this experience, unfortunately, and up to 4.5% of tracheostomies in children may be associated with severe infectious complications[366–369]. Studies of the local effects of tracheostomy on the tracheal tissues have clearly demonstrated early evidence of inflammation and subsequent development of scar tissue[322,324,371,372].

It has also been noted after tracheostomy in adults that the trachea soon becomes colonized with multiple organisms, especially *Enterobacteriaceae, P. aeruginosa,* and aerobic/facultative Gram-positive cocci in bacterial counts similar to those in patients with clinical pneumonia (10^7/ml). Upper airway saliva and throat cultures taken simultaneously demonstrated little correlation with those from the trachea, with a much greater prevalence of anaerobic organisms[373,374]. *Enterobacteriaceae* and *Pseudomonas* colonize the pediatric tracheostomy as well, but there may be a much higher incidence of anaerobic oral organisms in tracheal cultures[375]. Whether this represents a true difference related to the host or to the tubes used, or is an artifact of culturing techniques is not known. Group A β-hemolytic streptococci, *S. pneumoniae,* and *H. influenzae* may also colonize the pediatric tracheostomy[375].

Colonization versus Tracheitis versus Pneumonia

Differentiating between these conditions is often not an easy task. The previous sections have dealt with the enormous pressures on the airway flora in the sick patient and the changes in the flora of the oropharynx and trachea in the patient who is intubated or who has a tracheostomy. Any use of antibiotics will alter this flora, at least transiently, usually with the growth of more pathogenic organisms. Therefore, it is imprudent to treat the results of cultures obtained from the chronically instrumented airway unless there has been a clinical and radiographic change in parenchymal pulmonary status, such as pneumonia. If cultures of the airway have been performed, then knowledge of organisms colonizing the trachea may guide therapy when pneumonia develops. For example, a child who has had growth of *Pseudomonas* in the tracheal aspirate culture for 2 weeks develops fever, leukocytosis, and a definite infiltrate on a chest radiograph. Gram's stain of the tracheal secretions reveals predominantly Gram-negative rods of a single variety (similar to those seen in previous Gram's stains) and numerous polymorphonuclear leukocytes. It is reasonable to treat this child for a Gram-negative pneumonia, including *Pseudomonas,* pending results of sputum and blood cultures. The presence of large numbers of squamous cells or organisms resembling mouth flora suggests considerable contamination. However, if a patient develops a new pneumonia, and the Gram's stain demonstrates a marked shift in flora, e.g., to predominantly Gram-positive cocci, initial therapy should reflect this shift. Any information that suggests clearly the symptoms and radiographic findings were caused by another process—pulmonary embolus, congestive heart failure—should lead to cautiously discontinuation or not even starting the antibiotic therapy.

A necrotizing form of bacterial tracheitis can develop following a primary viral respiratory infection[376], including measles[377] or as a complication of tracheal intubation[378] and is becoming better understood[379]. Antibiotic therapy is required even in the absence of pneumonia. This is a difficult diagnosis to make. Tracheal radiographs may show subglottic narrowing with irregularities in the contour of the tracheal mucosa[380]. Bronchoscopic examination and culture of the tracheal mucosa may be required. Because of the severe changes in the trachea, intubation of those not already on respiratory support may be necessary[381]. When diagnosed in outpatients, an obstructive dyspnea may be noted, which can be confused with croup, epiglottitis, retropharyngeal abscess and even severe reactive airway disease. Critically ill children already receiving respiratory support in a PICU may not exhibit these signs. Obviously, cultures should be done with strict attention to avoiding contamination. Initial management should be guided by Gram stains of tracheal secretions obtained at intubation, bronchoscopy, or after tracheostomy/endotracheal tube change as clinically indicated. Blood cultures as well may help delineate the cause of the pneumonia. *S. aureus, H. influenzae*, streptococci, *Branhamella catarrhalis* and other organisms have been reported in patients admitted with this condition. When this condition arises in hospitalized patients, organisms reflect the colonization of the airway[382–385].

NOSOCOMIAL URINARY TRACT INFECTIONS (UTI)

Of the roughly 40 million persons who are hospitalized in the United States on an annual basis[386], approximately 1.5% ultimately develop a nosocomial UTI, ranging from 1.82% on medical services and 1.75% on surgical services to 0.215% on pediatric services and 0.6% in newborn nurseries[387]. This figure represents 41% of all nosocomial infections[386]. Approximately 60% of surgical nosocomial UTIs are catheter related and may prolong hospitalization an average of 2.4 additional days[388–389]. Additionally, university and community teaching hospitals have overall nosocomial infection rates nearly double that of community hospitals[387].

UTIs are relatively common in pediatric practice. It is generally well accepted that preschool and school-age girls have a 1 to 2% incidence of bacteriuria and that the incidence in boys is about 0.03%. Moreover, as many as two-thirds of the females may have no symptoms[390,391]. The incidence of bacteriuria in newborns ranges have been found to be from 0.1 to 1.0% and may be as high as 10% in low-birth-weight infants[392–395]. In the newborn period, urinary infections in males outnumber those in females by as many as 3 to 1 to 6 to 1[393,396], and distinct symptoms are uncommon. In the PICU population, the cumulative risk of UTI in catheterized patients approaches 30%, but is higher for infants less than 1 yr old[397]; this compares favorably with the risks in adult patients[389].

The definition of what constitutes a UTI can elicit spirited discussion. The gold standard for UTI diagnosis is suprapubic aspiration; virtually any bacterial growth can be presumed to represent true infection. Although initially performed in adults for comparison with simultaneous cultures by other methods, it is not wholeheartedly accepted by most adults. However, it has become a mainstay of culture technique in groups of patients with neurogenic bladders. It is generally accepted that a midstream "clean caught" specimen with a colony count more than 10^5 of a single organism constitutes a bona fide infection[398,399], but it has also been shown that as many as 21% of women with recurrent UTI have colony counts fewer than 10^5[400]. Factors such as frequency of voiding, hydration, antimicrobial therapy, fastidious organisms, and the presence of the perineal cleansing solution contaminating the specimen are regarded as potential mechanisms, whereby an infected urine may have fewer than 10^5 colonies/ml[401]. The presence of symptoms and pyuria help improve accuracy in borderline instances. Although the use of brief catheterization is an excellent method for the diagnosis of UTI[399], with 10^4 to 10^5 colonies/ml representing infection[401], it carries a risk of actually introducing infection, ranging from 1% in young healthy patients to as high as 10% in bedridden women and 17% in healthy parturients[399,402,403]. The presence of an indwelling urinary catheter may actually complicate the diagnosis of UTI, however. The underlying illness may cause fever or symptoms that may mimic urinary infection or may render the patient unable to communicate any symptoms. The catheter itself may obscure the symptoms of dysuria or frequency, and may lead to pyuria secondary to mechanical irritation in the absence of infection[404]. Garibaldi et al.[405] have suggested that catheterized patients with symptoms and a colony count more than 10^3 be classified as having a definite UTI, without symptoms but with a colony count more than 10^3 as probable UTI, and symptoms with a colony count fewer than 10^3 (one species) or more than 10^3 (two species) as possible urinary infections[404, 405]. Other investigators have also implicated colony counts lower than 10^5 as indicative of catheter-associated infections[406]. More recent work suggests that colony counts as low as 10^2 are indicative of 90% eventual development to more than 10^5 within 3 days[407]. Additionally, evidence suggests that midstream collection and meatal cleansing may not significantly improve upon culture results in young girls[408] nor, possibly, in uncircumcised young boys[409].

Open drainage catheterization was associated with a 90 to 95% incidence of infection within 3 to 4 days. Because of this, in 1958 Beeson[410] editorialized "The Case against the Catheter" but was unaware that work done in the 1920s[411] clearly showed that changing from an open-drainage (still prevalent in the 1950s) to a closed-sterile system greatly lowered the incidence of catheter-induced infection. After nearly universal adoption of closed-system sterile drainage in the 1960s, the incidence of UTIs associated with catheterization has greatly decreased, but urinary infection associated with the manipulation of the urinary tract still accounts for the single largest group of nosocomial infections in adults. What is currently known about the nature of the physical barriers to infection and the means of entry of organisms into the urinary tract?

In 1956 Guze and Beeson[412] reported that, even after thorough cleansing of the urethral orifice, 6 of 13 catheter tips inserted merely into the urethral opening grew pathogens in culture media. They also showed that 4 of 12 urine cultures obtained by catheterization were positive, but bladder aspirations during laparotomy just minutes earlier were all negative[(412)]. Helmholz[(413)] studied 82 adult males with an elaborate urethral-cot-culturing system and found Gram-positive organisms in the outer four-fifths of 5 to 10% of urethras, Gram-negative organisms in the entire length of the urethra in 4%, and in the outer three-fifths of the urethra in 6 to 11%. Using a similar device in 52 females, Cox showed that 100% of distal urethras contained bacteria in the proximal one-fourth adjacent to the bladder[(414)]. In spite of this information, Turck et al.[(415)] showed that of 200 healthy, young, men and women with mental retardation who initially had sterile urine, only one woman developed a significant UTI of more than 10^5 after a single brief catheterization. They also studied 75 elderly patients and found that 5.5% of the men and 15% of the women developed a significant UTI after only a single brief catheterization[(415)].

Kass[(399)] reported in 1956 that 95% of adult patients catheterized with an open system were infected within 4 days because of direct access to the bladder through the open lumen. He also showed that direct application of an organism to the urethral opening with the catheter in direct proximity led within 2 to 4 days to recovery of that organism from the urine through the catheter, implying entry of the organism into the bladder in the space between the catheter and urethral wall[(416)]. A similar study showed that 85% of catheter-associated bacteriurias in adult men and women were with organisms first cultured at the urethral meatus[(417)]. It has been shown that 68% of subsequent bacteriurias in males about to undergo prostate surgery were secondary to organisms present in the meatus at the time of catheter insertion[(418)]. These data suggest that in the catheterized patient whose closed drainage system is rigorously maintained, the space between the catheter and the urethral mucosa is the main source of contamination and subsequent infection. Although Kunin and McCormack[(419)] demonstrated that, over a period of 30 days, cumulative bacteriuria could be reduced about 25% with the use of sterile closed drainage, they also showed that approximately 50% of both males and females became infected within 11 to 13 days, and virtually all patients had bacteriuria if they remained catheterized for 30 days. In patients who were catheterized less than 3.5 days, Kunin and Steele[(420)] have shown that urinary catheters removed from females are nearly four times more likely to be colonized with organisms than are catheters from males. The most common isolates are Gram-positive *(S. epidermidis* and *Streptococcus faecalis)* in both sexes. Gram-negative organisms gradually colonize over time, but were always fewer than the Gram-positive organisms and found less often in males than females. In spite of the small numbers, the Gram-negative organisms readily lead to UTI[(420)].

Condom catheters have also been studied. Hirsh et al.[(402)] noted that with daily aseptic changing of the condom catheter, no infections occurred in patients who were cooperative or otherwise unable to manipulate and obstruct the system. However, infections occurred in 53% of those who interfered with the proper functioning of the condom system[(421)].

Because the use of sterile closed-drainage systems has not eliminated the problem of catheter-associated UTI, many investigators have attempted to lower the number of infections by various methods. All have stressed strict technique in catheter care and noted an increase in the number of infections with increasing breaches in proper technique. Antibiotics have been extensively evaluated. Some investigators assert that these agents are ineffective and select for multiple-resistant organisms[(422,423)]. Others find that these agents may decrease infections for several days after catheter insertion but, thereafter, infection rates are the same, with a tendency for the antibiotic group to become infected with resistant or more pathogenic organisms[(405,424–426)]. Controlled studies of twice daily meatal cleansing with povidone-iodine[(427)], the use of antibiotic-impregnated catheters[(428)], and the application of antibiotic lubricants[(429)] and creams[(430)] show no beneficial effect on incidence of infection. The povidone-iodine study actually demonstrated a higher incidence of bacteriuria in patients receiving meatal care with either povidone-iodine or green soap and water[(427)]. One prospective study of transurethral-prostate surgery patients has shown that a daily hexachlorophene sitz bath with twice daily application of antibiotic spray to the perineum resulted in less colonization of the perineum and significantly fewer associated bacteriurias[(431)]. Hydrogen peroxide instilled into the catheter drainage system has been found to be ineffective in altering the incidence of catheter-related bacteriuria[(432)]. Antibiotic and disinfectant irrigation of the catheter system has also failed to provide beneficial results[(432,433)]. However, catheter systems with preconnected sealed junctions are associated with significantly fewer bacteriurias[(434)].

Acute spinal cord-injured patients are not uncommon in a PICU. The resultant neurogenic bladder poses a specific challenge of infection prevention, amelioration, and treatment. Much work on this problem has been done both in spinal cord-injured patients and in meningomyelocele infants and children. Most of these patients will have a lifelong risk of at least partial urinary stasis[(435)] and will be at extremely high risk of recurrent UTI. Until the 1970s, most patients incurred frequent infections and eventual renal failure or underwent some form of diversion surgery with a lower rate of infections. Lapides et al.[(436)] showed that nonsterile intermittent bladder catheterization by the patient or the caretaker dramatically reduced the incidence of infections. Follow-up on this work 10 years later demonstrated that only 3% of children without vesicoureteral reflux and 37% of children with vesicoureteral reflux had febrile UTIs, and that only 2.6% of kidneys at risk experienced damage. Most of the children were on nitrofurantoin, sulfamethoxazole, or trimethoprim/sulfamethoxazole (TMP/SMX). The researchers also noted that renal scarring did not appear in the absence of vesicoureteral reflux nor after reflux was surgically repaired, despite continued long-term intermittent urethral catheterization[437]. This group has published experience with intermittent catheterization in infant boys as young as 18 months old and in infant girls as young as 1 week of age, with transient problems in only two boys, which did not require the discontinuation of catheterizations[438]. Others have demonstrated similar findings[439–441]. Children maintained on clean intermittent catheterization have significantly less asymptomatic bacteriuria than do children with ileal loop diversions (both groups received urinary antiseptics or low-dose antibiotics)[442]. In a small study of sterile intermittent catheterization requiring entry into the study within 48 hours of cord injury, urinary infection was preceded by a transition of introital, urethral, and glans colonization from normal flora to *Enterobacteriaceae*[443].

When a sick infant or child enters the invasive world of the ICU, urinary instrumentation may be necessary for diagnostic or therapeutic purposes. Such measures as cystoscopy, nephrostomy, urethral dilatation, percutaneous suprapubic catheterization, and most commonly urethral catheterization all infringe on the normal barriers for preserving sterility. Nosocomial diarrhea has also been shown to predispose to the development of nosocomial UTI[444]. Therefore, one would expect a relatively higher risk of developing a nosocomial UTI in the PICU setting. A recent study noted that the prevalence of urinary tract infection is nearly twice as high in PICU patients as in ward patients (9.7 versus 5.3/1000 admissions), and that more than 90% of these infections are catheter related. However, 51% of these infections occurred in children undergoing only intermittent catheterization. Although nearly one-third of the patients were asymptomatic, fever was the most common finding in those with symptoms. Approximately 85% had only a single organism, most commonly a Gram-negative rod, but 15% were infected with coagulase-negative staphylococci[445]. Our own unit's data confirms this finding. Pediatric urologic and neurologic patients have, respectively, four and two times the number of UTIs than do general pediatric patients in the same ICU[446].

INFECTIONS WITH DEVICES FOR MONITORING INTRACRANIAL PRESSURE

Increased intracranial pressure (ICP) is a major problem in the delivery of pediatric intensive care. Infants, children, and young adults are at a high risk of accidental or deliberate injury, and severe head trauma is a major sequelae of many of these events[447–453]. They are also a high-risk group for various central nervous system (CNS) infections, metabolic disorders (e.g., Reye syndrome), and other conditions (e.g., pseudotumor cerebri, mass lesions) that can profoundly increase ICP and portend an unsatisfactory result[454,455]. In acute situations, the monitoring of ICP allows for more rational judgments to be made regarding the appropriateness of therapy and the demonstration of improvement in intracranial compliance. In addition, the level of ICP can be more objectively correlated with changes in the physical examination[455,456] **(Table 30.8).**

Although observations about ICP effects on the intact animal were made as early as 1824[457], and lumbar paracentesis was used in 1891 to treat increased ICP secondary to tuberculous meningitis[458], it was in the early 1950s that direct intraventricular draining in humans was reported[459] and approximately 1960 when it was thought to be a readily applied clinical tool[460]. Infectious complications were reported from the beginning. However, variations in incidence were presumably because of differences in technique, patient population, duration of follow-up, use of antibiotics and steroids, and definitions of infection. What follows is a general summary of the problem of infections associated first with intracranial surgery and second with implanted externalized short-term pressure monitoring devices, such as ventricular drains, subarachnoid screws, and epidural fiberoptic transducers.

Although Cushing[461] stated that "certainly [neurosurgical] infections cannot be attributed to the intervention of the devil but must be laid at the surgeon's door," he had an astonishingly low rate of wound infections: 0.002% in 1915. In 1939, Cairns and Adelaide[462] reported a 2.7% incidence of postoperative death as a result of infections complicating intracranial operations, but Poppen[463] in 1943 reported no evidence of infection in over 500 ventricular drainage procedures. Woodhall et al.[464] in 1949 reported a postoperative infection incidence of 1.0% in craniotomy surgery. More recently, Balch[465] reported a 2.6% incidence of infection complicating clean (not transsphenoidal) neurosurgical procedures. These infections included both intradural and extradural sites[465]. Wright[466] reported an overall infection incidence of 5.7% following craniotomy in 2148 clean cases. However, he noted that if the surgery was extradural, the rate was only 1.4%. But if surgery was intradural, the rate was 5.4 to 6.3% (posterior fossa or supratentorial). He also found a lower incidence in patients less than 10 years of age (2.8%) than in patients more than 60 years of age (8.4%)[466]. Others have noted that neurosurgical patients undergo the same changes in bacterial flora after hospitalization and surgery as have been noted in surgical, medical, and ICU patients[467,468]. Thus, the incidence of postoperative neurosurgical infections after clean procedures should clearly be less than 10% and, indeed, in many institutions, is less than 5%.

Pressure monitoring devices transit the skin and calvarium, and in the case of catheters, continue through meninges and brain to the ventricle. However, subarachnoid screws stop at the subdural space, and epidural devices stop external to the dural membrane. **Table 30–8** lists the major reviews of experience with ICP monitoring[459,460,469–480]. Only the 1984 study by Mayhall et al.[481] used rigorous definitions and was prospective; the others generally mention infectious complications along with other elements of ICP monitoring **(Table 30.9).**

Table 30.8. Reviews of ICP Monitoring Infections[a]

Reference	*No. of Patients/ No. of Procedures*	*Type of Monitor*	*Placed in OR*	*Prophylactic Antibiotics*	*Other Antibiotics*	*Steroids*	*Care of System*	*Duration of Monitoring*	*Infections Related to Device*	*Comments*
Bering[(440)]	26/29	V	NS	NST	NS	NS	NS	<19 days	10.3%	
Lundberg[(441)]	130/	V	NS	All	NS	NS	NS	av. = 4–14 days	13%	
White et al.[(450)]	33/51	V	NS	NST	NS	NS	SHV-RR, IR	3–176 days av. = 21.5	vent—0.5% local—1.5%	
Sundbarg et al.[(451)]	938/	V	NS	N	Y	NS	CS	1–69 days av. = 8 days	definite—1.1% suspect—3.7%	
Wyler and Kelly[(452)]	70/102	V	S	63%	NS	NS	RC	0.5–15 days	no proph—27% proph—9%	
Smith and Alksne[(453)]	56/65	V	S	95%	NS	NS	SC	0.5–9 days	definite—4.6% possible—6.2%	
Shaywitz et al.[(454)]	24P/	V	NS	All	NS	All	NS	3–16 days	0	All Reye syndrome
Mayhall et al.[(462)]	172/213	V	S	S	NS	NS	ST, IR	NS	8.9%	Prospective: irrigation of system correlated with infection
Rosner and Becker[(455)]	112/	V, SS, VS	NS	S	S	S	NS	av. = 8 days	wound—2.7% device—15.2%	70% Gram-positive
Narayan et al.[(456)]	207/	V, SS, VS	NS	NS	NS	All	NS	≥3 days	vent—6.3%V men—5.3%SS	85% of infections in devices in place >5 days
Bruce et al.[(457)]	50P/	V, SS, VS	NS	NS	NS	NS	NS	1.5–10 days	local—20.5%SS vent—7.6%V poss. vent—15.2%	
Winn et al.[(458)]	147/	SS, VS	41%	N	S	90%	SD, IR	1–20 days av. = 5 days	vent—0.6%	
Levin[(459)]	140/	EFT	S	NS	NS	NS	NS	3–32 days av. = 9.2 days	0	
Ivan et al.[(460)]	52/	EFT	All	Y	Y	NS	NS	<1–31 days av. = 8 days	0	

[a]Abbreviations: P = pediatric; V = ventriculostomy; SS = subarachnoid screw; VS = V & SS in same patient; EFT = epidural fiberoptic transducer; NS = not stated; S = some; NST = not standardized; N = no; Y = yes; SHV = Spitz-Holter valve; RR = Rickham reservoir; IR = irrigation; CS = closed system; RC = regular changes in systems; SC = stopcock in line; ST = skin tunnel; SD = sterile dressing; av. = average; vent = ventriculitis; men = meningitis; poss. = possible.

Most studies have neither stated their operative preparation nor postoperative care and manipulation of drains. However, it is clear that increasing the frequency of breaks in the system or flushing of the drain increases the risk of infection. Antibiotic prophylaxis has not been rigorously studied, and no definite conclusions can be drawn. Mayhall et al.[(481)] found nafcillin prophylaxis to be of no value in patients with ventriculostomies, and Rosner and Becker[(474)] came to the same conclusion in their series of patients with ventriculostomies (some with subarachnoid screws also). However, Wyler's and Kelly's[(471)] experience with ventriculostomies suggests that prophylaxis is useful, but it is a retrospective study. Smith and Alksne[(472)] recommend the use of antistaphylococcal prophylaxis, but their data does not support any position.

Common sense would seem to suggest that the longer a ventricular drain is in place, the greater likelihood it will become infected. However, the study by Smith and Alksne[(472)] had a shorter mean duration for infected cases than noninfected ones. The prospective study by Mayhall et al.[(481)] did find that duration of insertion was directly related to increasing infections and suggested that ICP drains be replaced every 5 days as an effective way to reduce this complication. No study answers the question of the relevance of ICP-dose steroids and subsequent risk of infectious complications. In a recent study, it was noted that CSF production may be decreased by Gram-negative and multiple organism infection[(482)].

Once a drain is in place, what criteria for infection[(481)] are known? Fever and peripheral leukocytosis are helpful but far from specific. It also appears that as many as 22% of proven bacterial drain infections will not develop a cerebrospinal fluid cellular response. In addition, approximately the same percentage of patients will develop a cerebrospinal fluid pleocytosis without subsequent positive cultures. Placement of ventriculostomy drains either in the operating room or in the ICU appears to have no relationship to subsequent infection. Irrigation of a ventriculostomy catheter is significantly associated with increased infection as is intracranialand intraventricular hemorrhage with an ICP greater than 20 mm Hg. Therapy of suspected or proven infection or ventriculitis should be guided by results of cultures and Gram's stains, the site of infection, and antibiotics of known penetration into cerebrospinal fluid. Organisms associated with ventriculitis in patients with ICP drains are included in **Table 30–9.**

NOSOCOMIAL PATHOGENS AND ANTIBIOTIC RESISTANCE

The problem of antibiotic resistance has been receiving increasing attention from the lay public and medical establishment. It is of particular concern within the intensive care setting, "where there is a high density of antimicrobial use and an increased risk of development of bacterial infections due to the presence of high-risk hosts and invasive supportive devices"[(483)]. Infections caused by antibiotic-resistant bacteria are of special concern because of the increased difficulty of treatment and negative influence on patient outcome[(484)]. Infections resulting from antibiotic-resistant bacteria are associated with increased mortality compared with similar infections caused by nonresistant bacteria[(485,486)]. The following sections provide an overview of the problem of antibiotic resistance for the most frequently encountered nosocomial pathogens. Prevalence rates and epidemiologic patterns of resistance vary from one health care center to another. Therefore, awareness of local epidemiologic trends of resistance is necessary to optimize the management of patients within the pediatric intensive care unit.

Staphylococcus Aureus

Staphylococcus aureus is the primary nosocomial pathogen in the United States. It is the most frequent cause of skin and wound infections as well as nosocomial bacteremia and the second most frequent cause of hospital-acquired pneumonia (including ventilator-associated pneumonia)[(487)]. Methicillin-resistant *S. aureus* (MRSA) emerged as a nosocomial pathogen in the early 1960s[(488)]. Methicillin-resistance among *S. aureus* results from the presence of a unique penicillin binding protein (PBP2a) with a low affinity for beta-lactam antibiotics[(489)], which has been linked to a chromosomal gene known as mec[(490)]. Rates of methicillin-resistance among nosocomial isolates of *S. aureus* have increased from 8% in 1986 to 40% in 1992 for large teaching hospitals[(487)]. More recently, the pathogen has spread to smaller hospitals and nursing homes where the prevalence is as high as 20%[(487)]. Similar data are not available from pediatric institutions. The majority of methicillin-resistant strains of *S. aureus* are resistant to most other antibacterial agents, leaving vancomycin as the only remaining therapeutic agent[(491)].

Table 30.9. Organisms Reported to Cause ICP Monitor Infections[a]

Gram-positive	
	Staphylococcus epidermidis
	Staphylococcus aureus
	α-Streptococci
Gram-negative	
	Pseudomonas
	Enterobacter
	Acinetobacter
	Escherichia coli
	Klebsiella
	Serratia
	Providentia

[a]Adapted from Winn HR, et al. Intracranial subarachnoid pressure recording: experience with 650 patients. Surg Neurol 1977;8:41. Ivan LP, et al. Intracranial pressure monitoring with the fiberoptic transducer in children. Childs Brain 1980;7:303. Smith RW, Alksne JF. Infections complicating the use of external ventriculostomy. J Neurosurg 1976;44:567.

Coagulase-Negative Staphylococci

Coagulase-negative staphylococci, such as *S. epidermidis*, *S. hemolyticus* and *S. hominis* have been increasingly recognized as important pathogens since the 1970s[(492)]. Coagulase-negative staphylococci are the most frequent cause of infections associated with intravascular catheters and prosthetic devices in both adults and children[(486)]. Sixty to 90% of the coagulase negative staphylococci are methicillin-resistant[(486)]. Coagulase negative staphylococci produce beta-lactamase, and similar to MRSA, many of them possess PBP2a[(492)] rendering these strains resistant to penicillin, methicillin, and cephalosporins. Therapy for resistant strains of coagulase negative staphylococci is currently limited to the use of vancomycin. Infection with *S. hemolyticus* is of special concern because it can be resistant to vancomycin[(493)].

Enterococci

Enterococci are now the third most common cause of nosocomial infections in the United States[(486)]. These bacteria are frequently associated with intraabdominal infections, urinary tract infections, and bacteremia. Infection in children is more common after abdominal surgery, including liver or intestinal transplantation. Enterococcal endocarditis is uncommon among pediatric patients. Enterococci are difficult to treat because they are naturally resistant to many antibiotics, including all cephalosporins, erythromycin, clindamycin, and aminoglycosides. More recently, ampicillin resistance has become extremely common and is associated with the production of beta-lactamases in *E. faecalis*[(494)] or the presence of penicillin- binding proteins with a low affinity for beta-lactams in *E. faecium*[(495)]. The widespread dissemination of these two mechanisms has essentially eliminated the utility of penicillins in the treatment of enterococcal infections. Vancomycin alone or in combination with aminoglycosides is often the only therapeutic choice for treatment of this pathogen. Unfortunately, the recent emergence and subsequent spread of vancomycin-resistance among enterococci has occurred at a very rapid pace. As of 1993, 14% of enterococcal isolates from patients in intensive care units within the United States were resistant to vancomycin.[486]. Eighty-eight per cent of these strains were also resistant to ampicillin. Outbreaks of vancomycin-resistant enterococci have been reported among children[496] and within intensive care units[497]. Analysis of outcome of infections with these multiple-resistant strains showed an increased mortality in patients with bacteremia because of vancomycin-resistant enterococci compared with bacteremia resulting from vancomycin-susceptible enterococci[487]. Combination therapy with a beta-lactam (e.g. penicillin, ampicillin or imipenem) and vancomycin has been shown to be effective for some but not all strains of ampicillin and vancomycin-resistant *E. faecium* in vitro[498] and in an animal model[499]. Thus, in vitro evaluation for the presence of synergy among these antibiotics as well as therapeutic use should be considered in patients infected with these multiple-resistant enterococci. Unfortunately, many strains of vancomycin-resistant enterococci are resistant to all known therapeutic regimens[486].

Escherichia Coli

Escherichia coli is the second most frequent pathogen (and the most frequent Gram-negative bacteria) associated with nosocomial infection. The most common infectious syndromes caused by this organism are cystitis, pyelonephritis, and bacteremia. As many as 30% of community-acquired isolates and 40 to 50% of hospital-acquired isolates of *E. coli* are resistant to amoxicillin[492]. *E. coli* may be resistant to other commonly used antimicrobials such as trimethoprim/sulfamethoxazole[492]. Recovery of strains of *E. coli* that contain one or more beta-lactamases, including extended spectrum beta-lactamases, is also on the rise[492,500,501]. The presence of an extended-spectrum beta-lactamase inactivates advanced generation cephalosporins, ceftazidime and cefotaxime, as well as the monobactam, aztreonam. However, this has been less frequently reported than with *Klebsiella*. More recently, increasing use of fluoroquinolones has been associated with the development of quinolone-resistance (e.g., ciprofloxacin and norfloxacin) among strains of *E. coli*[502,503]. Although this has been reported for both community-acquired and nosocomial isolates, the greatest risk appears to be in patients chronically exposed to quinolones as part of a regimen of prophylaxis or treatment for febrile, neutropenic cancer patients[502]. Initial treatment for infections resulting from *E. coli* within the pediatric critical care unit should be based on knowledge of local antibiotic susceptibility patterns. In the absence of a known problem with multiple-resistant strains, the use of either a third generation cephalosporin, cefotaxime, or an aminoglycoside, gentamicin, should be appropriate therapy.

Pseudomonas Aeruginosa

Pseudomonas aeruginosa is second to *E. coli* in occurrence as a cause of Gram-negative nosocomial infections. It is a particular problem in patients with neutropenia because of hematologic malignancy or chemotherapy as well as children with cystic fibrosis. Development of antibiotic resistance, an important problem in this pathogen, typically results from the combination of poor penetration of the antibiotic into the cell and the presence of enzymes that inactivate or modify the antibiotics[492]. Observations that failure to eradicate *P. aeruginosa* in clinical infections was associated with resistance during therapy have led to the long-standing practice of using combination antimicrobial therapy for treatment of these infections[504]. However despite this practice, resistance to ceftazidime, aminoglycosides, fluoroquinolones, and more recently imipenem has been reported with increasing frequency[486,492]. Initial treatment of infections caused by *P. aeruginosa* should be based on antibiotic-resistance patterns within each hospital with appropriate modifications made when results of antimicrobial susceptibility testing are available., Strains of antibiotic-resistant *P. aeruginosa* are not uncommon in patients with cystic fibrosis. The inability to treat such strains has led to the recommendation that the presence of resistant strains of *P. aeruginosa* is a relative contraindication to lung transplantation in children with end-stage lung disease with Cystic Fibrosis.

Enterobacter Species

Enterobacter species have replaced *Klebsiella pneumoniae* as the third leading cause of Gram-negative nosocomial infection behind *E. coli* and *P. aeruginosa*[492]. The increasing frequency and importance of infections because of these pathogens may be explained by the presence of a chromosomally located cephalosporinase in all *Enterobacter* species. This beta-lactamase is capable of hydrolyzing advanced generation of cephalosporins, including cefotaxime and ceftazidime. Although this enzyme is not normally expressed, expression may be triggered by exposure to cephalosporins with subsequent selection of mutants that produce the beta-lactamase even in the absence of cephalosporins[492]. Thus, widespread use of third-generation cephalosporins has been associated with outbreaks of *Enterobacter* infection as well as emergence of resistance to these agents on therapy[485]. Additionally, admission to an intensive care unit was identified as a risk for *Enterobacter* bacteremia in 49% of patients in one series[485]. *Enterobacter* species expressing this beta-lactamase are also resistant to beta-lactamase inhibitors, such as clavulanate or sulbactam. Third-generation cephalosporins should be avoided in the treatment of even susceptible strains of *Enterobacter* species[485]. Treatment of multiply-resistant *Enterobacter* strains is best limited to imipenem. The potential benefit of combination therapy (with either an aminoglycoside or a fluoroquinolone) has not been studied.

Klebsiella Pneumoniae

Klebsiella pneumoniae is the fourth most common cause of nosocomial infection resulting from Gram-negative pathogens and is among the most likely to be multiple-antibiotic resistant. Since the mid-1980s, the frequency of *K. pneumoniae* isolates containing extended-spectrum beta-lactamases has been rapidly increasing[501]. Recent surveys of nosocomial isolates of *K. pneumoniae* from Europe show that 14% to 16% of strains produce extended-spectrum beta-lactamases[501]. Many of these strains have associated resistance to aminoglycosides[492]. Similar experiences have been reported from within the United States[501,505]. Data from the Children's Hospital of Pittsburgh reveals a drop in susceptibility of *K. pneumoniae* to piperacillin from 80% to 40% in a five year period and from 98% to 78% for gentamicin in a 10-year period. The rapid spread of extended-spectrum beta-lactamases among *K. pneumoniae* in this hospital is demonstrated by the dramatic decline in activity of ceftazidime for *K. pneumoniae* from 97% to 73% in a single year. (unpublished data). Management of patients with infection because of *K. pneumoniae* is complicated by both the potential for and presence of antibiotic resistance. Some strains of extended-spectrum beta-lactamase containing *K. pneumonia* will be resistant to ceftazidime but susceptible to cefotaxime in vitro. However, the use of cefotaxime has not been uniformly successful in the treatment of infection from strains with this susceptibility pattern[501]. Accordingly, the use of imipenem should be considered for patients with infection caused by ceftazidime-resistant *K. pneumoniae,* particularly those who are not improving on cefotaxime despite being susceptible on in vitro testing. As with *Enterobacter* species, the role of combination antimicrobial therapy has not been sufficientyl studied.

Preventing the Spread of Antibiotic Resistance

The increasing prevalence and spread of multiple-drug resistant pathogens has prompted new recommendations aimed at preventing esculation of this problem. Lack of available antimicrobial agents for the treatment of vancomycin-resistant enterococci has led to the recent publication of practice guidelines by the Hospital Infection Control Practices Advisory Committee[506]. These recommendations include: (1) the prudent use of vancomycin, (2) education of hospital staff regarding the problem of vancomycin resistance, (3) early detection and prompt reporting of vancomycin-resistant enterococci, and (4) immediate implementation of appropriate infection control measures (including gown and glove isolation) to prevent person-to-person transmission[506]. Although the epidemiology of antibiotics among specific pathogens within a given population has not been thoroughly studied, similar recommendations to those developed for vancomycin-resistant enterococci can be applied to most multiple-drug resistant bacteria. To implement these guidelines, physicians who care for children within the critical care setting will need to work closely with infection control personnel to set up surveillance for multiple-drug resistant bacteria within their unit.

Empiric Antibiotic Coverage in the era of Antibiotic Resistance

The critically ill nature of patients in the intensive care setting often mandates the empiric use of antibiotic therapy when infection is suspected. However, the use of any antibiotic may contribute to the development and spread of antibiotic resistance. Accordingly, the clinician must balance concerns for emerging antibiotic resistance with the appropriate treatment for serious infections. The tendency to use antibiotics for prolonged periods without clear indications or endpoints must be avoided.

Patients should undergo a careful clinical assessment aimed at identifying the source of infection before empiric therapy is initiated. Bacterial cultures should be obtained from the blood—including cultures obtained from the central venous catheter and a peripheral sample for patients in whom empiric therapy will be initiated—urine, and endotracheal aspirates in patients with indwelling catheters. Additional cultures should be considered if a patient has signs of upper respiratory tract infection, respiratory syncytial virus, or gastroenteritis, such as rotavirusor *Clostridium difficile.* Other laboratory information that may support the diagnosis of infection includes a complete blood count, urinanalysis, and chest radiograph.

Once the culture and laboratory database have been established, consideration of empiric therapy is appropriate, particularly in the critically ill patient. The presence of central venous catheters warrants consideration of the use of vancomycin as part of the initial antimicrobial therapy. Additional antimicrobial agents may be added in patients at risk for Gram-negative infection, for example, recent abdominal surgery, presence of pyuria, clinical or radiographic evidence of pneumonia. The choice of empiric coverage for Gram-negative bacilli should be influenced by knowledge of local problems with resistance. Third-generation cephalosporins, ceftazidime and cefotaxime, have an excellent spectrum of activity and safety for most Gram-negative pathogens. However, avoidance of these agents would seem prudent in intensive care units where a substantial proportion of Gram-negative isolates have developed resistance to these advanced generation cephalosporins. Alternative choices include aminoglycosides or combination betalactam/beta-lactamase inhibitors (e.g., ticarcillin/clavulanic acid, piperacillin/tazobactam). In patients who are known to be colonized with multiple-drug resistant pathogens, empiric use of imipenem may be necessary to cover appropriately for all potential pathogens.

Once a pathogen is identified, the choice of an antibiotic typically should represent the most narrow spectrum agent that has activity against this pathogen. Accordingly, use of vancomycin should be discontinued in patients who are infected with Gram-negative pathogens or with Gram-positive pathogens susceptible to alternative agents. Similarly, Gram-negative coverage should be discontinued in patients infected with a Gram-positive pathogen. Selection of therapeutic agents should also reflect a consideration of antimicrobial choices that provide the minimal amount of antibiotic pressure for development of resistance. If no pathogen or obvious source of fever is identified, discontinuation of antimicrobial therapy should be encouraged.

SUMMARY

This chapter has dealt, albeit briefly, with the problem of nosocomial infections in the pediatric ICU setting. When data has been available, specific pediatric information has been presented. It is hoped that the reader will acquire an understanding of the incredible pressure of illness, invasive procedures, devices, and antibiotics on patient and environmental microbial flora, with the very real risk for subsequent serious infection. It is also hoped that the references listed will stimulate some to a more thorough examination of these problems and lead to PICU-orientated nosocomial infection research.

Appendix 1—Definitions of Nosocomial Infection[4]

The most recent compilation of criteria for the diagnosis of nosocomial infections from the Centers for Disease Control (CDC) is summarized below. For a complete reading, see: Garner JS, et al. CDC definitions for nosocomial infections, 1988. Am J Infect Control 16:128–140, 1988, from which this summary was taken. For those interested in a brief history of the evolution of these diagnostic criteria, see the following: Centers for Disease Control Definitions of Nosocomial Infections—adapted from Centers for Disease Control: National Nosocomial Infection Study (NNIS) Site Definitions Manual. Atlanta, GA: Centers for Disease Control, 1975:1–82; Garner JS, Bennett JV, Scheckler WE, et al. Surveillance of nosocomial infections. In: Proceedings of the International Conference on Nosocomial Infections, Centers for Disease Control, Atlanta, 1970. Chicago, IL: American Hospital Association, 1971:277–281; Centers for Disease Control. Guidelines for determining presence and classification of infection. Appendix II. In: Outline for Surveillance and Control of Nosocomial Infections. Washington, DC: U.S. Department of Health, Education, and Welfare, 1972:17–19.

Several requirements are necessary for the diagnosis of a nosocomial infection. First, the information necessary to make the diagnosis involves a combination of clinical, laboratory, and diagnostic tests. There must be a stated clinical diagnosis of infection, which may require the initiation of appropriate antibiotics. The infection must not have been present or incubating at the time of admission. However, infections acquired in the hospital but manifesting after discharge and newborn infections acquired vaginally are considered nosocomial. Infection associated with a complication or extension of an infection(s) present on admission (unless the organism changes), and transplacental infections are not considered nosocomial. Unless specifically mentioned, no particular time limitations are placed on the diagnosis of any specific nosocomial infection; evidence must be examined linking the infection to the hospitalization.

I. Urinary Tract Infections
  A. Asymptomatic:
    1. With indwelling catheter present within 7 days prior to culture: no symptoms; $\geq 10^5$ organisms/ml of no more than two species.
    2. No indwelling catheter—no symptoms; two cultures with $\geq 10^5$ organisms/ml of the same organisms and no more than two species.
  B. Symptomatic: one of the following criteria
    1. One of the following: symptoms (e.g., fever, urgency, frequency, dysuria or suprapubic tenderness) with positive culture of $\geq 10^5$ colonies/ml, with no more than two species.
    2. Two of the following: symptoms (see "1") and any of the ensuing:
    —positive dipstick for leukocyte esterase or nitrate
    —≥ 10 WBC/cc or ≥ 3 WBC/high power field of unspun urine
    —organisms on Gram's stain of unspun urine
    —two cultures with repeated isolation of the same uropathogen (e.g., Gram-negative bacteria or *Staphylococcus saprophyticus*) with $\leq 10^2$ colonies/ml in nonvoided specimens
    —urine culture with $\downarrow$ 10^5 colonies/ml of single uropathogen in patient on an appropriate antibiotic
    —physician's diagnosis
    —physician institutes appropriate antibiotic
    3. Patient ≤ 12 months with one of the following symptoms (i.e., fever, hypothermia, apnea, bradycardia, dysuria, lethargy or vomiting), *and* urine culture with $\leq 10^5$ colonies/ml with no more than two organisms
    4. Patient ≤ 12 months with symptoms as in "3" above, and any of the following: see "2"

II. Lower Respiratory Infections—Pneumonia: must meet one of the following criteria:
  A. Rales or dullness and any of the following:
  —new or changed-character sputum
  —positive blood culture
  —pathogen from transtracheal aspirate, bronchial brushing, biopsy
  B. CXR with new or worsening infiltrate, consolidation, cavitation, effusion *and* any of the following:
  —as in "A", plus
  —isolation of virus or detection of viral antigen in respiratory secretions
  —diagnostic single antibody (IgM) or 4X increase in paired serum IgG for pathogen
  —histopathologic evidence for pneumonia
  C. Patient ≤ 12 months with two of the following: apnea, tachypnea, bradycardia, wheezing, rhonchi, or cough, and any of the following:
  —increased production of respiratory secretions
  —as in "B"
  D. Patient ≤ 12 months with CXR showing new or

progressive infiltrate, consolidation, cavitation, effusion and any of the following:
—as in "C"

III. Lower Respiratory Tract (Excluding Pneumonia), i.e., bronchitis, tracheobronchitis, bronchiolitis, tracheitis, lung abscess, empyema
   A. Bronchitis, tracheobronchitis, bronchiolitis, tracheitis, without evidence of pneumonia
      1. Patient has no clinical or radiographic evidence of pneumonia *and* has two of the following: fever, cough, new or increased sputum, rhonchi, wheezing and either of the following:
      —positive deep tracheal aspirate or bronchoscopy culture
      —positive antigen test on respiratory secretions
      2. Patient ≤12 months with no clinical or X-ray evidence of pneumonia *and* has two of the following with no other recognized cause: fever, cough, new or increased sputum, rhonchi, wheezing, respiratory distress, apnea, bradycardia *and* any of the following:
      —as in "1"
      —diagnostic single IgM titer or 4X rise in paired serum IgG titers for pathogen
   B. Other infections of the lower respiratory tract—one of the following:
      1. Positive smear or culture of lung tissue or fluid, including pleural fluid
      2. Lung abscess or empyema seen at surgery or histopathologic examination
      3. Abscess cavity seen on radiograph

IV. Primary Bloodstream Infection

If an organism isolated from blood is thought to have originated from a nosocomial infection at another site, then it is classified as a *secondary* bloodstream infection. However, intravascular device-associated bloodstream infections are considered primary bloodstream infections, even if signs of infection are present at the site of insertion.

   A. Laboratory-confirmed bloodstream infection requires one of the following:
      1. Recognized pathogen isolated from blood and not related to infection at another site
      2. Symptoms (fever, chills, or hypotension) and any of the following:
      —common skin contaminant isolated from two blood cultures drawn on separate occasions *and* not related to infection at another site
      —common skin contaminant isolated from blood culture in patient with intravascular access device *and* physician instituted appropriate antibiotic(s)
      —positive antigen test on blood *and* organism not related to infection at another site
      3. Patient ≤12 months with one of the following: symptoms (fever, hypothermia, apnea, or bradycardia) *and* any of the following:
      —as in "2"
   B. Clinical sepsis: must meet either of the following criteria:
      1. One of the following clinical signs with no other recognized cause (fever, hypotension, oliguria) *and* all of the following:
      —blood culture not done or no organism or antigen detected in blood
      —no apparent infection at another site
      —appropriate antimicrobial therapy instituted
      2. Patient ≤12 months has one of the following symptoms, such as fever, hypothermia, apnea, and bradycardia *and* all of the following:
      —see "1"

V. Cardiovascular System Infection
   A. Artery or vein infection: must meet one of the following:
      1. Positive culture from surgical specimen *and* blood culture either not done or negative
      2. Evidence of infection of vessels at surgery or by histopathology
      3. One of the following: fever, pain, erythema, or heat at involved vascular site *and* both of the following:
      — 15 colonies from semiquantitative catheter tip culture
      —blood culture not done or negative
      4. Purulent drainage at involved vascular site *and* blood culture not done or negative
      5. Patient ≤12 months with one of the following: fever, hypothermia (>37), apnea, bradcardia, lethargy, pain, erthema, or heat at involved vascular site *and* both of the following:
      —as in "3"
   B. Endocarditis, either natural or prosthetic heart valve, must meet one of the following criteria:
      1. Positive culture from valve or vegetation
      2. Two of following with no other recognized cause: fever, new or changed murmur, embolic phenomena, skin manifestations, CHF, arrhythmias, *and* physician institutes appropriate antibiotics (i.e., antemortem) *and* any of the following:
      —organism from two blood cultures
      —organisms on Gram's stain of valve when culture is negative or not done
      —valvular vegetation seen during surgery or autopsy
      —positive blood or urine antigen test
      —evidence of new vegetation by echocardiogram
      3. Patient ≤12 months with two or more of the following with no other recognized cause: fever, hypothermia, apnea, bradycardia, new or changed murmur, embolic phenomena, skin manifestations, CHF, arrhythmias *and* physician begins appropriate antimicrobial therapy (i.e., antemortem) *and* any of the following:
      —as in "2"

C. Myocarditis, pericarditis, mediastinitis—see reference 4

VI. Surgical Wound Infection

A. Incisional—within 30 days of surgery; involves skin, subcutaneous tissue, or muscle located above the fascial layer and *any* of the following:
1. Purulent drainage from the incision or drain
2. Positive culture
3. Surgeon deliberately opens wound; or clinical diagnosis made of infection

B. Deep—within 30 days of surgery (within 1 year if nonhuman-derived foreign body implant present); involves tissues or spaces at or beneath fascial layer and *any* of the following:
1. Purulent drainage from drain
2. Spontaneous dehiscence or surgical opening of wound in symptomatic patient (fever >38, pain) unless cultures negative
3. Presence of abscess
4. Surgical diagnosis

VII. Central Nervous System Infection

A. Intracranial infection (brain abscess, subdural or epidural infection, encephalitis)
1. Organism isolated from brain tissue or dura
2. Abscess or evidence of intracranial infection seen at surgery or by histopathology
3. Two of the following with no other recognized cause: headache, dizziness, fever, localizing neurologic signs, changing level of consciousness, or confusion and any two of the following:
—organism seen on microscopic examination of brain or abscess tissue obtained by aspiration, surgical biopsy or at autopsy
—positive urine or blood antigen test
—radiographic evidence of infection
—diagnostic single IgM antibody titer, or 4X increase in paired IgG titers for the pathogen
4. Patient ≤12 months of age with two of the following and no other recognized cause: fever, hypothermia, apnea, bradycardia, localizing neurologic signs or changing level of consciousness *and* physician institutes appropriate antimicrobial (i.e., antemortem) *and* any of the following:
—as in "3"

B. Meningitis or ventriculitis—must meet one of the following:
1. Positive cerebrospinal fluid (CSF) culture
2. One of the following with no other recognized cause: fever, headache, stiff neck, meningeal signs, cranial nerve signs, or irritability *and* physician institutes appropriate antimicrobial (i.e., antemortem) *and* any of the following:
—increased white cells, elevated protein and/or decreased glucose in CSF
—positive CSF Gram's stain
—positive CSF culture
—positive CSF, urine, or urine antigen test
—diagnostic single IgM titer or 4X rise in paired serum IgG titers for pathogen
3. Patient ≤12 months with one of the following and no other recognized cause: fever, hypothermia, apnea, bradycardia, stiff neck, meningeal signs, cranial nerve signs, or irritability *and* physician institutes appropriate antimicrobial (i.e., antemortem), *and* any of the following:
—as in "2"

C. Spinal abscess without meningitis—abscess of the spinal epidural or subdural space without involvement of the CSF or adjacent bone—must meet one of the following:
1. Organism isolated from said space
2. Abscess in said space seen at surgery, autopsy or by histopathologic examination
3. One of the following with no other recognized cause: fever, back pain, focal tenderness, radiculitis, paraparesis, or paraplegia *and* physician institutes appropriate antimicrobial (i.e., antemortem) *and* either of the following:
—positive blood culture
—radiographic evidence of spinal abscess

VIII. Eye, Ear, Nose, Throat and Mouth Infection—see reference 4

IX. Gastrointestinal System Infection—see reference 4

X. Reproductive Tract Infection—see reference 4

XI. Skin and Soft Tissue Infection—see reference 4

XII. Bone and Joint Infection—see reference 4

Appendix 2—Important Organisms Organized by Gram's Stain Morphologic Characteristics

I. Gram-positive Organisms
  A. Cocci
    1. Streptococci
      Group A—*S. pyogenes*
      Group B—*S. agalactiae*
      Group D—Enterococci: *S. faecalis*
                                             S. faecium
      Nonenterococi: *S. bovis*
                              S. equinus
                              Viridans Streptococci
                              e.g., *S. salivarius, S. sanguis, S. mutans, S. mitior, S. milleri*
    2. Pneumococci
    3. Micrococcaceae
      a. *Staphylococcus*
        S. aureus
        S. epidermidis
        S. saprophyticus
      b. *Micrococcus*
      c. *Aerococcus*
    4. Anaerobic Cocci
      a. *Peptostreptococcus*
      b. *Peptococcus*
      c. *Veillonella*
  B. Bacilli
    1. Spore-forming—aerobic/facultative
      B. anthracis
    2. Spore-forming—anaerobic
      Clostridium
    3. Nonspore-forming—aerobic
      a. *Listeria*
      b. *Corynebacterium*
      c. *Nocardia*
      d. *Erysipelothrix*
    4. Nonspore-forming—anaerobic
      a. *Propionibacterium*
      b. *Lactobacillus*
      c. *Eubacterium*
      d. *Bifidobacterium*
      e. *Actinomyces*
      f. *Arachnia*

II. Gram-negative Organisms
  A. Cocci
    1. *Neisseria*
    2. *Branhamella*
  B. Bacilli
    1. *Enterobacteriaceae*
      a. *Escherichia*
      b. *Edwarsiella*
      c. *Citrobacter*
      d. *Salmonella*
      e. *Shigella*
      f. *Klebsiella*
      g. *Enterobacter*
      h. *Hafnia*
      i. *Serratia*
      j. *Proteus*
      k. *Yersinia*
      l. *Erwinia*
    2. Vibrionaceae
      a. *Vibrio*
      b. *Aeromonas*
      c. *Plesiomonas*
    3. Nonfermentative
      a. *Pseudomonas*
      b. *Comamonas*
      c. *Alcaligenes*
      d. *Achromobacter*
      e. *Acinetobacter*
      f. *Moraxella*
      g. *Kingella*
      h. *Flavobacterium*
      i. *Eikenella*
  C. Coccobacillary
    1. *Haemophilus*
    2. *Bordetella*
    3. *Pasturella*
    4. *Francisella*
    5. *Brucella*
  D. Curved Bacilli
    1. *Campylobacter*
    2. *Spirillum*
  E. Helically Coiled
    1. *Borrelia*
    2. *Treponema*
    3. *Leptospira*
  F. Nonspore-forming—anaerobes
    1. *Bacteroides*
    2. *Fusobacterium*
    3. Anaerobic vibrios

References

1. Stamm WE. Infections related to medical devices. Ann Intern Med 1978;4–69.
2. Wenzel RP, et al. Identification of procedure related nosocomial infections in high risk patients. Rev Inf Dis 1981;3:701–707.
3. Centers for Disease Control. National Nosocomial Infection Study (NNIS) Site Definitions Manual. Atlanta, GA: Centers for Disease Control, 1975.
4. Garner JS, Bennett JV, Scheckler WE, et al. Surveillance of nosocomial infections. In: Proceedings of the International Conference on Nosocomial Infections, Centers for Disease Control, Atlanta, 1970. Chicago: American Hospital Association, 1971:277.
5. Centers for Disease Control. Guidelines for determining presence and classification of infection. Appendix II. In: Outline for Surveillance and Control of Nosocomial Infections. Washington, DC: U.S. Department of Health, Education, and Welfare, 1972.
6. Garner JS, et al. CDC definitions for nosocomial infections, 1988. Am J Infect Control 1988;16:128–140.
7. McGowan JE, Finland M. Infection and antibiotic usage at Boston City Hospital: changes in prevalence during the decade, 1964–1973. J Infect Dis 1974;129:421.
8. Haley RW, et al. Nosocomial infections in U.S. Hospitals, 1975–76. Estimated frequency by selected characteristics of patients. Am J Med 1981;70:947.
9. Centers for Disease Control. Nosocomial infection surveillance, 1980–1982. In: Centers for Disease Control Surveillance Summaries, 1983;32(No. 4SS):1SS.
10. Maki DG. Epidemic nosocomial bacteremias. In Wenzel RP, ed. Handbook of hospital acquired infections. Boca Raton, FL: CRC Press, 1981:401.
11. Stevens RM, et al. Pneumonia in an intensive care unit: a 30-month experience. Arch Intern Med 1974;134:106.
12. Freeman J, McGowan JE. Risk factors in nosocomial infection. J Infect Dis 1978;138:811.
13. Centers for Disease Control. Nosocomial infection surveillance, 1984. In: Centers for Disease Control Surveillance Summaries, 1986;35(No. 1SS):17SS–29SS.
14. Caplan ES, Hoyt N. Infection surveillance and control in the severely traumatized patient. Am J Med 1981;70:638.
15. Donowitz TZ, et al. High risk of hospital-acquired infection in the ICU patient. Crit Care Med 1982;10:355.
16. Horn SD, Bulkey G, Sharkey PD, et al. Interhospital differences in severity of illness. N Engl J Med 1985;313:20–24.
17. Knaus WA, Zimmerman JE, Wagner, et al. APACHE-Acute physiology and chronic health evaluation: a physiologically based classification system. Crit Care Med 1981;9:591–97.
18. Teh TS, Pollack MM, Holbrook PR, et al. Assessment of pediatric intensive care: application of the therapeutic intervention scoring system. Crit Care Med 1982;10:497–500.
19. Daschner FD, et al. Nosocomial infection in intensive care wards. A multicenter prospective study. Intensive Care Med 1982;8:5.
20. Wenzel RP, et al. Hospital acquired infection in intensive care unit patients: an overview with emphasis on epidemics. Infect Control 1983;4:371.
21. Brown RB, et al. A comparison of infections in different ICUs within the same hospital. Crit Care Med 1985;13:472.
22. Hemming VG, et al. Nosocomial infection in a newborn intensive care unit: results of forty-one months of surveillance. N Engl J Med 1976;294:1310.
23. Goldman DA, et al. Nosocomial infections in a neonatal intensive care unit. J Infect Dis 1981;144:449.
24. Wenzel RP, et al. Identification of procedure related nosocomial infection in high risk patients. Rev Infect Dis 1981;3:701.
25. Jarvis WR, Edwards JR, Culver DH, et al. Nosocomial infection rates in adult and pediatric intensive care units in the United States. Am J Medicine 1991;91:185S–191S.
26. Pollock E, et al. Use of the pediatric mortality score to predict nosocomial infection in a pediatric intensive care unit. Crit Care Med 1991;19:160–65.
27. Donowitz LG. High risk of nosocomial infection in the pediatric critical care patient. Crit Care Med 1986;14:26.
28. Welliver RC, et al. Unique epidemiology of nosocomial infection in a children's hospital. Am J Dis Child 1984;138:131.
29. Bowen-Jones J, et al. Nosocomial colonization and infection in a paediatric respiratory intensive care unit. S Afr Med J 1992;82:309–313.
30. Microbial flora of the oral cavity. In Burnett GW, ed. Oral microbiology and infectious disease, ed 4. Baltimore: Williams & Wilkins, 1976, chap 17.
31. Torrey JC, Reese MK. Initial aerobic flora of newborn infants: selective tolerance of upper respiratory tract for bacteria. Am J Dis Child 1945;69:208–14.
32. McCarthy C, Snyder ML, Parker RB. The indigenous oral flora of man. I. The newborn to the 1-year-old infant. Arch Oral Biol 1965;10:61.
33. Socransky SS, Manganiello SD. The oral microbiota of man from birth to senility. J Peridontol 1971;42:485.
34. Sprunt K, Redman W. Evidence suggesting importance of the role of interbacterial inhibition in maintaining balance of normal flora. Ann Intern Med 1968;68:579.
35. Sanders E. Bacterial interference. I. Its occurrence among the respiratory tract flora and characterization of inhibition of group A streptococci by viridans streptococci. J Infect Dis 1969;126:698.
36. Rosenthal S. Tager IB. Prevalence of Gram-negative rods in the normal pharyngeal flora. Ann Intern Med 1975;83:355.
37. LaForce FM, et al. Human oral defenses against Gram-negative rods. Am Rev Respir Dis 1976;114:929.
38. Johanson WG, et al. Bacterial adherence to epithelial cells in bacillary colonization of the respiratory tract. Am Rev Respir Dis 1980;121:55.
39. Mackowiak PA, et al. Pharyngeal colonization by Gram-negative bacilli in aspiration-prone persons. Arch Intern Med 1978;138:1224.
40. Rosenthal S, et al. Prevalence or Gram-negative rods in the normal pharyngeal flora. Ann Intern Med 1975;83:355.
41. Harris H, et al. Endotracheal intubation and its relationship to bacterial colonization and systemic infection of newborn infants. Pediatrics 1976;58:816.
42. Sprunt K, et al. Abnormal colonization and infection in neonates. Pediatr Res 1974;8:429.
43. McCurdy RS, Neter E. Effects of penicillins and broad spectrum antibiotics on the emergence of a Gram-negative bacillary flora in the upper respiratory tract of infants. Pediatrics 1952;572.
44. Johanson WG, Pierce AK, Sanford JP. Changing pharyngeal bacterial flora of hospital patients. Emergence of Gram-negative bacilli. N Engl J Med 1969;281:1137.
45. Valenti WM, et al. Factors predisposing to oropharyngeal colonization with Gram-negative bacilli in the aged. N Engl J Med 1978;298:1108.
46. Weinstein L. The spontaneous occurrence of new bacterial infections during the course of treatment with streptomycin or penicillin. Am J Med Sci 1947;214:56.
47. Weinstein L, et al. Infections occurring during (antibiotic) chemotherapy. A study of their frequency, type and predisposing factors. N Engl J Med 1954;254:247.
48. Louria DB, Kaminski T. The effects of four antimicrobial drug regimens on sputum superinfection in hospitalized patients. Am Rev Respir Dis 1962;85:649.
49. Tillotson JR, Finland M. Bacterial colonization and clinical superinfection of the respiratory tract complicating antibiotic treatment of pneumonia. J Infect Dis 1969;119:597.
50. Weinstein L, Musher DM. Antibiotic-induced suprainfection (Editorial). J Infect Dis 1969;119:662.
51. McGowan JE, Finland M. Infection and antibiotic usage at Boston City Hospital: changes in prevalence during the decade 1964–1973. J Infect Dis 1974;129:421.
52. Selden R, et al. Nosocomial *Klebsiella* infection: intestinal colonization as a reservoir. Ann Intern Med 1971;74:657.
53. Faden H, et al. Changes in nasopharyngeal flora during otitis media of childhood. Pediatr Infect Dis J 1990;9:623–26.
54. Wenzel RP, Veazey JM, Townsend TR. Role of the inanimate environment in hospital-acquired infections. In Cundy KR, Ball W, eds. Infection control in health care facilities: microbiological surveillance. Baltimore: University Park Press, 1977:71.
55. Remington JS, Schimpff SC. Please don't eat the salads. N Engl J Med 1981;304:433.
56. Casewell M, Phillips I. Food as a source of *Klebsiella* species for colonization and infection of intensive care patients. J Clin Pathol 1978;31:845.
57. Favero MS, et al. *Pseudomonas aeruginosa:* growth in distilled water from hospitals. Science 1971;173:836.
58. Aisner J, et al. *Aspergillus* infections in cancer patients. Association with fire proofing materials in a new hospital. JAMA 1976;235:411.
59. Sanders CV, et al. *Serratia marcescens* infection from inhalation therapy medications: nosocomial outbreak. Ann Intern Med 1970;73:15.
60. Morse LJ, et al. Hand lotions—a potential nosocomial hazard. N Engl J Med 1968;278:376.

61. Sheth KJ, et al. *Pseudomonas aeruginosa* otitis externa in an infant associated with a contaminated infant bath sponge. Pediatrics 1986;77:920–921.
62. Forseter G, et al. Blood contamination of tourniquets used in routine phlebotomy. Am J Infection Control 1990;18:386–390.
63. Rutala DR, et al. Infection risks associated with spirometry. Infect Control Hosp Epidem 1991;12:89–92.
64. Simmons B, et al. The role of handwashing in prevention of endemic intensive care unit infections. Infect Control Hosp Epidem 1990;11:589–94.
65. Maki DG, et al. Relation of the inanimate environment to endemic nosocomial infection. N Engl J Med 1982;307:1562.
66. Maki DG. Infections associated with intravascular lines. In: Remington JS, Swartz MN, eds. Current clinical topics in infectious disease. New York: McGraw-Hill, vol 3, 1982:309.
67. Maki DG, Ringer M, Alvarado CJ. Prospective randomized trial of povidone-iodine for prevention of infections associated with central venous and arterial catheters. Lancet 1991;338:339–43.
68. Costerton JW, et al. Practical measures to control device related bacterial infections. Internat J Artificial Organs 1993;18(11):765–70.
69. Marples MJ. Life on the human skin. Sci Am 1969;218:108.
70. Pecora DV, et al. Location of cutaneous microorganisms. Surgery 1968;64:1114.
71. Evans CA, et al. Bacterial flora of the normal human skin. J Invest Dermatol 1950;15:305.
72. Hoshal VL, et. Fibrin sleeve formation on indwelling subclavian central venous catheters. Arch Surg 1971;102:353.
73. Maki DG, et al. Nationwide epidemic of septicemia caused by contaminated intravenous products. I. Epidemiologic and clinical features. Am J Med 1976;60:471.
74. Collins RN, et al. Risk of local and systemic infection with polyethylene intravenous catheters. A prospective study of 213 catheterizations. N Engl J Med 1968;279:340.
75. Lewis G, Hecker JF. Infusion thrombophlebitis. Br J Anaesth 1985;57:220.
76. Neuhof H, Seley GP. Acute suppurative phlebitis complicated by septicemia. Surgery 1946;21:831.
77. Phillips RW, Eyre JD. Septic thrombophlebitis with septicemia. N Engl J Med 1958;259:729.
78. Moncrief JA. Femoral catheters. Ann Surg 1958;166.
79. Bansmer G, Keith D, Tesluk H. Complications following use of indwelling catheters of inferior vena cava. JAMA 1958;167:1606.
80. Crane C. Venous interruption for septic thrombophlebitis. N Engl J Med 1960;262:947.
81. Druskin MS, Siegel PD. Bacterial contamination of indwelling intravenous polyethylene catheters. JAMA 1963;185:966.
82. Moran JM, et al. A clinical and bacteriologic study of infections associated with venous cutdowns. N Engl J Med 1965;272:554.
83. Smits H, Freedman LR. Prolonged venous catheterization as a cause of sepsis. N Engl J Med 1967;276:1229.
84. Zinner SH, et al. Risk of infection with intravenous indwelling catheters: effect of application of antibiotic ointment. J Infect Dis 1969;120:616.
85. Norden CW. Application of antibiotic ointment to the site of venous catheterization—a controlled trial. J Infect Dis 1969;120:611.
86. Peter G, Lloyd-Still JD, Lovejoy FH. Local infection and bacteremia from scalp vein needles and polyethylene catheters in children. J Pediatr 1972;80:78.
87. Lloyd-Still JD, Peter G, Lovejoy FJ. Infected "scalp-vein" needles. JAMA 1970;213:1496.
88. Lowenbraun S, et al. Infection from intravenous "scalp-vein" needles in a susceptible population. JAMA 1970;212:451.
89. Harbin RI, Schaffner W. Septicemia associated with "scalp-vein" needles. South Med J 1973;66:638.
90. Maki DG, Drinka PJ, Davis TF. Suppurative phlebitis of an arm vein from a "scalp-vein" needle. N Engl J Med 1975;292:1116.
91. Irwin GR, Hart RJ, Martin CM. Pathogenesis and prevention of intravenous catheter infections. Yale J Biol Med 1973;46:85.
92. Maki DG, Weise CE, Sarafin HW. A semiquantitative culture method for identifying intravenous-catheter-related infection. N Engl J Med 1977;296:1306.
93. Wing EJ, et al. Use of quantitative bacteriologic techniques to diagnose catheter-related sepsis. Arch Intern Med 1979;139:482.
94. Cleri DJ, Corrado ML, Seligman SJ. Quantitative culture of intravenous catheters and other intravascular inserts. J Infect Dis 1980;141:781.
95. Sitges-Sera A, et al. Catheter sepsis: the clue is the hub. Surgery 1985;97:355.
96. Cooper GL, Hopkins CC. Rapid diagnosis of intravascular catheter-associated infection by direct Gram staining of catheter segments. N Engl J Med 1985;312:1142.
97. McCarty JM, et al. Outbreak of primary cutaneous aspergillosis related to intravenous arm boards. J Pediatr 1986;108:721.
98. Barson WJ, et al. Palmar aspergillosis in immunocompromised children. Pediatr Infect Dis 1986;5:264.
99. Grossman MF, et al. Primary cutaneous aspergillosis in six leukemic children. J Am Acad Dermatol 1985;12:313.
100. Garland JS, et al. Infectious complications during peripheral intravenous therapy with Teflon catheters: a prospective study. Pediatr Infect Dis J 1987;6:918–921.
101. Cronin WA, et al. Intravascular catheter colonization and related bloodstream infection in critically ill neonates. Infect Control Hosp Epidemiol 1990;11:301–308.
102. Smith-Wright DL, et al. Complications of vascular catheterization in critically ill children. Crit Care Med 1984;12:1015.
103. Mortensen JD. Clinical sequelae from arterial needle puncture, cannulation, and incision. Circulation 1967;35:1118.
104. Samaan HA. The hazards of radial artery pressure monitoring. J Thorac Cardiovasc Surg 1971;12:342.
105. Campion BC, et al. Arterial complications of retrograde brachial arterial catheterization. Mayo Clinic Proc 1971;46:589.
106. Bedford RF, Wollman H. Complications of percutaneous radial-artery cannulation: an objective prospective study in man. Anesthesiology 1973;38:228.
107. Ryan JF, et al. Arterial dynamics of radial artery cannulation. Anesth Analg 1973;52:1017.
108. Gardner RM, et al. Percutaneous indwelling radial-artery catheters for monitoring cardiovascular function. Prospective study of the risk of thrombosis and infection. N Engl J Med 1974;290:1227.
109. Wyatt R, Glaves I, Cooper DJ, et al. Proximal skin necrosis after radial-artery cannulation. Lancet 1974;1:1135.
110. Todres ID, Rogers MC, et al. Percutaneous catheterization of the radial artery in the critically ill neonate. J Pediatr 1975;87:273.
111. Goetzman BW, et al. Thrombotic complications of umbilical artery catheters: a clinical and radiographic study. Pediatrics 1975;56:374.
112. Miyasaka K, et al. Complications of radial artery lines in the pediatric patient. Can Anaesth Soc J 1976;23:9.
113. Prian GW. Complications and sequelae of temporal artery catheterization in the high-risk newborn. J Pediatr Surg 1977;12:829.
114. Russel JA, et al. A prospective evaluation of radial and femoral artery catheterization sites in critically ill patients (Abstract). Crit Care Med 1981;9:144.
115. Gaan D, et al. Cerebral damage from declotting Scribner shunts. Lancet 1969;2:77.
116. Matthews JI, Gibbons RB. Embolization complicating radial artery puncture. Adv Intern Med 1971;75:87.
117. Lowenstein E, et al. Prevention of cerebral embolization from flushing radial-artery cannulas. N Engl J Med 1971;285:1414.
118. Adams JM, et al. Bacterial colonization of radial artery catheters. Pediatrics 1980;65:94.
119. Ducharme FM, et al. Incidence of infection related to arterial catheterization in children: a prospective study. Crit Care Med 1990;16:272–276.
120. Michaelson ED, Walsh RE. Osler's node—a complication of prolonged arterial cannulation. N Engl J Med 1970;283:472.
121. Band JD, Maki DG. Infections caused by arterial catheters used for hemodynamic monitoring. Am J Med 1979;67:735.
122. Ersoz CJ, et al. Prolonged femoral arterial catheterization for intensive care. Anesth Analg 1970;49:160.
123. Soderstrom CA, et al. Arterial monitoring catheters: a prospective study of use and complications (Abstract). Crit Care Med 1981;9:203.
124. Russel JA, et al. A prospective evaluation of radial and femoral artery catheterization sites in critically ill patients (Abstract). Crit Care Med 1981;9:144.
125. Grassmick B, et al. Infection and colonization rates of femoral and non-femoral intravascular catheters in the intensive care unit (Abstract). Crit Care Med 1990;18:S208.
126. Thomas F, et al. The risk of infection related to radial vs femoral sites for arterial catheterization. Crit Care Med 1983;11:807.
127. Ducharme FM, et al. Incidence of infection related to arterial catheterization in children: a prospective study. Crit Care Med 1990;16:272–276.
128. Marshall AG, et al. Percutaneous arterial cannulation in children. Anaesthesia 1984;39:27.
129. Glenski JA, et al. A prospective evaluation of femoral artery monitoring in pediatric patients. Anesthesiology 1987;66:227.

130. Graves PW, et al. Femoral artery cannulation for monitoring in critically ill children: prospective study. Crit Care Med 1990;18:1363.
131. Lawless S, Orr R. Axillary arterial monitoring of pediatric patients. Pediatrics 1989;84:2735.
132. Cantwell GP, et al. Percutaneous catheterization of the axillary artery in the pediatric patient. Crit Care Med 1990;18:880–881.
133. Maki DG, et al. Septic endarteritis due to intra-arterial catheters for cancer chemotherapy. I. Evaluation of an outbreak. II. Risk factors, clinical features and management. III. Guidelines for prevention. Cancer 1979;44:1228.
134. Stamm WE, et al. Indwelling arterial catheters as a source of nosocomial bacteremia. An outbreak caused by *Flavobacterium* species. N Engl J Med 1975;292:1099.
135. Walton JR, et al. *Serratia* bacteremia from mean arterial pressure monitors. Anesthesiology 1975;43:113.
136. Weinstein RA, et al. Pressure transducers as a source of bacteremia after open heart surgery. Report of an outbreak and guide for prevention. Chest 1976;69:338.
137. Maki DG, et al. Endemic rate of fluid contamination and septicemia in arterial pressure monitoring. Crit Care Med 1981;9:144.
138. Donowitz LG, et al. *Serratia marcescens* bacteremia from contaminated pressure transducers. JAMA 1979;242:1749.
139. Tenold R, et al. Infection potential of nondisposable pressure transducers prepared prior to use. Crit Care Med 1987;15:582–583.
140. Paulus DA. Disposable transducers. In: Eighth Annual Meeting of Society of Cardiovascular Anesthesiologists (Abstract), 1986:29.
141. Luskin RL, et al. Extended use of disposable pressure transducers. JAMA 1986;255:916.
142. Portner PM, et al. Implantable electrical left ventricular assist system: bridge to transplantation and the future. Ann Thorac Surg 1989;47: 142–150.
143. Farrar DI, et al. Thoratec VAD system as a bridge to heart transplantation. J Heart Transplant 1990;9:415–423.
144. Joyce LD, et al. Results of te first 100 patients who received symbion total artificial hearts as a bridge to cardiac transplantation. Circulation 1989;80 (Supp III):192–201.
145. Miller CA, Pae WE, Pierce WS. Combined registry for the clinical use of mechanical ventricular assist pumps and the total artificial heart in conjunction with heart transplantation. Fourth official report J Heart Transplantation 1989;9:453–458.
146. McBride LR, et al. Device related infections in patients supported with mechanical circulatory support devices for greater than 30 days. ASAID 1991;37:M258–9.
147. Smith BE, et al. Complications of subclavian vein catheterization. Arch Surg 1965;90:228.
148. Christensen KH, et al. Complications of percutaneous catheterization of the subclavian vein in 129 cases. Acta Chir Scand 1967;133:615.
149. Henzel JH, DeWeese MS. Morbid and mortal complications associated with prolonged central venous cannulation. Awareness, recognition, and prevention. Am J Surg 1971;121:600.
150. Rosen M, Latto IP, Ng WS. Handbook of percutaneous central venous catheterization. Philadelphia: WB Saunders, 1981.
151. Bernard RW, et al. Subclavian vein catheterizations: a prospective study. II. Infectious complications. Ann Surg 1971;173:191.
152. Mogensen JV, et al. Subclavian vein catheterization and infection. A bacteriological study of 130 catheter insertions. Scand J Infect Dis 1972;4:31.
153. Michel L, et al. Microbial colonization of indwelling central venous catheters: statistical evaluation of potential contaminating factors. Am J Surg 1979;137:745.
154. Getzen LC, Pollak EW. Short-term femoral vein catheterization. A safe alternative venous access. Am J Surg 1979;138:875.
155. Poole JL. Subclavian vein catheterization for cardiac surgery in children. Anaesth Intensive Care 1980;8:81–83.
156. Eichelberger MR, et al. Percutaneous subclavian venous catheters in neonates and children. J Pediatr Surg 1981;16:547–553.
157. Venkataraman ST, et al. Percutaneous infraclavicular subclavian vein catheterization in critically ill infants and children. J Pediatr 1988;113:480–485.
158. Kanter RK, et al. Central venous catheter insertion by femoral vein: safety and effectiveness for the pediatric patient. Pediatrics 1986;77:842–847.
159. Pruitt BA, et al. Diagnosis and treatment of cannula-related intravenous sepsis in burn patients. Ann Surg 1980;191:546.
160. Saski TM, et al. Burn wound manipulation-induced bacteremia. J Trauma 1979;19:46.
161. Scheld WM, Sande MA. Endocarditis and intravascular infections. In: Mandell GL, Douglas RG, Bennett JE, eds. Principles and practice of infectious diseases. New York: John Wiley & Sons, 1985:520.
162. Berkowitz FE, et al. Suppurative thrombophlebitis: a serious nosocomial infection. Pediatr Infect Dis J 1987;6:64–67.
163. Katz JD, et al. Pulmonary artery flow-guided catheters in the perioperative period. Indications and complications. JAMA 1977;237:2832.
164. Kin YL, et al. Thrombocytopenia associated with Swan-Ganz catheterization in patients. Anesthesiology 1980;53:261.
165. Miller JJ, et al. Comparison of the sterility of long-term central venous catheterization using single lumen, triple lumen, and pulmonary artery catheters. Crit Care Med 1984;12:634.
166. Applefeld JJ, et al. Assessment of the sterility of longterm cardiac catheterization using the thermodilution Swan-Ganz catheter. Chest 1978;74:377.
167. Elliott CG, et al. Complications of pulmonary artery catheterization in the care of critically ill patients. A prospective study. Chest 1979;176:647.
168. Michel L, et al. Infection of pulmonary artery catheters in critically ill patients. JAMA 1981;245:1032.
169. Kelly CS, et al. Sepsis due to triple lumen central venous catheters. Surg Gynecol Obstet 1986;163:14.
170. Guidet B, et al. Skin versus hub culture to predict colonization and infection of central venous catheters in intensive care patients. Infection 1994;22:43–48.
171. Damen J, et al. Positive tip cultures and related risk factors associated with intravascular catheterization in pediatric cardiac patients. Crit Care Med 1988; 16:221–228.
172. Garrison P, Freedman LR. Experimental endocarditis. I. Staphylococcal endocarditis in rabbits resulting from placement of a polyethylene catheter in the right side of the heart. Yale J Biol Med 1970;42:394.
173. Greene JF, et al. Aseptic thrombotic endocardial vegetations. A complication of indwelling pulmonary artery catheters. JAMA 1973; 225:1525.
174. Greene JF, et al. Aseptic endocarditis and indwelling pulmonary artery catheters. JAMA 1975;233:891.
175. Pace NL, Horton W. Indwelling pulmonary artery catheters. Their relationship to aseptic thrombotic endocardial vegetations. JAMA 1975;233:893.
176. Lange HW, et al. Local complications associated with indwelling Swan-Ganz catheters: Autopsy study of 36 cases. Am J Cardiol 1983;52:1108.
177. Ducatman BS, et al. Catheter induced lesions of the right side of the heart. A one year prospective study of 141 autopsies. JAMA 1985;253:791.
178. Ehrie M, et al. Endocarditis with the indwelling balloon-tipped pulmonary artery catheter in burn patients. J Trauma 1978;18:664.
179. Rowley KM, et al. Right-sided infective endocarditis as a consequence of flow-directed pulmonary-artery catheterization. A clinicopathological study of 55 autopsied patients. N Engl J Med 1984;311:1152.
180. Noel GA, et al. Neonatal *Staphylococcus epidermidis* right-sided endocarditis: description of five catheterized infants. Pediatrics 1988; 82:234–239.
181. Damen J, et al. Microbiologic risk of invasive hemodynamic monitoring in patients undergoing open-heart operations. Crit Care Med 1985; 13:548.
182. Allen JR. The incidence of nosocomial infection in patients receiving total parenteral nutrition. In: Johnston IDA, ed. Advances in parenteral nutrition. Lancaster: MTP Press, 1978, chap 23.
183. Cohen IT, et al. Peripheral total parenteral nutrition employing a lipid emulsion (Intralipid): complications encountered in pediatric patients. J Pediatr Surg 1977;12:837.
184. Ziegler M, et al. Route of pediatric parenteral nutrition: proposed criteria revision. J Pediatr Surg 1980;15:472.
185. Andolina AS. Septic complications. In: Kerner JA, ed. Manual of pediatric parenteral nutrition. New York: John Wiley & Sons, 1983, chap 14.
186. Sanders RA, Sheldon GF. Septic complications of total parenteral nutrition. A five year experience. Am J Surg 1976;132:214.
187. McKee KT, et al. Gram-negative bacillary sepsis associated with use of lipid emulsion in parenteral nutrition. Am J Dis Child 1979;133:649.
188. Jarvis WR, et al. Polymicrobial bacteremia associated with lipid emulsion in a neonatal intensive care unit. Pediatr Infect Dis 1983;2:203.
189. Ashcraft KW, Leape LL. *Candida* sepsis complicating parenteral feeding. JAMA 1970;212:454.
190. Curry CR, Quie PG. Fungal septicemia in patients receiving parenteral hyperalimentation. N Engl J Med 1971;285:1221.
191. Helmuth WV, et al. The effects of protein hydrolysate monosaccharide infusion on low-birth-weight infants. J Pediatr 1972;81:129.

192. Montgomerie JZ, Edwards JE. Association of infection due to *Candida albicans* with intravenous hyperalimentation. J Infect Dis 1978;137:197.
193. Henderson DK, et al. Hematogenous *Candida* endophthalmitis in patients receiving parenteral hyperalimentation fluids. J Infect Dis 1981;143:655.
193a. Pockros PJ, Silberman H. Parenteral nutrition complicated by candidiasis (Letter to the Editor). J Infect Dis 1982;145:592.
194. Sanders RA, Sheldon GF. Septic complications of total parenteral nutrition. A five year experience. Am J Surg 1976;132:214.
195. Sitges-Serra A, et al. Catheter sepsis due to *Staphylococcus epidermidis* during parenteral nutrition. Surg Gynecol Obstet 1980;151:481.
196. Armstrong CW, et al. Infectious complications of hyperalimentation (Abstract 861). In: Twenty-First Interscience Conference on Antimicrobial Agents and Chemotherapy, Chicago, November 1981.
197. Prince A, et al. Management of fever in patients with central vein catheters. Pediatr Infect Dis 1986;5:20.
198. Flynn PM, et al. In situ management of confirmed central venous catheter-related bacteremia. Pediatr Infect Dis J 1987;6:729–734.
199. Hoshal VL, et al. Fibrin sleeve formation on indwelling subclavian central venous catheters. Arch Surg 1971;102:353.
200. Bailey MJ. Reduction of catheter-associated sepsis in parenteral nutrition using low-dose intravenous heparin. Br Med J 1979;1:1671.
201. Brismar B, et al. Reduction of catheter-associated thrombosis in parenteral nutrition by intravenous heparin therapy. Arch Surg 1982; 117:1196.
202. Alpan G, et al. Heparinization of alimentation solutions administered through peripheral veins in premature infants: a controlled study. Pediatrics 1984;74:375.
203. Broviac JW, et al. A silicone rubber arterial catheter for prolonged parenteral alimentation. Surg Gynecol Obstet 1973;136:602.
204. Hickman RO, et al. A modified right atrial catheter for access to the venous system in marrow transplant recipients. Surg Gynecol Obstet 1979;148:871.
205. Clift RA, et al. Infectious complications of marrow transplantation. Transplant Proc 1974;6:389.
206. Winston DJ, et al. Infectious complications of human bone marrow transplantation. Medicine 1979;58:1.
207. The European Organization for Research on Treatment of Cancer, International Antimicrobial Therapy Project Group. Three antibiotic regimens in the treatment of infection in febrile granulocytopenic patients with cancer. J Infect Dis 1978;137:14.
208. Lowder JN, et al. Bacteremias and fungemias in oncologic patients with central venous catheters. Changing spectrum of infection. Arch Intern Med 1982;142:1456.
209. Shapiro Ed, et al. Broviac catheter-related bacteremia in oncology patients. Am J Dis Child 1982;136:679.
210. Johnson PR, et al. Frequency of Broviac catheter infections in pediatric oncology patients. J Infect Dis 1986;154:570.
211. Trooskin SZ, et al. Prevention of catheter sepsis by antibiotic binding. Surgery 1985;97:547.
212. Armstrong CW, et al. Clinical predictors of infection of central venous catheters used for total parenteral nutrition. Infect Control Hosp Epidemiol 1990;11:71–78.
213. Brothers TE, et al. Experience with subcutaneous infusion ports in three hundred patients. Surg Gynecol Obstet 1988;166:295–301.
214. Wallace J, et al. Benefits, complications and care of implantable infusion devices in 31 children with cancer. J Pediatr Surg 1987;22: 833–838.
215. Ross HN, et al. Comparison of totally implanted reservoirs with external catheters as venous access devices in pediatric oncologic patients. Surg Gynecol Obstet 1988;167:141–144.
216. Morris JB, et al. Totally implantable vascular access devices in cystic fibrosis: a four-year experience with fifty-eight patients. J Pediatr 1990;117:82–85.
217. Kahn ML, Barboza RB, Kling GA, Heisel JE. Initial experience with percutaneous placement of the PAS port implantable venous access device. JVIR 1992;3:459–61.
218. Carey PC, et al. Long-term circulatory access via a peripheral implantable port. Br J Surg 1993;80:600–601.
219. Dato VM, et al. Candidemia in children with central venous catheters: role of catheter removal and amphotericin B therapy. Pediatr Infect Dis J 1990;9:309–314.
220. Raucher HS, et al. Quantitative blood cultures in the evaluation of septicemia in children with Broviac catheters. J Pediatr 1984;104:29–33.
221. Wing EJ, et al. Use of quantitative bacteriologic techniques to diagnose catheter-related sepsis. Arch Intern Med 1979;139:482–483.
222. Nichols WK. Vascular access. In VanStone JC, ed. Dialysis and the treatment of renal insufficiency. Chap 7. New York: Grune & Stratton, 1983:143.
223. Bell PRF, Wood RFM. External arteriovenous shunts. In: Bell PRF, Wood RFM, eds. Surgical aspects of haemodialysis. Chap 4. London: Churchill Livingstone, 1985:18.
224. Raja RM, et al. Subclavian vein and femoral vein catheterization for hemodialysis—one year comparison. Trans Am Soc Artif Intern Organs 1982;28:58.
225. Cheesbrough JS, et al. A prospective study of the mechanisms of infection associated with hemodialysis catheters. J Infect Dis 1986; 154:579.
226. Wagnild JP, et al. *Pseudomonas aeruginosa* bacteremia in a dialysis unit. II. Relationship to reuse of coils. Am J Med 1977;62:672.
227. Kuehnel EG. Outbreak of *Pseudomonas cepacia* bacteremia in a dialysis unit related to contaminated reused coils (Abstract). Clin Res 1975;23:466A.
228. Goetz A, et al. *Pseudomonas stutzeri* bacteremia associated with hemodialysis. Arch Intern Med 1983;143:1909.
229. Blagg CE, et al. Microbial contamination of water used for hemodialysis. Nephron 1975;15:81.
230. Favero MS, et al. Factors that influence microbial contamination of fluids associated with hemodialysis machines. Appl Environ Microbiol 1974;28:822.
231. Kidd EE. Bacterial contamination of dialysis fluid of artificial kidney. Br Med J 1964;1:880.
232. Jones DM, et al. Bacteriological studies of the modified Kiil dialyser. Br Med J 1970;3:135.
233. Maher JF, Schreiner GE. Hazards and complications of dialysis. N Engl J Med 1965;273:370.
234. Cossart YE, et al. Infection risks of haemodialysis—some preventive aspects. A report to the public health laboratory service by the working party on haemodialysis units. Br Med J 1968;3:454.
235. Hindman SJ, et al. Pyrogenic reactions during haemodialysis caused by extramural endotoxin. Lancet 1975;2:732.
236. Raij L, et al. Endotoxemia in febrile reactions during hemodialysis. Kidney Int 1973;4:57.
237. Uman SJ, et al. *Pseudomonas aeruginosa* bacteremia in a dialysis unit. I. Recognition of cases, epidemiologic studies and attempts at control. Am J Med 1977;82:667.
238. Nsouli KA, et al. Bacteremic infection in hemodialysis. Arch Intern Med 1979;139:1255.
239. Kaslow RA, Zellner SR. Infection in patients on maintenance haemodialysis. Lancet 1972;2:117.
240. Leone MR, MeEnery PT. Infection in the child receiving therapy from ESRD. In: Fine RN, Gruskin AB, eds. End stage renal disease in children. Philadelphia: WB Saunders, 1984:416.
241. Martin AM, et al. The aetiology and management of shunt infections in patients on intermittent haemodialysis. In: Dialysis and renal transplantation. Proceedings of the European Dialysis and Transplant Association. Vol 4, 1967:67.
242. Kuruvila KC, Beven EG. Arteriovenous shunts and fistulas for hemodialysis. Surg Clin North Am 1971;51:1219.
243. Curtis JR, et al. Maintenance hemodialysis. Q J Med 1969;149:49.
244. Byrne JP, et al. Advantages of surgical arteriovenous fistulas for hemodialysis. Arch Surg 1971;102:359.
245. McIntosh CS, et al. Maintenance of Silastic-Teflon shunts for intermittent haemodialysis. Br Med J 1969;4:717.
246. Farooki MS, et al. External arteriovenous shunts for intermittent long-term hemodialysis: five years' experience. Can Med Assoc J 1970; 103:1371.
247. Franzone AJ, et al. Hemodialysis in children. Experience with arteriovenous shunts. Arch Surg 1972;102:592.
248. Ralston AJ, et al. Infections of Scribner and Brescia arteriovenous shunts. Br Med J 1971;3:408.
249. Barcenas CG, et al. Staphylococcal sepsis in patients on chronic hemodialysis regimens. Intravenous treatment with vancomycin given once weekly. Arch Intern Med 1976;136:1131.
250. Foran RF, et al. Quinton-Scribner cannulas for hemodialysis. Review of four years' experience. Calif Med (West J Med) 1970;112:8.
251. Zeitlin J, et al. Graft infection and bacteremia with *Listeria monocytogenes* in a patient receiving hemodialysis. Arch Intern Med 1982;142:2191.
252. Cross AS, Steigbigel RY. Infective endocarditis and access site infections in patients on hemodialysis. Medicine 1976;55:453.
253. Francioli P, et al. Complications of *Staphylococcus aureus* bacteremia. Occurrence in patients undergoing long-term hemodialysis. Arch Intern Med 1982;142:1655.

254. Leonard A, et al. Bacterial endocarditis in regularly dialyzed patients. Kidney Int 1973;4:407.
255. Kirmani N, et al. *Staphylococcus aureus* carriage rate of patients receiving long-term hemodialysis. Arch Intern Med 1978;138:1657.
256. Yu VL, et al. *Staphylococcus aureus* nasal carriage and infection in patients on hemodialysis. N Engl J Med 1986;315:91.
257. Reed WP, et al. Bacterial colonization of Hemasite access devices. Surgery 1986;99:308.
258. Dobkin JF, et al. Septicemia in patients on chronic hemodialysis. Ann Intern Med 1978;88:28.
259. Bartlett RH. Extracorporeal life support for cardiopulmonary failure. Curr Probl Surg 1990;27:623–704.
260. Cornish JD, et al. Complications of neonatal extracorporeal membrane oxygenation. J Pediatr 1990;116: 1005–1006.
261. O'Rourke PP, et al. The effect of extracorporeal membrane oxygenation on the survival of neonates with high-risk congenital diaphragmatic hernia: 45 cases from a single institution. J Pediatr Surg 1991;26:147–152.
262. Stolar CJ, et al. Extracorporeal membrane oxygenation and neonatal respiratory failure: experience from the extracorporeal life support organization. J Pediatr Surg 1991;26:563–571.
263. Wetterberg T, et al. Total extracorporeal lung assist—a new clinical approach. Intensive Care Med 1991;17:73–77.
264. Berry FA, et al. A comparison of bacteremia occurring with nasotracheal and endotracheal intubation. Anesth Analg 1973;52:873.
265. McShane AJ, et al. Prevention of bacterial endocarditis: nasal intubation warrants prophylactic antibiotics. In: Eighth Annual Meeting of Society of Cardiovascular Anesthesiologists, 1986:83 (Abstract).
266. Berry FA, et al. Transient bacteremia during dental manipulation in children. Pediatrics 1973;51:476.
267. LeFrock JL, et al. Transient bacteremia associated with nasotracheal suctioning. Clin Res 1974;22:646.
268. Burman SO. Bronchoscopy and bacteremia. J Thorac Cardiovasc Surg 1960;40:635.
269. Arens JF, et al. Maxillary sinusitis: a complication of nasotracheal intubation. Anesthesiology 1974;40:415.
270. Gallagher TJ, Civetta JM. Acute maxillary sinusitis complicating nasotracheal intubation: a case report. Anesth Analg 1976;55:885.
271. Pope TL, et al. Maxillary sinusitis after nasotracheal intubation. South Med J 1981;74:610.
272. Caplan ES, Hoyt NJ. Nosocomial sinusitis. JAMA 1982;247:639.
273. Berman SA, et al. Otitis media in the neonatal intensive care unit. Pediatrics 1978;62:198.
274. Bos AP, et al. Sinusitis: hidden source of sepsis in post-operative pediatric intensive care patients. Crit Care Med 1989;17:886–888.
275. Evans FO, et al. Sinusitis of the maxillary antrum. N Engl J Med 1975;293:735.
276. Hamory BH, et al. Etiology and antimicrobial therapy of acute maxillary sinusitis. J Infect Dis 139:197.
277. Wald ER, et al. Acute maxillary sinusitis in children. N Engl J Med 1981;304:749.
278. Ommelslag D, et al. Eye infections caused by respiratory pathogens in mechanically ventilated patients. Crit Care Med 1987;15:80.
279. Veazey JM. Hospital acquired pneumonia. In Wenzel RP, ed. Handbook of hospital acquired infections. Boca Raton, FL: CRC Press, 1981:341.
280. Sanford JP, Pierce AK. Lower respiratory tract infections. In: Bennett JV, Brachman PS, eds. Hospital infections. Boston: Little, Brown, 1979:255.
281. Graybill JR, et al. Nosocomial pneumonia. A continuing problem. Am Rev Respir Dis 1973;108:1130.
282. Andrews CP, et al. Diagnosis of nosocomial bacterial pneumonia in acute diffuse lung injury. Chest 1981;80:254.
283. Stevens RM, et al. Pneumonia in an intensive care unit. A 30 month experience. Arch Intern Med 1974;134:106.
284. Donowitz LG, et al., ed. Hospital-acquired infection in the pediatric patient. Baltimore: Williams & Wilkins, 1988.
285. Centers for Disease Control. Measles surveillance, Report #11, 1977–1981:28 (issued 9/82).
286. LeClair JM, et al. Airborne transmission of chicken pox in a hospital. N Engl J Med 1980;302:450.
287. Morens DM, et al. An outbreak of varicella zoster virus infections among cancer patients. Ann Intern Med 1980;93:414.
288. Wenzel RP, et al. Hospital-acquired viral respiratory illness on a pediatric ward. Pediatrics 1977;60:367.
289. Kapila R, et al. A nosocomial outbreak of influenza A. Chest 1977;71:576.
290. Meibalane R, et al. Outbreak of influenza in a neonatal intensive care unit. J Pediatr 1977;91:974.
291. Hall CB, Douglas RG. Nosocomial influenza infection as a cause of intercurrent fever in infants. Pediatrics 1975;55:673.
292. Hall CB, Nosocomial viral respiratory infections: perennial weeds on pediatric wards. Am J Med 1981;70:670.
293. MacDonald NE, et al. Respiratory syncytial virus infection in infants with congenital heart disease. N Engl J Med 1982;307:397.
294. Hall CB, et al. Modes of transmission of respiratory syncytial virus. J Pediatr 1981;99:100.
295. Sims DG, et al. Hospital cross-infection on children's wards with respiratory syncytial virus and the role of adult carriage. Acta Pediatr Scand 1975;64:541.
296. Hall CB, et al. Control of nosocomial respiratory syncytial viral infections. Pediatrics 1978;62:728.
297. Glezen WP. Viral pneumonia as a cause and result of hospitalization. J Infect Dis 1983;147:765.
298. Gardner PS, et al. Virus cross-infection in pediatric wards. Br Med J 1973;2:571.
299. Rose HD, et al. Meningococcal pneumonia. A source of nosocomial infection. Arch Intern Med 1981;141:575.
300. Riley RL, et al. Infectiousness of air from a tuberculosis ward. Am Rev Respir Dis 1962;84:511.
301. Kurt TL, et al. Spread of pertussis by hospital staff. JAMA 1972; 221:264.
302. Feigin RD, Stechenberg BW. Diphtheria. In: Feigin RD, Cherry JD, eds. Textbook of pediatric infectious diseases. Philadelphia: WB Saunders, 1981:852.
303. Singer C, et al. *Pneumocystis carinii* pneumonia: a cluster of 11 cases. Ann Intern Med 1975;82:772.
304. Ruebush JK, et al. An outbreak of *Pneumocystis* pneumonia in children with acute lymphocytic leukemia. Am J Dis Child 132:143, 1978.
305. Pifer L, et al. *Pneumocystis carinii* infection: evidence for high prevalence in normal and immunosuppressed children. Pediatrics 1978;61:35.
306. England AC, et al. Sporadic and epidemic nosocomial legionellosis in the United States. Epidemiologic features. Am J Med 1981;70:707.
307. Kirby BD, et al. Legionnaires disease: report of sixty-five nosocomially acquired cases and reviews of the literature. Medicine (Baltimore) 1980;59:188.
308. Melish ME. Staphylococcal infections. In: Feigin RD, Cherry JD, eds. Textbook of pediatric infectious diseases. Philadelphia: WB Saunders, 1981:968.
309. Jacobs Rf. Nosocomial pneumonia in children. Infection 1991;19: 64–72.
310. Winterbauer HR, et al. New diagnostic approaches to the hospitalized patient with pneumonia. Semin Respir Infect 1987;2:57–66.
311. Barzilay Z, et al. Nosocomial bacterial pneumonia in ventilated children: clinical significance of culture-positive peripheral bronchial aspirates. J Pediatr 1988;112:421–24.
312. McDonald IH, Stocks JG. Prolonged nasotracheal intubation: a review of its development in a pediatric hospital. Br J Anaesth 1965;37:161.
313. Markham WG, et al. Prolonged nasotracheal intubation in infants and children. Can Anaesth Soc J 1967;14:11.
314. Abbott TR. Complications of prolonged nasotracheal intubation in children. Br J Anaesth 1968;40:347.
315. Allen TH, Steven IM. Prolonged endotracheal intubation in infants and children. Br J Anaesth 1965;37:566.
316. Harrison GA, Tonkin JP. Prolonged (therapeutic) endotracheal intubation. Br J Anaesth 1968;40:241.
317. Mattila MA, et al. Prolonged endotracheal intubation or tracheostomy in infants and children. J Pediatr Surg 1969;4:674.
318. Atherton ST, White DJ. Stomach as the source of bacteria colonizing respiratory tract during artificial ventilation. Lancet 1978;2:968.
319. Schwartz SN, et al: Sources of Gram-negative bacilli colonizing the trachea of intubated patients. J Infect Dis 1978;138:227.
320. Pugin J, et al. Oropharyngeal decontamination decreases incidence of ventilator-associated pneumonia. A randomized, placebo-controlled, double-blind clinical trial. JAMA 1991;265:2704–2710.
321. Bernhard WN, et al. Intracuff pressures in endotracheal and tracheostomy tubes. Chest 1985;87:720.
322. Friedberg SA, et al. Histologic changes in the trachea following tracheostomy. Ann Otol Rhinol Laryngol 1965;74:787.
323. Way WL, Sooy RA. Histologic changes produced by endotracheal intubation. Ann Otol Rhinol Laryngol 1965;74:799.
324. Lindholm CE. Prolonged endotracheal intubation. Acta Anaesthesiol Scand (Suppl) 1969;33:1.
325. Rubbo SD, et al. Source of *Pseudomonas aeruginosa* infection in premature infants. J Hyg Camb 1966;64:121.

326. Becker AH. Infection due to *Proteus mirabilis* in a newborn nursery. Am J Dis Child 1962;104:69.
327. Fierer J, et al. *Pseudomonas aeruginosa* epidemic traced to delivery room resuscitators. N Engl J Med 1967;276:991.
328. Klick JM, et al. An oxygen analyzer as a source of *Pseudomonas.* Anesthesiology 1978;49:293.
329. Ringrose RE, et al. A hospital outbreak of *Serratia marcescens* associated with ultrasonic nebulizers. Ann Intern Med 1968;69:719.
330. Moffett HL, Allan D. Colonization of infants exposed to bacterially contaminated mists. Am J Dis Child 1967;114:21.
331. Grieble HG, et al. Fine particle humidifiers: source of *Pseudomonas aeruginosa* infections in a respiratory disease unit. N Engl J Med 1970;282:531.
332. Sanders CV, et al. *Serratia marcescens* infections from inhalation therapy medications: nosocomial outbreak. Ann Intern Med 1970;73:15.
333. Mertz JJ, et al. A hospital outbreak of *Klebsiella* pneumoniae from inhalation therapy with contaminated aerosol solutions. Am Rev Respir Dis 1966;94:454.
334. Pierce AK, Sanford JP. Bacterial contamination of aerosols. Arch Intern Med 1973;131:156.
335. Rewarz JA, et al. The potential role of inhalation therapy equipment in nosocomial pulmonary infection. J Clin Invest 1965;44:831.
336. Pierce AK, et al. Long-term evaluation of decontamination of inhalation therapy equipment and the occurrence of necrotizing pneumonia. N Engl J Med 1970;282:528.
337. Meeks CH, et al. Sterilization of anesthesia apparatus. JAMA 1967;199:276.
338. Craven DE, et al. Contamination of mechanical ventilators with tubing changes every 24 or 48 hours. N Engl J Med 1982;306:1505.
339. Teres D, et al. Sources of *Pseudomonas aeruginosa* infection in a respiratory surgical intensive-therapy unit. Lancet 1973;1:415.
340. Deane RS, et al. Antibacterial action of copper in respiratory therapy apparatus. Chest 1970;58:573.
341. Craven DE, et al. Contaminated medication nebulizers in mechanical ventilator circuits: Source of bacterial aerosols. Am J Med 1984; 77:834.
342. Hess D, et al. Weekly ventilator circuit changes. A strategy to reduce costs without affecting pneumonia rates. Anesthesiology 1995;82: 903–911.
343. Salzman TC, et al. Hand contamination of personnel as a mechanism of cross-infection in nosocomial infections with antibiotic-resistant *Escherichia coli* and *Klebsiella-Aerobacter.* Antimicrob Agents Chemother 1967;7:97.
344. Knittle MA, et al. Role of hand contamination of personnel in the epidemiology of Gram-negative nosocomial infections. J Pediatr 1975;86:433.
345. Rosendorf LL, et al. Sources of Gram-negative infection after open-heart surgery. J Thorac Cardiovasc Surg 1974;67:195.
346. Casewell M, et al. Hands as route of transmission for *Klebsiella* species. Br Med J 1977;2:1315.
347. Doebbeling BN, et al. Comparative efficacy of alternative hand washing agents in reducing nosocomial infections in intensive care patients. NEJM 1992;327:88–93.
348. Morse LJ, et al. Septicemia due to *K. pneumoniae* originating from a handcream dispenser. N Engl J Med 1967;277:472.
349. Payne RW. Severe outbreak of surgical sepsis due to *Staphylococcus aureus* of unusual type and origin. Br Med J 1967;4:17.
350. Meers PD, Foster CS, Churcher GM, et al. Cross infection with *Serratia marcescens.* Br Med J 1978;1:328.
351. Buxton AE, et al. Nosocomial respiratory tract infection and colonization with *Acinetobacter calcoaceticus:* epidemiologic characteristics. Am J Med 1978;65:507.
352. Albert RK, Condie F. Hand-washing patterns in medical intensive care units. N Engl J Med 1981;304:1465.
353. Ramphal R, et al. Adherence of *Pseudomonas aeruginosa* to tracheal cells injured by influenza infection or by endotracheal intubation. Infect Immun 1980;27:614.
354. Goodwin Sr, Graves SA. Aspiration in intubated premature infants. Pediatrics 1985;75:85.
355. Browning DH, Graves SA. Incidence of aspiration with endotracheal tubes in children. J Pediatr 1983;102:582.
356. DuMoulin GC, et al. Aspiration of gastric bacteria in antacid-treated patients: a frequent cause of post-operative colonization of the airway. Lancet 1982;1:242.
357. Craven DE, et al. Nosocomial pneumonia in the 1990's: Update of epidemiology and risk factors. Sem Resp Infect 1990;5:157–72.
358. Craven DE, Steger KA, Barber TW. Preventing nosocomial pneumonia: state of the art and perspectives for the 1990's. AM J Med 1991;91: 44S–53S.
359. Frost EAM. Tracing the tracheostomy. Ann Otol 1976;85:618.
360. Snow N, et al. Management of necrotizing tracheostomy infections. J Thorac Cardiovasc Surg 1981;82:341.
361. Bryant LR, et al. Bacterial colonization profile with tracheal intubation and mechanical ventilation. Arch Surg 1972;104:647.
362. Meade JW. Tracheostomy—its complications and their management: a study of 12 cases. N Engl J Med 1961;265:519.
363. Chew JY, et al. Tracheostomy. Complications and their management. Arch Otolaryngol 1972;96:538.
364. Gotsman MS, et al. Respiratory infection following tracheostomy. Thorax 1964;19:89.
365. Skaggs JA, et al. Tracheostomy management, mortality, complications. Am J Surg 1969;35:393.
366. Oliver P, et al. Tracheostomy in children. N Engl J Med 1962;267:631.
367. Stool SE, et al. Tracheostomy in children: the use of plastic tubes. J Pediatr Surg 1968;3:402.
368. Reading P. Some postoperative hazards in tracheostomy on infants. J Laryngol Otol 1958;72:785.
369. Glover WJ. Nasotracheal intubation and tracheostomy in intensive care in infants. Acta Anaesthesiol Scand (Suppl) 1970;37:62.
370. Aberdeen E. Downes JJ. Artificial airways in children. Surg Clin North Am 1974;54:1155.
371. Stiles PJ. Tracheal lesions after tracheostomy. Thorax 1965;20:517.
372. Aass AS. Complications to tracheostomy and long term intubation: a follow-up study. Acta Anaesthesiol Scand 1975;19:127.
373. Bartlett JG, et al. Quantitative tracheal bacteriologic and cytologic studies in patients with long-term tracheostomies. Chest 1978;74:635.
374. Niederman MS, et al. Respiratory infection complicating long-term tracheostomy: the implication of persistent Gram-negative tracheobronchial colonization. Chest 1984;85:39.
375. Brook I. Bacterial colonization, tracheobronchitis and pneumonia following tracheostomy and long-term intubation in pediatric patients. Chest 1979;76:420.
376. Donnelly BW, McMillan JA, Weiner LB. Bacterial tracheitis: report of 8 new cases and review. Rev Inf Dis 1990;12(5):729–35.
377. Conley SF, et al. Measles-associated bacterial tracheitis. Ped Inf Dis J 1993;12:414–15.
378. Farber HJ, Berg RA. Bacterial tracheitis as a complication of endotracheal intubation. Ped Pulmonology 1991;11:87–89.
379. Walker P, Crysdale WS. Croup, epiglottis, retropharyngeal abscess, and bacterial tracheitis: evolving patterns of occurrence and care. International Anesthesia Clinics 1992;30:57–70.
380. Rojas J, Flanigan TH. Post intubation tracheitis in the newborn. Ped Inf Dis 1986;5:714–15.
381. Sofer S, Dagan R, Tal A. The need for intubation in serious upper respiratory tract infection in pediatric patients. Infection 1991;129: 131–34.
382. Sofer S, et al. Bacterial tracheitis: an old disease rediscovered. Clin Pediatr 1983;22:407–11.
383. Dudin AK, et al. Bacterial tracheitis among children hospitalized for severe obstructive dyspnea. Pediatr Infect Dis J 1990;9:293–295.
384. Ernst TN, et al. Bacterial tracheitis caused by *Branhamella catarrhalis.* Pediatr Infect Dis J 1987;6:574.
385. Park JW. Bacterial tracheitis caused by *Streptococcus agalactiae.* Pediatr Infect Dis J 1990;6:450–451.
386. Centers for Disease Control. National Nosocomial Infections Study Report. Annual Summary 1976, February 1978.
387. Centers for Disease Control. National Nosocomial Infection Study Report. Annual Summary 1979, March 1982.
388. Givens CD, Wenzel RP. Catheter-associated urinary tract infections in surgical patients: a controlled study on the excess morbidity and costs. J Urol 1980;24:646.
389. Martinez OV, et al. Bacteriuria in the catheterized surgical intensive care patient. Crit Care Med 1986;14:188.
390. Dodge WF, West EF, Travis LB. Bacteriuria in school children. Am J Dis Child 1974;127:364.
391. Kunin CM, Deutscher R, Paquin A. Urinary tract infection in school children: an epidemiologic, clinical and laboratory study. Medicine 1964;143:91.
392. Edelman CM, Ogwo JE, Fine BP, Martinez AG. The prevalence of bacteriuria in full-term and premature newborn infants. J Pediatr 1973;82:125.
393. Maherzi M, Guignard J, Torrado A. Pediatrics 1978;62:521.
394. Stamey TA. Pathogenesis and treatment of urinary tract infections. Baltimore: Williams & Wilkins, 1980:290.

395. Remington JS, Klein JO. Infectious diseases of the fetus and newborn infant. Philadelphia: WB Saunders, 1983:771.
396. Littlewood JM, Kite P, Kite BA. Incidence of neonatal urinary tract infection. Arch Dis Child 1969;44:617.
397. Kasian GF, et al. Bacteriologic surveillance of indwelling urinary catheters in pediatric intensive care unit patients. Crit Care Med 1988;16:679–682.
398. Stamey TA, Govan DE, Palmer JM. The localization and treatment of urinary tract infections: the role of bactericidal urine levels as opposed to serum levels. Medicine 1965;44:1.
399. Kass EH. Asymptomatic infections of the urinary tract. Trans Assoc Am Physicians 1956;69:56.
400. Kraft JK, Stamey TA. The natural history of symptomatic recurrent bacteriuria in women. Medicine 1977;56:55.
401. Stamey TA. Pathogenesis and treatment of urinary tract infections. Baltimore: Williams & Wilkins, 1980:7.
402. Turck M, Goffe B, Petersdorf RG. The urethral catheter and urinary tract infection. J Urol 1962;88:834.
403. Kaye M, de Vries J, MacFarlane KT. The initiation of urinary tract infection following a single bladder catheterization. Can Med Assoc J 1962;86:9.
404. Wenzel RP. CRC handbook of hospital acquired infections. Boca Raton, FL: CRC Press, 1981:513.
405. Garibaldi RA, Burke JP, Dickman ML, Smith CB. Factors predisposing to bacteriuria during indwelling urethral catheterization. N Engl J Med 1974;291:215.
406. Platt R. Polk BF, Murdock B, Rosner B. Outcome of low density microbial growth during indwelling bladder catheterization (Abstract 196). In: Program and Abstracts of the Twenty-Second Interscience Conference on Antimicrobial Agents and Chemotherapy. Chicago, 1982:100.
407. Stark RP, Maki DG. Bacteriuria in the catheterized patient. What quantitative level of bacteriuria is relevant? N Engl J Med 1984;311:560.
408. Lohr JA, et al. Bacterial contamination rates in voided urine collections in girls. J Pediatr 1989;114:91–93.
409. Saez-Llorens X, et al. Bacterial contamination rates for non-clean-catch and clean-catch midstream urine collections in uncircumcised boys. J Pediatr 1989; 114:934–995.
410. Beeson PB. The case against the catheter. Am J Med 1958;24:1.
411. Dukes C. Urinary infections after excision of the rectum: their cause and prevention. Proc R Soc Med 1928;22:1.
412. Guze LB, Beeson PB. Observations on the reliability and safety of bladder catheterization for bacteriologic study of the urine. N Engl J Med 1956;255:474.
413. Helmholz HF. Determination of the bacterial content of the urethra: a new method, with results of a study of 82 men. J Urol 1950;64:158.
414. Cox CE. The urethra and its relationship to urinary tract infection: the flora of the normal female urethra. South Med J 1966;59:621.
415. Turck M, Goffe B, Petersdorf RG. The urethral catheter and urinary tract infection. J Urol 1962;88:834.
416. Kass EH, Schneiderman LJ. Entry of bacteria into the urinary tracts of patients with inlying catheters. N Engl J Med 1957;256:566.
417. Garibaldi RA, et al. Meatal colonization and catheter-associated bacteriuria. N Engl J Med 1980;303:316.
418. Bultitude MI, Eykyn S. The relationship between the urethral flora and urinary infection in the catheterised male. Br J Urol 1973;45:678.
419. Kunin CM, McCormack RC. Prevention of catheter-induced urinary tract infections by sterile closed drainage. N Engl J Med 1966; 274:1155.
420. Kunin CM, Steele C. Culture of the surfaces of urinary catheters to sample urethral flora and study the effect of antimicrobial therapy. J Clin Microbiol 1985;21:902.
421. Hirsh DD, Fainstein V, Musher DM. Do condom catheter collecting systems cause urinary tract infection? JAMA 1979;242:340.
422. Sanford JP. Hospital acquired urinary-tract infections. Ann Intern Med 1964;60:903.
423. Petersdorf RG, et al. A study of antibiotic prophylaxis in unconscious patients. N Engl J Med 1957;257:1001.
424. Schaberg DR, Weinstein RA, Stamm WE. Epidemics of nosocomial urinary tract infection caused by multiply resistant Gram-negative bacilli: epidemiology and control. J Infect Dis 1976;133:363.
425. Kunin CM, McCormack RC. Prevention of catheter-induced urinary tract infections by sterile closed drainage. N Engl J Med 1966; 274:1155.
426. Butler HK, Kunin CM. Evaluation of specific systemic antimicrobial therapy in patients while on closed catheter drainage. J Urol 1968; 100:567.
427. Burke JP, et al. Prevention of catheter-associated urinary tract infections. Efficacy of daily meatal care regimens. Am J Med 1981;70:655.
428. Butler HK, Kunin CM. Evaluation of polymyxin catheter lubricant and impregnated catheters. J Urol 1968;100:560.
429. Kunin CM, Finkelberg Z. Evaluation of an intraurethral lubricating catheter in prevention of catheter-induced tract infections. J Urol 1971;106:982.
430. Classen DC, et al. Daily meatal care for prevention of catheter-associated bacteriuria: results using frequent applications of polyantibiotic cream. Infect Control Hosp Epidemiol 1991;12:157–162.
431. Brehmer B, Madsen PO. Route and prophylaxis of ascending bladder infection in male patients with indwelling catheters. J Urol 1972; 108:719.
432. Thompson RL, et al. Catheter-associated bacteriuria. Failure to reduce attack rates using periodic instillations of a disinfectant into urinary drainage systems. JAMA 1984;251:747.
433. Dudley MN, Barriere SL. Antimicrobial irrigations in the prevention and treatment of catheter-related urinary tract infections. Am J Hosp Pharm 1981;38:59.
434. Platt R, et al. Reduction of mortality associated with nosocomial urinary tract infection. Lancet 1983;1:893.
435. Merritt JL. Residual urine volume: Correlate of urinary tract infection in patients with spinal cord injury. Arch Phys Med Rehabil 1981;62:558.
436. Lapides J, Diokno AC, Lowe BS, Kalish MD. Followup on unsterile, intermittent self-catheterization. J Urol 1974;111:184.
437. Kass EJ, Koff SA, Diokno AC, Lapides J. The significance of bacilluria in children on long-term intermittent catheterization. J Urol 1981; 126:223.
438. Kass EJ, McHugh T, Diokno AC. Intermittent catheterization in children less than 6 years old. J Urol 1979;121:792.
439. Donovan WH, et al. Bacteriuria during intermittent catheterization following spinal cord injury. Arch Phys Med Rehabil 1978;59:351.
440. Anderson RU. Prophylaxis of bacteriuria during intermittent catheterization of the acute neurogenic bladder. J Urol 1980;123:364.
441. Krebs M, Halvorsen RB, Fishman IJ, et al. Prevention of urinary tract infection during intermittent catheterization. J Urol 1984;131:82.
442. Ehrlich O, Brem AS. A prospective comparison of urinary tract infections in patients treated with either clean intermittent catheterization or urinary diversion. Pediatrics 1982;70:665.
443. Moloney PJ, Doyle AA, Robinson BL, et al. Pathogenesis of urinary infection in patients with acute spinal cord injury on intermittent catheterization. J Urol 1981;125:672.
444. Lima NL, et al. A retrospective cohort study of nosocomial diarrhea as a risk factor for nosocomial infection. JID 1990;161:948–52.
445. Lohr JA, et al. Hospital-acquired urinary tract infection. Pediatrics 1989;83:193–199.
446. Merritt WT. Nosocomial infections in the pediatric intensive care unit. In: Rogers MC, ed. Textbook of pediatric intensive care. Chap 25. Baltimore: Williams & Wilkins, 1987: see Table 25–6.
447. Lansky LL, Wolcott GJ. Trauma to brain and spinal cord. In: Swaiman KF, Wright FS, eds. The practice of pediatric neurology. St. Louis: CV Mosby, 1975:775.
448. MMWR 1982;31:488.
449. MMWR 1984;33:13.
450. MMWR 1984;33:698.
451. Vaughn VC, McKay RJ, Behrman RE. The field of pediatrics. In: Nelson's textbook of pediatrics. ed 11. Philadelphia: WB Saunders, 1979;6.
452. Beger MS, et al. Outcome from severe head injury in children and adolescents. J Neurosurg 1985;62:194.
453. Colombani PM, et al. One year experience in a regional pediatric trauma center. J Pediatr Surg 1985;20:8.
454. Trauner DA. Reye's syndrome. Clin Prob Pediatr 1982;12:1.
455. Bruce DA, Berman WA, Schut L. Cerebrospinal fluid pressure monitoring in children: physiology, pathology and clinical usefulness. Adv Pediatr 1970;24:233.
456. Marshall LF, Smith RW, Shapiro HM. The influence of diurnal rhythm in patients with intracranial hypertension. Implications for management. Neurosurgery 1978;2:100.
457. Copper PR. Lectures on the principles and practices of surgery with additional notes, and cases by Frederick Tyrell. Vol 1. London: T & G Underwood, 1824:282.
458. Wynter WE. Four cases of tubercular meningitis in which paracentesis of the theca vertebralis was performed for relief of fluid pressure. Lancet 1:981, 1891.
459. Bering ED. A simplified apparatus for constant ventricular drainage. J Neurosurg 1951;8:450.

460. Lundberg NG. Continuous recording and control of ventricular fluid pressure in neurosurgical practice. Acta Psychiatr Scand 1960; 149(Suppl 36):1.
461. Cushing H. Concerning the results of operations for brain tumor. JAMA 1915;64:189.
462. Cairns H, Adelaide BS. Bacterial infections during intracranial operations. Lancet 1939;1:1193.
463. Poppen JL. Ventricular drainage as a valuable procedure in neurosurgery. Report of a satisfactory method. Arch Neurol Psychiatry 1943;50:587.
464. Woodhall B, Neill RG, Dratz HM. Ultraviolet radiation as an adjunct in the control of post-operative neurosurgical infection. II. Clinical experience, 1938–1948. Ann Surg 1949;129:802.
465. Balch RE. Wound infections complicating neurosurgical procedures. J Neurosurg 1967;26:41.
466. Wright RL. A survey of possible etiologic agents in postoperative craniotomy infections. J Neurosurg 1966;25:125.
467. Romig DA, et al. Bacterial flora and infection in patients with brain injury. J Neurosurg 1973;38:710.
468. Johanson W. Pierce AK, Sanford JP. Changing pharyngeal flora of hospitalized patients. Emergency of Gram-negative bacilli. N Engl J Med 1969;281:1137.
469. White RJ, et al. Temporary control of cerebrospinal fluid volume and pressure by means of an externalized valve-drainage system. J Neurosurg 1969;30:264.
470. Sundbarg G, et al. Complications due to prolonged ventricular fluid pressure recording in clinical practice. In Brock M, Dietz H, eds. Intracranial pressure, experimental and clinical aspects. Berlin: Springer Verlag, 1972:348.
471. Wyler AR, Kelly WA. Use of antibiotics with external ventriculostomies. J Neurosurg 1972;37:185.
472. Smith RW, Alksne JF. Infections complicating the use of external ventriculostomy. J Neurosurg 1976;44:567.
473. Shaywitz BA, et al. Monitoring and management of increased intracranial pressure in Reye's syndrome: results in 29 children. Pediatrics 1980;66:198.
474. Rosner MJ, Becker DP. ICP monitoring: complications and associated factors. In: Keener EB, ed. Clinical neurosurgery, chap 37. Baltimore: Williams & Wilkins, 1976:494.
475. Narayan RK, et al. Intracranial pressure: to monitor or not to monitor? A review of our experience with severe head injury. J Neurosurg 1982;56:650.
476. Bruce DA, et al. The role of intracranial pressure monitoring in a pediatric intensive care unit. In: Beks JWF, Bosch DA, Brock M, eds. Intracranial pressure. Berlin: Springer Verlag, 1976:323.
477. Winn HR, et al. Intracranial subarachnoid pressure recording: experience with 650 patients. Surg Neurol 1977;8:41.
478. Levin AB. The use of a fiberoptic intracranial pressure monitor in clinical practice. Neurosurgery 1977;1:266.
479. Ivan LP, et al. Intracranial pressure monitoring with the fiberoptic transducer in children. Childs Brain 1980;7:303.
480. Fleisher AS, et al. Continuous monitoring of intracranial pressure in severe closed head injury without mass lesions. Surg Neurol 1976;6:31.
481. Mayhall CG, et al. Ventriculostomy-related infections. A prospective epidemiologic study. N Engl J Med 1984;310:553.
482. Drake JM, et al. Cerebrospinal fluid flow dynamics in children with external ventricular drains. Neurosurgery 1991;28:242–250.
483. Kollef MH. Antibiotic use and antibiotic resistance in the intensive care unit: Are we curing or creating disease. Heart & Lung 1994; 23: 363–367.
484. Jacoby GA, Mederios AA. More extended-spectrum beta-lactamases. Antimicrob Agents Chemother 1991;35:1697–1704.
485. Chow JW, Fine MJ, Shlaes DM, et al. Enterobacter bacteremia: clinical features and emergence of antibiotic resistance during therapy. Ann Intern Med 1991;115:585–590.
486. Tomasz A. Multipe-antibiotic-resistant pathogenic bacteria. A report on the Rockefeller University Workshop. N Eng J Med 1994;330:1247–1251.
487. Emori TG, Gaynes RP. An overview of nosocomial infections, including the role of the microbiology laboratory. Clin Microbiol Rev 1993;6:428–42.
488. Mulligan ME, Murray-Leisure KA, Ribner BS, et al. Methicillin-resistant Staphylococcus aureus: A consensus review of the microbiology, pathogenesis and epidemiology with implications for prevetntion and management. Am J Med 1993;94:313–328.
489. Utsui Y, Yakota T. Role of an altered penicillin-binding protein in methicilklin and cephem-resistant Staphylococcus aureus. Antimicrob Agents Chemother 1985;28:397–403.
490. Hackbath CJ, Chambers HF. Methicillin-resistant staphylococci: genetics and mechanisms of resistance. Antimicrob Agents Chemother 1989;33:991–994.
491. Col NF, O'Connor RW. Estimating worldwide current antibiotic use: report of Task Force 1. Rev Infect Dis 1987;9:suppl 3:S232–S243.
492. Neu HC. The crisis in antibiotic resistance. Science 1992;257:1064–1078.
493. Schwalbe RS, Stapleton JT, Gilligan PH. Emergence of vancomycin resistance in coaguluase negative staphylococci. N Eng J Med 1987; 316:927–931.
494. Murray BE, Mederski-Samoraj B. Transferable beta-lactamase. A new mechanism for in vitro penicillin resistance in Streptococcus faecalis. J Clin Invest 1983;72:1168–1171.
495. Herman DJ, Gerding DN. Antimicrobial resistance among enterococci. Antimicrob Agents Chemother 1991;35:1–4.
496. Rubin LG, Tucci V, Cercenado E, Eliopoulos G, Isenberg HD. Vancomycin-resistant Enterococcus faecium in hospitalized children. Infect Control Hosp Epidemiol 1992;13:700–705.
497. Karanfil LV, Murphy M, Josephson A, Gaynes R, Mandel L, Hill BC, Swenson JM. A cluster of vancomycin-resistant Enterococcus faecium in an intensive care unit. Infect Control Hosp Epidemiol 1992;13: 195–200.
498. Green M, Barbadora K, Wadowsky RM. Simple test for synergy of ampicillin and vancomycin resistant strains of Enterococcus faecium. J Clin Microbiol 1994;32:2837–2839.
499. Caron FC, Carbon C, Guttman L. Triple combination penicillin-vancomycin-gentamicin for experimental endocarditis caused by a moderately penicillin and highly glycopeptide resistant isolate of Enterococcus faecium. J Infect Dis 1991;164:888–893.
500. Sanders CC. Beta-lactamases of Gram-negative bacteria: New challenges for new drugs. Clin Infect Dis 1992;14:1089–1099.
501. Medeiros AA. Nosocomial outbreaks of multiresistant bacteria: extended-spectrum beta-lactamases have arrived in North America. Ann Intern Med 1993;119:428–430.
502. Kern WV, Andriof E, Oethinger M, Kern P, Hacker J, Marre R. Emergence of fluoroquinolone-resistant Escherichia coli at a cancer center. Antimicrob Agents Chemother 1994;38:681–687.
503. Pena C, Albareda JM, Pallares R, Pujol M, Tubau F, Ariza J. Relationship between quinolone use and emergence of ciprofloxacin-resistant Escherichia coli in bloodstream infections. Antimicrob Agents Chemother 1995;39:520–524.
504. Pechere JC. Antibiotic resistance is selected primarily in our patients. Infect Control Hosp Epidemiol 1994;15:472–477.
505. Meyer KS, Urban C, Eagan JA, Berger BJ, Rahal JJ. Nosocomial outbreak of Klebsiella infection resistant to late-generation cephalosporins.
506. Hospital Infection Control Practices Advisory Committee. Recommendations for preventing the spread of vancomycin resistance. Infect Control Hosp Epidemiol 1995;16:1905–113.

Overwhelming Sepsis 31

Joshua P. Needleman
Alice D. Ackerman

INTRODUCTION

This chapter highlights diseases of infectious nature that may have such severe expression as to require admission of the patient to a critical care area. For the most part, these disorders carry a high risk of mortality if unrecognized and untreated. They are illnesses that also tend to result in an unfavorable outcome even when specific antimicrobial therapy is appropriately administered.

Pertinent aspects of pathophysiology are covered as they relate to expression of microbial disease in the critically ill child. Although some of the involved microbiological principles are reviewed as they apply to the organisms of interest, no attempt has been made to make this chapter a complete treatise on the field of infectious diseases. It concentrates on information essential to the intensive care practitioner when faced with a child who requires critical care and who appears to have an infectious disease. The peculiar aspects of infections as they relate to children of various ages are explored, and an approach to diagnosis and therapy of the common and not-so-common syndromes is included.

The chapter begins with a discussion of the general approach to life-threatening infections, and initial antibiotic choices, followed by a description of overwhelming sepsis and how the syndrome varies according to the age group encountered. Major pathogens that affect the neonate, infant, and child are explored in depth. Infections primarily affecting the central nervous system are discussed in Chapter 32. Other infections of particular interest to the intensive care specialist are discussed in Chapter 33. The pathophysiology of the shock syndromes and the use of monoclonal antibody and other antimediator therapies are discussed in Chapter 16.

APPROACH TO LIFE-THREATENING INFECTIONS

The basic principles of intensive care are the same whether one encounters a patient who has sepsis, cardiogenic shock, or severe trauma. Treatment of the life-threatening aspects of any disease process must always take precedence over specific therapy aimed at the underlying illness. Naturally, the early administration of disease-directed therapy (i.e., antibiotics) may prevent development of shock or respiratory failure, but the job of early recognition and initial intervention often rests with the emergency or ward physician. Therefore, the intensive care specialist must often forego, for a short time, the detailed consideration of a differential diagnosis and proceed to therapy that will salvage the failing vital functions of a critically ill child. The responsibility of making an etiologic diagnosis and instituting specific therapy must follow or be concurrent with establishment of an adequate airway, gas exchange, and cardiac output, for these are the processes that will potentially save the patient's life. The diagnosis and therapy of respiratory and hemodynamic failure have been explored elsewhere in this volume and will not be examined here.

Once a modicum of stability is established, a quick examination must be performed and highlights of the patient's history must be gathered; this should enable the physician to make a presumptive diagnosis and choose reasonable antimicrobial agents if an infection is suspected. The findings of fever, rash (petechial or otherwise), sudden hemodynamic collapse, meningeal or peritoneal signs, and altered mental status should indicate an infection. Presence of a cough or other respiratory signs, lymphadenopathy, or joint swelling may further establish the need for antibiotic therapy. Based on the information gathered in this limited fashion, broad categories of infections can be considered, and wide-spectrum antimicrobiologic coverage provided. Over the next several hours, further historic information may be elucidated, including recent travel to an area endemic for a particular parasitic or viral disease, history of recent or ongoing menses or tampon use, an animal or insect bite, and the status of the child's immunizations. Routine laboratory data will be gathered and a decision will be made, based on considerations discussed in the following section, whether to perform a lumbar puncture. Many of the signs and symptoms of sepsis may be mimicked by other disease entities, and an appropriate search for other causes of deterioration must be sought. Especially in the comatose child, a search for possible drugs and toxins must be made.

The practitioner of pediatric intensive care is faced with the unenviable task of evaluating patients that span a wide age range. The particular susceptibilities of the neonate differ from those of the older infant, child, and adolescent, and the pediatric intensive care specialist must be familiar with each group and their idiosyncrasies. Some of the age-related factors predisposing to particular infections were considered in Chapter 28. In addition, the wide range of underlying disease processes and levels of immune competence make assessment of the potentially infected critically ill pediatric patient far from simple. Nonetheless, certain principles (covered in the following section) can help the practitioner make a rational choice of initial broad-spectrum antibiotics. The exciting new area of monoclonal antibodies and other adjunctive therapies is growing at a rapid rate. Some of these agents may become part of the routine first-line therapy in the child with septic shock. These are described in Chapter 16.

Choice of Antibiotics

The initial antibiotics chosen for the treatment of overwhelming sepsis are dictated by the likely offending organism. This, in turn, depends primarily on (a) the patient's age, (b) the coexistence of any premorbid condition leading to impaired immune defenses, and (c) the presenting signs and symptoms. For example, a septic 7-yr-old child with leukemia and diffuse abdominal discomfort requires far different management than does a 3-day-old neonate with respiratory distress. In this section, various initial antibiotic regimens are based, in large part, on patient age and premorbid condition. It is neither the goal of the chapter nor is it feasible to provide an exhaustive review of appropriate antibiotics based on different foci of infection. Moreover, it should be emphasized here that the regimens outlined simply reflect the authors' current preferences. They cannot be applied to all situations. Local patterns of antibiotic resistance by common infecting organisms must also be considered. Individual preferences lead to the use of alternative, equally effective antibiotics. Furthermore, in this age of rapid antibiotic development, better drugs may be available within a few years. However, in all cases the overriding objective is to use the antibiotic or antibiotic combination most likely to eradicate the infection while minimizing the risks of superinfection or emergence of resistant organisms. Finally, the recommendations assume that after the first dose of antibiotic, the child will be further assessed, renal or hepatic impairment may be noted, and the advice of infectious disease consultants will be sought. Thus, the ongoing therapy may differ from that recommended here. Nonetheless, what follows represents a reasonable starting point.

In considering antibiotic choices for the septic neonate, it is easiest to divide the newborn period into an early and a later segment. During the first 7 days, the common offending organisms are group B streptococcus (GBS) and *Escherichia coli.* Less commonly, *Listeria monocytogenes, Staphylococcus aureus,* or *Streptococcus epidermidis* may cause sepsis[1,2]. Finally, as discussed later in the chapter, herpes simplex virus (HSV) may cause a fulminant sepsis-like pattern. In view of this constellation of potential infections, we use ampicillin and gentamicin often with the addition of cefotaxime as our initial therapy for the septic young neonate. Cefotaxime cannot be used as a single agent in this age group because is not effective against *L. mono-*

Table 31.1. Initial Antibiotics for Sepsis in Neonates Who Are Less Than 7 Days of Age

Focus	*Antibiotics*	*Dose*
Not relevant at this age	Ampicillin	100 mg/kg/day divided q 12 hr
	Gentamicin or tobramycin	2.5 mg/kg/dose given q 12–24 hr depending upon gestational age
	Cefotaxime	100 mg/kg/day divided q 12 hr
	Acyclovir[a]	30 mg/kg/day divided q 8 hr

[a]Only to be used if HSV infection is suspected, see text.

Table 31.2. Initial Antibiotics for Sepsis in Neonates Who Are More Than 7 Days of Age

Focus	*Antibiotics*	*Dose*
None, respiratory or CNS in previously healthy baby	Ampicillin and one of the following:	200 mg/kg/day divided q 8–12 hr
	Gentamicin or	2.5 mg/kg/dose given q 8–18 hr depending on gestational age and renal function (follow levels)
	Ceftriaxone or	100 mg/kg load, then 100 mg/kg/day divided q 12 hr
	Cefotaxime	100 mg/kg/day divided q 12 hr
None, respiratory or CNS in baby with central line	Add vancomycin to above	10–15 mg/kg/dose given q 8–18 hr (follow levels)
As above, but with endotracheal tube	Consider Ticarcillin/Clavulanate	300 mg/kg/day divided q 8 hr
Suspected necrotizing enterocolitis	Add Metronidazole or	15 mg/kg load, then 7.5 mg/kg/dose given q 8 hr
	Clindamycin	15–40 mg/kg/day divided q 6–8 hr

cytogenes. Resistance of *Enterobacter cloacae* to the drug has been reported[3,4], and gentamicin is known to be synergistic with beta-lactam antibiotics against Listeria and GBS. *Therefore, the use of cefotaxime without an aminoglycoside cannot be recommended.* Amikacin or tobramycin is often substituted for gentamicin. If there is a positive history of maternal HSV infection, acyclovir is added to the above regimen **(Table 31.1).**

In the older neonate, other considerations also become important. In a normal, full-term infant with no prior illness, the possibilities of late-onset GBS disease or *L. monocytogenes* infection are high, and therapy with ampicillin, gentamicin and cefotaxime or ceftriaxone are appropriate **(Table 31.2).** However, if the baby has been in the intensive care unit, the likely infecting organisms include both those that would be found in a previously healthy neonate and those common to critically ill children of all ages. For example, the presence of central lines raises the possibility of *S. aureus* or *S. epidermidis* infections, endotracheal intubation predisposes to various infections including *Pseudomonas aeruginosa,* and previous treatment with broad-spectrum antibiotics increases the risk of fungal superinfection. Finally, in the child with risk factors for necrotizing enterocolitis, anaerobic as well as aerobic enteric organisms must be considered[1,2,5].

Beyond the first month of life, the likely organisms causing overwhelming sepsis change little during childhood. Again, the major factors determining which organisms are responsible for a particular infection are the focus of that infection and the presence or absence of a premorbid condition, such as malignancy, or prolonged intravascular catheterization.

Consider first the previously healthy child **(Table 31.3).** *Streptococcus pneumoniae, Neisseria meningitidis* and *Haemophilus influenzae* are the three most common causes of bacterial meningitis and pneumonia in children. Thus, if a child presents with sepsis and a respiratory or central nervous system (CNS) focus, therapy with a third-generation cephalosporin, such as ceftriaxone, is reasonable. As resistant *S. pneumoniae* become more common, many centers are treating bacterial meningitis and other possible pneumococcal infections with vancomycin in addition to ceftriaxone until identification and antibiotic sensitivity are available. However, when deciding on initial antibiotic therapy in the child without either a respiratory or CNS focus, the possibility of a urinary tract infection with an enteric organism must be considered. Whenever Gram-negative sepsis is strongly entertained, the patient must be treated with two synergistic antibiotics. This is usually accomplished with the addition of an aminoglycoside to the previously described regimen. Finally, with either gastrointestinal or gynecological foci, the possibility of anaerobic as well as aerobic enteric organisms must be entertained. It is particularly important to remember the possibility of anaerobic infection in the child with a ruptured appendix[7]. In the septic child with an abdominal focus, we use an initial combination of ampicillin, gentamicin, and metronidazole or clindamycin to cover most organisms pending culture results. Some clinicians substitute cefoxitin for ampicillin in suspected abdominal infections.

The empiric management of the septic child with malignant disease is discussed in detail in Chapter 41. In brief, antibiotic coverage depends on the degree of neutropenia. If the neutrophil count exceeds 1000/μl, then the child may be managed as outlined in the previous discussion. If the count is under 1000/μl, then broad-spectrum therapy with

Table 31.3. Initial Antibiotics for Sepsis in Previously Healthy Children

Focus	*Antibiotic*	*Dose*
None, respiratory, or UTI	Ceftriaxone	100 mg/kg load, then 100 mg/kg/day divided q 12 hr
CNS	Add Vancomycin to the above if resistant *S. pnuemoniae* is a possibility	15 mg/kg dose q 8–18 hr (follow levels)
GU or GI	Add metronidazole to the above regimen	15 mg/kg load, then 7.5 mg/kg/dose given 6 hr (max 4 gram/day)

Table 31.4. Initial Antibiotics for Sepsis in Previously Ill Children

Focus	*Antibiotics*	*Dose*
None, in an immunocompromised host	Ceftazadime or	150 mg/kg/day divided q 8 hr
	Ticarcillin /Clavulanate	300 mg/kg divided q 4–6 hr
	and Gentamicin or	2.5 mg/kg/dose q 8 hr
	Amikacin and	15 mg/kg/day divided q 8 hr
	Nafcillin	150–200 mg/kg/day divided q 4–6 hr
None, but with a central line	same as in **Table 31.3**, but add Nafcillin or vancomycin	

Please see Chapter 41 for discussion of neutropenic hosts.

a combination such as vancomycin, ticarcillin clavulonate, and amikacin[8] or ceftazidime and amikacin[9] are initiated. Conditions other than malignancy may prompt the physician to initiate a broader spectrum of antibiotics for overwhelming sepsis while awaiting culture results **(Table 31.4).** For example, children with central lines are at increased risk of nosocomial infection with *S. epidermidis* or *S. aureus* as well as other organisms[10] (see also the discussion in Chapter 41). We tend to use vancomycin in the initial management of catheter sepsis when a methicillin-resistant staphylococcal organism is suspected. Disruption of the normal barriers to infection with urinary catheters and endotracheal tubes also predisposes to unusual and serious infections, particularly in patients who are relatively malnourished or who have been previously treated with broad-spectrum antibiotics. The difficulty in managing these patients is determining how to treat sepsis resulting from a nosocomial infection effectively without predisposing them to yet more resistant or dangerous infections. Our usual approach is to broaden therapy to cover for *Pseudomonas* or other organisms recently identified as colonizing either the child in question or other children in the unit. This approach usually leads us to a combination of either ticarcillin\lavulonate or Ceftazidime with an aminoglycoside and nafcillin or vancomycin depending on the likelihood of catheter sepsis. Ceftazidime alone should be avoided because the likelihood of resistant organisms developing is quite high[11,12].

If the child described previously is already being treated with this broad-spectrum regimen and is deteriorating or the organism is resistant to the usual broad spectrum antibiotics then some of the other, expanded spectrum antibiotics may be useful. The imipenem cilastatin combination has proven to be effective in these circumstances. It is effective against Gram-negative rods including *Enterobacter* and *Klebsiella* species and *P. aeruginosa* as well as various Gram-positive organisms and some anaerobes like *Bacteroides*[13,14]. We currently reserve it for patients who have developed sepsis while being treated with broad-spectrum antibiotics or who are unresponsive to the usual broad-spectrum regimen. In the patient being treated with such broad-spectrum antibiotics, it is important to maintain vigilance for superinfection with resistant organisms, care must be taken to culture all sites frequently, and to be acutely alert for fungal superinfection which can prove disastrous.

OVERWHELMING SEPSIS

Neonate

Although the pediatric intensive care specialist may see relatively few premature neonates, he or she will still encounter specific problems of this age group from time to time and must be attuned to presenting signs and symptoms as well as to the likely infectious agents. It is also necessary that he or she be aware of the spectrum of nosocomial illnesses seen in the neonatal ICU. Babies colonized with multiple-resistant Gram-negative organisms in the NICU may excrete them for up to a year following neonatal ICU discharge[1,15]. This presents a threat to other patients in the PICU through cross-infection, as discussed in Chapter 30.

The symptoms and signs of sepsis in the neonate are nonspecific, because the newborn possesses few means through which to manifest illness. The primary signs are respiratory distress, apnea, abdominal distention, vomiting, diarrhea, jaundice, loss of tone, lethargy, seizures, and abnormal body temperature, either fever or hypothermia[16]. Specific skin lesions, such as petechiae or pustules, may be present, but mottling as a result of decreased perfusion and changes in both cardiac output and peripheral vascular resistance are more commonly seen. The presentation of these signs may be subtle or fulminant. Fulminant signs usually indicate that an infectious disease is a diagnostic possibility. When only one or two of the signs are present, and the baby looks well, it is possible to overlook a potentially fatal microbiologic disease.

Numerous attempts to refine diagnostic evaluation of sick neonates have employed a variety of specific laboratory tests[17–24]. Although a markedly elevated white blood count (WBC) or an increased ratio of band forms to more mature neutrophils may be helpful in diagnosing bacterial disease, it is the septic babies with normal or low leukocyte counts who have the poorest outcomes, presumably because of a limited bone marrow reserve. Therefore, a normal WBC is not necessarily reassuring. Other factors, such as an elevated erythrocyte sedimentation rate or C-reactive protein, are nonspecific and are also relatively insensitive. A platelet count of less than 80,000 and findings of toxic granulations within polymorphonuclear leukocytes also provide indirect, suggestive evidence of infection. A large number of WBCs and bacteria in the gastric aspirate may be indicative of amnionitis, and examination of the Gram's stain may provide a clue to the predominant organism, but does not differentiate the bacteremic newborn from one without systemic infection.

In short, there are no hard and fast diagnostic criteria of sepsis in the neonate. Therefore, the practitioner must depend on a high level of suspicion and proceed to make a specific etiologic determination by obtaining samples of blood, urine, and spinal fluid for culture. The availability of rapid bacterial diagnostic testing such as latex agglutination or countercurrent immune electrophoresis has made this process somewhat easier and less time-consuming(25). Between 1 and 10 babies of every 1000 live births will acquire a bacterial infection(26), and between 20% and 75% of those infected will die or have long-term neurologic damage. Therefore, good neonatal medical practice will likely entail a fair amount of overtreatment.

Neonatal sepsis has been classified into categories of early-onset and late-onset disease, depending on whether presentation occurs during or after the first week of life, respectively. Although this classification is most useful with regard to the group B β-hemolytic streptococci as discussed in the following section, it is applicable to neonatal sepsis in general. Early-onset sepsis most commonly presents in the first 24 hours of life and is related to maternal risk factors(27) such as prolonged rupture of membranes, premature labor, chorioamnionitis, and occurrence of maternal fever in the immediate postpartum period. It has a high mortality, in some studies greater than 50%, and generally presents in a fulminant fashion(28,29). It is frequently associated with pneumonia. The organisms implicated in early-onset sepsis are generally related to contaminants of the maternal birth canal.

Late-onset disease that is of community origin (not nosocomial) does not correlate with maternal risk factors. The baby is usually infected with organisms that colonize the mother. Later onset of sepsis generally carries a lower risk of mortality, ranging from 10 to 20%, although a higher percentage of these babies have associated meningitis(30). Premature babies who remain hospitalized beyond the first week of life are at high risk to develop nosocomial infections(31).

In the past half century, the predominant organisms responsible for neonatal septicemia have changed several times(26,32–41), with a cycling pattern of infections caused by *Staphylococcus aureus* and hemolytic streptococcus. The predominant cause of puerperal fever, β-hemolytic streptococci, was nearly eradicated by the widespread use of penicillin in the late 1940s and early 1950s. At that time, *S. aureus* emerged as the major pathogen in epidemics of neonatal sepsis, but was significantly limited by widespread measures aimed at its eradication, the most important of which appeared to be washing of newborn babies with hexachlorophene products(34). Unfortunately, at the concentrations used, this preparation produced significant neurotoxicity in premature infants, and the bathing policy was abandoned. Although the hemolytic staphylococcus was restricted for several years by the bathing practices as well as the use of penicillinase-resistant penicillins, enteric Gram-negative organisms (especially *E. coli*) emerged as important neonatal microorganisms. Development of aminoglycosides then seemed to make way for a reemergence of β-hemolytic streptococci in the 1970s. In the 1980s, *S. aureus* (often methicillin-resistant) seemed to be making a comeback, at least in some institutions.

Recent reports have separated endogenously acquired from nosocomial infections. Group B streptococci and *E. coli* are the most common perinatal infections(2), whereas *S. epidermidis* and *S. aureus* are the most common nosocomial pathogens(2,5). *S. epidermidis* is the most commonly implicated organism in neonatal indwelling catheter colonization(42). *Pseudomonas,* other Gram-negative rods, and *Candida* also account for a significant number of episodes of nosocomial neonatal sepsis. Appropriate initial antibiotics were indicated in the previous discussion.

Reports of outbreaks of other organisms, such as *H. parainfluenzae*(43–46), *L. monocytogenes*(47–55), and *Flavobacterium meningosepticum* (56–58), are a reminder that although statistical information is useful, it cannot replace information regarding local patterns of microbiologic disease. HSV is an important cause of neonatal sepsis syndrome and is considered in detail in a following section. Immune compromise should be considered in the baby who fails to respond to appropriate therapy for the most common pathogens, an unusual organism, or a new pattern of antimicrobial resistance. A discussion of some specific neonatal pathogens follows.

Group B β-Hemolytic Streptococci

In 1887, streptococcal organisms were first implicated as a cause of bovine mastitis(59). Although occasional reports of streptococci in humans trickled through the literature, it was not until after 1933(60), when Lancefield had categorized the streptococcal organisms into the groups that are still in use today, that the group B streptococcus (GBS) was identified in the vaginas of pregnant and parturient women(61,62), some of whom were septic. The specific name *Streptococcus agalactiae* emphasizes the role this organism is believed to play among domesticated livestock. The significance of GBS as a neonatal pathogen was not fully appreciated until increasingly frequent reports appeared in the late 1950s. However, it was not until 1973, after two comparatively large series of GBS disease were reported, that the bimodal pattern of neonatal infection was recognized, and the early-onset and late-onset syndromes were described(63,64). Numerous subsequent studies have added important information regarding epidemiology, characterization of the organism, risks of nosocomial transmission, perinatal risk factors, clinical and laboratory evaluation, treatment, and outcome(65–84). A 1990 multistate surveil-

Table 31.5. Group B Streptococcal Disease Among Infants < 90 Days Old—Selected U.S. Counties[a]

	Early-onset Disease		*Late-onset Disease*		*Total Disease*	
	No.	*Rate(%)*	*No.*	*Rate (%)*	*No.*	*Rate (%)*
Incidence						
White	129	1.1	23	0.19	152	1.3
Black	92	2.0	31	0.67	123	2.7
All races	247	1.4	59	0.32	306	1.7
Deaths						
White	3	2.4	0		3	2.1
Black	7	8.6	3	13.0	10	9.0
All races	13	5.7	3	6.0	16	5.8
Gestational age						
<34 weeks	16	12.0	4	22.0	20	13.0
34–36 weeks	19	14.0	4	22.0	23	15.0
≥37 weeks	99	74.0	10	56.0	109	72.0

[a] *From MMWR 1992;41:25-32, with permission.*

lance study by the Centers for Disease Control (CDC) reported an incidence of GBS in infants less than 90 days old of 1.7/1000 live births. The description of GBS disease is separated into early-onset and late-onset groups because the presentation, natural history, epidemiology, bacteriology, and outcome differ according to the time of presentation. The overwhelming majority of GBS disease occurs in the first week of life (75–80%), with the majority of those occurring in the first 48 hours of life (approximately 50% of the total). The incidence over the succeeding 3 months of life is fairly constant, although some workers have noted a somewhat increased incidence at 3 to 4 weeks. GBS disease is rare beyond 3 months of age **(Table 31.5).**

Early-onset Disease

Neonates who develop GBS in the first several days of life most often have a fulminant acute course, characterized by apnea, respiratory distress, hypotension, poor perfusion, and other nonspecific signs of neonatal illness **(Table 31.6).** It is primarily a disease of premature babies of less than 35 weeks' gestation and weighing less than 2500 g at birth. In a recent multistate case-control study, increased risk of early onset disease was correlated with young maternal age, maternal rupture of membranes longer than 12 hours, intrapartum fever, prematurity, and a history of urinary tract infection during pregnancy[(85)]. Other risk factors associated with development of early-onset disease include twin gestation and low Apgar scores at 1 and 5 min. One study has shown persistent antepartum tachycardia to be an additional independent predictor of neonatal GBS sepsis[(86)]. Other factors that correlate with development of disease include heavy colonization of infants (growth of GBS from at least three separate surveillance sites, such as auditory canal, umbilicus, nose or throat, and anus) at or shortly after birth, and finding Gram-positive cocci on a stained smear of gastric aspirate. Studies that examined predictive assessments have included the evaluation of WBCs, percentage of band forms, and granulocyte reserves in analyses of bone marrow aspirates. Attempts to compare maternal antibody titers against the organism to risk of neonatal disease acquisition have also been made.

Table 31.6. Early-onset GBS Disease

	Clinical Characteristics
Age at onset	Less than 7 days; majority first 48 hr
Presentation	Apnea usually
Clinical appearance	Severely ill Cardiovascular collapse Persistent fetal circulation Persistent apnea Lung disease indistinguishable from RDS[a] Low birth weight (<2,500 g) Low Apgar scores
Associated maternal obstetrical complications	Maternal fever Premature labor (≤35 weeks) Ruptured membranes >12 hr Twin gestation
Mortality	Approximately 50%

[a] *RDS = respiratory distress syndrome.*

In another study[(72)], 12.5% of 2317 babies cultured at birth grew GBS from at least one site. However, only 4 were heavily colonized (growth from three or four sites). The mothers of the babies in this study were also cultured. It was found that only 3% of all babies who had early evidence of colonization were born to culture-negative mothers. Eight percent of heavily colonized babies developed GBS disease, in each case within 48 hours after birth. All of the late-onset infections in this study occurred in infants who were culture-negative at birth. The incidence rates of early-onset disease among colonized babies was 76.9/1000 heavily colonized infants and 5.0/1000 lightly colonized neonates. There were no early-onset infections among 2027 infants who were culture-negative at birth **(Table 31.7).**

Although the data on colonization are interesting and are able to predict 96% of those who became clinically infected, they do not assist in the early evaluation of the potentially septic neonate because a relatively large number of patients who have early-onset disease presents at or within several hours of birth. Therefore, rates of maternal colonization have been evaluated[(63,64,66,67,72,87)]. When selective culture media are used, and multiple sites are sampled, asymptomatic

Table 31.7. Incidence of GBS Septicemia and/or Meningitis in Prospectively Studied Infants[a]

		Early-onset Infections		*Late-onset Infections*		*Total*	
Newborn Population	*No.*	*No.*	*Rate/1000*	*No.*	*Rate/1000*	*No.*	*Rate/1000*
Total life births	2407	9	3.7	4	1.7	13	5.4
Infants cultured at birth	2317	8	3.5	3	1.3	11	4.7
Culture-negative infants	2027			3	1.5	3	1.5
Culture-positive infants	290	8	27.5			8	27.6
1–2 positive sites	199	1	5.0			1	5.0
3–4 positive sites	91	7	76.9			7	76.9

[a]*From Pass MA, Gray BM, Khare S, Dillon HC Jr. Prospective studies of group B streptococcal infections in infants. J Pediatr 1979;95:437.*

vaginal or rectal carriage is found in 25 to 35% of women at the time of delivery. Approximately three-quarters of the babies born to colonized mothers grow GBS from superficial cultures. The accurate recovery of organisms in the neonate also depends on culturing multiple sites. The most frequently colonized area in the neonate is the ear. Because the same strains are almost invariably recovered in any single mother-infant pair, vertical transmission of the organism before, during, or immediately after birth has been assumed. Approximately one-third of isolates are from each of the three types of GBS (type Ia, b, or c, type II, type III), indicating that there is no predilection for colonization based on type of GBS. Although some studies have listed a higher incidence[(72)], the majority of reports have indicated that 1 in 100 colonized babies will develop sepsis and/or meningitis because of GBS in the first few days of life. When all forms of early-onset disease are considered, there is no one type of GBS organism that predominates. However, in the 30% of cases complicated by meningitis, type III is isolated more than 80% of the time, indicating a specific tropism of type III for the meninges.

Studies that have attempted to quantify the expected mortality from early onset disease have reported a wide rage of results. This is likely resulting from a wide range of factors including available treatment, differences in patient populations, and the method by which the data was sampled. The CDC multistate surveillance data indicate a case fatality of 5.8%[(84)]. Other studies, most of which have looked at individual hospital data, have reported much higher rates of 25 to 50%[(88)]. The mortality in university hospitals appears to be twofold to threefold higher than that in community hospitals[(76)]. Babies with additional neonatal problems, such as prematurity and respiratory distress syndrome, are much more likely to die. In these infants, the mortality rate may reach 80%. Factors found to correlate poorly with survival in one study[(77)] were significant delay in instituting antibiotic therapy, prematurity, low 5-minute Apgar score, presence of shock, leukopenia, and rupture of membranes more than 12 hours before delivery **(Table 31.8).** The infants who died were significantly younger than those who survived, with a gestational age of 33.1 ± 2.9 weeks. More than 70% of those with fatal outcome presented with shock and had antibiotic therapy delayed by at least 12 hours from the time of onset of symptoms. The total WBC was lower (mean = 6400 ± 4600) as was the percent of granulocytes (mean = 23 ± 23). Of the mothers of these babies, 41% had ruptured membranes longer than 12 hours before delivery. One-quarter of all the neonates in this study were asymptomatic at the time the bacteremia was demonstrated. These babies were older (39 ± 2.7 weeks) with good Apgar scores (8.1 ± 1.6), had normal WBCs (16,200 ± 6200), and had a higher percentage of granulocytes than those who were overtly ill. More than 60% of these asymptomatic babies had prolonged rupture of membranes. In most cases, the presence of ruptured membranes for more than 12 hours was the reason blood cultures were obtained in the asymptomatic group.

On the basis of the previously mentioned findings, Lannering and colleagues[(75)] devised a scoring system to predict short-term outcome in early-onset disease. The vari-

Table 31.8. Severity of Early-onset GBS Disease Related to Patient Characteristics[a]

	Severity			
Characteristic	*Died*	*Assisted Ventilation*	*Supplemental Oxygen*	*Asymptomatic*
Gestational age (weeks)	33.1 ± 2.9	35.4 ± 3.5	37.9 ± 2.6	39.0 ± 2.7
Birth weight (g)	1969 ± 672	2311 ± 637	3068 ± 823	3158 ± 566
ROM > 12 hr (%)[b]	41	10	18	64
5-minute Apgar score	6.2 ± 2.5	7.6 ± 1.6	7.1 ± 1.8	8.1 ± 1.6
Granulocytes (%)	23 ± 23	46 ± 20	56 ± 26	63 ± 15
Total WBC (×1000)	6.4 ± 4.6	6.9 ± 4.2	11.2 ± 6	16.2 ± 6.2
Antibiotics delayed (%)	70	37	14	
Shock (%)	78	26	0	
No. of patients	29	29	24	28

[a] *From Lannering B, Larson LE, Rojas J, Stahlman MT. Early onset group B streptococcal disease: seven year experience and clinical scoring system. Acta Paediatr Scand 1983;72:597.*

[b] *ROM = rupture of membranes.*

Table 31.9. Discriminant Analysis: Weighting Coefficients and Relative Discriminating Power for Early-onset GBS Disease[a]

Variables	*Weighting Coefficient*	*Relative Discriminating Power*	*Code*
Gestational age	1.64	1.0	Weeks
Presence of shock	−10.82	0.93	Yes = 1: no = 0
WBC count	5.37	0.87	≥6000 = 2 5999 to 3000 = 1 ≤3000 = 0
ROM (>12 hr)[b]	−8.34	0.77	Yes = 1; No = 0
Delayed treatment (>12 hr)	−8.30	0.71	Yes = 1; No = 0
5-min Apgar score	1.66	0.67	Same

[a] *From Lannering B, Larson LE, Rojas J, Stahlman MT. Early onset group B streptococcal disease: seven year experience and clinical scoring system. Acta Paediatr Scand 1983;72:597.*
[b] *ROM = rupture of membranes.*

ables and relative discriminating power and weighting coefficients are listed in **Table 31.9.** Scores are calculated by adding the products of each of the six variables and their respective weighting coefficients. Figure 31.1 shows the discriminant score plotted against the probability of death. Because this is a smooth curve, the severity score may be a reasonable estimate of likelihood of survival or death in early-onset disease. These investigators documented a fall over the 7 years of the study in the mortality due to GBS and were able to relate it to the only other alteration they could identify: that of the rapidity with which antibiotic therapy was instituted. Therefore,they concluded that rapid establishment of appropriate antimicrobial therapy, especially in premature neonates with other risk factors for GBS, may help reduce mortality.

Variable numbers of babies with early-onset GBS are reported to have associated pneumonia. Although there may not be obvious roentgenographic findings in all cases, the majority of babies who die of the disease and are autopsied have Gram-positive organisms in the alveoli, and many have a cellular infiltrate characteristic of diffuse pneumonitis; they may also have development of hyaline membranes unrelated to respiratory distress syndrome.

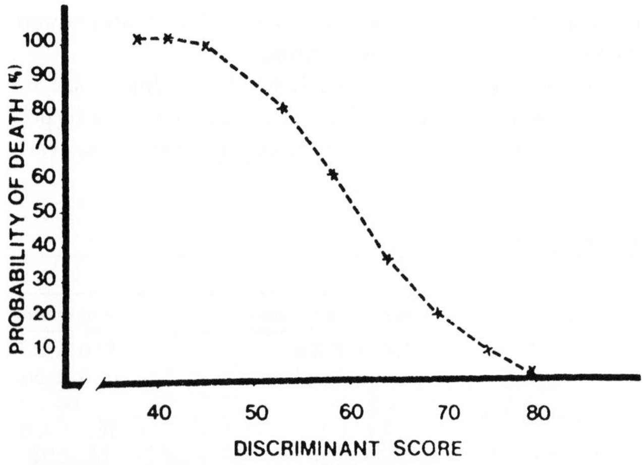

Figure 31.1. Discriminant score of Lannering et al (see Table 31.8) plotted against mortality at each interval. The *points* and *interpolated segments* provide an approximate relationship between discriminant score and probability of death in early-onset GBS infections. (From Lannering B, Larson LE, Rojas J, Stahlman MT. Early onset group B streptococcal disease: seven year experience and clinical scoring system. Acta Paediatr Scand 1983;72:597.)

Most babies with early-onset GBS will require intensive therapy. Obviously, those who are premature and in the high-risk, poor prognostic group will require the highest levels of support. At least 50% of babies with early-onset disease require ventilatory assistance for hypoxemia, or apnea not responsive to stimulation, and at least another 25% require supplementary oxygen. More than 35% of symptomatic babies develop hypotension, requiring fluid administration or pressor agents, although the details of the types of therapies required are not included in most of the reports. Babies with low 5-minute Apgar scores will require the usual intensive care approach given to the postischemic infant. Thrombocytopenia may be accompanied by frank disseminated intravascular coagulation (DIC) and clinical evidence of bleeding, requiring platelets, fresh frozen plasma, or cryoprecipitate, as described in Chapter 41.

Nearly 30% of infants with early-onset GBS develop meningitis[67], of whom 30% are reported to have seizures[80]. Further, in some cases, GBS organisms have been documented in the meningeal space on autopsy, when they had normal cerebrospinal fluid during life. This is particularly true of the babies with overwhelming infection that occurs immediately after birth.

Late-onset Disease

The incidence of late-onset GBS ranges from 0.2 to 1.5/1000 live births. For those who develop disease, there is no strong correlation between maternal colonization or perinatal complications. Premature infants who develop late-onset disease generally have been home, eating, gaining weight, and developing nicely when they become ill. The onset is less fulminant, and the mortality is lower (6 to 20%). When death occurs, it does so later in the hospital course than for babies with early-onset GBS (50 hours versus 15 hours). There is a high incidence of purulent meningitis, affecting about 75% of neonates with late-onset disease, and most infants have high cerebrospinal fluid protein (200 mg/dl), low glucose, and elevated white blood cells. Ninety-five percent of late-onset disease is caused by GBS type III, which has been postulated to have a special tropism for the meninges. It may be that somehow the interaction between this microorganism and the host allows better localization of disease, because bacteremia may also be accompanied by other forms of focal infection, such as septic arthritis, osteomyelitis, pleural empyema, cellulitis, breast abscess, and others[84,89].

The mechanism by which infants with late-onset disease become infected is not clear, since most of the mothers do not harbor the organism. Because the colonization rate rises in the nursery from nearly one-quarter of infants cultured on the first day of life to over 60% of those cultured at dis-

Table 31.10. Definition of Long-term Sequelae Resulting from GBS Meningitis[a]

Major Sequelae (N = 11)	*Mild or Moderate Sequelae (N = 8)*
Global mental retardation (7)	Unilateral sensorineural deafness (2)
Relapse of GBS meningitis (1)	Borderline mental retardation (2)
Uncontrolled seizures (6)	Spastic or flaccid monoparesis (3)
Cortical blindness (6)	Hydrocephalus, arrested (2)
Microcephalus (3)	Seizure disorder, controlled (1)
Hydrocephalus (3)	Expressive or receptive speech and language delay (2)
Spastic or flaccid quadriparesis (3)	Porencephalic cyst (1)
Central diabetes insipidus (1)	Mild frontal cortical atrophy (1)
Mild mental retardation (3)	Deficit in visual and auditory memory (1)

[a] *From Edwards MS, Rench MA, Haffar AAM, et al. Long-term sequelae of group B streptococcal meningitis in infants. J Pediatr 1985;106:717. Numbers in parentheses are number of patients.*

charge 3 days later, nosocomial transmission has been postulated. Personnel in nurseries and on obstetric units have a much higher rate of colonization with GBS than do their counterparts on medical-surgical units. Although nosocomial colonization quite clearly occurs, it is not obvious whether acquisition of disease at 1 month of life is in any way related to the organisms acquired before discharge from the nursery.

As with early-onset disease, the percentage of survivors has increased over the past decade. Unfortunately, the neurologic outcome for survivors of GBS meningitis has not improved as markedly. When the survivors of one study(79) were evaluated 3 years later, approximately 50% were reportedly normal, 21% had mild to moderate impairment, and 29% had severe neurologic deficit **(Table 31.10).** Factors predictive of poor prognosis (death or severe neurologic morbidity) included the presence of coma at hospital admission, an absolute neutropenia (less than 1000/ml3), cerebrospinal fluid protein greater than 300 mg/100 ml, and poor peripheral perfusion. The variables generally contributing to poor outcome in meningitis are discussed in the chapter on central nervous system (CNS) infections (Chapter 32).

Diagnosis

Since there are no specific physical signs or symptoms of GBS sepsis, the diagnosis cannot be based on clinical grounds alone. Likewise, routine laboratory tests are not helpful when trying to differentiate GBS from other causes of overwhelming sepsis in the neonate or infant. The differential diagnosis of the 10- to 14-day old baby who presents in shock with metabolic acidosis also includes noninfectious entities, such as coarctation of the aorta. If femoral pulses are absent or diminished, the infant should be treated with a continuous prostaglandin infusion, in addition to antimicrobial agents, until a definitive diagnosis is made.

Although the gold standard of diagnosis remains isolation of bacteria in culture, the development of rapid diagnostic methods for differentiating the predominant neonatal organisms has aided clinical judgment a great deal. The sensitivity of Latex agglutination to test for GBS antigen in concentrated urine samples approaches 100% in bacteremic patients. In patients with negative blood and cerebrospinal fluid cultures but evidence of GBS disease, measurements of sensitivity range from 67 to 88%. Specificity of the test has been measured at 93%. Typing of the GBS organisms is important, because this process can give helpful epidemiologic information.

Therapy

Although once thought to be universally sensitive to penicillin drugs, information is accruing that indicates GBS may be more difficult to treat than initially appreciated. There are several factors that in their interplay help regulate the relative sensitivity of the microorganism to penicillin in the living host, the most important of which is probably the individual's organism load.

One test commonly employed to assess the relative sensitivity of an organism for a particular antibiotic is determination of the minimal inhibitory concentration (MIC) of the antibiotic of interest against the particular strain of microorganism. The MIC of penicillin for GBS usually ranges from 0.03 to 0.12 μg/ml, which is easily achieved in the serum and spinal fluid. However, the test is usually performed with a standard inoculum of approximately 10^5 organisms. Some neonates have much higher concentrations of organisms (10^6 to 10^8 organisms per milliliter of cerebrospinal fluid have been documented). If the same test is performed with the highest concentration of bacteria, the MIC may be found to be 2 to 4 μg/ml(67). This level is not as easily reached in cerebrospinal fluid with routine doses of penicillin. Another variable that may explain difficulty treating this organism is the fact that some strains of GBS have become penicillin-tolerant, such that although the MIC is in the usual range, the minimal bactericidal (MBC) concentration may be more than 32 times the MIC(90). This is the case for 4 to 6% of strains evaluated(91) and may be responsible for some documented instances of treatment failure or recurrence(92,93).

The initial antibiotic therapy of the sick neonate generally consists of ampicillin and an aminoglycoside. This combination is effective against the majority of organisms encountered in the first month of life. In addition, ampicillin is nearly as good as penicillin if GBS is present, although there may be a twofold difference in their MICs. Also some evidence suggests that the ampicillin/gentamicin combination has a synergistic killing effect against the GBS organism. The group B streptococci, including those tolerant to penicillin, are usually sensitive to cefotaxime and ceftriaxone but not to moxalactam. Because *Listeria* is not sensitive to the third- generation cephalosporins, cefotaxime or ceftriaxone cannot be used alone in the initial therapy. The use of ampicillin and either cefotaxime or ceftriaxone is probably appropriate, but a possible negative interaction has been identified, in that the killing time of GBS is slightly delayed when the combination is used in vivo[82]. The addition of chloramphenicol to ampicillin is of no benefit in the treatment of GBS; in fact, this combination has been shown to be antagonistic because of the bacteriostatic effects of the former drug[94].

In addition to the general life-supportive measures and antibiotic administration required by babies infected with GBS, a number of adjunctive measures may be useful for the critically ill neonate who has shock and is at risk for dying within the first several hours of hospitalization. These approaches have been devised because of the relative inability of the neonate's immune system to handle GBS. Most specifically, the neonate is unable to opsonize the organism effectively. This is partly because of a deficiency of complement and lack of type-specific anti-GBS immunoglobulins G and M, as well as to the tendency for these sick babies to be granulocytopenic, with little or no bone marrow stores of myeloid precursors.

A small number of sick neonates have been treated with granulocyte transfusions with an apparent improvement in short-term outcome[95,96]. A similar response has been noted after double-volume exchange transfusions with whole blood that has been collected less than 24 hours previously. This procedure is thought to provide complement, antibody, and other plasma components in addition to white blood cells. One of the plasma products provided in this way is fibronectin, a glycoprotein that helps maintain vascular integrity and enhances phagocytic opsonization. Simple blood transfusion has also been associated with improved survival[97,98]. There is ongoing research with granulocyte colony-stimulating factor and granulocyte-macrophage colony-stimulating factor in GBS sepsis that may prove promising[99,100]. Intravenous immunoglobulin, hyperimmune globulin, and human anti-GBS monoclonal antibody[101–106] have all been evaluated in the therapy of this disease, as described previously. The finding that most babies with GBS are born to mothers who do not possess antibody against the infecting strain[69] and that opsonization is essential in the killing of encapsulated bacteria, including GBS[107–109], indicate that the passive immunization techniques have a great potential to change the outcome of this often catastrophic neonatal infection. However, their present effectiveness and utility remain to be confirmed.

Protective measures such as active or passive immunization of pregnant women[110], or chemoprophylaxis of colonized mothers and/or babies holds some promise[111], but will probably not be as effective as the combination of aggressive antimicrobial and adjunctive therapy of the infected neonate.

Listeria Monocytogenes

The bacterium *L. monocytogenes* is a facultative anaerobic Gram-positive rod. It primarily causes disease in various nonhuman species and has been associated with syndromes of meningoencephalitis and habitual abortion in goats, sheep, cows, and other animals[38,46,112]. No animal reservoir for human infection has ever been proven[112]. The first cases of neonatal listerial sepsis/meningitis documented in the literature were reported by Burn[49] in 1936. Almost 50 years before these four cases, Henle reported two neonatal cases of miliary granulomatosis, which were probably caused by *Listeria*[113]. It was not identified or named until 1926, when Murray et al.[114] isolated what they termed *Bacterium monocytogenes* from rabbits with a bacterial disease that caused a mononuclear leukocytosis. Three years later, the same bacterium was isolated from the blood of a man who had a mononucleosis-like syndrome[115]. In the 1930s, the organism was known as *Listerella,* and, finally in 1940, the official genus name became *Listeria*[55]. *Monocytogenes* refers to the prevalence of mononuclear cells in the bloodstream of most animal species infected with the organism and to the fact that, in some cases, organisms are found within the mononuclear cells.

Over the years, confusion has surrounded this microorganism, because it has several characteristics that allow it to be mistaken for other bacteria. The finding of a Gram-positive coccobacillary form in blood or cerebrospinal fluid is sometimes interpreted as a contaminating diphtheroid and, therefore, ignored. Because *Listeria* causes a small area of β-hemolysis when grown on sheep blood agar plates, it may be mistaken for a β-hemolytic streptococcal organism. The longer the organism stays in culture, the more coccoid the morphology becomes. Therefore, it is essential that the clinician specify his or her interest in isolating *Listeria* when disease is possible from this bacterium.

Reports of human disease have stressed the relatively high frequency among neonates and pregnant women[47–55,112,113,116]. Other groups who are at risk are the elderly and immune-compromised hosts[47,117]. Patients with reticuloendothelial malignancies and those who are receiving exogenous corticosteroids, are especially at risk. *Listeria* infection in previously healthy adults has been reported[118]. Disease in adults almost always presents as meningitis, often with associated sepsis. Mortality worsens with advancing patient age and debilitated preinfection status. For more information, the reader is referred to several reviews of *Listeria* in the adult population[47,117].

Infection in neonates has a bimodal presentation similar to that of GBS. Most disease appears to be sporadic, with occasional outbreaks and epidemics recorded in the literature[116,119–124]. Many cases of so-called early-onset disease may actually represent congenital infection with the offending organism, because some reports of early-onset listeriosis have been incidents of in utero death, such as stillbirth or spontaneous abortion. Nonetheless, since the majority of the literature specifies early-onset and late-onset disease, we will continue such designation here.

Early-onset Listerial Sepsis

Early-onset disease generally occurs within the first 3 days of life[47,48,50,52–55,116,119]. In 1985, Evans and colleagues[116] reported an outbreak of early-onset listeriosis caused by what may have been a particularly severe strain of the organisms. Of 15 cases of perinatal infection that occurred in a 5-month period at one institution in Nova Scotia, there were seven deaths. Four of the victims were stillborn between 20 and 30 weeks' gestation. The mother of each of the stillborn babies had a flu-like illness for a variable period of time preceding the fetal wastage. Symptoms in the mothers consisted of fever, headache, and other signs of illness such as abdominal pain, myalgias, or diarrhea. Diagnosis of fetal death was made between 4 hours and 4 days before delivery. Physical examination in the three babies in whom it was described included a rash noted to be of an extensive pustular and petechial nature and widespread over a large area of skin surfaces. Autopsy findings in this group of patients consisted of prominent granuloma formation in the skin, bronchi, liver, gastrointestinal tract, heart, kidneys, adrenals, bone marrow, and leptomeninges. Not all areas were involved in all patients. None of the mothers had ruptured membranes before fetal death.

The three neonates who succumbed shortly after delivery were also premature with gestational ages between 23 and 36 weeks. The mothers of these babies were also symptomatic, but none had prolonged rupture of membranes. The most immature baby died about 1 hour after delivery, and presented with a rash and respiratory distress. The other two babies died between 63 and 67 hours following delivery, and had low Apgar scores at birth and respiratory failure. All three had diffuse granulomatosis documented on autopsy.

Four of the remaining babies with severe disease survived, and four who had mild disease also survived. Those with severe disease all had respiratory distress, three had fever, and two had apnea and a rash. Two babies had meningitis and a residual spastic diplegia. These babies also were premature with gestational ages between 27 and 36 weeks. The four babies with mild disease ranged in age from 35 to 41 weeks. Two were healthy with no obvious evidence of systemic infection; the other two had fever and either respiratory distress or apnea.

The mean age of onset for the 15 patients discussed in this report was less than 1 hour after birth, which is significantly earlier than the mean age at onset of 1.4 days previously reported by the Centers for Disease Control (CDC)[48]. Since the CDC data represented endemic disease (19 cases in a 2-year period), it is possible that the particular type 4b strain, which caused the reported epidemic, was more devastating than previous sporadic infections. However, it is possible that some cases of *Listeria* are missed when they cause fetal death during a nonepidemic period. The overall mortality for the described series was 47%, which is higher than the CDC figures (33%), but in the range of previously reported[47–55] mortality figures for various series (25–70%). Sixty percent of babies had passed meconium into the amniotic fluid before delivery.

Other reports have described a similar set of circumstances surrounding perinatal infection, namely the presence of a febrile illness in approximately two-thirds of mothers; premature labor occurring 2 days to 2 weeks after the onset of maternal illness; meconium-stained amniotic fluid; and, in several cases, physical examination or autopsy findings consistent with disseminated infection in utero. In approximately 85%, findings of placental involvement with the microorganisms have been noted as well. Clinically, most babies with severe disease have a rash, hepatosplenomegaly, and fever.

In 1986, Boucher and Yonekura reported the results of a retrospective review aimed at identifying risk factors for early onset Listerial sepsis[125]. They concluded that a high maternal leukocyte count in combination with fetal tachycardia and diminished heart rate variability were indicative of a neonate at risk for a complicated course with *Listeria* sepsis.

Laboratory findings in neonates with early-onset disease have not been consistently reported. An associated anemia is found in 60% of patients. Leukopenia has been noted 20% of the time, but the WBC is elevated in 50% of affected newborns[55]. In the series reported by Lennon et al.[119], infected babies with totally normal leukocyte counts at birth developed few symptoms. Thrombocytopenia has been noted in 20 to 30%.

Babies with respiratory symptoms generally have abnormal chest roentgenograms, most showing patchy areas of pulmonic consolidation. It has been suggested that listerial pneumonitis may be caused by aspiration in utero of infected amniotic fluid[54]. Since many of the babies probably aspirate meconium, lung disease would be expected on that basis alone. None of the neonatal series has made a significant effort to separate the respiratory effects of the meconium aspiration syndrome from those of infection. In the report by Halliday and Hiratu[54], at least two of the three deaths were probably secondary to untreated (no tracheal suction at birth) meconium aspiration. Meningitis occurs in fewer than 30% of neonates with early-onset disease.

Investigators have looked for evidence of maternal vaginal colonization with the bacterium, in an effort to delineate the epidemiology of neonatal disease. Although vaginal cultures were overwhelmingly negative[119] (only 1 of 750 vaginal cultures in asymptomatic pregnant women, performed during the course of an outbreak of neonatal disease), there was a small but significant number of women who demonstrate rectal carriage (25 of 750 or 3%). Rates of rectal colonization were higher in certain geographic areas of the city in which the investigation took place, as well as among specific ethnic groups. It was speculated that variation in the rate of raw shellfish consumption may have been related to the increased rate of colonization and disease among the Polynesian group in Auckland. A recent CDC survey detected gastrointestinal carriage in 21% of household contacts of patients with invasive listeriosis[126].

Listeria outbreaks have been linked to contaminated food sources in the United States and in Europe. A multistate surveillance study by the CDC found that patients who had listeriosis were more likely than controls to have eaten soft cheeses and food purchased in delicatessens. Food from patients' refrigerators was cultured and *Listeria* was grown in

64% of the cases[127]. In Denmark, *Listeria* infection was linked to the consumption of unpasteurized milk and several types of cheeses[128].

Late-onset Listerial Disease

Late-onset disease is less common, occurs primarily in healthy full-term babies, is associated with meningeal infection, has a better prognosis, and is more often caused by type 4b[48–55]. Mean age at onset is 1 to 2 weeks, with almost all cases occurring by 30 days of age[48]. Mothers of affected babies are generally asymptomatic, although other family members may have a mild febrile illness. The mechanism of infection is not known but appears to be through fecal-oral spread. Nosocomial acquisition has not been reported, and rates of colonization among health care workers are not known. Long-term sequelae of late-onset infection appear to be infrequent, although postmeningitic hydrocephalus has been noted[48].

There are no specific clinical or laboratory findings that separate neonatal listerial meningitis from that caused by GBS, *E. coli*, or other pathogens. Only a small proportion of the patients have a mononuclear predominance of cells in the cerebrospinal fluid at presentation, although this probably changes with duration of infection, and the babies may or may not have organisms demonstrable on Gram's stain of the fluid[55]. Bacteremia is usually present. Other manifestations of disease may include pneumonitis, otitis media, or oculoglandular infection with purulent conjunctivitis. Rash is not a prominent finding in late neonatal infections; likewise, hepatosplenomegaly and evidence of miliary disease are usually lacking.

Immune Response to Listeria

Host resistance and response to listerial infection depends primarily on cell-mediated factors. Macrophages play an essential role in the host response to this organism and are critical in the development of a specific T-cell response. Lymphokines (especially interferon-γ and IL-2) are released by T cells and stimulate further macrophage activity. Of these factors, interferon-γ has been shown to be of greatest importance[129]. Neonatal T cells exhibit diminished production of interferon-γ. This is probably related to the immature relationship between monocytes (macrophages) and T cells, as described in Chapter 28. Animal species that have been tested do not reproducibly develop elevated antibody titers to the organism; the same situation is true for humans. There is no reliable serologic test to either look for evidence of recent infection or document immunity. Rodents respond to immunization and challenge with listerial organisms with proliferation of specific sets of T cells[130].

Therapy and Prevention

Evidence suggests that antimicrobial therapy of the mother at the onset of febrile illness is effective in either preventing overt disease in the neonate or in significantly limiting its severity[131]. Maternal disease is usually self-limited, with resolution of symptoms at or shortly after delivery, whether or not antibiotics are administered[54]. Postnatal treatment of the severely affected neonate may not be effective, since disease is generally widespread with disseminated granuloma formation (granulomatosis infantisepticum) at the time of delivery. As described previously, a number of those infected in utero are stillborn.

Ampicillin is the drug of first choice for most listerial infections[132]. In vitro studies indicate synergism of gentamicin with ampicillin, and most experts recommend initial therapy with the combination for 10 to 14 days, followed by another 7 days of ampicillin alone, if the organism is sensitive. *L. monocytogenes* is almost universally sensitive to tetracycline, but the antimicrobial agent is contraindicated during gestation and infancy because of well-described adverse effects on developing teeth and bones. The use of chloramphenicol, alone or in combination with penicillin or ampicillin, has resulted in high mortality in adults and is, therefore, contraindicated[117]. Trimethoprim-sulfamethoxazole (TMP-SMX) is a bactericidal drug that has been used successfully in adults[133]. It has excellent CNS penetration and has acceptable MICs against most strains of *Listeria*. Third-generation cephalosporins are not active against the organism[134,135].

Because cytokine production is diminished in neonates, as described previously, administration of interferon-γ or TNF-α may prove useful in the future. It is not clear whether administration of intravenous immunoglobulin (IVIG) would be efficacious.

Summary

The pediatric intensive care specialist is more likely to see late-onset disease with *Listeria*, since the majority of those at greatest risk for early-onset disease will probably be admitted to the newborn ICU (meconium aspiration and/or prematurity). Therefore, most of the babies treated in the PICU will have meningitis, but may also present with pulmonary problems. The actual incidence of late-onset disease is not known, but seems to vary according to location; therefore, it is impossible to predict the frequency with which any individual will have the opportunity to treat such a baby. In some areas, *Listeria* may make up as much as 20% of all cases of neonatal sepsis or meningitis[46]. It was the fifth most frequent cause of meningitis among all age groups in New York City[117]. Initial ICU therapy should reflect the common goals of initial assessment of the critically ill, followed by support of respiratory and cardiac functions, preservation of neurologic function, and specific antimicrobial therapy. Since there are no rapid diagnostic aids (with the exception of finding the presumptive organism on Gram's stain), the initial therapy must be broad spectrum and aimed at all likely causes of sepsis or purulent meningitis. Survival of babies with late-onset disease is to be anticipated; long-term sequelae of uncomplicated disease are unlikely.

Disseminated Herpes Simplex Virus (HSV) Infection

Introduction and Epidemiology

Although HSV types 1 and 2 are the etiologic agents in most human disease reported to be herpes, there are four other members of the human herpes virus group. These include cytomegalovirus (CMV), Epstein-Barr virus (EBV), varicella zoster virus (VZV), and human herpes virus type 6 (HHV-6, formerly known as roseola). All of these agents are capable of causing significant disease in humans of all ages, but because of the significance of HSV in the neonate we will concentrate on HSV-1 and HSV-2 illness in this section.

The reported frequency of HSV infections of the newborn doubled in the 1970s, so that by the early 1980s, the incidence was estimated at 1 in every 3750 live births(136). The neonate may have widely disseminated disease, with multiorgan system involvement, including but not limited to the CNS(137,138). The disease carries a high mortality rate, and a large percentage of survivors suffer significant neurologic sequelae(139,140).

The disease may be acquired prenatally or postnatally, but contraction of infection during delivery (natal infection) is the most common(137). The majority of infections in which a source is identified are related to maternal genital infection at the time of delivery(141,142). Likelihood of the neonate contracting disease in this manner is correlated with rupture of membranes of longer than 6 hours in a mother with active genital infection. Premature babies are more likely to become infected, although it may be that active infection predisposes to premature onset of labor. Babies born to women with a primary herpes infection are at a much greater risk than those born to women with reactivation of the disease. Delivery of babies by cesarean section less than 4 hours following rupture of membranes is to a great extent protective(140). Although 50 to 86%(140) of neonates born by either the vaginal or the cesarean route more than 6 hours after rupture of membranes contract disease, only 6% of babies delivered by cesarean section within 4 hours following rupture of membranes become infected. Approximately 70% of isolates from infected neonates are type 2(140). Isolation of type 1 virus does not exclude infection through the genital route, because 10 to 20% of adult genital disease may be caused by type 1(143).

In 1991, Brown and colleagues reported the results of a large prospective study of asymptomatic pregnant women in early labor(144). Of 15,923 cultured women, HSV was recovered from only 56. Of these, only 18 had serologic evidence of a recent primary infection. The remainder (65%) had reactivation of HSV. Although only 3% of infants born to women with reactivation of HSV developed neonatal herpes infection, 33% of those born to women with primary infection contracted the disease. Of the ten infants in this study who developed HSV infection, eight had fetal scalp electrodes for monitoring, nine were delivered by the vaginal route, and three were born to mothers with negative cultures, but with histories and serologies consistent with prior HSV infections. Seven of the neonates had type 2 disease. These infants had more severe disease, and only two of them recovered intact. Of the three infants with HSV-1, all recovered with intact neurodevelopmental status.

Postnatal acquisition also occurs and may result from contact of the neonate with infected maternal secretions, as well as contact with hospital personnel and others who are actively shedding virus in their saliva or carrying live virus on their hands. A 1978 case report(143) documented transmission of HSV type 1 from a physician to a neonate at delivery during oral endotracheal suctioning of the neonate because of meconium-stained amniotic fluid.

Clinical Manifestations

Neonatal HSV disease generally presents within the first week of life, but an incubation period of up to 21 days has been documented(145). The early course of disseminated infection is similar to that of acute bacterial sepsis and cannot be distinguished on clinical grounds. Mucosal or skin vesicular lesions are present in only 20 to 30% of affected babies. Meningoencephalitis occurs in approximately 50%, but cerebrospinal fluid analysis may be normal in the early stages of disease. When actively sought, the virus is generally recoverable by culture or fluorescent antibody technique in secretions from the trachea, nasopharynx, and gastrointestinal and genitourinary tracts and from the bloodstream(141). Recently, the polymerase chain reaction has been used to isolate HSV DNA from cerebrospinal fluid and serum of patients(146–149). Although not commonly available at present, this technique may prove valuable in diagnosis. Unfortunately, the identification of HSV in the neonate often occurs when the baby is close to death, since viral studies are not often done unless there is clinical reason to suspect infection based on maternal history or presence of vesicles in the baby.

Several case reports(150–153) have demonstrated fatal neonatal pneumonia in babies subsequently shown to be infected with the virus. The most recent of these was a 6-day-old baby who had a respiratory illness, subsequently requiring intubation for respiratory failure. He had a bilateral interstitial infiltrate on the initial chest radiograph. Liver transaminases were normal initially and on repeat examination. Examination of the cerebrospinal fluid did not suggest infection. The baby was noted to have an ammonia greater than 1000 μmol/liter, for which hemodialysis and subsequent continuous arteriovenous hemofiltration were employed, in conjunction with sodium benzoate and sodium phenylacetate. Evaluation for inborn errors was unrevealing. The baby expired 76 hours after the onset of the illness, despite therapy with broad-spectrum antibiotics, acyclovir, and IVIG. HSV type 2 was recovered from cultures of blood, lung, tracheal secretions, and conjunctivae. On autopsy, the only organ with significant disease was the lungs. The cause of the hyperammonemia was not clear, but was postulated to be related to severe hypoxemia during the course of the respiratory failure.

Table 31.11. Clinical Features and Mortality Rates of Neonatal HSV Disease

Disease	*Clinical Features*
Disseminated HSV	Apnea Respiratory distress Liver failure Hypotension DIC Superinfection common Mortality 92%
CNS disease	Seizures Lethargy or coma Elevated intracranial pressure Mortality 40%

Therefore, HSV should be suspected in any baby who has symptoms suggestive of sepsis. Associated findings in disseminated disease include acute adrenal hemorrhage and necrosis with shock, as well as ischemic and fatty changes in the liver. These babies are often apneic, develop respiratory distress and failure, and have clinical evidence of liver failure (jaundice, elevated transaminase levels) and severe hypotension requiring inotropic support(154). DIC, which often accompanies sepsis, may be difficult to treat and may lead to clinically significant bleeding. Seizures usually occur in patients with acute encephalitis. Bacterial superinfection of the debilitated baby is not uncommon.

Prognosis for babies with disseminated infection is poor;(134) this group of infants has a 92% mortality. When CNS involvement accompanies disseminated infection, the mortality is somewhat lower (72%), but the majority of survivors (57%) have serious neurologic sequelae(134). Mortality of localized CNS disease is 40%, with sequelae in 70% of survivors. Disease apparently localized to the skin, eye, or mouth is rarely fatal, but does carry some risk of neurologic consequences in up to 50% of cases. Primary pulmonary HSV has a reported mortality of between 67% and 89%(150–152,155,156). Pneumonitis associated with coagulopathy has been reported to have a 100% mortality rate in a recent review of mortality and morbidity predictors in this disease(156). Babies who have disseminated disease resulting from infection with HSV-2 have a poorer outcome than those infected with type 1 virus, potentially related to the apparently increased rate of pneumonitis and DIC associated with type 2. Another reason potentially worsening the outcome for those with HSV-2 is that it is less susceptible to treatment with acyclovir. **Table 31.11** lists clinical features and associated rates of mortality.

Prevention and Therapy

Such a grim outlook for this infection makes prevention essential, and early recognition and initiation of therapy are of paramount importance. As mentioned previously, cesarean section in the first few hours following rupture of membranes may be effective in preventing the majority of perinatally acquired infections when the mother has active genital herpes. There is no evidence that mothers with genital lesions need to be isolated from their babies postnatally, because no transmission has been demonstrated through genital secretions. However, good hygienic measures should be employed, and mothers should be instructed in frequent hand washing(142,143). In the presence of active oral lesions, proper procedures are less clear, but it may be wise to separate the mother and neonate until viral shedding has stopped(157). Virus may be shed until the skin has returned to normal. It is not known whether maternal use of a mask during handling or breast feeding is adequate. Nosocomial spread of the virus may occur, so neonates with suspected or proven infection should be isolated, and personnel providing close care must wear gloves and engage in vigorous hand washing after contact with the infants' secretions.

Specific therapy of HSV with an antiviral agent is essential. Currently, the drug of choice is acyclovir (ACV), which has recently been demonstrated to be as efficacious as vidarabine(158) when given at a dose of 30 mg/kg/day in three divided doses, administered every 8 hours. Although there is agreement that babies with documented disease or the presence of active lesions are indication for therapy with ACV, less agreement exists with regard to presumptive therapy of babies at risk. On the basis of clinical experience and from available information in the medical literature, this author recommends that any neonate with sepsis be treated with ACV if he or she fails to respond to empiric bacterial coverage, or if there is evidence of disseminated disease or isolated pneumonitis(159).

Adjunctive measures are not well documented. However, since passive immunization seems to be effective in animals, and babies who have received a high titer of maternal antibody are less likely to become infected, the use of human serum immunoglobulin, which is relatively rich in anti-HSV antibodies, may be of use. Evaluation of available IVIG preparations indicates that better efficacy will probably be achieved with the use of hyperimmune serum(160,161). No evidence exists to suggest that white cell transfusions are helpful, or that plasma components are useful except to halt the bleeding problems associated with DIC. At present, there are no commercially available monoclonal antibody preparations, nor is hyperimmune HSV globulin prepared.

Care of the sick infant with HSV is not different from that of the baby with overwhelming bacterial sepsis, and requires meticulous attention to the details of respiratory, hemodynamic, and CNS support and resuscitation discussed elsewhere in this volume. Specific issues related to the care of the patient with meningoencephalitis are discussed in Chapter 32.

Older Infant and Child

Beyond the first month of life, the spectrum of etiologic agents responsible for overwhelming sepsis changes. Gram-negative enteric organisms drop out of the picture in the immune competent host, and are replaced by *S. pneumoniae, N. meningitidis,* and *H. influenzae* type b. Sepsis resulting from β-hemolytic streptococcus and *S. aureus* is uncommon, except in certain situations that are defined in a later section.

Table 31.12. Pathogenic Bacteria Isolated from Children Seen in an Outpatient Department[a]

Organism	*No. of Patients*	*% with Positive Cultures*	*% of all 708 Patients with Cultures*
S. pneumoniae	19	61.3	2.68
H. influenzae type b	6	19.4	0.85
S. aureus	2	6.5	0.28
S. pyogenes	1	3.2	0.14
Microaerophilic streptococcus	1	3.2	0.14
N. meningitidis	1	3.2	0.14
Salmonella sp.	1	3.2	0.14
Total	31	100.0	4.37

[a] *From McGowan JE Jr, Bratton L, Klein JO, Finland M. Bacteremia in febrile children seen in a "walk-in" pediatric clinic. N Engl J Med 1973;288:1309. Reprinted by permission of the* New England Journal of Medicine.

Infants and children less than 2 years of age are often febrile, and may develop occult bacteremia(162–166). The problems involved in evaluation and therapy of such children need not be dealt with here, other than to mention that the mere presence of bacteria in the bloodstream (most often pneumococci) does not usually lead to overwhelming sepsis or the need for intensive care. Organisms isolated in a representative study of this problem are listed in **Table 31.12**(164). Many children with occult pneumococcal bacteremia are cured by the time the blood culture becomes positive, and, therefore, some may not require parenteral antimicrobial agents.

Of greater interest to the pediatric critical care practitioner is symptomatic bacteremia, which results in serious systemic manifestations of disease. Sepsis in the immune-deficient host is considered in Chapter 42. Overwhelming sepsis in the normal host may be primary (with no apparent localized source) or secondary to infection at a particular site. It is the primary bacteremias we will discuss here, which may present in a fulminant manner, and which may also lead to or have concomitant infection at other sites.

Meningococcemia is the classic infection in children without a source, and may be particularly fulminant, leading to death in a short time; it will be the major subject of discussion here. *H. influenzae* type b, although most often associated with meningitis, is in reality a blood-borne disease that may result in localized infection in a number of areas and, therefore, will also be addressed in this section. Other bacteria, as well as rickettsia and some viruses, can cause a similar picture of overwhelming sepsis in the older infant and child but are not as common as the first two microorganisms mentioned. They include *S. aureus*, β-hemolytic streptococcus, tularemia, brucellosis, plague, Rocky Mountain spotted fever, and viral hemorrhagic fevers. Some of these disease entities are discussed in Chapter 33.

Meningococcemia

Bacteriology

N. meningitidis is a Gram-negative coccus that usually grows in pairs or tetrads. It is aerobic, but may also grow as a facultative anaerobe, and prefers to grow with carbon dioxide enhancement on blood or chocolate agar. It is catalase- and oxidase-positive. All of the pathogenic strains have a polysaccharide capsule, the presence of which correlates with invasiveness. The chemical composition of the capsule determines the sero group to which the organism belongs. Clinically recognized sero groups are A through D, X, Y, Z, Z′, and W-135. Further classification is made on the basis of protein antigens found in the cell wall. Sero groups B and C make up the majority of clinical isolates. The type 2 protein antigen is associated with at least 50% of type B isolates and a significant percentage of type C organisms as well.

Epidemiology

The relative frequency of isolation of various serotypes varies with geographic location, as well as with time. An epidemiologic review of meningococcal disease in New York City(167) revealed an increasingly frequent isolation of some of the more recently recognized serotypes, with a substantial percentage of disease caused by serotypes Y and W-135 in addition to the classic groups A to C. Reasons for these epidemiologic variations are unknown, but they have been postulated to be related to either a natural cycling tendency of the meningococcus, or a response to increased immunity to serotypes A, B, and C produced by widespread immunizations in some areas. Additionally, it is clear that a number of previously untypable strains were actually W-135(168).

Disease caused by *N. meningitidis* is usually endemic, but there have been reports of epidemics, especially among military personnel. The epidemic nature of the disease was well demonstrated during World War II, when it was responsible for more deaths because of infection than any other single microorganism(169).

Over the past several decades, evaluation of endemic disease because of *N. meningitidis* has revealed an overall incidence of approximately two cases per 100,000 population per year. Ninety percent of disease occurs in children less than 2 years of age. In one study from Scandinavia(170), the incidence in infants less than 1 year of age was 15/100,000/yr. Data from the United States are similar, with an incidence in the same age group of 14.4/100,000/yr(168). Disease is rare in infants less than 1 month of age, although reports of neonatal meningococcemia have appeared from time to time(166,160–174). Although neonatal infection has generally been considered a more benign form of disease than that which occurs later in infancy, some cases in the first month of life have been described as fulminant, resulting in death shortly after diagnosis(162–174). Attack rates fall dramatically in the 4- to 9-year-old age group (Fig. 31.2).

In recent years, there have been several reports indicating an increasing occurrence of epidemics resulting from *N. meningitidis* serogroup C both in the United States(175,176) and in Canada(177). These cases tended to occur in older patients (more than 5 years) and had a higher mortality. In Canada, the predominant organism was a strain of serogroup C known as ET-15. The case fatality for ET-15 was 17.8% compared to 8.1% for all other invasive menin-

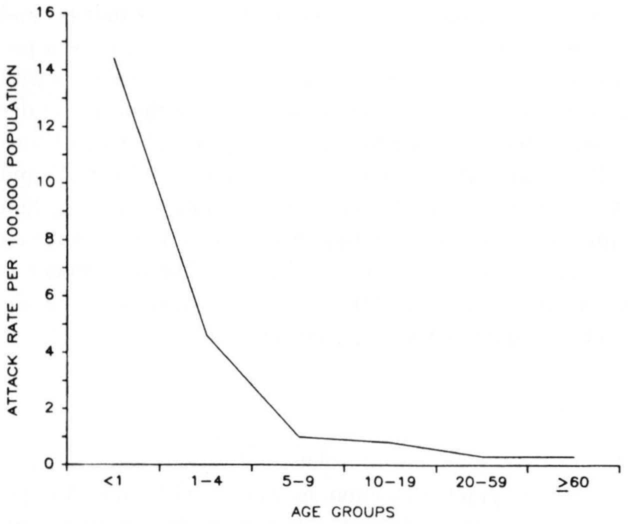

Figure 31.2. Meningococcal disease attack rates in the United States by age, 1975 to 1980. (From Band JD, Chamberland ME, Platt T, Weaver RE, Thornsberry C, Fraser DW. Trends in meningococcal disease in the United States, 1975–80. J Infect Dis 1983;148:754.)

gococcal disease[177]. In Los Angeles, an isolate of serogroup C known as ET-22 was responsible for a marked increase in the incidence of meningococcal disease in the late 1980s[175]. Overall, twenty-one outbreaks of serogroup C meningococcal disease were reported in the United States from 1980 to 1993. Eight of these outbreaks occurred in the last two years, indicating that epidemic serogroup C disease was becoming more prevalent at the same time as more virulent strains are emerging[176].

Nonepidemic systemic infection with *N. meningitidis* occurs sporadically, but is more prevalent in the late winter and early spring. Prior infection with influenza A or B has been associated with increased susceptibility to meningococcemia, and therefore, may explain the observed clustering of cases in some instances[178]. Varying sex ratios have been reported, but overall, infection is more common in males. In some series, males make up at least 60% of those affected[179–181]. Interestingly, the ratios are reversed when considering acute fulminating meningococcemia with females, making up as much as 70% of this hyperacute form of disease.

Carriage of the organism in the nasopharynx is common, and most individuals who are exposed become colonized[170]. Development of clinical infection correlates with lack of serum antibody. An elevation of the carriage rate occurs during epidemics, where spread is mostly among household contacts. The rate of carriage in the family group is much higher when the index case is an infant, compared to that of an older child or adult (38%, 17.5%, and 6.9%, respectively). Upper respiratory symptoms may accompany development of the carrier state and may be related to low-grade infections, or to preceding infections by influenza or ECHO viruses, which may then result in an accelerated rate of carriage as well as increased risk of actual infection by the meningococcus.

Clinical Manifestations

N. meningitidis causes a wide range of clinical disease. Noninvasive forms of infection may cause genitourinary and gastrointestinal disease, as well as purulent conjunctivitis, which may be easily confused with gonorrheal conjunctival disease. Meningococcal pharyngitis has also been reported, but true infection is difficult to separate from colonization[182].

Categorization of invasive systemic disease depends on whether the infection predominantly causes septicemia or meningitis. This may be a useful classification, and, as will be shown later, has implications regarding therapy and prognosis. The two groups of serious meningococcal infection truly represent a continuum in the spectrum of disease, since both groups have similar epidemiology, yet vary with regard to severity and outcome.

Initial symptoms of systemic infection usually consist of upper respiratory complaints, fever, joint pains, myalgias, rash, headache, and vomiting. Physical findings include high fever (greater than 40°C in 60%); rash that may be macular, petechial, or purpuric; and meningeal signs when meningitis predominates. Objective diffuse muscle tenderness is generally present. Signs of shock, such as hypotension, tachycardia, diminished perfusion, and cool skin in the presence of elevated core temperature are present in the cases of fulminant bacteremia. When petechiae are present (50 to 60%), they are more pronounced on the trunk and extremities. When purpura develops, the lesions are distinct from the petechiae and are usually a harbinger of severe disease. In the 80% of patients who have signs of meningeal involvement, alterations in level of consciousness and abnormal pupillary responses may occur, suggesting the presence of elevated intracranial pressure.

Laboratory findings vary with the severity of disease and have been correlated with prognosis in some situations. A study of factors useful in determining prognosis among pediatric patients with meningococcal infection was reported by Stiehm and Damrosch[183] in 1966. They reviewed 63 cases with an overall mortality rate of 19% and were able to set up a scoring system to predict those at highest risk of death. They found five factors that, when present, indicated an unfavorable prognosis **(Table 31.13).** If three or more factors were present at admission, the child had a

Table 31.13. Unfavorable Prognostic Features in Meningococcal Infections as Defined by Stiehm and Damrosch and Used to Determine the Prognostic Score[a]

1. Presence of petechiae for less than 12 hr prior to admission
2. Presence of shock (blood pressure 70 systolic or below)
3. Absence of meningitis (less than 20 WBC/mm^3) in cerebrospinal fluid
4. Blood leukocyte count normal or low (less than 10,000 WBC/mm^3)
5. Erythrocyte sedimentation rate normal or low (less than 10 mm/hr)

[a] *From Stiehm ER, Damrosch DS. Factors in the prognosis of meningococcal infection. J Pediatr 1966;68:457.*

Table 31.14. Relation of Prognostic Score to Fatality Rate in 63 Cases of Meningococcal Infections from Reference 125[a] and 15 Cases from Pediatric Literature

	Prognostic Score (Total of Unfavorable Prognostic Features)[b]	Total Cases	Died	Fatality Rate (%)
Reference 125 (63 cases)	0	21	1	4.7
	1	26	2	7.7
	2	6	0	0
	3	7	6	85.7
	4	2	2	100.0
	5	1	1	100.0
Cases from pediatric literature				
	1	4	1	25.0
	2	6	1	16.6
	3	5	4	80.0

[a] *From Stiehm ER, Damrosch DS. Factors in the prognosis of meningococcal infection. J Pediatr 1966;68:457.*
[b] *Defined in Table 31.13.*

greater than 85% chance of dying. If two or fewer factors were noted, the mortality rate was less than 10% **(Table 31.14).**

These poor prognostic factors relate both to the virulence of the organism and to host resistance factors, and their presence in the sickest patients can be explained on the basis of failure of the patient to respond adequately to and/or localize the infection. The absence of meningeal reaction (defined by Stiehm and Damrosch as fewer than 20 WBC/mm^3 of cerebrospinal fluid) and low leukocyte count may represent failure of the host's neutrophils to mount an appropriate response. Because the primary determinant of the sedimentation rate is fibrinogen, a low erythrocyte sedimentation rate in the presence of an infectious disease usually represents low levels of fibrinogen, which may indicate ongoing DIC. The interval, in terms of duration of petechiae before admission, relates to the rapidity with which the child's symptoms lead the parent to seek medical care. The presence of shock on admission indicates a high level of circulating endotoxin causing cardiovascular collapse.

In another study of prognostic factors, Niklasson et al.[(184)] looked at a population that included adults and were able to define six factors predictive of poor outcome that are similar to those of Stiehm and Damrosch but include thrombocytopenia and presence of temperature greater than 40°C. They did not evaluate the significance of the erythrocyte sedimentation rate **(Tables 31.15 and 31.16).**

Table 31.15. Unfavorable Prognostic Factors in Meningococcal Disease per Niklasson et al.[a]

1. Absence of meningitis (less than 100 WBC/mm^3 in cerebrospinal fluid).
2. Presence of low blood pressure (less than 70 in children less than 14 yr of age)
3. Presence of petechiae for less than 12 hr prior to admission
4. Presence of marked hyperpyrexia (rectal temperature 40°C or above)
5. Absence of marked leukocytosis (less than 15,000 WBC/mm^3 of blood)
6. Presence of thrombocytopenia (less than 100,000 platelets/mm^3 of blood)

[a] *Adapted with permission from Niklasson P, Lundbergh P, Strandell T. Prognostic factors in meningococcal disease. Scand J Infect Dis 1971;3:17.*

Table 31.16. Relation of Prognostic Score to Fatality Rate in 80 Patients with Meningococcal Disease[a]

Score	Total No.	Deaths	Fatality Rate (%)
A (N = 80)			
0	47	0	0
1	16	1	6
2	7	0	0
3	3	2	67
4	7	6	86
B (N = 77)			
0	32	0	0
1	27	0	0
2	10	1	10
3	3	1	33
4	2	1	50
5	3	3	100
C (N = 25)			
0	6	0	0
1	8	0	0
2	4	0	0
3	4	0	0
4	1	1	100
5	1	1	100
6	1	1	100

[a] *From Niklasson P, Lundbergh P, Strandell T. Prognostic factors in meningococcal disease. Scand J Infect Dis 1971;3:17. Part A includes only the first 4 prognostic factors given in Table 31.15; part B the first 5 factors; and part C all 6 factors. N = number of individuals.*

More recently, Wong and colleagues were able to identify a number of poor prognostic indicators among a group of 100 children with meningococcemia[(181)]. These included hypothermia, seizures or shock on presentation, total peripheral WBC less than 5000/mm^3, platelet count less than 100,000/mm^3, and the development of purpura fulminans.

The Glasgow Meningococcal Septicemia Prognostic Score is a prognostic score based totally on clinical parameters, except for inclusion of the arterial base deficit. It was recently validated by Thomson and colleagues in the United Kingdom **(Table 31.17)**[(185)]. A score of more than 8 predicts death 73% of the time, and a score of more than 10

Table 31.17. Glasgow Meningococcal Septicemia Prognostic Score[a]

Parameter	Points
BP < 75 mm Hg systolic, age <4 yr; <85 mm Hg systolic, age >4 yr	3
Skin/rectal temperature difference >3°C	3
Modified coma scale score <8 or deterioration of ≤3 points in 1 hr	3
Deterioration in hour before scoring	2
Absence of meningism	2
Extending purpuric rash or widespread ecchymoses	1
Base deficit (capillary or arterial) >8.0	1
Maximum score	15

[a] *With permission from Thomson APJ, Sill JA, Hart CA. Validation of the Glasgow Meningococcal Septicemia Prognostic Score: a 10-year retrospective survey. Crit Care Med 1991;19:26–30.*

predicts death 87.5% of the time. However, this scoring system could not predict death with a 100% certainty, so therapy should be undertaken for all patients regardless of score. Similar scoring systems have been developed by other investigators[186,187].

Other factors have also been found to be related to poor prognosis, but in a less predictive way. These include presence of eosinophils and low levels of 17-hydroxycorticoids (both representing relative failure of adrenocortical function), the meningococcal serotype (B and C more likely to cause death), age (less than 2 years of age more likely to have fatal outcome), levels of the circulating cytokines TNFα, IL-1, and interferon-γ[188], and the presence of circulating endotoxin[189].

The purpose of identifying which patients are most likely to die in the face of conventional therapy is to make the clinician more aware of the need for rapid therapeutic action in patients who present with an unfavorable score. The intensive care specialist will be more likely to institute invasive monitoring techniques and support of vital functions in anticipation of potential acute deterioration. In addition, applying a score to each patient allows evaluation and comparison of newer forms of therapy, over time and among various institutions.

Death from meningococcal disease is generally caused by intractable shock, even in patients with meningitis. Acute fulminating meningococcemia usually results in death in a matter of hours from the time of admission. Mean duration of survival was 9 hours, with a range of 2 to 20 hours in the study by Niklasson et al.[184]. The pathogenesis of the severe cardiovascular collapse has been a matter of debate and is discussed more fully in the following section. There is also a group of patients who die of profound neurologic deterioration, postulated by some authors to represent elevated intracranial pressure, with or without herniation[169]. Although numerous reports of intensive care therapy of patients with meningococcal meningitis are available, papers that include actual measurement of intracranial pressure are scarce. In the report by Nugent et al.[190], the authors maintain that continuous monitoring of intracranial pressure allowed more consistent control of the intracerebral pressure, and guided the therapeutic approach, in a way that could not have been achieved in the absence of intracranial pressure monitoring. The ease with which such monitoring is accomplished in the ICU setting and the rarity of adverse sequelae, especially with the use of a subarachnoid screw, make it a reasonable technique in patients with serious disease accompanied by loss of consciousness, presence of posturing or flaccidity, or evidence of third-nerve involvement, which may indicate compression of the brainstem by the uncal portion of the temporal lobe. Third-nerve dysfunction may also represent a localized inflammatory response to the organism, and the decision to monitor intracranial pressure must take into account the entire physical examination. Occasionally, documentation of diffuse cerebral edema on CT scan may reinforce the decision to monitor intracranial pressure. The absence of obvious edema, however, should not be taken as a reason not to institute monitoring if clinical signs and symptoms suggest elevated intracranial pressure. We should point out that ICP monitoring in this disease has not been studied formally, and its potential impact on outcome has not been substantiated.

Fulminant Meningococcemia (Waterhouse-Friderichsen Syndrome)

Cases of fulminant disease associated with bilateral adrenal hemorrhage documented on autopsy have been given the eponym Waterhouse-Friderichsen syndrome. Because this is a pathologic diagnosis, and because neither Waterhouse[191] nor Friderichsen[192] contributed significantly to the understanding of this syndrome, which was initially described by others, it is probably unreasonable to perpetuate the use of this term. Instead, we will use the term fulminant meningococcemia.

Fulminant meningococcemia is nearly always fatal and represents a hyperacute form of disease. Petechiae are universally present, purpura generally develops, and the patient's shock may or may not respond to the fluids and pressor agents generally employed[170,183,193,194]. Mercier and colleagues looked at the hemodynamic patterns of 18 children with meningococcal sepsis over a 5-year period[195]. They compared the hemodynamic profiles of survivors versus nonsurvivors, although nine of their patients died within 3 to 4 hours of reaching the PICU and, therefore, could not be studied. Both groups of patients required large infusions of fluid to remedy intravascular depletion. In the nonsurvivors, the wedge pressures remained low, despite receiving approximately 11 ml/kg/hr over the first 12 hours of their stay in the PICU. This was postulated to be caused by persistent capillary leak syndrome. Although cardiac function (cardiac index, stroke volume, and shortening fraction on echocardiogram) was low in both groups at the onset of monitoring, it improved over the first day or so in the survivors, whereas it remained unchanged in those destined to die of the disease, despite the use of inotropic agents. No one inotropic agent has emerged as clearly superior in this study. Other reports have referred to the use of pulmonary artery or central venous catheters but have not specifically documented hemodynamic effects of various therapeutic modalities[196,197].

Primary myocardial failure is an attractive explanation of failure of the patient to respond to many therapies generally employed in shock caused by other organisms. The finding of polymorphonuclear infiltrates in the myocardium in every autopsy case from a series by Bohm[198] in 1982 gives substantial support to the presence of a dysfunctional myocardium and perhaps reveals the cause of death among some patients who undergo sudden unexpected death from this disease.

The finding of bilateral adrenal hemorrhage in a large percentage of autopsied cases initially led to the belief that the intractable shock was related to adrenal cortical failure. Early attempts at treating this infection with exogenous corticosteroids were promising[199,200]. Larger studies have failed to demonstrate an effect on mortality[201–205], but sporadic reports of success[206] continue to appear in the literature. Evaluations of adrenocortical function have yielded variable results[207,208]. In many cases, some function is demonstrated, but it is not possible to know whether this function is adequate for the stress of the situation. In some cases, stimulation tests with ACTH have resulted in poor response. Replacement therapy, or administration of very large doses of hydrocortisone (40 to 50 mg/kg) or methylprednisolone, has not resulted in reversal of shock. Therefore, even if some adrenocortical insufficiency exists, it does not appear to be the sole cause of the shock.

Several authors have interpreted the pathologic findings in fulminant meningococcemia as consistent with the Schwartzman reaction, which is an experimental condition produced in rabbits exposed to endotoxin and which takes two different forms, local and systemic. In the local Schwartzman reaction, the animal is primed with subcutaneously administered endotoxin, followed 24 hours later by intravenous administration of the same substance. Such treatment results in hemorrhagic necrosis at the site of local injection. In the systemic Schwartzman reaction, both sublethal injections are by the intravenous route and result in bilateral cortical necrosis in the kidneys. Although several authors have attempted to relate the clinical and pathologic findings in fulminant meningococcemia to those seen in the Schwartzman reaction, such arguments have been inconsistent and inconclusive.

The current consensus of medical opinion regarding the pathophysiology of cardiovascular collapse in this disease is that it represents primary response to endotoxin. Indeed, intravenous injection of large doses of meningococcal endotoxin in most animal species results in a syndrome similar to that of fulminant meningococcemia, with significant vasomotor disturbance, high fever or hypothermia, leukopenia, hypoglycemia, and petechial hemorrhage with focal necrosis[209,210]. Unfortunately, it is not clear why the meningococcal endotoxin produces a more rapidly fatal disease than endotoxin derived from the enteric Gram-negative organisms, or why skin lesions and focal areas of coagulation and bleeding are more prominent in this disease. Pathologically, the areas of bleeding that are seen may be related to underlying coagulation in capillaries and venules, and may also be related to the severity of DIC produced by the organism[211,212]. However, Bohm[198] maintains the lesions, especially as detected in the skin, adrenals, and myocardium, are more consistent with direct endotoxigenic damage to endothelial and surrounding tissue. He postulates that death is caused by overwhelming toxemia that may be further complicated by adrenal failure and DIC. These findings were corroborated by Mittermayer et al.[213]. The pathophysiologic mechanisms relating to cardiovascular failure in endotoxic shock are described fully in Chapter 16 on cardiovascular physiology and shock, and will not be considered further here.

Differential Diagnosis

The differential diagnosis of acute meningococcemia includes endotoxin-producing bacterial diseases, such as *E. coli,* as well as others that can cause general prostration and meningitis, such as *H. influenzae* type b. Patients infected with enteroviruses may have fever and petechiae. Even in the absence of an obvious tick bite, the petechiae and purpura of Rocky Mountain spotted fever must make that entity a consideration as well. Noninfectious diseases, such as Henoch-Schönlein purpura, are also possible. Any disease or drug ingestion resulting in inadequacy of platelet number or function may be accompanied by intradermal bleeding. Such disorders include DIC of any cause, idiopathic thrombocytopenic purpura, and all the infectious causes listed in **Table 31.18.** Other bacterial diseases that may prove rapidly fatal include the Gram-negative rods, with *Pseudomonas* being the most likely.

Diagnostic testing must proceed rapidly and concurrently with initiation of therapy (described in the following section), if the patient has the greatest chance to survive. Evaluation for possible bacterial pathogens is imperative. This should include blood cultures, and the use of rapid antigen diagnostic testing (countercurrent immune electrophoresis or Latex agglutination) when available. The demonstration of Gram-negative diplococci on blood smear or buffy coat smear has been noted since 1944[214] in the disease and may be helpful, as may be the finding of organisms in scrapings from purpuric lesions. Appropriate laboratory tests include WBC with differential, erythrocyte sedimentation rate, platelet count, and evaluation for possible DIC with determination of prothrombin time, partial thromboplastin time, fibrinogen, and fibrin degradation products.

The remainder of the patient's evaluation should follow usual intensive care procedures. The patient's airway may be inadequate if the mental status is diminished. Additionally, oxygenation may be impaired by adult respiratory distress syndrome, pulmonary edema, or pneumonia. Increased metabolic demand of the patient in shock may make an otherwise normal level of gas exchange inadequate for the situation. For these reasons, arterial blood gases and chest radiographs must always be part of the initial and on going

Table 31.18. Infectious Diseases Associated with Petechiae

N. meningitidis
H. influenzae type b
N. gonorrhoeae
S. pneumoniae
S. pyogenes
Enteroviruses
Rubella
Rickettsiae
Mycoplasma
Epstein-Barr virus
Cytomegalovirus
Colorado tick fever
Arboviruses
Rat-bite fever
Y. pestis

evaluations. Indications for intubation and assisted ventilation in the setting of overwhelming sepsis are discussed in Chapters 2 and 9.

Detailed evaluation of the CNS is essential. The cause of an abnormal mental status must be determined. Although it is important to examine the cerebrospinal fluid for evidence of meningeal irritation, and to obtain cultures, other causes of altered neurologic function should be considered, some of which preclude the performance of a lumbar puncture. Neurologic dysfunction in a child with meningococcemia may be caused by direct effects of local infection and inflammation, diffuse cerebral edema with intracranial hypertension, or diminished cerebral perfusion resulting from the generalized shock state. If the child's Glasgow Coma Scale score is 7 or less, ongoing bedside measurement of intracranial pressure should be considered, and if indicated, should be instituted before the lumbar puncture is performed. If the child's condition allows it, a computed axial tomography (CAT) scan should be obtained before placement of an intraventricular catheter or subarachnoid screw. If the patient cannot be safely moved to the radiology department, a subarachnoid screw may be placed based on clinical findings alone. A spinal tap may then be performed if the intracranial pressure reading is less than 20 mm Hg, and there is no evidence of mass effect on CAT scan or physical examination. If the pressure is high, but the ventricles are visible on the scan, a ventricular catheter may be substituted for the screw, and a sample of cerebrospinal fluid obtained in that manner. Treatment of impending herniation should proceed as discussed in Chapter 18. Other contraindications to a lumbar puncture in these children include markedly abnormal clotting studies, thrombocytopenia, irreversible shock, and/or an unstable airway.

Therapy

Of all cases of meningococcemia, 10 to 20% may be classified as fulminant, with an 80 to 100% mortality among this group. As previously mentioned, death in this set of patients occurs rapidly, often within hours of hospital admission. Therefore, therapy must be specific, appropriate, and administered without delay, especially in those patients with a prognostic score (per Stiehm and Damrosch) of 3 or greater. Specific antibiotic therapy has traditionally consisted of high-dose penicillin. Recently, there have been reports of isolates of *N. meningitidis* that are relatively resistant to penicillin[(215)]. Since identification of the organism and antibiotic sensitivities are not available at the time of admission, it is inappropriate to use penicillin alone in the treatment of sepsis. A single daily dose of ceftriaxone (100 mg/kg/day) appears to be safe, efficacious, and without significant side effects, even when used for a short course (4 days)[(216,217)]. There is no evidence that simultaneous use of an aminoglycoside is harmful, so if there is any reason to suspect an enteric Gram-negative organism, the addition of gentamicin should be considered. In addition, if *Pseudomonas* is a strong possibility, an antipseudomonal cephalosporin should be considered.

There is no definitive evidence that corticosteroids are of benefit in changing the outcome of this disease. Administration of systemic corticosteroids can potentiate the Schwartzman reaction, but this adverse effect is only theoretical[(207,209)] and has not been shown to apply to the human with bona fide meningococcal infection. Therefore, there is no strong contraindication to the use of steroids and some theoretical benefit to supporting possibly borderline adrenal function in the presence of circulatory failure. The pathogen will not be known in the initial hours of therapy. Therefore, it is reasonable to use very high septic shock doses of methylprednisolone (30 mg/kg) followed by maintenance doses of steroids once meningococcemia is documented because there may be adrenocortical insufficiency, which may contribute to the hypotension and may be reversible[(206)].

Some researchers think heparin is of value because the hemorrhagic findings of purpura fulminans are associated with abnormal coagulation. Although benefit has not been conclusively demonstrated[(172,211)], anecdotal reports suggest widescale trials are indicated[(218,219)].

The efficacy of various inotropic and antihypotensive medications has not been documented in shock states related to meningococcal infection. The most widely used drug initially was norepinephrine, which has been sporadically beneficial[(194)] even when adrenocortical extract was not. Clinical trials with dopamine, dobutamine, epinephrine, or isoproterenol have not been performed; therefore, no information is available on which to recommend therapy with any particular agent. Although it is reasonable to suspect that amrinone, with its combined inotropic and afterload reducing effects might be of significant benefit in this disease, its use for meningococcal shock in children has not been reported. Many patients would not be candidates for amrinone therapy because of thrombocytopenia. In many of the published case reports, inotropic agents used singly or in various combinations have not altered the inevitable fatal outcome for some of these patients[(192,196,197,220)]. It is thought by some[(180)] that, despite all of the advances in critical support of the child made in the last decade, mortality has not been significantly reduced. It is not known whether the antiendotoxin monoclonal antibody will be useful in meningococcemia.

Most authors agree that plasma expansion is the first order of business, and that large volumes may be necessary in the presence of endotoxic shock[(193,196,197,220)] as it occurs in meningococcal infection. Beyond that, especially with the knowledge that some degree of myocarditis usually exists, it is clear that an inotropic agent may be of benefit. Afterload reduction may be useful in the presence of myocardial failure and diminished peripheral perfusion. It is possible that the combination of dobutamine for inotropy and nitroprusside for afterload reduction, with maintenance of adequate preload through the use of volume expansions, may be effective. However, in the patient with elevated intracranial pressure, nitroprusside infusion is relatively contraindicated, because it leads to preferential cerebral vasodilation and may diminish perfusion pressure by increasing intracranial pressure and, potentially, by diminishing arterial blood pressure. (See Chapter 18 on intracranial pressure monitoring and management.)

Appropriate therapy for cardiovascular perturbations will be more readily achieved with the aid of invasive hemodynamic monitoring through placement of a pulmonary artery catheter. This allows the clinician to measure central venous and pulmonary capillary occlusion pressures, as well as cardiac output. Adequacy of therapy may be assessed by calculating oxygen delivery and consumption. The decision to initiate invasive monitoring may be guided by determining the prognostic score at presentation. Because the death rate is low for children with a severity score of 0, 1, or 2 (per Stiehm and Damrosch, 183), routine monitoring potentially including an arterial line and central venous catheter should be sufficient, when coupled with conventional therapeutic measures. Those who are more severely ill have a much higher likelihood of succumbing to their infection and its complications and will need specific aggressive therapy aimed at correcting their particular hemodynamic abnormalities.

Since the majority of deaths in the poor prognostic group occur early in the hospital course, it is relatively easy to judge whether a particular intervention has altered the otherwise almost uniformly fatal outcome. For many, it will continue to be too late to change the course of their disease, because the hyperacute nature of the infection may put them very close to death on admission to the hospital. Therefore, emphasis must be placed on earlier recognition, treatment, and prevention, with multivalent immunizations in high-risk populations.

Pulmonary edema occurs with varying frequency in septicemic individuals. It may be severe and require intubation[(221)] and high levels of end-expired pressure. The cause of the edema may be either acute myocardial failure or adult respiratory distress syndrome. Because of the bleeding tendency of many of these children, any procedure, but especially intubation, should be approached with extreme care. The patient must be appropriately sedated or paralyzed to reduce the risk of trauma to soft tissues and subsequent bleeding complications. When possible, the procedure should be completed by an experienced anesthetist or intensive care specialist. Additionally, it is probably wise to avoid the nasotracheal route, with its increased hazards of bleeding from adenoidal beds in patients with DIC. Overzealous attempts at placing nasogastric tubes should likewise be avoided.

Therapy of elevated intracranial pressure may be necessary. If acute changes suggestive of impending uncal herniation are present, therapy may need to commence before the pressure can be measured. As discussed in Chapter 18, this therapy consists of acute hyperventilation through an endotracheal tube, administration of furosemide and/or mannitol, fluid restriction, and the potential addition of high-dose barbiturates. Because some of these maneuvers may not be possible in the patient who also has concomitant septic shock, knowledge of intracranial pressure, perfusion pressure, and the left atrial filling pressures is essential to guide rational management decisions. Therefore, the patient who appears at risk for elevated intracranial pressure in this setting should have the airway controlled, have a subarachnoid screw or intraventricular catheter, and a central venous or more preferably a pulmonary artery catheter in place. There is no evidence to suggest that the presence of any of these monitoring devices will make the infection more difficult to treat.

The use of continuous sympathetic block through caudal or lumbar epidural catheters has been reported in children with purpura fulminans[(222,223)]. Local vasodilation may be more efficacious than systemic afterload reduction in the child with marginal cardiovascular status, and has not led to hypotension in the children in whom it has been reported. Many untreated cases associated with significant purpura result in loss of the affected limb(s) because of progressive ischemia and eventual gangrene.

Complications

Patients who survive the first several days of the infection remain at risk for certain complications of meningococcemia, namely arthritis[(224)], deafness, gastroenteritis[(219)], pneumonia[(221)], and pericarditis-myocarditis[(225,226)]. The last named are the most important to the pediatric intensive care specialist. Generally, clinically evident myocarditis occurs at 4 to 7 days into the course of the illness, is probably a hypersensitivity reaction, and is noted in 3 to 5% of all patients. Some autopsy series have reported a much higher figure of myocarditis and have suggested the associated myocardial failure may relate directly to bacterial and leukocyte infiltration of the myocardium and conducting system. Such myocardial involvement may lead to sudden death from a dysrhythmia[(198,213,225,226)].

Pericarditis may be associated with effusion but rarely causes tamponade or needs therapeutic drainage. It may also cause dysrhythmias but does not appear to have as adverse an effect on myocardial function as does frank myocarditis. Development of either myocarditis or pericardial inflammation is not related to severity of sepsis or development of other complications. The pathogenesis is unknown.

Pneumonia may be severe, requiring respiratory support, and may coexist with pulmonary edema. Pleural effusions may develop, suggesting a possible immunologic reaction in this complication as well.

Arthritis and deafness are important to the patient, but do not present any specific problems to the intensive care specialist except with regard to discussion with the parents, as well as interpretation of neurologic data.

It is uniformly agreed that rifampin prophylaxis of household and day care center contacts is indicated[168]. The dose is 20 mg/kg/day given twice daily for 2 days. Many pharmacies will make a special suspension for use in young children. This recommendation may change as rifampin resistance emerges. It has been reported in outbreaks in Israel[227]. Other antibiotics are currently being evaluated, ofloxacin has been used in adults with promising results[228] but is not approved for pediatric use.

Summary

In summary, meningococcemia is a bacterial disease that has the capacity to cause devastating illness in young children and infants and requires initiation of antimicrobial and systemic supportive measures without delay. More data is needed with regard to the specific hemodynamic abnormalities and the methods of treating them, as well as information on the incidence of increased intracranial pressure and its effect on outcome in this disease.

Haemophilus Influenzae

Before the availability of the *H. influenzae* type b (Hib) conjugate vaccine, this organism was the most common cause of bacterial meningitis among children less than 5 years of age[229]; the relationship of this organism to the meningitic syndrome is discussed in Chapter 32. *H. influenzae* (type b as well as other types) causes a number of nonmeningitic, potentially life-threatening illnesses, including epiglottitis, pneumonia, and sepsis. Other clinical entities that do not usually require intensive care include osteomyelitis, septic arthritis, and facial or periorbital cellulitis. The nontypable strains are frequently implicated in cases of otitis media.

Bacteriology

The *H. influenzae* bacterium is a Gram-negative pleomorphic coccobacillus. It is a strict parasite, is aerobic and facultatively anaerobic, and has special growth-factor requirements. To achieve adequate growth in culture, the organism needs both factors X (hemin) and V (nicotinamide dinucleotide). Therefore, it grows well on chocolate agar as well as Levinthal or Fildes media[230].

H. influenzae was originally known as Pfeiffer's bacillus, after the man who, in 1892, originally identified the organism in sputum of influenza victims. Although it was later disproved to be the cause of influenza, the official name chosen in 1920 continued to reflect an association with the viral disease, as well as the bacterium's nutritional requirements for blood-containing media[231].

By 1931, a distinction had been made between encapsulated and nonencapsulated forms, and subsequently, immunologic methods were devised by which six strains were recognized on the basis of specific antigens contained in the polysaccharide capsule[232]. As with other bacteria that may be encapsulated, the presence of the capsule correlates well with invasiveness. The nonencapsulated strains of *H. influenzae* are known to cause surface infections of the ear, nose, throat, or lower respiratory tract, or may be carried asymptomatically, but are not generally implicated in bacteremia or other serious infections of the normal host. Additionally, the type b organisms cause a greater percentage of serious infection than other encapsulated types. Throughout this chapter, information regarding the organism will refer specifically to Hib unless otherwise indicated.

Epidemiology

The epidemiology of Hib infection has changed markedly since the introduction of the Hib conjugate vaccine[233–239]. The incidence of invasive Hib disease in the United States in patients younger than 5 years dropped from 41 per 100,000 in 1987 to 2 per 100,000 in 1993. During this time, the national incidence of invasive Hib disease in persons older than 5 years remained stable at 0.25 to 0.5 per 100,000[239]. Despite the tremendous success of the immunization program, the pediatric intensive care specialist is still likely to see occasional cases of Hib infection and, therefore, must maintain a high degree of suspicion.

H. influenzae is transmitted by person-to-person spread and is carried in the nasopharynx. Isolation of the infected patient is essential, as is treatment of the index case and all close contacts with rifampin to reduce carriage. It has been documented that immunization does not rapidly diminish carriage and, therefore, does not obviate prophylaxis and isolation[240]. Nosocomial spread to adult hospital staff has been reported[238].

Clinical Manifestations

The most common clinical presentation of *H. influenzae* type b is as acute meningitis, the diagnosis and therapy of which are discussed in Chapter 32. Epiglottitis is the second most common clinical syndrome produced by Hib, **(Table 31.19)** and its acute management as referable to the upper airway obstruction is covered in Chapter 2. Pneumonia caused by *H. influenzae* type b is not dramatically different from that caused by other microorganisms and requires the same general approach as any other acute lower respiratory infection.

Acute sepsis secondary to Hib may produce some confusion to the clinician in that it may mimic meningococce-

Table 31.19. Correlation of Levels of *H. influenzae* Bacteremia ≥1000 CFU per Milliliter of Blood with the Development of Epiglottitis in 64 Patients[a]

Diagnosis	*No. of Patients*	*Geometric Mean (CFU/ml of Blood)*	*No. of Patients with ≥1000 CFU/ml of Blood (%)*
Epiglottitis	23	123 ± 3.04[b]	0[b]
Meningitis	41	2,203 ± 7.9[b]	30 (73)[b]
Total	64	776 ± 40.0	30 (47)

[a] *From LaScolea LJ Jr, Rosales SV, Welliver RC, Ogra PL. Mechanisms underlying the development of meningitis or epiglottitis in children after* Haemophilus influenzae *type b bacteremia. J Infect Dis 1985;151:1162.*

[b] $p < 0.001$ *when comparing groups with epiglottitis and meningitis. CFU = colony-forming units.*

Table 31.20. Demographic Data for Patients with Apparent Meningococcemia: Comparison of Those with Proven *N. meningitidis* with Those with *H. influenzae*[a]

	N. Meningitidis (N = 30)	*H. Influenzae* (N = 12)
Age (months)	23.6 ± 4.7 (16.5)[b]	14.9 ± 3.3 (14.5)
Sex (M/F)	22/8	6/6
Season		
Winter	12	1
Spring	8	3
Summer	6	3
Fall	4	5
Interval between admission and onset of:		
Symptoms	2.5 ± 0.6 days (8 hr to 14 days)	1.7 ± 1.2 days (8 hr to 14 days)
Lesions	0.5 ± 0.3	0.6 ± 0.1
Antecedent illness (upper respiratory tract infection)	13	4 1 (tonsillitis)
Antecedent therapy	2 (1-penicillin G, 1-amoxicillin)	1 (erythromycin)
History of exposure to index case	1	0

[a] *From Jacobs RF, Hsi S, Wilson CB, et al. Apparent meningococcemia: clinical features of disease due to* Haemophilus influenzae *and* Neisseria meningitidis. *Pediatrics 1983;72:469. Reproduced by permission of* Pediatrics.
[b] *Values are means ± SE; range is shown in parentheses.*

mia[241,242]. A review of all children who had culture-proven overwhelming sepsis[243] in a hospital in Seattle documented that symptoms of *H. influenzae,* such as lethargy, shock, DIC, and a rash, are indistinguishable from that seen in meningococcemia **(Tables 31.20–31.22).** Adrenal hemorrhage was present in 55% of the fatal cases of Hib versus 67% of those who died from meningococcemia (not statistically different). The mortality rate for those with meningococcemia was 10% compared to 75% for those with *H. influenzae.* Additionally, the mean time from admission to death was shorter for those with Hib (20.7 hours compared to 120 hours for meningococcemia). The deaths seen in *H. influenzae* type b overwhelming sepsis were caused by intractable hypotension and progressive cardiac dysfunction unresponsive to therapy. Over half of the patients who died with Hib sepsis were treated with penicillin alone because of the clinical impression of meningococcal disease. This may have contributed to the higher early mortality rate. Secondary sites of involvement were not significantly different between infections caused by the two organisms; namely, there was a similar incidence of meningitis, myocarditis, pneumonia, otitis media, and osteomyelitis. The authors indicate that, from their data, there were no absolute clinical clues on which to base a microbiologic diagnosis in the patient who has petechiae or purpura accompanying fever and shock. The Gram's stain may be helpful, as may be determination of a presumed diagnosis by rapid antigen detection. However, there has been a report of a false-positive rapid antigen test in a patient recently immunized[244]. Consequently, until the bacteriologic diagnosis is confirmed, the patient with overwhelming sepsis must be treated expectantly for both meningococcemia and *H. influenzae* type b.

Therapy

Initial therapy of overwhelming sepsis caused by Hib is not different from that of meningococcemia, and the reader is referred to the previous section for a description of the general approach to this life-threatening infectious disease.

Little more need be added regarding treatment, except as it relates to specific antimicrobial therapy. At least 25% of all Hib isolates throughout the United States are resistant to ampicillin[245]. Resistance is caused by ability of the microorganism to produce β-lactamase and inactivate the ampicillin. The current drug of choice is a third-generation cephalosporin such as ceftriaxone. Chloramphenicol is also efficacious, and may be useful in the child with combined penicillin-cephalosporin allergy. There have been occasional reports of chloramphenicol-resistant *H. influenzae* type b, primarily from the United Kingdom[246]. Multiple-resistant strains also exist[247].

Prevention

Successful immunization is the most effective prevention available. In addition, close household and day care center contacts should receive chemoprophylaxis with rifampin at a dose of 20 mg/kg/day for 4 days. This should be provided regardless of results of nasopharyngeal cultures, because numerous reports have documented the failure of one-time

Table 31.21. Comparison of Clinical Presentation and Outcome in Patients with *N. meningitidis* and *H. influenzae* Who Presented with Apparent Meningococcemia[a]

	N. Meningitidis (N = 30)	*H. Influenzae* (N = 12)
Fever (≥38°C)	30	12
Irritable but alter	15	2
Lethargy or coma	15[b]	10
Vomiting	14	4
Headache	6	1
Rash	30/30	10/12
Petechial	2	4
Purpuric	3	4
Both	25[c]	2
Maculopapular	1[d]	2[e]
None	0	2
Shock	11	6
DIC	12	5
Adrenal hemorrhage	2/3[f]	5/9
Death	3/30[g]	9/12[h]
Time to death (hr) (mean ± SE)	120 ± 74/4[b]	20.7 ± 4.0

[a] *From Jacobs RF, Hsi S, Wilson CB, et al. Apparent meningococcemia: clinical features of disease due to* Haemophilus influenzae *and* Neisseria meningitidis. *Pediatrics 1983;72:469. Reproduced by permission of* Pediatrics.
[b] $p < 0.05$ *compared with* H. influenzae *cases.*
[c] *Six children required skin grafts.*
[d] *Petechiae were also present.*
[e] *Both were also purpuric.*
[f] *Denominator is number of patients examined postmortem.*
[g] $p < 0.005$ *compared with* H. influenzae: *1/14 with meningitis; 2/16 without meningitis.*
[h] *Six of nine with meningitis, 3/3 without meningitis.*

Table 31.22. Laboratory Findings and Therapy of Patients with *N. meningitidis* and *H. influenzae* Who Presented with Apparent Meningococcemia[a]

	N. Meningitidis (N = 30)	*H. influenzae* (N = 12)
Microbiology		
Blood		
Culture	22	6
Gram Stain[b]	5/9	NC[c]
Cerebrospinal fluid		
Culture	14[d]	9[d]
Gram stain	10/14	7/8
Skin lesion		
Culture	3/13	ND
Gram Stain	8/13	ND
Secondary sites of involvement:		
Meningitis	14	9
Myocarditis	6	2
Other	pneumonia, 2; otitis media, 1; osteomyelitis, 1; panophthalmitis, 1	Pneumonia, 2; otitis media, 2; osteomyelitis, 1; septic arthritis, 1; pericarditis, 1
Initial therapy	Penicillin, 11; ampicillin, 19	Penicillin, 5; ampicillin, 7
Complications	Seizures, 2; postmeningitis hydrocephalus, 1; renal failure, dialysis-dependent, 1	Pulmonary hemorrhage, 1

[a] *From Jacobs RF, Hsi S, Wilson CB, et al. Apparent meningococcemia: clinical features of disease due to* Haemophilus influenzae *and* Neisseria meningitidis. *Pediatrics 1983;72:469. Reprinted by permission of* Pediatrics.
[b] *Buffy coat Gram's stain.*
[c] *ND = not done.*
[d] *Includes each of the patients with sterile blood cultures.*

cultures to detect all carriers accurately. Adult members should probably be prophylaxed as well as children. The index case deserves rifampin therapy as well, since systemic administration of ampicillin and/or chloramphenicol does not eradicate nasopharyngeal carriage of the organism[(248)]. In numerous studies, rifampin reduces the carriage rate[(249,250)] and in at least one report reduces the rate of secondary infection[(250)]. It also alters chloramphenicol levels, and so it is reasonable to administer rifampin at the conclusion of the acute course of therapy, if the patient is being treated with chloramphenicol.

SUMMARY

This chapter discussed issues of overwhelming sepsis in children of different ages. A general approach to the critically ill potentially infected patient has been described. Appropriate initial antibiotic choices have been described, and adjunctive therapies, both available and experimental, have been mentioned. Infections of specific etiologies have been considered, with treatment recommendations made accordingly. The reader is referred to the listed references for further detailed information.

References

1. Goldmann DA. Bacterial colonization and infection in the neonate. Am J Med 1981;70:417.
2. Yu VYH. Neonatal sepsis and infection control policies in Australia. J Paediatr Child Health 1990;26:252–256.
3. Chadwick EG, Yogev R, Shulman ST. Combination antibiotic therapy in pediatrics. Am J Med 1986;80:166–171.
4. Modi N, Damjanovic V, Cooke RWI. Outbreak of cephalosporin resistant *Enterobacter cloacae* infection in a neonatal intensive care unit. Arch Dis Child 1987; 62:148–151.
5. Leonard EM, van Saene HKF, Shears P, Walker J, Tam PKH. Pathogenesis of colonization and infection in a neonatal surgical unit. Crit Care Med 1990;18:264–269.
6. Schaad UB. The cephalosporin compounds in severe neonatal infection. Eur J Pediatr 1984;141:143–146.
7. Lau WY, Fan ST, Yip WC, et al. Acute appendicitis in children. Aust NZ J Surg 1987;57:927–931.
8. Schenep JL, Hughes WT, Roberson PK, et al. Vancomycin, ticarcillin, and amikacin compared with ticarcillin-clavulanate and amikacin in the empirical treatment of febrile neutropenic children with cancer. N Engl J Med 1988;319:1053–1058.
9. The EORTC International Antimicrobial Therapy Cooperative Group. Ceftazidime combined with short or long course of amikacin for empirical therapy of gram-negative bacteremia in cancer patients with granulocytopenia. N Engl J Med 1987;317:1692–1698.
10. Olson TA, Fischer GW, Lupo MC, et al. Antimicrobial therapy of broviac catheter infections in pediatric hematology oncology patients. J Pediatr Surg 1987;22:839–842.
11. Bragman S, Sage R, Booth L, Noone P. Ceftazidime in the treatment of serious *Pseudomonas aeruginosa* sepsis. Scand J Infect Dis 1986; 18:425–429.
12. Johnson MP, Ramphal R. β-Lactam-resistant *Enterobacter* bacteremia in febrile neutropenic patients receiving monotherapy. J Infect Dis 1990;162:981–983.
13. Moellering RC, Eliopoulos GM, Sentochnik DE. The carbapenems: new broad spectrum β-lactam antibiotics. J Antimicrob Chemother 1989; 24:(Suppl A)1–7.
14. Bonatti H, Guggenbichler JP, Hager J. Treatment of nosocomial infections in children undergoing antimicrobial chemotherapy. Infection 1990;18:302–306.
15. Damato JJ, Eitzman DV, Baer H. Persistence and dissemination in the community of R-factors of nosocomial origin. J Infect Dis 1974;129:205.
16. Wientzen RL, McCracken GH Jr. Pathogenesis and management of neonatal sepsis and meningitis. Curr Probl Pediatr 1977;8:22.
17. Philip AGS, Baker CJ. Cerebrospinal fluid C-reactive protein in neonatal meningitis. J Pediatr 1983;102:715.
18. Clarke D, Cost K. Use of C-reactive protein in differentiating septic from aseptic meningitis in children. J Pediatr 1983;102:718.
19. Crain EF, Shelov SP. Febrile infants: predictors of bacteremia. J Pediatr 1982;101:686.
20. Voora S, Srinavson G, Lilien LD, Pildes RS. Fever in full-term newborns in the first four days of life. Pediatrics 1982;69:40.
21. Philip AGS, Hewitt JR. Early diagnosis of neonatal sepsis. Pediatrics 1980;65:1036.
22. Sabel KG, Wadsworth C. C-reactive protein (CRP) in early diagnosis of neonatal septicemia. Acta Paediatr Scand 1979;68:825.
23. Smith AL. The febrile infant. Pediatrics 1979;1:35.
24. McCracken GH. Controversies in pediatrics: what tests are indicated for the child under 2 with fever? Pediatr Rev 1979;1:51.
25. Thore M, Faxelius G, Hedin G, Johnsson H, Ringertz S, Schröder S, Schwan A, Thid S, Öhrner Y. The role of a commercial latex agglutination test in the diagnosis of group B streptococcal infection in neonates. Acta Paediatr Scand 1991;167–172.
26. Siegel JD, McCracken GH Jr. Medical progress: sepsis neonatorum. N Engl J Med 1981;304:642.
27. Klein JO, Dashefsky B, Norton CR, Mayer J. Selection of antimicrobial agents for treatment of neonatal sepsis. Rev Infect Dis 1983;5 (Suppl):S55.
28. Gluck L, Wood HF, Fousek MD. Septicemia of the newborn. Pediatr Clin North Am 1966;13:1131.
29. Freedman RM, Ingram DL, Gross I, et al. A half-century of neonatal sepsis at Yale 1928 to 1978. Am J Dis Child 1981;135:140.
30. Maguire GC, Nordin J, Myers MG, et al. Infections acquired by young infants. Am J Dis Child 1981;135:693.
31. Townsend TR, Wenzel RP. Nosocomial bloodstream infections in a newborn intensive care unit. Am J Epidemiol 1981;114:73.

32. Bennet R, Eriksson M, Zetterstrom R. Increasing incidence of neonatal septicemia: causative organisms and predisposing risk factors. Acta Paediatr Scand 1981;70:207.
33. Smith DH. Epidemics of infectious diseases in newborn nurseries. Clin Obstet Gynecol 1979;22:409.
34. Kaslow RA, Dixon RE, Martin SM, et al. Staphylococcal disease related to hospital nursery bathing practices—A nationwide epidemiologic investigation. Pediatrics 1973;51 (Suppl):S418.
35. Crosson F Jr, Feder H Jr, Bocchini A Jr, et al. Neonatal sepsis at the Johns Hopkins Hospital 1969–75. Bacterial isolates and clinical correlates. Johns Hopkins Med J 1977;140:37.
36. Dunham E. Septicemia in the newborn. Am J Dis Child 1933; 45:229.
37. Gotoff S, Behrman R. Neonatal septicemia. J Pediatr 1970;76:142.
38. McCracken G, Shinefeld H. Changes in the pattern of neonatal septicemia and meningitis. Am J Dis Child 1966;112:33.
39. Nyhan W, Fousek M. Septicemia of the newborn. Pediatrics 1978;22:268.
40. Ehrenkranz N. Bacterial colonization of newborn infants and subsequent acquisition of hospital bacteria. J Pediatr 1970;76:839.
41. Baumgart S, Hall SE, Compose JM, Polin RA. Sepsis with coagulase-negative staphylococci in critically-ill newborns. Am J Dis Child 1983;137:461.
42. Cronin WA, Germanson TP, Donowitz LG. Intravascular catheter colonization and related bloodstream infection in critically ill neonates. Infect Control Hosp Epidemiol 1990;11:301–308.
43. Nakamura KT, Beal DW, Koontz FP, Bell EF. Fulminant neonatal septicemia due to *Haemophilus parainfluenzae.* Am J Clin Pathol 1984;81:388.
44. Holt RN, Taylor CD, Schneider HJ, Hallock JA. Three cases of *Haemophilus parainfluenzae* meningitis. Clin Pediatr 1974;13:666.
45. Schreyer A, Mogilner BM. Septicemia and meningitis due to *Haemophilus parainfluenzae* in a newborn infant. Harefuah 1979;96:483.
46. Zinner SH, McCormack WM, Lee YH et al. Puerperal bacteremia and neonatal sepsis due to *Haemophilus parainfluenzae:* report of a case with antibody titers. Pediatrics 1972;49:612.
47. Bojsen-Moller J. Human listeriosis: diagnostic, epidemiological and clinical studies. Acta Pathol Microbiol Immunol Scand [B] 1972;229 (Suppl):1.
48. Albritton WL, Wiggins GL, Feeley JC. Neonatal listeriosis: distribution of serotypes in relation to age at onset. J Pediatr 1976;88:481.
49. Burn C. Clinical and pathological features of an infection caused by a new pathogen of the genus *Listerella.* Am J Pathol 1936;12:341.
50. Finegold S, Bradley S, Campbell M. *Listeria monocytogenes* meningitis: summation of literature and report of two new cases. Arch Intern Med 1954;93:515.
51. Maguire B, Relez H. Infections due to *Listeria monocytogenes* in infants and children. Am J Med Sci 1967;254:421.
52. Spilkin E, Rachmaninoff N, Climie A. *Listeria monocytogenes* meningitis. Report of two cases and review of the literature. Am J Clin Pathol 1968;49:671.
53. Lavetter A, Leedom J, Mathias A, et al. Meningitis due to *Listeria monocytogenes:* a review of 25 cases. N Engl J Med 1971;285:598.
54. Halliday H, Hiratu T. Perinatal listeriosis. A review of 12 patients. Am J Obstet Gynecol 1979;133:405.
55. Buchner L, Schneerson S. Clinical and laboratory aspects of *Listeria monocytogenes* infections: with a report of 10 cases. Am J Med 1968;45:904.
56. Thong ML, Puthucheary SD, Lee EL. *Flavobacterium* meningosepticum infection: an epidemiological study in a newborn nursery. J Clin Pathol 1981;34:429.
57. Hazuka BT, Dajani AS, Talbot K, Keen BM. Two outbreaks of *Flavobacterium* meningosepticum type E in a neonatal intensive care unit. J Clin Microbiol 1977;6:450.
58. Sabel KG, Brandberg A. Treatment of meningitis and septicemia in infancy with a sulphamethoxazole/trimethoprim combination. Acta Paediatr Scand 1975;64:25.
59. Nocard M. Sur une mammite contagieuse des vaches laitieres. Ann Inst Pasteur Microbiol 1887;1:109.
60. Lancefield RC. A serological differentiation of human and other groups of hemolytic streptococci. J Exp Med 1933;57:571.
61. Lancefield RC, Hare R. The serological differentiation of pathogenic and non-pathogenic strains of hemolytic streptococci from parturient women. J Exp Med 1935;61:335.
62. Fry RM. Fatal infections by hemolytic streptococcus group B. Lancet 1938;1:199.
63. Franciosi RA, Knostman JD, Zimmerman RA. Group B streptococcal neonatal and infant infections. J Pediatr 1973;82:707.
64. Baker CJ, Bennett FF, Gordon RC, Yow MD. Suppurative meningitis due to streptococci of Lancefield group B: a study of 33 infants. J Pediatr 1973;82:724.
65. Barton LL, Feigin RD, Lins R. Group B beta hemolytic streptococcal meningitis in infants. J Pediatr 1973;82:719.
66. Aber RC, Allen N, Howell JT, et al. Nosocomial transmission of group B streptococci. Pediatrics 1976;58:346.
67. Baker CJ. Summary of the workshop on perinatal infections due to group B streptococcus. J Infect Dis 1977;136:137.
68. Anthony BF, Okada DM. The emergence of group B streptococci in infections of the newborn infant. Annu Rev Med 1977;28:355.
69. Wilkinson H. Group B streptococcal infections in humans. Annu Rev Microbiol 1978;32:41.
70. Baker CJ, Kaspter DL. Correlation of maternal antibody deficiency with susceptibility to neonatal group B strep infection. N Engl J Med 1976;294:753.
71. Davis JP, Gutman LT, Higgins MV, et al. Nasal colonization of infants with group B streptococci associated with intrauterine pressure transducers. J Infect Dis 1978;138:804.
72. Pass MA, Gray BM, Khare S, Dillon HC Jr. Prospective studies of group B streptococcal infections in infants. J Pediatr 1979;95:437.
73. Ingram DL, Pedergrass EL, Bromberger PI, et al. Group B streptococcal disease. Am J Dis Child 1980;134:754.
74. Manos JP. Group B streptococcal infection in the neonate. Ann Clin Lab Sci 1982;12:239.
75. Lannering B, Larson LE, Rojas J, Stahlman MT. Early onset group B streptococcal disease: seven year experience and clinical scoring system. Acta Paediatr Scand 1983;72:597.
76. Mulder CJJ, Zanen HC. Neonatal group B streptococcal meningitis. Arch Dis Child 1984;59:439.
77. Ross PW: Group B streptococcus: profile of an organism. J Med Microbiol 1984;18:139.
78. Christensen RD, Rothstein G, Hill HR, Hall RT. Fatal early onset group B streptococcal sepsis with normal leukocyte count. Pediatr Infect Dis 1985;4:242.
79. Edwards MS, Rench MA, Haffar AAM, et al. Long-term sequelae of group B streptococcal meningitis in infants. J Pediatr 1985;106:717.
80. Chin KC, Fitzhardinge PM. Sequelae of early onset group B hemolytic streptococcal neonatal meningitis. J Pediatr 1985;106:819.
81. Christensen KK, Christensen P. Intravenous gamma-globulin in the treatment of neonatal sepsis with special reference to Group B streptococci and pharmacokinetics. Pediatr Infect Dis 1986;5:S189–S192.
82. Hoogkamp-Korstanje JAA. Activity of cefotaxime and ceftriaxone alone and in combination with penicillin, ampicillin and piperacillin against neonatal meningitis pathogens. J Antimicrob Chemother 1985;16: 327–334.
83. Bohnsack JF, Hawley MM, Pritchard DG, Egan ML, Shigeoka AO, Yang KD, Hill HR. An IgA monoclonal antibody directed against type III antigen on Group B streptococci acts as an opsonin. J Immunol 1989;143:3338–3342.
84. Zangwill KM, Schuchat A, Wenger JD. Group B Streptococcal disease in the United States, 1990: Report from a multistate active surveillance system. MMWR 1992;41(SS-6):25–32.
85. Schuchat A, Deaver-Robinson K, Plikaytis BD, Zangwill KM, Mohle-Boetani J, Wenger JD. Multistate case-control study of maternal risk factors for neonatal Group B streptococcal disease. Pediatr Infect Dis J 1994;13:623–629.
86. Spaans WA, Knox AJ, Koya HB, Mantell CD. Risk factors for neonatal infection. Aust NZ J Obstet Gynaecol 1990;30:327–330.
87. Steere AC, Aber RC, Warford LR, et al. Possible nosocomial transmission of group B streptococci in a newborn nursery. J Pediatr 1975;87:784.
88. Synnott MB, Morse DL, Hall SM. Neonatal meningitis in England and Wales: a review of national data. Arch Dis Child 1994;71:F75–F80.
89. Howard JB, McCracken GH Jr. The spectrum of group B streptococcal infections in infancy. Am J Dis Child 1974;128:815.
90. Siegel J. Prevention and treatment of group B streptococcal infections. Pediatr Infect Dis 1985;4 (Suppl):S33.
91. Siegel JD, Shannon KM, DePasse BM. Recurrent infection associated with penicillin-tolerant group B streptococci: a report of two cases. J Pediatr 1981;99:920.
92. Portnoy D, Wink I, Richards GK. Bursitis and cellulitis due to penicillin-tolerant group B streptococci. Can Med Assoc J 1982; 127:138.

93. Steinbrecker UP. Serious infection in an adult due to penicillin tolerant group B streptococcus. Arch Intern Med 1981;141:1714.
94. Baker CN, Thornsberry C, Facklam RR. Synergism, killing kinetics and antimicrobial susceptibility of group A and B streptococci. Antimicrob Agents Chemother 1981;19:716.
95. Cairo MS, Rucker S, Bennett GA, et al. Improved survival of newborns receiving leukocyte transfusions for sepsis. Pediatrics 1984;74:887.
96. Christensen RD, Rothstein G, Anstall HB, Bybee B. Granulocyte transfusions in neonates with bacterial infection, neutropenia, and depletion of mature marrow neutrophils. Pediatrics 1982;70:1.
97. Shigeoka AO, Hall RT, Hill HR. Blood transfusions in group B streptococcal sepsis. Lancet 1978;1:636.
98. Courtney SE, Hall RT, Harris DJ. Effect of blood transfusion on mortality in early onset group B streptococcal septicemia. Lancet 1979;2:462.
99. Cairo MS, Plunkett JM, Nguyen A, Van de Ven C. Effect of stem cell factor with and without granulocyte colony-stimulating factor on neonatal hematopoesis: In vivo induction of newborn myelopoiesis and reduction of mortality during experimental group B streptococcal sepsis. Blood 1992;80:96–101.
100. Wheeler JG, Givner LB. Therapeutic use of recombinant human granulocyte-macrophage colony-stimulating factor in neonatal rats with type III group B streptococcal sepsis. J Infect Dis 1992;165:938–41.
101. Fischer GW, Weisman LB, Hemming VG, London WT, Hunter KW Jr, Bosworth JM Jr, Sever JL, Wilson SR, Curfman BL. Intravenous immunoglobulin in neonatal group B streptococcal disease. Am J Med 1984;77:117.
102. Harris MC, Douglas SD, Kolski GB, Polin RA. Functional properties of anti-group B streptococcal monoclonal antibodies. Clin Immunol Immunopathol 1982;24:342.
103. Santos JI, Shigeoka AO, Rote NS, Hill HR. Protective efficacy of a modified immune serum globulin in experimental group B streptococcal infection. J Pediatr 1981;99:873.
104. Weisman LE, Stoll BJ, Kueser TJ, Rubio TT, Frank CG, Heiman HS, Subramanian KNS, Hankins CT, Anthony BF, Cruess DF, Hemming VG, Fischer GW. Intravenous immune globulin therapy for early onset sepsis in premature infants. J pediatr 1992;121:434–43.
105. Givner LB, Nagaraj SK. Hyperimmune human IgG or recombinant human granulocyte-macrophage colony-stimulating factor as adjunctive therapy for group B streptococcal sepsis in newborn rats. J Pediatr 1993;122:774–9.
106. Schreiber JR, Berger M. Intravenous immune globulin therapy for sepsis in premature neonates. J Pediatr 1992;122:401–2.
107. Anthony BF. Immunity to group B streptococci: interaction of serum and macrophages with types Ia, Ib, and Ic. J Exp Med 1976;143:1186.
108. Klesius PH, Zimmerman RA, Matthews JH, Krushak DH. Cellular and humoral immune response to group B streptococci. J Pediatr 1973; 83:926.
109. Baltimore RS, Kasper DL, Baker CJ, Goroff DK. Antigenic specificity of opsonophagocytic antibodies in rabbit antisera to group B streptococci. J Immunol 1977;118:673.
110. Morell A, Sidiropoulos D, Herrmann U, Christensen KK, Christensen P, Prellner K, Fey H, Skvaril F. IgG subclasses and antibodies to Group B streptococci, pneumococci, and tetanus toxoid in preterm neonates after intravenous infusion of immunoglobulin to the mothers. Pediatr Res 1986;20:933–936.
111. Patel DM, Le Blanc MH, Morrison JC, Graves GR, Glick CG, Martin JN, Rhodes PG, Chauhan SP. Postnatal penicillin prophylaxis and the incidence of group B streptococcal sepsis in neonates. Sou Med J 1994;87:1117–1120.
112. Rivera-Alsina MD, Saldana LR, Kohl S, Arias JW. *Listeria monocytogenes:* an important pathogen in premature labor and intrauterine fetal sepsis. J Reproduc Med 1983;28:212.
113. Henle A. Pseudotuberkulose bei neugeborenen. Zwillingen Arb a d Pathol Institut a Gottingen 143, 1883.
114. Murray EGD, Webb RA, Swann MBR. A disease of rabbits characterized by a large mononuclear leukocytosis, caused by a hitherto undescribed bacillus, Bacterium monocytogenes (h. sp.). J Pathol Bacteriol 1926;29:407.
115. Nyfeldt A. Etiologie de la mononucleose infectieuse. C R Soc Biol 1929;101:590.
116. Evans JR, Alexander CA, Stinson DA, Bortolussi R, Peddle LJ. Perinatal listeriosis: report of an outbreak. Pediatr Infect Dis 1985;4:237.
117. Cherubin CE, Marr JS, Sierra MF, Becker S. *Listeria* and Gram-negative bacillary meningitis in New York City, 1972–1979, frequent causes of meningitis in adults. Am J Med 1981;71:199.
118. Hearmon CJ, Ghosh SK. *Listeria monocytogenes* meningitis in previously healthy adults. Postgrad Med J 1989;65:74–78.
119. Lennon D, Lewis B, Colin M, et al. Epidemic perinatal listeriosis. Pediatr Infect Dis 1984;3:30.
120. Levy E, Nassau E. Experience with listeriosis in the newborn: an account of a small epidemic in a nursery ward. Ann Pediatr 1960;194:321.
121. Jacobs MR, Stein H, Budwane A, et al. Epidemic listeriosis: report of 14 cases detected in 9 months. S Afr Med J 1978;54:389.
122. Becroft DMO, Farmer K, Seddon RJ, et al. Epidemic listeriosis in the newborn. Br Med J 1971;3:747.
123. Niels Le Souef P, Walter BNJ. Neonatal listeriosis: a human outbreak. Med J Aust 1981;2:188.
124. Schlech WF, Lavigne PM, Bortolussi RA, et al. Epidemic listeriosis: evidence for transmission by food. N Engl J Med 1983;308:203.
125. Boucher M, Yonekura ML. Perinatal listeriosis (early-onset): correlation of antenatal manifestations and neonatal outcome. Obstet Gynecol 1986;68:593–597.
126. Schuchat A, Deaver K, Hayes PS, Graves L, Mascola L, Wenger JD. Gastrointestinal carriage of Listeria monocytogenes in household contacts of patients with listeriosis. J Infect Dis 1993;167:1261–2.
127. Centers for Disease Control. Foodbourne Listeriosis—United States, 1988–1990. JAMA 1992;267:2446–7.
128. Jensen A, Frederiksen W, Gerner-Smidt P. Risk factors for Listeriosis in Denmark, 1989–1990. Scand J Infect Dis 1994;26:171–178.
129. Wilson CB, Lewis DB. Basis and implications of selectively diminished cytokine production in neonatal susceptibility to infection. Rev Infect Dis 1990;12:S410–S420.
130. Chen-Woan M, McGregor DD. The mediators of acquired resistance to *Listeria monocytogenes* are contained within a population of cytotoxic T cells. Cell Immunol 1984;87:538.
131. Zervoudakis AL, Cederquist LL. Effect of *Listeria monocytogenes* septicemia during pregnancy on the offspring. Am J Obstet Gynecol 1976;48:335.
132. Gordon RC, Barrett FF, Clark DJ. Influence of several antibiotics singly and in combination on the growth of *Listeria monocytogenes.* J Pediatr 1972;80:667.
133. Spitzer PG, Hammer SM, Karchmer AW. Treatment of *Listeria monocytogenes* infection with trimethoprim-sulfamethoxazole: case report and review of the literature. Rev Infect Dis 1986;8:427–430.
134. Tessin I, Trollfors B, Thiringer K, Thörn Z, Larsson P. Concentrations of ceftazidime, tobramycin and ampicillin in the cerebrospinal fluid of newborn infants. Eur J Pediatr 1989;148:679–681.
135. Neu HC. Cephalosporins in the treatment of meningitis. Drugs 1987;34 (Suppl):135–153.
136. Committee on Fetus and Newborn, Committee on Infectious Diseases. American Academy of Pediatrics. Perinatal herpes simplex virus infections. Pediatrics 1980;66:147.
137. Overall JC. Viral infections of the fetus and the neonate. In: Feigin RD, Cherry JD, eds. Textbook of pediatric infectious disease. Philadelphia: WB Saunders, Chap 21, 1981:684.
138. Whitley RJ Neonatal Herpes Simplex virus infections. J Med Virol Suppl 1993;1:13–21.
139. Stuart-Harris C. The epidemiology and clinical presentation of herpes virus infections. J Antimicrob Chemother 1983;12 (Suppl B):1.
140. Nahmias AJ, Visintine A. Herpes simplex. In: Remington JS, Klein JO, eds. Infectious diseases of the fetus and newborn infant. Philadelphia: WB Saunders, 1976:156.
141. Francis DP, Herrmann KL, McMahon JR, et al. Nosocomial and maternally acquired herpes hominis infections. A report of four fatal cases in neonates. Am J Dis Child 1975;129:889.
142. Light IJ. Postnatal acquisition of herpes simplex by the newborn infant. A review of the literature. Pediatrics 1979;63:480.
143. Linneman CC Jr, Light IJ, Buchman TG, Ballard JL, Roizman B. Transmission of herpes simplex virus type 1 in a nursery for the newborn. Identification of viral isolates by DNA "fingerprinting." Lancet 1978;1:964.
144. Brown ZA, Benedetti J, Ashley R, Burchett S, Selke S, Berry S, Vontver LA, Corey L. Neonatal herpes simples virus infection in relation to asymptomatic maternal infection at the time of labor. N Engl J Med 1991;324:1247–1252.
145. Overall JC Jr. Dermatologic diseases. In: Galasso GJ, Merigan TC, Buchanan RA, eds. Antiviral agents and viral diseases of man. New York: Raven Press, 1979:305.
146. DeVicenzo JP, Thorne G, . Mild herpes simplex encephalitis diagnosed by polymerase chain reaction: a case report and review. Pediatr Infect Dis J 1994;13:662–664.

147. Schlesinger Y, Storch GA. Herpes simplex meningitis in infancy. Pediatr Infect Dis J 1994;13:141–4.
148. Uren EC, Johnson PDR, Montanaro J, Gilbert GL, Herpes simplex virus encephalitis in pediatrics: diagnosis by detection of antibodies and DNA in cerebrospinal fluid. Pediatr Infect Dis J 1993;12:1001–6.
149. Kimura H, Aso K, Kuuzushima K, Hanada N, Shibata M, Morishima T. Relapse of Herpes simplex encephalitis in children. Pediatrics 1992;89:891–894.
150. Van Dyke HB, Spector SA. Transmission of herpes simplex virus type 1 to a newborn infant during endotracheal suctioning for meconium aspiration. Pediatr Infect Dis 1984;3:153.
151. Mascola L, Cable DC, Walsh P, Guinan ME. Neonatal herpes simplex virus death manifested as rapidly progressive pneumonia. Clin Pediatr 1984;7:400.
152. Green G, King D, Ramansky S, Marble R. Primary herpes simplex pneumonia in a neonate. Am J Dis Child 1983;137:463.
153. Schutze GE, Edwards MS, Adham BI, Belmont JW. Hyperammonemia and neonatal herpes simplex pneumonitis. Pediatr Infect Dis J 1990;9:749–750.
154. Pugh RCB, Newns GH, Dudgeon JA. Hepatic necrosis in disseminated herpes simplex. Arch Dis Child 1954;29:60.
155. Hubbell C, Dominguez R, Kohl S. Neonatal herpes simplex pneumonitis. Rev Infect Dis 1988;10:431–438.
156. Whitley R, Arvin A, Prober C, Corey L, Burchett S, Plotkin S, Starr S, Jacobs R, Powell D, Nahmias A, Sumaya C, Edwards K, Alford C, Caddell G, Soong S-J. Predictors of morbidity and mortality in neonates with herpes simplex virus infections. N Engl J Med 1991;324:450–454.
157. Schreiner RL, Kleiman MB, Gresham EL. Maternal oral herpes: isolation policy. Pediatrics 1979;63:247.
158. Whitley R, Arvin A, Prober C, Burchett S, Corey L, Powell D, Plotkin S, Starr S, Alford C, Connor J, Jacobs R, Nahmias A, Soong S-J. A controlled trial comparing vidarabine with acyclovir in neonatal herpes simplex virus infection. N Engl J Med 1991;324:444–449.
159. Overall JC. Empiric therapy with acyclovir for suspected neonatal herpes simplex virus infection. Pediatr Infect Dis J 1989;8:808–809.
160. Kohl S, Loo L-S, Rench MA, Noya FJD, Feldman S, Baker CJ. Effect of intravenously administered immune globulin on functional antibody to herpes simplex virus in low birth weight neonates. J Pediatr 1989;115:135–139.
161. Whitley RJ. Neonatal herpes simplex virus infections: is there a role for immunoglobulin is disease prevention and therapy? Pediatr Infect Dis J 1994;13:432–9.
162. McCarthy PL. Controversies in pediatrics: what tests are indicated for the child under 2 with fever. Pediatr Rev 1979;1:51.
163. McCarthy PL, Grundy GW, Spiesel SZ, Dolan TF Jr. Bacteremia in children: an outpatient clinical review. Pediatrics 1976;57:861.
164. Teele DW, Pelton SI, Grant MJA, et al. Bacteremia in febrile children under 2 years of age: results of cultures of blood of 600 consecutive febrile children seen in a "walk-in" clinic. J Pediatr 1975;87:227.
165. Deleted
166. McGowan JE Jr, Bratton L, Klein JO, Finland M. Bacteremia in febrile children seen in a "walk-in" pediatric clinic. N Engl J Med 1973;288:1309.
167. Galaid EI, Cherubin CE, Marr JS, Schaefler S, Barone J, Lee W. Meningococcal disease in New York City, 1973 to 1978. JAMA 1980; 244:2167.
168. Band JD, Chamberland ME, Platt T, Weaver RE, Thornsberry C, Fraser DW. Trends in meningococcal disease in the United States, 1975–80. J Infect Dis 1983;148:754.
169. Daniels WB. Cause of death in meningococcic infection. Am J Med 1950;8:468.
170. Olcen P, Barr J, Kjellander J. Meningitis and bacteremia due to *Neisseria meningitidis:* clinical and laboratory findings in 69 cases from Orebro County 1965 to 1977. Scand J Infect Dis 1979;11:111.
171. Stiehm ER, Damrosch DS. Neonatal meningococcal meningitis: report of a case acquired in the nursery. J Pediatr 1966;68:654.
172. Sunderland WA, Harris HH, Spence DA, et al. Meningococcemia in a newborn infant whose mother had meningococcal vaginitis. J Pediatr 1972;81:856.
173. Jones RN, Slepack J, Eades A. Fatal neonatal meningococcal meningitis: association with maternal cervical-vaginal colonization. JAMA 1976;236:2652.
174. Clegg HW, Todres ID, Moylan FMB, Klein DE, Shannon DC. Fulminant neonatal meningococcemia. Am J Dis Child 1980;134:354.
175. Thomas JC, Bendana NS, Waterman SH. Meningococcal disease in Los Angeles County, 1981 through 1990. AM J of Public Health 1993;83:1790–1.
176. Jackson LA, Schuchat A, Reeves MW, Wenger JD. Serogroup C meningococcal outbreaks in the United States, an emerging threat. JAMA 1995;273:383–389.
177. Whalen CM, Hockin JC, Ryan A, Ashton F. The changing epidemiology of invasive meningococcal disease in Canada, 1985 through 1992, emergence of a virulent clone of Neisseria meningitidis. JAMA 1995;273:390–394.
178. Harrison LH, Armstrong CW, Jenkins SR, Harmon MW, Ajello GW, Miller GB, Broome CV. A cluster of meningococcal disease on a school bus following epidemic influenza. Arch Intern Med 1991;151: 1005–1009.
179. Manios SG, Kanakoudi F, Maniati E. Fulminant meningococcemia. Scand J Infect Dis 1971;3:127.
180. Havens PL, Garland JS, Brook MM, Dewitz BA, Stremski ES, Troshynski TJ. Trends in mortality in children hospitalized with meningococcal infections, 1957 to 1987. Pediatr Infect Dis J 1989;8:8–11.
181. Wong VK, Hitchcock W, Mason WH. Meningococcal infections in children: a review of 100 cases. Pediatr Infect Dis J 1989;8:224–227.
182. Glode MP, Smith AL. Meningococcal disease. In: Feigin RD, Cherry JD, eds. Textbook of pediatric infectious disease. Philadelphia: WB Saunders, 1981:916.
183. Stiehm ER, Damrosch DS. Factors in the prognosis of meningococcal infection. J Pediatr 1966;68:457.
184. Niklasson P, Lundbergh P, Strandell T. Prognostic factors in meningococcal disease. Scand J Infect Dis 1971;3:17.
185. Thomson APJ, Sills JA, Hart CA. Validation of the Glasgow meningococcal seticemia prognostic score: a 10-year retrospective survey. Crit Care Med 1991;19:26–30.
186. Tesoro LJ, Selbst SM. Factors affecting outcome in meningococcal infections. Am J Dis Child 1991;145: 218–220.
187. Emparanza JI, Aldamiz-Echevarria L, Perez-Yarza EG, Larranãga P, Jiminez JL, Labiano M, Ozcoidi I. Prognostic score in acute meningococcemia. Crit Care Med 1988;16:168–169.
188. Girardin E, Grau GE, Dayer J-M, Roux-Lombard P, the J5 Study Group, Lambert P–H. Tumor necrosis factor and interleukin-1 in the serum of children with severe infectious purpura. N Engl J Med 1988;319: 397–400.
189. Brandtzaeg P, Kierulf P, Gaustad P, Skulberg A, Bruun JN, Halvorsen S, Srensen. Plasma endotoxin as a predictor of multiple organ failure and death in systemic meningococcal disease. J Infect Dis 1989; 159:195–204.
190. Nugent SK, Bausher JA, Moxon ER, Rogers MC. Raised intracranial pressure: its management in *Neisseria meningitidis* meningoencephalitis. Am J Dis Child 1979;133:260.
191. Waterhouse R. A case of suprarenal apoplexy. Lancet 1911;1:577.
192. Friderichsen C. Nebennierenapoplexie bie kleinen kindern. Jahrb Kinderh 1918;87:109.
193. Perrotin D, Choutet P, Ginies G, Lamisse F. Hemodynamic study in a case of fulminant meningococcemia. Intensive Care Med 1980; 6:203.
194. Uhl HSM. Norepinephrine in the treatment of acute meningococcemia with shock (Waterhouse-Friderichsen syndrome) and an evaluation of adrenocortical function. N Engl J Med 1953;249:229.
195. Mercier J-C, Beaufils F, Hartmann J-F, Azéma D. Hemodynamic patterns of meningococcal shock in children. Crit Care Med 1988;16: 27–33.
196. Shneerson JM, Fawcett IW. The complications and management of meningococcal meningitis. Intensive Care Med 1979;5:5.
197. Bjorvatn B, Bjertnaes L, Fadnes HO, et al. Meningococcal septicemia treated with combined plasmapheresis and leucapheresis or with blood exchange. Br Med J 1984;288:439.
198. Bohm N. Adrenal, cutaneous and myocardial lesions in fulminating endotoxemia. Pathol Res Pract 1982;174:92.
199. Jahn JP, Boling L, Meagher TR, et al. The combination of ACTH, cortisone, hydrocortisone with antibiotics in the management of overwhelmingly severe infections. J Pediatr 1950;44:640.
200. Griffin JW, Daeschner CW. Meningococcal infections; with particular reference to fulminating meningococcemia (Waterhouse-Friderichsen syndrome) treated with cortisone and norepinephrine. J Pediatr 1954;45:264.
201. Koch R, Carson MJ. Meningococcal infections in children. N Engl J Med 1958;258:639.
202. Kass EH, Finland M. Corticosteroids and infections. Adv Intern Med 1958;9:45.
203. Margaretten W, McAdams J. An appraisal of fulminant meningococcemia with reference to the Schwartzman phenomenon. Am J Med 1958;25:868.

204. Tobin JL. Complications of meningococcus infection in a series of sixty-three consecutive sporadic cases. Am J Med Sci 1956;231:241.
205. Lepper MH, Spies HW. A clinical study of the use of cortisone, hydrocortisone, and corticotropin in the treatment of seriously ill patients with infections. Antibiot Annu 1956–1957:447, 1957.
206. Bosworth DC. Reversible adrenocortical insufficiency in fulminant meningococcemia. Arch Intern Med 1979;139:823.
207. Migeon CJ, Kenney FM, Hung W, Voorhees M. Study of adrenal function in children with meningitis. Pediatrics 1967;40:163.
208. May CD. Circulatory failure (shock) in fulminant meningococcal infection. Pediatrics 1960;25:316.
209. Davis CE, Arnold K. Role of meningococcal endotoxin in meningococcal purpura. J Exp Med 1974;40:159.
210. Ferguson JH, Chapman OD. Fulminating meningococcic infections and the so-called Waterhouse-Friderichsen syndrome. Am J Pathol 1948;24:763.
211. Fox B. Disseminated intravascular coagulation and the Waterhouse-Friderichsen syndrome. Arch Dis Child 1971;46:680.
212. Winkelstein A, Songster CL, Caras TS, Berman HH, West WL. Fulminant meningococcemia and disseminated intravascular coagulation. Arch Intern Med 1969;124:55.
213. Mittermayer C, Riede UN, Sandritter W. Rare manifestations of shock in man. Pathol Res Pract 1979;165:289.
214. Boger WP. Fulminating meningococcemia. Demonstration of intracellular and extracellular meningococci in direct smears of the blood. N Engl J Med 1944;231:385.
215. Woods CR, Smith AL, Wasilauskas BL, Campos J, Givner LB. Invasive disease caused by Neisseria meningitidis relatively resistant to penicillin in North Carolina. J Infect Dis 1994;170:453–6.
216. Martin E, Hohl P, Guggi T, Kayser FH, Fernex M, et al. Short course single daily ceftriaxone monotherapy for acute bacterial meningitis in children: results of a Swiss multicenter study. Part I. clinical results. Infection 1990;18:70–77.
217. Tuncer AM, Gür I, Ertem U, Ece A, Türkmen S, Deniz B, Gürman I, Tuncer S. Once daily ceftriaxone for meningococcemia and mengococcal meningitis. Pediatr Infect Dis J 1988;7:711–713.
218. Isaacman SH, Heroman WM, Lightsey AL. Purpura fulminans following late-onset group B beta-hemolytic streptococcal sepsis. Am J Dis Child Pediatr 1984; 138:915–916.
219. Kuppermann N, Inkelis SH, Saladino R. The role of heparin in the prevention of extremity and digit necrosis in meningococcal purpura fulminans. Pediatr Infect Dis J 1994; 13:867–873.
220. Little JR, Jost RG, Anderson CB, Wedner HJ, Kuhn C. Fulminant sepsis and death in a 33 year old immuno-compromised woman. Am J Med 1984;76:868.
221. Hopkins RL, Levine SD. Severe pulmonary edema in meningococcemia. Clin Pediatr 1983;22:452.
222. Tobias JD, Haun SE, Helfaer M, Nichols DG. Use of continuous caudal block to relieve lower-extremity ischemia caused by vasculitis in a child with meningococcemia. J Pediatr 1989;115:1019–1021.
223. Anderson CTM, Berde CB, Sethna NF, Pribaz JJ. Meningococcal purpura fulminans: treatment of vascular insufficiency in a 2-yr-old child with lumbar epidural sympathetic blockade. Anesthesiology 1989;71:463–464.
224. Vega LA. Acute meningococcemia with DIC, septic shock complicated by hypersensitivity monoarthritis. W Va Med J 1984;80:6.
225. Detsky AS. Complete heart block in meningococcemia. Ann Emerg Med 1983;12:391.
226. Moze JR, Oretsky MI, Hudson JA. Pericarditis as a complication of meningococcal meningitis. Ann Intern Med 1971;74:212.
227. Almog R, Block C, Gdalevich M, Lev B, Wiener M, Ashkenazi S. First recorded outbreaks of meningococcal disease in the Israel Defence Force: three clusters due to serogroup C and the emergence of resistance to rifampicin. Infection 1994;2:9–11.
228. Gilja OH, Halstensen A, Digranes A, Mylvaganam H, Aksnes A, Hoiby EA. Use of single-dose oflozxacin to eradicate tonsillopharyngitis carriage of Neiseria meningitidis. Antmicrob Agents and Chemo 1993;37:2024–2026.
229. Sell S. The clinical importance of *Haemophilus influenzae* infections in children. Pediatr Clin North Am 1970;17:415.
230. Hirschmann JV, Everett ED. Haemophilus influenzae infections in adults: report of nine cases and review of the literature. Medicine 1979;58:80.
231. Winslow CEA, Broadhurst J, Buchanan RE, et al. The families and genera of the bacteria. Final report of the Society of American Bacteriologists on characterization and classification of bacterial types. J Bacteriol 1920;5:191.
232. Pittman M. Variation and type specificity in the bacterial species: *Haemophilus influenzae.* J Bacteriol 1947;53:499.
233. Rathore MH, Dick M, Buckner P, Ayoub EM. Haemophilus influenzae type b invasive disease in urban and rural children. Sou Med J 1994;87:1083–1087.
234. Teare EL, Fairley CK, White J, Begg NT. Efficacy of Hib vaccine. The Lancet 1994;344:828–829.
235. Farley MM, Stephens DS, Brachman PS, Harvey C, Smith JD, Wenger JD. Invasive Haemophilus influenza disease in adults. Ann Int Med 1992;116:806–812.
236. Melville CAS, Laurenson IF, Augrove JA. Invasive Disease due to Haemophilus influenzae infection. BMJ 1994;309:58.
237. Kostman R, Sherry BL, Fligner CL, Egaas S, Sheeran P, Baker L, Bauwens JE, Clausen C, Sherer DM, Plorde JJ, Stull TL, Mendelman PM. Invasive Haemophilus influenzae infections in older children and adults in Seattle. Clin Infect Dis 1993;17:389–96.
238. McGechie DB. Nosocomial bacteremia in hospital staff caused by Haemophilus influenzae type B. J Hosp Infect 1992;21:159–160.
239. Centers for Disease Control. Progress toward Elimination of Haemophilus influenzae type b disease among infants and children—United States, 1987-1993. MMWR 1994;43:144–148.
240. Barbour ML, Mayon-White RT, Coles C, Crook DWM, Moxon ER. The impact of conjugate vaccine on carriage of Haemophilus influenzae type b. J Infect Dis 1995;171:93–8.
241. Beach RC, Clayden GS, Eyken SJ. Waterhouse-Friderichsen syndrome caused by Haemophilus Influenzae type b. BMJ 1979;2:1111.
242. Sjursen H, Hofstad T, Fugksang P, et al. Waterhouse-Friderichsen syndrome caused by *Haemophilus influenzae* type b in an adult. Infection 1981;9:300.
243. Jacobs RF, Hsi S, Wilson CB, et al. Apparent meningococcemia: clinical features of disease due to *Haemophilus influenzae* and *Neisseria meningitidis.* Pediatrics 1983;72:469.
244. Perkins M. False positive latex agglutination test in cerebrospinal fluid after immunization for haemophilus influenzae type b. Pediatr Infect Dis J 1993;12:614–615.
245. Jacobson JA, McCormick JB, Hayes P, et al. Epidemiologic characteristics of infections caused by ampicillin-resistant *Haemophilus influenzae.* Pediatrics 1976;58:388.
246. Kinmonth AL, Storrs CN, Mitchell RG. Meningitis due to chloramphenicol resistant *Haemophilus influenzae* type b. Br Med J 1978;1:694.
247. Mendelman PM, Doroshow CA, Gandy SL, et al. Plasmid-mediated resistance in multiply resistant *Haemophilus influenzae* type b causing meningitis: molecular characterization of one strain and review of the literature. J Infect Dis 1984;150:30.
248. Horner DB, McCracken GH Jr, Ginsberg CM, et al. A comparison of three antibiotic regimens for eradication of *Haemophilus influenzae* type b from the pharynx of infants and children. Pediatrics 1980;66:136.
249. Shapiro ED, Wald ER. Efficacy of rifampin in eliminating pharyngeal carriage of *Haemophilus influenzae* type b. Pediatrics 1980;66:5.
250. Band JD, Fraser DW, Ajello G, et al. Prevention of *Haemophilus influenzae* type b disease. JAMA 1984;251:2381.

Meningitis, Infectious Encephalopathies, and Other Central Nervous System Infections

32

Ivor D. Berkowitz
Frank E. Berkowitz
Charles Newton
R. Willoughby
Alice D. Ackerman

INTRODUCTION

The central nervous system (CNS) can be affected by many kinds of infectious processes that are caused by a multitude of organisms. This chapter does not attempt to cover the wide range of infectious disease processes that may involve the CNS. Instead, the discussion concentrates on those that are most common not only in the United States but also worldwide that are most devastating to the child. A discussion of bacterial meningitis and viral encephalitis follows with special reference to herpetic encephalitis, brain abscess, cerebral subdural empyema, and cerebral malaria. Although not directly affecting the brain, spinal epidural abscess is included in this chapter because of the significant neurologic signs displayed by the patients and the catastrophic nature of the disease.

BACTERIAL MENINGITIS

Of all cases of bacterial meningitis, it has been estimated that at least 75% occur in children less than 15 years of age[1]. Meningitis is the most common form of bacterial infection of the nervous system in children[2], and it is one of the most commonly faced life-threatening situations for pediatricians, general practitioners, and emergency room providers engaged in the care of infants and children. Most children with meningitis who are admitted to a pediatric intensive care unit have acute hematogenous meningitis, but patients with meningitis complicating shunt infections, neurosurgery, and tuberculosis are also cared for by pediatric intensive care specialists.

Epidemiology and Bacteriology

The overall incidence of acute hematogenous meningitis in the United States is about 5 per 100,000 persons with a higher incidence in infants[1,2]. The incidence may rise considerably during epidemics of meningococcal infection. *Streptococcus pneumoniae, Neisseria meningitidis,* and *Haemophilus influenzae* type b are the predominant organisms causing acute hematogenous meningitis in children between 2 months and 4 years of age[2,3]. The predominant organisms in different age groups are outlined in **Table 32.1.** These three encapsulated organisms account for at least 80% of culture-proven cases. Anatomic abnormalities, surgical procedures, neurologic trauma, or immune deficiency often underlie meningitis caused by other agents **(Table 32.2).** The bacteriology of these infections varies over time and according to geographic location. For example, in the United States group B streptococcus *(Streptococcus agalactiae)* became the predominant neonatal pathogen in the 1970s, whereas enteric rods had been the usual etiology. The widespread introduction of *Haemophilus influenzae* type b immunization has led to a reduction of invasive hemophilus disease[4]. Tuberculous (TB) meningitis is rare in the child, but with the resurgence of tuberculosis, TB meningitis is increasing in incidence.

Any of the other organisms listed in **Tables 32.1 and 32.2** must be considered, especially in the child with underlying risk factors, or the previously healthy youngster who fails to respond as expected to the administered antibiotics. It is unwise to dismiss the finding of any bacterium

Table 32.1. Usual Causes of Acute Hematogenous Bacterial Meningitis in Children in Different Age-Groups.

Age	*Organism*
0–2 months	*Streptococcus agalactiae* (Group B) Enteric bacilli *(Escherichia coli, Klebsiella Proteus, Citrobacter)* *Listeria monocytogenes*
2–4 months	*Streptococcus agalactiae* *Streptococcus pneumoniae* *Haemophilus influenzae* type b *Neisseria meningitidis*
4 months–5 years	*Streptococcus pneumoniae* *Neisseria meningitidis* *Haemophilus influenzae* type b
> 5 years	*Streptococcus pneumoniae* *Neisseria meningitidis*

Table 32.2. Common Microbial Causes of Meningitis Associated With Different Underlying Conditions.

Underlying Condition	*Organism*
Basilar skull fracture	*Streptococcus pneumoniae* *Haemophilus influenzae* type b *Neisseria meningitidis* *Staphylococcus aureus* *Streptococcus pyogenes* (Group A) Gram-negative bacilli
Post neurosurgery	Coagulase-negative *staphylococci* *Staphylococcus aureus* Gram-negative bacilli
Cerebrospinal fluid shunt	Coagulase-negative *staphylococci* *Staphylococcus aureus* Gram-negative bacilli coryneforms (diphtheroids) *Propionibacteria acnes* *Bacillus* species
Nosocomial (not post surgery)	*Staphylococcus aureus* *Candida* species Gram-negative bacilli
Immune Deficiencies	
hyposplenism (e.g. sickle cell disease)	*Streptococcus pneumoniae* *Haemophilus influenzae* *Neisseria meningitidis*
cell-mediated deficiency	*Listeria monocytogenes* *Salmonella* species *Nocardia* species *Cryptococcus neoformans* Dimorphic fungi (e.g. *Histoplasma capsulatum, Coccidioides immitis)*
neutropenia	*Streptococcus pneumoniae* *Listeria monocytogenes* Gram-negative bacilli enteric bacilli *Pseudomonas aeruginosa*
terminal complement component deficiencies	*Neisseria meningitidis*

as a contaminant in the child with suspected meningitis, especially if no other etiologic agent is identified. Multiple organisms may be involved in meningitis in a single patient, but this is more true for the neonate or for the older child with a foreign body, such as a ventriculoperitoneal shunt[5,6].

Pathogenesis

In order to induce meningitis—an infection of the subarachnoid space—the infecting organism must accomplish the following sequential pathogenic steps: (1) colonization and penetration of the nasopharyngeal epithelium, (2) vascular invasion, (3) intravascular survival, (4) attachment to cerebral microvessels and meningeal invasion of the CSF, and (5) induction of subarachnoid space inflammation[7,8]. The presence of bacteria in the CSF triggers an inflammatory cascade that produces the characteristic inflammatory CSF findings of bacterial meningitis as well as contributes to the primary pathophysiologic events that are responsible for the neurologic damage of this potentially devastating disease[7,8]. These events include alterations in cerebral blood flow, cerebral edema, elevated intracranial pressure, and possible alterations in central nervous system metabolism.

Attachment of bacteria to nasopharyngeal epithelial cells depends on the presence of bacterial virulence factors. Pili and fimbriae, filamentous-like bacterial appendages, mediate the epithelial adhesion of *H. influenzae* and *N. meningitidis* [9]. Carbohydrate adhesins play this role with *S. pneumoniae.* Invasive bacteria either penetrate or pass between nasopharyngeal epithelial cells and enter the systemic circulation where they must overcome a host-defense system, primarily that of complement-mediated, polymorphonuclear leukocyte phagocytosis[7]. The common bacteria causing hematogenous meningitis in children *(H. influenzae, N. meningitidis, S. pneumoniae, S. agalactiae,* and *E. Coli K-1)* possess a potent virulence factor that is a polysaccharide capsule and inhibits complement-mediated polymorphonuclear phagocytosis. Nonencapsulated strains of these organisms have lost the ability to cause invasive disease. Activation of the alternative complement pathway may partially counteract the antiphagocytic capsular polysaccharide of some strains of *S. pneumoniae.* Because the spleen removes nonopsonized material from the circulation, it plays an important host-defense role in individuals without antibody. Therefore, individuals who lack a functional spleen—resulting from congenital asplenia, splenectomy or sickle-cell disease—are at particular risk for overwhelming sepsis and meningitis caused by these encapsulated bacteria. The alternative complement pathway is also impaired in patients with sickle-cell disease.

The mechanisms whereby circulating bacteria penetrate the blood-brain barrier and seed the cerebrospinal fluid remains unclear. Numerous studies have demonstrated both in experimental models and in patients that a high-grade persistent bacteremia is necessary for meningeal seeding[10]. The neurotropic properties and virulence factors of the meningitis-causing bacteria that enable them to attach to brain structures are being unraveled. These factors include the presence of bacterial fimbriae, which bind the invading bacteria to host receptors on the choroid plexus and cerebral capillary endothelial cells facilitating transendothelial passage into the CSF[11]. Bacteria may also enter the CSF having been phagocytosed by circulating macrophages and associated with normal macrophage cell trafficking.

After penetration of the blood brain barrier and entrance into the subarachnoid space, bacterial multiplication proceeds quickly in a CSF environment of relative host immune deficiency[12,13]. Humorally mediated opsonic and bactericidal activity is poor because of a lack of or low concentration of specific antibody and complement and the capsular polysaccharides are intensely antiphagocytic. In addition, neutrophils are poorly phagocytic in the liquid medium of the CSF (impaired surface phagocytosis)[7].

Mechanisms of Subarachnoid Space Inflammation

The inflammatory response engendered by the presence of bacteria within the CSF is initiated by the subcapsular components of the infecting bacterial cell wall: lipo-oligosaccharides and peptidoglycans together with lipoteichoic acid in the case of *H. influenzae* and *S. pneumoniae* meningitis, respectively[14–16]. Implicit in this mechanism is the possibility that antibiotic treatment of meningitis with resultant bacteriolysis and release of cell wall fragments might indeed accentuate subarachnoid space inflammation and inflammation-dependent pathophysiologic events. Indeed studies of experimental and clinical meningitis have demonstrated increased concentrations of cell wall components as well as enhanced indices of inflammation, e.g., CSF leukocyte count, protein, and lactate concentration after antibiotic administration[17,18].

The mechanisms whereby bacterial cell wall indices induce inflammation is complex and not entirely clear[8,19]. The delay of several hours in the CSF inflammatory space response after experimental bacterial or cell wall component intracisternal administration, implicates a second messenger system involving one or more host derived inflammatory mediators[19]. Extensive research has focused on the role of members of the cytokine family in mediating this inflammation. In experimental animals, intracisternal administration of lipo-oligosaccharide and lipoteichoic acid is followed by an increase in CSF concentration of IL-1 and TNF-α as well as increased indices of CSF inflammation[20–23]. In clinical cases of meningitis, CSF concentrations of IL-1 and TNF-α are elevated at diagnosis and fall with appropriate antibiotic therapy[24,25]. The pathophysiologic significance of these cytokines is further supported by the experimental demonstration of increased concentration of CSF leukocytes and protein as well as blood-brain barrier disruption and brain edema after intrathecal IL-1 and TNF-α administration. Intrathecal administration of antibodies directed at IL-1 and TNF-α reduces this inflammatory response[23,26,27]. The sites of intracerebral cytokine production include meningeal macrophages, endothelial cells, and astroglia[19].

Other mediators that are involved in the development of CSF inflammation in bacterial meningitis include prostaglandins[28,29], interferon, macrophage inhibitory proteins (MIP-1 and MIP-2)[30], platelet activating factor (PAF)[25,31], and even oxygen free radicals and nitric oxide[32]. However, these inflammatory mediators have not been as extensively investigated as the cytokines, TNF-α and IL-1. PAF is another cytokine that induces enhanced blood-brain barrier permeability and cerebral edema without substantial CSF leukocytosis. Treatment with PAF antagonists significantly reduces cerebral edema in experimental meningitis caused by *S. pneumoniae* but not *H. influenzae*, suggesting an important pathophysiologic role only in pneumococcal disease[31]. In addition, elevated concentrations of PAF are present in the CSF of children with bacterial meningitis suggesting a pathogenic and pathophysiologic role[25].

Accumulating evidence indicates that increased production and release of cytokines (TNF-α, IL-1) are important determinants of leukocyte recruitment from blood into CSF. The adhesion to vascular endothelial cells and transendothelial migration of leukocytes is mediated by interaction between glycoprotein adhesion molecules and receptors on the endothelium and leukocytes. Three families of glycoproteins contribute to the process of adhesion and migration: (1) immunoglobulin super family, e.g. intercellular adhesion molecule (ICAM), (2) selections, e.g. leukocyte adhesion molecules (LAM, ELAM), and (3) integrins, e.g. CD11/CD18. Indeed, several cytokines either induce enhanced synthesis of or increase the binding affinity of these cellular adhesion molecules[19,33,34].

Having crossed the blood-brain barrier and entered the CSF, leukocytes participate in the inflammatory reaction with the release of toxic mediators, such as nitric oxide, oxygen free radicals, and prostaglandins. As will be discussed later, these mediators modulate cerebral blood flow, contribute to cerebral edema, perhaps alter cerebral metabolism and, no doubt, contribute in a variety of ways to neurologic sequelae of meningitis[8,19,34]. Recently, investigators have demonstrated that systemic administration of monoclonal antibodies directed at the CD11/18 leukocyte-endothelial adhesion molecule reduced the CSF leukocyte count as well as the degree of cerebral edema in experiment bacterial meningitis[35,36]. This data suggests that leukocytes contribute significantly to important pathophysiologic events in this disease.

The concept that inflammatory mediators and neutrophils, components of the over zealous host response induced by the release of bacterial cell wall components may contribute to the neurologic sequelae is a crucial advance in our understanding of the pathogenesis and pathophysiology of meningitis. This suggests that adjunctive anti-inflammatory therapies may modulate the damaging host response and may improve the outcome of bacterial meningitis.

Pathophysiology

The pathophysiologic events that result in the clinical manifestations and complications of meningitis and determine its neurologic sequelae are multiple and include (1) alterations in cerebral blood flow and its control, (2) cerebral vasculitis, (3) elevation of intracranial pressure, and (4) alterations in cerebral metabolism.

Cerebral Blood Flow in Meningitis

Cerebral blood flow (CBF) in meningitis is determined both by cerebral perfusion pressure and cerebrovascular resistance, factors potentially perturbed by pathophysiologic events in bacterial meningitis. Reduced cerebral blood flow potentially contributes to neurologic sequelae by limiting substrate delivery to brain tissue with resultant ischemia and even infarction, whereas cerebral hyperemia could increase cerebral blood volume and thereby elevate intracranial pressure[7,19]. Indeed, both experimental studies and investigation of clinical cases revealed significant alterations in cerebral blood flow and vascular pathology.

Experimental studies of different animal models of meningitis caused by a variety of organisms have demonstrated conflicting results of cerebral blood flow measurements. In experimental pneumococcal meningitis models, the cerebral blood flow changes are biphasic with an early phase, the first 6 hours, characterized by cerebral hyperemia[37–39]. With progressive infection, total cerebral blood flow falls to a level of approximately 25% of baseline values within 16 to 20 hours and is associated with a decrease in cerebral metabolic rate for oxygen ($CMRO_2$). In contrast, in *H. influenzae* type b meningitis in rabbits hyperemia persists for up to 16 hours with a normal $CMRO_2$, which is an example of luxury perfusion[40]. In infant Rhesus monkeys with *H. influenzae* type b meningitis, cerebral blood flow falls by approximately 60 to 70% after 7 to 12 days of infection[41]. In the rat and rabbit models, intracranial pressure progressively rises with the duration of infection and is elevated even in the early phase when it is associated with cerebral hyperemia and presumed increase in cerebral blood volume[38,40]. Although it has always been assumed that increased CSF lactate concentration is caused by cerebral ischemia and secondary anaerobic glycolytic metabolism, CSF lactate concentration increases even with normal cerebral blood flow and $CMRO_2$.

The mechanisms of cerebral arteriolar dilation responsible for the falling cerebral vascular resistance and cerebral hyperemia are multifactorial and appear related to the production of oxygen free radicals and nitric oxide, both potent cerebral vasodilators. Administration of either superoxide dismutase, an oxygen free radical scavenger, or inhibitors of nitric oxide synthase prevents this early phase of cerebral hyperemia[32,38,42]. The sites of production of these pathophysiologically significant free radicals are not defined but include leukocytes, vascular smooth muscle and endothelium, and glial cells. CSF lactic acidosis, increased CSF TNF α, and granulocytes may also play a role in the cerebral hyperemia.

The mechanisms of decreased cerebral blood flow associated with progressive infection are unclear but are likely to be multifactorial in nature. Elevated intracranial pressure is a major determinant of cerebral blood flow, and elevated intracranial pressure certainly develops in the well-characterized animal meningitis models in which a good correlation is found between elevated intracranial pressure and decreased cerebral blood flow[37]. A detailed discussion of elevated intracranial pressure in meningitis will follow. Preliminary evidence suggests that in addition to elevated intracranial pressure, host humoral factors may be responsible for the decreased cerebral blood flow in bacterial meningitis. In the rabbit pneumococcal model there is a close correlation between decreased cerebral blood flow and elevated TNF-α concentrations, suggesting a role for TNF as a cerebral vasoconstrictor[43]. It is unclear whether this is a primary event or secondary to decreased $CMRO_2$ and close linking of blood flow with metabolism. Recent studies have also suggested that endothelin may play a role in the induction of cerebral hypoperfusion in bacterial meningitis[44]. The reduction in regional cerebral blood flow is probably also related in some part to vasospasm, vasculitis, and vascular thrombosis with luminal narrowing. These vascular factors are discussed in detail in the following section.

Despite the high morbidity and mortality of meningitis, there is a relative paucity of clinical cerebral blood-flow data in patients with meningitis, particularly in children. Paulson demonstrated decreased regional cerebral blood flow of 30 to 40% using intra-arterial $Xe13^{133}$ in several patients with pneumococcal but not meningococcal disease[45]. In addition, he demonstrated impairment of autoregulation and CO_2 responsiveness in these patients. Several studies using transcranial Doppler sonographic techniques in both children and adults[46–48] with bacterial meningitis have demonstrated increase in flow velocity in the anterior cerebral artery (in children) and in basilar cerebral arteries (in adults) that peaks at day 3 to 4 of disease. Values that rise to 100% that of baseline day of diagnosis values return to normal within 14 to 21 days[48]. These Doppler changes are frequently not accompanied by clinical or radiologic evidence of focal CNS abnormalities. These Doppler findings are interpreted as evidence of blood vessel narrowing, although increased cerebral blood flow is also a possible explanation for this increase in cerebral blood flow velocity. The underlying vascular pathologic conditions that account for this possible vascular narrowing include vasculitis, vasospasm, and vascular compression from cerebral edema[47,48].

Ashwal examined total and regional cerebral blood flow by stable xenon-computed tomography in 20 seriously ill children who had acute bacterial meningitis[49]. In 65% of cases, total cerebral blood flow was normal but marked local variability of flow was seen. In 25% total CBF was significantly reduced. The flow reduction was greater in white matter than in gray matter. CO_2 responsiveness was also evaluated and remained intact in almost all the children.

Vasculitis

In both children and adults with bacterial meningitis, investigators have demonstrated that structural changes occur with focal vascular narrowing, which reflects vasculitis, thrombus formation, and possibly vasospasm affecting large intracerebral arteries, e.g. carotid, middle and anterior cerebral arteries (Fig. 32.2). These findings are frequently associated with clinical evidence of focal deficits secondary to cerebral infarction. The presence of these large vessels over the surface of the brain, surrounded and bathed by CSF containing activated white cells, bacteria, and inflammatory mediators, makes these vessels particularly susceptible to vascular damage. Such evidence of cerebral-vascular involvement in addition to cerebral blood-flow measurements in animals and humans has become evident from (1) autopsy studies demonstrating arteritis, thrombophlebitis, and sinus thrombosis[50,51]; (2) angiographic demonstration of arterial pathology including narrowing, focal dilation, thrombosis, and possible vasospasm (Figure 32.1)[52,53]; and (3) CT studies demonstrating focal intracranial infarction (Figure 32.2)[54,55]. The incidence of cerebral infarction in

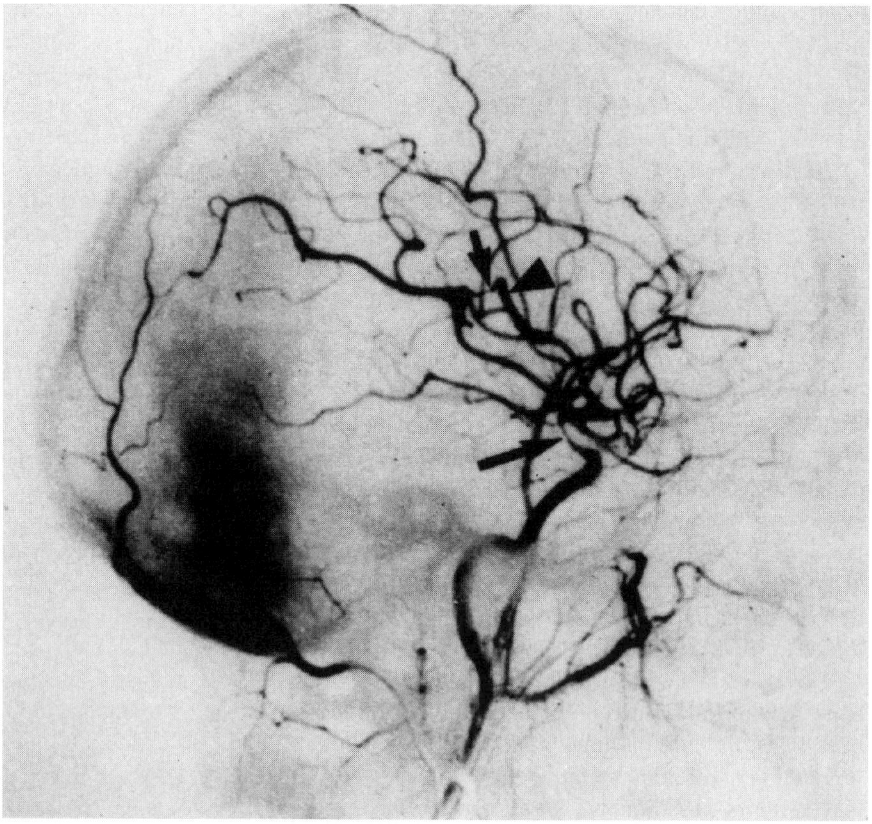

Figure 32.1. Lateral subtraction angiographic view in an adult with bacterial meningitis demonstrating severe narrowing in the supra clinoid portion of the right internal carotid artery (long arrow), ectatic (triangle) and narrowed (short arrow) segments in the middle cerebral artery distribution. From Pfister HW, Borasio GD, Dirnagle U, Bauer M, Einhäupl KM. Cerebrovascular complications of bacterial meningitis in adults. Neurology 1992;42:1497–1504.

children ranges from 3 to 12%, which usually follows a major vascular distribution. Most of the clinical reports of cerebrovascular complications involve children with *H. influenzae* type b meningitis. Pfister et al. demonstrated in a prospective angiographic study of adults with bacterial meningitis of varying causes and with focal clinical signs a 50% incidence of infarction and focal vascular changes, including vascular narrowing, vessel wall irregularities, and thrombosis affecting not only large arteries at the base of the brain, but also medium size arteries, small pial and intraparenchymal vessels and major sinuses and cortical veins[53]. Lipopolysaccharide and endogenous mediators,

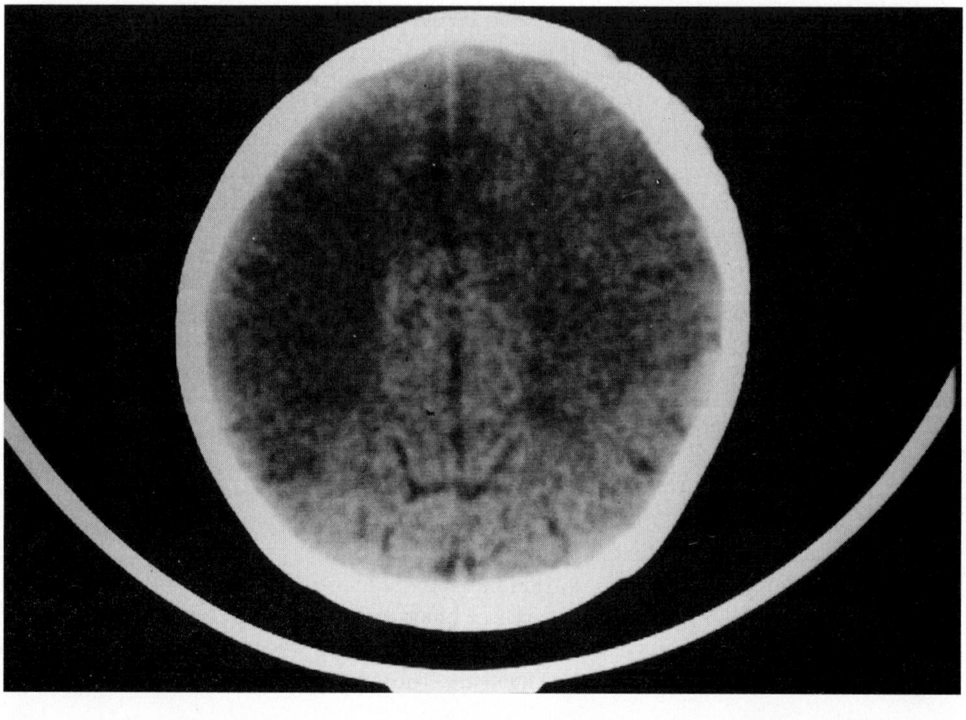

Figure 32.2. Brain CT scan of a child with *Haemophilus influenzae* meningitis, showing bilateral cerebral hemisphere infarcts.

such as Il-1, TNF, and PAF, may cause the pathologic conditions of vasculitis and thrombosis[19].

Autoregulation

The normal intact cerebrovascular system is able to maintain constant cerebral blood flow over a wide range of cerebral perfusion pressures by its ability to vary cerebrovascular resistance, which is known as autoregulation. Impairment of autoregulation in meningitis with purely pressure passive cerebral blood flow could make the brain particularly vulnerable to cerebral ischemia (with reduced cerebral perfusion pressure) and cerebral hyperemia as well as increased cerebral blood volume and elevated intracranial pressure (with elevation of systemic blood pressure and increased cerebral perfusion pressure). The experimental evidence evaluating autoregulation is conflicting. In a rabbit model of *S. pneumoniae* meningitis, autoregulation is clearly impaired[37]; however, autoregulation remains intact in a rabbit[56] but not in a rat model of *H. influenzae* meningitis[57]. Clinical evaluations of autoregulation are difficult because investigators are reluctant to subject patients with serious intracranial abnormalities to either pharmacologically induced hypertension or hypotension. Paulson (in the only appropriate study of this issue) has demonstrated autoregulatory impairment in a few patients with pneumococcal and meningococcal meningitis[45]. In spite of the paucity of clinical data evaluating autoregulation, clinical studies have demonstrated a correlation between low cerebral perfusion and poor outcome, although this is not necessarily a consequence of impaired autoregulation. Goiten demonstrated a poor outcome in children with meningitis when the cerebral perfusion was less than 30 mm Hg[58]. Other studies have demonstrated similar findings[59,60].

Elevated Intracranial Pressure

Intracranial pressure is a crucial determinant of cerebral perfusion pressure and is important in the outcome of bacterial meningitis in children. Several clinical studies using continuous intracranial pressure monitoring demonstrated that morbidity and mortality was highest in children with cerebral perfusion less than 30 mm Hg[58,60]. Analysis of these studies suggests that a decrease in cerebral perfusion pressure was related more to elevation of intracranial pressure than reduction in arterial blood pressure. Several studies in adults and children demonstrate that ICP is frequently elevated in patients with clinical meningitis, and the elevated intracranial pressure is usually maximally elevated within the first 24 to 48 hours after diagnosis[46,58,60–62]. Indeed, in the study by Mimm et al., the ICP was elevated in 33 of 35 children at the time of diagnosis of the disease[62].

In addition to the clinical observations that elevated ICP frequently accompanies the diagnosis of meningitis, substantial experimental evidence suggests that elevated ICP develops in all experimental models of meningitis. In some models, ICP is significantly elevated even within 21/2 hours of cisternal inoculation of bacteria[38,40].

The major causes of elevated intracranial pressure in bacterial meningitis are several and include cerebral edema, hydrocephalus, and cerebral hyperemia. Other complications that can contribute to increased intracranial pressure include subdural effusions and empyema, brain abscess, and cerebral infarction[7,63].

Cerebral Edema

Cerebral edema may occur because of vasogenic, cytotoxic, and interstitial mechanisms[64]. Vasogenic edema, distributed mainly in cerebral white matter, is characterized by increased permeability of the capillary endothelial cells. Increase in blood-brain barrier permeability has been demonstrated in experimental models of bacterial meningitis in response to both inoculation of bacteria, cell wall components, and cytokines[16,26,50,65,66]. Cytotoxic edema is caused by cellular swelling secondary to cell injury. This affects neurons, glial and endothelial cells and reflects failure of ATP-ase-dependent sodium exchange. Although it is unclear as to their precise site of action in edema formation, mediators of inflammation include oxygen free radicals[38], nitric oxide[32], PAF[67], arachidonic acid metabolites[29], leukocytes, and even bacterial toxins. Interstitial edema is caused by increased CSF hydrostatic pressure associated with hydrocephalus that often accompanies bacterial meningitis.

Hydrocephalus

Hydrocephalus with ventricular dilation and enlargement of the subarachnoid space demonstrated on CT or MRI scan is a common neuroradiographic finding and is present in up to 80% of children with bacterial meningitis (Figure 32.3)[55]. Serial scanning of these patients demonstrates that CSF volume is greatest within the first 72 hours after hospitalization, which is the period of greatest ICP elevation. The relative contribution of increased CSF volume to elevated ICP is unclear but it is likely that it has some significant role, particularly when accompanied by cerebral edema and cerebral hyperemia.

In experimental pneumococcal meningitis, hydrocephalus is caused by increased resistance to CSF outflow. This resistance represents either an obstruction to CSF flow in the supracortical subarachnoid space or at the arachnoid villi presumably from plugging by inflammatory debris[68]. Dexamethasone but not methylprednisolone pretreatment will attenuate this demonstrated increase in CSF outflow resistance.

Cerebral Hyperemia

Cerebral blood volume is an important yet not well-appreciated contributor to intracranial volume and pressure. Although measurements of cerebral blood volume in bacterial meningitis are not available, the early phase of bacte-

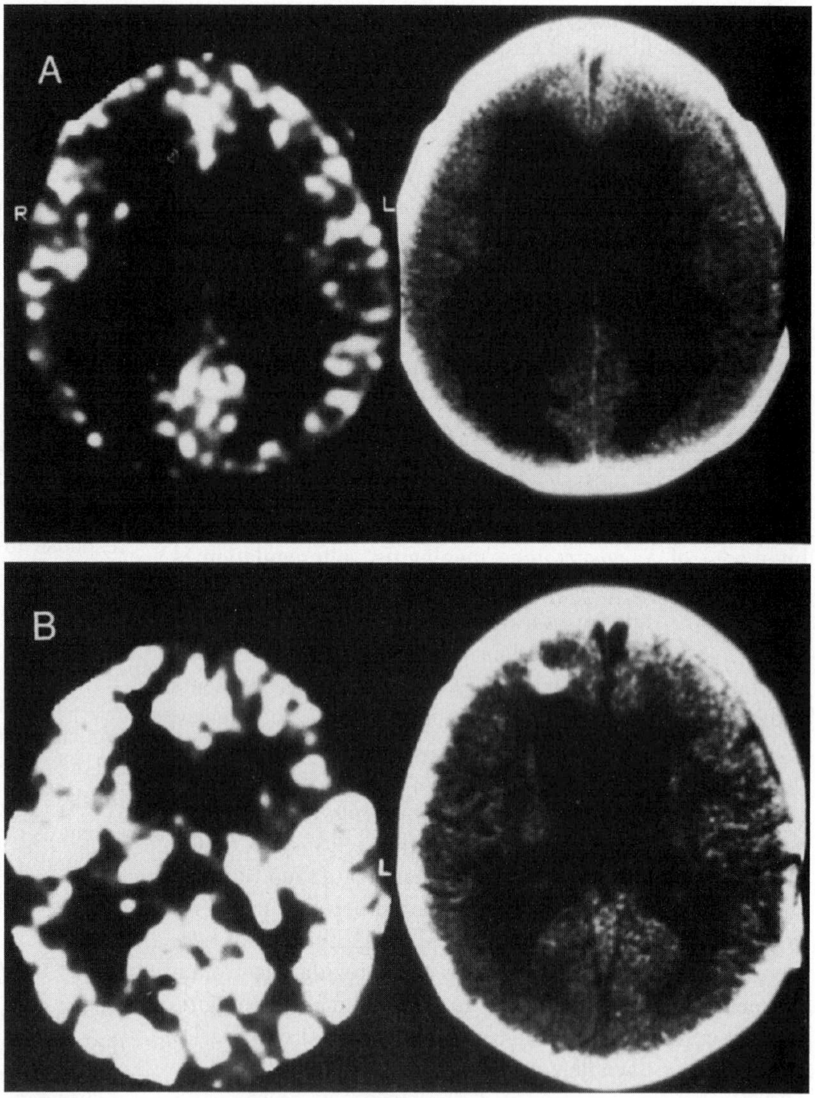

Figure 32.3. A) Stable Xe CBF map (left) in a child with bacterial meningitis and acute hydrocephalus demonstrating reduced total CBF. B) CBF increased by 35% after ventriculostomy. Note area of infarction in the left thalamus on the CT scan (right). From Ashwal S, Perkin RM, Thompson JR, Schneider S, Tomasi LG. Bacterial meningitis in children: Current concepts of neurologic management. Advances in Pediatrics 1993;40:185–215.

rial meningitis is characterized by cerebral hyperemia and profound pial arteriolar dilation. This suggests an increase in cerebral blood volume that probably contributes to elevated intracranial pressure[38,40,42,57]. In addition, cerebral hyperemia and pial arteriolar dilation potentially increase intraluminal microvascular pressure that could increase blood brain barrier leakage and interstitial edema.

Alterations of Cerebral Metabolism in Bacterial Meningitis

Profound alterations in cerebral metabolism, particularly affecting oxygen, lactate, glucose and excitatory amino acids, characterize bacterial meningitis and may potentially play a role in the pathophysiologic events responsible for neurologic damage[19,63].

Elevated CSF lactate concentration is a characteristic marker of abnormal brain metabolism in bacterial meningitis. CSF lactate concentration at the time of diagnosis of bacterial meningitis is usually several times higher than normal[69]. The origin and site of synthesis of the elevated lactate observed is unclear and controversial. For many years, the generally accepted explanation was that elevated intracranial pressure reduced cerebral perfusion pressure and cerebral blood flow with subsequent decrease in oxygen delivery, resulting in cerebral ischemia and anaerobic cerebral metabolism with lactate accumulation[8]. However, more recent studies demonstrated normal or even increased cerebral blood flow and normal $CMRO_2$ (suggesting luxury cerebral perfusion) is nevertheless still associated with increase in CSF lactate concentration. Lindquist and Moxon have demonstrated elevated CSF and brain lactate concentrations without evidence of biochemical ATP depletion in rabbits and rat models of bacterial meningitis[70,71]. To support this data, magnetic resonance spectroscopy study of a comatose patient with pneumococcal meningitis revealed normal brain intracellular pH and normal concentration of high-energy phosphates, suggesting normal brain energetics[72]. In addition, Anderson demonstrated in an experimental pneumococcal meningitis model that brain pH was decreased only in the superficial cortex, and that pH became normal as a pH electrode was advanced deeper into the brain tissues. This suggests that lactate diffuses from the CSF into the brain. Activated leukocytes were proposed as the site of lactate synthesis[73]. This hypothesis is controversial since there is other experimental evidence that shows no difference in CSF lactate concentrations when an experimental meningitis group is rendered neutropenic. Microdialysis studies of rabbits with bacterial meningitis demonstrated increased lactate production from brain, suggesting that infection primarily altered central nervous system metabolism in the direction of anaerobic pathways even in the presence of adequate CNS oxygen delivery[74].

The pathologic significance of increased CSF lactate is unclear. Increased lactate may contribute to enhanced cerebral blood flow particularly cortical blood flow, because decreased pH is a potent pial arteriolar vasodilator and an important determinant of cortical flow. CNS lactate accumulation could also cause the development of cerebral edema[63]. Whether elevated CSF lactate levels even contribute to the pathophysiologic abnormalities is controversial since there is both support of a correlation and lack thereof between elevated CSF lactate and morbidity and mortality[75,76].

Hypoglycorrhachia is almost an essential element of bacterial meningitis, yet the understanding of its development is unclear. Proposals have included increased glucose consumption by leukocytes and bacteria, but alteration in blood brain barrier transport is the most likely explanation[77].

Excitatory amino acids through interaction with glutamate receptors play a significant role in neuronal death in cerebral ischemia, another paradigm of CNS injury. Whether this pathway is involved as a mechanism of neuronal damage in meningitis is unclear, but several experimental studies have demonstrated an increased glutamate concentration in both CSF and brain microdialysis fluid[74]. The clinical significance of these findings in unknown.

Clinical Manifestations

Clinical presentation of acute bacterial meningitis is variable and differs according to infectious etiology, age, and resistance factors of the host, as well as length of time between onset of illness and first evaluation by a physician. The topic has been the subject of several reviews[78–80].

In general, most patients have fever, irritability, and mental status changes, usually associated with vomiting and loss of appetite. Headache is a common complaint in the older child, followed by development of neck rigidity approximately 12 to 24 hours into the illness. Neonates and infants less than 4 months of age may not reproducibly show signs of meningismus, but generally have nonspecific signs of systemic illness, which may include apnea and convulsions as well as other signs of sepsis as described in Chapter 31.

Older children may also develop seizures as an early manifestation of disease. For some, this is the reason for seeking medical attention[81]. The convulsions may be confused with febrile seizures if the spinal fluid is not evaluated for presence of cells or microorganisms. Convulsions occur in at least 30% of patients with meningitis at some point in their illness and may be focal or generalized. Focal seizures are more likely to occur with a localized infarction or in the presence of a subdural effusion. Generalized seizures may be the result of diffuse irritation from inflammation, diffuse ischemia, or hyponatremia that accompanies the development of the syndrome of inappropriate secretion of antidiuretic hormone (SIADH) (see the following discussion). Convulsions that are limited to the first 48 to 72 hours of illness generally have a better prognosis and are less likely to require long-term anticonvulsant therapy than those that occur later in the course of disease.

The duration and progression of symptoms depend on the peculiarities of the infecting organisms. As described in the preceding chapter, meningococcal sepsis and meningitis are often rapidly progressive and, in some cases, result in death several hours after the onset of illness. Although some cases of *H. influenzae* type b meningitis are fulminant in the same manner as *N. meningitidis*[61], most cases of haemophilus meningitis take a somewhat less rapid course. Pneumococcal meningitis may begin as bacteremia, and the child who is destined to develop acute bacterial meningitis is difficult to distinguish in the initial phases of illness from the child who may be considered to have benign or "occult" pneumococcal sepsis.

Evaluation of the child with suspected meningitis begins, as in most of medicine, with a history. In this case, factors of historical importance include exposure to another child with meningococcal or haemophilus meningitis, because these diseases tend to cluster. In addition, day-care arrangements should be explored fully, because children who attend day-care centers, where relatively large numbers of children are less than 5 years of age and are much more likely to develop haemophilus meningitis even in the absence of a documented case[82]. This is true presumably because nasopharyngeal disease spreads readily among these children. Of course, day care and household information is important once the diagnosis is made to determine the need for chemoprophylaxis of contacts. If a child has been fully immunized against *H. influenzae* type b, meningitis caused by this organism is very unlikely[4].

The diagnostic subtleties may not be so pronounced for the pediatric intensive care specialist as for the emergency or primary care physician. If the child requires intensive care, he or she generally will be comatose, be having seizures, or be in a state of hemodynamic instability. In such cases, the diagnostic possibilities include those entities listed in Chapter 21 on coma, the many causes of status epilepticus, and those implicated in generalized sepsis with endotoxic shock.

As always, the most critical aspects of the physical examination are evaluation of the patient's vital functions, with specific attention given to the basic ABCs of life support, before a search is made for etiologic clues. Abnormalities clearly present on the physical examination usually include meningismus, or pain associated with neck flexion, and limitation of movement of the neck, as evidenced by eliciting the Kernig and Brudzinski signs. Pathophysiologic correlation of the presence of these signs is presumed to be meningeal irritation resulting from inflammation, but abnormalities have been observed in the absence of striking pleocytosis. In addition, these signs may sometimes disappear with progression of illness and development of deep coma.

Examination of the pupils and retinae are important. As mentioned previously, abnormalities in the pupillary response to light may occur because of direct irritation of the third cranial nerve as it leaves the base of the brain. Limitations of ocular movement may result from irritation of the third and sixth nerves. Fourth-nerve involvement is less common but does occur. It is important to determine the cause of such findings, because the subsequent course will be much different if the signs are actually caused by elevated ICP, rather than localized inflammation. Papilledema is not a reliable sign in determining the presence or absence of elevated ICP, but if it is observed, chances are greater that intracranial hypertension exists. It may also be a helpful sign in the differential diagnosis, since papilledema that develops within the first day or two of illness is more likely caused by a ruptured brain abscess, subarachnoid extension of an intracranial extradural abscess, or other mass-type lesion[83]. Patients who have tuberculous and cryptococcal meningitis are more likely to have focal signs and papilledema than patients with meningitis caused by the usual bacteria. The retinae should be evaluated for the presence of possible hemorrhages, because their presence may be helpful in making the diagnosis of cortical vein and sagittal sinus thrombosis, abnormalities of blood clotting mechanisms, and certain types of trauma and child abuse leading to coma or seizure activity. In young infants, elevated ICP may be manifested by a bulging fontanelle. Anterior fontanelle herniation of brain tissue has been reported[84].

Differential Diagnosis

The clinical differential diagnosis of acute bacterial meningitis is listed in **Table 32.3.** The differential diagnosis varies with age and other host factors. It includes conditions that cause changes in mental status and those that cause pain on neck flexion.

Table 32.3. Differential Diagnosis of Meningitis According to the Patients Clinical Syndrome

Clinical Syndrome	*Differential Diagnosis*
Encephalopathy (disturbed level of consciousness, seizures)	Hypoglycemia, electrolyte disturbance, hypoxia, intoxication, head injury, stroke, vasculitis, inborn error of metabolism, focal intracranial suppuration, encephalitis, Reye syndrome
Raised intracranial pressure	Intracranial hemorrhage, focal intracranial suppuration, tumor, hydrocephalus
Neurological signs with neck-stiffness	Posterior fossa tumor, herniation
Fever with neck-stiffness	Pneumonia (especially right upper lobe), neck infections, cervical lymphadenitis, retropharyngeal abscess, cervical arthritis, spinal epidural abscess

Indications for Admission to the Pediatric Intensive Care Unit

The majority of patients with suspected bacterial meningitis are evaluated in the emergency department where the diagnosis is considered, and initial therapy is instituted. These children are usually sleepy, lethargic, or irritable, but arousable, and are generally admitted to an isolation room on the general pediatric ward. As noted, however, the clinical presentation may vary significantly, and some individuals will require intensive care. This is the case for the infant or child who arrives comatose with abnormal motor response to stimulation, abnormalities of the pupillary response to light, obvious cranial nerve involvement, or other signs potentially indicative of elevated ICP, such as bradycardia and hypertension. Likewise, the youngster who manifests signs of poor perfusion, obvious shock, cutaneous manifestations of disseminated intravascular coagulation (DIC), such as petechiae or purpura, or irregularities of respiratory pattern should be admitted to an area where he or she can have constant vigilant nursing care with close monitoring of vital signs. Laboratory data including significant metabolic acidosis, hypoxemia, hypercapnia, neutropenia, significant hyponatremia, anemia, or evidence of renal or liver dysfunction indicate that the particular patient has a more serious illness than most and requires observation in an ICU.

Although the individual does not appear critically ill, if circumstances on a general pediatric floor would potentially limit the level of observation, the child should be brought to the ICU, even if only for an overnight admission. The child whose course has been particularly rapid prior to presentation also deserves special observation and monitoring, because he or she is more likely to develop signs of septic shock or intracranial hypertension and to require higher levels of support than generally available on the usual pediatric floor.

Therefore, we recommend that in any case in which the course is complicated or severe, whether from a systemic or neurologic aspect, the child be admitted to the ICU at least until the course can be determined, the first several doses of antibiotics administered, and a tentative bacteriologic diagnosis made. It is only through early recognition of complications, such as shock or elevated ICP, that effective therapy can be initiated in a timely fashion and can potentially alter the outcome of fulminant meningitis.

Lumbar Puncture in the Critically Ill Child

The definitive diagnosis of meningitis is made by recovery of organisms from culture of the CSF, but the lumbar puncture (LP) procedure is not without risks. Contraindications to this procedure include cardiorespiratory instability, raised intracranial pressure, coagulopathy, and skin infection in the lumbar area.

The child with fever, headache, and mild lethargy who is evaluated in the emergency department for possible meningitis is not in the same category as the patient in the pediatric ICU. This child is combative, may have seizures, potentially is hemodynamically unstable, and is, therefore, at risk for significant cardiorespiratory compromise while being positioned for the spinal tap. In such a situation, the clinician must weigh the relative risks involved and decide whether to initiate therapy before or after the LP has been performed. In the setting of unstable vital signs, it is always better to postpone the tap.

Another situation in which LP is potentially hazardous is in the patient with severely elevated ICP in whom removal of fluid from the lumbar space may result in cerebral herniation(85). This may occur up to several hours after the spinal tap. This is particularly so when signs of elevated intracranial pressure are associated with signs either suggestive of a mass lesion or chronic ear or sinus infection, which are suggestive of a possible brain abscess. A spinal tap is contraindicated in the presence of a brain abscess with elevated intracranial pressure because of the high risk of herniation. If elevated intracranial pressure is highly suspected (based on clinical and CT scan findings) then the spinal fluid sample may more safely be obtained through ventricular puncture, during placement of a ventricular catheter to measure ICP, and should follow administration of antibiotics. It must be emphasized that intracranial hypertension is rare in the first few hours, although some patients will have malignant intracranial hypertension(61). Those cases in which a tap must be deferred because of potential herniation will not be many. Indeed, the presence of elevated ICP early in the course should encourage the physician to search for another cause of intracranial abnormality.

Lumbar puncture should also be avoided in the child with active DIC because of the risk of developing a spinal epidural hematoma, a catastrophic complication. For the patient who manifests abnormal clotting parameters, fresh-frozen plasma (FFP) or platelets can be administered immediately before the procedure.

When a lumbar puncture is contraindicated in a patient strongly suspected of having bacterial meningitis, antimicrobial therapy should be instituted immediately in the absence of a definitive diagnosis. Since most cases of community-acquired acute bacterial meningitis occurs because of a limited number of different bacteria, empiric antimicrobial therapy directed against the most likely organisms can be instituted (see the following discussion). If a lumbar puncture is performed subsequently the CSF might be sterile. However, a microbiological diagnosis might be made from the blood culture, which frequently yields the pathogen, or by antigen detection. The empiric therapy of nosocomial meningitis is much more difficult because there is a much greater variety of potential pathogens and of antimicrobial resistance patterns.

The critical care physician is often faced with accepting, in transfer, a child with suspected meningitis and mental status abnormalities from another institution. The question is often raised of whether the tap must be done before transfer. The same guidelines discussed previously apply to patients in whom a tap is contraindicated. In addition, any procedure that delays the administration of antibiotics or transfer of the child to an appropriate facility should be deferred and completed at the receiving hospital if the child is stable on arrival. Administration of antibiotics should *never* be postponed because of a proposed transfer from one institution to another, regardless of the ability of the referring physician or hospital to obtain appropriate cultures.

An opening pressure (OP) must be measured when a lumbar puncture is performed in patients with suspected meningitis. The normal OP in the adult and older child is up to 180 mm H_2O. For the neonate, the normal value is assumed to be between 90 and 110 mm H_2O(85–87), a value derived from noninvasive fontameter readings that have been correlated with direct intraventricular pressure measurements. The determination of OP must be made with the infant or child in a horizontal position and with his or her back relatively straight.

Laboratory Diagnosis

The definitive diagnosis of meningitis is made by recovery of organisms from the CSF. Since culture results may take 24 to 48 hours for the common organisms and even longer for more fastidious agents, other information derived from CSF examination is more helpful in making a presumptive diagnosis of bacterial meningitis within an hour or two. The appearance of the spinal fluid is the first readily appreciated characteristic, after measurement of the opening pressure. Meningitis is suspected if the fluid is grossly cloudy, and antibiotic therapy should be instituted immediately. A leukocyte count must be completed in a counting chamber, and a differential cell count done on a smear of cytocentrifuged specimens. Even when the spinal fluid appears clear, determination of the cell count is essential. Normal CSF findings in infants and children are a maximum of 5 WBCs/mm^3, all of which should be mononuclear(88,89). The normal CSF cell count values for neonates are noted in **Table 32.4.** In newborn babies, polymorphonuclear leukocytes may comprise up to 60% of the total white cell population and still be considered normal.

In meningitis, the CSF white cell count is generally elevated. Spinal fluid will continue to appear clear with up to 500 WBCs/mm^3 and does not become grossly turbid until very large numbers of cells are present. Infrequently, in the early stages of meningitis, CSF leukocytosis may not occur in spite of a positive CSF culture(90). In bacterial meningitis, granulocytes usually predominate, making up 80 to 90% of the total number of leukocytes. **Table 32.5** outlines the range of CSF values occurring in various forms of meningitis.

In acute meningitis, the CSF glucose and protein con-

Table 32.4. Composition of Normal Cerebrospinal Fluid According to Patient Age

	Total WBC/mm³ Count		*ANC*		*% of Neutrophils*		*Glucose (mg/d)*		*CSF-Blood Glucose Ratio*		*Protein (mg/dl)*	
	Mean	*Range*	*Mean*	*Range*	*Mean*	*Range*	*Mean*	*Range*	*Mean*	*Range*	*Mean*	*Range*
Premature Newborn	9.0	0–29	NR	NR	7.0	0–66	50	24–63	0.74	0.55–1.05	115	65–150
Term Newborn	8.2	0–22	NR	NR	61	NR	52	34–119	0.81	0.44–2.48	90	20–170
0–4 Weeks	11.0	0–50	0.40	0–7.5	2.2	0–15	46	36–61	NR	NR	84	35–189
4–8 Weeks	7.1	0–50	0.18	0–2.1	2.9	0–42	46	29–62	NR	NR	59	19–121

NR, not reported
ANC, absolute nucleated cell count/mm³
From Bonadio WA. The cerebrospinal fluid: physiologic aspects and alterations associated with bacterial meningitis. Pediatr Infect Dis J 1992;11:423–432.

centrations are typically deranged. The glucose value is generally much lower than the accepted normal of 50 to 60% of the serum glucose (in newborns, the norm is considered to be at least 75% of serum value), and in many instances, the absolute value is as low as 0 to 20 mg/dl (**Table 32.4** outlines normal ranges of CSF glucose in neonates). Because most of the normal data regarding glucose concentration have been reported as percentages of serum values, a blood glucose determination must be obtained. The timing of this test is crucial for valid results, yet the best interval between determination of blood and CSF glucose values is not clear. It is apparent that some period of equilibration is necessary for the CSF concentration to reflect serum values. This may be as long as 2 hours[91,92]. Therefore, glucose values are difficult to interpret in a patient who recently experienced an acute change in serum glucose, such as a seizure, or intravenous glucose administration for hypoglycemia. Under any circumstances, CSF glucose less than 40 mg/dl is considered hypoglycorrhachia unless the preceding hypoglycemia was very severe[93]. Although the association of hypoglycorrhachia with acute suppurative meningitis has been long established, its cause remains unclear. The proposed mechanisms include increased glucose consumption by brain, spinal cord, and possible phagocytosing leukocytes. Inhibition of glucose transport from blood across the blood-brain barrier has been proposed.

CSF protein concentration is elevated in bacterial meningitis usually to concentrations greater than 100 mg/dl. However, normal CSF protein values also vary with age. In the adult and older child, values of spinal fluid protein up to 45 mg/dl are accepted as being within the normal range, Table 32.4 outlines the range for full-term and premature infants. The presence of erythrocytes may raise the protein concentration by approximately 15 mg/dl for every 1000 RBCs/mm³ of spinal fluid.

A sample of CSF must also be sent to the microbiology laboratory for Gram's stain, culture, and sensitivity determination. The Gram's stain is the simplest, quickest, and most useful rapid test for confirming a diagnosis of bacterial meningitis. Although its sensitivity is only approximately 80%, its great benefit is that it can be performed rapidly within only a few minutes. Occasionally the CSF may be turbid, not because of large numbers of leukocytes, but because of large numbers of bacteria present. In addition to the pitfalls of false-negative and false-positive Gram's stains, there are potential pitfalls in the interpretation of the organisms seen. For example, Gram-negative bacilli may be confused with pneumococci, which are elongated and may appear pink in an overdecolorized preparation. *Acinetobacter,* a cause of nosocomial infection, may have the appearance of the meningococcus[94].

The bacterial culture represents "the gold standard" for the diagnosis of bacterial meningitis. The CSF should be cultured on solid media that will support the growth of the common pathogens, in addition to a suitable liquid medium. Various other tests of CSF have been developed to assist in the rapid differentiation between bacterial and viral meningitis. These include the Limulus amebocyte lysate test for the presence of endotoxin, and determination of C-reactive protein, fibronectin and lactate concentrations. These proposed tests are inadequately specific to accomplish their goal.

The antigen detection tests constitute a group of tests which are of value in specific circumstances only. Currently most of these tests utilize latex agglutination as the method for detection of bacterial antigen. Tests are available for antigens from *S. agalactiae; S. pneumoniae; H. influenzae* type

Table 32.5. Usual Cerebrospinal Fluid Findings in Different Types of Meningitis

Meningitis Type	*Leukocyte Count (cells/mm³)*	*Protein Concentration (mg/dl)*	*Glucose Concentration (mg/dl)*
Acute bacterial	Hundreds—thousands, neutrophils predominate	100–500	5–40
Viral	Up to few hundred, initially neutrophils then lymphocytes predominate	< 100	Normal
Tuberculous	25–100, rarely >500, lymphocytes predominate	100–200 or even higher	Reduced
Cryptococcal	< 50, lymphocytes predominate	20–500	Reduced
Syphilis	Average 500, lymphocytes predominate	100 (mean)	Normal

Adapted from Fishman RA. Cerebrospinal fluid in diseases of the nervous system 1992; 2nd ed., W.B Saunders Co. Philadelphia pp 253–343.

b; *N. meningitidis;* serogroups A, C, W 135; and *E. coli* type K1. Their potential value lies in their theoretical ability to demonstrate evidence of bacterial infection when the CSF analysis suggests such infection but when the Gram's stain and cultures are negative. This most likely occurs in patients who have been treated with antibiotics before obtaining the CSF[95–97]. Their sensitivity and specificity are inadequate for complete clinical reliability. Because patients with meningitis should be treated with antibiotics against all the likely pathogens until the culture results are available, the antigen detection tests that are costly should not influence initial therapy. If the cultures subsequently prove to be negative, these tests might be appropriate if it can be predicted that the results will influence the patient's management.

Nonspecific Laboratory Findings

Laboratory findings not related to spinal fluid abnormalities in the patient with meningitis generally reflect the bacterial nature of the disease. Most patients exhibit a striking leukocytosis with shift to the "left." Although, as is the case with overwhelming sepsis (see Chapter 31), neutropenia may occur, especially in the neonate. The WBC response may not be striking early in the course of disease, so a normal count, without a predominant concentration of polymorphonuclear leukocytes, should not dissuade the clinician from making the presumptive diagnosis of bacterial meningitis.

Other laboratory abnormalities depend on the severity of the infection and systemic and intracranial complications such as septic shock, elevated ICP, seizures, coma, and respiratory compromise. Expected findings in such a situation are not different from those encountered in sepsis and include metabolic acidosis, increased lactic acid level, hypocapnia or hypercapnia, hypoxemia, alteration of liver and cardiac enzymes, abnormalities of blood urea nitrogen and creatinine, and changes in electrolyte concentrations reflecting the presence of dehydration, SIADH, or diabetes insipidus (DI). Hyperglycemia may reflect response to acute stress, whereas hypoglycemia may represent inadequate stores of glycogen or inability to mobilize such stores, especially likely in a sick neonate.

Patients with concomitant meningitis and bacteremia may exhibit evidence of pneumonia, sinusitis, or involvement of other areas with the offending microorganism that are demonstrable with the use of various radiologic and other laboratory examinations.

Results of blood cultures may be helpful in determining the specific cause of the infection, especially in those subjects in whom antibiotic treatment must begin before the lumbar puncture is done. Although anergy may predominate in disseminated or meningeal tuberculosis, the finding of a positive purified protein derivative (PPD) or tine test may be helpful, when that organism is included in the list of possible etiologic agents.

Diagnostic Problems in Meningitis

Bloody CSF

Differentiation may be difficult between a traumatic (bloody) tap and true bleeding into the CSF pathway resulting from an intraventricular or subarachnoid hemorrhage or bloody CSF associated with an infection, e.g., herpetic encephalitis. If the CSF appears blood stained, the CSF should be collected in three or more sequential tubes. If the blood becomes more dilute in successive tubes as determined by macroscopic examination, hemoglobin estimation or red cell count, this finding is most suggestive of a traumatic tap. Blood that does not clear is more suggestive of true pathologic bleeding into the CSF. Blood present in the CSF for more than about 4 hours (i.e. resulting from a pathologic CNS hemorrhage) will begin to lyse resulting in xanthochromia of the supernatant of a centrifuged specimen. Therefore, this test should be completed within a short period after the lumbar puncture. The CSF leukocyte to erythrocyte ratio may provide helpful information in distinguishing a bloody tap from pathologic CNS hemorrhage. The CSF leukocyte to erythrocyte ratio in a traumatic tap is much the same as that in a peripheral blood sample obtained concurrently[98]. This can be calculated based on the respective counts of these cells in the peripheral blood. (This ratio is usually between 1:500 to 1:1000). A leukocyte to erythrocyte ratio significantly higher in the CSF than in the peripheral blood suggests a CSF pleocytosis supporting a diagnosis of meningitis. In a traumatic tap, the expected number of CSF leukocytes equals the number of CSF erythrocytes × (number of blood leukocytes/number of blood erythrocytes)[89]. A ratio or CSF leukocyte count significantly higher than expected suggests CSF pleocytosis.

Partially Treated Meningitis

The child who receives antibiotics before the lumbar puncture is completed raises some interesting issues of diagnosis that are worth considering. It has been estimated that as many as 50% of children with meningitis receive antibiotics in some form before diagnosis. Several studies have sought to define the manner in which indices of CSF inflammation are altered if prediagnosis antibiotic therapy had been started, and many contradictory findings have been reported[99–103]. The majority of patients who are given antibiotics before diagnostic lumbar puncture receive them as outpatients because of presumed respiratory infection or possible occult pneumococcal bacteremia. These children are generally given some form of oral penicillin in a relatively low dose (compared with standard meningitis doses).

The major factors that are primarily affected by such treatment are the length of patient's illness before hospital admission or spinal tap and the number of bacteria present in the CSF. Because the ability to document CSF infection by Gram's stain depends on the number of bacteria present, rapid diagnosis by microscopy of CSF is also affected by pretreatment. Although some authors have found the CSF WBC count to be altered by oral antibiotics, such that it may more resemble aseptic meningitis, others have not found this to be the case. The majority of evidence indicates that most patients with purulent meningitis will still have a predominance of neutrophils, a low glucose level, and elevated protein. Meningococcus isthe only bacterium whose growth in culture appears to be significantly altered by prior administration of antibiotics because of its exquisite sensitivity to penicillin. Bacteriologic diagnosis of pneumococcal or *H. influenzae* meningitis does not appear to be adversely affected, at least by oral administration of penicillin or ampicillin[101,102]. This might be different when prior treatment had been in the form of intramuscular ceftriaxone, which has become a common practice.

Although diagnosis may not be hampered by prior treatment with antibiotics, neither clinical course nor outcome is improved. Patients have the same number of complications and long-term sequelae whether they are pretreated with oral antibiotics[104]. The symptoms and extent of illness at admission are unchanged.

It is interesting to note that no major studies have been designed to examine prediagnosis antibiotic therapy in the hospitalized patient who develops nosocomial meningitis, other than those reporting disease in patients with head trauma and intraventricular foreign bodies, as discussed in Chapter 30 on nosocomial infections in the pediatric ICU. The effect on CSF laboratory data is not known in the patient in whom broad-spectrum high-dose antibiotics are begun parenterally, with deferment of the spinal tap for 6, 12, or 24 hours because of hemodynamic instability, severe neurologic deterioration, or bleeding diathesis. It is certainly possible that several hours after a dose of an effective antibiotic is administered, bacterial growth in the spinal fluid may be inhibited. This may affect Gram's stain results and bacterial colony counts, but with the possible exception of *N. meningitidis,* the fluid should not be sterile very soon after antibiotic administration. Cell count and glucose and protein values will not be changed early in the course of antibiotics, and enough clues should remain to point the clinician in the appropriate direction.

To improve the likelihood of an etiologic diagnosis, a latex agglutination test (see previous discussion) may be performed on CSF, blood, and especially urine[102] to detect antigen from the bacterial capsule. Antigen does not disappear rapidly, even with killing of the bacteria, and may persist for up to 5 days in the presence of adequate therapy.

Complications

Complications of meningitis are diverse and vary according to a number of factors including age of the patient, infecting organism, rapidity and adequacy of antibiotic therapy, and other parameters not yet defined. Adverse effects of disease may be acute and temporary or may result in permanent residua. Children may have profound or mild mental impairments, visual and auditory defects, persistent convulsions, communicating hydrocephalus, behavioral abnormalities and impairment of hypothalamic function, or long tract signs such as hemiparesis or quadriparesis[105].

Temporary problems include development of SIADH, DIC, septic shock, acutely elevated ICP, cerebral vasculitis, and recurrent fevers. Of course, there is some overlap in the two groups of complications, with some problems, such as seizures, hypothalamic injuries, as well as raised ICP, causing acute management problems and long-lasting sequelae. Seizures and increased ICP have been discussed previously. SIADH in meningitis has received much publicity. Consequently, the standard recommendation for fluid therapy in young children and infants with meningitis is to provide approximately two-thirds of calculated maintenance water requirements while providing a normal sodium intake. This issue remains controversial. Indeed, Powell has recently demonstrated in a controlled study of fluid management of meningitis that the elevated AVP concentration in many patients is not inappropriate and is due to hypovolemia[108]. The actual incidence of SIADH is unknown but has been noted in at least 4%[106] to 88%[107] of patients at the time of hospital admission. The syndrome is clinically defined as serum hyponatremia and hypo-osmolality in the presence of normovolemia, with a less than maximally dilute urine, and excessive urinary sodium loss in the absence of renal disease. Not every child with low serum sodium will have SIADH; such an assumption may lead to inappropriate restriction of volume in some patients[108]. A complete discussion of the diagnostic and general therapeutic approach to SIADH is presented in Chapter 38 on metabolic disturbances.

Although the pathogenesis of antidiuretic hormone (ADH) oversecretion is not clearly understood in this syndrome, it is presumed to be on the basis of inflammation in the area of the anterior pituitary. An alternative explanation is that it represents ischemia resulting from vasculitis in the presence of meningitis. Regardless of the specific cause, an exaggerated production of ADH has the potential to create several problems for any patient with meningeal infection. Retention of free water leads to hyponatremia, which may cause acute seizures and worsen the existing cerebral edema.

Other forms of dysfunction of the hypothalamic-pituitary axis may complicate meningitis, but with much lower frequency than SIADH. Such abnormalities include diabetes insipidus (DI), loss of temperature control, hyperphagia, and precocious puberty. Of these, the only entity of major concern during the acute stages of meningitis is DI. The excretion of large amounts of very dilute urine creates problems to the opposite extreme as those of SIADH. The patient with DI may rapidly become hypovolemic, with marked hypernatremia and seizures on that basis. The pathogenesis involves severe ischemia to the hypothalamus or pituitary and generally occurs only in severely ill patients with a poor prognosis[109]. Therapy of DI is described in Chapter 38 and consists of replacement of urine water losses when the disorder is mild, proceeding to supplementation of ADH as a continuous infusion, titrated to control urine output and serum sodium and osmolality values.

Disseminated intravascular coagulopathy (DIC) and septic shock may occur in meningitis, depending on the bacterial etiology. Both generally develop only in patients who are bacteremic. This happens most commonly in meningococcemia and, to a lesser extent, in *H. influenzae* meningitis and pneumococcal meningitis. Neonates with any form of bacterial meningitis are likely to develop DIC and septic shock. See the discussions on overwhelming sepsis (Chapter 31), on shock (Chapter 16), and on hematologic emergencies (Chapter 40). Therapy for these problems when they occur in meningitis does not differ from that for the patient with isolated sepsis. As noted in the prior discussion regarding systemic bacterial infections in infants and children, patients with meningitis alone have a better prognosis within each individual etiologic group than do patients in whom sepsis predominates. This is especially true in meningococcemia. Aggressive therapy of sepsis and associated DIC is essential in the meningitic patient, even when this means certain diagnostic studies, such as the LP, must be postponed, as indicated previously.

Focal neurologic signs, including hemiparesis or quadriparesis, may develop in the first few days of illness but are more common later in the course. Although numerous causes for localization of the neurologic examination need to be considered, including effects of vasculitis, vasospasm, and inflammation, evaluation of the child is essential for conditions that may require acute neurosurgical intervention. Such problems include subdural effusions and brain abscesses. Subdural effusions most likely occur beyond the first week of illness but may be noted at any time, including on admission. Effusions usually resolve spontaneously, without specific interventions(110). Indications for drainage of a subdural effusion include the presence of significant and persistent neurologic symptoms such as seizures, paresis, elevated ICP, and evidence of subdural empyema.

Subdural effusions are more common in *H. influenzae* type b meningitis than in infection because of other bacteria, but do occur regardless of the specific bacteriologic agent. In some series, up to 30 to 50% of infants and children have been noted to develop this complication(111–113). The pathogenesis has not been clearly delineated, but one group has postulated that subdural effusions form more frequently when a large volume of CSF is withdrawn during the diagnostic LP, resulting in shearing of bridging veins secondary to collapse of the brain away from the dura(114). However, such a theory does not explain the presence of effusions in some children at presentation. The pathogenesis of effusions seems more likely to be a combination of effects of the purulent infection in the subarachnoid space, including cerebral vasculitis with enhanced capillary leakage; relative cerebral ischemia with changes in cerebral blood flow, blood volume, and metabolism; and elevated ICP, all with subsequent transudation of fluid into the subdural space(115,116).

Intracerebral abscess must also be considered in a child with worsening focal signs, usually with persistent fever. An abscess develops subsequent to cerebritis, usually in an area of compromised vascular supply. Pathogenesis, diagnosis, and therapy of cerebral abscess and subdural empyema are discussed in a later section of this chapter.

Other causes of hemiparesis or other focal signs include development of stroke, or relative ischemia, caused by vasculitis, arterial spasm, or venous thrombosis, which may lead to an infarction(49,50,54,55).

The evaluation of focal neurologic signs in the course of pyogenic meningitis must include careful documentation of the changing neurologic examination. Neurologic and neurosurgical consultation is recommended with evidence of progression, worsening of signs or symptoms, presence of papilledema, elevated ICP, decline in Glasgow Coma Scale score, or unexplained cause of the symptoms. CT scan or MRI neuroimaging studies are most helpful in evaluating the causes of focal neurologic signs (infarction, effusion, abscess). More recently, Doppler studies have been helpful in defining flow abnormalities in major cerebral vessels even in adult patients(46–48). Angiography is rarely indicated. At any age, a radionuclide scan can provide information relating to blood flow and presence of discrete lesions, such as abscesses, infarctions, or effusions but has been largely replaced by the previously mentioned neuroimaging techniques. Electrophysiologic studies, such as electroencephalography (EEG), generally reveal diffuse evidence of cerebral involvement when neurologic signs are worrisome but are not helpful regarding the cause of the lesion.

The duration of fever varies a great deal during antibiotic therapy for bacterial meningitis. Fever that lasts beyond the 10th day is generally considered persistent or prolonged, whereas fever that recurs after at least 24 hours of apyrexia is considered a secondary or recurrent fever. The percentage of children who remain febrile or develop a secondary fever varies from 16 to 47%(117–119). The hospital day when patients first become afebrile depends on the bacterial agent. On the fifth day of appropriate antibiotic therapy, more than 85% of children with *S. pneumoniae* or *N. meningitidis* will be afebrile, but only 68% of those with *H. influenzae* meningitis will be free of fever. In addition, up to 80% of children with *H. influenzae* type b will develop a secondary febrile episode.

The most common cause of recurrent fever is nosocomial in origin and caused by phlebitis at an intravenous or cutdown site or to a hospital-acquired viral respiratory infection. The differential diagnosis of nosocomial illness in a child whose treatment in the pediatric ICU has included assisted ventilation or ICP monitoring must include acute ventriculitis, sinusitis, and mastoiditis. Subdural effusions make up another large category. Other causes include drug fevers and subdural empyemas. Disseminated foci of disease may occur and lead to septic arthritis, osteomyelitis, or pericarditis, especially in children with Hib and group B streptococcus infection. It is unusual for fever to be caused by actual persistence of the organism in the leptomeninges. But antibiotic failure does occur particularly with the emergence of antibiotic resistant bacteria and may result in persistent meningitis or the development of an intracerebral abscess.

In patients in whom fever persists beyond the 10th hospital day, the most likely cause is subdural effusion, followed by drug fever (most often in response to ampicillin), arthritis, brain abscess, and nosocomial infections, in descending order of frequency.

The clinical approach to a child with persistent or recurrent fever must take into account the previously described potential complications. The physician should begin evaluation of this problem first by ensuring that the initial diagnosis was correct and then by reviewing culture and sensitivity information regarding the original organism. It is reasonable to double-check the child's weight and calculation of antibiotic dosages. Consideration should be given to repeating the LP to review progress in clearing of the spinal fluid since the initial examination, as well as to document sterility and, possibly, to measure antibiotic levels or inhibitory or killing powers in the CSF. This should be considered in most patients with Gram-negative bacillary meningitis other than Haemophilus meningitis, and in meningitis caused by cefotaxime-resistant pneumococcal meningitis. Other studies of the CNS must be dictated by neurologic signs and symptoms, but given the frequency with which subdural effusions are implicated as a cause of fever in this setting, a CT scan is not unreasonable to perform, especially in the absence of any other definable site of infection. This assumes that a thorough physical examination has been completed, and a diligent attempt has been made to locate a possible source of nosocomial infection, as described fully in Chapter 30 on nosocomial infection in the pediatric ICU. Chest roentgenogram, WBC count, urinalysis, tracheal aspirate or sputum culture, sinus films, and viral cultures should be considered. Blood cultures are essential., Switching to an alternative drug, to which the bacterium is sensitive, may be made if drug fever is thought likely. Thirty percent to 50% of fevers have no etiology determined. It is only by carefully eliminating the most likely or the most potentially devastating complications that therapy can be completed in a rational way.

Therapy

Nonspecific Supportive Care

The level of supportive care provided for the neonate, infant, or child with meningitis will obviously vary with the severity of illness exhibited by the patient. For the child in the PICU with acute suppurative meningitis, the necessary care may entail the most sophisticated levels of support, including assisted ventilation, invasive hemodynamic monitoring and control, measurement and therapy of elevated ICP, therapy of any acute seizure activity, and complicated manipulations of fluids and electrolytes. In addition, the youngster will require high levels of nursing care, with meticulous attention paid to the neurologic examination and Glasgow Coma Scale, control of fever, and provision of a comfortable environment and soothing atmosphere. The child with suspected or proven bacterial meningitis requires respiratory isolation for 24 hours of antibiotic therapy after which time he or she is considered to be noninfectious (see previous discussion).

The approach to the neurocritical care-oriented therapy for the critically ill child with bacterial meningitis is presented in this chapter based on an understanding of the pathophysiology of the disease. Four major categories of therapy that will be discussed are (1) maintenance of cerebral perfusion, (2) management of elevated intracranial pressure, (3) antimicrobial therapy, and (4) adjunctive agents that modulate inflammation.

Maintenance of Cerebral Perfusion

The impairment of cerebral autoregulation in meningitis places the cerebral circulation at risk of hypoperfusion with cerebral ischemia from even a modest decrease in cerebral perfusion pressure, caused either by hypotension or increased intracranial pressure, both potential complications of meningitis[37,45]. Although systemic hypotension is not a particularly common presenting finding in children with acute bacterial meningitis, these patients are potentially at risk of hemodynamic instability because of either septic shock or hypovolemic shock. Impaired consciousness with decreased oral intake, vomiting, high fever, and an increase in insensible water loss places these patients at risk for dehydration. Rarely, a patient will have overwhelming sepsis, Waterhouse-Friderichsen syndrome with massive adrenal hemorrhage, and acute adrenal failure, not a common cause of hypotension. Management of dehydration and shock must be rapidly initiated with adequate volume replacement of either crystalloid or colloid if necessary guided by invasive hemodynamic monitoring. Much attention has been given toward the issue of the syndrome of inappropriate ADH release (SIADH) and its therapy by fluid restriction[106,107]. However, it is mandatory that hypovolemia and dehydration be corrected and that hypotension be avoided before fluid restriction is considered in the management of meningitis[108]. Restoring a normal blood pressure with careful fluid administration is more important than the concern of aggravating cerebral edema with volume infusion.

Management of Elevated Intracranial Pressure

It is apparent from several clinical studies noted previously that intracranial pressure is elevated to varying degrees in most patients with bacterial meningitis. However, some patients will have life-threatening intracranial hypertension with potential for cerebrovascular compromise and cerebral herniation[61]. Although ICP monitoring is certainly not routinely instituted in children with meningitis, and the criteria for ICP measurement are controversial and not uniformly accepted, monitoring should be considered when there are clinical signs or neuroimaging signs of moderate or severe elevation in intracranial pressure[58,120].

The conventional modalities for management of elevated

ICP in meningitis include mannitol, other diuretics, hyperventilation, barbiturates, and CSF drainage. The principles of their use are noted in Chapter 8. However, few specific studies document the efficacy of these various modalities in meningitis therapy and much of the therapy remains based on general physiologic principles.

MANNITOL AND OTHER DIURETICS. Mannitol is effective in reducing elevated intracranial pressure in conventional doses in bacterial meningitis[62,121]. Its efficacy may be reduced because of blood-brain barrier disruption and the passage of mannitol into the brain interstitium, reducing the interstitial to intravascular osmotic gradient. Studies in a rabbit model of haemophilus meningitis demonstrated the efficacy of mannitol in decreasing ICP, even though the effects disappeared within 4 hours[122]. Mannitol can be expected to decrease intracranial hypertension when it is due to edema, hyperemia, or even hydrocephalus. The mechanisms of action of mannitol in reducing elevated ICP are several and include acting as an osmotic diuretic; reducing blood viscosity, which causes cerebral microvascular constriction and reduces cerebral blood volume; and having a role as oxygen free radical scavenger.

HYPERVENTILATION. The rationale for the efficacy of hyperventilation in the management of elevated intracranial pressure is the cerebral vasoconstrictive effects of hypocapnia that results in decreased cerebral blood volume and a reduced intracranial pressure. However, this modality is only effective if the cerebral vasculature retains its responsiveness to hypocarbia. Since autoregulation is impaired, CO_2 responsiveness may be similarly compromised. In experimental *H. influenzae* meningitis in rabbits, CO_2 responsiveness remains intact[40]. Ashwall determined CO_2 responsiveness in children with meningitis using xenon tomography to measure cerebral blood flow[49]. The degree of CO_2 responsiveness varied among patients and in different areas of the brain but remained relatively intact. The authors raise concerns that indeed in some patients, hyperventilation (P_aCO_2 of 25 to 30 mm Hg) reduced flow to below the ischemic threshold. Hyperventilation must be used selectively, particularly in children with evidence of elevated intracranial pressure in whom neuroimaging studies reveal infarction. Hyperventilation in these patients, by reducing cerebral blood flow to levels that can induce ischemia, could potentially extend the area of vascular compromise[63]. Other ICP therapeutic modalities, e.g., mannitol, barbiturates, or hypothermia, might play a role in decreasing intracranial hypertension without extending the area of the infarct in these patients. However, such therapies have not proven valuable and indeed may present risks themselves[63].

REDUCTION OF CSF VOLUME. Patients with increased ventricular and subarachnoid space fluid without evidence of intracranial pressure elevation require no specific therapy since these changes respond with medical management of meningitis. CSF drainage must be considered if clinical or neuroradiographic evidence indicates elevated intracranial pressure, and ventriculostomy may be necessary because removal of CSF by the lumbar route is hazardous.[63]. Increased CSF fluid can be medically managed with drugs that decrease CSF production (acetazolamide, digoxin), but their efficacy is unproven[63].

STEROIDS. The role of steroids in reducing intracranial pressure is discussed in the following section.

FLUIDS. The conventional approach to fluid management in the patient who has meningitis was alluded to previously. In anticipation of possible SIADH, the well-hydrated child is often placed on a restricted water intake of two-thirds maintenance fluids made up in a solution containing approximately half-normal saline and dextrose as needed. This management plan is controversial since it has not been demonstrated that fluid restriction will actually prevent SIADH. Indeed, some investigators suggest that maintenance fluids be given based on sophisticated measurements of intravascular fluid volume as well as measurements of AVP[108]. Close monitoring with measurements of serum sodium, urine osmolality, and urine output must be continued carefully to detect SIADH. A 10% dextrose containing solution may be warranted with close attention paid to serum glucose values because many young infants are hypoglycemic, and the majority have hypoglycorrhachia. However, it is especially important to avoid inducing hyperglycemia because this may worsen outcome of states associated with cerebral ischemia. Consequently, the blood glucose level must be carefully watched, and the amount of administered glucose must be altered appropriately.

ANTICONVULSANTS. The child who had at least one seizure during the course of his or her early therapy, although potentially at low risk for ongoing seizures, is best treated with an anticonvulsant drug such as phenobarbital while in the ICU. The child whose neurologic or cardiorespiratory status is tenuous should be spared the additional metabolic demands and ischemic insults that may accompany seizures.

OTHER. All of the principles of neurointensive care must be followed in these patients, including ensuring optimal oxygenation and ventilation, or hyperventilation when intracranial hypertension is documented or suspected, and appropriate positioning of the patient to permit maximal drainage of venous outflow. Also, sedation is appropriate for the level of the child's perception of pain, discomfort, or agitation, and other apects of medical and nursing care of the patient with neurologic dysfunction as described in Chapter 18.

Antimicrobial Therapy

Although host defenses play a major role in the pathogenesis of bacterial meningitis, they play a very limited role in eliminating the infection. Therefore, bactericidal antibiotics are necessary for accomplishing this goal. In experimental meningitis in animals, it has been shown that the concentration of antibiotic in the CSF should exceed the minimal bactericidal concentration (MBC) of the organism for the drug by at least tenfold for adequate therapy[123,124].

Table 32.6. Cerebrospinal Fluid (CSF) Concentrations and CSF:Serum Ratios for Different Antimicrobial Agents

Drug	*CSF Conc. (μg/ml)*	*CSF/Serum Conc (%)*
ampicillin	3.6–16	39
amikacin	3.9–7.0	
azlocillin	42–125	30
aztreonam	2.1–20.8	2–18
cefotaxime	0.3–27.2	31–63
ceftazidime	7–23	10–20
ceftriaxone	5.4–20	3–25
chloramphenicol	5.4–11.5	45–99
ciprofloxacin	0.39–0.96	25–145
gentamicin	0.2–2.9	
imipenem	0.5–3.7	15–22
mezlocillin	20–90	16–43
nafcillin	1.2–10.3	30
penicillin	1.0	10
rifampin	0.3	5–20
sulbactam	12	3–134
ticarcillin	26–172	39–56
TMP/SMX	1.0/13.8	23–53/3–36
vancomycin	1.0–12.3	7.1–36.5

Adapted from Ristuccia AM, LeFrock JL. Cerebrospinal fluid penetration of antimicrobials. Antibiot Chemother 1992;45:118–152 and Barling RWA, Selkon JB. The penetration of antibiotics in the cerebrospinal fluid and brain tissue. J Antimicrob Chemother 1978;4:203–227.

The properties of antibiotics that favor their entry into the CSF include small molecular composition, high lipid solubility, and low degree of protein-binding. The entry of some is improved by the presence of inflammation, and the concentration of some, e.g. penicillin, is elevated by blockade of the CSF-blood exit pump by probenecid. The concentrations of different antibiotics usually attained in the CSF and their CSF to serum ratios are shown in **Table 32.6.**

Once the causative organism has been identified and its antimicrobial susceptibilities have been determined, antimicrobial therapy is relatively simple if the drugs are active against the organism and enter the CSF in adequate concentrations. Unfortunately this is not always the case.

The evolution of antimicrobial therapy of bacterial meningitis over the past two decades reflects the emergence of antibiotic resistance among the common microbial causes of the infection, especially *Haemophilus influenzae* and *Streptococcus pneumoniae.* As soon as resistance to a particular drug is recognized, although resistance may be extremely uncommon, two important questions must be asked: (1) What is the probability of this isolate being resistant? (2) At what probability of resistance (e.g. 1% or 5%) before the availability of antimicrobial susceptibility test results, is the physician prepared to treat the patient with antibiotics to which the causative organism may not be sensitive? Considering the potentially devastating effects of ineffective and delayed treatment of meningitis, the answer to the second question must surely be at a very low level.

The empiric treatment of patients with meningitis should be directed against the likely organisms, taking into account their possible resistance patterns. A combination of ampicillin and cefotaxime is recommended for neonates (see the following discussion). For infants, toddlers, and older children a combination of a third-generation cephalosporin (cefotaxime or ceftriaxone, but not ceftazidime) and vancomycin is recommended. Recommendations for treatment of patients with meningitis caused by an organism of known identity and antimicrobial susceptibility are shown in **Tables 32.7 and 32.8** [80,125–132]. The following discussion analyzes the evolution of these recommendations.

In the early 1970s, ampicillin was widely used as empiric therapy for meningitis in young children because it was active against *Haemophilus influenzae, Streptococcus pneumoniae,* and *Neisseria meningitidis.* Following the emergence of ampicillin resistance in *H. influenzae* in the mid-1970s, chloramphenicol was used in addition to ampicillin. Currently, approximately 30% of *H. influenzae* type b isolates in the United States are resistant to ampicillin[133]. Although chloramphenicol resistance has been reported, its prevalence has remained low[133]. Although it is a very effective agent and well absorbed from the gastrointestinal tract, physicians are reluctant to prescribe chloramphenicol because of potential adverse effects, namely aplastic anemia and gray-baby syndrome. In the United States, the drug has been largely replaced by third-generation cephalosporins such as cefotaxime and ceftriaxone, which are very active against *H. influenzae.* Fortunately these drugs are also highly active against *N. meningitidis,* and, until recently, were universally active against *S. pneumoniae.*

The usual therapy for pneumococcal meningitis was penicillin or ampicillin until the late 1970s, when penicillin strains of this organism emerged. Chloramphenicol and vancomycin were used for the treatment of patients infected with such strains until the third-generation cephalosporins became available. However, chloramphenicol therapy fail-

Table 32.7. Recommended Antimicrobial Therapy for Meningitis

Microorganism	*Therapy*	*Alternative Therapy*
Haemophilus influenzae	Cefotaxime, ceftriaxone, ampicillin*	Chloramphicol
Neisseria meningitidis	Penicillin	Cefotaxime, chloramphenicol
Streptococcus pneumoniae	Penicillin*, cefotaxime* vancomycin (see text)	Imipenem
Streptococcus agalactiae	Penicillin or ampicillin +/− gentamicin	Vancomycin, cefotaxime
Enteric bacilli	Cefotaxime, ceftriaxone, ceftazidime	Imipenem ciprofloxacin, aminoglycoside
Listeria monocytogenes	Ampicillin +/− gentamicin	Vancomycin, TMP/SMX
Pseudomonas aeruginosa	Ceftazidime or piperacillin + aminoglycoside	
Staphylococci	Nafcillin* or oxacillin* +/− rifampin, vancomycin +/− rifampin	

* *can be used alone only if susceptibility demonstrated*

Table 32.8. Daily Dosages of Antimicrobial Agents for Treatment of Meningitis in Pediatric Patients*

	Neonates		
Drugs	*0–7 days*	*8–28 days*	*Infants and Children*
Amikacin +‡	15–20 div q 12 h	20–30 div q 8 h	20–30 div q 8 h
Ampicillin	100–150 div q 12 h	150–200 div q 8 h or q 6 h	200–300 div q 6 h
Cefotaxime	100 div q 12 h	150–200 div q 8 h or q 6 h	200 div q 8 h or q 6 h
Ceftriaxone $			80–100 div q 12 h or q 24 h
Ceftazidime	60 div q 12 h	90 div q 8 h	125–150 div q 8 h
Chloramphenicol ‡	25 once daily	50 div q 12 h	75–100 div q 6 h
Gentamicin +‡	5 div q 12 h	7.5 div q 8 h	7.5 div q 8 h
Methicillin or nafcillin	100–150 div q 12 h or q 8 h	150–200 div q 8 h or q 6 h	200 div q 6 h
Penicillin G	100,000–150,000 div q 12 h	150,000–200,000 div q 8 hr or q 6 h	250,000 div q 6 h or q 4 h
Ticarcillin	150–225 div q 12 h r q 8 h	225–300 div q 8 h or q 6 h	300 div q 6 h
Tobramycin +‡	4 div q 12 h	6 div q 8 h	6 div q 8 h
Vancomycin +‡	20 div q 12 h	30 div q 8 h	40–60 div q 6 h

** In milligrams per kilogram (units per kilogram for penicillin G) per day divided (div), every (q) 12, 8, 6, or 4 hours(h).*
+ Smaller doses and longer intervals of administration especially for aminoglycosides and vancomycin, for very low birth weight neonates may be advisable.
‡ Monitoring of serum concentration is recommended to ensure safe and therapeutic values.
$ Use in neonates is not recommended because of inadequate experience for neonatal meningitis
From: Feigin RD and McCracken GH Jr., Klwin JO. Diagnosis and management of meningitis. Pediatr Infect Dis J 1992;11:784–814.

ures have been reported because of borderline susceptibility of the organism[134]. Unfortunately, strains of pneumococcus resistant to third-generation cephalosporins (as well as to penicillin) have emerged[125–127,130]. Although such strains are still relatively rare, patients with proven or suspected pneumococcal meningitis should be treated as if they could be infected with such a strain, until the causative organism has been isolated and its antimicrobial susceptibilities determined. Such therapy should consist of vancomycin in addition to cefotaxime or ceftriaxone until the susceptibility to penicillin and the third-generation cephalosporins is known[131]. The combination of rifampin and ceftriaxone might also be appropriate[129–135]. Experimental evidence indicates that even in strains resistant to third-generation cephalosporins, these cephalosporins exert a synergistic effect with vancomycin against resistant pneumococci[128]. Vancomycin-resistant strains of pneumococci have not yet been described, but this is possible considering that vancomycin resistance has spread to enterococci.

There has been some controversy as to the MICs at which pneumococcal resistance to the third-generation cephalosporins should be defined[125,127]. The current definition of susceptibility and resistance of pneumococci to cefotaxime and ceftriaxone (not ceftazidime) are as follows: MIC $\leq$ 0.5 μg/ml, susceptible; MIC 1 μg/ml, intermediate susceptibility; MIC $\geq$ 2 μg/ml, resistant[131]. Although patients whose isolates had MICs greater than 1 μg/ml were successfully treated with cefotaxime or ceftriaxone, failures of this therapy in patients whose isolates had the same MICs have been reported[131].

If a patient with pneumococcal meningitis either does not respond to therapy or yields an isolate that is shown to be resistant to cefotaxime or ceftriaxone, a lumbar puncture should be performed. Patients with such resistant isolates should be treated for at least 10 days with the previously mentioned combination[131].

The usual therapy for meningitis caused by *N. meningitidis* has been penicillin. Strains with reduced susceptibility to penicillin, MICs greater than 0.06 μg/ml, have been reported from many countries, including the United States, Canada, Spain, Israel, and Sweden[136–139]. Such strains have remained highly susceptible to third-generation cephalosporins[137].

Although resistance of *H. influenzae* to ampicillin is, in most cases, mediated by a β-lactamase, this is not the case in pneumococci and meningococci. In these organisms, the mechanism of resistance is alteration in the penicillin-binding proteins, the molecular targets of β-lactam antibiotics. These differences in mechanisms of antibiotic resistance have a possible therapeutic implication, namely that combinations of a β-lactam and a β-lactamase inhibitor might have activity against organisms in which resistance is mediated by a β-lactamase, but not in those in which resistance is mediated by a change in the penicillin-binding proteins.

DURATION OF ANTIMICROBIAL THERAPY. A scientific basis for recommendations for the optimal duration of therapy for meningitis would require a comparison of relapse rates in patients treated with the same drug for different durations. The findings for one organism and one drug would not necessarily be applicable to another organism or another drug. Radetsky has reviewed the history of practices in this regard illustrating the lack of information on which these practices have been based[140]. In a unique study, Lin et al. showed that in children with meningitis caused mostly by *H. influenzae* or pneumococcus, ceftriaxone therapy was as effective when given for 7 days as for 10 days[141]. Helwig has suggested the following minimum durations of therapy according to causative organism: *H. influenzae*, 7 days; *S. pneumoniae*, 7 days; and *N. meningitidis*, 4 days[142]. However, these recommendations are not universally accepted and other clinicians will treat these patients for longer periods. As organisms become more resistant to the agents used, more prolonged therapy may become necessary.

Adjunctive Agents That Modulate Inflammation

In spite of the clinical introduction of highly bactericidal antibiotics with excellent CSF penetration, the morbidity and mortality of bacterial meningitis remains high. Based on our current understanding of the mechanisms of inflammation and the pathophysiology of the neurologic damage of meningitis, this may not be surprising. At the time of clinical diagnosis of meningitis, the inflammatory cascade is well advanced with the release of cytokines, leukocyte activation, and increased production of other inflammatory mediators. The administration of highly bactericidal antibiotics kills bacteria and sterilizes the CSF, but in doing so results in the release of cell wall fragments that augment the deleterious inflammatory response. It now appears that advances in the treatment of meningitis corresponds to attenuation of CSF inflammation. Currently, only corticosteroids have undergone clinical trials and are in use in clinical practice. But other therapeutic modalities have demonstrated efficacy in animal meningitis models and these potential agents will also be briefly reviewed.

CORTICOSTERIODS. Corticosteroids are well-known, anti-inflammatory agents mediating this property by phospholipase A_2 inhibition, inhibition of TNF-α and IL-1 synthesis, and nitric oxide synthase inhibition[(19)]. In experimental animal models of either *S. pneumoniae* or *H. influenzae* meningitis, pretreatment with dexamethasone attenuates many pathophysiologic events. Steroid therapy reduces CSF outflow obstruction[(68)], cerebral edema, and cerebral hyperemia that occurs in the early phases of bacterial meningitis and elevated intracranial pressure[(38)]. Indices of inflammation such as elevated CSF leukocyte count, elevated protein, lactate and cytokine levels are also attenuated by steroid therapy in both experimental and clinical studies when compared with antibiotic treatment alone[(143)]. Since corticosteroids inhibit cytokine synthesis at a messenger RNA translation level rather than a gene transcription level, it can be understood why the potential benefit of corticosteroid administration is best achieved when these drugs are given simultaneously or before antibiotic administration.

Only dexamethasone as adjunctive therapy has been studied in clinical trials in patients[(143–146)]. Their findings and conclusions have been the subject of considerable controversy. These controlled double-blind trials examined the frequency of hearing loss and other neurologic sequelae of bacterial meningitis in children older than 2 to 3 months who were treated with dexamethasone or placebo in addition to antimicrobial therapy. The studies by Lebel[(144)], Odio[(143)], and Schaad[(145)] demonstrated a significantly decreased frequency of hearing loss in those receiving dexamethasone. In addition, those studies of Odio and Schaad revealed a decreased frequency of other neurologic sequelae. These beneficial effects were most striking when the drug had been administered 15 to 20 minutes before the antibiotic was administered. It is important to note that the benefits of dexamethasone could be shown only for cases of meningitis caused by *H. influenzae,* since there were inadequate number of cases caused by other organisms for any outcome conclusions to be drawn. The study by Wald et al. did not show these beneficial effects of dexamethasone[(146)]. A study by Girgis et al. demonstrated a significantly improved outcome in patients with pneumococcal meningitis treated with dexamethasone. A retrospective study reported by Kennedy et al. showed a trend toward a better outcome in patients with pneumococcal meningitis who received dexamethasone when compared with the control group[(148)]. Kanra et al. demonstrated that patients with pneumococcal meningitis treated with dexamethasone had a lower rate of hearing loss than those not receiving this agent[(148a)].

Several factors should be considered when the use of dexamethasone is contemplated and involve a consideration of the balance between the potential benefits of dexamethasone use and the possible side effects. In areas of the world where *H. influenzae* type b conjugate vaccines are widely used, meningitis caused by this organism is uncommon, and most cases of hematogenous meningitis are now caused by *S. pneumoniae* or *N. meningitidis.* Since penicillin-resistant and third-generation cephalosporin-resistant strains of *S. pneumoniae* are becoming more prevalent, vancomycin should be used in the empiric therapy of bacterial meningitis (see previous discussion). Of potential concern is in experimental meningitis dexamethasone reduces the CSF concentration of vancomycin, but not that of ceftriaxone[(132,149,150)] presumably by reducing inflammation and blood-brain barrier permeability. However, in a study of CSF samples of children treated with ceftriaxone, vancomycin, and dexamethasone for bacterial meningitis, Klugman et al. showed that CSF levels of vancomycin ranging from 2 to 5.9 μg/ml (mean 3.3 ± 1.1) were attained[(135)]. (The MICs of pneumococci to vancomycin are 0.5 to 1.0 μg/ml.) This study was not designed to determine whether vancomycin alone was effective in treating these patients, but it did suggest that levels of vancomycin greater than the MIC of pneumococci to vancomycin are achieved in patients with meningitis treated with steroids. If dexamethasone interferes with the entry of vancomycin into the CSF in humans, this could have a deleterious effect on the outcome of the infection[(132,149,150)].

Concern has been raised that steroids might have an adverse effect on the outcome of children with viral meningitis incorrectly diagnosed as having bacterial meningitis after preliminary evaluation of the CSF. Studies have revealed no adverse effects of such treatment[(151)]. A complication of steroid use in meningitis is gastrointestinal hemorrhage, but this is an uncommon event[(143)].

Recommendations for dexamethasone therapy in bacterial meningitis are as follows: (1) In patients with meningitis likely caused by *H. influenzae*—those not immunized against this organism, or those whose CSF shows Gram-negative bacilli—dexamethasone should be administered at the same time as or shortly after the first dose of antibiotic. The dosage is 0.15 mg per kg per dose, intravenously, and every 6 hours for four days[136]. (2) Although dexamethasone appears to be beneficial in patients with pneumococcal meningitis in some studies, its use might be detrimental in patients in whom attaining a high level of vancomycin in the CSF is critical. The weight of the potential benefits versus the probability of this disadvantage will vary from case to case. This question remains highly controversial in recent publications[131,152–154].

OTHER ANTI-INFLAMMATORY AGENTS. Nonsteroidal, anti-inflammatory agents inhibiting prostaglandin synthesis by cyclooxygenase inhibition ameliorate some pathophysiologic events in meningitis. The results of the nonsteroidal, anti-inflammatory drug oxindac, an indomethacin treatment in experimental *H. influenzae* and *S. pneumoniae* meningitis, are conflicting and controversial. In some studies, indices of inflammation are attenuated as are measurements of cerebral edema and elevated intracranial pressure but these effects are not demonstrated in all studies[29,155,156]. Indomethacin treatment also attenuates cerebral hyperemia in the early phase of bacterial meningitis[38]. Human studies using these agents have not yet been performed but may hold promise.

Platelet-activating factor (PAF) contributes to CSF leukocytosis and cerebral edema in bacterial meningitis. In experimental animals, intracisternal but not intravenous administration of a PAF inhibitor, L-659,989 attenuates the CSF inflammatory response and prevents cerebral edema in experimental pneumococcal but not *H. influenzae* meningitis[31]. Further laboratory research is needed before initiating clinical studies.

Pentoxifylline is a methylxanthine phosphodiesterase inhibitor with several anti-inflammatory properties that include inhibition of TNF-α production and the impairment of neutrophil activation by lipopolysaccharide and cytokines. In experimental hemophilus meningitis, pretreatment with pentoxifylline reduces the indices of CSF inflammation[157,158]. Further studies in which other pathophysiologic variables are measured must be instituted before clinical use.

Monoclonal antibodies directed at leukocyte-endothelium cell adhesion molecules are the most promising new agents for meningitis therapy. Since CSF leukocytosis and leukocyte transmigration through cortical vessels is such a prominent feature of the pathology of acute bacterial meningitis, these cells could represent a final common effector of tissue damage in bacterial meningitis. Monoclonal antibodies directed at the molecules responsible for leukocyte-endothelial adhesion can be used as a tool to evaluate the potential role of neutrophils as agents of CSF damage in meningitis and also as possible therapeutic agents. In experimental models of both *H. influenzae* and *S. pneumoniae* meningitis, intravenous administration of IB 4, a monoclonal antibody directed at the CD 18 integrin receptor complex, dramatically reduces CSF leukocytosis and other indices of CSF inflammation as well as the degree of cerebral edema[35,36]. When administered with antibiotics, the rate of bacterial killing within the CSF is not impaired despite the virtual absence of CSF leukocytes. The combination of dexamethasone and IB 4 antibody therapy produces a greater reduction in CSF inflammatory indices than either agent alone[36]. Clinical trials of the anti-CD 18 antibody are anticipated to begin by publication[34].

Immunotherapy

Certain bacterial organisms in some groups of children may be more effectively treated by adding passive immunization in the form of human intravenous immunoglobulin or (when available) monoclonal antibodies. This type of adjunctive therapy is particularly important for children who have immunoglobulin deficiencies and neonates whose immunologic capacities are limited. The value of such therapy depends to a great extent on the type of immune response generally evoked by the organism to kill the bacteria effectively. The best example of potential usefulness of immunotherapy is in the baby with group B streptococcus meningitis. This therapeutic approach is fully discussed in the section of Chapter 31 that deals with adjunctive approaches to the patient with sepsis. With advancement of recombinant deoxyribonucleic acid (DNA) techniques, monoclonal antibodies may become a useful tool in therapy of the infected child in the ICU, but much work needs to be done before such recommendations can be made.

Infection Control

Patients with meningitis caused by *H. influenzae* or *N. meningitidis* should be placed in respiratory isolation until they have received effective antimicrobial therapy for 24 hours[159,160]. The close contacts of patients with hemophilus infections should be offered chemoprophylaxis with rifampin, depending on the ages of the children in the family, and their immunization status. A dosage of 10 to 20 mg/kg (maximum of 600 mg) daily for 4 days should be used. Individuals given rifampin should be informed of adverse effects, drug interactions, and contra-indications[159]. All close contacts of patients with meningococcal infections should be offered chemoprophylaxis with rifampin either 10 mg/kg (maximum of 600 mg) per dose every 12 hours, for 2 days, or according to the same schedule as recommended for prophylaxis against hemophilus infection[160]. It is important to emphasize to contacts that chemoprophylaxis is not a guarantee against infection, and that they should see a physician if symptoms develop.

Outcome

The clinical course, rapidity of diagnosis, adequacy of therapy, and individual characteristics of host and disease determine the outcome and long-term sequelae for patients with purulent meningitis. Untreated cases are almost universally fatal, whereas with current methods of diagnosis and therapy, the mortality ranges from 5 to 10% for *H. in-*

fluenzae[161] and meningococcal[162] meningitis, up to 20% for pneumococcal, and between 15 and 20% for TB[162] meningitis in some forms of neonatal disease[123]. Long-term sequelae, including hydrocephalus, deafness, cortical or optic nerve blindness, hemiparesis or quadriparesis, or intellectual impairment, occur in 30 to 50% of survivors. Clearly, many of the deaths and some of the morbidity are related to effects of intracranial hypertension, some degree of cerebral ischemia, and responses to cerebral inflammation. It is not known how much reduction of morbidity and mortality may be accomplished by adopting a more consistently aggressive approach to the diagnosis and monitoring of, and the therapy for, elevated cerebral pressure in this disease. However, it is reasonable to make a sincere effort in this regard and then to reevaluate the outcome, once the various aspects of neurologic intensive care have been applied to this rather common, sometimes fulminant, and often fatal pediatric problem.

Other Forms of Meningitis and Their Antibiotic Management

Neonatal Meningitis

Meningitis in the neonate is frequently caused by bacteria acquired from the mother's birth canal, namely by *Streptococcus agalactiae,* enteric bacilli such as *Escherichia coli,* and *Listeria monocytogenes.* However, many cases are also hospital-acquired, especially in premature infants receiving intensive care management. The causative organisms include enteric bacilli, such as *Citrobacter* and *Enterobacter,* other Gram-negative bacilli—*Pseudomonas aeruginosa* and *Flavobacterium meningosepticum*—enterococci and staphylococci, all of which may be resistant to antimicrobial agents.[80,163,164].

The recommendations for antimicrobial therapy are based on the following susceptibilities **(Tables 32.7 and 32.8).** *Streptococcus agalactiae* is very susceptible to penicillin, ampicillin, and cephalosporins. Although tolerance in this organism is described (MBC ≥ 32-fold MIC), this is unusual and of debatable significance. However, the combination of a penicillin and gentamicin is bactericidal in vitro in this circumstance, which is of unclear clinical significance[165]. The enteric bacilli are usually susceptible to the third-generation cephalosporins such as cefotaxime, ceftriaxone, and ceftazidime, and to aminoglycosides such as gentamicin, tobramycin, or amikacin, but are nowadays frequently resistant to ampicillin. Consequently, the susceptibility patterns of these organisms in the specific intensive care unit should be taken into account. *Listeria monocytogenes* is susceptible to ampicillin and penicillin but is resistant to cephalosporins.

Therefore, empiric therapy of a neonate with meningitis should consist of ampicillin or penicillin plus a third-generation cephalosporin or an aminoglycoside[163,123,164]. Baker et al. recommend higher doses of ampicillin (300 to 400 mg/kg/day) or penicillin (500,000 units /kg/day) than are outlined in **Table 32.8** [165]. Because aminoglycosides have a narrow therapeutic index and may not attain therapeutic levels in body fluids, administration of a cephalosporin in cases of meningitis is frequently preferred. However, use of cephalosporins for all cases of suspected neonatal sepsis is not recommended because this practice may lead to third-generation, cephalosporin-resistant enteric bacilli by providing intense selective pressure in the limited space of a neonatal nursery[166].

Although imipenem-cilastatin is not generally recommended for the treatment of meningitis in neonates resulting from the high incidence of seizures associated with its use in this circumstance, it may be necessary in the treatment of patients with infections caused by highly resistant organisms. The dose is 20 to 25 mg/kg/dose every 12 hours[167–169]. Ciprofloxacin should also not be used routinely for treating patients with meningitis, but may be indicated in certain circumstances, such as infection caused by *Flavobacterium meningosepticum.* A dose of 5 to10 mg/kg/day divided every 12 hours in premature infants, and 15 to 20 mg/kg/dose every 12 hours in full-term neonates has been used[170,171].

Antibiotics should be given intravenously. The role of intraventricular administration of gentamicin in addition to intravenous therapy in cases of Gram-negative bacilla in neonates was evaluated during the 1970s. Intraventricular therapy was associated with a higher fatality than intravenous therapy alone[172]. Therefore this is not practiced routinely.

Chronic Meningitis

Chronic meningitis should be suspected in any individual with global or multifocal neurological deficits, or who has symptoms of meningitis for more than a few days. Although untreated acute bacterial meningitis may become chronic, chronic meningitis is usually caused by infections or diseases that are chronic by nature. Important causes of chronic meningitis include tuberculosis, syphilis, Lyme disease, and fungi, in particular cryptococcal infection. Of these, the most important is tuberculous meningitis because it is rapidly fatal if untreated, and its diagnosis has important public health implications. Tuberculous meningitis is difficult to diagnose because its progression is insidious[173]. The early symptoms are malaise, anorexia, vomiting, headache, and fever (stage I). Neurologic signs develop as it progresses. These include disturbed level of consciousness, cranial nerve palsies, including abnormal pupillary responses, papilledema, and long tract signs (stage II). Stage III is characterized by coma[175,176]. Because tuberculous meningitis causes significant pathology of the basal meninges, vascular involvement and hydrocephalus are common complications[177,178]. The diagnosis of tuberculous meningitis depends on physical findings, contact history, chest radiograph, Mantoux test, and characteristic abnormalities in the CSF **(Table 32.5).**

Antituberculous therapy should not be dependent on the demonstration of *Mycobacterium tuberculosis* on smear or by culture.

The mainstay of therapy is antituberculous chemotherapy[179–181]. This consists of isoniazid (10 mg/kg/day, maximum of 300 mg) rifampin (10 mg/kg/day, maximum of 600 mg), pyrazinamide (35 mg/kg/day, maximum 2 g), and streptomycin (20 to 40 mg/kg/day, maximum of 1 g). All four drugs are used for 2 months, after which the second two are discontinued. Although the usual duration of antituberculosis treatment is for 6 months, the recommended duration for tuberculous meningitis is 12 months. Alternative therapy is required in cases of drug-resistant tuberculosis.

The use of corticosteroids in tuberculous meningitis is somewhat controversial, but they are frequently used[181]. CSF shunting procedures for hydrocephalus are frequently necessary.

Nosocomial Meningitis

Although most patients with community-acquired meningitis are diagnosed in the emergency room, many patients with hospital-acquired meningitis develop the infection in the intensive care unit. Most cases of nosocomial meningitis develop as complications of neurosurgical procedures such as craniotomy[182], ventriculostomy[183], CSF shunting procedure, CNS reservoir insertion, subarachnoid bolt insertion, or transsphenoidal surgery[184]. Nosocomial meningitis may also follow head or face trauma with a basilar or skull fracture and CSF leak. It is more likely to develop in cases of CSF rhinorrhea than in CSF otorrhea, particularly if the leak persists for longer than 1 week. Nevertheless, meningitis may develop years after the initial trauma if a subclinical leak is present. Meningitis may develop as a complication of lumbar puncture for spinal anesthesia or myelography. It is most important to investigate the epidemiology of such cases thoroughly because such investigation may reveal a source of infection, e.g., contaminated skin disinfectants or poor operator technique. Occasionally nosocomial bacteremia will be complicated by hematogenous meningitis. This may occur in any patient with high-grade bacteremia but is more likely to occur in neonates. Occasionally meningitis will develop in a hospitalized immunocompromised patient. **Table 32.2** outlines the most common microbiologic causes of meningitis acquired in the previously mentioned circumstances.

The diagnosis and management of nosocomial meningitis are particularly difficult for several reasons. The neurologic examination, which provides important clinical information for diagnosing meningitis, often cannot be adequately performed because the patient is heavily sedated or even paralysed. The physical examination cannot be reliably interpreted because many neurosurgic patients have abnormal baseline neurologic findings. Neurosurgery can result in CSF pleocytosis in the absence of infection, complicating the interpretation of CSF examination. However, hypoglycorrhachia does not usually occur in this circumstance[182,185]. Raised intracranial pressure may be present that would contraindicate a lumbar puncture and CSF sampling. In this circumstance, a ventricular tap must be considered if meningitis is strongly suspected. It is important to make a microbiological diagnosis because the variety of possible causative microorganisms is wide, and they are likely to be resistant to multiple antibiotics. The infection may be associated with the presence of foreign material, e.g., ventriculoperitoneal shunt, which renders antimicrobial therapy less likely to be effective.

Ventricular Shunt Infections

Most cerebrospinal fluid shunts are ventriculo-peritoneal (VP) or, less commonly, ventriculoatrial (VA). The frequency of shunt infections varies from 2% to 30% and is influenced by numerous factors[188,189] such as age and skin flora.

The most common microbial causes of shunt infections are coagulase-negative staphylococci. Other causes include *Staphylococcus aureus*, coryneforms, enterococci, and, less commonly, Gram-negative bacilli. The infection is usually introduced at the time of surgery, although infection of the peritoneal end of VP shunts by bowel organisms, especially Gram-negative bacilli, may account for some cases.

The presenting clinical features are often nonspecific, such as fever and irritability; however, some of the apparently nonspecific features of infection might represent evidence of shunt malfunction. These include lethargy, anorexia, and vomiting. Because infected VP shunts discharge organisms into the peritoneal cavity, resulting in peritonitis and the formation of adhesions, patients with these infections may have abdominal pain[188–190] or features of shunt obstruction. Inflammation may be evident at the surgical wound or along the track of the shunt. Patients with VP shunt infections usually have symptoms within two weeks of shunt insertion, but may have symptoms weeks or months later.

Because infections of VA shunts are not usually associated with shunt malfunction, patients with these infections tend to have symptoms later, and often with nonspecific features of infection and features similar to those of subacute infective endocarditis, such as splenomegaly, hematuria, and arthralgia[189].

The diagnosis of these infections may be very difficult. VA shunt infections are sometimes associated with bacteremia, whereas this is rarely the case in VP shunt infections. Examination of ventricular fluid is the usual method by which VP shunt infections are diagnosed, but this fluid may be normal even in the presence of infection. Physicians may be reluctant to remove fluid from the shunt for fear of introducing infection. However, this fear does not appear to be justified[191]. CSF eosinophilia is frequently associated with shunt infections, and its persistence is associated with an increased risk of a requirement for shunt revision[192,193].

The management regimens of these infections are varied because there are no comparative trials of different forms of management. Initial shunt removal is advocated by some authors, whereas others advocate this only if the infection is severe or refractory to initial management[189,194]. Because these patients require CSF diversion, shunt removal necessitates external ventricular drainage. The external drain may also be used for the instillation of intraventricular antibiotics, such as vancomycin (10 to 20 mg daily)[189,195]. External drainage is associated with the potential for a new infection, which becomes progressively more likely with increased duration of external drainage[189]. Frame et al. advocate instillation of antibiotics into the ventricles through the reservoir and systemic administration of antibiotics, without shunt removal[196]. However, they externalize the peritoneal end of the shunt and allow it to drain into a closed system, obviating the need for an external drain. When the infection has resolved, they revise the peritoneal end of the shunt[195].

Yogev compared several reports in which different methods of management had been used and concluded that shunt removal with external drainage, followed by shunt replacement, provides the greatest chance of successful outcome[188]. He suggests an algorithm for management of shunt infections. If the infection is mild, therapy with intravenous antibiotics should be attempted. If the shunt has not been sterilized within 3 days, it should be removed and replaced only after it is demonstrably sterile 3 days after a 10-day course of antibiotics has been completed. He recommends intraventricular antibiotics only if the ventricular fluid can not be sterilized after shunt removal and recommends initial shunt removal if the infection is severe[188].

Considering that the most common microbial causes of shunt infections are coagulase-negative staphylococci, and that these are frequently resistant to methicillin, initial antibiotic therapy should consist of vancomycin (60 mg/kg/24 hours, divided every 6 to 8 hours, intravenously). If the shunt is not removed, the addition of rifampin (20 mg/kg/24 hours, divided every 12 hours orally) should be considered[188]. If the Gram-stain or cultures of the CSF reveal other causes, alternative therapy should be used, such as a third-generation cephalosporin for Gram-negative bacillary infections.

VIRAL ENCEPHALITIS

Epidemiology

Encephalitis is an infrequent disease, occurring predominantly in children, elderly and immunocompromised hosts. The incidence is highest in the second year of life (17 per 100,000 child-years) and declines to 1.0 per 100,000 child-years by age 15[197]. Epidemic encephalitis has declined as a result of improvements in living conditions and vector control, as well as the advent of vaccines against many of the childhood exanthems[198]. Mortality from encephalitis has not declined proportionately because agents that cause the majority of severe cases of encephalitis, such as herpes simplex virus and varicella zoster virus, remain endemic.

Table 32.9. Frequent Causes of Neonatal Encephalitis and Differential Diagnosis

	Diagnosis		
	Culture	*Serology available*	*PCR*[4]
Acute Infections			
Herpes simplex virus	Y	Y	Y
Enterovirus[1]	Y		Y
Adenovirus	Y		
Meningitis[2]	Y		
Congenital Infections			
Cytomegalovirus	Y	Y	Y
Toxoplasmosis		Y	
Syphilis		Y	
Herpes simplex virus	Y	Y	Y
Rubella	Y	Y	
Metabolic Disorders[3]			
Primary CNS Disorders			
Ischemia			
Hemorrhage			
Neuronal migration disorder			

[1]*Includes aseptic meningitis*
[2]*Especially Group B streptococcus, Listeria monocytogenes,* Citrobacter spp.
[3]*Propionic acidemia, methylmalonic acidemia, urea cycle defects, maple syrup urine disease*
[4]*Polymerase chain reaction often available in larger clinical microbiology laboratories*

Etiology

Neonatal Encephalitis

Although the brain is usually the only site of infection in the older child and adult with encephalitis, encephalitis in the neonate is often part of a multi-organ disease with features that resemble other systemic diseases, e.g. inborn error of metabolism[197]. This may explain, in part, the lower success rate in elucidating the cause of encephalitis in the first year of life[197,198].

Herpes simplex virus (HSV) encephalitis is the most common cause encephalitis in neonates (see discussion that follows) and is usually caused by HSV type 2 virus[199]. Neonatal encephalitis caused by enterovirus or adenovirus often occurs as part of a disseminated infection in the first week of life[200]. Enteroviruses can also cause encephalitis with aseptic meningitis. Congenital infections *with* cytomegalovirus, rubella virus, varicella-zoster virus, herpes simplex virus, human herpesvirus 6, and *Toxoplasma gondii* can cause structural brain damage and neurologic symptoms at birth. **Table 32.9** outlines the causes of neonatal encephalitis-encephalopathy.

Encephalitis in Infancy and Childhood

Encephalitis in the older infant or child can be infectious or reflect an aberrant immunologic response to a prior infection (post-infectious encephalitis)[201]. **Tables 32.10 and 32.11** outline the common and rare causes of encephalitis, respectively, in childhood. Infectious encephalitis is usually mild and often occurs in association with viral aseptic meningitis. Enteroviruses[200–202] and some arthropod-borne viruses (arboviruses)[203] are the most com-

Table 32.10. Common Etiologies of Acute Encephalitis in Childhood

	Frequency		*Diagnosis*		
	Infectious	*Post-infectious*	*Culture*	*Serology Available*	*PCR*[5]
Virus					
Enterovirus	++++[3]		Y		Y
Arthropod borne viruses	++++			Y	
Herpes simplex virus	+++		Y	Y	Y
Epstein-Barr virus	++			Y	Y
Adenovirus	+		Y		
HIV-1	+		Y	Y[4]	Y
Measles[1]	+	+		Y	
Mumps[1]	+	+		Y	
Rubella[1]	+	+		Y	
Varicella-zoster virus	+	++		Y	Y
HHV-6	+	++		Y	Y
Influenza virus	+	+			
Non-specific respiratory or gastrointestinal disease	+++				
Bacteria[2]					
Borrelia burgdorferi	++			Y	Y
Bartonella henselae	++				
Rickettsia rickettsii	++			Y	
Mycoplasma pneumoniae	+	+++		Y	
Vaccines		+			

[1]*Rare in U.S. vaccinated population*
[2]*Consider pyogenic bacteria, tuberculosis*
[3]*++++ frequent; +++ common; ++ infrequent; + rare*
[4]*Insensitive during seroconversion*
[5]*Polymerase chain reaction may be available in larger clinical microbiology laboratories.*

mon causes of mild encephalitis **(Table 32.10).** Herpes simplex virus infection is the leading cause of severe encephalitis throughout infancy and childhood[(201)]. Encephalitis is an infrequent complication of many common bacterial or viral infections. Adenovirus, Epstein-Barr virus (EBV)[(204)] and *Bartonella henselae* (the etiologic agent of cat scratch fever disease) cause sporadic cases[(205)].

Post-infectious encephalitis accounts for a significant proportion of clinical encephalitis after the first year of life[(201,206)]. Peak incidence is at 5 to 6 years of age. Post-infectious encephalitis often follows respiratory or intestinal tract infections and is associated with influenza virus, *Mycoplasma pneumoniae*[(207)], measles[(208)], mumps, varicella-zoster virus[(209)], and human herpes virus 6 **(Table 32.10).** Encephalitis following measles infection occurs once per thousand cases[(210)]. The incidence of post-infectious encephalitis has declined precipitously in countries following implementation of vaccination against measles, mumps, and rubella[(198)]. Encephalitis following chickenpox (0.3 per 1000 cases) may similarly decline with the advent of a vaccine against varicella[(198)]. Historically, immunizations have been associated with post-infectious encephalitis; in the United States, measles vaccination is estimated to cause fewer than one episode of encephalitis per one million doses administered.

Arbovirus encephalitis in North America occurs in the late summer and fall and is heralded by encephalitis in farm animals. Despite the potential for epidemics, most cases occur sporadically. St. Louis encephalitis virus is distributed throughout most of the United States and causes major epidemics that peak later than other arboviruses. Most infections are asymptomatic, and less than 1% have overt neurologic disease. Western equine encephalitis is the usual cause of arbovirus encephalitis in the western United States. Disease is concentrated in infants and the elderly. Eastern equine encephalitis and California encephalitis viruses occur in the central and eastern United States and cause diseases with a fulminant and mild course, respectively[(201,203)].

Tick-borne bacterial diseases also occur during warm months. Rocky Mountain spotted fever, which occurs primarily in the eastern United States, is complicated by meningoencephalitis in one third of cases and by coma in 10%.

Table 32.11. Rare Causes of Encephalitis

Viruses	**Fungi**
Mumps virus	*Cryptococcus*
Parainfluenza virus	*Histoplasma capsulatum*
Influenza virus	*Blastomyces dermatitidis*
Respiratory syncytial virus	*Coccidioides immitis*
Hepatitis A virus	**Protozoa**
Hepatitis B virus	*Naeglaria fowleri*
Rabies	*Plasmodium falciparum*
Bacteria	
Treponema pallidum	
Leptospira spp.	
Brucella spp.	
Myocobacterium tuberculosis	
Nocardia spp.	
Listeria monocytogenes	
Whipple's disease	

Ehrlichia causes encephalitis much less commonly. Lyme disease occurs in the East, the upper Midwest, and the Pacific Northwest, although its geographic range is spreading. The majority of infections are asymptomatic. About 15% of untreated patients can develop late neurologic sequelae, including meningitis, encephalitis, chorea, or neuritis.

Herpes simplex encephalitis is the most common cause of severe encephalitis throughout childhood (this entity is discussed in the following section in detail). The majority of encephalitis beyond the neonatal period is caused by HSV-1[(199,201)]. It is important to differentiate herpes encephalitis, caused primarily by HSV-1, from the aseptic meningitis syndrome complicating genital infections caused by HSV-2. Most cases of HSV encephalitis are believed to be caused by reactivation of latent virus. There is no correlation between the isolation of HSV from sites extrinsic to the CNS, such as oropharynx or genitalia, and the cause of a concurrent encephalitis[(211)]. Human herpes virus 6 can cause focal encephalitis in older children and adolescents in 6% of cases of presumed HSV encephalitis[(212)].

Infection with human immunodeficiency virus (HIV) results in neurologic disease in a large proportion of cases. Encephalitis can occur during seroconversion. Degenerative encephalopathy complicates late stage disease in up to 90% of HIV-infected children.

Rabies is rare in the United States, averaging one case each year. Half of human rabies occurs in children; history of exposure is unusual today[(213)].

Hemorrhagic shock with encephalopathy affects infants from 2 to 10 months of age; peak incidence is at 3 to 4 months. There is an infectious prodrome in 60% of cases, although there is no clustering of cases[(214)]. Reye syndrome generally occurs in children 2 to 12 years of age, several days after varicella, influenza, or a gastrointestinal illness. Salicylates have also been associated with Reye syndrome and are no longer indicated for routine antipyresis in children[(215)]. Although influenza and gastrointestinal illness are not true examples of encephalitis in that brain histology does not reveal inflammation, their clinical presentation is very similar to that of encephalitis and they must be considered in the differential diagnosis.

Pathogenesis

Encephalitis can be caused by several pathogenic mechanisms, depending on the virulence and cell tropism of the infectious agent and the exuberance of the host response. Infectious encephalitis is the result of direct invasion of any cell type in the brain or spinal cord. Infection by different agents can cause transient cellular dysfunction or result in rapid cytolysis. Infectious agents can enter the brain by the hematogenous route; this implies tropism of the agent for vascular endothelium as well as brain. The hematogenous route is believed to explain the generalized distribution of neonatal herpes encephalitis. Viruses can also enter the brain by neuronal tracts, causing focal encephalitis. Frontal and temporal localization is characteristic of herpes simplex encephalitis beyond the neonatal period. This localization is explained by direct extension of the virus through olfactory neurons or by retrograde spread of virus from the site of latency in the trigeminal ganglion to dendrites innervating the base of the brain.

Table 32.12. Encephalitis and Immunodeficiency

Immunodeficiency	*Culture*	*Serology Available*	*PCR*[7]	*Blood Metabolites*
Humoral				
Chronic enteroviral meningoencephalitis	Y		Y	
CMI (Including transplantation)[1]				
PML[2]			Y	
Subacute HSV encephalitis	Y	Y	Y	
Subacute measles panencephalitis		Y		
Progressive rubella panencephalitis	Y	Y		
Cytomegalovirus	Y	Y	Y	
Toxoplasma gondii		Y	Y	
Adenovirus	Y	Y		
Varicella-zoster virus	Y	Y	Y	
Human herpesvirus 6		Y	Y	
Reaction to OKT3 infusion[3]				
AIDS[4]				
Toxoplasma gondii		Y	Y	
Cytomegalovirus	Y	Y	Y	
Cryptococcus neoformans	Y	Y		Y[5]
HIV-1 encephalopathy	Y	Y	Y	Y[6]

[1]Cell-mediated immunity
[2]Progressive multifocal leukoencephalopathy (JC virus)
[3]Anti-lymphocyte globulin and anti-thymocyte globulin
[4]Acquired immunodeficiency syndrome
[5]D-arabinotol
[6]Quinolinic acid
[7]Polymerase chain reaction may be available in larger clinical microbiology laboratories

Many hematogenous pathogens cause direct endothelial damage to arteries, arterioles and capillaries, resulting in vasculitis, hemorrhage, and thrombosis. Systemic vasculitis caused by systemic lupus erythematosus or rheumatoid arthritis can similarly affect the brain.

Post-infectious encephalitis is an autoimmune process characterized by a perivenulitis with contiguous demyelination. It is uncommon under one year of age. With post-infectious encephalitis following measles, there is a T-lymphocyte response to myelin basic protein. Dysregulation of immune function, which commonly occurs in measles, may be partially contributory[(210)]. An extreme variant of post-infectious encephalitis is acute necrotizing hemorrhagic leukoencephalitis.

In immunodeficient patients, the course of infectious encephalitis is frequently subacute or chronic **(Table 32.12).**

Clinical Manifestations and Differential Diagnosis

Neonatal Encephalitis

Encephalitis should be considered in any infant with fever and signs of poor feeding, irritability, lethargy, or sepsis. Seizures or apnea can occur[(216)]. History of maternal fever in the peripartum may presage enterovirus or adenovirus infection in the neonate. History of maternal genital herpes is sought, although it is present in only 20 to 27% of infants with herpes infection[217]. Skin lesions can point to the diagnosis but are absent in 37% of cases of HSV encephalitis at presentation[217]. Evaluation of suspected neonatal sepsis should include cerebrospinal fluid culture for both bacteria and viruses. Abnormal liver function tests, consumptive coagulopathy, and acidosis are clues to disseminated disease. Usually acyclovir is given empirically to ill infants with a compatible history and signs of neonatal herpes infection. Management of less ill infants is individualized. Prolonged vomiting, hypoglycemia, and either severe acidosis or alkalosis with hyperammonemia in a young infant should lead to prompt evaluation and treatment for metabolic disorders[218].

Encephalitis in Infants and Children

Clinical manifestations of the inflammatory response are initially subtle and diverse. Specific neurologic findings vary according to which areas of the brain parenchyma are most severely affected and also with the degree of raised ICP. Although some features of acute encephalitis are similar to those found in aseptic meningitis and include headache, stiff neck, photophobia, fever, vomiting, and irritability, the hallmark of the disease is alteration of higher cerebral function, evidenced by change in level of consciousness, with psychiatric and behavioral abnormalities, or seizure activity. Predominant cortical involvement may lead to disorientation and confusion, basal ganglia involvement to movement disorders, and brainstem involvement to cranial nerve dysfunction. In some cases, spinal cord involvement (myelitis) may accompany the encephalitis, and flaccid paraplegia with abnormalities of the deep tendon reflexes may be the presenting signs of the illness. The various types of encephalitides cannot be distinguished on the basis of clinical signs or laboratory findings alone in most cases, although the presence of neurologic signs that localize to the temporal or frontal areas is suggestive of herpes simplex encephalitis (see the following discussion).

The presence of fever is helpful in distinguishing encephalitis from many encephalopathies due to toxins or inborn errors of metabolism. Infectious encephalitis frequently begins with a prodrome of fever, headache, personality change, or irritability lasting from hours to days. Lethargy follows and is the extent of progression in most cases. In more severe cases of encephalitis, lethargy may progress rapidly to autonomic instability, coma and, in some cases, death. In evaluating an infant or older child with encephalitis, the prodrome and rate of progression of the illness should be carefully established. In contrast to infectious encephalitis, the onset of post-infectious encephalitis is characteristically sudden. Convulsions, focal neurologic deficits, ataxia, movement disorders, and meningismus (with little pleocytosis) occur with both. Diagnosis of post-infectious encephalitis is more likely when onset of symptoms occurs one or more weeks after an upper respiratory illness or as fever or an exanthem subsides. However, infectious and post-infectious encephalitis usually cannot be distinguished by clinical findings. Usually, the infectious stimulus is subclinical or obscure.

The diagnostic distinction between infectious and post-infectious encephalitis may be difficult when the infectious agents can cause both forms of encephalitis. Mumps encephalitis can precede parotitis by several days; infectious or post-infectious encephalitis can occur as parotitis wanes.

An antecedent respiratory illness, exanthem, or vaccination suggests the possibility of post-infectious encephalitis. History of severe pharyngitis and fatigue in the older child may indicate EBV encephalitis. Exposure to kittens suggests *Bartonella henselae* (cat scratch) encephalitis[205]. Encephalitis in warm months raises the possibility of Rocky Mountain spotted fever, Lyme disease, or encephalitis caused by an enterovirus or arbovirus. History of travel or contact with ticks or mosquitoes should be sought. Local health departments may have knowledge of respiratory virus activity or arbovirus activity in sentinel animals. Foreign travel may expose the patient to many other infectious causes of encephalitis, and the advice of an infectious disease expert is recommended in such instances.

A careful physical examination is mandatory. Neurologic evaluation includes global assessment, such as Glasgow coma scale, as well as examination of focal sensory, motor, and cerebellar function. Prominent bulbar involvement can be suggestive of rabies infection. Documentation of specific findings should replace generalities such as lethargy. Infectious and post-infectious encephalitis may predominantly involve the brainstem. Discrete, localized involvement (Miller-Fisher syndrome or Birkenstaff's encephalitis) may be so extensive as to mimic brain death transiently. Post-infectious encephalitis typically involves multiple levels of the CNS, and the patient may have symptoms that demonstrate predominantly as cerebellar ataxia (especially after chickenpox), transverse myelitis, or optic neuritis. Lyme disease, which may include optic neuritis, cranial nerve palsies, and radiculitis, also involves multiple areas of the nervous system. *Listeria monocytogenes* rarely causes acute brainstem encephalitis without meningitis[219]. Careful examination of the skin may reveal a suggestive rash as is found in cases of Rocky Mountain spotted fever, Lyme disease, enteroviral, arboviral, and varicella infections. The rash of Rocky Mountain spotted fever is frequently subtle and present at the wrists, ankles, and axillae; rash of the palms and soles is an inconstant finding. Herpetic skin or mouth lesions in a child with encephalitis does not necessarily indicate causation. Parotitis, pharyngitis, or lymphadenopathy may suggest specific viralorigins. Respiratory signs are present in less than 50% of patients with mycoplasma encephalitis[207].

Hemorrhagic shock with encephalopathy is an idiopathic syndrome of cerebral edema and encephalopathy, profound shock, coagulopathy, and diarrhea. There is substantial overlap of the syndrome with heat stroke and malignant hyperthermia. Rectal temperature is usually greater than 39°C, and the onset of the encephalopathy is sudden. Brain infarction may occur. The coagulopathy appears after the hypotension; diarrhea may become bloody[(214)]. The diagnosis requires the exclusion of septic shock, toxic shock syndrome, Reye syndrome, and hemolytic-uremic syndrome. The patient who has Reye syndrome may have a prodrome of nausea and vomiting, followed by encephalopathy. Patients are usually afebrile and have hepatomegaly. Elevated blood ammonia is present in the majority of cases, but hypoglycemia and elevated liver transaminase levels are more variable. Although hemorrhagic shock with encephalopathy and Reye syndrome are not true examples of encephalitis, they must be considered in the differential diagnosis **(Table 32.13).**

Laboratory Diagnosis

In general, there is little correlation of cerebrospinal fluid (CSF) abnormalities with clinical or histologic severity of encephalitis. Analogous to the scenario of determining the cause of pneumonia by sampling pleural fluid, detecting the agent causing encephalitis by analyzing CSF is successful in only 15 to 50% of cases. Generally, the CSF is clear and colorless but it may be xanthochromic when blood has been present in the CSF for some time. CSF cell count and protein are frequently normal or slightly elevated, and the glucose concentration remains normal. In the early phase of infection there is often a mixed pleocytosis consisting of both polymorphonuclear and mononuclear cells. Although the CSF pleocytosis generally becomes more lymphocytic with time, in some types of infection, notably Eastern equine encephalitis, a polymorphonuclear predominance persists throughout the illness. Evaluation of the CSF early in the course of acute encephalitis may yield few or no cells[(220)]. Such a finding does not eliminate the diagnosis, and a repeat lumbar puncture after 1 to 2 days is often helpful in subsequently demonstrating pleocytosis. Vasculitis or tissue necrosis causes extravasation of red blood cells into CSF and elicits CSF leukocytosis with increased polymorphonuclear cells. The presence of red blood cells in the CSF is a late and inconstant indicator of HSV encephalitis. Consideration must also be given to subarachnoid hemorrhage from occult trauma or a vascular malformation.

Table 32.13. Differential Diagnosis of Acute Encephalitis

Infectious
Bacterial meningitis
Viral meningitis
Tuberculosis meningitis
Crytococcal meningoencephalitis
Rocky Mountain spotted fever
Brain abscess
Toxic
Drug intoxication
Lead encephalopathy
Carbon monoxide poisoning
Pertussis
Shigellosis[1]
Metabolic
Reye syndrome
Hepatic coma
Uremia
Hypoglycemia
Hypo, hyperosmolar states
Organic acidemias
Amino acidopathies
Urea cycle defects
Fat oxidation defects[2]
MELAS syndrome[3]
Acute intermittent porphyria
Primary brain abscess
First presentation of epilepsy
Neoplasms
Cerebrovascular accidents
Vasculitis
Systemic lupus erythematosis
Polyarteritis nodosa
Other
Pseudotumor cerebri
Trauma
Acute confusional migraine
Postinfectious encephalopathies

[1] *also caused by* Campylobacter jejuni, Salmonella *spp.,* Yersinia *spp.*
[2] *medium and long chain acyl-CoA dehydrogenase deficiency*
[3] *mitochnodrial encephalopathy, lactic acidosis, stroke syndrome*

Making a specific etiologic diagnosis requires confirmation by viral isolation, identification of viral agents by rapid diagnostic technology, or by demonstration of a rise in specific antibody titer. In only 15 to 70% of cases is an etiologic agent identified. The disease is often inferred from the isolation of pathogens at anatomic sites other than the CNS or by serology. Most HSV isolates from CSF are identified by tissue culture in 2 to 3 days. Isolation of enteroviruses, CMV, or other viruses may be significantly slower. However, many agents remain difficult to culture. Rapid diagnostic technology augments diagnosis by tissue culture. For example, shell vial assay with fluorescent antibody staining may detect CMV within 24 hours with a sensitivity of approximately 60% of the standard tissue culture. Molecular genetic assays such as PCR that identifies organism specific DNA sequences are likely to enhance specific diagnosis significantly. PCR assays currently available at large clinical microbiology laboratories can detect DNA from HSV[(221)], enterovirus, cytomegalovirus, Ebstein Barr virus, varicella-zoster virus[(222)], JC polyoma virus, *B. burgdorferi,* and *B. henselae.* Interpretation of PCR results must include an awareness of the potential for false positives by cross-contamination of laboratory specimens as well as false negatives, caused by either the anatomic distance of the infectious encephalitis process from the meninges and CSF or the presence of inhibitory factors in CSF[(221)]. Viral genomic material remains in the CSF from weeks to months, a potentially helpful factor in the elucidation of the cause of post-infectious encephalitis[(222)].

The presence of myelin basic protein in the CSF, in the absence of brain necrosis, indicates damage to oligodendrocytes. Elevated levels of myelin basic protein suggest demyelinating injury compatible with post-infectious encephalitis. The sensitivity of this test in the diagnosis of post-infections is approximately 60%. The presence of antibody (globulin) in CSF is indicative of local immune response and is assessed as a globulinto albumin ratio in CSF and serum. Total CSF immunoglobulins and antibodies to specific pathogens have been studied as diagnostic tests in viral encephalitis. The minimum time from onset of disease to detection of antibody is usually 4 to 5 days, limiting usefulness as an early test for infectious encephalitis. Intrathecal antibody levels are low in post-infectious encephalitis, in contrast to chronic viral infections of the CNS such as subacute sclerosing panencephalitis, a complication of measles infection, and subacute rubella encephalitis.

The specific cause of most cases of encephalitis is determined retrospectively, by demonstrating a rise in titer to the offending organism by measuring acute and convalescent antibody titers in sera or CSF. Such an antibody response generally takes 3 to 6 weeks and is therefore of no diagnostic assistance in the early stages of disease. Interpretation is confounded by lack of specificity of IgM assays, cross-reactive antibodies, and polyclonal production of intrathecal antibodies during CNS infection and in the case of mycoplasma encephalitis, the cross reaction of the organism with brain tissue[207]. **Table 32.14** outlines the laboratory evaluation of acute encephalitis.

Before clinical introduction of acyclovir, a drug without serious side effects, brain biopsy for histological examination, viral culture, and fluorescent antibody staining was a diagnostic option. This procedure is now rarely undertaken for the specific diagnosis of encephalitis.

Magnetic resonance imaging (MRI) is the most sensitive imaging modality for infectious encephalitis and detects brain inflammation and edema in the cerebral cortex, gray-white matter junction, basal ganglia, or cerebellum[223].

Table 32.14. Laboratory Evaluation of Acute Encephalitis

Lumbar Puncture
Opening pressure
Routine studies
CSF culture: virus, bacteria
Consider PCR panel
Consider specific antibody tests
Consider myelin basic protein
Other cultures
Blood culture: bacteria
Virus isolation: nasopharynx and stool
Consider virus isolation: blood buffy coat, urine
Metabolic screen
Serum electrolytes, calcium
Blood glucose
Blood pH[1]
Plasma ammonia[1] and amino acids
Urine organic acid
Toxicology screen: urine, serum
MRI
Consider EEG if HSV encephalitis suspected
Collect acute serum specimen
Consider cold agglutinins
Contact local health epidemiologist

[1]Plasma for amino acids and urine for organic acids are collected and frozen immediately, and sent for assay if blood pH or ammonia are abnormal.

Post-infectious encephalitis is associated with foci of demyelination in the semilunar white matter, basal ganglia, brainstem, or spinal cord. Demyelination is best detected in T2-weighted images. Post-infectious encephalitis often involves multiple areas of the brain and spinal cord, and tends to be symmetric. Lyme disease and multiple sclerosis may also involve diverse areas of brain, brainstem, and spinal cord. Use of gadolinium contrast improves the sensitivity of MRI for vasculitis and cerebral abscesses. Gadolinium also confirms that the multifocal areas of demyelination in post-infectious encephalitis are all of the same stage. However, this is in contrast to multiple sclerosis, which rarely appears explosively in children.

MRI may be insensitive in detecting encephalitis early, especially in neonates with higher brain water content. The sensitivities of CT and MRI for HSV encephalitis outside of the neonate are 60 and 80%, respectively (Figure 32.4). EEG is equally sensitive as MRI (80%); the information is complementary to neuroimaging. CT scanning is superior to other methods for detecting intracranial calcifications caused by congenital CMV and toxoplasmosis, HIV infection, and some metabolic diseases.

Therapy

Most children with evidence of acute encephalitis severe enough to alter the state of consciousness significantly should be admitted to the ICU for initial evaluation and supportive care. This is true especially in the early phases when the differential diagnosis includes other possibilities, such as cerebrovascular accidents and poisoning, as described previously. Moreover, it is essential to monitor the course closely and to follow the neurologic examination meticulously. Severe encephalitis can lead to extensive areas of perivascular infiltrates and diffuse cerebral edema with elevation of ICP and cerebral herniation. Encephalitis may lead to seizures that can be exceedingly difficult to control, and in some cases, actual neuronal destruction particularly of the brainstem may lead to respiratory compromise or hemodynamic instability. Because intensive supportive therapy may be required for these patients, it is recommended that the first 24 to 48 hours be spent in an intensive care area.

Indications for initiation of assisted ventilation are similar to those discussed elsewhere in this volume. The clinician should avoid the use of long-acting neuromuscular blocking agents for intubation and during mechanical ventilation, if possible, because of the high incidence of seizures in patients with encephalitis. Failure to recognize and to treat ongoing seizure activity in the paralyzed child may lead to profound metabolic acidosis, cerebral ischemia, and brain damage. If neuromuscular blockade is necessary, then continuous EEG or cerebral function monitoring should be employed while the patient remains paralyzed. The patient should be allowed to develop some spontaneous movements

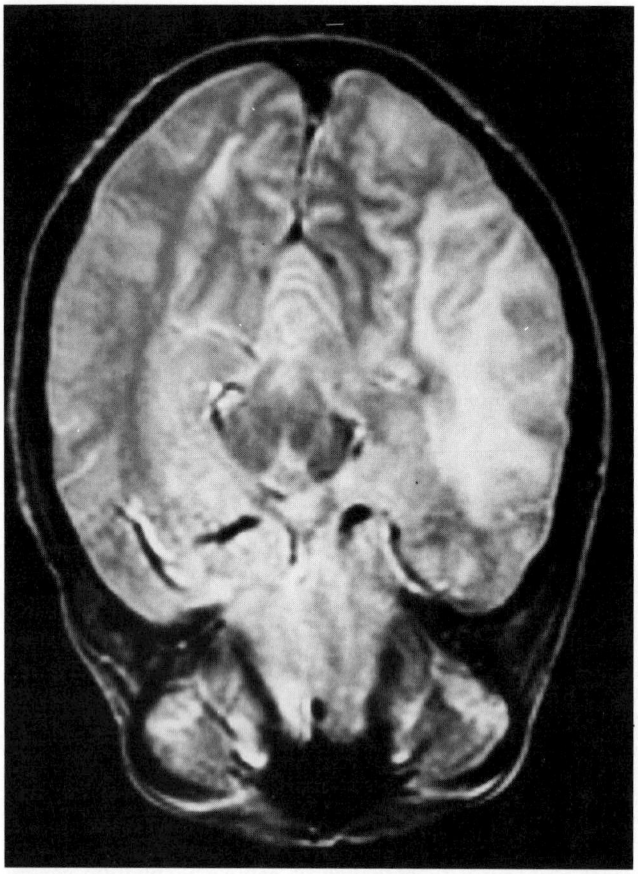

Figure 32.4. MRI depicting temporal encephalitis caused by HSV-1. Courtesy of R.R. Lee, Dept. of Radiology and Radiological Science, Johns Hopkins School of Medicine.

before administration of each dose of the neuromuscular blocking agent. Another drawback to use of neuromuscular blocking agents in patients with impairment of consciousness is that it does not permit repetitive performance of the neurologic examination. Thus, the development of raised ICP may not become clinically apparent until intracranial hypertension is of such magnitude as to cause the typical Cushing response and possible herniation. For these reasons, one must consider electively monitoring the ICP of any patient with acute encephalitis who requires continued neuromuscular blockade. Patients with a Glasgow Coma Scale of less than 8 are also candidates for ICP monitoring.

When elevated ICP is documented, therapeutic measures of hyperventilation, dehydration, and routine positioning should be employed. The use of corticosteroids is of no documented value and may prove harmful by causing dissemination of herpes simplex virus. No recommendations can be given concerning the use of barbiturate coma as an adjunctive measure to control intracranial hypertension in this disease because no systematic studies of this problem have been reported.

Specific antiviral therapy has been of documented benefit only in therapy for herpes simplex infections and is discussed later in the section on that disease entity.

Herpes Simplex Encephalitis

Herpes simplex encephalitis (HSE) is one of the most devastating of all CNS infections, with an untreated immediate mortality of over 65%(201). The majority of cases are caused by the type 1 strain, except in the neonate, where type 2 predominates. Herpes simplex is the most common cause of fatal sporadic viral encephalitis in the United States(201). It does not occur in epidemic form.

Clustering by season has been noted(224), but there is no evidence for contagion. Although HSE most often strikes adults, one-third of the cases occur in children and teenagers(226). In addition to its high mortality, untreated herpes encephalitis is associated with nearly uniformly devastating neurologic damage in the survivors, and even treated herpes encephalitis continues to be associated with high rates of mortality and morbidity. This is, at least in part, probably resulting from the difficulties in making a definitive diagnosis. There is little controversy over the fact that the outcome of the disease depends on the speed with which the diagnosis is made and appropriate therapy is instituted. However, even with early administration of acyclovir, a good outcome cannot be ensured. In the discussion that follows, an overview of herpes encephalitis in the neonate and older children is presented with particular attention directed to recent advances in diagnosis.

Neonatal Herpes Encephalitis

In the United States, neonatal HSV infection occurs with an incidence of approximately 1 per 3500 to 1 per 5000 deliveries, an incidence slightly less than that of group b streptococcal meningitis(201,226). Neonatal involvement with HSV can range from mild localized infection to fatal disseminated disease. Three different forms of the disease develop in neonates: (1) skin, eye, and mouth disease (45%); (2) encephalitis (35%); and (3) disseminated disease (20%). Overall, 50% of infants with neonatal HSV infection will have encephalitis as a component of their disease.

Neonatal HSV is usually acquired by vertical transmission from the genitally infected mother to the fetus or neonate. Infection is either acquired in utero (congenital infection) or during the birth process by contact with infected genital secretions (85% of cases). The remaining small percentage of cases is acquired by postnatal contact with the HSV. Most cases of neonatal HSV infection occur with identifiable risk factors for maternal transmission(217). The transmission rate from mother to infant is 30 to 40% when genital infection is primary and 3% for reactivated herpes infection. Thirty percent of women shedding HSV in labor had primary infection(226). The mean age at onset for HSV encephalitis is 11 days, later than the 6 days for cutaneous or systemic disease(227). The pathogenesis of the CNS disease in disseminated HSV infection is different from that of localized isolated herpes encephalitis. The CNS infection of infants with disseminated disease is usually diffuse, implying blood-borne spread to the brain. In contrast, in infants with encephalitis alone, the brain disease is initially often localized to one or both temporal lobes. Accession of HSV to brain with isolated encephalitis is considered to be through the intraneuronal spread(228).

Neonates with disseminated disease have a clinical picture similar to that of bacterial sepsis and cannot be distinguished on clinical grounds. Seventy-five percent of neonates with disseminated disease will have encephalitis. Mucosal or skin vesicular lesions are present in approximately 20 to 30% of infected infants. Neonates with disseminated disease have symptoms at approximately 6 days after birth. In contrast, neonates with isolated encephalitis (30% of neonatal HSV infections) have lesions at an average age of 2 weeks.

The clinical diagnosis of HSV infection in the neonate is difficult unless skin vesicles are present. Cultures of conjunctivae, nasopharynx, and rectum (obtained by single swab, in this order) at 48 to 72 hours of age may detect early infection of an exposed infant. Laboratory evidence of hepatocellular disease or coagulopathy may indicate disseminated viral sepsis. The increased brain water content in early infancy and poor localization of the virus after hematogenous infection reduce the sensitivity of an MRI or CT scan for the diagnosis of HSV encephalitis. EEG findings of a multifocal, periodic pattern discharges may be present, but are insensitive and nonspecific(229). Herpes simplex virus can be isolated from the CSF in approximately 50% of neonates with encephalitis or HSV sepsis, whereas isolation of the virus from older children and adults is uncommon(201).

Acyclovir and vidarabine are equally effective in treating neonatal HSV encephalitis(227). Cerebral necrosis may continue for several days after virologic cure. Virologic failures complicate 2% of cases. Relapses may occur in 8% of patients after 10 days of acyclovir therapy at a dose of 30 mg/kg/d(227). Many experts currently consider treatment with acyclovir at a dose of 45 mg/kg/d of acyclovir for 3 weeks. Anecdotal cases of recurrent irritability or progressive neurologic decline in association with cutaneous relapses of HSV-2 have prompted some experts to consider oral prophylaxis with acyclovir for 3 to 6 months after neonatal infection(230,231). The 15 to 30% oral bioavailability of acyclovir requires large oral doses administered four to five times daily. Famciclovir, a more bioavailable agent with longer half-life may be useful in the future in settings of prolonged therapy or secondary prophylaxis. Ganciclovir and foscarnet are active against herpes simplex, and new antiviral agents are now in clinical trials.

For HSV-infected infants with disseminated sepsis, mortality is 50 to 60%, with 60% of survivors developing normally after one year. With isolated encephalitis, 14% of infants die, and 29% develop normally after one year(227). The risk of death is increased with disseminated disease, coma, disseminated intravascular coagulopathy (DIC), and prematurity. The prognosis for HSV-2 CNS infections of the newborn is worse than for similar infections caused by HSV-1. Morbidity is more frequent in infants with encephalitis, disseminated disease, seizures, or infection with HSV-2(230).

Herpes Encephalitis in Infancy and Childhood

Pathogenesis

Pathogenesis of HSV encephalitis in older children remains unclear. It may result from both primary and recurrent HSV infection. Approximately 70% of HSV encephalitis cases are the result of reactivation, whereas the remaining 30% represent primary infection.

The route of spread of virus to the CNS in humans with primary disease is controversial but is probably through olfactory or even trigeminal nerve tracts. In cases of recurrent infection leading to HSV, encephalitis virus may be reactivated within the brain but peripheral reactivation in the olfactory bulb or trigeminal ganglia with neuronal spread is more likely(201).

Clinical Manifestations

The clinical course in older children is similar to that in adults. In young children and infants, historic information does not generally result in strong support for the specific viral agent, unless gingivostomatitis or skin lesions are also present. Encephalitis may begin suddenly or after a brief influenza-like prodrome. The youngsters are generally febrile with headache, vomiting, behavioral changes, and speech difficulty. Consciousness decreases with progression. Seizures may be generalized, but focal seizures are prominent. Stiffness of the neck is often noted. Focal neurologic signs develop in a majority of patients(263) and are thought to represent selective involvement of the temporal or frontal lobes(201). In one series, all patients with biopsy-proven HSV encephalitis had evidence of focal CNS disease by either clinical or neurodiagnostic assessment. Brainstem abnormalities develop that reflect effects of inflammation or cerebral edema and may be accompanied by papilledema and other signs of elevated ICP, including transtentorial herniation and cardiorespiratory instability.

The clinical syndrome consistent with herpes encephalitis may also be caused by human herpes virus 6(212), enteroviruses(231), metabolic disorders such as MELAS syndrome(232), acute hemorrhagic leukoencephalitis, or systemic vasculitis.

HSV encephalitis does not appear to be more common in immunosuppressed individuals. In some patients, the course is more indolent, with a paucity of inflammation and progression of neurologic deficits over weeks(233). Despite the high prevalence of seropositivity to HSV, CNS dysfunction in AIDS is correlated with CMV disease or other causes(234).

Laboratory Diagnosis

Laboratory findings in herpes encephalitis are nonspecific. Routine blood studies such as complete blood count and differential may be totally normal or may reflect the presence of an acute infectious process. When SIADH occurs, these patients may have hyponatremia[235], but otherwise, the electrolyte pattern is unremarkable.

Evaluation of CSF is essential, although on occasion (less than 5%) CSF examination may be totally normal. More often, however, abnormalities are encountered that are consistent with the diagnosis of encephalitis. These include pleocytosis of variable degree, usually consisting of less than 200 WBC total, which in the first 24 to 48 hours of illness is generally polymorphonuclear and progresses to a predominantly mononuclear cell count beyond that time. Fluid may be xanthochromic or may contain elevated numbers of RBCs, a finding thought to be caused by the necrotizing nature of the disease, consistent with release of blood into the subarachnoid space[236]. An erythrocyte count of more than 50 mm^3 was present 42% of cases[237]. The protein may be mildly elevated with mean protein concentration of 80 mg, sensitivity 82%, levels not usually exceeding 200 mg/100 ml, and the glucose content is generally, but not always[238,239], normal. The laboratory findings in the CSF may remain abnormal for several months[238,239]. Opening pressure should be measured but will probably be low initially. A sample of spinal fluid should be sent for bacteriologic as well as viral culture, although it is exceedingly unlikely that herpes simplex will be isolated from the CSF, even during the acute phase of infection.

The particular predilection of the virus for the temporal or frontal lobes has been used in employment of various ancillary diagnostic studies, which include EEG, CT scan, radionuclide brain scan, MRI scan, and brain biopsy.

The EEG demonstrates temporal region localization in approximately 80% of patients with characteristic paroxysmal localizing epileptiform discharges (PLEDS) in 65% of biopsy proven cases. Only approximately 50% of patients exhibit the classic EEG findings[242]. Others may have nonspecific electrical activity on admission with lateralization occurring later in the course[243,244]. Similar EEG findings may also occur in nonherpetic encephalitides, such as that resulting from infectious mononucleosis[245]. Therefore, EEG may provide evidence to support the diagnosis or point to an area of focal damage that could be biopsied, but it is not specific for HSV encephalitis.

Focal abnormalities may also be noted in approximately 50% of cases with sodium pertechnetate Tc 99m brain scan[246] and CT scan[237,247–249]. Characteristic findings on CT scan are unilateral low-density lesions or the suggestion of a mass effect in the medial temporal lobe or, in some cases, the insular cortex. When hemorrhage is associated with the lesion, there is streaked contrast enhancement. Although nearly all adult patients with biopsy-proven herpes develop abnormal CT scan findings, they are present on admission in only 64 to 92% and, sometimes, the scan is normal until the fifth day of illness. Therefore, the CT scan is also only a suggestive diagnostic study. It may be most useful in the early stages to eliminate diseases of a surgical nature, such as abscess or hemorrhage, which require immediate intervention. It is also a valuable tool when serial examinations are performed throughout the early course of disease to watch for progression of disease in the temporal lobes. MRI scan is more sensitive than the nuclear brain scan or CT scan for the diagnosis of HSV encephalitis[224] but has not been compared with PCR as regards diagnostic accuracy.

Immunologic methods to evaluate CSF and serum for the presence of herpes simplex antibody have been investigated but are not particularly useful for diagnosis because of poor sensitivity and specificity. In addition, the antibody response in the CSF does not appear before the fifth day of illness and is often low in severe cases[249]. Increasing experience with and a widening availability of PCR suggests that this test will be useful for the diagnosis of HSV encephalitis. Using primers from an HSV DNA sequence that were common to both HSV-1 and HSV-2 (either HSV DNA polymerase or glycoprotein domain) several investigators have reported successful identification of HSV DNA in the CSF of proven herpes encephalitis cases[201,251]. This test appears to have a sensitivity of more than 95% at the time of diagnosis and a specificity close to 100%.

Brain biopsy for tissue histology and culture is the definitive test for diagnosis of encephalitis. Routine brain biopsy for encephalitis has been advocated in adults, who have a lower incidence of encephalitis and a higher incidence of alternate, treatable diagnoses. The utility of routine biopsy in children is more controversial[252,253]. Because of improved neuroimaging and low adverse effects of current antiviral therapy, empiric therapy is the usual practice. Biopsy is reserved for patients with atypical features or disease that progresses despite empiric therapy. The relative roles for biopsy and PCR diagnosis of encephalitis remain to be elucidated.

Therapy

Early aggressive treatment of encephalitis may reduce mortality and neurologic sequelae. The risk of death from HSV encephalitis is greater with deep coma (GCS <6) and with a duration of disease greater than 4 days before treatment. Supportive aspects of care of the child with suspected or proven HSE are not different from those of patients with other acute CNS infections. Appropriate attention must be given to overall care of the airway and cardiorespiratory system, as well as to those aspects of neurointensive care previously discussed. Because of the necrotizing and often focal nature of herpes encephalitis, focal or generalized seizures may be a prominent aspect of disease as exhibited in the PICU, and may require extreme measures to achieve a seizure-free state. In addition, cerebral edema, elevated ICP, and herniation are common occurrences in patients with herpetic encephalitis. Therefore, when signs and symptoms are consistent with intracranial hypertension, rational treatment choices may be made more feasible through the use of ICP monitoring.

Acyclovir is currently the treatment of choice for HSV encephalitis in patients older than 6 months[254]. Treatment (30 mg/kg/d for 10 days) reduced mortality to approximately 30% from approximately 70% in untreated individuals. Relapse may occur in up to 5% of patients. Vidarabine (15 mg/kg/d for 10 days) reduces mortality to 44-54%; limited solubility of vidarabine requires its administration in fluid volumes of at least twice the daily basal metabolic requirement for water potentially complicating the management of cerebral edema and elevated intracranial pressure. Ganciclovir is active against most human herpes viruses but is associated with more toxicity. Acyclovir, ganciclovir, vidarabine, and famciclovir are all pro-drugs requiring virion-mediated phosphorylation for activation. Foscarnet and vidarabine do not require virion-enhanced phosphorylation for activity, and may be useful in rare instances or resistant (TK^-) viruses.

It is unclear whether corticosteroid or other immunomodulatory therapies attenuate the disease process of post-infectious encephalitis.

Outcome

The overall risks of death and morbidity from encephalitis are 3 to 4% and 7 to 10%, respectively. The incidence of complications is correlated inversely with the age at onset; children under one year of age have mortality of 40 to 50% in several retrospective series.

Cerebral edema, inappropriate antidiuretic hormone secretion, and vasomotor instability are frequent complications, which may result in rapid decline and death. In self-limited cases, lethargy or coma can last from a few days to more than a week; improvement occurs from days to weeks. Focal deficits can resolve over a period of months. Severe neurologic residua may include changes in personality, behavior disorders, mental retardation, blindness, movement disorders, paretic syndromes, spasticity, and persistent ataxia. Signs at presentation predictive of sequelae from infectious encephalitis frequently include lethargy or coma, focal motor deficits, and, in the case of arbovirus encephalitis, convulsions. In contrast, there is no correlation of the severity of the clinical presentation and outcome for most post-infectious encephalitis. Post-infectious encephalitis following measles infection results in death from 15 to 20% of cases and neurologic residua in 25%. Mycoplasma has been associated with severe sequelae in 25% of cases.

Infectious encephalitis can be followed by post-infectious encephalitis within a period of days to weeks. The clinician is challenged to distinguish virologic relapse, post-infectious encephalitis, or repeated episodes of a noninfectious neurologic or metabolic disorder.

Neonatal HSV encephalitis, when treated, is associated with a mortality of 14% for encephalitis and 50 to 60% for disseminated disease. Outcome is worse for infants with HSV-2 infection. In older children, mortality from HSV encephalitis is 28%. Forty to 50% of survivors have major neurologic sequelae. After a 10-day course of acyclovir therapy, 5 to 8% of patients with HSV encephalitis have a relapse within one month. Most patients with virologic relapse are cured with a second course of therapy. Cutaneous relapses occur in 20% of neonates within one month of cessation of acyclovir therapy[228].

California virus group encephalitis has a mortality of less than 1%, with seizure disorders in 10% of survivors. Eastern equine encephalitis results in death in 50 to 75% of cases, with neurologic damage in most survivors. In contrast Western equine encephalitis and St. Louis encephalitis groups have a fatality rate of 2 to 20%, respectively. Morbidity occurs in 10 to 25% of St. Louis virus group survivors and 13 to 56% of Western equine encephalitis cases.

Brain Abscess

Although meningitis is the most common symptom of bacterial infection within the intracranial vault, two additional entities need to be considered, namely brain abscess and subdural empyema. Both entities share the common denominators of bacterial infection of the CNS, potential mass effect with edema and herniation, and a need for expedient diagnosis to achieve a suitable outcome. Empyemas are discussed in a subsequent section.

Although not common, brain abscesses are the most frequently encountered form of localized intracranial infection in children[255]. About 25% of all brain abscess occur in children less than 15 years of age. Only recently has the almost uniformly fatal nature of the disease process been halted by a combination of new neurodiagnostic methods, rational use of antimicrobial agents, and appropriate surgical intervention. Death usually results from rupture of the abscess into the ventricular system with ensuing pyogenic ventriculitis or transtentorial herniation secondary to the mass effect of abscess and surrounding edema.

Pathogenesis

The infecting organism causing brain abscess may gain access to the CNS by one of several routes: (1) direct spread from a contiguous-infected extracranial site, (2) hematogenous spread from an extracranial site of infection, (3) inoculation of organism into brain parenchyma by penetrating trauma, and (4) spread from meningitis[256,257]. **Table 32.15** outlines the conditions predisposing to brain abscess in children, noting changes in epidemiology over the past 50 years. During the past 30 years, cyanotic congenital heart disease has replaced suppurative otic and sinus infection as the most common predisposing factor. Beyond the neonatal period, meningitis is a rare cause of brain abscess in developed countries. Overall, a predisposing factor can be determined in approximately 85% of all patients with brain abscess. Abscess may develop in almost every

Table 32.15. Conditions Predisposing to Brain Abscess in Children

Predisposing Condition	*Western Countries*		*Developing Nations*
	*Mid–1940's to 1960**	*1960's to Present+*	*1960's to Present++*
Congenital cyanotic heart disease	14.5%	35.5%	25.8%
Ear, nose, throat infection	43.9	23.1	23.9
Ear infection	36.2	9.3	21.6
Sinusitis	7.6	12.6	6.1
Head trauma	9.0	6.6	7.6
Neurosurgery	NR	3.3	1.7
Ventricular shunt	NR	2.6	2.2
Pulmonary infection	3.6	0.7	2.0
Dental infection	0.5	0.7	0.8
Bacterial meningitis	1.4	2.2	13.5
Tuberculosis	NR	1.5	NR
Other	11.3	9.5	4.8
Unknown	15.6	14.3	24.2

From Woods CR. Brain abscess and other intracranial suppurative complications. Adv Pediatr Infect Dis 1995;10:41–80.
** n=221,+ n=273,++ n=356 cases from several published series NR, not reported in these series*

area of the brain but is most common in the frontal and temporal lobes followed by the parietal lobe, cerebellum, and occipital lobes[(258)]. The parietal, frontal, and temporal lobe each represent the site of about 25% of brain abscesses.

Both the causative organism and the specific location of the abscess generally reflects the etiologic factors related to the abscess formation **(Table 32.16).** Therefore, abscess formation in the temporal lobe or ipsilateral cerebellar hemisphere is usually the result of chronic otitis or mastoiditis, whereas the patient with chronic sinusitis usually develops an abscess in the frontal lobe. Multiple abscesses may form from hematogenous spread. In children with cyanotic heart disease, abscesses most often form in the distribution of the middle cerebral artery[(259–261)].

Contiguous Spread

The incidence of intracranial suppuration complicating otogenic infection has declined dramatically in recent years in developed countries, presumably reflecting improved health care and the availability of antibiotics. Chronic otitis media is many times more likely to be complicated by a brain abscess than acute otitis media.

Brain abscess complicating chronic ear infections are usually solitary. More than 50% are located in the temporal lobe and 20% to 30% are found in the cerebellum[(258,262)]. In contrast, the frontal lobe is the predominant site for abscess complicating sinus infection, which is usually frontal and/or ethmoidal rather than maxillary. These infections tend to occur in older children, reflecting the late development of the frontal sinus. Brain abscess may rarely complicate cavernous sinus thrombosis. When infection spreads from an extracranial site, such as sinusitis or otitis, into the cranial cavity it is usually through a contiguous area of osteomy-

Table 32.16. Relationship of Predisposing Condition to Site of Brain Abscess and Microbial Isolates

Predisposing Condition	*Site of Abscess*	*Usual Microbial Isolates*
Contiguous site		
Otitis media or mastoiditis	Temporal lobe or cerebellum	Streptococci (anaerobic or aerobic), *Staphylococcus aureus*, *Bacteroides fragilis*, *Proteus* spp., and other Enterobacteriaceae, *Haemophilus* spp., *Pseudomonas aeruginosa*
Frontoethmoidal sinusitis	Frontal lobe	Predominantly streptococci; also *Bacteroides*, Enterobacteriaceae, *S. aureus*, *Haemophilus* spp.
Sphenoidal sinusitis	Frontal or temporal lobe	Same as frontoethmoidal sinusitis
Dental infection	Frontal lobe	Mixed *Fusobacterium* spp., *Bacteroides* spp., streptococci
Primary infection		
Penetrating cranial trauma or postsurgical infection	Related to the site of the wound or surgery	*S. aureus*, streptococci (including pneumococci), Enterobacteriaceae, *Clostridium* spp.
Distant infection site		
Congenital cyanotic heart disease (CCHD)	Middle cerebral artery distribution common, can occur at any site; multiple abscesses common	Viridans, anaerobic, and microaerophilic streptococci, *Haemophilus* spp.
Lung abscess, other pulmonary lung infections	Same as in CCHD	*Fusobacterium*, *Antinomyces*, and *Bacteroides* spp., streptococci, *Nocardia* spp.
Bacterial endocarditis	Same as in CHHD	*S. aureus*, streptococci
Compromised hosts	Same as in CHHD	*Toxoplasma gondii*, *Nocardia* spp., fungi, Enterobacteriaceae

Adapted from Wispelwey B, Dacey RG, Scheld WM: Brain abscess, in Sheld WM, Whitley RJ, Durack DT: Infections of the Central Nervous System. New York, Raven, 1991, p 459.
From Woods CR. Brain abscess and other intracranial suppurative complications. Adv Pediatr Infect Dis 1995;10:41–80.

elitis or through retrograde thrombophlebitis of emissary veins[258].

Hematogenous Spread

Brain abscesses formed by hematogenous seeding tend to develop at the junction of gray and white matter and usually in the distribution of the middle cerebral artery; hence the predominant location in temporal and parietal lobes[258]. Cyanotic congenital heart disease is the most common underlying condition that predisposes to hematogenously spread brain abscesses in children[263–267]. Children with any right-to-left intracardiac shunt are at risk for developing a brain abscess, but tetralogy of Fallot accounts for more than 60% of cyanotic congenital heart disease related abscesses, probably because it is a relatively common heart lesion. The increased blood viscosity associated with the compensatory polycythemia of cyanotic congenital heart disease or microembolism from the right-to-left shunt bypassing the pulmonary filter, probably results in a cerebral microinfarction which may then become seeded during subsequent bacteremia[257,268]. Brain abscess is rarely a complication of the chronic, low-grade bacteremia of subacute bacterial endocarditis. In contrast, the course of acute endocarditis with higher grade bacteremia and a greater likelihood of septic embolization is more frequently complicated by the development of brain abscess[257]. Miscellaneous acute suppurative infections as well as chronic pyogenic pulmonary infections such as bronchiectasis, lung abscess, and rarely infection in patients with cystic fibrosis may be the focus for hematogenous seeding of a brain abscess. Patients with syndromes associated with arteriovenous shunts, e.g., hereditary hemorrhagic telangiectasia, are at increased risk of developing brain abscess usually in adulthood[256,269]. Recently, cases of brain abscess that develop after esophageal dilation have been described[270]. However, the pathogenesis of this complication remains undefined.

Cranial Penetration

Brain abscess occasionally complicates neurosurgical procedures or penetrating brain injuries, and the risk relates to the extent of the underlying injury. Congenital malformations, e.g., encephaloceles and dermal sinuses, may rarely be complicated by brain abscess formation.

Meningitis

Brain abscess formation rarely complicates the course of bacterial meningitis in children beyond the neonatal age. In contrast Gram-negative meningitis when caused by *Proteus mirabilis* or *Citrobacter diversus* is complicated by abscess formation in 40 to 70% of patients[271]. These abscesses are usually multiple, frequently involve the frontal lobes, and may reach a very large size before being diagnosed[272–274].

Bacteriology

Brain abscesses are caused by an array of bacteria, fungi, and parasites. The specific organisms will depend to a great extent on the underlying cause of the abscess and immune status of the patient. With the exception of the neonatal period when *Citrobacter diversus* and *Proteus mirabilis* are the most common etiologic agents, the microbiology of brain abscess in children and adults are similar. Approximately 30% of brain abscesses are polymicrobial in nature[258,265,275,276]. Anaerobes, either as sole pathogens or mixed with aerobes, are present in approximately 30% of cases[275–277] and include *Bacteroides* species (most commonly *Bacteroides fragilis*), *Fusobacterium, Clostridium* species, *Actinomyces,* and anaerobic streptococci. Aerobic or microaerophilic streptococci account for approximately half of the aerobic isolates[257]. The most frequently isolated streptococci are those belonging to the *Streptococcus milleri* group. α-Hemolytic streptococci are the most common organisms isolated from brain abscess in patients with cyanotic congenital heart disease. *S. aureus* is most frequently isolated from trauma related brain abscesses. Aerobic gram negative organisms frequently isolated are *Proteus* species, *E. coli, Klebsiella* species, *Enterobacter* species, and *Pseudomonas aeruginosa.* The microbial etiology of brain abscess in immunocompromised patients is noted in **Table 32.16.**

Pathology

Because normal brain parenchyma is highly resistant to invasion by microorganisms, abscess formation seems to occur only in an area of underlying focal ischemia or necrosis. Poor vascular supply in the white matter, or at the gray-white matter interface makes these the most likely areas to be affected[278].

The progression of the pathologic changes observed in brain abscess is well described and occurs in four stages[279] as defined histopathologically and by CT scan. The first phase of abscess formation is that of early focal cerebritis characterized histopathologically by petechial hemorrhage, cerebral edema, leukocytic infiltrate, and tissue softening. The early phase of cerebritis generally lasts 1 to 3 days. In the phase of late cerebritis that may develop in the fourth to ninth days of illness, liquefaction necrosis occurs and the necrotic center reaches it maximum size. It is surrounded by an area of neovascularization, which contains fibroblasts that form the very early beginnings of a capsule. The third phase is that of early capsule formation in which the necrotic center shrinks, and some degree of resolution of cerebritis is seen. Late capsule formation usually occurs beyond 14 days and is characterized by a dense fibrous capsule surrounded by brain parenchyma in which there are reactive astrocytes and glial cells, marked neovascularization, and surrounding cerebral edema. In general, a total of 4 to 6 weeks may be required from the onset of focal cerebritis to late capsule formation[280]. This general histologic pattern of abscess formation may vary depending on the virulence of the organism and the host's immune system and predisposing condition[256]. Abscesses that develop from hematogenous spread tend to have less well-formed capsules than those arising from contiguous spread[257].

There are variations of this progression. Some patients may move rapidly from the stage of cerebritis to rupture into the ventricle, because capsule development may lag behind the progression of the bacterial disease. It has been noted that patients who have signs of a cerebral abscess often have a better outcome if their course was indolent; this would suggest that patients in whom a capsule develops may have a more benign course.

Cerebral blood flow, already altered by the presence of the infectious process, may be further compromised by the development of cerebral edema and elevated ICP. The intracranial hypertension further limits blood flow and may contribute to antimicrobial failure, as well as to death and neurologic sequelae of infection.

Clinical Manifestations

The clinical course of brain abscess before diagnosis is varied and depends upon the disease-causing organism, the pathogenic mechanism, the location of the abscess, and the presence or absence of meningitis or ventricular rupture.

The progression of the disease may be insidious, lasting many weeks or even months, or else relatively fulminant with rapid deterioration particularly if there is a rupture into the ventricular system with ventriculitis and meningitis. Most brain abscesses are diagnosed within 2 weeks of the onset of symptoms[256]. The clinical manifestations include symptoms and signs of infection, raised intracranial pressure, and focal neurologic symptoms and signs that depend on the site of the abscess. **Table 32.17** lists the clinical manifestations of brain abscess summarized from 13 reported series of brain abscess in children.

Older children usually have headache, fever, and vomiting. Headache develops in two-thirds of the patients, whereas fever and vomiting are features in approximately 50% of patients. Altered mental status is common and may range from lethargy to coma. Meningism suggests meningitis or abscess rupture into the ventricular system. Seizures that are more frequently generalized than focal may occur at any stage. Focal neurologic findings develop in about half of the patients, and their nature depends on the site of the abscess. Some children develop a hemiparesis or homonymous hemianopsia, and cranial nerve palsies are common. Papilledema may represent diffuse cerebral swelling, and sixth nerve palsy also caused by diffuse elevation of intracranial pressure may be falsely interpreted as a localizing sign. Cerebellar signs may predominate when the abscess is in the posterior fossa. Cranial nerve dysfunction, long tract signs, and meningismus may accompany brainstem abscess. Herniation in patients with cerebral abscess may occur spontaneously or after diagnostic lumbar puncture. Bleeding into the abscess may occur, and when combined with rupture into the ventricle represent catastrophic events. Fewer than 50% of patients have the typical triad of fever, headache, and focal neurologic findings[257,275].

Table 32.17. Signs and Symptoms of Children With Brain Abscess: Compilation From 13 Series of Pediatric Patients Encountered From 1945 to 1990

Manifestion	*Percent*
Headache	65
Fever	55
Vomiting	53
Papilledema	48
Focal neurologic deficit	47
Mental status changes	43
Meningeal signs	36
Seizure	34

From Woods CR. Brain abscess and other intracranial suppurative complications. Adv Pediatr Infect Dis 1995;10:41–80.

Table 32.18. Differential Diagnosis of Brain Abscess[a]

Infectious	**Vascular disorders**
Meningitis	Venous thrombosis
Bacterial	Cerebral hemorrhage
Viral	Subarachnoid hemorrhage
Tuberculosis	Cerebral infarction
Encephalitis	Migraine headache
Empyema	**Others**
Subdural	Collagen-vascular disease
Epidural	Multiple sclerosis
Cranial osteomyelitis	Cholesteatoma
Mycotic aneurysms	Cerebral contusion
Brain tumors	Congenital hydrocephalus
Primary	Subdural effusion
Metastatic	

[a]Information derived from Kaplan (288), Jadavji et al. (265) and Schurr (280).

The clinical manifestations of brain abscess in neonates are different from those in older children. Since brain abscess in neonates usually originates as a complication of meningitis, this entity should be suspected when the course of meningitis, particularly when caused by *Proteus mirabilis* or *Citrobacter diversus,* is complicated by persistently positive CSF cultures, enlarging head circumference, evidence of increased ICP of focal neurologic findings.

The differential diagnosis of brain abscess includes bacterial meningitis, viral encephalitis, brain tumor, vascular disorders, traumatic space-occupying lesions, and miscellaneous disorders with focal neurologic signs, such as collagen vascular diseases and multiple sclerosis **(Table 32.18).**

Laboratory and Radiologic Diagnosis

Routine laboratory studies are usually not particularly helpful in eliminating or confirming the diagnosis of brain abscess. The WBC count is elevated in the majority of cases, as is the erythrocyte sedimentation rate. Blood cultures are usually sterile unless the abscess is a complication of acute endocarditis. CSF findings are nonspecific, with pleocytosis, elevated protein, and even a low CSF glucose concentration. Gram's stain is negative in the absence of ventriculitis or meningitis[264,281], as is the bacterial culture. The CSF is normal in about 15% of patients with brain abscess. Since intracranial pressure is elevated in most patients with brain abscess and information gleaned from CSF examination is of little diagnostic or therapeutic use, a *spinal tap should not be performed* before neuroimaging studies if abscess is strongly considered. Approximately 25% of brain abscess patients develop signs of transtentorial herniation within several hours following a tap[282].

Definitive diagnostic studies are CT scanning[283,284] MRI, and radionuclide scanning of the brain, which have replaced arteriography and ventriculography for brain abscess diagnosis[285]. Rarely will a skull radiograph demonstrate air within a cavity, a pathognomonic finding for abscess. Radionuclide scans using sodium ^{99m}Tc-pertechnetate are capable of localizing areas of focal cerebritis, the early stage in the formation of a brain abscess, and thus, a particularly sensitive study for excluding a brain abscess[258,265]. CT scanning permits serial examinations of a patient with a brain abscess, allowing the clinician to follow the course of the disease and to optimize therapy[286]. The classic picture of an abscess depicted by CT scan is a hypodense area surrounded by a ring of contrast enhancement. Mass effect with midline shift may be seen and ependymal enhancement may be present with complicating ventriculitis. In addition, the CT scan is helpful in evaluating middle ear, mastoid, and paranasal sinuses. The CT scan may be unable to differentiate the early cerebritis stage from normal areas of the brain and is also limited by its inability to detect extremely small lesions. However, the high degree of sensitivity of the CT scan (more than 95%) is not paralleled by similar specificity. Infarction, granulomas, and neoplasm may present similar appearances. MRI is more sensitive than CT scan in detecting cerebritis and the extent of edema around the abscess. Therefore, the MRI may more easily detect early satellite lesions or extraparenchymal extension[257,285].

Therapy

The optimal management of most patients with pyogenic brain abscess requires both antibiotic and surgical drainage or excision. Surgical drainage of associated sinus or otologic suppurative disease may also be required.

Antimicrobial Agents

The choice of antibiotics is empiric since there have been no controlled antibiotic trials to guide the practitioner. The choice of antibiotics reflects both the likelihood of specific organisms in a given clinical setting and the ability of various antibiotics to penetrate the abscess. Penicillin has been used for many years in the treatment of brain abscess in combination with either chloramphenicol or metronidazole[272,287]. Penicillin penetrates the abscess cavities well and is bactericidal for most nonenterococcal streptococci and most anaerobes except *B. fragilis.* Chloramphenicol also has good abscess penetration and apart from *S. aureus* and Enterobacteriaceae, is bactericidal against most abscess causing organisms. Nafcillin or vancomycin, which have good abscess penetration, is indicated for *S. aureus* infections. Metronidazole is highly active against anaerobes. Third-generation cephalosporins are drugs of choice for most Enterobacteriaceae. In general, aminoglycosides are not drugs of first choice because of poor penetration into abscess cavities and inactivation by low pH in pus.

No single antibiotic can be recommended with assurance for the initial therapy of brain abscess. Generally, a broad-spectrum combination of agents must be employed[288]. Two widely used combinations are (1) penicillin and chloramphenicol, and (2) metronidazole and cefotaxime. For any antibiotic chosen, the highest recommended dose should be employed in the therapy of brain abscess, and continued for 6 to 8 weeks. More specific antistaphylococcal therapy with a semisynthetic penicillin such as nafcillin or vancomycin, if methicillin resistance is suspected, should be used in patients whose abscess follows surgical or accidental trauma. Patients who are immunosuppressed should be evaluated for the presence of fungi or parasites, and antifungal therapy may be started if clinical response to broad-spectrum antibiotics fails. **Table 32.19** lists suggested initial empirical regimens for brain abscess therapy according to predisposing underlying disease[273,289].

Corticosteroids

The adjunctive use of corticosteroids is controversial. Although they are efficacious in reducing edema surrounding the abscess and may be lifesaving when there is elevated intracranial pressure and clinical deterioration, steroids may decrease antibiotic penetration into the abscess cavity.

Table 32.19. Suggested Initial Empirical Antimicrobial Regimens for Brain Abscess in Children According to Predisposing Condition

Underlying Condition	*Antimicrobial Regimen*
Congenital cyanotic heart disease[a]	Penicillin + chloramphenicol
Sinusitis or head trauma	Nafcillin[b] + chloramphenicol
Otitis/mastoiditis	Nafcillin[b] + ceftazidime + metronidazole
Ventricular shunt infection	Vancomycin + ceftazidime
Meningitis	Third-generation cephalosporin ± aminoglycoside
Unknown	Nafcillin[b] + third-generation cephalosporin + metronidazole
Immunocompromised host	Nafcillin[b] + ceftazidime + metronidazole with consideration of amphotericin B

From Woods CR. Brain abscess and other intracranial suppurative complications. Adv Pediatr Infect Dis 1995;10:41–80. Adapted from Sáez-Llorens XJ, Umaña MA, Odio CM, et al: Pediatric Infect Dis J 8:455, 1989.

[a]Children with brain abscess and congenital cyanotic heart disease who have recently undergone corrective heart surgery should probably be treated similarly to children with ventriculoperitoneal shunt-related infections.

[b]Vancomycin should be substituted for nafcillin or other semisynthetic antistaphylococcal penicillins if a gram-positive organism with significant potential for resistance to these agents is suspected. A vancomycin dosage of up to 60 mg/kg/day given intravenously is indicated for intracranial infections. Peak concentrations should be monitored to ensure efficacy.

However, there is no evidence of delayed bacteriologic response to antibiotics when steroids are used[290].

Surgical Drainage

Surgical intervention provides the definitive treatment of cerebral abscess, but must be timed appropriately to achieve optimal results. Aspiration of the abscess or excision are the surgical techniques available and debate continues as to their relative roles. Opinions for each of these techniques is supported in the literature but neither technique has been proven superior. The advantages of aspiration that appears to be used more often than excision as an initial procedure in children[266,275,290] include low morbidity and mortality from brain injury and the ability to obtain specimens for culture, staining, and histology. Aspiration is usually performed with stereotactic CT guidance. Multiple aspirations may be required to drain some abscesses. Clinical deterioration or failure of aspiration and antibiotic therapy may indicate the need for surgical excision. Fungal abscesses usually require excision. Antibiotic therapy alone has been an effective therapeutic regimen in some cases[291–293]. This approach should probably only be attempted with cerebritis, small abscesses, identification of an etiologic agent in CSF, blood or aspirate, and the absence of elevated intracranial pressure. Medical therapy may be necessary when abscesses are multiple and because of location not amenable to drainage. However, CT-guided stereotactic aspirations permit access to almost any brain location.

The brain abscess patient with depressed neurologic state requires admission to a neurointensive care environment. Measurement of ICP in the child with hydrocephalus accompanying the abscess or who has significant edema surrounding the abscess may help guide therapy directed toward reducing intracranial hypertension and diminish the risk of herniation.

Outcome

The outcome of cerebral abscesses has been dismal in the past, with mortality as high as 70% in some series. Despite the use of broad-spectrum antibiotics, the actual rate of death had not decreased over the years, until the advent of the CT scan. Earlier diagnosis is possible with CT scans and MRI, and this may explain recent reports that demonstrate a markedly improved outcome for brain abscesses since the widespread availability of these diagnostic tools[286]. The mortality of children with brain abscess in the United States after the introduction of CT scanning is less than 6%[266,294,295], but 40% of patients remain with neurologic sequelae, including seizures, focal deficits, behavioral changes, and learning disability.

The outcome of cerebral abscess is related to the neurologic status of the patient on admission. Once the patient demonstrates decreased levels of consciousness, the mortality rises precipitously. It is obvious that the clinician should not wait for neurologic findings to appear before entertaining the diagnosis of the disorder. Mortality may also be increased in patients with underlying cyanotic congenital heart disease[268,296]. This may reflect the tendency for these patients to have multiple lesions. By maintaining a high index of suspicion, and with judicious use of scanning techniques, the outcome of this disease will continue to improve.

Rupture of a brain abscess into the ventricular system is a life-threatening event with a mortality that exceeds 50%[256] and with high morbidity. Manifestations of rupture include shock, high fever, altered sensorium, and meningeal signs. CSF examination usually demonstrates extremely marked CSF leukocytosis in excess of 50,000 cells/mm^3 and with severe hypoglycorrhagia. Therapy must include surgical drainage and antibiotic therapy[256].

SUBDURAL EMPYEMA

The presence of pus in the subdural space is an acute life-threatening emergency constituting approximately 20% of focal suppurative intracranial lesions, and carries a mortality of 10 to 20%. Some authors claim it is the most neglected and least understood of the focal intracranial infections[297,298], and all agree it represents an important neurosurgical emergency[299].

Pathogenesis

The pathogenesis of subdural empyema varies with the age of the child. In infants, the disease is generally preceded by acute meningitis[300] and therefore caused by the organisms commonly implicated in that disease process, most notably *H. influenzae, S. pneumoniae,* and Gram-negative rods. Subdural empyema complicates about 2% of cases of meningitis[300,301]. In older children and young adults, the subdural space is most often infected by direct spread of infection from the middle ear or paranasal sinuses[302]. Involvement of the subdural space may occur by spread of infection through the emissary veins, which are thin-walled and valveless and thereby allow unchecked connection between the dura and surrounding structures. Other ways in which the subdural space may become infected include direct extension of purulent material from an osteomyelitis of the skull, sinus, or adjacent abscess[256]. Chronic otitis media, mastoiditis, and previous head trauma may all predispose to development of subdural empyema, as can the presence of a chronic subdural effusion that subsequently becomes infected. Unlike the epidural space, the subdural space is not limited by attachment of the dura to the skull sutures allowing extension and spread of the empyema over wide areas of the hemisphere[256].

The majority of empyemas form on the convexity of the brain surface, over the cerebral hemispheres, with a smaller percentage occurring in the parafalcine region[303,304]. The potential subdural space is restricted at the base of the brain, so involvement there is rare. The majority of patients have unilateral involvement, although bilateral empyemas may occur in infants following purulent meningitis. Death may occur from severe elevation of ICP with herniation, cortical venous thrombosis, or extensive involvement of the brain parenchyma.

Clinical Manifestations

Subdural empyema may take an acute or subacute course, and generally the patient has signs of intracranial hypertension, meningismus, and cerebral dysfunction—symptoms in the older child that are similar to those of brain abscess.

Headache, vomiting, obtundation, and herniation may occur in rapid succession, and these symptoms are usually accompanied by fever and stiff neck. Most patients exhibit focal neurologic signs consisting of hemiparesis, hemiplegia, or seizures. Other patients may have ocular, brainstem, or cerebellar signs. Head size may increase in young infants, who generally exhibit bulging fontanelle, generalized signs such as irritability, lethargy, poor feeding, and vomiting, as early indications of disease[(256)].

The organisms responsible for the localized parameningeal infectious process are similar to those causing brain abscesses and depend on the pathogenic mechanisms and the age of the child. In the child and young adult, the most common organisms are the various aerobic streptococci, especially *S. pneumoniae. Staphylococcus epidermidis* and *S. aureus* follow closely. In the infant, the organisms most closely resemble the spectrum of agents seen in neonatal and infantile meningitis.

Laboratory and Radiologic Diagnosis

Laboratory findings are similar to those of brain abscess. The total WBC count is generally elevated as is the erythrocyte sedimentation rate. It may be difficult to differentiate subdural empyema from acute purulent meningitis when neck stiffness is present. Focal neurologic signs, clinical evidence of intracranial hypertension, or the findings of papilledema should make the clinician strongly suspicious of a parameningeal infection. In these cases, a spinal tap should be deferred because nearly 50% of such patients with subdural empyema may herniate within several hours of the lumbar puncture[(305)]. When completed, the results are variable, generally demonstrating mixed pleocytosis with lymphocytic or polymorphonuclear predominance, elevated protein, normal glucose and sterile cultures, findings more suggestive of a parameningeal focus of infection than meningitis.

CNS neuroimaging studies are diagnostic methods of choice. The CT scan usually defines the subdural process[(306)] but may occasionally fail to document the presence of the infected mass[(307,308)]. The usual appearance on CT scan is that of crescent-shaped lesion, which is hypodense, occasionally with visible loculations, and mass effect with shift of midline structures away from the side of the mass. Enhancement of the area immediately adjacent to the dura often occurs when contrast is injected. Sometimes parenchymal enhancement is also seen[(408,411)]. MRI is now the diagnostic imaging procedure of choice. Advantages of MRI over CT scan include the lack of bone artifact, the ability to detect smaller extracranial fluid collections, and the improved ability to differentiate extracranial collection of fluid from cerebritis, cerebral edema, and venous thrombosis[(256)]. MRI can also detect the density difference from elevated protein concentration and distinguish subdural abscess from sterile collections, such as subdural effusion.

Regardless of the method chosen to document the presence of the subdural empyema, the diagnosis must first be suspected in any infant with a known diagnosis of meningitis, or in an older child following penetrating head trauma, chronic otitis, sinusitis, mastoiditis, or cerebral abscess. Only through prompt suspicion, recognition, and diagnosis can the otherwise dismal outcome be altered.

Therapy

Eradication of the infectious focus requires a combined medical and surgical approach. However, the most appropriate or efficacious surgical intervention remains unclear in infants with subdural empyema complicating meningitis diagnostic paracentesis and possibly repeated subdural taps and antibiotic therapy is usually adequate.

When the empyema is secondary to otic or sinus infection, the empyema is usually grossly purulent and requires surgical drainage either through burr holes or more usually through craniotomy. Whatever surgical approach is taken, medical management, consisting of high-dose antibiotic therapy, control of intracranial hypertension, and miscellaneous supportive measures must be part of the ongoing care provided in the PICU. Antibiotics are continued for 3 to 6 weeks, and the progression of the lesion should be followed with serial CT or MRI scans.

The choice of antibiotics before obtaining cultures and sensitivity results will depend on the source of the infection. The appropriate treatment for meningitis (see previous discussion) can continue if the empyema complicates meningitis. This will usually consist of a third-generation cephalosporin. Empirical antimicrobial therapy for other forms of subdural empyema is the same for brain abscess **(Table 32.19).**

Outcome

Before the development of effective antibiotics, and even with surgical therapy, subdural empyema carried a mortality of at least 65%[(308,309)], which fell to 25 to 40% in the early antibiotic era. Currently, the rate is between 10% and 20% with advanced diagnostic methods and development of sophisticated neurointensive care techniques[(310,311)]. The most common problems following therapy are cerebral atrophy, seizures, and hemiparesis. Cortical dysfunction appears to be uncommon.

Spinal Epidural Abscess

Acute spinal epidural abscess is a distinctly uncommon entity, particularly in children[312,313]. Although the disease is rare and diagnosis is difficult, the complications of the disease are tragic and extreme because the victim may become paraplegic. Prompt diagnosis and treatment is crucial since the outcome is good if the diagnosis is made and therapy initiated before paralysis is complete. For this reason, we include the entity in this textbook.

Pathogenesis

Acute spinal epidural abscess may develop either from hematogenous dissemination from a distant site of infection or from local extension of an adjacent site of infection. Spinal trauma is also associated with spinal epidural abscess but its relevance is difficult to confirm in children. Perhaps a small traumatic epidural hematoma develops in these cases and is subsequently infected by transient bacteremia. In approximately 25 to 50% of patients, infection of the epidural space appears to arise from hematogenous spread usually from a skin or soft tissue site. Focal extension from an adjacent site of infection, e.g., vertebral osteomyelitis or diskitis, is a frequent pathogenic mechanism in adults with spinal epidural abscess but is uncommon in children[314]. Only rarely is spinal epidural abscess a complication of spinal anesthesia, diagnostic myelogram or lumbar puncture. *S. aureus* is the usual infecting organism (80% of cases). *S. viridans, S. pneumoniae* and *Salmonellae* each accounts for fewer than 5% of cases. Most cases (60%) of spinal epidural abscess are located in the thoracic or lumbar area and usually involve the posterior aspect of the epidural space[315].

Pathophysiology

The pathophysiology of acute spinal epidural abscess is more complex than it might appear. Probably the most important aspect in the progression of the disease is actual compression of the spine, with resultant ischemia. In addition, granulation tissue forms around the epidural abscess, and this tissue may compress the spine. Inflammation of the blood vessels may lead to thrombosis. Whether the paraplegia is due to ischemia and infarction secondary to thrombosis and venous thrombophlebitis, rather than cord compression[316], remains open to question, and autopsy data would suggest a combination of factors are involved[317].

Clinical Manifestations

The clinical presentation of spinal epidural abscess is related to patient age. Typically, in the first of four classically described phases, the adult develops back pain and severe spinal tenderness and generally seeks medical attention within 1 to 2 days of onset of these symptoms. In the second phase, nerve root involvement develops, producing hyperesthesias and other sensory deficits in a dermatomal distribution that may mimic sciatica, or even an acute abdomen[318]. Subsequently, limb paresis and sphincter disturbances may occur, implying impaired cord function. The final phase of the disease is characterized by total paraplegia[318]. The interval between the stage of absent or minimal neurologic abnormality and complete paraplegia may be as short as a few hours[319] but is usually several days.

In pediatric patients, particularly in infants and young children, the typical progression is not necessarily followed[318]. The usual clinical picture is that of fever, back pain, spine tenderness with a reluctance to lie prone progressing to weakness and paralysis. Root pain is only present in 20% of children with spinal epidural abscess[315]. Because of the difficulty in making the diagnosis in children, findings of neurologic deficits are already often present at the time of diagnosis. Physical examination reveals fever, possibly rigors and sometimes paraspinal and spinal swelling, induration, and tenderness. Irritation of dorsal nerve roots or T8–L1, which innervate the abdomen, may give rise to confusing abdominal findings that can mimic appendicitis[320] or even septic hip arthritis[314]. Meningismus may be present.

Infants present with fever and irritability but because of the nonspecificity of the symptoms and the difficulty in making the diagnosis, are usually admitted with established severe neurologic deficits[315]. **Table 32.20** outlines the common signs and symptoms of 55 pediatric cases of spinal epidural abscess collected from the literature[315]. Even in older children, many patients have evidence of neurologic compromise, including abnormal deep tendon reflexes, abnormalities of sensation, bladder and bowel incontinence, and extremity weakness and paralysis.

The differential diagnosis of spinal epidural abscess should include vertebral osteomyelitis, diskitis, herniated disk, spinal cord tumor, transverse myelitis, and even meningitis.

Table 32.20. Signs and Symptoms in 55 Cases of Spinal Epidural Abscess

Signs and Symptoms	%
Fever	64
Back pain	54
Paralysis	45
Rigor	44
Sphinteric disturbance	38
Paresis	33
Spinal tenderness	27
Sensory level	24
Radicular pain	20
Irritability	16
Paraspinous mass	16
Headache	11
Nausea and vomiting	9
Lethargy	5
Paresthesia	5
Papilledema	2

From Rubin G, Michowiz SD, Ashkenasi A, Tadmor R, Rappaport ZH. Spinal epidural abscess in the pediatric age group: case report and review of the literature. Pediatr Infect Dis J 1993;12:1007–1011.

Laboratory and Radiologic Diagnosis

White blood cell count is usually elevated as is the erythrocytic sedimentation rate. A lumbar puncture is frequently attempted in these patients because meningitis is suspected rather than spinal epidural abscess. In some of these cases, the abscess has been inadvertently tapped and frank pus aspirated. In others, there were less overt signs of meningeal infection with mild CSF leukocytosis, elevated protein concentration and/or hypoglycorrhagia[315]. Occasionally only the CSF protein was elevated. If spinal epidural abscess is suspected, spinal tap should not be performed for the following reasons: (1) there is a risk of inoculating the subarachnoid space with pus from the abscess, and (2) if there is a total spinal block, CSF drainage below the block may induce neurologic deterioration by causing downward spinal herniation[321].

Plain radiographs are usually unremarkable unless there is evidence of osteomyelitis or diskitis but occasionally paravertebral swelling may be noted. In the past, contrast myelography was the standard test. This procedure could demonstrate the location of the block but not the extent of the abscess. MRI and CT scanning are now the preferred diagnostic tests. MRI is the imaging modality of choice particularly with gadolinium contrast to enhance the images[322,323]. If an MRI scan is not available a CT scan may be helpful but is only diagnosis in 30% of cases[324]. The entire spine should be imaged because occasionally multiple abscesses are present.

Treatment

Surgical decompression with laminectomy with/without an epidural drain is the treatment of choice supplemented by appropriate antibiotic administration. Performing a laminectomy over many levels may cause concern because of the risk of instability and spinal deformity[315]. Appropriate cultures of pus are made at the time of drainage, and antibiotics therapy should be tailored to the culture results. Because of the high incidence of *S. aureus* as the cause of spinal epidural abscess, initial therapy should consist of a penicillinase-resistant penicillin together with a third-generation cephalosporin for Gram-negative coverage. Antibiotic therapy should be continued for at least 4 weeks.

Outcome

It is widely believed that early diagnosis and treatment are crucial for a good outcome. Early series describing spinal epidural infections reported high mortality, but many of these deaths were undoubtedly due to complications of paraplegia and sepsis. With modern-day management of this disease, including emergent laminectomy and antibiotic coverage, death is uncommon and the main issues of prognosis relate to the neurologic recovery to be expected in these patients. Huesner[318] suggested that if paralysis was present for less than 24 hours, prognosis for complete or partial recovery was good; however, paralysis for greater than 36 hours was associated with a poor prognosis. This has been corroborated in subsequent series[319,325,326]. The outcome in children is largely dependent on their neurologic condition at the time of hospitalization. In virtually all cases children who are symptomatic but without abnormal neurologic signs and children who have paresis can be expected to make a full recovery[315]. Of children who are paralyzed, approximately one-third will recover completely[315]. In a series of pediatric cases collected from the literature since 1980[315], 7% died, 14% were left with neurologic damage, and 80% were normal, outcomes that probably reflect the greater difficulty of diagnosis in children than in adults. Therefore, the outcome of this disease is largely related to the skill with which the clinician diagnoses the disease, a skill that consists primarily of an awareness of the entity and diagnostic speed.

Cerebral Malaria

Cerebral malaria is a clinical syndrome characterized by CNS dysfunction associated with *Plasmodium falciparum* infection. Although it is one of the major causes of death in children in sub-Saharan Africa, it is rarely seen in developed countries. However, with the increase in international travel, the incidence of severe falciparum malaria, including cerebral malaria, in developed countries is likely to increase[327].

Parasitology

Malaria is caused by protozoan parasites, of which only four species infect humans: *P. falciparum, P. ovale, P. vivax,* and *P. malariae. P. falciparum* is responsible for almost all the life-threatening disease, although *P. vivax* is rarely associated with splenic rupture[328]. The parasites are transmitted by female Anopheline mosquitos, which usually bite at night. Sporozoites enter into the bloodstream during feedingand undergo a stage of development in the liver, before invading the erythrocytes. In the erythrocytes, the parasites undergo a 48-hour cycle, growing from a ring stage, through trophozoite stages to schizonts, which burst and release merozoites into the blood stream. The erythrocytic stages are responsible for producing clinical symptoms. The cause of *P. falciparum* virulence is unknown, but a number of factors may contribute: it has a shorter pre-erythrocytic stage, prepatent period (interval between infection and appearance of parasites in the erythrocytes), and incubation period[329]. *P. falciparum* also produces more merozoites, which invade red cells of any age. Since more than one merozoite can infect a single red cell, multiple infections are common. All of these factors culminate in a parasitemia of 20 to 500,000/μl, which is a log order greater than infections with the other plasmodial parasites. Furthermore, *P. falciparum* is unique among plasmodial species that infect humans because the late trophozoites and schizonts are sequestered in the microcirculation of vital organs. Sequestration enhances the survival of the parasite, since it promotes growth in the relatively hypoxic environment of the venous circulation and permits the late erythrocytic stages to evade clearance by the spleen. However, sequestration may obstruct blood flow and impair metabolism of surrounding parenchymal cells and thereby cause the severe complications of falciparum malaria such as cerebral involvement[(330)], which is not found in the other types of human malaria.

Pathology

The pathologic hallmark of cerebral malaria is engorgement of the cerebral capillaries and venules with parasitized erythrocytes. This feature is not pathognomic, since it is also present in patients with noncerebral malaria[(331)], but the degree of sequestration is much greater in cerebral malaria. Macroscopically, the brain appears swollen with flattened gyri and ventricular compression. Cerebral edema is a common finding postmortem, but is rarely detected by computerized tomography during life. The cut surface of the brain is slate gray with multiple petechial hemorrhages scattered throughout parenchyma. The sequestration of erythrocytes containing mature stages of *P. falciparum* in the microvasculature of the brain is attributed to cytoadherence, the specific binding of the parasitized red cell to the endothelial cells of the vessels[(332)]. The binding appears to be mediated by parasite-derived proteins that form 'knobs' on the red cell surface, which attach to receptors, e.g., CD 36 and intracellular adhesion molecule (ICAM-1), on the luminal surface of the endothelial cells. Cytoadherence is promoted by low shear stress, possibly explaining the predilection of sequestration in the post capillary venules. Parasitized red cells also bind to uninfected cells to form rosettes, which may also play a role in the pathophysiology.

Pathogenesis

The pathogenesis of cerebral malaria is unknown, and the mechanisms of neurologic dysfunction are likely to be multifactorial. The most favored underlying hypotheses are the mechanical obstruction of the microvasculature by the sequestered parasites and/or the effect of toxic substances. Obstruction of blood flow through microvessels could reduce the delivery of oxygen and other substrates, causing a reduction in metabolism and level of consciousness. Cerebral lactate production is increased[(333)], possibly as a result of anaerobic glycolysis in the brain secondary to hypoxia. However, global ischemiais not a feature, since cerebral blood flow is not decreased[(333)] and most patients survive without sequelae.

Toxins are produced by parasitized erythrocytes, but their biologic functions have not been determined. However, plasmodial infections have been shown to stimulate monocytes to produce cytokines, principally TNFα, IL-1, and IL-6. TNF production significantly increases with schizont rupture and TNF is probably the mediator of fever associated with schizogony[(334)]. TNF stimulates the synthesis of nitric oxide, which in turn has been proposed as a central mediator in the pathogenesis of cerebral malaria[(335)], since it interferes with neuronal transmission by inhibiting glutamate induced excitatory synaptic activity. Furthermore, nitric oxide is a potent vasodilator, which may increase the cerebral blood volume. Circulating TNFα, IL-1 and IL-6 levels are high in African children with falciparum malaria and although there is considerable overlap in the TNFα concentrations, significantly higher concentrations were found in those with severe malaria compared with nonsevere malaria. The highest concentrations were associated with young age, hyperparasitemia, severe anemia, hypoglycemia, and death[(334)]. Besides coma, cytokines may be responsible for other manifestation of severe falciparum malaria, such as hypoglycemia, dyserythropoiesis and metabolic acidosis[(336)].

Pathophysiology

The pathophysiology of severe falciparum malaria in nonimmune individuals appears to be different from that in African children who are exposed to the parasites from birth[(328,337)]. Hypoglycemia, lactic acidosis, and severe anemia occur in both groups, but superinfections, pulmonary edema, and renal failure are much more common in nonimmune individuals. Most of the clinical studies were conducted in nonimmune adults, with little data published on nonimmune children.

Cerebral Hemodynamics

ICP is elevated in almost all African children with cerebral malaria[(338)]. Severe intracranial hypertension is associated with neurologic sequelae, transtentorial herniation, and death[(338–340)]. However, in nonimmune adults, transtentorial herniation is not a common postmortem feature, and opening lumbar puncture pressures are normal in most patients[(341)].

Raised ICP is probably caused by an increase in cerebral blood volume, secondary to an increase in cerebral blood flow and/or from the sequestration of cells within the cerebral microvasculature[(339)]. Cerebral blood flow is normal in adults, but cerebral vascular resistance appears to be increased[(333)]. In African children, CBF velocity is increased, particularly in association with seizures[(339)]. Cerebral edema does not appear to play a major role in raising the ICP in most immune and nonimmune patients; however, cytotoxic edema is associated with severe intracranial hypertension[(342)]. The blood-brain barrier appears to be intact in most patients, because the CSF protein is usually normal and cerebral edema is not detected on the CT scans of adults[(343)] or African children[(342)]. Furthermore, studies using radiolabeled albumin in adults found no difference in the entry of albumin to the CSF while the patients were unconsciousness or when they recovered[(341)].

Seizures

Seizures are an important presenting feature of cerebral malaria, especially in African children, and are associated with a poor outcome. Focal motor and generalized tonic-clonic convulsions are most commonly seen, but subclinical seizures that are only evident on electroencephalography are also present. The level of consciousness in some children improves with the administration of anticonvulsants suggesting that seizures are responsible for the depression of consciousness. The cause of the seizures in cerebral malaria is unclear, but is probably multifactorial. Seizures are unlikely to be simple febrile convulsions, since they occur more frequently than febrile convulsions in other groups of children and often have localizing features. Hypoglycemia and hyponatremia may be contributory factors. No association exists between intracranial hypertension and seizures.

Hypoglycemia

Hypoglycemia is a common complication of severe falciparum malaria, particularly cerebral malaria. In African children, it is significantly associated with neurologic sequelae and death[344]. The pathogenesis of hypoglycemia in nonimmune adults appears to be different to that in African children. In nonimmune adults, nonketotic hypoglycemia is caused by hyperinsulinemia, particularly during pregnancy and after the administration of quinine[345]. Although quinine administration also increases insulin secretion in African children, the hypoglycemic effect is not as marked, and when quinine is infused with 5% dextrose, it does not cause severe hypoglycemia[346]. In African children, hypoglycemia appears to be caused by impaired hepatic gluconeogenesis, resulting from either reduced hepatic blood flow[347], or lactate inhibiting the uptake of amino acids by the liver[344]. In addition, there may be an increase in utilization of glucose by the parasitized erythrocytes and hypoxic tissue aggravated by an enhanced basal metabolic rate. Hypoglycemia is not the cause of coma in these children, since the level of consciousness rarely improves after the administration of 50% glucose.

Lactic Acidosis

Lactic acidosis is a prominent feature of cerebral malaria in both nonimmune adults and African children. Lactic acid concentrations are increased in CSF and blood, with higher concentrations measured in fatal cases compared with survivors[348]. In African children, lactic acidosis is more common in younger children, those with deep coma, hypoglycemia, or severe anemia[349]. Both in African children and nonimmune adults, admission CSF lactate concentrations are a good predictor of outcome in cerebral malaria.

Lactate may be produced by anaerobic glycolysis of the parasitized erythrocytes and/or the human host. Most lactate is probably derived from the human host, for even with generous estimates of parasite burden, humans would be able to metabolize the lactate produced by the parasites[350]. Lactic acidosis may contribute to the pathophysiology of cerebral malaria, since it promotes cytoadherance and impairs gluconeogenesis and cardiac output.

Anemia

Hemolytic anemia resulting from the destruction of parasitized erythrocytes is an inevitable consequence of a falciparum malaria infection. Severe anemia is one of the life-threatening complications of *P. falciparum* in African children, either in the presence or absence of cerebral malaria or acidosis. Besides destruction of the parasitized erythrocytes by the spleen[351], anemia may be caused by failure of the bone marrow to produce erythrocytes manifesting as dyserythropoiesis[352] and immune-mediated intravascular hemolysis of both parasitized and nonparasitized red blood cells. In children with cerebral malaria, the lowest hematocrit is reached within the first 24 hours after treatment[353]. It is during this time that the fall in hemoglobin will have the most profound effects on the cardiovascular system, frequently requiring life-saving blood transfusions.

Clinical Manifestations

The direct CNS involvement of *P. falciparum* is difficult to define, since there are no pathognomonic pathologic features and CNS manifestations such as seizures, drowsiness, or flaccidity may be induced by the systemic effects of the falciparum infection (e.g., fever or hyponatremia). Thus, the World Health Organization[328] has adopted strict criteria for the diagnosis of cerebral malaria. These criteria include: (1) a patient is unable to localize a painful stimulus (such as pressure on the sternum) at least one hour after last seizure; (2) asexual parasites are present in the peripheral blood; and (3) other causes of encephalopathy (e.g., meningitis, encephalitis, or hypoglycemia) are excluded. Although this definition is suitable for research purposes, any child with *P. falciparum* infection and disturbed consciousness should be treated for cerebral malaria.

Cerebral malaria should be suspected in any child who has visited or even transiently landed at an airport in an endemic area and develops CNS symptoms such as headache and mental status changes. Currently, the risk of acquiring the infection from blood transfusions is very low. Congenital malaria occurs in infants born to nonimmune mothers who have a parasitemia during the later stages of pregnancy, particularly at the time of parturition.

Children with malaria usually have a history of fever, headache, irritability, restlessness, or drowsiness. They may refuse food, but are initially often very thirsty. Vomiting and to a lesser extent diarrhea are common, but are seldom so severe as to cause dehydration or electrolyte depletion. Children may also complain of abdominal pain and some are constipated.

Fever is usually present, although its absence does not exclude the diagnosis. In most children, the temperature is greater than 39°C, often continuous or irregular, and without any definite pattern. Mild icterus is common. Meningism may be present such that cerebral malaria cannot be differentiated clinically from bacterial meningitis[354]. Seizures are common and often precipitate the lapse into unconsciousness. Brainstem signs including dysconjugate eye movement and decerebrate posturing also occur. Retinal hemorrhages may be present, but papilledema is rare. The liver is often enlarged and may be slightly tender. Splenic enlargement, which may not be present on admission, usually occurs a few days into the illness. Spontaneous bleeding from the gastrointestinal tract occurs in nonimmune individuals.

Laboratory Features

The parasite count in severe falciparum malaria varies considerably, ranging from a barely detectable parasitemia to greater than 20% erythrocytes parasitized. Although children with higher parasitemias tend to be sicker than those with low parasitemias, some children are very ill even with a low degree of parasitemia. The lack of a detectable parasitemia does not exclude the diagnosis of cerebral malaria, since the parasites may be sequestered within the deep vascular beds, or chemoprophylaxis may have suppressed the parasitemia. Thus, blood smears need to be examined every 6 hours for 48 hours to exclude this infection.

Anemia, usually with evidence of hemolysis (raised unconjugated bilirubinemia, low haptoglobin concentration) is almost always present. Severe anemia (hemoglobin < 5.0 g/dl) can occur in up to a third of nonimmune patients with cerebral malaria. Thrombocytopenia is common, but rarely severe enough to cause bleeding. Fibrin degradation products are raised, but laboratory features of frank disseminated intravascular coagulation are uncommon.

Hypoglycemia and a lactic acidosis are the major metabolic complications. Hypoxemia is associated with pulmonary edema and infections. Renal impairment is common. Hyponatremia is mainly caused by salt depletion, but some cases may be caused by inappropriate ADH secretion. Hypoalbuminemia is also common and may result in low plasma calcium concentrations. Hypophosphatemia is a feature of severe malaria and may be exacerbated by glucose therapy.

CSF is usually acellular and other diagnoses such as encephalitis should be entertained if a pleocytosis is found, but cerebral malaria cannot be excluded. CSF lactate concentrations are raised, but protein and glucose concentrations are usually normal. Blood cultures may reveal an occult septicemia, particularly caused by Gram-negative organisms and urine cultures should be done to detect concurrent urinary tract infections. Tracheal aspirates and a chest roentgenogram are required for the detection of chest infections.

Clinical Course

Nonimmune individuals tend to remain unconscious for a median of 48 hours after the onset of treatment. Seizures may occur in about 50%. Neurologic sequelae that include cranial nerve lesions, extrapyramidal tremor, polyneuropathy, epilepsy, or psychiatric manifestations occur in about 5% of nonimmune individuals[328,355]. In African children, sequelae are more common and more severe. Hemiparesis, ataxia, epilepsy and cortical blindness are the most common sequelae, but some children are left in a vegetative state[356]. The mortality in nonimmune individuals ranges from 15to 26%, with patients usually dying within the first 4 days of the illness from renal failure or pulmonary edema. In African children, the mortality is similar, but most children die within 24 hours of admission with brainstem signs suggestive of herniation, metabolic acidosis, severe hypoglycemia, or anemia.

Treatment

Any child with severe falciparum malaria should be admitted to the intensive care unit (See **Table 32.21**). The management of a child with cerebral malaria should be considered in three phases: the management of a child with impaired level of consciousness, antimalarial therapy, and treatment of the complications. The management of an unconscious child is discussed in Chapter 21. This section deals with a specific antimalarial therapy and the treatment of the complications.

Antimalarial Therapy

Treatment of severe falciparum malaria is complicated by the emergence of parasites that are resistant to various antimalarial drugs and the difficulty of obtaining specific antimalarial drugs in various countries. Any child with features of severe falciparum malaria, should be treated with a parental antimalarial therapy **(Table 32.22).** At present, the drugs of choice for treatment of severe falciparum malaria are the cinchinoid alkaloids, quinine, and its diastereomer quinidine[357,358]. Since quinine for intravenous administration is unavailable in the United States, quinidine is the agent of choice for parenteral use in the country. These drugs are effective against the latter erythrocytic stages, decreasing the parasitemia after about 12to 24 hours of therapy. Most authorities recommend a loading dose to rapidly achieve high therapeutic levels[328,358,359], but this should be avoided in the children who have been given cinchinoids or mefloquine within the last 24 hours. Mild side effects are common, particularly cinchonism (tinnitus, hearing loss, nausea, restlessness, and blurred vision). Se-

Table 32.21. Indications for Admission of a Patient With Cerebral Malaria to the ICU

Any perturbation of consciousness, more than 1 hour after a seizure
Parasitemia > 5% erythrocytes
Hb < 5.0 g/dl or massive intravascular hemolysis
Repeated episodes of hypoglycemia
Severe metabolic acidosis: pH < 7.2
Spontaneous bleeding
Renal failure
Pulmonary edema

Table 32.22. Antimalarial Therapy

Primary antimalarial therapy	
Quinidine (6.2 mg base = 10 mg gluconate salt)	6.2 mg base/kg IV infusion over 1–2 hours, followed by 0.012 mg/kg/min for 72 hours or until patient can swallow.
Quinine (12.5 mg base = 15 mg dihydrochloride salt)	12.5 mg base/kg (loading dose) diluted in isotonic fluid by IV infusion over 2 hours, then 8.4 mg/kg over 2 hours until patient can swallow.
Drugs used to achieve complete cure	
Quinine sulfate	25 mg/kg/day tid for 3–7 days.
Sulfadoxine + pyrimethamine (Fansidar ®)	Single dose of: < 1 yr: ¼ tablet 1–3 yr: ½ tablet 4–8 yr: 1 tablet 9–14 yr: 2 tablets >14 yr: 3 tablets
Clindamycin	20–40 mg/kg/day tid for 3 days.

rious cardiovascular side effects, such as hypotension and cardiac arrhythmias, may occur if the drugs are administered undiluted and too rapidly. The Q-T interval should be monitored during the infusion. Hypoglycemia is an important complication of drug therapy in nonimmune individuals[345]. Since cinchinoid drugs can also cause severe CNS toxicity such as blindness, coma, and convulsions, their levels should be monitored, if possible.

Currently, other antimalarial drugs should be used as adjuncts against parasites that are relatively resistant to the cinchinoids, to shorten the course of therapy, or for the treatment of nonsevere falciparum malaria. Halofantrine is an effective drug with limited resistance. However, cardiovascular toxicity and a lack of a parental formula limit its use in severe falciparum malaria. Mefloquine is also effective in most areas but cannot be given parentally, and its bioavailability is reduced in patients with cerebral malaria when it is administered in a nasogastric tube. Chloroquine is an effective blood schizonticide, but the spread of chloroquine-resistant strains of *P. falciparum* has severely limited its use, and it should not be used in the treatment of severe falciparum malaria. The sulfonamides (sulfadoxine, sulfalene, and cotrimoxazole) used in combination with other drugs (pyrimethamine) can be used for presumptive treatment but should not be used for the treatment of severe falciparum malaria. The biquanides (proguanil and chlorproguanil) are useful prophylactic drugs. Antibiotics (tetracycline, doxycycline, clindamycin, and fluoroquinolones) are effective against the blood stages, but should not be used as primary antimalarial drugs, although they can be used to achieve a clinical cure of infection caused by strains that are refractory to the cinchinoids. The peroxide antimalarial drugs (artesunate, artemether, and arteether) are fast-acting and act against all blood stages, reducing the time to parasite clearance and fever resolution in comparison to the cinchinoid alkaloids. The peroxide drugs are undergoing clinical trials and are not yet universally available, but may become effective alternatives to the cinchinoids for the treatment of severe malaria.

Supportive Treatment

Children with severe falciparum malaria should be monitored closely. Blood glucose and fluid balance should be measured every 6 hours, parasitemia and hematocrit every 12 hours. Electrolytes, tests of renal function, albumin, calcium, phosphate, and blood gases should be performed at least daily during the acute stages.

Hyperpyrexia should be treated with standard modalities for lowering temperature. Seizures must be treated promptly with a benzodiazepine drug, and a prophylactic anticonvulsant such as phenytoin or phenobarbital should be used if they recur. Stomach contents should be aspirated through a nasogastric tube to reduce the risk of aspiration pneumonia. Elective endotracheal intubation is indicated for progressive obtundation (Glasgow coma scale 8 or less). A CT or MRI scan should be completed to exclude brain swelling before a lumbar puncture is performed. If brain swelling is detected, ICP monitoring should be considered. Raised ICP may be controlled by mannitol[339], but the role of hyperventilation is unclear. Steroids appear to be deleterious, increasing the incidence of bleeding without any beneficial effect on outcome[355]. Other treatments such as heparin, prostacyclin, dextran, or epinephrine have been advocated without adequate evidence and are not recommended[328].

Blood transfusions should be considered when the hematocrit falls toward 20%, or the child has evidence of cardiovascular compromise. The role of exchange transfusions in the management of cerebral malaria is controversial. Exchange transfusions may reduce the parasitemia more rapidly than chemotherapy alone and may also remove harmful metabolites, toxins, and restore normal red cell mass platelets guarding factors albumin and other depleted substances[360]. The advantages must be balanced against the dangers of this procedure, and as yet there have been no control trials demonstrating the benefit of this procedure[358]. However, most authorities recommend exchange transfusion in patients who have parasitemias in excess of 10% or who are deteriorating in spite of conventional treatment. Vitamin K and cryoprecipitate should be administered if a patient has a bleeding diathesis.

Blood glucose concentration needs to be monitored frequently and checked if the patient deteriorates. A therapeutic trial of 50% glucose 0.6 ml/kg by intravenous bolus injection should be administered if hypoglycemia is suspected, and should be followed by a continuous infusion of 10% dextrose if episodes of hypoglycemia recur. If repeated doses of hypertonic dextrose for the treatment of the hyperinsulinemic hypoglycemia aggravate the electrolyte disturbances or fluid overload, then a somatostatin analogue sandrostatin SMS201-995 can be tried as a single subcutaneous dose of 50 μg[361]. Lactic acidosis is treated by correcting hypovolemia and improving oxygenation. Sodium bicarbonate appears to be of little value, and although dichloracetate improves lactic acidosis[362], this drug has not been shown to improve the outcome.

Dehydration must be cautiously corrected, since fluid overload may precipitate fatal pulmonary edema. Renal function needs to be carefully monitored because acute renal failure is a common cause of death in nonimmune patients. Indications for dialysis or hemofiltration include hyperkalemia, uremia, metabolic acidosis, and pulmonary edema. Massive intravascular hemolysis is also an indication for dialysis to avoid fluid overload during the life-saving blood transfusions. Patients with pulmonary edema or adult respiratory distress syndrome require supplemental oxygen and positive pressure ventilation, with positive end expiratory pressure to maintain adequate oxygenation, and diuretics or hemofiltration to correct the fluid overload.

Secondary bacterial infections should always be suspected. Blood, urine, and CSF should be sent for culture, and repeated examinations of the chest should be performed since aspiration or hypostatic pneumonia are common. Broad spectrum antimicrobial treatment should be started as soon as a complicating infection is suspected.

Severe falciparum malaria is a multisystem disease and advice from hematologists, infectious disease specialists, and nephrologists may be needed. A reference center, such as the Center for Disease Control (CDC) in Atlanta, should be contacted for current information about antimalarial therapy.

SUMMARY

This chapter has covered many issues pertaining to infections of bacterial and viral and protozoal origin that primarily affect the CNS. Pathogenesis and pathophysiology of these disorders as well as diagnostic methods and approaches to therapy have been stressed. Understanding expected perturbations of cerebral physiology allows the pediatric intensive care specialist to develop a comprehensive approach to treatment for children who have these infections, and provide an appropriate level of intensive care aimed at preserving CNS function while treating the underlying disorder. If the outcome of some of these problems is to be improved, sophisticated methods of controlling intracranial hypertension and preserving cerebral blood flow must be employed in a rational and consistent manner.

References

1. Schech WF. The epidemiology of bacterial meningitis antibiotics. Antibiotics and Chemotherapy 1992;45:5–17.
2. Wenger JD, Hightower AW, Facklam RR, Gaventa S, Broome CV and the Bacterial Meningitis Study Group. Bacterial meningitis in the United States, 1986; Report of a multistate surveillance study. J Infect Dis 1990;162:1316–1323.
3. Phillips CF. Epidemiology of bacterial meningitis. Pediatric Annals 1994;23:67.
4. U.S. Public Health Service: Progress toward elimination of Haemophilus influenzae type b disease among infants and children - United States, 1993-–994. Morbid Mortal Weekly Report 1995;44:545–6.
5. Gromisch DS, Gordon SG, Bedrosian L, Sall T. Simultaneous mixed bacterial meningitis in an infant. Am J Dis Child 1970;119:284.
6. Herweg JC, Middlekamp JN, Hartmann AF. Simultaneous mixed bacterial meningitis in children. J Pediatr 1963;63:76.
7. Tunkel AR, Sheld WM. Pathogenesis and pathophysiology of bacterial meningitis. Ann Rev Med 1993;44:103.
8. Sáez-Llorens X, Ramilo O, Mustafa MM, Mertsola J, McCracken GH. Molecular pathophysiology of bacterial meningits: current concepts and therapeutic implications. J Pediatr 1990;116:671–684.
9. Weber A, Harris R, Lohrke S, Forney L, Smith AL. Inability to express fymbrial results in impaired ability of *Haemophilus influenzae* b to colonize the nasopharynx. Infect Immun 1991;59:4724–4728.
10. Moxon ER, Smith AL, Averill DR, Smith DH. *Haemophilus influenzae* meningitis in infant rats after intranasal innoculation. J Infect Dis 1974;129:154–162.
11. Parkkinen J, Korhonen TK, Pere A, Hacker J, Soinila S. Binding sites in the rat brain for *Escherichia coli* S. fimbriae associated with neonatal meningitis. J Clin Invest 1988;81:860–865.
12. Simberkoff MS, Moldover NH, Rahal JJ Jr. Absence of detectable bactericidal and opsonic activities in normal and infected human cerebrospinal fluids: a regional host defense deficiency. J Lab Clin Med 1980;95:362–372.
13. Rahal JJ, Simberkoff MS. Host defense and antimicrobial therapy in adult gram-negative bacillary meningitis. Ann Intern Med 1982; 96:468–474.
14. Tuomanen E, Liu H, Hengstler B, Zak O, Tomasz A. The induction of meningeal inflammation by components of the pneumococcal cell wall. J Infect Dis 1985;151:859–868.
15. Tomasz A, Saukkonen K. The nature of cell wall-derived inflammatory components of pneumococci. Pediatr Infect Dis J 1989;8:902–903.
16. Wispelwey B, Lesse AJ, Hansen EJ, Scheld WM. *Haemophilus influenzae* lipopolysaccharide-induced blood brain barrier permeability during experimental meningitis in the rat. J Clin Invest 1988;82: 1339–1346.
17. Täuber MG, Shibl AM, Hackbarth CJ, Larrick JW, Sande MA. Antibiotic therapy, endotoxin concentration in cerebrospinal fluid, and brain edema in experimental *Escherichia coli* meningitis in rabbits. J Infect Dis 1987;156:456–462.
18. Arditi M, Ables L, Yogev R. Cerebrospinal fluid endotoxin levels in children with *H. influenzae* meningitis before and after administration of intravenous ceftriaxone. J Infect Dis 1989;160:1005–1011.
19. Townsend GC, Scheld WM. Adjunctive therapy for bacterial meningitis: Rationale for use, current status, and prospects for the future. Clin Infect Dis 1993;17(Suppl 2):S537–S549.
20. Waage A, Halstensen A, Shalaby R, Brandtzaeg P, Kierulf P, Espevik T. Local production of tumor necrosis factor α, interleukin 1, and interleukin 6 in meningococcal meningitis: relation to the inflammatory response. J Exp Med 1989;170:1859–1867.
21. Quagliarello V, Scheld WM. Bacterial meningitis: pathophysiology and progress. N Engl J Med 1992;327:864–872.
22. Mustafa MM, Ramilo O, Olsen KD, et al. Tumor necrosis factor in mediating experimental *Haemophilus influenzae* type b meningitis. J Clin Invest 1989;84:1253–1259.
23. Saukkonen K, Sande S, Cioffe C, Wolpes, Sherry B, Cerami A, Tuomanen E. The role of cytokines in the generation of inflammation and tissue damage in experimental gram-positive meningitis. J Exp Med 1990;171:439–448.
24. Mustafa MM, Lebel MH, Ramilo O. Correlation of interleukin-1β and cachectin concentration in cerebrospinal fluid and outcome from bacterial meningitis. J Pediatr 1989;115:208–213.
25. Arditi M, Manogue KR, Caplan M, Yogev R. Cerebrospinal fluid cachectin/tumor necrosis factor-α and platelet-activating factor concentrations and severity of bacterial meningitis in children. J Infect Dis 1990;162:139–147.
26. Quagliarello VJ, Wispelwey B, Long Wj Jr, Scheld WM. Recombinant human interleukin-1 induces meningitis and blod-brain barrier injury in the rat: characterization and comparison with tumor necrosis factor. J Clin Invest 1991;87:1360–1366.
27. Ramilo O, Sáez-Llorens X, Mertsola J, et al. Tumor necrosis factor α/cachectin and interleukin 1β initiate meningeal inflammation. J Exp Med 1990;172:497–507.
28. Mustafa MM, Ramilo O, Sáez-Llorens X, Olsen KD, Magness RR, McCracken GH Jr. Cerebrospinal fluid prostaglandins, interleukin 1β, and tumor necrosis factor in bacterial meningitis: clinical and laboratory cor-

relation in placebo-treated and dexamethasone-treated patients. Am J Dis Child 1990;144:883–887.
29. Tureen JH, Tauber MG, Sande MA. Effect of indomethacin on the pathophysiology of experimental meningitis in rabbits. J Infect Dis 1991;163:647–649.
30. Saukkonen K, Sande S, Coiffe C, et al. The role of cytokines in the generation of inflammation and tissue damage in experimental gram-positive meningitis. J Exp Med 1990;171:439–448.
31. Cabellos C, MacIntyre DE, Forrest M, Boroughs M, Prasad S, Tuomanen E. Differing roles of platelet activating factor during inflammation of the lung and subarachnoid space. J Clin Invest 1992;90:612–618.
32. Koedel U, Bernatowicz A, Paul R, Frei K, Fontana A, Pfister HW. Experimental pneumococcal meningitis: cerebrovascular alterations, brain edema, and meningeal inflammation are linked to the production of nitric oxide. Ann Neurol 1995;37:313–323.
33. Springer TA. Adhesion receptors of the immune system. Nature 1990;346:425–434.
34. Spellerberg B, Tuomanen EI. The pathophysiology of pneumoccal meningitis. Ann Med 1994; 26:411–418.
35. Tuomanen EI, Saukkonen K, Sande S, Cioffe C, Wright SW. Reduction of inflammation, tissue damage and mortality in bacterial meningitis in rabbits treated with monoclonal antibodies against adhesion - promoting receptors of leukocytes. J Exp Med 1989;170:959–969.
36. Sáez-Llorens X, Jafari HS, Severien C. Enhanced attenuation of meningeal inflammation and brain edema by concommitant administration of anti-CD 18 monoclonal antibodies and dexamethasone in experimental Haemophilus meningitis. J Clin Invest 1991;88:2003–2011.
37. Tureen JH, Dworkin RJ, Kennedy SL, Sachdeva M, Sande MA. Loss of cerebrovascular autoregulation in experimental menigitis in rabbits. J Clin Invest 1990;85:577–581.
38. Pfister HW, Koedel U, Haberl Rl, et al. Microvascular changes during the early phase of experimental bacterial meningitis. J Cereb Blood Flow Metab 1990;10:914–922.
39. Tureen JH. Cerebral blood flow and metabolism in experimental meningitis. Pediatr Infect Dis J 1989;8:917–919.
40. Slater AJ, Berkowitz ID, Wilson DA, Traystman RJ. Cerebrovascular responsiveness to CO_2 in *Haemophilus influenzae* type b meningitis in rabbits. Am J Physiol 1994;266(Heart Circ Physiol 35):H1755–H1761.
41. Smith AL, Daum RS, Scheifele D, Syriopolou V, Averill DR, Roberts MC, Stull TL. Pathogenesis of haemophilus influenzae meningitis. In: *Haemophilus influenzae.* Epidemiology, Immunology, and Prevention of Disease, edited SH Sell and PF Wright. New York: Elsevier Biomedical, 1982, 89–109.
42. McKnight AA, Keyes WG, Hudak ML, Jones MD. Oxygen free radicals and the cerebral arteriolar response to group B streptococci. Pediatr Res 1992;31:640–644.
43. Pfister HW, Fontana A, Tauber M, Tomasz A, Scheld MW. Mechanisms of brain injury in bacterial meningitis: Workshop summary. Clin Infect Dis 1994;19:463–479.
44. Tureen JH, Kartalija M, Liu Q. Attenuation of cerebral pathophysiologic antibodies by anti-tumor necrosis factor-alpha monoclonal antibody in experimental pneumococcal meningitis in the rabbit. Abst of the 34th ICAAC 1994;B66.
45. Paulson OB, Hansen EL, Kristensen HS, Brodersen P. Cerebral blood flow, cerebral metabolic rate of oxygen and CSF acid-base parameters in patients with acute pyogenic meningitis and with acute encephalitis. Acta Neurol Scand 1972;28 (Suppl 51):407.
46. McMenamin JB, Volpe JJ. Bacterial meningitis in infancy: effects on intracranial pressure and cerebral blood flow velocity. Neurology 1984;34:500.
47. Goh D, Minns RA. Cerebral blood flow velocity monitoring in pyogenic meningitis. Arch Dis Child 1993;68:111–119.
48. Haring H-P, Rötxer H-K, Reindl H, Berek K, Kampfl A, Pfausler B, Schmutzhard E. Time course of cerebral blood flow velocity in central nervous system infections. Arch Neurol 1993;50:98–101.
49. Ashwal S, Stringer W, Tomasi L, Schneider S, Thompson J, Perkin R. Cerebral flood flow and carbon dioxide reactivity in children with bacterial meningitis. J Pediatr 1990;117:523–530.
50. Adams RD, Kubik CS, Bonner FJ. The clinical and pathological aspects of influenzal meningitis. Arch Pediatr 1948;65:354–376;408–441.
51. Cairns H, Russell DS. Cerebral arteritis and phlebitis in pneumococcal meningitis. J Pathol Bacteriol 1946;58:649–665.
52. Yamashima T, Kashihara K, Ikeda K, Kubota T, Yamamoto S. Three phases of cerebral arteriopathy in meningitis: vasospasm and vasodilatation followed by organic stenosis. Neurosurgery 1985;16:546–553.
53. Pfister HW, Borasio GD, Dirnaglu U, Bauer M, Einhäupl KM. Cerebrovascular complications of bacterial meningitis in adults. Neurology 1992;42:1497–1504.
54. Stovring J, Snyder RD. Computed tomography in children bacterial meningitis. J Pediatr 1980;96:820–823.
55. Cabral DA, Flodmark O, Farrell K, Speert DP. Prospective study of computed tomography in acute bacterial meningitis. J Pediatr 1987; 111:201–205.
56. Slater AJ, Berkowitz ID, Wilson DA, Traystman RJ. Cerebrovascular autoregulation in *H. influenzae* type b meningitis in rabbits. FASEB J 1993;7:A3077.
57. Berkowitz ID, Jones MD, Hayden WR, Traystman RJ. *Haemophilus influenzae* type b impairment of microvascular autoregulation in rats. Pediatr Res 1993;33:48–51.
58. Goitein KJ, Tamir I. Cerebral perfusion pressure in central nervous system infections of infancy and childhood. J Pediatr 1983;103:40.
59. Gaussorgues P, Guerin C, Boyer F, et al. Intracranial hypertension in comatose bacterial meningitis. Presse Med 1987;16:1420–1423.
60. Rebaud P, Berthier JC, Hartemann E, Floret D. Intracranial pressure in childhood central nervous system infections. Intensive Care Med 1988;14:522–525.
61. MacDonald NE, Keene DL, Mackenzie AMR, Humphreys P, Jefferies AL, Ivan LP. Fulminating *Haemophilus influenzae* b meningitis. Can J Neurol Sci 1984;11:78.
62. Minns RA, Engleman HM, Stirling H. Cerebrospinal fluid pressure in pyogenic meningitis. Arch Dis Child 1989;64:814–820.
63. Ashwal S, Tomasi L, Schneider S, Perkin R, Thompson J. Bacterial meningitis in children: pathophysiology and treatment. Neurology 1992;42:6739–748.
64. Fishman RA. Brain Abscess. N Engl J Med 1975;293:708.
65. Quagliarello VJ, Long WK, Scheld MW. Morphologic alterations of the blood brain barrier with experimental meningitis in the rat: temporal sequence and role of encapsulation. J Clin Invest 1986;77:1084–1095.
66. Patrick D, Betts J, Frey R, Prameya R. *Haemophilus influenzae* lipopolysaccharide disrupts confluent monolayers of Bovine brain endothelial cells via a serum dependent cytotoxic pathway. J Infect Dis 1992;165:865–872.
67. Frerichs KU, Lindsberg PJ, Hallenbeck JM, Feurstein GZ. Platelet-activating factor and progressive brain damage following focal brain injury. J Neurosurg 1990;73:223–233.
68. Scheld WM, Dacey RG, Winn HR, Welsh JE, Jane JA, Sande MA. Cerebrospinal fluid outflow resistance in rabbits with experimental meningitis: alterations with penicillin and methylprednisolone. J Clin Invest 1980;66:243–253.
69. Bland RD, Lister RC, Ries JP. Cerebrospinal fluid lactic acid level and pH in meningitis. Am J Dis Child 1974;128:151–156.
70. Moxon ER, Smith AL, Averill DR, Brain carbohydrate metabolism during experimental *Haemophilus influenzae* meningitis. Pediatr Res 1979;13:52–59.
71. Lindquist RW, Lundbergh P, Hultman E. Experimental meningitis in the rabbit. II. Cerebral energy metabolism in relation to increased cerebrospinal fluid concentrations of lactate. Acta Neurol Scand 1987;75:405–409.
72. Matthews PM, Shoubridge E, Arnold DL. Brain phosphorus magnetic resonance spectroscopy in acute bacterial meningitis. Arch Neurol 1989;46:994–996.
73. Anderson NEO, Gyring J, Hansen AJ, Laursen H, Siesjo BK. Brain acidosis in experimental pneumococcal meningitis. J Cereb Blood Flow Metab 1989;9:381–387.
74. Guerra-Romero L, Tureen JH, Fournier MA, Makrides V, Täuber MG. Amino acids in cerebrospinal and brain interstitial fluid in experimental pneumococcal meningitis. Pediatr Res 1993;33:510–513.
75. Rutledge J, Benjamin D, Hood L, Smith A. Is the CSF lactate measurement useful in the management of children wih suspected bacterial meningitis? J Pediatr 1981;98:20—24.
76. Giampaolo C, Scheld WM, Savory J, Sande MA, Wills MA, Boyd JC. A multivariate approach to prognostication in experimental bacterail meningitis. Am J Clin Pathol 1981;76:442–449.
77. Cooper AJ, Beaty HN, Oppenheimer SI, Goodner CJ, Petersdorf RG. Studies on the pathogenesis of meningitis VII glucose transport and spinal fluid production in experimental pneumococcal meningitis. J Lab Clin Med 1968;71:473–482.
78. Isenberg H. Bacterial meningitis: Signs and symptoms. Antibiotics and Chemotherapy 1992;45:79–95.
79. Lipton JD, Schafermeyer RW. Evolving concepts in pediatric bacterial meningitis - Part 1: Pathophysiology and diagnosis. Ann Emerg Med 1993;22:1602–1615.

80. Feigin R, McCracken GH, Klein JO. Diagnosis and management of meningitis. Pediatr Infect Dis J 1992;11:785–814.
81. Handrick W, Wasser ST. Seizures during bacterial meningitis. Antibiotics and Chemotherapy 1992;45:239–253.
82. Granoff DM, Daum RS. Spread of *Haemophilus influenzae* type b: recent epidemiologic and therapeutic considerations. J Pediatr 1980; 97:854.
83. Bell WE, McCormick WF. Neurologic infection in children. Philadelphia: WB Saunders, 1981:3.
84. Cueva JP, Egel RT. Anterior fontanel herniation in Group B Streptococcus meningitis in newborns. Pediatr Neurology 1994; 10:332–5.
85. Horwitz SJ, Boxerbaum B, O'Bell J. Cerebral herniation in bacterial meningitis in childhood. Ann Neurol 1980;7:524.
86. Salmon JH, Hajjar W, Bada HS. The fontogram: a noninvasive intracranial pressure monitor. Pediatrics 1977;60:721.
87. Vidyasagar D, Raju TNK, Chiang J. Clinical significance of monitoring anterior fontanel pressure in sick neonates and infants. Pediatrics 1978;62:996.
88. Naidoo BT. The cerebrospinal fluid in the healthy newborn infant. S Afr Med J 1968;42:933.
89. Bonadio WA, Smith DS, Goddard S, Burroughs J, Khaja G. Distinguishing cerebrospinal fluid abnormalities in children with bacterial meningitis and traumatic lumbar puncture. J. Infect Dis 1990;162:251–4.
90. Polk DB, Steele RW. Bacterial meningitis presenting with normal cerebrospinal fluid. Pediatr Infect Dis J 1987;6:1040–42.
91. Myers GG, Netsky MG. Relation of blood and cerebrospinal fluid glucose. Experiments in the dog. Arch Neurol 1962;6:18.
92. Grayzel HG, Orent ER. Blood and cerebrospinal fluid sugar. Am J Dis Child 1927;34:1007.
93. Kelley AG. Sugar findings in normal and pathological spinal fluids. South Med J 1923;16:407.
94. Berkowitz FE. Acinetobacter meningitis: a diagnostic pitfall. A report of 3 cases. S Afr Med J 1982;61:448.
95. Bhisitkul DM, Hogan AE, Tanz RR. The role of bacterial antigen detection tests in the diagnosis of bacterial meningitis. Pediatr Emerg Care 1994;10:67–71.
96. Maxson S, Lewno MJ, Schutze GE. Clinical usefulness of cerebrospinal fluid bacterial antigen studies. J Pediatr 1994; 125:235–8.
97. Thomas JG. Routine CSF antigen detection for agents associated with bacterial meningitis: another point of view. Clin Microbiol Newsletter 1994;16:89–95.
98. Fishman RA. Cerebrospinal fluid in diseases of the nervous system. 1992;2nd edition, WB Saunders Co. Philadelphia, pp 253–343.
99. Harter DH. Preliminary antibiotic therapy in bacterial meningitis. Arch Neurol 1963;9:343–347.
100. Winkelstein JA. The influence of partial treatment with penicillin on the diagnosis of bacterial meningitis. J Pediatr 1970;77:619.
101. Lewin EB. Partially treated meningitis. Am J Dis Child 1974;128:145.
102. Feldman WE. Effect of prior antibiotic therapy on concentrations of bacteria in CSF. Am J Dis Child 1978;132:672.
103. Blazer S, Berant M, Alon U. Effect of antibiotic treatment on cerebrospinal fluid. Am J Clin Pathol 1983;80:386–7.
104. Bohr V, Rasmussen N, Hansen B, et al. 875 cases of bacterial meningitis: diagnostic procedures and the impact of preadmission antibiotic therapy. Part III of a three-part series. J Infect 1983;7:193.
105. Kobani A, Jadavji I. Sequelae of acute bacterial meningitis in children. Antibiotics and Chemotherapy 1992;45:209–217.
106. Prince AS, Neu HC. Fluid management in *Haemophilus influenzae* meningitis. Infection 1980;8:5–7.
107. Feigin RD, Stechenberg BW, Chang MJ, et al. Prospective evaluation of treatment of *Haemophilus influenzae* meningitis. J Pediatr 1976;88:542–548.
108. Powell KR, Sugarman IL, Eskenazi AE, Woodin KA, Kays MA, McCormick KL, Miller ME, Sladek CD. Normalization of plasma arginine vasopressin concentrations when children with meningitis are given mainenance plus replacement fluid therapy. J Pediatr 1990;117: 515–522.
109. Lam A, Sibbald WJ, Boone J. Transient diabetes insipidus as a complication of *Haemophilus meningitis.* Pediatrics 1978;61:785.
110. Benson P, Nyhan WL, Shimizu H. The prognosis of subdural effusions complicating pyogenic meningitis. J Pediatr 1960;57:679.
111. Smith MHD, Dormont RE, Prather GW. Subdural effusions complicating bacterial meningitis. Pediatrics 1951;7:34.
112. Platou R, Rinker A, Derrick J. Acute subdural effusions and late sequelae of meningitis. Pediatr 1959;23:962–971.
113. Snedeker JD, Kaplan SL, Dodge PR, Holmes SJ, Geigin RD. Subdural effusion and its relationship with neurologic sequelae of bacterial meningitis in infancy: A prospective study. Pediatr 1990;36:163–170.
114. Williams JM, Stevens H. Postmeningitic subdural effusions. J Int Coll Surg 1957;27:590.
115. Feigin RD, Dodge PR. Bacterial meningitis: newer concepts of pathophysiology and neurological sequelae. Pediatr Clin North Am 1976;23:541–556.
116. Gitlin D. Pathogenesis of subdural collections of fluid. Pediatrics 61:272, 1978.
117. Lin TY, Nelson JD, McCracken GH. Fever during treatment for bacterial meningitis. Pediatr Infect Dis 1984;3:319.
118. Balagtas RC, Levin S, Nelson KE, Gotoff SP. Secondary and prolonged fevers in bacterial meningitis. J Pediatr 1970;77:957.
119. Lipiridou O, Lazaridou S, Manios S. Recurrent and persistent fever in bacterial meningitis with adequate response to antimicrobial therapy. Scand J Infect Dis 1973;5:23.
120. Tasker RC, Matthew DJ, Kendall B. Computed tomography in the assessment of raised intracranial pressure in non-traumatic coma. Neuropediatrics 1990;21:91–96.
121. Minns RA, Engleman HM. The use of CSF pressure recordings in acute bacterial meningitis. Zeitschrift fur Kinderchirurgie 1988;43 Suppl 2:28–29.
122. Syrogiannopoulos GA, Olsen KD, McCracken GH Jr. Mannitol treatment in experimental *Haemophilus influenzae* type b meningitis. Pediatr Res 1987;22:118–122.
123. Sable CA, Scheld WM. Theoretical and practical considerations of antibiotic therapy for bacterial meningitis. Antibiot Chemother 1992;45:96–117.
124. Ristuccia AM. Cerebrospinal fluid penetration of antimicrobials. Antibiotics and Chemotherapy 1992;45:118–152.
125. John CC. Treatment failure with use of a third-generation cephalosporin for penicillin-resistant pneumococcal meningitis: case report and review. Clin Infect Dis 1994;18:188–93.
126. Catalan MJ, Fernandez JM, Vazquez A, de Seijas EV, Suarez A, de Quiros JCLB. Failure of cefotaxime in the treatment of meningitis due to relatively resistant *Streptococcus pneumoniae.* Clin Infect Dis 1994;18:766-9.
127. Tan TQ, Schutze GE, Mason EO, Kaplan SL. Antibiotic therapy and acute outcome of meningitis due to *Streptococcus pneumoniae* considered intermediately susceptible to broad-spectrum cephalosporins. Antimicrob Agents Chemother 1994;38:918–923.
128. Friedland IR, Paris M, Ehrett S, Hickey S, Olsen K, McCracken GH Jr. Evaluation of antimicrobial regimens for treatment of experimental penicillin- and cephalosporin-resistant pneumococcal meningitis. Antimicrob Agents Chemother 1993;37:1630–6.
129. Friedland IR, McCracken GH Jr. Management of infections caused by antibiotic-resistant *Streptococcus pneumoniae.* N Engl of Med 1994;331:377–82.
130. Leggiadro RJ. Penicillin - and cephalosporin-resistant *Streptococcus pneumoniae:* an emerging microbial threat. Pediatr 1994;93: 500–503.
131. Paris M, Ramilo O, McCracken GH Jr. Management of meningitis caused by penicillin-resistant *Streptococcus pneumoniae.* Antimicrob Agents Chemother 1995;39:2171-5.
132. Paris MM, Hickey SM, Uscher MI, Shelton S, Olsen KD, McCracken GH Jr. Effect of dexamethasone on therapy of experimental penicillin- and cephalosporin-resistant pneumococcal meningitis. Antimicrob Agents Chemother 1994;38:1320–24.
133. Jorgensen JH. Update on mechanisms and prevalence of antimicrobial resistance in *Haemophilus influenzae.* Clin Infect Dis 1992;14: 1119–23.
134. Friedland IR, Klugman KP. Failure of chloramphenicol therapy in penicillin-resistant pneumococcal meningitis. Lancet 1992;339:405–8.
135. Klugman KP, Friedland IR, Bradley JS. Bactericidal activity against cephalosporin-ressitant *Streptococcus pneumoniae* in cerebrospinal fluid of children with acute bacterial meningitis. Antimicrob Agents Chemother 1995;39:1988–91.
136. Committee on Infectious Diseases. Dexamethasone therapy for bacterial meningitis in infants and children. In:1994 Red Book. American Academy of Pediatrics, Elk Grove, Illinois, pp 558–559.
137. Block C, Davidson Y, Melamed E, Keller N. Susceptibility of *Neisseria Meningitidis* in Israel to penicillin and other drugs of interest. J Antimicrob Chemother 1993;32:166–8.
138. Woods CR, Smith AL, Wasilauskas BC, Campos J, Givner LB. Invasive disease caused by *Neisseria meningitidis* relatively resistant to penicillin in North Carolina. J Infect Dis 1994;170:453–6.
139. Backmann A, Danielsson D, Olcen P. Plasmid carriage and antibiotic

susceptibility of *Neisseria meningitidis* strains isolated in Sweden 1981–1990. Eur J Clin Microbiol Infect Dis 1993;12:683–9.
140. Radetsky M. Duration of treatment in bacterial meningitis: a historical inquiry. Pediatr Infect Dis J 1990;9:2–9.
141. Lin T-Y, Chrane DF, Nelson JD, McCracken GH Jr. Seven days of ceftriaxone therapy is as effective as ten days' treatment for bacterial meningitis. JAMA 1985;253:3559–63.
142. Helwig H. Duration of treatment of bacterial meningitis. Antibiotics and Chemotherapy 1992;45:153–160.
143. Odio CM, Faingezicht I, Paris M, Nassar M, Baltodano A, Rogers J, Saez-Llorens, Olsen KD, McCracken GH Jr. The beneficial effects of early dexamethasone administration in infants and children with bacterial meningitis. N Engl J Med 1991:324:1525–31.
144. Lebel MH, Freij BJ, Syrogiannopoulos GA, Chrane DF, Hoyt MJ, Stewart SM, Kennard BD, Olsen KD, McCracken GH Jr. Dexamethasone therapy for bacterial meningitis: results of two double-blind, placebo controlled trials. N Engl J Med 1988;319–964–71.
145. Schaad UB, Lips U, Gnehm HE et al. Dexamethasone therapy for bacterial meningitis in children. Lancet 1993;342:457–61.
146. Wald ER, Kaplan SL, Mason EO, Sabo D, Ross L, Arditi M, Wiedermann BL, Barson W, Kim KS, Yogev R, Hofkosh D; for the Meningitis Study Group. Dexamethasone therapy for children with bacterial meningitis. Pediatrics 1995;95:21–28.
147. Girgis NI, Farid Z, Mikhail IA, Farrag I, Sultan Y, Kilpatrick ME. Dexamethasone treatment for bacterial meningitis in children and adults. Pediatr Infect Dis J 1989;8:848–51.
148. Kennedy WA, Hoyt MJ, McCracken GH Jr. The role of corticosteroid therapy in children with pneumococcal meningitis. Am J Dis Child 1991;145:1374–8.
148a. Kanra GY, Ozen H, Secmeer G, Ceyhan M, Ecevit Z, Belgin E. Beneficial effects of dexamethasone in children with pneumonococcal meningitis. Pediatr Infect Dis J 1995;14:490–4.
149. Cabellos C, Martinez-Lacasa J, Martos A, Tubau F, Fernandez A, Viladrich PF, Gudiol F. Influence of dexamethasone on efficacy of ceftriaxone and vancomycin therapy in experimental pneumococcal meningitis. Antimicrob Agents Chemother 1995;39:2158–60.
150. Gaillard J-L, Abadie V, Cheron G, Lacaille F Mahut B, Silly C, Matha V, Coustere C, Lokiec F. Concentrations of ceftriaxone in cerebrospinal fluid of children with meningitis receiving dexamethasone therapy. Antimicrob Agents Chemother 1994;38:1209–10.
151. Wagner DC, Kennedy WA, Hoyt MJ, McCracken GH Jr. Lack of adverse effects of dexamethasone therapy in aseptic meningitis. Pediatr Infect Dis J 1990;9:922–923.
152. Lebel M. Dexamethasone therapy of bacterial meningitis. Antibiot Chemother 1992;45:169–183.
153. Prober CG. The role of steroids in the management of children with bacterial meningitis. Pediatrics 1995;95:29–31.
154. Schaad UB, Kaplan SL, McCracken GH Jr. Steroid therapy for bacterial meningitis. Clin Infect Dis 1995;20:685–90.
155. Tuomanen E, Hengstler B, Rich R, Bray MA, Zak O, Tomasz A. Nonsteroidal anti-inflammatory agents in the therapy for experimental pneumococcal meningitis. J Infect Dis 1987;155:985–990.
156. Tureen JH, Stella FB, Clyman RI, Mauray F, Sande MA. Effect of indomethacin on brain water content, cerebrospinal fluid white blood cell response and prostaglandin E_2 levels in cerebrospinal fluid in experimental pneumococcal meningitis in rabbits. Pediatr Infect Dis J 1987;6:1151–1153.
157. Sáez-Llorens X, Ramilo O, Mustafa MM, et al. Pentoxifylline modulates meningeal inflammation in experimental bacterial meningitis. Antimicrob Agents Chemother 1990;34:837–843.
158. Sable CA, Aubin MA, Scheld WM. Pentoxifylline effect on *Haemophilus influenzae* type b (Hib)-induced alteration in blood-brain barrier permeability (BBBP) in experimental meningitis [abstract no. 920]. In: Program and abstracts of the 31st Interscience Conference on Antimicrobial Agents and Chemotherapy. Washington, DC: American Society for Microbiology, 1991.
159. Committee on Infectious Disease. Haemophilus influenzae infections. In 1994 Red Book. American Academy of Pediatrics, Elk Grove, Illinois, pp 205–207.
160. Committee on Infectious Diseases. Meningococcal infections. In 1994 Red Book. American Academy of Pediatrics, Elk Grove, Illinois, pp 323–6.
161. McGowan JE Jr, Klein JO, Bratton L, Barnes MW, Finland M. Meningitis and bacteremia due to *Haemophilus influenzae:* occurrence and mortality at Boston City Hospital in 12 selected years, 1935 to 1972. J Infect Dis 1974;130:119.
162. Goldacre MJ. Acute bacterial meningitis in childhood. Incidence and mortality in a defined population. Lancet 1976;1:28.
163. de Louvois J. Acute bacterial meningitis in the newborn. J Antimicrob Chemother 1994;34 Suppl A:61–73.
164. Klein JO, Marcy SM: Bacterial sepsis and meningitis. In: Remington JS, Klein JO (eds): Infectious diseases of the fetus and newborn infant. 4th edition, WB Saunders, Philadelphia, 1995, pp 835–90.
165. Baker CJ, Edwards MS. Group B streptococcal infection: In: Remington JS, Klein JO (eds): Infectious diseases of the fetus and newborn infant. 4th edition, 1995, WB Saunders, Philadelphia, pp 980–1054.
166. Bryan CS, John JF Jr., Pai MS et al Gentamicin vs cefotaxime for therapy of neonatal sepsis: Relationship to drug resistance. Am J Dis Child 1985;139:1086–9.
167. Reed MD, Kliegman RM, Yamashita TS, Myers CM, Blumer JL. Clinical pharmacology of imipenem and cilastatin in premature infants during the first week of life. Antimicrob Agents Chemother 1990; 34:1172–7.
168. Sáez-Lloren X, McCracken GH Jr. Clinical pharmacology of antibacterial agents. In: Remington JS, Klein JO (eds): Infectious diseases of the fetus and newborn infant. 4th edition, WB Saunders, Philadelphia, pp 1287–1336.
169. Stuart RL, Turnidge J, Grayson ML. Safety of imipenem in neonates. Pediatr Infect Dis J 1995;14:804–805.
170. Gocen SDR, Ilunga F, Cheesbrough JS, Tillotson GS, Hichens M, Felmingham D. The treatment of neonatal meningitis due to Gram-negative bacilli with ciprofloxacin: evidence of satisfactory penetration into the cerebrospinal fluid 1993:26:253–6.
171. Bannon MJ, Stutchfield PR, Weindling AM, Damjanovic V: Ciprofloxacin in neonatal Enterobacter cloacae septicaemiae. Arch Dis Child 1989;64:1388–91.
172. McCracken GH Jr., Mize SG, Threlkeld N. Intraventricular gentamicin therapy in Gram-negative bacillary meningitis of infancy. Report of the Second Neonatal Meningitis Cooperation Study Group. Lancet 1980;1:787–91.
173. Roberts FJ. Problems in the diagnosis of tuberculous meningitis. Arch Neurol 1981;38:319–20.
174. Peacock WJ, Deeny JE. Improving the outcome of tuberculous meningitis in childhood. S Afr Med J 1984;66:597–8.
175. Idriss ZH, Sinno AA, Kronfol NM. Tuberculous meningitis in Childhood. Am J. Dis Child 1976;130:364–7.
176. Humphries MJ, Lam WK, Teoh R. Nonrespiratory tuberculosis. In: Davies PDO (ed). Clinical tuberculosis Chapman and Hall Medical, London, 1994, pp 102–107.
177. Leiguarda R, Berthier M, Starkstein S, Nogues M, Lylyk P. Ischemic Infarction in 25 children with tuberculous meningitis. Stroke 1988;19:200–204.
178. Waecker NJ, Connor JD. Central nervous system tuberculosis in children: a review of 30 cases. Pediatr Infect Dis J 1990;9:539–43.
179. Committee on Infectious Diseases: Tuberculosis. In:1994 Red Book. American Academy of Pediatrics; Elk Grove, Illinois, 1994, pp 480–500.
180. Holdiness MR. Management of tuberculous meningitis. Drugs 1990;39:224–233.
181. Kasik JE. Central nervous system tuberculosis. In: Schlossberg D (ed): Tuberculosis. 3rd edition. Springer-Verlag, NY, 1994;pp129–141.
182. Tenney JH. Bacterial infections of the central nervous system in neurosurgery. Neurologic Clinics 1986;4:91–14.
183. Mayhall CG, Archer NH, Lamb A, Spadora AC, Baggett JW, Ward JD, Narayan RK. Ventriculostomy-related infections. A prospective epidemiologic study. N Engl J Med 1984;310:553–9.
184. Haile-Mariam T, Laws E, Tuazon CU. Gram-negative meningitis associated with transsphenoidal surgery: case reports and review. Clin Infect Dis 1994;18:553–6.
185. Stephens JL, Peacock JE. Uncommon infections: eye and central nervous system. In (ed) Wenzel RP: Prevention and control of nosocomial infections. 2nd edition. Williams and Wilkins, Baltimore, 1993, pp 746–775.
186. Ready LB, Helfer D. Bacterial meningitis in parturients after epidural anesthesia. Anesthesiology 1989;71:988–90.
187. Gelfand MS, Abolnik IZ. Streptococcal meningitis complicating diagnostic myelography: three cases and review. Clin Infect Dis 1995;20:582–7.
188. Yogev R. Cerebrospinal fluid shunt infections: a personal view. Pediatric Infect Dis J 1985;4:113–147.
189. Bayston R. Hydrocephalus shunt infection. J Antimicrob Chemother 1994;34 Suppl A: 74–84.

190. Odio C, McCracken EH Jr., Nelson JD. CSF shunt infections in pediatrics. A seven-year experience. Am J Dis Child 1984;138:1103–8.
191. Noetzel MJ, Baker RP. Shunt fluid examination: risks and benefits in the evaluation of shunt malfunction and infection. J Neurosurg 1984;61:328–32.
192. Tung H, Raffel C, McComb JG. Ventricular cerebrospinal fluid eosinophilia in children with ventriculoperitoneal shunts. J. Neurosurg 1991;75:541–4.
193. Vinchon M, Vallee L, Prin L, Desreumaux P, Dhellemmes P. Cerebrospinal fluid eosinophilia in shunt infections. Neuropediatrics 1992;23:235–40.
194. Morissette I, Gourdeau M, Francoeur J. CSF shunt infections: a fifteen-year experience with emphasis on management and outcome. Canad J Neurological Sciences 1993;20:118–22.
195. McLaurin RL, Frame PT. Treatment of infections of cerebrospinal fluid shunts. Rev Infect Dis 1987;9:595–603.
196. Frame PT, McLaurin RL. Treatment CSF shunt infections with intrashunt plus oral antibiotics therapy. J Neurosurg 1984;60:354–60.
197. Koskiniemi M, Rautonen J, Lehtokoski-Lehtiniemi E, Vaheri A. Epidemiology of encephalitis in children: a 20-year survey. Ann Neurol 1991;29:492.
198. Koskiniemi M, Vaheri A. Effect of measles, mumps, rubella vaccination on pattern of encephalitis in children. Lancet 1989;1:31.
199. Whitley RJ, Lakeman F. Herpes simplex virus infections of the central nervous system: Therapeutic and diagnostic considerations. Clin Infect Dis 1995;20:414–420.
200. Rotbart H. Enteroviral infections of the central nervous system. Clin Infect Dis 1995;20:971–981.
201. Whiley RJ. Viral encephalitis. N Engl J Med 1990;323:242–250.
202. Modlin JF, Dagan R, Berlin LE, Virshup DM, Yolken RH, Menegus M. Focal encephalitis with enterovirus infections. Pediatrics 1991;88: 841–845.
203. Johnson RT. Arboviral encephalitis. In: Tropical and Geographical Medicine, 2nd ed., Warren KX, Mahmoud AAF. New York: McGraw-Hill 1989:691–700.
204. Whiley RF, Cobbs CG, Alford CA Jr, et al. Diseases that mimic herpes simplex encephalitis: diagnosis, presentation, and outcome. JAMA 1989;262:234–239.
205. Wright A, Moffit J, Evans OB. Cat scratch encephalopathy. J Missip St Med Assoc 1986;27:29–31.
206. Johnson RT, Griffen De, Gendelman HE. Postinfectious encephalomyelitis. Semin Neurol 1985;5:180–190.
207. Lehtokoski-Lehtiniemi E, Koskiniemi M-L. *Mycoplasma pneumoniae* encephalitis: a severe entity in children. Pediatr Infect Dis J 1989;8:651.
208. Johnson RT. Slow infection of the central nervous system caused by conventional viruses. Ann N Y Acad Sci 1994;724:6–13.
209. Whitley RJ. Varicella-Zoster virus infections. In: Galasso GJ, Whitley RJ, Merigan TC, eds. Antiviral agents and viral disease of man. 3rd ed. New York: Raven Press, 1990:235–263.
210. Johnson RT, Griffin DE, Hirsch RL, et al. Measles encephalomyelitis - clinical and immunologic studies. N Engl J Med 1984;310:137.
211. Whitley R, Lakeman AD, Nahmias A, Roizman B. DNA restriction-enzyme analysis of Herpes simplex virus isolates obtained from patients with encephalitis. N Engl J Med 1982;307:1060.
212. McCullers JA, Lakeman FD, Whitley RJ. Human herpes virus 6 is associated with focal encephalitis. Clin Infect Dis 1995;21:571.
213. Baer GM, Bellini WJ, Fishbein DB. Rhabdoviruses. In:Fields BN, Knipe DM, eds. Fields virology. 2nd ed. Vol.1. New York: Raven Press, 1990:883–930.
214. Bacon CJ, Hall SM. Haemorrhagic shock encephalopathy syndrome in the British Isles. Arch Dis Child 1992;67:985.
215. Committee on Infectious Diseases . Aspirin and Reye syndrome. Pediatrics 1982;69:810.
216. Whitley RJ. Herpes simplex virus infections. In: Remington JS, Klein JO, eds. Infectious diseases of the fetus and newborn infant. Philadelphia: W.B. Saunders, 1990:282–305.
217. Whitley RJ, Corey L, Arvin A, et al. Changing presentation of Herpes simplex virus infection in neonates. J Infect Dis 1988;158:109.
218. Brusilow SW, Valle DL, Arn P. Symptomatic inborn errors of metabolism. Curr Ther Neonat Perinat Med 1990;2:164.
219. Uldry P-A, Kuntzer T, Bogousslavsky J, et al. Early symptoms and outcome of Listeria monocytogenes rhombencephalitis: 14 adult cases. J Neurol 1993;240:235.
220. Whitley RJ, Soong SJ, Linneman C Jr, Liu C, Pazin G, Alford CA. Herpes simplex encephalitis: clinical assessment. JAMA 1982;247: 317–320.
221. Lakeman FD, Whitley RJ, National Institute of Allergy and Infectious Diseases Collaborative Antiviral Study Group. Diagnosis of herpes simplex encephalitis: application of polymerase chain reaction to cerebrospinal fluid from brain-biopsied patients and correlation with disease. J Infect Dis 1995;171:857.
222. Puchhammer-Stockl E, Popow-Kraupp T, Heinz FX, Mandl CW, Kunz C. Detection of varicella-zoster virus DNA by polymerase chain reaction in the cerebrospinal fluid of patients suffering from neurological complications associated with chicken pox or herpes zoster. J Clin Microbiol 1991;29:1513.
223. Smith RR. Neuroradiology of intracranial infection. Pediatr Neurosurg 1992;18:92.
224. Whitley RJ, Soong SJ, Dolin R, et al. Adenine arabinoside therapy of biospy-proved herpes simplex encephalitis: National Institute of Allergy and Infectious Disease Collaborative Antiviral Study. N Engl J Med 1977;297:289.
225. Cohen JI. Clinical conference at the Johns Hopkins Hospital: herpes simplex encephalitis. Johns Hopkins Med J 1980;147:157.
226. Brown ZA, Benedetti J, Ashley R, et al. Neonatal Herpes simplex virus infection in relation to asymptomatic maternal infection at the time of labor. N Engl J Med 1991;324:1247.
227. Whitley R, Arvin A, Prober C, et al. A controlled trial comparing vidarabine with acyclovir in neonatal Herpes simplex virus infection. N Engl J Med 1991;324:444.
228. Johnson RT. The pathogenesis of acute viral encephalitis and post infectious encephalomyelitis. J Infect Dis 1987;155:359–364.
229. Mikati MA, Feraru E, Krishnamoorthy K, Lombroso CT. Neonatal herpes simpliex meningoencephalitis: EEG investigations and clinical correlates. Neurol 1990;40:1433.
230. Whitley R, Arvin A, Prober C, et al. Predictors of morbidity and mortality in neonates with Herpes simplex virus infections. N Engl J Med 1991;324:450.
231. Modlin JF, Dagan R, Berlin LE, Virshup DM, Yolken RH, Menegus M. Focal encephalitis with enterovirus infections. Pediatrics 1991; 88:841.
232. Johns DR, Stein AG, Wityk R. MELAS syndrome masquerading as herpes simplex encephalitis. Neurol 1993;43:2471.
233. Price R, Chernik NL, Horta-Barbosa L, Posner JB. Herpes simplex encephalitis in an anergic patient. Am J Med 1973;54:222. 234.Fox JD, Brink NS, Zuckerman MA, et al. Detection of herpes virus DNA by nested polymerase chain reaction in cerebrospinal fluid of human immunodeficiency virus-infected persons with neurologic disease: a prospective evaluation. J Infect Dis 1995;172:1087.
234. Fox JD, Brink NS, Zuckerman MA, et al. Detection of herpes virus DNA by nested polymerase chain reaction in cerebrospinal fluid of human immunodeficiency virus-infected persons with neurologic disease: a prospective evaluation. J Infect Dis 1995;172:1087.
235. Rovit RL, Sigler MH. Hyponatremia with herpes simplex encephalitis. Arch Neurol 1964;10:595.
236. Miller JK, Hesser F, Tompkins VN. Herpes simplex encephalitis. Ann Intern Med 1966;64:92.
237. Whitley RJ, Soong S-J, Linneman C,Jr., et al. Herpes simplex encephalitis. Clinical assessment. JAMA 1982;247:317.
238. Morrison RE, Miller MH, Lyon LW, et al. Adult meningoencephalitis caused by Herpesvirus hominis type 2. Am J Med 1974;56:540.
239. Sarubbi FA Jr, Sparling PF, Glezen WP. Herpes virus hominis encephalitis. Virus isolation from brain biopsy in seven patients and results of therapy. Arch Neurol 1973;29:268.
240. Gutman LT, Wilfert CM, Eppes S. Herpes simplex virus encephalitis in children: analysis of cerebrospinal fluid and progressive neurodevelopmental deterioration. J Infect Dis 1986;154:415.
241. Koskiniemi M, Vaheri A, Manninen V, et al. Herpes simplex virus encephalitis. New diagnostic and clinical features and results of therapy. Arch Neurol 1980;37:763.
242. Nolan DC, Carruthers MM, Lerner AM. Herpesvirus hominis encephalitis in Michigan. N Engl J Med 1970;282:10.
243. Ch'ien LT, Boehm RM, Robinson H, et al. Characteristic early electroencephalographic changes in herpes simplex encephalitis. Clinical and virologic studies. Arch Neurol 1977;34:361.
244. Smith JB, Westmoreland BF, Reagan TJ, Sandok BA. A distinctive clinical EEG profile in herpes simplex encephalitis. Mayo Clin Proc 1975;50:469.
245. Greenberg DA, Weinkle DJ, Aminoff MJ. Periodic EEG complexes in infectious mononucleosis encephalitis. J Neurol Neurosurg Psychiatry 1982;45:648.
246. Karlin CA, Robinson RG, Hinthorn DR, et al. Radionuclide imaging in herpes simplex encephalitis. Radiology 1978;126:181.

247. Enzmann DR, Ranson B, Norman D, Talberth E. Computed tomography of herpes simplex encephalitis. Radiology 1978;129:419.
248. Davis JM, Davis KR, Kleinman GM, et al. Computed tomography of herpes simplex encephalitis with clinicopathological correlation. Radiology 1978;129:409.
249. Koskiniemi M, Piiparinen H, Leikola M, Färkkilä M, Vaheri A, Study Group . Poor antibody production in fatal herpes encephalitis. J Infect Dis 1995;171:1692.
250. Rowley A, Whitley RJ, Lakeman FD, Wolinsky SM. Rapid detection of herpes-simplex-virus DNA in cerebrospinal fluid of patients with herpes simplex encephalitis. Lancet 1990;335:440–441.
251. Aurelius E, Johansson B, Sköldeberg B, Staland A, Forgren M. Rapid diagnosis of herpes simplex encephalitis by nested polymerase chain reaction of cerebrospinal fluid. Lancet 1991;337:189–192.
252. Kohl S, James AR. Herpes simplex virus encephalitis during childhood: importance of brain biopsy diagnosis. J Pediatr 1985;107:212.
253. Whitley R, Cobbs CG, Alford CA, et al. Diseases that mimic herpes simplex encephalitis. Diagnosis, presentation, and outcome. JAMA 1989;262:234.
254. Whitley RJ, Alford CA, Hirsch MS, et al. Vidarabine versis acyclovir therapy in Herpes simplex encephalitis. N Engl J Med 1986;314:144.
255. Fischer EG, McLennan JE, Suzuki Y. Cerebral abscess in children. Am J Dis Child 1981;135:746.
256. Woods CR. Brain abscess and other intracranial suppurative complications. Advances Pediatr Infect Dis 1995;10:41–79.
257. Wispelwey B, Scheld WM. Brain Abscess. Sem Neurol 1992; 12:273–278.
258. Nielsen H. Cerebral abscess in children. Neuropediatrics 1983;14: 76–80.
259. Matson DD, Salam M. Brain abscess in congenital heart disease. Pediatrics 1961;27:772.
260. Fischbein CA, Rosenthal A, Fischer EG, et al. Risk factors for brain abscess in patients with congenital heart disease. Am J Cardiol 1974;34:97.
261. Raimondi AJ, Matsumoto S, Miller RA. Brain abscess in children with congenital heart disease. J Neurosurg 1965;23:588.
262. Teed RW. Meningitis from the sphenoid sinus. Arch Otolaryngol 1938;28:589–619.
263. Kagawa M, Takeshita M, Yato S, et al. Brain abscess in congenital cyanotic heart disease. J Neurosurg 1983;58:913.
264. Hirsch JF, Roux FX, Sainte-Rose C, et al. Brain abscess in childhood. Childs Brain 1983;10:251.
265. Jadavji T, Humphreys RP, Prober CG. Brain abscesses in infants and children. Pediatr Infect Dis 1985;4:394.
266. Moss SD, McLone DG, Arditi M, et al. Pediatric cerebral abscess. Pediatr Neurosci 1988;14:291–296.
267. Fischer EG, McLennan JE, Suzuki Y. Cerebral abscess in children. Am J Dis Child 1981;135:746–749.
268. Patrick CC, Kaplan SL. Current concepts in the pathogenesis and management of bran abscesses in children. Pediatr Clin North Am 1988;35:625–636.
269. Gelfand MS, Stephens DS, Howell EI, et al. Brain abscess: Association with pulmonary arteriovenous fistula and hereditary hemorrhagic telangiectasia: Report of three cases. Am J Med 1988;85:718–720.
270. Leahy WR, Toyka KV, Fischbeck KH. Cerebral abscess in children secondary to esophageal dilatation. Pediatrics 1977;59:300–301.
271. Kline MW. Citrobacter meningitis and brain abscess in infancy: Epidemiology, pathogenesis, and treatment. J Pediatr 1988;113: 430–434.
272. Dodge PR, Pomeroy SL. Parameningeal infectious (including brain abscess, epidural abscess, subdural empyema), in Feigin RD, Cherry JD: Textbook of Pediatric Infectious Diseases, ed 3. Philadelphia, WB Saunders, 1992, pp455–462.
273. Renier D, Flandin C, Hirsch E, et al. Brain abscesses in neonates. A study of 30 cases. J Neurosurg 1988;69:877–882.
274. Vogel LC, Ferguson L, Gotoff SP. *Citrobacter* infections of the central nervous system in early infancy. J Pediatr 1978;93:86.
275. Sáez-Llorens XJ, Umaña MA, Odio CM, et al. Brain abscess in infants and children. Pediatr Infect Dis J 1989;8:449–458.
276. Brook I. Bacteriology of intracranial abscess in children. J Neurosurg 1981;54:484–488.
277. Theophilo F, Markakis E, Theophilo L, et al. Brain abscess in childhood. Child Nerv Syst 1985;1:324–328.
278. Garvey G. Current concepts of bacterial infections of the central nervous system: bacterial meningitis and bacterial brain abscess. J Neurosurg 1983;59:735.
279. Brutt RH, Enzmann DR, Yeager AS. Neuropathological and computerized tomographic findings in experimental brain abscess. J Neurosurg 1981;55:590.
280. Schurr P. Brain abscess in childhood. Dev Med Child Neurol 1965;7:433.
281. Harrison MJG. The clinical presentation of intracranial abscesses. Q J Med 1982;204:461.
282. Samson DS, Clark K. A current review of brain abscess. Am J Med 1973;54:201.
283. Weisberg LA. The role of CT in the evaluation of patients with intracranial CNS infections—Inflammatory disorders. Comput Radiol 1984;8:29.
284. Stevens EA, Norman D, Kramer RA, et al. Computed tomographic brain scanning in intraparenchymal pyogenic abscesses. AJR 1978; 130:111.
285. Smith RR. Neuroradiology of intracranial infection. Pediatr Neurosurg 1992;18:92–104.
286. Rosenblum ML, Hoff JT, Norman D, et al. Decreased mortality from brain abscesses since advent of computerized tomography. J Neurosurg 1978;49:658.
287. Whispelwey B, Dacey RG, Scheld WM. Brain abscess. In Scheld WM, Whitley RJ, Durack DT. Infections of the Central Nervous System. New York, Raven, 1991:457–486.
288. Kaplan K. Brain abscess. Med Clin North Am 1985;69:345.
289. Weidermann BL. Subdural, epidural, and subgaleal infections. In Kaplan ST. Current Therapy in Pediatric Infectious Disease, ed 3. St. Louis, Mosby, 1993:152–153.
290. Tekkök IH, Erbengi A. Management of brain abscess in children: Review of 130 cases over a period of 21 years. Child Nerv Syst 1992;8:411–416.
291. Berg B, Franklin G, Cuneo R, et al. Nonsurgical cure of brain abscess: Early diagnosis and follow-up with computerized tomography. Ann Neur 1978;3:474–478.
292. Rennels MB, Woodard CL, Robinson WL, et al. Medical cure of apparent brain abscesses. Pediatrics 1983;72:220–224.
293. Keren G, Tyrell DL. Nonsurgical treatment of brain abscesses: Report of two cases. Pediatr Infect Dis J 1984;3:331–334.
294. Idriss ZH, Gutman LT, Kronfol NM. Brain abscesses in infants and children. Clin Pediatr (Phila) 1978;17:738–746.
295. Buonaguro A, Colangelo M, Daniels B. Neurological and behavioral sequelae in children operated on for brain abscess. Child Nerv Syst 1989;5:153–155.
296. Kagawa M, Takeshita M, Yato S, et al. Brain abscess in congenital cyanotic heart disease. J Neurosurg 1983;58:913–917.
297. Renaudin JW, Frazee J. Subdural empyema—Importance of early diagnosis. Neurosurgery 1980;7:477.
298. Courville CB, Blomquist OA. Traumatic pachymeningitis internal and subdural abscess: with special reference to pathogenesis and pathology. Arch Surg 1941;42:890.
299. LeBeau J, Creissard P, Harispe L, et al. Surgical treatment of brain abscesses and subdural empyema. J Neurosurg 1973;38:198.
300. Farmer TW, Wise GR. Subdural empyema in infants, children and adults. Neurology 1973;23:254.
301. Jacobson PL, Farmer TW. Subdural empyema complicating meningitis in infants: Improved prognosis. Neurology 1981;31:190–193.
302. Silverberg AL, DiNubile MJ. Subdural empyema and cranial epidural abscess. Med Clin North Am 1985;69:361.
303. Bhandari YS, Sarkari NB. Subdural empyema. A review of 37 cases. J Neurosurg 1970;32:35.
304. Wega S, Morooka Y, Yamamoto Y, et al. Interhemispheric subdural empyema with enlarged meningeal arteries. Surg Neurol 1979;11:175.
305. Kaufman DM, Miller MH, Steigbigel NH. Subdural empyema: analysis of 17 recent cases and review of the literature. Medicine 1975;54:485.
306. Cornell SH, Chiu LC, Christie JH. Diagnosis of extracerebral fluid collections by computed tomography. AJR 1978;131:107.
307. Baddour LM. Limitations of the computed tomographic scan in the diagnosis of subdural empyema. J Tenn Med Assoc 1982;75:668.
308. Dunker RO, Khakoo RA. Failure of computed tomographic scanning to demonstrate subdural empyema. JAMA 1981;246:1116.
309. Kubik CS, Adams RD. Subdural empyema. Brain 1943;66:18.
310. Borzone M, Capuzzo T, Rivano S, et al. Subdural empyema: fourteen cases surgically treated. Surg Neurol 1980;13:449.
311. Hockley AD, Williams B. Surgical management of subdural empyema. Childs Brain 1983;10:294.
312. Baker CJ. Primary spinal epidural abscess. Am J Dis Child 1971;121:337.
313. Bullock R. Unusual presentation of pyogenic spinal epidural abscess: a case report. S Afr Med J 1981;59:723.

314. Jacobsen FS, Sullivan B. Spinal epidural abscess in children. Orthopedics 1994;17:1131–1138.
315. Rubin G, Michowiz SD, Ashkenasi A, Tadmor R, Rappaport ZH. Spinal epidural abscess in the pediatric age group: case report and review of the literature. Pediatr Infect Dis J 1993;12:1007–1011.
316. Hulme A, Dott NM. Spinal epidural abscess. Br Med J 1954;1:64.
317. Russell NA, Vaughan R, Morley TP. Spinal epidural infection. J Can Sci Neurol 1979;6:325.
318. Heusner AP. Nontuberculosis spinal epidural infections. N Engl J Med 1948;239:845–854.
319. Phillips GE, Jefferson A. Acute spinal epidural abscess. Observations from fourteen cases. Postgrad Med J 1979;55:712.
320. Tyson GW, Grant A, Strachan WE. Spinal epidural abscess presenting as acute abdomen in a child. Br J Surg 1979;66:3.
321. Hollis PH, Malis LI, Zappulla RA. Neurological deterioration after lumbar puncture below complete spinal subarachnoid block. J Neurosurg 1986;64:253–256.
322. Post MJD, Sze G, Quencer RM, Eismont FJ, Green BA, Gahbauer H. Gadolinium-enhanced MR in spinal infection. J Comput Assist Tomogr 1990;14:721–729.
323. Leys D, Lesoin F, Viaud C, et al. Decreased morbidity from acute bacterial spinal epidural abscesses using computed tomography and nonsurgical treatment in selected patients. Ann Neurol 1985;17:350–355.
324. Danner RL, Hartman BJ. Update on spinal epidural abscess: 35 cases and review of the literature. Rev Infect Dis 1987;9:265–274.
325. Hakin Rn, Burt AA, Cook JB. Acute spinal epidural abscess. Paraplegia 1979;17:330–338.
326. Yang SY. Spinal epidural abscess. NZ Med J 1982;95:302f.
327. McCaslin RI, Pikis A, Rodriquez WJ. Pediatric *Plasmodium falciparum* malaria: a ten-year experience from Washington DC. Pediatr Infect Dis J 1994; 13:709–715.
328. Warrell DA, Molyneux ME, Beales PF. Severe and complicated malaria. Trans R Soc Trop Med Hyg 1990; 84(suppl 2):1–65.
329. Anonymous. Bruce-Chwatt's Essential Malariology. 3rd ed. London: Edward Arnold, 1993:
330. White NJ, Ho M. The pathophysiology of malaria. Adv Parasit 1992; 31:83–173.
331. MacPherson GG, Warrell MJ, White NJ, Looareesuwan S, Warrell DA. Human cerebral malaria. A quantitative ultrastructural analysis of parasitized erythrocyte sequestration. Am J Pathol 1985; 119:385–401.
332. Ockenhouse CF, Ho M, Tandon NN, et al. Molecular basis of sequestration in severe and uncomplicated Plasmodium falciparum malaria: differential adhesion of infected erythrocytes to CD36 and ICAM-1. J Infect Dis 1991; 164:163–169.
333. Warrell DA, White NJ, Veall N, et al. Cerebral anaerobic glycolysis and reduced cerebral oxygen transport in human cerebral malaria. Lancet 1988; 2:534–538.
334. Kwiatkowski D, Hill AV, Sambou I, et al. TNF concentration in fatal cerebral, non-fatal cerebral, and uncomplicated Plasmodium falciparum malaria. Lancet 1990; 336:1201–1204.
335. Clark IA, Rockett KA, Cowden WB. Possible central role of nitric oxide in conditions clinically similar to cerebral malaria. Lancet 1992; 340:894–896.
336. Clark IA, Chaudhri G, Cowden WB. Roles of tumour necrosis factor in the illness and pathology of malaria. Trans R Soc Trop Med Hyg 1989; 83:436–440.
337. Marsh K, Forster D, Waruiru C, et al. Life-threatening malaria in African children: Clinical spectrum and simplified prognostic criteria. N Engl J Med 1995; 332 (21):1399–1404.
338. Newton CR, Kirkham FJ, Winstanley PA, et al. Intracranial pressure in African children with cerebral malaria. Lancet 1991; 337:573–576.
339. Mendis I, Carter R. Clinical disease and pathogenesis of malaria. Parasitology Today 1995; 11(5):PTI1–16.
340. Walker O, Salako LA, Sowunmi A, Thomas JO, Sodeine O, Bondi FS. Prognostic risk factors and post mortem findings in cerebral malaria in children. Trans R Soc Trop Med Hyg 1992; 86:491–493.
341. Warrell DA, Looareesuwan S, Phillips RE, et al. Function of the blood-cerebrospinal fluid barrier in human cerebral malaria: rejection of the permeability hypothesis. Am J Trop Med Hyg 1986; 35:882–889.
342. Newton CRJC, Peshu N, Kendall B, et al. Brain swelling and ischaemia in Kenyans with cerebral malaria. Arch Dis Child 1994; 70:281–287.
343. Looareesuwan S, Warrell DA, White NJ, et al. Do patients with cerebral malaria have cerebral oedema? A computed tomography study. Lancet 1983; 1:434–437.
344. Taylor TE, Molyneux ME, Wirima JJ, Fletcher A, Morris K. Blood glucose levels in Malawian children before and during the adminstration of intravenous quinine for severe falciparum malaria. N Engl J Med 1988; 319:1040–1047.
345. White NJ, Warrell DA, Chanthavanich P, et al. Severe hypoglycemia and hyperinsulinemia in falciparum malaria. N Engl J Med 1983; 309:61–66.
346. Molyneux ME, Taylor TE, Wirima JJ, Harper G. Effect of rate of infusion of quinine on insulin and glucose responses in Malawian children with falciparum malaria. BMJ 1989; 299:602–603.
347. Molyneux ME, Looareesuwan S, Menzies IS, et al. Reduced hepatic blood flow and intestinal malabsorption in severe falciparum malaria. Am J Trop Med Hyg 1989; 40(5):470–476.
348. White NJ, Warrell DA, Looareesuwan S, Chanthavanich P, Phillips RE, Pongpaew P. Pathophysiological and prognostic significance of cerebrospinal-fluid lactate in cerebral malaria. Lancet 1985; 1:776–778.
349. Krishna S, Waller DW, ter Kuile F, et al. Lactic acidosis and hypoglycaemia in children with severe malaria: pathophysiological and prognostic significance. Trans R Soc Trop Med Hyg 1994; 88:67–73.
350. Lynk A, Gold R. Review of 40 children with imported malaria. Pediatr Infect Dis J 1989; 8:745–750.
351. Looareesuwan S, Ho M, Wattanagoon Y, et al. Dynamic alteration in splenic function during acute falciparum malaria. N Engl J Med 1987; 317:675–679.
352. Phillips RE, Pasvol G. Anaemia of Plasmodium falciparum malaria. Baillieres Clin Haematol 1992; 5:315–330.
353. Molyneux ME, Taylor TE, Wirima JJ, Borgstein A. Clinical features and prognostic indicators in paediatric cerebral malaria: a study of 131 comatose Malawian children. Q J Med 1989; 71 (265):441–459.
354. Wright PW, Avery WG, Ardill WD, McLarty JW. Initial clinical assessment of the comatose patient: cerebral malaria vs. meningitis. Pediatr Infect Dis J 1993; 12:37–41.
355. Warrell DA, Looareesuwan S, Warrell MJ, et al. Dexamethasone proves deleterious in cerebral malaria. A double-blind trial in 100 comatose patients. N Engl J Med 1982; 306:313–319.
356. Kawo NG, Msengi AE, Swai AB, Chuwa LM, Alberti KG, McLarty DG. Specificity of hypoglycaemia for cerebral malaria in children. Lancet 1990; 336:454–457.
357. Phillips RE, Warrell DA, White NJ, Looareesuwan S, Karbwang J. Intravenous quinidine for the treatment of severe falciparum malaria: clinical and pharmacokinetic studies. N Engl J Med 1985; 312:1273–1278.
358. Miller KD, Greenberg AE, Campbell CC. Treatment of severe malaria in the United States with continous infusions of quinidine gluconate and exchange transfusion. N Engl J Med 1989; 321:65–70.
359. White NJ, Looareesuwan S, Warrell DA, et al. Quinine loading dose in cerebral malaria. Am J Trop Med Hyg 1983; 32:1–5.
360. Looareesuwan S, Phillips RE, Karbwang J, White NJ, Flegg PJ, Warrell DA. Plasmodium falciparum hyperparasitaemia: use of exchange transfusion in seven patients and a review of the literature.. Q J Med 1990; :227:471–481.
361. Phillips RE, Looareesuwan S, Molyneux ME, Hatz C, Warrell DA. Hypoglycaemia and counterregulatory hormone responses in severe falciparum malaria: treatment with Sandostatin. Q J Med 1993; 86:233–240.
362. Krishna S, Supanaranond W, Pukrittayakamee S, et al. Dichloroacetate for lactic acidosis in severe malaria: a pharmacokinetic and pharmacodynamic assessment. Metabolism 1994; 43 (8):974–981.

Specific Infectious Diseases of Interest to the Intensivist

33

Alice D. Ackerman

INTRODUCTION

It is impossible to include in this chapter a discussion of all of the infections the pediatric intensivist may be called upon to treat, since infection with almost any organism, including those that are usually benign, may lead to life-threatening diseases or complications under special circumstances. This chapter describes a selection of diseases of particular interest to the pediatric intensivist. The author acknowledges that certain diseases of special interest to some intensivists have been omitted and apologizes to those readers who may be disappointed at not finding a certain microorganism described. The following sections are arranged and presented in an arbitrary order, which is not meant to convey a particular importance of one over another.

TETANUS

Historical Background

Tetanus has been known for centuries as a terrible scourge and producer of great pain and contortion before inevitable death. It was first described by Hippocrates[1] in 400 BC, when he wrote about a ship's captain who hurt his right index finger on an anvil. A foul discharge from the wound was followed by inability to speak and trouble with his tongue. On the third day, opisthotonos and sweating developed, and the patient finally died on the sixth day.

Arataeus portrayed the natural history as well as the emotional distress of the patient with untreated tetanus in the second century AD. His description is as clear and vivid as any before or since[1]: "Tetanus, in all its varieties, is a spasm of an exceedingly painful nature, very swift to prove fatal, but neither easy to be removed. . . ."

In the early 19th century, the Scottish surgeon Charles Bell provided a clear visual description[2] of the disorder by drawing a portrait of a British soldier with severe tetanus from wounds received in the Peninsula War (Fig. 33.1).

The modern history of tetanus begins in the late 19th century. The disease's infectious cause was shown by Carle and Rattone[3] in 1884, who were able to produce disease in rabbits inoculated with human pus, and, further, to transmit it from diseased to healthy rabbits. The following year, Nicolaier discovered the organism in soil and was able to

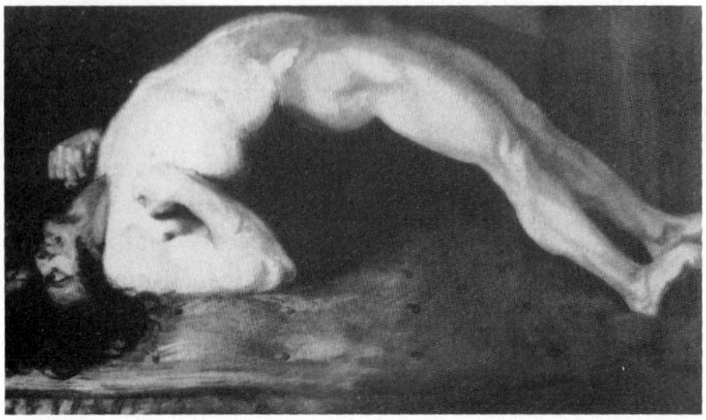

Figure 33.1. Portrait by Sir Charles Bell of British soldier with tetanus. (From Finegold SM. Anaerobic bacteria in human disease. New York: Academic Press, 1977.)

produce clinical disease in animals by inoculating them with soil samples. In 1889, *Clostridium tentani* was isolated by Kitasato[4].

In 1890, Faber showed that a toxin and not a whole bacterium was involved in production of disease. In the same year, Von Behring and Kitasato[5] identified and isolated the antitoxin and showed that long-term immunity in the serum of animals was bactericidal. Nocard first showed the protective effect of antitoxin in humans in 1897. By the start of World War I, bovine and equine tetanus antitoxins were commercially available, and their prophylactic use by the British Army helped diminish the death rate from tetanus.

The first formaldehyde inactivation of toxin, which forms a harmless toxoid, was accomplished independently by Glenny and Ramon in 1920. In 1926, Descoby proved that inactivation of toxin with both heat and formaldehyde yielded a safe toxoid that retained its immunogenicity. Alum precipitation of toxoid was reported by Glenny and colleagues[6], also in 1926; such treatment was found to greatly enhance the antigenicity of the inactivated toxoid. No major changes in the vaccine have been made since that time.

Bacteriology

C. tetani is the organism that causes tetanus. It is a Gram-positive, obligate, anaerobic bacillus that exists in two forms. The vegetative forms contain numerous flagellae, are motile, and form spores that are located in only one end of the bacterium, which gives it a characteristic drumstick appearance (Fig. 33.2). Although the vegetative forms are susceptible to antiseptics and heat, the spores formed are very resistant and may persist for many years in a contaminated area, such as soil. The spores are adversely affected by direct sunlight. Laboratory growth occurs best at 37°C under anaerobic conditions on blood agar. There are 10 identified serotypes, all of which produce similar toxins, and immunization with one is effective against all types. The organisms are ubiquitous in nature.

Two exotoxins are produced by *C. tetani,* but only one, called tetanospasmin, is implicated in the pathogenesis of disease. It is second in potency, among toxins, only to botulinal toxin. As little as one-half pound of tetanus toxin may be sufficient to kill the entire human population of the world. In humans, a lethal dose of toxin is much less than the immunizing dose, so that natural immunity does not occur. The other exotoxin, called tetanolysin, produces hemolysis but has no known clinical importance.

Tetanus is a major cause of disease and death worldwide, despite the fact that immunization provides almost complete protection. More than 500,000 deaths are estimated to occur annually from tetanus, and about half of these deaths are in neonates[7]. Newborns, especially those born at home, of nonimmunized mothers are particularly susceptible—more so when unsanitary conditions prevail. Many neonatal deaths secondary to umbilical tetanus occur in the absence of medical care, and the actual incidence of such situations may be much higher than is reported or appreciated.

Alum-absorbed tetanus toxoid has been available in the United States since the 1920s, and the incidence of disease has steadily declined with widespread immunization. The infection was first made a reportable disease by the Centers for Disease Control and Prevention (CDC) in 1965, when an active surveillance system was initiated. The number of cases and deaths has fallen steadily since that time[8]. Between 1985 and 1990, 365 total cases were reported to the CDC, 92.6% of cases were in adults[9].

The overall mortality rate from tetanus averages about 45% but varies from 18% to nearly 100% in some studies. Mortality is highest among neonates and elderly persons, in whom poor immunologic status, diminished nonspecific resistance to disease, and underlying illness contribute to susceptibility. However, as a result of the increasing availability of neonatal critical care services in Mexico, the death rate from neonatal tetanus there fell from 46% (1970 to 1980) to 12.9% (1980 to 1990)[10]. Heroin addicts have a higher death rate from tetanus than the general population[2].

Epidemiologically, tetanus has been divided into types

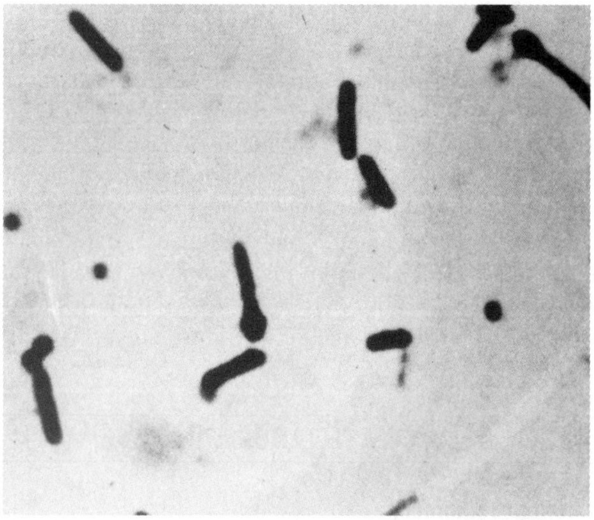

Figure 33.2. Typical drumstick appearance of *C. tetani* from patient with tetanus. (From Finegold SM. Anaerobic bacteria in human disease. New York: Academic Press, 1977.)

based on the method or source of contamination. By far, the most common type is accidental tetanus. Other types include umbilical or neonatal, obstetrical, otogenic, and surgical[11]. In up to 20% of cases, the source is never identified. Such cases may include unsuspected wounds or injuries that appear minor or have healed before the onset of symptoms.

Accidental tetanus occurs following contamination of a wound with *C. tetani* spores. Under appropriate anaerobic conditions, facilitated by the formation of pus or an abscess, a retained foreign body, or diminished blood flow to the area, the spores germinate into the vegetative forms capable of producing toxin. Although deep wounds heavily contaminated with dirt or organic material may be more likely to develop clinical tetanus, any wound, abrasion, infection, burn, or ulceration must be considered suspect. Dental infections are relatively frequent but often overlooked sources of infection.

In the United States, most tetanus cases occur in the south central and southeastern states. More cases occur in the spring and summer, presumably because an increase in outdoor work causing increased exposure to the organism. Persons who have never been immunized are at greater risk than those whose immunization status has become inadequate through lack of regular immunization.

Action of Tetanus Toxin

Pathophysiology

Tetanospasmin, the toxin that produces disease, is secreted only by vegetative forms of the organism. *C. tetani* exists in soil and animal excreta in the spore form. Generation of toxin requires induction of the vegetative state, which occurs only when the organism is introduced into tissue that has a low oxidation-reduction potential and low partial pressure of oxygen. These conditions exist in tissue that has been damaged by injury, foreign body, or local production of pus. Toxin, thus produced, must then travel to the central nervous system (CNS). The nature of this transport has been much debated in the literature.

The current understanding is that in local tetanus, the toxin is absorbed from motor endplates in the afflicted muscle, with subsequent retrograde flow by means of axonal transport to the ventral horns of the spinal cord[12]. In these cases, the area of injury is the first affected. The toxin may then traverse the spinal cord, producing disease in other areas. This is known as the *local neural pathway*. Such a scenario clearly does not explain transmission in the 75% of cases that present with trismus (lockjaw), regardless of the site of inoculation.

Toxin transport in generalized tetanus is by means of the perineuronal lymphatic system into the bloodstream via the thoracic duct. In addition, some toxin is absorbed directly from the muscle into the blood[13]. Direct involvement of the CNS from the bloodborne toxin is not possible because the blood-brain barrier is impervious to the toxin, which is a protein of about 67,000 daltons[14]. Most likely, bloodborne toxin is distributed to peripheral muscles, where it is taken up by motor neurons. Retrograde transmission occurs, both through the axon and the perineuronal spaces to the cell body. No symptoms appear until the toxin crosses the synaptic space and is taken up by the presynaptic membrane in the interneuron, the anterior horn cells of the spinal cord, or the motor nuclei of the cranial nerves. Intraaxonal transport of toxin occurs at the rate of 3.35 mm/hr[11]. Transmission through the cranial nerves and motor neurons of the neck (because of their relatively short length and greater levels of activity) is most rapid, thereby explaining the early findings of trismus and risus sardonicus that often herald the onset of disease. Some toxin also enters sensory and autonomic (sympathetic and parasympathetic) neurons and has been found in dorsal and lateral horn cells of the spinal cord as well as in surrounding brainstem nuclei, especially in the medulla.

The toxin binds to the cell membrane via the *carboxyl* terminus of the heavy chain. The amino terminus then mediates internalization of the toxin[15]. The underlying mechanism of action of tetanospasmin is inhibition of release of neurotransmitter from the presynaptic membrane[16–20], which appears to be mediated by the light chain[15]. Although inhibitory neurons are predominantly affected, resulting in generalized disinhibition, the condition is not a static one, as evidenced by the alternating nature of many of the symptoms. Effector neurons are also involved. Tetanus toxin has been found to act in four separate areas: the brain, spinal cord, motor endplates, and the autonomic nervous system.

In the brain and spinal cord, tetanospasmin binds to cerebrosides and gangliosides, interferes with transmission in polysynaptic pathways, and dramatically decreases transmission in the inhibitory interneurons, resulting in unchecked excitation. Tetanospasmin accumulates in the presynaptic terminals and inhibits transmitter release, but does not block uptake at postsynaptic membranes. Toxin preferentially accumulates in glycinergic terminals, resulting in predominant disinhibitory effects. Accumulation in γ–aminobutyric acid (GABA) terminals in the brain may result in generalized disinhibition; this helps explain the development of the tetanic convulsions that occur as the disease progresses.

In the motor endplate, release of acetylcholine is inhibited, and the transmitter accumulates in the presynaptic terminal. Certain stimuli have been shown experimentally to induce rhythmic release of transmitter from the endplate, resulting in sustained contraction.

Disinhibition of the autonomic nervous system also occurs, resulting in unchecked but intermittent sympathetic activity and alterations in bladder function and intestinal motility[21]. Tetanospasmin also binds to thyrotropin receptors on thyroid cells, resulting in increased release of iodine, stimulation of certain thyroid functions, and elevation in resting sympathetic tone[11]. Destructive lesions of the brainstem have been noted in fatal cases. These presum-

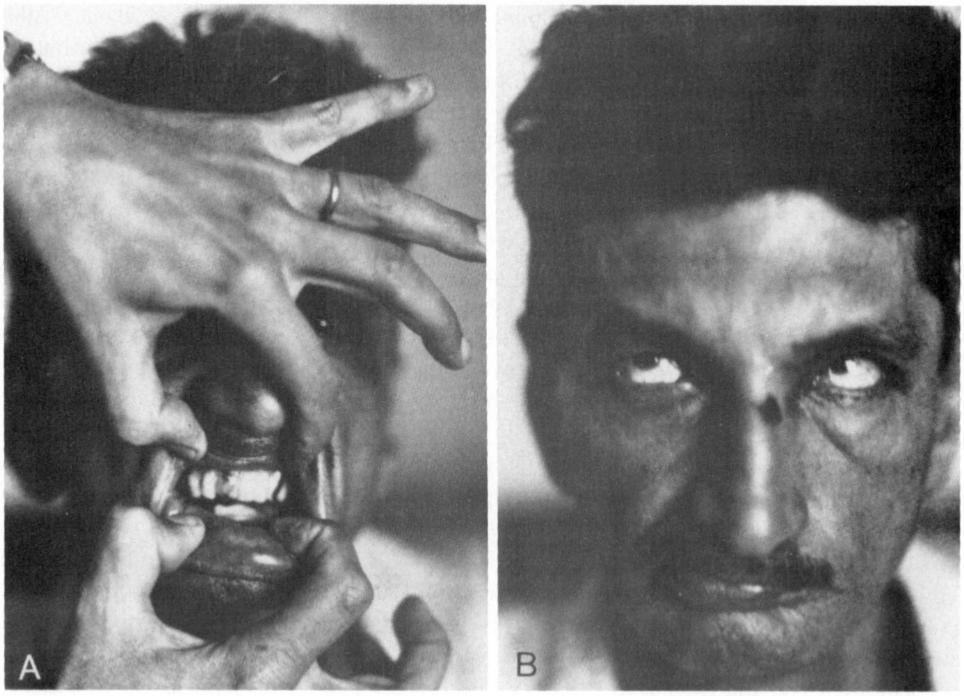

Figure 33.3. Trismus in patient with tetanus. (From Veronesi R, ed. Tetanus: important new concepts. Princeton, NJ: Excerpta Medica, 1981.)

ably play a role in the development of autonomic nervous system hyperactivity[15].

Clinical Presentation

Symptoms of tetanus develop after an incubation period that ranges from 24 hours to several months after injury; however, the incubation period is commonly from 3 to 21 days[22]. Initial symptoms may consist of stiffness and crampy pain in the wounded muscle, but this finding may be completely absent. Often the first symptomatic expression of disease is a stiffness in the neck and jaw; trismus (lockjaw) is present in about 75% of cases[11]. In other patients, tetanus may present as backache, muscular rigidity, or lower extremity pain. Facial paralysis may accompany cephalic tetanus. Sometimes, there are premonitory symptoms of unexplained irritability and sensory changes. In some cases of cephalic tetanus, when the cortical gray matter becomes involved before the signs of generalized tetanus manifest, psychological disturbances and mental status changes may predominate[11].

The patient with trismus has difficulty opening the mouth because of masseter spasm (Fig. 33.3) and is, therefore, unable to chew. As other facial muscles become hypertonic, facial features become somewhat contorted into the classic risus sardonicus (Fig. 33.4). Muscles of the trunk are next to become involved, leading to rigidity in the paravertebral muscles, which results in thoracic kyphosis and lumbar lordosis. Involvement of these muscles may result in opisthotonus. The tension of abdominal muscles makes it difficult to rule out peritonitis or an abdominal source of the infection by means of clinical examination. The limb muscles are next to be affected. The upper limbs flex, and the lower limbs extend. As the disease progresses, after a period of generalized hypertonia the patient has tetanic convulsions, which are actually rhythmic spasms, sometimes of frightening intensity, that may be painful. Depending upon the severity of the disease, such spasms may occur from several times a day to as often as once a minute. Finally, the muscles of respiration are affected. When the spasms involve the glottis and respiratory muscles, apnea occurs and death may be imminent if apnea does not resolve rapidly or is not treated aggressively with muscle relaxants and respiratory support. Pharyngeal spasms result in severe dysphagia, making eating impossible for these patients, and they may not be able to handle their secretions.

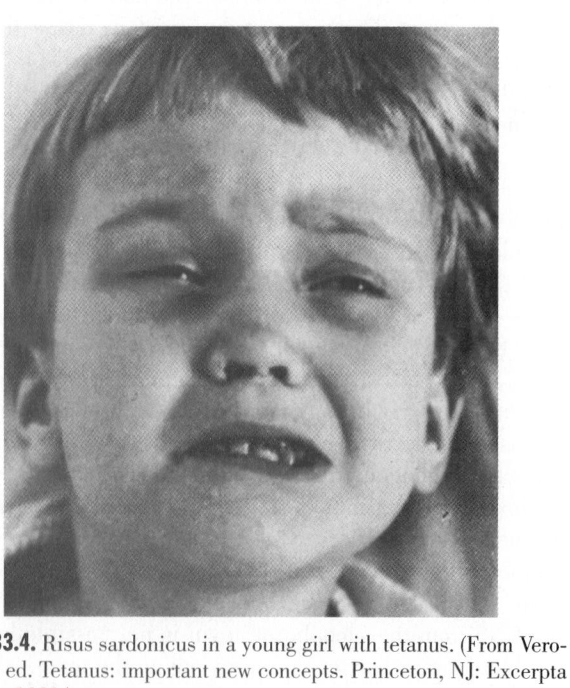

Figure 33.4. Risus sardonicus in a young girl with tetanus. (From Veronesi R, ed. Tetanus: important new concepts. Princeton, NJ: Excerpta Medica, 1981.)

Prognosis has been related to many factors[23–27]. Patients whose disease has a short incubation period (less than 7 days) are at greatest risk of developing severe tetanus, which bears a high rate of mortality. A short time between injury and onset of symptoms correlates with a large volume of inoculum and circulating toxin. An even more sensitive prognostic indicator is the length of time between initial onset of symptoms and development of tetanic spasms. When this period is less than 48 hours in duration, the prognosis is grave. Development of fever has also been noted to be a poor prognostic sign, as have tachycardia and spasms of severe intensity. Clinically, tetanus has generally been divided into three grades: benign, moderate, and severe **(Table 33.1)**[11].

Neonatal tetanus is almost always generalized, related to contamination of the umbilical stump, and particularly severe[7,11,22,28,29]. The median age at onset is 6 to 7 days. The first symptom is often difficulty sucking and swallowing because of stiffness of the jaw and pharyngeal muscles. The disease progresses rapidly to generalized hypertonicity and then to tetanic spasms. Apnea commonly results from spasm of the respiratory muscles. Vomiting occurs because of increased abdominal tone, often leading to pulmonary aspiration of gastric contents. If the child survives, the spasms generally subside by the end of the second week of illness. The ability to swallow returns by the end of the fourth week, and relaxation of the hypertonic muscles may require another 2 weeks.

Diagnosis and Differential Diagnosis

The diagnosis of tetanus is made completely on clinical grounds. There are no serologic tests, and results of bacteriologic cultures are often negative[11]. Diagnosis can be aided by obtaining data regarding the nature of a preceding injury as well as history of previous immunization. In cases in which the diagnosis is not certain, infected material from the patient's wound may be withdrawn and injected into the hind leg of a rodent. The animal may then be watched for signs and symptoms of local tetanus[8].

Nonspecific laboratory findings may include elevated total white blood cell count with leukocytosis and lymphopenia; alterations in the serum protein electrophoretic pattern, with elevation in the α_2–globulin and γ–globulin fractions; and decreased concentrations of α_1–globulin and β–globulin. There is a generalized increase in circulating levels of epinephrine and norepinephrine, as well as a high rate of excretion of metabolites of these compounds in urine. Plasma creatine phosphokinase levels are elevated, presumably owing to the intensity of muscular contractions. Serum cholinesterase levels are decreased, which has no apparent impact on the disease, its course, or prognosis[30].

Diagnosis is often difficult or delayed in the patient with very early tetanus, who presents with no clear evidence or history of injury and with localized neck stiffness or trismus. Meningitis is easily ruled out because, at this stage, fever is not generally present, and the child has no mental status changes. Analysis of cerebrospinal fluid (CSF) may be mildly abnormal, commonly with an elevation in protein content[31]. The causes of trismus are many, and children who arrive in the emergency department unable to open their mouths are most likely to have peritonsillar abscess, temporomandibular joint disease, or abscess of the alveolar ridge. In patients suffering from an acute phenothiazine reaction, torticollis is present in addition to trismus.

Other diseases that may mimic tetanus are hypocalcemic tetany (in which low serum calcium levels and typical posture of the hands and feet make the diagnosis clear), strychnine poisoning, and rabies. In rabies, CNS involvement along with altered mental status occurs early, and there is prominent early respiratory embarrassment and dysphagia. In strychnine poisoning, symptoms advance very rapidly, trismus occurs late, and hypertonia alternates with hypotonia.

Results of a study of tetanus in Finland, published in 1990, revealed that half of 106 patients of all ages (not neonates) who presented with acute tetanus also had a delayed diagnosis, including two patients in whom the diagnosis was only made after death[31]. The alternative diagnoses considered initially in 47 of the patients are presented in **Table 33.2.**

Complications

Respiratory

Before the development of modern methods of intensive respiratory care, most patients with severe tetanus died of respiratory failure. Insufficient respiration may occur be-

Table 33.1. Grades of Tetanus Severity

	Grade		
Factor	*Benign*	*Moderate*	*Severe*
Incubation period	>20 days	10 to 20 days	<10 days
Spasms	Absent	Present	Frequent and severe
Fever	Absent	Present	>39°C
Dysphagia	Absent	Present	Severe
Muscle rigidity	Mild: generalized or localized	Intense: upper body most affected	Intense: generalized without relief
Other signs		Cough: inhibited	Apnea, sympathetic overactivity, tissue hypoxia
Therapy	Observation ± sedation	Sedation ± neuromuscular blockade	Sedation, paralysis ± treatment of autonomic dysfunction

Data are from Reference 11.

Table 33.2. Alternative Diagnosis of 47 Patients with Tetanus at the First Visit to a Doctor

Diagnosis	*Number of Patients*
Pharyngitis, common cold	7
Undefined neurologic disease	6
Side effect of phenothiazine	4
Disease of the esophagus	4
Epilepsy	3
Psychogenic symptoms	3
Stomatitis	2
Disease of the temporomandibular joint	2
Encephalitis	2
Facial paresis	2
Other	12
Total	47

Modified with permission from Luisto M. Tetanus in Finland: diagnostic problems and complications. Ann Med 1990; 22:15–19.

cause of spasm of the inspiratory muscles or acute laryngospasm. Early intervention combining muscle relaxation, airway control with an endotracheal tube or tracheostomy, and assisted ventilation along with induction of total or partial neuromuscular blockade has become the mainstay of tetanus therapy in the ICU and is responsible for diminution of the mortality rate.

There are some controversial issues surrounding respiratory care of the tetanus patient, which are discussed in Chapter 8. Regardless of which agents are chosen to achieve sedation, relaxation, and adequate air exchange, protection of the airway is of paramount importance, and neuromuscular blockade combined with heavy sedation must be initiated if spontaneous respiratory efforts are inadequate or if mechanical ventilation cannot overcome tetanic spasms of the chest wall muscles and diaphragm.

Even with optimal airway management, patients with tetanus continue to be at risk for pulmonary infections, owing to prolonged mechanical ventilation, inspissation of secretions, and intermittent inhibition of respiratory excursions. Some of these infections may prove fatal. Patients on ventilators have an increased risk of developing conjunctivitis or other ocular problems[31].

Autonomic Nervous and Cardiovascular Systems

The cardiovascular complications of tetanus carry the greatest risk of death in today's ICU environment[22,32,33]. Involvement of the autonomic nervous system occurs primarily in patients with severe disease (based on prognostic factors already described) who require mechanical ventilation, most of whom are receiving sedative drugs, muscle relaxants, and paralytics. Both sympathetic and parasympathetic disinhibition occur, although syndromes of sympathetic overactivity have been more consistently described.

Symptoms of sympathetic overactivity generally occur in the second to third week of illness[21], but may be present earlier in particularly severe cases. The syndrome is heralded by alterations of heart rate and blood pressure level, which vary in a hectic fashion, unrelated to generation of spasms (Fig. 33.5). These changes are accompanied by increased cardiac output, elevation of peripheral vasomotor tone, and elevated venous pressure, findings which are associated with rapid fluctuations in systemic vascular resistance and evidence of myocardial dysfunction[34]. Peripheral vasoconstriction may be intense enough to cause ischemia and pallor of the skin in a stocking-glove distribution[35]. Profuse sweating of the face and thorax may occur along with peripheral constriction and in the absence of hyperpyrexia, although occasionally, high fevers are also present. Although the most common electrocardiographic finding is sinus tachycardia, other rhythm disturbances, such as supraventricular tachycardia, multifocal premature

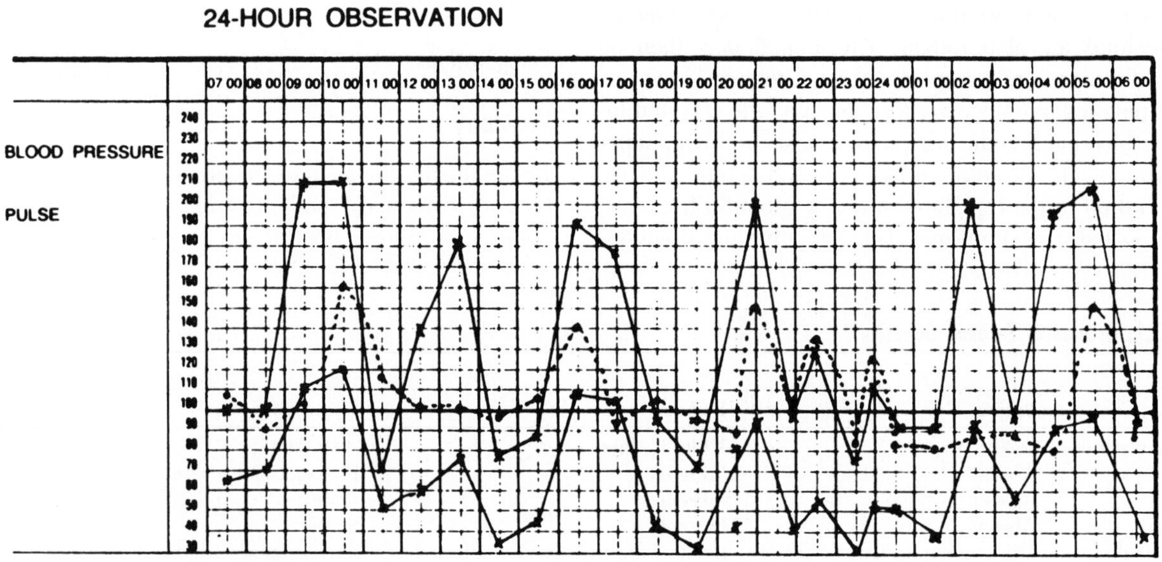

Figure 33.5. Graphic representation of marked cardiovascular disturbances in a patient with severe tetanus, on day 7 of hospitalization, before treatment with magnesium sulfate. X——X = blood pressure; ··· = pulse rate. (From James MFM, Manson EDM. The use of magnesium sulfate infusions in the management of very severe tetanus. Intensive Care Med 1985;11:5.)

atrial contractions, and premature ventricular contractions have been noted. The constellation of symptoms may occur spontaneously or in response to even minor stimuli, as is the case with tetanic spasms. Symptoms cannot be alleviated with analgesia or sedation.

When catecholamine levels and metabolites are measured[36], elevations of epinephrine and norepinephrine levels are consistently documented. Evening cortisol levels[37] are elevated, but this may result more from an altered diurnal pattern or a response to being in the ICU than from the effect of the toxin. The significance of elevated catecholamine levels goes beyond symptomatic sympathetic overdrive. At least one series[38] has reported autopsy results in patients with elevated catecholamine levels and tetanus and has documented widespread myocardial damage that cannot be distinguished from that caused by inadvertent catecholamine overdose or the catecholamine excess seen in pheochromocytoma. What was once postulated to be a direct myocardial depressant effect of the toxin[22] is now believed to more likely be caused by excessively high levels of circulating catecholamines. Sympathetic overactivity may end with profound and untreatable hypotension and bradycardia, accompanied by evolving and progressive myocardial failure and associated alterations in ST segments and T waves that are suggestive of cardiac ischemia.

Parasympathetic overactivity may lead to severe preterminal bradycardia, sinus arrest, and increased bronchial and salivary secretions. Patients may respond to endotracheal suctioning with marked bradycardia. Direct damage to the vagal nucleus has been implicated in addition to potential local damage to the sinus node and to reflex excessive vagal tone.

Treatment of autonomic dysfunction has been approached in a number of ways. Induction and maintenance of general anesthesia with nitrous oxide or halothane[33] has resulted in resolution of symptoms, but therapy was abandoned because of documented or theoretical side effects of the agents involved. Administration of magnesium sulfate has been effective without major adverse effects on cardiac function[35,39]. James and Manson[35] demonstrated that the use of magnesium sulfate by constant infusion, adjusted by monitoring blood magnesium levels, reduced the extreme variability of vital signs (Fig. 33.6), diminished the requirements for neuromuscular blockade and sedation, and allowed better overall control of severely ill patients. Patients were carefully monitored by means of pulmonary artery balloon catheters, and the investigators were able to prove that the infusion did not adversely affect stroke volume or cardiac output. Systemic vascular resistance, pulmonary artery pressure, and pulmonary capillary wedge pressure did not change markedly. The treated patients experienced no decrease in blood pressure to unacceptable levels.

Attempts to control heart rate and blood pressure through β–blockade may be successful, but a case has been reported in which a 7-year-old child developed tachycardia and subsequent cardiac arrest following oral propranolol administration[40]. Simultaneous administration of α–blocking agents, such as phentolamine, has increased the efficiency with which propranolol lowers blood pressure. Successful therapy with labetalol[41,42] has been reported. This drug is both an α–antagonist and β–antagonist. The treatment of hypertension with direct β–blocking agents may be particularly dangerous in patients in whom sympathetic overload is intermittent and who may depend on some degree of β-stimulation to maintain cardiac output.

If pure β-antagonist agents are used, they should be given in small doses intravenously and titrated for effectiveness. The use of enteral administeration of propranolol is contraindicated if the the drug can be administered parenterally, because the alterations in gastrointestinal motility may make absorption erratic and response unpredict-

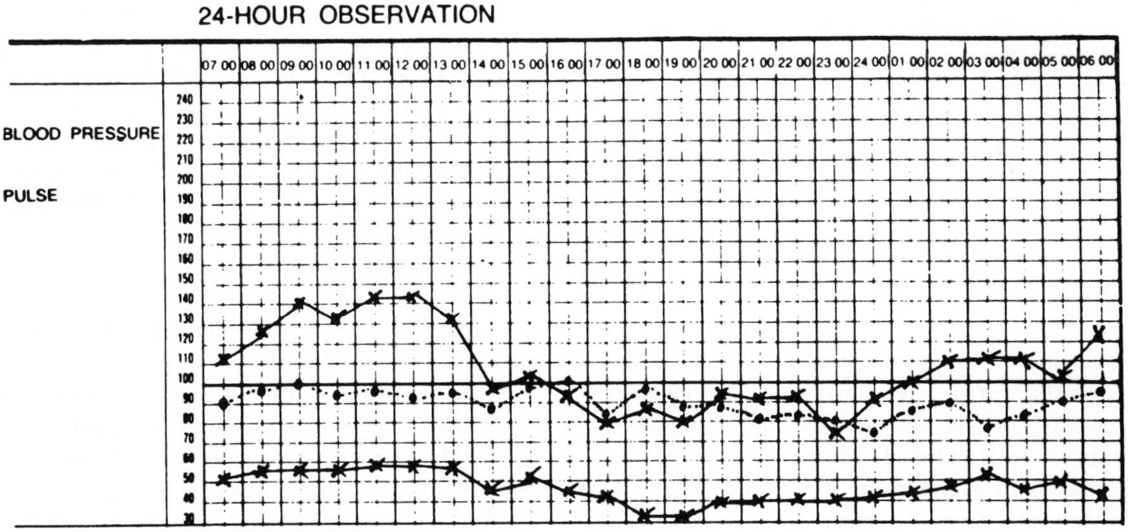

Figure 33.6. Twenty-four hr record of the same patient as represented in Figure 33.5 2 days after commencement of magnesium therapy. X——X = blood pressure; ··· = pulse rate. (From James MFM, Manson EDM. The use of magnesium sulfate infusions in the management of very severe tetanus. Intensive Care Med 1985;11:5.)

able. Agents with short half-lives (e.g., esmolol) may be preferable[43].

In light of the current state of knowledge concerning autonomic instability in tetanus, a prudent approach to management to achieve full control of the respiratory system first is recommended (see Chapters 8 and 9), thereby also achieving control of painful muscle spasms. If wide swings in blood pressure or heart rate occur with any degree of frequency, further reduction of stimulation should be sought, if possible, and additional pain relief should be provided with a narcotic agent. Additional therapy should aim to depress the CNS further if tolerated (e.g., high-dose barbiturates). Infusions of magnesium sulfate may be attempted by those who are familiar with its use. Only if all of this is unsuccessful at controlling the episodes of hypertension should an attempt be made to treat it with combined α–blockade and β–blockade. Labetalol may be an appropriate drug in the adult, and enough experience in its use has been accumulated in children to recommend it as a safe alternative to pure β–blockers. When possible, patients should be monitored invasively. Cardiac output and peripheral vascular resistance, as well as oxygen consumption, should be closely monitored.

Metabolic

Metabolic complications may have the most far-reaching effects in patients who survive the acute episodes of tetanus[44–46]. A significantly increased metabolic rate along with marked nitrogen wasting is a result both of increased muscle activity and metabolism secondary to spasms in those patients who are not paralyzed and also a result of high levels of catecholamines. The patient remains in a generally catabolic state. Attempts to provide large numbers of calories usually result in severe elevation of serum glucose levels, and these patients usually require insulin administration with their enteral or parenteral nutrition. Enteral feeding may result in adverse effects such as emesis and aspiration when abdominal muscles contract, especially in the presence of ileus. A recent report[47] suggests that metabolic rates of patients appropriately sedated are within 10% of predicted basal rates, and can remain relatively stable with ongoing control of sympathetic activity.

Other Complications

Other complications that have been noted include gastrointestinal hemorrhage from stress ulcers, diaphragmatic paralysis, thromboembolism, and persistent orthopedic abnormalities caused by fractured thoracic vertebrae. Myositis ossificans may occur at the site of a previously contracted muscle, presumably from intramuscular hemorrhage and subsequent calcification. Limb deformities secondary to muscle contractures are not uncommon.

Death

Respiratory failure continues to lead the list of causes of death, followed by hemodynamic instability, hemorrhage, and sepsis as a result of superinfection of the lung or urinary tract. While the death rate directly attributable to tetanus has dropped dramatically since the advent of intensive care, deaths due to iatrogenic and other complications have become more frequent.

In the absence of modern intensive care facilities, 65% of tetanus deaths occur in the first 48 hours; over 95% of deaths occur by the end of the first week of illness[8]. Almost all patients (nearly 100%) die from respiratory muscle spasm. Because the symptoms of sympathetic overactivity are often not present until the second or third week of illness, most patients who have severe tetanus and for whom intensive care is not available expire before they exhibit such complications. This may be why neonates have not been noted to have a prominent component of sympathetic overactivity; in the places where tetanus neonatorum is prevalent, pediatric intensive care facilities are not.

Therapy

The only uniformly effective approach to tetanus is prevention of disease by active immunization with alum-absorbed tetanus toxoid and maintenance of the fully immunized state[9,48,49]. Full immunization is the responsibility of health departments and government agencies, but all physicians should encourage and help enforce rules regarding immunization in schools and workplaces. An often-ignored segment of the population are those in late middle age and elderly persons, who are at greatest risk of dying from the disease if they become infected.

The goals of acute therapy of tetanus are to support the vital functions and provide pain relief and muscle relaxation. Diazepam, morphine, chlorpromazine, dantrolene, and propofol[50–55] are all drugs that have been used to achieve some degree of muscle relaxation. Pancuronium bromide and other nondepolarizing neuromuscular blocking agents, including atracurium besylate, have been used to achieve adequate ventilation and to stop tetanic convulsions[56–58], often for prolonged periods. Tracheostomy versus nasotracheal intubation for specific airway control is a debated issue[59]. For neonates, nasotracheal intubation, with care to avoid accidental extubations, may be preferable to tracheostomy for this self-limited disease. Intrathecal administration of baclofen may relieve symptoms of contractures and paroxysms but may also lead to CNS and respiratory depression if doses are repeated[60]. The means to provide respiratory system support must therefore be available. The adjunctive use of corticosteroids has reduced the mortality rate from severe tetanus as well as the need for mechanical ventilation and tracheostomy[61].

When the injury is still apparent, especially if there is

any chance of a retained foreign body, the wound should be explored and debrided. Tetanus hyperimmune globulin should be administered immediately; if possible, an hour or so before surgical debridement. The value of antitoxin therapy is limited, in that it is without effect on toxin that has already bound to nervous tissue[11] and can only inactivate free toxin in the bloodstream. The administration of penicillin or chloramphenicol inhibits growth of *C. tetani* in the wound and, therefore, prevents generation of more toxin but does not change the natural progress of the disease.

The general principles of intensive care must be followed, especially with regard to appropriate caloric provisions, physical therapy to limit contractures, and psychological support. In addition, because these patients seem more at risk for thrombotic complications (possibly from vascular spasm caused by catecholamine excess), some authors recommend the use of low-dose heparin prophylactically[2,50].

Natural immunity to tetanus does not occur, so patients with tetanus must receive active immunization to prevent recurrence of disease. Immunization should begin during the acute stage in hospital. The primary immunization series should be given over a 6-month period. Patient education is exceedingly important. If the public is permitted to become complacent, or if the physician assumes a laissez-faire attitude toward immunization, the pediatric intensivist is likely to see an increasing number of cases of this potentially devastating disease.

BOTULISM

Introduction

Botulism is caused by a neurotoxin elaborated by the bacterium *Clostridium botulinum,* an anaerobic Gram-positive bacillus that forms heat-resistant spores. The organism is widely distributed in nature. Germination of spores and subsequent multiplication of organisms in a suitable environment results in production of a heat-labile toxin that is the most deadly substance known, able to cause death in extremely small doses[62,63]. Three specific forms of disease have been described: food-borne, wound, and infant botulism. An unclassified disease category includes victims more than one year old in whom a vehicle of infection cannot be identified[64].

Seven types of botulinal toxin have been identified, designated by the letters A through G. The majority of disease in humans is caused by types A, B, and E and the minority by type F. Types C and D are most often implicated in botulism in animals and birds, occasionally affecting humans, and type G has been identified in soil[65] but has not been associated with human disease. Type A toxin has been developed for use as a therapeutic agent in certain conditions involving involuntary muscle spasm[66].

Action of the Toxin

All of the identified botulinal toxins act via the same mechanism, i.e., by blocking release of acetylcholine from nerve endings. The toxin's effects have been demonstrated at four different levels of the peripheral nervous system: the neuromuscular junction, parasympathetic nerve endings, autonomic ganglia, and acetylcholine-releasing sympathetic nerve endings. The effects on the neuromuscular junction have been most extensively studied and are considered the most important[67]. The pathogenesis of disease involves initial binding of toxin to nerve endings. However, binding alone is not sufficient to induce paralysis: the molecule (or part of it) must be transported into the nerve cell in a process known as translocation, the specific mechanism of which remains obscure[62]. The toxin must also be lysed before it can become activated; the activated portion then, probably, binds to a site within the target cell where it may remain for months. The level of blockade of acetylcholine release is thought to be inhibition of calcium-mediated acetylcholine granule exocytosis from terminal axons[66,68]. Toxin is rapidly absorbed from the gastrointestinal tract, transported by blood and lymphatic systems, and bound to peripheral neural tissue. Action of pancreatic enzymes, especially trypsin, is important in the activation of certain toxin types, especially type E.

In wound botulism, native toxin produced by *C. botulinum* is released directly into the bloodstream. Type E has never been implicated in production of wound botulism[69], suggesting that toxins able to cause wound botulism must be released in activated form.

Clinical Syndromes

Infant Botulism

Infant botulism is a rare disease. It was first recognized in 1976[70]. It is caused by *C. botulinum* toxin produced within the gastrointestinal tract of the young patient, rather than preformed in contaminated foods as is classic food-borne botulism. The first known case occurred in 1931, although it was only recognized as such[71] after Pickett's description in 1976[63]. Factors that allow germination of spores, colonization of the gut, and intraintestinal production of toxin in infants but not in older children or adults are not fully elucidated. Studies in immature animals and fowl[72–75] have suggested that the presence of a normal mature pattern of enteric microflora may be important in preventing disease in older people.

Epidemiology

The occurrence of infant botulism is typically limited to patients between 1 and 12 months of age, although cases occurring earlier have been reported[76]. A 3-year-old child was found to have infant botulism following bone marrow transplantation[77]. Prevalence does not change in regard to

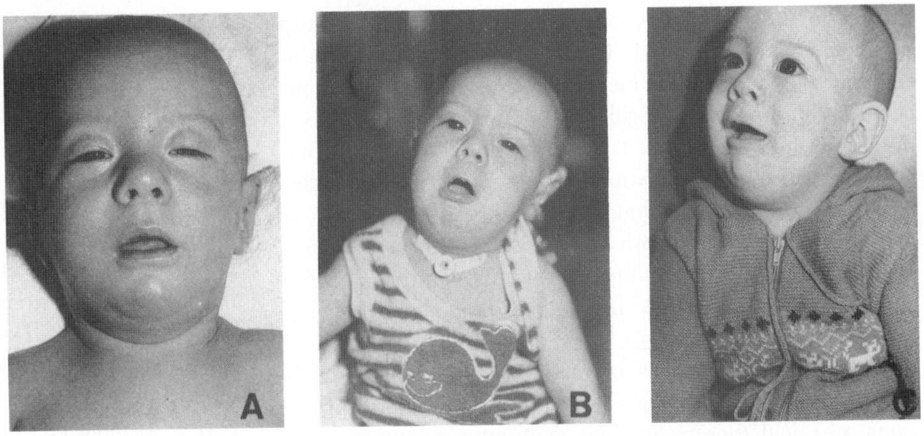

Figure 33.7. Typical case of infant botulism. **A.** On admission, baby had bilateral ptosis and facial diparesis. **B.** Same infant 4 weeks later with tracheostomy in place because of persistence of inadequate protective airway reflexes, multiple cranial nerve involvement, and poor head control. **C.** Nine weeks after admission; complete recovery. (From Brown LW. Infant botulism. Pediatr Ann 1984; 13:135.)

race or gender. More cases have been identified in California than anywhere else. This finding may represent results of aggressive surveillance methods, but more probably reflects an uneven geographic distribution of botulism spores, as suggested by an epidemiologic survey of infant botulism in Pennsylvania(78).

One potentially avoidable food source that has been associated with some cases of infant botulism is honey, which is implicated in about 35% of cases. *C. botulinum* spores, but not toxin, have been found in honey fed to these patients(79,80). It is therefore recommended that children less than 1 year old not be fed honey(81). Consumption of corn syrup has also been identified in some studies as a risk factor(82). Other environmental sources have been identified(80,83). Formula-fed babies are at greater risk for severe disease than those who consume breast milk in the month preceding onset of illness, but exclusive breast feeding has been associated with increased risk of disease in infants more than 2 months old(82,84). Iron supplements in both formula–fed and breast–fed infants may predispose them to particularly severe disease(85). Iron fortification of both whey-based and casein-based infant formulas alters the intestinal flora, decreasing colonization by staphylococci and bacteroides, and increasing the growth of clostridia and enterococci(86). In most cases, however, no source of spores is ever identified(85).

Clinical Features

The clinical spectrum of infant botulism ranges from asymptomatic "carriage" of *C. botulinum*(87) to a hyperacute form of disease in which a previously healthy baby is found dead in bed and appears to have been the victim of sudden infant death syndrome (SIDS)(87–89). The majority of infants studied have disease of moderate to severe intensity and require hospitalization. In most of these babies, constipation is the first sign (but is often only recognized retrospectively). The child is subsequently listless and lethargic with decreased appetite. Neuromuscular paralysis follows in a descending pattern, with involvement of the cranial nerves (resulting in bulbar palsies) progressing to involvement of the muscles of respiration (Fig. 33.7). General muscle weakness and hypotonia usually precede the onset of respiratory insufficiency. Not all cases progress to respiratory muscle paralysis, and the diagnosis of botulism, if not considered, may be overlooked. Some physical findings may be helpful in the early diagnosis of infant botulism **(Table 33.3)** in addition to general signs and symptoms **(Table 33.4).** There may be findings consistent with pneumonia and metabolic abnormalities accompanying dehydration, which may confuse the clinical picture(90). Administration of aminoglycosides may worsen the progression of paralysis(91) because these antibiotics decrease release of acetylcholine from nerves of the diaphragm. The progression of symptoms in infant botulism is comparable to symptoms elicited in awake adults who are given small sequential doses of competitive muscle relaxants **(Table 33.5)**(92). As in patients who are partially paralyzed by nondepolarizing agents, flexion of the neck may result in acute airway obstruction and apnea(92). The most commonly entertained diagnosis in babies with early infant botulism is sepsis. Other entities to be considered are listed in **Table 33.6.**

The course and severity of disease in any particular baby is impossible to predict. However, once weakness becomes apparent, the disease generally progresses over several days to the maximal extent it will reach in that patient, remains in a relatively constant state for at least 2 weeks, and then gradually improves. Infants who progress to respiratory failure may require assisted ventilation for several months(93). Tracheostomy may be necessary before recovery has proceeded to the point where airway control and protective reflexes have returned to a safe level. Tracheostomy, however, may lengthen hospitalization(94) and should be undertaken only if absolutely necessary. The majority of infants with this disease do not have significant airway complications despite prolonged intubation(95).

Diagnosis

Presumptive diagnosis can be made on the basis of the signs, symptoms, and course of presentation. Definitive diagnosis requires a finding of toxin in the blood or of the organism, toxin, or spores in the stool. Such laboratory diagnosis is cumbersome and time-consuming and requires that specimens be sent to a reference or research laboratory(96). A rapid enzyme immunoassay developed in the

Table 33.3. Physical Findings That May Be Helpful in the Diagnosis of Infant Botulism[a]

Test	*Findings*	*Interpretation*
1. Shine a bright light in the eye and observe the briskness of the pupillary light reflex. Once the iris constricts, remove the light. As soon as the iris dilates, again shine the light in the eye. Continue for 1–3 min without interruption.	Pupillary constriction, which may initially be brisk, eventually becomes sluggish. An initially midposition pupil may become dilated at rest as the test continues.	Fatigability when repetitive muscle contraction is required is one hallmark of botulism. Infection—a most important consideration in the differential diagnosis at presentation—does not impair the pupillary light reflex (unless CNS infection).
2. Shine the light along the optical axis so that it falls directly on the fovea. Keep the light continuously on the fovea for 1–3 min, even if the infant tries to deviate the eyes. Observe the infant's efforts and ability to deviate the eyes. Observe the vigor and purposefulness of the infant's efforts to avoid the light.	Latent ophthalmoplegia may be elicited. Efforts to push away the examiner's hand or to squirm away from the light may be feeble or not purposefully continued.	A sustained bright light on the fovea is most uncomfortable, and an infant with normal motor ability uses it to avoid the sensation.
3. Place a clean fifth finger in the infant's mouth (but be certain that doing so does not compromise adequate air flow). Note the strength and especially the duration of the reflex sucking efforts. If the infant has an empty stomach, advance the finger and manually gauge the briskness and strength of the gag reflex. (Feeling the gag reflex regularly is also a useful way to follow the infant's recovery.)	The suck is weak and of short duration. The gag reflex is diminished.	Fatigability, as in 1 above.

[a] *From Arnon SS. Infant botulism. Annu Rev Med 1980;31:541.*

1980s[97,98] may provide the clinician with the ability to make a diagnosis shortly after admission in suspected cases. Supportive evidence is provided in many cases by electrodiagnostic studies[99]. Electromyography detects brief duration, small amplitude, and overly abundant motor endplate action potentials. With high rates of repetitive nerve stimulation, a staircase phenomenon is observed in which there is an excessive incremental response (Fig. 33.8). These studies, however, are not 100% reliable[100], and "negative" results in a patient with signs and symptoms consistent with botulism should not eliminate the disease from consideration.

Table 33.4. Signs and Symptoms in Hospitalized Patients with Infant Botulism

Autonomic dysfunction
- Constipation
- Neurogenic bladder
- Hypertension

Hypotonia and weakness
- Decreased resistance to passive motion
- Lack of spontaneous motor activity
- Motor response to noxious stimuli diminished
- Poor head control

Cranial nerve dysfunction
- Decreased suck and swallow ability
- Weak cry
- Facial diplegia
- External ophthalmoplegia
- Sluggishly reactive pupils

Absent or diminished deep tendon reflexes

Respiratory insufficiency
- Associated with progressive weakness and cranial nerve dysfunction
- Provoked by postural manipulation for procedures

From Brown LW. Infant botulism. Adv Pediatr 1981;28:141.

Treatment

Babies in whom infant botulism is suspected and in whom any signs of muscle weakness are manifested should be carefully observed, and monitored for apnea and bradycardia, preferably in an intensive or intermediate care unit. If gag and cough reflexes are suppressed, no attempts should be made to feed the patient by mouth. Assessment of respiratory mechanics and reserve should be made and, if respiratory insufficiency seems imminent, intubation of the tra-

Table 33.5. Comparison of Symptom Progression in Patients with Infant Botulism and Those Undergoing Competitive Neuromuscular Blockade

Infant Botulism	*Competitive Blockade*
Constipation, tachycardia	Blurred vision, tachycardia
↓	↓
Loss of head control[a] Difficulty feeding[a] Weak cry[a] Depressed gag reflex[a]	Loss of head lift[a] Weakness in jaw muscles Decreased hand grip (sustained)[a] Bulbar weakness
↓	↓
Peripheral motor weakness	Peripheral motor weakness
↓	↓
Diaphragmatic weakness	Diaphragmatic weakness

[a] Repetitive muscle activity.
From L'Hommedieu C, Polin RA. Progression of clinical signs in severe botulism: therapeutic implications. Clin Pediatr 1981;20:90.

Table 33.6. Differential Diagnosis of Infant Botulism

Systemic
Sepsis/meningitis
Electrolyte/mineral imbalance
Metabolic encephalopathy
Reye's syndrome
Intoxication—organophosphates, heavy metals
Hypothyroidism
Subacute necrotizing encephalomyelitis
Organic acidurias
Neuromuscular
Poliomyelitis
Infantile spinal muscular atrophy
Acute polyneuropathy—Guillain-Barré syndrome, diphtheria
Tick paralysis
Congenital myasthenia gravis
Muscular dystrophy—"congenital," myotonic dystrophy
Congenital myopathy

From Brown LW. Infant botulism. Adv Pediatr 1981;28:141.

chea or tracheostomy and assisted ventilation as needed are indicated. A detailed discussion of the respiratory aspects of botulism is found in Chapter 8.

Affected infants do not require treatment with antitoxin, nor have antibiotics (parenteral or oral) been proven to be effective, except for therapy of associated infectious complications(101). Treatment with human botulism immune globulin may be effective(77). As mentioned above, aminoglycoside antibiotics may potentiate the neuromuscular blockade, precipitating acute respiratory failure. If such preparations must be used, they should be given in the intensive care unit (ICU) under the supervision of a physician trained in the care of the infant airway.

Although theoretically beneficial in removing the source of toxin, the use of purgatives and emetics has not been proven effective and is potentially dangerous in the impaired child. Because organisms and, more importantly, toxin may be excreted in the stool for several months after onset of the infection(101), caregivers must be instructed in methods by which they may avoid exposure. Likewise, all specimens sent to the laboratory should be labeled with the possible diagnosis and transported in biohazard containers.

The syndrome of inappropriate secretion of antidiuretic hormone has been present in a number of children with infant botulism, most(84), but not all(102), of whom have been receiving mechanical ventilation. The short-term outcome is excellent in infants in whom the diagnosis is considered early in the course of disease and who receive appropriate supportive care(90). Long-term outcome has not been assessed.

Food-Borne Botulism

Botulism that occurs after ingestion of preformed toxin in contaminated food is the most common of all forms of the disease. More than 2000 cases and 760 outbreaks have been recorded(64). Type A toxin has been implicated most often in outbreaks in which a specific type is identified. The food products most often associated with disease are home-

Table 33.7. Botulism: Five Cardinal Features as Defined by CDC

Absence of fever except in presence of complicating infection
Normal mental status
Pulse rate normal or slow
Absence of numbness, paresthesias, and sensory deficit
Neurologic manifestations usually symmetrical

Data are from Reference 58.

canned vegetables, fruits, and meat products. Type E toxin has caused outbreaks of botulism after ingestion of contaminated seafood(103).

Symptoms of botulism include cranial nerve dysfunction, diplopia, dysarthria, and dysphagia. These symptoms begin some time after the onset of gastrointestinal distress, which includes nausea, vomiting, diarrhea, and abdominal cramps. Constipation becomes prominent later on. There is an incubation period of several hours to 8 days after ingestion of the toxin-containing food; most commonly, 18 to 36 hours(104) elapse before onset of symptoms. In general, the shorter the incubation period, the more severe and protracted the disease(63,105). Muscle weakness occurs in a descending fashion and may be more pronounced in the proximal limbs(106). Dryness of mucous membranes is common, and urinary retention occurs in some patients. Tachycardia is not a prominent finding in this form of botulism. The pupils may be either normal or fixed and dilated, and reflexes are usually depressed but symmetric. The cardinal features of botulism as defined by the CDC(64) are listed in **Table 33.7.**

The differential diagnosis includes numerous diseases, mostly noninfectious **(Table 33.8).** As in infant botulism, definitive diagnosis depends on the presence of toxin in the patient's stool or serum, although this is not always possible to determine(107). Suspect food should also be examined, if available. Electromyographic findings similar to those in infant botulism are helpful in diagnosis of food-borne botulism.

Treatment consists of induced vomiting and catharsis,

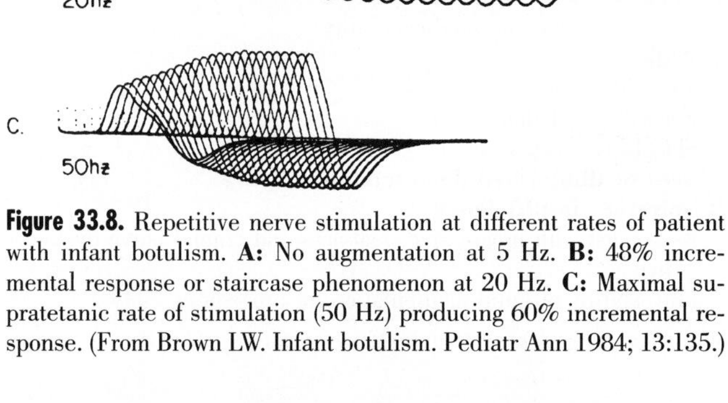

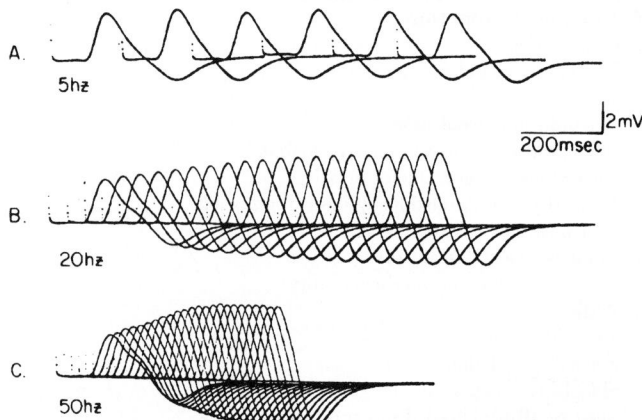

Figure 33.8. Repetitive nerve stimulation at different rates of patient with infant botulism. **A:** No augmentation at 5 Hz. **B:** 48% incremental response or staircase phenomenon at 20 Hz. **C:** Maximal supratetanic rate of stimulation (50 Hz) producing 60% incremental response. (From Brown LW. Infant botulism. Pediatr Ann 1984; 13:135.)

and careful observation of the patient. Emesis should not be induced if the airway reflexes are impaired or if consciousness is depressed. In such cases, controlled intubation of the trachea with a cuffed endotracheal tube followed by gastric lavage may be an alternative. Supportive care, including assisted ventilation, is lifesaving. Administration of antitoxin is effective only if provided early in the course of the disease because it inactivates free serum toxin. Botulinal toxin is irreversibly bound to nerve endings, so antitoxin has no effect once binding has occurred. Toxin may circulate in serum up to 30 days after the onset of disease[(58)]. The decision to use antitoxin is not a simple one, as there are great risks, such as anaphylaxis and serum sickness, associated with administration of the drug, which is a horse serum product. Nonetheless, the CDC recommends immediate administration of trivalent (ABE) antitoxin to patients who have botulism[(108)]. The agent may be obtained by calling the CDC at (404) 639-2888.

Adjunctive therapeutic measures include administration of drugs, such as guanidine, that increase the amount of acetylcholine released at the nerve terminals[(109)]. These agents have not been proven definitively effective[(110)] and have a long list of potential adverse effects. The recommended dose of guanidine hydrochloride is 35 mg/kg/day[(111)]. Administration of penicillin has been advocated by some, but no data support this viewpoint, and such antibiotic use may contribute to the development of nosocomial pneumonia[(112)].

Wound Botulism

Wound botulism is rare and consists of development of signs and symptoms of botulism after an injury but in the absence of an identifiable food source of disease and evidence of gastrointestinal disease. It is a known complication of intravenous drug abuse[(113,114)]. Wound botulism has also occurred after chronic intranasal cocaine abuse[(115)] and tooth abscess[(116)]. Many cases are not recognized on initial presentation. This disease carries a 10% mortality rate[(114)]. In addition to supportive care and antitoxin therapy, patients should undergo emergent wound debridement to remove the source of toxin.

Table 33.8. Differential Diagnosis of Food-Borne Botulism

Other types of food poisoning:
Staphylococcus, Salmonella, Shigella, chemical
Guillain-Barré syndrome
Carbon monoxide poisoning
Cerebrovascular accident
Viral encephalitis
Neuropsychiatric disorders
Phenothiazine drug reaction
Myasthenia gravis
Alcohol or other chemical intoxication
Diphtheria
Tick paralysis

STAPHYLOCOCCAL AND STREPTOCOCCAL TOXIC SHOCK SYNDROMES

Superantigens

Both staphylococcal and streptococcal toxic shock syndromes are mediated by toxins now commonly known as superantigens. Superantigens are bacterially and/or virally derived compounds which interact with the major histocompatibility class II proteins and activate T cells by binding to the variable region of the beta (V-beta) chain of the T cell receptor[(117)]. Stimulation leads to polyclonal T cell activation which results in massive release of lymphokines, such as TNF-alpha and IL-6[(118)], which are most likely the elements responsible for the shock and multiorgan dysfunction seen in these diseases[(117,118)]. The polyclonal activation generally results in reversible reduction in the number of circulating CD4+ lymphocytes[(119)] and variable changes in other T cell subpopulations. Superantigens differ from conventional antigens chiefly in the manner in which they are processed and presented to the T cell receptor.

The specific toxins related to the diseases discussed in this section, which are toxic shock syndrome 1 (TSST-1) and the streptococcal superantigens (streptococcal pyrogenic exotoxins A,B,C, and F, streptococcal superantigen [SSA], and the M proteins) represent a small subset of this increasingly important class of immune mediators. Superantigens are now believed to be potentially involved in a variety of other disorders, including Kawasaki disease, HIV infection, and certain autoimmune processes[(120–122)]. Analysis of the molecular structure of the superantigens has revealed a close homology between the amino termini of the streptococcal and staphylococcal toxins capable of causing toxic shock syndrome. Such homology suggests that the molecular biologic approach to the treatment of all superantigen–related diseases may be similar, and this may offer hope of success in avoiding the often fatal multiple organ system failure that so often accompanies these diseases.

Staphylococcal Toxic Shock Syndrome

Staphylococcal toxic shock syndrome (TSS) is a recently described illness[(123)] that existed a long time before it was finally recognized as a specific toxin-mediated clinical entity in the mid–1970s[(124–129)]. The disease is caused by coagulase-positive staphylococci that liberate an exoprotein known as TSST-1 toxin[(130)]. Although some patients have evidence of *S. aureus* bacteremia[(130–132)] or deep tissue infection[(123,130–132)], simple colonization of a wound or mucous membrane with a TSST-1 toxin liberating strain is enough to cause severe disease[(133–136)]. The majority of cases identified between 1978 and the mid–1980s were in menstruating women with coagulase-positive staphylococci isolated from vaginal-cervical cultures[(137–139)]. The syndrome also occurs in burned or scalded children[(140)], in postoperative patients[(141,142)], and in patients with AIDS[(142)]. In the menstrual cases, the majority of isolated organisms produce TSST-1, whereas a variety of toxins are isolated from patients with other types of the disease. Some of the nonmenstrual cases have involved infection or colonization of the vagina or cervix, occurring postpartum or after therapeutic abortion[132], and some have also been associated with use of contraceptive diaphragms[143–145]. The relative noninvasiveness of the infecting organism and the failure of the host to form antibodies to the toxin for at least 2 years after infection[146] may help explain the recurrent nature of disease, especially in menstrual cases.

The incidence of TSS increased until the mid-1980s, and has fallen consistently since that time[130,147,148]. While the incidence of menses-associated cases has decreased, the incidence of nonmenstrual TSS has not, resulting in an increased percentage of nonmenstrual cases[148]. Menstrual cases occur overwhelmingly in Caucasian women (97%), most of whom are between 15 and 34 years of age[130]. In the first 21 weeks of 1995, 84 cases of confirmed TSS were reported to the CDC[149]. Case fatality rates dropped from 10% for cases with onset before 1980, to 2.6% for cases with onset after 1983. Fatality rates are higher in males (8.8%) than in females (4.4%).

There is no rapid diagnostic test available for definitive diagnosis. Therefore, the CDC developed a set of diagnostic criteria based on clinical and laboratory findings **(Table 33.9).** The criteria have subsequently been amended to include blood cultures positive for *S. aureus.* Laboratory isolation of *S. aureus* capable of producing TSST-1 lends further credence to the diagnosis. An alternative diagnostic scheme has been proposed for children **(Table 33.10)**[150], but has not been adopted by the CDC.

While variable in intensity, the order in which clinical manifestations develop is relatively constant and does not differ significantly between those patients with menstrual and nonmenstrual TSS (Fig. 33.9). However, some differences have been noted between children and adults with the syndrome. While only a small number of adults have had a prominent prodromal illness, nearly all children have between 1 and 6 days of symptoms preceding illness, including fever, mucosal and/or conjunctival hyperemia, erythroderma, vomiting, diarrhea, myalgias, and dizziness[131]. Whereas the majority of adults admitted to the hospital have overt hypotension[137], this finding is not prominent at admission in children, although it usually develops later.

Toxic shock syndrome is a multisystem disease mediated by superantigen–induced cytokine release **(Table 33.9).** The final common pathway involves effects of the cytokines released by T-cell V-beta stimulation, which are tumor necrosis factor-alpha (TNF-α) and interleukin-1 (IL-1). When circulating in large quantities, these cytokines result in massive vasodilation with extravasation of fluid and serum proteins. The most common manifestations are hypotension, oliguria with acute tubular necrosis, low central venous pressures, pulmonary and peripheral edema, and low serum albumin levels with hypocalcemia. It has not been possible to exclude direct effects of the toxin on liver, kidney, or myocardium, because pathologic changes seen in these organs are not totally consistent with ischemia or hypoperfusion.

Complications of the syndrome may include rhabdomyolysis (increased urine and serum myoglobin values), hy-

Table 33.9. Toxic Shock Syndrome Case Definition[a]

Criteria A

Fever—Temperature ≥38.9°C (102°F)

Rash—Diffuse or palmar erythroderma progressing to subsequent peripheral desquamation (hands and feet)

Mucous membrane—Nonpurulent conjunctival hyperemia, or oropharyngeal hyperemia, or vaginal hyperemia, or discharge

Hypotension—Systolic blood pressure <90 mm Hg for an adult (>16 yr) or <5th percentile for age of child; or orthostatic hypotension as shown by a drop in diastolic blood pressure ≥15 mm Hg from recumbent to sitting; or history of orthostatic dizziness

Multisystem involvement (≥4 of the following):

- Gastrointestinal—History of vomiting or diarrhea at onset of illness
- Muscular—CPK, ≥2 × ULN 4–20 days after onset
- CNS—Disorientation or alteration in consciousness without focal signs when patient is not in shock or hyperpyrexic
- Renal—BUN or serum creatinine clearance, ≥2 × ULN, and abnormal findings on urinalysis (≥5 WBC per high power field; ≥1 RBC per high power field; protein, ≥1+); or oliguria defined as urine output <1 ml/kg/hr for 24 hr
- Hepatic—Total serum bilirubin level ≥1.5 × ULN; or SGPT ≥2 × ULN.
- Hematologic—Thrombocytopenia (platelets <100,000/mm^3)
- Cardiopulmonary—Adult respiratory distress syndrome; or pulmonary edema; or new onset 2° or 3° heart block; or ECG criteria for myocarditis decreased voltage and ST-T–wave changes; or heart failure shown by new onset of gallop rhythm or by increase in size of cardiac silhouette from one chest roentgenogram to another during the course of the illness, or diagnosed by cardiologist
- Metabolic—Serum calcium level, ≤7.0 mg/dl with serum phosphate level, ≤2.5 mg/dl, and total serum protein level, ≤5.0 mg/dl

Evidence for absence of other causes:

- When obtained: negative blood, throat, urine, or CSF cultures[a]
- When obtained: absence of serologic evidence of leptospirosis, rickettsial disease, or rubeola
- Evidence for absence of Kawasaki syndrome: no unilateral lymphadenopathy or fever lasting >10 days

Criteria B

At least two episodes meeting criteria for fever, rash, mucous membrane, hypotension, and one of the situations under multisystem involvement

[a] *Blood cultures positive for* S. aureus *are accepted.*
From Chesney PJ, Davis JP, Purdy WK, et al. Clinical manifestations of toxic shock syndrome. JAMA 1981;246:741.
CPK = creatine phosphokinase; ULN = upper limits of normal for laboratory; BUN = blood urea nitrogen; WBC = white blood cell(s); RBC = red blood cell(s); SGPT = serum glutamic pyruvic transaminase.

Table 33.10. Proposed Simplified Diagnostic Criteria for Toxic Shock Syndrome in Children[a]

Pyrexia ≥39°C
Lymphopenia
Rash
Shock
Diarrhea and/or vomiting
Irritability

[a] *Modified with permission from Cole RP, Shakespeare PG. Toxic shock syndrome in scalded children. Burns 1990;16:221–224.*

pophosphatemia, metabolic acidosis, hypoventilation secondary to severe muscle weakness, and adult respiratory distress syndrome requiring mechanical ventilation. Children appear more likely to require respiratory support than adults(131). Tachydysrhythmias potentially requiring drug or countershock therapy have been described(137). In fatal cases, the cause of death is irreversible systemic effects of disease: shock, respiratory failure, cardiac dysrhythmias, untreatable coagulopathy, or severe cerebral ischemia resulting in brain death(131,134,135,151,152).

The mainstay of therapy consists of supportive care aimed at preservation of vital organ function. Massive fluid administration is generally required to return the central venous pressure to an adequate level and to restore urine output. Because hypoalbuminemia may worsen peripheral edema, colloid administration may be of benefit. Caution should be used, however, since infusions of albumin in patients with diffusely leaky capillaries may result in worsening of pulmonary edema. Specific data concerning amount and type of fluid resuscitation performed in these patients have not been reported, so no specific recommendations can be given. Some patients require dopamine or other pressor agents to normalize blood pressure when response to fluid administration is inadequate, depending on results of assessment with invasive hemodynamic monitoring.

The need for inotropic support has been observed most consistently in patients who present with elevated serum creatinine levels (more than 3 mg/dl); this finding predicts a prolonged hospital course. Postulated reasons for the link between acute renal failure and lengthy disease course include: (1) the patients who require dopamine have the most severe disease and, therefore, would be expected to have a prolonged period of recovery and (2) that the possibly impaired renal clearance of the toxin may contribute to ongoing disease. With regard to the latter theory, it would be interesting to see if initiation of peritoneal dialysis or hemodialysis would result in a more rapid abatement of symptoms. Plasmapheresis has been proposed as a possible treatment, based on a single case report of a patient who was mistakenly thought to have a pulmonary embolus and was placed on cardiopulmonary bypass, with almost immediate and nearly complete resolution of hemodynamic instability(151).

Systemic administration of a β-lactamase-resistant antistaphylococcal antibiotic is recommended. Although such treatment may not have a profound effect on the short-term outcome(137), antibiotic therapy does appear to reduce recurrence. Endotoxin-neutralizing monoclonal antibody has been demonstrated to be of value in an animal model(153). No data support or refute the use of corticosteroids or naloxone(154). An effort should be made to remove any potentially infected material, such as retained tampons, and to irrigate the vagina or any suspicious wounds to reduce further production and release of toxin. Even clean-looking wounds may be infected, as there is generally no purulent response(132). Diseases that mimic toxic shock syndrome **(Table 33.11)** should be ruled out.

Long-term sequelae consist of prolonged muscle weakness and fatigue, loss of fingers or toes, abnormal renal function, behavioral changes or memory impairment, and reversible hair and nail loss(137,154,155).

Streptococcal Toxic-Shock Syndrome

The mid-1980s saw the resurgence of group A betahomolytic streptococci (GAS) as a causative agent in lifethreatening disease. The streptococcal TSS is one form of severe GAS disease. **Table 33.12** lists a recently proposed classification of GAS infections(156). The Working Group on Severe Streptococcal Infections of the Respiratory Disease

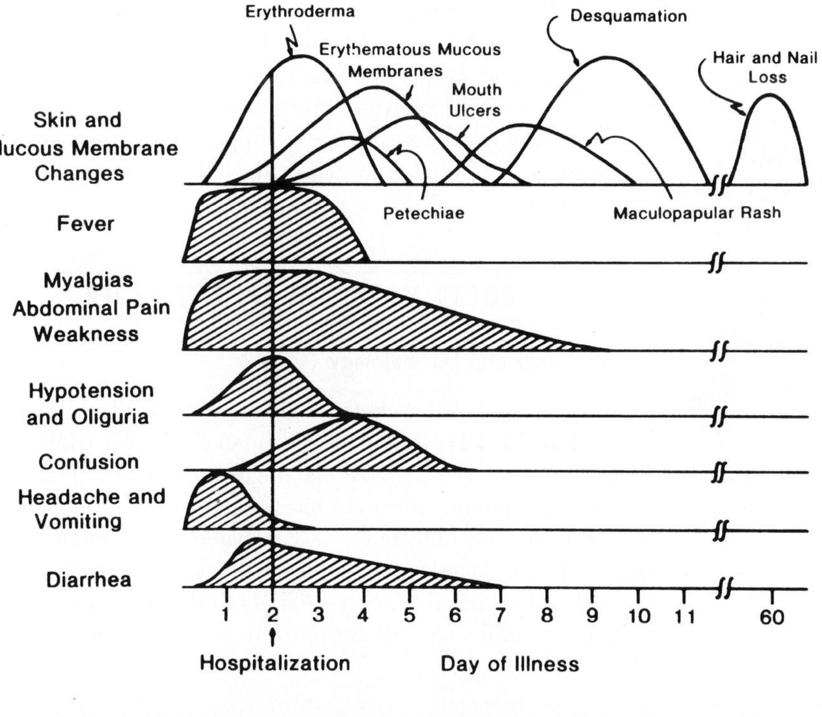

Figure 33.9. Composite drawing of major systemic, skin, and mucous membrane manifestations of TSS. (From Chesney PJ, Davis JP, Purdy WK, et al. Clinical manifestations of toxic shock syndrome. JAMA 1981;246:741.)

Table 33.11. Differential Diagnosis of Toxic Shock Syndrome

Infections	
	Rash-associated viral syndromes
	Rocky Mountain spotted fever
	Kawasaki disease
	Scaled skin syndrome
	Streptococcal scarlet fever
	Overwhelming sepsis
	Leptospirosis
	Tick typhus
	Legionnaires' disease
	Gastroenteritis
	Pelvic inflammatory disease
Noninfectious (or postinfectious)	
	Acute rheumatic fever
	Hemolytic uremic syndrome
	Lupus
	Adverse drug reactions

Branch of the CDC has developed a proposed case definition for streptococcal Toxic Shock Syndrome (STSS), **(Table 33.13)** [156]. Such case criteria should help to expand knowledge of the epidemiology, clinical course, and outcome of the disease.

Diagnosis rests on isolation of GAS from a site which is either normally sterile (i.e., blood) or normally nonsterile (i.e., nasopharynx) plus fulfillment of other criteria listed in **Table 33.13.** When the isolate is from a normally sterile site, the case is considered definite, if from a normally nonsterile site the case is probable.

Hoge and colleagues[157] reported, in a retrospective population-based study published in 1993, an overall mortality rate of 20%, with higher mortality in the youngest (age 5 or younger, 40%) and oldest (age 65 or younger, 31%) age groups. Although these investigators substantiated an increase in toxic and shock-like symptoms related to GAS infection since 1985, they did not find an absolute increase in necrotizing fasciitis/myositis in the study population during the period of study. Therefore, the epidemic of "flesh-eating" bacteria popularized in the lay press and on television news programs is most likely overstated.

Treatment is not substantially different from that for staphylococcal TSS. Antibiotic choice is governed by results of sensitivity testing. Systemic support therapy is dictated by the specific organ systems affected and the severity of dysfunction.

Table 33.12. Classification of Group A Streptococcal Infection[a]

I. Streptococcal TSS (Defined by criteria in 33.9)
II. Other invasive infections: defined by isolation of group A streptococci from a *normally sterile site* in patients not meeting criteria for streptococcal TSS
   A. Bacteremia with no identified focus
   B. Focal infections with or without bacteremia, including meningitis, pneumonia, peritonitis, puerperal sepsis, osteomyelitis, septic arthritis, necrotizing fasciitis, surgical wound infections, erysipeas, and cellulitis
III. Scarlet fever: defined by a scarlatina rash with evidence of group A streptococcal infection, most commonly pharyngotonsillitis
IV. Noninvasive infections: defined by the isolation of group A streptococci from a nonsterile site
   A. Mucous membrane: including pharyngitis, tonsillitis, otitis media, sinusitis, vaginitis
   B. Cutaneous: impetigo
V. Nonsuppurative sequelae: defined by specific clinical findings with evidence of a recent group A streptococcal infection
   A. Acute rheumatic fever
   B. Acute glomerulonephritis

Reproduced from The Working Group on Severe Streptococcal Infections. Defining the group A streptococcal toxic shock syndrome. JAMA 1993;269:390–391.
[a] *Examples of conditions in each category are not inclusive.*

Table 33.13. Definition of Streptococcal Toxic Shock Syndrome[a]

I. Isolation of group A streptococci *(Streptococcus pyogenes)*
   A. From a normally sterile site (eg, blood; cerebrospinal, pleural, or peritoneal fluid; tissue biopsy; surgical wound; etc.)
   B. From a nonsterile site (eg, throat, sputum, vagina, superficial skin lesion, etc.)
II. Clinical signs of severity
   A. Hypotension: systolic blood pressure ≤90 mm Hg in adults or ≤5th percentile for age in children, and
   B. ≥2 of the following signs
      1. Renal impairment: creatinine level ≥177 μmol/L (≥2 mg/dL) for adults or ≥2 times the upper limit of normal for age in children. In patients with preexisting renal disease, ≥2-fold elevation over the baseline level
      2. Coagulopathy: platelet count of $\leq 100 \times 10^9$/L (≤100, 000/mm^3) or disseminated intravascular coagulation defined by prolonged clotting times, low fibrinogen level, and the presence of fibrin degradation products
      3. Hepatic involvement: alanine aminotransferase (SGOT) and asparate aminotransferase (SGPT) twice the upper limit of normal for age. In patients with preexisting liver disease, a ≥2-fold elevation over the baseline level
      4. Adult respiratory distress syndrome: acute onset of diffuse pulmonary infiltrates and hypoxemia in the absence of cardiac failure, or evidence of diffuse capillary leak manifested by acute onset of generalized edema, or pleural or peritoneal effusions with hypoalbuminemia
      5. A generalized erythematous macular rash that may desquamate
      6. Soft-tissue necrosis, including necrotizing fasciitis or myositis, or gangrene

[a] *An illness fulfilling criteria I.A. and II, A. and B. can be defined as a* definite *case. An illness fulfilling criteria I.B. and II. A. and B. can be defined as a* probable *case if no other etiology for the illness is identified.*
Reproduced from: The Working Group on Severe Streptococcal Infections. Defining the Group A Streptococcal toxic shock syndrome JAMA 1993;269:390–391.

ROCKY MOUNTAIN SPOTTED FEVER

Overview and Epidemiology

Of the numerous rickettsial diseases that affect humans **(Table 33.14),** Rocky Mountain spotted fever (RMSF) is the most important affecting the United States. Pediatric medical care providers are most affected, because children are commonly infected[158]. The name is misleading, because significantly more cases occur each year in areas east of the Mississippi River, especially in the southeastern and south central states. *Rickettsia rickettsii,* the causative agent,

Table 33.14. Rickettsial Diseases That Affect Humans

Organism	*Disease*	*Geographic Location*	*Vector*
R. ricketsii	Rocky Mountain spotted fever	Western hemisphere	Ticks
R. conorii	Boutonneuse fever, African and Indian tick fevers	Africa, Europe, India, Middle East	Ticks
R. australis	Queensland tick typhus	Australia	Ticks
R. sibirica	North Asia tick-borne rickettsiosis	Siberia, Mongolia	Ticks
R. akari	Rickettsial pox	North America, Europe	Mite
R. prowazekii	Epidemic typhus	Worldwide	Body louse
R. mooseri	Endemic typhus	Worldwide	Flea
R. tsutsugamushi	Scrub typhus	Asia, Australia, Pacific Islands, Malaysia	Thrombiculid mite
Coxiella burnetii	Q fever	Worldwide	Ticks
Rochalimaea quintana	Trench fever	Worldwide	Body louse
Ehrlichia chafeensis	Human ehrlichiosis	United States	Ticks

is an obligate intracellular parasite that resides in several species of ticks: the eastern dog tick, *Dermacentor variabilis* in the eastern states; the western wood tick, *Dermacentor andersoni*, in the western. Other species of tick have been found to carry the disease(159,160). Adult female ticks pass the disease to their offspring without detriment, so the tick acts as the reservoir as well as the vector of infection. Small mammals, especially rodents, are a source of disease if they are bitten by a tick during the rickettsemic phase of their illness(128). Humans are only incidentally involved when bitten by an adult tick. Transmission of the agent takes some time, perhaps several hours, so prompt recognition and removal of ticks may prevent infection. Transmission may also occur if a breach in the skin is contaminated with a crushed tick; care should therefore be used when removing a tick attached to another person. The remover may acquire the disease while the bitten person escapes without infection(161). Transmission has occurred in a laboratory setting in which infected particles have been inhaled(162–164), as well as through needle stick(165) and blood transfusion(166).

RMSF increased in incidence through the 1970s, reaching a peak in 1977. Since that time, the incidence has fallen from an overall median of 0.48 cases per 100,000 population per year(158) for the years 1981–1983 to an incidence of 0.26 per 100,000 population in 1990(167). Higher attack rates have been reported in endemic areas: up to 2.7 cases per 100,000 in Oklahoma(168) and 6.5 cases per 100,000 population per year in parts of New York State(169). Case-fatality ratios vary according to age; persons age 30 and older have an 8.4% chance of succumbing to the disease; whereas, in those younger than age 30, the case-fatality ratio is only 2.2%. More than 15% of elderly victims die of the disease or its complications(158). The highest incidence of disease is among children in the age 5 to 9 range. More than half of all cases occur in persons younger than age 19(158). Presumably, this is because of the prevalence of *R. rickettsii* in the eastern dog tick and the close association of children and their dogs. In the west, more disease occurs among older people who work out of doors and are exposed to ticks that feed on small wild mammals and rodents. Because transmission of RMSF requires the activity of ticks, the incidence is seasonal and peaks in the warm weather months. In the first 21 weeks of 1995, 56 confirmed cases were reported to the CDC(149).

Clinical Aspects

The incubation period of RMSF is 2 to 14 days, with a mean of 7 days between tick bite and onset of symptoms(161). Less severe disease tends to be associated with longer incubation periods. The first symptom noted by most patients is fever, often accompanied by headache and generalized malaise, soon followed by vomiting, myalgias, and photophobia(158,161,170–175). The fever increases with spikes as high as 105° to 106°F(160). There is generally a hectic pattern to the febrile state, and body temperature may decrease to nearly normal in the morning, only to rise again in the afternoon. As the disease progresses, headache increases in intensity and may be accompanied by stiffness of the neck. Some children have shaking chills, abdominal pain, or diarrhea. Mental status eventually becomes clouded, and the youngster may be listless, lethargic, apathetic, or frankly comatose.

The rash generally appears 2 to 4 days after the onset of fever and has been noted in nearly all children with RMSF(170), although it may be variable in nature or not occur at all(176). The rash is often the first clue to the cause of a seemingly undifferentiated febrile illness. The eruption begins as discrete erythematous macules, first observed on the ankles and feet and shortly thereafter on the wrists and hands. The rash gradually progresses, with involvement of the limbs and finally of the abdomen. In some children, it may start on the trunk and move outward to involve the extremities(159). Regardless of its progression, the rash is almost always most pronounced over the extremities and almost always involves the palms and soles. In quality, what starts as a rash of discrete blanching macules of several millimeters in diameter becomes morbilliform, then papular, and then darkens in hue. Over the succeeding several days, it gradually becomes petechial and, sometimes, frankly purpuric. This purpura is related to underlying coagulopathy and may become so severe as to result in overt gangrene of ear lobes, scrotum, digits or, in particularly severe cases, more than one limb(177). In some children, petechiae and purpura do not develop and the rash remains maculopapular or morbilliform, making the diagnosis less apparent. Mucous membranes may become involved, conjunctivitis is often present, and nonpitting edema of the limbs and periorbital areas is prominent.

Associated findings may include isolated splenomegaly[(172)] or hepatosplenomegaly with mild transient elevation of serum transaminases. Acute tubular necrosis may occur because of hypovolemia; sometimes renal vasculitis and interstitial nephritis complicate the clinical picture[(178,179)]. Interstitial pneumonitis and myocarditis may occur but are generally without clinical importance. Hemodynamic collapse may occur acutely and is most often related to inadequate intravascular volume. When hypotension fails to respond to fluid administration, myocardial failure secondary to myocarditis should be suspected.

Neurologic abnormalities may be prominent and severe in some cases. Cortical blindness and deafness may occur but are usually transient. Cranial nerve dysfunction often results in oculomotor palsies. Vascular involvement of the retina and optic nerve may lead to papilledema without an elevation in intracranial pressure. The neurologic course may resemble that of acute encephalitis or meningitis, with neck stiffness, lethargy, confusion, disorientation, and coma.

If untreated, the disease reaches its peak of severity in the middle of the second week after initial appearance of the rash. Severe cases progress to deep coma, hemodynamic collapse, respiratory failure, progressive thrombocytopenia, and disseminated intravascular coagulation (DIC) with overt bleeding into the CNS, lungs, or gastrointestinal tract. Before the development of specific antibiotics, the mortality rate was 20 to 30%[(180)].

Laboratory evaluation usually reveals leukocytosis (with an increased number of band forms), mild anemia, thrombocytopenia with hypofibrinogenemia, and an elevated level of fibrin degradation products. Electrolyte abnormalities are common, primarily hyponatremia and hypochloremia. Serum albumin level is often low, blood urea nitrogen and creatinine levels are elevated, as are hepatic enzyme levels. Examination of the CSF may show normal results or may reveal a lymphocytic pleocytosis with elevated protein levels but normal glucose concentration and no organisms on Gram's stain.

A complement fixation titer of at least 16 or indirect fluorescent antibody titer of 64 or more confirms disease, as does a fourfold rise in either titer. A Weil-Felix reaction test, which detects cross-reaction with *Proteus* OX-19 or OX-2 antigens, also shows a fourfold rise in unequivocal cases. Other tests that may be helpful include latex agglutination, microagglutination, and indirect hemagglutination procedures. Each of these should demonstrate a fourfold rise or an absolute titer of 128. None of these tests are helpful in the acute period of infection, as antibody titers do not peak until 2 to 4 weeks into the illness. Immunoperoxidase staining of tissue may be useful when applied retrospectively[(181)]. Experience with polymerase chain reaction (PCR) testing has been disappointing because of lack of sensitivity requiring reamplification[(182)], and monoclonal enzyme immunoabsorbant assay has shown some potential in a research laboratory setting[(183)].

Considering and making a presumptive diagnosis is essential. Specific antibiotic therapy initiated early in the course of disease may avert death[(161)]. A springtime or summer febrile illness and unexplained neurologic disease with accompanying rash should spark the clinician to consider, treat, and seek *R. rickettsii.* Muscle biopsy may be a useful evaluative tool and would be expected to show perivascular lymphocyte infiltration. Results of testing of the specimen by direct immunofluorescence may be positive. The tissue should be Giemsa-stained, which may reveal the presence of coccobacillary forms not observed on Gram's stain or hematoxylin–eosin stain.

Differential diagnosis includes the diseases listed in **Table 33.15.** Many of these entities have a prominent vasculitic component, as does RMSF. Indeed, most findings correlate with underlying disseminated thrombovasculitis. The vasculitis may be caused by direct invasion of arterioles and capillaries by *R. rickettsii,* leading to proliferation of endothelial components and perivascular inflammation[(184,185)]. The result is a diffuse vasculitis affecting many organ systems. Origin of the often-observed thrombocytopenia and DIC is not clearly understood, nor is the microbial proliferation in the brain often seen at autopsy understood[(186)]. A 4-year-old child with RMSF and an acquired coagulation inhibitor was reported in 1987[(187)]. A more recent study of patients with confirmed Rocky Mountain spotted fever[(188)] revealed that 50% of patients expressed endothelium-associated immunoglobulin in serum (IgM or IgG or both) and 21% had antibodies that bound to phos-

Table 33.15. Differential Diagnosis of Rocky Mountain Spotted Fever

Other rickettsial diseases
Murine typhus
Typhoid fever
Colorado tick fever
Ehrlichiosis
Bacterial and spirochetal diseases
Meningococcemia
Disseminated streptococcal sepsis
Tularemia
Leptospirosis
Rat-bite fever
Viral diseases
Atypical measles
Enteroviruses
Epstein-Barr virus
Others
Juvenile arthritis
Systemic lupus erythematosis
Henoch-Schönlein purpura
Thrombotic thrombocytopenic purpura
Hemolytic uremic syndrome
Kawasaki disease

pholipids, and were, therefore, suspected of having antibodies that could stimulate a coagulopathy, potentially by activation of protein C. Oxidant injury to endothelial cells may also contribute to vascular findings[189]. Additional work in this area may augment our ability to treat the vasculitis and coagulopathy complications of this disease.

The newest entity in the differential diagnosis of RMSF is human ehrlichiosis, a tickborne disease that has been increasing since the mid-1980s. Ehrlichiosis is endemic in the mid–Atlantic and South Central regions of the United States. Its presentation is similar to that of RMSF, except that the rash is somewhat less prominent and leukopenia is a common finding. Fever, chills, headache, malaise, and thrombocytopenia are prominent findings in children[190,191]. It may present as a disease indistinguishable from TSS[190].

The diagnosis, once suspected, may be confirmed by serologic testing, PCR,[192] or Western blot analysis.

Treatment of RMSF and ehrlichiosis consists of specific antimicrobial therapy and supportive care. Most children in whom either disease is recognized early and in whom appropriate antibiotics are administered, do not require the services of the ICU.

Antibiotics of choice are chloramphenicol (75 to 100 mg/kg/day) or tetracycline (100 mg/kg/day). Chloramphenicol is preferred in children. Serum chloramphenicol levels should be monitored throughout the therapeutic course, because clearance rates appear to change with duration of therapy[193]. The recommended length of therapy varies, but most experts believe treatment should continue for 6 to 7 days beyond defervescence. When such treatment is initiated early, the disease is often aborted, the patient becomes afebrile in 24 to 48 hours, and symptoms gradually improve. When antibiotics are not given until later in the disease or when the course of illness has progressed very rapidly, the fever may last a week or longer after therapy begins. In the preantibiotic era, patients who did not die of RMSF began to improve after 2 to 3 weeks of fever and rash.

Critical care support of advanced disease may include assisted ventilation necessitated by pulmonary edema resulting from vasculitis and hypoalbuminemia; treatment of pleural effusions or empyema; invasive hemodynamic monitoring and support, especially when the hypotensive patient also experiences renal failure; hemodialysis or peritoneal dialysis for acute renal failure; replacement of plasma, platelets, blood, and clotting factors; possible heparinization if thrombotic complications are overwhelming; and neurologic, nutritional, and physical therapy support of comatose patients. As in any disorder involving thrombocytopenia and DIC, care should be employed during any procedure such as central line insertion, lumbar puncture, and endotracheal intubation. As discussed in regard to meningococcemia, the nasotracheal approach to intubation should probably be avoided. There does not appear to be a role for corticosteroid therapy in any phase of the infection, although this issue has not been adequately studied.

Long-term sequelae of mild disease are minimal. When complications such as convulsions, CNS hemorrhages, or amputations occur, prolonged or permanent disability should be expected.

Summary

Rocky Mountain spotted fever is easily treatable but sometimes difficult to recognize. The infection primarily affects children in the summer months. Because the key to prevention of mortality and serious morbidity lies in prompt institution of specific antibiotics, the physician must be aware of both the common and rare manifestations of disease. Therapy should never be withheld while awaiting definitive diagnosis. Appropriate support of vital systems should be provided while waiting for the antimicrobial agents to exert an effect. Occasionally, a patient will have a progressive and fatal course, despite early, appropriate, and aggressive therapy[161].

LEGIONNAIRES' DISEASE

Legionnaires' disease was first recognized in 1976 after an outbreak of pneumonia in Philadelphia[194]. The causative agent was subsequently identified and named *Legionella pneumophila*, thereby defining an entirely new family (Legionellaceae), genus, and species of bacteria[195]. Evaluation of frozen specimens containing previously unidentified bacteria indicated that the bacterium had existed and caused disease as long ago as 1947[196]. It causes acute pulmonary disease, mostly among adult males, but has also been noted in infants and children[197–204]. An acute febrile illness, known as Pontiac fever, that resembles influenza but occurs in the absence of pneumonia is also caused by *L. pneumophilia*. The organism accounts for up to 15% of adult community-acquired pneumonias[205], and prevalence of elevated titers in children is quite high in some communities. It has caused outbreaks in hospitals and adult critical care units. A 1993 report from Saudi Arabia indicated that *Legionella* species were responsible for 2% of all cases of pneumonia requiring admission to the ICU over a 16-month period[206]. Classic disease involves multiple organ systems. Presenting complaints are usually fever, nonproductive cough, encephalopathy, and seizures. Cerebellar signs may be markedly severe. Three children were reported to have acute cerebellar ataxia; each had a fourfold rise in antibody titer[204]. Hepatic and renal abnormalities are often noted. The disease may be fatal, especially in immunocompromised patients. The lung disease is usually lobar, but may show nearly any pattern. Diagnosis is generally confirmed by identification of *Legionella* organisms by DPA, isolation in culture, latex agglutination test, enzyme-linked immunosorbent assay, (ELISA) or radioimmunosorbent assay (RIA) techniques. Serologic diagnosis is possible during convalescence[207].

Specific therapy consists of administration of erythromycin for at least 3 weeks, either alone or in combination with rifampin. Treatment is not always successful, perhaps because erythromycin is only inhibitory for *Legionella* species[208]. The macrolide antibiotic clarithromycin has been demonstrated to be effective in vitro[208].

Infection-related problems are usually resolved with therapy, but chronic lung disease may result[197]. Except for the very rare baby with progressive respiratory failure, or the immunocompromised child, the pediatric intensivist is unlikely to be called upon to treat this disease. Most children manifest a rise in antibody titer associated with mild upper respiratory infection or undifferentiated febrile illness. In the outbreak of nosocomial legionnaires' disease at the Children's Hospital of Columbus, four of seven children required mechanical ventilation[204]. Disease may be particularly severe in the immunocompromised host, although it remains an uncommon cause of pneumonia in patients with HIV infection[209], and has not been reported in patients receiving *Pneumocystis carinii* pneumonia prophylaxis with trimethoprim-sulfamethoxazole. The physician must, however, consider legionnaires' disease in an immunodepressed child with fever and pneumonia that are unresponsive to the usual antibiotics. The organism is often found to be contaminating water supplies and subsequently disseminating via pulmonary aspiration from air conditioning or ingestion of contaminated potable water[210].

SUMMARY

This chapter reviews important aspects of infectious diseases that intensivists may be called upon to treat. Particular issues surrounding diagnosis, therapy, and prevention have been stressed. The wide range of infections primarily affecting the CNS have not been discussed in this chapter, but they are dealt with at length in Chapter 32.

References

1. Major RH. Classic descriptions of disease. Springfield, IL: Charles C Thomas, 1945;91.
2. Finegold SM. Anaerobic bacteria in human disease. New York: Academic Press, 1977;487.
3. Carle R. Studio esperimentale sull'eziologia del tetano. G Acad Med Torino 1884;32:174.
4. Kitasato S. Ueber den Tetanus Bacillus. Z Hyg Infektr 1889;7:225.
5. Von Behring E, Kitasato S. Ueber des zus tande kommen der diphtherie-immunitat und der tetanus-immunitat bei teiren. Dtsch Med Wochenichr 1890;16:1113.
6. Glenny AT, Pope CG, Waddington H. The antigenic value of the toxin-antitoxin precipitate of Ramon. J Pathol Bacteriol 1926;29:31.
7. Stoll BJ. Tetanus. Pediatr Clin North Am 1979;26:415.
8. Dowell VR, Jr. Botulism and tetanus: selected epidemiologic and microbiologic aspects. Rev Infect Dis 1984:6 (Suppl):S202.
9. Centers for Disease Control and Prevention. Successful strategies in adult immunization. MMWR 1991;40:700–703, 709.
10. Saltigeral SP, Macias PM, Mejia VJ, et al. Neonatal tetanus experience at the National Institute of Pediatrics in Mexico City. Pediatr Infect Dis J 1993; 12:722–725.
11. Veronesi R, Focaccia R. The clinical picture. In: Veronesi R, ed. Tetanus: important new concepts. Princeton, NJ: Excerpta Medica, 1981;183.
12. Roofe PG. Role of the axis cylinder in transport of tetanus toxin. Science 1947;105:180.
13. Abell JJ, Kror WM, Chalaen W. Researchers on tetanus. Bull Johns Hopkins Hosp 1938;63:373.
14. Friedman U, Zuger G, Hollander A. Investigations on the pathogenesis of tetanus, I and II. J Immunol 1939;36:473.
15. Wright DK, Lalloo UG, Nayiager S, et al. Autonomic nervous system dysfunction in severe tetanus: current perspectives. Crit Car Med 1989;17:371–375.
16. Brooks VB, Curtis DR, Eccles JC. Mode of action of tetanus toxin. Nature 1955;175:120.
17. Davies JR, Morgan RS, Wright EA, et al. The effect of local tetanus intoxication on the hind limb reflexes of the rabbit. Arch Int Physiol 1954;62:248.
18. Kaeser HE, Sander A. Tetanus toxin, a neuromuscular blocking agent. Nature 1969;223:842.
19. Laurence DR, Webster RA. Pathologic physiology, pharmacology, and therapeutics of tetanus. Clin Pharmacol Ther 1963;4:36.
20. Zacks SI, Shef MF. Tetanus toxin: fine structure and localization of binding site in striated muscle. Science 1968;159:643.
21. Kerr JH, Corbett JL, Prys-Roberts C, et al. Involvement of the sympathetic nervous system in tetanus. Lancet 1968;2:236.
22. Alfery DD, Rauscher A. Tetanus: a review. Crit Car Med 1979;7:1176.
23. Faust RA, Vickers OR, Cohn I Jr. Tetanus: 2449 cases in 68 years at Charity Hospital. J Trauma 1976;16:704.
24. Habte-Gabr E, Mengistu M. Tetanus in Gondar Public Health College Hospital, Ethopia: a review of 72 cases. Ethiop Med J 1978;16:53.
25. Kerr J. Current topics in tetanus. Intensive Care Med 1979;5:105.
26. Tillman DB. Tetanus. West J Med 1978;129:107.
27. Veronesi R. Clinical observations on 712 cases of tetanus subject to four different methods of treatment: 18.2% mortality rate under a new method of treatment. Am J Med Sci 1956;232:629.
28. Adams JM, Kenny JD, Rudolph AJ. Modern management of tetanus neonatorum. Pediatrics 1979;64:472.
29. Khoo BH, Lee EL, Lam KL. Neonatal tetanus treated with high dosage diazepam. Arch Dis Child 1978;53:737.
30. Porath A, Acker M, Perel A. Serum cholinesterase in tetanus. Anaesthesia 1977;32:1009.
31. Luisto M. Tetanus in Finland: diagnostic problems and complications. Ann Med 1990;22:15–19.
32. Tseuda K, Oliver PB, Richter RW. Cardiovascular manifestations of tetanus. Anesthesiology 1974;40:588.
33. Prys-Roberts C, Kerr JH, Corbett JL, et al. Treatment of sympathetic overactivity in tetanus. Lancet 1969;1:542.
34. Udwadia FE, Sunavala JD, Jain MC, et al. Haemodynamic studies during the management of severe tetanus. Quart J Med 1992; 83:449–60.
35. James MFM, Manson EDM. The use of magnesium sulfate infusion in the management of very severe tetanus. Intensive Care Med 1985;11:5.
36. Keilty SR, Gray RC, Dundee JW, et al. Catecholamine levels in severe tetanus. Lancet 1968;2:195.
37. Levell MJ, Stitch SR, Dykes JRW, et al. Adrenal cortical function in patients with tetanus. Br J Anaesth 1970;42:531.
38. Rose AG. Catecholamine-induced myocardial damage associated with pheochromocytomas and tetanus. S Afr Med J 1974;48:1285.
39. Lipman J, James MFM, Erskine J, et al. Autonomic dysfunction in severe tetanus: magnesium sulfate as an adjunct to deep sedation. Crit Car Med 1987;15:987–988.
40. Buchanan N, Smit L, Cane RO, et al. Sympathetic overactivity in tetanus: fatality associated with propranolol. Br Med J 1979;2:274.
41. Dundee JW, Morrow WFK. Labetalol in severe tetanus. Br Med J 1979;1:1121.
42. Hanna W, Grell GAC. Labetalol in hypertensive emergencies. Br Med J 1978;3:772.
43. King WW, Cave DR. Use of esmolol to control autonomic instability of tetanus. Am J Med 1991; 91:425–428.
44. Femi-Pearse D. Blood gas tensions, acid-base status, and spirometry in tetanus. Am Rev Respir Dis 1974;110:390.
45. Femi-Pearse D, Afonja AO, Elegebeleye OO, et al. Value of determination of oxygen consumption in tetanus. Br Med J 1976;1:74.
46. O'Keefe SJD, Wesley A, Jialal I, et al. The metabolic response and problems with nutritional support in acute tetanus. Metabolism 1984;33:482.
47. Linton DM, Wells Y, Potgieter PD. Metabolic requirements in tetanus. Crit Car Med 1992; 20:950–952.
48. Centers for Disease Control and Prevention. Diphtheria, tetanus, and

pertussis: guidelines for vaccine prophylaxis and other preventive measures. MMWR 1985;34:405.
49. Eriksson E, Ullberg-Olson K. Guidelines for prevention of tetanus. (Addendum) In: Veronesi R, ed. Tetanus: important new concepts. Princeton, NJ: Excerpta Medica, 1981:264.
50. Christensen NA. Treatment of the patient with severe tetanus. Surg Clin North Am 1969;49:1183.
51. Femi-Pearse D. Experience with diazepam in tetanus. Br Med J 1966;2:862.
52. Hendrickse RG, Sherman PM. Tetanus in childhood: report of a therapeutic trial of diazepam. Br Med J 1966;2:860.
53. Phatak AT, Shah SH. Diazepam as adjuvant therapy in childhood tetanus. Clin Pediatr 1970;9:573–576.
54. Farquhar I, Hutchinson A, Curran J. Dantrolene in severe tetanus. Intensive Care Med 1988;14:249–250.
55. Borgeat A, Opovic V, Schwander D. Efficiency of a continuous infusion of propofol in a patient with tetanus. Crit Car Med 1991;19: 295–297.
56. Roizen M, Feeley TW. Pancuronium bromide. Ann Intern Med 1979;88:64.
57. Duvaldestin P, Gilbert C, Henzel D, et al. Pancuronium blood level monitoring in patients with tetanus. Intensive Care Med 1979;5:111.
58. Peat SJ, Patter DR, Hunter JM. The prolonged use of atracurium in a patient with tetanus. Anaesthesia 1988;43:962–963.
59. Pather M, Hariparsad D, Wesley AG. Nasotracheal intubation versus tracheostomy for intermittent positive pressure ventilation in neonatal tetanus. Intensive Care Med 1985;11:30.
60. Saissy JM, Demaziere J, Vitris M, et al. Treatment of severe tetanus by intrathecal injections of baclofen without artificial ventilation. Intensive Care Med 1992;18:241–244.
61. Chandy ST, Peter JV, John L, et al. Betamethasone in tetanus patients: an evaluation of its effect on the mortality and morbidity. J Assoc Physicians India 1992;40:373–376.
62. Sugiyama H. *Clostridium botulinum* neurotoxin. Microbiol Rev 1980;44:419.
63. Koenig MG, Drutz DJ, Mushlin AI, et al. Type B botulism in man. Am J Med 1967;42:208.
64. Centers for Disease Control and Prevention. Botulism in the United States, 1899–1977. In: Handbook for epidemiologists, clinicians, and laboratory workers. May, 1979.
65. Giminez DF, Ciccarelli AS. Another type of *Clostridium botulinum.* Zbl Bakt I Abt Orig 1970;215:221.
66. Hambleton P. *Clostridium botulinum* toxins: a general review of involvement in disease, structure, mode of action, and preparation for clinical use. J Neurol 1992;239:16–20.
67. Simpson L. Pharmacological studies on the cellular and subcellular effects of botulinum toxin. In: Lewis GE Jr, ed. Biomedical aspects of botulism. New York: Academic Press, 1981;35.
68. Kao I, Drachman DB, Price DL. Botulinum toxin: mechanism of presynaptic blockade. Science 1976;193:1256.
69. Schaffner W. Botulism: perspective on the conference. In: Lewis GE Jr, ed. Biomedical aspects of botulism. New York: Academic Press, 1981;359.
70. Pickett J, Berg B, Chaplin E, et al. Syndrome of botulism in infancy: clinical and electrophysiologic study. N Engl J Med 1976;295:770.
71. Arnon SS, Werner SB, Faber HK, et al. Infant botulism in 1931: discovery of a misclassified case. Am J Dis Child 1979;133:580.
72. Mills DC, Sugiyama H. Comparative sensitivities of infant and adult mice to botulinum toxin (Abstract #P11). Annual meeting of the American Society of Microbiologists, Los Angeles, 1979.
73. Moberg LJ, Sugiyama H. Microbial ecologic basis of infant botulism as studied with germ-free mice. Infect Immunol 1979;25:653.
74. Miyazaki S, Sakaguchi G. Experimental botulism in chickens: the cecum as the site of production and absorption of botulinum toxin. Jpn J Med Sci Biol 1978;31:1.
75. Sugiyama H, Mills DC. Intraintestinal toxin in infant mice challenged intragastrically with *Clostridium botulinum* spores. Infect Immunol 1978;21:59.
76. Hurst DL, Marsh WW. Early severe infantile botulism. J Pediatr 1993;122:909–911.
77. Shen WP, Felsing N, Lang D, et al. Development of infant botulism in a 3-year-old female with neuroblastoma following autologous bone marrow transplantation: potential use of human botulism immune globulin. Bone Marrow Transplant 1994;13:345–347.
78. Long SS. Epidemiologic study of infant botulism in Pennsylvania: report of the infant botulism group. Pediatrics 1985;75:928.
79. Midura TF, Snowden S, Wood R, et al. Isolation of *Clostridium botulinum* from honey. J Clin Microbiol 1979;9:282.
80. Arnon SS, Midura TF, Damus K, et al. Honey and other environmental risk factors for infant botulism. J Pediatr 1979;94:331.
81. Brown LW. Infant botulism and the honey connection. J Pediatr 1979;94:337.
82. Spika JS, Shaffer N, Hargrett-Bean N, et al. Risk factors for infant botulism in the United States. Am J Dis Child 1989;143:828–832.
83. Chin J, Arnon SS, Midura TF. Food and environmental sources of infant botulism in California. Rev Infect Dis 1979;1:693.
84. Schreiner MS, Field E, Ruddy R. Infant botulism: a review of 12 years' experience at the children's hospital of Philadelphia. Pediatrics 1991;87:159–165.
85. Arnon SS. Infant botulism. Annu Rev Med 1980;31:541.
86. Balmer SE. Wharton BA. Diet and faecal flora in the newborn: iron. Arch Dis Child 1991;66:1390–1394.
87. Arnon SS, Chin J. The clinical spectrum of infant botulism. Rev Infect Dis 1979;1:614.
88. Peterson DR, Eklund MW, Chinn NM. The sudden infant death syndrome and infant botulism. Rev Infect Dis 1979;1:630.
89. Arnon SS, Midura TF, Damus K, et al. Intestinal infection and toxin production by *Clostridium botulinum* as one cause of sudden infant death syndrome. Lancet 1978;1:1273.
90. Brown LW. Infant botulism. Pediatr Ann 1984;13:135.
91. Brown LW. Infant botulism. Adv Pediatr 1981;28:141.
92. L'Hommedieu C, Polin RA. Progression of clinical signs in severe botulism: therapeutic implications. Clin Pediatr 1981;20:90.
93. Wolfe JA, Pasquariello P, Rowe LD, et al. Tracheotomy for infant botulism. Ann Otol 1979;88:861.
94. Schreiner MS, Field E, Ruddy R. Infant botulism: a review of 12 years' experience at the Children's Hospital of Philadelphia. Pediatrics 1991;87:159–165.
95. Wohl DL, Tucker JA. Infant botulism: considerations for airway management. Laryngoscope 1992;102:1251–1254.
96. Hatheway CL. Laboratory procedures for cases of suspected infant botulism. Rev Infect Dis 1979;1:647.
97. Dezfulian M, Yolken R, Bartlett J. Rapid diagnosis of a case of infant botulism by enzyme immunoassay. Pediatr Infect Dis 1985;4:399.
98. Dezfulian M, Bartlett JG. Detection of *Clostridium botulinum* type A toxin by ELISA using antibodies produced in immunologically tolerant animals. J Clin Microbiol 1984;19:645.
99. Schrager GO, Diamond M, Rosnowski SZ, et al. Electrodiagnosis in the evaluation of progressive hypotonia in infancy with particular reference to infant botulism. J Med Soc NJ 1982;79:125.
100. Graf WD, Hays RM, Astley SJ, et al. Electrodiagnosis reliability in the diagnosis of infant botulism. J Pediatr 1992;120:747–749.
101. Johnson RO, Clay SA, Arnon SS. Diagnosis and management of infant botulism. Am J Dis Child 1979;133:586.
102. Kurland G, Seltzer J. Antidiuretic hormone excess in infant botulism. Am J Dis Child 1987;141:1227–1229.
103. Geiger JC. An outbreak of botulism. JAMA 1942;117:22.
104. Meyer KF. Botulism. Calif Med 1964;48:100–101.
105. Koening MG, Spickard A, Cardella MA, et al. Clinical and laboratory observations of type E botulism in man. Medicine 1964;43:517.
106. Cherington M. Botulism: ten year experience. Arch Neurol 1974;30:432.
107. Dowell VR, McCroskey LM, Hatheway CL, et al. Coproexamination for botulinal toxin and *Clostridium botulinum.* JAMA 1977;238:1829.
108. Peter G, Halsey NA, Marcuse EK, Pickering LK, eds. 1994 red book: report of the committee on infectious diseases. 23rd ed. Elk Grove, IL: American Academy of Pediatrics, 1994;160–162.
109. Otsuka M, Endo M. The effect of guanidine on neuromuscular transmission. J Pharmacol Exp Ther 1960;128:273.
110. Faich GA, Graebner RW, Sato S. Failure of guanidine therapy in botulism A. N Engl J Med 1971;285:773.
111. Roblot P, Roblot F, Fauchere JL, et al. Retrospective study of 108 cases of botulism in Poitiers, France. J Med Microbiol 1994;40:379–384.
112. Barrett DH. Endemic food-borne botulism: clinical experience, 1973-1986 at Alaska Native Medical Center. Alaska Med 1991;33: 101–108.
113. Burningham MD, Walter FG, Mechem C, et al. Wound botulism. Ann Emerg Med 1994;24:1184–1187.

114. Mechem CC, Walter FG. Wound botulism. Vet Hum Toxicol 1994; 36:233–237.
115. Richter RW. Infections other than AIDS. Neurol Clin 1993;11:591–603.
116. Weber JT, Goodpasture HC, Alexander H, et al. Wound botulism in a patient with a tooth abscess: case report and review. Clin Infect Dis 1993;16:635–639.
117. Irwin MJ, Gascoigne NR. Interplay between superantigens and the immune system. J Leukoc Biol 1993;54:495–503.
118. Norrby-Teglund A, Pauksens K, Norgren M, et al. Correlation between serum TNFα and IL6 levels and severity of group A streptococcal infections. Scand J Infect Dis 1995;27:125–130.
119. Michie C, Scott A, Cheesbrough J, et al. Streptococcal toxic shock–like syndrome—evidence of superantigen activity and its effects on T lymphocyte subsets in vivo. Clinical & Experimental Immunology 1994;98:140–144.
120. Akiyama T, Tamauchi H, Nakazato K, et al. Possible role of *Streptococcus pyogenes* in mucocutaneous lymph node syndrome. XI. Immunoelectron microscopic observation of protoplast-like "spherical bodies" detected in peripheral blood of MCLS patients. Acta Paediatr Jpn 1991;33:292–299.
121. Akiyama T, Yashiro K. Probable role of *Streptococcus pyogenes* in Kawasaki disease. Eur J Pediatr 1993;152:82–92.
122. Kotzin BL, Leung DY, Kappler J, et al. Superantigens and their potential role in human disease. Adv Immunol 1993;54:99–166.
123. Todd J, Fishaut M, Kapral M, et al. Toxic-shock syndrome associated with phage-group I staphylococci. Lancet 1978;2:1116.
124. McCloskey RV. Scarlet fever and necrotizing fasciitis caused by coagulase-positive hemolytic *Staphylococcus aureus* phage type 85. Ann Intern Med 1973;78:85.
125. Dunnet WN, Schallibaum EM. Scarlet-fever–like illness due to staphylococcal infection. Lancet 1960;2:1227.
126. Aranow H Jr, Wood WB. Staphylococcal infection simulating scarlet fever. JAMA 1942;119:1491.
127. Stevens FA. The occurrence of *Staphylococcus aureus* infection with a scarletiniform rash. JAMA 1927;88:1957.
128. Schlievert PM, Shands KM, Dann BB, et al. Identification and characterization of an exotoxin from *Staphylococcus aureus* associated with toxic shock syndrome. J Infect Dis 1980;143:509.
129. Bergdoll MS, Crass BA, Reiser RF, et al. A new staphylococcal enterotoxin, enterotoxin F, associated with toxic-shock syndrome *Staphylococcus aureus* isolates. Lancet 1981;1:1017.
130. Reingold AL. Epidemiology of toxic-shock syndrome, United States, 1960–1984. MMWR 1984;33:19SS.
131. Wiesenthal AM, Todd JK. Toxic shock syndrome in children aged 10 years or less. Pediatrics 1984;174:112.
132. Reingold AL, Hargrett NT, Dann BB, et al. Nonmenstrual toxic shock syndrome: a review of 130 cases. Ann Intern Med 1982;96:871.
133. Bartlett P, Reingold Al, Graham DR, et al. Toxic shock syndrome associated with surgical wound infections. JAMA 1982;247:1448.
134. Paris AL, Herwaldt LA, Blum D, et al. Pathologic findings in twelve fatal cases of toxic shock syndrome. Ann Intern Med 1982;96:852.
135. Larkin SM, Williams DN, Osterholm MT, et al. Toxic shock syndrome: clinical, laboratory, and pathologic findings in nine fatal cases. Ann Intern Med 1982;96:858.
136. Lentino JR, Rytel MW, Davis JP. Serologic evidence of non-invasive nature of *Staphylococcus aureus* infection in the toxic-shock syndrome. N Engl J Med 1981;305:641.
137. Chesney PJ, Davis JP, Purdy WK, et al. Clinical manifestations of toxic shock syndrome. JAMA 1981;246:741.
138. Davis JP, Chesney PJ, Wand PJ, et al. Toxic-shock syndrome: epidemiologic features, recurrence, risk factors, and prevention. N Engl J Med 1980;303:1429.
139. Shands KN, Schmid GP, Dan BB, et al. Toxic-shock syndrome in menstruating women. Association with tampon use and *Staphylococcus aureus* and clinical features in 52 cases. N Engl J Med 1980;303:1436.
140. McAllister RM, Mercer NS, Morgan BD, et al. Early diagnosis of staphylococcal toxaemia in burned children. Burns 1993;19:22–25.
141. Miller SD. Postoperative toxic shock syndrome after lumbar laminectomy in a male patient. Spine 1994;19:1182–1185.
142. Strausbaugh LJ. Toxic shock syndrome. Are you recognizing its changing presentations? Postgrad Med 1993;94:107–118.
143. Hyde L. Toxic shock syndrome associated with diaphragm use. J Fam Pract 1983;16:616.
144. Baehler EA, Dillon WP, Cumbo TJ, et al. Prolonged use of a diaphragm and toxic shock syndrome. Fertil Steril 1982;38:248.
145. Lee RV, Dillon WP, Baehler E. Barrier contraceptives and toxic shock syndrome. Lancet 1982;1:221.
146. Stolz SJ, Davis JP, Vergeront JM, et al. Development of antibody to staphylococcal enterotoxin F in Wisconsin toxic-shock patients: implications for recurrences. Proceedings of the 22nd International Conference on Antimicrobial Agents and Chemotherapy (Abstract #371), Miami Beach, FL, 1982.
147. Schuchat A, Broome CV. Toxic shock syndrome and tampons. Epidemiol Rev 1991;13:99–112.
148. Reingold AL. Toxic shock syndrome: an update. Am J Obstet Gynecol 1991;165:1236–1239.
149. Summary-cases of specified notifiable diseases, United States, cumulative, week ending May 27, 1995 (21st week). MMWR 1995;44:406.
150. Cole RP, Shakespeare PG. Toxic shock syndrome in scalded children. Burns 1990;16:221–224.
151. Farber BF, Broome CV, Hopkins CC. Fulminant hospital-acquired toxic shock syndrome. Am J Med 1984;77:331.
152. Smith DB, Gulindon J. Fatal cerebral edema complicating toxic shock syndrome. Neurosurgery 1988;22:598–599.
153. Priest BP, Schlievert PM, Dunn DL. Treatment of toxic shock syndrome with endotoxin-neutralizing antibody. J Surg Res 1989;46:527–531.
154. Chesney PJ, Crass BA, Polyak MB, et al. Toxic-shock syndrome: management and long-term sequelae. Ann Intern Med 1982;96:847.
155. Rosene KA, Copass MK, Kastner LS, et al. Persistent neuropsychological sequelae of toxic shock syndrome. Ann Intern Med 1982;96:865.
156. The working group on severe streptococcal infections. Defining the group A streptococcal toxic shock syndrome. JAMA 1993;269: 390–391.
157. Hoge CW, Schwartz B, Talkington DF, et al. The changing epidemiology of invasive group A streptococcal infections and the emergence of streptococcal toxic shock-like syndrome. JAMA 1993;384–389.
158. Fishbein DB, Kaplan JE, Bernard KW, et al. Surveillance of Rocky Mountain spotted fever, United States, 1981–1983. MMWR 1984; 33:15SS.
159. Peterson JC, Overall JC, Shapiro JL. Rickettsial diseases of childhood. J Pediatr 1947;30:495.
160. Harrell GT. Rocky Mountain spotted fever. Medicine 1949;28:333.
161. Riley HD. Rickettsial diseases and Rocky Mountain spotted fever, (part 1). Curr Probl Pediatr 1981;11:4.
162. Oster CN, Burke DS, Kenyon RH, et al. Laboratory-acquired Rocky Mountain spotted fever: the hazard of aerosol transmission. N Engl J Med 1977;297:863.
163. Calia FM, Bartelloni PJ, McKinney RW. Rocky Mountain spotted fever: laboratory infection in a vaccinated individual. JAMA 1970;211:2111.
164. Johnson JE III, Kadull PJ. Rocky Mountain spotted fever acquired in a laboratory. N Engl J Med 1967;277:842.
165. Sexton DJ, Gallis HA, McRae JR, et al. Possible needle-associated Rocky Mountain spotted fever. N Engl J Med 1975;292:645.
166. Wells GM, Woodward TE, et al. Rocky Mountain spotted fever caused by blood transfusion. JAMA 1978;239:2763.
167. Rocky Mountain spotted fever—United States, 1990. MMWR 1991;40:451–453, 459.
168. Kirk JL, Fine DP, Sexton DJ, et al. Rocky Mountain spotted fever: a clinical review based on 48 confirmed cases, 1943–1986. Medicine 1990;69:35–45.
169. White DJ, Flynn MK. Rocky Mountain spotted fever in New York state. Ann NY Acad Sci 1990;590:248–255.
170. Bradford WD, Hawkins HK. Rocky Mountain spotted fever in childhood. Am J Dis Child 1977;131:1228.
171. Sexton DJ, Banks PM, Weig S, et al. Late appearance of skin rash and abnormal serum enzymes in Rocky Mountain spotted fever. J Pediatr 1975;87:580.
172. Haynes RE, Sanders DY, Cramblett HG. Rocky Mountain spotted fever in children. J Pediatr 1970;76:685.
173. Hazard GW, Ganz RN, Nevin RW. Rocky Mountain spotted fever in the eastern United States: thirteen cases from the Cape Cod area of Massachusetts. N Engl J Med 1969;280:57.
174. Rubio T, Riley HD, Nida JR, et al. Thrombocytopenia in Rocky Mountain spotted fever. Am J Dis Child 1968;116:88.
175. Atkin MD, Strauss HS, Fisher GU. A case report of "Cape Cod" Rocky Mountain spotted fever with multiple coagulation disturbances. Pediatrics 1965;36:627.
176. Sexton DJ, Corey GR. Rocky Mountain "spotless" and "almost spot-

less" fever: a wolf in sheep's clothing. Clin Infect Dis 1992; 15: 439–448.
177. Kirkland KB, Marcdom PK, Sexton DJ, et al. Rocky Mountain spotted fever complicated by gangrene: report of six cases and review. Clin Infect Dis 1993;16:629–634.
178. Green WR, Walker DH, Cain BG. Fatal viscerotropic Rocky Mountain spotted fever. Am J Med 1978;64:523.
179. Walker DH, Mattern WD. Acute renal failure in Rocky Mountain spotted fever. Arch Intern Med 1979;139:443.
180. Peters AH. Tick-borne typhus (Rocky Mountain spotted fever). Epidemiologic trends, with particular reference to Virginia. JAMA 1971;216:1003.
181. White WL, Patrick JD, Miller LR. Evaluation of immunoperoxidase techniques to detect *Rickettsia rickettsii* in fixed tissue sections Am J Clin Pathol 1994;101:747–752.
182. Sexton DJ, Kanj SS, Wilson K, et al. The use of a polymerase chain reaction as a diagnostic test for Rocky Mountain spotted fever. Am J Trop Med Hyg 1994;50:59–63.
183. Radulovic S, Speed R, Feng HM, et al. EIA with species-specific monoclonal antibodies: a novel seroepidemiologic tool for determination of the etiologic agent of spotted fever rickettsiosis. J Infect Dis 1993;168:1292–1295.
184. Hand WL, Miller DH, Reinarz JA, et al. Rocky Mountain spotted fever. Am J Med 1978;64:523.
185. Woolbach SB. Studies on Rocky Mountain spotted fever. J Med Res 1919;41:1.
186. Miller JQ, Price TR. The nervous system in Rocky Mountain spotted fever. Neurology 1972;22;561.
187. Scimeca PG, Weinblatt ME, Kochen JA. Acquired coagulation inhibitor in association with Rocky Mountain spotted fever. Clin Pediatr 1987;26:459–463.
188. Walker TS, Triplett DA. Serologic characterization of Rocky Mountain spotted fever. Am J Clin Pathol 1991;95:725–732.
189. Santucci LA, Gutierrez PL, Silverman DJ. *Rickettsia rickettsii* induces superoxide radical and superoxide dismutase in human endothelial cells. Infect Immun 1992;60:5113–5118.
190. Fichtenbaum CJ, Peterson LR, Weil GJ. Ehrilichiosis presenting as a life-threatening illness with features of the toxic-shock syndrome. Am J Med 1993;95:351–357.
191. Harkess JR, Ewing SA, Brumit T., et al. Ehrlichiosis in children. Pediatrics 1991;87:199–203.
192. Anderson BE, Sumner JW, Dawson JE, et al. Detection of the etiologic agent of human ehrlichiosis by polymerase chain reaction. J Clin Microbiol 1992;30:775–780.
193. Coakley JC, Hudson I, Shann F, et al. A review of therapeutic monitoring of chloramphenicol in patients with *Haemophilus influenzae* meningitis. J Paediatr Child Health 1992;28:249–253.
194. Fraser DW, Psai TR, Orenstein W, et al. Legionnaires' disease: description of an epidemic of pneumonia. N Engl J Med 1977;297:1189.
195. Brenner DJ, Steigerwalt AG, McDade JE. Classification of the legionnaires' disease bacterium: *Legionella pneumophila*, genus novum, species nova, of the family Legionnellaceae, familia nova. Ann Intern Med 1979;90:656.
196. McDade JE, Brenner DJ, Bozeman FM. Legionnaires' disease bacterium isolated in 1947. Ann Intern Med 1979;90:659.
197. Beyer P, Kahn D, Horbach J, et al. Unusual progression of a *Legionella pneumophila* infection in a young child. Eur J Pediatr 1984;141:173.
198. Nigro G, Pastoris MC, Fantasia MM, et al. Acute cerebellar ataxia in pediatric legionellosis. Pediatrics 1983;72:847.
199. Cutz E, Thorner PS, Rao P, et al. Disseminated *Legionella pneumophila* infection in an infant with severe combined immunodeficiency. J Pediatr 1980;100:760.
200. Anderson RD, Lauer BA, Fraser DW, et al. Infections with *Legionella pneumophila* in children. J Infect Dis 1981;143:386.
201. Muldoon RL, Jaeker DL, Kiefer HK. Legionnaires' disease in children. Pediatrics 1981;67:329.
202. Orenstein WA, Overturf GD, Leedom JM, et al. The frequency of *Legionella* infection prospectively determined in children hospitalized with pneumonia. J Pediatr 1981;99:403.
203. Anderson R, Bergan T, Halvorsen K, et al. Legionnaires' disease combined with erythema multiforme in a 3-year-old boy. Acta Paediatr Scand 1981;70:427.
204. Brady MT. Nosocomial legionnaires disease in a children's hospital. J Pediatr 1989;115:46–50.
205. Kayser FH. Changes in the spectrum of organisms causing respiratory tract infections: a review. Postgrad Med J 1992;68:517–523.
206. Dahmash NS, Chowdhury MNH. Re-evaluation of pneumonia requiring admission to an intensive care unit: a prospective study. Thorax 1994;49:71–76.
207. Roig J, Carreres A, Domingo C. Treatment of legionnaire's disease: current recommendations. Drugs 1993;46:63–79.
208. Reda C, Quaresimat T, Pastoris MC. In-vitro activity of six intracellular antibiotics against *Legionella pneumophilia* strains of human and environmental origin. J Antimicrob Chemother 1994;33:757–764.
209. Blatt SP, Dolan MJ, Hendrix CW, et al. Legionnaires' disease in human immunodeficiency virus–infected patients: eight cases and review. Clin Infect Dis 1994;18:227–232.
210. Blatt SP, Parkinson MD, Pace E, et al. Nosocomial legionnaires' disease: aspiration as a primary mode of disease acquisition. Am J Med 1993;95:16–22.

Molecular Biology and Genetic Analysis 34

Deborah A. Schwangel

INTRODUCTION

Intensivists, traditionally specialists in the physiology of organ systems, are now recognizing the need to understand the submicroscopic components of the cell's nucleus and to apply the principles of molecular medicine to the treatment of intensive care unit (ICU) patients. Understanding the whole human organism is ultimately facilitated by studying its most fundamental components, DNA and RNA. Genetic analysis is the process of resolving genetic material into these component parts. Molecular biology is the term used to describe the study of molecules (including DNA and RNA) in biological processes. The specific study of the biology of DNA is called molecular genetics. Many of the complex disorders common to intensive care practice have not been pathophysiologically defined because complete understanding of them has required principles of science heretofore unknown. Technological advances in molecular biology and genetic analysis are now allowing some of the most challenging medical questions to be answered. Eventually, treatments for previously untreatable disorders will be available. Bringing molecular biology and genetics into the intensive care unit will result in a greater knowledge of physiology. The marriage of the two may be called molecular physiology, a basic science specialty for future intensivists. Intensivists should thus prepare themselves to be fluent in the language of molecular medicine in order to use these new technologies for the therapeutic and ethical advantages of patients.

This chapter is intended to be a tool by which critical care physicians can begin to learn molecular language and related technology, including definitions, introductory discussions, descriptions of techniques, applications to clinical medicine, and some prospects for the future. A glossary and list of suggested readings are found at the end of the chapter.

HISTORY AND TECHNOLOGICAL PROGRESS

More than 100 years ago, the Austrian monk Gregor Mendel described the principles of heredity through his classic experiments with peas; thus began the science of genetics. Although these beginnings were humble, the fundamental principles Mendel stated are strong and have been confirmed many times in the 130 years since their description. Mendel's work initially went unrecognized by his contemporaries, and it was not until the early twentieth century that others made supportive observations. In 1944, Avery reported that DNA carried genetic information[(1)]. Sickle cell anemia was the first disorder determined to be caused by a molecular defect[(2)]. After Linus Pauling's description of the molecular basis of sickle cell anemia in 1949[(2)], the β-globin gene was the first human gene to be isolated[(3)], and the amino acid substitution that causes sickle cell anemia was described[(3)]. The double helix structure of DNA was revealed in 1953 by Watson and Crick[(4,5)], which made the establishment of the complete genetic code possible by 1966[(6,7)]. During the 60s and 70s the work of geneticists was largely focused on bacterial models. Gene sequencing techniques were discovered and perfected[(8,9)], which led to more rapid identification of genes and genetic mutations. Progress in human genetics was steady until it exploded in 1985, shortly after the description of the polymerase chain reaction (PCR)[10]. The last decade has yielded an active and productive human genome project, the identification of more than 3000 human genes, and preliminary data that suggests future success with human gene therapy.

The growing catalog of the human genome may be accessed by computer with an Internet connection. The Genome Data Base (GDB) catalogs genes that have been mapped or otherwise described, and it gives information on chromosomal location, DNA sequence, and primers and probes to study particular genes. Online Mendelian Inheritance in Man (OMIM), by Dr. Victor McKusick, is an online, up-to-date version of Mendelian Inheritance in Man that describes the morbid anatomy of the human genome. GDB and OMIM can be accessed on the Internet through Gopher (Figure 34.1). The human genome project is a worldwide coordinated effort to characterize the human genome (all of the human genetic material), so that all human genes are discovered and accessible for further study. By 2010, every human gene may be mapped to a specific chromosomal location. Subsequent study should lead to sequencing of these genes and knowledge of their mutations, polymorphisms, and protein products, and ultimately their etiology in disease.

```
login:
password:

> gopher ↵

> 3.  Basic science research resources/ ↵

> 3.  Databanks - Sequences, structures, gene mapping, etc./ ↵

> 3.  Genome and gene mapping data/ ↵

> 3.  Human genome data/ ↵

>        1.  The Genome Data Base (GDB)/ ↵
         2.  Online Mendelian Inheritance in Man (OMIM) <?>
         3.  Other human genome data

>        1.  About these searches
         2.  GDB forms and third party software
         3.  Search loci in GDB <?>
         4.  Search citations in GDB <?>
         5.  Search polymorphisms in GDB<?>
         6.  Search mutations in GDB <?>
         7.  Search probes in GDB <?>
         8.  Search map information in GDB <?>
         9.  Search contacts in GDB <?>
         10.  Search libraries in GDB <?>
         11.  Search cell lines in GDB <?>
         12.  OMIM-On line Mendelian Inheritance in Man
```

⇒

Question: What is the chromosomal locus of the cystic fibrosis gene?

-access GDB
-choose # 3 "search loci in GDB" ↵
-type cystic fibrosis ↵
-choose # 1 "locus: GOO-120-584:CFTR"

This information will come on screen:

GDB ID: GOO-120-584
symbol: CFTR
type: gene
aliases: CF
locus name: cystic fibrosis transmembrane conductance regulator
cyto location: 7q31.3
assign. modes: linkage/family studies
MIM: 219700
etc.

Answer: chromosome 7, long arm at locus 31.3

⇓

Question: What is the disease pathogenesis of cystic fibrosis?

-go to OMIM ↵
-at prompt type cystic fibrosis ↵
-choose # 1: 219700 cystic fibrosis ↵

The screens to follow will show the fully referenced text including a description of the disorder, pathophysiology, pathogenesis, genetics and known mutations.

Figure 34.1. Using the Internet to search the Genome Data Base and Online Mendelian Inheritance in Man.

STRUCTURE AND FUNCTION OF THE HUMAN GENOME

Anatomy

The human genome consists of 3 billion base pairs of DNA, distributed on 22 pairs of autosomes (i.e., chromosomes 1 to 22) and the pair of sex chromosomes (i.e., XX or XY). The nucleotides, adenine (A), guanine (G), thymine (T) and cytosine (C), are attached to a sugar phosphate backbone to form a single DNA strand. RNA strands are composed of two pyrimidines, cytosine and uracil (U), and two purines, adenine and guanine. The nucleotides on one DNA strand form hydrogen bonds with nucleotides on a complementary DNA strand to form the double helix. DNA complementary pairs are A-T, C-G. RNA-DNA or RNA-RNA complementary pairs are A-U, C-G. Each chromosome is a single DNA molecule that carries the coding strands, or blueprints, for thousands of proteins. The sequence of DNA that codes for and regulates the function and replication of a single protein is called a gene. Each gene is composed of exons (i.e., coding regions) and introns (i.e., noncoding regions).

An estimated 100,000 human genes are contained within the human genome. The chromosomes are numbered according to size and characteristic shape. Each has a short arm and a long arm, designated as p and q respectively. The naming of chromosomal loci is done by numbering them in ascending order from the centromere to the telomere on either the p or q arm. Specific genes are given names, and research markers are given numbers that have nothing to do with chromosomal loci numbers. Once mapped, genes or markers are given a reference map location such as 7q31.3 for the cystic fibrosis gene, or cystic fibrosis transmembrane receptor (CFTR) (Figure 34.2).

In addition, a mitochondrial genome exists that can be thought of as another human chromosome. The mitochondrial genome is circular, descended from and resembling a bacterial genome. Each mitochondrion contains about 10 identical copies of this chromosome, each of which is made up of 16,569 nucleotides, 0 introns, and 37 genes[11]. The mitochondrial genes code for 22 transfer RNAs (tRNA), 2 ribosomal RNAs (rRNA), and 13 peptides that are subcomplexes involved in oxidative phosporylation[11–12].

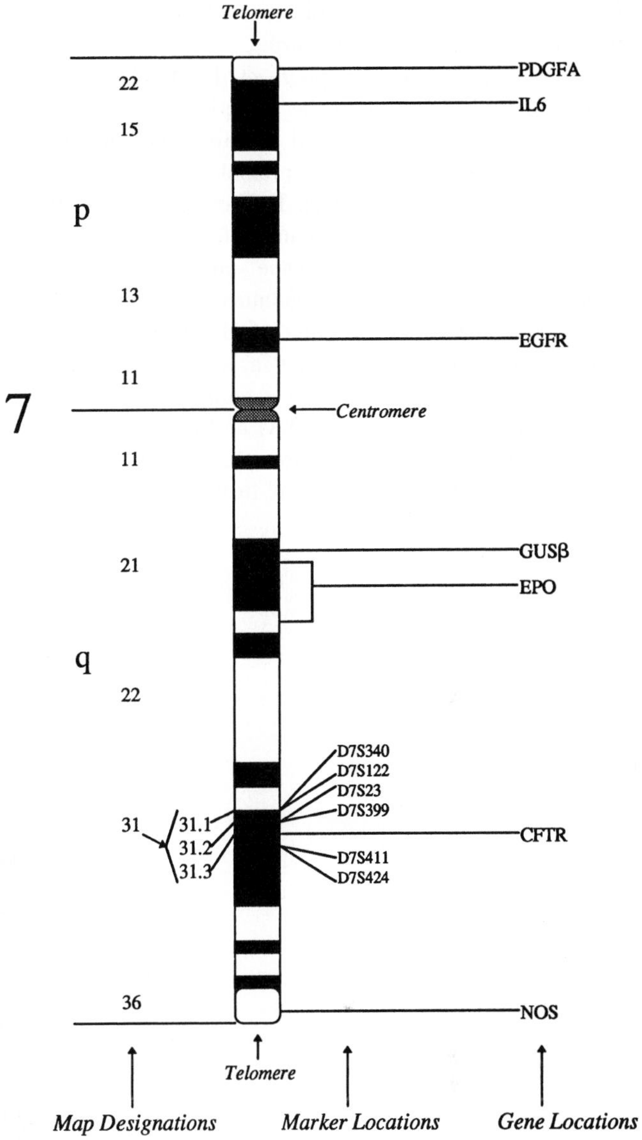

Figure 34.2. Depiction of a map of chromosome 7. Map designations are on left-hand side of figure. Short arm of chromosome is designated p; long arm, q. Loci on either p or q are numbered in ascending order from centromere to telomere. Marker and gene locations are shown on right side of figure. When exact map location of a gene is not known, it may be designated as a range, e.g., EPO. The genes listed are only a small sampling of the genes that have been mapped to chromosome 7. The CFTR gene is located at 7q31.3, and flanking markers are shown at 7q31. PDGFA, platelet-derived growth factor, alpha polypeptide; IL6, interleukin-6; EGFR, epidermal growth factor receptor; GUSB, glucuronidase, β; EPO, erythropoietin; CFTR, cystic fibrosis transmembrane receptor; NOS, nitric oxide sythase 3. From: McKusick VA. Mendelian inheritance in man. 11th ed. Baltimore: The Johns Hopkins University Press, 1994:xxiii–xxiv.

Chemistry and Physiology

All hereditary information is transmitted from parents to offspring via DNA packaged as chromosomes. For the purposes of replication, the strands of DNA separate (denature), allowing polymerases to catalyze the formation of new complementary strands of DNA or RNA. The hydrogen bonds that link strands of DNA are relatively easily broken (i.e., denatured by thermal or chemical means), but the covalent bonds that attach the nucleotides to the sugar phosphate backbone are not. When denaturation occurs, the double helix unwinds and the strands separate. Denaturation is reversible (i.e., renaturation) when the conditions that initiated it are stopped; renaturation re-forms the double helix. This process occurs either with the original complementary DNA strand or a new or altered complementary strand. The ability to renature with any complementary strand makes possible the laboratory techniques known as *in situ* hybridization and polymerase chain reaction (both described later). Thus, the replication chemistry of DNA is important both *in vivo* and *in vitro.*

Replication and transcription of DNA always takes place in one direction, from the 5′ end to the 3′ end of a gene (Figure 34.3). The 5′ end contains nucleotides that serve as initiating sequences, promoters, and enhancers for transcription (Figure 34.4). Promoters and enhancers influence rates of transcription and determine tissue specificities. The 3′ end of a gene contains termination sequences and also some regulatory elements. Coding regions of DNA exist in units of 3 consecutive bases called codons, each coding for a specific amino acid **(Table 34.1).** The DNA forms a template for transcription onto messenger RNA (mRNA) and subsequent translation into protein, which requires tRNA and rRNA. The regulatory elements of a gene may turn its own expression on or off; alternatively, other genes may regulate each other's expression.

Normal function of the human genome includes regulation of the cell cycle. Genetic regulation suppresses unchecked passage through the cell cycle, which can result in the runaway growth characteristic of malignant cells. Other regulators of the cell cycle may result in apoptosis, which is programmed cell death (sometimes referred to as cellular suicide). Apoptosis normally plays a role in the development and regression of primordial tissues and in the protection of the organism against cancer growth and viral infections.

Pathology and Pathophysiology

Many different pathologic alterations in the human genome have been reported and are referred to as mutations (i.e.,

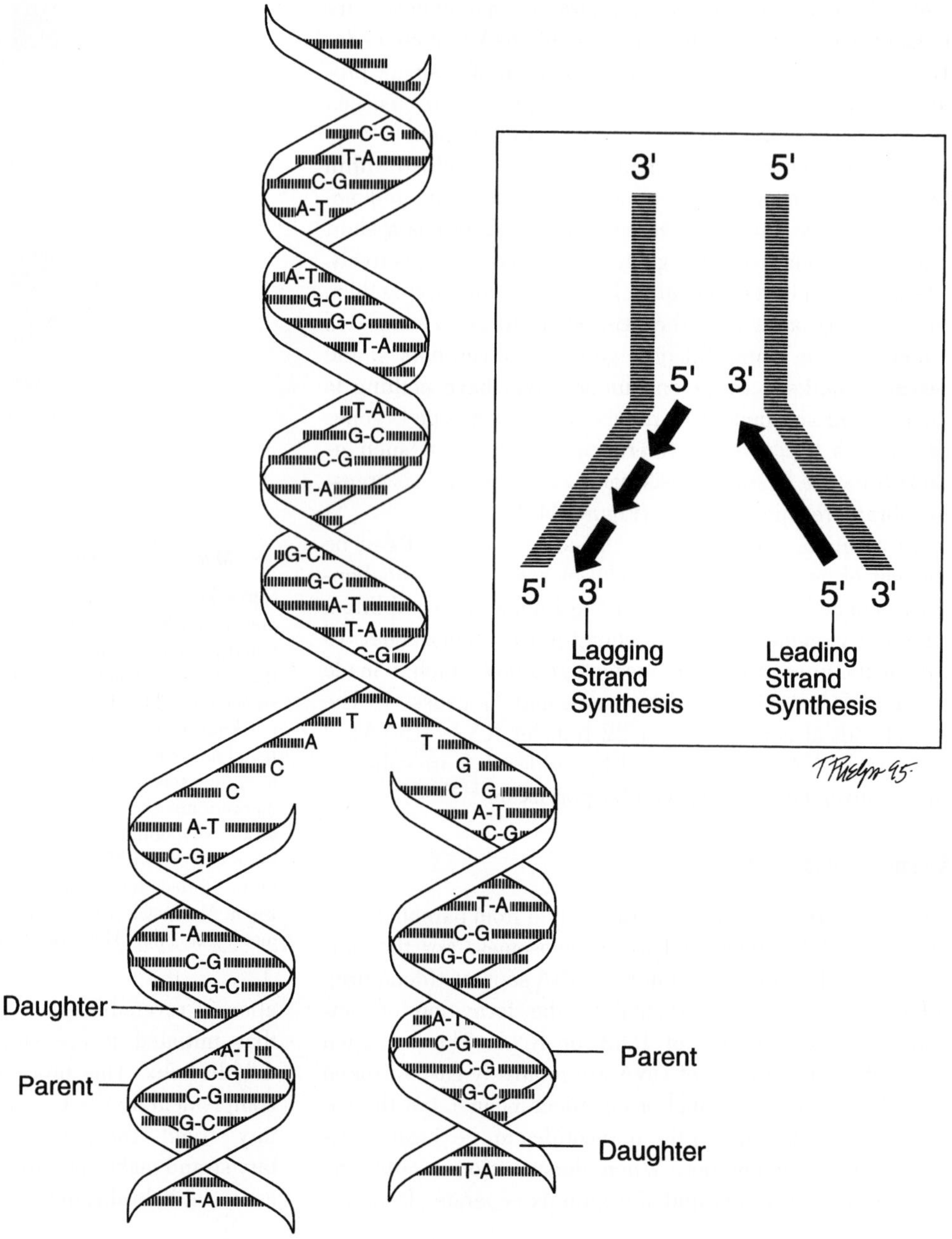

Figure 34.3. DNA replication follows unwinding of double helix. Two new strands are synthesized from parent strands. Process always occurs in 5′ → 3′ direction. Reproduced with permission from Clayton, DA. Structure, replication, and transcription of DNA. In: Leder P, Clayton DA, Rubenstein E. Introduction to Molecular Medicine. New York: Scientific American 1994;32.

variations from the normal genetic sequence). Mutations should be distinguished from polymorphisms, which are differences in DNA sequence that do not result in disease. Polymorphisms exist in regulatory regions or noncoding regions and do not create an abnormal protein product, and are responsible for normal inter-individual variations. Mutations may be either spontaneous or induced, gametic or somatic. They can take several forms, including point mutation, trinucleotide expansion, whole or partial gene deletion, partial chromosomal deletion, rearrangement, or addition. A point mutation (single base-pair change) is caused by a deletion, substitution, or addition that changes the code or reading frame affecting protein synthesis. An example of such a mutation is the A→T substitution, which changes GAG, the code for glutamic acid, to GTG, the code for valine. This single amino acid change results in the creation of hemoglobin S, the protein that causes sickle cell anemia.

A trinucleotide expansion mutation causes disorders such as Huntington's disease, fragile X syndrome, and myotonic dystrophy **(Table 34.2).** The gene of an unaffected person contains a small number of copies of the trinucleotide sequence, but an affected person has many more copies. Fragile X patients have more than 200 copies of a GCC repeat at Xq28 on the long arm of the X chromosome; normally there are 6 to 25 copies[13]. Myotonic dystrophy is genetically characterized by a CTG repeat which normally consists of 5 to 27 copies; mildly affected persons have at least 50 repeats; and the most severely affected, those with congenital disease, have 1500 to 6000 copies of the trinucleotide[14,15]. Parents of affected patients have an intermediate number of copies, so that geneticists can predict that offspring will be affected. This is the molecular basis for anticipation, or the tendency of some diseases to appear at earlier onset ages and with increasing severity in successive generations (Figure 34.5). Trinucleotide expansions cause decreased or absent protein production or gains in function.

Mutations may be inherited or acquired. Environmental influences, such as x-irradiation or free radical species, may induce mutations. These influences are of special interest to cancer geneticists because environmental agents can cause activation of a proto-oncogene or loss of a tumor-suppressor gene. Proto-oncogenes normally function to promote cell division; they must be switched off to stop cell division. When left switched on by mutation, tumor production is the result. The mutated proto-oncogene is called an oncogene. In contrast, tumor-suppressor genes normally function to slow or stop passage through the cell cycle. When all function of a tumor-suppressor gene is lost, tumor development results from uncontrolled cellular proliferation. The retinoblastoma and Wilms' tumor genes are examples of tumor-suppressor genes. The cell cycle is normally regulated by a number of checkpoints. Alterations in any checkpoint may result in abnormal cell proliferation or cell death. The p53 gene, known to be mutated in a variety of human cancers[16], codes for a protein that serves as a regulator of the cell cycle. Environmental agents can mutate this gene; molecular evidence of p53 mutagenesis exists for tobacco and alcohol in head and neck cancers[17].

Table 34.1. The Genetic Code

Amino Acid	Codon(s)
Alanine	GCA, GCC, GCG, GCT
Arginine	CGA, CGC, CGG, CGTAG A, AGG
Asparagine	AAC, AAT
Aspartic acid	GAC, GAT
Cysteine	TGC, TGT
Glutamic acid	GAA, GAG
Glutamine	CAA, CAG
Glycine	GGA, GGC, GGG, GGT
Histidine	CAC, CAT
Isoleucine	ATA, ATC, ATT
Leucine	CTA, CTC, CTG, CTTTA, TTG
Lysine	AAA, AAG
Methionine	ATG
Phenylalanine	TTC, TTT
Proline	CCA, CCC, CCG, CCT
Serine	TCA, TCC, TCG, TCTAGC, AGT
Threonine	ACT, ACC, ACG, ACT
Tryptophan	TGG
Tyrosine	TAC, TAT
Valine	GTA, GTC, GTG, GTT
	TAG, TAA, TGA[a]

[a]*Stop Codes*

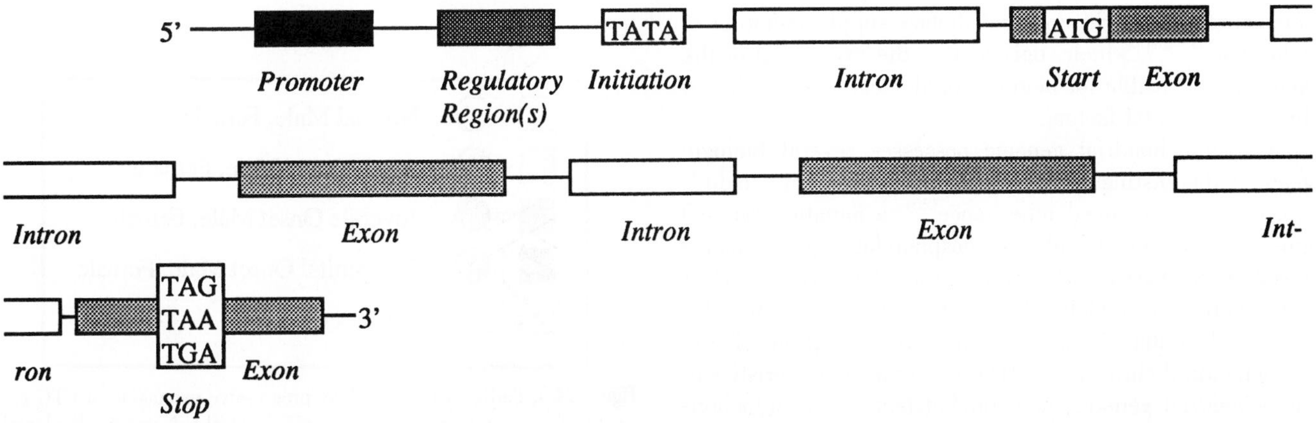

Figure 34.4. Cartoon representation of gene anatomy. Components of a gene include coding regions (exons), noncoding regions (introns), regulatory and promoter sequences, and start and stop signals.

Table 34.2. Disorders Resulting from the Trinucleotide Expansion Mutation

Disease	*Mode of Inheritance*	*Repeat Sequence*	*Normal Number of Repeats*	*Disease Number of Repeats*
Fragile X syndrome	X-linked recessive	CGG	6–52	50–>1000
Spinal and bulbar muscular atrophy	X-linked sex-limited	CAG	12–33	40–62
Myotonic dystrophy	Autosomal dominant	CTG	5–40	50–>3000
Huntington's disease	Autosomal dominant	CAG	9–30	40–121
FRAXE mental retardation	X-linked recessive	CGG	6–25	100–>1000
Dentatorubral pallidoluysian atrophy	Autosomal dominant	CAG	9–23	49–75
spinocerebellar ataxia type 1	Autosomal dominant	CAG	9–39	41–81

Adapted from Monckton DG, Caskey CT. Unstable triplet repeat diseases. Circulation 1995;91:514.

Classically inherited mutations are those that appear in subsequent generations according to the laws of Mendel; the patterns follow dominant or recessive models. Not all disorders are inherited according to Mendelian law; examples are imprinting, uniparental disomy, and negative complementation. Imprinting is defined as a difference in gene expression from that of the parent of origin. Uniparental disomy is the inheritance of both copies of a particular chromosome (or a portion thereof) from only one parent. Negative complementation refers to interfering interactions between alleles.

One region of the genome that illustrates imprinting is the proximal long arm of chromosome 15 (15q). One gene in that region is imprinted (inactive) on the maternal copy and a neighboring gene is imprinted on the paternal copy. If offspring have maternal disomy for chromosome 15q or if the paternal locus is deleted or inactivated by mutation, Prader-Willi syndrome results[18]. If offspring have paternal disomy or inactivation of the maternal copy of chromosome 15q, Angelman syndrome is the result[19,20].

Single gene disorders may be strongly influenced by the environment. Disorders such as glucose-6-phosphate dehydrogenase (G6PD) deficiency or malignant hyperthermia are not recognizable until persons with a faulty gene are exposed to certain environmental triggering agents. There are also many multifactorial genetic disorders, such as congenital heart disorders, cleft lip and palate, and genitourinary anomalies; each of these are recognized to run in families but do not follow classic patterns of Mendelian inheritance. Neural tube defects also run in families, but several investigators have shown a reduction in the incidence of these anomalies with periconceptual dietary supplementation of folic acid[21–24], which suggests that the expression of the gene(s) responsible for neural tube defects may be altered by environmental factors.

The mitochondrial genome possesses several biologic features that distinguish it from the nuclear genome, including strictly matrilineal inheritance[25], a mutation rate 10 times that of nuclear oxidative phosphorylation genes, manifestation of disease with advancing age because of declining numbers of mitochondria, and the possibility of mitochondrial mutations present in only a portion of the mitochondrial chromosome. These unique characteristics of mitochondrial genetics help predict features of mitochondrial genetic disorders[26–29]. Disorders due to mutations in mitochondrial DNA include many neurologic disorders: some epilepsies, blindness, and deafness[29]. Aminoglycoside-induced deafness is one specific example, which occurs in certain Asian populations[30–32] whose families show a pattern transmitted exclusively through females[31] and a mutation that favors aminoglycoside binding[32]. The mutation occurs in a region where aminoglycosides are known to bind and leads to tissue-specific impairment of the mitochondrial translation system, impaired adenosine triphosphate (ATP) production in the cochlea, and deafness[30,33]. Susceptible persons differ from others in that deafness occurs with nontoxic levels of aminoglycosides.

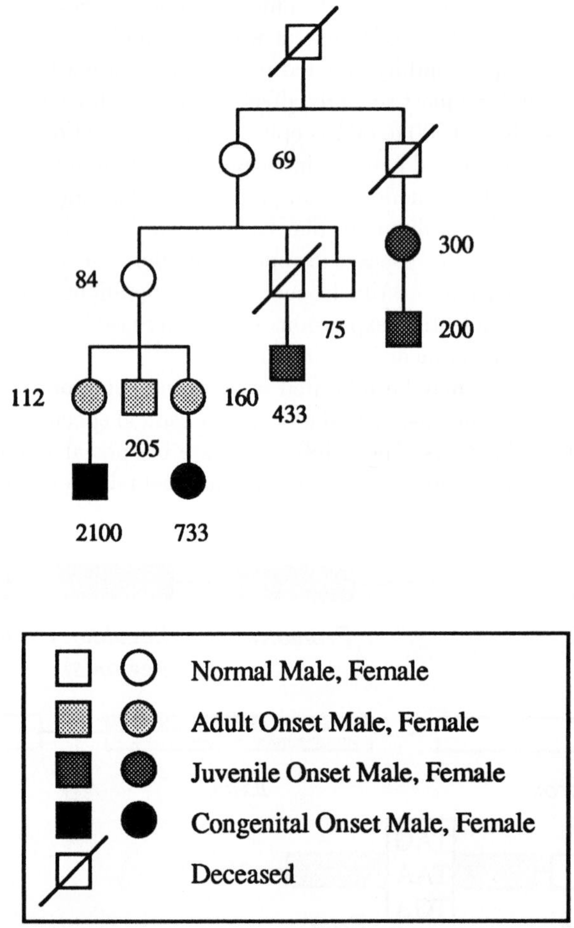

Figure 34.5. Pedigree that displays progressive expansion of CTG repeat in family members with myotonic dystrophy. Numbers displayed indicate how many copies of CTG repeat are present in each individual. Reproduced with permission from Monckton DG, Caskey CT. Unstable triplet diseases. Circulation 1995;91:515.

Table 34.3. Partial List of Triggers of Apoptosis

Physiologic	
	TNF[a]
	Glutamate
	Dopamine
	N-methyl-D-aspartate
	Calcium
	Glucocorticoids
Damage-related Inducers	
	Heat shock
	Viral infection
	Bacterial toxins
	Oncogenes
	p53
	Free radicals
	Cytolytic T cells
	Nutrient deprivation
Therapeutic Agents	
	Anthracyclines
	Cisplatin
	Methotrexate
	Vincristine
	Nitrogen mustard
	Gamma radiation
	UV radiation
Toxins	
	Ethanol
	β-amyloid peptide

Partial list of factors which can induce apoptosis.
[a]TNF = tumor necrosis factor. List adapted from Thompson CB. Apoptosis in the pathogenesis and treatment of disease. Science 1995;267:1457.

Apoptosis, or cellular self-destruction, is a fascinating part of the mechanism of homeostasis in organs and multicellular organisms. It is responsible for developmental modeling of the growing human and prevention of unchecked cellular proliferation throughout life. Teleologically, normal apoptosis has functional importance in morphology and probably also in host defense against viral attack[34]. Apoptosis is controlled by genes involved in regulation of the cell cycle. This type of cell death is pathologically distinguished from necrosis by microscopic evidence of cell shrinkage rather than the swelling and extrusion of cellular contents characteristic of necrotic cell death (Figure 34.6). The dying apoptotic cell maintains the integrity of its cell membrane. Neighboring phagocytes are signalled to engulf it, and there is no induction of an inflammatory response. A variety of environmental signals may inhibit or induce apoptosis **(Tables 34.3 and 34.4).** Exaggerated apoptosis and failed apoptosis are mechanisms that result in abnormal tissue growth and atrophy, respectively (Figure 34.7). Inhibition of apoptosis is a key factor in the development of malignancies[35]. The p53 gene product, important in the development of some cancers, is required for cells to initiate apoptosis in response to environmental triggers[36]. A gene called BCL2, when overexpressed, prevents stimulated cells from initiating apoptosis[37], resulting in tissue overgrowth. Therapeutic regulation of the cell cycle in dysregulated cancer cells is one way in which chemotherapy and radiation therapy help cancer patients[35,38]. Altering the apoptotic threshold by inhibiting cell surface receptors that trigger cell death may also be possible. Inhibiting agents may include the Fas receptor or tumor necrosis factor (TNF) antibodies[39,40].

Evidence from animal studies suggests that apoptosis plays a role in the pathology of autoimmune disorders[35]. Apoptosis may also be a host defense against viral infection, down-regulating cellular machinery to prevent proliferation of the viral genome. Alternatively, viruses can prevent apoptosis to establish viral latency. Such pathologic processes have been shown for the Epstein-Barr virus[41]. Exaggerated apoptotic cell death is characteristic of infection with human immunodeficiency virus (HIV); the onset of AIDS is correlated with the apoptotic death of uninfected T cells[42,43]. Many other disorders are also thought to be perpetuated by apoptotic cell death **(Table 34.5).** Cerebral and myocardial

Table 34.4. Partial List of Inhibitors of Apoptosis

Physiologic	
	Growth factors
	CD40 ligand
	Neutral amino acids
	Zinc
	Estrogen
	Androgens
	Extracellular matrix
Viral	
	Adenovirus
	Baculovirus
	EBV[a]
	Herpes γ1 34.5
	African swine fever
	Cowpox
Pharmacologic	
	Calpain inhibitors
	Cysteine protease inhibitors
	Phenobarbital
	α-hexachlorocyclohexane

[a]EBV, Epstein-Barr virus. Adapted from Thompson CB. Apoptosis in the pathogenesis and treatment of disease. Science 1995;267:1457.

Table 34.5. Disorders Associated with Increased or Decreased Apoptosis

Inhibited Apoptosis	
	Lymphomas
	Carcinomas with p53 mutations
	Breast cancer
	Prostate cancer
	Ovarian cancer
	SLE[a]
	Immune-mediated glomerulonephritis
	Herpesvirus infections
	Poxvirus infections
	Adenovirus infections
Increased Apoptosis	
	AIDS
	Alzheimer's disease
	Parkinson's disease
	Amyotrophic lateral sclerosis
	Retinitis pigmentosa
	Cerebellar degeneration
	Aplastic anemia
	Myocardial infarction
	Stroke
	Alcohol-induced liver disease

[a]SLE, systemic lupus erythematosis. Adapted from Thompson CB. Apoptosis in the pathogenesis and treatment of disease. Science 1995;267:1458.

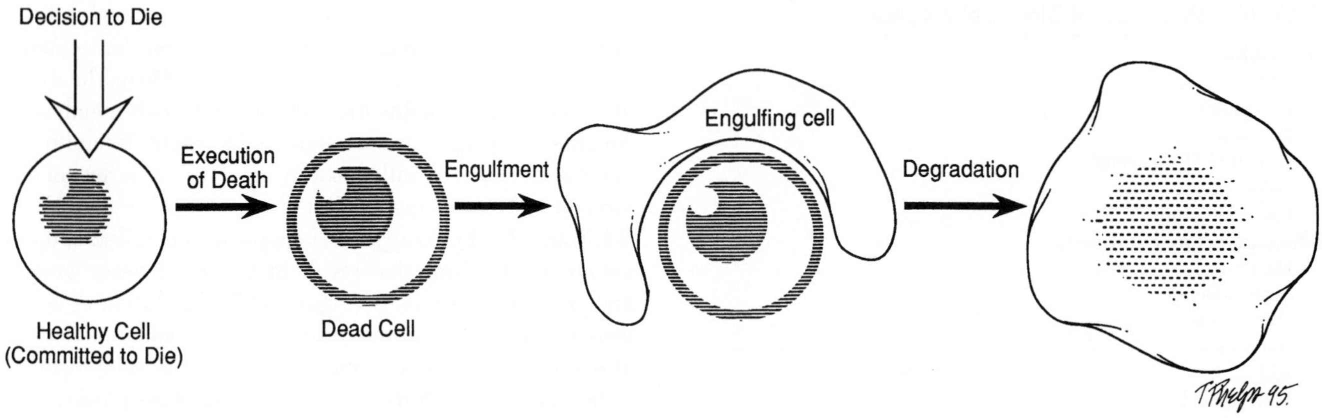

Figure 34.6. Apoptosis: cellular death that does not invite an inflammatory reaction. Adapted from Steller, H. Mechanisms and genes of cellular suicide. Science 1995;267:1445.

infarctions share both necrotic and apoptotic forms of cell death(44). Normal and abnormal consequences of apoptosis in the human heart are reviewed by James(45) and include normal postnatal remodeling of the conduction system, evidence for apoptotic cell death in various conduction disturbances, and nonnecrotic degeneration in cardiomyopathies.

TECHNIQUES USED IN THE STUDY OF DNA

There are now many ways to study DNA and inherited disorders. The first step is to determine the existence of a disorder and to define its characteristics, or phenotype. Studying family pedigrees helps establish the pattern of inheritance of a disorder, which may be, for example, present in every generation or in every other generation, in males only or in both males and females. If the disorder is not multifactorial or the phenotype is not strongly influenced by differences in penetrance, it may be possible to determine if inheritance follows Mendelian law and to classify it as autosomal dominant or recessive, or sex-linked (Figure 34.8).

Cytogenetics, the microscopic study of chromosomes, may identify certain disorders. For many years, cytogeneti-

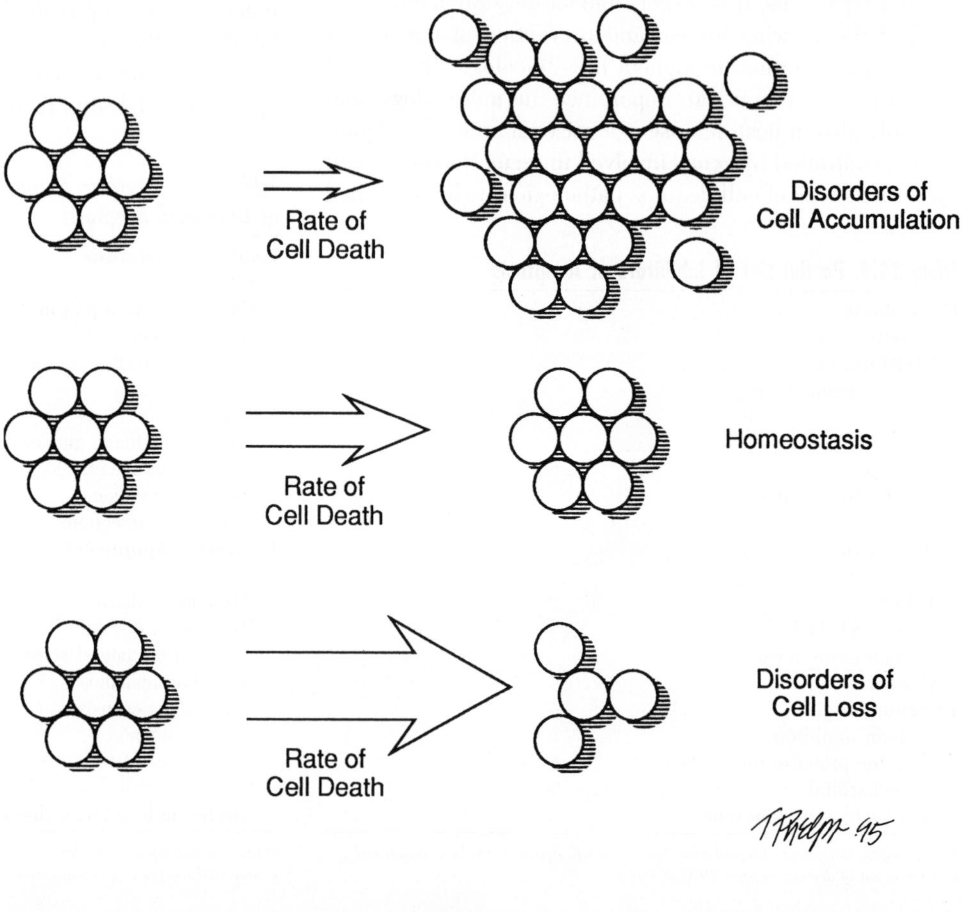

Figure 34.7. Apoptosis and homeostasis. Adapted from Thompson CB. Apoptosis in the pathogenesis and treatment of disease. Science 1995;267:1457.

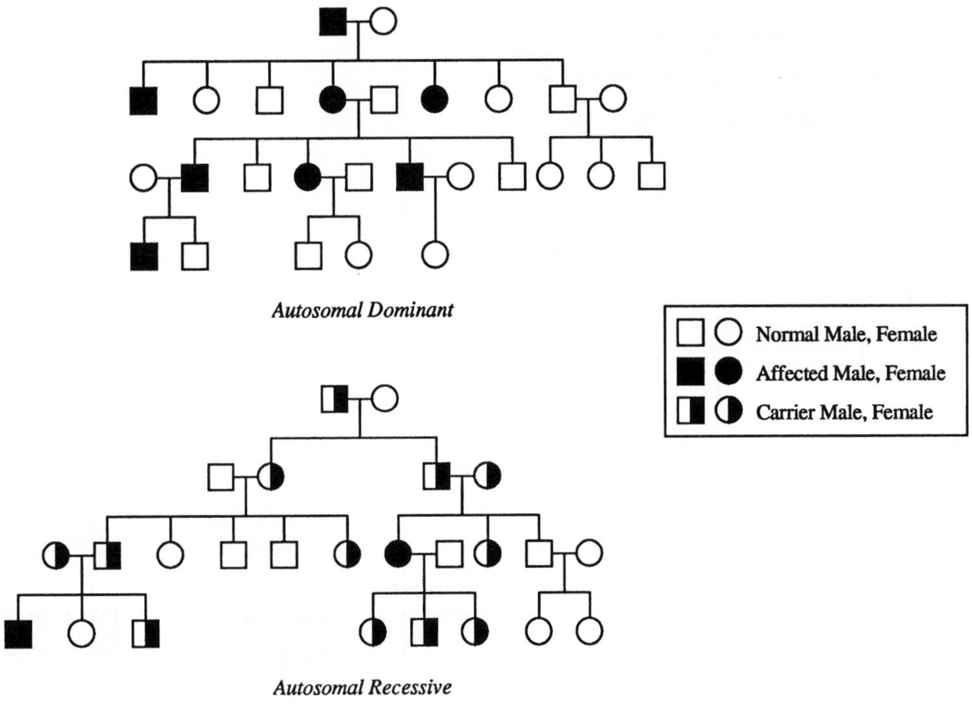

Figure 34.8. Autosomal dominant and autosomal recessive inheritance patterns as illustrated by pedigrees.

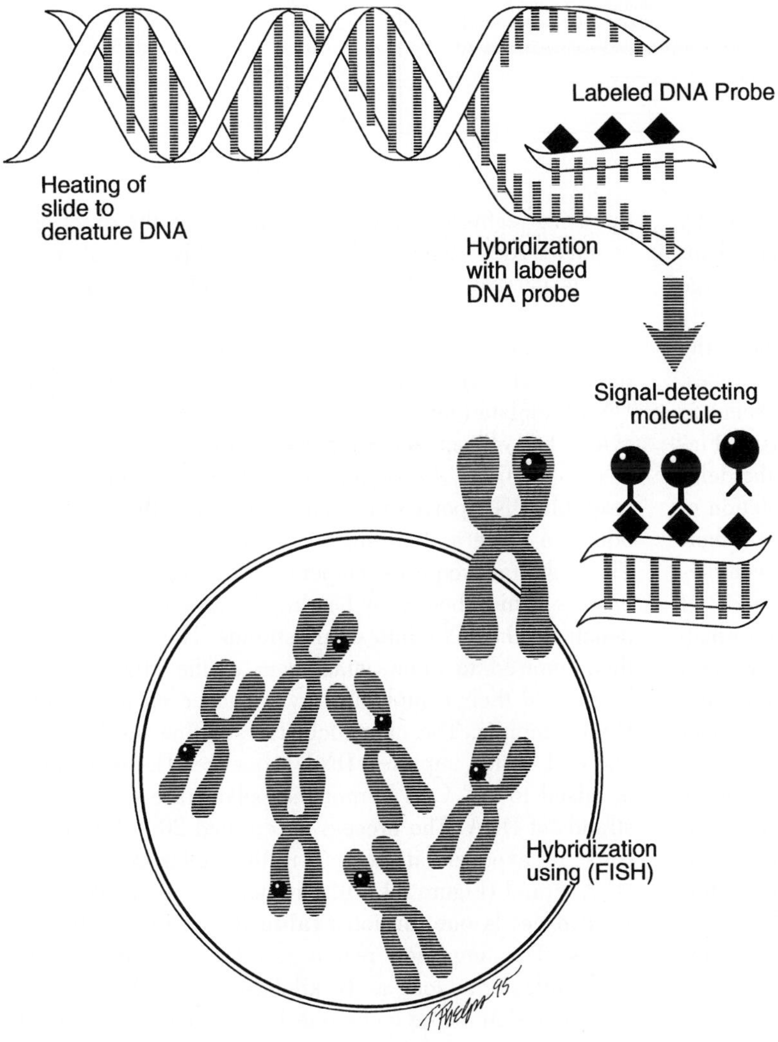

Figure 34.9. Process of *in-situ* hybridization involving binding of labeled nucleic acid probe to DNA under study. Signal-detecting molecule, which can be fluorescent molecule or other molecule detectable by microscopy, shows where probe has bound to study DNA. FISH = fluorescent *in-situ* hybridization.

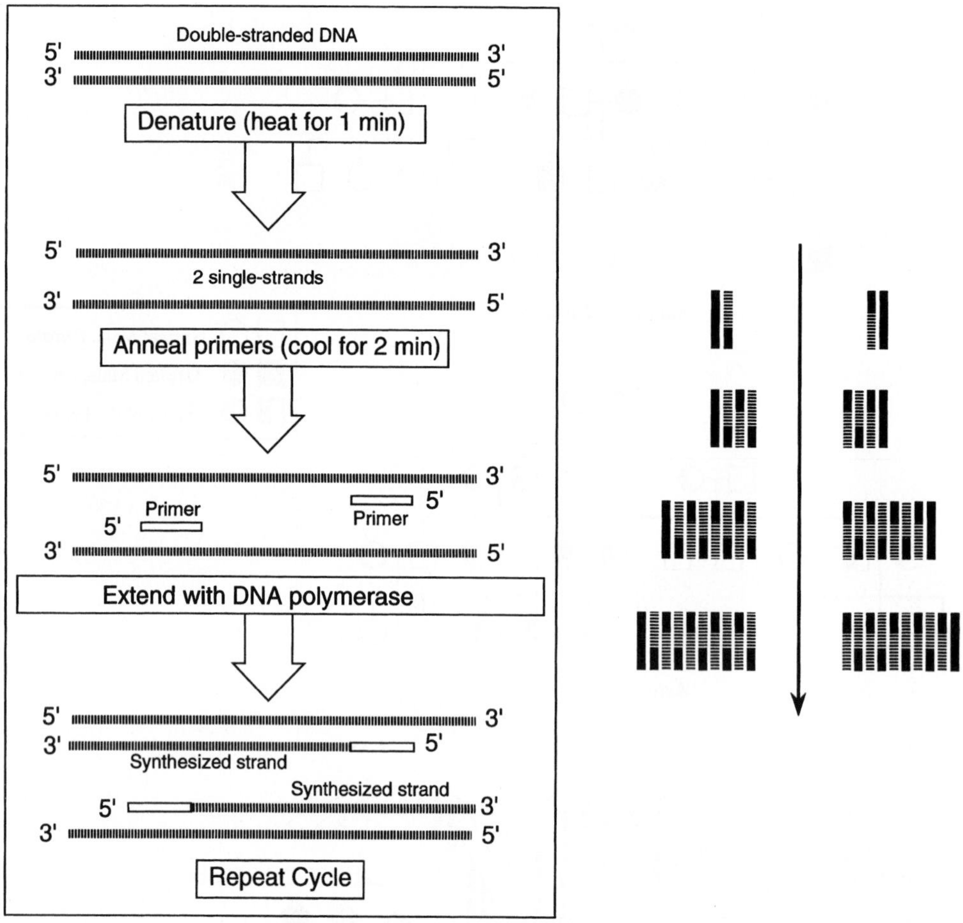

Figure 34.10. Mechanism of amplification of DNA by PCR. Each newly synthesized strand serves as template for DNA synthesis in next cycle; each cycle doubles number of DNA strands.

cists were primarily involved in evaluation of karyotypes by means of standard light microscopy, a useful method for identifying trisomies, large chromosomal deletions, or large translocations. Technological advancements have greatly improved resolution of cytogenetic techniques, through the use of fluorescent-labeled or radioisotope-labeled probes. This technique, called *in situ* hybridization (fluorescent *in situ* hybridization [FISH] if fluorescent labeling is used (Figure 34.9), identifies chromosomal defects such as the deletion of 13q14.11 in retinoblastoma cells or the deletion of 11p13 in Wilms' tumor cells. A labeled probe is a short segment of a known DNA sequence that binds to its complement when allowed to anneal (bind) to a specimen of genomic DNA. Since the probe sequence is known to map to a particular chromosomal location, finding the probe's signal on another chromosome indicates a translocation and failure to bind could indicate deletion of the chromosomal segment in question.

Higher resolution techniques are also available. When a single gene is studied, it is sometimes necessary to look at a single portion of that gene to establish a genotype. Toward this goal, the specific portion of the gene is amplified. Amplification is done by cloning or by PCR, as described below. Cloning is the process of copying a specified portion of DNA through the use of bacterial machinery. Once the specified DNA segment has been amplified, sequencing techniques are used to determine the exact order of nucleotides along the DNA chain. This level of resolution is needed to identify point mutations or the genetic code.

PCR is a technique used to amplify a specific DNA sequence. The reaction components include the subject's DNA template (genomic DNA, usually derived from leukocytes), two oligonucleotide primers (about 20 base pairs of DNA specific to the portion of DNA under study), a thermostable DNA polymerase, and a supply of the four nucleotides to serve as building blocks for a new DNA strand. The technique requires temperature cycling of the reaction mixture, which begins by heating the sample to 94° C; this denatures the DNA into single strands. The temperature is then lowered to allow attachment of the oligonucleotide primers to their complementary sequence on the genomic DNA template. The oligonucleotides define the beginning and end of the amplified DNA sequence. The temperature is raised to 72° C to permit the polymerase to build new strands of DNA. The process is repeated 20 to 30 times to cause an exponential increase in the copies of the desired DNA strand (Figure 34.10). The number of copies synthesized exceeds one million **(Table 34.6)** in less than 30 cycles. The amplified region can be as short as a few nucleotides or as long as 10 kilobases (10,000 base pairs). The limitation of the technique is that some portion of the

Table 34.6. Exponential Nature of Amplification Achieved by PCR

Cycle Number	*Number of Product Strands*
1	0
2	0
3	2
4	4
5	8
6	16
7	32
8	64
9	128
10	256
11	512
12	1024
13	2048
14	4096
15	8192
16	16,384
17	32,768
18	65,536
19	131,072
20	262,144
21	524,288
22	1,048,576
23	2,097,152
24	4,194,304
25	8,388,608
26	16,777,216
27	33,544,432
28	67,108,864
29	134,217,728
30	268,435,456
31	536,870,912
32	1,073,741,824

genomic DNA sequence must be known in order to make the flanking oligonucleotide primers. If genomic DNA is not available, mRNA can sometimes be used to provide the needed template. The product of RNA PCR is complementary DNA (cDNA), which is obtained by using the enzyme reverse transcriptase to catalyze the reaction. Reverse transcriptase is a viral enzyme found in retroviruses. (HIV is a particularly complex retrovirus.) Retroviruses are RNA viruses that use reverse transcriptase to convert the viral RNA genome into a DNA copy that can be integrated into a host-cell genome. The viral genome is then replicated each time the host-cell replicates its genome. Retroviruses may be used as vectors in the laboratory or possibly *in vivo* for gene therapy. Reverse transcriptase may be used in the laboratory for cloning and to obtain comparisons of cDNA from normal and abnormal tissue; such comparisons can reveal differences in gene expression or gene splicing.

PCR is used in the search for disease-producing genes in a process called linkage analysis. Genotypes are compared to phenotypes in families with disorders that follow inheritance patterns, such as autosomal dominant or recessive. A determination of linkage is made if the probability of linkage exceeds that of no linkage. Genotypes are obtained through the study of polymorphisms in the human genome; polymorphisms are defined as multiple (more than two) alleles occurring at one particular genetic locus throughout a population of individuals. There are now numerous known polymorphic locations, called markers, which are spread throughout the human genome and are available for linkage studies. Some disease genes that have

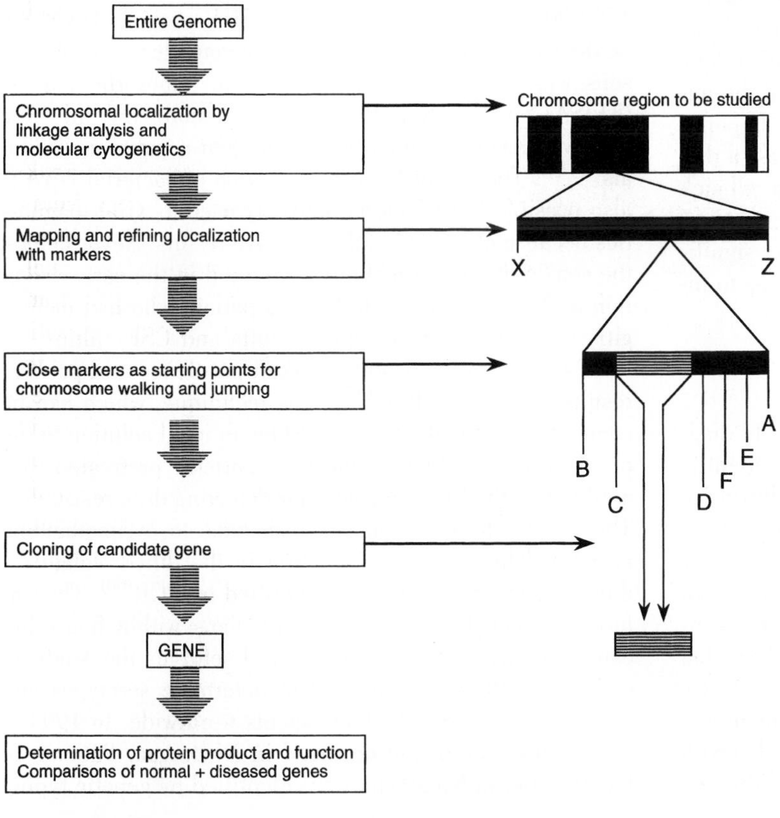

Figure 34.11. Flowchart Summary of process involved in conducting genome search.

been identified using linkage analysis techniques include the cystic fibrosis gene[46,47], the Huntington's disease gene[48], and the first breast cancer gene[49]. The process of finding a gene is graphically represented in Figure 34.11.

APPLICATIONS OF BASIC MOLECULAR GENETICS AND MOLECULAR BIOLOGY TO CLINICAL MEDICINE

Genetic Diseases in PICU Populations

Genetic disease accounted for the primary diagnosis of 11 to 16% of patients admitted to pediatric teaching hospitals in 1978[50]. Estimates of causes of infant mortality in the United States suggest that congenital malformations account for the largest group[51]. Heritable conditions also account for many patients in the ICU population. Cunniff and colleagues[52] determined that heritable conditions were diagnosed in 19% of patients who died in one pediatric intensive care unit (PICU) over a 5-year period. Of patients determined to have heritable conditions, 16% had chromosomal abnormalities, 33% had a recognized syndrome, 29% had a single defect in development and, 22% had an unrecognized syndrome. In addition, 41% of deaths were erroneously classified on death records, resulting in underestimation, in this study, of the impact of genetic disorders on PICU populations[52]. The term heritable is not defined by the authors but should be defined as a nonlethal genetic change that is passed on to descendants[53]. The figures published by Cunniff[52] may include lethal mutations or disorders of unknown etiology. The authors also indicated that asthma, epilepsy, and diabetes were not considered heritable, despite the existing body of knowledge that shows clearly inherited forms or components of these disorders. This is a second way that the study underestimated the impact of heritable, or genetic, disorders on the PICU population. It may seem reasonable to assume that unless a disorder is acquired, such as injury or acute infection, all sick patients have an inherited disorder. Nevertheless, Cunniff[52] showed that genetic disorders contribute significantly to mortality in pediatric patients, readmissions to intensive care units, and health care costs.

Diagnosis

The techniques of molecular genetics can be used to diagnose many conditions. For example, in an effort to identify a specific infectious agent, the gold standard is culturing of microorganisms. However, results are sometimes not available for days, and false negatives are possible, especially in the cases of viruses or fastidious bacteria. Two principal molecular techniques used in the detection of microorganisms are nucleic acid hybridization and DNA amplification using PCR. Nucleic acid hybridization is the binding of a probe to a target specimen of DNA (Figure 34.9). The probe, in this case, is a short segment of DNA usually labeled with a detectable substance, such as a radioisotope or a fluorescent end. A probe must be specific for sequences in the genome of the microbe and must not bind to host DNA. The bound products are transferred to a membrane after gel electrophoresis and may then be detected by autoradiography or other detection systems. This technique of probing is called Southern blotting (Northern blotting if RNA is being detected, or Western blotting if an antibody probe is used to detect protein). Both blotting techniques and PCR have been used successfully to identify viruses from heart muscle in cases of myocarditis and cardiomyopathies[54–56]. Kandolf and colleagues[57] found that in 24% of patients with clinically suspected acute myocarditis, enteroviral RNA was present in endomyocardial biopsy samples. Hyypiä and associates[58] developed a set of primers and probes that can be used to identify and discriminate between enteroviruses and rhinoviruses.

PCR is a sensitive technique, requiring only minute amounts of template (i.e., DNA) from almost any type of sample. Nearly 100 organisms have been detected by PCR. This technology is extremely helpful when there are too few organisms present to be detected by other means. An example is *Borrelia burgdorferi*, the organism causing Lyme disease, in which the range of symptoms and the limited diagnostic methods available often delay diagnosis[59]. Cinque and colleagues[60] used PCR to detect the presence of viruses other than HIV in the cerebrospinal fluid (CSF) of patients who died of AIDS; they estimated their detection limits to be 20 cytomegalovirus (CMV) DNA molecules, 4 Epstein-Barr virus (EBV) DNA molecules and 10 Jacob Creutzfeld virus (JCV) DNA molecules. Others have found the limit of detection of HIV molecules to be 10 per μg of human DNA (i.e., one HIV DNA molecule in 100,000 to 150,000 mononuclear cells)[61,62]. HIV proviral DNA can be detected by PCR in peripheral mononuclear cells of persons with disparate enzyme-linked immunosorbent assay (ELISA) and Western blot results[63], and HIV infection positivity has been diagnosed in antigen-negative individuals[64–66]. The use of PCR for detection of bacterial DNA is also possible but is not as routinely used as viral diagnostics because of possible false-positive results. Nevertheless, the sensitivity of the technique resulted in the early detection of *Neisseria* meningitidis in a patient who had meningitis and whose Gram's stain results and CSF culture results were negative despite marked purulence and positive results on blood culture[67]. This technique, which can be completed in 2 to 4 hours, could be an ideal solution to the problem of microbial diagnosis in patients pretreated with antibiotics. PCR is also useful for detecting drug resistance. The genetic basis of malaria resistance to pyrimethamine is defined by a specific mutation in the dihydrofolate reductase gene, which can be identified by PCR[68]. This information can be available to clinicians within hours because culturing is not necessary. Useful to the study of epidemics, PCR can be used to determine serotypes and track movement of infectious agents worldwide. In 1994, a dengue fever epidemic occurred in Nicaragua. Patients in Panama and in Nicaragua were identified by genetic typing

Table 34.7. Existing PCR Systems for Enteric Pathogens

Campylobacter sp.
Entamoeba histolytica
Enteric adenovirus
Enterohemorrhagic *E. coli*
Enteroinvasive *E. coli/shigella* sp.
Enterotoxigenic *E. coli*
Helicobacter pylori
Listeria monocytogenes
Norwalk virus
Rotavirus
Salmonella sp.
Staphylococcus aureus sp.
Vibrio cholera O1
Yersinia sp.

E. coli = Escherichia coli. *List adapted from Ecchevaria P, Sethabutr O, Serichantalergs O. Modern diagnosis (with molecular tests) of acute infectious diarrhea. Gastroenterology Clin N Am 1993;87:682.*

to have the same serotype that caused an epidemic in India and Sri Lanka from 1989 to 1992[69].

The sensitivity of PCR can lead to false-positive results, a drawback when used for microbial diagnosis; minute amounts of DNA present in the laboratory from other samples can contaminate equipment, reagents, or specimens. The scale of the problem is well-illustrated by the following: One drop of product from a PCR test mixed with the volume of water in an Olympic-sized swimming pool may be reamplified during a subsequent PCR test and yield a false-positive result[70]. Also, PCR detects the presence of nonviable organisms, which may result in identification of an organism successfully eradicated with therapy or one that is not the cause of infection. Problems of contamination should be preventable with strict adherence to careful laboratory technique[71] or at least detectable if negative controls are run with every assay. PCR sensitivity requires proper sample preparation, which may be time-consuming, depending on the source of the DNA or RNA. Reagent assembly is also time-consuming, unless kits are purchased. Commercially available PCR kits (containing pre-packaged reagents) increase the ease of PCR testing and minimize preparation time, but they also add to cost. Because of the risks of false-positive results and ongoing development of kits, PCR is not yet routinely used for bacterial diagnostics. PCR kits for *Legionella* and *Chlamydia* species and HIV are commercially available, and PCR systems have been developed for the enteric pathogens listed in **Table 34.7.**

In addition to microbiologic applications, PCR has been used in many investigations, from forensics, linkage studies, or gene mapping to determination of human evolutionary patterns. Specimens have been taken from archival (fixed pathology) specimens[72,73], hairs[74], and ancient mummies[75,76]. Oncology is another field for application of PCR technology. Although the chromosomal characteristics of leukemias can be defined by probing techniques, PCR detection is faster and simpler and sensitive even if only few residual cells are present after therapy[77–79]. PCR is a highly automatable technique, leading to faster, more cost-effective diagnostics. Developments in PCR technology that uses fluorescently labeled oligonucleotides are accelerating the automation process. Fluorescent labels are advantageous in many ways; they are nontoxic, stable, may be stored for years, and allow multiple samples to be run concurrently because the labels show up as different colors. In addition, Schwengel and colleagues[80] reported the detection of fluorescently labeled products to be as accurate or more accurate than standard autoradiographic techniques.

Gene Therapy

Somatic Gene Therapy

The introduction of a normal recombinant gene (one that has been re-engineered to replace disease-producing mutations with normal segments of DNA) into cells of a person who has inherited a specific mutant gene is theoretically curative. Candidates for such interventions are patients with single-gene disorders, such as inborn errors of metabolism. The normal gene is preferably placed into the cells of the affected organ system, such as the hematopoietic system in diseases like thalassemia or sickle cell anemia. Since the targeted tissues are only those needed to achieve normal or near-normal function, the rest of the body continues to carry the abnormal DNA with which the patient was born. The germline is not affected, and, therefore, the risk of disease transmission to succeeding generations is not changed. (Germline gene therapy is discussed later in this chapter.)

Virtually any gene can be transferred into another cell, which will then express the normal gene product. The first successful *in vitro* correction of an enzymatic deficiency was in cells of persons with Lesch-Nyhan syndrome. Treated cells, grown in culture, were able to produce hypoxanthine phosphoribosyltransferase, which is absent in cells of patients with the syndrome[81,82]. Numerous other gene products have subsequently been successfully produced after gene transfer *in vitro.*

There are a variety of gene transfer procedures, most of which are inefficient and not practical for use *in vivo.* Successful gene therapy *in vivo* requires transfer of the DNA into the host cell and then both transcription (DNA copied onto mRNA) and translation (mRNA translated into a protein). In addition, it may be important that the transferred gene is only expressed in certain tissues or that the regulation of expression is normal. Viral vectors for gene transfer are the most promising vehicles for gene therapy *in vivo.* Either DNA or RNA viruses may be used. DNA viruses which have shown the most promise are the adenoviruses and the parvoviruses[83]. Failure to incorporate the vector's genome into the host cell sometimes occurs because of the obstacles shown in Figure 34.12.

The retroviruses are RNA viruses that infect cells by injecting their RNA genome into the host[84,85]. The genetic information is then incorporated into the host cell and reverse transcriptase copies it into DNA. The DNA enters the cell nucleus and is incorporated into the chromosomal DNA of the host. This is a highly efficient process, and the ret-

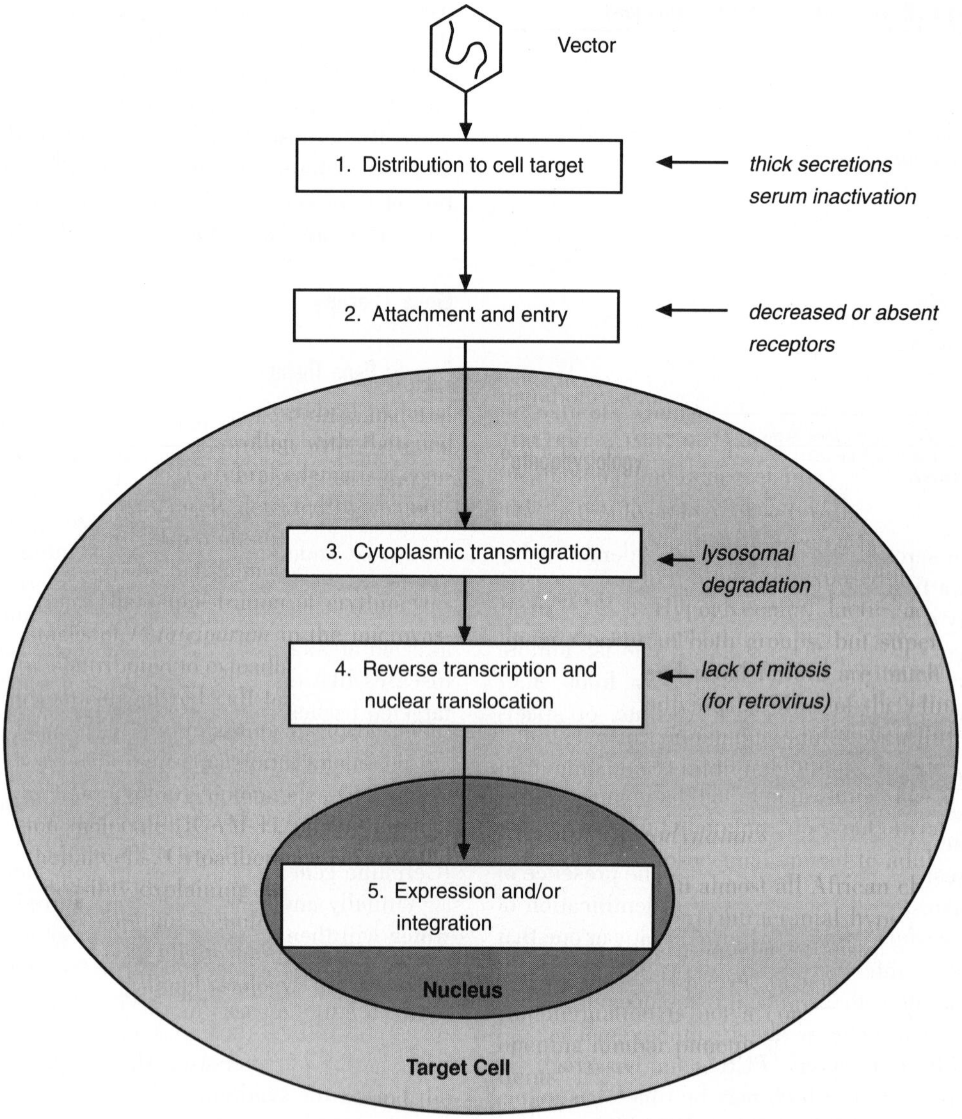

Figure 34.12. Steps and obstacles involved in delivery of vector DNA to host cell. Obstacles are designated by arrows next to delivery steps. Reproduced with permission from Afione SA, Conrad CK, Flotte TR. Gene therapy vectors as drug delivery systems. Clin Pharmacokinet 1995;28:181.

roviruses have little tissue specificity[84]. Retroviruses are preferred over other viruses because human genes can be inserted into the retroviral genome, creating a chimeric genome that can be efficiently integrated into the genome of the host[86,87]. These retroviruses can be engineered to contain corrective human genes while lacking the genetic material that codes for malignant or viral transformation[88,89]. These are two advantages of using retroviruses rather than DNA viruses in gene therapy.

There are some potential dangers in the use of retroviruses, however. First, disease-producing viruses may be created if the therapeutic retrovirus recombines with an endogenous virus[90]. Second, recombination may occur with proto-oncogenes, activating their malignant potential[91]. Third, the retrovirus could integrate into the middle of a functioning host gene, which may then be inactivated or made dysfunctional by insertional mutagenesis[92]. Another problem of gene therapy *in vivo* is that transgene expression generally does not last more than 3 weeks[93], possibly because of vector degradation by T lymphocytes, since subsequent exposures lead to antibody-mediated reduction in gene expression[94]. Nevertheless, transient expression may prove sufficient to achieve the desired effect in certain applications, such as prevention of arterial restenosis[95].

Methods for extending gene therapy to animals or humans are still under investigation, but several approaches are available. Cells from bone marrow, fibroblasts, skin, liver, or pancreas may be transformed in culture and then transplanted into live hosts. Alternatively, whole hosts may be infected with the recombinant viral vector, or specific systems may be targeted. Nabel and associates[96] established the feasibility of using catheter techniques to transfer foreign DNA to the arterial wall[96,97]. Subsequent animal experiments confirmed that gene transfer may

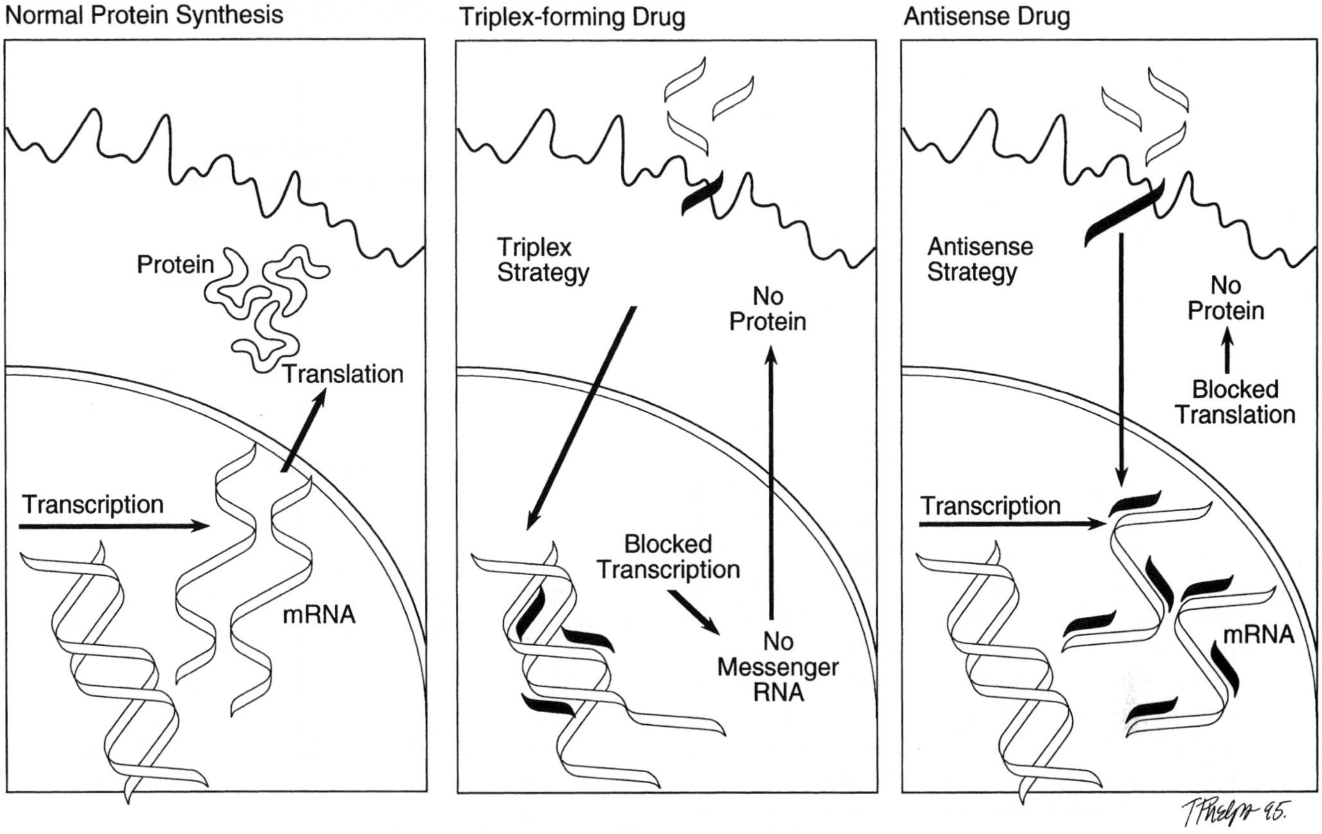

Figure 34.13. Mechanisms by which triplex and antisense drugs block protein production.

successfully be applied to atherosclerotic arteries[98] and achieve therapeutic effects[99]. A 1995 report[100] also describes the use of the retinoblastoma gene (whose product inhibits cell cycle progression) applied via adenovirus vector to arterial walls in several animals. The authors report successful regulation of smooth-muscle cell proliferation after injury and suggest not only a possible form of gene therapy but draw comparisons between molecular mechanisms of vascular repair and carcinogenesis[100].

The following experimental steps are prerequisites for human gene therapy trials: Identification of a disease-causing gene; creation of a transgenic animal model to prove that the gene in question indeed causes the disease; and use of gene therapy in an animal model to successfully treat the disease[101].

Germline Therapy

Germline therapy is meant to change the DNA of sperm, ova, or early-stage embryos, thus changing the DNA of all of the host's cells and also that of progeny. Several descriptions of techniques for germline changes have been published. DNA sequences have been injected into one-cell fertilized eggs of laboratory animals and have achieved successful integration of up to 30%[102,103]. Transgenic mice have been created by microinjection or retroviral infection of embryos at the one-cell to eight-cell stage[104–107]. In one experiment, sperm treated with exogenous DNA successfully integrated with the new sequences[108]. Limitations for use of these techniques in humans are the difficulty of diagnosis of a genetic defect at the embryonic stage and the possibility of insertional mutagenesis of normal genes causing developmental malformations[109,110]. In addition, sociological and ethical issues in germline therapy are complicated.

Genetic Medicines

Researchers are attempting to design new drugs that bind to nucleic acids and alter protein production of a targeted normal gene, as opposed to gene therapy, which aims to permanently reconfigure an abnormal gene. DNA or RNA may be selected as new drugs used to alter protein synthesis in two ways: First, as a triplex agent that selectively inhibits transcription of a gene; second, as an antisense strategy that impedes translation (Figure 34.13)[111]. Because the new drugs will be short segments of DNA or RNA, they will be unique sequences of nucleotides able to bind only with a complementary nucleotide sequence. The nucleotide segment, or oligomer, will have absolute specificity to the gene targeted for decreased protein production. Since the oligomer is not a complete gene sequence, it cannot code for protein itself.

Early laboratory experiments with these new drugs have been successful and shown no signs of toxicity[111]. Trials are underway using oligomers to prevent replication of the human papillomavirus and HIV[111]. Antisense therapies have been successful for treating Kaposi's sarcoma[112] in laboratory animals and in blocking heart allograft rejection in mice(113). Liu and associates(114) have used a c-*fos* antisense oligomer to disrupt expression of the c-*fos* gene in the brain. This gene may be induced by ischemia and may be a proto-oncogene. It is an early response gene that, when induced, results in a cascade of cellular activity. This work on blocking expression of the c-*fos* gene may help foster the genetic study of both the normal and the ischemic brain.

Genetic Regulation

Oxygen as a Gene Regulator

Regulation of gene expression is a complicated process that occurs by means of the interaction among regulatory sequences within gene exons (coding sequences) or introns (noncoding sequences) and the multiple substances that influence either DNA replication or protein production. Many genes are likely to be regulated by oxygen. Hypoxia increases the expression of erythropoietin (EPO) mRNA, and the oxygen sensor for the regulation of EPO production is a heme protein. When oxygen tension falls, the heme protein is in the reduced conformation, which triggers increased expression of the EPO gene(115). Another gene inducible by hypoxia is the tyrosine hydroxylase (TH) gene in the carotid body. In a demonstration of increased TH mRNA after hypoxia, Millhorn and colleagues(116) showed that a reduction in oxygen tension rather than hemoglobin desaturation is the effective stimulus. In addition, hypercapnia did not result in increased TH gene expression(116). Hyperoxia is also a regulator of gene function, but increases expression of genes such as those coding for enzymes that protect cells from free radical damage. Little is known about the effects of hypoxia or hyperoxia on pulmonary endothelial-cell gene expression. Certain oxygen-regulated genes are turned on or off at birth. Which genes these are and what effect premature birth has on them has yet to be described. Mechanisms of lung repair during hypoxia or hyperoxia should be explored. An area rich for research is the role of oxygen therapy on gene expression and lung repair in patients with bronchopulmonary dysplasia (BPD) or adult respiratory distress syndrome (ARDS)(117).

In various states of oxidant stress (referring to the presence of reactive oxygen species), characteristic patterns of cellular and DNA damage are seen. Such lesions include DNA breaks and chromosomal aberrations(118) and have been associated with mutation and malignant transformation in experiments(119,120) (Figure 34.14). Neutrophils in patients with chronic granulomatous disease (deficient NADPH oxidase/0_2 synthetase) have decreased mutagenic capability compared with neutrophils of healthy persons(121). Free-radical scavengers may inhibit oxyradical nucleic acid damage. Superoxide dismutase (SOD) is a metalloprotein that exists to detoxify superoxides. SOD has been shown to protect against pulmonary oxygen toxicity from toxic oxygen species in mouse models(122,123). As a result, induction of genes coding for (or exogenous administration of) SOD or glutathione peroxidase may become available therapies for disorders such as ARDS. Exogenous administration may be less successful because SOD may not reach the microenvironment where the damage has been (or is being) done. Induction of the MnSOD (manganese SOD) gene has been accomplished by tracheal instillation of interleukin-1 (IL-1) in rats(124). Other sources of oxyradical production may be amenable to intervention: for example, prostaglandins titrate levels of neutrophil activation; allopurinol inhibits xanthine oxidase; arachidonic acid metabolism is potentially controllable at many different pathway points. Strategies of dealing with the generation of oxyradicals are likely to be less successful(125).

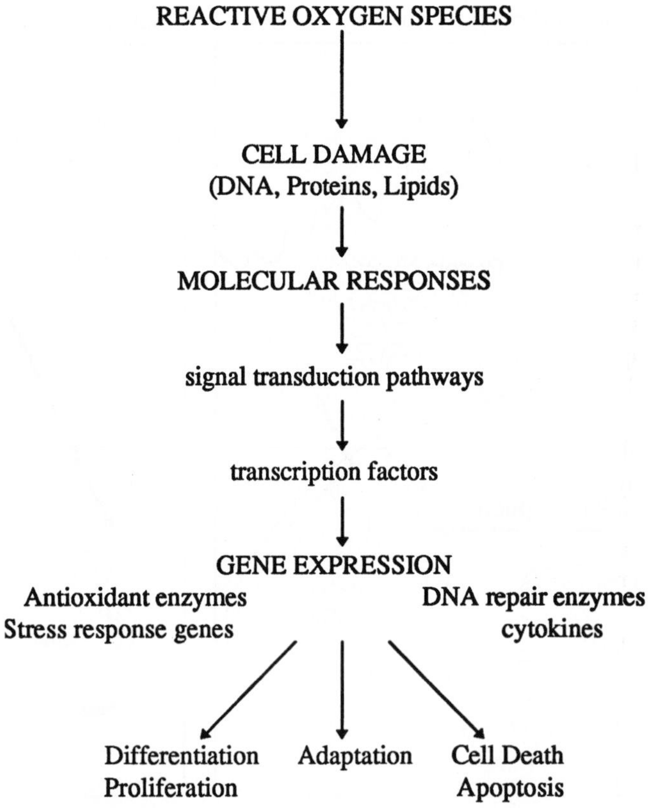

Figure 34.14. Reactive oxygen species and gene expression. Reproduced with permission from Camhi SL, Lee P, Choi AMK. The oxidative stress response. New Horizons 1995;3:170.

Other interesting mechanisms of altering gene expression pertaining to the heart have been studied. There is evidence that pressure overload changes expression of genes coding for the contractile apparatus. Quantitative changes resulting in increased tissue mass lead to hypertrophy, but qualitative changes also occur. In rodent models, adult myocin heavy-chain gene expression is suppressed and fetal myocin heavy-chain gene expression is turned on(126,127). Reexpression of fetal phenotypes in the heart and other tissues (e.g., liver, bone marrow) may reflect a common consequence of growth signals in states of regeneration. As Parker states: "Thus, fetal gene expression in cardiac hypertrophy may simply reflect common regulatory pathways for growth, rather than adaptation, and experimentally serves as a useful end-point for the study of trophic signalling"[128].

Cellular Stress Responses

Intensivists are accustomed to dealing with stress response on the level of the whole organism, but every cell has a repertoire of four different responses to stress: heat-shock response, oxidative stress response, ultraviolet stress response, and the acute-phase response[129]. These four stressors can be damaging to DNA and protein. The stress responses are characterized by changes in gene expression that overlap each other, because few stress-activated transcription factors exist and a particular cell cannot execute all of the stress responses simultaneously[130]. Cells primed by a first, relatively minor, stress become resistant to a second stress that is more severe[131,132]. This phenomenon is called stress tolerance and has been correlated with the expression of heat-shock proteins[133].

Sepsis

Hemodynamic derangements during sepsis are mediated by the effects of endotoxin, TNF, IL-1 and other mediators[134,135]. Stress induces heat-shock protein-70 (HSP-70) mRNA. The major role of HSP-70 is preventing premature folding and denaturation of damaged protein. It also acts as a chaperone in other protein-protein interactions. *In vitro* data support protection of cells from lysis by TNF as a result of the presence of heat shock proteins[136–138]. It is possible that down-regulation of heat-shock protein expression and synthesis is a major factor in the high rate of mortality associated with sepsis[139,140]. Heat-shock proteins can be induced by treatment with heat[141] or a variety of different chemical agents[142]. Some clinically relevant inducers of the heat-shock response are shown in **Table 34. 8.** If fever is a hyperthemic stress[143], then induction of heat-shock proteins may be a mechanism by which fever brings about beneficial effects and clinical use of antipyretics may be disadvantageous to patients with early sepsis. It may also be possible to pharmacologically induce heat-shock protein expression to modulate the inflammatory process[144]. Studies of endotoxemia in rats have shown increased survival after induction of heat-stress proteins by either thermal or chemical means[141,145]. Endotoxin exposure increases expression of genes, including the MnSOD gene[146], prostaglandin G/H synthase, which generates prostanoids[147,148]. Generation of TNF is also increased in response to endotoxin[149,150]. TNF gene expression can be increased by γ-interferon or decreased by corticosteroids, pentoxifylline, amrinone, cyclosporine A and other agents[151]. Polymorphisms in the TNFα-promoter region, which is close to the human leukocyte antigen (HLA) loci, may explain why some haplotypes are associated with a high rate of TNF production and others with a low rate of production[152].

Table 34.8. Inducers of Heat Shock Response

Type of Stress	*Agent*
Environmental	Temperature
	Heavy metals
	Ethanol
	Oxygen free radicals
	Oxygen peroxide
Metabolic	Glucose starvation
	Tunicamycin
	Calcium ionophores
	Amino acid analogs
Clinical	Ischemia/reperfusion
	Shock
	Anoxia
Pathogenic	Endotoxin[a]
	Viruses
	Bacteria

[a]*Only in enterocytes. Adapted from De Maio A. The heat shock response. New Horizons 1995;3:200.*

Disorders such as the systemic inflammatory response syndrome (SIRS) and multiple organ dysfunctions syndrome (MODS) are truly disorders for which the ICU is meant. Etiologic investigations have led intensivists to consider these disorders exaggerations of normal host-defense systems[153]. Do these disorders arise because of a redundancy of inflammatory mediators or because of abnormal intracellular signal-processing that results in pathologically sustained inflammatory mediator release[101]? TNFα, a cytokine known to have beneficial effects, is also a mediator of shock and MODS[154–156]. The human TNFα gene is located on the short arm of chromosome 6. Its 3′ region is known to contain polymorphisms[157], which exist in or near promoter regions of the gene, that have not yet led to proof of predilection for disease. However, Han and Beutler[158] reported that a sequence of the TNFα 3′ region causes a decrease in translational efficiency of the gene, which is overcome when stimulated with lipopolysaccharide[158,159]. Such findings suggest that polymorphisms in TNFα genes may be associated with TNFα-mediated diseases.

Genetics in Industry and Clinical Medicine

Industrial applications of recombinant technologies have allowed large-scale production of proteins that are otherwise in short supply because the only available sources are human beings or animals. Animal sources sometimes result in drugs with allergic potential to human patients, and some animal proteins, such as animal-derived growth hormones, are ineffective in humans. Proteins from animal or human sources are also potential infection risks to recipients and are usually much more expensive than recombinant proteins. Recombinant systems may use bacteria, yeast, cultured insect cells, or mammalian cells. The first licensed recombinant drug was human insulin[160]. Subsequently, the human growth hormone, tissue plasminogen activator, erythropoietin, monoclonal antibodies, and a hepatitis B virus vaccine have been engineered by such systems **(Table 34.9)**[161]. Recombinant apolipoprotein A-I Milano, which has shown therapeutic potential in decreasing arterial plaque in rabbits, may be available for human applications in the future[162].

Table 34.9. A Partial List of Biologic Agents Approved by the U.S. Foot and Drug Administration, 1993–1995

Agent	*Indication*
Alpha interferons	Hairy-cell leukemia
	Kaposi's sarcoma
	Genital warts
	Non-A, non-B hepatitis
Beta interferon	Multiple sclerosis
Chicken pox vaccine	Prevention of chicken pox
DNase	Secretion management in cystic fibrosis
Erythropoietin	Anemia of chronic renal failure
	Anemia of AIDS
Factor VIII	Hemophilia A
Gamma interferon	Chronic granulomatous disease
Granulocyte colony-stimulating factor	Chemotherapy-induced granulocytopenia
Hepatitis A virus vaccine	Prevention of hepatitis A
Hepatitis B virus vaccine	Prevention of hepatitis B
Human growth hormone	Growth hormone deficiency
Human insulin	Diabetes mellitus
Indium-labeled murine monoclonal antibody	Detection of colon cancer
Interleukin-2	Renal cell carcinoma
OKT3	Acute renal allograft rejection
Tissue plasminogen activator (TPA)	Acute myocardial infarction

ETHICS

Much has been written about the ethical use of genetic technologies and therapies. Debates are fueled by the press, films, television, and literary works (such as Huxley's *Brave New World*[163]). Conscientious scientists and physicians anticipate the potential conflicts that might arise from the introduction of new drugs or methods. Such debates were stirred when growth hormone was produced with recombinant-DNA technology. The increased supply of this drug raised the question of who is entitled to treatment with growth hormone: Should it be offered to children who do not have disease but may be of short stature when this would be a handicap in the eyes of the parents? There is no reason to believe that height is an index of happiness[164].

The ethics debate regarding human genetic manipulation is much more complex than the growth hormone debate. It is also much more emotionally charged, because it involves topics such as abortion and eugenics. The ethical debates regarding genetics can be divided into the following six issues:

1. Identification of disease-causing genes and persons at risk. Comparatively little debate arises about the identification of genes that cause disease. However, identification of persons at risk can make those persons uninsurable. In addition, not everyone wants to know about their level of risk.
2. Somatic gene therapies that may result in an altered germline. Most somatic gene therapies target disease states, which is considered an ethical application of these therapies. A small possibility of altering the germline may exist in some of these applications[103]. Experiments with animals have resulted in insertional mutagenesis whereby introduction of a normal DNA segment has disrupted native gene function and caused death or cancer in the progeny[165,166]. However, in a successful application of germline therapy, the future offspring would benefit by prenatal repair of the disease-producing gene mutation.
3. Consent cannot be obtained from persons for treatment with germline therapies. In medical practice, patients commonly give implied or explicit consent for therapies or procedures. Hence, some would find the concept of germline therapy to be unethical because of lack of consent by offspring. However, parents are legally given the right to provide proxy consent for treatment of their offspring. It is assumed (not always correctly) that, in conceiving, bearing, and raising children, parents have considered the best interests of their children.
4. Identification of the "abnormal" embryo may lead to abortion. The abortion question continues to be sociologically unresolved. Those opposing abortion are against it in any or almost any case. The proponents of choice on the abortion issue may find genetic reasons for termination acceptable. However, even to those willing to consider abortion, the definition of what constitutes abnormality varies among people and may also vary over time. Technologically, the selection of healthy embryos (as is done in the case of *in vitro* fertilization) will be simpler than any attempt to perform germline therapy.
5. Alteration of the germline for the improvement of offspring. This issue has perhaps the most vehement opposition because of the "slippery-slope" argument and the risks of practicing eugenics. What prevents the unethical application of technology in such a way as abused by Hitler? Is it acceptable to "play God" and engineer a superhuman race? Even if the technology is acceptable for use in patients with pathologic states, how do we define pathology?

As Rifkin states: "Once we decide to begin the process of human genetic engineering, there is really no logical place to stop. If diabetes, sickle cell anemia, and cancer are to be cured by altering the genetic makeup of an individual, why not proceed to other disorders, myopia, color blindness, left handedness? Indeed, what is to preclude a society from deciding that a certain skin color is a disorder[167]?"

Ledley writes: "To avoid even accidental usurpation of genetic technologies for eugenic purposes, each application of genetics to medicine must clearly identify an individual whose affliction is the target of therapy, specific individual liberties which are reinforced by each genetic intervention, and evidence that the assent of the individual has been obtained[168]."

Berger adds: "A second major concern is that 'eliminating so-called bad genes will lead to a dangerous narrowing of the diversity in the gene pool' and attempts to cleanse the germline over tens or hundreds of years will lose traits that we later realize are important[169]."

Danks warns: "It requires an extraordinary combination of arrogance and ignorance to propose that we will soon understand these matters well enough to indulge in genetic manipulation to 'improve the human race'[(170)]."

6. How will the human genome project and recombinant technologies affect the cost and distribution of health care resources? In the current climate of health care reengineering we are reminded daily about limitations in resources. Yet, if a drug or technology exists to treat a disorder, society believes that everyone has equal rights to health and should have access to necessary treatments. Genetic technologies are expensive, but sometimes early diagnosis and early intervention can be cost-saving.

SUMMARY

Genetic technologies are becoming widely used; therefore, it is only a matter of time before clinicians will feel compelled to study this science as it affects their practice of medicine. The intensive care unit is uniquely suited to applying some of the biotechnologies discussed in this text. Critically ill patients may be recipients of genetic medicines or gene therapies to treat either acquired acute illnesses or inherited disorders. Critical illness may be a good target for gene therapy because of the high rate of mortality and need for only transient treatment. In addition, future study may elucidate the causes of such disorders as ARDS, MODS, BPD, and retinopathy of prematurity. We may be able to predict who will die with exposure to endotoxin and define how gene expression can be changed to result in treatment of a disorder. All of these changes should be accomplished during the age of shrinking health care dollars. Ironically, the high initial cost of biotechnologies may result in lower long-term cost because of improved efficiency, earlier diagnosis, and more effective treatment. Societies must also continue to struggle with the ethical application of new capabilities in diagnosis or treatment.

Glossary

allele One of two or more alternate forms of a gene at one particular chromosomal location (locus).
aneuploidy An abnormal chromosomal number (e.g., monosomy, trisomy).
annealing The portion of the polymerase chain reaction (PCR) process during which relative cooling allows binding of primers to the complimentary DNA template.
anticipation The appearance of a disease in successive generations at earlier ages and with increasing severity, caused by the phenomenon of trinucleotide expansion.
base pair Two nitrogenous bases that pair to form a double-stranded DNA or RNA molecule.
cDNA Complementary DNA is DNA synthesized from an RNA template using the enzyme reverse transcriptase.
centromere The site of attachment of chromosomes to reproductive spindles. The location of the centromere determines the shape of the chromosome.
chimera A mosaic individual organism that has mutated or has been grafted to contain two or more forms of DNA sequence. Chimeric DNA is a recombinant DNA molecule containing sequences from more than one organism.
chromosome A single DNA molecule containing numerous genes.
clone A population of cells or organisms derived from a single parent cell or organism by the process of mitosis.
codon A triplet of DNA or RNA nucleotides that forms the blueprint of a single amino acid or signals the start or stop of the genetic message is complementary to codon.
cytogenetics The study of genetics in the context of cytology, which involves the structure and behavior of chromosomes.
disomic Having two homologous (identical) chromosomes; said of an individual organism or cell.
DNA Deoxyribonucleic acid.
eugenics The improvement of the human species by selective breeding or selective alteration of the germline to enhance a positive gene or negate a deleterious gene; referred to, respectively, as positive and negative eugenics.
exon The segment of a gene that is transcribed and translated into protein.
3′ end The downstream portion of a gene, which contains stop sequences and regulatory regions.
5′ end The upstream end of a gene, which contains starting sequences, promoters, and regulators.
gene The basic unit of inheritance, which is a segment of DNA coding for a protein or RNA, or which may not be transcribed itself but which regulates transcription of other genes.
genetic code The total of 64 DNA triplets, each of which is the blueprint for one of 20 amino acid or start or stop signals. Each amino acid is coded for by 2 to 4 codons.
genetic analysis The resolution of the genetic material into its component parts.
genome The entire complement of hereditary factors (i.e., genes, chromosomes).
genotype The particular genetic or allelic constitution of an individual or organism.
germline Genetic material ancestral to the gametes (i.e., primordial oocytes and spermatozoa).
haploid Having a single set of unpaired chromosomes.
haplotype The set of alleles from closely linked loci that are carried by an individual organism.
imprinting Different expression of the same gene depending on the parent of origin.
***in situ* hybridization** The localization of a DNA sequence; achieved by binding with a nucleic acid probe.
intron A genetic sequence interposed between exons that does not code for amino acids.
karyotype An individual organism's DNA chromosomal complement defined by number and morphology as it exists during metaphase.
linkage The tendency of certain genes to be inherited together when they are neighbors on a chromosome.
locus (pl. loci) The location on a chromosome of a gene or marker.
map A diagram or representation of the relative locations of genes and their estimated distances from each other on a particular chromosome.
marker A polymorphic segment of DNA sequence having a known chromosomal location, which can be used to determine an individual's genotype.
molecular biology A branch of biology in which biological processes are studied at the level of interactions of molecules.
mRNA Messenger RNA; the RNA molecule onto which DNA is copied. mRNA moves the transcript from the nucleus to the cytoplasm, where translation occurs.
mutation 1) The process of changing a gene (verb). 2) heritable alteration of a gene (noun).
nucleotide Any of the purine or pyrimidine building blocks of DNA.
oligonucleotide Any short (about 20 nucleotides) segment of DNA, which can be used as a probe or primer for *in situ* hybridization or PCR.
oncogene Genes whose products have the ability to trans-

form eukaryotic cells so that they grow in a manner analogous to tumor cells.
p Designates the short arm of a chromosome.
penetrance The frequency with which a genotype manifests itself in the phenotype of the carriers.
phenotype The observable expression of a genotype.
polymerase An enzyme which catalyzes the replication of DNA.
polymerase chain reaction (PCR) A technique for *in vitro* DNA amplification.
polymorphism The regular occurrence of two or more alleles at a given locus in a single population.
primer A short DNA or RNA sequence used to initiate DNA synthesis.
probe A defined DNA or RNA sequence used to bind to (and therefore detect) complementary sequences of study DNA.
promoter A DNA sequence that directs transcription of genes.
proto-oncogene A normal gene that can combine with the product of an oncogene to induce malignant activity.
q Designates the long arm of a chromosome.
recombinant DNA A novel DNA sequence formed by *in vitro* combination of two different DNA molecules.
recombination A normal process of genetic information exchange that occurs during meiosis between homologous DNA strands.
reverse transcriptase An RNA-directed DNA polymerase by which cDNA may be obtained.
RNA Ribonucleic acid.
rRNA Ribosomal RNA; the RNA molecules that are the structural subunits of the ribosomes.
sequence The order and exact content of nucleotides in a DNA or RNA molecule.
stop sequences Those nucleotides that signal the end of transcription (i.e., UAA, UAG, UGA).
telomere The terminal segment of a chromosome.
transcription The process of copying DNA onto mRNA, the first step in production of a protein molecule.
transgenic Containing a foreign gene, said of an organism or cell changed by means of gene transfer. The new genetic information is transferred to successive generations.
translation The second step in protein production, in which mRNA codes for specific amino acids.
translocation Chromosomal structural change, characterized by the moving of chromosomal segments to an abnormal position.
trisomy The presence of an extra chromosome.
tRNA Transfer RNA; the molecule involved in the translation of mRNA into amino acids.
tumor suppressor gene A gene whose product can suppress cell division or tumorigenesis.

Sources

Klug WS, Cummings MR. Concepts of Genetics. 4th ed. New York: MacMillan, 1994.
Lewin B. Genes V. New York: Oxford University Press, 1994.
Rieger R, Michaelis A, Green MM. Glossary of Genetics. 5th ed. Berlin: Springer-Verlag, 1991.

SUGGESTED READINGS

General Genetics

Klug WS, Cummings MR. Concepts of Genetics. 4th ed. New York: MacMillan, 1994.
Leder P, Clayton DA, Rubenstein E. Introduction to Molecular Medicine. New York: Scientific American, 1994.
Lewin B. Genes V. New York: Oxford University Press, 1994.
Watson JD, Gilman M, Witkowski J, Zoller M. Recombinant DNA. 2nd ed. New York: Scientific American, 1992.

Apoptosis and the Cell Cycle

Hartwell LH, Kastan MB. Cell cycle control and cancer. Science 1994;266:1821-1828.
James TN. Normal and abnormal consequences of apoptosis in the human heart. Circ 1994;90:556-573.
Thompson CB. Apoptosis in the pathogenesis and treatment of disease. Science 1995;267:1456-1462.

Clinical Applications

Buchman TG, Zehnbauer BA. Molecular biology in the intensive care unit: a framework for interpretation. New Horizons 1995;3:139-145.
Naber SP. Molecular pathology—diagnosis of infectious disease. N Eng J Med 1994;331:1212-1215.

Regulation of Gene Expression

Camhi SL, Lee P, Choi AMK. The oxidative stress response. New Horizons 1995;3:170-182.
Parker TG. Molecular biology of myocardial hypertrophy and failure: gene expression and trophic signaling. New Horizons 1995;3:288-300.
Ribeiro SP, Villar J, Slutsky AS. Induction of the stress response to prevent organ injury. New Horizons 1995;3:301-311.
Williams G, Giroir BP. Regulation of cytokine gene expression: tumor necrosis factor; interleukin-1; and the emerging biology of cytokine receptors. New Horizons 1995;3:276-287.

Gene Therapy

Afione SA, Conrad CK, Flotte TR. Gene therapy vectors as drug delivery systems. Clin Pharmacokinet 1995;28:181-189.
Ledley FD. Somatic gene therapy for human disease: background and prospects. Part 1. J Pediatr 1987;110:1-8.
Tizzano EF, Buchwald M. Cystic fibrosis: beyond the gene to therapy. J Pediatr 1992;120:337-349.

Triplex and Antisense Therapies

Cohen JS, Hogan ME. The new genetic medicines. Scientific American 1994;271:76-82.

Ethics

Allen DB, Fost NC. Growth hormone therapy for short stature: panacea or Pandora's box? J Pediatr 1990;117:16-21.
Berger EM, Gert BM. Genetic disorders and the ethical status of germ-line gene therapy. J Med Philos 1991;16:667-683.

References

1. Avery OT, MacLeod CM, MacCarty M. Studies on the chemical nature of the substance inducing transformation of pneumococcal types. J Exp Med 1944;79:137–158.
2. Pauling L, Itano HA, Singer SJ, et al. Sickle cell anemia: a molecular disease. Science 1949;110:543–548.
3. Ingram VM. Gene mutations in human hemoglobin: the chemical difference between normal and sickle cell hemoglobin. Nature 1957;180:326–328.
4. Watson JD, Crick FHC. Molecular structure of nucleic acids: a structure for deoxyribose nucleic acid. Nature 1953;171:737–738.
5. Watson JD, Crick FHC. Genetical implications of the structure of deoxyribonucleic acid. Nature 1953;171:964–967.
6. Crick FHC, Barnett CL, Brenner S, et al. General nature of the genetic code for proteins. Nature 1961;192:1227–1232.
7. Nishimura S, Jones DS, Khorana HG. The in vitro synthesis of a copolypeptide containing two amino acids in alternating sequence dependent upon a DNA-like polymer containing two nucleotides in alternating sequence. J Mol Biol 1965;13:302–324.
8. Sanger F, Nicklen S, Coulson AR. DNA sequencing with chain-terminating inhibitors. Proc Natl Acad Sci-USA 1977;74:5463–5467.
9. Maxam AM, Gilbert W. A new method of sequencing DNA. Proc Natl Acad Sci-USA 1977;74:560–564.
10. Saiki RK, Scharf SJ, Faloona F, et al. Enzymatic amplification of beta-globin sequences and restriction site analysis for diagnosis of sickle cell anemia. Science 1985;230:1350–1354.
11. Anderson S, Bankier AT, Barrell BG, et al. Sequence and organization of the mitochondrial genome. Nature 1981;290:457–465.
12. McKusick VA. Mendelian inheritance in man. 11th ed. Baltimore: The Johns Hopkins University Press, 1994;xxiii–xxiv.
13. Knight SJ, Flannery AV, Hirst MC, et al. Trinucleotide repeat amplification and hypermethylation of a CpG island in FRAXE mental retardation. Cell 1993;16:127–134.
14. Brook JD, McCurrach ME, Harley HG, et al. Molecular basis of myotonic dystrophy: expansion of a trinucleotide (CTG) repeat at the 3′ end of a transcript encoding a protein kinase family member. Cell 1992;68:799–808.
15. Harley HG, Rundle SA, MacMillan JC, et al. Size of the unstable CTG repeat sequence in relation to phenotype and parental transmission in myotonic dystrophy. Am J Hum Genet 1993;52:1164–1174.
16. Hollstein M, Sidransky D, Vogelstein B, et al. p53 mutations in human cancers. Science 1991;253:49–53.
17. Brennan JA, Boyle JO, Koch WM, et al. Association between cigarette smoking and mutation of the p53 gene in squamous-cell carcinoma of the head and neck. N Engl J Med 1995;332:712–717.
18. Nicholls RD, Knoll JHM, Butler MG, et al. Genetic imprinting suggested by maternal heterodisomy in nondeletion Prader-Willi syndrome. Nature 1989;342:281–285.
19. Knoll JH, Nicholls RD, Magenis RE, et al. Angelman and Prader-Willi syndromes share a common chromosome 15 deletion but differ in parental origin of the deletion. Am J Med Genet 1989;32:285–290.
20. Williams CA, Zori RT, Stone JW, et al. Maternal origin of 15q11–13 deletions in Angelman Syndrome suggest a role for genomic imprinting. Am J Med Genet 1990;35:350–353.
21. Mulinare J, Cordero JF, Erickson JD, et al. Periconceptual use of multivitamins and the occurrence of neural tube defects. JAMA 1988;260:3141–3145.
22. Milunsky A, Jick H, Jick SS, et al. Multivitamin/folic acid supplementation in early pregnancy reduces the risk of neural tube defects. JAMA 1989;262:2847–2852.
23. Bower C, Stanley FJ. Dietary folate as a risk factor for neural-tube defects: evidence from a case-control study in Western Australia. Med J Aust 1989;150:613–619.
24. Czeizel AE, Dudás I. Prevention of the first occurrence of neural-tube defects by periconceptual vitamin supplementation. N Eng J Med 1992;327:1832–1835.
25. Hutchison CA III, Newbold JE, Potter SS, et al. Maternal inheritance of mammalian mitochondrial DNA. Nature 1974;251:536–538.
26. Fine PEM. Mitochondrial inheritance and disease. Lancet 1978;2: 659–662.
27. Shoffner JM, Wallace DC. Mitochondrial genetics: principles and practice. Am J Hum Genet 1992;51:1179–1186.
28. Wallace DC. Mitochondrial genetics: a paradigm for aging and degenerative diseases? Science 1992;256:628–632.
29. Wallace DC, Lott MT, Shoffner JM, et al. Mitochondrial DNA mutations in epilepsy and neurological disease. Epilepsia 1994;35 Suppl 1:S43–50.
30. Fischel-Ghodsian N, Prezant TR, Bu X, et al. Mitochondrial ribosomal RNA gene mutation in a patient with sporadic aminoglycoside ototoxicity. Am J Otolaryngol 1993;14:399–403.
31. Hu DN, Qui WQ, Wu BT, et al. Genetic aspects of antibiotic induced deafness: mitochondrial inheritance. J Med Genet 1991;28:79–83.
32. Hutchin T, Haworth I, Higashi K, et al. A molecular basis for human hypersensitivity to aminoglycoside antibiotics. Nucleic Acids Res 1993;21:4174–4179.
33. Prezant TR, Agapian JV, Bohlman MC, et al. Mitochondrial ribosomal RNA mutation associated with both antibiotic-induced and non-syndromic deafness. Nature Genet 1993;4:289–294.
34. Vaux DL, Haecker G, Strasser A. An evolutionary perspective on apoptosis. Cell 1994;76:777–779.
35. Thompson CB. Apoptosis in the pathogenesis and treatment of disease. Science 1995;267:1456–1462.
36. Lowe SW, Schmitt EM, Smith SW, et al. p53 is required for radiation-induced apoptosis in mouse thymocytes. Nature 1993;362:847–849.
37. Hockenbery D, Nunez G, Milliman C, et al. Bcl-2 is an inner mitochondrial membrane protein that blocks programmed cell death. Nature 1990;348:334–336.
38. Ohmori T, Podack ER, Nishio K, et al. Apoptosis of lung cancer cells caused by some anti-cancer agents (MMC, CPT-11, ADM) is inhibited by bcl-2. Biochem Biophys Res Commun 1993;192:30–36.
39. Cheng J, Zhou T, Liu C, et al. Protection from Fas-mediated apoptosis by a soluble form of the Fas molecule. Science 1994;263:1759–1762.
40. Clement MV, Stamenkovic I. Fas and tumor necrosis factor receptor-mediated cell death: similarities and distinctions. J Exp Med 1994;180:557–567.
41. Henderson S, Rowe M, Gregory C, et al. Induction of bcl-2 expression by Epstein-Barr virus latent membrane protein 1 protects infected B cells from programmed cell death. Cell 1991;65:1107–1115.
42. Meyaard L, Otto SA, Jonker RR, et al. Programmed death of T cells in HIV-1 infection. Science 1992;257:217–219.
43. Ameisen JC, Capron A. Cell dysfunction and depletion in AIDS: the programmed cell death hypothesis. Immunol Today 1991;12:102–105.
44. Cohen JJ. Apoptosis: the physiologic pathway of cell death. Hosp Pract 1993;28:35–43.
45. James TN. Normal and abnormal consequences of apoptosis in the human heart. Circ 1994;90:556–573.
46. Rommens JM, Iannuzzi MC, Kerem B, et al. Identification of the cystic fibrosis gene: chromosome walking and jumping. Science 1989; 245:1059–1065.
47. Riordan JR, Rommens JM, Kerem B, et al. Identification of the cystic fibrosis gene: cloning and characterization of complementary DNA. Science 1989;245:1066–1073.
48. MacDonald ME, Ambrose CM, Duyao MP, et al. A novel gene containing a trinucleotide repeat that is expanded and unstable on Huntington's disease chromosomes. Cell 1993;72:971–983.
49. Miki Y, Swensen J, Shattuck-Eidens D, et al. A strong candidate for the breast and ovarian cancer susceptibility gene BRCA1. Science 1994;266:66–71.
50. Hall JG, Powers EK, McIlvaine RT, et al. The frequency and financial burden of genetic disease in a pediatric hospital. Am J Med Genet 1978;1:417–436.
51. Sever L, Lynberg MC, Edmonds LD. The impact of congenital malformations on public health. Teratology 1993;48:547–549.
52. Cunniff C, Carmack JL, Kirby RS, et al. Contribution of heritable disorders to mortality in the pediatric intensive care unit. Pediatrics 1995;95:678–681.
53. Rieger R, Michaelis A, Green MM. Glossary of Genetics. 5th ed. Berlin: Springer-Verlag, 1991.
54. Bowles NE, Richardson PJ, Olsen EGJ, et al. Detection of coxsackie-B-virus specific RNA sequences in myocardial biopsy samples from patients with myocarditis and dilated cardiomyopathy. Lancet 1986;1:1120–1123.
55. Jin O, Sole MJ, Butany JW, et al. Detection of enterovirus RNA in myocardial biopsies from patients with myocarditis and cardiomyopathy using gene amplification by polymerase chain reaction. Circulation 1990;82:8–16.
56. Zoll GJ, Melchers WJG, Kopecka H, et al. General primer-mediated polymerase chain reaction for detection of enteroviruses: application for diagnostic routine and persistent infections. J Clin Microbiol 1992;30:160–165.
57. Kandolf R, Klingel K, Mertsching H, et al. Molecular studies on en-

teroviral heart disease: patterns of acute and persistent infections. Eur Heart J 1991;12(Supp D):49–55.
58. Hyypiä T, Auvinen P, Maaronen M. Polymerase chain reaction for human picornaviruses. J Gen Virol 1989;70:3261–3268.
59. Naber SP. Molecular pathology—diagnosis of infectious disease. N Eng J Med 1994;331:1212–1215.
60. Cinque P, Brytting M, Vago L, et al. Diagnosis of virus-associated opportunistic diseases of the central nervous system in patients with HIV infection by polymerase chain reaction on cerebrospinal fluid. Ann NY Acad Sci 1994;724:170–172.
61. Loche M, Mach B. Identification of HIV-infected seronegative individuals by a direct diagnostic test based on hybridization to amplified viral DNA. Lancet 1988;2:418–421.
62. Edwards JR, Ulrich PP, Weintrub PS, et al. Polymerase chain reaction compared with concurrent viral cultures for rapid identification of human immunodeficiency virus infection among high-risk infants and children. J Pediatr 1989;115:200–203.
63. Schochetman G, Ou C-Y, Jones WK. Polymerase chain reaction. J Infect Dis 1988;158:1154–1157.
64. Imagawa DT, Lee MH, Wolinsky SM, et al. Human immunodeficiency virus type I infection in homosexual men who remain seronegative for prolonged periods. N Engl J Med 1989;320:1458–1462.
65. Pezzella M, Rossi P, Lombardi V, et al. HIV viral sequences in seronegative people at risk detected by in situ hybridization and polymerase chain reaction. Br Med J [Clin Res] 1989;298:713–716.
66. Loche M, Mach B. Identification of HIV-infected seronegative individuals by a direct diagnostic test based on hybridization to amplified viral DNA. Lancet 1988;2:418–421.
67. Kristiansen B, Ask E, Jenkins A, et al. Rapid diagnosis of meningococcal meningitis by polymerase chain reaction. Lancet 1991; 337:1568–1569.
68. Wellems TE. Molecular genetics of drug resistance in *Plasmodium falciparum* malaria. Parasitology Today 1991;7:110–112.
69. Centers for Disease Control and Prevention. Dengue Type 3 infection—Nicaragua and Panama, October-November 1994. MMWR 1995;44: 21–24.
70. Wilson SM. Application of nucleic acid-based technologies to the diagnosis and detection of disease. Trans Royal Soc Tropical Med Hygiene 1993;87:609–611.
71. Kwok S, Higuchi R. Avoiding false positives with PCR. Nature 1989;339:237–238.
72. Shibata D, Martin WJ, Arnheim N. Analysis of DNA sequences in forty-year-old paraffin-embedded thin-tissue sections: a bridge between molecular biology and classical histology. Cancer Res 1988;48:4564–4566.
73. Impraim CC, Saiki RK, Erlich HA, et al. Analysis of DNA extracted from formalin-fixed, paraffin-embedded tissues by enzyme amplification and hybridization with sequence-specific oligonucleotides. Biochem Biophys Res Commun 1987;142:710–716.
74. Higuchi R, von Beroldingen CH, Sensabaugh GF, et al. DNA typing from single hairs. Nature 1988;332:543–546.
75. Pääbo S, Giffor JA, Wilson AC. Mitochondrial DNA sequences from a 7000-year-old brain. Nucleic Acids Res 1988;16:9775–9787.
76. Pääbo S. Ancient DNA: extraction, characterization, molecular cloning, and enzymatic amplification. Proc Natl Acad Sci-USA 1989;86:1939–1943.
77. Gunther KE, Cohn RJ, Mendelow BV. Polymerase chain reaction in cancer diagnosis. S Afr Med J 1993;83:514–516.
78. Lee MS, Chang KS, Cabanillas F, et al. Detection of minimal residual cells carrying the t(14:18) by DNA sequence amplification. Science 1987;237:175–178.
79. Lee MS, Chang KS, Freireich EJ, et al. Detection of minimal residual bcr/abl transcripts by a modified polymerase chain reaction. Blood 1988;72:893–897.
80. Schwengel DA, Jedlicka AE, Nanthakumar EJ, et al. Comparison of fluorescence-based semi-automated genotyping of multiple microsatellite loci with autoradiographic techniques. Genomics 1994;23:46–54.
81. Brennand J, Konecki DS, Caskey CT. Expression of human and Chinese hamster hypoxanthine-guanine phosphoribosyl transferase cDNA recombinants in cultured Lesch-Nyhan and Chinese hamster fibroblasts. J Biol Chem 1983;258:9593–9596.
82. Jolly DJ, Okayama H, Berg P, et al. Isolation and characterization of a full length, expressible cDNA for human hypoxanthine phosphoribosyltransferase. Proc Natl Acad Sci-USA 1983;80:477–481.
83. Afione SA, Conrad CK, Flotte TR. Gene therapy vectors as drug delivery systems. Clin Pharmacokinet 1995;28:181–189.
84. Weiss R, Teich N,Varmus H, et al. RNA tumor viruses. Cold Spring Harbor, NY:Cold Spring Harbor Laboratory, 1984.
85. Bishop JM. The molecular biology of RNA tumor viruses: a physician's guide. N Engl J Med 1980;303:675–682.
86. Tabin CJ, Hoffman JN, Goff SP, et al. Adaptation of a retrovirus as a eukaryotic vector transmitting the herpes simplex virus thymidine kinase gene. Mol Cell Biol 1982;2:426–436.
87. Hwang LH, Gilboa E. Expression of genes introduced into cells by retroviral infection is more efficient than that of genes introduced into cells by DNA transfection. J Virol 1984;50:417–424.
88. Mann R, Mulligan RC, Baltimore D. Construction of a retrovirus packaging mutant and its use to produce helper free defective retroviruses. Cell 1983;33:153–159.
89. Cepko CL, Roberts BE, Mulligan RC. Construction and applications of a highly transmissible murine retrovirus shuttle system. Cell 1984;37:1053–1062.
90. Goldfarb MP, Weinberg RA. Generation of novel, biologically active Harvey sarcoma viruses via apparent illegitimate recombination. J Virol 1981;38:136–150.
91. Hayward WS, Neel BG, Astrin SM. Activation of a cellular oncogene by promoter insertion in ALV induced lymphoid leukosis. Nature 1981;290:475–480.
92. King W, Patel MD, Lobel LI, et al. Insertion mutagenesis of embryonal carcinoma cells by retroviruses. Science 1985;228:554–558.
93. Steg PG, Feldman LJ, Scoazec J-Y, et al. Arterial gene transfer to rabbit endothelial and smooth muscle cells using percutaneous delivery of an adenoviral vector. Circulation 1994;90:1648–1656.
94. Kozarsky KF, McKinley DR, Austin LL, et al. In vivo correction of low-density lipoprotein receptor deficiency in the Watanabe heritable hyperlipidemic rabbit recombinant adenoviruses. J Bil Chem 1994;269:13695–13702.
95. Isner JM, Feldman LJ. Gene therapy for arterial disease. Lancet 1994;344:1653–1654.
96. Nabel EG, Plautz G, Boyce DM, et al. Recombinant gene expression in vivo within endothelial cells of the arterial wall. Science 1989;244:1342–1344.
97. Nabel EG, Plautz G, Nabel GJ. Site-specific gene expression in vivo by direct gene transfer into the arterial wall. Science 1990;249:1285–1288.
98. Leclerc G, Gal D, Takeshita S, et al. Percutaneous arterial gene transfer in a rabbit model: efficiency in normal and balloon-dilated atherosclerotic arteries. J Clin Invest 1992;90:936–944.
99. Ohno T, Gordon D, San H, et al. Gene therapy for vascular smooth muscle cell proliferation after arterial injury. Science 1994;265: 781–784.
100. Chang MW, Barr E, Seltzer J, et al. Cytostatic gene therapy for vascular proliferative disorders with a constitutively active form of the retinoblastoma gene product. Science 1995;267:518–522.
101. Buchman TG, Zehnbauer BA. Molecular biology in the intensive care unit: a framework for interpretation. New Horizons 1995;3:139–145.
102. Making mice with designer genes. J NIH Res I 1989:107.
103. Lappé M. Ethical issues in manipulating the human germ line. J Med Philos 1991;16:621–639.
104. Palmiter RD, Brinster RL. Transgenic mice. Cell 1985;41:343–345.
105. Gordon JW, Ruddle FH. Gene transfer into mouse embryos: production of transgenic mice by pronuclear injection. Methods Enzymol 1983;101:411–433.
106. Van der Putten H, Botteri FM, Miller AD, et al. Efficient insertion of genes into mouse germ line via retroviral vectors. Proc Natl Acad Sci-USA 1985;82:6148–6152.
107. Jahner D, Haase K, Mulligan R, et al. Insertion of the bacterial gpt gene into the germ line of mice by retroviral infection. Proc Natl Acad Sci 1985;82:6927–6931.
108. Barinagg M. Making transgenic mice: Is it really that easy? Science 1989;245:590–591.
109. Harbers K, Kuehn M, Delius H, et al. Insertion of retrovirus into the first intron of alpha-1 collagen gene to embryonic lethal mutation in mice. Proc Natl Acad Sci-USA 1984;81:1504–1508.
110. Woychik RP, Stewart TA, Davis LG, et al. An inherited limb deficiency created by insertional mutagenesis in a transgenic mouse. Nature 1985;318:36–40.
111. Cohen JS, Hogan ME. The new genetic medicines. Scientific American 1994;12:76–82.
112. Ensoli B, Markham P, Kao V, et al. Block of AIDS-Kaposi's sarcoma (KS) cell growth, angiogenesis, and lesion formation in nude mice by antisense oligonucleotide targeting basic fibroblast growth factor. J Clin Invest 1994;94:1736–1746.
113. Stepkowski SM, Tu Y, Condon TP, et al. Blocking of heart allograft rejection by intercellular adhesion molecules-1 antisense oligonucleo-

tides alone or in combination with other immunosuppressive modalities. J Immunol 1994;153:5336–5346.
114. Liu PK, Salimen A, He YY, et al. Suppression of ischemia-induced fos expression and AP-1 activity by an antisense oligodeoxynucleotide to *c-fos* mRNA. Ann Neurol 1994;36:566–576.
115. Goldberg MA, Dunning SP, Bunn HF. Regulation of the erythropoietin gene: Evidence that the oxygen sensor is a heme protein. Science 1988;242:1412–1415.
116. Millhorn DE, Czyzyk-Krzeska M, Bayliss DA, et al. Regulation of gene expression by hypoxia. Sleep 1993;16:S44–S48.
117. Fanburg BL, Massaro DJ, Gerutti PA, et al. Regulation of gene expression by O_2 tension. Am J Physiol 1992;262:L235–L241.
118. Spragg RG. DNA strand break formation following exposure of bovine pulmonary artery and aortic endothelial cells to reactive oxygen products. Am J Respir Cell Mol Biol 1991;4:4–10.
119. Cerutti PA. Prooxidant states and tumor promotion. Science 1985;227:375–381.
120. Imlay JA, Linn S. DNA damage and oxygen radical toxicity. Science 1988;240:1302–1309.
121. Weitzman SA, Weitberg AB, Clark EP, et al. Phagocytes as carcinogens: malignant transformation produced by human neutrophils. Science 1985;227:1231–1233.
122. White CW, Avraham KB, Shanley PF, et al. Transgenic mice with expression of elevated levels of copper-zinc superoxide dismutase. J Clin Invest 1991;87:2162–2168.
123. Wispe JR, Warner BB, Clark JC, et al. Human Mn-superoxide dismutase in pulmonary epithelial cells of transgenic mice confers protection from oxygen injury. J Biol Chem 1992;267:23937–23941.
124. White JE, Tsan M-F. Induction of pulmonary Mn superoxide dismutase mRNA by interleukin-1. Lung Cell Mol Physiol 1994;266:L664–L671.
125. Zimmerman JJ. Oxyradical species and their relationship to pathophysiology in pediatric critical care illness. Crit Car Clin 1988;4:645–661.
126. Izumo S, Lompre AM, Matsuoka R, et al. Myosin heavy chain messenger RNA and protein isoform transitions during cardiac hypertrophy: Interaction between hemodynamic and thyroid hormone-induced signals. J Clin Invest 1987;79:970–977.
127. Schwartz K, Lecarpentier Y, Martin JL, et al. Myosin isoenzyme distribution correlates with speed of myocardial contraction. J Mol Cell Cardiol 1981;13:1071–1075.
128. Parker TG. Molecular biology of myocardial hypertrophy and failure: gene expression and trophic signalling. New Horizons 1995;3:288–300.
129. Buchman TG. Manipulation of stress gene expression: A novel therapy for the treatment of sepsis? Crit Care Med 1994;22:901–903.
130. Buchman TG, Cabin DE. Molecular biology of circulatory shock III. HepG2 cells demonstrate two patterns of shock-induced gene expression which are independent, exclusive and prioritized. Surgery 1990;108:902–911.
131. Li GC, Werb Z. Correlation between synthesis of heat shock proteins and development of thermotolerance in Chinese hamster fibroblasts. Proc Natl Acad Sci 1982;79:3218–3222.
132. Landry J, Chretien P. Relationship between hyperthermia-induced heat shock proteins and thermotolerance in Morris hepatoma cells. Biochem Cell Biol 1983;61:428–437.
133. Li GC. Elevated levels of 70,000 dalton heat shock protein in transiently thermotolerant Chinese hamster fibroblasts and in their stable heat resistant variants. Int J Radiat Oncol Biol Phys 1985;11:165–177.
134. Morrison DC, Ryan JC. Endotoxin and disease mechanisms. Annu Rev Med 1987;38:417–432.
135. Giroir BP. Mediators of septic shock: New approaches for interrupting the endogenous inflammatory cascade. Crit Care Med 1993; 21:780–789.
136. Jäättelä M, Saksela K, Saksela E. Heat shock protects WEHI 164 target cells from the cytolysis by tumor necrosis factors α β . Eur J Immunol 1989;19:1413–1417.
137. Gromgowski S, Yagi J, Janeway CA Jr. Elevated temperature regulates tumor necrosis factor-mediated immune killing. Eur J Immunol 1989;19:1709–1714.
138. Kusher DI, Ware CF, Gooding LR. Induction of the heat shock response protects cells from lysis by tumor necrosis factor. J Immunol 1990;145:2925–2931.
139. Villar J, Ribeiro SP, Mullen JB, et al. Induction of the heat shock response reduces mortality rate and organ damage in a sepsis-induced acute lung injury model. Crit Care Med 1994;22:914–921.
140. Gething MJ, Sambrook J. Protein folding in the cell. Nature 1992;355:33–45.
141. Villar J, Edelson JD, Post M, et al. Induction of heat stress proteins is associated with decreased mortality in an animal mode of acute lung injury. Am Rev Resp Dis 1993;147:177–181.
142. Ribeiro SP, Villar J, Downey GP, et al. Sodium arsenite induces heat shock protein-72 kilodalton expression in the lungs and protects rats against sepsis. Crit Care Med 1994;22:922–929.
143. Kluger MJ, O'Reilly B, Shope TR, et al. Further evidence that stress hyperthermia is a fever. Physiol Behav 1987;39:763–766.
144. Morimoto RI. Cells in stress: Transcriptional activation of heat shock genes. Science 1993;259:1409–1410.
145. Ryan AJ, Flanagan SW, Moseley PL, et al. Acute heat stress protects rats against endotoxin shock. J Appl Physiol 1992;73:1517–1522.
146. Brigham KL, Canonico AE, Conary JT. Mediator gene expression in sepsis: Implications for therapy. In: Vincent JL, ed. Mediators of sepsis. Update in Intensive Care and Emergency Medicine. Berlin: Springer-Verlag, 1992;16:393–405.
147. Conary JT, Canonico AE, Parker RE, et al. Expression of a CMV promoter driven ovine prostaglandin G/H synthase gene in the lungs of rabbits. Am Rev Resp Dis 1992;145:A850.
148. Conary JT, Brown DL, Shepherd VE, et al. Expression of a CMV promoter driven ovine prostaglandin G/H synthase gene in cultured lung endothelial cells. Am Rev Resp Dis 1992;145:A839.
149. Johnson J, Brigham KL, Meyrick B. Morphological changes in lungs of anesthetized sheep following intravenous infusion of recombinant human tumor necrosis factor alpha. Am Rev Resp Dis 1992;144:179–186.
150. Wheeler AP, Jesmok G, Brigham KL. Tumor necrosis factor's effects on lung mechanics, gas exchange, and airway reactivity in sheep. J Appl Physiol 1990;68:2542–2549.
151. Tracey KJ, Cerami A. Tumor necrosis factor: An updated review of its biology. Crit Care Med 1993;21:S415–S422.
152. Jongeneel CV, Briant L, Udalova I, et al. Extensive genetic polymorphism in the human tumor necrosis factor region and relation to extended HLA haplotypes. Proc Natl Acad Sci-USA 1992;88:9717–9721.
153. Buchman TG. Multiple organ failure. Curr Opin Gen Surg 1993;1: 26–31.
154. Tracey KJ, Beutler B, Lowry SF. Shock and tissue injury induced by recombinant human cachectin. Science 1986;234:470–474.
155. Damas P, Reuter A, Gysen P, et al. Tumor necrosis factor and interleukin-1 serum levels during severe sepsis in humans. Crit Care Med 1989;17:975–978.
156. Marano MA, Fong Y, Moldawer LL, et al. Serum cachectin/tumor necrosis factor in critically ill patients with burns correlates with infection and mortality. Surg Gynecol Obstet 1990;170:32–38.
157. Beutler B, Brown T. Polymorphism of the mouse TNF-α locus: sequence studies of the 3′-untranslated region and first intron. Gene 1993;129:279–283.
158. Han J, Brown T, Beutler B. Endotoxin-responsive sequences control cachectin/tumor necrosis factor biosynthesis at the translational level. J Exp Med 1990;171:465–475.
159. Han J, Beutler B. The essential role of the UA-rich sequence in endotoxin-induced cachectin/TNF synthesis. Eur Cytokine Netw 1990;1:71–75.
160. Goeddel DV, Kleid DG, Bolivar F, et al. Expression of chemically synthesized genes for human insulin. Proc Natl Acad Sci-USA 1979;76:106–110.
161. Watson JD, Gilman M, Witkowski J, Zoller M. Recombinant DNA. 2nd ed. New York: Scientific American, 1992.
162. Ameli S, Hultgardh-Nilsson A, Cercek B, et al. Recombinant apolipoprotein 1-A Milano reduces intimal thickening after balloon injury in hypercholesterolemic rabbits. Circ 1994;90:1935–1941.
163. Huxley A. Brave New World. New York: Harper & Row, 1932.
164. Allen DB, Fost NC. Growth hormone for short stature: Panacea or Pandora's box? J Pediatr 1990;117:16–21.
165. Wagner EF, Covarrubias L, Stewart TA, et al. Prenatal lethalities in mice homozygous for human growth hormone sequences integrated in the germ line. Cell 1983;36:647–655.
166. Marx JL. The case of the misplaced gene. Science 1982;218:983–985.
167. Rifkin J. Algeny. New York: Viking Press, 1983.
168. Ledley FD. Distinguishing genetics and eugenics on the basis of fairness. J Med Ethics 1994;20:157–164.
169. Berger EM, Gert BM. Genetic disorders and the ethical status of germ-line therapy. J Med Philos 1991;16:667–683.
170. Danks DM. Germ-line gene therapy: No place in treatment of genetic disease. Hum Gene Ther 1994;5:151–152.

Nutrition and Gastrointestinal Emergencies

Section Six

Section Editor:

James C. Fackler

Nutrition and Metabolism in the Critically Ill Child

35

Barbara A. Haber and Clifford S. Deutschman

INTRODUCTION

Malnutrition has long been recognized as an important disease entity in children. Numerous studies in the 1950s and 1960s documented the widespread nature of this problem in developing countries, and a great deal of effort was directed toward the classification of childhood malnutrition[1]. During the same period, Cuthbertson in Great Britain[2] and Moore[3] in Boston were investigating the metabolic response to injury. It was not until later that interactions between the consequences of decreased intake and increased demand began to be appreciated[4]. Both ultimately result in inappropriate loss of body cell mass, which is, by definition, protein-energy malnutrition (PEM). Until recently it was thought that only severe malnutrition resulted in increased mortality. However, meta-analysis of 28 studies demonstrates that when anthropometric data and survival curves are normalized, increased mortality is demonstrated in moderate and mild as well as severe malnutrition[5]. Although none of these studies was carried out in the intensive care unit (ICU) setting, the data are applicable and should influence clinical management.

The critically ill pediatric patient is particularly prone to the development of PEM. Substrate deprivation, accelerated demand brought on by injury/disease, and the increased metabolic needs associated with growth may contribute to the development of PEM. In children, this can be expected to have a particularly devastating effect. The child is a growing organism with little metabolic reserve to combat serious illness, trauma, or infection. As would be predicted, Steinhorn and Green found that the severity of illness correlates with alteration in energy metabolism[6]. Unlike adults, who can survive for long periods of time in the face of severe limitations of intake, it may be expected that children are acutely dependent on substrate supply even in the absence of disease.

Because the nutritional needs of critically ill children have not been extensively investigated, certain assumptions will be made in our approach. First, despite the lack of firm scientific evidence to support the notion, it is assumed that appropriate nutritional support is of benefit to the critically ill child. The question is, therefore, not whether to feed the critically ill child but what to feed. This is the area in which the most new information has recently developed. Second, given the absence of investigations into the metabolic derangements associated with critical illness in children, much of the data cited is derived from adults.

The specific questions to be addressed are (a) What are the normal metabolic requirements of the child? (b) What are the metabolic consequences of decreased intake in the absence of other disease processes? (c) What are the effects of acute inflammatory processes on metabolism? (d) How does one detect the presence and degree of nutritional depletion? and (e) How can nutritional support be rationally used?

NORMAL METABOLIC REQUIREMENTS IN THE CHILD

Derivation of Energy

Fuel requirements for cellular processes are met by the degradation of high-energy phosphate compounds, especially adenosine triphosphate (ATP). These compounds are highly reactive, and therefore are not amenable to storage. At any given time, the entire human body contains only enough ATP to provide energy for several minutes. Therefore, metabolism is geared toward the continuous synthesis of sufficient ATP or ATP-like compounds to ensure that deficits do not occur.

Three classes of substrate that are amenable to storage provide energy (as well as serving other functions) for the continuous synthesis of ATP (Fig. 35.1). Oxidation of carbohydrate primarily involves glucose entry into the Emden-Meyerhoff pathway, although other sugars and starches can be metabolized to glucose or glycolytic intermediaries. ATP can be generated by anaerobic metabolism of glucose-derived pyruvate to lactate or conversion of pyruvate to acetyl coenzyme A (CoA) for entry into the tricarboxylic acid (TCA) cycle. Similarly, β-oxidation of fatty acids to acetyl CoA and malonyl CoA provides for entry of these substrates into the Krebs cycle. Fats can also be converted to the ketone bodies acetoacetate, β-hydroxybutyrate, and acetone. These can be metabolized to form acetyl CoA for entry into the TCA cycle. Some amino acids can serve as precursors to acetyl CoA, while others enter the TCA cycle as α-ketoglutarate, succinyl CoA, fumarate, or oxaloacetate. Finally, a number of amino acids provide substrate for hepatic and renal gluconeogenesis. Metabolism of carbohydrate, protein, and fat to completion yields energy in the quantities noted in **Table 35.1.**

Glucose is stored as glycogen, which is found primarily in muscle and liver. Glycogen, in turn, is a polymer of

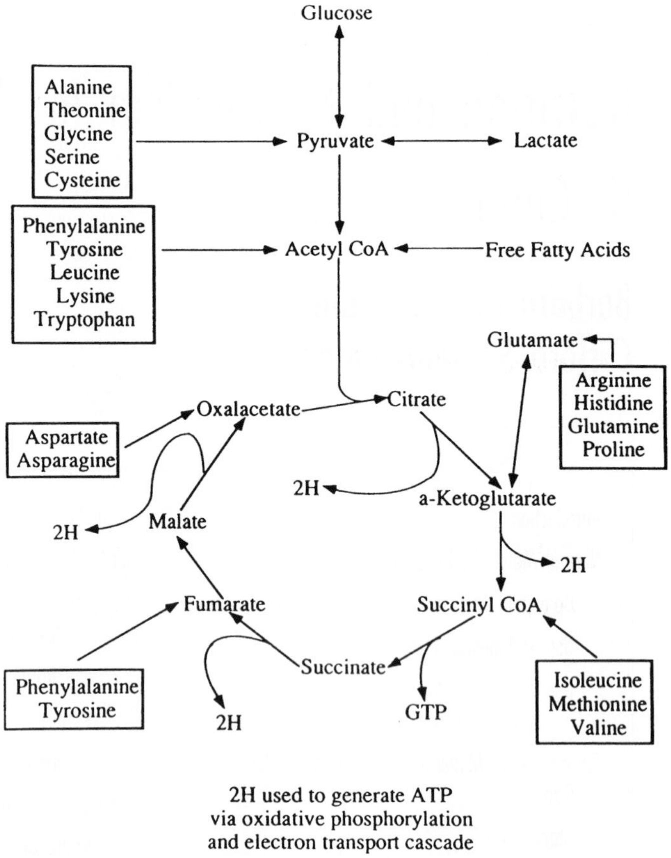

Figure 35.1. Pathways to ATP. Glucose, fatty acids, and many amino acids can be hydrolyzed to yield hydrogen species that ultimately are used to generate ATP. Additionally, certain amino acids can be converted to glucose while glucose can be converted to fat. Free fatty acids, however, cannot be converted to glucose.

glucose-1-phosphate residues linked by a 1- to 4-phosphate bridge. In muscle, breakdown of glycogen leads to production of glucose-1-phosphate that is isomerized to glucose-6-phosphate and then enters the oxidative pathway. In hepatocytes, glucose-6-phosphate can be dephosphorylated to glucose; muscle lacks the enzyme to catalyze this step. Thus, breakdown of hepatic glycogen can provide substrate for the entire organism, while muscle glycogen is available only for use within the muscle itself and cannot be released systemically. Breakdown of glycogen is stimulated by a number of hormones, especially epinephrine[7].

Fat is stored in a number of tissues and may constitute as much as 20% of gross body weight in normal infants. Release of intracellular fat is catalyzed by a series of hormone-sensitive lipases found on the cellular side of blood vessels or within the membranes of adipocytes themselves[8,9]. The actions of these enzymes result in the re-

Table 35.1. Energy Production per Gram of Substrate Metabolized

Substrate	*Kcal/gram*
Carbohydrate	4–5
Protein	4–5
Fat	9

Table 35.2. Essential Amino Acids and Fatty Acids

Essential Amino Acids	*Essential Fatty Acids*
Arginine	Linoleic acid
Histidine	Linolenic acid
Isoleucine	
Leucine	
Lysine	
Methionine	
Phenylalanine	
Threonine	
Tryptophan	
Valine	
Semiessential amino acids	Semiessential fatty acids
Synthesized only from essential precursors	Synthesized only from essential fatty acids
Cysteine	Arachidonic acid
Tyrosine	

lease of free fatty acids and glycerol from cells. Breakdown, uptake, and reesterification of triglycerides to glycerol and free fatty acids by cells is promoted by the hormone lipoprotein lipase, which is concentrated on the lumenal side of blood vessels(10). Hormone-sensitive lipases are stimulated by epinephrine, glucagon, and cortisol(9) and are inhibited by insulin(9,11), while lipoprotein lipase is stimulated by insulin(12) and heparin(13) and is inhibited by tumor necrosis factor (TNF)(14). Hepatic synthesis of the ketone bodies is directly inhibited by insulin(15).

Amino acids are stored as somatic protein in muscle, as smooth muscle in many tissues, and as circulating and intracellular compounds. The fact that these proteins are constantly being degraded and resynthesized provides a mobile pool of nitrogenous compounds for synthetic purposes. In the face of a decline in serum glucose levels, secretion of epinephrine, cortisol, and glucagon rises(16). This stimulates proteolysis and hepatic gluconeogenesis. Insulin directly inhibits skeletal muscle breakdown but has no such effect on visceral smooth muscle(4,17).

Use of Ingested Foodstuffs

Precursors of storage compounds are generated by either the absorption of ingested material or by breakdown and alteration of endogenous compounds. In the face of carbohydrate deficiency, fat is broken down to fatty acids and ketones and metabolized, while protein provides substrate for hepatic and renal gluconeogenesis. On the other hand, the body lacks the capacity to synthesize several fats and amino acids. These are, therefore, termed essential. There are two essential fats (linoleic, from which arachadonate is derived, and linolenic acids), and 10 essential and two semiessential amino acids **(Table 35.2).** The body is dependent on exogenous sources for these compounds.

Ingested protein (Fig. 35.2) is hydrolyzed in the gut by a number of brush border enzymes to constituent amino acids or oligopeptides. These smaller compounds are then transported across the lumen by another series of enzymes and then directed to liver, muscle, or other organs. Some amino acids are directly used by enterocytes to turn over

Table 35.3. Daily Nitrogen Losses

Urine	2 mg N per basal kcal
Feces	20% of urinary losses
Skin	10 mg/kg

brush border or transport enzymes and to synthesize compounds involved in the maintenance of mucosal integrity(18). Absorbed amino acids not used for protein synthesis can be deaminated (to yield urea), and their carbon skeletons can be used for gluconeogenesis. Alternatively, they can be converted to other amino acids via various synthetic pathways. Since protein is constantly turned over, to some extent, protein requirements can be estimated via quantification of daily nitrogen losses **(Table 35.3).**

Fat (Fig. 35.3) is ingested as triglycerides and forms chylomicrons within the gut lumen. These, in turn, enter mesenteric lymphatics and, eventually, the systemic circulation via the thoracic duct. These can then either be used by the liver or stored.

Ingested polysaccharides (Fig. 35.4) are broken down within the gut to oligosaccharides and monosaccharides. Absorbed sugars are further hydrolyzed and transported

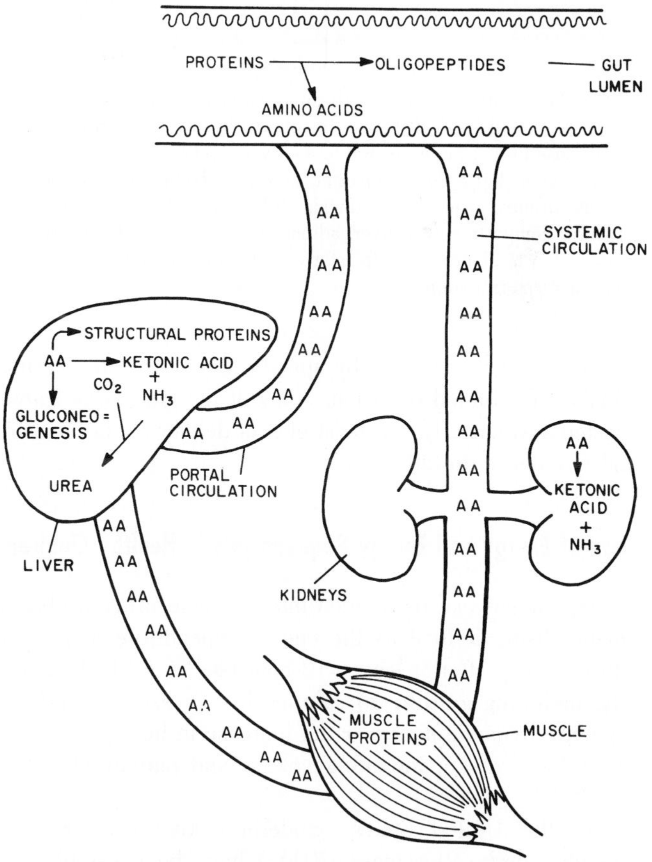

Figure 35.2. Pathway of utilization of ingested protein. Certain amino acids can be converted to glucose. The direct combustion of most amino acids for energy requires formation of the corresponding α keto acid. Free amino groups are, in general, transferred to glutamate. Alternatively, ammonia generated by this process can be eliminated directly or converted to urea.

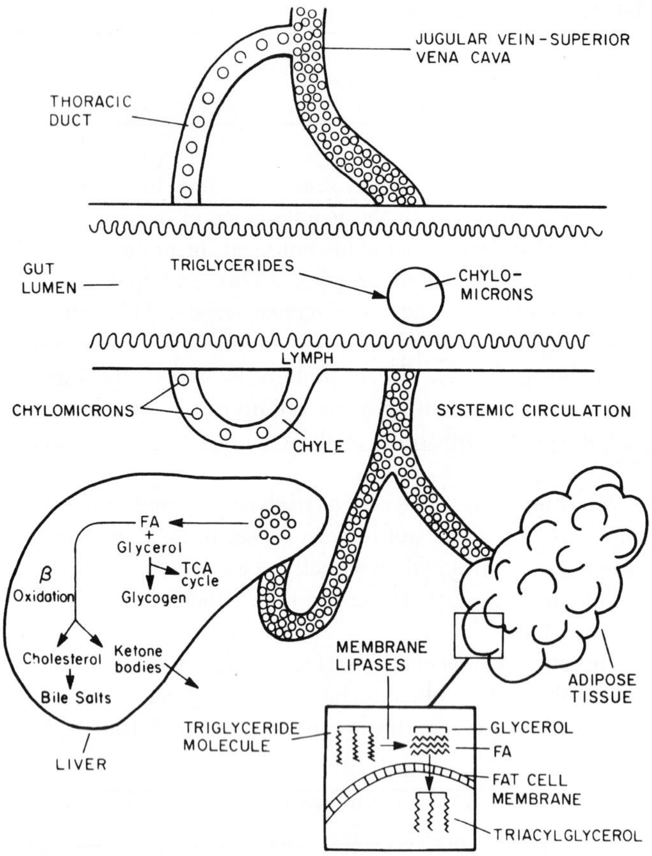

Figure 35.3. Pathways of fat utilization. Chylomicrons absorbed from the gut enter the blood via the lymphatic system and can be stored in adipose tissue. Fat delivered to the liver can be β-oxidized to yield acetyl- or malonyl-CoA, converted to ketone bodies for transport to remote tissues, or used to synthesize bile salts. Transfer to the intracellular compartment, in liver, adipose tissue, or elsewhere requires conversion to glycerol and free fatty acids, followed by either oxidation or reesterification.

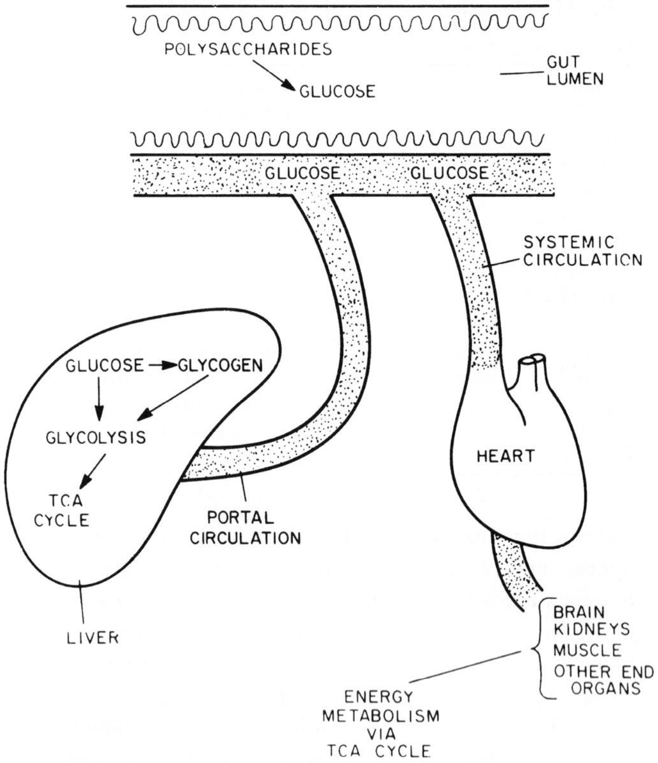

Figure 35.4. Pathways of glucose utilization. Absorption of oligo- and monosaccharides across the intestinal border is facilitated by a Na^+-linked ATPase storage in muscle or liver involves polymerization of glucose to glycogen. Oxidation can occur under anaerobic conditions, yielding 45 kcal/mole of glucose with lactate as the end product, or via the Krebs cycle under aerobic conditions, resulting in the release of 686 kcal/mole of glucose.

across the brush border by specific enzymes and sodium/ATPase-facilitated diffusion. Some of the glucose is transported systemically, but most of it is delivered via the portal circulation to the liver.

Use of Energy and Energy Requirements in Healthy Children

Energy needs can be divided into four categories: (a) basal metabolism, defined as the energy expenditure at rest or during sleep after at least a 12-hour fast[19]; (b) body activity, including growth; (c) calories lost in excreta; and (d) specific dynamic action or the increase in heat production after food intake, including enteral and parenteral nutrition[20].

In the United States, guidelines known as recommended daily allowances (RDAs) have been established by the Food and Nutrition Board of the National Academy of Sciences[21]. These are based on the average needs of healthy individuals and add a 30 to 50% excess to meet the requirements of individuals on the far end of the normal range. The energy needs of infants and children by age and sex are noted in **Table 35.4.** Current recommendations by the Committee on Nutrition of the American Academy of Pediatrics is that 30 to 40% of these needs be composed of fat in infants and young children[22]. Protein requirements based on age are noted in **Table 35.5,** while fat requirements are detailed in **Table 35.6.**

Table 35.4. Mean Heights and Weights and Recommended Energy Intake in Infants and Children

Age	*Weight (kg)*	*Height (cm)*	*Energy Needs (Kcal) (Range)*
Infants:			
0–6 months	6	60	kg × 115 (95–145)
7–12 months	9	71	kg × 105 (80–135)
Children:			
1–3 years	13	29	1300 (900–1800)
4–6 years	20	112	1700 (1300–2300)
7–10 years	28	132	2400 (1650–3300)
Males:			
11–14 years	45	157	2700 (2000–3700)
15–18 years	66	176	2800 (2100–3900)
Females:			
11–14 years	46	157	2200 (1500–3000)
15–18 years	55	163	2100 (1200–3000)

From: Committee on Dietary Allowance, Food and Nutrition Board, National Research Council. Recommended Dietary Allowances, ed. 9. Washington, DC: National Academy of Sciences, 1980:23.

Table 35.5. Protein Requirements in Infants and Children

Age	*Protein (g)*
Infants:	
0–6 months	kg × 2.2
7–12 months	kg × 2.0
Children:	
1–3 years	23
4–6 years	30
7–10 years	34
Males:	
11–14 years	45
15–18 years	56
Females:	
11–14 years	46
15–18 years	46

PROTEIN-ENERGY MALNUTRITION—STARVATION VERSUS STRESS

By definition, PEM is the inappropriate loss of body cell mass secondary to intake or use of substrate in a manner that is inadequate to meet metabolic demands. After a heated debate in the literature(23,24), it was generally agreed that PEM in children presents as a spectrum of disease perhaps best described by the nutritional pyramid of Jelliffe(25). In this classification, progressive deviation from normal is observed as the severity of PEM increases from mild to moderate to severe. With the recognition that PEM was potentially a common problem in hospitalized adults(26,27), the issue has been reexamined in greater depth(28,29). It is evident from this reappraisal that marasmus, the predominant form of childhood malnutrition in developing countries, is associated with inadequate food intake and/or absorption, while kwashiorkor, once thought to result from insufficient protein intake, is most likely due to carbohydrate excess in the face of an inflammatory process, such as measles. A review of the metabolic processes underlying starvation and inflammatory hypermetabolism will demonstrate why such a distinction is of consequence.

Starvation

Starvation, or the acute cessation of macronutrient intake, involves no direct injury. Metabolism is directed toward decreased energy expenditure, conservation of endogenous energy sources, and provision of adequate substrate to tissues in quantities sufficient to permit essential function(30). As a consequence, most energy use is by the central nervous system (CNS). Initially, this demand is met by glucose.

Glucose is stored in humans as glycogen. Cahill has estimated that glycogen equivalent to about 1000 kcal is stored in liver and muscle(31). Only that stored in liver is available for transport to the CNS; muscle glycogen must be used locally. Hepatic glycogenolysis can provide a 70-kg adult with about 720 kcal, which will last less than 24 hours. Serum glucose levels will then decrease. To compensate, epinephrine, cortisol, and glucagon are released, muscle is catabolized, and amino acids are made available for hepatic and renal gluconeogenesis(30,32). Additionally, as the glucose level falls, insulin levels decrease. This, in turn, leads to lipolysis and ketonemia(33). Ketonemia inhibits pyruvate dehydrogenase and blocks glucose-derived substrate from entering the Krebs cycle(34). Acetyl-CoA, derived from fat and ketones, becomes the primary fuel for most tissues. During the first 24 hours of fasting, about 300 kcal of protein and 1600 kcal of fat stores are consumed(31). If catabolism continued at this rate, the approximately 141,000 kcal stored in fat and 24,000 in muscle in a 70-kg adult would be consumed in under 3 months. Adjustments, therefore, are made to conserve fuel stores further and to reduce the dependence on glucose.

While serum glucose and insulin levels decrease and free fatty acid levels increase for several days after the onset of fasting, ultimately, a plateau is reached(32–36). Ketone levels continue to rise, as does serum glucagon. Gluconeogenesis peaks at about 1 week(36) and is associated with nitrogen losses of 10 to 12 g/day. With continuation of the starvation process, nitrogen excretion falls (ultimately to less than 3 g/day), gluconeogenesis declines(37), and alanine release from muscle is attenuated(37). This, to a large extent, reflects adaptation of the brain to ketone use(38,39). Other glucose-dependent tissues (fibroblasts, phagocytic cells, red blood cells, and the renal medulla) use glucose but metabolize it only to pyruvate and lactate. These compounds can be taken up by the liver and resynthesized to glucose (the Cori cycle, Fig. 35.5)(37).

When exogenous substrate is provided in any form, the system responds appropriately. For example, glucose administration raises insulin secretion, decreases counterregulatory hormone levels, and impairs gluconeogenesis, proteolysis, and ketosis(30,31). When the need for increased skeletal muscle activity arises, this is met by primary metabolism of branched-chain amino acids(30), increased production of lactate and pyruvate to enter the Cori cycle, and release of gluconeogenic amino acids to be synthesized to glucose via the alanine cycle(40). The above mechanisms render metabolic rate responsive to tissue demand and substrate availability. Thus, low levels of neuroendocrine modulation are required. Eventually, a clinical picture similar to marasmus is observed, with proportional loss of body fat and muscle mass(23,24,28,29). Tissue and water are also lost in proportion to one another(41,42).

Table 35.6. Fat Requirements in Infants and Children

	Dietary Fat (g/kg)
Infants	4–5
Children	3–4
Adolescents	2–3

Starvation and Stress Hypermetabolism

Significant differences exist between the states of isolated starvation and stress-induced hypermetabolism, despite the fact that both ultimately result in an inappropriate loss of

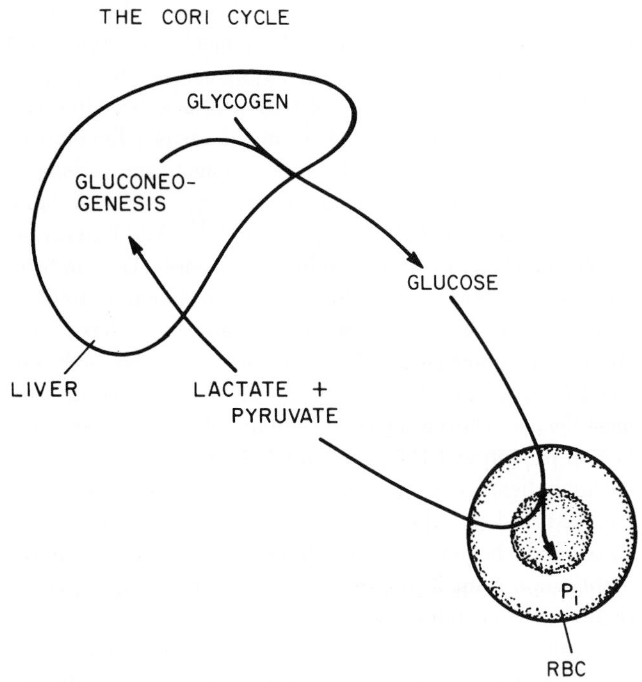

Figure 35.5. The Cori cycle in erythrocytes. The same process can occur in other glucose-dependent tissues as well as any cell respiring anaerobically.

body cell mass **(Table 35.7)**. Cuthbertson originally described the response to trauma as consisting of two phases an initial *ebb phase,* which is equivalent in modern terminology to shock, and a subsequent *flow phase,* which corresponds to the period of hypermetabolism[43]. Ebb phase, which is associated with a decrease in metabolic rate[44], may be transitory or persistent, depending on the magnitude of the insult and the speed with which blood volume is restored[43]. Flow phase begins with the restoration of perfusion and may persist for days to weeks[43]. Moore and Ball[45,46] have subdivided flow phase into *catabolic* and *anabolic* components. The first involves the cannibalization of endogenous tissue to provide for the demands of hypermetabolism, while the latter involves restitution when the demands of hypermetabolism have resolved.

Table 35.7. Comparison of Starvation and Stress Hypermetabolism

	Starvation	*Stress Hypermetabolism*
Resting energy Expenditure	Decreased	Increased
Respiratory quotient	Low (0.65)	High (0.85)
Mediator activation	—	+++
Regulatory Responsiveness	++++	+
Primary fuels	Fat	Mixed
Proteolysis	+	+++
Branched chain	+	+++
Oxidation	—	—
Hepatic protein	+	+++
Synthesis	—	—
Ureagenesis	+	+++
Urinary nitrogen loss	+	+++
Gluconeogenesis	+	+++
Ketone body production	++++	+

Patients fall in a continuum between the extremes of starvation and stress hypermetabolism (175).

Table 35.8. Effects of Flow-Phase Stressed Metabolism on End-Organ Function

Cardiovascular
Increased cardiac output
Peripheral vasodilatation
Capillary leak
Expansion of vascular compartment
Pulmonary
Increased dead space
Ventilation/perfusion mismatch
Increased minute ventilation
Increased respiratory rate
Renal
Salt and water retention
Impaired concentrating ability
Hepatic
Gluconeogenesis
Lipid oxidation
Acute phase protein synthesis
Impaired Bile Excretion
Gastrointestinal
Ileus
Depletion of brush border enzymes
Loss of mucosal barrier integrity
Stress ulceration and bleeding
Skeletal muscle
Proteolysis
Adipose tissue
Lipolysis

It is convenient to think of the hypermetabolic phase of the inflammatory response as being initiated by some signal that acts as an *activator*. Activation initiates a systemic response that is controlled by *mediators*, which, in turn, modify the *end-organ response*, that is, the behavior of components of homeostatic function that are clinically recognizable[47]. The activators are perhaps least well understood but involve any process that leads to tissue destruction or mimics this process. Thus, surgery and trauma as well as sepsis, endothelial injury, or the resolution of a large hematoma can activate the response. Studies indicate that aspects of a hypermetabolic response may even result after respiratory insufficiency or uncomplicated myocardial infarction[48].

Three general classes of mediators participate in the propagation of the stress response. These include afferent and efferent neural pathways, endocrine mediators, and compounds synthesized and released by white cells (humoral component). In turn, the end-organ effects involve a global increase in metabolic rate and effects on specific organ systems **(Table 35.8)**. The increase in metabolic rate is proportional to the magnitude of the insult (Fig. 35.6)[49]. In response to tissue injury, cellular migration to the area of damage occurs in a temporally ordered sequence. Initially, platelets and neutrophils are sequestered to effect hemostasis, debridement, and infection control. Macrophages and lymphocytes then enter the area and specifically en-

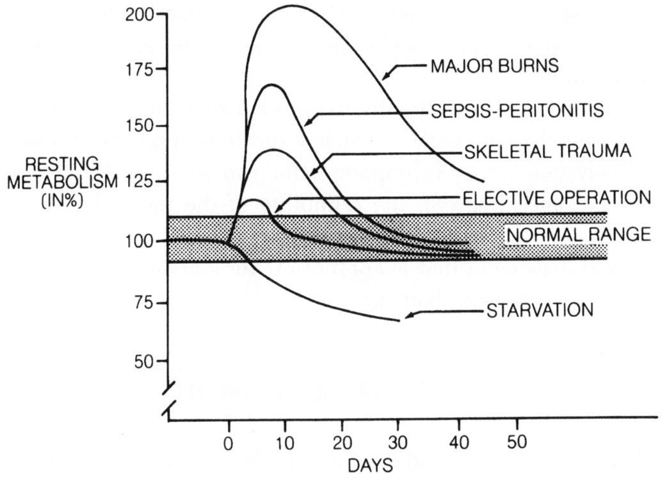

Figure 35.6. Changes in resting energy expenditure (REE) over time as a function of level of stress. (From Long CL, et al. J Parenter Enteral Nutr 1979;3:452.)

hance wound healing and aid in control of infection. Finally, fibroblasts, epithelial cells, and endothelial cells are responsible for scar formation, coverage, and angiogenesis[50]. Metabolically, these cells are primarily dependent on glucose (and, to some degree, glutamine)[50]; this dependence may be of key importance in explaining why the hypermetabolic state is necessary and occurs.

Organ system function reflects the overall increase in metabolic activity and is designed to effect substrate delivery. Cardiac output and especially heart rate increase, and peripheral resistance declines[51]. Capillary leak occurs, and new capillaries are recruited. Minute ventilation, especially respiratory rate[52], and carbon dioxide production are increased as is dead space, yielding a ventilatory equivalent that may be as much as 75% higher than in normal individuals[53]. Renal mechanisms that facilitate fluid and salt retention are activated and provide volume to fill the dilated vascular system[54]. In addition, isotopic studies have demonstrated transfer of intracellular fluid into the vascular and interstitial compartments[55–57]. This, to some degree, accounts for the loss of body cell mass that is the hallmark of the malnourished state[57].

Hepatic, somatic muscle, and adipose tissue alterations associated with the hypermetabolic state are interlinked. The liver responds to the insult with increased protein synthesis, particularly of acute phase reactants, such as antiproteases and procoagulants[58]. Synthesis of nonessential substances, such as albumin and other transport proteins, is decreased[59]. Gluconeogenesis is increased, with the substrate primarily coming from smooth and skeletal muscle[56,60]. Lipolysis provides a major energy source[55].

Initiation of the systemic mediator response appears to reside in the CNS, which probably constitutes the initial afferent component of the stress response. Hume and Egdahl demonstrated that denervation of a limb prior to injury blocked the increase in the excretion of cortisol metabolites noted in the injured state[61]. Other workers have noted that catecholamine and vasopressin responses to injury can be attenuated by regional anesthesia or by spinal cord injury[62–66]. Using radiolabeling techniques, Hilsted et al. showed that elevations in norepinephrine after surgery were due to increased secretion by the sympathetic nervous system[67]. Pain also appears to affect the response; epidural morphine has been shown to attenuate the catechol response to aortic reconstructive surgery[68]. Thus, the CNS appears to play an important role in mediation of the stress response.

Endocrine mediators believed to be of importance include catecholamines, cortisol, ADH/vasopressin, glucagon, aldosterone, and perhaps renin/angiotensin. Levels of epinephrine rise transiently after elective surgery[68] but are more profoundly elevated in critical illness[55,60]. Cortisol is increased after surgery and in critical illness[69], and the response of the adrenal cortex to ACTH is doubled[70]. Vasopressin levels may increase 50-fold after surgery and may remain elevated for up to 5 days[71]. Glucagon elevations are dependent on the magnitude of the insult; thus, changes may be undetectable in procedures of small magnitude, such as elective hernia repair, but may be markedly elevated after more extensive surgery or trauma[72]. Aldosterone secretion is increased and may be, in part, responsible for salt and water retention[73].

White cell products, along with histamine, bradykinin, serotonin, and complement, are important mediators of the stress response. The major importance of these mediators, however, is not local but the effects that are noted with their systemic release[47,55]. Alternatively, these mediators may be carried by white cells to target organs remote from injury or fixed-tissue leukocytes (i.e., hepatic macrophages or Kupffer cells) may be stimulated to release their products. Macrophage products of importance in the mediation of hypermetabolism include interleukin-l (IL-1)[74], TNF, and IL-6[75].

Hyperglycemia and glucose intolerance are hallmarks of stressed metabolism[50]. Hepatic glucose production is elevated[76] and is relatively unsuppressed by infused glucose or insulin[77]. Overall, glucose use is increased[78], but serum glucose levels are mildly to severely elevated, reflecting gluconeogenesis. Hyperglycemia results in hyperinsulinemia[76,79]. The elevated insulin levels inhibit ketosis[79]. Therefore, the brain remains highly dependent on glucose. Glucose uptake and oxidation also reflect use by infiltrating cells in wound tissue. Uptake of glucose is largely insulin independent; in most tissues, extremely high insulin levels are required to alter glucose uptake[77]. However, when glucose levels in critically ill patients are elevated to a point at which an insulin response of more than 30 μU/ml (a concentration sufficient to enhance glucose uptake by muscle and adipose tissue under normal conditions) is elicited, uptake of glucose by muscle is not markedly increased[77]. Similarly, achieving euglycemia in critically ill patients requires five times the amount of infused insulin as controls[80]. Uptake and oxidation of glucose by hepatocytes is diminished[81] and may result in conversion of partially oxidized glucose to fatty acids[82]. Hepatic steatosis may, therefore, occur.

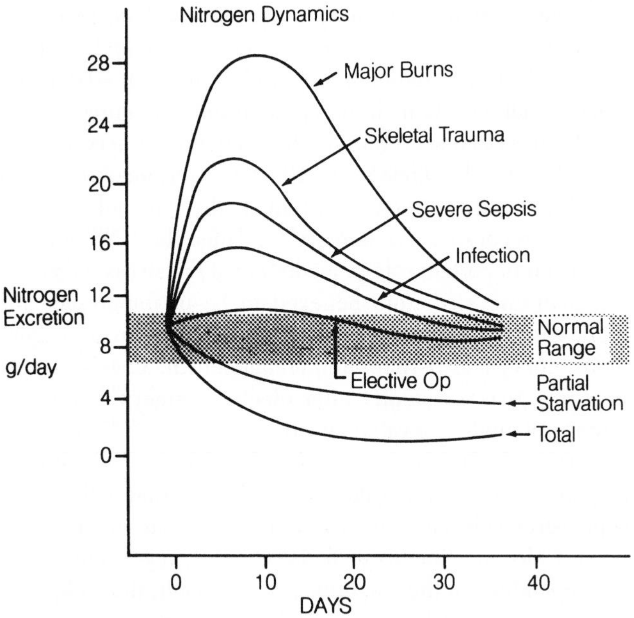

Figure 35.7. Nitrogen excretion over time as a function of level of stress. (From Long CL, et al. J Parenter Enteral Nutr 1979;3:452.)

Lipolysis is enhanced in the face of stress[82–85]. This increased mobilization is unsuppressed by glucose[85] or insulin[86]. Peripheral oxidation of lipids is markedly increased[86]. Hepatic use of long-chain fatty acids may reach maximal levels in the face of increased delivery[86]. Ultimately, this results in intrahepatic reesterification and fatty liver[87].

Protein breakdown is enhanced to a degree proportional to the magnitude of stress[88–92] (Fig. 35.7) and seems to occur mainly to provide carbon skeletons for use in gluconeogenesis. In fact, the rate of elevation of resting energy expenditure (REE) may correlate with the excretion of the nitrogenous byproducts of gluconeogenesis from amino acids[91,93]. Protein turnover, in general, is increased in severe stress, although this does not appear to be so in elective surgery, and the rate of degradation appears to exceed the rate of synthesis[89].

The changes in overall metabolism and substrate mobilization reflect the effects of endogenous mediators. Protein breakdown reflects the effects of catecholamines, cortisol, glucagon, IL-1[89], and TNF[75]. In an animal model, use of β-2 antagonists blocked the proteolytic effects of burn injury[55]. Lipolysis, mediated primarily by the hormone-sensitive lipase system present in adipocytes, is responsive to norepinephrine, glucagon, and, to a lesser degree, corticosteroids and growth hormone[82], which appear to exert permissive effects. Insulin inhibits these enzymes[8]. Triglyceride uptake by adipose tissue is dependent on the enzyme lipoprotein lipase, localized to the capillary endothelium[10]. This compound is directly inhibited by TNF[73]. The hormonal control of oxidation of fat within tissues has not been studied. Finally, gluconeogenesis is directly stimulated by catecholamines, glucagon, cortisol, and perhaps growth hormone[77]. The high levels of insulin have the effect of blocking, to some degree, the mobilization of amino acids from skeletal muscle and increasing reliance on visceral stores[90].

The discussion of the differences between starvation and hypermetabolism, both of which result in inappropriate loss of body cell mass, is important for two reasons. First, as will become apparent, the reliability of the tools of nutritional assessment depends on the mechanism of depletion. Second, treatment that is appropriate for starvation may not be so for hypermetabolism.

NUTRITIONAL ASSESSMENT

Identification and quantitation of PEM is particularly difficult in the pediatric ICU (PICU) patient because many of the standard modes of nutritional assessment are frought with difficulties. Isotope techniques are neither clinically feasible nor compatible with the multiple measurements needed to follow progression. Indirect alternatives exist but may have pitfalls, of which the clinician must be aware. A review of the various indirect measures of nutritional status follows.

Anthropometrics

In the evaluation of first-degree PEM, only standard growth curves, the most rudimentary of assessment tools, are necessary. The child who suddenly or progressively deviates from an established pattern is at high risk for depletion. Weight is more likely to be affected by acute changes, while deviation from the height curve perhaps reflects long-standing caloric deprivation. In evaluating more severe changes, Waterlow has classified PEM into four stages based on the ratio of actual weight to the 50th percentile of weight for height (**Table 35.9**)[94]. Pollack et al. have used this weight/height index for the initial assessment of PICU admissions[95]. In addition, these workers have used height indexed to the height of the 50th percentile. This is useful in assessing chronic changes, but its value in acute illness is not clear.

Body fat can be assessed from measurements of triceps and subscapular skinfold thickness; head, chest, arm, thigh, and calf circumferences; arm length; and crown-rump length[96,97]. This calculation is illustrated in **Table 35.10.** In infants, 10% of body weight should be fat; by 5 to 10 months of age, this should be up to 20%. Arm muscle size has been calculated from arm circumference and triceps

Table 35.9. Waterlow Stages

Stage	*WHI*[a]	*LLI*	
0	>0.9	>0.9	Normal
1	0.8–0.9	0.9–0.95	At risk
2	0.7–0.79	0.85–0.89	At risk
3	<0.7	<0.85	PCM

[a]*WHI, weight-height index; LLI, length-length index; PCM, protein-calorie malnutrition.*

Table 35.10. Calculations for Determining Value for Total Body Fat by the Method of Dauncey et al[a,b]

Trunk volume of fat = (crown-rump length − diameter of head) * T_{trunk}, where T_{trunk} is subscapular skinfold thickness − 2 mm (factor for skin thickness)
Upper limb volume of fat = (length of upper arm + length of lower arm) * circumference of upper arm * T_{trunk}, where T_{trunk} is triceps skinfold thickness − 2 mm.
Lower limb volume of fat = (supine length − crown-rump length) * ½ (circumference at midthigh + circumference at midcalf) * T_{leg}, where T_{leg} is triceps skinfold thickness − 2 mm.
Total body fat weight = 0.9 (trunk volume + 2 * arm volume + 2 * leg volume), where 0.9 is a factor representing the density of human fat.

[a]*In infants with normal stores, fat should represent 10% of weight. By 5–10 months, fat should represent 20% of weight.*
[b]*From Dauncey MJ, Gandy G, Gairdner D: Assessment of total body fat in infancy from skinfold measurements. Arch Dis Child 52:223, 1977.*

skinfold and should be useful in assessing the depletion of lean body mass.

There are several important caveats in the use of anthropometrics. The data available are population based and may not be applicable to individual patients[29,98]. Furthermore, the edema and ecchymoses often encountered in the ICU setting interfere with accurate determinations. Acute fluid shifts and changes in circulating albumin influence weight, arm circumference, and skinfold thickness determinations.

Biochemical Changes

Because of the problems associated with anthropmetrics, a number of other measurements are used in conjunction both for establishing the initial nutritional status and for monitoring changes. Four visceral proteins—albumin, transferrin, prealbumin (transthyretin), and retinol-binding protein are used[99–107]. The plasma half-life of each protein is noted in **Table 35.11;** shorter half-life proteins correlate better with acute changes, and the longer-lived proteins are better for the evaluation of chronic problems. As with anthropometrics, each of these values may be inaccurate in certain settings. For example, isolated starvation does not alter plasma protein concentrations until severe depletion is present[108–112]; this reflects the uniform loss of water and cellular mass. On the other hand, hypermetabolism leads to a decrease of protein concentrations without severe loss of body cell mass, reflecting factors noted in **Table 35.12**[113–115]. Protein determinations may be either falsely elevated or depressed depending on hydration status, leakage into the lumen of the gastrointestinal (GI) tract, leakage into interstitial tissues, and/or lack of catabolism by the kidneys in renal failure. Nevertheless, several workers have demonstrated an impressive correlation between low albumin levels and poor outcome in adult surgical patients[116,117].

Table 35.11. Plasma Proteins Used for Nutritional Assessment and Their Half-Lives

Plasma Protein	*t½*
Transferrin	8 days
Albumin	20 days
Prealbumin	2 days
Retinol-binding protein	10 hours

Table 35.12. Factors Altering Plasma Protein Concentrations in Stress

Decreased synthesis
Increased metabolism
Expanded extravascular space
Extravasation into soft tissues

An alternative to specific protein determinations is measurement of nitrogen balance. Nitrogen balance reflects the interplay of catabolism and anabolism and is a useful and accurate assessment tool in the adult population. All patients with PEM are, by definition, in negative nitrogen balance[118], and the magnitude of the negative balance may be used in determining energy expenditure. Hypermetabolic patients, who are catabolizing tissue for gluconeogenesis, have a more negative balance[88]. In contrast, the conservative state imposed by chronic starvation leads to an only slightly negative balance[31,88]. Nitrogen balance, in the absence of exogenous support, can be estimated from urinary urea nitrogen excretion over a 24-hour period. This will constitute about 93% of total urinary nitrogen losses. There are a number of limitations in the applicability of nitrogen balance measurements to the PICU patient. Administration of amino acid containing solutions and drainage of protein containing fluid from body cavities may lead to nitrogen loss and alter nitrogen balance. More importantly, obtaining complete urine collections is difficult, as often the patient does not have a urinary catheter in place, and urinating into a container may be difficult for young patients.

Cell-Mediated Immunity and Lymphopenia

Total lymphocyte[119] counts and impaired cell-mediated immunity[120] have been correlated with nutritional status. These may be difficult to interpret in children, given the variable response of an immature immune system. Additionally, numerous other factors, including cancer, collagen vascular diseases, uremia, hepatic dysfunction, and drug administration may impair cell-mediated immunity[121–123]. Quantification of T-lymphocyte subpopulations, with particular reference to killer cells, may be more specific[124].

Given the difficulties associated with nutritional assessment techniques, what is the practitioner, in the hospital with a critically ill patient, to do? Several authors advocate the use of a careful history and physical examination, coupled with the knowledge of the disease process, as the most effective means of assessing nutritional status[125–128]. Jeejeebhoy and Meguid have advocated the use of peripheral muscle strength as a useful tool[121]. Perhaps the most useful tool of all, particularly over the course of hospitalization, is metabolic assessment based on the combination of nitrogen balance and indirect calorimetry.

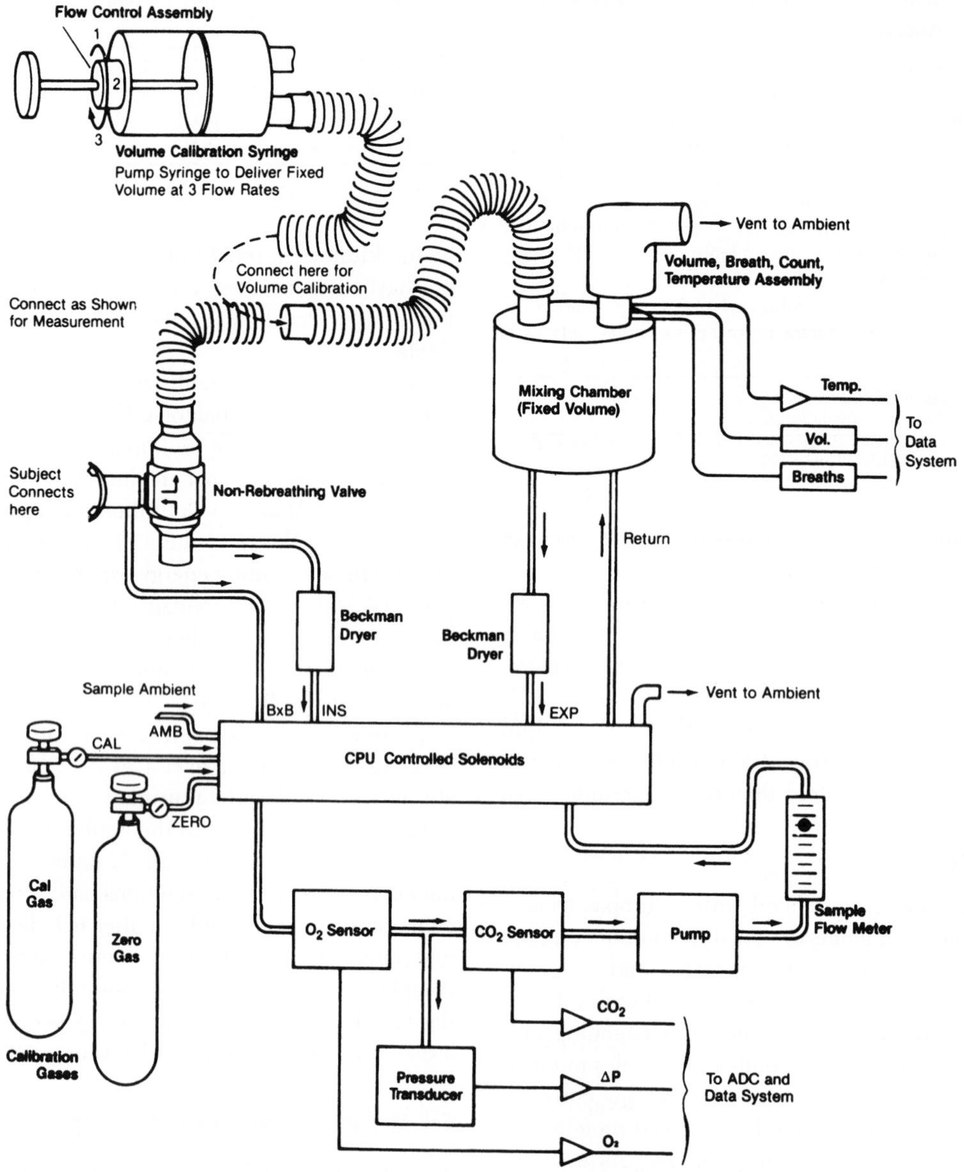

Figure 35.8. Schematic diagram of the portable indirect calorimeter. Samples are taken at six sites: *EXP*, dried expired gas from the mixing chamber; *INS*, dried inspired gas; *BxB*, undried breath-by-breath sample from patient's mouth; *CAL*, calibration gas; and *ZERO*, zero calibration gas. The pump draws the sample across the O_2 and CO_2 sensors at a rate specified by the flowmeter. The pressure differences in the sample cells (ΔP) are also recorded and corrected for by the microprocessor data system. *ADC*, alphanumeric display console; *CPU*, central processing unit. (From Norton, AC. Development and testing of a microprocessor-controlled system for measurement of gas exchange and related variability in man during rest and exercise. Sensor Medics Corp., Anaheim, CA, reprint 025, 1985:1.)

Indirect Calorimetry and Normal Energy Expenditure

Indirect calorimetry[129] is based on the recognition that the body is a chemical furnace and, like all physical entities, must follow the basic laws of thermodynamics. In combustion, the use of energy involves the consumption of oxygen (VO_2) and the production of carbon dioxide (VCO_2), nitrogenous waste, and water in a stoichiometric fashion. Further, according to the first law of thermodynamics, energy can be neither consumed nor created, but can merely change forms. When matter is converted by the body to heat, measurement of VO_2 and VCO_2 will indirectly reflect the basal metabolic expenditure involved.

Indirect calorimetry also circumvents many of the problems associated with other modes of nutritional assessment. Since the method directly measures the conversion of energy to heat, there is no need to apply population based data to individual patients.

Alterations in tissue composition also will not obscure the meaning of the data. Starvation is associated with a decrease in overall metabolism, while hypermetabolic states result in increased metabolism. Thus, following a patient over time will allow recognition of the nature of the metabolic problem and tailoring of support to meet individual needs.

Table 35.13. Various Fuels and Their Respiratory Quotients

Fuel	*Respiratory Quotients*
Carbohydrate	1.0
Fat	0.7
Protein	0.8

Most commercially available indirect calorimeters are the open type (Fig.35.8). In this system, the patient breathes through a valve system that separates inspired and expired gases. Inspired gas has a known concentration of oxygen, $C0_2$, and nitrogen. The volume of exhaled gas is measured, and a sample is collected and analyzed, either by mass spectrometry or by polarographic/paramagnetic oxygen electrodes and near-infrared $C0_2$ spectrometry. $V0_2$ and $VC0_2$ can then be calculated using the following equations:

$$V0_2 = V_I(F_I0_2) - V_E(F_E0_2)$$
$$VC0_2 = V_I(F_IC0_2) - V_E(F_EC0_2)$$

and the respiratory quotient (RQ) can be calculated:

$$RQ = VC0_2/V0_2$$

The RQ reflects whole body substrate use. The relationship between fuel and RQ is noted in **Table 35.13.**

Physiologically, RQ represents an instantaneous summary of the interplay between oxidation and synthesis of various metabolic substrates. The ratio can vary from 0.7 to 1.2. Excess carbohydrate calories, however, can result in net fat synthesis. This involves high levels of $C0_2$ production (Fig. 35.9).

Basal energy expenditure can be obtained from tables derived from age- and sex-matched controls[130]. Alternatively, since patients in an ICU environment are rarely in a basal state, Kinney et al. have defined REE as the measured energy expenditure in a quiet supine individual[131]. REE is a function of sex, age (A, in years), height (H, in cm), and weight (W, in kg) and can be calculated using the Harris-Benedict equation[132]. This is an empirically derived formula devised from pooled data obtained from normal healthy subjects.

For men:

$$\text{REE (kcal/day)} = 66.5230 + 13.7516\,W + 5.0033\,H - 4.775\,A$$

For women:

$$\text{REE (kcal/day)} = 655.0955 + 9.6534\,W + 1.8946\,H - 4.756A$$

Alternatively, REE can be derived from metabolic cart measurement using the following formulae:

$$\text{REE (kcal/min)} = (3.0)(VO_2) + (1.1)(VCO_2)$$
$$\text{REE (kcal/day)} = \text{kcal/min} \times 1440$$

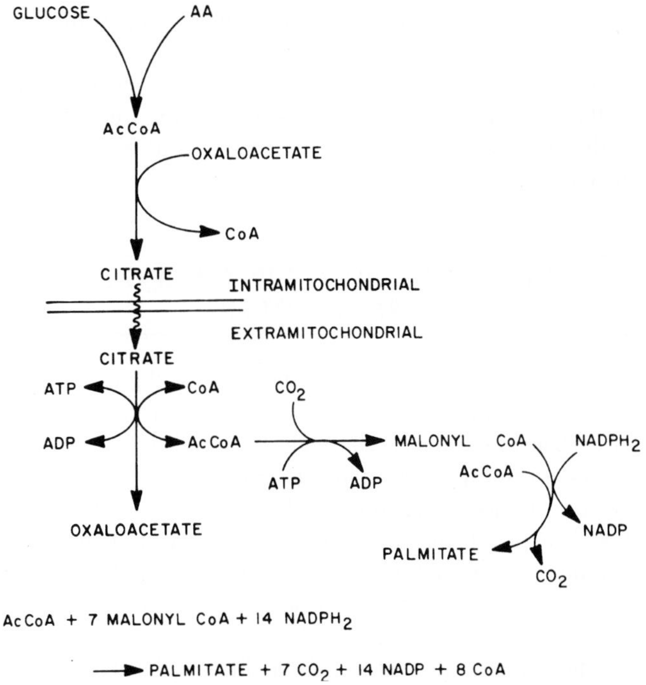

Figure 35.9. Conversion of carbohydrates and amino acids to fatty acids. Since 1 mole of glucose produces 2 moles of acetyl-CoA, the synthesis of palmitate from acetyl-CoA and malonyl-CoA results in the release of $14CO_2$ molecules (the RQ for this process is 7).

The major limitation of this procedure in the pediatric population is that a cuffed endotracheal tube is required. Typically, only the older patient's tube is cuffed. Furthermore, the equations pertaining to respiratory quotient are inaccurate when the inspired oxygen fraction is above 40%. Lastly, leaks in the line can introduce further errors, as can rapid variation in flow areas.

If the patient has a cuffed endotracheal tube and is not receiving significant oxygen support, then using these formulae is an accurate way to monitor metabolic parameters and response to nutritional support.

NUTRITIONAL SUPPORT

Autocannibalism, resulting from stressed metabolism, is the major metabolic consequence of critical illness in adults. The same may not, however, be true for children. A 1989 report documented a high level of abnormalities of various nutritional indices in children admitted to a PICU[98]. Nonetheless, the exact metabolic response to critical illness has not been investigated in the pediatric population. One may expect the response to be exaggerated, given the overall increase in metabolic demand imposed by the need for growth and development and the limited reserve available to the child. Children are less capable than adults of withstanding the effects of unstressed starvation; the requirements imposed by hypermetabolism are likely to be even more poorly tolerated. We will briefly review the general application of parenteral and enteral nutritional support in critical illness.

The major changes that have occurred recently pertain to the selection of alimentation solutions, the trend toward early feedings, and the use of food not only as nutrition but also as therapy.

NUTRITIONAL THERAPY IN THE SEVERELY STRESSED PATIENT

The major effect of stressed metabolism is the occurrence of autocannibalism which is unresponsive to the provision of carbohydrate alone. The body breaks down its own reserves to supply energy and precursors for the synthesis of glucose. It has been estimated that after use of 80% of the fuel reserves, the organism dies. Since autocannibalism can continue undetected, substrate supply may rapidly become insufficient to support both local organ and overall energy needs. Organ failure may result.

The pediatric patient has the additional disadvantage of requiring a certain number of calories for growth. If this quantity of energy is not available, growth ceases. The infant and child may not have the caloric reserve to meet this need[133]. For example, the 1000-g premature infant contains about 1% fat and 8.5% protein. If all of this fat and protein (about 400 kcal) are used to meet metabolic demand, and if we assume that the stressed caloric requirement for such an infant is on the order of 57 to 100 kcal/kg/day, endogenous substrate is available for only 4 days. A full-term infant has a reserve of approximately 2000 kcal or 20 to 25 days, and the 1-year old child has a reserve of about 40 to 50 days (compared with the adult reserve of 2 to 3 months). These figures underscore the urgency of early initiation of metabolic support.

Modes of Nutritional Repletion

Two routes are available for the administration of nutrients: enteral and parenteral.

Enteral Route

Enteral nutrition is always preferable when the intestine is functional, accessible, and safe to use. There are a number of reasons for following the dictum "If the gut is available, use it." Selected studies indicate that enteral feeding reduces the incidence of intra-abdominal and pulmonary sepsis after major trauma[134]. Conversely, total parenteral nutrition (TPN) has been associated with an increase in septic morbidity, higher costs, and the induction of immunologic derangements which may actually magnify the inflammatory response associated with injury and sepsis. Thus, there is an increased trend toward the use of enteral over parenteral support.

Enteral nutrition also supports maintenance of the gut barrier and may prevent bacterial invasion. This is achieved by luminal supply of adequate nutrients to the mucosa[135] and the induction of trophic hormones. These combine to provide the energy required to support the high turnover of enteric cells[136–139]. The fuels used by the small bowel are glutamine and ketones[140], while short-chain fatty acids derived from metabolism of dietary fiber by endogenous flora nourish the colonic mucosa[135]. Gut trophic hormones, which stimulate growth and cell turnover, are released as a result of luminal nutrient provision[136,141]. Absence of luminal nutrients from starvation[142], prolonged parenteral nutrition[137], or defunctionalization[143] leads to an atrophic intestinal mucosa and reduces bacterial counts in the colon[135]. In the face of critical illness, gut mucosal integrity may be even further compromised. Glutamine is released from catabolized skeletal muscle in stress, and enterocyte consumption is markedly increased[144]. Since glutamine, a nonessential amino acid, is not present in most parenteral nutrition formulations, the gut is acutely dependent on endogenous stores, which may become exhausted. Mucosal atrophy may occur very quickly. One potential consequence of mucosal atrophy and loss of mucosal integrity is bacterial translocation[145]. In comparing the effects of parenteral and enteral nutrition on bacterial translocation, Alverdy et al. noted that TPN was associated with a 66% incidence of translocation, elemental enteral feeding a 33% incidence, and complex oral feedings were *not* associated with translocation[146].

Three basic kinds of enteral feeding formulae are available for use at the present time: elemental, nonelemental, and modular.

The elemental formulae, e.g., Peptamen, Neochate One Plus, and Vivonex, contain nitrogen as free amino acids or peptides; carbohydrates as oligosaccharides, maltodextrins, or hydrolyzed corn starch; and lipids as safflower oil, corn oil, or medium-chain triglycerides. Each is available in a pediatric form that is apppropriate for the child over the age of 1 year. In the first year of life, when a different balance of nutrients and a lower osmolality is needed, available alternatives include Alimentum, Nutramigen, Neochate, and Pregestimil. Each is designed for ease of nutrient absorption. There are numerous nonelemental formulas, which will not be compared here. The major differences are in concentration, palatability, and manufacturer. The modular formulae are designed so that supplementation can be used to satisfy the specific needs of a patient. The carbohydrate reduced formulae are useful for the patient with severe upper GI mucosal damage with loss of the carbohydrate metabolizing enzymes or patients with specific inborn errors of carbohydrate metabolism. The protein reduced diets are used for patients with specific metabolic problems (e.g., ornithine transcarbamylase [OTC] deficiency).

Two major changes have occurred in the development of enteral feeds. The first relates to nitrogen source. Most elemental diets contain free amino acids. However, recent studies demonstrate that peptides, obtained by the enzymatic hydrolysis of whey protein, are more equally and uniformly absorbed than free amino acids[134]. Absorption is magnified in diseases of the small intestine, such as celiac sprue. Other benefits include improved growth, lower ureagenesis, greater production of growth factors, and improved support of hepatic function in the critically ill patient.

The second change involves alternative fat sources. Conventional lipids have been implicated in a variety of iatrogenic side effects in critically ill patients, while long-chain triglycerides of the omega-6 family may be detrimental to immune function. Some authors believe that excessive long-chain fats are associated with increased infections and mortality. Alternative lipids (fish oils, medium-chain triglycerides, and structured lipids) have been proposed as substitutes for conventional long-chain, polyunsaturated omega-6 fatty acids. Fish oils contain long-chain polyunsaturated omega-3 fatty acids which appear to be anti-inflammatory[(147)]. Unlike long-chain triglycerides, medium-chain triglycerides are rapidly cleared from the blood and are completely oxidized. However, medium-chain triglycerides contain no essential fatty acids. Structured lipids, which contain a combination of long-chain and medium-chain side chains similar to the structure of omega-3 fatty acids and omega-6 fatty acids, offer the advantages of long-chain triglycerides (essential fatty acids) and of medium-chain triglycerides (rapid clearance and oxidation).

Routes of Feeding

Enteral feeding may be administered directly into the stomach or small intestine by nasal/oral routes. Small-bowel feedings are useful if the stomach is dysfunctional (poor emptying or obstructed) or reflux is an issue. However, delivery of hyperosmolar solutions into the small bowel may be poorly tolerated. The stomach is an excellent osmoregulator, and acid delivery into the small intestine initiates a physiologic pancreatic response. There are numerous small, soft feeding tubes available for nasoenteric feeding that need infrequent replacement. Jejunal tubes may be used even for a short time after gastric surgery since small intestine peristalsis is maintained postoperatively.

Complications of Enteral Nutrition

Technical complications of enteral nutrition involving misplacement of feeding tubes are, unfortunately, quite common[(98,148)]. Tubes can enter the cranium, the tracheobronchial tree, the pleural space, or the lung parenchyma. They can also cause esophagitis, esophageal ulceration, mediastinal perforation, gastric ulceration, and rupture of varices. Reflux and pulmonary aspiration is a complication of intragastric feeding in critically ill patients[(149–152)], which can be avoided by feeding distal to the ligament of Treitz[(149,150,153)]. Diarrhea resulting from either hyperosmolar formulae or malabsorption secondary to depleted brush border enzymes can usually be controlled with bulking agents, feeding glucose polymers rather than a lactose- or sucrose-based diet. In some cases, choosing a modular formula with a reduced carbohydrate content is necessary[(154)]. Severe villous atrophy and loss of brush border enzymes in stressed states or after prolonged gut rest may necessitate the use of elemental feedings[(150)]. Elemental feedings have occasionally been associated with elevated transaminase enzymes and hyperbilirubinemia[(155,156)], although this is a rare complication compared to that associated with parenteral nutrition. As with TPN, high-caloric enteral formulae can increase VCO_2 and adversely affect ventilatory function. If feeding via the enteral route is not possible, the alternative is parenteral nutrition.

Parenteral Route

Historically, from the time it was recognized that ingested nutrients are absorbed into the bloodstream, physicians reasoned that direct administration of nutrients into a vein would prove beneficial[(157)]. A 1944 case report detailing an infant boy who demonstrated nutritional improvement after receiving a glucose, casein hydrolysate, and lecithin-olive oil homogenate mixture for 5 days represents the first pediatric case report of parenteral nutrition support[(158)]. In the 1960s, Dudrick and coworkers[(159)], at the Massachusetts General Hospital, reported successful use of long-term TPN to support growth. Today parenteral nutritional therapy involves the administration of a hypertonic solution of glucose, amino acids, trace elements, and vitamins in an isotonic lipid emulsion.

The current widespread use of parenteral nutrition can be attributed to a general increase in awareness of the importance of nutritional therapy, and several modifications developed over the years have improved efficacy and safety: (1) Crystalline amino acid mixtures have replaced protein hydrolysates, (2) safe parenteral lipid emulsions have developed, (3) trace mineral and vitamins have been added, and (4) catheters and infusion pumps have improved[(157)].

Route of Delivery

Parenteral nutrition can be delivered either centrally or peripherally. The advantages of peripheral nutrition is that delivery is via a conventional intravenous catheter. However, the delivery of calories is limited by acceptable tonicity. The upper limit of tonicity tolerated by peripheral veins is usually considered to be about 700 mOsm, and therefore the administration of maintenance calories by this route may not be possible. As the tonicity of the solution increases, problems such as phlebitis and tissue damage from infiltration of the hypertonic solution occur with increased frequency. Peripheral parenteral nutrition is most useful either as a supplement to enteral feedings or as a stop-gap measure until a central line can be placed to administer TPN. With central TPN, solutions above 700 mOsm can be used, and thus adequate calories can be delivered. This advantage must be weighed against the complications associated with central venous access.

Continuous Versus Cyclic Infusion of TPN

Cyclic TPN was developed in order to mimic normal feeding behavior. Since continuous TPN is analogous to an unremitting fed state, with persistently elevated insulin and glucose levels and circulation to the pancreas without initial hepatic metabolism, both carbohydrate and lipid metabolism may be deranged. By supplying nutrients over a portion of a 24-hour period, a number of complications may be avoided. Cyclic administration of dextrose is associated with higher rates of lipid oxidation and lower rates of lipid storage. Furthermore, high circulating glucose suppresses release of the essential fatty acid, linoleic acid, into plasma. Thus the usual fat accumulation in the liver due to increased hepatic lipogenesis and plasma essential fatty acid deficiency caused by failure of free fatty acid mobilization from adipose tissue may be eliminated[(160)].

Effects of TPN During Stressed Starvation

In critically ill individuals, the effects of stress are of paramount importance. We will try to rationally approach the effects of delivery of carbohydrate, lipid, and protein in stressed starvation, in the hope of arriving at reasonable recommendations.

Carbohydrate

The goal of glucose administration in stressed patients is to provide energy and to spare lean body mass maximally without causing untoward side effects. Burke et al.[(161)], using burn patients (average of 31.1% of body surface area), and Elwyn et al.[(162)], using patients after severe trauma, explored the effects of glucose infusions on energy production and nitrogen balance. These investigators found that (a) glucagon and catecholamine secretion were not suppressed by high glucose loads, with catecholamine secretion increasing in proportion to the quantity of glucose infused; (b) serum fatty acid concentration did not decrease with glucose infusion; (c) glucose turnover and glycogen deposition were markedly increased, despite high circulating levels of glucagon and catecholamines; (d) protein synthesis was unaffected by glucose infusion; and (e) fat oxidation may also be impaired. Elwyn et al. claimed that gluconeogenesis from alanine could be completely suppressed at very high glucose loads (500 to 600 g/70 kg/day) but Burke et al. found that protein breakdown was resistant to suppression by glucose with higher infusion rates.

Although glucose infusion may be nitrogen sparing, the limitations noted above are important for the critically ill patient, and furthermore, excessive glucose substantially contributes to CO_2 production. According to Askanazi et al., glucose loads increase VCO_2 and, hence RQ, by at least two mechanisms: (a) a thermogenic effect yielding increased REE[(163)], and (b) conversion of glucose into fat[(164)]. Both effects can be minimized if half of nonprotein calories are administered as fat and not glucose[(164,165)]. Carpentier et al.[(83)] showed that in TPN containing only glucose and amino acid, the insulin response to TPN did not inhibit the breakdown of triglycerides but did decrease formation of ketone bodies. Finally, as pointed out by Bistrian[(4)], high glucose levels increase insulin secretion. This, in turn, is associated with preferential cannibalization of smooth muscle for gluconeogenesis since insulin inhibits skeletal muscle proteolysis. Therefore, while it would appear that some glucose is necessary for metabolic processes, after a point one sees diminishing returns. Overadministration does not increase oxidation or spare protein but may increase fever, CO_2 production, hepatic steatosis, and smooth muscle breakdown. This, in turn, may result in respiratory, hepatic, GI, and wound healing failure.

Lipid

Parenteral soybean oil emulsion first became available for use in the United States in the mid-1970s. Since then, several soybean oil emulsions and soybean/safflower oil emulsions have developed[(157)]. A reasonably small dose of either, approximately 0.5 g/kg/day, prevents development of essential fatty acid deficiency, a particularly important advantage for small infants, in whom this abnormality can develop[(166)]. The metabolism of parenteral lipid is similar to enteral metabolism. However, instead of entering the circulation as chylomicrons via the lymphatic system, parenteral lipid emulsions enter the blood stream directly as chylomicron- or very low density lipoprotein-like particles. Before these particles can be hydrolyzed, they must incorporate apoprotein-C-II which is necessary for activation of lipoprotein lipase and subsequent metabolism[(157)]. In the critically ill patient these processes may be altered.

In septic patients, levels of serum triglycerides and free fatty acids are frequently elevated. Impaired lipid metabolism is attributed to decreased activity of lipoprotein lipase[(167,168)] secondary to elevations of growth hormone, relative deficiency of insulin, increased corticosteroids, and TNF. Elevated insulin levels may also increase esterification, an effect magnified by high glucose levels which can lead to inappropriate fat deposition in tissues, especially in the liver.

Proper use of lipids can benefit the patient by being nitrogen sparing. The benefits are dependent on the patient's metabolic state and the proportion of lipids in the diet. Nordenstrom et al.[(169)], using $^{14}CO_2$-labeled Intralipid, demonstrated increased plasma clearance of lipids in patients with trauma and sepsis. Glucose infusion further increased lipid clearance[(170)]. Thus, despite net total body fat synthesis, exogenous lipid is oxidized and can serve as a caloric source. Although Long et al.[(171)] and Woolfson et al.[(172)] found no nitrogen sparing when lipids were administered to stressed patients, Jeejeebhjoy et al.[(173)] and Bark et al.[(174)] found that above a minimal carbohydrate load, lipid emulsions and glucose were equal in their nitrogen-sparing ability. The current dictum is that carbohydrate and lipids spare nitrogen equally once glucose infusions reach the level of 200 g/70 kg/day; below that level, glucose is superior[171,175].

Complications of Lipid Infusion

The major controversies associated with lipid preparations involve reduced pulmonary diffusion capacity in animals and adult volunteers, decreased oxygenation in low-birth-weight infants, and hypoxemia in premature infants. All are associated with administration of large bolus doses of the soybean emulsions[98,176,177]. Mechanisms postulated include fatty microemboli[178] and/or elaboration of vasodilator prostaglandins[179] that modify hypoxic pulmonary vasoconstriction and increase venous admixture[180]. More importantly, lipid emulsions may yield pulmonary hypertension independent of hypoxemia. Lipids also interfere with immune function. Leukocytes function abnormally in the presence of fat emulsion, an effect which is attributed to a high content of linoleic acid and a high production of PGE_2, an immunosuppressive prostanoid[138]. Lipid deposits in the RES throughout the body have been noted at postmortem examinations of infants receiving parenteral lipid prior to death. High levels of lipid oxidation may impair glucose use and increase hepatic steatosis[82]. Along the same lines, long-chain fatty acids move intercellularly via a carnitine carrier which is saturable[181]. This can result in ectopic lipid deposition. Patients receiving the 10% rather than the 20% soy emulsion for any period of time have hyperphospholipidemia, hypercholesterolemia, and in some cases hypertriglyceridemia[182].

Protein

Protein requirements change with age in the pediatric population. During the first month of life, Fomon calculates the estimated needs at 2 g/kg/day. By 4 to 5 months, this drops to 1.2 g/kg/day, while for the preterm infant, this requirement exceeds 2 g/kg/day[183,184]. Despite these predictions, the requirements for the specific patients are much more complex. Caloric requirements are influenced by source of amino acid, need for catch-up growth, losses, and increased metabolic demands[157].

Losses can vary greatly. Those patients receiving complete TPN have minimal loss of nitrogen in their stool, and factors such as infection, stress, and surgery can each lead to increased urinary nitrogen losses. Injured or septic patients excrete more unchanged nitrogen than unstressed subjects[92]. In adults, the protein requirement may increase by as much as 300%; pediatric studies have shown similar increases[185]. This increase reflects the use of the carbon skeletons of amino acids as substrate for the TCA cycle or gluconeogenesis, as well as synthesis of acute phase proteins. While increasing nitrogen intake will improve nitrogen balance, this effect will plateau at some point. Specific nitrogen intake is used more completely if accompanied by a higher rather than a lower concomitant energy intake; however, there is a level beyond which further increases do not improve utilization. The recommended energy:protein ratio is at least 84 kJ/g amino acid[157]. Overadministration of protein in the face of severe catabolism may lead to prerenal azotemia due to nitrogen generated by deamination. One approach taken in the adult population is to administer protein to the depleted or hypercatabolic patient until serum BUN increases to about 100 mg/dl[98]. Dialysis may be needed at this point to prevent osmotic diuresis, pericardial restriction or uremic encephalopathy.

Composition of Amino Acid Intake

Recent investigations into the provision of nitrogenous compounds in stress have been concerned less with how much to give than with what to give. Early infant formulas containing soy protein which is low in methionine content were associated with lower rates of weight gain and nitrogen retention[186]. Modern soy preparations are now supplemented with this amino acid. Similarly, taurine, cystine, and tyrosine are thought to be needed in larger proportions in infants[157]. The amino acid composition of available parenteral solutions vary and must be considered. A number of mixtures are specially designed for the pediatric population.

A number of formulations designed to be disease specific have been developed. Solutions high in branched-chain amino acids are used for hepatic encephalopathy and metabolic stress. In 1976 Fischer and coworkers reported increased nitrogen retention and improvement in hepatic encephalopathy in patients treated with an amino acid formula deficient in sulfur-containing and aromatic amino acids and rich in branched-chain amino acids (isoleucine, leucine and valine)[187]. Other workers have investigated the use of branched-chain formulae in various stress states[188–195]. Results have been promising for hepatic encephalopathy[196] but mixed in other settings. Furthermore, it is not clear if the value in liver failure lies in the increased branched-chain content or in the low levels of potentially toxic (phenylalanine, tyrosine, cysteine, methionine) amino acids. No analogous studies have been performed in the pediatric population[197]. Because of the ambiguous data and lack of pediatric studies, it is probably only minimally indicated to use these formulae.

Glutamine has already been cited as an important fuel for the GI tract in stress[198]. Many TPN formulations do not contain glutamine. Animal studies using glutamine-supplemented TPN[199–204] have indicated improvements in gut mass, gut nitrogen retention, gut mucosal height and liver fatty infiltration. Two small studies in adult patients have demonstrated that glutamine-enriched TPN improved nitrogen retention but did not ultimately affect outcome[205,206]. The amount of glutamine needed for optimal care is unknown. However, glutamine may become an essential amino acid in stress since it is a precursor for the synthesis of nucleotides such as adenosine triphosphate, purines, and pyrimidines and functions as a fuel source for enterocytes and colonocytes. Arginine, although a nonessential amino acid, is thought to promote wound healing and enhance immune function in stress[157,175]. Therefore, some authors have advocated increased administration of this amino acid to stressed patients. Last, a number of nonprotein parenteral modifications are being investigated, including short-chain fatty acids, omega-3 fatty acids, and dietary nucleosides for the same reasons as discussed in the enteral nutrition section[138].

Protein synthesis is an energy-storing process. As such, the administration of amino acids alone can result in depletion of fat stores. Administration of glucose and lipid to the level of zero-energy balance may be needed, along with amino acid infusions, to allow for the maintenance of body energy stores. Elwyn et al.[207] demonstrated in unstressed starvation that even with high nitrogen loads, negative energy balance did not produce an increase in REE or result in positive nitrogen balance. During positive energy balance, however, a high nitrogen load was associated with increased REE and an increase in tissue mass consisting of 63% fat and 27% lean body mass. If energy stores are maintained, the nitrogen balance can be improved.

The most important principle is that nutrition needs to be provided in a balanced fashion. Theoretically, an inadequate intake of any nutrient required for metabolism limits the extent to which protein is deposited as new tissue. The best example of this phenomenon is the study by Rudman et al., who demonstrated that withdrawal of electrolytes from an otherwise balanced solution resulted in decreased retention of nitrogen and a lower rate of weight gain[208].

Use of Insulin with TPN

Use of insulin with TPN has been shown to be of little benefit. TPN plus insulin was originally used to counteract the hyperglycemia of injury. The hyperglycemia was not entirely due to decreased glucose tolerance but was also due to increased gluconeogenesis that was unresponsive to exogenously administered calories. It was hoped that added insulin would help stop gluconeogenesis and promote the storage of fat. Burke et al.[161] examined the effects of insulin on protein breakdown in burn patients and found that there was slightly increased incorporation of 14C-leucine with insulin but that this effect was not statistically significant. The addition of insulin had no effect on glucagon or catecholamine concentration in plasma. Insulin may specifically impair skeletal muscle proteolysis[4].

Thus, since insulin has no proven benefit, it is probably wiser not to use it except in cases of extreme hyperglycemia resulting in osmotic diuresis.

Effect of TPN on Body Water

Protein-calorie malnutrition and the flow phase of trauma and sepsis are accompanied by an increase in extracellular fluid[108,209–211]. Because of the increased capillary leak and microvascular injury that accompany the flow phase, the volume of distribution of albumin is increased to include the extravascular compartment. Serum levels may remain in the low to normal range. Starker[115] demonstrated, in stressed patients, expansion of the extracellular space after initiation of TPN, even with positive nitrogen balance. Contraction of the extracellular space did not occur until after the microvascular injury had healed, the albumin pool had contracted, and diuresis had begun. Ongoing stress, as in chronic sepsis, can prevent the normalization of extracellular fluid when TPN[115,212] is initiated. Larca and Greenbaum[213] studied patients on ventilators and found that those who had a rise in plasma protein during TPN could be weaned from ventilatory support, while those who did not have a rise could not be weaned, perhaps indicating that the latter patients underwent diuresis and had some increase in protein synthesis.

Rational Metabolic Support

Nutritional formulae should ideally be administered to meet measured or calculated energy expenditures. For children, the energy cost of many stressed conditions has not yet been determined. Souba and Wilmore[214] describe a simple method for estimating energy requirements that is readily applicable to children, if one assumes the availability of data for basal metabolic rate (BMR)[130,215]. The energy requirement for weight maintenance is calculated according to the following formula:

$$\text{Energy (kcal/day)} = \text{BMR} \times \text{stress factor} \times 1.25$$

BMR may be derived from **Table 35.4.** The stress factor may be estimated from Figure 35.7. The factor of 1.25 takes into account the 25% increase in energy requirements associated with hospital activity or stress related to treatment. The value obtained from the *BMR × stress factor* term should give a reasonable estimate of REE. Alternatively, REE can be measured by indirect calorimetry[129]. The additional fluid required to administer the TPN may be prohibitory in small children or in patients with primary cardiac or pulmonary disease. Judicious use of diuretics may play a role.

Many routes of central venous cannulation for the purpose of administering TPN have been used. The most popular route is the subclavian vein. Other routes include the internal and external jugular, the femoral[150], the saphenous[216], and the inferior epigastric veins[217]. For long-term TPN, tunneled silastic catheters with Dacron felt cuffs may be appropriate. The cuffs permit ingrowth of fibroblasts and thus help prevent the tracking of infectious organisms down the catheter length. With careful maintenance, these lines have remained in place for as long as 1 year without complications in oncologic patients receiving chemotherapy.

Mechanical or Technical Complications Related to Venous Access

Technical complications associated with placement of catheters for parenteral alimentation are listed in **Table**

Table 35.14. Technical Complications of Parenteral Nutrition

Pneumothorax	Thoracic duct injury
Air embolism	Brachial plexus injury
Subcutaneous emphysema	Phrenic nerve injury; arrhythmias
Arterial laceration	Ventricular perforation
Hemothorax	Cardiac tamponade
Mediastinal hematoma	Venous thrombosis
Hydrothorax	Catheter sepsis

35.14[149,218,219]. Perhaps the most important is catheter-related sepsis[221–224], which usually results from migration of organisms through the dermal tunnel formed during catheter insertion[219,220]. The incidence of infection increases with the length of time that the catheter is in place[150], and is more common with polyvinyl chloride catheters[150,218]. Uncommonly, improperly prepared or contaminated solutions can contain organisms and result in bacteremia[221].

Complications Related to Total Parenteral Nutrition

Complications related to infusion of hyperalimentation vary according to amino acid, dextrose, fatty acid, and electrolyte composition. Crystalline amino acid solutions generally have little toxicity. Although Grant implicated a tryptophan breakdown product in the development of abnormal liver function in some patients receiving TPN[222], this finding has not been substantiated by other investigators and more likely represents an effect of gut rest. Wilmore and coworkers implicated glutamine deficiency in the loss of intestinal mucosal integrity and believe this has implications for the development of septic complications in stressed patients[18]. Deamination of infused amino acids can result in prerenal azotemia[150].

Administration of pure carbohydrate formulae increases VCO_2 more than balanced nutritional regimens and can result in ventilatory insufficiency in marginally compensated individuals[223]. If glucose is administered in excess of the body's ability to use this substrate, hepatic steatosis and elevated levels of very-low-density lipoproteins may result[224,225]. This complication can usually be avoided by using fat as a partial source of calories. Hyperglycemia occurs frequently during glucose administration in stressed patients[150,226]. While usually easily reversed with insulin administration, use of insulin during stress metabolism may be associated with previously mentioned problems. Excess insulin can cause hypoglycemia when TPN infusion is slowed or discontinued[218].

Infusion of long-chain fatty acids can cause febrile reactions with associated chills, nausea, vomiting, and hypotension. This response, however, is rarely observed during infusions of modern soy and safflower-based formulations[227]. Thrombocytopenia occurs with fat administration, but abnormal bleeding has not been reported[228]. Hypertriglyceridemia can occur, and fat preparations should be avoided in patients with abnormal triglyceride clearance[150,218,226]. Fat-induced reduction of neutrophil chemotaxis and impairment of bacterial clearance have been reported in experimental animals[229–232]. If fat is not included in TPN formulations, essential fatty acid deficiency may result in dermatitis, alopecia, thrombocytopenia, and impaired wound healing[150,218]. The amount of lipid to give the pediatric patient is controversial. Excess lipid infusions (greater than 3.0 g/kg/day) may cause cholestatic jaundice in the adult[233]. Rapid lipid infusions can cause the arterial partial pressure of oxygen to fall by a mechanism involving increased prostanoid production from infused arachidonate[234]. These complications are weighed against the benefits of caloric delivery and nutritional repletion. Most typically, pediatric patients are given 3.0 to 3.5 g/kg/day of lipid.

Hypokalemia, hypophosphatemia, hypomagnesemia, and other electrolyte abnormalities can develop early in the course of nutritional repletion and can result in seizures, respiratory and cardiac failure, and death[150,235–239]. These abnormalities are thought to occur secondary to calciuria that is responsive to phosphate administration[240]. Unless elemental trace minerals are replaced, deficiencies may develop. Selenium deficiency is associated with abnormal PMN and T-cell function secondary to its role in the antioxidant glutathione peroxidase[241,242]. Zinc deficiency can result in diarrhea, mental depression, dermatitis, poor wound healing, platelet clumping, and impaired chemotaxis[243]. Chromium deficiency is associated with glucose intolerance and peripheral neuropathy[244]. Copper deficiency results in hypochromic anemia, leukopenia, and reduced levels of superoxide dismutase, a scavenger of superoxide free radicals[245,246].

Intravenous hyperalimentation in adults is associated with periportal fat infiltration, canalicular plugging, centrilobular cholestasis, and pigment accumulation within hepatocytes[247,248]. Elevated gamma-glutamyl-transferase, alkaline phosphatase, and hyperbilirubinemia generally reflect gallbladder sludge formation and/or cholelithiasis[240,248]. A similar pattern of transient enzyme elevation is occasionally observed when enteral feedings are begun after long periods of gut rest; this probably represents clearance of sludge as cholecystokinin release is stimulated[249].

The possibility also exists that susceptibility to infection may be directly affected by the administration of TPN. Nugent[250] found delayed clearance of *Staphylococcus aureus* from the peritoneal macrophages incubated with Intralipid. Loo et al.[251] found that Intralipid interferes with leukocyte cellular cytotoxicity for herpes simplex virus. Palmblad et al.[252], however, found no effect of TPN either with or without Intralipid on neutrophil migration or phagocytic function; Shamberger et al.[253] determined that TPN, either with or without Intralipid, had no effect on recovery from chemotherapy induced myelosuppression.

Parenteral Nutrition and Hepatic Dysfunction in Children

TPN-associated hepatic dysfunction appears to occur more commonly in infants and children[133,254–258] than in adults[240,259]. The degree of hepatic dysfunction can range from mild elevation of bilirubin or transaminases[254] to frank hepatic failure[255]. The incidence ranges in premature infants from 23 to 50%[254,260], with the highest rates occurring in infants weighing less than 1000 g at birth (50%)[259], or in those with severe surgical disease of the abdomen or peritonitis[255,256]. In most cases, TPN-associated liver disease is manifested by cholestasis with elevated serum levels of direct-reacting bilirubin and either mild[260] or no[254] elevation of alkaline phosphatase, although no features are pathognomonic[260]. Hyperkalemia and elevation of serum levels of bile salts have been noted to precede the occurrence of physiologic hyperbilirubinemia and jaundice[261] in both premature and full-term neonates[262]. Cholelithiasis has also been reported both in infants[257] and in adults[240]. TPN-related cholestasis is considered to be benign, with resolution usually occurring within 1 to 4 months after cessation of TPN[260]. The appearance of cholestatic jaundice has been reported to occur in as short a time as 5 days in low-birth-weight infants (1500 g)[254], and the risk probably increases with the duration of therapy[254,258]. In one series, all infants receiving TPN for longer than 50 days developed cholestasis[256]. Dahms and Halpin[263] performed serial liver biopsies in a series of TPN patients and found persistence of mild cholestasis, the appearance of periportal fibrosis, and collagen deposition on the spaces of Disse after following clinical recovery from jaundice after TPN was stopped. A study by Vileisis et al.[264] implicated amino acid intake as a possible factor favoring the development of cholestatic jaundice in premature infants; infants with higher amino acid intakes (4 g/kg/day) developed more severe cholestatic jaundice earlier than infants given smaller amounts of amino acid (2.6 g/kg/day). Other investigators[265,266] have focused on the dextrose intake, hypothesizing that dextrose overload results in hepatic lipogenesis and intrahepatic bile obstruction. These workers proposed that cholestasis can be reversed by decreasing the dextrose calorie to nitrogen ratio[266]. This association has led to the recommendation that infants be given TPN in which the nonprotein calorie:nitrogen ratio does not exceed 200 : 1[267]. Merritt et al.[268] found that intraperitoneally administered tryptophan produces elevations in serum bile acid concentrations in rat pups. As yet, the causes of TPN-associated cholestasis remain ill defined[269], and the diagnosis remains one of exclusion. Potential therapies include discontinuation of TPN[269], use of cholecystokinin[270], daily enteral stimulation to induce bile-duct contracture, metronidazole to prevent bacterial overgrowth[271], ursodeoxycholic acid to promote bile flow and change the polar to nonpolar ratio of bile acids, and taurine to stimulate conjugation of bile salts[272].

CONCLUSION

There are compelling reasons for the institution of early metabolic support in the critically ill child. These relate to the exquisite dependence of the growing organism on adequate nutritional intake and the smaller endogenous metabolic reserves available to children. It is incumbent upon the astute clinician to be aware of the potential for metabolic depletion, to assess the needs of the patient, and to institute such therapy as may seem appropriate. A framework for assessment has been presented. Whether or not this approach can alter outcome in critically ill children needs to be evaluated in the future. Nutrition, once thought to be only supportive, has now proven to be therapeutic. The recent trends focus on the early provision of metabolic support and the use of formulations designed to prevent iatrogenic complications. The utility of these approaches, however, requires scientific assessment.

References

1. Gomez F, Ramos-Galvan R, Frenk S, et al. Mortality in third degree malnutrition. J Trop Pediatr 1956;2:77.
2. Cuthbertson DP. Observations on the disturbance of metabolism produced by injury to the limbs. Q J Med 1932;1:233.
3. Moore FD. The metabolic care of the surgical patient. Philadelphia: WB Saunders, 1959.
4. Bistrian BR. Interaction of nutrition and infection in the hospital setting. Am J Clin Nutr 1977;30:1228.
5. Pelletier DL. The potentiating effects of malnutrition on child mortality: Epidemiologic evidence and policy implications. Nutrition Reviews 1994;52:409.
6. Steinhorn DM. Starvation in the PICU. Arch Surg 1981;116:158.
7. Vester JW, Rudney H. Carbohydrates. In: Fisher JE, ed. Surgical Nutrition. Boston, Little, Brown, 1983:165.
8. Steinberg D, Khoo JC. Hormone sensitive lipase of adipose tissue. Fed Proc 1977;36:1986.
9. Blackburn GL, Phinny SD. Lipid metabolism in injury. In: Burke JF, ed. Surgical physiology. Philadelphia, WB Saunders, 1983:98.
10. Eckel RH. Lipoprotein lipase: a multifunctional enzyme relevant to common metabolic diseases. N Engl J Med 1989;320:1060.
11. Butcher RW, Baird CE, Sutherland EW. Effects of lipolytic and antilipolytic substance on adenosine 3',5-monophosphate levels in isolated fat cells. J Biol Chem 1968;243:397.
12. Garfinkle AS, Nilsson-Ehle P, Schotz MC. Regulation of lipoprotein lipase induction by insulin. Biochim Biophys Acta 1976;424:264.
13. Boberg J, Carlson LA, Normell L. Production of lipolytic activity by the isolated perfused dog liver in response to heparin. Life Sci 1964;3:1011.
14. Semb H, Peterson J, Tavernier J, et al. Multiple effects of tumor necrosis factor on lipoprotein lipase in vivo. J Biol Chem 1987;262:8390.
15. Garber AJ, et al. Hepatic ketogenesis and gluconeogenesis in humans. J Clin Invest 1974;54:981.
16. Owen OE, et al. Energy expenditure in feasting and fasting. J Clin Invest 1969;48:574.
17. Ryan NT, Blackburn GL, Clowes GHT, Jr. Differential sensitivity to elevated endogenous insulin levels during experimental peritonitis in rats. Metabolism 1974;23:1081.
18. Wilmore DW, Smith RJ, O'Dwyer ST, et al. The gut: a central organ after surgical stress. Surgery 1988;104:917.
19. Gump FE, Martin P, Kinney JM. Oxygen consumption and caloric expenditure in surgical patients. Surg Gynecol Obstet 1973;137:499.
20. Askanazi J, Rosenbaum SH, Michelsen CB, Elwyn DH, et al. Increased body temperature secondary to total parenteral nutrition. Crit Care Med 1980;8:736.
21. Wilson MH. Feeding the healthy child. In: Oski F, ed. Principles and procedures in pediatrics. Philadelphia, J.B. Lippincott, 1990:533.
22. Committee on Nutrition, American Academy of Pediatrics. Prudent life-style for children: dietary fat and cholesterol. Pediatrics 1986;78:521.
23. McLaren DS. The great protein fiasco. Lancet 1974;2:83.
24. McLaren DS. A fresh look at protein-calorie malnutrition. Lancet 1966;2:485.
25. Jelliffe DB. Protein-calorie malnutrition in tropical preschool children: a review of recent knowledge. J Pediatr 1959;54:227.

26. Bistrian BR, Blackburn GL, Hallowell E, et al. Protein status of general surgical patients. JAMA 1974;230:858.
27. Bistrian BR, Blackburn GL, Bitale J, et al. Prevalence of malnutrition in general medical patients. JAMA 1976;235:1567.
28. McLaren SS, Meguid MM. Nutritional assessment at the crossroads. J Parenter Enteral Nutr 1983;7:575.
29. McLaren DS. A fresh look at protein-energy malnutrition in the hospitalized patient. Nutrition 1988;4:1.
30. Levenson SM, Seifter E. Starvation: metabolic and physiologic responses. In: Fischer JE, ed. Surgical Nutrition. Boston, Little, Brown, 1983:423.
31. Cahill GF, Jr. Starvation in man. N Engl J Med 1970;282:668.
32. Owen OE, Felig P, Morgan AP, et al. Liver and kidney metabolism during prolonged starvation. J Clin Invest 1969;48:574.
33. Garber AJ, Menzel PH, Boden G, et al. Hepatic ketogenesis and gluconeogenesis in humans. J Clin Invest 1974;54:981.
34. McGarry FD, Foster DW. Regulation of ketogenesis and clinical aspects of the ketotic state. Metabolism 1972;21:471.
35. Cahill GF, Jr., Herrera MG, Morgan AP, et al. Hormone fuel interrelationships during fasting. J Clin Invest 1966;45:751.
36. Cahill GF Jr, Aoki TT. Conditions with abnormal energy balance: partial and total starvation. In: Kinney JM, ed. Assessment of energy metabolism in health and disease. Columbus, OH, Ross Laboratories, 1980:129.
37. Cahill GF, Jr., Felig P, Marliss EB. Some physiological principles of parenteral nutrition. In: Fox CL, Nahans GG, eds. Body fluid replacement in surgical patients. New York, Grune & Stratton, 1979:286.
38. Gjedde A, Crone C. Induction processes in blood-brain transfer of ketone bodies during starvation. Am J Physiol 1975;229:1165.
39. Owen OE, Morgan AP, Kemp HG, Sullivan JM, et al. Brain metabolism during fasting. J Clin Invest 1967;46:1589.
40. Elia M, et al. Energy metabolism during exercise in normal subjects undergoing total starvation. Hum Nutr Clin Nutr 1984;38:355.
41. Kinney JM, Weissman C. Forms of malnutrition in stressed and unstressed patients. Clin Chest Med 1986;7:19.
42. Viart P. Blood volume(51Cr) in severe protein calorie malnutrition. Am J Clin Nutr 19;29:2576.
43. Cuthbertson DP. The disturbance of metabolism produced by long bone non-bony injury, with notes on certain abnormal conditions of bone. J Biochem 1930;24:1244.
44. Ryan NT. Metabolic adaptions for energy production during trauma and sepsis. Surg Clin North Am 1976;56:1073.
45. Moore FD, Ball MR. The metabolic response to surgery. Springfield, IL: Charles C Thomas, 1952.
46. Moore FD. Bodily changes in surgical convalescence. Ann Surg 1953;137:289.
47. Fath JJ, Meguid MM, Cerra FB. Hormonal and metabolic responses to surgery and stress. In: Goldsmith HM, ed. Practice of surgery. New York, Harper and Row, 1985.
48. Klein S, Peters EJ, Shangraw RE, Wolfe RR. Lipolytic response to metabolic stress in critically ill patients. Crit Care Med 1991;19:776.
49. Long CL, Spencer JL, Kinney JM. Carbohydrate metabolism in man: effects of elective operation and major injury. J Appl Physiol 1971;31:110.
50. Cadwell MD. Importance of cellular metabolism in the inflammatory response to tissue injury. In: Bihari DJ, Cerra FB, eds. Multiple organ failure. Fullerton,CA, Society of Critical Care Medicine, 1989:37.
51. Cerra FB, Seigel JH, Border JR, et al. Correlations between metabolic and cardiopulmonary measurements in patients after trauma, general surgery and sepsis. J Trauma 1979;19:621.
52. Askanazi J, Silverberg PA, Hyman AI, Rosenbaum SH, et al. Patterns of ventilation in postoperative and acutely ill patients. Crit Care Med 1979;7:41.
53. Kinney JM, Askanazi J, Gump FE, Foster RJ, et al. Use of the ventilatory equivalent to separate hypermetabolism from increased dead space ventilation. J Trauma 1980;20:111.
54. Moore FD. Endocrine changes after anesthesia, surgery and unanesthetized trauma in man. Rec Prog Hormone Res 1957;13:511.
55. Popp MB, Brennan MF. Metabolic response to trauma and infection. In: Fischer JE, ed. Surgical Nutrition. Boston, Little, Brown, 1983:479.
56. Moore FD, et al. The body cell mass and its supporting environment. Philadelphia, WB Saunders, 1963.
57. Forse RA, Shizgal HM. The assessment of malnutrition. Surgery 1980;88:17.
58. Perlmutter DH. Distinct mediators and mechanisms regulate human acute phase gene expression. In: Liss AR, ed. Stressed induced proteins. New York, 1989.
59. Fleck A. The acute phase response: implications for nutrition and recovery. Nutrition 1988;4:109.
60. Wilmore DW, Long JM, Mason AD. Catecholamines: mediator of the hypermetabolic response to thermal injury. Ann Surg 1974;180:653.
61. Hume DM, Egdahl RH. The importance of the brain in the endocrine response to injury. Surg Forum 1959;150:697.
62. Hume DM. The secretion of epinephrine, norepinephrine, and corticosteroids in the adrenal venous blood of the dog flowing single and repeated trauma. Surg Forum 1957;8:111.
63. Ukai M, Moran WH Jr., Zimmerman B. The role of visceral afferent pathways on vasopressin secretion and urinary excretory patterns during surgical stress. Ann Surg 1968;168:1.
64. Newsome HH, Rose JC. The response of human adrenocorticotrophic hormone and growth hormone to surgical stress. J Clin Endocrinol Metab 1971;33:481.
65. Bromage RR, Shabata HR, Willoughby HW. Influence of prolonged epidural blockade on blood sugar and cortisol response to operations upon the upper part of the abdomen and the thorax. Surg Gyncol Obstet 1971;132:1051.
66. Hume DM. The endocrine and metabolic response to injury. In: Schwartz SI, ed. Surgery. New York, McGraw-Hill, 1969:2.
67. Hilsted J, Christensen JN, Madsbad S. Whole-body clearance of norepinephrine. J Clin Invest 1983;71:500.
68. Breslow MJ, et al. Epidural morphine decreases post-operative hypertension by attenuating sympathetic nervous system hyperactivity. JAMA 1989;261:3577.
69. Sandberg AA, et al. The effects of surgery on the blood levels and metabolism of 17-hydroxy-corticosteroids. J Clin Invest 1954;33:1509.
70. Udelsman RA, et al. Responses of the hypothalamic-pituitary-adrenal and renin-angiotensin axes and the sympathetic nervous system during controlled surgical and anesthetic stress. J Clin Endocrinol Metabol 1987;64:986.
71. Bormann BV, et al. Influence of epidural fentanyl on stressed induced elevations of plasma vasopressin (ADH) after surgery. Anesth Analg 1983;62:727.
72. Matsubara Y, Iwafuchi M, Muto T, et al. Plasma glucagon changes in surgical patients. Jpn J Surg 1979;9:327.
73. Breslow MJ. Neuroendocrine response to surgery. In: Breslow MJ, Miller CF, Rogers MC, eds. Perioperative management. St. Louis, CV Mosby, 1990:180.
74. Roh MS, Moldawer LL, Ekman LG, et al. Stimulatory effect of interleukin-1 upon hepatic metabolism. Metabolism 1986;35:419.
75. Beutler BV, Cerami A. Cachectin (tumor necrosis factor): a macrophage hormone governing cellular metabolism and inflammatory response. Endocrine Rev 1988;9:57.
76. Gump FE, Long C, Killian P, Kinney JM. Studies of glucose intolerance in septic injured patients. J Trauma 1974;14:387.
77. Wolfe RR. Carbohydrates metabolism in critically ill patients. Crit Care Med 1987;3:11.
78. Wolfe RR, Allsop JR, Burke JF. Glucose metabolism in man: metabolic responses to intravenous glucose infusion. Metabolism 1979;28:210.
79. Gil KM, Askanazi J, Human AI. Substrate utilization in the acutely ill: implications for nutritional support. In: Shoemaker WC, ed. Critical care medicine: state of the art. Fullerton, CA, Society of Critical Care Medicine, 1984.
80. Wolfe RR, Durkot MJ, Allsop JR, et al. Glucose metabolism in severely burned patients. Metabolism 1979;28:1031.
81. Meszaros K, Bojta J, Bautista AP, et al. Glucose utilization by Kupffer cells, endothelial cells and granulocytes in endotoxemic rat liver. Am J Physiol 1991;260:C7.
82. Weiner M, Rothkopf MM, Rothkopf G, et al. Fat metabolism in injury and sepsis. Crit Care Clin 1987;3:25.
83. Carpentier YA, Askanazi J, Elwyn DH, et al. Effects of hypercaloric glucose infusion on lipid metabolism in injury and sepsis. J Trauma 1979;19:649.
84. Carpentier YA, Askanazi J, Elwyn DH, et al. The effect of carbohydrate intake on the lipolytic rate in depleted patients. Metabolism 1980;29:974.
85. Nordenstrom J, Carpentier YA, Askanazi J, et al. Metabolic utilization of intravenous fat emulsion during total parenteral nutrition. Ann Surg 1982;196:221.
86. Galster AD, Bier DM, Cryer PE, et al. Plasma palmitate turnover in subjects with thermal injury. J Trauma 1984;24:938.
87. Kaminski DL, Adams A, Jellinek M. The effect of hyperalimentation on hepatic lipid content and lipogenic enzyme activity in rats and man. Surgery 1980;88:93.

88. Long CL, Schaffel N, Geiger JW, et al. Metabolic response to injury and illness: estimation of energy and protein needs from indirect calorimetry and nitrogen balance. J Parenter Enteral Nutr 1979;3:452.
89. Elwyn DH. Protein metabolism and requirements in critically ill patients. Crit Care Clin 1987;3:57.
90. Kien CL, Young RV, Rohrbaugh DR, Burke JF. Increased rates of whole body protein synthesis and breakdown in children recovering from burns. Ann Surg 1978;187:833.
91. Birkhahn RH, Long CL, Fitkin D, Geiger JW, et al. Effects of major skeletal trauma on whole body protein turnover in man measured by L-(1, 14C)-leucine. Surgery 1980;88:294.
92. Long CL, Jeevanandam M, Kim BM, Kinney JM. Whole body protein synthesis and metabolism in septic man. Am J Clin Nutr 1977;30:1340.
93. Duke JH Jr, Jorgenson SB, Broell JR, Long CL, et al. Contribution of protein to caloric expenditure following injury. Surgery 1970;68:168.
94. Waterlow JC. Classification and definition of protein-calorie malnutrition. Br Med J 1972;3:566.
95. Pollack MM, Wiley JS, Holbrook PR. Early nutritional depletion in critically ill children. Crit Care Med 1981;9:580.
96. Dauncey MJ, Gandy G, Gairdner D. Assessment of total body fat in infancy from skinfold thickness measurements. Arch Dis Child 1977;52:223.
97. Frisancho AR. Triceps skinfold and upper arm muscle size norms for assessment of nutritional status. Am J Clin Nutr 1974;27:1052.
98. Deutschman CS. Protein-energy malnutrition in the perioperative period. In: Breslow MJ, Miller CF, Rogers MC, eds. Perioperative management. St. Louis, CV Mosby, 1989.
99. McFarlane H, Ogbeide S, Reddy K, Adock J, et al. Biochemical assessment of protein-calorie malnutrition. Lancet 1969;1:392.
100. Ingebleek Y, DeVisscher M, DeNayer P. Measurement of prealbumin as index of protein-calorie malnutrition. Lancet 1972;2:106.
101. Sirisinha S, Suskind R, Edelman R, Charupaiana C, et al. Complement and C3-proactivator levels in children with protein-calorie malnutrition and effect of dietary treatment. Lancet 1991;1:101673.
102. Young GA, Chen C, Hill GL. Assessment of protein-calorie malnutrition in surgical patients from plasma proteins and anthropometric measurements. Am J Clin Nutr 1978;31:429.
103. Rothschild MA, Oratz M, Schreiber SS. Albumin synthesis. N Engl J Med 1972;286:748.
104. Whitehead RG, Coward WA, Lunn PG. Serum albumin concentration and onset of kwashiorkor. Lancet 1973;1:63.
105. Awai M, Brown EB. Studies of the metabolism of I^{131} labelled human transferrin. J Lab Clin Med 1963;61:363.
106. Ingenbleek Y, Vanden Schrieck G, DeNayer P, DeVisscher M. Albumin, transferrin, and the thyronine-binding prealbumin/retinol-binding protein (TBPA-RBP) complex in assessment of malnutrition. Clin Chim Acta 1975;63:61.
107. Peterson PA. Demonstration in serum of two physiological forms of the human retinol binding protein. Eur J Clin Invest 1971;1:437.
108. Deo MG, Ghan AK, Ramalingaswani V. Metabolism of albumin and body fluid compartments in protein deficiency: an experimental study in rhesus monkeys. J Nutr 1986;5:63.
109. Broom J, Fraser MH, McKenzie K. The protein metabolic response to short-term starvation in men. Clin Nutr 1986;5:63.
110. Jones WPT, Hay AM. Albumin metabolism: effect of nutritional state and dietary protein intake. J Clin Invest 1979;47:1958.
111. Keys A, et al. The biology of human starvation. Minneapolis: University of Minnesota Press, 1950.
112. Roza AM, Tuitt D, Shizgal HM. Transferrin-A poor measure of nutritional status. J Parenter Enteral Nutr 1984;8:523.
113. Fleck A. The acute phase response: implications for nutrition and recovery. Nutrition 1988;4:109.
114. Golden MHN. Transport proteins as indices of nutritional status. Am J Clin Nutr 1982;35:1159.
115. Starker PM. Serum albumin levels as an index of nutritional support. Surgery 1982;91:194.
116. Buzby GP. Prognostic nutritional index in gastrointestinal surgery. Am J Surg 1980;139:160.
117. Harvey KB. Biological measures of the formulation of a hospital prognostic index. Am J Clin Nutr 1981;34:2013.
118. Mickell JJ. Urea nitrogen excretion in critically ill children. Pediatrics 1982;70:949.
119. Bistrian BR, Blackburn GL, Scrimshaw NS, Flatt J. Cellular immunity in semistarved states in hospitalized adults. Am J Clin Nutr 1975;28:1148.
120. Meakins JL. Delayed hypersensitivity: indicator of acquired failure of host defenses in sepsis and trauma. Ann Surg 1977;186:241.
121. Jeejeebhoy KN, Meguid MM. Assessment of nutritional status in the oncologic patient. Surg Clin North Am 1986;66:1077.
122. Miler CL. Immunological assays as measurements of nutritional status: a review. J Parenter Enteral Nutr 1978;2:554.
123. Twomey P, Ziegler D, Rombeau J. Utility of skin testing in nutritional assessment: a critical review. J Parenter Enteral Nutr 1982;6:50.
124. Abbott WC, et al. The effect of nutritional support on T-Lymphocyte subpopulations in protein calorie malnutrition. J Am Coll Nutr 1986;5:577.
125. Baker JP, et al. Nutritional assessment: a comparison of clinical judgment and objective measurements. N Engl J Med 1982;206:969.
126. Detsky AS, et al. Evaluating the accuracy of nutritional assessment techniques applied to hospitalized patients: methodology and comparisons. J Parenter Enteral Nutr 1984;8:153.
127. MacBurney M, Wilmore DW. Decision-making in nutritional care. Surg Clin North Am 1981;61:571.
128. Ottow RT, Bruining HA, Jeekel J. Clinical judgement versus delayed hypersensitivity skin testing for the prediction of postoperative sepsis and mortality. Surg Gynecol Obstet 1984;159:475.
129. Bursztein S, Elwyn DH, Askanazi J. Energy metabolism, indirect calorimetry and nutrition. Baltimore: Williams & Wilkins, 1989.
130. Consolazio CF, Johnson RE, Pecora LJ. Physiological measuremennt of metabolic functions in man. New York: McGraw-Hill, 1963:
131. Kinney MM, Zarem HA, Rogers RL. Energy expenditure and utilization of carbohydrate, fat, and protein in hospitalized patients. J Clin Invest 1959;38:1017.
132. Harris JA, Benedict TG. In: Biometric studies of basal metabolism in man. Publication 279. Washington, DC, Carnegie Institute, 1919.
133. Peden V, Witzleben C, Skelton M. Total parenteral nutrition. J Pediatr 1971;78:180.
134. Kudsk KA. Clinical applications of enteral nutrition. Nutr Clin Practice 1994;9:165.
135. Zaloga GP. Nutrition and the prevention of systemic infection. In: Taylor RW, Shoemaker WC, eds. Critical care: state of the art. Fullerton, CA, Vol. 12. Society of critical care medicine, Fullerton, CA 1991.
136. Ryan GP, Dudrick SJ, Copeland EM, et al. Effects of various diets on colonic growth in rats. Gastroenterology 1979;77:658.
137. Johnson LR, Copeland EM, Dudrick SJ, et al. Structural and hormonal alterations in the gastrointestinal tract of parenterally fed rats. Gastroenterology 1975;68:1177.
138. Levine GM, Deren JJ, Steiger E, et al. Role of oral intake in maintenance of gut mass and disaccharidase activity. Gastroenterology 1974;67:975.
139. Thompson JS, Vaigam WP, Forst CF, et al. The effect of nutrient delivery on gut structure and diamine oxidase levels. J Parenter Enteral Nutr 1987;11:28.
140. Windmueller HG. Glutamine utilization by the small intestine. Adv Enzymol 1982;53:201.
141. Lickley HHLA, Track NS, Vranic M, et al. Metabolic response to enteral and parenteral nutrition. Am J Surg 1978;135:172.
142. Steiner M, Bourges HS, Freeman LS. Effect of starvation on the tissue composition of the intestine in the rat. Am J Physiol 1969;215:75.
143. Gleeson MH, Dowling RH, Peters TJ. Biochemical changes in intestinal mucosa after experimental small bowel by-pass in the rat. Clin Sci 1972;43:743.
144. Souba WW, Wilmore DW. Postoperative alterations of arteriovenous exchange of amino acids across the gastrointestinal tract. Surgery 1984;84:342.
145. Deitch EA, Wintertron J, Li MA. The gut is a portal of entry for bacteremia. Ann Surg 1987;205:681.
146. Alverdy JC, Aoys E, Moss GS. Total parenteral nutrition promotes bacterial translocation from the gut. Surgery 1988;104:185.
147. Bell SJ, Mascioli EA, Bistrian BR, Babayan VK, et al. Alternative lipid sources for enteral and parenteral nutrition: Long- and medium-chain triglycerides, structured triglycerides, and fish oils. Journal of the American Dietetic Association 1991;91:74.
148. Materese LE. Enteral Nutrition. In: Fischer JE, ed. Surgical Nutrition. Boston: Little, Brown, 1983.
149. Cerra FB, ed. Pocket manual of surgical nutrition. St. Louis: C.V. Mosby, 1984.
150. Schlichtig R, Ayres SM. Nutritional support of the critically ill. Chicago: Year Book, 1988.
151. Byrne WJ, Euler AR, Ashcraft E. Gastroesophageal reflux in the severely retarded who vomit: criteria for the results of surgical intervention in twenty-two patients. Surgery 1982;91:95.
152. Mollitt DL, Golladay ES, Seibert JJ. Symptomatic gastroesophageal re-

flux following gastrostomy in neurologically impaired patients. Pediatrics 1985;75:1124.
153. Grant JP, Curtas MS, Kelvin KM. Fluoroscopic placement of nasojejunal feeding tubes with immediate feeding using a non-elemental formula. J Parenter Enteral Nutr 1983;7:299.
154. Kelly TW, Patrick MR, Hillman KM. Study of diarrhea in critically ill patients. Crit Care Med 1983;11:7.
155. Nelson LM, Russell RI. Influence of the intake and composition of elemental diets on bile acid metabolism and hepatic lipids in the rat. J Parenter Enteral Nutr 1986;10:399.
156. Zarchy TM, Lipman TO, Finkelstein JD. Elevated transaminases associated with an elemental diet. Ann Intern Med 1978;89:221.
157. Heird WC. Amino acid and energy needs of pediatric patients receiving parenteral nutrition. In: Gaull GE, ed. Pediatric clinics of North America. Philadelphia, W.B. Saunders, 1995:765.
158. Helfrick FW, Abelson NM. Intravenous feeding of a complete diet in a child: A report of a case. J Pediatr 1944;25:400.
159. Dudrick SJ, Wilmore DW, Vars HS. Long-term total parenteral nutrition with growth, development, and positive nitrogen balance. Surgery 1968;64:134.
160. Gramlich LM, Bistrian BR. Cyclic parenteral nutrition: Considerations of carbohydrate and lipid metabolism. Nutrition in Clinical Practice 1994;9:49.
161. Burke JF, Wolfe RR, Mullany CJ, Mathews DE, et al. Glucose requirements following burn injury. Ann Surg 1979;190:274.
162. Elwyn DH, Kinney JM, Jeevanandam M. Influence of increasing carbohydrate intake on glucose kinetics in injured patients. Ann Surg 1979;32:117.
163. Askanazi J, Rosenbaum SH, Michelsen CB, Elwyn DH, et al. Increased body temperature secondary to total parenteral nutrition. Crit Care Med 1980;8:736.
164. Askanazi J, Nordenstrom J, Rosenbaum SH, et al. Nutrition for the patients with respiratory failure: glucose vs. fat. Anesthesiology 1981;54:373.
165. Nordenstrom J, Jeevanandam M, Elwyn DH. Increasing glucose intake during total parenteral nutrition increases norepinephrine excretion in trauma and sepsis. Clin Physiol 1981;1:525.
166. Friedman Z, Danon A, Stahlman MT, et al. Rapid onset of essential fatty acid deficiency in the newborn. Pediatrics 1978;58:640.
167. Kaufmann RL, Matson CF, Rowberg AH, Beisel WR. Defective lipid disposal mechanisms during bacterial infection in rhesus monkeys. Metabolism 1976;25:615.
168. Robin AP, Askanazi J, Greenwood MRC. Lipoprotein lipase activity in surgical patients: influence of trauma and infection. Surgery 1981;90:401.
169. Nordenstrom J, Askanazi J, Elwyn DH. Nitrogen balance during total parenteral nutrition: Glucose vs. fat. Ann Surg 1983;197:27.
170. Robin AP, Nordenstrom J, Askanazi J, et al. Plasma clearance of fat emulsion in trauma and sepsis: use of a three-stage lipid clearance test. J Parenter Enteral Nutr 1980;4:505.
171. Long JM III, Wilmore DW, Mason AD Jr. Effect of carbohydrate and fat intake on nitrogen excretion during total intravenous feeding. Ann Surg 1977;185:417.
172. Woolfson AMJ, Heatley RV, Allison SP. Insulin to inhibit protein catabolism after injury. N Engl J Med 1979;300:14.
173. Jeejeebhoy KM, Anderson GH, Nakhooda AF. Metabolic studies in total parenteral nutrition with lipid in man: comparison with glucose. J Clin Invest 1976;57:125.
174. Bark S, Holm I, Hakansson I, Wretlind A. Nitrogen sparing effect of fat emulsion compared with glucose in the postoperative period. Acta Chir Scand 1976;142:423.
175. Barton RG. Nutrition support in critical illness. Nutr Clin Prac 1994;9:127.
176. Greene HL, Hazlett O, Demaree R. Relationship between intralipid-induced hyperlipemia and pulmonary function. Am J Clin Nutr 1976;29:127.
177. Sundstrom G, Zauner GW, Arborelius M. Decrease in pulmonary diffusing capacity during lipid infusion in healthy men. J Appl Physiol 1973;34:816.
178. Wiener L, Forsyth D. Pulmonary pathophysiology of fat embolism. Am Rev Respir Dis 1965;92:113.
179. McKeen CR, Brigham KL, Bowers RE, Harris TR. Pulmonary vascular effects of fat emulsion infusion in unanesthetized sheep: prevention by indomethacin. J Clin Invest 1978;62:129.
180. Inwood RJ, Gora P, Hunt CE. Indomethacin inhibition of intralipid-induced lung dysfunction. Prostaglandins Med 1981;6:503.
181. Brass EP, Hoppel CL. Carnitine metabolism in the fasting rat. J Biol Chem 1978;253:2588.
182. Haumont D, Deckelbaum RJ, Richelle M, et al. Plasma lipid and plasma lipoprotein concentrations in low birth weight infants given parenteral nutrition with 20% compared to 10% Intralipid. J Pediatr 1989;115:787.
183. Fomon SJ. Requirements and recommended dietary intake of protein during infancy. Pediatr Res 1991;30:391.
184. Fomon SJ, Bell EF. Energy. In: Fomon SJ, ed. Nutrition of Normal Infants. St. Louis, C.V. Mosby, 1995:103.
185. Knutrud O. The water and electrolyte metabolism in the newborn child after major surgery. Oslo, Norway: Universitets Forlaget, 1965.
186. Fomon SJ, Ziegler EE, Filer LJ, et al. Methionine fortification of soy protein formula fed to infants. Am J Clin Nutr 1979;32:2460.
187. Fischer JE, Rosen HM, Eveid A, James JH, et al. The effect of normalization of plasma amino acids on hepatic encephalopathy in man. Surgery 1976;81:77.
188. Daly JM, Mihranian MH, Kehoe JE. Effects of post-operative infusion of branched chain amino acids on nitrogen balance and forearm muscle substrate flux. Surgery 1983;94:151.
189. Bonau RA, Jeevanandam M, Moldawer L. Muscle amino acid flux in patients receiving branched-chain amino acid solutions after surgery. Surgery 1987;101:400.
190. Abumnrad NN, Robinson RP, Goochi BR. The effect of leucine infusion on substrate flux across the human forearm. J Surg Res 1982;32:453.
191. Aoki T, Brennan MF, Fitzpatrick GF. Leucine meal increases glutamine and total nitrogen release from forearm muscle. J Clin Invest 1981;68:1522.
192. Cerra FB, Mazuski J, Teasley K. Nitrogen retention in critically ill patients is proportional to the branched chain amino acid load. Crit Care Med 1983;11:775.
193. Bonau RA, Aug SD, Jeevanadam M. High branched chain amino acid solutions: relationship of composition to efficacy. J Parenter Enteral Nutr 1984;8:622.
194. Freund H, Hoover HC, Atamian S. Infusion of the branched chain amino acids in postoperative patients. Ann Surg 1979;190:18.
195. Cerra F, Hirsh J, Mullen K. The effect of stress level, amino acid formula, and nitrogen dose on nitrogen retention in trauma and septic stress. Ann Surg 1986;205:282.
196. Cerra FB, Chung NK, Fischer JE. Disease specific amino acid infusion (F080) in hepatic encephalopathy: a prospective randomized double blind controlled trial. J Parenter Enteral Nutr 1985;9:288.
197. Matarese LE. Rationale and efficacy of specialized enteral nutrition. Nutr Clin Practice 1994;9:58.
198. Windmueller HG, Spaeth AE. Uptake and metabolism of plasma glutamine by the small intestine. J Biol Chem 1974;249:5070.
199. Klimberg VS, Souba WW, Sitren H. Glutamine-enriched total parenteral nutrition supports gut metabolism. Surg Forum 1989;15:175.
200. Hwang TL, O'Dwyer ST, Smith RJ. Preservation of small bowel mucosa using glutamine-enriched parenteral nutrition. Surg Forum 1987;38:56.
201. Grant JP, Snyder PJ. Use of L-glutamine in total parenteral nutrition. J Surg Res 1988;44:506.
202. Meritt J, Witkowski TA, Nagele R. Glutamine and smooth muscle morphology of the gut in rats on total parenteral nutrition. J Am Coll Nutr 1989;8:537.
203. O'Dwyer ST, Scott T, Smith RJ. 5-Fluorouracil toxicity on small intestine mucosa but not white blood cells is decreased by glutamine. Abstr Clin Res 1987;35:369A.
204. O'Dwyer ST, Smith RJ, Kripke SA. New fuels for the gut. In: Rombeau JL, Caldwell MD, eds. Clinical nutrition: enteral and tube feeding. Philadelphia, W.B. Saunders, 1990:540.
205. Stehle P, Zander J, Mertes N. Effect of parenteral glutamine peptide suppplements on muscle glutamine loss and nitrogen balance after major surgery. Lancet 1989;1:231.
206. Hammargvist F, Wernerman J, Ali R, et al. Addition of glutamine to total parenteral nutrition after elective abdominal surgery spores free glutamine in muscle, counteracts the fall in muscle protein synthesis and improves nitrogen balance. Ann Surg 1989;209:455.
207. Elwyn DH, Grump FE, Munro HN. Changes in nitrogen balance of depleted patients with increasing infusions of glucose. J Clin Nutr 1979;32:1597.
208. Rudman D, et al. Elemental balances during intravenous hyperalimentation of under-weight adult subjects. J Clin Invest 1975;55:94.
209. Barac-Nicto M, Spurr GB, Lotero H, Maksud MG, et al. Body composition during nutritional repletion of severely undernourished man. Am J Clin Nutr 1979;32:981.

210. Sherwin RS. Effect of starvation on the turnover and metabolic response to leucine. J Clin Invest 1978;61:1471.
211. Elwyn DH, Bryan-Brown CW, Shoemaker WC. Nutritional aspects of body water dislocations in postoperative and depleted patients. Ann Surg 1975;182:76.
212. Shizgal HM. Effect of malnutrition on body composition. Surg Gynecol Obstet 1981;152:22.
213. Larca L, Greenbaum DM. Effectiveness of intensive nutritional regimes in patients who fail to wean from mechanical ventilation. Crit Care Med 1982;10:297.
214. Souba WW, Wilmore DW. Planning total parenteral nutrition. Clin Anaesth 1983;633:
215. Denedic FG, Talbot FB. The gaseous metabolism of infants. 210th ed. Washington, D.C.: 1914:168.
216. LaSala PA, Starker PM, Askanazi J. The saphenous system for long-term parenteral nutrition. Crit Care Med 1983;11:378.
217. Donahoe PK, Kim SH. The inferior epigastric vein as an alternate site for central venous hyperalimentation. Pediatr Surg 1980;15:737.
218. Fischer JE, Freund HR. Central alimentation. In: Fischer JE, ed. Surgical nutrition. Boston, Little, Brown, 1983.
219. Syndman DR. Total parenteral nutrition related infections: prospective epidemiological study using semi-quantitative methods. Am J Med 1984;73:695.
220. Linares J, Sitges-Serra A, Garau J. Pathogenesis of catheter sepsis: a prospective study with quantitative and semiquantitative cultures of catheter hub and segments. Clin Microbiol 1985;21:357.
221. Harris JA, Cobb CG. Persistent Gram-negative bacteremia: observations in twenty patients. Am J Surg 1983;125:705.
222. Grant JP. Serum hepatic enzyme and bilirubin elevations during parenteral nutrition. Surg Gynecol Obstet 1977;145:573.
223. Askanazi J, Rosenbaum SH, Hyman AI. Respiratory changes induced by the large glucose loads of total parenteral nutrition. JAMA 1980;243:1444.
224. McDonald ATJ, Phillips MJ, Jeejeebhoy KN. Reversal of fatty liver by intralipid in patients on total parenteral alimentation. Gastroenterology 1973;64:885.
225. Meguid MM, et al. Reduced metabolic complications in total parenteral nutrition: pilot study using fat to replace one third of glucose calories. J Parenter Enteral Nutr 1984;5:304.
226. Cerra FB. Hypermetabolism, organ failure and metabolic support. Surgery 1987;101:1.
227. Jeejeebhoy KN, Marliss EB. Energy supply in total parenteral nutrition. In: Fischer JE, ed. Surgical nutrition. Boston, Little, Brown, 1983.
228. Gibson JC, Simons LA, Raik E, Barton L. Haematological and biochemical abnormalities associated with intralipid hyperalimentation. Anaesth Intensive Care 1978;6:350.
229. Fischer JW, et al. Diminished bacterial defenses with intralipid. Lancet 1980;2:819.
230. Hamaway KJ, Moldawer LL, Georggieff M. The effects of lipid emulsions on reticuloendothelial system function in the injured animal. J Parenter Enteral Nutr 1985;9:559.
231. Shennib H, et al. Depression and delayed recovery of alveolar macrophage function during starvation and refeeding. Surg Gynecol Obstet 1984;158:535.
232. Sobrado J, et al. Lipid emulsions and reticuloendothelial system function in healthy and burned guinea pigs. J Clin Nutr 1985;42:855.
233. Allerdyee DB. Cholestasis caused by lipid emulsions. Surg Gynecol Obstet 1982;154:641.
234. Hageman JR, Hunt CE. Fat emulsions and lung function. Clin Chest Med 1986;7:69.
235. Agusti ASGN, et al. Hypophosphatemia as a cause of failed weaning: the importance of metabolic factors. Crit Care Med 1984;12:142.
236. Iseri LT, Freed J, Bures AT. Magnesium deficiency and cardiac disorders. Am J Med 1985;58:837.
237. Knochel JP. The pathophysiology and clinical characteritics of severe hypophosphatemia. Ann Intern Med 1977;137:203.
238. Molloy DW, et al. Hypomagnesemia and respiratory muscle power. Am Rev Respir Dis 1984;129:497.
239. Silvas SE, Paragas PD. Paresthesias, weakness, seizures and hypophosphatemia in patients receiving hyperalimentation. Gastroenterology 1972;62:513.
240. Messing B, et al. Does total parenteral nutrition induce gall bladder sludge formation in lithiasis. Gastroenterology 1983;84:1012.
241. Baker SS, Cohen JH. Altered oxidative metabolism in selenium deficient rat granulocytes. J Immunol 1983;130:2856.
242. Shils ME, Jacobs DH, Cunningham-Rundles S. Selenium deficiency and immune function in home TPN patients. Am J Clin Nutr 1983;37:716.
243. Prasad AS. Clinical, endocrinological and biochemical effects of zinc deficiency. Clin Endocrinol Metabol 1985;14:567.
244. Jeejeebhoy KN, et al. Chromium deficiency, glucose intolerance and neuropathy reversed by chromium supplementation in a patient receiving long-term total parenteral nutrition. Am J Clin Nutr 1977;30:531.
245. Bozzetti F, Inglese MG, Terno G. Hypocupremia in patients receiving total parenteral nutrition. J Parenter Enteral Nutr 1983;7:563.
246. Shike M. Cooper in parenteral nutrition. Bull NY Acad Med 1984;60:132.
247. King WWK, et al. Nutritional efficacy and hepatic changes during intragastric, intravenous and prehepatic feeding in rats. J Parenter Enteral Nutr 1983;7:443.
248. Sheldon GF, Peterson ST, Saunders R. Hepatic dysfunction during hyperalimentation. Arch Surg 1978;113:504.
249. Duetschman CS, et al. Transient elevation of hepatic enzymes following resumption of gut feedings in ICU patients. Nutr Int 1987;3:42.
250. Nugent KM. Intralipid effects on reticuloendothelial function. J Leukocyte Biol 1984;36:123.
251. Loo LS, Tang JP, Kohn S. Inhibition of cellular cytotoxicity of leukocytes for herpes simplex virus-infected cells in vitro and in vivo by intralipid. J Infec Dis 1982;146:64.
252. Palmblad J, Brostrom O, Lahnborg G. Neutrophil functions during total parenteral nutrition and Intralipid infusion. Am J Clin Nutr 1982;35:1430.
253. Shamberger RC, Pizzo PH, Goodgame JT. The effect of total parenteral nutrition on chemotherapy-induced myelosuppression. Am J Med 1983;74:40.
254. Beale EF, Nelson RM, Bucciarelli RL. Intrahepatic cholestasis associated with parenteral nutrition in premature infants. Pediatrics 1979;64:342.
255. Hodes JE, Grosfeld JL, Weber TR. Hepatic failure in infants on total parenteral nutrition (TPN): clinical and histopathologic observation. J Pediatr Surg 1982;17:463.
256. Benjamin DR. Hepatobiliary dysfunction in infants and children associated with long-term total parenteral nutrition. A clinico-pathologic study. Am Soc Clin Pathol 1981;76:276.
257. Akierman A, Elliott PD, Gall DG. Association of cholelithiasis with total parenteral nutrition and fasting in a preterm infant. Can Med Assoc J 1984;131:122.
258. Pereira GR, Sherman MS, DiGiacomo J. Hyperalimentation-induced cholestasis. Am J Dis Child 1981;135:842.
259. Thompson JS, Madison Hodges R.E.. The incidence and prevention of complications of total parenteral nutrition. Nebr Med J 1983;68:321.
260. Sinatra FR. Cholestasis in infancy and childhood. Curr Probl Pediatr 1982;12:3.
261. Manginello FP, Javitt NB. Parenteral nutrition and neonatal cholestasis. J Pediatr 1979;94:296.
262. Barnes S, Berkowitz G, Hirschowitz BI. Postnatal physiological hypercholemia in both premature and fullterm infants. J Clin Invest 1981;68:775.
263. Dahms BB, Halpin TC. Serial liver biopsies in parenteral nutrition-associated cholestasis of early infancy. Gastroenterology 1981;81:136.
264. Vileisis RA, Inwood RJ, Hunt CE. Prospective controlled study of parenteral nutrition-associated cholestatic jaundice: effect of protein intake. Pediatrics 1980;96:893.
265. Parsa MN, Habif DV, Gerrer JM. Indications technique and complication. Bull NY Acad Med 1972;48:920.
266. Sheldon GF, Peterson SR, Sanders R. Hepatic dysfunction during hyperalimentation. Arch Surg 1978;113:504.
267. Cohen IT. Special considerations in the paediatric patients. Clin Anaesthesiol 1983;1:669.
268. Merritt RJ, Sinatra RR, Henton D, Neustein H. Cholestatic effect of intraperitoneal administration of tryptophane to suckling rat pups. Pediatr Res 1984;18:904.
269. Seashore JH. Metabolic complications of parenteral nutrition in infants and children. Surg Clin North Am 1980;60:1239.
270. Doty JE, Pitt HA, Porter-Fink V, Denbestein L. Cholecystokinin prophylaxis of parenteral nutrition-induced gall-bladder disease. Ann Surg 1984;201:76.
271. Capron JP, Herve MA, Gineston JL, Braillon A. Metronidazole in prevention of cholestasis associated with total parenteral nutrition. Lancet 1983;1:446.
272. Guertin F, Toy CC, Lepiji G, et al. Effects of taurine on total parenteral nutrition-associated cholestasis. J Parenter Enteral Nutr 1991;15:247.

Gastrointestinal and Hepatic Failure in the Pediatric Intensive Care Unit

36

Glenn T. Furuta,
Elizabeth L. Rogers, and
Alan M. Leichtner

INTRODUCTION

The gastrointestinal (GI) tract serves as the portal of entry for both nutrients and potential pathogens. Diseases of the GI tract may themselves necessitate admission of a patient to the intensive care unit (ICU) or may complicate disorders of other systems. Some GI complications are avoidable, most are treatable, but all are potentially lethal. Children admitted to the ICU, regardless of their primary illness, may have their course complicated by bleeding, ileus, diarrhea, or pancreatitis. Optimal outcome depends on careful repeated monitoring, appropriate diagnostic testing, and rapid intervention when required.

HOST DEFENSE MECHANISMS

The GI tract serves as not only a digestive organ but also as the largest immune organ in the body. During a lifetime, the gut is exposed to more than 100 tons of foodstuffs. The adult GI tract reaches a length of over 7 meters and spans a surface area of 400 m^2. The GI lumen and brush border

Table 36.1. Nonimmune and Immune Elements of the Gastrointestinal Tract

NONIMMUNE
Saliva
Gastric acid
Proteolytic enzymes
Bile
Cryptdins
Epithelial tight junctions
Peristalsis
IMMUNE
B cells
T cells
Helper T cells
Suppresor T cells
Macrophages
Neutrophils
Mast cells
Eosinophils
Immunoglobulins
Cytokines

contain digestive mediators such as hydrochloric acid, lipase, bile, proteolytic enzymes, and disaccharidases. To maintain the patient's nutritional state, these agents digest fat, protein, and carbohydrates, so that nutrients may be absorbed and transported to the liver to be used as energy and biosynthetic substrates. Despite its importance, the gut is one of the first major organs affected by shock and one of the last to regain tissue oxygenation and blood flow[1]. In order to protect the body from its constant exposure to microbes, toxins, and other antigenic stimuli, the gut has developed an intricate array of defense **(Table 36.1).**

Nonimmune defense elements include chemical and mechanical barriers such as saliva, gastric acid, proteolytic enzymes, bile, cryptdins, and the epithelial tight junctions[2,3]. Saliva contains peroxidase, which inhibits the growth of bacteria, and lysozyme, which lyses bacteria and enhances phagocytosis. The mucous layer provides a barrier separating bacteria from the villous surface of the small intestine. The bile acids, chenodeoxycholic and cholic acids, possess antibacterial qualities. Cryptdins are low molecular weight proteins that are derived from the Paneth cells in the crypts of Lieberkuhn. Preliminary findings suggest that cryptdins may form an antimicrobial barrier in the intestinal tract.

The gut contains more than 10^{10} immunologically active cells that constitute more than half of the lymphoid cells of the body. These cells produce a variety of soluble mediators, such as immunoglobulins and cytokines, which participate in both the protection of the intestine from chronic exposure to foreign particles and the processing of antigen if these should penetrate the mucosal surface[4,5]. Secretory immunoglobulin A (IgA) binds to bacteria in the lumen, thus preventing the microrganisms from attaching to mucosa. Antigens that penetrate the nonimmune defenses and avoid contact with IgA may break through the epithelium, thus encountering resident T cells, B cells, mast cells, eosinophils, and monocytes. In concert with their mediators, these cells protect the host from potential insult from antigens. For instance, the heterogeneous mast cell population that resides in the mucosa and submucosa may participate in an immediate type hypersensitivity response to foreign antigen. Histamine release from the mast cells may stimulate intestinal fluid secretion and peristalsis and thus potentially remove the antigen[6].

GASTROINTESTINAL BLEEDING

Definition

Upper or lower GI bleeding may be the primary reason for admission to the ICU, or it may represent a complication of a critically ill patient's primary disease. By definition, upper GI tract bleeding originates proximal to the ligament of Trietz and presents with hematemesis, bloody gastric aspirates, or rectal bleeding. Nasal bleeding or hemopytsis should be excluded as sources. Lower GI tract bleeding is the result of mucosal disruption distal to the ligament of Trietz and may present as either melena or hematochezia. Melena is defined as black, tarry stools containing denatured blood; hematochezia is bright red blood from the rectum. Currant jelly stool is a descriptive term for a mixture of mucus and blood seen in patients with ischemic injury.

Two factors are unique to establishing the cause of bleeding in pediatric patients. First, the patient's age can serve as a guide in establishing the cause of bleeding. For example, a neonate may have hematochezia from milk protein allergy, whereas this symptom would be very unusual in an adult patient. Second, several congenital and hereditary vascular or polypoid disorders may be more apt to manifest with GI bleeding in the pediatric age range **(Table 36.2).**

Presentation

Massive upper GI bleeding, i.e., bleeding severe enough to produce hypotension or require transfusion, is an unusual occurrence in pediatric patients. Causes include peptic ulcer disease, esophageal or gastric varices, and vascular malformations[7,8]. Massive lower intestinal bleeding may occur in patients with Crohn's disease, ulcerative colitis, Meckel's diverticulum, intussusception, Schönlein-Henoch purpura, vascular malformations, intestinal duplications, ischemic injury, or hemolytic uremic syndrome[9–11]. Gastritis, or gastric and duodenal ulcers, may be secondary to acid injury, medication toxicity, or *Helicobacter pylori* infection[12]. Medications that may cause damage to the gastric mucosa include aspirin, nonsteroidal antiinflammatory drugs (NSAIDs), and high-dose corticosteroids. Gastritis caused by *H. pylori* infection is characterized by a mixed infiltrate of plasma cells, lymphocytes, and polymorphonuclear cells in association with urease-producing flagellated gram-negative organisms. *H. pylori* is the leading cause of duodenal and gastric ulcers in adults. Diagnostic tests include serologic measurements of *H. pylori*-specific IgG, breath tests for urea production, endoscopic biopsies

Table 36.2. Causes of Gastrointestinal Bleeding

	Upper Gastrointestinal Bleeding	
Newborns and infants	Toddlers	Children and adolescents
Swallowed maternal blood	Esophagitis	Esophagitis
Esophagitis	Mallory-Weiss syndrome	Mallory-Weiss syndrome
Gastritis	Gastritis	Gastritis
Ulcer	Ulcer	Ulcer
Vascular malformation	*Helicobacter pylori* infection	*H. pylori* infection
Vitamin K deficiency	Arteriovenous malformations	Hemobilia
	Esophageal or gastric varices	Arteriovenous malformations
		Esophageal or gastric varices
	Lower Gastrointestinal Bleeding	
Newborns and infants	Toddlers	Children and adolescents
Swallowed maternal blood	Polyps	Infectious enteorcolitis
	Hereditary	
Upper GI hemorrhage	Juvenile	Inflammatory bowel disease
Protein allergy	Intussusception	Arteriovenous malformation
Necrotizing enterocolitis	Antibiotic-associated enterocolitis	Polyps
		Hereditary
Hirschprung's disease–associated enterocolitis	Infectious enterocolitis	Hemolytic uremic syndrome
Malrotation and volvulus	Meckel's diverticulum	Antibiotic-associated enterocolitis
Infectious enterocolitis	Intestinal duplication with gastric lining	
	Hemolytic uremic syndrome	
	Schöenlein-Henoch purpura	

and culture. Treatment with a variety of antibiotic protocols is effective[13–15]. Although serologic evidence of infection has been documented in asymptomatic pediatric patients[16], the association of *H. pylori* with peptic ulcer disease in children is probably similar to that in adults[17].

Therapy

The management of massive GI hemorrhage includes treatment of hypovolemic shock, pharmacologic efforts to prevent further bleeding, and identification of the source of bleeding. The details of management of hypovolemic shock may be found in Chapter 16. A large amount of bleeding may occur within the bowel lumen, thus hidden from direct observation. Therefore, close monitoring of vital signs is essential to predict luminal blood loss in patients at risk. Large-bore intravenous access should always be maintained. Room temperature (rather than iced) gastric lavage, using tap water or saline solution, should be administered to remove clots. The use of room temperature lavage fluid reduces the risk of hypothermia in the small pediatric patient.

In some cases, control of bleeding may be attained by intravascular injection of vasoactive medications such as vasopressin or somatostatin. Vasopressin reduces both splanchnic arterial blood flow and portal venous pressure. Continuous infusion of vasopressin at a dose of 0.2 to 0.4 units/1.73 m^2/minute is effective in patients with stress-induced gastritis, Mallory-Weiss tears, and prehepatic portal hypertension[18]. Side effects include oliguria, hypertension, arrhythmias, and seizures[19]. The continuous infusion of somatostatin has fewer side effects. Somatostatin's effects are thought to be caused by a reduction in gastric blood flow and inhibition of gastric acid secretion, and gastrin production. When the patient is hemodynamically stable, efforts should be made to identify the source of bleeding as described in the next section. Thermal or laser coagulation by endoscopy may be applied directly to the lesion. Local injection of epinephrine provides hemostasis and may improve results when used with endoscopic electrocoagulation. If bleeding is caused by varices, sclerotherapy or variceal banding may be used, as described later in the section on hepatic failure.

Stress Gastritis

Definition

Unique to patients with acute illness, stress gastritis is characterized by diffuse inflammation of the gastric mucosa. The possibility of stress gastritis developing becomes greater if the reason for admission to the ICU is head trauma, major organ failure with hypotension, burns, liver failure, or illness from cancer chemotherapy or antiinflammatory medications **(Table 36.3).**

Pathophysiology

Stress gastritis occurs when normal mucosal integrity is impaired. The integrity of the mucosal cell membrane and the adjacent tight junctions are of prime importance in prevent-

Table 36.3. Factors Predisposing Patients to Stress-Induced Gastritis

Antiinflammatory agents
Bile reflux
Burn injury
Ethanol
Head trauma
Hypotension and ischemia
Liver failure
Major organ failure

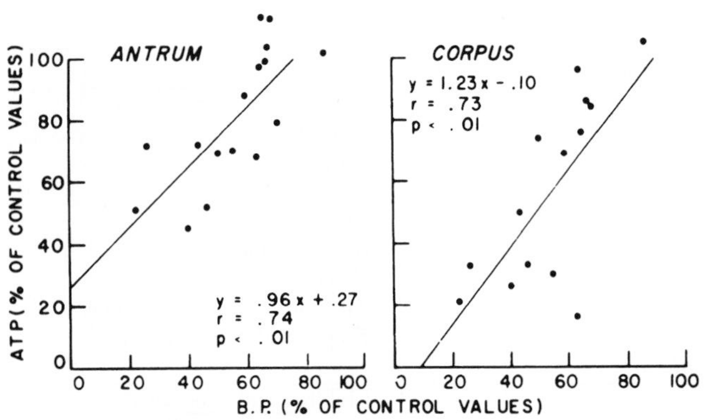

Figure 36.1. Relationship between mean arterial blood pressure (BP) (percentage of control level) and ATP level (percentage of mean control level) in mucosa of antrum and corpus of rabbits subjected to a single bleed. Data collected at 15 and 60 minutes after withdrawal of blood are pooled. From Menguy R, Master YF. Mechanism of stress ulcer: effects of hemorrhagic shock on energy metabolism in the mucosa of the antrum, corpus, and fundus of the rabbit stomach. Gastroenterology 1974;66:1172.

ing stress gastritis[20]. Hypoxia and decreased mucosal blood flow impair that integrity. The mucous layer on the mucosa plays a major role in preventing the diffusion of hydrogen ions backward from the gastric juice through the gastric epithelium. During hypoxia or reduced blood flow, the gastric mucosa loses its ability to produce sufficient amounts of mucus. Menguy and Master[21] have postulated that shock induces stress erosions by means of a profound gastric mucosal energy deficit evidenced by a reduction in adenosine triphosphate (ATP) levels in the gastric mucosa (Fig. 36.1). This energy deficit results in cell death, breakdown of tight cell junctions, or inhibition of cellular metabolism, enabling backward diffusion of acid and mucosal injury. Bile acids such as taurocholate break the mucosal barrier, uncouple oxidative phosphorylation of gastric mucosal mitochondria, and inhibit gastric mucosal adenosine triphosphatase (ATPase), thus increasing the damage to the mucosal cell after shock[22].

Ischemia makes the mucosa more susceptible to damage by acid[23]. Acid pH levels also markedly augment the damaging effects of bile salts on mucosal integrity[24]. High fasting concentrations of salt, alcohol, aspirin, or anti-inflammatory agents such as indomethacin, phenylbutazone, or naproxen[25] also decrease the integrity of the cell wall. This leads to hydrogen ions seeping from the lumen[26] through or between epithelium to the submucosa. Measurement of intramural pH level confirms that stress ulceration occurs in patients whose intramural pH level is less than the low limit of normal[27]. Once hydrogen ions have penetrated the epithelium, they may stimulate the release of histamine from mast cells resulting in inflammation, edema, disruption of the upper layer of the mucosa, and, ultimately, an acute erosion. If the process is allowed to continue, injury penetrates the mucosa and muscularis mucosa and produces an acute ulcer.

Stress gastritis may be a result of disruption in the interrelationships among the GI mucosa, hormone-releasing factors, hormones, and the excitatory and inhibitory responses of the peripheral and central nervous system. The discovery of neuropeptides within the gastric and intestinal tissues and the observation that some of these may have ulcerogenic properties or mediate ulcerogenic processes has led to great interest in this theory. The stimulatory effect of acetylcholine in the release of histamine is one example of this relationship. Hernandez and others have summarized these findings[28].

Recognition

Stress lesions can present with hematemesis, melena, hematochezia, or a slow decrease in hematocrit. Abdominal pain and tenderness on physical examination may occur. Nasogastric aspirate contains coffee-ground material or bright red blood. The rate of bleeding is variable but may be rapid enough to result in exsanguination.

The incidence of significant upper GI bleeding as a result of stress gastritis in the pediatric ICU setting is difficult to establish because studies have examined different subsets of critically ill patient populations and the definition of upper GI hemorrhage is not standardized. In one of the largest prospective studies, Lacroix and associates used blood in nasogastric aspirates or hematemesis as evidence of upper GI bleeding[29]. They found less than 1% of patients had bleeding severe enough to cause hypotension or to require transfusion[29]. A significant number of these patients received enteral nutrition and acid prophylaxis. In a retrospective study that excluded patients with high risk factors for GI bleeding such as GI tract surgery, abdominal trauma, peptic ulcer disease, GI tract infection, and ethanol ingestion, Cochran and colleagues examined emesis, gastric aspirates, and stool for gross evidence of blood[30]. They found that 25% of patients had macroscopic evidence of bleeding and that there were no clinical sequelae from this blood loss. Risk factors for GI bleeding in this group included shock, neurosurgical and cardiovascular surgery lasting longer than 3 hours, and trauma. Nasogastric aspirates and vital signs were examined as indicators of gastric bleeding by Lopez-Herce and others[31]. In this prospective study, they determined that 86% of critically ill pediatric patients with a modified Zinner score (indicating severity of illness) greater than three, had macroscopic evidence of upper GI bleeding and that 9.3% of patients had bleeding sufficient to result in a 15% decrease in hematocrit. Upper GI bleeding after thermal burns has been prospectively studied in adults by Czaja and others[32]. In this series, lesions occurred within 72 hours in 74% of patients; gastric ulceration was found in 22% and duodenal ulceration occurred in 28%. In adult patients without risk factors for head injury, burns over more than 30% of the body, peptic ulcer disease, organ transplantation, or recent hemodynamically significant GI bleeding, Cook and associates[33] determined that less than 2% of patients admitted to the ICU had clinically important bleeding. Coagulopathy and respiratory failure requiring at least 2 days of mechanical ventilation were defined as risk factors in this narrowly defined group of patients. In summary, the exact incidence of clinically significant upper GI bleeding secondary to stress gastritis is difficult to determine but appears to correlate with the presence of shock and acidosis, previous GI disease, trauma and burn injuries, organ transplantation, glucocorticoid administration, coagulopathy, and intracranial disease.

Prevention

The frequency of stress gastritis complications in critically ill children and adults has been shown to decrease when careful control of the gastric intraluminal pH level is achieved. Although data suggests caution because of the possibility of an increased potential of nosocomial infection[34,35], the gastric pH level should be maintained at more than 4.0 to decrease morbidity and mortality from stress ulcers[36,37]. By increasing the gastric pH level to at least 4.0, backward diffusion of hydrogen ions is reduced. Hastings and others demonstrated the effectiveness of antacid therapy in maintaining gastric acid neutralization and preventing GI hemorrhage in critically ill patients[38]. Effectiveness of antacids in preventing gastric bleeding and mucosal lesions has been shown by others[39,40], but the frequency of antacid doses, the time required to measure gastric pH level, and the incidence of antacid side effects has resulted in the use of H_2-receptor antagonists and sucralfate by some clinicians. Effective acid suppression, as defined by a gastric pH level of more than 4.0, is obtained with H_2-receptor antagonist agents[41], and these agents are effective in reducing the incidence of stress gastritis. They should be given by continuous infusion rather than intermittent dosing to ensure maximum pH control[42,43]. Sucralfate, through its ability to stimulate epidermal growth factor, bicarbonate and mucous secretion, binding of bile acids, and increase of mucosal blood flow, protects the mucosa from the effects of ulcerogenic properties of acid and gastric bleeding[31,44,45]. Eddleston and associates performed endoscopic examinations to evaluate stress ulcerations in mechanically ventilated adult patients who received sucralfate or placebo[46]. Upon admission to the ICU, 5 of 23 patients had stress erosions, but none had ulcer formation. Three days later, one patient treated with sucralfate and 5 treated with placebo had endoscopic evidence of gastric ulceration. Thus, in this small number of patients, sucralfate appeared effective in preventing stress gastritis. In adults, sucralfate appears to be a safe medication, and side effects related to nosocomial pneumonia or aluminum toxicity do not appear to be clinically significant[47]. A comparison of patients treated prophylactically with sucralfate or cimetidine did not show differences in rates of nosocomial pneumonia, gastrointestinal hemorrhage, or mortality[48].

Adult patients with gastric lesions induced by use of NSAIDS respond promptly to traditional H_2-receptor antagonists if the NSAID is discontinued. If the NSAID must be continued, administration of prostaglandin (PG) analogs such as enprostil has been shown to be more effective than placebo in treating gastritis. Intravenous preparations of PG analogs for gastrointestinal bleeding are not available, and side effects include diarrhea, dysmennorhea, and vaginal spotting[49].

Table 36.4. Treatment of Bleeding in the ICU

Hemodynamic resuscitation
Convene treatment team
Nasogastric lavage
Endoscopy to determine cause and treat
Treatment specific to cause

Early attention to nutrition may play a role in preventing stress-induced bleeding. In a nonrandomized retrospective study, Choctaw and others used enteral feeding of an elemental diet to decrease the incidence of bleeding in patients with severe burns[50]. In their experience, elemental feeding resulted in a decrease in mortality rate from 55% to 38%, a decreased rate of major bleeding from 30% to 3%, and a decreased rate of minor bleeding from 44% to 20%[50]. There are several mechanisms by which enteral feeding may be beneficial in the prevention of GI bleeding. The normal turnover of the gastric mucosal lining cells is quite rapid, with a half-life of 12 to 14 hours. Where stress has damaged the mucosa, rapid renewal of cells becomes imperative for avoiding backward diffusion of acid. Enteral administration of protein has been shown to release gastrin, a potent stimulator of cell turnover. Additionally, elemental diets buffer gastric acid and, during infusion, maintain gastric pH levels of more than 4.0[51].

Therapy

Table 36.4 reviews the approach to treatment of GI bleeding in the ICU. After bleeding is recognized, hemodynamic stabilization is the initial therapeutic goal. Intravenous fluids consisting of colloid, packed red blood cells, and/or fresh frozen plasma should be given until tachycardia and orthostasis are resolved. A nasogastric tube is essential to monitor the severity of bleeding and to deliver lavage fluid. Intravenous H_2-receptor antagonists are often administered to prevent further bleeding, but data indicating that intravenous H_2-receptor antagonists or enteral antacids stop bleeding faster than lavage alone are not convincing.

A team approach provides the best treatment for the child with stress-induced bleeding, and it should consist of the physician primarily responsible for the child's care, a gastroenterologist, a surgeon, and, often, a radiologist. Endoscopy should be quickly performed to identify the site of the bleeding. If a discrete ulcer or bleeding site is found, endoscopic therapy with electrical or laser cautery or application of topical coagulants may be indicated.

When endoscopy is unsuccessful in locating the site of the upper intestinal hemorrhage, arteriography should be undertaken. Isotope-labelled red blood cell scans may help in localizing the bleeding site(s) before angiography. Upper GI series are not indicated in this condition because the yield is low and the presence of barium in the GI tract precludes the use of arteriography later.

Usually, stress gastritis stops bleeding in response to lavage and correction of underlying hemodynamic problems, but sometimes bleeding is brisk and persists. Intraarterial vasopressors or thromboembolic agents are especially useful in suppressing severe bleeding[52–55]. Rarely, patients with stress gastritis bleed so quickly and continuously that hemodynamic stability cannot be maintained. When this occurs, surgical intervention with vagotomy (not always permanently successful), vessel identification and ligation, or total gastrectomy (successful but carrying high mortality and morbidity rates) should be considered.

PARALYTIC ILEUS AND PSEUDOOBSTRUCTION

Pathophysiology

Postoperative ileus, defined as the functional inhibition of propulsive bowel activity after surgery, irrespective of pathogenetic mechanism, is common especially after abdominal laparotomy, and severity is inversely related to the child's age. Livingston and Passaro define two kinds of postoperative ileus; the first is uncomplicated ileus that resolves spontaneously within 2 to 3 days, and the second is postoperative paralytic ileus that lasts more than 3 days[56]. Postoperative ileus is thought to result from temporary inhibition of the extrinsic regulation of motility. Alteration of sympathetic neuronal hyperactivity in patients who have undergone surgery not involving the intestines may result in decreased motility caused by suppression of the migrating bursts of action potentials from the stomach through the small intestine and the colon. In these cases, postoperative inhibition of intestinal activity is most profound and most persistent in the colon, less so in the small intestine, and least in the stomach. Surgery involving opening of the peritoneum are thought to result in inhibition of local and intrinsic nervous systems as well as contractile systems. Although ileus has been shown to be more severe with laparotomy than with other procedures, the role that handling or direct manipulation of the gut plays in the development of ileus appears to be less than previously thought. The colon is the portion of the gut most sensitive to inhibition of motility caused by anesthesia because it is the part of the gut most dependent on neural control mechanisms to achieve motility. Postoperative ileus has been attributed to inhibition by stress-related catecholamines, release of neurohumoral agents such as vasopressin, sympathetic extrinsic pathway stimulation, parasympathetic fiber inhibition, decreased release of acetylcholine, release of endogenous opiates, or inhibition by anesthetic agents themselves. Catecholamine levels are high in the postoperative period and reduce gut motility. Vasopressin is secreted during laparotomy and is believed to decrease small bowel contractility, although the mechanism has not been defined. Although morphine inhibits small bowel propulsion and endogenous opiates have been proposed as one of the causes of postoperative ileus, reversal of postsurgical ileus with naloxone has not been successful.

Table 36.5. Factors Associated with Paralytic Ileus

Metabolic factors
Infections
Cardiac failure
After surgery (abdominal or other)
Parkinsonism
Fractures
Alcoholism
Pancreatitis or cholecystitis
Urinary tract disease
Cancer

Factors associated with paralytic ileus are shown in **Table 36.5.** Metabolic disturbances, such as hypokalemia, hyponatremia, hypomagnesemia, and decreased osmolarity, may contribute to the perpetuation of ileus. Hypokalemia is thought to exert its effects by interfering with acetylcholine release when serum potassium is less than 2.5 mg/dL.

Anoxic damage affects the especially sensitive intramural intestinal ganglia, and thus hypoxia may cause intestinal paralysis. In shock, disproportionate shunting of blood away from GI tract to the brain, heart, and kidneys occurs. Localized areas of hypoxia in the small bowel may occur, resulting from dilatation of the bowel, loss of peristalsis, and functional obstruction. If the anoxic event is prolonged, permanent destruction of the mesenteric ganglia may be seen[57].

Localized ileus may occur in conjunction with intraperitoneal inflammation seen in cholecystitis, pancreatitis, urinary tract infections, appendicitis, abscesses, or lower lobe pneumonias. Franken and others[57] postulated that infection causes inflammation of afferent nerves, which, in turn, evokes reflex inhibition of peristalsis. Additionally, conditions that alter the parasympathetic (excitatory) to sympathetic (inhibitory) ratio of gut stimulation may result in ileus. This is the presumed mechanism of ileus after retroperitoneal hemorrhage, as well as in posterior neoplasms and spinal cord disease. Likewise, certain drugs cause functional obstruction by altering the parasympathetic to sympathetic ratio. Anticholinergic activity is responsible for the constipation and ileus seen with the phenothiazine-like antidepressants, such as chlorpromazine and amitriptyline[58]. Ganglionic blockers, benztropine, anti-cholinergic agents, morphine, meperidine, methadone, and other opioids are also often the cause of functional obstruction[58]. Verapamil and cyclosporine also have been associated with constipation. A thorough drug history, therefore, is mandatory for patients with idiopathic ileus.

Recognition

Patients with postoperative ileus may have abdominal distention, nausea, vomiting, delayed defecation, and decreased bowel sounds[59]. Patients with localized functional obstruction, however, may have abdominal pain, nausea, and vomiting with normal, decreased, or hyperactive bowel

Table 36.6. First-line Treatment of Ileus

NPO.
Nasogastric or intestinal decompression
Discontinue narcotics and smooth muscle relaxants (if possible)
Colonic decompression with rectal tube

sounds. A dilated terminal ileum and transverse colon accompanied by no air in the descending colon or rectum is seen in mechanical obstruction but can occasionally be seen in functional obstruction. When plain films of the abdomen show multiple air-filled loops, the precise cause of the obstruction can be difficult to identify. This clinical picture can usually be differentiated from mechanical obstruction by water-soluble contrast media or metrizamide enema or colonoscopy. Metrizamide is used to enhance bowel images in neonates and young children when barium is contraindicated because of suspected perforation and when water-soluble contrast media is of concern because of its hypertonicity[(60)]. Real-time ultrasonography has been used to evaluate the cause of mechanical obstruction in children and has been especially useful in patients with intussusception[(61)]. Lastly, manometric evaluation of postoperative patients may provide valuable information for both accuracy of diagnosis and effectiveness of therapy[(62)].

Not all postoperative ileus is functional. Prolonged ileus, or ileus that recurs 1 to 3 weeks after surgery, may be mechanical obstruction secondary to intussusception[(63,64)] or adhesions. Ein and Ferguson described 10 children who developed intussusception after laparotomy[(63)]. Diagnosis is difficult because most of the usual symptoms of obstruction are missing or obscured by nasogastric suction and analgesic medication given after surgery. Postoperative intussusceptions are usually ileoileal, appear within 8 days of surgery, and require surgical correction[(63)]. Intestinal adhesions as a cause of postoperative obstruction tend to occur more than 2 weeks after surgery.

Complications that may arise from chronic ileus include small-bowel overgrowth with subsequent steatorrhea and fat-soluble vitamin malabsorption and caloric deprivation.

Therapy

Table 36.6 reviews the intial approach to patients with ileus. For clinically evident ileus, nasointestinal intubation remains the only therapy proven to be effective[(56)]. Ileus usually resolves with decompression; correction of underlying metabolic, infectious, or inflammatory processes; and intravenous nutritional support. Bowel sounds and the passage of flatus followed by bowel movements usually marks the end of ileus. Symptoms of partial small-bowel mechanical obstruction may also be relieved in some cases by nasogastric suction[(65)]. If the cecum has dilated to more than 12 cm in diameter, the danger of perforation increases[(66)] even if there is no mechanical reason for the obstruction. If nasogastric decompression fails to reduce the cecal dilation, decompression with a colonoscope may be successful. If the cecal dilation cannot be quickly decreased, cecostomy is indicated because perforation carries with it a 35 to 75% mortality rate. When functional obstruction is suspected, narcotics, smooth muscle relaxants, and parasympathomimetic agents should be avoided, because these agents may increase the chance of bowel perforation.

Pharmacologic agents evaluated in clinical trials but not yet successful in the treatment of postoperative ileus are listed in **Table 36.7.** Although phentolamine and propranolol prevent postoperative suppression of gastric contractions, they do not prevent small-bowel ileus. Edrophonium is more effective than neostigmine in restoring small-bowel function in uncontrolled trials, but the use of these agents is limited because of their systemic side effects. Alpha-adrenergic blockade and intraperitoneal instillation of anesthetic agents to block the release of inhibitory mediators have been used, but controlled trials are yet to be performed. Opiate receptor blockade has not been proven to be useful. A relationship may exist between increased PGE_2 levels and ileus. Indomethacin has been administered with varying results, but PGE_2 has been found to increase peristalsis in one limited study[(67)]. Gastric inhibitory peptide was shown to have only minimal effect on colonic pseudoobstruction[(68)]. Metoclopramide stimulates gastric and small-bowel motility but does not stimulate colonic motility; Davidson and colleagues showed that it was not helpful for postoperative ileus[(69)]. Cerulein has been shown to stimulate small-bowel motility, but its practicality has not yet been demonstrated in controlled studies of ileus. During the last several years, there has been an increased interest in two medications with gastrointestinal pro-kinetic properties. Cisapride, an agent used in the treatment of gastroesophageal reflux and functional constipation, has been used in the patient with postoperative ileus; in some series, earlier

Table 36.7. Postoperative Ileus: Proposed treatments but not proven effective

Adrenergic modulation:
Phentolamine
Edrophonium
Neostigmine
Alpha-adrenergic blockade
Propranolol
Opiate receptor blockade
Anesthetic blockade
Intraperitoneal
Spinal
Adrenergic neuron
Parasympathetic stimulation
Prostaglandin antagonists
Indomethacin
PGF2
Metachlorpropamide
Neurohumoral activation
Gastric inhibitory peptide
Cerulein
Gastrointestinal pacing
Transpercutaneous electrical nerve stimulation
Cisapride
Motilin receptor stimulation
Erythromycin

return of bowel sounds, flatus, and stool production were seen[70], although in others, these effects were not so clearly shown[71]. Cisapride also conferred a small benefit in the alteration of postoperative small-bowel motility as measured by intestinal intraluminal manometry[62]. Erythromycin, an antibiotic in the macrolide family, accelerates gastric emptying in diabetic gastropathy and chronic intestinal pseudoobstruction and has been shown to be beneficial in the transpyloric passage of naso- or oro-duodenal tubes[72]. Erythromycin is thought to increase intestinal contractions by binding to the gut motilin receptor[73]; its role in the treatment of postoperative ileus, however, has not been established.

Alternative modes of therapy are being explored for this perplexing problem. Since reflex sympathetic inhibition is one of the theoretical causes of postoperative ileus, early attempts at treating ileus focused on the use of spinal anesthesia to obliterate reflex pathways synapsing in the spinal cord and were apparently successful[56]. In controlled studies, neither adrenergic neuronal blockade nor parasympathetic stimulation, however, has been found to be useful. Studies of GI pacing in humans have not been promising[68]. Direct electrical stimulation of the lumbosacral region, however, increases intestinal peristalsis. Transcutaneous electrical nerve stimulation (TENS) has been tried in reflex ileus accompanying acute spinal cord injury and in neurologically impaired patients with chronic ileus[74]. The production of bowel movements or diarrhea and the ability of the patient to tolerate oral feedings occurred 2 to 8 days after neurostimulation. The potential usefulness of TENS in the postoperative patient for prevention of ileus has been suggested by Hymes and associates[75]. The value of TENS in the routine postoperative patient has yet to be proven, and controlled clinical trials are needed.

Other Disorders of Motility

Several other conditions affecting digestive tract motility may cause severe illness in the pediatric patient. These include chronic idiopathic intestinal pseudoobstruction (CIIP), toxic megacolon accompanied by ulcerative colitis, and Hirschsprung's disease.

CIIP is a recurring condition characterized by functional bowel obstruction without organic, mechanical, or pathologic cause[76,77]. The clinical course in children is characterized by intermittent episodes of abdominal distension, vomiting, abdominal pain, diarrhea, constipation, and malnutrition. Radiographic studies are the mainstay of diagnosis; they show abnormal esophageal motility, delayed gastric emptying, dilated loops of small intestine, and disturbed colonic motility. Since many children with pseudoobstruction have esophageal dysmotility, esophageal manometric studies aid diagnosis. The patient with CIIP may require intensive care secondary to acute episodes of functional obstruction necessitating nasogastric suction and fluid and electrolyte support.

Toxic megacolon, a complication of chronic ulcerative colitis, may also be life-threatening. The clinical presentation may be superimposed on that of fulminant colitis[78]; the condition is characterized by rapid deterioration with abdominal distension, disappearance of bowel sounds, and toxemia. Precipitating factors include potassium deficiency, opiate treatment, barium enema or colonoscopy procedures, and mechanical obstruction. Plain films of the abdomen show colonic distension. Since toxic megacolon has a high rate of mortality, the condition demands intensive medical therapy, decompression of the small intestine by intubation, and consultation with surgical staff.

Enterocolitis associated with Hirschprung's disease or aganglionosis coli may be life-threatening. Hirschprung's disease usually presents during infancy with constipation. Alternatively, patients may have enterocolitis either before or after colostomy placement. Enterocolitis is characterized by voluminous watery stools, fever, sudden circulatory collapse, and severe mucosal necrosis and ulceration; a high rate of mortality is typical of this illness[79]. Although *Clostridium difficile* has been suggested as a potential pathogen, no specific infectious agents have been determined to be causative. The patient must receive fluid and electrolyte support and broad-spectrum antibiotic therapy.

DIARRHEA

Definition

Diarrhea is defined as an increase in the number, fluidity, water content, or volume of stools, resulting from alterations in the digestive, absorptive, or secretory functions of the intestinal tract. A stool weight of more than 10 g/kg/day in an infant or more than 200 g/day in an older child may be defined as diarrhea[80]. In the postoperative or critically ill child, diarrhea occurs principally because of drug therapy, infection, or malabsorption **(Table 36.8).** Young children are at great risk for infectious diarrhea and resulting dehydration.

Pathophysiology

Inability to assimilate nutrients results from disruption of the intraluminal processes of digestion, injury to small-bowel mucosa, disruption of transport mechanisms across the epithelium, or inability to transport nutrients away from the small bowel by means of blood or lymph. Intraluminal processes requiring pancreatic lipase and bile salts are particularly critical to the digestion of fat. Thus, steatorrhea may develop in the infant or child with disruption of pancreatic function because of inadequate lipolysis. Severe liver disease may result in bile salt concentrations below the critical micellar concentration in the intestinal lumen, which impairs the ability of lipids to gain the aqueous solubility required for their absorption. Intestinal stasis in the postoperative patient or in the child with a dysmotility syndrome, such as pseudoobstruction, also impairs fat assimilation by permitting accumulation of colonic bacteria in the small intestine. This condition, known as bacterial over-

Table 36.8. Causes of Diarrhea

Malabsorption
Intraluminal dysfunction
Pancreatic insufficiency
Liver failure
Bacterial overgrowth secondary to dysmotility, antibiotic use, or hypochlorhydria
Enterocyte damage or brush-border enzyme depletion
Postinfection
Hypoxia
Necrotizing enterocolitis
Surgical resection
Inflammatory bowel disease
Congenital microvillus atrophy
Congenital absence of disaccharidase
Lymphatic obstruction
Infection
Viruses
Rotavirus
Adenovirus
Calicivirus
Astrovirus
Bacterial
Salmonella sp.
Shigella sp.
Campylobacter jejuni
Escherichia coli 0157:H7
Clostridium difficile
Yersinia sp.
Parasites
Aeromonas sp.
Giardia lamblia
Cryptosporidium sp.
Agents
Antibiotics
Antacids
Chemotherapeutic agents
Colchicine
Digitalis preparations
Nutritional formula feedings
Lactulose
Potassium supplements
Propranolol
Quinidine

growth, may result in deconjugation of bile acids. Such deconjugated bile acids are ineffective in forming micelles[81] and compromise digestion.

Although the mucosal phase of absorption is critical to all nutrients, injury or dysfunction of the intestinal mucosa becomes clinically evident primarily by its effect on carbohydrate absorption. Malabsorption of carbohydrates, in turn, causes an osmotic diarrhea. In addition, bacterial fermentation of a portion of the nonabsorbed carbohydrate reaching the colon results in the formation of short-chain fatty acids. This further contributes to the osmotic load presented to the colon and limits water resorption. In addition, short-chain fatty acids stimulate peristalsis. Abdominal distention ensues because of the large fluid loads in the lumen and the production of gaseous products of fermentation[82].

Complete digestion and absorption of sugars require the action of brush-border carbohydrases including lactase, sucrase-alpha dextrinase, trehalase, and glucoamylase. Injury to the villous surface on which these enzymes reside impairs sugar absorption[83], resulting in osmotic retention of water in the intestinal lumen[84]. Depletion of carbohydrases may occur as a result of a variety of viral, bacterial, or parasitic injuries (Fig. 36.2). Enzyme depletion is also noted in the critically ill child who is significantly malnourished.

More information regarding the effect of impaired blood flow and inadequate oxygenation on the function of the enterocyte is needed. The ability of the small intestine to sustain oxygen delivery is somewhat less than that of skeletal muscle[85]. In the small bowel, oxygen delivery is least to the villous tip because of the countercurrent system of blood vessel flow. Normally, the delivery of luminal stimuli, i.e., food, to the small-bowel mucosa results in increased jejunal blood flow or functional hyperemia. Microsphere studies of blood flow in experimental animals indicate that the postprandial increase in intestinal blood flow is not mediated solely by the local presence of nutrients in the lumen. Rather, the presence of food in the stomach and upper small intestine causes a diffuse decrease in vascular resistance along the entire extent of the bowel[86] and may be mediated by hormones or the nervous system.

Studies of the effect of asphyxia on organ blood flow in newborn piglets show that blood flow to the stomach and to the small and large intestines is decreased under conditions of inadequate oxygenation[87]. Furthermore, the changes in blood flow over a 90-minute period were associated with dilation of segments of the small and large intestines. If such dilation occurs under clinical conditions, small-bowel bacterial overgrowth may occur. Bacterial overgrowth, in turn, has a major effect on digestion of fat, as was previously described, and results in considerable impairment of sugar absorption[88]. Carbohydrate malabsorption has been reported in conditions associated with impairment of blood flow and gut hypoxia. For example, monosaccharide intolerance, characterized by the inability to absorb glucose, has been reported over the first several months of life after severe anoxia[89].

The mucosal phase of absorption is also compromised by intestinal resection. Postoperative diarrhea in the infant or child who has had major resection of the small intestine

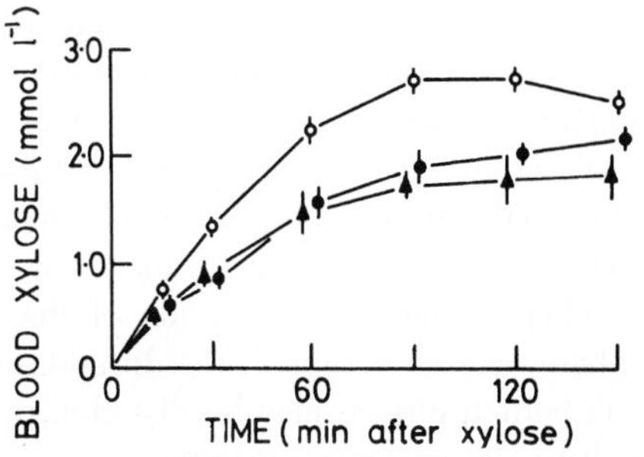

Figure 36.2. Depression of blood xylose concentrations after 25 g of oral xylose in patients with acute and chronic infections compared with controls. From Cooke GC. Influence of systemic infections on xylose absorption. Acta Trop (Basel) 1981;38:176.

results principally from the decreased absorptive surface area available to luminal contents. Diarrhea may be worsened in these patients by *(a)* gastric acid hypersecretion, *(b)* entry of bile salts into the colon causing a cholorrheic enteropathy with contraction of the bile salt pool, and *(c)* abnormalities in GI motor activity[90].

Postoperative diarrhea may also ensue if lymphatic flow from the mesentery is impeded by the surgical procedure. In addition to steatorrhea, obstruction of lymphatic flow from the intestine causes protein-losing enteropathy, with resulting hypoalbuminemia and lymphopenia.

Necrotizing Enterocolitis

Necrotizing enterocolitis (NEC) is a clinicopathologic disorder of insidious or acute onset characterized by feeding intolerance, abdominal distension, bloody stools, and disseminated intravascular coagulation that predominantly, although not exclusively, affects premature infants. Pneumatosis intestinalis is the pathognomonic radiologic finding. Mortality rate ranges from 18 to 40% and appears to increase if infants are of low birth weight, develop other perinatal complications, or require surgical procedures to evaluate or treat complications of NEC[91,92]. Pathologic features include focal or diffuse ulceration and necrosis of the distal bowel or colon and, in some cases, the upper intestinal tract. The cause is not certain but infection, toxin, early enteral feedings, increased permeability of the immature intestine, maternal cocaine use, and/or hypoxia are associations. Hypoxic injury to the intestinal mucosa is critical to most etiologic theories[85,93]. Data indicate that hypoxia in experimental animals may affect transport of simple sugars. Weanling rats exposed to environments high in nitrogen suffer a loss of intestinal transport capacity for carbohydrate by sodium-dependent mechanisms in the absence of changes in histology, ultrastructure of the small intestinal mucosa, or disaccharidase levels[94]. In other animal models, pathologic changes of NEC included intestinal ischemia and vascular hyperviscosity[95,96].

Infectious Causes of Diarrhea

Infectious causes of diarrhea in the intensive care patient are common **(Table 36.8).** Nosocomial infection is a likely cause of diarrhea in the ICU harboring rotavirus, and rotavirus-like infection have been particularly incriminated[97,98]. Viral infections result in diarrhea caused by absorption impairment as well as stimulation of water and electrolyte secretion from the mucosa to the lumen. Secretion may be mediated by the release of prostaglandins, receptor-mediated activation of cyclic adenosine monophosphate, adenylate cyclase, or activation of the guanosine monophosphate cyclase system[99,100]. In addition, the infected brush-border surface may be distorted, with reduction of brush-border enzymatic activity.

Diarrhea may also be caused by *C. difficile* infection[101]. *C. difficile* elaborates toxins that result in mucosal inflammation and fluid secretion. Antibiotic use may be a predisposing factor, but this infection can develop in patients not exposed to these agents. Viscidi and Bartlett[102] have reported 10 cases occurring in children less than 4 years old. The most common antibiotics causing pseudomembranous enterocolitis, which is the most severe form of *C. difficile*-induced disease, are penicillins, cephalosporins, and clindamycin[102]. Antibiotics disrupt the normal colonic flora, allowing colonization with *C. difficile.* The clinical implications of this colonization, however, in pediatric patients are not always clear. A large proportion of asymptomatic neonates and infants shed *C. difficile* toxin or have evidence of the organism in their stool[103,104], and most often this organism is associated with diarrhea, not colitis. Despite these facts, *C. difficile* infection should always be sought in patients with diarrhea, especially bloody diarrhea, as it is a treatable cause[105,106]. This is particularly important in hospitalized patients because of the possibility of nosocomial spread of this pathogen.

Other pathogens causing diarrhea include community-acquired infectious agents, such as *Salmonella* species, *Giardia lamblia* and *Escherichia coli* 0157.H 7[60].

Table 36.9. Evaluation of Diarrhea

Document increased stool frequency and volume
Gross stool examination
Seek symptoms suggesting cause
Examination for infectious or inflammatory particles
Fecal examination
Blood, leukocytes, ova, and parasites
Culture for enteric pathogens
ELISA for viral pathogens
C. difficile toxin
Sigmoidoscopy
Evaluation for malabsorption
Stool pH, fat, alpha-1-antitrypsin levels
Breath hydrogen test
D-Xylose test
Small-bowel radiographic imaging series
Small-bowel biopsy

Diagnosis

The first step in evaluation of diarrhea is to carefully document the stool frequency and characteristics **(Table 36.9).** Vomiting often accompanies diarrhea in viral gastroenteritis. Fever suggests either a bacterial or viral cause; *Shigella* species-caused dysentery, for example, is often seen with a high temperature and febrile convulsions. Abdominal pain and tenesmus accompany bacterial infection in the colon by *Yersinia enterocolitica, C. jejuni, Shigella* species, and enteropathogenic *E. coli*[107]. Stool examination can be very useful: Infections involving the small bowel usually result in watery diarrhea, while infectious colitis results in stool containing blood, with or without mucus[107].

Fecal Blood

The presence of visible blood in diarrheal stools should trigger further investigation for enteric pathogenic species such as *Shigella, Yersinia, Campylobacter, E. coli* H7.0157, *Aeromonas,* or *amebiasis.* Alternatively, the presence of bright red blood in the stool may indicate Crohn's colitis, ulcerative colitis, allergic colitis, or ischemic injury. Infants with NEC may have visible blood in the stool. Stools containing no visible blood should be tested for occult blood. A variety of methods, including guaiac-impregnated filter paper (Hemoccult) are available for this purpose.

Fecal Leukocytes

Examination of the diarrheal stool for white cells is useful in identifying infectious or inflammatory causes of diarrhea. A stool sample should be smeared on a glass slide and stained with methylene blue or Wright's stain. The presence of neutrophils in the stool suggests *Shigella, Yersinia, Campylobacter,* or invasive *E. coli* species as possible causes. The presence of leukocytes generally eliminates viral or toxigenic bacterial causes of diarrhea. Eosinophils may be an indicator of allergic disease.

Stool Culture

If bacteria are suspected as the cause of the patient's diarrhea, stool culture for enteric pathogens is appropriate. Laboratories differ in the assays they use, and each specimen must be fresh and transported immediately. The presence of *C. difficile* can be detected by culture or by assay for *C. difficile* toxin. Stool-cytotoxin bioassays are sensitive (94 to 100%) and specific (99%)[106]. Stool toxin may also be identified by enzyme-linked immunosorbent assay (ELISA).

Virus Identification

Viral causes of diarrhea may be detected by ELISA for viral antigens. ELISA for rotavirus is extremely sensitive[97]. The rotazyme also detects adenovirus.

Screening Tests for Carbohydrate Malabsorption

Screening tests for carbohydrate malabsorption, using freshly passed feces, are meaningful only if the child being tested is currently being fed a potentially offending carbohydrate. These fecal screening tests include the measurement of fecal pH level and reducing substances in the stool. Release of organic acids by bacterial fermentation of malabsorbed sugar forms the basis for using fecal pH level as a screening test for carbohydrate malabsorption[108]. The test is performed by dipping Nitrazine paper into the most liquid part of a fresh stool. The resulting color on the paper is compared with the reference chart provided. A fecal pH level of 5.5 or below is abnormal. Reducing sugars that escape small-bowel absorption and are excreted in the stool may be detected by placing a small amount of fecal material in a test tube and diluting it with twice its volume of water. Fifteen drops of the resulting suspension are then placed in a second test tube with a Clinitest tablet. The color of the reaction is compared with a reference chart provided in the Clinitest kit used for testing of urine. Positive results are 0.5% of total volume or greater. A result of 0.25% of volume is considered equivocal. Since sucrose is not a reducing sugar, an accurate test for sucrose malabsorption requires the use of 1 normal hydrochloric acid (N HCl) instead of water.

Breath Hydrogen Test

Excretion of hydrogen in the breath results when carbohydrate that escapes small-bowel absorption is fermented by colonic bacteria. A fixed portion of the hydrogen produced is absorbed into the portal circulation and excreted in breath. The choice of sugar substrate for testing is dependent on the nature of the carbohydrate malabsorption suspected: Thus, lactose is the substrate used when lactose malabsorption is suspected. The test is commonly performed after an overnight fast, but fasting time may be shortened in the smaller infant. Antibiotics may alter the results of testing and cause false-negative results. Elevated levels of breath hydrogen before ingestion of carbohydrate may indicate small-bowel bacterial overgrowth. Methods for breath hydrogen testing for malabsorbtion of lactose and other sugars are described by Perman and others[109].

Sigmoidoscopy

Sigmoidoscopic examination is valuable if Crohn's disease, ulcerative colitis, or pseudomembranous colitis is suspected. Flexible sigmoidoscopy, with limited introduction of air, can be performed even in small children, and biopsies can easily be obtained. Pseudomembranous colitis is characterized by excrescences and raised yellow pseudomembranes with areas of ulceration. Pseudomembranous colitis induced by *C. difficile* is only one end of the spectrum of *C. difficile*-induced disease. In fact, the most common clinical presentation of this infection is self-limited diarrhea. Biopsy samples are often critical in defining whether inflammatory lesions are acute or chronic. Acute infiltration with polymorphonuclear cells is suggestive of a recent infection, whereas chronic inflammation with a mixture of mononuclear polymorphonuclear cells and signs of regeneration and crypt distortion are consistent with chronic colitis, such as Crohn's disease or ulcerative colitis. In addition, granulomas in the pathologic specimen suggest Crohn's disease.

Therapy

Acute self-limited diarrhea such as that caused by viral agents may necessitate a short period of clear liquid diet, followed by early introduction of more complex carbohydrate feedings. If evidence of severe mucosal damage or secretory diarrhea is present, more intensive supportive care may be necessary to correct fluid and electrolyte disturbances. Infants are at higher risk than adults for dehydration and malnutrition.

Assessment of hydration status may be made by physical examination as well as with monitoring of urine volume and central venous pressure. Fluid replacement should be modified according to the child's normal daily fluid requirement, electrolyte deficit, and ongoing fluid and electrolyte losses as estimated by measuring volume of stool, vomitus, and urine[107]. Vomiting is not a contraindication for oral rehydration therapy unless ileus, obstruction, or an acute abdomen is present. Even in diarrhea associated with injury to the absorptive surface of the intestines, enough absorptive capacity often remains for diarrheal losses to be replaced with oral nutrient supplement electrolyte solutions[110]. In the child with severe dehydration, rapid restitution should be made, with 20 to 30 mL/kg of isotonic saline containing 5% dextrose in water administered intravenously[107]. Children with hypernatremic dehydration should have their electrolytes normalized over 2 to 3 days to avoid cerebral edema[107].

Malabsorptive conditions require modification of the child's enteral feedings. Whenever possible, changes in feedings should be made on the basis of identification of the nutrients malabsorbed by the patient. Therapy of severe intestinal injury and short bowel syndrome often may necessitate intravenous hyperalimentation. Total parenteral nutrition (TPN) has dramatically improved survival after massive small-bowel resection and may permit normal infant growth and development[111]. Short bowel syndrome may gradually improve as the bowel adapts by dilation of the bowel lumen, lengthening of villi, and slowing of motility. During this adaptive time, tube feedings of defined constituent or modular formulas should be administered to the degree tolerated. Early enteral administration of specialized formulas may increase enterocyte hyperplasia while improving the negative nitrogen balance of the patient and repleting missing nutrients[112]. Nutritional therapy is discussed further in Chapter 35.

There is no evidence that "antidiarrheal" agents, such as Lomotil or Kaopectate, help cure infectious diarrhea. In fact, evidence suggests that these agents may prolong and worsen the severity of the disease, especially in *Shigella* and *C. jejuni* infections[113]. Additionally, antidiarrheal compounds interfere with identification of enteropathogens in stool specimens and have a high overdose potential in children[114]. The use of these agents, therefore, should be avoided.

Guidelines for therapy of specific bacterial infections may be obtained from a variety of sources[108,115,116] and depend on identification of the offending agent. Invasive *Salmonella* infection can be treated with ampicillin, trimethoprim-sulfamethoxazole, cefotaxime, or chloramphenicol. *Giardia* infection can be treated with metronidazole and other similar agents. Compounds such as the fluoroquinolones, which are effective in the treatment of acute infectious diarrhea in adults, are not approved for use in children because of their potential side effects[114]. Nonspecific modalities for the treatment of *C. difficile* colitis include discontinuation of the inciting antimicrobial agent, avoidance of antiperistaltic drugs, and supportive care to correct dehydration and electrolyte disturbances. Metronidazole is the drug of choice for *C. difficile* infection. Enteral administration is preferred, but if contraindicated, intravenous administration results in bactericidal levels in the bowel lumen through biliary excretion and colonic exudation. Enteral vancomycin is also effective therapy but is expensive. Intravenous administration of vancomycin is not excreted into the GI lumen and therefore should not be used. Diarrhea caused by recurrent *C. difficile* is usually secondary to incomplete eradication of spores and not to organism resistance. Therefore recurrent disease does not necessarily necessitate a change in the antibiotic, but it may require prolonged therapy. A variety of other treatment approaches for recurrent disease have been attempted, including tapering antibiotic therapy, or using rifampin, cholestyramine, or bacteriotherapy with fecal enemas, but which is the best method is not known[106].

GASTROINTESTINAL DISEASE IN HIV-INFECTED AND IMMUNOCOMPROMISED PATIENTS

The gastrointestinal mucosa is a large target organ for opportunistic infections and disease in patients with acquired immunodeficiency syndrome (AIDS). Mucosal ulcerations, diarrhea, pancreatitis, and malnutrition are found in 30 to 70% of pediatric patients with AIDS[117,118].

In the patient infected with human immunodeficiency virus (HIV), esophageal or GI inflammation or ulceration is associated most commonly with *Candida albicans* infection or acid injury. Because of continuous antibiotic use and hypochlorhydria, these patients are predisposed to oral or esophageal *C. albicans* infection. Hypochlorhydria can result from the use of H_2-receptor antagonists or from AIDS-related gastropathy. Severe esophageal disease can occur in the absence of oral thrush. Other infectious causes include Epstein-Barr virus (EBV), cytomegalovirus (CMV), and herpes simplex virus. Stress and ulcerogenic medications also contribute to this mucosal inflammation.

Diarrhea develops in 20 to 40% of pediatric HIV-infected patients. In addition to the pathogens seen in immunocompetent patients with diarrhea, *Cryptosporidum* and *Mycobacterium avium* complex should be sought as infectious causes. In fact, *Cryptosporidium* species may be the most common infectious pathogen isolated from AIDS patients with diarrhea[119], and the clinical severity of the diarrhea may be directly correlated with the number of cryptosporidia present in the stool[120]. Although alterations in the secretory immune response of patients with AIDS have been suggested as one of the predisposing factors for these mucosal infections, a pathogen-specific secretory IgA response to *Cryptosporidium* infection has been shown[121]. Infectious causes for diarrhea are listed in **Table 36.10.** Up to six stool samples, rectal biopsy, and/or duodenal biopsy may be required to make a diagnosis, and pathogen-negative diarrhea is still often reported[118]. Antimicrobial treatment of identified enteric pathogens in HIV-infected patients is indicated.

Pancreatitis is a common problem in HIV-infected pediatric patients. In one series, 17% of 53 HIV-infected patients were affected[122]. Factors associated with the development of pancreatitis were CD4 counts of less than 100

Table 36.10. Infectious Causes of Diarrhea Found in AIDS Patients

Protozoan	
	Cryptosporidium sp.
	Isospora belli
	Entamoeba histolytica
Viruses	
	HIV
	Herpes simplex
	Cytomegalovirus
	Epstein-Barr virus
Mycobacterium	
	Mycobacterium avium-intracellulare
Fungus	
	Candida sp.

cells/mm^3 and the use of aerosolized pentamidine isothionate. The majority of these patients died within 8 months after diagnosis. Other causes of pancreatitis include *Mycobacteria* species, adenovirus, and CMV, and medications such as trimethoprim-sulfamethoxazole, dideoxyinosine, isoniazid, rifampin, pyrazinamide, and ethioamide[(123)].

Malnutrition occurs often and is secondary to many factors[(124,125)]. Patients have decreased caloric intake because of oropharyngeal, esophageal, or gastric ulceration, nausea, or anorexia. Nutritional requirements may be increased because of infections or multiorgan dysfunction. Mucosal damage from repeated infections, small-bowel overgrowth secondary to repeated antibiotic use, and AIDS gastropathy or enteropathy, may result in carbohydrate, protein, or fat malabsorption.

Patients with malignant tumors or primary immunodeficiencies or those receiving immunosuppressive therapy are also at risk for GI disease. Diarrhea may be caused by either infectious gastroenteritis, graft versus host disease (GVHD), or toxic effects of medications. Infections most commonly isolated include coxsackie virus, astrovirus, rotavirus, echovirus and adenovirus, *C. difficile,* and *Giardia.* In some bone marrow transplant units, infection is the most common cause of acute diarrhea, whereas GVHD is seen more often in others[(126)]. Skin biopsies of lesions are often useful in diagnosis of GVHD, but intestinal biopsy can also be diagnostic. Of 150 episodes of acute diarrhea in adult patients after bone marrow transplant, 48% were caused by GVHD and 13% by infectious organisms. Intestinal biopsy identified GVHD in 14 patients who previously had had skin biopsies that were not diagnostic[(126)].

Typhlitis was initially described as necrotizing colitis involving the cecum ("typhlon" in Greek) that occurred in patients with acute leukemia[(127)]. Since then, this entity has been recognized in not only patients with advanced malignant tumors but also in patients with immunodeficiencies. A review of 33 pediatric patients with this potentially life-threatening condition identified common findings of abdominal pain, bloating, and/or GI bleeding, fever, neutropenia, and thrombocytopenia[(128)]. Radiographic abnormalities ranged from a dilated cecum and small bowel to right colonic pneumatosis intestinalis . The medical management includes discontinuation of oral intake, administration of parenteral nutrition and antibiotics, and maintenance of an adequate coagulation state[(129,130)].

Table 36.11. Congenital Anomalies Associated with Pancreatitis

Anomalous insertion of the common bile duct
Choledochal cysts
Congenital stenosis of the ampulla of Vater
Duodenal diverticulum
Intrapancreatic ductal duplications
Pancreas divisum
Periampullary duodenal duplication
Stricture of the common duct

PANCREATITIS

Definition

Acute pancreatitis is a clinical condition characterized by sudden onset of abdominal pain with an elevation of serum pancreatic enzyme levels that occurs in both pediatric[(131,132)] and adult patients[(133)]. Pathologic specimens display a range of findings, from pancreatic interstitial edema and peripancreatic fat necrosis to extensive pancreatic parenchymal necrosis, edema, and hemorrhage. In the pediatric age group, pancreatitis is associated with a variety of conditions, including infections, trauma, congenital malformations of the pancreatic ducts, drugs and toxins, metabolic disorders, and hepatitis[(131,132,134)]. Mumps, coxsackie virus, EBV, and enterovirus have been accompanied by acute pancreatic inflammation. Obstruction of the pancreatic duct caused by congential anomalies **(Table 36.11)** or ascarides infection has been reported. In some series, child abuse, bicycle injury, or hereditary pancreatitis have been listed as the most common causes of pancreatitis[(135)]. Pancreatitis may complicate metabolic diseases, such as cystic fibrosis, amino acid dyscrasias, and hyperlipoproteinemias[(136)].

Recognition

Pancreatitis should be suspected in the child with an acute onset of abdominal pain, nausea, vomiting, and localized ileus **(Table 36.12).** Although the pain of pancreatitis occurs in the epigastrium, it differs from the pain of peptic

Table 36.12. Recognition of Pancreatitis

Band-like epigastric pain
Radiation through to back
Nausea
Vomiting
Low-grade fever
Tachycardia
Tachypnea
Moderate leukocytosis
Hyperamylasemia
Hypocalcemia
Hypoglycemia
Localized ileus on plain films

ulcer disease in that it is usually band-like rather than crampy, with referral straight through to the back[137]. If the tail of the pancreas is involved, there may be localized inflammation of the diaphragm and phrenic nerve, with pain referred to the left shoulder. Occasionally, left shoulder pain may be more severe than the abdominal discomfort, which may distract physicians from the cause of the disease process.

Fever is common, ranging from 100 to 103° F, and tachycardia and tachypnea often occur. Usually blood pressure is normal, although profound orthostatic hypotension may be seen. The abdomen is mildly to moderately tender, rarely with board-like stiffness or rebound tenderness. Bowel sounds are decreased but present in all but the most severe cases.

Diagnosis

Serum amylase has a half-life of approximately 2 hours[138]. In pancreatitis, levels are usually elevated, although the height of elevation does not correlate with the severity of the clinical disease process. Other processes associated with hyperamylasemia include parotitis, esophageal perforation, acute renal failure, pregnancy, and bowel infarction[133]. In the absence of a clear elevation of amylase level or when other causes of hyperamylasemia exist, other enzyme measurements may assist in the diagnosis. Serum lipase level tends to be elevated for a longer time and is increased in most cases of pancreatitis. Pancreatic trypsinogen is a cationic protein that can be measured by immunoassay: serum levels rise early in the course of pancreatitis and remain elevated for up to 5 days[139]. Other often noted laboratory findings include leukocytosis (12,000 to 18,000 cells/mm^3) and hemoconcentration.

Laboratory findings that suggest a poor prognosis in adults **(Table 36.13)** include a serum calcium level of less than 7.5 mg/dl, leukocytosis of more than 20,000/mm^3, Po_2 of less than 60 mm/Hg, and azotemia. The cause of hypocalcemia of fatal pancreatitis is probably multifactorial, including extraskeletal calcium sequestration, hypersecretion of glucagon, hypomagnesemia, and saponification of fatty acids[140]. Other laboratory parameters that are useful in staging the severity of pancreatitis include levels of serum cyclic adenosine monophosphate, albumin, methemalbumin, serum ribonuclease, and C-reactive protein. However, these laboratory values are not of universal value in clinical management[141]. Prognostic factors have not been established in pediatric patients.

During pancreatitis, any organs that come in direct contact with the pancreas may exhibit dysfunction secondary to localized inflammation. Thus, localized areas of ileus in loops of bowel that come in contact with the pancreas are often seen. This leads to radiographic findings of a "sentinel loop" if the small bowel is involved, and a "colon cutoff sign" if the transverse colon and descending colon are affected. Through a similar mechanism, red and white blood cells may be seen on urinalysis if the inflamed tail of the pancreas impinges on the the left kidney. When the head of the pancreas is swollen and edematous and there is inflammation of the common bile duct, mild cholestasis may be seen. At these times, the alkaline phosphatase or 5′-nucleotidase may be two to four times normal levels, and the serum bilirubin may be 2 to 5 mg/dL.

Table 36.13. Ominous Findings in the Patient with Pancreatitis

Serum calcium < 7.5 mg/dL
WBC > 20,000/mm^3
PO_2 < 60 mm/Hg
BUN > 20 mg/dL

Therapy

"Pancreatic rest" is the mainstay of therapy for pancreatitis. Therefore, patients should be given nothing by mouth (NPO). Fat and protein must be kept out of the proximal bowel: These nutrients cause the release of cholecystokinin, which, in turn, leads to pancreatic enzyme release and further destruction of the inflamed pancreas.

Intravenous fluids can be lifesaving, as the accumulation of fluid in the surrounding tissue can be a major problem. Fluid and colloid should be given quickly and in sufficient amounts to decrease tachycardia and to correct orthostasis. Central venous or pulmonary artery pressure monitoring may be necessary because of combined hypovolemia and pulmonary complications. Careful restitution of serum calcium, magnesium, and potassium levels is necessary in the more severe cases.

Abdominal pain can be severe: patients may require narcotic analgesics for relief. This is especially necessary to recognize in older children who have abused drugs and are viewed with skepticism when complaining of pain.

In patients with gastric atony secondary to localized inflammatory response, large volumes of gastric secretion accumulate. These patients feel more comfortable with nasogastric decompression.

There are theoretical reasons why Trasylol, a chemotrypsin activation inhibitor, might be useful[142], but double-blind studies have varied in showing a conclusively beneficial effect. Likewise, glucagon has been suggested as a method of suppressing pancreatitis, but controlled studies have been inconclusive[143]. The routine use of somatostatin, or its analog octreotide, in patients with acute or chronic pancreatitis is not indicated, but in some patients the use of these medications has been shown to decrease the severity of pain and incidence of complications[144,145]. The beneficial effects are thought to be due to the agents' ability to inhibit pancreatic exocrine secretion. Several laboratory models of pancreatitis have been used to examine the effects of antioxidant therapy in prevention of an inflammatory reaction. In chemically induced acute hemorrhagic pancreatitis, pretreatment with free radical ablation therapy reduced tissue damage and serologic evidence of pancreatic inflammation[146]. Patients with idiopathic chronic pancreatitis ingest fewer antioxidants, such as selenium and vitamins E and C, than sex and age matched controls, suggesting that deficiencies of these nutrients may be associated with disease. Case reports also suggest that prophylactic therapy with antioxidants may be useful in preventing recurrent attacks[147–150].

Patients with severe pancreatitis should be continued on NPO orders for 3 to 4 days after the abdominal discomfort, fever, leukocytosis, and hyperamylasemia disappear. Careful refeeding involves a trial of carbohydrate solids. If tolerated, the diet can be changed slowly by adding small amounts of protein and low-fat foods. In the more protracted cases, elemental feedings have been used. Intake should be stopped immediately if abdominal discomfort, fever, or leukocytosis recurs.

While the child is under NPO restrictions, nutritional status may be maintained by peripheral parenteral nutrition as long as the child was not malnourished to begin with and the pancreatitis appears to be resolving quickly. If the child is malnourished, consideration should be given to early initiation of central venous parenteral nutrition to correct nitrogen balance more quickly.

Complications

Pancreatitis usually has a low rate of morbidity and mortality, but in 10 to 20% of patients, potentially serious complications occur **(Table 36.14)**. Complications may result when pancreatic enzymes, such as phospholipase A, lipase, and elastase, are activated and released, causing necrosis of the pancreas and surrounding organs[151]. Fluid can collect as pancreatic ascites, pancreatic pseudocysts, pleural effusion, or pericardial effusion.

Since the advent of ultrasonography, 40 to 60% of patients with acute pancreatitis were found to have pseudocysts or a collection of pancreatic enzymes beyond the usual confines of the pancreas, i.e. after rupture of the pancreatic duct with extravasation of pancreatic juices. The escaping secretions eventually cause development of a capsule composed of granulation and fibrous tissue that lacks a true epithelial lining, thus the use of the prefix "pseudo." Pseudocysts are usually asymptomatic and disappear with the resolution of the pancreatitis. Prolonged hyperamylasemia, recurrent pain with refeeding, and persistent ileus should raise the suspicion of a larger-than-usual pseudocyst.

In addition to slowing the recovery from pancreatitis, pseudocysts themselves may result in further complications. The "walls" of pseudocysts may be any structure adjacent to the fluid collection, including the lesser sac[152], stomach wall, small intestine, colon, biliary system, or vascular system. If the enzymatic proteins in this cyst become activated, digestion of the capsule may occur, resulting in perforation of a viscus, severe cholangitis, thrombosis of a major vein such as the splenic vein, or perforation into a major artery with exsanguination[133]. Also, inflammation in the perirenal space can lead to right-sided hydronephrosis.

Large or rapidly expanding pseudocysts are considered ominous in combination with acute pancreatitis. Surgical intervention should be considered for patients with acute pancreatitis who are receiving appropriate therapy but have an acutely expanding or large pseudocyst that appears to be compromising the vascular or biliary systems. Large asymptomatic pseudocysts that are found serendipitously after a bout of acute pancreatitis may be followed for weeks. If cysts do not resolve spontaneously, they can be surgically drained, but percutaneous or endoscopic drainage of pancreatic fluid collections is effective in most patients, making the need for laparotomy less frequent.

Infected pancreatitis may be suspected when there is higher than usual fever or leukocytosis or involuntary abdominal guarding or rigidity. Pancreatic abscess is a fairly uncommon complication, but if untreated, carries a 50 to 90% mortality rate. Indications for computed tomography (CT) include acute pancreatitis that is not responding to conservative management, pancreatitis with enlarging pleural effusions, and a clinical deterioration after initial improvement[151]. Although prophylactic antibiotics have not been shown to be cost effective, antibiotics effective against gut flora should be started as soon as pancreatic abscess is suspected. Additionally, percutaneous or surgical drainage should be considered. With multiple percutaneous catheters, cure rates from 60 to 90% have been reported[151]. Stanten and Frey have reported a mortality rate of less than 15% in necrotizing pancreatitis and pancreatic abscess when a comprehensive management plan as suggested in **Table 36.15** is followed[153].

Although pulmonary complications are often underappreciated, they can occur in as many as 40% of patients with pancreatitis[154]. When pulmonary effusion occurs, it is usually on the left side, although bilateral sympathetic effusions have been seen. The loss of intrapulmonary surfactant after release of pancreatic lipase and phospholipase

Table 36.14. Complications of Pancreatitis

Pancreatic abscess
Pancreatic pseudocyst
Pancreatic effusions
Ascites
Pleural
Pericardial
Gastric hemorrhage
Right-sided hydronephrosis
Splenic infarction or hematoma
Hypocalcemia
Hyperglycemia
Coagulopathy
Subcutaneous fat nodules
Respiratory distress syndrome
Shock

Table 36.15. Management of Pancreatic Abscess

Rapid assessment of physiologic derangement
Prompt enhanced CT scan for anatomic evaluation
Early institution of hemodynamic monitoring
Adequate fluid resuscitation
Percutaneous aspiration to identify septic foci
Aggressive surgical debridement

into serum may result in severe atelectasis. In certain cases, endotracheal intubation and positive end-expiratory pressure are indicated.

Other systemic complications include coagulopathy secondary to circulating proteases, subcutaneous nodules caused by metastatic fat necrosis, and metabolic abnormalities such as hyperglycemia and hypocalcemia. Hyperglycemia results from decreased insulin levels and release of glucagon. Replacement with fresh frozen plasma, intravenous calcium, or insulin may be indicated.

LIVER FAILURE IN THE PEDIATRIC INTENSIVE CARE UNIT

Essential to the care of children with hepatic failure is an understanding of the anatomic and physiologic basis of normal hepatic function. The complications of liver failure and the effect of therapeutic interventions on the liver may then be interpreted in terms of their relationship to hepatic pathophysiology.

Anatomic and Physiologic Considerations

The liver synthesizes a large number of proteins, most of which are exported, and excretes metabolic products. Hepatic functions also include the storage and breakdown of glycogen, oxidative phosphorylation, oxidation of fatty acids, synthesis of cholesterol and bile acids, conjugation of bilirubin, and the metabolism of pharmacologic agents. Hepatocytes are rich in enzymes including NAPDH, cytochrome P-450, and cytochrome reductase systems. Proper functioning of the liver requires adequate blood flow to deliver nutrients and oxygen to the metabolically active cells and an efficient, low-pressure biliary excretion system. Approximately 20 to 40% of cardiac output passes through the liver. Less than 25% of blood entering the liver comes through the hepatic artery; the vast majority comes through the portal venous system. Thus, factors that alter blood flow to the portal vein are the major determinants of hepatic blood flow. Increase of splanchnic blood flow from eating results in a threefold increase in hepatic blood flow. Decrease of splanchnic blood flow during exercise, hypovolemia, or sympathetic stress causes a dramatic decrease in hepatic blood flow[(155)].

A number of conceptual frameworks have been developed to describe the fundamental anatomic units of the liver. One of the proposed anatomic concepts is that of the lobule. In the middle of the lobule is the central vein. Extending out to the periphery are cords of hepatocytes. The outer boundary is surrounded by portal triads, which are composed of a portal vein, hepatic artery and a bile duct. The acinus is the other anatomic description of the hepatic microscopic structure, perhaps better used to explain the hepatic microcirculation. In this scheme, the portal triad is in the central position, and the hepatocytes surround it in concentric zones. At the periphery are the hepatic veins. Blood from the portal vein and hepatic artery mixes within the liver in hepatic sinusoids and flows through the sinusoids adjacent to hepatocytes. Between the blood and the hepatocytes are the fenestrated sinusoidal wall and the space of Disse. Cells in the sinusoidal wall include fenestrated endothelial cells that provide channels between the plasma and the hepatocytes; the Kupffer cell, a macrophage that becomes more numerous with increasing antigen load; and the Ito cell, or fat cell, that is thought to participate in fibrogenesis. The blood then flows to the terminal central veins to exit the liver through the hepatic veins[(155)]. Oxygen tension decreases as the blood approaches the hepatic vein. Any increase in pressure within the usually low-pressure hepatic vein system, such as with congestive heart failure, causes decreased outflow from the liver, ischemia of those hepatocytes closest to the hepatic veins, and passive congestion of the liver. Eventually, there is increased lymphatic pressure, increased resistance to portal inflow, and sequestration or third spacing of blood volume.

Hepatocytes exhibit polarity with sinusoidal and canalicular surfaces. When two or three hepatocytes come together, there is differentiation of their adjoining cell membranes with the development of tight junctions and a bile canalicular membrane with microvilli. Conjugated products of metabolism are then excreted through the microvilli into the bile canaliculus and flow through the biliary ductules, the bile ducts, and the common bile duct. Bile flows through the common bile duct, which connects with the main pancreatic duct at the ampulla and enters the second portion of the duodenum.

Definitions and Causes

Fulminant hepatic failure (FHF) is defined as the development of hepatic encephalopathy within 2 to 8 weeks of initial symptoms in someone who has no previous history of liver disease. Hepatic failure describes the loss of liver function resulting from an acute or chronic hepatic disease[(155)].

Viral infections and drug toxicity are the most common causes of FHF. Hepatitis B is the most common viral infection causing FHF[(156)]. Persons exposed to hepatitis B virus who then develop FHF tend to have both an enhanced antibody response, because there is earlier appearance of antibodies to the hepatitis B surface antigen (anti-HBs) and the e antigen (anti-HBe), and more rapid clearance of hepatitis B surface antigen than is found in patients who do not have fulminant hepatitis[(157)]. During infancy, fulminant hepatic failure may develop as a result of congenital viral infections such as CMV, herpes virus, enterovirus, or hepatitis B virus. In toddlers and older children EBV and hepatitis A, B, and D are more common. Hepatitis D is acquired either through coinfection with hepatitis B or as a result of superinfection of HBsAg-positive carriers. Experimental evidence suggests that if hepatitis D occurs as a result of

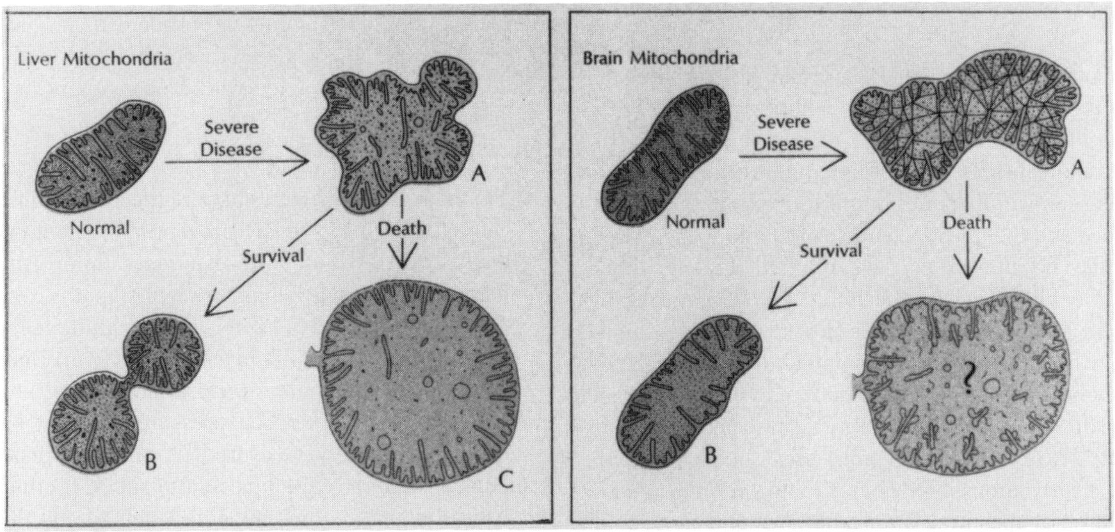

Figure 36.3. Liver mitochondria in severe disease (left, A) often assume a pleomorphic form and show less of dense bodies and expanded matrix space. In survivors (left, B), most mitochondria appear quite normal except for increased fission. Nonsurvivors (left, C) present expanded matrix, protein disorganization, and membrane rupture. In the brain, mitochondrial changes are less well studied, but substantial matrix expansion may occur in severe disease (right, A), although "web-work" may remain intact. In one patient who survived (right, B), expanded matrix, "broken" protein, and membrane ruptures were shown. Changes in fatal cases are unknown. From Haller JS. The enigmatic encephalopathy of Reye's syndrome. Hosp Pract 1975;10:93.

superinfection of HBsAg-positive carriers, hepatic disease is more severe than in patients who are infected with hepatitis B and D simultaneously.

Drug-induced FHF may be related to toxic effects or may be immune-mediated. Hepatic necrosis is associated with acetaminophen, phenytoin, valproic acid, isoniazid, halothane, and carbon tetrachloride ingestion. Halothane-induced hepatitis may present with either mild elevation of levels of transaminases or with hepatic failure. The latter form is rare, especially in the pediatric patient, and causes significant mortality[(158)]. The pathogenesis of halothane-induced hepatitis is thought to be immune-mediated. Many patients have serum antibodies specific for halothane-altered hepatic microsomal proteins[(159)]. These proteins have been isolated from the livers of animals and humans who have been exposed to halothane[(160)]. A systemic hypersensitivity reaction characterized by fever, rash, arthralgias, and hepatocellular damage may be seen resulting from treatment with sulfamethoxazole, sulfasalazine, carbamazepine, and phenytoin. Ingestion of toxic amounts of iron, acetaminophen, and vitamin A may all cause acute hepatic failure.

Children who present with hepatic failure may have end-stage chronic liver disease or previously undiagnosed liver disease. Patients with biliary atresia may have hepatic failure before or after portoenterostomy. A variety of metabolic diseases, such as tyrosinemia, alpha-1 antitrypsin deficiency, Wolman's disease, errors in fatty acid oxidation defects, Wilson's disease, Niemann-Pick disease, hereditary fructose intolerance, and cystic fibrosis, may result in hepatic failure[(155)].

Other miscellaneous causes include Budd-Chiari syndrome, cancer, and hemangioma and Reye's syndrome. Reye's syndrome was first reported in 1929 but was described in detail by Reye, Morgan, and Baral in 1963[(161)]. This clinicopathologic diagnosis describes acute sporadic encephalopathy of unknown cause in association with panlobular microvesicular fat accumulation in the liver and is commonly found with hepatic failure[(155)]. Clinical symptoms are pronounced nausea, usually followed by protracted vomiting, confusion, and coma. Unlike hepatic failure of other causes, jaundice is conspicuously absent in Reye's syndrome. Although liver failure itself can be profound, the most frequent cause of death in children with Reye's syndrome is cerebral edema. If the child does not die of acute liver failure or of the associated complications, recovery may be complete, as there is rapid regeneration of the injured hepatic tissue after toxic damage. Reye's syndrome is a disease process that affects the mitochondrial system of the body[(162)]. Figure 36.3 depicts an artist's perception of the mitochondrial alteration seen in the liver and brain of patients with Reye's syndrome[(163)]. Reye's syndrome most often affects children aged 6 to 12 years, usually appearing as a sequel of an acute viral syndrome. There often is a history of treatment with aspirin. Since this association has been made, efforts to prevent the use of aspirin, especially during varicella and influenza infection, have been associated with a marked decrease in the incidence to as low as 0.1 per 100,000 patients less than 18 years of age[(164–168)]. Although the mechanism behind the relationship of Reye's syndrome to aspirin is not well understood, a suggestion has been made that the syndrome and aspirin may both result in uncoupling of oxidative phosphorylation, resulting in decreased ATP production.

Recognition

Mild to moderate nausea, anorexia, and fatigue are common in acute hepatitis. Protracted vomiting, altered behavior, increased bruisability, or the presence of, or increase in, ascites indicate the onset of hepatic failure. Behavioral alterations seen with hepatic failure range from euphoria to belligerence and the unexpected use of foul language. Sleep patterns may be altered, e.g., sleeping all day and awake all night. Confusion may range from altered spatial orientation (the reason for the Reitan trail test or the five-pointed star test) to slurred speech and complete disorientation. Asterixis may be present. Hyperventilation, hyperthermia, and hyperreflexia signal significant central nervous system involvement[(169)]. As the disease progresses, the child may be lethargic, poorly arousable, unarousable, or may demonstrate decerebrate posture. Throughout the course, the depth of hepatic encephalopathy is one of the most reliable means of assessing the severity of the hepatic failure[(169)].

Liver function tests are usually drawn at the time of admission. Transaminase levels become elevated, with altered hepatocellular membrane integrity. The exact value of transaminase levels does not correlate with severity of the disease; however, levels are usually elevated tenfold to 100-fold above levels normal in FHF. In metabolic diseases, this elevation may not be as marked. The pattern of change in transaminase levels with time can be useful in following the activity of the disease as long as the liver is still capable of producing transaminases. In acute hepatic failure, sometimes such rapid destruction of hepatocytes occurs that the serum transaminase levels seem to fall precipitously as a premoribund event.

Since alkaline phosphatase is produced in the bile canaliculus in response to increased canalicular pressure, alkaline phosphatase of liver origin increases with any extrahepatic or intrahepatic obstruction to bile flow. Inflammation, hydropic degeneration of hepatocytes, or hepatocytes enlarged by fat or metabolites may be intrahepatic causes for alkaline phosphatase level elevation in acute hepatic failure. Because alkaline phosphatase levels are expected to be high in children because of bone growth, measurement of 5′-nucleotidase, an alkaline phosphatase more specific to the liver, may be useful to differentiate bone from liver alkaline phosphatase and works better than heat fractionation for this purpose. Gamma-glutamyl transpeptidase is an enzyme distributed throughout the hepatobiliary tree that may be increased in biliary tract disease. It also is present in many other organs including the pancreas, seminal vesicles, lungs, kidney, and heart.

Neither serum transaminase nor alkaline phosphatase levels define liver function, however. Liver function can be quantified by carefully monitoring serum albumin level prothrombin time, or individual coagulation factor levels, all of which require active hepatocyte metabolism and, thus, reflect "function"[(170)]. With severe deterioration of liver function, a mixed hyperbilirubinemia arises in the range of 15 to 40 mg/dL; albumin level decreases to less than 3.0 mg/dL, and prothrombin time is more than 3 seconds beyond control. Hypoglycemia, which is defined as 1g/kg/hour, has been associated with a poor prognosis[(171)].

Therapeutic Guidelines

Care should be taken to support the patient until hepatic regeneration can occur, by preventing or treating the complications of GI bleeding, respiratory failure, hepatorenal syndrome, infection, hepatic encephalopathy, and cerebral edema. See **Table 36.16** for general guidelines.

Basic monitoring should consist of hourly observations of blood pressure, pulse, respiration, mental status, urine output, and central venous pressure. Arterial blood gases should be routinely measured. A single toxicology panel should be ordered on admission to rule out other treatable causes of coma. Serum ammonia levels (preferably arterial) are useful in confirming a hepatic origin of coma and in monitoring progress, although correlation with degree of encephalopathy is variable. Likewise, serial electroencephalograms may be useful. Intracranial pressure monitoring is done in some ICUs when grade III encephalopathy ensues.

The mainstays of therapy are to keep the patient normovolemic and maintain normal electrolyte levels. Profound hypoglycemia is found in as many as 40% of children with acute hepatic failure and must be vigorously treated. Significant alterations often occur in serum sodium and potassium levels. Patients with acute hepatic failure may require large doses of intravenous potassium solution to maintain a normal serum level because of the kaliuresis associated with secondary hyperaldosteronism. Because of a variety of complex factors, including altered glomerular flow and increased vasopressin and aldosterone concentrations, the renal excretion of water and sodium is impaired. Therefore, sodium should be given with caution even when the serum concentration of sodium is low.

Adequate caloric intake is essential. Since children with acute hepatic failure may have severe hepatic encephalopathy, if oral nutrition cannot be safely maintained TPN should be started at once. Hypertonic glucose administration is usually necessary because the ability of the liver to store glycogen has been impaired. Protein administration should be sufficient to prevent endogenous protein breakdown without increasing ammonia production. Branched-chain amino acid administration has been suggested to correct relative deficiency and to decrease muscle catabolism,

Table 36.16. Management of Children with Fulminant Hepatic Failure

Admit to an ICU, preferably a liver failure unit
Develop a team approach for patient's projected needs
Distinguish between FHF and exacerbation of chronic liver disease
Establish cause: diagnostic serologic and drug testing
Carefully control fluid and electrolyte status
Provide prophylaxis against stress-induced bleeding and encephalopathy
Monitor for infection and encephalopathy
Consider for transplantation

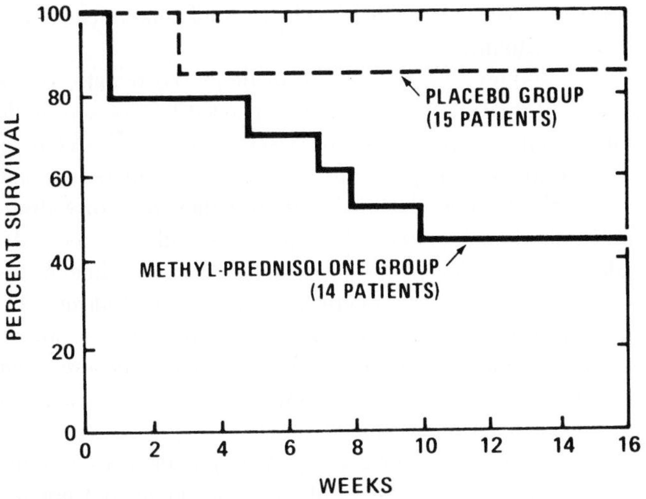

Figure 36.4. Survival curves for two treatment groups during the 16-week study period. Reprinted with permission from Gregory PB, Knaver CM, Kempson RL, Miller R. Steroid therapy in severe viral hepatitis: A double-blind randomized trial of methylprednisolone vs. placebo, N Engl J Med 1976;294:683.

thus decreasing the production of aromatic amino acids and ammonia(172). Analogs of branched-chain amino acids have also been used to displace nitrogen from glutamine, to act as a nutritional source, and to clear encephalopathy.

Although fatty acid emulsions are usually given to patients on TPN as a convenient method for delivering calories and essential fatty acids, this may not be tolerated in patients with liver disease who cannot metabolize the fatty acids quickly. Intrahepatic accumulation of fatty acids may further compromise hepatic function, and nonesterified fatty acids may compete with tryptophan for binding on albumin, thereby increasing the chance for encephalopathy(172).

There are no specific medications to improve liver failure. Adrenocorticosteroids have been used for some types of FHF. However, some investigators have shown that steroids are not helpful and may be mildly deleterious in patients with fulminant viral hepatitis(173). Figure 36.4 shows the relative 16-week survival of patients treated with the steroid methylprednisolone versus those receiving placebo.

Insulin and glucagon administration were proposed by Farivar and colleagues(174) to stimulate hepatic regeneration. Although this approach has been successful in murine hepatitis in mice, its usefulness in humans has been limited. A randomized, controlled therapeutic trial in 38 patients with FHF failed to show that the combination of insulin and glucagon therapy had any benefit related to morbidity or mortality(175).

Hepatic growth factor, also termed macrophage stimulating factor, is a serum protein synthesized by hepatocytes that appears to stimulate hepatic DNA synthesis and phagocytosis by macrophages. Serum levels in patients with FHF are 36 times higher than in patients with acute hepatitis. The clinical significance of these measurements, however, has yet to be determined(176–178).

PGE is produced by the hepatocyte, and its biologic effects include vasodilation, hypotension, increased cardiac output, brochodilation, intestinal hypermotility, inhibition of interleukin-2 (IL-2) production, and induction of neutrophil chemotaxis. PGE may protect the hepatocyte from hypoxia and drug-induced, viral, and immune-mediated injury. Clinical trials of intravenous PGE1 have demonstrated some benefit in patients with drug-induced and viral FHF(179), but the side effects of diarrhea, fever, and hypotension may obviate the routine use of this agent(180).

Specific antiviral therapy is limited and usefulness in children is not certain, but as vaccination against hepatitis B virus becomes more common a decrease in hepatic disease caused by this organism is likely(181).

Prognosis

Mortality rates for FHF depend on the cause and severity of illness. The case fatality rate in the Viral Hepatitis Surveillance Program, was 0.2 to 2.5%, with the highest fatality rate in non-A, non-B infections. Mortality rate was higher in patients more than 50 years old and less than 5 years old(156). In contrast, a 60% mortality rate was seen in the Fulminant Hepatic Failure Surveillance Study: this rate rose to 80% when grade IV encephalopathy was present(182). Others have presented similar findings(175). Survival depends in part on continuous attention to detail and cautious intervention designed to keep patients' metabolic state as normal as possible. Although the more severe grades of encephalopathy occur in cases of more severe hepatic failure with a poorer prognosis, recovery from FHF can be complete and often without permanent neurologic sequelae.

Complications

Gastrointestinal Bleeding

As many as 70% of patients with FHF may experience GI bleeding, and as many as 30% of those die from this complication. Bleeding occurs primarily because of stress-induced gastritis and complications of portal hypertension, which are exacerbated by the coagulopathy of liver disease and sequestration of platelets in an enlarged spleen.

The incidence of stress gastritis in patients with hepatic failure can be reduced by maintaining the pH level of the gastric contents at 4.5 or more(34,35). In adults, this measure has meant a decrease in severe bleeding from 54% of cases to 4% and a related decrease in mortality rate(183). There is no evidence that one H_2-receptor antagonist agent is better than another in preventing stress gastritis in hepatic failure. Cimetidine, however, is associated with mild alterations in both hepatic blood flow, hepatic metabolism, and encephalopathy in some patients. Therefore, many ICUs now prefer ranitidine.

Complications of portal hypertension include esophageal or gastric varices or portal hypertensive gastropathy. Varices of the esophagus or stomach are sometimes asymptomatic but may manifest with massive GI bleeding. In a series of 76 pediatric patients awaiting liver transplantation, 19 sustained bleeding from varices[184]. Portal hypertensive gastropathy (PHG), or congestive gastropathy, describes dilation of the gastric submucosal capillaries and ectasia of the mucosal venules and capillaries in patients with intrahepatic or extrahepatic portal hypertension. This lesion occurs in both adult and pediatric patients, but the incidence of bleeding from PHG is difficult to determine since the diagnosis of PHG is often made at the time of endoscopy for bleeding esophageal varices[8].

When bleeding begins, therapy focuses on the maintenance of hemodynamic stability and prevention of further bleeding. Initial measures include intravenous administration of fresh frozen plasma, normal saline, and plasma expanders, as well as nasogastric lavage. Even though sodium retention may cause increasing ascites, maintaining adequate flow to the kidneys is paramount, so saline administration should not be withheld if central venous pressure begins to fall. Nasogastric suction should be applied carefully since high vacuum pressures may result in mucosal denuding. Often, the initial bleeding responds acutely to supportive measures of blood volume restoration. Coagulopathy develops secondary to inadequate synthesis of factors V, VII, and X. Vitamin K administered in a dosage of 0.2 mg/kg up to 10 mg/day for 3 days should be administered, although the coagulopathy may not respond. Diffuse intravascular coagulopathy may also exist in patients with acute or chronic liver disease, with exacerbations during stress that are induced by bleeding or infection. As described earlier, vasopressin or somatostatin may be useful in the pharmacologic treatment of bleeding.

Rebleeding or persistent bleeding are indications for more invasive therapy, including sclerotherapy, balloon compression, endoscopic variceal ligation, transjugular intrahepatic portosystemic shunts[185,186], and surgical decompression or ligation. Endoscopic sclerotherapy has provided effective hemostasis and has been the traditional therapy for bleeding varices. It has been used successfully for decades in adults and children. Successful eradication is possible but recurrence is not unusual[187]. Complications of sclerotherapy include retrosternal discomfort, transient pyrexia, esophageal ulceration, mediastenitis, and esophageal stricture. Rebleeding can occur in one-third of patients, presumably due to reformation of esophageal varices or presence of gastric varices. In adult patients, endoscopic placement of rubber clips around esophageal varices (termed variceal banding) is a recent addition to the treatment options for bleeding vessels. This alternative approach has also proved beneficial in pediatric patients with bleeding varices[188]. Shunt surgery is often effective, but associated with a high rate of shunt thrombosis in the pediatric age group.

Ascites

Ascites is a common complication of acute and chronic liver disease. It may exacerbate respiratory or renal failure or serve as a medium for the development of spontaneous bacterial peritonitis.

Ascites develops as a result of increased hepatic resistance, decreased oncotic pressure caused by low serum albumin, and altered aldosterone secretion[189,190]. As liver disease worsens, hepatic vascular resistance increases and ascitic fluid accumulates. This fluid is thought to arise from either the hepatic sinusoids or the intestinal capillaries. In addition, albumin synthesis is decreased, resulting in decreased intravascular oncotic pressure. Activation of arterial receptors by the decreasing intravascular volume stimulates water and sodium retention. Increased renin secretion stimulates production of aldosterone and angiotensin II and further sodium and water retention.

With new-onset ascites, diagnostic paracentesis is indicated to assure that the fluid is a transudate and not infected. Treatment of ascites focuses on sodium restriction, spironolactone administration, and slow diuresis. Patients should receive less sodium than they excrete in their urine. Therapeutic paracentesis was often used until the 1950s, when it was abandoned because of the development of useful diuretics and the risk of precipitating intravascular collapse, sepsis, electrolyte derangement, or hepatorenal syndrome. More recently, safer therapeutic paracentesis has been reported with the addition of albumin infusion and close monitoring of intravascular status. Therapeutic paracentesis is most often indicated in situations of respiratory embarassment.

Respiratory Failure

Neurogenic pulmonary edema, fluid overload from the antidiuretic-like activity with liver failure, and intrapulmonary shunting caused by the release of vasoactive products in liver failure may be responsible for the hypoxia seen in 40 to 60% of patients with hepatic failure. Increasing the concentration of inspired oxygen may be all that is necessary in some patients to correct the hypoxia; others may benefit from positive end-expiratory pressure. Although theoretical risks of ischemic liver injury exist with intubation and mechanical ventilation, this therapeutic intervention not only provides access for the provision of tissue oxygenation but also protects the airway from aspiration in patients with worsening hepatic encephalopathy.

Hepatorenal Syndrome

Hepatorenal syndrome occurs when previously normal kidneys decompensate in the presence of hepatic failure. Pathologic abnormalities of the kidney are minimal and, in fact, if these kidneys are transplanted, they sustain normal function. Although the exact cause is not known, this syndrome appears to result from both a redistribution in renal blood flow and change in glomerular filtration rate. Most patients have a decreased effective intravascular volume secondary to impaired protein formation by the liver. The cirrhotic liver increases intrahepatic vascular resistance, thus decreasing venous return and subsequent cardiac output. Although most patients with liver disease seem to be volume overloaded and have both inappropriate aldosterone-like activity and inappropriate antidiuretic hormone-like activity, much of the volume load does not recirculate because of portal hypertension. Decreased hepatic metabolism of bacterial endotoxins and substance P favor peripheral vasodilation[191]. The balance between PG formation and degradation is altered[190]. There appears to be a relative increase of PGs with renal vasoconstrictive properties, such as the eicosanoids thromboxane B2 and leukotriene E2, and decrease of vasopressin, causing medullary interstitial dilation. Other contributing factors include the effect of increased serum bile acids on renal membrane function[192]. Evidence of renal failure occurs in as many as 70% of patients with acute hepatic failure.

The diagnosis of hepatorenal syndrome should be suspected in patients with significant liver disease and oliguria, elevated blood urea nitrogen (BUN), normal urinary sedimentation, hyperosmolar urine, high urine to plasma creatinine ratio, and a very low urine sodium level (less than 10 mEq/L)[193]. Central venous pressure monitoring becomes crucial in patients with potential hepatorenal syndrome. A central venous pressure of 3 to 8 mm Hg allows sufficient volume to perfuse the kidneys without impeding hepatic vein overflow. If hepatorenal syndrome is suspected, a fluid load should be given to raise the central venous pressure to 10 mm Hg quickly, using salt-poor albumin and fluid. Additional volume or an increase of central venous pressure to more than 10 mm Hg may lead to decreased portal flow and greater hepatic damage. In patients who require exquisitely sensitive fluid management and, particularly, in patients with pulmonary edema, a pulmonary artery catheter may be used instead of a central venous catheter. Hepatorenal syndrome may be associated with overaggressive diuresis and administration of antiinflammatory agents or aminoglycosides. Nonsteroidal antiinflammatory drugs can reduce renal plasma flow and glomerular filtration rate, resulting in water retention, dilutional hyponatremia, renal failure, and ascites that is resistant to diuretics. Great care should be taken to prevent precipitous drops in intravascular volume that may invoke hepatorenal syndrome. This includes avoiding large-volume paracentesis and strong diuretics, which could decrease intravascular volume.

The protective effects of intravenous mannitol have been shown perioperatively in patients with obstructive jaundice. Mannitol causes volume expansion and retains renal blood flow despite low perfusion pressures. It also may play a role in preventing endothelial cell swelling and tubular obstruction. Therefore, in the absence of pulmonary edema, addition of a plasma expander such as mannitol plus concomitant furosemide may increase diuresis, as long as the central venous pressure is maintained by minute-to-minute observation at a range of 3 to 10 mm Hg. Excessive diuresis with a drop of central venous pressure may result in irreversible renal shutdown.

The use of dopamine, other catecholamines, or corticosteroids has not proven effective in patients with hepatorenal syndrome. Reinfusion of ascites back into the superior vena cava by using standard intravenous tubing and pumping systems has been proposed. Similar results may also be expected from a LeVeen shunt, although a large controlled trial is not yet complete. Unfortunately, such shunts often clog when used in children.

Infections

Patients with chronic liver disease are immunocompromised, and bacteremia develops significantly more often in them than other hospitalized patients[194]. This may be caused by impaired hepatic reticuloendothelial phagocytosis or diminished bactericidal and opsonic activity[195–197]. Four types of infection commonly seen in children with liver disease are (a) bacteremia by gut organisms as a result of poor hepatic clearing of organisms seeded from the edematous bowel of portal hypertension; (b) spontaneous bacterial peritonitis; (c) urinary tract infections; and (d) aspiration pneumonias. Gram positive organisms such as *Streptococcus pneumoniae*, *Staphylococcus aureus*, and group A β-hemolytic streptococci are the most common cause of bacteremia and peritonitis, and *E. coli* is the most common gram-negative infectious organism. Worsening of encephalopathy, sudden onset of hepatorenal syndrome, or the development of fever or leukocytosis, however, should raise suspicion of infection. Hygienic precautions, attention to avoiding activities likely to cause sepsis (such as drawing blood from the femoral area), and expeditious administration of antibiotics (if signs of infection appear) may contribute to increased survival. There is ample evidence that intravenous prophylactic antibiotics are not of value, but selective intestinal decontamination with poorly absorbed enteral antibiotics, such as neomycin, colistin, and nytstatin, has been shown to be beneficial in the prevention of infection with enterobacteria[198].

Hepatic Encephalopathy

Hepatic encephalopathy is a multifactorial syndrome characterized by symptoms ranging from drowsiness to coma. A great deal of research has been devoted to further understanding of this complex problem, often with conflicting or nonreproducible results. Two theories suggest that encephalopathy results from either diminished hepatic synthesis of a substance other than glucose that is necessary for normal brain function or diminished hepatic metabolism of a gut-derived substance that is either directly neurotoxic or that promotes neural inhibition[199].

Ammonia intoxication has been long suspected as one of the major problems in hepatic encephalopathy. Increased serum ammonia levels are found in many, but not all, patients with hepatic encephalopathy. The height of the ammonia level does not correlate with the grade of encephalopathy. If the ammonia level is elevated in a patient with encephalopathy, however, the ammonia level tends to rise as the encephalopathy worsens and decrease as the encephalopathy improves. Likewise, interventions that increase ammonia levels, such as increased ingestion of nitrogen-containing products, are associated with worsening enceph-

Table 36.17. Controlled Trials of Branched-chain Amino Acid Therapy in Hepatic Coma

Investigator	*Number of Patients*	*Test solution*[a]	*Control*	*Results*[a]
Mendenhall	57	Oral branched chain amino acid (BCAA)	Hospital diet	Improved nutrition in BCAA group; no difference in coma
Egberts	22	Oral BCAA	Casein	Improved psychometric tests, but no difference in "ability to drive" for BCAA group
Michel	70	IV BCAA	Amino acids	No difference between groups
Cerra	70	IV FO80	Neomycin/dextrose	BCAA superior; only 13 of 35 survived control therapy
Wahren	50	IV BCAA	Glucose	No difference in encephalopathy; more deaths in BCAA group

[a] BCAA = branched-chain amino acid.

alopathy. Therapeutic interventions that decrease ammonia levels, such as trapping of ammonia in the gut (with lactulose) or decreasing the urea-producing gut organisms (with antibiotics and lactulose), are associated with concomitant improvement in encephalopathy. Arterial ammonia level correlates better with the degree of encephalopathy than does venous ammonia level.

The mechanism by which ammonia may precipitate encephalopathy is not well understood. One theory is that ammonia converts glutamate, a powerful neuroexcitatory compound, to glutamine, a compound lacking or blocking effective excitatory transmission(200). Ammonia is also thought to depress cerebral blood flow and oxygen consumption and may have a direct effect on the neuronal cell membrane. In contrast, animal studies have shown that during alkalemia, cerebrospinal fluid ammonia concentrations increase, and this hyperammonemic state is associated with increased blood flow(201).

Alteration of neurotransmission may be a more likely explanation of the accompanying reversible central neurologic deficits. Ammonia, amino acids, short-chain fatty acids, octopamine, and other compounds that interfere with the normal flow of information from one neuron to the next have been implicated in encephalopathy. Acetylcholine, norepinephrine, dopamine, and serotonin are the "classic" neurotransmitters(200). The more recently described gut peptides, vasoactive intestinal polypeptide (VIP), somatostatin, bombesin, and the enkephalins, can also act as neurotransmitters. Agents that interfere with transmission, or bind, or displace neurotransmitters from receptor sites may be thought of as "false" neurotransmitters. Octopamine, for example, has been shown to be taken up and released by neurons that normally store norepinephrine and dopamine(200). In one study, the degree of encephalopathy correlated with the degree of elevation of plasma octopamine level(202).

In the case of false neurotransmitters, it is the intracellular and intravesicular synaptic levels or receptor site levels that are important, so that pharmacologic interventions may not prove or disprove their presence. Large doses of octopamine have not caused coma, despite decreasing brain catecholamine levels. Likewise, pharmacologic doses of l-dopa and bromocriptine have failed to improve survival from hepatic encephalopathy in controlled trials(200).

Serum amino acid profiles show abnormal results in patients with hepatic failure(203); however, the correlation between the degree of abnormality and the degree of encephalopathy is variable from study to study. Aromatic and straight-chained amino acid levels are elevated in patients with hepatic failure, whereas branched-chain amino acids are relatively decreased. This results in increased levels of glutamine, methionine, phenylalanine, tyrosine, and tryptophan. The clinical utility of this finding is not certain. Investigators have failed to show improved cerebral function or decreased mortality in patients with hepatic encephalopathy treated with branched-chain amino acids(204). Analysis of the literature by Ericksson and Conn **(Table 36.17)** suggests that in controlled trials that compared branched-chain amino acids with nonspecific therapy, such as glucose or conventional amino acids, there were no statistically significant differences in encephalopathy or mortality(205). Interestingly, treatment outcomes with branched-chain amino acids were also no different than treatment outcomes with lactulose; thus, branch-chain amino acids appear to be no more effective than conventional antihepatic coma therapy. Specifically, Ericksson and Conn conclude that branched-chain amino acid therapy does not result in improvement of acute, chronic, or subclinical hepatic encephalopathy, despite correction of the plasma amino acid abnormalities. Branched-chain amino acids may, however, be better tolerated in some patients with cirrhosis as a supplement to dietary protein than other forms of protein. Studies on the use of keto-analogs of the branched-chain amino acids have had conflicting results(205). Correction of mental status without alteration of plasma amino acid profiles has also been reported(206), once again corroborating the fact that many factors may be involved.

Gamma aminobutyric acid (GABA) is synthesized in neurons by decarboxylation of glutamate. The concentration of GABA is high in the brain, found in 25 to 45% of all nerve endings: GABA is the principal inhibitory neurotransmitter of the mammalian brain(200). Inhibitory neurotransmitters increase the permeability of neurons to anions such as chloride, which makes excitable membranes more resistant to depolarization(207). The neuroinhibitory actions of benzodiazepines and barbiturates are mediated by the GABA neurotransmitter receptor system(200). Preliminary studies in humans with hepatic encephalopathy indicate that GABA plasma levels are elevated, perhaps suggesting increased formation or increased release from neurons. In addition, GABA penetrates the intact blood-brain barrier during FHF[208]. Schafer and Jones have shown that GABA is also a product of enteric bacteria[209], thus potentially explaining why patients with encephalopathy improve with antibiotic therapy effective against gut flora. Other studies, however, have failed to correlate serum levels of GABA with clinical stages of encephalopathy[210]. Hepatic encephalopathy resembles encephalopathies induced by drugs that potentiate GABA-aminergic neurotransmission. Animals with hepatic encephalopathy show increased sensitivity to benzodiazepine and GABA-receptor agonists, while therapy with substances that inhibit binding of benzodiazepines[211], such as the benzodiazepine-receptor antagonists (flumazenil), shows some reversible improvement in the degree of experimental encephalopathy . Other substances that competitively bind to GABA-like receptors have been found in the brain and cerebrospinal fluid of patients with encephalopathy[212]. These may have agonist properties that contribute to hepatic encephalopathy.

Arginine, a branched-chain amino acid of which levels are low in patients with liver failure, is important in the detoxification of hyperammonemia. It has been postulated that the addition of arginine to the serum of patients with encephalopathy may decrease the degree of encephalopathy by reducing the ammonia load.

Methionine, and its metabolic product mercaptan, have long been suspected of worsening encephalopathy. Methionine inhibits brain microsomal (Na, K)-ATPase. Blood mercaptans may correlate better than ammonia levels with the severity of encephalopathy[175]. It has been postulated that the administration of branched-chain amino acids lowers the penetration of methionine through the blood-brain barrier by competing for a common transport mechanism[213]. Some researchers, however, believe that methionine and mercaptans are unlikely to be of major pathogenic importance[214].

As liver failure increases, the stage of hepatic encephalopathy increases. Precipitating factors that also worsen encephalopathy include excessive protein load, respiratory alkalosis[202], hyponatremia, hypokalemia, hypoglycemia, infection, upper intestinal bleeding, azotemia, hypoxia, and administration of medications that suppress the sensorium[215,216].

Methods to monitor patients with hepatic encephalopathy include repeated physical examinations and electroencephalograms. A system for classifying encephalopathy uses a scheme of 0 to IV (**Table 36.18**)[169]. The clinical findings of increased muscular tone, brisk deep tendon reflexes, and tremor during hepatic encephalopathy resemble those of patients with extrapyramidal dysfunction and suggest depression of dopaminergic central activity[205].

Table 36.18. Clinical Staging System for Hepatic Encephalopathy

Grade O:	No disease
Grade I:	Altered spatial orientation, sleep patterns, and affect; tremor
Grade II:	Drowsy, lethargic, agitated, slurred speech, confusion, asterixis, increased muscle tone, dysarthric, hyperreflexive, hyperventilation
Grade III:	Stuporous, but arousable by voice; sleepy most of the time; intention tremor; incoherent
Grade IV:	Unarousable; no spontaneous movements; irregular respiration; sluggish pupils; possible decorticate or decerebrate posturing

Electroencephalography showing slow waves and triphasic waves are confirmatory but neither diagnostic nor easily quantifiable. Visually evoked potentials have been used in a rabbit model of hepatic encephalopathy[217,218]and may become a method for assessing patients because of its ease of use and sensitivity[219].

Metabolic abnormalities found in patients with hepatic encephalopathy include reduced affinity of hemoglobin for oxygen, nonspecific alteration in cerebral glucose metabolism, increased serum levels of substance P[220], and decreased ketone production. Fatty acids depress membrane enzymes, interfere with disposition of ammonia, and augment the coma-causing potential of ammonia and mercaptans.

Treatment of hepatic encephalopathy includes the prevention and therapy of processes known to precipitate encephalopathy, i.e., reduction in protein intake and reduction of serum ammonia levels by the treatment with neomycin plus a laxative or lactulose[221,222]. Neomycin has been successfully used as an antibiotic that is poorly (less than 1%) absorbable and effective at least acutely against urea-splitting gut flora. Lactulose or lactitol, nonabsorbable synthetic disaccharides, cause a watery osmotic diarrhea of low pH. This results in loss of the normal urea-splitting colonic flora and overgrowth of lactobacilli organisms. The low pH may also prevent the absorption of ammonia and aromatic amino acids. Although lactulose is more expensive than neomycin, it has become the standard therapy for hepatic encephalopathy because of its low toxicity. Hypernatremia is a complication of lactulose therapy. Lactitol may have fewer side effects then lactulose. Lactose enemas also reduce encephalopathy[223].

Addition of branched-chain amino acids to intravenous hypertonic (20%) glucose may help improve nutritional status[224] and reduce the concentration of aromatic amino acids[225] but has not been consistently shown to improve cerebral function better than the conventional therapy described earlier[226,227] and is costly. Use of GABA-antagonists has been advocated by a number of centers. In a study of 14 patients with hepatic encephalopathy complicating cirrhosis, Bansky and others reported a rapid, distinct but transient improvement in the mental status of 71%[228] after intravenous administration of flumazenil.

Cerebral Edema

Cerebral edema is the apparent cause of death in 25 to 81% of adult and pediatric patients with hepatic failure[229-234]. Also, it is found on autopsy in 80% of patients who die of FHF[156]. The cause of cerebral edema is as poorly understood as the cause of encephalopathy, but both appear to be related because patients who enter progressively deeper levels of encephalopathy eventually have cerebral edema if the process is not stopped. One mechanism may be altered

Table 36.19. Neurologic Signs Associated with Increased Intracranial Pressure

Increased muscle tone
Increased deep tendon reflexes
Abnormal pupillary reflexes
Hyperventilation

permeability of the blood-brain barrier caused by ammonia, octanoate, mercaptans, and *E. coli* endotoxin[235]. Cerebral edema results from the inability to maintain intracellular water and electrolyte homeostasis. Many of the toxic substances that accumulate during FHF are known to inhibit membrane Na^+K^+-APTase. Any reduction in brain Na^+K^+-ATPase activity is likely to impair neurotransmission and potentially cause glial cell swelling[236]. The degree of enzyme activity reduction, however, correlates more closely with the degree of encephalopathy than with the development of cerebral edema[236]. Inappropriate pathologic cerebral vasodilation has also been proposed as an avoidable cause of increased intracranial pressure (ICP) in the brains of patients with hepatic encephalopathy[204].

Table 36.19 reviews the neurologic signs associated with high ICP. According to Ede, one of the earliest signs is an increase in muscle tone in the extremities; hyperventilation is usually marked[236]. Pupillary responses are a reliable sign of increased ICP, for the pupils become dilated and react sluggishly to light. Clinical signs appear when an ICP of 30 mm Hg is reached[236]. As ICP increases further, decerebrate posturing occurs with trismus and opisthotonus. Bilateral dilated fixed pupils are usually indicative of irreversible brainstem compression[236].

The monitoring of ICP is generally a safe and valuable tool in the patient with FHF[156]. It provides a more reliable measure of cerebral edema than clinical signs and computerized tomography and provides valuable information with which to guide the clinical management of the patient in stage III or IV encephalopathy. However, it has not been proven that measurements of ICP improve survival. Elevated ICP is usually treated once it has reached a persistent level of 30 mm Hg **(Table 36.20).** Steps to vigorously reduce ICP are similar to those discussed in Chapter 18 and include proper positioning of the child, elective intubation and hyperventilation, and osmotic diuresis. Any manipulation of the patient may result in sudden increases of ICP, so attention must be paid to maintaining the patient's thorax position at 45° to the horizontal and avoiding head turning. To be effective, these techniques must be initiated early enough in the course of the disease so that fixed neurologic changes from cerebral edema have not occurred. Because the level of consciousness correlates with the degree of respiratory alkalosis[202], some researchers have recommended initiating ICP monitoring when PCO_2 is more than 25 torr, i.e., the level that is associated with cerebral vasodilation. ICP monitoring may also be indicated when PCO_2 is less than 20 torr, i.e., the level that has been correlated with inadequate cerebral blood flow[237]. One study has shown the use of ICP monitoring in selecting patients for orthotopic liver transplantation[238]. When the cerebral perfusion pressure was less than 40 mm Hg for more than 2 hours, a 100% mortality rate occurred after transplant. If cerebral perfusion pressure was more than 50 mm Hg, all patients survived.

Table 36.20. First-step Approach to Increased Intracranial Pressure

Elevation of head of bed to 45°
Avoid turning head, which increases resistance to venous flow in neck
Hyperventilate mechanically
Administer mannitol plus furosemide if indicated
Maintain cerebral perfusion pressure > 30 mm Hg

Mannitol has been used, at least in part, to induce an osmolar gradient between brain cells and the intravascular system so that fluid can be drawn out of the brain. By achieving an intravascular osmolarity of 300 to 350 mOsm, there is a reduction of the amount of water volume in the brain and ICP is reduced. The use of mannitol in FHF has resulted in significantly greater survival in one controlled study[239]. The synergistic effect of using furosemide plus mannitol has allowed for the reduction of ICP at lower serum osmolarities than are required with use of mannitol alone[237]. To be effective, however, osmotic diuresis must be started before significant elevations in ICP occur. It also must be used with caution in the presence of renal impairment, since fluid overload may increase ICP. Appropriate rapid infusion of mannitol at 0.5 mg/kg may decrease ICP a mean of 22 mm Hg and reverse early clinical signs of cerebral edema. Glycerol has also been used to induce an osmotic gradient; however, once glycerol is metabolized to glucose, it no longer acts as an osmolar sump pump.

"Brain resuscitation" by decreasing the metabolic demands of the brain using hypothermia or barbiturates has been reported. Both techniques may also reduce blood flow and blood volume in the brain, thereby reducing ICP. Evidence that hepatic encephalopathy is significantly decreased or that mortality rate is decreased in FHF because of these maneuvers, however, is lacking.

Although corticosteroids are of use in patients with increased ICP from tumors, controlled studies have failed to prevent cerebral edema or to increase survival in patients with FHF, but rather result in increased mortality rates[173].

Special Techniques

Charcoal hemoperfusion[240], peritoneal dialysis, polyacrylonitrile membrane hemodialysis[241], and exchange transfusion procedures have been tried in an effort to support the patient until hepatic regeneration occurs. Each of these techniques has resulted in temporary arousal of children or adults from deep stages of encephalopathy. Despite initial enthusiasm, however, increased survival rates have not occurred with these techniques[242]. Although hemoperfusion has been reported to reverse coma transiently, its usefulness in increasing survival in humans has been limited[243].

Table 36.21. Charcoal Hemoperfusion Trial: Overall Survival in 137 Patients by Cause

Etiology	*n*	*Survival (%)*
Paracetamol overdose	85	52.9
Hepatitis A	6	66.7
Hepatitis B	18	38.9
Hepatitis, non-A non-B	20	20.0
Drug-induced	8	12.5

William's report of 137 patients treated with charcoal hemoperfusion is shown in **Table 36.21**[157]. Animal and human studies suggest that better results may be achieved if hemoperfusion is begun early and performed often[240]. Plasmapheresis transiently improves hepatic encephalopathy and may be useful in patients before liver transplantation[244–247].

Artificial hepatic support systems are being developed that can remove toxic substances and resupply activated factors while the damaged liver recovers[157,241,248,249]. These systems are composed of porcine hepatocytes, which are grown on membranes in synthetic casings. The casings are grafted to the patient's vascular system and function as an artificial liver until a transplanted liver becomes available or the patient's liver recovers.

In patients with a poor prognosis with FHF, liver transplantation should be considered early to allow as much time as possible for a donor organ to become available. Transplantation for FHF is increasing in frequency, with survival rates higher than any other mode of therapy[250]. Recent reports indicate a 60 to 70% survival rate for children and adults with FHF who undergo liver transplantation. Discouraging, however, is the evidence that more than 25% of the patients die before an organ becomes available[251]. By the time grade IV encephalopathy and ventilator dependence ensue, it may be too late to initiate transplantation[252]. Indications for transplantation and the use of part of living related-donor livers for children with chronic liver disease have also increased as they have become accepted in transplant centers[253–255]. This new technique may improve survival in some patients.

Many of the decisions regarding transplant for FHF depend on the cause of liver disease and its clinical course. Rapid deterioration is often a signal to contemplate transplant. Children with chronic liver disease who may have a poor prognosis, such as those with non-A, non-B hepatitis, also should be considered early, before irreversible complications occur.

Further information on liver transplantation can be found in Chapter 37.

SUMMARY

Patients may require admission to the intensive care unit because of GI bleeding, paralytic ileus, diarrhea, pancreatitis, liver failure, or a GI complication of their primary disease. Each GI illness carries a significant morbidity and/or mortality rate. Although our understanding of these illnesses is still limited, technologic advances and the novel use of pharmacologic agents have offered improved methods for diagnosis and treatment: Recent advances permit the clinician to provide better care. More laboratory data and clinical trials are needed to determine the utility of new ideas in the treatment of pediatric patients with GI and hepatic failure in the ICU.

References

1. Hartmann M, Montgomery A, Jonsson K, et al. Tissue oxygenation in hemorrhagic shock measured as transcutaneous oxygen tension, subcutaneous oxygen tension, and gastrointestinal intramucosal pH in pigs. Crit Care Med 1991;19:205–210.
2. Char S, Farthing MJG. Bacteria and gut immunity. Curr Op Gastroenterol 1994;10:659–663.
3. Lehrer RI, Lichtenstein AK, Ganz T. Defensins:antimicrobial and cytotoxic peptides of mammalian cells. Annu Rev Immunol 1993;11:105–128.
4. Fiocchi C, Binion BG, Katz JA. Cytokine production in the human gastrointestinal tract during inflammation. Curr Op Gastroenterol 1994; 2:639—644.
5. Wershil BK, Strober W. Cytokines and immune regulation: An overview. In: Walker WA, Harmatz PR, Wershil BK. ed. Immunophysiology of the Gut, San Diego: Academic Press 1993:87–95.
6. Gall DG. Gastrointestinal anaphylaxis: effect on gastric and intestinal function. In: Walker WA, Hermatz PR, Wershil BK ed. Immunophysiology of the Gut. San Diego: Academic Press 1993:59–68.
7. Nord KS. Peptic ulcer disease in the pediatric population. Pediatric Clin North Am 1990;35:117–140.
8. Hyams JS, Treem WR. Portal hypertensive gastropathy in children. J Ped Gastroenterol Nutr 1993;17:13–18.
9. Roberts JR, Sachar DB ,Greenstein AJ. Severe gastrointestinal hemorrhage in Crohn's disease. Ann Surg 1991;213:207–211.
10. St-Vil D, Brandt ML, Panic S, et al. Meckel's diverticulum in children: a 20 year review. J Ped Surg 1991;26:1289–1292.
11. Vinton NE. Gastrointestinal bleeding in infancy and childhood. Gastroenterology Clin North Am 1994;23:93–122.
12. Sherman PM. Peptic ulcer disease in children. Gastroenterology Clin North Amer 1994;23:707–725.
13. Bayerdorffer E, Miehlke S, Mannes GA, et al. Double blind trial of omeprazole and amoxicillin to cure *Helicobacter pylori* infection in patients with duodenal ulcer. Gastroenterology 1995;108:1412–1417.
14. Heldenberg D, Wagner Y, Heldenberg E, et al. The role of *Helicobacter pylori* in children with recurrent abdominal pain. Am J Gastroenterol 1995;90:906–909.
15. Sonnenberg A ,Townsend WF. Costs of duodenal ulcer therapy with antibiotics. Arch Int Med 1995;155:922–928.
16. Blecker U, Hauser B, Lanciers S, et al. The prevalence of *Helicobacter pylori*-positive serology in asymptomatic children. J Pediatr Gastroenterol Nutr 1993;16:252–256.
17. Drumm B, Sherman P, Cutz E, et al. Association of *Campylobacter pylori* on the gastric mucosa with antral gastritis in children. N Engl J Med 1987;316:1557.
18. Berry R, Perrault J. Gastrointestinal bleeding. In: Walker WA, Rune PR, Hamilton JR, et al. ed., Pediatric Gastrointestinal Disease. Philadelphia: B.C. Decker 1991:111–145.
19. Resnick RH. Intraarterial vasopressin:a continuing challenge. Gastroenterology 1975;68:411–412.
20. Konturek SJ, Konturek JW. Gastric adaptation: basic and clinical aspects. Digestion 1994;55:131–138.
21. Menguy R, Master Y. Mechanism of stress ulcer: effects of hemorrhagic shock on energy metabolism in the mucosa of the antrum, corpus, and fundus of the rabbit stomach. Gastroenterology 1974;66:1168.
22. Menguy R, Masters Y. Mechanism of stress ulcer: influence of sodium taurocholate on gastric mucosal energy metabolism during hemorrhagic shock and on mitochondrial respiration and ATPase in gastric mucosa. Dig Dis 1976;21:1001.
23. Skillman J, Gould S, Chung R, et al. The gastric mucosal barrier: clinical and experimental studies in critically ill and normal man, and in the rabbit. Ann Surg 1974;172:564.

24. Eastwood G. Effect of pH on bile salt injury to mouse gastric mucosa: a light and electron-microscope study. Gastroenterology 1975;68:1456.
25. Smith B, Skillman J, Edwards B, et al. Permeability of the human gastric mucosa: alteration by acetylsalicylic acid and ethanol. N Engl J Med 1971;285:716.
26. Cooke A. The role of mucosal barrier in drug-induced gastric ulceration and erosions. Dig Dis 1976;21:155.
27. Fidden-Green R, McGough E, Pittenger G, et al. Predictive value of intramural pH and other risk factors for massive bleeding from stress ulceration. Gastroenterology 1983;85:613.
28. Hernandez DE. Neuroendocrine mechanisms of stress ulceration: Focus on thyrotropin-releasing hormone. Lif Sci 1986;39:279–296.
29. Lacroix J, Nadeau D, Laberge S, et al. Frequency of upper gastrointestinal bleeding in a pediatric intensive care unit. Crit Care Med 1992;20:35–42.
30. Cochran EB, Phelps SJ, Tolley EA, et al. Prevalence of and risk factors for upper gastrointestinal tract bleeding in critically ill pediatric patients. Crit Care Med 1992;20:1519–1523.
31. Lopez-Herce J, Dorao P, Elola P, et al. Frequency and prophylaxis of upper gastrointestinal hemorrhage in critically ill children: a prospective study comparing the efficacy of almagate, ranitidine, and sucralfate. Crit Care Med 1992;20:1082–1089.
32. Czaja A, McAlhany J, Pruitt BJ. Acute gastroduodenal disease after thermal injury: an endoscopic evaluation of incidence and natural history. N Engl J Med 1974;291:925.
33. Cook DJ, Fuller HD, Guyatt GH, et al. Risk factors for gastrointestinal bleeding in critically ill patients. N Engl J Med 1994;330:377–381.
34. Tryba M. The gastropulmonary route of infection—fact or fiction? Am J Med 1991;91:135S–146S.
35. Kappstein I, Schlugen G, Friedrich T, et al. Incidence of pneumonia in mechanically ventilated patients treated with sucralfate or cimetidine as prophylaxis for stress bleeding: bacterial colonization of the stomach. Am J Med 1991;91:125S–131S.
36. Silen W. Stress ulcers. Viewpoints Dig Dis 1971;3:5.
37. Curtis L, Simonian S, Buerck C, et al. Evaluation of the effectiveness of controlled pH in management of massive upper gastrointestinal bleeding. Am J Surg 1973;125:474.
38. Hastings PR, Skillman JJ, Bushnell LS, et al. Antacid titration in the prevention of acute gastrointestinal bleeding: a controlled randomized trial in 100 critically ill patients. N Engl J Med 1978;298:1041–1045.
39. Vergin H, Kori-Linder C. Putative mechanism of cytoprotective effect of certain antacids and sucralfate. Dig Dis Sci 1990;35:1320–1327.
40. Derrida S, Nury B, Slama R, et al. Occult gastrointestinal bleeding in high-risk intensive care unit patients receiving antacid prophylaxis: frequency and significance. Crit Care Med 1989;17:122–125.
41. Lacroix J, Infante-Rivard C, Gauthier M, et al. Upper gastrointestinal tract bleeding acquired in a pediatric intensive care unit: prophylaxis trial with cimetidine. J Pediatr 1986;108:1015–1018.
42. Peura D, Koretz R. Prophylactic therapy of stress-related mucosal damage: why, which, who, and so what? Am J Gastroenterol 1990;85:935.
43. Burgess P, Larson GM, Davidson P, et al. Effect of ranitidine on intragastric pH and stress related upper gastrointestinal bleeding in patients with severe head injury. Dig Dis Sci 1995;40:645–650.
44. Truba M. Stress bleeding prophylaxis with sucralfate; pathophysiologic basis and clinical use. Scand J Gastroenterol 1990;25:S173.
45. Borrero E, Bank S, Margolis I, et al. Comparison of antacid and sucralfate in the prevention of gastrointestinal bleeding in patients who are critically ill. Amer J Med 1985;79:62–64.
46. Eddleston JM, Pearson RC, Holland J, et al. Prospective endoscopic study of stress erosions and ulcers in critically ill adult patients treated with either sucralfate or placebo. Crit Care Med 1994;22:1949–1954.
47. Tryba M, Kurz-Muller K, Donner B. Plasma aluminum concentration in long term mechanically ventilated patients receiving stress ulcer prophylaxis with sucralfate. Crit Care Med 1994;22:1769–1773.
48. Ryan P, Dawson J, Teres D, et al. Nosocomial pneumonia during stress ulcer prophylaxis with cimetidine and sucralfate. Arch Surg 1993;128:1353–1357.
49. Shaw-Stiffel TA, Roberts EA. Treatment of acid-peptic disease. In: Walker WA, Rune PR, Hamilton JR, et al. ed. Pediatric Gastrointestinal Disease. Philadelphia: B.C. Decker, 1991:1702–1715.
50. Choctaw W, Fujita C, Zawacki B. Prevention of upper gastrointestinal bleeding in burn patients. Arch Surg 1980;115:1073.
51. Solem L, Strate R, Fischer R. Antacid therapy and nutritional supplementation in the prevention of Curling's ulcer. Surg Gynecol Obstet 1979;148:367.
52. Rahn N III, Tishler J, Han S, et al. Diagnostic and interventional angiography in acute gastrointestinal hemorrhage. Diag (Berl) Radiol 1982;143:361.
53. Athanasoulis C, Waltman A, Novelline R, et al. Angiography—its contribution to the emergency management of gastrointestinal hemorrhage. Radiol Clin North Am 1976;14:265.
54. Waltman A. Transcatheter embolization versus vasopressin infusion for the control of arteriocapillary gastrointestinal bleeding. Cardiovasc Intervent Radiol 1980;3:289.
55. Reuter S, Chuag V, Bree R, et al. Selective arterial embolization for control of massive upper gastrointestinal bleeding. AJR 1975;125:119.
56. Livingston E, Passaro E. Postoperative ileus. Dig Dis Sci 1990;35(1):121.
57. Franken EJ, Smith W, Smith J. Paralysis of the small bowel resembling mechanical intestinal obstruction. Gastrointest Radiol 1980;5:161.
58. Davis J, Nusbaum M. Chlorpromazine therapy and functional large bowel obstruction. Am J Gastroenterol 1973;60:635.
59. Schippers E, Holscher A, Ballschweiler E, et al. Return of interdigestive motor complex after abdominal surgery. Dig Dis Sci 1991;36:621.
60. Cohen M, Weber T. Metrizamide in neonatal and childhood small bowel obstruction. AJR 1982;139:689.
61. Bowerman R, Silver T, Jaffe M. Real-time ultra-sound diagnosis of intussusception in children. Radiology 1982;143:527.
62. Benson MJ, Roberts JP, Wingate DL, et al. Small bowel motility following major intra-abdominal surgery: the effects of opiates and rectal cisapride. Gastroenterology 1994;106:924–936.
63. Ein H, Ferguson J. Intussusception—the forgotten postoperative obstruction. J Pediatr Surg 1971;6:16.
64. Raudkivi P, Smith H. Intussusception: analysis of 98 cases. Br J Surg 1981;68:645.
65. Peetz D, Gamelli R, Pilcher D. Intestinal intubation in acute, mechanical small-bowel obstruction. Arch Surg 1982;117:334.
66. Adams J. A dynamic ileus of the colon: an indication for cecostomy. Arch Surg 1974;109:503.
67. Fiedler L. PGF2a—a new therapy for paralytic ileus? In: Samuelson B, Paoletti R, eds. Advances in prostaglandin and thromboxane research. New York: Raven Press, 1980:1609.
68. Nadrowski L. Paralytic ileus: Recent advances in pathophysiology and treatment. Curr Surg 1983;40:260.
69. Davidson ED, Hersh T, Brinner RA, et al. The effects of metoclopramide on postoperative ileus. Ann Surg 1979;190:27.
70. Pescatori M. Effect of cisapride on clinical parameters in post-operative ileus. Progr Med 1987;43:111–114.
71. Hallerback, Bergmen B, Bong H, et al. Cisapride in the treatment of postoperative ileus. Aliment Pharmacol Therap 1991;5:503–511.
72. Kawamura O, Sekiguchi T, Kusano M, et al. Effect of erythromycin on interdigestive gastrointestinal contractile activity and plasma motilin concentration in humans. Dig Dis Sci 1993;38:870–876.
73. Catnach SM, Fairclough PD. Erythromycin and the gut. Gut 1992;33:397–401.
74. Richardson RR, Cerullo LJ. Transabdominal neurostimulation in treatment of neurogenic ileus. Appl Neurophysiol 1979;42:375.
75. Hymes AC, Yonehiro EG, Raab DE. Electrical surface stimulation for treatment and prevention of ileus and atelectasis. Surg Forum 1974;25:222.
76. Byrne WJ, Cipel L, Euler AR, et al. Chronic idiopathic pseudo-obstruction in children—clinical characteristics and prognosis. J Pediatr 1977;90:585.
77. Krishnamurthy S, Schuffler MD. Pathology of neuromuscular disorders of the small intestine and colon. Gastroenterology 1987;93:819–834.
78. Werlin SL, Grand RJ. Severe colitis in children and adolescents: diagnosis, course and treatment. Gastroenterology 1977;73:828.
79. Bill AH, Chapman ND. The enterocolitis of Hirschsprung's disease—its natural history and treatment. Am J Surg 1962;103:70–74.
80. Rhoads JM, Powell DW. Diarrhea. In: Walker WA, Rune PR, Hamilton JR, et al. Pediatric Gastrointestinal Disease, Philadelphia: B.C. Decker, 1991:62–78.
81. Hill MJ, Drasar BS. Degradation of bile salts by human intestinal bacteria. Gut 1968;9:22.
82. Perman JA. Carbohydrate intolerance and the enteric microflora. In: Carbohydrate intolerance in infancy. Lifshitz F, ed. New York: Marcel Dekker, 1982:137.
83. Cooke GC. Influence of systemic infections on xylose absorption. Acta Trop (Basel) 1981;38:173.
84. Wright TL, Heyworth MF. Maldigestion and malabsorbtion. In: Sleisenger MH, Fordtran JS, ed. Gastrointestinal disease: pathophysiology, diagnosis and management. Philadelphia: W.B. Saunders, 1989:263–282.

85. Granger DN, Richardson PDI, Kvietys PR, et al. Intestinal blood flow. Gastroenterology 1980;78:837.
86. Bond JH, Prentiss RA, Levitt MD. The effects of feeding on blood flow to the stomach, small bowel, and colon of the conscious dog. J Lab Clin Med 1979;93:594.
87. Alward CT, Hook JB, Helmrath TA, et al. Effect of asphyxia on cardiac output and organ blood flow in the newborn piglet. Pediatr Res 1978;12:824.
88. Perman JA. Contaminated small bowel syndrome. In: Hoekelman RA, ed. Principles of pediatrics: health care of the young. New York: McGraw-Hill, 1978:808.
89. Akesode F, Lifshitz F, Hoffman KM. Transient monosaccharide intolerance in a newborn infant. Pediatrics 1973;51:891.
90. Remington M, Malagelada JR, Zinsmeister A, et al. Abnormalities in gastrointestinal motor activity in patients with short bowels: effect of a synthetic opiate. Gastroenterology 1983;85:629.
91. Lemelle JL, Schmitt M, Miscault Gd, et al. Neonatal necrotizing enterocolitis: a retrospective and multicentric review of 331 cases. Acta Paediatr Suppl 1994;396:70–73.
92. Santulli TV, Schullinger JN, Herd WC. Acute necrotizing enterocolitis in infancy: a review of 64 cases. Pediatrics 1975;5:376.
93. Amoury RA. Necrotizing enterocolitis: a continuing problem in the neonate. World J Surg 1993;17:363–373.
94. Lifshitz F, Wapnir RA, Pergolizzi R, et al. Hypoxia effects on carbohydrate transport. Pediatr Res 1976;10:356.
95. Israel E. Necrotizing enterocolitis. In: Walker WA, ed. Pediatric Gastrointestinal Disease. Philadelphia: BC Decker, 1991:639–646.
96. Israel EJ. Neonatal necrotizing enterocolitis, a disease of the immature mucosal barrier. Acta Paediatr Suppl 1994;396:27–32.
97. Yoken RH, Bartlett JG, Leister F. Enzyme-linked immunosorbent assay (ELISA) for detection of human reovirus-like agent of infantile gastroenteritis. Lancet 1977;2:263.
98. Willoughby RE, Wee SB, Yolken RH. Non-group A rotavirus infection associated with severe gastroenteritis in a bone marrow transplant patient. Pediatr Infect Dis J 1988;7:133–135.
99. Kimberg DV. Cyclic nucleotides and their role in gastrointestinal secretion. Gastroenterology 1974;67:1023.
100. Field M. Intestinal secretion. Gastroenterology 1974;66:1063.
101. Tedesco FJ. Pseudomembranous colitis: pathogenesis and therapy. Med Clin North Am 1982;66:655.
102. Viscidi RP, Bartlett JG. Antibiotic-associated pseudomembranous colitis in children. Pediatrics 1981;67:381.
103. Tullus K, Aronsson B, Marcus S, et al. Intestinal colonization with *Clostridium difficile* in infants up to 18 months of age. Eur J Clin Microbiol Infect Dis 1989;150:390–393.
104. Donta ST, Myers MG. *Clostridium difficile* toxin in asymptomatic neonates. J Pediatr 1982;100:431–434.
105. Wolfhagen MJHM, Meijer K, Fluit AC, et al. Clinical significance of *Clostridium diffficile* and its toxins in faeces of immunocompromised children. Gut 1994;35:1608–1612.
106. Kelly CP, Pothoulakis C, LaMont JT. *Clostridium difficile* colitis. N Engl J Med 1994;330:257–262.
107. Leung AKC, Robson WLM. Acute diarrhea in children; what to do and what not to do. Postgrad Med 1989;86(8):161.
108. Silverman A, Roy CC. Pediatric clinical gastroenterology. St. Louis: CV Mosby, 1983:893.
109. Perman JA, Barr RG, Watkins JB. Sucrose malabsorption in children: non-invasive diagnosis by interval breath hydrogen determination. J Pediatr 1978;93:17.
110. Field M, Rao MC, Chang EG. Intestinal electrolyte transport and diarrhea disease. N Engl J Med 1989;321:879.
111. Wilmore DW, Dudrick SJ. Growth and development of an infant receiving all nutrients exclusively by vein. JAMA 1968;203:860.
112. Votik AJ, Echave V, Brown AR, et al. Use of elemental diet during the adaptive stage of short gut syndrome. Gastroenterology 1973;65:419.
113. Nolan CM, Johnson KE, Coyle MB, et al. *Campylobacter jejuni* enteritis: efficacy of antimicrobial and antimotility drugs. Am J Gastroenterol 1983;78:621.
114. Pickering LK. Therapy for acute infectious diarrhea in children. J Pediatr 1991;118(4):S118.
115. Peters G, ed. Red book: Report of the committee on infectious diseases. 23rd ed. Elk Grove: American Academy of Pediatrics, 1994.
116. Feigin RD, Cherry JD. Textbook of Pediatric Infectious Diseases. 3rd ed. Philadelphia: WB Saunders, 1993.
117. Lewis JD, Winter HS. Intestinal and hepatobiliary diseases in HIV-infected children. Gastroenterology Clin North Amer 1995;24:119–132.
118. Gazzard BG. Practical advice for the gastroenterologist dealing with symptomatic HIV disease. Gut 1990;31:733.
119. Gerberding JL. Diagnosis and management of HIV-infected patients with diarrhea. J Antimicrob Chemother 1989;23 (Suppl A):83.
120. Goodgame RW, Kimball K, Ou C, et al. Intestinal function and injury in acquired immunodeficiency syndrome-related cryptosporidiosis. Gastroenterology 1995;108:1075–1082.
121. Benhamou Y, Kapel N, Hoang C, et al. Inefficacy of intestinal secretory immune response to *Cryptosporidium* in acquired immunodeficiency syndrome. Gastroenterology 1995;108:627–635.
122. Miller TL, Winter HS, Luginbuhl LM, et al. Pancreatitis in pediatric human immunodeficiency virus infection. J Pediatr 1992;120:223–227.
123. Butler KM, Venson D, Henry N, et al. Pancreatitis in human immunodeficiency virus-infected children receiving dideoxyosine. Pediatrics 1993;91:747–751.
124. Miller TL, Orav EJ, Martin SR, et al. Malnutrition and carbohydrate malabsorption in children with vertically-transmitted human immunodeficiency virus-1 infection. Gastroenterology 1991;100:1296–1302.
125. Internal Pediatric Intestinal HIV Study Group. Intestinal malabsorption of HIV-infected children: relationship to diarrhoea, failure to thrive, enteric micro-organisms and immune impairment. AIDS 1993;7:1435–1440.
126. Cox GJ, Matsui SM, Lo RS, et al. Etiology and outcome of diarrhea after marrow transplantation: a prospective study. Gastroenterology 1994;107:1398–1407.
127. Wagner ML, Rosenberg HS, Fernbach DJ, et al. Typhilitis: a complication of leukemia in childhood. Am J Roentgenol Radium Ther Nucl Med 1970;109:341–350.
128. Katz JA, Wagner ML, Gresik MV, et al. Typhilitis: an 18-year experience and postmortem review. Cancer 1990;65:1041–1047.
129. Shamberger RC, Weinstein HJ, Delorey MJ, et al. The medical and surgical management of typhlitis in children with acute nonlymphocytic (myelogenous) leukemia. Cancer 1986;57:603–609.
130. Yeager AM, Kanof ME, Kramer SS, et al. Pneumatosis intestinalis in children after allogenic bone marrow transplantation. Pediatr Radiol 1987;17:18–22.
131. Weizman Z, Durie PR. Acute pancreatitis in childhood. J Pediatr 1988;113:24–29.
132. Haddock G, Coupar G, Youngson GG, et al. Acute pancreatitis in children: a 15 year review. J Pediatr Surg 1994;29:719–722.
133. Steinberg W, Tenner S. Acute pancreatitis. N Engl J Med 1994; 330:1198–1210.
134. Roberts IM. Disorders of the pancreas in children. Gastroenterol Clin North Amer, 1990;19:963–973.
135. Perrault P. Hereditary pancreatitis. Gastroenterol Clin North Amer, 1994; 19:743–752.
136. Kahler SG, Sherwood WG, Woolf D, et al. Pancreatitis in patients with organic acidemias. J Pediatr 1994;124:239–243.
137. Rogers EL. Can you spot the pain of acute pancreatitis? Mod Med 1980;48:28.
138. Peiper-Bigelow C, Strocchi A ,Levitt MD. Where does serum amylase come from and where does it go? In Gastroenterol Clin North Amer, 1990: W.B. Saunders: Philadelphia. 793–810.
139. Durie PR. Pancreatitis. In: Walker WA, ed. Pediatric Gastrointestinal Disease. Philadelphia: BC Decker, 1991:1209–1236.
140. Weir GC, Lesser PB, Droop LJ, et al. The hypocalcemia of acute pancreatitis. Ann Intern Med 1975;83:185.
141. Ferguson CM, Bradley CL. Can markers for pancreatic necrosis be used as indicators for surgery? Am J Surg 1990;160:459.
142. Trapnell JE, Rigby CC, Talbot CH, et al. A controlled trial of trasylol in the treatment of acute pancreatitis. Br J Surg 1974;61:177.
143. Olazabal A, Fuller R. Failure of glucagon in the treatment of alcoholic pancreatitis. Gastroenterology 1978;74:489.
144. Buchler MW, Binder M, Friess H. Role of somatostatin and its analogues in the treatment of acute and chronic pancreatitis. Gut 1994;35:515–519.
145. Debas HT. Somatostatin: physiologic and clinical potential. View Dig Dis 1988;20:13–17.
146. Schoenberg MH, Buchler M, Younes M, et al. Effect of antioxidant treatment in rats with acute hemorrhagic pancreatitis. Dig Dis Sci 1994;39:1034–1040.
147. Braganza JM, Thomas A, Robinson A. Antioxidants to treat chronic pancreatitis in childhood? Case report and possible implications for pathogenesis. Int J Pancreatol 1988;3:209–216.
148. Bragnza JM, Jeffrey IJ, Foster J, et al. Recalcitrant pancreatitis: eventual control by antioxidants. Pancreas 1987;2:489–494.

149. Uden S, B Ilton B, Guyan PM, et al. Rationale for antioxidant therapy in pancreatitis and cystic fibrosis. Adv Exp Med Biol 1990;264:555–572.
150. Uden S, Bilton D, Nathan L, et al. Antioxidant therapy for recurrent pancreatitis:placebo-controlled trial. Aliment Pharmacol Ther 1990; 4:357–371.
151. VanSkonnenberg E, Casola G, Varney RR, et al. Imaging and interventional radiology for pancreatitis and its complications. Radiol Clin North Am 1989;27(1):65.
152. Meyers MA, Evans JA. Effects of pancreatitis on the small bowel and colon: spread along mesenteric planes. AJR 1973;119:151.
153. Stanton R, Frey CF. Comprehensive management of acute necrotizing pancreatitis and pancreatic abscess. Arch Surg 1990;125:1269.
154. Rovner AJ, Westcott JL. Pulmonary edema and respiratory insufficiency in acute pancreatitis. Radiology 1976;118:513.
155. Mowat AP. Liver disorders in childhood. 2nd ed. London: Butterworths, 1987:408.
156. Hoofnagle JH, Carithers RL, Shapiro C, et al. Fulminant hepatic failure: summary of a workshop. Hepatology 1995;21:240–252.
157. Williams R. Management of acute liver failure. Postgrad Med J 1988;64:769–777.
158. Kenna JG, Neuberger J, Mieli-Vergani G, et al. Halothane hepatitis in children. BMJ 1987;294:1209–1211.
159. Martin JL, Kenna JG, Martin BM, et al. Halothane hepatitis patients have serum antibodies that react with protein disulfide isomerase. Hepatology 1993;18:858–863.
160. Pohl JR. Drug-induced allergic hepatitis. Seminars in liver disease. 1990;10:305–315.
161. Reye RDK, Morgan G, Baral J. Encephalopathy and fatty degeneration of the viscera: a disease entity in childhood. Lancet 1963;2:749–752.
162. Bove KE, McAdams AJ, Partin JC, et al. The hepatic lesion in Reye's syndrome. Gastroenterology 1975;69:685.
163. Haller JS. The enigmatic encephalopathy of Reye's syndrome. Hosp Pract 1975;10:91.
164. Starko KM, Ray CG, Dominguez LB, et al. Reye's syndrome and salicylate use. Pediatrics 1980;66:859–864.
165. Khan AS, Kent J, Schonberger LB. Aspirin and Reye's syndrome. Lancet 1993;341:968.
166. Glasgow JFT, Moore R. Reye's syndrome 30 years on. BMJ 1993;307:950–951.
167. Davis DL, Buffler T. Reduction in deaths after labelling for risk of Reye's syndrome. Lancet 1992;340:1042.
168. Reye's syndrome surveillance—United States, 1987 and 1988. MMWR 1989;38:325–327.
169. Rogers EL, Rogers MC. Fulminant hepatic failure and hepatic encephalopathy. Pediatr Clin North Am 1980;27:701.
170. Pereira LM, Langley PG, Hayllar KM, et al. Coagulation factor V and VIII/V ratio as predictors of outcome in paracetamol induced fulminant hepatic failure: relation to other prognostic indicators. Gut 1992;33:98–102.
171. Davis MA, Peters TL, Redeker AG, et al. Appraisal of the mortality in acute fulminant viral hepatitis. N Engl J Med 1968;278:1248–1253.
172. Bernardini P, Fischer JE. Amino acid imbalance and hepatic encephalopathy. Ann Rev Nutr 1982;2:419.
173. Gregory PB, Knauer CM, Kempson RL, et al. Steroid therapy in severe viral hepatitis: a double-blind, randomized trial of methylprednisolone vs. placebo. N Engl J Med 1976;294:682.
174. Farivar M, Wands JR, Isselbacher KJ, et al. Effect of insulin and glucagon on fulminant murine hepatitis. N Engl J Med 1976;295:1517.
175. Woolf GM, Redeker AG. Treatment of fulminant hepatic failure with insulin and glucagon; a randomized, controlling trial. Dig Dis Sci 1991;36(1):92.
176. Gohda E, Tsubouchi H, Nakayama H, et al. Human hepatocyte growth factor in blood of patients with fulminant hepatic failure—basic aspects. Dig Dis Sci 1991;36:785–790.
177. Tsubouchi H, Hirono S, Gohda E, et al. Human hepatocyte growth factor in blood of patients with fulminant hepatic failure. Part 1: Clinical aspects. Dig Dis Sci 1991;36:780–784.
178. Shiota G, Okano J, Umeki K, et al. Serum hepatocyte growth factor in acute hepatic failure in comparison to acute hepatitis. Res Commun Mol Pathol Pharm 1994;85:157–162.
179. Sinclair SB, Levy GA. Treatment of fulminant viral hepatic failure with prostaglandin E—a preliminary report. Dig Dis Sci 1991;36:791–800.
180. Sheiner P, Sinclair S, Greig P. A randomized control trial of prostaglandin E1 in the treatment of fulminant hepatic failure. Hepatology 1992;16:88A.
181. Romero R, Lavigne JE. Viral hepatitis in children. Seminars in liver disease 1994;14:289–302.
182. Trey C, Smith CA. Acute hepatic failure in the critically ill child. Philadelphia: WB Saunders, 1972:104.
183. Meguid MM, Campos AC, Hammond WG. Nutritional support in surgical practice Part 2. Am J Surg 1990;159:427.
184. Sokal EM, Van Hoorebeek N, Van Obbergh L, et al. Upper gastrointestinal tract bleeding in cirrhotic children candidates for liver transplantation. Eur J Pediatr 1992;151:326–328.
185. Heyman MB, LaBerge JB, Somberg KA, et al. Transjugular intrahepatic portosystemic shunts in children. Gastroenterology 1995;108: A1084.
186. LaBerge JM, Somberg KA, Lake JR, et al. Two-year outcome following transjugular intrahepatic portosystemic shunt for variceal bleeding: results in 90 patients. Gastroenterology 1995;108:1143–1151.
187. Hassall E, Berquist WE, Ament ME, et al. Sclerotherapy for extrahepatic hypertension in childhood. J Pediatr 1989;115:69–74.
188. Fox VL, Carr-Locke DL, Conners PJ, et al. Endoscopic ligation of esophageal varices in children. J Pediatr Gastroenterol Nutr 1995; 20:202–208.
189. Dudley FJ. Pathophysiology of ascites formation. Gastroenterol Clin NA, 1992;21:215–235.
190. Gentilini P, Laffi G. Pathophysiology and treatment of ascites and the hepatorenal syndrome. Baillieres Clin Gastroenterol 1992;6:581–607.
191. Lang F, Gerok W, Haussinger D. New clues to the pathophysiology of hepatorenal failure. Clin Investig 1993;71:93–97.
192. Wilkinson SP, Gazzard BG, Arroyo V, et al. Relation of renal impairment and hemorrhagic diathesis to endotoxemia in fulminant hepatic failure. Lancet 1974;1:521.
193. Epstein M. Hepatorenal syndrome: emerging perspectives of pathophysiology and therapy. J Am Soc Nephrol 1994;4:1735–1753.
194. Gradual N, Milman N, Kirkegaard E, et al. Bacteremia in cirrhosis of the liver. Liver 1986;6:297–301.
195. Rimola A, Soto R, Bory F, et al. Reticuloendothelial system phagocytic activity in cirrhosis and its relation to bacterial infection and prognosis. Hepatology 1984;4:53–58.
196. Wyke RJ, Rajkovic IA, Williams R. Opsonisation by serum from patients with chronic liver disease. Clin Exp Immunol 1983;51:91–98.
197. Fieror J, Finley F. Deficient serum bactericidal activity against *Escherichia coli* in patients with cirrhosis of the liver. J Clin Invest 1979;63:912–921.
198. Salmeron JM, Tito L, Rimola A, et al. Selective intestinal decontamination in the prevention of bacterial infection in patients with acute liver failure. J Hepatol 1992;14:280–285.
199. Jones EA, Skilnick P, Gammal SH, et al. NIH conference: the gamma-aminobutyric acid A receptor complex and hepatic encephalopathy. Ann Intern Med 1989;110(7):532.
200. Schafer DF, Jones EA. Potential neural mechanisms in the pathogenesis of hepatic encephalopathy. Prog Liver Dis 1982;7:615.
201. Weigle CG, Koehler RC, Brusilow SW, et al. Arterial pH modulation of regional cerebral blood flow during hyperammonemia in dogs. Am J Phys 1990;269:H34–41.
202. Cangiano C, Farber MO, Cardelli-Cangiano P, et al. Plasma levels of false neurotransmitters across the brain in portal-systemic encephalopathy. Eur J Clin Invest 1982;12:15.
203. Fischer JE, Funovics JM, Aguirre A, et al. The role of plasma amino acids in hepatic encephalopathy. Surgery 1975;78:276.
204. Wahren J, Denis J, Desurmont P, et al. Is intravenous administration of branched chain amino acids effective in the treatment of hepatic encephalopathy? A multicenter study. Hepatology 1983;3:475.
205. Ericksson LS, Conn HB. Branched-chain amino acids in the management of hepatic encephalopathy: an analysis of variants. Hepatology 1989;10:228.
206. Weber FLJ, Reiser BJ. Relationship of plasma amino acids to nitrogen balance and portal-systemic encephalopathy in alcoholic liver disease. Dig Dis Sci 1982;27:103.
207. Roberts E. The gamma-aminobutyric acid (GABA) system and hepatic encephalopathy. Hepatology 1984;4:342.
208. Basset ML, Mullen KD, Scholz B, et al. Increased brain uptake of GABA in a rabbit model of hepatic encephalopathy. Gastroenterology 1990;98:747–757.
209. Schafer DF, Jones EA. Hepatic encephalopathy and the gamma-aminobutyric-acid neurotransmitter system. Lancet 1982;2:18.
210. Ferenci P, Kleinberger G, Schafer DF, et al. Serum levels of gamma-aminobutyric-acid like activity in acute and chronic hepatocellular disease. Lancet 1983;1:811.

211. Bosman DK, van den Buijs CA, de Haan JG, et al. The effects of benzodiazapine-receptor antagonists and partial inverse agonist on acute hepatic encephalopathy in the rat. Gastroenterology 1991; 101:772–781.
212. Basile AS, Hughes RD, Harrison PM, et al. Elevated brain concentrations of 1,4-benzodiazepines in fulminant hepatic failure. N Engl J Med 1991;325:473–478.
213. Smith AR, Rossi-Fanelli F, Freund H, et al. Sulfur-containing amino acids in experimental hepatic coma in the dog and monkey. Surgery 1979;85:677.
214. Mardini HA, Bartlett K, Record CO. Blood and brain concentrations or mercaptans in hepatic and methanethiol induced coma. Gut 1984; 25:284.
215. Schenker S, Breen KJ, Hoyumpa AMJ. Hepatic encephalopathy: current status. Gastroenterology 1974;66:121.
216. Crossley IR ,Williams R. Progress in the treatment of chronic portasystemic encephalopathy. Gut 1984;25:85.
217. Schafer DF, Pappas SC, Brody LE, et al. Visual evoked potentials in a rabbit model of hepatic encephalopathy. Part 1. Sequential changes and comparisons with drug-induced comas. Gastroenterology 1984;86:540.
218. Pappas SC, Ferenci P, Schafer DF, et al. Visual evoked potentials in a rabbit model of hepatic encephalopathy. Part 2. Comparison of hyperammonemic encephalopathy, postictal coma, and coma induced by synergistic neurotoxins. Gastroenterology 1984;86:546.
219. Zeneroli ML, Pinelli G, Gollini G, et al. Visual evoked potential: a diagnostic tool for the assessment of hepatic encephalopathy. Gut 1984;25:291.
220. Hortnagl H, Singer EA, Lenz K, et al. Substance P is markedly increased in plasma of patients with hepatic coma. Lancet 1984;1:480.
221. Butterworth RF. Pathogenesis and treatment of portal-systemic encephalopathy: an update. Dig Dis Sci 1992;37:321–327.
222. Orlandi F, Freddara U, Candelaresi MT, et al. Comparison between neomycin and lactulose in 173 patients with hepatic encephalopathy. a randomized clinical study. Dig Dis Sci 1981;26:498.
223. Uribe M, Berthier JM, Lewis H, et al. Lactose enemas plus placebo tablets vs neomycin tablets plus starch enemas in acute portal systemic encephalopathy. Gastroenterology 1981;81:101.
224. Keohane PP, Attrill H, Grimble G, et al. Enteral nutrition in malnourished patients with hepatic cirrhosis and acute encephalopathy. J Parenter Enteral Nutr 1983;7:346.
225. Striebel JP, Holm E, Lutz H, et al. Parenteral nutrition and coma therapy with amino acids in hepatic failure. J Parenter Enteral Nutr 1979;3:240.
226. Rossi-Fanelli F, Riggio O, Cangiano C, et al. Branched-chain amino acids vs lactulose in the treatment of hepatic coma. A controlled study. Dig Dis Sci 1982;27:929.
227. Sieg A, Walker S, Czygan P, et al. Branched-chain amino acid-enriched elemental diet in patients with cirrhosis of the liver. A double-blind crossover trial. Z Gastroenterol 1983;21:644.
228. Bansky G, Meier PJ, Riedere E, et al. Effects of the benzodiazepine receptor antagonist flumazenil in hepatic encephalopathy in humans. Gastroenterology 1989;97:744.
229. Psacharopoulos HT, Mowat AP, Davies M, et al. Fulminant hepatic failure in childhood: and analysis of 31 cases. Arch Dis Child 1980; 55:252–258.
230. Ware AJ, D'Agostino A, Combes B. Cerebral edema: a major complication of massive hepatic necrosis. Gastroenterology 1971;61:877–884.
231. Pirola RC, Ham JM, Elmslie RG. Management of hepatic coma complicating virus hepatitis. Gut 1969;10:898–903.
232. Silk DBA, Trewby PN, Chase RA, et al. Treatment of fulminant hepatic failure by polyacrylonitrile membrane hemodialysis. Lancet 1977;2:1–3.
233. Ede RJ, Gimson AES, Bihari D, et al. Controlled hyperventilation in the prevention of cerebral edema in fulminant hepatic failure. J Hepatol 1986;2:43–51.
234. Devictor D, Tahiri C, Rousset A, et al. Management of fulminant hepatic failure in children. An analysis of 56 cases. Crit Care Med 1993;21:S349.
235. Zaki AEO, Wardle EN, Canalese J, et al. Potential toxins of acute liver failure and their effects on blood-brain barrier permeability. Experientia 1983;39:988.
236. Ede RJ, Williams R. Hepatic encephalopathy and cerebral edema. Sem Dig Dis 1986;6(2):107.
237. Haller J. Intracranial pressure monitoring in Reye's syndrome. Hosp Pract 1980;15:101.
238. Inagaki M, Shaw B, Schafer D. Advantages of intracranial pressure monitoring in patients with fulminant hepatic failure. Gastroenterology 1992;102:A826.
239. Canalese J, Gimson AES, Davis C, et al. Controlled trial of dexamethasone and mannitol for the cerebral oedema of fulminant hepatic failure. Gut 1982;23:625.
240. Papadopoulou ZL, Novello AC. The use of hemoperfusion in children. Pediatr Clin North Am 1982;29:1039.
241. Denis J, Opolon P, Nusinovici V, et al. Treatment of encephalopathy during fulminant hepatic failure by haemodialysis with high permeability membrane. Gut 1978;19:787.
242. Zieve L. Hepatic encephalopathy: summary of present knowledge with an elaboration on recent developments. Prog Liver Dis 1979;6:327.
243. Chamuleau RAF, Popken RJ, Beyerbracht EC, et al. Problems in treating experimentally induced acute hepatic failure by hemoperfusion or cross circulation. Hepatology 1983;3:696.
244. Splendiani G, Tancredi M, Daniele M, et al. Treatment of acute liver failure with hemodetoxification techniques. Int J Artif Organs 1990; 13:370–374.
245. Riviello JJ, Halligan GE, Dunn SP, et al. Value of plasmapheresis in hepatic encephalopathy. Pediatr Neurol 1990;6:388–390.
246. Larsen FS, Hansen BA, Jorgensen LG, et al. High-volume plasmapheresis and acute liver transplantation in fulminant hepatic failure. Transpl Proc 1994;26:1788.
247. Winikoff S, Gasmann MS, Spivak W. Plasmapheresis in a patient with hepatic failure awaiting liver transplantation. J Pediatr 1985;107: 547–549.
248. Rozga J, Posesta L, LePage E, et al. Bioartifical liver to treat severe acute liver failure. Ann Surg 1994;219:538–544.
249. Jauregui HO, Mullon CJ, Trenkler D, et al. In vivo evaluation of a hollow fiber liver assist device. Hepatology 1995;21:460–469.
250. Starzl TE, Putnam CW, Corman JL. Transplantation of the liver. Indications for hepatic transplantation. J Pediatr 1982;100:681.
251. Pappas SC. Fulminant hepatic failure and the need for artificial liver support. Mayo Clin Proc 1988;63:198.
252. Starzl TE, Demetris AJ. Liver transplantation: a 31 year perspective. Curr Probl Surg 1990;27(4):202.
253. Whitington PF, Balistreri WF. Liver transplantation in pediatrics: indications, contraindications, and pretransplant management. J Pediatr 1991;118(2):169.
254. Broelsch CE, Burdelski M, Rogiers X, et al. Living donor for liver transplantation. Hepatology 1994;20:49S–55S.
255. Tanaka K, Uemoto S, Tokunaga Y, et al. Living related liver transplantation in children. Am J Surg 1994;168:41–48.

Liver Transplantation 37

Charles L. Schleien
G. Patricia Cantwell
Andreas G. Tzakis

HISTORY

Orthotopic liver transplantation (OLT) was first performed in 1963. The first successful transplants were in a large series of mongrel dogs given nonrelated livers: Many of the dogs survived for more than 4 months[(1)]. The usual immunosuppressive regimen at that time and throughout the 1960s consisted solely of azathioprine and corticosteroids. Many of these dogs lived for long periods; one dog died of old age more than 10 years after surgery[(2)]. This ultimately led to an operation in 1967 on a 19-month-old female child with a large primary hepatoma. She died 13 months later of metastases from the original tumor; but the first evidence of prolonged survival after liver transplantation was provided[(3)].

The great breakthrough for successful OLT occurred in 1980 with the introduction of cyclosporine for postoperative immunosuppression. The 1-year survival rate for liver transplantation before that time was 30 to 40%, and the 5-year survival rate was 25 to 30%[(4)]. Since the beginning of the "cyclosporine era," the 1-year survival rate has gradually increased to more than 80%, and the 5-yr survival rate to more than 70%[(5–7)]. Other recent refinements of liver transplantation methods include newer immunosuppressive agents, including FK 506 and monoclonal and antilymphocyte antibodies, advances in surgical technique, and changes in the process of organ procurement. Today, the greatest challenge facing the transplant team is to increase public awareness regarding issues of organ donation and to facilitate the allocation of this scarce and precious resource to patients who need it.

INDICATIONS

With continuing improvement in the survival rate after OLT, the scope of indications also continues to broaden. Now, with such wide application of the technique, the principal problem for transplantation systems is the limited availability of donors. This problem has been alleviated somewhat by the use of reduced-size livers and split-liver grafting.

Patients who are classified as requiring OLT include

those who have[1] progressive hepatic failure, such as biliary atresia, fulminant hepatic failure secondary to infection, toxin or drug ingestion, and metabolic diseases, such as Wilson's disease;[2] nonprogressive liver disease with a higher morbidity rate than that of transplantation (i.e., Alagille syndrome);[3] systemic disease with primary or secondary hepatic involvement, such as cystic fibrosis, and metabolic diseases, including α_1-antitrypsin deficiency; and[4] a primary hepatic malignant tumor **(Table 37.1).**

The most common indication for liver transplantation in children is biliary atresia[8]. In the United States, this disease occurs at a frequency estimated between 1 in 8,000 to 25,000 live births; 400 to 600 new cases of biliary atresia occur every year[9]. Most of these patients have had surgery before transplant, including one or more portoenterostomy, or the Kasai procedure, consisting of a portoenterostomy via a Roux-en-Y jejunal limb to drain small bile ducts within the porta hepatis. The procedure is successful when increased bile production, decreased jaundice, and signs of normal physical and mental development ensue; but this occurs in only 30 to 50% of cases[10,11] and may delay the need for transplantation beyond age 5[12–16]. Of patients in whom one or more Kasai procedure has failed, at least 90% die before they reach the age of 5, typically reaching end-stage liver failure between age 9 and 18 months[17,18]. Even those who have successful Kasai operations usually die after a number of years; few patients survive to enjoy normal teen or adult life. Thus, early transplantation is usually warranted after an unsuccessful Kasai procedure during infancy. The role of the Kasai operation continues to be re-evaluated because the number of procedures before transplant decrease the survival rate[19].

Table 37.1. Indications

Conditions likely to progress to hepatic failure
Biliary atresia
Fulminant hepatic failure: infection, toxin, drug
Chronic active hepatitis—hepatitis B or C
Metabolic diseases (e.g. Wilson's disease)
Cryptogenic cirrhosis
Progressive cholestasis
Byler disease
Nonprogressive liver disease
Intrahepatic cholestasis
Alagille's syndrome
Neonatal hepatitis
Systemic disease with hepatic involvement
Cystic fibrosis
α_1-Antitrypsin deficiency
Tyrosinemia
Crigler-Najjar syndrome
OTC deficiency
Wilson's Disease
Familial hypercholesterolemia
Glycogen Storage Disease Types III and IV
Perinatal Hemochromatosis-iron storage disease
Hepatic malignancy
Primary malignancy
Disease with secondary hepatic malignancy
Tyrosinemia
α_1-Antitrypsin deficiency
Glycogen storage disease type I

The diagnosis of cirrhosis represents a spectrum of disease that may be compatible with OLT. Indications for OLT in children with cirrhosis include chronic active hepatitis caused by hepatitis B or C; fulminant hepatic failure caused by a virus, toxin, or drug; idiopathic neonatal hepatitis; congenital hepatic fibrosis; secondary biliary fibrosis; and metabolic diseases, which include α_1-antitrypsin deficiency, tyrosinemia, glycogen storage diseases types III and IV, Wilson's disease, and perinatal hemochromatosis (iron storage disease). Hepatitis C is the leading viral cause of chronic active hepatitis necessitating transplant. Patients with liver-based inborn errors of metabolism are treated by providing a phenotypically normal liver: This has been successful in a number of patients with various metabolic diseases **(Table 37.1)**[20–23].

In young adults with a diagnosis of postnecrotic cirrhosis, the 5-year survival rate in patients not receiving OLT is 70%, equal to those receiving OLT[24]. Thus, a number of factors may influence the decision to offer a transplant to a patient with cirrhosis, including the cause, other primary or secondary systemic problems, nutritional status, and immunologic status. Because the cirrhotic liver has little ability to regenerate, decompensation accompanied by, for example, coagulopathy, encephalopathy, weight loss, and progressive ascites is an indication for immediate OLT[25]. Many criteria have been used to assist physicians in making the earliest possible decision for OLT so that the patient is in optimal condition to tolerate surgery and its associated problems. For example, the Child criteria, a commonly used way to score liver dysfunction severity in adults, are based on the patient's extent of ascites, grade of encephalopathy, serum albumin and bilirubin levels, and severity of coagulopathy. These criteria have been used to grade the functional status of patients with cirrhosis[24]. Functional severity scores have also been used in a limited fashion in children and infants with cirrhosis[26].

Children with nonprogressive primary liver disease include patients with intrahepatic cholestasis, such as Alagille syndrome (arteriohepatic dysplasia),[27] and idiopathic neonatal hepatitis[28]. Alagille syndrome is an autosomal dominant disorder with variable modes of expression, characterized by facial features such as a broad forehead and pointed chin; vertebral defects; pulmonary artery stenosis; and cholestasis. In these patients, symptoms usually may be managed medically, although at times the disease progresses to incapacitation[29]. When this occurs, OLT is probably warranted. Tzakis and associates reported a 57% survival rate with normal liver function (a mean of 4.4 years after surgery) in 23 children with Alagille syndrome and end-stage liver disease who underwent liver transplantation. Death was caused by cardiovascular failure secondary to cardiopulmonary disease[30].

The prognosis after OLT for patients with symptomatic hepatocellular carcinoma is poor; there is a 43% recurrence rate. The results are somewhat better with hepatoblastomas and incidental hepatomas than with large primary hepatomas[31]. Further increase in survival depends on medical anticancer therapy before and after surgical removal of the carcinoma as well as more effective immunosuppressive and chemotherapeutic regimens[31–33].

CONTRAINDICATIONS

Presently, there are only a few contraindications for OLT in children and infants. The list has decreased as survival rate increases, and as our understanding of perioperative principles, including immunosuppression, nutrition, and management of other organ systems, improves. Criteria for exclusion of OLT in the past included advanced cardiac, pulmonary, or renal disease; severe hypoxemia; sepsis; and portal vein thrombosis[34]. In a recent review, however, none of these exclusion criteria were thought to be absolute[25]. Relative contraindications for OLT are *(a)* acceptable alternative medical therapy, *(b)* expected suboptimal outcome, *(c)* impairment of other organ systems that would compromise function of the graft, *(d)* major systemic infection, and *(e)* cancer with a high postsurgical recurrence rate[25]. Absolute contraindications for OLT are uncontrollable extrahepatic sepsis and the presence of an unresectable hepatic malignant tumor.

When other organ systems are involved, OLT must be considered on an individual basis. Patients with biliary atresia and Alagille syndrome have a high incidence of complex congenital heart disease. These patients should undergo a thorough cardiac evaluation before transplantation. Similarly, patients with pulmonary compromise from intrapulmonary shunting secondary to hepatic disease should be assessed with pulmonary angiography. In these patients, hypoxemia may be reversible after OLT[35–37]. Patients with associated organ involvement, including renal and gastrointestinal (GI) disease, should be evaluated by the appropriate subspecialist. The presence of hepatorenal syndrome is not a contraindication for transplantation, since it typically resolves postoperatively[38]. Patients with other systemic diseases, such as cystic fibrosis, who receive OLT have a reasonable survival rate (more than 60%): The longest period of survival in this group is 5 years[25]. The major vascular anomalies associated with biliary atresia are no longer regarded as contraindications for surgery. Even patients with absence of the portal vein can be successfully treated with transplantation[39].

Systemic infection is considered a contraindication to surgery, except when it is chronic. For example, ascending cholangitis associated with biliary atresia may be refractory to medical management. Allowing liver failure to progress while trying to manage a chronic or refractory infection is unwise and often results in surgery in a seriously ill and unstable patient. This is also true for the other complications of liver failure such as coagulopathy and encephalopathy. Allowing these medical conditions to advance before transplantation is performed decreases the ultimate rate of survival.

Patients with metastatic disease may not be good candidates for OLT because of the high rate of recurrence[40]. Other cancers of the liver, such as sarcoma, also mean a poor long-term outcome after OLT. However, patients with metabolic diseases associated with a high rate of cancer (i.e., tyrosinemia) should receive OLT before a neoplasm develops.

PREOPERATIVE MANAGEMENT OF THE DONOR

After the declaration of brain death, meticulous management of physiologic parameters in the donor is imperative to avoid unnecessary loss of donor organs **(Table 37.2).** The basic principles of intensive care should be followed, with close monitoring of vital functions, i.e., blood pressure, heart rate, body temperature, urine volume, arterial blood gas determination, and electrocardiographic data.

Typically, intravascular volume should be maintained at normal levels by closely measuring mean arterial blood pressure, central venous pressure, and even pulmonary capillary wedge pressure in the labile patient. Following brain death, fluid administration often needs to be liberalized,

Table 37.2. Donor—Preoperative Management

Respiratory
Optimize arterial blood gases
Maintain pulmonary physiotherapy
Avoid respiratory alkalosis
Anticipate pulmonary edema (neurogenic, fluid overload, cardiogenic, aspiration)
Cardiovascular
Monitor BP, heart rate, ECG
Monitor central venous pressure and pulmonary artery pressure as indicated
Maintain urine output (≥1 ml/kg/hr)
Renal
Avoid consequences of excessive diuresis
Hyperosmolality
Hypokalemia
Hypernatremia
Endocrine
Treat diabetes insipidus
Free water replacement
Exogenous vasopression
Treat hyperglycemia
Avoid effects of hypothermia
EEG changes
ECG abnormalities
Arrhythmias
↓Cardiac contractility
↓GFR
Coagulopathy
Altered cellular metabolism
Infection
Appropriate antibiotics
CNS
Treat autonomic instability (BP ↑ or ↓, HR ↑ or ↓)
Often secondary dehydration → liberalize fluids

as the patient with closed head trauma usually is dehydrated as a consequence of treatment for cerebral edema. In addition, many patients continue to have autonomic nervous system instability, manifested by labile blood pressure and heart rate. When these problems occur, they should be managed with fluids and appropriate vasoactive drug therapy. Care should be taken to ensure that adequate organ perfusion is maintained when vasoconstrictors are needed to stabilize the blood pressure. Urine volume should be maintained at normal or above normal levels (at least 1 mL/kg/hour). Often, low-dose dopamine is used to maintain renal blood flow. Diabetes insipidus is a common sequela to head trauma or brain death and should be managed with a vasopressin infusion or arginine vasopression and fluid replacement. Specific vasodilation may be necessary in patients with persistent hypertension. Serum sodium, potassium, ionized calcium, arterial blood gas, and pH levels should be kept at normal by making adjustments in the type and quantity of crystalloid administered. Ventilator parameters should be adjusted to optimize arterial blood gas levels. Antibiotic therapy may be necessary to treat local infections (i.e., urinary tract infection). The donor should not receive a drug to which the recipient is allergic.

DONOR OPERATION

The first consideration regarding use of the donor organ is size. A liver graft, in order to be implanted, has to be similar in size to the diseased liver being removed[41,42]. The shortage of pediatric donors and the great variability in the size of liver needed has led to the use of reduced-size grafts[43–48]. Liver fragments formed from hepatectomies include the results of a right hepatectomy, right trisegmentectomy, and left lateral segmentectomy. The disadvantages of the use of a liver segment include hemorrhage, biliary fistula, and infections of the raw surface. However, the larger size of the donor artery decreases the incidence of hepatic artery thrombosis.

The decision as to whether a donor organ is acceptable is typically made by means of evaluation of the liver by the donor's surgeon. The use of perfect donors with hemodynamic stability and normal blood biochemistry values does not ensure a great advantage in graft survival. Insistence on these ideal donor conditions results in a waste of an already scarce resource.

The liver is harvested as part of a multiple organ procurement, which usually involves liver, renal, and thoracic teams working in harmony. When the donor's condition is stable, a preliminary dissection of all the organs to be removed is performed, and at this time the anatomy is defined. Then the organs are cooled in situ by the rapid infusion of a chilled solution into the aorta. For the liver, additional perfusion is provided through a separate cannula inserted through the splenic vein or other major side branch of the portal vein. When the donor is unstable, cooling through the aorta is performed urgently before careful dissection is performed.

The liver is preserved in special solutions. The solution developed by University of Wisconsin provides safe preservation of the liver for at least 12 to 16 hours, compared with 6 to 8 hours for previously used solutions[49,50]. This increased length of preservation has allowed longer distances between donor and recipient, permitted the procedure to be done less urgently, and facilitated better surgical preparation of the operative field and back table procedures, especially for reduced-size liver transplants.

PREOPERATIVE MANAGEMENT OF THE RECIPIENT

A number of issues related to the transplant candidate must be resolved by the time the patient presents for preoperative management. These issues include: *(a)* confirmation of the diagnosis, consisting of full anatomic definition of the portal circulation and biliary tree; *(b)* staging of the patient's condition; *(c)* determination of possible contraindications to OLT; *(d)* evaluation of other organ system dysfunction that may complicate the perioperative period; and *(e)* financial and social arrangements **(Table 37.3).**

The role of the intensivist in the preoperative period de-

Table 37.3. Preoperative Evaluation of Potential Liver Transplant Recipient

History and physical examination
Previous medical/surgical history
Body weight and height
Nutritional status
Laboratory evaluation:
CBC, platelets
Electrolytes, BUN, creatinine, glucose, calcium (total & ionized), magnesium, phosphorus, uric acid
Protein electrophoresis
Bilirubin, γ-glutamyl transpeptidase (GGTP), amylase, ammonia
PT, PTT
Arterial blood gas/pH
Hepatitis A and B screen
Blood, urine, sputum, ascitic fluid cultures as needed
Blood typing, HLA type, cytotoxic antibody screen
Other evaluation
Ceruloplasmin
α_1-Antitrypsin level and phenotype
Antimitochondrial, antithyroid, and antinuclear antibodies
Iron, iron binding capacity, ferritin
Quantitative immunoglobulins
Radiologic imaging
Chest
Abdominal ultrasound
Abdominal CT
Cholangiography (if indicated)
Arteriography (if indicated)
Ancillary evaluation
Upper GI panendoscopy
Colonoscopy (as indicated)
ERCP (as indicated)
Ophthalmologic evaluation
Neuropsychiatric evaluation
EEG
Psychosocial services

pends on the condition of the patient. In patients with end-stage liver disease, consultation with the intensivist may be needed only to address issues of nutritional support and pulmonary physiotherapy. On the other hand, the patient with encephalopathy may require the full range of skills of the intensivist, including intracranial pressure (ICP) monitoring and therapy; cardiovascular support; and dialysis, plasmapheresis, or continuous arteriovenous hemofiltration to prevent primary renal insufficiency and fluid overload. Ventilator support should be instituted early in comatose patients to hyperventilate for purposes of ICP management, airway protection in the patient with an absent gag reflex or bleeding varices, and for pulmonary physiotherapy, including enhanced oxygen delivery in the patient with intrapulmonary shunting secondary to cirrhosis. Thus, preoperative patient management is aimed at optimizing organ function before going to the operating room. The potential for altered physiologic variables caused by altitude effects, should air transport be required, must also be carefully considered(51).

INTRAOPERATIVE MANAGEMENT

The overwhelming majority of patients undergoing hepatic replacement therapy receive an orthotopic transplant, with the native liver entirely removed and a whole or partial organ surgically implanted in another (orthoptic) position(17,52,53). Some centers use segmental auxiliary transplantation in patients with metabolic deficiencies without removing the native liver(54). This discussion of intraoperative technique and complications after OLT is confined to orthotopic transplants **(Table 37.4).**

A team approach is critical for a successful outcome. Communication among the surgeon, anesthesiologist, and perfusionist is important for a smooth operation. Before making the incision, careful positioning and preparation of the patient is necessary to maintain temperature control and to prevent pressure ulceration during a long procedure. In the pediatric patient, vascular access must be obtained above the diaphragm to ensure that fluids and drugs reach the central circulation. Appropriate-sized sheath introducers are useful for both the placement of a Swan-Ganz catheter for cardiac monitoring as well as delivery of large volumes of blood products and fluids. Arterial access for monitoring blood gases and continuous measurement of blood pressure is imperative. Patients often have a markedly elevated cardiac output and, as mentioned above, may have significant pulmonary shunts(35). Correction of fluid deficits and optimization of cardiovascular and coagulation status may be necessary in the period before anesthetic induction.

Table 37.4. Surgery

Before incision
Vascular access—large bore catheters
Arterial access
Correct dehydration
Optimize cardiovascular and coagulation status
Proper positioning
First phase: recipient hepatectomy
Dissect liver
Complications:
Adhesions
Portal hypertension/bleeding
Anatomic abnormalities
Pneumothorax
Second phase: anhepatic stage
Clamps placed
Establish veno-veno bypass (>25 kg)
Remove liver
Superior vena cava anastomosis
Inferior vena cava anastomosis
Portal vein anastomosis
Complications:
Air embolus
Third phase: reperfusion stage
Remove clamps
Hemostasis established
Hepatic artery anastomosis
Biliary reconstruction
Complications:
Hypotension/bradycardia
Surgical bleeding

SURGICAL TECHNIQUE

The operation itself involves three phases: the recipient hepatectomy phase, the anhepatic phase, and the reperfusion phase **(Table 37.4).** Each phase has its own inherent problems and complications that must be anticipated. The recipient hepatectomy phase may be lengthy, depending on the number of previous Kasai operations and the presence of adhesions as well as on the severity of portal hypertension and the level of neovascularization that has occurred in the area of the liver. In addition, the recipient may have anatomic abnormalities such as situs inversus, a preduodenal portal vein, or an absent inferior vena cava that may require careful intraoperative assessment and reconstruction(55). Patients with coagulopathy may require factor replacement during the hepatectomy stage to avoid an exsanguinating hemorrhage. The hilum is generally exposed first, and the liver is freed from its attachments to the diaphragm and the retroperitoneum. The hepatic artery and common bile duct are transected, which is followed by venous clamping. Care is taken to prevent early ligation of the portal vein to avoid venous congestion and increased bleeding from portal hypertension.

The anhepatic phase begins after placement of vascular clamps on the hepatic artery, portal vein, and suprahepatic and intrahepatic inferior vena cava (IVC) and subsequent removal of the liver (Fig. 37.1). In patients who weigh less than 15 to 20 kg and are not undergoing venovenous bypass during the anhepatic phase, test clamping is performed before hepatectomy to assess the vascular response to decreased venous return. Fluid boluses may be needed to provide central venous pressure adequate to maintain cardiac output and blood pressure. If the patient tolerates the test clamping for 5 minutes, the clamps are placed and the liver is removed. Piggyback liver transplantation may be helpful

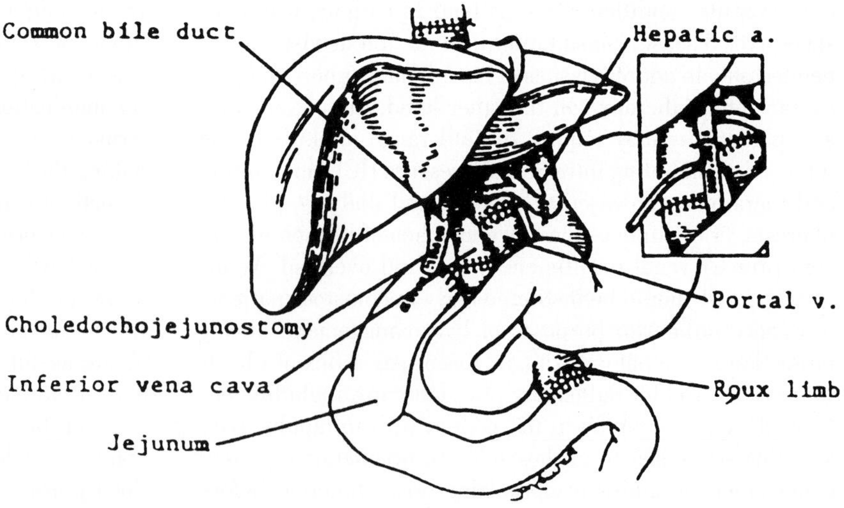

Figure 37.1. Orthotopic liver transplantation (liver replacement). Biliary tract is usually reconstructed with choledochojejunostomy (to a Roux limb) or (inset) with a choledochocholedochostomy, which is stented with a T tube. From Starzl TE, Demetris AJ. Liver transplantation: a 31-year perspective. Part 1. In: Wells SA Jr, ed. Current problems in surgery. Pittsburgh: Year Book Medical Publishers, 1990:56.

when venovenous bypass is not possible and is used routinely in our institution[56]. It allows the recipient's vena cava to remain intact throughout the procedure. The liver is stripped off the vena cava, and an ostium is created to receive venous outflow from the graft. In patients weighing more than 15 to 20 kg, venovenous bypass is often used (Fig. 37.2). Both techniques serve to decrease intraoperative bleeding and intestinal venous congestion and pressure, resulting in an increase of mesenteric and renal perfusion. Venovenous bypass involves inserting a cannula into the portal vein and the subhepatic IVC by way of the femoral vein to return venous blood to the suprahepatic circulation via the axillary vein. Venous cannulae comprised of heparin-bonded tubing are connected by a centrifugal pump that returns the bypassed blood to the right atrium. The use of venovenous bypass has dramatically reduced intraoperative blood loss in older patients[57].

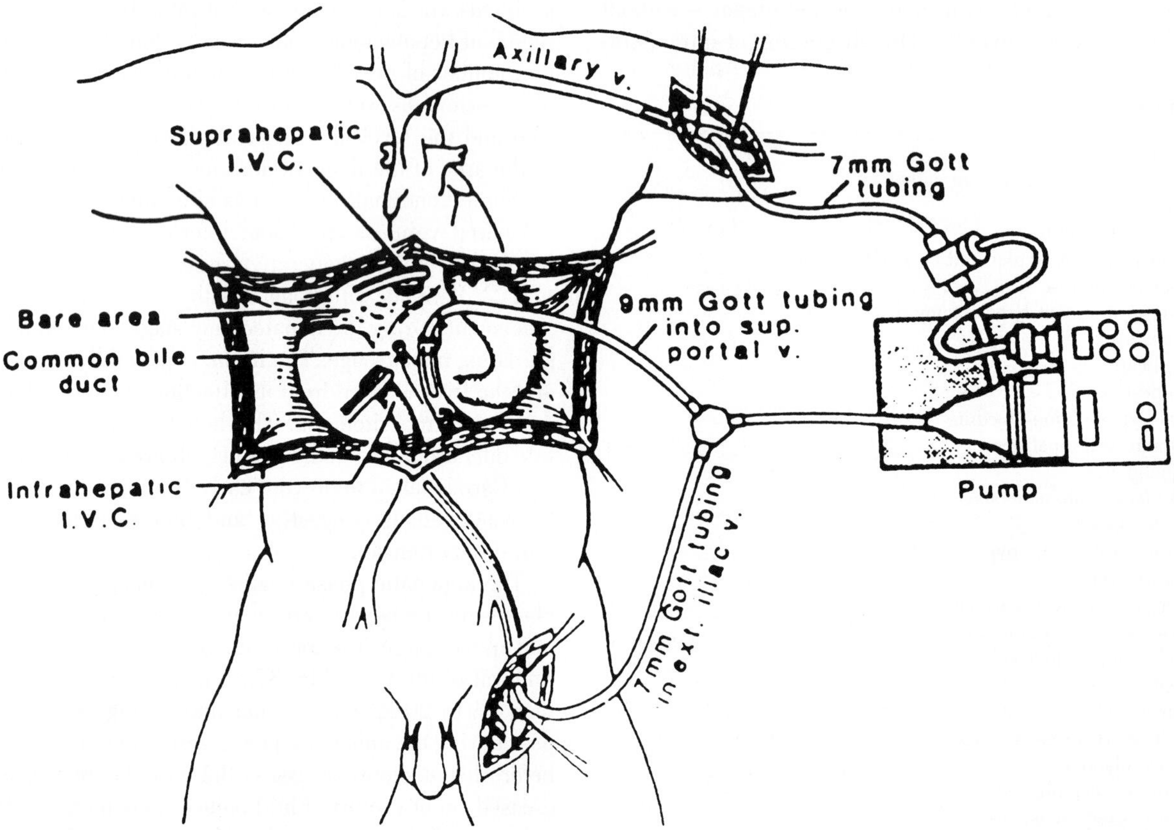

Figure 37.2. Pump-driven venovenous bypass, which allows decompression of splanchnic and systemic venous beds with return of blood to axillary vein without need for heparinization. From Starzl TE, Demetris AJ. Liver transplantation: a 31-year perspective. Part 1. In: Wells SA Jr, ed. Current problems in surgery. Pittsburgh: Year Book Medical Publishers, 1990:73.

During the anhepatic phase, the superior and then the inferior vena caval anastomoses are performed, and the donor liver is perfused with cold Ringer's lactate solution to remove the potassium-containing preservation solution as well as any air from the vascular tree. Following the vena caval anastomoses, the portal vein anastomosis is performed. When it is completed, the liver is reperfused. The vascular clamps are removed, and any bleeding is controlled by direct suture ligation.

The reperfusion phase begins upon release of the vascular clamps. As the liver fills with blood, there is washout of small amounts of potassium-containing residual perfusion solution and release of congested blood from within the portal system and IVC. This may result in transient hypotension and bradycardia, necessitating administration of vasopressors such as phenylephrine and ephedrine, atropine, and agents to buffer the increased acid and potassium load. In addition, the reperfusion phase may be characterized by surgical bleeding from any of the anastomoses or branches of the vena cavae, portal vein, or hepatic artery that have not been ligated during organ retrieval. The cut edge of the segmental liver transplant may be a major source of surgical bleeding that must be controlled directly. During the reperfusion phase, as the liver begins to function, the patient's coagulopathy typically diminishes. In infants, because of the risk of vascular thrombosis (usually of the hepatic artery), the administration of coagulation factors generally is avoided unless significant bleeding persists. During the early reperfusion phase and following adequate hemostasis, the arterial anastomosis is performed. Significant variations in donor and recipient arteries exist in one-third of cases, so many variations of arterial reconstruction may be performed. Following the arterial anastomosis, the biliary reconstruction is performed using a direct duct-to-duct anastomosis with a T tube for biliary drainage in older patients. A Roux-en-Y choledochojejunostomy is performed in infants and in other patients with biliary atresia[(58)]. In children, the Roux-en-Y technique is required in more than 90% of cases.

Intraoperative Complications

Complications that may occur during the surgical procedure include hemodynamic instability, metabolic disturbances, intestinal and renal ischemia, and pulmonary insufficiency. Hemodynamic instability, usually a result of hypovolemia secondary to bleeding, may also be caused by myocardial depression associated with hypocalcemia, acidosis, or other factors released following reperfusion of the liver. Metabolic disturbances include hypoglycemia, hypocalcemia, and citrate intoxication from transfused blood; hyperkalemia; metabolic acidosis; and late metabolic alkalosis. Air embolism may occur during venovenous bypass or because of inadequate flushing of the liver during implantation. Pulmonary complications include pneumothorax, pleural effusion, and atelectasis. Abdominal closure may be difficult, resulting in increased intra-abdominal pressure that causes hypotension and high venous mesenteric and renal pressures that cause intestinal and renal ischemia. This occurs most often in smaller patients with a donor liver that is too large. Infrequently, a silo or fascial patch is necessary to close the abdomen to minimize abdominal pressure and allow normal ventilation.

POSTOPERATIVE CARE OF THE LIVER

In many respects, the success of OLT hinges on the management of the patient, both in the operating room and in the first few days following surgery. During the postoperative period, rapid changes in liver function as well as extrahepatic dysfunction require the skills of the many subspecialty services forming the multidisciplinary critical care team.

Postoperative Care and Monitoring

Children undergoing liver transplantation require extensive postoperative monitoring of arterial blood pressure, central venous pressure, heart rate, electrocardiogram (ECG) tracings, respiratory rate, oxygen saturation, body temperature, urinary output, abdominal drain output, and bile output. A pulmonary artery catheter is useful in patients with congestive heart failure, cardiac dysfunction, or pulmonary hypertension. Abdominal girth and body weight should be measured twice daily. Hourly neurologic checks are imperative during the early postoperative course. Upon arrival at the ICU, the patient may be hypothermic because of temperature loss during surgery or transport from the operating room. Active warming should be undertaken, using warmed and humidified inspired ventilator gases, warmed fluid and blood products, and warming blankets. Routine intensive care should also include respiratory and ventilator management; attention to fluid, electrolytes, and nutrition; and all of the modalities available in pediatric intensive care units (ICUs). The subsequent text highlights management of problems unique to the liver transplant patient.

Hepatic Complications: Diagnosis and Management

A number of primary hepatic complications occur after liver transplantation. Many of these complications result in loss of graft function and may ultimately necessitate retransplantation **(Table 37.5).** Retransplantation rates vary from 5 to 30% of first-time recipients, depending on the institution and characteristics of the donor graft.

Primary Nonfunction

Primary nonfunction is the failure of the graft to synthesize clotting factors, to metabolize ammonia, and to excrete bile in the immediate postoperative period despite adequate blood flow. Primary nonfunction is the most common reason for retransplantation[(59)]: It occurs most often when the

Table 37.5. Evaluation of Liver Dysfunction—Posttransplant

	Primary Nonfunction	*Acute Rejection*	*Hepatic Artery Thrombosis*	*Portal Vein Thrombosis*	*Biliary Leak/obstruction*	*Infection*
Clinical symptoms	Hypoglycemia Coma Renal Failure Metabolic acidosis Cardiogenic shock Hyperammonemia	Fever Encephalopathy	Fever	Fever Intestinal swelling Ascites GI bleeding	Fever Peritonitis	Fever Malaise Anorexia
Lab						
AST/ALT	+/+++	+/+++ (3–7 days)	+/+++ (3–7 days)	+/+++ (3–7 days)	0/+	+/++
GGT	+	+	+	+	+++	+
Bilirubin	+/+++	+/+++	+/+++	+/+++	+/+++	0/++
Coagulation profile	+/+++	+/+++	+/+++	+/+++	0/+	0/+
WBC	0/+	+/+++	+/+++	+/+++	0/+	+/+++
Cultures	Negative	Negative	+/−	+/−	+/−	+
Ancillary tests						
Ultrasonography	Normal blood flow	Echogenicity	Absent flow/ infarction	Absent flow/ infarction	Dilated bile ducts	Abscess
KUB			Intrahepatic air			
CT			Occluded vessel Infarction Bowel/biliary disruption, extrinsic compression (hematoma, biloma, intrahepatic abscess)	Occluded vessel Infarction Bowel/biliary disruption	Dilated bile ducts Biloma Extrinsic compression of common duct	Abscess ileus Abscess
Angiography			↓/Absent flow	↓/Absent flow		Parenchymal defect
Radionuclide scan	Delayed ejection	↓ Uptake Delayed excretion	Delayed excretion	Delayed excretion	Abnormal T-tube cholangiogram	
Biopsy		Portal inflammatory infiltrate Portal/central vein Endothelialitis Bile duct damage	Severe necrosis	Severe necrosis	Dilated ducts	Inflammatory infiltrates Inclusion bodies +Cultures Viral stains

liver used is from infant donors who had sustained hypoxic injury[60]. Primary nonfunction remains a clinical problem, despite methods to improve liver function in the donor before organ retrieval.

Primary nonfunction typically presents with rising liver transaminase levels, profound hypoglycemia, coagulopathy despite attempts at correction, progressive coma, renal failure, severe metabolic acidosis, and cardiogenic shock. The recipient with evidence of primary nonfunction should be placed on the list for emergency retransplantation. During the critical period of diminished liver function, exquisite fluid balance must be maintained, often with dialysis or slow, continuous ultrafiltration. Fluid administration must be minimized, since patients may be oliguric and often require coagulation factors via administration of blood products. To prevent progressive neurologic damage and cerebral edema, the patient must have another transplant as soon as possible.

Vascular Occlusion

Vascular occlusion with accompanying graft loss, most often encountered in infants, occurs in 5 to 20% of pediatric transplants[58,61–63]. The vena cava, portal vein and, most commonly, the hepatic artery become occluded in the early postoperative period. Vascular occlusion is caused by intramural thrombus formation or, less commonly, by extrinsic compression or vessel kinking. Venous anastomotic stenoses complicating liver transplantation have been successfully treated with percutaneous transluminal angioplasty[64]. The transplanted liver is exquisitely sensitive to hypoxia or hypotension, and vascular occlusion results in severe hepatic dysfunction necessitating retransplantation. The risk of arterial thrombosis is higher if the vessels are smaller than 3 mm in diameter, a revision of the anastomosis was required, or aortic or iliac grafts were needed as conduits to the hepatic artery[65]. Less than 10% of patients with a hepatic artery occlusion survive without retransplantation.

Unfortunately, there are no definitive signs or symptoms of hepatic artery thrombosis. Most occur within hours or days of transplantation; they may occur even 1 to 2 weeks after transplantation. Signs and symptoms consist of fulminant liver failure with increased liver transaminase and bilirubin levels, and worsening coagulopathy. Other possible signs are biliary complications, such as bile leak or biliary stricture, or episodes of bacteremia with fever and leukocytosis. Hepatic artery thrombosis may be heralded by the appearance of intrahepatic air on an abdominal plain film. The absence of a pulse over the artery on Doppler ultrasonography lends further credence to the diagnosis, which should be confirmed by selective arteriography[(66)].

Portal vein thrombosis may present with fulminant necrosis, intestinal swelling, or massive ascites[(67)]. It usually occurs when the recipient splanchnic venous bed has been altered by a portal-systemic shunt, a splenectomy, or other operation[(67)]. Portal vein thrombosis has also been associated with protein C deficiency[(68)]. After the first postoperative month, portal vein thrombosis may result in upper GI bleeding from esophageal varices as a result of recurrent portal hypertension. The necessary evaluation is similar to that for hepatic artery thrombosis and should include a Doppler flow study of the portal vein and venous portography or a venous-phase superior mesenteric artery arteriogram. Portal vein thrombosis may resolve spontaneously[(69)], or result in recanalization[(70)] or collateralization. Late portal vein thrombosis resulting in variceal bleeding may require sclerotherapy, a distal splenorenal shunt, and retransplantation[(67)].

Thrombosis of the suprahepatic or intrahepatic IVC is rare, occurring in less than 1% of patients[(71)]. Occlusion of the IVC may present with lower trunk and extremity edema and renal insufficiency.

When a portal vein or hepatic artery occlusion is diagnosed by means of Doppler ultrasound and arteriography[(66)], the patient should undergo immediate thrombectomy with revascularization. Because of the high rate of reocclusion, the patient should be listed for immediate retransplantation[(72,73)]. While awaiting retransplantation, management includes administering supplemental oxygen and antibiotic therapy to prevent infection with gram-negative bacteria, anaerobes, and enterococci. Serial abdominal ultrasound scans or computed tomographic (CT) scans are used to rule out extrinsic vessel compression by an intrahepatic abscess, hematoma, or biloma.

Intravascular volume and hepatic perfusion pressure should be maintained at normal levels in the immediate posttransplant period to prevent vascular occlusion. Correction of a coagulopathy should be avoided in patients who are not actively bleeding[(17,65)]. Coagulopathy at this time is caused by a number of factors, including decreased clotting factors, thrombocytopenia, and decreased ionized calcium levels caused by citrate binding. Thrombocytopenia is common and occurs secondary to decreased circulating platelet half-life or increased uptake of platelets into the graft[(74)]. Typically, factor or platelet replacement is administered only when active bleeding occurs or the platelet count falls below 20,000/mm^3. Coagulation parameters are allowed to normalize without transfusion over the first 2 to 3 days after surgery.

Biliary Complications

In the early postoperative period, a bile leak resulting in peritonitis or abscess formation means another operation[(75)]. Hepatic artery thrombosis is suspected whenever a biliary complication occurs because the principal blood supply of the graft bile duct is the hepatic artery. Favorable results have been reported regarding use of ursodeoxycholic acid to prevent biliary cirrhosis after hepatic artery thrombosis[(76)]. The biliary tree anastomosis may leak or become disrupted, stenotic, or occluded[(77)]. In addition, bile may leak from the cut edge of a segmental graft. The occurrence of biliary tract complications occurs at a rate of 10 to 20%[(78)]. The diagnosis of bile leak, or biliary tract obstruction, is made by ultrasonography, CT scan, or T tube cholangiogram[(79,80)]. Strictures of the bile ducts can, at times, be opened by transhepatic stenting, dilation, or biliary drainage[(81)]. Percutaneous transhepatic drainage has been used to decompress a dilated intrahepatic biliary tree. Ultrasound or CT guidance may be useful in percutaneous drainage of a bile collection. If these procedures are unsuccessful, repeated surgery is necessary[(82)]. Biliary fluid collections must be cultured to isolate potential pathogens. If the biliary anastomosis becomes completely disrupted, reoperation with Roux-en-Y choledochojejunostomy drainage is recommended[(4,48,82,83)].

Hemorrhage

Bleeding in the early postoperative period is a relatively common complication requiring another operation in 5 to 10% of patients[(84)]. The coagulopathy that occurs following reperfusion of the donor liver associated with multiple vascular anastomoses and the cut edge of segmental grafts provides the setting for postoperative bleeding. When increasing bleeding from surgical drains persists in spite of normalization of clotting factors, the patient should undergo an exploratory laparotomy to achieve hemostasis. A large hematoma is often found in the perihepatic area without a discrete bleeding site. The removal of the hematoma results in decreased consumption of clotting factors and often suffices to control the hemorrhage.

Acute Rejection

Acute rejection occurs commonly in the first few weeks after transplantation. Various immunosuppressive regimens are used, but despite them, as many as 80% of recipients have at least one early episode of rejection, usually 3 to 70 days after transplant[(85)]. The first rejection episode occurs an average of 23 days after transplant in children (15 days in adults)[86]. Acute rejection is usually heralded by fever, increased bilirubin and liver enzyme levels, encephalopathy, and decreased uptake of tracer agent during nuclear radioisotope scan[87]. The section on immunosuppressive therapy outlines treatment of rejection.

Graft vs. Host Disease

The liver graft is capable of mounting an immunologic reaction against the host, resulting in graft versus host disease (GVHD), which may manifest in two ways. It may arise from a humoral cause in which the donor is of a compatible but unidentified major blood group (e.g., O to A). Rarely, cellular GVHD may be seen, including involvement of skin, GI tract, lungs, and hematopoietic elements.

Diagnosis of Hepatic Complications

Severe complications may occur early in the postoperative course, resulting in graft loss and the need for retransplantation. Frequent assessment of liver function, including measurement of total and direct bilirubin levels; transaminase levels, i.e., aspartase transaminase (AST), alanine transaminase (ALT), gamma-glutamyl transferase (GGT); and alkaline phosphatase level is routine. When postoperative complications do not occur, liver enzymes typically reach peak levels within 72 hours and rapidly fall to normal levels thereafter. Persistent or increasing elevation of liver enzymes may indicate primary nonfunction. Between postoperative days 3 and 7, rising levels of liver enzymes may indicate vascular occlusion or acute rejection. Specifically, elevation of bilirubin and alkaline phosphatase levels may indicate cholestasis from liver injury, biliary leak, or infection of the biliary tree. A GGT level greater than 500 IU/L is usually a sign of acute rejection or biliary tract obstruction[83].

To further discriminate among the causes of liver dysfunction synthetic and metabolic function should be assessed. Prothrombin time (PT), partial thromboplastin time (PTT), and fibrinogen level are measured daily and should normalize over the first 72 hours after surgery. A sudden change in level of clotting function signifies graft dysfunction caused by vascular occlusion or acute rejection. The serum ammonia level may rise in the first week after surgery, indicating severe graft dysfunction.

In addition to clinical examination and liver function tests, a number of diagnostic studies are useful in following the patient in the early postoperative period. The most useful examination is color Doppler ultrasonography, which assesses flow through the hepatic artery, portal vein, hepatic veins, and vena cava as well as fluid collections in the perihepatic area[88,89]. This test is usually performed within 36 hours after surgery to gather baseline information and, later in the course, when any complication ensues. Diagnosis of a vascular thrombosis by ultrasonography may be confirmed by selective arteriography[90].

The biliary tract is assessed on the fifth to seventh day following surgery. The older patient who has a duct-to-duct anastomosis with a T tube, should have a T tube cholangiogram to assess healing of the biliary tract and provide evidence of obstruction or leak. Patients with a Roux-en-Y choledochojejunostomy routinely receive a 99mTc-DISIDA scan in the first postoperative week to assess uptake and excretion of radioactive tracer into the intestinal tract. Delayed uptake of tracer is associated with an improperly preserved donor liver, vascular compromise, or rejection. The delay of excretion into the biliary system may indicate hepatocellular damage from rejection, ischemia, or viral infection[86,91]. When liver function test results are normal, a liver biopsy is useful to test for early rejection. A biopsy is routinely performed following reperfusion of the liver and on posttransplant days 7 and 30: Results are used to refine immunosuppressive management. An abdominal CT scan is useful in searching for the presence of an intra-abdominal fluid collection[88], which may be a source of infection and should be drained percutaneously or by laparotomy. In the long run, rejection remains the most common cause of graft loss after liver transplantation.

IMMUNOSUPPRESSION

Types of Rejection

Three forms of rejection are described: *(1)* humoral or hyperacute, *(2)* cellular or acute, and *(3)* chronic.

Humoral rejection typically occurs only hours or days after transplantation; hence, the term hyperacute refers to rejection of the donor organ by preformed antibodies. These antigraft antibodies are isoagglutinins of both IgG and IgM classes, which can cause clots that plug the liver microvasculature. Other cytotoxic antibodies, although less of a problem with liver transplants compared with heart or kidney grafts, may cause hyperacute rejection. Pathologic findings in these cases include immunoglobulin deposits, arteritis, and ischemic necrosis of the graft. Practically, even though the early graft failure rate may reach 30% when carrying out transplantation with a positive lymphocytotoxic crossmatch, most surgeons do not allow a positive crossmatch to deter transplantation if there is an overriding need.

Cellular rejection occurs acutely usually days or weeks after transplantation. The pathologic findings are characterized by mononuclear-cell infiltration of the liver concentrated in the portal triads. The intrahepatic bile ducts are most affected, and there is some inflammatory attack of arteries and portal veins. Consequently, a decreased total liver blood flow is characteristic on Doppler ultrasonographic examination. The central veins can also be invaded, leading to obliterative endophlebitis and subsequent outflow block, as in the Budd-Chiari syndrome. These pathologic findings also result clinically in graft edema, intrahepatic cholestasis, and parenchymal damage with biochemical changes. Successful treatment may resolve all of these problems if instituted before graft destruction occurs or chronic rejection ensues.

Chronic rejection, usually seen months or years after transplant, has been observed as soon as 3 or 4 weeks after transplant. It is heralded by occlusive arterial disease, disappearance of intrahepatic bile ducts, and parenchymal fibrosis. A sparse cellular infiltrate in the portal tracts is characteristic. Clinically, chronic rejection is manifested by obstructive jaundice progressing over time to liver failure. Preservation of synthetic and other parenchymal function are early findings.

Pharmacology

Corticosteroids

The agents with the longest clinical use are the nonspecific agents, corticosteroids and azathioprine. High-dose corticosteroids, used in the initial management and treatment of rejection in combination with other immunosuppressant agents, work via a direct lymphocytotoxic effect. In moderate doses, corticosteroids affect lymphocyte and macrophage activation and proliferation as well as cytokine production. Corticosteroids probably inhibit cell membrane activation by inhibiting the activity of phospholipase A_2, which is involved in prostaglandin synthesis. Complications of corticosteroid therapy include salt and water retention, hypertension, and GI hemorrhage. Long-term problems include stunting of growth, and cosmetic deformation including moon facies, buffalo hump, striae, and bone abnormalities.

Azathioprine

Azathioprine works via its active metabolite, 6-mercaptopurine. This antimetabolite competitively inhibits the synthesis of DNA by inhibiting purine nucleotidase. Azathioprine has a direct effect on all lymphocyte subsets and suppresses the bone marrow production of all cell lines. It is also used in combination with other immunosuppressants for the prevention, but not the reversal, of rejection. Side effects of azathioprine therapy are principally related to bone marrow suppression with decreased white blood cell count, red cell mass, or platelet count. Dosage adjustment is required for significant leukopenia or other evidence of bone marrow suppression.

Cyclosporine

The clinical availability of the fungal peptide cyclosporine, produced from *Streptomyces tsukubaensis,* made an immediate impact on the success of liver and all other organ transplantation. At immunosuppressive doses, cyclosporine selectively inhibits T-helper lymphocytes, sparing B lymphocyte, macrophage, and bone marrow function. At the cellular level, cyclosporine inhibits T-helper cell production of cytokines, particularly interleukin-2 (IL-2), required for T-lymphocyte proliferation. Cyclosporine also inhibits the elaboration of the high affinity IL-2 receptor by the cytotoxic T cell. The IL-2 receptor is a marker of cytotoxic T cell maturation and is required for IL-2 responsiveness and proliferation. The suppressor T cell is spared by cyclosporine. The noninhibition of the suppressor T cell may result in tolerance to the drug, observed in animal models of rejection[(92)]. At the subcellular level, cyclosporine interferes with activation signal transduction from the cell membrane to the nucleus. Membrane events are unaffected. Nuclear events, such as messenger RNA and DNA synthesis, are not directly affected. Cytoplasmic signals are blocked, preventing nuclear activation of oncogenes and inducible genes for IL-2 and other cytokines. Calcium-dependent signals via calmodulin, phospholipase A_2, and protein kinase C are inhibited[(92–94)]. Other specific binding proteins for cyclosporine, including cyclophilin, a cis-trans peptidyl prolylisomerase, have been identified[(95,96)]. Use of cyclosporine requires an awareness of many potential drug interactions **(Table 37.6).** Complications of cyclosporine therapy include hypertension, renal dysfunction, and hirsutism. Significant renal dysfunction requires a dosage reduction. Other milder complications include hyperuricemia, mild hyperglycemia, and neurologic dysfunction characterized by tremors and, occasionally, by seizures[(94)].

FK 506

The newer macrolide antibiotic, FK 506, functions by inhibiting IL-2 production and IL-2 receptor expression. Calcium-dependent signals are principally inhibited[(97)]. A specific binding protein for FK506 has been identified[(98)]. Both the FK-binding protein and cyclophilin possess cis-trans propylprolyl isomerase activity. Enzyme activity of the binding proteins and their inhibition by cyclosporine or FK 506, is not, however, required for immunosuppressive activity of drugs and their derivatives[(99)]. These binding proteins may serve as transport proteins or facilitate binding of drugs to the immunosuppressive receptor.

The complications attributed to FK 506 include toxicities also associated with cyclosporine, such as nephrotoxicity with hypertension, hyperglycemia, and neurotoxicity. The incidence of nephrotoxicity is similar to that with cyclosporine, but usually accompanied by less severe hyper-

Table 37.6. Cyclosporine Drug Interactions

Drugs that ↑ cyclosporine levels
Cimetidine
Erythromycin
Ketoconazole
High-dose methylprednisolone
Nonsteroidal anti-inflammatory agents
Drugs that ↓ cyclosporine levels
Phenobarbital
Phenytoin
Rifampin
Isoniazid
Trimethoprim (intravenous)
Drugs that potentiate nephrotoxicity
Aminoglycosides
Amphotericin B
Acyclovir

tension. Hyperglycemia may require the chronic use of insulin. Neurologic toxicity is manifested by agitation, tremors, insomnia, and seizures. The hirsutism and coarsening of facial features seen with cyclosporine are not observed with FK 506[100,101].

The major advantage to date of FK 506 compared with cyclosporine is the ability to use it as a single agent, thus avoiding the toxicity of drugs such as corticosteroids and azathioprine. Typically it is used as a sole agent for up to 3 months after transplant. Among patients who are alive with their primary graft and receiving FK 506, 93% are corticosteroid-free; of those who had successful rescue therapy, 82% are corticosteroid-free[100].

Another devastating complication secondary to FK 506 and cyclosporine is lymphoproliferative disease, usually of the B-cell type associated with Epstein-Barr virus and epithelial or hematopoietic malignant tumors[102–104]. When a pathologic diagnosis is made, immunosuppressive drugs are usually stopped in order to treat the cancer: Chemotherapy may be instituted in these instances.

Antilymphocyte Globulins

Antilymphocyte globulins (ALG) are polyclonal or monoclonal antilymphocyte antibodies designed to eliminate lymphocytes from the circulation and lymphoid depots of the transplant recipient. ALGs are used either to treat rejection or as prophylaxis[105]. They are prepared in animals (i.e., horse, rabbit, goat) by the injection of human lymphocytes (or lymphoblasts)[106]. Theoretically, these drugs are T-cell–specific, yet clinically they affect both B and T cells, since they represent a polyclonal response of the immune apparatus of the immunized animal. Polyclonal antibodies may be used several times without creating resistance.

Antithymocyte globulin (ATG) is a polyclonal sheep or horse immunoglobulin active against human T lymphocytes. It specifically binds to mature T lymphocytes and inactivates or destroys them in association with complement or macrophages. Although ATG is highly purified, serious systemic reactions occur, including fever, chills, skin rash, and serum sickness secondary to antibody complexes in the transplant recipient.

A more sophisticated ALG, OKT3 is a murine antihuman T-lymphocyte monoclonal antibody. The CD3 receptor on mature T-lymphocytes is closely related to the T3 receptor that specifically binds antigen in association with class I or II major histocompatibility antigens. This monoclonal antibody is the first in a series of specific anti–T-lymphocyte compounds. Binding of OKT3 to mature T-lymphocytes may eliminate them from their role in rejection by blocking the T-cell receptor or by specifically killing the T lymphocyte. OKT3 is highly effective in stopping established rejection episodes and has been used to prevent rejection in the early transplant period[107]. The effectiveness of the monoclonal antibody may be eliminated by formation of blocking antimurine antibodies.

Complications associated with OKT3 therapy include a capillary leak syndrome causing pulmonary edema and resulting in hypoxemia, fever, and occasionally, neurologic symptoms characterized by headache and meningismus.

Drug Regimens

Immunosuppressive regimens vary widely among institutions[108]. It is essential for the intensivist to have a comprehensive understanding of the possible side effects of different immunosuppressive agents **(Table 37.7).** The recent trend in therapy has been toward the use of methylprednisolone and FK 506 in the early postoperative period[109–114]. FK 506 is typically begun at a dose of 0.15 mg/kg/day given as a single slow intravenous infusion. When oral doses are tolerated, 0.15 mg/kg is given twice

Table 37.7. Immunosuppressive Drugs—Side Effects

Corticosteroids
Hypertension
Na/H_2O retention
Hyperglycemia
GI bleeding
Muscle weakness
Personality changes
Infection
Azathioprine
Bone marrow suppression
Infection
Nausea, vomiting
Mucosal ulceration
Cyclosporine
Hypertension
Renal dysfunction
Hirsutism
Hyperuricemia
Neurologic dysfunction—tremors, seizures
Hyperglycemia
Muscle weakness
Personality changes
Infection
Na/H_2O retention
FK506
Renal dysfunction
Hyperglycemia
Hyperuricemia
Neurotoxicity—tremors, agitation, insomnia, seizures
Hypertension
OKT-3
Fever
Headache
Pulmonary edema
Meningismus/headache
Antithymocyte globulin (ATG)
Anaphylaxis
Serum sickness
Infection
Lymphopenia
Antihuman lymphoblast globulin (ALG)
Thrombocytopenia
Lymphopenia
↑ BUN, creatinine
Anaphylaxis
Serum sickness
Chills, rashes, dyspnea

per day[115]. Methylprednisolone or prednisone are started immediately postoperatively and discontinued when graft function is stable.

The dose is usually increased in cases of rejection if the trough level is less than 2 ng/mL and there is no nephrotoxicity. The dose is decreased in the absence of rejection if the trough level is more than 3 ng/mL or if there are signs of nephrotoxicity.

In cases of rejection, FK 506 doses are in the high therapeutic range, and corticosteroids are pulsed intravenously. OKT3 is typically used in steroid-resistant rejection episodes.

NONHEPATIC MANAGEMENT

Fluids, Electrolytes, Nutrition, GI Tract

Fluid status, electrolyte balance, coagulation status, and liver and kidney function can all be assessed using the aforementioned monitoring techniques. Hematocrit, platelet count, PT, PTT, electrolyte levels (including ionized calcium and bicarbonate), and arterial blood gas levels should be monitored every few hours for the first 2 days after surgery. Blood urea nitrogen (BUN), creatinine, calcium, phosphorus, total and direct bilirubin, SGOT (AST), SGPT (ALT), alkaline phosphatase, γ-GGT, ammonia, amylase, albumin, and FK 506 or cyclosporine levels are followed on a daily basis unless the clinical course mandates tighter monitoring **(Table 37.8).**

Postoperative fluid management is challenging and requires frequent alterations. Generally, the postoperative patient is fluid overloaded in such a way that fluids are given initially at 80% of maintenance requirements. Nasogastric and abdominal drain outputs are replaced by an isotonic crystalloid or colloid solution. Other physiologic parameters should be followed closely to maintain a high-normal central venous pressure (7 to 10 mm Hg), urine output of 1 to 2 mL/kg/hour, and a normal mean arterial blood pressure. Low-dose dopamine, 0.5 to 3.0 μg/kg/minute, may be administered to enhance kidney and mesenteric perfusion. Hypovolemia is catastrophic to graft function and must be avoided.

Table 37.8. Laboratory Assessment Following Liver Transplantation

Frequent (every 6–8 hr)
Hematocrit, platelets
PT/PTT
Electrolytes
Arterial blood gas/pH
Ionized calcium
Daily
CBC
BUN
Creatinine
Total and ionized calcium
Phosphorus
Total and direct bilirubin
SGOT (AST)
SGPT (ALT)
Alkaline phosphatase
GGT
Ammonia
Amylase
Total protein/albumin
Immunosuppressive drug level (e.g. cyclosporine/FK 506)
Chest radiograph

Electrolyte imbalances are common. Hyponatremia usually is caused by excess free water administration and is corrected by fluid restriction. Vigorous use of diuretics also results in hyponatremia. Low levels of serum ionized calcium are common, especially when large blood transfusions have been administered. Calcium chloride (given as a 10 to 20 mg/kg dose intravenously every 4 to 6 hours for three to four doses) is the preferred agent after liver transplantation, since calcium gluconate must be metabolized by the liver to mobilize calcium. Calcium should be given through a central venous catheter since extravasation of calcium can lead to calcification of subcutaneous tissue. Hypomagnesemia may be corrected with magnesium sulfate (given as a 25 to 50 mg/kg dose intravenously every 4 to 6 hours for three to four doses). Since magnesium is protein-bound, total magnesium levels are related to the albumin level. Low calcium and magnesium levels must be treated expeditiously to avoid coagulation and central nervous system complications.

Hypokalemia also occurs secondary to aggressive diuresis and should be treated with intravenous infusions of potassium chloride; the dose is 0.3 mEq/kg/hour for patients with a serum potassium level of less than 3.0 mEq/L. The intravenous potassium chloride maintenance infusion may be increased from 20 to 60 mEq/L when the serum potassium level is 3.0 to 3.5 mEq/L.

Hyperkalemia results from renal dysfunction and graft necrosis. This disorder is managed by stopping all potassium-containing fluids and administering sodium polystyrene (Kayexalate) enemas. Severe hyperkalemia is treated with calcium chloride (20 mg/kg intravenously), sodium bicarbonate (1 to 2 mEq/kg intravenously over 3 to 5 minutes), and an infusion of glucose (0.5 g/kg intravenously), and insulin (0.3 u/g in a glucose intravenously). Ultimately, dialysis may be required if these measures are not successful in lowering the potassium level.

Hypophosphatemia results from inadequate vitamin D absorption, elevated parathormone levels, increased renal phosphate excretion caused by high-dose corticosteroid administration, increased phosphate uptake by the liver, and decreased total body phosphate stores secondary to malnutrition. Hypophosphatemia may lead to decreased erythrocyte levels of 2,3-DPG, causing increased affinity of hemoglobin for oxygen and, therefore, tissue hypoxia, and poor neutrophil chemotactic and phagocytic activity. Other clinical manifestations of hypophosphatemia include paresthesias, weakness or ataxia, seizures, coma, decreased myocardial contractility, hemolysis, and diminished platelet aggregation. Hypophosphatemia may present as an inability to wean the patient from the ventilator. It is treated with sodium or potassium phosphate, 0.3 to 0.6 mmol/kg intravenously over 6 hours. Calcium supplementation may be required to avoid hypocalcemic tetany.

It is imperative that the patient's nutritional status be assessed carefully(116). Nutritional markers include total protein, albumin, prealbumin, cholesterol, triglyceride, retinal-binding protein, and transferrin. Patients with preexisting cirrhosis, biliary atresia, or cancer are typically profoundly deficient in protein calories in the postoperative period. Intravenous hyperalimentation usually is instituted on the second postoperative day. Since postoperative ileus generally resolves by the third to fourth postoperative day, enteral feedings may be initiated at that time. A silastic feeding tube may be placed beyond the pylorus if the patient is unable to take adequate oral feedings(117). Refeeding bile into the GI tract increases the capacity to absorb fat and also may protect against endotoxemia and renal failure.

Glucose intolerance, manifested by hyperglycemia and glucosuria, is commonly associated with high doses of corticosteroids along with FK 506 and cyclosporine. Transient hyperglycemia also results early in the postoperative course from the release of glucose from dead donor-hepatocytes or from an elevated glucagon level(118). In patients with hyperglycemia, an insulin infusion allows adequate caloric intake until glucose tolerance improves. Intravenous lipids should not be administered until the triglyceride level falls below 200 mg/dL. Severe hypoglycemia is associated with primary graft failure and should be treated with a glucose infusion until retransplantation.

A nasogastric tube, usually placed during surgery, is maintained at low continuous suction. An antacid (at a dose of 0.5 to 1.0 mL/kg) is administered via the nasogastric tube every 2 to 4 hours to maintain the gastric pH level at more than 5.0(119). When normal bowel function returns during the first postoperative week, nasogastric suction can be discontinued. The use of H_2-receptor antagonists following liver transplantation is controversial: they may cause reversible elevation of liver transaminase levels(120–123). Elevated aminotransferase levels generally occur in patients receiving large doses of intravenous H_2-blockers. Cimetidine and ranitidine have both been implicated in causing hepatitis (cholestatic, mixed cholestatic-hepatocellular, or pure hepatocellular pattern), although this complication is rare(123). Hepatic blood flow is probably not markedly altered by the use of H_2-blockers(121–129). Ranitidine has less of an effect on the metabolism of other drugs compared with cimetidine(130). The dosage of cimetidine is 30 mg/kg/day given in four divided doses and that of ranitidine is 1 to 2 mg/kg/day in divided doses every 8 hours. During the postoperative period, it remains imperative to maintain an index of suspicion for surgical complications including GI perforation(131,132).

Pulmonary Management

The thrust of initial respiratory care is directed toward ventilator weaning and tracheal extubation, which usually may be accomplished within 36 hours of the operation. Routine criteria for weaning from mechanical ventilation are used. However, despite meticulous attention to pulmonary status, some patients require extended periods of ventilatory support. Malnourished and very young infants often require a protracted course of mechanical ventilation because of generalized weakness or abnormal chest wall mechanics. Most cases of delayed tracheal extubation are caused by a depressed respiratory drive secondary to oversedation, prolonged paralysis, impaired hepatic recovery, or pain.

Table 37.9. Respiratory Complications

Depressed respiratory drive
Oversedation
Prolonged paralysis
Impaired hepatic recovery: hyperammonemia
Pain
Pulmonary edema
Atelectasis
Restrictive effect of large donor liver
Pneumonia
Pleural effusion, commonly right-sided
Diaphragmatic paralysis—phrenic nerve injury
Absent gag reflex
Inability to handle secretions—associated with hepatic encephalopathy
Metabolic alkalosis
Electrolyte disorder (hypophosphatemia, hypocalcemia, hypokalemia)

Other pulmonary complications following transplantation include pulmonary edema, atelectasis, adult respiratory distress syndrome (ARDS), pleural effusion, metabolic alkalosis, diaphragmatic paralysis, and abdominal distention **(Table 37.9).** Daily chest radiographs allow diagnosis of these complications in addition to observation of the position of indwelling tubes and intravascular catheters. Pulmonary edema occurs secondary to fluid overload, but is generally controlled simply with diuretics, fluid restriction, and positive end-expiratory pressure (PEEP). PEEP is maintained at 5 cm H_2O unless higher levels are required to maintain the PaO_2 at more than 70 mm Hg despite an fraction of inspired oxygen (F_IO_2) of 0.5. Excessive PEEP should be avoided because of its potential to decrease cardiac output and hepatic blood flow(133–137). Hemodynamic monitoring may be used to assist in maintaining cardiac output with volume and inotropes so that adequate PEEP is used to minimize the shunt fraction to less than 15 to 20%(138). Aggressive chest physiotherapy is used, including frequent suctioning, turning, clapping, postural drainage, incentive spirometry, and early mobilization. Symptoms of atelectasis are pain, general anesthesia, decreased movement, abdominal distention, and pneumonia. Bronchoscopy is a useful therapeutic tool with persistent atelectasis. Sepsis or pneumonia should be treated in the presence of ARDS. Following transplantation, pneumonia or sepsis is associated with cytomegalovirus (CMV), *Pneumocystis carinii, Streptococcus faecalis, Pseudomonas aeruginosa, Aspergillus fumigatus,* and streptococcal pneumonia(58,139). Pleural effusions are usually right-sided and are often associated with ascites or fluid overload. The pleural effusion is attributed to trauma induced by inadvertent clamping of a small section of the right hemidiaphragm as the suprahepatic vena cava is clamped. A coexisting phrenic nerve palsy with temporary paralysis of the right hemidiaphragm may also be seen. Diuretics may be used to lessen the ascites and pleural effusion. Pleural drainage is indicated when respiratory compromise is present. This procedure should be undertaken with caution in the presence of coagulopathy and because of the numerous collateral vessels that are present secondary to the preexisting liver disease.

Normal respiratory movements may be hindered by high intra-abdominal pressures caused by a large donor liver or by ascites. If the pressure is secondary to ascites, drainage by peritoneal dialysis catheter may be done. A donor liver that is larger than the recipient's native liver may cause pulmonary compromise by decreasing the total lung volume, restricting diaphragmatic movement, and causing ventilation/perfusion ($\dot{V}/\dot{Q}$) mismatching from atelectasis.

Hypokalemic metabolic alkalosis may cause difficulty in weaning the patient from mechanical ventilation. It occurs after the transfusion of large volumes of banked blood because the ensuing metabolism of citrate to bicarbonate is exacerbated with the subsequent use of diuretic therapy and nasogastric suction. Generally, the alkalosis is mild and resolves without treatment within 36 hours after surgery. However, respiratory compensation may be significant with P_aCO_2 values of more than 55 mm Hg. In these cases, it may be difficult to wean the patient from mechanical ventilation because of a lack of spontaneous respirations. Acetazolamide or a dilute hydrochloric acid infusion may be needed to return the blood pH to normal.

Cardiovascular Management

Preoperatively, hepatic failure is associated with increased cardiac output, left ventricular dilation and hypertrophy, low systemic and pulmonary vascular resistance, and systemic and pulmonary shunting because of arteriovenous malformations. Following transplantation, the systemic vascular resistance normalizes and the cardiac output decreases. The low diastolic pressure in the pretransplant patient, owing to decreased systemic and pulmonary vascular resistance, is usually not a problem after surgery. Postoperatively, fluid overload may result in decreased left ventricular compliance and decreased contractility. When myocardial dysfunction exists, it should be managed with inotropic agents or afterload reducing agents, such as nitroprusside or nitroglycerin[85]. Many patients are selenium-deficient or have an occult cardiomyopathy.

Hypertension is often encountered in the immediate postoperative period, and is usually attributed to pain[58]. Morphine, 0.1 mg/kg, or fentanyl, 1 to 2 μg/kg may be effective in achieving postoperative analgesia, or patient-controlled analgesia may be used. Typically, there is a relatively low need for analgesia after transplant[140]. If there is no response to appropriate doses of analgesics, hypertension may be secondary to intravascular volume overload. Hypertension may also be attributed to other factors, including elevated renin and catecholamine levels,[141] and may be exacerbated by renal toxicity caused by corticosteroids, FK 506, cyclosporine, or other drugs. When systemic hypertension does not respond to pain control or diuresis, medications such as nitroprusside, a calcium channel blocker (e.g., nifedipine), or hydralazine should be used. The hypertension is generally transient and usually does not require treatment beyond the first month after transplant.

Hematologic Management

Hematologic disorders after transplantation include hemolytic anemia, aplastic anemia[142], and coagulation disorders. Hemolytic anemia may occur in ABO-compatible, nonidentical recipients[143]. The donor's B lymphocytes recognize the recipient's ABO antigens as foreign and produce antiblood type antibody (graft versus host response). Usually, this is seen within the first month after transplantation and is typically self-limited, lasting approximately 2 to 4 weeks[144]. Signs of a graft versus host response encompass hemoglobinuria, a sudden increase in total bilirubin level, minimal hepatic parenchymal enzyme changes, a decreased serum hemoglobin level, an increased reticulocyte count, and evidence of an unobstructed biliary tract on abdominal ultrasound examination. Measurement of serum haptoglobin level is not useful in the evaluation, since it may be decreased as a result of liver dysfunction. Serial reticulocyte counts are the most useful tool in following the progression of hemolysis. When evidence of hemolysis persists, the patient should receive type O blood.

Typically, following transplantation, PTT decreases to control levels within 2 days, and PT normalizes by 5 to 7 days[145]. Postoperative coagulopathy is manifested by prolonged PT and PTT and thrombocytopenia. The coagulopathy is usually responsive to appropriate component therapy: It should be corrected only if active bleeding is present or if the coagulation tests are more than twice their control level. Graft dysfunction is associated with a lack of response to therapy with fresh frozen plasma or platelets. The degree of ongoing liver dysfunction, preoperative aspirin use, and large amounts of blood transfusion contribute to a clinically apparent coagulopathy. When repeated packed red blood cell transfusions are needed to maintain the hematocrit above 25 to 30%, surgical reexploration may be necessary to establish hemostasis.

Renal Management

The combination of FK 506, cyclosporine, corticosteroids, and an increase in serum renin level prevents the kidneys from responding appropriately to salt and volume overload with adequate diuresis and natriuresis. Therefore, appropriate postoperative therapy should include salt restriction[146], liberal use of diuretics, and angiotensin-converting enzyme inhibitors for patients with a low creatinine excretion index[141].

Acute renal failure most often occurs in patients who have preexisting renal disease, including hepatorenal syndrome, FK 506 or cyclosporine toxicity, other drug toxicity, or acute tubular necrosis. Good graft function usually results in prompt resolution of preexisting hepatorenal syndrome[(38)]. Refractory postoperative renal failure, even in patients with preexisting hepatorenal syndrome, is suggestive of systemic infection or graft dysfunction. Venovenous bypass significantly reduces the incidence of acute renal failure after liver transplantation in adults[(147)]. However, venovenous bypass, which decompresses the mesenteric venous system and IVC resulting in enhanced renal perfusion, is generally not used in children who weigh less than 15 kg. In these patients, the suprarenal vena cava is occluded during the implantation of the new liver, resulting in a decrease in urine output. Mannitol may be given in an effort to increase urine output and to minimize renal injury resulting from caval cross-clamping. Acute tubular necrosis is generally attributed to perioperative hypotension and massive intraoperative transfusions. FK 506 or cyclosporine levels must be meticulously monitored because of their propensity to cause acute tubular necrosis[(110,112)]. The combination of hypovolemia and FK 506 administration increases the incidence of postoperative renal failure.

Metabolic acidosis, when it occurs in the immediate postoperative period, is secondary to hepatic or renal failure. When severe, it may be controlled with continuous arteriovenous hemofiltration and predilution with sodium bicarbonate.

Infection Management

Infection is a common cause of death in the postoperative phase. Distinguishing between infection and rejection is necessary, since infection requires a decrease in the dosage of immunosuppressive drugs while rejection usually necessitates an increase in dosage. Surveillance cultures should be obtained from the throat, endotracheal tube, urine, blood, stool, and bile. A lumbar puncture should also be done to rule out central nervous system (CNS) infection, if warranted by the clinical examination. Samples must be cultured for aerobes, anaerobes, viruses, and fungi. An index of suspicion should also be maintained for reactivation of tuberculosis, *Legionella* species, and hepatitis B virus (HBV). Hepatitis B infection in liver transplant patients usually results from reinfection from a chronic infection[(148)]. Although hepatitis C virus is a primary cause of liver injury after transplantation in adults, the prevalence of hepatitis C infections in infants and children is substantially less[(149)]. Children who have an enterostomy in place from a previous Kasai procedure are at increased risk for wound infections and, for this reason, the enterostomy should be closed before the transplant.

Protective isolation is not mandatory in the postoperative period. However, strict hand washing should be enforced to limit the spread of infection by hospital personnel. The patient's own GI flora is the greatest threat of infection. Various posttransplant infectious agents have been reported[(150–154)].

Appropriate antibiotics effective against biliary pathogens (*Klebsiella* species, *Escherichia coli,* and enterococcus) should be continued postoperatively. The combination of ampicillin and cefotaxime is an effective regimen. Mycostatin oral suspension given four times a day via nasogastric tube and mycostatin vaginal suppositories (for adolescent girls) given three times a day help minimize the incidence of oral and vaginal candidiasis. Selective bowel decontamination may be used to eliminate an endogenous source of gram-negative and fungal organisms from the GI tract[(139,155)]. Treatment consists of a solution of gentamicin (80 mg), polymyxin E (100 mg), and nystatin (2,000,000 U) administered through a nasogastric tube or orally, as tolerated. The solution can also be applied to the oral cavity while the patient is still tracheally intubated[(139)].

Bacterial pneumonia is relatively uncommon as a cause of infection after surgery. It is most often seen in immunosuppressed children with an underlying disease such as cystic fibrosis, α_1-antitrypsin deficiency, or chronic bronchitis. The antibiotic regimen may be altered in accordance with results of surveillance cultures. Fiberoptic bronchoscopy with bronchoalveolar lavage may be helpful in specific cases of pneumonia. In the event of a new pulmonary infiltrate, erythromycin and trimethoprim-sulfamethoxazole (TMP-SMX) provide adequate coverage for *Legionella* and *P. carinii* infection before culture results are available. Other bacterial infections include cholangitis and intra-abdominal abscesses. Cholangitis may be associated with mechanical obstruction of the biliary tree; therefore, biliary obstruction must be excluded[(156)].

CMV, herpes simplex virus (HSV), and Epstein-Barr virus (EBV) are the most common viral infections seen after transplantation[(157)]. Adenovirus has been associated with overwhelming pneumonitis and hepatitis[(158)]. CMV titers may be elevated because of a new infection or reactivation of a previous infection. Asymptomatic shedding of CMV is detected by isolation of the virus in the urine or pharynx in the absence of clinical illness or an increase in the anti-CMV–IgM titer. When symptoms of active infection are not present, the patient should be treated for rejection. Whenever possible, CMV-positive donors are used in CMV-positive recipients. In one study, four of 12 CMV-negative recipients received a liver from a CMV-positive donor, and only one patient ultimately survived the transplant[(159)]. Another group also had a higher survival rate (100%) in patients who remained CMV-negative after transplant compared with those who had primary posttransplant CMV infection (78%)[(160)]. Of the six patients who were CMV-positive before transplant, only one received an organ from a CMV-positive donor; none of the six patients had symptomatic disease after transplantation, although all of the patients had asymptomatic viruria for months[(159)]. Some institutions have reported a decrease in the number of primary CMV infections in CMV-seronegative transplant recipients with a seronegative donor when prophylactic treatment and CMV-negative blood products are employed[(161–164)]. Prophylaxis with intravenous CMV immune globulin has not triggered a decreased incidence of posttransplant infections[(165)]. In a retrospective review of 26 pediatric liver transplant patients, King and coworkers report a 54% incidence of CMV infection (14 patients) and note that the major risk factor for severe CMV disease was a seropositive donor[166].

A CMV infection may be heralded by fever, malaise, anorexia, abnormal results on liver function tests (levels of bilirubin and transaminases), leukopenia, pneumonitis (interstitial pulmonary infiltrates and positive results on culture of bronchoalveolar lavage), and enteritis (abdominal pain, nausea, vomiting, GI hemorrhage, diarrhea, and mucosal ulcerations that are positive for CMV seen at endoscopy)[167]. Severe cases may result in hepatitis, pneumonitis, colitis, sepsis, and cerebritis[159,161]. Evidence of viral infection is occasionally found on liver biopsy, usually with evidence of concomitant rejection. Primary infection is associated with a more severe clinical course than does a reactivation-associated infection[165].

Severe CMV infection is treated by decreasing the dose of immunosuppressive agents and adding gancyclovir to the patient's regimen[168]. In severe cases of hepatitis, pneumonitis, duodenitis, gastritis, or colitis, immunosuppressive agents may have to be discontinued. Patients with severe CMV infection and concomitant rejection have been successfully treated with a combination of OKT3 and gancyclovir.

Acyclovir is used to treat any sign of herpes infection. Topical therapy is used for cutaneous lesions; invasive infection requires systemic therapy[157]. Herpes encephalitis is usually fatal despite prompt institution of acyclovir therapy and withdrawal of immunosuppressive drugs.

EBV infections range from an asymptomatic, isolated rise in viral titers to mononucleosis or lymphoma[169]. Acyclovir is used to treat EBV infections. Lymphoma is secondary to immunosuppressive drug use; therefore, it is managed by withdrawal of immunosuppressive drugs rather than with chemotherapy. Breinig and coworkers reported a 57% incidence of EBV infection by means of serologic testing with only 12% of cases being symptomatic[157]. Of the patients with primary EBV infections, 14% contracted an EBV-associated lymphoproliferative syndrome between 2 months and 2 years after the infection[157].

As noted previously, *Candida albicans* is often encountered in the immunocompromised host. *Aspergillus* species cause the next most frequent fungal infection, which is usually fatal. Other risk factors for fungal infections include a prolonged operation and the use of relatively high doses of antibiotics and immunosuppressive agents. Positive results on blood cultures should be taken seriously and not merely attributed to central line colonization. Specimens from indwelling venous and arterial catheters must be cultured often. Amphotericin B should be strongly considered if fungemia is suspected. Ketoconazole is not recommended for use in transplant recipients because of its high rate of hepatotoxicity and its effect of increasing the immunosuppressive level[170]. The dose of amphotericin B should be adjusted cautiously in the presence of altered renal function[171,172].

The most life-threatening nonviral infection in the transplant recipient is *P. carinii* pneumonia. When pneumocystic infection is suspected, prompt institution of TMP/SMX therapy is warranted. The diagnosis may be facilitated by examination of samples from bronchoalveolar lavage[173,174]. In the event of a resistant infection or an allergy to sulfa drugs, pentamidine isethionate may be used. The incidence of *P. carinii* infection in the immunocompromised patient may be reduced by using TMP/SMX prophylaxis.

Neurologic Management

Neurologic function may be depressed after liver transplantation because of the lingering effects of anesthetics, narcotics, and neuromuscular blocking agents. Compromised liver or kidney function may prolong the excretion of many of these drugs and lengthen the period of neurologic derangement. The majority of patients become responsive within the first postoperative day. Patients who had preoperative encephalopathy may take many days to recover normal CNS function.

CNS complications include seizures, strokes, peripheral neuropathy, and "dulled mentation"[175–178]. Seizures are usually grand mal, and evaluation generally reveals negative results on head CT scan and lumbar puncture. Nevertheless, the possibility of an intracranial hemorrhage, infarct due to clot or air embolism, or metabolic disorder, such as hyponatremia, hypoglycemia, FK 506 or cyclosporine toxicity, should be ruled out[179,180]. Other factors associated with seizures are fluid retention, hypertension, high-dose corticosteroid therapy[181], hypomagnesemia[182,183], graft dysfunction, and demyelination[184]. Reduction of the FK 506 or cyclosporine dosage is advisable in cases of suspected toxicity. Cyclosporine-induced CNS toxicity has also been seen in association with a low serum cholesterol level[185]. It has been suggested that cyclosporine administration is related to demyelination and neurologic toxicity. Berden and coworkers reported normalization of white matter on CT scan as well as electromyographic evidence of axonal degeneration after cessation of cyclosporine therapy[176]. The majority of seizures may be controlled with phenobarbital[186]. When anticonvulsant therapy is instituted, it is important to monitor FK 506 or cyclosporine levels, since both phenobarbital and phenytoin are associated with decreasing plasma levels of these agents[170].

Cerebral edema, either vasogenic or cytotoxic, may complicate management both before and after transplant. ICP monitoring may be prudent, although placement of a monitoring device may be problematic in respect to a coincident profound coagulopathy. At this point, there is scant literature regarding the value of ICP monitoring to guide specific interventional therapy in liver transplant recipients.

Psychosocial Management

Social and financial management are important aspects of successful transplantation. Some of the social problems encountered are related to finances, chronic disease, interpersonal relationships within the family, age of the patient, and sophistication of caretakers. Children usually do well in readapting to a normal life and continuing with school achievements[187,188]. Motor development may be adequate, although growth may be impeded[189,190]. The majority of children go home 1 month after transplantation. Routine pediatric care may be continued by their general pediatrician who, in concert with the transplant center, monitors liver function and immunosuppression. An annual liver biopsy is performed to aid in adjustment of immunosuppressive therapy.

Table 37.10. Survival[a]

	1 Yr	*3 Yr*	*5 Yr*	*No. of patients*
Hanover, Germany[118]	82%	57%		35
Toronto[117]	61%	61%		18
Dallas[119]	75%	73%		80
Boston[144]	60%	60%		23
UCLA[143]	79%	70%		38
Pittsburgh[142]	70%	70%	69%	265
Belgium[14]	76%	74%		139

[a]*Reference numbers in parentheses.*

PROGNOSTIC FACTORS AND OUTCOME

Before 1980, when azathioprine was used as the main immunosuppressive drug, OLT had a 30 to 40% rate of survival for 1 year. With the introduction of cyclosporine in 1980[191], the 1-year survival rate improved to 60 to 80%[192] **(Table 37–10).** Recent (1993) data obtained regarding the use of FK 506 reveal 1-year survival rates of 80 to 90% (Figure 37.3) [193]. Pediatric patients have a slightly higher survival rate than adult patients[192]. There is only a minimal change between the 1-year to 3 to 5 year survival rates.

The rate of retransplantation ranges from 10%[194] to 17%[159] and results from a variety of causes, including acute rejection of the liver, primary nonfunction of the liver, and acute vascular complications. Infants may be at a higher risk for retransplantation than other age groups[18,195].

As the number of transplants performed in pediatric patients increases, a number of high-risk factors have been established, which include young age, diagnosis, recipient anatomy, and preoperative coma. In a review of infants less than 1 year old who received an OLT, Sokal and colleagues reported a 65% actuarial 1-year survival rate, compared with 76% for all transplant patients, and a 3-yr actuarial survival rate of 50% for this group of infants[18]. Another group reported a primary graft nonfunction rate of 39% in infants[196]. This rate is comparable to a 60% survival rate in infants reported from Pittsburgh[192]. Recent evidence shows a possible trend towards improved survival (77%) in small infants[195]. The perioperative problems that occur more often in infants include hepatic artery thrombosis necessitating retransplanation (in 15 to 25% of infants)[18,192,197], defects of biliary tract reconstruction, and intestinal problems from previous portoenterostomies[192]. In addition, complications such as diaphragmatic paralysis, which occurred in 31% of patients in one study, are tolerated less well in infants[194].

Superina and associates report a number of high-risk factors, including young age, extrahepatic biliary atresia (typically correlated with previous surgery in infants), portal vein atresia or thrombosis, and preoperative hepatic coma[159]. Only 54% of the patients with at least one of those factors were alive 3 to 23 months after OLT. The presence of pretransplant encephalopathy, particulary when severe, is associated with a poor outcome. More than 50% of these patients do not recover neurologic function after surgery[25]. The decision to operate should ideally be made before neurologic deterioration progresses. Severe clinical dysfunction occurs because of cerebral edema or decreased cerebral blood flow caused by hyperammonemia, other metabolites, or gamma aminobutyric acid

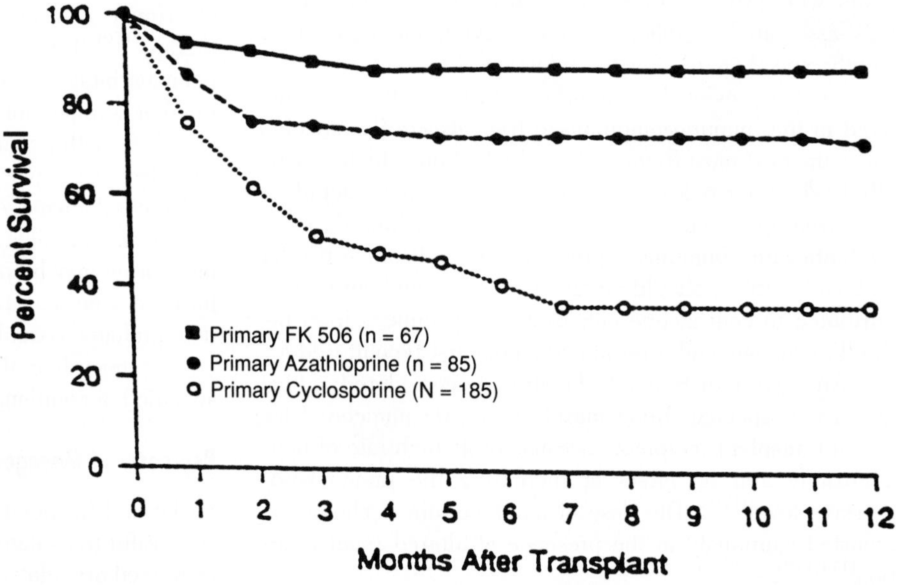

Figure 37.3. Pediatric liver transplantation recipient survival; FK 506 vs. azathioprine vs. cyclosporine. From Tzakis AG, Starzl TE. Liver transplantation. In: Aschraft KW, Holder TM eds. Pediatric Surgery. Philadelphia: WB Saunders, 1992:520.

(GABA)–ergic agonists[198]. The risk of CMV infection in patients who are CMV-negative before surgery is high and carries an increased risk of postoperative complications and death.

Postoperative factors that bode well for survival include normalization of a previously abnormal coagulation profile, maintenance of metabolic substrates such as serum glucose and amino acids[83], and the absence of lactic acidosis[199–201]. High factor V levels are associated with relatively fewer postoperative bleeding complications[202]. Furthermore, bile drainage through a T tube is an encouraging sign early in the postoperative course[4].

Multivisceral transplants including the liver have been used in treatment of patients with failure of more than one visceral organ system[5,203]. Intestinal transplantation, whether accomplished alone or in combination with other intraabdominal organs, under FK 506 immunosuppression yields results comparable to those obtained from commonly performed organ transplants[204–207].

SUMMARY

In conclusion, the intensive care management of patients undergoing liver transplantation is challenging and must encompass many medical disciplines. The problems encountered are caused by the patient's underlying disease and may be magnified by dysfunction of other organ systems. Many of the technologic advances in diagnosis and pharmacotherapy available should be used to manage the array of complications, both hepatic and nonhepatic, that may occur in the posttransplant patient. As immunosuppressive therapy continues to improve, resulting in less rejection and less toxicity; as surgical technique and organ preservation become more refined; and as diagnostic modalities become more sophisticated, survival rates will continue to improve. Organ procurement, however, remains a critical problem.

References

1. Starzl TE, Marchioro TL, Porter KA, et al. Surgery 1965;58:131.
2. Starzl TE. Experience in hepatic transplantation. Philadelphia: WB Saunders, 1969.
3. Starzl TE, Groth CG, Brettschneider L, et al. Orthotopic homotransplantation of the human liver. Ann Surg 1968;168:392.
4. Starzl TE, Iwatsuki S, Van Thiel DH, et al. Evolution of liver transplantation. Hepatology 1982;2:614.
5. Tzakis AG, Starzl TE. Liver transplantation. In: Pediatric Surgery. 2nd ed. Ashcraft KW, Holder TM, ed. Philadelphia, WB Saunders Company, 1992;505–524.
6. Eckhoff DE, D'Alessandro AM, Knechtle SJ, et al. 100 consecutive liver transplants in infants and children: an 8-year experience. J Pediatr Surg 1994;29:1135.
7. Gordon RD, Fung J, Tzakis AG, et al. Liver transplantation at the University of Pittsburgh, 1984 to 1990. Cl Transplants 1991:105.
8. Belle SH, Beringer KC, Detre KM. Trends in liver transplantation in the United States. Cl Transplants 1993:19.
9. Alagille D. Extrahepatic biliary cirrhosis. NIH consensus development conference on liver transplantation. Bethesda, MD: NIH, 1982:17.
10. Kasai M. Watarabe I, Oni R. Follow-up studies of long-term survivors after hepatic portoenterostomy for "noncorrectable" biliary atresia. J Pediatr Surg 1975;10:173.
11. Barkin RM, Lilly JR. Biliary atresia and the Kasai operation: continuing care. J Pediatr 1980;96:1015.
12. Lilly JR, Karrer FM, Hall RJ, et al. The surgery of biliary atresia. Ann Surg 1989;210:289.
13. Grosfeld JL, Fitzgerald JF, Predaina R, et al. The efficacy of hepatoportoenterostomy in biliary atresia. Surgery 1989;106:692.
14. Houwen RHJ, Zwierstra RP, Severijnen RS, et al. Prognosis of extrahepatic biliary atresia. Arch Dis Child 1989;64:214.
15. Kobayashi A, Itabashi F, Ohbe Y. Long-term prognosis in biliary atresia after hepatic portoenterostomy: analysis of 35 patients who survived beyond 5 years of age. J Pediatr 1984;105:243.
16. Kasai M, Mochizuki I, Ohkohchi N, et al. Surgical limitation for biliary atresia: indication for liver transplantation. J Pediatr Surg 1989;24:851.
17. Esquivel CO, Koneru B, Karrer F, et al. Liver transplantation before 1 year of age. J Pediatr 1987;110:545.
18. Sokal EM, Veychemans F, de Ville de Goyet J, et al. Liver transplantation in children less than 1 year of age. J Pediatr 1990;117;205.
19. Shah HA, Spivak W. Neonatal cholestasis. New approaches to diagnostic evaluation and therapy. Pediatr Cl North America 1994;41:943.
20. Jan D, Laurent J, Lacaille F, et al. Unite de transplantation pediatrique, Hopital des Enfants Malades, Paris, France. Transplantation Proceedings 1995;27:1706.
21. Todo S, Starzl TE, Tzakis A, et al. Orthotopic liver transplantation for urea cycle enzyme deficiency. Heptatol 1992;15:419.
22. Touraine JL, Laplace S, Rezzoug F, et al. The place of fetal liver transplantation in the treatment of inborn errors of metabolism. J Inherited Metab Dis 1991;14:619.
23. Kelly DA. Organ transplantation for inherited metabolic disease. Arch Dis Childhood 1994;71:181.
24. Keating JJ, Johnson RD, Williams R. Clinical course of cirrhosis in young adults and therapeutic potential of liver transplantation. Gut 1985;26:1359.
25. Whitington PF, Balistreri WF. Liver transplantation in pediatrics: indications, contraindications, and pretransplant management. J Pediatr 1991;118:169.
26. Malatack JJ, Schaid DJ, Urbach AH, et al. Choosing a pediatric recipient of orthotopic liver transplantation. J Pediatr 1987;111:479.
27. Marino JR, ChapChap P, Esquivel CO, et al. Liver transplantation for arteriohepatic dysplasia (Alagille's syndrome). Transplant Intl 1992;5:61.
28. Adrian-Casavilla F, Reyes J, Tzakis A, et al. Liver transplantation for neonatal hepatitis as compared to the other two leading indications for liver transplantation in children. J Hepatol 1994;21:1035.
29. Balistreri WF. Neonatal cholestasis. J Pediatr 1985;106:171.
30. Tzakis AG, Reves J, Tepetes K, et al. Liver transplantation for Alagille's syndrome. Arch Surg 1993;128:337.
31. Selby R, Kadry Z, Carr B, et al. Liver transplantation for hepatocellular carcinoma. World J Surg 1995;19:53.
32. Iwatsuki S, Starzl TE, Sheahan DG, et al. Hepatic resection versus transplantation for hepatocellular carcinoma. Ann Surg 1991;214:221.
33. Esquivel CO, Gutierrez C, Cox KL, et al. Hepatocellular carcinoma and liver cell dysplasia in children with chronic liver disease. J Pediatr Surg 1994;29:1465.
34. Perlmutter D, Vacanti J, Donahoe P, et al. Liver transplantation in pediatric patients. Chicago: Mosby Year Book, 1985.
35. McCloskey JJ, Schleien CL, Schwarz K, et al. Severe hypoxemia and intrapulmonary shunting resulting from cirrhosis reversed by liver transplantation in a pediatric patient. J Pediatr 1991;118:902.
36. Barbe T, Losay J, Grimon G, et al. Pulmonary arteriovenous shunting in children with liver disease. J Pediatr 1995;126:571.
37. Grimon G, Andre L, Bernard O, et al. Early radionuclide detection of intrapulmonary shunts in children with liver disease. J Nuclear Med 1994;35:1328.
38. Wood RP, Ellis D, Starzl TE. The reversal of the hepatorenal syndrome in four pediatric patients following successful orthotopic liver transplantation. Ann Surg 1987;205:415.
39. Woodle ES, Thistlethwaite JR, Emond JC, et al. Successful orthotopic liver transplantation in congenital absence of the portal vein. Surgery 1990;107:475.
40. Ringe B, Wittekind C, Bechstein WO, et al. The role of liver transplantation in hepatobiliary malignancy. Ann Surg 1989;209:88.
41. Yokoyama I, Tzakis AG, Imventarza O, et al. Pediatric liver transplantation from neonatal donors. Transplant Intl 1992;5:205.
42. Urata K, Kawasaki S, Matsunami H, et al. Calculation of child and adult standard liver volume for liver transplantation. Hepatol 1995;21:1317.
43. Broelsch CE, Emond JC, Whitington TF, et al. Application of reduced-

size liver transplants as split grafts, auxiliary orthotopic grafts, and living related segmental transplants. Ann Surg 1990;212:368.
44. Jurim O, Csete M, Gelabert HA, et al. Reduced-size grafts—the solution for hepatic artery thrombosis after pediatric liver transplantation? J Pediatr Surg 1995;30:53.
45. Slooff MJ. Reduced size liver transplantation, split liver transplantation, and living related liver transplantation in relation to the donor organ shortage. Transplant Intl 1995;8:65.
46. Bilik R, Greig P, Langer B, et al. Survival after reduced-size liver transplantation is dependent on pretransplant status. J Pediatr Surg 1993;28:1307.
47. Jurim O, Shackleton CR, McDiarmid SV, et al. Living-donor liver transplantation at UCLA. Am J Surg 1995;169:529.
48. Cacciarelli TV, So SK, Egawa H, et al. Impact of reduced-size liver transplantation on rejection and liver allograft outcome in the pediatric population. Transplantation Proceedings 1995;27:1239.
49. Belzer FO, Soutard JH. Principles of solid-organ preservation by cold storage. Transplantation 1988;45:673.
50. Belzer FO, D'Alessandro AM, Hoffmann RM, et al. The use of UW solution in clinical transplantation. A 4-year experience. Ann Surg 1992;215:579.
51. Waisman Y, Klein BL, Rachmel A, et al. In-flight esophageal variceal bleeding en route for liver transplantation: a case report and review of the literature. Pediatr Emerg Care 1991;7:157.
52. Iwatsuki S, Shaw BW, Starzl TE. Liver transplantation for biliary atresia. World J Surg 1978;2:571.
53. Otte JB, de Ville de Goyet J, Sokal E, et al. Size reduction of the donor liver is a safe way to alleviate the shortage of size-matched organs in pediatric liver transplantation. Ann Surg 1990;211:146.
54. Houssin D, Franco D, Berthelot P, et al. Heterotopic liver transplantation in end-stage HBS-Ag positive cirrhosis. Lancet 1980;1:1990.
55. Rayner SC, Weed RP, Shaw B, et al. Liver transplantation in a patient with abdominal situs inversus. Transplantation 1988;45:661.
56. Tzakis AG, Reyes J, Nour B, et al. Temporary end to side portacaval shunt in orthotopic hepatic transplantation in humans. Surg Gynecol Obstet 1993;176:181.
57. Griffith BP, Shaw BW Jr, Hardesty RL, et al. Veno-venous bypass without systemic anticoagulation for transplantation of the human liver. Surg Gynecol Obstet 1985;160:271.
58. Gartner JC Jr, Zitelli B, Malatack JJ, et al. Orthotopic liver transplantation in children: two-year experience with 47 patients. Pediatrics 1984;74:140.
59. Millis JM, Brems JJ, Hiatt JR, et al. Orthotopic liver transplantation for biliary atresia: evolution of management. Arch Surg 1988;123:1237.
60. Bilik R, Yellen M, Superina RA. Surgical complications in children after liver transplantation. J Pediatr Surg 1992;27:1371.
61. Todo S, Makowka L, Tzakis AG, et al. Hepatic artery in liver transplant. Transplant Proc 1987;19:2406.
62. Hesselink EJ, Klompmaker IJ, Pruim J, et al. Hepatic artery thrombosis after orthotopic liver transplantation—a fatal complication or an asymptomatic event. Transplant Proc 1989;21:2462.
63. Tzakis AG, Gordon RD, Shaw BW Jr, et al. Clinical presentation of hepatic artery thrombosis after liver transplantation in the cyclosporine era. Transplantation 1985;40:667.
64. Zajko AB, Sheng R, Bron K, et al. Percutaneous transluminal angioplasty of venous anastomotic stenoses complicating liver transplantation: intermediate-term results. J Vasc Intervent Radiol 1994;5:121.
65. Mazzafferro V, Esquivel CO, Makowka L, et al. Hepatic artery thrombosis after pediatric liver transplantation: medical or surgical event? Transplantation 1989;47:971.
66. Segel MC, Zajko AB, Bron KM, et al. Doppler ultrasound as a screen for hepatic artery thrombosis after liver transplantation. Transplantation 1986;41:539.
67. Wozney P, Zajko AB, Bron KM, et al. Vascular complications after liver transplantation: a 5-year experience. AJR 1986;147:652.
68. Harper PL, Edgar PF, Luddington RJ, et al. Protein C deficiency and portal thrombosis in liver transplantation in children. Lancet 1988;2:924.
69. Burke GW, Ascher NL, Hunter D, et al. Orthotopic liver transplantation: non-operative management of early, acute portal vein thrombosis. Surgery 1988;104:924.
70. Helling TS. Thrombosis and recanalization of the portal vein in liver transplantation. Transplantation 1985;40:446.
71. Lerut J, Tzakis AG, Bron K, et al. Complications of venous reconstruction in human orthotopic liver transplantation. Ann Surg 1987;205:404.
72. Tzakis AG. The dearterialized liver graft. Semin Liver Dis 1985;5:375.
73. Shaw BW Jr, Gordon RD, Iwatsuki S, et al. Hepatic retransplantation. Transplant Proc 1985;17:264.
74. Plevak DJ, Halma GA, Forstrom LA, et al. Thrombocytopenia after liver transplantation. Transplant Proc 1988;20(Suppl 1):630.
75. Esquivel CO, Jaffe R, Gordon RD, et al. Liver rejection and its differentiation from other causes of graft dysfunction. Semin Liver Dis 1985;5:369.
76. Bilik R, Superina RA, Phillips J, et al. Prevention of biliary cirrhosis following hepatic arterial thrombosis after liver transplantation in children by using ursodeoxycholic acid. J Pediatr Surg 1995;30:49.
77. Neuhaus P, Brolsch CH, Ringe B, et al. Results of biliary reconstruction after liver transplantation. Transplant Proc 1984;16:1225.
78. Peclet MH, Ryckman FC, Pedersen SH, et al. The spectrum of bile duct complications in pediatric liver transplantation. J Pediatr Surg 1994;29:214.
79. Zajko AB, Campbell WL, Logsdon GA, et al. Cholangiographic findings in hepatic artery occlusion after liver transplantation. Am J Radiol 1987;149:485.
80. Zajko AB, Campbell WL, Bron KM, et al. Cholangiography and interventional biliary radiology in adult liver transplantation. Am J Radiol 1985;144:127.
81. Zajko AB, Sheng R, Zetti GM, et al. Transhepatic balloon dilation of biliary strictures in liver transplant patients: a 10 year experience. J Vasc Interven Radiol 1995;6(1):79-83.
82. Sherlock S. Hepatic transplantation. South Med J 1987;80:357.
83. Van Thiel D. Liver transplantation. Pediatr Ann 1985;14:474.
84. Ascher NL, Najarian JS. Liver transplantation in children. In: Blumgart LH, ed. Surgery of the liver and biliary tract. Edinburgh: Churchill Livingstone, 1988.
85. Stock PG, Payne WD. Liver transplantation. Crit Care Clin 1990;6:911.
86. Stock PG, Snover D, Payne WD, et al. Biopsy-guided immunosuppressive therapy in the treatment of liver transplant rejection: an individualized approach. Clin Trans 1987;1:179.
87. Snover DC, Sibley RK, Freese DK, et al. Orthotopic liver transplant rejection: a sequential liver biopsy study. Transplant Proc 1985;17:272.
88. Zegel HG, Cole-Beuglet C, Carpenter G. Pre- and postoperative hepatic transplant evaluation by ultrasound and computerized tomography. J Clin Ultrasound 1981;9:101.
89. Segel MC, Zajko AB, Bowen A, et al. Hepatic artery thrombosis after liver transplantation radiologic evaluation. Am J Radiol 1986;146:137.
90. Don S. Selected topics in hepatobiliary imaging. Seminars Pediatr Surg 1992;1:260.
91. Cahill CJ, Pain JA, Bailey ME. Bile salts, endotoxin and renal function in obstructive jaundice. Surg Gynecol Obstet 1987;165:519.
92. Colombani PM, Robb A, Hess AD. Cyclosporine A binding to calmodulin: a possible site of action on T-lymphocytes. Science 1985;228:337.
93. Colombani PM, Hess AD. T-lymphocyte inhibition by cyclosporine: potential mechanisms of action. Biochem Pharmacol 1987;36:3789.
94. Kahan BD. Drug therapy—cyclosporine. N Engl J Med 1989;321:1725.
95. Handschumacher RE, Harding MW, Rice J, et al. Cyclophilin: a specific cytosolic binding protein for Cyclosporin A. Science 1984; 226:544.
96. Foxwell BM, Mackie A, Ling V, et al. Identification of the multidrug resistance-related P-glycoprotein as a cyclosporine binding protein. Mol Pharmacol 1989;36:543.
97. Dumont FJ, Staruch MJ, Koprak SK, et al. Distinct mechanism of suppression of murine T-cell activation by the related macrolides FK506 and rapamycin. J Immunol 1990;144:251.
98. Harding MW, Galat A, Uehling DE, et al. A receptor for the immunosuppressant FK506 is a cis trans peptidyl-prolyl isomerase. Nature 1989;341:758.
99. Sigal NH, Dumont F, Durette P, et al. Is cyclophilin involved in the immunosuppressive and nephrotoxic mechanism of action of Cyclosporin A? J Exp Med 1991;173:619.
100. Tzakis AG, Reyes S, Todo B, et al. Two-year experience with FK 506 in pediatric patients. Transplant Proc 1993;25:619.
101. Egawa H, Esquivel CO, So SK, et al. FK506 conversion therapy in pediatric liver transplantation. Transplantation 1994;57:1169.
102. Reyes J, Tzakis A, Green M, et al. Posttransplant lymphoproliferative disorders occurring under primary FK 506 immunosuppression. Transplant Proc 1991;23:3044.
103. Cox KL, Lawrence-Miyasaki LS, Garcia-Kennedy R, et al. An increased incidence of Epstein-Barr virus infection and lymphoproliferative dis-

order in young children on FK506 after liver transplantation. Transplantation 1995;59:524.
104. Lones MA, Mishalani S, Shintaku IP, et al. Changes in tonsils and adenoids in children with posttransplant lymphoproliferative disorder: report of three cases with early involvement of Waldeyer's ring. Human Pathol 1995;26:525.
105. Belitsky P, MacDonald AS, Cohen AD, et al. Comparison of antithymocyte globulin and continuous IV Cyclosporin A as induction immunosuppression for cadaver kidney transplant. A prospective randomized study. Transplant Proc 1991;23:999.
106. Heyworth F. Clinical experience with antilymphocyte serum. Immunol Rev 1982;65:79.
107. Busuttil RW, Colonna JO II, Hiatt JR, et al. The first 100 liver transplants at UCLA. Ann Surg 1987;206:387.
108. Bumgardner GL, Roberts JP. New immunosuppressive agents. Gastroenterol Clin N Am 1993;22:421.
109. McDiarmid SV, Klintmalm G, Busutil RW. FK 506 rescue therapy in liver transplantation: outcome and complications. Transplant Proc 1991;23:2996.
110. Tzakis AG, Reyes J, Todo S, et al. FK 506 versus cyclosporine in pediatric liver transplantation. Transplant Proc 1991;23:3010.
111. Jain AB, Fung JJ, Tzakis AG, et al. Comparative study of cyclosporine and FK 506 dosage requirements in adult and pediatric orthotopic liver transplant patients. Transplant Proc 1991;23:2763.
112. McDiarmid SV, Busutil RW, Ascher NL, et al. FK506 (tacrolimus) compared with cyclosporine for primary immunosuppression after pediatric liver transplantation. Results from the U.S. Multicenter Trial. Transplantation 1995;59:530.
113. Todo S, Fung JJ, Starzl TE, et al. Single-center experience with primary orthotopic liver transplantation with FK 506 immunosuppression. Ann Surg 1994;220:297.
114. Jain AB, Fung JJ, Todo S, et al. One thousand consecutive primary orthotopic liver transplants under FK 506: survival and adverse events. Transplant Proc 1995;27:1099.
115. McDiarmid SV, Colonna JO II, Shaked A, et al. Differences in oral FK506 dose requirements between adult and pediatric liver transplant patients. Transplantation 1993;55:1328.
116. Becht MB, Pedersen SH, Ryckman FC, et al. Growth and nutritional management of pediatric patients after orthotopic liver transplantation. Gastroenterol Clin N Am 1993;22:367.
117. Wicks C, Somasundaram S, Bjarnason I, et al. Comparison of enteral feeding and total parenteral nutrition after liver transplantation. Lancet 1994;344:837–840.
118. DeWolf AM, Kang YG, Todo S, et al. Glucose metabolism during liver transplantation in dogs. Anesth Analg 1987;66:76.
119. Hastings PR, Skilman JJ, Bushnell LS, et al. Antacid titration in the prevention of acute gastrointestinal bleeding: a controlled randomized trial in 100 critically ill patients. N Engl J Med 1978;298:1041.
120. Brogden RN, Carmine AA, Heel RC, et al. Ranitidine: a review of its pharmacology and therapeutic use in peptic ulcer disease and other allied diseases. Drugs 1982;24:267.
121. Grant SM, Langtry HD, Brogden RN. Ranitidine: an updated review of its pharmacodynamic and pharmacokinetic properties and therapeutic use in peptic ulcer disease and other allied diseases. Drugs 1989;37:801.
122. Lewis JH. Hepatic effects of drugs used in the treatment of peptic ulcer disease. Am J Gastroenterol 1987;82:987.
123. Feldman M, Burton ME. Histamine 2-receptor antagonists. Standard therapy for acid-peptic diseases (Part 1). N Engl J Med 1990; 323:1672.
124. Feely J, Wilkinson GR, Wood AJJ. Reduction of liver blood flow and propranolol metabolism by cimetidine. N Engl J Med 1981;304:692.
125. Daneshmend TK, Ene MD, Parker G, et al. Effects of chronic oral cimetidine on apparent liver blood flow and hepatic microsomal enzyme activity in man. Gut 1984;25:125.
126. Jackson JE. Reduction of liver blood flow by cimetidine. N Engl J Med 1981;305:99.
127. Dunk AA, Jenkins WJ, Burroughs AK, et al. The effect of ranitidine on the plasma clearance and hepatic extraction of indocyanine green in patients with chronic liver disease. Br J Clin Pharmacol 1983;16:117.
128. Donn KH, Powell JR, Rogers JF, et al. Lack of effect of histamine H_2-receptor antagonists on indocyanine green disposition measured by two methods. J Clin Pharmacol 1984;24:360.
129. Ohnishi K, Nakayama T, Saito M, et al. Effects of cimetidine and ranitidine on splanchnic hemodynamics in patients with chronic liver disease. Am J Gastroenterol 1985;80:290.
130. Somogyi A, Gugler R. Drug interactions with cimetidine. Clin Pharmacokinet 1982;7:23.
131. Marujo WC, Stratta RJ, Langnas AN, et al. Syndrome of multiple bowel perforations in liver transplant recipients. Am J Surg 1991;162:594.
132. Yamanaka J, Lynch SV, Ong TH, et al. Posttransplant gastrointestinal perforation in pediatric liver transplantation. J Pediatr Surg 1994; 29:635.
133. Pollack MM, Fields AI, Holbrook PR. Cardiopulmonary parameters during high PEEP in children. Crit Care Med 1980;8:372.
134. Kumar A, Falke KJ, Geffin B, et al. Continuous positive-pressure ventilation in acute respiratory failure. N Engl J Med 1970;283:1430.
135. Powers SR, Mannal R, Neclerio M, et al. Physiologic consequences of positive end-expiratory pressure (PEEP) ventilation. Ann Surg 1973;178:265.
136. Suter PM, Fairley HB, Isenberg MD. Optimum end-expiratory airway pressure in patients with acute pulmonary failure. N Engl J Med 1975;292:284.
137. Robotham JL, Lixfield W, Holland L, et al. The effects of positive end-expiratory pressure on right and left ventricular performance. Am Rev Respir Dis 1980;121:677.
138. Gallagher TJ, Civetta JM, Kirby RR. Terminology update: optimal PEEP. Crit Care Med 1978;6:323.
139. Plevak DJ, Southorn PA, Narr BJ, et al. Intensive-care unit experience in the Mayo liver transplantation program: the first 100 cases. Mayo Clin Proc 1989;64:433.
140. Eisenach JC, Plevak DJ, Van Dyke RA, et al. Comparison of analgesic requirements after liver transplantation and cholecystectomy. Mayo Clin Proc 1989;64:356.
141. Lawless S, Ellis D, Thompson A, et al. Mechanisms of hypertension during and after orthotopic liver transplantation in children. J Pediatr 1989;115:372.
142. Cattral MS, Langnas AN, Markin RS, et al. Aplastic anemia after liver transplantation for fulminant liver failure. Hepatol 1994;20:813.
143. Gordon R, Iwatsuki S, Esquivel C, et al. Liver transplantation across ABO blood groups. Surgery 1986;100:342.
144. Ramsey G, Nusbacher J, Starzl TE, et al. Isohemagglutinins of graft origin after ABO-unmatched liver transplantation. N Engl J Med 1984;311:1167.
145. Martin LK, Kang Y, DeWolf AM. Coagulation changed immediately following liver graft reperfusion. Transplant Proc 1991; 23:1946.
146. Curtis J, Luke R, Jones P, et al. Hypertension in cyclosporine-treated renal transplant recipients is sodium dependent. Am J Med 1988;85:134.
147. Shaw B, Martin D, Marquez J, et al. Advantages of venous bypass during orthotopic transplantation of the liver. Semin Liver Dis 1985;5:344.
148. Demetris AJ, Lasky S, Van Thiel D, et al. Recurrent hepatitis B in liver allograft recipients. Differentiation between viral hepatitis B and rejection. Am J Pathol 1986;125:161.
149. Nowicki MJ, Ahmad N, Heubi JE, et al. The prevalence of hepatitis C virus (HCV) in infants and children after liver transplantation. Digestive Dis Sci 1994;39:2250.
150. Green M, Tzakis A, Reyes J, et al. Infectious complications of pediatric liver transplantation under FK 506. Transplant Proc 1991;23:3038.
151. Green M, Wald ER, Tzakis A, et al. Aspergillosis of the CNS in a pediatric liver transplant recipient: case report and review. Rev Infec Dis 1991;13:653.
152. George DL, Arnow PM, Fox A, et al. Patterns of infection after pediatric liver transplantation. Am J Dis Children 1992;146:924.
153. Uemoto S, Tanaka K, Fujita S, et al. Infectious complications in living related liver transplantation. J Pediatr Surg 1994;29:514.
154. Mazariegos GV, Green M, Reyes J, et al. Rubella infection after orthotopic liver transplantation. Pediatr Infec Dis J 1994;13:161.
155. Smith SD, Jackson RJ, Hannakan CJ, et al. Selective decontamination in pediatric liver transplants. A randomized prospective study. Transplantation 1993;55:1306.
156. D'Alessandro AM, Kalayoglu M, Pirsch JD, et al. Biliary tract complications after orthotopic liver transplantation. Transplant Proc 1991;23:1956.
157. Breinig MK, Zitelli B, Starzl TE, et al. Epstein-Barr virus, cytomegalovirus, and other viral infections in children after liver transplantation. J Infect Dis 1987;156:273.
158. Michaels MG, Green M, Wald ER, et al. Adenovirus infection in pediatric liver transplant recipients. J Infec Dis 1992;165:170.

159. Superina RA, Pearl RH, Roberts EA, et al. Liver transplantation in children: the initial Toronto experience. J Pediatr Surg 1989;24:1013.
160. Burdelski M, Schmidt K, Hoyer PF, et al. Liver transplantation in children: the Hanover experience. Transplant Proc 1987;19:3277.
161. Andrews WS, Wanek E, Fyock B, et al. Pediatric liver transplantation: a 3 year experience. J Pediatr Surg 1989;24:77.
162. Stratta RJ, Shaefer MS, Cushing KA, et al. Successful prophylaxis of cytomegalovirus disease after primary CMV exposure in liver transplant recipients. Transplantation 1991;51:90.
163. Boudreaux JP, Hayes DH, Mizrahi S, et al. Decreasing incidence of serious cytomegalovirus infection using gancyclovir prophylaxis in pediatric liver transplant patients. Transplant Proc 1993;25:1872.
164. Green M, Reyes J, Nour B, et al. Randomized trial of gancyclovir followed by high-dose oral acyclovir vs gancyclovir alone in the prevention of cytomegalovirus disease in pediatric liver transplant recipients: preliminary analysis. Transplant Proc 1994;26:173.
165. Rakela J, Wiesner RH, Taswell HF, et al. Incidence of cytomegalovirus infection and its relationship to donor-recipient serologic status in liver transplantation. Transplant Proc 1987;19:2399.
166. King SM, Petric M, Superina R, et al. Cytomegalovirus infections in pediatric liver transplantation. Am J Dis Child 1990;144:1307.
167. Sakr M, Hassanein T, Gavaler J, et al. Cytomegalovirus infection of the upper gastrointestinal tract following liver transplantation—incidence, location, and severity in cyclosporine- and FK506-treated patients. Transplantation 1992;53:786.
168. Harbison MA, De Girolami PC, Jenkins RL, et al. Gancyclovir therapy of severe cytomegalovirus infections in solid-organ transplant recipients. Transplantation 1986;46:82.
169. Hanto DW, Friaaera G, Gajk-Peczalska KJ, et al. Epstein-Barr virus, immunodeficiency, and B-cell lymphoproliferation. Transplantation 1985;39:461.
170. Cockburn I. Cyclosporin A: a clinical evaluation of drug interactions. Transplant Proc 1986;18:50.
171. Ringden O, Andstrom E, Remberger M, et al. Safety of liposomal amphotericin B (AmBisome) in 187 transplant recipients treated with cyclosporin. Bone Marrow Transplant 1994;14:S10.
172. Tollemar J, Hockerstedt K, Ericzon BG, et al. Liposomal amphotericin B prevents invasive fungal infections in liver transplant recipients. A randomized, placebo-controlled study. Transplantation 1995;59:45.
173. Stover DE, Zaman MB, Hajdu SI, et al. Bronchoalveolar lavage in the diagnosis of diffuse pulmonary infiltrates in the immunocompromised host. Ann Intern Med 1984;101:1.
174. Young JA, Hopkin JM, Cuthbertson WP. Pulmonary infiltrates in immunocompromised patients: diagnosis by cytological examination of bronchoalveolar lavage fluid. J Clin Pathol 1984;37:390.
175. Adams DH, Ponsford S, Gunson B, et al. Neurologic complications following liver transplantation. Lancet 1987;1:949.
176. Berden JH, Hotsma AJ, Merx JL, et al. Severe central nervous system toxicity associated with cyclosporine. Lancet 1985;1:219.
177. Stein DP, Lederman RJ, Vogt DP, et al. Neurological complications following liver transplantation. Ann Neurol 1992;31:644.
178. Menegaux F, Keeffe EB, Andrews BT, et al. Neurological complications of liver transplantation in adult versus pediatric patients. Transplantation 1994;58:447.
179. Starzl TE, Schneck SA, Mazzoni G, et al. Acute neurological complications after liver transplantation with particular reference to intraoperative cerebral air embolus. Ann Surg 1978;87:236.
180. Wijdicks EF, de Groen PC, Weisner RH, et al. Intracerebral hemorrhage in liver transplant recipients. Mayo Clin Proc 1995;70:443.
181. Durrant S, Chipping PM, Palmer S, et al. Cyclosporin A, methylprednisolone, and convulsions. Lancet 1982;2:829.
182. Allen RD, Hunnisett AG, Morris PJ. Cyclosporin and magnesium. Lancet 1985;1:1283.
183. Thompson CB, June CH, Sullivan KM, et al. Association between cyclosporine neurotoxicity and hypomagnesemia. Lancet 1984;2:1116.
184. Vogt DP, Lederman RJ, Carey WD, et al. Neurologic complications of liver transplantation. Transplantation 1988;45:1057.
185. de Groen PC, Aksamit AJ, Rakela J, et al. Central nervous system toxicity after liver transplantation: the role of cyclosporine and cholesterol. N Engl J Med 1987;317:861.
186. Wood RP, Shaw BW, Starzl TE. Extrahepatic complications of liver transplantation. Semin Liver Dis 1985;5:377.
187. Windsorova D, Stewart SM, Lovitt R, et al. Emotional adaptation in children after liver transplantation. J Pediatr 1991;119:880.
188. Zamberlan KE. Quality of life in school-age children following liver transplantation. Maternal-Child Nurs J 1992;20:167.
189. Paradis KJG, Freese DK, Sharp HL. A pediatric perspective on liver transplantation. Pediatr Clin N Am 1988;35:409.
190. Codoner-Franch P, Bernard O, Alvarez F. Long-term follow-up of growth in height after successful liver transplantation. J Pediatr 1994;124:368.
191. Starzl TE, Klintmalm GB, Porter KA, et al. Liver transplantation with use of cyclosporin A and prednisone. N Engl J Med 1981;305:266.
192. Starzl TE, Esquivel C, Gordon R, et al. Pediatric liver transplantation. Transplant Proc 1987;19:3230.
193. Kocoshis SA, Tzakis A, Todo S, et al. Pediatric liver transplantation, history, recent innovations, and outlook for the future. Cl Pediatr 1993;32:386.
194. Hiatt JR, Ament ME, Berquist WJ, et al. Pediatric liver transplantation at UCLA. Transplant Proc 1987;19:3282.
195. Dunn SP, Weintraub W, Vinocur CD, et al. Is age less than 1 year a high-risk category for orthotopic liver transplantation? J Pediatr Surg 1993;28:1048.
196. Vacanti JP, Lillehei RL, Jenkins RL, et al. Liver transplantation in children: the Boston center experience in the first 30 months. Transplant Proc 1987;19:3261.
197. Tan KC, Yandza T, de Hemptinne B, et al. Hepatic artery thrombosis in pediatric liver transplantation. J Pediatr Surg 1988;23:927.
198. Basile AS, Hughes RD, Harrison PM, et al. Elevated brain concentrations of 1,4-benzodiazepines in fulminant hepatic failure. N Engl J Med 1991;325:473.
199. Fath JJ, Estrin J, Belani K, et al. Lactate metabolism during hepatic transplantation: evidence for a perfusion-sensitive patient population. Transplant Proc 1985;17:284.
200. Fath JJ, Ascher NL, Konstantinides FN, et al. Metabolism during hepatic transplantation: indications of allograft function. Surgery 1984;96:664.
201. Jenkins RL, Clowes GH Jr, Bosari S, et al. Survival from hepatic transplantation: relationship of protein synthesis to histological abnormalities in patient selection and postoperative management. Ann Surg 1986;204:364.
202. Stock PG, Estrin JA, Payne W. Prognostic perioperative factors in outcome following liver transplantation. Transplant Proc 1987;19:2427.
203. Starzl TE, Todo S, Tzakis A, et al. Multivisceral and intestinal transplantation. Transplant Proc 1992;24:1217.
204. Tzakis AG, Todo S, Starzl TE. Intestinal transplantation. Ann Rev Med 1994;45:79.
205. Tzakis AG, Todo S, Reyes J, et al. Piggyback orthotopic intestinal transplantation. Surg Gynec Obst 1993;176:297.
206. Tzakis AG, Todo S, Reyes J, et al. Intestinal transplantation in children under FK5-6 immunosuppression. J Pediatr Surg 1003;28:1040.
207. Tzakis AG, Todo S, Reyes J, et al. Clinical intestinal transplantation: focus on complications. Transplant Proc 1992;24:1238.

Renal, Endocrine, and Metabolic Disorders

Section Seven

Section Editor

James C. Fackler

Renal Disorders in Pediatric Intensive Care 38

Matthew M. Hand
Michael L. McManus
William E. Harmon

INTRODUCTION

Renal failure or insufficiency often complicates the care of critically-ill patients and contributes substantially to overall morbidity and mortality. Patients with chronic renal failure require frequent hospitalization and admission to the intensive care unit (ICU) for a variety of reasons and often continue to do so after receiving kidney transplantation. Even more commonly, previously healthy persons who are experiencing a serious acute illness or injury may sustain renal injury as a primary or secondary event.

Acute renal failure (ARF), the sudden cessation of kidney function with or without oliguria, results in the gradual accumulation of waste substances and fluids that would normally be excreted. Without treatment or recovery, acid loading, perturbation of electrolyte balance, and fluid retention occur. Fluid retention produces tissue edema that may spread to compromise function in other organs. Because contemporary critical care measures typically necessitate administration of fluid volumes far in excess of basal requirements, the loss of renal function necessarily effects many aspects of care. For example, in the absence of satisfactory renal function, measures such as transfusion, parenteral nutrition, or antibiotic administration may gradually produce severe fluid overload and become more life-threatening than life-saving.

Renal failure may be caused by a variety of insults, including ischemia, nephrotoxins, and a range of primary renal diseases. A comprehensive list of conditions that may lead to renal failure is provided in **Table 38.1.** This chapter is intended to provide an overview of renal physiology and pathophysiology as it applies to the care of critically ill children. Rather than focusing upon specific disease processes unique to the kidney, an understanding of basic physiology is used as a basis for suggesting management strategies for problems commonly encountered in the ICU. Discussions include fluid and electrolyte therapy, ARF and its complications, hemolytic uremic syndrome (HUS), hypertension, renal transplantation, and hepatorenal syndrome (HRS).

RENAL PHYSIOLOGY

Renal physiology may be divided into three areas (a) renovascular function, (b) tubular function, and (c) humoral mechanisms.

Renal Blood Flow and Vascular Anatomy

The primary unit of the kidney is the nephron. Each kidney contains approximately 1 million nephrons. The nephron is composed of two primary structures, a glomerulus and a tubule, with each further divided into segments of differing structures and functions. The kidneys receive 20% of the cardiac output and, when compared by weight, enjoy blood flow that is fourfold that of the liver and eightfold that of coronary blood flow[1,2].

Blood enters the kidney via the renal artery and branches into numerous interlobar arteries. The interlobar arteries divide further into interlobular arteries that subsequently form the afferent arterioles. Blood flows through the afferent arteriole into the glomerulus. In the renal cortex, blood exits the glomerulus via the efferent arteriole and enters the peritubular capillaries. In the juxtamedullary region, efferent arterioles enter the medulla and elongate to form the basic unit of the countercurrent capillary system, the vasa recta. Blood returns to the systemic circulation sequentially via the interlobular, interlobar, and renal veins[1,2].

Regulation of Renal Blood Flow

Renal blood flow is autoregulated. In the adult kidney, a constant rate of renal perfusion is maintained over mean arterial pressures with a range of from approximately 80 to 160 mm Hg[1]. In the neonatal period, renal blood flow increases, in the same way as pulmonary blood flow, soon after birth, doubling in the first 2 weeks of life, tripling by 1 year, and approaching adult levels (on a per M^2 basis) in the preschool years[3]. Experimental data show that autoregulation similar to that of the adult kidney occurs across a much lower blood pressure range in infants and children[3,4].

The means by which renal blood flow autoregulation occurs are only partly understood. Although several potential mechanisms have been described, it appears that no single factor completely controls renovascular tone. Nonetheless,

Table 38.1. Causes of Renal Failure in Children

Prerenal/Hypoperfusion
Hemorrhage
Dehydration
Septic shock
Surgery
Diabetes mellitus
Diabetes insipidus
Burns
Decreased cardiac function
Anatomic
Obstruction (posterior urethral valves, tumor, blood clots)
Congenital renal disease
Multicystic dysplastic kidneys
Autosomal recessive polycystic kidney disease
Renal agenesis/hypoplasia
Papillary necrosis
Toxins
Organic solvents (ethylene glycol, methanol)
Metals (lead,mercury, gold, bismuth)
Chelating agents
Radiocontrast dyes
Myoglobin (rhabdomyolysis, crush injuries, malignant hyperthermia)
Hemoglobin (transfusion reaction, venomous bites)
Uric acid
Oxalate
Immunologic/Vasculitis
Hemolytic uremic syndrome
Acute postinfectious glomerulonephritis
Rapidly progressive glomeruloneophritis
Systemic lupus erythematosus
Goodpasture's syndrome
Wegener's granulomatosis/ANCA–positive vasculitis
Membranoproliferative glomerulonephritis
Henoch-Schönlein purpura
Nephrotic syndrome
Infectious
Bacterial
Viral
Mycoplasma
Bacterial endocarditis
Drugs
Antibiotics
Aminoglycosides
Penicillin
Amphotericin B
Angiotensin converting enzyme inhibitors
Acyclovir
Nonsteroidal antiinflammatory drugs (indomethacin, ibuprofen)
Anesthetic agents (methoxyflurane)
Vascular
Bilateral renal artery/vein thrombosis

an appreciation of the known mechanisms participating in the control and support of renal blood flow is critical to an understanding of acute renal failure.

The Renin-Angiotensin System and Prostaglandins

The renin-angiotensin system has been studied extensively with regard to its effect on renal blood flow. The afferent and efferent arterioles have been shown to be principle sites for renin release in response to decreases in renal perfusion pressure, increases in sympathetic nerve stimulation, and decreases in sodium chloride (NaCl) delivery to the macula densa[2,5–8]. Release of renin subsequently leads to an increase in circulating angiotensin-2 (A2). Renin cleaves angiotensinogen (produced in the liver) to angiotensin-1 (A1) which, in turn, is converted to A2 by the action of pulmonary angiotensin-converting enzyme (ACE). A2 causes vasoconstriction in both the afferent[7] and efferent arterioles[9]; its major effect appears to be in the efferent arteriole[10]. A2 maintains intraglomerular pressure by increasing efferent arteriole vascular resistance and thus preserving the glomerular filtration rate (GFR). In addition, A2 also stabilizes normal intravascular volume by enhancing release of both aldosterone and antidiuretic hormone (ADH) (Figure 38.1) to promote retention of sodium and water.

Prostaglandins (such as PGE2 and PGI) play an important role in maintaining renal blood flow through afferent and efferent vasodilatation. Vasoconstriction with inhibition of afferent blood flow may decrease intraglomerular pressure and precipitate renal failure. In recent years, prostaglandins have been shown to play a much larger and more complicated role in regulation of both blood flow and tubular function than previously recognized. Several studies have shown that, particularly hypovolemic patients, prostaglandins are responsible for maintaining renal blood flow[11–13]. In their absence, vasoconstrictor mechanisms are unopposed and may precipitate ischemic injury that progresses to renal insufficiency or failure.

Together, the described mechanisms account for 60% of renal blood flow autoregulation[13]. Appreciation of this becomes critical when ACE inhibitors or nonsteroidal antiinflammatory drugs (NSAIDS) are used. In conditions involving intravascular depletion, such as congestive heart failure or postoperative capillary leak, or in conditions such as renal artery stenosis, when renal blood flow is dependent upon one or both of these mechanisms, the addition of ACE inhibitors or prostaglandin inhibitors may rapidly precipitate renal failure.

Nitric Oxide and Endothelin

Nitric oxide (NO), also known as endothelium-derived relaxation factor (EDRF), is produced by three (possibly four) different synthetase isozymes[14]. At least three forms of nitric oxide synthetase (NOS) have been found in kidney tissue at both the vascular and tubular levels[14–17]. NO has potent vasodilatory properties[18–22], and inhibition of NOS by blockers such as N-nitro-L-Argininemethylester increases naturesis[23,24], suggesting that NO is also involved in sodium reabsorption. The macula densa contains abundant NOS[17,25]. At least three possible functions for renal NO have been postulated thus far (1) as a mediator of renin release from the afferent arteriole, (2) as modulator of tubuloglomerular feedback, and (3) as a controller of mesangial cell contraction and thus of ultrafiltration coefficient[14,17,25].

Endothelin is a 21-amino acid peptide that is known to be an extremely potent vasoconstrictor[26,27]. It is produced by many different tissue types and cell lines, but the specific function of endothelin in control of renal blood flow is unclear[28]. Endothelin appears to play a major role in ARF, producing both increased renal vascular resistance and depressed GFR[29]. Under the influence of endothelin, an increase in mesangial cell contraction occurs. This response is likely the mechanism causing a reduction in the glomerular capillary ultrafiltration coefficient. Atrial natriuretic

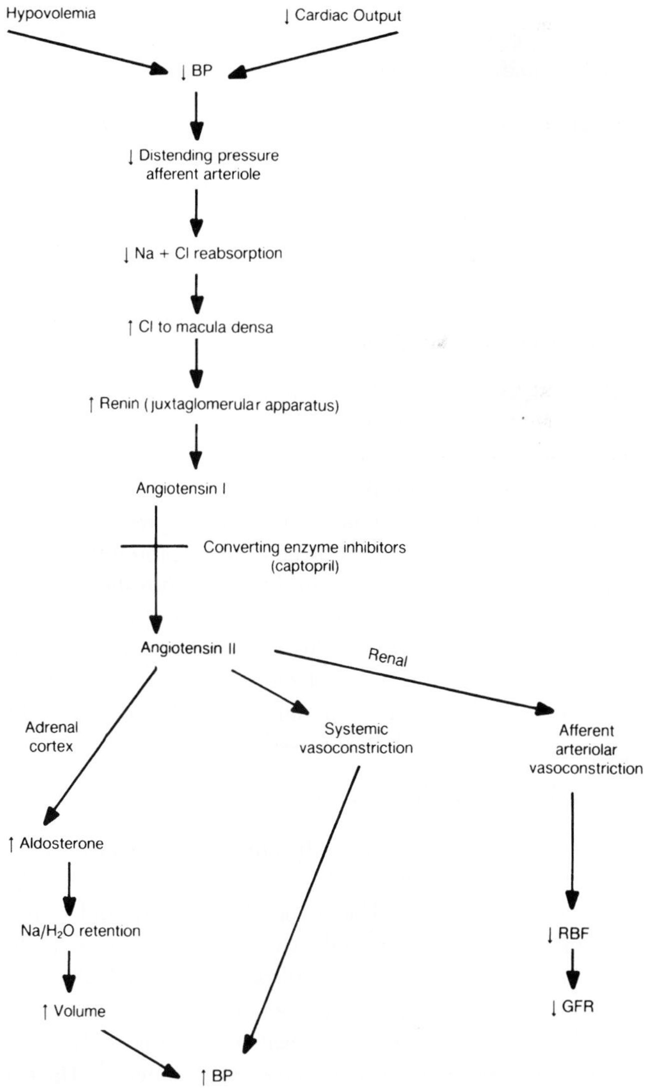

Figure 38.1. Role of renin-angiotensin system in elevation of blood pressure. *BP* = blood pressure, *RBF* = renal blood flow.

peptide (ANP) release appears to be directly stimulated by endothelin and may be partially responsible for increased urinary flow and sodium excretion when low-dose (nonpressor) endothelin is administered[30–32]. Antiendothelin antibodies have been shown to markedly decrease the severity of ARF in some experimental models[33].

Dopamine

Dopamine receptors in the afferent arteriole have been shown to have varying effects, depending on the degree of dopaminergic stimulation[34]. At low doses, dopamine dilates the renal vasculature and, at higher doses, causes renal vasoconstriction[35–37]. Dopamine also possesses a natriuretic effect at the tubular level, which may be the primary source of the diuresis often observed with infusions[38,39]. Increasing sodium chloride delivery to the medullary thick ascending limb (mTAL) of the loop of Henle and the macula densa affects the juxtaglomerular apparatus (JGA) and vascular flow. However, although infusions on the order of 2.5 to 5 $\mu g/kg^{-1}/minute^{-1}$ have traditionally been employed as "renal doses" to augment urine flow, plasma levels of dopamine correlate poorly with infusion rates in pediatric patients.

Neural Control

Neuronal innervation of the vascular bed has been shown to control vascular tone but is not the primary regulator. The denervated kidney retains its ability to autoregulate blood flow.

Glomerular Filtration Rate

GFR is determined by the hydrostatic and oncotic pressure within the nephron. The hydrostatic pressure within the glomerulus is greater than the hydrostatic pressure within the tubule (Bowman's capsule), forcing filtrate out of the capillary bed and into the tubule. The oncotic pressure within the glomerulus is generated by nonfiltered proteins (primarily albumin) and helps to retain filtrate within the vascular space[40–42]. As filtrate is generated, the oncotic pressure increases across the glomerulus and is greater in the efferent arteriole than the afferent arteriole. Increased oncotic pressure is particularly important for reabsorption in the vasa recta. GFR can be expressed as follows:

$$GFR = Kf\ (\text{hydrostatic pressure-oncotic pressure})$$

where Kf is the filtration coefficient of the glomerulus[1].

Filtration across the capillary endothelium is dependent on a number of factors. The endothelium is surrounded by a basement membrane and podocytes. Foot processes branching off of the podocytes form filtration slits that allow for passage of the ultrafiltrate. The foot processes and basement membrane are composed of negatively charged glycoproteins that repel other negatively charged particles[43]. The net result is limited filtration of large particles with negative charges. Structures with a molecular weight of less than 5000 daltons are freely filtered, whereas large particles (such as albumin, with a weight of 69,000 daltons) are minimally filtered[1,43,44]. In certain conditions, such as nephrotic syndrome, the foot processes are effaced, the negative charge is lost, and significant proteinuria occurs. Protein binding also limits filtration of certain substances (such as medications or calcium) by the above mechanism.

Tubular Function

The renal tubules function to maintain fluid and electrolyte status, along with controlling toxin excretion. The majority of reabsorption occurs in the proximal tubule. Final control of solute excretion occurs in the distal tubule.

The Proximal Tubule

The proximal tubule receives the ultrafiltrate directly from the glomerulus. Fluid within the proximal tubule is isotonic with plasma and remains so amidst reabsorption of sodium, anions, and water in this portion of the nephron. Thus, upon leaving the proximal tubule, the osmolarity of the ultrafiltrate is approximately the same as plasma.

Reabsorption along the proximal tubule is dependent on Na^+-K^+ adenosine triphosphatase (ATPase) activity resident in the basolateral membrane[45–47]. As sodium is pumped from tubule cells to the interstitium, the resultant gradient draws sodium from the tubular lumen. Sodium pumped into the interstitium subsequently diffuses into the peritubular capillaries. All other solute and water reabsorption in the proximal tubule is driven by the gradients produced through action of the Na^+-K^+ ATPase pump. Approximately 67 to 70% of all sodium entering the proximal tubule is reabsorbed[1,48]. Sodium reabsorption is increased by angiotensin and glucocorticoids[1,48].

Regardless of ultrafiltrate production, the percentage of sodium reabsorption in the proximal tubule is relatively constant. Anion resorption is coupled with and driven by sodium reabsorption. In the first half of the proximal tubule, sodium reabsorption is coupled with that of bicarbonate, amino acids, glucose, phosphate, and lactate. As chloride concentration increases in the second half of the tubule, Cl^- becomes the predominant anion reabsorbed with sodium. Glucose, lactate, and amino acids typically are completely absorbed in the proximal tubule[1,49,50].

The Loop of Henle

After leaving the proximal tubule, the ultrafiltrate enters the loop of Henle. There, only approximately 20% of filtered Na, K, and Cl is resorbed. The principle function of the loop of Henle is urine concentration and dilution, and this is accomplished through the osmotic gradient provided by the countercurrent multiplier. The maximal concentration gradient, occurring at the turn of the loop, is approximately 1200 mOsm[1]. The venous system which surrounds the loop of Henle is the vasa recta. By increasing and decreasing *oncotic* pressure as they pass through the medulla, the vasa recta remove fluid and solute from the tubular lumen. The descending tubule is permeable to water but relatively impermeable to sodium. The ascending tubule is relatively impermeable to water but actively reabsorbs sodium[(51)]. The macula densa of the JGA resides in this region. Urine flow rate and GFR are partially regulated by Cl, prostaglandins, adenosine, and urine volume presented to the macula densa[(52)].

Of particular importance, particularly in acute renal failure, is the Na^+-K^+ ATPase resident in the mTAL. This section of the nephron is critical for urinary dilution, with ADH stimulating Na^+ reabsorption in this area[(52)]. Oxygen delivery to the mTAL is tenuous, making it uncommonly sensitive to ischemia. Furosemide inhibits the Na-K-2Cl ATPase, and its use may diminish tubular oxygen demands and ameliorate the severity of ARF[(53)].

The Distal Tubule

The distal tubule reabsorbs approximately 12% of the total Na^+ and Cl^- resorbed in the tubule. Unlike previous sections of the nephron, the distal tubule secretes K^+ and bicarbonate. The proximal segment of the distal tubule is impermeable to water; therefore, it is critical for urine dilution. The distal segment of the distal tubule (cortical collecting duct) is made of two cell types, principal and intercalated cells; these cells secrete K^+ and bicarbonate (or hydrogen ions), respectively[(1,54)].

The Collecting Duct

The collecting duct is particularly sensitive to hormonal effects and functions to regulate the final urinary concentration. Aldosterone receptors of the principal cells enhance Na^+ uptake and K^+ excretion[(52,55–57)]. ADH enhances water reabsorption. In the absence of ADH, the collecting duct is relatively impermeable to water, yet ADH dramatically increases water permeability[(55,51)]. Urea is passively reabsorbed in the inner medullary collecting duct (IMCD). Movement of urea depends on urea concentration in the tubule relative to the medullary interstitium. The reabsorption of urea is critical for maintaining the medullary interstitial concentration gradient.

FLUID AND ELECTROLYTE MANAGEMENT

Basal Requirements

The amount of fluid and electrolytes needed to replace typical losses from the body and to maintain homeostasis under usual circumstances is often termed the "maintenance" requirement. A variety of approximations have been suggested for such requirements, the most popular being based upon predicted caloric expenditure as estimated by the child's surface area or weight[(58)]. In using such approximations, "maintenance" fluid therapy calculations should be recognized as rough estimates, which are *indirectly* based upon measured requirements during *typical* caloric expenditure.

Table 38.2. Caloric Expenditure/kg of Body Weight

1–10 kg	100 kcal/kg/day
10–20 kg	1000 kcal + 50 kcal/kg over 10 kg/day
>20 kg	1500 kcal + 20 kcal/kg over 20 kg/day

In 1957, caloric expenditures per kilogram of body weight were described by Holiday and Seger[(59)], who noted that relative caloric expenditure decreases as body weight increases **(Table 38.2).** Therefore, fluid requirements per kilogram of body weight are much greater in infants than in children and adults. Additionally, patients with increased energy expenditure beyond a basal metabolic state have greater fluid requirements. Fever, for example, increases basal requirements by about 12.5% for every degree of temperature more than 38°C[(58)].

In addition to metabolic changes, renal function is also a critical factor in determining whether typical maintenance fluid calculations apply to a specific patient. Urine output represents approximately two-thirds of the maintenance intake calculated by caloric expenditure. These calculations are based upon the assumption that the kidneys are able to excrete isotonic urine (i.e., urine with a specific gravity of 1.010 and an osmolality of 290 mOsm/L)[(58)]. The remaining third of the fluid requirement is replacement for that lost via insensible losses, including respiration and evaporation from the skin. Both normal homeostatic compensatory mechanisms and pathologic renal function greatly alter urine output and maintenance requirements. Congestive heart failure, for example, elicits mechanisms aimed to support plasma volume through retention of salt and water, thereby resulting in diminished urine output. Similarly, in renal failure or the syndrome of inappropriate antidiuretic hormone (SIADH), urine output is altered and fluid management must be adjusted accordingly. In such conditions, careful estimation of initial hydration state, using weight, physical examination, and related factors, followed by careful tabulation of overall output and intake directs initial therapy.

Standard maintenance electrolyte therapy involves primarily sodium and potassium. Empiric calculations suggest that 3 to 5 mEq of sodium and 2 to 3 mEq potassium per 100 mL of maintenance fluid is sufficient **(Table 38.3).**

Table 38.3. "Maintenance" Fluid and Electrolyte Requirements[a]

Fluid Requirements by Body Weight:	
1–10 kg	100 mL/kg/day
10–20 kg	1000 mL + 50 cc/kg over 10 kg/day
>20 kg	1500 mL + 20 cc/kg over 20 kg/day
Electrolyte Composition of Solutions:	
Sodium	3–5 mEq/100 mL
Potassium	2–4 mEq/100 mL
Chloride	2–3 mEq/100 mL

[a] *Patients with normal renal function*

Table 38.4. Composition of Body Fluids

	Electrolyte (mEq/Liter)		
Fluid	*Na*	*K*	*Cl*
Gastric	20–80	5–20	100–150
Pancreatic	120–140	5–15	40–80
Biliary	120–140	5–15	80–120
Small intestinal	100–140	5–15	90–130
Ileostomic	45–135	3–15	20–115
Diarrheal	10–90	10–80	10–110

Replacement

The basis of fluid replacement therapy is the return to the patient of the same composition and volume of fluid that has been lost. In the ICU setting, particularly for a patient with ARF, it is preferable to measure or estimate fluid and electrolyte losses and replace them proportionately rather than depending on estimates of maintenance fluid requirements. In the ICU, insensible losses are approximated and all other losses are measured. Appropriate volumes and composition of replacement fluids are provided. Fluid and electrolytes are lost via urine, insensible losses (i.e., respiratory tract, sweat, evaporation), pathologic states such as vomiting and diarrhea, and through external drains such as nasogastric tubes. Urine replacement is a simple matter determined by the volume of ongoing output and its electrolyte composition, as determined by measurement of urine electrolytes. The volume of insensible losses depend on the clinical setting and may be more complex to calculate. As a general estimate, basal insensible losses are 300 mL/M^2/day. Ventilated patients have decreased respiratory losses. Febrile patients have increased insensible losses as discussed above. Perhaps the most dramatic examples of increased insensible losses are seen in burn patients, whose requirements for fluid and electrolyte replacement are massive, owing to both metabolic changes and fluid translocation. The composition of replacement fluids for insensible losses is generally free water. The replacement fluids for other losses are variable, yet generally should be isotonic **(Table 38.4).**

If the patient is euvolemic, replacement fluid volumes can be set to match output. In the ICU, where patients may have multiple intravenous catheters, insensible losses may be replaced at a constant infusion rate, while a second intravenous solution may replace other fluid losses at a rate calculated to match the previous 1 to 4 hours' output. Thus, the patient may have several intravenous infusates, replacing urine, insensible, and other outputs simultaneously but separately.

ACUTE RENAL FAILURE

Renal failure is defined as the cessation of kidney function *with or without changes in urine volume.* Anuria is arbitrarily defined as urine output of less than 0.5mL/kg/hour, while oliguria is urine output of more than 1 mL/kg/hour[60]. The incidence of acute renal failure in pediatric intensive care units is highly variable[61–63]. In pediatric patients undergoing cardiac surgery, an 8% incidence of renal failure has been reported[63]. Of the 3,235 patients admitted to the cardiac intensive care unit of Children's Hospital in Boston between 1992 and 1994, 2.3 % had clinically significant renal failure. Although correlation of renal failure with mortality scores (i.e., PRISM, APACHE) is not absolute, there is clearly an increased risk of mortality in patients with renal failure[64–69].

Nonoliguric Versus Oliguric Renal Failure

Of all cases of acute renal failure, approximately 70% are nonoliguric and 30% are oliguric. Nonoliguric renal failure has been reported to occur more often in patients with nephrotoxic insults than in patients with ischemic injury, and the overall insult to the kidneys is believed to be less in nonoliguric renal failure[70–74]. Experience with adult patients has led Rahman and Cogner to conclude that residual GFR accounts for the variations in urine output observed in nonoliguric ARF[72]. These authors have also reported that, even in ischemic injury, the incidence of nonoliguric ARF is greater than that of oliguric ARF. These findings are also supported by data derived elsewhere[75,76].

Unfortunately, scant corroborative data are available for the pediatric population. With little question, however, patient outcome is better and management easier in patients with nonoliguric renal failure[77,78]. Fluid management and nutritional support are much less problematic, and invasive therapies, such as ultrafiltration, are unnecessary when the patient has adequate urine output[70,71,73,74].

Overall, the critical issue is maintenance of adequate urine output and prevention of further renal injury. Because of the better outcome in patients with nonoliguric renal failure, many investigators have attempted to "convert" oliguric to nonoliguric renal failure[79–85]. Interpretation of data from such trials is difficult, however, since outcomes may be related to differences in severity of the original renal insult[86]. Specifically, overall recovery rates may be skewed in favor of conversion to nonoliguric failure because fundamental insults associated with nonoliguria generally are less severe. Regardless, the management of most patients is simplified by increased urine output, and many clinicians choose this course.

Diagnostic Studies

The diagnosis of ARF can usually be made with results of urinalysis and a few simple laboratory tests. Determination of the cause of ARF is usually possible by history alone, yet occasionally requires more extensive evaluation, such as radiologic or nuclear studies.

Renal failure is often separated into three major categories: prerenal, renal (intrinsic), and postrenal. In point of fact, each condition can progress to another, and ARF is often multifactorial in nature.

Prerenal azotemia generally does not involve intrinsic renal damage and can be distinguished from true renal failure by the kidney's response to the underlying insult. In prerenal azotemia, renal blood flow is decreased. In response, the kidney attempts to maintain intravascular volume via several mechanisms. First, the afferent arteriole, through autoregulation, constricts as part of a systemic response to support blood pressure; yet, in so doing, a decreased renal perfusion results. At the same time, the efferent arteriole also constricts to maintain intraglomerular filtration pressure and GFR[87,88]. As discussed above, there is an increase in renin secretion and in production of A2[87]. As GFR decreases, the amount of glomerular filtrate also decreases. In the proximal tubule, the percentage reabsorption of sodium and chloride continues at a constant rate[89]. In the distal tubule, under the effects of aldosterone, there is an increase in sodium reabsorption. Tubuloglomerular feedback at the distal tubule (macula densa) produces a decrease in glomerular blood flow. Urea, unlike creatinine, can be reabsorbed in the tubule. With a decrease in filtrate volume, an increase in relative concentration of urea in the filtrate occurs, leading to increased reabsorption. As a result, in prerenal azotemia the fractional excretion of sodium is low and the serum blood urea nitrogen level (BUN) to creatinine level ratio is more than 20. The fractional excretion of sodium (FE_{Na}) is calculated as follows:

$$U_{Na}/P_{Na} \times P_{cr}/U_{cr} \times 100 = FE_{Na}$$

Where the U_{Na} is urinary sodium, P_{cr} is plasma creatinine, P_{Na} is plasma sodium, and U_{cr} is urinary creatinine, all from simultaneously obtained "spot" blood and urine samples. Values in neonates and infants differ slightly from those in older children because of their greater urinary losses of sodium. In the presence of loop diuretics, such as furosemide, the FE_{Na} is artificially high and not particularly useful. In such cases, when diuretics must be given, the fractional excretion of urea (calculated similarly) may be used.

The renal failure index (RFI) is based on similar variables. Like the FE_{Na}, the numbers are slightly different for neonates. RFI is calculated as follows:

$$RFI = (U_{Na} \times 100)/U_{cr}/S_{cr}$$

Where S_{cr} is the serum creatinine and other variables are as above.

A comparison of the laboratory values and calculated indices in prerenal and intrinsic renal failure is shown in **Table 38.5.**

Ultrasound examinations can be helpful in the diagnosis of ARF. Classic ultrasonographic findings in acute tubular necrosis (ATN) include poor corticomedullary differentiation and increased Doppler resistive index ([systolic peak-diastolic peak]/systolic peak)[60]. These findings are consistent with increased vascular tone and medullary venous pooling. Ultrasonography is particularly helpful in diagnosis of obstructive and congenital forms of renal failure, such as multicystic dysplastic kidneys, polycystic kidney disease, hydroureter, and hydronephrosis. Color Doppler imaging of the renal vessels can assist in diagnosis of vascular thrombosis and is specific but not sensitive for the diagnosis of renal artery thrombosis. Intravenous pyelogram (IVP) is rarely indicated or helpful in the diagnosis of ARF in children.

Nuclear medicine scans are available to evaluate renal function and anatomy. There are three primary nuclear medicine renal scans: DMSA (technetium-99m dimercaptosuccinic acid) scan, a static image, shows anatomy and may demonstrate cortical scarring or injury[90]; DTPA (technetium-99m diethylenetriamine pentaacetate)[90] and MAG3 (technetium-99m mercaptoacetyltriglycine) scans [91], which are dynamic, show renal function, urinary excretion, and upper tract outflow[91]. Also, DTPA and MAG3 may be useful in evaluating ureteral or urethral obstruction and may help to distinguish prerenal azotemia from intrinsic renal dysfunction. More recently, the GFR scan, using tracers such as MAG3 or iothalamate, has been used to assess glomerular filtration. This exam may become important in evaluating patients with long-standing renal disease or in patients in whom collection of timed urine specimens for calculation of GFR is difficult.

For the most part, nuclear medicine exams are not necessary in diagnosis of ARF, but may aid in identifying its cause[92]. Renal scans are also particularly useful in evaluating renal transplant recipients in the postoperative period.

Pathophysiology

The pathophysiology of ARF primarily involves renal perfusion and tubular dysfunction. Injury to the kidney can result from hypoperfusion and ischemia, from nephron damage caused by toxins, or from inflammation. Not uncommonly in the ICU, several causes are combined; for example, sepsis treated with aminoglycosides often leads to ARF.

Ischemia of the kidneys can take on many forms but has the same endpoint. The clinical scenario determines the cause of renal ischemia. Total obstruction of renal blood flow may be apparent, as in arterial thrombosis, or a global decrease in perfusion may be seen with hypotension or vasculitis. In the well-perfused kidney, approximately 90% of blood flow goes to the renal cortex. During an ischemic event, there appears to be an increase in blood flow to the

Table 38.5. Urine and Serum Laboratory Values in Prerenal and Intrinsic Renal Failure

	Prerenal	*Renal*
BUN/Cr	>20	<20
FENa	<1%	>2%
Renal Failure Index	<1%	>1%
U_{Na}	<20mEq/L	>40mEq/L
Specific Gravity	>1.020	<1.010
U_{osm}	>500mOsm/L	<350mOsm/L
U_{osm}/P_{osm}	>1.3	<1.3

medulla[93]. It is not clear whether this alteration in blood distribution is caused by an alteration in perfusion or to "pooling" of blood in the medulla. Brezis and Rosen have shown that decreased perfusion to the medulla and subsequent lower partial pressure of oxygen to the 10 to 20 mm Hg range (as compared to 50 mm Hg in the cortex) places the medulla and (primarily) the mTAL at risk for ischemia[53]. These investigators have also shown that when combined with an increasing work load of the tubule, ischemia to the mTAL worsens tubular damage[53,94]. Increasing perfusion and oxygen presentation to the tubule or decreasing work load of the tubule (as seen with furosemide administration and blocking of the Na-K-2Cl transporter) lessened tubular damage. Taken together, these findings suggest that renal ischemia, like myocardial ischemia, may be conceptualized as the result of an energy supply/demand imbalance[53].

The eventual outcome of ischemia is cell damage and death. Cellular destruction is most evident in the tubules. The initial reports of ARF described necrosis of the tubules, and ATN rapidly became synonymous with ARF. Ischemic injury results first in loss of the brush border on the luminal (apical) side of the tubule[95]. Subsequently, there is cell swelling and loss of polarity of the Na^+-K^+ ATPase[95–98]. Molitoris found that this loss of polarity occurred within 10 minutes of ischemia[96–98]. With more advanced insults, cells begin to form vacuoles and to detach from the basement membrane. Cell swelling narrows the tubular lumen and cell death produces large amounts of debris that may mechanically obstruct the lumen as well[95,99]. Obstruction of the tubule and breakdown of the tubule's integrity sets the stage for tubular back-leak, which causes an increase in intraluminal pressure and, in turn, a decrease of GFR. Other, undescribed factors are also at work, since studies have shown that tubular back-leak alone is not sufficient to fully account for the decrease in GFR seen in ATN.

General Prevention Strategies

Many studies have attempted to determine the optimal methods of preventing ARF and its effects[79–85]. Such studies are typically centered on one of three clinical goals: The first is to recognize the patients at risk for ARF and to provide aggressive therapy to avoid renal insults; the second is to prevent progression from prerenal azotemia to ARF; the third is to prevent oliguria.

Many patients in the ICU are at risk for renal failure. As previously discussed, renal blood flow is autoregulated and relies upon a number of mechanisms to maintain renal perfusion. However, when renal blood flow decreases, GFR also decreases and the patient has prerenal azotemia despite these mechanisms. With a prolonged or severe decrease of renal blood flow, autoregulation is eventually lost. Numerous clinical scenarios (e.g., sepsis, cardiac disease, dehydration, hemorrhage, capillary leak, renal artery disease) cause decreases in renal perfusion that exceed autoregulatory capabilities.

Patients with chronic renal failure or those with previous renal insults are at particular risk. Preservation of renal perfusion in these patients is critical, and the therapeutic approach is relatively straightforward. Maintenance of isovolemia, adequate cardiac output, and normal blood pressure is essential. Avoidance of nephrotoxins (such as aminoglycosides, NSAIDS, amphotericin B), drugs that may diminish renal blood flow (such as ACE inhibitors), and further volume depletion may help to avoid further renal damage. However, these measures may be exceedingly difficult (or impossible) to implement in patients with total body fluid overload, capillary leak, and edema. Despite total body salt and water overload, such patients routinely present with intravascular volume depletion. In such "prerenal" states, aggressive diuresis or ultrafiltration would likely cause further renal compromise and either precipitate or exacerbate ARF. Similarly, maintenance of adequate oncotic pressure with provision of colloid and nutrition while striving for isovolemia is a difficult, yet appropriate, goal. This is especially true for patients with multiple drains (i.e., chest tubes, peritoneal drains) and particularly large protein losses. On the other hand, when faced with a patient with fluid overload and progressive organ failure, fluid removal becomes the prime concern and aggressive diuresis or ultrafiltration is required. In such circumstances, the clinician and patient are forced to accept the likelihood of progressive renal dysfunction.

Preservation of renal function and urine output has been attempted by numerous investigators. We review these therapeutic options and their proposed efficacy.

Diuretics, particularly furosemide, have been used to ameliorate or prevent renal failure and oliguria. The rationale for loop diuretic therapy is based on two principles. First, Brezis and Rosen have shown that furosemide blocks the Na-K-2Cl transporter in the thick ascending limb, thus reducing oxygen consumption and cell damage[53]. These investigators further showed that furosemide helped preserve renal function in rats exposed to indomethacin and radiocontrast media[94]. This effect was enhanced in rats receiving normal saline. Second, reduction in tubular reabsorption increases urine flow and reduces tubular obstruction and back-leak. Consequently, large doses of diuretics may help preserve renal function and urine output if initiated early in ARF.

Mannitol functions as an osmotic diuretic that is freely filtered by the glomerulus. There are four potential mechanisms by which mannitol might prevent acute renal failure: (1) Increased urine flow through the tubules preventing tubular obstruction; (2) Osmotic action decreasing endothelial cell swelling and damage; (3) Decreased blood viscosity with enhanced renal perfusion; (4) Free radical scavenging. Thus far, administration of mannitol has been shown to increase urine output, but improvement of renal function has not been conclusively demonstrated in clinical settings[86].

"Renal-dose" dopamine (2.5 to 5 μg/kg/minute) has been used for years in attempts to prevent or reduce renal failure. Dopamine enhances sodium excretion and maintains urine output. Studies have been conducted to evaluate the efficacy of dopamine in ARF. Most of these studies have shown that dopamine enhances urine output but does not change the incidence of renal failure[100–103]. The natriuretic effect of dopamine enhances sodium and chloride flow to the macula densa and increases the work load for the mTAL. The increased oxygen requirement of the tubule cells and possible impairment of the tubuloglomerular feedback mechanism are theoretical risks. Despite the widespread use of this practice, there is no scientific evidence that renal-dose dopamine is beneficial. As a pressor and inotrope, however, dopamine is effective for maintaining blood pressure and may be helpful in maintaining renal perfusion. At very high doses (more than 20 μg/kg/minute), vasoconstrictive effects may overwhelm other hemodynamic effects and compromise renal blood flow.

Endothelin, a potent vasoconstrictor, causes decreased renal perfusion and can induce renal failure. In animal experiments, antiendothelin antibodies reduce renal failure and improve renal function[33]. Elevated levels of endothelin have been reported in patients with hemolytic-uremic syndrome, and endothelin levels may participate in a variety of renal pathologies. To date, there have been no human trials of antiendothelin antibody therapy for ARF.

Thyroxine (T4) has also been studied in ARF[104]. In animal models of ischemic renal failure, a more rapid improvement in renal function occurred in animals that received thryroxine than in others. The mechanism is not clear but is believed to be caused by either increased uptake of adenosine diphosphate (ADP) to form adenosine triphosphate (ATP) or stabilization of tubule cell membranes. In a similar set of experiments, ATP-$MgCl_2$ infusions also produced decreased histologic damage and improved renal recovery[105].

ANP has been studied in both animals and humans[106,107]. Infusions of ANP with and without dopamine have been shown to improve renal function and to reduce the duration of renal insufficiency. Further clinical studies are needed to determine the benefit of ANP in ARF.

Finally, theophylline has also been used as an adenosine antagonist to prevent a reduction in glomerular filtration. One study demonstrated preservation of glomerular filtration in humans with contrast-induced renal insufficiency[108]. As with ANP and thyroxin, further studies are needed to clarify theophylline use in ARF.

Specific Prevention Strategies

Three clinical scenarios deserve special consideration, because renal damage may be prevented if specific treatment is undertaken early. Hemoglobinuria, myoglobinuria, and uric acid nephropathy may often be predicted and renal damage limited.

Hemoglobinuria

Hemoglobinuria is seen in patients with red blood cell lysis (as in transfusion reaction, hemolytic uremic syndrome, ethanol sclerotherapy, extracorporeal circulation). The precise mechanism of hemoglobin nephropathy is not clear; proposed causes include: (1) dissociation of hemoglobin (or myoglobin) to ferrihemate, a tubular toxin, in acidic urine; (2) tubular obstruction by precipitated heme pigments; and, (3) inhibition of glomerular flow by prostaglandin inhibition or increased renin activation[109]. In massive hemolysis, the stromal component of the red blood cell likely causes mechanical obstruction and has a greater nephrotoxic effect than hemoglobin[110]. Treatment of hemoglobin nephropathy focuses on preventing and inhibiting the toxic mechanisms. Increasing urine flow by aggressive hydration decreases tubular obstruction. Alkalinization of the urine increases hemoglobin solubility and decreases the toxic effect of hemoglobin[111]. The urine pH level may be raised by bicarbonate infusion and carbonic anhydrase inhibitors. Mannitol and furosemide increase urine flow and reduce tubular obstruction[109]. In refractory cases, exchange transfusion or plasmapheresis lowers serum hemoglobin levels.

Myoglobinuria

Myoglobin-induced nephrotoxicity occurs in patients with muscle injuries, such as electrocution, malignant hyperthermia, crush injuries, and other causes of rhabdomyolysis. The mechanism of tubular damage is believed to be the same as for hemoglobin injury[112]. Myoglobin is a smaller molecule than hemoglobin and is more freely filtered. Thus, myoglobin may pose a greater risk for nephrotoxity than hemoglobin. Preventing renal damage is the goal in susceptible patients. The hallmark of myoglobinuria is urine that tests positive for blood without the presence of red blood cells. The diagnosis is confirmed by an elevated serum creatine phosphokinase (CPK) level. Myoglobinuria associated with rhabdomyolysis involves extensive muscle damage and creatinine release. With rhabdomyolysis, the serum creatinine level may increase by more than 2 mg/dL/day early in the course[109]. The BUN/creatinine ratio is typically less than 10. The massive tissue destruction usually involved can lead to significant hyperkalemia[113]. Treatment of myoglobin nephropathy is the same as for hemoglobin-induced nephropathy. Aggressive hydration, diuresis, and alkalinization[111] (to a urine pH level of more than 7) are essential.

Uric Acid Nephropathy

Uric acid is the product of purine turnover and, when significantly elevated, may cause ARF. The typical patient at risk has tumor lysis syndrome as a result of the initiation of chemotherapy for solid tumors or acute lymphoproliferative diseases with high cell turnover rates. Cell lysis after chemotherapy results in elevation in serum uric acid levels and subsequently in uric acid excretion. Uric acid precipitates in acidic urine, intratubular obstruction, and renal failure then occur[114]. Treatment involves aggressive hydration to produce high urine flow rates, bicarbonate infusion to alkalinize the urine, and treatment with xanthine oxidase inhibitors before chemotherapy is started[114]. If renal failure develops, even with aggressive therapy, dialysis is indicated.

Management of Renal Failure

Fluid Therapy

Standard "maintenance fluids" are appropriate for patients with normal renal function under normal clinical conditions. In the situation of ARF, provision of "maintenance" fluid can cause fluid overload, hypertension and pulmonary edema. In polyuric states, these fluids may lead to dehydration. Proper management of the patient in renal failure involves replacing losses. As discussed above, fluid losses include insensible losses, urine output, and other losses (i.e., surgical drains, nasogastric tubes, diarrhea). Insensible losses are calculated generally at 300 mL/M^2/day. Other losses should be measured. Electrolyte concentrations of replacement solutions should be guided by the concentration found in lost fluids. The standard concentrations of body fluids are indicated in table 38.4. Urine replacement is calculated using urine electrolytes. While the patient has ARF, no potassium should be given until normal serum potassium concentration is attained and some potassium is excreted. If the patient has substantial urine output, significant potassium depletion could occur. Daily measurement of body weight (occasionally twice a day) and frequent assessment of serum electrolyte levels are essential for determining the accurate composition of fluid and electrolyte replacement.

Electrolytes Therapy

Sodium

The usual sodium abnormality in ARF is hyponatremia caused by water retention[58]. In patients with hyponatremia and volume overload, restriction of free water intake to less than the volume of output allows for hypotonic fluid loss and leads to correction of hyponatremia. Serum sodium should be viewed as a reflection of total body water, whereas urine sodium is often an indicator of total body sodium.

The patient with hyponatremia and dehydration generally has a very low serum sodium level and requires fluid and sodium replacement. The sodium deficit is calculated by the following formula[58]:

$$\text{Sodium deficit} = (\text{normal serum sodium level} - \text{actual serum sodium level}) \times 0.6 \times (\text{body weight in kg})$$

This formula describes the total cation deficit, but it is safe to assume that the losses are sodium. Normal serum sodium level should be 135 mEq/L.

Symptomatic hyponatremia (i.e., obtundation and seizures) may be treated with 3% saline infusions. In an emergency, standard (1 mEq/mL) $NaHCO_3$ solution, available with resuscitative medications, may be used. The sodium deficit formula is used for calculation of the amount of sodium that must be replaced. Although hyponatremic seizures are difficult to control using anticonvulsants, they respond well to relatively modest rises in serum sodium level. Rapid return to normonatremia, however, may precipitate neurologic injury. For this reason, in cases of symptomatic hyponatremia, it is most prudent to use lower goals (such as 125 mEq/L) as for target serum sodium level. 3% saline contains 513 mEq/L of sodium, is extremely hypertonic, and should be administered with extreme caution.

Potassium

Patients with ARF accumulate potassium because the kidney is responsible for elimination of 85 to 90% of daily potassium excretion. The remaining 10 to 15% is removed by the gastrointestinal tract. Patients with chronic renal failure may compensate by increasing their gastrointestinal losses, but similar compensation in patients with ARF is unlikely.

Many patients not only have decreased potassium excretion but also have increased potassium generation. Patients with rhabdomyolysis, hemolysis, tissue necrosis, and other cellular damage experience a large release of intracellular potassium. When a decrease in excretion and an increase in generation are combined with acidosis, commonly occurring in the critically ill child, serum potassium levels can increase dramatically. For each 0.1 unit decline in pH level, K^+ increases by 0.5 mEq/L.

Hyperkalemia is life-threatening because of the importance of the intracellular potassium gradient in regulation of cardiac action potential generation and conduction. The transmembrane resting potential of −90 mV is maintained through the functioning of the ATP-dependent Na^+/K^+ pump. The triggering of the cardiac action potential, however, once this gradient has been established, is dependent not on the action of the pump but on changes in permeability of the membrane to potassium. Elevation of extracellular potassium causes a decrease in the negativity of the transmembrane potential, which is predicted by the Nernst equation. The speed with which the ions traverse the membrane is dependent upon the magnitude of the gradient; therefore, an elevation in extracellular potassium and a less negative transmembrane potential leads to a slower potassium flux across the membrane. In the pacemaker cells, there is normally a slow spontaneous depolarization during diastole that is caused by a slow leakage of sodium into the cell at the time when permeability to potassium is diminished. When the threshold level is reached (−70mV), sodium channels open and sodium floods into the cell. When the resting potential is less negative with respect to the threshold, fewer sodium channels open, and the amplitude and slope of phase 0 are diminished. The result is a prolonged P-R interval. The atrioventricular node cells are particularly sensitive to this effect. Atrioventricular block may occur, resulting from impaired conduction. The initial suspicion of hyperkalemia on the electrocardiogram (ECG) is peaked or "tenting" T waves. Subsequently the P wave may flatten, the P-R interval may be prolonged, and the QRS complex may widen. Ventricular fibrillation or asystole eventually occurs.

Because the consequences of hyperkalemia are severe, aggressive therapy is warranted. Treatment should be started when the serum K^+ is more than 6 mEq/L or at lower levels if the serum K^+ is rising rapidly. Therapy involves protection of the myocardium, shift of K^+ from extracellular to intracellular sites, and removal of K^+ via the gastrointestinal tract or dialysis. In urgent situations, the myocardium may be protected from the effects of hyperkalemia by infusion of calcium (10 mg/kg elemental Ca^{++} as CaCl or calcium gluconate). Calcium increases potassium conductance and calcium entry through calcium channels. The potential effect is to increase conductance and contractility.

In emergencies, intracellular movement of potassium is enhanced by administration of glucose, bicarbonate, and insulin. One protocol suggests administration of 0.25 units regular insulin per gram of glucose. Movement of K^+ to intracellular locations restores the transmembrane potential and conductance.

Reduction of total body potassium is necessary for long-term stabilization and may be accomplished by administration of a cation exchange resin or by dialysis. Kayexalate is a sodium polystyrene sulfonate resin that exchanges K^+ for Na^+ in the intestine. The colon is the primary area of K^+ excretion from the GI tract, and therefore, Kayexalate can be given orally, via nasogastric tube, or as an enema. Often, Kayexalate can be combined with sorbitol to increase GI output. The dose of Kayexalate is 1 gm/kg of body weight, and enemas can be repeated hourly.

If dialysis is necessary, Kayexalate should be continued until serum K^+ levels return to normal. Potassium levels should not be measured sooner than 4 hours after completion of dialysis, since serum potassium levels decrease significantly during dialysis, yet subsequently rise to reach a new equilibrium concentration within 4 hours. Typically, in hyperkalemia, a potassium-free dialysate is used. If peritoneal dialysis or continuous venovenous hemofiltration (CVVH) are the only available treatment modalities, Kayexalate should be continued throughout the course of the treatment, because K^+ clearance with peritoneal dialysis or CVVH is substantially less than with hemodialysis. Treatment for hyperkalemia is outlined in **Table 38.6.**

Nutrition Therapy

Patients with ARF are initially in a catabolic state[115]. There are 4 primary goals in managing the nutritional needs of patients in ARF: (1) Maintaining adequate caloric intake, (2) avoiding excessive protein intake to control the rise in BUN, (3) minimizing potassium and phosphate intake, and, (4) reducing fluid intake[116].

Maintaining adequate caloric intake can be difficult in patients with ARF. This is particularly true in patients who are oliguric because of the volume required for total daily caloric intake. Central venous access is often needed to deliver concentrated parenteral nutrition. Potassium should be removed from all fluids during the initial phase of ARF. In the patient who can receive enteral nutrition, high-calorie formulas may be delivered in small volumes. Formula containing 50 to 60 kcal per ounce can be produced[117,117a]. This is not simply a concentrated formula: The formula initially has to be diluted to avoid excessive potassium and phosphate intake. Calories are added to the recipe by means of concentrated carbohydrates and lipids. Amino acid intake is essential for improvement of patient outcome[115,118–120]. The goal is to decrease urea generation and therefore the need for dialysis, while continuing to deliver amino acids. Protein intake should be 1 to 1.5 gm/kg/day. A number of formulas are composed of only essential amino acids to decrease urea production. If only 1 to 1.5 gm/kg/day of protein is delivered to the patient, these formulas are usually unnecessary. Investigators have shown that provision of essential amino acids, with or without nonessential amino acids, improves the outcome in patients with ARF.

If appropriate nutritional support cannot be attained because of fluid restriction, ultrafiltration with or without dialysis is necessary. If urea generation is excessive in the catabolic patient, dialysis is necessary. Peritoneal dialysis, chest tubes, and peritoneal drains may result in removal of large amounts of protein. These protein losses can be calculated by measuring the protein concentration in the fluid.

Table 38.6. Treatment of Hyperkalemia

Drug or Method	*Dose & Route*	*Onset (Duration)*	*Mode of Action*	*Comments*
Calcium gluconate (100 mg/mL)	10 mg/kg over 5 minutes; may repeat ×2	Immediate (30–60 minutes)	Counteracts electrophysiologic effects of hyperkalemia	Monitor ECG for bradycardia; stop infusion if pulse < 100/minute
Sodium bicarbonate (1mEq/mL)	1–2 mEq/kg I.V. bolus or infusion over 20 minutes	20 min (1–4 hours)	Causes movement of K+ intracellularly	Assure adequate ventilation; do not give simultaneously with calcium
Glucose & Insulin	1–2 g/kg and 0.3 unit/kg together over 1–2 hours	15–30 min (3–6 hours)	Causes movement of K+ intracellularly	Monitor blood sugar
Kayexalate	1 gm/kg in 30% sorbitol P.R. or in 70% sorbitol P.O.	15–30 minutes	Removes K+ from body	Removes 1 mEq K+/gm resin; exchanges Na+equimolarly with K+
Dialysis	Hemodialysis is most rapid	Immediate	Removes K+ from body	Do not ignore first 4 steps while preparing for dialysis

The protein loss can then be replaced with albumin or fresh frozen plasma.

Renal Replacement Therapy

A number of factors influence the need for renal replacement therapy. Acute dialysis is needed when conservative medical management is unable to maintain fluid and electrolyte balance, control acid-base balance, maintain a BUN level of less than 150 mg/dL, or treat symptomatic uremia. See **Table 38.7.**

Renal replacement therapy is available via a large number of modalities. All the therapies are based on principles of solute mass transfer and ultrafiltration (fluid removal). The choice depends on the clinical scenario and the experience at individual centers.

The principles of thermodynamics describe mass balance resulting from the application of dialysis and guide the clinical application of dialysis and hemofiltration. The amount of a solute removed by the procedure is described as mass transfer. The amount of solute transfer is dependent on the dialyzer clearance for the solute, the duration of the treatment, the volume of distribution of the solute, and thus the concentration gradient across the dialysis membrane. In most clinical situations, there exists a dynamic equilibrium and overall mass balance depends on the relationship of generation of a particular solute and its rate of removal, which is the product of its clearance and concentration (Figure 38.2). In hemodialysis, clearance is dependent on the dialyzer permeability-surface area product and the flow rates of dialysate and blood. In peritoneal dialysis, clearance is dependent on peritoneal membrane function, dwell time, volume of dialysate, and duration of "exchanges".

Hemodialysis

Hemodialysis results in removal of solutes from a patient's serum. Two mechanisms permit this removal of solute: diffusion and convection. Diffusion is dependent on a concentration gradient to "force" the solute from one area of distribution to another, typically from the patient's serum to the dialysate. Convection results in "dragging" the solute across a membrane along the solvent (ultrafiltrate). Diffusion is the predominant mechanism for effective clearance in hemodialysis. Clearance of a solute is dependent on the type and size of the dialyzer, blood flow through the dialyzer, and dialysate flow. Mass transfer is dependent on the clearance, the duration of treatment, and volume of distribution of the solute. Using these variables, expected change in the concentration of a solute can be calculated with the following formula[121].

$$C_t/C_0 = e^{-KT/V}$$

Where C_t is the final concentration at time t, C_0 is the initial concentration, K is the clearance of the dialyzer at a particular blood flow, T is the duration of the treatment, V is the volume of distribution of the solute. Most often, urea is the molecule on whose clearance acute dialysis treatments are modeled. Accurate urea clearance can be calculated for any dialysis treatment.

Ultrafiltration is the removal of fluid (ultrafiltrate). Ultrafiltration can be performed independent of solute transfer with modern dialysis machines, and extremely accurate control of ultrafiltration can be accomplished. Ultrafiltration is controlled independent of blood flow and is regulated by a transmembrane pressure applied by the dialysis machine.

Central access is essential for adequate acute hemodialysis. A continuous circuit from "arterial" to "venous" site is required. Three techniques are used. First, separate access lines may be placed, one arterial and one venous. Rarely, however is an arterial catheter used for hemodialysis. Second and more commonly, a single catheter with two ports is placed in a large vein. There is a distal port, the "venous" port, and a proximal "arterial" side port. The dialysis pump pulls blood from the "arterial" port and after passing through the dialyzer, returns it to the patient via the "venous" port. Unfortunately, the proximity of the catheter ports permits approximately 15% "recirculation" of blood (i.e., blood returning to the patient is sucked back

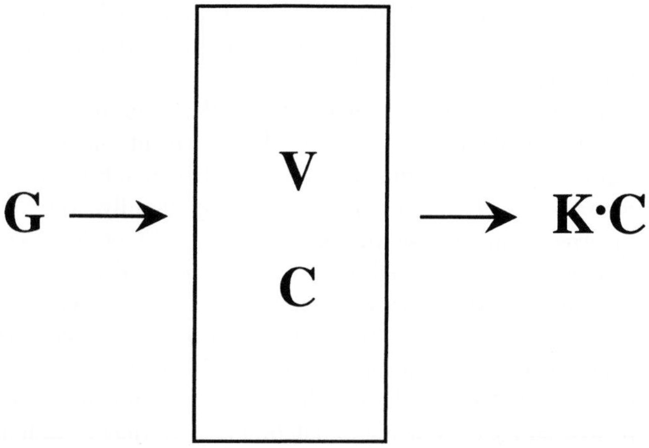

Figure 38.2. The mass balance dynamic equilibrium represented as a single pool model. G = generation rate (mg/min) of a solute (for example, urea) into the body space. The total amount of solute in the body space is the product of the solute's volume of distribution in that space, V (mL), and the solute concentration, C (mg/mL). Mass transfer out of the space (mg/min) = solute clearance, K (mL/min) times solute concentration, C (mg/mL).

Table 38.7. Indications for Acute Dialysis or Hemofiltration

Intractable acidosis
Fluid overload, pulmonary edema
BUN > 150 mg/dL
Symptomatic uremia (encephalopathy, pericarditis)
Hyperkalemia (serum K+ >7 mEq/L)
Hyperammonemia
Ultrafiltration for nutritional support, transfusions
Exogenous toxins (lithium, salicylate, ethanol, methanol, ethylene glycol, aminoglycosides, bromide, theophylline, phenobarbital)
Hyponatremia or hypernatremia

Table 38.8. Temporary and Permanent Hemodialysis Catheters for Pediatric Patients

Type	*Manufacturer*	*External Diameter*	*Length*	*Indication*
Temporary	MedComp	7F	4 in	Newborn-infant subclavian
	MedComp	7F	6 in	Newborn-infant femoral
	MedComp	7F	8 in	Newborn-infant femoral
	MedComp	7F	12 in	Newborn-infant femoral
	MedComp	9F	4 ¾in	Toddler subclavian
	MedComp	9F	6in	Toddler femoral
	MedComp	9F	8in	Toddler femoral
	Quinton	10F	4 ¾in	Child, small adult
	Quinton	11F	5in	Child subclavian/femoral
	Quinton	11F	7in	Adult subclavian
Permanent	MedComp	8F	18cm	Infant
	MedComp	8F	24cm	Infant/Child
	Quinton	10F	28cm	Child
	MedComp	11.5F	28cm	Adult
	Quinton	12F	36cm	Adult
	Quinton	12F	40cm	Adult

into the dialyzer without first circulating in the patient). Recirculation decreases clearance but can be compensated for by increasing the duration of the dialysis treatment. Third, a single-lumen catheter can be used with special equipment that permits "single-needle" dialysis. This equipment includes special clamps and pumps that alternate pumping blood into the patient and removing it sequentially through the same catheter. Recirculation is extensive with this method, and it is therefore not often used.

Large-bore catheters are required for dialysis because the blood flow can be a limiting factor. Catheter size is dictated by patient size[122]. Suitable dual-lumen catheters are available now for infants. **Table 38.8** lists appropriate central venous access catheters for different sized patients. Preferred sites of insertion include left subclavian, right internal jugular, and femoral veins. For adequate flows via femoral catheters, ports must reside in an inferior vena cava that is free from clots and external compression.

Dialysis disequilibrium syndrome and other symptoms occurring during dialysis are generally related to osmotic shifts during the treatment. To avoid these sequelae, dialysis should be initiated before BUN level exceeds 150 mg/dL. The initial treatment should decrease BUN level by 20 to 30%. Urea clearance can then be increased by 25% per day. Therefore, dialysis is often performed on three consecutive days increasing gradually to a maximum of 75% reduction of BUN level. Treatments are then changed to an alternate day schedule unless urea generation is excessive or daily ultrafiltration is necessary. Complications of hemodialysis are listed in **Table 38.9.** Mannitol can be used to maintain serum osmolarity in patients who are likely to experience difficulty with osmotic shifts, specifically those with cerebral edema. In these cases, mannitol should be infused at a constant rate, G, calculated by the equation shown in Figure 38.2. In this case, G = KC where K is the dialysis mannitol clearance (about the same as creatinine clearance) and C is the desired steady-state serum mannitol concentration (about 400 mg/dL). Furthermore, many dialysis machines have a sodium "step program" that gradually decreases dialysate sodium concentration to avoid rapid sodium fluctuations. Sodium "step" programs have been shown to improve patient tolerance and reduce morbidity[123–125]. Along with frequent low-clearance dialysis treatments, they decrease complications caused by osmotic shifts during hemodialysis therapy.

Tabl 38.9. Complications of Hemodialysis

Hypotension
Bleeding
Muscle cramps
Embolism
Disequilibrium syndrome
Catheter infection
Complement activation

Hypotension is another complication of hemodialysis, which is usually associated with rapid ultrafiltration and subsequent intravascular depletion. To avoid large shifts in extracorporeal blood volume, no more than 10% total blood volume should be in the tubing and dialyzer. If the tubing and dialyzer volume requires more than 10% of total blood volume or the patient is hemodynamically compromised, the tubing should be primed with albumin and packed red blood cells (prbc). The hematocrit of the prime should be 40 to 45%. The following formula is used to calculate the amount of blood and albumin to prime the line.

$$(\text{Vpr} \times \text{Hctprbc}/\text{Phct}) - \text{Vpr} = \text{Valb}$$

Where Vpr is the volume of prbcs for the prime (typically 100mL), Hctprbc is the hematocrit of the prbc, Phct is the desired hematocrit of the prime and Valb is the volume of 5% albumin added to Vpr for the prime. Albumin (5%) alone can be used to prime the dialysis tubing in a patient who is hypoalbuminemic. Hypotension during dialysis is treated by stopping or slowing ultrafiltration and by using colloid or crystalloid infusion for volume replacement.

The mortality rate is higher in patients with ARF who require dialysis than in those who do not[126]. Studies in animals indicate that leukocyte infiltrate in the kidney may influence recovery from renal failure. Complement activation potential by the dialysis membrane influences renal recovery in animals. Recently, Hakim and colleagues showed an improved outcome in adults with ARF receiving dialysis with "biocompatible" membranes[126].

Peritoneal Dialysis

Peritoneal dialysis necessitates placement of a catheter, surgically or percutaneously, into the intraperitoneal space and instillation of dialysate for mass transfer of solute and for ultrafiltration. Urea clearance is not as efficient as in hemodialysis but does maintain a more gradual and steady urea clearance. Peritoneal dialysis may be easier to administer, particularly in infants. Similar principles pertain to peritoneal dialysis and hemodialysis. Mass transfer is dependent upon diffusion and convection. Unlike in hemodialysis, blood flow or dialysis size cannot be changed in peritoneal dialysis. Dialysate volume and frequency of dialysate exchanges may be increased or decreased to effect solute clearance. A number of techniques have been used to measure the dialysis efficiency in chronic peritoneal dialysis[121]. Unfortunately, there is no conclusive test of the effectiveness of peritoneal dialysis. In ARF, the need for extensive calculations of peritoneal dialysis kinetics is rare. The dialysis prescription is derived from the patient's clinical status and metabolic status as well as by the need for ultrafiltration[121].

Ultrafiltration in peritoneal dialysis is obtained through the use of dextrose as an osmotic agent in the dialysate. Increasing the dextrose concentration increases ultrafiltrate removal: The standard concentrations are 1.5%, 2.5%, and 4.25%. The solutions may be combined to produce intermediate concentrations.

Relative contraindications to peritoneal dialysis are found in patients with intraperitoneal drains and bowel rupture, diaphragmatic hernia, diaphragm surgery, or communication between the abdominal and the thoracic cavities.

Complications of peritoneal dialysis include peritonitis, dialysate leakage, catheter blockage, hyperglycemia, decreased vital capacity, pleural effusions, hypotension, protein loss, and visceral rupture. Meticulous care is required with handling of the catheter and the catheter site. Sterile technique must always be used. To prevent leakage, surgical placement with tunneling of a cuffed catheter improves closure around the catheter.

Once the catheter is placed, the proper dialysate volume is critical for adequate dialysis and patient tolerance of the procedure. After three successive, rapid flushes to assure catheter patency, dialysis is begun with 10mL/kg of dialysate. Initially, 1.5% dextrose concentration dialysate is used to avoid excessive ultrafiltration. As the patient adapts to the intraperitoneal volume, the dialysate volume is increased by 10 mL/kg/dwell to a maximum of 40 to 50 mL/kg/dwell. Clearance is increased by administering short, frequent dwells. Ultrafiltrate is increased by increasing dextrose concentration and dwell frequency. Dwell times vary from 30 minutes to 6 hours. Peritoneal dialysis cyclers can be used to instill and drain dialysate and are particularly useful for treatment of infants.

Catheter obstruction can limit instillation and draining of the dialysate. The obstruction may be caused by fibrin deposition, infection, omentum around the catheter, or by abdominal organs impinging on the catheter. If infection or fibrin depostion is suspected, urokinase instillation and removal may clear the obstruction. The appropriate dosage of urokinase is unknown; 5,000 to 20,000 U has been used. Positioning of the patient may help relieve some obstructions.

Peritonitis is a notable complication of peritoneal dialysis. Typically, the causative bacterial organism is skin flora. Enteric flora, fungus, and other gram-negative rods, such as *Pseudomonas* species, may cause peritonitis, particularly in infants and malnourished patients. Clinical findings include fever, abdominal pain, vomiting, cloudy dialysate, catheter obstruction, and hypotension. Occasionally, urea clearance and ultrafiltration decrease in patients with peritonitis. Evaluation of suspected peritonitis includes complete blood count (CBC) and peritoneal fluid cell count and culture. If peritonitis is suspected, therapy should be instituted before culture results are available. There are two principle therapies for peritonitis: (1) intraperitoneal antibiotics and (2) aggressive dialysis. Vancomycin and gentamicin are added to the dialysate and instilled. The initial concentration of vancomycin is 500 mg/L. Subsequent dwells contain 20 mg/L vancomycin. Gentamicin is instilled at a concentration of 8 mg/L. Frequent exchanges help clear the infection and maintain urea clearance. Third generation cephalosporins can be used instead of gentamicin. Urokinase has been used to aid in treating peritonitis but its full benefit has not been determined.

Hemofiltration

Continuous venoveous hemofiltration (CVVH) and continuous arteriovenous hemofiltration (CAVH) are alternative methods of renal replacement therapy. Hemofiltration is the process of passing blood over a membrane and allowing hydrostatic force to generate an ultrafiltrate. Clearance is minimal in these modalities because there is no dialysate flow to generate a diffusion gradient. Solvent drag (convection) results in low levels of clearance. CVVH and CAVH are used primarily for ultrafiltration, (i.e., fluid removal)[127–133].

CONTINUOUS VENOVENOUS HEMOFILTRATION. CVVH requires central venous access, a blood pump, an ultrafiltrate pump, and a suitable hemofilter. The central venous access is the same as for hemodialysis. A single catheter with dual lumens or two separate venous sites may be used. In the single catheter technique, the distal port is the "venous" port and the proximal port is the "arterial" port. Blood flow is controlled by the blood pump. Blood flows from the "arterial" side through the hemofilter and returns to the body via the venous side. Ultrafiltrate flow rate can be controlled by an intravenous pump. CVVH does not rely on the patient's blood flow or cardiac output to maintain hemofiltration. CVVH is pump-driven and, therefore, is suitable for patients with marginal perfusion pressure. Modern CVVH machines can control all aspects of the treatment.

Complications of CVVH include bleeding, hypotension, catheter infections, and decreased intravascular volume. In the patient with marginal renal functions (i.e., GFR less than 50 to 75%) removal of intravascular volume may result in decreased renal perfusion and worsened renal insufficiency. This situation is particularly difficult in the patient with total body fluid overload and intravascular depletion. Heparin is required to avoid clotting of the filter and tubing. The goal of heparinization is an activated clotting time of 120 to 150 seconds. Patients who cannot tolerate systemic anticoagulation may not be suitable for hemofiltration. Also, small patients may be "chilled" by the procedure unless some type of blood warmer is utilized.

CONTINUOUS ARTERIOVENOUS HEMOFILTRATION. CAVH is another form of hemofiltration in which blood flow through the filter is dependent on the patient's perfusion pressure. CAVH is not driven by a mechanical pump and therefore is difficult to perform in the hypotensive patient. The blood flow circuit is similar to CVVH, but there are significant differences. Two access sites are required: An arterial site is needed to generate blood flow and a venous site for blood return. Ultrafiltrate generation is dependent on blood flow. The ultrafiltrate flow may be controlled by intravenous pumps as in CVVH. If a patient has poor perfusion pressure, blood flow is slow and therefore ultrafiltrate generation is low. To some extent, this safeguards against excessive ultrafiltration but may be the rate-limiting factor in patients who need fluid removal.

As in hemodialysis, the extracorporeal blood volume required to prime the tubing should not be more than 10% of the patient's total blood volume, particularly for pediatric patients. To avoid hemodynamic compromise or worsening of hemodynamic instability, the tubing is primed with prbcs and albumin. The priming hematocrit should be 40 to 45%. The patient who requires dopamine, epinephrine, or norepinephrine often needs the dosage increased when initiating hemofiltration or hemodialysis. This may result from either dilution from the tubing prime or clearance from the filter.

HEMOFILTRATION WITH DIALYSIS. CVVHD combines CVVH with continuous dialysis, and the blood flow circuit is the same as for CVVH. There are two dialysate ports on the Amicon filter. Peritoneal dialysate is pumped countercurrent to the blood flow through the filter. The dialysate generally has a 1.5% glucose concentration and uses lactate as a buffer, which may restrict the use of this modality in patients who cannot convert lactate as a buffer. The dialysate removed from the filter is controlled by a pump, which filter controls not only the dialysate flow but also the ultrafiltrate volume. Urea clearance is dependent principally on dialysate flow rate.

A particularly important aspect of hemofiltration, hemodialysis, and peritoneal dialysis is the ultrafiltrate composition. Ultrafiltrate is isotonic: The electrolyte urea and creatinine concentrations are isotonic to serum. As ultrafiltrate volume increases, particularly in small patients, large sodium losses may occur and appropriate fluid and electrolyte replacement is required.

HEMOLYTIC UREMIC SYNDROME

Diagnosis and Pathophysiology

HUS was first described in 1955 by Conrad Gasser, a Swiss hematologist. Gasser detailed five fatal cases in children presenting with acquired hemolytic anemia, renal failure, and thrombocytopenia. Pathologic examination of the kidney revealed cortical necrosis and thrombotic microangiopathy. In some of the children, similar microangiopathic changes were present in other organs. Subsequently, sporadic reports of similar cases began to accumulate worldwide, growing to include epidemic clusters, usually in association with a prodromal diarrheal illness.

Clinical findings of HUS include pallor, anuria or oliguria, and tachycardia. Mild neurologic symptoms such as irritability, ataxia, tremors, or behavioral changes are common, and central nervous system (CNS) involvement is sometimes the presenting complaint. Laboratory evaluation reveals anemia, uremia, thrombocytopenia, and a blood smear showing microangiopathic hemolysis. Pathologic characteristics of HUS include widespread endothelial damage and thrombotic microangiopathy with infarction[134].

Causes

HUS is now recognized as both a multisystem disease of the microcirculation and a common cause of renal failure. Familial forms with both autosomal dominant and recessive patterns have been described, as has association with drugs including oral contraceptives, antimicrobials[135], and chemotherapeutic agents. HUS is also known occasionally to complicate bone marrow transplantation, pregnancy, and human immunodeficiency virus (HIV) infection.

While many noninfectious causes of HUS are recognized, in children the syndrome most commonly accompanies enteric infection with *Escherichia coli* serotype 0157:H7. Typically, signs and symptoms of HUS develop during the resolution phase of a diarrheal illness; toxigenic *E. coli* is often recoverable from the stool. Surface endotoxin and elaborated Shiga-like toxins (SLTs) are thought to act synergistically in production of endothelial injury, vasculopathy, and organ damage[136,137]. Other proposed pathogenetic mechanisms include abnormalities in prostacyclin (PG12)[138] or endothelin production, alterations in coagulation and fibrinolysis[139], and production of ultra large von Willebrand factor multimers[140].

Outcome

With initiation of short-term dialysis, the mortality rate from HUS is now generally less than 5%. Experience from our institution suggests that most early mortality is the result of neurologic involvement, and such involvement remains the primary indication for admission to our ICU. Other serious complications of HUS include hemorrhagic colitis, sepsis, myocarditis/pericarditis, pericardial effusion with tamponade, and ventricular dysfunction.

Aside from permanent neurologic damage, morbidity from HUS is primarily determined by the extent of recoverable renal function. Reported rates of progression to chronic renal failure vary widely, yet are generally on the order of 5%. The need for more than 2 weeks of dialysis carries a worse prognosis for full recovery[141]. Data gathered by Fitzpatrick and colleagues suggest that many children who leave the hospital with apparent full recovery go on to experience subtle forms of chronic nephropathy[142]. In a 5-year followup, 30% of children had urine albumin/ urine creatine (UA/UC) more than 2 standard deviations above the mean, 18% had a significantly decreased GFR, and the cohort as a whole had mean blood pressures significantly higher than normal[142].

Patients progressing to chronic renal failure are typically considered for transplantation. Although recurrence in patients who received transplants has been described in several case reports, the precise risk is difficult to ascertain. It appears, however, that the risk is low, even in living-related donor organs. In contrast, chronic graft rejection may be slightly higher in patients receiving transplants for HUS than for other primary diseases[143].

Treatment

Currently, therapeutic interventions for severe HUS are controversial. By analogy to adult thrombotic thrombocytopenic purpura (TTP), plasma infusion and plasmapheresis have been advocated by some authors yet have not proved beneficial in large controlled trials[144,145]. Identification of high antibody titers to *E. coli* O157:H7 LPS in sera from HUS patients as well as the presence of antibody to SLTs in commercial immune globulin preparations has fueled speculation that the presence of circulating anti-SLT and O157-LPS antibodies may influence disease severity. This being so, it has been suggested that some protection might be conferred by immune globulin administration[146,147]. Thus far, administration of immunoglobulin preparations to children with HUS has met with mixed results. Preliminary data from a trial of high-dose gamma globulin infusion showed substantial improvement in treated patients[148], yet Robson and associates[149] were able to demonstrate clear benefit in only one of nine children similarly treated. Variables including severity of disease, length of illness, concurrent therapies, and precise antibody content of infused globulin preparations pose significant challenges to definitive trials of immunoglobulin therapy for HUS.

HYPERTENSION

Hypertension in children is defined as an average blood pressure greater than the 95th percentile for age and gender; normal blood pressure is less than the 90th percentile for age and gender. Blood pressures between the 90th and 95th percentile are borderline hypertension. Normal blood pressures are shown in **Table 38.10.**

Hypertension is either essential or secondary. Essential hypertension is hypertension for which no obvious source is found; secondary hypertension is caused by underlying organ damage or disease process. The rule of thumb for pediatric hypertension is the younger the patient and the higher the blood pressure, the greater probability of secondary hypertension. Secondary hypertension is discussed in this section.

Mechanisms

Many mechanisms have been proposed for hypertension. Secondary hypertension may be placed in one of five categories: (1) volume-related, (2) renal, (3) neuronal, (4) vascular, or (5) humoral (endocrine or neoplastic).

Volume-related hypertension occurs in patients with renal disease and fluid retention. Sodium intake worsens fluid retention and hypertension. Hypertension from volume overload is a particular problem in the oliguric patient. Fluid overload can lead to heart failure, pulmonary edema, and anasarca. When there is an increase in intravascular volume, baroreceptors in the carotid arteries, glomerular arterioles, central nervous system, and right atrium respond by attempting to excrete free water and sodium. ADH levels decrease, aldosterone levels are suppressed, and atrial natriuretic factor (ANF) is released. In the functioning kidney, free water and sodium is excreted. The patient with renal disease is unable to increase free water clearance, leading to fluid overload and hypertension. Volume overload is treated by aggressive diuresis or ultrafiltration.

The renin-angiotensin system (RAS) is one of the principle mechanisms of blood pressure control. Renin is released from the JGA and stimulates angiotensin produc-

Table 38.10. Range of Blood Pressure in Children

	95th Percentile		*99th Percentile*	
Age Group	*Systolic*	*Diastolic*	*Systolic*	*Diastolic*
≤ 7 days	96		106	
8–30 days	104		110	
1–24 months	112	74	118	82
3–5 years	116	76	124	84
6–9 years	122	78	130	86
10–12 years	126	82	134	90
13–15 years	136	86	144	92
16–18 years	142	92	150	98

tion[150]. Angiotensin is converted by ACE in the lung to A2, which is a potent vasoconstrictor causing increased systemic vascular resistance (SVR) and afterload. When intravascular volume decreases, renin is released and SVR increases. Aldosterone secretion is also stimulated by the RAS with increased sodium reabsorption and fluid retention. Renal parenchymal damage or decreased renal perfusion, as in renal artery stenosis, increases renin release and subsequently hypertension[151].

ANF is released from the right atrium (RA)[150]. The stimulus for ANF release is stretching of the RA by increased preload. ANF has a number of possible actions; in the kidney, ANF stimulates sodium excretion and diuresis. ANF has also been been shown to cause vasodilatation and inhibit aldosterone.

A digitalis-like factor, also called "third factor", has been found to inhibit Na-K-ATPase and increase blood pressure. Although the effect on the kidney is natriuresis and diuresis, this factor increases vascular tone and blood pressure. "Third factor" is released from the hypothalamus, and its full implications in hypertension have not been characterized[150,152].

Calcium plays an important role in control of blood pressure. Intracellular calcium is essential for muscle tone in vascular cells[153]. Calcium is also important for receptor actions on cell membranes and cell responses[153,154].

In unusual situations, hypertension may be caused by endocrine or hormonal secretions. Adrenal secretion of glucocorticoids or excessive secretion of catecholamines, as in pheochromocytoma or neuroblastoma, may cause hypertension.

Evaluation and Causes

When the diagnosis of hypertension is made in the pediatric ICU, secondary causes must be evaluated. Unlike the adult population, in whom essential hypertension is common, essential hypertension is less likely in children. Although there are many causes of hypertension, renal disease must be ruled out.

The clinical history and physical examination are critical in determining the cause of hypertension. Past history of hypertension, family history of hypertension or renal disease, and medications or illicit drug use are important in reviewing the patient's history. The physical examination may give clues to the cause of hypertension. Cafe au lait spots, abdominal bruits (although only 30% of patients with documented renal artery stenosis have an abdominal bruit), abdominal masses, diminished femoral pulses, or elfin facies suggest renovascular disease or cystic renal disease. Blood pressure must be measured in all four extremities. A cushingoid appearance is associated with corticosteroid excess. Papilledema can be seen with severe hypertension or increased CNS pressure. Fluid intake greater than output with increased weight gain and edema suggest volume overload. Hypertension associated with general anesthesia, sweating, and flushing point to pheochromocytoma.

Laboratory and radiologic investigation of hypertension focuses on the kidneys. Urinalysis testing for hematuria, red blood cell casts, and proteinuria must be obtained. Serum electrolytes, BUN, and creatinine levels need to be obtained. If the diagnosis is not apparent by the previous evaluation, a plasma renin activity and aldosterone level are obtained. Renal ultrasonography is necessary to visualize the renal parenchyma and collecting system. Also, blood flow through the renal arteries can be evaluated for renal artery stenosis or thrombus[90]. Ultrasound is specific but not sensitive for renal artery stenosis: A definitive diagnosis is made by arteriography[90]. More recently, magnetic resonance angiography and ACE inhibitor renal scans have been used, but arteriography is still the gold standard. If the clinical setting suggests mineralocorticoid excess, measurement of aldosterone level may be indicated. Pheochromocytomas are rare, but if suggested by the clinical picture, urinary and serum catecholamine levels may be measured. CT scan and ^{131}I metaiodobenzylguanidine (MBIG) scan should be performed when a pheochromocytoma is suspected, because there is a possibility of multiple tumors[90]. Renal scans are not usually necessary in the ICU unless the patient has a history of frequent urinary tract infections or vesicoureteral reflux. In this situation, a renal scan may show areas of scarring that may be the cause of hypertension.

Treatment in the ICU

After the diagnosis of hypertension is made and the cause is discerned, therapy may be initiated. In a hypertensive crisis or emergency, immediate intervention is necessary. In the ICU, treatment is usually started in patients with severe hypertension, with blood pressure greater than the 95th percentile for age. Patients with borderline hypertension generally do not require immediate therapy. A list of antihypertensive agents is provided in **Table 38.11.**

Medications

Diuretics

Diuretics are often used in the ICU for patients with fluid overload. The patient with hypertension with volume overload who still can generate adequate urine output may benefit from diuretic use. Diuretics are also helpful in decreasing fluid retention that occurs with vasodilators.

Loop diuretics, such as furosemide, work at the level of the loop of Henle[94]. The mechanism of action is blockage of the Na-K-2Cl transporter. Loop diuretics typically produce a brisk diuresis and, in doing so, may have a number of adverse effects. The side effects include hypokalemia, dehydration, metabolic alkalosis, nephrocalcinosis, and ototoxicity. Furosemide can be administered orally or intravenously (as a bolus or continuous drip).

Thiazide diuretics block sodium reabsorption in the distal tubule[1]. When combined with loop diuretics, thiazides can cause significant sodium loss and hyponatremia. Thiazides have little use in acute hypertension but, like loop

Table 38.11. Treatment of Hypertension in Children

Agent	*Dose*	*Onset (Duration)*	*Comments*
Parenteral Agents			
α-Blocker			
Phentolamine (Regitine) (5 mg powder supplied with 1 mL diluent-further dilute to 10 mL for 0.5 mg/mL)	0.05–0.2 mg/kg IV	<30 sec (15–30 min)	For diagnosis of pheochromocytoma; may cause marked tachycardia, hypotension, arrhythmias from unopposed β effect
β-Blockers			
Propranolol (Inderal) (1 mg/mL vial-dilute to 10 mL with saline 0.1 mg/mL)	Test dose of 0.005 mg/kg IV, then 0.01 mg/kg IV; may repeat every 10 min to effect	2–4 min (3–6 hr)	Contraindication: myocardial disease, asthma; useful adjunct to vasodilator therapy to control tachycardia; may cause AV block, bradycardia, hypoglycemia; infants may be relatively resistant to blockade; do not give if heart rate <90, if age <3, if cardiac output is HR dependent.
Labetalol (Normodyne, Trandate) (5 mg/mL vial)	1–3 mg/kg/hr	Within minutes	β and α blocker, rare cases of hepatocellular injury
Direct vasodilators			
Diazoxide (Hyperstat) (15 mg/mL–20 mg vial)	1 mg/kg IV bolus (5 mg/kg maximum) may repeat in 5 min	1–5 min (up to 12 hr)	Hyperglycemia, sodium + water retention—may need concomitant diuretic therapy; contraindications: diabetes, marked tachycardia, thiazide sensitivity
Hydralazine (Apresoline) (20 mg/mL vial)	0.1–0.2 mg/kg every 1–2 hr IV 0.2–0.5 mg/kg IM every 3–4 hr	10–20 min/3–4 hr	Lupus-like syndrome
Nitroprusside (Nipride) (50 mg lyophilized powder): dilute [3 × body weight (kg)] = mg in 100 mL for 1 mL/hr = 0.5 µg/kg/min; protect from light-photodegradation (wrap in foil)—change solution every 24 hr	0.5–8 µg/kg/min titrated to blood pressure	Immediate (diseases on termination of infusion)	a. Monitor with arterial line b. Administer with controlled infusion pump c. Administer through central line if possible d. Positioning with head up may potentiate hypotensive effect e. Monitor blood thiocyanate if: 1. used > 24 hr 2. rate > 10µg/kg/min for > 6 hr 3. discontinue if thiocyanate level > 10 mg/dL Thiosulfate is antidote Monitor arterial blood gases for: 1. Metabolic acidosis-cyanide toxicity 2. ↓PO_2 caused by intrapulmonary shunting: May increase intracranial pressure
Calcium channel blocker			
Verapamil (Calan/Isoptin) (5 mg/2-mL vial)	Test dose of 0.01 mg/kg IV then 0.05–0.2 mg/kg	2–4 min (1–2 hr)	May cause high-grade AV block if given along with propranolol; not used widely in children
ACE Inhibitor			
Enalaprilat	5–28 µg/kg/day divided every 8–24 hrs	5–15 minutes (6 hours)	May cause oliguria, hyperkalemia, acute renal failure
Enteral agents			
α-Blockers			
Prazosin (Minipress) capsules: 1, 2, 5 mg	1 mg first dose 0.05–0.1 mg/kg every 8–12 hr, maximum 0.4 mg/kg/24 hr		Hypotension frequent after first dose
β-Blockers			
Propranolol (Inderal) Tablets: 10, 20, 40, 60, 80 mg	0.5 mg/kg every 6–12 hr; may increase every 3–6 days		Contraindications; heart failure, asthma, AV block, pheochromocytoma before blockade, liver disease; may mask sympathetic response to shock, hemorrhage; may cause bradycardia, atrioventricular block, CNS depression
Metoprolol (Lopressor) tablets: 50, 100 mg	1 mg/kg every 12 hr; may increase every 7 days		β_1-selective (less bronchospasm, otherwise same as propranolol); tablet size limits use in young children
Aetnolol (Tenormin) tablets: 50, 100 mg	1 mg/kg every 24 hr		Same as metoprolol; renal elimination ($T_{1/2}$ 6–9 hr if CrCl normal), if CrCl 15–35 mL/min/1.73 m^2, $T_{1/2}$ = 16–27 hr; if CrCl <15, $T_{1/2}$ > 27hr
Labetalol (Trandate) tablets: 100, 200 mg	1 mg/kg every 8 hours		β and α_1 blocker, not studied in children

Table 38.11. Treatment of Hypertension in Children Parenteral Agents (continued)

Agent	*Dose*	*Onset (Duration)*	*Comments*
Calcium channel blocker			
Nifedipine (Procardia) 10/20 mg capsules Sustained release tablets: 30, 60, 90 mg	Acute: 0.25–0.5 mg/kg S.L./P.O. Repeat q 30–60 min Chronic: 1 mg/kg/d divided every 6–24 hr	Capsule 5–20 min (4–12 hr) Sustained release (12–24 hr)	Side effects: Flushing, headache, hypotension, edema, tachycardia, constipation
Vasodilators			
Hydralazine (Apresoline) tablets: 10, 25, 50, 100 mg	1–2 mg/kg every 4–6 hr, maximum 8mg/kg/24 hr, increase every 3–4 days		Lupus-like syndrome is side effect
Minoxidil (Loniten)	0.1–0.2 mg/kg every day (duration 12–14 hr), maximum 1–mg/kg/24 hr, increase every 3 days		Sodium retention; use with diuretic, hypertrichosis, fluid retention; discontinue gradually; may cause pericardial effusion
Central α-agonist			
α-Methyldopa (Aldomet) tablets: 125, 250, 500 mg: suspension: 250 mg/5mL	25–50 mg/kg every 6–8 hr, increase every 2 days		Can cause liver function abnormalitis; contraindication in liver disease—follow liver function tests; Coombs-positive hemolytic anemia, sedation
Clonidine (Catapres) tablets: 0.1, 0.2, 0.3 mg	0.01–0.03 mg/kg b.i.d., maximum 0.06 mg/kg/24 hr, increase every 2–4 days		Discontinue gradually to avoid rebound hypertension, dry mouth/sedation; follow fundus examination for retinal degeneration, used infrequently in children.
Angiotensin converting enzyme (ACE) inhibitors			
Captopril (Capoten) tablets: 25, 50, 100 mg (scored)	0.5–1 mg/kg t.i.d., maximum dose: CrCl Normal 6 mg/kg/day CrCl 40–80 4 mg/kg/day CrCl 20–40 2 mg/kg/day CrCl 10–20 1 mg/kg/day CrCl <10 0.5 mg/kg/day		Give 1 hr before meals—food inhibits absorption 20–40%, can cause decline in renal function: rash, eosinophilia, leukopenia 0.3% (in patients on immunosuppressants or those with autoimmune disease), proteinuria 1%, monitor for hyperkalemia, taste disturbance; renal excretion
Enalopril tablets: 2.5, 5, 10, 20 mg	0.15 mg/kg b.i.d. or q.d.		Give 1 hr before meals—food inhibits absorption 20–40%, can cause decline in renal function: rash, eosinophilia, leukopenia 0.3% (in patients on immunosuppressants or those with autoimmune disease), proteinuria 1%, monitor for hyperkalemia, taste disturbance; renal excretion

diuretics, may help to decrease fluid retention associated with vasodilators.

Carbonic anhydrase inhibitors have little use in the treatment of acute hypertension in the ICU.

Aldosterone antagonists such as spironolactone inhibit aldosterone in the cortical collecting duct[1]. Although their use is limited in acute hypertension, these agents are often used in patients with elevated aldosterone levels, such as patients with liver failure. Aldosterone inhibitors may be beneficial in patients with primary hyperaldosteronism-induced hypertension. These patients typically present with hypokalemia and metabolic alkalosis. Elevated serum aldosterone levels and low plasma renin activity help confirm the diagnosis.

ACE Inhibitors

ACE inhibitors block conversion of A1 to A2 in the pulmonary vasculature. As previously discussed, renin is produced in the renal vessel and at the JGA. Renin stimulation of the liver increases the production of A1 precursors. A2 is a potent vasoconstrictor. Blockage of ACE inhibits conversion to A2 and thus decreases systemic vascular resistance. A number of ACE inhibitors have been developed: Three are particularly important in pediatrics, largely because of their mode of administration.

Captopril, enalapril, and intravenous enalaprilat are commonly used ACE inhibitors. Captopril may be crushed and given in suspension form, which is often necessary in children. Intravenous enalaprilat is particularly useful in patients who are not taking anything orally or for whom very small volumes of captopril would be difficult to administer, such as in neonates.

Side effects of ACE inhibitors include reversible renal insufficiency, hyperkalemia, cough, and angioedema[155]. In the neonatal ICU, captopril has been associated with refractory hypotension and stroke. Patients with renal artery stenosis are at particular risk for renal failure. A2s primary action is vasoconstriction of the efferent arteriole. If renal blood flow is decreased from renal artery stenosis and vasoconstriction at the efferent arteriole is released, intraglomerular pressure drops and renal failure ensues[156,157]. Thus, in patients with bilateral or unilateral renal artery stenosis, ACE inhibitors should be avoided.

Calcium Channel Blockers

Calcium channel blockers inhibit calcium influx in vascular smooth muscle[158]. Calcium is important in smooth muscle contraction, and inhibition of calcium channels causes vascular relaxation and thus decreases SVR. Nifedipine is often used for pediatric hypertension, because its action is primarily on the vascular bed and not on myocardial conductance[159]. Verapamil, on the other hand, has more cardiac conductance activity and has been associated with sudden cardiac death in infants. Nifedipine is available as a gel cap and in a long-acting form. The gel cap can be punctured and the suspension aspirated for sublingual administration. The onset of action is rapid and useful in patients not taking anything orally when administered sublingually, but the duration of action is decreased. The primary side effects of nifedipine are tachycardia, headache, flushing, ankle edema, and hypotension.

Beta and Alpha Blockers

Beta blockers have two mechanisms of action, a decrease in cardiac ionotropy and chronotropy and a decrease in renin release[160,161]. Beta blockers are available in long and short acting forms. The major side effects are primarily bradycardia, cardiac failure, bronchospasm, and CNS effects (e.g., agitation, drowsiness, sleep disturbances).

Alpha blockers, such as prazosin, may be used for hypertension. Prazosin blocks the alpha-1 receptor at the postsynaptic sites of the peripheral vessels. Unfortunately, orthostatic hypotension and tachycardia limit the use of prazosin. Clonidine, on the other hand, is an alpha-2 receptor agonist; the principal side effects are dry mouth and sedation. Clonidine is available as a patch and can be used in patients with CNS-induced hypertension and adrenergic stimulation. The patch takes at least 3 days to work, therefore blood pressure management by other medications is necessary in the interim.

Vasodilators

Vasodilators include nitroprusside, diazoxide, minoxidil, and hydralazine. Their mechanism of action, although not completely understood, lead to vasodilatation and decreased blood pressure. Nitroprusside is used as a intravenous drip for severe hypertension. It has a rapid onset of action and short half-life, allowing for precise control of the blood pressure. An important toxicity of nitroprusside is its conversion to thiocyanate[162]. Thiocyanate is excreted in the urine, and therefore patients with renal insufficiency are at particular risk for thiocyanate toxicity. Patients with liver disease are unable to convert cyanide to thiocyanate and are at risk for cyanide toxicity. Serum levels of thiocyanate and cyanide should be measured in patients who require prolonged administration of nitroprusside or who have renal or liver insufficiency. Hydralazine is a vasodilator that may be given orally or intravenously. The primary side effects include tachycardia, hypotension, tachyphylaxis, headache, pancytopenia, and a lupus-like syndrome (uncommon in children).

Minoxidil is a potent oral vasodilator. The side effects of minoxidil include hypertrichosis, tachycardia, and fluid retention.

Diazoxide is a potent intravenous vasodilator. It is highly protein bound and therefore has a long half-life. Diazoxide has a rapid onset of action and is used primarily for hypertensive crisis[163,164]. The side effects include hypotension and hyperglycemia[165]. Hypotension may be avoided if smaller, more frequent boluses are given, such as 1 mg/kg times five doses. Furosemide should be given after diazoxide to decrease fluid and sodium retention.

When choosing which antihypertensive medication to use in a hypertensive patient, the following criteria should be considered: (1) severity of hypertension, (2) route of administration, (3) risk of bronchospasm limiting beta blocker use, and (4) a history or suspicion of renal artery stenosis contraindicating ACE inhibitor use.

Hypertensive Emergency

Hypertensive emergencies require blood pressure management within hours. They include hypertension-induced cardiac failure or pulmonary edema, hypertensive encephalopathy, hypertension from pheochromocytoma, hypertension with intracranial hemorrhage, or hypertension induced blindness[166]. Hypertensive encephalopathy can occur when the mean arterial pressure exceeds autoregulation capability of the cerebral vessels[167]. The differential diagnosis of hypertensive encephalopathy includes consideration of encephalitis, intracranial hemorrhage or thrombosis, tumor, and pseudotumor cerebri. Evaluation of a hypertensive emergency is similar to evaluating other forms of hypertension. A renal cause needs to be ruled out immediately. Disorders of the CNS should be examined. An ECG or echocardiogram can discern cardiac complications from hypertension.

Therapy for hypertensive emergency needs to be initiated immediately. The patient should be monitored in the ICU. Frequent automated blood pressures should be available or an arterial line may be necessary. One author recommends decreasing the blood pressure by one-third of the planned reduction in the first 6 hours, by one-third over the next 12 to 36 hours, and by the final third over the next 48 hours.[167a]

Nitroprusside is one of the first-line drugs for hypertensive crisis. A continuous infusion beginning at 0.5 μg/kg/minute to a maximum of 8 to 10 μg/kg/minute. As previously stated, thiocyanate levels need to be measured if a prolonged course of nitroprusside is required. Nitroprusside has a rapid onset and is effective for only minutes, allowing for accurate control of blood pressure.

Labetalol is a combined alpha and beta blocker. Although often effective in moderate blood pressure disturbances, potency is usually insufficient for severe, sustained hypertension. Labetalol is given first in loading doses of 0.25 mg/kg, repeated incrementally to a total of 1 mg/kg. A continuous intravenous infusion at a rate of 1 to 3 mg/kg/hour is then convenient until blood pressure control is obtained. Labetalol has a gradual onset and may be well controlled. Side effects include dizziness, gastrointestinal upset, headaches, and urinary retention. Like all beta blockers, labetalol may precipitate bronchospasm in asthmatic patients. Bradycardia may be reversed by atropine.

Diazoxide is usually very effective in treating hypertensive emergencies. Administration of diazoxide requires rapid intravenous infusion. Hypotension, a side effect of diazoxide, can be avoided if smaller amounts, such as 1 mg/kg, are given repeatedly.

Intravenous enalaprilat has been effective in treating hypertensive emergencies in adults. There does not appear to be any increased benefit to using an ACE inhibitor in this clinical situation. Phentolamine is an alpha blocker that is administered intravenously. It has a short but rapid onset of action, and is particularly useful for patients with a suspected pheochromocytoma.

Nifedipine[(168)] and hydralazine have both been shown to be effective in hypertensive crisis. A limitation of nifedipine is that oral or sublingual administration does not allow for accurate dosing or control of the rate of blood pressure reduction. The dosage limitation is particularly marked in smaller children.

RENAL TRANSPLANTATION

Renal Transplantation in Infants and Children

Renal transplantation has long been recognized as the treatment of choice for children with chronic renal failure[(169)]. Although there have been marked improvements in the technique of chronic dialysis, this form of treatment remains an incomplete therapy for children with end-stage renal disease. Neither hemodialysis nor peritoneal dialysis provides a continuously normal metabolic state for these children. Furthermore, despite marked improvements in these treatments provided by the recent addition of recombinant human erythropoietin[(170)] and recombinant human growth hormone[(171)], children receiving chronic dialysis generally do not grow and develop normally[(172,173)]. Thus, dialysis is generally regarded as a bridge to transplantation. The majority of children with chronic renal failure undergo a course of treatment with chronic dialysis before receiving a renal transplant[(173)]. Nonetheless, virtually all of these children ultimately are considered candidates for renal transplantation.

End-stage renal disease is uncommon in children, with the annual incidence estimated at about 2.5 new cases in children under 18 years of age per million base population[(174)]. Thus, less than 1,000 children have end-stage renal disease in the United States annually. The causes of chronic renal failure are substantially different for children than they are for adults and vary by age. Approximately 25% of end-stage renal disease cases are in children less than 5 years old[(173)]. Among these children, congenital disorders, such as obstructive uropathy, renal dysplasia, other structural abnormalities, and congenital nephrotic syndrome comprise the leading diagnoses[(173)]. In the older patients, acquired renal diseases, such as focal segmental glomerulosclerosis, chronic glomerulonephritis, and reflux nephropathy, predominate. Approximately 60% of all pediatric renal transplant recipients are boys, probably because the causes of end-stage renal disease are more common in young males[(173)].

Although infants and very young children comprise only a small percentage of pediatric renal transplants, their treatment requires special attention[(175)]. Mortality rates for both dialysis and renal transplantation are substantially higher for children less than 2 years of age[(173)]. The reasons for increased morbidity and mortality are probably related to their susceptibility to particular infections, as well as to the technical complications of the procedures themselves[(175)].

The use of living donors provides important advantages in patient and graft survival, particularly for young infants[(173,175,176)]. Since living donors are typically parents, the donor is generally adult. Even if a cadaver donor is used, there are reasons to avoid young donors, particularly for small infants[(177)]; thus, the usual donor for a young infant is an adult. In addition to the obvious technical problems of simply fitting an adult kidney into the abdomen of an infant, mismatches in blood flow to the transplanted graft, compared with what it had received in the donor, produces an opportunity for graft dysfunction, hypertension, and possibly graft thrombosis. Appropriate postoperative care in these patients requires special consideration and experience.

Pediatric recipients of renal transplants are at particular risk for loss of graft function from acute irreversible rejection episodes[(178)] and from graft thrombosis[(179)]. In older children and adults, the incidence of acute rejection is at least 50%, but most of these episodes are treatable and reversible. In children less than 2 years of age, between 25 and 50% of acute rejection episodes are irreversible, and in those aged 2 to 5, up to 10% are irreversible[(178)]. Reasons for poor outcome of acute rejection episodes in children may be related to the immune reactivity of children[(180)], the severity of the rejection episodes, or perhaps to delays in diagnosis and treatment. Furthermore, thrombosis is a unique cause of graft failure in young children. It rarely occurs in adult recipients but may represent up to 15% of graft failures, particularly in young recipients[(179,181)].

More complete descriptions of the transplant process, techniques, and outcome can be found in other sources[(182)]. The remainder of this section deals with only those components of transplant that are provided in the ICU, including the immediate perioperative treatment of the pediatric transplant recipient and the care of children with serious posttransplant infections.

Perioperative Treatment

Fluid and Electrolyte Management

Adequate perfusion of the transplanted graft is an essential component of successful posttransplant management of the pediatric recipient, particularly of infants. As indicated above, the risk of thrombosis of the transplanted organ is substantial, particularly when either the donor or recipient is young[(179)]. Thus, careful monitoring of blood pressure and central venous pressure are extremely important[(181,183)]. Blood pressure should be maintained at least at the upper limits of normal for age. Central venous pressure is typically maintained between 8 to 12 mm Hg.

Fluid management is generally provided by separate replacement solutions for different sources of output. For example, calculated insensible losses can be replaced by 5% dextrose solutions. Urine output is generally replaced initially by half normal saline. Subsequent changes in concentration can be guided by frequent assessment of urinary electrolyte concentrations. Generally, a 1 : 1 replacement of urine volume is maintained for at least the first 2 to 3 days postoperatively. Nasogastric output is replaced as usual. Drainage from other sources, particularly surgical drains, must also be replaced. Patients who had previously been treated with chronic peritoneal dialysis often continue to have substantial losses from the peritoneal space, particularly if it was disrupted by the transplant surgery, such as in the case of infants. Peritoneal losses must be replaced by at least isotonic solutions and perhaps by albumin. Assessment of the patient is achieved by frequent monitoring of serum electrolytes, osmolality, and body weight. Frequently, total body water is expanded by 10% in the first few days postoperatively.

Subsequent management in patients who have regained good renal function permits slow removal of this excess fluid over several days. Typically, this is achieved by replacing only a fraction of the urine output to keep the patient in a negative balance each day. When this is undertaken, the patient must not be allowed to lose an excessive amount of fluid each day. For example, a 10 kg child who received an adult kidney may be producing 5 liters of urine on the second postoperative day. Replacement of three-fourths of this urine output may produce a negative fluid deficit of 1.25 liters in a single day. That volume would represent more than a 10% decrease in total body weight, which may be excessive.

Some patients do not have immediate graft function after surgery. The incidence of acute tubular necrosis is higher in cadaveric than in living donor transplantation[(173)]. The incidence rises substantially when the cold ischemia time exceeds 24 hours[(173)]. Also, young infants, in whom vascular anastomosis may be difficult and for whom, therefore, warm ischemia time is excessive, are also at high risk. In these cases, postoperative dialysis may be necessary for several days or weeks. The usual indications and techniques of dialysis are applicable, but excessive ultrafiltration must be avoided to reduce the risk of poor perfusion to the graft. If patients have had pretransplant peritoneal dialysis, the peritoneal catheter is often not removed, particularly if there is a high risk of acute tubular necrosis. Peritoneal dialysis may be continued, using the same techniques that had been used before transplant. Complications may arise in small infants because of the large mass of the transplanted kidney and because of pain associated with the surgical incision. Hemodialysis is also possible in all infants, using dual-lumen catheters[(122,184)]. Particular attention must be directed at avoiding hypotension resulting from either high blood flow rates or excessive ultrafiltration during dialysis. As is the case with all infants, the use of ultrafiltration controlling devices is mandatory in these circumstances[(122,184)]. CVVH may be used for gentle ultrafiltration but, as indicated previously, the risk of bleeding secondary to continuous heparinization is increased in the postoperative patient. During all of these procedures, infusion of normal saline or albumin may be necessary when hypotension occurs.

Immunosuppression

All transplant patients require substantial immunosuppression to prevent or treat acute rejection episodes. The immunosuppression delivered in the first 1 to 2 weeks after transplant is often referred to as "induction" therapy. Most patients receive high-dose induction therapy and then have gradual reduction in doses of many medications to reach "maintenance" levels of immunosuppression several months later. Currently, maintenance immunosuppression generally consists of prednisone, azathioprine, and cyclosporine. Several new drugs, including FK506[(185)] and mycophenolate mofietel[(186)], are just being introduced for renal transplant recipients.

Antibodies directed towards human leukocyte antigens have often been used as induction therapy for renal transplantation. The use of "antibody induction" has been controversial, and few controlled trials have occurred, despite widespread use. Substantial benefits of antibody induction therapy, particularly in young infants, have been suggested from retrospective analysis of pediatric registry data. Nonetheless, carefully controlled trials have only recently begun. Multiple preparations have been used in the past. Many of these have been comprised of horse antihuman lymphocyte globulin[(183)] ("Minnesota ALG", "ATGAM"). These are polychronal antibodies that are derived from injection of human lymphocytes into horses. The serum is harvested from the horses, and the globulin preparation is purified. Other sources, such as rabbit antithymocyte serum, have also been used[(187)]. Although many preparations seem to be highly effective, lot-to-lot variation has produced variable results. Complications, such as anemia or thrombocytopenia caused by concurrent presence of antibodies to these elements, have also limited usefulness of these substances.

A monoclonal antibody directed against the T3 antigen on mature human peripheral lymphocytes, known as OKT3, has been used for both prophylactic and antirejection therapy in organ transplant recipients[(188,189)]. The precise mechanism of OKT3 in causing immunosuppression is somewhat controversial, since the antibody does not seem to result in lysis of the target cells. Nonetheless, its effectiveness in causing striking levels of temporary immunosuppression is not disputed. OKT3, however, does have complications. The most serious for the intensivist is the "first-use" reaction[190]. Administration of OKT3, particularly to patients with a substantial percentage of primed circulating lymphocytes, often provokes release of multiple lymphokines from these cells. This results in a shock-like state, including hypotension, high fever, and pulmonary edema. Thus, particular attention to respiratory status and avoidance of severe fluid overload in patients receiving the first several doses of OKT3 is imperative. Often, patients who are receiving prophylactic OKT3 receive the first dose intraoperatively while they are still intubated. Careful attention to pretreatment control of respiratory status has lessened the frequency of serious first-dose reaction substantially[190,191]. Subsequent doses of this agent have few immediate side effects. When antibody induction therapy is provided, concurrent treatment with azathioprine and cyclosporine is often delayed, but prednisone is usually provided concurrently.

Alternatively, many programs use cyclosporine[192] or FK506[185] rather than antibody induction in the first few days. In these cases, intravenous infusion of the agents is often necessary because oral administration may be unsuccessful as a result of postoperative ileus and poor absorption. In these cases, avoidance of a high serum level of these agents is important, since each of them is nephrotoxic. Protocols using constant low-dose infusion are often used. Although there is some concern about increased incidence or severity of nephrotoxicity related to intravenous administration, there is little substantial evidence for this phenomenon. Provision of concurrent calcium channel blockers such as nifedipine seem to ameliorate nephrotoxicity[192].

Although most acute rejection episodes can be successfully treated and reversed, prevention is preferable. Provision of immunosuppression drugs must be consistent, and careful monitoring of their efficacy is important. Lack of sufficient administration of cyclosporine and FK506 may be assessed by frequent monitoring of trough blood levels. Total peripheral lymphocyte counts can be assessed when antilymphocyte preparations are provided. Assessment of circulating T3 positive cells is important if OKT3 preparations are used.

Newer monoclonal antibodies directed at other specific targets are currently under investigation, but information about their efficacy, particularly in children, is lacking.

Many of the immunosuppressant agents have immediate complications, which also must be monitored. Corticosteroid medications often cause hypertension, sodium retention, and hyperglycemia. Cyclosporine and FK506 administration have been associated with hyperkalemia, decreased GFR, and hypertension. Careful monitoring and treatment of these complications is necessary, but decreasing doses [or elimination] of the drugs because of the complications should be avoided.

Treatment of Rejection Episodes

Despite adequate prophylactic immunosuppression, the majority of pediatric transplant patients have at least one acute rejection episode[173]. These episodes are associated with the infiltration of lymphocytes into the graft. In the immediate posttransplant period, the clinical symptoms include fever, swelling of the graft, tenderness over the graft site, decreased urine output, and rising serum creatinine levels, associated with diminished graft function. In these circumstances, multiple tests are often obtained, such as renal ultrasound or renal nuclear medicine scan. These studies are designed to detect causes for these symptoms other than rejection, such as obstruction of the graft, urinary leak, and others. None of these tests, however, produce clear evidence of rejection. Thus, diagnosis of rejection is often based on the clinical signs and symptoms and sometimes is confirmed by percutaneous graft biopsy. Rejection must always be included in differential diagnosis of posttransplant fever. In the pediatric patient, particularly very small infants who receive an adult kidney, decreases in renal function are often difficult to ascertain in the early stages of rejection. Thus, heightened suspicion must be maintained to avoid having a rejection episode remain untreated for a long period. Unfortunately, rejection episodes in young infants are more often irreversible than in older patients. The reasons for this irreversible nature of rejection episodes are not clear but may be related to delays in diagnosis.

As indicated, rejection episodes are most often reversible if diagnosed quickly. Treatment with either pulse corticosteroids (Solumedrol, 25 mg /kg daily for 3 days) or antilymphocyte preparations, such as ATGAM or OKT3. In most of these cases, provision of antirejection therapy leads to a rapid decrease in symptoms such as fever and graft tenderness. Depending on the severity of the rejection episode, the graft may suffer acute tubular necrosis, and recovery of renal function is often delayed. Assessment of whether the rejection episode has been reversed in these cases is sometimes difficult. Repeated or therapeutically unresponsive rejection episodes are sometimes treated by changes to other immunosuppressant medication such as FK506.

Graft Thrombosis

Graft thrombosis is, unfortunately, much more common in pediatric renal transplant recipients than in adults[179]. It accounts for 13% of graft failures in pediatric recipients. Overall, primary nonfunction, vascular thrombosis, or miscellaneous technical causes occur in 4.4% of pediatric transplants[179]. Despite increasing knowledge about the risk of graft thrombosis, the incidence does not seem to have changed substantially in the past decade.

For pediatric cadaver donor transplants, the incidence of graft thrombosis is principally related to young donor age[179]. A recent change in the United States allocation system has led to a decreased use of young donors, particularly for young recipients[193]. For living donor transplant recipients, the young recipient age seems to be associated with a much higher incidence of graft thrombosis[179]. The precise causes for thrombosis in these patients remain unclear. The large mismatch, however, between the cardiac output of the young recipient and the usual blood flow expected by an adult kidney probably are related to this phenomenon. Patients at highest risk are those who become volume-depleted or hypotensive during or after the transplant procedure; those patients who have acute tubular necrosis and subsequent swelling and increased pressure within the graft; and those for whom perfusion of the graft may be compromised. In this latter group, young infants who retain their own native kidneys or those who have high urine output from the kidneys may be at particular risk. Lack of pretransplant donor nephrectomy has not been associated with increased risk of graft thrombosis, but those who did not have any pretransplant dialysis may be at a higher risk[179].

Avoidance of young cadaver donors for infant recipients seems to be particularly important in preventing graft thrombosis. Meticulous attention to fluid and electrolyte management, maintenance of adequate perfusion of the graft, and avoidance of procedures that may compromise perfusion of the graft are key. Anticoagulation, in the form of low-dose heparin infusions, is currently being tested in some transplant programs. Unfortunately, once graft thrombosis has occurred, recovery of renal function is almost never achieved.

Posttransplant Infections

Immunosuppressed renal transplant recipients are at particularly high risk for opportunistic infections, which are the reason for 26% of the hospitalizations of pediatric recipients in the first 6 months after transplant and approximately 10% to 15% thereafter[173]. Infection represents approximately 40% of the causes of mortality in pediatric transplant recipients. Three infections deserve particular comment.

Cytomegalovirus (CMV) infection has serious sequelae in immunocompromised hosts. For renal transplant recipients, the most severe disease is found in recipients who had never been exposed to the virus before transplant and who receive a graft from a donor who had previously been infected with it. The CMV-negative recipient/CMV-positive donor group is at highest risk for occurrence of posttransplant CMV disease and has the most severe symptoms and the highest mortality[194]. Pediatric recipients, who would be more likely to be CMV-negative, may be at much higher risk, particularly if they receive grafts from adult donors. Multiple approaches have been proposed to prevent severe CMV disease. The provision of high titer CMV gammaglobulin to CMV-negative recipients of CMV-positive grafts has been shown to be safe and effective[195]. Generally, this procedure does not prevent disease but ameliorates its severity. The use of oral acyclovir in these patients may also prevent disease, but there is significant controversy about its efficacy[196,197]. Provision of intravenous ganciclovir, particularly at the time of treatment with antilymphocyte antibody preparations, is currently under study. Treatment of severe CMV disease with intravenous ganciclovir has been shown to be efficacious in most recipients[198,199]. This treatment is often given to leukopenic patients who have high fevers, but it is clearly indicated in patients with visceral involvement, including those with pneumonia, hepatitis, or enteritis.

Varicellavirus infection is generally mild in normal children but may be severe or even fatal in children receiving immunosuppressant medications[200]. Children who have not had chicken pox before transplantation should receive varicella zoster immune globulin (VZIG) at the time of any exposure if they are receiving immunosuppression. Provision of oral acyclovir to these patients during the incubation period is currently under study. Treatment with intravenous acyclovir is currently warranted if patients have clinical disease[201]. Unfortunately, even aggressive and early treatment is sometimes insufficient for patients who present with visceral varicella disease[200]. The efficacy of pretransplant varicella vaccine is not yet known, but susceptible patients probably should be appropriately vaccinated before immunosuppression.

Pneumocystis carinii pneumonia occurs in about 3% of all renal transplant recipients, including children. This disease usually has an onset 2 to 6 months after transplantation. Patients typically present with fever, tachypnea, and moderately severe hypoxia without cough or dyspnea. Diagnosis is often suspected on the basis of characteristic x-ray findings and can be verified by bronchial washing or even analysis of sputum[202,203]. Treatment consists of intravenous trimethoprim-sulfamethoxazole or pentamidine[204] and is usually successful. Most renal transplant recipients receive trimethoprim-sulfamethoxazole prophylaxis in the first several months after transplantation. Prophylaxis can be achieved with aerosolized pentamidine, but this form of prevention is generally not applicable to young infants.

HEPATORENAL SYNDROME

Pathophysiology

Renal failure following liver failure has been described for many years[205]. Hepatorenal syndrome (HRS) is renal failure with liver failure when no other source of renal insufficiency can be found, such as in acute tubular necrosis, prerenal azotemia, or obstructive nephropathy. The cause of hepatorenal syndrome remains elusive, but more recent advances have helped identify the pathologic mechanisms.

The typical clinical scenario of hepatorenal syndrome is a patient with cirrhosis, ascites, and progressive renal insufficiency. Unfortunately, renal disease is not uncommon in patients with liver disease, and distinguishing between HRS and other causes of renal insufficiency may be difficult. Commonly, the patient who has HRS sustained a precipitating event resulting in decreased intravascular volume (e.g., gastrointestinal bleeding, aggressive diuresis, paracentesis) or nephrotoxin exposure[206]. However, HRS can occur without a precipitating event[206].

The hallmarks of HRS are an intense, functional vasoconstriction of the renal vasculature and decreased renal perfusion with preservation of tubular function. Renal vasoconstriction has been revealed with labeled xenon washout and selected renal arteriograms[(207)]. In the HRS, there is a reduction in xenon washout and marked renal vasoconstriction, particularly to cortical nephrons. Postmortem renal arteriogram shows a return of renal vasculature architecture. Doppler ultrasound typically demonstrates an increased intrarenal resistive index in patients with HRS[(205)]. The vasoconstriction is described as functional because as the liver disease is repaired, the renal insufficiency improves. A patient who receives a functioning liver transplant may experience improvement of their renal disease[(208)]. Also, a kidney transplanted from a patient with HRS may function normally in a patient without HRS[(209)]. Patients with HRS avidly reabsorb sodium and water; urine is often concentrated. The plasma renin and aldosterone levels are often elevated. A low urine sodium level and high urine specific gravity or osmolarity in patients with HRS may be helpful in distinguishing between HRS and ATN[(206)].

Several mechanisms have been described for HRS[(205,206)]. Two principal theories are currently entertained. A variation or combination of both concepts occurs in most patients with HRS. The first is the "underfill" theory. Patients with HRS are believed to be relatively depleted in intravascular volume. The term "relative" refers to not only the intravascular volume decrease but also a decrease in peripheral vasoconstriction and SVR. The intravascular depletion and decrease in SVR lead to a decrease in renal perfusion and subsequently in renal vasoconstriction. As would be expected, patients with HRS have high plasma renin, A2, aldosterone, and endothelin levels. The decrease in SVR may be caused by a number of factors, none of which have been completely defined. Endotoxin, nitric oxide, vasoactive intestinal peptide, prostacyclin, and bradykinin may play a role in lowering SVR in patients with HRS. Regardless, avid sodium reabsorption begins before ascites appears and suggests that a decrease in the SVR occurs before volume depletion[(206)].

The second hypothesis is the "overflow" theory, in which avid sodium and water reabsorption occur. Abnormal Starling forces in the portal venous bed and a decreased oncotic pressure combined with an expanded intravascular volume from sodium reabsorption result in ascites. Also, there is an increase in sympathetic renal nerve activity resulting in renal vasoconstriction.

Differential Diagnosis

Distinguishing HRS from ATN and prerenal azotemia may be difficult. Patients with HRS have the characteristic laboratory findings of volume depletion and renal vasoconstriction, which are low urine sodium, high urine osmolality, high urine-to-plasma osmolality, and high BUN to creatinine ratio. These results are in contrast to ATN, in which the urine sodium is elevated (>30 mEq/L); urine osmolality is similar to serum osmolality; and there is a low urine-to-plasma osmolality and low BUN to creatinine ratio (less than 20:1). Unfortunately, prerenal azotemia has the same urinary and serum findings as HRS. Prerenal azotemia usually responds to volume repletion, whereas HRS may not. Volume repletion may not be accurate in distinguishing HRS from prerenal azotemia because often patients with liver failure and altered Starling forces in their intravascular space require large-volume colloid replacement to adequately improve their volume status.

Renal vasoconstriction is mediated by the following mechanisms: the RAS[(210,211)], renal prostaglandins[(212,213)] and thromboxane[(214,215)], endothelin[(216)], sympathetic nerve activity[(217)], and nitric oxide[(218)]. The pathogenesis of HRS depends on these humoral and neuronal factors combined with intravascular depletion and depressed SVR. Patients with HRS often have a decreased urinary prostaglandin-to-thromboxane ratio[(215)], elevated plasma renin level[(210)], elevated endothelin level[(216)], and increased sympathetic nerve activity[(217)]. Endotoxin release from the gastrointestinal tract and nitric oxide production cause peripheral vasodilatation and subsequently decrease renal perfusion and renal vasoconstriction. All of these mechanisms have been implicated in HRS.

Treatment

Attempts to improve outcome in HRS have been dismal; the syndrome is considered universally fatal[(205,206)]. Two aspects of therapy are particularly important. First is prevention. Prevention of volume depletion (by avoiding aggressive diuresis, paracentesis, or hemorrhage) and avoidance of nephrotoxic agents may decrease progression to HRS. Patients with cirrhosis are particularly sensitive to NSAIDS and may have significant worsening of their renal function from taking these medications[(206)]. Monitoring volume status with central venous access is critical to proper fluid management. Second, orthotopic liver transplantation and improvement of liver disease improves HRS. Other attempts to improve outcome in HRS have not been found to be practical or successful. Peritoneovenous shunts may improve central venous pressure and intravascular volume, but long-term outcome is not improved[(219,220)]. Dialysis may be used in patients in whom improvement of liver disease is expected, as in patients expecting liver transplantation. Head-out water immersion may improve urine output and renal perfusion but are not practical as a long-term modality[(206)]. Prevention and liver transplantation remain the mainstay of therapy.

References

1. Rose B. Renal physiology, Part 2. In: Rose B, ed. Clinial physiology of acid-base and electrolyte disorders. 2nd ed. New York: McGraw-Hill, 1984:45.
2. Spitzer A. Renal physiology and functional development. In: Edelmann C, ed. Pediatric kidney disease. Boston: Little, Brown, 1978:25–128.
3. Jose PA, Slotkoff LM, Montgomery S, et al. Autoregulation of renal blood flow in the puppy. Am J Physiol 1975;229:983.
4. Chevalier RL, Kaiser DL. Autoregulation of renal blood flow in the rat: effects of growth and uninephrectomy. Am J Physiol 1983;244.

5. Peart WS. Renin-angiotensin system. [Review]. N Engl J Med 1975;292:302.
6. Haber E. The renin-angiotensin system and hypertension. [Review]. Kidney Int 1979;15:427.
7. Casellas D, Carmines PK, Navar LG. Microvascular reactivity of in vitro blood perfused juxtamedullary nephrons from rats. Kidney Int 1985;28:752.
8. Navar LG, Rosivall L. Contribution of the renin-angiotensin system to the control of intrarenal hemodynamics. Kidney Int 1984;25:857.
9. Douglas JG. Angiotensin receptor subtypes of the kidney cortex. [Review]. Am J Physiol 1987.
10. Denton KM, Fennessy PA, Alcorn D, et al. Morphometric analysis of the actions of angiotensin II on renal arterioles and glomeruli. Am J Physiol 1992;262:F367–372.
11. Chevalier RL, Carey RM, Kaiser DL. Endogenous prostaglandins modulate autoregulation of renal blood flow in young rats. Am J Physiol 1987;253:F66–75.
12. Schnermann J, Briggs JP. Participation of renal cortical prostaglandins in the regulation of glomerular filtration rate. [Review]. Kidney Int 1981;19:802.
13. Schnermann J, Briggs JP, Weber PC. Tubuloglomerular feedback, prostaglandins, and angiotensin in the autoregulation of glomerular filtration rate. Kidney Int 1984;25:53.
14. Bachmann S, Mundel P. Nitric oxide in the kidney: synthesis, localization, and function. [Review]. Am J Kidney Dis 1994;24:112.
15. Bachmann S, Bosse HM, Mundel P. Topography of nitric oxide synthesis by localizing constitutive NO synthases in mammalian kidney. Am J Physiol 1995;268:F885–98.
16. Tojo A, Gross SS, Zhang L, et al. Immunocytochemical localization of distinct isoforms of nitric oxide synthase in the juxtaglomerular apparatus of normal rat kidney. J Am Soc Nephrol 1994;4:1438.
17. Wilcox CS, Welch WJ, Murad F, et al. Nitric oxide synthase in macula densa regulates glomerular capillary pressure. Proc Nat Acad Sci–USA 1992;89:11993.
18. Baylis C, Harton P, Engels K. Endothelial derived relaxing factor controls renal hemodynamics in the normal rat kidney. J Am Soc Nephrol 1990;1:875.
19. King AJ, Brenner BM. Endothelium-derived vasoactive factors and the renal vasculature. [Review]. Am J Physiol 1991.
20. King AJ, Brenner BM, Anderson S. Endothelin: a potent renal and systemic vasoconstrictor peptide. Am J Physiol 1989;256:F1051–8.
21. Luscher TF, Bock HA, Yang ZH, et al. Endothelium-derived relaxing and contracting factors: perspectives in nephrology (editorial). (Review). Kidney Int 1991;39:575.
22. Lahera V, Salom MG, Fiksen OM, et al. Mediatory role of endothelium-derived nitric oxide in renal vasodilatory and excretory effects of bradykinin. Am J Hypertens 1991.
23. Radermacher J, Klanke B, Kastner S, et al. Effect of arginine depletion on glomerular and tubular kidney function: studies in isolated perfused rat kidneys. Am J Physiol 1991.
24. Radermacher J, Klanke B, Schurek HJ, et al. Importance of NO/EDRF for glomerular and tubular function: studies in the isolated perfused rat kidney. Kidney Int 1992;41:1549.
25. Mundel P, Bachmann S, Bader M, et al. Expression of nitric oxide synthase in kidney macula densa cells. Kidney Int 1992;42:1017.
26. Yanagisawa M, Kurihara H, Kimura S, et al. A novel potent vasoconstrictor peptide produced by vascular endothelial cells. Nature 1988;332:411.
27. Yanagisawa M, Masaki T. Endothelin, a novel endothelium-derived peptide. Pharmacological activities, regulation and possible roles in cardiovascular control. (Review). Biochem Pharmacol 1989;38:1877.
28. Pernow J, Hemsen A, Lundberg JM. Tissue specific distribution, clearance and vascular effects of endothelin in the pig. Biochem Biophys Res Comm 1989;161:647.
29. Shibouta Y, Suzuki N, Shino A, et al. Pathophysiological role of endothelin in acute renal failure. Life Sciences 1990;46:1611.
30. Zeidel ML, Brady HR, Kone BC, et al. Endothelin, a peptide inhibitor of Na(+)-K(+)-ATPase in intact renaltubular epithelial cells. Am J Physiol 1989;257:1101-1107.
31. Fukuda Y, Hirata Y, Yoshimi H, et al. Endothelin is a potent secretagogue for atrial natriuretic peptide in cultured rat atrial myocytes. Biochem Biophys Res Comm 1988;155:167.
32. Fukuda Y, Hirata Y, Taketani S, et al. Endothelin stimulates accumulations of cellular atrial natriuretic peptide and its messenger RNA in rat cardiocytes. Biochem Biophys Res Comm 1989;164:1431.
33. Gellai M, Jugus M, Fletcher T, et al. Reversal of postischemic acute renal failure with a selective endothelinA receptor antagonist in the rat. J Clin Invest 1994;93:900.
34. Brodde OE. Vascular dopamine receptors: Demonstration and characterization by in vitro studies. (Review). Life Sciences 1982; 31:289.
35. Goldberg LI. Dopamine—clinical uses of an endogenous catecholamine. (Review). N Eng J Med 1974;291:707.
36. Goldberg LI. Cardiovascular and renal actions of dopamine: potential clinical applications. (Review). Pharmacol Rev 1972;24:1.
37. Kapusta DR, Robie NW. Plasma dopamine in regulation of canine renal blood flow. Am J Physiol 1988;255:R379–87.
38. Siragy HM, Felder RA, Howell NL, et al. Evidence that intrarenal dopamine acts as a paracrine substance at the renal tubule. Am J Physiol 1989;257:F467–77.
39. Seri I, Kone BC, Gullans SR, et al. Locally formed dopamine inhibits Na+-K+-ATPase activity in rat renal cortical tubule cells. Am J Physiol 1988;255:F666–73.
40. Maddox DA, Deen WM, Brenner BM. Dynamics of glomerular ultrafiltration. VI. Studies in the primate. Kidney Int 1974;5:271.
41. Deen WM, Troy JL, Robertson CR, et al. Dynamics of glomerular ultrafiltration in the rat. IV. Determination of the ultrafiltration coefficient. J Clin Invest 1973;52:1500.
42. Brenner BM, Humes HD. Mechanics of glomerular ultrafiltration. N Eng J Med 1977;297:148.
43. Brenner BM, Hostetter TH, Humes HD. Molecular basis of proteinuria of glomerular origin. N Eng J Med 1978;298:826.
44. Renkin EM, Robinson RR. Glomerular filtration. (Review). N Eng J Med 1974;290:785.
45. Rector FJ. Sodium, bicarbonate, and chloride absorption by the proximal tubule. (Review). Am J Physiol 1983;244.
46. Grantham JJ. The renal sodium pump and vanadate. (Review). Am J Physiol 1980;239.
47. Katz AI. Renal Na-K-ATPase: its role in tubular sodium and potassium transport. Am J Physiol 1982;242.
48. Cogan MG. Disorders of proximal nephron function. (Review). Am J of Med 1982;72:275.
49. Kurtzman NA, Pillay VK. Renal reabsorption of glucose in health and disease. Arch Intern Med 1973;131:901.
50. Carone FA, Peterson DR. Hydrolysis and transport of small peptides by the proximal tubule. (Review). Am J Physiol 1980;238.
51. Jones DP, Chesney RW. Tubular Function. In: Holliday MA, Barratt TM, Avner ED, eds. Pediatric Nephrology. 3rd ed. Baltimore: Williams and Wilkins, 1994:117.
52. Celsi G, Aperia A. Sodium, chloride, and water excretion. In: Holliday MA, Barratt TM, Avner ED, eds. Pediatric Nephrology. 3rd ed. Baltimore: Williams and Wilkins, 1994:99.
53. Brezis M, Rosen S. Hypoxia of the renal medulla—its implications for disease. (Review). N Eng J Med 1995;332:647.
54. Schwartz GJ. General principles of acid-base physiology. In: Holliday MA, Barratt TM, Avner ED, eds. Pediatric Nephrology. 3rd ed. Baltimore: Williams and Wilkins, 1994:222.
55. Rocha AS, Kudo LH. Water, urea, sodium, chloride, and potassium transport in the in vitro isolated perfused papillary collecting duct. (Review). Kidney Int 1982;22:485.
56. Stokes JB, Ingram MJ, Williams AD, et al. Heterogeneity of the rabbit collecting tubule: localization of mineralocorticoid hormone action to the cortical portion. Kidney Int 1981;20:340.
57. Stokes JB. Ion transport by the cortical and outer medullary collecting tubule. [Review]. Kidney Int 1982;22:473.
58. Winters RW. Maintenance Fluid Therapy. In: Winters RW, ed. The body fluids in pediatrics. 1st ed. Boston: Little, Brown, 1973:113.
59. Holliday MA, Segar WE. Maintenance need for water in parenteral fluid therapy. Pediatrics 1957;19.
60. Guido KM, Devarajan P, Boydstun II, et al. Acute renal failure. In: Holliday MA, Barratt TM, Avner ED, eds. Pediatric nephrology. 3rd ed. Baltimore: Williams and Wilkins, 1994:1176.
61. Gomez CF, Maroto AE, Galinanes M, et al. Acute renal failure associated with cardiac surgery. Child Nephrol Urol 1988;9:138.
62. Shaw NJ, Brocklebank JT, Dickinson DF, et al. Long-term outcome for children with acute renal failure following cardiac surgery. Int J Cardiol 1991;31:161.
63. John EG, Levitsky S, Hastreiter AR. Management of acute renal failure complicating cardiac surgery in infants and children. Crit Care Med 1980;8:562.

64. Woodrow G, Turney JH. Cause of death in acute renal failure. Nephrol Dial Transplant 1992;7:230.
65. Bullock ML, Umen AJ, Finkelstein M, et al. The assessment of risk factors in 462 patients with acute renal failure. Am J Kidney Dis 1985;5:97.
66. Corwin HL, Teplick RS, Schreiber MJ, et al. Prediction of outcome in acute renal failure. Am J Nephrol 1987;7:8.
67. Chew SL, Lins RL, Daelemans R, et al. Outcome in acute renal failure. (Review). Nephrol Dial Transplant 1993;8:101.
68. Hakim RM, Wingard RL, Parker RA. Effect of the dialysis membrane in the treatment of patients with acute renal failure. N Eng J Med 1994;331:1338.
69. Maher ER, Robinson KN, Scoble JE, et al. Prognosis of critically-ill patients with acute renal failure: APACHE II score and other predictive factors. Quart J Med 1989;72:857.
70. Anderson RJ, Linas SL, Berns AS, et al. Nonoliguric acute renal failure. N Eng J Med 1977;296:1134.
71. Anderson RJ, Linas SL, Berns AS, et al. Nonoliguric acute renal failure. N Engl J Med 1968;206:891.
72. Rahman SN, Conger JD. Glomerular and tubular factors in urine flow rates of acute renal failure patients. Am J Kidney Dis 1994;23:788.
73. Rasmussen HH, Ibels LS. Acute renal failure. Multivariate analysis of causes and risk factors. Am J Med 1982;73:211.
74. Hou SH, Bushinsky DA, Wish JB, et al. Hospital-acquired renal insufficiency: a prospective study. Am J Med 1983;74:243.
75. Myers BD, Moran SM. Hemodynamically mediated acute renal failure. (Review). N Eng J Med 1986;314:97.
76. Dixon BS, Anderson RJ. Nonoliguric acute renal failure. (Review). Am J Kidney Dis 1985;6:71.
77. Chevalier RL, Campbell F, Brenbridge AN. Prognostic factors in neonatal acute renal failure. Pediatrics 1984;74:265.
78. Grylack L, Medani C, Hultzen C, et al. Nonoliguric acute renal failure in the newborn: a prospective evaluation of diagnostic indexes. Am J Dis Child 1982;136:518.
79. Kjellstrand CM. Ethacrynic acid in acute tubular necrosis. Indications and effect on the natural course. Nephron 1972;9:337.
80. Kleinknecht D, Ganeval D, Gonzalez-Duque LA, et al. Furosemide in acute oliguric renal failure: a controlled trial. Nephron 1976;17:51.
81. Luke RG, Linton AL, Briggs JD, et al. Mannitol therapy in acute renal failure. Lancet 1965;1:980.
82. Luke RG, Briggs JD, Allison ME, Kennedy AC. Factors determining response to mannitol in acute renal failure. Am J Med Sci 1970;259:168.
83. Cantarovich F, Fernandez JC, Locatelli A, et al. Furosemide in high doses in the treatment of acute renal failure. Postgrad Med J 1971;47:13–7 Suppl.
84. Cantarovich F, Galli C, Benedetti L, et al. High dose furosemide in established acute renal failure. Br Med J 1973;4:449.
85. Cantarovich F, Galli C, Benedetti L, et al. High dose furosemide in established acute renal failure. Br Med J 1973;4:449.
86. Levinsky NG, Berbard DB, Johnston PA. Mannitol and loop diuretics in acute renal failure. In: Brenner BM, Lazarus JM, eds. Acute renal failure. Philadelphia: WB Saunders, 1983:712.
87. Henrich WL, Berl T, McDonald KM, et al. Angiotensin II, renal nerves, and prostaglandins in renal hemodynamics during hemorrhage. Am J Physiol 1978;235.
88. Henrich WL, Anderson RJ, Berns AS, et al. The role of renal nerves and prostaglandins in control of renal hemodynamics and plasma renin activity during hypotensive hemorrhage in the dog. J Clin Invest 1978;61:744.
89. Stein JH, Osgood RW, Boonjarern S, et al. Segmental sodium reabsorption in rats with mild and severe volume depletion. Am J Physiol 1974;227:351.
90. Siegel MJ, St AT, Siegel BA. Imaging techniques in the evaluation of pediatric hypertension. (Review). Ped Nephrol 1987;1:76.
91. Gordon I. Imaging the kidneys and urinary tract. In: Holliday MA, Barratt TM, Avner ED, eds. Pediatric nephrology. 3rd ed. Baltimore: Williams and Wilkins, 1994:421.
92. Rudnick MR, Bastil CP, Elfinbein IB, et al. The differential diagnosis of acute renal failure. In: Brenner BM, Lazarus JM, eds. acute renal failure. Philadelphia: WB Saunders, 1983:176.
93. Passmore JC, Baker CH. Intrarenal blood flow distribution in irreversible hemorrhagic shock in dogs. J Trauma 1973;13:1066.
94. Heyman SN, Brezis M, Greenfeld Z, et al. Protective role of furosemide and saline in radiocontrast-induced acute renal failure in the rat. Am J Kidney Dis 1989;14:377.
95. Bonventre JV. Mechanisms of ischemic acute renal failure (clinical conference). Kidney Int 1993;43:1160.
96. Molitoris BA, Falk SA, Dahl RH. Ischemia-induced loss of epithelial polarity. Role of the tight junction. J Clin Invest 1989;84:1334.
97. Molitoris BA, Nelson WJ. Alterations in the establishment and maintenance of epithelial cell polarity as a basis for disease processes. (Review). J Clin Invest 1990;85:3.
98. Molitoris BA, Geerdes A, McIntosh JR. Dissociation and redistribution of Na+,K(+)-ATPase from its surface membrane actin cytoskeletal complex during cellular ATP depletion. J Clin Invest 1991; 88:462.
99. Mason J, Olbricht C, Takabatake T, et al. The early phase of experimental acute renal failure. I. Intratubular pressure and obstruction. Pflugers Archiv Euro J Physiol 1977;370:155.
100. Duke GJ, Bersten AD. Dopamine and renal salvage in the critically ill patient. (Review). Anaes Int Care 1992;20:277.
101. Duke GJ, Briedis JH, Weaver RA. Renal support in critically ill patients: low-dose dopamine or low-dose dobutamine? Crit Care Med 1994;22:1919.
102. Flancbaum L, Choban PS, Dasta JF. Quantitative effects of low-dose dopamine on urine output in oliguric surgical intensive care unit patients. Crit Care Med 1994;22:61.
103. Baldwin L, Henderson A, Hickman P. Effect of postoperative low-dose dopamine on renal function after elective major vascular surgery. Ann Int Med 1994;120:744.
104. Sutter PM, Thulin G, Stromski M, et al. Beneficial effect of thyroxin in the treatment of ischemic acute renal failure. Ped Nephrol 1988;2:1.
105. Gaudio KM, Siegel NJ. New approaches to the treatment of acute renal failure. (Review). Ped Nephrol 1987;1:339.
106. Conger JD, Falk SA, Hammond WS. Atrial natriuretic peptide and dopamine in established acute renal failure in the rat. Kidney Int 1991;40:21.
107. Rahman SN, Kim GE, Mathew AS, et al. Effects of atrial natriuretic peptide in clinical acute renal failure. Kidney Int 1994;45:1731.
108. Erley CM, Duda SH, Schlepckow S, et al. Adenosine antagonist theophylline prevents the reduction of glomerular filtration rate after contrast media application. Kidney Int 1994;45:1425.
109. Flamenbaum W, Gehr M, Gross M, et al. Acute renal failure associated with myoglobinuria and hemoglobinuria. In: Brenner BM, Lazarus JM, eds. Acute Renal Failure. Philadelphia: WB Saunders Company, 1983:269.
110. Lowenstein J, Faulstick DA, Yiengst MJ, et al. The glomerular clearance and renal transport of hemoglobin in adult males. J Clin Invest 1961;40:1172.
111. Eneas JF, Schoenfeld PY, Humphreys MH. The effect of infusion of mannitol-sodium bicarbonate on the clinical course of myoglobinuria. Arch Int Med 1979;139:801.
112. Corwin HL, Schreiber MJ, Fang LS. Low fractional excretion of sodium. Occurrence with hemoglobinuric- and myoglobinuric-induced acute renal failure. Arch Int Med 1984;144:981.
113. Grossman RA, Hamilton RW, Morse BM. Nontraumatic rhabdomyolysis and acute renal failure. N Eng J Med 1974;291.
114. Martinez-Maldonado M, Benabe JE, Lopez-Novoa JM. Acute renal failure associated with tubulointerstitial disease, including papillary necrosis. In: Brenner BM, Lazarus JM, eds. Acute renal failure. Philadelphia: WB Saunders Company, 1983:434.
115. Feinstein EI, Blumenkrantz MJ, Healy M, et al. Clinical and metabolic responses to parenteral nutrition in acute renal failure. A controlled double-blind study. Medicine 1981;60:124.
116. Takala J. Nutrition in acute renal failure. (Review). Crit Care Clin 1987;3:155.
117. Spinozzi NS, Grupe WE. Nutritional implications of renal disease. IV. Nutritional aspects of chronic renal insufficiency in childhood. J Am Dietetic Assoc 1977;70:493.
117a. Spinozzi, NS: Chronic Renal Disease. In: Queen, PM and Lang, CE (eds) Handbook of Pediatric Nutrition, 1993. Gaithersburg, MD. Aspen Publishing, 471–482.
118. Abel RM, Beck CH Jr, Abbott WM, et al. Improved survival from renal failure after treatment with intravenous essential L-amino acids and glucose. N Engl J Med 1973;288:695.
119. Feinstein EI, Kopple JD, Silberman H, et al. Total parenteral nutrition with high or low nitrogen intakes in patients with acute renal failure. Kidney Int (Suppl) 1983;16:5319–23.
120. Leonard CD, Luke RG, Siegel RR. Parenteral essential amino acids in acute renal failure. Urology 1975;6:154.

121. Alexander SR, Harmon WE, Jabs K. Dialysis in children. In: Henrich WL, ed. Principles and practice of dialysis. Baltimore: Williams and Wilkins, 1994:393.
122. Sadowski RH, Harmon WE, Jabs K. Acute hemodialysis of infants weighing less than five kilograms. Kidney Int 1994;45:903.
123. Sadowski RH, Allred EN, Jabs K. Sodium modeling ameliorates intradialytic and interdialytic symptoms in young hemodialysis patients. J Am Soc Nephrol 1993;4:1192.
124. Aguilera D, Diab N, Faivre JM. Influence of sodium dialysate variation on hemodynamic stability. Kidney Int (Suppl) 1988;25:5187–9.
125. Jenson BM, Dobbe SA, Squillace DP, et al. Clinical benefits of high and variable sodium concentration dialysate in hemodialysis patients. Anna J 1994;21:115.
126. Hakim RM, Breillatt J, Lazarus JM, et al. Complement activation and hypersensitivity reactions to dialysis membranes. N Eng J Med 1984;311:878.
127. Yorgin PD, Krensky AM, Tune BM. Continuous venovenous hemofiltration. Ped Nephrol 1990;4:640.
128. Canaud B, Garred LJ, Christol JP, et al. Pump assisted continuous venovenous hemofiltration for treating acute uremia. Kidney Int (Suppl) 1988;24:5145–6.
129. Bellomo R, McGrath B, Boyce N. Effect of continuous venovenous hemofiltration with dialysis on hormone and catecholamine clearance in critically ill patients with acute renal failure. Crit Care Med 1994;22:833.
130. Bellomo R, Parkin G, Love J, et al. A prospective comparative study of continuous arteriovenous hemodiafiltration and continuous venovenous hemodiafiltration in critically ill patients. Am J Kidney Dis 1993;21:400.
131. Schneider NS, Geronemus RP. Continuous arteriovenous hemodialysis. Kidney Int (Suppl) 1988;24:5159–62.
132. Macias WL, Mueller BA, Scarim SK, et al. Continuous venovenous hemofiltration: an alternative to continuous arteriovenous hemofiltration and hemodiafiltration in acute renal failure. Am J Kidney Dis 1991;18:451.
133. Latta K, Krull F, Wilken M, et al. Continuous arteriovenous haemofiltration in critically ill children. Ped Nephrol 1994;8:334.
134. Habib R. Pathology of the hemolytic-uremic syndrome. In: Kaplan B, Trompeter R, Moake J, eds. Hemolytic-uremic syndrome and thrombotic thrombocytopenic purpura. New York: Marcel Dekke, 1992:315.
135. Powell H, Davidson P, McCredie D, et al. Haemolytic-uraemic syndrome after treatment with metronidazole. Med J Aus 1988;49:222.
136. Louise CB, Obrig TG. Shiga toxin-associated hemolytic-uremic syndrome: combined cytotoxic effects of Shiga toxin, interleukin-1 beta, and tumor necrosis factor alpha on human vascular endothelial cells in vitro. Infect Immun 1991;59:4173.
137. Louise CB, Obrig TG. Shiga toxin-associated hemolytic uremic syndrome: combined cytotoxic effects of shiga toxin and lipopolysaccharide (endotoxin) on human vascular endothelial cells in vitro. Infect Immun 1992;60:1536.
138. Remuzzi G, Marchesi D, Mecca G, et al. Haemolytic-uraemic syndrome: deficiency of plasma factor(s) regulating prostacyclin activity? Lancet 1978;ii:871.
139. Bergstein JM, Riley M, Bang NU. Role of plasminogen-activator inhibitor type 1 in the pathogenesis and outcome of the hemolytic uremic syndrome. N Eng J Med 1992;327:755.
140. Rose P, Struthers G, Robertson M, et al. Factor III von Willebrand protein in haemolytic-uraemic syndrome and systemic vasculitides. Lancet 1990;335:500.
141. Trompeter RS, Schwartz R, Chantler C, et al. Haemolytic-uraemic syndrome: an analysis of prognostic features. Arch Dis Child 1983;58:101.
142. Fitzpatrick MM, Shah V, Trompeter RS, et al. Long term outcome of childhood haemolytic uraemic syndrome. Br Med J 1991;303:489.
143. Hebert D, Mauer SM. Hemolytic-uremic syndrome and transplantation. In: Kaplan B, Trompeter R, Moake J, eds. Hemolytic-uremic syndrome and thrombotic thrombocytopenic purpura. New York: Marcel Dekke, 1992:179.
144. Loirat C, Sonsino E, Hinglais N, et al. Treatment of the childhood haemolytic uraemic syndrome with plasma. Ped Nephrol 1988;2:279.
145. Rizzoni G, Claris-Appiani A, Edefonti A, et al. Plasma infusion for hemolytic-uremic syndrome in children: Results of a multicenter controlled trial. J Pediatr 1988;112:284.
146. Bitzan M, Moebius E, Ludwig K, et al. High incidence of serum antibodies to Escherichia coli O157 lipopolysaccharide in children with hemolytic-uremic syndrome. J Pediatr 1991;119:380.
147. Ashkenazi S, Cleary TG, Lopez E, et al. Anticytotoxin-neutralizing antibodies in immune globulin preparations: potential use in hemolytic-uremic syndrome. J Pediatr 1988;113:1008.
148. Sheth K, Gill J, Leichter H. High-dose intravenous gamma globulin infusions in hemolytic-uremic syndrome: a preliminary report. Am J Dis Child 1990;144:268.
149. Robson WLM, Fick GH, Jadavji T, et al. The use of intravenous gammaglobulin in the treatment of typical hemolytic uremic syndrome. Pediatr Nephrol 1991;5:289.
150. Bailie MD, Rasoulpour M. Renal and cellular mechanisms that modify blood pressure. In: Loggie JM, ed. Pediatric and adolescent hypertension. Boston: Blackwell Scientific, 1992:8.
151. Dillon MJ, Smellie JM. Peripheral plasma renin activity, hypertension and renal scarring in children. Contrib Nephrol 1984;39:68.
152. Buckalew VJ, Gruber KA. Natriuretic hormone. (Review). Ann Rev Physiol 1984;46:343.
153. Exton JH. Calcium signalling in cells—molecular mechanisms. (Review). Kidney Int (Suppl) 1987;23:568–81.
154. Exton JH. Mechanisms of action of calcium-mobilizing agonists: some variations on a young theme. (Review). Faseb J 1988;2:2670.
155. Williams GH. Converting-enzyme inhibitors in the treatment of hypertension. (Review). N Eng J Med 1988;319:1517.
156. Curtis JJ, Luke RG, Whelchel JD, et al. Inhibition of angiotensin-converting enzyme in renal transplant recipients with hypertension. N Engl J Med 1983;308:377.
157. Zusman RM. Renin- and non-renin-mediated antihypertensive actions of converting enzyme inhibitors. Kidney Int 1984;25:969.
158. Vanhoutte PM. Calcium-entry blockers, vascular smooth muscle and systemic hypertension. (Review). Am J Cardiol 1985;55.
159. Lerner GR, Gruskin AB. Calcium Channel Antagonists and ACE inhibitors. In: Loggie JM, ed. Pediatric and adolescent hypertension. Boston: Blackwell Scientific, 1992:159.
160. Sinaiko AR. Influence of adrenergic nervous system on vasodilator-induced renin release in the conscious rat. Proc Soc Exper Biol Med 1981;167:25.
161. Sinaiko AR. Drugs affecting the adrenergic nervous system. In: Loggie JG, ed. Pediatric and adolescent hypertension. Boston: Blackwell Scientific, 1992:138.
162. Kreye VA. Direct vasodilators with unknown modes of action: the nitro-compounds and hydralazine. (Review). J Cardio Pharmacol 1984;6 suppl 4:5646–55.
163. McCrory WW, Kohaut EC, Lewy JE, et al. Safety of intravenous diazoxide in children with severe hypertension. Clin Pediatr 1979;18:661.
164. Welch TR, Strife CF. The vasodilators. In: Loggie JM, ed. Pediatric and adolescent hypertension. Boston: Blackwell Scientific, 1992:150.
165. Charles MA, Danforth EJ. Nonketoacidotic hyperglycemia and coma during intravenous diazoxide therapy in uremia. Diabetes 1971;20:501.
166. Koch WJ. Hypertensive emergencies. (Review). N Eng J Med 1974;290:211.
167. Ledingham JG, Rajagopalan B. Cerebral complications in the treatment of accelerated hypertension. Quart J Med 1979;48:25.
167a. Arhus GS, Farihe M. Management of Hypertensive Emergencies in Children. In Loggie JM, ed. Pediatric and Adolescent Hypertension. Boston: Blackwell Scientific 1992:369–377.
168. Dilmen U, Caglar MK, Senses DA, et al. Nifedipine in hypertensive emergencies of children. Am J Dis Child 1983;137:1162.
169. Fine RN. Renal transplantation for children—the only realistic choice. Kidney Int (Suppl) 1985;17:S15.
170. Jabs K, Harmon W. Recombinant human erythropoietin therapy in children on dialysis. Adv Renal Repl Therapy 1996:(in press).
171. Fine RN, Kohaut EC, Brown D, et al. Growth after recombinant human growth hormone treatment in children with chronic renal failure: report of a multicenter randomized double-blind placebo-controlled study. Genentech Cooperative Study Group. J Pediatr 1994;124:374.
172. Alexander SR, Sullivan EK, Harmon WE, et al. Maintenance dialysis in North American children and adolescents: a preliminary report. North American Pediatric Renal Transplant Cooperative Study (NAPRTCS). Kidney Int (Suppl) 1993;43:S104.
173. Avner ED, Chavers B, Sullivan EK, et al. Renal transplantation and chronic dialysis in children and adolescents: the 1993 annual report of the North American Pediatric Renal Transplant Cooperative Study. Pediatr Nephrol 1995;9:61.
174. US Renal Data System 1995 Annual Data Report. NIH, NIDDK, Bethesda: 1995:109.

175. Harmon WE. Treatment of children with chronic renal failure. (Review). Kidney Int 1995;47:951.
176. Briscoe DM, Kim MS, Lillehei C, et al. Outcome of renal transplantation in children less than two years of age. Kidney Int 1992;42:657.
177. Harmon WE, Alexander SR, Tejani A, et al. The effect of donor age on graft survival in pediatric cadaver renal transplant recipients—a report of the North American Pediatric Renal Transplant Cooperative Study. Transplantation 1992;54:232.
178. Tejani A, Stablein D, Alexander S, et al. Analysis of rejection outcomes and implications—a report of the North American Pediatric Renal Transplant Cooperative Study. Transplantation 1995;59:500.
179. Harmon WE, Stablein D, Alexander SR, et al. Graft thrombosis in pediatric renal transplant recipients. A report of the North American Pediatric Renal Transplant Cooperative Study. Transplantation 1991;51:406.
180. Ettenger RB, Blifeld C, Prince H, et al. The pediatric nephrologist's dilemma: growth after renal transplantation and its interaction with age as a possible immunologic variable. J Pediatr 1987;111:1022.
181. van Lieburg AF, de Jong MC, Hoitsma AJ, et al. Renal transplant thrombosis in children. J Pediatr Surg 1995;30:615.
182. Yadin O, Grimm P, Ettenger R. Renal transplantation in children: clinical aspects. In: Holliday M, Barratt T, Avner E, eds. Pediatric nephrology. Baltimore: Williams & Wilkins, 1993:1390–1408.
183. Najarian JS, Frey DJ, Matas AJ, et al. Renal transplantation in infants. Ann Surg 1990;212:353.
184. Knight F, Gorynski L, Bentson M, et al. Hemodialysis of the infant or small child with chronic renal failure. Anna J 1993;20:315.
185. Ellis D, Shapiro R, Jordan ML, et al. Comparison of FK-506 and cyclosporine regimens in pediatric renal transplantation. Pediatr Nephrol 1994;8:193.
186. Ettenger R, Mentser M, Potter D, et al. Mycophenolate mofetil in pediatric renal transplantation: A report of the pediatric mycophenolate study group. Am Soc Transpl Physicians (abstract) 1995:181.
187. Levey RH, Parkman R. Whole antilymphocyte serum: a potent safe immunosuppressive agent for intravenous use in man. Transplant Proc 1977;9:1019.
188. Norman DJ, Kahana L, Stuart F, Jr., et al. A randomized clinical trial of induction therapy with OKT3 in kidney transplantation. Transplantation 1993;55:44.
189. Abramowicz D, Norman DJ, Goldman M, et al. OKT3 prophylaxis improves long-term renal graft survival in high-risk patients as compared to cyclosporine: combined results from the prospective, randomized Belgian and US studies. Transplant Proc 1995;27:852.
190. Norman DJ, Kimball JA, Barry JM. Cytokine-release syndrome: differences between high and low doses of OKT3. Transplant Proc 1993;25:35.
191. Robinson ST, Barry JM, Norman DJ. The hemodynamic effects of intraoperative injection of muromonab CD3. Transplantation 1993;56:356.
192. Suthanthiran M, Haschemeyer RH, Riggio RR, et al. Excellent outcome with a calcium channel blocker-supplemented immunosuppressive regimen in cadaveric renal transplantation. A potential strategy to avoid antibody induction protocols. Transplantation 1993;55:1008.
193. Davies DB, Breen TJ, Guo T, et al. Waiting times to pediatric transplantation: an assessment of the August 1990 change in renal allocation policy. Transplant Proc 1994;26:30.
194. Pollard RB. Cytomegalovirus infections in renal, heart, heart-lung and liver transplantation. (Review). Pediatr Infect Dis J 1988;7:S97.
195. Snydman DR, Werner BG, Heinze-Lacey B, et al. Use of cytomegalovirus immune globulin to prevent cytomegalovirus disease in renal-transplant recipients. N Engl J Med 1987;317:1049.
196. Wong T, Lavaud S, Toupance O, et al. Failure of acyclovir to prevent cytomegalovirus infection in renal allograft recipients. Transpl Int 1993;6:285.
197. Balfour H Jr, Chace BA, Stapleton JT, et al. A randomized, placebo-controlled trial of oral acyclovir for the prevention of cytomegalovirus disease in recipients of renal allografts. N Engl J Med 1989;320:1381.
198. Harbison MA, De Girolami PC, Jenkins RL, et al. Ganciclovir therapy of severe cytomegalovirus infections in solid-organ transplant recipients. Transplantation 1988;46:82.
199. Paya CV, Hermans PE, Smith TF, et al. Efficacy of ganciclovir in liver and kidney transplant recipients with severe cytomegalovirus infection. Transplantation 1988;46:229.
200. Lynfield R, Herrin JT, Rubin RH. Varicella in pediatric renal transplant recipients. Pediatrics 1992;90:216.
201. Nyerges G, Meszner Z, Gyarmati E, et al. Acyclovir prevents dissemination of varicella in immunocompromised children. J Infect Dis 1988;157:309.
202. Tuazon CU, Delaney MD, Simon GL, et al. Utility of gallium 67 scintigraphy and bronchial washings in the diagnosis and treatment of *Pneumocystis carinii* pneumonia in patients with AIDS. Am Rev Respir Dis 1985;132:1087.
203. Masur H, Gill VJ, Ognibene FP, et al. Diagnosis of *Pneumocystis* pneumonia by induced sputum technique in patients without AIDS. Ann Intern Med 1988;109:755.
204. Siegel SE, Wolff LJ, Baehner RL, et al. Treatment of *Pneumocystis carinii* pneumonitis. A comparative trial of sulfamethoxazole-trimethoprim v pentamidine in pediatric patients with cancer: report from the Children's Cancer Study Group. Am J Dis Child 1984;138:1051.
205. Amend WJ. Pathogenesis of hepatorenal syndrome. (Review). Transplant Proc 1993;25:1730.
206. Epstein M. Hepatorenal syndrome: emerging perspectives of pathophysiology and therapy (editorial). (Review). J Am Soc Nephrol 1994;4:1735.
207. Epstein M, Berk DP, Hollenberg NK, et al. Renal failure in the patient with cirrhosis. The role of active vasoconstriction. Am J Med 1970;49:175.
208. Iwatsuki S, Popovtzer MM, Corman JL, et al. Recovery from "hepatorenal syndrome" after orthotopic liver transplantation. N Eng J Med 1973;289:1155.
209. Koppel MH, Coburn JW, Mims MM, et al. Transplantation of cadaveric kidneys from patients with hepatorenal syndrome. Evidence for the functional nature of renal failure in advanced liver disease. N Eng J Med 1969;280:1367.
210. Epstein M, Levinson R, Sancho J, et al. Characterization of the renin-aldosterone system in decompensated cirrhosis. Circ Res 1977;41:818.
211. Schroeder ET, Eich RH, Smulyan H, et al. Plasma renin level in hepatic cirrhosis. Relaton to functional renal failure. Am J Med 1970;49:186.
212. Boyer TD, Zia P, Reynolds TB. Effect of indomethacin and prostaglandin A1 on renal function and plasma renin activity in alcoholic liver disease. Gastroenterology 1979;77:215.
213. Epstein M. Renal prostaglandins and the control of renal function in liver disease. (Review). Am J Med 1986;80:46.
214. Zipser RD, Kronborg I, Rector W, et al. Therapeutic trial of thromboxane synthesis inhibition in the hepatorenal syndrome. Gastroenterology 1984;87:1228.
215. Zipser RD, Radvan GH, Kronborg IJ, et al. Urinary thromboxane B2 and prostaglandin E2 in the hepatorenal syndrome: evidence for increased vasoconstrictor and decreased vasodilator factors. Gastroenterology 1983;84:697.
216. Moore K, Wendon J, Frazer M, et al. Plasma endothelin immunoreactivity in liver disease and the hepatorenal syndrome. N Eng J Med 1992;327:1774.
217. Bichet DG, Van PV, Schrier RW. Potential role of increased sympathetic activity in impaired sodium and water excretion in cirrhosis. N Eng J Med 1982;307:1552.
218. Vallance P, Moncada S. Hyperdynamic circulation in cirrhosis: a role for nitric oxide? Lancet 1991;337:776.
219. Linas SL, Schaefer JW, Moore EE, et al. Peritoneovenous shunt in the management of the hepatorenal syndrome. Kidney Int 1986;30:736.
220. Stanley MM, Ochi S, Lee KK, et al. Peritoneovenous shunting as compared with medical treatment in patients with alcoholic cirrhosis and massive ascites. Veterans Administration Cooperative Study on Treatment of Alcoholic Cirrhosis with Ascites. N Eng J Med 1989;321:1632.

Endocrine, Mineral, and Metabolic Disease in Pediatric Intensive Care

39

Daniel S. Kohane
Joseph R. Tobin
and Isaac S. Kohane

INTRODUCTION

This chapter reviews endocrinologic disease, diagnosis, and management as relevant to care of children in the ICU. We provide detail of the underlying pathophysiologies, to the extent that they help clarify diagnostic or therapeutic decision making.

Some sections of this chapter have a subsection titled "Anesthesia, Intubation, and the Perioperative Period," which focuses on special considerations relating to airway management, control of circulation, and perioperative care. The special implications of intensive care pharmacotherapy (particularly anesthetics, pressors, and muscle relaxants) to the disease state are discussed. Intraoperative (operating room) anesthetic management is not germane to this chapter. In all situations the airway, breathing, and circulation are the most important issues and should be addressed first, in that order. Everything else is secondary.

DISORDERS OF THE ADRENAL CORTEX

Since at least 1856, when Brown-Sequard[1] noted that the "adrenals were essential for life," it has been recognized that adrenal disease can be fatal. Since then, regulation of the entire hypothalamic-pituitary-adrenal (HPA) axis has been studied, in the resting state and under stressful conditions characteristic of the intensive care unit (ICU).

In this section, we review adrenal physiology and function and several pathologically reduced-function and excess-function states. At the end, we return to the central questions of relevance to critical care: What is the normal response of the HPA axis to stress and what are the risks associated with abnormal responses?

Embryology

By about 2 months of gestation, the fetal adrenal glands have organized from mesenchymal cells. Migration of neuroectodermal cells into these developing glands form the adrenal medulla. The fetal adrenal glands continue to grow through at least the early third trimester of gestation. The fetal adrenal gland is relatively deficient in 3-beta hydroxylase activity; consequently dehydroepiandrosterone (DHEA) and DHEA sulfate are the major adrenal products. They are used by the placental enzymatic machinery to produce several steroid hormones, including estrogens, that are important for normal gestation. During the second trimester, a rim of tissue

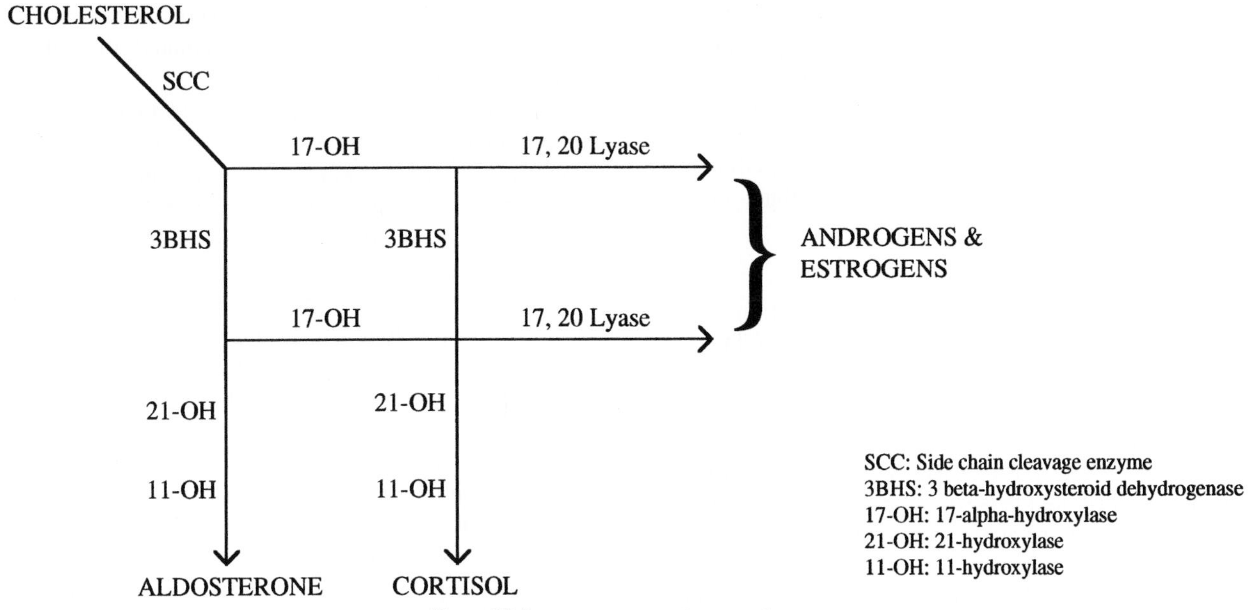

Figure 39.1. Steroid biosynthetic pathways.

comprising the "definitive zone" or adult adrenal gland appears. The remainder of the fetal adrenal degenerates rapidly after birth and disappears by the end of the first year of life.

At the end of the first year of life, the definitive zone has become the adult adrenal cortex with three histologically distinct zones. The outermost, the zona glomerulosa, is principally responsible for mineralocorticoid synthesis. Beneath the glomerulosa is the fasciculata and the innermost layer the reticularis. The last two layers are responsible for glucocorticoid synthesis and also for synthesis of weak androgens (e.g., DHEA). These highly vascular structures receive their blood supply from the plexus of several small arteries that feed a panglandular sinusoidal network. Venous outflow drains into a single large vein for each gland.

Overview of Adrenal Steroidogenesis

Thorough understanding of steroid biosynthetic pathways is crucial for effective diagnosis and treatment of many of the inherited disorders of the adrenal gland. Recognizing the major pathways of mineralocorticoid and glucocorticoid synthesis, diagrammed in Figure 39–1, is helpful in understanding various adrenal enzymatic deficiencies. Only the major enzymes and hormonal end products are included, but a standard endocrinologic text may be consulted for a more detailed discussion. The numbers attached to the enzyme names refer to carbon positions on the steroid common structures. For reference, a steroid skeleton annotated with carbon positions is provided in Figure 39–2.

Free cholesterol is maintained in a small pool within the adrenal gland. Conversion of cholesterol to pregnenolone is the rate-limiting step for steroidogenesis, catalyzed by side-chain cleave enzyme. This intramitochondrial conversion is the step at which steroid synthesis is controlled by adrenocorticotropin (ACTH) and angiotensin II, the latter being most important in the glomerulosa. Subsequently, as outlined in Figure 39–1, androgens and estrogens are produced by 17-hydroxylation, followed by cleavage of the 17,20 carbon-carbon bond (going from left to right on the diagram).

The mineralocorticoid synthetic pathway converts pregnenolone to aldosterone by the successive actions of 3-beta-hydroxylation, 21-hydroxylation, 11-hydroxylation, and then 18-hydroxylation and 18-oxidation (going from top to bottom on the left of the diagram). Similarily, the

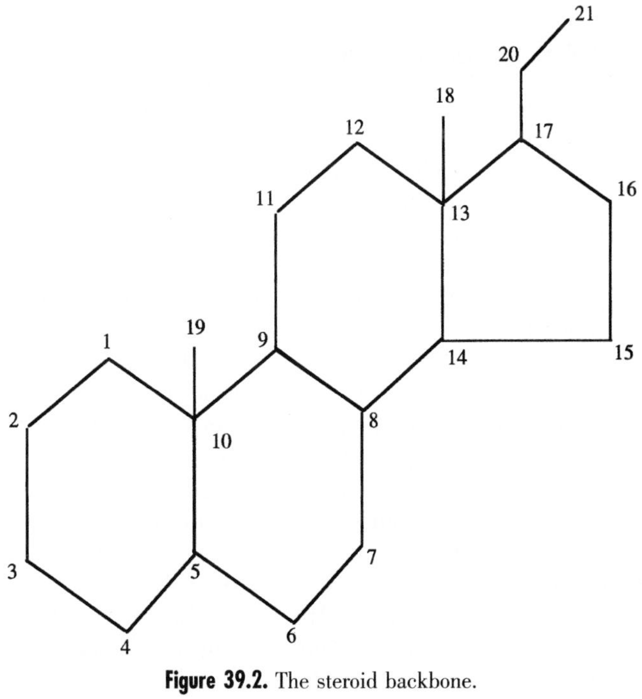

Figure 39.2. The steroid backbone.

glucocorticoid synthetic pathway produces cortisol by successive 3-beta-hydroxylation, 21-hydroxylation, and 11-hydroxylation. Severe deficiencies of these enzymes lead to inadequate production of the hormones further down the pathway and accumulation of steroid precursors prior to enzyme deficiency. The constellation of clinical and laboratory findings and treatment are covered in sections that follow.

Adrenocorticotropin

Adrenocorticotropin (ACTH) is the principal stimulus for glucocorticoid synthesis in the adrenal gland. ACTH synthesis and secretion are stimulated by corticotropin-releasing hormone (CRH) via cAMP-linked CRH receptors. Arginine vasopressin (AVP) also stimulates ACTH release and acts synergistically with CRH. Excitatory and inhibitory input is contributed by several parts of the brain to the CRH-secreting neurons of the paraventricular nucleus of the hypothalamus. Excitatory input is transduced by cholinergic, serotoninergic, and noradrenergic neurotransmission as well as by interleukin (IL) 1 and 6. The latter two cytokines may play a role in the hypothesized immune-endocrine feedback loop[(2)]. Inhibitory inputs include gamma-aminobutyric acid, norepinephrine, and glucocorticoids.

ACTH is a 39-amino-acid peptide synthesized as part of a much larger peptide, pro-opiomelanocortin (POMC). The POMC gene, on chromosome 2, undergoes tissue-specific posttranslational processing. In the intermediate lobe of the pituitary gland, one of the cleavage products is alpha-melanocyte-stimulating hormone. In the anterior pituitary lobe, it is cleaved into beta-lipotropin (the amino-terminal peptide), ACTH, and joining peptide. Since production of these cleavage products is directly proportional to the amount of POMC synthesized, differences in their serum concentrations are due to differences in clearance rates.

Control of Cortisol and Androgen Production

The zona fasciculata and reticularis cell respond to ACTH binding to the cell membrane, which is enhanced in the presence of extracellular calcium. ACTH activates adenylate cyclase, producing a rise in intracellular cyclic adenosine monophosphate (cAMP). cAMP activates protein kinase A, which accelerates conversion of cholesterol to pregnenolone by the side chain cleavage enzyme (the rate-limiting step), resulting in enhanced cortisol production. This induction of steroidogenesis by ACTH happens within minutes. Chronic exposure to ACTH causes many of the adrenal synthetic enzymes to increase in activity and also promotes gland hypertrophy and hyperplasia.

Glucocorticoids provide long-loop negative feedback inhibition of ACTH synthesis in the pituitary corticotrope cells and of hypothalamic synthesis of CRH and AVP. Inhibition appears to be mediated through both type I (mineralocorticoid) and type II receptors, which bind both the glucocorticoid ligand and specific regulatory gene sites. Latency of these mechanisms varies from a few seconds[(3)] to 2 hours. The rapid response feedback (seconds to minutes) appears to be mediated through nongenomic mechanisms.

A significant stressor (e.g., surgery) can cause sufficient secretion of CRH and/or AVP to overcome feedback inhibition, even in the presence of large amounts of glucocorticoids. "Stress" in this context denotes a variety of stimuli that are directly or indirectly noxious, a significant perturbation of the physiologic milieu, or even a state of mind (e.g., fear). The HPA axis can increase its usual steroid output threefold to tenfold[(4)] in response to psychological[(5)] or physical[(6)] stress. In surgery, activation of the HPA axis peaks not at the time of incision but with the reversal of anesthesia[(7)].

In view of the magnitude of the stress response and the many functions attributed to glucocorticoids, it might seem that physiologic serum glucocorticoid levels and a generous glucocorticoid stress response would be absolutely necessary for daily life as well as for survival of extreme situations typical of the ICU. However, there is a growing body of evidence that reveals a more circumscribed role for glucocorticoids. Studies of homologous recombinant ("gene knockout") mice homozygous for CRH deficiency[(8)] have revealed that a very low level of glucocorticoid (produced by the adrenal gland) is sufficient for most daily activity. Further, these mice appear to tolerate the stress of anesthesia (with ether) and of surgery just as well as controls. Even though these results are quite interesting, it is not clear whether they can be generalized to humans. Therefore, glucocorticoid supplementation near the time of surgery continues to be a prudent measure in patients with insufficient glucocorticoid production.

The other important products of the fasciculata/reticularis unit are the androgens, whose secretion is also stimulated by ACTH, with a circadian rhythm. DHEA and DHEA sulfate constitute the largest portion of adrenal androgen output. A smaller quantity consists of androstenedione. Testosterone is not produced in any significant quantity by the adrenal glands but is the product of peripheral tissue conversion of the three main adrenal androgens, chiefly androstenedione. In the adult male, of course, the main source of androgen is testicular tissue.

Studies of the interactions between the HPA axis and the immune system have suggested that these two systems act in concert to respond to stress and microbiologic invasion with reciprocal feedback mechanisms. For example, cytokines associated with inflammation, such as IL-1, can cause release of CRH and ACTH[(9)]. IL-6 also stimulates release of ACTH and glucocorticoids[(9)]. The glucocorticoids in turn have multiple effects on the immune system that generally act to reduce the mobility of cells of the immune system. They inhibit release of histamine and production of cytokines, such as IL-6 and IL-1[(10,11)]. Whether these effects are relevant to normal physiology or are merely due to administration of pharmacologic doses of cytokine or hormone remains unclear.

Control of Aldosterone Production

The zona glomerulosa produces aldosterone in response to many factors, including ACTH, hyperkalemia, arterial hypotension, and hyponatremia. The latter two, which reflect extracellular fluid (ECF) depletion, affect aldosterone in the following manner. Juxtaglomerular cells located in the wall of the afferent arteriole of the renal glomerulus respond to decreases in arterial pressure or sodium concentration by increasing renin secretion. Renin cleaves angiotensinogen to angiotensin I (a decapeptide), which is further broken down to angiotensin II (a heptapeptide) by angiotensin-converting enzyme in the lung. Angiotensin II is the principal stimulus to aldosterone secretion. Angiotensin II binds to a G-protein-coupled receptor in zona glomerulosa cells, initiating a cascade of events that raise the concentration of intracellular calcium, increasing aldosterone synthesis[12]. The increase in aldosterone preserves ECF volume by enhancing renal conservation of sodium.

ACTH acts on the glomerulosa to increase aldosterone output just as it acts on the reticularis/fasciculata unit to increase cortisol output. After several days of ACTH stimulation, however, the glomerulosa "escapes" or becomes resistant, and aldosterone output falls (perhaps due to sodium and/or fluid retention, with subsequent decreased renin and/or angiotensin).

Hyperkalemia is a major direct stimulus for aldosterone production. Aldosterone output is increased threefold by a rise in serum potassium of 0.5 mEq/L, even though hyperkalemia inhibits renin production. Aldosterone induces kaliuresis and renal sodium conservation.

Actions of Aldosterone

The important actions of aldosterone are confined to the kidney. Nonrenal effects on enhanced sodium retention and potassium excretion from the gut, sweat glands, and salivary glands are insignificant in terms of body sodium and potassium balance. The principal site of action for aldosterone, at least for extracellular volume control, is the distal renal tubule, where aldosterone binds the type I glucocorticoid receptor (also known as the mineralocorticoid receptor) and triggers production of proteins that are involved in the structure and function of the sodium channel and in generation of ATP. Stimulation of ATP may itself increase production of proteins required for sodium channel function. The type I glucocorticoid receptor has roughly equal affinity for aldosterone and cortisol. This lack of specificity is surprising, given that cortisol has much less mineralocorticoid activity than aldosterone. Cortisol actually does not bind to the type I receptor in vivo, because 11-beta-hydroxysteroid dehydrogenase converts cortisol to cortisone (which does not bind this receptor) before it can bind. (This was recently elucidated in work on the syndrome of apparent mineralocorticoid excess, described later in the section on endocrine hypertension. It appears to be caused by a deficiency in the activity of 11-beta-hydroxysteroid dehydrogenase.)

Active sodium reabsorption commences within 2 hours of starting an infusion of aldosterone, with water and chloride accompanying the sodium passively. Potassium excretion seems to be enhanced by increased sodium reabsorption in the distal tubule, which is presumed to create a luminal negative charge favoring cation entry. Sodium depletion allows nearly complete sodium reabsorption in the proximal tubule, so that aldosterone can have little further effect in the distal tubule; hence, kaliuresis is impeded. Sodium loading, on the other hand, results in increased distal tubular aldosterone-dependent sodium resorption with accentuated kaliuresis. Aldosterone-induced sodium resorption results in increased negativity of distal renal tubular urine, causing increased excretion of other cations, including hydrogen, magnesium, and ammonium ions. In this way, metabolic alkalosis can result from aldosterone excess as long as sodium supply is maintained.

All these effects of aldosterone may be inhibited by substances that compete for the distal tubular binding sites. Such agents include spironolactone, progesterone, and 17-hydroxyprogesterone (which is elevated in the most common form of congenital adrenal hyperplasia). Triamterene (a potassium-sparing diuretic) appears not to compete with aldosterone binding but interferes with aldosterone function, thereby promoting sodium excretion and potassium reabsorption.

Actions of Cortisol

Cortisol represents 90% of the glucocorticoid output of the adrenal glands. In blood, 90% to 97% of cortisol is bound to corticosteroid-binding globulin and albumin, with the binding system saturating at a cortisol level of about 25 μg/dL. The roughly 5% to 10% unbound fraction (higher when corticosteroid-binding globulin is saturated) of cortisol appears to be the metabolically active pool, since it is the only form available to cell receptors. Protein binding decreases due to stress, shock, and severe trauma, which results in a higher free-cortisol concentration in these states[13,14].

Cortisol passes easily through cell membranes, binding to a cytosolic receptor protein[15]. The binding complex then enters the cell nucleus, where the steroid-receptor complex attaches to specific regulatory DNA sequences called glucocorticoid response elements (GREs). How GRE-glucocorticoid complexes affect transcriptional processes remains unclear.

There is some evidence that glucocorticoids accelerate glycogenolysis in the liver directly by stimulating glucose 6-phosphatase and indirectly by increasing hepatic sensitivity to glucagon and the action of catecholamines at the α-adrenergic receptor. Precursors of gluconeogenesis are increased, both by protein catabolism and by glycerol production via glucocorticoid-induced lipolysis. There is some controversy as to whether glucocorticiods increase glycogenolysis[16,17].

Lipolysis is increased by glucocorticoids, even in cushingoid patients with characteristic moon facies and buffalo hump. However, these patients have a voracious appetite and hyperinsulinemia and so overcompensate for the lipolytic effect of glucocorticoids. Hyperinsulinemia presumably arises from glucocorticoid excess, which inhibits peripheral tissue glucose uptake. This decreased use of glucose, coupled with increased proteolysis, lipolysis, and gluconeogenesis, results in elevated blood glucose. This hyperglycemia, in turn, increases insulin secretion.

Glucocorticoids can improve renal blood flow and glomerular filtration rate and so can increase urinary output. They are necessary for normal excretion of water load. In glucocorticoid deficiency there are both direct renal tubular effects(16) and increased AVP levels(18), suggesting a role for glucocorticoids in release of AVP.

Excess glucocorticoids reduce intestinal calcium absorption and increase calciuria and phosphaturia. Serum calcium is maintained by increased parathyroid hormone, which mobilizes calcium from bone. This can result in pronounced osteopenia, which is potentiated by direct stimulation of osteolysis by excess glucocorticoids and by bone protein catabolism(17).

Cortisol causes an increase in cardiac output and systemic resistance. Intracytoplasmic glucocorticoid receptors have been identified in myocardial and vascular tissue as well as in most nucleated cells. Peak myocardial performance is achieved only when specific myocardial cytoplasmic receptors are occupied(19). These receptors are specific for glucocorticoids, and aldosterone has no effect. Prolonged cortisol deficiency reduces myocardial mass.

Glucocorticoids also appear to improve the integrity of the vascular system. This has prompted trials of supraphysiologic steroid supplementation for patients in shock(20,21). Results have been disappointing(22,23). Nontheless, physiologic glucocorticoid levels are required for cardiovascular response to stress.

As mentioned, it has been shown that CRH, ACTH, and cortisol production rise dramatically in response to stressors, including major trauma, surgery, and psychological stress. Consequently, the conventional wisdom has been that patients unable to generate "stress" levels of glucocorticoid are at risk and therefore should receive supplemental glucocorticoid. Although it is advisable to continue to treat patients accordingly, recent discoveries, detailed in the following section, call this widely held practice into question.

Adrenal Disease

The pathophysiology of adrenal disorders can be categorized into hyperfunction and hypofunction and further classified as primary or secondary (i.e., to hypothalamus or pituitary disease) disorders. Nevertheless, because of the diagnostic approach to these disorders, classification is functional and anatomic for some disorders (e.g., Cushing's syndrome) and biochemical for others (e.g., many congenital adrenal hyperplasias).

Adrenal Hypofunction

Adrenal insufficiency can be primary, secondary, or tertiary. Primary insufficiency can result from one or more defects in production of mineralocorticoids and/or glucocorticoids or from global adrenal failure (Addison's disease). Secondary insufficiency results from disorders of the pituitary (ACTH deficiency) and tertiary insufficiency from disorders of the hypothalamus (CRH deficiency). Presentation and treatment of specific types of adrenal hypofunction depend on the underlying disorder.

Primary Adrenal Insufficiency (Addison's Disease)

In primary adrenal insufficiency, all three adrenal cortical layers are destroyed or inactive. Acute adrenal crisis is uncommon in the pediatric ICU but can be catastrophic **(Table 39–1).** Clinical manifestations include those of both inadequate mineralocorticoid and glucocorticoid effects. The mineralocorticoid lack is responsible for disordered electrolytes (hyponatremia, hyperkalemia, hypercalcemia, acidosis) and for loss of ECF volume, presenting as weight loss, dehydration, hypotension, or frank shock. Quadriplegia has been reported in association with hyperkalemia. The shock (or preshock) state has some unusual features, in that it may be poorly responsive to volume and catecholamine infusions. This is likely due to the glucocorticoid deficit(24,25).

The most frequently seen cause, up to 90% of cases in some series(26), is autoimmune adrenalitis, occurring in isolation or part of polyglandular autoimmune endocrinopathy. The most common associated autoimmune endocrine diseases are Hashimoto's thyroiditis (25%), Graves' disease (10%), diabetes mellitus (10% to 20%), hypogonadism (10%), and hypoparathyroidism (5%). Five decades ago, granulomatous diseases (e.g., tuberculosis) and fungal diseases may have accounted for the majority of cases of Addison's disease. Currently, it may account for 10% to 15% of cases. Increasingly, opportunistic infections in patients infected with HIV have been found in association with necrotizing adrenalitis or more subtle blunting of the normal

Table 39.1. Treatment of the Patient with Suspected Adrenal Crisis

1. Establish a secure intravenous line and withdraw blood for determination of baseline cortisol, electrolytes, blood urea nitrogen, glucose, and Ca^{2+}. Do Chemstrip test.
2. Give 2 mL of 25% dextrose in water per kilogram intravenously unless glucose is known to be normal.
3. Start 5% dextrose in normal saline solution at double the usual maintenance rate. For shock, infuse 20 mL of normal saline or lactated Ringer's solution per kilogram as rapidly and as often as is needed to reverse shock.
4. Give 0.2 mg dexamethasone (or 1 mg methylprednisolone) per kilogram intravenously.
5. Give 250 μg ACTH intravenously.
6. Repeat the plasma cortisol determination (30 to 60 minutes) after the administration of ACTH.
7. Begin intravenous hydrocortisone replacement.

adrenal output. Adrenal insufficiency in these patients is worsened by the use of ketoconazole, which inhibits several steroidogenic enzymes, and rifampin, which increases cortisol clearance. Infiltration of the adrenal gland by tumor is far more rare in pediatric patients than in adults.

Adrenoleukodystrophy is increasingly recognized as a potential cause of Addison's disease. In this disorder, very-long-chain fatty acids accumulate in several neural tissues as well as in the adrenal gland. Diagnosis is made by urine or serum assays for the presence of very-long-chain fatty acids. Adrenoleukodystrophy can present first as Addison's disease before any neurologic findings are seen. Therefore, it should be considered in the patient with Addison's disease of unknown cause.

Severe systemic illness can cause adrenal hypofunction. Poor adrenal perfusion due to shock can reduce corticosteroid output[27], although more recent data demonstrate that the adrenal medulla is protected during shock[28] and the adrenal cortex and medulla are protected during hypoxia[29]. The Waterhouse-Friderichsen syndrome (which can present at any age) represents acute hemorrhage into the adrenal glands as the result of coagulopathy associated with sepsis (classically meningococcemia).

In the neonate, several disorders of adrenal enzymes may result in inefficient or absent production of both mineralocorticoid and glucocorticoid. They are classified as types of congenital adrenal hyperplasia (CAH) because cortisol insufficiency leads to stimulation of the adrenal enzymatic machinery, with glandular hypertrophy and hyperplasia. Details of diagnosis and management of these rare disorders are beyond the scope of this chapter, but they merit brief mention. The most common CAH is 21-hydroxylase deficiency, with an incidence of around 1 in 20,000[30]. This rate is sufficiently high for several states to run pilot neonatal screening programs for 17-hydroxyprogesterone[31], which is markedly elevated in this disorder. CAH presents typically as a "salt-wasting" crisis between days 5 and 15 of life. Girls with 21-hydroxylase deficiency are often easier to diagnose because of the virilization that results from excessive adrenal androgen production. Much less common forms, of CAH, causing combined deficiency of adrenal steroid synthesis, include 3-beta-hydroxylase deficiency and deficiency of side chain cleavage enzyme. In these last two forms, androgen production in the testes and adrenal gland is so compromised that boys have incomplete or even absent virilization (i.e., pseudohermaphroditism).

Even more rare than CAH are several forms of inadequate or absent development of the adult adrenal gland, which are lumped under the rubric of congenital adrenal hypoplasia. These include X-linked hypoplasia (located at Xp21, near Duchenne's muscular dystrophy and glycerol kinase deficiency), an autosomal recessive form, a sporadic form, and another X-linked variant associated with hypogonadotropic hypogonadism.

PRESENTATION. Clinical presentation of Addison's disease is determined by deficiency of glucocorticoid and mineralocorticoid and a resulting rise in ACTH, CRH, renin, and angiotensin II. These secondary elevations in response to the primary deficiency may contribute to the discomfort and nausea experienced by patients with Addison's disease. Symptoms on presentation invariably include weakness, fatigue, and anorexia. Nausea and other gastrointestinal (GI) symptoms occur in over half of patients. Salt craving and muscle and joint pain occur in a minority of patients. Hypoglycemia in children, especially after a prolonged fast, is not uncommon.

Pigmentation of the skin and mucosa is increased, particularly at skin folds, in sun-exposed areas, and at scars. It is not clear which of the POMC-derived molecules are responsible for this pigmentation. Weight loss and hypotension are also present in most patients at the time of diagnosis.

Laboratory abnormalities include hyponatremia and hyperkalemia. Hyponatremia is due in part to aldosterone deficiency but also to changes in the set-point of AVP and in renal free-water clearance caused by the decrease in glucocorticoid activity. The hyperkalemia can be life-threatening, and should be treated immediately to prevent fatal dysrhythmias. Hypercalcemia is sometimes associated with Addison's disease. Complete blood cell count typically reveals eosinophilia, lymphocytosis, and mild normocytic, normochromic anemia.

TREATMENT. "Stress" hydrocortisone administration in patients in adrenal crisis is usually begun at intravenous daily doses equivalent to 28 to 56 mg/m^2. This recommended dosage is about four to eight times the nonstressed physiologic daily dose of 7 mg/m^2[32]. When the child's condition is stable, the dose can be tapered within a day to the physiologic range. Slower tapering is necessary only if glucocorticoids are being used for an underlying disease (e.g., asthma, cerebral edema) that could worsen with rapid tapering. When converted to oral maintenance therapy, the dose should be 14 mg/m^2 daily (double the intravenous dose) because of inactivation in the GI tract and first-pass hepatic metabolism.

In hyponatremia, salt can be replaced by normal saline infusion or in tablets, depending on the severity of the hyponatremia and the mental status of the patient. The mineralocorticoid action of cortisol is often sufficient when used in these stress doses. Mineralocorticoid replacement with 9-alpha-fluorocortisol typically is only instituted as the patient becomes ready for transfer from the ICU to the floor and is only available as an enteric preparation.

Central Adrenal Insufficiency

Several disorders of the HPA axis result in insufficient ACTH or ACTH effect. Although ACTH can acutely stimulate mineralocorticoid production, aldosterone is adequately controlled by the renin-angiotensin system in its absence. Only glucocorticoid and androgen production are significantly affected by the absence of ACTH or ACTH effect.

Secondary Adrenal Insufficiency

Insufficient ACTH production can be caused by any destructive process in the pituitary. Pituitary tumors, craniopharyngiomas, autoimmune hypophysitis, granulomatous disease, and trauma to the sella have all been reported in association with decreased ACTH secretion as well as other pituitary deficiencies. A CRH challenge in a patient with secondary insufficiency results in minimal ACTH response, in contrast to the marked response in tertiary insufficiency[(33)]. Diagnosis and management of secondary adrenal insufficiency in the ICU is similar to that of tertiary insufficiency.

Tertiary Adrenal Insufficiency

Perhaps the most common cause of adrenal insufficiency in the ICU is tertiary adrenal insufficiency caused by prior administration of glucocorticoids. When they are administered in high doses, particularly with long-acting glucocorticoids or with multiple doses per day, the HPA axis is suppressed in a characteristic sequence. First, CRH secretion is suppressed, and consequently, stores of ACTH in corticotrope cells decrease and much less ACTH is secreted. With chronic lack of ACTH stimulation, the zona fasciculata atrophies and has a minimal to subnormal glucocorticoid response to short, acute challenges with ACTH. Although the length of the glucocorticoid exposure required to achieve this suppression is controversial, it appears to be between 1 and 3 weeks and is likely to be dose- and preparation-related[(34)].

Recovery from glucocorticoid-induced HPA suppression follows the reverse sequence. Morning ACTH levels gradually rise, presumably in response to reactivation of CRH activity. Subsequently the zona fasciculata increases its output. This recovery process can take as long as 6 to 12 months[(35)].

If a patient has been treated with high-dose glucocorticoid for more than a week, it is prudent to assume tertiary adrenal insufficiency is present and to administer stress-dose levels of glucocorticoids in a critically ill patient, even though there have been few documented deaths from glucocorticoid-induced HPA failure[(36)]. One explanation for the apparent low mortality of this condition may be that anticipation and aggresive treatment are successful in preventing such deaths. Alternatively, it may be that HPA failure is under-recognized because of difficulties in documenting its presence in situations where corrective therapy is readily available.

Wide variability in patient susceptibility to HPA suppression has resulted in widely differing conclusions regarding the optimal regimen of long-term steroid use and the need for "stress" coverage. The multiplicity of recommendations may also be due to the possibility that glucocorticoids are not as necessary for the survival of surgical or life-threatening stress as had been previously thought, a hypothesis congruent with the aforementioned experience with mice that have had CRH gene disruption.

Other causes of tertiary adrenal insufficiency include tumors or surgery that affects the hypothalamus. Radiation can also cause deficiency, although the central components of the HPA axis appear to be much more resistant to ablation than other hypothalamic and pituitary hormones. Current central nervous system (CNS) radiation doses for malignant tumor rarely lead to HPA insufficiency.

Free-water clearance is decreased by decreased levels of glucocorticoid, probably both by effects on AVP release from the posterior pituitary and by direct effects on the distal renal tubule. Consequently, if adrenal insufficiency has been profound and of long duration, transient diuresis may be noted during the initial period of treatment with stress levels of glucocorticoids.

Before administering replacement stress levels of glucocorticoids, administering a few simple tests can help determine if the patient has a suppressed HPA axis. Also, the information is useful in formulating a treatment plan after the acute episode: A random or morning cortisol level greater than 20 μg/dL suggests adequate function, whereas a level less than 5 μg/dL suggests some suppression or insufficiency.

Also, a cortisol level of 20 μg/dL after a test intravenous bolus of ACTH suggests adequate adrenal function, although it does not rule out recent suppression of CRH that has yet to cause adrenal atrophy. Differentiation between pituitary and hypothalamic hypofunction may be accomplished by administering an intravenous bolus of corticotropin-releasing factor (CRF) of 1 μg/kg IV, which produces a brisk (30-minute) rise in plasma ACTH levels in patients with an intact pituitary gland. Nevertheless, no critically ill child should await performance and results of a stimulation test if adrenal insufficiency is contributing to a life-threatening situation. Stress glucocorticoids should be administered and the stimulation test aborted or delayed until the child's condition is more stable.

Isolated Mineralocorticoid Deficiency

Any disruption of the renin-angiotensin-aldosterone axis can potentially result in isolated mineralocorticoid deficiency. The typical presentation includes hyperkalemia, hyponatremia, and sometimes hypotension.

Adrenal Enzymatic Defects

Two enzymatic actions are responsible for catalyzing the reactions converting corticosterone to aldosterone. These have been referred to as corticosterone 18-methyl oxidase I (CMO I) and corticosterone methyl oxidase II (CMO II). Both enzymatic activities are part of the same protein complex coded by CYP11B2 (which is also responsible for 11-hydroxylase activity in the zona glomerulosa). Mutations causing deficient CMO II activity lead to inadequate aldosterone production and a salt-losing state[(37)]. Laboratory profile includes high plasma renin activity (PRA), low aldosterone levels, and high 18-hydroxycorticosterone. Treatment includes salt supplementation (NaCl starting at 2 g/day in infants) and 9-alpha-fluorocortisol (0.05-1 mg/day).

Pseudohypoaldosteronism

Pseudohypoaldosteronism is characterized by deficient mineralocorticoid effect despite hyperreninemia and hyperaldosteronism. It may be acquired or congenital. The acquired form is found in association with obstructive uropathy and/or urinary tract infections[(38,39)] and presents as a salt-wasting crisis with high PRA and aldosterone levels. The salt-wasting state resolves spontaneously, as does the hyperaldosteronemia, often with treatment of the underlying disorder. Congenital pseudohypoaldosteronism can be inherited in an autosomal-recessive pattern. In infants, it presents as a salt-losing state that is unresponsive to treatment with exogenous mineralocorticoids. It is thought to be due to a variety of qualitative and quantitative mineralocorticoid receptor defects, none of which have been identified[(40)]. Severity of the salt-wasting appears to attenuate with age[(41)].

Acquired Hypoaldosteronism

In hyporeninemic hypoaldosteronism, renin is not secreted in response to the usual stimuli (low systemic arterial pressure, low sodium and high potassium levels) and therefore the mineralocorticoid response is inadequate. The underlying disorder is not known in most cases, although there is a strong association with diabetes mellitus. One possible explanation is autonomic neuropathy with decreased catecholamine secretion and responsiveness[(42)]. Many of these patients are asymptomatic, with only mild to moderate hyperkalemia. In the ICU, administration of heparin may exacerbate relative hypoaldosteronism by inhibiting its synthesis and thereby precipitate significant salt wasting and volume loss. The diagnosis of hyporeninemic hypoaldosteronism can often be made in the setting of chronicity of hyperkalemia in association with hyperreninemia in volume-depleted states.

Anesthesia, Intubation, and the Perioperative Period

Of principal concern are patients who are acutely hypocortisolemic and inadequately treated. The provision of stress-dose steroids is recommended. Further interventions and monitoring needs are determined by the patient's clinical status. Dehydration and electrolyte abnormalities (hyponatremia, hyperkalemia, hypercalcemia, acidosis) should be corrected. Hyperkalemia is a contraindication to the use of succinylcholine. Patients in shock may require little or no anesthesia.

Intubation should be prompt in unstable or obtunded patients. Nausea and vomiting associated with glucocorticoid deficiency and hypotension may place the patient at risk of aspiration. Which anesthetic agents and pressors (if any) are used must be dictated by the anticipated depressed cardiac output and decreased responsiveness to catecholamines seen in glucocorticoid deficiency. If etomidate is considered in these patients, resultant depression of the adrenal cortical stress response inhibiting 17-alpha-hydroxylase and 11-beta-hydroxylase and the cholesterol side chain cleavage enzyme[(44)] for 5 to 8 hours must be recognized[(43)]. Production of cortisol, 17-hydroxyprogesterone, aldosterone, and corticosterone are reduced. Thiopental[(45)], propofol[(45)], and midazolam[(46)] do not depress the adrenocortical response to stress, but some of these drugs inhibit steroidogenic enzymes in vitro[(47)].

The need for muscle relaxants may be reduced if the patient has muscle weakness.

Cushing's Syndrome

Cushing's syndrome refers to the set of clinical findings that develop as the result of chronic exposure to glucocorticoids. Nevertheless, some causes of Cushing's syndrome also demonstrate androgen and mineralocorticoid excess. Other forms of adrenal hyperfunction that primarily affect mineralocorticoid function are described later in the section on endocrine hypertension.

Causes

Probably the most common cause of hypercortisolism is administration of glucocorticoids, typically to treat chronic inflammatory disease. In this case, the history will be informative, making diagnosis simple.

Endogenous causes of hypercortisolism present diagnostic challenges. These are classified as either ACTH-dependent (secondary adrenal hyperfunction) or ACTH-independent (primary adrenal hyperfunction). In children under age 7[(48,49)], ACTH-independent Cushing's syndrome is more common. In older children, ACTH-dependent causes account for 80% to 90% of cases, most of which are due to pituitary disorders (i.e., Cushing's disease), 10% to 20% to ectopic synthesis of ACTH, and a very small number to ectopic CRH production. Sites for ectopic ACTH synthesis include oat cell carcinoma, thymic and bronchial carcinoid, pancreatic islet cell tumor, pheochromocytoma, and various other carcinomata and carcinoids.

About one third of cases of ACTH-independent Cushing's syndrome are due to adrenal adenoma and two thirds to adrenal carcinoma. Rarely, the patient may have micronodular adrenal disease.

Clinical Presentation

In the pediatric ICU, the earliest and most suggestive signs of Cushing's syndrome are missed unless a careful history is taken, including a growth curve. Children typically have a decrease in their height centile with acceleration or maintenance of their weight centile.

Centripetal obesity (truncal obesity with thin or even

wasted extremities), which is very common in adults with Cushing's syndrome, is atypical in children. Instead, uniformly distributed (generalized) obesity is usual. Accumulation of adipose tissue in the face produces the moon facies. Similar accumulation occurs in the supraclavicular fossae and on the neck, producing the buffalo-hump appearance.

Glucose intolerance, hypertension, proximal muscle weakness, and oligomenorrhea are also frequent manifestations. Again, unlike in adult patients, hypertension is rarely accompanied by heart failure. Striae appear, typically on the abdomen, due to atrophy of the skin, which reveal underlying blood vessels and tissues and so are more purple than striae of children with idiopathic obesity (i.e., stretch marks). Hirsutism and acne may be present in up to half of pediatric patients.

Less commonly, patients have increased bruising, hypokalemic alkalosis, and/or avascular necrosis of the hip. In cases of Cushing's syndrome due to hypersecretion of ACTH, hyperpigmentation may be noted on gums, intertriginous folds, and scars. Psychological disorders occur in up to 50% of patients in some series[5]. Manifestations include mania, depression, insomnia, and hyperactivity.

Diagnosis

Making the biochemical diagnosis of Cushing's syndrome is difficult in the ICU. The usual screening studies (8 A.M. serum cortisol level checked after 15 μg/kg of dexamethasone given the previous night or 24-hour urinary free-cortisol excretion) are likely to be positive if only because the stress of critical illness is likely to stimulate the HPA axis. Consequently, in the ICU, diagnosis is made on clinical grounds using features of the history and physical examination.

Further workup is also best performed after the patient is out of the ICU. Liddle's test, the low dose-high dose dexamethasone suppression test, consists of 2 days of 0.5 mg oral dexamethasone (30 μg/kg) every 6 hours followed by 2 mg (120 μg/kg) every 6 hours for 2 days. If urinary free cortisol is suppressed by more than 90% by the end of the test, an ACTH-independent cause is suggested. Increasingly, the ovine CRH stimulation test is being used. A rise in ACTH and cortisol from baseline by at least 20% suggests ACTH-dependent Cushing's syndrome. However, false-positive results in Liddle's test and ovine CRH tests do occur. Other tests, such as bilateral inferior petrosal sinus sampling, are best done in a clinical research center, under well-controlled conditions and in the hands of experienced operators.

Anesthesia, Intubation, and the Perioperative Period

Children who have been exposed to high doses of endogenous or exogenous steroids are susceptible to pathological fractures. Therefore, great care should be taken during positioning for procedures and even during seemingly innocuous activities such as physical therapy. There may be coexisting muscle weakness; neuromuscular blocking drugs should be used judiciously.

Serum electrolyte and glucose levels may be abnormal (hyperglycemia, hypokalemia, alkalosis). In general, it is best to return serum levels to normal, although data to back this practice are often weak. For example, there are conflicting clinical studies on the association between ventricular ectopy and hypokalemia, and no increase in ectopy has been demonstrated in hypokalemic patients undergoing anesthesia[50]. Furthermore, it is not clear what effect hypokalemia has on dosing of muscle relaxants[51,52].

Postoperative care after adrenalectomy is routine for an abdominal procedure, but patients may require supplemental steroids.

Synthetic Corticosteroids

The preceding general discussion of glucocorticoid and mineralocorticoid effects can be applied to the broad array of synthetic adrenocorticosteroids available to clinicians. To use these adrenocorticosteroids sensibly, however, clinicians must understand the differences between them in terms of potency and proportion of glucocorticoid and mineralocorticoid effects.

In many ICU patients, the intravenous route is the only effective means of administration of drugs. This prevents the the use of several steroids, including prednisone and cortisone, which require hepatic hydroxylation to become active. In fact, only four commercially available intravenous corticosteroids are of concern here: hydrocortisone (cortisol), prednisolone, methylprednisolone, and dexamethasone **(Table 39–2).** The synthetic steroids have lower binding affinity to the corticosteroid binding globulin than cortisol, so most of the synthetic glucocorticoids circulate weakly bound to albumin, with about one third unbound.

Despite an increased free fraction, the half-lives of synthetic glucocorticoids are longer than that of cortisol. Synthetic glucocorticoids also bind the type II glucocorticoid receptor more avidly than cortisol. The combination of higher affinity and longer half-life contributes to the increased potency of these steroids. Glucocorticoid potency itself is hard to quantify, because it has multiple dimensions, such as measures of eosinophil suppression, glycogen deposition, and suppression of the HPA axis.

The important differences among the four intravenous steroids pertain to their mineralocorticoid effects. Hydrocortisone (cortisol) has the greatest sodium-retaining prop-

Table 39.2. Intravenous Adrenocorticosteroids

Steroid	*Glucocorticoid Potency*	*Mineralocorticoid Potency*
Hydrocortisone	1	1
Prednisolone	4	0.8
Methylprednisolone	5	0.5
Dexamethasone	25	0

Adapted from Haynes RJ, Murad F. Adrenocorticotropic hormone; adrenocortical steroids and their synthetic analogs; inhibitors of adrenocortical steroid biosynthesis. In: Gilman A, Goodman L, Rall T, et al, eds. The pharmacologic basis of therapeutics. New York: Macmillan, 1985:1459.

erties, dexamethasone has none, and prednisolone and methylprednisolone have intermediate properties. For patients in shock from adrenal insufficiency, the balanced effects of hydrocortisone are appropriate. However, when glucocorticoid effect (i.e., anti-inflammatory property) and hypovolemia are desired, as in patients with intracranial hypertension from a brain tumor, dexamethasone is the appropriate drug.

The plasma half-lives of the intravenous steroids are about 80 minutes for cortisol (hydrocortisone), 3.5 hours for prednisolone, and 4.7 hours for dexamethasone. Their biologic half-lives are about one and a half to two times as long[53,54]. Degradation occurs in both hepatic and extrahepatic sites, followed by renal excretion of the metabolites. Liver disease or uremia, therefore, prolong the effects of administered glucocorticoids[53,55].

HYPERTENSION

Hypertension in the pediatric ICU is rarely caused by primary endocrine disease. This should only be considered and evaluated after the more common causes are ruled out. More often, hypertension has an iatrogenic cause, such as fluid and/or solute overload, medication administration, or increased intracranial pressure (ICP).

Pathophysiology and Etiology

Endocrine causes of hypertension are mostly associated with disorders of the renin-angiotensin-adrenal (RAA) system. Miscellaneous other endocrine-related disorders with hypertension are briefly reviewed at the end of this section. Endocrinopathies causing hypertension can be classified as those with high PRA and those with low PRA. In the former, the pathologic condition is thought to be in the kidney and in the latter in the adrenal gland. Although this classification scheme is convenient, its diagnostic validity is not proven.

The principal steroid responsible for salt retention and therefore many causes of endocrine hypertension is aldosterone. Regulation of the RAA axis has been reviewed in preceding text.

Whether the hypertension is caused by a primary renal disorder or an adrenal disorder, the end result is increased aldosterone activity, which causes increased Na/K exchange at the distal tubule. Consequently, in both cases, the patient has a high urinary potassium level and may demonstrate varying degrees of hypokalemia.

High-PRA Hypertension

When a cause can be found, childhood hypertension (presenting outside the ICU) is most likely to be due to renal, cardiovascular (coarctation), or renovascular factors[56] (which only secondarily result in endocrinopathy). The high renin state associated with these renal diseases results in hypertension. These renal diseases are covered in a separate chapter. A renin-secreting tumor is a very rare cause of high PRA hypertension[57], with an incidence of 8 per 30,000 cases of hypertension in one series. The tumors are small, averaging about 2.5 cm, and are well visualized on computed tomography (CT).

Low PRA with Elevated Mineralocorticoid Activity

Two adrenal enzyme deficiencies that cause decreased production of cortisol and hence congenital adrenal hyperplasia also result in hypertension. Deficiency of 17-alpha-hydroxylase (gene on chromosome 10) prevents efficient synthesis of both glucocorticoids and sex steroids, with resulting accumulation of intermediate compounds in the mineralocorticoid synthetic pathway (which have intrinsic mineralocorticoid activity). Therefore, patients may present with undervirilization[58,59], hypertension, and hypokalemia. Their steroid profile includes elevations of most steroids in the mineralocorticoid pathway (18-OH-deoxycorticosterone, corticosterone), except for aldosterone, which is low because of suppressed PRA. The same enzyme also catalyzes cleavage of the 17-20 carbon-carbon bond (previously referred to as 17,20 lyase activity), which is required for sex steroid synthesis. Hypertension is treated with replacement glucocorticoids that suppress ACTH production and consequently also suppress accumulation of the mineralocorticoid intermediate compounds.

Reduced activity of 11-hydroxylase also impairs cortisol production. However, as can be seen in Figure 39–1, it does not impede androgen production. Rather, glucocorticoid precursors are shunted toward androgen synthesis. Therefore, girls may have significant virilization and may first present as pseudohermaphrodites. Accumulation of steroids with mineralocorticoid activity, such as deoxycorticosterone, is associated with hypertension even though aldosterone activity is reduced. The role of deoxycorticosterone in producing hypertension is unclear; there have been cases of 11 hydroxylase deficiency presenting with salt wasting[60]. Also, deoxycorticosterone levels in this condition are sometimes comparable to levels in nonhypertensive salt-wasting conditions[41].

It was previously thought that the same enzyme coded for 11 hydroxylase activity in the zona glomerulosa and zona fasciculata. Two isozymes for 11 hydroxylase have since been identified, coded for by genes on chromosome 8[61]. CYP 11B1 codes for the isozyme that predominates in the zona fasciculata and CYP 11B2 codes for the isozyme in the zona glomerulosa. Patients with the presentation described here have been found to have mutations of CYP 11B1[62].

Glucocorticoid-suppressible hyperaldosteronism (GSH) is an autosomal dominant form of hypertension characterized by high levels of aldosterone, 18-oxo-cortisol, and 18-hydroxycortisol, which rapidly responds to treatment with glucocorticoids. In GSH, aldosterone is elevated despite low PRA. The mechanism underlying GSH is an unequal cross-over event that creates a fusion gene, in which the CYP

11B1 gene is fused with the promoter of aldosterone synthase[63,64]. This chimeric gene causes synthesis of aldosterone to be tightly coupled to ACTH production and not to angiotensin II. The hypertension responds to suppression of ACTH with dexamethasone, typically within 1 to 2 days.

Another familial form of severe hypertension, the syndrome of apparent mineralocorticoid excess (AME)[65], presents with normal serum aldosterone and cortisol levels but elevated ratios of urinary metabolites of cortisol to metabolites of cortisone. A brief discussion of the mineralocorticoid receptor may aid in understanding the pathophysiology of this interesting disease.

Cortisol has an affinity for the mineralocorticoid receptor that is approximately equal to that of aldosterone. Cortisol is usually prevented from acting as a potent mineralocorticoid through conversion of cortisol to cortisone (which does not bind the receptor) at the distal collecting tubule by the enzyme 11-betahydroxysteroid dehydrogenase (11BHSD) before it can bind to the mineralocorticoid receptor[66]. In several kindreds with AME, mutations have been found in the gene that codes for one of the 11BHSD isozymes: 11BHSD2[67,68]. Diagnosis is made by finding high ratios of cortisol to cortisone urinary metabolites. Treatment with dexamethasone suppresses cortisol production and can relieve the hypertension. Often a mineralocorticoid antagonist, such as spironolactone, is more effective. AME can be reproduced by licorice, which poisons 11BHSD2.

Primary hyperaldosteronism is very rare in children, and there is considerable variation in the reported proportion of adrenal adenoma versus bilateral adrenocortical hyperplasia[69–72]. Relative risk appears to be increased in females. Workup for primary hyperaldosteronism is unlikely to proceed in the ICU because it involves testing the response of the RAA axis to a saline load after discontinuation of medication (e.g., glucocorticoids, angiotensin-converting enzyme [ACE] inhibitors). Workup for aldosterone-secreting adrenal adenomas includes CT or magnetic resonance imaging (MRI) of the adrenal glands.

Other endocrine disorders associated with hypertension include hypercalcemia and perhaps hyperparathyroidism through direct effects on the renin-angiotensin systems[73]. Acromegaly is associated with hypertension[74] in as many as half of cases, possibly because of its effect on sodium transport. Hyperthyroidism is associated with systolic hypertension. Hypothyroidism can also be associated with hypertension, but the mechanism remains unclear[75].

PHEOCHROMOCYTOMA

Pheochromocytoma is one of the less common causes of endocrine hypertension in children. Diagnostic workup and management pose particular challenges, particularly in the perioperative period.

Pathophysiology

During organogenesis, some neural crest cells differentiate into pheochromoblasts and then into chromaffin cells. The chromaffin cells penetrate the developing adrenal cortex to form the medulla and also become distributed throughout the embryo, particularly in ganglia. Control of the secretory functions of chromaffin cells is the result of complex and incompletely understood interactions between the various CNS centers, the peripheral sympathetic system, hormonal signaling, and the local metabolic milieu. Chromaffin cells in these various locations can synthesize catecholamines, but in most chromaffin cells outside the adrenal medulla, catecholamine synthesis does not proceed beyond norepinephrine. Epinephrine is synthesized from norepinephrine by a glucocorticoid-dependent enzyme, phenylethanolamine-N-methyl transferase.

Catecholamines released into the blood stream by the adrenal medulla are mostly epinephrine, 10% to 20% norepineprhine. Catecholamines are metabolized, largely by the liver, through the actions of catechole-o-methyl transferase (COMT) and monoamine oxidase (MAO). Dopamine is metabolized by COMT and MAO to homovanillic acid. Norepinephrine and epinephrine are metabolized by COMT to normetanephrine and metanephrine and then to 3-methoxy-hydroxymandelic acid by MAO.

Distribution and Associations

Pheochromocytomas are rare catecholamine-secreting tumors of chromaffin origin. However, together with ganglioneuromas and neuroblastomas, they represent the most common abnormalities of the adrenal medulla in the pediatric population. They can be located in any tissue in which chromaffin tissue might be located (e.g., bladder wall, organ of Zuckerkandl). According to some classification schemes, tumors of chromaffin-tissue origin occurring within the adrenal gland are pheochromocytomas and those outside are paragangliomas. Most tumors present before age 14[76]. Adrenal tumors in children are more likely to be bilateral than in adults. Also, in childhood pheochromocytoma, norepinephrine is likely to be the predominant secretory product (in adults, both norepinephrine and epinephrine are likely to be elevated). Although they are rarely fatal by invasion or metastatic spread, these tumors can have hemodynamic consequences that cause significant morbidity and mortality[77].

Pheochromocytoma can occur in association with phakomatoses including Sturge-Weber syndrome, von Hippel-Landau, neurofibromatosis, and the autosomal dominant familial multiple endocrine neoplasia II (MEN II). Pheochromocytoma occurs in 50% of cases of MEN IIa, in association with medullary thyroid cancer and hyperparathyroidism[78]. It also occurs in 50% of MEN IIb, in association with medullary thyroid cancer, mucosal neuromas, and a marfanoid body habitus. In both forms of MEN II, medullary thyroid cancer typically presents before pheochromocytoma. Even so, it is considered prudent practice to screen yearly for pheochromocytoma with catecholamine screening tests, starting at about age 4. MEN IIa is of particular interest because of its association with the recently identified RET proto-oncogene, located near the centromeric region of chromosome 10. Mutations of the RET proto-oncogene have been mapped in families with MEN IIa[76,79,80]. The molecular probe for the RET proto-oncogene enables the search for tumors to be focused solely on family members carrying the mutation.

Clinical Presentation

Children present with sustained rather than paroxysmal symptoms. The classical adult symptom triad of paroxysmal sweating, palpitations, and headache are unusual in children. Characteristic sustained childhood signs and symptoms include hypertension, headache, sweating, nausea, vomiting, disturbed vision, emotional liability, and weight loss. Orthostatic hypotension may be seen in older children, presumably due to volume contraction[81]. Constipation, growth failure, tremor, tachycardia, polydipsia, polyuria, enuresis, and acrocyanosis are sometimes seen. Children may be polycythemic due to volume contraction, and hematocrit may be greater than 50%.

Unsuspected sustained severe hypertension may eventually bring a child to medical attention because of hypertensive encephalopathy or cardiac failure. These are emergencies that must be managed expeditiously but cautiously, because aggressive therapy may be detrimental. Pheochromocytomas can also synthesize hormones other than catecholamines, including vasoactive intestinal polypeptide, somatostatin, and calcitonin, which can further exacerbate the presentation. Also, high epinephrine output can have substantial effects on other metabolic systems (e.g., increased gluconeogenesis and lipolysis).

Diagnosis

Diagnostic testing begins with assaying random samples or 24-hour collections of urine for total catecholamines, 3-methoxy-hydroxymandelic acid, metanephrine, normetanephrine, and creatinine. If testing reveals an elevated metabolite, follow-up should include measurement of urinary epinephrine and norepinephrine excretion. Total catecholamine output is likely to be greater than 200 μg/24 hours in the presence of a tumor. However, conditions under which measurements are obtained should be carefully considered. If the patient is in a life-threatening state, elevations of catecholamine output are difficult to interpret. Similarly if the patient is receiving a catecholamine infusion for hemodynamic support, the usual reference ranges are not applicable.

If there are paroxysmal symptoms, an attempt should be made to obtain a urine sample during an episode. Urinary epinephrine and norepinephrine assays serve as confirmatory tests and offer more information if epinephrine proves to be the predominant hormone. High epinephrine excretion suggests an intramedullary site for the tumor and predicts an increased risk (compared with predominantly norepinephrine-secreting neoplasms) for tachydysrhythmias.

Localization

After biochemical evidence of a catecholamine-secreting tumor has been collected, subsequent steps are directed toward safe resection of the neoplasm. The first step is to locate the site of the tumor. CT and MRI are the least invasive and safest techniques and should be used first[82–87]. Ultrasonography is less sensitive than other imaging studies but is adequate, particularly with younger, nonobese children. Metaiodobenzylguanidine is taken up preferentially by chromaffin tissue; therefore radiolabeled metaiodobenzylguanidine provides an effective scanning technique for pheochromocytoma localization, particularly for whole-body radionuclide scanning. Often it is used in conjunction with another imaging technique.

If these measures fail to provide sufficient information, venography and arteriography may be considered. Venography is safer than arteriography, but interpretation of catecholamine levels at various venous sites may be misleading (e.g., an episodically secreting tumor may be missed)[88,89]. Arteriography is more risky, especially since dye injection may induce the pheochromocytoma to secrete catecholamines and produce an acute hypertensive crisis. For this reason, a candidate for arteriography should receive sympathetic blockade, as for surgery itself. Also, because of risks involved and the possibility of misinterpretation, these invasive techniques should only be conducted by experienced personnel.

Treatment

Surgical excision is the treatment for pheochromocytoma. Further details relevant to ICU care are described in the next section.

In patients with inoperable or malignant pheochromocytoma, the tyrosine hydroxylase inhibitor metyrosine can be used to decrease catecholamine synthesis and palliate the endocrinologic effects of the tumor.

A cautionary note is warranted with regard to acute therapy for chronic severe hypertension. The lower limit of the autoregulatory curve for cerebral blood flow appears to be shifted upward in chronically hypertensive adults (as well as in animal models)[90–97]. Although there are no such data on chronically hypertensive children, it seems likely that they, too, may begin to experience diminished cerebral blood flow when mean blood pressure falls to a point perhaps 20 or 30 mm Hg above the usual deflection point of about 50 mm Hg. With gradual and sustained treatment, the autoregulatory curve should return to normal.

Anesthesia, Intubation, and the Perioperative Period

Alpha-adrenergic blockade is the cornerstone of preoperative preparation of patients with pheochromocytoma and has lead to a massive decline in perioperative mortality. Goals are to prevent paroxysmal release of catecholamines and to alleviate the chronically vasoconstricted state so that the intravascular volume can be repleted. The latter goal helps avert having to give pressors (which can trigger the pheochromocytoma) on induction of anesthesia and may prevent or mitigate hypotension when the tumor is removed. Repletion with intravenous saline solution should be accomplished during the final 1 or 2 preoperative days. Use of a pulmonary artery catheter has been reported to be helpful in this regard[(98)] but is not considered standard unless the patient has significant cardiomyopathy. Alpha blockade also counteracts the tendency toward hyperglycemia caused by the tumor.

Two alpha blockers are commonly used in this context. Phenoxybenzamine is an alpha-1 antagonist and a weaker alpha-2 antagonist. It is longer acting than phentolamine and can be taken by mouth, making it a better choice for preoperative control.

Phentolamine is both an alpha-1 and an alpha-2 antagonist. Alpha-2 antagonism may cause increased norepinephrine levels in the heart, leading to tachycardia. It is given intravenously, either as a bolus or as an infusion. Its onset of action is within 2 to 5 minutes, and it is relatively short acting. These characteristics make it ideal for intraoperative alpha blockade.

Adrenergic blockade begins at least 2 weeks before arteriography or surgery and always with an α-adrenergic blocking agent. The alpha-blocking agent of choice is oral phenoxybenzamine, begun at 5 mg every 12 hours for young children or 10 mg every 12 hours for older children. This dosage should be increased twice weekly until normotension is achieved or until side effects (nasal congestion, GI irritation, orthostatic hypotension) appear.

Baroreceptor reflex and other reflexes are hindered by alpha blockade; consequently, patients often have orthostatic hypotension. Alpha blockade also causes nasal stuffiness, which may complicate nasal intubation.

Oral clonidine does not suppress plasma catecholamine levels in patients with pheochromocytoma[(99,100)], unlike the suppression seen in patients with essential hypertension. Some authors advocate only partial alpha-adrenergic blockade to allow unsuspected multiple tumors to be detected by the blood pressure spikes resulting from their manipulation during surgery[(101)].

Pure beta blockade should not be undertaken in patients with pheochromocytomas; the unopposed alpha effects of the serum catecholamines lead to vasoconstriction in the face of depressed cardiac output, possibly precipitating heart failure. However, beta blockade (in conjunction with alpha blockade) is useful in preventing or controlling dysrythmias (e.g., in epinephrine-secreting tumors). Propranolol may be the first-line beta-blocking agent, although under some circumstances it may be ideal to use agents that are shorter acting (e.g., in perioperative or ICU care) or more beta$_1$ specific (e.g., in bronchospasm). Propranolol can be used acutely in a dose of 0.01 to 0.1 mg/kg by slow intravenous push (maximum dose, 1 mg at a time) with concurrent electrocardiographic (ECG) monitoring. The oral regimen consists of 5 to 10 mg every 6 to 8 hours initially, which is increased cautiously to produce the desired results. Heart failure is the chief drawback to be anticipated[(88)] (see the corresponding subsection under hyperthyroidism for more on beta blockers and their toxicity). Beta blockade is continued until surgery. Optionally, one might switch to a shorter-acting agent, such as esmolol[(102)], during times when hemodynamic lability is expected (e.g., at intubation or intraoperatively).

Catecholamine cardiomyopathy does occur in children with pheochromocytomas[(103)], so cardiac evaluation should be performed to rule it out. Preoperative resolution of symptoms and normalization of blood pressure predict an uncomplicated outcome; there is suggestion that aggressive volume administration leads to cardiopulmonary complications, such as congestive heart failure and pulmonary edema[(103)]. Use of a pulmonary artery catheter may be helpful if there is evidence of cardiac dysfunction. Data suggest that right atrial filling pressure may not accurately reflect pulmonary capillary wedge pressure in some patients with this condition[(104)]. Invasive monitoring of arterial and central venous pressure are also useful in any setting where a patient with this tumor may be expected to have rapid, marked changes in blood pressure and intravascular volume, including treatment of a hypertensive crisis, induction of anesthesia (whether for surgery or for some other emergency), and postoperative care.

Sedation and ample local anesthesia are desirable preceding procedures, including placement of invasive monitors, since anxiety may lead to catecholamine release. However, oversedation may cause hypercapnia, which also leads to catecholamine release. Choice of drugs is geared to minimizing sympathetic stimulation. Morphine causes histamine release, which can lead to catecholamine release[(105)]. Fentanyl does not cause histamine release and generally induces bradycardia via increased central vagal tone[(106,107)]. Oral or intravenous benzodiazepines and scopolamine are also useful. Scopolamine causes minimal if any changes in heart rate even though it is an anticholinergic agent, but some investigators believe that it causes excessive behavioral changes in children. Regional anesthesia may be very helpful in patients with a pheochromocytoma who need a peripheral procedure (e.g., reduction of an open wrist fracture) or for pain relief postoperatively.

Anticholinergics are best avoided unless absolutely necessary (although the tachycardia associated with glycopyrrolate is minimal).

Intubation is a potentially hazardous procedure, since laryngoscopy causes a potent sympathetic reaction. If a patient presents for emergency surgery or intubation and cannot receive the usual course of preoperative alpha-adrenergic blockers, administration of phentolamine and/or nitroprusside or other antihypertensive agents may be necessary, and such agents should be at hand. Nitroprusside is very effective in lowering blood pressure but may cause reflex tachycardia (which responds to beta blockers). Trimethaphan causes histamine release and therefore should be avoided.

Induction of anesthesia is performed with any agent except ketamine (which causes a central sympathetic outpouring). The patient should be deeply anesthetized prior to intubation, either by intravenous or inhalational agents (about 1.3 times the minimum alveolar concentration (MAC) is usually needed to blunt sympathetic responses). Fentanyl (1 to 3 μg/kg) (or other short-acting opioid) and/or lidocaine (1.5 mg/kg) may attenuate the sympathetic response to intubation.

Intravascular volume is replenished with the goals of alleviating orthostatic hypotension and normalizing the hematocrit level.

Muscle relaxant drug selection should exclude those that cause histamine release (atracurium, mivacurium, curare, and metocurine) or are vagolytic (pancuronium and gallamine). Vecuronium is a good selection in this respect. Doxacurium and pipecuronium are also acceptable from a hemodynamic standpoint but may be of limited usefulness for emergency intubation because of their long onset of action and duration. Succinylcholine may induce catecholamine release from the pheochromocytoma by a number of mechanisms: Histamine release, ganglonic (nicotinic) stimulation, and abdominal wall fasciculation[108]. Still, its use may be necessary in the context of a rapid sequence induction, particularly since a consistent triggering effect on pheochromocytomas has not been demonstrated.

Rocuronium[109,110], a new nondepolarizing muscle relaxant, may prove to be optimal. It provides intubating conditions in less than 60 seconds at doses of 0.6[111] to 1.2 mg/kg[112] and has mild cardiovascular effects. Dosing may be different in very small children, since volume distribution seems to be relatively large at younger ages[110]. Rocuronium has a duration similar to vecuronium[112,113], about 20 to 35 minutes. Regardless of the agent used, nondepolarizing neuromuscular blockade can be reversed in the usual manner if necessary.

The key aspects of postoperative care are monitoring and treating hypotension and hypoglycemia. Hypotension can occur at any time after ligation of the venous drainage of the tumor. Nevertheless, about half of patients are still hypertensive immediately postoperatively. Persistence of hypertension for more than 1 to 2 days may raise the suspicion that residual tumor remains. A catecholamine-mediated hypertensive crisis may share features with other conditions, including malignant hyperthermia, as discussed in the section on hyperthyroidism. Patients who have had bilateral adrenalectomy need replacement steroids (e.g., oral hydrocortisone, 14 mg/m^2 daily.

Vomiting is a prominent symptom of pheochromocytomas[114]. Unfortunately, use of some antiemetic agents can have untoward effects. Droperidol can trigger a hypertensive crisis in some patients with pheochromocytoma. Suggested mechanisms have included inactivation of a dopaminergic inhibitory system, which normally prevents adrenal catecholamine release[115], and blockade of presynaptic alpha adrenoceptors[116]. Metoclopramide also is not recommended in pheochromocytoma[117], because it causes increased catecholamine secretion[118]. In fact, metoclopramide is used as a diagnostic test to screen for pheochromocytomas[119]. Other drugs should therefore be considered for perioperative nausea and vomiting. Ondansetron may provide a safe alternative, although there is little experience with this drug in pheochromocytomas at present.

DISORDERS OF GLUCOSE METABOLISM

Diabetic Ketoacidosis

Diabetic ketoacidosis (DKA) is certainly among the most frequently discussed[120–140], if not the most frequently seen, metabolic disorders in ICUs. Despite advancing knowledge of the pathophysiology and treatment of diabetes mellitus, DKA remains a significant source of morbidity and mortality in all age groups and in locations as diverse as Korea and Denmark[141,142]. In Pittsburgh, the prevalence of insulin-dependent diabetes mellitus (IDDM) is 1.4 in 1000 and the incidence is 16 in 100,000[143]. From Rochester, Minnesota, comes a report of 13 episodes of DKA per 1000 IDDM patient-years[144]. The mortality rate for DKA ranges from 3% to 17%[140,142,145] and is especially high in the elderly, with children representing 1.6% of all DKA deaths[146].

Pathophysiology of Diabetic Ketoacidosis

Diabetes mellitus arises from inadequate insulin effects and, in children, almost always from inadequate amounts of insulin. Insulin acts on several metabolic pathways, including carbohydrate and lipid metabolism, nitrogen balance, and many regulatory systems.

Insulin

Insulin must be considered in terms of both its facilitative and inhibitory effects. Insulin stimulates anabolism and, therefore, storage of glycogen, protein, and fat in muscle, liver, and adipose tissue. Insulin also enhances cell uptake of ketone bodies[147]. Conversely, it inhibits glycogenolysis, gluconeogenesis, proteolysis, lipolysis, and ketogenesis[148–151]. Insulin exerts its effects by two means: by rapidly changing the kinetics of key enzymes through phosphorylation and by slowly changing the quantity of these enzymes.

Normal adult insulin secretion is about 40 to 50 U/day, with surges in secretion occurring in response to food consumption. Direct stimuli include glucose, mannose, leucine, and vagal stimulation. Glucose-induced insulin release may be increased by arginine, β-adrenergic input, and GI hormones or may be decreased by somatostatin, α-adrenergic input, and use of certain drugs, such as phenytoin, diazoxide, and vinblastine[148].

In the liver, insulin stimulates formation of glycogen, protein, and triglycerides, whereas it inhibits breakdown of glycogen. Insulin also promotes glycolysis and impedes gluconeogenesis and ketogenesis in the liver[148–151]. Insulin deficiency, therefore, allows unchecked hepatic ketogenesis and gluconeogenesis, with additional glucose release through unimpeded glycogenolysis[152]. After the first few hours of insulin deficiency, glucose production declines significantly[153]; therefore, impaired glucose utilization and slowed urinary excretion (from hypovolemia and low glomerular filtration rate [GFR][154] are the important reasons for continued increasing hyperglycemia.

In muscle, insulin accomplishes three essential anabolic functions: it enhances cellular entry of glucose, promotes glycogen synthesis, and promotes amino acid transport and protein synthesis. In diabetes, these processes are impaired so that glucose fails to enter the cells, glycogen is depleted (although its depletion is not linked to glucose export from muscle), and protein catabolism is unbalanced[148].

In fat, insulin inhibits intracellular lipolysis, enhances lipoprotein cleavage to allow fat absorption, and enhances glucose entry to provide for production of glycerol in order to form triglycerides. With insulin deficiency, lipolysis continues unabated, while fat absorption and triglyceride synthesis are blocked[148].

At least six glucose transport proteins have been identified, all with a shared motif of 12 transmembrane domains. Of the six, GLUT4 has been thought to be critical in glucose homeostasis because it is the major transporter in tissues where glucose transport is thought to be insulin dependent[155]. Insulin appears to stimulate translocation of the GLUT4 transporter from an intracellular site to the cell membrane. However, recent studies[156] suggest that the role of GLUT4 has not been completely elaborated. In mice in which the GLUT4 transporter gene has been disrupted, glucose metabolism is abnormal, but the mice are not overtly diabetic.

Counterregulatory Hormones

Glucagon and insulin have an intricate metabolic relationship that is central to the pathogenesis of DKA[157,158]. The liver is the main target organ for glucagon, where it stimulates glycogenolysis, gluconeogenesis (from glycerol and amino acid precursors), and production of ketone bodies (from fatty acids). These effects follow the induction of several enzymes by an increase in the relative proportion of glucagon to insulin.

Release of glucagon is enhanced by hypoglycemia. This effect is inhibited by β-hydroxybutyrate (i.e., by ketones). Glucagon levels also rise in response to increased levels of amino acids. Release of glucagon is inhibited by hyperosmolality[159]. Glucagon-inhibitory effects (including that of somatostatin, mentioned later) are probably not very important, since the absolute concentration of glucagon is often normal in DKA[160,161].

The effects of glucagon on ketogenesis are mediated in two ways. Glucagon increases the formation of carnitine, which is essential for fatty acid entry into mitochondria. Glucagon also inhibits formation of malonylcoenzyme A (malonyl-CoA), a compound that normally inhibits the esterification of fatty acids with carnitine. The net result is thus unimpaired entry of fatty acids into the β-oxidation pathway[152,162]. Acetoacetate and β-hydroxybutyrate are produced in abundance. The relative lack of insulin allows lipolysis to continue excessively, providing substrate for formation of ketones.

Ketogenesis is accompanied by glycogenolysis and gluconeogenesis. These processes are enhanced by a rising glucagon/insulin ratio in portal venous blood. Of the counterregulatory hormones, only glucagon has a clearly established pivotal role in the genesis of hyperglycemia and ketosis in humans[163]. When its release is inhibited by somatostatin, ketosis is prevented.

Cortisol, growth hormone, epinephrine, and norepinephrine are all present in excess in patients in DKA[128,129,160–164], but it is impossible to separate whether the increased serum hormone levels are due to precipitating stress (infectious, emotional, traumatic) or DKA itself. Although the increased blood levels of these "stress hormones" are quite possibly secondary effects of DKA, they probably also facilitate its progression. Growth hormone appears to enhance lipolysis and block glucose uptake by muscle. Cortisol enhances gluconeogenesis, blocks glucose uptake by muscle, and supports lipolysis. Epinephrine impedes insulin release, promotes lipolysis and glycogenolysis, blocks glucose uptake by muscle, and diminishes hepatocellular fructose 2,6-diphosphate (fructose 2,6-P2), thus promoting gluconeogenesis and inhibiting glycolysis. (Alpha-adrenergic receptors stimulate hepatic glycogenolysis and gluconeogenesis, and decrease insulin production; beta adrenergic receptors also stimulate hepatic glycogenolysis and gluconeogenesis but decrease insulin production.)

In addition, increased levels of vasopressin, plasma renin activity, and aldosterone, as well as depressed levels of atrial natriuretic factor, have been reported in patients in DKA[165–168]. The vasopressin response seems to be appropriate to the volume depletion and hypertonic state and is no doubt enhanced by the nausea experienced by many patients. It has been suggested that elevated vasopressin levels play a role in increasing the risk of cerebral herniation in patients receiving aggressive rehydration[169].

Hyperglycemia with ketosis has been observed during prostaglandin E1 infusion[170]. Prostaglandins may stimulate glucagon release, inhibit insulin release, and have other effects on glucose homeostasis that have not yet been clarified. Prostacyclin may play a role in the reduced vascular tone seen in DKA, and other eicosanoids may also have functions in that disturbed cardiovascular state[171–174].

Metabolic Derangements in Diabetic Ketoacidosis

Lipemia and Ketosis

Insulin suppresses ketogenesis and lipolysis at lower levels than are required to increase glucose transport. In the absence of insulin, a number of metabolic events shift fatty acid metabolism to the inner mitochondrial membrane, where the fatty acid chains undergo beta oxidation to ketone bodies. The pivotal step in this transfer is carnitine palmitoyl transferase I (CPTI). CPTI catalyses the reaction of fatty acyl coA with carnitine to create fatty acyl carnitine, which then enables the fatty acid to be transported to the inner membrane, where it is converted back to the fatty acyl coA in a reaction catalyzed by carnitine palmitoyl transferase II. The fatty acid is then available for beta oxidation, which results in ketogenesis.

Malonyl coA inhibits CPTI. In insulin-deficient states, malonyl coA levels are reduced (because acetyl coA carboxylase activity is deceased, impeding the generation of acetyl coA from pyruvate). The decrease in malonyl coA causes increased CPTI activity and subsequent ketogenesis. This process is further accelerated by the increased fatty acid substrate resulting from increased lipolysis. Acetyl coA carboxylase is further inhibited by fatty acids and glucagon, both of which are elevated in insulin deficiency.

An important hallmark of DKA is the acidosis due to elevated plasma concentrations of the ketoacids acetoacetate and β-hydroxybutyrate. Depressed insulin levels permit lipolysis to accelerate in adipose tissue, releasing long-chain fatty acids. In the liver, these fatty acids are shunted toward β-oxidation and ketone production rather than being transported out as triglycerides; this path is determined by the increased glucagon/insulin ratio. Ketones normally stimulate insulin release and thereby inhibit lipolysis; the lack of this feedback in insulin deficiency permits extreme lipemia and ketonemia and prevents triglyceride synthesis in adipose tissue[(152)]. This hypertriglyceridemia may be responsible for a rise in immunoreactive somatostatin[(175)], and hypertriglyceridemia has been reported to be severe enough to produce dramatic masking of hyperglycemia[(176)]. Nonenzymatic decarboxylation of acetoacetate also produces elevated acetone concentrations in plasma[(177)].

In rare cases, patients with diabetic ketosis present without acidemia. DKA has been seen with a pH of 7.7 (presumably due to excessive use of diuretics)[(178)].

The commonly used tests for serum ketones employ the nitroprusside reaction, which reflects acetoacetate levels well and acetone less well (about 20 moles of acetone react the same as 1 mole of acetoacetate)[(130)]. Hydroxybutyrate does not react at all. This fact is important for correct interpretation of reported ketone levels, since the relative proportions of the three compounds may vary greatly, influenced by acid-base and redox states. Normally, the β-hydroxybutyrate/acetoacetate ratio is about 3:1, but it may reach 15:1 in severe DKA, and acetone may represent one and one-half to four times the molar concentration of acetoacetate[(130,177,179)].

An important method of removing excess acid in DKA is through nonenzymatic conversion of acetoacetate to acetone and carbon dioxide. Acetone is then excreted in breath and urine (in a 5:1 ratio). This mechanism removes about one-fourth of the H+ generated by hepatic ketogenesis. Relative hypoxia, by shifting acetoacetate toward β-hydroxybutyrate, reduces the body's ability to eliminate ketoacids by the acetone route[(177)].

Lactic Acidosis

Lactic acid in DKA may arise, in part, from anaerobic glycolysis in hypoperfused tissues during hypovolemia caused by osmotic diuresis. This anaerobic state increases the ratio of NADH to NAD, favoring formation of lactate as the hydroxy acid of pyruvate. Likewise, a greater proportion of acetoacetate is converted to its hydroxy acid, β-hydroxybutyrate[(179)]. Measuring lactate and acetoacetate gives a crude indication of the relative proportions of ketoacids.

Non-Anion Gap Acidosis

Hyperchloremic acidosis in DKA has been reported by several investigators[(179–182)]. In one carefully documented case, this was found to result from excessive urinary losses of the salts of β-hydroxybutyrate[(182)]. Other reports[(180,181)] suggest that although hyperchloremic acidosis may be present on admission for DKA, it is more common during initial therapy. The proposed mechanism is based on the observation that patients with an increased anion gap present with greater prerenal azotemia[(180)].

Presumably, acute volume depletion with the onset of DKA results in acidosis with the expected increased unmeasured anions. If, however, the patient is able to maintain salt and water intake for a significant period of time, urinary losses of the sodium and potassium salts of β-hydroxybutyrate allow wasting of bicarbonate, resulting in acidosis out of proportion to the measured anion gap. Aggressive intravenous fluid resuscitation with solutions containing large amounts of chloride (e.g., normal saline) may potentiate this effect and may be further increased by differences in the volumes of distribution of bicarbonate and ketones[(179)]. Thus, patients presenting with DKA and a small anion gap recover from acidosis more rapidly if acetate is used in place of chloride in the administered intravenous fluid.

Hyperosmolality

The hyperosmolar state induced by insulin deficiency is as harmful as ketoacidosis. Osmolality can be measured in the laboratory or can be estimated:

Formula 1: Osmolality = [glucose (mg/dL)/18] + [BUN (mg/dL)/2.8] + 2[Na (mEq/L) + K (mEq/L)]

Thus, both hyperglycemia and dehydration contribute to hyperosmolality. In fact, the values generally reported suggest that in a typical child with DKA, glucose is elevated by about 400 mg/dL, and urea nitrogen (BUN) by about 15 mg/dL, therefore contributing about 22 and 5 mOsm/L, respectively. The volume of fluid loss for this typical child in DKA represents 15% of body weight.

The fluid loss is due to osmotic diuresis induced by glucose. When fluid loss is severe enough to impair GFR, excretion of excess glucose is slowed and hyperglycemia accelerates. The combination of rapidly rising glucose and BUN results in extreme hyperosmolality. Hyperosmolality has been noted to correspond with levels of obtundation and with electroencephalogram (EEG) abnormalities better than other laboratory measurements in DKA[183,184].

Derangements in Serum Electrolytes and Minerals in Diabetic Ketoacidosis

Sodium, Chloride, and Water

Loss of water through osmotic diuresis is, arguably, the most dangerous process brought about by DKA. Cardiorespiratory function can remain adequate to sustain life even at the extremes of pH and osmolality seen in DKA, but shock invariably occurs when dehydration is severe.

Estimation of the degree of dehydration is best made by known body weight. Unfortunately, this is usually not possible, so estimates are made based on physical findings, which are based on ECF volume. Extracellular volume is maintained by plasma hyperosmolality, so the deficit in total body water is easily underestimated in these patients. Indices obtainable by invasive monitoring (e.g., central venous pressure, pulmonary capillary wedge pressure) can give useful information on volume status but are rarely necessary.

As discussed earlier, chloride is retained in exchange for ketone salts, especially in patients maintaining large volumes of fluid and salt intake during development of DKA. The resultant hyperchloremia may be worsened, prolonging recovery from acidosis, if normal saline is used in large volumes during resuscitation. An effective solution in this situation will contain 10% to 30% of sodium as acetate or bicarbonate. The common practice of supplying potassium as a 50/50 mixture of chloride and phosphate salts is also beneficial in this situation.

Hyponatremia is usually reported by the laboratory when sera from DKA patients are analyzed, and often the reportedly low value is an artifact. Extreme lipemia can decrease the measured sodium value simply by decreasing the aqueous phase of blood, in which sodium is found. A correction formula has been proposed[185]:

Formula 2: True (aqueous phase) serum sodium (mEq/L) = [reported sodium (mEq/L)][0.021 (triglycerides (g/dL) + 0.994)]

Another important shift in sodium measurement is produced by hyperglycemia. However, this is not an artifact in the sense that the measured sodium correctly reflects the dilutional effects of water flowing into the vascular compartment due to the osmotic gradient. As the amount of glucose rises in the ECF, water shifts there from intracellular fluid (ICF), thus lowering the concentration of other solutes, including sodium. The classic formula of adding 2.8 mEq/L to the measured sodium for every elevation of blood glucose of 100 mg/dL assumes that water influx has brought ECF to isoosmolality, clearly not a valid assumption in DKA. The shift in sodium concentration is closer to 1.6 mEq/L for every elevation in glucose concentration of 100 mg/dL, producing the following formula for predicted serum sodium if the patient was rendered euglycemic (corrected):

Formula 3: Sodium (mEq/L) predicted = [reported sodium (mEq/L) + 0.016 (glucose (mg/dL)]

With use of formulas 2 and 3, the sodium concentration that would be measured if hyperglycemia and lipemia were cleared can be approximated:

Formula 4: Sodium (mEq/L) predicted if euglycemic and eutriglyceridemic = (reported sodium (mEq/L))(0.021 (triglycerides (g/dL)) + 0.994) + 0.016 (glucose (mg/dL))

Some intensivists believe that this calculated correction of sodium concentration provides a useful guideline for hydration. However, the measured serum sodium level is the "real" actual sodium concentration in blood. The corrected sodium level is a theoretical calculation.

Potassium

Hyperkalemia is commonly found at presentation with DKA[186,187] and is the product of several factors[188–192]. Hyperkalemia is commonly believed to be the result of the elevated extracellular hydrogen ions being exchanged for the major intracellular cation, potassium. According to theory, the protons from the increased amount of ketoacids travel down their concentration gradient into the ICF. This then alters the transmembrane electrical potential, to favor release of cations from the ICF. Potassium, as the major ICF cation, moves down this electrical gradient into the ECF. This may not be a mechanism of great importance in DKA. Hyperosmolality and low insulin concentrations and decreased renal tubular potassium secretion appear to be more important. Hyperkalemia correlates with BUN and with pH, and the mechanism for decreased potassium secretion is unclear[186,193–195].

Hyperosmolality probably produces two important effects: Potassium redistributes from ICF to ECF. Progressive diuresis leads to dehydration and, eventually, diminished glomerular filtration, with resultant decreased potassium excretion.

The effectiveness of glucose and insulin in combination in treatment of hyperkalemia is well known; potassium's entry into muscle cells is facilitated. In the absence of insulin, a glucose load produces hyperkalemia, which can be reversed by insulin.

Oral intake of potassium is often poor in these patients, and continued osmotic diuresis results in progressive depletion of body potassium stores. Consequently, when insulin is infused, hypokalemia is likely to result unless potassium is supplied early in treatment. In DKA, serum potassium levels do not correlate well with either lactic acidosis or ketoacidosis.

Phosphate, Calcium, and Magnesium

Profound hypophosphatemia and depressed levels of red blood cell (RBC) 2,3-diphosphoglycerate (2,3-DPG) have been described in DKA by numerous investigators[196–199]. Presumably these are due to osmotic diuresis and competition with glucose for reabsorption at the renal tubules. During the first 24 hours of treatment of DKA, the phosphate concentration falls further, and 2,3-DPG remains depressed[197] unless phosphate is supplied with resuscitation fluids.

The clinical significance of these deficiencies is unclear. It has been suggested by many that the low levels of RBC 2,3-DPG serve to decrease the P50 of oxyhemoglobin (the PO_2 at which hemoglobin is 50% saturated with oxygen), thus decreasing peripheral release of oxygen from hemoglobin. Acidosis initially counter balances this by increasing the P50. Phosphate levels can be improved, but with no clear benefit[200]. Some researchers have reported a beneficial effect of 2,3-DPG, but phosphate repletion had not been found to have any significant effect on 2,3-DPG[199] or P50[198] in a randomized study until recently. Even then, a statistically significant rise in P50 (from 20.5 to 22.5 torr) with phosphate replacement[201] is of uncertain clinical importance. The grave consequences of chronic hypophosphatemia, such as rhabdomyolysis, hemolysis, and poor leukocyte function, have not been reported in DKA. Hypophosphatemia has been found to cause insulin resistance[202], but the clinical relevance of this to DKA is unclear.

In short, phosphate replacement is of theoretical benefit only. Its use must be approached with caution, and careful monitoring of calcium and magnesium levels is warranted. The chief advantage to using potassium phosphate may be in reducing the amount of chloride delivered and thereby helping avoid hyperchloremic acidosis during therapy.

During treatment of DKA, exuberant replacement of phosphate can result in depressed serum levels of calcium and magnesium[203,204]. In spite of this, tetany is rarely seen. Results of a prospective, controlled study in children with DKA[205] showed only a slight diminution of total serum calcium, and potassium phosphate administration had no effect on serum ionized calcium. Furthermore, this study failed to demonstrate that phosphate infusion had any beneficial effect on phosphorus homeostasis. Magnesium may be deficient in diabetic children[206], and extreme hypomagnesemia can be seen in DKA, where it is believed to inhibit the response of parathyroid hormone to hypocalcemia. No benefit has been demonstrated for routine replacement of magnesium in DKA.

The sections on calcium, magnesium, and phosphorus metabolism provide further details on disturbances in these electrolytes.

Clinical Presentation of Diabetic Ketoacidosis

DKA is present when serum glucose concentration is more than 300 mg/dL, a serum nitroprusside test is positive at 1:2 dilutions or greater, the blood pH is below 7.3 (although the pH may be falsely elevated by other variables), and the serum bicarbonate concentration is below 15 mEq/L[130]. Approximately 30% of newly diabetic children present with DKA[144], and 10% of patients with DKA are admitted in a comatose state[140,145,184,207]. The mortality rate for all patients with DKA is about 9%; it is higher in the elderly[144,145]. There are about 75 deaths from DKA yearly among 100,000 diabetics under age 15 in the United States; neurologic collapse from cerebral edema is a common cause of death[129,141,142,146,208–213].

Children with DKA often present with a familiar history (i.e., polyuria, polydipsia, polyphagia, and weight loss). These symptoms are followed by headache, abdominal pain, vomiting, lethargy, and hyperpnea. Initial contact often reveals an acutely ill child with lethargy, dehydration, hyperpnea, and occasionally the smell of acetone on the breath. If the history is vague or unavailable and the child is unresponsive, differential diagnosis, unfortunately, is broad and includes intoxication (especially with salicylates and alcohol), Reye's syndrome, inborn errors of metabolism, sepsis, meningoencephalitis, nonketotic hyperglycemic coma, or hypoglycemic coma in addition to DKA,.

The child with DKA who arrives in the emergency department with a clear sensorium and good peripheral circulation may not require admission to the ICU[125]. However, the presence of profound shock, coma, respiratory failure, or dysrhythmias (or suspicion that the child is at risk for any of these) indicates a need for prompt ICU admission. As in all situations, treatment priorities follow the "ABCs": first the airway, then breathing, then circulation.

Evaluation of Patients with Diabetic Ketoacidosis

Initial laboratory evaluation may include various tests to exclude other entities in the differential diagnosis. Initial tests specifically needed to begin monitoring the course of therapy for DKA should include blood gases, pH, electrolytes, BUN, glucose, creatinine, osmolality, ketones, lactate, calcium, magnesium, and phosphate. Hourly determinations should follow for pH, PCO_2, Na^+, K^+, glucose, and ketones, with the interval lengthened only when stable control has been achieved. The full initial panel should be repeated every 4 to 6 hours during the first 24 hours of treatment. For patients with mild DKA, fewer laboratory tests and interventions may be needed[125]; effective use of such a low-cost approach has been documented[214].

The ECG should be continuously monitored and displayed. Additionally, a lead II strip should be run and saved hourly at first, to aid in detecting severe alteration in K^+

and Ca^{2+}. Urine output must be carefully followed, and patients in shock should have a bladder catheter placed. Neurologic status should be assessed at least hourly, and in obtunded patients, a method of quantification (such as the Glasgow Coma Scale) is helpful. Clearly, such patients require individualized care and frequent monitoring of vitals by a nurse skilled in pediatric intensive care.

Shock

Children with shock from DKA severe enough to warrant admission to the ICU should have continued aggressive fluid therapy. Careful monitoring is essential. An arterial catheter should be placed both to permit continuous measurement of blood pressure and to provide a means for rapid blood sampling for monitoring acid base, electrolyte, and glucose status. A central venous pressure line may be helpful in following volume status. A urinary bladder catheter is essential to monitor ongoing losses and promptly detect renal failure from the antecedent hypoperfused state.

Adequate vascular access for volume resuscitation is crucial. This requirement may be complicated by the need to have one intravenous line dedicated to an insulin infusion, another to infusions of other drugs (e.g., pressors), and so on.

Cerebral Edema

Despite improvements in management of DKA in the past 25 years, mortality due to cerebral edema remains unchanged. Estimates of the incidence of clinically apparent cerebral edema have a wide range (0.1% to 1.0%), probably because of different interpretations of what significantly constitutes the problem. The outcome of cerebral edema is poor: Mortality is 60% to 80%, 13% to 26% have long-term neurologic morbidity, and only 7% to 10% are free of complications. Very few predictors of which children are at risk for significant cerebral edema have withstood the test of time. However it does appear that children under age 5 with a new diagnosis of IDDM and with a prolonged period of untreated DKA are at increased risk.

It is widely believed that cerebral edema is a result of treatment of DKA, specifically rehydration. One study found that rates of hydration greater than 4 L/m^2 carried a higher risk of cerebral edema[(169)]. Yet this association, obtained retrospectively, does not prove causality and remains contested. In fact, specific risk factors for cerebral edema have been elusive and controversial.

The rationale behind concern about vigorous rehydration is that in order to maintain adequate cell volume, brain cells autoregulate their osmotic gradients by generating intracellular idiogenic osmoles (possible candidates for these osmoles include taurine, sorbitol, fructose, and glutamine). It has been hypothesized that these idiogenic molecules are slowly metabolized and therefore cause a relatively large influx of water during rehydration, causing overexpansion of neurons. A related hypothesis[(215)] suggests that as ketoacids and free fatty acids diffuse into CNS cells, the cells' Na/H exchanger acts to normalize intracellular pH by shifting H^+ out, thereby increasing intracellular sodium, which in turn increases cell volume during rehydration. It has yet to be shown that a significant quantity of the organic acids generated in DKA (e.g., acetoacetate) do actually diffuse into brain cells.

Some studies suggest that AVP, which is appropriately elevated in the context of intravascular depletion in DKA, does not always drop back down when treatment of DKA restores normal osmolality[(169)]. Therefore, the patient may become rapidly hypo-osmolar, and the brain, enclosed in a fixed space, cannot safely accommodate the resulting influx of water into cells. Insulin also contributes to the influx of sodium, potassium, and water into CNS cells. In experimental studies with rabbits and rats, cerebral edema could not be demonstrated in the absence of insulin.

Still, some observations and questions remain unanswered concerning the pathogenesis of cerebral edema. There have been several cases of radiographically demonstrated cerebral edema[(216)] and a reported death from cerebral edema[(217)] prior to initiation of treatment. It is also not clear why adults with DKA are less suseptible to cerebral edema. Nonetheless, despite the controversy and lack of definitive answers, it is prudent to hydrate vigorously only as required to maintain hemodynamic stability and subsequently to complete volume repletion over a 48-hour period.

The indications for lumbar puncture and ICP monitoring in DKA are unclear but should be carefully considered in each case. In children, especially infants, with DKA who have fever and clouded sensorium, concerns should always be raised about sepsis or meningoencephalitis and whether a lumbar puncture should be performed to prove the existence of infected cerebrospinal fluid (CSF) before antimicrobial therapy is initiated. Contraindications are twofold: First, positioning the child with preexisting shock and acidosis for lumbar puncture may embarass both chest excursion and venous return to the heart. Second, the child may have significant cerebral edema, and a sudden withdrawal of lumbar CSF could produce downward herniation of the intracranial contents. For these reasons, in a child with DKA in whom meningoencephalitis is considered likely, antibiotics should be given during the initial resuscitation. Lumbar puncture can be performed later, if still deemed important, and may reveal Gram stain or antigenic evidence of common bacterial infections.

Endotracheal intubation for airway protection should be strongly considered in children in DKA in coma (Glasgow Coma Score of 7 or less). ICP monitoring need not be instituted for most children with DKA who present in coma. In the majority, the sensorium clears with correction of the metabolic abnormalities. If the patient's neurologic status worsens or fails to improve once hyperglycemia is corrected, CT scanning and ICP monitoring are needed. (The anesthetic drugs used for intubation may cloud neurologic examination, at least transiently.) CT scan should precede ICP monitoring, because coma may be due to CNS infarction from hyperviscosity or other unsuspected intracranial pathologic conditions[218,219]. At all stages, caution is essential to avoid overly rapid correction of serum hyperosmolality or acidosis (at least with bicarbonate). Either event could theoretically potentiate cerebral edema. Once ICP monitoring has been established, treatment of cerebral edema is the same as that in other CNS cytotoxic states: Elevation of the head of the bed, keeping the head in the midline, hyperventilation, drugs to reduce ICP (refer to Chapter 18).

Aggressive management of elevated ICP in a child treated for DKA may be unsuccessful, but it may offer some chance for good recovery in an as yet poorly identified subset of children[212,218].

Pulmonary Edema

Another unusual finding in DKA, possibly related in part to osmolality changes, is pulmonary edema. The observation of increasing oxygen requirements with or without radiographic changes consistent with pulmonary edema has been made by several authors. Abundant theories are available as explanations, including myocardial failure[140], low plasma oncotic pressure[207], and increased pulmonary capillary permeability[220,221]. Since raised ICP is seen in DKA, a neurogenic basis for this pulmonary edema may also be a reasonable explanation[222]. Of course, vomiting and blunted consciousness suggest aspiration of gastric contents as a reasonable explanation for development of opacification on chest radiograph.

Care should be taken to ensure that adequate arterial blood oxygenation continues in order to avoid further tissue injury (especially CNS) and prolonged acidosis. Low plasma oncotic pressure should be avoided, and any potential neurogenic cause for pulmonary edema should be promptly treated. The standard blood gas indicators for intubating the patient with acute respiratory failure (e.g., $Paco_2$ greater than 50 torr, Sao_2 less than 90% with FIo_2 greater than 0.60) are not strictly applicable in DKA. In the face of metabolic acidosis, respiratory failure may occur well before $Paco_2$ rises to 50 torr. Poor cardiac output makes otherwise "borderline" Pao_2 and Sao_2 values wholly inadequate for tissue oxygenation. Sustained hyperpnea results in fatigued respiratory muscles, and development of electrolyte disturbances potentiates this. Deepening coma is a strong indication for establishing a controlled airway.

For these and other reasons, intubation of the child in DKA must be considered early and in anticipation of rapid multisystem failure. If positive end-expiratory pressure (PEEP) of more than 5 cm H_2O is employed, the clinician needs to consider that the cardiac output suffers most from PEEP in the hypovolemic patient. This is particularily important in the presence of coma, which implies elevated ICP. PEEP decreases cardiac output (which reduces cerebral perfusion pressure [CPP]) and increases central venous pressure (which impedes venous return from the head, leading to increased ICP and hence decreased CPP). A pulmonary artery (Swan-Ganz) catheter may help in titration of PEEP, central venous pressure, and cardiac output with respect to each other and to ICP.

Cardiac Dysrhythmias

Life-threatening disturbances in cardiac rhythm can be caused by hyperkalemia, hypokalemia, or hypocalcemia, all of which can occur in patients being treated for DKA. On admission of a child with DKA to the emergency department, ECG monitoring should be started and continued until the child is clearly responding to therapy with normalizing blood chemistries and neurologic status. Early in the course of treatment, an ECG may provide the earliest evidence of hyperkalemia (peaked T-waves)[187,223,224]. Lead II provides reliable information in patients of all ages, whereas in small children, T-wave morphology in the precordial leads may be misleading.

Management of Diabetic Ketoacidosis

Physicians direct the care of the critically ill child in DKA most effectively when they have a clear set of priorities forming the framework for therapeutic plans **(Table 39–3).** In descending order of importance, these priorities are:

1. Establishment of the airway, breathing, and circulation
2. Consideration of differential diagnosis
3. Provision of insulin
4. Fine tuning of biochemistry
5. Care to avoid complications of therapy

After ensuring that the airway and breathing are adequate, the circulating blood volume should be optimized. Intravenous access is obtained, and an infusion of normal saline solution or Ringer's lactate (both readily available and isotonic) is started immediately. Volumes of 10 to 20 mL/kg are administered as rapidly as possible and as often as necessary until blood pressure and evidence of skin and organ perfusion are seen. A blood sample is taken for complete blood cell count, glucose, BUN, electrolytes, calcium, magnesium, phosphate, osmolality, Pco_2, and pH. A few drops are withdrawn for a reagent strip glucose determination and a capillary-tube hematocrit, which provides rapid evidence of hemoconcentration and allows gross examination for lipemic serum.

If the diagnosis is not clear at this point or if further data is needed to clarify suspected precipitants to the DKA, blood might be sent for toxicology screening, prothrombin time, ammonia, liver enzymes, or culture. Lactate and ketones rarely are obtained, since they provide little additional information than the calculation of the anion gap.

After shock has been corrected, and as the measured sodium approaches the corrected sodium, the crystalloid is changed to 0.45% NaCl, since this more closely mimics the fluid lost in DKA. The infusion rate is then calculated to correct the estimated water deficit over about 48 hours, which keeps the rate well within the modest limits currently recommended[120,214,225,226]. In the absence of hyperkalemia, potassium is added, 40 mEq/L, as the chloride and/or

Table 39.3. Initial Treatment for Suspected Diabetic Ketoacidosis

Goal	*Time*	*Approach*
1. ABCs	First minutes	Intubate if patient is comatose and ensure adequate breathing and circulation
2. Differential diagnosis and begin monitoring	First minutes	Brief history Venipuncture (large bore IV) and complete blood cell count, blood urea nitrogen, glucose, electrolytes, osmolality, pH, Pco_2, Ca^{2+}, Mg^{2+}, PO_4, and spun hematocrit; Do Chemstrip test ECG: monitor and check rhythm strip (check T-waves)
3. Volume repletion	First minutes	Assess blood pressure, heart rate, and skin perfusion Give normal saline or lactated Ringer's solution 10 mL/kg repeatedly as needed to reverse shock
4. Reverse hyperglycemia and ketosis	After Step 2 is in progress, give regular insulin of 0.1	U/kg per hr intravenously
5. Fine-tune biochemistry	After Steps 2 and 3 are in progress, change volume replacement to 0.45% saline solution with 25 mEq KCl and 20 mEq K_2HPO_4/L	Adjust solution according to monitored ECG, electrolytes, and pH
6. Avoid hypoglycemia	When glucose ≤300 mg/dL, add 5% dextrose to intravenous fluid	Increase to 10% dextrose if necessary

phosphate salt. Bicarbonate is probably best avoided unless acidosis is extreme and is thought to be causing dangerous myocardial dysfunction.

Following the initial phase of fluid resuscitation in which shock is reversed, fluid therapy is planned for the ensuing 48 hours, allowing for maintenance needs, ongoing losses (vomiting, osmotic diuresis), and correction of the estimated deficit. This deficit, generally equal to at least 15% of body weight, is partly made up by resuscitation fluids and is completely replaced over a period of 48 hours. As noted earlier, measurements of serum electrolytes are often misleading until hyperglycemia and lipemia have cleared.

One note of caution: A child with known diabetes who presents with obtundation may not be in DKA, but may in fact be hypoglycemic (e.g., from an overdose of insulin). Therefore, if hyperglycemia cannot be documented promptly, the child should receive intravenous dextrose at a dose of 0.5 g/kg (2 mL of 25% dextrose [D25W] in water per kilogram). D50W should always be diluted with an equal volume of water. Risk (even if the patient really is hyperglycemic) is minimal, and benefits to a potentially hypoglycemic brain may be enormous.

As soon as hyperglycemia and ketosis are confirmed, a continuous intravenous infusion of regular insulin is established at a rate of 0.1 U/kg per hour through a separate intravenous line. There is no established need for an initial intravenous bolus of 0.1 U/kg insulin[227–230]. When the serum glucose decreases to 300 mg/dL, 5% dextrose is added to the intravenous fluids.

It is a commonly held belief that a low-dose continuous infusion is the best method of insulin delivery in treating DKA. However, there are also other effective methods. Since the discovery of insulin in 1922[231], physicians have also used large subcutaneous doses and high-dose infusions (up to 100 U/hr)[232]. Although no reproducible statistically significant difference has been found in the biochemical response of children with DKA treated with constant intravenous low-dose insulin infusion rather than with large-dose subcutaneous injections, investigators found universal appeal in the ability to use smaller amounts of insulin. They also cited, as advantages of the constant-infusion method, the predictably steady fall in glucose concentrations and the ability to alter therapy quickly[233–241].

The use of sodium bicarbonate in children with DKA remains controversial, largely because the putative benefits and risks remain unproved. When acidosis is severe (pH < 7.1), bicarbonate therapy has been proposed to improve myocardial function, reduce the potential for dysrhythmia, diminish insulin resistance, reduce the work of breathing, hasten recovery from coma, and avoid the hyperchloremic state that can prolong acidosis. Stated risks include increased hemoglobin-oxygen affinity (thus risking increased tissue hypoxia), paradoxically increasing CNS acidosis (by more rapid diffusion of CO_2 than HCO_3 across the blood-brain barrier), reducing the ionized fraction of calcium, and producing hypokalemia. Not one of these concerns has been demonstrated by prospective reproducible study to be of practical significance in children with DKA[242,243].

If bicarbonate is to be given, rapid injection should be avoided. The best method of infusion of bicarbonate is to include it in the crystalloid solutions that are given in the first few hours, at a concentration of 25 to 50 mEq/L. Since one of the stated concerns about bicarbonate is its ability to produce "paradoxical" CNS acidosis by making CO_2 available to cross the blood-brain barrier, an alternative to consider might be tris(hydroxymethyl)aminomethane (THAM). It has been demonstrated to offer promise in reducing brain tissue acidosis in an animal model of traumatic brain injury[244] and to increase brain cellular lactate export in a preliminary report on a model of global brain ischemia[245].

Anesthesia, Intubation, and the Perioperative Period

Diabetics in DKA present a number of difficulties, the most serious being acidosis, obtundation, and hypovolemia. Supplemental oxygen should be provided and the airway should be protected, particularly in the context in the context of changes in mental status or hemodynamic instability.

Induction of anesthesia to facilitate intubation may precipitate cardiovascular collapse in severely hypovolemic patients. It may be helpful to insert an intraarterial catheter to monitor rapid changes in blood pressure during induction. The arterial line also may be very useful in monitoring acid-base and glucose status. The patient's volume status should be optimized prior to induction if possible. In the context of cardiovascular compromise, ketamine—which stimulates the sympathetic system[(246)]—may be useful[(247)], although it is associated with disorientation and hallucinations or dreams[(247)]. Etomidate also causes minimal cardiovascular depression[(248–252)] but may not be a wise choice given the possibility of concurrent adrenal dysfunction in diabetes (see section on adrenal insufficiency). Induction with good hemodynamic stability can also be achieved with 1 to 2 μg/kg of fentanyl with 0.05 to 0.1 mg/kg midazolam. The bradycardia from fentanyl may be detrimental in a patient whose cardiac output is dependent on heart rate. However, this effect, which is centrally mediated via the vagus nerve[(106,107)], is easily treated or prevented with an anticholinergic drug.

Other options include a ketamine-midazolam combination[(247)] or as much as 0.3 mg/kg midazolam. Midazolam has the advantage of providing antegrade amnesia and of mitigating the undesirable psychological effects of ketamine. In fact, any agent can be used to induce anesthesia provided dosing is done carefully, with close monitoring of vital signs (although it may be best to avoid thiopental and propofol in situations where hemodynamic stability is critical). Regardless of the method employed, pharmacologic means of raising blood pressure and heart rate should be available.

The obtunded patient (Glasgow Coma Scale < 7–8) may need little, if any, anesthesia for intubation; muscle relaxation may suffice. Sedating a drowsy child is probably an excessive risk except immediately before intubation, since sedation can lead to complete obtundation and/or hypoventilation with respiratory acidosis. The latter aggravates the existing metabolic acidemia. In addition, hypercarbia causes increased cerebral blood flow[(253)] and increased ICP. If the child has cerebral swelling, this may be poorly tolerated.

A child with cerebral swelling should be intubated with extreme care taken to avoid hypercarbia and swings in blood pressure. Invasive blood pressure monitoring and ICP monitoring may be helpful in these situations, since the hemodynamic effects of treatment of other problems (e.g., correction of hypovolemia or hypotension) may have deleterious effects on ICP and vice versa. Furthermore, it is desirable for the child to be deeply anesthetized before laryngoscopy to avoid increases in ICP[(254,255)]. It is particularly important to avoid coughing and bucking; muscle relaxants help achieve this goal. Children with increased ICP are at increased risk for nausea and vomiting, and consequently aspiration. A rapid sequence induction[(256)], or at least application of cricoid pressure during intubation, should be considered, especially if the child is already obtunded. Ketamine is not an ideal choice in the context of cerebral edema; it increases cerebral blood flow and hence ICP[(257–259)]. However, it may still be the drug of choice in hypotensive patients, since maintaining blood pressure generally takes precedence over neurologic issues.

Muscle relaxants are commonly used to facilitate intubation, particularily in the context of rapid sequence induction. Succinylcholine has always been the drug of choice for emergency intubations, but DKA presents two relative contraindications to its use. Succinylcholine induces a rise of 0.5 to 1 mEq/L in healthy patients, which could induce cardiac arrest in a patient who is already hyperkalemic. Thus, this is a strong contraindication. Succinylcholine also raises ICP mildly. This consideration, though real, is probably of secondary importance to the crucial issue of airway protection. Some have advocated a "defasciculating" dose of pancuronium (0.01 mg/kg IV) to blunt these two effects[(260)], but this method is probably not reliable. Rocuronium[(109,110)] is a new rapid-onset nondepolarizing muscle relaxant that shows some promise in this situation. (See the subsection under pheochromocytoma for further details.)

Elective preoperative care of diabetic children differs from adults because children rarely have the end-organ damage seen in adults (e.g., coronary artery disease, peripheral vascular disease, renal damage, autonomic neuropathy, including diabetic gastroparesis)[(261)]. Children with long-standing diabetes may have mild limited joint mobility due to tightness of the skin, but this rarely presents problems when positioning the patient for procedures such as laryngoscopy, as is sometimes experienced in adults. Similarly, the increased predisposition to infection is less marked in diabetic children (but appropriate attention to aseptic technique is still warranted). Nonetheless, there are ample reports (often from parts of the world where medical care is less accessible) of end-organ dysfunction in the children. Even in developed countries, there are conflicting reports regarding the incidence and severity of left ventricular dysfunction, nephropathy, and other conditions in children with diabetes.

One study of potential relevance to intubation of diabetic children reports delayed gastric emptying of solids and postprandial antral hypomotility[(262)]. This may present an aspiration risk, particularly with the nausea and vomiting seen in evolving DKA.

Insulin therapy on the morning of surgery is tailored to prevent hyperglycemia without provoking hypoglycemia while the patient is taking nothing by mouth. Ideally, elective surgery should be scheduled early in the day to simplify glycemic management. Preoperative evaluation should include serum glucose and electrolytem evaluation as well as a measure of the patient's degree of ketosis, if any (urine ketones).

There are many perioperative regimens and methods of controlling DKA[(263–271)]. The specific protocol used probably does not matter as much as close monitoring of serum glucose levels. The following is a fairly typical preoperative protocol.

In the morning, an intravenous infusion of 5% dextrose solution is started at a maintenance rate. Serum glucose is checked prior to insulin administration to prevent hypoglycemia. One half of the patient's total morning dose of insulin is given as subcutaneous intermediate-acting insulin. Dosing should be modified according to the serum glucose level and adjusted for the amount of "sliding scale" insulin received overnight, if any. Alternatively, insulin can be given by continuous infusion. This is reported to result in better intraoperative control, but there is little experience with this method in children[236,241,272,273].

Oral hypoglycemic agents should be continued until the day of surgery. Management is otherwise similar to treatment of IDDM (glucose infusion and monitoring of serum glucose), except that insulin is generally not necessary.

DKA and other medical problems (e.g., sepsis) should be corrected prior to surgery if possible. If surgery cannot wait for medical optimization, insulin requirements of children in such catabolic states may be higher than in well-controlled patients[274].

Diabetic patients can have postoperative hypoglycemia or hyperglycemia. Hypoglycemia can result from administration of an excess of insulin over glucose.

One final consideration is the increased susceptibility of patients taking NPH insulin to allergic reactions to protamine sulfate, with potentially devastating consequences when the drug is used to reverse heparin[275,276].

Transition from Pediatric ICU to Ward

During the initial presentation of DKA, the ICU specialist is unlikely to have to use any insulin other than regular insulin. However, as planning begins for transition of the patient to ward care, subcutaneous dosing with a mixed insulin regimen is often started. We briefly review here the available insulin preparations and their use.

When acidosis has resolved, mental status is normal, and interest in food returns, the patient may be advanced to oral feeding and subcutaneous insulin. Since intravenous insulin has a half-life of only a few minutes, it is an error to discontinue intravenous insulin before subcutaneous insulin has been given. Subcutaneous insulin should be given only when a meal both precedes it and stays in the patient. The proper sequence, therefore, is to allow a meal or snack at an appropriate time, give regular insulin (subcutaneously) at a dose of 0.25 U/kg (or more or less as indicated by the preceding drip requirements), and discontinue the intravenous drip of insulin. Then, it is appropriate to discontinue any central venous or arterial catheters and arrange to transfer the patient out of the pediatric ICU.

Most patients with new-onset diabetes mellitus are started on human insulin obtained by DNA recombinant techniques. Purefied beef, beef-pork, and pork insulins are increasingly being phased out by manufacturers, and there are few indications for their use over human analogues. Animal insulins may have slightly longer half-lives, but if this is desired, a similar result can be accomplished with combinations of human short- and long-acting insulins. Insulin preparations typically come in a vial at a concentration of U100 (100 U/mL). This is a convenient concentration for most children. However, in infants, where 0.5 or 0.25 U can make a big change in the daily dose, a more dilute insulin (U10, 10 U/mL) is available to allow for more accurate dosing. If this is not available, most insulin manufacturers can provide a diluent solution to allow preparation of U10 from U100.

The starting dose of subcutaneous insulin can be calculated in a number of ways. The intravenous rate can be used and multiplied by 24 to give a total daily dose. Alternatively, the following guidelines can be used: a prepubertal patient who presented in DKA requires 0.5 to 1.0 U/kg per day, with the upper end of the range most applicable in patients who had moderate to severe ketoacidosis and therefore are more likely to be transiently insulin resistant. Pubertal adolescents are likely to require 1.0 to 1.5 U/kg per day. The total daily dose is given as two to four injections per day. The regimen selected depends on the age of the patient, the common practice of pediatric endocrinologists in the area who will be following the patient's long-term care, and an assessment of what regimen the patient's family will be able to maintain.

The total daily dose is given as a combination of short- and long-acting insulins. Short-acting (regular) insulins typically have onset of action within 0.5 hours, peak action at 1 to 2 hours, and duration of action of approximately 3 to 6 hours. Intermediate-duration (lente, NPH) insulins have onset of action 2 to 3 hours after injection with peak action at 5 to 6 hours and a duration of 12 to 20 hours. Long-acting (ultralente, PZI) insulins have a modest peak action at 6 to 12 hours and provide continued activity for 18 to 16 hours, and therefore are rarely given until insulin requirements are well established.

A common initial regimen is obtained by first calculating the total daily dose and then splitting the total dose into two thirds to be taken in the morning before breakfast and one third in the evening before dinner. Each premeal dose is also split into two thirds intermediate-duration insulin and one third short-acting insulin.

For example, a child who weighs 36 kg may be started at 36 U/day: the morning dose of 24 U composed of 16 U NPH and 8 U regular insulin, and the evening's 12 U consisting of 8 U of NPH and 4 U of regular insulin. Since even the short-acting insulins take at least half an hour to act, if the patient is receiving insulin infusion in the ICU, the infusion should be discontinued only half an hour after the subcutaneous injection. Also, before administering the injection, it should be verified that a meal is available to the patient within half an hour and that the patient is sufficiently alert and interested in eating.

Hyperosmolar Hyperglycemic Nonketotic Coma

Hyperosmolar hyperglycemic nonketotic coma (HHNC) is an extremely unusual occurrence in childhood, characterized by marked hyperglycemia with resultant hyperosmolality, dehydration, and a lowered level of consciousness in the absence of ketosis or acidosis. The usual definition includes serum osmolality in excess of 350 mOsm/L[219,277,278].

The important differences in pathogenesis and treatment between HHNC and DKA are due to negligible ketoacid production in the former. The absence of ketosis is due to a normal insulin/glucagon ratio. The causes of HHNC can be lumped into three broad categories: lack of water, excess of glucose, and excess of counterregulatory hormones (glucagon is elevated, but not in relation to insulin).

The syndrome is much more common in the elderly, but causes for increased risk with age are not known[219,279]. The greater risk in blacks than whites may be due to social factors rather than race per se[277]. The mortality rate (at least in adults) is quite high (40% to 60%)[219,280]. HHNC has been seen in children with diabetes mellitus, sometimes as the presenting symptom. It has also been seen in nondiabetic children with hyperosmolar dehydration[281,282], in a child receiving epinephrine for asthma[283], and in children following suprasellar surgery[284].

Potential causes at any age include severe trauma, infection, hyperalimentation, exogenous corticosteroids, catecholamines, phenytoin, diazoxide, loxapine, amoxapine, and thiazide diuretics. Limited access to fluid is often a significant factor in the genesis of HHNC[219,280,285–287].

Fluid replacement is the central issue in treatment and consists initially of boluses of 20 mL/kg of normal saline solution infused as rapidly and as frequently as is needed to reverse shock. In the absence of hyperkalemia (or peaked T waves on ECG), potassium is added to the initial intravenous fluids in a concentration of 10 to 20 mEq/L. The need for phosphate replacement is even less clear in pediatric HHNC than in DKA; hence, phosphate is best left out of intravenous fluids initially.

Once shock has been treated effectively, intravenous fluid is converted, usually to 5% dextrose/0.45% NaCl (vide infra) to continue cautious correction of the hyperosmolar state. Potassium chloride supplementation is continued and may be increased as indicated by serial measurements. The rate of infusion, as in DKA, is calculated to replace the presenting deficit over 24 to 48 hours, plus allowances for maintenance needs and replacement of continuing losses.

Insulin is used with great caution in HHNC, since serum glucose can fall precipitously. An initial continuous intravenous infusion of 0.05 U/kg per hour may be adequate and is adjusted based on closely monitored reagent-strip and laboratory blood glucose measurements. When the blood glucose reaches 300 mg/dL, 5% dextrose is added to intravenous fluids. If the blood glucose level continues to fall, the insulin drip should be reduced or stopped before hypoglycemia ensues[277,281,288].

The initial differential diagnosis and laboratory screening tests are the same for HHNC and DKA. Close monitoring of osmolality, glucose, sodium, potassium, chloride, calcium, phosphate, and magnesium is continued through the first 24 hours of treatment.

The cause of HHNC in any child should be investigated carefully. Special attention should be given to over supply of glucose, restriction of fluid, and administration of any of the medications mentioned, either accidentally or as a manifestation of child abuse.

Hyperglycemia in the Head-Injured Child

Hyperglycemia in the head-injured child is common, although it may not be severe enough to qualify as HHNC. The pathogenesis probably relates to increased endogenous catecholamines and corticosteroids from the stress of injury. Their effects are potentiated iatrogenically by the administration of pressors and inotropes (sympathomimetic agents), corticosteroids (given by some to minimize cerebral edema), and intravenous dextrose administration. Serum glucose is further elevated when urine losses in a patient with diabetes insipidus are replaced with a solution containing 5% glucose (1% to 2.5% dextrose in a balanced salt solution may be sufficient).

Hyperglycemia has been shown to correlate with the severity of brain injury[288], although there is controversy as to whether hyperglycemia really is a poor prognostic sign[289]. An especially effective way to exacerbate this problem is to replace urine losses from diabetes insipidus with solutions containing 5% dextrose, when 1% to 2.5% dextrose (in large volumes of hypotonic salt solutions) may be more than adequate.

The hazards of hyperglycemia to the injured brain have been demonstrated clinically and in animal experiments. Ischemic brain injury occurring in hyperglycemic rats is significantly worse than ischemic injury in normoglycemic ones[290]. Retrospective studies have shown that ischemic brain injury is worse in patients with hyperglycemia during recovery than in patients with normoglycemia[291]. Plum, in reviewing work from his own group and others, theorized that in the ischemic brain, the harmful effects of increased glucose are mediated by elevated lactic acid levels, resulting in enhanced damage to both neurons and astrocytes[292].

Experimental data suggest that the deleterious effects of hyperglycemia on the ischemic brain occur if high glucose levels exist before ischemia occurs. This does not mean that hyperglycemia is not to be feared after the ischemic insult (stroke, near drowning, shock, trauma) has happened, since brain ischemia may recur in the pediatric ICU (e.g., from intracranial hypertension, systemic hypotension). Furthermore, adult patients receiving glucose shortly after head injury have been found to have increased brain lactate production when compared with controls given no glucose[293]. In addition, hyperosmolality induced by extremes of hyperglycemia affect global CNS function as noted in earlier sections. Adequate nutrition is also impeded by hyperglycemia, in that glucose delivery must be restricted, thus allowing tissue catabolism to continue. Volume status is affected via osmotically induced diuresis.

There are two approaches to hyperglycemia in the brain-injured patient, and neither can presently be proven to improve outcome. One approach is to withhold dextrose initially (from a few hours to a few days, with careful monitoring of blood glucose), under the assumption that the risks to the brain of giving glucose outweigh the benefits to the rest of the body. The other approach is to continue dextrose in the nutritional support and to use insulin when hyperglycemia is a problem. A continuous infusion of insulin starting at 0.05 U/kg per hour provides more exact and smooth control over blood glucose than does intermittent subcutaneous insulin and may improve tissue anabolism while the potentially harmful effects of high blood glucose levels on the injured brain are avoided. An over supply of carbohydrates can be problematic, even if blood glucose is normal. If over supply of carbohydrates allows for fat deposition, the respiratory quotient may exceed 1.0; the increase in CO_2 production necessitates an increase in minute ventilation and can make hyperventilation or weaning from mechanical ventilation difficult. The increase in CO_2 may also lead to a rise in ICP, which may be undesirable in a child with head trauma.

Hypoglycemia

This section contains an overview of the pathophysiology of hypoglycemia, which has been described in detail in excellent reviews and standard texts[(157,294–298)]. Special attention is paid to the different aspects of hypoglycemia at different ages.

All mentions of blood glucose in this section refer to measurements derived from whole blood. Whole blood yields glucose values that are 10% to 15% lower than measurements obtained from serum or plasma. Glucose measurements can be artifactually lowered if the sample contains excessive numbers of leukocytes (as in leukemia) or nucleated RBCs[(299)]. Bedside glucose measurements can be taken by various means, with the glucose oxidase reagent strip method demonstrating the best accuracy[(300)].

The brain accounts for 20% of the body's total metabolic demands. Since it cannot utilize fatty acids, it presents a large fixed demand for glucose and ketones. Indeed, all the complex countermeasures against hypoglycemia can be seen as the body's attempts to continue to ensure the fuel supply to the CNS. In fasting, hepatic glycogenolysis is the initial fuel source, but it can supply only a few hours' worth of glucose. After hepatic glycogen is depleted, glucose must be created from amino acids, lactate, and the glycerol moiety of triglycerides. The ketones produced by hepatic oxidation of fatty acids, favored by a low insulin/glucagon ratio, also constitute an important energy source for the brain during fasting.

CNS hypoglycemia provides the stimulus for activation of mechanisms that elevate blood glucose. The blood glucose threshold at which this occurs is generally higher in the context of cerebral hypoperfusion or a rapid fall in glucose concentration and is lower in the neonate[(294,296)]. The most important antihypoglycemic measure appears to be release of glucagon and epinephrine; their effects seem to be additive. Inadequate levels of these two hormones leave the patient with little defense against insulin-induced hypoglycemia[(157,301)]. Growth hormone, adrenal corticosteroids, and catecholamines other than epinephrine play supportive roles in the response to hypoglycemia[(294,296,297)]. Their effects are summarized in the preceding discussion of DKA.

In the child with normal alimentary function and metabolic pathways, normoglycemia represents a balance between the factors causing hypoglycemia (fasting, insulin, and glucose utilization) and the hyperglycemic factors described. Hyperglycemic effects are more physiologically complex and act to increase brain glucose supply: insulin release is inhibited, glycogenolysis and gluconeogenesis are stimulated, and muscle cell use of glucose is impeded. In addition, cardiac output and total systemic vascular resistance are increased, presumably increasing cerebral blood flow and, therefore, glucose delivery to the brain tissue[(294)].

Neonatal Period

Glucose homeostasis is balanced more tenuously in neonates than in adults. The normal-term neonate, in the fed state, shows a decline in blood glucose from maternal levels to 50 mg/dL at 2 hours of age, rising to about 70 mg/dL by the third day of life. Blood glucose levels are normally lower in premature neonates. In neonates weighing less than 2500 g, hypoglycemia is said to exist when the blood glucose is less than 20 mg/dL. For term infants above 2500 g, hypoglycemia is defined by a blood glucose level below 30 mg/dL in the first 72 hours and below 40 mg/dL thereafter[(302,303)].

In the normal fasted term neonate, hepatic glycogen stores are sufficient to meet glucose demands for 8 to 12 hours, after which glucose from gluconeogenesis, fats, and ketones become important sources of energy[(296)]. Hepatic glycogen stores fall by 90% in the first 2 to 3 postnatal hours. As this glucose source is depleted, the neonate begins to utilize more fat, so the respiratory quotient falls from 0.9 to 1.0 to 0.7[(297)].

Neonatal hypoglycemia is usually transient, occurring in the first 48 hours after birth, and the cause is usually unclear. Hypoglycemia may be asymptomatic or may produce any part of a broad spectrum of symptoms, including tremulousness and poor feeding, hypotonia, temperature instability, periodic breathing, apnea, cyanosis, convulsions, and coma[(304)]. These are nonspecific symptoms and should be ascribed to hypoglycemia only if correction of low blood glucose resolves the symptoms. Commonly known causes of transient hypoglycemia include maternal diabetes, neonatal hypothermia, asphyxia, polycythemia, infections, respiratory distress syndrome (RDS), adrenal hemorrhage, and small size. Prompt recognition of hypoglycemia is aided by careful observation of newborns at risk and may be avoided by ensuring oral or intravenous (as 10% dextrose) glucose supply in the first few hours of life.

The preferred method of administration of intravenous dextrose for neonates is as a 10% to 20% solution supplying 4 to 8 mg/kg per minute continuously after an initial bolus of 0.5 to 2.0 g of dextrose/kg in a 25% solution. Fifty percent dextrose is not used in neonates because of its extremely high osmolality (about 2800 mOsm/L), which may cause significant local tissue damage. Central venous access may be necessary in order to deliver these high-osmolality solutions. An umbilical artery line can also be used, with the caveat that if the tip of the catheter is near the take-off of the superior mesenteric artery (at T11 or T12) or celiac (T10) artery from the aorta, the pancreas may receive arterial blood that is very rich in glucose. The pancreas may thus sense hyperglycemia and increase insulin release, even in the presence of systemic hypoglycemia.

Asymptomatic transient hypoglycemia that is successfully treated early carries a good prognosis[302]. Persistent neonatal hypoglycemia reflects a more serious disorder and may be more difficult to treat. Causes include hereditary disorders of carbohydrate metabolism, such as the glycogen storage disorders, galactosemia, hereditary fructose intolerance, or fructose-1,6-diphosphatase deficiency. Hereditary defects in amino acid, such as maple syrup urine disease, propionic acidemia, tyrosinosis, or methylmalonic aciduria, can also cause hypoglycemia. Persistently depressed serum glucose results from insulin excess due to many causes, including Beckwith-Wiedemann syndrome, erythroblastosis fetalis, trisomy 13, and the islet cell dysmaturation syndrome[305], which includes β-cell hyperplasia, or islet cell hyperplasia. Deficient human growth hormone, cortisol, or ACTH may also be a cause[296,304,306,307]. Further discussion of diagnosis and treatment of all these specific potential causes is beyond the scope of this chapter but may be found in standard texts of neonatology and metabolic disease.

Initial steps in managing neonates with persistent hypoglycemia are the same as those used in managing patients with transient hypoglycemia. Other treatment methods, including hydrocortisone use (5 mg/kg per day in two doses) or prednisone (1 mg/kg per day), may be of help. Diazoxide (10 to 15 mg/kg per day orally in three doses) may decrease insulin release and aid in achieving normoglycemia. Repeated random collections of blood for simultaneous insulin and glucose level testing may reveal relative hyperinsulinemia.

If the infant has hyperinsulinism and medical therapy is failing to maintain normoglycemia, laparotomy may be indicated for resection of tumor or, in the absence of tumor, for subtotal pancreatectomy[308,309]. Continuous subcutaneous infusion of somatostatin (8.3 mg/kg per hour) and glucagon (5.4 mg/kg per hour) has been used successfully as a temporizing measure and offers theoretical advantages over maintaining continuous intravenous infusions[310].

Infancy to Adolescence

Two thirds of cases of hypoglycemia in infants older than 1 month are idiopathic; within this group are included unclassified cases (20%), cases of leucine-sensitive hypoglycemia (30%), and cases of ketotic hypoglycemia (50%). The other one third of the cases of hypoglycemia are due to a wide variety of disorders **(Table 39–4)**[296].

In the ICU setting, the main concerns regarding hypoglycemia are neuroglycopenia leading to seizures or coma[311], and/or the primary illness of which hypoglycemia is a manifestation.

Treatment of childhood hypoglycemia (blood glucose < 45 mg/dL) begins with intravenous dextrose, 0.5 g/kg. This can be given as a 25% solution to a child of any age; the 50% solution is best reserved for adolescents whose veins are large enough to tolerate the osmolality. The bolus of dextrose should be followed by a constant intravenous infusion of 10% dextrose.

Glucagon, in a dose of 0.1 to 0.3 mg/kg (up to 1 mg maximum)[296], may be given intravenously or intramuscularly. This agent generates its immediate effect by glycogenolysis and therefore is ineffective in disorders in which glycogen is absent (starvation, ketotic hypoglycemia), glycogen storage or lysis is abnormal (the glycogenoses), or liver function is inadequate (e.g., Reye's syndrome, hepatitis)[302]. Furthermore, glucagon should be accompanied by a supply of dextrose to avoid depletion of carbohydrate stores.

Glucagon has other pharmacologic uses, such as in treating low-cardiac-output states after cardiopulmonary bypass surgery or from congestive myocardial infarction, congestive heart failure, and beta-adrenergic blocker toxicity. However, it is expensive, causes hypokalemia and hyperglycemia, and commonly causes nausea and vomiting in awake patients.

Unlike glucagon, diazoxide acts by impeding the release of insulin and thus is useful only in hyperinsulinemic patients. Hyperinsulinism is identified by persistence of nonketotic hypoglycemia despite dextrose replacement and is documented by insulin levels. The dosage of diazoxide is 10 mg/kg per day divided into two or three enteral doses. The intravenous route can be used, but the extremely potent hypotensive effect of diazoxide, even at 1 mg/kg, makes this a less desirable route of administration and dictates a slow infusion with careful monitoring of blood pressure. Hydrocortisone, 5 mg/kg per day, or its glucocorticoid equivalent may be a useful adjunct in persistent hypoglycemia (refer to the section on hypoadrenalism)[296]. Epinephrine has also been suggested as an adjunct, but the potent cardiovascular effects and subsequent lactic acidosis make this a poor choice. As mentioned earlier, continuous infusion of glucagon and somatostatin subcutaneously may hold promise for safe and effective temporizing treatment of hypoglycemia due to hyperinsulinism.

Treatment of hypoglycemia should begin promptly, particularly in infants or young children who have been fasting and stressed (a common occurrence in the pediatric ICU) and then given an inadequate supply of dextrose and calories. Perioperatively, neonates may need 20 mg/kg per minute of dextrose[312]. Concentrated glucose solutions may be necessary to avoid excessive fluid loads. A hypoglycemic child should not be restricted to a nothing-by-mouth diet without an adequate intravenous dextrose supply. The critically ill child is always at risk for hypoglycemia and must have a secure intravenous line in place at all times.

Should the intravenous line fail, it should be replaced immediately.

The differential diagnosis should be addressed once treatment is under way. Other causes of hypoglycemia may be recalled with the mnemonic HECK: Hepatomegaly, endocrinopathy, chemicals, ketosis.

Hepatomegaly suggests the possibility of the glycogenoses, hereditary fructose intolerance, fructose-1,6-diphosphatase deficiency, galactosemia, phosphoenolpyruvate carboxykinase deficiency, carnitine deficiency, hepatitis, Reye's syndrome, tumor, or hepatotoxins.

Endocrinopathies associated with hypoglycemia (aside from pancreatic ones discussed later) include hypopituitarism and hypoadrenalism.

Chemicals (medications and toxins) whose use may lead to hypoglycemia include aspirin, acetaminophen, ethanol, sulfonylureas, hypoglycin (from the unripe ackee fruit), and of course, insulin[296,302].

Ketosis must be ruled out when hypoglycemia is unaccompanied by any of the other clues listed. The presence of ketones suggests an intact ketogenic system. The insulin/glucagon ratio must be decreased, leading to fatty acid mobilization from adipose tissue, as well as adequate carnitine and cofactors allowing for fatty acid β-oxidation in the liver. Ketotic hypoglycemia may occur in a normal infant or young child after prolonged fasting but is seen within as little as 24 hours of fasting in thin infants and toddlers with ketotic hypoglycemia. This, the most common form of childhood hypoglycemia, may simply represent the extreme case of all small children who have relatively diminished substrate for gluconeogenesis as a result of having little muscle mass and relatively large brains with high glucose demand or it may represent mild and as yet characterized disorders of gluconeogenesis[313–318].

Hypoglycemia without ketosis is due to hyperinsulinemia or a failure of hepatocellular ketogenesis. Hyperinsulinemia is further suggested by persistent hypoglycemia despite intravenous dextrose and is proven by measuring simultaneous serum insulin and glucose levels. The most common cause of hyperinsulinemia is exogenous over sup-

Table 39.4. Causes of Hypoglycemia

- Lack of available glucose or its precursors
- Inadequate caloric intake
- Low-birth-weight infants
  - Kwashiorkor
  - Low-phenylalanine diet
  - Starvation
- Impaired absorption or excessive loss
  - Chronic diarrhea
    - Intestinal disaccharidase deficiency
    - Monosaccharide malabsorption
  - Renal glycosuria
- Increased peripheral glucose utilization
- Hyperinsulinism
  - Infants of diabetic mothers
  - Infants with erythroblastosis
  - Beckwith syndrome
  - Nesidioblastosis
    - β-cell hyperplasia, idiopathic
    - Leucine-sensitive hypoglycemia
  - Islet cell adenoma
  - Subclinical diabetes mellitus
- Extrapancreatic tumors
  - Mesenchymal tumors
  - Hepatoma
  - Adrenocortical carcinoma
  - Pseudomyxoma
  - Teratomas
  - Epithelial tumors
  - Congenital neuroblastoma
  - Wilms' tumor
- Deficiency in hepatic glucose formation and release
- Enzymatic defects
  - Glycogen synthetase deficiency
  - Glycogen storage diseases
  - Type I (glucose-6-phosphatase deficiency)
  - Type III (amylo-1,6-glucosidase or debranching enzyme deficiency)
  - Type IV (hepatophosphorylase deficiency)
  - Galactosemia (galactose-1-phosphate uridylyltransferase deficiency)
  - Hereditary fructose intolerance (fructose-1-phosphate aldolase deficiency)
  - Fructose-1,6-diphosphatase deficiency
  - Deficiencies in hormonal regulation
  - Growth hormone deficiency
- Adrenocortical insufficiency
  - Addison's disease
  - Congenital adrenal hyperplasia
  - ACTH deficiency
  - ACTH unresponsiveness
- Catecholamine deficiency
- Glucagon deficiency
- Inborn errors of amino acid metabolism
  - Maple syrup urine disease
  - Propionicacidemia
  - Tyrosinosis
  - Metylmalonic aciduria
  - Isovaleric acidemia
- Liver disease
  - Hepatitis
  - Cirrhosis
  - Fatty degeneration of the liver (Reye's syndrome)
- Idiopathic hypoglycemia
- Neonatal hypoglycemia
  - Small-for-gestational-age infants
  - Infants of mothers with toxemia
  - Infants with CNS hemorrhage or infection
  - Infants with respiratory distress syndrome
  - Abrupt cessation of intravenous hypertonic glucose solutions
- Onset after 2 months of age
  - Leucine-sensitive hypoglycemia
  - Ketotic hypoglycemia
  - Unclassified (unknown) types
- Miscellaneous
- Pharmacologic or toxic
  - Salicylate
  - Alcohol
  - Oral hypoglycemia agents (biguanides, sulfonylureas)
  - Insulin
  - Unripe ackees (hypoglycin) (Jamaican vomiting sickness)
  - THAM-TRIS (hydroxymethyl)aminomethane
  - Phosphorus
- Defects in regulatory function of CNS
  - Tumors, hemorrhage, injury infection
  - Cold

Adapted from Kogut M. Hypoglycemia: pathogenesis, diagnosis, and treatment. In: Gluck L, Cone T, Dodge P, eds. Current problems in pediatrics. Chicago: Year Book, 1974:3.

ply. There are many reports of hypoglycemia in the juvenile diabetic population[319–324].

Other causes of hyperinsulinism range from the structurally defined islet cell hyperplasia, nesidioblastosis, adenomatosis, and adenoma to the functionally defined leucine-sensitive hypoglycemia (synonymous with postprandial hypoglycemia in children)[325–329]. The leucine-sensitive hypoglycemic child probably has nesidioblastosis. In most cases of hyperinsulinemia, medical management as described earlier is effective, but surgery may be necessary for some to maintain adequate blood glucose control[330–340].

Hypoglycemia associated with failure of ketogenesis can occur despite normal insulin and glucagon levels, because of defects in the hepatic processing of fatty acids. Deficiencies of carnitine and fatty acylcoenzyme A (acyl-CoA) dehydrogenase have been reported as causes of nonketotic hypoglycemia[341–344].

Anesthesia, Intubation, and the Perioperative Period

Anesthetics can mask signs and symptoms of hypoglycemia, such as irritability and seizures (neuroglycopenia). Apnea due to hypoglycemia obviously does not occur in patients who are intubated and mechanically ventilated. The only signs of hypoglycemia may be changes in heart rate or blood pressure caused by sympathetic arousal or substrate depletion. Therefore, it is important for the intensivist to maintain a high index of suspicion for this potentially serious yet readily treatable condition.

DISORDERS OF WATER HOMEOSTASIS

Introduction

Cell structure and function are critically dependent on homeostasis of water and ion concentrations. Consequently, multiple regulatory systems with redundant sensing and effector arms serve to maintain this homeostasis within a narrow range. These systems include interdependent regulation of vasopressin and renal function and thirst. Safe and prompt treatment of disorders of water metabolism rests on understanding the normal physiology of these regulatory systems.

AVP, commonly referred to as the antidiuretic hormone (ADH), is synthesized in neurons of the supraoptic nucleus and paraventricular nucleus, which also synthesize oxytocin.

Vasopressin is transported from the hypothalamic nuclei within the axonal processes of the neurons that synthesized them. Unmyelinated axonal fibers from magnocellular neurons of the supraoptic nucleus and paraventricular nucleus terminate in the posterior pituitary. Other axons originating in the parvicellular neurons of the paraventricular nucleus terminate in the median eminence. The significance of this innervation is that if the pituitary stalk is transected inferiorly there may still be intact axons that terminate above the incision sufficient in number to preserve adequate AVP release.

During axonal transport, AVP is packaged in secretory vesicles in association with cystine-rich proteins termed "neurophysins." There are several neurophysins, but each appears to be specific to a hormone. The AVP neurophysin is synthesized by the same gene that codes for AVP, located on chromosome 20[345]. Posttranslational processing produces both molecules from a prohormone. The biologic significance of neurophysins is unclear, but disorders of these molecules may result in disorders of AVP synthesis and secretion. Several kindreds have been identified, in which autosomal dominant familial diabetes insipidus is associated with a mutation affecting neurophysin[346–349].

Release of AVP from storage in the posterior pituitary and median eminence is regulated by an osmosensor located near the anterior hypothalamus, which helps to maintain blood osmolality in its normal range of 280 to 290 mOsm/kg[350]. Changes in osmolality change the size and shape of cells of the osmosensor, which then signals, via neurotransmitters, the AVP-containing neurons. When AVP-containing neurons are stimulated, they release AVP into nearby capillaries, and AVP is transported by blood to the site of its effects. Most people have a lower threshold, the osmotic threshold, below which they do not have measurable amounts of AVP (i.e., less than 1 pg/mL). Typically the osmotic threshold is about 283 mOsm/kg, and above it there is a linear increase in AVP concentration that reaches a plateau of approximately 20 pg/mL at an osmolality of 320 mOsm/kg.

Water balance is also sensed through a variety of barosensors that measure pressure and, indirectly, blood volume. These barosensors are located in the left atrium, carotid sinus, and aortic arch. Decreased output from these sensors (e.g., in hypovolemia) causes release of AVP and possibly stimulates thirst. These pressure and volume sensors are much less sensitive than the osmosensor (which can sense changes as small as 1%) and typically stimulate vasopressin release only after a change of 10% to 15%. However, the stimulus to vasopressin release is much greater in response to hemodynamic stimuli and can result in vasopressin levels measuring 100 pg/mL or greater.

Vasopressin acts through three receptors discovered to date: V1, V2, and V3. All receptors are G-protein-coupled transmembrane proteins[351]. They trigger different intercellular messaging systems. V1 is principally found in blood vessels and the liver.

Binding of the V1 receptor causes release of intracellular calcium and activation of the protein kinase C system. Receptor binding causes vasoconstriction and hepatic glycogenolysis.

In the renal medullary and cortical collecting duct cells, AVP binds to the V2 receptor and stimulates adenylate cyclase. The subsequent increase in cAMP produces an increase in the luminal cell membrane permeability to water, allowing the return of water from tubular lumen to plasma. The maximal effect of AVP is to produce a urine osmolality approaching 1200 mOsm/L and a urine flow as low as 0.5 mL/kg per hour. In the absence of AVP, the kidney permits urine osmolality approaching 50 mOsm/L and flows of 15 to 20 mL/kg per hour(352–355).

The V3 receptor has been identified on the anterior pituitary(356), where it mediates AVP-triggered release of ACTH (i.e., V3 is responsible for vasopressin-driven activation of the pituitary-adrenal axis).

Normally, people with free access to fluids and food drink about half their total daily water requirement and obtain the remaining half from the water content of solid foods. Normal water losses from an infant after the first month of life include approximately 1000 mL of urine (about 60% of total water losses), 400 mL (about 25%) through the skin, 250 mL (about 15%) through the lungs, and 50 mL (about 3%) in the feces, per square meter of body surface area. For neonates, the total water requirements per square meter increase with decreasing age and greater prematurity, approaching 70 mL/m^2 per hour in the neonate of 27 weeks' gestational age(357). If water intake lags behind water loss, a water deficit begins to appear.

Control of thirst becomes increasingly important as the water intake falls towards the minimum necessary (approximately 1 L/m^2) or exceeds the maximum excretable load (approximately 15 to 20 L/m^2, as elaborated in the following text). The thirst sensor may exist in the same location as the osmosensor, although this is not known definitively. Previously it had been thought that the set point for thirst was 0 to 15 mOsm/kg higher than the osmotic set point so that drinking would be stimulated only once vasopressin had been released to conserve water. Recent studies(358) suggest that the two set points are at the same osmolarity.

Control of Water Metabolism in the ICU

The intensivist cannot assume that any of the regulatory systems preserving water balance are operational in the critically ill child and must be ready to intervene to maintain homeostasis of this crucial physiologic system. Obviously, if the patient is unconscious, thirst control is no longer relevant. As described later, many surgical and pharmacologic interventions in the ICU further compromise control of water balance. Furthermore, AVP release can be affected by common nonosmotic or nonhemodynamic events, such as nausea, emesis, and hypoglycemia, which may shift the set point or alter the slope of the relationship between osmolality and AVP release(359,360).

For the large class of clinical settings in which AVP is released despite adequate osmolality, this release is deemed inappropriate (i.e., the syndrome of inappropriate secretion of antidiuretic hormone [SIADH]).

Syndrome of Inappropriate Secretion of Antidiuretic Hormone

SIADH is a common problem in the pediatric ICU and presents as relative hypersthenuria with hyponatremia. In patients presenting with hyponatremia, a low urinary output, a high urinary specific gravity, and high urinary sodium excretion, a disorder of inappropriately excessive secretion of ADH, leading to decreased free water clearance, should be suspected. However, to seriously indicate the diagnosis of SIADH, measured serum osmolality should be low while urinary osmolality is high. Serum osmolality less than 280 mOsm/kg can be considered low and urinary osmolality greater than 600 mOsm/kg is inappropriately high in the presence of a low serum osmolality. Although the threshold numbers can be argued and there are cases of SIADH with higher serum osmolality and lower urine osmolality than these thresholds, the vast majority of cases meet these criteria.

The name for the diagnosis itself may be considered inappropriate in the sense that the body is sometimes responding normally to perceived hypovolemia (ECF depletion). However, by convention, the appropriateness of AVP secretion is determined with respect to plasma osmolality or sodium concentration alone(361). Consequently, we continue to use that name to refer to situations in which nonosmotic control of AVP appears to be in effect and hyponatremia results. It is worth considering, however, that the inappropriate secretion of AVP in the vast majority of cases of SIADH discussed in the clinical literature was assumed, not proven, since AVP was rarely measured in clinical practice before radioimmunoassay kits for AVP became widely available. In addition, there are many conditions with sodium and water metabolism similar to SIADH, including hypothyroidism, edematous conditions associated with hyponatremia (e.g., failure of the heart, kidneys, and liver), primary polydipsia, and depletional hyponatremia. Even though these conditions may feature hyponatremia and hypersthenuria, they are excluded from the diagnosis.

As mentioned earlier, there are well-described nonosmotic stimuli for AVP release, and they are potent enough to "reset the osmostat" to a lower level of serum sodium. For example, a child on a positive pressure ventilator has decreased cardiac transmural pressure, which stretch receptors misinterpret as reduced ECF. This then leads to increased AVP release, which can lead to relative hypersthenuria and hyponatremia (i.e., SIADH). Excessive AVP release certainly precedes development of hyponatremia, as excessive free water retention takes a significant period of time, allowing alert clinicians to diagnose SIADH, in the face of a normal serum sodium level, when a euvolemic patient has hypersthenuric oliguria(362).

Concomitant Conditions

Clinicians should anticipate development of SIADH in a wide variety of clinical situations, such as nausea and vomiting, head injury and subarachnoid hemorrhage(363), pituitary surgery(364), scoliosis repair(365), cardiac surgery(366), meningoencephalitis(367), chemotherapy (vincristine[368], cytosine arabinoside[369]), burns(370,371), respiratory infections(372), respiratory failure as the result of various causes[373–375], and measles and malaria[376]. Many disorders associated with SIADH[377] are listed in **Table 39–5.**

SIADH occurring after hypothalamic or pituitary surgery is worthy of special mention, because if its sudden appearance is not promptly recognized, significant morbidity can result. If there has been transection of axons emanating from the preoptic or paraventricular neurons and terminating in the posterior pituitary, there follows a characteristic triphasic time course of diabetes insipidus followed by SIADH and then again by diabetes insipidus. The first phase is due to the lack of secretion of AVP; the second is due to the unregulated release of AVP because of retrograde degeneration of the AVP secreting neurons. The last phase occurs if insufficent neurons survive to release an adequate amount of AVP. The first phase lasts 1 to 4 days and the second up to 10 days; the last phase is permanent. Daily monitoring of specific gravity, serum sodium, and fluid balance provide adequate warning of the transition from one phase to another. Daily weights are also helpful in this regard.

Table 39.5. Disorders Associated with the Syndrome of Inappropriate Secretion of Antidiuretic Hormone

Central nervous system disorders
Infection
Tuberculosis
Bacterial meningitis
Encephalitis
Trauma
Hypoxia/ischemia
Psychosis
Tumor
Guillain-Barré
Ventriculoatrial shunt block
Acute intermittent porphyria
Cavernous sinus thrombosis
Subarachnoid hemorrhage
Multiple sclerosis
Anatomical abnormalities
Vasculitis
Chest infection
Tuberculosis
Bacterial pneumonia
Bacterial empyema
Mycoplasma pneumoniae
Viral
Fungal
Positive pressure ventilation
Decreased left atrial pressure
Pneumothorax
Asthma
Cystic fibrosis
Mitral valve commissurotomy
Patent ductus arteriosus ligation
Malignancy
Drugs
Increase arginine vasopressin secretion
Vincristine
Cyclophosphamide
Carbamazepine
Morphine
Phenothiazine
Ara-A
Potentiate renal effect of arginine vasopressin
Acetaminophen
Indomethacin
Other infections
Bacterial lymphadenitis
Bacterial arthritis
Bacterial abscess
Bacterial sepsis
Rickettsial
Diabetic ketoacidosis
Idiopathic

Adapted from Kaplan S, Feigin R. Syndromes of inappropriate secretion of antidiuretic hormone in children. Adv Pediatr 1980;27:247.

Conditions that may mimic SIADH in producing excessive urinary sodium losses in the face of hyponatremia include adrenal insufficiency, diuretic use, renal tubular dysfunction, and hypothyroidism[378–380].

In the past few years, increasing numbers of cases of cerebral salt wasting have been reported[381,382]. These patients present after head trauma or cranial surgery. Without close attention to fluid status, their pathophysiology can be confused with that of SIADH. In cerebral salt wasting, as in SIADH, hyponatremia can be marked and occurs in association with normokalemia. Urinary sodium is inappropriately high in both situations. Vasopressin is also elevated in cerebral salt wasting, but it represents an appropriate response to volume depletion caused by the diuresis. Unlike in SIADH, urinary output is not particularly low and volume restriction is not effective in restoring eunatremia. Instead, large amounts of salt supplementation are required to restore normal sodium concentrations.

The pathophysiology underlying cerebral salt wasting remains somewhat unclear. The leading hypothesis is that one of the many natriuretic peptides is secreted in abnormal amounts, possibly the brain natriuretic peptide, which is found in both the CNS and heart. This natriuretic peptide causes aldosterone suppression, diuresis, and natriuresis[383]. At least four natriuretic peptides have been identified, and the assays used in most clinical laboratories react only with atrial natriuretic peptide. Therefore, most studies to date have not included measurements of the brain natriuretic peptide, which might have greater relevance to cerebral salt wasting.

Therapy

SIADH is rarely the reason for admission to the pediatric ICU. Rather, it is seen in association with a serious primary illness and usually resolves as the triggering problem improves. Therapy for SIADH is best begun as an anticipatory action rather than as a corrective reaction. The disorder is common enough that a child with an illness known to cause SIADH might undergo fluid restriction provided he or she is hemodynamically stable. An alternative may be to supply normal sodium and water maintenance amounts and to follow serum sodium levels closely. AVP levels have been shown to fall when this approach has been used in children with meningoencephalitis[384].

Fluid restriction is safest when accompanied by an understanding of the quantitative requirements for water balance. The following example makes reasonable assumptions about renal concentrating capacity and osmotic loads. If these differ greatly for a given patient, the same calculation can be repeated with the different parameters.

The maximum concentrating ability of the kidney (i.e., under the effect of AVP on the V2 receptor) is approximately 1200 mOsm/kg. A fasting patient has an obligate osmotic load to be excreted of approximately 300 mOsm/m^2. With intravenous feeding, this load can easily rise to 600 mOsm/m^2. Therefore, 600 mOsm can be excreted in 0.5 kg of water per square meter (= 0.5 L/m^2).

Insensible water losses vary with patient temperature and ventilator status but often reach 0.5 L/m^2. In addition, the patient's metabolism generates approximately 0.25 L/m^2 of water.

In summary, to maintain water balance, the patient should be supplied with 0.5 L/m^2 (to excrete osmotic load) plus 0.5 L/m^2 (to make up for insensible losses) minus 0.25 L/m^2 (supplied by the patient metabolism), for a total of 0.75 L. Fluid supplementation in a patient subject to maximal antidiuresis at a rate greater than 0.75 L/m^2 daily results in hyponatremia.

A child with symptomatic hyponatremia requires more aggressive therapy. Symptoms relate to the lowering of plasma osmolality and are primarily neurologic, from malaise to obtundation, coma, and seizures. In symptomatic hyponatremic patients, 3% saline is given in an amount calculated to restore serum sodium to a conservative target of 125 mEq/L over a few hours. The number of milliequivalents needed can be calculated easily:

$$\text{Formula 5: Sodium deficit (mEq)} = 0.6 \times \text{BW (in kg)} \times (125 - \text{measured Na}^+)$$

Since 3% saline contains 0.513 mEq of sodium per milliliter, the volume to infuse is easily calculated. The solution contains about 1000 mOsm/L and, consequently, is irritating to veins and potentially injurious to tissues into which it might extravasate. To rapidly correct the osmolar deficit, however, it must be given undiluted. However, too rapid correction may be dangerous and risks the onset of pontine myelinolysis. Therefore, the replacement dose should be calculated to increase the serum sodium concentration at no more than 0.6 to 1 mEq/hr. Again, sodium supplementation should be used only in an acute emergency (to avoid precipitating acute volume overload); SIADH is best treated with strict fluid restriction in most cases.

Urea infusions may offer an alternative acute measure[(385)], although use of loop diuretics has been more widely reported[(386–388)]. Use of these diuretic agents presumes that the physician is replacing urinary electrolyte losses, orally or intravenously; for more rapid correction, 3% saline solution with added potassium chloride may be used. Urinary losses are measured and replaced hourly until the desired serum sodium concentration is reached.

The preceding discussion relates to therapy for euvolemic patients with SIADH. Clearly, if a child is significantly hypovolemic as well as hyponatremic, blood volume must be corrected (and the diagnosis of SIADH may be suspected unless there is some obvious reason for hypovolemia, such as hemorrhage). Fluid restriction is contraindicated in this case, at least until an adequate blood volume is restored[(389)], preferably with normal saline solution or blood products. Long-term therapy for SIADH, including treatment with lithium[(390–392)], demeclocycline[(393)], and phenytoin[(394)], is generally out of place in the pediatric ICU.

Diabetes Insipidus

Classification and Pathophysiology

Diabetes insipidus (DI) is a syndrome seen in a variety of rare situations in the pediatric ICU. It consists of two broad categories: vasopressin sensitive (central) and vasopressin insensitive (nephrogenic).

In vasopressin-sensitive DI, hypotonic polyuria responds to exogenous administration of AVP, and renal mechanisms for concentration of urine are intact. The defect is inadequate secretion of AVP for the given state of hyperosmolality. This reflects an absence or disorder of neurons capable of producing AVP. This state may arise as an idiopathic or familial disorder. Genetic disorders leading to central DI include mutations in the prepro-arginine-vasopressin-neurophysin II gene (prepro-AVP-NPII)[(347,348)], which is inherited in an autosomal dominant pattern. This form of DI does not present at birth and is thought to be associated with degenerative disease of the supraoptic nucleus and paraventricular nucleus. Wolfram's syndrome, also known by the initials of its most frequent manifestations (diabetes insipidus, diabetes mellitus, optic atrophy, and deafness, DIDMOAD), is another form of DI, inherited in autosomal recessive pattern; DI presents in one third to half of cases. Diabetes mellitus often precedes the onset of DI.

DI may also arise as the consequence of injury to the neurons synthesizing AVP or to the axons along which AVP is ferried to the posterior pituitary. This may be seen with local injuries, such as those caused by local granulomas, tumors, cysts, histiocytosis, and suprasellar surgery. In global brain injuries (e.g., severe cerebral ischemia, infections, trauma), the anterior hypothalamus is also injured, thereby producing DI during recovery from the global insult[(352,395–402)].

When the ability of the kidney to concentrate urine fails and hypotonic polyuria develops, vasopressin-insensitive (or nephrogenic) DI is said to have occurred. In several families, this lesion is congenital. This includes many mutations of the V2 vasopressin receptor, inherited in an X-linked pattern. Mutations in the aquaporin-2 water channel also result in congenital nephrogenic DI, inherited in an autosomal recessive pattern[(349)]. In other disorders, the defect appears to result from a primary aberration in the concentration gradient of the medullary tubule. Other reported causes of nephrogenic DI include pyelonephritis, polycystic kidney disease, obstructive uropathy, acute tubular necrosis, radiation nephritis, lithium, demeclocycline, hypokalemia, hypercalcemia, sickle cell anemia, Sjögren's syndrome, protein starvation, and "gradient washout" from massive diuresis or primary polydipsia[352,354,355,403,404].

Diagnosis

The hallmark of diagnosis is an excessive flow of dilute urine. Urine osmolality generally is less than 200 mOsm/L, which corresponds approximately to a specific gravity of less than 1.005. However, since water reabsorption in the proximal tubule is intact, urine osmolality may reach 400 in the context of severe dehydration.

In either form of DI, plasma osmolality may be normal but becomes elevated if water losses are not being aggressively and accurately replaced. Therefore, accurate and detailed records of patient intake and output are mandatory. If urine osmolality is <300 mOsm/L when the plasma osmolality is ≤295 mOsm/L, the patient has DI, assuming he or she has not received an osmotic diuretic (glucose, mannitol, glycerol, X-ray contrast agents). All that remains for diagnosis is to demonstrate whether the patient responds to AVP[405].

Differential diagnosis should include nonoliguric renal failure, excessive fluid intake, and osmotic diuresis. When seen in the pediatric ICU, either of the latter two disorders is likely to be the consequence of medical therapy. Whenever infusions of fluid provide free water greatly in excess of ongoing losses, the result is a state of hypotonic polyuria accompanying plasma hypoosmolality. This is not DI, in that the patient with an excessive fluid intake has hypoosmolar plasma and responds to a reduction of free-water supply by normal concentration of urine.

Osmotic diuresis is, at times, produced deliberately by infusions of such agents as mannitol and radiographic contrast media, but it may also be produced by hyperglycemia. The key differentiating feature is that urine osmolality remains close to that of plasma.

Children with nonoliguric renal failure are usually distinguishable by the fractional excretion of sodium, defined as the ratio of sodium clearance over creatinine clearance, expressed as a percentage:

$$\text{Forumla 6: } [(\text{Urine Na}^+) \times (\text{plasma creatinine})] \div [(\text{urine creatinine}) \times (\text{plasma Na}^+)] \times 100$$

This can be remembered as the percentage of filtered sodium that is excreted and is usually less than 1%.

Given these considerations, there is seldom if ever an indication in the critically ill child to proceed through a classical diagnostic workup with water deprivation or to measure plasma levels of AVP. If, in the pediatric ICU, the patient has hypotonic polyuria with hypertonic plasma, then he or she has DI. The only remaining diagnostic test is a trial of intranasal desmopressin (DDAVP) or intravenous AVP to tell whether the patient has AVP-responsive DI. Details of the use and risks of AVP analogues are described under Treatment.

Prognostic Importance in the Pediatric ICU

In patients undergoing suprasellar surgery, DI is neither surprising nor indicative of any grave global brain injury. DI can be expected to begin within hours of surgery, to continue for 2 or 3 days, and then resolve. However, if more than 80% of the AVP containing hypothalamoneurohypophyseal tracts are damaged, DI recurs in 2 or 3 days and is permanent[352,395,400,401].

A more worrisome situation is global brain injury accompanied by DI. Small retrospective reviews of patients with DI occurring in a variety of global cerebral insults suggest that death almost universally follows development of DI in 1 to 5 days[396–398]. There have been numerous reports, on small groups of children, describing high rates of central DI in brain-dead children[406–410]. Presumably, this grave prognostic sign merely reflects a cerebral insult that is truly global.

Therapy

The most controlled situation in which DI is likely to occur in the pediatric ICU is after intracranial suprasellar surgery, where its onset is anticipated. Often, however, DI is not anticipated and arises in a patient already ill from trauma, infection, or massive brain ischemia. Volume losses may be sizable in children who can ill afford any hemodynamic instability. For patients in shock, initial fluid replacement consists of large volumes of isotonic solutions. A dose of 20 mL/kg of body weight should be given as often and as rapidly as is necessary to reverse shock.

Once shock has been treated, the fluid administered should be hypotonic. Given that patients with DI can have urine osmolality as low as 50 mOsm/kg, replacing fluid losses with fluid that has a tonicity greater than this low urine osmolality will likely lead to increasing serum hypertonicity.

Ideally, solutions should not contain more than about 37 mEq of sodium per liter (one fourth normal saline) to avoid excessive sodium loading. It becomes necessary, therefore, to add dextrose to maintain an osmolality of infusate above 200 mOsm/L (each gram of dextrose per liter (0.1%) of infusate adds about 6 mOsm/L). Large volumes of an approximately correct solution can be made by adding equal volumes of 5% dextrose in water and 0.45% normal saline, yielding 2.5% dextrose in 0.2% normal saline solution. These intravenous fluids may result in hyperglycemia when given at high rates, particularly in patients in life-threatening situations who have high levels of counterregulatory hormones (particularly cortisol and epinephrine, which lead to increased gluconeogenesis and insulin resistance). Patients given large doses of glucocorticoids (e.g., high-dose dexamethasone) during and after neurosurgery are particularly at risk. Hyperglycemia leads to osmotic diuresis if the glucose level exceeds the renal threshold (of approximately 180 mg/dL). To avoid this situation, it may be necessary to reduce the dextrose load or institute a continuous infusion of insulin, with careful attention to blood glucose values.

Matching of intravenous infusion rates to urine output should be reassessed at hourly intervals and followed very carefully, with plasma and urine osmolalities determined every 2 to 4 hours and serum sodium concentrations determined as frequently. As in any hypernatremic state, correction should occur over about 48 to 72 hours[403,404,411]. Often, appropriate fluid administration is all that is necessary for management of DI.

In theory, one could calculate a patient's fluid requirements based on his or her expected urine output (insensible losses are minor in comparison), as was done in the calculation for fluid replacement in SIADH. For example, if the patient's urine osmolality is 100 mOsm/kg and the obligate daily osmotic load (fasting) is 300 mOsm/m^2, a patient in DI produces a urine output of at least 3 L/m^2. Unfortunately, osmotic loads are highly variable and hard to measure, so an empirical approach is adopted instead.

Urine output is matched with hypotonic fluids up to a maximum of 4 L/m^2 per day (a lesser rate may lead to too rapid correction of hypernatremia). The reason for this ceiling is that the kidneys promptly excrete whatever volume the patient is given. Capping the urine replacement causes modest volume contraction, so fluid reabsorption in other parts of the nephron is stimulated. Thus, even if infused fluids are hypotonic, the patient is likely to have net fluid losses before reaching equilibrium. For this reason, it is not unusual to see the serum sodium of patients with central DI managed solely with fluids reach the mid-150 mEq/L range.

Continuous infusion of aqueous AVP for treatment of central DI is a rational alternative to fluid management alone. DDAVP (1-desamino-8-D-arginine vasopressin) therapy, administered by intranasal or subcutaneous route, is not as safe. DDAVP is a V2-selective analog to AVP, which makes it free of cardiovascular and CNS side effects and therefore a favored regimen for outpatient therapy. When DDAVP is given to a patient who is not fully alert and therefore cannot regulate his or her thirst, administration of fluids can lead to significant and life-threatening hyponatremia. This is less of an issue with aqueous AVP infusion, which can be turned off with rapid return of diuresis (provided, of course, that the patient is being watched closely). The ability to rapidly modulate urine output can be very useful (e.g., in the care of a brain-dead patient with DI who has become a beating-heart cadaveric kidney donor, and in whom increased urine output is desired).

In patients with vasopressin-sensitive DI, AVP infusions may obviate the need for large volumes of fluid and avoid the risk of inducing osmotic diuresis and of rapid electrolyte shifts. However, it bears repetition that patients receiving aqueous AVP drip should be treated as if they have achieved full antidiuresis and consequently must continue appropriate fluid restriction.

The optimum rate of infusion of AVP has not been well established, but 1.5 mU/kg per hour is used at many critical care centers. There is no shortage of alternate dosage schemes[353,412–418]. The infusion rate can be increased (doubled every 30 minutes) or decreased, but it is likely that there is a ceiling to the effectiveness of AVP. It should rarely be necessary to infuse more than 10 mU/kg per hour (435 pg/kg per minute).

AVP is a potent vasoconstrictor, and experimentally this effect is most extreme in severe CNS injury[353]. Although myocardial infarction from generalized vasoconstriction is of lesser concern in children than in adults, other harmful effects may be seen from massive systemic vasoconstriction. Generalized tissue ischemia can result in profound lactic acidosis. Local effects may include actual infarction of skin over the extremities. For these reasons, extremely high rates of AVP infusion should be used only with great caution.

DDAVP is available in both intranasal and intravenous forms, but its significantly longer half-life makes it less suitable than AVP for rapidly titratable control of water balance in the critically ill child[419,420].

DISORDERS OF CALCIUM, MAGNESIUM, AND PHOSPHATE METABOLISM

Calcium

Calcium plays a major role in many biochemical reactions and is a messenger within and between cells. Calcium is also a major component of the skeleton, which serves as a large calcium reservoir. Derangements of calcium flux and concentration are not uncommon in the critical care setting. They usually are of relatively brief duration and so rarely result in skeletal abnormalities even though they can cause significant physiologic disturbances.

Calcium's central role in all aspects of metabolism means that its absence or excess can have widespread and serious effects. Calcium excess is unusual in the pediatric ICU and is less problematic than hypocalcemia.

Homeostasis and Metabolism

Calcium homeostasis is achieved through the actions of three hormones: parathyroid hormone, 1,25-dihydroxycholecalciferol (1,25$(OH)_2D$), and calcitonin. These hormones act in concert to maintain calcium homeostasis by affecting three organ systems: the gut (source), bone (reservoir), and kidneys (excretion).

Parathyroid hormone is an 84-amino acid polypeptide produced and stored in the parathyroid glands. The prohormone, pre-pro-parathyroid hormone, is synthesized from the gene located at 11p15.2-p15.1 and undergoes two cleavage steps, the second of which occurs in the endoplasmic reticulum where the hormone if finally stored in secretory granules. Its secretion is stimulated by a decrease in serum concentration of ionized calcium. After its release from the chief cell, the peptide is cleaved again, to a 34 amino acid N-terminal fragment, which produces most of parathyroid hormone's effects. The parathyroid hormone receptor is coded for by a gene at 3p22-p21.1 and is a G-protein-linked receptor acting via membrane-bound adenylate cyclase to increase cyclic AMP.

Through this mechanism, parathyroid hormone causes increased renal tubular reabsorption of calcium and magnesium and decreased distal tubular reabsorption of bicarbonate and phosphate. In bone, parathyroid hormone causes increased resorption of calcium and phosphate. Therefore, if parathyroid hormone is elevated, there may be significant hypophosphatemia and metabolic acidosis.

The recent cloning and characterization of a calcium sensor gene[421] has provided insight into the regulation of parathyroid hormone by calcium. Binding of extracellular calcium to the "calcium binding pocket" of the sensor molecules of parathyroid chief cells causes a change in conformation that is transduced, by the G-proteins component of the sensor into phospholipase-C activation. This triggers a cascade of intracellular reactions, which include synthesis and release of parathyroid hormone. Several inherited disorders of the calcium sensor have been identified[421], but they are likely to be rare causes of perturbed calcium metabolism in critically ill patients.

Acute hypomagnesemia has a similar effect on parathyroid hormone, although prolonged hypomagnesemia also inhibits parathyroid hormone secretion. Parathyroid hormone secretion is also stimulated by catecholamines, histamine, and prostaglandins.

Parathyroid hormone's effects on calcium metabolism are both direct and indirect. Its direct action is upon the skeleton. In response to parathyroid hormone binding to its receptors on the osteoblast, cells release humoral factors that then stimulate increased osteoclast activity. Its indirect effects are through vitamin D.

Vitamin D is produced in the skin (D3) or is ingested (D2) and undergoes unregulated hepatic 25-hydroxylation and renal 1-hydroxylation to $1{,}25(OH)_2D$. 1-hydroxylation is stimulated by hypophosphatemia and hypocalcemia. Parathyroid hormone increases $1{,}25(OH)_2D$ production indirectly by first inducing hypophosphatemia. This activated form of vitamin D then increases intestinal absorption of calcium and phosphate by first opening calcium transport channels (in minutes to seconds) and also stimulating production of calbindin in the GI tract to increase facilitated transport[422] (in minutes to hours).

Calcitonin is a 32-amino acid polypeptide produced in thyroid parafollicular cells, and its secretion is stimulated by an increase in serum ionized calcium (as well as by alcohol, glucagon, and β-adrenergic agonists). Calcitonin inhibits bone resorption and enhances urinary excretion of phosphate and calcium. However, calcitonin's role in calcium physiology remains unclear. Children with congenital athyreosis or who have had total thyroidectomy do not appear to have disordered calcium metabolism.

Physiology

Ionized calcium (Ca^{2+}) is the important, physiologically active form of this electrolyte, both inside and outside the cell. The remaining 99% of the body's calcium (in bone, or bound to proteins or cations) acts as a metabolically inactive reservoir.

The common clinical laboratory evaluation of calcium measures total concentration in serum. The normal range in older children and adults is about 9.0 to 10.6 mg/dL (4.3 to 5.3 mEq/L). However, calcium levels vary with age, particularly in the neonatal period. The normal range for calcium in the newborn period is significantly lower (7.6 to 11.4 mg/dL). At physiologic pH (pH 7.4), 40% is bound to albumin (at pH 7.4); 10% is complexed to bicarbonate, phosphate, or citrate; and the remaining 50% is free ionized calcium (Ca^{2+}), with a normal range of about 2 to 2.5 mEq/L.

A commonly employed rule of thumb is that an increment of 1 g/dL in serum albumin causes an increment of 0.8 mg/dL (0.4 mEq/L) in total calcium and that a pH increment of 0.1 U causes a 10% decrement in Ca^{2+}[389]. Estimating the Ca^{2+} concentration from known total calcium, albumin, and pH has been demonstrated to be misleading[423–426].

However, direct measurement of Ca^{2+}, though ideal, is also problematic. Blood must be collected anaerobically, since CO_2 loss (into an air bubble) alters pH, therefore binding to albumin. RBCs must be quickly removed to avoid acidosis from lactate production. Some anticoagulants form complexes with Ca^{2+} and should be avoided in sample collection. Nevertheless, in the ICU, this is often the calcium measurement of choice.

In the myocardium, Ca^{2+} plays a central role in both generation of the action potential and the excitation-contraction process. The action potential of pacemaker cells begins as a steady slow depolarization due to Ca^{2+} influx (hence, the effectiveness of calcium channel blockers in reducing arrhythmias). The subsequent rapid depolarization of pacemaker and of nonpacemaker cells is due to sodium influx. Ca^{2+} entry is largely responsible for the subsequent plateau phase of depolarization and for initiation of myocardial cell contraction.

Ca^{2+} entry appears to be through two "gates," one opened by sufficient membrane depolarization (the voltage-dependent gate) and the other opened by β-adrenergic receptor stimulation, which increases cAMP (the phosphorylation-dependent gate)[16].

Myocardial cell contraction takes place after initial Ca^{2+} entry causes a secondary flux of Ca^{2+} from stores in the sarcoplasmic reticulum and across the cell membrane. The increased intracellular Ca^{2+} binds to one component of troponin (a regulatory Ca^{2+}-binding protein found in cardiac and skeletal myocytes). This binding causes a structural change in troponin, resulting (in the presence of ATP) in tropomyosin-actin cross-bridging and contraction.

After contraction, Ca^{2+} is removed from the troponin complex, returned to the sarcoplasmic reticulum, and pumped out of the cell (by ATPase pumps). Ca^{2+} also exits from cells in exchange for sodium traveling into cells down the concentration gradient. This exchange is impaired when intracellular sodium concentration rises (reducing the electrochemical drive for sodium to enter cells), such as occurs when the sodium-potassium ATPase pump is "poisoned" by cardiac glycosides. The higher intracellular Ca^{2+} that results allows for more forceful contraction[427].

Ca^{2+} release and reuptake in the myocardium are relatively slow, partly because the sarcoplasmic reticulum is less extensive than in skeletal muscle. Cardiac contraction is enhanced by factors that enhance intracellular Ca^{2+} concentration (Ca^{2+} infusions, cardiac glycosides, β-adrenergic agonists) and is impaired by influences that lower Ca^{2+} inside the myocyte (hypocalcemia, Ca^{2+} channel blocking drugs, ATP depletion by ischemia, or phosphate depletion).

Skeletal muscle similarly relies on Ca^{2+} to allow contraction. The mechanisms for intracellular calcium homeostasis are similar to those of the heart. However, in skeletal muscle, the sarcoplasmic reticulum is more extensive and reuptake of released Ca^{2+} is quicker. For this reason, a single stimulus only causes a submaximal contraction (a twitch), since Ca^{2+} is removed before maximal force is achieved. Repetitive stimuli summate, allowing saturating Ca^{2+} concentrations to develop and the muscle to develop maximal force[16]. Thus, in skeletal muscle, where Ca^{2+} flux is rapid and of large magnitude, the determining factor of force of contraction is the presence of effective repetitive stimuli from the neuromuscular junction.

Calcium is important at the neuromuscular junction, where it is essential for presynaptic release of acetylcholine. When neuronal depolarization reaches the end plate, Ca^{2+} permeability increases, allowing ingress of Ca^{2+}. The calcium ions bind with acetylcholine vesicles, allowing them to fuse with the end plate membrane, releasing acetylcholine at the synapse[16].

Within the nervous system, Ca^{2+} is involved in functioning of many enzyme systems. Calmodulin, a Ca^{2+}-binding protein, mediates the effects of Ca^{2+} on various intracellular enzyme systems. These enzymes include adenylate cyclase, phosphodiesterase, phospholipase A2, plasma membrane Ca^{2+}-ATPase, and protein kinases involved in neurotransmitter release. Calmodulin has also been found in brain postsynaptic densities[428]. Given the complexity implicit in these findings, it is not surprising that abnormally high or low Ca^{2+} concentrations in ECF result in profound CNS derangements, including hypercalcemic coma and hypocalcemic seizures.

The effects of calcium on vascular smooth muscle are also important. Calmodulin is the Ca^{2+} receptor (not the troponin of myocardial and skeletal muscle). The Ca^{2+}-calmodulin complex activates myosin kinase, resulting in actin-myosin coupling and cell contraction (vasoconstriction). In these cells, β-adrenergic transmitters stimulate cAMP both to deactivate myosin kinase (directly resulting in vasodilatation) and to enhance Ca^{2+} efflux. α-Adrenergic agonists enhance Ca^{2+} influx, resulting in vessel constriction.

Hypercalcemia

Hypercalcemia is encountered less often than is hypocalcemia in the pediatric ICU. This is because the two disorders that most frequently cause elevated Ca^{2+} concentration in adults, namely hyperparathyroidism[429,430] and cancers of breast, lung, kidney, head, and neck and myeloma[431], are less common in children[432]. Even more rare is the humoral hypercalcemia of malignancy that is usually associated with parathyroid hormone-related peptide. More commonly, hypercalcemia due to malignancy in childhood is caused by direct bony invasion or metastasis by tumor[433] or tumor lysis[434].

The immobile skeleton of a child in an ICU is not subject to the usual daily stimulation of the piezoelectric forces generated by stress on the skeleton during nomal ambulation. In the absence of such stimulation, there is a marked change in the calcium exchange between the skeleton and the extracellular fluid. The resulting increase in calcium outflow from the skeleton can lead to hypercalcemia[432,435–438]. The effect is more pronounced in children than adults because of their higher rate of bone turnover. The hypercalcemia of immobilization can be distinguished from hyperparathyroidism and hypervitaminosis D because serum levels of parathyroid hormone and calcitriol are suppressed.

Granulomatous diseases, such as sarcoidosis and tuberculosis, are associated with hypercalcemia. This is presumably due to calcidiol being activated by 1-alpha-hydroxylase activity in the macrophages associated with the granulomatous state[439].

William syndrome (peripheral pulmonic stenosis, or supravalvar aortic stenosis, "elfin facies") is associated with idiopathic infantile hypercalcemia. The hypercalcemia usually resolves by age 1 or 2 years.

Familial hypocalciuric hypercalcemia[440] is caused by a mutant calcium sensor gene (described previously), usually in the heterozygote state. The sensor is present on renal tubular cells as well as on parathyroid chief cells, which explains the increased renal tubular calcium resorption in familial hypocalciuric hypercalcemia. The disease rarely becomes clinically significant except in the homozygous state, where it presents as neonatal hyperparathyroidism.

Primary hyperparathyroidism (other than disorders of the calcium sensor gene) has also been reported. Hyperplasia or tumor growth of the gland can be associated with multiple endocrine neoplasia and usually is found only in older children. In multiple endocrine neoplasia I, hyperparathyroidism is associated with pituitary and pancreatic tumors. In multiple endocrine neoplasia IIa, hyperparathyroidism is associated with thyroid medullary carcinoma and pheochromocytoma and has been linked to mutations in the RET proto oncogene[(79)].

Tertiary hyperparathyroidism is the autonomous production of parathyroid hormone by the parathyroid glands after a prolonged period of stimulation (e.g., in chronic uremia).

Hypercalcemia in children may also arise from hyperthyroidism, pheochromocytoma[(441)], hypervitaminosis A or D, thiazides, furosemide, or milk-alkali syndrome.

Hypercalcemia may present with general malaise, fatigue, failure to thrive, polyuria, vomiting, decreased renal function, constipation, abdominal pain, and occasionally, hypertension. (Onset of unexplained hypertension in a patient in the pediatric ICU should remind the clinician of the child's immobility and prompt evaluation of serum calcium concentration.) If hypercalcemia is associated with hypercalciuria (i.e., urinary calcium-creatinine ratio 0.2 or total urinary calcium output 4 mg/kg in 24 hr)[(442)], the child is at risk for nephrocalcinosis.

Treatment

Measures for directly reducing serum Ca^{2+} concentration include hydration with saline solution (10 mL/kg per hour) with furosemide (1 mg/kg every 6 hours)[(443,444)] to induce brisk calciuresis. Other beneficial measures include restriction of Ca^{2+} intake and avoidance of vitamin D, thiazides, and Ca^{2+}-containing antacids. Digitalis preparations should also be reduced, in view of the effects of hypercalcemia in potentiating digitalis-related rhythm and conduction disturbances.

When hydration and diuresis are insufficient to achieve eucalcemia, or if eucalcemia cannot be maintained, other modes of therapy can be used.

Calcium may be lowered by agents that form complexes with it. Intravenous agents include phosphates (0.15 to 0.30 mmol/kg over 12 hours) and etidronate (EHDP, a biphosphonate that is an effective inhibitor of osteoclastic activity, 15 to 50 mg/kg over 4 hours)[(436,445,446)]. Oral and rectal phosphates (0.5 to 1 mmol/kg per day) may also be used. In all of these methods, risks include hypocalcemia, metastatic calcification, hypotension, renal failure, and heart failure. These intravenous agents may bring about the desired result quickly but may also risk precipitous hypocalcemia. This method of therapy requires prehydration and careful monitoring of electrolytes and should not be used in the face of hyperphosphatemia and/or renal impairment. The product of the concentrations of calcium and phosphorus ($Ca^{2+} \times P$) (in mg/dL) should be kept below 60, and the patient should be monitored for metastatic calcification (by slit-lamp examination and soft tissue radiographs).

When excessive bone resorption is significant (malignancy, immobility), drugs inhibiting this process may be of help. Calcitonin (4 to 8 U/kg intravenously over 24 hours), mithramycin (10 to 25 g/kg intravenously for 2 to 21 days), glucocorticoids (prednisone, 1 to 2 mg/kg per day intravenously divided into four doses; or hydrocortisone, 1 to 5 mg/kg four times a day), and indomethacin (1 mg/kg per day) have been used in adults and may be useful in children, although such experience has not been extensively reported[(447–450)].

Of these drugs, calcitonin is by far the least toxic. It is more effective in children than in adults in lowering calcium[(451)], probably because of the high rate of bone turnover in children. Nevertheless, it is not uniformly effective and, even when effective, only works for 1 to 6 days (longer if used with prednisone, 1 mg/kg per day). Glucocorticoids are reasonably safe and inhibit osteoclastic activity and gut absorption of Ca^{2+}. Indomethacin acts only when bone resorption is due to prostaglandin-secreting tumors, which is rare. Propranolol, used to treat hyperthyroidism, may be effective for the hypercalcemia seen with that disorder. Mithramycin is an extremely toxic antibiotic that inhibits osteoclastic activity but also depresses the functions of the liver, kidney, and bone marrow. If hyperparathyroidism is suspected, mithramycin should be avoided in view of the severe marrow suppression it can cause, since neck explorations are hazardous enough without the added risk of thrombocytopenia.

Anesthesia, Intubation, and the Perioperative Period

Hypercalcemia should be corrected before elective surgery, if possible. If surgery must proceed, hydration with normal saline is critical. There are no specific problems with intubation and related drugs, but one should be aware of the possibility of organ dysfunction, including cardiac (ECG changes bradycardia, heart block), renal (polyuria and inability to concentrate urine), CNS (sedation), muscular (muscle weakness), and GI (nausea and vomiting) problems. Choice of drugs may be affected by these. Consequently, monitoring with continuous ECG (though shortening of the QTc may not be a reliable indicator of serum calcium level[[452]]), a urinary bladder catheter, and other methods are warranted. pH status should be followed closely during intubation and while the patient is mechanically ventilated, because acidosis exacerbates hypercalcemia. However, hyperventilation may not be desirable; while it may decrease ionized calcium, it also decreases plasma potassium concentration.

Effects of hypercalcemia on requirements for muscle relaxants are unpredictable. If the patient has muscle weakness, he or she may need less muscle relaxant. On the other hand hypercalcemia has been shown to increase the requirement for muscle relaxants in hyperparathyroidism[(453)], although other data suggest that it is only an important effect at high serum calcium levels[(454)], if at all[(455)].

Hypocalcemia

Causes of hypocalcemia can be considered in three broad categories: Parathyroid hormone deficiency, vitamin D deficiency, and chelation or depletion.

Parathyroid hormone deficiency states can be induced

by direct injury to (or absence of) the parathyroids due to idiopathic disease, trauma, radiation, infiltration, or surgery. Excision, ischemia, or necrosis of the parathyroid glands after thyroid surgery is not uncommon. Parathyroid function can also be suppressed by severe bodily injury (trauma, burns, sepsis), pancreatitis, maternal hyperparathyroidism, drugs, and severely low magnesium concentrations. Hypomagnesemia may inhibit release of parathyroid hormone as well as impair end-organ response to parathyroid hormone. Vitamin D activity may be affected by decreased uptake from the gut (dietary lack, malabsorption), by decreased activation (liver disease, renal disease, pseudohypoparathyroidism, rhabdomyolysis, lack of sunlight), or by increased loss of vitamin D (nephrosis, anticonvulsant use). In many countries, including the United States, vitamin D2 supplementation in many foodstuffs, including milk, has made nutritional rickets very rare. The inherited forms of vitamin D deficiency are similarly rare. These include pseudo-vitamin D deficiency, which is linked to a mutation of the 1-alpha-calcidiol hydroxylase gene on 12q. Also, a mutation of the calcitriol receptor gene on 12q12-q14 has been linked to end-organ resistance to vitamin D.

Ca^{2+} may be chelated and depleted by a great number of processes. Massive infusion of blood products (for shock, cardiopulmonary bypass, hemodialysis, or exchange transfusion) causes hypocalcemia via chelation to citrate and ionized hypocalcemia from alkalosis. Repeated transfusions can also result in hypoparathyroidism due to iron overload[(456)]. Phosphates and can cause hypocalcemia[(457,458)]. Respiratory alkalosis can dramatically reduce total calcium and phosphate, as well as ionized calcium[(459)]. Mechanisms for many of the known causes of hypocalcemia may well be mixed[(204,300,460–486)].

Differential diagnosis of hypocalcemia changes with the age of the patient. Early neonatal hypocalcemia (birth to 4 or 5 days old) is most common in premature infants, those with severe neonatal cardiorespiratory distress, and those with diabetic mothers. Causes of this phenomenon are not fully elucidated but probably include prolonged suppression of the parathyroid glands by the relatively hypercalcemic fetal environment, insufficient calcium delivery in the early neonatal diet, and decreased mobilization of skeletal calcium due to elevated levels of stress hormones. Also, insufficiency of the vitamin D system, particularly the 1-alpha-hydroxylation of calcidiol, can be present during this period. Late neonatal hypocalcemia (5 or 6 days and onwards) can be caused by an increased phosphorus load, which shifts the calcium-phosphorus equilibrium toward mineralization in bone and also inhibits synthesis of calcitriol.

Increased phosphorus levels can result from a diet of unmodified cow's milk, cell lysis (e.g., massive hemolysis), and decreased renal function (leading to decreased phosphate clearance).

Hypoparathyroidism can also occur in this period. Presentations include transient hypoparathyroidism due to maternal hypercalcemia and embryologic disorders of the parathyroids, such as DiGeorge's syndrome, which can include immunological disorders, congenital heart disease, and a variety of qualitative or quantitative defects in the synthesis of parathyroid hormone[(487)]. Many cases of DiGeorge's syndrome appear to be associated with deletions in chromosome 22q11[(488)].

An increasing number of reports have appeared documenting hypocalcemia in older, critically ill children in the absence of any obvious cause. Proposed causes include intracellular magnesium depletion, elevated levels of calcitonin, and blunted release of parathyroid hormone in the stressed state. All of these hypotheses are contested[(427,489)].

Measurements of serum calcium levels are, obviously, central to diagnosis. As mentioned, total serum calcium is of less interest, physiologically, than the level of Ca^{2+} concentration. This fact is well illustrated by the observation that a healthy person can hyperventilate to produce tetany. The total calcium is hardly affected, while the ionized calcium is greatly reduced, accounting for the symptoms.

The ideal, then, is to monitor ionized calcium levels, daily at least, in all pediatric ICU patients. Because this is not a universally available test, other strategies have been evolved for estimating Ca^{2+} concentrations. The ECG has been proposed as a tool for assessing (by Q-T interval) physiologic evidence of low Ca^{2+} but has not been demonstrated to be reliable. One might attempt to calculate Ca^{2+} by reasoning that total calcium is usually approximately twice the concentration of free ionized Ca^{2+}, and correcting for pH and albumin concentration. Results are at best an inaccurate guess.

Tetany is the symptom most readily attributed to hypocalcemia; familiar manifestations are the Chvostek and Trousseau signs (however, eliciting Trouseau's sign can be very uncomfortable for an awake child). Interestingly, tetany is not due to increased muscle excitability; muscular excitability is actually depressed. Hypocalcemia impedes acetylcholine release at neuromuscular junctions and depletes cellular stores needed for effective muscular contraction. However, in the presence of low Ca^{2+}, neurons show decreased thresholds of excitation (i.e., easier to excite), have repetitive responses to a single stimulus, and have reduced accommodation. This increase in neuronal excitability overrides the inhibitory effects of hypocalcemia on the neuromuscular junction and myocyte.

Neuronal excitability occurs in both sensory and motor nerves, so that hypocalcemia produces a spectrum of peripheral and CNS effects, from mild paresthesias to tetany (including hands, arms, feet, larynx, and bronchioles), psychiatric changes, papilledema, and seizures[(490)]. The actual intracellular mechanisms responsible for the uninhibited neuronal physiology in hypocalcemia have not been established. Presumably, the Ca^{2+}-calmodulin complex normally activates one or more enzymes that inhibit membrane excitability. This complex may become dysfunctional in hypocalcemia.

An underlying disorder (neck mass injuries, pancreatitis, hepatomegaly, anasarca) may increase the index of suspicion for hypocalcemia. A recent hospital course may reveal possible causes, such as cardiopulmonary bypass, transfusions, chemotherapy, aminoglycosides, infusions of phosphate or bicarbonate, acute respiratory alkalosis, heart failure(491–493), cardiac dysrhythmias(494,495), infantile apnea(496), urinary retention(497), hypotension(498), ineffective digitalization(499), papilledema, seizures(500,501), prolonged curarization(502), and, of course, tetany.

Laboratory data can yield clues. Hypomagnesemia suggests inadequate intake of Mg^{2+} or excessive losses, while hypermagnesemia suggests excess intake or decreased renal excretion. Hyperphosphatemia suggests excessive supply, rhabdomyolysis, chemotherapy, or renal failure. If Mg^{2+} is normal and phosphorus is low or normal, serum immunoreactive parathyroid hormone may be measured (or parathyroid hormone infused[503]) to distinguish hypoparathyroidism inadequate vitamin D activity or pseudohypoparathyroidism. In the latter cases, serum immunoreactive parathyroid hormone is high and the serum calcium does not rise in response to a parathyroid hormone challenge.

For patients in the pediatric ICU, hypocalcemia should be treated unless it is boderline and asymptomatic (depending on the underlying disorder)(504–507). However, patients with impending neuromuscular or cardiovascular collapse require prompt restoration of serum ionized calcium(508–510). At least one study has demonstrated a more predictable rise in Ca^{2+} with calcium chloride than with the gluconate or gluceptate salts. A reasonable approach is to give, intravenously, 0.1 mL of 10% $CaCl_2$/kg over 5 to 10 minutes. The advantage of this salt over the other salts is probably very slight(511–513). All calcium salt solutions are capable of causing tissue damage with extravasation and should be given through use of a secure catheter in a large vein, if possible. Calcium salts precipitate in bicarbonate, so the two should never be given in the same line. Calcium infusions should be given with great caution to patients taking digitalis, since hypercalcemia potentiates glycoside toxicity. Rapid infusion of calcium salts can be dysrhythmogenic, even if the patient is not taking digitalis. Specifically, bradycardia and asystole can result from intravenous Ca^{2+} infusion. Patient should have contiuous ECG monitoring, and atropine should be readily available before a calcium bolus is infused intravenously. Once the patient is asymptomatic, intravenous boluses of calcium should be replaced, if possible, with oral supplements (or added to intravenous infusions).

Normocalcemia may be difficult to sustain in the presence of hypomagnesemia, hypoparathyroidism, or inadequate vitamin D. Hypomagnesemia is best treated with 0.3 to 1 mEq of magnesium chloride per kilogram over 12 to 24 hours. Magnesium sulfate is less desirable, since sulfates complex with calcium. Hypoparathyroidism, pseudohypoparathyroidism, and vitamin D deficieny are all managed by adding vitamin D in an appropriate form to Ca^{2+} supplementation.

Anesthesia, Intubation, and the Perioperative Period

Hypocalcemia should be suspected whenever large volumes of blood are transfused (citrate chelates calcium, and the alkalosis from large transfusions may further lower ionized calcium levels). Hypocalcemia from transfusion(464) is more likely when metabolism or elimination of citrate is impaired (hypothermia, hepatic dysfunction, renal failure) or when the transfusion is given rapidly. Continuous monitoring of the QT interval on ECG may be useful, but it is not always altered in hypocalcemia.

Sudden hypocalcemia may first come to clinical attention because of laryngospasm or spasm of other muscles (tetany). Laryngospasm from hypocalcemia has been described in a wide variety of conditions, including renal failure(514) and celiac disease(515). Treatment includes airway management and prompt intravenous delivery of calcium. Intubation may also be necessary if hypocalcemia-induced CNS toxicity proceeds to severe confusion and seizures.

Hypocalcemia should be corrected prior to surgery when possible.

Magnesium

Magnesium is an essential cofactor for enzymatic processes using adenosine triphosphate (ATP). Thus, magnesium-dependent processes include oxidative phosphorylation, DNA transcription, protein synthesis, and cell membrane pumps. Fortunately, the element is so common in food and water sources that it is virtually unavoidable. Magnesium uptake occurs chiefly in the ileum. About 25% of the 25 to 30 mEq of elemental Mg^{2+} taken in daily is absorbed normally; in magnesium deficiency up to 60% is absorbed. Excessive intake of magnesium rarely presents a problem, since renal excretion readily prevents hypermagnesemia, but hypomagnesemia develops relatively easily(516,517).

Adult body stores of magnesium total about 28 mEq/kg. Fifty percent of this is in bone, 25% in muscle, 1% in ECF, and 24% in the rest of the body's soft tissues. Within cells, most magnesium is complexed with phosphate, citrate, adenosine phosphates, and other anions. About 30% of the bone fraction is freely diffusible (70% is bound to hydroxyapatite).

Magnesium losses from stool, skin, and urine are normally about 0.3 mEq/kg daily. Renal tubular reabsorption of magnesium occurs mostly in the loop of Henle and to a lesser extent in the proximal convoluted tubule. In most children body stores of magnesium depend on the amount reabsorbed in the kidney, provided dietary assumption of this mineral is normal.

Most cellular functions that are dependent on magnesium require normal intracellular magnesium stores. Therefore, signs and symptoms of magnesium excess or deficit mostly reflect tissue stores. Unfortunately, serum levels correlate poorly with tissue stores, makings diagnosis of these relatively infrequent disorders challenging.

Normally, total plasma magnesium concentration is 1.4 to 2.0 mEq/L (1.7 to 2.4 mg/dL). Plasma magnesium is 65% to 80% bound to proteins. Little is published about the relative value of measuring total versus ionized plasma magnesium. Total body stores of magnesium can be evaluated by measuring the amount excreted after an intravenous load (described in the section on hypomagnesemia).

Magnesium has therapeutic uses, including as an antihypertensive or anticonvulsant agent and recently as treatment for asthma (bronchodilator).

Hypermagnesemia

Hypermagnesemia is extremely uncommon. In fact, while one study found 9% of serum samples from hospitalized patients to contain excessive magnesium, none of the samples yielded values above 4.0 mEq/L[(518)]. Since ECG changes occur with values above 5 mEq/L and symptoms generally occur with values above 10 mEq/L, the study supports the view that clinically significant hypermagnesemia is rare.

Hypermagnesemia occurs chiefly in either massively increased intake or impaired renal excretion. The most common cause of symptomatic hypermagnesemia in children may be induced maternal hypermagnesemia, since magnesium sulfate is given in pharmacologic doses in treating preeclampsia and eclampsia, which can produce paralysis in the neonate (vide infra). The other major cause is renal insufficiency. Other reported causes include Addison's disease, hypothyroidism, lithium intoxication, excessive use of magnesium-containing antacids or enemas in the presence of renal failure, excessive magnesium in dialysate, milk-alkali syndrome, and viral hepatitis[(516,519)]. Also, magnesium renal clearance is decreased in situations of increased parathyroid hormone activity, including familial hypocalciuric hypercalcemia and primary hyperparathyroidism, and can lead to hypermagnesemia. Cell death can also provide an increased load of magnesium, as occurs in tumor lysis or ketoacidosis.

Premonitory symptoms of hypermagnesemia include decreased deep tendon reflexes, nausea, vomiting, and skin flushing. Later clinical manifestations include hypocalcemia (due to depression of parathyroid hormone secretion and of its peripheral effectiveness), neuromuscular blockade, ECG changes (prolonged P-R, QRS, and Q-T intervals, atrioventricular block), myocardial depression, bradycardia (possibly due to suppression of sinoatrial node conduction), and asystole. Neuromuscular blockade appears to be due to decreased acetylcholine release, diminished end plate sensitivity to acetylcholine, and an increased axonal threshold for excitation.

Treatment of isolated hypermagnesemia should consist simply of restricting intake and inducing diuresis. If the hypermagnesemia is producing symptoms, more aggressive treatment is warranted. As a rapid temporizing measure, calcium may be given intravenously. Neonatologists commonly administer 100 mg of calcium gluconate per kilogram (equivalent to 30 mg of calcium chloride per kilogram) or about 10 mg of elemental calcium per kilogram. The adult literature suggests a 5- to 10-minute infusion of 100 mg of elemental calcium as either salt. For children, therefore, about 10 mg of calcium chloride per kilogram is appropriate, followed with diuresis or, if necessary, dialysis (both peritoneal and hemodialysis are effective).

While calcium partially reverses the deleterious effects of magnesium, it also reverses any therapeutic effects. This is worth bearing in mind when dealing with patients with seizures or preeclampsia; calcium reverses the anticonvulsant properties of magnesium.

Anesthesia, Intubation, and the Perioperative Period

As stated, magnesium limits acetylcholine release, decreases the depolarizing effect of acetylcholine, and reduces membrane excitability at the neuromuscular junction (as in the CNS). Consequently, even in the therapeutic range, magnesium causes increased sensitivity to depolarizing and nondepolarizing muscle relaxants[(455,520–522)], although there are some conflicting data on this matter[(523)]. The maintenance dose and/or dosing interval should be altered accordingly. However, in emergency situations, the intubating dose should probably not be reduced, since the goal is to achieve adequate intubating conditions as quickly as possible. Duration of blockade is a secondary concern. Magnesium also potentiates the muscle-relaxing properties of general anesthetics, as well as their negative inotropic effects. Interestingly, magnesium may mitigate the rise in serum potassium seen with succinylcholine[(523)].

Magnesium crosses the placenta, although maternal concentrations in the therapeutic range rarely result in neonatal depression. Neonatal signs of toxicity include decreased muscle tone, respiratory depression, and apnea.

Standard ICU monitoring is recommended. Neuromuscular monitors may be useful, particularly if muscle relaxants are used. A urinary bladder catheter is necessary if saline and/or diuretics are used to reduce the serum magnesium concentration. Acidosis should be prevented, either with bicarbonate or by ensuring adequacy of ventilation, in order to avoid an increase in the serum ionized magnesium.

Hypomagnesemia

Hypomagnesemia occurs in 11% of hospitalized patients, in comparison with the 9% with hypermagnesemia[(518)]. Studies in ICUs have found 20% to 50% of patients to be hypomagnesemic, with the lowest incidence in the patient group with the poorest renal function (i.e., the lowest renal magnesium loss)[(519,524,525)].

Presumably, the chief cause of hypomagnesemia is inadequate supply to the critically ill patient receiving no enteral feeding. If this lack of supply is accompanied by increased losses, symptomatic hypomagnesemia may result. Increased GI losses can be due to malabsorption states[(526)], laxative use, bowel fistulas, small bowel disease or resection, or prolonged nasogastric suction. Renal losses may be due to drugs, such as diuretics, aminoglycosides[527,528], chemotherapeutics[529], vitamin D, calcium, digitalis, amphotericin B[530], insulin, or theophylline[531]. They may also be caused by alcohol[532], transfusions, cardiopulmonary bypass[533,534], intrinsic renal disease (nephritis, nephrosclerosis, renal tubular disease, acute tubular necrosis), or may be stimulated by other disorders, such as DKA, hypophosphatemia, hypercalcemia, possibly hypokalemia, hyperparathyroidism, hyperaldosteronism, or hyperthyroidism.

Excessive losses in sweat and breast milk have also been noted, and pancreatitis is believed to be associated with hypomagnesemia (which may, in turn, contribute to hypocalcemia in pancreatitis)[519,535–538]. Familial hypomagnesemia may involve both poor gut absorption and defective renal reabsorption[539,540].

Despite the poor correlation between tissue magnesium stores and serum levels, hypomagnesemia is usually not evident until the serum level drops below 1.5 to 1.0 mg/dL. If the level is higher and there is still a suspicion of hypomagnesemia, tissue levels can be measured indirectly by measuring urinary excretion of the mineral after a test load of magnesium. If tissue is replete, typically 80% of the load is excreted; less excretion suggests tissue depletion. However, the load excreted may not accurately reflect tissue stores if there is abnormal renal reabsorption of magnesium or if there are other abnormal magnesium losses. Previously, it was thought that erythrocyte intracellular magnesium concentrations might reflect tissue stores, but recent studies cast doubt on the validity of this measure[541].

The literature is rather confusing on the clinical manifestations of hypomagnesemia, since early reports did not differentiate true effects of hypomagnesemia from those of the hypocalcemia frequently seen with hypomagnesemia. In one recent report, 9 of 33 hypomagnesemic adult ICU patients had hypocalcemia that was corrected with magnesium replacement. An additional two patients were normomagnesemic but hypocalcemic and became normocalcemic with magnesium therapy[524]. Hypocalcemia is apparently due to failure of magnesium-dependent adenylate cyclase in the parathyroids and bone, so that parathyroid hormone levels are low (due to decreased parathyroid responsiveness to hypocalcemia) and end-organ response to parathyroid hormone infusion is subnormal[542,543].

The effects of hypomagnesemia on the neuromuscular system are the same as are those seen in hypocalcemia. However, at least one report of normocalcemic hypomagnesemic tetany is available to defend the view that hypomagnesemia is a potentially independent cause of CNS symptoms[544,545]. Muscular wasting and weakness are also described in magnesium deficiency[546].

The cardiovascular manifestations of hypomagnesemia also overlap with those of hypocalcemia and hypokalemia (and may, at least in part, be due to the latter two secondary disorders). These changes include ECG changes (increased P-R and Q-T intervals, flat broad T-waves), ventricular tachydysrhythmias, and increased susceptibility to digitalis toxicity[547,548].

Other electrolyte disturbances seen in association with hypomagnesemia include hypokalemia, hyponatremia, hypophosphatemia, and distal renal tubular acidosis. The hypokalemia is presumed to be due to failure of the renal tubular Na^+-K^+-ATPase pump. Similarly, hypomagnesemia may impair the ATP-dependent sodium, potassium, hydrogen, and phosphate pumps in the renal tubular cells, thus accounting for the excess urinary losses of these electrolytes. Since magnesium reabsorption is coupled with renal reabsorption of calcium and sodium, the increased renal losses of sodium and calcium result in increased magnesium loss.

Treatment

Causes of increased loss of magnesium must be identified and treated appropriately, within the context of the current renal function. If GFR is reduced, magnesium replacement may result in hypermagnesemia. Also, if the patient has not been fed for an extended period of time, tissue stores are probably depleted unless intravenous fluid contains maintenance amounts of magnesium (as do most total-parenteral-nutrition solutions).

Owing to the large bone pool of diffusible magnesium that must equilibrate with the serum pool, it may take 4 or 5 days to achieve equilibrated normomagnesemia. For patients with normal renal function and no increased losses of magnesium, supplying the normal daily magnesium requirement of 0.3 to 0.4 mEq/kg per day intravenously should suffice. Up to 1 mEq/kg per day is probably safe, if necessary, in patients with normal renal function. These intravenous infusions are best delivered in the maintenance-fluid solution rather than as a bolus. The renal threshold for excretion of magnesium is at plasma concentrations of 1.5 to 2.0 mg/dL, so that high peak concentrations due to rapid magnesium infusions can result in a relatively high degree of renal excretion, giving a poor clinical response. Again, the serum magnesium level should be followed closely, especially in patients with poor renal function[516,519,549,550].

Anesthesia, Intubation, and the Perioperative Period

Hypomagnesemia can present problems related to dysrhythmias (digoxin toxicity, torsades de pointes, supraventricular tachycardia) or neurologic and neuromuscular dysfunction, including weakness, stridor (laryngospasm), and seizures. Replacement therapy is curative (at least transiently), but caution should be taken not to give magnesium too rapidly intravenously in order to avoid toxicity. Magnesium can be given intramuscularly, but uptake is unreliable and the injection is painful. There are no specific anesthetic-related considerations, but there is the possibility of related electrolyte abnormalities, especially of sodium, potassium, and calcium.

Phosphate

Phosphorus exists in the body in the form of phosphates—the salts of phosphoric acid (H_3PO_4). In the biologic pH range, phosphates exist as HPO_4^{2-} and $H_2PO_4^{2-}$ in a molar ratio of 2:1 to 6:1 (average, 4:1). The average phosphate valence, then, is about -1.8. Rather than report phosphates in milliequivalents or amounts of $H_2PO_4^-$ and HPO_4^{2-} in millimoles per liter, clinical laboratories in the United States report either milligrams of phosphorus per deciliter or the equivalent in inorganic (i.e., not complexed to organic molecules) phosphate, generally abbreviated as PO_4 with no stated valence. This convention is used in this chapter.

Total body phosphate (PO_4) varies with age. The full-term newborn has about 5.6 g of phosphorus (0.18 mole of PO_4) per kilogram of fat-free tissue. The typical 70-kg adult who is 15% fat has 12 g of phosphorus (0.39 mole of PO_4) per kilogram of fat-free tissue, which amounts to about 700 g or 23 moles of PO_4. Of this, 99% is intracellular, and 80% of that pool is in bone. The serum pool is 12% to 15% protein-bound, with the remainder being free phosphates. The rate of exchange between these pools may be influenced by insulin, glucose, pH, degree of hypophosphatemia, and probably by many other factors. This makes the volume of distribution for infused PO_4 unpredictable as well(551). Serum values for PO_4, (as for Mg^{2+}, Ca^{2+}, and all predominantly intracellular ions) are at best a rough approximation of body stores. The normal range for serum phosphate also varies with age. The high phosphate levels seen in early childhood are a reflection of the extensive bone remodeling in progress during growth.

Phosphate homeostasis is achieved by balancing its renal excretion with the generous intake that occurs due to its abundance in all natural food sources. The normal adult intake of phosphate is 800 to 1200 mg of phosphorus per day, which is approximately equal to the sum of the 700 to 1000 mg of urinary losses and 100 to 300 mg of fecal losses. Eighty percent of the ingested PO_4 is absorbed in the small bowel, with half of the absorption dependent on vitamin D-stimulated transport and half dependent on passive means. Phosphate is the major anion accompanying calcium intake. The intake of phosphate is sufficient so that deficiency caused by poor nutritional intake is rare(552,553). However, in profuse diarrhea or chronic administration of aluminum-containing antacids (which prevent phosphate absorption), phosphate levels may be impaired.

Phosphate homeostasis is heavily dependent on filtration and reabsorption in the kidney. More than 90% of the plasma pool of PO_4 is filtered in the kidney, and most is reabsorbed in the proximal tubule so that only 5% to 15% of the filtered load of PO_4 is excreted. Most of this reabsorption occurs in the proximal renal tubule by an active pH and sodium-dependent process. This mechanism for PO_4 reabsorption is saturated at a maximal threshold rate. The maximal threshold rate is reduced (i.e., phosphaturia increased) by aminohippurate sodium, amino acids, glucose and sodium (by competition for a common resorption mechanism), acetoacetate, sodium bicarbonate, acidosis (both respiratory and metabolic), thyroid hormone, estrogen, digoxin, corticosteroids, hypomagnesemia, hypokalemia, renal tubular defects, and, most importantly, by parathyroid hormone (via adenylate cyclase).

Conversely, the maximal threshold rate is increased (i.e., phosphaturia decreased) by growth hormone, vitamin D, and PO_4 depletion. The antiphosphaturic effect of PO_4 depletion is potent enough to override the phosphaturic parathyroid hormone effect.

Serum phosphate concentration is also influenced by shifts between ECF and ICF. Most of the disorders responsible for such shifts do so by causing increased glycolysis. The reasons for this are twofold. First, PO_4 accompanies glucose into cells. Second, glycolysis requires PO_4 at nearly every step. Stimuli for glycolysis include alkalosis, insulin and epinephrine, recovery from protein-caloric malnutrition, hypothermia, burns, and DKA(554). The flux between ECF and ICF can cause significant hypophosphatemia within minutes to hours.

The metabolic roles of phosphate are far too numerous to discuss here in any detail. For the scope of this chapter, it is sufficient to consider four categories of phosphate metabolism: Those involving ATP, 2,3-DPG, membrane phospholipids, and bone. PO_4 is essential for the regeneration of ATP. Depletion of 2,3-DPG is contributory to this energy deficit, since reduced 2,3-DPG results in a lowered P50 for oxyhemoglobin. (From a normal PaO_2 of 27, it can drop to near 16 torr.) The result of this deficit is reduced oxygen release from hemoglobin and relative tissue hypoxia. Lack of PO_4 results also in osteomalacia and pathologic fractures.

Hyperphosphatemia

Excessive serum phosphorus concentrations essentially are clinically silent, except insofar as they cause hypocalcemia. When serum PO_4 rises, increased chelation with Ca^{2+} ensues, rapidly lowering serum levels of the calcium cation. The binding of Ca^{2+} and PO_4 results in metastatic (soft tissue) calcification when the product of the concentrations (in milligrams per deciliter) of total calcium and inorganic phosphorus exceeds 60. The falling Ca^{2+} level stimulates parathyroid hormone secretion and inhibits renal formation of $1,25(OH)_2D$. Phosphaturia then follows as a result of the effects of both the increased parathyroid hormone and the hyperphosphatemia itself on reducing the maximal threshold rate. As the Ca^{2+} concentration falls, the patient may begin to exhibit signs of tetany, which may become profound(555).

Causes of hyperphosphatemia consist of three categories: Excessive phosphate intake, inadequate excretion, and ICF-to-ECF shifts. Intake must be fairly massive in order to overwhelm the normally effective renal excretory mechanism. Such intake generally results from massive intravenous infusions or from oral or rectal phosphate overuse. Other exogenous sources of phosphorus include the "white phosphorus" in incendiary bombs, which can be absorbed through skin burn wounds.

Inadequate excretion of PO_4 occurs when the maximal threshold rate/GFR ratio rises. Hence, any cause for a decrease in GFR (e.g., renal failure, volume depletion, myocardial failure) or an increase in maximal threshold rate (by growth hormone, vitamin D, hypoparathyroidism, pseudohypoparathyroidism) reduces phosphate excretion. The hyperphosphatemia that occurs may be sufficient to push the calcium-phosphate product well above 60 and result in metastatic calcifications. It is thought that this is the reason for the calcification of the cornea and basal ganglia seen in many patients with hypoparathyroidism or pseudohypoparathyroidism.

Shifts of PO_4 from ICF to ECF are seen in a variety of clinical situations in which cell lysis is prominent, such as oncotherapy[(434)], rhabdomyolysis, and shock. For the same reason, RBC breakage during blood drawing may produce spurious hyperphosphatemia.

When the cause is unclear, measurement of GFR and of daily urinary PO_4 loss may clarify the nature of the problem. (Normal phosphorus urinary excretion is $<$ 1500 mg/day in adults.)

Treatment

Therapy for hyperphosphatemia depends, of course, on the cause. In general, maneuvers include elimination of excess intake, use of aluminum hydroxide antacids (1 mL/kg every 6 hours helps, even in the absence of enteral PO_4 intake), and restoration of plasma volume with saline solution. Insulin and glucose administration can also help acutely reduce phosphorus levels. Dialysis is effective, if necessary. Note that symptomatic hypocalcemia, if present, receives the highest priority for treatment.

Hypophosphatemia

Abnormally low serum PO_4 concentrations are seen in a wide variety of clinical situations that are the converses of the categories cited for hyperphosphatemia: Reduced intake, increased excretion, and shifts from ECF to ICF[(553,555)]. Some disease states, such as DKA, may involve all three mechanisms. Excess urinary losses of phosphate in DKA arise from a tendency of glycosuria (by competing for the PO_4 reabsorption mechanism), ketonuria, and acidosis to lower the maximal threshold rate. The problem is excacerbated by osmotic diuresis and diminished dietary intake as the child becomes ill. Insulin drives the serum PO_4 (along with glucose and potassium) into cells, further aggravating hypophosphatemia.

Other disorders that reduce serum PO_4 levels by means of lowering the maximal threshold rate include renal tubular disorders (congenital, recovery from acute tubular necrosis or renal transplantation), acidosis, pregnancy, heavy-metal poisoning, hypokalemia, paint and glue sniffing[(556)], Wilson's disease, glycosuria (i.e., even without DKA), lack of or resistance to vitamin D, hyperparathyroidism, and possibly by this mechanism, Reye's syndrome[(557)]. The maximal threshold rate/GFR ratio can also be decreased, with resultant hyperphosphaturia and hypophosphatemia, by an increase in GFR. Thus, correction of a state of low cardiac output by saline-solution infusion or administration of pressors may result in increased urinary loss of PO_4 as GFR improves.

Inadequate phosphate intake alone is an unusual cause of hypophosphatemia. However, hospitalized patients with no enteral feeding are clearly at risk. Fluid intake consisting entirely of carbohydrate-containing, phosphate-free, intravenous solutions results in phosphate depletion. Patients with persistent gut dysfunction (emesis, diarrhea, malabsorption, prolonged nasogastric suctioning) must be considered at risk, and intravenous phosphate must be supplied in the maintenance fluids (vide infra).

Phosphate-binding antacids can increase the loss of body PO_4, leading to significant hypophosphatemia. Intracellular shift of phosphate is a problem seen during recovery from various widespread cellular insults, such as hypothermia, burns[(558)], starvation ("refeeding syndrome"), sepsis, toxic shock syndrome[(559)], and DKA. As noted in the earlier discussion of phosphate homeostasis, it is increased glycolysis, occurring during recovery from these disorders, that is responsible for the ICF uptake of PO_4. Acute alkalosis itself triggers glycolysis and so also produces intracellular PO_4 shift.

The physiologic consequences of hypophosphatemia have been alluded to in the earlier section dealing with phosphate metabolism. To recapitulate, phosphate depletion has been associated with rickets, reduced 2,3-DPG in RBCs, and widespread cellular ATP depletion. Rickets is especially likely to develop in rapidly growing infants supported by total parenteral nutrition without adequate phosphate[(398)]; however, it can also occur well into adolescence[(399)]. The observed 2,3-DPG changes in RBC have not proven to be clinically significant, nor has phosphate replacement in DKA been well demonstrated to be of more than theoretical benefit.

ATP depletion appears to be the final common pathway for many of the clinical manifestations of hypophosphatemia. These include depressed leukocyte phagocytosis, increased RBC and platelet destruction[(560)], muscular weakness, respiratory failure[(561)], depressed myocardial function[(562)], rhabdomyolysis, CNS dysfunction (from mood changes to seizures and coma), and liver failure[(552,554)].

Treatment

Treatment of hypophosphatemia ideally begins in anticipation of, rather than in response to, a falling concentration of serum PO_4. If the serum phosphorus level is less than 1.0 mg/dL, intravenous correction is appropriate. For phosphorus values of 0.5 to 1.0 mg/dL, suggested infusion doses range from 0.05 to 0.25 mmol of PO_4 per kilogram given intravenously over 4 to 12 hours. Patients with a serum phosphorus concentration below 0.5 mg/dL should receive PO_4 at 0.09 to 0.5 mmol/kg over 4 to 12 hours[199,281,551,563–565]. Known risks of PO_4 infusion include hyperkalemia (the potassium salt of PO_4 is usually used), hypocalcemia, metastatic calcification, hypomagnesemia, hyperphosphatemia, hypotension, hyperosmolality, and renal failure. The lower end of the dosage ranges should be used in the presence of hypocalcemia or renal failure, and PO_4 should not be given if hypercalcemia is present.

Oral forms of phosphate are not well tolerated because they have a bad taste and cause diarrhea. Results are better when the phosphate is given in several divided doses, every 4 to 6 hours, and the dose is started at the low end of the range and gradually increased.

DISORDERS OF THE THYROID

Embryology

The thyroid gland progenitor cells originate in the epithelium of the pharyngeal floor. This epithelium forms a diverticulum, which then travels caudally, steadily acquiring its bilobed mature form. Initially, it remains connected to the floor of the pharynx by means of a long duct, which usually disappears during gestation but may on occasion persist as the thyroglossal duct. Anomalies in this migration can leave some or all functioning thyroid tissue anywhere along the path from the pharynx to the central regions of the fourth pharyngeal pouch. Therefore, prior to the removal of such structures, care should be taken to ensure that the ectopic tissue does not represent the entire functioning gland.

The thyroid gland is capable of significant iodine concentration and synthesis of thyroxine (T_4) by about 9 to 11 weeks. Thyrotropin (TSH) secretion starts to rise in weeks 14 to 16, presumably due to increased thyrotropin-releasing hormone (TRH) secreted by the fetal hypothalamus (fetal gut secretion of TRH also plays a role[566]).

Transplacental TSH passage is minimal. However, transplacental passage of T_4 and triiodothyronine (T_3) does occur, despite high outer-ring deiodinase activity of the placenta. This may account for the preservation of neurologic development in athyreotic fetuses treated soon after birth. Propylthiouracil also crosses the placenta and can inhibit fetal and newborn thyroid function. Maternal thyroid stimulating immunoglobulins and thyroid-binding inhibitory immunoglobulins can also cross the placenta. Therefore, in newborn children of mothers with a history of thyroid autoimmunity, particularly Graves' disease, the incidence of neonatal disorders of thyroid function can be as high as 1 out of 70 (almost 60 times the incidence of congenital hypothyroidism from athyreosis or thyroid ectopy). Neonates with this maternal history should be watched closely for signs of thyroid disorders. If there is any clinical suspicion, thyroid-hormone-binding ratio, T_4, and TSH levels should be measured, and titers of the aforementioned immunoglobulins should be ascertained.

Pathophysiology

The regulation of thyroid function falls under both hypothalamic-pituitary control and intrathyroidal autoregulation. The hypothalamus produces TRH, which reaches the anterior pituitary by portal veins, releasing TSH. TSH acts via a receptor on thyroid follicular cells, facilitating secretion of thyroid hormones. TRH decreases the sensitivity of the anterior pituitary to the negative feedback effect of T_3 on secretion of TSH (T_4 has minimal feedback effect).

TRH is a tripeptide found in numerous tissues as well as the hypothalamus. Serum TRH levels probably reflect mostly the output of nonhypothalamic sources. Thus, serum TRH levels are not useful in understanding thyroid control. The roles of TRH as a potential neurotransmitter and in other non-TSH-releasing capacities are under investigation.

The details of thyroid hormone synthesis are outside the scope of this chapter. However, a few comments are helpful in understanding thyroid hormone levels and their perturbations in disease.

T_4 is composed of an inner and outer ring derived from two coupled tyrosyl residues of a thyroid protein, thyroglobulin. Each ring caries two iodine atoms. T_3 only has one iodine atom on its outer ring. T_4 is secreted in much larger quantities than T_3. In the adult thyroid gland, approximately 90 μg of T_4 and 30 μg of T_3 are secreted daily. However, most T_3 is generated by peripheral conversion of T_4 to T_3 (mostly in the liver) by the enzyme thyroxine 5' deiodinase. T_3 is the biologically active hormone and has multiple effects. Effects of T_3 appear to act principally through binding of nuclear receptors, which bind to the regulatory elements of multiple genes and modify the expression of these genes.

T_3 receptors are members of the superfamily[567] of nuclear receptors that includes retinoic acid, steroids (including estrogen), and vitamin D. The T_3 receptor genes alpha and beta are located on chromosome 17 and 3, respectively. Alternate splicing for each gene generates at least two receptor subtypes for each gene: Alpha-1, alpha-2 and beta-1, beta-2. All except beta-2 are expressed in most tissues. However, there is considerable variation from one tissue to another in the amount of each receptor and the amount of receptor mRNA protein. Furthermore the expression of these receptors responds differently to T_3 in different tissues. In chronic, severe illness, the amount of T_3 receptors increases, at least in monocytes[568], in peripheral blood and in hepatocytes.

Less than 1% of either T_4 or T_3 is free in the serum to bind receptors. T_4 is 99.97% bound and T_3 is 99.7% bound. The higher binding affinity of T_4 gives it a smaller volume of distribution and longer half-life than T_3. In adults, T_4 has a half-life of approximately 1 week, with daily turnover of approximately 10%. T_3 has a half-life of 1 day, with a daily turnover of approximately 75%. In neonates the half-life can be as low as 50% of the adult value.

The principal binding proteins are, in decreasing order of affinity, thyroid-binding globulin, thyroid-binding prealbumin, and albumin. Since most commonly used assays for thyroid hormones measure total thyroid hormone concentration, indirect measures of free thyroid concentration are often obtained with the total measurements.

The most common of these, the T_3 uptake test, is a measure of how much radiolabeled T_3 tracer incubated with the patient's serum sample can be recovered. If a lot of tracer is recovered (i.e., a high T_3 uptake) there must be few available free T_3 binding sites on serum proteins of the sample. This suggests either a decreased amount of binding protein or an increased amount of free hormone competing with the tracer T_3 for the available binding sites. Conversely, if very little tracer is recovered, it must have remained bound to the serum sample proteins, indicating a large number of available binding sites. This suggests that there is either an excess of binding proteins or decreased free hormone levels. Although several laboratories report T_3 uptake as a percentage, increasingly it is reported as a normalized number, a ratio comparing the sample T_3 uptake against a reference sample from the American Thyroid Association. Using this method, a low uptake with reference to the ATA sample is less than 1 and a high uptake is greater than 1. This normalized number is variously referred to as thyroid-hormone-binding ratio or the thyroxine binding globulin index.

Although many of the mechanisms responsible for the cellular effects of thyroid hormones remain unclear, the effects can be summarized: Oxygen consumption is increased at rest, and all tissues except brain, spleen, and testis contribute to the increase. Thyroid hormone increases adrenergic receptor sites in myocardial cells and glucocorticoid receptors in lung tissue and may increase catecholamine effects at postreceptor sites. Chronotropic and inotropic effects of thyroid hormone can be reversed by β-adrenergic blockade, but this does not influence oxygen consumption[(569)], providing evidence that thyroid hormone action is not exclusively through adrenergic mechanism activation. Some of these effects may be mediated by T_3's effect on enhanced production of alpha myosin heavy chain and depression of the production of myosin beta heavy chain[(570)]. Thyroid hormone accelerates metabolism of various hormones (e.g., insulin, cortisol), bone turnover (resulting at times in hypercalcemia)[(571–573)], and hematopoiesis[(574)]. Glucose intolerance may be due to increased glucagon level and effect[(575)]. Thyroid hormone is needed for normal hypoxic and hypercapnic drives and for various endocrine functions, such as normal luteinizing hormone, follicle-stimulating hormone, growth hormone, adrenal hormone activity, parathyroid hormone activity[(576)], and maturation of many systems in the early neonatal period[(577)].

Thyroid hormone has several effects on lipid metabolism. T_3 stimulates both lipogenesis and lipolysis associated with T_3-stimulated thermogenesis. In hypothyroidism, low-density lipoprotein cholesterol is increased, and the number of available low-density lipoprotein receptors is decreased. In rats, thermogenesis is stimulated in brown fat in response to high caloric intake, cold stress, in the presence of uncoupling protein (so-called because of its effect on oxidative phosphorylation), and T_3 and beta$_3$ adrenergic stimulation. Humans typically have minimal brown fat deposits after the neonatal period, but T_3 may play a similar role in deep white fat deposits. T_3 also stimulates Na/K ATPase in multiple tissues, which may also cause increased thermogenesis.

Thyroid hormone appears to have significant effects on human growth and growth hormone (GH), with reductions in both GH pulsatility and insulin-like growth factor-1 (IGF-1) in hypothyroid states[(578–580)].

Controversy exists in the adult and pediatric literature regarding thyroid function tests as predictors of mortality[(581–584)]. Until further delineation of the nature of these changes is forthcoming, we reserve comment.

Thyroid Storm

Thyrotoxic crisis (thyroid storm) is a rare manifestation of juvenile thyrotoxicosis, itself an uncommon disorder[(585)]. Despite its rarity, thyroid storm is a topic of considerable interest in the pediatric ICU for two reasons. First, it represents a unique form of acute multisystem failure in children. Second, it is a disorder not easily recognized and carries a high morality rate unless diagnosed early and treated aggressively. Here we briefly review the pathophysiology of hyperthyroidism, provide a description of the clinical presentation and diagnostic evaluation of the child in thyrotoxic crisis, and outline a course of therapy for thyroid storm.

Pathophysiology

Graves' disease, the most common cause of thyrotoxicosis, has a genetic basis and an autoimmune pathogenesis. It appears to be associated in white patients with the histocompatibility antigens HLA-B8 and DW3 and in Oriental patients with DKA-BW35. However, the mode or modes of inheritance have not been fully elucidated[(576,586)]. The immunologic basis for the disorder appears to be that T-lymphocytes become sensitized to thyroid antigens and cause B-lymphocytes to produce antibodies against these antigens. The most important of these immunoglobulins, pathophysiologically, is the one identified as thyroid-stimulating immunoglobulin (TSI). This antibody, once called a long-acting thyroid stimulator, is found in virtually all patients with Graves' disease. TSI is capable of producing increased thyroid growth and function, at least partly through occupancy of the TSH receptor.

Clinical Presentation

Thyrotoxicosis has a nonspecific presentation in the critically ill patient, causing such effects as tachycardia, nervousness, and muscle weakness. In children, eye findings (e.g., exopthlamos) and goiter may not be prominent, and therefore, presentation can be less than obvious. Most helpful in such circumstances is the history. If the patient is a neonate, a maternal history of autoimmune thyroid disease is relevant. Otherwise, a history of prior thyroid disease or a diagnosis of one of the syndromes or disorders known to be associated with thyrotoxicosis is helpful.

Usually, there is some precipitating event that triggers the thyrotoxic crisis, such as infection, trauma, surgery, DKA, or radiation, and onset is usually abrupt[576,587]. Thyrotoxicosis has also been reported secondary to exogenous thyroid hormone ingestion, such as in isolated cases and epidemiologic investigations of food processing contamination[588,589], toxic adenoma of the thyroid[590], and following haloperidol use[591] or iodide ingestion. Thyrotoxic crisis shares features with sepsis, malignant hyperthermia, anticholinergic poisoning, transfusion reaction, and adrenal crisis (more fully discussed in the section on Anesthesia, Intubation, and the Perioperative period).

Severity of symptoms is not related to the concentration of T_3 or T_4. Indeed, T_4 and T_3 levels in a thyrotoxic crisis are often in the same range as in cases of moderate thyrotoxicosis that do not even even require hospitalization (as in cases of thyroid hormone overdose)[592,593].

Given the effects of thyroid hormone, one could correctly anticipate that an excess would produce signs and symptoms referable to a hypermetabolic state, with a particularly stimulated cardiovascular system. In fact, the most common reported findings in childhood thyrotoxicosis are, in descending order, goiter, tachycardia, nervousness[594], increased pulse pressure, proptosis, increased appetite, tremor, weight loss, and heat intolerance[595]. Dysrhythmias and congestive heart failure have been reported (although high-output failure is rare except in the severely compromised neonate or the older adolescent). Shock, psychosis, coma, and seizures[596] have also been reported.

Symptoms are generally insidious in onset and, at first, are frequently assumed to be normal signs of adolescence. The disorder in children is found in association with diabetes mellitus[597], juvenile rheumatoid arthritis, Down's syndrome, McCune-Albright syndrome, Addison's disease, myasthenia gravis, Hashimoto's thyroiditis, and possibly, systemic lupus erythematosus, chronic active hepatitis, and the nephrotic syndrome. Any child known to have an endocrinopathy or autoimmune disease should be considered at risk for thyroid disease. Fever, cutaneous flushing, diaphoresis, weakness, lethargy, confusion, and extreme tachycardia occur and may be accompanied by hepatomegaly, jaundice, nausea, and vomiting. Untreated, the illness progresses to extreme hyperpyrexia, coma, and death[595].

Serum should be sent for determination of the levels of T_4, free T_4, T_3, and free T_3, if available. Resin T_3 uptake yields the reciprocal of thyroid hormone-binding sites available. Thus, resin T_3 uptake multiplied by T_3 or T_4 gives a free T_3 index or free T_4 index, rough indicators of the actual free T_3 and free T_4 levels. For a child who is critically ill, further testing is ill advised in most cases, and treatment should begin promptly. If the severity of illness warrants placement of a pulmonary artery catheter, confirmation of the hypermetabolic state is found in elevation of the cardiac index and oxygen consumption index. Echocardiography can provide similar information noninvasively[598].

Neonatal thyrotoxicosis may be seen more frequently in neonatal ICUs, but symptoms may become apparent only after discharge of the newborn from the hospital following birth. Mothers with Graves' disease may have transplacental passage of TSIs. Some drugs cross the placenta, so if the mother is being medically treated, the infant may appear euthyroid at birth. As the levels of these antithyroid drugs fall in the bloodstream, the child becomes progressively more hyperthyroid. Symptoms may reach a crisis by 1 to 2 weeks of age, and the infant appears febrile, irritable, and potentially septic. Infants may also demonstrate failure to thrive, diarrhea, feeding intolerance, hepatosplenomegaly, thrombocytopenia, and seizures, for which other diagnoses must be considered, including infection (congenital and acquired neonatal), predelivery drug abuse in the mother, and congenital heart disease (presenting as congenital heart failure)[599].

Treatment

Therapy for the child in thyroid storm is directed at the triggering illness, at the hyperdynamic cardiovascular state, at the effects of the accelerated metabolic state, and at the thyroid gland itself. Attention is first given to the airway (see section on Anesthesia, Intubation and the Perioperative Period). A large-bore intravenous catheter is secured, and hypovolemia is corrected rapidly (20 mL of normal saline or lactated Ringer's solution per kilogram as rapidly and as often as necessary). Fever is reduced with use of a cooling blanket and antipyretics.

Salicylates should be avoided, because they displace thyroid hormone from protein-binding sites. Intravenous propranolol (0.01 mg/kg) is given by slow push every 10 minutes until the hyperdynamic cardiovascular state is improved or a total of 5 mg is given. Propylthiouracil given by nasogastric tube, at 20 to 30 mg/kg per day in four divided doses, stops organification of iodide and reduces intrathyroidal and peripheral conversion of T_4 to T_3. One hour after administration of propylthiouracil, sodium iodide can be infused intravenously at 1 to 2 g/day. Glucocorticoids may reduce serum T_3 levels. Dexamethasone, 0.1 mg/kg given every 6 hours, should be more than sufficient[595]. The oral radiocontrast agents sodium ipodate and iopanoic acid have been used as potent inhibitors of peripheral conversion of T_4 to T_3[497,504]. Surgery and use of radioiodine are not part of the acute therapy for thyroid storm[600].

Although treatment has been initiated, careful monitoring is continued (see section on Anesthesia, Intubation and the Perioperative Period). Once the patient is stable, propranolol can be continued orally at 4 mg/kg per day in four divided doses, with a 10-mg dose generally being adequate (although some adolescents may require up to a 60-mg dose). Clinical improvement should be seen within 24 hours, and resolution of the crisis should be achieved within a week.

Anesthesia, Intubation, and the Perioperative Period

This section applies to both hyperthyroid patients who require intensive care for some unrelated reason (e.g., motor vehicle accident) and to children in thyroid storm. The principles of care are the same in either case; the difference is the degree to which they are applied.

Patient assessment should begin with the airway, as in any critical situation. Supplemental oxygen should be provided as necessary. Most hyperthyroid children are awake and alert and can maintain their airway without intervention. However, if intubation becomes necessary, the patient with a goiter may have a distorted or obstructed airway, making intubation challenging. In addition, a goiter may make it difficult to position the head ideally for laryngoscopy.

Further assessment via radiologic techniques may be helpful, and preparation for a difficult intubation may be warranted, such as having a fiberoptic laryngoscope[601] or laryngeal mask airway at hand. (There is considerable experience with both airway-management tools in this setting[602,603], usually for airway evaluation, although they are rarely necessary[604] for intubation). In these cases, the problem may not be in visualization of the vocal cords on laryngoscopy, but rather in advancing the tube; tracheal obstruction may impede advancement of the tube, even if the tube is in "the right place." A selection of smaller tubes should be available in case it is necessary to advance beyond the obstruction. An armored (Tovell) tube may be necessary to prevent tube kinking. If the airway is considered very difficult, particularly with an intrathoracic or subglottic obstruction, an awake induction or induction with an inhalational anesthetic in the operating room may be considered, so as to preserve spontaneous ventilation until the airway is secured.

Ectopic thyroid tissue (e.g., lingual thyroid) may provide an unusual and unexpected cause of difficult intubation[605] or airway obstruction. It may be prudent to arrange a surgical backup plan in case the airway cannot be secured from above. If airway obstruction is not imminent, an attempt can be made to shrink the ectopic thyroid tissue by administering thyroid hormones (which suppress TSH and thus remove a stimulus to growth of the tissue). Radionuclide scanning can demarcate the extent of the problem prior to surgery.

Appropriate monitoring is important and should include continuous ECG (to detect tachycardia and dysrhythmias) and monitoring of body temperature. External and internal means of treating hyperthermia should be readily available (cooling blankets and cooled intravenous fluids). Antipyretics are also useful, but use of aspirin and salicylates should be avoided because they displace thyroid hormones from protein-binding sites[606,607]. Invasive monitoring may be necessary in hemodynamically unstable patients.

Patients are often hypovolemic. Large-bore intravenous access should be obtained and fluid resuscitation performed as indicated, with the caveat that these patients may be in high-output failure.

Endotracheal intubation and other procedures should be done with the least possible stimulation of sympathetic reflexes. Premedication with a benzodiazepine or similar agent to sedate the patient is useful. Beta-antagonists (e.g., esmolol), narcotics (e.g., fentanyl), or lidocaine (1.0 to 1.5 mg/kg intravenously, or 120 mg [adult dose] by inhalation) help blunt the sympathetic response to laryngoscopy[608–611]. Newer, shorter-acting beta-antagonists are probably easier to use than propanolol, because they have shorter durations[612,613] and (in the case of esmolol) are $beta_1$-specific[614].

The use of beta blockers entails several risks: Excessive blockade, hypotension, bradycardia, heart block, hypoglycemia (particularly in children), and mental status changes[615], including drowsiness, dizziness, loss of consciousness, hallucinations, and seizures[615]. Treatment of beta-blocker toxicity[615–617] includes administration of beta-agonists (although huge doses may be necessary), atropine (although some researchers question its effectiveness), and glucagon. Severe bradycardia that is refractory to these treatments may respond to external or transvenous pacing. It is important to maintain intravascular volume and adequate ventilation. There is no role for forced diuresis.

Anticholinergic drugs, such as atropine and glycopyrrolate, which are sometimes used before intubation, are probably best avoided in hyperthyroid patients, because they can cause tachycardia. In addition, they reduce sweating and thus exacerbate hyperpyrexia. If an anticholinergic agent is absolutely necessary, glycopyrrolate may be a better selection since it causes less tachycardia[618].

Exaggerated sensitivity of the sympathetic system[75,619,620] should also be considered when treating hypotension. A direct-acting vasopressor (e.g., phenylephrine) may be preferable to an indirect-acting agent, such as ephedrine, whose activity is partly due to the release of endogenous norepinephrine[621]. The latter may provoke an exaggerated response. Epinephrine-containing solutions (e.g., local anesthetics with epinephrine) should be used with caution.

Most anesthetics are suitable for laryngoscopy in hyperthyroid patients, with the exception of ketamine, which has potent sympathetic stimulant effects[622] and has been associated with alarming reactions even when given to hypothyroid patients who have been rendered euthyroid[623]. Thiopental has the theoretical advantage of having a molecular structure similar to propylthiouracil. It has also been shown to inhibit the hydrogen peroxide-generating system of the thyroid gland[624], an action shared by halothane and enflurane but not by local anesthetics and tranquilizers. Clinically, this is probably not significant; the ability of an induction agent to impair thyroid function in some respect does not necessarily mean that it is useful in hyperthyroidism. For example, ketamine, thiopental, and midazolam have all been shown to reduce production of thyroglobulin (by inhibiting cAMP production) and T_3 (by inhibiting 5′-deiodinase)[625]. However, one would not chose to use ketamine in a hyperthyroid patient, as discussed above. Regardless of the agent used, it is important that the patient be deeply anesthetized at the time of intubation to minimize the degree of sympathetic stimulation from laryngoscopy.

Control of the airway should be achieved expeditiously, since hypercarbia could result in unwanted stimulation of the sympathetic system[(626)]. For the same reason, spontaneous ventilation is probably best avoided in the anesthetized patient.

There is a time-honored hypothesis that hypermetabolic conditions increase the amount of anesthetic required to achieve adequate anesthesia for a given procedure[(627)], although this view is contested in the literature[(628)]. Similarly, it was long believed that the anesthetic requirement is increased in hyperthyroidism, but studies have shown that the anesthetic requirement is not changed in dogs rendered hyperthyroid or hypothyroid[(629)], possibly because cerebral metabolic oxygen consumption is unchanged[(628,630)].

However, secondary effects of thyroid illness may affect the rate and depth of induction of anesthesia. Hyperthermia or hypothermia may affect the anesthetic requirements[(631–634)]. In general the minimum alveolar concentration of an inhalation anesthetic (the dose required to prevent movement in 50% of patients upon incision) is increased by about 5% for every 1°C rise in temperature; hypothermia has the opposite effect. In addition, induction with inhalational agents may be slowed (in hyperthyroidism) or accelerated (in hypothyroidism) because of secondary changes in cardiac output[(635,636)]. This probably accounts for the clinical sense that anesthetic demand is altered in these conditions.

Care should be taken not to abrade or compress the eyes during intubation of patients who have exopthalmos. This care should be maintained as long as the patient is sedated and/or paralyzed. Eye lubricants, artificial tears, and taping the eyes shut are helpful in this matter.

Muscle relaxation, if required, should be achieved with agents that have minimal cardiovascular effects (e.g., using vecuronium rather than pancuronium, which has vagolytic properties). However, other considerations may take precedence (e.g., the use of succinylcholine in an emergency intubation). It is also possible that histamine-releasing muscle relaxants (d-tubocurarine, metocurine, atracurium, and mivacurium) may stimulate the sympathetic system, although their net clinical effect usually is mild hypotension.

Reversal of nondepolarizing neuromuscular blockade, if necessary, is achieved with a combination of a cholinesterase inhibitor and an antimuscarinic drug (which is given to prevent excessive muscarinic side effects from the anticholinesterase). As mentioned, glycopyrrolate causes less tachycardia than atropine[(618)] and therefore is probably a better selection.

The incidence of myasthenia gravis is increased among adults with thyroid disorders. The same is true in children, although to a lesser extent[(637)]. This, together with the tendency toward muscular weakness, suggest reduction of the dose of muscle relaxants and the use of a twitch monitor to guide continued dosing.

Thyroid storm is a rare event in children, particularly in the perioperative period[(638)]. When it occurs in the perioperative period in adults, it is usually 6 to 18 hours after surgery. However, other conditions can present in a similarly dramatic manner during or after surgery. Thyroid storm may be difficult to distinguish from malignant hyperthermia[(639)], which is a lethal condition if untreated and so must be recognized and attended to promptly. Pheochromocytoma can also have a presentation similar to malignant hyperthermia[(640)] and thyroid storm[(641)]. The distinction is not academic, since treatment of these diseases is very different and misdiagnosis can be harmful.

For example, beta-blockers are the treatment of choice for thyroid storm but would cause unopposed alpha-adrenergic action in pheochromocytomas. Similarly, if malignant hyperthermia is misdiagnosed as one of the other conditions, the patient may not receive dantrolene, a lifesaving medication. Several characteristics can help distinguish malignant hyperthermia from the other conditions:

1. Muscle rigidity is a feature of malignant hyperthermia.
2. The endocrine conditions do not respond to treatment with dantrolene.
3. Malignant hyperthermia and pheochromocytoma usually (but not always) present intraoperatively, while thyroid storm typically presents postoperatively.
4. $PaCO_2$ and end-tidal CO_2 are elevated in malignant hyperthermia and thyroid storm[(642)] but not in pheochromocytoma.

Differential diagnosis is further complicated by entities such as sepsis, transfusion reactions, intraventricular hemorrhage[(643)], and neuroleptic malignant syndrome[(644)], a condition very similar to malignant hyperthermia triggered by neuroleptic drugs. Rhabdomyolysis is common in both malignant hyperthermia and neuroleptic malignant syndrome[(645)] and has been reported in pheochromocytoma[(646)] and thyroid storm[(647)]. It is also possible for a patient to have two of these diseases simultaneously (e.g., pheochromocytoma and hyperthyroidism[(641)]).

Treatment of thyroid storm is supportive, with particular attention to dehydration (volume resuscitation), hyperthermia (cooling), tachycardia (drugs to control heart rate), high-output heart failure, and obtundation (airway management). The principal management methods have been outlined in the preceding text.

The congestive heart failure seen in thyroid storm may be refractory to digitalis preparations. Furthermore, beta-antagonists may present problems when used in patients in heart failure or in whom some other contraindication exists, such as bronchospasm. Selective beta1 antagonists, such as esmolol, may be useful if the patient has bronchospastic disease (which is exacerbated by $beta_2$ blockade). In extremis, plasmapheresis[(648,649)] or dialysis[(649)] can be used to remove T_4 from the circulation before emergency surgery, but the usefulness of both techniques has often been questioned[650,651]. Reserpine[652], guanethedine[653], and lithium[654] have also been used to control the symptoms of hyperthyroidism. Hydrocortisone has been reported to be of use in thyroid storm, even in the absence of concurrent adrenal suppression[655].

Another consideration in hyperthyroidism is the possibility of altered drug metabolism[656]. For example, the activity of hepatic mixed function oxidases is increased in hyperthyroidism[657]. However, what impact this might have on clinical practice is unclear.

Elective surgeries and procedures should be delayed until the patient has been rendered euthyroid and is no longer hyperdynamic. Various perioperative regimens have been used, which generally emphasize the role of beta-blockers, antithyroid drugs, and iodine[658–667]. One approach is to treat the patient with propylthiouracil or methimazole for 2 to 3 months prior to surgery. Potassium iodide can be introduced 10 days before surgery. Another approach uses 7 to 14 days of beta blockers and potassium iodide. In the event of an emergency, beta-blockers and similar drugs must be used to control the circulation acutely; antithyroid drugs are not of immediate use, but getting them "on board" may ease the subsequent clinical course.

Thyroid surgery is associated with a variety of well-recognized complications[668]. The patient should be evaluated for airway obstruction throughout the postoperative period. While stridor may be due to garden-variety postintubation subglottic stenosis, which usually responds to humidified gases and racemic epinephrine, there are many other possible causes. The patient may have a neck-wound hematoma, necessitating immediate surgical consultation for possible wound reopening[669]. Immediate reintubation may be necessary and may be technically challenging. Postoperative tracheomalacia or neck edema can present similar problems. Vocal cord paralysis can occur, resulting from transection of one or both recurrent laryngeal nerves. Unilateral recurrent layngeal nerve damage causes ipsilateral vocal cord paralysis and hoarseness. Bilateral damage causes aphonia and can result in airway obstruction on inspiration.

The function of the vocal cords can be ascertained by laryngoscopy or by asking the patient to say "e." Complete airway obstruction requires emergency intubation followed by tracheostomy. Hypocalcemia results from inadvertent parathyroidectomy, but other variables have been associated with postoperative hypocalcemia in the absence of parathyroidectomy. These include the free T_4 level and the presence of substernal thyroid disease or of carcinoma[670]. Usually, patients do not become symptomatic for 1 or 2 days, but symptoms can occur much earlier, even in the recovery room. Stridor or laryngospasm may be the first manifestation of hypocalcemic tetany. The serum ionized calcium level is diagnostic, and intravenous administration of calcium is therapeutic.

Given the potential risks, patients who have undergone thyroidectomy should only be extubated under optimal conditions (i.e. fully awake, neuromuscular blockade fully reversed, etc.). ICU physicians should also be on the lookout for air in subcutaneous tissue, the pleura, or mediastinum.

Nonthyroid Illness (Sick Euthyroid Syndrome)

In the ICU, nonthyroidal illness is the most common cause of abnormal thyroid hormone levels. Therefore physicians should understand the pathophysiology of nonthyroidal illness and be able to distinguish it from less common causes of perturbations of serum levels of thyroid hormone.

Although there is considerable variation in the thyroid hormone levels in nonthyroidal illness, it typically involves depression of T_3, variably associated with depression of T_4 (typically in more severe and prolonged critical illness) without elevation of TSH. As patients recover from their critical illness, T_3 and T_4 return to the normal range, sometimes accompanied by a rise of TSH to the range found in hypothyroid patients. In adult patients, the severity of disease and mortality correlate inversely with T_4 and T_3 levels[581,582]. Of note, attempts to improve mortality rates in these patients with use of supplemental T_4 or T_3 has either failed to show benefit or has been inconclusive at best[671].

In nonthyroidal illness, the activity of peripheral deiodinases is depressed, particularly the 5′ (outer ring) deiodinase, which is responsible for converting T_4 to T_3 and reverse T_3 to T_2. The net result is usually a drop in T_3 levels and a reciprocal rise in rT3. T_3 and T_4 may well drop into the hypothyroid range. However, even in neonates, the free T_4 is rarely below the lower limits of normal[672]. One hypothesis to explain this is that the total T_4 is lower due to decreased TBG levels or decreased binding affinity of T_4 to TBG, while the free T_4 level is normal. Consequently, reverse T_3 and free T_4 levels may be helpful in distinguishing nonthyroidal illness from other causes of hypothyroidism.

In the ICU, there are many factors that can affect thyroid hormone levels: Many of the medications used can affect thyroid hormone function tests. T_4 to T_3 conversion can be reduced by several classes of drugs (e.g., glucocorticoids, propanolol, propylthiouracil), resulting in a decrease in T_3 and a slight rise in free T_4. The anticonvulsants phenytoin and carbamezipine tend to lower T_4 and T_3 levels[673,674], both by increasing hepatic metabolism (the major effect) and by displacing T_4 from binding proteins. Dopamine, somatostatin, opioids, and dexamethasone can cause blunting of TSH level and can prevent the rise in TSH seen in early hypothyroidism. Furosemide and salicylates in high doses displace T_4 and T_3 from binding proteins and thereby cause a transient increase of free T_4 and free T_3 but a lower total T_3 and total T_4 at equilibrium. Exposure to povidone-iodine (skin preparation used before surgery) may cause abnormalities in thyroid function tests in newborns[675,676].

During critical illness, there are changes both in measured peripheral thyroid hormone concentration and conversions and in thyroidal axis regulation and responses[677,678]. Total T_4 and T_3 levels are often found to be low and are the result of several mechanisms. First, there is decreased secretion of T_4 from the thyroid. Second, decreased thyroid hormone protein binding occurs, so the free T_4 level may be normal or high. It has been suggested that free T_4 still exerts inhibitory feedback on T_4 release or TSH release, which partly accounts for the low total T_4 and normal (i.e., relatively low) TSH levels. The total T_3 is also low, which may also be due to decreased protein binding, or to impaired peripheral conversion from T_4 and T_3, as described.

Furthermore, even after these abnormalities in thyroid function test are discovered, interpretation of results is difficult. Attempting to differentiate patients with sick euthyroid syndrome from truly hypothyroid patients by TRH stimulation test or TSH response is problematic. Hypothyroid patients would be expected to have an exaggerated TSH response to TRH stimulation because of lack of inhibition by peripheral thyroid hormones. Sick euthyroid patients should have a blunted (or normal) TSH response to TRH stimulation, presumably because of an "appropriate" (for their condition) level of T_4 and T_3 in the circulation. Unfortunately, truly hypothyroid patients may also have a blunted TSH response to TRH if they are receiving a dopamine infusion, have fasted longer than 60 hours, are acutely hyperpyrexic, or are hyperpyrexic immediately following surgery. Currently, the free thyroidal index and repeated complete axis testing are the most useful tests to follow thyroidal function in nonthyroidal illness.

Hypothyroidism

Hypothyroidism in patients in the ICU is more often a coexisting illness than a primary or life-threatening problem requiring the intensivist's expertise. Most infants with congenital hypothyroidism are identified by mandatory newborn screening in the United States. This screening, performed on a small quantity of blood dried on filter paper and sent to a reference laboratory, has documented an incidence of congenital primary hypothyroidism (due to ectopic gland or athyreosis) approaching 1 out of 3500. These infants are asymptomatic or minimally symptomatic, and the diagnosis is easily missed[(679)] until permanent neurologic impairment has occurred.

Some screening programs use elevated TSH (approximately 20 μU/mL or greater) to detect congenital primary hypothyroidism. Increasingly, screening programs include both T_4 and TSH, identifying many of the 1 in 80,000 infants with central (tertiary or secondary) hypothyroidism as well as those infants with a delayed rise in their TSH.

Routine thyroid screening is not performed until 48 to 72 hours because of fluctuations in thyroid hormone levels during the first 48 hours of life. In some centers, testing is repeated at 2 weeks of age. The timing of the screen is done to accommodate testing of other inborn errors of metabolism that become more easily diagnosed after 48 hours of enteral nutrition (usually including a protein source and lactose). Although the normal range is slightly altered compared with testing in older patients, the interpretation of test results for primary (glandular) or secondary (pituitary) failure are similar.

Several factors in the pediatric ICU may thwart the screening programs, depending on how they are implemented. For example, hypothyroid infants who are receiving dopamine or a pharmacologic dose of dexamethasone may have a suppressed TSH response in the presence of a marginal T_4 level and therefore have normal results on neonatal screening. Blood transfusion or cardiopulmonary bypass may falsely normalize the results (a false-negative test). If possible, the patient should be screened before blood-product exposure; if this is not possible, testing should be postponed to a later date. Further examples of situations that confound interpretation of thyroid function tests can be found in the section on nonthyroidal illness.

Acquired hypothyroidism may coexist in patients with other autoimmune diseases or may result from thyroid or pituitary surgery or craniospinal irradiation. Patients with diabetes mellitus that is difficult to control may have acquired hypothyroidism or adrenal insufficiency. An added difficulty for the intensivist is that acute diabetic ketoacidosis alters thyroid function. During these acute decompensations there are decreases in TSH, T_4, and T_3 and an increase in reverse T_3[(680–683)]. This indicates an alteration in control mechanisms of thyroid hormone secretion and peripheral conversion to the more active T_3. Further investigations are currently being done to further the understanding of these findings.

Patients who have undergone transsphenoidal hypophysectomy or who have sellar or suprasellar tumor should be carefully evaluated for panhypopituitarism, including secondary hypothyroidism. Patients who have received craniospinal irradiation for CNS tumors or as part of multimodal therapy for leukemia have been found to have thyroid function abnormalities[(684)].

The thyroid gland has a nonmonotonic response to iodine exposure. Initially, increasing iodine augments thyroid hormone production and release. However, with further increases, several synthetic processes, including organification, are inhibited. The mature thyroid gland is capable of controlling (autoregulating) the amount of iodine transported across the membrane of the follicular cell and can therefore escape from inhibition of thyroid hormone production from chronically high levels of iodine. Neonates, especially if premature, have immature autoregulation of this transport mechanism. As a result, they can become profoundly hypothyroid from iodine exposure[(685,686)].

In the ICU, such exposure includes topical use of iodine-containing antiseptics and iodine-containing radio-opaque intravenous dyes (e.g., for intravenous pyelograms or cardiac catheterizations). There is a 1- to 2-week latency period (partly due to the long half-life of T_4) before hypothyroidism induced by iodine exposure has an impact on the measured hormone concentrations. Consequently, hypothyroidism caused by this mechanism is not detected by neonatal screening. Only a minority of infants with significant iodine exposure may become hypothyroid. Unfortunately, to date, how to reliably identify patients at the greatest risk is not known, except that perhaps, extreme prematurity is a risk factor(687).

Tertiary (hypothalamic) hypothyroidism can also cause results in thyroid function tests similar to those of the far more common nonthyroidal illness (sick euthyroid syndrome) in the ICU (described previously); that is, the T_4 level is low and TSH is not elevated. If a patient is suspected to have tertiary hypothyroidism, a reverse T_3 level or a measured free T_4 level (not one calculated from total T_4 and thyroid-hormone-binding ratio) can be obtained and should be low (reverse T_3 is high in nonthyroidal illness and free T_4 is normal). Also, most patients with tertiary hypothyroidism have abnormal TSH responses to a TRH-stimulation test. The TSH peak is delayed (later than 30 to 45 minutes after TRH infusion) and does not return to baseline within the usual 2 to 3 hours. Before pursuing an expensive workup in the critically ill child whose T_4 is low and TSH is not elevated, consider that the incidence of tertiary hypothyroidism is approximately 1 in 80,000. Unless strongly suspected (e.g., because of other pituitary or hypothalamic deficits), this evaluation may await the end of the critical illness, at which point TSH and T_4 can be reevaluated.

Myxedema is the most severe presentation of hypothyroidism and is extremely rare in children. All the symptoms of a severe hypometabolic state (bradycardia, mental sluggishness, hypothermia, constipation) may be present. Additionally, coma with congestive heart failure with tachycardia and pericardial effusion may be present. Myxedema may also have coexistent SIADH and hypocortisolism. For emergency treatment, the rules of airway, breathing, and circulation apply. The euthyroid state is then achieved slowly with T_3 or T_4 replacement and, for potential occult hypocortisolism, cortisol replacement.

Anesthesia, Intubation, and the Perioperative Period

The concerns in the hypothyroid patient, who is typically hypometabolic, are in some respects the opposite of those in the hyperthyroid patient. For example, ketamine may be of benefit by virtue of its stimulation of the sympathetic system, and the antimuscarinic effects of pancuromium may be useful. There is a very widely held clinical belief that hypothyroid patients are more susceptible to the cardiovascular depressant effects of most anesthetic drugs and are prone to prolonged or accentuated effects from them(688). While there are some reports in the literature that support this notion(689,690), objective data to confirm these impressions are scant, and animal studies have failed to show an increased sensitivity to inhalational anesthetics(629). Nevertheless, it is best to be careful when using such drugs in these patients. Furthermore, altered body temperature may affect sensitivity to some anesthetics, and decreased metabolism may slow the clearance of narcotics and other drugs(656,657,688,691).

Hypothyroid patients can receive sedative premedication for procedures, as well as appropriate medication for pain relief and anxiolysis, with the caveat that they may be more sensitive to drugs than expected. Symptomatically hypothyroid patients may have depressed ventilatory responses to hypoxia and hypercarbia(688,692), which may be exacerbated by these drugs. The use of nonopioid analgesics, or of regional anesthetics when appropriate, may be helpful. Some advocate administering a corticosteroid before surgery in case the patient also has depressed adrenal function.

Intubation can be facilitated by any induction agent, although ketamine may present some advantages, as mentioned. One should remain aware of the fact that cardiac output(688) and baroreceptor activity may be decreased(693) and that these patients are vasoconstricted and hypovolemic(688). Consequently, there is the possibility of severe hypotension following induction with vasodilating drugs. Induction agents, such as thiopental, should be given incrementally with appropriate monitoring.

Muscle relaxation can be achieved with succinylcholine or a nondepolarizing drug, but it might be prudent to avoid drugs that can cause hypotension, particularly when administering the agent in rapid boluses (curare and metubine by histamine release and ganglionic blockade, atracurium and mivacurium by histamine release). Hypothyroid patients have muscle weakness, including weakness of the respiratory muscles(694), and may have increased sensitivity to muscle relaxants. Reversal of neuromuscular blockade with a cholinesterase inhibitor and anticholinergic drug does not present any particular problems, except that the response to peripheral nerve stimulation is depressed in severe hypothyroidism(695), thus making it difficult to gauge the depth of pharmacologic paralysis. Extubation should wait until the patient is euthermic and fully alert.

Gastric emptying time is affected by thyroid status(696); precautions to prevent pulmonary aspiration should be taken in the context of hypothyroidism.

Elective surgery should be postponed until the patient's thyroid status has been optimized with medications, particularly if he or she is symptomatic. While this recommendation makes sense, it is by no means clear that there is an increased risk of surgery in mild to moderate hypothyroidism(697), though the incidence of several perioperative complications (e.g., intraoperative hypotension) is increased(697). It is also not obvious that the conclusions derived from most studies, which involve adult patients, are directly applicable to children.

The postoperative hypothyroid patient is likely to have a long wake-up period, during which time special attention must be paid to prolonged respiratory depression. Hypothermia should be avoided because of its tendency to cause apnea, metabolic acidosis, bradycardia, and coagulopathy and its potentiation of neuromuscular blockade and general anesthesia(698).

ENDOCRINE THERAPY OF CATABOLIC STATES

Critically ill children are at risk for the effects of prolonged catabolism. Multiple hormones (e.g., cortisol, epinephrine) are stimulated under the stress of severe illness, leading to lipolysis, muscle catabolism, and bone resorption. In addition, the nutrition of children in the ICU, even when receiving parenteral nutrition, can be insufficient and thereby accelerate the catabolism. When recovery from the disease state would require considerable anabolism (e.g., in burns), prolonged catabolism can contribute to long hospitalizations, difficulty in weaning from ventilators, and increased mortality.

Hyperalimentation is reviewed in another chapter. Here we briefly review the physiology of growth hormone (GH) and insulin-like growth factor 1 (IGF-1) and how they have been or can be used to promote improved outcomes through increased and more timely anabolic activity.

GH is synthesized in the pituitary, mostly as a 191 amino acid peptide with two intermolecular disulfide bonds. Alternate gene splicing leads to a second GH of lower molecular weight that is produced in much smaller quantities. GH is tightly regulated by secretion of growth hormone releasing hormone and somatostatin. The former stimulates GH synthesis whereas the latter inhibits GH release. GH inhibits it own secretion. Many of GH's actions are mediated though IGF-1, which is synthesized in the liver (in several tissues, it is synthesized independently of GH) upon stimulation by GH. IGF-1 also inhibits GH production. Stress states usually stimulate GH, but in catabolic illness (in the ICU), GH is often found to be at low levels[(699)], possibly due to the suppressive effect of the high concentrations of intravenous glucose typically administered in this setting.

Other studies have found the basal levels of GH in critically ill patients to be elevated, but with decreased pulsatile activity[(700)]. Metabolic effects of GH include stimulation of protein anabolism, lipolysis, and insulin resistance. Among the complications in the use of GH in critically ill patients is development of hyperglycemia (at higher doses). This can lead to significant caloric loss, dehydration, and further catabolism. For this reason, IGF-1 is being evaluated for use in promoting wound healing and anabolism in the ICU[(701)].

IGF-1 is a 70 amino acid polypeptide whose prohormone is coded for on the long arm of chromosome 12. IGF-1 acts through a receptor that bears some shared motifs with the insulin receptor, including its tetrameric structure and tyrosine kinase activity. IGF-1 appears to stimulate hyperplasia in many tissues and to potentiate the effect of several other hormone systems; for example, it enhances the effect of ACTH on the adrenal cortex[(702)]. Unlike GH, IGF-1 has a hypoglycemic effect when administered intravenously[(703)].

Promising results with GH include findings in a study of burned children, which demonstrated improved wound healing[(704)]. It has been demonstrated that GH administration over a week can significantly reduce catabolism and spare nitrogen wasting in critical care and surgical settings[(705,706)]. The anabolic effects require concurrent intensive hyperalimentation[(707)]. Also in adults, GH treatment of patients with chronic obstructive pulmonary disease has been shown to improve nitrogen balance and pulmonary function[(708)]. However, these results should be considered preliminary, and some studies have not shown improved nitrogen balance in GH-treated patients[(709)]. Treatment of children with GH in the ICU should therefore be limited to approved clinical trials.

CARCINOID SYNDROME

Carcinoid tumors are a group of very rare, highly differentiated neuroendocrine neoplasms, which usually occur in the gut. The appendix is the most common location in children. Their presentation is usually similar to appendicitis, and appendectomy is usually curative since the malignant potential of carcinoid tumors is very low. These tumors release a variety of hormones and mediators. The most common are serotonin, histamine, and kinins (bradykinin, kallikrein).

Mediators are usually metabolized by the liver and/or lung, provided the carcinoid tumor has not metastasized (an even more rare event), thus bypassing those organs. The symptom complex that the carcinoid tumor causes (carcinoid syndrome) depends on the mediator or mediators it is producing. Serotonin is the most important one; measurement of blood levels of serotonin and urine levels of its metabolites are crucial to the diagnosis. It causes vasoconstriction, secretory diarrhea, and increased intestinal tone. Kallikrein causes vasodilation and bronchoconstriction. Histamine causes vasodilation, dysrhythmias, and bronchoconstriction. Marked lability of blood pressure is common. Hyperglycemia or hypoglycemia can occur. Right-sided heart disease due to plaque formation on the valves and myocardium is a famous complication of long-standing disease.

The principal differential diagnostic entities are mastocytosis, medullary carcinoma of the thyroid, and pheochromocytoma.

Anesthesia, Intubation, and the Perioperative Period

Since the symptoms experienced by a given patient relate to the particular mediator released by the tumor, one might expect the preoperative history to yield clues as to the problems to expect. However, a large proportion of patients in whom intraoperative bronchospasm develops have not had it before. Therefore, treatment of each patient must be adjusted to symptoms. Hemodynamic and cardiac status, intravascular volume, serum electrolytes, and nutrition (especially hyperglycemia or hypoglycemia) should be optimized. Dysrhythmias (usually supraventricular) should be treated. Octreotide can be used to stabilize the patient with bronchoconstriction[(710)] or diarrhea[(711)] or in carcinoid crisis (severe hypotension or severe hypertension with tachycardia)[(712)].

Acute management is geared toward avoidance of triggering pernicious mediators from the tumor; octreotide is very effective[(712)]. Mediator release can be induced by direct pressure on the tumor but also by palpation or even surgical preparation of the abdomen. Succinylcholine is believed to induce mediator release via abdominal-wall fasciculation, among other mechanisms. Sympathetic stimulation also triggers mediator release. The factors to avoid in this regard include hypercarbia, hypothermia, hypotension, and drugs that enhance histamine release (e.g., curare) or stimulate the sympathetic system directly (e.g., ketamine). (See the sections on hyperthyroidism and pheochromocytomas for a full discussion of avoidance of sympathetic stimulation.) Hypotension should be treated with volume expansion rather than catecholamines or sympathomimetic agents if possible. Angiotensin may also be useful in this circumstance(713).

Antagonists of serotonin (methysergide, cyproheptadine, ketanserin), kinins (corticosteroids, aprotinin), and histamine (H_1 and H_2 blockers) may be useful (although the advent of octreotide[714] may have rendered many of these drugs obsolete in the treatment of carcinoid tumors). Prophylactic use of some of these agents may also be indicated. Consultation with an endocrinologist will be helpful.

Monitoring should be matched to the clinical condition. An arterial line is extremely useful in the presence of blood pressure fluctuations or if pressors or vasodilators are to be used. A bladder catheter and central venous pressure line are commonly placed for intraoperative care. A pulmonary artery line may be helpful if there is cardiac involvement.

Another consideration is the location of the tumor. Bronchial carcinoids are the most frequently seen pulmonary neoplasm of childhood(715–717), and patients commonly present with wheezing, atelectasis, cough, fever, hemoptysis, and pneumonitis. Children with these conditions are potentially at risk for airway obstruction, reactive airways, and difficulties with positive-pressure ventilation. They commonly require bronchoscopy and biopsy for diagnosis. Treatment often involves thoracotomy and pulmonary resection, or laser resection.

It is difficult to make firm treatment recommendations for perioperative treatment. The literature on the perioperative or ICU care of this rare condition is not particularily helpful. Much of it consists of case reports or institutional experiences rather than large, well-designed studies. Furthermore, most of the published experience is in the adult population.

INBORN ERRORS OF METABOLISM

There is an amazing variety of the rare conditions that make up inborn errors of metabolism. Many of them have impressively polysyllabic scientific names (e.g., galactosylceramide lipidosis), and some have interesting but uninformative eponyms (e.g., Krabbe disease) that are not particularly helpful to the uninitiated. Many have more than one name. For example, the same entity is referred to as Batten disease, Jansky-Bielschowsky disease, and the late infantile amaurotic idiocy form of neuronal ceroid lipofuscinosis (not to be confused with the juvenile form, Spielmeyer-Sjogren disease). While acute care of patients with these illnesses is usually fairly generic (i.e., supportive), their management occasionally involves drugs that are seldom used in any other context (e.g., sodium benzoate and sodium phenylacetate). Consequently, it is usually advisable to involve an expert as soon as an inborn error of metabolism is suspected.

Most commonly, intensivists care for these patients in the context of an operative procedure (e.g., tracheostomy), intercurrent illness (e.g., aspiration pneumonia), or metabolic imbalance (e.g., hyperammonemic crisis) in a child with a known diagnosis. However, on occasion, a child comes to the ICU who is extremely sick, and only later is he or she found to have a metabolic disorder, often after a prolonged and extensive workup. Therefore, it is important for the intensivist to keep the possibility of these diseases in mind, in the correct setting (chance favors the prepared mind). In the following section, signs and symptoms that may alert the vigilant physician are reviewed, and a brief overview of the workup is given. The highlights of a number of conditions with special ICU-related considerations are provided.

Antenatal diagnosis and neonatal screening can detect many of these illnesses. Some of the more commonly screened diseases include phenylketonuria, maple syrup urine disease, galactosemia, and congenital adrenal hypoplasia. Many other tests are available (e.g., biotinidase deficiency). The particular panel used in newborns varies from state to state.

Many metabolic illnesses present early in life, often in association with the introduction of protein to the diet (e.g., urea cycle disturbances), hypoglycemia (e.g., glutaric acidemia type II), or hypotonia (e.g., Pompe disease). Other diseases present later in life, often with insidious signs, such as slowing or loss of developmental milestones or failure to thrive. Vomiting, lethargy or obtundation, a syndrome resembling Reye's syndrome, hyperventilation or apnea, seizures (especially if intractable), and muscular abnormalities are characteristic.

Physical findings may include jaundice or hepatomegaly (seen in many of these conditions), cataracts (e.g., galactosemia), macrocephaly (e.g., glutaric acidemia type I), cardiomyopathy (e.g., long chain fatty acid oxidation defects), and a list of others. The urine may have a characteristic odor (e.g., "mousey" in phenylketonuria) or color (e.g., black in alkaptonuria). The family history may provide useful information (consanguinity, previous neonatal deaths, previous child with metabolic disease).

Suggestive biochemical abnormalities **(Table 39–6)** include metabolic acidosis with an increased anion gap, hyperammonemia, ketoacidosis (from one of a number of alpha-ketoacids of abnormally metabolized amino acids), and hypoketotic hypoglycemia. Some of these presentations may be easily mistaken for sepsis in a sick infant. (Sepsis is also not uncommon in galactosemia and propionic and methylmalonic acidemia.)

The initial approach once an inborn error of metabolism

Table 39.6. Characteristic Biochemical Abnormalities of Some Inborn Errors of Metabolism

Disease	*Defect*
Urea cycle defects	Hyperammonemia, primary respiratory alkalosis
Organic acidemias	Hyperammonemia, metabolic acidosis with increased anion gap, neutropenia, thrombocytopenia
Amino acidopathies	Ketosis
Disorders of carbohydrate metabolism	Nonglucose reducing substances in urine, lactic acidosis, hypoglycemia

is suspected is to stop all enteral feeding and to start an intravenous glucose/electrolyte solution. There are a number of laboratory tests **(Table 39–7)** that are commonly used, both to evaluate the presence of an inborn error of metabolism and to rule out infection, acquired metabolic disorders (e.g., poisoning), nutritional abnormalities, and other acquired illnesses. These should be performed during the acute phase of illness, not after treatment is under way.

Eventually, the final specific laboratory test will be done (e.g., muscle biopsy, fibroblast assays). Again it is important to emphasize that the intensivist's most important goal is to suspect and then support the child with these conditions. The specifics of workup and management of the illness are best left to the experts. There are many excellent reviews of the decision trees involved in diagnosing these conditions[718].

Anesthetic Implications

This subsection provides a very general overview of the major issues pertinent to the management of some of these conditions. Given the rarity of these diseases, the recommendations are generally made on the basis of theoretical concerns and common sense rather than strong documentation from clinical studies.

Some basic considerations are of importance to the induction of anesthesia or perioperative management, and these issues are often not obvious a priori:

Table 39.7. Screening Workup for Metabolic Disorders

Blood
Arterial blood gas, ammonia, and calcium
Arterial or venous glucose, creatinine, electrolyte levels (and anion gap), blood urea nitrogen, creatinine, uric acid
Liver function tests, particularly in the presence of hyperammonemia (e.g., prothrombin time, partial thromboplastin time, aminotransferases, albumin)
Freeze sample for further analysis (e.g., amino acids, carnitine)
Complete blood cell count
Blood culture
Urine
Urinalysis (reagent strip, including reducing substances, glucose, ketones, pH)
Save an aliquot for further analysis (e.g., amino acids and organic acids, carbohydrates, orotic acid, glycosaminoglycans)
Urine culture
Cerebrospinal fluid
If obtained, hold an aliquot in the freezer for further testing (e.g., amino acids, lactate, pyruvate)

1. Significant metabolic abnormalities (e.g., hypoglycemia, hyperammonemia)
2. Airway abnormalities (e.g., macroglossia in some glycogen storage diseases, "gargoylism" in the mucopolysaccharidoses) or other issues that make safe intubation difficult (e.g., cervical spine laxity in Morquio disease)
3. Organ dysfunction (e.g., cardiac problems in Pompe disease, seizures in maple syrup urine disease)
4. Special disease-specific problems (e.g., drugs to avoid in acute intermittent porphyria; conditions requiring avoidance of succinylcholine)

These problems should be optimized prior to induction. If the airway is problematic, availability of special equipment should be considered (e.g., fiberoptic bronchoscope, Bullard laryngoscope, laryngeal mask airway). Intubation in the operating room with a surgeon on hand to perform a tracheostomy if necessary may also be prudent.

General principles of anesthesia should be applied to each problem. For example, if a syndrome involves severe cardiac dysfunction, invasive monitoring may be helpful and other drugs rather than thiopental for intubation may be considered. In a syndrome featuring muscle weakness, muscle relaxants should be used sparingly. If abdominal distention is prominent (e.g., severe hepatomegaly), if the patient is prone to vomiting, or if the mental status is altered, airway protection should receive special consideration. Potentially epileptogenic drugs (e.g., methohexital, ketamine) should be avoided in conditions predisposing to seizures.

Clearly, reviewing the details of the patient's disease from an appropriate reference is a good idea if there is time to do so; this practice will assist in minimizing or avoiding unpleasant surprises.

Glycogen Storage Disease I (von Gierke)[719,720]

Metabolic error: glucose-6-phosphatase deficiency.

Clinical characteristics: massive hepatomegaly, severe lactic acidosis and hypoglycemia, short stature, bleeding diathesis, hyperuricemia, and some patients have a Fanconi-like nephropathy.

Comments: patients should be treated as if they had a "full stomach" because of hepatomegaly. A glucose-containing infusion should be maintained, and serum glucose and pH should be monitored. A bleeding time should be obtained if surgery is anticipated (coagulation studies are generally normal, even in the presence of increased bruising and epistaxis).

Glycogen Storage Disease II (Pompe)[721,722]

Metabolic error: alpha glucosidase deficiency; there are infantile, juvenile, and adult forms.

Clinical characteristics: hypotonia, muscle weakness, macroglossia, cardiomyopathy, recurrent pneumonia, and hepatomegaly.

Comments: cardiac function can be poor. Typically, there is left-axis deviation on the ECG, along with a short P-R interval and inverted T-waves. Cardiac arrest and ventricular fibrillation have been reported following induction of anesthesia. A thorough cardiac evaluation is indicated. Drugs with minimal cardiac depressant effects (e.g., etomidate) may be best.

Macroglossia may make intubation difficult. In addition, muscular weakness predisposes the patient to atelectasis and mucous plugging.

Succinylcholine may be contraindicated.

Galactosemia[723]

Metabolic error: galactose-1-phosphate uridyl transferase deficiency.

Clinical characteristics: failure to thrive, vomiting, dehydration, hypoglycemia, jaundice and hepatomegaly, cirrhosis, coagulopathy, and predisposition to gram-negative sepsis in the newborn period.

Comments: management of fluids, electrolytes, and glucose are the principal acute concerns. Lactose is to be avoided. Metabolic abnormalities and other perturbations (e.g., coagulopathy) correct relatively quickly once lactose is withdrawn from the diet.

Phenylketonuria[724]

Metabolic error: phenylalanine hydroxylase deficiency.

Clinical characteristics: mental retardation, seizures, hypopigmentation, mousey odor, eczema.

Comments: no specific issues aside from the need for a phenylalanine-free diet. Aspartame, which is in many oral medications, is also to be avoided.

Homocystinuria[725]

Metabolic error: cystathionine beta-synthase deficiency.

Clinical characteristics: optic lens dislocation, mental retardation, seizures, arterial and venous thrombi and thromboemboli, osteoporosis, and other skeletal abnormalities.

Comments: thromboses, which are due to increased platelet adhesiveness (from activation of clotting factor XII by homocystine), and perhaps abnormal vasculature can occur in any vascular bed and are usually the cause of death. Preoperative evaluation of the CNS (detailed neurologic examination), heart (ECG), and possibly other organs is warranted. Conditions predisposing to thrombosis should be avoided (dehydration, vascular stasis, hypothermia, prolonged dependent position of any body part). Wrapping the legs with bandages or using pressurized boots may reduce the incidence of thrombosis. A low-molecular-weight plasma expander may be helpful.

Maple Syrup Urine Disease[724,726]

Metabolic error: defective branched chain ketoacid dehydrogenase, leading to accumulation of those amino acids and their alpha-keto acids.

Clinical characteristics: mental retardation, seizures, metabolic acidosis, liver failure, thromboembolism.

Comments: management of glucose and pH is most important.

Mucopolysaccharidosis Type I (Hurler's syndrome)[727–731]

Metabolic error: alpha-L-iduronidase deficiency. A type of lysosomal enzyme disorder.

Clinical characteristics: short stature, coarse facies, macroglossia, abnormal teeth, short thick neck, deposition of mucopolysaccharide in the larynx and trachea leading to airway narrowing, meningeal thickening leading to hydrocephalus, corneal clouding, mental retardation, contractures with decreased joint mobility, restrictive lung disease, pulmonary infections, abdominal hernias, cardiomyopathy, coronary artery disease, and valvular heart disease. Cardiac manifestations are commonly the cause of death.

Comments: presents challenges in a variety of organ systems. The airways in these children are notoriously difficult to intubate. Pulmonary and cardiac reserve is often very limited. Congestive heart failure and pulmonary hypertension may be present.

Other Mucopolysaccharidoses[727,729,731–734]

Comments: the spectrum of problems is similar to what is seen in Hurler's syndrome, although they are usually less extensive and less severe. Atlantoaxial instability due to odontoid hypoplasia is seen in types IV (Morquio), VI (Maroteaux-Lamy), and VII (Sly). Fiberoptic or lighted-stylet intubation may be advisable in order to avoid causing neurologic damage. Many of these diseases have their own important characteristics (e.g., aortic valve involvement in Morquio and Sly diseases).

Urea Cycle Disturbances[735–737]

Metabolic error: ornithine transcarbamylase deficiency, carbamyl phosphate synthetase deficiency, and others.

Clinical characteristics: lethargy, hypotonia, vomiting, coma (possibly requiring ventilatory support), seizures, hyperammonemia, increased glutamine and alanine, and increased orotic aciduria (except in carbamyl phosphate synthetase deficiency). The hyperammonemia may be associated with severe cerebral edema and hyperventilation.

Comments: severity of symptoms correlates with the degree of hyperammonemia. Consequently, the disease is exacerbated by an intercurrent illness or large protein load (feeding, GI bleeding). Treatment is geared toward improving nitrogen elimination, whether by drug administration (sodium benzoate, sodium phenylacetate, L-arginine) or by dialysis. Nitrogen-free parenteral nutrition (e.g., 20% dextrose) reduces plasma nitrogen by helping to reduce protein catabolism.

Gaucher Disease (glucocerebrosidosis, glucosylceramide lipidosis)

Metabolic error: glucocerebrosidase deficiency; a type of sphingolipidosis, which is a subtype of lysosomal enzyme disorder.

Clinical characteristics: type I, the most common, does not affect the nervous system. Involvement of the reticuloendothelial system causes hepatosplenomegaly and pancytopenia. Bony degeneration is common and can lead to pathologic fractures (particularly of the vertebrae), aseptic necrosis of the femoral head, and bone pain. Pulmonary disease may be present.

Type II is neurovisceral with a rapid, devastating onset. It has the classic triad of trismus, strabismus, and retroflexion of the head. Patients have difficulty handling secretions and have recurrent aspirations. Hepatosplenomegaly is prominent. These patients may have spasticity and seizures.

Type III incorporates features of Types I and II but is slower in onset.

Comments: hematologic abnormalities should be addressed, although not necessarily treated, prior to surgery. The potential for or presence of fractures may make patient positioning difficult. The trismus and retroflexed head position can make intubation difficult. Patients may be at increased risk for aspiration due to poor airway reflexes.

Lesch-Nyhan Syndrome[738]

Metabolic error: hypoxanthine-guanine phosphoribosyl transferase deficiency (a disorder of purine metabolism).

Clinical characteristics: hyperreflexia, dystonia, chorea, athetosis, seizures, self-mutilation, aggresive behavior, subcutaneous uric acid tophi, renal calculi, nephropathy, regurgitation, vomiting, and an increased serum uric acid level.

Comments: sedation may be crucial in a child with this condition. Benzodiazepines are a good selection, although in some circumstances intramuscular ketamine (for the uncontrollable child) or rectal barbiturates (preoperatively) may be better (despite their epileptogenic potential). Use of measures to mitigate the probability of aspiration (antacids, H_2 blockers, "rapid sequence induction") may be advisable. Intubation may be rendered difficult if the child's pica has caused perioral scarring. Drugs that are cleared through the kidneys should be used with caution. Succinylcholine is perhaps best avoided in this spastic skeletal muscle disorder.

There may be increased sensitivity to narcotics, and the sympathetic response to stress and exogenous catecholamines may be abnormal.

Porphyrias[739–743]

Metabolic error: a variety of defects in porphyrin synthesis. There are two main types, hepatic and erythropoietic, depending on where the defect is principally expressed.

Clinical characteristics (of acute intermittent porphyria): abdominal pain, seizures, SIADH, psychosis, cranial nerve paresis, autonomic dysfunction, peripheral neuropathy, and hypoventilation (from intercostal and phrenic nerve involvement).

Comments: the erythropoeitic forms are mainly expressed in childhood and the hepatic types from adolescence onward. The main point of importance for our purposes is that some drugs are known to trigger acute intermittent porphyria. These include barbiturates, ethanol, dilantin, diazepam, local anesthetics, pentazocine, corticosteroids, imipramine, and tolbutamide. These drugs are also hazardous in variegate porphyria and hereditary coproporphyria.

References

1. Brown-Sequard C. Recherches experimentales sur la physiologie et la pathologie des capsules surrenales. Arch Gen Med 1856;5:385.
2. Falaschi P, Martocchia A, Proietti A, et al. Immune system and the hypothalamus-pituitary-adrenal axis: common words for a single language. Ann NY Acade Sci 1994;741.
3. Hua SY, Chen YZ. Membrane receptor-mediated electrophysiological effects of glucorticoid on mammalian neurons. Endocrinol 1989; 124:687.
4. Levine A, Cohen D, Zadik Z. Urinary free cortisol values in children under stress. J Pediatr 1994;125:853.
5. Fava GA. Affective disorders and endocrine disease: new insights from psychosomatic studies. Psychosomatics 1994;35:341.
6. Udelsman R, Holbrook NJ. Endocrine and molecular responses to surgical stress. Curr Probl Surg 1994;31:653.
7. Yeh FC, Chang CL. Acute neuroendocrine and metabolic stress responses of anesthesia and surgery. Ma Tsui Hsueh Tsa Chi Anaesthesiologica Sinica 1992;30:125.
8. Muglia L, Jacobson L, Dikkes P, Majzoub J. Corticotropin-releasing hormone deficiency reveals major fetal but not adult glucocorticoid need. Nature 1995;373:427.
9. Spath-Schwalbe E, Born J, Schrezenmeier H, et al. Interleukin-6 stimulates the hypothalamus-pituitary-adrenocortical axis in man. J Clini Endocrinol Metab 1994;79:1212.
10. van den Brink HR, van Wijk MJ, Geertzen RG, et al. Influence of corticosteroid pulse therapy on the serum levels of soluble interleukin 2 receptor, interleukin 6 and interleukin 8 in patients with rheumatoid arthritis. J Rheumatol 1994;21:430.
11. Arzt E, Sauer J, Pollmacher T, et al. Glucocorticoids suppress interleukin-1 receptor antagonist synthesis following induction by endotoxin. Endocrinol 1994;134:672.
12. Burnay M, Python C, Vallotton M, et al. Role of the capacitative calcium influx in the activation of steroidogenesis by angiotensin-II in adrenal glomerulosa cells. Endocrinol 1994;135:751.
13. Savu L, Zouaghi H, Carli A, Nunez E. Serum depletion of corticosteroid binding activities, an early marker of human septic shock. Biochem Biophys Res Commun 1981;102:411.
14. Zouaghi H, Savu L, Delorme J, et al. Loss of serum transcortin in human shock associated with severe infection by Candida albicans. Acta Endocrinol 1983;102:277.
15. Ballard P, Ballard R. Cytoplasmic receptor for glucocorticoids in lung of the human fetus and neonate. J Clin Invest 1974;53:477.
16. Genuth S. The endocrine system. In: Berne RML, ed. Physiology. St Louis:CV Mosby, 1983:893.
17. Tyrell J, Aron D, Forsham P. Glucocorticoids & adrenal androgens. In: Greenspan F, ed. Basic and clinical endocrinology. Norwalk, CT: Appleton & Lange, 1991:323.
18. Raff H. Glucocorticoid inhibition of neurohypophysial vasopressin secretion. Am J Physiol 1987;21:R635.
19. Schmidt T, Diehl E. The in vitro activation of rat cardiac glucocorticoid antagonist- versus agonist-receptor complexes. Biochim Biophys Acta 1988;970:212.
20. Lucas C, Ledgerwood M. The cardiopulmonary response to massive doses of steroids in patients with septic shock. Arch Surg 1984;119:537.
21. Sprung C, Caralis P, Marcial E, et al. The effects of high-dose corticoids in patients with septic shock: a prospective controlled study. N Engl J Med 1984;311:1137.
22. Bone R, Fisher CJ, Clemmer T, et al. A controlled trial of high-dose methylprednisolone in the treatment of severe sepsis and septic shock. N Engl J Med 1987;317:653.
23. Veterans Administration Systemic Sepsis Cooperative Study G: effect of high-dose glucocorticoid therapy in patients with clinical signs of systemic sepsis. N Engl J Med 1987;317:659.
24. Fritz I, Levine R. Action of adrenal cortical steroids and norepinephrine on vascular responses of stress in adrenalectomized rats. Am J Physiol 1951;165:456.
25. Ramey E, Goldstein M, Levine R. Action of norepinephrine and adre-

nal cortical steroids on blood pressure and work performance of adrenalectomized dogs. Am J Physiol 1951;165:450.
26. Kong M, Jeffcoate W. Eighty-six cases of Addison's disease. Clin Endocrinol 1994;41:757.
27. Herman A, Mack E, Egdahl R. The relationship of adrenal perfusion to corticosteroid secretion in prolonged hemorrhagic shock. Surg Gynecol Obstet 1971;132:795.
28. Breslow M, Mennen A, Koehler R, et al. Adrenal medullary and cortical blood flow during hemorrhage. Am J Physiol 1986;250.
29. Nishijima M, Breslow M, Raff H, et al. Regional adrenal blood flow during hypoxia in anesthetized, ventilated dogs. Am J Physiol 1989;256.
30. New M, Speiser P. Genetics of adrenal steroid 21-hydroxylase deficiency. Endocrine Revi 1986;7:331.
31. Allen DB. Newborn screening for congenital adrenal hyperplasia in Wisconsin. Wisconsin Med J 1993;92:75.
32. Esteban N, Loughlin T, Yergey A, et al. Daily cortisol production rate in man determined by stable isotope dilution/mass spectrometry. J Clin Endocrinol Metabolism 1991;72:39.
33. Petersen DD, Magnuson MA, Granner DK. Location and characterization of two widely separated glucocorticoid response elements in the phosphoenolpyruvate carboxykinase gene. Molec Cell Biol 1988;8:96.
34. Danowski TS, Bonessi JV, Sabeh G, et al. Probablities of pituitary-adrenal responsiveness after steroid therapy. Ann Intern Med 1964;61:11.
35. Kendall J, Egans M, Stott A, et al. The importance of stimulus intensity and duration of steroid administration in suppression of stress-induced ACTH secretion. Endocrinol 1972;90:525.
36. Christy N. HPA failure and glucocorticoid therapy. Hosp Pract 1984;77:77.
37. Globerman H, Rosler A, Theodor R, et al. An inherited defect in aldosterone biosynthesis caused by a mutation in or near the gene for steroid 11-hydroxylase. N Engl J Medicine 1988;319:1193.
38. Kuhnle U, Guariso G, Sonega M, et al. Transient pseudohypoaldosteronism in obstructive renal disease with transient reduction of lymphocytic aldosterone receptors: results in two affected infants. Hormone Res 1993;39:152.
39. Burgos CE, Cid JL-H, Juaniz IS, et al. Salt-losing tubulopathy secondary to urinary infection: a form of transitory pseudohypoaldosteronism. Anales Espanoles de Pediatria 1989;30:404.
40. Arai K, Tsigos C, Suzuki Y, et al. No apparent mineralocorticoid receptor defect in a series of sporadic cases of pseudohypoaldosteronism. J Clin Endocrinol Metab 1995;80:814.
41. Rosler A. The natural history of salt-wasting disorders of adrenal and renal origin. J Clin Endocrinol Metab 1984;59:689.
42. Tuck ML, Sambhi MP, Levin L. Hyporeninemic hypoaldosteronism in diabetes mellitus: studies of the autonomic nervous system's control of renin release. Diabetes 1979;28:237.
43. Fragen RJ, Shanks CA, Molteni A, et al. Effects of etomidate on hormonal response to surgical stress. Anesthesiol 1984;61:652.
44. Wagner RL, White PF. Etomidate inhibits adrenocortical function in surgical patients. Anesthesiol 1984;61:647.
45. Fragen RJ, Weiss HW, Molteni A. The effect of propofol on adrenocortical steroidogenesis: a comparative study with etomidate and thiopental. Anesthesiol 1987;66:839.
46. Crozier TA, Beck D, Schlaeger M, et al. Endocrinological changes following etomidate, midazolam or methohexital for minor surgery. Anesthesiol 1987;66:628.
47. Robertson WR, Reader SC, Davidson B, et al. On the biopotency and site of action of drugs affecting endocrine tissues with specific reference to the antisteroidogenic effect of anesthetic agents. Postgrad Med J 1985;61:145.
48. Mindermann T, Wilson CB. Pediatric pituitary adenomas. Neurosurg 1995;36:259.
49. Ross NS. Epidemiology of Cushing's syndrome and subclinical disease. Endocrinolo Metabo Clin North Am 1994;23:539.
50. Wong KC, Schafer PG, Schultz JR. Hypokalemia and anesthetic implications. Anesthes Analges 1993;77:1238.
51. Hill GE, Wong KC, Shaw CL, et al. Acute and chronic changes in intra- and extracellular potassium and responses to neuromuscular blocking agents. Anesthes Analges 1978;57:417.
52. Miller RD, Roderick LL. Diuretic-induced hypokalemia, pancuronium neuromuscular blockade and its antagonism by neostigmine. Brit J Anaesthes 1978;50:541.
53. Haynes RJ, Murad F. Adrenocorticotropic hormone; adrenocortical steroids and their synthetic analogs; inhibitors of adrenocortical steroid biosynthesis. In: Gilman A, Goodman L, Rall T, et al, eds. The pharmacologic basis of therapeutics. New York: Macmillan, 1985:1459.
54. Meikle A, Tyler F. Potency and duration of action of glucocorticoids. Am J Med 1977;63:200.
55. Berorem H. The influence of uremia on pharmacokinetics and protein binding of prednisolone. Acta Med Scand 1983;213:333.
56. O'Neill J. Renovascular hypertension. Sem Pediatr Surg 1994;3:114.
57. Haab F, Duclos J, Guyenne T, et al. Renin secreting tumors: diagnosis, conservative surgical approach and long-term results. J Urol 1995;153:1781.
58. Biglieri EG, Herron MA, Brust N. 17-alpha hydroxylase deficiency in men. J Clin Invest 1966;45:1946.
59. Yanase T, Simpson E, Waterman MR. 17-alpha hydroxylase/17-20 lyase deficiency: from clinical investigation to molecular definition. Endocr Rev 1991;12:91.
60. Zachmann M, Tassinari D, Prader A. Clinical and biochemical variability of congenital adrenal hyperplasia due to 11 beta-hydroxylase deficiency: a study of 25 patients. J Clin Endocrinol Met 1983; 56:222.
61. Mornet E, Dupont J, Vitek A, et al. Characterization of two genes encoding human steroid 11-beta-hydroxylase (p450 11B). J Biol Chem 1989;264:961.
62. White PC, Dupont J, New MI, et al. A mutation in CYP11B1 (Arg-448 ≥ His) associated with steroid 11 beta-hydroxylase deficiency in Jews of Moroccan origin. J Clin Invest 1991;87:1664.
63. Lifton RP, Dluhy RG, Powers M, et al. A chimeric 11beta-hydroxylase/aldosterone synthase gene causes glucocorticoid-remediable aldosteronism and human hypertension. Nature 1992;355:262.
64. Pascoe L, Curnow K, Slutsker L, et al. Glucocorticoid-suppressible hyperaldosteronism results from hybrid genes created by unequal crossover between CYP 11B1 and CYP 11B2. Proc Natl Acad Sci USA 1992;89:8327.
65. Ulick S, Ramirez L, New M. An abnormality in reductive metabolism in a hypertensive syndrome. J Clin Endocrinol Metabolism 1977; 44:799.
66. Funder J, Pearce P, Smith R, et al. Mineralocorticoid action: target-tissue specificity is enzyme not receptor mediated. Science 1988;242:583.
67. Wilson R, Harbison M, Krozowski Z, et al. Several homozygous mutations in the gene for 11-beta-hydroxysteroid dehydrogenase type 2 in patients with Apparent Mineralocorticoid Excess. J Clin Endocrinol Metab 1995 (in press)
68. Mune T, Rogerson F, Nikkila H, et al. Human hypertension caused by mutations in the kidney isozyme of 11-beta-hydroxysteroid dehydrogenase. Nature Genet 1995;10:394.
69. Thomas CG Jr, Smith AT, Griffith JM, et al. Hyperadrenalism in childhood and adolescence. Ann Surg 1984;199:538.
70. Morales L, Rovira J, Rottermann M, et al. Adrenocortical tumors in childhood: a report of four cases. J Pediatri Surg 1989;24:276.
71. Cibas ES, Medeiros LJ, Weinberg DS, et al. Cellular DNA profiles of benign and malignant adrenocortical tumors. Am J Surg Pathol 1990;14:948.
72. Perry RR, Nieman LK, Cutler GB Jr, et al. Primary adrenal causes of Cushing's syndrome: diagnosis and surgical management. Ann Surg 1989;210:59.
73. Grant FD, Mandel SJ, Brown EM, et al. Interrelationship betwwen the renin angiotensin-aldosterone and calcium homeostatic systems. J Clin Endocrinol Metab 1992;75:988.
74. Ezzat S, Forster M, Berchtold P, et al. Acromegaly: clinical and biochemical features in 500 patients. Medicine 1994;73:233.
75. Saito I, Saruta T. Hypertension in thyroid disorders. Endocrinol Metabolism Clini North Am 1994;23:379.
76. Caty M, Coran A, Geagen M, et al. Current diagnosis and treatment of pheochromocytoma in children: experience with 22 consecutive tumors in 14 patients. Arch Surg 1990;125:978.
77. Ram C. Pheochromocytoma. Cardiol Clin 1988;6:517.
78. Raue F, Frank-Raue K, Grauer A. Multiple endocrine neoplasia Type 2. Endocrinol Metab Clin North Am 1994;23:137.
79. Chew SL, Lavender P, Jain A, et al. Absence of mutations in the MEN2A region of the ret proto-oncogene in non-MEN 2A phaeochromocytomas. Clini Endocrinol 1995;42:17.
80. Beldjord C, Desclaux-Arramond F, Raffin-Sanson M, et al. The RET protooncogene in sporadic pheochromocytomas: frequent MEN 2-like mutations and new molecular defects. J Clin Endocrinol Metab 1995;80:2063.
81. Bravo EL. Evolving concepts in the pathophysiology, diagnosis, and treatment of pheochromocytoma. Endocr Rev 1993;15:356.
82. Lefkowitz R, Caron M, Stiles G. Adrenergic receptors. N Engl J Med 1984;310:1570.

83. Adams JE, Johnson RJ, Rickards D, et al. Computed tomography in adrenal disease. Clin Radiol 1983;34:39.
84. Atuk N. Pheochromocytoma: diagnosis, localization, and treatment. Hosp Pract 1983;187:187.
85. Bravo E, Gifford R. Pheochromocytoma: diagnosis, localization and management. N Engl J Med 1984;311:1298.
86. Falke T, te Strake L, Shaff M, et al. MR imaging of the adrenals: correlation with computed tomography. J Comput Assist Tomogr 1986;10:242.
87. Shapiro B, Fig L, Gross M, et al. Radiochemical diagnosis of adrenal disease. Crit Rev Clin Lab Sci 1989;27:265.
88. Voorhess M. Disorders of the adrenal medulla; multiple endocrine adenomatosis syndromes. In: Kaplan S, ed. Clinical pediatric and adolescent endocrinology. Philadelphia: WB Saunders, 1982:207.
89. Allison D, Brown M, Jones D, et al. Role of venous sampling in locating a phaeochromocytoma. Br Med J 1983;286:1122.
90. Reed G, Devous M. Cerebral blood flow autoregulation and hypertension. Am J Med Sci 1985;289:37.
91. Vorstrup S, Barry D, Jarden J, et al. Chronic antihypertensive treatment in the rat reverses hypertension-induced changes in cerebral blood flow autoregulation. Stroke 1984;15:312.
92. Fujishima M, Sadoshima S, Ogata J, et al. Autoregulation of cerebral blood flow in young and aged spontaneously hypertensive rats (SHR). Gerontology 1984;30:30.
93. Barry D, Strandgaard S, Graham D, et al. Cerebral blood flow in rats with renal and spontaneous hypertension: resetting of the lower limit of autoregulation. J Cereb Blood Flow Metab 1982;2:347.
94. Barry D, Strandgaard S, Graham D, et al. Effect of diazoxide-induced hypotension in cerebral blood flow in hypertensive rats. Eur J Clin Invest 1983;13:201.
95. Barry D, Strandgaard S, Graham D, et al. Cerebral blood flow during dihydralazine-induced hypotension in hypertensive rats. Stroke 1984;15:102.
96. Gifford RWJ. Effect of reducing elevated blood pressure on cerebral circulation. Hypertension 1983;5:17.
97. Hoffman W, Miletich D, Albrecht R. The influence of antihypertensive therapy on cerebral autoregulation in aged hypertensive rats. Stroke 1982;13:701.
98. Pinaud M, Desjars P, Tasseau F, et al. Preoperative acute volume loading in patients with pheochromocytoma. Crit Care Med 1985;13:460.
99. Manger WM, Gifford RW Jr. Pheochromocytoma: current diagnosis and management. Cleveland Clin J Medicine 1993;60:365.
100. Sjoberg RJ, Simcic KJ, Kidd GS. The clonidine suppression test for pheochromocytoma: a review of its utility and pitfalls. Arch Intern Med 1992;152:1193.
101. Teply JF, Lawrence GH. Pheochromocytoma. Am J Surg 1980;140:107.
102. Nicholas E, Deutschman C, Allo M, et al. Use of esmolol in the intraoperative management of phaeochromocytoma. Anesth Analg 1988; 67:1114.
103. Turner MC, Lieberman E, DeQuattro V. The perioperative management of pheochromocytoma in children. Clin Pediatr 1992;31:583.
104. Mihm FG. Pulmonary artery pressure monitoring in patients with pheochromocytoma. Anesthes Analges 1983;62:1129.
105. Hamaji M, Oka N, Tashiro C. Anaesthetic management with morphine in phaeochromocytoma. Can Anaesthes Soc J 1984;31:681.
106. Reitan JA, Stengert KB, Wymore MC, et al. Central vagal control of fentanyl induced bradycardia during halothane anesthesia. Anesthes Analges 1978;75:31.
107. Laubie M, Schmit H, Vincent M. Vagal bradycardia produced by microinjection of morphine-like drugs into the nucleus ambiguus in anesthetized dogs. Europ J Pharmacol 1979;59:287.
108. Hull CJ. Phaeochromocytoma: diagnosis, preoperative preparation and anesthetic management. Brit J Anaesthes 1986;58.
109. Vuksanaj D, Fisher DM. Pharmacokinetics of rocuronium in children aged 4–11 years. Anesthesiol 1995;82:1104.
110. O'Kelly B, Fiset P, Meistelman C, et al. Pharmacokinetics of rocuronium in paediatric patients. Europ J Anesthesiology (Suppl) 1994;9:57.
111. Tryba M, Zorn A, Thole H, et al. Rapid-sequence orotracheal intubation with rocuronium: a randomized double-blind comparison with suxamethonium-preliminary communication. Eur J Anesthesiol (Suppl) 1994;9:44.
112. Magorian T, Flannery KB, Miller RD. Comparison of rocuronium, succinylcholine, and vecuronium for rapid-sequence induction of anesthesia in adult patients. Anesthesiol 1993;79:913.
113. Huizinga AC, Vandenbrom RH, Wierda JM, et al. Intubating conditions and onset of neuromuscular block of rocuronium (ORG 9426): a comparison with suxamethonium. Acta Anaesthesiol Scand 1992;36:463.
114. Couzigou P, Richard-Molard B, Fleury B, et al. Chronic vomiting disclosing pheochromocytoma. Gastroenterologie Clinique et Biologique 1984;8:88.
115. Montiel C, Artalejo AR, Bermejo PM, et al. A dopaminergic receptor in adrenal medulla as a possible site of action for the droperidol-evoked hypertensive response. Anesthesiol 1986;65:474.
116. Oh TE, Turner CW, Ilett KF, et al. Mechanism of the hypertensive effect of droperidol in pheochromocytoma. Anaesthes Intens Care 1978;6:322.
117. Ponte CD, Nappi JM. Review of a new gastrointestinal drug-metoclopramide. Ame J Hosp Pharm 1981;38:829.
118. Oishi S, Shimada T, Sato T. Case of intrathoracic pheochromocytoma occuring 9 years after resection of intraabdominal paraaortic pheochromocytoma: effect of metoclopramide and sulpiride on catecholamine secretion in vitro. Folia Endocrinologica Japonica 1983;59:1608.
119. Hsu TS, Lee CP, Kuo CT. Diagnostic use of metoclopramide in hypertension caused by pheochromocytoma. Internat J Cardiol 1993;42:79.
120. Ellis EN. Concepts of fluid therapy in diabetic ketoacidosis and hyperosmolar hyperglycemic nonketotic coma. Pediatr Clin North Am 1990;37:313.
121. Hanley RM. 'Diabetic' emergencies: they happen with or without diabetes. Postgrad Med 1990;88:90.
122. Israel RS. Diabetic ketoacidosis. Emerg Med Clin North Am 1989;7:859.
123. Reitano G. Diabetic ketoacidosis in children. J Endocrinol Invest 1989;12:105.
124. Sanson TH, Levine SN. Management of diabetic ketoacidosis. Drugs 1989;38:289.
125. Bonadio WA, Gutzeit MF, Losek JD, et al. Outpatient management of diabetic ketoacidosis. Am J Dis Child 1988;142:448.
126. Chapman J, Wright AD, Nattrass M, et al. Recurrent diabetic ketoacidosis. Diabetic Med 1988;5:659.
127. Kitabchi AE, Murphy MB. Diabetic ketoacidosis and hyperosmolar hyperglycemic nonketotic coma. Med Clin North Am 1988;72:1545.
128. Krane EJ. Diabetic ketoacidosis: biochemistry, physiology, treatment, and prevention. Pediatr Clin North Am 1987;34:935.
129. Kreisberg RA. Diabetic ketoacidosis: an update. Crit Care Clin 1987;3:817.
130. Sperling M. Diabetic ketoacidosis. Pediatr Clin North Am 1984;31:591.
131. Fulop M. The treatment of severely uncontrolled diabetes mellitus. Adv Intern Med 1984;29:327.
132. Barrett E, DeFronzo R. Diabetic ketoacidosis: diagnosis and treatment. Hosp Pract 1984;89:89.
133. Yri-Jarvinen H. Diabetic ketoacidosis [Editorial]. N Engl J Med 1984;310:199.
134. Schade D, Eaton R. Diabetic ketoacidosis-pathogenesis, prevention and therapy. Clin Endocrinol Metab 1983;12:321.
135. Kandel G, Aberman A. Selected developments in the understanding of diabetic ketoacidosis. Can Med Assoc J 1983;128:392.
136. Hillman K. Resuscitation in diabetic ketoacidosis. Crit Care Med 1983;11:53.
137. Kreisberg R. Diabetic ketoacidosis: new concepts and trends in pathogenesis and treatment. Ann Intern Med 1978;88:681.
138. Drash A. The treatment of diabetic ketoacidosis. J Pediatr 1977;91:858.
139. Felig P. Diabetic ketoacidosis. N Engl J Med 1974;250:1360.
140. Beigelman P. Severe diabetic ketoacidosis (diabetic "coma"): 482 episodes in 257 patients. Experience of three years. Diabetes 1971;20:490.
141. Lee HK, Oh YS, Chung YH, et al. Epidemiological characteristics of ketoacidosis among Korean diabetic patients. J Korean Med Sci 1987;2:7.
142. Snorgaard O, Eskildsen PC, Vadstrup S, et al. Diabetic ketoacidosis in Denmark: epidemiology, incidence rates, precipitating factors and mortality rates. J Intern Med 1989;226:223.
143. Drash A. The epidemiology of diabetes mellitus in children and adolescents. Pediatr Ann 1983;12:629.
144. Johnson D, Palumbo P, Chu C. Diabetic ketoacidosis in a community-based population. Mayo Clin Proc 1980;55:83.
145. Faich G, Fishbein H, Ellis S. The epidemiology of diabetic acidosis: a population-based study. Am J Epidemiol 1983;117:551.
146. Holman R, Herron C, Sinnock P. Epidemiologic characteristics of mortality from diabetes with acidosis or coma, United States, 1970. Am J Public Health 1983;73:1169.
147. Keller U, Lustenberger M, Stauffacher W. Effect of insulin on ketone

body clearance studied by a ketone body "clamp" technique in normal man. Diabetologia 1988;31:24.
148. Karam J, Salber P, Forsham P. Pancreatic hormones & diabetes mellitus. In: Greenspan F, ed. Basic and clinical endocrinology. Norwalk, CT: Appleton & Lange, 1991:592.
149. Ehrlich R. Diabetes mellitus in childhood. Clin Endocrinol Metab 1982;11:195.
150. Sperling M. Diabetes mellitus. In: Kaplan SA, ed. Clinical pediatric and adolescent endocrinology. Philadelphia: WB Saunders, 1982:131.
151. Cahill G. Physiology of insulin in man. Diabetes 1971;20:785.
152. Foster D, McGarry J. The metabolic derangements and treatment of diabetic ketoacidosis. N Engl J Med 1983;309:159.
153. Miles J, Gerich J. Glucose and ketone body kinetics in diabetic ketoacidosis. Clin Endocrinol Metab 1983;12:303.
154. Miltenyi M, Szabo A, Tulassay T, et al. Reduced glomerular filtration and elevated urinary protein excretion in diabetic ketoacidosis. Acta Paediatr Scand 1990;79:444.
155. Kraegen E, Sowden J, Halstead M, et al. Glucose transporters and in vivo glucose uptake in skeletal and cardiac muscle: fasting, insulin stimulation and immunoisolation studies of GLUT1 and GLUT4. Biochem J 1993;295:287.
156. Katz EB, Stenblt AE, Hatton K, et al. Cardiac and adipose tissue abnormalities but not diabetes in mice deficient in GLUT4. Nature 1995;377:151.
157. Cryer P. Glucose counterregulation in man (Review). Diabetes 1981;30:261.
158. Unger R, Raskin P, Srikant C, et al. Glucagon and the A cells. Recent Prog Horm Res 1976;33:477.
159. Kawai K, Ohmori H, Okuda Y, et al. Effects of 3-hydroxybutyrate and hyperosmolarity on glucagon release from isolated perfused canine pancreas. Endocrinol Jpn 1989;36:501.
160. MacGillivray M, Bruck E, Voorhees M. Acute diabetic ketoacidosis in children: role of the stress hormones. Pediatr Res 1981;15:99.
161. Malchoff C, Pohl S, Kaiser D, et al. Determinants of glucose and ketoacid concentrations in acutely hyperglycemic diabetic patients. Am J Med 1984;77:275.
162. McGarry J, Foster D. Hormonal control of ketogenesis; biochemical considerations. Arch Intern Med 1977;137:495.
163. Gerich J, Lorenzi M, Bier D. Prevention of human diabetic ketoacidosis by somatostatin: evidence for an essential role of glucagon. N Engl J Med 1975;292:985.
164. Schade D, Eaton R. The controversy concerning counterregulatory hormone secretion: a hypothesis for the prevention of diabetic ketoacidosis? Diabetes 1977;26:596.
165. Charlton JA, Thompson CJ, Baylis PH. Possible mechanisms responsible for the rise in plasma vasopressin associated with diabetic ketoacidosis in the rat. J Endocrinol 1988;116:343.
166. Durr JA, Hoffman WH, Hensen J, et al. Osmoregulation of vasopressin in diabetic ketoacidosis. Am J Physiol 1990;259.
167. Ishikawa S, Saito T, Okada K,et al. Prompt recovery of plasma arginine vasopressin in diabetic coma after intravenous infusion of a small dose of insulin and a large amount of fluid. Acta Endocrinol 1990;122:455.
168. Tulassay T, Rascher W, Korner A, et al. Atrial natriuretic peptide and other vasoactive hormones during treatment of severe diabetic ketoacidosis in children. J Pediatr 1987;111:329.
169. Duck SC, Wyatt DT. Factors associated with brain herniation in the treatment of diabetic ketoacidosis. J Pediatr 1988;113:10.
170. Cohen M, Nihill M. Postoperative ketotic hyperglycemia during prostaglandin E1 infusion in infancy. Pediatrics 1983;71:842.
171. Miltenyi M, Tulassay T, Szabo A,et al. Urinary prostaglandins in hyperglycaemic ketoacidosis of type I diabetes mellitus. Pediatr Nephrol 1990;4:44.
172. Mourits AT, Jensen IW, Nielsen LK, et al. Plasma 6-keto-PGF1 alpha, thromboxane B2 and PGE2 during diabetic ketoacidosis. Prostaglandins Leukotr Essent Fatty Acids 1990;40:39.
173. Parker J, Lane J, Axelrod L. Cooperation of adipocytes and endothelial cells required for catecholamine stimulation of PGI2 production by rat adipose tissue. Diabetes 1989;38:1123.
174. Quyyumi AA, Iaffaldano R, Guerrero JL, et al. Prostacyclin and pathogenesis of hemodynamic abnormalities of diabetic ketoacidosis in rats. Diabetes 1989;38:1585.
175. Binimelis J, Webb SM, Serrano J, et al. Plasma immunoreactive somatostatin is elevated in diabetic ketoacidosis and correlates with plasma non-esterified fatty acid concentration. Diabetic Med 1987;4:221.
176. Rumbak MJ, Hughes TA, Kitabchi AE. Pseudonormoglycemia in diabetic ketoacidosis with elevated triglycerides. Am J Emerg Med 1991;9:61.
177. Owen O, Trapp V, Skutches C. Acetone metabolism during diabetic ketoacidosis. Diabetes 1982;31:242.
178. Cronin J, Kroop S, Diamond J, et al. Alkalemia in diabetic ketoacidosis. Am J Med 1984;77:192.
179. Halperin M, Bear R, Hannaford M, et al. Selected aspects of the pathophysiology of metabolic acidosis in diabetes mellitus. Diabetes 1981;30:781.
180. Adrogue H, Wilson H, Boyd A. Plasma acid-base patterns in diabetic ketoacidosis. N Engl J Med 1982;307:1603.
181. Oh M, Carroll H, Goldstein D, et al. Hyperchloremic acidosis during the recovery phase of diabetic ketosis. Ann Intern Med 1978;89:925.
182. Hammeke M, Bear R, Lee R. Hyperchloremic metabolic acidosis in diabetes mellitus: a case report and discussion of the pathophysiologic mechanisms. Diabetes 1978;27:16.
183. Tsalikian E, Becker D, Crumrine P. Electroencephalographic changes in diabetic ketosis in children with newly and previously diagnosed insulin-dependent diabetes mellitus. J Pediatr 1981;98:355.
184. Fulop M, Rosenblatt A, Kreitzer S, et al. Hyperosmolar nature of diabetic coma. Diabetes 1975;24:594.
185. Goldman M, Kashani M. Spurious hyponatremia in diabetic ketoacidosis with massive lipid elevations. J Med Soc N J 1982;79:591.
186. Fulop M. Serum potassium in lactic acidosis and ketoacidosis. N Engl J Med 1979;300:1087.
187. Gaal L, Leeuw I. Hyperkalemia in diabetic ketoacidosis (Editorial). Diabetes Care 1981;4:576.
188. Cox M, Sterns R, Singer I. The defense against hyperkalemia: the roles of insulin and aldosterone. N Engl J Med 1978;299:525.
189. Goldfarb S, Cox M, Singer I, et al. Acute hyperkalemia induced by hyperglycemia: hormonal mechanisms. Ann Intern Med 1976;84:426.
190. Makoff D, DaSilva J, Rosenbaum B. On the mechanism of hyperkalaemia due to hyperosmotic expansion with saline or mannitol. Clin Sci 1971;41:383.
191. Morena M, Murphy C, Goldsmith L. Increase in serum potassium resulting from the administration of hypertonic mannitol and other solutions. J Lab Clin Med 1969;73:291.
192. Seldin D, Tarail R. Effect of hypertonic solutions on metabolism and excretion of electrolytes. Am J Physiol 1949;159:160.
193. Fulop M. Hyperkalemia in diabetic ketoacidosis. Am J Med Sci 1990;299:164.
194. Uribarri J, Oh MS, Carroll HJ. Hyperkalemia in diabetes mellitus. J Diabetic Complications 1990;4:3.
195. West ML, Magner PO, Richardson RM, et al. A renal mechanism limiting the degree of potassium loss in severely hyperglycemic patients. Am J Nephrol 1988;8:373.
196. Bohannon NJ. Large phosphate shifts with treatment for hyperglycemia. Arch Intern Med 1989;149:1423.
197. Kanter Y, Gerson A, Bessman A. 2,3-Diphosphoglycerate, nucleotide phosphate, and organic and inorganic phosphate levels during the early phases of diabetic ketoacidosis. Diabetes 1977;26:429.
198. Fisher J, Kitabchi A. A randomized study of phosphate therapy in the treatment of diabetic ketoacidosis. J Clin Endocrinol Metab 1983;57:177.
199. Keller U, Berger W. Prevention of hypophosphatemia by phosphate infusion during treatment of diabetic ketoacidosis and hyperosmolar coma. Diabetes 1980;29:87.
200. Wilson H, Keuer S, Lea S. Phosphate therapy in diabetic ketoacidosis. Arch Intern Med 1982;142:517.
201. Clerbaux T, Reynaert M, Willems E, et al. Effect of phosphate on oxygen-hemoglobin affinity, diphosphoglycerate and blood gases during recovery from diabetic ketoacidosis. Intensive Care Med 1989;15:495.
202. DeFronzo R, Lang R. Hypophosphatemia and glucose intolerance: evidence for tissue insensitivity to insulin. N Engl J Med 1980;303:1259.
203. Winter R, Harris C, Phillips L, et al. Diabetic ketoacidosis induction of hypocalcemia and hypomagnesemia by phosphate therapy. Am J Med 1979;67:897.
204. Zipf W, Bacon G, Spencer M, et al. Hypocalcemia, hypomagnesemia, and transient hypoparathyroidism during therapy with potassium phosphate in diabetic ketoacidosis. Diabetes Care 1979;2:265.
205. Becker D, Brown D, Steranka B, et al. Phosphate replacement during treatment of diabetic ketosis. Am J Dis Child 1983;137:241.
206. Ewald U, Gebre-Medhin M, Tuvemo T. Hypomagnesemia in diabetic children. Acta Paediatr Scand 1983;72:367.

207. Sprung C, Rackow E, Fein I. Pulmonary edema: a complication of diabetic ketoacidosis. Chest 1980;77:687.
208. Alberti KG. Diabetic emergencies. Br Med Bull 1989;45:242.
209. Gordon D, MacCuish AC. Cerebral oedema in diabetic ketoacidosis. Scott Med J 1988;33:212.
210. Hamblin PS, Topliss DJ, Chosich N, et al. Deaths associated with diabetic ketoacidosis and hyperosmolar coma. Med J Aust 1973;151:441.
211. Molitch ME. Diabetes mellitus: pathophysiology and current trends in management. J Am Optom Assoc 1988;59:842.
212. Rogers B, Sills I, Cohen M, et al. Diabetic ketoacidosis: neurologic collapse during treatment followed by severe developmental morbidity. Clin Pediatr 1990;29:451.
213. Scibilia J. Why do children with diabetes die? Acta Endocrinol (Suppl) 1986;279:326.
214. Moss JM. Diabetic ketoacidosis: effective low-cost treatment in a community hospital. South Med J 1987;80:875.
215. van der Meulen JA, Klip A, Grinstein S. Possible mechanism for cerebral oeema in diabetic ketoacidosis. Lancet 1987;2:306.
216. Krane EJ, Walman JK, Wolfsdorf JI. Subclinical brain swelling in children during treatment of diabetic ketoacidosis. N Eng J Med 1985;316:857.
217. Glascow AM. Devastating cerebral edema in diabetic ketoacidosis before therapy. Diabetes Care 1991;14:77.
218. Rosenbloom AL. Intracerebral crises during treatment of diabetic ketoacidosis. Diabetes Care 1990;13:22.
219. Mather H. Management of hyperosmolar coma. J R Soc Med 1980;73:134.
220. Brun-Buisson C, Bonnet F, Bergeret S. Recurrent high-permeability pulmonary edema associated with diabetic ketoacidosis. Crit Care Med 1985;13:55.
221. Powner D, Snyder J, Grenvik A. Altered pulmonary capillary permeability complicating recovery from diabetic ketoacidosis. Chest 1975;68:253.
222. Malik A. Mechanisms of neurogenic pulmonary edema. J Am Heart Assoc 1985;57:1.
223. Soler N, Bennett M, Fitzgerald M, et al. Electrocardiogram as a guide to potassium replacement in diabetic ketoacidosis. Diabetes 1974; 23:610.
224. Malone J, Brodsky S. The value of electrocardiogram monitoring in diabetic ketoacidosis. Diabetes Care 1980;3:543.
225. Adrogue HJ, Barrero J, Eknoyan G. Salutary effects of modest fluid replacement in the treatment of adults with diabetic ketoacidosis: use in patients without extreme volume deficit. JAMA 1989;262:2108.
226. Hillman K. Fluid resuscitation in diabetic emergencies: a reappraisal. Intens Care Med 1987;13:4.
227. Fort P, Waters S, Lifshitz F. Low-dose insulin infusion in the treatment of diabetic ketoacidosis: bolus versus no bolus. J Pediatr 1980;96:36.
228. Kitabchi A, Matteri R, Murphy M. Optimal insulin delivery in diabetic ketoacidosis (DKA) and hyperglycemic, hyperosmolar nonketotic coma (HHNC). Diabetes Care 1982;5:78.
229. Hofeldt F, Kelly M. Low-dose insulin regimens in the management of diabetic ketoacidosis: efficacy and pitfalls. Minn Med 1983;66:25.
230. Carroll P, Matz R. Uncontrolled diabetes mellitus in adults: experience in treating diabetic ketoacidosis and hyperosmolar nonketotic coma with low-dose insulin. Diabetes Care 1983;6:579.
231. Banting F, Best C. The internal secretion of the pancreas. J Lab Clin Med 1922;7:251.
232. Page M, Alberti K, Greenwood R. Treatment of diabetic coma with continuous low-dose infusion of insulin. Br Med J 1974;2:687.
233. Nyhan W. Diabetic ketosis and acidosis: the continuous infusion of low doses of insulin. J Pediatr 1975;87:846.
234. Drop S, Duval-Arnould B, Gober A. Low-dose intravenous insulin infusion versus subcutaneous insulin injection: a controlled comparative study of diabetic ketoacidosis. Pediatrics 1977;59:733.
235. Lightner E, Kappy M, Revsin B. Low-dose intravenous insulin infusion in patients with diabetic ketoacidosis: biochemical effects in children. Pediatrics 1977;60:681.
236. Edwards G, Kohaut E, Wehring B, et al. Effectiveness of low-dose continuous intravenous insulin infusion in diabetic ketoacidosis: a prospective comparative study. J Pediatr 1977;91:701.
237. Tamborlane W, Genel M. Discordant correction of hyperglycemia and ketoacidosis with low-dose insulin infusion. Pediatrics 1978;61:125.
238. Heber D, Molitch M, Sperling M. Low-dose continuous insulin therapy for diabetic ketoacidosis. Arch Intern Med 1977;137:1377.
239. Martin AL, Martin MM. Continuous infusion of insulin vs repeated sc injections in the treatment of diabetic ketoacidosis in children. Acta Diabetol Lat 1978;15:81.
240. Kappy M, Lightner E. Low-dose intravenous insulin in the treatment of diabetic ketoacidosis. Am J Dis Child 1979;133:523.
241. Perkin R, Marks J. Low-dose continuous intravenous insulin infusion in childhood diabetic ketoacidosis. Clin Pediatr 1979;18:540.
242. Munk P, Freedman M, Levison H, et al. Effect of bicarbonate on oxygen transport in juvenile diabetic ketoacidosis. J Pediatr 1974;84:510.
243. Lever E, Jaspan J. Sodium bicarbonate therapy in severe diabetic ketoacidosis. Am J Med 1983;75:263.
244. Yoshida K, Marmarou A. Effects of tromethamine and hyperventilation on brain injury in the cat. J Neurosurg 1991;74:87.
245. Schurmann W, Lindner K, Pfenninger A, et al. Tromethamine for cerebral resuscitation. Crit Care Med 1991;19.
246. Silvay G. Ketamine. Mt Sinai J Med 1983;50:300.
247. White PF. Comparative evaluation of intravenous agents for rapid sequence induction: thiopental, ketamine, and midazolam. Anesthesiology 1982;57:279.
248. Bruckner JB, Gethmann JW, Patschke D, et al Investigations in the effects of etomidate in the human circulation. Anaesthetist 1974;23:322.
249. Colvin MP, Savege TM, Newland PE, et al. Cardiorespiratory changes following induction of anesthesia with etomidate in patients with cardiac disease. Brit J Anaesthes 1979;51:551.
250. Kettler D, Sonntag H, Donath V, et al. Haemodynamics, myocardial function, oxygen requirements and oxygen supply of the human heart after administration of etomidate. In: Doenicke AE, ed. Etomidate: an intravenous hypnotic agent. New York: Springer, 1977:81.
251. Criado A, Maseda J, Navarro E, et al. Induction of anaesthesia with etomidate: haemodynamic study of 36 patients. Br J Anaesthes 1980;52:803.
252. Patschke D, Bruckner JB, Gethmann JW, et al. Comparison of the immediate effects of etomidate, propanidid and thiopentone on haemodynamics, coronary blood flow and myocardial oxygen consumption. Acta Anaesthesiologica Belgica 1975;26:112.
253. Michenfelder JD. Anesthesia and the brain. New York: Churchill Livingstone, 1988:94.
254. Millar C, Bissonette B. Awake intubation increases intracranial pressure without affecting cerebral blood flow velocity in infants. Can J Anesthes 1994;41:281.
255. Kofke WA, Dong ML, Bloom M, et al. Transcranial Doppler ultrasonography with induction of anesthesia for neurosurgery. J Neurosurg Anesthesiol 1994;6:89.
256. Stoelting RK, Miller RD. Intravenous anesthetics: basics of anesthesia. New York: Churchill Livingstone, 1994:61.
257. Gardner AE, Dannemiller FJ, Dean D. Intracranial cerebrospinal fluid pressure in man during ketamine anesthesia. Anesthes Analges 1972;51:741.
258. Wyte SR, Shapiro HM, Turner P, et al. Ketamine-induced intracranial hypertension. Anesthesiol 1972;36:174.
259. Schulte AM, Esch J, Pfeifer G, et al. The influence of intravenous anaesthetic agents on primarily increased intracranial pressure. Acta Neurochirurgica 1978;45:15.
260. Gregory G. Induction of anesthesia. In: Gregory G, ed. Pediatric anesthesia. New York: Churchill Livingstone, 1989:539.
261. Ockert DB, Hugo JM. Diabetic complications with special anaesthetic risk. S Afr J Surg 1992;30:90.
262. Reid B, DiLorenzo C, Travis L, et al. Diabetic gastroparesis due to postprandial antral hypomotility in childhood. Pediatrics 1992;90:43.
263. Hirsch IB, Gill JBM, Cryer PE, et al. Perioperative management of surgical patients with diabetes mellitus. Anesthesiology 1991;74:346.
264. Woodruff RE, Lewis SB, McLeskey CH, et al. Avoidance of surgical hyperglycemia in diabetic patients. JAMA 1980;244:166.
265. Podolsky S. Management of diabetes in the surgical patient. Med Clin North Am 1982;66:1361.
266. Meyers EF, Alberts D, Gordon MO. Perioperative control of blood glucose in diabetic patients: a two-step protocol. Diabetes Care 1986;9:40.
267. Walts LF, Miller J, Davidson MB, et al. Perioperative management of diabetes mellitus. Anesthesiology 1981;55:104.
268. Meyer EJ, Lorenzi M, Bohannon WV, et al. Diabetic management by insulin infusion during major surgery. Am J Surg 1979;137:323.
269. Jaspers CA, Elte JW, Olthof G. Perioperative diabetes regulation with the help of a standard protocol. Neth J Med 1994;44:122.
270. Pezzarossa A, Taddei F, Cimicchi MC, et al. Perioperative management of diabetic subjects. Subcutaneous versus intravenous insulin administration during glucose-potassium infusion. Diabetes Care 1988;11:52.

271. Husband DJ, Thai AC, Alberti KG. Management of diabetes during surgery with glucose-insulin-potassium infusion. Diabetic Med 1986;3:69.
272. Martin MM, Martin AA. Continuous low-dose infusion of insulin in the treatment of diabetic ketoacidosis in children. J Pediatr 1976;89:560.
273. Weber ME, Abbasi V. Continuous intravenous insulin therapy in severe diabetic ketoacidosis: variations in dosage requirements. J Pediatr 1977;91:755.
274. Mizock BA. Alterations in carbohydrate metabolism during stress: a review of the literature. Am J Medi 1995;98:75.
275. Sharath MD, Metzger WJ, Richerson HB, et al. Protamine-induced fatal anaphylaxis: prevalence of antiprotamine immunoglobulin E antibody. J Thor Cardiovasc Surg 1985;90:86.
276. Stewart WJ, McSweeney SM, Kellett MA, et al. Increased risk of severe protamine reactions in NPH insulin-dependent diabetics undergoing cardiac catheterization. Circulation 1984;70:788.
277. Knight G, Leatherdale B. The role of race and environment in the development of hyperosmolar hyperglycaemic non-ketotic coma. Postgrad Med J 1982;58:351.
278. Kern E, Simmons D, Martin D. Diabetic ketoacidosis and hyperglycemic nonketotic coma. In: Chernow B, ed. Endocrine aspects of acute illness. New York: Churchill Livingstone, 1985:285.
279. Cahill GJ. Hyperglycemic hyperosmolar coma: a syndrome almost unique to the elderly. J Am Geriatr Soc 1983;31:103.
280. Leske J. Hyperglycemic hyperosmolar nonketotic coma. J Emerg Nurs 1984;10:145.
281. Kingston M, Al-siba IM. Treatment of severe hypophosphatemia. Crit Care Med 1985;13:16.
282. Boulware SD, Tamborlane WV. Not all severe hyperglycemia is diabetes. Pediatrics 1992;89:330.
283. Hoffman W. Hyperglycaemic hyperosmolar non-ketotic coma in a non-diabetic child (Editorial). Diabetologia 1983;25:531.
284. Freidenberg G, Kosnik E, Sotos J. Hyperglycemic coma after suprasellar surgery. N Engl J Med 1980;303:863.
285. Asplund K, Eriksson S, Hagg E. Hyperosmolar non-ketotic coma in diabetic stroke patients. Acta Med Scand 1982;212:407.
286. Collins B, Nelson J. Hyperosmolar non-ketotic diabetic coma precipitated by Leptospira hebdomadis infection. Isr J Med Sci 1983;19:359.
287. Tollefson G, Lesar T. Nonketotic hyperglycemia associated with loxapine and amoxapine: case report. J Clin Psychiatry 1983;44:347.
288. Merguerian P, Perel A, Wald U, et al. Persistent non-ketotic hyperglycemia as a grave prognostic sign in head-injured patients. Crit Care Med 1981;9:838.
289. Parish RA, Webb KS. Hyperglycemia is not a poor prognostic sign in head-injured children. J Trauma 1988;28:17.
290. Pulsinelli W, Waldman S, Rawlinson D, et al. Moderate hyperglycemia augments ischemic brain damage: a neuropathologic study in the rat. Neurology 1982;32:1239.
291. Pulsinelli W, Levy D, Sigsbee B, et al. Increased damage after ischemic stroke in patients with hyperglycemia with or without established diabetes mellitus. Am J Med 1983;74:540.
292. Plum P. What causes infarction in ischemic brain? The Robert Wartenberg lecture. Neurology 1983;33:222.
293. Robertson C, Goodman J, Narayan R, et al. The effect of glucose administration on carbohydrate metabolism after head injury. J Neurosurg 1991;74:43.
294. Young C, Karam J. Hypoglycemic disorders. In: Greenspan F, ed. Basic and clinical endocrinology. Norwalk, CT: Appleton & Lange, 1991:651.
295. Schwartz R. Diabetic ketoacidosis and coma. In Smith C, ed. The critically ill child. Philadelphia: WB Saunders 1977:230.
296. Kogut M. Hypoglycemia: pathogenesis, diagnosis, and treatment. In: Gluck L, Cone T, Dodge P, eds. Current problems in pediatrics. Chicago: Year Book, 1974:3.
297. Senior B, Wolfsdorf J. Substrate, gluconeogenesis, and hypoglycemia in children. Pediatr Clin North Am 1979;26:171.
298. Lovinger R. Emergency treatment of hypoglycemia in children. VA Med 1983;110:50.
299. Macaron C, Kadri A, Macaron Z. Nucleated red blood cells and artifactual hypoglycemia. Diabetes Care 1981;4:113.
300. Chernow B, Diaz M, Cruess D. Bedside blood glucose determinations in critical care medicine: a comparative analysis of two techniques. Crit Care Med 1982;10:463.
301. Linde J, Nilsson L, Barany F. Diabetes and hypoglycemia in chronic pancreatitis. Scand J Gastroenterol 1977;12:369.
302. Kliegman R, Behrman R. Diseases of the newborn infant: premature and full-term. In: Behrman R, Vaughan, eds. Nelson textbook of pediatrics. Philadelphia: WB Saunders, 1987:385.
303. Cornblath M, Poth M. Hypoglycemia. In: Kaplan S, ed. Clinical pediatric and adolescent endocrinology. Philadelphia: WB Saunders, 1982:366.
304. Eriksson M, Zetterstrom R. Neonatal convulsions; incidence and causes in the Stockholm area. Acta Paediatr Scand 1979;68:807.
305. Case Records of the Massachusetts General Hospital. N Engl J Med 1978;299:241.
306. Shermeta D, Mendelsohn G, Haller J. Hyperinsulinemic hypoglycemia of the neonate associated with persistent fetal histology and function of the pancreas. Ann Surg 1980;191:182.
307. Kauschansky A, Genel M, Smith G. Congenital hypopituitarism in female infants. Am J Dis Child 1979;133:165.
308. Moazam F, Rodgers B, Talbert J, et al. Near-total pancreatectomy in persistent infantile hypoglycemia. Arch Surg 1982;117:1151.
309. Campbell J, Rivers S, Harrison M, et al. Treatment of hypoglycemia in infants and children: surgical considerations. Am J Surg 1983; 146:21.
310. Bougneres P, Landier F, Garnier P, et al. Treatment of insulin excess by continuous subcutaneous infusion of somatostatin and glucagon in an infant. J Pediatr 1985;106:792.
311. Carter WJ Jr. Hypothermia: a sign of hypoglycemia. Jacep 1976;5:594.
312. Mercer S, Bass J. Hypoglycemia associated with pediatric surgical procedures. Can J Surg 1983;26:246.
313. Haymond M, Pagliara A. Ketotic hypoglycaemia. Clin Endocrinol Metab 1983;12:447.
314. Wolfsdorf J, Sadeghi-Nejad A, Senior B. Hypoalaninemia and ketotic hypoglycemia: cause or consequence? Eur J Pediatr 1982;138:28.
315. Wilensky J, Goldberg M, Ziyai F, et al. Infantile cataracts, Coats' disease, and ketotic hypoglycemia. J Pediatr Ophthalmol 1976;13:75.
316. Catlett J. Ketotic hypoglycemia. W 1983:126.
317. Dahlquist G, Gentz J, Hagenfeldt L. Ketotic hypoglycemia of childhood: a clinical trial of several unifying etiological hypotheses. Acta Pediatr Scand 1979;68:649.
318. Haymond MW. Hypoglycemia in infants and children. Endocrinol Metab Clin North Am 1989;18:211.
319. Scott R, Scandrett M. Nocturnal cortisol release during hypoglycemia in diabetes. Diabetes Care 1981;4:514.
320. Goldstein D, England J, Hess R. A prospective study of symptomatic hypoglycemia in young diabetic patients. Diabetes Care 1981;4:601.
321. Polonsky K, Bergenstal R, Pons G. Relation of counterregulatory responses to hypoglycemia in type I diabetics. N Engl J Med 1982;307:1106.
322. White N, Skor D, Cryer P. Identification of type I diabetic patients at increased risk for hypoglycemia during intensive therapy. N Engl J Med 1983;308:485.
323. Hillson R. Hypoglycemia and hypothermia (Editorial). Diabetes Care 1983;6:211.
324. Haumont D, Dorchy H, Pelc S. EEG abnormalities in diabetic children. Clin Pediatr 1979;18:750.
325. Ran A, Anderson R. The diagnosis of postprandial hypoglycemia. Diabetes 1981;30:996.
326. Roe T, Kogut M. Idiopathic leucine-sensitive hypoglycemia syndrome: insulin and glucagon responses and effects of diazoxide. Pediatr Res 1982;16:1.
327. Johnson D, Dorr K, Swenson W, et al. Reactive hypoglycemia. JAMA 1980;243:1151.
328. Buss R, Kansal P, Roddam R. Mixed meal tolerance test and reactive hypoglycemia. Horm Metab Res 1982;14:281.
329. Foa P, Dunbar J, Klein S. Reactive hypoglycemia and A-cell ('pancreatic') glucagon deficiency in the adult. JAMA 1980;244:2281.
330. Hansen I, Levy M, Kerr D. Differential diagnosis of hypoglycemia in children by responses to fasting and 2-deoxyglucose. Metabolism 1983;32:960.
331. Hansen I, Levy M, Kerr D. The 2-deoxyglucose test as a supplement to fasting for detection of childhood hypoglycemia. Pediatr Res 1984;18:490.
332. Hansen K, Duck S. Teledyne sleep sentry: evaluation in pediatric patients for detection of nocturnal hypoglycemia. Diabetes Care 1983;6:597.
333. Tonghua L, Zianjiu Z, Yu Z, et al. Hypoglycemia: insulinoma or islet hyperplasia? Chin Med J 1980;93:545.

334. Simmons P, Telander R, Carney J. Surgical management of hyperinsulinemic hypoglycemia in children. Arch Surg 1984;119:520.
335. Nathan D, Axelrod L, Proppe K. Nesidioblastosis associated with insulin-mediated hypoglycemia in an adult. Diabetes Care 1981;4:383.
336. Dahms B, Landing B, Blaskovics M, et al. Nesidioblastosis and other islet cell abnormalities in hyperinsulinemic hypoglycemia of childhood. Hum Pathol 1980;11:641.
337. Rosenbloom A, Hunt S. Prognosis of impaired glucose tolerance in children with stress hyperglycemia, symptoms of hypoglycemia, or asymptomatic glucosuria. J Pediatr 1982;101:340.
338. Wolfsdorf J, Sadeghi-Nejad A, Senior B. Ketonuria does not exclude hyperinsulinemic hypoglycemia. Am J Dis Child 1984;138:168.
339. Weidenheim K, Hinchey W, Campbell WJ. Hyperinsulinemic hypoglycemia in adults with islet-cell hyperplasia and degranulation of exocrine cells of the pancreas. Am J Clin Pathol 1983;79:14.
340. White N, Warrell D, Chanthavanich P. Severe hypoglycemia and hyperinsulinemia in falciparum malaria. N Engl J Med 1983;309:61.
341. Winterer J. Carnitine and neonatal ketosis. J Pediatr 1982;99:840.
342. Slonim A, Borum P, Tanaka K. Dietary-dependent carnitine deficiency as a cause of nonketotic hypoglycemia in an infant. J Pediatr 1981;99:551.
343. Teijema H, van Gelderen H, Gieskberts M. Hypoketosis as a cause of symptoms in childhood hypoglycemia. Eur J Pediatr 1980;134:51.
344. Stanley C, Hale D, Coates P. Medium-chain acyl-CoA dehydrogenase deficiency in children with non-ketotic hypoglycemia and low carnitine levels. Pediatr Res 1983;17:877.
345. Schmale H, Heinsohn S, Richter D. Structural organization of the rat gene for the arginine vasopressin-neurophysin II precursor. EMBO J 1983;2:763.
346. Bahnsen U, Oosting P, Swaab DF, et al. A missense mutation in the vasopressin-neurophysin precursor gene cosegregates with human autosomal dominant neurohypophyseal diabetes insipidus. EMBO J 1992;11:19.
347. Nagasaki H, Ito M, Yuasa H, et al. Two novel mutations in the coding region for neurophysin-II associated with familial central diabetes insipidus. J Clin Endocrinol Metab 1995;80:1352.
348. Repaske DR, Browning JE. A de novo mutation in the coding sequence for neurophysin-II (Pro24—Leu) is associated with onset and transmission of autosomal dominant neurohypophyseal diabetes insipidus. J Clin Endocrinol Metab 1994;79:421.
349. Fujiwara TM, Morgan K, Bichet DG. Molecular biology of diabetes insipidus. Ann Rev Med 1995;46:331.
350. Mazjoub JA. Disorders of the posterior pituitary. In: Kelly W, ed. Textbook of internal medicine. New York: Lippincott, 1992:1987.
351. Carmichael M, Kumar R. Molecular biology of vasopressin receptors. Semin Nephrol 1994;14:341.
352. Ramsay D. Posterior pituitary gland. In: Greenspan F, ed. Basic and clinical endocrinology. Norwalk, CT: Appleton & Lange, 1991:177.
353. Guyton A, Hall J. Vasopressin and cardiovascular regulation. In: Guyton A, Hall J, eds. Cardiovascular physiology. Baltimore: University Park Press, 1982.
354. Moses A. Diabetes insipidus and ADH regulation. Hosp Pract 1977;37:37.
355. Miller M. New tools for diagnosing and treating disorders of water metabolism. Res Staff Phys 1979;37:37.
356. Keyzer Yd, Auzan C, Lenne F, et al. Cloning and characterization of the human V3 pituitary vasopressin receptor. FEBS Letters 1994;356:215.
357. Friis-Hansen B. Water: the major nutrient. Acta Paediatr Scand Suppl 1982;299:11.
358. Phillips EM, Butler T, Baylis P. Osmoregulation of vasopressin and thirst: comparison of 20% mannitol wtih 5% saline as osmotic stimulants in healthy man. Clin Endocrinol 1994;21:207.
359. Baylis PH. Osmoregulation and control of vasopressin secretion in healthy humans. Am J Physiol 1987;253:R671.
360. Thompson CJ, Freeman J, Record CO, et al. Hypernatraemia due to a reset osmostat for vasopressin release and thirst, complicated by nephrogenic diabetes insipidus. Postgrad Med J 1987;63:979.
361. Streeten DHP, Moses AM, Miller M. Disorders of the neurohypophysis. In: Braunwald E, Isselbacher KJ, Petersdorf RG, et al, eds. Harrison's Principles of Internal Medicine. 11 ed. New York: McGraw-Hill, 1987:1729.
362. Househam K, Vermeulen J, Klein M. Early clinical diagnosis of the syndrome of inappropriate secretions of antidiuretic hormone. S Afr Med J 1983;63:498.
363. Doczi T, Bende J, Huszka E, et al. Syndrome of inappropriate secretion of antidiuretic hormone after subarachnoid hemorrhage. Neurosurg 1981;9:394.
364. Cusick J, Hagen T, Findling J. Inappropriate secretion of antidiuretic hormone after transsphenoidal surgery for pituitary tumors. N Engl J Med 1984;311:36.
365. Burrows F, Shutack J, Crone R. Inappropriate secretion of antidiuretic hormone in a postsurgical pediatric population. Crit Care Med 1983;11:527.
366. Ting S, Eshaghpour E. Inappropriate secretion of antidiuretic hormone after open heart surgery. Am J Dis Child 1980;134:873.
367. Menon R, Sharma V, Siddiqui H, et al. Syndrome of inappropriate secretion of antidiuretic hormone (SIADH) in children with meningoencephalitis. Indian J Med Res 1983;77:373.
368. Tomita M, Suzuki H, Matsuoka Y, et al. Increased renal kallikrein secretion in SIADH after vincristine therapy. Endocrinol Jpn 1981;28:637.
369. Rudnick S, Cadman E, Capizzi R, et al. High dose cytosine arabinoside (HDARAC) in refractory acute leukemia. Cancer 1979;44:1189.
370. Stark H, Weinberger A, Ben-Bassat M. Persistent hyponatremia and inappropriate antidiuretic hormone secretion in children with extensive burns. J Pediatr Surg 1979;14:149.
371. Shirani K, Vaughan G, Robertson G, et al. Inappropriate vasopressin secretion (SIADH) in burned patients. J Trauma 1983;23:217.
372. Rivers R, Forsling M, Olver R. Inappropriate secretion of antidiuretic hormone in infants with respiratory infections. Arch Dis Child 1981;56:358.
373. Szatalowicz V, Goldberg J, Anderson R. Plasma antidiuretic hormone in acute respiratory failure. Am J Med 1982;72:583.
374. Bahna S, Kaushik S. Water and electrolyte status in children with acute asthma. J Asthma 1984;21:73.
375. Nutman J, Wilunsky E, Avni A, et al. Syndrome of inappropriate antidiuretic hormone secretion in newborn infants with respiratory problems. Isr J Med Sci 1981;17:1009.
376. Ogunye O, Gbadebo A. Syndrome of inappropriate antidiuretic hormone (SIADH) in measles and malaria infections. Trop Geogr Med 1981;33:165.
377. Bode H. Disorders of the posterior pituitary. In: Kaplan S, ed. Clinical pediatric and adolescent endocrinology. Philadelphia: WB Saunders, 1982:366.
378. Kaplan S, Feigin R. Syndromes of inappropriate secretion of antidiuretic hormone in children. Adv Pediatr 1980;27:247.
379. Hochberg Z, Benderly A. Normal osmotic threshold for vasopressin release in the hyponatremia of hypothyroidism. Horm Res 1983; 17:128.
380. Robson W, Arbus G, Balfe J. Bartter's syndrome; differentiation into two clinical groups. Am J Dis Child 1979;133:636.
381. Diringer M, Ladenson PW, Borel C, et al. Sodium and water regulation in a patient with cerebral salt wasting. Arch Neurol 1989;46:928.
382. Ganong CA, Kappy MS. Cerebral salt wasting in children. The Need for recognition and treatment. Am J Dis Child 1993;147:167.
383. Espiner EA, Richards AM, Yandle TG, et al. Natriuretic hormones. Endocrinol Metab Clin North Am 1995;24:481.
384. Powell KR, Sugarman LI, Eskenazi AE, et al. Normalization of plasma arginine vasopressin concentrations when children with meningitis are given maintenance plus replacement fluid therapy. J Pediatr 1990; 117:515.
385. Decaux G, Brimioulle S, Genette F, et al. Treatment of the syndrome of inappropriate secretion of antidiuretic hormone by urea. Am J Med 1980;69:99.
386. Decaux G, Waterlot Y, Genette F,et al. Treatment of the syndrome of inappropriate secretion of antidiuretic hormone with furosemide. N Engl J Med 1981;304:329.
387. Decaux G. Treatment of the syndrome of inappropriate secretion of antidiuretic hormone by long loop diuretics. Nephron 1983;35:82.
388. Hantman D, Rossier BZ, Schrier R. Rapid correction of hyponatremia in the syndrome of inappropriate secretion of antidiuretic hormone: an alternative treatment to hypertonic saline. Ann Intern Med 1973;78:870.
389. Rose B. Clinical physiology of acid-base and electrolyte disorders. New York: McGraw Hill, 1984.
390. Baker R, Hurley R, Feldman W. Treatment of recurrent syndrome of inappropriate secretion of antidiuretic hormone with lithium. J Pediatr 1977;90:480.

391. White M, Fetner C. Treatment of the syndrome of inappropriate secretion of antidiuretic hormone with lithium carbonate. N Engl J Med 1975;292:390.
392. Finsterer U, Beyer A, Jensen U, et al. The syndrome of inappropriate secretion of antidiuretic hormone (SIADH)-treatment with lithium. Intens Care Med 1982;8:223.
393. De Troyer A, Demanet J. Correction of antidiuresis by demeclocycline. N Engl J Med 1975;293:915.
394. Tanay A, Yust I, Peresecenschi G, et al. Long-term treatment of the syndrome of inappropriate antidiuretic hormone secretion with phenytoin. Ann Intern Med 1979;90:50.
395. Scanarini M, de'Avella D, Zuccarello M, et al. Neurogenic disorders of ADH secretion: clinical and neuropathological correlations. Acta Neuropathol 1981;7:403.
396. Keren G. Diabetes insipidus indicating a dying brain. Crit Care Med 1982;10:798.
397. Glauser F. Diabetes insipidus in hypoxemic encephalopathy. JAMA 1976;235:932.
398. Rothschild M, Shenkman L. Diabetes insipidus following cardiorespiratory arrest. JAMA 1977;238:620.
399. Stuart C, Neelon F, Lebovitz H. Disordered control of thirst in hypothalamic-pituitary sarcoidosis. N Engl J Med 1980;303:1078.
400. Balestrieri F, Chernow B, Rainey T. Postcraniotomy diabetes insipidus: who's at risk? Crit Care Med 1982;10:108.
401. Bucher H, Zapf J, Torresani T, et al. Insulin-like growth factors I and II, prolactin, and insulin 19 growth hormone-deficient children with excessive, normal, or decreased longitudinal growth after operation for craniopharyngioma. N Engl J Med 1983;309:1142.
402. Czernichow P, Pomarede R, Basmaciogullari A, et al. Diabetes insipidus in children: III. Anterior pituitary dysfunction in idiopathic types. J Pediatr 1985;106:41.
403. Bacon G, Spencer M, Hopwood N, et al. Diabetes insipidus and inappropriate antidiuretic hormone secretion. In: Bacon G, Spencer M, Hopwood N, et al, eds. A practical approach to pediatric endocrinology. Chicago: Year Book, 1982:252.
404. Weitzman R, Kleeman C. The clinical physiology of water metabolism: III. The water depletion (hyperosmolar) and water excess (hyposmolar) syndromes. West J Med 1980;132:16.
405. Sterns R, Spital A. Disorders of water balance. In: Kokko J, Tannen R, eds. Fluids and electrolytes. Philadelphia: WB Saunders, 1990:139.
406. Outwater K, Rockoff M. Diabetes insipidus accompanying brain death in children. Neurology 1984;34:1243.
407. Fiser D, Jiminez J, Wrape V, et al. Diabetes insipidus in children with brain death. Crit Care Med 1987;15:551.
408. Barzilay Z, Somekh E. Diabetes insipidus in severely brain damaged children. J Med 1988;19:47.
409. Kissoon N, Frewen T, Bloch M, et al. Pediatric organ donor maintenance: pathophysiologic derangements and nursing requirements. Pediatrics 1989;84:688.
410. Howlett T, Keogh A, Perry L, et al. Anterior and posterior pituitary function in brain-stem-dead donors. Transplantation 1989;47:828.
411. Shalhoub R. Correcting disorders of serum sodium concentration. Drug Ther 1979;59:59.
412. Mohring J, Glanzer K, Maciel J, et al. Greatly enhanced pressor response to antidiuretic hormone in patients with impaired cardiovascular reflexes due to idiopathic orthostatic hypotension. J Cardiovasc Pharm 1980;2:367.
413. Cowley A. Vasopressin and cardiovascular regulation. In: Guyton A, Hall J, eds. Cardiovascular physiology. Baltimore: University Park, 1982:189.
414. Chanson P, Jedynak CP, Dabrowski G, et al. Ultralow doses of vasopressin in the management of diabetes insipidus. Crit Care Med 1987;15:44.
415. Revzani I, Artman H, Garibaldi L, et al. Continuous infusion of aqueous pitressin for treatment of central diabetes insipidus (DI). Endocr Soc Program Abstracts 1979;95:95.
416. Gruskin A, Baluarte H, Prebis J, et al. Serum sodium abnormalities in children. Pediatr Clin North Am 1982;29:907.
417. Marks J. Central diabetes insipidus. In: Levin D, Morriss F, Moore G, eds. A practical guide to pediatric intensive care. St Louis: CV Mosby, 1984:313.
418. McDonald J, Martha P, Kerrigan J, et al. Treatment of the young child with postoperative central diabetes insipidus. Am J Dis Child 1989;143:201.
419. Cobb W, Spare S, Reichlin S. Neurogenic diabetes insipidus: management with DDAVP (1-desamino-8-D-arginine vasopressin). Ann Intern Med 1978;88:183.
420. Ziai F, Walter R, Rosenthal I. Treatment of central diabetes insipidus in adults and children with desmopressin: a synthetic analogue of vasopressin. Arch Intern Med 1978;138:1382.
421. Brown E, Pollak M, Hebert S. Molecular mechanisms underlying the sensing of extracellular Ca^{2+} by parathyroid and kidney cells. European Journal of Endocrinology 1995;132:523.
422. Johnson J, Kumar R. Renal and intestinal calcium transport: roles of vitamin D and vitamin D-dependent calcium binding proteins. Semin Nephrol 1994;14:119.
423. Broner C, Stidham G, Westenkirchner D, et al. Hypermagnesemia and hypocalcemia as predictors of high mortality in critically ill pediatric patients. Crit Care Med 1990;18:921.
424. Pittinger C, Chang P, Faulkner W. Serum ionized calcium: some factors influencing its level. South Med J 1971;64:1211.
425. Sorell M, Rosen J. Ionized calcium: serum levels during symptomatic hypocalcemia. J Pediatr 1957;87:67.
426. Szyfelbein S, Drop L, Martyn J. Persistent ionized hypocalcemia in patients during resuscitation and recovery phases of body burns. Crit Care Med 1981;9:454.
427. Zaloga G. Hypocalcemia in critically ill patients. Crit Care Med 1992;20:251.
428. Cheung W. Calmodulin plays a pivotal role in cellular regulation. Science 1980;207:19.
429. Allo M, Thompson N, Harness J. Primary hyperparathyroidism in children, adolescents, and young adults. World J Surg 1982;6:771.
430. Kelly T. Primary hyperparathyroidism; a personal experience with 242 cases. Am J Surg 1980;140:632.
431. Mundy G, Ibbotson K, D'Souza S, et al. The hypercalcemia of cancer: clinical implications and pathogenic mechanisms. N Engl J Med 1984;310:1718.
432. Lee D, Zawada E, Kleeman C. The pathophysiology of clinical aspects of hypercalcemic disorders. West J Med 1978;129:278.
433. Al-Rashid R, Cress C. Hypercalcemia associated with neuroblastoma. Am J Dis Child 1979;133:838.
434. Cohen L, Balow JM. Acute tumor lysis syndrome. Am J Med 1980;68:486.
435. Bergstrom W. Hypercalciuria and hypercalcemia complicating immobilization. Am J Dis Child 1978;132:553.
436. Lawrence G, Loeffler R, Martin L, et al. Hypercalcemic disorders. J Bone Joint Surg 1973;55:55.
437. Rosen J, Wolin D, Finberg L. Immobilization hypercalcemia after single limb fractures in children and adolescents. Am J Dis Child 1978; 132:560.
438. Zuiden L, Anquist K, Schachar N, et al. Pathophysiology of immobilization hypercalcemia. Can J Surg 1982;25:646.
439. Adams J. Vitamin D metabolite-mediated hypercalcemia. Endocrinol Metab Clin North Am 1989;18:765.
440. Law W, Heath H. Familial benign hypercalcemia (hypocalciuric hypercalcemia). Ann Intern Med 1985;102:511.
441. Stewart A, Hoecker J, Mallette L, et al. Hypercalcemia in pheochromocytoma. Ann Intern Med 1985;102:776.
442. Lemann J, Worcester E, Gray R. Hypercalciuria and stones. Am J Kidney Dis 1991;17:386.
443. Bilezikian J. Management of acute hypercalcemia. N Engl J Med 1992;326:1196.
444. Mimouni F, Tsang RC. Parathyroid and vitamin D-related disorders. In: Kaplan SA, ed. Clinical pediatric endocrinology. Philadelphia: Saunders, 1990:442.
445. Walton R, Russell R, Smith R. Changes in the renal and extrarenal handling of phosphate induced by disodium etidronate (EHDP) in man. Clin Sci Mol Med 1975;49:45.
446. Haag E, Eklund M, Torring O. Disodium etidronate in hypercalcaemia due to immobilization. Br Med J 1984;288:607.
447. Ellas E, Reynoso G, Mittleman A. Control of hypercalcemia with mithramycin. Ann Surg 1972;175:431.
448. Godfrey T, Loma L. Mithramycin for hypercalcemia of malignant disease. West J Med 1971;115:1.
449. Stewart A. Therapy of malignancy-associated hypercalcemia. Am J Med 1983;74:475.
450. West T, Joffe M, Sinclair L, et al. Treatment of hypercalcemia with calcitonin. Lancet 1971;1:675.
451. Kaul S, Sockalosky J. Human synthetic calcitonin therapy for hypercalcemia of immobilization. J Pediatr 1995;126:825.

452. Gunst MA, Drop LJ. Chronic hypercalcaemia secondary to hyperparathyroidism: a risk factor during anaesthesia? Br J Anaesthes 1980;52:507.
453. Roland EJ, Wierda JM, Eurin BG, et al. Pharmacodynamic behaviour of vecuronium in primary hyperparathyroidism. Can J Anaesthes 1994;41:694.
454. Kirita A, Iwasaki H, Fujita S, et al. Vecuronium-induced neuromuscular blockade in two patients with hyperparathyroidism and a patient with hypoparathyroidism. Jpn J Anesthesiol 1992;41:136.
455. Okamoto T. Effects of magnesium and calcium on muscle contractility and neuromuscular blockade produced by muscle relaxants and aminoglycoside. Jpn J Anesthesiol 1992;41:1910.
456. Sanctis VD, Vullo C, Bagni B, et al. Hypoparathyroidism in beta-thalassemia major: clinical and laboratory observations in 24 patients. Acta Haematologica 1992;88:105.
457. Grosskopf I, Graff E, Charach G, et al. Hyperphosphataemia and hypocalcaemia induced by hypertonic phosphate enema: an experimental study and review of the literature. Human Exp Toxicol 1991;10:351.
458. De Vizia B, Mansi A. Calcium and phosphorus metabolism in full-term infants. Monatsschrift Kinderheilkunde 1992;140:S8.
459. Watchko J, Bifano E, Bergstrom W. Effect of hyperventilation on total calcium, ionized calcium, and serum phosphorus in neonates. Crit Care Med 1984;12:1055.
460. Auffant R, Downs J, Amick R. Ionized calcium concentration and cardiovascular function after cardiopulmonary bypass. Arch Surg 1981;116:1072.
461. Chan J, Young R, Hartenberg M, et al. Calcium and phosphate metabolism in children with idiopathic hypoparathyroidism or pseudohypoparathyroidism: effects of 1,25-dihydroxy vitamin D3. J Pediatr 1985;106:421.
462. Chesney R, Rosen J, DeLuca H. Disorders of calcium metabolism in children. In: Collu R, ed. Recent progress in pediatric endocrinology. Vol 5. New York: Raven, 1983:5
463. Chesney R, McCarron D, Haddad J, et al. Pathogenic mechanisms of the hypocalcemia of the staphylococcal toxic-shock syndrome. J Lab Clin Med 1983;101:576.
464. Denlinger J, Nahrwold M, Gibbs P, et al. Hypocalcaemia during rapid blood transfusion in anaesthetized man. Br J Anaesth 1976;48:995.
465. Freedman D, Shannon M, Dandona P, et al. Hypoparathyroidism and hypocalcaemia during treatment for acute leukaemia. Br Med J 1982;284:700.
466. Fox G. Hypocalcemia complicating bicarbonate therapy for salicylate poisoning. West J Med 1984;141:108.
467. Finsterer U, Betz J, Braun S, et al. Metabolism of phosphate and calcium after severe accidental trauma. Scand J Clin Lab Invest 1983;165:117.
468. Fairris G, Mason P, Fairris N. Hypocalcaemia in pernicious anaemia. Br Med J 1984;288:607.
469. Guberman A, Jaworski Z. Pseudohypoparathyroidism and epilepsy: diagnostic value of computerized cranial tomography. Epilepsia 1979;20:541.
470. Goldsmith M, Parry D. Heparin-induced hypocalcaemia in rabbits. Nature 1966;210:1286.
471. Heubi J, Partin J, Schubert W. Hypocalcemia and steatorrhea: clues to etiology. Dig Dis Sci 1983;28:124.
472. Hayes F, Green A, Senzer N, et al. Tetany: a complication of cis-dichlorodiamineplatinum (II) therapy. Cancer Treat Rep 1979;63:547.
473. Harrigan C, Lucas C, Ledgerwood A. Significance of hypocalcemia following hypovolemic shock. J Trauma 1983;23:488.
474. Johnston CCJ, Grinnan E, Wilson H, et al. Protamine-induced hypocalcemia. Endocrinol 1970;87:1211.
475. John H, Wills M, Marcus R. Changes in plasma calcium concentration following subtotal thyroidectomy. Br J Surg 1966;53:685.
476. Kruse K, Bartels H, Ziegler R, et al. Parathyroid function and serum calcitonin in children receiving anticonvulsant drugs. Eur J Pediatr 1980;133:151.
477. Matsuda I, Takekoshi Y, Tanaka M, et al. Pseudohypoparathyroidism type II and anticonvulsant rickets. Eur J Pediatr 1979;132:303.
478. Olinger G, Hottenrott C, Mulder D. Acute clinical hypocalcemic myocardial depression during rapid blood transfusion and postoperative hemodialysis. J Thorac Cardiovasc Surg 1976;71:503.
479. Piechowiak G, Grobner W, Kremer H, et al. Pseudohypoparathyroidism and hypocalcemia "myopathy"; a case report. Klin Wochenschr 1981;59:1195.
480. Robertson G, Moore E, Switz D, et al. Inadequate parathyroid response in acute pancreatitis. N Engl J Med 1976;294:512.
481. Reyes H, Wright J, Rosenfield R. Prevention of hypocalcemia in children due to parathyroid infarction after thyroidectomy. Surg Gynecol Obstet 1979;148:76.
482. Reedy J, Zwiren G. Enema-induced hypocalcemia and hyperphosphatemia leading to cardiac arrest during induction of anesthesia in an outpatient surgery center. Anesthesiol 1983;59:578.
483. Stamp T. Effects of long-term anticonvulsant therapy on calcium and vitamin D metabolism. Proc R Soc Med 1974;67:64.
484. Tieder M, Modai D, Samuel R, et al. Hereditary hypophosphatemic rickets with hypercalciuria. N Engl J Med 1985;312:611.
485. Taylor B, Sibbald W, Edmonds M, et al. Ionized hypocalcemia in critically ill patients with sepsis. Can J Surg 1978;21:429.
486. Taitz L, Wales J, Spitz L. Hypocalcaemic seizures following gastrectomy. Eur J Pediatr 1983;141:36.
487. Greenberg F. DiGeorge syndrome: an historical review of clinical and cytogenetic features. J Med Genet 1993;30:803.
488. Driscoll D. Genetic basis of DiGeorge and velocardiofacial syndromes. Curr Opinions Pediatr 1994;6:702.
489. Gallardo J, Fardella P, Pumarino H, et al. Plasma calcium levels in critical patients with and without sepsis. Revista Medica de Chile 1991;119:262.
490. Arnaud C, Kolb F. The calcitropic hormones & metabolic bone disease. In: Greenspan F, ed. Basic and clinical endocrinology. Norwalk, CT: Appleton & Lange, 1991:247.
491. Giles T, Iteld B, Rives K. The cardiomyopathy of hypoparathyroidism. Chest 1981;79:225.
492. Murros J, Luomanmaki K. A case of hypocalcemia, heart failure and exceptional repolarization disturbances. Acta Med Scand 1980; 208:133.
493. Troughton O, Singh S. Heart failure and neonatal hypocalcaemia. Br Med J 1972;4:76.
494. Griffin J. Neonatal hypocalcemia and complete heart block. Am J Dis Child 1965;110:672.
495. Johnson J, Jennings R. Hypocalcemia and cardiac arrhythmias. Am J Dis Child 1968;115:373.
496. Gershanik J, Levkoff A, Duncan R. The association of hypocalcemia and recurrent apnea in premature infants. Am J Obstet Gynecol 1972;113:646.
497. Knapp M, Gough K. An unusual neurological manifestation of hypocalcemia. Lancet 1967;1:475.
498. Chaimovitz C. Hypocalcemia hypotension. JAMA 1972;222:86.
499. Chopra D, Janson P, Sawin C. Insensitivity to digoxin associated with hypocalcemia. N Engl J Med 1977;296:917.
500. Clarke P, Carre I. Hypocalcemia, hypomagnesemic convulsions. J Pediatr 1967;70:806.
501. Grant D. Papilloedema and fits in hypoparathyroidism with a report of three cases. Q J Med 1953;22:243.
502. McKie B. Hypocalcaemia and prolonged curarization; a case report. Br J Anaesth 1969;41:1091.
503. Hochberg Z, Moses A, Richman R. Parathyroid hormone infusion test in children and adolescents. Miner Electrolyte Metab 1984;10:113.
504. Collier V, Mitch W. Accelerated progression of chronic renal insufficiency after parathyroidectomy. JAMA 1980;244:1215.
505. Lapatsanis P. Calcium and phosphorus disturbances in children. Paediatrician 1982;11:110.
506. Pettifor J, Ross P, Moodley G, et al. The effect of dietary calcium supplementation on serum calcium, phosphorus, and alkaline phosphatase concentrations in a rural black population. Am J Clin Nutr 1981;34:2187.
507. Wells DAJ, Ross A, Dale J, et al. Transplantation of the parathyroid glands: current status. Surg Clin North Am 1979;59:167.
508. Henrich W, Hunt J, Nixon J. Increased ionized calcium and left ventricular contractility during hemodialysis. N Engl J Med 1984;310:19.
509. Mirro R, Brown D. Parenteral calcium treatment shortens the left ventricular systolic time intervals of hypocalcemia neonates. Pediatr Res 1984;18:71.
510. Redding J, Haynes R, Thomas J. Drug therapy in resuscitation from electromechanical dissociation. Crit Care Med 1983;11:681.
511. Drop L, Cullen D. Comparative effects of calcium chloride and calcium gluceptate. Br J Anaesth 1980;52:501.
512. Drop L, Laver M. Low plasma ionized calcium and response to calcium therapy in critically ill man. Anesthesiology 1975;43:300.
513. White R, Goldsmith R, Rodriguez R, et al. Plasma ionic calcium levels

following injection of chloride, gluconate, and gluceptate salts of calcium. J Thorac Cardiovasc Surg 1978;71:609.
514. Young HA, Ferguson IT. Laryngeal tetany: an unusual presentation of chronic renal failure. J Laryngol Otol 1977;91:373.
515. Waeber G, Pralong G, Breitenstein E, et al. Laryngospasm: unusual manifestation of celiac disease. Schweizerische Medizinische Wochenschrift 1993;123:432.
516. Balestrieri F. Magnesium metabolism in the critically ill patient. In: Chernow B, Geelhoed G, eds. Endocrine aspects of acute illness. New York: Churchill Livingstone, 1985:217.
517. Cronin R. Magnesium disorders. In: Kokko J, Tannen R, eds. Fluids and electrolytes. Philadelphia: WB Saunders, 1990:631.
518. Wong E, Rude R, Singer F, et al. A high prevalence of hypomagnesemia and hypermagnesemia in hospitalized patients. Am Soc Clin Pathol 1983;79:348.
519. Rude R, Singer F. Magnesium deficiency and excess. Annu Rev Med 1981;32:245.
520. Fuchs-Buder T, Wilder-Smith OH, Borgeat A, et al. Interaction of magnesium sulfate with vecuronium-induced neuromuscular block. Br J Anaesthes 1995;74:405.
521. Sinatra RS, Philip BK, Naulty JS, et al. Prolonged neuromuscular blockade with vecuronium in a patient treated with magnesium sulfate. Anesthesi Analges 1985;64:1220.
522. Ghoneim MM, Long JP. The interaction between magnesium and other neuromuscular blocking agents. Anesthesiology 1970;32:23.
523. James MF, Sinatra RS. Succinylcholine pretreatment with magnesium sulfate. Anesthes Analges 1986;65:373.
524. Ryzen E, Wagers P, Singer F, et al. Magnesium deficiency in a medical ICU population. Crit Care Med 1985;13:19.
525. Reinhart R, Desbiens N, et al. Hypomagnesemia in patients entering the ICU. Crit Care Med 1985;13:506.
526. Houston B, Turner T. Severe electrolyte abnormalities in a pregnant patient with a jejunoileal bypass. Arch Intern Med 1978;138:1712.
527. Patel R, Savage A. Symptomatic hypomagnesemia associated with gentamicin therapy. Nephron 1979;23:50.
528. Nanji A, Denegri J. Hypomagnesemia associated with gentamicin therapy. Drug Intell Clin Pharm 1984;18:596.
529. Thomas F, Mucha M, Rush I, et al. Hypomagnesemia: higher risk using total parenteral nutrition in the treatment of patients with malignancies. J Surg Oncol 1980;13:35.
530. Barton C, Pahl M, Vaziri N, et al. Renal magnesium wasting associated with amphotericin B therapy. Am J Med 1984;77:471.
531. Hall K, Dobson K, Dalton J, et al. Metabolic abnormalities associated with intentional theophylline overdose. Ann Intern Med 1984;101:457.
532. Randall B. Fatty liver and sudden death. Hum Pathol 1980;11:147.
533. McLellan B, Reid S, Lane P. Massive blood transfusion causing hypomagnesemia. Crit Care Med 1984;12:146.
534. Sclarra M, Marana E, Cavaliere F, et al. Changes of serum magnesium ions in open heart surgery. Resuscitation 1983;10:253.
535. Agus Z, Wasserstein A, Goldfarb S. Disorders of calcium and magnesium homeostasis. Am J Med 1981;72:473.
536. Flink E. Magnesium deficiency: etiology and clinical spectrum. Acta Med Scand 1981;647:125.
537. Juan D. Clinical review: the clinical importance of hypomagnesemia. Surgery 1982;91:510.
538. Ryzen E, Rude RK. Low intracellular magnesium in patients with acute pancreatitis and hypocalcemia. Western J Med 1990;152:145.
539. Stromme J, Johnsen J, Harnaes K, et al. Familial hypomagnesemia-a follow-up examination of three patients after 9-12 years of treatment. Pediatr Res 1981;15:1134.
540. Duran M, Borst G, Osburne R, et al. Concurrent renal hypomagnesemia and hypoparathyroidism with normal parathormone responsiveness. Am J Med 1984;76:151.
541. Arnold A, Tovey J, Mangat P, et al. Magnesium deficiency in critically ill patients. Anaesthesia 1995;50:203.
542. Garty R, Alkalay A, Bernheim J. Parathyroid hormone secretion and responsiveness to parathyroid hormone in primary hypomagnesemia. Isr J Med Sci 1983;19:345.
543. Miller R, Krebs R, Neal B, et al. Hypomagnesemia: suppression of secondary hyperparathyroidism in chronic renal failure. JAMA 1979;241:722.
544. Wacker W, Moore F, Ulmer D, et al. Normocalcemic magnesium deficiency tetany. JAMA 1962;180:161.
545. Saul R, Selhorst J. Downbeat nystagmus with magnesium depletion. Arch Neurol 1981;38:650.
546. Dhingra S, Solven F, Wilson A, et al. Hypomagnesemia and respiratory muscle power. Am Rev Respir Dis 1984;129:497.
547. Suresh S, Sainani G. Prolonged repolarization and hypomagnesemia. Am Heart J 1978;96:702.
548. Levine S, Crowley T, Hai H. Hypomagnesemia and ventricular tachycardia. Chest 1982;81:244.
549. Chernow B, Smith J, Rainey T, et al. Hypomagnesemia: implications for the critical care specialist. Crit Care Med 1982;10:193.
550. Johansson B. Magnesium infusion in decompensated hypomagnesemic patients. Acta Pharmacol Toxicol 1984;54:125.
551. Lentz R, Brown D, Kjellstrand C. Treatment of severe hypophosphatemia. Ann Intern Med 1978;89:941.
552. Gertner J, Broadus A, Anast C, et al. Impaired parathyroid response to induced hypocalcemia in thalassemia major. J Pediatr 1979;95:210.
553. Lau K. Phosphate disorders. In: Kokko J, Tannen R, eds. Fluids and electrolytes. Philadelphia: WB Saunders, 1990:505.
554. Knochel J. The pathophysiology and clinical characteristics of severe hypophosphatemia. Arch Intern Med 1977;137:203.
555. Stoff J. Phosphate homeostasis and hypophosphatemia. Am J Med 1982;72:489.
556. Streicher Z, Gabow P, Moss A, et al. Syndromes of toluene sniffing in adults. Ann Intern Med 1981;94:758.
557. Carroll J, Kanter R. Hypophosphatemia and Reye's syndrome. Crit Care Med 1985;13:480.
558. Lennquist S, Lindell B, Nerdstrom H, et al. Hypophosphatemia in severe burns. Acta Chir Scand 1979;145:1.
559. Chesney R, Chesney P, Davis J, et al. Renal manifestations of the staphylococcal toxic-shock syndrome. Am J Med 1981;71:583.
560. Borghi L, Canali M, Sani E. Erythrocyte sodium transport in acute hypophosphatemia in man. Miner Electrolyte Metab 1984;10:26.
561. Varsano S, Shapiro M, Taragan R, et al. Hypophosphatemia as a reversible cause of refractory ventilatory failure. Crit Care Med 1983;11:908.
562. O'Connor L, Wheeler W, Buthune J. Effect of hypophosphatemia on myocardial performance in man. N Engl J Med 1977;297:901.
563. Andress D, Vannatta J, Whang R. Treatment of refractory hypophosphatemia. South Med J 1982;75:766.
564. Vannatta J, Whang R, Papper S. Efficacy of intravenous phosphorus therapy in the severely hypophosphatemic patient. Arch Intern Med 1981;141:885.
565. Lloyd CW, Johnson CE. Management of hypophosphatemia. Clin Pharm 1988;7:123.
566. Grasso S, Buffa R, Martino E, et al. Gastrin (G) cells are the cellular site of the gastric thyrotropin-releasing hormone in human fetuses and newborns: a chromatographic, radioimmunological, and immunocytochemical study. J Clini Endocrinol Metabo 1992;74:1421.
567. Evans R. The steroid and thyroid hormone receptor superfamily. Science 1988;240:889.
568. Williams G, Franklyn J, Neuberger J, et al. Thyroid hormone receptor expression in the "sick euthyroid" syndrome. Lancet 1989;2:1477.
569. Klein I, Levey G. New perspectives on thyroid hormone, catecholamines, and the heart. Am J Med 1984;76:167.
570. Dillmann W. Biochemical basis of thyroid hormone action in the heart. Am J Med 1990;88:626.
571. Burman K, Monchik J, Earll J, et al. Ionized and total serum calcium and parathyroid hormone in hyperthyroidism. Ann Intern Med 1976;84:668.
572. Manicourt D, Demeester-Mirkine N, Brauman H, et al. Disturbed mineral metabolism in hyperthyroidism: good correlation with triiodothyronine. Clin Endocrinol 1979;10:407.
573. Daly J, Greenwood R, Himsworth R. Serum calcium concentration in hyperthyroidism at diagnosis and after treatment. Clin Endocrinol 1983;19:397.
574. How J, Davidson R, Bewsher P. Red cell changes in hyperthyroidism. Scand J Haematol 1979;23:323.
575. Kabadi U, Eisenstein A. Glucose intolerance in hyperthyroidism: role of glucagon. J Clin Endocrinol Metab 1980;50:392.
576. Greenspan F, Rappaport B. Thyroid gland. In: Greenspan F, ed. Basic and clinical endocrinology. Norwalk, CT: Appleton & Lange, 1991:188.
577. Morishige W. Thyroid hormone influences glucocorticoid receptor levels in the neonatal rat lung. Endocrinology 1982;111:1017.
578. Chernausek SD, Underwood LE, Utiger RD, et al. Growth hormone secretion and plasma somatomedin-C in primary hypothyroidism. Clin Endocrinol 1983;19:337.
579. Iwatsubo H, Omori K, Okada Y, et al. Human growth hormone secre-

tion in primary hypothyroidism before and after treatment. J Clin Endocrinol Metab 1967;27:1751.
580. Katz HP, Youlton R, Kaplan SL, et al. Growth and growth hormone: III. Growth hormone release in children with primary hypothyroidism and thyrotoxicosis. J Clin Endocrinol 1969;29:346.
581. Kaptein E, Weiner J, Robinson W, et al. Relationship of altered thyroid hormone indices to survival in nonthyroidal illness. Clin Endocrinol 1982;16:565.
582. Slag M, Morley J, Elson M, et al. Hypothyroxinemia in critically ill patients as a predictor of high mortality. JAMA 1981;245:43.
583. Uzel N, Neyzi O. Thyroid function in critically ill infants with infections. Pediatr Infect Dis 1986;5:516.
584. Zucker A, Chernow B, Fields A, et al. Thyroid function in critically ill children. J Pediatr 1985;107:552.
585. Buckingham B, Costin G, Roe T, et al. Hyperthyroidism in children. Am J Dis Child 1981;135:112.
586. Thomas J, Leclere J, Hartemann P, et al. Familial hyperthyroidism without evidence of autoimmunity. Acta Endocrinol 1982;100:512.
587. Jacobs R. Acute hyperthyroidism precipitated by trauma. South Med J 1979;72:890.
588. Hedberg C, Fishbein D, Janssen R, et al. An outbreak of thyrotoxicosis caused by the consumption of bovine thyroid gland in ground beef. N Engl J Med 1987;316:993.
589. Cohen JI, Ingbar S, Braverman L. Thyrotoxicosis due to ingestion of excess thyroid hormone. Endocr Rev 1989;10:113.
590. Lepre F, Cameron D, Hartley L. Toxic adenoma in childhood: case report. Aust Paediatr J 1983;19:258.
591. Hoffman W, Chodoroff G, Piggott L. Haloperidol and thyroid storm. Am J Psychiatry 1978;135:484.
592. Wiener J. Value of the free triiodothyronine index in the diagnosis of hyperthyroidism. Eur J Nucl Med 1980;5:119.
593. Litovitz T, White J. Levothyroxine ingestions in children. Am J Emerg Med 1985;3:297.
594. Rockey P, Griep R. Behavioral dysfunction in hyperthyroidism. Arch Intern Med 1980;140:1194.
595. Clayton G, Foley T, LaFranchi S, et al. Disorders of the thyroid. In: Kaplan S, ed. Clinical pediatric and adolescent endocrinology. Philadelphia: 1982:69.
596. Aiello D, DuPlessis A, Pattishall EI, et al. Thyroid storm: presenting with coma and seizures. Clin Pediatr 1989;28:571.
597. Cooppan R, Kozak GP. Hyperthyroidism and diabetes mellitus. Arch Intern Med 1980;140:370.
598. Lester L, Sodt P, Rich B, et al. Cardiac abnormalities in children with hyperthyroidism. Pediatr Cardiol 1982;2:215.
599. Neal P, Jansen R, Lemons J, et al. Unusual manifestations of neonatal hyperthyroidism. Am J Perinatol 1985;2:231.
600. Stockigt J, Topliss D. Diagnosis and management of hyperthyroidism. Med J Aust 1986;145:278.
601. Scherlitz A, Peters J. A guidewire as a reintubation aid: translaryngeal fiberoptic insertion of a guidewire into the trachea to assist fiberoptic reintubation in patients difficult to intubate. Anaesthetist 1994;43:618.
602. Shaha A, Alfonso A, Jaffe BM. Acute airway distress due to thyroid pathology. Surgery 1987;102:1068.
603. Greatorex RA, Denny NM. Application of the laryngeal mask airway to thyroid surgery and the preservation of the recurrent laryngeal nerve. Ann Roy Coll Surg Engl 1991;73:352.
604. McHenry CR, Piotrowski JJ. Thyroidectomy in patients with marked thyroid enlargement: airway management. Am Surg 1994;60:586.
605. Lammer H, Mitterschiffthaler G, Fischer F. The lingual thyroid, an unexpected and rare intubation difficulty. Anaesthetist 1989;38:206.
606. Munro SL, Lim CF, Hall JG, et al. Drug competition for thyroxine binding to transthyretin (prealbumin): comparison with effects on thyroxine-binding globulin. J Clin Endocrinol Metab 1989;68:1141.
607. Lim CF, Bai Y, Topliss DJ, et al. Drug and fatty acid effects on serum thyroid hormone binding. J Clin Endocrinol Metab 1988;67:682.
608. Chung KS, Sinatra RS, Halevy JD, et al. A comparison of fentanyl, esmolol, and their combination for blunting the haemodynamic responses during rapid-sequence induction. Can J Anaesth 1992;39:774.
609. Sklar BZ, Lurie S, Ezri T, et al. Lidocaine inhalation attenuates the circulatory response to laryngoscopy and endotracheal intubation. J Clin Anesth 1992;4:382.
610. Vucevic M, Purdy GM, Ellis FR. Esmolol hydrochloride for management of the cardiovascular stress responses to laryngoscopy and tracheal intubation. Br J Anaesth 1992;68:529.
611. Helfman SM, Gold MI, DeLisser EA, et al. Which intubation drug prevents tachycardia and hypertension associated with tracheal intubation: lidocaine, fentanyl, or esmolol. Anesth Analg 1991;72:482.
612. Wiest DB, Trippel DL, Gillette PC, et al. Pharmacokinetics of esmolol in children. Clin Pharmacol Therapeut 1991;49:618.
613. Cuneo BF, Zales VR, Blahunka PC, et al. Pharmacodynamics and pharmacokinetics of esmolol, a short-acting beta-blocking agent, in children. Pediatr Cardiol 1994;15:296.
614. Volz-Zang C, Eckrich B, Jahn P, et al. Esmolol, an ultrashort-acting, selective beta 1-adrenoceptor antagonist: pharmacodynamic and pharmacokinetic properties. Europ J Clin Pharmacol 1994;46:399.
615. Eibs HG, Oberdisse U, Brambach U. Intoxication with beta-receptor blockers. Deutsche Medizinische Wochenschrift 1982;107:1139.
616. Taboulet P, Cariou A, Berdeaux A, et al. Pathophysiology and management of self-poisoning with beta-blockers. J Toxicol [Clin] 1993;31:531.
617. Critchley JA, Ungar A. The management of acute poisoning due to beta-adrenoceptor antagonists. Med Toxicol Adverse Drug Exper 1989;4:32.
618. Sengupta A, Gupta PK, Pandey K. Investigation of glycopyrrolate as a premedicant drug. Br J Anaesthes 1980;52:513.
619. Martin WH, Spina RJ, Korte E. Effect of hyperthyroidism of short duration on cardiac sensitivity to beta-adrenergic stimulation. J Am Coll Cardiol 1992;19:1185.
620. Polikar R, Burger AG, Scherrer U, et al. The thyroid and the heart. Circulation 1993;87:1435.
621. Weiner N. Norepinephrine, epinephrine, and the sympathomimetic amines. In: Gilman AG, Gilman LS, Gilman A, eds. The pharmacological basis of therapeutics. 6th Edn. New York: Macmillan, 1980:163.
622. Zsigmond EK, Kelsch RC, Kothary SP. Rise in plasma free norepinephrine during anesthetic induction with ketamine. Behav Neuropsych 1975;6:81.
623. Kaplan JA, Cooperman LH. Alarming reactions to ketamine in patients taking thyroid medication treatment with propanolol. Anesthesiology 1971;35:229.
624. Kotake Y. In vitro effects of anesthetics on hydrogen peroxide generating system of the thyroid gland. Masui–Jpn J Anesthesiol 1993;42:1820.
625. Massart C, LeTellier C, Malledant Y, et al. Modulation of the functional properties of human thyrocytes in monolayer of follicle culture: effects of some anaesthetic drugs. J Molec Endocrinol 1991;7:57.
626. Brofman JD, Leff AR, Munoz NM, et al. Sympathetic secretory response to hypercapnic acidosis in swine. J Applied Physiol 1990;69:710.
627. Guedel AE. Metabolism and reflex irritability in anesthesia. JAMA 1924;83:1736.
628. Munson ES, Hoffman JC, DiFazio CA. The effects of acute hypothyroidism and hyperthyroidism on cyclopropane requirements in rats. Anesthesiology 1968;29:1094.
629. Babad AA, Eger EI 2d. The effects of hyperthyroidism and hypothyroidism on halothane and oxygen requirements in dogs. Anesthesiology 1968;29:1087.
630. Barker SB, Klitgaard HM. Metabolism of tissues excised from thyroxine-injected rats. Am J Physiol 1952;170:81.
631. Munson ES, Eger EI 2d. The effects of hyperthermia and hypothermia on the rate of induction of anesthesia: calculations using a mathematical model. Anesthesiology 1970;33:515.
632. Vitez TS, White PF, Eger EI 2d. Effects of hypothermia on halothane MAC and isoflurane MAC in the rat. Anesthesiology 1974;41:80.
633. Eger EI, Johnson BH. MAC of I-653 in rats, including a test of the effect of body temperature and anesthetic duration. Anesthes Analges 1987;66:974.
634. Antognini JF. Hypothermia eliminates isoflurane requirements at 20 degrees C. Anesthesiology 1993;78:1152.
635. Munson ES, Eger EI 2d, Bowers DL. The effects of changes in cardiac output and distribution on the rate of cerebral anesthetic equilibration: calculations using a mathematical model. Anesthesiology 1968;29:533.
636. Eger EI 2d, Bahlman SH, Halsey MJ, et al. The effect of distribution of increased cardiac output on the pulmonary exchange of halothane, nitrous oxide, and methoxyflurane. Anesthes Analges 1973;52:625.
637. Rodriguez M, Gomeez MR, Howard FM Jr, et al. Myasthenia gravis in children: long-term follow-up. Ann Neurol 1983;13:504.
638. Lawless ST, Reeves G, Bowen JR. The development of thyroid storm in a child with McCune-Albright syndrome after orthopedic surgery. Am J Dis Child 1992;146:1099.
639. Peters KR, Nance P, Wingard WW. Malignant hyperthyroidism or malignant hyperthermia? Anesthes Analges 1981;60:613.
640. Allen GC, Rosenberg H. Phaeochromocytoma presenting as acute malignant hyperthermia: a diagnostic challenge. Can J Anesthes 1990; 37:593.

641. Ambesh SP. Occult pheochromocytoma in association with hyperthyroidism presenting under general anesthesia. Anesthes Analges 1993;77:1074.
642. Tan WC, Cheah JS. The role of sympathomimetic amines in the dyspnoea of thyrotoxicosis. Ann Acad Med (Singapore) 1983;12:462.
643. Serlin S. Intraoperative hyperthermia associated with intraventricular hemorrhage. J Clin Anesthes 1991;3:153.
644. Caroff SN. The neuroleptic malignant syndrome. J Clin Psychiatry 1980;41:79.
645. Heiman-Patterson TD. Neuroleptic malignant syndrome and malignant hyperthermia: important issues for the medical consultant. Med Clin North Am 1993;77:477.
646. Shemin D, Cohn PS, Zipin SB. Pheochromocytoma presenting as rhabdomyolysis and acute myoglobinuric renal failure. Arch Intern Med 1990;159:2384.
647. Bennett WR, Huston DP. Rhabdomyolysis in thyroid storm. Am J Med 1984;77:733.
648. DeRosa G, Testa A, Menichella G, et al. Plasmapheresis in the therapy of hyperthyroidism associated with leukopenia. Haematologica 1991;76:72.
649. Binimelis J, Bassas L, Marruecos L, et al. Massive thyroxine intoxication: evaluation of plasma extraction. Intens Care Med 1987;13:33.
650. Sakata S, Komaki T, Kojima N, et al. The effect of double filtration plasmapheresis on thyroid hormone economy and thyroid function. Jpn J Med 1986;25:246.
651. Carter JN, Eastman CJ, Kilham HA, et al. Rational therapy for thyroid storm. 1975;5:458.
652. Anaissie E, Tohme JF. Reserpine in propanolol-resistant thyroid storm. Arch Intern Med 1985;145:2248.
653. Mazzaferri EL, Skillman TG. Thyroid storm: a review of 22 episodes with special emphasis on the use of guanethidine. Arch Intern Med 1969;124:684.
654. Tsunoda T, Mochinaga N, Eto T, et al. Lithium carbonate in the preoperative preparation of Graves' disease. Jpne J Surg 1991;21:292.
655. Mackin JF, Canary JJ, Pittman CS. Thyroid storm and its management. N Engl J Medi 1974;291:1396.
656. Prange AJ Jr, Lipton MA, Shearin RB, et al. The influence of thyroid status on the effects and metabolism of pentobarbital and thiopental. Biochemic Pharmacol 1966;15:237.
657. Saenger P, Rifkind AB, New MI. Changes in drug metabolism in children with thyroid disorders. J Clin Endocrinol Metab 1976;42:155.
658. Baeza A, Aguayo J, Barria M, et alG. Rapid preoperative preparation in hyperthyroidism. 1991.
659. Feek CM, Sawers JS, Irvine WJ, et al. Combination of potassium iodide and propanolol in preparation of patients with Graves' disease for thyroid surgery. N Engl J Med 1980;302:883.
660. Lennquist S, Jortso E, Anderberg B, et al. Beta blockers compared with antithyroid drugs as preoperative treatment in hyperthyroidism: drug tolerance, complications, and postoperative thyroid function. Surgery 1985;98:1141.
661. Thorne AC, Bedford RF. Esmolol for perioperative management of thyrotoxic goiter. Anesthesiology 1989;71:291.
662. Stehling LC. Anesthetic management of the patient with hyperthyroidism. Anesthesiology 1974;41:585.
663. Lee KS, Kim K, Hur KB, et al. The role for propanolol in the preoperative preparation of patients with Graves' disease. Surg Gynecol Obstet 1986;162:365.
664. Lumosky GI, Ivanova NA, Kabanova GM. Preoperative treatment of patients with thyrotoxicosis. Am J Surg 1984;147:263.
665. Peden NR, Gunn A, Browning MC, et al. Nadolol and potassium iodide in combination in the surgical treatment of thyrotoxicosis. Br J Surg 1982;69:638.
666. Dial P, Hastings PR. The use of a selective beta-adrenergic receptor blocker for the preoperative preparation of thyrotoxic patients. Ann Surg 1982;196:633.
667. Adlerberth A, Stenstrom G, Hasselgrom PO. The selective beta 1-blocking agent metoprolol compared with antithyroid drug and thyroxine as preoperative treatment of patients with hyperthyroidism. Results from a prospective, randomized study. Ann Surg 1987; 205:182.
668. Netterville JL, Aly A, Ossoff RH. Evaluation and treatment of complications of thyroid and parathyroid surgery. Otolaryngol Clin North Am 1990;23:529.
669. Shaha AR, Jaffe BM. Practical management of post-thyroidectomy hematoma. J Surg Oncol 1994;57:235.
670. McHenry CR, Speroff T, Wentworth D, et al. Risk factors for postthyroidectomy hypocalcemia. Surgery 1994;116:641.
671. Brent GA, Hershman JM. Thyroxine therapy in patients with severe non-thyroidal illness and low serum thyroxine concentration. J Clini Endocrinol Metab 1986;63:1.
672. Wilson D, Hopper A, McDougall I, et al. Serum free thyroxine values in term, premature, and sick infants. J Pediatr 1982;101:113.
673. Yuksel A, Yalcin E, Cenani A. Influence of long-term carbamazepine treatment on thyroid function. Acta Paediatrica Japonica 1993;35:229.
674. Isojarvi JI, Pakarinen AJ, Myllyla VV. Thyroid function with antiepileptic drugs. Epilepsia 1992;33:142.
675. Lyen K, Finegold D, Orsini R, et al. Transient thyroid suppression associated with topically applied povidone-iodine. Am J Dis Child 1982;136:369.
676. L'Allemand D, Gruters A, Heidemann P, et al. Iodine-induced alterations of thyroid function in newborn infants after prenatal and perinatal exposure to povidone iodine. J Pediatr 1983;102:935.
677. Zaloga G, O'Brian J. Euthyroid sick syndrome. Am Fam Physician 1985;31:236.
678. Zaloga G, Chernow B. Thyroid function in acute illness. In: Chernow B, Geelhoed G, eds. Endocrine aspects of acute illness. New York: Churchill Livingstone, 1985:67.
679. Willi S, Moshang TJ. Diagnostic dilemmas: results of screening tests for congenital hypothyroidism. Pediatr Clinic North Am 1991;38:555.
680. Ahmad N, Cohen M. Thyroid storm with normal serum triiodothyronine level during diabetic ketoacidosis. JAMA 1981;245:2516.
681. Bernasconi S, Vanelli M, Nori G, et al. Serum TSH, T4, T3, FT4, FT3, rT3, and TBG in youngsters with non-ketotic insulin-dependent diabetes mellitus. Horm Res 1984;20:213.
682. Chiarelli F, Tumini S, Verrotti A, et al. Effects of ketoacidosis and puberty on basal and TRH-stimulated thyroid hormones and TSH in children with diabetes mellitus. Horm Metab Res 1989;21:494.
683. Chiarelli F, Verrotti A, Tumini S, et al. Fibronectin and thyroid hormones in children with diabetic ketoacidosis. Acta Paediatr Scand 1987;76:665.
684. Livesey E, Brook C. Thyroid dysfunction after radiotherapy and chemotherapy of brain tumors. Arch Dis Child 1989;64:593.
685. Pennington JA. A review of iodine toxicity reports. J Am Diet Assoc 1990;90:1571.
686. L'Allemand D, Gruters A, Beyer P, et al. Iodine in contrast agents and skin disinfectants is the major cause for hypothyroidism in premature infants during intensive care. Horm Res 1987;28:42.
687. Smerdely P, Boyages S, Wu D, et al. Topical iodine-containing antiseptics and neonatal hypothyroidism in very-low-birthweight infants. Lancet 1989:661.
688. Murkin JN. Anesthesia and hypothyroidism: a review of thyroxine physiology, pharmacology, and anesthetic implications. Anesthes Analges 1982;61:371.
689. White VA, Kumagai LF. Preoperative endocrine and metabolic considerations. Medi Clin North Am 1979;63:1321.
690. Kim JM, Hackman L. Anesthesia for untreated hypothyroidism: report of three cases. Anesthes Analges 1977;56:299.
691. Kato R, Takanaka A, Takahashi A. Effect of thyroid hormone on the substrate interaction with P-450 in the oxidation of drugs by liver microsomes. J Biochem 1970;68:613.
692. Duranti R, Gheri RG, Gorini M, et al. Control of breathing in patients with severe hypothyroidism. Am J Med 1993;95:29.
693. McBrien DJ, Hindle W. Myxoedema and heart failure. Lancet 1963;1:1066.
694. Siafakas NM, Salesiotou V, Filaditaki V, et al. Respiratory muscle strength in hypothyroidism. Chest 1992;102:189.
695. Miller LR, Benumof JL, Alexander L, et al. Completely absent response to peripheral nerve stimulation in an acutely hypothyroid patient. Anesthesiology 1989;71:779.
696. Szilagyi A, Lerman S, Barr RG, et al. Reversible lactose malabsorption and intolerance in Graves' disease. Clin Investig Med 1991;14:188.
697. Ladenson PW, Levin AA, Ridgway EC, et al. Complications of surgery in hypothyroid patients. Am J Med 1984;77:261.
698. Vacanti FX, Ryan JF. Temperature regulation. In: Cote CJ, Ryan JF, Todres ID, et al, eds. A practice of anesthesia for infants and children. Philadelphia: Saunders, 1993:
699. Ward HC, Halliday D, Sims AJ. Protein and energy metabolism with biosynthetic human growth hormone after gastrointestinal surgery. Ann Surg 1987;206:56.
700. Ross R, Miell J, Holly J, et al. Levels of GH binding activity, IGFBP-1,

insulin, blood glucose and cortisol in intensive care patients. Clini Endocrinol 1991;35:361.
701. Clemmons DR, Underwood LE. Role of insulin-like growth factors and growth hormone in reversing catabolic states. Hormone Res 1992;38:37.
702. Veldhuis JD, Rogers RJ, Dee A, et al. The insulin-like growth factor, somatomedin-C, induces the synthesis of cholesterol side-chain cleavage P-450 and adrenodoxin in ovarian cells. J Biol Chem 1986;261:2499.
703. Froesch ER, Guler HP, Schmid C, et al. Therapeutic potential of insulin-like growth factor. I. Trends Endocrinol Metab 1990;1:254.
704. Herndon DN, Barrow RE, Kunkel KR, et al. Effects of recombinant human growth hormone on donor-site healing in severely burned children. Ann Surg 1990;212:424.
705. Koea JB, Douglas RG, Shaw JH, et al. Growth hormone therapy initiated before starvation ameliorates the catabolic state and enhances the protein-sparing effect of total parenteral nutrition. Br J Surg 1993;80:740.
706. Hammarqvist F, Stromberg C, von der Decken A, et al. Biosynthetic human growth hormone preserves both muscle protein synthesis and the decrease in muscle-free glutamine, and improves whole-body nitrogen economy after operation. Ann Surg 1992;216:184.
707. Ziegler TR, Rombeau JL, Young LS, et al. Recombinant human growth hormone enhances the metabolic efficacy of parenteral nutrition: a double-blind, randomized controlled study. J Clin Endocrinol Metab 1992;74:865.
708. Pape GS, Friedman M, Underwood LE, et al. The effect of growth hormone on weight gain and pulmonary function in patients with chronic obstructive lung disease. Chest 1991;99:1495.
709. Roth E, Valentini L, Semsroth M, et al. Resistance of nitrogen metabolism to growth hormone treatment in the early phase after injury of patients with multiple injuries. J Trauma 1995;38:136.
710. Quinlivan JK, Roberts WA. Intraoperative octreotide for refractory carcinoid-induced bronchospasm. Anesthes Analges 994;78:400.
711. Debas HT, Gittes G. Somatostatin analogue therapy in functioning neuroendocrine gut tumors. Digestion 1993;54:68.
712. Warner RR, Mani S, Profeta J, et al. Octreotide treatment of carcinoid hypertensive crisis. Mt Sinai J Med 1994;61:349.
713. Buckley FP. Anesthesia and obesity and gastrointestinal disorders. In: Barash PG, Cullen BF, Stoelting RK, eds. Clinical Anesthesia. 2d ed. Philadelphia: Lippincott, 1992:1181.
714. Roy R, Carter RF, Wright PD. Somatostatin, anaesthesia and the carcinoid syndrome: peri-operative administration of a somatostatin analogue to suppress carcinoid tumour activity. Anaesthesia 1987; 42:627.
715. Wang LT, Wilkins EW Jr, Bode HH. Bronchial carcinoid tumors in pediatric patients. Chest 1993;103:1426.
716. Hancock BJ, DiLorenzo M, Youssef S, et al. Childhood primary pulmonary neoplasms. J Pediatr Surg 1993;28:1133.
717. Hause DW, Harvey JC. Endobronchial carcinoid and mucoepidermoid carcinoma in children. J Surg Oncol 1991;46:270.
718. Ward JC. Inborn errors of metabolism of acute onset in infancy. Pediatr Rev 1990;11:205.
719. Edelstein G, Hirshmann CA. Hyperthermia and ketoacidosis during anesthesia in a child with glycogen-storage disease. Anesthesiology 1980;52:90.
720. Cox JM. Anesthesia and glycogen-storage disease. Anesthesiology 1968;29:1221.
721. Rosen KR, Broadman LM. Anesthesia for diagnostic muscle biopsy in an infant with Pompe's disease. Can Anaes Soc J 1986;33:790.
722. McFarlane HJ, Soni N. Pompe's disease and anesthesia. Anaesthesia 1986;41:1219.
723. Hsia DJ. Galactosemia. Springfield, Ill.: Charles C. Thomas, 1969.
724. Nyhan WL. Abnormalities in amino acid metabolism in clinical medicine. Norwalk, CT: Appleton-Century-Crofts, 1984.
725. Parris WC, Quimby CW Jr. Anesthetic considerations for the patient with homocystinuria. Anesthes Analges 1982;61:708.
726. Delaney A, Gal TJ. Hazards of anesthesia and operation in maple-syrup-urine disease. Anesthesiology 1976;44:83.
727. Herrick IA, Rhine EJ. The mucopolysaccharidoses and anesthesia: a report of clinical experience. Can J Anaesthes 1988;35:67.
728. Wilder RT, Belani KG. Fiberoptic intubation complicated by pulmonary edema in a 12-year old child with Hurler sydrome. Anesthesiology 1990;72:205.
729. Baines D, Keneally J. Anaesthetic implications of the mucopolysaccharidoses: a fifteen-year experience in a children's hospital. Anaesthes Intens Care 1983;11:198.
730. Renteria VG, Ferrans VJ, Roberts WC. The heart in the Hurler syndrome: gross, histologic and ultrastructural observations in five necropsy cases. Am J Cardiol 1976;38:487.
731. Kempthorne PM, Brown TC. Anesthesia and the mucopolysaccharidoses: a survey of techniques and problems. Anaesthes Intens Care 1983;11:203.
732. Birkinshaw KJ. Anaesthesia in a patient with an unstable neck: Morquio syndrome. Anaesthesia 1975;30:46.
733. Jones AEP, Croley TF. Morquio syndrome and anesthesia. Anesthesiology 1979;51.
734. Hopkins R, Watson JA, Jones JH, et al. Two cases of Hunter's sydrome: the anaesthetic and operative difficulties in oral surgery. Br J Oral Surg 1973;10:286.
735. Batshaw ML, Brusilow S, Waber L, et al. Treatment of inborn errors of urea synthesis: activation of alternative pathways of waste nitrogen synthesis and excretion. N Engl J Med 1982;306:1387.
736. Batshaw M, Monahan P. Treatment of urea cycle disorders. Enzyme 1987;38:242.
737. Batshaw ML, Hyman SL, Coyle JT, et al. Effect of sodium benzoate and sodium phenylacetate on brain serotonin turnover in the ornithine transcarbamylase-deficient sparse-fur mouse. Pediatr Res 1988;23:368.
738. Larson LO, Wilkins RG. Anesthesia and the Lesch-Nyhan syndrome. Anesthesiology 1985;63:197.
739. Dundee JW, McCleery WNC, McLoughlin G. The hazard of thiopental anesthesia in porphyria. Anesthes Analges 1962;41:567.
740. Mustajoki P, Heinonen J. General anesthesia in "inducible" porphyria. Anesthesiology 1980;55:15.
741. Rizk SF, Jacobson JH 2d, Silvay G. Ketamine as an induction agent for acute intermittent porphyria. Anesthesiology 1977;46:305.
742. Famewo CE. Induction of anaesthesia with etomidate in a patient with acute intermittent porphyria. Can Anaes Soc J 1985;32:171.
743. Mitterschiffthaler G, Theiner A, Hetzel H, et al. Safe use of propofol in a patient with acute intermittent porphyria. Br J Anaesthes 1988;60:109.

Poisoning and the Critically Ill Child

40

Alan D. Woolf
Ivor D. Berkowitz
Erica Liebelt
Mark C. Rogers

INTRODUCTION

Childhood poisoning is a common clinical problem encountered by the pediatric intensive care specialist. Although intense educational efforts by health care providers and the use of childproof medication containers since 1972 have continued to reduce the morbidity and mortality from poisoning[1], approximately 100 children in the United States who are less than 5 years of age still die annually from poisoning, and many thousands of critically ill poisoned children are admitted to pediatric intensive care units throughout the country[2].

In general, poisoning in children who are less than 5 years of age is accidental and accounts for about 85% to 90% of pediatric poisoning[3,4]. The exploratory behavior of children in this age category together with the lack of close supervision, particularly in psychologically and economically stressed families[5,6], may allow the child access to medication and other noxious household agents. Less frequently, intentional poisoning—a form of child abuse—occurs in young children[7,8,9].

Poisoning in the child who is older than 5 years is generally considered intentional and comprises the remaining 10% to 15% of childhood poisonings. Alcohol and street drugs are popular with teenagers to produce mood changes, and unintentional overdoses will occasionally ensue. Suicide attempts or suicide gestures account for most hospital admissions of poisoned teenagers[10]. **Table 40.1** lists the agents most frequently responsible for severe poisoning in children. Accidental intoxication in young children is usually caused by the ingestion of a single product. Conversely, suicidal adolescents frequently ingest multiple drugs, potentially making both the diagnosis and the management of intoxication in such patients more complicated and difficult.

CLINICAL APPROACH TO THE POISONED CHILD

Immediate Evaluation and Diagnosis

Since respiratory failure with hypoxia, hypotension, arrhythmias, and seizures are the most life threatening systemic manifestations of drug intoxication, emergency cardiorespiratory stabilization and basic life support must precede any

Table 40.1. Drugs Involved in Serious Childhood Poisonings[a]

Drugs	*Others*
Acetaminophen	Alcohols (ethyl, isopropyl, methyl)
Antiarrhythmics	Ethylene glycol
Anticonvulsants	Caustics
Antihistamines	Herbicides
Antihypertensives	Organophosphates
Aminophylline	Other Pesticides
Aspirin	Petroleum distillates
β-Blockers	
Calcium channel blockers	
Digoxin	
Hallucinogens	
Iron	
Opioids	
Oral hypoglycemic agents	
Theophylline	
Tricyclic antidepressants	

[a]From Kilham HA. Hospital management of severe poisoning. Pediatr Clin North Am 1980;27:603.

diagnostic steps in the poisoned child, in either the emergency room or the pediatric intensive care unit[11]. It is desirable that a "team approach" to the poisoned child be taken. The most skilled team member should initially evaluate the patient and initiate the emergency stabilization phase, while other members obtain a history and diagnostic and therapeutic information from a poison control center or other resources.

Respiratory

Respiratory failure can complicate other symptoms of intoxication such as upper airway obstruction, central nervous system depression, continuous convulsions, neuromuscular blockade, increased oral and airway secretions, aspiration, and pulmonary edema[11]. Ensuring the adequacy of the patient's airway is the first priority. This can be accomplished by chin lift or jaw thrust maneuvers, or by the placement of an oral or nasopharyngeal airway or an endotracheal tube. Only endotracheal intubation will protect the airway of a comatose patient, whose gag reflex is absent, from the hazards of aspiration. After airway patency is ensured, the adequacy of ventilation is assessed and, if necessary, manually or mechanically assisted. Supplemental oxygen should be administered.

Cardiovascular

Cardiovascular stabilization requires close monitoring of the blood pressure, heart rate, electrocardiogram, and urine output, as well as the adequacy of peripheral perfusion by clinical examination, blood gases, and even blood lactate determinations. Adequate intravenous access must be secured. Emergency blood tests can be obtained with the placement of an intravenous line.

Hypotension in the poisoned child is usually associated with absolute or relative hypovolemia, either due to arteriolar or venous vasodilatation or due to capillary leakage with third-space fluid loss[12,13]. This hypotension is usually responsive to rapid intravenous fluid administration of isotonic crystalloid solution. There should be no reluctance to insert a central venous line or even a Swan-Ganz catheter for further hemodynamic evaluation and management if the hypotension is resistant to volume infusion. Hypotension may also be temporarily reversed by the application of military antishock trousers (MAST suit). Since arrhythmias and myocardial depression are less frequent contributing factors to hypotension[11], antiarrhythmics and vasoactive drugs such as dopamine or epinephrine are only occasionally required to restore a normal blood pressure.

The detection of arrhythmias depends upon continuous electrocardiographic monitoring. The specific therapy of complicating arrhythmias is best accomplished after the identity of the intoxicating agent is known, but emergency therapy is often needed before a specific poisoning is diagnosed. Potentially aggravating factors such as hypotension, hypoxia, and electrolyte and acid-base abnormalities should be appropriately treated. The management of specific arrhythmias that complicate particular intoxications is discussed in their respective sections later in this chapter.

The following comments are only a brief overview of the acute management of some drug-induced arrhythmias. The most classic arrhythmias of concern in intoxicated pediatric patients are frequent ventricular ectopic beats and ventricular tachycardia. These are initially treated with lidocaine or bretylium, the same drugs that are usually used for managing these arrhythmias in nonpoisoned patients. However, in the case of intoxication with membrane depressant drugs such as the tricyclic antidepressants (TCAs), some conventional antiarrhythmics such as procainamide or quinidine are contraindicated[13]. These TCA-related arrhythmias generally respond to administration of sodium bicarbonate, although Lidocaine may also be used, and if necessary, a secondary drug such as phenytoin should be considered. Sinus or junctional bradycardia may respond to intravenous atropine. Complete atrioventricular (AV) block may require a transvenous pacemaker.

Neurologic

If there is any suspicion of concomitant head trauma, the cervical spine should be immobilized until a thorough radiographic examination has excluded cervical spine injury. Seizures developing in an intoxicated patient may be caused directly by drug toxicity or may reflect hypoxia, hypoglycemia, or electrolyte disturbances. Vigorous attempts must be made to correct any underlying metabolic disturbance, as well as to control these seizures with anticonvulsants such as diazepam, lorazepam, midazolam, phenobarbital, or phenytoin.

After initial cardiorespiratory stabilization and treatment of seizures, general supportive care must be instituted. Attention must be directed toward optimizing fluid, electrolyte, acid-base, glucose, and temperature homeostasis, as well as toward establishing a diagnosis.

Diagnosis

The diagnosis of poisoning may be obvious when, for example, a young child is found with an empty drug bottle in hand or with a mouth full of pill fragments. In many cases, however, the diagnosis is difficult or not even considered, either because an older patient purposefully falsifies the medical history or because the patient, due to insufficient age or confused mental status, is unable to provide accurate information.

Since there are some poisonings, albeit only a few, where the administration of a specific antidote may be lifesaving, it is paramount for the clinician always to consider the possible diagnosis of poisoning. This is especially the case when a child in the "at risk" group of less than 5 years old has developed acute symptoms of disturbed consciousness, abnormal behavior, seizures, coma, an unusual odor, respiratory distress, shock, arrhythmias, metabolic acidosis, severe vomiting and diarrhea, cyanosis, unresponsiveness to oxygen (methemoglobinemia), or other puzzling multisystem disorders[15].

In addition, underlying drug and ethanol intoxication should be considered in adolescent and adult victims of accidental trauma. Laboratory tests may be necessary to rule out the presence of "silent" or co-ingested toxins present with no symptoms such as acetaminophen. Local poison control centers can be of assistance in making a diagnosis in an unknown poisoning, developing a management strategy, and locating exotic antidotes[16].

History

During the stabilization period, information should be obtained either from the patient's parents, family members, or friends, or from paramedics who have accompanied the patient to the hospital, about the possible intoxicating agents, the mode of intoxication, the maximum potential dose, and the time since exposure[15]. If poisoning is suspected but the history is not confirmative, information about available drugs in the home should be obtained by asking about illnesses of the patient or of other family members. Knowledge of the initial clinical symptomatology prior to arrival at a facility is certainly helpful. Poisoning as a form of child abuse should be considered if the history does not appear consistent with the physical and laboratory findings[7] (Dine).

Physical Examination

A physical examination is particularly important for any patient with a questionable exposure to a toxic agent[15]. Specific physical findings may be elicited that can either suggest a diagnosis of poisoning by a particular agent or group of drugs **(Table 40.2)**[14] or else indicate that an underlying medical disease rather than an intoxication is the cause of the clinical problem.

The initial assessment will include noting vital signs. Blood pressure, heart rate and rhythm, respiratory pattern and rate, and body temperature can be altered by certain poisonings. Hypertension is a prominent feature of intoxication with sympathomimetic agents, particularly phenylpropanolamine, phencyclidine, and amphetamines. Narcotics, sedative hypnotics, TCAs, calcium channel blockers, and β-blocker overdoses frequently produce hypotension. Clonidine may present with either hypotension or hypertension.

Severe poisoning with alcohol, narcotics, barbiturates, and the sedative hypnotics are marked by depressed respiration. Tachypnea and Kussmaul respirations are symptoms frequently associated with salicylate poisoning, metabolic acidosis related to ethylene glycol ingestion, methanol ingestion, and cyanide poisoning.

Examination of the oral mucous membrane is important. A dry mouth is typical of anticholinergic intoxication. Excess salivation is an easily recognized sign of exposure to organophosphate and carbamate insecticides. Oral burns are often present after ingestion of corrosive agents, such as alkalis, acids, and paraquat. Specific odors of certain agents on the patient's breath can provide vital diagnostic information. For instance, the smell of bitter almonds is associated with cyanide, and a garlic odor with arsenic or organophosphate poisoning.

Close attention must be paid to the physical examination of the skin, which includes observation of skin color and temperature, noting the presence or absence of sweating, and a search for skin lesions. Cyanosis unresponsive to oxygen is indicative of methemoglobinemia. Sweating is a feature of sympathomimetic or organophosphate poisoning and dry, warm skin can be indicative of anticholinergic poisoning.

The cardiac and electrocardiographic examination may suggest specific intoxications. Bradycardia is a prominent feature of digitalis, cholinergic, clonidine, and β-blocker intoxication. Supraventricular tachycardia is frequently associated with aminophylline, phencyclidine (PCP), TCA, phenothiazine, and other anticholinergic drug intoxication. Ventricular premature beats and life-threatening ventricular tachyarrhythmias may complicate intoxication with digitalis, tricyclics and other anticholinergics, cocaine, phenylpropanolamine, and other over-the-counter sympathomimetics. Hypoxia, especially when caused by carbon monoxide or cyanide intoxication, may also precipitate these serious arrhythmias. A prolonged Q-T interval and widened QRS complexes are seen with either TCA or phenothiazine intoxication. A prolonged Q-T interval alone is suggestive of hypocalcemia that may accompany ethylene glycol intoxication. Chemical asphyxiants, such as cyanide, carbon monoxide, and hydrogen sulfide, may also cause acute S-T segment elevations, suggesting diffuse myocardial injury.

Examination of the lungs can also provide unexpected clues related to the nature of a poisoning. Wheezing is typical of organophosphate poisoning. Rales are suggestive of pulmonary edema, a feature of narcotic intoxication, or pneumonia, a symptom of hydrocarbon intoxication, as well as aspiration.

The abdominal examination, in particular the assessment of bowel sounds, may be helpful. Hyperperistalsis is noted with cholinergic poisons, and decreased bowel sounds are characteristic of narcotic and anticholinergic drugs. The presence of macroscopic or occult blood in the stool might suggest aspirin, iron, or phosphorus ingestion.

Level of consciousness and behavioral changes must be frequently assessed in the intoxicated child. Coma, a nonspecific finding, is caused by many drugs in overdose, such as the anticholinergics, sedative hypnotics, and the alcohols. Eye examinations must include the measurement of pupillary size, evaluation of the optic disc, and evaluation of extraocular muscle function. The presence of abnormal movements, such as muscle fasciculations, myoclonus, and seizures, can suggest certain poisons. Organophosphates typically produce muscle fasciculations and weakness. Myoclonus is associated with anticholinergic, phenothiazine, and haloperidol overdoses.

Table 40.2. Clinical Manifestations of Poisonings[a]

Sign or Symptom	*Poison*
Odor	
Bitter almond	Cyanide
Acetone	Isopropyl alcohol, methanol, acetylsalicylic acid
Pungent aromatic	Ethchlorvynol
Oil of wintergreen	Methyl salicylate
Pear	Chloral hydrate
Garlic	Arsenic, phosphorus, thallium, organophosphates, selenium
Alcohol	Ethanol, methanol
Petroleum	Petroleum distillates
Skin	
Cyanosis (unresponsive to oxygen—methemoglobinemia)	Nitrates, nitrites, phenacetin, benzocaine
Red flush	Carbon monoxide, cyanide, boric acid, anticholinergics
Sweating	Amphetamines, LSD, organophosphates, cocaine, barbiturates
Dry	Anticholinergics
Bullae	Barbiturates, carbon monoxide
Jaundice	Acetaminophen, mushrooms, carbon tetrachloride, iron, phosphorus
Purpura	Aspirin, warfarin, snakebite
Temperature	
Hypothermia	Sedative hypnotics, ethanol, carbon monoxide, phenothiazines, TCAs, clonidine
Hyperthermia	Anticholinergics, salicylates, phenothiazines, TCAs, cocaine, amphetamines, theophylline
Blood pressure	
Hypertension	Sympathomimetics (especially phenylpropanolamine in over-the-counter cold remedies) organophosphates, amphetamines, PCP
Hypotension	Narcotics, sedative hypnotics. TCAs, phenothiazines, clonidine, β-blockers, calcium channel blockers
Pulse Rate	
Bradycardia	Digitalis, sedative hypnotics, β-blockers, ethchlorvynol, calcium channel blockers
Tachycardia	Anticholinergics, sympathomimetics, amphetamines, alcohol, aspirin, theophylline, cocaine, TCAs
Arrhythmias	Anticholinergics, TCAs, organophosphates, phenothiazines, digoxin, β-blockers, carbon monoxide, cyanide, theophylline
Mucous Membranes	
Dry	Anticholinergics
Salivation	Organophosphates, carbamates
Oral lesions	Corrosives, paraquat
Lacrimation	Caustics, organophosphates, irritant gases
Respiration	
Depressed	Alcohol, narcotics, barbiturates, sedative/hypnotics
Tachypnea	Salicylates, amphetamines, carbon monoxide
Kussmaul	Methanol, ethylene glycol, salicylates
Wheezing	Organophosphates
Pneumonia	Hydrocarbons
Pulmonary edema	Aspiration, salicylates, narcotics, sympathomimetics
Central nervous system	
Seizures	TCAs, cocaine, phenothiazines, amphetamines, camphor, lead, salicylates, isoniazid, organophosphates, antihistamines, propoxyphene, strychnine
Pupils, miosis	Narcotics (except Demerol and Lomotil), pheothiazines, organophosphates, diazepam, barbiturates, mushrooms (muscarine types)
Mydriasis	Anticholinergics, sympathomimetics, cocaine, TCAs, methanol, glutethimide, LSD
Blindness, optic atrophy	Methanol
Fasciculation	Organophosphates
Nystagmus	Diphenylhydantoin, barbiturates, carbamazepine, PCP, carbon monoxide, glutethimide, ethanol
Hypertonus	Anticholinergics, strychnine, phenothiazines
Myoclonus, rigidity	Anticholinergics, phenothiazines, haloperidol
Delirium/psychosis	Anticholinergics, sympathomimetics, alcohol, phenothiazines, PCP, LSD, marijuana, cocaine, heroin, methaqualone, heavy metals
Coma	Alcohols, anticholinergics, sedative hypnotics, narcotics, carbon monoxide, tricyclic antidepressants, salicylates, organophosphates, barbiturates
Weakness, paralysis	Organophosphates, carbamates, heavy metals
Gastrointestinal System	
Vomiting, diarrhea, abdominal pain	Iron, phosphorus, heavy metals, lithium, mushrooms, fluoride, organophosphates, arsenic

[a]From Guzzardi L, Bayer MJ. Emergency management of the poisoned patient. In: Bayer M, Rumack BH, Wanke LA, eds. Toxicologic emergencies. Bowie, MD: Robert J. Brady, 1984.

Table 40.3. Toxidromes[a]

Drug Involved	*Clinical Manifestations*
Anticholinergics (atropine, scopolamine, TCAs, phenothiazines, antihistamines, mushrooms)	Agitation, hallucinations, coma, extrapyramidal movements, mydriasis, flushed, warm dry skin, dry mouth, tachycardia, arrhythmias, hypotension, hypertension, decreased bowel sounds, urinary retention
Cholinergics (organophosphates and carbamate insecticides)	Salivation, lacrimation, urination, defecation, nausea, and vomiting, sweating, miosis, bronchorrhea, rales and wheezes, weakness, paralysis, confusion and coma, muscle fasciculations
Opiates	Slow respirations, bradycardia, hypotension, hypothermia, coma, miosis, pulmonary edema, seizures
Sedative/hypnotics	Coma, hypothermia, central nervous system depression, slow respirations, hypotension, tachycardia
Tricyclic Antidepressants	Coma, convulsions, arrhythmias, anticholinergic manifestations
Salicylates	Vomiting, hyperpnea, fever, lethargy, coma
Phenothiazines	Hypotension, tachycardia, torsion of head and neck, oculogyric crisis, trismus, ataxia, anticholinergic manifestations
Sympathomimetics (amphetamines, phenylpropanolamine, ephedrine, caffeine, cocaine, aminophylline)	Tachycardia, arrhythmias, psychosis, hallucinations, delirium, nausea, vomiting, abdominal pain, piloerection
Alcohols, Glycols (methanol, ethylene glycol) also **Salicylates, Paraldehyde, Iron, Isoniazid, Phenformin**	Elevated anion gap metabolic acdoisis

[a]From Motenson NC, Greensher J. The unknown poison. Pediatrics 1974;54:337.

Certain poisonings are associated with prominent clinical findings and can be grouped into "toxidromes" as an aid to the diagnosis of intoxication in a patient with unknown ingestion[(14,17)]. Several such toxidromes are illustrated in **Table 40.3.**

Laboratory Diagnosis

Simple, readily available clinical laboratory tests can play an important role in the diagnosis and management of a poisoned patient. Electrolytes, glucose, arterial blood gas, measured osmolality, and urinalysis can suggest the diagnosis of a specific intoxication, particularly in a comatose patient **(Table 40.4).**

Metabolic acidosis with an increased "anion gap" indicates an elevated plasma concentration of an unmeasured anion. Such anions include the acidic metabolites of methanol, ethylene glycol, paraldehyde, and toluene; lactate (as a result of tissue hypoxia or ischemia) or carbon monoxide, and cyanide poisoning; and the mixed organic acids associated with iron and aspirin intoxication. Using the equation Na − (Cl + HCO_3), the normal anion gap has been determined to be 12 ± 4 mEq/l[(18)]; however, a recent study has demonstrated that the range for a normal anion gap has decreased to 7 ± 4 mEq/l as a result of a change in lab instrumentation and higher chloride values[(19)]. A low anion gap results from an increase in unmeasured cations or a decrease in unmeasured anions and can be seen in lithium, iodine, and bromide intoxications[(20)]. Mixed ingestions may yield a "normal" gap[(21)].

An "osmolar gap" is defined as the difference between the calculated osmolarity and measured osmolality and can be a useful adjunct in diagnosing poisoning by the alcohols[(22,23)]. Under normal physiologic conditions, the serum osmolality, as calculated by the formula: serum osmolality = (2 × Na) + blood urea nitrogen/2.8 + glucose/18 closely approximates the measured osmolality if determined by the "freezing point" method: 285 mOsm/kg H_2O. If, how-

Table 40.4. Routinely Available Labortory Tests That May Suggest Poisoning

Test	*Poison*
Decreased hemoglobin saturation with normal or increased PO_2 (measured not calculated hemoglobin saturation)	Carbon monoxide, agents causing methemoglobinemia (nitrates, nitrites, benzocaine, dapsone, pyridium, sulfonamides)
Elevated anion gap, metabolic acidosis	Methanol, ethanol, ethylene glycol, salicylates, isoniazid, paraldehyde, iron, phenformin
Low anion gap	Lithium, iodine, bromide
Elevated osmolar gap	Ethanol, methanol, isopropyl alcohol, ethylene glycol, acteone, propylene glycol
Hyperkalemia	Potassium, digoxin, lithium, fluoride
Hypokalemia	Theophylline, barium, caffeine, diuretics (chronic), toluene (chronic)
Hypoglycemia	Insulin, ethanol, isopropyl alcohol, salicylates, oral hypoglycemia agents, propanolol
Hyperglycemia	Salicylates, theophylline, Vacor, caffeine, iron
Hypocalcemia	Ethylene glycol, salicylates
Urinalysis	Oxalic acid crystalluria
	Ethylene glycol
	Ketonuria
	Isopropyl alcohol, ethanol, salicylates

ever, the serum contains a significant concentration of a small molecular weight, osmotically active compound, such as methanol, ethanol, isopropyl alcohol, mannitol, or glycerol, there will be a large difference between the measured and calculated osmolality—the so-called osmol gap. A normal osmol gap is defined as less than 10 mOsm. The alcohol level in the blood can subsequently be calculated by using a conversion factor specific for each alcohol (for example, for ethanol, each 1 mOsm increase corresponds to a blood ethanol increment of 4.3mg/dL).

The osmolar gap analysis has several limitations. Normal values may range from -5 to $+15$, demonstrating large population variability[24]. Therefore, a small or "normal" osmol gap does not exclude toxic alcohol ingestion. Second, it is imperative that the freezing point depression method be used to measure the osmolarity. A falsely low measured osmolarity may result from using a vapor pressure method because the alcohols will boil off before the boiling point of water is reached. Finally, a low or nonexistent osmol gap may be associated with a significant toxic alcohol poisoning. After the alcohols undergo metabolism, their acid metabolites (except isopropanol) will not contribute to the osmol gap[25].

Bedside screening tests can provide the physician with immediate information that is both clinically useful and cost effective. The addition of 10% ferric chloride solution to urine will turn it purple in the presence of salicylates, although it is only a qualitative test and cannot distinguish between therapeutic and toxic levels. A positive test can also be noted in the presence of acetacetic acid and phenylpyruvic acid. The Ames Phenistix® reagent strips turn purple-brown in the presence of salicylates or phenothiazines.

The presence of calcium oxalate crystals in the urine may indicate ethylene glycol poisoning. Also, urine examination under ultraviolet light or Wood's lamp of a patient who ingested antifreeze containing ethylene glycol may reveal bright fluorescence because of the presence of fluorescein that is routinely added to antifreeze[26]. However, the absence of these crystals or fluorescence cannot exclude ethylene glycol poisoning.

When blood appears dark or chocolate brown it is indicative of methemoglobinemia. This is best observed by placing a drop of blood on white filter paper.

Radioopaque densities on plain abdominal radiographs may confirm the ingestion of iron tablets, chloral hydrate, enteric coated tablets, arsenic, mercury, lead, some phenothiazines, and some heroin and cocaine drug packages[27].

Hospital and commercial laboratories use the term "toxicology screen" to denote their unique selection of toxic substances to be tested. The value of the routine toxicology screen in the initial evaluation and management of the poisoned patient is limited[28]. First, the turnaround time for results is usually several hours for a complete screen, during which time the poisoned patient should already be receiving decontamination and supportive care measures.

Second, these screens may look only at a limited number of drugs depending on the epidemiology of drug intoxication in a particular area. It is unrealistic for physicians to expect a clinical laboratory to be able to identify each of many hundreds or even thousands of available drugs and toxins rapidly and with a high degree of sensitivity and specificity. Also, there are numerous drugs and toxins not commonly included in toxicology screening **(Table 40.5).** Therefore, a negative screen does not always rule out poisoning.

Third, these screens use methods with broad specificity to detect many drugs and sensitivity may be poor for many drugs, increasing the number of analytical false negative results. On the other hand, therapeutic drug concentrations may be detected during a screen in a clinically asymptomatic patient, contributing to increases in false positive results.

For toxicology screens to be useful and cost-effective, they must identify in a timely fashion any substances for which quantitative determination is necessary to initiate therapeutic modalities. Examples of specific antidotal therapy would include N-acetylcysteine therapy for acetaminophen intoxication and hemoperfusion for theophylline intoxication[29]. Toxicology screens may also be useful in establishing or confirming a clinical diagnosis, determining prognosis of a patient, determining whether a withdrawal reaction may occur, and confirming brain death.

Each clinician should be familiar with the particular hospital's toxic screen to know what drugs can and cannot be detected. To make the most efficient use of the toxicology laboratory, the physician should provide the lab with information about the suspected agents and clinical manifestations of the intoxication. Furthermore, it is important for the physician to communicate with the laboratory when specific drug quantitation must be done on an emergency basis so that prompt therapeutic interventions can be made. Toxicology screens will generally detect narcotics, analgesics, barbiturates, some cyclic antidepressants, sedative-hypnotics, alcohols (except ethylene glycol), and drugs of abuse. In most laboratories, urine is the specimen of choice

Table 40.5. Drugs and Toxins Not Included in Routine Toxicology Screening[a]

Antiarrhythmic agents
Antihypertensives
Benzodiazepines (alprazolam, midazolam, clonazepam)
Beta Blockers
Calcium Channel Blockers
Cyanide
Digoxin
Ethylene glycol
Fentanyl and other synthetic opiates
Hypoglycemic agents
Isoniazid
Lithium
LSD
Monoamine Oxidase Inhibitors
Organophosphates
Plant toxins
Solvents and hydrocarbons

[a] *some of these are available as separate specific tests*

for the initial qualitative screening for many drugs and substances of abuse, while quantitative levels of drugs, volatile alcohols, and confirmation of positive urine tests should be done on blood samples.

TREATMENT

Decontamination

Surface Decontamination

Once the patient has been stabilized, steps to prevent further intoxication should proceed. Skin contact with external poisons, such as organophosphate insecticides and corrosive agents, is halted by removing contaminated clothing and washing the skin with large quantities of water. Ocular exposure must be halted by irrigating the eyes with copious amounts of saline or water. Never apply any neutralizing chemical to the skin or instill it into the eye.

Dilution

In the past, dilution has been recommended as an initial step in gastrointestinal decontamination in the hope that this would dilute and thereby delay absorption of the poison. Although this may be efficacious after the ingestion, several studies have demonstrated enhanced gastrointestinal absorption of ingested poisons; therefore, this treatment is not recommended for noncaustic ingestions[30]. Oral dilution of an ingested alkaline or weak acid caustic with milk or water may be beneficial in decreasing tissue damage if it is performed immediately after exposure[31].

Gastrointestinal Tract Decontamination

Gastrointestinal decontamination measures for the suspected or known poisoned patient have generated a great deal of controversy in the past several years because previous concepts have been challenged by new clinical studies. Recent studies demonstrating the relatively small benefit of gastric emptying[32,33] and the effectiveness of activated characoal alone without gastric emptying[34] have changed the thinking about gastrointestinal decontamination. When a physician treats a child with a known or suspected toxic ingestion, it is important to develop a rational approach to GI decontamination that is individualized based on the patient's age, the substance ingested, time since ingestion, and presence of coingestants, as well as to understand each decontamination intervention and its limitations.

In deciding whether gastrointestinal decontamination is needed, the physician must consider three factors: (1) the risk to the patient caused by the ingestion; (2) the likelihood that gastric emptying will remove a clinically significant amount of the ingestion; and (3) whether the benefits of removing the amount of agent outweigh the risks of gastric emptying[35].

Emesis

Although the role of ipecac-induced emesis in poison management has significantly diminished in the past decade, it remains a useful method of gastric emptying for selected patients. Ipecac stimulates vomiting by both peripheral and central mechanisms[36]. Stimulation of local gastric receptors that are centrally conducted via the autonomic nervous system is responsible for early vomiting. Vomiting which occurs after 30 minutes is caused by the action of systemically absorbed ipecac on the central chemoreceptor trigger zone.

Syrup of Ipecac, in the dose of 10 ml for infants 6 months to 1 year of age, 15 mL for young children, and 30 mL for adolescents and adults, is the drug of choice for inducing emesis. It is highly effective, producing emesis in less than 30 minutes in at least 90% of children. Ipecac usually produces an average of three episodes of emesis within 30 to 60 minutes after administration[37]. The administration of water following the ipecac is of little benefit. The dose of ipecac may be repeated once if emesis does not occur within 30 minutes.

Syrup of Ipecac may be indicated for home use to begin treatment for potentially toxic ingestions. In addition, it may play a role in the emergency department when gastric emptying is needed for substances that may not pass through a large lavage tube like plant or mushroom fragments, adherent masses of pills, or large pills or pill fragments, particularly enteric-coated and sustained release tablets.

Contraindications to the use of ipecac syrup include:

- a child less than 6 months of age;
- a nontoxic ingestion;
- a lethargic or comatose patient;
- the ingestion of caustic agents;
- seizures associated with the intoxication;
- a compromised gag reflex;
- the concomitant ingestion of sharp, solid substances;
- children with hemorrhagic diathesis; or
- the ingestion of a large quantity of drug that might rapidly produce seizures or coma, such as TCAs or propoxyphene.

Finally, ipecac-induced emesis is contraindicated when vomiting will delay administration of an oral antidote.

There have been no reports of direct ipecac toxicity when it has been administered in the recommended doses. Ipecac toxicity after an overdose is characterized by nausea, vomiting, diarrhea, cardiac arrhythmias, hypotension, and neurologic manifestations of tremor, weakness, and seizures[38]. Chronic ipecac intoxication may result in dehydration, electrolyte abnormalities (especially hypokalemia), myopathy, and cardiomyopathy[39,40].

Gastric Lavage

Currently, no controlled study has shown either emesis or lavage to be clearly superior in drug removal. When gastric emptying is indicated, gastric lavage is preferable to ipecac-induced emesis in the majority of potentially life-threatening poisonings.

Lavage is best accomplished through a large-bore orogastric tube after the aspiration of gastric contents. The patient should be lying on his or her left side, head slightly lower than feet, and the largest orogastric lavage tube that can be reasonably and safely passed should be used, for example, a 16 to 28 French tube in children, 36 to 40 Fr in adolescents. A smaller caliber nasogastric or feeding tube may be used for liquid toxins. Lavage should be undertaken with water or 0.45% saline in aliquots of 150 to 200 ml for adolescents and 50 to 100 mL in young children until the return is clear, a total volume of 1 to 2 liters in children and adolescents and 500 mL to 1 liter in toddlers. In young children a 0.45% or normal saline solution is preferable to prevent hyponatremia.

Gastric lavage is most effective when performed within 1 to 2 hours after the toxic ingestion. However, since opioids, phenothiazines and TCAs may delay gastric emptying time, substantial quantities of such drugs may be removed by gastric decontamination for a few hours after ingestion. Gastric lavage is contraindicated with strong acid or alkali ingestion, ingestion of sharp materials, drug packets, and when the ingestion is deemed nontoxic.

Activated Charcoal

Activated charcoal has been shown to adsorb many different drugs effectively, thereby decreasing their systemic absorption from the gastrointestinal tract. A fine, black powder that is both odorless and tasteless, charcoal's small particle size and the existence of a pore network provide a very large surface area that approximates 1000 m^2/g of compound. Activated charcoal is best administered mixed with water as a slurry, in a dose of 10 times the estimated weight of the compound ingested because in vitro, optimal binding of several drugs is produced at a charcoal:drug ratio of 10:1[41]. Clinically, when the dose of the ingested drug is unknown, a dose of 1 g/kg for children and 50 to 100 g for adults is recommended.

A single dose of activated charcoal should be administered after nearly all suspected toxic ingestions. Activated charcoal has been demonstrated to be more effective than gastric emptying in preventing drug absorption[42] and just as effective as gastric emptying and charcoal in a selected sample of poisoned patients[15,16]. Substances poorly or not adsorbed by charcoal include iron, lithium, alcohols, mineral acids or bases, most solvents, and most water-insoluble compounds including hydrocarbons[43]. However, a history of ingesting a substance unlikely to be adsorbed to activated charcoal should not preclude its use, since the history obtained is many times incomplete or inaccurate, and coingestion of substances well adsorbed to charcoal is common. Since absorption in the gastrointestinal system of anticholinergic drugs, narcotics, and sustained release and enteric coated preparations is prolonged, activated charcoal should be administered even 12 to 24 hours after these drugs are ingested.

Activated charcoal is generally safe and has few contraindications. The use of charcoal after ingestion of caustic substances is not indicated. Charcoal is also not recommended for ingestions of pure petroleum distillates and other agents not well adsorbed to charcoal but that do carry a high risk of pulmonary aspiration. Therapeutic doses do not effectively adsorb either alkalis or mineral acids, and the fine black powder may interfere with the endoscopic examination of the esophagus and stomach[44].

Adverse effects of charcoal include nausea, vomiting and constipation. Pulmonary aspiration of charcoal is the most serious complication, sometimes resulting in fatalities; therefore, it is necessary to stress the importance of adequate airway protection before its administration[45–49].

Cathartics

Cathartics are administered to patients with orally induced intoxications to reduce drug absorption by shortening intestinal transit time. The mechanism of their action is not precisely known, but the osmotic gradient created increases the passage of fluid from mucosa to lumen, enhancing gastrointestinal motility. Other suggested mechanisms related to the action of cathartics include the release of cholecystokinin that inhibits electrolyte and water reabsorption and increases intestinal motility[50].

Saline cathartics administered alone are not as effective as activated charcoal in reducing drug absorption[51]. Various studies have suggested that a single dose of charcoal with a cathartic may be equally efficacious[52,53], more efficacious[54], or less efficacious[55] than charcoal alone in preventing drug absorption. Although there are no studies demonstrating that cathartics actually reduce the total amount of drug absorbed, their use is probably still warranted as an additional technique to evacuate the gastrointestinal tract as treatment for some specific ingestions.

Cathartics may be more effective in poisoning by drugs such as narcotics and TCAs, which slow intestinal motility. Cathartics are not warranted in the routine management of low risk ingestions in children.

There is some evidence that sorbitol and higher doses of magnesium citrate produce shorter times to the first charcoal stool, although the clinical significance of these findings in terms of reducing drug absorption and decreasing morbidity are not known[56,57]. Magnesium citrate is administered at a dose of 4 mL/kg with a maximum dose of 300 ml, magnesium sulfate at 250 mg/kg up to a total dose of 30 grams. The dose of sorbitol is 0.5 g/kg of 70% concentration (10 to 20 ml in children, up to 50 to 100 mL in adolescents). Sorbitol is recommended for children aged 1 to 12 years and adolscents aged 13 to 19 years. Sorbitol should not be administered to children under 1 year of age due to the risk of severe fluid shifts and electrolyte abnormalities. It is important to be aware that many charcoal preparations come premixed with sorbitol and should not be routinely administered on a repetitive basis to children. Mineral oil or stimulant cathartics like castor oil are not recommended because of the risk of aspiration and enhanced toxin absorption.

Contraindications to the use of cathartics include a dynamic ileus, diarrhea, abdominal trauma, and intestinal obstruction. The administration of magnesium sulfate or citrate is contraindicated in patients with renal failure.

Administration of a single dose of a cathartic agent has not been associated with adverse effects when there are no contraindications to its use and it is appropriately dosed. Case reports have shown that cathartic-induced hypermagnesemia can occur in patients with normal renal function in accidental overdoses or after multiple doses of magnesium cathartics[58–60]. Hypocalcemia, hyperphosphatemia, and hypokalemia have been reported after use of hypertonic phosphate enemas[61,62]. Young children are at particular risk for the severe fluid and electrolyte abnormalities, intravascular volume depletion, hypernatremia, shock, and acidosis which have been reported after excessive sorbitol dosing[63].

Whole Bowel Irrigation

Whole bowel irrigation (WBI) is based on a technique initially described for preoperative bowel preparation. Isotonic polyethylene glycol electrolyte solutions such as CoLyte® or Golytely® are used to flush out the gastrointestinal tract without causing fluid and electrolyte shifts, with the theoretical advantage of reducing the bioavailability of the drug or toxin by decreasing the time available for drug absorption. The initial successful experiences with WBI were reported in the treatment of iron poisonings in patients with radiographic evidence of residual iron in the GI tract[64]. Subsequent studies have shown WBI to be beneficial after ingestion of ampicillin, lithium, and enteric coated salicylates[65–67].

Whole bowel irrigation is potentially indicated for life-threatening ingestions of drugs poorly adsorbed to activated charcoal such as lithium, iron, and lead chips, drugs too massive for activated charcoal alone such as sustained release theophylline and calcium channel blockers, or ingested drug packets or vials[68–71]. The dose is 1 to 2 L/hour in adolescents and adults and 0.5 L/hour in children. WBI should be used for 4 to 6 hours or until the rectal effluent is clear.

Contraindications to WBI include ileus and abdominal perforation or obstruction. Adverse effects include rectal itching and vomiting, especially with rapid administration. WBI is not a substitute for activated charcoal, which should be administered before or during WBI solution if a charcoal-adsorbable drug is involved. The overall role of WBI in managing poisonings is still being evaluated.

Other GI Decontamination Modalities

Both human volunteer and animal studies have shown that sodium polystyrene sulfonate (Kayexalate)® is effective in preventing gastrointestinal absorption of lithium and increasing its elimination[72–74]. Cholestyramine has been demonstrated to enhance the elimination of organochlorine pesticides such as Lindane and Kepone[75,76].

Surgical gastrointestinal decontamination may be indicated for a few select situations. Surgical intervention is necessary for mechanical bowel obstruction or bowel ischemia due to heroin or cocaine drug packets[77,78]. If drug packets containing large amounts of cocaine rupture, immediate surgical removal of the remaining drug may be warranted following appropriate medical stabilization due to the lack of an antidote and the potential life-threatening toxicity of cocaine[79]. Finally, massive iron ingestions with iron remaining on radiographs despite aggressive attempts at gastric emptying and whole bowel irrigation may warrant surgical gastrotomy if serious systemic toxicity persists or gastrointestinal bleeding occurs[80].

Antidotes

The use of either a pharmacologic antagonist or chelating agent should always be considered as a possible therapeutic modality in the care of a critically ill poisoned child[11,15,81,82,83]. Unfortunately, however, only a small proportion of poisoned patients are amenable to such therapy **(Table 40.6),** and in only a few poisonings is antidotal therapy urgent. These antidotes must be available in emergency rooms and intensive care units and include:

- oxygen or hyperbaric oxygen for carbon monoxide poisoning;
- naloxone for narcotic respiratory depression;
- amyl nitrite;
- sodium nitrite;
- sodium thiosulfate for cyanide poisoning;
- methylene blue for methemoglobinemia-inducing agents; and
- atropine for organophosphate and carbamate poisonings.

Most recently, flumazenil has been commercially available as a specific receptor antagonist to the respiratory and neurologic depressant effects of benzodiazepines[84–87]. Flumazenil has also been used successfully to reverse periodic apnea in a neonate associated with maternal benzodiazepine use during pregnancy[88]. For most cases of intoxication, supportive care, not the administration of an antidote, is the backbone of effective therapy and care.

Hastening the Elimination of Poisons

Although it would certainly seem logical to stress therapeutic modalities that might enhance the elimination of poisons, enthusiasm must be tempered by the admonition of Locket, that the therapy of a poisoned patient must be directed toward supportive care and not toward "collecting the poison"[89,90].

Although there is certainly much evidence documenting the efficacy of diuresis, hemoperfusion, dialysis, and other techniques **(Table 40.7)** in enhancing the excretion of

Table 40.6. Specific Intoxications and Their Antidotes[a]

Poison	*Antidote*	*Dosage*
Acetaminophen	*N*-Acetylcysteine (Mucomyst)	140 mg/kg orally, initial dose, then 70 mg/kg every 4 hr for 17 doses (68 hr)
Anticholinergics	Physostigmine	Adult: 2.0 mg Child: 0.5 mg, i.v., i.m., s.c.: repeat 5-min intervals until desired effect achieved to maximum of 2 mg, not for use in tricyclic antidepressant poisoning
β-Blocking agents	Glucagon	Adult: 3 mg bolus, followed by mg/hr infusion Child: 0.05 mg/kg bolus, followed by 0.07 mg/kg infusion
	Isoproterenol, dopamine, epinephrine	Infusions titrate to effect
Carbon monoxide	Oxygen	100% O_2 consider hyperbaric oxygen
Cyanide	Amyl nitrite, sodium nitrite	Adult: Amyl nitrate inhalation pending administration of i.v. sodium nitrite 300 mg (3% solution) then sodium thiosulfate 12.5 g (25% solution) Child: (For children who weigh less than 25 kg, sodium nitrite and sodium thiosulfate doses are dependent on the hemoglobin concentration, since an overdose can cause fatal methemoglobinemia):

Hemoglobin (g/100 ml)	**Initial Dose 3% Na Nitrite** (ml/kg i.v.)	then	**Initial Dose 25% Sodium Thiosulfate** (mg/kg i.v.)
8	0.22 (6.6 mg/kg)		1.10
10	0.27 (8.3 mg/kg)		1.35
12	0.33 (10 mg/kg)		1.65
14	0.39 (11.6 mg/kg)		1.95

Ethylene glycol	Ethanol	Loading dose Adult: 0.6 g/kg i.v. Child: 0.7 g/kg (Loading dose to achieve blood level of 100 mg/dL) Maintenance dose Child/Adult: 125 mg/kg/hr Infuse the sum of the loading dose and first hour's maintenance dose over the first hour: infusions adjusted to maintain blood levels 100 mg/dL
Iron salts	Deferoxamine	Deferoxamine 15 mg/kg/hr i.v. until urine color is normal or iron level less than 100 μg/dL
Isoniazid	Pyridoxine (vitamin B6)	When the dose of isoniazid is known, administer an equivalent amount of i.v. pyridoxine: if supplies are limited or the dose unknown, administer 5 g: repeat dose if no response: cumulative dose is 20 g in children and 40 g in adults
Lead	DMSA, penicillamine	250 mg/m^2/dose i.m. q4h
	Calcium disodium edetate (EDTA)	83 mg/m^2/dose i.m. q4h
	British Antilewisite (BAL)	
Methanol	Ethanol	For dosage: see under ethylene glycol
Methemoglobin-producing agents (nitrites, nitrates, phenacetin, phenazopyridine)	Methylene blue	1–2 mg/kg i.v. (0.1–0.2 mL/kg of a 1% solution over 5–10 min) (contraindicated in methemoglobinemia secondary to sodium nitrite administration for cyanide poisoning)
Narcotics	Naloxone	Adult: 0.4 mg i.v.: repeat at 10 times dose if no response and findings are consistent with narcotic overdose Child: 0.1 mg/kg i.v.
Organophosphate insecticides	Atropine	Adult: 2–5 mg i.v. Child: 0.05 mg/kg i.v. Repeat every 10–30 min to achieve adequate atropinization
	Pralidoxine	Only after atropine Adult: 1 g i.v. Child: 25 mg/kg i.v. Repeat after 1 hr if weakness and fasciculations persist
Phenothiazines (occulogyric crisis)	Diphenhydramine	0.5–1.0 mg/kg i.v. or i.m. (not to exceed 50 mg)

[a]From Henretig FM, Cupit GC, Temple AR. Toxicologic emergencies. In: Fleisher G, Ludwig S, eds. Textbook of pediatric emergency medicine. Baltimore: Williams & Wilkins, 1983.

Table 40.7. Techniques of Hastening the Removal of Poisons from Blood and Tissues[a]

Urinary pH control ("ion trapping")
Hemodialysis, peritoneal dialysis
Hemoperfusion
Gastric suctioning
Activated charcoal ("gastrointestinal dialysis")
Exchange transfusion
Plasmapheresis
Drug antibodies

[a] From Pond SM. Diuresis, dialysis, hemoperfusion. Indications and benefits. Emerg Clin North Am 1982;2:29.

many poisons, there is a paucity of randomized, prospective, controlled clinical studies to demonstrate that these therapeutic modalities are effective in reducing the mortality and morbidity from poisoning[90–92]. Since this is particularly so in the pediatric age group, many of the suggested indications for these procedures have been extracted from anecdotal pediatric case reports or from the adult literature without true clinical validation in children. Proponents of hemoperfusion have stressed that this modality will shorten the duration of coma in some poisoned patients, thereby lessening the duration of required artificial ventilation and its associated morbidity[93–96]. Although this may well be an important factor in reducing mortality in adult patients with underlying cardiorespiratory disease, it may not be so in otherwise healthy, young children.

Although the following general guidelines have been suggested when the techniques of hemoperfusion and hemodialysis to enhance the active removal of intoxicating compounds in adults are considered, the indications for employing these techniques in children are not well defined:

1. Signs of severe or progressive clinical intoxication, particularly when unresponsive to aggressive medical therapy: Such examples might include hypotension that is unresponsive to volume replacement, arrhythmias or seizures refractory to conventional treatment, severe persistent metabolic acidosis in spite of the administration of large doses of sodium bicarbonate, or deep coma, when mortality rates in adults are known to exceed 10%.
2. Ingestion and absorption of a potentially lethal dose of a toxin, even though the patient may not be symptomatic at that time: Examples include the ingestion of large doses of paraquat or ethylene glycol.
3. Blood concentrations of a drug that indicate potentially serious intoxication: Many studies have demonstrated the relationship between the blood level of some drugs and the severity of clinical poisoning. Examples are poisoning with salicylates, ethylene glycol, methanol, TCAs, theophylline, paraquat, and lithium.
4. Impaired normal route of elimination of the drug: This may be due to underlying disease or drug-induced damage of the organ primarily responsible for drug elimination or detoxification. Such examples are the institution of dialysis for acetylsalicylic acid or ethylene glycol intoxication because of renal failure. Organ injury is not, however, the only mechanism whereby drug elimination is compromised. Although many drugs exhibit first-order elimination kinetics, the metabolic pathways for others like theophylline and salicylates become saturated at high serum concentrations, limiting the rate of metabolism and subsequent elimination; therefore, clearance decreases as the dose ingested and the plasma concentration increase.
5. Development of complications of coma, e.g., pneumonia, adult respiratory distress syndrome, or the presence of an underlying condition that might predispose to such complications.

Since the clinical superiority of some of these methods over conservative, supportive care alone is not always well established in children, the adage of "primum non nocere" must be the overall guide, and the decision to employ these techniques must be made after weighing the risks and complications of the procedure against the potential benefits. **Table 40.8** lists the recommended techniques for accelerating the removal of drugs in some common poisonings.

Diuresis With or Without Alteration of Urine pH

Many drugs are excreted from the body by the kidney by one or more of three processes: 1) filtration by the glomerulus of a drug that is not protein bound; 2) secretion of some drugs by active transport systems into the proximal convoluted tubules; and 3) passive bidirectional diffusion of lipid soluble, un-ionized drug along a concentration gradient that occurs down the length of the nephron. As water and sodium are reabsorbed along the nephron, the concentration

Table 40.8. Choice of Techniques for Removal of Common Toxins in which Eliminative Therapy may be Indicated[a]

	Levels Above Which Enhanced Elimination Techniques May Be Indicated (μg/ml)	*Technique[a]*
Barbiturates phenobarbital	100	HP, HD, D, HP_b
Choral Hydrate (trichloroethanol)	50	HD, HP
Ethanol	500 mg/dL	HD
Ethchlorvynol	150	HP
Ethylene glycol	50 mg/dL	HD
Glutethimide	40	HP
Isopropanol	400 mg/dL	HD
Meprobamate	100	HP
Methanol	50 mg/dL	HD
Methaqualone	40	HP
Methotrexate		HP
Paraquat		HP
Salicylates	100 mg/dL	HD
Theophylline	50	HP

[a]From Wanke LA, Bennett WM. Enhancement of elimination diuresis, peritoneal dialysis, hemodialysis, and hemoperfusion. In: Bayer MJ, Rumack BH, Wanke LA, eds. Toxicol emergencies. Bowie, MD; Robert J. Brady. 1984.
[a]D = diuresis; HD = hemodialysis; HP = hemoperfusion, in order of preference.

of intraluminal drug increases, and the gradient that is established favors reabsorption rather than excretion. Insuring an adequate urine flow (2 to 5 cc/kg/hour) reduces the concentration of the drug in the distal segment, and, by reducing the concentration gradient, reduces reabsorption, thereby enhancing excretion.

Diuresis is sometimes combined with techniques to change urinary pH. Enhancing excretion by altering pH is based on the principle that efficient reabsorption across the renal tubular epithelium occurs only when the compound is un-ionized and relatively lipid soluble. The proportion of drug that exists in the ionized and un-ionized forms depends on the pK of the drug and the pH of the solution. A drug that is a weak acid or base will become ionized by gaining or donating a hydrogen ion. By altering the pH of the urine, the proportion of ionized or nonpolar drug can be enhanced, "trapping" this poorly resorbed compound in the tubular lumen, reducing reabsorption and enhancing excretion. Since the pK of salicylate is 3, the ratio of the ionized to the un-ionized form is 1:1 at a pH of 3. At a pH of 7.4, the ratio is 25,000:1. Thus at a physiologic blood pH (e.g. 7.40), most of the salicylate is in ionized form and unable to cross cell membranes (e.g. into neuronal cells) where it could do harm. If the urine is alkalinized to a pH 7.5–8.0, most of the salicylate in the renal tubular lumen will be in ionized form and will be excreted, as opposed to being reabsorbed into the blood by renal tubular processes.

Based on this discussion, it can be seen that several criteria should be met before diuresis with pH alteration can be considered as a therapeutic modality[(97)]:

- The drug must have a predominantly renal route of excretion. Highly lipid-soluble drugs or drugs excreted primarily by the liver cannot be efficiently removed by this technique.
- The drug must be poorly protein bound to allow for adequate glomerular filtration.
- The pK of the drug must be such that, by altering urinary pH, enough ionization can occur to ensure adequate trapping.

Drugs with pK values in the range of 3.0 to 7.2 such as isoniazid, salicylate, and phenobarbital are amenable to enhanced excretion by alkaline diuresis. The excretion of drugs with pK values in the range of 7.2 to 9.5 such as quinidine, PCP, fenfluramine, and amphetamine can be enhanced by acid diuresis, although the potential risks associated with acidification rarely make the benefits acceptable. Acid diuresis can increase the excretion of weak bases, but clinically, this modality plays little role in the management of poisoned patients.

Diuresis is accomplished by the administration of intravenous fluids at one to three times maintenance requirements to establish a urine output of 2 to 5 ml/kg/hr. Bladder catheterization allows the accurate measurement of urine output. Since some infants with salicylate intoxication may be considerably dehydrated, rapid rehydration may be necessary before diuresis can be accomplished. Diuretics such as mannitol and furosemide can be added to ensure high urine flow rates.

Alkalinization of the urine to pH 7.0 or greater is achieved by adding sodium bicarbonate in concentrations of 50 to 75 mEq/L to the intravenous fluids. Hypokalemia, whether preexistent or induced by the bicarbonate administration, may make the patient relatively resistant to attempts at producing urinary alkalinization. Aggressive potassium supplementation will correct this situation.

Acetazolamide, a carbonic anhydrase inhibitor, was previously used to achieve urinary alkalinization because of its ability to enhance urinary bicarbonate excretion. However, the systemic metabolic acidosis that is induced may worsen salicylate toxicity by increasing the proportion of un-ionized, lipid-soluble serum salicylate, thereby enhancing its penetration into the central nervous system[(98)]. Thus, this treatment modality is no longer recommended.

Complications of diuresis include fluid overload with cerebral edema, pulmonary edema, hyponatremia, and water intoxication. Alkalemia and hypokalemia can complicate sodium bicarbonate use. Urine pH values and serum sodium, potassium, and acid-base parameters must be frequently monitored when these techniques are employed.

Hemodialysis

Hemodialysis describes the movement of solutes through a semipermeable membrane along a concentration gradient. In hemodialysis, the artificial membrane is contained within the dialysis coil. Only a brief discussion of some of the physicochemical and toxicokinetic principles that are important in understanding the use of dialysis in the intoxicated patient is made below. These factors include the size, lipid-water solubility, volume of distribution (V_D), and protein binding properties of the intoxicating drug, as well as certain physical characteristics of the dialysis membrane

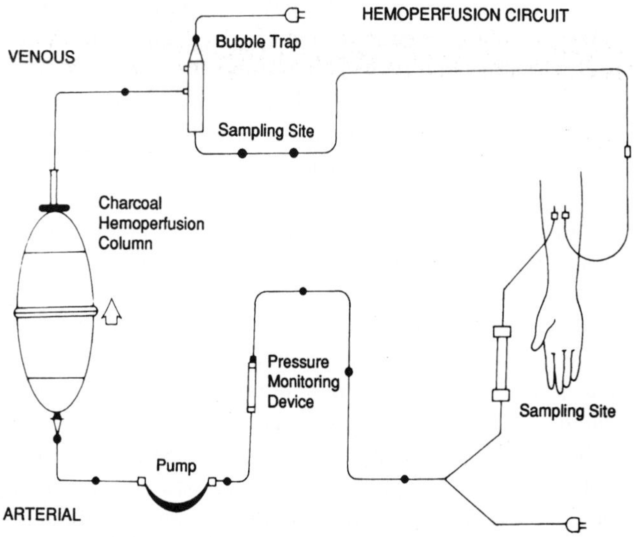

Figure 40.1. Clinical hemoperfusion circuit. (From Gelfand MC, Winchester JF, Knepshield JH, et al. Charcoal hemoperfusion in severe drug overdosage. Trans Am Soc Artif Intern Organs 1977;23:599.)

and of the dialysate[92,97,99]. Although the above factors are easily realized, no single factor determines the dialyzability of any drug. This is determined by the complex interactions of these different factors.

Solutes with a low molecular weight cross dialysis membranes more readily than larger size compounds. Those with molecular weights of greater than 500 are dialyzed progressively less well.

The V_D is important in determining the efficacy of dialysis. It is one of the factors that determines the accessibility of the drug for removal by dialysis. This parameter defines that fraction of the ingested dose of a drug that is contained within the plasma compartment, compared with that contained within other fluid compartments. It is only the plasma component that is available for immediate removal.

The V_D of a solute is dependent on lipid solubility, protein binding, active transport, and pH gradients. It is large with very lipid-soluble or highly protein-bound drugs. If the apparent volume of distribution of a solute is greater than 1 L/kg, only a small proportion of the drug burden will be contained in the plasma and be dialyzable. Even though the dialysis may be very efficient with a high clearance rate, only the small amount contained within the plasma, a small fraction of the total amount of drug ingested, will be removed.

The degree of binding to proteins also determines the efficacy of dialysis. All drugs are bound to varying extents to circulating plasma proteins. Since these do not cross the dialysis membrane, it is only the free, unbound drug that determines the concentration gradient from blood to dialysate. The poorer the protein binding, the greater will be its dialyzability. Generally, solutes that are greater than 90% protein-bound are poorly dialyzed. All the above considerations also apply to a drug's metabolites, if they, too, are toxic. Unfortunately, much of the toxicokinetic data regarding drug metabolites are not yet available.

The degree of water solubility, as measured by lipid-water partition coefficients, will also determine the dialyzability of drugs and their distribution. Drugs poorly soluble in water are less well dialyzed into aqueous dialysates. In addition, these compounds are widely distributed in body fat, producing a reservoir that is not readily accessible for decontamination.

Other physical factors that affect the clearance of solutes by dialysis are the characteristic properties of both the dialysis membrane, such as surface area, pore size, and permeability, and the properties of the dialysate. These include its flow rate, volume, temperature, and chemical composition, which are important in determining the concentration gradient along which dialysis occurs.

In general, drugs that are effectively dialyzed are poorly protein-bound, are highly water soluble, and have a low V_D. They have a molecular structure and physical characteristics that enable rapid diffusion across the dialysis membranes. Methanol is an ideal candidate for removal by dialysis. It is a small molecular weight (32 daltons), poorly protein-bound, highly water soluble compound that has a low V_D of 0.6 L/kg. In addition, it is metabolized to toxic metabolites that are themselves dialyzable. In comparison, TCAs are poorly removed by dialysis. They are lipid soluble and greater than 90% protein-bound, with a large V_D of 20 l/kg.

Hemoperfusion

Hemoperfusion is the process whereby compounds are cleared from the blood as it comes into direct contact with an adsorbent material contained in a cartridge in an extracorporeal circuit[92,93,99,100]. Hemoperfusion was first used clinically in the 1960s[91,101]. Early use, with activated charcoal granules as the adsorbent, was complicated by the destruction of blood elements and charcoal particle embolization. Microencapsulation of activated charcoal, initially with a collodion-albumin[102] coating and subsequently with acrylic hydrogel, albumin cellulose nitrate, and cellulose acetate, resulted in several commercially available systems with improved biocompatability (Hemocol, Adsorba cartridges). Charcoal embolization was prevented and the severity of the thrombocytopenia was reduced. The fixed-bed charcoal system, in which activated charcoal granules were adhered to a sheet of chlorosulfonated polyethylene that was then rolled into a column, was another attempt to prevent these early complications—the Becton-Dickinson system.

Although these techniques have eliminated charcoal embolization, the application of the various coating polymers has somewhat reduced the adsorptive capability of these charcoal cartridges. Diffusion through this coating must take place prior to adsorption. Since the membrane thickness varies from 0.02 to 3.5 m in the ACAC and Hemocol columns, respectively, the significance of this diffusion barrier will vary.

More recently, a group of uncoated, uncharged polystyrene resins—Amberlite XAD-2 and the newer, more efficient XAD-4—have been introduced as the adsorptive phase in hemoperfusion cartridges. They consist of insoluble resin beads made of fused polystyrene microspheres which have extremely large surface areas. Each gram of Amberlite XAD-2 and XAD-4 has a surface area of 330 and 750 m^2/g, respectively[103].

Charcoal can adsorb both polar and nonpolar compounds, and it is the adsorbent of choice for polar compounds, such as salicylates[99]. Amberlite XAD-4 is superior to other hemoperfusion adsorbents for removing lipid-soluble drugs, such as barbiturates, glutethimide, methaqualone, ethchlorvynol, meprobamate, TCAs, theophylline, and digoxin[118]. In fact, extraction of many of these drugs from the perfusing blood is almost complete, and the clearance often equals the blood flow rate through the coil.

The gradual reduction in drug clearance during charcoal hemoperfusion that probably results from the deposition of cellular debris and plasma proteins on the adsorbent material necessitates changing the charcoal cartridge every 2 to

4 hours. There is a much slower reduction of clearance when Amberlite XAD-4 cartridges are used, and they usually do not require changing during the course of hemoperfusion.

Many of the physicochemical and toxicokinetic factors that limit the applicability of dialysis in a particular intoxication are not of significance during hemoperfusion.[92–94]. Molecular weight, water solubility, and the degree of plasma protein binding are not limiting factors in hemoperfusion because of the high adsorbent area that comes directly into contact with the blood[103]. Whereas drugs with molecular weights of greater than 500 are progressively less dialyzable, drugs with molecular weights ranging from 100 to as high as 40,000 can be removed by hemoperfusion.

Hemoperfusion is effective in removing many polar, water-soluble compounds such as salicylic acid, as well as nonpolar, lipid-soluble drugs, such as methaqualone and meprobamate, that are poorly dialyzed[103]. For efficient dialysis, the compound must be poorly bound to plasma proteins. Drugs highly bound may, however, be effectively removed by hemoperfusion, as long as the affinity of the adsorbent for the drug is greater than that of the plasma proteins.

The V_D, however, remains important in determining the clinical usefulness of hemoperfusion. It does not affect the clearance or extraction ratio. Drugs with large V_Ds may be completely extracted from the blood as they pass through the cartridge, but if only a small amount of ingested drug is present in the plasma compartment only a small total amount, a small fraction of the ingested dose, may be removed from the body. The rate-limiting factors in hemoperfusion become the affinity of the adsorbent for the drug, the rate of flow through the cartridge, and the rate of equilibration of the drug from peripheral tissues to blood. The indications for employing hemoperfusion in intoxicated patients have been discussed earlier in this chapter. **Table 40.8** lists some intoxications for which hemoperfusion may be indicated.

In the past, the use of hemoperfusion in children was limited because of the large size of the available adsorption cartridges[93,104,105]. However, infants weighing less than 5 kg have undergone successful hemoperfusion with use of the standard cartridges[106,107]. Smaller cartridges with priming of volumes of 100 ml have recently become commercially available in the United States. Their use will facilitate hemoperfusion in small children.

The clinical use of hemoperfusion requires the technical and clinical expertise, as well as equipment, that is needed to perform hemodialysis[104]. Suitable vascular access using a double-lumen catheter placed in the subclavian or femoral vein must be obtained for establishing the extracorporeal circuit (Fig. 40.1). Such a technique is suitable for children as small as 10 kg. The umbilical artery and vein can be used for vascular access in the newborn. For children beyond the newborn period but weighing less than 10 kg, two separate venous sites must be cannulated because the double-lumen catheters are generally too large to be placed in these infants.

The adsorptive column is flushed with saline prior to use to remove particles that may have accumulated during transport and storage. The circuit is then primed with saline or heparinized whole blood. The amount of blood removed from the patient into the extracorporeal circuit should not exceed 10% of the blood volume to prevent cardiovascular instability and hypotension. Clotting within the circuit is prevented by maintaining the Lee White clotting times at 40 to 50 min with heparin. The blood is pumped in an antigravity direction at high flow rates—between 2 and 10 mL/kg—to take advantage of the extraction efficiency of the columns.

The most frequent complications during hemoperfusion are the development of hypotension and thrombocytopenia. Platelet counts usually return to normal after 24 to 48 hours and bleeding complications are uncommon. Other complications include hypocalcemia[99], hypoglycemia, and hypothermia. Some authorities have placed a hemodialyzer in series with the hemoperfusion circuit when performing hemoperfusion in small infants[106] to minimize hypothermia and electrolyte disturbances that might be more severe with the use of the relatively large columns. Blood glucose and calcium concentrations should be monitored during the perfusion. The risk of particle embolization, a previously common complication, has been almost entirely eliminated with the newer columns.

Activated Charcoal "Gastrointestinal Dialysis"

In addition to its use in absorbing ingested drugs in the gut lumen and reducing their systemic absorption, several investigators have demonstrated that orally administered activated charcoal increases the nonrenal clearance of drugs such as phenobarbital[108,109], aminophylline[110,111], carbamazepine[112], salicylate[113], and digitoxin[114], even if they have been administered parenterally. In one study, the biologic half-life ($t_{1/2}$) of phenobarbital was decreased on average from 110 to 45 hours during charcoal administration[109]. By effectively adsorbing the drug in the gut lumen, charcoal converts the gut to an "infinite sink"[109]. This enhances the diffusion of drug from the systemic circulation across the gut mucosa into the lumen.

At present, this therapeutic modality is recommended for phenobarbital, digoxin, carbamazepine, and theophylline intoxication. Activated charcoal in a dose of 1 g/kg in a child, or 50 to 100 g in an adult, should be orally administered every 2 to 4 hours. Some concerns have been raised regarding this modality. The large amount of material in the stomach may be aspirated in obtunded patients unless intubated. Charcoal prepared in osmotic cathartics may produce dramatic fluid shifts in young children when given in multiple doses or in excess[115].

Plasmapheresis

Plasmapheresis, a process of plasma removal by continuous centrifugation, has been used in drug intoxications to facilitate the removal of such highly protein-bound drugs as theophylline[116] and the digoxin-antibody fragment complex[117]. It has also been successfully used in chromic acid and chromate poisoning[118] but has largely been replaced, when indicated, by hemoperfusion.

Exchange Transfusion

Exchange transfusion has been used as a therapeutic modality in drug intoxications, especially in very small infants and particularly in those intoxications complicated by intravascular hemolysis and methemoglobinemia[118]. In addition to removing the intoxicating drug, fragmented and methemoglobin-containing cells are replaced by intact erythrocytes. In general, drug clearances are disappointing with this technique.

Immunotherapy

Advances in immunology over the past two decades have created the opportunity to use antibodies in the intoxicated patient to bind to drugs, reverse their toxicity, and enhance their elimination[119,120]. Antibody therapy has been used with dramatic results in children with severe digoxin intoxication unresponsive to conventional therapy[121].

Early investigators demonstrated the efficacy of intact, 150,000-dalton, antidigoxin antibodies, consisting of one Fc and two Fab fragments, in reversing the effects of severe digoxin poisoning. The intact antibody, however, produced an antigen-antibody complex too large to be excreted by the kidneys. In spite of the reduction of toxicity, the use of this intact antibody raised the question of the possibility of antigen-antibody dissociation and recurrent toxicity. Papain cleavage of the intact antibody produced 50,000-dalton Fab fragments that retained immunologic affinity and specificity. This drug-Fab complex can be filtered by the glomerulus and excreted by the kidney. Immunopharmacology therapy of drug overdoses is at present limited to digoxin and colchicine intoxication, although expansion to other drugs is under study[122,123].

The following sections of this chapter will discuss the details of the pharmacology, toxicology, pathophysiology, clinical manifestations, and therapy of some specific drugs and chemical agents that cause serious poisoning of children.

ACETAMINOPHEN INTOXICATION

The widespread availability of acetaminophen in over-the-counter preparations has resulted in large numbers of both accidental and suicidal intoxications. It is a safe drug when used in recommended doses, but striking hepatic dysfunction can develop with an acute ingestion of more than 7.5 g in adults or 140 mg/kg in children[124].

Pharmacology

Acetaminophen (*N*-acetyl-*p*-aminophenol) is a mild analgesic and effective antipyretic when administered in recommended therapeutic doses. It is available in tablet, capsule, liquid, and suppository forms, either alone or in combination with anticholinergics, antihistamines, muscle relaxants, narcotics, and sympathomimetics, and is a constituent of several hundred prescription and over-the-counter analgesic, cough, and cold preparations.

Acetaminophen is rapidly absorbed after a therapeutic dose and peak levels are achieved within 1 to 2 hours. Protein binding of acetaminophen is less than 20% even in overdose situations. The V_D is 0.9 to 1.0 l/kg[124,125,126]. It is rapidly taken up and concentrated by the liver, the primary site of metabolism. Here, greater than 90% of acetaminophen is conjugated with sulfate and glucuronate to form inactive, nontoxic, polar compounds that are excreted by the kidney. The sulfate and glucuronate conjugates are the predominant metabolites in infants and adults, respectively. There is a gradual maturation of these pathways until the adult pattern of conjugation develops at approximately 9 to 12 years of age[127]. Under therapeutic circumstances, less than 2% of acetaminophen is excreted unchanged in the urine and approximately 4% is conjugated with glutathione by the cytochrome P-450-dependent mixed-function oxidase enzyme system to form renally excreted mercapturic acid and cysteine conjugates (Fig. 40.2).

Pathophysiology

It is along this pathway to the mercapturic acid conjugate that the considered toxic intermediate of acetaminophen metabolism is formed. A small fraction of the dose of acetaminophen is metabolized by the hepatic cytochrome P-450-dependent mixed-function oxidase enzyme system to yield a highly reactive electrophilic arylating metabolite, possibly *N*-acetyl-benzoquinonimine, that binds to intracellular hepatic macromolecules and produces cell necrosis and damage[128,129,130,131] (Fig. 40.2). Under therapeutic circumstances, the small amount of this compound formed is rapidly inactivated by conjugation with glutathione to form mercapturic acid and the cysteine conjugate of acetaminophen. Metabolism via this pathway is reflected by the amount of mercapturic acid and cysteine conjugates excreted in the urine[132,133]. These metabolites comprise less than 1% of acetaminophen conjugates in the urine under therapeutic circumstances, but they constitute 35 to 40% in the severely poisoned patient.

After a toxic dose, hepatic glutathione stores can be depleted by binding the increased amount of the reactive intermediate that is produced[128,129,131,134]. The detoxification capacity of the liver is exceeded when the level of glutathione is depleted by approximately 70%. There is a direct relationship between the extent of glutathione depletion and hepatic dysfunction[128,129,135]. Histologically, the brunt of the hepatic cellular changes is borne by the

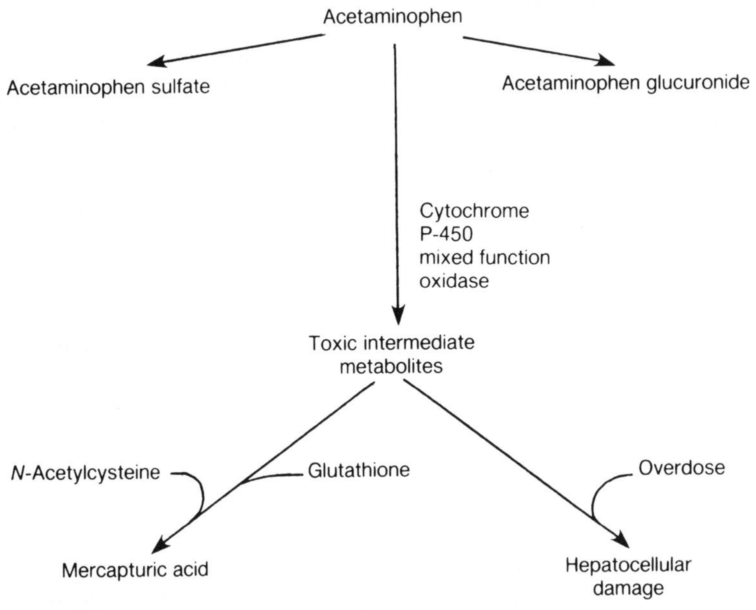

Figure 40.2. Metabolism of acetaminophen. (From Agran PF, Zenk KE, Romansky SG. Acute liver failure and encephalopathy in a 15-month-old infant. Am J Dis Child 1983;137:1112.)

centrilobular zones, the areas of greatest P-450 enzyme activity.

Experimentally, inducers of cytochrome P-450 activity aggravate the acetaminophen-induced hepatotoxicity. Depletion of glutathione stores will similarly worsen hepatic damage(131). New evidence suggests that excessive fasting, both by depleting glutathione and reducing the extent of glucuronide conjugation of acetaminophen in the liver, may increase the susceptibility of patients taking the drug chronically to hepatic injury(136).

As noted above, hepatic toxicity is caused by the reactive intermediates that accumulate, causing glutathione depletion and thereby producing cellular necrosis. Therapeutically, exogenous glutathione should be the ideal agent but it does not readily enter hepatocytes(135). Over the past decade several glutathione precursors, e.g., cysteine(137), *N*-acetylcysteine(138,139), methionine, and other sulfhydryl donors, such as cysteamine(140) and *S*-adenosylmethionine, have experimentally reduced the extent of acetaminophen-induced glutathione depletion and thereby lessened the severity of the hepatic damage. N-acetylcysteine, now regarded as the treatment of choice, is discussed in later in this section under the heading "Treatment."

Clinical Manifestations

The clinical course of significant acetaminophen intoxication in adolescents and adults can be divided into four stages(125,131,134,139,141):

- *Stage 1:* The first 12 to 24 hours are remarkable for nausea, anorexia, and vomiting. Some patients may, however, remain entirely asymptomatic. Central nervous system, respiratory, and cardiac manifestations are not features during this early phase, and their presence should alert one to the possible ingestion of additional drugs.
- *Stage 2:* This stage is marked clinically by the resolution of the early gastrointestinal symptoms, but the clinician should not be reassured, since the resolution of these symptoms is of no prognostic importance. Most patients will become asymptomatic for a period even if severe liver dysfunction subsequently appears. Biochemical evidence of hepatic dysfunction with elevation of transaminases, bilirubin, and prothrombin time will begin to appear approximately 36 hours after ingestion.
- *Stage 3:* Liver function abnormalities reach their peak on the third and fourth day. This is associated with a recrudescence of nausea, vomiting, and anorexia—symptoms of hepatitis. The extraordinarily high levels of transaminases that may exceed 10,000 IU/mL do not necessarily herald liver failure. Fulminant liver failure, with jaundice, encephalopathy, and bleeding, is an infrequent occurrence and does not inevitably complicate untreated acetaminophen poisoning. Other known complications of severe intoxication include renal failure(142,143), pancreatitis(144), and myocardial injury(145).
- *Stage 4:* This is the recovery stage and lasts approximately 7 to 8 days. Chronic hepatitis is not a feature of acetaminophen intoxication, and liver function tests and liver biopsy and histology of patients who survive return to normal.

The clinical manifestations and the course of acetaminophen intoxication in infants and young children are somewhat different from that described above. With rare exceptions, children who have ingested acetaminophen in doses well in excess of the toxic range for adults and adolescents

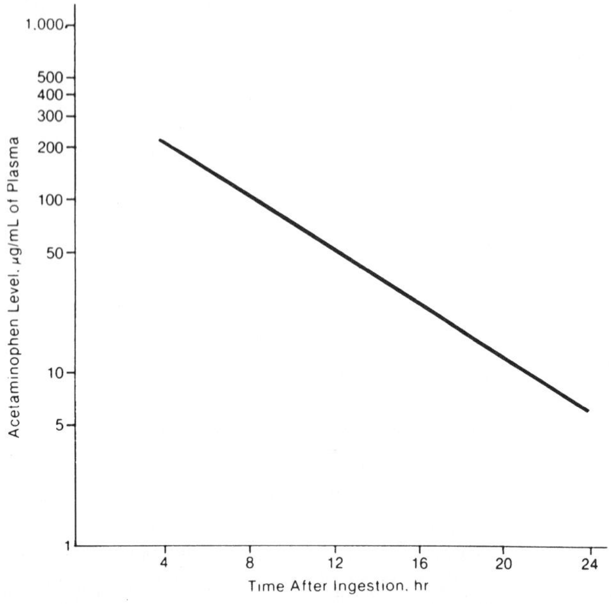

Figure 40.3. Acetaminophen toxicity nomogram. *Area above line* indicates probable hepatotoxic reaction. *Area below line* indicates no hepatotoxic reaction. (From Rumack BH, Peterson RC, Koch GC, et al. Acetaminophen overdose. Arch Intern Med 1981;141:380.)

appear strikingly resistant to its toxic effects[(138,146,147)]. Overwhelming liver failure is extremely rare. The precise mechanisms responsible for the young child's tolerance to acetaminophen intoxication are not precisely known, but some suggestions have been proposed.

The fairly consistent early emesis after acetaminophen ingestion in young children may account for the fact that serum levels of young children are only infrequently in the toxic range in spite of large doses ingested. Yet, if toxic levels are achieved, these young children display relative resistance to the hepatotoxic effects of acetaminophen. Maturational differences in acetaminophen metabolism may account for the difference in susceptibility to toxicity[(126,127,148)]. The age-related differences in glucuronidation and sulfation were noted above. In addition, preliminary observations have suggested that the less severe hepatotoxicity may be accounted for by the metabolism of a smaller fraction of the acetaminophen dose by the P-450 mixed-function oxidase enzyme system than occurs in adults.

A few cases of acetaminophen intoxication in young infants have been described[(126,149,150)]. They have been caused by both acute and chronic administration. The clinical presentation of these children is different from that noted earlier for adults and adolescents and includes hypothermia, shock, encephalopathy, severe hypoglycemia, and biochemical evidence of liver dysfunction. The differential diagnosis of this presentation should include Reye's syndrome, metabolic liver disease, and sepsis. In some of these cases described in the literature, there was rapid clinical improvement following intravenous fluid and glucose administration and general supportive care.

Prediction of Toxicity

The assessment of the risk for hepatic damage after a toxic ingestion of acetaminophen has become important in establishing guidelines for the institution of therapy with the specific antidotes now available. Because of the wide range of hepatic glutathione stores and P-450 mixed function oxidase enzyme system activity, there is only a rough correlation between the dose ingested and hepatic toxicity. As a rough guide, an ingestion of 150 mg/kg in a child and 7.5 g in an adult should be considered potentially toxic. Liver damage is very uncommon with ingestions of less than 125 mg/kg, but severe damage will occur in about 50% of adults with intoxications of 250 mg/kg and in almost 100% of those with a 350 mg/kg ingestion[(124)].

The wide range of factors that influence toxicity after an ingestion necessitates the correlation of serum levels with the potential to produce liver damage. Studies by Rumack and others[(134,138,139,151)] resulted in the formulation of a nomogram (Fig. 40.3) that defines, with good correlation, the risk of hepatic damage in terms of serum levels and duration of time since ingestion. Clinically significant liver damage is generally defined as an SGOT (aspartate aminotransferase) level of greater than 1000 IU/L. In these studies, therapy was given only up to 24 hours after ingestion. The untreated group, therefore, constituted both patients who declined therapy and those who sought medical attention after 24 hours. Liver damage in patients with serum levels above the treatment line occurred in 7%, 29%, and 62% of patients depending on whether they had received therapy less than 10 hours, between 10 and 16 hours, and more than 16 hours after ingestion, respectively. The risk of hepatic damage for patients with serum levels below the treatment line was only 1%. The higher the serum level and the later the treatment was begun the greater was the liver dysfunction. The nomogram that begins at 4 hours postingestion and ends at 24 hours applies only to acute intoxication. Values obtained before 4 hours do not yet reflect peak serum levels. After 24 hours, hepatocellular damage has already occurred.

Treatment

The initial stage of treatment should consist of emesis or lavage and cathartics. If other drugs have been ingested in addition to acetominophen, activated charcoal should be administered as well. The treatment of acetominophen toxicity complicated with other agents is discussed later in this section.

N-Acetylcysteine is the only antidotal agent available in the United States for the treatment of acetaminophen poisoning. When administered less than 16 hours, and even up to 24 hours, after ingestion, it has the profound effect of lowering both morbidity and mortality[(138,139,151,152)]; while both intravenous[(152,153)] and oral preparations of the drug are efficacious, the oral form is the therapy of choice in the United States[(138)].

The precise mode of action of *N*-acetylcysteine is unclear, but after being taken up by the liver cells, it is metabolized to cysteine, a precursor of glutathione that binds the reactive toxic intermediate of acetaminophen metabolism. A less significant interaction is the direct reaction of *N*-acetylcysteine with the toxic intermediate and its excretion in the urine.

If, on the basis of the 4-hour postingestion level plotted on the nomogram, the patient appears at risk for hepatic toxicity, therapy with *N*-acetylcysteine should begin with a loading dose of 140 mg/kg. The commercially available 20% solution (Mucomyst)®, is unpalatable, and must be mixed with three parts of soda or grapefruit juice to make a drinkable 5% solution that reduces vomiting to a minimum. A maintenance dose of 70 mg/kg should follow every 4 hours for 17 doses. A dose should be repeated if vomiting occurs within 1 hour of administration. If activated charcoal has been previously administered, it may be removed by nasogastric lavage prior to *N*-acetylcysteine administration, although the effect is negligible(154). If persistent vomiting prevents oral administration, the drug can still be given via a duodenal tube. Antiemetics such as metaclopramide and ondansetron have also been helpful in reducing emesis during *N*-acetylcysteine therapy(155).

Therapy should be started up to 24 hours after ingestion. *N*-Acetylcysteine is an extremely safe drug and even relatively delayed administration will not worsen liver failure should it develop. If liver function abnormalities are already present, *N*-acetylcysteine treatment is still recommended and, reportedly, is helpful and safe(156,157,158,159).

There is new evidence that *N*-acetylcysteine may be effective in reducing the incidence of cerebral edema and hypotension in those patients who have already developed acetaminophen-induced fulminant hepatic failure with encephalopathy(157,158,159). Intravenous *N*-acetylcysteine also seemed to improve the survival of patients in hepatic failure when it was administered until the patient recovered from the encephalopathy.

If acetaminophen blood levels are not readily available on an emergency basis, a blood specimen should be obtained, and the decision to begin *N*-acetylcysteine therapy should be made on the basis of a suggestive history. Treatment can then be stopped if the reported level is nontoxic.

Although there have been claims that charcoal hemoperfusion is efficacious in the therapy of patients who present more than 10 hours after acetaminophen ingestion(160,161), data in the literature do not support this, and this therapeutic modality cannot be recommended.

ALCOHOLS

Isopropyl Alcohol Intoxication

Isopropyl alcohol is widely used in industry and is also found in many products used in the home. These include hair tonics, rubbing alcohol, aftershave lotions, perfumes, skin lotions, and antifreeze compounds(162,163). The epidemiology of isopropyl alcohol poisoning is similar to that of methanol and ethylene glycol. These compounds are ingested either accidentally by young children or intentionally as alcohol [ethanol] substitutes by adolescents or adults. They are frequently used as suicidal agents. Ingestion is the prime route of exposure, but inhalation of isopropyl vapor has been implicated as the mechanism of exposure in infants poisoned during sponging for fever(164). Skin absorption is apparently negligible.

Pharmacology and Pathophysiology

The toxic dose is approximately 1 ml/kg of 70% isopropyl alcohol. More than one swallow should be considered potentially toxic in children. Isopropanol is approximately twice as toxic as ethanol but less toxic than methanol(162). It is rapidly absorbed after oral ingestion and, because of its high lipid solubility and low molecular weight, is distributed throughout the total body water compartment ($V_D = 0.62 - 0.7$ L/kg)(164). Approximately 20% of an ingested dose is metabolized by hepatic alcohol dehydrogenase to acetone that is excreted by both lung and kidney together with a large proportion of unaltered isopropyl alcohol.

Clinical Manifestations

The signs and symptoms of isopropyl toxicity closely resemble those of ethanol overdose. The neurologic manifestations include lethargy, dizziness, ataxia, confusion, and coma. Nystagmus is common. Miosis is usual but pupil size may be variable. An early stage of excitement seen with ethanol toxicity is, however, lacking. Gastrointestinal symptoms of vomiting, abdominal pain, and even hematemesis from gastritis are prominent. With severe intoxication, deep coma develops that may be associated with hypotension, pulmonary edema, hypoventilation, respiratory arrest, and hypothermia. The slow excretion of isopropyl alcohol and the fact that acetone, its metabolite, is itself a CNS depressant, may account for the prolonged CNS symptoms that frequently last longer than 24 hours. Arrhythmias and renal and liver dysfunction are infrequent. Hypoglycemia occurs, particularly in young children.

Attempts have been made to correlate the severity of the clinical manifestations with blood levels of isopropanol, but no close correlation has been demonstrated(163,165). Coma is generally present, however, with levels greater than 100 to 200 mg/dL. Determinations of pH and blood gases, electrolytes, blood urea nitrogen, glucose, osmolality, and ketone must be made(165).

Laboratory Tests

The laboratory findings of patients with isopropyl alcohol intoxication are discussed later in this chapter, together with those of patients poisoned by other alcohols.

Treatment

Therapy consists of general supportive care together with gastric decontamination, either by ipecac-induced emesis or by gastric lavage. The efficacy of charcoal and cathartics is unknown. Cardiorespiratory support may be required for a severely intoxicated child. Hypotension usually responds to volume infusion. In contrast to methanol and ethylene glycol intoxication, ethanol therapy plays no role in the management of isopropanol poisoning.

The most controversial aspect of therapy is that of dialysis and the indications for its use. Hemodialysis is clearly effective in removing isopropanol from the body(163,166,167). Conservative supportive management alone is advocated even for the comatose patient, since the mortality rate of the group in the absence of hypotension is virtually nil. Since the combination of severe hypotension and coma enhances the mortality rate to greater than 30%, some authorities suggest that dialysis be reserved for this group of patients alone. Other suggested indications for dialysis include a blood level of greater than 400 to 500 mg/dL, because these levels usually imply very severe poisoning(162).

Methanol Intoxication

Methanol is a chemical with widespread use in industry as a solvent. In the home, it is used as a major component of gas-line antifreeze compounds, windshield washers, and solid can fuel, as fuel for model airplanes, and as a paint remover(162). Most nonindustrial accidents in adults occur from accidental or intentional ingestion of methanol as an ethanol substitute(168,169,170). Most childhood poisonings are due to accidental ingestion of methanol-containing compounds carelessly left around the home.

Usually methanol poisoning is due to oral ingestion, but cases caused by inhalation of methanol vapor and by skin absorption(171) have been reported. There is no safe dose. Amounts as little as 5 ml are lethal to a toddler and can cause blindness in an adult. For an adult, 1 mL/kg can be lethal.

Pharmacology And Toxicology

After oral ingestion, methanol is rapidly absorbed from the gastrointestinal tract and is rapidly distributed throughout the total body water compartment. Peak blood levels are achieved within 30 to 90 min. Approximately 30% of an ingested dose is excreted unchanged by the lungs, 5% excreted in the urine, and the largest component slowly metabolized to toxic byproducts, particularly by the liver(162).

The degradative pathway of methanol metabolism is noted in Figure 40.4. Methanol is oxidized to formaldehyde by alcohol dehydrogenase, primarily in the liver and kidney. Formaldehyde is subsequently oxidized to formic acid in a reaction requiring single carbon fragments donated by folic acid compounds(162,172).

The clinical symptomatology of methanol poisoning is biphasic. Initial symptoms are those of CNS depression and are secondary to the direct action of methanol on the CNS. The more classical delayed manifestations of acidosis and visual disturbances are due to the effects of the byproducts of methanol metabolism.

There are conflicting data regarding the pathogenesis of the elevated anion gap metabolic acidosis that occurs in methanol poisoning. Several studies have demonstrated that the rise in formate concentration is adequate to account for the elevated anion gap in mildly or moderately acidotic patients(173). Other researchers have demonstrated that elevated formate levels account for only 50% of the increase in the anion gap(174,175,176). In addition, some investigators have noticed elevated lactate levels in more severely acidotic patients(177,178). This increase in lactate levels may be due to increased hepatic lactate production that occurs as a result of the reversal of normal oxidation of lactate to pyruvate because of the trapping of NAD^+ as NADH that is secondary to the oxidation of methanol to formic acid(176,177).

Recently, experimental work with a primate model of methanol-induced optic papillitis and retinal disease has suggested that locally produced formate rather than formaldehyde accumulates in the retina to produce ocular damage(175). The acidosis plays no role in the ocular damage(175).

Primates are most susceptible to methanol poisoning because of a relative deficiency of folate cofactors necessary for formic acid metabolism. Rats metabolize methanol without toxic effect(177,179). Folate-deficient rats, however, develop metabolic acidosis and ocular damage(180). Folate or 5-formyltetrahydrofolate administration to primates will prevent ocular damage and the development of metabolic acidosis after a methanol challenge(179).

Clinical Manifestations

The initial phase of toxicity is that of mild inebriation and drowsiness due to the direct effect of methanol on the CNS. The subsequent characteristic clinical symptoms caused by methanol metabolites follow an asymptomatic period of 6 to 24 hours after ingestion(162,172,181). They include restlessness, headache, vertigo, CNS depression, nausea, vomiting, and abdominal pain. The mechanism of the gastrointestinal symptoms is unclear but may be due to the coexistent pancreatitis, an entity that is frequently present. Photophobia, blurring of vision, and the appearance of "snowflakes" in the visual field are typical visual symptoms. Kussmaul-type breathing, a formaldehyde odor on the breath, hyperemia of the optic discs, retinal edema, and fixed dilated pupils are classic findings. Coma, convulsions, and apnea are poor prognostic signs and are indicative of large overdoses. Death is caused by circulatory collapse or respiratory arrest.

Permanent sequelae include blindness secondary to optic atrophy and rarely, in adults, a Parkinson's disease-like syndrome with hypokinesis, tremor, and spasticity, the result of infarction of the putamen, a lesion recently documented by computerized axial tomography(182,183).

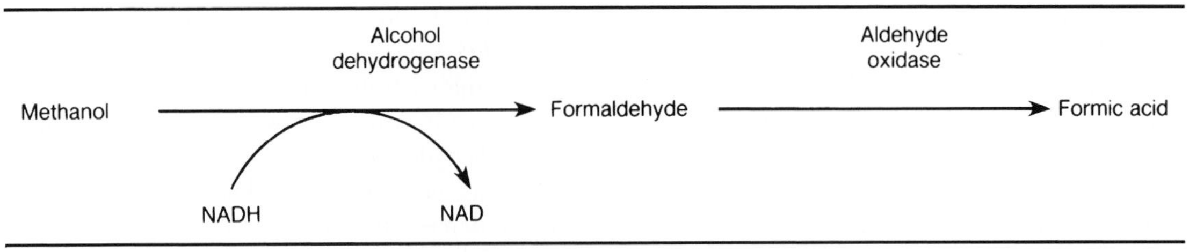

Figure 40.4. Metabolism of methanol.

Treatment

Routine general supportive measures should be instituted immediately, and emesis with ipecac or gastric lavage initiated. Charcoal administration is usually recommended, but there are no data confirming its efficacy.

The metabolic acidosis is frequently severe and the pH and base deficit must be immediately and repeatedly assessed with blood gas determinations. Large amounts of sodium bicarbonate may be needed to restore the buffer base. Dialysis, as discussed below, will aid in the correction of both the acidosis and the hypernatremia that can complicate the administration of large amounts of sodium bicarbonate. Treatment of the acidosis and normalization of serum pH per se will not, however, prevent ocular damage[(184)].

Because toxicity is largely due to the accumulation of formic acid and other metabolites[(173,174)] and not to methanol itself, the most crucial aspects of specific therapy of methanol poisoning are: (1) the administration of ethanol to slow the production of formaldehyde and formic acid[(185,186)], and (2) dialysis to remove both methanol and its toxic byproducts[(187,188,189)].

Since alcohol dehydrogenase has a much higher affinity for ethanol than for methanol, the administration of ethanol blocks methanol metabolism, with a subsequent reduction in the level of toxic formic acid and formaldehyde, and allows the unaltered excretion of methanol from the body by respiratory and renal routes. An ethanol blood level of 100 to 150 mg/dl will saturate alcohol dehydrogenase and achieve this goal[(185,186)]. Based on the 0.6 L/kg (adult) and 0.7 L/kg (child) volume of distribution (V_D) of ethanol, a loading dose of 600 mg/kg and 700 mg/kg will produce the desired plasma concentration (Cp) in adults and children, respectively ($Cp = dose/V_D \times$ body weight). Since ethanol is metabolized at approximately 125 mg/kg/hr in nonalcoholics with normal liver function, an infusion of this amount is required to maintain therapeutic levels[(190)].

Ethanol may be administered either orally or intravenously. It should be noted for dose calculations that the specific gravity of ethanol is 0.790, 10% ethanol for intravenous administration—a convenient dilution made in 5% dextrose in water—and 95% ethanol for oral administration. The intravenous loading dose of 10% ethanol is, therefore, 7.5 mL/kg or 8.75 mL/kg for adults and children, respectively[(190)]. The 125 mg/kg/hr maintenance dose can be administered intravenously as approximately 1.50 ml/kg/hr of a 10% ethanol solution. Since ethanol is removed by dialysis, either supplementaldoses must be administered[(185)], or ethanol should be added to the dialysate[(170)]. Frequent blood alcohol determinations are necessary to ensure therapeutic levels. Frequent glucose determinations are mandatory because hypoglycemia frequently complicates alcohol administration in children.

Hemodialysis is the definitive treatment modality for reducing formate and methanol levels in poisoned patients[(181,187,191,192,193)]. Indications for dialysis include blood methanol levels of greater than 50 mg/dL, severe metabolic acidosis, and neurologic or visual symptomatology[(162,172,191)]. Formate levels may also be determined to guide therapy[(194)].

Advances in the understanding of the pathogenesis of methanol toxicity have led to several experimental therapeutic modalities. Pyrazoles are potent inhibitors of alcohol dehydrogenase. 4-Methylpyrazole has been successful in the therapy of methanol poisoning in experimental primates[(195,196)]. 5-Formyltetrahydrofolic acid enhances the conversion of formate to carbon dioxide and water in primates and has experimentally prevented methanol toxicity in monkeys. There are as yet no recommendations for the use of these agents in humans[(179)].

Ethylene Glycol Intoxication

Ethylene glycol is toxicologically the most important of a group of widely used glycols. Whereas ethylene glycol and methanol intoxications in adults are usually due to their ingestion as alcohol substitutes, ethylene glycol poisoning in children is most frequently caused by the accidental ingestion of any of a range of household products. Ethylene glycol is widely used in industry but is also found around the home in cosmetic preparations and as a major component of automobile radiator antifreeze solution[(162)]. Ethylene glycol has also been implicated as an agent used in the intentional poisoning of children[(197)].

Pharmacology and Pathophysiology

Ethylene glycol is a sweet-tasting, colorless, odorless liquid that is rapidly and almost completely absorbed after oral ingestion. Transcutaneous and inhalational absorption is negligible. After absorption, it is rapidly distributed throughout the total body water compartment with an estimated V_D of 0.65 to 0.83 liter/kg. Approximately 25% of an ingested dose is excreted unchanged in the urine. The remainder is rapidly metabolized, largely by liver and kidney, to toxic metabolites. The minimum lethal dose of ethylene glycol is approximately 1.4 to 1.6 mL/kg[162,172,198]. In a recent Swedish series of 36 severely poisoned adults patients, the mortality rate was 17%[199].

The major clinical manifestations of ethylene glycol intoxication include severe neurotoxicity, metabolic acidosis, nephrotoxicity, and cardiorespiratory failure[162,198,199]. These are largely caused by the accumulation of toxic metabolic byproducts. An understanding of its metabolism, therefore, is central to an appreciation of the pathophysiology and therapy of intoxication with this compound.

The $t_{1/2}$ of ethylene glycol in the absence of alcohol is approximately 3 hours. This is dramatically prolonged to approximately 17 hours by ethanol by virtue of its competitive inhibition of alcohol dehydrogenase[200], a point of therapeutic importance that is discussed later in this chapter.

Ethylene glycol is oxidized to glycoaldehyde by alcohol dehydrogenase. Glycoaldehyde is subsequently metabolized to glycolic acid and then to glyoxylic acid. Glyoxylic acid is subject to several degradative pathways that yield oxalomalate, formate, glycine, and oxalate, as well as hydroxyketoadipate and hydroxyketoglutarate (Fig. 40.5)[198].

The pathogenesis of the neurologic dysfunction is complex. The aldehydes—glycoaldehyde, glycolate, and glyoxylate—inhibit a wide spectrum of CNS biochemical reactions and, because the peak of their production coincides with the development of CNS symptoms, they have been implicated in exerting a direct toxic effect on the CNS and play an important role in the pathogenesis of the CNS disturbances that occur 6 to 12 hours after ingestion[198,201]. Cerebral edema complicating cellular damage may enhance cerebral dysfunction. Ethylene glycol per se may also contribute to the early phase of inebriation.

Calcium oxalate crystal deposition in the meninges, perivascular spaces, and cerebral vessel walls is part of the pathologic findings in patients who have died of ethylene glycol poisoning and has been implicated in the pathogenesis of the CNS disturbances[202]. However, in experimental studies in which rats were administered the metabolites glycoaldehyde and glycolic and glyoxylic acids, CNS manifestations of toxicity developed without calcium oxalate crystal deposition, further implicating the aldehyde metabolites, and not calcium oxalate, as a causative factor of the CNS disorder[203].

A severe elevated anion gap metabolic acidosis is the characteristic laboratory abnormality of ethylene glycol intoxication. Clinically a blood pH as low as 6.46 has been documented in a patient who subsequently recovered from ethylene glycol poisoning[204]. The anions that contribute to the acidosis are largely glycolic and lactic acids[205,206].

Oxalic acid was initially believed to be responsible for the metabolic acidosis but is now considered of minimal importance. In experimental studies with ethylene glycol poisoning in monkeys, glycolic acid alone is present in adequate concentrations to account for the degree of metabolic acidosis. However, lactic acid is important in human cases of ethylene glycol intoxication, and other organic acids may also contribute to this metabolic acidosis[207].

During the oxidation of ethylene glycol to glycoaldehyde and glycolate by alcohol dehydrogenase and aldehyde oxidase, respectively, large amounts of NADH are formed that, by altering the NADH:NAD ratio, result in the production of increased amounts of lactic acid. In addition, the products of glyoxylate metabolism, by inhibiting the Krebs cycle, will further increase lactate and pyruvate production[208].

Oxalic acid chelates serum calcium and is deposited as calcium oxalate crystals in many tissues. The resultant hypocalcemia may produce the clinical manifestations of tetany and myocardial dysfunction.

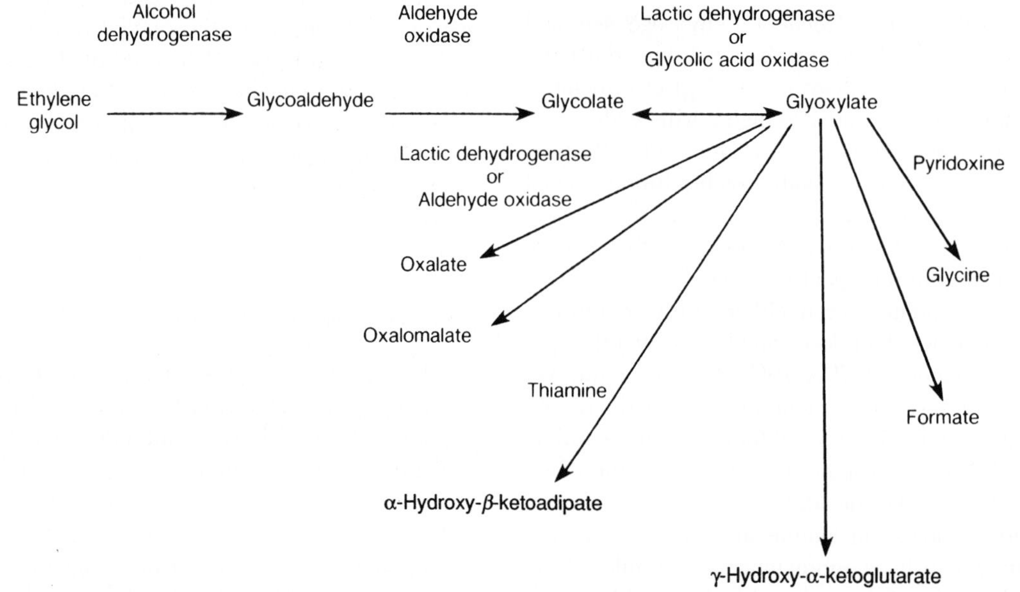

Figure 40.5. Metabolism of ethylene glycol. (From Parry MF, Wallach R. Ethylene glycol poisoning. Am J Med 1974;57:143.)

Clinical Manifestations

The clinical manifestations of severe poisoning by ethylene glycol have been classified into three sequential stages[(198,201,209)]. The first phase occurs between 30 minutes and 12 hours after ingestion and is characterized by CNS manifestations that include slurred speech, ataxia, confusion, somnolence, nausea, and vomiting. The patient appears drunk but without the smell of ethanol on the breath. In severe intoxication, coma and seizures may develop.

Other neurologic features include nystagmus, papilledema, ophthalmoplegias, strabismus, myoclonic jerks, hypocalcemic tetany, and focal or generalized seizures[(198,210)]. Isolated cranial nerve deficits have been noted in some cases[(211)]. If a lumbar puncture is performed, the cerebrospinal fluid displays the findings consistent with a meningoencephalitis, with pleocytosis, and with an elevated protein concentration[(201)]. The elevated anion gap metabolic acidosis typically becomes manifest during this early phase, as does the oxalate crystalluria.

If the patient survives the first 12 to 18 hours, the onset of the second stage is marked by the development of cardiorespiratory failure with pulmonary edema, tachypnea, tachycardia, and cyanosis[(198)]. The pathophysiology of the cardiopulmonary failure is unclear but may be related to the effects of toxic intermediary metabolites of ethylene glycol as well as to the effects of the widespread deposition of calcium oxalate crystals in the lungs and heart[(202)].

The third phase of intoxication is characterized by the development of renal failure. This develops in the survivors between 1 and 3 days after ingestion and is clinically characterized by flank pain and oliguric renal failure with hematuria and proteinuria. The pathogenesis of the renal failure is unclear but probably multifactorial in origin.

Although the observation of calcium oxalate crystals is an important diagnostic finding in the urine of patients with suspected ethylene glycol poisoning (Fig 40.6), the intrarenal deposition of these crystals is not the primary cause of renal failure, as was initially considered[(202,212)]. In experiments, primates intoxicated with small doses of ethylene glycol develop renal failure and mild glomerular lesions but in the absence of intrarenal crystal deposition. In addition, sequential renal biopsies demonstrate healing even in the presence of calcium oxalate crystals[(213,214)].

The cytotoxic effects of the metabolic products of ethylene glycol, such as glycoaldehyde and glycolic and glyoxylic acid, are the most likely cause of the renal damage. Tubular damage develops in monkeys after administration of these compounds[(212)]. The renal lesion of ethylene glycol intoxication is characterized by acute tubular necrosis and interstitial nephritis. Calcium oxalate crystals, arranged in sheaves, rosettes, or prisms within the tubules and occasionally within proximal tubular cells, are typical histologic findings. Glomerular changes are minimal[(214)].

Renal function will return to normal or near normal in a majority of patients, although oliguria may occasionally be greatly prolonged and last up to 50 days. Infrequently, interstitial fibrosis will progress to cause chronic renal insufficiency.

Laboratory Tests

The laboratory findings of patients with ethylene glycol intoxication are discussed, together with those poisoned by other alcohols, later in this chapter. With aggressive management, including ethanol administration and hemodialysis, patients have survived blood concentrations of ethylene glycol as high as 146.1 mmol/L[(215)].

Treatment

As with the management of intoxication caused by the other alcohols, emergency therapy consists of general supportive care together with gastric decontamination. The efficacy of charcoal in absorbing ethylene glycol is undocumented.

The metabolic acidosis must be aggressively treated with sodium bicarbonate; the amount to be given is determined by repeated pH and blood gas determinations[(201)]. Hypernatremia is a potential complication of the massive doses of sodium bicarbonate that may be required, and this may be another factor suggesting the early use of dialysis. Hypocalcemia should be corrected with intravenous calcium gluconate. High urine flow rates have been recommended to enhance renal clearance of ethylene glycol and its me-

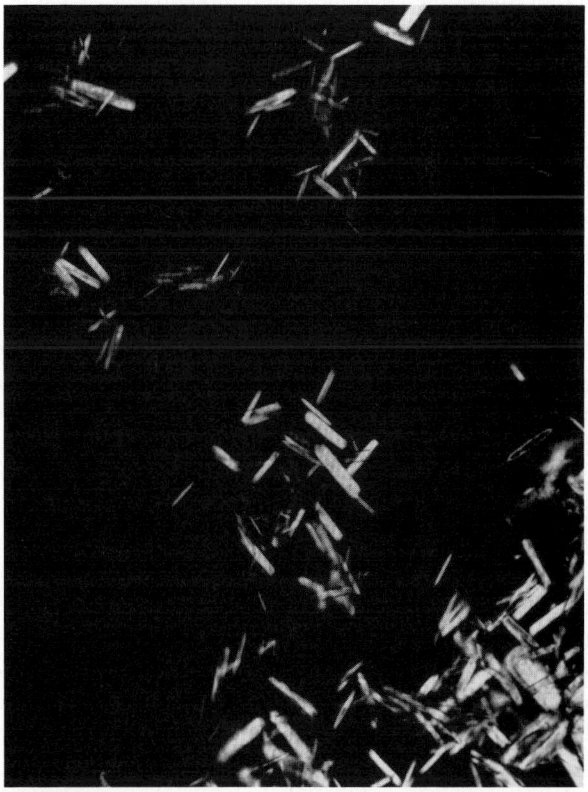

Figure 40.6. Calcium oxalate monohydrate crystals in the urine of a patient with ethylene glycol intoxication (From Godolphin W. Meagher EP, Sanders HD, et al. Unusual calcium oxalate crystals in ethylene glycol poisoning. Clin Toxicol 1980;16:479.chester JF, Knepshield JH, et al.)

tabolites, and furosemide or mannitol administration has been recommended by some investigators[198,216]. As in the case of methanol poisoning, it is the metabolic derivatives of ethylene glycol, rather than ethylene glycol per se, that are toxic.

Ethanol is a competitive inhibitor of the oxidation of ethylene glycol by alcohol dehydrogenase, thereby slowing the rate of production of metabolites and allowing the excretion of unmetabolized ethylene glycol by the kidneys[200,217]. Developing renal damage may limit this therapy as a sole therapeutic regimen.

Since ethylene glycol is rapidly metabolized, with a $t_{1/2}$ of approximately 3 hours, ethanol therapy must rapidly be instituted. Enzyme blocking with ethanol can lengthen the $t_{1/2}$ of ethylene glycol to 17 hours[215]. If there is a strong suspicion of ethylene glycol poisoning based on consistent clinical manifestations and supported by the laboratory abnormalities of an elevated anion gap metabolic acidosis and elevated osmolar gap, then ethanol therapy should commence, pending the result of a serum ethylene glycol determination. Other indications for beginning ethanol therapy include acidemia regardless of the ethylene glycol level and a peak serum level of greater than 20 mg/dL, irrespective of the symptomatology[162,172].

A protocol for the intravenous or oral administration of ethanol to achieve the optimal blood levels of 100 to 150 mg/dL is fully described above in the section discussing the management of methanol intoxication[190]. Ethanol therapy should be continued until the ethylene glycol level has declined to zero, even though this may take several days. Although the desired ethanol level of 100 to 150 mg/dL is often quoted as that required to saturate alcohol dehydrogenase, it should be noted that substantially lower serum concentrations will still cause considerable inhibition of this enzyme. The enzyme is 50% inhibited at an ethanol concentration of 20 mg/dL and more than 90% inhibited at 50 mg/dL, whereas a concentration of ethylene glycol of greater than 300 mg/dL is required to only 50% saturate the enzyme[217].

Hemodialysis is highly effective in removing both ethylene glycol before it can be metabolized and its toxic metabolites: Glycoaldehyde, glycolate, glyoxylate, and oxalic acid[205,216,218]. Although both peritoneal and hemodialysis are effective, hemodialysis is preferred because of its greater efficiency[219]. Kinetic studies by Peterson et al[200] have demonstrated a reduction in the $t_{1/2}$ of ethylene glycol from 17 hours with ethanol treatment alone, to 2.5 hours with concurrent ethanol therapy and hemodialysis. Sodium bicarbonate and not sodium acetate should be used as the dialysate buffer[201]. Indications for initiating hemodialysis include persistent metabolic acidosis that is not rapidly correctable with sodium bicarbonate, a blood ethylene glycol level of greater than 50 mg/dL irrespective of symptoms, and the presence of renal failure or marked oxaluria[162,172,191,193,219]. Hemoperfusion has been used in patients with ethylene glycol intoxication but is not recommended[220].

Knowledge of the pathophysiology of ethylene glycol poisoning has led to the development and use of experimental therapeutic agents. Pyridoxine supplementation has been suggested as part of the therapy of ethylene glycol intoxication but its efficacy is unproven. Pyridoxal phosphate is a cofactor in the conversion of glyoxylate to glycine by the glyoxylate transaminase. Pyridoxine may enhance the production of glycine at the expense of oxalate production (Fig. 40.8), with possible reduction in calcium oxalate tissue deposition. In a similar fashion, thiamine pyrophosphate, a cofactor in the reaction producing hydroxy-ketoadipate (Fig. 40.9), has also been recommended to reduce the amount of glyoxylic acid converted to oxalate[198].

Pyrazoles are inhibitors of alcohol dehydrogenase. 4-Methylpyrazole has been shown in experimental animals to ameliorate ethylene glycol poisoning[221], and may be useful in human poisoning[222,223]. In one mentally retarded adult patient who accidentally ingested 100 grams of ethylene glycol, administration of 4-methylpyrazole prevented neurologic and renal damage from occurring and avoided the need for hemodialysis[224].

Differential Diagnosis and Laboratory Findings in Ethanol, Methanol, Isopropanol, and Ethylene Glycol Intoxication

The accurate diagnosis of poisoning by these agents is of critical importance because of the necessity for ethanol therapy, a specific antidote to prevent the delayed, potentially lethal toxicity of methanol and ethylene glycol. It must be emphasized that since the initial clinical manifestations of poisoning by these compounds are so similar and may closely resemble those produced by other intoxications, such as salicylates, as well as by other medical illnesses, such as Reye's syndrome and diabetic ketoacidosis, the laboratory diagnosis takes on extreme importance. **Table 40.9** notes the clinical and laboratory findings that are of help in the differential diagnosis of poisoning by these various alcohols and glycols.

An elevated osmolar gap is characteristic of poisoning by these agents[218,225,226,227], although occasionally misleading[228]. The magnitude of the contribution of these agents toward serum osmolarity is noted in **Table 40.10.** Patients with salicylate intoxication or diabetic ketoacidosis will show no increase in the osmolar gap.

Severe metabolic acidosis with an elevated anion gap and without major ketonemia or ketonuria is characteristic of poisoning with methanol and ethylene glycol[162,181], although a normal anion gap may be misleading in patients with mixed ingestions. Isopropanol and ethanol poisoning, in contrast, produce only mild to moderate metabolic acidosis, also with an elevated anion gap but with ketosis. Whereas the ketosis of isopropanol intoxication is due to acetone alone, the ketosis associated with ethanol and seen primarily in chronic adult alcoholics is due to β-hydroxybutyrate and acetoacetate. All three ketone bod-

Table 40.9. Comparative Features of Toxicity with Common Alcohols and Glycols[a]

Feature	*Ethanol*	*Methanol*	*Isopropyl Alcohol*	*Ethylene Glycol*
Toxic dose[b]	0.72 ml/kg 600 mg/kg	0.14 ml/kg 120 mg/kg	0.3 ml/kg 300 mg/kg	0.11 ml/kg 120 mg/kg
Breath odor	Ethanol	Methanol formaldehyde	Isopropyl alcohol, acetone	None
More specific clinical features	Gastritis	Retinal edema, fixed dilated pupils	Gastritis, hematemesis	Renal failure
Metabolic acidosis (increased anion gap)	Mild-moderate (with chronic abuse in adults)	Marked (formate and lactate)	None—mild (acetone)	Marked (glycolate, glyoxalate, oxalate)
Osmolar gap	Present	Present	Present	Present
Onset	30–60 min	CNS symptoms rapid acidosis, visual symptoms late (12–24 hr)	30–60 min	CNS symptom rapid, acidosis, renal failure late (24–48 hr)
Toxic entity	Ethanol	Methanol—CNS depression Formate—acidosis, ocular damage	Isopropyl alcohol, acetone	Ethylene glycol—CNS depression Oxalate—renal damage
Other laboratory findings	Hypoglycemia	Elevated amylase, decreased mean cell volume, hypocalcemia	Hypoglycemia	Elevated blood urea nitrogen creatinine, hypocalcemia
Ketosis	Alcohol ketoacidosis (chronic alcoholic, adult) (actoacetate and β-hydroxybutyrate)	Absent	Marked acetone	Absent
Specific antidote	None	Ethanol	None	Ethanol

[a] From Kulig K, Duffy JP, Linden CH, et al. Toxic effects of methanol, ethylene glycol and isopropyl alcohol. Top Emerg Med 1984;6:14.
[b] The amount of pure solution that, on ingestion, would produce a peak blood level of 20 mg/100 ml for methanol and ethylene glycol 50 mg/100 for isopropyl alcohol, and 100 mg/100 ml for ethanol, assuming a volume of distribution of 0.6 liter/kg.

ies are present in diabetic ketoacidosis. Significant ketonemia without severe acidosis suggests isopropanol intoxication[(229)].

Other blood tests can produce helpful clues. Hypoglycemia is a common occurrence in isopropanol and ethanol intoxication[(162)]. Hypocalcemia is a frequent finding in patients with severe ethylene glycol and methanol poisoning. The hypocalcemia associated with ethylene glycol poisoning is produced by the chelation of serum calcium by oxalate, with subsequent deposition of calcium oxalate in the tissues. Amylase levels may be indicative of pancreatitis secondary to methanol ingestion. Elevated BUN and creatinine levels as well as other chemical features of acute renal failure may be present later in the course of ethylene glycol intoxication.

Urinalysis may yield critical information, particularly in the case of ethylene glycol poisoning. In ethylene glycol intoxication, oxalate crystals appear in urine as early as 4 hours after ingestion, although this finding may be delayed by many hours. The octohedral "envelope" dihydrate form of calcium oxalate is typically found, although the prismatic "hemp seed" monohydrate form is also frequently seen[(230,231,232)] (Fig. 40.6). The presence of both forms of dimorphic crystal in the same urine is pathognomonic for calcium oxalate. Proteinuria and hematuria may also be detected.

The definitive diagnosis of poisoning by any of the above agents is made by identification of the offending agent by the toxicology laboratory. Gas chromatography must be used because the enzymatic techniques using alcohol dehydrogenase will not distinguish between the different alcohols. A special request for ethylene glycol determination must be made since it will not be detected by the same methods used to detect the other alcohols.

ANTICHOLINERGIC INTOXICATION

The availability of hundreds of drugs with anticholinergic properties has made anticholinergic poisoning, whether from intentional overdose or accidental ingestion, a common clinical problem. Experimentation with the mood-altering properties of anticholinergic drugs, as well as of some common plants and mushrooms, has resulted in an increase in the number of accidentally intoxicated adolescents and young adult patients.

Table 40.10. Effect of Alcohols and Glycols on Serum Osmolality[a]

For each 1 mg of:	Serum osmolality (mOSm/KgH$_2$O) will increase:
Ethanol	0.22
Methanol	0.34
Ethylene glycol	0.20
Isopropyl alcohol	0.17
The increase in serum osmolality of 1 mOsm/kg H$_2$O caused by:	Corresponds with a change in concentration of __mg/100ml
Ethanol	4.3
Methanol	2.6
Ethylene glycol	5.0
Isopropyl alcohol	5.9

[a] From Kulig K, Duffy JP, LInden CH, et al. Toxic effects of methanol, ethylene glycol and isopropyl alcohol. Top Emerg Med 1984;6:14.

Pharmacology and Pathophysiology

Acetylcholine functions as a neurotransmitter at certain sites within the CNS;

- parasympathetic and sympathetic ganglia and neuromuscular junctions acting through nicotinic receptors; and
- parasympathetic nerve endings and sympathetic nerve endings to sweat glands acting through muscarinic receptors.

Anticholinergic drugs block the action of acetylcholine by competitive inhibition at these muscarinic receptors as well as at various CNS cholinergic receptors to produce the anticholinergic syndrome.

Tables 40.11 and 40.12 lists the vast array of pharmaceuticals, plants, and mushrooms that possess anticholinergic properties. For some of these compounds, the anticholinergic effects are desired, as in gastrointestinal antispasmodics. With other classes of drugs, e.g., the TCAs or phenothiazines, the anticholinergic properties are undesirable side effects.

Table 40.11. Pharmaceutical Drugs, Plants, and Mushrooms with Anticholinergic Properties

Antihistamines
Diphenhydramine (Benadryl)
Dimenhydrinate (Dramamine)
TCAs
Amitriptylin (Elavil)
Nortriptyline (Pamelor)
Imipramine (Tofranil)
Desipramine (Norpramin)
Doxepin (Sinequan)
Phenothiazines
Chlorpromazine (Thorazine)
Thioridazine (Mellaril)
Trifluoperazine (Stelazine)
Antiparkinsonian drugs
Benztropine mesylate (Congentin)
Trihexyphenidyl (Artane)
Belladonna Alkaloids and related drugs
Atropine
Glycopyrrolate
Scopolamine
Homatropine
Hyocyamine
Muscle Relaxants
Carisoprodol (Soma)
Cyclobenzaprine (Flexeril)
Orphenadrine (Norflex)
Antispasmodics
Dicyclomin (Bentyl)
Hyoscyamine (Levsin)
Trihexyphenidyl (Artane)
Plants
Jimsonweed
Deadly nightshade
Bittersweet
Jerusalem cherry
Black henbane
Mushrooms
Amanita muscaria
Amanita pantherina

Table 40.12. Examples of Plants Containing Anticholinergic Alkaloids[a]

Name	*Toxic Alkaloid*
Datura stramonium (jimsonweed, locoweed)	Hyoscyamine, hyoscine
Hyoscyamus niger (black henbane)	Hyoscyamine, hyoscine
Atropa belladona (deadly nightshade)	Hyoscyamine
Cestrum nocturnum (night-blooming jessamine)	Atropine
Lycium halimifolium (matrimony vine)	Hyoscyamine
Aminita muscaria (fly agaric)	
Amanita panterina (panther mushroom)	
Solanum dulcamara (bittersweet)	Solanine
Solanum nigrum (black nightshade)	Hyoscyamine
Solanum pseudocapsium (Jerusalem cherry)	Solanine, solanidine, solanocapsine

From Kulig K, Rumack BH. Anticholinergic poisoning. In: Haddad LM, Winchester JF, eds. Clinical management of poisoning and drug overdose. Philadelphia, WB Saunders, 1983.

The plants causing anticholinergic poisoning **(Table 40.12)** contain tropane alkaloids which include atropine (a mixture of D- and L-hyoscyamine), solanine, madragorine and scopolamine (L-hyoscine). The alkaloid content of various parts of these plants may vary enormously depending on climatic factors but usually the seeds have the highest content. The unknown amount of active alkaloid in these seeds and leaves predisposes patients who ingest these products to particularly severe anticholinergic poisoning. Jimson weed has become popular again in the 1990s among adolescents and young adults experimenting with the plant for its hallucinogenic properties[(233,234)].

Clinical Manifestations

The signs and symptoms of anticholinergic poisoning can be divided into the peripheral effects on muscarinic receptors and central manifestations, and can be easily remembered by recalling the lines, "Hot as a Hare, Blind as a Bat, Dry as a Bone, Red as a Beet, Mad as a Hatter." The peripheral anticholinergic effects include tachycardia—the earliest and most consistent finding—hypertension, dry mucous membranes, flushed, warm skin without perspiration, elevated temperature, mydriasis, blurred vision, decreased bowel sounds, constipation, and urinary retention. Arrhythmias, apart from sinus tachycardia, are uncommon with most pure anticholinergics, and their presence suggests either a TCA or phenothiazine intoxication. Ingestions of large amounts of diphenydramine may result in a prolonged QT interval[(235,236)].

The central anticholinergic syndrome is characterized by confusion, memory loss, agitation, hallucinations, delirium, seizures, and, occasionally, coma. The notable absence of sweat in an agitated patient is a clinical feature and may result in significant hyperthermia and rhabdomyolysis due to the body's decreased ability to dissipate heat[(237)]. Although the patient may be agitated and uncontrollable, self-mutilation and violent behavior are rare. The presence of peripheral anticholinergic findings may be the key to making the diagnosis of anticholinergic syndrome when the broad differential diagnosis of acute psychosis must be entertained in a psychotic patient.

Laboratory Tests

There is no laboratory test to confirm the diagnosis of anticholinergic poisoning. The diagnosis is made clinically based on a history of ingestion and typical physical findings. Electrolytes and blood glucose level should be obtained on any patient with altered mental status. Acetaminophen and salicylates are commonly found in many of the over-the-counter antihistamine products with anticholinergic properties; thus, quantitative levels should be obtained in intentional overdoses and large accidental ingestions. An ECG should be obtained in patients with suspected anticholinergic poisoning for QT and QRS interval measurements and detection of ventricular dysrhythmias.

Treatment

Aggressive supportive care with attention to airway establishment, cardiac monitoring and IV access should be initiated in the patient presenting with suspected anticholinergic poisoning. Serial assessments of vital signs and mental status should be performed to detect rising temperature or pulse rate.

Since gastric emptying may be markedly delayed by many anticholinergic drugs, gastric lavage may be indicated even if the ingestion has occurred 24 to 48 hours prior to presentation. Activated charcoal should be administered to all patients. Agitated, delirious patients may require endotracheal intubation prior to gastric decontamination.

Extreme agitation, hallucinations, and psychosis should be treated with intravenous benzodiazepines or physostigmine. Benzodiazepines should be administered until the patient's agitation is controlled to prevent the development of hyperthermia and rhabdomyolysis. Seizures should be treated with benzodiazepines and/or phenobarbital. Ventricular dysrhythmias may respond to standard doses of lidocaine. Torsades de pointes may be treated with magnesium sulfate and/or overdrive pacing.

The use of physostigmine as antidotal treatment for the patient with anticholinergic intoxication is controversial. Physostigmine is a short acting, nonspecific cholinesterase inhibitor. Because of its tertiary ammonium structure, it can traverse the blood-brain barrier and reverse the coma, confusion, hallucinations and seizures characteristic of central anticholinergic toxicity. Complications from its use include induction of cholinergic crisis and precipitation of seizures, bradyarrhythmias, and asystole which are seen when physostigmine is used in the management of cyclic antidepressant toxicity and non-anticholinergic poisonings.

Prior to using physostigmine, one must weigh the benefits of its use in the particular clinical setting with its potential risks. For physostigmine to be used safely, the patient should have both peripheral and central anticholinergic signs, a narrow QRS complex on ECG, and no history of exposure to other toxins that may cause intraventricular conduction delays such as cocaine, quinidine, procainamide, mesoridazine, thioridazine, and TCAs. Clinical indications may include CNS depression, severe agitation, hallucinations, and/or supraventricular tachycardia with hemodynamic instability or ischemic chest pain. The clinical effect of physostigmine lasts only 20 to 60 minutes. Thus, its utility is limited because most patients can be managed supportively[238].

The recommended dose for children is 0.5 mg intravenously administered over several minutes and repeated at 5 to 10 minute intervals until 2.0 mg have been given or reversal of toxic effects is noted. In adults, 1.0 mg is the initial dose which can be repeated until the desired effect is achieved or 4.0 mg has been given. The cardiac rhythm should be monitored during administration and atropine readily available in case cholinergic toxicity occurs.

Some investigators have used the administration of physostigmine as a diagnostic test—a rapid reversal of signs and symptoms allegedly confirming anticholinergic poisoning, thereby obviating the need for CT scans and lumbar punctures. This conclusion is open to dispute, however, since physostigmine causes nonspecific arousal and has awakened patients from intoxications caused by many other drugs[239]. Since the diagnosis of anticholinergic poisoning can usually be made on the basis of clinical findings, this diagnostic trial is probably unnecessary.

CAUSTICS

Product Types

Despite safe packaging and a reduction in the concentration of caustics in some household products, children are still frequently injured by exposure to corrosives. Corrosives should be distinguished from products containing only gastrointestinal irritants like many dishwashing liquids, which can result in some mild symptoms but never any significant burns.

Alkaline caustics include lye (sodium hydroxide), ammonia in greater than 5% solutions, industrial strength sodium hypochlorite in greater than 5% solutions, powdered laundry detergents containing sodium carbonate, other detergents that contain sodium tripolyphosphate, and such household chemicals as drain openers (sodium hydroxide) and mildew removers (concentrated sodium hypochlorite). Button batteries also contain potassium hydroxide, which can result in corrosive injury if the integrity of the battery has been breached[240]. Commercial alkalis used for cleaning drains, pipelines, and steel storage tanks on farms are a particular hazard to children living in rural areas[241,242].

Acid products include rust removers and cement cleaners (hydrofluoric acid), metal cleaners (oxalic or sulfamic acids), toilet bowl cleaners (muriatic acid, hydrochloric acid), slate and swimming pool cleaners, and oven cleaners (sulfuric acid). Automotive batteries contain sulfuric acid.

Some tablet or powdered reagents—Clinitest® tablets for urine glucose testing, for instance, contain copper sulfate, sodium carbonate, sodium hydroxide, and citric acid—are comprised of caustic chemicals that can result in severe, penetrating focal burns[(243)].

Pathophysiology

Ingestion of caustic products can result in two types of injury. Alkaline products typically produce *liquefaction necrosis* by saponification of cellular fats with protein degradation, rapidly resulting in deep injury often limited to the oropharynx and proximal segment of the esophagus. Ingestion of an acid is more likely to produce a superficial *coagulation necrosis* with excessive heat production and eschar formation, extending down the length of the esophagus into the stomach. In in vitro experiments, both acids and alkalis at concentrations less than 10% produced severe damage to a cat's esophagus after as short an exposure as 30 seconds[(244)].

Inflammation and tissue damage can be rated by the appearance of tissues at endoscopy:

- grade 0: No damage;
- grade 1: Superficial erythema, edema and mucosal desquamation only;
- grade 2: Areas of blistering, placque formation, ulceration and deeper tissue damage that may extend into the esophageal wall in contiguous but not circumferential regions;
- grade 3: Tissue sloughing that extends transmurally through the submucosa into periesophageal tissues and is circumferential in at least some areas.

Esophageal regions of highest vulnerability to caustic injury appear to be anatomic areas of narrowing and stagnation of movement, specifically the cricopharyngeal area, the impression of the aortic arch and left bronchus, and the lower esophageal sphincter[(245)].

Clinical Manifestations

Corrosive chemicals differ in their potency depending on their molar strength, dissociation constant (pH), and other chemical properties. The potential for injury varies with not only the specific chemicals involved, but also their quantity and concentration, the duration of contact, whether they are liquid or solid, other diluents present, and the vulnerability of the tissues involved.

Dermal or mucous membrane exposures can result in extensive and/or deep burns. Inhalation of fumes or powdered detergents may precipitate the corrosive chemicals on mucous membranes, in the oropharynx, and in the airway, resulting in tearing, burning of the eyes and nose, sore throat, bronchospasm, cough, and shortness of breath. Clinicians should be aware that a caustic ingestion may also cause respiratory damage[(246,247)]. In one study, over 40% of children had upper airway lesions at direct laryngoscopy after a caustic ingestion[(248)]; those with severe esophagitis were at a particularly high risk for developing airway burns[(248)]. A splash during the ingestion can also cause dermal or ocular injury. A careful physical exam is paramount.

Severe poisoning is characterized by nausea, vomiting, oropharyngeal placques, burns and swelling, dysphagia and throat pain, and refusal to eat or drink[(249)]. Systemic signs include fever, respiratory distress, cardiovascular collapse, hypocalcemia (hydrofluoric acid only), and acidosis (seen with ingestion of acids). Abdominal pain, subcutaneous emphysema, pneumothorax, pneumomediastinum, or peritonitis signal perforation.

Diagnosis

It is controversial as to whether or not severe esophageal lesions—grade 2 or 3—can be seen in a child in the absence of oral findings such as mucosal burns, edema, stridorous breathing, drooling, and refusal to eat or drink[(250,251,252,253)]. Some children can have remarkably few symptoms of caustic poisoning despite evident esophageal lesions at endoscopy. In one study, 30% of children with significant esophageal or gastric injury had no oropharyngeal burns[(252)]. Another retrospective study could identify no swallowing or abdominal complaints in 12% of children with grade 2 esophageal burns[(253)].

Treatment

Initial managment of caustic injury includes extensive washing and diluting of dermal or ocular exposures, fresh air and oxygen for inhalations, and wiping and flushing as much debris out of the mouth as possible in the case of ingestion of a solid caustic product. Swallowed button batteries are best tracked by serial radiography; those in the esophagus must be removed immediately[(240,254,255)]. The majority of batteries in the stomach or intestines remain intact and pass via the rectum uneventfully; however, a cathartic may be administered.

For ingestion of liquid caustics, giving the patient nothing by mouth is probably the safest initial management. Ipecac, gastric lavage, and activated charcoal should all be avoided. Intravenous fluids, an arterial line for monitoring blood pressure and gases, and airway control are often instituted early after the patient's arrival. Cautious suction and then cold water dilution through a small nasogastric or orogastric tube in a controlled environment has occasionally been attempted in serious acid or Clinitest® tablet ingestions[(243,256)], but is of uncertain benefit. Neutralization of a caustic is dangerous and contraindicated; the resulting exothermic reaction can exacerbate tissue destruction[(256)].

Endoscopy is recommended for patients within the first 24 hours after the ingestion in order to assess and stage any damage. Endoscopy delayed beyond 48 hours after the poisoning risks perforation, since injury to the esophagus will produce maximal weakness to its integrity at about that time[(249)]. Steroids have been recommended for patients suffering grade 2 esophageal lesions in order to reduce inflammation, granulation, and later stricture formation, although controlled studies have not demonstrated a clear benefit[257]. Steroids may be helpful in the patient with airway edema or bronchospasm. Antibiotics are recommended only for patients who have evidence of bacterial esophagitis or other secondary infection[249].

Complications

In the acute period, hemorrhage, esophageal perforation, mediastinitis, pneumothorax, peritonitis, and gastric perforation have all been documented, often with disastrous consequences. Emergent gastrectomy has been necessary for some patients with extensive corrosive injury to the stomach[256,258]. Oropharyngeal edema may result in airway compromise and respiratory distress, requiring emergency intubation.

Late complications include infection, pyloric stenosis, stricture formation, and chronic esophageal dysmotility or gastric deformity[259]. Of 60 children found to have burns upon initial endoscopy in one study, 35% went on to stricture formation and 18% required esophageal replacement[257]. Severely affected patients may require a period of esophageal rest; a gastrostomy and total parenteral nutrition may be necessary. Later functional assessments include morphologic grading by repeat endoscopy, dynamic studies of motility and reflux, radiographic evaluations, and manometric measurements of intraluminal pressures[259]. Bougienage is indicated for those patients with chronic swallowing difficulties and esophageal strictures; colonic interposition has been required in some patients with a completely dysfunctional esophagus[257]. An increased risk of esophageal or gastric carcinoma has been documented in survivors of a serious corrosive ingestion[245].

COCAINE POISONING

Epidemiology

Cocaine continues to be one of the most commonly abused drugs in the United States, exacting an enormous toll in terms of human suffering, health care utilization, and economic losses. More than 30 million Americans are estimated to have experimented with cocaine at least once; 5 million reportedly use it regularly[260]. Infants, children, and adolescents are also exposed[261]. As many as 2.4% of children visiting the pediatric emergency department of a large inner city hospital were found in one study to have urine samples positive for cocaine[262]; a separate study in a different urban setting found the pediatric urine positivity rate to be 5.4%[263].

Cocaine has well established legitimate medical uses as a local anesthetic and vasoconstrictor. However the hydrochloride salt is also used illegally, most commonly by nasal insufflation (snorting) or by intravenous injection. A more available, more addicting, and less costly form of cocaine, 'crack', first became a problem in the United States in 1983[264]. The alkaloidal base, made by mixing the salt with ammonia with or without sodium bicarbonate, is known as crack because of the popping sound the crystals make when they are burned. As opposed to cocaine hydrochloride, which decomposes when heated, crack can be smoked, with rapid absorption through the lungs to achieve an immediate 'high', equivalent to that reached by intravenous injection of the drug.

Ingestion of cocaine bags in order to smuggle them into countries has also previously been described[265,266,267,268]. These so-called 'body packers' seal the drug well inside condoms or other packaging materials before ingesting them; they take care not to allow leakage of the cocaine into the intestines, which might have life-threatening medical consequences. Patients who hurriedly ingest bags or vials of cocaine to avoid capture by police, known as 'body stuffers', cannot secure the packaging of the drugs as well, and thereby run a much greater risk of developing serious symptoms.

Infants and children may be exposed to cocaine either passively by the absorption of cocaine in breast milk[269], by inhaling smoke in rooms where crack is being smoked, or by active ingestion of cocaine mistakenly left within their reach.

Pharmacology

Cocaine acts as a neurologic and cardiovascular stimulant via its effects on sympathetic tone. It blocks reuptake of norepinephrine at preganglionic sympathetic nerve endings, resulting in excess norepinephrine in the synaptic cleft. In the heart, this local excess of norepinephrine increases both pulse and cardiac automaticity while decreasing nodal refractoriness and accelerating conduction velocity throughout the His-Purkinje conduction system.

Cocaine has other pharmacologic effects. It also triggers the release of epinephrine and is associated with an increase in dopamine concentrations in affected tissues. Cocaine also acts on the cellular membrane directly to produce an anesthetic effect. In the heart, this membrane-stabilizing effect is not unlike that of quinidine. Cocaine also alters membrane permeability, affecting calcium transport in vascular smooth muscle cells and provoking vasospasm[270].

Cocaine is readily absorbed through nasal mucous membranes, reaching peak blood concentrations within 5 to 10 minutes. Local nasal vasoconstriction caused by the drug itself delays absorption and peak effects achieved via this route. However, when cocaine is injected intravenously, its peak effects are felt almost immediately. Also, when the freebase is smoked, the large surface area of the lungs becomes the vehicle of absorption, such that peak drug concentrations are reached in the blood almost immediately and the euphoric 'rush' experienced is similar to that reached with intravenous cocaine use[264]. The pharmacokinetics of cocaine metabolism and elimination are very individualized; there is great variation both intra- and interindividually.

Cocaine undergoes both enzymatic and nonenzymatic degradation in the blood and liver. It is degraded by liver and plasma cholinesterase isoenzymes with a plasma half-life of less than one hour. Enzymatic esterification produces a less active ecgonine methyl ester metabolite. Cocaine is also hydrolyzed nonenzymatically to produce benzoylecgonine and ethyl-methyl ecgonine metabolites. Finally, a small amount of cocaine is demethylated in the liver to produce norcocaine, which is itself a potent neurotoxin.

Clinical Effects

Cocaine abuse, and particularly crack smoking, is a rapidly addicting behavior. Patients experience giddiness and euphoria, feelings of self-satisfaction, increased perceptions, increased strength, and decreased fatigue. These pleasurable sensations are quickly replaced by a dysphoria; in crack smoking, the 'high' may last only 10 to 20 minutes. The dysphoria may lead to self-recrimination, agitation, anxiety, or symptoms of clinical depression[(271)].

Through its release of catechols into the blood, cocaine may cause an adrenergic storm with stimulatory CNS, cardiovascular, and respiratory effects. Consequently, seizures, vasoconstrictive hypertension, and hyperthermia may lead to ischemic cardiac complications, CNS bleeding and infarction, and other end-organ failure, any combination of which may result in cardiovascular collapse, coma, and death. Oral doses of 1 to 3 grams of cocaine can be lethal; about 750 to 800 mg by IV may be lethal. There is, however, a wide latitude of interindividual dose ranges of tolerance to the effects of cocaine[(272,273)].

There is a wide range of CNS effects caused by cocaine. Patients may exhibit bizarre behaviors and delirium acutely, consistent with a toxic psychosis. Frequently, central stimulant effects cause patients to seem progressively more agitated, dizzy, anxious, and irritable. The user's demeanor is notable for restlessness, jitteriness, and hyperalertness. Stereotypical movements, bruxism, and tics may be apparent, and impaired judgment and risk-taking behaviors are common. Paranoid delusional thinking may be reflected in unpredictable outbursts of anger or aggression. Homicides, suicides, traffic accidents, and falls can follow intoxication by cocaine; as many as 27% of violent deaths among young adults in New York City were associated with prior cocaine use[(274)].

Other serious neurologic consequences of cocaine use are seen in children as well as adults[(275,276,277)]. Mott has found seizures to be the most common neurologic complication of pediatric cocaine exposures[(277)]. Cocaine may cause seizures through a variety of mechanisms—direct irritation of epileptogenic foci, production of a focal cerebral vasculitis, or by the actions of adulterants such as amphetamine, ephedrine, lidocaine, phencyclidine, and strychnine used to dilute the concentration of cocaine sold on the street[(278)]. Chronic cocaine use may saturate neuronal tissues with concentrations that result in pharmacologic 'kindling', the gradual progressive recruitment of susceptible neurons into paroxysmal electrical discharge[(278)].

Seizures can also be seen as a secondary phenomenon in patients who experience focal cerebral ischemia or subarachnoid hemorrhage due to vasospasm and/or hypertensive crisis[(279)]. Cardiac dysrhythmias, through the production of thrombosis or hypotension, can lead to cerebral hypoperfusion, increasing susceptibility to seizures. Finally, hyperthermia induced by cocaine can itself precipitate seizure activity.

Cerebral arterial vasospasm and hypertension can also cause focal cerebral subarachnoid, intraparenchymal, and intraventricular hemorrhages, resulting in lateralizing neurologic signs, seizures, coma, and cerebral infarction[(276,279,280)]. Spinal infarction has also been described in adults after cocaine use[(276)]. Both hemorrhagic and ischemic strokes are postulated in association with cocaine use[(279)]. Abrupt onset of global headache shortly after cocaine use is a common clinical symptom. Neonates are also at high risk for seizures, cerebral hemorrhage, and vertebral infarction following maternal use of cocaine in pregnancy[(281,282)].

The cardiovascular and respiratory effects of cocaine are related to its predictable effects on pulse, blood pressure, and tissue oxygen consumption. Hypertension, sometimes severe, and tachycardia are commonly seen. Rapid respirations, dyspnea, palpitations, and chest pain are common findings and can be explained by several different etiologies[(283)]. Coronary arterial vasospasm has been documented after cocaine administration, both in animal subjects as well as in humans. Anginal ischemia and myocardial infarction are both associated with cocaine use[(273)]. Such cardiac effects can be seen following intranasal use, inhalation of crack smoke, or after intravenous injection of the drug; they are not necessarily related either to route of use or dose and may be seen in patients without a previous history of heart disease[(284)]. In one study, 17% of 359 adults presenting to four different emergency departments for treatment of chest pain had cocaine metabolites detectable in their urine[(285)].

Other etiologies of chest pain after cocaine use include pneumothorax or pneumomediastinum, cardiac arrhythmias such as ventricular tachycardia or fibrillation, and the onset of cocaine-induced myocarditis. Pulmonary complications include rales, rhonchi, cough, sputum production, and shortness of breath[(283)]. Cocaine-induced asthma has been described.

Chronic cocaine effects on the central nervous system include tactile hallucinations, often called 'cocaine bugs' or 'snow lights,' and difficulties with mentation and memory. Other effects of cocaine include hyperthermia, with extremely high body temperatures produced by three separate mechanisms[(272)]:

- Cocaine acts on the central thermoregulatory mechanism in the hypothalamus as an exogenous pyrogen.
- It raises body temperature through its mediation of strong muscular contractions and increased tonus.
- Through its vasoconstrictive actions, cocaine prevents natural body cooling mechanisms such as dissipation of heat through dilated peripheral vascular beds.

Rhabdomyolysis is a common complication of the hyperthermia syndrome associated with cocaine use, although it may also be seen in acute cocaine toxicity without temperature elevation[286]. Roth has noted that rhabdomyolysis, when accompanied by acute renal failure, liver dysfunction, and disseminated intravascular coagulation, has a high mortality rate[286].

Miscellaneous clinical effects of cocaine include appetite disturbances and weight loss, abdominal pain and bowel ischemia, known as 'cocaine colitis'. Intravenous use of cocaine may also cause a local cellulitis.

Laboratory Diagnosis

Ecgonine metabolites may be detectable in urine for up to 72 to 96 hours after cocaine use, whereas blood cocaine concentrations usually fall to nondetectable levels within 30 to 60 minutes of use[287]. In chronic heavy cocaine users, ecgonine metabolites may be detected in the urine for up to 2 weeks after the most recent use. Commercial EMIT cocaine assays are very specific and sensitive to urine concentrations of less than 200 μg/L[288]. The adolescent cocaine user may be simultaneously using opiates or other sedative-hypnotics to 'take the edge off' the euphoria or to achieve combined effects[271]. Therefore, a toxic screen of blood and urine for other drugs of abuse is recommended[283].

Other useful studies in the cocaine-intoxicated patient include ECG monitoring and a chest x-ray, especially in the patient with chest pain. Blood creatinine kinase isoenzyme fractions may be helpful in ruling out either myocardial infarction or significant rhabdomyolysis. Renal function tests are important in patients with significant rhabdomyolysis. Abdominal films may confirm ingestion in patients who are suspected of swallowing bags of cocaine.

Pathological Diagnosis

Cocaine use sometimes produces pathological changes in heart tissues, although a normal heart does not rule out chronic cocaine use. Endomyocardial biopsies performed on seven adult patients who admitted previous cocaine use showed multifocal myocardial necrosis, focal myocarditis, and a dilated cardiomyopathy[289]. Extensive loss of myofibrils suggested a pathogenesis of eventual multifocal interstitial fibrosis and heart failure. Focal patches of eosinophilic myocarditis were found in some chronic cocaine users by Isner[284].

A typical contraction band necrosis has been found in the hearts of some cocaine abusers at autopsy[290]. Such contraction bands may be the result of direct catechol-mediated changes in myocardial calcium homeostasis, which results in myofibril damage and fibrosis. Contraction bands may mediate fatal re-entrant arrhythmias postulated as the mechanism of cocaine-related death in some patients[291]. One case control study found contraction bands in 93% of autopsied hearts from patients in whom death was attributed to cocaine, as opposed to being present in 45% of autopsied controls, who had died of causes unrelated to cocaine[291].

Treatment

Treatment of the cocaine intoxicated child or adolescent involves supportive care for the patient and monitoring in an intensive care setting as long as there are new-onset neurologic events, continuing chest or abdominal pain, or cardiovascular lability. The agitated patient may require moderate amounts of a benzodiazepine, such as diazepam, for sedation. The use of phenothiazines to control agitation may be harmful, since these agents can lower the seizure threshold of the patient[273].

Adequate hydration with intravenous fluids is important, especially in the patient who develops significant rhabdomyolysis. Swallowed cocaine should be treated with activated charcoal. Treatment of body packers or stuffers depends upon the number of bags swallowed, the length of time elapsed, the presence or absence of symptoms, and the likelihood that a bag will leak or rupture. Signs of bowel obstruction, bowel ischemia, or significant cocaine toxicity may indicate a need for early surgical intervention; however, if the patient is asymptomatic, conservative management with activated charcoal and gentle catharsis is adequate. Some have advocated whole bowel irrigation using an isotonic polyethylene glycol solution given in large quantities to greatly speed up transit of bags through the intestines.

Cocaine-associated hypertensive crisis is one of the most common medical problems facing the practitioner. Subarachnoid hemorrhage is an important complication of such rapid blood pressure elevations, such that immediate pharmacologic intervention to lower blood pressure is advisable. Sedation with an agent such as a benzodiazepine will help to alleviate such hypertension. Phentolamine given at 5 to 10 mg intravenously, a specific alpha-blocking antihypertensive agent, is the antihypertensive drug of choice. Alternatively, clinicians have had success managing cocaine-induced hypertension with sublingual nifedipine or a direct vasodilator such as sodium nitroprusside or nitroglycerin. Verapamil, given at a dose of 10 mg intravenously, was able to alleviate cocaine-induced coronary arterial vasospasm and reduce blood pressure in one volunteer study of 15 adults who were given cocaine while undergoing cardiac catheterization[270].

Traditional beta blockers such as propranolol are not recommended for cocaine-induced malignant hypertension, since unopposed alpha-agonist effects may exacerbate the patient's condition[292,293]. However, labetalol, with both alpha and beta blocking capabilities, has been suggested also as an alternative antihypertensive agent[273].

Seizures usually respond to benzodiazepines such as diazepam or lorazepam[294]. In this regard, it should be noted that the benzodiazepine antagonist flumazenil is relatively contraindicated for use in the patient suffering adverse effects of a polydrug overdose that may include both cocaine and a benzodiazepine. In this situation, flumazenil may unmask seizures induced by cocaine but previously suppressed by the concomitant abuse of a benzodiazepine. In an animal experiment, rats given 100 mg/kg cocaine + 5 mg/kg diazepam intraperitoneally simultaneously had no seizures and only a 50% death rate as opposed to a 90% seizure rate and 100% death rates in rats given the cocaine-diazepam mixture followed by intravenous flumazenil[294].

Cocaine-induced hyperthermia syndrome is a life-threatening toxic reaction and requires aggressive therapy with antipyretics, cooling blankets, and iced saline lavage[272,286]. Muscle paralysis with a nondepolarizing agent and intubation may be necessary in some patients to reduce contractions contributing to hyperthermia. Careful serial monitoring of core temperature is advisable in all patients with cocaine toxicity admitted to intensive care.

Nitroglycerin was found to be effective in over half of those patients experiencing cocaine-induced myocardial ischemia and chest pain[295]. Lidocaine, given as 1 mg/kg IV push, may be required to suppress ventricular ectopy.

Symptomatic patients will require close monitoring in an intensive care setting, although the toxic effects of acute exposures to cocaine, if uncomplicated by secondary hemorrhage or seizures, will usually abate within 6 to 12 hours after exposure.

CYANIDE INTOXICATION

Although acute cyanide poisoning is an uncommon occurrence, it is of toxicologic importance because of its rapidly lethal action and the fact that antidotal therapy may be life saving.

Cyanide salts are widely used in the electroplating, steel, rubber, and mining industries[296]. In the past, hydrogen cyanide gas, the volatile form of the free acid (HCN), and its derivatives such as cyanogen chloride, as well as acrylonitrile and cyanamide, were widely used as fumigants and in industry[296]. Childhood exposure to hydrogen cyanide gas may occur in household fires in which the combustion of various polymers such as polyvinylchloride, polyurethane, nitrocellulose, paper, wool, silk, nylon, and polyacrylnitrile yields hydrogen cyanide[297,298,299]. Acetonitrile, used in cosmetics, has proven to be a lethal source of cyanide in children[300,301]. Hydrogen cyanide is absorbed by inhalation as well as transdermally. Laboratory reagents are occasionally the source of cyanide used as suicidal agents by chemists and pharmacists. Other cyanide-containing compounds are available in the home in silver polishes, rodenticides, and insecticides.

During the past decade, numerous reports of cyanide poisoning in adults and children have occurred as a result of the ingestion of cyanogenic glycosides[302,303]. These compounds, of which amygdalin is the best known, are found in over a thousand plant species. Amygdalin is found in high concentration in the pits of many fruits and berries, including wild cherries, plums, peaches, and lima and cassava beans. It is present in especially high concentrations in the pits of apricots and bitter almonds. Apricot pits contain up to 400 mg of cyanide per 100 g of moist seeds[304]. They are sold as vitamin B_{17} in health food stores and have been responsible for cases of severe cyanide poisoning[305] and even death.

Laetrile, the principal component of which is amygdalin, contains 6% cyanide by weight and is also a potentially lethal cause of cyanide intoxication when ingested in large doses[306]. One child died after ingesting between one and five 500 mg laetrile tablets[307]. Amygdalin is not toxic until broken down by either emulsin, an enzyme within the kernel, or by β-galactosidase, a microbial enzyme present within intestinal flora, to produce glucose and mandelonitrile[308,309]. This compound is further degraded to hydrogen cyanide and benzaldehyde. This process explains the fact that laetrile is toxic only when ingested or administered rectally[310] and does not readily produce cyanide intoxication when administered parenterally because of the absence of the necessary cleaving enzymes in nonintestinal tissues.

Cyanide intoxication is also a potential complication of the use of sodium nitroprusside[311,312,313]. The widespread use of this agent in operating rooms and intensive care units has been accompanied by increasing number of reports of cyanide intoxication and even deaths[312,314,315,316,317,318]. The nitroprusside molecule contains five cyanide groups per molecule and is 44% cyanide by weight. The mechanism whereby the cyanide moieties are released from the nitroprusside molecule is complex and incompletely understood[318,319]. Recent studies have suggested that nitroprusside can be broken down by a nonenzymatic reaction with hemoglobin to yield methemoglobin and an unstable nitroprusside radical. This decomposes to release five cyanide ions, one of which combines with the methemoglobin to produce cyanmethemoglobin. The remaining four cyanide ions either are converted to thiocyanate or mediate toxic effects by interaction with cytochrome oxidase if the detoxification pathways are overwhelmed[311,313]. Nitroprusside has also been blamed for delayed CNS toxicity from cyanide[320].

Finally, cyanide has also been an agent used in product tampering cases (i.e., intentional, malicious contamination of over the counter remedies) which have resulted in both injury and death[321].

Pathophysiology

Cyanide inhibits the final steps of oxidative phosphorylation by binding reversibly with the ferric iron of cytochrome oxidase—specifically, in the cytochrome a-a_3 complex, the terminal oxidase of the mitochondrial electron transport chain, which halts the aerobic metabolism and blocks the major pathway of high energy phosphate production[309,322,323]. In rats given intravenous KCN, cerebral cytochrome oxidase activity is depressed, with corresponding decreases in cerebral glycogen and ATP and increases in cerebral lactate and ADP levels[323]. The result is histotoxic anoxia.

Glycolysis continues with further pyruvate production. Since the pyruvate can no longer be incorporated in the tricarboxylic acid cycle, it is reduced to lactate that rapidly accumulates, producing a systemic lactic acidosis—an important laboratory finding in cyanide intoxication. The iron of hemoglobin is in the ferrous state and does not react with cyanide. Cyanide poisoning is characterized by an inability to use oxygen at the cellular level—"internal asphyxia." There is no compromise of either oxygen transport to tissues or of its dissociation from hemoglobin[(324)].

Although the inhibition of cytochrome oxidase is probably central to the pathophysiology of cyanide intoxication, it should be noted that, in most cases of cyanide poisoning, cyanide is present in concentrations far in excess of the amount necessary to inhibit cytochrome oxidase[(309)]. With such excess, other enzyme systems are also inhibited. In fact, several other enzymes are as sensitive or even more sensitive to inhibition by cyanide than cytochrome oxidase[(309)].

Cyanide Antagonism

Low levels of cyanide are normally present in vivo, and it is only when the physiologic detoxification mechanisms are overwhelmed that clinical poisoning develops. Although this is a field of research that is being intensively investigated, the classes of compounds therapeutically available for cyanide antagonism and their use were initially described 50 to 150 years ago[(309)]. They consist of compounds that will: *(a)* enhance the biotransformation of cyanide, and *(b)* bind cyanide. These are the nitrites and cobalt compounds, as well as drugs that encourage cyanohydrin formation.

Cyanide Biotransformation

The physiologic biotransformation and detoxification of cyanide occurs in mitochondria in reactions catalyzed by two sulfur transferases—rhodanase and mercaptopyruvate sulfur transferase[(325)]. The rhodanase-catalyzed reaction is the better known detoxification mechanism, but recent work has, in addition, suggested a significant role for mercaptopyruvate sulfur transferase. Rhodanase catalyzes a reaction involving the transfer of a sulfane sulfur from thiosulfate to form an enzyme complex and the subsequent reaction of the complex with cyanide to yield thiocyanate, a relatively nontoxic compound, that is then excreted in the urine. The importance of this rhodanase reaction is its irreversibility.

Mercaptopyruvate sulfur transferase is also capable of converting cyanide to thiocyanate. In addition, rhodanase is responsible for the interconversion of several sulfane compounds, in which an ionized sulfur is bonded to another sulfur. These exist in a pool, possibly complexed with serum albumin[(325)], and are the source of thiosulfate used in the detoxification reaction[(325)]. Such compounds include thiosulfate, persulfides, polythionates, and most important, mercaptopyruvate, which can be converted by mercaptopyruvate sulfur transferase to thiosulfate or combine with cyanide to form thiocyanate[(309,325)].

Clinically, sodium thiosulfate is administered as an antidote to prevent the depletion of the endogenous sulfane pool, to ensure adequate substrate for the rhodanase-catalyzed formation of thiocyanate from the reaction of cyanide and cyanmethemoglobin with sulfane donors[(309)].

Cyanide Binding

The chemical binding of cyanide can be induced by nitrites, cobalt compounds, and cyanohydrin formation. Hemoglobin has a low affinity for cyanide, but by oxidizing the ferrous iron to the ferric form, sodium nitrite produces a large pool of methemoglobin. Methemoglobin has a high degree of affinity for cyanide and, by the law of mass action, can strip the cyanide molecule from its bond with cytochrome oxidase, reactivating the electron transport system and yielding cyanmethemoglobin. The cyanide is then removed from this compound by rhodanase and combined with thiosulfate to form thiocyanate[(309)]. It is for this reason that sodium nitrite and sodium thiosulfate should be administered together; either alone is not as effective as their combined use. These drugs have been the mainstay of cyanide antidotal regimens since their original use by Chen et al in 1933[(326)].

The understanding of this mechanism of cyanide detoxification has led to the development of new, more rapid methemoglobin inducers, such as 4-dimethylaminophenol (DMAP)[(327)]. In spite of the rapid rate of methemoglobin formation with DMAP, many investigators still consider sodium nitrite superior because the longer $t_{1/2}$ of methemoglobin, induced by sodium nitrite in animals, prevented a subsequent relapse of cyanide poisoning that occurred with the release of cyanide from cyanmethemoglobin that was formed with the more rapid methemoglobin inducers[(328)]. The reason for the more prolonged methemoglobinemia induced by nitrites is unclear, but it may be related to the nitrite-induced inhibition of methemoglobin reductase[(328)].

In spite of the known mechanism of action of methemoglobin and its formation by sodium nitrite, the mechanism of action of sodium nitrite in cyanide poisoning may be more complex and may not be related only to its ability to produce methemoglobin[(309,329,330)]. This was initially suggested by studies that demonstrated that, in spite of the slow generation of methemoglobin by sodium nitrite, its antidotal effect is very rapid. Recent studies have demonstrated that, under experimental circumstances when methemoglobin formation is prevented by pretreatment with methylene blue, sodium nitrite will still prevent cyanide toxicity[(330)]. The alternative mechanism of action of sodium nitrite is under intense investigation at present.

It has been known for more than 50 years that the cobalt ion can form a stable complex with cyanide, but its use as an antidote in cyanide poisoning has been limited by its known toxicity[(309)]. Interest in cobalt as an antidote was restored when hydroxycobalamin was reported to be an effective cyanide antidote[(331)]. Of the several cobalt-containing compounds that have been tested as cyanide antidotes, dicobalt ethylenediaminetetraacetic (cobalt-EDTA) acid has been most widely studied in animals and in man[332,333]. The rapid combination of cobalt with cyanide, compared with the slow production of methemoglobin by sodium nitrite, and the absence of the risk of excess methemoglobin production are suggested advantages of these compounds.

Cyanide can react with various carbonyl side chains to form cyanohydrin intermediates[309]. Recent work has shown that sodium pyruvate, by reacting with cyanide to form a cyanohydrin, can ameliorate the toxic effect of cyanide poisoning in intact animals[334] and in cell cultures. In animal studies, sodium pyruvate alone is not as effective as sodium nitrite as an antidote, but it does enhance the protective effect of sodium thiosulfate. The addition of sodium pyruvate alone is not as effective as sodium nitrite as an antidote, but it does enhance the protective effect of sodium thiosulfate. The addition of sodium pyruvate to the sodium nitrite-sodium thiosulfate regimen further enhances the antidotal action of these drugs. This line of research is being actively pursued at present.

Clinical Manifestations

The onset of symptoms will vary depending on the route of administration of cyanide. Inhaled hydrogen cyanide gas can prove lethal within seconds. Enteric or cutaneous absorption of a cyanide salt may take minutes to hours to produce clinical poisoning. The signs and symptoms of cyanide poisoning are nonspecific and are manifestations of cellular hypoxia, particularly of the CNS and myocardium[296,309].

Dizziness, headache, palpitations, tachypnea, and hypertension—signs and symptoms that resemble acute anxiety—are the earliest findings and rapidly progress to confusion, convulsions, and death. Nausea and vomiting are due to gastrointestinal irritation, but frequently CNS depression and coma develop before the gastrointestinal irritation is manifest.

Inhibition of carotid body metabolism is responsible for the initial hyperpnea, but medullary center depression produces subsequent respiratory depression. Myocardial ischemia is clinically manifest by arrhythmias, pulmonary edema, and hypotension. Bradycardia is a typical early finding. Cyanosis is conspicuously absent early in the clinical course. Examination of the fundus may reveal both red retinal arteries and veins, a dramatic demonstration of the decreased arterial-venous oxygen content difference that results from decreased cellular oxygen utilization. Lactic acidosis is an important laboratory finding.

Diagnosis

Since antidotal treatment must be instituted rapidly, prior to a blood cyanide determination, the diagnosis of cyanide poisoning must be based on a high index of suspicion of exposure to cyanide together with a consistent catastrophic clinical presentation[335]. The classic pathognomonic smell of bitter almonds is sometimes present, but the ability to smell this compound is genetically determined and present in only 20% to 40% of people. Supportive laboratory data include an elevated anion gap metabolic acidosis, a decrease or even equivalence of the arterial-mixed venous oxygen content difference, and a normal arterial PO_2 and measured oxygen saturation[336]. A plasma lactate concentration greater than 10 mmol/L was a sensitive indicator of cyanide intoxications in victims of fire-related smoke inhalation[297].

Whole blood cyanide determinations are not part of a routine drug screen and should be specially requested if indicated. Because of the rapid course of cyanide poisoning and the emergent need for antidotal treatment, blood cyanide determinations play no role in the acute diagnosis and management of cyanide poisoning. Such determinations are only useful for the retrospective confirmation of a clinical diagnosis. The value of blood thiocyanate levels in patient management is unknown, since thiocyanate levels do not correlate well with a patient's clinical appearance or with simultaneously drawn blood cyanide levels[296].

Normal blood cyanide values for nonsmokers are less than 0.2 μg/mL, with smokers demonstrating levels up to 0.8 μg/mL. Stupor and agitation may be evident at blood levels of 1.0 to 2.5 μg/mL; cyanide levels greater than 2.5 μg/mL are associated with coma and are potentially fatal[296]. Since some blood specimen tubes contain cyanide as an enzyme inhibitor, it is important to ensure that the blood sample tubes are cyanide-free prior to their use. The minimum lethal dose for a 70-kg individual receiving no medical care is 200 to 300 mg cyanide salts, although persons ingesting up to 3 grams have survived with good medical treatment[296].

Iatrogenic cyanide intoxication as a complication of the intraoperative or intensive care use of sodium nitroprusside must be considered in the face of a metabolic acidosis or increasing dose requirements, particularly when more than 10 μg/kg/min are being infused or when a total of 0.5 to 3.5 mg/kg has been administered. Other investigators have suggested that toxicity is unlikely if less than 3 μg of nitroprusside per kilogram per minute has been infused for a period of less than 72 hours. Cyanide and thiocyanate levels may be obtained if toxicity is considered, to confirm the diagnosis retrospectively.

Treatment

The therapy of the patient with cyanide poisoning is a true medical emergency and is unique in that antidotal therapy is probably life-saving. Resuscitation, decontamination, supportive care, and the prevention of further cyanide intoxication of the patient must proceed hand in hand with concomitant antidotal administration. Prolonged advanced life support should not prevent the patient's rapid transfer to a medical facility with available cyanide antidotes, although supportive care alone occasionally has been reported as successful[337].

Prevention of further exposure to cyanide entails the removal of clothing and washing of the skin if there has been external exposure. Rescuers may require special breathing apparatus if hydrogen cyanide gas is responsible. After cyanide ingestions, gastric lavage should be performed without delay. Emesis is inappropriate since the patient, even if initially alert, may rapidly become comatose and then may be at risk of pulmonary aspiration. Activated charcoal and saline cathartics should follow the lavage, even though cyanide is only slightly bound to activated charcoal and this modality has not been proven effective.

Supportive therapy must initially consist of maintenance of the airway, respiration, and cardiovascular stability. Oxygen at 100% concentration should be administered to all patients. If the inhibition of cytochrome oxidase is the only mechanism of cyanide lethality, there would be no rational basis for oxygen therapy—oxygen utilization and not supply or delivery is the central lesion of cyanide poisoning. Nevertheless, there are many experimental data in animals that demonstrate striking amelioration of the signs of cyanide toxicity[338,339], particularly when combined with sodium nitrite and sodium thiosulfate administration. The role of hyperbaric oxygen is less defined but may be considered in the patient who does not appear to improve with conventional treatment or in whom endogenous metabolism of cyanide-generating chemicals may continue to expose the patient to additional doses of cyanide for hours[322,340,341,342].

The acidosis should be treated with sodium bicarbonate. Pulmonary edema is treated with diuretics, artificial ventilation, and positive end-expiratory pressure and, if necessary, by the administration of inotropic agents to improve cardiac function. Arrhythmias are managed with conventional antiarrhythmic agents. The value of supportive care must be emphasized.

In spite of the reported cases of complete recovery of patients with potentially lethal levels of blood cyanide who were managed by general supportive measures alone[337], the efficacy of the sodium nitrite-sodium thiosulfate regimen, developed more than 50 years ago by Chen et al[326], is still the recommended therapy for patients with cyanide intoxication.

The Eli Lilly Cyanide Antidote Kit No. M-76 is the most widely available antidote in the United States. The initial step consists of breaking the amyl nitrite pearls onto a gauze pad and allowing the patient to inhale the vapors by placing the gauze over the patient's nose or over the Ambu bag intake valve for 15 to 30 seconds of each minute. Since this agent will produce only approximately 5% methemoglobin, it is a temporizing measure to be adopted until intravenous access is obtained and intravenous sodium nitrite can be administered. The initial sodium nitrite adult dose is 300 mg administered as 10 mL of a 3% solution at a rate of 2.5 to 5.0 mL/min. This is immediately followed by 12.5 g of sodium thiosulfate intravenously as 50 mL of a 25% solution. An additional half of the original dose may be repeated if there is no clinical improvement.

Berlin[343] has proposed a pediatric dosage schedule for sodium nitrite and sodium thiosulfate based on both body weight and hemoglobin concentration in an attempt to prevent toxic methemoglobinemia **(Table 40.13).** Hall et al have described the kinetics of this antidotal therapy[344].

It must be emphasized that the sodium nitrite and thiosulfate therapy is not without hazard. Preparation must be made to treat the hypotension that almost invariably occurs. Volume infusion and vasopressors may be needed. Since methemoglobin does not transport oxygen, the accumulation of excessive concentrations of methemoglobin is potentially toxic. The aim of sodium nitrite therapy should be to achieve a methemoglobin concentration of approximately 30%. Signs of tissue hypoxia will appear with greater than 40% methemoglobin. This will occur at even lower concentrations of methemoglobin in the case of combined cyanide and carbon monoxide poisoning when the overall concentration of oxygen-carrying hemoglobin is even further reduced by the presence of carboxyhemoglobin.

Several of the newer cyanide antidotes are not yet available for clinical use in the United States but either have been effective in laboratory tests or are clinically in use in several European countries. Dimethylaminophenol is a more rapid inducer of methemoglobin than sodium nitrite, but whether, in combination with sodium thiosulfate, it is more effective than the classic antidotal combination is unclear[327,328,332,345,346]. Cobalt-EDTA is available in Europe as Kelocyanor and is administered as a 300- to 600-mg intravenous dose to adults. It is not, however, without potential side effects that include hypotension, arrhythmias, and gastrointestinal irritation.

Hydroxycobalamin (vitamin B_{12a}) was originally proposed as a cyanide antidote in 1952. It combined with cyanide to form cyanocobalamin (vitamin B_{12}). Although studies of sodium nitroprusside toxicity have suggested a moderate protective effect when hydroxycobalamin is administered as a prophylactic agent[316,317], only preliminary data are available to advocate its use in severe cyanide poisoning[347]. Experimentally, 5 grams of hydroxocobalamin have been given intravenously initially followed by 12.5 grams of sodium thiosulfate, each infused over 30 minutes. α-Ketoglutaric acid has also been demonstrated effective in cyanide intoxicated animals[348,349,350].

Table 40.13. Variation of Sodium Nitrite Dose with Hemoglobin Concentration*

Hemoglobin (gm/100 ml)	*Initial Dose $NaNO_2$ mg/kg*	*Initial Dose 3% $NaNO_2$ Solution ml/kg*	*Initial Dose 25% Sodium Thiosulfate ml/kg*
7.0	5.8	0.19	0.95
8.0	6.6	0.22	1.10
9.0	7.5	0.25	1.25
10.0	8.3	0.27	1.35
11.0	9.1	0.30	1.50
12.0	10.0	0.33	1.65
13.0	10.8	0.36	1.80
14.0	11.6	0.39	1.95

**The initial dose of sodium nitrite will produce 26.8% methemoglobinemia. The sodium thiosulfate dose is based on the adult ratio: 5 cc 25% sodium thiosulfate to 1 cc 3% sodium nitrite.*

HYDROCARBON POISONING

Hydrocarbon ingestions account for a significant number of accidental ingestions in children less than 6 years of age. In 1993, AAPCC reported 55,903 exposures to hydrocarbons including turpentine and pine oil; 52% of these exposures were in children less than 6 years of age. About 22% of exposures in this age cohort involved gasoline exposures resulting in four deaths[351]. These products are often attractively packaged, scented, and colored, e.g., Old English Red Furniture Polish and green kerosene lamp oil. In addition, they are often poured into drinking glasses, soda bottles, or coffee cups for easier dispensing, making them much more attractive and accessible for the inquisitive toddler to drink. Solvent abuse via inhalation of some halogenated hydrocarbons is becoming increasingly prevalent among the adolescent population and responsible for many deaths each year.

Physical Properties and Toxicity

Hydrocarbons responsible for human poisoning can be classified into four groups. Three of these groups are petroleum distillates (crude oil by-products): straight chain aliphatic compounds, halogenated compounds, and aromatic compounds. The fourth group is pine wood distillates. The physical properties of hydrocarbons determine the risk of aspiration and potential for toxicity.

Viscosity is the resistance to flow through a calibrated orifice and provides the best estimate of the aspiration potential. It is measured in Saybolt Seconds Universal (SSU) with substances less than 60 SSU having high aspiration potential and those with greater than 100 SSU having minimal aspiration risk.

Volatility is the ability of a substance to vaporize, or exist in a gaseous form. Highly volatile hydrocarbons displace alveolar oxygen when aspirated, leading to transient hypoxia. Surface tension is the cohesiveness of the molecules on a liquid's surface. Reduced surface tension allows the rapid spread of a substance from the mouth to the trachea. Petroleum distillates with low surface tension and low viscosity are serious aspiration hazards. The most viscous products are usually nontoxic.

Aliphatic petroleum distillates, such as gasoline, naphtha, mineral spirits, kerosene, and mineral seal oil are used in products such as fuels, degreasers, lacquer thinner, charcoal lighter fluid, and furniture polish. They are poorly absorbed from the GI tract. Gasoline and naphtha have high volatilities, causing primary CNS depression by fume inhalation in the absence of pulmonary toxicity[352]. Mineral spirits, kerosene, and mineral seal oil cause aspiration pneumonitis because of their low volatility and low viscosity. Mineral oil, motor oil, transmission fluid, and petroleum jelly are essentially nontoxic; however, direct aspiration of mineral oil may occur in very young infants, sometimes causing lipoid pneumonia.

Mineral seal oil is found in 20% to 99% concentration in furniture polish such as Old English Red Furniture Polish® and warrants emphasis because of its unusually severe and protracted pulmonary manifestations[353]. It probably has the greatest risk among hydrocarbons for aspiration pneumonia although its viscosity of 47 SSU is actually greater than kerosene, naphtha, and turpentine, whose viscosities range from 30 to 33 SSU. Three explanations have been proposed to account for the more severe clinical course caused by these furniture polishes[354]:

1. Larger volumes may be ingested because of the bright red color, flat taste, and less mucous membrane irritation;
2. Production of lipoid pneumonia in addition to chemical pneumonitis; and
3. Colorizing and odorizing additives (oil of cedarwood, camphor, lemon, wintergreen, and aniline dye) may contribute to the pulmonary toxicity as well.

Halogenated hydrocarbons include primarily chlorine-substituted compounds. Methylene chloride is found in paint strippers, fumigants, and degreasers and is metabolized, in part, to carbon monoxide, producing symptoms of this toxic gas. Carbon tetrachloride is used as a solvent and refrigerant and can cause severe liver toxicity (centrilobular hepatic necrosis), as can trichloroethylene and trichloroethane. Trichloroethylene, found in typewriter correction fluid, paint and spot removers, and degreasants, is responsible for a significant number of deaths and near deaths of adolescents secondary to inhalation abuse[355,356]. Fluorinated and chlorinated hydrocarbons (freons), used as refrigerants and propellants, are also commonly abused hydrocarbon solvents resulting in deaths secondary to inhalation[357–359].

Aromatic hydrocarbons—benzene, toluene, and xylene—are highly volatile substances that are readily absorbed after inhalation and well absorbed from the GI tract. These hydrocarbons are used as solvents, degreasers, and additives in pesticides. Abuse of toluene and xylene sometimes involves inhalation by "huffing" through a soaked cloth or "bagging" after vaporization in a plastic bag. Otherwise, toxic effects are usually secondary to chronic exposure.

Turpentine is a distillate of pine wood, containing different terpenes, and used as a paint thinner and household solvent. Pine oil is used in household cleaners, polishes, and disinfectants and contains a mixture of terpene hydrocarbons and alcohols. Both are readily absorbed from the GI tract. Turpentine and pine oil both can cause aspiration pneumonitis as a result of low viscosity[360–362]. Unlike aliphatic hydrocarbons, both can cause neurological symptoms because of systemic absorption. **Table 40.14** displays the relative toxicities of various hydrocarbons.

Pathophysiology

Hydrocarbons are believed to solubilize the lipid surfactant layer leading to alveolar instability, distal airway closure, ventilation/perfusion mismatches, and subsequent hypox-

Table 40.14. Toxicity of Hydrocarbons

Hydrocarbon	*Uses*	*Pulmonary Aspiration*	*CNS Toxicity (Mechanism)*	*Systemic Toxicity*	*GI Decontamination*
ALIPHATIC PETROLEUM DISTILLATES					
High volatility, Low viscosity					
Gasoline	Fuel	±	+ (Inh)	Low	No
Naphtha	Lighter fluid	±	+ (Inh)	Low	No
Low volatility, Low viscosity					
Mineral spirits	Solvent, paint thinner	++	± (Inh)	Low	No
Kerosene	Fuel, lighter fluid	++	± (Inh)	Low	No
Mineral seal oil	Furniture polish	++	± (Inh)	Low	No
Low volatility, High viscosity					
Mineral oil	Baby oil, laxative	+[a]	—	None	No
Heavy gas oil	Motor oil, transmission fluid	±	—	None	No
Lubricants	Petroleum jelly, paraffin	—	—	None	No
CHLORINATED HYDROCARBONS					
Methylene chloride	Solvent, paint strippeer	—	+ (Inh, Sys)	High	Yes
Carbon tetrachloride	Solvent, refrigerant	—	+ (Inh, Sys)	High	Yes
Trichloroethylene	Typewriter correction fluid, spot removers	+	+ (Inh, Sys)	High	Yes
AROMATIC HYDROCARBONS					
Benzene	Solvent, synthesizer in dyes, rubber, adhesives	+	++ (Inh, Sys)	High	Yes
Toluene	Solvent for paint, lacquers, glues	+	++ (Inh, Sys)	High	Yes
Xylene	Solvent, degreaser	+	++ (Inh, Sys)	High	Yes
PINE WOOD DISTILLATES					
Turpentine	Solvent, paint thinner	++	+ (Sys)	Intermed[bc]	
Pine oil	Disinfectants, cleaners	+	+ (Sys)	Intermed[bc]	

Low viscosity = <60 SSU; High viscosity = >100 SSU
GI Decontamination = gastric evacuation and activated charcoal. See text for further details.
++ = significant + = present ± = equivocal — = absent; Inh = Inhalation; Sys = systemic toxicity
[a] *Lipoid pneumonia*
[b,c] *When ingested in large quantities or high concentrations. See text for further details.*
Adapted from Goldfrank LR. Hydrocarbons. In: Goldfrank's Toxicologic Emergencies. 5th ed. Norwalk CT: Appleton & Lange, pp. 1238, 1239, 1240.

emia[363,364]. Hydrocarbon pneumonitis is characterized histopathologically by interstitial inflammation, atelectasis, hyperemia, vascular thrombosis, bronchial and bronchiolar necrosis, intraalveolar hemorrhage, edema, polymorphonuclear exudate, and formation of hyaline membranes thought to occur secondary to direct alveolar and capillary damage by the hydrocarbon[365].

Clinically, this injury is manifested as dyspnea, tachypnea, rhonchi, rales, wheezing, cyanosis, and fever. These changes may progress to hemorrhagic bronchopneumonia, pulmonary edema, and adult respiratory distress syndrome (ARDS) rapidly within a 24 hour period. Later pulmonary complications also reported with hydrocarbon pneumonitis include pleural effusion, pneumothorax, pneumomediastinum, and pneumatoceles. Mineral oil and heavy lubricants can produce a lipoid pneumonia that is more localized and less inflammatory than the pneumonitis produced by low viscosity petroleum distillates like mineral seal oil and kerosene[366].

Clinical Presentation

Hydrocarbon poisoning primarily affects the pulmonary, CNS, and gastrointestinal systems. Gasping, coughing, gagging, and choking are presumptive evidence of aspiration, although these transient symptoms as well as initial cyanosis may occur immediately because of hydrocarbon volatilization. Most patients will exhibit some respiratory symptoms—tachypnea, persistent cough, rales, rhonchi, wheezing—within 2 hours of a significant aspiration[363]. Symptoms may progress over 24 hours but usually resolve by the second or third day.

The majority of CNS toxicity secondary to hydrocarbons is due to aspiration-induced hypoxia. Some toxicity may also be related to volatilization on ingestion with displacement of oxygen or the presence of aromatic impurities or other toxic additives, such as nitrobenzene or insecticides which may cause direct CNS toxicity. CNS symptoms include lethargy, irritability, dizziness, confusion, excitement, stupor, and coma. Children with signs and symptoms of serious aspiration pneumonias usually present with concommitant signs of CNS depression. Poor GI absorption limits the CNS toxicity of most petroleum distillate products.

Gastrointestinal symptoms are common but usually minor. As a result of a direct toxic effect to mucous membranes, they cause burning of the mouth and oropharynx, nausea, vomiting, and abdominal pain. Hematemesis may be seen with toluene, benzene, pine oil, and turpentine ingestions[367]. Spontaneous vomiting is a significant risk factor for the development of aspiration pneumonitis.

Myocardial injury is rare after acute hydrocarbon ingestions; however, James et al reported ECG evidence of myocardial injury after mineral seal oil ingestion in a child[368]. Sensitization of the myocardium to endogenous catecholamines resulting in ventricular dysrhythmias has been demonstrated in animal studies with aromatic and halogenated hydrocarbons but only hypothesized to occur similarly in humans[357,358]. Deaths secondary to inhalation abuse of freon (fluorinated) and chlorinated solvents have been attributed to this sensitization phenomenon, although coronary vasospasm and simple asphyxia have also been suggested[359,369].

Fever is present in about 30% of patients with aspiration pneumonitis, probably secondary to direct pulmonary tissue damage. Most fevers appear within the first 24 hours and subsequently resolve. Persistent fever beyond 48 to 72 hours suggests bacterial infection. Other clinical symptoms may be present due to mixed ingestions of hydrocarbon solvents and other substances such as pesticides.

Chronic exposure to benzene may present with aplastic anemia or leukemia[370]. Chronic inhalation of toluene can result in a characteristic renal tubular acidosis and CNS symptoms of cerebellar ataxia and chronic encephalopathy[371,372].

Turpentine ingestions can result in similar GI symptoms of nausea, vomiting, abdominal pain, and diarrhea, as well as respiratory symptoms secondary to aspiration. It can also cause hemorrhagic cystitis, glomerulonephritis, hematuria, and albuminuria and imparts an odor of violets to the urine[373]. In severe ingestions, CNS effects may include ataxia, dizziness, excitement, seizures, stupor, or coma.

Similarly, pine oil can cause mucous membrane irritation with resultant vomiting, epigastric pain, hemorrhagic gastritis, and diarrhea. Systemic absorption may lead to somnolence, delirium, and ataxia, independent of co-ingested alcohols[374,375]. In the majority of cases of pine oil ingestions, intoxication is limited even with large ingestions[376]. Unlike petroleum distillates, there is some evidence that pulmonary complications due to pine oil result from systemic absorption and deposition of pine oil in lungs via the bloodstream[377].

Laboratory Findings

Hydrocarbon levels in the blood are neither useful nor practical in the immediate management period. An arterial blood gas may demonstrate hypoxemia secondary to ventilation/perfusion mismatch and/or hypercarbia secondary to progressing respiratory failure. A carboxyhemoglobin level should be obtained on any patient exposed to methylene chloride.

Leukocytosis is commonly present during the first 48 hours not related to bacterial infection. Intravascular hemolysis has been reported in children with gasoline, kerosene, and dry cleaning fluid (perchloroethylene) ingestions[352,378].

Chest x-ray abnormalities can appear as early as 20 to 30 minutes and as late as 24 hours after aspiration. Bilateral basilar infiltrates, right basilar infiltrates, and fine perihilar densities are the most commonly reported patterns of hydrocarbon aspiration[360]. Segmental atelectasis and localized air trapping are commonly seen while pleural effusions, areas of consolidation, pneumomediastinum, and pneumothorax are much less common. Asymptomatic pneumatoceles may appear in a small number of children 3 to 15 days postingestion, resolving in several weeks to months without any complications. Most patients who have immediate clinical symptoms of aspiration will have some abnormalities, although minor, on an initial chest x-ray even though their symtoms may rapidly resolve. Although radiographic abnormalities may be delayed, most patients who will eventually have an abnormal x-ray will have abnormalities within 2 hours after the ingestion[379]. However, a normal chest x-ray immediately after ingestion does not mean that clinical symptoms will resolve. Virtually all patients who remain clinically symptomatic 6 hours postingestion will have abnormal radiographs.

Management

The majority of children who accidentally ingest hydrocarbon products have no initial symptoms, require no further medical evaluation, and can be safely observed at home for the development of respiratory symptoms. Any child who has inital symptoms suggestive of pulmonary aspiration immediately following the ingestion, such as coughing, choking, or gasping, should be evaluated in a health care facility. Basic supportive care should be provided for all symptomatic patients whether from inhalation, aspiration, or ingestion. ECG monitoring and pulse oximetry should be initiated. A chest x-ray should be obtained on any child who had initial respiratory symptoms.

The role of decontamination measures, primarily gastric evacuation after aliphatic hydrocarbon ingestions, has been controversial because of the fundamental clinical question about the extent of gastrointestinal absorption of hydrocarbons and whether this absorption plays a significant role in producing pneumonitis versus aspiration directly. Also, there was concern that inducing vomiting or placing an orogastric lavage tube would further increase a child's risk of hydrocarbon aspiration. Well-designed animal studies have demonstrated that GI absorption of aliphatic hydrocarbons such as kerosene and naphtha does not contribute to development of aspiration pneumonitis and that CNS toxicity does not occur in the absence of aspiration[380–383]. Further support for the concept that pulmonary toxicity is related to aspiration, not absorption, comes from the finding of heterogeneous and focal pulmonary lesions on chest radiographs compatible with direct pulmonary injury.

Reports of human intravenous hydrocarbon injections have demonstrated more diffuse, homogeneous chemical pneumonitis, which reaffirms previous animal data that the first capillary bed encountered exhibits the most toxic injury from hydrocarbons[380,381,384,385]. The relative risk of spontaneous aspiration as compared with iatrogenic aspiration during induced emesis or lavage is not known. Human clinical studies attempting to determine whether ipecac-induced emesis or gastric lavage contributed or protected children from development of aspiration pneumonitis do not provide unequivocal support for either decision[360,386].

Rational decisions concerning gastric evacuation after hydrocarbon ingestion depend on the particular substance ingested and its intrinsic toxicity, the amount of substance ingested, whether it was accidental or intentional, and the child's mental status. Accidental ingestions of highly viscous petroleum distillates with poor GI absorption—mineral oil, lubricants, home fuel oil, and diesel fuel oil—and highly volatile petroleum distillates with minimal GI absorption—mineral seal oil and naphtha—do not require stomach evacuation. If the child's mental status and airway are normal, emesis may be indicated when there is no spontaneous vomiting and a toxic hydrocarbon known to produce systemic toxicity is ingested, such as halogenated and aromatic hydrocarbons, or hydrocarbons with a toxic additive such as heavy metals or pesticides. Ipecac-induced emesis is not indicated for turpentine and pine oil ingestions because of the rapidity of CNS toxicity as well as mucous membrane irritation.

Gastric lavage should be performed when removal of a liquid substance is indicated but ipecac-induced emesis is contraindicated, when there is concomitant ingestion of another drug or toxin in which lavage is indicated, or when rapid onset of a toxin's activity, particularly CNS depression, is expected, as with camphor and pine oil. Large volumes of turpentine require gastric lavage. Pine oil ingestions rarely require gastric decontamination except when large amounts or high concentrations (greater than 20%) are ingested. A nasogastric tube may be used for the removal of liquid substances.

Activated charcoal is not indicated in nontoxic hydrocarbon ingestions because hydrocarbons are poorly adsorbed. Although its effects in preventing [intestinal] absorption are limited, charcoal may be indicated if the hydrocarbon has a toxic additive or a toxic drug or toxin is concomitantly ingested.

Aspiration pneumonitis is treated with supportive care measures, primarily supplemental oxygen and bronchodilators for wheezing. Prophylactic or therapeutic steroids as well as prophylactic antibiotics have not been found to improve clinical outcome(387,388). Continuous positive airway pressure (CPAP) and mechanical ventilation with PEEP may be necessary in severe cases of hydrocarbon pneumonitis to maintain adequate oxygenation(389). Extracorporeal membrane oxygenation (ECMO) has been used in severe cases of hydrocarbon pneumonitis refractory to standard mechanical ventilation(390,391). High frequency jet ventilation has been reported as a successful alternative to ECMO and conventional ventilation(392). Theoretically, early administration of surfactant may be helpful because of hydrocarbon's ability to destroy surfactant although no animal or clinical studies have demonstrated this benefit.

Epinephrine and isoproterenol theoretically may induce ventricular dysrhythmias because of halogenated hydrocarbon's sensitization of myocardium and should probably be avoided unless required for basic resuscitation. Severe methylene chloride poisoning should be treated with 100% oxygen and, possibly, hyperbaric oxygenation(393). Hyperbaric oxygenation has been advocated for severe carbon tetrachloride poisoning(394).

Disposition of the child with hydrocarbon ingestion or aspiration depends on presence of initial clinical symptoms, persistence of symptoms, and substance ingested. Anas et al developed criteria for hospitalizing and discharging children after reviewing 950 cases of hydrocarbon ingestions. These criteria have continued to be supported by clinical experience(395).

Symptomatic children with abnormal initial chest x-rays, children with massive ingestions, hypoxic children despite normal x-ray, and children with significantly abnormal initial chest x-rays should all be hospitalized. Six-hour observation in an emergency department or acute care setting may be warranted for children with potentially insignificant ingestions or children with initial symptoms upon presentation which resolve. After this six-hour period, admission is needed if asymptomatic patients develop symptoms during this period or mildly symptomatic patients with a normal chest x-ray do not improve. Asymptomatic children with a normal chest x-ray and asymptomatic children with a mildly abnormal chest x-ray who do not develop symptoms during the observation period may be discharged to home(396).

IRON INTOXICATION

Acute iron intoxication remains a common and potentially lethal cause of poisoning in children. Of the approximately 5000 cases of iron poisoning that are reported to national poison control centers in the United States, approximately 7% will require hospitalization(397). Several factors account for the high incidence of iron poisoning. Iron-containing compounds, either as iron tablets or iron-fortified vitamins, are easily available and widely used in households, primarily as nutritional supplements during pregnancy and childhood. Their frequent candy-like appearance makes them clearly attractive to young children. In addition, iron supplements are usually regarded by the lay community as health-promoting compounds and not as potentially lethal drugs.

The severity of iron intoxication is directly related to the amount of elemental iron that has been ingested(400). An estimation of this may provide a rough guide to the potential severity of the intoxication. These estimations are, however, notoriously unreliable. When calculating the ingested dose, one must realize that the amount of contained elemental iron will depend on the particular iron compound ingested. The iron content of the ferrous gluconate, sulfate, and fumarate salts is 12%, 20%, and 33%, respectively. It is generally considered that ingestions of elemental iron of less than 20 mg/kg will be insignificant. Mild toxicity is likely after ingestion of 20 to 60 mg/kg. Moderate to severe intoxications may occur with ingestion of more than 60 mg/kg. An ingestion of greater than 200 mg/kg is potential lethal, unless the patient is rapidly and appropriately treated(397).

Pathophysiology

Under physiologic circumstances, only 10 to 15 mg of dietary iron is absorbed daily from the gastrointestinal tract. The functional mucosal barrier to iron absorption is, however, completely overwhelmed after a massive iron ingestion when iron is absorbed by first-order kinetics. Iron is absorbed as the ferrous form in the duodenum and jejunum and converted to ferric iron in the gastrointestinal mucosal cells. From there, it enters the blood where it is bound to transferrin, an iron-specific, β_1-globulin carrier protein, that transports it to the bone marrow for hemoglobin synthesis, and to the reticuloendothelial system and liver cells for storage as ferritin and hemosiderin.

Normally, 35 ± 15% saturated transferrin circulates in a concentration of 200 to 400 μg/dl. The normal circulating serum iron concentration is 50 to 150 μg/dL, reflecting a transferrin saturation of 20 to 50%. In acute iron intoxication, the total serum iron concentration may exceed the total iron binding capacity of transferrin, such that free, toxic iron circulates.

Apart from the loss of 1 to 2 mg of iron per day in sweat, bile, urine, and replaced gastrointestinal and epidermal cells, there is no physiologic mechanism for enhancing iron excretion after an acute overdose.

The effects of the increased circulating, unbound iron are observed most noticeably on the gastrointestinal tract and the cardiovascular, coagulatory, hepatic, and central nervous systems with widespread disruption of intermediary metabolism[(398,399,400,401,402)].

The vomiting, diarrhea, and abdominal pain that occasionally progress to lethal hemorrhagic gastroenteritis are attributed to the direct corrosive and toxic effects of the ingested iron salts on the mucosal surfaces of the gastrointestinal tract[(403)]. Acute, focal, gut necrosis that complicates vascular thrombosis may lead to perforation and peritonitis[(404,405)]. Healing by fibrosis produces areas of stenosis and obstruction. Initial gut damage is not a prerequisite for severe iron intoxication. Markedly elevated serum iron levels may develop in the absence of mucosal damage.

The pathogenesis of shock and cardiovascular depression is unclear. There are scant hemodynamic data on humans with iron intoxication and only a limited number of animal studies. It has been suggested that the high concentration of circulating iron or ferritin produces venous pooling. This, together with the generalized capillary leak and "third space" loss of fluid as well as blood loss from the gut, results in hypovolemia, hemoconcentration, decreased preload and reduced cardiac output, and decreased tissue perfusion[(400,406)].

Several factors are involved in the metabolic acidosis associated with severe iron poisoning. Shock and hypotension result in reduced tissue perfusion, anaerobic metabolism, and lactic acidosis. Large amounts of hydrogen ion are released into the circulation with the conversion of ferrous iron to its ferric form and its subsequent hydration. In addition, organic acids such as lactate and citrate accumulate as a result of the iron-induced, mitochondrial damage and alteration in Krebs cycle function[(405,407)].

The hepatocyte is the primary site of free iron uptake once the Kupffer cells have become saturated, and it is the mitochondria that become the primary intracellular target. Electron microscopic studies in experimental iron intoxication have demonstrated the localization of iron in the mitochondrial cristae, the site of the electron transport system and high-energy phosphate synthesis[(407,408,409)]. Iron-induced lipid peroxidation of the mitochondrial membrane has been associated with disturbances of the electron transport system and Krebs cycle function. In addition, it has been suggested that the increased intramitochondrial concentration of iron that exists in the intoxicated state might be creating an electron sink result in the shunting of electrons away from the cytochrome system, impairing ATP production, and causing cell damage and death[(407)].

Coagulopathy is the hallmark of severe iron poisoning in humans and laboratory animals. This is multifactorial, with disseminated intravascular coagulation, depressed synthesis of hepatic coagulation factors, and iron-induced alteration of factors of both the intrinsic and extrinsic coagulation cascades playing a role[(406)]. The coagulopathy is characterized by prolongation of the prothrombin, thrombin, and partial thromboplastin times. In vitro studies have demonstrated that the predominant abnormality is an iron-mediated interference with activated thrombin as well as other enzyme systems of the intrinsic cascade—a manifestation of the general susceptibility of serum proteases to nontransferrin-bound, ferric iron[(410,411,412)].

Clinical Manifestations

The clinical manifestations of iron intoxication have been divided into four phases[(398)]. The initial phase, attributed primarily to the direct effects of iron on the stomach and ileum, is characterized by nausea, vomiting, diarrhea, and abdominal pain. Severe iron poisoning does not develop in the absence of these gastrointestinal symptoms. With severe intoxication, these manifestations may progress to a severe hemorrhagic gastroenteritis with hematemesis and melena. Fever and leukocytosis may also reflect mucosal damage when intoxication is severe. In severe poisoning, shock and encephalopathy may develop during this very early stage. Approximately 25% of deaths from iron poisoning occur during this early phase[(397,398,399,400,401)].

The second phase, one of temporary recovery after the initial successful resuscitative measures, occurs between 6 and 12 hours after the ingestion. It is one of deceptive quiescence, lasting from 6 hours to several days. It is characterized by amelioration of the gastrointestinal and neurologic symptoms and, with intensive appropriate therapy, even the restoration of hemodynamic stability. Some patients will, in fact, completely recover from this point.

For others, this improvement is short-lived. They progress to the third phase, with recrudescence of gastrointestinal symptoms, the metabolic acidosis, the shock, and the CNS depression with lethargy and coma. The liver dysfunction is characterized by jaundice, elevated bilirubin and serum transaminases, profound hypoglycemia, and coagulopathy[413]. Renal failure may also develop. Some patients will progress to this phase of severe multisystem failure without experiencing the quiescent second phase[397,398,399,400] and, indeed, indicators of severe dysfunction may only be obvious in the second phase when looked for carefully.

The fourth phase of iron intoxication is occasionally experienced 4 to 6 weeks after ingestion by those who have survived severe iron poisoning. It is characterized by pyloric, gastric, or intestinal stenosis, the result of the healing and scarring of the gastrointestinal tract lesions[414].

Prediction of Toxicity

The prediction of toxicity is important in deciding who should be treated for toxicity and how rapidly and aggressively this should be carried out. As noted earlier, the amount of iron ingested is useful in predicting the likelihood of serious poisoning. The estimation of the ingested amount, however, is frequently inaccurate and unreliable.

The serum iron concentration has repeatedly been shown to correlate with the severity of iron intoxication (**Table 40.15**) [397,415,416]. Serum iron levels peak between 2 and 6 hours after a large ingestion. This is the optimal time to obtain a serum iron level. After 6 hours, the serum iron has been rapidly cleared from the serum, especially by the liver. A level drawn after this time may be normal even if there has been a potentially lethal ingestion. Even if serum iron determinations are immediately available, iron binding capacity measurements are frequently not available and are not needed for acute management.

Recent data have questioned the accuracy of most methods of measuring iron binding capacity in the face of acute intoxication[417,418,419]. Iron levels that are less than 300 μg/dL produce only mild, if any, symptoms. Moderate gastrointestinal toxicity may occur with levels between 300 and 500 μg/dL although such levels may not require specific antidotal therapy[420]. Progressive toxicity is observed when levels exceed 500 μg/dL and potentially lethal toxicity exists when levels exceed 1000 μg/dL[397].

Although serum iron levels are fairly predictive of the severity of iron poisoning, they are not always available on an emergency basis. In addition, since there have been cases of serious iron poisoning with serum levels of less than 300 μg/dL, normal serum iron levels do not rule out potentially serious intoxication. Several semiquantitative tests that estimate the presence of free, circulating iron, such as the Fischer[415] or Cooper tests, have been devised, but their accuracy has been questioned.

Studies have, however, demonstrated that certain clinical findings as well as simple laboratory tests are also useful in selecting those patients who are more likely to have significant toxicity[421]. Vomiting and diarrhea that develop in the 6 hours after ingestion, hyperglycemia—blood glucose concentration greater than 150 mg/dL, leukocytosis—white cell count greater than 15,000 cells/mm^3, and an abdominal radiograph that demonstrates the presence of radiopaque material are each highly predictive of and specific for a serum iron level of greater than 300 μg/dL. Of these findings, vomiting has the highest sensitivity and predictive value. The development of serious toxicity is unlikely after an asymptomatic period of more than 6 hours after an ingestion[421].

Table 40.15. Assessment of the Potential Severity of Acute Iron Intoxication Based on the Serum Iron Level[a]

Iron Level (μg/dL)	*Potential Severity*
<100	Toxicity unlikely
100–300	Minimal toxicity
300–500	Moderate toxicity
500–1000	Severe toxicity
>1000	Potentially lethal toxicity

[a]From Henretig FM, Temple AR. Acute iron poisoning. Emerg Med Clin North Am 1984;2:121.

Laboratory Tests

The importance of the rapid determination of serum iron has been stressed above. The serum glucose should be repeatedly followed. Hyperglycemia early in the course may be followed by severe hypoglycemia. White blood cell counts have predictive values and anemia may develop from gut blood loss. Blood gas determinations are important in assessing the severity of the metabolic acidosis. Coagulation studies will detect clotting abnormalities and liver function tests should be followed. The stools may turn black from either the ingested iron or altered intestinal blood and must be tested for the presence of occult blood.

Diagnosis

Vomiting, diarrhea, and hemorrhagic gastroenteritis with shock and CNS depression are typical of severe iron poisoning. Other poisonings with prominent gastrointestinal symptoms include those of arsenic, phosphorus, mercury, organophosphate insecticides, laxatives, and mushrooms. It must be emphasized that the determination of serum iron levels is not part of the routine toxicology screening tests. This test must be specifically requested.

Treatment

Prompt gastric emptying by ipecac-induced emesis is the initial step in gastric decontamination in the alert patient with an intact gag reflex. Gastric lavage via a large bore orogastric hose must be performed after airway protection is ensured if there is any question about the ability of the patient to protect the airway. This procedure may be performed following emesis for potentially serious iron poisoning if the ingested dose exceeds 60 mg/kg or when the post-emesis abdominal roentgenogram demonstrates persistent radiopaque material[397,400]. Alkalinization of the stomach contents precipitates iron as relatively insoluble ferrous bicarbonate and hydrous iron oxide although the clinical utility of this approach is questionable. Disodium phosphate lavage solutions that convert iron to ferrous phosphate have been used as lavage solutions, but have fallen into disfavor because of severe hyperphosphatemia, hypocalcemia, tetany, and hypernatremic dehydration that have occasionally followed their use[422,423].

Other reports have recommended gastric lavage with deferoxamine solutions to reduce iron absorption, but this remains controversial. There are no clinical studies that document the efficacy of either deferoxamine lavage or its enteral administration. If, in spite of vigorous gastric lavage, abdominal radiographs continue to demonstrate the presence of gastric iron-containing aggregates, consideration must be given to the removal of the drug mass by gastrotomy[424] or whole bowel irrigation.

Specific Chelation Therapy

Deferoxamine, an avid iron-binding ligand, is a safe and effective chelating agent for the therapy of iron intoxication[425,426]. Deferoxamine chelates free iron, as well as iron in storage as ferritin and hemosiderin, to form water soluble, renally excreted ferrioxamine. Although transferrin-bound iron is only minimally removed, hemoglobin- and cytochrome-bound iron are not chelated. Since the urinary elimination of ferrioxamine does not appear to account entirely for the drug's effectiveness, investigators have suggested that deferoxamine may also exert a protective effect at the cellular level by making iron unavailable to intracellular binding sites where its toxic effects are mediated[400].

Indications for initiation of deferoxamine include estimated ingestions of greater than 100 mg/kg of iron, severe gastroenteritis, a serum iron of greater than 500 μg/dL, or a serum iron between 300 and 500 μg/dL at 4 to 6 hours when accompanied by hyperglycemia, acidosis, hemodynamic instability, or lethargy[420]. Six hours after ingestion, treatment should be guided by clinical symptoms and history rather than the serum iron if it is low.

Deferoxamine therapy should be instituted as an intravenous infusion at 15 mg/kg/hr to prevent tachycardia and hypotension. Deferoxamine should be administered until the urine no longer exhibits a vin rose color, or until the serum iron is less than 100 μg/dL. Deferoxamine appears to be relatively nontoxic. Tachycardia and severe hypotension have been noted after too rapid an infusion[397] and renal function may be altered by even recommended infusion rates[427]. General supportive care and close monitoring are of crucial importance in the severely intoxicated patient. The development of shock must be anticipated. Adequate intravenous access should be established, and "third space" and intestinal fluid loss must be rapidly replaced, if necessary, guided by central venous pressure monitoring, to maintain urine output and ferrioxamine clearance. Blood transfusion may be necessary to replace substantial enteric blood loss.

Expected complications, which include metabolic acidosis, CNS depression, hypoglycemia, liver failure, and bleeding dyscrasia, will require appropriate monitoring and therapy. Rare cases of *Yersinia enterocolitica* sepsis have been reported from siderophore-induced stimulation of bacterial growth[428].

Although free iron is not dialyzable, iron bound as ferrioxamine can be removed by either peritoneal dialysis, hemodialysis or continuous arteriovenous hemofiltration[429], should acute renal failure ensue.

If the pathophysiologic events of iron poisoning involve the iron-induced generation of free radicals and subsequent membrane peroxidation, then therapy with either free radical scavengers or antioxidants might be effective. At the present time, however, there are insufficient data to recommend the use of any such agent for the treatment of iron poisoning[400].

OPIOID INTOXICATION

The opioids include a broad spectrum of compounds that interact with several subspecies of neural opioid receptors—the μ, κ, and δ receptors. The exogenous opioids are either natural alkaloids of opium (morphine, codeine), semisynthetic derivatives (heroin, hydromorphone, oxycodone, oxymorphone), or completely synthetic derivatives (e.g., butorphanol, fentanyl, levorphanol, meperidine, methadone, propoxyphene, and pentazocine). Dextramethorphan is an opioid with antitussive but no analgesic or addictive properties. Diphenoxylate is an opioid that is combined with atropine (Lomotil)® as a treatment for diarrhea. These agents are primarily prescribed for the relief of severe pain and some are also important as anesthetic, antidiarrheal, and antitussive agents.

Opioid intoxication in children occurs under several circumstances. It is frequently the result of the accidental or suicidal ingestion of potent opioids, such as methadone, prophoxyphene, or pentazocine, or by a large overdose of cough mixtures and pain medications. The residual respiratory depressive effects of narcotics used for anesthesia are frequently observed in the intensive care unit. Iatrogenic overdose after parenteral opioid administration for sedation or pain relief is occasionally observed in the hospital setting. Opioid intoxication by intravenous abuse is uncommon in pediatric patients.

In spite of the large number of available opioid drugs, the clinical manifestations of intoxication and the appropriate therapies for the management of intoxication are so similar that they will be discussed as a single class of drugs.

Pharmacology and Pathophysiology

Although the pharmacokinetics of many of the opioids of all three classes have been studied under therapeutic circumstances, much less is known about the pharmacokinetics of these agents in the intoxicated patient. Opioids are generally well absorbed after oral, intranasal, subcutaneous, or intramuscular administration. Oral administration results in lower serum levels than an equal amount of parenterally administered drug, because of first-pass hepatic extraction and metabolism. Small amounts of most opioids are excreted unchanged in the urine. The large remainder undergoes hepatic biotransformation by several reactions including conjugation with glucuronic acid, hydrolysis, hydroxylation, *N*-demethylation, and oxidation[(430)].

Extensive research over the past 20 years has suggested that the action of the exogenously administered opioids is mediated by their interaction with three different stereospecific, saturable receptors in the CNS—the μ, κ, and δ receptors. Different opioids bind with different affinities to these receptors to exhibit variable agonistic or antagonistic actions. On the basis of their variable interactions with these receptors, the exogenous opioids may be classified as agonists, antagonists, or mixed agonist-antagonist for particular receptors **(Table 40.16).** An opioid may, therefore, act as an agonist at one receptor but as an antagonist at another—an example of receptor dualism.

An appropriate understanding of the pathophysiology of opioid intoxication is predicated on the knowledge of the pharmacologic effects of the various opioids. Central nervous system effects include analgesia, mental clouding, sedation, dysphoria, and depression of the cough reflex. Increasing doses produce lethargy, sleep, and coma. Most important, from a toxicologic point of view, is the potential for profound respiratory depression that results from a reduction in the sensitivity of the medullary respiratory centers to a rising PCO_2. Opioids also depress the brainstem centers that control breathing rhythmicity. Typically, the reduced minute ventilation is caused by a reduction in respiratory rate, but with severe intoxication, tidal volume is also decreased. Central nervous system excitation is manifest by nausea, vomiting, and miosis, an almost pathognomonic finding in opioid intoxication. Seizures can be seen with propoxyphene and meperidine intoxication.

Analgesic and even anesthetic doses of most opioids produce little cardiac depression in healthy patients. The arteriolar and venous dilation produced by morphine and related opioids is partly responsible for the hypotension of narcotic intoxication. This vasodilatation is caused by both the release of histamine and the central inhibition of adrenergic tone. Hypoxia substantially exacerbates this opioid-induced hypotension. Finally, opioids can cause decreased gastrointestinal motility which has implications for GI decontamination.

Table 40.16. Central Nervous System Receptor System[a]

Receptor	*Agonist*	*Antagonist*	*Postulated Clinical Effects*
μ	Morphine	Pentazocine	Analgesia
	Codeine	Cyclazocine	Euphoria
	Heroin	Nalorphine	Respiratory depression
	Dihydromorphinone	Naloxone	Miosis
	Oxycodeine	Naltrexone	
	Fentanyl		
K	Pentazocine	Naloxone	Analgesia
	Nalorphine	Naltrexone	Sedation
	Morphine-like analgesics		Miosis
	Levallorphan		
	Fentanyl		
δ	Pentazocine	Naloxone	Dysphoria
	Cyclazocine	Naltrexone	Delusions
	Nalorphine		Hallucinations
	Levallorphan		

[a]From Bradberry C, Raebel MA. Continuous infusion of naloxone in the treatment of narcotic overdose. Drug Intell Clin Pharm 1981;15:945.

Clinical Manifestations

In general, the clinical manifestations of opioid drug poisoning in children are similar irrespective of the particular drug ingested. The differences are due mostly to the time course of toxicity. The triad of respiratory depression, miosis, and impaired consciousness is characteristic of opioid intoxication. The ingestion of other hypnotic, sedative, or psychotropic drugs in overdose may also produce severe CNS and respiratory depression, but since these drugs usually produce pupillary dilation, the presence of miosis helps to distinguish between these two classes of drugs. Mydriasis with opioid intoxication can occur with severe hypoxia and may also be seen with the ingestion of Lomotil®—a fixed combination preparation of the opioid diphenoxylate and atropine. The clinical manifestations of intoxication with this compound are the results of either the sequential or combined manifestations of anticholinergic poisoning (flushing, fever, lethargy, tachycardia, ileus, and urinary retention) and those of narcotic intoxication[(431)].

Hypotension and bradycardia are often seen in patients with opioid overdoses. Most opioids do not cause arrhythmias with the exception of propoxyphene. Norpropoxyphene, a metabolite of propoxyphene, is cardiotoxic, causing intraventricular conduction delays, heart block, bigeminy, and nonspecific ST-T wave abnormalities. Norpropoxyphene's cardiotoxic effects are not reversed by naloxone[(432,433)]. Noncardiogenic pulmonary edema is a complication of heroin and methadone overdoses. This may follow either parenteral, nasal, or oral administration of the opioids. The onset is usually rapid following intravenous heroin use, but may be delayed up to 24 hours. Possible mechanisms include anaphylaxis, hypoxia, and capillary injury secondary to street adulterants used to "cut" the opioid[(434)]. Direct CNS stimulation by opioids has been suggested by some to produce neurogenic pulmonary edema—a form of noncardiogenic pulmonary edema. The pulmonary edema is clinically manifest by hypoxemia, cyanosis, respiratory distress, tachycardia, rales, and respiratory and metabolic acidosis. Radiologically, it is demonstrated by bilateral, fluffy, perihilar infiltrates. Aspiration and infectious pneumonia may also complicate opioid overdoses and resemble opioid-induced pulmonary edema.

Seizures, in the absence of hypoxia, may occur following meperidine and propoxyphene overdoses. Normeperidine is the active metabolite of meperidine with twice the convulsant activity. In patients with sickle cell disease, neoplasms, or renal disease, the half-life of normeperidine is markedly prolonged[435].

Rhabdomyolysis secondary to deep coma and pressure necrosis of muscle occasionally complicates severe narcotic intoxication and may result in renal failure[436].

The rapidity of onset of the above described signs and symptoms of opioid intoxication varies with the particular narcotic and the route of administration. Of the orally ingested agents, propoxyphene is alarmingly rapid in its actions and can result in profound CNS depression in considerably less than an hour.

Designer fentanyls deserve special mention due to their extreme potency and irregularities as a result of drug dilution, resulting in brief epidemics of deaths and respiratory arrests[437]. "China white" and "Tango and Cash" are street names of fentanyls which include 3-methylfentanyl, parafluorofentanyl, and alpha methylacetylfentanyl, which may be hundreds to thousands of times more potent than morphine or heroin. They lead to CNS depression and respiratory arrest within minutes of intravenous injection.

Laboratory Tests

The qualitative detection of opioids or their metabolites in urine is available in most clinical laboratories to confirm the clinical diagnosis of opioid intoxication. Quantitative assays are technically difficult and play no role in the diagnosis or management of those intoxications. The laboratory can play a vital role in the determination of coingestants, or drugs, such as acetaminophen, that are present in fixed combinations with some opioids, such as propoxyphene or codeine.

Treatment

Initial management must be directed toward maintenance of an airway, adequate ventilation, oxygenation, and circulation. This may necessitate immediate endotracheal intubation and mechanical ventilation.

Naloxone (*N*-allylnoroxymorphone) is an opioid receptor antagonist capable of reversing the effects of exogenous and endogenous opioids. Naloxone is an antagonist at all three opioid receptors, and since it is devoid of any agonistic action, it will not add to any preexistent respiratory depression—a finding observed with the older partial antagonists. Naloxone reverses the respiratory and CNS depression, miosis, analgesia, dysphoria, euphoria, gastrointestinal stasis, and bradycardia caused by opioids. Naloxone does not reverse the cardiotoxic effects of norpropoxyphene. Although animal studies have demonstrated that opioid anatagonists prevent convulsions from meperidine and propoxyphene, this has not been demonstrated in human clinical experience[438].

The use of naloxone can be both diagnostic and therapeutic. It has always been considered that a response to naloxone in a comatose patient with respiratory depression and miosis confirms the diagnosis of opioid intoxication. However, naloxone has been shown to reverse the CNS depression caused by ethanol[439], clonidine[440], valproic acid[441], and diazepam[442] intoxication. Although subcutaneous, intramuscular, endotracheal, and sublingual routes can be used, intravenous naloxone administration is preferred because of its more rapid and reliable onset of action.

The dose of naloxone required to reverse the opioid effect is a function of receptor affinity and the quantity of opioid involved. The appropriate reversal dose of naloxone for adults and children has been widely debated. The American Academy of Pediatrics recommends an initial dose of 0.1 mg/kg for neonates as well as for children 1 month to 5 years (or < 20 kg). In older children, a minimum dose of 2.0 mg is recommended[443]. If there is no clinical response, another 2.0 mg is recommended every 2 to 3 minutes until at least 10 mg is given without a response. If there is no response observed after 10 mg, the diagnosis of narcotic-induced coma should be questioned; alternatively, a mixed drug overdose may be present. Larger doses, up to 10 mg, are recommended for acute methadone, propoxyphene, pentazocine, diphenoxylate, or codeine overdoses[444]. Patients in the hospital setting who develop CNS toxicity or respiratory depression from opioid administration may be given smaller amounts of naloxone initially to reverse the toxic effects while allowing the analgesic effect to persist.

Since the duration of action of most narcotics that are responsible for intoxication is significantly longer than that of naloxone ($t_{1/2}$ of several hours versus $t_{1/2}$ of 1 hour), additional doses of naloxone may be necessary to prevent the recurrence of CNS and respiratory depression. These repeated doses may be necessary for more than 24 hours, particularly after intoxication with very long-acting opioids such as methadone.

To maintain adequate reversal by maintaining high brain levels of naloxone and to obviate the need for frequent, intermittent doses, several reports have proposed and demonstrated the efficacy of a continuous naloxone infusion[445,446]. Controlled studies have not yet demonstrated an improved outcome when a continuous naloxone infusion has been used compared with repeated bolus administration. The required infusion dose will vary depending on the implicated opioid and the intoxicating dose. The dose must be titrated according to the patient's clinical response.

Goldfrank et al[447] have provided a dosing nomogram based on naloxone's pharmacokinetics, which proposes giving two thirds of the bolus dose that resulted in reversal as the hourly rate. A continuous infusion is, however, no substitution for continuous monitoring, close observation, and frequent clinical evaluation. The patient must be very closely observed after the infusion is discontinued. The appearance of any signs of deterioration are treated with a repeat bolus dose of naloxone and reinstitution of the infusion.

Naloxone is a particularly safe drug, and even massive doses of approximately 4 mg/kg have been administered without undue side effects. Hypertension, hypotension, atrial and ventricular arrhythmias, pulmonary edema and cardiac arrest have been reported in the anesthesiology literature when naloxone was used to reverse narcotic depression postoperatively(448,449,450). These patients had underlying organic heart disease, hypertension, or narcotic addiction and underwent major surgical procedures. It is hypothesized that abrupt and massive catecholamine release contributed to these effects. Thus, it is recommended that naloxone be used judiciously in small incremental doses of 0.1 or 0.2 mg in postoperative surgical patients(444). The use of naloxone as a diagnostic and therapeutic agent for unconscious patients in the emergency setting is not analogous to its use after surgery. Naloxone plays an important role in management of suspected or known opioid overdose. The only significant adverse effect reported when naloxone has been used in acutely poisoned patients has been the precipitation of opiate withdrawal, an uncommon scenario in the pediatric population.

GI decontamination is warranted for opioid ingestions after initial stabilization. Emesis must not be induced in anyone who is not alert and must be carefully considered if a patient has ingested a large dose of a rapidly acting drug such as propoxyphene. Since gastric emptying may be delayed due to inhibition of gastric motility, lavage may be indicated many hours after ingestion. If there is any concern about the ability of the patient to protect the airway, lavage should be performed only after the passage of an endotracheal tube, to ensure airway protection. Activated charcoal and a saline cathartic should subsequently be given. Multiple dose activated charcoal has been shown to increase the elimination of propoxyphene and diphenoxylate because of enterohepatic circulation(451,452).

Neither dialysis nor forced diuresis enhances the clearance of the opioids, and these therapeutic modalities play no role in the management of opioid-intoxicated patients.

Supplemental oxygen and the use of mechanical ventilation with positive end-expiratory pressure are central to the management of pulmonary edema. Diuretics play little role because, in the face of low cardiac filling pressures, they may precipitate hypotension and aggravate hypoxemia by increasing the intrapulmonary shunt. Optimizing both preload and positive end-expiratory pressure in a severely ill patient with noncardiogenic pulmonary edema is best achieved with the hemodynamic information gained by the placement of a Swan-Ganz catheter.

Seizures should be aggressively treated with intravenous benzodiazepines. Preexisting respiratory depression may be aggravated by this therapy, and one should be prepared to manage the airway with endotracheal intubation and artificial ventilation. Naloxone has not been demonstrated to terminate seizures in humans.

All children with a history of Lomotil® ingestion should be admitted to the hospital for 24-hour observation and monitoring. This recommendation results from the reports of children whose initial symptoms, especially coma and respiratory depression, were prolonged up to 30 hours and reports of the recurrence of respiratory and CNS depression 12 to 24 hours after the ingestion, presumably from the accumlation of the active long-acting opioid metabolite difenoxine. The lowest toxic doses reported to be associated with signs and symptoms of opioid/atropine poisoning in children are one half to two tablets. Furthermore, there is no correlation between dose ingested and severity of toxicity, warranting close monitoring for any child with a history of Lomotil® ingestion(453).

ORGANOPHOSPHATE AND CARBAMATE INSECTICIDE INTOXICATION

Two major classes of insecticides used for agricultural and domestic purposes are organophosphates and carbamates. Their popularity is due to their effectiveness as insecticides, as well as to the fact that these compounds do not accumulate in nature and are relatively rapidly decomposed after application. In 1993 there were over 19,000 reported exposures to organophosphates and/or carbamates with over 7000 occurring in children less than 6 years of age(351). There is a spectrum of relative toxicity of these compounds. The most highly toxic compounds include the nerve gases, sarin, soman, and tabun, as well as the industrial insecticides TEPP, parathion, mevinphos (Phosdrin)®, azinphos-methyl (Guthion)®, and disulfoton (Di-Syston)®. Insecticides with intermediate toxicity include coumaphos (Co-Ral), trichlorfon (Dylox)®, and chlorpyrifos (Dursban)®. The least toxic organophosphates are those for domestic use and include malathion (Cythion)®, dichlorvos (Vapona)®, and diazinon (Spectracide). The carbamate insecticides are a group of diverse chemicals derived from carbamic acid and are widely used both as agricultural and household garden insecticides. Aldicarb, carbaryl, and propoxur are examples of commonly used carbamates(454).

The organophosphate insecticides are rapidly absorbed through the skin, gastrointestinal tract, conjunctiva, and respiratory tract. Poisoning in children occurs as a result of accidental ingestion and/or skin/inhalation exposure from playing in areas recently treated with insecticides(455). In adults, poisoning occurs from occupational exposure and intentional suicidal ingestions.

Pathophysiology

The neurotransmitter acetylcholine is present in the terminal endings of all postganglionic parasympathetic nerves (muscarinic receptors), parasympathetic and sympathetic ganglia (nicotinic receptors), neuromuscular junction (nicotinic receptors), and certain sites within the central nervous system. After release from nerve endings and effecting action potentials at these synapses or the neuromuscular junction, acetylcholine is hydrolyzed to inactive choline and acetic acid by the enzyme acetylcholinesterase.

The phosphate moiety of the organophosphate insecticide binds irreversibly to acetylcholinesterase to form a stable, inactive, phosphorylated enzyme complex. Acetylcholinesterase has an affinity for organophosphates approximately 106 times more than for acetylcholine. Unhydrolyzed acetylcholine subsequently accumulates at the sites of acetylcholine synaptic transmission, causing overstimulation and disruption of transmission in both the peripheral and central nervous systems. Clinical manifestations are the result of muscarinic, nicotinic, and CNS receptor stimulation **(Table 40.17).**

The pathophysiology of carbamate poisoning differs from organophosphate poisoning in two important respects. First, the carbamates only transiently inactivate acetylcholinesterase with subsequent rapid enzyme reactivation. Second, carbamates do not effectively penetrate the CNS, resulting in limited CNS toxicity. Thus, the clinical manifestations of carbamate poisoning resemble those of organophosphate poisoning but are of shorter duration and lack the signs and symptoms of CNS involvement.

Clinical Manifestations

The dose, route of exposure, potency, and lipid solubility of the particular organophosphate determine the rapidity of onset and the sequence of development of signs and symptoms. Onset of symptoms may develop within minutes of massive ingestions or inhalation. In most cases of poisoning, the symptoms and signs are almost always observed within 12 hours of exposure, except with the more recently developed, highly fat-soluble organophosphates (fenthion, chlorfenthion) in which clinical manifestations may develop after several days[456].

The signs and symptoms of organophosphate poisoning can be classified into three categories based on receptors type. Muscarinic effects are *s*alivation, *l*acrimation, *u*rination, *d*efecation, *g*astrointestinal distress,and *e*mesis as reflected in the acronym SLUDGE. Nicotinic effects include muscle fasciculations, weakness, paralysis, areflexia, hypertension, tachycardia, pupillary dilation and pallor. Central nervous system manifestations include restlessness, emotional lability, headache, tremor, drowsiness, confusion, slurred speech, ataxia, generalized weakness, delirium, psychosis, coma, seizures, and cardiorespiratory depression[457].

The spectrum of clinical severity depends on the degree of acetylcholinesterase inhibition. Mild poisoning is usually manifested by fatigue, headache, nausea, vomiting, cramps, diarrhea, sweating, and salivation. Severely poisoned patients are comatose, hypotonic, weak, or paralyzed with respiratory difficulty, cyanosis, fasciculations, and copious oral and bronchial secretions. Tachycardia or bradycardia may be present depending on the relative balance of nicotinic and muscarinic stimulation. An electroencephalogram is useful in differentiating persistent, severe fasciculations from true seizures[458]. Many organophosphates have a characteristic garlic odor which may be useful in establishing the diagnosis.

Death in severely poisoned patients is due to cardiorespiratory failure. The mechanism of respiratory failure complicating severe poisoning is multifactorial. Hypoventilation may be due to muscular weakness, seizures, CNS respiratory center depression, or upper airway obstruction from accumulated secretions and hypotonic weakened pharyngeal musculature. Inability to oxygenate and ventilate also results from excessive bronchial secretions, bronchospasm, aspiration, atelectasis, and pulmonary edema. ARDS has been reported after severe organophosphate poisoning[459]. Hydrocarbon aspiration can aggravate the respiratory failure as hydrocarbons are common solvents for organophosphates.

The initial phase of cardiac involvement is manifested by tachycardia and hypertension—signs of nicotinic receptor stimulation. This is followed by muscarinic receptor stimulation and parasympathetic discharge with sinus bradycardia and varying degrees of AV block[460,461]. Studies have suggested that a third phase of cardiac involvement is characterized by prolongation of the Q-T interval alone or with T-U waves, premature ventricular beats, or pleomorphic ventricular tachycardia (Torsades de Pointes)[462,463]. This malignant arrhythmia may occur early or late in the clinical course, up to several days after intoxication, and may be a cause of the delayed deaths due to organophos-

Table 40.17. Clinical Manifestations of Organophosphate and Carbamate Poisoning

Anatomic Site	*Manifestation*
Central nerevous system effects	Headache, restlessness, emotional lability, dizziness, tremor, slurred speech, ataxia, confusion, lethargy, coma, seizures, respiratory and cardiovascular depression
Nicotinic effects	
Skeletal muscle	Fasciculations, cramps, weakness, areflexia, paralysis
Sympathetic ganglia	Tachycardia, hypertension, arrhythmias, pallor, mydriasis
Muscarinic effects	
Cardiac	Bradycardia, hypotension, heart block, arrhythmias
Respiratory	Bronchorrhea, bronchoconstriction (wheezing), dyspnea, cyanosis, pulmonary edema
Gastrointestinal	Anorexia, cramps, vomiting, nausea, diarrhea, tenesmus, fecal incontinence
Salivary glands	Excess salivation
Sweat glands	Increased sweating
Eyes	Miosis, lacrimation, blurred vision
Bladder	Urinary incontinence
Miscellaneous	Garlic odor, fever

[a]Modified from Haddad LM. The organophosphate insecticides. In: Haddad LM, Winchester JF, eds. Clinical management of poisoning and drug overdose. Philadelphia: WB Saunders, 1983.

phates. The mechanism of this third form of cardiotoxicity is unknown but appears unrelated to the use of therapeutic agents, hypoxia, acidosis, or electrolyte imbalance. Other electrocardiographic abnormalities observed include S-T segment and T-wave depression and supraventricular arrhythmias.

Delayed neurotoxicity from organophosphate exposure typically presents 1 to 3 weeks after exposure and may be manifested as peripheral neuropathies, such as lower extremity paresthesias, weakness and ataxia progressing to upper extremities, sometimes resulting in flaccid paralysis; memory impairment; personality changes; depression; and cognitive and thought disorders[464,465]. An "intermediate syndrome," occurring 1 to 4 days after an acute cholinergic phase, has been described in humans[466]. This syndrome is characterized by muscle weakness, particular in neck flexors and proximal muscles, cranial nerve palsies, diarrhea, diminished or absent ankle or knee reflexes, and sudden respiratory arrest. It is unclear whether this intermediate syndrome represents the later phase of toxicity from highly lipid-soluble organophosphates or undertreated organophosphate poisoning.

The clinical manifestations of carbamate insecticide poisoning differ from those of organophosphate in two important ways. Since the inactivation of acetylcholinesterase is short lived, the clinical manifestations are usually milder and of shorter duration. In addition, since the carbamates have poor CNS penetration, the prominent CNS manifestations of organophosphate poisonings are conspicuously absent[455,467], although late manifestations have been reported[468].

Laboratory Tests

The specific diagnosis of organophosphate poisoning can be confirmed by laboratory measurement of red blood cell acetylcholinesterase and plasma pseudoacetylcholinesterase. The levels of these enzymes reflect the degree of inactivation of synaptic acetylcholinesterase. Depressed red cell cholinesterase levels are more specific in the diagnosis of organophosphate poisoning, but this assay is more difficult and less available.

Cholinesterase levels can be difficult to interpret. For a result to provide meaningful information, a baseline level should be available for comparison. Laboratory "normals" must be used with caution because of individual variability of enzyme levels and their relationship to lab normals. Low serum pseudocholinesterase levels are less specific, since they may also be present in patients who are pregnant or who have malnutrition, liver disease, and various genetic deficiencies of the enzyme.

Although clinical manifestations do not always parallel the degree of acetylcholinesterase activity, mild poisoning is usually associated with greater than 20% activity, moderate poisoning with 10% to 20% of normal activity, and severe poisoning with less than 10% activity[469,470]. The blood for red cell acetylcholinesterase determination must be drawn before the administration of oxime enzyme reactivators, since normal levels may then be measured, in spite of clinical organophosphate poisoning. Pseudocholinesterase levels are unaffected by the oxime agents, and they remain low in the face of reactivator therapy.

Specific laboratory diagnosis can be made by the determination of organophosphate compounds in gastric contents or in urine by gas or thin-layer chromatography. Also, *p*-nitrophenol, a metabolic product of some commonly used organophosphates, can easily be measured in urine and is a nonspecific diagnostic test for exposure to the organophosphates.

The differential diagnosis of organophosphate poisoning can be complicated by the fact that some patients present with unusual features detracting from the true diagnosis. Mydriasis rather than miosis is not an uncommon finding and may be accompanied early in the clinical course by tachycardia and hypertension, signs of intense sympathetic ganglia and postganglionic adrenal medulla stimulation. Hyperglycemia, glycosuria, and coma may initially suggest diabetic ketoacidosis[471,472], but ketonuria and ketoacidosis are absent. Mild poisoning with wheezing, cough, fever, and leukocytosis can mimic respiratory tract infection. A low grade fever may persist for many days after intoxication. The bradycardia and heart block may even suggest intoxication with digoxin, β-blocker, or calcium channel blocker drug.

Treatment

Therapy of patients with organophosphate poisoning will depend on the severity of the poison. Observation alone may be all that is required in the mildest cases, but aggressive cardiorespiratory support may be urgently needed for the most seriously intoxicated patients.

Initial supportive care must be directed toward the maintenance of an adequate airway that can be easily compromised by muscular weakness, excessive secretions, emesis, and seizures—typical features of severe poisoning. Intubation and artificial ventilation must be instituted for respiratory failure. Predictably, the action of succinylcholine as an adjunct to intubation will be greatly prolonged[473]. Continuous electrocardiographic monitoring is necessary due to the proclivity toward arrhythmias.

Immediate decontamination is crucial. All clothing must be removed, and skin and hair should be thoroughly washed with soap and water. Gastrointestinal decontamination and activated charcoal are needed for recent accidental or intentional ingestions.

Atropine and the oximes are the classic organophosphate poisoning antidotes, although scopolamine and glycopyrrolate have also been advocated[474,475]. Atropine alone blocks the effects of acetylcholine in the CNS and at muscarinic receptors but has no effect on the neuromuscular junction. The recommended initial pediatric dose of atropine is 0.05 mg/kg intravenously; the adult dose 2 mg. Doses should be repeated at 5- to 10-minute intervals until adequate decrease and drying of oral and bronchial secretions is achieved. Pupillary dilation should not be used as a therapeutic endpoint. Tachycardia is not a contraindication to atropine and may be the result of hypoxia and continuing autonomic stimulation. Once adequate atropinization has been achieved, repeat doses should be given every 30 to 60 minutes because of the relatively short $t_{1/2}$ of atropine.

Some authors have suggested that control of clinical symptoms is best achieved by the use of a continuous infusion of atropine at 0.02 to 0.08 mg/kg/hr, depending on the degree and stage of intoxication[(476)]. Enormous doses of atropine, which may exceed 0.5 mg/kg/day, may be required over the course of treatment. Hundreds of milligrams of atropine have been administered to some patients within the first 24 hours of therapy.

Depending on the organophosphate involved, atropine administration may be required for many days. Signs of improvement after 12 to 24 hours are indications to begin the gradual tapering of atropine doses. Medical observation for at least 24 hours is mandatory if atropine has been administered[(477,478)]. Prolonged ileus may develop as a consequence of the administration of these high doses of atropine and may necessitate parenteral nutrition.

Pralidoxime (2-PAM) is an acetylcholinesterase reactivator and is the only such drug available for clinical use in the United States. Since the inactivation of acetylcholinesterase by organophosphates is essentially irreversible, restoration of enzyme function in the untreated patient is dependent upon de novo synthesis. Pralidoxime hastens the restoration of enzyme activity by competing with acetylcholine for the phosphate moiety of the organophosphate insecticide, thereby releasing the intact functional enzyme. Since the benefit of pralidoxime action is most striking at nicotinic receptors, weakness, paralysis, and muscle fasciculations are indicators for its administration. Improvement in strength may be observed within 10 minutes of administration.

Although pralidoxime is a quaternary ammonium compound and would not be expected to cross the blood-brain barrier, there is still some clinical evidence to suggest that it does have a CNS effect. Pro-2-PAM is an experimental dihydropyridine derivative of 2-PAM, synthesized to improve the CNS effect of pralidoxime[(479,480)]. It acts as a precursor drug, allowing in vivo oxidation to convert it to 2-PAM once it has crossed the blood-brain barrier.

Since the degree of irreversible inactivation of acetylcholinesterase by organophosphates increases with time, many investigators have stressed the need to administer pralidoxime within 48 hours after exposure for the drug to be effective. Treatment with 2-PAM is more effective if started early and used with acute rather than chronic organophosphate poisoning. Pralidoxime and atropine are synergistic and should be used together. If a patient requires atropine for muscarinic symptoms, then use of pralidoxime is also indicated.

Pralidoxime is administered intravenously over 30 minutes, at a dose of 20 to 40 mg/kg up to 1 gram, the adult dose. Rapid IV bolus administration should be avoided because of reports of respiratory and cardiac arrest. The dose may be repeated after 1 hour if weakness and fasciculations persist. Some patients may require multiple doses of pralidoxime before a clinical response is noted. Large amounts of pralidoxime may be required for prolonged periods in severely poisoned patients. Continuous infusions of up to 0.5 g/hour in adults have been effective[(481,482)]. Poisoning with newer fat soluble organophosphates such as fenthion or chlorfenthion may necessitate administration of atropine and 2-PAM for much longer periods of time[(483)].

The role of oximes in the treatment of carbamate poisoning is controversial. Human clinical studies have not confirmed whether oximes are beneficial for carbamate poisoning. Animal studies using pralidoxime alone or with atropine have showed an increase in carbaryl toxicity[(484,485)]. These studies have contributed to the recommendation that oximes are contraindicated in carbamate poisoning. One recent study demonstrated that oxime administration in children with aldicarb and methomyl poisoning did not worsen the condition of the patients, nor did it contribute to their recovery[(486)]. The use of pralidoxime is recommended whenever the pesticide is unknown or is known to contain a mixture of organophosphate and carbamates. Atropine is still needed as an antidote in carbamate poisoning.

PHENCYCLIDINE (PCP) INTOXICATION

In 1957, PCP was introduced as an experimental nonnarcotic, nonbarbiturate general anesthetic agent. It was, however, withdrawn for human use in 1965 because of its disturbing hallucinogenic and psychotomimetic side effects. In 1967, it was reintroduced commercially as the veterinary anesthetic, Sernylan. In that year it also appeared as a street drug-the "PeaCe Pill" in the Haight-Ashbury district of San Francisco. Unpredictable side effects and frequent "bad trips" led to an only transient appearance. In the early 1970s, because of the ease of manufacture in clandestine drug kitchens and home laboratories, PCP reappeared largely in urban ghettos where it was frequently misrepresented as other more expensive and glamorous drugs, such as cocaine, LSD, tetrahydrocannabinol, psilocybin, and mescaline. It became widely known and used as a primary drug of abuse, assuming street names that included, "angel dust," "mist," "hog," "PCP," "rocket fuel," and many others[(487,488)].

The mode of exposure to PCP is either by smoking (frequently with marijuana), snorting, oral ingestion, or rarely, and then usually only in the most chronic abusers, by intravenous abuse. The potency of PCP-laced cigarettes varies widely, from as little as 0.1 mg to as much as 160 mg per cigarette. When PCP is smoked or snorted, the dose is usually self-titrated. Oral ingestion of an unsuspected large dose or intravenous use is more likely to produce very severe intoxication.

PCP intoxication of pediatric patients occurs under several circumstances. Adolescents become intoxicated by purposefully experiencing the mood-altering properties of PCP, or they may be given PCP-laced drugs or cigarettes by their peers without their knowledge[(489)]. Infants and young children are exposed by accidental ingestion of PCP, by passive inhalation of ambient, PCP-tainted cigarette smoke[(490,491,492)], or occasionally, by intentionally being administered PCP—a form of child abuse.

Pharmacology and Toxicology

PCP is a white crystalline powder; approximately 30 of its analogs are arylcyclohexylamines. PCP is a weak base with a pK of 8.5. This property accounts for the relatively large amounts of PCP that are secreted and ion-trapped in the stomach, as well as for its enhanced renal elimination in acidified urine. PCP is a highly lipophilic drug that is rapidly absorbed from the alkaline contents of the small intestine. Clinical manifestations develop within a few minutes of inhalation, insufflation, or intravenous use. Oral bioavailability is about 72%[(493)]; ingestion produces symptoms within 20 to 60 minutes. PCP's volume of distribution in adults averages 6.2 L/kg[(493)]. The free fraction of PCP in blood averages about 22%, with 78% of the drug bound to plasma proteins[(494)]. Its high lipid solubility accounts for a large volume of distribution as well as its strong affinity for adipose and neural tissue. These factors, together with its participation in an enterogastric recirculation pathway, account in some part for the prolonged and fluctuating clinical course of intoxication.

PCP is largely hydroxylated by hepatic enzymes to inactive monohydroxy compounds that are excreted in the urine as the glucuronidated conjugates together with a small fraction of unmetabolized PCP. The mean elimination half-life ($t_{1/2}$) of PCP in volunteers who ingested PCP or smoked PCP-laced cigarettes ranged from 21 to 24 ± 7 hours[(493,495)].

Analogs of PCP, such as PHP, PCC, TCP, or PCE, may contaminate or replace its illicit laboratory synthesis. The clinical manifestations produced by these drugs resemble those of PCP intoxication. Detection of some of these compounds in toxicology laboratory screening tests is problematic and makes the diagnosis of intoxication by these agents difficult.

The mechanisms of action of PCP have undergone intense investigation, but the pathophysiology of the intoxication is still unclear. The prominent sympathomimetic effects of PCP intoxication have been attributed to both β- and adrenergic-agonistic and anticholinergic actions[(496,497)]. The neurologic and psychotomimetic manifestations have been variously associated with anticholinergic and dopaminergic antagonistic actions. PCP may increase both the firing rate and burst activity of dopamine neurons as well as preventing dopamine reuptake[(498)]. Recently, phencyclidine receptors have been characterized within the N-methyl D-aspartate (NMDA) protein complex, perhaps the most important modulator of excitatory neurotransmission within mammalian neurologic systems[(499,500)]. NMDA-associated PCP receptors have been located in the hippocampus, neocortex, basal ganglia, and limbic system; PCP's antagonism of the NMDA complex may account for some of its psychotomimetic effects[(499,500,501)].

Finally PCP potentiates the pressor response to epinephrine, norepinephrine, and serotonin. It inhibits reuptake of catechols at alpha-adrenergic receptors, which may account in part for the production of hypertension[(502)]. It also has been shown to be a direct myocardial depressant[(502)].

Clinical Manifestations

PCP intoxication is characterized by a wide array of clinical manifestations affecting several organ systems[(487,503,504,505,506)]. The pharmacologic effects of PCP intoxication are generally dose-related. Several investigators have classified the clinical presentation of adults with PCP intoxication into those with low-dose, moderate-dose, or high-dose intoxication[(487,488,504,506)]. Less than 10 mg of PCP generally produces low-dose intoxication. These patients usually present with the psychiatric, behavioral, and other neurologic and cardiovascular manifestations of PCP intoxication. Patients with high-dose intoxication caused by greater than 100 mg of PCP are usually comatose with the more marked neurologic findings noted below.

The hemodynamic findings of PCP intoxication are characteristically those of mild systolic and diastolic hypertension. Occasionally, severe hypertension may be associated with intracerebral hemorrhage.

Ventilation is well maintained in most low- and moderate-dose PCP-intoxicated patients, a feature that promoted its early use as an anesthetic agent. Hypoventilation and apnea may develop with massive overdoses. Laryngeal and pharyngeal reflexes are typically hyperactive with the potential risk of laryngospasm with laryngeal or pharyngeal manipulation. Flushing, diaphoresis, and increased bronchial secretions are other features of the autonomic nervous system stimulation that are occasionally seen.

The CNS manifestations of PCP intoxication are profound and best known. Nystagmus, which may be either vertical, horizontal, or rotary, is present in more than 50% of patients[(505)]. The pupils are typically midsize or miotic, and reactive. Dilated pupils are an infrequent finding. The characteristic motor disturbances of PCP intoxication include hyperactive reflexes, muscle rigidity, catalepsy, opisthotonus, localized dystonic reactions, purposeless facial grimacing, myoclonus, athetosis, and ataxia. Seizures are not infrequently a complication in large overdoses[(487,505)].

Rhabdomyolysis with myoglobinuria and even acute renal failure may complicate the muscle contractions associated with the dystonic motor activity in as many as 1% of patients intoxicated with PCP[(507)]. This can occur with isometric muscle contraction even in the absence of convulsions[(508,509)].

Moderate hyperthermia was a feature in 2.6% of cases in one study of 1,000 cases of PCP intoxication[(505)]. It may or may not be accompanied by rhabdomyolysis. While altered myoplasmic calcium transport in tense skeletal muscles may be one explanation for increased heat production, central neural mechanism(s) may also underlie the fever. In some patients hyperthermia from PCP exposure has has been followed by submassive liver necrosis and death[510].

Coma is a feature of moderate- or high-dose intoxication it was present in 10% of McCarron's series of 1,000 patients[505]. It may last for hours or many days in the most severe intoxications. Patients may be completely unresponsive but remain with open eyes. Characteristic electroencephalographic patterns of PCP intoxication include rhythmic activity sometimes interrupted by periodic slow or sharp wave complexes[511,512].

Sensory anesthesia may be part of the associated neurologic findings in intoxicated patients. They may remain quite unaware of sustained lacerations, contusions, or fractures.

The psychiatric manifestations of PCP intoxication are frequent and varied. Changes in behavior with a spectrum ranging from catatonia to bizarre, violent, and aggressive actions are seen. Prominent body image distortion is frequently present as are frank visual and auditory hallucinations. The patient's affect may vary from mania to marked dysphoria. Delusions of superhuman strength are characteristic of PCP intoxication, and such distortions have led to violent and traumatic deaths. Intoxicated patients have jumped off cliffs or have been killed because they believed they could stop oncoming vehicles. PCP's dissociative effects may lead to bizarre self-mutilation incidents with no accompanying pain or discomfort; as an example, one delusional man bit his own forearms almost to the bone[513].

With the exception of the prominent psychiatric symptoms, the clinical manifestations of PCP intoxication in the infant and young child are characterized by a spectrum of findings similar to those observed in the adults[491,492,514,515]. In mildly intoxicated children, who are not obtunded and who respond to pain, a dull trance-like stare, hallucinations, cerebellar signs with nystagmus, and lethargy alternating with periods of agitation are the most frequently observed signs. Miosis, hypersalivation, opisthotonus, hypertonia and hyperreflexia, choreoathetoid movements, and mild hypertension are the most frequently observed findings. Obtundation, sometimes even with an eye-open stare, is the most prominent feature of severe intoxication.

Seizures may also occur in both severely and mildly intoxicated children, unlike adults who develop seizures only when they are severely intoxicated[491]. These seizures are usually generalized and of short duration. Apnea and respiratory depression are also occasionally observed in young children.

Deaths due to PCP intoxication are usually the result of accidents associated with behavioral disturbances and risk-taking activities. Occasionally, fatalities are caused by uncontrolled seizures, intracranial bleeding, and respiratory depression[516,517,518].

Diagnosis

In contrast with intoxication produced by other psychedelic drugs, such as LSD or mescaline, the physical examination of the PCP-intoxicated patient provides clinical clues that help in the diagnosis in the absence of either the laboratory support or history of PCP intoxication. Low-dose PCP intoxication can be distinguished from other psychedelic drug intoxications by the presence of nystagmus, ataxia, blank stare, sensory anesthesia, hypertension, and the absence of mydriasis. Patients with moderate or severe PCP intoxication may clinically resemble cases of sedative-hypnotic overdose. Hypertension, hyperreflexia, abnormal posturing, and the absence of significant respiratory depression will support the diagnosis of PCP intoxication[487].

Laboratory Findings

Several chromatographic and enzyme immunoassay techniques of varying sensitivities are available for the detection of PCP in urine, blood, and other body fluids. Quantitative determinations are not of particular importance, since there is no constant relationship between the serum or urine levels of PCP and the severity of intoxication. Serum concentrations as high as 1879 mg/mL have been associated with survival[519]. Since PCP is lipophilic, and may be detectable in urine for prolonged periods after a rapid decline in blood level, urine remains the specimen of choice to be screened for PCP in the patients suspected of intoxication. In chronic PCP abusers, urinary excretion for as long as 30 days after the last exposure has been reported[520]. Other sporadically detected, nonspecific laboratory abnormalities include an elevation of the SGOT and SGPT and hypoglycemia. An elevation of the CPK and myoglobinuria are present with rhabdomyolysis.

Treatment

Since most adolescents and adults are intoxicated by snorting or smoking PCP, inducing emesis and the routine administration of activated charcoal and cathartics are not indicated unless exposure is by ingestion. In the comatose patient where the mode of exposure is unknown, gastric lavage through an orogastric hose, and the administration of intragastric activated charcoal and a cathartic should be performed after airway protection is ensured. Airway reflexes are hyperactive and particular care should be taken to prevent laryngospasm with the passage of a nasogastric or orogastric tube. Repeated doses of activated charcoal may be efficacious in binding PCP that continues to be secreted by the stomach. Continuous gastric suctioning has been recommended for the same reason, although electrolytes must be closely monitored in this circumstance[487,491].

General supportive care is the key to successful treatment in the PCP-intoxicated patient. The mildly intoxicated patient should be observed in a quiet, darkened environment devoid of extraneous auditory, visual, or tactile stimuli. Patients must be continuously observed and prevented from injuring themselves. The technique of "talking down" patients, sometimes successfully used for the management of the agitated patient intoxicated with other hallucinogens, is frequently unsuccessful with the PCP-intoxicated patient[(487,515)]. Patients who are combative should be sedated with diazepam, lorazepam or haloperidol. Phenothiazines may potentiate the anticholinergic side effects and reduce the seizure threshold for PCP.

Seizures are usually easily controlled with intravenous diazepam. Severe hypertension is uncommon, but hydralazine, diazoxide, nitroprusside, and propranolol may be used. The use of verapamil remains controversial[(521,522)]. Rhabdomyolysis with myoglobinuria should be managed with intravenous fluids and a diuretic such as mannitol or furosemide to ensure a diuresis. Urinary alkalinization, the usual therapy for rhabdomyolysis in other clinical circumstances, is controversial in the setting of PCP intoxication, because of its action in enhancing the renal absorption of this drug.

Severe muscle rigidity, hyperthermia, or status epilepticus may require neuromuscular blockade and mechanical ventilation. Hyperthermia should also be treated with aggressive core cooling; the efficacy of dantrolene is not well documented in the context of PCP intoxication.

Techniques to enhance the elimination of PCP from intoxicated patients have been proposed[(523)], but their efficacy remains unproven. Hemodialysis has not been shown to enhance the secretion of PCP, although it may be necessary in those patients with prolonged renal failure secondary to PCP-induced rhabdomyolysis. PCP-specific antibody Fab fragments have been recently developed and shown to change the kinetics of PCP's disposition in animals[(524,525)], but have so far been used only for investigational purposes[(526)].

SALICYLATE INTOXICATION

For many years, aspirin was the leading cause of both accidental poisoning and deaths due to poisoning in children. The increased use of acetaminophen, the use of child resistant containers, and changes in drug safety legislation that restricted the number of flavored children's aspirin tablets in a container to 45 g (thirty six 1.25 g tablets)—an amount that would produce only mild intoxication in a 10 kg child—dramatically reduced the incidence of acute accidental poisoning and deaths in young children. Since the early 1970s, aspirin has no longer been the leading cause of childhood poisoning[(527)].

Although declining in incidence, acute salicylate poisoning that occurs either accidentally in a young child or intentionally as a suicidal overdose in an adolescent or adult is still the most frequently considered form of salicylate intoxication. A more common, yet probably less well recognized form of salicylate poisoning is chronic salicylate poisoning. This occurs as a result of excessive administration over a prolonged period, usually longer than 12 to 24 hours. The aspirin is usually being administered as part of a therapeutic regimen but with parental, patient, or physician misunderstanding of appropriate dosage.

The decline in incidence of acute intoxication has not been paralleled by a similar decline in the incidence of chronic intoxication. Chronic poisoning is now the most frequently encountered form of aspirin poisoning and certainly accounts for most of the deaths due to salicylate intoxication[(528,529)].

Pharmacology

Aspirin (acetylsalicylic acid, ASA) is available in tablets, capsules, and suppositories, as well as in combination with antihistamines, sympathomimetics, anticholinergics, narcotics, and acetaminophen in various proprietary preparations. Over 200 aspirin-containing compounds are available in the United States. Salicylic acid is the active toxic metabolite of ASA. Other therapeutically used potentially toxic salicylic acid salts include sodium salicylate, magnesium salicylate, choline salicylate, and bismuth subsalicylate. Salicylamide, another salicylate and a component of several over the counter sleeping preparations, is also potentially toxic. Topical salicylic acid, a topical keratolytic[(530)] and homomethyl salicylate, a sunscreen compound, are also potentially toxic, either by cutaneous or gastrointestinal absorption.

Methyl salicylate, though an infrequent cause of salicylate poisoning, poses the threat of severe, rapid-onset salicylate toxicity because of its liquid, concentrated form. Sources of methyl salicylate include topical liniments and lotions such as Ben Gay Extra Strength Arthritis Rub® and Icy Hot Cream® which contain 30% methyl salicylate and oil of wintergreen—used both as a liniment and food flavoring additive—which contains 98% to 100% methyl salicylate[(531)].

The absorption of aspirin is dependent on the gastric emptying rate and the release characteristics of the varying salicylate preparations. Absorption of most conventional tablets or capsules is rapid, but prolonged, incomplete, and erratic with enteric coated preparations[(532)]. Liquid preparations are more rapidly absorbed than tablets. Large doses can delay gastric emptying and may be absorbed over a prolonged period exceeding 24 hours. Delayed absorption may also be caused by salicylate-induced pylorospasm[(533)] or bezoar formation[(534)].

Since aspirin is a weak acid, with a pK of 3.5, about 50% of the salicylate appears in the un-ionized form in the stomach and hence is rapidly absorbed. Absorption occurs

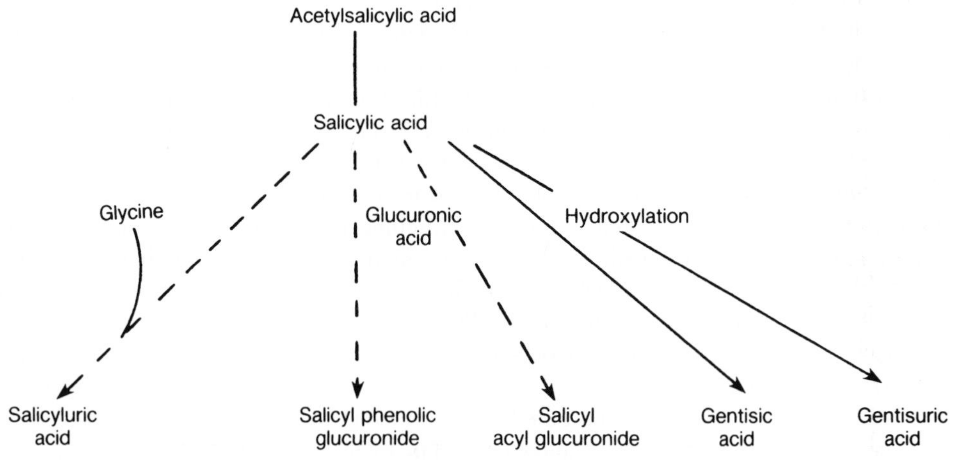

Figure 40.7. Metabolism of acetyl salicylic acid. (---) Zero-order kinetics at toxic levels. (—) first-order kinetics at toxic levels.

in the alkaline small intestine because of the large surface area despite the higher pH. The stomach and blood hydrolyze acetylsalicylic acid to salicyclic acid and acetic acid. Circulating salicylic acid is 50% to 90% protein bound with the remainder in plasma in the active, ionized state[535]. At toxic salicylate levels, protein binding decreases to less than 75%, increasing the availability of the free fraction of drug. The apparent V_D is approximately 0.1 to 0.2 L/kg under therapeutic circumstances and can increase up to 0.6 L/kg under toxic circumstances in the face of acidosis. Acetylsalicylic acid is responsible for the antiplatelet effects of aspirin, but it is salicylic acid, its major metabolite, that is responsible for its antiinflammatory and antipyretic properties, and is the toxic compound in salicylate overdose.

Salicylic acid is excreted from the body by the kidney after conversion by several hepatic biotransformation pathways to five inactive conjugated metabolites (Fig. 40.7)[536]. With low therapeutic doses of aspirin, approximately 70% of salicylic acid is conjugated with glycine to yield salicyluric acid—the major metabolite. Smaller amounts of salicylic acid are converted to salicyl phenolic or salicyl acyl glucuronide, hydroxylated to gentisic acid and gentisuric acid, or excreted unchanged as salicylic acid by glomerular filtration and tubular secretion. Except in renal failure, the metabolites of salicylic acid are excreted as rapidly as they are formed and are of no toxicologic importance[536].

The metabolic pathways for the synthesis of the two quantitatively most important metabolites—salicyluric and salicyl phenolic glucuronide-display Michaelis-Menten elimination kinetics—(zero-order kinetics) at high therapeutic and toxic plasma levels and first-order kinetics at therapeutic levels. The other metabolic pathways obey first-order kinetics. Knowledge of aspirin metabolism can thus explain the short, 15 to 20 minute t_{half} of aspirin, the 2 to 3 hour t_{half} of salicylic acid after a single therapeutic dose, the 6 to 12 hour $t_{1/2}$ with therapeutic serum levels, but the prolonged $t_{1/2}$ of greater than 20 hours after toxic ingestions. Chronic salicylate intoxication can occur because zero-order elimination kinetics are operative when high therapeutic serum levels from repeated doses are achieved. At this point, a small increase in dose can cause a much larger increase in serum salicylate level than would be observed if the same dose was administered in the presence of a lower serum concentration[536,537].

Under normal therapeutic circumstances, hepatic biotransformation pathways are largely responsible for salicylic acid detoxification. Only 5% to 10% of salicylic acid is excreted unchanged in the urine at low aspirin doses, with the remainder being metabolized by the liver. The renal excretion of salicylic acid, however, becomes of paramount importance during salicylate intoxication, when the major hepatic metabolic pathways for the elimination of salicylic acid become saturated[536]. Under these circumstances, 50% or more of unmetabolized salicylic acid is excreted by the kidney. This is of primary importance in understanding the rationale for using alkaline diuresis as a therapeutic modality.

Clinical Manifestations and Pathophysiology

Salicylate poisoning is characterized by a wide range of clinical symptoms and signs that characteristically include tinnitus in older children and adults, fever, sweating, tachycardia, hyperventilation, nausea, vomiting, dehydration, and CNS signs of lethargy, coma, and seizures[527,537,538]. An understanding of the clinical state of salicylate poisoning and its appropriate therapy must be based on a thorough appreciation of the pathophysiologic changes induced by toxic doses of salicylates. The primary pathophysiologic effects of salicylates include the uncoupling of oxidative phosphorylation and the interference in carbohydrate, lipid, and amino acid metabolism[538]. It is the secondary and tertiary effects of these events that produce the clinical picture of salicylate intoxication that is discussed below.

Fever is a common feature of salicylate intoxication in children. It is primarily due to the potent metabolic stimulant effect of salicylates that uncouples oxidative phosphorylation in a manner similar to that of 2,4-dinitrophenol, depleting the tissues of intracellular high energy phosphates. This enhances total body oxygen consumption, carbon dioxide production, basal metabolic rate, and heat production—biochemical events that are clinically manifest by fever, flushed skin, sweating, and signs of a hyperdynamic circulation. Dehydration, so frequent a finding in salicylate intoxication, reduces physiologic sweating, further aggravating the pyrexia[539].

Acid-base disturbances that consist of either respiratory alkalosis, metabolic acidosis, or a mixed acid-base disturbance of metabolic acidosis and respiratory alkalosis frequently accompany salicylate intoxication in both children and adults[540,541]. From a pathophysiologic point of view, these disturbances are caused by a combination of three processes: *(a)* increased alveolar ventilation; *(b)* increased carbon dioxide production; and *(c)* increased endogenous acid production. The relative contribution of each of these components to the overall acid-base disturbances is dependent on both the severity and duration of the intoxication and the age of the patient.

Salicylates directly stimulate the medullary respiratory centers to increase alveolar ventilation, reducing arterial PCO_2 to produce a respiratory alkalosis. This effect is independent of the increase in oxygen consumption or carbon dioxide production. There is an increase in renal bicarbonate excretion with depletion of buffer reserve as a metabolic compensatory response to the respiratory alkalosis.

As a result of the salicylate-induced uncoupling of oxidative phosphorylation, carbon dioxide production is increased. This tends to reduce the magnitude of the respiratory alkalosis, but the primary hyperventilation is the dominant factor, and a respiratory acidosis component does not develop unless alveolar ventilation is compromised by pulmonary complications, such as pulmonary edema or aspiration, or by coingested CNS depressant drugs.

The etiology of the metabolic acidosis is complex[537,538]. In spite of the fact that salicylates are weak acids, they are not present in high enough concentrations, even in severe intoxications, to entirely account for a significant acidosis (Fig. 40.8). The metabolic acidosis is largely due to the metabolic disruption that occurs with salicylate intoxication and that affects primarily carbohydrate and lipid metabolism.

Salicylates uncouple oxidative phosphorylation and also inhibit several enzymes of the Krebs cycle, particularly alpha-keto-dehydrogenase and succinic acid dehydrogenase, with subsequent accumulation of pyruvate, lactate, and other Krebs cycle intermediates. Enhanced metabolism, in turn, stimulates lipolysis with the increased production of ketone bodies, β-hydroxybutyrate, and acetoacetate. Inhibition of hepatic aminotransferases by salicylates elevates blood amino acid levels and results in aminoaciduria. Together, the accumulation of these unmeasured organic acids is largely responsible for the metabolic acidosis of salicylate intoxication[542].

In addition, the increase in renal bicarbonate excretion

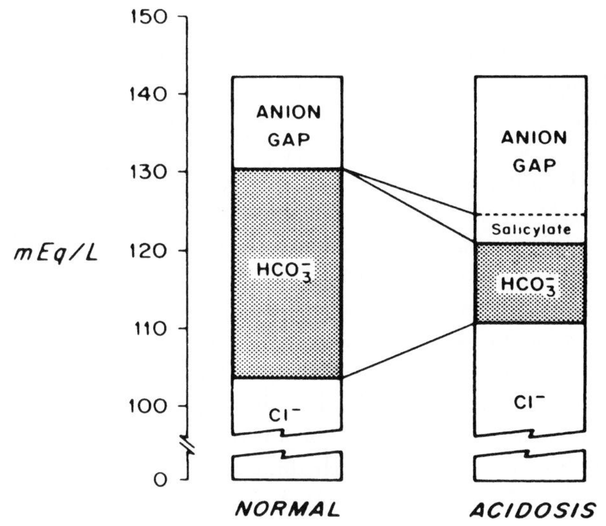

Figure 40.8. Patterns of extracellular anion composition in normal children and in children with salicylate-induced acidosis. (From Harrington JT, Cohen JJ. Metabolic acidosis. In: Cohen JJ, Kassirer JP, eds. Acid-base. Boston: Little, Brown, 1982.)

that occurs early, as a compensatory mechanism to the initial respiratory alkalosis, depletes the buffering capacity of the extracellular fluid and contributes to the later generation of a metabolic acidosis caused by the metabolic disturbance noted above. Renal failure, if it develops, will also contribute to the metabolic acidosis.

A respiratory alkalosis, metabolic acidosis, or a mixed acid-base disorder of respiratory alkalosis-metabolic acidosis may all occur in salicylate intoxication. It appears that both the age of the patient and the chronicity of the intoxication are the prime determinants of the predominant acid-base disturbance[540,541].

Respiratory alkalosis is only transient in young children and usually occurs simultaneously with a significant metabolic acidosis. In young children, persistent respiratory alkalosis is uncommon. A pure metabolic acidosis is often seen after an acute ingestion rather than a mixed acid-base disturbance with a normal pH, which predominates as the presenting acid-base disorder especially when the intoxication is chronic[528]. Respiratory alkalosis is more frequently observed in older children, adolescents, and adults. Thus, the mixed acid-base disturbance of respiratory alkalosis and metabolic acidosis is the more common initial presentation in the older child and adolescent. However, the concomitant ingestion of CNS depressants such as alcohol, barbiturates, benzodiazepines, or TCAs may blunt the respiratory stimulatory effects of salicylates, unmasking the metabolic acidosis and even producing a respiratory acidosis[541,230].

In addition to its influence on acid-base metabolism, the effects of salicylates on carbohydrate metabolism are also reflected in abnormalities of blood glucose concentration. Hyperglycemia and glycosuria are common, particularly early in the course of acute intoxication, mimicking diabetes mellitus. This hyperglycemia probably reflects both an increase in the rate of absorption of glucose from the intestine and the inability of the tissues to utilize delivered glucose adequately. Small children, particularly those with chronic salicylate intoxication, as well as those late in the course of acute intoxication, may develop life-threatening hypoglycemia.

Disturbances of water and electrolyte metabolism frequently accompany salicylate intoxication[537,538,539]. Dehydration is an almost universal feature of severe salicylate intoxication and is multifactorial in its etiology. Fever, perspiration, and hyperventilation enhance insensible water loss from the skin and lungs. The decreased oral intake and vomiting, as well as the increase in obligatory water and electrolyte loss necessitated by the enhanced renal solute load of organic acids, further aggravate the dehydration and electrolyte loss. Hypernatremic dehydration is frequently observed because of the marked increase in insensible water loss.

Dehydration, with its accompanying reduction in urine output, compromises the renal pathway of salicylic acid elimination. This is of critical importance since, in the intoxicated state, the hepatic enzymes for salicylic acid metabolism become saturated and cannot further increase the metabolic breakdown of salicylate, making the kidneys the primary organ of elimination. Hyponatremia may occasionally be associated with the syndrome of inappropriate release of antidiuretic hormone (SIADH)[543].

Potassium metabolism is also frequently disturbed. Total body potassium is depleted by the obligatory urine loss associated with the organic aciduria. Hypokalemia may also occur during the phase of the initial respiratory alkalosis as a result of both the compensatory excretion of sodium and potassium bicarbonate in the urine and the shift of potassium from the extracellular to the intracellular compartment. Hypokalemia may also complicate the iatrogenic metabolic alkalosis as a result of urinary alkalinization. Hypocalcemia can be precipitated by either respiratory or iatrogenic metabolic alkalosis from alkalinization.

CNS toxicity is manifest clinically in moderate and severe toxicity by restlessness, agitation, delirium, and lethargy that progress to coma and seizures. These findings of severe toxicity are more frequently observed in young children in whom a severe metabolic acidosis is usually present. CNS disturbances in adults also occur more frequently in the face of acidosis.

Experimental studies of salicylate intoxication in animals provide an explanation for the association between the metabolic acidosis and the severity of CNS toxicity. Working with salicylate-intoxicated rats, Hill[544] demonstrated that bicarbonate infusions raised blood pH and lowered brain and muscle salicylate concentrations. Acetazolamide lowered blood pH and raised tissue salicylate concentrations and the mortality rate[544,545].

Studies in children have shown a close correlation between the degree of acidosis reflecting the severity of toxicity and the blood/cerebrospinal fluid salicylate ratio[546]. Since salicylate is a weak acid, the distribution of salicylate between extracellular and intracellular compartments will be determined by the relative pH values of the respective spaces. A decrease in pH will increase that proportion of the drug that exists in the nonionized form, i.e., the lipid soluble state, allowing its diffusability across cell membranes. A fall in pH from 7.4 to 7.2 will double the concentration of nonionized salicylate, thereby increasing the V_D of aspirin by enhancing salicyclate transfer into tissues, particularly the brain.

Therapeutic alkalinization will promote its ionization, trapping salicylate in the extracellular fluid and preventing its movement into cells[547]. Seizures occasionally complicate salicylate intoxication and may be caused by high fever, hypernatremia, cerebral edema, hypocalcemia, or decreased cerebral and cerebrospinal fluid glucose concentrations, even with normal blood levels.

Although the altered level of consciousness associated with salicylate intoxication is usually present at the time of diagnosis, when the salicylate level is at its peak, these changes may also be delayed, occurring 24 to 48 hour after the initial presentation[548]. These delayed CNS manifestations are usually due to the development of cerebral edema.

The pathogenesis of cerebral edema in salicylate intoxication is unclear but probably multifactorial in origin. Occasionally, it may be attributed to rapidly developing hyponatremia with SIADH[543]. The entry of salicylate into the brain under circumstances of severe metabolic acidosis[544–547] and the possibility of low CNS concentrations of glucose that result from brain glucose utilization in excess of supply have been implicated in the development of cerebral edema[549]. Rarely, cerebral edema may be associated with hepatic failure either with or without the association of Reye's syndrome.

The hemorrhagic complications associated with salicylate intoxication are uncommon in acute intoxication and are usually associated only with severe, chronic poisoning. Decreased platelet adhesiveness and hypoprothrombinemia due to the inhibition of vitamin K-dependent synthesis of factor VII contribute to the coagulopathy[550].

Noncardiogenic pulmonary edema has been reported in children and adults with severe salicylate poisoning[551], although it is usually seen in older adults with levels greater than 40 mg/dL or in the setting of chronic intoxication. The normal or low filling pressures suggest that the edema is noncardiogenic in origin and is due to alveolar capillary leakage[552,553]. The exact pathogenesis of salicylate-induced alveolar capillary permeability is unclear, although hypoxia has been suggested as an important factor[552,553]. Also, salicylates may increase permeability by their interaction with platelets or by affecting prostaglandin synthesis. By their profound actions on the CNS, salicylates have the potential to precipitate neurogenic pulmonary edema, a form of noncardiogenic pulmonary edema.

The effects of salicylates on renal function are not prominent. Celluria, the shedding of renal tubular cells, and proteinuria occur with intoxication, but these do not necessarily reflect acute tubular necrosis that occasionally complicates severe dehydration. Oliguria is usually secondary to dehydration.

Occasionally, severe salicylate intoxication is associated with reversible elevation of hepatic transaminases, evidence of drug-induced hepatitis.

Diagnosis

Usually, the clinical diagnosis of acute salicylate intoxication is not difficult. A child who earlier was found with a mouthful of pill fragments or an open medicine container presents with the typical signs and symptoms described above. Adolescents are so uncomfortable because of the tinnitus, nausea, vomiting, and hyperventilation that they are only too willing to identify the drug they have ingested.

The diagnosis of chronic, therapeutic salicylate intoxication is more difficult. Presenting signs and symptoms may include hearing loss and tinnitus, nausea, vomiting, dyspnea, tachycardia, hyperthermia, and mental status changes such as confusion, agitation, hyperactivity, slurred speech, hallucinations, seizures, and coma(554). The features of fever, vomiting, and hyperventilation may well be attributed to the underlying disease and, if the diagnosis of salicylate intoxication is not considered, these persistent symptoms may well prompt further aspirin administration. Although these signs and symptoms are seen in acute toxicity, their slower onset and perhaps less severe appearance may delay recognition of toxicity. Patients with chronic salicylism may be misdiagnosed as having delirium, dementia, sepsis, diabetic ketoacidosis, respiratory failure, or cardiopulmonary disease.

The administration of aspirin during intercurrent viral infections, such as varicella or influenza B infections, has been implicated as a causative factor of Reye's syndrome(555). Salicylates are frequently detected in the serum of patients with this disease when first hospitalized. The hyperglycemia, glycosuria, metabolic acidosis, and ketonuria of salicylate intoxication resemble the laboratory findings of diabetic ketoacidosis. The clinical presentation and severe ketoacidosis of acetoacetylcoenzyme A thiolase deficiency can similarly resemble salicylate intoxication as well as producing a false-positive salicylate blood test(556). Neonatal salicylate toxicity secondary to third trimester maternal aspirin use may present with symptoms similar to sepsis and thus go unrecognized(557).

The clinical diagnosis of salicylate intoxication is easily confirmed by the laboratory determination of the plasma salicylate concentration, a rapid, easily performed colorimetric test that is available in all hospital laboratories. This test measures the concentration of both salicylic acid and its metabolites. Chromatographic techniques are available in some laboratories to measure salicylic acid as opposed to its metabolites. A rapid preliminary diagnosis can be made by the use of the ferric chloride or the Phenistix® test. When ferric chloride is added to urine it will turn the sample purple in the presence of salicylate. The Phenistix® turns brown when salicylates are present in the urine or serum.

Assessment of the Severity of Intoxication

An assessment of the severity of intoxication will guide the clinician in predicting the subsequent course, as well as in deciding on appropriate therapy. The amount of drug ingested in a single acute ingestion can be used to predict the subsequent degree of toxicity(538) **(Table 40.18).** These guidelines do not apply to chronic salicylate intoxication. It has, however, been suggested that chronic toxicity is likely when greater than 100 mg/kg/day of salicylate have been administered for 2 or more days.

One ml of 98% methyl salicylate is equivalent to 1.4 gram of aspirin in salicylate potency and action. Thus, one teaspoon of oil of wintergreen is equivalent to approximately 7000 mg of salicylate or 21.7 adult (325 mg) aspirin tablets(531). Ingestions of as little as 1 to 2 teaspoons of oil of wintergreen have been fatal in children(558). One should consider any ingestion of these products a potentially serious poisoning. Pepto Bismol® contains 8.7 mg of salicyclic acid/ml; thus consumption of large quantities (200 to 300 mL) which are recommended for traveler's diarrhea may result in exposure to large amounts of salicylates(559).

Although symptoms of salicylate poisoning are uncommon at concentrations less than 30 mg/dL, clinical toxicity correlates poorly with serum levels. Absorption of salicylate from ingested enteric-coated aspirin preparations is erratic and peak levels may only be reached after more than 24 hours.

Although disturbances in acid-base status do not necessarily correlate with the level of serum salicylates, the severity of acidosis is considered by some to reflect the severity of poisoning since the degree of acidosis largely determines the amount of salicylate that enters the brain and other target organs. Clinical studies have demonstrated that there is a correlation between the degree of acidosis and the blood/cerebrospinal fluid salicylate ratio, a measure of intracerebral salicylate concentration(546). While CSF salicylate levels may be more predictive of severe toxicity, their use in clinical management is not practical.

The clinical findings, in both acute and chronic intoxication, reflect the severity of intoxication. Mild intoxication is characterized by mild hyperpnea, some lethargy, vomiting, and tinnitus. Hyperpnea and prominent neurologic disturbances with depressed consciousness but without coma or convulsions suggest moderate poisoning. Severe intoxication is marked by severe hyperpnea, hyperthermia, coma, and convulsions(527,538). Studies have confirmed the clini-

Table 40.18. Assessment of the Severity of Acute Salicylate Intoxication Based on the Estimated Dose Ingested[a]

Ingested dose (mg/kg)	*Estimated severity*
<150	No toxic reaction expected
150–300	Mild-to-moderate toxic reaction
300–500	Severe toxic reaction
>500	Potentially lethal toxic reaction

[a]From Temple AR. Acute and chonric effects of aspirin toxicity and their treatment. Arch Intern Med 1981;141:364.

cal impression that more severe cases of salicylate poisoning occur in association with chronic rather than acute intoxication. At each of three different blood salicylate concentration ranges, symptoms of hyperventilation, dehydration, and severe CNS manifestations occurred with a much greater frequency in the chronically intoxicated group of patients than in the acute group(528). The delay in making the diagnosis and the more severe acidosis, as well as the saturation elimination kinetics that characterize repeated doses of salicylate, account for more severe disease.

Treatment

As with all intoxications, initial therapy is directed toward ensuring ventilation, oxygenation, and cardiovascular stability. Prevention of further absorption can be accomplished by ipecac-induced emesis or gastric lavage, followed by activated charcoal and cathartic administration. Since salicylates delay gastric emptying time, lavage may be indicated even 12 to 24 hours after ingestion to remove residual pill fragments.

Activated charcoal adsorbs aspirin effectively, reducing peak salicylate concentrations 40% to 50% when given one half to one hour postingestion(561). It also effectively binds enteric-coated and sustained release preparations. However, aspirin desorption from the charcoal complex over time may diminish its impact on total absorption(562). Repetitive doses of activated charcoal may prevent desorption of aspirin as well as inhibit further absorption from enteric-coated or sustained release preparations(563,564). Multiple doses of charcoal may also reduce serum salicylate concentrations by enhancing postabsorptive elimination through GI dialysis(565,566). Some recent studies have questioned the effectiveness of multiple-dose charcoal for acute salicylate poisonings(567,568). However, both were limited by small sample sizes and subtoxic doses of aspirin.

Whole bowel irrigation with activated charcoal theoretically may diminish the time for potential salicylate desorption as well as enhance the intestinal elimination of sustained release preparations or aspirin bezoars(569). However, one clinical study failed to show an increase in salicylate elimination using this combination(570). Endoscopic manipulation may be necessary to break up and remove concretions.

Serum salicyclate levels should be obtained 2 and 6 hours after ingestion of immediate release preparations. In potentially large overdoses, salicylate levels should be monitored every 2 to 4 hours until a peak level is obtained. Suspected toxic ingestion of sustained release or enteric-coated preparations mandates monitoring of the salicyclate levels for at least 24 hours. More frequent salicylate determinations may be warranted to assess the efficacy of treatment and possible need for hemodialysis in a severely intoxicated child. For methyl salicylate ingestions, a level should be obtained immediately upon presentation and then at 2 hours because of its rapid absorption and rapid onset of toxicity.

Supportive general care is of particular importance in salicylate intoxication because of the multisystem involvement that potentially affects lungs, gastrointestinal tract, liver, kidney, and nervous system. Severe dehydration frequently accompanies severe intoxication and rapid fluid replacement with large volumes of isotonic solution such as normal saline or Ringer's lactate may be necessary to restore the circulating blood volume, correct hypotension, improve peripheral perfusion, and restore urine flow. Subsequent fluid replacement will depend upon the degree of dehydration. Saline (0.45%) with 35 to 70 mEq sodium bicarbonate per liter is a suitable replacement solution for a dehydrated acidotic child. Dextrose should be added to the solution as needed.

Close monitoring of the concentration of electrolytes, glucose, and calcium, are mandatory. Frequent blood gas monitoring is necessary to monitor the efficacy of alkalinization therapy and provide a framework for interpretation of salicylate levels. Hypernatremia must be gradually corrected to prevent cerebral edema from developing. The addition of potassium chloride, in concentrations of 20 to 80 mEq/L, may be necessary to correct the hypokalemia so that urinary alkalinization can be effective. Calcium supplementation may be necessary for the management of hypocalcemia. Hyperpyrexia is managed by external cooling with a cooling blanket or ice.

Systemic metabolic acidosis must be treated aggressively. Its role in enhancing the passage of salicylates from the extracellular space into the cells, especially the brain, where disruption of mitochondrial function and intermediary metabolism can occur has been discussed above. Sodium bicarbonate is the alkalinizing agent of choice. Since it is almost solely an alkalinizer of the extracellular space, it increases the intracellular-to-extracellular gradient of diffusible, nonionized drug, enhancing the trapping of salicylate in the extracellular plasma. Tromethamine (THAM) is an intracellular as well as an extracellular buffer and by diminishing the diffusing gradient may trap salicylate in the brain. Its use is not recommended for correcting acidosis due to salicylates.

Acidosis may be treated by initial intravenous bolus of sodium bicarbonate (1 to 2 mEq/kg) followed by bicarbonate infusion consisting of 88 to 100 mEq of $NaHCO_3$ in 1 liter of D5 0.25% NaCl (1/4 NS) to run at 1.5 to 2 times the maintenance fluid rate until good urine flow is obtained. Blood gases should be monitored to guide the frequency and quantity of sodium bicarbonate administration. Intravenous alkalinization dramatically increases the ionized fraction of salicylic acid, decreases renal reabsorption, and decreases salicylate entry into the brain and other tissues. Control of ventilation through endotracheal intubation may assist in the management of patients with acidemia by hyperventilation and subsequent respiratory alkalosis; however, this should never be considered an alternative for urinary alkalinization.

Enhancing salicyclate elimination is best accomplished through urinary alkalinization and extracorporeal methods for severely intoxicated children. Salicylates are ionized and therefore less diffusable in a more alkaline environment because salicylic acid is a weak acid. When the urine pH increases from 5 to 8, the renal clearance of salicylate increases 10 to 20 times (Figure 40.9)[571]. Urinary alkalinization for salicylate poisoning demonstrates the concept of ion trapping—it enhances the excretion of ionized form of salicylate in the alkaline urine (Fig. 40.10). After volume resuscitation and initial rehydration, maintenance fluid administration for urinary alkalinization can be given as D5W with 44 to 132 mEq/L of bicarbonate plus 20 to 40 mEq/L of KCl. Additional $NaHCO_3$ should be added to maintain a urine pH between 7 and 8. This urinary pH achieves maximum ion trapping and salicylate excretion.

The concomitant serum and urine alkalinization with sodium bicarbonate will prevent salicylates from entering the brain as well as enhancing their excretion from the body. Acetazolamide, a non-competitive carbonic anhydrase inhibitor, should not be used because it causes a systemic metabolic acidosis despite its ability to form alkaline urine. Alkalinization should be considered for patients with acute toxicity whose levels exceed 35 mg/dL and for patients manifesting moderate to severe salicylism—usually secondary to chronic intoxication—despite levels less than 35 mg/dL.

Alkalinization is not without hazards. Sodium bicarbonate administration may aggravate hypernatremia and hypokalemia. It may also precipitate hypocalcemia and subsequent seizures. The increased sodium administration may also aggravate pulmonary edema. Because of the high solute load, it should not be instituted in patients with congestive heart failure, renal failure, or cerebral edema. These patients should receive earlier treatment with hemodialysis.

Forced alkaline diuresis is no longer recommended for severe aspirin poisoning. The renal excretion of salicyclate

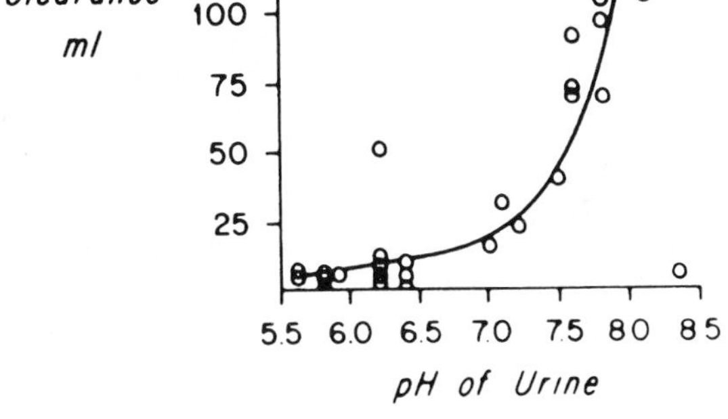

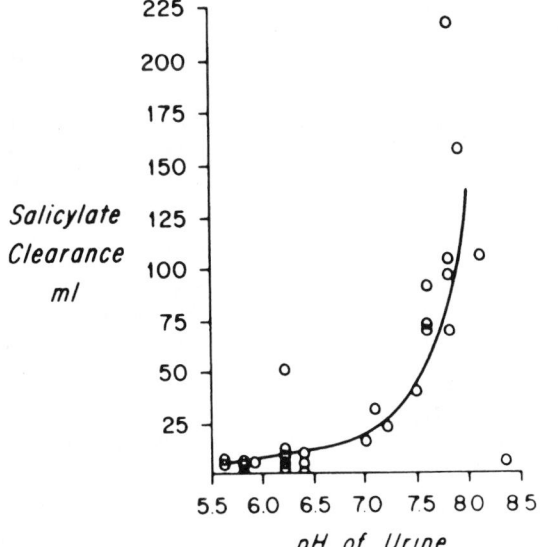

Figure 40.9. Influence of urine pH on the renal clearance of salicylate. (From Harrington JT, Cohen JJ. Metabolic acidosis. In: Cohen JJ, Kassirer JP, eds. Acid-base. Boston: Little, Brown, 1982.)

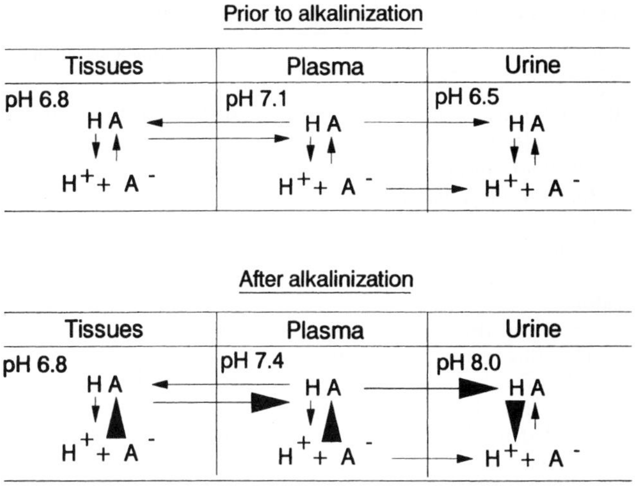

Figure 40.10. Rationale for alkalinization. (From Flomenbaum NE, Goldfrank LR. Salicylates. In: Goldfrank's Toxicologic Emergencies. 5th ed. Goldfrank LR, Flomenbaum NE, Lewin NA et al, eds. Norwalk CT: Appleton & Lange, 1994;504. Adapted from Temple AR: Acute and chronic effects of aspirin toxicity and their treatment. Arch Intern Med 1981;141:367. Used with permission).

is more dependent on urine pH than on flow rate. The use of forced diuresis alone with diuretics, osmotic agents, or fluid volumes has not been proven effective for enhancing salicylate elimination[572]. Furthermore, cerebral and pulmonary edema may be exacerbated from overhydration and electrolyte imbalances and alkalosis may worsen from this therapy.

Hemoperfusion and hemodialysis are both efficient extracorporeal techniques for enhancing salicylate elimination from the blood. Charcoal hemoperfusion results in better salicylate clearance (57 to 116 mL/min) than hemodialysis (35 to 80 mL/min)[573]. However, hemodialysis is considered the extracorporeal method of choice because it allows for rapid correction of fluid and electrolyte abnormalities and acid-base disturbances uncorrectable by hemoperfusion in addition to enhancing a salicylate clearance. General indications for hemodialysis are a salicylate level greater than 100 mg/dL in acute overdose, renal failure, noncardiogenic pulmonary edema, persistent CNS disturbances, progressive deterioration in vital signs, congestive heart failure, severe acid-base or electrolyte imbalances despite appropriate treatment, and hepatic compromise with coagulopathy[573].

THEOPHYLLINE INTOXICATION

Theophylline is a methylxanthine derivative used for the treatment of asthma, bronchospasm, and neonatal apnea. Theophylline compounds are available as liquid, tablets, and beaded capsules. Aminophylline is the ethylenediamine salt of theophylline which contains approximately 85% anydrous theophylline. **Table 40.19** lists currently available sustained release preparations which have become a popular form of prescribed theophylline because of their

Table 40.19. Sustained-Release Theophylline Products

Brand	*Theophylline Content (mg)*
Capsules	
Slo-Bid Gyrocaps (Rhone-Poulenc Rorer)	50, 75, 100, 125, 200, 300
Slo-Phyllin Gyrocaps (Rhone-Poulenc Rorer)	60, 125, 250
Theoclear L.A. (Central)	130, 260
Theo-Dur Sprinkle (Key)	50, 75, 125, 200
Theophyl-SR (McNeil)	125, 250
Tablets	
Quibron-T/SR (Roberts)	300
Respbid (Boehringer Ingelheim)	250, 500
Theo-Dur (Key)	100, 200, 300, 450
Theolari-SR (3M)	200, 250
Theo-X Extended Release (Carnrick)	100, 200, 300
T-PHYL (Purdue Frederick)	200
Uniphyl (Purdue Frederick)	400
24-Hour Preparation	
Theo-24 Extended Release Capsules (Whitby)	100, 200, 300, 400

once or twice a day dosing; however, they have also contributed to increasing incidence of chronic theophylline poisoning. Although theophylline use has declined over the past several years due to increasing use of beta agonists and corticosteroids, it continues to be prescribed frequently. Theophylline's narrow therapeutic index and wide availability contribute to persistent acute and chronic intoxication in the pediatric population.

Pharmacology

Theophylline is rapidly and completely absorbed after oral administration of conventional solution or plain uncoated tablets, with peak serum levels reached within two hours. Enteric coated or sustained release preparations may cause delayed or prolonged toxicity due to continued release of theophylline[574,575,576]. These formulations vary in the completeness, rate, and consistency of absorption. Sustained release preparations increase the duration of drug levels by increasing the absorption half-life, sometimes over 12 to 24 hours, rather than altering the clearance. Therefore, a single early serum theophylline determination may not reflect the severity of intoxication because the onset of severe toxicity may be delayed for hours.

After absorption, distribution is rapid throughout the extracellular space with a volume of distribution of approximately 0.45 l/kg—a value that is constant in both adults and children. Less than 10% of the ingested dose is excreted unchanged in the urine. Theophylline is metabolized by hepatic mixed function oxidases (cytochrome P_{450}) to renally excreted metabolites 1-methyluric acid, 1,3-dimethyluric acid, and 3-methylxanthine (Fig. 40.11). 3-methylxanthine is the most active metabolite, displaying 30 to 70% of the pharmacologic activity of theophylline, but usually is not present in pharmacologically significant concentrations. In neonates, unlike older children and adults, theophylline is methylated to form caffeine[577].

The pharmacokinetics and toxicokinetics of theophylline are complex and responsible for many accidental and iatrogenic intoxications. Furthermore, there is significant interindividual variability in the elimination kinetics of theophylline even under therapeutic circumstances. Although the volume of distribution remains relatively constant in different age groups, the clearance of theophylline is highly variable and depends on the efficiency of the hepatic biotransformation, interaction with other drugs, and the individual's age[577,578].

Theophylline clearance increases with age from the neonatal period, reaching maximum rates during early childhood and then gradually decreasing until adult values are

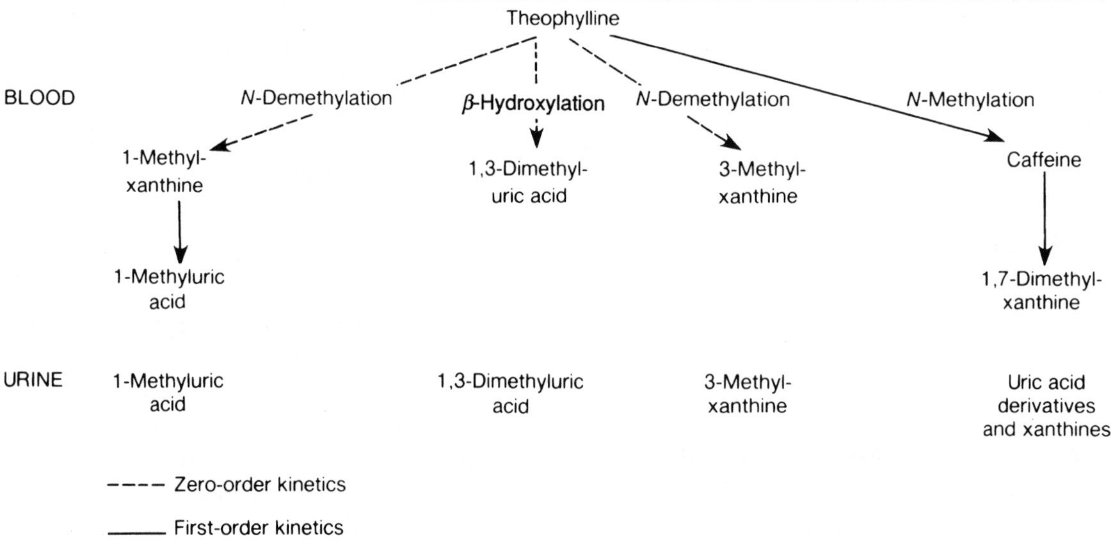

Figure 40.11. Metabolism of theophylline. (From Weinberger M. The pharmacology and therapeutic uses of theophylline. J Allergy Clin Immunol 1984;73:525.)

Table 40.20. Relationship Between Age and Theophylline Elimination[a]

Age	*Clearance mean ± SD (mL/kg/min)*	*Half-life mean ± SD (hr)*
Premature infants	0.29 ± 0.01	30 ± 6.5
Infants		
<24 wk		13 ± 4.7
>24 wk		6.8 ± 2.2
Young children, 1–4 yr	1.7 ± 0.6	3.4 ± 1.1
Older children		
4–12 yr	1.5 ± 0.4	—
6–17 yr	1.4 ± 0.6	3.7 ± 1.1
13–15 yr	0.8 ± 0.2	—
Adults (healthy, nonsmoking asthmatics	0.65 ± 0.19	8.7 ± 2.2

[a]*From Weinberger M, Hendeles L, Ahens R. Drugs used for asthma. Pediatr Clin North Am 1981;28:47.*

achieved in late adolescence **(Table 40.20).** Thus, neonates have significantly longer elimination half-lives compared to children and adolescents. In addition, liver dysfunction, congestive heart failure, acute viral illnesses with high fever in children, and the coadministration of several drugs, such as erythromycin and cimetidine, decrease the hepatic clearance of theophylline and prolong the half-life, potentially precipitating theophylline toxicity. Cigarette and marijuana smoking, as well as phenobarbital and diphenylhydantoin administration, enhance theophylline's metabolism, thereby increasing its clearance.

Theophylline demonstrates Michaelis-Menten elimination kinetics which is a mixture of first- and zero-order elimination. At therapeutic concentrations, theophylline follows first-order elimination kinetics—a constant *percentage* of drug is eliminated per unit of time (concentration dependent). At toxic concentrations, this pattern changes to zero-order or saturable elimination—a constant *quantity* of drug is eliminated per unit of time. It represents the physiologic saturation of a capacity-limited enzyme system. Thus, small dosage increases may result in disproportionately higher serum levels and toxicity. Saturation or zero-order kinetics and the prolonged absorption from the ingestion of sustained release theophylline preparations account for the dramatically prolonged $t_{1/2}$ and the reduced clearance that frequently characterize the theophylline intoxicated state. An appreciation of all of these factors is important both in preventing toxicity and in understanding the pathogenesis of theophylline intoxication.

Pathophysiology

The biochemical pathophysiology of theophylline toxicity remains unclear but is under investigation. Evidence supports the hypothesis that the metabolic and cardiovascular manifestations of the intoxicated state are due to excessive stimulation of the β-adrenergic system. Theophylline increases circulating levels of epinephrine and norepinephrine by enhancing release both from adrenergic nerve terminals and the adrenal medulla[579–581]. Although phosphodiesterase inhibition by theophylline is minimal at therapeutic concentrations, this action is likely operative at toxic levels of the drug. By increasing intracellular cyclic AMP concentrations, the drug may enhance or mimic the effects of beta-receptor agonism by catecholamines. Pharmacologically, this results in smooth muscle relaxation, peripheral vasodilation, myocardial stimulation, and CNS excitation.

Metabolic disturbances characteristic of severe acute theophylline toxicity—hypokalemia, hyperglycemia, elevated concentrations of free fatty acids, hypophosphatemia, metabolic acidosis, and leukocytosis—are due to β-adrenergic stimulation[582,583]. Hyperglycemia is caused by stimulatory effects of elevated catecholamine concentrations and cyclic AMP on hepatic glucose production. Metabolic acidosis may be secondary to hypotension or seizures as well as an effect of catecholamine stimulation. Hypokalemia results from intracellular shifts of potassium, not renal losses. These metabolic disturbances, especially hypokalemia and metabolic acidosis, may exacerbate the cardiac toxicity from theophylline, but probably do not affect clinical outcome. However, they have potential diagnostic value in distinguishing the type of intoxication when a detailed history is unavailable.

Hypotension is due to β-adrenergic-mediated peripheral vasodilation and may be worsened from volume depletion secondary to vomiting. Further support for the pathophysiologic role of circulating catecholamines derives from the use of beta blockers in experimental animal models of theophylline intoxication whereby propanolol, a beta blocker, ameliorated the hypotension and tachycardia as well as the hypokalemia, hypophosphatemia, and hyperglycemia[584,585].

Recent theories suggest that theophylline acts as an antagonist at adenosine receptors found on bronchial smooth muscle, the myocardium, and central nervous system[586]. The exact etiology of theophylline-induced seizures is unclear, but cerebral vasoconstriction and central adenosine antagonism have been proposed[587]. Furthermore, cardiac dysrhythmias may be caused in part by adenosine antagonism in addition to beta-agonist stimulation.

Clinical Manifestations

Theophylline toxicity is characterized by multisystem manifestations that include the gastrointestinal, cardiovascular, and central nervous system. The clinical manifestations differ according to the type of intoxication-acute toxicity, chronic toxicity, or acute-on-chronic toxicity (an acute overdose in a patient chronically receiving theophylline)[588,589]. It is important to distinguish between these types of intoxications because risk of life-threatening toxicity and thresholds for management interventions differ depending on the chronicity of toxicity.

Acute toxicity is the result of a single overdose, either as a result of an accidental childhood ingestion or a suicide attempt. Usual manifestations include nausea, vomiting, sometimes hematemesis, tremor, anxiety, and sinus tachycardia. Hypokalemia, hypophosphatemia, hyperglycemia, leukocytosis, and metabolic acidosis are seen during acute toxicity. Studies have demonstrated that major signs of acute theophylline toxicity—seizures, hypotension and ventricular dysrhythmias—may be predicted by a theophylline level greater than 80 to 100 μg/mL[(588,590)]. However, one pediatric study reported four acutely intoxicated children who experienced seizures with theophylline levels less than 70 μg/mL[(591)]. Theophylline-induced seizures place a patient at higher risk for further morbidity and mortality and may be refractory to conventional drug therapy.

The most common theophylline-induced dysrhythmias are sinus tachycardia and supraventricular tachycardia. Other dysrhythmias reported with acute intoxication include premature ventricular contractions, bigeminy, ventricular tachycardia, and ventricular fibrillation[(592)]. Hypotension is also an ominous sign with severe theophylline poisoning. A widened pulse pressure is a common finding in patients with severe acute toxicity.

Chronic intoxication can result from intentional or unintentional repetitive drug administration over a period of time, a prescribing error, decrease in hepatic clearance of the drug, or drug interaction as described above. The usual group susceptible to this type of poisoning are very young infants, adolescents, or elderly patients. Signs of chronic toxicity may be subtle and include anorexia, nausea, palpitations, or vomiting. However, seizures may be the initial clinical presentation with levels as low as 40 μg/mL[(593)]. In one study of children chronically overdosed with theophylline, peak theophylline level did not predict major toxicity[(589)]. Children with chronic toxicity who had life-threatening events were significantly younger than those who remained well (1.6 versus 8.0 years). Metabolic abnormalities are not present in chronic intoxication. Tachycardia may be seen but hypotension is rare.

Children chronically receiving theophylline who acutely overdose (acute-on-chronic toxicity) usually manifest clinical signs and symptoms of acute toxicity and should be treated in the same manner.

Laboratory Findings

Laboratory assessment should include electrolytes, glucose, and serum theophylline level. Theophylline levels are essential for diagnosis and determination of emergency management. Levels are helpful in predicting major toxicity in acute overdoses. Children with acute exposure generally tolerate levels less than 80 to 100 μg/mL while those with chronic exposure may be intolerant of levels greater than 40 μg/mL. In acute overdoses, levels should be repeated every 2 hours until a decrease is demonstrated by two successive levels and then every 4 to 6 hours until the level is less than 20 μg/mL. Single levels are not sufficient because continued absorption from sustained release preparations may result in peak levels 12 to 24 hours after ingestion. In addition, the magnitude of the rise in theophylline concentration is prognostic and signals the need for more aggressive intervention. An increasing level or persistently high level may also be an indication of inadequate decontamination with persistent absorption or the presence of a bezoar.

Treatment

Emergency management of theophylline intoxication must begin with rapid assessment of vital signs and a serum theophylline level. GI decontamination is important and must proceed emergently after stabilization of the patient's airway and circulation. Decisions regarding the use of ipecac, lavage, charcoal, and whole bowel irrigation depend on the chronicity of intoxication, when the ingestion occurred, and whether symptoms are present.

Ipecac-induced emesis may be used at home if the ingestion occurred within 30 minutes. It should be avoided in the hospital setting because it often leads to protracted vomiting, limiting the ability to administer activated charcoal—an integral component of treatment. If spontaneous vomiting has not occurred, orogastric lavage should be performed.

Activated charcoal is an essential component of GI decontamination because of its effective adsorbency of theophylline and its ability in enhancing theophylline elimination[(594)]. Multiple doses of activated charcoal enhance theophylline clearance by gastrointestinal dialysis—enhancing the back diffusion of theophylline from the blood into the intestinal lumen and preventing the absorption of remaining drug in the GI tract. Several studies have demonstrated the efficacy of repetitive doses of charcoal in decreasing theophylline's elimination half-life and increasing its clearance[(595–598)]. Charcoal should be administered in a dose of 0.5 to 1.0 g/kg every 2 hours until the theophylline level declines on two successive levels, and then every 4 hours until the level is less than 20 μg/mL.

Antiemetics should be administered aggressively to permit charcoal retention. Metoclopramide, droperidol, and ondansetron have been used successfully[(599)]. Theoretically, phenothiazines should not be used because they may lower the seizure threshold. Continuous nasogastric instillation of charcoal may also be effective if the patient has refractory vomiting[(600)].

Whole bowel irrigation should be considered in patients with increasing theophylline levels despite adequate GI decontamination and/or to enhance elimination of sustained release preparations.

Extracorporeal techniques are highly effective in enhancing theophylline elimination and are recommended for severe theophylline toxicity. Estimated theophylline clearance with hemodialysis is 0.4 to 1.2 ml/min/kg; however, charcoal hemoperfusion can increase theophylline elimination four- to sixfold to a clearance of 2.4 ml/min/kg and is the preferred procedure[(601–605)]. Indications for charcoal hemoperfusion or hemodialysis in otherwise healthy children are a theophylline level of 80 to 100 μg/mL in a patient with acute poisoning, theophylline level of 70

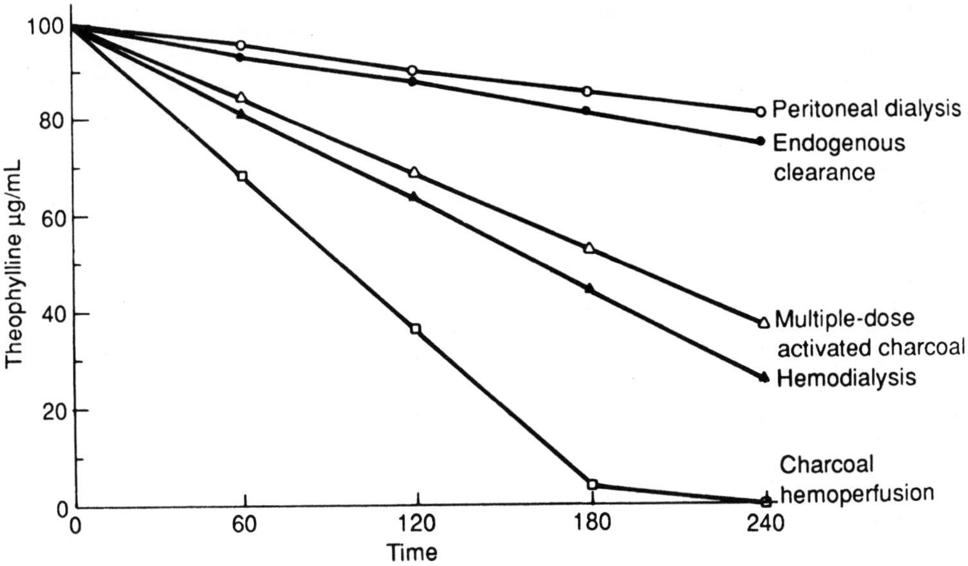

Figure 40.12. A comparison of theophylline clearance rates for peritoneal dialysis, hemodialysis, charcoal hemoperfusion, and multiple-dose activated charcoal. To approximate total body clearance, the endogenous clearance should be added to each of the processes. (From Weisman RS, Goldfrank LR, Howaland MA. Theophylline. In: Goldfrank's Toxicologic Emergencies. 5th ed. Goldfrank LR, Flomenbaum NE, Lewin NA et al, eds. Norwalk CT: Appleton & Lange, 1994;570. Used with permission.)

µg/mL 4 hours after ingestion of a sustained release preparation, theophylline level of 40 µg/mL in a patient with chronic poisoning, or severe toxicity—seizures, refractory hypotension, ventricular dysrhythmias—regardless of the serum concentration.

Complications from charcoal hemoperfusion include thrombocytopenia and hypocalcemia. Because charcoal hemoperfusion is not widely available, hemodialysis is an acceptable alternative. Repetitive doses of activated charcoal should be continued throughout the time of hemoperfusion and subsequently until the theophylline concentration is less than 20 µg/mL and major symptoms have resolved. Continuous arteriovenous hemoperfusion has been reported to be effective in substantially enhancing theophylline clearance in severe acute poisoning[606,210], while exchange transfusion may be an alternative in a neonate where hemodialysis or perfusion is not feasible[607] (Fig. 40.12).

Initial therapy for seizures should include benzodiazepines followed by barbiturates[608]. Phenytoin has been shown not to be effective. Theophylline-induced seizures may be refractory to conventional therapy and require general anesthesia with neuromuscular blockade and ventilatory support.

No treatment is necessary for supraventricular tachycardia if the patient is hemodynamically stable and has no chest pain. If pharmacological therapy is needed, short acting beta-adrenergic antagonists (such as esmolol) or verapamil (in children over 1 year of age) may be used[584,608,609]. Ventricular tachycardia can be treated with standard doses of lidocaine. Hypotension is treated initially with crystalloid fluid boluses followed by predominantly alpha adrenergic vasopressors. Although beta adrenergic antagonists have been shown to reverse hypotension, they must be used cautiously in patients with asthma[609].

Vital signs and ECG monitoring should continue until symptoms have resolved and the serum theophylline level is less than 20 µg/mL. Since hypokalemia is caused by intracellular shift of potassium and does not reflect total body deficit, it usually resolves spontaneously without aggressive treatment. All patients who meet criteria for charcoal hemoperfusion, demonstrate any signs of major toxicity, or have rapidly rising theophylline levels should be referred to a tertiary care medical facility for intervention and monitoring.

TRICYCLIC ANTIDEPRESSANT INTOXICATION

Cyclic antidepressants, particularly tricyclic antidepressants (TCAs), continue to be a leading cause of death in reported poisonings involving pharmaceutical agents in the United States. There are two groups of acutely poisoned patients noted in the pediatric population—accidental ingestions by toddlers and intentional ingestions by adolescents. Cyclic antidepressants are being prescribed with increasing frequency to pediatric patients with depression, chronic pain syndrome, enuresis, and, recently, as an alternative to stimulants for children with attention deficit hyperactivity disorder[610].

Pharmacology and Pharmacokinetics

Cyclic antidepressants (CA) can be categorized into first- and second-generation antidepressants, as shown in **Table 40.21**[611]. The first-generation cyclic antidepressants are the classic TCAs, popularized in the 1950s because of their mood elevating properties and characterized by their three-ring chemical structure. The second generation cyclic antidepressants, were developed in the 1980s and 1990s with the intent to reduce the severe toxicity and adverse effect profile being reported with TCA use.

Amoxapine is a dibenzooxapine cyclic antidepressant whose toxic profile is characterized by a very high incidence

Table 40.21. Cyclic Antidepressant Pharmacologic and Toxicologic Properties

	Amine Reuptake Activity						
Drug	*Norepinephrine*	*Serotonin*	*Dopamine*	*Anticholinergic*	*Prolonged QRS Complex*	*Hypotension*	*Seizures*
First-generation							
Amitriptyline	++	++++	0	++++	++++	++++	++++
Clomipramine	++	++++	0	++++	++++	++++	++++
Doxepin	+	++	0	+++	++++	++++	++++
Trimipramine	+	+	0	++++	++++	++++	++++
Deslpramine	++++	+	0	++	++++	+++	++++
Nortriptyline	+++	++	0	+++	++++	+++	++++
Protriptyline	+++	++	0	+++	++++	++++	++++
Imipramine	+++	+++	0	+++	++++	++++	++++
Second-generation							
Amoxapine	+++	++	[1]+	+++	+	+	++++
Bupropion	0	0	++	+	0	+	++++
Fluoxetine	0	++++	0	0	0	0	0
Maprotiline	+++	+	0	+++	++++	++++	++++
Trazodone	0	+++	0	0	0	+	0
Sertraline	+	++++	0	+	0	0	0

0 = none; + = very low; ++ = low; +++ = moderate; ++++ = high; 1 = blocks dopamine receptors

of seizures and less cardiotoxicity than TCAs[612]. Maprotiline is a tetracyclic compound causing symptoms similar to those of conventional TCAs with a very high incidence of seizures, cardiac dysrhythmias, and prolonged coma[613]. Bupropion is a unicyclic antidepressant in which seizures have been associated with chronic ingestions of greater than 450 mg/day but no CNS or cardiac toxicity in a small number of acute overdoses[614,615].

The development of selective serotonin reuptake inhibitors (SSRI)—fluoxetine, trazadone, sertraline, and paroxetine—has resulted in the reduction of significant cardiac and central nervous system toxicity. Reported toxicity to this class of drugs has been limited to CNS depression (primarily lethargy), sinus tachycardia, and gastrointestinal symptoms[616–620]. However, when combined with other drugs which modify neurotransmitter activity, for instance, MAO inhibitors, SSRIs have the potential to cause serious toxicity—the hyperserotonergic syndrome.

Cyclic antidepressants are rapidly and almost completely absorbed from the GI tract. Their anticholinergic properties cause markedly slow gastric emptying, prolonging the absorption in the overdose setting. CAs are highly lipophilic drugs and have large volumes of distribution (10 to 50 L/kg). Tissue levels are many times higher than serum levels. Myocardial concentrations of TCAs, in particular, may reach 40 to 200 times those of serum. They are extensively bound to proteins (85 to 95%), making extracorporeal removal of little benefit[621].

Metabolism occurs in the liver by demethylation and hydroxylation. Both parent compound and metabolite retain their pharmacologic activity. CAs undergo enterohepatic and enterogastric circulation as a result of biliary and gastric secretion and subsequent reabsorption of parent compound and metabolites. A small percentage of the parent compound is renally excreted. The half-life of these drugs ranges from 4 hours (trazadone) to 93 hours (nortriptyline) in therapeutic doses; however, after toxic ingestions, these times may increase dramatically.

The pharmacologic mechanisms of cyclic antidepressants are due to:

1. inhibition of neurotransmitter reuptake at central presynaptic terminals;
2. central and peripheral anticholinergic effects;
3. membrane depressant effects on the sodium channels of the distal conduction system in the heart;
4. alpha-adrenergic blockade; and
5. inhibition of central sympathetic reflexes[622].

The CAs express these different pharmacological actions in varying degrees as shown in **Table 40.21.**

Ten to twenty mg/kg of most TCAs will cause moderate to severe toxicity (therapeutic dose is 2 to 4 mg/kg/day). To put this amount into perspective for clinical use, as little as two 50 mg imipramine tablets may cause significant toxicity in a toddler weighing 10 kilograms. SSRIs appear to have a much higher toxicity threshold from limited reports[619,620].

Clinical Manifestations and Pathophysiology

Cyclic antidepressant toxcity is characterized by a combination of peripheral anticholinergic, central nervous system, and cardiovascular effects depending on the neurotransmitters most affected. The progression of toxicity is rapid and unpredictable for TCA overdoses. A child who presents awake and alert with apparent trivial signs of poisoning may clinically deteriorate within 30 to 60 minutes.

Peripheral anticholinergic effects include dry mucous membranes; dry, flushed skin; mydriasis; blurred vision; tachycardia; hypertension; decreased GI motility; and urinary retention. These signs and symptoms occur frequently and early after ingestion.

Central nervous system effects are characterized by a clinical spectrum varying from confusion, agitation and lethargy in milder cases to delirium, seizures, respiratory depression, and coma in more severely intoxicated patients.

Seizures due to CA toxicity are caused by a complex interaction of cholinergic, serotonergic, and adrenergic neurotransmitters. CAs have been shown to inhibit the chloride channel on the GABA receptor complex which correlates with seizure frequency[623].

Most seizures from CAs are brief, generalized tonic-clonic, and self-limited, occurring within 12 hours of ingestion and most commonly within 2 hours after ingestion[624]. Of course, the concomitant ingestions of drugs such as cocaine and/or benzodiazepines may exacerbate or retard seizure manifestations. Seizures may be preceded by a normal mental status and may lead to abrupt cardiovascular deterioration.

Recurrent seizures or status epilepticus may be resistant to several modes of therapy, especially those due to amoxapine. Furthermore, seizures and their accompanying hypoxia and acidosis may aggravate CA-induced arrhythmias and hypotension by increasing binding to myocardial sodium channels. Twitching, myoclonic jerks, and choreoathetosis are also sometimes seen with CA toxicity.

Cardiovascular complications of TCA toxicity are responsible for their significant morbidity and mortality. Even in therapeutic doses, sinus tachycardia, conduction delays, and orthostatic hypotension may be present[622].

The anticholinergic effects of CAs are responsible for the sinus tachycardia which is almost universally present in all ingestions as well as therapeutic doses. Mild transient hypertension seen early in the course is also a result of the anticholinergic effects.

Blockade of norepinephrine reuptake by adrenergic neurons potentiates the effects of norepinephrine on the cardiovascular system. This enhances the sinus tachycardia produced by the anticholinergic mechanisms, aggravates hypertension, and precipitates arrhythmias by activating latent pacemaker cells. Persistent blockade of norepinephrine reuptake may eventually lead to catecholamine depletion with decreased contractility, decreased vasomotor tone, and hypotension.

The direct quinidine-like myocardial depressant action of TCAs is responsible for the most serious cardiac manifestations of TCA intoxication. TCAs block rapid sodium channels during phase 0 of the action potential in the distal His-Purkinje conduction system of the heart. It is this local anesthetic effect that causes intraventricular conduction delays, reentrant ventricular dysrhythmias, and hypotension. Conduction delays are manifested by prolongation of the PR, QRS, QTc intervals, and various degrees of heart block[625]. The prolonged QRS complex may be manifested as a right bundle branch block with a rightward shift of the QRS axis. Ventricular dysrhythmias include ventricular extrasystoles, bigeminy, severe bradycardia, ventricular tachycardia, fibrillation, and asystole. The wide, bizarre QRS, complexes of ventricular tachycardia may be monomorphic or polymorphic like Torsades de pointes[625,626].

Conduction changes on the electrocardiogram (ECG) reflect the pathophysiology of TCA poisoning at the cellular level; it would be logical that similar electrophysiological changes are occurring in the CNS, predisposing the patient to seizures. Various authors have investigated the utility of the ECG in predicting ventricular dysrhythmias and seizures in patients with acute TCA ingestions. Boehnert and Lovejoy reported that 33% of their study population who had a QRS interval of 100 milliseconds or longer developed seizures and 14% developed ventricular dysrhythmias[627]. However, a subsequent study failed to support this relationship between QRS duration and occurrence of seizures and dysrhythmias[628].

A terminal 40 millisecond frontal plane QRS axis (T40-ms) between 120 and 270 degrees has been reported to be associated with TCA toxicity[629] and in one study, was found to be a more sensitive indicator of general toxicity than the QRS interval alone[630]. However, the T40-ms axis is not easily measured in the absence of specialized computer-assisted analysis, limiting its practical utility. It can be estimated by looking at the terminal QRS deflection in Leads 1 and aVR.

Liebelt et al[631] prospectively studied 79 patients with acute TCA overdoses and demonstrated that the terminal R wave and R wave/S wave ratio in Lead aVR were significantly greater in those patients who developed seizures and ventriclar dysrhythmias. An R wave in lead aVR of 3 mm was the only ECG variable that significantly predicted seizures and/or dysrhythmias. The terminal R wave and R/S ratio are easily quantifiable measurements that can be made from a routine ECG.

Hypotension is a prominent cardiovascular sign of CA intoxication. The pathophysiology is multifactorial including loss of peripheral vascular tone due to alpha-adrenergic blockade and probably more importantly, decreased myocardial contractility due to the quinidine-like membrane stabilizing effects.

Patients with CA overdoses frequently develop secondary complications. Rhabdomyolysis may result from excessive seizure activity. Pulmonary complications include noncardiogenic pulmonary edema and aspiration pneumonia[632].

Laboratory Tests

Rapid quantitative determination of CA plasma concentration is neither clinically useful nor readily available. Although CA levels exceeding 1000 ng/mL are observed in patients with significant clinical toxicity—coma, seizures and dysrhythmias, life-threatening toxicity is also observed in patients with levels less than 1000 ng/mL[633,634]. The minimal correlation between clinical toxicity and serum concentration is due to the large volume of distribution of CAs with subsequent high tissue:serum ratio; thus, the serum concentration does not accurately reflect the total body burden of the drug.

Quantitative and/or qualitative determinations may be useful in documenting the presence or absence of the ingestion. This information can be used in conjunction with the patient's clinical course and ECG to guide management and disposition.

Routine laboratory studies including glucose and electrolytes should be obtained for any child presenting with altered mental status. An arterial blood gas should be obtained to assess the degree of acidosis and guide alkalinization therapy if needed. Urinalysis can help diagnose rhabdomyolysis. A 12 lead electrocardiogram should be obtained on all patients. Serial ECGs are indicated to follow conduction disorders and dysrhythmias.

Treatment

Any child with a suspected or known ingestion of a CA requires immediate evaluation and treatment. After stabilization of the airway, ventilation, blood pressure, and peripheral perfusion, gastric decontamination must be performed. Given the unpredictability of clinical deterioration and rapid onset of CNS depression and seizures, the use of ipecac syrup is contraindicated. Gastric lavage is indicated for most cases of suspected or known CA ingestions due to the potential serious toxicity. Since the anticholinergic actions of some CA, particularly TCAs, may dramatically delay gastric emptying, attempts at gastric lavage even 12 to 24 hours after ingestion may yield unabsorbed drug. Patients who are obtunded or seizing require lavage, but only after intubation to protect the airway.

An initial dose of activated charcoal with cathartic should be administered to all patients. Multiple doses of charcoal without a cathartic may be indicated because of the CA enterohepatic circulation; there is some evidence to support its ability to enhance the rate of CA elimination[(635)]. However the evidence is not overwhelming to support more than an additional one or two doses. Furthermore, it is important to monitor for the development of an ileus to prevent abdominal complications.

Management of Central Nervous System Toxicity

Adequate airway protection with intubation should be considered in any comatose patient or patient with a depressed mental status. Unlike naloxone, the routine use of flumazenil in the patient with altered mental status is not indicated, especially those with a known or suspected CA ingestion. The benzodiazepine receptor, like the cyclic antidepressants, is also part of the GABA receptor complex. Administration of flumazenil may further inhibit the chloride channel like CAs, thereby increasing the risk of seizures[(636)].

Physostigmine is a short-acting cholinesterase inhibitor which can potentially reverse both CNS and peripheral anticholinergic effects. This drug was used in the past to reverse the CNS toxicity of CA. However, physostigmine may increase the risk of cardiac toxicity and has been shown to cause bradycardia and asystole as well as precipitate seizures in CA-poisoned patients[(637,638)].

Recurrent seizures and status epilepticus need prompt treatment to prevent worsening acidosis, hypoxia, and the development of hyperthermia and rhabdomyolysis. Benzodiazapines are effective as first line therapy for seizures. If this therapy fails, barbiturates should be administered and, finally, neuromuscular paralysis should be induced with general anesthesia with continuous EEG monitoring.

The role for phenytoin as an anticonvulsant for CA-induced seizures is less clear. Some data demonstrate beneficial effects while other data question its efficacy. Furthermore, there are some animal studies suggesting it may potentiate ventricular dysrhythmias[(639)]. Continuous infusions of the short-acting benzodiazpine midazolam and general anesthetic propofol have been used successfully for the control of refractory seizures[(640,641)].

Management of Cardiovascular Toxicity

Isolated sinus tachycardia due to CAs does not require any specific therapy. Serum alkalinization with sodium bicarbonate is the therapeutic intervention indicated for cardiac conduction delays, dysrhythmias, and hypotension. Substantial evidence for the efficacy of hypertonic sodium bicarbonate therapy has been collected in animal models[(642,643)].

The mechanism of action for the therapeutic effect of alkalinization is probably multifactorial. First, the sodium channel blockade caused by CA may be overcome by increasing the extracellular concentration of sodium. Second, alkalinization increases the concentration of nonionized drug, facilitating its egress from the sodium channel receptor site. Alkalinization may increase the protein binding of CAs in the serum, thereby decreasing free, unbound pharmacologically active drug, although this mechanism probably does not contribute significantly to the effect of alkalinization as much as the two former ones. Sodium bicarbonate therapy appears to be more effective than hyperventilation alone or administration of hypertonic saline in animal models[(643,644)]. A recent study has shown the effectiveness of hypertonic saline and dextran solution in reversing hypotension and QRS prolongation[(645)]. Consistent guidelines for alkalinization with sodium bicarbonate for CA-induced cardiac toxicity are not available.

Sodium bicarbonate should be administered initially as a bolus of 1 to 2 mEq/kg (Figs. 40.13a–c). A continuous bicarbonate infusion with 100 to 150 mEq of sodium bicarbonate in 1 l of 5% dextrose in water should be titrated over the next 4 to 6 hours to achieve a blood pH of 7.45 to 7.55. The endpoint for alkalinization is not well-established. Most authors advocate continuing alkalinization at least 24 hours after the ECG has normalized in conjunction with improvement in the patient's overall clinical status. Sodium bicarbonate infusion can be used in conjuntion with hyperventilation (pCO_2 of 30 to 40 mmHg) if the patient is intubated. No studies have been performed looking at the role of prophylactic alkalinization in preventing cardiac toxicity and probably should not be done since it involves risks like hyperosmolarity, cerebral vasoconstriction, and decreased ionized calcium concentrations.

In addition to serum alkalinization, lidocaine is the antiarrhythmic agent recommended for CA-induced dysrhythmias, although there are no controlled studies documenting its efficacy. Because lidocaine has membrane stabilizing properties that may impair conduction and contractility,

A

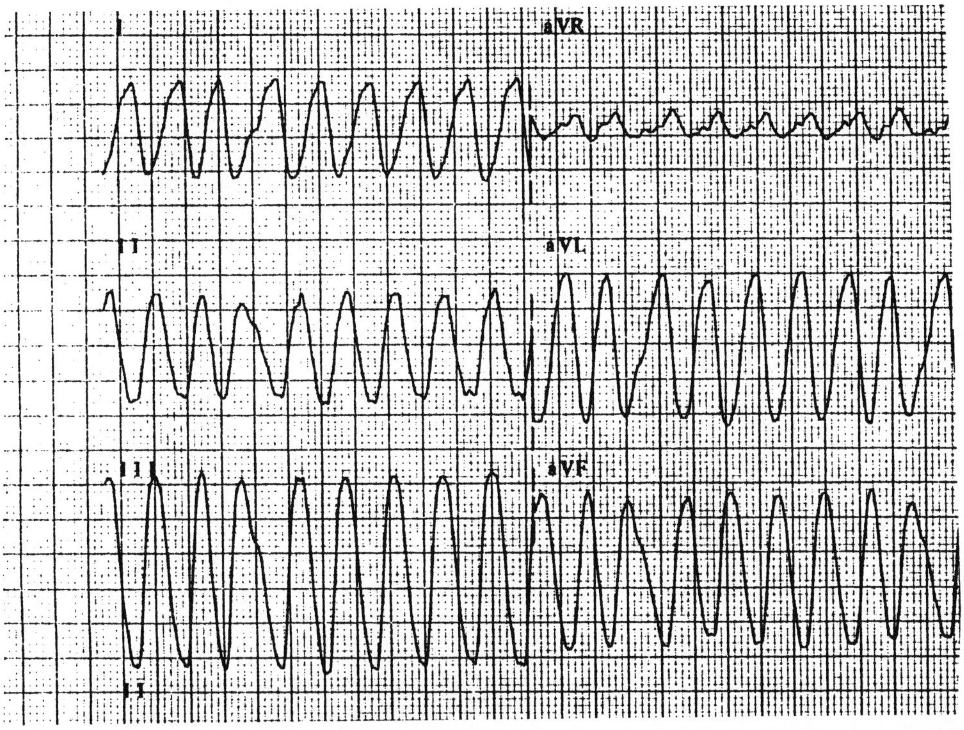

Figure 40.13a. Initial ECG of a 2 ½ year old female who presented after an accidental ingestion of 75 mgs (7.5 mg/kg) of a neighbor's desipramine. ECG shows a wide complex tachycardia. She initially presented awake and alert and then had a generalized tonic-clonic seizure within the first 10 minutes.

B

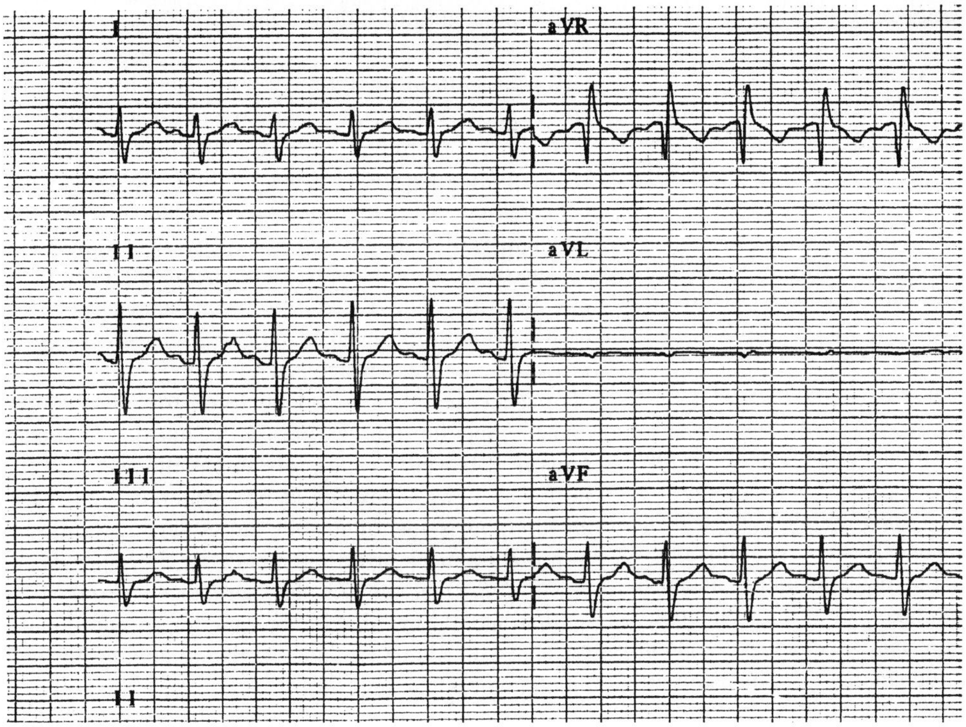

Figure 40.13b. ECG 30 minutes after arrival. Interim treatment included 1 mEq/kg $NaHCO_3$ and 1 mg/kg lidocaine. ECG shows narrowing of the QRS complex (duration of 140 msec), R wave amplitude in lead aVR of 6.0 mm, and R/S ratio of 1.2.

some authors argue against its use in CA poisoning[646]. Because of its antiarrhythmic properties, magnesium sulfate may be beneficial in the treatment of ventricular dysrhythmias[647], although its role in CA toxicity needs further evaluation.

Type IA antiarrhythmics (quinidine, procainamide, disopyramide) and Type Ic antidysrhythmics (flecainide, encainide, and propafenone) are contraindicated in CA-induced dysrhythmias because of the similar quinidine-like effects they exert on the myocardium. The use of phenytoin for CA-induced dysrhythmias is controversial. The proposed antiarrhythmic mechanism of phenytoin is improvement of conduction velocity and membrane responsiveness, theoretically making it a reasonable choice for CA-induced dysrhythmias. Several animal and human studies have advocated its success in preventing or reversing conduction abnormalities although they were not well-controlled studies and had very small numbers[648–650]. Other studies suggest phenytoin may have a proarrhythmogenic effect in the presence of CA[639].

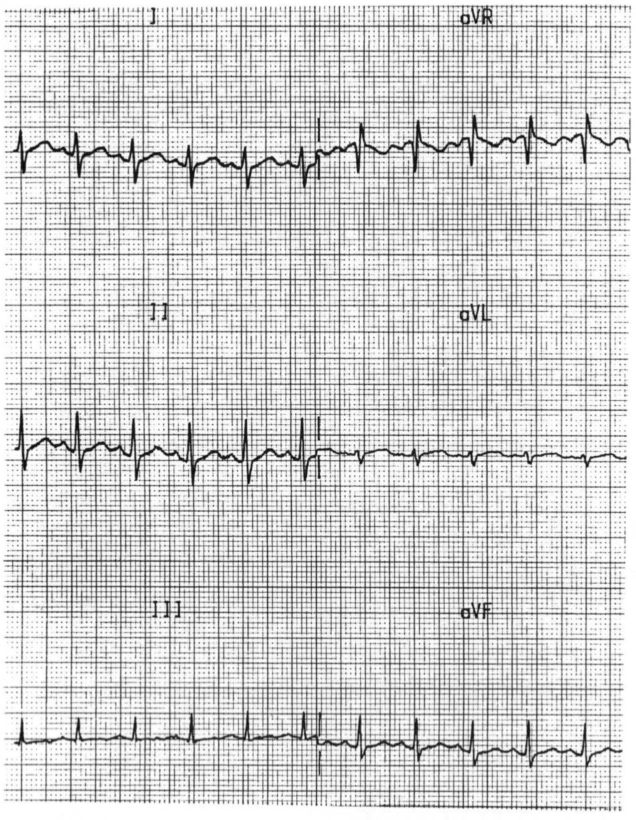

C

Figure 40.13c. ECG about 9 hours later. Patient was on a sodium bicarbonate drip. No further lidocaine was given. ECG shows further narrowing of QRS interval and decrease in amplitude of the R wave in lead aVR.

Hypotension should be treated initially with crystalloid infusions, up to 30 ml/kg, with the patient in Trendelenburg position. If fluid administration fails to correct hypotension, vasoactive agents should begin. Central venous pressure or pulmonary artery catheterization may be necessary to guide the choice of vasopressor or inotropic agents, depending on the measured cardiac output and systemic vascular resistance.

Theoretically, direct-acting alpha-adrenergic agonists such as norepinephrine are more effective than dopamine, which is a partially indirect acting catecholamine. Because CAs prevent neuronal reuptake of catecholamines, norepinephrine-depleted neurons may be unable to respond to indirectly-acting agents like dopamine[651]. This theoretical advantage has not been substantiated by well-designed studies. High dose dopamine may be as effective as norepinephrine for hypotension[652]. Dobutamine should be selected if hypotension is a result of low cardiac output due to loss of inotropy. Practically speaking, in severe CA overdoses with refractory hypotension, a combination of vasopressors and inotropes should be used.

Other Treatment Modalities

Because of the CA large volume of distribution and protein binding, neither hemodialysis nor hemoperfusion are effective modalities for enhancing elimination. In severely poisoned patients, cardiopulmonary bypass may have a role in improving survival, although further controlled studies are needed[653].

Research involving immunotherapy with CA-specific antidbodies has not been clinically applicable as of yet due to the large amount of antibody required to achieve toxicity reversal and the large number of structurally different CAs, necessitating numerous CA-specific antibodies and limiting their clinical utility[654].

Monitoring/Disposition

All patients who present with a known or suspected CA ingestion should receive continuous cardiac monitoring. Whether *all* patients should be admitted for medical monitoring is a point of discussion. Several retrospective studies appear to support an algorithm which takes into account presenting signs and symptoms. If the patient is asymptomatic at presentation, undergoes gastrointestinal decontamination, and remains asymptomatic in the health care facility for a minimum of 6 hours, the patient may be medically cleared for psychiatric evaluation or discharged home[655,656]. If any major signs of toxicity are present on initial presentation—altered mental status, conduction disturbances (QRS interval of 100 msec, R wave of 3 mm, and rightward shift of the terminal QRS axis), hypotension, seizures, or dysrhythmias—admission to a monitored bed is mandatory. Certainly if there are any concerns about the accuracy of the ingestion history, psychosocial issues, or other concomitant drugs ingested with the potential for delayed toxicity, medical admission is warranted.

The duration of intensive care monitoring is another area of controversy. Older literature recommends 48 to 72 hours of ICU monitoring even in mild CA ingestions due to reports of late-onset cardiac and CNS effects; however, review of these cases shows inadequate gastric decontamination and therapeutic interventions. Late, unexpected complications in CA overdoses are rare in patients who had little or no major signs of toxicity at presentation[657]. If appropriate therapy is instituted, new onset seizures and conduction disturbances or arrhythmias after 24 hours do not occur[658,659]. Once the ECG has normalized, serial ECGs and cardiac monitoring should continue for an additional 12 to 24 hours off alkalinization therapy, assuming the patient's mental status has improved.

References

1. Walton WW. An evaluation of the poison prevention act. Pediatrics 1982;69:363.
2. Lacroix J, Gaudreault P, Gauthier M. Admission to a pediatric intensive care unit for poisoning: a review of 105 cases [see comments]. Crit Care Med 1989;17:748.
3. Maragos GD. Epidemiology of childhood poisoning update. Pediatrician 1979.
4. Woolf AD, Lovejoy FH Jr. Epidemiology of drug overdose in children. Drug Safety 1993;9:291.
5. Deeths TM, Margolis J. Repetitive poisoning in children—a statistical study of 1057 cases. J Pediatr 1971;78:299.
6. Margolis JA. Psychosocial study of childhood poisoning: a five year follow up. Pediatrics 1971;47:439.
7. Dine MS, McGovern ME. Intentional poisoning of children—an over-

looked category of child abuse. Report of seven cases and review of the literature. Pediatrics 1982;70:32.
8. Fischler R. Poisoning: a syndrome of child abuse. Am Fam Pract 1983;28:103.
9. Woolf AD, Wynshaw-Boris A, Rinaldo P, Levy HL. Intentional ethylene glycol poisoning presenting as an inherited metabolic disorder. J Pediatr 1992;120:421.
10. Garfinkel BD, Froese A, Hood J. Suicide attempts in children and adolescents. Am J Psychiatry 1982;139:1257.
11. Kilham HA. Hospital management of severe poisoning. Pediatr Clin North Am 1980;27:603.
12. Benowitz NL, Rosenberg J,Becker CE. Cardiopulmonary catastrophes in drug-overdosed patients. Med Clin North Am 1979;63:267.
13. Benowitz NL, Goldschlager N. Cardiac disturbances in the toxicologic patient. In: Haddad LM, Winchester JF, eds. Clinical management of poisoning and drug overdose. Philadelphia: WB Saunders, 1983.
14. Mofenson HC, Greensher J. The unknown poison. Pediatrics 1974;54:336.
15. Woolf AD. Poisoning in children and adolescents. Pediatrics in Review 1993;14:411.
16. Lovejoy FH, Robertson W, Woolf AD. Poison centers, poison prevention and the pediatrician. Pediatrics 1994;94:220.
17. Woolf AD, Anderson A. The diagnosis and initial management of pediatric poisonings. Emerg Care Q 1990;6:7.
18. Witte DL, Rodgers JL, Barrett DA. The anion gap: its use in quality control. Clin Chem 1976;22:643.
19. Winter SD, Pearson R, Gabow PA, et al. The fall of the serum anion gap. Arch Intern Med 1990;150:311.
20. Goldstein RJ, Lichtenstein NS, Souder D. The myth of the low anion gap. JAMA 1980;243:1737.
21. Heckerling PS. Ethylene glycol poisoning with a normal anion gap due to occult bromide intoxication. Ann Emerg Med 1987;16:1384.
22. Smithline N, Gardner KD. Gaps: anionic and osmolal. JAMA 1976;236:1594.
23. Gennari FJ. Serum osmolality: uses and limitations. N Engl J Med 1984;310:102.
24. Hoffman RS, Smilkstein MJ, Howland MA, Goldfrank LR. Osmol gaps revisited: normal values and limitations. J Toxicol Clin Toxicol 1993;31:81.
25. Steinhard B. Case reports: severe ethylene glycol intoxication with normal osmolal gap—"a chilling thought." J Emerg Med 1990;8:583.
26. Winter ML, Ellis MD, Snodgrass WR. Urine fluorescence using a Wood's lamp to detect the antifreeze additive sodium fluorescein: a qualitative adjunctive test in suspected ethylene glycol ingestions. Ann Emerg Med 1990;19:663.
27. Savitt DL, Hawkins HH, Roberts JR. The radiopacity of orally ingested medications. Ann Emerg Med 1981;16:331.
28. Kellerman AL, Fihn SD, LoGerfo JP, et al. Impact of drug screening in suspected overdose. Ann Emerg Med 1987;16:1206.
29. Bailey DN. The role of the laboratory in treatment of the poisoned patient: laboratory perspective. J Anal Toxicol 1987;6:136.
30. Dean BL, Peterson R, Garrettson LK, et al. American Association of Poison Control Centers Policy Statement. Gastrointestinal dilution with water as a first aid procedure for poisoning. J Toxicol Clin Toxicol 1982;19:531.
31. Homan CS, Maitra SR, Lane BP, Geller ER. Effective treatment of the rat esophagus with early saline dilution therapy. Ann Emerg Med 1993;22:178.
32. Kulig KW, Bar-Or D, Cantrill SV, et al. Mangement of acutely poisoned patients without gastric emptying. Ann Emerg Med 1985;14:562.
33. Merigan KS, Woodward M, Hedges JR, et al. Prospective evaluation of gastric emptying in the self-poisoned patient. Am J Emerg Med 1990;8:479.
34. Curtis RA, Barone J, Giacona N. Efficacy of ipecac and activated charcoal and cathartic: prevention of salicylate absorption in a simulated overdose. Arch Intern Med 1984:144:48.
35. Smilkstein MJ, Flomenbaum NE. Techniques used to prevent absorpiton of toxic compounds. In: Goldfrank LR, Flomenbaum NE, Lewin NA, et al, eds. Goldfrank's toxicologic emergencies. 5th ed. Norwalk: Appleton & Lange, 1994:47.
36. Stewart JJ. Effects of emetics and cathartic agents on the gastrointestinal tract and the treatment of toxic ingestion. J Toxicol Clin Toxicol 1983:20:199.
37. Corby DG, Decker WJ, Moran MJ, et al. Clinical comparision of pharmacologic emetics in children. Pediatrics 1968;42:361.
38. Manno BR, Manno JE. Toxicology of ipecac: a review. Clin Toxicol 1977;10:221.
39. Schiff R, Wurzel C, Brunson S, et al. Death due to chronic syrup of ipecac in patients with major eating disorders. N Engl J Med 1985;313:1457.
40. Isner JM. Effects of ipecac on the heart. N Engl J Med 1986;314:1253.
41. Boehm JJ, Oppenheim RC. An in vitro study of the adsorption of the various drugs by activated charcoal. Aust J Pharmacol Sci 1977:4:107.
42. Tenenbein M, Cohen S, Sitar DS. Efficacy of ipecac-induced emesis, orogastric lavage, and activated charcoal for acute drug overdose. Ann Emerg Med 1987;16:838.
43. Kornberg AE, Dolgin J. Pediatric ingestions: charcoal alone versus ipecac and charcoal. Ann Emerg Med 1991;20:648.
44. Knopp R. Caustic ingestions. J Am Coll Emerg Physician 1979;8:329.
45. Harsch H. Aspiration of activated charcoal. N Engl J Med 1986;314:318.
46. Givens T, Holloway M, Wason S. Pulmonary aspiration of activated charcoal: a complication of its misuse in overdose management. Ped Emerg Care 1992;8:137.
47. Elliot CG, Colby TV, Kelly TM, et al. Charcoal lung: bronchiolitis obliterans after aspiration of activated charcoal. Chest 1989;96:672.
48. Menzies DG, Busuttel A, Prescott LF. Fatal pulmonary aspiration of oral activated charcoal. Br Med J 1988;297:459.
49. Silbermann H, Davis SM, Lee A. Activated charcoal aspiration. NC Med J 1990;51:79.
50. Steward J. Effects of emetic and cathartic agents on the gastrointestinal tract and the treatment of toxic ingestions. J Toxicol Clin Toxicol 1983;20:199.
51. Chin L, Picchioni A, Gillespie T. Saline cathartics and saline cathartics plus activated charcoal as antidotal treatments. Clin Toxicol 1981;18:865.
52. Al-Shareef AH, Buss DC, Allen EM, Routledge PA. The effects of charcoal and sorbitol (alone and in combination) on plasma theophylline concentration after a sustained release formulation. Hum Exp Toxicol 1990;9:179.
53. McNamara R, Aaron C, Gemborys M. Sorbitol catharsis does not enhance efficacy of charcoal in simulated acetominophen overdose. Ann Emerg Med 1988;17:243.
54. Keller R, Schwab R, Krenzelok E. Contribution of sorbitol combined with activated charcoal in prevention of salicylate absorption. Ann Emerg Med 1990;19:654.
55. Van de Graff W, Thompson L, Sunshine I, et al. Absorbent and cathartic inhibition of enteral drug absorption. J Pharmacol Exp Ther 1982;221:656.
56. Sue YJ, Woolf A, Shannon M. Efficacy of magnesium citrate cathartic in pediatric toxic ingestions. Ann Emerg Med 1994;24:709.
57. Phillips L, Nichols M, King W. A comparison of cathartics in pediatric ingestions (abstract). Vet Hum Tox 1994;36:377.
58. Jones J, Heiselman D, Doughert J, et al. Cathartic-induced magnesium toxicity during overdose management. Ann Emerg Med 1986;15:1214.
59. Mofenson H, Caraccio T. Magnesium intoxication in a neonate from oral magnesium hydroxide laxative. J Toxicol Clin Toxicol 1991;29:215.
60. Smilkstein M, Steedle D, Kulig K. Magnesium levels after magnesium containing cathartics. J Toxicol Clin Toxicol 1988;26:51.
61. Martin R, Lisehora G, Braxton M, et al. Fatal poisoning from sodium phosphate enema: a case report and experimental study. JAMA 1987;257:2190.
62. Sotos J, Cutler E, Finkel M, et al. Hypocalcemic coma following two pediatric phosphate enemas. Pediatrics 1977;60:305.
63. Farley TA. Severe hypernatremic dehydration after use of an activated charcoal-sorbitol suspension. J Pediatr 1986;109:719.
64. Tenenbein M. Whole bowel irrigation in iron poisoning. J Pediatr 1987;111:142.
65. Tenenbein M, Cohen S, Sitar DS. Whole bowel irrigation as a decontamination procedure after acute drug overdose. Arch Intern Med 1987;147:905.
66. Smith SW, Ling LJ, Halstenson CE. Whole bowel irrigation as a treatment for acute lithium overdose. Ann Emerg Med 1991;20:536.
67. Kirshenbaum LA, Mathews SC, Sitar DS, et al. Whole bowel irrigation versus activated charcoal in sorbitol for the ingestion of modified-release pharmaceuticals. Clin Pharmacol Ther 1989;46:264.
68. Burkhart KK, Wuerz RC, Donovan JW. Whole-bowel irrigation as adjunctive treatment for sustained-release theophylline overdose. Ann Emerg Med 1992;21:1316.
69. Hoffman RS, Smilkstein MJ, Goldfrank L. Whole bowel irrigation and

the cocaine body packer: a new approach to a common problem. Am J Emerg Med 1990;8:523.
70. Everson GW, Bertaccini EJ. Use of whole bowel irrigation (WBI) in an infant following iron overdose. Am J Emerg Med 1991;9:366.
71. Roberge RJ, Martin TG. Whole bowel irrigation in an acute oral lead intoxication. Am J Emerg Med 1992;10:577.
72. Linakis JG, Eisenberg MS, Lacouture PG, et al. Multiple-dose sodium polystyrene sulfonate in lithium intoxication: an animal model. Pharmacol Toxicol 1992:70:38.
73. Tomaszewski C, Musso C, Pearson JR. Lithium absorption prevented by sodium polystyrene sulfonate in volunteers. Ann Emerg Med 1992;21:1308.
74. Belanger DR, Tierney MG, Dickinson G. Effect of sodium polystyrene sulfonate on lithium bioavailability. Ann Emerg Med 1992; 21:1312.
75. Cohn WJ, Boylan J, Blanke RV, et al.Treatment of chlordecone (Kepone) toxicity with cholestyramine. N Engl J Med 1978;298:243.
76. Kassner JT, Maher TJ, Hull KM, Woolf AD. Cholestyramine as an adsorbent in acute lindane poisoning: a murine model. Ann Emerg Med 1993;22:1392.
77. Utecht MJ, Stone AF, McCarron MM. Heroin body packers. J Emerg Med 1993;11:33.
78. Caruana DS, Weinbach B, Goerg D, et al. Cocaine-packet ingestion: diagnosis, management, and natural history. Ann Inter Med 1084;100:73.
79. Suarez CA, Arango A, Lester JL. Cocaine-condom ingestion: surgical treatment. JAMA 1977;238:1391.
80. Foxford R, Goldfrank L. Gastrotomy: a surgical approach to iron overdose. Ann Emerg Med 1985;14:1223.
81. Goldfrank L, Cohen L, Flomenbaum N, et al. Newer antidotes and controversies in antidotal therapy. Emerg Med Annu 1984;3:223.
82. Litovitz TL. Anecdotal antidotes. Emerg Med Clin North Am 1984; 2:145.
83. Gelman C, Conner CS. Rational use of antidotes in toxicology. In: Bayer MJ, Rumack BH, Wanke LA, eds. Toxicologic emergencies. Bowie, MD: Robert J. Brady, 1984.
84. Brogden RN, Goa KL. Flumazenil—a reappraisal of its pharmacological properties and therapeutic efficacy as a benzodiazepine antagonist. Drugs 1991;42:1061.
85. Hojer J, Baehrendtz S. A placebo-controlled trial of flumazenil given by continuous infusion in severe benzodiazepine overdosage. Acta Anaesthesiol Scand 1991;35:584.
86. Klotz U, Kanto J. Pharmacokinetics and clinical use of flumazenil (Ro 15–1788). Clin Pharmacokin 1988;14:1.
87. Ritz R, Zuber M, Elsasser S. Use of flumazenil in intoxicated patients with coma. Intensive Care Med 1990;16:242.
88. Richard P, Autret E, Bardol J. The use of flumazenil in a neonate. Clin Toxicol 1991;29:137.
89. Locket S. Evaluation of various forms of treatment administered in poisoning. Practitioner 1973;210:709.
90. Todd JW. Do measures to enhance drug removal save life? Lancet 1984;1:331.
91. Cherskov M. Extracorporeal detoxification: still debatable. JAMA 1982;247:3047.
92. Blye E, Lorch J, Cortell S. Extracorporeal therapy in the treatment of intoxication. Am J Kidney Dis 1984;3:321.
93. Gelfand MC. Charcoal hemoperfusion in treatment of drug overdose. Dial Transplant 1977;6:8.
94. Gelfand MC, Winchester JF. Hemoperfusion in drug overdosage: a technique when conservative management is not sufficient. Clin Toxicol 1980;17:583.
95. Bismuth C, Conso F, Wattel F, et al. Coated activated charcoal hemoperfusion: experience of French antipoison centers: about 60 cases. Vet Hum Toxicol 1979;21:2.
96. Volans GN, Vale JA, Crome P, et al. The role of charcoal hemoperfusion in the management of acute poisoning by drugs. In: Kenedi RM, Courtney J, Craylor JDS, et al., eds. Artificial organs. Baltimore: University Park Press, 1976.
97. Pond SM. Diuresis, dialysis and hemoperfusion. Indications and benefits. Emerg Med Clin North Am 1984;2:29.
98. Hill JB. Experimental salicylate poisoning: observations on the effects of altering pH or tissue and plasma salicylate concentrations. Pediatrics 1971;47:658.
99. Winchester JF. Dialysis and hemoperfusion of poisons and drugs. Trans Am Soc Artif Intern Organs 1977;23:762.
100. Wanke LA, Bennett WM. Enhancement of elimination: diuresis, peritoneal dialysis, hemodialysis, and hemoperfusion. In: Bayer MJ, Rumack BH, Wanke LA, eds. Toxicologic emergencies. Bowie, MD: Robert J. Brady, 1984.
101. Yatzidis H. A convenient hemoperfusion micro-apparatus over charcoal for the treatment of endogenous and exogenous intoxications: its use as an effective artificial kidney. Proc Eur Dial Transplant Assoc 1964;1:83.
102. Chang T. Removal of endogenous and exogenous toxins by microencapsulated adsorbent. Can J Physiol Pharmacol 1969;47:1043.
103. Pond S, Rosenberg J, Benowitz NL, et al. Pharmacokinetics of hemoperfusion for drug overdose. Clin Pharmacokinet 1981;4:329.
104. Papadopoulou ZL, Novello AC. The use of hemoperfusion in children. Past, present and future. Pediatr Clin North Am 1982;29:1039.
105. Gelfand MC, Colon AR, Knepshield JH, et al. Successful management of stage IV hepatic coma in a child by hemocarboperfusion. In: Kenedi RM, Courtney JM, Gaylor JDS, et al., eds. Artificial organs. London: Macmillan, 1977.
106. Chavers BM, Kjellstrand CM, Wiegand C, et al. Technique for use of charcoal hemoperfusion in infants: experience in two patients. Kidney Int 1980;18:386.
107. Mauer SM, Chavers BM, Kjellstrand CM. Treatment of an infant with severe chloramphenicol intoxication using charcoal column hemoperfusion. J Pediatr 1980;96:136.
108. Berg MJ, Berlinger WJ, Goldberg JM, et al. Acceleration of the body clearance of phenobarbital by oral activated charcoal. N Engl J Med 1982;307:642.
109. Levy G. Gastrointestinal clearance of drugs with activated charcoal. N Engl J Med 1982;307:676.
110. Berliner WJ, Spector R, Goldberg MJ, et al. Enhancement of theophylline clearance by oral activated charcoal. Clin Pharmacol Ther 1983;33:351.
111. Shannon M, Amitai Y, Lovejoy FHJ. Multiple dose activated charcoal for theophylline poisoning in young infants. Pediatrics 1987;80:368.
112. Neuvonen PJ, Elonen E. Effect of activated charcoal on absorption and elimination of phenobarbitone, carbamazepine, and phenylbutazone in man. Eur J Clin Pharmacol 1980;17:51.
113. Kirshenbaum LA, Mathews SC, Sitar DS, et al. Does multiple-dose charcoal therapy enhance salicylate excretion? Arch Intern Med 1990; 150:1281.
114. Pond SM, Jacobs M, Marks J, et al. Treatment of digitoxin overdose with oral activated charcoal. Lancet 1981;2:1177.
115. Farley TA. Severe hypernatremic dehydration after use of an activated charcoal-sorbitol suspension. J Pediatr 1986;109:719.
116. Laussen P, Shann F, Butt W, et al. Use of plasmapheresis in acute theophylline toxicity. Crit Care Med 1991;19:288.
117. Rabetoy GM, Price CA, Findlay JW, et al. Treatment of digoxin intoxication in a renal failure patient with digoxin-specific antibody fragments and plasmapheresis. Am J Nephrol 1990;10:518.
118. Yarbrough BE. Current management of the poisoned patient. South Med J 1988;81:892.
119. Colburn WA. Specific antibodies and Fab fragments to alter the pharmacokinetics and reverse the pharmacologic toxicologic effect of drugs. Drug Metab Rev 1980;11:223.
120. Smith TW, Haber E, Yeatman L, et al. Reversal of advanced digoxin intoxication with Fab fragments of digoxin-specific antibodies. N Engl J Med 1976;294:797.
121. Woolf A, Wenger T, Smith TW, Lovejoy FH. Use of digoxin-specific Fab fragments for severe pediatric digitalis poisoning: report of a multicenter experience. N Engl J Med 1992;326:1739.
122. Baud FJ, Sabouraud A, Vicaut E, et al. Brief report: treatment of severe colchicine overdose with colchicine-specific Fab fragments. N Engl J Med 1995;332:642.
123. Hursting MJ, Opheim KE, Raisys VA, et al. Tricyclic antidepressant-specific Fab fragments alter the distribution and elimination of desipramine in the rabbit: a model for overdose treatment. J Toxicol Clin Toxicol 1989;27:53.
124. Linden CN, Rumack BH. Acetaminophen overdose. Emerg Med Clin North Am 1984;2:103.
125. Rumack BH. Acetaminophen. In: Haddad LM, Winchester JF, eds. Clinical management of poisoning and drug overdose. Philadelphia: WB Saunders, 1983.
126. Peterson RG, Rumack BH. Pharmacokinetics of acetaminophen in children. Pediatrics 1978;62:877.
127. Peterson RG, Rumack BH. Age as a variable in acetaminophen overdose. Arch Intern Med 1981;141:390.

128. Mitchell JR, Thorgeirsson SS, Potter WZ, et al. Acetaminophen-induced hepatic injury; protective role of glutathione in man and rationale for therapy. Clin Pharmacol Ther 1974;16:676.
129. Mitchell JR, Jollow DJ, Potter WZ, et al. Acetaminophen-induced hepatic necrosis. IV. Protective role of glutathione. J Pharmacol Exp Ther 1973;187:211.
130. Miner DJ, Kissinger PT. Evidence for the involvement of *N*-acetyl-*p*-quinonimine in acetaminophen metabolism. Biochem Pharmacol 1979;28:3285.
131. Prescott LF, Critchley J. The treatment of acetaminophen poisoning. Annu Rev 1983;23:87.
132. Davis M, Simmons CJ, Harrison NG, et al. Paracetamol overdose in man: relationship between pattern of urinary metabolites and severity of liver damage. Q J Med 1981;45:181.
133. Jollow DJ, Thorgeirsson SS, Potter WZ, et al. Acetaminophen induced hepatic necrosis. II. Metabolic disposition of toxic and nontoxic doses of acetaminophen. Pharmacology 1974;12:251.
134. Rumack BH, Matthew H. Acetaminophen poisoning and toxicity. Pediatrics 1975;55:871.
135. Prescott LF, Newton RW, Swainson CP, et al. Successful treatment of severe paracetamol overdosage with cysteamine. Lancet 1974;1:588.
136. Whitcomb DC, Block GD. Association of acetaminophen hepatotoxicity with fasting and ethanol use. JAMA 1994;272:1845.
137. Strubelt O, Siegirs CP, Schutt A. The curative effect of cysteamine cysteine and dithiocarb in experimental paracetanol poisoning. Arch Toxicol 1974;33:55.
138. Rumack BH, Peterson RG. Acetaminophen overdosage: incidence, diagnosis and management in 46 patients. Pediatrics 1978;62:898.
139. Rumack BN, Peterson RG, Koch CG, et al. Acetaminophen overdose: 662 cases with evaluation of oral acetylcysteine treatment. Arch Intern Med 1981;141:380.
140. Prescott LF, Park J, Sutherland GR, et al. Cysteamine, methionine, and penicillamine in the treatment of paracetamol poisoning. Lancet 1976;2:109.
141. Hamilyn AN, Douglas AP, James O. The spectrum of paracetamol (acetaminophen) overdose: clinical and epidemiological selectives. Postgrad Med J 1978;54:400.
142. Brown R. Hepatic and renal dosage with paracetamol overdosage. J Clin Pathol 1968;21:273.
143. Boyer TD, Rouff SL. Acetaminophen induced hepatic necrosis and renal failure. JAMA 1976;218:440.
144. Mofenson HC, Caraccio TR, Nawaz H, et al. Acetaminophen induced pancreatitis. J Toxicol Clin Toxicol 1991;29:223.
145. Sanerkin NG. Acute myocardial necrosis in paracetamol poisoning. Br Med J 1971;3:478.
146. Rumack BH. Aspirin versus acetaminophen. A comparative view. Pediatrics 1978;62:943.
147. Henretig FM, Selbst SM, Forrest C, et al. Repeated acetaminophen overdosing causing hepatotoxicity in children. Clinical reports and literature review. Clin Pediatr (Phila) 1989;28:525.
148. Alam SN, Roberts RJ, Fisher LJ. Age related differences in salicylamide and acetaminophen conjugation in man. J Pediatr 1977;90:130.
149. Greene JW, Craft L, Ghishan F. Acetaminophen poisoning in infancy. Am J Dis Child 1983;137:386.
150. Agram PF, Zenk KE, Romansky SG. Acute liver failure and encephalopathy in a 15 month old infant. Am J Dis Child 1983;137:1107.
151. Smilkstein MJ, Knapp GL, Kulig KW, Rumack BH. Efficacy of oral *N*-acetylcysteine in the treatment of acetaminophen overdose. N Engl J Med 1988;319:1557.
152. Prescott LF, Illingworth RN, Critchley J, et al. Intravenous *N*-acetylcysteine: the treatment of choice for paracetamol poisoning. Br Med J 1979;2:1097.
153. Smilkstein MJ, Bronstein AC, Linden C, Augenstein WL, Kulig KW, Rumack BH. Acetaminophen overdose: a 48-hour intravenous *N*-acetylcysteine treatment protocol. Ann Emerg Med 1991;20:1058.
154. Ekins BR, Ford DC, Thompson MI, et al. The effect of activated charcoal on *N*-acetylcysteine absorption in normal subjects. Am J Emerg Med 1987;5:483.
155. Reed MD, Marx CM. Ondansetron for treating nausea and vomiting in the poisoned patient. Ann Pharmacother 1994;28:331.
156. Parker D, White JP, Paton D, et al. Safety of late acetylcysteine treatment in paracetamol poisoning. Hum Exp Toxicol 1990;9:25.
157. Harrison PM, Keays R, Bray GP, Alexander GJM, Williams R. Improved outcome of paracetamol-induced fulminant hepatic failure by late administration of acetylcysteine. Lancet 1990;335:1572.
158. Harrison PM, Wendon JA, Gimson AES, Alexander GJM, Williams R. Improvement by acetylcysteine of hemodynamics and oxygen transport in fulminant hepatic failure. N Engl J Med 1991;324:1852.
159. Keays R, Harrison PM, Wendon JA, Forbes A, Gove C, Alexander GJM, Williams R. Intravenous acetylcysteine in paracetamol induced fulminant hepatic failure: a prospective controlled trial. Brit Med J 1991;303:1026.
160. Helliwell M, Vale A, Goulding R. Haemoperfusion in "late" paracetamol poisoning. Hum Toxicol 1981;1:25.
161. Helliwell M, Essex E. Hemoperfusion in "late" paracetamol poisoning. Clin Toxicol 1981;18:1225.
162. Kulig K, Duffy KP, Linden CH, et al. Toxic effects of methanol, ethylene glycol and isopropyl alcohol. Topic Emerg Med 1984;6:14.
163. Lacouture PG, Wason S, Abrams A, et al. Acute isopropyl alcohol intoxication. Diagnosis and management. Am J Med 1983;75:680.
164. McFadden SW, Haddow JF. Coma produced by topical application of isopropanol. Pediatrics 1969;43:622.
165. Kelner M, Bailey DN. Isopropanol ingestion: interpretation of blood concentrations and clinical findings. J Toxicol Clin Toxicol 1983;20:497.
166. Freireich AW, Cinque TJ, Xanthaky EA. Hemodialysis for isopropanol poisoning. N Engl J Med 1969;277:699.
167. King LH, Bradley DP, Shires DL. Hemodialysis for isopropyl alcohol poisoning. JAMA 1970;211:1855.
168. Becker CE. Acute methanol poisoning—"the blind drunk." Medical staff conference University of California, San Francisco. West J Med 1981;135:122.
169. Bennett IV, Cary FH, Mitchell GL, et al. Acute methyl alcohol poisoning—a review based on experiences in an outbreak of 323 cases. Medicine 1953;32:431.
170. Swartz RD, Millman RP, Billi JE, et al. Epidemic methanol poisoning. Chemical and biochemical analysis of a recent episode. Medicine 1981;60:373.
171. Kahn A, Blum D. Methyl alcohol poisoning in an 8-month old boy: an unusual route of intoxication. J Pediatr 1979;94:841.
172. Wanke LA. Methanol and ethylene glycol poisoning. In: Bayer MJ, Rumack BH, Wanke LA, eds. Toxicologic emergencies. Bowie, MD: Robert J. Brady, 1984.
173. Sejersted OM, Jacobsen D, Ovrebo S, et al. Formate concentrations in plasma from patients poisoned with methanol. Acta Med Scand 1983;213:105.
174. McMartin KE, Ambre JJ, Tephly TR. Methanol poisoning in human subjects. Role of formic acid accumulation in the metabolic acidosis. Am J Med 1980;68:414.
175. McMartin KE, Makar AB, Martin AG, et al. Methanol poisoning. I. The role of formic acid in the development of metabolic acidosis in the monkey and the reversal by 4-methylpyrazole. Biochem Med 1975; 13:319.
176. Clay KL, Murphy RC, Watkins WD. Experimental methanol toxicity in the primate: analysis of metabolic acidosis. Toxicol Appl Pharmacol 1975;34:49.
177. Editorial. Methanol poisoning. Lancet 1983;1:910.
178. Smith SR, Smith S, Buckley BM. Combined formate and lactate acidosis in methanol poisoning. Lancet 1981;2:1295.
179. Nocker PE, Eells JT, Tephly TR. Methanol toxicity: treatment with folic acid and 5-formyl tetrahydro folic acid. Alcohol Clin Exp Res 1980;4:378.
180. Makar AB, Tephyl TR. Methanol poisoning in folate deficient rats. Nature 1976;261:715.
181. Jacobsen D, McMartin KE. Methanol and ethylene glycol poisonings—mechanism of toxicity, clinical course, diagnosis, and treatment. Med Toxicol 1986;1:309.
182. McLean DR, Jacobs H, Mielke BW. Methanol poisonings: a clinical and pathological study. Ann Neurol 1980;8:161.
183. LeWitt PA, Martin SD. Dystonia and hypokinesis with putaminal necrosis after methanol intoxication. Clin Neuropharmacol 1988;11:161.
184. Potts AM, Proglin S, Farkas L, et al. Additional observations on methanol poisoning in the primate test object. Am J Ophthalmol 1955;40:76.
185. McCoy HG, Cipolle RJ, Ehlers S, et al. Severe methanol poisoning. Application of a pharmacokinetic model for ethanol therapy and hemodialysis. Am J Med 1979;67:804.
186. Peterson CD. Oral ethanol dose in patients with methanol poisoning. Am J Hosp Pharm 1981;38:1024.
187. Keyvan LH, Tannenberg AM. Methanol intoxication. Comparison of peritoneal dialysis and hemodialysis treatment. Arch Intern Med 1976;134:293.

188. Tobin M, Lianos E. Hemodialysis for methanol poisoning. J Dial 1979;3:97.
189. Gonda A, Gault H, Churchill D, et al. Hemodialysis for methanol intoxication. Am J Med 1978;64:749.
190. Aronow R, ed. Handbook of common poisonings in children. 2nd ed. Evanston, IL: American Academy of Pediatrics, 1983.
191. Kruse JA. Methanol poisoning. Intensive Care Med 1992;18:391.
192. Jacobsen D, Bredesen JE, Eide I, et al. Anion and osmolal maps in the diagnosis of methanol and ethylene glycol poisoning. Acta Med Scand 1982;212:17.
193. Suit PF, Estes ML. Methanol intoxication: clinical features and differential diagnosis. Cleveland Clin J Med 1990;57:464.
194. Osterloh JD, Pond SM, Grady S, et al. Serum formate concentrations in methanol intoxication as a criterion for hemodialysis. Ann Intern Med 1986;104:200.
195. Blomstrand R, Ostling WH, Lof A, et al. Pyrazoles as inhibitors of alcohol oxidation and as important tools in alcohol research. An approach to therapy against methanol poisoning. Proc Natl Acad Sci USA 1979;7:3499.
196. McMartin KE, Hedstrom KG, Tolf B, et al. Studies on the metabolic interactions between 4-methyl-pyrazole and methanol using the monkey as an animal model. Arch Biochem Biophys 1980;199:606.
197. Woolf AD, Wynshaw-Boris A, Rinaldo P, Levy HL. Intentional infantile ethylene glycol poisoning presenting as an inherited metabolic disorder. J Pediatr 1992;120:421.
198. Parry MF, Wallach R. Ethylene glycol poisoning. Am J Med 1974;57:143.
199. Karlson-Stiber C, Persson H. Ethylene glycol poisoning: experiences from an epidemic in Sweden. Clin Toxicol 1992;30:565.
200. Peterson DC, Collins AJ, Himes J, et al. Ethylene glycol poisoning. Pharmacokinetics during therapy with ethanol and hemodialysis. N Engl J Med 1981;304:21.
201. Frommer JP, Ayus JC. Acute ethylene glycol intoxication. Am J Nephrol 1982;2:1.
202. Pons CA, Custer RP. Acute ethylene glycol poisoning. A clinicopathologic report of 18 fatal cases. Am J Med Sci 1946;211:544.
203. Bove KE. Ethylene glycol toxicity. Am J Clin Pathol 1966;45:46.
204. Blakeley KR, Rinner SE, Knochel JP. Survival of ethylene glycol poisoning with profound acidemia. N Engl J Med 1993;328:515.
205. Jacobsen D, Ovrebo S, Ostborg J, et al. Glycolate causes the acidosis in ethylene glycol poisoning and is effectively removed by hemodialysis. Acta Med Scand 1984;216:409.
206. Gabow PA, Clay K, Sullivan JB, et al. Organic acids in ethylene glycol intoxication. Ann Intern Med 1986;105:16.
207. Clay KL, Murphy RC. On the metabolic acidosis of ethylene glycol intoxication. Toxicol Appl Pharmacol 1977;39:39.
208. Bachman E, Goldberg L. Reappraisal of the toxicology of ethylene glycol. III. Mitochondrial effects. Food Cosmet Toxicol 1971;9:39.
209. Moriarty RW, McDonald RH. The spectrum of ethylene glycol poisoning. Clin Toxicol 1974;7:583.
210. Ahmed MM. Ocular effects of antifreeze poisoning. Br J Ophthalmol 1971;55:854.
211. Palmer BF, Eigenbrodt EH, Henrich WL. Cranial nerve deficit: a clue to the diagnosis of ethylene glycol poisoning. Am J Med 1989;87:91.
212. Roberts JA, Seibold HR. Ethylene glycol toxicity in the monkey. Toxicol Appl Pharmacol 1969;15:624.
213. Flanagan P, Libcke JH. Renal biopsy observations following recovery from ethylene glycol nephrosis. Am J Clin Pathol 1964;41:171.
214. Berman LB, Schneiner GE, Feys L. The nephrotoxic lesions of ethylene glycol. Ann Intern Med 1957;46:611.
215. Curtin L, Kraner J, Wine H, Savitt D, Abuelo JG. Complete recovery after massive ethylene glycol ingestion. Arch Intern Med 1992; 152:1311.
216. Underwood F, Bennett WM. Ethylene glycol intoxication. Prevention of renal failure by aggressive management. JAMA 1973;226:1453.
217. Freed CR, Bobbitt WJ, Williams RM, et al. Ethanol for ethylene glycol poisoning. N Engl J Med 1981;304:976.
218. Jacobsen D, Ostby N, Bredesen JE. Studies on ethylene glycol poisoning. Acta Med Scand 1982;212:11.
219. Rothman A, Normann SA, Manoguerra A, Bastian JF, Griswold WR. Short-term hemodialysis in childhood ethylene glycol poisoning. J Pediatr 1986;108:153.
220. Sangster B, Prenen J, Degroot A. Ethylene glycol poisoning. N Engl J Med 1980;302:465.
221. Chou JY, Richardson KE. The effect of pyrazole in ethylene glycol toxicity and metabolism in the rat. Toxicol Appl Pharmacol 1978;43:33.
222. Baud FJ, Bismuth C, Garnier R, et al. 4-Methylpyrazole may be an alternative to ethanol therapy for ethylene glycol intoxication in man. J Toxicol Clin Toxicol 1986;24:463.
223. Baud FJ, Galliot M, Astier A, et al. Treatment of ethylene glycol poisoning with intravenous 4-methylpyrazole. N Engl J Med 1988;319:97.
224. Harry P, Turcant A, Bouachour G, Houze P, Alquier P, Allain P. Efficacy of 4-methylpyrazole in ethylene glycol poisoning: clinical and toxicokinetic aspects. Human Exp Toxicol 1994;13:61.
225. Stokes JB, Amerson F. Prevention of organ damage in massive ethylene glycol ingestion. JAMA 1980;243:2065.
226. Cadnapaphornchai P, Taheo S, Bhathena D, et al. Ethylene glycol poisoning—Diagnosis based on high osmolal and anion gaps and crystalluria. Ann Emerg Med 1981;10:94.
227. Brown CG, Trumbull D, Klein SW, et al. Ethylene glycol poisoning. Ann Emerg Med 1983;12:501.
228. Eisen TF, Lacouture PG, Woolf AD. Serum osmolality in alcohol ingestions. Am J Emerg Med 1989;7:256.
229. Agarwal SK. Non acidotic acetonemia: a syndrome due to isopropyl alcohol intoxication. J Med Soc NJ 1979;76:914.
230. Terlinsky AS, Grochowski J, Gedy KL, et al. Identification of typical calcium oxalate crystalluria following ethylene glycol ingestion. Am J Clin Pathol 1981;76:223.
231. Godolphin W, Meagher EP, Sardes HD, et al. Unusual calcium oxalate crystals in ethylene glycol poisoning. Clin Toxicol 1980;16:479.
232. Jacobsen D, Akesson I, Shefter I. Urinary calcium oxolate monohydrate crystals in ethylene glycol poisoning. Scand J Clin Lab Invest 1982;42:231.
233. Vanderhoff BT, Mosser KH. Jimsonweed toxicity: management of anticholinergic plant ingestion. Am Fam Physician 1992;46:526–530.
234. Klein-Schwartz W, Oderda GM. Jimsonweed intoxication in adolescents and young adults. Am J Dis Child 1984;138:737–739.
235. Rinder CS, D'Amato SL, Rinder HM. Survival in complicated diphenydramine overdose. Crit Care Med 1988;16:1161–1162.
236. Hestand HE, Teske DW. Diphenhydramine hydrochloride intoxication. J Pediatr 1977;90:1017–1018.
237. Frankel D, Dolgin J, Murray BM. Non-traumatic rhabdomyolysis complicating antihistamine overdose. J Tox Clin Tox 1993;31:493–496.
238. Rodgers GC, Von Kanel RL. Conservative treatment of jimsonweed ingestion. Vet Hum Tox 1993;35:32–33.
239. Nattel S, Bayne L, Ruedy J. Physostigmine in coma due to drug overdose. Clin Pharmacol Ther 1979;25:96–102.
240. Thompson N, Lowe-Ponsford F, Mant TGK, Volans GN. Button battery ingestion: a review. Adv Drug React Acute Pois Rev 1990;9:157–182.
241. Edmonson MB. Caustic alkali ingestions by farm children. Pediatrics 1987;79:413–6.
242. Neidich G. Ingestion of caustic alkali farm products. J Pediatr Gastroent Nut 1993;16:75–77.
243. Lacouture PG, Gaudreault P, Lovejoy FH. Clinitest tablet ingestion: an *in vitro* investigation concerned with initial emergency managment. Ann Emerg Med 1986;15:143–6.
244. Ashcraft KW, Padula RT. The effect of dilute corrosives on the esophagus. Pediatrics 1974;53:226–32.
245. Rothstein FC. Caustic injuries to the esophagus in children. Pediatr Clin North Am 1986;33:665–74.
246. Einhorn A, Horton L, Altieri M, Ochsenschlager D, Klein B. Serious respiratory consequences of detergent ingestions in children. Pediatrics 1989;84:472–4.
247. Vergauwen P, Moulin D, Buts JP, Veyckemans F, Hamoir M, Hanique G. Caustic burns of the upper digestive and respiratory tracts. Eur J Pediatr 1991;150:700–3.
248. Moulin D, Bertrand J, Buts J, Nyakabasa M, Otte J. Upper airway lesions in children after accidental ingestion of caustic substances. J Pediatr 1985;106:408–10.
249. Friedman EM, Lovejoy FH. The emergency management of caustic ingestions. Emerg Clin North Am 1984;2:77–86.
250. Previtera C, Giusti F, Guglielmi M. Predictive value of visible lesions (cheeks, lips, oropharynx) in suspected caustic ingestion: may endoscopy reasonably be omitted in completely negative pediatric patients? Pediatr Emerg Care 1990;6:176–78.
251. Gorman RL, Khin-Maung-Gyi MT, Klein-Schwartz W, Oderda GM, Benson B, Litovitz T, et al. Initial symptoms as predictors of esophageal injury in alkaline corrosive ingestions. Am J Emerg Med 1992; 10:189–94.

252. Crain EF, Gershel JC, Mezey AP. Caustic ingestions—symptoms as predictors of esophageal injury. Am J Dis Child 1984;138:863–65.
253. Gaudreault P, Parent M, McGuigan MA, Chicoine L, Lovejoy FH. Predictability of esophageal injury from signs and symptoms: a study of caustic ingestion in 378 children. Pediatrics 1983;71:767–70.
254. Litovitz T, Butterfield AB, Holloway RR, Marion LI. Button battery ingestion: assessment of therapeutic modalities and battery discharge state. J Pediatr 1984;105:868–73.
255. Litovitz T. Battery ingestions: product accessibility and clinical course. Pediatrics 1985;75:469–76.
256. Penner GE. Acid ingestion: toxicology and treatment. Ann Emerg Med 1980;9:374–9.
257. Anderson KD, Rouse TM, Randolph JG. A controlled trial of corticosteroids in children with corrosive injury of the esophagus. New Engl J Med 1990;323:637–40.
258. Allen RE, Thoshinsky MJ, Stallone RJ, Hunt TK. Corrosive injuries of the stomach. Arch Surg 1970;100:409–13.
259. Cadranel S, DiLorenzo C., Rodesch P, Piepsz A, Ham HR. Caustic ingestion and esophageal function. J Pediatr Gastroent Nutr 1990;10:164–8.
260. National Institute of Drug Abuse. National Household Survey on Drug Abuse. Population estimates, 1991; revised November, 1992. DHHS publication 4# (ADM) 92–1887, 1992.
261. Shannon M, Lacouture PG, Roa J, Woolf A. Cocaine exposure among children seen at a pediatric hospital. Pediatrics 1989;83:337.
262. Kharasch SJ, Glotzer D, Vinci R, Weitzman M, Sargent J. Unsuspected cocaine exposure in young children. Am J Dis Child 1991;145:204.
263. Rosenberg NM, Meert KL, Knazik SR, Yee H, Kauffman RE. Occult cocaine exposure in children. Am J Dis Child 1991;145:1430.
264. Anonymous. "Crack." Med Lett 1986;28:69.
265. Caruana DS, Weinbach B, Goerg D, Gardner LB. Cocaine-packet ingestion—diagnosis, management, and natural history. Ann Intern Med 1984;100:73.
266. McCarron MM, Wood JD. The cocaine "body packer" syndrome. JAMA 1983;250:1417.
267. Roberts JR, Price D, Goldfrank L, et al. The bodystuffer syndrome: a clandestine form of drug overdose. Am J Emerg Med 1986;4:24.
268. Suarez CA, Arango A, Lester JL. Cocaine condom ingestion: surgical treatment. JAMA 1977;278:1391.
269. Chasnoff IJ, Lewis DE, Squires L. Cocaine intoxication in a breast-fed infant. Pediatrics 1987;80:836.
270. Negus BH, Willard JE, Hillis LD, Glamann DB, Landau C, Snyder RW, Lange RA. Alleviation of cocaine-induced coronary vasoconstriction with intravenous verapamil. Am J Cardiol 1994;73:510.
271. Estroff TW, Schwartz RH, Hoffman NG. Adolescent cocaine abuse-addictive potential, behavioral, and psychiatric effects. Clin Pediatr 1989;28:550.
272. Gay GR. Clinical management of acute and chronic cocaine poisoning. Ann Emerg Med 1982;11:562.
273. Lathers CM, Tyau LSY, Spino MM, Agarwal I. Cocaine-induced seizures, arrhythmias, and sudden death. J Clin Pharmacol 1988;28:584.
274. Marzuk PM, Tardiff K, Leon AC, et al. Fatal injuries after cocaine use as a leading cause of death among young adults in New York City. N Engl J Med 1995;332:1753.
275. Garland JS, Smith DS, Rice TB, Siker D. Accidental cocaine intoxication in a nine-month old infant: presentation and treatment. Pediatr Emerg Care 1989;5:245.
276. Mody CK, Miller BL, McIntyre HB, Cobb SK, Goldberg MA. Neurologic complications of cocaine abuse. Neurology 1988;38:1189.
277. Mott SH, Packer RJ, Soldin SJ. Neurologic manifestations of cocaine exposure in childhood. Pediatrics 1994;93:557.
278. Holland RW, Marx JA, Earnest MP, Ranniger S. Grand mal seizures temporally related to cocaine use: clinical and diagnostic features. Ann Emerg Med 1992;21:772.
279. Levine SR, Brust JCM, Futrell N, Ho KL, Blake D, Millikan CH, Brass LM, Fayad P, Schultz LR, Selws JF, Welch KMA. Cerebrovascular complications of the use of the "crack" form of alkaloidal cocaine. N Engl J Med 1990;323:699.
280. Feinman BN. Neurologic sequelae of cocaine. Hosp Pract 1989:97.
281. Chasnoff IJ, Bussey ME, Savich R, Stack C. Perinatal cerebral infarction and maternal cocaine use. J Pediatr 1986;108:456.
282. Volpe J. Effect of cocaine use on the fetus. N Engl J Med 1992;326:399.
283. Brody SL, Slovis CM, Wrenn KD. Cocaine-related medical problems: consecutive series of 233 patients. Am J Med 1990;88:325.
284. Isner JM, N Engl J Med 1986;315:1438.
285. Hollander JE, Todd KH, Green G, Heilpern KL, Karras DJ, Singer AJ, et al. Chest pain associated with cocaine: an assessment of prevalence in suburban and urban emergency departments. Ann Emerg Med 1995;26:671–676.
286. Roth D, Alarcon FJ, Fernandez JA, Preston RA, Bourgoignie JJ. Acute rhabdomyolysis associated with cocaine intoxication. N Engl J Med 1988;319:673.
287. Woolf AD, Shannon MW. Clinical toxicology for the pediatrician. Pediatr Clin North Am 1995;42:317.
288. Lewin NA, Goldfrank LR, Hoffman RS. Cocaine. In: Goldfrank LR, Flomenbaum NE, Lewis NA, Weisman RS, Howland MA, Hoffman RS, eds. Goldfrank's toxicologic emergencies. 5th ed. Norwalk, CT: Appleton & Lange, 1994.
289. Peng S, French WJ, Pelikan PCD. Direct cocaine cardiotoxicity demonstrated by endomyocardial biopsy. Arch Pathol Lab Med 1989; 113:842.
290. Karch SB, Billingham ME. The pathology and etiology of cocaine-induced heart disease. Arch Pathol Lab Med 1988;112:225.
291. Tazelaar HD, Karch SB, Stephens BG, Billingham ME. Cocaine and the heart. Hum Pathol 1987;18:195.
292. Lange RA, Cigarroa RG, Flores ED, McBride W, Kim AS, Weells PJ, Bedotto JB, Dansiger RS, Hollis LD. Potentiation of cocaine-induced coronary vasoconstriction by beta-adrenergic blockade. Ann Intern Med 1990;112:897.
293. Hollander JE, Hoffman RS, Gennis P, Fairweather P, DiSano MJ, Schumb DA, Feldman JA, Fish SS, Dyer S, Wax P, Whelan C, Schwarzwald E. Nitroglycerin in the treatment of cocaine associated chest pain—clinical safety and efficacy. Clin Toxicol 1994;32:243.
294. Derlet RW, Albertson TE. Diazepam in the prevention of seizures and death in cocaine-intoxicated rats. Ann Emerg Med 1994;23:494.
295. Hollander JE, Hoffman RS, Gennis P, Fairweather P, DiSano MJ, Schumb DA, Feldman JA, Fish SS, Dyer S, Whelan C, Schwarzwald E. Prospective multicenter evaluation of cocaine-associated chest pain. Acad Emerg Med 1994;1:330.
296. Kulig KW, Ballantyne B. Case Studies in Environmental Medicine: Cyanide Toxicity. Agency for Toxic Substances & Disease Registry (ATSDR). U.S. DHHS. November, 1991.
297. Baud FJ, Barriot P, Toffin V, et al. Elevated blood cyanide concentrations in victims of smoke inhalation. N Engl J Med 1991;325:1761.
298. Jellinek H, Takata K. Toxic gas evolution from polymers: evolution of hydrogen cyanide from polyurethanes. J Polymer Sci 1977;15.2269.
299. Symington IS. Cyanide exposure in fires. Lancet 1978;2:91.
300. Caravati EM, Litovitz TL. Pediatric cyanide intoxication and death from an acetonitrile-containing cosmetic. JAMA 1988;260:3470.
301. Rainey PM, Roberts WL. Diagnosis and misdiagnosis of poisoning with the cyanide precursor acetonitrile: nail polish remover or nail glue remover? Am J Emerg Med 1993;11:104.
302. Lasch E, ElShawa R. Multiple cases of cyanide poisoning by apricot hemels in children from Gaza. Pediatrics 1981;68:5.
303. Shragg TA, Albertson TE, Fisher CJ. Cyanide poisoning after bitter almond ingestion. West J Med 1982;136:65.
304. Holzbecher MD, Moss MA, Ellenberger HA. The cyanide content of laetrile preparations, apricot, peach and apple seeds. Clin Toxicol 1984;22:341.
305. Morse DL, Harrington J, Heath CW. Laetrile, apricot pits and cyanide poisoning. N Engl J Med 1976;295:1264.
306. Dorr RT, Paximos J. The current status of laetrile. Ann Intern Med 1978;89:389.
307. Braico KT, Humbert JR, Terplan KL, et al. Laetrile intoxication. Report of a fatal case. N Engl J Med 1979;300:238.
308. Beamer WC, Shealy RM, Prough DS. Acute cyanide poisoning from laetrile ingestion. Ann Emerg Med 1983;12:7.
309. Way JL. Cyanide intoxication and its mechanism of antagonism. Annu Rev Pharmacol Toxicol 1984;24:451.
310. Ortega JA, Creek JE. Acute cyanide poisoning following administration of laetrile enemas. J Pediatr 1978;93:1059.
311. Cohn JN, Burke LP. Nitroprusside. Ann Intern Med 1979;91:752.
312. Linakis JG, Lacouture PG, Woolf A. Monitoring cyanide and thiocyanate concentrations during infusion of sodium nitroprusside in children. Pediatr Cardiol 1991;12:214.
313. Tinker JH, Michenfelder JD. Sodium nitroprusside: pharmacology, toxicology and therapeutics. Anesthesiology 1976;43:340.
314. Atkins D, West D, Smith F, et al. Cyanide toxicity following nitroprusside induced hypotension. Can Anaesth Soc J 1977;24:651.
315. Davies DW, Kadar D, Steward DJ, et al. A sudden death associated

with the use of sodium nitroprusside for induction of hypotension during anesthesia. Can Anaesth Soc J 1975;22:547.
316. Cottrell JE, Casthely P, Bordie JD, et al. Prevention of nitroprusside induced cyanide toxicity with hydroxycobalamin. N Engl J Med 1978;298:809.
317. Krapez JR, Vesey CJ, Adams L, et al. Effects of cyanide antidotes used with sodium nitroprusside infusions. Sodium thiosulfate and hydroxycobalamin given prophylactically to dogs. Br J Anaesth 1981;53:793.
318. Vesey CJ, Cole PV, Simpson PJ. Cyanide and thiocyanate concentrations following sodium nitroprusside infusions in man. Br J Anaesth 1976;48:651.
319. Smith RK. Nitroprusside produces cyanide poisoning via a reaction with hemoglobin. J Pharmacol Exp Ther 1974;191:557.
320. Ram Z, Spiegelman R, Findler G, et al. Delayed postoperative neurological deterioration from prolonged sodium nitroprusside administration. Case report. J Neurosurg 1989;71:605.
321. Centers for Disease Control, Mortality & Morbidity Weekly Report (MMWR). Cyanide poisonings associated with over the counter medication. Washington, 1991;40:161.
322. Gonzales J, Sabatini S. Cyanide poisoning: pathophysiology and current approaches to therapy. Int J Artif Organs 1989;12:347.
323. MacMillan VH. Cerebral energy metabolism in cyanide encephalopathy. J Cereb Blood Flow Metab 1989;9:156.
324. Robin ED. Dysoxia. Abnormal tissue oxygen utilization. Arch Intern Med 1977;137:905.
325. Westley J, Adler A, Westley L, et al. The sulfur transferase. Fund Appl Toxicol 1983;3:377.
326. Chen KK, Rose CL, Clowes G. Methylene blue, nitrites, and sodium thiosulfate against cyanide poisoning. Proc Soc Exp Biol Med 1933; 31:250.
327. Kiese M, Weger NS. Formation of ferric haemoglobin with aminophenols in the human for the treatment of cyanide poisoning. Eur J Pharmacol 1969;7:97.
328. Kruszyna R, Kruszyna H, Smith R. Comparison of hydroxylamine, 4-dimethyl aminophenol and nitrite protection agonist cyanide poisoning in mice. Arch Toxicol 1982;49:191.
329. Holmes RK, Way JL. Mechanism of cyanide antagonism by sodium nitrate. Pharmacologist 1982;24:182.
330. Way JL. Cyanide antagonism. Fund Appl Toxicol 1983;3:383.
331. Mushett CW, Kelley KL, Bosier GE, et al. Antidotal efficacy of vitamin B_{12} (hydroxycobalamin) in experimental cyanide poisoning. Proc Soc Exp Biol Med 1952;81:234.
332. Marrs TC, Swanston DW, Bright JE. 4-Dimethylaminophenol and dicobalt edetate (Kelocyanor) in the treatment of experimental cyanide poisoning. Hum Toxicol 1985;4:591.
333. Nagler J, Provoust RA, Parizel G. Hydrogen cyanide poisoning treatment with cobalt EDTA. J Occup Med 1978;20:414.
334. Schwartz C, Morgan RL, Way L, et al. Antagonism of cyanide intoxication with sodium pyruvate. Toxicol Appl Pharmacol 1979;50:437.
335. Vogel SN, Sultan TR, Teneyck RP. Cyanide poisoning. Clin Toxicol 1981;18:367.
336. Johnson RP, Mellors JW. Arteriolization of venous blood gases: a clue to the diagnosis of cyanide poisoning. J Emerg Med 1988;6:401.
337. Graham DL, Laman D, Theodore J, et al. Acute cyanide poisoning complicated by lactic acidosis and pulmonary edema. Arch Intern Med 1959;137:1051.
338. Cope C. The importance of oxygen in the treatment of cyanide poisoning. JAMA 1961;175:1061.
339. Burrows GE, Way JL. Cyanide intoxication in sheep. Therapeutic value of oxygen or cobalt. Am J Vet Res 1977;38:223.
340. Litovitz TL, Larkin RF, Myers RA. Cyanide poisoning treated with hyperbaric oxygen. Am J Emerg Med 1983;1:94.
341. Scolnick B, Hamel D, Woolf AD. Successful treatment of life-threatening propionitrile exposure with sodium nitrite/sodium thiosulfate followed by hyperbaric oxygen. J Occup Med 1993;35:577.
342. Ivanov KP. The effect of elevated oxygen pressure of animals poisoned with potassium cyanide. Pharmacol Toxicol 1959;22:476.
343. Berlin CM. The treatment of cyanide poisoning in children. Pediatrics 1970;46:793.
344. Hall AH, Doutre WH, Ludden T, et al. Nitrite/thiosulfate treated acute cyanide poisoning: estimated kinetics after antidote. J Toxicol Clin Toxicol 1987;25:121.
345. Vick JA, Froehlich H. Treatment of cyanide poisoning. Military Med 1991;156:330.
346. Weger NP. Treatment of cyanide poisoning with 4-dimethylaminophenol (DMAP)—experimental and clinical overview. Middle East J Anesthesiol 1990;10:389.
347. Hall AH, Rumack BH. Hydroxycobalamin/sodium thiosulfate as a cyanide antidote. J Emerg Med 1987;5:115.
348. Dalvi RR, Sawant SG, Terse PS. Efficacy of α-ketoglutaric acid as an effective antidote in cyanide poisoning in dogs. Vet Res Commun 1990;14:411.
349. Yamamoto H. Protection against cyanide-induced convulsions with alpha-ketoglutarate. Toxicol 1990;61:221.
350. Norris JC, Utley WA, Hume AS. Mechanism of antagonizing cyanide-induced lethality by alpha-ketoglutaric acid. Toxicol 1990;62:275.
351. Litovitz TL, Clark LR, Soloway RA. 1993 Annual Report of the American Association of Poison Control Centers Toxic Exposure Surveillance System. Am J Emerg Med 1994;12:546–584.
352. Banner W, Wilson PD. Systemic toxicity following gasoline aspiration. Am J Emerg Med 1983;3:292–294.
353. Litovitz T. Hydrocarbon ingestions. Ear, Nose, & Throat Journal 1983;62:45–55.
354. Griffin JW, Daeschner CS, Collins VP, et al. Hydrocarbon pneumonitis following furniture polish ingestion. J Pediatr 1954;45:13–26.
355. King GS, Smialek JE, Troutman WG. Sudden death in adolescents resulting from the inhalation of typewriter correcting fluid. JAMA 1985;253:1604–1606.
356. Gerace RV. Near fatal intoxication by 1,1,1 trichloroethane. Ann Emerg Med 1981;10:533–534.
357. Bass M. Sudden sniffing death. JAMA 1970;212:2075–2079.
358. Reinhardt CF, Azar A, Maxfield ME, et al. Cardiac arrhythmias and aerosol "sniffing." Arch Environ Health 1971;22:265–279.
359. Taylor GJ, Harris WS. Cardiac toxicity of aerosol propellants. JAMA 1970;214:81–85.
360. Beamon RF, Siegel CJ, Landers G, et al. Hydrocarbon ingestion in children: a six-year retrospective study. JACEP 1976;5:771–775.
361. Jacobziner H, Raybin HW. Turpentine poisoning. Arch Pediatr 1961;78:357–364.
362. Victoria MS, Nangia BS. Hydrocarbon poisoning: a review. Ped Emerg Care 1987;3:184–186.
363. Marandian MH, Youssefian H, Saboury M, et al. Intoxication accidentelle par ingestion de petrole chez l'enfant: etude clinique, radiologique, biologique et anatomopathologique, a propos de 3462 cas. Ann Pediat 1981;28:601–609.
364. Giammaona ST. Effects of furniture polish on pulmonary surfactant. Am J Dis Child 1963;113:658–663.
365. Eade NR, Taussig LM, Marks MI. Hydrocarbon pneumonitis. Pediatr 1974;54:351–357.
366. Beerman B, Christensson T, Moller P, et al. Lipoid pneumonia: an occupational hazard of fire-eaters. Br J Med 1984;289:1728–1729.
367. Goldfrank LR. Hydrocarbons. In: Goldfrank LR, Flomenbaum NE, Lewin NA, et al., eds. Goldfrank's toxicologic emergencies. 5th ed. Norwalk, CT: Appleton & Lange, 1994:1231–1244.
368. James FW, Kaplan S, Benzing G III. Cardiac complications following hydrocarbon ingestion. Am J Dis Child 1971;121:431–433.
369. Nierenberg DW, Horowitz MG, Harris KM, James DG. Mineral spirits inhalation associated with hemolysis, pulmonary edema and ventricular fibrillation. Arch Intern Med 1991;151:1437–1440.
370. Rinsky RA, Smith AB, Horning R. Benzene and leukemia: an epidemiologic risk assessment. N Engl J Med 1987;316:1044–1050.
371. Taher SM, Anderson RJ, McCarthy R, et al. Renal tubular acidosis associated with toluene sniffing. N Engl J Med 1974;290:765–768.
372. Hormes JT, Filley CM, Rosenberg NL. Neurologic sequelae of chronic solvent vapor abuse. Neurology 1986;36:698–702.
373. Klein FA, Hackler RH. Hemorrhagic cystitis associated with turpentine ingestion. Urology 1980;16:187.
374. Brook MP, McCarron MM, Mueller JA. Pine oil cleaner ingestion. Ann Emerg Med 1989;18:391–395.
375. Hill RM, Barer J, Hill LL, et al. An investigation of recurrent pine oil poisoning in an infant by the use of gas chromatographic-mass spectrometric methods. J Ped 1975;87:115–118.
376. Erickson T, Popiel R, Hryhorczuk DO, Raba JM. Pine oil cleaners in prison (letter). Ann Emerg Med 1990;19:445.
377. Tobin, T Swerczek TW, Blake JW. Pine oil toxicity in the horse: drug detection, residues and pathological changes. Res Com Chem Path Pharm 1976;15:291–301.
378. Algren JT, Rodgers GC. Intravascular hemolysis associated with hydrocarbon poisoning. Ped Emerg Care 1992;8:34–35.

379. Daeschner CW, Blattner RJ, Collins VP. Hydrocarbon pneumonitis. Pediatr Clin North Am 1957;4:243–253.
380. Wolfsdorf J. Kerosene intoxication: an experimental approach to the etiology of the CNS manifestations in primates. J Pediatr 1976;88:1037–1040.
381. Bratton L, Haddow JE. Ingestion of charcoal lighter fluid. J Pediatr 1975;87:633–636.
382. Wolfe BN, Brodeur AE, Shields JB. The role of gastrointestinal absorption of kerosene in producing pneumonitis in dogs. J Pediatr 1970;76:867–873.
383. Dice WH, Ward G, Kelley J, et al. Pulmonary toxicity following gastrointestinal ingestion of kerosene. Ann Emerg Med 1982;11:138–142.
384. Wason S, Greiner PT. Intravenous hydrocarbon abuse. Am J Emerg Med 1986;4:543–544.
385. Neeld EM, Limacher MC. Chemical pneumonitis after the intravenous injection of hydrocarbon. Radiology 1978;129:36.
386. Ng RC, Darwish H, Stewart DA. Emergency treatment of petroleum distillate and turpentine ingestion. Can Med Assoc J 1974;111:537–538.
387. Steele RW, Conklin RH, Mark HM. Corticosteroids and antibiotics for the treatment of fulminant hydrocarbon aspiration. JAMA 1972;219:1434–1437.
388. Marks MI, Chicoine L, Legere G et al. Adrenocorticosteroid treatment of hydrocarbon pneumonia in children—a cooperative study. J Pediatr 1972;81:366–369.
389. Zucker AR, Berger S, Wood LDH. Management of kerosene-induced pulmonary injury. Crit Care Med 1986;14:303–304.
390. Scalzo AJ, Weber TR, Jaeger RW, et al. Extracorporeal membrane oxygenation for hydrocarbon aspiration. Am J Dis Child 1990;144:867–871.
391. Weber TR, Tracy TF, Connors R, et al. Prolonged extracorporeal support for nonneonatal respiratory failure. J Ped Surg 1992;27:1100–1104.
392. Bysani GK, Rucoba RJ, Noah ZL. Treatment of hydrocarbon pneumonitis. High frequency jet ventilation as an alternative to extracorporeal membrane oxygenation. Chest 1994;106:300–303.
393. Stewart RD, Fisher TN, Hosko MJ, et al. Experimental human exposure to methylene chloride. Arch Environ Health 1972;25:342–348.
394. Truss CS, Killenberg PG. Treatment of carbon tetrachloride poisoning with hhyperbaric oxygen. Gastroenterology 1982;82:767–769.
395. Anas N, Namasonthi V, Ginsburg CM. Criteria for hospitalizing children who have ingested products containing hydrocarbons. JAMA 1981;246:840–843.
396. Ellenhorn MJ, Barceloux DG, eds. Hydrocarbon products. In: Medical toxicology; diagnosis and treatment of human poisoning. New York: Elsevier, 1988:940–947.
397. Henretig FM, Temple AR. Acute iron poisoning in children. Emerg Med Clin North Am 1984;2:121.
398. Covey TJ. Ferrous sulfate poisoning—a review, case summarizes and therapeutic regimine. J Pediatr 1964;64:218.
399. Greengard J. Iron poisoning in children. Clin Toxicol 1975;8:575.
400. Robotham JL, Lietman PS. Acute iron poisoning—a review. Am J Dis Child 1980;134:875.
401. Jacobs J, Greene H, Gendel BR. Acute iron intoxication. N Engl J Med 1965;273:1124.
402. Stein M, Blayney D, Feit T, et al. Acute iron poisoning in children—University of California, San Diego and University Hospital San Diego (specialty conference). West J Med 1976;125:289.
403. Gezernik W, Schmaman A, Chappell JS. Corrosive gastritis as a result of ferrous sulfate ingestion. S Afr Med J 1980;57:151.
404. Roberts RJ, Nayfield S, Soper R, et al. Acute iron intoxication with intestinal infarction managed in part by small bowel resection. Clin Toxicol 1975;8:3.
405. Knott LN, Miller RC. Acute iron intoxication with intestinal infarction. J Pediatr Surg 1978;13:720.
406. Whitten CF, Brough AJ. The pathophysiology of acute iron poisoning. Clin Toxicol 1971;4:585.
407. Robotham JL, Troxler RF, Lietman PS. Iron poisoning: another energy crisis. Lancet 1974;2.664.
408. Ganote CE, Nahara G. Acute ferrous sulfate hepatotoxicity—rats: an electron microscopic and biochemical study. Lab Invest 1973;28:426.
409. Witzleben CL. An electron microscopic study of ferrous sulfate-induced liver damage. Am J Pathol 1966;49:1053.
410. Evensen SA, Forde R, Opedal I, et al. Acute iron intoxication with abruptly reduced levels of vitamin K-dependent coagulation factors. Scand J Haematol 1982;29:25.
411. Hendriksson P, Nilsson L, Nilsson IM, et al. Fatal iron intoxication with multiple coagulation defects and degradation of factor VIII and factor XIII. Scand J Haematol 1979;22:235.
412. Rosenmund A, Haeberli A, Straub PW. Blood coagulation and acute iron toxicity: reversible iron-induced inactivation of serine proteases in vitro. J Lab Clin Med 1984;103:524.
413. DeCatro FJ, Jaeger R, Gleason WA. Liver damage and hypoglycemia in acute iron poisoning. Clin Toxicol 1977;10:287.
414. Reynolds LG, Klein M. Iron poisoning—a preventable hazard of childhood. S Afr Med J 1985;67:680.
415. Fischer DS, Parkman R, Finch SC. Acute iron poisoning in children. The problems of appropriate therapy. JAMA 1971;218:1179.
416. Temple AR. Correlation of toxicologic manifestations of iron poisoning and serum iron levels. Their value as a prediction of severity (abstr). Vet Hum Toxicol 1979;21:136.
417. Bentur Y, St LP, Klein J, et al. Misinterpretation of iron-binding capacity in the presence of deferoxamine. J Pediatr 1991;118:139.
418. Burkhart KK, Kulig KW, Hammond KB, et al. The rise in the total iron-binding capacity after iron overdose. Ann Emerg Med 1991;20:532.
419. Tenenbein M, Yatscoff RW. The total iron-binding capacity in iron poisoning. Is it useful? Am J Dis Child 1991;145:437.
420. Bosse GM. Conservative management of patients with moderately elevated serum iron levels. Clin Toxicol 1995;33:135.
421. Lacouture PG, Wason S, Temple AR, et al. Emergency assessment of severity in iron overdose by clinical and laboratory methods. J Pediatr 1981;99:89.
422. Bachrach L, Correa A, Levin R, et al. Iron poisonings: complications of hypertonic phosphate lavage therapy. J Pediatr 1979;94:147.
423. Geffner MF, Opas LU. Phosphate poisoning complicating treatment of iron ingestion. Am J Dis Child 1980;134:509.
424. Peterson CD, Fifield CG. Emergency gastrotomy for acute iron poisoning. Ann Emerg Med 1980;9:262.
425. Henretig FM, Karl SR, Weintraub WH. Severe iron poisoning treated with enteral and intravenous desferoxamine. Ann Emerg Med 1983;12:306.
426. McEnery JT, Greengard J. Treatment of acute iron ingestion with desferoxamine in 20 children. J Pediatr 1966;68:773.
427. Koren G, Bentur Y, Strong D, et al. Acute changes in renal function associated with deferoxamine therapy. Am J Dis Child 1989;143:1077.
428. Milteer RM, Sarpong S, Poydras U. *Yersinia enterocolitica* septicemia after accidental oral iron overdose. Pediatr Infect Dis J 1989;8:537.
429. Banner W, Vernon D. Continuous arterio-venous hemofiltration in experimental iron intoxication. Crit Care Med 1989.
430. Jaffe JH, Martin WR. Opioid analgesics and antagonists. In: Goodman Gilman A, Rall TW, Nies AS, et al., eds. Goodman and Gilman's the pharmacologic basis of therapeutics. New York: McGraw-Hill, Inc., 485–521.
431. McCarron MG, Challoner KR, Thompson GA. Diphenoxylate-atropine (Lomotil) overdose in children: an update (report of eight cases and review of the literature). Pediatr 1991;87:694–700.
432. Gary N, Maher JF, De Myttenaere MH, et al. Acute propoxyphene hydrochloride intoxication. Arch Intern Med 1968;121:453–457.
433. Holland DR, Steinberg MI. Electrophysiologic properties of propoxyphene and norpropoxyphene in canine conductive tissue in vitro and in vivo. Toxicol Appl Pharmacol 1979;47:123–133.
434. Goldfrank LR, Weisman RS. Opioids. In: Goldfrank LR, Flomenbaum NE, Lewin NA, et al., eds. Goldfrank's toxicologic emergencies. Norwalk, CT: Appleton & Lange, 769–783.
435. Szeto HH, Inturrisi CE, Howde R, et al. Accumulation of normeperidine, an active metabolite of meperidine, in patients with renal failure or cancer. Ann Intern Med 1977;86:738–740.
436. Blain PG, Lane R, Rawlins MD. Opiate induced rhabdomyolysis. Hum Toxicol 1985;4:71.
437. Hibbs J, Perper J, Winek CL. An outbreak of designer drug related deaths in Pennsylvania. JAMA 1991;265:1011–1013.
438. Bonfiglio MF, Mauro VF. Naloxone in the treatment of meperidine induced seizures. Drug Intell Clin Pharm 1987;21:174–175.
439. Jefferys DB, Volans GN. An investigation of the role of the specific opioid antagonist naloxone in clinical toxicology. Hum Toxicol 1983;2:227–231.
440. Kulig K, Duffy J, Rumack BH, et al. Naloxone for treatment of clonidine overdose. JAMA 1982;247:1697.
441. Alberto G, Erickson T, Popiel R, et al. Central nervous system manifestations of a valproic acid overdose responsive to naloxone. Ann Emerg Med 1989;18:889–891.

442. Bell EF. The use of naloxone in the treatment of diazepam poisoning. Pediatrics 1975;87:803–804.
443. American Academy of Pediatrics Committee on Drugs. Naloxone dosage and route of administration for infants and children: addendum to emergency drug doses for infants and children. Pediatrics 1990; 86:484–485.
444. Kunkel DB. Narcotic antagonist update. Emerg Med 1987;19:97–108.
445. Gourlay GK, Coulthard K. The role of naloxone infusions in the treatment of overdoses of long half-life narcotic agonists: application to normethadone. Br J Clin Pharmacol 1983;15:269.
446. Lewis JM, Klein SW, Benson BF, et al. Continuous naloxone infusion in pediatric narcotic overdose. Am J Dis Child 1984;138:944.
447. Goldfrank LR, Weisman RS, Errick JK, et al. A Dosing nomogram for intinuous intravenous infusion naloxone. Ann Emerg Med 1986; 15:566–570.
448. Azar I, Turndorf H. Severe hypertension and multiple atrial premature contractions following naloxone administration. Anesth Analg 1979;58:524–525.
449. Flacke JW, Flacke WE, Williams GD. Acute pulmonary edema following naloxone reversal of high-dose morphine anesthesia. Anesthesiology 1977;47:376–378.
450. Michaelis LL, Hickey PR, Clark TA, et al. Ventricular irritability associated with the use of naloxone. Ann Thorac Surg 1974;18:608–614.
451. Karim A, Ranney RE, Evensen KL, et al. Pharmacokinetics and metabolism of diphenoxylate in man. Clin Pharmacol Ther 1972;13: 407–419.
452. Karkkainen S, Neuvonen P. Effect of oral charcoal and urine pH on dextropropopxyphene pharmacokinetics. Int J Clin Pharmacol Ther Toxicol 1985;23:219–225.
453. Curtis J, Goel K. Lomotil poisoning in children. Arch Dis Child 1979;54:222–225.
454. Mortensen ML. Managment of acute childhood poisinings caused by selected insecticides and herbicides. Pediatr Clin North Am 1986;33:421.
455. Zwiener RJ, Ginsburg CM. Organophosphate and carbamate poisoning in infants and children. Pediatrics 1988;81:121–126.
456. Davies JE, Barquet AB, Freed VH, et al. Human pesticide poisonings by a fat soluble organophosphate insecticide. Arch Environ Health 1975;30:608.
457. Namba T, Nolte CT, Jackrel J, Grob D. Poisoning due to organophosphate insecticides. Am Med J 1971;50:475–492.
458. Rieger H, Okonek S. The EEG in alkylphosphate poisoning. Electroencephalogr Clin Neurophysiol 1975;39:555.
459. Kass R, Kochar G, Lippman M. Adult respiratory distress syndrome from organophosphate poisoning. Am J Emerg Med 1991;9:32.
460. Kiss Z, Fazekas T. Arrhythmias in organophosphate poisoning. Acta Cardiol 1979;34:323–330.
461. Namba T, Greenfield M, Grob D. Malathion poisoning: a fatal case with cardiac manifestations. Arch Environ Health 1970;21:533.
462. Ludomirsky A, Klein HO, Sarell P, et al. QT prolongation and insecticide poisoning. Am J Cardiol 1982;49:1654.
463. Brill DM, Maisel AS, Prabhu R. Polymorphic ventricular tachycardia and other complex arrhythmias in organophosphate insecticide poisoning. J Electrocardiol 1984;17:97.
464. Rosenstock L, Keifer M, Daniell WE, McConnell, Claypoole K, et al. Chronic central nervous system effects of acute organophosphate pesticide intoxication. Lancet 1991;338:223–227.
465. Aiuto LA, Pavlakis SG, Boxer RA. Life-threatening organophosphate-induced delayed polyneuropathy in a child after accidental chlorpyrifos ingestion. J Pediatr 1993;122:658–660.
466. Senanayake N, Karalliedde L. Neurotoxic effects of organophosphorus insecticdes: an intermediate syndrome. N Engl J Med 1987;316: 761–763.
467. Sofer S, Tal, A, Shahak E. Carbamate and organophosphate poisoning in early childhood. Ped Emerg Care 1989;5:222–225.
468. Dickoff DJ, Gerber O, Turobsky Z. Delayed neurotoxicity after ingestion of carbamate pesticide. Neurology 1987;37:1229.
469. Coye MJ, Barnett PG, Midtling JE, Velasco AR, Romero P, Clements CL, et al. Clinical confirmation of organophosphate poisoning by serial cholinesterase analyses. Arch Intern Med 1987;147:438–442.
470. Midtling JE, Barnett PG, Coye MJ, et al. Clinical management of field worker organophosphate. West J Med 1985;142:514–518.
471. Meller D, Fraser I, Kryger M. Hyperglycemia in anticholinesterase poisoning. Can Med Assoc J 1981;124:745.
472. Zadik Z, Blachar Y, Barak Y, et al. Organophosphate poisoning presenting as diabetic ketoacidosis. J Toxicol Clin Toxicol 1983;20:381.
473. Selden BS, Curry SC. Prolonged succinycholine-induced paralysis in organophosphate insecticide poisoning. Ann Emerg Med 1987;16: 215–217.
474. Bardin PG, Van ESF. Organophosphate poisoning: grading the severeity and comparing treatment between atropine and glycopyrrolate. Crit Care Med 1990:18:956.
475. Kanto J, Klotz U. Pharmacokinetic implications for the clinical use of atropine, scopolamine and glycopyrrolate. Acta Anaesthesiol Scand 1988;32:69.
476. LeBlanc FN, Benson BE, Gilg AD. A severe organophosphate poisoning requiring the use of an atropine drip. J Toxicol Clin Toxicol 1986;24:69.
477. Sidell FR, Borak J. Chemical warfare agents: II. Nerve agents. Ann Emerg Med 1992;21:865–871.
478. diKart WL, Kiestra SH, Sangster B. The use of atropine and oximes in organophosphate intoxication: a modified approach. J Toxicol Clin Toxicol 1988;26:199–208.
479. Bodor N, Shek E. Higuchi T. Delivery of a quaternary pyridinium salt across the blood-braine barrier by its dihydropyridine derivative. Science 1975;190:155.
480. Rumps S, Faff J, Borkowska G, et al. Central therapeutic effects of dihydro derivative of pralidoxime (Pro 2-pam) in organophosphate intoxication. Arch Int Pharmacodyn Ther 1978;232:321.
481. Farrar Hc, Wells TG, Kearns GL. Use of continuous infusion of pralidoxime for treatment of organophosphate poisoning in children. J Pediatr 1990;116:658.
482. Thompson DF. Pralidoxime chloride continuous infusions (letter). Ann Emerg Med 1987;16:831.
483. Merrill DG, Mihm FG. Prolonged toxicity of organophosphate poisoning. Crit Care Med 1982;20:550.
484. Natoff IL, Reiff B. Effect of oximes on the toxicity of anticholine esterase carbamates. Toxicol Appl Pharmacol 1973;25:569–575.
485. Harris LW, Talbot BG, Lennox WJ, et al. The relationship between oxime induced reactivation of carbamylated acetylcholinesterase and antidotal efficacy against carbamate intoxication. Toxicol Appl Pharmacol 1989;98:128–133.
486. Lifshitz M, Rotenberg M, Sofer S, Tamiri T, Shahak E, Almog S. Carbamate poisoning and oxime treatment in children: a clinical and laboratory study. Pediatrics 1994;93:652–655.
487. Milhorn HT. Diagnosis and management of phencyclidine intoxication. AFP 1991;43:1293.
488. Tong TG, Benowitz NL, Becker CE, et al. Phencyclidine poisoning. JAMA 1975;234:512.
489. Schwartz RH, Hoffmann NG, Smith D, et al. Use of phencyclidine among adolescents attending a suburban drug treatment facility. J Pediatr 1987;110:322.
490. Schwartz RH, Einhorn A. PCP intoxication in seven young children. Pediatr Emerg Care 1986;2:238.
491. Karp HN, Kaufman ND, Anand SK. Phencyclidine poisoning in young children. J Pediatr 1980;97:1006.
492. Welch MJ, Correa GA. PCP intoxication in young children and infants. Clin Pediatr 1980;19:510.
493. Cook CE, Brine DR, Jeffcoat AR, et al. Phencyclidine disposition after intravenous and oral doses. Clin Pharmacol Ther 1982;31:625.
494. Giles HG, Corrigall WA, Khouw V, et al. Plasma protein binding of phencyclidine. Clin Pharmacol Ther 1982;31:77.
495. Cook CE, Brine DR, Quin GD, et al. Phencyclidine and phenylcyclohexene disposition after smoking phencyclidine. Clin Pharmacol Ther 1982;31:635.
496. Lillrank SM, O'Connor WT, Saransaari P, et al. In vivo effects of local and systemic phencyclidine on the extracellular levels of catecholamines and transmitter amino acids in the dorsolateral striatum of anaesthetized rats. Acta Physiol Scand 1994;150:109.
497. Maayani S, Weinstein H, Ben-Zvi N, et al. Psychotomimetics as anticholinergic agents I. Biochem Pharmacol 1974;23:1263.
498. French ED. Phencyclidine and the midbrain dopamine system: electrophysiology and behavior. Neurotoxicol Teratol 1994;16:355.
499. MacDonald JF, Bartlett MC, Mody I, et al. The PCP site of the NMDA receptor complex. Adv Exp Med Biol 1990;268:27.
500. Sircar R, Li CS. PCP/NMDA receptor-channel complex and brain development. Neurotoxicol Teratol 1994;16:369.
501. Paul IA. Angel dust and other antagonists. New Biol 1990;2:139.
502. Showalter CV, Thornton WE. Clinical pharmacology of phencyclidine toxicity. Am J Psychiatr 1977;134:1234.
503. Barton CN, Sterling ML, Vaziri ND, et al. Phencyclidine intoxication;

clinical experience in 27 cases confirmed by urine assay. Ann Emerg Med 1981;10:243.
504. Rappolf RT, Gay GR, Farris RD. Phencyclidine (PCP) intoxication: diagnosis in stage and algorithms of treatment. Clin Toxicol 1980;16:509.
505. McCarron MM, Schultze BW, Thompson GA, et al. Acute phencyclidine intoxication: incidence of clinical findings in 1,000 cases. Ann Emerg Med 1981;10:237.
506. McCarron MM, Schulze BW, Thompson GA, et al. Acute phencyclidine intoxication: clinical patterns, complications and treatment. Ann Emerg Med 1981;10:290.
507. Patel R, Connor G. A review of thrity cases of rhabdomyolysis-associated acute renal failure among PCP users. J Toxicol Clin Toxicol 1986;23:547.
508. Akmal M, Valdin JR, McCarron MM, et al. Rhabdomyolysis with and without acute renal failure in patients with phencyclidine intoxication. Am J Nephrol 1981;1:91.
509. Patch R, Das M, Palazzolo M, et al. Myoglobinuric acute renal failure in phencyclidine overdose: report of observations in eight cases. Ann Emerg Med 1980;9:549.
510. Armen R, Kanel G, Reynolds T. Phencyclidine-induced malignant hyperthermia causing submassive liver necrosis. Am J Med 1984;77:167.
511. Meyer JS, Griefenstein F, DeVault M. A new drug causing symptoms of sensory deprivation: neurological, electroencephalographic and pharmacological effects of Sernyl. J Nerv Ment Dis 1959;129:54.
512. Stockard J. Electroencephalographic findings in phencyclidine intoxication. Arch Neurol 1976;33:200.
513. Grove VE. Painless self-injury after ingestion of "angel dust." JAMA 1979;242:655.
514. Liden CB, Lovejoy FH, Costello CE. Phencyclidine (Sernylan) poisoning. J Pediatr 1973;88:844.
515. Liden CB, Lovejoy FH, Costello CE. Phencyclidine—nine cases of poisoning. JAMA 1975;234:513.
516. Kessler GF, Demers LM, Berlin C, et al. Phencyclidine and fatal status epilepticus. N Engl J Med 1974;291:979.
517. Bessen HA. Intracranial hemorrhage associated with phencyclidine abuse. JAMA 1982;248:585.
518. Eastman JW, Cohen SN. Hypertensive crisis and death associated with phencyclidine poisoning. JAMA 1975;231:1270.
519. Young JD, Crapo LM. Protracted phencyclidine coma from an intestinal deposit. Arch Intern Med 1992;152:859.
520. Simpson GM, Khajawall AM, Alatorre E, et al. Urinary phencyclidine excretion in chronic abusers. J Toxicol Clin Toxicol 1982;19:1051.
521. McCann DJ, Smith CM, Winter JC. A caution against use of verapamil in phencyclidine intoxication (letter). Am J Psychiatry 1986;143:679.
522. Price WA, Giannini AJ, Krishen A. Management of acute PCP intoxication with verapamil. J Toxicol Clin Toxicol 1986;24:85.
523. Aronow R, Done AK. Phencyclidine overdose. An emerging concept of management. J Am Coll Emerg Physician 1978;7:56.
524. McClurkan MB, Valentine JL, Arnold L, et al. Disposition of a monoclonal anti-phencyclidine Fab fragment of immunoglobulin G in rats. J Pharmacol Exp Ther 1993;266:1439.
525. Owens SM, Mayersohn M. Phencyclidine-specific Fab fragments alter phencyclidine disposition in dogs. Drug Met Disp 1986;14:52.
526. Casalotti SO, Kozikowski AP, Fauq A, et al. Monoclonal antibodies against a phencyclidine derivative are used to investigate protein-ligand interactions. Eur J Pharmacol 1993;247:209.
527. Dove A. Aspirin overdosage: incidence, diagnosis and management. Pediatrics 1978;62.
528. Gaudreault P, Temple AR, Lovejoy FN. The relative severity of acute versus chronic salicylate poisoning in children: a clinical comparison. Pediatr 1982;70:566.
529. McIntyre MS, Angle CR. Aspirin fatalities—the new taxonomy. Pediatr 1982;69:249.
530. Davies MG, Vella BD, Greaves MW. Systemic toxicity from topically applied salicylic acid. Br J Med 1979;1:661.
531. Liebelt EL, Shannon MW. Small doses, big problems: a selected review of highly toxic common medications. Ped Emerg Care 1993;9:292.
532. Wortzman DG, Grunfeld A. Delayed absorption following enteric coated aspirin overdose. Ann Emerg Med 1987;16:434.
533. Harris FC. Pyloric stenosis: holdup of enteric-coated aspirin tablets. Br J Surg 1973;60:979.
534. Bogazc K, Caldron P. Enteric coated aspirin bezoar: elevation of serum salicylate level by barium study. Am J Med 1981;83:783.
535. Levy G. Clinical pharmacokinetics of salicylates: a reassessment. Br J Clin Pharmacol 1980;10:285S.
536. Levy G. Clinical pharmacokinetics of aspirin and acetaminophen. Pediatr 1978;62:867.
537. Temple AR. Pathophysiology of aspirin toxicity with implications for management. Pediatr 1978;141:364.
538. Temple AR. Acute and chronic effects of aspirin toxicity and the treatment. Arch Intern Med 1981;141:364.
539. Snodgrass W, Rumack BH, Peterson RG, et al. Salicylate toxicity following therapeutic doses in young children. Clin Toxicol 1981;18:247.
540. Winters RW, White JS, Hughes MC, et al. Disturbances of acid-base equilibrium in salicylate intoxication. Pediatr 1959;23:260.
541. Gabow PA, Anderson RJ, Potts DE, et al. Acid-base disturbances in the salicylate-intoxicated adult. Arch Intern Med 1978;138:1481.
542. Schwartz R, Landy G. Organic acid excretion in salicylate intoxication. J Pediatr 1965;66:638.
543. Temple AR, George DJ, Done AK, et al. Salicylate poisoning complicated by fluid retention. Clin Toxicol 1976;9:61.
544. Hill JB. Experimental salicylate poisoning: observations on the effects of altering pH or tissue and plasma salicylate concentrations. Pediatrics 1971;47:658.
545. Buchanan N, Kundig H, Eyberg C. Experimental salicylate intoxication in young baboons. J Pediatr 1975;86:225.
546. Buchanan N, Rabinowitz L. Infantile salicylism—a reappraisal. J Pediatr 1974;84:391.
547. Hill JB. Salicylate intoxication. N Engl J Med 1973;288:1110.
548. Dove DJ, Jones T. Delayed coma associated with salicylate intoxication. J Pediatr 1982;100:493.
549. Bray PF, Gardiner AY. Salicylism and severe brain edema. N Engl J Med 1977;297;1235.
550. Pearson HA. Comparative effects of aspirin and acetaminophen on hemostasis. Pediatr 1978;62:926.
551. Fischer CH, Albertson TE, Foulke GE. Salicylate induced pulmonary edema. Clinical characteristics in children. Am J Emerg Med 1985;3:33.
552. Heffner J, Starkey T, Anthony P. Salicylate induced noncardiogenic pulmonary edema. West J Med 1979;130:263.
553. Hormaechea E, Carlson RW, Rogove H, et al. Hypovolemia, pulmonary edema and protein changes in severe salicylate poisoning. Am J Med 1979;66:1046.
554. Gabow PA. How to avoid overlooking salicylate intoxication. J Crit Illness 1986;1:77.
555. Starko KM, Mullick FG. Hepatic and cerebral pathology findings in children with fatal salicylate intoxication: further evidence for a casual relation between salicylate and Reye's syndrome. Lancet 1983;1:326.
556. Robinson BN, Sherwood WG, Taylor J, et al. Acetoacetyl CoA thiolase deficiency: a cause of severe ketoacidosis in infancy simulating salicylism. J Pediatr 1979;95:228.
557. Buck ML, Grebe TA, Bond GR. Toxic reaction to salicylate in a newborn infant: similarities to neonatal sepsis. J Pediatr 1993;122:955.
558. Howrie DL, Moriarty R, Breit R. Candy flavoring as a source of salicylate poisoning. Pediatr 1985;75:869.
559. Feldman S, Chen SL, Pickering LK. Salicylate absorption from bismuth subsalicylate preparation. Clin Pharmacol Ther 1981;29:788.
560. Done AK. Salicylate intoxication: significance of measurements of salicylate in blood in cases of acute ingestion. Pediatr 1960;26:800.
561. Levy G, Tsuchiya T. Effect of activated charcoal on aspirin absorption in man. Part I. Clin Pharmacol Ther 1972;13:317.
562. Fillippone G, Fish S, LaCouture P, et al. Reversible adsorption (desorption) of aspirin from activated charcoal. Arch Intern Med 1987;147:1390.
563. Barone J, Raia J, Chain Y. Evaluation of the effects of multiple dose activated charcoal on the absorption of orally administered salicylate in a simulated toxic ingestion model. Ann Emerg Med 1988;17:34.
564. Hillman RJ, Prescott LF. Treatment of salicylate poisoning with repeated oral charcoal. Br Med J 1986;291:1472.
565. Mofenson HC, Caraccio TR, Greensher J, et al. Gastrointestinal dialysis with activated charcoal and cathartic in the treatment of adolescent intoxications. Clin Pediatr 1985;24:678.
566. Vertrees JE, McWilliams BC, Kelly HW. Repeated oral administration of activated charcoal for treating aspirin overdose in young children. Pediatr 1990;85:594.
567. Kirshenbaum LA, Mathews SC, Ditar DS, Tenenbein M. Does multiple-dose charcoal therapy enhance salicylate excretion? Arch Intern Med 1990;1281.
568. Ho JL, Tierney MG, Dickinson GE. An evaluation of the effect of re-

peated doses of oral activated charcoal on salicylate elimination. J Clin Pharmacol 1989;29:366.
569. Tenenbein M. Whole bowel irrigation as a gastrointestinal decontamination procedure after acute poisoning. Med Toxicol 1988;3:77.
570. Mayer AL, Sitar DS, Tenenbein M. Multiple-dose charcoal and whole bowel irrigation do not increase clearance of absorbed salicylate. Arch Intern Med 1992;152:393.
571. Morgan AG, Polak A. The excretion of salicylate in salicylate poisoning. Clin Sci 1971;41:475.
572. Prescott LF, Balali-Mood M, Critchley JA, et al. Diuresis or urinary alkalinization for salicylate poisoning. Br Med J 1982;285:1383.
573. Flomenbaum NE, Goldfrank LR. Salicylates. In: Goldfrank LR, Flomenbaum NE, Lewis NA, et al., eds. Goldfrank's toxicologic emergencies. 5th ed. Norwalk, CT: Appleton & Lange, 1994:501.
574. Minocha A, Spyker DA. Acute overdose with sustained release drug formulations: perspectives in treatment. Med Toxicol 1986;1:300.
575. Roberson NJ. Fatal overdose from a sustained release theophylline preparation. Ann Emerg Med 1985;14:154.
576. Bernstein G, Jehle D, Bernaski E, Braen GR. Failure of gastric emptying and charcoal administration in fatal sustained-release theophylline overdose: pharmacobezoar formation. Ann Emerg Med 1992;21:1388.
577. Gaudreault P, Guay J. Theophylline poisoning: pharmacological considerations and clinical management. Med Tox 1986;1:169.
578. Ogilvie RI. Clinical pharmacokinetics of theophylline. Clin Pharmacokinet 1978;3:267.
579. Bestal RE, Eiriksson CE, Musser B, et al. Effect of intravenous aminophylline on plasma levels of catecholamines and related cardiovascular and metabolic responses in man. Circulation 1983;67:162.
580. Kearney TE, Manoguerra AS, Curtis GP, et al. Theophylline toxicity and the beta-adrenergic system. Ann Intern Med 1985;102:766.
581. Curry SC, Vance MV, Requa R, et al. The effects of toxic concentrations of theophylline on oxygene consumption, ventricular work, acid-base balance and plasma catecholamine levels in the dog. Ann Emerg Med 1985;14:554.
582. Sawyer WT, Caravati M, Ellison MJ, et al. Hypokalemia, hyperglycemia, and acidosis after intentional theophylline overdose. Am J Emerg Med 1985;3:408.
583. Shannon M, Lovejoy FH. Hypokalemia after theophylline intoxication: the effects of acute vs chronic poisoning. Arch Intern Med 1989;149:2725.
584. Gaar GG, Banner W, Laddu. The effects of esmolol on the hemodynamics of acute theophylline toxicity. Ann Emerg Med 1987;16:1334.
585. Biberstein MP, Ziegler MG, Ward DM. Use of beta-blockade and hemoperfusion for acute theophylline poisoning. West J Med 1984; 141:485.
586. Fredholm BB. Theophylline action on adenosine receptors. Eur J Respir Dis 1980;180(suppl);29.
587. Morgan PF, Deckert J, Jacobson KA, et al. Potentent convulsant actions of adenosine receptor antagonist, xanthine amine confener (XAC). Life Sci 1989;45:719.
588. Olson KR, Benowitz NL, Woo OF, Pond SM. Theophylline overdose: acute single ingestion versus chronic repeated overmedication. Am J Emerg Med 1985;3:386.
589. Shannon M, Lovejoy FH. Effect of acute versus chronic intoxication on clinical features of theophylline poisoning in children. J Pediatr 1992;121:125.
590. Shannon M. Predictors of major toxicity after theophylline overdose. Ann Intern Med 1993;119:1161.
591. Baker MD. Theophylline toxicity in children. J Pediatr 1986;109:538.
592. Henderson A, Wright DM, Pond SM. Mangement of theophylline overdose patients in the intensive care unit. Anaesth Intens Care 1992;20(1):56.
593. Zwillich CW, Sutton FD, Neff TA, et al. Theophylline-induced seizures in adults. Ann Intern Med 1975;82:784.
594. Sintek C, Hendeles L, Weinberger M. Inhibition of theophylline absorption by activated charcoal. J Pediatr 1979;94:314.
595. Shannon M, Amitai Y, Lovejoy FH. Multiple dose activated charcoal for theophylline poisoning in young infants. Pediatr 1987;80:368.
596. Gal P, Miller A, McCue JD. Oral activated charcoal to enhance theophylline elimination in an acute overdose. JAMA 1984;251:3130.
597. Mahutte CK, True RJ, Michiels TM, et al. Increased serum theophylline clearance with orally administered activated charcoal. Am Rev Respir Dis 1983;128:820.
598. Kulig KW, Bar-Or D, Rumack BH. Intravenous theophylline poisoning and multiple-dose charcoal in an animal model. Ann Emerg Med 1987;16:842.
599. Roberts JR, Carney S, Boyle SM, Lee DC. Ondansetron quells drug-resistant emesis in theophylline poisoning. Am J Emerg Med 1993;11(6):609.
600. Ohning BL, Reed MD, Blumer JL. Continuous nasogastric administration of activated charcoal for the treatment of theophylline intoxication. Ped Pharmacol 1986;5:241.
601. Levy G, Gibson TP, Whitman W, et al. Hemodialysis clearance of theophylline. JAMA 1977;237:1466.
602. Woo OF, Pond SM, Benowitz NL, et al. Benefit of hemoperfusion in acute theophylline intoxication. Clin Toxicol 1984;22:411.
603. Heath A, Knudsen K. Role of extracorporeal drug remoal in acute theophylline poisoning. A review. Med Toxicol Adverse Drug Exp 1987;2:294.
604. Park GD, Spector R, Roberts RJ, et al. Use of hemoperfusion for treatment of theophylline intoxication. Am J Med 1983;74:961.
605. Russo ME. Management of theophylline intoxication with charcoal-column hemoperfusion. N Engl J Med 1979;300:24.
606. Lin JL, Lim PS. Continuous artreriovenous hemoperfusion in acute poisoning. Blood Purif 1994;12(2):121.
607. Shannon M, Wernovsky G, Morris C. Exchange transfusion in the treatment of severe theophylline poisoning. Pediatr 1992;89:145.
608. Goldberg MJ, Spector R, Miller G. Phenobarbital improves survival in theophylline-intoxicated rabbits. J Toxicol Clin Toxicol 1986;24:203.
609. Seneff M, Scott J, Friedman B, et al. Acute theophylline toxicity and the use of esmolol to reverse cardiovascular instability. Ann Emerg Med 1990;19:671.
610. Singer HS, Brown J, Quaskey S, Rosenberg LA, Mellits ED, Denckla MB. The treatment of attention-deficit hyperactivity disorder in Tourette's syndrome: a double-blind placebo-controlled study with clonidine and desipramine. Pediatr 1995;95:74–81.
611. Cohen H, Hoffman RS, Howland MA. Cyclic antidepressant poisoning: a review and case report. J Pharm Pract 1993;6:89–102.
612. Kulig K, Rumack BH, Sullivan JB, et al. Amoxapine overdose: coma and seizures without cardiotoxic effects. JAMA 1982;248:1092–1094.
613. Wedin BP, Oderda GM, Klein-Schwartz W. Relative toxicity of cyclic antidepressants. Ann Emerg Med 1986;15:797–804.
614. Davidson J. Seizures and bupropion: a review. J Clin Psychiatry 1989;50:256–261.
615. Wellbutrin product summary. Research Triangle Park, NC: Burroughs Wellcome, January 1991.
616. Spiller HA, Morse S. Fluoxetine ingestion: a one year retrospective study. Vet Hum Toxicol 1990;32:153–155.
617. Borys DJ, Setzer SC, Ling LJ. The effects of fluoxetine in the overdose patient. Clin Toxicol 1990;28:331–340.
618. Lesar T, Kingston R, Dahn R, et al. Trazodone overdose. Ann Emerg Med 1983;12:221–223.
619. Klein-Schwartz W, Anderson B. Analysis of bertraline only overdoses (abstract). Vet Human Tox 1994;36:378.
620. Myers LB,Dean BS, Krenzelok EP. Paroxetine (Paxil): overdose assessment of a new selective serotonin reuptake inhibitor (abstract). Vet Hum Tox 1994;36:370.
621. Frommer DA, Kulig KW, Marx JA, Rumack B. Tricyclic antidepressant overdose: a review. JAMA 1987;257:561–526.
622. Marshall JB, Forker AD. Cardiovascular effects of tricyclic antidepressant drugs: therapeutic usage, overdose, and management of complications. Am Heart J 1982;103:401–413.
623. Malatynska E, Knapp RJ, Ikeda M, et al. Antidepressants and seizure-interactions at the GABA-receptor chloride-ionophore complex. Life Sci 1988;43:303–307.
624. Ellison DW, Pentel PR. Clinical features and consequences of seizures due to cyclic antidepressant overdose. Am J Emerg Med 1989;7:5–10.
625. Langou RA, Van Dyke C, Tahan SR, et al. Cardiovascular manifestations of tricyclic antidepressant overdose. Am Heart J 1980;100: 458–464.
626. Peters RW, Buser GA, Kim HJ, Gold MR. Tricyclic overdose causing sustained monomorphic ventricular tachycardia. Am J Card 1992;70:1226–1228.
627. Boehnert MK, Lovejoy FH. Value of the QRS duration versus the serum drug level in predicting seizures and ventricular arrhythmias after an acute overdose of tricyclic antidepressants. N Engl J Med 1985;313:474–479.
628. Foulke GE, Albertson TE. QRS interval in tricyclic antidepressant over-

dosage: inaccuracy as a toxicity indicator in emergency settings. Ann Emerg Med 1987;16:160–163.
629. Niemann JT, Bessen HA, Rothstein RJ, Laks MM. Electrocardiographic criteria for tricyclic antidepressant cardiotoxcity. Am J Cardiol 1986;57:1154–1159.
630. Wolfe TR, Caravati EM, Rollins DE. Terminal 40-ms frontal plane QRS axis as a marker for tricyclic antidepressant overdose. Ann Emerg Med 1989;18:348–351.
631. Liebelt EL, Francis PD, Woolf AD. ECG lead aVR versus QRS interval in predicting seizures and arrhythmias in acute tricyclic antidepressant toxicity. Ann Emerg Med 1995;26:195–201.
632. Shannon M, Lovejoy FH. Pulmonary consequences of severe tricyclic antidepressant ingestion. Clin Toxicol 1987;25:443–461.
633. Petit JM, Spiker DG, Ruwitch JF, et al. Tricyclic antidepressant plasma levels and adverse effect after overdose. Clin Pharmacol Ther 1977;21:47–51.
634. Lavoie FW, Gansert GG, Weiss RE. Value of initial ECG findings and plasma drug levels in cyclic antidepresant overdose. Ann Emerg Med 1990;19:696–700.
635. Swartz CM, Sherman A. The treatment of tricyclic antidepressant overdose with repeated charcoal. J Clin Psychopharmacol 1984;4:336–340.
636. Spivey WH. Flumazenil and seizures: analysis of 43 cases. Clin Therap 1992;14:292–305.
637. Pentel P, Peterson CD. Asystole complicating physostigmine treatment of tricyclic antidepressant overdose. Ann Emerg Med 1980;9: 588–590.
638. Newton RW. Physostigmine salicylate in the treatment of tricyclic antidepressant overdosage. JAMA 1975;231:941–943.
639. Callaham M, Shumaker H, Pentel P. Phenytoin prophylaxis of cardiotoxicity in experimental amitriptyline poisoning. J Pharmacol Exp Ther 1988;245:216–220.
640. Kumar A, Bleck TS. Intravenous midazolam for the treatment of refractory status epilepticus. Crit Care Med 1992;20:483–488.
641. Merigian KS, Browning RG, Leeper KV. Successful treatment of amoxapine-induced refractor status epilepticus with Propofol (Diprivan). Acad Emerg Med 1995;2:128–133.
642. Sasyniuk BI, Jhamandas V. Mechanism of reversal of toxic effects of amitriptyline on cardiac purkinje fibers by sodium bicarbonate. Ann Emerg Med 1986;15:1052–1059.
643. Pentel P, Benowitz N. Efficacy and mechanism of action of sodium bicarbonate in the treatment of desipramine toxicity in rats. J Pharmacol Exp Ther 1984;230:12–19.
644. Pentel PR, Benowitz NL. Tricyclic antidepressant poisoning: management of arrhythmias. Med Toxicol 1986;1:101–121.
645. McCabe JL, Menegazzi JJ. Recovery from severe cyclic antidepressant overdose with hypertonic saline/dextran in a swine model. Acad Emerg Med 1994;1:111–115.
646. Ahmad S. Management of cardiac complications in tricyclic antidepressant poisoning. J Royal Soc Med 1980;73:79.
647. Knudsen K, Abrahamsson J. Effects of magnesium sulfate and lidocaine in the treatment of ventricular arrhythmias in experimental amitriptyline poisoning in the rat. Crit Care Med 1994;22:494–498.
648. Hagerman GA, Hanashiro PK. Reversal of tricyclic-antidepressant-induced cardiac conduction abnormalities by phenytoin. Ann Emerg Med 1981;10:82–86.
649. Mayron R, Ruiz E. Phenytoin: does it reverse tricyclic-antidepressant-induced cardiac conduction abnormalities? Ann Emerg Med 1986; 15:876–880.
650. Kulig K, Bar-or D, Marx J, Wythe E, Rumack B. Phenytoin as treatment for tricyclic antidepressant cardiotoxicity in a canine model (abstract).Vet Hum Toxicol 1984;26:399.
651. Buchman AL, Dauer J, Geiderman J. The use of vasoactive agents in the treatment of refractory hypotension seen in tricyclic antidepressant overdose. J Clin Psychopharmacol 1990;10:409–413.
652. Vernon DD, Banner W, Garrett JS, Dean JM. Efficacy of dopamine and norepinephrine for treatment of hemodynamic compromise in amitriptyline intoxication. Crit Care Med 1991;19:544–549.
653. Larkin GL, Graeber GM, Hollingsed MJ. Experimental amitriptyline poisoning: treatment of severe cardiovascular toxicity with cardiopulmonary bypass. Ann Emerg Med 1994;23:480–486.
654. Pentel PR, Keyler DE, Brunn GJ, et al. Redistribution of tricyclic antidepressants in rats using a drug-specific monoclonal antibody: dose-response relationship. Drug Metab Dispos 1991;19:24–28.
655. Callaham M, Kassel D. Epidemiology of fatal tricyclic antidepressant ingestion: implications for management. Ann Emerg Med 1985;14:1–9.
656. Foulke GE, Albertson TE, Walby WF. Tricyclic antidepressant overdose: emergency department findings as predictors of clinical course. Am J Emerg Med 1986;4:496–500.
657. Stern TA, O'Gara PT, Mulley AG, Singer DE, Thibault GE. Complications after overdose with tricyclic antidepressants. Crit Care Med 1985;13:672–674.
658. Shannon MW. Duration of QRS disturbances after severe tricyclic antidepressant intoxication. Clin Toxicol 1992;30:377–386.
659. Fasoli RA, Glauser FL. Cardiac arrhythmias and ECG abnormalities in tricyclic antidepressant overdose. Clin Toxicol 1981;18:155–163.

Hematologic and Oncologic Conditions

Section Eight

Section Editor

Alice D. Ackerman

Hematologic Disorders in the Pediatric Intensive Care Unit

41

Allen E. Eskenazi
Mark L. Bernstein
John B. Gordon

INTRODUCTION

The hematologic issues of most concern in the pediatric intensive care unit (PICU) are often secondary to other disease processes, such as cancer, trauma, and infection. Consequently, many hematologic disorders are discussed in other chapters. Similarly, issues such as oxygen transport and the influence of 2,3-diphosphoglycerate (2,3-DPG) are covered in the cardiovascular section. In this chapter, we have chosen to emphasize some specific hematologic topics not discussed in detail elsewhere in this text.

RED CELL DISORDERS IN THE PEDIATRIC INTENSIVE CARE UNIT

Anemia is undoubtedly the most common red cell disorder in pediatric intensive care. In most instances the anemia is secondary to bleeding and treatment is not complicated—the source of bleeding must be identified and treated while red blood cells are transfused as needed. In the absence of identifiable bleeding, the clinician must determine whether the anemia is due to inadequate production (e.g., conditions resulting in marrow replacement or aplastic crises in patients with chronic hemolytic anemias) or accelerated destruction (e.g., hemolytic-uremic syndrome). Two conditions which the intensivist will frequently encounter, sickle cell disease (SCD) and severe hemorrhage necessitating massive transfusion, will be discussed in some detail in this chapter.

Sickle Cell Disease

SCD refers to those hemoglobinopathies characterized by the formation of sickled red cells in response to deoxygenation. This autosomal recessive disorder is caused by the substitution of valine for glutamine at the sixth amino acid position of the beta chain of hemoglobin. The heterozygous state, hemoglobin AS (sickle cell trait), occurs in about 8% of American blacks, while homozygosity occurs in 0.4%[(1)]. Sickle cell anemia (hemoglobin SS) is the most common cause of SCD[(2–7)]. Whites, particularly those of Mediterranean origin, are occasionally affected. Individuals of Middle Eastern origin are also affected, although the phenotypic expression is often less severe. The other common causes of the SCD phenotype are hemoglobin SC and hemoglobin S-beta thalassemia. These, as well as other mixed hemoglobinopathies, can cause varying degrees of sickling[(1–7)]. Although the phenotypic diagnosis of SCD can usually be made on the basis of the clinical findings and the peripheral blood smear examination, the precise type of hemoglobinopathy is established by hemoglobin chromatography or electrophoresis[(1–7)]. DNA analysis may also be undertaken, particularly for prenatal diagnosis[(8)].

The most frequent clinical manifestations of SCD are (a) vaso-occlusive events involving any vascular bed, (b) splenic sequestration, (c) acute aplasia, and (d) splenic dysfunction[(2–7)]. These may lead to life-threatening complications requiring admission to the PICU, such as stroke and acute chest syndrome, acute anemia, and sepsis. Another cause of PICU admission in this population is the need for close monitoring during partial exchange transfusions. In the following pages, the pathophysiology of the disorder will be briefly reviewed; then the critical complications of SCD and their therapy will be presented.

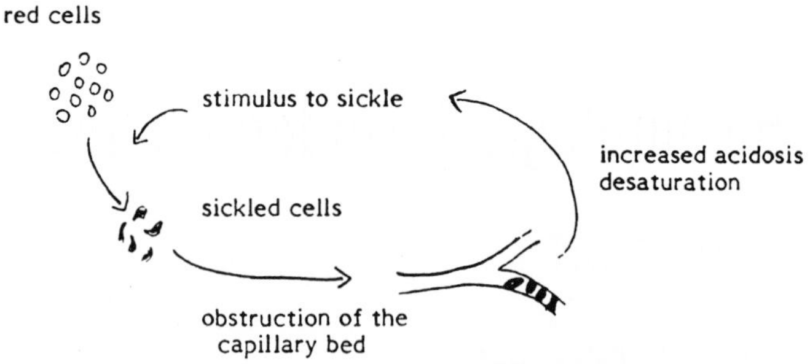

Figure 41.1. The "vicious" cycle of progressive sickling causing intravascular occlusion.

Pathophysiology of SCD

The complications seen in patients with SCD are ultimately due to the sickling of red blood cells, leading to vascular occlusion and a resulting inability to deliver oxygen to the target organ. Upon partial or total deoxygenation, hemoglobin S (Hb S) reversibly polymerizes into paracrystalline polymers, called gels, inside the cell. These polymers exist in a spectrum of forms ranging from aggregated hemoglobin tetramers to highly ordered fiber aggregates that fill and distort the red blood cell[(9)]. Perturbations in oxygen saturation, temperature, pH, ionic strength, 2,3-DPG, carbon monoxide, and the presence of non-sickle hemoglobin affect the formation of Hb S gels. The development of gelled hemoglobin leads to distortion of cell morphology, changes in cellular viscosity, and ultimately vascular sludging, resulting in organ infarction. Patients who become hypoxic, acidotic, dehydrated, and febrile are likely to develop manifestations of vaso-occlusive disease. However, in the presence of higher amounts of Hb F or Hb A_2, the polymerization process is inhibited and complications are less common.

The classical view of a vaso-occlusive crisis is that a "vicious cycle" is established[(1–7,10)] in which flow slows (perhaps because of hypotension or increased adherence of red cells with narrowing of the vascular lumen), causing local hypoxemia and acidosis with consequent sickling of red cells. Viscosity then increases, giving rise to even slower flow with eventual sludging in the capillary bed (Fig. 41.1). Factors that may promote sickling are listed in **Table 41.1.** As will be noted later, the vicious cycle theory probably does not apply to all vaso-occlusive crises; however, it likely explains the pathogenesis of bony and abdominal crises.

Table 41.1. Factors That May Promote Sickling

1. Pressure related
   a. Hypotension
   b. Pulmonary hypertension
2. Resistance related
   a. Vasoconstriction
   b. Increased hematocrit (>35%)
3. Desaturation related
   a. Hypoxemia
   b. Acidosis

How, given the above theoretical considerations, could the vicious cycle be prevented or interrupted?

Therapy that prevents gelation in a cell fully hemoglobinized with Hb S (carbon monoxide, cyanide) has not been clinically useful [1], in part because of its inacceptability to patients[11]. Similarly, agents that decrease viscosity (urea, mannitol, etc.) cause diuresis (hence, increased viscosity) when given in the doses required to lower viscosity in vitro[1,11]. Increased cell hydration interferes with sickling. This has been shown in vitro by use of membrane active agents such as cetiedil[12,13], although there is not uniform agreement concerning efficacy[14]. Altering the hemoglobin content of sickle cells has also been attempted through the use of the chemotherapeutic agents 5-azacytidine and hydroxyurea[15–18]. These agents enhance fetal hemoglobin synthesis, which, as mentioned earlier, results in interference with the stearic forces necessary for gel formation. The chronic use of hydroxyurea in adults has resulted in increased fetal hemoglobin synthesis and a reduction in the number of vaso-occlusive crises. However, the potential mutagenic and carcinogenic effects of these drugs have thus far precluded their use in pediatric patients[19].

Since there is no therapy that can effectively and safely inhibit gelation and subsequent sickling in children, current management of the sickle cell patient focuses on minimizing precipitants and the complications of SCD. The first of these discussed here is the vaso-occlusive crisis. The acute vaso-occlusive crisis can be functionally defined as an ischemic insult resulting from vascular occlusion due to sickled cells. The precise mechanism of the occlusion is not always clear. The vicious cycle theory discussed earlier probably applies in the case of bony or abdominal crises involving small vessels. However, pulmonary infarcts and strokes may be caused by other mechanisms, including marrow emboli[20] in the case of the former and, perhaps, spontaneous platelet aggregation[21,22] or endothelial damage with intimal hyperplasia in the case of the latter[23,24].

Regardless of pathogenesis, various conditions such as hypoxia, hypotension, and viral or bacterial respiratory infections **(Table 41.2)** have been associated with vaso-occlusive crises. Unfortunately, no obvious precipitant can be identified in many instances of vaso-occlusive crisis; nonetheless, the first step in managing the child with SCD involves prevention of those precipitating events if possible. These measures presume that the child with SCD has been identified at or shortly after birth and that the child has been enrolled in a comprehensive care program. As long as the child has been identified and his or her parents have been trained to recognize early signs and symptoms, dehydration with subsequent hypotension can be prevented and early aggressive treatment of lung disease will minimize hypoxemia. Moreover, the use of both prophylactic penicillin and vaccination reduce the incidence of pneumococcal infection[25–27] and hence some of the morbidity and mortality seen in this disorder.

Table 41.2. Clinical Precipitants of a Vaso-occlusive Crisis

1. Pressure related
   a. Hypotension
      i. Dehydration
      ii. Shock
      iii. Anesthetics
      iv. Other drugs
      v. Tourniquets
   b. Increased central venous pressure
      i. Pericardial disease
      ii. Heart failure
2. Resistance related
   a. Vasoconstriction
      i. Shock
      ii. Cold
   b. Increased viscosity (increased hematocrit)
      i. Dehydration
      ii. Transfusion (excessive)
3. Miscellaneous
   a. Infection
      i. Viral
      ii. Bacterial
   b. Overexertion
   c. Hypoxia
      i. Pneumonia
      ii. High altitude

Transfusion Therapy of SCD

In many instances, it becomes necessary to transfuse the patient with SCD. In most situations this is not done to correct the anemia per se, since this is a lifelong, chronic process, but instead to reduce or eliminate the number of sickle cells in the circulation, thus preventing some of the complications from these sickle RBCs. In these situations, the patient's RBCs are exchanged for sickle-negative RBCs, thereby reducing the number of cells capable of producing vaso-occlusion. In all circumstances, it is necessary to screen the donor blood for sickle hemoglobin. Furthermore, the risks of blood transfusion must be weighed against the benefits in every situation. In essence, the benefits are an increase in the hematocrit and a decrease in the Hb S concentration, providing better oxygen delivery and reducing the risk of vaso-occlusion. The risks include infection, aloimunization, transfusion reaction, hemochromatosis, and, rarely, death[28–30]. Various prophylactic and therapeutic indications for transfusion therapy are outlined in **Table 41.3** and are discussed in more detail below.

Over the past number of years, the advances in perioperative management of the child with SCD have effectively diminished mortality and morbidity[31,32]. Preoperatively, the child must be carefully assessed for signs and symptoms of infection that, if present, dictate cancellation of elective cases. It is essential that good hydration be maintained at all times. Furthermore, hypoxia both intraoperatively and postoperatively must be prevented. To this end, administration of O_2 by mask and vigorous postoperative encouragement to cough, deep-breathe, and perform incentive spirometry must be employed. Careful attention should also

Table 41.3. Indications for Transfusion Therapy in Sickle Cell Disease

1. Prophylactic
   a. Preoperative
   b. Poststroke
   c. ?Pregnancy (The use of prophylactic transfusions in pregnancy is controversial)
2. Therapeutic
   a. Acute chest syndrome
   b. Stroke
   c. Spinal cord infarct
   d. Persistent priapism
   e. Aplastic crisis
   f. Sequestration crisis
   g. Multiple trauma
   h. Uncontrollable (nonresolving) crisis

be paid to other factors that might precipitate a crisis in the operating room, such as hypothermia and prolonged use of tourniquets[31–34]. Whether patients with SCD need preoperative reduction in the percent of sickle RBCs is the subject of a current multi-institutional study. Until the results of this study are available, it is generally advisable to prepare the patient in advance of surgery, so that the percentage of HbS RBCs is less than 30%[31–35]. For elective surgery, repeated simple transfusion in the clinic every 2 weeks may be used to keep the hematocrit at approximately 35% and the reticulocytes below 1%, thus inhibiting endogenous sickle erythrocyte production. Due to the shortened survival of the patient's own sickle cells, their number will gradually decrease, and that of the transfused cells, increase. After 4 to 6 weeks, the percentage of Hb S will be less than 30%, so that surgery may be safely undertaken. In more urgent cases, large volume partial exchange transfusion using simultaneous withdrawal and infusion of red blood cells may be employed.

A relatively simple exchange transfusion regimen that we often employ requires a venous catheter for infusion and an arterial catheter for removal of the child's blood. In older children, a large-bore venous catheter may be substituted for the arterial line. Removal of 20 cc/kg of the patient's blood is performed while 15 cc/kg of packed sickle-negative blood is infused. This procedure is performed over 1-½ to 2 hours and is repeated 24 hours later. The percentage of HbS cells will be reduced to approximately 30% by this procedure[36]. If more rapid reduction in sickle hemoglobin is needed (e.g., cerebral ischemia), an alternative approach is to exchange twice the patient's red cell volume for packed red blood cells (PRBCs). As long as the patient's initial hematocrit is less than 25%, the final hematocrit will usually be less than 36%. We usually accomplish the exchange over 4 to 6 hours and verify the hematocrit every 2 hours. If it exceeds 35% at any point, we add fresh frozen plasma (FFP) to the PRBCs infused during the remainder of the partial exchange transfusion.

Vaso-occlusive Crises

The molecular basis of sickling and the pathogenesis of the sickling process have been discussed. The diagnosis and treatment of established vaso-occlusive crises is reviewed in this section. A general approach is presented, followed by a discussion of the management of specific types of crises. The diagnosis of any crisis is made on the basis of the general complaints of fever, malaise, anorexia, and the specific complaints of pain or other symptoms and signs related to the organ involved[2–7]. Therapy (outlined in **Table 41.4**) is aimed at (a) removing the precipitating cause, (b) treating the complications of the crisis, and (c) preventing further vaso-occlusion. Hydration, infection control, and pain control are the mainstay of therapy in all cases[2–7]. Supplemental oxygen should be supplied if the patient is hypoxemic due to lung disease or hypoventilation. Supplemental oxygen in nonhypoxemic patients will not enhance delivery of oxygen to areas of vaso-occlusion and therefore does not provide additional therapeutic benefit. Patient-controlled analgesia is the optimal choice of pain control, although its use in very young children may be difficult. High-dose intravenous methylprednisolone therapy (15 mg/kg/day for 2 days, maximum daily dose 1000 mg) has recently been shown to be a useful adjunct to pain management[37]. Although there is evidence that fibrin and thrombin formation are increased in steady state SCD, antiplatelet and anticoagulant agents have not been found to be therapeutically effective[38] and may in fact cause bleeding into the area of infarction[39].

Acute Chest Syndrome

The acute chest syndrome (ACS) is characterized by fever, pleuritic chest pain, tachypnea, cough, hypoxemia, an infiltrate on chest x-ray, and a drop in baseline hemoglobin[39–42]. Pleural effusions may also be present. Many patients are initially admitted for other reasons, typically bone pain, and develop signs of ACS during their hospitalization. The cause of the syndrome is often not identified. There are reports of bone marrow emboli[20], in situ thromboses[43], and asthma[44]. In perhaps 25% of cases, bacterial pneumonia, often *Streptococcus pneumoniae,* is identified[42]. One report indicated that 13% of patients with ACS had *Chlamydia pneumoniae* infection[45]. Recently, blood phospholipase A_2 levels have been found to be increased, probably secondary to release of bone marrow fat. This in turn leads to

Table 41.4. General Approach to Management of Vaso-occlusive Crises

1. Diagnosis
   a. History (is it a typical crisis?)
   b. Physical examination
   c. Laboratory tests
      i. Complete blood count and reticulocyte count
      ii. Ancillary tests (see text)
2. Treatment
   a. Oxygen if hypoxemic
   b. Hydration at 1.5 × maintenance
   c. Analgesics (narcotics and anti-inflamatory agents)
   d. Antibiotics
   e. ?steroids (steroid prescription is controversial)

the release of free fatty acids and lysophospholipids, which may then result in lung inflammation[46].

Although it is often unclear whether the cause of ACS is infection or infarction, it is essential that the patient be treated as if both are occurring. Infection leads to localized acidosis and hypoxia, which promote intravascular sickling. Infarction results in pain and hypoventilation, which may then promote a secondary pulmonic infection. We therefore do not advocate the use of ventilation-perfusion scans to distinguish infectious from thrombotic causes since therapy must be directed toward alleviating both processes.

Therapy of the ACS follows the general principles outlined earlier. Pain relief is essential to allow effective cough and pulmonary toilet. The advantages and risks of continuous infusion of narcotics have been discussed[47]. Currently, we favor patient-controlled analgesia devices, but fixed-rate infusions of short-acting narcotics such as fentanyl (1 to 2 μg/kg/hr) may be required. We initiate antibiotic therapy in any febrile child with ACS, whether an organism has been identified or not. The consequences of untreated pneumococcal disease or other bacterial infections are devastating in this population[40–42]; recent evidence suggests that *Mycoplasma* or *Chlamydia* can also cause ACS[45]. Therefore, we begin therapy with ceftriaxone and erythromycin. Any child who is at risk for unusual organisms (e.g., airway intubation or long hospital stay) is treated with antistaphylococcal and antipseudomonas agents (e.g., nafcillin and ceftazadime with or without an aminoglycoside). Supplemental oxygen may be of benefit to hypoxemic patients, although it will not correct arterial hypoxemia in the face of severe ventilation-perfusion mismatch. We routinely administer O_2 via mask or nasal prongs in an effort to maintain arterial pO_2 over 90 mm Hg and hemoglobin saturation above 98%. In the child with severe ACS and the development of acute respiratory distress syndrome (ARDS) unresponsive to simple supplemental oxygen, intubation is often required in addition to the exchange transfusion. Further issues in the treatment of ARDS are discussed in Chapter 7.

The decision to perform a partial exchange transfusion depends on the child's condition. Partial exchange transfusion of children with relatively mild signs and symptoms of ACS is recommended by many hematologists with a view to minimizing the progression of the disorder. This approach may obviate the need for intubation, since the ACS often promptly resolves after transfusion. Obviously, if severe hypoxemia is present (e.g., P_aO_2 under 100 mm Hg with an F_iO_2 over 0.6), then an exchange transfusion is needed. Similarly, if the patient presents with severe, advanced ACS with widespread infarction and an x-ray picture indistinguishable from ARDS, an urgent exchange transfusion is required. Details on performing an exchange transfusion have been discussed. The viscosity of blood in the patient with Hb S rises considerably when the hematocrit is greater than 35%, resulting in decreased oxygen delivery[48]. Therefore exchange transfusion is preferable to simple red blood cell transfusion, with the goal of reducing the percentage of Hb S to less than 30%.

Stroke

The second vaso-occlusive crisis that frequently results in intensive care admissions is stroke. A prospective cohort study performed in Jamaica reported a prevalence of 7.8% by age 14[49]. Approximately 70 to 80% of strokes are infarcts, with less than 10% of patients having a preceding transient ischemic attack[50,51]. The diagnosis of stroke is made on the basis of the usual clinical signs. In most cases there are no warning signs. Focal seizures may precede the onset of ischemic symptoms and should be considered presumptive evidence of cerebrovascular disease[50]. Headaches are common in SCD and are not reliable indicators of vascular disease[24]. Upon admission of a child with neurologic signs suggesting stroke, computed tomography (CT) or magnetic resonance imaging (MRI) must be emergently performed to define any abnormalities as well as rule out treatable lesions such as subdural bleeding. Where available, magnetic resonance angiography (MRA) is useful in defining abnormalities in the central nervous system (CNS) vasculature[52]. If there are no signs of increased intracranial pressure, a lumbar puncture should be performed to exclude the unlikely, but possible, coexistence of an infectious process. It is also worth noting that occasionally a patient will exhibit stroke-like signs or other neurologic signs (seizure, confusion, encephalopathy) due to lead toxicity. Thus, obtaining a lead level may be appropriate in the initial assessment of the child[53].

The etiology and pathogenesis of thrombotic stroke in children with SCD remain controversial. The large caliber of an undamaged artery eliminates the possibility of sickled cells clogging the circulation. Angiographic and pathologic studies demonstrate proximal intracranial arterial stenosis, particularly the internal carotid artery. Histologically there is segmental thickening of the vessel walls and intimal hyperplasia. Occlusion of the vessel may result from the intimal hyperplasia alone, superimposed thrombosis, and/or distal thromboembolization[38]. There is also a subset of patients in whom small-vessel disease can be demonstrated. These lesions may precede symptomatic stroke or may cause cognitive deficits in these patients[54]. It has been hypothesized that infarcts of the vasa vasorum might cause endothelial damage, with subsequent intimal hyperplasia and thrombus formation; however, the vasa vasorum are present only in extracranial vessels[23], so an alternate mechanism for intimal hyperplasia must be found. The apparent predilection of intimal hyperplasia for sites of arterial bifurcation suggest that endothelial injury at sites of high flow turbulence may be a key factor[38]. Interestingly, while most strokes in children are due to infarcts, as many as one-third of strokes in adults are hemorrhagic[24]. It is postulated that the repeated insults to the intracerebral arterial endothelium that occur during childhood may weaken it, leading to aneurysm formation, and these may later rupture[24,50].

The most important intervention in the child exhibiting stroke is an immediate exchange transfusion aimed at pre-

Table 41.5. Sites of Vaso-occlusive Crises

1. Bone
   a. Marrow
   b. Cortex (long bones)
   c. Dactylitis (hands and feet)
2. Abdomen
3. Chest
4. Brain
   a. Infarction
   b. Hemorrhage
5. Miscellaneous
   a. Penis (priapism)
   b. Spinal cord
   c. Orbit (apex syndrome)

venting progression of the stroke. Beyond that, therapy for the child with stroke is supportive, as outlined before. If a large infarct has occurred, it is necessary to observe the child for possible intracranial hypertension. Anticoagulant therapy is contraindicated. Prompt institution of physical therapy will aid in long-term management. The natural history of untreated stroke in SCD is one of recurrent infarcts and progressive arterial occlusion[23,24,50,55–59]. It has been found that chronic transfusion therapy aimed at maintaining the hematocrit over 35% and the Hb S below 30%, thus avoiding sickling episodes, is effective in preventing evolution of the vascular lesions seen on an angiogram and preventing subsequent strokes[23,24,50,55–59]. More recent evidence suggests that maintenance of Hb S levels less than 50% is effective for the prevention of recurrent stroke and significantly reduces blood requirements[60]. The transfusions are required indefinitely, since cessation of transfusion has been associated with recurrent strokes[24,55,57]. Chelation therapy with desferoxamine will, therefore, be necessary to slow iron overload and its attendant complications.

Other Crises

ACS and stroke are the most devastating vaso-occlusive crises commonly leading to ICU admission of the pediatric population. However, they are not the most common crises overall. Since children admitted to the ICU with SCD are prone to other crises **(Table 41.5)**, it is well to briefly review them here. The classical vicious cycle theory of the pathogenesis of sickling probably applies to all of these vaso-occlusive crises. The precipitant of the crisis in many cases is not identified but may include infection, dehydration, overexertion, or hypoxia, as mentioned above **(Table 41.2)**.

Bony crises may involve marrow (long bones, vertebrae) or the cortex itself[61,62]. In children younger than 2 years of age, the small bones of the hands and feet are most frequently involved[63], giving rise to the hand-foot syndrome, or dactylitis. In all cases, pain, fever, and leukocytosis are common. Rarely, marrow involvement will cause aplasia or embolism[20]. Usually, however, pain is the principal problem and resolves with general supportive care. In the case of cortical involvement, pain, redness, and swelling over the affected area are seen, making the differentiation from osteomyelitis difficult[61,62]. The white blood cell count and differential are not helpful in distinguishing infection from infarction. Children with SCD are prone to infection and may develop osteomyelitis. For differentiating the two conditions, diagnostic procedures, including culture of the blood and of the lesion, are needed. Examination of the fluid obtained from a needle aspirate of the affected area may reveal the causative organism. A combination of bone and marrow scanning may be helpful in distinguishing between osteomyelitis and a bony infarct[61]. Despite the relative rarity of infection compared with a bony vaso-occlusive crisis, if redness and swelling are present, particularly over only one bone, initial therapy should include antibiotics effective against the typical organisms *Salmonella* and *Staphylococcus aureus*[64,65]. When culture results are available, the antibiotics can then be appropriately adjusted.

Abdominal crises are characterized by pain, fever, malaise, anorexia, and occasionally nausea. On examination, absent or sparse bowel sounds and abdominal tenderness are common. The abdominal crises arise from occlusion of mesenteric vessels or the vessels of some of the viscera (e.g., spleen, kidney)[66]. The major differential diagnosis in the case of abdominal crises, particularly if severe, is between vaso-occlusive crisis and a surgical condition. It has been said that children with SCD frequently undergo unnecessary laparotomy[66]. A good history and physical examination may obviate the need for laparotomy. If the pain is typical of previous crises, it is likely again a crisis; if not, other causes must be excluded. Of the surgical conditions, cholecystitis is probably most common[34,66]. The excessive hemolysis associated with SCD results in gallstones. Fortunately, up to 71% of gallstones are radiopaque and thus may be seen on plain x-ray; ultrasound of the gallbladder may identify stones or gallbladder abnormalities if the x-ray does not[67]. Therapy of the abdominal crisis follows the general principles noted above. It is critical to maintain adequate hydration. Furthermore, pain control will prevent the pulmonary atelectasis that often occurs because of splinting of the abdomen. If an attack does not resolve over 3 to 6 days, a surgical condition must be suspected[66] and more vigorously sought.

There are a few other complications of vaso-occlusive crises that, although rare, may require admission to the ICU. These include intractable priapism[2–7], orbital infarction[68], and spinal cord infarction[69]. All may require exchange transfusion therapy in addition to general supportive measures.

Aplastic and Sequestration Crises

Although vaso-occlusive crises are the most common causes of ICU admission for children with SCD, they are not the only ones. Anemia, infection, and chronic organ failure also lead to admission. In addition to the chronic moderate anemia of SCD, acute drops in hemoglobin may occur. These are due either to aplasia or, in younger children, to sequestration crises[2–7,70–73]. The most commonly identified cause of an aplastic crisis is infection with parvovirus B19[74]. Aplastic crises are characterized by a rapid decrease in the baseline Hb without an appropriate reticulocyte response. Because the patient continues to have severe hemolysis due to the underlying SCD, the Hb falls rapidly. The period of marrow aplasia usually only lasts a few days. The degree of anemia and cardiovascular compromise will dictate the clinician's response. Simple PRBC transfusions (as opposed to exchange transfusions) are typically employed to bring the patient's Hb level back to baseline.

A more dramatic and potentially fatal form of severe anemia is the acute sequestration crisis (ASC)[2–7,70,71,75]. This is the leading cause of death in Jamaican children with SCD[75], although a less common cause elsewhere. It is defined as an acute drop in hemoglobin by over 2 g/dl associated with splenomegaly, reticulocytosis, and signs of intravascular volume depletion. Acute shock associated with a decrease in hemoglobin of over 4 g/dl is fatal in 35% of cases. It has been shown that a relatively minor episode of ASC with hemoglobin drops of only 2 to 4 g/dl must be carefully noted, since 20 to 50% of children will have a recurrence. In the Jamaican population, mortality was 20% during the second or third attack. The crises occur in children between 10 and 27 months of age and virtually never after 5 years of age[70,71]. This is presumably because autosplenectomy has occurred by 5 years of age in patients with Hb SS. In patients with the variant sickle cell syndromes Hb SC or Hb S-beta thalassemia, complete autosplenectomy is delayed and may not occur. Therefore, there is a continued risk of sequestration in these children.

Clinically, the child with an ASC appears pale, is irritable, and may be in shock. Therapy consists principally of restoring circulating blood volume. Initially, Ringer's lactate or normal saline may be used to reverse shock; however, prompt blood transfusion is essential. Interestingly, in some instances, the transfusion will result not only in resolution of shock but also in a return of the sequestered blood to the circulation. Thrombocytopenia and leukopenia secondary to hypersplenism may also be seen in acute sequestration. The long-term management of the child who has had ASC is difficult. There is a significant risk of recurrence, so in countries where health care services may be limited in availability, or in situations where close follow-up care of the child is impossible, splenectomy is recommended after one episode of ASC[72]. If good health care is available and the parents can be instructed in how to monitor the spleen size and observe the child for symptoms of sequestration, then observation, rather than splenectomy, may be appropriate. In view of the infectious risks to the young child after splenectomy—even one with impaired splenic function, as is the case in anemia—avoiding splenectomy seems the best approach if prompt attention to crises can be provided.

Sepsis

Bacterial infection has been the most common cause of death in children with SCD. The institution of newborn screening programs, early use of prophylactic penicillin, and the aggressive treatment of febrile children with SCD has reduced the morbidity and mortality from infection[76,77]. These children are at increased risk of sepsis, primarily from encapsulated organisms (e.g., *Streptococcus pneumoniae, Neisseria meningitidis, and Hemophilus influenzae* type B), because of impaired splenic function[78] and decreased opsonic activity[79]. Treatment of bacterial sepsis is similar to that in non-sickle cell patients with prompt initiation of antibiotics and supportive care as outlined elsewhere in this text. We advocate that any child with SCD and a temperature over 38.5° C be treated with antibiotics, whether he looks "well" or not. If good follow-up is not possible as an outpatient, the child should be admitted to the hospital. Any child who looks septic should be treated regardless of his or her temperature[80,81].

Other Complications

In addition to vaso-occlusive crises, anemia, and infection, repeated infarction can result in failure of various organs. For example, anatomic[82] and functional abnormalities of the kidney may occur, resulting in chronic renal failure. Dialysis or transplantation may be needed[83], though this is quite unusual in the pediatric age group. Chronic anemia, with or without actual myocardial infarctions, leads to cardiac dysfunction[84] and, in the face of volume overload or sepsis, severe congestive heart failure may occur. Similarly, chronic respiratory disease may lead to heightened susceptibility to acute respiratory failure when another insult is superimposed. Finally, older patients with SCD often also develop cor pulmonale[85].

It is clear from this brief review that the current management of SCD is restricted to treating the consequences of the disorder, not the underlying pathophysiology. Over the next few years, advances in prenatal diagnosis, bone marrow transplantation[86], and gene therapy[87] may result in a cure for the disease. However, as noted by many authors, the gap between discovering the molecular basis of the disease and establishing a cure has not shrunk appreciably in the past 50 years.

Hemorrhage

General Approach

The approach to a bleeding child presented here is a subjective one that reflects the authors' conception of how to concentrate on the obvious while not forgetting the obscure in formulating a differential diagnosis and treatment plan. Other approaches have been proposed and may be equally useful, but this one, which combines the overall clinical picture (i.e., "sick"-looking versus "well"-looking child) with the simple laboratory screening tests of hemostatic function (e.g., platelet count, hematocrit, prothrombin time [PT], partial thromboplastin time [PTT], and fibrin/fibrinogen degradation products [FDP]), allows an effective and simple classification of hemorrhage in the ICU setting. Reviews of both

Table 41.6. Etiologic Classification of Hemorrhage[a]

1. Vessel related
   a. Trauma
   b. Surgery
   c. Vasculitis
2. Platelet related
   a. Thrombocytopenia
   b. Thrombocytopathy
3. Plasma phase related
   a. Congenital factor deficiency
   b. Liver disease
   c. Disseminated intravascular coagulopathy

[a]*Major categories and illustrative examples.*

similar and different approaches to the bleeding child or adult are presented in several publications[88–91].

The first step in any approach to the bleeding child is to obtain a thorough history and physical examination. This, more than anything else, will separate the children into a "sick" versus "well" grouping. The history, particularly as it relates to bleeding, can help the physician place the child into one of the general etiologic categories of bleeding **(Table 41.6).** Obviously, a child with profuse bright red bleeding after trauma or surgery most likely has a "mechanical" cause of bleeding that is most quickly remedied by locating and clamping the disrupted vessel. On the other hand, the child who has been "well" but developed petechiae and now demonstrates a suggestion of an intracranial mass lesion most likely has isolated platelet deficiency caused by idiopathic thrombocytopenic purpura. In contrast to these two situations of "well" children demonstrating hemorrhage, consider the "sick" child who has a history of fever and lethargy followed by the development of purpura. Examination reveals a septic child with easy bleeding, suggesting the diagnosis of disseminated intravascular coagulation (DIC).

The history guides one to an initial appreciation of whether the bleeding is isolated or part of a larger illness. It also determines the chronicity of the situation. Similarly, the physical examination should explore these two issues. It is particularly important to determine the clinical severity of the hemorrhage, i.e., is shock present or imminent? As discussed elsewhere in this text, this requires assessment of the cardiovascular, respiratory, renal, and cerebral function **(Table 41.7).** Once it has been established that shock is present and appropriate initial therapy has been instituted **(Table 41.8),** a more extensive physical examination can be performed to search for clues to the cause of hemorrhage. In particular, purpura and petechiae may suggest platelet dysfunction or the loss of vascular integrity, while purpura and oozing from venous puncture sites may point to a defect in the plasma phase of coagulation. The head and neck examination should note whether icterus is present, retinal hemorrhages are seen, or adenopathy is prominent. The abdominal examination may reveal hepatosplenomegaly. Finally, the general picture may suggest sepsis. In the traumatized child, occult bleeding sites (e.g., abdomen, thigh) must be sought.

The history and physical examination will thus suggest the likely cause (or at least the etiologic category) and will aid in identifying the severity of the hemorrhage. A few laboratory tests will usually suffice to narrow the differential diagnosis to one or two possibilities. Obviously, these will include nonhematologic tests if renal, liver, or other systemic diseases are suspected. However, only the hematology tests will be emphasized here **(Table 41.9).** Of the tests listed here, the platelet count, PT, PTT, and FDP are the most widely available and useful in establishing a diagnosis. With them and the clinical examination, the category of illness can be identified and therapy can often be initiated.

Therapy for the bleeding child can be divided into three phases: (a) initial resuscitation if in shock, (b) restoration of hematocrit to normal (or acceptable) levels, and (c) correction (if possible) of the underlying disorder. The care of the child in shock is discussed in Chapter 16. In this segment of this chapter, transfusion therapy is discussed; in the next section, disorders of coagulation are considered.

Table 41.7. Stages of Pediatric Blood Volume Loss (Shock) and Associated Clinical Signs[a]

Blood Volume Loss	*Clinical Signs*
<20%	CV: Tachycardia: weak, thready pulses Skin: Cool to touch, capillary refill 2–3 sec Renal: Slight decrease in urine output, increase in specific gravity CNS: Irritable, may be combative
25%	CV: Tachycardia: weak, thready distal pulses Skin: Cold extremities, cyanosis and mottling Renal: Decrease in urine output CNS: Confusion, lethargy
40%	CV: Frank hypotension: tachycardia may progress to bradycardia Skin: Pale, cold Renal: No urine ouput CNS: Comatose

CV = cardiovascular; CNS = central nervous system.
[a]*From Rasmussen GE, Grande CM. Int Anesth Clin 1994;32:83, with permission.*

Transfusion of Blood Products

Blood for Replacement

Most blood banks now fractionate their units into PRBCs, FFP, platelet concentrates, and cryoprecipitate. The vari-

Table 41.8. Initial Therapy for the Child with Significant Hemorrhage

1. Without shock
   a. Oxygen by mask
   b. Large-bore peripheral intravenous catheters
   c. Ringer's lactate at twice maintenance
   d. Cross-match
   e. Draw diagnostic tests
2. With shock
   a. Oxygen by mask or endotracheal tube
   b. Large-bore peripheral intravenous catheters and/or central line
   c. Ringer's lactate 20 cc/kg infused over 5 minutes and repeated as needed
   d. Draw diagnostic tests
   e. Insert urinary catheter

Table 41.9. Routine Tests of Hemostasis

Test	*Normal Value*	*Abnormal Disease State*
Platelet count	150,000–300,000/μl	Thrombocytopenia 2° to increased destruction or decreased production
Bleeding Time	<9 minutes	von Willebrand's disease, abnormal platelet function, collagen-vascular disease
PT	11.0–14.0 sec	Factor deficiency (VII, X, V, II, I), coumadin therapy
PTT	24–36 sec	Factor deficiency (XII, XI, IX, VIII, X, V, II, I), factor inhibitors (e.g., lupus anticoagulant), von Willebrand's disease, heparin therapy
Fibrinogen	>150 mg/dl	Hypofibrinogenemia (DIC, liver disease, primary fibrinogenolysis), dysfibrinogenemia
Thrombin time	<17 sec	Dysfibrinogenemia, hypofibrinogenemia, heparin therapy
Reptilase Time	<24 sec	Dysfibrinogenemia, hypofibrinogenemia, heparin therapy
FDP	Absent	DIC, intravascular thromobosis, primary fibrinogenolysis

ous blood products and their uses are shown in **Table 41.10.** Under usual circumstances, the specific replacement blood product is administered. However, the benefits of an increased hemoglobin with its improved oxygen-carrying capacity or improved coagulation due to increased clotting factors or platelet count must be weighed against the risks of transfusing blood products. The dangers include microaggregates, anaphylaxis, hemolysis, coagulopathy, metabolic derangements, infection, alloimmunization, and graft-versus-host disease (GVHD)[92,93]. During massive transfusion, many of the blood components may be given, exposing the recipient to multiple donors, thus increasing the risks of adverse reaction. Consequently, some authors[94] have recommended the use of ultrafresh whole blood, drawn within 4 hours of administration. Others[95], however, have found this unnecessary and use only fractionated products.

Alterations in Blood as a Result of Storage

Most blood for transfusion is collected from volunteer donors and then fractionated into components—PRBC, platelet concentrates, FFP, and cryoprecipitate—within 6 hours of collection to enable component specific replacement. The red blood cells are stored in flexible plastic bags at 4° C to decrease their metabolic demands and so improve shelf-life[96–99]. Platelets agglutinate when refrigerated and so are kept at room temperature[100]. Plasma and cryoprecipitate are kept frozen.

Red blood cells undergo significant alteration during storage, accumulating the "lesions of storage"[97,101,102]. Much of the damage is due to loss of membrane surface area and flexibility[97,101,102]. Red cell damage is best correlated with declining adenosine triphosphate (ATP) levels, although the relationship is imperfect. Newer preservation solutions attempt to preserve ATP levels with higher concentrations of dextrose and adenine. Some also contain mannitol to prevent osmotic lysis. The additional volume of the additive results in a final hematocrit of approximately 55%, which improves the flow rate during transfusion. However, the toxicity of the additive solution, particularly the adenine component, is unknown, particularly in neonates requiring large volume transfusion, as well as in patients with renal impairment, since adenine is excreted via the kidney[103,104].

Even with better preservation, up to 1% of cells may undergo osmotic lysis during storage from failure of the sodium-potassium adenosine-triphosphatase (ATPase)-dependent pump. These lysed cells release free hemoglobin and potassium[97]. Moreover, up to 30% of the transfused erythrocytes may be excessively fragile and, therefore, destroyed in the reticuloendothelial system[105]. Furthermore, particulate debris, consisting of red cell, leucocyte, and platelet fragments, as well as fibrin, forms in the buffy coat layer primarily over the first 7 days of storage. Much of this debris is less than 164 μm in diameter[106,107] and is not filtered by standard 170-μm filters. The consequences of infusing these microaggregates are discussed later.

Blood for Massive Transfusion

A consideration of the techniques involved in and the consequences of massive transfusion will serve as an overview of the problems inherent in transfusion therapy. Massive transfusion is usually defined as the replacement of at least one blood volume, estimated as 75 ml/kg for children younger than 1 year of age and for burned children and as 70 ml/kg for all others[108–110]. In pediatrics, the most common problems requiring massive transfusion are orthopedic surgery or surgery for malignant disease, massive trauma, cardiopulmonary bypass surgery, and extracorporeal membrane oxygenation (ECMO). It is important to note that in children the signs of volume loss are often more subtle than in adults. In particular, blood pressure may be preserved, whereas tachycardia may be prominent (see **Table 41.7**)[111].

A seriously ill, hemorrhaging patient may require large volumes of blood products, particularly PRBC, in a short time. In the trauma patient, there will be no blood already cross-matched, and the patient's blood type may not be known. Since a full cross-match takes 45 minutes to an hour, blood is often required before a full cross-match can be completed. Two different strategies may be employed. The United States military approach in both the Korean and the Vietnam wars was to stockpile group O blood containing a low titer of anti-A and anti-B antibody[112]. This diminishes the risk of inducing hemolysis in a group A or group B recipient. Such hemolysis remains a possibility; typing a recipient whose blood volume has been replaced by group O red cells (and plasma in the case of whole blood (WB) transfusion) may be difficult[95]. Switching to type-specific blood after beginning the transfusion with group O WB has been reported to lead to hemolysis due to passively transfused anti-A and anti-B antibodies[112]. Nonetheless, group O PRBC have been extensively used as the initial blood for replacement by the Maryland Institute of Emergency Medical Services Systems, most commonly in the setting of several severely traumatized patients presenting simultaneously[95]. They believe that errors in administration are consequently minimized and report neither hemolysis nor typing difficulties as problems, with only 5 of 170 non-group-O recipients demonstrating serologic evidence of incompatibility after transfusion that averaged 6 units per patient for the group as a whole. Physicians at the University of Pennsylvania similarly recommend uncrossmatched type O blood[113].

An alternative strategy is to begin resuscitation with

Table 41.10. Summary of Blood Components

Components:	Red blood cells
Major indications:	Symptomatic anemia: decreased red cell mass
Action:	Restoration of blood volume, restoration of oxygen-carrying capacity
Not indicated for:	Pharmacologically treatable anemia, coagulation deficiency
Special precautions:	Must be ABO-compatible
Hazards:	Hepatitis, allergic reactions, febrile reactions, HIV
Rate of infusion:	Within 2 hr; for massive loss, fast as patient can tolerate
Components:	Red blood cells, leukocytes removed
Major indications:	Febrile reactions from leukocyte antibodies in patients who require red blood cells
Action:	(See under "Red blood cells" above)
Not indicated for:	Pharmacologically treatable anemia, coagulation deficiency
Special precautions:	Must be ABO-compatible
Hazards:	Hepatitis, HIV
Rate of infusion:	(See under "Red blood cells" above)
Components:	Red blood cells, washed deglycerolized
Major indications:	As above, also IgA sensitization
Action:	(See under "Red blood cells" above)
Not indicated for:	Pharmacologically treatable anemia, coagulation deficiency
Special precautions:	Must be ABO-compatible
Hazards:	Hepatitis, HIV
Rate of infusion:	(See under "Red blood cells" above)
Components:	Whole Blood
Major indications:	Hypoxia with volume deficit, massive transfusion
Action:	Restoration of blood volume and oxygen-carrying capacity
Not indicated for:	Condition responsive to specific component
Special precautions:	Must be ABO-identical; labile coagulation factors deteriorate 24 hr after collection
Hazards:	Hepatitis, allergic reactions, febrile reactions, circulatory overload, HIV
Rate of infusion:	Fast as patient can tolerate for massive loss
Components:	Fresh Frozen Plasma (FFP)
Major indications:	Deficit of plasma coagulation factors
Action:	Source of labile and nonlabile plasma factors
Not indicated for:	Condition responsive to specific concentrate
Special precautions:	Must be ABO-compatible
Hazards:	Allergy, infections (hepatitis, cytomegalovirus, HIV)
Rate of infusion:	Approximately 0.5 ml/kg/min
Components:	Cryoprecipitated antihemolytic factor
Major indications:	Hemophilia A, von Willebrand's disease, hypofibrinogenemia, factor XIII deficiency
Action:	Provides factor VIII, fibrinogen
Not indicated for:	Coagulation defect not defined
Special precautions:	Rapid infusion and frequent repeat doses may be necessary
Hazards:	Hepatitis, HIV
Rate of infusion:	Approximately 10 ml/min
Components:	Platelets
Major indications:	Bleeding from thrombocytopenia or platelet function abnormality
Action:	Improves hemostasis
Not indicated for:	Plasma coagulation deficits, conditions with rapid platelet destruction
Special precautions:	Do not use microaggregate filters
Hazards:	Hepatitis, allergic reactions, febrile reactions, HIV
Rate of infusion:	One unit (from WB) every 10 min (platelet packs obtained by pheresis require longer transfusion times)
Components:	Granulocytes
Major indications:	Neutropenia and infection
Action:	Provides circulating granulocytes
Not indicated for;	Infection responsive to antibiotics
Special precautions:	Do not use microaggregate filters; must be ABO-compatible
Hazards:	Hepatitis, allergic reactions, febrile reactions
Rate of infusion:	One pheresis unit over 2- to 4-hr period; closely observe for reactions

Table 41.11. Various Causes of Bleeding After Cardiopulmonary Bypass[a]

Common (95–99%)
Defective surgical hemostasis
Acquired transient platelet dysfunction
Uncommon (1–5%)
Drug-induced platelet dysfunction (aspirin)
Thrombocytopenia (drug-induced or heparin-induced antibodies, sepsis, posttransfusion purpura, fat emboli)
Vitamin K-dependent factor deficiencies (warfarin, liver dysfunction)
Consumptive coagulopathy (sepsis, cardiogenic shock)
Inherited clotting factor deficiencies or platelet dysfunction
Doubtful significance
Primary fibrinolysis
Heparin (inadequate neutralization, rebound)
Protamine excess

[a]*From Woodman RC and Harker LA, Blood 1990;76:1681, with permission.*

crystalloid solutions (perhaps including hypertonic saline[114,115] and plasma protein fraction or albumin before the blood type of the patient is obtained. The blood type can be determined within 5 minutes if a blood bank technician is immediately available. Gervin and Fisher[116] transfused 875 units of type-specific uncross-matched blood into 160 severely hypovolemic trauma patients who could not be adequately resuscitated with crystalloid solutions alone. No major transfusion reactions were observed, and no incompatibilities were noted on subsequent cross-match even in the 8% of patients who had previously been transfused. If slightly more time is available, or after the initial units have been transfused, an immediate spin saline cross-match may be performed. This will detect almost all clinically significant antibodies[117,118] and can usually be completed within 15 minutes. Advances in electronic technology may soon provide a third alternative. A central laboratory may provide blood types on blood donors and patients previously tested, allowing almost instantaneous verification of donor and recipient blood groups, assuming the recipient has had a blood type performed (e.g., at the time of blood donation)[119].

Once administered, the complications associated with massive transfusion are the result of (a) differences in the transfused blood products compared with those of the patient's unshed blood, (b) dilutional coagulopathies, (c) abnormalities resulting from the underlying disease process, and (d) in the case of cardiopulmonary bypass and ECMO, changes induced by the pump and/or oxygenator itself. Each of these complications is discussed in further detail later in this chapter.

Cardiopulmonary Bypass and ECMO

Cardiopulmonary bypass demands, in essence, a massive transfusion, especially in infants and young children in whom the pump is primed with blood. A number of specific metabolic and hematologic complications are of particular concern to the intensivist: citrate toxicity, microaggregates, and the coagulopathy induced by the pump.

Abbott[120] has shown markedly decreased ionized calcium concentrations during pump perfusion, with citrate levels as high as five times normal even 5 hours after surgery in children in whom blood was used to prime the pump. He suggests decreased citrate clearance due to hypothermia. Because decreased ionized calcium may interfere with contractility, and the postoperative myocardium is often poorly contractile, ionized calcium determinations may be useful in the postoperative period. In their absence, an infusion of calcium chloride (0.3 ml/kg of a 10% solution, maximum 10 ml) can be given as a therapeutic trial in the face of low cardiac output or hypotension. Although the pathologic role of microaggregates on the lung is unclear, in patients on bypass the lung filter is not present. Therefore, microembolic phenomena would affect the systemic vasculature. Such embolization has been postulated as the cause of the confusional state postbypass and 40-μm microaggregate filters are recommended[106].

The hemostatic defects created by cardiopulmonary bypass have been well reviewed[121] and are summarized in **Table 41.11.** A dilutional coagulopathy occurs during bypass that may persist for up to 48 hours, particularly affecting platelet number, fibrinogen, and factor V levels[121]. Neonates may be especially susceptible to this dilutional coagulopathy[122]. Overall, however, most but not all authors agree that the most important change is decreased platelet function resulting from activation while traversing the bypass pump[121,123], with bubble oxygenators causing more damage than the membrane type[124,125]. This results in granule release and poor platelet adhesion and aggregation[123,125–127]. More recently, Kestin et al.[124] suggested that heparinization and its interference with the thrombin-platelet interaction is the primary, and extrinsic, cause of platelet dysfunction after cardiopulmonary bypass. In contrast, Ferraris et al. demonstrated an intrinsic platelet unresponsiveness to thrombin stimulation[128]. Most agree that, whatever the exact mechanism, platelet dysfunction is the primary nonsurgical cause of postoperative bleeding. If bleeding does occur, 1 unit of platelets for each 5 to 7 kg of body weight should be administered[121,127] **(Table 41.12).** A recent trial of fresh blood replacement compared with reconstituted component replacement after cardiopulmonary bypass in children showed decreased blood loss in young children (younger than 2 years of age) who underwent complex cardiac repairs and were given blood less

Table 41.12. Management of Bleeding After Cardiopulmonary Bypass

1. Site
   a. If localized (especially mediastinal tubes), consider local (surgical) source
   b. Several bleeding sites, especially oozing from punctures, suggests systemic coagulopathy
2. Replacement
   a. Platelets: 1 unit per 5–7 kg body weight
   b. If still oozing, consider:
      Fresh frozen plasma 10–15 cc/kg
      Cryoprecipitate 1 unit/3 kg
      More platelets
   c. If available, consider fresh (<48 hr old) whole blood

than 48 hours old[129]. The authors postulate improved platelet function in the fresh blood compared with older platelet concentrate as the reason for the decreased blood loss. They caution, however, that the fresh blood must undergo routine thorough screening for safety and should be irradiated prior to administration to prevent GVHD.

Platelet dysfunction may be ameliorated by the intraoperative use of prostacyclin, which has been shown to also diminish heparin requirements and blood loss[130–133]. Platelet factor 4 and β-thromboglobulin levels, both markers of platelet activation, are lower in prostacyclin-treated patients[132]. While vasodilation and hypotension responsive to volume may occur, they have not been problematic[130,132]. A controlled study of prostacyclin in adult men undergoing cardiopulmonary bypass showed a limited benefit; however, other authors recommend against its routine use[133]. A newer analog, ZK-36, that does not cause hypotension has been shown experimentally to preserve platelet number and prevent myocardial platelet deposition after induced global ischemia and cardiopulmonary bypass and may have greater utility[134]. In another study, the use of the serine proteinase inhibitor aprotinin has also been shown to preserve platelet adhesiveness due to preservation of glycoprotein Ib receptors[135].

Less important mechanisms leading to hemorrhage include primary fibrinolysis and unneutralized heparin (either from too low a dose of protamine or from heparin "rebound" due to the shorter half-life of protamine)[127]. Gundry and colleagues have called into question the existence of this latter phenomenon and cautioned against the empiric and possibly excessive use of protamine in the postoperative period[136]. Moreover, more precise heparinization and protamine reversal may be possible using newer monitoring technology[137]. Furthermore, heparin-coated bypass systems may further decrease the need for systemic heparinization with its attendant risks[138]. Other therapeutic interventions include desmopressin acetate (DDAVP), which was initially reported to reduce blood loss in patients undergoing cardiac surgery[139]. However, other studies show no benefit and even suggest increased loss in the DDAVP-treated group[140,141]. Finally, as mentioned above, the serine proteinase inhibitor aprotinin has been shown to reduce significantly transfusion requirements after cardiopulmonary bypass[135,142–144]. Several small pediatric trials have not demonstrated significant utility in decreasing postoperative blood loss despite variable dosage regimens and have raised the concern of induced renal tubular dysfunction[145,146]. A potential adjunctive therapy in managing postoperative bleeding is topical application of fibrin glue[147].

ECMO is increasingly used in pediatrics, particularly for neonatal pulmonary disease, as discussed elsewhere in this textbook. Thrombotic and bleeding complications are important causes of ECMO-associated morbidity and mortality. Again, platelet activation in the extracorporeal circuit with subsequent platelet dysfunction is an important contributor to these problems[121,123]. Meticulous control of heparinization, perhaps through the use of activated clotting times, may help limit the risk[148]. Thromboresistant circuits using heparin-bonded tubing, thus decreasing or eliminating the need for systemic heparinization, have been used in Europe[149,150] and Japan[151] and will be undergoing trial in North America[152]. Deficiencies of multiple clotting factors during the initiation of ECMO may also contribute to the bleeding diathesis in these patients[153].

Complications of Blood Transfusion

HEMOLYSIS. The most catastrophic complication after red blood cell transfusion is a major hemolytic transfusion reaction. This is most commonly due to an ABO mismatch. In a review of 70 fatal transfusion reactions, Honig and Bove[154] found 44 that were due to acute hemolysis. Forty-two were most likely due to antibody-mediated red cell destruction. Thirty-eight of the 44 cases (86%) were due to ABO incompatibility and 37 of the 44 cases were associated with human error. The most common was clerical error, accounting for 33 of the 37 cases. Of the clerical errors, failure to identify adequately the recipient prior to starting the transfusion occurred in 17 of the 37 incidents (45%)-most frequently in locations where two or more people requested blood for different patients. More recent reviews[155,156] confirm clerical error leading to ABO or, less commonly, Rh-antigen mismatch as the most frequent cause of fatal transfusion reaction. Establishing a system requiring "obsessional" attention to positive identification of the blood specimen, the blood obtained for transfusion and the patient to be transfused can decrease error[155,156]. Other antibodies that have been associated with fatal transfusion reactions include anti-Kell, and probably anti-JKa (Kidd system) antibodies[154,156,157]. Additional hemolytic antibodies include anti-Le (Lewis system) and anti-Fya (Duffy system)[156,158]. Overall, however, blood transfusion has been remarkably safe, with an estimated immediate mortality rate from all causes of 1/422,000 units transfused[154].

METABOLIC ABNORMALITIES. A variety of metabolic abnormalities can be induced by transfused blood. The red cells are commonly depleted of 2,3-DPG[96,97,99] and so have enhanced oxygen affinity. Thus, oxygen unloading to tissues may be impaired[105]. In the situation of massive transfusion, Sohmer and Scott[95] found the most deleterious metabolic effect to be hypothermia. This may be prevented by warming the blood to above 32° C prior to administration[94,115,159]. Hyperkalemia is a potential risk due to the high plasma concentration of potassium in stored blood[95,160]. However, in a patient not already in renal failure, delayed hypokalemia is more likely as the transfused red blood cells regain their normal metabolic function and increase the intracellular concentration of potassium[94,95].

The citrate in the preservative must be metabolized by the tissues, especially the liver. Before it is eliminated, it may chelate covalent cations such as calcium and magnesium[99,159] and so decrease the ionized fractions needed for normal enzyme function. This rarely presents a clinical problem, however, and hypercalcemia has been reported from overly vigorous calcium supplementation[159]. Many transfusionists now recommend the use of calcium only if the ionized calcium is determined to be low or if electrocardiographic changes are seen[94,95,159]. Magnesium deficiency (0.5 mg/dl; normal range, 1.7 to 2.5) has been reported[161], but this occurred in a patient who received 92 units of PRBC, 62 units of platelets, 98 units of FFP, and 36 units of cryoprecipitate from the time of her admission in shock after a motor vehicle accident to her death 44 hours later.

Jaundice may also be seen after massive transfusion, most likely as a result of the large volumes of damaged red cells infused (up to 30% of the total volume), with an underperfused, somewhat poorly functional liver[94]. The free hemoglobin present due to hemolysis during storage must also be cleared[95].

As discussed previously, newer RBC preservation solutions contain additional adenine, a potentially nephrotoxic compound. While this has proven safe for small volume transfusions in neonates[162], the safety of adenine in larger-volume transfusions (such as exchange transfusion or bypass, including ECMO) is unknown. Consequently, the Pediatric Hemotherapy Committee of the American Association of Blood Banks has recommended centrifuging the unit of RBCs, removing the additive, and replacing it at the time of transfusion with another solution such as normal saline or FFP, depending on the clinical circumstances[160].

INFECTION AND GRAFT-VERSUS-HOST DISEASE. Infectious agents may also be transmitted through blood transfusion. Bacterial contamination is rare, but hepatitis B, hepatitis C, cytomegalovirus (CMV), malaria, and the human immunodeficiency virus (HIV) may also be transmitted by transfusion[157,163,164]. The risks of the latter are diminished with the current blood bank screening techniques. In the case of immunocompromised patients, including neonates, oncology patients, and children undergoing or likely to undergo organ transplantation, CMV-negative blood should be sought if the patient is known to be CMV-negative.

Immunocompromised patients are also at risk for GVHD. Before transfusing these children with any blood product likely to contain lymphocytes, the product should be irradiated to kill the lymphocytes. Moreover, because of the high risk of GVHD after transfusion, all directed donor blood products from first-degree relatives should be irradiated, regardless of the immunologic status of the recipient[165,166].

MICROAGGREGATES. Storage of WB or PRBC leads to the accumulation of debris composed of leukocytes, platelets, and fibrin, mostly during the first week[95,106,107]. These particles are mostly in the range of 20 to 170 μm and so are not removed by standard 170-μm filters[107]. Using an optical scattering technique, Reynolds and Simon[107] found the numbers of microaggregates to be similar in units of PRBC and WB. Buffy-coat-depleted RBC units were produced by inverted centrifugation and contained significantly fewer microaggregates. In clinical practice, buffy-coat-poor cells are prepared by a washing technique that requires their use within 24 to 48 hours of preparation. Consequently, they are rarely available in an emergency, nor are they routinely prepared for elective surgery, to diminish wastage if they are not needed. A newer technique involves the filtration of blood at the time of collection[167]. This may decrease not only the risk of alloimmunization and febrile transfusion reactions, but also the risk of transmission of CMV[167–169] and the extent of microaggregate formation, possibly by decreasing the available amount of neutrophil enzymes, such as elastase, in the stored product[167]. These filtration techniques are, however, not readily available at this time.

The clinical importance of microaggregates is controversial. Theoretically, these small clumps can obstruct small vessels in the first capillary bed they traverse, which (except for cardiopulmonary bypass) is the pulmonary vasculature. This could lead to ventilation of unperfused lung (increased dead space) or to severe ventilation-perfusion mismatch if increased lung water accumulates. This was postulated as the cause of death in two soldiers in Vietnam who had received 97 and 27 units of blood, respectively, after nonpulmonary injury and who died of respiratory failure. Autopsy showed multiple pulmonary emboli consisting of amorphous and cellular debris[170]. Subsequent animal studies have shown conflicting results[106]. While some studies have shown increased pulmonary capillary permeability, possibly from humoral factors (e.g., serotonin)[171,172] or microembolism[173], others[174] have shown the importance of concomitant sepsis or the effect of shock alone in generating local microthrombi[106]. Collins et al.[175] showed the importance of concomitant pulmonary injury in a retrospective study of Vietnam combat casualties. Those who had only peripheral injuries showed no difficulties in oxygenation despite massive transfusion, often with old blood given through filters sometimes used until gross clots were visible in the line. There was no difference in arterial oxygen partial pressure (P_aO_2) in those receiving less than 5 units and those receiving over 10 units (average, 24.5 units). Patients with pulmonary injury developed marked hypoxemia, and those with abdominal injury interestingly showed a modest impairment in oxygenation. Thus, transfused microaggregates may play an additive role in subclinical pulmonary injury. Such a supportive role was also seen by Pepe et al.[176], who analyzed factors predicting the development of ARDS. They found an independent role for transfusion of more than 22 units of blood over 12 hours and an augmentation when concomitant sepsis, aspiration, or pulmonary contusion was present.

Overall, these data suggest that it may be prudent to use 40-μm microfilters or washed red blood cells (if available) in patients who have concomitant lung disease or a sepsis syndrome. The importance of microaggregate filtration in patients with SCD with the chest syndrome, probably a combination of infection and infarction[40–42], remains to be defined. It should be noted that microaggregate filters may shed microaggregates during continued use[107,177,178]. Furthermore, forcing blood through a commercially available 20-μm stainless steel mesh micropore filter led to hemolysis of the transfused unit, with death of one infant and near death of another due to what was essentially an iatrogenic massive hemolytic reaction[179]. Newer filters may be more efficient[180,181] without overly slowing the transfusion rate. Nonetheless, they may become blocked if used for multiple transfusions. One group recommends changing filters after approximately 6 units of packed red blood cells[182].

TRANSFUSION-ASSOCIATED LUNG INJURY. In addition to possible lung injury from microaggregates, rarely, ARDS may develop shortly after the transfusion of blood products, most commonly whole blood or fresh frozen plasma. The mechanism appears to be leucoagglutination with subsequent pulmonary sequestration of neutrophils caused by antibodies in the donor plasma. The donors are usually multiparous women. Management is supportive[183,184].

COAGULOPATHY. Stored WB or RBC concentrates contain few functional platelets and decreased levels of coagulation factors, especially the labile factors V and VIII[94,95]. Massive transfusion can, therefore, lead to a dilutional coagulopathy. Cote et al.[109] showed an exponential decay of percent platelet number versus blood volumes replaced (with PRBC and frozen red cells). They also showed recruitment of platelets, since calculation of standard washout curves would have resulted in much lower counts than those observed. The only children who showed abnormal bleeding had fewer than 100,000 platelets per microliter. Prophylactic transfusions of sufficient FFP to maintain normal PT and activated PTT were given, so the role of plasma factors could not be assessed. They recommended transfusion of 0.3 units of platelets per kilogram body weight in surgical patients with platelet counts of less than 100,000 per microliter. Counts et al.[185], in a study of adult trauma patients, supported the importance of the platelet count in predicting abnormal bleeding, particularly when more than 1½ blood volumes were transfused. They found little relation between volume infused and plasma phase coagulation. Mannucci et al.[186] found that the platelet count was correlated with the number of units of WB or PRBC transfused and that the PT and fibrinogen were also correlated, although they were less frequently abnormal. Routine administration of 1 unit of FFP per 3 units of WB and/or PRBC, or of 3 platelet concentrates and 2 FFP for 10 units of WB and/or PRBC yielded no group differences in coagulation parameters or volume of blood replacement required, possibly due to individual variability in the severity of coagulopathy. Therefore, they recommended monitoring the coagulation status during replacement and treating detected abnormalities on an individual basis rather than using predetermined replacement protocols.

Although they also demonstrated a dilutional coagulopathy, unlike Mannucci et al.[186], Hewson et al.[187] showed the major determinant of a prolonged PTT at more than 4 hours from the time of surgery to be the duration of closely antecedent hypotension, presumably a reflection of an induced consumption coagulopathy. They, likewise, recommended careful monitoring of parameters. However, particularly in patients with head injuries, they suggested replacement with PRBC and FFP on a one-to-one basis to prevent dilutional coagulopathy. They did not discuss the use of prophylactic transfusion of platelet concentrates. Faringer et al.[188] found a relatively high incidence of coagulopathy in 44 adult patients who received, within a 24-hour period, more than 10 units of PRBCs preserved with one of the newer storage solutions (AS-1). They have adopted a replacement policy of transfusing platelets for counts less than 100,000/μl, fresh frozen plasma for a prothrombin time more than 1.5 times the normal control, and cryoprecipitate for a fibrinogen concentration less than 100 mg/dl. They feel this is particularly important in the brain-injured patient, although they recognize the controversy in the literature. It is of note that consumption coagulopathy may also be induced during scoliosis surgery[189], because of either bony decortication or extensive tissue injury[190]. Furthermore, albumin given during resuscitation has been shown to decrease levels of fibrinogen, factor VIII, prothrombin, and antithrombin III without increasing FDP, possibly due to decreased liver synthesis[191,192].

When the liver itself is diseased, abnormal coagulation results, since the liver synthesizes fibrinogen, prothrombin, protein C, protein S, antithrombin III, alpha$_2$-macroglobulin, plasminogen, and factors V, VII, IX, X, XI, and XII. This is particularly true in hepatocellular (as opposed to biliary tract) disease. In addition, poor clearance of plasminogen activators and underproduction of inhibitors, mainly alpha-2 antiplasmin and type I plasminogen activator inhibitor, lead to enhanced fibrinolysis[193]. Liver transplantation is being increasingly used as a therapy in end-stage liver disease. During the operation, a median dose of 24 units of PRBC was given to a series of adults[194,195], i.e., a massive transfusion of greater than 2 blood volumes. Blood loss and patient survival have been correlated with preoperative coagulation abnormalities[195], suggesting that preoperative correction may improve outcome. During the procedure itself, increased fibrinolysis was found in the anhepatic phase[194]. Reperfusion of the liver was accompanied by significant worsening of coagulation parameters. Kang et al.[194] postulated that dilution by the perfusion solution, metabolic acidosis, hypothermia, and decreased ionized calcium levels could all be contributory. Careful monitoring and correction with the use of a thromboelastograph decreased the total fluid volume infused from a mean of 31 liters in unmonitored patients to 20 liters in the monitored group. However, the total number of blood product units was similar—about 70 in each group. More units of platelets and cryoprecipitate and fewer units of PRBC and FFP were used in the monitored group[194]. In a series of 200 children, Carlier et al.[196] found similar preoperative, anhepatic, and reperfusion stages compared with those described in adults, although the intraoperative changes in the children were less dramatic than those in adults. In addition, preoperative coagulopathies did not seem to play an important role in predicting the amount of bleeding. Rather, previous abdominal surgery, often related to the cause of the underlying liver disease (e.g., biliary atresia) or to the need for reexploration, was most important. Aprotinin, a serine proteinase inhibitor, has been used with variable success to decrease intraoperative blood loss during hepatic transplantation[(197)].

ANAPHYLAXIS. Anaphylaxis after transfusion is rare and usually occurs in IgA-deficient patients with high-titer anti-IgA antibodies[(157)]. Several previously described cases of noncardiogenic pulmonary edema ascribed to anaphylaxis[(198,199)] may actually represent the transfusion associated lung injury discussed earlier.

Alternatives to Donor Blood Products

The possible hazards of microaggregates, the definite risks of administration errors and transmitted infections, and the myriad other potential complications discussed above have forced a reappraisal of when blood should be administered and have encouraged research into non-blood-replacement therapy. Obviously, there are situations when blood is life saving and the lack of blood will certainly lead to death. However, various recent studies call into question the commonly employed practice of transfusing patients at an arbitrarily set hematocrit or hemoglobin concentration. The "transfusion triggers" commonly used for transfusion of preoperative or critically ill patients are a hematocrit of 30% or an oxygen extraction ratio (i.e., oxygen consumption/oxygen delivery) of 50%[(92,200)]. However, in a group of 32 adult patients with septic or cardiogenic shock who had undergone initial fluid resuscitation with non-blood-containing solutions, transfusion of red blood cells caused an increase in Hb concentration from 8.3 to 10.5 g/dl but did not alter oxygen consumption or lactate concentrations[(201)]. Similarly, in a study of adult baboons, acute hemodilution causing a decrease in hematocrit from 33.2 to 14.9% did not alter oxygen consumption[(202)]. In both of these studies, the key appears to have been the maintenance of euvolemia that permitted an increase in cardiac output sufficient to permit adequate oxygen delivery. Moreover, in the baboon study, an oxygen extraction ratio of 60% was achieved with no increase in lactate production. The authors therefore questioned whether a 50% extraction ratio should be used as an absolute indication for transfusion[(201)]. On the other hand, in a study of 1-month-old lambs, Heusser and colleagues found that although anemic lambs could increase their cardiac output to maintain oxygen delivery under baseline conditions, when they were acutely stressed by decreasing the cardiac output, the most anemic lambs demonstrated a decrease in oxygen consumption with a rise in lactate concentration at a higher cardiac output than did the lambs with higher hematocrits[(203)]. While this is not surprising, it illustrates very well the fact that increased oxygen extraction above 50% leaves little room for additional stresses on the patient. Thus, we are still faced with the dilemma of weighing the risks of transfusion against the increased margin of safety provided by a higher hematocrit. At present, there seems to be no absolute answer in the unstable patient, but in the stable, volume-replete child, the routine transfusion at a hematocrit of 30% would seem inappropriate. Future studies are needed to determine whether and under what conditions the trigger can be safely lowered to a hematocrit of 20%[(92,93,200)].

How low the hematocrit can be safely lowered has also become a major ethical and legal issue regarding patients with religious interdictions to transfusion, such as the Jehovah's Witnesses. Members of this group believe that receiving transfusions of blood products violates the biblical proscription against ingesting blood. Members who are transfused are believed to have sinned and are excommunicated[(204)]. Some courts have upheld the wishes of competent adult Jehovah's Witnesses, and physicians have been forced to allow a patient to die rather than receive a transfusion[(204,205)]. In the case of a child, the court will usually overrule the wishes of the parents if the child's life is in danger. However, comprehensive care of the child demands that we should attempt to follow the requests of the parents if at all possible. Therefore, in this group of patients, determining the lowest safe "transfusion trigger" is particularly important, and the search for a blood transfusion alternative takes on even greater importance. Further consideration of the legal and ethical issues surrounding the care of pediatric Jehovah's Witnesses is beyond the scope of this chapter and has been reviewed in recent articles[(205,206)].

One approach to avoiding donor blood transfusion in the nonemergency situation is acute limited normovolemic hemodilution. This technique involves reducing the patient's hematocrit to about 20% by withdrawal of blood while simultaneously infusing Ringer's lactate. The withdrawn blood can later be reinfused[(207)]. Strict attention must be paid to maintaining normovolemia[(208)]. In addition, while usually safe for young patients, conditions that increase the risk of myocardial ischemia, such as aortic stenosis, must be kept in mind[(208,209)]. Blood incompatibility and transmitted infections could also be averted through transfusion of the patient's own shed blood lost during surgery. In the context of massive transfusion, this entails the use of surgical suction techniques and scavenging devices that can safely harvest shed blood and prepare it for reinfusion by removing contaminating organisms, air, and microemboli while minimizing hemolysis[(210–212)]. A final alternative to the risks of blood transfusion, and perhaps, to the objections of Jehovah's Witnesses, is the use of blood substitutes. These alternatives are polymerized free hemoglobin, encapsulated hemoglobin solutions, and perfluorochemical emulsions[(213,214)]. While some of these show promise, none has yet been of demonstrated clinical benefit without significant toxicity or potential toxicity. However, ongoing research will likely result in improved products of clinical utility[(213–218)].

Miscellaneous

Before leaving the topic of transfusion therapy, mention should be made of the striking hypotension seen occasionally (by us and others) during rapid infusion of FFP in postoperative cardiac and burn patients. Whether this represents activation of various kinins[(219)], acute binding of ionized calcium, or an as-yet not understood mechanism, it has led us to adopt the practice of infusing plasma (and platelets) relatively slowly (i.e., over more than 20 minutes) in these patients. If rapid volume infusion is required, a crystalloid or 5% albumin solution is infused.

PATHOPHYSIOLOGY OF HEMOSTASIS AND THROMBOSIS

The clinician in the ICU is often faced with perturbations in the delicate balance between hemostasis and thrombosis. When a blood vessel is damaged, subendothelial collagen and tissue factor are exposed, leading to recruitment of platelets to form a hemostatic plug. The platelet plug serves as a surface for blood coagulation reactions triggered by tissue factor, leading to the stepwise activation of the fluid phase of coagulation to produce a fibrin clot. This complex cascade process is held in check by anticoagulants, including protein C, protein S, and antithrombin III. The clot is ultimately lysed by the fibrinolytic system as repair to the vessel and extravascular tissue occurs. This section will deal with the separate components of the hemostatic process—the blood vessel, the cellular phase (platelets), and the fluid phase (coagulation factors) in healthy individuals and will address several specific pathophysiologic conditions that the ICU physician is likely to encounter.

Vessel Wall

The endothelial cell wall is not a passive conduit to blood flow but is an active responder to cytokines in the circulation and an active secretor of both procoagulant and anticoagulant proteins. Endothelial cells (ECs) are the major site of synthesis of bioactive molecules involved in hemostasis—collagen, laminin, fibronectin, and von Willebrand's factor (VWF) which provide sites of attachment for platelets and leukocytes. Abnormalities in these proteins, such as Ehlers-Danlos disease or von Willebrand's disease (VWD) may result in serious bleeding. ECs also express a number of anticoagulant properties. They inhibit platelet adherence and aggregation through prostacyclin production (PGI_2)[(220,221)]. They provide binding sites for thrombin that allow thrombin to be inactivated by antithrombin III[(222)], thus preventing intravascular thrombosis. They have cell surface cofactor sites for antithrombin III that catalyze the inactivation process for circulating thrombin[(223)]. They express a thrombin receptor (thrombomodulin) that, in addition to inactivating the clot-promoting activities of thrombin, forms a complex that activates protein C[(224)], a potent inhibitor of plasma phase coagulation. Protein C, when attached to a surface by protein S[(225–227)], inactivates factors V and VIII. Finally, the endothelial cell enhances clot dissolution by endothelial cell-mediated tissue plasminogen activator (tPA) release.

Platelets

Platelets are small (3 to 4 μm in diameter and 1 μm in depth), discoid-shaped, anuclear cells derived from megakaryocytes in the bone marrow[(228)]. Maturation time is approximately 4 to 5 days, and they circulate for approximately 10 days under normal conditions. Newly formed platelets are larger and more hemostatically active than older ones.

The role of platelets has been extensively reviewed[(229–231)]. Briefly, when vascular integrity is disrupted, collagen is exposed. Collagen is a very potent stimulus for platelet adhesion, and in the presence of VWF, adhesion of platelets to the disrupted area occurs. As they adhere, the platelets swell and become sticky. The exogenous adenosine diphosphate (ADP) available then leads to the primary aggregation response. Subsequently, the "release reaction" occurs, in which the contents of the granules within platelets are extruded. The dense granules contain endogenous ADP, serotonin, and other stimulants of aggregation that lead to a secondary wave of irreversible aggregation. Of particular importance is the role of thromboxane A_2 in stimulating this secondary aggregation. Thromboxane A_2 is a metabolite of the cyclo-oxygenase pathway of arachidonic acid metabolism. It and serotonin both promote vascular constriction as well as platelet aggregation. Cyclo-oxygenase inhibitors and prostacyclin (produced by the endothelium) oppose this constriction and aggregation[(232)]. However, usually, the release reaction and secondary aggregation lead to an amplification of the hemostatic response until a clot is formed. Clot consolidation then occurs through the interaction of platelets and endothelium with the coagulation cascade. Finally, clot retraction occurs.

The platelet membrane is exceedingly important for its extracellular interactions and as a target of immunologic destruction. For example, glycoprotein Ib is the main receptor for adhesion to VWF. Fibrinogen binds to glycoprotein IIb-IIIa and acts as a bridge between adjacent platelets. Deficiencies of these surface glycoproteins (Bernard-Soulier syndrome and Glanzmann's thrombasthenia, respectively) results in platelet functional disorders[(228)]. Two diallelic platelet antigen systems have been identified on the surface—the PL^{A1} and PL^{B1} antigens. Of these, PL^{A1} is of greater clinical importance, since it is maternal sensitization to this antigen that leads to the majority of cases of neonatal isoimmune thrombocytopenia[(233)]. Finally, the human lymphocyte antigen (HLA) system is thought to be responsible for up to 75% of cases of alloimmunization seen in patients requiring frequent transfusions[(234)].

Platelet disorders leading to inadequate hemostasis can be considered in terms of insufficient numbers (thrombocy-

Table 41.13. Etiology of Thrombocytopenia

1. Decreased production
   a. Bone marrow suppression
      i. Chemotherapy
      ii. Radiation therapy
      iii. Other drugs
   b. Aplastic anemia
   c. Malignancy
   d. Congenital amegakaryocytosis
   e. HIV
2. Accelerated destruction or loss (nonimmune)
   a. Congenital
      i. TORCH (toxoplasmosis, rubella, CMV, herpes) infections
      ii. Giant hemangioma (Kasabach-Merritt syndrome)
   b. Acquired
      i. HUS, TTP
      ii. Infection
      iii. DIC
      iv. Necrotizing enterocolitis
      v. Massive transfusion
      vi. Hypersplenism
      vii. Hypothermia
3. Accelerated destruction or loss (immune)
   a. Infection
   b. Idiopathic thrombocytopenia purpura
   c. Neonatal passive immunization
   d. Autoimmune disorders
   e. Drug-induced

topenia) or defective action (thrombocytopathy). Thrombocytopenia can be due to inadequate production or accelerated loss or destruction of platelets. A platelet count between 50,000 and 100,000/μl is often sufficient to permit normal hemostasis during a surgical procedure. If the count is between 20,000 and 50,000/μl, hemostasis is less likely to be achieved during surgery, although it may be if most of the circulating platelets are young. Finally, if the count is less than 20,000/μl, the risk of spontaneous bleeding becomes significant. The causes of thrombocytopenia are numerous **(Table 41.13).** Inadequate production may be due to malignancy, chemotherapy, or aplasia. Accelerated destruction or loss may be due to immune or nonimmune mechanisms.

Defective platelet function is a less common cause of significant bleeding in children requiring intensive care, except for the problems seen after cardiopulmonary bypass or ECMO, as discussed earlier. There are many causes of acquired thrombocytopathy. Of these, drug-induced defects must be emphasized **(Table 41.14),** since many of the drugs implicated are administered to critically ill children. Because children in ICUs are often at risk for bleeding, these drugs may aggravate the situation.

The diagnosis of defective hemostasis resulting from platelet inadequacies is made on the basis of clinical and laboratory findings. Clinically, petechiae, purpura, and easy bleeding and bruising suggest the diagnosis. Historically, symptoms of a more generalized disorder, such as malignancy or renal failure, may point to the cause. Similarly, the physical examination may differentiate between multisystem disease and a specific platelet disorder. Laboratory investigation should include a complete blood count and examination of the blood smear. Tests for PT, PTT, and FDP should be performed to exclude DIC.

Decreased platelet number suggests a production failure or enhanced destruction. In the absence of a known underlying marrow-infiltrating disorder such as leukemia, immune destruction is most likely in the general pediatric population (i.e., outside the ICU setting). In the neonate, this is most frequently due to transplacentally transferred anti-PL^{A1} or anti-HLA IgG antibody (alloimmune destruction)[235,236]. In the older child, the autoimmune destruction is due to idiopathic thrombocytopenic purpura. A bone marrow aspiration, and occasionally a bone marrow biopsy, may be necessary to confirm adequate megakaryocyte numbers, thus excluding marrow failure. In the ICU setting, decreased production from secondary effects of illness or medication and enhanced destruction due to consumption, often from sepsis-related DIC, are more prominent. Again, bone marrow aspiration and/or biopsy is occasionally required to confirm adequate production, especially if the enhanced destruction of DIC or other disorders like hemolytic uremic syndrome (HUS) cannot be otherwise confirmed. Confirmation of alloimmune destruction in the neonate may often be possible by determination of maternal, paternal, and infant PL^{A1} type, and by a search for anti-PL^{A1} antibody. In the absence of anti-PL^{A1}, anti-HLA antibody should be sought[237–239]. If no antibody is detected, a bone marrow examination is necessary to exclude congenital amegakaryocytosis.

In the face of a normal platelet count and a normal PT and PTT with a negative FDP assay, a bleeding time should be determined to confirm the suspicion of thrombocytopathy. An abnormally long bleeding time may result from abnormal blood vessels (seen occasionally in the heritable connective tissue disorders), decreased platelet numbers

Table 41.14. Drugs That Inhibit Platelet Function[a]

Nonsteroidal anti-inflammatory drugs	Aspirin, ibuprofen, indomethacin, naproxen, and others
Antibiotics	Penicillins, cephalosporins, nitrofurantoin
Cardiovascular drugs	Dipyridamole, diltiazem, propranolol, sodium nitroprusside, verapamil, nifedipine, nitroglycerin
Anticoagulant, fibrinolytic, and antifibrinolytics	Epsilon aminocaproic acid, heparin, protamine, alteplase
Anesthetics and narcotics	Benzocaine, cocaine, lidocaine, procaine, tetracaine, halothane, heroin
Psycotropic drugs	Amitriptyline, haloperidol, imiprimine, nortriptyline, chlorpromazine
Chemotherapy	L-asparaginase, vincristine, carmustine, daunorubicin
Antihistamines	Chlorpheniramine, diphenhydramine
Other drugs	Guaifenesin, dextran, pseudoephedrine

[a]*Adapted from George JN and Shattil SJ, N Engl J Med 1991;324:31.*

below 50,000/μl, or deficient platelet function. A prolonged bleeding time with normal platelet numbers thus suggests platelet dysfunction or a microvascular defect[(229,230)]. In the ICU, platelet dysfunction will most commonly be due to medication (e.g., salicylates, antibiotics). von Willebrand's disease (VWD), a decrease or dysfunction of the factor VIII antigen (VIII:Ag) and its multimeric aggregates (the ristocetin cofactor activity, Rcof), may also lead to a prolonged bleeding time because ristocetin cofactor binds platelet to platelet and platelet to vessel wall by attaching to glycoprotein Ib, and possibly, the IIb/IIIa complex, on the platelet surface. The diagnosis is made by determination of factor VIII coagulant levels (VIII:C), factor VIII:Ag, and ristocetin cofactor and, occasionally, by crossed immunoelectrophoresis or sodium dodecyl sulfate (SDS) gel electrophoresis. Family history is helpful, since classic VWD is inherited as an autosomal dominant disorder[(240)]. Intrinsic platelet defects, such as those seen in thrombasthenia, storage pool disease, Bernard-Soulier syndrome, and the Grey platelet syndrome, are much less common. They require aggregation studies and, occasionally, platelet electron microscopy for diagnosis[(241)].

Platelet Transfusion

In most instances, platelets are prepared for transfusion from a single unit of whole blood. Current collection procedures recover approximately 85% of the platelets in a single unit of whole blood. The platelets are suspended in 50 to 70 mL of donor plasma and are stored for up to 5 days at 22° C (platelet concentrate). In some instances, a large quantity of platelets can be harvested from a single individual by apheresis. A typical apheresis product contains the approximate equivalent of 6 units of platelet concentrate. For young children or patients in congestive heart failure, the platelets can be further concentrated, but with a potential 5 to 10% decrease in the number of platelets available for transfusion[(242)].

A rough guide to the dosage of platelets to be transfused in the nondestructive setting is one unit of random donor platelets per 5 to 7 kg of body weight or 5 units per m^2 of body surface area. This will raise the platelet count within 15 minutes upon completion of the transfusion by 50,000/μl[(242)]. A platelet count obtained at this time (when the tubing is being disconnected) will be an accurate measure of the efficacy of the transfusion. A count significantly lower than that expected must raise the possibility of alloimmunization (discussed below) or other causes of platelet destruction. Clinical situations that may result in posttransfusion platelet counts lower than expected are listed in **Table 41.15.** In practice, many clinicians will transfuse one unit per 5 to 7 kg of body weight in patients requiring multiple transfusions in an attempt to decrease the frequency of transfusions.

There are multiple potential complications from platelet transfusions. The risks of infectious complications is generally greater than those from RBC transfusions because the typical patient receiving platelet transfusions is being exposed to multiple donors per transfusion. Transfusion reactions are not uncommon and can be classified as either febrile or allergic. Febrile reactions are caused by alloreactive antibodies in the recipient's plasma that react with antigens on transfused platelets or accompanying white blood cells[(243,244)]. Pretreatment with antipyretics and leukocyte depletion of future transfusions is usually successful in blocking further febrile reactions. Allergic reactions manifested by skin rash, pruritus, hives, or even anaphylaxis are caused by previous sensitization of the recipient to plasma protein components in the transfusion. If an allergic reaction begins to develop, the platelet transfusion should be held until antihistamines (diphenhydramine) and, if needed, steroids are administered. The infusion may be resumed once the patient stabilizes. Leukocyte depletion will not prevent this problem, but premedication with steroids and antihistamines will be successful in most patients. The platelets may be washed free of plasma, but with some loss of platelet number.

One cause of poor response to platelet transfusions that deserves special mention is alloimmunization in the multiply transfused patient. Patients who have been pregnant or exposed to multiple blood products may develop antibodies to HLA class I antigens that are expressed on platelets and white blood cells that contaminate platelet and red blood cell transfusions. Patients who are immunosuppressed are less likely to develop alloantibodies, but often these are the patients who receive the most transfusions (e.g., oncology patients) and may therefore still develop alloantibodies. Use of single-donor platelets and leukocyte depletion filters may help delay the development of alloimmunization[(234)]. Ultraviolet irradiation of platelet products, which reduces the HLA antigen stimulus to alloantibody production[(245)], is being examined in a prospective study. Cross-matching of platelets is available only at a limited number of institu-

Table 41.15. Variables Resulting in Decreased Posttransfusion Platelet Count[a]

Platelet Component
Donor platelet count
Technique of platelet collection
Platelet component age
Storage conditions
Infusion time
Blood filter type
Leukocyte removal
Reducing platelet plasma volume
Washing platelets
Clinical Condition
Fever
Sepsis
DIC
Hepatosplenomegaly
Alloantibodies
Massive blood loss
HUS/TTP
Necrotizing enterocolitis

[a]*From Nugent DJ. In: Nathan DG and Oski FA. Hematology of infancy and childhood. Philadelphia: WB Saunders, 1993:1784.*

tions on an experimental basis. Treatment of the patient with alloimmunization requires judicious use of blood products and the use of platelets obtained from HLA class I compatible donors.

Treatment of Selected Thrombocytopenias and Thrombocytopathies

Malignancy

The most common causes of inadequate platelet production in children are malignant diseases and their treatment. In the ICU setting, the child with malignant disease is often at risk for bleeding—indeed, bleeding is one of the most common causes of death. The child may bleed spontaneously, resulting in intracranial disaster, pulmonary hemorrhage, or life-threatening gastrointestinal bleeding[(88)], or the child may bleed because of an invasive procedure (e.g., endotracheal intubation, urinary catheterization). In view of these risks, some centers prophylactically transfuse all nonalloimmunized children in the effort to maintain their platelet count over 20,000/μl. This approach is not universally employed[(246–248)] because of the risk of alloimmunization and the questionable long-term benefit. Even if prophylactic therapy is not used routinely, we believe platelet infusions prior to central venous catheterization or lumbar puncture should be employed. Children with brain tumors or recent CNS surgery should have their platelet count maintained at a level of 50,000/μl to prevent spontaneous intracranial bleeding. Furthermore, there is little debate that significant bleeding in this patient population warrants immediate platelet transfusion[(249)]. The recent identification and cloning of a cytokine to stimulate marrow production of platelets (thrombopoietin) should lead to the development of a clinically available agent to ameliorate thrombocytopenia in patients with deficient production and hopefully decrease the transfusion requirements of these patients[(250)].

Dilutional Thrombocytopenia

As discussed earlier, thrombocytopenia can develop after massive transfusion needed for surgery or trauma. In these patients, it is essential to exclude a surgically treatable cause of bleeding even if thrombocytopenia is present. Furthermore, correction of abnormalities in the plasma phase of coagulation is often needed (i.e., FFP administration). In the postoperative period, platelet transfusion is usually administered if the platelet count is less than 50,000/μl. If the count is between 50,000 and 100,000/μl, transfusion is not needed unless the child is actively bleeding. As discussed earlier, bleeding can occur in postoperative cardiac surgical patients as a result of platelet dysfunction even if the actual count exceeds 100,000/μl.

Infection and Thrombocytopenia

Another nonimmune cause of thrombocytopenia that may result in bleeding responsive to platelet infusion is excessive destruction due to infection. The disorders of platelets seen in infectious disease arise from a number of mechanisms[(251–253)]. These include activation of the coagulation cascade, direct platelet damage, immune mechanisms, and deposition due to collagen exposure. Platelet infusion may correct the thrombocytopenia, although this effect will be short-lived and can only be considered as an interim measure until the infection is controlled.

Miscellaneous

Some nonimmune mechanisms of destructive thrombocytopenia that are unlikely to be responsive to platelet infusions include the microangiopathic anemias, such as HUS and thrombotic thrombocytopenic purpura (TTP)[(254,255)]. Consumption in a giant hemangioma (Kasabach-Merritt syndrome) or sequestration in an enlarged, overactive spleen (hypersplenism) may also result in only a brief response to platelet infusion.

Idiopathic Thrombocytopenic Purpura

Patients with immune-mediated thrombocytopenias are unlikely to demonstrate an increase in their platelet counts in response to platelet infusion[(235,236,238,256–258)]. Of these, the most common disorder in children is ITP. Acute ITP is typically seen in children aged 2 to 6 years during the colder months. The cause is uncertain, although the disorder often follows a viral infection. Clinically, the child usually exhibits petechiae and oozing from the mucous membranes. Signs and symptoms of bone marrow infiltrative disorders, such as fever, bone pain, lymphadenopathy, and hepatosplenomegaly should be absent. Given this constellation of signs and symptoms, some authors question the need for bone marrow examination, but others feel an aspiration must be performed to exclude malignancy or aplastic anemia, however unlikely[256,258 259)]. ITP is usually self-limited, resolving within 1 month[(235,257,258)].

Acute ITP of childhood is usually caused by the production of autoantibodies which bind to platelets, resulting in their destruction by the reticuloendothelial system. ITP rarely requires any therapy other than observation, much less an ICU admission. While gingival bleeding and mild hematuria are common, serious bleeding is rare. For example, the incidence of serious intracranial hemorrhage was previously estimated at 1 to 5%, but more recently it has been suggested that the incidence is less than 1%[(258,260,261)]. In view of the low risk of intracranial hemorrhage, prophylactic therapy has been increasingly questioned. Nonetheless, many hematologists still advocate the use of steroids or intravenous immunoglobulin therapy for children with acute ITP and platelet counts under 20,000/μl[(256,258,262)]. Both prednisone (4 mg/kg/day) and intravenous gamma-globulin treatment result in fewer days with a platelet count less than 20,000/μl compared with patients receiving no treatment[(263)]. High-dose intravenous methylprednisolone therapy (30 mg/kg/day for 3 days) has also been shown to be effective in rapidly increasing the platelet count[(264)]. The advantage of steroids over intravenous IgG is principally that the former are much cheaper and easier to administer. However, since corticosteroids are an integral part of therapy for leukemia, it is essential to rule out leukemia by bone marrow examination before instituting steroid therapy.

Rarely, bleeding will be of such a magnitude that it becomes critical. Serious bleeding in acute ITP is a problem, since a simple platelet infusion is ineffective in raising the count for any significant period(249,265,266), and therapy with IgG or high-dose steroids may not have a sufficiently rapid effect on the platelet count. In the event of life-threatening bleeding, all these measures, including transfusion, should be employed. Emergency splenectomy may be performed in cases of serious bleeding, since the spleen is the site of destruction of the antibody-coated platelets. After splenectomy, platelet survival is prolonged and hemostasis can be secured. However, splenectomy raises the long-term risks of serious infection and thus should not be undertaken unless absolutely essential.

Neonatal Thrombocytopenia

The neonate merits special consideration in any discussion of thrombocytopenia. Nonimmune mechanisms of thrombocytopenia include giant hemangioma and congenital infection **(Table 41.13).** The immune mechanisms that must be considered are (a) passive immunization acquired from the mother with ITP or other forms of immune thrombocytopenia and (b) isoimmunization of these infants that arises because a PL^{A1}-negative mother has been previously sensitized to PL^{A1}-positive platelets, and the infant has PL^{A1}-positive platelets. This latter disorder resembles red cell alloimmunization(267–270), although it is more likely to occur with the first pregnancy than is, for example, Rh hemolytic disease. Therapy of isoimmune neonatal thrombocytopenia includes transfusion of PL^{A1}-negative platelets. Antenatal treatment with steroids and intravenous gamma globulin may be helpful in preventing neonatal intracranial hemorrhage(267). Passive immune thrombocytopenia is most often treated expectantly, although steroids and intravenous IgG have been used(236,271).

Thrombocytopathy

As pointed out earlier, thrombocytopenia is a more common cause of hemorrhage than is thrombocytopathy. Nonetheless, it is important to note that there are congenital disorders of platelet function, such as Bernard-Soulier syndrome and Glanzmann's thrombasthenia(241), as well as acquired causes, particularly drugs **(Table 41.14).** Patients with congenital disorders may require platelet transfusions in spite of having a normal platelet count. The acquired defects include renal disease, which can also cause accelerated destruction(272). Antibiotics are well known to cause hemostatic defects(273–275), as are some anticonvulsant medications(276,277). Of greatest importance are the cyclo-oxygenase inhibitors, such as aspirin and indomethacin(229,230,278). Therapy for bleeding in these cases is most often directed at identifying and removing the offending drug. If the drug causes irreversible platelet defects, such as defects in cyclo-oxygenase inhibition produced by aspirin, and if bleeding is severe, platelet transfusion may be required.

von Willebrand's Disease

VWD is the most common inherited bleeding disorder, with approximately 0.01% of the population having symptomatic disease and 1% of the population having detectable abnormalities in the VWD protein(279). Although VWD is actually a defect in the fluid phase of coagulation, it is grouped here with platelet disorders because of the platelet dysfunction that occurs due to abnormalities in the von Willebrand's factor (VWF). As mentioned previously, VWF is responsible for the adherence of platelets to damaged endothelium, primarily due to its interaction with the platelet membrane glycoprotein Ib. It is also involved with platelet-platelet aggregation via the platelet membrane protein glycoprotein IIb/IIIa(280). Classification of VWD is based on partial quantitative deficiency of VWF (Type 1), qualitative defects (Type 2), or near complete deficiency of VWF (Type 3)(279). VWF circulates as a noncovalent complex in blood with factor VIII and is responsible for the production and survival of factor VIII(281). Thus, laboratory studies of patients with VWD will show a prolonged bleeding time (due to defective platelet adherence to subendothelial collagen), and prolongation of the PT and PTT (due to decreased levels of factor VIII). Specific assays for VWD involve the measurement of VWF activity using the antibiotic ristocetin and agarose gel electrophoresis of VWF.

The range of clinical bleeding seen in VWD is quite broad. Many patients have no clinical bleeding and are diagnosed because of prolongation of the bleeding time or PTT during preoperative evaluations. Others have significant bleeding which is primarily mucosal-epistaxis, menorrhagia, and postoperative. Treatment is based on providing adequate levels of functional VWF. Approximately 80% of patients with VWD will achieve normal hemostasis with infusion of desmopressin acetate (DDAVP, 0.3 μg/kg IV over 15 to 30 minutes in isotonic saline)(282). This response is due to the ability of DDAVP to stimulate release of VWF/factor VIII complex from endothelial stores and is therefore useful for patients with Type 1 disease (mild quantitative deficiency) and avoids the use of blood-derived protein. In patients with Type 2 or Type 3 VWD, DDAVP is not likely to provide adequate hemostasis. These patients have traditionally been treated with FFP or cryoprecipitate. However, these products continue to carry a significant risk of transmission of viral diseases, and most hematologists prefer to treat patients with significant VWD with purified factor VIII products that contain high titers of functional VWF (e.g., Humate-P). The usual dose is 50 U/kg IV every 24 hours in patients at prolonged risk of extensive bleeding. Epsilon aminocaproic acid (Amicar), an inhibitor of fibrinolysis, is

Table 41.16. Nomenclature of Coagulation Factors

Factor	*Synonym*
I	Fibrinogen
II	Prothrombin
III	Tissue thromboplastin
IV	Calcium
V	Proaccelerin
VII	Proconvertin
VIII:C	Antihemophilic factor A
IX	Christmas factor
X	Stuart-Prower factor
XI	Plasma thromboplastin antecedent
XII	Hageman factor
XIII	Fibrin-stabilizing factor

a useful perioperative adjunct for patients with VWD, particularly those undergoing oral and genitourinary procedures.

Plasma Phase of Coagulation

Coagulation

The formation of a platelet plug will temporarily stop bleeding. This plug is then solidified by the generation of a fibrin clot through the combined action of the coagulation factors, which are listed in **Table 41.16.** A cascade of enzymatic reactions by the coagulation proteins is triggered, resulting in the generation of thrombin and a fibrin mesh network that combines with the platelets, resulting in the stable clot. The cascade classically has been divided into two pathways: (a) the surface-activated intrinsic system consisting of factors XII, XI, IX, and VIII, which is tested in the laboratory by the activated partial thromboplastin time (PTT), and (b) the tissue factor-activated extrinsic system, tested by the PT (Fig. 41.2).

Regardless of the method of activation, the product of the clotting cascade is thrombin, which is produced by cleavage of prothrombin through the joint action of Xa, V, and calcium, which normally act at the platelet surface. Once thrombin (factor IIa) is generated from prothrombin, it accelerates the clotting process by activating factors V and VIII and by stimulating platelet aggregation[283].

Thrombin cleaves fibrinopeptides A and B from fibrinogen, leaving fibrin monomer. Fibrin monomers then spontaneously polymerize into large fibers. These fibers are cross-linked by activated factor XIII (XIIIa), which may also further the binding of fibrin to fibronectin and then to collagen, anchoring the clot to connective tissue. Factor XIII is itself activated by thrombin, so that thrombin catalyzes both the formation and the stabilization of the fibrin clot. Various vasoactive fibrinopeptides are also released and stimulate vasoconstriction. The normal clot protects itself from dissolution by the release of plasminogen activator inhibitors from activated platelets and by binding alpha$_2$-antiplasmin to the clot surface[283].

It is important to point out that vitamin K is critical, since it is needed for the activation of several synthesized coagulation proteins by carboxylating critical amino acids. Prothrombin (factor II) as well as factors VII, IX, X, protein C, and protein S must undergo vitamin K dependent processing into functional zymogens. Vitamin K deficiency is therefore associated with a hemorrhagic diathesis. Furthermore, most factors, with the exception of VIII, are synthesized in the liver, so that coagulation will be deranged in severe liver disease.

Fibrinolysis

Without a system of fibrinolysis after clot formation, there would be no possibility of blood resuming its normal flow. Fortunately, normal plasma contains substances that inhibit both thrombin and factor Xa. Moreover, there is a complete

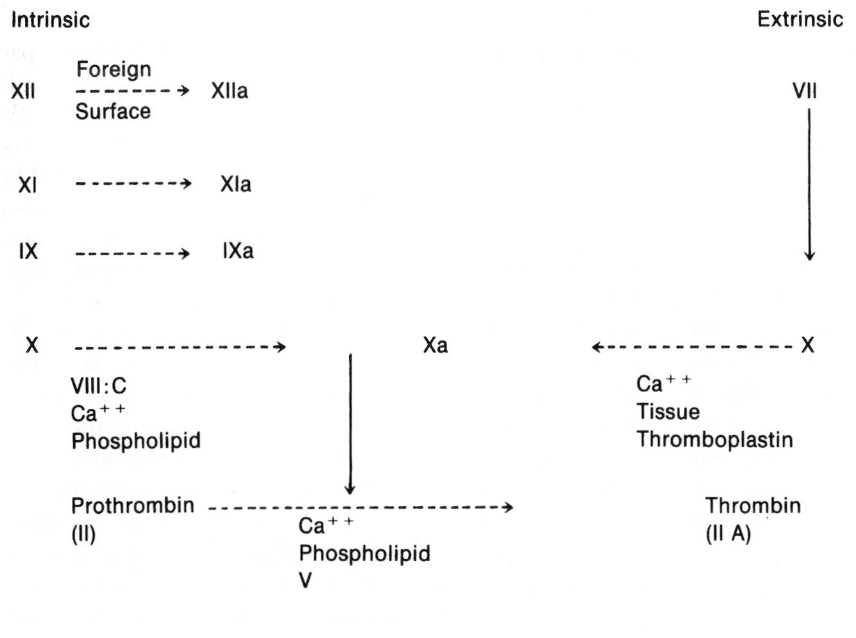

Figure 41.2. During clot formation, intrinsic and extrinsic pathways activate factor X (phase I) prior to the formation of thrombin (phase II).

fibrinolytic process by which the body actively dissolves clots, in which the normal endothelial cell plays a crucial role. When thrombin is bound to the endothelial receptor, thrombomodulin, it loses its ability to cleave fibrinogen, aggregate platelets, and activate factor V[(224,284)]. It will instead activate a glycoprotein, protein C[(224,225,227,283)]. Activated protein C may then bind to lipid surfaces through the action of another vitamin K-dependent glycoprotein, protein S, where it will inactivate activated factors V (Va) and VIII:C (VIII:Ca)[(225)]. Moreover, activated protein C indirectly elevates levels of tissue plasminogen activator, promoting fibrinolysis[(224,227)].

The endothelial cell also elaborates heparin-like molecules which bind antithrombin III (ATIII)[(285)]. ATIII accounts for about 75% of the antithrombin activity of plasma, primarily by its inhibition of Xa. Heparin causes a conformational change of ATIII such that, after binding of heparin to ATIII, the anticoagulant activity is immediate[(286,287)]. This ATIII/heparin complex inhibits all the vitamin K-dependent proteins, except for VIIa.

Finally, at the site of a clot, the endothelial cell elaborates tPA[(285,288)]. The tPA cleaves plasminogen into plasmin—a nonspecific peptidase—that lyses the fibrin clot. Plasminogen circulates throughout the body; however, tPA is particularly efficient at producing plasmin in the presence of fibrin rather than fibrinogen; thus, fibrinolysis is localized to the clot surface. The action of plasmin is itself limited by a fast-acting inactivator, alpha$_2$-antiplasmin, that normally is bound to a fibrin clot by XIIIa[(283,289)].

Disseminated Intravascular Coagulation

Disseminated intravascular coagulation (DIC) is the most dramatic example of derangement of this delicately balanced system. Critically ill children in the ICU may develop the catastrophic thrombotic and hemorrhagic syndrome of DIC as a final common pathway complicating their underlying illness. We will discuss the pathophysiology of the syndrome, focusing on acute, hemorrhagic, sepsis-induced DIC, the most common manifestation of the syndrome in children. We will then outline an approach to management, emphasizing control of the etiologic disorder but also describing some of the newer antithrombin agents.

Pathophysiology

DIC is an acquired thrombohemorrhagic disorder that is the consequence of a great variety of underlying disorders. The central feature is the concomitant activation of both the coagulation and fibrinolytic cascades, resulting in the paradoxical clinical situation of simultaneous thrombus deposition and hemorrhagic diathesis[(290–292)]. Regardless of the underlying disorder, the central feature of DIC is the generation of thrombin in the systemic circulation. Once thrombin is formed, there is cleavage of fibrinogen into fibrin monomers which polymerize into fibrin clot throughout the microcirculation of multiple organs. As fibrin is deposited, platelets are attracted, become trapped, and thrombocytopenia results. Red blood cells may be damaged as they attempt to navigate through the intravascular thrombi, resulting in microangiopathic hemolytic anemia.

There is simultaneous release of tissue plasminogen activator (tPA), which activates the fibrinolytic system via the conversion of plasminogen to plasmin. Plasmin circulates systemically and begins to lyse the fibrin clots that have been deposited in the circulation. It cleaves fibrinogen and fibrin into fragments labeled X, Y, D, and E, which are collectively termed fibrin degradation products (FDPs). These FDPs further aggravate the bleeding diathesis by interfering with platelet aggregation. In addition to degrading fibrinogen and fibrin, plasmin also degrades multiple clotting factors and activates the complement pathway. The presence of activated complement results in red blood cell and platelet lysis, as well as increase in vascular permeability which may lead to hypotension and shock[(290–292)].

Clinical Features

The clinical signs of DIC are somewhat variable, but usually consist of fever, hypoxia, hypotension, acidosis, CNS dysfunction, petechiae and purpura, and oozing from surgical or traumatic wounds[(290–292)]. The signs of organ dysfunction (CNS, pulmonary, and renal) have classically been attributed to fibrin deposition in the microcirculation, but such features may be in large part due to hypotension and tissue ischemia secondary to the process instigating the DIC[(293)]. Because of the overt nature of bleeding, hemorrhage is more frequently noted than occult thromboses, but cutaneous infarctions and acral gangrene may be evident. Thrombosis alone is not common, except in patients with chronic DIC secondary to malignancy (Trousseau's syndrome)[(292)]. There is some evidence that the relative balance of thrombosis versus hemorrhage is different depending upon the underlying disorder[(294)], but these findings are probably more useful from a laboratory and therapeutic perspective than from a diagnostic perspective.

Laboratory Findings

The laboratory abnormalities characteristic of DIC reflect the combination of excess thrombosis and fibrinolysis. However, no single study is pathognomonic for DIC. As expected from the pathophysiology, the PT and PTT are usually prolonged, secondary to plasmin degradation of fibrinogen and other clotting factors. However, prolongation of the PT and PTT are present only in 50 to 75% of patients with DIC, and thus normal values do not exclude the diagnosis[(290)]. Fibrinogen is usually depleted, but since it is an acute phase reactant, a normal level may actually suggest ongoing destruction. Furthermore, since fibrinogen is produced in the liver, a low plasma level may be due to liver disease rather than DIC. Thrombocytopenia is a common feature; FDPs are elevated in 85 to 100% of patients. However, since FDPs are a consequence of plasmin activity, they do not give an indication of the extent of thrombotic activity[(290)]. Since FDPs are cleared by the reticuloendothelial

Table 41.17. Causes of Disseminated Intravascular Coagulation

1. Infection
   a. Gram-negative
      i. Endotoxin
   b. General mechanisms
      i. Direct endothelial damage
      ii. Antigen-antibody complexes
         (1) Platelet activation
      iii. Direct platelet activation
      iv. Venous/vascular stasis
2. Tumor
   a. Leukemia
      i. Acute promyelocytic leukemia
   b. Solid tumors (Trousseau's syndrome)
3. Obstetric
   a. Abruption
   b. Retained dead fetus
4. Neonatal
   a. Necrotizing enterocolitis
   b. Respiratory distress syndrome
5. Hemolytic uremic syndrome
6. Giant hemangioma
7. Trauma
   a. Severe head injury
   b. Crush injuries
   c. Burns
8. Miscellaneous
   a. Shock (anaphylaxis, heat stroke, etc.)
   b. Snake venom
   c. Transfusion reactions

system, elevated FDPs can be seen in liver disease and are not diagnostic of DIC. Fragmented RBCs may be seen on a peripheral blood smear, but only 50% of patients with DIC will have evident schistocytes, and their absence does not exclude DIC[(291)].

Many other tests have been used to diagnose DIC. Measurement of the activity of specific coagulation factors is usually not helpful, and other assays, such as euglobulin lysis time, ethanol gelation, and protamine sulfate precipitation tests, are generally too insensitive, nonspecific, or time-consuming to be useful in most clinical situations[(290,293)]. Newer assays for D-dimer (one of the specific fibrin degradation products) or prothrombin fragment 1 + 2 (generated as a byproduct of thrombin formation) are more sensitive and specific for the diagnosis of DIC[(290)], but are available clinically in only a few institutions. From a practical standpoint, measurement of the PT, PTT, fibrinogen, FDPs, CBC, and liver function studies in a patient with a condition known to predispose to DIC, should be sufficient to make the diagnosis.

Clinical Syndromes

Please see **Table 41.17** for a list of the causes of DIC.

SEPSIS. Any sepsis syndrome may lead to DIC, and a wide variety of organisms have been implicated. Most characteristic, however, are Gram-negative infections associated with endotoxin release. Endotoxin can directly injure the vessel wall, exposing the subendothelium. The exposed subendothelial surface can initiate contact activation of the coagulation cascade[(283)]. Further, endotoxin can directly activate factor XII[(295)], with the ensuing derangements discussed above. Pathologic overactivation of the contact system may also lead to neutrophil activation and release, furthering tissue injury[(296)]. In addition, endotoxin directly binds to a specific platelet receptor, causing the release reaction and furthering both pathologic thrombosis and subsequent platelet depletion[(251)]. Endotoxin also stimulates the synthesis of tissue factor activity by monocytes, which can then activate factor X in the presence of factor VIIa[(251)].

Both Gram-negative bacteria and other infectious organisms can induce DIC through mechanisms other than endotoxin-mediated effects. These include direct endothelial damage, which is worsened by generalized vascular stasis in shock states or by locally decreased flow in organs injured by the accumulation of organisms and inflammatory cells. The leukocytes may further cause damage by releasing mediators, including proteolytic granular enzymes, superoxides, and sulfated mucopolysaccharides, that further damage the endothelium[(291)]. Antigen-antibody complexes may form, leading to platelet injury. In fact, organisms may attach to the platelet surface, leading to direct platelet injury. Sometimes, the attachment of the organisms is followed by specific antibody binding and platelet destruction. Nonspecific lymphocyte stimulation may lead to autoantibody production. While these mechanisms may further the thrombocytopenia in DIC, they may also lead to an isolated decrease in the platelet count[(251)].

Overall, sepsis-related DIC is a fulminant process whose predominant clinical manifestation is hemorrhage[(297,298)]. Nonetheless, it is important to remember that widespread microthrombosis leading possibly to organ ischemia is an ongoing process. This is dramatically evident in purpura fulminans. Intravascular occlusion of the terminal arterioles in the skin gives rise to sharply demarcated areas of hemorrhagic necrosis, which may coalesce if larger vessels are subsequently occluded[(297)]. Digit or even limb gangrene may supervene. Renal damage varying from glomerular injury to cortical necrosis may also occur, and a confusional state, convulsions, or coma may be furthered by microvascular occlusion in what may be an underperfused brain. Pulmonary injury and gastrointestinal ulceration may also result from clots in small vessels[(297)].

DIC ASSOCIATED WITH TUMOR. In adults, DIC associated with cancer is most often a chronic, low-grade, primarily thrombotic process seen most frequently in adenocarcinomas (Trousseau's syndrome). In acute promyelocytic leukemia (APL), the abnormal granules have tissue factor activity[(299)]. The cells may also have fibrinolytic capacity. Hemorrhage is a frequent presenting manifestation of APL and may worsen with the initiation of therapy, when the disrupted cells release their abnormal granules.

More general studies aimed at determining the incidence of coagulopathy in childhood leukemias found laboratory abnormalities of the clotting system to be common, although clinical thrombosis or bleeding was rare[(300,301)]. Abnormalities were more common in acute myeloid leukemia (AML) than in acute lymphocytic leukemia (ALL) and were especially frequent in monocytic and myelomonocytic variants of AML.

SEVERE HEAD INJURY. Brain tissue is known to be a potent thromboplastin. In fact, it is the thromboplastin used in the laboratory evaluation of the classic extrinsic pathway determined by the PT. Severe brain injury may, therefore, release thromboplastic substances into the circulation, where they initiate coagulation. In 16 brain-injured patients who died within 24 hours of admission, there was histopathologic evidence of DIC in 14 when such evidence was carefully sought[302]. Large thrombi were found most frequently in the brain and spinal cord, liver, lungs, kidneys, and pancreas, while microthrombi were found most frequently in the liver, pituitary, pancreas, thymus, brain and spinal cord, large intestine, kidneys, and lungs (both are listed in descending order of frequency). Concomitant hypotension, respiratory impairment, or both were common. In a study of 87 children evaluated within 2 hours of injury, Miner et al.[303] found the severity of injury to correlate with the presence of DIC (defined by abnormalities in three of the following five: tests for PT, PTT, and FDP; platelet count; and fibrinogen level). Moreover, the prognosis was worse for those with DIC even within the same clinical and radiologic category of severity, reflecting either underestimation of the extent of injury or the worsening of that injury by microthrombus formation. Unfortunately, no evaluation of autopsy material was included. The laboratory abnormalities corrected rapidly, although this may have been speeded by replacement with cryoprecipitate, platelets, and FFP.

OBSTETRIC ACCIDENTS. Tissue thromboplastic material may also be released into the circulation after a dead fetus has been retained for longer than 2 weeks. In placenta abruptio, clotting factors may be consumed at the site of the retroplacental clot, but thromboplastic material from degenerating placental tissue may also enter the circulation[297].

NEONATAL ILLNESS. Birth depression (defined as a 1-minute Apgar score of less than 3 and a 5-minute Apgar score of less than 7) and sepsis are the most common causes of DIC in the newborn[304]. Necrotizing enterocolitis, a syndrome of intestinal mucosal injury most closely related to infection but also related to ischemic bowel injury, which disproportionately affects the small premature infant, may also lead to either thrombocytopenia or DIC[270,305]. The release of thromboplastic material from the injured bowel wall may be etiologic. Certainly, in those cases associated with infection, sepsis-associated thrombocytopenia or DIC may supervene. The respiratory distress syndrome may occasionally be complicated by DIC. Obstetric problems such as toxemia and third-trimester bleeding figure prominently in neonatal as well as maternal DIC. As always, the small premature (less than 1500 g, 32 weeks' gestation) is at increased risk[304].

HEMOLYTIC UREMIC SYNDROME. Hemolytic Uremic Syndrome (HUS) is a triad of uremia, microangiopathic hemolytic anemia, and thrombocytopenia, which most frequently affects children after gastroenteritis. Verotoxin-producing *Escherichia coli* may be the causative organism in many of these enteritis-associated cases, and neuramidase-producing organisms have been implicated also[306,307]. Other causes of the syndrome include shigellosis, familial prostacyclin deficiency, and inherited C2 deficiency[255,308]. Thrombocytopenia is usually more prominent than DIC, and thrombosis, particularly in the renal microvasculature and perhaps in the brain also, is more important than hemorrhage. The verotoxin, in particular, may act by inducing a plasma factor that causes platelet aggregation by use of glycoproteins IIb and IIIa[307]. Microvascular occlusion in cerebral vessels is particularly pronounced in TTP, a closely related if not identical syndrome in adults.

MISCELLANEOUS. Any shock state can lead to sufficient tissue injury to activate the coagulation mechanism in a widespread fashion. Antibody-mediated hemolytic transfusion reactions can induce DIC. Red cell stroma or hemoglobin alone is not sufficient: antibody must be bound to the red cell surface as well[309]. In the Kasabach-Merritt syndrome, consumption of coagulation factors occurs within the confines of a giant hemangioma. Fibrinolysis induced by the abnormal endothelium may play a role, and thrombocytopenia is often prominent[310]. In certain parts of the world, snake bite can lead to DIC[311]. Finally, tissue injury from trauma or burns are well recognized causes of DIC[290,291].

Therapy

There is perhaps no other situation in medicine where the therapy is so controversial. The only clear agreement is that the underlying condition that precipitated the DIC must be controlled. A dramatic example of the efficacy of such therapy is in obstetric disorders, in which evacuation of the uterine contents removes the thrombotic stimulus and allows for rapid normalization of hemostasis[297]. Elimination of the thrombotic initiators is more difficult in sepsis or other shock states, in which there may be diffuse vascular damage. Careful attention to the maintenance of adequate tissue perfusion, adequate oxygenation, and correction of metabolic derangements are essential. There are no good prospective, randomized, controlled studies of different therapeutic interventions in DIC, in part because of the myriad of precipitating diseases, the broad range of ages, and diverse clinical statuses.

As previously mentioned, the generation of thrombin is central to the pathophysiology of DIC. Antithrombin therapy would therefore seem to be the logical treatment. Therapy with heparin has been advocated, but no consistent benefit has been demonstrated in most clinical situations[291,292,312]. However, some authors continue to advocate heparin therapy to prevent continued microvascular thrombus formation[290,297]. Heparin accelerates the activity of antithrombin III (AT III). Since AT III levels are quite variable in patients with DIC, the effect of heparin can be unpredictable and thus exacerbate hemorrhage. This has led some to advocate low-dose, subcutaneous heparin rather than higher-dose, intravenous heparin[290].

Nonetheless, there are at least two specific indications for heparin therapy. In purpura fulminans, fibrin deposition in small vessels is of major pathologic significance, and heparin therapy clearly improves outcome[297,312,313]. Significant dermal or acral ischemia with patchy decreased skin perfusion but without full blown purpura fulminans is also an indication for heparinization[312]. Evidence of venous or arterial thromboembolism is another relatively clear indication for heparin therapy. End-organ dysfunction, such as kidney, heart, or lung dysfunction, that is due, at least in part, to microthrombi, is a more controversial indication for heparinization[290,297,312]. Heparinization in acute promyelocytic leukemia is similarly controversial[312]. Heparin therapy has not been shown to improve clinical manifestations or affect ultimate outcome in patients in whom DIC is due to snake venom, heat stroke, massive head trauma, or hemolytic transfusion reactions[312]. Heparin is contraindicated in patients who have excessive bleeding in closed spaces (intracranial, intraspinal, or pericardial)[312]. Newer therapies, including low molecular weight heparin[314] and antithrombin III concentrates[315] have shown some efficacy, but their routine use must still be considered investigational.

Factor replacement therapy is indicated in patients with low fibrinogen and/or factor levels and thrombocytopenia who have active bleeding[312]. Although theoretically possible, "fuelling the fire" by giving the patient more prothrombin has only rarely been proven to occur[312] and should not dissuade the clinician from administering platelets and FFP or cryoprecipitate to patients who are actively bleeding. FFP in a dose of 10 to 15 ml/kg supplies all factors in limited concentration. One unit of platelets per 5 kg of body weight is estimated to raise the platelet count 50,000/μl. One unit of cryoprecipitate per 5 kg of body weight will raise the fibrinogen concentration about 75 mg/dl. Postinfusion platelet counts and fibrinogen levels should be monitored to determine transfusion needs.

The use of antifibrinolytic agents such as epsilon aminocaproic acid or tranexamic acid is not routinely indicated[290,312], because inhibition of fibrinolysis may lead to microvascular fibrin deposition, resulting in organ dysfunction. In rare instances, they may be used to control excessive bleeding but should probably not be used without the concomitant administration of heparin to prevent microvascular thrombi.

Liver Disease

Severe liver failure profoundly affects the coagulation cascade and fibrinolytic system and their inhibiting proteins. The liver synthesizes fibrinogen and the vitamin K-dependent factors II (prothrombin), VII, IX, X, protein C, and protein S, as well as factors V, XI, XII and XIII. In addition, an abnormal fibrinogen may be synthesized in patients with a variety of hepatic disorders, particularly chronic active hepatitis, cirrhosis, and acute liver failure[316]. This acquired abnormality impairs fibrin polymerization, resulting in poor clot formation. The synthesis of factors V and VII is especially dependent upon liver synthesis; measurements of their levels are particularly sensitive indicators of liver synthetic function. However, factor assays are not always rapidly available clinically, so measurement of the PT is often a very useful, albeit indirect, measure of hepatic protein synthesis[317].

Thrombocytopenia is common and is most often due to hypersplenism with sequestration of platelets. Platelet function is also impaired, with resultant prolongation of the bleeding time. This is probably secondary to poor clearance by the failing liver of FDPs, which are known to inhibit platelet activity[290].

The damaged liver may poorly clear plasminogen activators and may synthesize decreased amounts of alpha$_2$-antiplasmin[318]. Accelerated fibrinolysis may, therefore, contribute to the hemostatic defect in liver failure and may be more frequent than DIC in the absence of complicating infection. The distinction between these two conditions may be difficult. Relative preservation of platelet numbers, with negative assays for fibrinopeptide A and D-dimer, low levels of FDP, and shortened clot lysis times would support a diagnosis of fibrinolysis rather than DIC.

Hemophilia

Inherited deficiencies of plasma coagulation factors will occasionally require ICU management. The most common deficiency is that of factor VIII (hemophilia A), followed by factor IX deficiency (hemophilia B). Other factor deficiencies are quite rare and will not be discussed in detail here. Both factor VIII and factor IX deficiency are X-linked, so that the severe expression is limited to the hemizygous male[319–321]. The factor activity present in a patient's plasma is expressed as a percentage of normal activity. According to Lyon's hypothesis, occasional heterozygous females will inactivate enough of the normal X chromosome in precursor cells to have an activity level lower than the predicted 50%, although that level is not often less than 20%[322]. Bleeding manifestations vary with the factor level, with severely affected patients having activities usually less than 1%; moderately-severe patients have activities between 1 and 5%. Moderately affected patients have activities between 5 and 15%, and mildly affected patients have values between 15 and 25%. Patients with values greater than 25% rarely bleed excessively, except with major traumatic or surgical stress[319–321]. The overall incidence of both hemophilias is variably quoted as 1:10,000 males or 1:10,000 population, with VIII:C deficiency being about four times as common as IX deficiency[319–321,323].

Most bleeding episodes involve the muscles and

joints[319–321,324,325] and, more rarely, mucosal surfaces, perhaps because muscles and joints are relatively deficient in tissue factor activity and so require the augmentation pathway of factor VIII and factor IX for factor X activation. These bleeds rarely require intensive care and so will not be further discussed here.

Bleeding in the hemophiliac may be life-threatening either because of quantitative loss or because of location. Volume loss and the oxygen-carrying capacity (red cells) should be replaced in accordance with the general principles of patient management in these situations. In addition, factor replacement therapy is required. If the bleeding disorder is not yet specifically diagnosed but has been suspected because of excessive bleeding in relation to the extent of injury, a screening PT and PTT should be performed. In VIII and IX deficiency, the PT is normal but the PTT is prolonged, usually at least 60 seconds in patients with severe deficiencies. FFP contains both factors and should be administered in a dose of at least 15 ml/kg in a patient with excessive bleeding, a normal PT, and a prolonged PTT. An emergency factor assay can usually be performed within 1 hour and can give an idea as to which factor is deficient. The level after a bleed may be lower than the patient's usual level, due to consumption of limited stores. Once a determination as to which factor is deficient has been made, more definitive replacement therapy can be given. One unit of VIII:C activity per kilogram will raise the VIII:C level about 2%[319,320,324]. FFP contains 1 unit/ml, so that a large volume is required for adequate replacement. Cryoprecipitate contains 60 to 80 units of VIII:C activity per bag, and each bag is usually about 10 ml in volume. The lyophilized VIII:C concentrates vary by batch. As an example, a vial of a current batch contains about 280 units per bottle, requiring 10 ml of normal saline for reconstitution prior to administration[319,320,324]. The multiplicity of donors required to prepare the concentrates raises the risks of infection, particularly HIV. Initial attempts to prevent this included heat treatment, which destroys HIV but not hepatitis viruses. Subsequently, factor VIII:C preparations have been heated in solution, or organic solvent extracted, and so rendered hepatitis virus free. High-purity concentrates achieved through the use of monoclonal antibodies and effective viral killing procedures are now available, although the resultant product is more expensive. Recombinant factor VIII:C is also now available[319,320,324,325]. For major bleeding, correction to at least 70% and perhaps to 100% activity (50 units/kg) is recommended[319,320,324]. In factor IX-deficient patients, 1 unit of factor IX per kilogram will raise the activity only slightly more than 1%. Replacement to greater than 80% would, therefore, require the administration of 80 units of lyophilized IX concentrates per kilogram, which are heat-treated as are the VIII:C concentrates. Blood precautions should be observed both when drawing up the concentrate and when performing the venipuncture. The concentrate may be administered either through a filtered needle or Soluset. In patients with mild to moderate classic hemophilia who have suffered a relatively minor injury, DDAVP, a vasopressin analog, may be administered in a dose of 0.3 μg/kg, diluted in normal saline, intravenously over 20 minutes, since it raises the VIII:C levels twofold to threefold by stimulating release from endogenous stores[319,324,326,327].

Bleeding may also be life threatening due to location. The CNS and the airway are the two most common potentially lethal areas of bleeding in the hemophiliac[320,328–330]. Gilchrist et al.[330] estimated the risk of intracranial bleeding as being between 2.0 and 3.5% per year. Overall, intracranial bleeds account for approximately 25% of hemorrhagic deaths in hemophiliacs[320]. After all but the most minor head trauma, replacement therapy to levels of 100% activity should be given. However, if brain swelling is suspected, DDAVP should not be used since it may lead to water retention, although water intoxication has not been reported at this dose. A CT scan of the brain should be performed to rule out intracranial bleeding. However, a negative result should not be overly reassuring, since the bleeding may be delayed. Therefore, a repeat CT scan should be done if the patient clinically deteriorates[320,329,330].

Airway bleeding[328] may follow local trauma, including prolonged dental work. Again, replacement to levels of 100% activity should be given.

Of patients with VIII:C deficiency, 10 to 15% develop anti-VIII:C antibodies or inhibitors[331–333]. Management of these patients remains a clinical challenge[333,334]. In patients with low-titer inhibitors (less than 5 Bethesda units), the antibody may be overwhelmed with large doses of VIII:C followed by a continuous VIII:C infusion. This will cause an anamnestic antibody rise in 4 to 5 days and so is reserved for life-threatening situations[331,335]. In patients with higher titer inhibitors, IX concentrates or activated IX concentrates are given. Factor VIII:C bypassing activity is present in IX concentrates, perhaps reflecting activated factor X (Xa) activity. Activated complexes, which presumably contain more of this activity, are commercially available, although expensive (e.g., FEIBA, Autoplex). They are titered for IX levels, not for bypassing activity levels, so the dose recommended for bleeding, 80 units/kg, is an empirical one[336–338]. The Xa may cause a low-grade state of DIC through widespread thrombin activation, so that fibrinolytic inhibitors such as tranexamic acid or epsilon-aminocaproic acid (Amicar) must be avoided when IX complexes are given[339]. An alternative approach is to use porcine factor VIII. Porcine factor VIII prepared from slaughterhouse-derived pork plasma is often active in patients with antihuman factor VIII:C inhibitors. Many of these patients have low or no antiporcine factor VIII inhibitors. Porcine factor VIII:C is able to support normal hemostasis and has even been used repeatedly in some patients with no loss of efficacy[340]. A recombinant activated factor VII is also available. It bypasses the factor VIII:C blockade and avoids some of the thromboembolic complications seen with activated complexes. Both plasma-derived and recombinant factor VIIa have been used successfully in a number of patients with inhibitors[333,340,341].

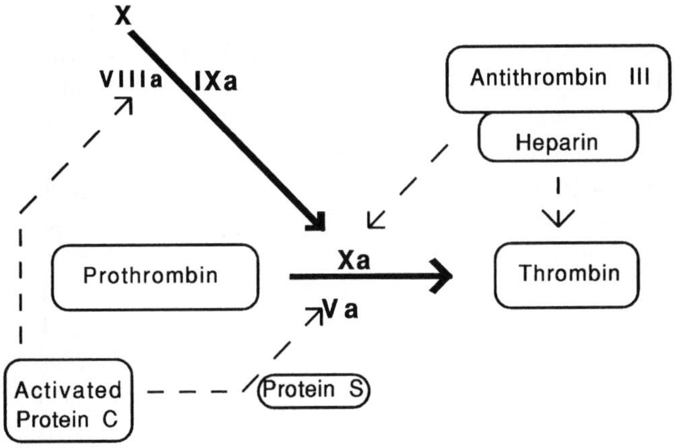

Figure 41.3. Physiologic Anticoagulants. Dashed lines represent inhibitory activity. (Adapted from Bauer KA and Rosenberg RD, Semin Hematol 1991;28:10–18.)

Thrombosis

Mechanisms and Causes of Thrombosis

Loss of vascular integrity, stasis of the blood, and increased coagulability were identified as the precipitants of thrombosis by Virchow over a century ago. As noted in the fibrinolysis section above, the endothelium plays a critical role in the modulation of clot formation necessary to maintain normal blood flow. The endogenous anticoagulants include thrombomodulin, protein S, protein C, antithrombin III, heparin cofactor II, and others (Fig. 41.3), while the fibrinolytic system (Fig. 41.4) is composed of tissue plasminogen activating factor, alpha-2 macroglobulin, and plasminogen[(342)]. Thus, it can readily be appreciated that vascular abnormalities resulting from intravascular line insertion, trauma, or inflammation, may lead to thrombus formation. In addition, stasis due to hypovolemia, hyperviscosity, immobility, injury or intravascular catheters is not an uncommon cause of thrombosis in the PICU. Finally, congenital or acquired abnormalities of coagulation other than those associated with endothelial dysfunction may lead to a hypercoagulable state **(Table 41.18)**[(343)].

Congenital abnormalities of the proteins modulating co-

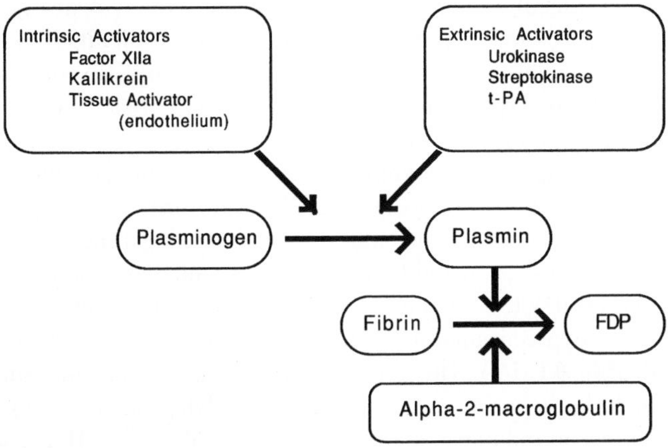

Figure 41.4. Fibrinolysis.

Table 41.18. Causes of Increased Coagulability[a]

Physiologic Alteration	*Clinical Condition*
Blood flow	
Hypovolemia	Shock, dehydration
Hyperviscosity	Polycythemia, leukocytosis, thrombocytosis, SCD
Mechanical stasis	Immobilization after surgery
Foreign bodies	Catheters, cardiac prostheses
Vessels	
Anatomic defects	Congenital heart disease, vascular abnormalities
Endothelial disorders	Vasculitis, inflammation
Blood Coagulation	
Increased and/or abnormal procoagulants	Cancer, pregnancy, dysfibrinogenemias, inflammatory bowel disease
Decreased anticoagulants	AT III deficiency, protein S or C deficiency
Decreased fibrinolysis	Hereditary defects
Increased platelet-vessel reactivity	Coronary artery disease, diabetes mellitus, transient ischemic attacks
Mixed or idiopathic	HUS, TTP, oral contraceptives, nephrotic syndrome, recurrent idiopathic DVT

[a]*Adapted from Hathaway WE, Am J Dis Child 1984:138:301–304.*

agulation can have devastating effects. For example, deficient or dysfunctional protein C leads to recurrent thrombosis[(344)] and in the homozygous state has been associated with purpura fulminans[(226)]. Moreover, since vitamin K antagonists like warfarin cause a decrease in protein S and C concentrations, loading with high doses may lead to thrombosis[(226,345)]. It is of note that protein C levels are lower in newborns, leading to speculation that infants may be at higher risk of abnormal coagulation[(346)]. Protein S deficiency can also cause thrombosis[(345,347)], particularly in adults[(348)]. An inhibitor of activated protein C has been found, but its significance is not certain[(349)]. Congenital antithrombin III deficiency is also associated with a thrombotic tendency[(350,351)], as is plasminogen deficiency, although the latter appears to be associated more with thrombosis in late adolescence and adulthood[(342)].

Acquired deficiencies of protein C and protein S have been described with varicella[(352)], and deficiencies of antithrombin III have been seen with nephrotic syndrome[(353)] and L-asparaginase administration[(354,355)]. Finally, a miscellaneous group of disorders associated with defective coagulation and increased thrombosis have been described, including systemic lupus erythematosus[(356)], inflammatory bowel disease[(357)], antiphospholipid syndrome[(358,359)], and homocyteinuria[(360)].

Deep Vein Thrombosis

Epidemiology and Etiology

Reports in the adult literature estimate that as many as 900,000 patients have deep venous thromboses (DVT) each year in the United States. Of these, some 300,000 to 600,000 will suffer pulmonary embolism, with a mortality rate of 140,000 to 200,000 per year[361]. The factors thought to predispose adults to DVT include congestive heart failure, lung and abdominal cancers, trauma, pregnancy, paralysis or immobility, and old age[361–363]. These disease conditions are relatively infrequently seen in children, and spontaneous DVT, particularly with pulmonary embolism, is rare[364–367]. However, both arterial and venous thrombosis leading to significant morbidity and mortality are seen in children with acquired and congenital defects of the normal control of procoagulant and fibrinolytic processes[342,344–346,348,352,353,356,368–370]. Moreover, diseases leading to decreased blood flow, such as immobilization and shock or altered vascular endothelial integrity such as occurs in vasculitis, can also enhance the risk of thrombosis[356,357]. Finally, the advent of liver transplantation has introduced yet another cause of altered vascular integrity with thrombosis[371].

Although the incidence of spontaneous DVT is very low in children, there has been a marked increase in the incidence of iatrogenic arterial and venous thrombosis as the use of intravascular catheters for invasive monitoring and/or intravenous therapy has become more and more prevalent in neonatal and pediatric ICUs and in pediatric cardiology. For example, Berman and colleagues identified a total of 37 children and infants in their pediatric and neonatal ICUs who developed thrombosis of great veins or right atrium related to intravascular catheters over a 5-year period[372]. Of these patients, eight died as a consequence of the thrombosis. The total number of admissions to the ICUs was approximately 5000, so the actual incidence of catheter-related thrombosis may appear low. However, since not all patients admitted to the ICUs had catheters, and thromboses are not always recognized, the authors suggest that the incidence of hemodynamically significant venous thrombosis might be as high as 5 to 10%. Other studies of neonatal ICUs suggest that the incidence of thrombosis is 11 to 16%, although hemodynamic complications are lower[373–376]. In a study of femoral venous lines in children, 35% had thrombosis, although only in one patient was the diagnosis clinically evident[377]. Particular risk factors for DVT in these studies included small size, high hematocrit levels, low blood pressure, increased coagulability, and home parenteral nutrition[378]. Finally, in cancer patients with long-term indwelling catheters, the combination of thrombosis and infection has been well described[379,380].

Diagnosis and Therapy

Management of the child with suspected DVT includes (a) urgent confirmation of the presence or absence of thrombosis and assessment of the risk (or presence) of pulmonary embolism or other critical event, (b) a search for possible predisposing factors, and (c) institution of appropriate therapy. Because of its relative rarity in the pediatric population, the diagnosis of DVT requires a high degree of suspicion. Certain historical features of the case may help. For example, a family history of hypercoagulability, a history of nephrotic syndrome, or an injury leading to prolonged immobilization are all associated with increased risk of DVT. Physical findings such as an obstructed intravascular catheter; pain and swelling of the extremity distal to the site of suspected DVT; or the constellation of marked swelling, blue discoloration, and tenderness of one leg after femoral venous catheterization suggest a DVT. However, the reliability of simple clinical diagnosis of DVT with pulmonary embolus has been notoriously poor in adults, so further laboratory investigations are warranted[381].

A variety of tests may be employed to confirm the diagnosis of DVT. These include venography, impedance plethysmography, ultrasonography, thermography, and I-125 fibrinogen leg scanning[382–386]. Of these, venography is the "gold standard" but has the disadvantages of (a) not always being readily available, (b) a significant false-negative rate, and (c) the risks associated with the injection of radiopaque dyes. Other techniques, such as impedance plethysmography and ultrasonography, appear very useful for femoral and pelvic DVT, but less so for calf thromboses. However, since only proximal DVTs appear to lead to a significant risk of pulmonary embolus[381,387], then this may not be particularly important. A combination of techniques (e.g., duplex ultrasonography and venography) has been advocated by some authors as an efficient approach to the diagnosis[383], but ultrasonography alone may be sufficient[386], particularly in children with suspected great vein or atrial thrombus[372,388].

If a significant DVT is identified, a ventilation/perfusion scan may be desirable to exclude pulmonary embolism. However, the incidence of angiographically proven pulmonary embolism in the face of intermediate or low likelihood ventilation/perfusion scans is significant[381,389]. Therefore, if an embolus is suspected and the scan is inconclusive, then a decision to either investigate further with angiography or embark upon empiric therapy is warranted. The decision to treat a patient with anticoagulants or fibrinolytics is relatively easy to make if a large proximal DVT is present with or without pulmonary embolus. This is particularly true if there are no factors predisposing the patient to severe hemorrhage. However, the decision to treat a critically ill child with high risk of gastrointestinal, intracerebral, or other bleeding in the face of inconclusive evidence for thrombosis or pulmonary embolus is more difficult. Nonetheless, it has been suggested that if the findings are equivocal, the real question is not why should one treat, but what are the grounds for withholding therapy[381].

If therapy is to be employed, initial hematologic studies should include a cross-match, PT, PTT, fibrinogen concentration, platelet count, and activated clotting time (ACT). In the case of a child exhibiting a spontaneous or unexplained DVT, a search for factors predisposing him or her to a hypercoagulable state should also be undertaken **(Table 41.19).** The usual antithrombotic armamentarium includes heparin, warfarin, and thrombolytics such as streptokinase, urokinase, and recombinant tPA[390–395]. Heparin is most commonly employed in the therapy of distal DVT,

Table 41.19. Laboratory Work-up of Hypercoagulable States

Studies	*Disorder*
Basic hematologic tests	
CBC and platelet count	
PT, PTT	
Tests for decreased endogenous anticoagulant activity	
Antithrombin III activity	AT III deficiency or dysfunction
Protein S and C activity	Protein S or C deficiency
Heparin cofactor II	Heparin cofactor II deficiency
Tests of altered fibrinolytic function	
Plasminogen activity	Plasminogen deficiency or dysfunction
Tests of abnormal coagulants	
Reptilase or thrombin time	Dysfibrinogenemia
Fibrinogen activity	Dysfibrinogenemia
Anticardiolipin antibodies	Antiphospholipid syndrome

while proximal DVT or established pulmonary embolism are treated with heparin by some(390,391,396,397) and with thrombolytics by others(395,398,399). Therapeutic anticoagulation or fibrinolytic therapy are relatively contraindicated in patients with likely bleeding sources (e.g., intracranial bleed, gastrointestinal hemorrhage) and during the early postoperative period. However, the effects of heparin can be quickly reversed with protamine and the effects of fibrinolytics reversed by the cessation of the infusion and administration of FFP. Thus, the risks of bleeding must be weighed against the risks of the thrombosis.

Heparin has been used both as a continuous intravenous infusion and by intermittent subcutaneous injection(390,391), but the former seems decidedly better. In adults, an initial intravenous dose of 5000 units or 50 units/kg is followed by a continuous infusion rate of 15 to 25 units/kg/hr, with a goal of achieving an ACT of 150 to 190 sec(391) or a PTT twice normal. In newborns and older infants, McDonald and Hathaway noted that higher infusion rates (e.g., 20 to 35 units/kg/hr) were sometimes needed(396). More recently, Andrew et al. found that in infants under 1 year of age, a bolus dose of 75 U/kg followed by 28 U/kg/hr was necessary to achieve adequate anticoagulation(400). The obvious adverse effect of heparin therapy is bleeding, but this risk can be minimized by closely monitoring after the ACT or measuring the PTT regularly and keeping it in the 1.5 to 2 times control range (usually 55 to 85 sec). **Table 41.20** provides an algorithm for adjusting the heparin infusion rate after the initial bolus. After acute anticoagulation has been achieved with heparin, oral therapy with warfarin sodium is initiated if chronic anticoagulation is indicated. The international normalized ratio (INR) has been established to provide a uniform standard for warfarin anticoagulation. Warfarin therapy for established thrombi should be adjusted to achieve an INR of 2.0 to 3.0.

Table 41.20. Postbolus Intravenous Heparin Dose Titration Nomogram[a]

aPTT (sec)	*Rate Change*	*Additional Action*
≤45	+15%	Repeat aPTT in 4–6 hr
46–54	+7%	Repeat aPTT in 4–6 hr
55–85	0	Repeat aPTT every 4–6 hr for the first 24 hr, then every 12 hr
86–110	−7%	Stop heparin infusion for 1 hour. Repeat aPTT 4–6hr after resuming infusion
>110	−15%	Stop heparin infusion for 1 hour. Repeat aPTT 4–6 hr after resuming infusion

[a]*Adapted from Hull RD, et al., Arch Intern Med 1992;152:1591.*

In contrast to heparin, which acts as a cofactor with antithrombin III to prevent coagulation, the plasminogen activators urokinase, streptokinase, and tPA increase fibrinolysis, thereby lysing the clot. Thus, thrombolysis therapy intuitively seems better than heparin therapy, and it has become popular in treating large proximal venous thromboses and acute pulmonary embolism (as well as coronary artery obstruction) in adults. However, whether it is truly more efficacious is unclear(397). In children, fibrinolytic therapy has been used in great vein and atrial thromboses(372,401,402), in renal vein thromboses(403), for occlusion of grafts(404), and in cases of arterial thrombosis(405–407). The advantages of urokinase over streptokinase are mainly that there is a lower incidence of allergic reactions to the former. On the other hand, urokinase is more expensive. Both urokinase and streptokinase activate circulating and bound plasminogen, resulting in degradation of fibrinogen and other clotting factors as well as lysis of the clot. Recombinant tPA has the advantage of little antigenicity and activates only bound plasminogen; however, it has not been clearly shown to be more effective than other fibrinolytics.

The dose range of streptokinase reported for use in neonates and children was 1000 to 4000 units as a loading dose followed by 1000 units/hr in three studies(406,408,409) and 50 to 100 units/kg/hr in another(404). In most studies, the dose was raised by 500 to 1000 IU/kg/hr if there was no response to the initial therapy. The urokinase doses are in the range of 4000 to 4400 IU/kg as a loading dose over 20 minutes followed by 4000 to 6000 IU/kg/hr(372,392). Finally, tPA dosing with alteplase was 0.5 mg/kg/hr for the first hour followed by 0.25 mg/kg/hr until clot lysis in postcardiac catheterization patients(405). It should be noted that the fibrinolytic therapy will be of little use in the face of severe plasminogen deficiency associated with some congenital defects. In addition, the lower plasminogen levels of newborns may account for the failures of fibrinolytic therapy sometimes seen in this population(410–412). It is possible that supplemental plasminogen administered with FFP may be helpful in infants and other patients with depressed plasminogen levels who require lytic therapy. The duration of therapy with streptokinase or urokinase is usually brief (24 to 72 hours), by which time the clot will have lysed if the therapy is effective. Plasminogen activators are generally administered for less than 24 hours. It should be noted that fibrinogen levels will usually fall, and these and clotting functions can be used to monitor excessive plasminogen activator administration. After clot lysis has occurred, heparin therapy may be required to prevent rethrombosis. Subsequently, oral anticoagulation may be required.

Arterial Thrombosis

Arterial thrombosis has also become a major problem in the NICU, PICU, and cardiac catheterization laboratory. In a report by Caplan and colleagues, 29 neonates with aortic thrombosis were identified over a 5-year period(413), and the literature is now replete with articles extolling the virtues of different approaches (e.g., fibrinolytic, heparin, and surgery) to arterial thrombosis in both intensive care and post-catheterization infants and children(405,406,408,409,414–416).

Arterial thrombosis in children and neonates is usually the result of retrograde cardiac catheterization for diagnosis of congenital heart disease or insertion of a femoral artery or umbilical artery catheter for monitoring. The signs of obstructed arterial flow are quite clear. The distal extremities become pale and pulseless, or, in the case of aortic thrombosis, there is decreased urine output, with the eventual appearance of signs of gut ischemia. If decreased perfusion is noted, the line should be removed if at all possible and the limb observed to establish whether the obstruction was due to thrombosis or spasm. Spasm may be relieved by the injection of small amounts of lidocaine. If the signs of obstruction do not resolve within a few hours of removal of the intra-arterial line, a thrombus must be considered. Again, the options available are heparin, which is advocated by some, or plasminogen activators. The dose ranges used are similar to those mentioned above. The treatment regimen we favor for suspected arterial thrombosis is a modification of that proposed by Wessel and colleagues: (a) a period of observation of 4 hours to exclude the possibility of simple vasospasm; (b) if the pulse is still absent after 4 hours, the child is heparinized with 50 U/kg of heparin, and then an infusion of heparin aimed at maintaining the PTT at 1.5 to 2 times normal is continued; and (c) if after 12 to 24 hours there is still no pulse, streptokinase or urokinase therapy is initiated 4 hours after the heparin is stopped(409). It is of note that younger neonates appear to be more resistant to thrombolytic therapy, possibly because of lower plasminogen concentrations. Thus, concomitant administration of FFP or cryoprecipitate has been advocated by some, although this may not improve the fibrinolytic activity of the drug(372).

With either venous or arterial thrombosis, failure of medical management may lead to surgical intervention. Ligation of the inferior vena cava or placement of a filter may be life saving in the patient with a proximal DVT unresponsive to heparin or lytic therapy. Similarly, thrombectomy has been used in treating aortic thrombosis, although the efficacy of this approach in young infants has been limited(415,416). Obviously, with thrombosis—as with so many disorders in the PICU—prevention is more efficacious than treatment. However, with the exception of selected surgical patients and perhaps in immobilized trauma patients, prophylaxis with pneumatic stockings and low-dose heparin will not prevent most thromboses seen in the PICU.

References

1. Dean J, Schechter AN. Sickle-cell anemia: molecular and cellular bases of therapeutic approaches. 1–3. N Engl J Med 1978;299:752–63, 804–11, 863–70.
2. Charache S. The treatment of sickle cell anemia. Arch Intern Med 1974;133:698–705.
3. McIntosh S. Hematologic and oncologic complications in the critically ill child. Yale J Biol Med 1984;57:199.
4. Mills ML. Life-threatening complications of sickle cell disease in children. JAMA 1985;254:1487–1491.
5. Powars DR. Natural history of sickle cell disease—The first ten years. Semin Hematol 1975;12:267–285.
6. Scott RB. Advances in the treatment of sickle cell disease in children. Am J Dis Child 1985;139:1219–1222.
7. Vichinsky EP, Bertram HL. Suggested guidelines for the treatment of children with sickle cell anemia. Hemat/Oncol Clin North Am 1987;1:483–501.
8. Benz EJ. Molecular genetics of the sickling syndromes: evolution of new strategies for improved diagnosis. Am J Pediatr Hematol Oncol 1984;6:59–66.
9. Eaton WA, Hofrichter J. Sickle hemoglobin polymerization. In: Embury SH, Hebbel RP, Mohandas N, Steinberg MH, eds. Sickle Cell Disease: Basic Principles and Clinical Practice. New York: Raven Press, Ltd., 1994.
10. Berger SA, King WS. Diffusion and convection in the capillaries in sickle-cell disease. Blood Cells 1982;8:153.
11. Kraus AP, Robinson H, Cooper RM. Clinical trial of therapy for sickle cell vaso-occlusive crises. JAMA 1974;228:1120.
12. Berkowitz LR, Orringer EP. Effect of cetiedil, an in vitro antisickling agent, on erythrocyte membrane cation permeability. J Clin Invest 1981;68:1215–1220.
13. Schmidt WF, Asakura T, Schwartz E. Effect of cetiedil on cation and water movement in erythrocytes. J Clin Invest 1982;69:589–594.
14. Chang H, Ewert SM, Bookchin RM, Nager RL. Comparative evaluation of fifteen anti-sickling agents. Blood 1983;61:693–704.
15. Dover GJ, Charache S, Nora R, Boyer SH. Progress toward increasing fetal hemoglobin production in man: experience with 5-azacytidine and hydroxyurea. Ann NY Acad Sci 1985;445:218.
16. Charache S, Dover GJ, Smith K, Talbot CCJ, Moyer M, Boyer S. Treatment of sickle cell anemia with 5-azacytidine results in increased fetal hemoglobin production and is associated with nonrandom hypomethylation of DNA around the alpha and beta globin gene complex. Proc Natl Acad Sci USA 1983;80:4842–4846.
17. 17. Ley TJ, DeSimone J, Noguchi C, et al. 5-Azacytidine increases globin synthesis and reduces the proportion of dense cells in patients with sickle cell anemia. Blood 1983;62:370–380.
18. Platt OS, Orkin SH, Dover GJ, Beardsley GP, Miller B, Nathan DG. Hydroxyurea enhances fetal hemoglobin production in sickle cell anemia. J Clin Invest 1984;74:652–656.
19. Charache S, Terrin ML, Moore RD, et al. Effect of hydroxyurea on the frequency of painful crises in sickle cell anemia. N Engl J Med 1995;332:1317–22.
20. Shapiro MP, Hayes JA. Fat embolism in sickle cell disease. Arch Intern Med 1984;144:181–182.
21. Mehta P, Mehta J. Circulating platelet aggregates in sickle cell disease patients with and without vaso-occlusion. Stroke 1979;10:464–466.
22. Mehta P, Mehta J. Abnormalities of platelet aggregation in sickle cell disease. J Pediatr 1980;96:209–213.
23. Jeffries BF, Lipper MH, Kishore PRS. Major intracerebral arterial involvement in sickle cell disease. Surg Neurol 1980;14:291–295.
24. Pavlakis SG. Neurologic complications of sickle cell disease. Adv Pediatr 1989;36:247–276.
25. Buchanan GR, Smith SJ. Pneumococcal septicemia despite pneumococcal vaccine and prescription of penicillin prophylaxis in children with sickle cell anemia. Am J Dis Child 1986;140:428–432.
26. Ahonkhai VI, Landesman SH, Fikrig SM. Failure of pneumococcal vaccine in children with sickle-cell disease. N Engl J Med 1979;301:26.
27. Pearson HA. A neonatal program for sickle cell anemia. Adv Pediatr 1986;33:381–400.
28. Orlina AR, Unger PJ, Koshy M. Post-transfusion alloimmunization in patients with sickle cell disease. Am J Hematol 1978;5:101–6.
29. Vichinsky EP, Earles A, Johnson RA, Hoag MS, Williams A, Lubin B. Alloimunization in sickle cell anemia and transfusion of racially unmatched blood. N Engl J Med 1990;322:1617–21.

30. Charache S. Problems in transfusion. N Engl J Med 1990;322:1666.
31. Bentley PG, Howard ER. Surgery in children with homozygous sickle cell anemia. Ann R Coll Surg Eng 1979;61:55–59.
32. Burrington JD, Smith MD. Elective and emergency surgery in children with sickle cell disease. Surg Clin North Am 1976;56:55–71.
33. Janik J, Seeler RA. Perioperative management of children with sickle hemoglobinopathy. J Pediatr Surg 1980;15:117–120.
34. Malone BS, Werlin SL. Cholecystectomy and cholelithiasis in sickle cell anemia. Am J Dis Child 1988;142:799–800.
35. Morrison JC, Whybrew MS, Bucovaz ET. Use of partial exchange transfusion preoperatively in patients with sickle cell hemoglobinopathies. Am J Obstet Gynecol 1978;132:59–63.
36. Lanzkowsky P, Shende A, Karayalcin G, Kim Y-J, Aballi AJ. Partial exchange transfusion in sickle cell anemia. Am. J. Dis. Child. 1978;132:1206–1208.
37. Griffin TC, McIntire D, Buchanan GR. High-dose intravenous methylprednisolone therapy for pain in children and adolescents with sickle cell disease. N Engl J Med 1994;330:733–737.
38. Francis RB, Johnson CS. Vascular occlusion in sickle cell disease: current concepts and unanswered questions. Blood 1991;77:1405–1414.
39. Bromberg PA. Pulmonary aspects of sickle cell disease. Arch Intern Med 1974;133:652–657.
40. Haupt HM, Moore GW, Bauer TW, M. HG. The lung in sickle cell disease. Chest 1982;81:332–337.
41. Young RC, Castro O, Baxter RP, et al. The lung in sickle cell disease: a clinical overview of common vascular, infectious, and other problems. J Natl Med Assoc 1981;73:19–26.
42. Davies SC, Luce PJ, Win AA, Riordan JF, Brozovic M. Acute chest syndrome in sickle cell disease. Lancet 1984;1:36.
43. Walker BK, Ballas SK, Burka ER. The diagnosis of pulmonary thromboembolism in sickle cell disease. Am J Hematol 1979;7:219–232.
44. Perin RJ, McGeady SJ, Travis SF, Mansmann HC. Sickle cell disease and bronchial asthma. Ann Allergy 1983;50:320–322.
45. Miller ST, Hammerschlag MR, Chirgwin K, et al. Role of Clamydia pneumonia in acute chest syndrome of sickle cell disease. J Pediatr 1991;118:30–33.
46. Styles L, Schalkwijk C, Vichinsky E, Lubin BH, Kuypers FA. Dramatically increased phospholipase A2 in sickle cell disease associated with acute chest syndrome (ACS). Blood 1994;84:219a.
47. Cole TB, Sprinkle RH, Smith SJ, Buchanan GR. Intravenous narcotic therapy for children with severe sickle cell pain crisis. Am J Dis Child 1986;140:1255–1259.
48. Schmalzer EA, Lee JO, Brown AK, Usami S, Chien S. Viscosity of mixtures of sickle cells and normal red cells at varying hematocrit levels: implications for transfusion. Transfusion 1987;27:228–233.
49. Balkaran B, Char G, Morris JS, Thomas PW, Serjeant BE, Serjeant GR. Stroke in a cohort of patients with homozygous sickle cell disease. J. Pediatr. 1992;120:360–366.
50. Powars D, Wilson B, Imbus C, Pegelow C, Allen J. The natural history of stroke in sickle cell disease. Am J Med 1978;65:461–471.
51. Frempong KO. Stroke in sickle cell disease: demographic, clinical and therapeutic considerations. Semin Hematol 1991;28:213–219.
52. Kogutt MS, Goldwag SS, Gupta KL, Kaneko K, Humbert JR. Correlation of transcranial Doppler ultrasonography with MRI and MRA in the evaluation of sickle cell disease patients with prior stroke. Pediatr Radiol 1994;24:204–6.
53. Nelson MS, Chisolm JJ. Lead toxicity masquerading as sickle cell crisis. Ann Emerg Med 1986;15:748–750.
54. Adams RJ. Neurologic complications. In: Embury SH, Hebbel RP, Mohandas N, Steinberg MH, eds. Sickle Cell Disease: Basic Principles and Clinical Practice. New York: Raven Press, Ltd., 1994.
55. Wang WC, Kovnar EH, Tonkin IL, et al. High risk of recurrent stroke after discontinuance of five to twelve years of transfusion therapy in patients with sickle cell disease. J Pediatr 1991;118:377–382.
56. Wilimas J, Goff JR, Anderson HR, Langston JW, Thompson E. Efficacy of transfusion therapy for one to two years in patients with sickle cell disease and cerebrovascular accidents. J Pediatr 1980;96:205–208.
57. Seeler RA, Royal JE. Commentary: sickle cell anemia, stroke, and transfusion. J Pediatr 1980;96:243–244.
58. Russell MO, Goldberg HI, Reis L, et al. Transfusion therapy for cerebrovascular abnormalities in sickle cell disease. J Pediatr 1976;88: 382–387.
59. Wood DH. Cerebrovascular complications of sickle cell anemia. Stroke 1978;9:73–75.
60. Cohen AR, Martin MB, Silber JH, Kim HC, Frempong KO, Schwartz E. A modified transfusion program for prevention of stroke in sickle cell disease. Blood 1992;79:1657–1661.
61. Rao S, Solomon N, Miller S, Dunn E. Scintigraphic differentiation of bone infarction from osteomyelitis in children with sickle cell disease. J Pediatr 1985;107:685–688.
62. Keeley KK, Buchanan GR. Acute infarction of long bones in children with sickle cell anemia. Pediatrics 1982;101:170–175.
63. Stevens MCG, Padwich M, Sergeant GR. Observation on the natural history of dactylitis in homozygous sickle cell disease. Clin Pediatr 1981;20:311–317.
64. Adeyokunnu AA, Hendrickse RG. Salmonella osteomyelitis in childhood. Arch Dis Child 1980;55:175–184.
65. Givner LB, Luddy RE, Schwartz AD. Etiology of osteomyelitis in patients with major sickle hemoglobinopathies. J Pediatr 1981;99: 411–413.
66. Kudsk KA, Tranbaugh RF, Sheldon GF. Acute surgical illness in patients with sickle cell anemia. Am J Surg 1981;142:113–117.
67. Holt RW, Wagner R. Ultrasonic evaluation of the gallbladder in sickle cell disease. J Natl Med Assoc 1979;71:1027–1028.
68. Blank JP, Gill FM. Orbital infarction in sickle cell disease. Pediatrics 1981;67:879–881.
69. Rothman SM, Nelson JS. Spinal cord infarction in a patient with sickle cell anemia. Neurology 1980;30:1072–1076.
70. Topley JM, Rogers DW, Stevens MCG, Sergeant GR. Acute splenic sequestration and hypersplenism in the first five years in homozygous sickle cell disease. Arch Dis Child 1981;56:765–769.
71. Mann JR, Cotter KP, Walker RA, Bird GWG, Stuart J. Anaemic crisis in sickle cell disease. J Clin Pathol 1975;28:341–344.
72. Emond AM, Morais P, Venugopal S, Carpenter RG, Serjeant GR. Role of splenectomy in homozygous sickle cell disease in childhood. Lancet 1984;1:88–91.
73. Blacklock HA, Mortimer PP. Aplastic crisis and other effects on the human parvovirus infection. Clin Haematol 1984;13:679–691.
74. Rao SP, Miller ST, Cohen BJ. Transient aplastic crisis in patients with sickle cell disease. Am J Dis Child 1992;146:1328–1330.
75. Thomas AN, Pattison C, Serjeant GR. Causes of death in sickle-cell disease in Jamaica. Br Med J Clin. Res. Ed. 1982;285:633–635.
76. John AB, Ramlal A, Jackson H, Maude GH, Sharma AW, Serjeant GR. Prevention of pneumococcal infection in children with homozygous sickle cell disease. Br Med J 1984;288:1567–1570.
77. Gaston MH, Verter JI, Woods G, et al. Prophylaxis with oral penicillin in children with sickle cell anemia. A randomized trial. N. Engl. J. Med. 1986;314:1593–1599.
78. Pearson HA, Spencer RP, Cornelius EA. Functional asplenia in sickle-cell anemia. N Engl J Med 1969;281:923–926.
79. Bjornson AB, Lobel JS. Direct evidence that decreased serum opsonization of *Streptococcus pneumoniae* via the alternative complement pathway in sickle cell disease is related to antibody deficiency. J Clin Invest 1987;79:388–398.
80. Rogers ZR, Morrison RA, Vedro DA, Buchanan GR. Outpatient management of febrile illness in infants and young children with sickle cell anemia. J Pediatr 1990;117:736–739.
81. Wilimas JA, Flynn PM, Haris S, et al. A randomized study of outpatient treatment with ceftriaxone for selected febrile children with sickle cell disease. N Engl J Med 1993;329:472–476.
82. Buckalew VM, Someren A. Renal manifestations of sickle cell disease. Arch Intern Med 1974;133:660–669.
83. Gonzalez-Carrillo MG, Rudge CJ, Parsons V, Bewick M, White JM. Renal transplantation in sickle cell disease. Clin Nephrol 1982;18: 209–210.
84. Lindsay J, Meshel JC, Patterson RH. The cardiovascular manifestations of sickle cell disease. Arch Intern Med 1974;133:643–651.
85. Collins FS, Orringer EP. Pulmonary hypertension and cor pulmonale in the sickle hemoglobinopathies. Am J Med 1982;73:814–821.
86. Thomas ED. Marrow transplantation for nonmalignant disorders. N Engl J Med 1985;312:44–47.
87. Bank A, Markowitz P, Lerner N. Gene transfer. Ann NY Acad Sci 1989;565:37.
88. Kempin S, Gould-Rossbach P, Howland WS. Disorders of hemostasis in the critically ill cancer patient. In: Howland WS, Carlton GC, eds. Critical care of the cancer patient. Chicago: Year Book, 1985: 211–260.
89. Kanter RC, Oski FA. The acutely bleeding child. In: Shoemaker WC,

Ayres S, Grenvik A, Thompson WL, Holbrook PR, eds. Textbook of critical care. Philadelphia: WB Saunders, 1989: 898–902.
90. Montgomery RR, Hathaway WE. Acute bleeding emergencies. Pediatr Clin North Am 1980;27:327.
91. Buchanan G. Neonatal coagulation: normal physiology and pathophysiology. Clin Haematol 1978;7:85.
92. Stehling L, Simon TL. The red blood cell transfusion trigger: physiology and clinical studies. Arch Pathol Lab Med 1994;118:429.
93. Blanchette VS, Hume HA, Levy GJ, Luban NL, Strauss RG. Guidelines for auditing pediatric blood transfusion practices. Am J Dis Child 1991;145:787–796.
94. Isbister JP. Haemotherapy for acute haemorrhage. Anaesth Intensive Care 1984;12:217.
95. Sohmer PR, Scott RL. Massive transfusion. Clin Lab Med 1982;2:21.
96. Rock G, Tocchi M, Ganz PR, Tackaberry ES. Incorporation of plasticizer into red cells during storage. Transfusion 1984;24:493–498.
97. Sohmer PR, Moore GL, Beutler E, Peck CC. In vivo viability of red blood cells stored in CPDA-2. Transfusion 1982;22:479.
98. Moore GL, Peck CC, Sohmer PP, Zuck TF. Some properties of blood stored in anticoagulant CPDA-1 solution. A brief summary. Transfusion 1981;21:135.
99. Moore GL, Ledford ME, Merydith A. The biochemical effects on CPDA-2-drawn red blood cells of delayed refrigeration prior to component preparation. Transfusion 1982;22:485.
100. Murphy S, Gardner FH. Platelet preservation: effect of storage temperature maintenance of platelet viability— Deleterious effect of refrigerated storage. N Engl J Med 1969;280:1094.
101. Wolfe L. The red cell membrane and the storage lesion. Clin Haematol 1985;14:259.
102. Wolfe LC. The membrane and the lesions of storage in preserved red cells. Transfusion 1985;25:185.
103. Goodstein MH, Locke RG, Wlodarczyk D, Goldsmith LS, Rubenstein SD, Herman JH. Comparison of two preservation solutions for erythrocyte transfusions in newborn infants. J Pediatr 1993;123:783–788.
104. Luban NLC, Strauss RG, Hume HA. Commentary on the safety of red cells preserved in extended-storage media for neonatal transfusions. Transfusion 1991;31:229–35.
105. Sohmer PR, Dawson RB. The significance of 2,3-DPG in red blood cell transfusions. CRC Crit Rev Clin Lab Sci 1979;11:107.
106. Snyder EL, Bookbinder M. Role of microaggregate blood filtration in clinical medicine. Transfusion 1983;23:460.
107. Reynolds LO, Simon TL. Size distribution measurements of microaggregates in stored blood. Transfusion 1980;20:669.
108. Collins JA. Hemorrhage, shock, and burns: pathophysiology and treatment. In: Petz LD, Swisher SN, eds. Clinical practice of blood transfusion. New York: Churchill Livingstone, 1981:425.
109. Cote CJ, Liu LM, Szyfelbein SK, Goudsouzian NG, Daniels AL. Changes in serial platelet counts following massive blood transfusion in pediatric patients. Anesthesiology 1985;62:197–201.
110. Furman EB, Roman DG, Lemmer LA, Hairabet J, Jasinska M, Laver MB. Specific therapy in water, electrolyte, and blood volume replacement during pediatric surgery. Anesthesiology 1975;42:187–193.
111. Rasmussen GE, Grande CM. Blood, fluids, and electrolytes in the pediatric trauma patient. International Anesthesiology Clinics 1994;32:79–101.
112. Camp FR, Shields CE. Military blood banking—Identification of the group O, universal donor for transfusion of A, B, and AB recipients—An enigma of two decades. Milit Med 1967;132:426.
113. Phillips GR, Kauder DR, Schwab CW. Massive blood loss in trauma patients: The benefits and dangers of transfusion therapy. Postgraduate Med 1994;95:61–72.
114. Brimacombe J, Berry A. Hypertonic solutions in massive hemorrhage (letter). Br J Anaesth 1993;70:705.
115. Hamilton SM. The use of blood in resuscitation of the trauma patient. Can J Surg 1993;36:21–27.
116. Gervin AS, Fisher RP. Resuscitation of trauma patients with type-specific uncrossmatched blood. J Trauma 1984;24:327.
117. Meyer EA, Shulman IA. The sensitivity and specificity of the immediate—spin crossmatch. Transfusion 1989;29:99.
118. Shulman IA, Nelson JM, Saxena S, et al. Experience with the routine use of an abbreviated crossmatch. Am J Clin Pathol 1984;82:178–181.
119. Judd WJ. Are there better ways than a cross-match to demonstrate ABO incompatibility? Transfusion 1991;31:192.
120. Abbott TR. Changes in serum calcium fractions and citrate concentrations during massive blood transfusions and cardiopulmonary bypass. Br J Anaesth 1983;55:753.
121. Woodman RC, Harker LA. Bleeding complications associated with cardiopulmonary bypass. Blood 1990;76:1680.
122. Kern FH, Morana NJ, Scars JJ, Hickey PR. Coagulation defects in neonates during cardiopulmonary bypass. Ann Thorac Surg 1992;54:541–6.
123. Addonizio VP. Platelet function in cardiopulmonary bypass and artificial organs. Hematol/Oncol Clin North Am 1990;4:145.
124. Kestin AS, Valeri CR, Khuri SF, et al. The platelet function defect of cariopulmonary bypass. Blood 1993;82:107–117.
125. Nilsson L, Bagge L, Nystrom SO. Blood cell trauma and postoperative bleeding: comparison of bubble and membrane oxygenators and observations on coronary suction. Scand J Thorac Cardiovasc Surg 1990;24:65–69.
126. Harker LA, Malpass TW, Branson HE, et al. Mechanism of abnormal bleeding in patients undergoing cardiopulmonary bypass: acquired transient platelet dysfunction associated with selective alpha-granule release. Blood 1980;56:824–834.
127. Bick RL. Hemostasis defects associated with cardiac surgery, prosthetic devices, and other extracorporeal circuits. Semin Thromb Hemost 1985;11:249.
128. Ferraris VA, Rodriguez E, Ferraris SP, et al. Platelet aggregation abnormalities after cardiopulmonary bypass. Blood 1994;83:299–301.
129. Manno CS, Hedberg KW, Kim HC, et al. Comparison of the hemostatic effects of fresh whole blood, stored whole blood, and components after open heart surgery in children. Blood 1991;77:930–936.
130. Longmore DB, Bennett JG, Hoyle PM, et al. Prostacyclin administration during cardiopulmonary bypass in man. Lancet 1981;1:800–804.
131. Weston MJ. Prostacyclin and extracorporeal circulation. Br Med Bull 1983;39:285.
132. Aren C, Feddersen K, Radegran K. Effects of prostacyclin infusion on platelet activation and postoperative blood loss in coronary bypass. Ann Thorac Surg 1983;36:49.
133. Fish KJ, Sarnquist FH, van Steennis C, et al. A prospective randomized study of the effects of prostacyclin on platelets and blood loss during coronary artery bypass operations. J Thorac Cardiovasc Surg 1986;91:436–442.
134. Huddleston CB, Hammon JWJ, Wareing TH, et al. Amelioration of the deleterious effects of platelets activated during cardiopulmonary bypass: comparison of a thromboxane synthetase inhibitor and a prostacyclin analogue. J Thorac Cardiovasc Surg 1985;89:190–195.
135. van Oeveren W, Harder MP, Roozendaal KJ, Eijsman L, Wildevuur CR. Aprotinin protects platelets against the initial effect of cardiopulmonary bypass. J Thorac Cardiovasc Surg 1990;99:788–796.
136. Gundry SR, Drongowski RA, Klein MD, Coran AG. Postoperative bleeding in cardiovascular surgery. Am Surg 1989;55:162–165.
137. Hill AG, et al. More precise heparin and protamine management during cardiopulmonary bypass. Proc Am Acad Cardiovasc Perf 1990;11:12.
138. von Segesser LK, Turina M. Cardiopulmonary bypass without systemic heparinization for 24 hours. Am SECT Proceed 1989;76–82.
139. Salzman EW, Weinstein MJ, Weintraub RM, et al. Treatment with desmopressin acetate to reduce blood loss after cardiac surgery: a double blind randomized trial. N Engl J Med 1986;314:1402–1406.
140. LoCicero F, Massad M. Any value for desmopressin acetate (DDAVP) in cardiopulmonary bypass operations? J Thorac Cardiovasc Surg (letter) 1990;99:945.
141. Seear MD, Wadsworth LD, Rogers PC, Sheps S, Ashmore PG. The effect of desmopressin acetate (DDAVP) on postoperative blood loss after cardiac operations in children. J Thorac Cardiovasc Surg 1989;98:217–219.
142. Rocha E, Hidalgo F, Llorens R, Melero JM, Arroyo JL, Paramo JA. Randomized study of aprotinin and DDAVP to reduce postoperative bleeding after cardiopulmonary bypass surgery. Circulation 1994;90:921–7.
143. Royston D, Bidstrup BP, Taylor KM, Sapsford RN. Effect of aprotinin on the need for blood transfusion after repeat open-heart surgery. Lancet 1987;2:1289–1291.
144. Bidstrup BP, Royston D, Sapsford RN, Taylor KM. Reduction in blood loss and blood use after cardiopulmonary bypass with high dose aprotinin (Trasylol). J Thorac Cardiovasc Surg 1989;97:364–372.
145. Ranucci M, Corno A, Pavesi M, et al. Renal effects of low dose aprotinin in pediatric cardiac surgery. Minerva Anestesiologica 1994;60:361–6.
146. Boldt J, Knothe C, Zickmann B, Wege N, Dapper F, Hempelmann G. Comparison of two aprotinin dosage regimens in pediatric patients having cardiac operations. Influence on platelet function and blood loss. J Thorac Cardiovasc Surg 1993;105:705–11.

147. Cribble JW, Nes PM. Fibrin glue: the perfect operative sealant? Transfusion 1990;30:741.
148. Green TP, Isham-Schopf B, Steinhorn RH, Smith C, Irmiter RJ. Whole blood activated clotting time in infants during extracorporeal membrane oxygenation. Crit Care Med 1990;18:494–498.
149. Peters J, Radermacher P, Kuntz ME, et al. Extra-corporeal $C0_2$-removal with a heparin coated artificial lung. Intens Care Med 1988;14: 578–584.
150. Bindslev L, Eklund J, Norlander O, et al. Treatment of acute respiratory failure by extra-corporeal carbon dioxide elimination performed with a surface heparinized artificial lung. Anesthesiology 1987;67:117–120.
151. Tsuno K, Terasaki H, Otsu T, Okamoto T, Sakanashi Y, Morioka T. Newborn extracorporeal lung assist using a novel double lumen catheter and a heparin-bonded membrane lung. Intens Care Med 1993;19:70–2.
152. Klein MD, Whittlesey GC. Extra-corporeal membrane oxygenation. Pediatr Clin N Am 1994;41:365–384.
153. McManus ML, Kevy SV, Bower LK, Hickey PR. Coagulation factor dificiencies during initiation of extracorporeal membrane oxygenation. J Pediatr 1995;126:900–904.
154. Honig CL, Bove JR. Transfusion-associated fatalities: review of Bureau of Biologics reports 1976–1978. Transfusion 1984;20:653.
155. Linden JV, Kaplan HS. Transfusion errors: Causes and effects. Transfusion Med Rev 1994;8:169–183.
156. Nicholls MD. Transfusion: Morbidity and mortality. Anaesth Intens Care 1993;21:15–19.
157. Dahlke MB. Red blood cell transfusion therapy. Med Clin North Am 1984;68:639.
158. Greenwalt TJ. Pathogenesis and management of hemolytic transfusion reactions. Semin Hematol 1981;18:84.
159. Collins JA. Massive blood transfusion. Clin Haematol 1976;5:201.
160. Wolfe LC. Oxidative injuries to the red cell membrane during conventional blood preservation. Semin Hematol 1989;307:26.
161. McLennan BA, Reid SR, Lane PL. Massive blood transfusion causing hypomagnesemia. Crit Care Med 1984;12:146.
162. Card RT. Red cell membrane changes during storage. Trans Med Rev 1988;2:40.
163. Perkins HA. Transfusion-associated AIDS. Am J Hematol 1985;19:307.
164. Curran JW, Lawrence DN, Jaffe H, et al. Acquired immunodeficiency syndrome (AIDS) associated with transfusions. N Engl J Med 1984;310:69–75.
165. Sanders MR, Graeber JE. Posttransfusion graft-versus–host disease in infancy. J Pediatr 1990;117:159–163.
166. Anderson KC, Weinstein HJ. Transfusion-associated graft-versus-host disease. N Engl J Med 1990;323:315–321.
167. Davey RJ, Carmen RA, Simon TL, et al. Preparation of white cell depleted red cells for 42 day storage using an integral in-line filter. Transfusion 1989;29:496–499.
168. Gilbert GL, Hayes K, Hudson IL, James J. Prevention of transfusion-acquired cytomegalovirus infection in infants by blood filtration to remove leukocytes. Lancet 1989;1:1228–1231.
169. de Graan-Hentzen YC, Gratama JW, Mudde GC, et al. Prevention of primary cytomegalovirus infection in patients with hematologic malignancies by intensive white cell depletion of blood products. Transfusion 1989;29:757–760.
170. Moseley RV, Doty DB. Death associated with multiple pulmonary emboli soon after battle injury. Ann Surg 1970;171:336.
171. Berman IR, Illiescu H, Ranson JHC, Eng K. Pulmonary capillary permeability—A transfusion lesion. J Trauma 1976;16:41.
172. Mayer JE, Kerstein TE, Humphrey EW. Effects of transfusion of emboli and aged plasma on pulmonary capillary permeability. J Thorac Cardiovasc Surg 1981;82:358.
173. Brown C, Dhurandhar HN, Barrett J, Litwin MS. Progression and resolution of changes in pulmonary function and structure due to pulmonary microembolism and blood transfusion. Ann Surg 1977;185:92–99.
174. Esrig BC, Fulton RL. Sepsis, resuscitated hemorrhagic shock and "shock lung": an experimental correlation. Ann Surg 1976;182:218.
175. Collins JA, James PM, Bredenberg CE, Anderson RW, Heisterkamp CA, Simmons RL. The relationship between transfusion and hypoxemia in combat casualties. Ann Surg 1978;188:513–520.
176. Pepe PE, Potkin RT, Reus DH, Hudson LD, Carrico CJ. Clinical predictors of the adult respiratory distress syndrome. Am J Surg 1982;144:124–130.
177. Durtschi MB, Haisch CE, Reynolds L. Effect of micropore filtration on pulmonary function after massive transfusion. Am J Surg 1979;138:8.
178. Linko K. A comparison of six microaggregate blood filters: filtration efficiency, capacity and hemolysis in vitro. Vox Sang 1980;39:52.
179. Schmidt WF, Kim HC, Tomassin N, Schwartz E. RBC destruction caused by a micropore blood filter. JAMA 1982;248:1629.
180. Sirchia G, Wenz B, Rebulla P, Parravicini A, Carnelli V, Bertolini F. Removal of white cells from red cells by transfusion through a new filter. Transfusion 1990;30:30–33.
181. Sirchia G, Rebulla P, Parravicini A, Carnelli V, Gianotti GA, Bertolini F. Leukocyte depletion of red cell units at the bedside by transfusion through a new filter. Transfusion 1987;27:402–405.
182. Donaldson MDJ, Scaman MJ, Park GR. Massive blood transfusion. Br J Anaesth 1992;69:621–630.
183. Malouf M, Glanville AR. Blood transfusion related adult respiratory distress syndrome. Anaesth Intens Care 1993;21:44–49.
184. Popovsky MA, Chaplin HC, Jr., Moore SB. Transfusion-related acute lung injury: a neglected, serious complication of chemotherapy. Transfusion 1992;32:589–592.
185. Counts RB, Haisch C, Simon TL, Maxwell NG, Heimbach DM, Carrico CJ. Hemostasis in massively transfused trauma patients. Ann Surg 1979;190:91–99.
186. Mannucci PM, Federici AB, Sirchia G. Hemostasis testing during massive blood replacement. Vox Sang 1982;42:113.
187. Hewson JR, Neame PB, Kumar N, et al. Coagulopathy related to dilution and hypotension during massive transfusion. Crit Care Med 1985;13:387–391.
188. Faringer PD, Mullins RJ, Johnson RL, Trunkey DD. Blood component supplementation during massive transfusion of AS-1 red cells in trauma patients. J Trauma 1993;34:481–487.
189. Raphael BG, Lackner H, Engler GL. Disseminated intravascular coagulation during surgery for scoliosis. Clin Orthop 1982;162:41.
190. Mayer PJ, Gehlsen FA. Coagulopathies associated with major spinal surgery. Clin Orthop Rel Res 1989;245:83.
191. Johnson SD, Lucas CE, Gerrick SJ, Ledgerwood AM, Higgins RF. Altered coagulation after albumin supplemented for treatment of oligemic shock. Arch Surg 1979;114:379–383.
192. Lucas CE, Ledgerwood AM, Mammen EF. Altered coagulation protein content after albumin resuscitation. Ann Surg 1982;196:198.
193. Paramo JA, Rocha E. Hemostasis in advanced liver disease. Sem Thromb Hemost 1993;19:184–190.
194. Kang YG, Martin DJ, Marquez J, et al. Intraoperative changes in blood coagulation and thromboelastograph monitoring in liver transplantation. Anesth Analg 1985;64:888–896.
195. Bontempo FA, Lewis JH, Van Thiel DH, et al. The relation of preoperative coagulation findings to diagnosis, blood usage, and survival in adult liver transplantation. Transplantation 1985;39:532–536.
196. Carlier M, Van Obbergh LJ, Veyekemans F, et al. Hemostasis in children undergoing liver transplantation. Sem Thromb Hemost 1993;19:218–222.
197. Groh J, Welte M, Azad SC, Anthuber M, Haller M, Kratzer MA. Does aprotinin really reduce blood loss in orthotopic liver transplantation? Sem Throm Hemost 1993;19:306–308.
198. Hashim SW, Kay HR, Hammond GL, Kopf GS, Geha AS. Noncardiogenic pulmonary edema after cardiopulmonary bypass: an anaphylactic reaction to fresh frozen plasma. Am J Surg 1984;147:560–564.
199. O'Connor PC, Erskine JG, Pringle TH. Pulmonary oedema after transfusion with fresh frozen plasma. Br Med J 1981;282:379.
200. Carson JL, Willett LR. Is a hemoglobin of 10 g/dl required for surgery? Med Clin N Am 1993;77:335–47.
201. Dietrich KA, Conrad SA, Hebert CA, Levy GL, Romero MD. Cardiovascular and metabolic response to red blood cell transfusion in critically ill volume-resuscitated nonsurgical patients. Crit Care Med 1990;18:940–944.
202. Levine E, Rosen A, Sehgal L, Gould S, Sehgal H, Moss G. Physiologic effects of acute anemia: implications for a reduced transfusion trigger. Transfusion 1990;30:11–14.
203. Heusser F, Fahey JT, Lister G. Effect of hemoglobin concentration on critical cardiac output and oxygen transport. Am J Physiol 1989;256:H527–32.
204. Fontanarosa PB, Giorgio GT. The role of the emergency physician in the management of Jehovah's Witnesses. Ann Emerg Med 1989;18:1089–1095.
205. Layon AJ, D'Amico R, Caton D, Mollet CJ. And the patient chose: medical ethics and the case of the Jehovah's Witness. Anesthesiology 1990;73:1258–1262.
206. Macklin R. The inner workings of an ethics committee: latest battle over Jehovah's Witnesses. Hastings Center Report 1988;Feb/March: 15–20.
207. Grubbs PE, Marini CP, Fleischer A. Acute hemodilution in an anemic

Jehovah's Witness during extensive abdominal wall resection and reconstruction. Ann Plast Surg 1989;22:448–451.
208. Gillon J. Controversies in transfusion medicine: acute normovolemic hemodilution in elective major surgery: con. Transfusion 1994;34:269–271.
209. Stehling L, Zauder HL. Controversies in transfusion medicine: perioperative hemodilution: pro. Transfusion 1994;34:265–268.
210. Kharasch SJ, Millham F, Vinci RJ. The use of autotransfusion in pediatric chest trauma. Pediatr Emerg Care 1994;10:109–112.
211. Jacobs LM, Hsieh JW. A clinical review of autotransfusion and its role in trauma. JAMA 1984;251:3283.
212. Isbister JP. Autotransfusion: an impossible dream? Anaesth Intensive Care 1984;12:236.
213. Odling-Smee W. Red cell substitutes. Br Med J 1990;300:599.
214. Kahn RA, Allan RW, Baldassare J. Alternate sources and substitutes for therapeutic blood components. Blood 1985;66:1.
215. Millard RW. Oxygen solubility, rheology and hemodynamics of perfluorocarbon emulsion blood substitutes. Artificial Cells, Blood Substitutes and Immobilization Biotechnology 1994;22:235–44.
216. Holman WL, McGiffin DC, Vicente WV, Spruell RD, Pacifico AD. Use of current generation perfluorocarbon emulsions in cardiac surgery. Artificial Cells, Blood Substitutes and Immobilization Biotechnology 1994;22:979–90.
217. Kumar R. Recombinant hemoglobins as blood substitutes: a biotechnology perspective. Proc Soc Exp Biol Med 1995;208:150–8.
218. Williamson L. Homologous blood transfusion: The risks and alternatives. Br J Haematol 1994;88:451–8.
219. Alving BM, Hojima Y, Pisano J, et al. Hypotension associated with prekallikrein activator (Hageman-factor fragments) in plasma protein fraction. N Engl J Med 1978;299:66–70.
220. Baenziger NL, Dillender MJ, Majerus PW. Cultured human skin fibroblasts and arterial cells produce a labile platelet inhibitory prostaglandin. Biochem Biophys Res Commun 1977;78:294.
221. Adelman B, Stemerman MB, Mennell D, Handin RI. The interaction of platelets and aortic subendothelium: inhibition of adhesion and secretion by prostaglandin I2. Blood 1981;58:198–205.
222. Lollar P, Owen WG. Clearance of thrombin from circulation in rabbits by high-affinity binding sites on endothelium. Possible role in the inactivation of thrombin by antithrombin III. J Clin Invest 1982;69:726.
223. Busch C, Owen WG. Identification in vitro of an endothelial cell surface cofactor for antithrombin. III. Parallel studies with isolated perfused rat hearts and microcarrier cultures of bovine endothelium. J Clin Invest 1982;69.
224. Esmon CT. Protein C: biochemistry, physiology, and clinical implications. Blood 1983;62:1155.
225. Walker FJ. Protein S and the regulation of activated protein C. Semin Thromb Hemost 1984;10:131.
226. Griffin JL. Clinical studies of protein C. Semin Thromb Hemost 1984;10:162.
227. Esmon CT, Esmon NL. Protein C activation. Semin Thromb Hemost 1984;10:122.
228. Tuffin DP. The platelet surface membrane: ultrastructure, receptor binding and function. In: Page CP, ed. The platelet in health and disease. Oxford: Blackwell Scientific Pulications, 1991: 10–60.
229. Weiss HJ. Platelet physiology and abnormalities of platelet function: I. N Engl J Med 1975;293:531.
230. Weiss HJ. Platelet physiology and abnormalities of platelet function: II. N Engl J Med 1975;293:580.
231. Plow EF, Ginsberg MH. Molecular basis of platelet function. In: Hoffman R, Benz EJ, Jr., Shattil SJ, Furie B, Cohen HJ, Silberstein LE, eds. Hematology: basic principles and practice. New York: Churchill Livingstone, 1995: 1524–1535.
232. Davies SC, Machin SJ. Prostacyclin (PGI2). Intensive Care Med 1983;9:49.
233. Mueller-Eckhardt C, Grubert A, Weisheit M, et al. 348 cases of suspected neonatal alloimmune thrombocytopenia. Lancet 1989;1: 363–366.
234. Schiffer CA. Prevention of alloimmunization against platelets. Blood 1991;77:1–4.
235. Bussel JB. Autoimmune thrombocytopenic purpura. Hematol/Oncol Clin North Am 1990;4:179.
236. Andrew M, Barr RD. Increased platelet destruction in infancy and childhood. Semin Thromb Hemost 1982;8:248.
237. Murphy S. In search of a platelet Coombs test. N Engl J Med 1983;309:490.
238. Moore SB. Immune thrombocytopenias and platelet antibodies. Mayo Clin Proc 1982;57:778.
239. Harmon JA, Miller WV. Platelet antibodies: their detection and significance. Am J Med Technol 1981;47:797.
240. Zimmerman TS, Ruggeri ZM. Von Willebrand's disease. Clin Haematol 1983;12:175.
241. Hardisty RM. Hereditary disorders of platelet function. Clin Haematol 1983;12:153.
242. Nugent DJ. Platelet transfusion. In: Nathan DG, Oski FA, ed. Hematology of infancy and childhood. Fourth ed. Philadelphia: W. B. Saunders, 1993:1781–1795.
243. de Rie MA, van der Plas-van Dalen CM, Engelfriet CP, von dem Borne AE. The serology of febrile transfusion reactions. Vox Sang. 1985;49:126–134.
244. Decary F, Ferner P, Giavedoni L, et al. An investigation of nonhemolytic transfusion reactions. Vox Sang. 1984;46:277–285.
245. Deeg HJ. Transfusions with a tan-prevention of allosensitization by ultraviolet irradiation. Transfusion 1989;29:547.
246. Kutti J, Zaroulis CG, Dinsmore RE, Reich L, Clarkson BD, Good RA. A prospective study of platelet-transfusion therapy administered to patients with acute leukemia. Transfusion 1982;22:44–47.
247. Ilett SJ, Lilleyman JS. Platelet transfusion requirements of children with newly diagnosed lymphoblastic leukaemia. Acta Haematol 1979; 62:86.
248. Murphy S, Litwin S, Herring LM, et al. Indications for platelet transfusion in children with acute leukemia. Am J Hematol 1982;12: 347–356.
249. Kelton JG, Blajchman MA. Platelet transfusions. Can Med Assoc J 1979;121:1353.
250. Foster DC, Sprecher CA, Grant FJ, et al. Human thrombopoietin: gene structure, cDNA sequence, expression, and chromosomal localization. Proc. Natl. Acad. Sci USA 1994;91:13023–13027.
251. Wilson JJ, Neame PB, Kelton JG. Infection-induced thrombocytopenia. Semin. Thromb. Hemost. 1982;8:217–233.
252. Semerano N, Lattanzio A. Interaction of platelets with bacterial endotoxins. Agents Actions 1983;13:461.
253. Clawson CC, White JG. Platelet interaction with bacteria. V. Ultrastructure of congenital afibrinogenemic platelets. Am J Pathol 1980;98:197.
254. Brain MC, Naeme PB. Thrombotic thrombocytopenic purpura and the hemolytic uremic syndrome. Semin Thromb Hemost 1982;8:186.
255. Drummond KN. Hemolytic uremic syndrome-then and now. N Engl J Med 1985;312:116–118.
256. Dubansky AS, Oski FA. Controversies in the management of acute idiopathic thrombocytopenic purpura: a survey of specialists. Pediatrics 1986;77:49.
257. Kelton JB, Gibbons S. Autoimmune platelet destruction: idiopathic thrombocytopenic purpura. Semin Thromb Hemost 1982;8:83.
258. Buchanan GR. Overview of ITP treatment modalities in children. Blut 1989;59:96.
259. Halperin DS, Doyle JJ. Is bone marrow examination justified in idiopathic thrombocytopenic purpura? Am J Dis Child 1988;142:508.
260. Humphreys RP, Hockley AD, Freedman MH, Saunders EF. Management of intracerebral hemorrhage in idiopathic thrombocytopenic purpura. J Neurosurg 1976;45:700–704.
261. Woerner SJ, Abildgaard CF, French BN. Intracranial hemorrhage in children with idiopathic thrombocytopenic purpura. Pediatrics 1981;67:453–460.
262. Ozsoylu S, Irken G, Karabent A. High dose intravenous methylprednisolone for acute childhood idiopathic thrombocytopenic purpura. Eur J Hematol 1989;42:431–435.
263. Blanchette VS, Luke B, Andrew M, et al. A prospective, randomized trial of high-dose intravenous immune globulin G therapy, oral prednisone therapy, and no therapy in childhood acute immune thrombocytopenia purpura. J Pediatr 1993;123:989–995.
264. van Hoff J, Ritchey AK. Pulse methylprednisolone therapy for acute childhood idiopathic thrombocytopenic purpura. J Pediatr 1988; 113:563–566.
265. Blajchman MA, Shepherd FA, Perrault RA. Clinical use of blood, blood components and blood products. Can Med Assoc J 1979;121:33–42.
266. Slichter SJ. Controversies in platelet transfusion therapy. Annu Rev Med 1980;31:509.
267. Bussel JB, Berkowitz RL, McFarland JG, Lynch L, Chitkara U. Antenatal treatment of neonatal alloimmune thrombocytopenia. N Engl J Med 1988;319:1374–1378.
268. Blanchette V, Andrew M, Perlman M, Ling E, Ballin A. Neonatal autoimmune thrombocytopenia: role of high dose intravenous immunoglobulin G therapy. Blut 1989;59:139–144.
269. Kelton JG, Blanchette VS, Wilson WE, et al. Neonatal thrombocytope-

nia due to passive immunization: prenatal diagnosis and distinction between maternal platelet alloantibodies and autoantibodies. N Engl J Med 1980;302:1401–1403.
270. Andrew M, Kelton J. Neonatal thrombocytopenia. Clin Perinatol 1984;11:359–391.
271. Kelton JG. Management of the pregnant patient with idiopathic thrombocytopenic purpura. Ann Intern Med 1983;99:796.
272. Lindsay RM, Clark WF. Platelet destruction in renal disease. Semin Thromb Hemost 1982;8:138.
273. Brown CH, Natelson EA, Bradshaw W, Williams TW, Jr., Alfrey CP, Jr. The hemostatic defect produced by carbenicillin. N Engl J Med 1974;291:265-270.
274. Alexander DP, Russo ME, Fohrman DE, Rothstein G. Nafcillin-induced platelet dysfunction and bleeding. Antimicrob Agents Chemother 1983;23:59–62.
275. Slonaker CE, Luper WE. Moxalactum-associated platelet dysfunction. JAMA 1983;250:729.
276. Morris N, Barr RD, Pai KR, Kelton JG. Valproic acid and thrombocytopenia. Can Med Assoc J 1981;125:63–64.
277. Loiseau P. Sodium valproate, platelet dysfunction and bleeding. Epilepsia 1981;22:141.
278. Corazza MS, Davis RF, Merritt TA, Bejar R, Cvetnic W. Prolonged bleeding time in preterm infants receiving indomethacin for patent ductus arteriosus. J Pediatr 1984;105:292–296.
279. Sadler JE, Gralnici HR. Commentary: A new classification for von Willebrand disease. Blood 1994;84:676–679.
280. Ruggeri ZM, Zimmerman TS. von Willebrand factor and von Willebrand disease. Blood 1987;70:895–904.
281. Kaufman RJ. Genetic engineering of factor VIII. Nature 1989;342:207.
282. de la Fuente B, Kasper CK, Rickles FR, Hoyer LW. Response of patients with mild and moderate hemophilia A and von Willebrand's disease to treatment with desmopressin. Annals of Internal Medicine 1985;103:6–14.
283. Lammle B, Griffin JH. Formation of the fibrin clot: the balance of procoagulant and inhibitory factors. Clin. Haematol. 1985;14:281.
284. Hemker HC, Lindhout TH. A clotting scheme for 1984. Nouv Rev Fr Hematol 1984;26:227.
285. Nawroth P, Kisiel W, Stern D. The role of endothelium in the homeostatic balance of heamostasis. Clin. Haematol. 1985;14:531.
286. Bennett JS. Blood coagulation and coagulation tests. Med Clin North Am 1984;68:557.
287. Rosenberg RD. Actions and interactions of antithrombin and heparin. N Engl J Med 1975;292:146.
288. Erickson LA, Schleef RR, Ny T, Loskuloff DJ. The fibrinolytic system of the vascular wall. Clin Haematol 1985;14:513.
289. Bick RL. The clinical significance of fibrinogen degradation products. Semin Thromb Hemost 1983;8:302.
290. Bick RL. Disseminated intravascular coagulation: objective criteria for diagnosis and management. Med Clin North Am 1994;78:511–543.
291. Gilbert JA, Scalzi RP. Disseminated intravascular coagulation. Emergency Med Clin North Am 1993;11:465–480.
292. Rubin RN, Colman RW. Disseminated intravascular coagulation: approach to treatment. Drugs 1992;44:963–971.
293. Edelman B, Heyman MR. Blood component therapy for trauma patients. In: Stene JK, Grande CM, eds. Trauma anesthesia. Baltimore: Williams and Wilkins, 1991: 144.
294. Takahashi H, Tatewaki W, Wada K, Hanano M, Shibata A. Thrombin vs. plasmin generation in disseminated intravascular coagulation associated with various underlying disorders. Am. J. Hematology 1990;33:90–95.
295. Aasen AO, Smith-Erichsen N, Amundsen E. Plasma kallikrein-kinin system in septicemia. Arch. Surg. 1983;118:343.
296. Carvalho AC. Activation of the contact system of plasma proteolysis in the adult respiratory distress syndrome. J. Lab. Clin. Med. 1988;112:270.
297. Marder VJ, Martin SE, Colman RW. Consumptive thrombohemorrhagic disorders. In: Colman RW, Hirsh J, Marder VJ, Salzman EW, eds. Hemostasis and thrombosis: basic principles and clinical practice. Philadelphia: JB Lippincott, 1982: 975–1025.
298. Colman RW, Marder VJ. Disseminated intravascular coagulation (DIC): pathogenesis, pathophysiology, and laboratory abnormalities. In: Colman RW, Hirsh J, Marder VJ, Salzman EW, eds. Hemostasis and thrombosis: basic principles and clinical practice. Philadelphia: JB Lippincott, 1982:654.
299. Gralnick HR. Cancer cell procoagulant activity. In: Donati MB, Davidson JF, Garattini S, eds. Malignancy and the hemostatic system. New York: Raven Press, 1981: 57.
300. Abshire TC, Gold SH, Odom LF, Carson SD, Hathaway WE. The coagulopathy of childhood leukemia. Thrombin activation or primary fibrinolysis? Cancer 1990;66:716–721.
301. Ribeiro RC, Pui PH. The clinical and biological correlates of coagulopathy in children with acute leukemia. J Clin Concol 1986;4:1212–1218.
302. Kaufman HH, Hui KS, Mattson JC, et al. Clinicopathological correlations of disseminated intravascular coagulation in patients with head injury. Neurosurgery 1984;15:34–42.
303. Miner ME, Kaufman HH, Graham SH, Haar FH, Gildenberg PL. Disseminated intravascular coagulation fibrinolytic syndrome following head injury in children: frequency and prognostic implications. J Pediatr 1982;100:687–691.
304. Woods WG, Luban NL, Hilgartner MW, Miller DR. Disseminated intravascular coagulation in the newborn. Am J Dis Child 1979;133:44–46.
305. Kliegman RM, Fanaroff AA. Necrotizing enterocolitis. N Engl J Med 1984;310:1093–1103.
306. Karmali MA, Petric M, Lim C, Fleming PC, Arbus GS, Lior H. The association between idiopathic hemolytic uremic syndrome and infection by verotoxin-producing *Escherichia coli* J Infect Dis 1985;151:775–782.
307. Rose PE, Armour JA, Williams CE, Hill FG. Verotoxin and neuraminidase induced platelet aggregating activity in plasma: their possible role in the pathogenesis of HUS. J Clin Pathol 1985;38:438–441.
308. Fong JSC, de Chadarevian J-P, Kaplan BS. Hemolytic uremic syndrome: current concepts and management. Pediatr Clin North Am 1982; 29:835.
309. Greenwalt TJ. Pathogenesis and management of hemolytic transfusion reactions. Semin Hematol 1981;18:84.
310. Warrell RP, Kempin SJ. Treatment of severe coagulopathy in the Kasabach-Merritt syndrome with aminocaproic acid and cryoprecipitate. N Engl J Med 1985;313:309–312.
311. Prentice CRM. Acquired coagulation disorders. Clin Haematol 1985;14:441.
312. Feinstein DI. Treatment of disseminated intravascular coagulation. Semin Thromb Hemost 1988;14:351–362.
313. Spicer T, Tan JM. Purpura fulminans. Am J Med 1976;61:566.
314. Sakuragawa N, Hasegawa H, Maki M, Nakagawa M, Nakashima M. Clinical evaluation of low-molecular-weight heparin (FR-860) on disseminated intravascular coagulation (DIC)—a multicenter co-operative double-blind trial in comparison with heparin. Thrombosis Research 1993;72:475–500.
315. Blauhut B, Kramar H, Vinazzer H, Bergmann H. Substitution of antithrombin III in shock and DIC: a randomized study. Thrombosis Research 1985;39:81–89.
316. Green G, Thomson JM, Dymock IW, Poller L. Abnormal fibrin polymerization in liver disease. Br J Haematol 1976;34:427.
317. Hathaway WE, Goodnight SH. Disorders of hemostasis and thrombosis, a clinical guide.New York: McGraw-Hill, Inc., 1993:211–216.
318. Francis RM, Feinstein DI. Clinical significance of accelerated fibrinolysis in liver disease. Haemostasis 1984;14:460.
319. Furie B, Limentani SA, Rosenfeld CG. A practical guide to the evaluation and treatment of hemophilia. Blood 1994;84:3–9.
320. Brettler DB, Kraus EM, Levine PH. Clinical aspects of and therapy for hemophilia A. In: Hoffman R, Benz EJ, Jr., Shattil SJ, Furie B, Cohen HJ, Silberstein LE, eds. Hematology: basic principles and practice. New York: Churchill Livingstone, 1995:1648–1663.
321. Roberts HR, Gray TF, III. Clinical aspects of and therapy for hemophilia B. In: Hoffman R, Benz EJ, Jr., Shattil SJ, Furie B, Cohen HJ, Silberstein LE, ed. Hematology: basic principles and practice. New York: Churchill Livingstone, 1995:1678–1685.
322. Miller CH. Genetics of hemophilia and von Willebrand's disease. In: Hilgartner MW, ed. Hemophilia in the child and adult. New York: Masson Publishing, 1982:29.
323. Kasper CK, Dietrich SL. Comprehensive management of haemophilia. Clin Haematol 1985;14:489.
324. Gill JC. Therapy of factor VIII deficiency. Semin Throbosis Hemostasis 1993;19:1–12.
325. Roberts HR. Factor VIII replacement therapy: issues and future prospects. Ann NY Acad Sci 1991;614:106.
326. Warrier AI, Luscher JM. DDAVP: a useful alternative to blood components in moderate hemophilia A and von Willebrand's disease. J Pediatr 1983;102:228.

327. Mannucci PM, Canciani MT, Rota L, Donovan BS. Response of factor VIII/von Willebrand factor to DDAVP in healthy subjects and patients with hemophilia A and von Willebrand's disease. Br J Haematol 1981;47:283–293.
328. Stanievich JF, Marshark G, Stool SE. Airway obstruction in a hemophiliac child. Ann Otol 1980;80:572.
329. Andes WA, Wulff K, Smith WB. Head trauma in hemophilia: a prospective study. Arch Intern Med 1984;144:1981.
330. Gilchrist GS, Piepgras DG, Roskos RR. Neurologic complications in hemophilia. In: Hilgartner MW, ed. Hemophilia in the child and adult. New York: Masson Publishing, 1982:99.
331. White GC, McMillan CW, Blatt PM, Roberts HR. Factor VIII inhibitors: a clinical overview. Am J Hematol 1982;13:335.
332. McMillan CW. Clinical patterns of hemophilic patients who develop inhibitors. In: Hoyer LW, ed. Factor VIII inhibitors. New York: Alan R. Liss, 1984:31.
333. Hedner U, Glazer S. Management of hemophilia patients with inhibitors. Hematology/Oncology Clinics of North America 1992;6: 1035–1046.
334. Kasper CK. Treatment of Factor VIII inhibitors. In: Coller BS, ed. Progress in hemostasis and thrombosis. Philadelphia: WB Saunders Co., 1989:57–86.
335. Abildgaard CF. Management of inhibitors in hemophilia. In: Hilgartner MW, ed. Hemophilia in the child and adult. New York: Masson Publishing, 1982:167.
336. Lusher JM, Blatt PM, Penner JA, et al. Autoplex versus proplex: a controlled, double-blind study of effectiveness in acute hemarthroses in hemophiliacs with inhibitors to factor VIII. Blood 1983;62:1135–1138.
337. Prentice CRM. Comparison of factor VIII and prothrombin complex concentrates in the treatment of inhibitor patients. In: Hoyer LW, ed. Factor VIII inhibitors. New York: Alan R. Liss, 1984: 197.
338. Itultin MB. Studies of factor IX concentrate therapy in hemophilia. Blood 1982;62:677.
339. Sullivan DW, Purdy LJ, Billingham M, Glader BE. Fatal myocardial infarction following therapy with prothrombin complex concentrates in a young man with hemophilia A. Pediatrics 1984;74:279.
340. Brettler DB, Forsberg AD, Levine PH, et al. The use of porcine factor VIII concentrate (Hyate:C) in the treatment of patients with inhibitor antibodies to factor VIII. A multicenter US experience. Arch Intern Med 1989;149:1381–1385.
341. Macik BG, Hohneker J, Roberts HR, Griffin AM. Use of recombinant activated Factor VII for treatment of a retropharyngeal hemorrhage in a hemophiliac patient with a high titer inhibitor. Am J Hematol 1989;32:23N234.
342. Bick RL. Hypercoagulability and thrombosis. In: Bick RL, ed. Disorders of Thrombosis and Hemostasis. Chicago: ASCP Press, 1992: 261–290.
343. Hathaway WE. Use of antiplatelet agents in pediatric hypercoagulable states. Am J Dis Child 1984;138:301–304.
344. Bordeaux DH, Abshire TC, Marlar RA. Dysfunctional protein C deficiency (Type II). Am J Clin Pathol 1993;99:677–686.
345. Walker FJ. Protein S and thrombotic disease. Proc Soc Exp Biol Med 1992;200:285–295.
346. Manco-Johnson MJ, Abshire TC, Jacobson LJ, Marlar RA. Severe neonatal protein C deficience: prevalence and thrombotic risk. J Pediatr 1991;119:793–798.
347. Comp PC, Esmon CT. Recurrent venous thromboembolism in patients with a partial deficiency of protein S. N Engl J Med 1984;311:1525.
348. Awidi AS, Abu-Khalaf M, Herzallah U, et al. Hereditary thrombophilia among 217 consecutive patients with thromboembolic disease in Jordan. Am J Hematol 1993;44:95–100.
349. Suzuki K, Nishioka J, Kusumoto H, Hashimoto S. Mechanism of inhibition of activated protein C by protein C inhibitor. J Biochem 1984;95:187–195.
350. Sie P, Dupouy D, Pichon J, Boneu B. Constitutional heparin cofactor II deficiency associated with recurrent thrombosis. Lancet 1985;2: 414–416.
351. Tran TH, Marbet GA, Duckert F. Association of hereditary heparin cofactor II deficiency with thrombosis. Lancet 1985;2:413.
352. Nguyen P, Reynaud J, Pouzol P, Munzer M, Richard O, Francois P. Varicella and thrombotic complications associated with transient protein C and protein S deficiencies in children. Eur J Pediatr 1994;153: 646–649.
353. Kaplan BS, Chesney RW, Drummond KN. The nephrotic syndrome and renal vein thrombosis. Am J Dis Child 1978;132:367–370.
354. Mitchell L, Hoogendoorn H, Giles AR, Vegh P, Andrew M. Increased endogenous thrombin generation in children with acute lymphoblastic leukemia: risk of thrombotic complications in L-asparaginase-induced antithrombin III deficiency. Blood 1994;83:386–91.
355. Shapiro AD, Clarke SL, Christian JM, Odom LF, Hathaway WE. Thrombosis in children receiving L-asparaginase. Determining patients at risk. Am J of Pediatr Hematol-Oncol 1993;15:400–5.
356. Bernstein ML, Sternbach M, Bellefleur M, Esseltine DW. Thrombotic and hemorrhagic complications in children with lupus anticoagulant. Am J Dis Child 1984;138:1132–1135.
357. Lloyd-Still JD, Tomasi L. Neurovascular and thromboembolic complications of inflammatory bowel disease in childhood. J Pediatr Gastroenterol Nutr 1989;9:461–466.
358. Jicha DL, Caty MG, Lillehei CW. Primary antiphospholipid syndrome in a child with lower extremity arterial thrombosis. J Pediatr Surg 1994;29:1519–20.
359. Khamashta MA, Cuadrado MJ, Mujic F, Taub NA, Hunt BJ, Hughes GR. The management of thrombosis in the antiphospholipid-antibody syndrome. N. Engl. J. Med. 1995;332:993–7.
360. Rees MM, Rodgers GM. Homocysteinemia: association of a metabolic disorder with vascular disease and thrombosis. Thrombosis Research 1993;71:337–59.
361. Benotti JR, Dalen JE. The natural history of pulmonary embolism. Clin Chest Med 1984;5:403–410.
362. Collins R, Scrimgeour A, Yusuf S, Peto R. Reduction in fatal pulmonary embolism and venous thrombosis by perioperative administration of subcutaneous heparin. N Engl J Med 1988;318:1162–1173.
363. Smith MD, Bressler EL, Lonstein JE, Winter R, Pinto MR, Denis F. Deep venous thrombosis and pulmonary embolism after major reconstructive operations on the spine. J Bone Joint Surgery 1994;76: 980–985.
364. Nguyen LT, Laberge JM, Guttman FM, Albert D. Spontaneous deep vein thrombosis in childhood and adolescence. J Pediatr Surg 1986;21:640–643.
365. Gorenstein A, Katz S, Levy P, Schiller M. Noniatrogenic deep vein thrombosis of lower extremities in children. Z Kinderchir 1986;41: 375–378.
366. Goldhagen J, Alford BA, Prewitt LH, Thompson L, Hostetter MK. Suppurative thrombophlebitis of the internal jugular vein: report of three cases and review of the pediatric literature. Pediatr Infect Dis 1988;7:410–414.
367. Matthew DJ, Levin M. Pulmonary thromboembolism in children. Intensive Care Med 1986;12:404–406.
368. Whitlock JA, Janco RL, Phillips JA. Inherited hypercoagulable states in children. Am J Pediatr Hematol/Oncol 1989;11:170–173.
369. Israels SJ, Seshia SS. Childhood stroke associated with protein C or S deficiency. J Pediatr 1987;111:562–564.
370. Ambruso DR, Jacobson LJ, Hathaway WE. Inherited antithrombin III deficiency and cerebral thrombosis in a child. Pediatrics 1980;65: 125–131.
371. Langnas AN, Marujo W, Stratta RJ, Wood RP, Shaw BW, Jr. Vascular complications after orthotopic liver transplantation. Am J Surg 1991;161:76–82.
372. Berman W, Fripp RR, Yabek SM, Wernly J, Corlew S. Great vein and right atrial thrombosis in critically ill infants and children with central venous lines. Chest 1991;99:963–967.
373. Pippus KG, Giacomantonio JM, Gillis DA, Rees EP. Thrombotic complications of saphenous central venous lines. J Pediatr Surg 1994;29:1218–1219.
374. Tanke RB, van Megen R, Daniels O. Thrombus detection on central venous catheters in the neonatal intensive care unit. Angiology 1994;45:477–480.
375. Mehta S, Connors AF, Jr., Danish EH, Grisoni E. Incidence of thrombosis during central venous catheterization of newborns: a prospective study. J Pediatr Surg 1992;27:18–22.
376. Gault DT. Vascular compromise in newborn infants. Arch Dis Child. 1992;67:463–467.
377. Talbott GA, Winters WD, Bratton SL, O'Rourke PP. A prospective study of femoral catheter-related thrombosis in children. Arch Pediatr Adolesc Med 1995;149:288–291.
378. Andrew M, Marzinotto V, Pencharz P, et al. A cross-sectional study of catheter-related thrombosis in children receiving total parenteral nutrition at home. J Pediatr 1995;126:358–363.
379. Rupar DG, Herzog KD, Fisher MC, Long SS. Prolonged bacteremia with catheter-related central venous thrombosis. Am J Dis Child 1990;144:879–882.
380. Raad II, Luna M, Khalil SA, Costerton JW, Lam C, Bodey GP. The re-

lationship between the thrombotic and infectious complications of central venous catheters. JAMA 1994;271:1014–6.
381. Grant BJB. Noninvasive tests for acute venous thromboembolism. Am J Respir Crit Care Med 1994;149:1044-1047.
382. Hull R, Hirsh J, Sackett DL, Powers P, Turpie AGG, Walker I. Combined use of leg scanning and impedance plethysmography in suspected venous thrombosis. N Engl J Med 1977;296:1497–1500.
383. Van der Meer J, Donker AJM. Diagnosis of deep venous thrombosis. Neth J Med 1984;27:298–304.
384. Clarke JC, McIlrath EM. The role of emergency venography in the diagnosis and management of deep venous thrombosis. Ulster Med J 1990;59:46–50.
385. Hull RD, Raskob GE, LeClerc JR, Jay RM, Hirsh J. The diagnosis of clinically suspected venous thrombosis. Clin Chest Med 1984;5: 439–456.
386. Heijboer H, Buller HR, Lensing AWA, Turpie AGG, Colly LP, ten Cate JW. A comparison of real-time compression ultrasonography with impedance plethysmography for the diagnosis of deep vein thrombosis in symptomatic outpatients. N Engl J Med 1993;329:1365–1369.
387. Moser KM, LeMoine JR. Is embolic risk conditioned by location of deep vein thrombosis? Ann Int Med 1981;94:439–444.
388. Hammerli M, Meyer RA. Doppler evaluation of central venous lines in the superior vena cava. J Pediatr 1993;122:S104–8.
389. Anonymous. Value of the ventilation/perfusion scan in acute pulmonary embolism. Results of the prospective investigation of pulmonary embolism diagnosis (PIOPED). The PIOPED Investigators. JAMA 1990;263:2753–2759.
390. Hyers TM. Antithrombotic therapy for venous thromboembolism. Clin Chest Med 1984;5:479–486.
391. Hull RD, Raskob GE, Hirsh J, et al. Continuous intravenous heparin compared with intermittent subcutaneous heparin in the initial treatment of proximal vein thrombosis. N Engl J Med 1986;315:1109–1114.
392. Schmidt B, Andrew M. Report of Scientific and Standardization Subcommittee on Neonatal Hemostasis Diagnosis and Treatment of Neonatal Thrombosis. Thrombosis & Haemostasis 1992;67:381–2.
393. Alkalay AL, Mazkereth R, Santulli T, Jr., Pomerance JJ. Central venous line thrombosis in premature infants: a case management and literature review. Am J Perinatol 1993;10:323–6.
394. Dillon PW, Fox PS, Berg CJ, Cardella JF, Krummel TM. Recombinant tissue plasminogen activator for neonatal and pediatric vascular thrombolytic therapy. J Pediatr Surg 1993;28:1264–8.
395. Anderson BJ, Keeley SR, Johnson ND. Caval thrombolysis in neonates using low doses of recombinant human tissue-type plasminogen activator. Anaesth Intens Care 1991;19:22–27.
396. McDonald MM, Hathaway WE. Anticoagulant therapy by continuous heparinization in newborn and older infants. J Pediatr 1982;101: 451–457.
397. Anderson DR, Levine MN. Thrombolytic therapy for the treatment of acute pulmonary embolism. Can Med Assoc J 1992;146:1317–1324.
398. Volgesang GB, Bell WR. Treatment of pulmonary embolism and deep vein thrombosis with thrombolytic therapy. Clin Chest Med 1984;5: 487–494.
399. Stiegler H, Arbogast H, Nees S, Halder A, Grau A, H. R. Thrombectomy, lysis, or heparin treatment: concurrent therapies of deep vein thrombosis: therapy and experimental studies. Semin Thromb Hemostas 1989;15:250–258.
400. Andrew M, Marzinotto V, Massicote P, et al. Heparin therapy in pediatric patients: a prospective cohort study. Pediatr Res 1994;35:78–83.
401. Doyle E, Britto J, Freeman J, Munro F, Morton NS. Thrombolysis with low dose tissue plasminogen activator. Arch Dis Child 1992;67:1483–4.
402. Rosenbaum T, Rammos S, Kniemeyer HW, Gobel U. Extended deep vein and inferior vena cava thrombosis in a 15-year-old boy: successful lysis with recombinant tissue-type plasminogen activator 2 weeks after onset of symptoms. Eur J Pediatr 1993;152:978–980.
403. Ricci MA, Lloyd DA. Renal venous thrombosis in infants and children. Arch Surg 1990;125:1195–1199.
404. LeBlanc JG, Culham JAG, Chan KW, Patterson MW, Tipple M, Sandor GG. Treatment of grafts and major vessel thrombosis with low-dose streptokinase in children. Ann Thorac Surg 1986;41:630–635.
405. Zenz W, Muntean W, Beitzke A, Zobel G, Riccabona M, Gamillscheg A. Tissue plasminogen activator (alteplase) treatment for femoral artery thrombosis after cardiac catheterisation in infants and children. Br Heart J 1993;70:382–5.
406. Brus F, Witsenburg M, Hofhuis WJD, Hazelzet JA, Hess J. Streptokinase treatment for femoral artery thrombosis after arterial cardiac catheterization in infants and children. Br Heart J 1990;63:291–294.
407. Giacoia GP. High-dose urokinase therapy in newborn infants with major vessel thrombosis. Clin Pediatr 1993;32:231–7.
408. Kirk CR, Qureshi SA. Streptokinase in the management of arterial thrombosis in infancy. Int J Cardiol 1989;25:15–20.
409. Wessel DL, Keane JF, Fellows KE, Robichaud H, Lock JE. Fibrinolytic therapy for femoral arterial thrombosis after cardiac catheterization in infants and children. Am J Cardiol 1986;58:347–351.
410. Corrigan JJ, Allen HD, Jeter M, Malone JM. Aortic thrombosis in a neonate: failure of urokinase therapy. Am J Pediatr Hemat/Oncol 1982;4:243–247.
411. Andrew M, Brooker L, Leaker M, Paes B, Weitz J. Fibrin clot lysis by thrombolytic agents is impaired in newborns due to a low plasminogen concentration. Thrombosis & Haemostasis 1992;68:325–30.
412. Ryan CA, Andrew M. Failure of thrombolytic therapy in four children with extensive thromboses. Am J Dis Child 1992;146:187–93.
413. Caplan MS, Cohn RA, Langman CB, Conway JA, Shkolnik A, Brouillette RT. Favorable outcome of neonatal aortic thrombosis and renovascular hypertension. J Pediatr 1989;115:291–295.
414. Evans DJ, Pizer BL, Moghal NE, Joffe HS. Neonatal aortic arch thrombosis. Arch Dis Child 1994;71:F125–7.
415. Uva MS, Serraf A, Lacour-Gayet F, et al. Aortic arch thrombosis in the neonate. Ann Thorac Surg 1993;55:990–992.
416. Chaikof EL, Dodson TF, Salam AA, Lumsden AB, Smith RB, 3d. Acute arterial thrombosis in the very young. J Vasc Surg 1992;16:428–35.

Management of the Child with Malignant Disease in the Pediatric Intensive Care Unit

42

Allen E. Eskenazi
Mark J. Mogul
Andrew M. Yeager
John B. Gordon

INTRODUCTION

The purpose of this chapter is to provide the intensivist with the theoretical and practical information necessary to administer comprehensive care to critically ill pediatric oncology patients. It is assumed that the intensivist will have access to consultative services from oncologists, infectious disease specialists, immunologists, and other specialists as needed. Nonetheless, the intensivist must understand enough about the patient's underlying condition both to appreciate the patient's needs and to interact effectively with the various consultants. Therefore, although this chapter emphasizes the diagnosis, pathophysiology, and therapy of life-threatening complications, the diagnosis and therapy of the most common childhood tumors will also be addressed.

Neoplastic disease is second only to trauma as the leading cause of death in the 1- to 15-year-old population[1–3].

Table 42.1. Distribution of Childhood Neoplasms (%)[a]

	Age (yr)		
Neoplasm	*0–4*	*5–9*	*10–15*
Leukemias	35–40	31–35	18–24
Central nervous system	12–14	25–26	17–20
Lymphomas	5	19–21	19–25
Neuroblastoma	13	2.2	<1
Kidney	9.2	6.1	2
Bone	<1	5	10.5
Soft tissue	3.7	3.5	6

[a] *From Sutow WW. General aspects of childhood cancer. In: Sutow WW, Fernbach DJ, Vietti TJ, eds. Clinical pediatric oncology. St. Louis: CV Mosby, 1984:1, and Altman AJ, Schwartz AD, eds. The cancer problem in pediatrics: epidemiologic aspects. In: Malignant diseases of infancy, childhood and adolescence. Philadelphia: WB Saunders, 1977:1.*

The leukemias are the most common malignancies of childhood, followed by brain tumors and the lymphomas. All other tumors together make up less than 40% of the total at any age. Most of these are sarcomas and neuroectodermal malignancies rather than the ectodermal or endodermal carcinomas more commonly seen in adults[(1–3)]. **Table 42.1** lists a sampling of the common childhood tumors and their relative frequency at different ages. It should be noted that although the term *malignant tumor* suggests a cancer capable of both local invasion and distant metastases, and *benign tumor* usually suggests a slowly growing, localized mass, both can lead to critical conditions. Therefore, in this chapter, the term malignant disease refers to either type of cancer.

ADMISSION TO THE INTENSIVE CARE UNIT

Indications for Admission

Despite the relatively high frequency of childhood malignancies and the myriad complications of the diseases and their treatment, until recently children with malignant disease have been infrequently admitted to pediatric intensive care units (PICUs). It was generally believed that little benefit was to be gained by subjecting cancer patients to the rigors of intensive care if the ultimate outcome of their disease was fatal. However, new developments in oncology, immunology, infectious disease, and intensive care are making recovery from cancer and its critical complications a possibility. In this section of the chapter, the issues of who should be admitted and what alterations to the usual PICU routine are required will be addressed.

Although it is relatively easy to identify those patients sick enough to require the machinery and personnel of the PICU, admission should also be determined by a reasonable likelihood of the patient surviving the acute illness, achieving remission from the cancer, and going on to a life of reasonable quality. Given the relative lack of data concerning likely outcome in the pediatric oncology population, the policy should be to apply the same general criteria for the admission of these children as are used with all children. Namely, there should be: (a) a life-threatening condition requiring the close observation or interventions best provided in the PICU and (b) the honest expectation that with the care available in the PICU, the child will recover. Which oncology patients are likely to need the PICU? There are three groups: (a) a small number of patients will come to the PICU at the time of diagnosis with a life-threatening complication of the tumor; (b) another group will require intense monitoring and close observation during or after high-risk procedures, and (c) most commonly, patients will be admitted with major complications due to either ongoing disease or the consequence of therapy. As the ability to provide intensive supportive care improves and the intensity of therapy increases, the number of children in the second group is growing[(4)].

In coming to a decision about admission to the PICU, it is important for the intensive care and oncology teams to discuss the child's therapy and prognosis carefully both among themselves and with the parents (and child). If it is believed that, with the resolution of an acute process, there is reasonable hope for cure of or remission from the underlying cancer, then the child should be admitted to the PICU and aggressive therapy pursued. Thus, most children in groups (a) and (b) above will warrant PICU admission. However, some children, particularly in group (c), have demonstrably little hope of recovery or cure. Failure to recognize and discuss the terminal nature of the child's condition will lead to needless pain and discomfort for the child, parents, and staff[(5–7)].

Alterations in the PICU Routine

Psychologic Needs of Patient and Staff

When a child with neoplastic disease is admitted to the PICU, it is critical that the PICU staff appreciate the unique features and needs—both psychologic and medical—of these oncology patients. Most often, the family and child have been in the hospital before, are familiar with the ward routine, and have bonded with the members of the oncology team[(5,8,9)]. The PICU staff can facilitate the transition to intensive care for the child and his or her parents by encouraging all members of the oncology team to remain closely involved with the child and family despite their possibly diminished direct responsibility for care in the PICU. This provides familiar faces for the patient during a very stressful period and provides excellent resources for PICU personnel. Furthermore, carefully explaining the PICU routine (visiting hours, etc.) and designating a primary nurse and physician for the patient will be helpful. Accurate and consistent communication is sometimes difficult in the setting of multiple caregivers and can lead to confusion and misconceptions on the part of both staff and patient. Frequent meetings of the entire treatment team (physicians, nurses, social workers, other support staff) to develop consistent care plans and goals are essential. Members of the team are encouraged to voice their concerns, displeasures, and thoughts on death and dying. Only in this way will the patient and family receive optimal medical, nursing, and psychologic care. Then the primary physician and nurse should communicate the problems and plans to the family. All consultants must speak with the primary physician or nurse prior to, or instead of, speaking with the parents and child. This approach can diminish (although it rarely totally eliminates) the all too frequent problems of confused and frustrated parents, children, and staff[5,8,9].

Infection Prevention

The major medical alterations in the PICU routine required in caring for the oncology patient, particularly if neutropenic, are related to the increased risk of infection in these children[10–13], although even nonneutropenic patients are at increased risk of infection[14]. Most often, the infecting organism is one with which the patient has been previously colonized[14]. If the child has been at home, the organism causing infection may be the normal body flora. In the hospital, however, the child may acquire resistant Gram-negative or -positive organisms, particularly in the PICU setting[15–18]. Furthermore, exposure to broad-spectrum antibiotics may predispose the patient to infection with fungal or more unusual opportunistic bacteria[10–12,15–18].

What alterations in the PICU routine can diminish the risks of infection? The total protective environment (laminar air flow rooms, masks, gowns and gloves, sterilized food, gut decontamination) has been shown to reduce the incidence of bacterial infection[19–23]. Nevertheless, overall survival may not be altered significantly for patients so protected, for many have died of viral infections, hemorrhage, or their primary malignancy[12]. The installation of laminar air flow rooms, as noted by Pizzo[21], is very cumbersome and expensive. A less expensive alternative is simple reverse isolation—gown, mask, and gloves. Although this seems an intuitively useful procedure, it is not of proven benefit in preventing either the spread of viral respiratory infection or bacterial infections[24,25]. However, it will serve to remind all staff of how compromised these patients are. Moreover, the need to gown and mask seems to reduce the number of personnel in contact with the patient, which may be of benefit in decreasing the risk of exposure to potentially harmful organisms[26], but it is vital that these precautions not interfere with the contact necessary to provide quality care. Since the spread of organisms that eventually colonize the patient occurs principally through staff-to-patient hand contact, strict hand washing must be enforced, particularly if a protective environment is not to be used[26–28]. The contribution of inanimate objects to the incidence of nosocomial infection is unclear[27,28]; however, frequent changing of ventilator tubing, humidifiers, etc., in the hope of preventing serious contamination of equipment in the PICU is probably of value[16].

In addition to reverse isolation, some other procedures may be of benefit to the patient. Clearly, avoidance of the indiscriminate use of broad-spectrum antibiotics for all patients in the PICU will reduce the emergence of highly resistant organisms[29]. All invasive procedures should be preceded by careful skin preparation. The routine blood testing should be minimized and finger-stick blood samples avoided if possible. Intravascular catheters require special caution and will be discussed in the infection section below. Despite the advances made in catheter technology and notwithstanding the techniques available to reduce the risk of catheter-related infection, it is important for the intensivist to weigh the benefits of invasive monitoring carefully against the risk of infection in children with neoplastic disease. Is a urinary catheter or an arterial line absolutely necessary? The question can be extended to some therapeutic procedures. Is it better to tolerate moderate hypoxemia with oxygen provided by face mask than to improve oxygenation with endotracheal intubation but increase the risk of pulmonary infection? There is no obvious answer to these questions, but a case-by-case approach rather than strict adherence to a policy is probably best.

COMPLICATIONS OF CANCER

Infectious Complications

Serious bacterial infection remains a major cause of PICU admission and death in cancer patients. In this section of the chapter, the normal host defenses to infection will be briefly reviewed, emphasizing how they are altered in the case of the oncology patient. Then issues of infection prophylaxis and prevention will be discussed, followed by an approach to the diagnosis and management of sepsis, viral infection, and fungemia in these patients.

Normal and Abnormal Host Defenses

Although the oncology patient is a very visible example of the immunocompromised host, most children admitted to intensive care suffer from some impairment of the normal host defenses, which include (a) barriers to infection, (b) cellular and humoral immunity, and (c) the phagocytes. Abnormalities of these host defenses may arise because of congenital deficiencies, age-dependent deficiencies, acquired diseases, or as a consequence of therapy as discussed in detail in Chapters 28 and 29.

Barriers to Infection

The primary defenses against infection are the barriers preventing access of the microorganisms to the host[30]. These include local physical, chemical, humoral, and phagocytic defenses **(Table 42.2)**. The respiratory system of the normal host is an excellent example of a well-equipped barrier against infection. The intact mucosa, the cilia, the mucus produced, and the cough reflex prevent the penetration of bacteria below the glottis. Should an organism overcome these defenses, local antibodies and phagocytes will neutralize the agent, preventing systemic infection and, often, even significant local disease. Similar defenses are avail-

Table 42.2. Barriers to Infection

Physical	
	Skin and mucosa
	Cell turnover and shedding
	Ciliary action, peristalsis, and cough
	Normal skin and mucosal flora
Chemical	
	Mucous
	pH (gut)
	Fatty acids produced by anaerobic bacteria
Humoral	
	Secretory antibodies
Phagocytic	
	Local macrophages
	Local neutrophils
	Local lymphocytes

able to all body surfaces in contact with the external environment[(30)].

Disorders of the barriers to infection are innumerable, with trauma (accidental and surgical) and burns being the most common in the PICU setting. In the oncology patient, it is the invasive and therapeutic procedures used in the PICU as well as the destructive effects of chemotherapy and radiation therapy to mucosal surfaces that lead most often to destruction of the normal barriers to infection. For example, endotracheal tubes defeat the normal role of the cilia and cough reflex; intravascular lines and implanted catheters provide an ideal portal of entry for infection. Finally, antibiotics alter normal skin and intestinal flora, making way for nosocomial infection[(30)].

Cellular and Humoral Immunity

Should an organism penetrate the initial barriers to infection, it is met by the immune system. While it may be convenient to think of cellular and humoral immunity as distinct entities, their interplay makes such divisions artificial. Nonetheless, for the sake of simplicity, we will consider first the lymphocytes and macrophages, then the immunoglobulins and complement system. The T cells make up 55 to 75% of the lymphocyte population. These cells have specific antigen receptors on their surfaces, and through complex interaction with the macrophages[(31–35)], they are activated and release a variety of lymphokines that stimulate B-cell production of antibody, clonal expansion of T cells, and increased hematopoiesis[(34,35)].

The B cells comprise most of the other lymphocytes. These cells, after proper stimulation, differentiate into plasma cells and produce antigen-specific immunoglobulins[(36)]. Five major classes of immunoglobulins exist (IgE, IgD, IgA, IgG, and IgM), and numerous subclasses have been identified. The latter three antibody classes are currently best understood in terms of host defenses. IgA, particularly secretory IgA, forms one of the barriers to infection mentioned before. IgG and IgM are potent bacterial opsonins, and both can activate the complement system via the classical pathway[(36)].

The complement system is made up of a number of circulating proteins that can be activated by a variety of stimuli[(36)]. Without stimulation, there is usually a balance between the activated factors and natural inhibitors present in the circulation. Figure 42.1 shows the classical and alternative complement pathways. The classical pathway is activated by IgG- or IgM-antigen complexes, while the alternative pathway is activated by bacterial cell wall components (and some other antigens) through interaction with the small amounts of C3b always circulating in the plasma. If this interaction occurs in the presence of the required cofactors, then the complex so formed, C3bBb, like the C4,2 complex, can activate more C3 and set off the cascade. The various activated complement proteins act in different ways. C3a and C5a are both chemotactic for neutrophils. C3b is a potent opsonin. C5 is critical in the control of fungal infection, while C6 − 9 are directly cytolytic and seem necessary for the control of *Neisseria* infections[(36)].

Many diseases and therapies can impair humoral immunity **(Table 42.3)**. Malnutrition is of particular importance in the intensive care setting and in the oncology patient[(37–40)]. In the pediatric population, it has been shown that not only does better nutrition decrease the frequency of sepsis, but it may improve the overall outcome of cancer patients and certainly improves the sense of well-being[(38–40)]. Therefore, an aggressive approach to nutrition should be adopted. As soon as the child has stabilized, enteral or parenteral nutrition should be instituted. In addition to malnutrition induced by illness and the anorexia associated with chemotherapy, cancers can cause depression

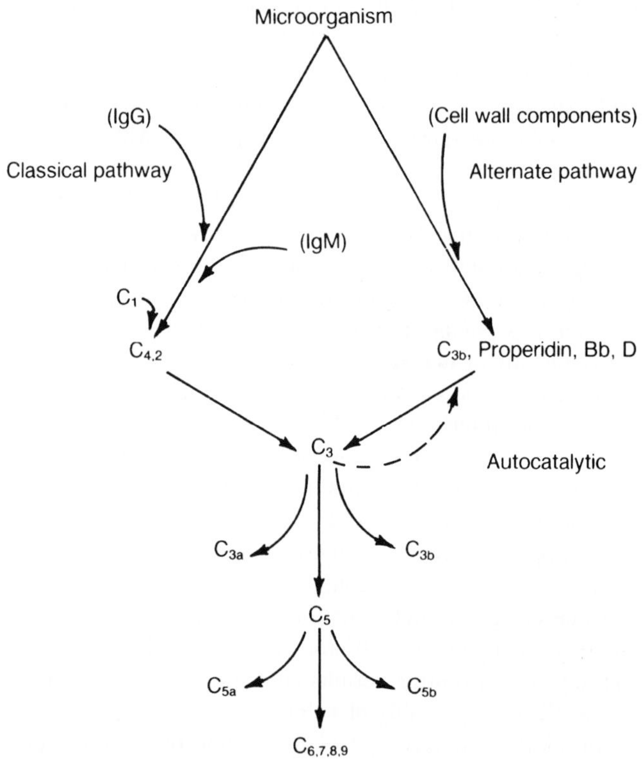

Figure 42.1. Complement cascade. From Winkelstein JA. The role of complement in the host's defense against *Streptococcus pneumoniae.* Rev Infect Dis 1981;3:289, with permission.

Table 42.3. Acquired Immunodeficiency

T cell
Malnutrition
Viral infections, including HIV
Tuberculosis
Steroids, chemotherapy, other immunosuppressive drugs
Uremia
Diabetes
Surgery
Burns
Parasitic infections
Sarcoidosis
Bone marrow transplantation
B cell (immunoglobulins)
Nephrotic syndrome
Leukemia/lymphoma
Burns
Splenectomy
Bone marrow transplantation
Complement
Hepatic failure
Burns
Steroids
Hemoglobinopathies (sickle cell related)
Autoimmune disorders
Severe infection (bacterial)
Splenectomy

of immune function. For example, the leukemias have been associated with poor B-cell function, even after apparent cure of the primary disease increasing predisposition to infection[41]. Finally, cancer therapy, particularly the use of steroids and other immunosuppressives, is associated with diminished lymphocyte function[14].

Phagocytes

The immune system readies the microbe for killing by opsonizing it and attracting phagocytes through chemotactic stimulation. The phagocyte then engulfs the organism and kills it by a variety of intracellular biochemical mechanisms[42]. The polymorphonuclear leukocytes (PMN) and, to a lesser extent, the macrophages are the major phagocytes. To respond to the immune system, the phagocyte must be able to migrate in response to the chemotactic stimulus, must be able to engulf the organism, and must have an intact respiratory burst mechanism and myeloperoxidase system with which to kill the organism. Most important in the context of this chapter, there must be an adequate number of phagocytes present.

Acquired diseases of the phagocytes are relatively rare and relate primarily to loss of numbers rather than function, generally as a consequence of chemotherapy. The degree of neutropenia (severe = less than 100/μl, moderate = 100−500/μl, mild = 500−1000/μl) is positively correlated with morbidity and mortality due to both bacterial infection and fungal disease[43]. Historically, the mortality rate was as high as 80% in patients with severe neutropenia of more than 3 weeks' duration. It is not surprising that infection remains a leading cause of death in these patients. The introduction of recombinant granulocyte colony-stimulating factor (G-CSF) and granulocyte-macrophage colony-stimulating factor (GM-CSF) have led to the amelioration of chemotherapy-induced neutropenia and a subsequent decrease in infection rates[44]. While involvement of the bone marrow by malignancies or destruction by chemotherapy are the major causes of acquired neutropenia, it is of note that a variety of bacterial and viral infections can cause neutrophil dysfunction[45].

In summary, both the cancer and its therapy cause the loss of normal host defenses. Physical barriers are disrupted by malignancies involving the skin or the mucosa and by therapy associated with mucositis, as well as by the invasive procedures often employed in the PICU. Humoral and cellular immunity are decreased in the leukemias and lymphomas and other malignancies involving the marrow and reticuloendothelial system. Debilitation and malnutrition and the frequent use of corticosteroids also lead to diminished immune function. Finally, cancers involving the bone marrow and chemotherapy often cause neutropenia with the ensuing decrease in phagocytic capacity.

Infection Prevention in the Child with Malignant Disease

Environment and Antibiotics

In the earlier discussion of alterations in the PICU routine, some of the techniques for avoiding infection in patients were mentioned. In particular, the success of total protective environments in preventing infection was discussed[19–23]. While laminar air flow rooms may not be possible for the critically ill oncology patient, isolation with the use of gowns, masks, and gloves by the staff can be easily accomplished and thorough hand washing is a must. Trimethoprim-sulfamethoxazole (TMP-SMX) is routinely used as prophylaxis against *Pneumocystis carinii*[46]. We favor the use of TMP-SMX for all children who have leukemia or lymphoma or have undergone either intensive chemotherapy or bone marrow transplantation. In view of the risk of *Candida* overgrowth associated with broad-spectrum antibiotic use, nystatin is often used, but its efficacy against *Candida albicans* even in doses of 1 million IU four to six times a day is limited[11]. The development of newer antifungal agents such as fluconazole for fungal prophylaxis[47] has reduced morbidity and mortality from this organism. The use of parenteral antibiotics for infection prophylaxis has been abandoned in view of the risk of superinfection with resistant organisms[19,43,48].

Immunization and Antiviral Prophylaxis

A number of methods of viral infection prevention have been used with varying success. Zoster-immune plasma is useful in the child who has been exposed to varicella[49,50]. Moreover, immunization of children with live attenuated varicella vaccine has been effective and carried few side effects[51]. Hepatitis B immunoglobulin may be helpful in cases of hepatitis exposure[52]. Cytomegalovirus (CMV) infection is a major concern in oncology patients, particularly

Table 42.4. Infection Prevention in the Pediatric Intensive Care Unit

Scrupulous hand washing by staff
Reverse isolation techniques (mask, gown, gloves)
Scrupulous oral, dental, skin hygiene for patient
Prompt insertion (in operating room) of central venous catheter if prolonged intravenous access is needed
Acyclovir or immune globulin for varicella prophylaxis after documented exposure

after bone marrow transplantation. Avoidance of CMV-positive blood may reduce the risk of developing the infection in patients who were previously seronegative, but activation of CMV in a CMV-positive child poses a major problem. Various approaches to prophylaxis include intravenous immune globulin, acyclovir, and ganciclovir as discussed later in this chapter[53–55]. Moreover, intravenous immunoglobulins have been associated with a decrease in the frequency of some bacterial infections in bone marrow transplant patients, and the risks of administration are low[53]. Bacterial vaccines, like pneumococcal vaccines, may not be as efficacious in this population as in normal hosts because of the oncology patient's poor immune function, as discussed earlier. **Table 42.4** summarizes some of the techniques of infection prevention discussed above.

Intravascular Catheters

A final topic that deserves mention in this section on infection prevention is care of intravascular lines. Peripheral venous and arterial lines should be repositioned every 2 to 4 days[56–58]. Central lines require particular care. If a central line is placed percutaneously under emergent conditions, it should be considered contaminated and should be changed as soon as the child's condition permits[58]. Once the child is stable, insertion of a longer-term Silastic catheter may be desirable. There is good evidence that the incidence of infection is higher in those patients with central lines than those without; however, in those children who require frequent chemotherapy, parenteral nutrition, and other medications, they are a necessity, and the incidence of infection with the Silastic catheters is acceptably low provided trained nurses use sterile techniques in changing solutions[59–63]. The types of long-term catheters available include the Broviac (single-lumen) and Hickman (double-lumen) externalized type and the implanted type (e.g., Infus-a-port). Of these, earlier studies suggested that the latter carries less risk of infection but requires surgical implantation and percutaneous access[60–62]. More recent prospective data suggest that there is no difference in infection rate between subcutaneously implanted versus externalized catheters[10]. Interestingly, the double-lumen catheters had no higher infection rate than did the single-lumen type,[63] and given the needs of the PICU patient, we therefore favor insertion of the double-lumen catheter.

Given the importance of central venous access in these children, one is faced with a dilemma when the oncology patient with a central line becomes febrile. If it is not essential, the line should be removed; peripheral catheters should be used for a couple of days, allowing time for the infection to clear, and then a new line inserted if needed. More often, the line is judged essential, so we institute antibiotic therapy through the line. The antibiotic(s) selected should include coverage against *Staphylococcus aureus* and *S. epidermidis* (the most common infecting organisms) and may need to include good Gram-negative coverage and antifungal agents (discussed below)[10,43]. Finally, in some patients, thrombosis with infection will occur (see also Chapter 41), leading to the need for both thrombolytic and antibiotic therapy[64].

Infection in the Child with Malignant Disease

Likely Causes

The child with neoplastic disease may have a critical infection at the time of diagnosis, particularly if leukemia or lymphoma is present, or if a normal barrier to infection has been disrupted. In patients with hematologic malignancies, the infection may be caused by Gram-positive or encapsulated Gram-negative organisms (e.g., *Streptococcus pneumoniae, Haemophilus influenzae*) because of the loss of both cellular and humoral immunity. If neutropenia is present, the cause of the infection may also include opportunistic or enteric Gram-negative organisms, *S. aureus,* or *S. epidermidis*[10,12,41,43,48,65,66].

Similarly, management of the child with a known malignancy who is admitted to the PICU for a suspected bacterial infection or develops one while in the PICU will largely depend on the presence or absence of neutropenia. In patients without neutropenia, the infection will often be due to common pathogens. In the hospitalized neutropenic child, however, the cause may be *S. aureus, S. epidermidis,* or a mixed aerobic and anaerobic infection[10,12,41,43,48,65,66]. Other factors, such as prolonged antibiotic administration, the presence of indwelling catheters, poor oral hygiene[67] or debilitation, and poor functional status before the onset of infection also increase the risk of severe nosocomial infection.

Signs and Symptoms

The early diagnosis of suspected bacterial infection and prompt initiation of therapy are essential in the child with neoplastic disease. Delay in therapy may lead to septic shock. However, since the diagnosis of infection may be difficult, both a high degree of suspicion and a low threshold for initiation of therapy are necessary. Various reviews[10,11,43,65] have outlined useful approaches to these patients. The patient with a normal leukocyte count may have the classic signs of infection, but the neutropenic patient (or one receiving steroids) will often have less obvious signs and symptoms. Fever is usually present but may be masked in patients receiving massive doses of steroids. From 55 to 70% of febrile episodes in oncology patients are of infectious origin[10,11,43,65]. Although a fever may be due to drugs, the underlying neoplastic disease, or other factors, its presence indicates infection until proven otherwise. On occasion, fever will be absent. Classic manifestations of systemic infection may be attenuated or absent[68]. For example, pneumonia may be present without rales or lobar consolidation[69]; meningitis or peritonitis may be severe, but the usual symptoms may be absent because of the lack of normal inflammatory responses. Equally important, phlebitis may be present with minimal erythema, induration, or purulent drainage.

In addition to fever, subjective complaints of feeling poorly, altered states of consciousness, or any complaints referable to a specific area of discomfort should lead to a careful search for occult or overt infection involving the ears, throat, sinuses, chest, abdomen, perianal area, skin, bones, and joints. Further assessment of the possibility of infection requires appropriate laboratory investigation, including a full sepsis work-up, and interpretation of the data in the context of a low leukocyte count. Chest x-rays, arterial blood gases, and other tests (e.g., chest and abdomen computed tomography [CT] studies) may be useful; however, in most cases, the initial diagnosis of infection will rest on clinical judgment that "the child looks septic."

Therapeutic Approach: Nonneutropenic Host

If a febrile child with malignant disease has a neutrophil count greater than 1000/μl, one can opt to await culture results before initiating antibiotic therapy. Alternatively, empiric therapy can be initiated. Empiric therapy in the nonneutropenic patient, particularly if the child has not been recently hospitalized or subjected to invasive procedures, should be aimed at the organisms likely to cause infection in a normal host. *S. pneumoniae* or *H. influenzae* are, for example, the likely causes of respiratory disease[70], and specific therapy with a single antibiotic, such as ceftriaxone, can be initiated. The decision to await cultures or use narrow antibiotic coverage should be rescinded if the infection is severe, the child appears seriously ill, or the neutrophil count is falling[10,11,43,65].

Therapeutic Approach: Neutropenic Host

In the neutropenic host, antibiotic therapy should be initiated immediately, even if the child "looks well." It is important that each institution develop a consistent set of criteria for the mandatory, rapid initiation of broad-spectrum antibiotics in the febrile, neutropenic host. The likely organisms were discussed above and are summarized in **Table 42.5.** Institutional prevalence and sensitivity patterns should be periodically examined to determine the best empiric therapy. A further hint as to the likely organism may be obtained from prior surveillance cultures obtained from hospitalized patients and clinical signs if present. Regardless of the likely organism(s), empiric broad-spectrum antibiotic coverage, often with multiple drugs, is indicated[10,43,65,66,71–73]. In general, initial empiric broad-spectrum therapy in the febrile neutropenic child may include ceftazidime alone[71] or with an aminoglycoside[74]. However, the frequent emergence of Gram-positive infections with ceftazidime monotherapy should prompt a low threshold for the addition of more extensive Gram-positive coverage with, for example, nafcillin[65]. A commonly employed alternative regimen is the combination of an anti-pseudomonas penicillin (ticarcillin or piperacillin) and an aminoglycoside (gentamicin, tobramycin, or amikacin)[72]. This latter combination, with or without addition of a cephalosporin, has been effective against many pathogens seen in these patients, including *Pseudomonas, Klebsiella,* and *Staphylococcus* species[10,43,65,66,71–73]. Nafcillin or vancomycin is often added for coverage against *Staphylococcus* species (e.g., *S. aureus, S. epidermidis*); vancomycin is recommended in situations where methicillin-resistant *Staphylococcus* is known to be prevalent[66] or if catheter-related sepsis is strongly suspected. However, emergence of multiply resistant *Enterococci* has made empiric addition of vancomycin less desirable[75]. Other agents are added or substituted as indicated by clinical response (or lack thereof), alteration in the primary focus of the infection, data from surveillance cultures, and microbiologic culture and sensitivity data from the fever work-up. For example, the addition of an agent effective against *Bacteroides fragilis* and other anaerobes, such as clindamycin or metronidazole, may be necessary in cases of intra-abdominal or gynecologic infections[10,11,43,65].

Table 42.5. Likely Organisms Causing Sepsis in Oncology Patients

Escherichia coli	Neutropenia, abdominal focus
Staphylococcus aureus, Staphylococcus epidermidis	Defective barriers against infection, neutropenia, poor functional status
Pseudomonas aeruginosa	Neutropenia, relapse of malignancy
Streptococcus pneumoniae	Leukemia, lymphoma, primary pulmonary focus, splenectomy
Klebsiella pneumoniae	Neutropenia, relapse of malignancy
Bacteroides fragilis	Neutropenia, abdominal focus, relapse of malignancy
Haemophilus influenzae	Leukemia, lymphoma, splenectomy

Two important questions that arise after initiating empiric therapy concern duration of treatment and whether to escalate antimicrobial therapy. The nonneutropenic child can be treated in much the same manner as any patient with suspected sepsis: initial antibiotics are continued until culture results are available. If results are positive, the antibiotics are adjusted appropriately and continued for 10 to 14 days (assuming that the neutrophil count is stable and not decreasing to neutropenic levels). If the cultures are negative,

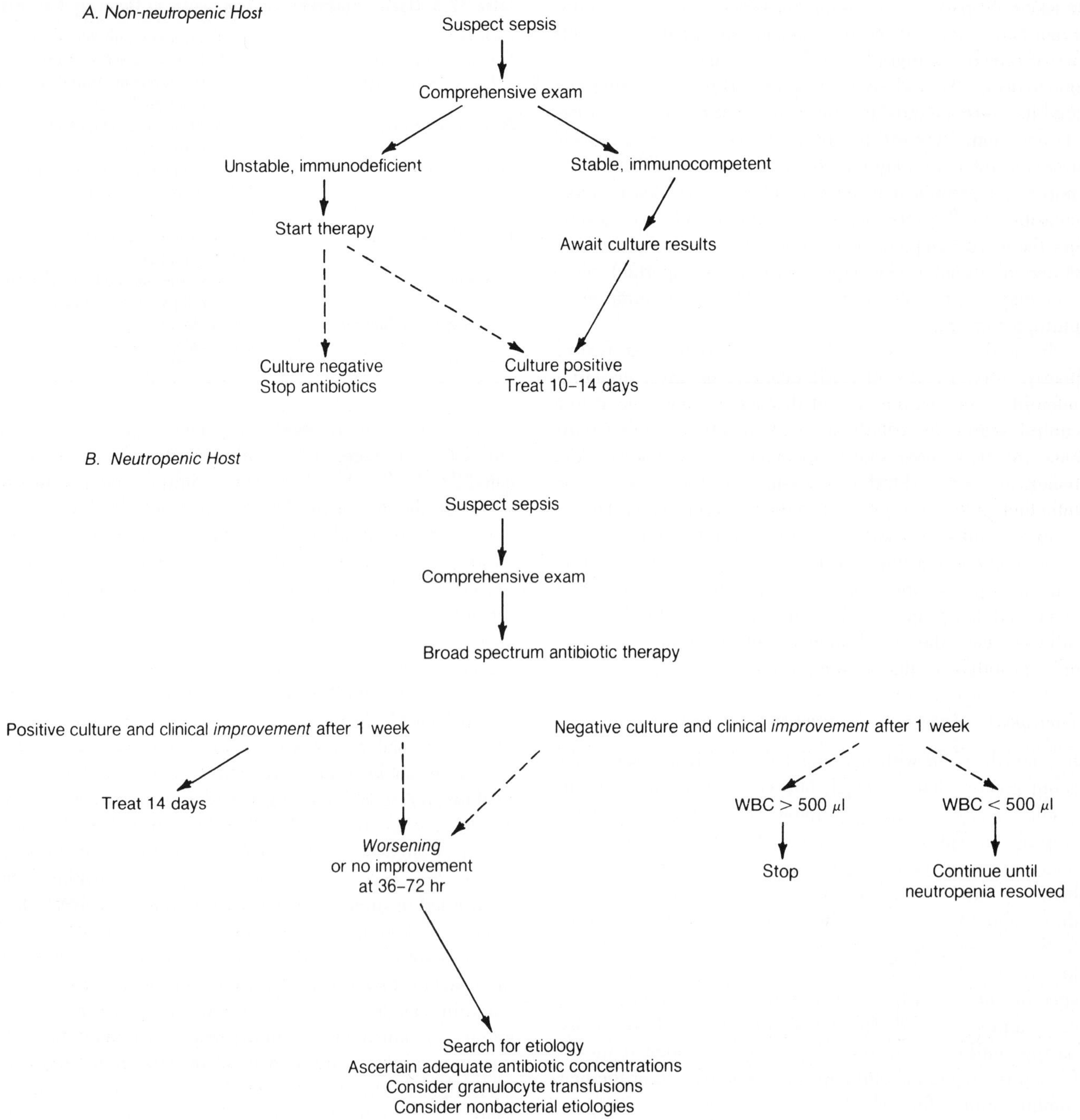

Figure 42.2. Approach to suspected bacterial infection.

then antibiotics may be stopped if the patient has a normal neutrophil count and the fever has resolved. In the latter case, if signs and symptoms of infection persist, further evaluation is indicated to look for nonbacterial causes of infection[10,11,43,65,72].

A more conservative approach is advocated for the neutropenic patient[72] (Fig. 42.2). Briefly, if a culture result is positive and the patient is doing well, then the antibiotics are appropriately adjusted and continued for at least 1 week or until the neutrophil count is over 500/μL. If, on the other hand, no positive culture result is obtained but the neutrophil count exceeds 500/μL 1 week after starting therapy, antibiotics are discontinued, as for the nonneutropenic host. The incidence of recurrent bacterial infection in these patients is low as long as the neutropenia is resolved[10,11]. However, if the child remains neutropenic after 7 days but the infection has apparently resolved (e.g., defervescence) after initiation of antibiotics, the risk of recurrent infection is high if antibiotics are withdrawn before the neutropenia resolves, so they are continued until the neutrophil count exceeds 500/μL.

The neutropenic child who remains persistently febrile despite first-line antibiotics belongs to a special group of patients. Like nonneutropenic patients who do not respond to antibiotics when treated for a suspected or documented infection, it is essential to ascertain that (a) the choice of antibiotics is appropriate, (b) the dose is appropriate, (c) serum drug concentrations are adequate, (d) a drug fever is unlikely, and (e) another infection is not present. If the child's condition worsens (e.g., persistent fever, hemodynamic instability) despite 36 to 72 hours of therapy, and no good explanation (points a to d above) exists for this deterioration, we empirically expand or switch the broad-spectrum antibiotic coverage. The addition of vancomycin and or clindamycin should be strongly considered.

Fungal Infection

If the deterioration has been rather gradual, the possibility of fungal infection must be considered. A variety of factors predispose the patient to fungal infection, including neutropenia, malnutrition, high-dose steroid administration, and prolonged antibiotic use[11,65,76,77]. Central venous catheters have also been associated with fungemia, and certainly any condition involving defective T-cell function has been associated with an increased incidence of fungemia (e.g., burns, immunosuppressive therapy, leukemia, lymphoma, graft-versus-host disease [GVHD], multiple surgical procedures)[11,65,76,77]. The organisms most commonly seen in children with neoplastic disease are *Candida albicans* and *Aspergillus* species; however, *Candida* species other than *albicans* (e.g., *tropicalis, krusei*), *Cryptococcus neoformans, Mucor* species, and other less common fungal pathogens have been noted, particularly as causes of unexplained persistent fever, brain abscesses, meningitis, multiple pulmonary infiltrates, or hepatic and splenic lesions[11,65,76,77].

The diagnosis of a fungal infection may be difficult. As most patients are colonized by *Candida* species, the skin, throat, and stool specimens may yield positive cultures that do not represent invasive disease; however, persistence of non-*albicans* species of *Candida*, even in surveillance cultures, may be indicative of aggressive fungal disease in the profoundly immunocompromised neutropenic host. *Candida* infections of the esophagus, urinary tract, trachea, and skin must also be considered in the patient with focal signs and symptoms and positive surveillance cultures[11,65,76,77]. For example, fungal emboli may be manifested as discrete cutaneous nodules, biopsy of which may demonstrate characteristic hyphal forms. Any evidence of CNS dysfunction or infection in the immunocompromised host should lead to a search for a fungal as well as a bacterial cause. Finally, pneumonia in these children may be due to a fungus (see below). CT studies of the chest may demonstrate characteristic nodular patterns of fungal pneumonia, especially *Aspergillus*[78], and intra-abdominal involvement, such as abscesses or granulomata in liver, spleen, and/or kidneys, may also be apparent on CT scans[79]. The difficult problem of deciding whether a febrile neutropenic patient with no signs of focal infection has fungemia is common[11,65,76,77]. Specific tests, such as blood cultures, may be positive in less than 50% of cases of serious disseminated fungal infection[11,76,77]. To increase the yield, bone marrow aspirates for culture have been advocated, and certainly, if a focus of infection is suspected, then biopsy of the lesion is indicated[11,76,77]. Antigen detection methods are disappointing for most fungal infections, but some newer biochemical methods are promising[80]. Some clinical clues that may point to fungal pathogens as the cause of infection are noted in **Table 42.6.**

Table 42.6. Clinical Clues of Fungemia

Endophthalmitis	Ocular pain, burning, etc., with colonies of *Candida* visible on the retina (may not be present in neutropenic host)
Cutaneous manifestations	Macules and/or nodular rash (punch biopsy may show organisms)
Pneumonitis	Pleuritic chest pain, wedge-shaped infiltrate on chest radiograph; abnormal CT scan
Endocarditis	Fever, emboli, heart murmur, etc. (nonspecific for fungus)
Esophagitis	Fever, dysphagia, raggedy esophagus on barium swallow, plaques on endoscopy
Disseminated infection	Diffuse myalgias; tenderness of muscles to palpation

The decision to start antifungal therapy is often based on the suspicion that fever, malaise, and other nonspecific complaints that persist despite antibiotics are due to fungemia. The drug of choice in empirical therapy is intravenous amphotericin B. A test dose of 1 mg is given to exclude the possibility of major allergic reactions, then full maintenance therapy (0.5 to 1.0 mg/kg/day administered over 1 to 6 hr) should be initiated[11,77]. Doses as high as 1.5 mg/kg/day may be required for treatment of *Aspergillus* infections[11]. Treatment is continued for at least 2 to 3 weeks or until a total dose of 1 to 2 g has been given; some patients with disseminated visceral infection (e.g., hepatosplenic candidiasis) may require a much more prolonged course of amphotericin therapy over several months[76]. Simply treating the child until blood cultures are negative is not advised in view of the difficulty culturing these organisms[11,77].

Amphotericin B causes a variety of adverse reactions[76,77]. Rigors and chills, the most common reaction to amphotericin administration, can be controlled by premedication with meperidine, 0.5 mg/kg IV, and acetaminophen, 10 to 15 mg/kg PO. Occasionally, steroids (e.g., hydrocortisone) are also needed to control the rigors associated with the infusion. Nausea and vomiting can be controlled with antiemetics. More serious are the problems of renal toxicity and potassium wasting; these side effects resolve within several weeks after cessation of therapy and are not indications to stop therapy. Liposomally encapsulated amphotericin appears to be associated with less renal toxicity and is currently undergoing multi-institutional trials[81]. Finally, the combination of amphotericin and leukocyte transfusion has been associated with pneumonitis. Despite these adverse effects, amphotericin B remains the best antifungal agent for empiric antifungal therapy in the febrile neutropenic patient.

Five other antifungal agents miconazole, 5-flucytosine (5-FC), ketoconazole, fluconazole, and itraconazolem-have recently achieved attention[82,83]. 5-FC is only available in an oral form; oral absorption is good, and the drug has relatively mild side effects. It is not recommended for use alone because resistance may rapidly develop; however, 5-FC works synergistically with amphotericin B, and this combination is especially useful in infection with *Candida* species other than *albicans* and invasive aspergillosis. However, leukopenia is a common side effect, limiting the usefulness of 5-FC in patients who are already neutropenic. Miconazole, a synthetic imidazole, is intravenously administered and has a number of minor side effects, including nausea; its spectrum of fungicidal activity limits its use for empiric therapy. Ketoconazole, a related structure, is also useful in some situations but may cause hepatic dysfunction and must be used with caution in patients with hepatic dysfunction. Fluconazole, a triazole compound, may be administered orally or parenterally for treatment of *Candida* pharyngitis and esophagitis and for cryptococcosis (but not cryptococcal meningitis); its major adverse effect is gastrointestinal distress, which usually does not interfere with treatment. Itraconazole is a well-tolerated oral azole with potential clinical efficacy against *Aspergillus, Candida,* and *Histoplasmosis,* among others. It appears to be as effective as amphotericin B in treating invasive aspergillosis and has fewer side effects. Until more experience is obtained in the treatment of fungal infection with these agents in febrile neutropenic children, amphotericin B is still recommended as the empirical antifungal drug of choice for these patients. If a known pathogen is identified, specific therapy is appropriate[11,65].

Viral Infection

Viral infections, particularly those caused by herpes viruses (herpes simplex, varicella zoster, and CMV), are common in bone marrow transplant (BMT) patients and children undergoing remission-induction therapy for acute leukemia[11,43,48,65,84]. The possibility of viral pneumonitis must be entertained in all cases of pulmonary dysfunction (discussed later). Historically, the case-fatality rate from pneumonitis due to CMV has been very high (60 to 80%) in immunocompromised individuals, especially BMT patients. Recently, the use of the antiviral agent ganciclovir in combination with either high-dose intravenous immunoglobulin or CMV hyperimmune globulin has been shown to affect favorably CMV pneumonitis in BMT recipients[85–87]. Mucocutaneous lesions caused by herpes simplex virus, varicella, and varicella zoster virus are amenable to therapy with acyclovir[88,89], and prophylactic administration of this agent may prevent reactivation of latent herpes simplex infection in patients undergoing intensive cytoreductive therapy (e.g., for acute myeloid leukemia) or BMT[90].

Protozoal Infection

In addition to fungal and viral causes of a poorly responding infection, protozoal infections, particularly pulmonary disease from *P. carinii,* must be considered in the leukemic and BMT patient[11,43]. Most authors suggest empirically adding trimethoprim-sulfamethoxazole (TMP-SMX) (20 mg/kg/day as TMP, divided every 6 hr) to the antibiotic regimen of a patient with suspected nonbacterial pneumonitis for at least 3 days prior to undertaking a lung biopsy[11,43]. Since as many as 50% of cases of nonbacterial pneumonitis are due to *P. carinii,* this approach has obviated the need for biopsy in many patients[91,92]. Bronchoscopy or bronchoalveolar lavage may be employed in an effort to make a diagnosis prior to initiating therapy, but these procedures carry significant risk and often require endotracheal intubation. Moreover, the value of bronchoscopy may be limited[93]. However, at lavage or biopsy, resistant *P. carinii* is identified in up to 15% of cases despite previous therapy with TMP-SMX, dictating a switch to or addition of pentamidine isethionate (4 mg/kg/day), so failure to respond to TMP-SMX indicates the need for a more invasive diagnostic approach. Since a response to therapy may not be evident for 4 to 5 days, progression during this time does not necessarily imply ineffective therapy[11].

Granulocyte Transfusion

Therapy of suspected sepsis, then, proceeds from antibacterial therapy to consideration of fungal, viral and/or protozoal causes, particularly if there is a primary pulmonary focus of the infection. If none of these possibilities is likely, or if the patient does not respond to any reasonable anti-infectious agent, then the use of granulocyte transfusions for neutropenic septic patients may be considered. Although granulocyte transfusions are associated with a number of risks, there is a definite role for them in granulocytopenic patients or patients with dysfunctional granulocytes (e.g., chronic granulomatous disease) who remain septic in spite of appropriate antimicrobial therapy[94]. The efficacy of the transfusions depends upon the ability to transfuse substantial numbers of granulocytes. A minimum of 10^{10} cells is recommended[94]. The adverse effects of granulocyte transfusion are myriad. White cells, even when obtained from family members, carry risks of allergic reaction and GVHD[95–97]. Repeated exposure to granulocyte transfusions may diminish the efficiency of platelet or granulocyte transfusion because of alloimmunization[96], and granulocyte survival is greatly diminished in the patient who is already alloimmunized against various platelet products. The use of multiple donors may make subsequent bone marrow transplantation more difficult because of alloimmunization against donor-specific (usually minor transplantation) antigens. GVHD after granulocyte transfusion can be prevented by irradiation of the leukocytes with 1500 to 3000 rads before transfusion[97,98]. Repeated transfusions are associated with an increased risk of introduction of CMV infection as well[99,100]. Pneumonitis, a serious complication of granulocyte infusion therapy, may not be avoidable[101]; it is more severe in patients receiving amphotericin B therapy after or concurrent with leukocyte transfusions[102,103]. However, pneumonitis per se is not a contraindication to granulocyte transfusions. The risk of hypoxemia must be part of the equation when deciding whether to use granulocytes, and pulmonary function must be carefully monitored in these patients. The frequent minor complications of granulocyte transfusions—fever, chills, and rigors—can be avoided by premedication with hydrocortisone (1 mg/kg IV), diphenhydramine (1 mg/kg IV), and acetaminophen (10 to 15 mg/kg PO).

Hematologic Complications

General Concepts

Patients receiving chemotherapy or with tumors infiltrating marrow frequently develop hypoproductive pancytopenia. This places the patient at risk for (a) neutropenia and the development of opportunistic infections, (b) severe anemia and its associated consequences of congestive heart failure and hypoxemia, and (c) thrombocytopenia and the risk of life-threatening hemorrhage. Myelosuppression typically occurs 7 to 14 days after the administration of most, but not all, chemotherapeutic drugs. Myelosuppression from the nitrosoureas (BCNU, CCNU) is typically late (4 to 6 weeks after administration), while the commonly used drugs vincristine, L-asparaginase, and steroids are generally not myelosuppressive[104,105]. The use of hematopoietic growth factors (e.g., G-CSF and GM-CSF) shorten the duration of leukopenia[44]. Chemotherapy and frequent use of broad-spectrum antibiotics may promote the development of coagulopathies with the risks of hemorrhage or thromboses. Many of these hematologic complications have been discussed in depth previously in this chapter and in Chapter 41. This section will focus on some of the hemorrhagic and thrombotic complications that the intensivist may encounter in these patients.

Hemorrhage is second to infection as a leading cause of death in children with leukemia and accounts for about 14% of deaths[106,107]. The causes of hemorrhage are thrombocytopenia, coagulopathy, or a combination of both. Thrombocytopenia may arise because of tumor involvement of the bone marrow, myelosuppression due to chemotherapy and/or radiotherapy, or increased destruction of platelets by immune or nonimmune mechanisms[105]. Several tumors may be associated with coagulopathies (e.g., promyelocytic leukemia), but these are uncommon in children[106,108]. More commonly, a clotting disorder in the child with neoplastic disease may result from chemotherapy administration, deficiency of vitamin K-dependent factors due to antibiotic-induced vitamin K deficiency or liver dysfunction, liver failure, or sepsis.

Investigation of abnormal bleeding demands a few tests of coagulation status as well as history and physical examination. These tests include prothrombin time (PT), partial thromboplastin time (PTT), fibrinogen concentration, and search for the presence of fibrin degradation products (FDP) as well as a complete blood count. With these tests, one can determine whether (a) simple thrombocytopenia is present, (b) a factor deficiency exists, or (c) a consumptive process seems more likely as indicated by elevated PT, PTT, and FDP with decreased fibrinogen and platelets.

Thrombocytopenia

Thrombocytopenia is most often of little clinical consequence if the platelet count is over 50,000/μL. Between 20,000 and 50,000/μL there is increased risk of abnormal bleeding during surgical procedures or with trauma. Historically, patients have been prophylactically transfused for platelet counts of 20,000/μL or less. This "20,000/μL trigger" was based on data obtained in the 1960s, when the use of aspirin was widespread. More recent data[109,110] suggests that the threshold for prophylactic transfusion can be set at 5,000/μL in patients without fever or bleeding and at 10,000/μL in patients with these signs. However, in an intensive care setting, it is likely that patients will have a number of circumstances that will necessitate the maintenance of a higher platelet count than would be necessary in other settings. Because of a higher incidence of spontaneous bleeding in patients with brain tumors, we recommend that the platelet count of these patients be maintained at a level of 50,000/μL or greater. Vomiting, coughing, the presence of an endotracheal tube, or retinal hemorrhages are warning signals that indicate the need for prophylactic platelet transfusions. Obviously, significant active bleeding requires platelet transfusions.

In a normal patient, 1 unit of transfused platelets for every 5 to 7 kg of body weight will increases the count by about 50,000/μL. This formula does not take into account either ongoing platelet consumption or the presence of alloimmunization. Determination of 10-minute posttransfusion platelet count is therefore important, and more frequent blood samples for assessment of platelet survival counts may be needed. The interval at which platelets are administered depends on the patient's response to each transfusion.

Platelet transfusions are generally safe. Allergic reactions occur, and the physician must be ready to treat these with diphenhydramine or epinephrine as required. Fever and chills may accompany a transfusion but are usually adequately managed with acetaminophen (10 to 15 mg/kg PO), diphenhydramine (1 mg/kg IV) or hydrocortisone (1 mg/kg IV); patients who have had documented febrile responses to platelets and other blood products may be premedicated 30 to 45 minutes before transfusion with acetaminophen.

Of concern is alloimmunization development of alloantibodies directed against specific human lymphocyte antigens (HLA), platelet antigens, or other blood-borne antigens. Patients alloimmunized against platelets have marked decreases in the platelet increment noted 10 minutes post-transfusion and by the shorter-than-usual life span of these platelets. Without alloantibodies, the half-life of platelets is 7 days; with significant alloimmunization, platelets may be destroyed within hours. To prevent alloimmunization, some suggest using single-donor and/or HLA-matched platelets[111], but sometimes this is impractical.

Coagulopathy

If bleeding is present but thrombocytopenia is not, there may be a deficiency of clotting factors. In particular, the child who has been receiving antibiotics and parenteral nutrition may be vitamin K-deficient. Thus, an elevated PT should be treated with vitamin K (1 to 5 mg IV). While we do not administer fresh frozen plasma (FFP) simply for abnormal coagulation tests, if bleeding is present in association with a coagulopathy, then the use of FFP is recommended. If fibrinogen concentrations are very low, cryoprecipitate infusions may be beneficial.

While thrombocytopenia and coagulation defects caused by either malignancy or chemotherapy are amenable to therapy, disseminated intravascular coagulation (DIC) with hemorrhage is more resistant to intervention, as discussed in Chapter 41. DIC usually occurs in association with sepsis and may also be seen in children with newly diagnosed or relapsed acute promyelocytic leukemia. The guiding principle of therapy of DIC is that treatment of the underlying cause[112–115]. Although not of proven benefit, we administer platelets, vitamin K, and FFP if significant bleeding occurs in the patient with DIC (see Chapter 41 for further discussion of DIC and other bleeding disorders).

One specific situation that deserves special mention in this section is the patient receiving L-asparaginase for lymphoid malignancies. L-asparaginase is an enzyme that depletes serum of the amino acid asparagine, which is essential for protein synthesis in leukemic cells. Synthesis of plasma coagulation factors (especially fibrinogen, factor IX, and factor X) and their inhibitors (notably protein C, protein S, and antithrombin III) is also reduced with the potential of an imbalance between coagulants and anticoagulants[116]. This may result in either thrombotic or hemorrhagic complications in these patients, estimated at 1 to 2% of patients receiving this drug[117]. The most devastating of these complications are CNS thromboses and hemorrhages, although with appropriate intervention, the outcome has generally been good[117,118]. Therapy is aimed at replacing deficient factors with FFP. Anticoagulation with heparin and then coumadin may be indicated.

Respiratory Complications

In this and the next few subsections of the chapter, the emphasis will be placed on a practical approach to the diagnosis and therapy of various life-threatening complications in the oncology patient. An organ-system-oriented approach will be employed, and those facets of diagnosis and therapy unique to the child with neoplastic disease will be considered in detail. Those aspects of general therapy that are pertinent will be briefly touched on, but more details are available in other chapters of this book. In considering each organ system, the cause of the complication will be identified as the tumor, its therapy, or the combined consequences of tumor and therapy.

Obstruction of the Airways

Airway obstruction from a mediastinal mass is a medical emergency because of potential compromise of respiratory and/or cardiac function. The need to obtain tissue for diagnostic studies must be weighed against the need to alleviate symptoms from the obstructing mass. It is essential that intensivists, medical oncologists, radiation oncologists, surgeons, radiologists, and anesthesiologists rapidly evaluate the child to plan the appropriate studies and interventions.

The mediastinum is anatomically divided into three regions, and tumors may arise in any of these regions. Malignant tumors of the anterior mediastinum, which are usually lymphomatous in origin, are either Hodgkin's or non-Hodgkin's lymphomas[119,120]; bronchial cysts, germ cell tumors, and teratomas may also be found in this region. Lymphomas may also affect lymph nodes in the middle mediastinum. Most tumors of the posterior mediastinum are neurogenic in origin and include neuroblastoma, ganglioneuromas, and others.

The diagnosis of airway obstruction is no more difficult in the oncology patient than in the normal child. Stridor, dyspnea, and anxiety all point to the diagnosis; however, it should be noted that the decrease in airway cross-sectional area usually exceeds 50% before significant symptoms appear. Moreover, the clinical distress may not correlate with the degree of obstruction[121]. Nonetheless, marked retractions, diminished air entry, and cyanosis on examination imply impending respiratory arrest and dictate emergent therapy. The cause of obstruction may be established with a history and physical examination. Chest radiographs will show a clinically significant mediastinal mass if present, and CT will allow full evaluation of the extent of the mass[120,122].

The management of the child with a mediastinal mass has been the source of some debate. While the noninvasive tests mentioned above will identify a mass and may suggest a cause, a tissue diagnosis is necessary to implement definitive therapy. The tissue may be available from a superficial lymph node or the bone marrow. However, in many instances, biopsy or complete excision of the mediastinal mass may be the only way to obtain tissue for a definitive diagnosis. Anesthesia and intubation of the trachea are more difficult in this patient population[119,121–124] because of the potential for exacerbation of extrinsic airway compression. Shamberger and colleagues suggest that the size

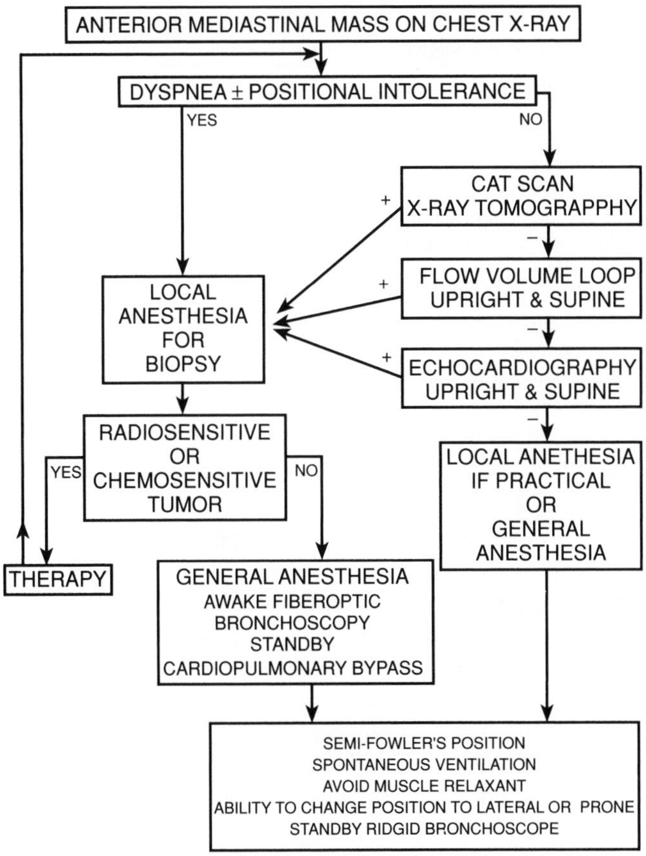

Figure 42.3. Flow chart describing the preoperative evaluation of the patient with an anterior mediastinal mass. +, positive finding; -, negative work-up. From Neuman, GG et al. The anesthetic management of the patient with an anterior mediastinal mass. Anesthesiology 1984;60:144–147, with permission.

of the trachea should be determined by CT scanning and, in any patient with a greater than 50% reduction in tracheal size, alternatives to intubation should be sought[(122)]. These include node biopsy, emergency radiotherapy, or, if a biopsy is critical, inhalational general anesthesia with a mask[(122)]. Pulmonary flow volume loop assessment may also be useful in the preanesthesia evaluation[(119,123,124)]. Figure 42.3 describes the preoperative evaluation of the child with a mediastinal mass. Halothane has been the preferred inhalational agent for induction of anesthesia in a child with a mediastinal mass and critical airway obstruction requiring intubation[(125)]. Sevoflurane, a new inhaled anesthetic with fewer hemodynamic effects and faster recovery time than halothane, will probably become the preferred agent in this setting[(126)]. A skilled bronchoscopist must be on hand for the intubation in the event that the endotracheal tube cannot be easily inserted. In the case of difficult intubation, an orotracheal or nasotracheal tube can be inserted over the bronchoscope. It should extend beyond the area of compression. Occasionally, an armored endotracheal tube may be helpful in getting beyond the obstruction. In rare cases, the risk of intubation is considered too great by the anesthetist or surgeon, and empirical therapy is initiated. A biopsy should be done as soon as feasible (i.e., within 1 to 2 days of initiating therapy)[(121)]. The therapy of a mediastinal mass depends on the tumor type but usually includes radiation and/or chemotherapy, as discussed in the final section of this chapter. With the initiation of therapy, there may be tumor and peritumor tissue swelling. Therefore, the degree of obstruction may actually increase over the first day or two of therapy.

Parenchymal Disease

Malignancies

Pulmonary parenchymal disease is much more common than airway obstruction. Primary pulmonary malignancies are unusual in children[(127)]. Parenchymal involvement is occasionally seen with histiocytosis X[(128,129)] and rarely with leukemia[(130)]. Metastatic pulmonary disease can be seen in patients with osteogenic and Ewing's sarcoma, Wilms' tumor, and other malignancies. However, the likely causes of respiratory failure and significant pulmonary parenchymal disease are infection, hemorrhage, chemotherapy, and radiation.

Infection

As discussed above in the Infectious Complications of the chapter, pulmonary infection in a nonneutropenic host, with no other factors putting the patient at risk for nosocomial infection, will most likely be caused by usual respiratory pathogens. However, if neutropenia exists, the child has been intubated, or a mass obstructs a bronchus, then Gram-negative organisms or *S. aureus* are more likely pathogens. The approach to pneumonitis is similar to that outlined for sepsis in general. Usually, the patient will have symptoms and signs of fever, cough, and respiratory embarrassment. As mentioned above, broad-spectrum antibiotics are usually initiated with the onset of fever and respiratory symptoms, after appropriate history and physical and laboratory examinations. However, if there is no convincing evidence of a bacterial infection, the possibility of viral, fungal, or protozoal organisms should be considered early in the course of the illness, particularly in the BMT patients[(11,43,86,91,93,131–135)]. Furthermore, noninfectious causes of pneumonitis, such as radiation and chemotherapy, are not uncommon in these children[(136)] **(Table 42.7).** If no cause is clearly implicated, most specialists start TMP-SMX (20 mg/kg/day, divided every 6 hr IV) in addition to the broad-spectrum antibiotics, because the high incidence of *P. carinii. P. carinii* infections are typically associated with fever, tachypnea, and bilateral infiltrates radiating from the hili on chest radiograph. However, in the oncology patient these typical findings may be absent. As mentioned earlier in this chapter, the empiric approach to pneumonitis of treating with TMP-SMX without a biopsy is successful in many instances. However, if the patient does not respond to this approach within 48 to 72 hours, a biopsy is warranted; for despite the risks, the lung biopsy has a higher yield in identifying potentially curable conditions, such as

Table 42.7. Differential Diagnosis of Diffuse Pulmonary Infiltrates (Pneumonitis) in the Child with Malignant Disease

Bacteria
Any Gram-negative or Gram-positive agent, including *Nocardia, Legionella, Listeria,* and *Mycobacterium*
Fungi
Aspergillus
Candida
Mucor
Cryptococcus
Viral
Herpes simplex
Varicella zoster
Cytomegalovirus
Measles
Epstein-Barr virus
Parasites
Pneumocystis carinii
Toxoplasma gondii
Miscellaneous
Radiation
Chemotherapy (methotrexate)
Leukemic infiltrate

fungal disease, resistant *P. carinii,* or rarely, malignancy, than do bronchoscopy and lavage[93]. Specialists at many centers will also add erythromycin to the antimicrobial regimen to treat possible *Mycoplasma* or *Legionella.*

Radiation and Chemotherapy

The consequences of chemotherapy and radiation on lung function are well established[136]. Pulmonary fibrosis is seen after treatment with a variety of agents **(Table 42.8).** Furthermore, dactinomycin and doxorubicin may potentiate radiation fibrosis. Although most patients remain asymptomatic, severely affected individuals may manifest dyspnea on exertion, cough, fever, or decreased exercise tolerance. Hypoxemia may be documented by blood gas analysis or pulse oxymetry. Radiographic changes consistent with fibrosis may be seen on chest x-ray, but chest CT scan is the preferred imaging modality. Pulmonary function testing demonstrates reduced maximum breathing capacity, decreased tidal volume, and decreased diffusion capacity[136].

A recent report by Morgan and Breit[137] elegantly reviews the mechanisms involved in radiation-induced lung injury. Classic radiation pneumonitis is a dose-related toxicity mediated by inflammatory cytokines and growth factors such as tumor necrosis factor-alpha and transforming growth factor-beta released by pulmonary macrophages in direct response to radiation. A second form of injury, which they have termed "sporadic radiation pneumonitis," is less common and is characterized by an alveolar lymphocytosis of activated T-helper cells. This appears to be similar in many respects to other hypersensitivity pneumonidities, such as farmer's lung disease and pigeon breeder's disease. This may be the same mechanism that is seen after methotrexate administration[138]. This latter form of lung injury is often responsive to steroids, with little permanent fibrosis, whereas classic radiation pneumonitis usually results in permanent lung impairment.

Table 42.8. Antineoplastic Therapies Associated with Pulmonary Fibrosis

Bleomycin
BCNU, CCNU
Busulfan
Cyclophosphamide
Methotrexate
Radiation

Table 42.9. Conditions Associated with Respiratory Failure in Children with Malignant Disease

Neuromuscular
Coma
Seizures
Malnutrition
Airway Disease
Extrinsic compression (e.g., lymphoma)
Pulmonary parenchymal disease
Infection
Noninfectious pneumonitis (drugs, radiation)
Pulmonary fibrosis
Shock lung
Congestive heart failure
Miscellaneous
Pleural effusion (malignant, infectious)
Abdominal tumors

Therapy of drug- or radiation-induced pulmonary disease is somewhat limited. Occasionally, the initial inflammatory response seen in the first days after radiation exposure or cyclophosphamide is severe, and supportive ventilatory therapy may be needed to treat the accompanying pulmonary edema (capillary leak). The more typical pulmonary fibrosis that develops insidiously over months does not seem to be reversible. As mentioned, steroids may be beneficial in some cases. Since the fibrosis seen after bleomycin therapy may be exacerbated by supplemental oxygen administration, probably due to increased production of oxygen free radicals, the use of supplemental oxygen in patients with fibrosis must be judicious[139].

Respiratory Failure

Table 42.9 lists some of the common causes of respiratory distress and/or failure in the children admitted to our PICU over the past few years. Children with neuromuscular disorders so severe that they are unable either to protect their airways or to maintain adequate ventilation obviously need intubation. While seizures and coma are more common causes of intubation and mechanical ventilation, malnutrition is not an unusual cause of inability to wean from mechanical ventilation[140], particularly in this population. Obstruction of the airway was discussed above. Parenchymal disease is the most common cause of respiratory failure. Acute respiratory distress syndrome, or shock lung, may occur with sepsis or other conditions[132,141]. A shock lung-type picture has been described in some children with leukemia and elevated blast counts leading to pulmonary leukostasis[142,143]. It may also be seen after radiation or chemotherapy, as mentioned earlier. Finally, pulmonary edema secondary to heart failure can occur in these patients, and pleural effusions occasionally are seen.

The treatment of respiratory failure is considered in detail in other chapters of this book, so its management will be only briefly considered here. The major differences between the oncology patient and the normal host are (a) the possibly debilitated premorbid condition, (b) the increased risk of infection and bleeding, and (c) the potential for enhanced oxygen toxicity as a consequence of previous chemotherapy or radiotherapy. Therefore, the risks of excessive tiring and sudden respiratory collapse in a malnourished child must be weighed against the likelihood of infection after intubation. The treatment of respiratory failure characterized by hypoxemia with or without hypercarbia poses various problems in these patients. General therapeutic measures include supplemental inspired oxygen by mask, the maintenance of the hemoglobin above 12 g/dl and cardiac output at appropriate levels. Diuresis may prove useful in maintaining the arterial oxygen tension in an acceptable range regardless of the primary pulmonary condition, since many causes of respiratory failure are associated with increased lung water. Finally, if a pleural effusion is present and causing significant compromise, thoracocentesis will improve the situation.

If, despite these measures, the oxygen saturation does not improve (i.e., the P_aO_2 remains below 50 to 60 mm Hg with an F_iO_2 of 0.4 to 0.5), or respiratory acidosis worsens, then intubation must be considered. Although there are significant risks with intubation and the invasive monitoring that often accompany it, we use these relatively conservative criteria as the cutoff point for elective intubation unless there are compelling reasons to believe that the severity of respiratory failure will not get worse. There are various reasons for this aggressive approach. First, oxygen toxicity may increase with higher inspired O_2[144]. Second, it becomes progressively harder to deliver an F_iO_2 above 0.4 to 0.5 by mask, particularly in young children (although high flow systems with reservoirs make it possible). Third, the arterial oxygen pressure (P_aO_2) less than 60 torr despite an F_iO_2 of 0.4 suggests that a large intrapulmonary shunt may be present, and increasing the F_iO_2 to 1.0 will not necessarily improve the saturation. Thus, the risks of severe hypoxemia and death during intubation will already be significant and will likely increase if one delays the intubation. Once the patient has been intubated, we attempt to maintain the F_iO_2 below 0.4 through the use of positive end-expiratory pressure (PEEP) and careful monitoring of pulse oximetry, blood gases, and oxygen delivery if necessary. There is no evidence that early PEEP will prevent progression of the primary lung disease; however, it may reduce the risk of O_2 toxicity[145,146].

Table 42.10. Common Cardiovascular Disorders in Critically Ill Pediatric Oncology Patients

Condition	*Etiology*
Myocardial dysfunction	Drug-induced cardiomyopathy Radiation-induced cardiomyopathy Primary or metastatic neoplasms
Miscellaneous cardiac conditions	Pericardial tamponade Septic shock
Vascular disorders	Superior vena cava syndrome Hypertension

Cardiovascular Complications

Effects of Malignancies

Numerous cardiovascular complications can arise as a consequence of neoplastic disease, chemotherapy, or radiotherapy in pediatric oncology patients **(Table 42.10).** As was the case in the pulmonary section, the emphasis here is on those features of diagnosis and therapy that are unique to pediatric oncology patients.

Primary cardiac tumors are extremely rare[147,148], and metastatic disease usually involves the pericardium rather than the myocardium[149]. Moreover, pericardial tamponade may be seen after initiation of radiotherapy or chemotherapy[147–149]. Thus, the malignant diseases per se rarely cause heart failure or shock.

Effects of Chemotherapy and Radiation

A variety of chemotherapeutics as well as radiotherapy **(Table 42.11)** can cause cardiomyopathy[147,150–153]. The most widely recognized agents capable of inducing a decrease in myocardial function are the anthracyclines (e.g., doxorubicin, daunomycin, idarubicin, mitoxantrone). Although myocyte injury increases linearly with increasing cumulative dose, the incidence of congestive heart failure begins to increase logarithmically at a cumulative doxorubicin dose of 550 mg/m^2[154]. Furthermore, young children may be more sensitive to anthracyclines than adults[155]; the cardiotoxic effects may be enhanced either by radiotherapy to the heart or mediastinum[156] or by drugs such as cyclophosphamide and ifosfamide[157,158]. Most patients who receive anthracyclines are asymptomatic, but damage to the myocardium is detectable even at low cumulative doses[151]. The long-term implications of these changes is not clear at this time. The pathologic lesions of anthracycline exposure are characterized by myofibrillar loss and cytoplasmic vacu-

Table 42.11. Cardiac Complications of Cancer Therapy

Cardiomyopathy	
Acute:	Cyclophosphamide (>100 mg/kg)
Chronic:	Doxorubicin, daunorubicin, mitoxantrone, idarubicin Radiation
Arrhythmia	
	Doxorubicin *m*-AMSA

olization, which starts as a localized process and later becomes diffuse. Cyclophosphamide may also cause direct cardiotoxicity in the absence of anthracycline exposure. Patients may develop heart failure 10 to 15 days after receiving high-dose cyclophosphamide. Unlike anthracycline toxicity, the pathologic lesion is hemorrhagic cardiac necrosis[147,159].

The mechanism of anthracycline-induced cardiomyopathy is not certain; however, since superoxide radicals are formed by the drug, a possible mechanism involving lipid peroxidation has been proposed. Attempts at prevention of the cardiomyopathy with vitamin E or coenzyme Q_{10} (both free radical scavengers) have had little or no benefit[160]. Other mechanisms involving platelet-activating factor, prostaglandins, histamine, anthracycline metabolites, and calcium have been proposed, but none provides a comprehensive, consistent explanation[160]. ICRF-187, a metal chelating agent, has been shown to protect experimental animals from anthracycline-induced cardiotoxicity, and is undergoing trials in humans[161].

Radiotherapy may cause adverse cardiac effects, including pericarditis with chronic effusion and myocardial fibrosis[150,154,162]. Histologically, interstitial fibrosis is seen with vascular narrowing, though the pathophysiology remains under active investigation[154]. Factors that influence the development of radiation injury include dosing techniques, volume, and specific region of the heart treated. It appears that doses up to 25 Gy are safe in children, and 40 Gy may be delivered to small regions without the development of cardiac dysfunction[154].

The physical findings of cardiomyopathy in the cancer patient are similar to those in the normal host. The history of chemotherapy and radiation should alert the intensivist to the possibility of cardiomyopathy when faced with a child with malignant disease and signs of congestive heart failure. In the asymptomatic child with a history of anthracycline use, echocardiography (systolic time interval, ejection fraction, shortening fraction) may point to diminished myocardial reserves as a consequence of cardiomyopathy and identify the child at risk of myocardial decompensation; however, a normal echocardiographic study does not necessarily preclude the presence of myocardial disease[147]. Moreover, the echocardiographic results will simply show decreased myocardial function and not identify the cause. Endocardial biopsy will potentially provide the tissue diagnosis in the case of a severe isolated anthracycline-induced cardiomyopathy.

Therapy of severe congestive heart failure associated with anthracyclines includes diuretics and dobutamine[163] and cessation of the offending chemotherapeutics. Chronic digoxin and diuretic therapy may benefit the patient[164], but in general the prognosis for late-onset congestive heart failure is poor, and cardiac transplantation should be considered[165]. Treatment with angiotensin converting enzyme (ACE) inhibitors such as enalapril appears promising[166] and will be studied in a multi-institutional protocol. However, in the PICU setting, there are usually multiple possible causes for the severe congestive heart failure and shock seen in the oncology patient, and therapy will usually include both inotropic and vasodilator support.

In addition to congestive heart failure, chemotherapy may induce other complications in children with neoplastic disease. The first of these is cardiac arrhythmias. Numerous reports show that doxorubicin may cause supraventricular arrhythmias acutely, particularly if the drug is administered quickly. Ventricular fibrillation is a rare complication, although it has been reported as a late complication related to anthracycline-induced myocardial fibrosis[167]. Another chemotherapeutic agent, m-AMSA, has been associated with ventricular tachycardia or fibrillation while it is being administered. Children receiving this drug should have electrocardiographic monitoring during the period of drug administration.

Another complication of therapy is pericardial effusion and/or tamponade. Lymphomatous pericardial involvement may cause a significant effusion. As mentioned, radiation may also cause constrictive pericarditis, which will become apparent months after treatment. The diagnosis of pericardial effusion or constrictive pericarditis in the oncology patient is confirmed as it is in the non-oncologic patient, with history, physical findings of tamponade, chest radiograph, electrocardiogram, and evidence of fluid or constriction on echocardiogram. Acutely, pericardiocentesis may be needed, while in the longer term either subxiphoid drainage or pericardiectomy may be necessary[154,168].

Shock in the Child with Malignant Disease

The diagnosis and treatment of shock in children with malignant disease is similar to that in a normal host (see Chapters 13 and 16). There is a tendency to assume that sepsis is the only cause of shock in oncology or immunocompromised patients. However, in addition to the cardiomyopathies discussed above, the oncology patient is also at risk for hemorrhagic and cardiogenic shock as well as critical pericardial tamponade. Thus, if a child shows signs of shock, one must establish the cause while resuscitation is initiated. The physical findings may well point to tamponade as opposed to hypovolemia or cardiogenic shock, but in any case, an electrocardiogram, a chest radiograph, and an echocardiogram will be of great assistance in making the diagnosis.

The therapy of shock in all cases begins with oxygen by mask and intravenous fluids. As discussed earlier, endotracheal intubation entails risks, but profound hypoxemia and hypotension increase the risks of fatal dysrhythmias, too. Thus, in the face of septic shock, early intubation should be seriously considered, particularly if the child has a history of radiation, chemotherapy, etc., that may increase the child's susceptibility to the pulmonary capillary leakiness seen with sepsis. The fluid management in shock is often complicated. Obviously, hemorrhage requires volume replacement in adequate amounts. However, the chemotherapy-induced myocardial dysfunction together with sepsis may result in poorer tolerance of fluid loading in the oncology patient than in the normal child. Hemodynamic monitoring with a thermodilution pulmonary artery catheter and arterial catheter may, therefore, be needed to help guide inotropic support. Since many oncology patients have received steroids in the recent past, we favor the use of stress doses of cortisone (25 to 50 mg/m^2/day, divided every 6 hr IV) in the face of shock to obviate any possibility of an Addisonian crisis(169). This is so even though the use of steroids in septic shock has not been shown to be of benefit in improving the outcome from shock itself(170,171). Another ancillary measure in the treatment of septic shock may be the use of antiendotoxin antibodies(172).

Vascular Disorders

Children with malignant disease may also develop other hemodynamic disorders. Two of these, although uncommon, deserve discussion: superior vena cava syndrome and pheochromocytoma. Superior vena cava syndrome arises most commonly as a consequence of venous stasis caused by a mediastinal mass, and more rarely because of invasion of the vein by neoplasm or intraluminal thrombosis. Typically, this obstruction of venous drainage will cause engorgement of the veins and plethora of the head, neck, and upper extremities, often with edema and induration of the soft tissues(173,174). The diagnosis is made by physical examination and chest radiograph followed by appropriate tests for a tissue diagnosis, as discussed earlier. Therapy of the mass lesion is essential to relieve the syndrome.

The other vascular condition to be considered is pheochromocytoma. This tumor is uncommon in childhood and has been reported to be malignant in 13% of cases(175). The tumor is most often found in the adrenal medulla, and symptoms and signs are related to the secretion of vasoactive catecholamines. The symptoms include headache, palpitations, weight loss, and irritability. Systolic hypertension is the most reliable sign. The diagnosis is suspected on the basis of clinical symptoms, elevation of urinary catecholamine metabolites (vanillylmandelic acid and total metanephrines), and the presence of a suprarenal mass(176). Metaiodobenzylguanidine (MIBG) scanning is a very effective imaging technique in this disease(177) and should be performed in all patients suspected of having pheochromocytoma. The diagnosis of pheochromocytoma is made at surgery. Preoperatively, the patient requires control of hypertension and other catecholamine-related phenomena. This is most often accomplished with a β-blocker such as propranolol and a vasodilator such as nitroprusside or an α-adrenergic blocker such as phentolamine(178). The hypertension is associated with low blood volume and, as the vasodilator therapy is started, the child may require considerable volume replacement. Anesthetic techniques must take into account the acute loss of catecholamine secretion that occurs with excision of the tumor and the potential for sudden surges of catecholamines while the tumor is manipulated. Postoperatively, the vasodilators and adrenergic blockers are withdrawn, and the children usually do well with adequate volume replacement.

Before concluding this section of the chapter, it would be worthwhile to review briefly the other common causes of hypertension seen in pediatric oncology patients or in PICU patients generally(179). Mild to moderate hypertension is seen in oncology patients who are in pain or are anxious—an easily treated but too often forgotten cause(180). It is particularly important to control pain and its associated agitation in the thrombocytopenic cancer patient, especially if the patient is intubated. More severe hypertension is usually due to (a) intracranial pathology or (b) renal disease. In either case, hypertensive encephalopathy and/or intracranial hemorrhage may occur consequent to the hypertension, especially if a bleeding diathesis exists. Significant hypertension, then, is a true emergency in these patients and requires prompt intervention. Nitroprusside, with or without a β-blocker, is very effective in the PICU setting. Subsequent therapy depends, in part, on the cause of the hypertension. If ongoing antihypertensive therapy is needed, hydralazine and a diuretic, with or without a β-blocker, are often effective.

Neurologic Complications

The child with neoplastic disease may acquire a variety of neurologic deficits related to the neoplasm, the therapy, or a combination of both. The most common neurologic complications that the intensivist is likely to encounter—seizures, coma, and strokes—will be discussed both as initial presenting features of a newly diagnosed malignancy and as findings in the child with a previously established malignancy.

Seizures

Most primary brain tumors in childhood are infratentorial(181,182) and thus not likely to cause seizures. However, children with supratentorial tumors are more prone to the development of seizures, and in fact, except for headaches, seizures are the most frequent presenting complaint in patients with supratentorial lesions(183). Similarly, while metastatic disease may cause seizures in adults, metastases to the brain are relatively uncommon in the childhood malignancies. Although some children with leukemias may have CNS disease, the more typical presentation in these patients is raised intracranial pressure or cranial nerve dysfunction(184). Nonetheless, malignancies metastatic to the brain cannot be excluded as a cause of seizure in children, for as survival of patients with malignancies prone to cerebral metastases improves, the incidence will likely increase(182). **Table 42.12** lists the common extracranial childhood malignancies associated with CNS involvement at some point in the illness.

Most often, the cause of seizures in a child with newly diagnosed or long-established neoplastic disease will be unrelated to the tumor. The more likely causes include hemorrhage or infection if myelosuppression is present, and metabolic abnormalities (hypocalcemia, uremia, hyponatre-

Table 42.12. Pediatric Tumors Metastatic to the Central Nervous System

Primary Lesion	*Frequency of Occurrence*
Leukemias (ALL, AML)	3–10% with CNS prophylactic therapy
Lymphomas	Rare with CNS prophylactic therapy
Retinoblastoma	Significant
Neuroblastoma	Rare, except local spinal column invasion
Wilms' tumor	Rare, except for rhabdoid and clear cell variants
Rhabdomyosarcoma (head and neck)	Common
Germ cell tumors	Rare

mia) if renal failure or a large tumor load is present[185,186]. One must also remember to exclude causes totally unrelated to the neoplasm, such as idiopathic epilepsy. Chemotherapy has also been associated with seizures. In particular, vincristine and high-dose cyclophosphamide can cause the syndrome of inappropriate antidiuretic hormone secretion (SIADH) with significant hyponatremia and seizures[187–189]. Treatment with intrathecal or high-dose methotrexate has also been associated with seizures[190,191]. Other systemically administered chemotherapeutics associated with seizures are L-asparaginase, cisplatin, and cytosine arabinoside[192–194].

Other possible causes of seizures in the child with an established neoplasm include bleeding and infections. Most often, the patient with a bleeding diathesis will have a large bleed causing a coma rather than seizures. The infectious possibilities include bacterial, viral, and fungal causes of encephalitis, meningitis, or brain abscess[195]. The bacterial causes include commonly seen agents of childhood (e.g., *S. pneumoniae, H. influenzae,* and *Neisseria meningitidis*) and agents seen in immunocompromised hosts, such as Gram-negative rods, *L. monocytogenes,* and *S. aureus,* as discussed in the infection section above. CNS infections may also be due to fungal or protozoal disease. Cryptococcal meningitis is seen in immunocompromised hosts, so it must always be considered in oncology patients particularly those with lymphomas and leukemia[195]. *Candida, Coccidioides,* and *Histoplasma* may also cause meningitis in these patients. In addition to meningitis, brain abscesses can present with seizures. The organisms causing these are similar to those responsible for meningitis; however, the Gram-negative enteric organisms *(Escherichia coli, Pseudomonas aeruginosa,* and *Proteus mirabilis),* are the most common bacterial pathogens, while *Aspergillus* and *Candida* species are responsible for fungal disease[195]. Finally, CNS toxoplasmosis may also lead to brain abscesses[195].

Table 42.13 outlines an approach to the child with seizures in terms of diagnosis and therapy. Control of the seizure must be a first priority. This is particularly true if the child is thrombocytopenic for, although the seizure may not be due to a CNS bleed, the seizure may certainly precipitate a subsequent intracranial bleed. Therapy includes oxygen by mask and diazepam or lorazepam intravenously. Subsequent to initial control of the seizure, we favor the use of phenytoin (15 to 20 mg/kg loading dose, then 5 to 8 mg/kg/day) for maintenance of seizure control. If this is ineffective, phenobarbital may be added; however, its sedative effect may obscure neurologic signs. Further discussion of the general principles of seizure control can be found in Chapter 22. Chemotherapy-related seizures that are due to SIADH, e.g., after vincristine or cyclophosphamide therapy, are usually treated with fluid restriction, although occasionally diuretics and/or hypertonic saline are needed. Cisplatin-induced seizures may be due to intracranial edema[193]; therefore, management should include osmotic diuresis. It is of note that cisplatin-induced seizures are unusual now that the children are often pretreated with mannitol or furosemide.

Coma

Coma may be caused by the primary brain tumors of childhood[181,182,196]. The infratentorial brain tumors often cause obstructive hydrocephalus leading to chronic intracranial hypertension **(Table 42.14)**. The diagnosis is usually made relatively early when the child presents with the signs and symptoms of gradually increasing intracranial hypertension, such as headache, vomiting, and papilledema. Occasionally, a patient may present with significant obtundation or signs of central or uncal herniation due to a neoplasm. If a child presents with impending herniation and papilledema is absent, other causes of coma must be considered. **Table 42.15** lists the common causes of stupor

Table 42.13. Approach to the Diagnosis of Seizures

1. Control the seizure, provide supportive care
2. History and physical to identify possible causes
   a. Metastases
   b. Bleeding
   c. Meningitis
   d. Abscess
   e. Drug-induced seizure
   f. Other
3. Laboratory tests and diagnostic procedures
   a. Complete blood count
   b. Electrolytes, calcium, glucose (magnesium if cisplatin is being administered)
   c. Blood, urine, etc., cultures if infection is likely
   d. Lumbar puncture if infection or metastatic process is suspected and *no* signs of intracranial hypertension are present
   e. CT scan if signs of intracranial hypertension exist or abscess, metastases, or bleed is suspected
4. Therapeutic procedures
   a. Tumor mass: Radiotherapy or chemotherapy and/or surgery
   b. Drug related: Identify cause, stop drug, provide antidote if possible
   c. Infection: Initiate antibiotics for likely bacteria; initiate amphotericin B if fungal agent is suspected; initiate acyclovir if herpes encephalitis is suspected (see Infectious Complications)
   d. Bleeding: If a bleeding focus is suspected or identified, emergent transfusion of platelets and FFP is needed (see Hematologic Complications)

Table 42.14. Historical and Physical Findings in Childhood Brain Tumors (Infratentorial)

Headache (particularly in morning)
Diplopia, ataxia
Vomiting
Lethargy and mood changes
Papilledema, nerve VI palsy
Hypertension
Coma/signs of impending herniation

and coma associated or unassociated with intracranial hypertension.

It can be seen from the table that there are a variety of possible causes for stupor and coma. Of greatest importance to the intensivist is determining whether intracranial hypertension accompanies coma. To this end, the initial objective of the history and physical examination is to determine the depth of coma and the stability of the neurologic and other vital signs. The presence or absence of signs of herniation must be quickly ascertained and the evidence of a focal lesion sought. As discussed in the section on seizures, evidence for infection or bleeding may be established by the history and physical examination. Bleeding, in particular, must be excluded on clinical grounds by noting the lack of significant petechiae, non-CNS bleeding, or conjunctival and retinal hemorrhages. After completing this initial assessment and providing emergency therapy, a CT or magnetic resonance imaging (MRI) scan is mandatory unless a non-mass-related cause can be clearly identified. The lumbar puncture is deferred until after the CT scan, but antibiotics should be started immediately if infection seems likely.

Treatment depends on a number of factors. If the patient is stuporous or comatose but has neither focal signs nor

Table 42.15. Causes of Stupor and Coma in Children with Neoplastic Disease

Cause	*Intracranial Hypertension*	*Herniation Syndrome*
Tumor		
Infratentorial	Yes	Central
Supratentorial	Yes	Uncal
Bleeding		
Subdural or epidural	Yes	Uncal
Intracerebral	Yes	Uncal or central
Infection		
Meningitis	Rarely	Central
Abscess	Rarely	Uncal
Therapy		
SIADH[a]	Yes	Central
Confusional states[b]	Possibly	
Somnolence syndrome[c]	No	
Others		
Postictal state	No	
Metabolic encephalopathy	Possible	Central
Sedative overdose	No	
Hypertensive encephalopathy	Possible	Central

[a] *Vincristine and cyclophosphamide.*
[b] *Cisplatin and L-asparginase.*
[c] *MTX/irradiation.*

Table 42.16. Immediate Therapy for Intracranial Hypertension

Intubation and hyperventilation
Osmotic and loop diuretics
Steroids
Platelet and FFP transfusions if bleeding suspected
Surgical decompression if indicated and feasible

signs of intracranial hypertension and the other vital signs are stable, one has the luxury of carefully investigating the various possibilities in an orderly fashion and starting therapy when a likely cause for the coma becomes apparent. An electroencephalogram may prove useful. If, on the other hand, the patient is deeply comatose, has signs of critical intracranial hypertension, or has unstable vital signs, a swifter approach is needed **(Table 42.16).** The patient should be initially managed for intracranial hypertension by hyperventilation with a bag and mask. Then oral-tracheal intubation with appropriate anesthesia can be undertaken. Osmotic or loop diuretics can be simultaneously administered. If bleeding is suspected, 1 unit of platelets per 5 kg of body weight should be infused as soon as they can be obtained. The patient should also receive 20 ml/kg of FFP (with a diuretic if necessary). Intracranial pressure monitoring and further therapy can then be instituted. If epidural or subdural bleeding is highly suspected on clinical grounds, then surgical decompression without a prior CT scan may be considered. However, since most often these patients are thrombocytopenic and platelets must be administered before craniectomy, there is usually time for a CT scan to be performed (see also Chapters 18 to 21).

Strokes, Spinal Cord Compression, and Other Disorders

Strokes may be seen in children with neoplastic disease either as a direct result of their tumor or as a consequence of therapy. Brain tumors, especially those of the brainstem, may compress or infilitrate vital structures, resulting in stroke[(196)]. The leukemias may infiltrate cranial nerves, resulting in paresis, or may accumulate in perivascular tissue, with subsequent compression of vessels, leading to ischemic damage, necrosis, and hemorrhage[(196)]. Leukemic patients with extremely high white blood counts either at presentation or at relapse are prone to the development of hyperviscosity, which may be manifested by altered mental status or thrombotic stroke[(197)]. Finally, thrombotic or hemorrhagic strokes may be caused by administration of L-asparaginase. This enzyme may disrupt the balance between coagulation proteins and endogenous anticoagulants, resulting in either a hypercoagulable state or a hemorrhagic diathesis[(117,118)].

Spinal cord compression may develop from primary CNS tumors or extramedullary tumors eroding the vertebral column[(196,198)]. Intramedullary tumors that may cause signs of compression (radicular pain, sensory loss, motor weakness) include primary astrocytomas, ependymomas, and drop metastases from medulloblastomas. Pediatric tumors that may cause extramedullary compression include benign lipomas

Table 42.17. Common Antineoplastic Agents and Their Adverse Neurologic Effects

	Nervous System		
Agent	*Central*	*Autonomic*	*Peripheral*
Methotrexate	Aseptic meningitis Arachnoiditis Demyelination Somnolence syndrome Chronic leukoencephalopathy		
Cyclophosphamide	SIADH		
Cisplatin	Ototoxicity Cerebral edema Seizures		Optic neuritis Sensory neuritis
Vincristine	SIADH	Ileus	Peripheral neuropathy
Cytosine arabinoside	Arachnoiditis Cerebellar dysfunction		
Procarbazine	Acute cerebellar ataxia		
L-Asparaginase	Encephalopathy Seizures Thromboses		
Radiation	Somnolence syndrome Necrosis Demyelination		

and neurofibromas and malignant neuroblastomas, lymphomas, and sarcomas[(196)]. Emergent CT scanning is essential, and in most instances surgical decompression is required. In many instances, emergent radiotherapy is also indicated. Occasionally, a patient with thrombocytopenia who has recently undergone a lumbar puncture (e.g., intrathecal therapy for leukemia) may develop a spinal dural bleed and signs of compression. Treatment in this case requires correction of the thrombocytopenia and perhaps surgical decompression.

Last, a number of therapeutic agents may alter central or peripheral nervous system function. Some of the more commonly employed agents and their toxicities are listed in **Table 42.17.** Therapy is generally supportive, although many of these toxicities, such as cytosine arabinoside-induced cerebellar dysfunction and cisplatin-induced ototoxicity, may be irreversible.

Renal and Metabolic Complications

Renal and metabolic complications, like those involving the respiratory, cardiovascular, and nervous systems, may arise from the malignancy, the therapy, or a combination of both. In this section of the chapter, the causes of renal failure will be reviewed, various metabolic disorders will be considered, and some aspects of therapy will follow. Prerenal failure may occur as a consequence of sepsis, hemorrhage, or other causes of intravascular depletion. Less commonly, it occurs because of extrinsic compression of renal vessels[(199,200)]. Intrinsic renal failure may arise as a consequence of tumor infiltration. Wilms' tumor rarely causes renal dysfunction; however, leukemic or lymphomatous involvement of the kidney may lead to azotemia and oliguria[(200,201)]. Finally, obstructive nephropathies may arise because of tumor compression of bladder or urethra. A wide range of chemotherapeutics[(202,203)] **(Table 42.18),** as well as radiation[(204)] and antibiotics[(205–207)], can cause acute or chronic renal failure. Clearly then, the disorders of renal function are due to multiple causes, including not only the cancer and its therapies, but also antibiotics, antifungal agents, and such systemic problems as septic shock.

The most dramatic disturbances are seen in patients with large tumor burdens and high growth fractions who develop the tumor lysis syndrome. It is most prominent in patients with Burkitt's lymphoma or T-cell leukemia/lymphoma, but it can also be seen in patients with other forms of leukemia. The syndrome consists of hyperuricemia, hyperkalemia, and hyperphosphatemia and is evident either at presentation or within 5 days of commencing effective chemotherapy or radiation therapy[(197,208,209)]. It occurs as a direct result of tumor cell breakdown, either spontaneously or secondary to therapy. Intracellular phosphate and potassium are released, and uric acid is derived from the

Table 42.18. Chemotherapeutic Agents Associated with Genitourinary Injury

Agent	*Injury*	*Preventive/therapeutic Measures*
Methotrexate	Renal tubular	Hydration Alkalinization
Cisplatin	Tubular necrosis	Mannitol Saline diuresis Electrolyte replacement
Cyclophosphamide	Hemorrhagic cystitis	Vigorous diuresis MESNA
Ifosfamide	Hemorrhagic cystitis Tubular necrosis (Fanconi-like syndrome)	Vigorous diuresis MESNA Electrolyte replacement

breakdown of nucleic acids. Uric acid or calcium-phosphate crystals may form and precipitate in the kidney, resulting in oliguria and azotemia. Therapy entails hydration, alkalinization of the urine, and allopurinol. Intravenous hydration consisting of 5% dextrose, 0.25N saline, and 30 to 100 mEq sodium bicarbonate per liter should be delivered at two to four times maintenance requirements to produce a urine pH of 7.0 to 7.5; potassium-containing fluids should be avoided. This will promote urinary phosphate and uric acid excretion. Urine that is more alkaline than pH 7.5 may promote the development of hypoxanthine stones or calcium phosphate precipitation in the renal tubules and is to be avoided[(208,209)]. Allopurinol (300 mg/m^2/day) is given to prevent the continued formation of uric acid. Levels of these metabolic breakdown products as well as urea nitrogen and creatinine levels must be monitored frequently.

If the child does not respond to the initial medical intervention, or if signs of azotemia or oliguria are present, then hemodialysis or peritoneal dialysis may need to be initiated prior to the start of cancer therapy. If one opts not to initiate early prophylactic dialysis in the child at risk, the patient must be carefully observed in terms of metabolic and fluid status and dialysis promptly instituted if medical management does not maintain metabolic homeostasis. Once the tumor load has decreased, the tumor lysis syndrome resolves. The objective until that time is to prevent permanent renal damage. The overall therapy of renal failure, with the exception of controlling the uric acid concentration, is similar to that in the nononcologic patient. Hemodialysis catheters should be removed as soon as possible to minimize the risk of infection. Other associated problems, such as hypertension, must be identified and appropriately treated.

The cause of renal failure not associated with the tumor lysis syndrome may be determined by history and physical examination, and laboratory investigations will define the severity of the metabolic disturbances **(Table 42.19).** More specific tests, including x-rays, sonograms, CT, and a biopsy may be needed to make a definite diagnosis of the cause of renal failure. Therapy of renal failure depends on the cause as well as the severity. Obviously, as outlined in Chapter 37, fluid intake must be judiciously limited, electrolytes maintained in the appropriate range, and the patient monitored for development of uremic complications. If uremic complications develop (e.g., fluid overload, uremic bleeding, acid-base disturbance), then dialysis or continuous arteriovenous hemofiltration must be considered. Furthermore, modification of chemotherapeutic schedules is necessary. Although the reviews by Bennett et al.[(210,211)] (drug therapy in renal failure) applies to adults, they do provide guidelines for treating children with renal failures.

Table 42.19. Laboratory Tests in Renal Failure

Urinalysis
24-hr creatinine clearance
Electrolytes, blood urea nitrogen, creatinine
Complete blood count
Blood gas (pH and bicarbonate)
Calcium, phosphorus, uric acid

In the absence of renal failure, the oncology patient may exhibit some peculiar fluid and electrolyte abnormalities[(212,213)]. Water and sodium balance is deranged most commonly by excessive water administration or SIADH. SIADH is seen with various malignancies, respiratory disease, and the chemotherapeutics discussed in the neurology subsection of this chapter. In all of these cases, the hyponatremia is best treated by fluid restriction, although occasionally diuretics or hypertonic saline is necessary. Oncology patients may receive excessive amounts of salt, leading to pulmonary edema, particularly if they are treated with high sodium content antibiotics and frequent plasma or albumin infusions. Fluid overload is treated with diuretics in these patients as in the nononcologic PICU population.

Although hyperkalemia is seen in the tumor lysis syndrome as discussed above, it is rarely a problem in oncology patients in the absence of renal failure. Potassium wasting may occur for unexplained reasons and is occasionally seen in children with advanced malignancies. Other possible causes include toxic tumor-related metabolites, chemotherapy, antibiotics, antifungal agents, and diuretics[(201,214)]. Hypercalcemia is seen with primary or metastatic tumors of bone[(215)]. Calcium concentrations in excess of 12 mg/dl are treated with furosemide and a forced saline diuresis. Mithramycin may be required for extreme hypercalcemia[(215)]. Hypocalcemia is seen with the tumor lysis syndrome and requires therapy only if the patient is symptomatic; however, we often treat prophylactically if the calcium concentration is below 6 mg/dl. It is of note that both hypocalcemia and hypomagnesemia have been documented as a result of cisplatin and ifosfamide therapy and should be monitored in patients receiving these drugs[(202,216,217)].

Gastrointestinal Complications

As with other organ systems, gastrointestinal complications may occur in the oncology patients as a consequence of the tumor itself or as a consequence of therapy. Many malignant diseases may involve the gastrointestinal tract through either direct invasion or extrinsic compression of the gut. In children, the latter problem is more common. Typical neoplasms causing either complication include lymphoma, neuroblastoma, rhabdomyosarcoma, and Wilms' tumor[(218)]. The child with a gastrointestinal tumor usually presents with weight loss, anorexia, and occasionally obstructive symptoms. A high index of suspicion for malignancy must be maintained in the patient with recurrent intussusception. Although the tissue diagnosis is made at surgery, the suspected cause may be established by radiologic and/or sonographic imaging preoperatively in conjunction with biochemical analysis[(218–220)].

The child with cancer is also susceptible to intestinal

infection and perforation. Since many patients are neutropenic, the inflamatory component of these complications may be blunted and may also be less well localized than in an otherwise healthy child[209]. Typhlitis, a combination of hemorrhagic and agranulocytic necrosis involving the cecum, usually seen after intensive antileukemic therapy, is a particularly serious complication, often leading to intestinal perforation[219,220]. If infection is suspected, a fungal cause must be included in the differential diagnosis, particularly if symptoms of esophagitis are present. If bacterial infection is suspected, broad-spectrum antibiotic coverage, including anaerobic coverage, should be initiated.

Thrombocytopenia and the presence of a coagulopathy predispose children to gastrointestinal hemorrhage, particularly in the PICU setting, where stress ulcers and bleeding are seen in children without bleeding diatheses. Major bleeding requires urgent platelet and FFP administration, as previously noted. Antacids or histamine H_2-antagonists may reduce the likelihood of hemorrhage. Multiple antineoplastic agents result in mucositis, including anthracyclines, methotrexate, cytosine arabinoside, 5-fluorouracil, and radiation therapy. Treatment is supportive fluids, analgesia, and topical care, until mucosal regrowth occurs. Leukovorin may help ameliorate methotrexate-induced mucositis[221]. Other specific side effects of chemotherapy that the intensivist should be cognizant of are paralytic ileus after treatment with the vinca alkaloids vincristine and vinblastine[222] and pancreatitis after L-asparaginase therapy[192]. Therapy consists of discontinuation of the agent and supportive measures similar to the nononcology patient.

Chemotherapy will commonly cause nausea and vomiting. Although this rarely leads to shock, the intensivist must appreciate the likelihood of this adverse effect. Premedication with antiemetics will relieve unnecessary misery for these children. The serotonin receptor antagonists ondansetron (0.45 mg/kg/day, maximum 32 mg/day) and granisetron (10 to 20 μg/kg/day, maximum 1.0 mg/day) are the drugs of choice for chemotherapy-induced nausea[223,224]. Chlorpromazine (up to 1 mg/kg IV every 4 to 6 hr), droperidol (up to 0.1 mg/kg IV every 4 to 6 hr), or metoclopramide (up to 1 mg/kg IV every 4 to 6 hr) are often useful adjuncts. They may cause dystonic reactions[225], so, although diphenhydramine is not an effective antiemetic when used alone, we favor its use (1 mg/kg every 4 hr) both for prophylaxis against extrapyramidal effects and for sedation.

Liver disease is another complication seen in the oncology patient. Primary tumors of the liver are rare in childhood; however, a variety of chemotherapeutics have been associated with cirrhosis and fibrosis, although the causal relationship has been somewhat difficult to establish. The nitrosoureas and antimetabolites may cause hepatic toxicity[221]. Topley et al.[226] noted that significant liver disease was unusual in leukemic patients, and Locasiulli et al.[227] showed that children with abnormal liver function tests had evidence of prior hepatitis B virus infection. The management of liver failure is considered elsewhere in this text (Chapter 36).

BONE MARROW TRANSPLANTATION

The child who has undergone BMT is at risk for most of the complications discussed earlier in the chapter and several other problems relatively limited to BMT patients; these problems often necessitate admission to the PICU[228]. BMT is undertaken in children with selected nonneoplastic diseases, including congenital immunodeficiency syndromes[229], severe aplastic anemia[230], some genetic storage diseases[231], and several hemoglobinopathies[232,233], but it is most commonly performed in patients with malignancies. The most common indications for BMT are acute myelocytic leukemia (AML) in first or second remission and acute lymphoblastic leukemia (ALL) in second remission, although in selected high-risk ALL cases BMT may be employed in first remission[234–236]. Allogeneic BMT necessitates identification of an HLA-compatible donor, most often a sibling; alternatively, an unrelated donor identified through national or international registries or a mismatched family donor can be used. The recipient is prepared for transplantation by administration of an intensive chemotherapy regimen with or without total body irradiation to eliminate residual tumor; this intensive therapy (called the preparative regimen) also eradicates normal marrow cells. To replace these normal stem cells, bone marrow is collected from the donor and infused intravenously into the recipient. The preparative regimen must, therefore, also provide sufficient immunosuppression to prevent graft rejection. Recently, there has been an increase in the use of autologous marrow transplantation for children with leukemia, lymphoma, and some solid tumors, in which the patient serves as his or her own marrow donor. This minimizes or obviates the difficulties arising from allogeneic transplantation (graft-versus-host disease, opportunistic viral infections, failure to engraft, etc.). The child's own marrow is collected, ideally when the patient is clinically tumor free (i.e., in complete remission). The marrow may be treated ex vivo with specific antitumor monoclonal antibodies, immunomagnetic microspheres, or selected chemotherapeutic agents (e.g., 4-hydroperoxycyclophosphamide or mafosfamide) and is then cryopreserved. After the patient receives the preparative regimen, the autologous marrow is thawed and infused intravenously. This technique has been especially useful in AML[237,238], lymphoma[239], and selected solid tumors such as neuroblastoma[240], and Ewing's sarcoma[241].

The complications of BMT account for death in 20 to 35% of allogeneic BMT patients[242]. Common causes of mortality and morbidity are acute and chronic graft-versus-host-diseases (GVHD), opportunistic infections, pulmonary dysfunction due to infectious or noninfectious pneumonitides, and venoocclusive disease (VOD). Acute GVHD occurs in 30% to more than 50% of allogeneic BMT recipients and is characterized by skin rash, hepatic dysfunction, and diarrhea[242]. Immunologic recovery is slow in patients with GVHD, and local (e.g., intestinal) immunity is also impaired; as a result, children with GVHD have increased susceptibility to opportunistic infections(242–244). As acute GVHD results from an immunologic attack by allogeneic donor cytotoxic T-lymphocytes against recipient organs, the problem is obviated in autologous transplantation, in which the patient serves as the donor. To prevent the development of acute GVHD in the allogeneic BMT recipient, cyclosporine (alone or in combination with steroids and/or low-dose methotrexate) is generally administered prophylactically for several months after BMT(245,246). Adverse effects of long-term cyclosporine administration have been reported, including hirsutism, tremors, hypertension, and renal insufficiency(247). Acute GVHD may develop despite prophylaxis and requires more intensive immunosuppression with corticosteroids in addition to higher doses of cyclosporine; other agents, such as antithymocyte globulin or thalidomide, may be needed in severe cases(242,248).

Even in the absence of GVHD, the BMT patient is at high risk for opportunistic infections. Immediately after BMT, granulocytopenia is profound, and the child is at risk for overwhelming bacterial or fungal sepsis. Two to six weeks after BMT, as myeloid engraftment proceeds, recovery of neutrophil counts above 0.5×10^9/l lessens the risk of these aplasia-associated infections. Both humoral and cellular immune function are impaired for several months after BMT, accounting for the high risk of viral, fungal, and protozoal infection in these children(84,248,249). Of particular concern is the development of CMV infection, which can lead to persistent fevers, hepatitis, rarely retinitis or enteritis, but most commonly (and most seriously) interstitial pneumonitis(86,250,251). Many clinical manifestations of CMV are the consequence of reactivation of latent virus from initial CMV infection, often years earlier, as indicated by presence of anti-CMV IgG antibodies in the patient's serum. In children without previous CMV infection, transfusion of blood products from CMV-positive donors particularly granulocytes and nonleukocyte depleted platelets may introduce this virus and lead to infection(251,252). Fortunately, the exclusive transfusion of CMV-seronegative blood products into CMV-negative patients and the prophylactic or therapeutic intravenous administration of the antiviral agent ganciclovir for those exposed to CMV has decreased the morbidity and mortality associated with CMV in the BMT patient(85).

Pneumonitis and pulmonary insufficiency is a third cause of morbidity and mortality in the BMT patient. There appear to be three distinct risk periods. During the first 2 weeks after transplantation, fungal or bacterial infection is most likely. Pulmonary edema is also common during that period, presumably secondary to a "capillary leak" syndrome caused by release of lymphokines such as tumor necrosis factor-α from activated monocytes(253). The child with pneumonitis and/or respiratory failure during this early phase is treated for suspected bacterial pneumonia with broad-spectrum antibiotics. In many cases, this syndrome can be prevented by maintaining patients at a stable goal weight for 2 to 3 weeks after BMT, preventing weight gain with fluid restriction and administration of diuretics such as furosemide. The second risk period is 6 to 12 weeks after BMT, when CMV infection can occur. Characteristically, an interstitial pneumonitis is seen on chest radiograph. The patients may benefit from a trial of TMP-SMX (if not receiving it prophylactically) for there is a small but definite risk of *P. carinii* at this stage, but this pathogen is more commonly seen 3 to 6 months after BMT. As discussed earlier in the chapter, bronchoalveolar lavage or an open lung biopsy may become necessary to determine viral, fungal, or other treatable causes of pneumonitis. A third and much less common risk period occurs from 6 to more than 12 months after BMT. Rarely, patients develop progressive respiratory failure characterized by both hypoxia and restrictive lung disease. Histologic examination of the lung reveals pulmonary fibrosis and/or bronchiolitis obliterans, usually in association with chronic GVHD(254). This condition may respond to treatment with high-dose methylprednisolone (5 to 10 mg/kg/day for 1 week, with rapid tapering to 2.0 to 2.5 mg/kg/day), but many patients with this uncommon complication develop progressive fatal hypoxemia. Treatment of underlying chronic GVHD is obviously important in these situations.

Last, regimen-related toxicity to the liver, termed veno-occlusive disease (VOD), can cause significant morbidity and mortality in the BMT patient. VOD is a clinical diagnosis that is marked by weight gain secondary to fluid retention, tender hepatomegaly, and jaundice(255,256). Two important risk factors for its development are preexisting liver dysfunction and the use of total body irradiation or busulfan as part of the preparative regimen. Histologically, VOD is characterized by localized intraluminal coagulation and intimal proliferation in small hepatic venules(257). Attempts to prevent or treat this disorder with a variety of anticoagulants and thrombolytics have inconsistently met with success(258–260). VOD typically occurs in the first several weeks after BMT in 10 to 60% of patients and presents with a wide clinical spectrum of severity(256). The overall case-fatality rate of VOD is 50%; virtually all patients with mild to moderate VOD (i.e., maximum serum bilirubin ≤ 10 mg/dl) recover, and more than 95% of patients with severe disease die as a result of multi-organ system failure(256,261). As mentioned above, an open discussion involving the transplant team, the PICU team, and the family should be held regarding the prognosis of this posttransplant complication and whether aggressive medical support should be initiated or continued for patients who incur severe VOD.

DIAGNOSIS AND THERAPY OF NEOPLASTIC DISEASE

Thus far, the emphasis of this chapter has been on the recognition, diagnosis, prevention, and therapy of life-threatening complications in children with neoplastic disease. This final section, which reviews a general approach

Table 42.20. Common Presenting Findings in Acute Leukemia of Childhood

Signs and Symptoms	*Laboratory Data*
Hemorrhage (petechiae, ecchymoses, purpura)	Anemia
Hepatosplenomegaly	Leukocytosis
Lymphadenopathy	Thrombocytopenia
Fever	Hyperuricemia
Pallor	Disseminated intravascular coagulopathy
Bone or joint pain	
Gingival hyperplasia	

to the diagnosis and therapy of the tumors themselves, should help the intensivist interact more fully and effectively with the consultant oncologist. Although specific chemotherapeutic regimens and protocols are not discussed, the agents are reviewed in terms of modes of action and notable toxicities.

Common Pediatric Malignancies

Leukemia, the most common childhood neoplasm, best serves as an example of an approach to the diagnosis and therapy of cancer in children. ALL accounts for 75 to 80% of cases, and AML makes up the remainder[2,3,262,263]. The common signs and symptoms of leukemia at initial diagnosis are noted in **Table 42.20,** and those problems that may lead to an intensive care admission are summarized in **Table 42.21.**

The diagnosis of leukemia is often obvious on clinical grounds. Bone marrow obtained by biopsy or aspirate is necessary to confirm the diagnosis and classify the leukemia by cell type in preparation for appropriate therapy. Assessment of organ involvement, metabolic status, and the presence or absence of infection is also important prior to initiating antileukemia therapy **(Table 42.22).**

The general approach to the lymphomas[264–267] or any of the solid nonhematologic tumors is similar to that for leukemia. The lymphomas are the third most common childhood neoplasm, and the causes for PICU admission are similar to those seen in leukemia; of particular note is the frequency of mediastinal masses that cause respiratory obstruction and the rare occurrence of the tumor lysis syndrome secondary to cell breakdown, causing renal failure. Diagnosis of lymphoma, much like leukemia, is confirmed by tissue analysis. Most often, biopsy of a superficial lymph node or the bone marrow will yield the necessary information, and imaging studies such as CT of chest and abdomen may be useful in staging extent of disease. In some instances, a mediastinal mass must be biopsied, with the attendant risks discussed earlier in the chapter. Although staging laparotomy is performed much less frequently for Hodgkin's disease, some patients may have had splenectomy as a result of this procedure. In non-Hodgkin's lymphomas of childhood, splenectomy is rarely indicated; it places the child at a high risk of infection and provides little additional information that would alter diagnosis or management.

Table 42.21. Complications That May Lead to ICU Admission of Children with Leukemia

Tumor-related	**Therapy-related**
Blast count >100,000/μl	High-risk procedures
Large tumor load	Myelosuppression
Hyperuricemia	Organ dysfunction
Renal dysfunction	**Specific disorders**
Mediastinal mass	Sepsis and shock
Myelosuppression	Hemorrhage and shock
	Respiratory failure

Table 42.22. Routine Laboratory Investigation in the Child Suspected of Having Leukemia

Hematologic
- Complete blood count
- Blood smear examination
- Bone marrow aspirate for morphologic, immunophenotypic, cytogenetic, and histochemical analyses

Biochemical
- Electrolyte panel
- BUN and creatinine
- Uric acid
- Calcium and phosphorus
- Liver function tests

Other studies
- Blood and/or surveillance cultures
- Urinalysis (culture if indicated)
- Chest radiograph
- Electrocardiogram and echocardiogram
- Lumbar puncture to rule out CNS leukemia

Brain tumors are the second most common malignancies of childhood; approximately two-thirds are infratentorial. The presenting symptoms often reflect intracranial hypertension secondary to hydrocephalus. Supratentorial lesions may be associated with focal neurologic signs and, in the case of craniopharyngioma, a characteristic combination of visual and endocrine deficits. The diagnosis of brain tumor is made by history, physical examination, and radiologic studies including CT and MRI scans. A tissue diagnosis is often necessary for confirmation and appropriate treatment. These patients may require intensive care for the management of intracranial hypertension and postoperative monitoring after posterior fossa exploration. The patient with a craniopharyngioma may also require a PICU stay for management of fluid and electrolyte imbalances related to posterior pituitary insufficiency.

Other malignancies of childhood are relatively uncommon and rarely require intensive care. The interested reader may wish to refer to general pediatric oncology texts[2,3] for additional information.

Therapy for Childhood Malignancies

The various modalities of therapy for the childhood malignancies include surgery, radiation, chemotherapy, and BMT;

Table 42.23. Classes of Chemotherapeutic Agents

Antimetabolites
Vinca alkaloids
Antibiotics
Alkylating agents
Miscellaneous compounds

Table 42.25. Vinca Alkaloids

Agent	*Administration*	*Precautions*	*Toxicity*
Vincristine	IV	Avoid extravasation	Neuro, GI (ileus), SIADH
Vinblastine	IV	Avoid extravasation	Marrow, GI

a comprehensive discussion of the approaches can be found in other sources[2,3]. Surgery is indicated for diagnosis, palliation, or total excision of childhood neoplasms. In the PICU setting, surgery may also be necessary for the acute relief of a life-threatening obstruction (e.g., hydrocephalus with intracranial hypertension). Similarly, radiation may be needed in the treatment of the neoplasm, particularly for acute therapy of an obstructing mediastinal mass or spinal cord compression[268,269]. The complications of radiotherapy include respiratory, myocardial, and renal dysfunction, as well as myelosuppression if large areas of marrow are exposed[270].

Chemotherapeutic agents form the mainstay of treatment for the childhood neoplasms. All of the agents act by disrupting some aspect of normal cell growth or division. Combinations of drugs allow increased efficacy at subtoxic doses and decrease the likelihood of drug resistance by tumor cells. Theoretical considerations of cell kinetics dictate the type and timing of the various drugs used in the empirical clinical studies that have led to the current therapy protocols. The disease-specific protocols will not be discussed here; most are updated and reviewed by multicenter clinical groups and are available if needed. In pediatric oncology, the only hormones regularly used fall into the glucocorticoid class. Most agents used are nonhormones that can be classified by mechanism of action **(Table 42.23).** Each class of agents will be discussed, then specific agents will be reviewed in terms of route of administration, special features, and particular toxicities. Gastrointestinal toxicity ranges from nausea and vomiting to marked stomatitis and ulceration. Marrow toxicity, when indicated, refers to significant neutropenia or thrombocytopenia. A variety of allergic reactions have been reported with almost any of the agents used in pediatric oncology, but our understanding of the pathogenesis of the nonallergic manifestations of drug toxicities is poor. The discussion accompanying each agent is far from exhaustive; interested readers are directed to selected texts for more detailed information[2,271].

The antimetabolites **(Table 42.24)** interact with various cellular enzymes, inhibiting some aspect of metabolism or replication depending on the particular drug. For example, methotrexate (MTX) competitively inhibits the activity of dihydrofolate reductase (DHFR). Interestingly, this inhibition can be blocked in normal cells by leucovorin (folinic acid), probably by bypassing DHFR. This approach has led to the use of supralethal doses of methotrexate followed by leucovorin rescue of normal cells in the treatment of some malignancies. Other antimetabolites, such as cytosine arabinoside (Ara-C), 6-mercaptopurine (6-MP), and 6-thioguanine (6-TG), inhibit DNA synthesis. The vinca alkaloids in common use, vincristine and vinblastine **(Table 42.25),** are derived from the periwinkle plant. Both of these agents inhibit microtubule function within the cell. This prevents the formation of normal spindle apparatus during metaphase, thus inhibiting cell division. Several antitumor agents are antibiotics, including the anthracyclines (daunorubicin and doxorubicin [Adriamycin]), actinomycin D, and bleomycin **(Table 42.26).** The anthracyclines and actinomycin D inhibit the synthesis of DNA in tumor cells by acting on a specific enzyme, DNA topoisomerase II[272]. Another antitumor antibiotic, bleomycin, directly inhibits DNA synthesis. These agents are noted for their cumulative organ toxicity; the anthracyclines cause cardiac toxicity, and bleomycin causes pulmonary fibrosis and enhances pulmonary oxygen toxicity.

The alkylating agents **(Table 42.27)** cause breaks in DNA strands, cross-linkage of the strands, and miscoding during replication. Nitrogen mustard (HN_2), L-phenylalanine mustard (L-PAM), chlorambucil, ifosfamide, and cyclophosphamide are the commonly used drugs in this class. The nitrosoureas, BCNU and CCNU, also act by alkylating DNA. Marrow toxicity is the dose-limiting toxicity of all these agents, although there is substantial variability in the timing, magnitude, and duration of marrow hypoplasia among these agents. Of note is the particularly late hematopoietic toxicity of the nitrosourea compounds, in which

Table 42.24. Antimetabolites

Agent	*Administration*	*Precautions*	*Toxicity*
Methotrexate (MTX)	IV, PO, intrathecal (IT)	With high dose (>240 mg/m^2) alkalinize urine and employ leukovorin rescue	GI, marrow, renal, hepatic
Cytosine arabinoside (Ara-C)	IV, SC, IT	Arachnoiditis with IT	GI, marrow, neuro
6-Mercaptopurine (6-MP)	IV (investigational), PO	Reduce 6-MP dose when allopurinol is used	Marrow (mild), hepatic, renal
6-thioguanine	IV, PO		GI, hepatic

Table 42.26. Antitumor Antibiotics

Agent	*Administration*	*Precautions*	*Toxicity*
Doxorubicin (Adriamycin)	IV	Avoid extravasation, verify hepatic function	Marrow, GI, cardiac, hepatic
Daunorubicin	IV	Avoid extravasation, verify normal hepatic function	Marrow, cardiac
Idarubicin	IV	Avoid extravasation, verify normal hepatic function	Marrow, GI, cardiac
Mitoxantrone	IV	Avoid extravasation	Marrow, GI, cardiac
Actinomycin D	IV	Verify normal hepatic function	Marrow, GI, hepatic
Bleomycin	IV	Cumulative dose <400 units	Pulmonary fibrosis, GI, skin

Table 42.27. Alkylating Agents

Agent	*Administration*	*Precautions*	*Toxicity*
Cyclophosphamide (Cytoxan)	IV, PO	Maintain good urine output, concurrent MESNA administration	Marrow, hemorrhagic cystitis, GI, pulmonary fibrosis, SIADH, cardiac (high dose)
Ifosfamide	IV	Maintain good urine output, concurrent MESNA administration	Marrow, hemorrhagic cystitis, renal, GI
Melphalan	IV, PO		Marrow, GI
Busulfan	PO	Seizure prophylaxis for high dose	Seizures (high dose), pulmonary fibrosis
BCNU (carmustine)	IV	Administer slowly	Marrow (delayed myelosuppression, renal, pulmonary fibrosis)
CCNU (lomustine)	PO		Marrow (delayed myelosuppression, renal, pulmonary fibrosis)
Cisplatin	IV	Maintain urine output with osmotic diuretic	Renal, ototoxicity, marrow, GI
Carboplatin	IV		Marrow

marrow suppression may be apparent 1 or more months after administration of these drugs.

The other commonly used drugs in pediatric oncology **(Table 42.28)** include the enzyme L-asparaginase, the podophyllotoxin derivatives etoposide (VP-16) and teniposide (VM-26), the platinum compounds cisplatin and carboplatin, amsacrine (m-AMSA), and the glucocorticoids. L-asparaginase blocks protein synthesis by depleting cells of the amino acid asparagine. Like some of the antitumor antibiotics, the podophyllotoxin derivatives and amsacrine inhibit DNA synthesis by inhibition of DNA topoisomerase II. The glucocorticoids are directly lymphocytotoxic to lymphoid leukemic and lymphoma cells.

CONCLUSION

Although great strides have been made in the diagnosis and treatment of childhood neoplastic disease, much remains unanswered. Hopefully, collaboration among clinical oncologists, basic investigators, and intensive care personnel will lead to a better understanding of pediatric oncology, its treatments, and its complications.

References

1. Neglia JP, Robison LL. Epidemiology of the childhood leukemias. Pediatr Clin North Am 1988;35:675–692.
2. Pizzo PA, Poplack DG, eds. Principles and practice of pediatric oncology. Philadelphia: J.B. Lippincott, 1993.
3. Fernbach DJ, Vietti TJ, eds. Clinical pediatric oncology. 4th ed. St. Louis: Mosby-Year Book, 1991.
4. Sculier JP, Ries F, Verboven N, Coune A, Klastersky J. Role of intensive care unit in a medical oncology department. Eur J Cancer Clin Oncol 1988;24:513–517.
5. Dahlquist LM. Principles of total care: psychosocial issues and interventions. In: Fernbach DJ, Vietti TJ, eds. Clinical pediatric oncology. St. Louis: Mosby-Year Book, 1991:273–83.
6. Holder AR. Parents, courts, and refusal of treatment. J Pediatr 1983;103:515.
7. Wanzer SH, Federman DD, Adelstein SJ, et al. The physician's responsibility toward hopelessly ill patients. A second look. N Engl J Med 1989;320:844–849.
8. Perin G, Manchester PB. Pediatric oncology nursing. In: Sutow WW, Fernbach DJ, Vietti TJ, eds. Clinical pediatric oncology. 3rd ed. St. Louis: CV Mosby, 1984:262.
9. Griffin JP, Comley C. Role of the oncology nurse when the patient with cancer is transferred to the critical care unit. Oncol Nurs Forum 1989;16:703–707.

Table 42.28. Miscellaneous Chemotherapeutic Agents Used in Pediatric Oncology

Agent	*Administration*	*Precautions*	*Toxicity*
L-Asparaginase	IM	Anaphylaxis	Pancreatitis, hemorrhagic or thrombotic diathesis, hypoproteinemia, seizures
VP-16 (etoposide)	IV, PO	Infusion rate-related hypotension, anaphylaxis	Marrow, GI
VM-26 (teniposide)	IV	Infusion rate-related hypotension, anaphylaxis	Marrow, GI
Corticosteroids	IV, PO		Multiple organ system toxicities, immunosuppression
Procarbazine	PO	Antabuse-like activity	Myelosuppression

10. Pizzo PA, Rubin M, Freifeld A, Walsh TJ. The child with cancer and infection. I. Empiric therapy for fever and neutropenia, and preventive strategies. J Pediatr 1991;119:679–694.
11. Pizzo PA, Rubin M, Freifeld A, Walsh TJ. The child with cancer and infection, II. Nonbacterial infections. J Pediatr 1991;119:845–857.
12. Mitchell CD. Management of infections in the neutropenic child with cancer. Pediatr Ann 1988;17:678–686.
13. Schimpff SC. Infection prevention during profound granulocytopenia. Ann Intern Med 1980;93:358.
14. Leventhal BG, Cohen P, Triem SC. Effect of chemotherapy on the immune response in acute leukemia. Isr J Med Sci 1974;10:866.
15. Donowitz LG, Wenzel RP, Hoyt JW. High risk of hospital-acquired infection in the ICU patient. Crit Care Med 1982;10:355.
16. Ronald AR. Nosocomial infections, infection control and critical care medicine. Ann R Coll Phys Surg Can 1984;17:473.
17. Cross A, Allen JR, Burke J, et al. Nosocomial infections due to Pseudomonas aeruginosa: review of recent trends. Rev Infect Dis 1983;5:S837–S845.
18. Martone WJ, Osterman CA, Fisher KA, Wenzel RP. Pseudomonas cepacia: implications and control of epidemic nosocomial colonization. Rev Infect Dis 1981;3:708–715.
19. Hann IM, Prentice HG. Infection prophylaxis in the patient with bone marrow failure. Clin Haematol 1984;13:523.
20. Buckner CD, Clift RA, Sanders JE, et al. The Seattle marrow transplant team. Protective environment for marrow transplant recipients. Ann Intern Med 1978;89:893.
21. Pizzo PA. The value of protective isolation in preventing nosocomial infections in high risk patients. Am J Med 1981;70:631.
22. Ribas-Mundo M, Granena A, Rozman C. Evaluation of a protective environment in the management of granulocytopenic patients: a comparative study. Cancer 1981;48:419.
23. Bodey GP, Rodriquez V, Murphy WK, Burgress MA, Benjamin RS. Protected environment-prophylactic antibiotic program for malignant sarcomas: randomized trial during remission induction chemotherapy. Cancer 1981;47:2422.
24. Donowitz LG. Failure of the overgown to prevent nosocomial infection in the pediatric intensive care unit. Pediatrics 1986;77:35–38.
25. Hall CB, Douglas RG. Nosocomial respiratory syncytial viral infections. Am J Dis Child 1981;135:512–515.
26. Goldmann DA, Durbin WA. Nosocomial infections in a neonatal intensive care unit. J Infect Dis 1981;144:449–459.
27. Maki DG. Control of colonization and transmission of pathogenic bacteria in the hospital. Ann Intern Med 1978;89:777.
28. Maki DG, Alvarado CJ, Hassemer CA, Zilz MA. Relation of the inanimate hospital environment to endemic nosocomial infection. N Engl J Med 1982;307:1562.
29. McGowan JE. Antimicrobial resistance in hospital organisms and its relation to antibiotic use. Rev Infect Dis 1983;5:1033–1048.
30. Abraham SN. Barrier defects. In: Patrick CC, ed. Infections in immunocompomised infants and children. New York: Churchill Livingstone, 1992:25–34.
31. Herrod HG. Cell-mediated immunity. In: Patrick CC, ed. Infections in immunocompromised infants and children. New York: Churchill Livingstone, 1992:63–74.
32. Rosenthal AS. Regulation of the immune response—Role of the macrophage. N Engl J Med 1980;303:1153.
33. Unanue ER. Cooperation between mononuclear phagocytes and lymphocytes in immunity. N Engl J Med 1980;303:977.
34. Dinarello CA, Mier JW. Lymphokines. N Engl J Med 1987;317: 939–945.
35. Bellanti JA, Kadlec JV, Escobar-Gutierrez A. Cytokines and the immune response. Pediatr Clin North Am 1994;41:597–621.
36. Virella G. Humoral immunity and complement. In: Patrick CC, ed. Infections in immunocompromised infants and children. New York: Churchill Livingstone, 1992:75–94.
37. Chandra RK. Interactions of nutrition, infection and immune response. Acta Pediatr Scand 1979;68:137–144.
38. Mauer AM, Burgess JB, Donaldson SS, et al. Special nutritional needs of children with malignancies: a review. J Paren Enter Nutr 1990;14:315–324.
39. Holcomb GW, Ziegler MM. Nutrition and cancer in children. Surg Ann 1990;22:129–142.
40. Chandra RK, Tejpar S. Review/commentary diet and immunocompetence. Int J Immunopharmacol 1983;5:175.
41. Allen JB, Weiner LB. Pneumococcal sepsis in childhood leukemia and lymphoma. Pediatrics 1981;67:292.
42. Tosi MF. Disorders of phagocyte function. In: Patrick CC, ed. Infections in immunocompromised infants and children. New York: Churchill Livingstone, 1992:35–62.
43. Albano EA, Pizzo PA. Infectious complications in childhood leukemias. Pediatr Clin North Am 1988;35:873–901.
44. Lieschke GJ, Burgess AW. Granulocyte colony-stimulating factor and granulocyte-macrophage colony-stimulating factor. N Engl J Med 1992;327:99–106.
45. Solomkin JS, Jenkins MK, Nelson RD, Chenoweth D, Simmons RL. Neutrophil dysfunction in sepsis. II. Evidence for the role of complement activation products in cellular deactivation. Surgery 1981;90:319.
46. Hughes WT, Kuhn S, Chaudhary S, et al. Successful chemoprophylaxis for *Pneumocystis carinii* pneumonitis. N Engl J Med 1977;297:1419–1426.
47. Milliken ST, Powles RL. Antifungal prophylaxis in bone marrow transplantation. Rev Infect Dis 1990;12:S374–S379.
48. Barson WJ, Brady MT. Management of infections in children with cancer. Hematol Oncol Clin North Am 1987;1:801–839.
49. Balfour HH, Groth KE. Zoster immune plasma prophylaxis of varicella: a follow-up report. J Pediatr 1979;94:743.
50. Orenstein WA, Heymann DL, Ellis RJ, et al. Prophylaxis of varicella in high-risk children: dose-response effect of zoster immune globulin. J Pediatr 1981;98:368.
51. Lawrence R, Gershon AA, Holzman R, Steinberg SP. The risk of zoster after varicella vaccination in children with leukemia. N Engl J Med 1988;318:543–548.
52. Perillo RP, Campbell CR, Strang S, Bodicky CJ, Costigan DJ. Immune globulin and hepatitis B immune globulin. Arch Intern Med 1984;144:81.
53. Berkman SA, Lee ML, Gale RP. Clinical uses of intravenous immunoglobulins. Semin Hematol 1988;25:140–158.
54. Meyers JD, Reed EC, Shepp DH, et al. Acyclovir for prevention of cytomegalovirus infection and disease after allogeneic marrow transplantation. N Engl J Med 1988;318:70–75.
55. Winston DJ, Ho WG, Lin CH, et al. Intravenous immune globulin for prevention of cytomegalovirus infection and interstitial pneumonia after bone marrow transplantation. Ann Intern Med 1987;106:12–18.
56. Tager IB, Ginsberg MB, Ellis SE, et al. An epidemiologic study of the risks associated with peripheral intravenous catheters. Am J Epidemiol 1983;118:839.
57. Band JD, Maki DG. Infections caused by arterial catheters used for hemodynamic monitoring. Am J Med 1979;67:735.
58. Norwood S, Ruby A, Civetta J, Cortes V. Catheter-related infections and associated septicemias. Chest 1991;99:968–975.
59. van Hoff J, Berg AT, Seashore JH. The effect of right atrial catheters on infectious complications of chemotherapy in children. J Clin Oncol 1990;8:1255–1262.
60. Mirro J, Rao BN, Kumar M, et al. A comparison of placement techniques and complications of externalized catheters and implantable port use in children with cancer. J Pediatr Surg 1990;25:120–124.
61. Ross MN, Haase GM, Poole MA, Burrington JD, Odom LF. Comparison of totally implanted reservoirs with external catheters as venous access devices in pediatric oncologic patients. Surg Gynecol Obstet 1988;167:141–144.
62. Wallace J, Zelter PM. Benefits, complications, and care of implantable infusion devices in 31 children with cancer. J Pediatr Surg 1987;22:833–838.
63. Shulman RJ, Smith EO, Rahman S, Gardner P, Reed T, Mahoney D. Single- vs. double-lumen central venous catheters in pediatric oncology patients. Am J Dis Child 1988;142:893–895.
64. Rupar DG, Herzog KD, Fisher MC, Long SS. Prolonged bacteremia with catheter-related central venous thrombosis. Am J Dis Child 1990;144:879–882.
65. Weinberger M, Pizzo PA. The evaluation and management of neutropenic patients with unexplained fever. In: Patrick CC, ed. Infections in immunocompromised infants and children. New York: Churchill Livingstone, 1992:335–356.
66. Rubin M, Hathorn JW, Marshall D, Gress J, Steinberg SM, Pizzo PA. Gram-positive infections and the use of vancomycin in 550 episodes of fever and neutropenia. Ann Intern Med 1988;108:30–35.
67. Heimdahl A, Mattson T, Dahloff G, Lonnquist B, Ringden O. The oral cavity as a port of entry for early infections in patients treated with

bone marrow transplantation. Oral Surg Oral Med Oral Pathol 1989;68:711–716.
68. Bartlett AV, Zusman J, Daum RS. Unusual presentations of *Haemophilus influenzae* infections in immunocompromised patients. J Pediatr 1983;102:55.
69. Favor LF, Tarpay M, Blackstock R. Septicemia in children with cancer. South Med J 1979;72:132.
70. Siber GR. Bacteremias due to *Haemophilus influenzae* and *Streptococcus pneumoniae*. Am J Dis Child 1980;134:668.
71. Pizzo PA, Hathorn JW, Hiemenz J, et al. A randomized trial comparing ceftazidime alone with combination antibiotic therapy in cancer patients with fever and neutropenia. N Engl J Med 1986;315:552–558.
72. Hughes WT. Guidelines for the use of antimicrobial agents in neutropenic patients with unexplained fever. J Infect Dis 1990;161:381–396.
73. Shenep JL, Hughes WT, Roberson PK, et al. Vancomycin, ticarcillin, and amikacin compared with ticarcillin-clavulanate and amikacin in the empirical treatment of febrile, neutropenic children with cancer. N Engl J Med 1988;319:1053–1058.
74. The EORTC. Ceftazidime combined with a short or long course of amikacin for empirical therapy of gram negative bacteremia in cancer patients with granulocytopenia. N Engl J Med 1987;317:1692–1698.
75. Rubin LG, Tucci V, Cercenado E, Eliopoulos G, Isenberg HD. Vancomycin-resistant Enterococcus faecium in hospitalized children. Infect Control Hosp Epidemiol 1992;13:700–5.
76. Pizzo PA, Walsh TJ. Fungal infections in the pediatric cancer patient. Semin Oncol 1990;17:6–9.
77. Brown AE. Overview of fungal infections in cancer patients. Semin Oncol 1990;17:2–5.
78. Kuhlman JE, Fishman EK, Burch PA, Karp JE, Zerhouni EA, Siegelman SS. CT of invasive pulmonary aspergillosis. AJR 1988;150:1015–1020.
79. Pastakia B, Shawker TH, Thaler M. Hepatosplenic candidiasis: wheels within wheels. Radiology 1988;166:417–421.
80. Walsh TJ, Hathorn JW, Sobel JD, et al. Detection of circulating Candida enolase by immunoassay in patients with cancer and invasive candidiasis. N Engl J Med 1991;324:1026–1031.
81. Ringden O, Meunier F, Tollemar J, et al. Efficacy of amphotericin B encapsulated in liposomes (AmBisome) in the treatment of invasive fungal infections in immunocompromised patients. J Antimicrob Chemother 1991;28(Suppl. B):73–82.
82. Como JA, Dismukes WE. Oral azole drugs as systemic antifungal therapy. N Engl J Med 1994;330:263–272.
83. Anonymous. Systemic antifungal drugs. Med Let Drugs Ther 1994;36:16–18.
84. Saral R, Burns WH, Prentice HG. Herpes virus infections: clinical manifestations and therapeutic strategies in immunocompromised patients. Clin Haemotol 1984;13:645.
85. Forman SJ, Zaia JA. Treatment and prevention of cytomegalovirus pneumonia after bone marrow transplantation: where do we stand? Blood 1994;83:2392–2398.
86. Emanuel D, Cunningham I, Jules-Elysee K, et al. Cytomegalovirus pneumonia after bone marrow transplantation successfully treated with the combination of ganciclovir and high-dose intravenous immunoglobulin. Ann Intern Med 1988;109:777–782.
87. Reed EC, Bowden RA, Dandliker PS, Lilleby KE, Meyers JD. Treatment of cytomegalovirus pneumonia with ganciclovir and intravenous cytomegalovirus immunoglobulin in patients with bone marrow transplants. Ann Intern Med 1988;109:783–788.
88. Prober CG, Kirk LE, Keeney RE. Acyclovir therapy of chickenpox in immunosuppressed children—A collaborative study. J Pediatr 1982;101:622.
89. Balfour HH, Jr. Intravenous acyclovir therapy for varicella in immunocompromised children. J Pediatr 1984;104:133.
90. Saral R, Burns WH, Laskin OL, Santos GW, Lietman PS. Acyclovir prophylaxis of herpes-simplex-virus infections. N Engl J Med 1981;305:63.
91. Hall TS, Hutchins GM, Baker RR. A critical review of the use of open lung biopsy in the management of the oncologic patient with acute pulmonary infiltrates. Am J Clin Oncol 1987;10:249–252.
92. Imoke E, Dudgeon DL, Colamboni P, Leventhal B, Buck JR, Haller JA. Open lung biopsy in the immunocompromised host. J Pediatr Surg 1983;18:918.
93. Stokes DC, Shenep JL, Parham D, Bozeman PM, Marienchek W, Mackert PW. Role of flexible bronchoscopy in the diagnosis if pulmonary infiltrates in pediatric patients with cancer. J Pediatr 1989; 115:561–567.
94. Strauss RG. Granulocyte transfusion therapy. Hematol Oncol Clin North Am 1994;8:1159–1166.
95. Dahlke MB, Keashen M, Alavi JB, Koch PA, Eisenstaedt R. Granulocyte transfusions and outcome of alloimmunized patients with gram-negative sepsis. Transfusion 1982;22:374.
96. Arnold R, Goldmann SF, Pflieger H. Lymphocytotoxic antibodies in patients receiving granulocyte transfusions. Vox Sang 1980;38:250.
97. Nikoskelainen J, Soderstrom KO, Rajamaki A, et al. Graft-versus-host reaction in 3 adult leukaemia patients after transfusion of blood cell products. Scand J Haematol 1983;31:403.
98. Anderson KC, Weinstein HJ. Transfusion associated graft-versus-host disease. N Engl J Med 1990;323:315.
99. Buckner CD, Clift RA. Prophylaxis and treatment of infection of the immunocompromised host by granulocyte transfusion. Clin Haematol 1984;13:557.
100. Barbara JAJ, Tedder RS. Viral infections transmitted by blood and its products. Clin Haemotol 1984;13:693.
101. Karp DD, Ervin TJ, Tuttle S, Gorgone BC, Lavin P, Yunis EJ. Pulmonary complications during granulocyte transfusions: incidence and clinical features. Vox Sang 1982;42:57.
102. Bow EJ, Schroeder ML, Louie TJ. Pulmonary complications in patients receiving granulocyte transfusions and amphotericin B. Can Med Assoc J 1984;130:593.
103. Wright DG, Robichaud KJ, Pizzo PA, Deisseroth AB. Lethal pulmonary reactions associated with the continued use of amphotericin B and leukocyte transfusions. N Engl J Med 1981;304:1186.
104. Balis FM, Holcenberg JS, Poplack DG. General principles of chemotherapy. In: Pizzo PA, Poplack DG, eds. Principles and practice of pediatric oncology. Philadelphia: J. B. Lippincott, 1993:197–245.
105. Hoagland HC. Hematologic complications of cancer chemotherapy. Semin Oncol 1982;9:95.
106. Steuber CP, Mahoney DH, Jr. Ogden AK. Acute myeloid leukemia and myeloproliferative disorders. In: Fernbach DJ, Vietti TJ, eds. Clinical pediatric oncology. St. Louis: Mosby-Year Book, 1991: 377–396.
107. Crist WM, Pullen DJ, Rivera GK. Acute lymphoid leukemia. In: Fernbach DJ, Vietti TJ, eds. Clinical pediatric oncology. St. Louis: Mosby-Year Book, 1991: 305–335.
108. Stone RM, Mayer RJ. The unique aspects of acute promyelocytic leukemia. J Clin Oncol 1990;8:1913–1921.
109. Gmur J, Burger J, Schanz U, Fehr J, Schaffner A. Safety of stringent prophylactic platelet transfusion policy for patients with acute leukaemia. Lancet 1991;338:1223–1226.
110. Beutler E. Platelet transfusions: the 20,000/μL trigger. Blood 1993;81:1411–1413.
111. Kutti J, Zaroulis CG, Dinsmore RE, Reich L, Clarkson BD, Good RA. A prospective study of platelet-transfusion therapy administered to patients with acute leukemia. Transfusion 1982;22:44.
112. Feinstein DI. Treatment of disseminated intravascular coagulation. Semin Thromb Hemost 1988;14:351–362.
113. Bick RL. Disseminated intravascular coagulation: objective criteria for diagnosis and management. Med Clin North Am 1994;78:511–543.
114. Gilbert JA, Scalzi RP. Disseminated intravascular coagulation. Emerg Med Clin North Am 1993;11:465–480.
115. Rubin RN, Colman RW. Disseminated intravascular coagulation: approach to treatment. Drugs 1992;44:963–971.
116. Bezeaud A, Drouet L, Leverger G, Griffin JH, Guillin M-C. Effect of L-asparaginase therapy for acute lymphoblastic leukemia on plasma vitamin K-dependent coagulation factors and inhibitors. J Pediatr 1986;108:698–701.
117. Ott N, Ramsay NKC, Priest JR, et al. Sequelae of thrombotic or hemorrhagic complications following L-asparaginase therapy for childhood lymphoblastic leukemia. Am J Pediatr Hematol Oncol 1988;10: 191–195.
118. Shapiro AD, Clarke SL, Christian JM, Odom LF, Hathaway WE. Thrombosis in children receiving L-asparaginase. Am J Pediatr Hematol Oncol 1993;15:400–405.
119. Pullerits J, Holzman R. Anaesthesia for patients with mediastinal masses. Can J Anaesth 1989;6:681–688.
120. King RM, Telander RL, Smithson WA, Banks PM, Han MT. Primary mediastinal tumors in children. J Pediatr Surg 1982;17:512–520.
121. Halpern S, Chatten J, Meadows AT, Byrd R, Lange B. Anterior mediastinal masses: anesthesia hazards and other problems. J Pediatr 1983;102:407.
122. Shamberger RC, Holzman RS, Griscom NT, Tarbell NJ, Weinstein HJ. CT Quantitation of tracheal cross-sectional area as a guide to the surgical and anaesthetic management of children with anterior mediastinal masses. J Pediatr Surg 1991;26:138–142.
123. Neuman GG, Weingarten AE, Abramowitz RM, Kushins LG, Abramson

AL, Ladner W. The anesthetic management of the patient with an anterior mediastinal mass. Anesthesiology 1984;60:144–147.
124. Victory RA, Casey W, Doherty P, Breatnach F. Cardiac and respiratory complications of mediastinal lymphomas. Anaesth Intens Care 1993;21:366–369.
125. Fisher DM, Robinson S, Brett CM, Perin G, Gregory GA. Comparison of enflurane, halothane and isoflurane for diagnostic and therapeutic procedures in children with malignancies. Anesthesiology 1985;63:647–650.
126. Piat V, Dubois M-C, Johanet S, Murat I. Induction and recovery characteristics and hemodynamic responses to sevoflurane and halothane in children. Anesth Analg 1994;79:840–844.
127. Epstein DM, Aronchick JM. Lung cancer in childhood. Med Pediatr Oncol 1989;17:510–513.
128. Carlson RA, Hattery RR, O'Connell EJ, Fontana RS. Pulmonary involvement by histiocytosis X in the pediatric age group. Mayo Clin Proc 1976;51:542.
129. Crystal RG, Bitterman PB, Rennard SI, Hance AJ, Keogh BA. Interstitial lung disease of unknown cause. N Engl J Med 1984;310:235.
130. Georgitis J, Eigen H, Provisor D, Baehner RL. Isolated pulmonary leukemia relapse following successful bone marrow transplant in a child with acute lymphoblastic leukemia. Pediatrics 1979;64:913.
131. Hull HF, Blumhagen JD, Benjamin D, Corey L. Herpes simplex viral pneumonitis in childhood. J Pediatr 1984;104:211.
132. Cordonnier C, Bernaudin J-F, Bierling P, Huet Y, Vernant J-P. Pulmonary complications occurring after allogeneic bone marrow transplantation. Cancer 1986;58:1047–1054.
133. Wingard JR, Mellits ED, Sostrin MB, et al. Interstitial pneumonitis after allogeneic bone marrow transplantation. Medicine 1988;67: 175–185.
134. Stokes DC, Bozeman PM. Sinopulmonary infections in immunocompromised infants and children. In: Patrick CC, ed. Infections in immunocompromised infants and children. New York: Churchill Livingstone, 1992:357–375.
135. Feldman S. Legionella. In: Patrick CC, ed. Infections in immunocompromised infants and children. New York: Churchill Livingstone, 1992: 467–473.
136. McDonald S, Rubin P, Phillips TL, Marks LB. Injury to the lung from cancer therapy: clinical syndromes, measurable endpoints, and potential scoring systems. Int J Radiation Oncol Biol Phys 1995;31:1187–1203.
137. Morgan GW, Breit SN. Radiation and the lung: a reevaluation of the mechanisms mediating pulmonary injury. Int J Radiation Oncol Biol Phys 1995;31:361–369.
138. White DA, Rankin JA, Stover DE, Gellene RA, Gupta S. Methotrexate pneumonitis: bronchoalveolar findings suggest an immunologic disorder. Am Rev Respir Dis 1989;139.
139. Gilson AJ, Sahn SA. Reactivation of bleomycin lung toxicity following oxygen administration. Chest 1985;88:304–306.
140. Rochester DF, Esau SA. Malnutrition and the respiratory system. Chest 1984;85:411.
141. Ingbar DH, White DA. Acute respiratory failure. Crit Care Clin 1988;4:11–40.
142. Lester TJ, Johnson JW, Cuttner J. Pulmonary leukostasis as the single worst prognostic factor in patients with acute myelocytic leukemia and hyperleukocytosis. Am J Med 1985;79:43–48.
143. Myers TJ, Cole SR, Klatsky AU, Hild DH. Respiratory failure due to pulmonary leukostasis following chemotherapy of acute nonlymphocytic leukemia. Cancer 1983;51:1808.
144. Deneke SM, Fanburg BL. Normobaric oxygen toxicity of the lung. N Engl J Med 1980;303:76.
145. Shapiro BA, Cane RD, Rand B, Harrison RA. Positive end-expiratory pressure therapy in adults with special reference to acute lung injury: a review of the literature and suggested clinical correlations. Crit Care Med 1984;12:127.
146. Pepe PE, Hudson LD, Carrico CJ. Early application of positive end-expiratory pressure in patients at risk for the adult respiratory distress syndrome. N Engl J Med 1984;311:281.
147. Ewer MS, Ali MK. Critical cardiologic considerations in the cancer patient. Crit Care Clin 1988;4:41–60.
148. Rozencweig M, Piccart M, Von Hoff DD. Cardiac disorders in cancer patients. In: Klastersky J, Staquet MJ, eds. Medical complications in cancer patient. New York: Raven Press, 1981:211.
149. Theologides A. Neoplastic cardiac tamponade. In: Yarbro JW, Bornstein PS, eds. Oncologic emergencies. New York: Grune & Stratton, 1981:1.
150. Brosius FC III, Waller BF, Roberts WC. Radiation heart disease. Analysis of 16 young (aged 15 to 33 years) necropsy patients who received over 3,500 rads to the heart. Am J Med 1981;70.
151. Lipshultz SE, Colan SD, Gelber RD, Perez-Atayde AR, Sallan SE, Sanders SP. Late cardiac effects of doxorubicin therapy for acute lymphoblastic leukemia in childhood. N Engl J Med 1991;324: 808–815.
152. Steinherz LJ, Steinherz PG, Tan CT, Heller G, Murphy ML. Cardiac toxicity 4 to 20 years after completing anthracycline therapy. JAMA 1991;266:1672–1677.
153. O'Connell TX, Berenbaum MC. Cardiac and pulmonary effects of high doses of cyclophosphamide and isophosphamide. Cancer Res 1974;34:1586–1691.
154. Truesdell S, Schwartz CL, Clark E, Constine LS. Cardiovascular effects of cancer therapy. In: Schwartz CL, Hobbie WL, Constine LS, Ruccione KS, eds. Survivors of childhood cancer. St. Louis: Mosby, 1994: 159–175.
155. Pratt CB, Ransom JL, Evans WE. Age-related Adriamycin cardiotoxicity in children. Cancer Treat Rev 1978;62:1381–1385.
156. Billingham ME, Bristow MR, Glatstein E, Mason JW, Masek MA, Daniels JR. Adriamycin cardiotoxicity: endomyocardial biopsy evidence of enhancement by irradiation. Am J Surg Pathol 1977;1:17–23.
157. Oberlin O, Habrand JL, Zucker JM, et al. No benefit of ifosfamide in Ewing's sarcoma: a nonrandomized study of the French Society of Pediatric Oncology. J Clin Oncol 1992;10:1407–1412.
158. Minow RA, Benjamin RS, Lee ET, Gottlieb JA. Adriamycin cardiomyopathy-risk factors. Cancer 1977;39:1397–1402.
159. Goldberg MA, Antin JH, Guinan EC, Rappeport JM. Cyclophosphamide cardiotoxicity: an analysis of dosing as a risk factor. Blood 1986;68:1114–1118.
160. Olson RD, Mushlin PS. Doxorubicin cardiotoxicity: analysis of prevailing hypotheses. FASEB J 1990;4:3076–3086.
161. Curran CF, Narang PK, Reynolds RD. Toxicity profile of dexrazoxane (Zinecard[R], ICRF-187, ADR-529, NSC-169780), a modulator of doxorubicin cardiotoxicity. Cancer Treat Rev 1991;18:241–252.
162. Hancock EW. Heart disease after radiation. N Engl J Med 1983;308:587.
163. Weber KT, Andrews V, Janicki JS. Cardiotonic agents in the management of chronic cardiac failure. Am Heart J 1982;103:639.
164. Goorin AM, Borow KM, Goldman A, et al. Congestive heart failure due to adriamycin cardiotoxicity: its natural history in children. Cancer 1981;47:2810.
165. Starnes V. Heart transplantation in children with cardiomyopathies. J Heart Lung Transplant 1991;10:815–819.
166. Leversha AM, Wilson NJ, Clarkson PM, Calder AL, Ramage MC, Neutze JM. Efficacy and dosage of enalapril in congenital and acquired heart disease. Arch Dis Child 1994;70.
167. Couch RD, Loh KK, Sugino J. Sudden cardiac death following adriamycin therapy. Cancer 1981;48:38.
168. Rinkevich D, Borovik R, Bendett M, Markiewicz W. Malignant pericardial tamponade. Med Pediatr Oncol 1990;18:287–291.
169. Byyny RL. Withdrawal from glucocorticoid therapy. N Engl J Med 1976;295:30–32.
170. Kass EH. High-dose corticosteroids for septic shock. N Engl J Med 1984;311:1176.
171. Sprung CL, Caralis PV, Marcial EH, et al. The effects of high-dose corticosteroids in patients with septic shock. N Engl J Med 1984;311:1137.
172. Ziegler EJ, Fisher CJ, Jr. , Sprung CL, et al. Treatment of gram-negative bacteremia and septic shock with HA-1A human monoclonal antibody against endotoxin. N Engl J Med 1991;324:429–436.
173. Abner A. Approach to the patient who presents with superior vena cava obstruction. Chest 1993;103:394S–397S.
174. Yellin A, Mandel M, Rechavi G, Neuman Y, Ramot B, Lieberman Y. Superior vena cava syndrome associated with lymphoma. Am J Dis Child 1992;146:1060–1063.
175. Ein SH, Weitzman S, Thorner P, Seagram CG, Filler RM. Pediatric malignant pheochromocytoma. J Pediatr Surg 1994;29:1197–1201.
176. Werbel SS, Ober KP. Pheochromocytoma. Update on diagnosis, localization, and management. Med Clin North Am 1995;79:131–53.
177. Gelfand MJ. Meta-iodobenzylguanidine in children. Semin Nucl Med 1993;23:231–242.
178. Pratilas V, Pratilas MG. Anaesthetic management of phaeochromocytoma. Can Anaesth Soc J 1979;26:253.
179. Monster M. Diagnosis and treatment of hypertension in children. Pediatr Clin North Am 1982;29:933.
180. Miser AW, Miser JS. The treatment of cancer pain in children. Pediatr Clin North Am 1989;36:979–999.

181. Pollack IF. Brain tumors in children. N Engl J Med 1994;331:1500–1507.
182. Van Eys J. Malignant tumors of the central nervous system. In: Fernbach DJ, Vietti TJ, eds. Clinical pediatric oncology. St. Louis: Mosby-Year Book, 1991:409–426.
183. Heideman RL, Packer RJ, Albright LA, Freeman CR, Rorke LB. Tumors of the central nervous system. In: Pizzo PA, Poplack DG, eds. Principles and practice of pediatric oncology. Philadelphia: J B Lippincott, 1993:633–681.
184. Bleyer WA. Central nervous system leukemia. Pediatr Clin North Am 1988;4:789–814.
185. Hildebrand J. Neurological disorders in cancer patients and their treatment. In: Klastersky J, Staquet MJ, eds. Medical complications in cancer patients. New York: Raven Press, 1981:51.
186. Carincross JG, Posner JB. Neurological complications of systemic cancer. In: Yarbro JW, Bornstein RS, eds. Oncologic emergencies. New York: Grune & Stratton, 1981:177.
187. Kaplan RS, Wiernik PH. Neurotoxicity of antineoplastic drugs. Semin Oncol 1982;9:103.
188. Robertson GL, Bhoopalam N, Zelkowitz LJ. Vincristine neurotoxicity and abnormal secretion of antidiuretic hormone. Arch Intern Med 1973;132:717–720.
189. Bressler RB, Huston DP. Water intoxication following moderate-dose intravenous cyclophosphamide. Arch Intern Med 1985;145:548–549.
190. Jaffe N, Takaue Y, Anzai T, Robertson R. Transient neurologic disturbances induced by high-dose methotrexate treatment. Cancer 1985;56:1356–1360.
191. Bleyer WA, Poplack DG, Simon RM. Neurotoxicity and elevated cerebrospinal fluid methotrexate concentration in meningeal leukemia. N Engl J Med 1973;289:770–773.
192. Cairo MS. Adverse reactions of L-asparaginase. Am J Pediatr Hematol Oncol 1982;4:335–339.
193. Mead GM, Arnold AM, Green JA, Macbeth FR, Williams CJ, Whitehouse JM. Epileptic seizures associated with cisplatin administration. Cancer Treat Rep 1982;66:1719.
194. Eden OB, Goldie W, Wood T, Etcubanas E. Seizures following intrathecal cytosine arabinoside in young children with acute lymphoblastic leukemia. Cancer 1978;42:53–58.
195. Yogev R. Central nervous system infections in the immunocompromised host. In: Patrick CC, ed. Infections in immunocompromised infants and children. New York: Churchill Livingstone, 1992:393–406.
196. Cohen ME, Duffner PK. Tumors of the brain and spinal cord including leukemic involvement. In: Swaiman KF, ed. Pediatric neurology: principles and practice. St. Louis: Mosby-Year Book, Inc., 1994:887–950.
197. Pimentel L. Medical complications of oncologic disease. Emerg Med Clin North Am 1993;11:407–419.
198. Byrne TN. Spinal cord compression from epidural metastases. N Engl J Med 1992;327:614–619.
199. Green DM, D'Angio GJ, Beckwith JB, et al. Wilms' Tumor (Nephroblastoma, Renal Embryoma). In: Pizzo PA, Poplack DG, eds. Principles and practice of pediatric oncology. Philadelphia: J. B. Lippincott, 1993: 713–737.
200. Garnick MB, Mayer RJ. Management of acute renal failure associated with neoplastic disease. In: Yarbro JW, Bornstein RS, eds. Oncologic emergencies. New York: Grune & Stratton, 1981: 247.
201. Kaplan BS, Gault MH, Knaack J. Nephropathy as a consequence of neoplasms or their treatment. In: Klastersky J, Staquet MJ, eds. Medical complications in cancer patients. New York: Raven Press, 1981:175.
202. Ries F. Nephrotoxicity of chemotherapy. Eur J Cancer Clin Oncol 1988;24:951–3.
203. Skinner R, Pearson AD, Coulthard MG, et al. Assessment of chemotherapy-associated nephrotoxicity in children with cancer. Cancer Chemother Pharmacol 1991;28:81–92.
204. Dewit L. Radiation injury in the human kidney: a prospective analysis using specific scintigraphic and biochemical endpoints. Int J Radiat Oncol Biol Phys 1990;19:977–983.
205. Appel GB, Neu HC. The nephrotoxicity of antimicrobial agents. I. N Engl J Med 1977;296:663.
206. Appel GB, Neu HC. The nephrotoxicity of antimicrobial agents. II. N Engl J Med 1977;296:722.
207. Appel GB, Neu HC. The nephrotoxicity of antimicrobial agents. III. N Engl J Med 1977;296:784.
208. Arrambide K, Toto RD. Tumor lysis syndrome. Semin Nephrol 1993;13:273–280.
209. Lange B, D'Angio G, Ross AJ III, O'Neill JA, Jr., Packer RJ. Oncologic emergencies. In: Pizzo PA, Poplack DG, eds. Principles and practice of pediatric oncology. Philadelphia: J. B. Lippincott, 1993: 951–972.
210. Bennett WM, Muther RS, Parker RA, et al. Drug therapy in renal failure: dosing guidelines for adults. I. Antimicrobial agents, analgesics. Ann Intern Med 1980;93:62.
211. Bennett WM, Muther RS, Parker RA, et al. Drug therapy in renal failure: dosing guidelines for adults. II. Sedatives, hypnotics, and tranquilizers; cardiovascular, antihypertensive, and diuretic agents; miscellaneous agents. Ann Intern Med 1980;93:286.
212. Kopec IC, Groeger JS. Life-threatening fluid and electrolyte abnormalities associated with cancer. Crit Care Clin 1988;4:81–105.
213. Flombaum CD. Acute renal failure and dialysis in cancer patients. Crit Care Clin 1988;4:61–79.
214. Kliger AS, Lovett DH. Electrolyte abnormalities in cancer patients. In: Yarbro JW, Bornstein RS, eds. Oncologic emergencies. New York: Grune & Stratton, 1981:215.
215. Ralston SH, Gallacher SJ, Patel U, Campbell J, Boyle IT. Cancer-associated hypercalcemia: morbidity and mortality. Ann Intern Med 1990;112:499–504.
216. Voute PA, de Kraker J. Ifosfamide in pediatric oncology. Semin Oncol 1992;19:2–6.
217. Vogelzang NJ. Nephrotoxicity from chemotherapy: prevention and management. Oncology 1991;5:97–112.
218. Ortega JA, Malogolowkin MH. Epithelial and neuroectodermal tumors of the gastrointestinal, genitourinary, and gynecological tracts. In: Fernbach DJ, Vietti TJ, eds. Clinical pediatric oncology. St. Louis: Mosby-Year Book, 1991:611–626.
219. Dewar I, Lim CN, Michalyshyn B, Akabutu J. Gastrointestinal complications in patients with acute and chronic leukemia. Can J Surg 1981;24:67.
220. Stellato TA, Shenk RR. Gastrointestinal emergencies in the oncology patient. Semin Oncol 1989;16:521–531.
221. Mitchell EP, Schein PS. Gastrointestinal toxicity of chemotherapeutic agents. Semin Oncol 1982;9:52.
222. Bender RA, Hamel E, Hande KR. Plant alkaloids. In: Chabner BA, Collins JM, eds. Cancer chemotherapy: principles and practice. Philadelphia: J B Lippincott, 1990:253–275.
223. Marty M, Pouillart P, Scholl S, et al. Comparison of the 5-hydroxytryptamine$_3$ (serotonin) antagonist ondansetron (GR38032F) with high-dose metoclopramide in the control of cisplatin-induced emesis. N Engl J Med 1990;322:816–821.
224. Craft AW, Price L, Eden OB, et al. Granisetron as antiemetic therapy in children with cancer. Med Pediatr Oncol 1995;25:28–32.
225. Terrin BN, McWilliams NB, Maurer HM. Side effects of metoclopramide as an antiemetic in childhood cancer chemotherapy. J Pediatr 1984;104:38.
226. Topley JM, Benson J, Squier MV, Chessells JM. Hepatotoxicity in the treatment of acute lymphoblastic leukaemia. Med Pediatr Oncol 1979;73:393.
227. Locasiulli A, Vergani GM, Uderzo C, et al. Chronic liver disease in children with leukemia in long-term remission. Cancer 1983;52:1080.
228. Afessa B, Tefferi A, Hoagland HC, Letendre L, Peters SG. Outcome of recipients of bone marrow transplants who require intensive-care unit support. Mayo Clin Proc 1992;67:117–122.
229. Lenarsky C, Parkman R. Bone marrow transplantation for the treatment of immune deficiency states. Bone Marrow Transplant 1990;6:361–369.
230. Storb R, Etzioni R, Anasetti C, et al. Cyclophosphamide with antithymocyte globulin in preparation for allogeneic marrow transplantation in patients with aplastic anemia. Blood 1994;3:941–949.
231. Krivit W, Shapiro EG. Bone marrow transplant for storage diseases. In: Desnick RJ, ed. Treatment of Genetic Diseases. New York: Churchill-Livingstone, 1991:203–221.
232. Lucarelli G, Clift RA. Bone marrow transplantation in thalassemia. In: Forman SJ, Blume KG, Thomas ED, eds. Bone Marrow Transplantation. Boston: Blackwell Scientific Publications, 1994:829–839.
233. Johnson FL, Mentzer WC, Kalinyak KA, Sullivan KM, Abboud MR. Bone marrow transplantation for sickle cell disease. The United States experience. Amer J Ped Hematol Oncol 1994;16:22–26.
234. Yeager AM. Bone marrow transplantation in children. Pediatr Ann 1988;17:694–714.
235. Bordigoni P, Vernant JP, Souillet G, et al. Allogeneic bone marrow transplantation for children with acute lymphocytic leukemia in first remission: A cooperative study of the Groupe d'Etude de la Greffe de Moelle Osseuse. J Clin Oncol 1989;7:747–753.
236. Barrett AJ, Horowitz MM, Ash RC, et al. Bone marrow transplantation

for Philadelphia chromosome-positive acute lymphocytic leukemia. Blood 1992;79:3067–3070.
237. Yeager AM, Kaizer H, Santos GW, et al. Autologous bone marrow transplantation in patients with acute nonlymphocytic leukemia, using ex vivo marrow treatment with 4-hydroperoxycyclophosphamide. N Engl J Med 1986;315:141–147.
238. Yeager AM, Rowley SD, Kaizer H, Santos GW. Ex vivo chemopurging of autologous bone marrow with 4-hydroperoxycyclophosphamide to eliminate occult leukemic cells: laboratory and clinical observations. Am J Pediatr Hematol Oncol 1990;12:245–256.
239. Weaver CH, Petersen FP, Appelbaum FR, et al. High-dose fractionated total body irradiation, etoposide, and cyclophosphamide followed by autologous stem-cell support in patients with malignant lymphoma. J Clin Oncol 1994;12:2559–2566.
240. Graham-Pole J, Casper J, Elfenbein G, et al. High-dose chemoradiation supported by marrow infusions for advanced neuroblastoma: a Pediatric Oncology Group study. J Clin Oncol 1991;9:152–158.
241. Burdach S, Jurgens H, Peters C, et al. Myeloablative radiochemotherapy and hematopoietic stem-cell rescue in poor-prognosis Ewing's sarcoma. J Clin Oncol 1993;11:1482–1488.
242. Vogelsang GB, Wagner JE. Graft-versus-host disease. Hematol Oncol Clin North Amer 1990;4:625–639.
243. Noel DR, Witherspoon RP, Storb R, et al. Does graft-versus-host disease influence the tempo of immunologic recovery after allogeneic human marrow transplantation? An observation on 56 long-term survivors. Blood 1978;51:1087–1105.
244. Beschorner WE, Yardley JH, Tutschka PJ, Santos GW. Deficiency of intestinal immunity with graft-vs-host disease in humans. J Infect Dis 1981;144:38–46.
245. Chao NJ, Schmidt GM, Niland JC, et al. Cyclosporine, methotrexate, and prednisone compared with cyclosporine and prednisone for prophylaxis of acute graft-versus-host disease. New Engl J Med 1993;329:1225–1230.
246. Nash RA, Pepe MS, Storb R, et al. Acute graft-versus-host disease: analysis of risk factors after allogeneic marrow transplantation and prophylaxis with cyclosporine and methotrexate. Blood 1992;80:1838–1845.
247. Myers BD, Ross J, Newton L, Luetscher J, Perloth M. Cyclosporin-associated chronic nephropathy. N Engl J Med 1984;311:699–705.
248. Santos GW, Tutschka PJ, Brookmeyer R, et al. Cyclosporine plus methylprednisolone versus cyclophosphamide plus methylprednisolone as prophylaxis for graft-versus-host disease: a randomized double blind study in patients undergoing allogeneic marrow transplantation. Clin Transplant 1987;1:21–28.
249. Winston DJ, Gale RP, Meyer DV, Young LS. Infectious complications of human bone marrow transplantation. Medicine 1979;58:1–31.
250. Young LS. An overview of infection in bone marrow transplant recipients. Clin Haematol 1984;13:661.
251. Betts RF. Cytomegalovirus infection in transplant patients. Prog Med Virol 1982;28:44–64.
252. Hersman J, Meyers JE, Thomas ED, Buckner CD, Clift R. The effect of granulocyte transfusions on the incidence of cytomegalovirus infection after allogeneic marrow transplantation. Ann Intern Med 1982; 9:149–152.
253. Holler E, Kolb HJ, Möller A, et al. Increased serum levels of tumor necrosis factor- precede major complications of bone marrow transplantation. Blood 1990;75:1011–1016.
254. Holland HK, Wingard JR, Beschorner WE. Bronchiolitis obliterans in bone marrow transplantation and its relationship to chronic graft-v-host disease and low serum IgG. Blood 1988;72:621–627.
255. McDonald GB, Sharma P, Matthew DE, Shulman HM, Thomas ED. Venoocclusive disease of the liver after bone marrow transplantation: diagnosis, incidence, and predisposing factors. Hepatology 1984;4: 116–122.
256. McDonald GB, Hinds MS, Fisher LD, et al. Veno-occlusive disease of the liver and multi-organ failure after bone marrow transplantation: a cohort study of 355 patients. Ann Int Med 1993;118:255–267.
257. Shulman HM, Gown AM, Nugent DJ. Hepatic venoocclusive disease after bone marrow transplantation. Immunohistochemical identification of the material within occluded central venule. Am J Pathol 1987;127:549–558.
258. Attal M, Huguet F, Rubie H, et al. Prevention of hepatic veno-occlusive disease after bone marrow transplantation by continuous infusion of low-dose heparin: a prospective, randomized trial. Blood 1992; 79:2834–2840.
259. Bearman SI, Hinds MS, Wolford JL, et al. A pilot study of continuous infusion heparin for the prevention of hepatic venoocclusive disease after bone marrow transplantation. Bone Marrow Transplant 1990;5:407–411.
260. Bearman SI, Shuhart MC, Hinds MS, McDonald GB. Recombinant human tissue plasminogen activator for the treatment of established severe hepatic venoocclusive disease of the liver after bone marrow transplantation. Blood 1992;80:2458–2462.
261. Jones RJ, Lee KSK, Beschorner WE, et al. Venoocclusive disease of the liver following bone marrow transplantation. Transplantation 1987;44:778–783.
262. Cassano WF, Eskenazi AE, Frantz CN. Therapy for childhood acute lymphoblastic leukemia. Curr Opin Oncol 1993;5:42–52.
263. Pui C-H, Crist WM. Biology and treatment of acute lymphoblastic leukemia. J Pediatr 1994;124:491–503.
264. Kurtzberg J, Graham ML. Non-Hodgkin's lymphoma. Biologic classification and implication for therapy. Pediatr Clin North Am 1991;38:443–56.
265. Donaldson SS, Link MP. Hodgkin's disease. Treatment of the young child. Pediatr Clin of North Am 1991;38:457–73.
266. White L, Siegel SE, Quah TC. Non-Hodgkin's lymphomas in children. I. Patterns of disease and classification. Crit Rev Oncol Hematol 1992;13:55–71.
267. White L, Siegel SE, Quah TC. Non-Hodgkin's lymphomas in children. II. Treatment. Crit Rev Oncol Hematol 1992;13:73–89.
268. Prosnitz LR, Kapp DS, Weissberg JB. Radiotherapy. I. N Engl J Med 1983;309:771.
269. Prosnitz LR, Kapp DS, Weissberg JB. Radiotherapy. II. N Engl J Med 1983;309:834.
270. Mandell LR, Wharam MD, Jr. Radiotherapy. In: Fernbach DJ, Vietti TJ, eds. Clinical pediatric oncology. St. Louis: Mosby-Year Book, 1991: 155–172.
271. Chabner BA, Collins JM. Cancer chemotherapy: principles and practice. Philadelphia: J. B. Lippincott, 1990.
272. Liu LF. DNA topoisomerase poisons as antitumor drugs. Ann Rev Biochem 1989;58:351–375.

Surgical and Anesthetic Considerations

Section Nine

Section Editor

William J. Greeley

Multiple Trauma in the Pediatric Patient 43

Joseph D. Tobias
Gail E. Rasmussen
Myron Yaster

INTRODUCTION

Multisystem trauma accounts for 50% of deaths occurring in children more than 1 year of age with nearly 23,000 lives lost per year. This compares with the adult population in which only 15% of deaths are traumatic in origin (150,000 deaths per year)[1–4]. An even greater issue is that for every pediatric patient that dies as a result of trauma, there are four survivors who are permanently disabled (approximately 100,000 per year).

Following trauma, the likelihood of death and the degree and duration of disability are influenced by both the promptness and the quality of emergency care received by the patient. In Maryland, since 1977, children less than 15 years of age have been preferentially transported to the state-wide regional pediatric trauma center at Johns Hopkins Hospital. This center is one component of the Maryland Institute for Emergency Medical Services Systems that is outlined in Figure 43.1. The system provides for initial evaluation and emergency care at the scene; communication via radio directly with the trauma or burn center; and subsequent transport by helicopter or ambulance to the definitive care facility for adult trauma, pediatric trauma, burns, hand injuries, or neonatal emergencies[5]. Such a system has substantially improved the outcome and prognosis

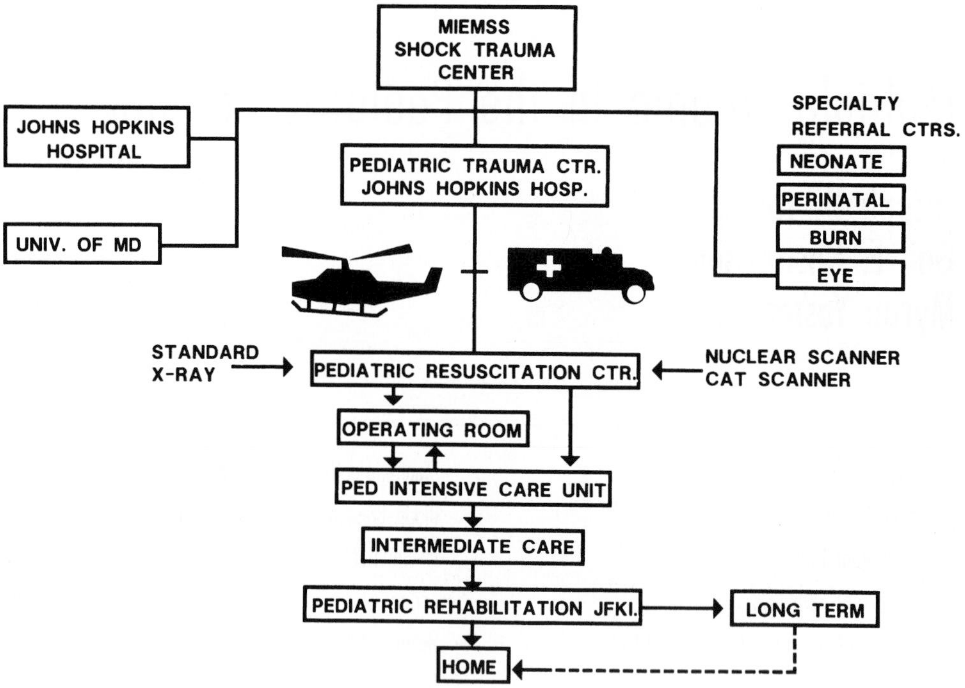

Figure 43.1. Organizational outline of the Maryland Institute for Emergency Medical Services Systems (MIEMSS) is shown. This system provides for emergency care and evaluation in the field followed by air or ground transportation to definitive care facilities. Within the pediatric resuscitation center, facilities exist for the initial assessment, resuscitation, and diagnosis of the injury as well as for definitive immediate and long-term care.

of the injured pediatric patient in Maryland. Mortality has been reduced to 7% of all patients who arrive in the emergency room, regardless of the severity or number of organ systems injured[5,6]. Additionally, because of close affiliation with The John F. Kennedy Institute for the Developmentally Handicapped, patients are evaluated and treated by various rehabilitative services almost immediately. This procedure may further minimize the consequences of serious injury and allow for the prompt institution of rehabilitative services.

This chapter will explore the pathophysiology that occurs following trauma and discuss a management scheme for the injured pediatric patient. This will be followed by a review of major organ system failure as it pertains to the care of the pediatric trauma patient. Obviously, multiple trauma may impact on every organ system. The reader is referred to other chapters in this book that discuss specific organ injuries in greater detail.

PATHOPHYSIOLOGY

Regardless of whether trauma results from an uncontrollable injury such as a motor vehicle accident or an intentional injury such as child abuse, a series of reflex responses are initiated in an attempt to maintain the body's internal milieu. Both neurally and humorally mediated reflexes occur to maintain effective circulatory volume and vital organ perfusion. Although these responses are essential for the immediate maintenance of blood pressure, cardiac output, and organ perfusion with short-term survival of the victim, the continued response may have significant detrimental physiologic effects that must be controlled to improve the chances of long term survival.

The physiologic derangements that occur as a result of multiple trauma activate several different afferent and efferent pathways (Figs. 43.2 and 43.3). The afferent pathways include input as a result of changes in effective circulating blood volume, central anticipation of pain or danger, and nociceptive input from the site of injury. The efferent limb of the reflex arc includes a neurohumoral response modulated by the pituitary and its hormones as well as neurally mediated responses via the autonomic nervous system. The latter may act either directly on vascular tone or indirectly through the release of endogenous catecholamines from the adrenal medulla. Additionally, the kidney responds to changes in perfusion pressure, serum osmolarity, and serum sodium concentrations to maximize fluid and sodium conservation to attempt to restore effective circulating volume.

Afferent Limb

The status of blood volume, cardiac filling pressures, and arterial blood pressure are continuously relayed to the brainstem via baroreceptors in the carotid sinus, aortic arch, and at the venoatrial junctions of the right and left atria[7–10] (Fig.43.2). These baroreceptors are specialized, slowly adapting stretch receptors, which reflect the degree of stretch as well as the rate of change of the stretch in vessel walls. This provides information on blood pressure and pulsatile flow. Fibers from these receptors travel via the vagus nerve and the sinus branch of the glossopharyngeal nerve to the region of the solitary nucleus in the medulla. These receptors exert a tonic inhibition on the cardiovascular center of the medulla resulting in the inhibition of sympathetic efferents to the heart and blood vessels[11]. When hemorrhage or extravascular sequestration of extracellular fluid at the site of injury results in a decrease in effective circulating blood volume, this is detected by the baroreceptors, resulting in the release of the medullary cardiovascular center from baroreceptor inhibition. This results in an increase in the efferent activity and sympathetic stimulation.

An additional component of the afferent limb is conducted by nociceptive pathways (Fig. 43.2). Tissue injury and local ischemia lead to the accumulation of anaerobic metabolites and the production of a diverse group of chemicals that includes kinins, histamine, serotonin, prostaglandins, and leukotrienes; all of which stimulate the nociceptive receptors[12] and cause profound systemic effects.

The above described chemicals stimulate the free nerve endings of first order neurons that transmit pain from the periphery to the spinal cord. Pain is conducted to the spinal cord by small myelinated (A delta) and unmyelinated (C) sensory fibers whose cell bodies are located in the dorsal root ganglia[13]. The axons of the first order neurons exit the dorsal root ganglia and travel rostrally and caudally in Lissauer's tract prior to synapsing with second order neurons in the dorsal horn of the spinal cord. Complex interactions occur within the dorsal horn of the spinal cord in the substantia gelatinosa thus modulating the nociceptive input. The integrated information then travels via the lateral spinothalamic (neospinothalamic) tract and the spinoreticulo-diencephalic (paleospinothalamic) tract[14,15]. The lateral spinothalamic tract synapses at the level of the thalamus with third order neurons that project to the sensory cortex allowing the perception and localization of pain. The spinoreticulo-diencephalic tract projects into the reticular activating system at the medulla, pons, and mesencephalon, and then terminates in the intralaminar nuclei of the thalamus and hypothalamus. These connections to the brainstem provide much of the afferent input for the reflex activity that occurs following trauma.

A final level of integration occurs within the thalamocortical projections. Neurotransmitters and neuromodulators act at many points along these pathways either to enhance or to inhibit the transmission of the nociceptive input. Modulation of pain transmission by endogenous endorphins explains the production of analgesia by brainstem stimulation as well as the analgesia produced by opioid agonists such as morphine[16,17]. Electrical stimulation of the periaqueductal-periventricular regions activates a descending inhibitory pathway that blunts nociceptive input at the spinal cord level. This descending pathway is also controlled via opioid receptors and opioid agonists such as morphine produce some analgesia through this pathway.

Efferent Pathways

In response to the afferent stimuli discussed above, profound responses occur via the efferent limb of the reflex arc. These responses are mediated through the autonomic nervous system (both parasympathetic and sympathetic outflow tracts) and the neuroendocrine system (hypothalamus-pituitary-peripheral hormones) as seen in Figure 43.3.

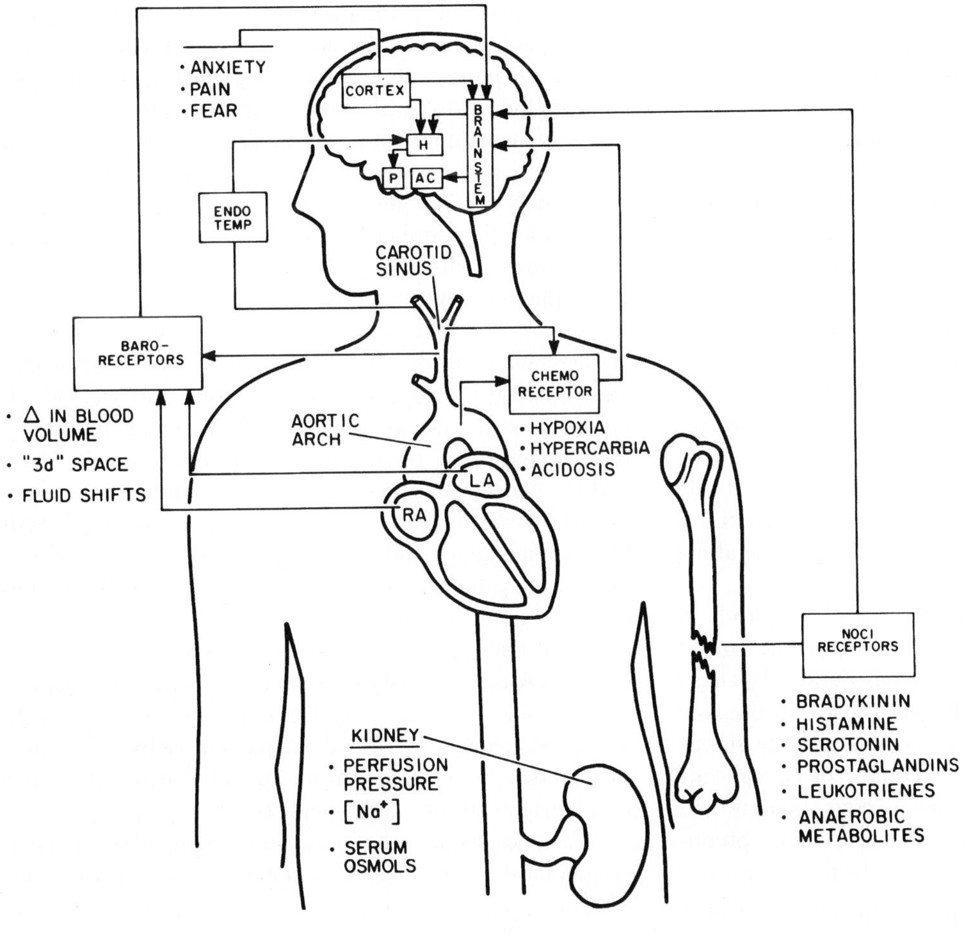

Figure 43.2. Neural and humoral afferent pathways that are activated following injury. These pathways are stimulated to protect and conserve the effective circulating blood volume and maintain adequate perfusion to the vital organs. Blood temperature, tissue metabolites, endotoxin *(ENDO)*, serum sodium *($[Na^+]$)*, and serum osmolarity may also be involved in these afferent pathways. The input is integrated in the brainstem, hypothalamus *(H)*, pituitary *(P)*, autonomic centers *(AC)*, and the kidney.

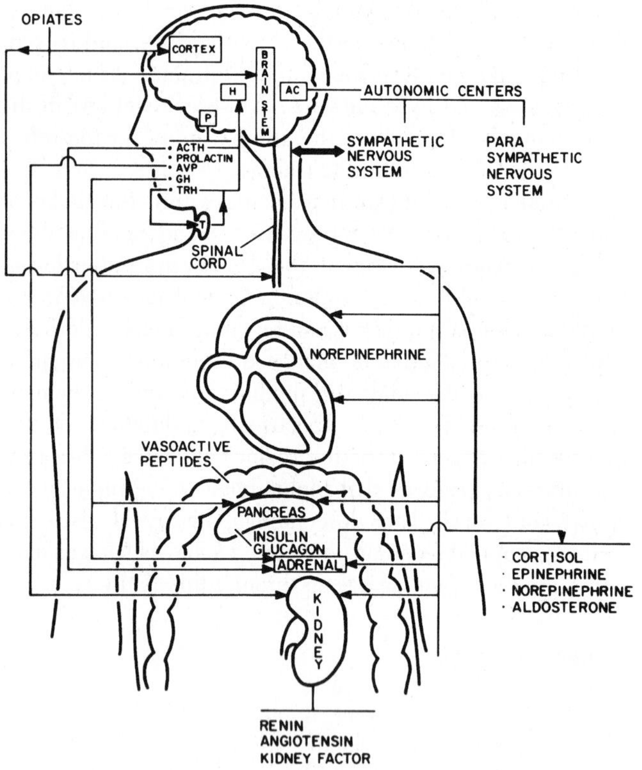

Figure 43.3. Efferent humoral and neural pathways that act to support intravascular volume and maintain perfusion to the vital organs following trauma. Abbreviations: *H* hypothalamus; *P* pituitary; *AC* autonomic centers; *T* thyroid gland; *AVP* arginine vasopressin; *GH* growth hormone; *TSH* thyroid-stimulating hormone.

The sympathetic nervous system innervates effector cells throughout the body. As they transverse the sympathetic chain, each preganglionic cell synapses on multiple postganglionic neurons in several different ganglia. In this fashion, an amplification and a diffuse discharge of the sympathetic system is possible. Firing of the ganglionic neurons (of which the chromaffin cells of the adrenal medulla can be considered) results in activation of the four different adrenergic receptors: $beta_1$, $beta_2$, $alpha_1$, and $alpha_2$[18]. Catecholamines can cause either excitation or inhibition of smooth muscle contraction, depending on the site, the dose, and the catecholamine present. Norepinephrine, for example, which is the principal endogenous catecholamine released by the adrenergic ganglion cells, is primarily an alpha and beta1 agonist and therefore causes smooth muscle contraction or vasoconstriction. Epinephrine, which is released from the adrenal medulla, stimulates both the alpha and $beta_{1,2}$ receptors.

Stimulation of the sympathetic nervous system leads to increased cardiac contractility[19], reduction in the size of the veins[20], and selective arteriolar constriction[21]. These effects serve to support arterial blood pressure in the face of a reduction in blood volume. Direct sympathetic stimulation and effects mediated via the release of endogenous catecholamines lead to an increase in both inotropy and chronotropy of cardiac muscle and pacemaker cells. Stimulation of the vascular smooth muscle results in vasoconstriction of the capacitance and resistance vessels. The increased sympathetic activity effects both the precapillary and the postcapillary sphincters. Precapillary constriction decreases capillary pressure and promotes fluid flux into the circulation while postcapillary constriction has the reverse effect. Following hemorrhage or injury, sympathetic activity favors precapillary vasoconstriction[22–24], which results in decreased capillary perfusion pressure and promotes the movement of protein-free fluid from the extracellular space into the capillaries. This results in a temporary restoration of circulating blood volume[25].

The second phase of reflex volume restitution occurs from an increase in extracellular fluid caused by a shift of fluid from the intracellular space to the interstitium. This latter effect is mediated by an increase in extracellular osmolality[8,26]. Following hemorrhage in humans[27] and in animals[28], the rise in osmolality is directly related to the plasma glucose concentration. However, this glucose-induced rise in osmolality is also dependent on the victim's nutritional state and the extent of hemorrhage[29].

With major blood loss and decrease in blood flow, the resultant hypoxia, ischemia, and acidosis result in a loss of tone of the precapillary sphincters with little or no effect on the postcapillary sphincters. The persistence of postcapillary contraction and precapillary relaxation results in increased capillary hydrostatic pressure that favors fluid movement from the vascular space into the interstitium. This results in the movement of fluid from the vascular space into the interstitium or the so-called "third space". The magnitude of third space loss is related to the extent of tissue injury and to the amount of blood loss.

Catecholamines also produce significant metabolic effects including hyperglycemia, hyperlipidemia, increased oxygen consumption, and hyperkalemia[30]. Beta adrenergic receptor stimulation results in hepatic glucose release via glycogenolysis and gluconeogenesis from lactate via the Cori cycle. In peripheral tissue, stimulation increases lipolysis in fat cells and glycogenolysis with decreased glucose uptake by muscle cells. Alpha adrenergic stimulation reduces insulin and glucagon secretion. The overall effect of catecholamines on the islet cells is to increase glucagon and decrease insulin secretion[18,30]. Both the sympathetic nervous system and the adrenal medulla are responsible for the hyperglycemic response following injury, which is crucial for the second phase of volume restitution[31,32]. Antidiuretic hormone, the release of which is stimulated directly by catecholamines and indirectly related to decreased cardiac filling volumes, further increases volume restitution by decreasing free water excretion[33].

Unfortunately, the prolonged elevation of blood glucose levels promotes catabolism, increased oxygen consumption, and an "energy crisis" that has many detrimental effects. The persistence of increased sympathetic activity and neuroendocrine tone changes from an initial beneficial effect to a detrimental effect if it persists.

While the changes that occur in the sympathetic nervous system have been categorized in adults, the magnitude and results of sympathetic stimulation are less well characterized during childhood. The functional integrity of the autonomic nervous system is unclear during early life. Autonomic responses are present but diminished in the newborn. In several species, the neonatal heart has reduced stores of catecholamine and incompletely developed neural connections suggesting a decreased ability to respond to direct sympathetic stimulation as well as to circulating catecholamines[34,35]. Thus, in newborns the baroreceptor response to volume change may be attenuated and their ability to respond to changes in circulating blood volume may be compromised[36].

Corticotropin-Releasing Factor—ACTH—Cortisol

Gann[8] and Pirkle and Gann[37,38] demonstrated that an elevation of plasma cortisol is essential to produce the increase in extracellular osmolality following hemorrhage which in turn is crucial in the movement of fluid from the intracellular space into the interstitium during the second phase of blood volume restitution. Dogs fasted following adrenalectomy and given basal cortisol replacement failed to exhibit an increase in osmolality following hemorrhage. Conversely, dogs subjected to adrenalectomy and given replacement cortisol at levels designed to mimic a physiologic response to hemorrhage showed an appropriate increase in osmolality.

Cortisol release is under neural control and if impulses from the injured area are prevented from reaching the central nervous system, cortisol release and other neuroendocrine responses do not occur[38,39]. In response to certain stimuli (injury, cold, stress), corticotropin-releasing factor (CRF) is released at neuronal endings in the median eminence of the hypothalamus and transported via the hypophyseal-portal vessels to the adenohypophysis where it stimulates secretion of adrenocorticotropic hormone (ACTH). ACTH acts in the adrenal cortex via specific receptors to activate adenylate cyclase and convert adenosine triphosphate (ATP) to cyclic adenosine monophosphate (cAMP). The increased intracellular concentration of cAMP activates specific protein kinases and promotes the production and release of both cortisol and aldosterone. The secretion of cortisol is subject to both negative and positive feedback control[40,41].

The mechanism(s) by which cortisol increases serum osmolality are not completely clear. It is known that cortisol stimulates gluconeogenesis, diminishes the peripheral utilization of glucose, and promotes protein catabolism and lipolysis. Glucocorticoids also inhibit the action of insulin and potentiate the effects of epinephrine and glucagon on glucose production[40,41].

Insulin-Glucagon

Insulin and glucagon are produced in the islets of Langerhans in the pancreas (Fig. 43.3)[42]. Insulin is produced in the beta cell whereas glucagon is produced in the alpha cell. The role of insulin is to promote the storage of all fuels while glucagon serves as a hormone of fuel mobilization. Insulin is essential for the transport of glucose across cell membranes; it promotes glycogen, fat, and protein synthesis, and inhibits protein degradation. Glucagon, on the other hand, promotes glycogenolysis, gluconeogenesis, and hepatic lipolysis. As mentioned previously, injury leads to suppression of insulin secretion via an alpha adrenergic-mediated response that is potentiated by glucocorticoids[43]. The net effect is an increase in serum glucose and substrate mobilization that increases serum osmolality and helps restore blood volume. In addition to its hormonal/metabolic effects, glucagon has positive inotropic and chronotropic activity. Unfortunately, its use as a therapeutic agent has so far been limited.

Antidiuretic Hormone (ADH)

The two principal physiologic stimuli for the secretion of antidiuretic hormone (ADH), also referred to as arginine vasopressin, are an increase in plasma osmolality or a decrease in extracellular fluid volume[44]. Vasopressin acts on the cells of the renal collecting system to increase permeability to free water[45]. It does this through a reflex loop that originates in the low-pressure baroreceptors located in the atria. The catecholamines also play a role in the pathway that mediates the osmotic and non-osmotic release of ADH[46]. The effect is dependent on which receptor is stimulated. Beta adrenergic stimulation decreases diuresis while alpha adrenergic stimulation promotes diuresis. The role of ADH following trauma is to conserve water and restore intravascular volume. Unfortunately, ADH secretion whether appropriate or inappropriate can lead to dilutional hyponatremia, low urine output, and the potential for the exacerbation of cerebral edema especially in the setting of closed head injury.

In addition to its effects on water homeostasis, ADH has direct effects on the contractile elements of smooth muscle. Generalized vasoconstriction occurs in the smooth muscle of the vasculature with an elevation of the mean arterial pressure. The vasoconstriction may not be beneficial since perfusion to the skin and gastrointestinal tract may be markedly reduced[47]. ADH has also been shown to play some role in the regulation of ACTH production[8,44].

Renin-Angiotensin-Aldosterone

The most potent of the humoral systems that is activated in shock is the renin-angiotensin-aldosterone system. The kidney and juxtaglomerular apparatus of the afferent arterioles perceive the low perfusion pressure, changes in serum sodium concentration/osmolarity, and changes in chloride concentration in the renal tubules[47]. A reflex response is initiated to promote salt and water conservation and increase intravascular volume.

Decreased renal perfusion or decreased chloride concentration of the fluid in the renal tubules promotes renin release by the juxtaglomerular cells. Renin release is mediated by both adrenergic and dopaminergic receptor stimulation as well as by a decrease in renal arteriolar pressure[48,49]. Renin is a low-molecular-weight enzyme that cleaves a beta$_1$ globulin from angiotensinogen to form angiotensin I. Angiotensin I is converted into its active form, angiotensin II, by angiotensin-converting enzyme, which is found throughout the body, especially in the pulmonary endothelium[45]. Angiotensin II is among the most potent vasoconstrictors found in the body. In addition to its direct vasoconstrictor properties, it also has direct chronotropic and inotropic properties. In the adrenal gland, it is a major stimulus to the production of aldosterone. Aldosterone acts on the ascending loop of Henle and in the collecting ducts of the kidney to increase sodium and water absorption.

Following angiotensin release, the initial response is an increase in peripheral vascular resistance to maintain blood pressure. If other factors do not occur (i.e. volume resuscitation), the vasoconstriction which is initially beneficial to maintain perfusion pressure, can be detrimental. Prolonged vasoconstriction can lead to ischemic renal tubular necrosis and peripheral hypoperfusion and profound alterations in vascular tone. These may lead to irreversible circulatory decompensation, which may contribute to the state of irreversible shock[50]. This is the physiologic basis for the suggested use of the angiotensin converting enzyme inhibitor, captopril, in shock[50]. Once again, the beneficial and at times life saving effects of the initial response may prove to be detrimental if they persist.

Opioid Peptides

The endogenous opioid peptides are important in normal and abnormal behavior, hormonal release, analgesia, thermoregulation, and control of respiratory function[51]. Endogenous opioids such as beta endorphin potentiate the release of many hormones including growth hormone, ADH, and ACTH[51]. Because endorphins are released by stress and exogenous opiates can cause hypotension, it has been hypothesized that the endogenous opioids contribute to the hypotension of shock. Based on this, it has been suggested that opioid receptor antagonism may be a useful therapeutic modality[52,53]. Although pharmacologic manipulation of the endogenous opioid system may hold great promise, many problems exist since antagonists such as naloxone augment traumatic pain.

INITIAL ASSESSMENT OF THE CHILD WITH LIFE-THREATING MULTIPLE ORGAN INJURIES

The successful initial management of the critically injured pediatric, multiple trauma patient depends on the expertise of physicians and emergency medical personnel and a systematic approach to trauma resuscitation management (Fig.43.4). Regardless of the situation, age of the patient, or circumstances surrounding the injury, within the first 60

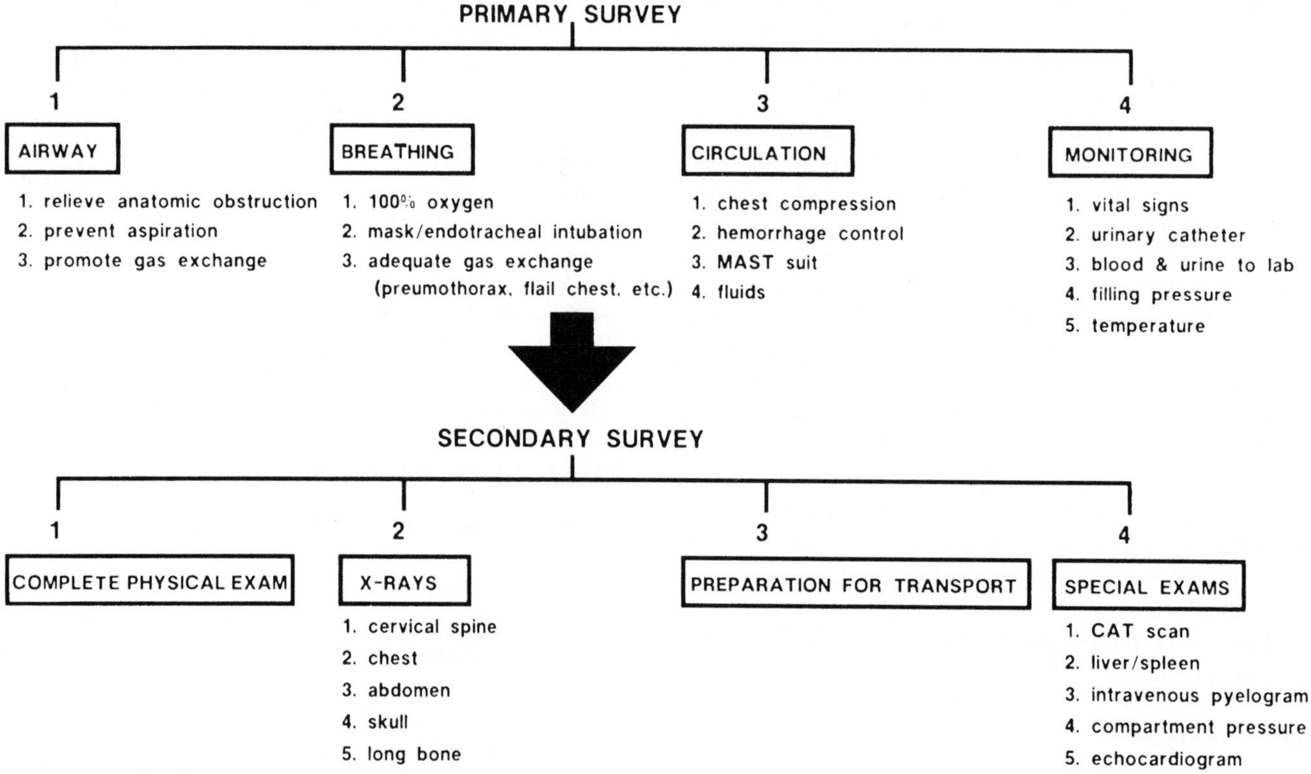

Figure 43.4. Protocol for the resuscitation, assessment, and diagnosis of the pediatric trauma patient. The approach to the patient is composed of a primary and secondary survey. The primary survey consists of the evaluation for life-threatening injuries and the initial resuscitation. This is followed by the secondary survey consisting of a complete physical examination, radiographic imaging/diagnostic studies, and preparation for transport.

seconds of the victim's presentation, one must assess the airway and cardiorespiratory function. There are several important questions:

1. Is the airway patent?
2. Is the patient breathing?
3. Are the respiratory efforts adequate?
4. Is stridor or cyanosis present?
5. Are breath sounds symmetrical?
6. Is the trachea in the midline?
7. Is there circulatory collapse?
8. Is there control of hemorrhage?
9. Is the patient conscious?

The first 20 to 30 minutes of evaluation and resuscitation will be a primary factor in most cases, of determining both whether the patient will survive and with what sort of sequelae. This time is divided into a primary survey with initial resuscitation and stabilization followed by a secondary survey which consists of a complete examination from head-to-toe and definitive care. The latter usually occurs in the pediatric ICU environment. The definitive care of a seriously ill child may require special facilities and specialists. Every institution should have a protocol for patient transfer following the initial resuscitation and stabilization. The latter may include control of the airway and resuscitation of the circulation.

Primary Survey

Airway

All else will fail and be futile if the first step of trauma management, airway control, is ineffective. The physician faced with the trauma patient must recognize that airway management in this setting is somewhat different from the non-trauma setting. The "A" of the ABC's of rescuscitation should be thought of as standing for airway and cervical spine stabilization. The three goals of airway management are: to relieve anatomic obstruction, to prevent the aspiration of gastric contents, and to promote adequate gas exchange. (A more complete discussion of airway management is given in Chapter 2). Supplemental oxygen by facemask is recommended for all trauma patients until the primary survey is completed.

Several factors predispose the trauma patient, especially children, to airway obstruction. Airway obstruction most commonly occurs because the tongue and/or pharyngeal soft tissues collapse into the airway. This is particularly true following injuries in which consciousness is lost either due to closed head injury or cardiovascular compromise with inadequate cerebral perfusion. In children, several factors increase the likelihood of anatomical obstruction of the upper airway. The proportionally larger head compared to the rest of the body promotes neck flexion and the oral cavity is relatively small while the tongue is relatively large. Simple measures to relieve anatomical obstruction include: proper positioning of the head, specifically avoidance of neck flexion; anterior displacement of the mandible (jaw thrust maneuver); or placement of an appropriately sized oral airway. These latter two are best avoided in combative or semiconscious patients because they may be poorly tolerated and sometimes lead to retching and vomiting. Of the three maneuvers to open a patient's airway (head tilt, jaw thrust, and chin lift), only the latter two are appropriate for the trauma patient. The head tilt is avoided because of the possibility of associated cervical spine injury. While soft tissue relaxation may be responsible for airway obstruction, the airway may also be blocked by a foreign body (vomitus, blood, gum, candy), severe maxillofacial injury, or injuries to the larynx and/or chest, which may lead to airway disruption or compression.

After relieving anatomical airway obstruction, one must assess the patient's state of consciousness and laryngeal reflexes. The absence or diminution of laryngeal reflexes may predispose to aspiration. All victims of trauma should be considered to have a full stomach, and to be at risk for pulmonary aspiration of gastric contents. This is the case regardless of when the victim last ate. Gastric emptying is delayed significantly by trauma, pain and fear[54].

Following major trauma, gas exchange may be compromised. Arterial hypoxemia is common and can be caused by airway obstruction (see above) or hypoventilation. The latter may be the result of central nervous system injury, increased abdominal pressure, an unstable chest wall, lung injury (pulmonary contusion, aspiration, barotrauma), or cardiovascular instability (direct myocardial injury, tamponade, hemorrhagic shock). Endotracheal intubation allows the delivery of high concentrations of oxygen, the use of positive end-expiratory pressure, internal stabilization of a flail chest, control of ventilation, as well as airway protection from aspiration. Other patients that may require urgent endotracheal intubation are those who have burns of the face and neck, are hemodynamically unstable, require sedation for diagnostic studies, or have a serious CNS injury.

Decisions regarding endotracheal intubation include the route (oral versus nasal) and awake versus anesthetized. The preferred route for endotracheal intubation in the pediatric trauma patient in all initial situations is oral[55]. Attempts at nasal intubation often lead to bleeding which can obstruct visualization and make further attempts impossible. Further problems may include gagging and vomiting or outright failure. Additionally, awake nasal intubation can lead to significant increases in intracranial pressure and is absolutely contraindicated in that setting. Nasal intubation is also contraindicated in patients with evidence of facial trauma, CSF leaks, or suggestion of basilar skull fracture (i.e Battle's sign, raccoon eyes, hemotympanum). There are reports of nasogastric tubes being advanced through fractures in the cribiform plate into the cranial vault and it is suspected that this could occur with an endotracheal tube.

Advocates of the nasal route suggest its use (i.e., blind nasal intubation) in the patient with suspected cervical spine injury as a means of limiting neck movement. However, significant degrees of cervical spine movement occur with nasal intubation and, to date, no studies have demonstrated a benefit of nasal versus oral intubation in patients with cervical spine trauma[(56,57)]. In fact, an increased incidence of adverse effects has been reported with nasal as compared to oral intubation.

Whenever intubation is necessary, preparation is an absolute requirement to ensure that it is accomplished in an expedient manner. Equipment should include an Ambu bag and oxygen source (it is important to always ensure that the oxygen flow is turned on), appropriate size masks, laryngoscope, endotracheal tubes, stylet, suction, and drugs. The appropriate equipment and drugs should be prepared prior to the patient's arrival.

The method(s) used for tracheal intubation will be dependent on an informed judgment as to one's own intubating skills, the patient's hemodynamic status, and the assessment of the normalcy of the patient's upper airway, larynx, and trachea[(55)]. Tracheal intubation may be difficult with injuries to the airway, face, and neck or if the patient has a short neck, receding jaw, small mouth, or large tongue.

The second issue with trauma victims is that they are at risk for aspiration during intubation. Because each trauma victim is considered to have a full stomach, techniques to minimize regurgitation of stomach contents are imperative. These techniques include: cricoid pressure (i.e., Sellick's maneuver)[(58)], rapid neuromuscular blockade with induction of anesthesia (rapid sequence induction). Decompression and emptying of the stomach with an orogastric tube is controversial. In an awake patient, this may be a useful technique; however, it may induce vomiting. It is certainly not indicated in patients with altered mental status. The use of a nonparticulate antacid, such as sodium citrate, is an important adjunct; by raising gastric pH, it reduces the pulmonary consequences if gastric contents are aspirated. Aspiration of gastric contents is most detrimental when the pH is low (less than 2.5) and the volume is high (greater than 0.4 mL/kg). Again, this will be of limited utility in patients with altered mental status.

More important than emptying the stomach or the administration of an antacid is the technique and drugs used for securing the airway. The goal of a rapid sequence intubation is to secure the airway while protecting the lungs from acid aspiration. Cricoid pressure[(58)] is a technique that prevents the passive regurgitation of stomach contents from entering the pharynx. The upper esophagus is compressed against the cervical vertebral column by applying anteroposterior pressure on the cricoid cartilage. The cricoid cartilage is the only complete ring of the trachea and can be used to occlude the esophagus without occluding the airway. Cricoid pressure is maintained until proper placement of the endotracheal tube is confirmed or until the patient fully reawakens if intubation is unsuccessful.

The second key to a successful intubation is the use of rapidly acting neuromuscular blocking agents. With rapid neuromuscular blockade and anesthesia, the possibility of vomiting at the time of intubation is also reduced. It also provides ideal conditions for tracheal intubation. Rapid sequence induction of anesthesia and paralysis should always be preceded by the administration of 100% oxygen via a tight-fitting face mask. Often imprecisely called preoxygenation, the purpose of 100% oxygen is to denitrogenate the lungs. With full denitrogenation, the typical adult can sustain approximately 4 minutes of apnea without hypoxia. However, infants may only tolerate 30 seconds of apnea, even if fully denitrogenated, because the infant's functional residual capacity is relatively smaller while oxygen consumption is larger than that of the adult. Denitrogenation is accomplished by 3 to 5 minutes of tidal breathing. If the need for endotracheal intubation is more emergent, another alternative that is equally as effective is 5 to 8 vital capacity breaths of 100% oxygen[(59)]. The use of a pulse oximeter during endotracheal intubation provides an added margin of safety and alerts the physician performing the intubation when the attempt should be aborted and bag-mask ventilation started.

Normal Airway

If the airway is normal, one may proceed with the use of neuromuscular blocking agents and sedative/analgesic agents for endotracheal intubation **(Tables 43.1 and 43.2).** Care must to taken to avoid exacerbating a cervical spine injury. As intubation is frequently performed prior to obtaining appropriate x-rays to rule out an injury, a technique must be used to avoid cervical spine injury. This can be accomplished by the application of manual in-line axial traction (Fig. 43.5). The choice of neuromuscular blocking agent includes either a depolarizing agent such as succinylcholine or a non-depolarizing agent (pancuronium, vecuronium). The advantages of succinylcholine include a rapid onset of action (30 to 45 seconds) and a short duration of action (4 to 5 minutes). The latter may be particularly important in patients with head trauma or suspected cervical spine injury so that immediate reassessment of their clinical status is possible. Rapid neuromuscular blockade is most commonly achieved with the depolarizing muscle relaxant succinylcholine (2 mg/kg). Succinylcholine has been considered contraindicated in patients with open globe injuries since the contraction of the extraocular muscles may lead to the expulsion of the vitreous[(60)]. Ex-

Table 43.1. Contraindications to Succinylcholine

1. Hyperkalemia
2. Muscular dystrophies
3. Burns
4. Metabolic acidosis
5. Paraplegia/quadraplegia
6. Denervation injury
7. Metastatic rhabdomyosarcoma
8. Parkinson's disease
9. Disuse atrophy
10. Polyneuropathy
11. Degenerative CNS diseases

Table 43.2. Intubating Drugs and Doses

Neuromuscular blocking agents	
succinylcholine	2 mg/kg
pancuronium	0.15 mg/kg
vecuronium	0.1–0.3 mg/kg
rocuronium	0.6–1.2 mg/kg
Amnestic/analgesic agents	
ketamine	0.5–2 mg/kg
pentothal	2–6 mg/kg
propofol	2–3 mg/kg
etomidate	0.2–0.3 mg/kg
midazolam	0.05–0.1 mg/kg
Miscellaneous medications	
lidocaine	1–1.5 mg/kg
atropine	0.01 mg/kg
glycopyrrolate	0.005–0.01 mg/kg

tensive burns, crush injuries, and various neurologic and neuromuscular diseases remain contraindications for succinylcholine[61] **(Table 43-1).** In this setting, an exaggerated hyperkalemic response may be seen. Its use in patients with increased intracranial pressure is controversial[62,63]. While it has been demonstrated that succinylcholine may cause a modest increase in intracranial pressure, the rapid neuromuscular blockade allows endotracheal intubation to occur sooner with improvements in oxygenation and ventilation which are more important determinants of cerebral blood flow and intracranial pressure. Additional adverse effects with succinylcholine include arrhythmias and bradycardia. In the trauma setting, regardless of the age of the patient, a small dose of an anticholinergic such as atropine (5 to 10 mcg/kg up to 0.4 mg) is suggested prior to the administration of succinylcholine.

It has been suggested that a small dose of a nondepolarizing muscle relaxant (e.g. pancuronium, 0.01 mg/kg) be administered before succinylcholine to prevent the skeletal muscle fasciculations associated with the latter's use. Reasons to avoid this practice include:

1. Children less than age 6 yr do not fasciculate[64]
2. The use of nondepolarizing muscle relaxants increases the dose requirement of succinylcholine necessary for complete paralysis[65]
3. It delays the onset of paralysis[65]It can, on occasion, cause significant neuromuscular paralysis of the patient with aspiration risk and respiratory insufficiency
4. It is generally recommended that the priming dose precede succinylcholine administration by at least 3 minutes

In conditions that contraindicate the use of succinylcholine, a non-depolarizing agent may be used. Options include pancuronium, vecuronium, and most recently rocuronium. Other non-depolarizing agents such as curare and atracurium are relatively contraindicated as they may induce histamine release and induce some degree of hypotension. Pancuronium (0.15 mg/kg) as an intravenous bolus produces relatively rapid paralysis. Succinylcholine will cause complete paralysis of a patient within 30 to 45 seconds of an intravenous bolus and the resultant paralysis will last for approximately 5 min. It does not require a reversal agent to terminate its effect. Pancuronium requires 90 to 120 seconds to provide neuromuscular blockade and the paralysis will last approximately 60 to 90 minutes. Pancuronium requires reversal of its neuromuscular blockade with anticholinesterases such as neostigmine (0.07 mg/kg) or edrophonium (1.0 mg/kg) plus antimuscarinics such as atropine (0.02 mg/kg).

Alternatives to pancuronium include vecuronium and rocuronium. As vecuronium is devoid of cardiovascular side effects, increased doses can be used to speed the onset of neuromuscular blockade. While the usual intubating dose of 0.1 mg/kg may take 120 seconds to produce conditions

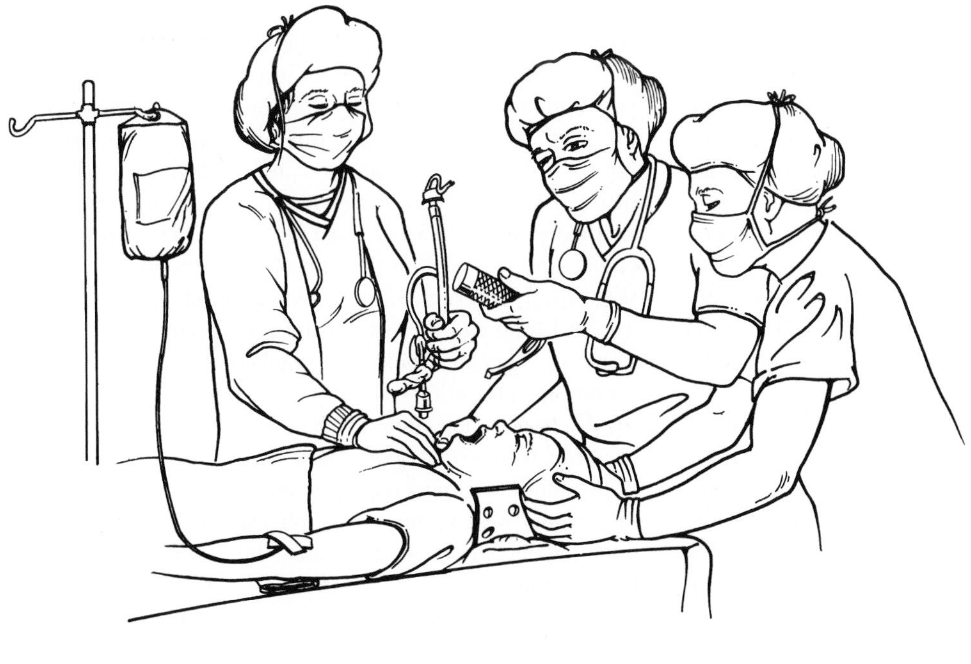

Figure 43.5. Technique for oral endotracheal intubation in the pediatric trauma patient using cricoid pressure and "manual in-line axial traction". The technique generally requires three individuals. The individual on the left is applying cricoid pressure while the individual on the right holds the patient's head in a neutral position with two hands using manual in-line traction. Prior to intubation and after in-line traction is applied, the anterior portion of cervical collar is removed.

suitable for endotracheal intubation, increasing the dose to 0.3 mg/kg will speed the onset of blockade to 60 to 90 seconds. However, with this larger dose, the duration of blockade will be 60 to 70 minutes. Priming may also be used to speed the onset of vecuronium. For this, 0.01 mg/kg is administered followed by the remainder of the intubating dose of 0.15 mg/kg. Again, as with the use of the defasiculating dose, the priming dose may induce significant amounts of neuromuscular blockade especially in the trauma patient and it is generally recommended that the intubating dose be given 2 to 3 minutes after the priming dose. Such a practice can significantly delay appropriate airway management.

The problem of the delayed onset with non-depolarizing muscle relaxants has been somewhat alleviated with the introduction of rocuronium. Like vecuronium, rocuronium has minimal cardiovascular effects. It has the most rapid onset of any of the non-depolarizing agents and will provide acceptable intubating conditions in most patients within 60 seconds[(66)].

The second decision pertains to the drugs and the dose used to induce anesthesia during rapid sequence induction **(Table 43.2).** Comatose patients should not be given any anesthetic drug for intubation. In the hemodynamically unstable patient, etomidate (0.2 to 0.3 mg/kg) or a small dose of ketamine (0.5 to 1 mg/kg) may be used to provide amnesia/analgesia without significantly affecting cardiovascular function. Ketamine is contraindicated in patients with significant head injury because it increases intracranial pressure, cerebral oxygen consumption, and cerebral blood flow[(67,68)]. When injury and blood loss are minor and intravascular volume has been restored, the usual dose of thiopental (4 to 6 mg/kg), propofol (2 to 3 mg/kg) or ketamine (1 to 2 mg/kg) can be given.

The stimulus of intubation is extreme and can significantly increase intracranial pressure. Therefore, endotracheal intubation should not be performed on an awake patient with serious closed head trauma. The increases in intracranial pressure can be blunted or eliminated completely with adequate anesthesia provided by thiopental (4 to 6 mg/kg), etomidate (0.2 to 0.3 mg/kg), propofol (2 to 3 mg/kg), or fentanyl (4 to 8 mcg/kg). Additionally, the administration of lidocaine (1 to 2 mg/kg), 60 seconds prior to intubation, may effectively blunt the rise in intracranial pressure[(69,70)]. Unfortunately, all anesthetic agents can produce hypotension, particularly in the hypovolemic patient. Patients who are conscious and whose hemodynamic status is marginal can still receive analgesia/amnesia during intubation. However, reduced doses should be used: thiopental (1 to 1.5 mg/kg), ketamine (0.5 mg/kg) or midazolam (0.05 mg/kg).

Once endotracheal intubation is accomplished, proper confirmation of tube placement is mandatory. Correct tube placement can be confirmed by one of several means including direct visualization of the tube passing through the vocal cords, auscultation, the presence of mist in the tube, the presence of carbon dioxide, fiberoptic documentation of tracheal rings and subsequent chest x-ray. The use of capnography or documentation of end-tidal CO_2 serves as a useful adjunct to endotracheal tube placement and should be considered routine in any setting in which endotracheal intubation occurs.

If the trachea cannot be intubated after paralysis and sedative agents have been given, an immediate decision must be made as to how to handle the failed intubation. A second attempt at intubation may be tried after changing the patient's head position, the laryngoscope blade, or adding pressure on the larynx to help visualize the glottis. If these maneuvers fail, 100% oxygen should be administered through a tight-fitting face mask and bag-mask ventilation. Cricoid pressure should not be removed until the patient awakens. As this point, the alternatives to be considered should follow the algorithm provided by American Society of Anesthesiologists for failed intubation (Fig. 43.6). If mask ventilation is successful, there is time to consider alternative routes of securing the airway. These may include fiberoptic intubation, performance of a tracheostomy using local anesthesia, or needle cricothyrotomy with a large-bore intravenous catheter. Needle cricothyrotomy is accomplished by inserting a 14- or 16-gauge intravenous catheter through the 14-gauge the cricothyroid membrane into the trachea (Fig. 43.7). To accomplish this, the catheter is advanced through the skin into the trachea with a syringe that is filled with air or air/saline. Constant pressure is maintained on the plunger as the syringe is advanced and air bubbles will be seen in the saline when the trachea is entered. The plastic catheter is then advanced into the trachea. An alternative means includes the use of a syringe and needle as previously described, but with the passage of a guidewire into the trachea followed by a dilator and a catheter. The latter may ensure that the catheter is not advanced off the needle into a false tract. This can be disastrous as jet ventilation may then result in subcutaneous emphysema and distort the anatomy for further airway maneuvers. Another option includes the attachment of an end-tidal carbon dioxide detector to the syringe or needle. As the trachea is entered, carbon dioxide will be sensed.

Once the catheter is placed in the trachea, oxygenation can then be maintained by intermittent jets from a high pressure system. An oxygen line and toggle valve originating at a 50 psi oxygen source can be attached with a lever fitting directly to the intravenous catheter. Alternatively, the small end of the 15 mm adapter from a 3.0 mm endotracheal tube will fit into the end of the intravenous catheter (Fig. 43.7). Alternatively, the small end of a 7.0 mm endotracheal tube can be inserted into the barrel of a 3 mL syringe and the luer lock end attached to the catheter. The 15 mm adapter allows connection to a supply of oxygen for insufflation at low flow (1 to 2 liters/min) or to a high-pressure (50 psi) oxygen source for bag or jet ventilation. Both insufflation and bag/jet ventilation may be hazardous in patients with upper airway obstruction because exhalation may be impeded and cause lung overdistention and barotrauma.

If bag/mask ventilation cannot be accomplished, one

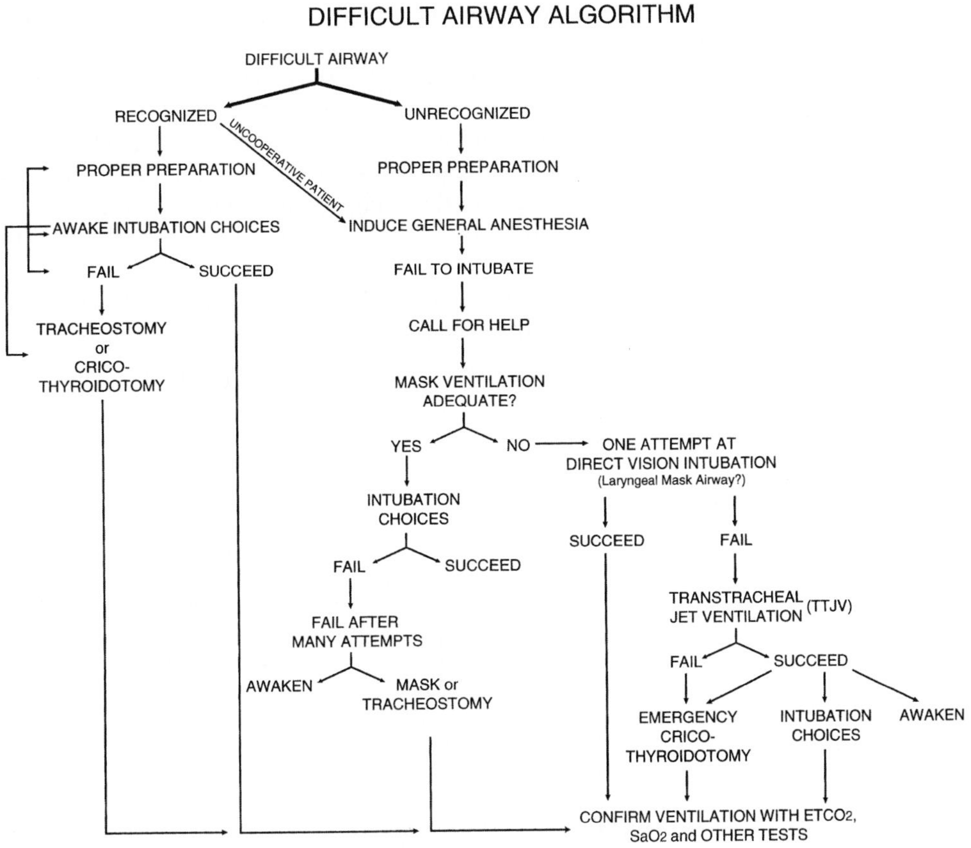

Figure 43.6. The difficult airway algorithm as suggested by the American Society of Anesthesiologists. The algorithm provides a step-wise plan for the management of the anticipated or more importantly, unanticipated difficult airway.

must move quickly along the ASA algorithm. A recent addition to airway management is the laryngeal mask airway[71,72] (Fig. 43-8). The laryngeal mask airway or LMA was introduced for clinical use in the United States in 1991. It is passed blindly into the oropharynx until resistance is felt. At that point, the cuff is inflated. The 15 mm adaptor is connected to an Ambu bag or the anesthesia circuit and either spontaneous or positive pressure ventilation is possible. In the trauma setting, the advantages of the LMA are that it can be passed blindly without neck movement. While it will have limited use in the trauma setting, it may have a role in the "can't intubate/can't ventilate" scenario prior to transtracheal jet ventilation. The LMA does not seal the airway and therefore the patient is still at risk for aspiration. It can be used with cricoid pressure. It should be used only as a temporizing measure in the pediatric trauma patient to re-establish ventilation and oxygenation while other methods of airway management are organized. Several sizes of the LMA are available **(Table 43.3).**

When endotracheal intubation fails, alternative means of airway management such as the LMA or transtracheal jet ventilation are used to maintain or re-establish oxygenation and ventilation so that definitive airway management can proceed in a relatively controlled situation. This may include surgical cricothyrotomy. An emergent tracheostomy should be avoided if at all possible. Emergency tracheostomy can be fraught with complications including complete loss of airway secondary to bleeding, bilateral pneumothoraces, permanent damage to the trachea, and overt operative failure. The procedure is best performed after the airway has been protected. Whenever possible, the best rule is to try to anticipate that the airway is going to be difficult so that tracheostomy, if necessary, is performed under a controlled situation. If necessary, it should be done with only local infiltration.

Complicated Airway

Occasionally, tracheal intubation is thought to be complicated in the initial assessment. When the midface, mandible, neck, or larynx is injured; bone fragments, hematoma, and/or edema can cause complete airway obstruction. In the presence of maxillofacial or airway injury, one should never risk sudden airway obstruction by using neuromuscular blocking or hypnotic agents. The endotracheal tube or indeed any tube should not be passed blindly. Blind nasal passage can lead to intubation of the nasal sinuses or the

Table 43.3. Description of the Different Sizes of Laryngeal Mask Airways

Mask Size	*Patient Weight (kg)*	*Internal Diameter (mm)*	*Cuff Volume (ml)*
1	less than 6.5	5.25	2–5
2	6.5–20	7.0	7–10
2.5	20–30	8.4	14
3	30–70	10	15–20
4	70–90	12	25–30
5	greater than 90	11.5	30–40

cranium or cause further dislodgement of bone and tissue. Blunt injuries of the neck can fracture and disrupt the airway and make passage of an endotracheal tube impossible. Such injuries are usually associated with cervical spine injury. These are best managed via tracheostomy under local anesthesia or needle cricothyrotomy.

Patients having neck, serious head, or deceleration injuries should be assumed to have cervical spine injury (refer to the heading "Acute Spinal Cord Injury" within this chapter). The primary goal of initial management is to prevent further injury by reducing external compression and preventing further displacement of the injured elements. When tracheal intubation is necessary before a traction device can be applied, longitudinal (axial) traction must be applied manually (Fig. 43.5). An assistant (preferably a neurosurgeon) stands at the head of the patient's bed, places his or her hands on the patient's mastoid processes, and applies a traction force in the cephalad direction, keeping the mastoid process in line with the axis of the head (Fig. 43.5). These maneuvers should prevent any extension or flexion of the cervical spine during laryngoscopy and tracheal intubation. If tracheal intubation is expected to be easy, an-

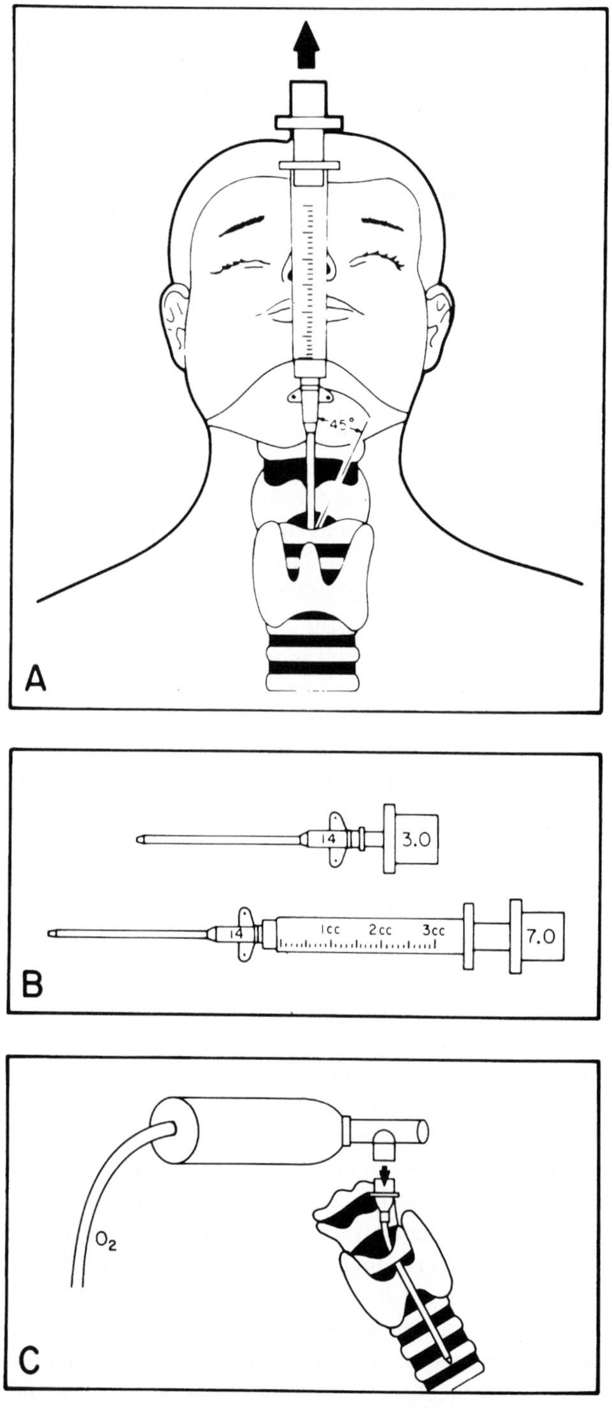

Figure 43.7. (A) Needle cricothyrotomy is performed by palpating the cricothyroid membrane in the midline. This membrane is located between the cricoid cartilage (inferiorly) the thyroid cartilage (superiorly). Needle cricothyrotomy is performed using a 14 or 16 gauge over-the-needle catheter technique. The catheter is held at a 45° angle to the skin, parallel to the trachea. As the needle and catheter are advanced, the attached syringe is constantly aspirated until the entry of air into the syringe is detected. This verifies the intratracheal position of the needle and catheter. Another technique includes the placement of a few mL's of saline into the syringe to provide an air/saline interface to permit the visualization of bubbles in the saline as air is aspirated. Once entry into the trachea is identified, the catheter is advanced and the needle withdrawn. The syringe is then reattached to the catheter to check for free aspiration of air to ensure an intratracheal position. (B) The small end of a 3.0 mm endotracheal tube connector will fit into the end of the 14 or 16 gauge catheter. Alternatively, the small end of a 7.0 mm endotracheal tube connector will fit into the barrel of a 3 mL syringe, which will fit into the end of the catheter. (C) The 15 mm end of the endotracheal tube connector can then be attached to an oxygen delivery system. This may include an anesthesia machine, a jet ventilator system, or a standard resuscitation bag.

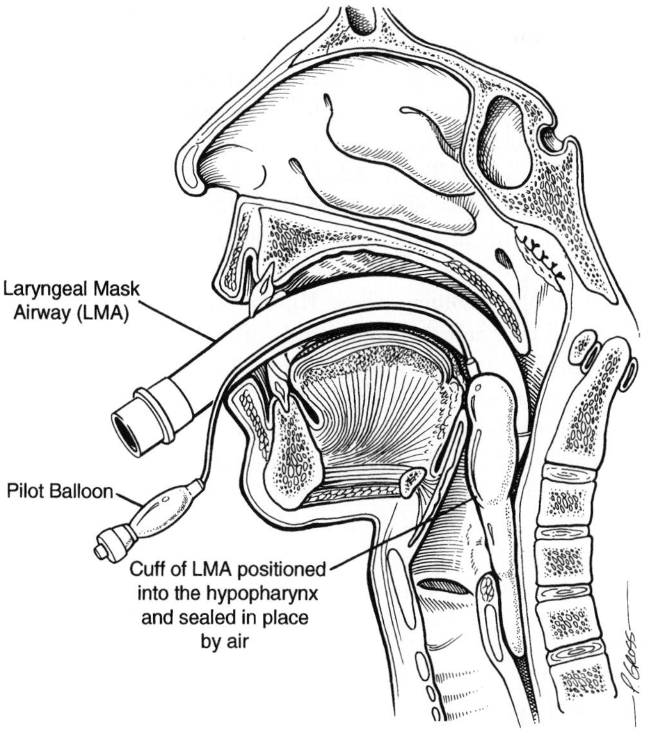

Figure 43.8. Diagram showing the correct positioning for a laryngeal mask airway. The mask is designed to be inserted blindly into the oropharynx and sit in the hypopharynx over the glottic opening. Inflation of the cuff forms a seal over the glottis allowing for either spontaneous or controlled ventilation.

esthesia can be induced using the rapid sequence induction technique described above (succinylcholine will not produce catastrophic hyperkalemia in the first 24 to 48 hours following a cervical spinal cord injury). If tracheal intubation cannot be accomplished without an acceptable degree of flexion or extension of the neck, an oral fiberoptic intubation, tracheostomy under local anesthesia or needle cricothyrotomy may be necessary. Once again, "blind" nasotracheal intubation in any pediatric trauma patient is not recommended. In the emergent situation, one should intubate in the most facile and routine manner possible, namely, via the oral route[(55)].

Respiratory Function (Breathing)

Once a patent airway is established, the next step of the evaluation is establishing the adequacy of ventilation. If apnea or hypoventilation are noted, assisted ventilation is immediately instituted with 100% oxygen. Ventilation is initiated with tidal volumes of 10 to 15 mL/kg and a rate dependent on the patient's age. Rates of 10 to 15 breaths/minute are generally sufficient for adults while neonates and infants may require rates as high as 40 to 60 breaths/minute. A minute ventilation of 150 mL/kg/min will usually produce arterial carbon dioxide pressures of around 40 mm Hg. In the patient with associated closed head trauma, the initial minute ventilation has traditionally been increased to lower arterial carbon dioxide pressure further in an attempt to control intracranial pressure. The efficacy of hyperventilation in the initial treatment of patients with closed head injury has recently been questioned[(73)].

If poor ventilation and abnormal pulmonary compliance is noted, an immediate evaluation is necessary. The first step should be ausculation of breath sounds to rule out mainstem intubation. This is more likely to be a problem in younger patients. A suction catheter should be passed through the endotracheal tube to ensure that the endotracheal tube is not kinked or that secretions or blood have not blocked the tube. If this is not the case, auscultation of breath sounds and a chest x-ray are indicated to rule out a pneumothorax. In the spontaneously breathing patient, an unstable chest wall from a flail segment may interfere with ventilation.

If a pneumothorax is suspected, either because of lack of movement of the chest wall or absence of breath sounds, needle aspiration should be carried out followed by thoracostomy tube placement if the pneumothorax is verified (refer to the heading "Chest Trauma" within this chapter). Oftentimes, there may not be time to obtain a chest film if the child's ventilatory or cardiovascular function is deteriorating. A flail chest wall is best managed by an endotracheal tube with positive end-expiratory pressure. This will stabilize the chest wall and allow for adequate ventilation.

In spite of an adequate airway and effective ventilation, there may still be hypoxia and arterial desaturation due to pathologic right-to-left shunting through damaged pulmonary tissue, or secondary to aspiration, pneumonia, or lung contusion. Although these latter problems will require subsequent evaluation and treatment (see below), the initial approach is the same: to secure the airway and maintain adequate ventilation with 100% oxygen.

Circulation

Following the establishment of an airway and effective gas exchange, attention is next directed to the circulation. Long-term patient outcome and the severity of subsequent sequelae is directly related to the speed with which shock is treated and corrected. The prompt correction of hypovolemia is the single most important factor in the prevention of post-traumatic sequelae such as acute renal failure or the development of "shock lung".

The basic steps in the management of hemorrhagic shock are:

1. Control of active hemorrhage
2. Placement of intravenous lines
3. Volume replacement

Although blood loss is easily recognized with external hemorrhage, fractures of the long bones or pelvis produce hidden blood loss that may reach 1 to 2 liters in adults. Control of obvious external hemorrhage is of paramount importance. In most situations, direct pressure over the site of hemorrhage will be successful. Tourniquet techniques are rarely advocated or used. Massive abdominal hemorrhage or hemorrhage following fracture of the long bones of the lower extremities can be controlled with a pressurized, pneumatic garment such as military anti-shock trousers (MAST), which is available in various pediatric sizes. In extreme situations, massive abdominal hemorrhage may be controlled by thoracotomy and cross-clamping of the descending aorta. However, the technique does not always achieve complete hemostasis and abdominal control of the bleeding must be accomplished rapidly to prevent abdominal visceral ischemia[74].

When the MAST is unavailable or control of hemorrhage requires immediate surgery, catecholamines such as epinephrine or norepinephrine may be needed to support the patient en route to the operating room. The definitive treatment of blood loss is to control hemorrhage followed by replacement with appropriate fluids including blood. Both epinephrine and norepinephrine may cause irreversible mucosal ischemia by shunting blood away from the gut and the periphery[75,76]. Inotropic agents should be used only as a temporizing agent and not instead of appropriate volume resuscitation.

Recent controversy has also been raised concerning the possible adverse effects of volume resuscitation in the trauma patient. The down side to immediate volume resuscitation include an increase in blood pressure which may disrupt hemostatic mechanisms as well as a dilution of coagulation factors. The practice of immediate volume resuscitation versus immediate surgical control followed by volume resuscitation is open for debate. The appropriate response may be to resuscitate to the point of achieving low, but normal blood pressure followed by immediate surgical intervention. Future studies are needed to address these issues, especially in the pediatric population.

Obtaining adequate venous access for resuscitation may be a difficult task in the pediatric patient. The triage and transport of children should not be delayed by attempting to obtain access in the field. These children are better served by immediate transportation to an emergency facility rather than spending time in the field. An alternative access route for younger patients (less than 6 to 8 years) is the intraosseous route. This route provides direct access to the central circulation and may be used for the administration of fluids, blood, inotropic agents, as well as drugs for endotracheal intubation[77].

Blood Volume

Blood volume is estimated based on the patient's ideal body weight[78,79]. Through age 14 years, the range is 6.5 to 8.0% of the total body weight (i.e., 65 to 80 ml/kg of optimal body weight). In newborns, the figure approaches 9 to 10% of the optimal body weight. The volume deficit is best evaluated by examination.

The most sensitive monitor of cardiac output and volume status in a child is the heart rate. The adequacy of circulation is assessed by noting the quality, rate, and regularity of the pulse and secondarily by obtaining the blood pressure. Young children vasoconstrict rapidly and may maintain a normal blood pressure even though they have lost as much as 25% of their circulating blood volume. Heart rate elevation is a much earlier sign of hypovolemia. A classification of hypovolemia and associated signs/symptoms is shown in **Table 43.4.**

With blood loss of 10 to 15% of the total blood volume (Class I), clinical symptoms most often include only an increase in pulse rate. With the loss of 20 to 25% of the circulating blood volume (Class II), there is a further increase in pulse rate and the appearance of tachypnea. The blood pressure responds with a narrowing of pulse pressure and a decrease in systolic arterial blood pressure. At this time, there are concomitant signs of peripheral vasoconstriction with pallor, cyanosis, and poor capillary refill. With a loss of 30 to 35% of the effective circulating blood volume (Class III), there is a marked decrease in urinary output, the pulse is thready, and mental confusion is evident. With loss of more than 40% of the circulating blood volume (Class IV), the clinical symptoms include coma and non-palpable blood pressure.

Fluid Replacement

The definitive therapy for blood loss and extracellular fluid loss is the appropriate administration of intravenous fluids and blood. The simplest, safest, and most rapid means of obtaining venous access is by percutaneous peripheral vein cannulation. At least one large intravenous line should be started as quickly as possible. Because of the smaller size of veins in children and the fact that veins usually collapse when a child is in shock, percutaneous peripheral cannulation may be difficult to perform and very time-consuming. In that situation, initial access to the circulation can be rapidly obtained by placement of an intraosseous cannula. The

Table 43.4. Advanced Trauma Life Support Classification of Shock

Class I:
15% acute blood volume loss or less
Blood pressure normal
Pulse increased 10–20%
No change in capillary refill
Class II:
20–25% loss of blood volume
Tachycardia greater than 150 beats/min
Tachypnea 35–40 breaths/minute
Capillary refill prolonged
Systolic blood pressure decreased
Pulse pressure decreased
Orthostatic hypotension of greater than 10–15 torr
Urine output greater than 1 ml/kg/hr
Class III:
30–35% blood volume loss
All of the above signs
Urine output less than 1 ml/kg/hr
Lethargic, clammy, vomiting
Class IV:
40–50% blood volume loss
Nonpalpable pulses
Obtunded

preferred site is the medial aspect of the tibia, 2 to 4 centimeters below the anterior tibial tuberosity. While there are several commercially available intraosseous needles, a 16- or 18-gauge spinal needle can also be used. Fluid resuscitation and several different medications can be administered through the intraosseous needle. This can be followed by either cutdown or central line placement for definite access. For cutdowns, the brachial vein of the upper extremity or, when the MAST is not in use, the saphenous vein of the lower extremity are usually easiest. Favored entry sites for central venous access include the internal jugular, external jugular, femoral, and subclavian veins. Access to the jugular system may be limited in patients with suspected cervical spine injury. The femoral veins should not be used in cases of suspected intra-abdominal injury since the fluid/blood/drugs administered may extravasate into the peritoneal space if there is a disruption of the intra-abdominal vessels. While speed is essential, sterile technique and proper positioning of the patient must not be neglected.

Shires, et al.[80,81] showed that the effective circulating volume was decreased following trauma and hemorrhage due to the loss of blood and a reduction in the interstitial fluid volume. Using radioactive sulfate, Shires, et al. demonstrated that water and salt from the interstitial fluid space refills the plasma water by the Starling law of fluid distribution across capillaries as well as by leaking into the intracellular fluid space. Furthermore, incidental to the trauma and blood loss, an internal sequestration of functional ECF occurs and is often referred to as third space losses. The magnitude of third space loss is related to the extent of tissue injury and the severity of blood loss. The fluid and salt within the third space act as sequestered fluid and is nonfunctional in terms of the duties of the ECF. Replenishment of this interstitial water and salt loss with balanced salt solutions (crystalloids) has been advocated by many as the primary fluid therapy following trauma[82].

The studies by Shires, et al.[80,82] have been criticized because the sulfate ion may inaccurately reflect the ECF volume. Other investigators have repeated the experiments of Shires, et al. and found no deficit in ECF beyond that accounted for by measured intravascular volume loss[83]. These authors claim that the primary problem in the reduced ECF is not the decrease in interstitial water, but rather the reduction in intravascular volume. After surgery or trauma, there is a shift of albumin from the plasma volume into the interstitial fluid volume with preferential binding of albumin to skin and muscle[84]. This results in decreased plasma oncotic pressure and hypovolemia. The decrease in plasma protein is further exacerbated by protein catabolism. Thus, replenishment of plasma protein with agents such as albumin or hydroxyethyl starch has been advocated[85,86] as the primary replacement fluid following trauma.

The most commonly used oncotically active fluids for volume replacement are 5% albumin, 6% hydroxyethyl starch, and low molecular weight dextran (Dextran 40). The latter agent is seldom used in the trauma setting as it induces platelet dysfunction, interferes with cross-matching of blood, and may be filtered by the renal tubules leading to renal failure.

Albumin is a naturally occurring plasma protein that provides approximately 80% of the intravascular colloid oncotic pressure in normal subjects[87]. The albumin molecule has a molecular weight of 69,000 and is relatively impermeable to the vascular membrane under normal circumstances. The vascular membrane may be disrupted with trauma allowing albumin to pass into the interstitial spaces. The intravascular half-life of albumin is 24 hours with hemodynamic improvement persisting for up to 36 hours after administration[88]. As albumin is heat treated, there are no infectious disease risks with its use. Another protein product derived from blood (plasma protein fraction or plasminate) is not recommended for trauma use as it can occasionally cause hypotension due to the presence of activated mediators of the kininogen pathway.

Hydroxyethyl starch is a synthetic colloid that consists of a hydroxyethyl-substituted, branched-chain amylopectin with a molecular weight of 69,000. Although its elimination half-time is 17 days, in clinical practice it expands the plasma volume for only 24 to 36 hours[89]. Adverse effects include inhibition of platelet aggregation following the administration of more than 15 to 20 mL/kg.

Although several different types of fluids have been suggested for the initial trauma resuscitation, there is no substitute for blood, particularly in Class III and IV patients. The debate concerning the use of colloids and crystalloids has raged in the literature and in clinical practice over the past two decades[83,85]. Studies have consistently shown that less than 25% of balanced salt solutions administered remain within the intravascular space following fluid resuscitation and the remainder fills the interstitial and intracellular fluid spaces[80,86]. This egress of fluid may initially be an advantage in resuscitation. Fluid shifts among the intracellular, interstitial, and intravascular compartments are governed by osmotic/oncotic gradients and hydrostatic pressure as described by Starling. A net loss of fluid and protein from the vascular compartment may result in pulmonary edema and an increased risk of developing the adult respiratory distress syndrome. Patients receiving colloid would be expected to have high colloid oncotic pressures, whereas patients receiving crystalloid would be expected to have low colloid oncotic pressure. Clinical studies[90,91] in critically ill adults have found strong correlations between decreased colloid oncotic pressure and an increased pulmonary wedge pressure and the subsequent development and severity of pulmonary edema. However, healthy patients who are victims of trauma do not seem to develop these problems. Indeed, studies in young trauma patients treated with colloids or crystalloids showed no differences in the development of pulmonary edema or in pulmonary dysfunction despite the lowered colloid oncotic pressure seen with crystalloid administration[92,93]. Finally, there is a marked cost reduction when using crystalloids compared with using colloids. The cost of 1 liter of 5% albumin is as much as 50 times that of a vasoactively equivalent amount (4 liters) of Ringer's lactate.

There also remains controversy as to which particular crystalloid is best **(Table 43.5).** Many prefer Ringer's lactate as the crystalloid solution because its chloride concentration (109 meq/L) closely resembles the plasma chloride while the lactate provides a source of buffer. The lactate of Ringer's lactate is converted by the liver into bicarbonate. One problem with Ringer's lactate is that the sodium concentration of 130 meq/L is somewhat hypotonic compared to normal plasma leading many to consider it a hypotonic fluid and somewhat inappropriate for use in patients with closed head injury.

In contrast, the infusion of large amounts of isotonic saline can result in a metabolic, hyperchloremic acidosis. While the sodium concentration of 154 meq/l is isotonic and appropriate for use in the head trauma patient or for fluid resuscitation, the high chloride concentration is responsible for the subsequent development of acidosis and hyperchloremia. A third alternative is Plasmalyte with a more physiologic concentration of sodium and chloride **(Table 43.5).** Its buffers include both gluconate and acetate.

Aside from the isotonic crystalloids, recent attention has shifted to the possible beneficial effects of hypertonic crystalloids with or without the addition of colloid. These agents were used in clinical practice as early as World War I. The idea behind the use of hypertonic crystalloids is to restore effective circulating blood volume with a lower volume of fluid (4 to 5 mL/kg). This is accomplished since the hypertonic saline increases serum osmolarity and promotes the movement of endogenous fluid into the intravascular space. Additional effects demonstrated in laboratory animals include an increase in inotropic function of the heart, constriction of capacitance vessels, decrease in resistance vessels, and dilatation of precapillary sphincters[94-96]. The initial clinical studies in humans have shown similar beneficial effects. Holcroft et al. and Vassar et al. have both demonstrated successful resuscitation of trauma patients with hypertonic saline (250 mL of 7.5% sodium chloride) without adverse effects except for transient hypokalemia[97,98]. These agents may have particular benefit for patients with associated closed head injuries. Clinical studies in adult trauma victims have demonstrated improved survival following resuscitation with hypertonic saline as compared with Ringer's lactate[99,100]. Hypertonic saline effectively restored intravascular volume while also decreasing brain water.

Although the ideal resuscitation fluid has not yet been clearly identified, the initial studies in adults support the superiority of hypertonic saline solutions (i.e., 7.5% NaCl). These solutions restore intravascular volume with a rapid mobilization of endogenous fluid, reduce vascular resistance, and improve myocardial contractility. The effects may be prolonged by the addition of colloid to the solution. These agents may be particularly beneficial in the patient with associated closed head injury. Additionally, these agents are inexpensive and have a long shelf life.

Table 43.5. Composition of Isotonic Crystalloids (Meq/L)

Fluid	*Na^+*	*Cl^-*	*K^+*	*Buffer*	*Ca^{++}*	*Mg^{++}*
Normal Saline	154	154	0	None	0	0
Plasmalyte	140	98	5	Acetate 27 Gluconate 23	0	3
Ringer's lactate	130	109	4	Lactate 28	3	0

Regardless of the fluid chosen, an initial 20 to 30 ml/kg of an isotonic crystalloid solution is given as quickly as possible. If systemic arterial blood pressure does not return to normal levels following fluid challenge, additional crystalloid and blood are infused and titrated against urine output, skin perfusion, heart rate, and blood pressure. If systemic arterial blood pressure and central venous pressure cannot be maintained with 50 mL/kg of balanced salt solution and blood, the MAST is applied. The most frequent error made in the immediate therapy of the trauma patient is slow or inadequate administration of fluid and blood and/or the failure to use MAST.

Balanced salt solutions are not intended as substitutes for blood. Blood must be administered to Class III or IV patients (blood loss in excess of 30% of the effective circulating volume). Fresh whole blood is the ideal blood product because of its ease of administration, the presence of clotting factors, normal 2,3-DPG levels, normal pH, and most importantly because it duplicates what is being lost. However, fresh whole blood is rarely, if ever, available. Whole blood that is more than a few days old has lost most of the labile clotting factors and offers no advantage over packed cells and blood products.

The hematocrit of a unit of packed red blood cells will depend on the anticoagulant used. With citrate phosphate dextrose (CPD) the average hematocrit is 65 to 75% while the more commonly used adenine anticoagulants (ADSOL) have hematocrits of 50 to 60%. An equal amount of crystalloid should be administered with packed red blood cells to prevent an increased hematocrit and high viscosity. Packed or red blood cells should be reconstituted with normal saline, plasmalyte, or 5% albumin.

In the emergent resuscitative phase of therapy in Class III and Class IV patients, time may not allow a full type and crossmatch to be accomplished before transfusion. When using uncrossmatched blood, it is best to obtain at least an ABO and Rh type and partial crossmatch. This is sometimes referred to as an incomplete or immediate phase crossmatch. The immediate phase crossmatch eliminates serious hemolytic reactions due to errors in the ABO typing. It will fail to detect only a few unexpected antibodies outside the ABO system, most of which are clinically insignificant. If time does not permit even a preliminary screen, ABO and Rh type-specific, uncrossmatched blood is still preferable (and more abundant) than type O negative, Rh negative uncrossmatched blood. For proper use of type-specific blood, the ABO and Rh type of the patient must be determined before transfusion. Of patients never exposed to blood, fewer than one in 1000 will have an unexpected antibody detected in the immediate phase crossmatch[87]. Type O negative, Rh negative blood can be used when type-specific blood is unavailable. Type O blood lacks both the A and B antigens on the red cell and is not hemolyzed by the anti-A, anti-B antibodies that may be present in the recipient's plasma. However, some O negative, Rh negative donors have anti-A and anti-B antibodies in their serum, and these antibodies can hemolyze the recipient red blood cells. Thus, type O negative, Rh negative crossmatched packed red blood cells should be used in preference to O negative, Rh negative whole blood[102].

Blood warmers should be used whenever possible especially if the volumes delivered are great or if the patient is small. Although of theoretical value, micropore filters (40 microns) are not routinely recommended. These filters are designed to filter out microaggregates of platelets, granulocytes, and stroma from ruptured red blood cells, but their efficacy has never been proven[103] and their use may interfere with the rapid administration of blood. Standard (170 micron) filters should be used.

Hemostasis

With the exception of factor V and factor VIII, all plasma coagulation factors are relatively stable in banked blood. With massive hemorrhage and transfusion (greater than 15 units of stored blood in adults[102,103] or more than 2 blood volumes in a child), hemostatic defects may occur. The hemostatic defects are related to a dilution or decrease of both platelet and circulating protein coagulation factors.

The level of platelets necessary for adequate hemostasis has been widely debated. Aside from the actual number of platelets present, the state of platelet function must also be adequate for proper hemostasis. Similarly, the actual number of platelets is not as important as the rapidity and rate at which the platelet count decreases. A slow descent to 10,000 platelets/mm^3 in thrombocytopenic patients (e.g., those with leukemia) may be well tolerated, whereas a precipitous decline from 250,000 to 50,000 platelets/mm^3 may not. Following massive transfusion, thrombocytopenia results from dilution after the administration of platelet-poor bank blood or crystalloid and colloid solutions[104,105]. When platelet levels fall below 50,000/mm^3 and there is clinical evidence of bleeding, it is appropriate to begin platelet transfusions. A general rule of thumb is to administer 6 units to an adult or 0.1 to 0.2 units/kg in a child.

With the trend toward the use of large volumes of crystalloid and red blood cell concentrates to treat hemorrhage, all coagulation factors, both labile (factors V and VIII) and stable, may be depleted[102,103]. This results in a prolongation of the partial thromboplastin time (PTT)[105]. The dilutional coagulopathy is rapidly corrected once perfusion is restored, but may be exacerbated by the development or persistence of hypotension[106]. Hewson, et al.[106] demonstrated that, regardless of the etiology, shock-related elevations of PTT are marked and persist when resuscitation does not restore blood pressure rapidly and permanently in victims of massive hemorrhage.

The treatment of a coagulation defect remains replacement of the appropriate factors or product responsible for the coagulopathy. Fresh frozen plasma (FFP) provides the equivalent clotting factors of a single unit of fresh whole blood. The administration of FFP should be considered when 200% of the calculated circulating blood volume has been replaced with crystalloid and red cell concentrates. At that point, an evaluation of the coagulation cascade is indicated. While routine laboratory tests such as PT and PTT may take a significant amount of time; the thromboelastogram, which is used primarily intraoperatively, if available, will not only provide information concerning the coagulation cascade, but also determine platelet function, and the presence of fibrinolysis.

Consideration for platelet administration begins when 100 to 150% of the calculated circulating blood volume has been replaced with crystalloid and red cell concentrates. Frequent monitoring of coagulation screening tests and platelet counts are necessary as well as aggressive correction of hypovolemia and reversal of shock to avoid further exacerbation of the coagulation defects (i.e. disseminated intravascular coagulation).

Military Anti-Shock Trousers (MAST)

When abdominal or lower extremity hemorrhage or shock is present, the use of MAST for transport and emergency resuscitation may be indicated[107,108]. MAST evolved from the compression suits used by pilots to prevent gravity-induced redistribution of peripheral blood flow. These pneumatic garments are available in sizes for children 4 years of age and older. Aside from supporting blood pressure, MAST is useful to stabilize pelvic, hip, and long bone fractures of the lower extremity as well as to tamponade lacerated arterial and venous injuries in these organs. The only absolute contraindication to MAST is in the patient with respiratory insufficiency, as inflation of the abdominal component may impede ventilatory function. The abdominal section should not be inflated in patients with abdominal trauma in which the viscera are protruding.

MAST increases mean arterial blood pressure with a redirection of blood flow to the brain and heart. Two effects have been suggested to account for the increase in mean arterial pressure including an increase in venous return by autotransfusion[109,110] and an increase in peripheral vascular resistance[107,111].

MAST may be used in patients with associated closed head injury. Studies in adults have shown that in the presence of hypovolemic shock, the application of antishock trousers does not raise intracranial pressure to any significant level. The increase in cerebral perfusion pressure may reduce cerebral ischemia in this setting[112,113].

MAST is composed of three separate air chambers, each of which fastens with Velcro closures. Each chamber can be individually inflated and deflated through a simple foot pump and ball-valve device. The chambers are deflated by an automatic relief valve which also acts as a "pop-off" to prevent over-pressurization. The trousers are inflated sequentially (leg components first) to provide just enough counterpressure to raise the arterial blood pressure to desired levels. Sudden removal or deflation can result in an immediate shift of fluid and blood to the lower half of the body with a precipitous drop in mean arterial pressure. Once inflated in the field for transport, MAST should not be deflated until arrival at the trauma center. Deflation should also be carried out sequentially. The abdominal portion is deflated first followed by each of the lower extremity compartments. If blood pressure cannot be maintained during deflation, additional volume is administered to return the pressure to predeflation values before another compartment is deflated.

Due to adverse effects, there is some controversy concerning the use of MAST. Prolonged inflation with high pressures can lead to ischemia of skin, soft tissue, and muscle. Rhabdomyolysis with acidosis and hyperkalemia from subsequent tissue necrosis has followed prolonged use. MAST is not a substitute for the rapid infusion of fluids to the trauma patient and has limited role for in-hospital use. However, it may be a valuable tool in the prehospital stabilization of patients.

Monitoring: Urinary Catheter

Although invasive monitoring is one of the hallmarks of modern intensive care, one must never forget the physical examination. Aside from the previously mentioned signs and symptoms, one should note the skin turgor, core skin temperatures, whether or not the eyes are sunken, and whether urine is present as well as its rate of production. The single most important monitor and guide to the adequacy of fluid replacement in the pediatric patient is the measurement of urine production. Urine production may cease completely following hemorrhagic shock and flows of at least 0.5 to 1.0 mL/kg/hour are considered the goals of fluid therapy. In addition to measuring urine output, the bladder catheter facilitates the diagnosis of urinary tract injury and rhabdomyolysis. The presence of microscopic or gross hematuria is strongly suggestive of urinary tract injury. Because the insertion of the urethral catheter itself can cause hematuria, the urine that is examined should ideally be a spontaneously voided specimen.

Rhabdomyolysis with myoglobin release and myoglobinuria is common following crush injuries[(114)] and electrical burns. It may also occur following prolonged localized trauma such as may occur in "march myoglobinuria"[(115)]. Prompt diagnosis is essential because renal failure (acute tubular necrosis), electrolyte abnormalities (increased plasma concentrations of potassium, phosphorus, and calcium) with resultant cardiac arrhythmias may result in mortality. The diagnosis is made by gross pigmentation of the urine or a positive urine dipstick for heme without associated red blood cells seen on microscopic examination. The positive heme test for myoglobin must be differentiated from other urinary pigments including hemoglobin and porphyria.

Both hemoglobin and myoglobin will produce positive reactions to benzidine reagents, orthotoluidine, and the commonly used urinary dipsticks for blood. Urine centrifugation with observation of supernatant color will differentiate pigmenturia from hematuria. Color may vary from pink to red to red-brown in hemoglobinuria. Myoglobinuria produces a color from brown to pink, and porphyria a burgundy color.

Hemoglobinuria produced by hemolysis will be associated with pink serum because haptoglobin forms complexes with free circulating hemoglobin. Only after haptoglobin binding sites have been saturated will free hemoglobin be filtered in the urine. Because haptoglobin does not bind myoglobin, serum haptoglobin levels are normal in myoglobinuria (and unmeasurably low in hemoglobinuria). Following rhabdomyolysis, leakage from damaged muscle cells leads to very high levels of circulating muscle enzymes such as creatinine phosphokinase (and also SGOT). These may be useful in the differential diagnosis

The risks of bladder catheterization in males, particularly in the presence of pelvic fractures, as well as the risks of infection are discussed more fully in the section on abdominal injury (see below). The incidence of adverse effects can be lessened if it is remembered that the bladder catheter should pass easily and the procedure should be stopped if resistance is encountered.

Blood Pressure and Filling Pressures

As mentioned previously, arterial blood pressure may be normal with as much as a 15 to 25% loss of total blood volume. Arterial blood pressure can be measured with several techniques:

1. Sphygmomanometer cuff and palpation, stethoscope, or Doppler
2. Automatic blood pressure monitoring devices
3. Direct intra-arterial pressure monitoring

The latter is the method of choice in seriously injured patients because it provides beat-to-beat monitoring capability as well as ready access for blood sampling.

When blood loss is significant and large amounts of crystalloid and blood are required, estimation of intravascular volume by central venous pressure (CVP) or pulmonary capillary wedge pressure (PCWP) monitoring is essential. Initially, right heart filling pressures provide useful information and in the absence of other disease states, provides an accurate estimation of left ventricular filling pressures. Certain circumstances may mandate the placement of a flow-directed, balloon-tipped pulmonary artery catheter, including circulatory instability with cardiovascular dysfunction, significant lung disease or the need to measure cardiac output determinations (e.g., to determine oxygen delivery/consumption).

Fluids are administered using Weil's "5 to 2" or "7 to 3" rule according to whether the monitor is the CVP or PCWP respectively[116]. The volume is infused based on the pressure response to a fluid challenge, not based on the pressures initially measured. If the CVP is less than 8 mm H_2O or the PCWP is less than 12 mm Hg, 10 to 20 mL/kg of an isotonic solution is infused over 10 minutes. If at any time during the infusion, the CVP increases by more than 5 cm H_2O or the PCWP increases by more than 7 mm Hg, the infusion is discontinued. Following the infusion, if the CVP has increased by less than 5 cm H_2O but more than 2 cm H_2O or the PCWP has increased by less than 7 mm Hg but more than 3 mm Hg, the patient is observed for a 10 minute interval. If during the interval of observation, the CVP is greater than 2 cm H_2O above the starting value or if the PCWP is 3 mm Hg above the starting value, no additional fluid is administered. If, on the other hand, the CVP or the PCWP falls below 2 cm H_2O or 3 mm Hg of the starting value, the fluid challenge is resumed. Fluids are administered until either the hemodynamic signs of shock are corrected or the "5 to 2" or "7 to 3" rule is violated. Spinal cord injury with spinal shock should be suspected in patients with unexplained, refractory shock, especially in the presence of good peripheral perfusion whose blood pressure does not respond to appropriate fluid administration. In these patients, the sympathectomy associated with the cervical spine injury can lead to a significant drop in systemic vascular resistance. In this setting, the use of agents with alpha adrenergic agonist effects such as phenylephrine or norepinephrine may be needed to restore circulatory function.

Environment

In the ABC's of resuscitation, "D" is considered diagnosis and "E" the environment. Completely undressing the patient is frequently mandatory for proper evaluation and resuscitation. However, when undressed and placed in a cold environment (even room temperature), children rapidly lose heat due to their fairly large body surface area relative to their body mass and due to their increased minute ventilation and its accompanying heat of vaporization. Additionally, the younger the child, the less subcutaneous tissue that is available for heat insulation. With heat loss, endogenous processes begin to increase heat production to prevent a decrease in body temperature. This places enormous metabolic demands on the patient. The injured, poorly perfused child may be unable to meet these demands. This underlines the necessity to monitor body temperature and prevent hypothermia. Three simple maneuvers to conserve heat in children include:

1. External heating lamps
2. Warming intravenous fluids and blood
3. Wrapping exposed body parts in materials that prevent heat loss such as plastic bags[117]. The latter technique prevents evaporative heat loss and is quite effective at heat conservation.

The last step in the primary survey includes a rapid neurologic evaluation. A key component of the neurologic evaluation is the assignment of a Glasgow Coma Scale score (GCS) (refer to the heading "Head Trauma" within this chapter). The neurologic examination should concentrate on the patient's level of consciousness, the GCS, and a search for signs of increased intracranial pressure that might necessitate endotracheal intubation. A more thorough examination is performed as part of the secondary survey.

The basic principle of resuscitation is to begin treatment of life-threatening organ injuries during resuscitation and not wait until after a complete evaluation of the child has occurred. While the physician team is addressing the ABC's, a senior trauma nurse should record the baseline findings, the fluids and drugs administered, and the ongoing responses of the patient to the therapy. By doing this, the trends toward improvement or deterioration can be detected and appropriate measures taken. The senior trauma nurse can also be helpful by providing baseline normal data and resuscitation dosages for children in the patient's age range.

Secondary Survey

Following the initial stabilization of the cardiorespiratory system and aggressive treatment of shock, a complete physical examination (including the child's back) should take place. This is referred to as the secondary survey. It should take place approximately 15 to 20 minutes into the period of primary resuscitation and is performed in a head-to-toe fashion.

The order of physical examination of the child's body may vary, but injuries should be evaluated in descending order of urgency. The pediatric trauma victim should be assessed using a protocol in which all body areas are evaluated systematically. Finding one injury, even if severe, should not interfere with the remainder of the evaluation. The evaluation should always be gentle with particular care taken to avoid manipulation of the spinal axis. Most importantly, vital signs should be frequently repeated. These can change dramatically and quickly in the trauma setting.

The secondary survey begins with an evaluation of the head. This starts with the eyes, including the conjunctiva, pupillary size and reaction to light, fundal appearance, and assessment of vision if the child is conscious. The face and scalp are then carefully examined. Maxillofacial trauma, including fractures and scalp lesions, should be palpated for, especially over bony prominences. Localized hematomas and ecchymoses, especially those located in the periorbital region ("raccoon eyes") and behind the ears ("Battle's sign") are indicative of basilar skull fractures. Similarly, the tympanic membrane and nose should be examined for blood and cerebrospinal fluid (CSF) as evidence of either basal skull fracture or meningeal tear. Fluid dripping from the nose should be checked for glucose to confirm that it is CSF. Finally, the scalp itself should be carefully examined for lacerations and underlying soft tissue injury.

Next, the neck is examined looking for subcutaneous emphysema, hematoma, or localized pain on examination. This is done only following the lateral cervical spine film. The cervical spine is palpated. The location of the trachea is assessed to ensure that it is in a midline position. The neck is examined for discoloration and the neck veins are inspected looking for distention which may indicate cardiac tamponade or tension pneumothorax.

Following the head and neck examination, the chest is examined. In addition to adequacy and rate of ventilation, any asymmetry in chest wall excursion or painful areas should be observed with particular attention to the presence of a flail segment. After observation, a more thorough pulmonary and cardiovascular examination is performed using auscultation, percussion, and palpation. At this point, the blood pressure should be rechecked. Specific aspects of thoracic injury, diagnosis, and management are discussed in greater detail in the following sections.

The examination of the abdomen is next. The specific diagnosis of an intra-abdominal injury is not necessary at this point. What needs to be determined is whether surgical intervention is urgent or emergent. The initial examination of the abdomen, which consists of inspection, careful palpation, and auscultation is begun and repeated at 15 to 20 minute intervals.

If the child is conscious, calmly asked questions and gentle palpation may identify areas of significant tenderness. A rapidly expanding abdominal girth is indicative of ongoing bleeding and is an urgent indication for further diagnostic studies which may include peritoneal lavage, computed tomography (CT) scan, or radionuclide scanning. An oral gastric tube should be passed in all patients with abdominal trauma. This removes air from the stomach and improves ventilation, empties liquid and particulate matter and decreases the likelihood of aspiration, and provides diagnostic information concerning the presence of blood in the upper gastrointestinal tract. The back is an important part of the abdominal examination and the patient should be turned for proper evaluation of the posterior part of the body.

Also included in the abdominal examination is an examination of the pelvis and rectum. The bony prominences of the pelvis are palpated for tenderness and instability. The perineum is examined for lacerations, hematomas, or active bleeding. If a pelvic fracture is suspected or seen on a radiograph, a rectal examination should be carried out to evaluate the possibility of bone fragment injury to pelvic structures. Occasionally, examination of other body areas may also suggest an abdominal injury. Shoulder pain is often seen and suggests diaphragmatic irritation. Possible causes include free air in the abdomen or splenic injury (particularly with left upper quadrant pain).

Although genitourinary tract injury is common, the majority of these injuries are subtle in nature. Any child with pelvic fracture, perineal swelling or discoloration, flank tenderness, rib fracture, or abdominal tenderness should be considered to have a genitourinary injury until proven otherwise. As mentioned above, if an injury to the genitourinary tract is suspected, a urinary catheter should be inserted. Bladder decompression via a bladder catheter provides a means to measure urine output, urine for examination, prevents urinary obstruction from blood clots in the bladder and provides a route for contrast radiograph studies.

The extremities are examined next looking for abrasions, contusions, or hematoma formation. Bony instability is noted and a neurovascular examination is performed to assess the presence of compromised blood flow and development of a "compartment" syndrome. Disruption of blood flow to an extremity results in pulselessness, pallor, paresthesia, and paralysis (the so-called "4 P's"). Nerve injuries at the time of trauma or secondary to motion during transport are usually of one of three types: neuropraxia (a temporary conduction deficit), axonal disruption or neuromesis (disruption of the entire nerve bundle, including the nerve sheath).

Inadequate concern or lack of recognition of an injury to a neurovascular bundle can lead to unnecessary morbidity. The blood vessels in injured limbs are vulnerable to compression or laceration. These blood vessels can continue to bleed and exacerbate hypovolemic shock or bleed into an intact fascial compartment and cause the "compartment syndrome." Bleeding and edema within an intact fascial compartment can lead to the development of increased pressure, muscle ischemia and death. While pulses may be intact distally with a compartment syndrome exists, one constant finding is severe pain even with passive motion. Muscle compartment pressures can be evaluated during the secondary survey using an 18 gauge needle and a water manometer. Compartment pressures of 40 cm H_2O should cause concern while pressures greater than 60 cm H_2O require fasciotomy.

Finally, a neurologic examination is performed. A thorough neurologic examination can be carried out in a stepwise fashion including assessment of the cranial nerves as well as peripheral motor and sensory evaluation. The Glasgow Coma Scale is a standardized examination developed by Jennett, et al.[118]. It has been modified for use in children[119,120] and should be documented for all head injured patients **(Table 43.6).** The parameters measured include eye opening, verbal responses, and motor responses following verbal and auditory stimuli. The coma scale is standardized in all patients so that repeated examinations, which form the foundation for appropriate management, will be the same even if performed by different examiners. The remainder of the neurologic examination as well as therapeutic interventions and modalities utilized in head trauma management are detailed in the portion of this chapter titled "Head Trauma".

Table 43.6. Pediatric Coma Scale

More than 1 Year	Less than 1 Year
Eye Opening:	
4 spontaneously	spontaneously
3 to verbal command	to shout
2 to pain	to pain
1 no response	no response
Best motor response:	
6 follows commands	————
5 localizes pain	localizes pain
4 flexion withdrawal	flexion withdrawal
3 flexion abnormal (decorticate)	flexion abnormal (decorticate)
2 extension (decerebrate)	extension (decerebrate)
1 no response	no response

More than 5 yr	2–5 years	0–23 months
Best verbal response:		
5 oriented and conversive	appropriate words and phrase	smiles, coos, cries appropriately
4 disoriented and conversive	inappropriate words	cries
3 inappropriate words	cries/screams	inappropriate crying/screaming
2 incomprehensible sounds	grunts	grunts
1 no response	no responses	no responses

History of Injury

The final step in the secondary survey is to obtain a history of the onset of the injury or illness. This can often be obtained from accompanying family members or from the emergency medical technicians. Knowledge of the forces of injury that are responsible for a child's trauma can be important in determining the extent of injury and help in management of those injuries.

The parents should be included in this phase of the management, especially if the child is conscious, because they can be an invaluable emotional support at this time. A review of the past medical history is in order because childhood illnesses and systemic diseases may complicate or change the management of the acute trauma.

At this stage in preparation for transfer either to the PICU or to the operating room, a high index of suspicion and awareness of early signs of deterioration or development of new complications must be maintained. One physician must be responsible for the whole child so that the individual patient is not divided up into organ systems with the overall picture lost as a consequence.

Definitive Care

At this stage, the child should be either hemodynamically stable with a controlled airway or rapidly on the way to the operating room because of instability. In the former situation, appropriate specialized radiologic studies including CT or radionuclide scanning will be in order before the child is taken to the PICU. In preparing the child for transport, the airway must be firmly controlled and there should be constant monitoring of the cardiorespiratory system. This should include continuous pulse oximetry, non-invasive blood pressure monitoring, and continuous electrocardiography. An additional monitor which is now manufactured by several companies in sizes small enough for transport and which may be invaluable during patient transport is end-tidal capnography. The latter not only allows control of carbon dioxide as a therapeutic measure for control of ICP, but also documents endotracheal tube location. Aside from monitoring, a full complement of resuscitative drugs and airway equipment should be brought during the transport. The carefully documented records of the resuscitative efforts should accompany the patient at all times.

The trauma nurse as well as the primary resuscitating physician should accompany the child to his or her next destination whether that is the operating room or the PICU. This improves not only the transport of the patient, but also allows the transfer of critically important data and a plan of management.

Protocol management is an enormous advantage to ensure the proper priorities of treatment and to ensure that the resuscitative measures necessary for the treatment of life-threatening trauma and illness is sequentially carried out. This emphasizes the necessity for a plan of unified management with a team captain constantly communicating with all team members and specialty consultants. Only under rare circumstances should the phase of initial assessment and management of the patient require more than 1 hour in the resuscitative area. Preferably, this phase should be accomplished in 20 to 30 minutes.

CHEST TRAUMA IN INFANTS AND CHILDREN

The intensive care of a child with serious chest trauma should begin immediately during the primary resuscitation phase in the emergency room. Chest trauma often causes severe hypoxemia and hypotension which allows little time for evaluation or consultation. This is especially true in children because their increased metabolic rate results in oxygen demands that are two to three times greater than those of an adult. The child's normal compensatory mechanism for this increased oxygen demand is an increased minute ventilation, which may be severely compromised following chest injury. On the other hand, pediatric patients generally have few, if any, systemic or chronic diseases and seem to have remarkable reserves to sustain them following injury. Almost all deaths from thoracic injury in children occur after the victim reaches the resuscitation center and most children can be treated successfully with prompt diagnosis and aggressive early management[(121,122)].

The incidence of chest trauma in the pediatric age group varies from 7 to 54% depending on the series and the criteria for inclusion[(122,123)]. In general, 15 to 20% of injured children will have an associated chest injury that requires immediate assessment and management. Mortality from chest trauma in the pediatric age group ranges between 7%

and 14%[124] with mortality increasing to 20% in children less than 5 years of age[125]. Approximately two-thirds of these deaths occur after the child reaches the hospital. Chest trauma contributes little to the late hospital mortality from trauma with virtually all deaths occurring early in the hospitalization. Thus, both the early diagnosis and management of the child with a chest injury may fall primarily to emergency room physicians, rather than on surgeons or intensivists.

The vast majority of thoracic injuries in children (85%) can be managed by standard pediatric emergency room procedures and are certainly within the capabilities of well-trained emergency physicians. These procedures rarely require major operative intervention. Penetrating injuries to the chest are most unusual in children and usually result from fractured ribs rather than from external missiles[124,126,127].

Blunt trauma accounts for at least 90 to 95% of the life-threatening chest injuries in the childhood age group. Most of these injuries are the result of motor vehicular injury (pedestrian more than occupant) and from falls[128]. As a result, there is a high incidence of associated injuries (greater than 50%) of the head, abdomen and extremities[126]. These associated injuries must be considered early on in the management. Head injury, in particular, is responsible for most of the mortality and morbidity.

There are several other reasons why the child differs from the adult with regard to chest injury. The more compliant chest of the child contributes to a low incidence of rib fracture and, as a result, serious intrathoracic injury may be present in the absence of obvious chest wall injury. The mediastinum of the child is likewise more mobile and this contributes to a low incidence of major vessel and airway injury.

Evaluation of Chest Trauma in Children

Following evaluation of the airway, breathing, and circulation, the acute care physician should next search for the most common life-threatening thoracic injuries in the childhood age group. Virtually all chest injuries can be diagnosed during the initial primary assessment or during the secondary survey of the chest. This may be done using the physical examination (particularly inspection and auscultation) supplemented by chest radiographs and the electrocardiogram (ECG). Several injuries are immediately life-threatening and present during the initial assessment period. These include airway obstruction, open pneumothorax, flail chest, tension pneumothorax, massive hemothorax, and cardiac tamponade. Several injuries are potentially life-threatening and are identified during the secondary survey when the chest radiograph and ECG are obtained. These include tracheobronchial tears, pulmonary contusion, myocardial contusion, ruptured diaphragm, esophageal rupture, or partial aortic transection.

The most acute emergency is cardiopulmonary arrest. If there is a respiratory arrest, immediate assisted bag/mask ventilation followed by intubation is indicated. As mentioned previously, the orotracheal route is preferable under almost all circumstances and mechanical ventilation with 100% oxygen should be started. Cardiac arrest from blunt chest trauma is nearly always associated with multiple-system injuries and results from hypovolemia either from external or internal blood loss. Rarely, this will result from cardiac tamponade or aortic rupture (see below). External cardiac massage is often successful unless the period of hypoxemia has caused irreversible injury. If the primary cause of a cardiorespiratory arrest is an intrathoracic injury, the child generally requires operative intervention as soon as the ABC's have been completed and initial resuscitation begun. Open thoracotomy in the emergency room is rarely indicated (see below) or successful[129,130].

Open Pneumothorax or Sucking Chest Wound and Tension Pneumothorax

Massive blunt trauma or a penetrating injury may cause a loss of a portion of the chest wall and result in a communication between the pleural space and the environment. This produces an immediate equilibration of intrathoracic and atmospheric pressures with collapse of the lung and shift of the mediastinum. If the opening is large, air passes freely in and out, but if the opening is small, there may be ingress during inspiration and obstruction during expiration with further shift of the mediastinum. The latter situation results in a tension pneumothorax. If the chest wall defect is large, there is essentially no ventilation from the lung on that side. There may also be a to-and-fro movement of the mediastinum that impedes venous return to the right heart.

The initial treatment is simple and direct. The defect in the chest wall is covered with a sterile-occlusive dressing, which converts the open pneumothorax to a closed pneumothorax. The dressing is taped securely in place and a chest tube is placed in the pleural space and connected to underwater drainage with a suction apparatus. Definitive treatment of the open chest wound requires surgical intervention and is best performed in the controlled atmosphere of the operating room. The initial management is to control the adverse physiologic effects of a tension pneumothorax.

Flail Chest

A flail chest is characterized by a chest wall segment that has lost continuity with the thorax and moves with changes in intrathoracic pressure. The movement is paradoxical: in with inspiration and out with expiration. This injury is the result of a high-velocity trauma and is usually associated with multiple rib fractures. It is rarely seen in children because high-velocity, direct-chest injury is uncommon. Additionally, rib fractures are less common in children than adults because children have very pliable ribs that are resistant to fracture[131,132].

The flail segment interferes with normal ventilatory physiology because the free segment of the chest wall moves inward with inspiration and outward with expiration. This paradoxical movement is pathognomonic of a flail chest. The nearer the defect is to the diaphragm, the more seriously it interferes with ventilation. The other pathophysiologic feature of a flail chest is the frequently associated contusion and/or penetrating injury of the lung parenchyma. This results in a diffusion abnormality and decreases the volume of pulmonary parenchyma available for respiration.

The diagnosis is made by the visual inspection of the paradoxical movement of the chest wall. Palpation will often reveal crepitus secondary to rib or cartilage fracture. The radiograph may show rib fractures, a mediastinal shift or the underlying pulmonary contusion. Immediate treatment includes stabilization of the flail segment. This is accomplished by hand or sandbag pressure over the flail segment. While this corrects the instability of the chest wall, the child will also generally require endotracheal intubation and positive pressure ventilation to achieve adequate oxygenation and ventilation. The initial therapy should also include humidified oxygen and a limitation of crystalloid resuscitation if the remainder of the injuries permit so that there will be a decrease in extravasation of fluid into the injured pulmonary parenchyma and a limitation of the secondary acute pulmonary edema.

Definitive treatment of the flail chest takes place in the PICU by controlled ventilation and positive end-expiratory pressure. The inflated lung acts as a splint, stabilizes the rib fractures and decreases pain associated with the chest wall injury. Analgesics should also be administered because of the pain associated with chest wall movement. This may include parenteral opioids or regional anesthetic techniques such as epidural or interpleural analgesia. Often, the severity of the underlying injury to the lung is more of a determinant in recovery than is the chest wall injury itself. In any event, prolonged ventilatory support may be necessary.

Cardiac Tamponade

Cardiac tamponade occurs relatively infrequently with blunt trauma in children. However, it may result from stab wounds or from penetration of a fractured rib into the heart. Gunshot wounds to the heart usually result in fatal hemorrhage rather than pericardial tamponade. Nevertheless, cardiac tamponade with hemopericardium is a life-threatening injury associated with trauma in children. The classic clinical presentation of "pulsus paradoxicus", severe hypotension and distended neck veins is seen in children as well as in adults. Neck vein distention may be difficult to identify in small infants. The detrimental physiologic effects of cardiac tamponade result from the impedance of right heart filling during diastole because of the pressure of blood within the contained pericardium. This causes a decrease in cardiac output and ultimately, lethal impairment of cardiac output. If the physical findings and signs suggest tamponade, a definitive diagnosis is made by pericardiocentesis using a large (14-gauge) catheter over-the-needle device. Once in place, it can also be used to temporize the situation until definitive repair can be accomplished.

Pericardiocentesis is performed by inserting the needle under the xiphoid at a 30° angle, aimed at the left shoulder. Constant aspiration is applied to the syringe as the needle is advanced. Virtually all children with pericardial tamponade will ultimately require surgical exploration in the operating room.

Secondary Survey of Thoracic Injuries

Following rapid exclusion or initial management of life-threatening thoracic injuries, the chest is re-evaluated for any visible signs of inadequate respiratory excursion, asymmetry of respiration, or local evidence of injury. Palpation and auscultation are essential components of this secondary evaluation of the chest.

The most common occult and potentially serious injuries to the chest and its contents should now be assessed. In order of frequency they are:

1. Pulmonary contusion
2. Pulmonary laceration
3. Pulmonary hematoma
4. Tracheobronchial tear
5. Myocardial contusion
6. Diaphragmatic rupture
7. Partial aortic or great vessel disruption
8. Esophageal perforation

Pulmonary Contusion

Hemoptysis or suctioning of blood from the endotracheal tube, subcutaneous emphysema in the base of the neck, or a persistent air leak following placement of a chest tube for pneumothorax are suggestive of pulmonary parenchymal injury in a child. Pulmonary contusion from blunt injuries to the chest is common and is frequently associated with both localized pulmonary edema and atelectasis. Pulmonary dysfunction may be compounded by aspiration of gastric contents, which is common with severe, blunt injuries to the thorax. If there is extensive involvement of pulmonary parenchyma by contusion and/or hemorrhage or acid aspiration, acute respiratory distress syndrome (ARDS) may develop.

The clinical findings of ARDS and pulmonary contusion are similar and may coexist. Symptoms of ARDS include respiratory distress (tachypnea, dyspnea, hypoxemia) with radiographic evidence of diffuse alveolar infiltrates, loss of lung volumes, and increased extraparenchymal lung water in the setting of normal cardiovascular function.

Pulmonary contusion similarly presents with respiratory distress, particularly hypoxemia, due to the right-to-left shunting through the contused, atelectatic, and underventilated pulmonary parenchyma. Radiographic evidence of pulmonary contusion includes early consolidation of lung parenchyma that may be focal in nature with resolution over 2 to 6 days. Overhydration of patients with pulmonary contusions must be avoided because fluid will sequester in the damaged lung tissue. Small areas of pulmonary contusion often require no active treatment, but patients with extensive involvement will usually require ventilatory support with positive end-expiratory pressure[133,134]. The extravasation of fluid and blood into the alveolar and interstitial spaces provides an excellent "culture medium" for bacterial infection, and abscess or empyema formation may follow.

Pulmonary Laceration

Tears into the pulmonary parenchyma may result from blunt trauma due to fractured ribs or compression of the chest wall even without fractures. A laceration obviously can occur from any type of penetrating injury as well. Minor peripheral parenchymal lacerations rarely cause major problems and are usually successfully treated by chest tube insertion for the associated pneumothorax with re-expansion of the lung against the chest wall. Major hemorrhage is rarely associated with peripheral parenchymal injuries and, therefore, re-expansion of the lung by tube thoracostomy is adequate treatment. Larger injuries or those located more centrally may require open thoracotomy and surgical repair.

Pulmonary Hematoma

Both a parenchymal contusion and parenchymal laceration may lead to contained bleeding or hematoma in the lung tissue. Although radiographic findings of pulmonary hematomas may be dramatic, they usually resolve in a few days without the need for surgical intervention. Although abscess formation due to secondary infection is uncommon in children, because of the potential seriousness of this complication, prophylactic antibiotics may be indicated.

Tracheobronchial Tears

While penetrating injuries resulting in tears to the trachea or major bronchi are usually obvious, problems related to blunt trauma are more common and more difficult to diagnose. At least half of the deaths associated with major tracheobronchial tears occur immediately after the injury and are usually the result of very large tears from extensive blunt or penetrating forces. The more common, less severe injuries to the tracheobronchial tree are suggested by coarse bronchi or stridor, indicative of partial airway obstruction. In the child with a strangulation injury, especially if there is subcutaneous emphysema in the cervical area, the diagnosis should be suspected.

When signs are present suggesting an injury to the tracheobronchial tree or when an injury is suspected, bronchoscopy to visualize the trachea and major bronchi is used to confirm the diagnosis. If there is a persistent large air leak following placement of a chest tube for pneumothorax, a tear of a major bronchus should be suspected. Under such circumstances, a second chest tube, and even a third, may be necessary to control the air leak. In these cases, early endoscopy and thoracotomy to control the air leak and to repair the bronchial tear is indicated. The indications for early thoracotomy are continued extensive air leak, compression of the tracheobronchial tree and expanding hematoma in the mediastinum or neck[135–137]. Respiratory management of these patients may be extraordinarily difficult because positive pressure ventilation primarily ventilates the path of least resistance, namely the fistula. Spontaneous ventilation, even in intubated patients, is more successful. In older patients, a double-lumen endotracheal tube can isolate the fistula and allow one-lung ventilation. In younger patients (less than 40 kg), this is not possible and other less practical techniques such as mainstem intubation or bronchial blockers are needed to allow for one lung ventilation.

High-frequency ventilation has also been used in this setting to allow for effective ventilation while minimizing peak inflating pressures. It may be effective even when conventional ventilation has failed[138]. When other measures fail to allow for effective ventilation, extracorporeal membrane oxygenation (venous-arterial or venous-venous) may allow for support of oxygenation and carbon dioxide removal until surgical repair of the defect can be accomplished.

Myocardial Contusion

Myocardial contusion results from a concussive injury to the chest. The direction of the force of the impact is typically anteroposterior. It is a relatively frequent finding in the adult victim of a motor vehicle accident because the patient is often the driver of the automobile and the chest is crushed against the steering column[139]. Myocardial contusion for other occupants of the automobile is much less common. In the pediatric age range, steering wheel and dashboard injuries and hence myocardial contusion are rare[139,140].

The signs and symptoms are relatively non-specific including chest pain. Dysrhythmias and myocardial dysfunction with congestive failure may occur in an isolated number of patients. Myocardial contusion should be entertained in the trauma patient who develops or remains persistently hypotensive despite appropriate volume resuscitation. In that setting, the usual findings of congestive heart failure such as increased cardiac silhouette and an elevated CVP with persistently low blood pressure should suggest the diagnosis and the need for further evaluation. The diagnosis of a myocardial contusion is made based on a series of tests including: electrocardiography, echocardiography, determination of cardiac enzymes, and radionuclide angiography. Treatment is primarily supportive. Severe cases may require invasive monitoring with a pulmonary artery catheter to appropriately determine fluid requirements and the use of inotropic agents. Because children with myocardial contusion are at risk for sudden and lethal dysrhythmias, even if the initial electrocardiogram is unremarkable, they require admission to a critical care unit and continuous cardiac monitoring.

Rupture of the Diaphragm

Traumatic rupture of the diaphragm results from compression forces over the lower chest and upper abdomen[141–143]. It has been recognized with increased frequency in the pediatric trauma patient following blunt trauma or with lap belt injuries. Rupture is more common on the left side, possibly because the right diaphragm is buttressed by the liver. A small tear in the diaphragm may not cause immediate symptoms, but eventually results in progressive herniation of abdominal contents through the diaphragmatic defect. Smaller injuries are frequently missed initially because the radiographic findings may be interpreted as an elevated diaphragm or atelectasis and/or pleural fluid in the lower chest[(144)]. The diagnosis should be suspected when the left diaphragm is not clearly visualized on the initial chest radiograph or when a hemo-pneumothorax does not clear completely with placement of a chest tube[(145)]. Rupture of the diaphragm may also be found at the time of abdominal exploration for severe intra-abdominal injury[(146)]. Treatment is operative repair.

Impending Thoracic-Aortic Disruption

Impending or partial aortic disruption as well as a tear of the great vessels is extremely uncommon in children because rarely is sufficient force brought to bear on the chest and mediastinal structures in this age group[(147)]. The injury is usually the result of a severe deceleration injury that can occur during a high speed motor vehicle accident or a fall from extreme heights. Aortic rupture occurs from blunt forces at sites of attachment of the aorta; therefore, the most frequent tears are at the origin of the left subclavian artery near the attachment of the ligamentum arteriosum. Tears of the thoracic aorta are fatal in 80 to 90% of adults, and this is probably also true in the rare instances in which it occurs in children. The high mortality is related both to the injury and the extent of the trauma necessary to cause it.

Patients with partial aortic disruptions are more likely to present for emergent care. Clinical signs and symptoms include cardiac murmur and back pain. These non-specific signs combined with a compatible injury should heighten one's level of suspicion. The diagnosis is further suggested by a widened mediastinum with loss of the aortic knob, deviation of the endotracheal tube or trachea to the right, or deviation of the esophagus (NG tube) to the left. The injury may be associated with fractures of the first and second ribs[(148)]. Due to its location, a fracture of the first rib implies a significant deceleration injury and is a frequent accompanying sign in patient's with aortic arch injuries. The diagnosis is confirmed by aortography or more recently MRI scanning. Treatment is emergent thoracotomy and surgical repair.

Traumatic Asphyxia

Traumatic asphyxia is a rare complication of blunt trauma to the chest in children[(150)], resulting from the sudden intense compression of the chest wall with a closed glottis. This sudden increase in intrathoracic pressure is transmitted to the large veins of the upper torso with rupture of fine capillaries in the skin and conjunctiva. The condition is diagnosed in a child with petechial hemorrhages in the sclerae, conjunctiva, and the skin of the upper extremities and head. Because these same capillary hemorrhages occur in the brain due to the greatly increased intracranial venous pressure, significant transient neurologic dysfunction can occur due to suffusion into the brain. Although dramatic in presentation, the hemorrhages will resolve over several days and may require nothing more than ventilatory support[(150)]. The primary significance of traumatic asphyxia is its recognition and its implication that there has been a severe, blunt traumatic injury to the chest wall.

Emergency Room Thoracotomy in Children

Emergency room thoracotomy is rarely needed in adults and is perhaps never indicated in children except for cardiopulmonary arrest that does not respond to external cardiac massage and ventilatory support. More importantly, emergency room thoracotomy is rarely, if ever, successful[(129)]. On the other hand, urgent thoracotomy in an operating room environment may be necessary for:

1. Massive, progressive hemothorax with continuing blood loss greater than 100 mL/hr through a chest tube
2. Major cardiac wounds with associated hemopericardium
3. Impending disruption of the thoracic aorta
4. Tracheobronchial rupture with persistent air leak

While these life-threatening injuries are being diagnosed, aggressive resuscitation with the basic ABC's of resuscitation should continue to get the patient in reasonable condition for an urgent thoracotomy in the operating room.

POST-TRAUMATIC RESPIRATORY FAILURE

Following trauma, a variety of factors may be responsible for respiratory failure including CNS dysfunction, airway problems, direct pulmonary parenchymal diseases, and/or neuromuscular problems. In the multiple trauma patient, the etiology may be multifactorial. The most frequent intrathoracic injuries include: flail chest, multiple rib fractures, hemo-pneumothorax, lung contusion, lung laceration, cardiac wounds, and diaphragmatic rupture[(151)]. The lung may be directly damaged by thermal or chemical substances with resultant bronchospasm, bronchitis, pneumonia, or pulmonary edema[(152)]. Finally, acute respiratory failure may be secondary to head or spinal cord injury. In the former situation, there is loss of consciousness and control of breathing, as well as loss of protective reflexes, which may lead to aspiration pneumonia. With spinal cord injury, loss of respiratory muscle innervation leads to respiratory insufficiency[(153)]. Respiratory failure may also be caused by direct injury to the lung and chest. The latter may manifest one or two days following the injury.

The lung has a limited number of ways of reacting to injury so that the different types of acute injury result in similar pathophysiologic responses. The common denominator is injury at the alveolar-capillary interface with altered permeability and the resultant leakage of proteinaceous fluid from the intravascular space into the interstitium and subsequently, the alveolar spaces themselves. The entire spectrum of injury is referred to by many synonyms, including adult respiratory distress syndrome (ARDS), pulmonary insufficiency syndrome (PIS), shock lung, and post-traumatic pulmonary insufficiency[154–156]. The principal denominators in the injuries leading to ARDS appear to be systemic hypotension and extensive tissue damage. Indeed, many of the therapeutic maneuvers taken to counteract the consequences of trauma and injury may contribute to aggravate the respiratory failure that ensues.

The clinical evolution of ARDS is delayed for some time after the injury (12 to 24 hours). The major clinical criteria for ARDS are: a catastrophic preceding event, hypoxemia, decreased pulmonary compliance, chest radiographic findings of diffuse bilateral alveolar infiltrates, a decrease in the functional residual capacity (FRC), and normal cardiac function. Clinical signs and symptoms include tachypnea, dyspnea, and hypoxemia. Carbon dioxide tensions are low early on in the course of ARDS and maintained at the expense of minute ventilation that is several-fold times normal values. If the disease process is not reversed, arterial hypoxemia becomes refractory to treatment, arterial carbon dioxide tension increases, and inadequate tissue perfusion and death may ensue.

The mechanisms leading to ARDS remain uncertain. ARDS may result from direct injury to the lung or be one manifestation of multi-system organ failure in a patient with a systemic illness such as sepsis. Regardless of the etiology, it is proposed that the injury leads to the release of endogenous compounds that alter the capillary membrane permeability of the lung. Several mediators that are locally produced at the site of injury, if permitted to enter the circulation, can exert profound effects on the lung and produce the increased permeability, pulmonary vasoconstriction, and airway constriction seen in ARDS. Among the nociceptive mediators that cause increased permeability are the leukotrienes, platelet activating factors, and activated complement in granulocytes[157,158]. Despite the identification of several humoral factors, the ones responsible for ARDS have not yet been identified.

Aside from the primary injury itself, many of the therapeutic maneuvers required to treat an injured patient may aggravate the pathophysiologic responses of the lung. Infusion of saline, plasma, and blood products used to restore the effective circulating volume following injury may enhance fluid leakage into the alveoli. The use of high concentrations of oxygen in treating ARDS may produce oxygen toxicity[159] and collapse of the most severely ventilation-perfusion mismatched alveoli via resorption of oxygen (resorption atelectasis). Finally, mechanical ventilation may result in baro/volutrauma and further exacerbate the disease process.

ABDOMINAL TRAUMA IN INFANTS AND CHILDREN

Abdominal injuries in infants and children result primarily from blunt, rather than penetrating forces, and are frequently accompanied by skeletal and/or head injuries[160]. The basic principle of evaluation of a child with a possible abdominal injury is the determination of whether operative intervention is necessary for an acute abdomen or control of hemorrhage[161]. The extent of intra-abdominal injury in a child may be difficult to determine because of an inadequate history, a presumed inconsequential injury, or the frequent absence of external clinical signs of internal injury[162]. The external evidence of blunt trauma are often not impressive. The usual association with head, skeletal, and other multiple-system injuries may also mislead or misdirect the unwary physician away from the abdominal process. The high incidence of abdominal injury in the unconscious child makes evaluation even more difficult[163]. Deaths related to intra-abdominal injuries are caused by either early hemorrhage or later peritonitis. During the initial abdominal examination, top priority is given to the question of whether intra-abdominal hemorrhage is the most immediate threat to life.

Penetrating Wounds

Penetrating wounds are usually caused by gunshot or stabbings and may cause injury to any or all of the abdominal viscera and vessels. For practical purposes, all penetrating wounds of the abdomen require operative intervention[164]. The initial ABC's of hemodynamic resuscitation and airway management are performed before operative intervention. If the primary care facility is not prepared to handle small children, including pediatric anesthesia and intensive care, the initial resuscitation should be focused on early stabilization, wound dressing, and transfer to an appropriate pediatric hospital.

Penetrating injuries result in either bleeding or perforation of hollow viscera, and therefore, frequently give early evidence of peritoneal irritation and/or hemorrhagic shock. If such internal injuries are not obviously present, a significant injury may still exist and therefore surgical exploration is still indicated. Occasionally, penetrating wounds result in evisceration of abdominal contents. The organs should not be replaced into the abdomen nor be allowed to twist or kink. The abdominal contents should be covered with moist, sterile dressings until operative repair can take place.

Blunt Trauma

As in all major trauma in children, blunt injuries account for at least 90% of major abdominal injuries[150,165]. Hemorrhage, due to blunt trauma to the spleen or liver or disruption of major vessels, is the main focus of attention as it is the most immediate threat to life[166]. The spleen and liver are the most commonly injured solid organs in the child[167,168]. The organs may be so severely injured with massive damage that immediate exploration is indicated as soon as the ABC's have been managed. The pancreas and the duodenum may also be injured, usually by high-speed deceleration, as occurs when a child crashes against the handlebars of a bicycle[169–172]. This may also occur as a result of blunt trauma from child abuse. The hollow viscera may also be lacerated by deceleration injuries and torn at their sites of attachment such as the ligament of Treitz and the ileocecal-valve area[170,173]. Other abdominal organs that are frequently injured are the kidneys, ureters, bladder, and mesentery. Associated injuries may involve the ribs, pelvis, and spine.

Secondary Survey

The primary purpose of the abdominal examination in the traumatized child is not to obtain a specific diagnosis of organ injury, but to determine the next course in management. Assessment may be difficult because the children are often apprehensive, unwilling to cooperate, semicomatose or unconscious. Relatively trivial, or apparently insignificant trauma may be responsible for major intestinal or pancreatic injuries as well as injuries to the liver and spleen.

Diagnostic Studies

Following the physical examination, appropriate laboratory and imaging studies are obtained. The serum amylase level may be a useful adjunct to the physical examination as it is elevated in pancreatic injury, bowel ischemia, or transection of the proximal intestine[174]. Other important laboratory tests include the type and crossmatch, the complete blood count, the PT/PTT and urinalysis which may demonstrate hematuria or myoglobinuria.

Although plain films may be the initial tests ordered in the evaluation of abdominal injuries, they are seldom helpful[175]. The most accurate diagnostic tools (aside from serial physical examination) are radionuclide scans, CT scans with contrast enhancement[176], intravenous pyelogram (IVP) with cystogram and urethrogram, and peritoneal lavage[177].

The majority of liver and spleen injuries can be diagnosed with a radionuclide scan[178,179]. The technique has the advantage of being noninvasive and reasonably rapid. It can be performed at the bedside in the intensive care unit.

CT scanning is also useful to document the extent of solid organ injury. CT scans can also be used to image the pancreas and kidney, as well as assess for the presence of free blood, fluid, and air in the abdomen[175]. In many centers, the abdominal CT scan has replaced the IVP for the evaluation of renal trauma. Problems with the CT scan include radiation exposure, transport of the seriously injured patient from the intensive care unit, and difficulty in patient monitoring while in the scanner.

The IVP, cystogram, and urethrogram are time-honored tools for evaluating genitourinary trauma. Rather than expose all children with renal trauma to the risk of a potentially serious reaction to the contrast agent, unnecessary radiation, and a delay in the diagnosis of other injuries, many recommend the use of the IVP only under certain circumstances:

1. When the urinalysis demonstrates gross hematuria with physical evidence of renal injury
2. If renal artery injury is suspected[180,181]

Finally, there is peritoneal lavage. Peritoneal lavage is the traditional standard for the intra-abdominal investigation for the presence of hemorrhage[182]. In most centers where radionuclide scanning or CT are used to evaluate abdominal trauma, peritoneal lavage is rarely used. However, it is still a useful test for assessing intra-abdominal bleeding and the need for surgical exploration of the abdomen. Because lavage irritates the peritoneum for 24 to 48 hours, it may obscure subsequent abdominal evaluation.

With the current trend of nonoperative treatment for intra-abdominal bleeding of moderate degree, fewer indications for peritoneal lavage are accepted in many regional pediatric trauma centers. Peritoneal lavage is no longer used to assess whether patients with hepatic and splenic injuries require surgical intervention. In this setting, the presence of blood used to be an indication for surgical intervention. The decision to operate is no longer based on the presence of intraperitoneal blood, but rather the ongoing transfusion requirements and serial abdominal examinations.

Peritoneal lavage may be carried out by the surgeon in the operating room when a child requires an operation (and general anesthesia) for another organ system injury. Because general anesthesia will make further examination of the abdomen practically impossible, peritoneal lavage may be used in this setting as a test to support an indication for exploration of the abdomen under the same general anesthetic.

Peritoneal lavage is performed by inserting a pediatric-sized peritoneal dialysis catheter under direct vision through the lower abdominal midline with infusion of 10 mL/kg of crystalloid solution (normal saline or Ringer's lactate) into the abdominal cavity. A simple peritoneal tap is no longer considered adequate for the evaluation of intra-abdominal bleeding. The fluid is left in place for 5 to 10 minutes. Peritoneal lavage is considered abnormal if the effluent obtained has greater than 100 red blood cells/mm^3.

Management

The diagnosis of specific intra-abdominal injuries is often difficult on initial examination and an aggressive diagnostic approach based upon an established protocol is mandatory. Meticulous physical examination, repeated as often as necessary, with maintenance of a high index of suspicion for abdominal injury is the basic guideline for successful treatment of blunt trauma to the abdomen. If the abdominal injuries result in significant blood loss that prevent successful re-establishment or maintenance of vital functions and indicate ongoing blood loss, the child should be taken immediately to the operating room for urgent laparotomy and resuscitation.

Experience in several children's trauma centers in the United States and Canada in the past decade has documented the remarkable observation that serious injuries to the spleen and liver may frequently be self-limiting and the child may only need volume replacement with crystalloid or blood without operative intervention[183–187]. The nonoperative treatment of proven injuries to the liver and spleen should be carried out in tertiary care facilities by pediatric specialists in an intensive care environment. It should never be attempted in community hospital environments because of the possibility of rapid deterioration. Observation is only indicated in patients that respond to initial volume resuscitation and remain hemodynamically stable. Progressive deterioration of cardiovascular function is a sign of ongoing blood loss and the need for surgical intervention.

HEAD TRAUMA

Significant head trauma (see also Chapter 24) occurs in 50% of children who have sustained blunt trauma[(188)]. More significantly, virtually all fatalities from trauma result from significant CNS injury. Aggressive management has produced survivors with good recovery without major motor or intellectual deficits[(189)]. This contrasts with the adult experience in which profound functional loss occurs in the majority of survivors[(190,191)].

Initial Management

Resuscitation of the head-injured patient is initially directed toward preserving or restoring cardiorespiratory functioning. Initial fluid resuscitation is carried out to restore cardiovascular function. However, overhydration may result in cerebral edema and increased ICP. Once effective circulating blood volume is restored, fluids should be minimized and should include only isotonic crystalloid. While young children are prone to hypoglycemia due to decreased glycogen stores, low serum glucose in the immediate trauma setting is exceedingly rare. Hyperglycemia may be detrimental during periods of relative cellular hypoxia due to the resultant shift to anaerobic metabolism and the production of greater amounts of intracellular lactate. As such, frequent monitoring of serum glucose is indicated in the trauma setting without the administration of glucose containing IV fluids. A similar plan should be followed in the setting of spinal cord injury (see below).

The primary damage to the CNS that occurs at the moment of injury is not reversible by any therapeutic intervention. Effective management of head injury depends on the prevention of the secondary insults of hypoxia and ischemia as well as prevention of progressive increases in intracranial pressure. Hypoxia may result from respiratory insufficiency or ischemic hypoxia from reduced cerebral blood flow secondary to cerebral edema, mass lesion, increased intracranial pressure, or systemic hypotension. Aggressive treatment of associated injuries is indicated to prevent cardiovascular, pulmonary, renal, or metabolic disturbances that may impede neurologic recovery.

Although epidural and subdural hematomas occur in children, the primary cause of mortality in children with head injury is diffuse cerebral swelling. This is manifested by obliteration of the intracranial CSF spaces and venous congestion. Several different mechanisms of injury may lead to CNS injury and resultant cerebral edema. "Coup" or "contrecoup" injuries cause contusions, lacerations, and multifocal parenchymal hematomas in children due to the vulnerability of the child's brain to the accelerative and decelerative forces compressing the brain against bony prominences and the calvarial walls. Shear forces from rapid rotary changes may produce deep parenchymal hemorrhages or edema within the brain[(192,193)]. In children who lose consciousness immediately at the time of injury, the injury pattern is one of diffuse injury involving the white matter of both cerebral hemispheres, periventricular area, midbrain, and pons. The presence of a lucid period following the injury suggests diffuse brain swelling or intracranial hematoma as the cause of the progressive decrease in mental status. Intracranial hematoma is rare in children. Contusions and lacerations of the brain, which are much more common, generally occur on the tips of the temporal lobes and the undersurface of the frontal lobes. Subdural or epidural hematomas, intracranial bleeding, or other intracranial pathology, such as contusion or lacerations, in the absence of a history of significant trauma such as a motor vehicle injury should be considered child abuse (refer to the heading "Child Abuse" in this chapter)[(194)]. Abuse remains the most common cause of serious head injury in children less than 1 year of age[(194)].

Structural damage to the calvarium may also occur associated with closed head injury. Basilar skull fractures are diagnosed on the basis of physical examination. "Raccoon eyes" or circumscribed unilateral or bilateral periorbital ecchymoses are due to intraorbital bleeding from fractures of the roof of the orbits. Bleeding from the ear represents a fracture through the lateral portion of the temporal bones. Battle's sign, an area of ecchymoses behind the pinna, represents blood dissecting to the skin from a mastoid fracture and usually presents 12 to 24 hours after an injury. Drainage of CSF through the nose or ear is a manifestation of meningeal disruption at the site of a basilar fracture and carries the risk of meningitis. Despite the risk of infection, prophylactic use of antibiotics is not recommend since this only tends to select out for resistant organisms[(195)]. However, an immediate evaluation and institution of antibiotic therapy is indicated if signs suggestive of infection are noted.

A rapid, but complete, neurologic examination provides an indication of the nature of the cerebral injury and establishes a baseline for determining patient improvement or deterioration. The Glasgow Coma Scale is invaluable for this purpose. The parameters of this scale are based on eye opening, motor response, and verbal response **(Table 43.6).** Scores of eight or less are suggestive of severe injury and indicate the need for immediate airway support and the invasive monitoring and treatment of ICP. Other components of the neurologic examination include: (a) pupillary size and reaction to light, (b) corneal reflex, (c) oculomotor-vestibular reflexes, (d) presence or absence of a gag response, (e) spontaneous respiration and respiratory pattern, and (f) spontaneous movement of the extremities including tone, reflexes, and abnormal posture. During trauma resuscitation, the oculovestibular response rather than the oculocephalic response is advised because it is inadvisable to rotate from side-to-side the head of a patient with potential cervical injury.

The function of the cranial nerves reflects the integrity of the brainstem and the afferent and efferent pathways along the cranial nerves. Examination of the eyes is one of the most critical parts of the neurologic examination in the comatose patient. The size and reactivity of the pupils as well as the corneal reflex tests cranial nerves II, III, V, and VII. A unilateral, fixed dilated pupil is one sign of herniation of the uncus through the tentorium cerebelli with compression of the third cranial nerve. Midbrain lesions produce pupils that are fixed in midposition. Lesions in the pons are associated with pinpoint, minimally reactive pupils. Various drugs can also produce the gamut of pupillary responses from fixed to dilated. The barbiturates, opioids, and benzodiazepines produce pinpoint pupils while anticholinergic agents such as atropine may result in large, minimally reactive pupils.

A useful test of brainstem function is the oculovestibular reflex (e.g., cold calorics). This test focuses on peripheral vestibular apparatus to the eighth nerve nucleus, medial longitudinal fasciculus, extraocular motor nuclei, and peripheral extraocular nerves and muscles. The test is performed by the instillation of cold water into the ear canal. It should not be performed unless the tympanic membrane is intact. In the awake patient, oculovestibular testing with cold water will produce nystagmus with the fast component away from the side that is irrigated. Since the rapid component of nystagmus is controlled by cortical function, it is absent in patients with altered mental status. As such, only the slow component operates resulting in tonic deviation of the eyes toward the side that is irrigated with cold water. An opposite response occurs with warm water.

Radiology

Following initial stabilization and resuscitation, CT scanning is the primary, and usually, the only diagnostic procedure performed in children with severe head injury. On the other hand, "mild head trauma" is an extremely common pediatric complaint and accounts for numerous visits to the emergency room. The need for radiologic investigation such as skull films and CT imaging has been confusing. The majority of patients with "mild head injury" do not develop intracranial pathology even if the injury results in skull fractures. Leonidas, et. al.[196] reviewed 354 pediatric skull films following head trauma and found a 4.2% incidence of fractures. With the exception of one child with a depressed skull fracture, treatment was not altered by detection of a fracture. Their criteria for skull films after head trauma are listed in **Table 43.7.**

Table 43.7. Criteria for Skull Films after Head Trauma

1.	Age less than 1 year
2.	Loss of consciousness for 3 minutes
3.	Skull penetration
4.	Previous craniotomy with shunt in place
5.	Palpable scalp hematoma
6.	Skull depression
7.	CSF from nose or ear
8.	Blood in middle ear
9.	Battle's sign
10.	Raccoon's eyes
11.	Lethargy, coma, stupor
12.	Focal neurologic signs

CT scanning is one of the most effective tools to diagnose both skull and brain injuries[197,198]. Adequate immobilization of the head is mandatory to avoid motion artifacts that may obscure intracranial pathology. In children or combative patients this may require sedation or general anesthesia. Therefore the decision must be made whether sedation is appropriate and safe or whether endotracheal intubation and control of the airway is indicated. The CT scan should be obtained in all patients with a depressed level of consciousness or any focal neurologic deficit. It is effective in demonstrating epidural or subdural hematoma and intracerebral trauma such as contusions, intracerebral hematoma, subarachnoid and intraventricular hemorrhage, cerebral swelling, pneumocephalus, and cerebral edema with midline shift. Based on the density, the CT scan may differentiate between hemorrhage, edema, infarct, foreign body, etc.

Intracranial Pressure (ICP) Management

Following completion of the CT scan, consideration should be given to the placement of an intracranial pressure monitoring system. All trauma patients with a Glasgow Coma Scale score of 8 or less should be monitored[120]. Unfortunately, there is no universal agreement regarding the most appropriate method for measuring ICP. The most commonly used devices include an intraventricular catheter, a subarachnoid bolt screw, and most recently, a fiberoptic device[199–203]. With these three devices, the catheter tip is placed in the ventricle, the subarachnoid space, or the parenchyma, respectively. All three are placed through a hole that is drilled in the skull. The intraventricular catheter is inserted directly into the lateral ventricle. The bolt is screwed into position with its tip lying 1 to 2 mm below the surface of the dura into the subarachnoid space. The subarachnoid bolt may be difficult or impossible to place in newborns and small infants. In these patients, the skull is thin, making it difficult to secure the device. A major advantage of the intraventricular drain, despite its higher complication rate (hemorrhage and infection) is the ability to drain CSF, which can immediately lower intracranial pressure. Unfortunately, in the worst cases when the ventricles are narrowed by massive edema, there is little CSF available for removal and placement of the intraventricular catheter is technically quite difficult. Because of the limitations with both the intraventricular catheter and the subarachnoid bolt, many institutions have switched to the intraparenchymal fiberoptic catheter to measure ICP.

The measurement and subsequent control of ICP is a crucial aspect in management of patients with closed head injury[204–206]. A thorough discussion of the pathophysiology, monitoring, and therapy of intracranial hypertension is presented in Chapters 18, 19, 20, and 24.

Post-Traumatic Seizures

Post-traumatic seizures may be divided into those occurring early on (less than 3 days) after the injury and those that persist or occur more than a week after the injury. Early onset seizures are relatively frequent in the pediatric population and generally do not require long term therapy. Due to the detrimental effects of seizures on cerebral blood flow and ICP, anticonvulsant agents are generally recommended for patients that develop early seizures even if they are brief and self-limited. The majority of these patients will have normal EEG's and do not require long term anticonvulsant therapy.

Late post-traumatic epilepsy is defined as one or more seizures occurring at least 1 week after head injury without any other obvious cause. The overall incidence is approximately 7 to 10% in most studies[207,208]. The relatively high incidence of post-traumatic seizures (both early and late) has led to the suggestion for the use of prophylactic anticonvulsants in head injury patients. The rationale is based on experimental work showing that the prophylactic administration of anticonvulsants has a suppressive effect on the development of an epileptogenic focus[208]. However, Young, et. al.[209] in a double-blinded, prospective study, demonstrated that phenytoin administration soon after head injury and continued for 15 months did not decrease the incidence of post-traumatic seizures when compared with placebo. Prophylactic anticonvulsant therapy does not seem warranted. However, if seizures occur, they should be treated aggressively with anticonvulsants. Seizures result in increased local metabolic requirements and a secondary increase in cerebral blood flow, cerebral blood volume, and ICP. Initial therapy includes a benzodiazepine (lorazepam 0.05 mg/kg) followed by either phenobarbital (20 to 30 mg/kg) and/or phenytoin (20 mg/kg) for long term treatment. While phenobarbital is generally effective, its sedative effects may make ongoing neurologic examination more difficult. Therefore, phenytoin is usually chosen as the first line drug. If the patient is receiving neuromuscular blocking agents for a protracted period of time, continuous EEG monitoring is recommended.

ACUTE SPINAL CORD INJURY

Acute spinal cord injury (see Chapter 24) occurs with an incidence of approximately 40 to 50 cases per million population in the United States or approximately 11,000 new cases per year[210–214]. Of these, 1 to 5% occur in children less than 15 years of age[215,216]. The cervical region is the most commonly injured part of the spine. The mechanism of injury varies according to the age group. In the first decade of life, motor vehicle trauma is the most common cause. In patients 11 to 15 years of age, the etiology is split equally between sports/recreational injuries and motor vehicular accidents. There is also an increased number of injuries related to gunshot wounds. The level of injury also varies according to the age of the patient. High cervical lesions (C_{1-3}) are more common in infants and toddlers while injury generally occurs at the C_{4-7} level in adolescents and adults.

Approximately 50% of the injured die before they reach the hospital or during their acute hospitalization. Unfortunately, the vast majority of survivors are severely disabled with permanent or complete paralysis. Spinal cord injuries are especially frustrating and frightening because emergency medical care and effective resuscitation preserve life, while virtually nothing can be done to restore lost function[217–219].

Pathophysiology

Following traumatic injury to the cord, small flame hemorrhages on the gray matter and pia mater are observed[220,221]. Over the next minutes, the hemorrhages seen in the gray matter spread to the white matter. Inflammatory cells, including polymorphonuclear leukocytes and fibroblasts increase dramatically in the cord tissue and herald various degrees of cellular necrosis. The release of lysosomal enzymes following spinal cord injury has been documented and may play a role in the pathogenesis of traumatic paralysis[222].

One of the most critical elements in the evolution of the biochemical and morphologic alterations following spinal cord trauma is the vascular blood flow to the cord[223,224]. As with the brain, spinal cord injury results in loss of autoregulation and changes in the arterial venous blood flow patterns of the cord. Decreased perfusion caused by narrowing or occlusion of cord microvessels produces tissue ischemia, anaerobic metabolism, accumulation of lactate, and breakdown of the adenosine triphosphate (ATP)-dependent sodium-potassium pump. Cellular damage to the sodium-potassium membrane transport can lead to tissue edema and necrosis[225]. The injury leads to a series of biochemical processes involving membrane phospholipid breakdown and the production of circulating prostaglandins along with stimulation of adenosine diphosphate (ADP). This produces platelet aggregation, thromboxane A_2 release, vasospasm and vasoconstriction, which may lead to further ischemia and tissue necrosis.

Management

Proper care of the potentially unstable spine begins at the scene of the injury and continues until the spine has been proven stable. All comatose patients and/or those with multiple trauma should be treated as though spinal cord injury has occurred. Gentle, manual traction to stabilize the neck and establish an airway is crucial. The soft cervical collars provide no significant protection[226]. In-line traction, using 5 lbs. of force and sandbags provides the best initial immobilization and cervical spine stabilization. Avoidance of maneuvers that may cause further damage are particularly important during airway manipulation and endotracheal intubation (see above).

Once the spine and cord have been protected from further damage, the patient must be resuscitated and injuries treated as indicated. With high thoracic or cervical injuries, a state of "spinal shock" occurs resulting from absent sympathetic tone distal to the level of injury. This results in significant hypotension due to the sudden decrease in systemic vasular resistance. The patient is usually hypotensive, bradycardic, and hypothermic. This results in multiple management problems. Moving and/or tilting a patient in this condition can be hazardous inasmuch as the normal compensatory mechanisms for postural changes are lost. If the problem is not suspected and recognized, massive fluid overload can occur from "knee-jerk" treatment of an assumed hypovolemic patient. Treatment should include volume resuscitation to deal with fluid/blood loss related to other injuries with the use of a direct acting vasoconstrictor such as phenylephrine to increase systemic vascular resistance.

The patient with a cervical spinal cord lesion is at risk to develop respiratory failure because of paralysis of some or all of the muscles of respiration. Even if diaphragmatic function is intact, fatigue and inability to clear secretions may occur due to the paralysis of abdominal and intercostal musculature with an inability to cough. This may result in progressive atelectasis with hypoxia and hypercapnia.

Because these patients have their head and neck stabilized and immobilized, the normal extension and flexion maneuvers involved in endotracheal intubation will not be possible. In the absence of associated closed head trauma, awake intubation or fiberoptic intubation may be possible in older, cooperative patients. In those unable or unwilling to cooperate, oral endotracheal intubation following general anesthesia and muscle paralysis with thiopental and succinylcholine paralysis should be used. The risk of succinylcholine-induced massive hyperkalemia begins three days after injury and may persist indefinitely following injury if there is residual paralysis.

The denervated bladder must be drained. Continuous catheter drainage is safest for the first few days following injury. Ileus and acute gastric distention are common and gastric decompression with a naso/orogastric tube is indicated.

Radiology

There is considerable confusion regarding the incidence of radiologic abnormalities in children with spinal cord injury. Several authors have emphasized the total absence of radiographic abnormalities in most cases of traumatic spinal cord injury in children[228,229]. This is referred to as SCIWORA or spinal cord injury without radiographic abnormality. This is the result of the increased laxity of ligaments in younger patients allowing for stretching of the vertebral column and spinal cord distraction without bony damage.

Initially, a cross-table lateral view of the spine is taken with the film just lateral to one shoulder with both shoulders depressed so that the entire cervical spine to the top of T_1 is visible. This is followed by an anterio-posterior film. The addition of oblique views do not significantly increase the sensitivity of x-ray evaluation of the cervical spine. CT scans greatly facilitate the evaluation of spinal trauma and do not require risky positioning for tomography, myelography, etc.[228]. Additionally, the CT scan provides a better view of the first two cervical vertebrae including the odontoid process.

The propensity for cervical injury and the confusion concerning radiologic examination in children may be due to the fact that the child's spinal canal can be stretched two inches while the cervical cord can be pulled only one-fourth of an inch before rupturing[230]. Further damage to the cord may be caused by bony fragments, an extruded disc, a subluxated vertebral body, or vertebral body fracture fragments.

An important, noninvasive tool that may be both diagnostic and prognostic is somatosensory-evoked potentials (SEP) monitoring[231]. The technique involves stimulation of a peripheral afferent sensory nerve with a reading obtained from a contralateral somatosensory cortex from a scalp electrode. Patients with a complete cord lesion have an absent SEP. The presence or return of the SEP may be an indication of improved prognosis and may precede clinical improvement.

Spinal Cord Resuscitation

The initial treatment of the multiple trauma patient with a spinal cord injury includes the usual airway management and cardiovascular resuscitation. Once the ABC's have been completed, there may be some role for pharmacologic agents to reverse or prevent further spinal cord injury.

Clinical treatments for acute spinal cord injury have not proven uniformly successful. However, a recent randomized trial showed a benefit to early administration of methylprednisolone[232]. Methylprednisolone was administered as a bolus dose of 30 mg/kg followed by an infusion of 5.4 mg/kg/hour for 23 hours. Improvement in eventual neurologic outcome occurred only in patients in whom the methylprednisolone was administered within eight hours of the injury. Although this trial excluded patients less than 13 years old, there seems good reason to adopt the practice[233]. With such therapy, monitoring and control of blood glucose is recommended as well as prophylaxis for peptic ulcer formation.

Other therapies such as osmotic diuretics[234] to decrease secondary edema and low-molecular-weight dextran to improve microcirculatory flow have not been shown to be effective. Hyperbaric oxygen, by increasing available oxygen to the ischemic cord, may be of value in acute compression injuries although its use has been limited in clinical practice. Finally, success has been reported with the use of spinal cord cooling within the first four hours of an injury[235,236]. This therapeutic approach involves the local perfusion of the spinal cord with large quantities of iced solutions to lower the cord temperature to 10° C or less. The basis for this therapy is that hypothermia lowers the metabolic and oxygen needs and thereby improves the local microcirculation and prevents metabolic acidosis. There are multiple technical problems involved with the technique including how to deliver the iced solution, how long the solution should be used, and in what clinical situations it should be started.

Sequelae of Spinal Cord Injury

Respiratory failure remains a major cause of mortality and morbidity in patients suffering from spinal cord injury. Following high cervical lesions, there is a loss of expiratory muscle control with loss of intercostal and abdominal innervation. Ventilation continues via innervation of the diaphragm (C_{3-5}) and accessory muscles (cranial nerve XI). The ability to cough is absent and even a simple upper respiratory tract infection can lead to progressive respiratory failure. Immediate supportive and therapeutic measures may include postural drainage, inhalation therapy, and antibiotics. Higher lesions (above C_{4-5}) require permanent mechanical ventilation.

Urinary tract infection is the other major cause of mortality in spinal cord-injured patients. As such, the prevention of urologic complications remains one of the most important objectives in successful rehabilitation. Intermittent catheterization should be started as early as possible[237]. Initial problems with incontinence between catheterizations may be the result of bladder spasm following the initial injury and may respond to antispasmodic agents. The goal of therapy is to prevent overdistention of the bladder with high residual volumes which can lead to ureteral reflux and an increased risk of infection.

The normal microbial inhabitants of the skin, colon, and vagina are the usual pathogens of infection. The common portal of entry is the external urethra[237]. Reinfection and relapse are common. Reinfection is usually due to high residual volume, poor perineal care, and poor catheter technique whereas relapse is most common with stones and kidney infections.

Following spinal cord injury, prolonged immobility leads to changes in calcium metabolism. Urolithiasis may occur and is attributed to immobility, hypercalciuria, hypercalcemia, urinary stasis, high urine pH, and urinary tract infection with urea-splitting organisms[239].

Hypercalcemia may also occur in the setting of immobilization following a spinal cord injury[240]. Its manifestations include vomiting, polydipsia, polyuria, anorexia, nausea, malaise, and listlessness. These symptoms may lead to the diagnosis of depression or an acute surgical abdomen. Hypercalcemia can have significant deleterious effects on renal function leading to decreased creatinine clearance, especially if serum calcium is greater than 12 mg%. Progressive nephrocalcinosis may lead to renal failure. Serum calcium levels this high can lead to irreversible kidney damage, especially if they persist for more than 6 months. Acute therapy includes furosemide and saline to abruptly lower serum calcium followed by chronic therapy with oral phosphates to decrease gastrointestinal calcium absorption.

CHILD ABUSE

The incidence of abuse is estimated at six to ten cases per 1000 population[241] with death occurring in approximately 5 to 20% of victims[241,242]. Most patients are less than 5 years of age with the majority being less than 2 years old. The antecedents of child abuse can be divided into risk factors pertaining to the parent or the child **(Table 43.8).**

The clinical signs of child abuse take many forms including bruises, welts, lacerations, abdominal injuries, burns, bone fractures, skull fractures, subdural hematoma, and venereal diseases[242]. Kempe, et al.[243] using these signs and symptoms, coined the phrase "the battered child syndrome." In 1974, Caffey[244] pointed out that the majority of abused infants presented without external evidence or history of trauma. He coined the phrase "infantile whiplash shaking syndrome" to describe a number of patients with intracranial and intraocular hemorrhages in the absence of external trauma to the head or fracture of the calvaria. These "shaking" injuries were thought to be the result of bleeding from the easily torn bridging veins of the infant's meninges. The infant's head and blood vessels are particularly vulnerable to shaking and whiplash because of: a relatively large head and weak neck muscles; the abundance of unmyelinated brain tissue which permits excessive stretching of the brain and vessels; and the increased pliability of the skull as compared to the rigidly fixed internal soft tissue structures such as the falx cerebri.

Distinguishing between deliberately inflicted and accidentally occurring trauma is not easy as both may produce similar types of injury[245,246]. Clues may be obtained from the history and the physical examination. Parents often relate a story that does not explain the clinical findings or change the story frequently during the initial hospital visit.

Table 43.8. Antecedents of Child Abuse

Parental Risk Factors:
1. Unwanted pregnancy
2. Disturbed family relationships
3. Parent who was abused
4. Poor self-esteem
5. Young age
6. Alcohol/drug problems
Child Risk Factors:
1. Low birth weight/premature
2. Recurrent or chronically ill
3. Hyperactive or aggressive child

The parents may appear reluctant to give information or they may be inconsistent about the dates of the injury (see below). A history of low birth weight or complicated neonatal course or a maternal illness leading to prolonged separation from the infant may be a clue to child abuse[247,248]. On physical examination, there may be signs of general neglect such as poor skin hygiene, malnutrition, or failure to thrive. There may be evidence of old, healed lesions such as burns (cigarettes, forced contact with heating devices such as radiators, hot plates), scalds (forced immersion, particularly buttocks and perineum), abrasions, and soft tissue swellings. Particular attention should also be directed at evidence of sexual abuse such as condylomata, perianal and genital hematoma, venereal disease (oral and genital), pain in anogenital area, and pregnancy.

The physical examination should document growth parameters, and it should include description of soft tissue injuries as well as photographs of all injuries. Estimation of the age of cutaneous contusions on an abused child is usually more often requested of the pediatrician and the intensivist than the pathologist. Wilson's summary[249] **(Table 43.9)** is an invaluable aid. The number of contusions should be enumerated and the pattern, shape, color, location, and size measured and catalogued. Color photographs are essential in further documenting the nature of these lesions.

The laboratory investigation may be essential in documenting and discerning the etiology of the child's problem. A hematocrit, platelet count, and coagulation profile should be obtained to rule out a bleeding diathesis. Electrolytes, blood urea nitrogen, liver function tests, and blood for toxicology will help establish or rule out causes of coma such as Reye's syndrome, renal failure, and poisoning. Additionally, urine is obtained for toxicology and evidence of renal trauma. Oral, genital, and anal cultures should be obtained for evidence of venereal disease. Finally, radiographic studies are mandatory. Studies should include posteroanterior and lateral skull and chest films (rib fractures), complete skeletal survey including hands, long bones, fingers, and toes, and when applicable, a CT scan.

Radiographic manifestation of child abuse include new and old injuries. Common findings include subperiosteal hemorrhages, epiphyseal separations, periosteal shearings, metaphyseal fragmentations, previously healed periosteal calcifications, and shearing of the metaphysis[250,251]. The CT scan is particularly important in assessing the child with an altered level of consciousness. Evidence of structural intracranial damage such as intracranial hemorrhage, subdural or epidural hematoma, contusions, or cerebral edema in the absence of major known trauma is diagnostic of child abuse. This view is supported by Billmire and Myers[194] and Helfer et al.[246] who reported that children who suffered accidental trauma such as falling from bed rarely, if ever, had intracranial injury worse than a concussion.

Table 43.9. Relationship Between Color and Age of Contusions*

Color	*Age*
Reddish-blue or purple	immediate/less than 24 hours
Blue-purple	1–5 days
Green	5–7 days
Yellow	7–10 days
Brown	10–14 days
Resolution	2–4 weeks

**Modified from Wilson EF. Estimation of the age of cutaneous contusion in child abuse (Pediatrics 1977;60:750).*

The diagnosis of child abuse is uncomfortable and even experienced physicians may be reluctant to entertain the possibility. Child abuse often becomes a diagnosis of exclusion and it is thought of only after more "acceptable" diagnoses are ruled out. Similarly, some[252] think that "the diagnosis of abuse demands absolute certainty to avoid conviction of innocent parents and unwarranted removal of children from their homes". However, the physician must be a patient advocate and the possibility of abuse must be investigated before children are put back in the home as well as to protect siblings who are still in the home. The investigation of abuse should be considered in the initial management plan. The "burden of proof" rests not on the physician, but on the local protective and law enforcement agencies. Involvement of social service and the state welfare departments allows the intensive care unit staff to attend to the child's medical problems while hospital and state authorities deal with the issues surrounding the possible abuse. The parents should be informed of the suspicions in such a way that antagonism between the medical team and the family is minimized.

Finally, one must be prepared to go to court to testify. Many physicians are intimidated by the adversarial nature of the legal system. Nevertheless, the physician's knowledgeable participation may be critical to the appropriate disposition of a child abuse case. The following tips may be helpful in carrying out testimonial responsibilities:

1. Know the details of the case. Review the medical record carefully and bring it (and your own summary note) with you to court.
2. Do not be intimidated. One of the attorneys will try to "rattle you", usually during the review of your credentials, perhaps calling you "Mister" rather than "Doctor." Do not take this personally; rather be firm and to the point. Most judges will not permit any significant harassment of a professional witness.
3. Take your time. Speak clearly and slowly and address the jury. It is useful to use a chalkboard or flip pad to diagram complex ideas in the courtroom.
4. Complex questions require complex answers. If you are unsure of what a question means, ask the lawyer to clarify it. If an attorney asks a complex question and demands a simple "Yes" or "No" response, it is your duty to state that the question cannot be appropriately answered that way. In our experience, the judge will inevitably allow a more comprehensive response.
5. Maintain a neutral position. Your responsibility is to tell the truth, not to take sides.
6. Make use of pretrial depositions. You have a right to review the process and content of your testimony as well

as that of other expert witnesses. Consult with the hospital's legal department to review testimony and the courtroom process.

References

1. "National Safety Council". Accident Facts. Chicago, National Safety Council, 1983.
2. Gallagher S, Finison K, Guyer B, et al. The incidence of injuries among 87,000 Massachusetts children and adolescents: results of the 1980–81 statewide childhood injury prevention program surveillance system. Am J Public Health 1984;74:1340.
3. Baker SP, O'Neil B, Karpf RS. The injury fact book. Lexington, MA: Lexington Books, 1984.
4. Division of Injury Control Centers for Disease Control. Childhood injuries in the United States. Am J Dis Child 1990;144:627.
5. Haller JA, Shorter N, Miller D, et al. Organization and function of a regional pediatric trauma center: does a system of management improve outcome? J Trauma 1983;23:691.
6. Haller JAJ, Buck JR. Trauma in the child: regional pediatric centers for life-threatening injuries. Progr Crit Care Med 1984;1:208.
7. Ead HW, Green JH, Neil E. A comparison of the effects of pulsatile and non-pulsatile flow through the carotid sinus on the reflexogenic activity of the sinus baroreceptors in the cat. J Physiol (Lond) 1952;118:509.
8. Gann DS. Endocrine control of plasma protein and volume. Surg Clin North Am 1976;56:1135.
9. Kircheim HR. Systemic arterial baroreceptor reflexes. Physiol Rev 1976;56:100.
10. Korner PI. Integrative neural cardiovascular control. Physiol Rev 1971; 51:312.
11. Mancia G, Donald DE, Sheppard JT. Inhibition of adrenergic outflow to peripheral blood vessels by vagal afferents from the cardiopulmonary region in the dog. Circ Res 1973;33:713.
12. Iggo A. Peripheral and spinal pain mechanisms and their modulation. In: Bonica JJ, Albe-Fassard DG, eds. Advances in pain research and therapy. New York: Raven Press, 1976:381.
13. Nashold BS, Ostadhl RH. Dorsal root entry zone lesions for pain relief. J Neurosurg 1979;51:59.
14. Wall PD, Dubner R. Somatosensory pathways. Am Rev Physiol 1972; 34:315.
15. Sato A, Schmidt RF. Somatosympathetic reflexes: afferent fibers, central pathways, discharge characteristics. Physiol Rev 1973;53:916.
16. Mayer DJ, Wolfe TL, Akil H, et al. Analgesia from electrical stimulation in the brainstem of the rat. Science 1971;174:1351.
17. Herz A, Albus K, Metys J, Schubert P, et al. On the central sites for the antinociceptive action of morphine and fentanyl. Neuropediatrics 1970;9:539.
18. Mayer SE. Neurohumoral transmission and the autonomic nervous system. In: Gilman AG, Goodman LS, Gilman A, eds. The pharmacological basis of therapeutics. New York: Macmillan, 1980.
19. Sarnoff SJ, Mitchell JH. The control of the function of the heart. In: Hamilton WF, Dow P, eds. Handbook of Physiology. Vol. II, Section 2, Circulation. Washington, DC: American Physiological Society, 1962.
20. Alexander RS. Venomotor tone in hemorrhage and shock. Circ Res 1955;3:181.
21. Green HO, Rapela CE, Conrad MC. Resistance (conductance) and capacitance phenomena in terminal vascular beds. In: Hamilton WF, Dow P, eds. Handbook of Physiology. Vol. II, Section. 2, Circulation. Washington, DC: American Physiological Society, 1963:935.
22. Landis EM, Pappenheimer JR. Exchange of substances through the capillary walls. In: Hamilton WF, Dow P, eds. Handbook of Physiology. Vol. II, Section 2, Circulation. Washington, DC: American Physiological Society, 1963:961.
23. Chien S. Role of sympathetic nervous system in hemorrhage. Physiol Rev 1967;47:214.
24. Chien S. Role of sympathetic nervous system in surviving acute hemorrhage. Am J Physiol 1964;26:21.
25. Shoemaker WC. Pathophysiology and therapy of shock syndromes. In: Shoemaker WC, Thompson WL, Holbrook PR, eds. Textbook of critical care. Philadelphia: WB Saunders, 1984:52.
26. Boyd DR, Mansberger ARJ. Serum water and osmolal changes in hemorrhagic shock: an experimental and clinical study. Am Surg 1968;34:744.
27. Carey LC, Lowery BD, Cloutier CT. Blood sugar and insulin response of humans in shock. Ann Surg 1970;172:342.
28. Jarhult J, Hillman J, Mellander S. Circulatory effects evoked by "physiological" increases of arterial osmolality. Acta Physiol Scand 1975;93:129.
29. Gann DS, Baertschi AJ, Ward DG, et al. Homeostasis of blood volume through hemodynamic control of ACTH and cortisol. In: James V, ed. Medica International Congress Series No.402, Endocrinology, Amsterdam: Excerpta Medica, Vol. I. 1976:245.
30. Young JB, Landsberg L. Catecholamines and intermediary metabolism. Clin Endocrinol Metab 1977;6:599.
31. Edwards AV. The glycogenolytic response to stimulation of the splanchnic nerves in adrenalectomized calves, sheep, dogs, cats and pigs. J Physiol (Lond) 1971;213:741.
32. Lautt WW, Cote MG. The effect of 6-hydroxydopamine-induced hepatic sympathectomy on the early hyperglycemic response to surgical trauma under anesthesia. J Trauma 1977;17:270.
33. Levi J, Coburn J, Kleeman CR. Mechanism of the antidiuretic effect of beta-adrenergic stimulation in man. Arch Intern Med 1976;136:25.
34. Friedman WF. Physiologic properties of the developing heart. Prog Cardiovasc Dis 1972;15:87.
35. Liebowitz EA, Novick JS, Rudolph AM. Development of myocardial sympathetic innervation in the fetal lamb. Pediatr Res 1972;6:887.
36. Waldman S, Kraus AN, Auld PAM. Baro-receptors in preterm infants: their relationship to maturity and disease. Dev Med Child Neurol 1979;21:714.
37. Pirkle JC Jr, Gann DS. Restitution of blood volume after hemorrhage: role of the adrenal cortex. Am J Physiol 1976;230:1683.
38. Pirkle JC Jr, Gann DS. Expansion of interstitial fluids is required for full restitution of blood volume after hemorrhage. J Trauma 1976; 16:937.
39. Hume DM, Edghal RH. The importance of the brain in the endocrine response to injury. Ann Surg 1959;150:697.
40. Haynes RCJ, Murad F. Adrenocorticotropic hormone: adrenocortical steroids and their synthetic analogs: inhibitors of adrenocortical steroid biosynthesis. In: Gilman AG, Goodman LS, Gilman A, eds. The pharmacological basis of therapeutics. New York: Macmillan, 1980.
41. Yates FE, Marsh DJ, Maran JW. The adrenal cortex. In: Mountcastle VB, ed. Medical physiology. Vol. II. St. Louis: CV Mosby, 1980:1558.
42. Larner J. Insulin and oral hypoglycemic drug: glucagon. In: Gilman AG, Goodman LS, Gilman A, eds. The pharmacological basis of therapeutics. New York: Macmillan, 1980.
43. Unger RH, Orci L. Physiology and pathophysiology of glucagon. Physiol Rev 1976;56:778.
44. Zimmerman EA, Stillman MA, Recht LD, et al. Vasopressin and corticotropin releasing factor: an axonal pathway to portal capillaries in the zona externa of the median eminence containing vasopressin and its interaction with adrenal corticoids. Ann NY Acad Sci 1977;297:405.
45. Gottschalk CW, Lassiter WE. Mechanisms of urine function. In: Mountcastle VB, ed. Medical Physiology. Vol. II. St. Louis: CV Mosby, 1980:1165.
46. Miller TR, Handelman WA, Arnold PE, et al. Effect of central catecholamine depletion on the osmotic and nonosmotic stimulation of vasopressin (antidiuretic hormone) in the rat. J Clin Invest 1979;64:1599.
47. Edmund R, West SP. A study of the effects of vasopressin on portal and systemic blood pressure. Surg Gynecol Obstet 1962;114:458.
48. Davis JP, Freeman RH. Mechanisms regulating renin release. Physiol Rev 1976;56:1.
49. Dinnerstein RJ, Vannice J, Henderson RC, et al. Histoflourescence technique provides evidence for dopamine containing neuronal elements in the canine kidney. Science 1979; 205: 497.
50. Fettman MJ, Hand MS, Chandrasina LG, et al. Effects of captopril on hemodynamic and metabolic parameters in awake endotoxemic Yucatan minipigs. Circ Shock 1984;12:25.
51. Morley JE. The endocrinology of the opiates and opioid peptides. Metabolism 1981;30:195.
52. Holaday JW, Loh HH. Endorphin-opiate interactions with neuroendocrine systems. Adv Biochem Psychopharmacol 1979;20:227.
53. Faden AI, Holaday JW. Opiate antagonists: a role in the treatment of hypovolemic shock. Science 1979;205:317.
54. Davies JAH, Howell TH. The management of anaesthesia for the full stomach case in the casualty department. Postgrad Med J 1973;49:58.
55. Hastings RH, Marks JD. Airway management for trauma patients with potential cervical spine injuries. Anesth Analg 1991;73:471.
56. Dronen SC, Merigian KS, Hedges JR, et al. A comparison of blind nasotracheal and succinylcholine-assited intubaiton in the poisoned patient. Ann Emerg Med 1987;16:650–652.

57. Layman PR. An alternative to blind nasal intubation. Anaesthesia 1983;38:165.
58. Sellick BA. Cricoid pressure to control regurgitation of stomach contents during induction of anaesthesia. Lancet 1961;2:404.
59. Gold MI, Duarte I, Muravchick S. Arterial oxygenation in conscious patients after 5 minutes and after 30 seconds of oxygen breathing. Anesth Analg 1981;60:313.
60. Meyers EF, Krupin T, Johnson M, et al. Failure of nondepolarizing neuromuscular blockers to inhibit succinylcholine-induced increased intraocular pressure, a controlled study. Anesthesiology 1978;48:149.
61. Gronert GA, Theye RA. Pathophysiology of hyperkalemia induced by succinylcholine. Anesthesiology 1975;43:89.
62. White PF, Schlobohm RM, Pitts LH, et al. A randomized study of drugs for preventing increases in intracranial pressure during endotracheal suctioning. Anesthesiology 1982;57:242.
63. Cottrell JE, Hartung J, Griffin JP, et al. Intracranial and hemodynamic changes after succinylcholine administration in cats. Anesth Analg 1983;62:1006.
64. Cook DR. Muscle relaxants in infants and children. Anesth Analg 1981;60:335.
65. Cullen DJ. The effect of pretreatment with nondepolarizing muscle relaxants on the neuromuscular blocking action of succinylcholine. Anesthesiology 1971;35:572.
66. Magorian T, Flannery KB, Miller RD. Comparison of rocuronium, succinylcholine, and vecuronium for rapid sequence induction of anesthesia in adult patients. Anesthesiology 1993;79:913–918.
67. Wyte SR, Shapiro HM, Turner P, et al. Ketamine-induced intracranial hypertension. Anesthesiology 1971;36:174.
68. Takeshita G, Okuda Y, Sari A. The effects of ketamine on cerebral circulation and metabolism in man. Anesthesiology 1972;36:69.
69. Bedford RF, Persing JA, Pobereskin L, et al. Lidocaine or thiopental for rapid control of intracranial hypertension. Anesth Analg 1980;59:435.
70. Yukioka H, Yoshimoto N, Nishimura K, et al. Intravenous lidocaine as a suppressant of coughing during tracheal intubation. Anesth Analg 1985;64:1189.
71. Pennant JH, White PF. The laryngeal mask: Its uses in anesthesiology. Anesthesiology 1993;79:144–163.
72. Pennant JH, Pace NA, Gajraj NM. Role of the laryngeal mask airway in the immobile spine. J Clin Anesth 1993;5:226–230.
73. Muizelaar JP, Marmarou A, Ward JD, et al. Adverse effects of prolonged hyperventilation in patients with severe head injury: a randomized clinical trial. J Neurosurg 1991;75:731–739.
74. Brotman S, Oster-Gromite M, Cox EF. Failure of cross clamping thoracic aorta to control intra-abdominal bleeding. Ann Emerg Med 1982;11:147.
75. Ming SC, Levitan R. Acute hemorrhagic necrosis of the gastrointestinal tract. N Engl J Med 1960;263:59.
76. Chernow B, Rainey TG. Endogenous and exogenous catecholamines in critical care medicine. Crit Care Med 1982;10:409.
77. Tobias JD, Nichols DG. Intraosseous succinylcholine for orotracheal intubation. Pediatr Emerg Care 1990;6:108–109.
78. Moore FS, McMurray JD, Parker HF, et al. Body composition: total body water and electrolyte; intravascular and extravascular phase volumes. Metabolism 1956;5:447.
79. Furman EB, Roman G, Lemmer LAS, et al. Specific therapy in water, electrolyte and blood volume replacement during pediatric surgery. Anesthesiology 1975;42:187.
80. Shires GT, Williams J, Brown F. Acute changes in extracellular fluids associated with major surgical procedures. Ann Surg 1961;154:803.
81. Shires GT, Carrico CT. Current status of the shock problem. In: Ravitch MM, ed. Current problems in surgery. Chicago: Year Book Medical Publishers, 1966.
82. Shires T, Collins D, Carrico J, et al. Fluid therapy in hemorhagic shock. Arch Surg 1964;88:688.
83. Shoemaker WC, Hauser CJ. Critique of crystalloid versus colloid therapy in shock and shock lung. Crit Care Med 1979;7:117.
84. Skillman JJ. The role of albumin and oncotically active fluids in shock. Crit Care Med 1976;4:55.
85. Poole GV, Meredith JW, Pennell T, et al. Comparison of colloids crystalloid in resuscitation from hemorrhagic shock. Surg Gynecol Obstet 1982;154:577.
86. Rackow EC, Falk JL, Fein A, et al. Fluid resuscitation in circulatory shock: a comparison of the cardiorespiratory effects of albumin, hetastarch, and saline solutions in patients with hypovolemic and septic shock. Crit Care Med 1983;11:839.
87. Tullis JL. Albumen. JAMA 1977;237:355.
88. Rothschild MA, Bauman A, Yalow RS, et al. Tissue distribution of I-131 labeled human serum albumin following intravenous administration. J Clin Invest 1955;34:1354.
89. Metcalf W, Papadopoulos A, Tufaro R, et al. A clinical physiologic study of hydroxyethyl starch. Surg Gynecol Obstet 1970;131:255.
90. Weil MH, Henning RJ, Morissetta M, et al. Relationship between colloid osmotic pressure and pulmonary artery wedge pressure in patients with acute cardiorespiratory failure. Chest 1982;82:433.
91. Rackow EC, Fein IA, Siege J. The relationships of colloid oncotic pressure and pulmonary artery pressure gradient to pulmonary edema and mortality in critically ill patients. Chest 1982;82:433.
92. Lowe RJ, Moss GS, Jilek J, et al. Crystalloid versus colloid in the etiology of pulmonary failure after trauma—a randomized trial in man. Crit Care Med 1979;7:107.
93. Moss GS, Lowe RJ, Jilek J, et al. Colloid or crystalloid in the resuscitation of hemorrhagic shock: A controlled clinical trial. Surgery 1981;89:434.
94. Wildenthal K, Mierzqiak DS, Mitchell JH. Acute effects of incrased serum osmolarity on left ventricular performance. Am J Physiol 1969;216:898–904.
95. Rowe GG, Mckenna DH, Corliss RJ, et al. Hemodynamic effects of hypertonic sodium chloride. J Appl Physiol 1972;32:182–184.
96. Lundvall J, Mellander S, White T. Hyperosmolarity and vasodilation in human skeletal muscle. Acta Physiol Scand 1969;77:224–233.
97. Holcroft J, Vassar M, Perry C, et al. Use of a 7.5% NaCl/6% destran 70 solution in the resuscitation of injured patients in the emergency room. Prog Clin Biol Res 1989;299:331–338.
98. Vassar M, Perry C, Holcroft J. Analysis of potential risks associated with 7.5% sodium chloride resuscitation of traumatic shock. Arch Surg 1990;125:1309–1315.
99. Holcroft J, Vassar M, Perry C, et al. 3% NaCl and 7.5% NaCl/ dextran-70 in the resuscitation of severely injured patients. Ann Surg 1987;206:279–288.
100. Holcroft J, Vassar M, Perry C, et al. Perspectives on clinical trials for hypertonic saline/dextran solutions for the treatment of traumatic shock. Braz J Med Biol Res 1989;22:291–293.
101. Brzica SM. Complications of transfusion therapy. Annual Refresher Course Lectures of the American Society of Anesthesiologists, 1984. Lecture 106, 1984 (unpub).
102. Miller RD, Robbins TO, Tong MJ, et al. Coagulation defects associated with massive blood transfusions. Ann Surg 1971;174:794.
103. Laks H, Handin RI, Martin V, et al. The effects of acute normovolemic hemodilution on coagulation and blood utilization in major surgery. J Surg Res 1976;20:225.
104. Miller RD. Complications of massive blood transfusions. Anesthesiology 1973;39:82.
105. Lucas CE, Ledgerwood AM. Clinical significance of altered coagulation tests after massive transfusion for trauma. Am Surg 1981; 47:125.
106. Hewson JR, Neame PB, Kuman N, et al. Coagulopathy related to dilution and hypotension during massive transfusion. Crit Care Med 1985;13:387.
107. Gaffney FA, Thal ER, Taylor WF, et al. Hemodynamic effects of medical anti-shock trousers. J Trauma 1981;21:931.
108. Mattox KL, Bickell W, Pepe PE, et al. Prospective MAST study in 911 patients. J Trauma 1989;29:1104.
109. Palafox BA, Johnson MN, McEwen DK, et al. ICP changes following application of the MAST suit. J Trauma 1981;21:55.
110. Bircher N, Safar P, Stewart R. A comparison of standard, "MAST"-augmented and open-chest CPR in dogs: a preliminary investigation. Crit Care Med 1980;8:147.
111. Kaback KR, Sanders AB, Meislin HW. MAST suit update. JAMA 1984;252:2598.
112. McSwain NE, Jr. G-suits and shock: a non-invasive transfusion technique. J Kans Med Soc 1976;77:438.
113. Lee HR, Blank WF, Massim WH, et al. Venous return in hemorrhagic shock after application of military anti-shock trousers. Am J Emerg Med 1983;1:7.
114. Robotham JL, Haddow JE. Rhabdomyolysis and myoglobinuria in childhood. Pediatr Clin North Am 1976;23:279.
115. Rowland LP, Penn AS. Myoglobinuria. Med Clin North Am 1972; 56:1233.
116. Weil MH. Patient evaluation,"vital signs" and initial care. In: Shoemaker WC, Thompson WL, eds. Critical care medicine, state of the art. Vol. I. Fullerton, CA: Society of Critical Care Medicine, 1980:1.
117. Rowe MI, Taylor M. Transepidermal water loss in the infant surgical patient. J Pediatr Surg 1981;16:878.

118. Jennett B, Teasdale G, Braakman R, et al. Prognosis of patients with severe head injury. Neurosurgery 1979;4:283.
119. Mayer T, Walker ML, Shasha I, et al. Effect of multiple trauma on outcome of pediatric patients with neurological injuries. Childs Brain 1981;8:189.
120. Bruce DA, Raphaely RC, Goldberg AI. Pathophysiology treatment and outcome following severe head injury in children. Childs Brain 1979;5:174.
121. Kirsh MM, Sloan H. Chest trauma—General principles of management. Boston: Little, Brown and Co., 1977.
122. Otherson HB: Cardiothoracic injuries: pediatric trauma. New York: John Wiley & Sons, 1978.
123. Haller JAJ, Shermeta DW. Major thoracic trauma in children. Pediatr Clin North Am 1975;222:341.
124. Bellinger SB. Penetrating chest injuries in children. Ann Thorac Surg 1972;14:635.
125. Meller JL, Little AG, Shermeta DW. Thoracic trauma in children. Pediatrics 1984;74:813.
126. Sinclair MC, Moore TC. Major surgery for abdominal and thoracic trauma in childhood and adolescence. Pediatr Surg 1974;9:155.
127. Simpson JS. Thoracic injuries. In: The surgical staff: care for the injured child. Toronto: The Hospital for Sick Children, 1975.
128. Colombani PM, Buck JR, Dudgeon DL, et al. One year experience in a regional pediatric trauma center. J Pediatr Surg 1985;20:14.
129. Beaver BL, Colombani PM, Buck JR, et al. Efficacy of emergency room thoracotamy in pediatric training. J Pediatr Surg 1987;22:19.
130. Rothenberg SS, Moore EE, Moore FA, et al. Emergency department thoracotomy in children—a critical analysis. J Trauma 1989; 29:1322.
131. Myllynen P, Kivioja A, Wilppula E, et al. Pathophysiology, treatment and prognosis. Ann Chir Gynaecol 1983;72.43.
132. Levy JL Jr. Management of crushing chest injuries in children. South Med J 1972;65:1040.
133. Fulton RL, Peter ET, Wilson JN. The pathophysiology and treatment of pulmonary contusions. J Trauma 1970;10:719.
134. Trinkle JK, Furman RW, Hinshaw MA, et al. Pulmonary contusion: pathogenesis and effect of various resuscitative measures. Ann Thorac Surg 1973;16:568.
135. Burke JF. Early diagnosis of traumatic rupture of the bronchus. JAMA 1962;181:682.
136. Ecker RR, Libertini RV, Ria WJ, et al. Injuries of the trachea and bronchi. Ann Surg 1971;11:289.
137. Myers WO, Leape LL, Holder TM. Bronchial rupture in a child with subsequent stenosis, resection and anastomosis. Ann Thorac Surg 1971;12:442.
138. Turnbull AD, Carlon G, Howland WS, et al. High frequency jet ventilation in major airway or pulmonary disruption. Ann Thorac Surg 1980;32:468.
139. Lasky II, Nahum AM, Siegel AW. Cardiac injuries incurred by drivers in automobile accidents. J Forensic Sci 1969;14:13.
140. Golladay ES, Donahoo JS, Haller JAJ. Special problems of cardiac injuries in infants and children. J Trauma 1979;19:526.
141. McCune RP, Roda CP, Eckert C. Rupture of diaphragm caused by blunt trauma. J Trauma 1976;16:531.
142. Dronen SC. Disorders of the chest wall and diaphragm. Emerg Med Clin North Am 1983;1:449.
143. Sharma LK, Kennedy RF, Heneghan WD. Rupture of the diaphragm resulting from blunt trauma in children. Can J Surg 1977;20:553.
144. Johnson CF, Reyes HM, Replogle R. Diaphragmatic hernia from penetrating thoracoabdominal injury in an infant. J Pediatr Surg 1970;5:572.
145. White JJ, Oh KS, Haller JA. Positive-contrast peritoneography for accurate delineation of diaphragmatic abnormalities. Surgery 1974; 76:398.
146. Meyers NA. Traumatic rupture of the diaphragm in children. Aust N Z J Surg 1964;34:123.
147. Castagna J, Nelson RJ. Blunt trauma to branches of the aortic arch. J Thorac Cardiovasc Surg 1975;69:521.
148. Kirsh MM, Crane JD, Kahn DR, et al. Roentgenographic evaluation of traumatic rupture of the aorta. Surg Gynecol Obstet 1970;131:900.
149. Haller JA, Donahoo JS. Traumatic asphxia in children: pathophysiology and management. J Trauma 1971;11:453.
150. Jones MJ, James EC. The management of traumatic asphxia: case report and literature review. J Trauma 1976;16:235.
151. Wilson RF, Gibson DG, Antomenko D. Shock and acute respiratory failure after chest trauma. J Trauma 1977;17:697.
152. Rapaport FT, Nemirovsky MS, Bacharoff R. Mechanisms of pulmonary damage in severe burns. Ann Surg 1973;177:472.
153. Petty TL. Acute respiratory failure after surgery or trauma. In: Petty TL, ed. Intensive and rehabilitative respiratory care. Philadelphia: Lea & Febiger, 1982:306.
154. Anderson RR, Holliday RL, Drieger AA, et al. Documentation of pulmonary capillary permeability in the adult respiratory distress syndrome accompanying human sepsis. Am Rev Respir Dis 1979;119:869.
155. Lyrene RK, Truog WE. Adult respiratory distress syndrome in a pediatric intensive care unit: Predisposing conditions, clinical course, and outcome. Pediatrics 1981;67:790.
156. Petty TL. The adult respiratory distress syndrome: confessions of a lumper. Am Rev Respir Dis 1975;111:713.
157. Said SI. Pulmonary metabolism of prostaglandins and vasoactive peptides. Annu Rev Physiol 1982;44:257.
158. Hammerschmidt DE, Weaver LJ, Hudson LD. Association of complement activation and elevated plasma C5a with adult respiratory distress syndrome. Lancet 1980;1:947.
159. Frank L, Massaro D. The lung and oxygen toxicity. Arch Intern Med 1979;139:347.
160. Touloukian RJ. Pediatric trauma. New York: John Wiley & Sons, 1978.
161. Haller JA, Jr. A new philosophy of pediatric splenic surgery: save our spleens. Surg Rounds 1980;3:23.
162. Philippart AI. Blunt abdominal trauma in childhood. Surg Clin North Am 1977;57:151.
163. Haller JA, Jr. Newer concepts on emergency care of children with major injuries. Pediatrics 1973;52:485.
164. Barlow B, Niemirska M, Gandhi RP. Ten years experience with pediatric gunshot wounds. J Pediatr Surg 1982;17:927.
165. Grosfeld JL. Symposium on childhood trauma. Pediatr Clin North Am 1975;22:269.
166. Polk HC, Flint LM. Intraabdominal injuries in polytrauma. World J Surg 1983;7:56.
167. Oakes DD. Splenic trauma. Curr Probl Surg 1981;6:346.
168. Hendren WH, Kim SH. Trauma of the spleen and liver in children. Pediatr Clin North Am 1975;22:349.
169. Graham JM, Pokorny WJ, Mattox KL, et al. Surgical management of acute pancreatic injuries in children. J Pediatr Surg 1978;13:693.
170. Grosfeld JL, Cooney DR. Pancreatic and gastrointestinal trauma in children. Pediatr Clin North Am 1975;22:365.
171. Otherson HB, Moore FT, Boles ETJ. Traumatic pancreatitis and pseudocyst in childhood. J Trauma 1968;8:535.
172. Stone HH. Pancreatic and duodenal trauma in children. J Pediatr Surg 1972;7:670.
173. Stewart DR, Byrd CL, Schuster SR. Intramural hematomas of the alimentary tract in children. Surgery 1970;68:550.
174. Olsen WR. The serum amylase in blunt abdominal trauma. J Trauma 1973;13:200.
175. Franken EAJ, Smith JA. Roentgenographic evaluation of infant and childhood trauma. Pediatr Clin North Am 1975;22:303.
176. Kane NM, Cronan JJ, Dorfman GS, et al. Pediatric abdominal trauma: evaluation by computed tomography. Pediatrics 1988;82:11.
177. Kuhn JP. Diagnostic imaging for the evaluation of abdominal trauma in children. Pediatr Clin North Am 1985;32:1427.
178. Lutzker LG, Chun KJ. Radionuclide imaging in the nonsurgical treatment of liver and spleen trauma. J Trauma 1981;21:382.
179. McConnell BJ, McConnell RW, Guiberteau MJ. Radionuclide imaging in blunt trauma. Radiol Clin North Am 1981;19:37.
180. Guice K, Oldham K, Elde B, et al. Hematuria after blunt trauma: when is pyelography useful? J Trauma 1983;23:305.
181. McAminch JW, Federle MP. Evaluation of renal injuries with computerized tomography. J Urol 1982;128:456.
182. Powell DC, Bivins BA, Bell RM. Diagnostic peritoneal lavage. Surg Gynecol Obstet 1982;155:257.
183. Stone HH, Ansley JD. Management of liver trauma in children. J Pediatr Surg 1977;12:3.
184. Sherman R. Perspectives in management of trauma to the spleen: 1979. Presidential Address. American Association for the Surgery of Trauma. J Trauma 1980;20:1.
185. Haller JA, Jr. Management of major abdominal trauma. In: Carter D, Polk H, Jr., eds. Trauma. Woburn, MA: Butterworth, 1981.
186. King DR, Lobe TE, Haase GM, et al. Selective management of injured spleen. Surgery 1981;90:677.
187. Wesson DE, Filler RM, Kin SB, et al. Ruptured spleen—When to operate? J Pediatr Surg 1981; 16:324.
188. Mayer T, Walker MC, Johnson DG, et al. Causes of morbidity and mortality in severe pediatric trauma. JAMA 1981;245:719.
189. Mahoney WJ, D'Souza BJ, Haller JA, Jr., et al. Long-term outcome of

children with severe head trauma and prolonged coma. Pediatrics 1983;71:756.
190. Jennett B, Teasdale G, Galbraith S, et al. Severe head injury in three countries. J Neurol Neurosurg Psychiatry 1977;40:291.
191. Jennett B, Carlin J. Preventable mortality and morbidity after head injury. Injury 1979;10:31.
192. Mitchell DE, Adams JH. Primary impact damage to the brainstem in blunt head injuries, does it exist? Lancet 1973;2:215.
193. Stritch SJ. The pathology of brain damage due to blunt head injury. In: Walker HE, Cavenas WF, Critchly M, eds. The late effects of head injury. Springfield, IL: Charles C Thomas, 1969:501.
194. Billmire ME, Myers PA. Serious head injury in infants: accident or abuse? Pediatrics 1985;75:340.
195. Patzakis MJ, Harvery P, Ivler D. The role of antibiotics in the management of open fractures. J Bone Joint Surg 1974;56A:532.
196. Leonidas JC, Ting W, Binkiewicz A, et al. Mild head trauma in children: when is a roentgenogram necessary? Pediatrics 1982;69:139.
197. Hershey BL, Zimmerman RA. Pediatric brain computed tomography. Pediatr Clin North Am 1985;32:1477.
198. Zimmerman RA, Bilaniuk LT. Computed tomography in pediatric head trauma. J Neuroradiol 1981;8:257.
199. Jennett WB, Teasdale G. Special investigations and methods of monitoring. In: Jennett WB, Teasdale G, eds. Management of head injuries. Philadelphia: F.A. Davis, 1981:111.
200. Mickell JJ, Reigel DH, Cook DR, et al. Intracranial pressure: monitoring and normalization therapy in children. Pediatrics 1977;59:606.
201. Haller J. Intracranial pressure monitoring in Reye's syndrome. Hosp Pract 1980;15:101.
202. Tasker RC, Matthew DJ. Cerebral intraparenchymal pressure monitoring in non-traumatic coma: clinical evaluation of a new fibreoptic device. Neuropediatrics 1991;22:47.
203. Chambers IR, Mendelow AD, Sinar EJ, et al. A clinical evaluation of the Camino subdural screw and ventricular monitoring kits. Neurosurgery 1990;26:421.
204. Marshall LF, Smith RW, Shapiro HM. The outcome with aggressive treatment in severe head injury. Part I: The significance of intracranial pressure monitoring. J Neurosurg 1979;50:20.
205. Miller JD, Butterworth JF, Gudeman SK, et al. Further experience in the management of severe head injury. J Neurosurg 1981;54:289.
206. Bruce DA, Schut L, Bruno LA, et al. Outcome following severe head injuries in children. J Neurosurg 1978;48:679.
207. Annegers JF, Grabow JD, Grover RV, et al. Seizures after head trauma: a population study. Neurology 1980;30:683.
208. Wada JH, Sato M, Wake A, et al. Prophylactic effects of phenytoin, phenobarbital and carbamazepine examined in kindling cat preparations. Arch Neurol 1976;33:426.
209. Young B, Rapp RP, Norton JA, et al. Failure of prophylactically administered phenytoin to prevent late posttraumatic seizures. J Neurosurg 1983;58:236.
210. Albin MS. Acute cervical spinal injury. Crit Care Clin 1985;1:267.
211. Trafton PG. Spinal cord injuries. Surg Clin North Am 1982;62:61.
212. Kraus JF, Franti CE, Riggins RS, et al. Incidence of traumatic spinal cord lesions. J Chronic Dis 1975;28:471.
213. Kalsbeek WD, McLaurin RC, Harris BSH, et al. The National Head and Spinal Cord Injury Survey: major findings. J Neurosurg 1980;53:519.
214. Bracken MD, Freeman DHJ, Hellenbrad K. Incidence of acute traumatic hospitalization of spinal cord injury in the US: 1970–1977. Am J Epidemiol 1981;113:615.
215. Burke DC. Injuries of the spinal cord in children. In: Vinken PJ, Bruyn GM, eds. Handbook of clinical neurology. Vol. 25. Amsterdam: North Holland Publishing Co., 1976:175.
216. Andrews LG, Jurg SK. Spinal cord injuries in children in British Columbia. Paraplegia 1979;17:442.
217. Feuer H. Management of acute spine and spinal cord injury, old and new concepts. Arch Surg 1976;111:638.
218. Green BA, Callahan RA, Klose KJ, et al. Acute spinal cord injury: current concepts. Clin Orthop 1981;154:125.
219. Yashon D. Pathogenesis of spinal cord injury. Orthop Clin North Am 1978;9:247.
220. Dohrmann GJ, Allen WE. Microcirulation of traumatized spinal cord: a corrrelation of microangiography and blood flow patterns in transitory and permanent paraplegia. J Trauma 1975;15:1003.
221. Assenmacher DR, Ducker TB. Experimental traumatic paraplegia. J Bone Joint Surg 1971;53A:671.
222. Naftchi NE, Demeny M, Decrescito V, et al. Biogenic amine concentrations in traumatized spinal cords of cats. Effects of drug therapy. J Neurosurg 1974;40:52.
223. Senter HJ, Venes JL, Kauer JS. Alteration of posttraumatic ischemia in experimental spinal cord trauma by a central nervous depressant. J Neurosurg 1979;50:207.
224. Senter HJ, Venes JL. Loss of autoregulation and posttraumatic ischemia following experimental spinal cord trauma. J Neurosurg 1979;50:198.
225. Eidelberg E, Sullivan J, Brigham A. Immediate consequences of spinal cord injury: Possible role of potassium in axonal conduction block. Surg Neurol 1975;3:317.
226. Hatchen HJ. Spinal cord injury in children and adolescents: diagnostic pitfalls and therapeutic consideration in the acute stage. Paraplegia 1977;15:55.
227. Burke DC. Traumatic spinal paralysis in children. Paraplegia 1974; 11:268.
228. Mace SE. Emergency evaluation of cervical spine injuries: CT versus plain radiographs. Ann Emerg Med 1985;14:973.
229. Kewalraani LS, Tori JA. Spinal cord trauma in children: neurologic patterns, radiologic features and pathomechanics of injury. Spine 1980;5:11.
230. Leventhal HR. Birth injuries of the spinal cord. J Pediatr 1960; 56:447.
231. Rowed DW, McLean JAG, Tator CH. Somatosensory evoked potentials in acute spinal cord injury: prognostic value. Surg Neurol 1978;9:203.
232. Bracken MB, Shepard MJ, Collins WF, et al. A randomized control trial of methylprednisolone or naloxone in the treatment of acute spinal cord injury. Results of the Second National Acute Spinal Cord Injury Study. N Engl J Med 1990;322:1405.
233. Jaffe D, Wesson D. Emergency management of blunt trauma in children. N Engl J Med 1991;324:1477.
234. De La Torre JC, Johnson CM, Goode DJ, et al. Pharmacologic treatment and evaluation of permanent experimental spinal cord trauma. Neurology 1975;25:508.
235. Merritt JL. Urinary tract infections, causes and management, with particular reference to the patient with spinal cord injury: a review. Arch Phys Med Rehabil 1976;57:365.
236. Albin MS, White RJ, Acosta-Rua G. Study of functional recovery produced by delayed localized cooling after spinal cord injury in primates. J Neurosurg 1968;29:113.
237. Tsubokawa T, Nakamura S, Hyashi N, et al. The circulatory disturbance of spinal cord injury and its response to local cooling therapy. Neurol Med Chir (Tokyo) 1975;15:87.
238. Guthman L, Frankel H. Value of intermittent catheterization in early management of traumatic paraplegia and teraplegia. Paraplegia 1966;4:63.
239. Tori JA, Kewalraani LS. Urolithiasis in children with spinal cord injury. Paraplegia 1978;16:357.
240. Maynard FM, Iman K. Immobilization hypercalcemia in spinal cord injury. Arch Phys Med Rehabil 1977;58:16.
241. Reece RM, Grodin MA. Recognition of nonaccidental injury. Pediatr Clin North Am 1985;32:41.
242. Kempe CH. Symposium on child abuse. Pediatrics 1973;51:773.
243. Kempe CH, Silverman FN, Steele BF. The battered child syndrome. JAMA 1962;181:105.
244. Caffey J. The whiplash shaken infant syndrome: manual shaking by the extremities with whiplash-induced intracranial and intraocular bleeding, linked with residual brain damage and mental retardation. Pediatrics 1974;54:396.
245. Klein DM. Central nervous system injuries. In: Ellestein NS, ed. Child abuse and neglect: a medical reference. New York: John Wiley & Sons, 1973:73.
246. Helfer RE, Slovis TL, Block M. Injuries resulting when small children fall out of bed. Pediatrics 1977;60:533.
247. Hunter RS, Kilstrom N, Kraybell EN, et al. Antecedents of child abuse and neglect in premature infants: a prospective study in a newborn intensive care unit. Pediatrics 1978;61:629.
248. Fontana VJ. The diagnosis of the maltreatment syndrome in children. Pediatrics 1973;51:780.
249. Wilson EF. Estimation of the age of cutaneous contusions in child abuse. Pediatrics 1977;60:750.
250. Akbarnia AK, Torg JS, Kirkpatrick J, et al. Manifestations of the battered-child syndrome. J Bone Joint Surg 1974;56A:1159.
251. Dorst JP. Child abuse. Radiologie 1982;22:335.
252. Hobbs CJ. Skull fracture and the diagnosis of abuse. Arch Dis Child 1984;59:246.

Neuroendocrine Response to Stress 44

Gregory Stidham
Mark C. Bugnitz

INTRODUCTION

The neuroendocrine response to stress is a topic that has been the subject of considerable recent interest. This chapter has three objectives: (a) to provide a general overview of the neuroendocrine response to stress as it is currently understood; (b) to illustrate how this response is generally adaptive, though it may dysfunction and compromise adaptation to and survival of the stressor; and (c) to highlight the small available amount of information pertaining to the specifics of the response in the pediatric patient.

OVERVIEW

The neuroendocrine response to stress is a complex interaction of multiple systems that follows a threat to the physiologic stability of the organism. Some examples include hemorrhage, sepsis, burns, and even psychologic threat. The integration of the several components of this response is so sophisticated that Gann and Lilly[1] described the response as a neuroendocrine "reflex."

The neuroendocrine response to stress, or the neuroendocrine reflex, consists of an afferent limb, central nervous system (CNS) sites of integration and modulation, and an efferent limb. The afferent limb consists of "sensors" that detect disturbances of or threats to physiologic stability, and of neural pathways that conduct signals initiated by these sensors to the CNS. Within the CNS, complex interactions occur between brainstem centers which then orchestrate the efferent response.

The efferent limb of the neuroendocrine response to stress consists of the sympathoadrenal (or sympathoendocrine) axis and the hypothalamic-pituitary axis. Earlier concepts of these two axes and their role in the stress response have had to be greatly expanded in recent years to include the growing appreciation for the added roles of endogenous opioids, prostaglandins, cytokines, and output of other endocrine organs as effectors of the response.

The direct consequences of the neuroendocrine response to stress include cardiovascular adaptations, adaptations in the regulation of water and electrolyte homeostasis, and metabolic adaptations, particularly oxygen consumption and substrate formation and utilization. Indirect consequences include prostaglandin activation and alterations in immunologic function.

AFFERENT LIMB

Cardiovascular Regulatory Receptors

Cardiovascular function is continuously monitored by neural sensors that detect changes in numerous circulatory parameters[2]. The carotid sinus, innervated by a branch of the glossopharyngeal (IXth cranial) nerve, is a dilatation in the wall of the internal carotid at its base where it joins the external carotid artery. The rich network of nerve fibers innervating these structures terminates in the connective tissue adventitia of the vessel walls, oriented so as to align them along the long axis of the vessel. These sensors respond to stretch in the vessel wall produced by increased intraluminal pressure.

Adjacent to the carotid sinuses are the carotid bodies, small clumps of polyhedral cells comprising a highly vascular structure containing a network of sinusoids. These are in close proximity to special sensory cells that respond to a variety of chemical stimuli. These sensors relay information about changes in circulatory state via the glossopharyngeal nerves to the nucleus tractus solitarius in the medulla.

The wall of the aorta in the region of the transverse arch, carotid artery, and subclavian artery is richly endowed with a network of branching nerve fibers that derive from the vagus (Xth cranial) nerve. The orientation of these fibers, which comprise the aortic baroreceptors, is similar to that of the nerves in the carotid sinus, and they also respond to changes in the vessels induced by local intraluminal pressure changes.

In addition to the pressure and stretch sensors in the aorta and its major branches, tissues that are sensitive to mechanical and chemical stimulation are found in the lungs, the walls of the atria and the ventricles, and in the junctions of the venae cavae and pulmonary veins with the right and left atria. These receptors communicate with the medulla via both myelinated and unmyelinated afferent fibers in the Xth cranial nerve.

The various cardiovascular regulatory receptors work in concert to detect minute changes in both intravascular pressure and volume. Signals generated by these receptors are carried by their respective pathways to centers that integrate this input and begin to orchestrate the efferent response. Some integration occurs outside the CNS (e.g., preganglionic sympathetic neuron mediated local vasoconstriction in response to a local cold stimulus), but the majority is integrated at the level of the medulla and the hypothalamus.

The interconnections and the interactions among the centers of integration are complex. Early understanding of numerous independent reflex arcs has given way to a much more complex concept involving modulation of afferent signals at several levels within the brain, as well as numerous interactions occurring at a variety of levels within the CNS modulating efferent responses.

Electrical stimulation of various sites in the floor of the fourth ventricle produce either vasoconstriction or vasodilatation responses. These "pressor" and "depressor" sites respond to input from the cardiovascular regulatory receptors. In addition, these centers receive neural input from higher centers, including hypothalamus, cerebral cortex, and from the nucleus tractus solitarius, creating a complexly interacting system regulating peripheral vascular tone.

The hypothalamus, when stimulated electrically, initiates either increases or decreases in both blood pressure and heart rate, depending on the exact site of stimulation. These same hypothalamic centers are responsive to changes in body temperature and control the vascular tone in cutaneous vessels involved in heat loss and conservation.

Nociceptive and Sensory Receptors

The role of sensory input in the afferent limb of the neuroendocrine response has become increasingly clear over the years. Gordon et al.[3], as well as others, have demonstrated that denervation of a limb eliminates the adrenal response to stimulation and injury to that limb. Similarly, humans undergoing abdominal surgery demonstrate marked blunting of the adrenocortical and growth hormone responses if they have received spinal anesthesia[4]. Other sensory input also undoubtedly plays a role in the response, with both visual and auditory, and conceivably, olfactory, stimuli producing the subjective state of anxiety and the neuroendocrine response seen with physiologic stress.

Nociceptive input reaches the CNS by way of both small myelinated and larger unmyelinated fibers, projecting rostrally and caudally to synapses in the substancia gelatinosa and dorsal columns in the spinal cord. Pain fibers then travel contralaterally, ascending in the lateral spinothalamic tract to the sensory nucleus of the thalamus. Neurons from these nuclei project to the cortex and are responsible for the conscious perception of pain.

Separate tracts ascend in the spinal cord to the medial reticular area by the spinoreticular pathways. It is here that direct anatomic connections are made to the medullary sympathetic center, as well as rostral projections to the medial thalamus and the hypothalamus.

EFFERENT LIMB

Overview

The efferent responses to the wide variety of complexly interacting afferent input are initiated primarily in two locations: the pituitary and the brainstem autonomic centers. The output of these components of the "reflex" is in the form of nerve stimulation in the sympathetic and parasympathetic nervous system, and the release of hormones. These hormones then act either directly on end-organs, or indirectly by stimulating the release of other hormones. Thus, the effectors may be considered to be one of either two types: those that are under pituitary hormone control (hypothalamic-pituitary axis) and those that are under sympathetic nervous system control (sympathoendocrine axis).

The stress response is characterized by elevations in cortisol, glucagon, and the catecholamines. Insulin levels are also elevated[5], as well as growth hormone[6,7], aldosterone[8], and vasopressin[9]. It is of interest that the patterns and magnitude of hormonal responses to physiologic stress predict outcome with an accuracy comparable to clinical and physiologic scoring systems[10–14].

Hypothalamic-Pituitary Axis

ACTH-Cortisol

Signals produced by nociceptive and circulatory stimuli travel from the medulla to the hypothalamus via three separate neural projections. Two facilitative pathways synapse in the ventromedial and suprachiasmatic nuclei and in the paraventricular nucleus of the hypothalamus. An inhibitory pathway ascends into the posterior hypothalamus. Input from all of these areas of the hypothalamus converges on the median eminence where corticotropin-releasing factor (CRF) is secreted. This compound is secreted into the vessels of the hypothalamohypophyseal portal system and into the anterior pituitary. Here, CRF acts on the chromophobe cells, causing their release of adrenocorticotropic hormone (ACTH). CRF release is influenced and modulated by other hormones, including angiotensin II[15] and local vasopressin[16,17], catecholamines[18], vasoactive intestinal peptide[18], and others.

ACTH itself is a derivative of a much larger molecule, pro-opiocortin. The other portions of this molecule are released simultaneously with ACTH, and include β-endorphin, β-lipotropin, and γ-melanocyte-stimulating hormone (γ-MSH).

ACTH released by the anterior pituitary reaches cells in the zona fasciculata of the adrenals, where adenylate cyclase activation and cyclic adenosine monophosphate (c-AMP) production activate protein kinases. These, in turn, catalyze the conversion of cholesterol into pregnenolone, with the ultimate production and release of cortisol.

Stress also affects the production and secretion of other steroid hormones. While cortisol levels increase in proportion to severity of burn, adrenal androgen dehydroepiandrosterone production is decreased[19]. Decreased testosterone levels are observed after surgery[20,21] and after myocardial infarction[22]. Critically ill women and men experience decreases in circulating plasma concentration of sex hormones[23], probably accounting for the frequently observed amenorrhea seen in critically ill women. These decreases in sex steroid production probably reflect a diversion of substrate to pathways involved in the increased cortisol synthesis, and may be mediated by decreased secretion of follicle-stimulating hormone (FSH) and luteinizing hormone (LH)[24] or due to decreased response of the pituitary to gonadotropin-releasing hormone (GnRH)[25]. The magnitude of the depressions in LH, FSH, and testosterone have been shown to correlate with predicted mortality in critically ill adult patients[26].

Arginine Vasopressin

Decreased circulating blood volume, detected by stretch and baroreceptors in the cardiovascular system, produces afferent signals projecting to the hypothalamus, probably via pathways similar or identical to those involved in stimulation of CRF release[2], leading to release of arginine vasopressin (ADH), an eight-amino acid peptide synthesized in the supraoptic and paraventricular nuclei of the hypothalamus. It is transported along nerve cell axons projecting into the median eminence and the posterior lobe of the pituitary, where depolarization of these nerve cells produces an exocytosis and release of the hormone. Increased plasma osmolality, as is seen after hemorrhage, is also sensed in the hypothalamus and produces secretion of ADH, but this osmolality response is overridden by responses to changes in circulating volume. (The control of and disorders of ADH secretion are discussed in Chapter 39.)

Growth Hormone

Increased levels of growth hormone have been demonstrated in stress, after surgery, and after traumatic injury. Neural inputs converge on the median eminence of the pituitary, originating from the ventromedial and arcuate nuclei of the hypothalamus and from the limbic system. In response to stimulation from these inputs, the pituitary secretes both releasing and inhibiting factors into the hypothalamohypophyseal portal vessels, which carry these hormones to the anterior pituitary. There, these hormones influence the secretion of growth hormone by the somatotrophic cells. Other hormones also influence this secretion, including glucagon, ADH, estrogens, and arginine, which promote growth hormone release by action on the ventromedial nucleus. Glucocorticoids inhibit the secretion of growth hormone.

The primary stimulus for growth hormone secretion is growth hormone-releasing factor. Somatostatin, a hormone also produced in the hypothalamus, is a potent inhibitor of growth hormone secretion, and is also a potent inhibitor of its own secretion by pancreatic δ-cells.

Thyroid Hormone

Thyroid-stimulating hormone (TSH) is the primary regulator of thyroid gland function. Production of this hormone is under hypothalamic control through the production by neurosecretory cells of thyrotropin-releasing hormone (TRH), which is secreted into the hypothalamohypophyseal portal circulation[2]. TRH binds to thyrotroph cells in the anterior pituitary, and by adenylate cyclase activation and c-AMP production, stimulates those cells to secrete TSH. TSH secretion, in turn, is limited by negative feedback related to circulating thyroid hormone levels, which also act to inhibit TRH release by the hypothalamus.

The thyroid hormones derive from thyroglobulin, a large

glycoprotein synthesized in the follicular cells of the thyroid gland. This large molecule is richly iodinated after adenosine triphosphate (ATP)-dependent active transport of iodide at the basal surface of the follicular cells, and contains about 26 atoms of iodide. The mature thyroglobulin is stored extracellularly as colloid in the lumen of the thyroid follicles.

When TSH binds to specific high-affinity receptors on the surface of thyroid cells, endocytosis of the thyroglobulin is stimulated, along with increased activity of all pathway steps in the synthesis of thyroid hormones. After reabsorption of thyroglobulin, the endocytic vesicles fuse with lysosomes where the thyroglobulin molecules are cleaved by lysosomal proteases, with the resultant secretion of T3 and T4. Each molecule of thyroglobulin yields an average of three to four residues of T4 and 0.2 of T3, with a ratio of about 10:1 T4:T3 secreted into the circulation.

Each T4 molecule contains four atoms of iodide and is subjected to degradation by either of two enzymes, one of which yields T3, the active thyroid hormone, the other rT3 (reverse T3), an inactive form. The relative activities of these two enzymes represent an important mechanism for regulating the amount of active hormone available for entry into cells and metabolic activity, as do the levels of circulating carrier proteins (thyroid-binding globulin, thyroid-binding prealbumin, and albumin).

Prolactin

Prolactin release occurs after both physical and emotional stress. The exact pathways involved in the control of prolactin release remain somewhat elusive but are thought to involve the inhibition of the tonic release of dopamine, which acts as a prolactin-inhibitor. In addition, these pathways may theoretically control the release of prolactin-releasing factor into the hypothalamohypophyseal portal circulation. Once stimulated, the anterior pituitary releases prolactin.

Sympathoendocrine Axes

Autonomic Nervous System

Activation of the sympathetic nervous system by circulatory and nociceptive stimuli is primarily mediated at the level of the medullary sympathetic vasomotor areas. The instantaneous sympathetic response to cardiovascular perturbations does not require input from higher centers, a direct reflex response thought to be operative in the sympathetic activation by hypoglycemia as well[2].

Medullary mediation of the sympathetic response to nociceptive and other stress stimuli is more complex. Although painful stimuli can elicit a generalized sympathetic nervous system response in the decerebrate animal[4], this response is greatly modified by input from rostral cortex and hypothalamus in the intact animal[27].

Catecholamines

Direct sympathetic nervous system innervation of vascular smooth muscle makes possible the rapid responses seen after small changes in circulating blood volume. More diverse effects result from the stimulation of the adrenal. The adrenal medulla is innervated by fibers emanating from the intermediolateral column of the spinal cord, which then travel via the splanchnic nerves to synapse directly on the chromaffin cells. Release of acetylcholine by these nerves causes depolarization of the cell membrane of the chromaffin cells, producing the exocytotic release of preformed catecholamines (epinephrine and norepinephrine).

Renin-Angiotensin-Aldosterone

The juxtaglomerular cells of the renal afferent arterioles receive sympathetic innervation via the renal nerves. These fibers, with both adrenergic and dopaminergic transmitters, stimulate renin secretion[2]. In addition to responding to the sympathetic stimulation, the macula densa also responds to decreases in renal arteriolar pressure detected by intrarenal baroreceptors and to decreases in distal tubular sodium delivery. Renin is secreted into the circulation, as well as directly and locally into the renal arteriole and the interstitium of the kidney.

Renin acts systemically by cleaving an hepatic-produced α1-globulin, angiotensinogen, forming angiotensin I. Angiotensin I, an inactive molecule, is converted to the active angiotensin II by the carboxydipeptidase, angiotensin-converting enzyme, found largely in the lung and kidney. Angiotensin II is the major active peptide, although a third form, angiotensin III, also acts on the zona glomerulosa cells of the adrenal cortex.

Angiotensin II is a potent vasoconstrictor, acting directly on arterial and arteriolar smooth muscle with a resultant increase in blood pressure. One affected vessel is the renal arteriole, where constriction reduces glomerular filtration and contributes to water conservation.

Both angiotensin II and III bind to specific receptors in the adrenal cortex, where they stimulate increased synthesis and secretion of aldosterone. This hormone, which also responds to small changes in serum potassium, serving to maintain potassium concentration within a very normal range, acts primarily on the distal tubule. Potassium and hydrogen ions are excreted in response to aldosterone stimulation, with sodium and water being reabsorbed and conserved.

Glucagon and Insulin

Glucagon and insulin are secreted by the pancreas. Their secretion is controlled primarily by three mechanisms: circulating blood glucose, CNS outflow, and other circulating hormones. Pancreatic islet cells receive significant sympathetic innervation. While sympathetic outflow may increase secretion of both, increased α activity will block release.

Insulin produced by the β-cells is released in response to increased blood glucose and vagal stimuli. Circulating catecholamines will suppress its release. Once released into the circulation, insulin has both paracrine (local) effects and endocrine (distant organ) effects. The first target cells reached by insulin are the α-cells in the periphery of the pancreatic islets. α-Cells produce glucagon and are inhibited when acted upon by insulin, the major paracrine effect of insulin[(28)].

Insulin's endocrine effects occur in three major areas: liver, muscle, and fat. In the liver, it promotes anabolism by increasing glycogen synthesis and storage and inhibiting gluconeogenesis by decreasing hepatocyte intracellular c-AMP concentration. Insulin also increases triglyceride synthesis and very low density lipoprotein (VLDL) formation by the liver. It inhibits catabolism by preventing glycogenolysis and ketogenesis in addition to the aforementioned inhibition of gluconeogenesis.

In muscle, insulin increases not only transport of glucose to the cells, but also amino acid transport, resulting in increased protein synthesis. Also, by enhancing the activity of glycogen synthetase and inhibiting glycogen phosphorylase, insulin promotes glycogen synthesis[(28)].

In fat, insulin's major effect is to increase triglyceride storage. It does so by decreasing lipolysis, inducing lipoprotein lipase, and increasing the transport of glucose into fat cells, thereby making it available for triglyceride synthesis.

Glucagon has effects that are opposite those of insulin. Its secretion is stimulated by hypoglycemia, ingestion of protein, infusion of amino acids, opiate peptides, growth hormone, exercise, glucocorticoids, gastrin, catecholamines, and stimuli that act to increase sympathetic nervous system outflow, i.e., nociceptive or hemodynamic input[(1,29,30)]. Glucagon is under negative feedback control, such that hyperglycemia suppresses its release. Insulin, and somatostatin, which is produced by δ-cells of the pancreatic islets, inhibit release of glucagon[(28)].

The liver is the major target organ for glucagon. Most of its effects there appear to depend upon activation of adenylate cyclase resulting in an increase in hepatocyte c-AMP[(30)]. Glucagon stimulates glycogen breakdown by activation of hepatocyte glycogen phosphorylase A. It also stimulates gluconeogenesis and ketogenesis from amino acid and fatty acid precursors, respectively[(28)]. Glucagon has not been proven to possess peripheral effects outside the liver in response to physiologic stimuli. However, there is some evidence that it stimulates lipase in adipose tissue and induces glycogenolysis in muscle[(1)]. The key to glucose homeostasis and, therefore, the balance between anabolism and catabolism appears to be the ratio of insulin to glucagon. The ratio of insulin and glucagon (I/G) presented to the liver determines this balance[(31)]. The I/G ratio varies inversely with the need for endogenous glucose production. In normal subjects, the I/G ratio after overnight fasting is approximately 3. After total starvation, it may drop below 0.5. However, when the need for endogenous glucose is blocked by glucose infusion, the I/G ratio may increase to greater than 15. The normal relationship of insulin and glucagon is often altered after trauma, sepsis, or burns. This will be discussed in more detail below.

Opiate Peptides

Since the discovery of enkephalins by Hughes et al. in 1975[(32)], there has been an intense amount of work done in an effort to elucidate the role of the morphine-like substances known as opiate peptides. Originally, these substances were believed to be involved primarily in pain physiology; however, in the past 20 years, experimental evidence has implicated them as major components of the stress response.

There are essentially three opiate peptide systems. The enkephalin system contains two pentapeptides—methionine enkephalin (metenkephalin) and leucine enkephalin (leuenkephalin). Metenkephalin has the sequence NH2-tyrosine-glycine-glycine-phenylalanine-methionine-COOH. Leuenkephalin has the same structure as metenkephalin except leucine replaces methionine. These enkephalins apparently reside in the same cell[(33)].

The active compound in the second system is β-endorphin, a 31-amino acid peptide whose N-terminal pentapeptide sequence is identical to the structure of metenkephalin. β-Endorphin is a fragment of the pro-opiocortin molecule, which is also the precursor of ACTH and β-lipotropin. The opiate peptides interact with a variety of receptors that are distributed widely throughout the CNS. Dynorphins are found in high concentration in the posterior lobe of the pituitary, the hypothalamus, and the cerebellum.

Enkephalins are found throughout the CNS and are especially concentrated in the limbic system and along pain pathways[(33)]. They are present primarily in nerve endings, an observation that is consistent with the theory that enkephalins act as neurotransmitters[(34)]. The distribution of enkephalin nerve terminals is in the substancia gelatinosa of the spinal cord, the amygdala, and the central thalamus. They have been found in the intramural ganglia of the gastrointestinal (GI) tract and are also present in peripheral nerves such as the vagus. Outside of the CNS, enkephalins have been identified in paracrine cells of the GI tract, salivary glands, and the adrenal medulla.

The distribution of β-endorphin is much different from that of the enkephalins. β-Endorphin is found in diffuse projections from the hypothalamus to the thalamic centra. Outside of the CNS, β-endorphin is found only in the pituitary, where it occurs in the same cells as ACTH[(33)]. It is released into the circulation from the anterior and intermediate lobes. Anterior lobe release is associated with ACTH release and is likely under similar control[(1)]. However, release from the intermediate lobe may be under dopaminergic control. Stimuli that cause release of ACTH will also cause release of β-endorphin and β-lipotropin. Recent data suggest that pharmacologic actions produced by β-endorphin are mediated by the release of enkephalins[35].

The physiology of the opioid peptide system is complex and not fully understood. It is evident from much experimental data that endorphins play an important role in the modulation of pain[36–38]. Much of their function in pain modulation appears to relate to antinociception[39–41]. The antinociception effect may occur through inhibition of substance P, an excitatory neurotransmitter involved in nociceptive pathways from sensory fibers. Enkephalins have been found to decrease substance P release from cultured sensory neurons. Opiate peptides may modulate nociception at the periphery, particularly in inflamed tissue[39].

Opiate peptides may also function as hormones, especially β-endorphin. Enkephalins are degraded very rapidly, and it is doubtful whether they could reach distant targets if released into the bloodstream. β-Endorphin, however, has a half-life of 10 minutes in blood and may reach receptors far from the area of synthesis[33]. As mentioned earlier, stimuli that lead to release of ACTH also release equal amounts of β-endorphin. In turn, β-endorphin has been shown to have the capability of generating a sympathetic nervous system response. Intracerebroventricular administration of β-endorphin in dogs causes a 30-fold increase in plasma epinephrine and a sixfold increase in plasma norepinephrine, leading to a 70% increase in plasma glucose[42] β-Endorphin has also been shown to inhibit insulin release from pancreatic islet cells[43], to stimulate release of dopamine from adrenal medullary cells[44], and to potentiate the excretion of prolactin and growth hormone[1]. It has been postulated by some[45] that β-endorphin may play an inhibitory role in the secretion of ACTH. At the same time, both ACTH and glucocorticoids have been shown to inhibit release of β-endorphin in humans[46].

Consistent with this hormone-like role is the localization of enkephalins in the intestine as well as the brain. This distribution resembles that of other peptides that appear to serve hormone-like roles in the intestine and act as neurotransmitters in the brain, such as somatostatin, gastrin, vasoactive intestinal peptide, and substance P[34]. Recent work has shown that opiate peptoids may act as mediators and modulators of the immune system. In vitro, β-endorphin enhances natural killer cell lymphocyte activity, an effect that is reversed by naloxone[30]. β-Endorphin also has the ability to regulate interleukin-1 production by bone marrow cells and to suppress activation of human B-lymphocytes[47]. Lymphocytes, once stimulated by CRF, have the ability to secrete β-endorphin[48]. From these data, it is evident there is a close link between the opiate peptides and the immune system.

Opiate peptides are also believed to play a role in cardiovascular hemodynamics[49], respiratory control[50], and blood pressure regulation[51]. Clinical evidence of their role in the neuroendocrine responses will be discussed later in this chapter.

EFFECTORS AND EFFECTS: THE STRESS RESPONSE

Catecholamines

After stimulation by sympathetic nerves, the adrenal medulla chromaffin cells undergo depolarization and release by calcium-dependent exocytosis of preformed chromaffin granules. These catecholamines circulate both as free and conjugated form, with the later representing 60 to 90% of the total[52]. In stress, total catecholamine levels increase rapidly, but the ratio between free and conjugated remains the same[52].

Circulating epinephrine represents adrenal medullary secretion, while circulating norepinephrine represents "spill-over" into the plasma of norepinephrine secreted by sympathetic nerve terminals. Most norepinephrine is cleared by immediate reuptake by the nerves. The remainder is cleared quickly from the plasma, with the lung being a primary organ of clearance[53]. Epinephrine is cleared by rapid uptake by most tissues and is quickly deactivated by O-methylation. The half-life of these circulating catecholamines is about 30 seconds[54].

Catecholamines exert their influence on end-organs by binding with specific receptors: α_1 and α_2, β_1 and β_2, and the dopaminergic receptors. This interaction results in intracellular second messenger modulation mediating, finally, the cell-specific effects.

The cardiac and peripheral vascular effects of catecholamine stimulation are discussed in detail in Chapter 39. In addition to the circulatory effects, the catecholamines play a pivotal role in the metabolic responses to stress.

Hepatic production of glucose is markedly accelerated through several catecholamine-mediated mechanisms. Glycogen phosphorylase-a is stimulated, while glycogen synthetase is inhibited, with the resultant breakdown of glycogen[2] and release of glucose. Lactate conversion to glucose is accelerated by stimulation of the Cori cycle. Hepatic ketogenesis also is increased. The result of all these actions is increased production of glucose.

Catecholamine effects on other peripheral tissues include increased glycogenolysis and decreased glucose uptake in muscle, and increased lipolysis in adipose tissue. Epinephrine, moreover, inhibits pancreatic insulin secretion in the stress response and promotes a peripheral insulin resistance[55–57], both of which contribute to the hyperglycemia of the stress response.

Massive catecholamine output is seen in all critical illness, including sepsis[58–61] and burns[62]. Persistent catecholamine elevation is associated with poor outcome in trauma, burns, and in infants after cardiac surgery[63,64]. This observation led some investigators to use adrenergic blocking agents[65–67], but with only equivocal results.

In summary, the noncardiovascular effects of the high circulating catecholamines in the stress response are the me diation of several mechanisms that promote hyperglycemia: glycogenolysis, hepatic gluconeogenesis, mobilization of gluconeogenic precursors primarily from skeletal muscle protein, lypolysis, inhibition of insulin secretion, and peripheral insulin resistance. In general, the hyperglycemia and increased availability of glucose substrate, particularly for cardiac and brain function, is an adaptive response. Some evidence suggests, however, that the sustained hypermetabolism which may ensue can ultimately be detrimental.

Cortisol

After ACTH stimulation, cortisol release occurs within 1 to 3 minutes[68]. Upon entry into the circulation, under normal circumstances, 75% of cortisol is bound to plasma proteins, principally transcortin, an α1-glycoprotein, also called cortisol-binding globulin. Approximately 15% is bound loosely to albumin[1]. The remaining 10% circulates unbound. It is this portion that acts upon cells. Normally, total cortisol levels are near 13 μg/dl. If the total cortisol level exceeds 20 μg/dl, all binding sites on cortisol-binding globulin are saturated, and any further increase leads to an increase in free cortisol. Unbound cortisol passes easily into cells, and there it is bound to specific receptors in the cytosol. This cortisol receptor complex enters the nucleus of the cell and interacts with DNA to modulate transcription of m-RNA[1]. Through this mechanism, cortisol exerts profound influence over enzyme activity and protein content throughout the body.

Cortisol is a strong stimulator of gluconeogenesis by increasing the activity of such enzymes as pyruvate carboxylase, phosphoenolpyruvate carboxylase, and glucose-6-phosphatase. It also inhibits several glycolytic enzymes. Cortisol increases proteolysis, especially in the muscle, leading to an increase in nitrogen loss[69]. At the same time, it inhibits protein synthesis in extrahepatic tissues[70]. Cortisol causes an increase in alanine synthesis, which is a major substrate for gluconeogenesis. It sensitizes adipose tissue to the action of growth hormone and catecholamines, both of which cause lipolysis. Rizza et al.[71] studied insulin dose-response characteristics for suppression of glucose production and stimulation of glucose utilization in six healthy volunteers in response to a cortisol infusion, giving serum levels comparable to those seen in moderate stress. Their results showed that cortisol led to a decrease in hepatic and extrahepatic sensitivity to insulin. These data implicated a postreceptor mechanism for this insulin resistance.

It is well known that circulating cortisol has a negative feedback on ACTH release from the anterior pituitary. There is also evidence that glucocorticoids may produce negative feedback on corticotropin-releasing hormone as well. Other evidence suggests the presence of glucocorticoid receptors on neurons diffusely located in the CNS and on corticotropin-releasing hormone secreting cells in the hypothalamus.

There is evidence that cortisol regulates the biosynthesis of catecholamines in the adrenal medulla through its effects on phenylethonalamine-N-methyl transferase (PNMT), the enzyme responsible for conversion of norepinephrine to epinephrine. Glucocorticoids are believed to be inhibitors of PNMT degradation[72]. During stress in rats, PNMT activity increases, with a subsequent increase in epinephrine secretion believed to be related to increased glucocorticoid secretion.

It has been shown frequently that adrenal secretion of cortisol increases after injury and surgery. Ganong[73] found that the magnitude and duration of cortisol increase in the perioperative period was proportional to the magnitude of stress. Similarly, burn patients sustain an increase in plasma cortisol level within 2 hours of injury, which is in direct proportion to the magnitude of burn. In the work of Barton et al.[74], this relationship held true in moderately burned patients, but the most severely burned had cortisol levels that were decreased both absolutely and in relation to ACTH levels, probably reflecting impairment of adrenal responsiveness to ACTH.

Other authors have also confirmed the relative hypoadrenalism in other states of critical illness. Baldwin and Allo[75] and Kidess et al.[76] have both reported small groups of critically ill patients with refractory hypotension or multiple system organ failure associated with low systemic vascular resistance (SVR) and low cortisol levels who responded rapidly and dramatically to stress doses of corticosteroids. These patients had low cortisol levels; however, patients in one series who were administered corticotropin had cortisol responses which were not consistent[75] with hypoadrenalism defined by normal values.

In a more carefully designed study, Reincke et al. examined the functional integrity of the hypothalamic-pituitary-adrenal axis in 53 critically ill adults and seven controls[77]. Patients were separately subjected to an overnight dexamethasone suppression test and a CRF stimulation test. All patients had elevated baseline cortisol and ACTH levels which were not fully suppressible. At the same time, CRF produced an increase in both ACTH and cortisol levels above the already elevated baseline. The authors speculate that these effects may be due to altered glucocorticoid feedback on ACTH secretion in critical illness, or to the presence of other peptides with CRF-like activity, such as vasopressin or cytokines.

Cortisol's role in the stress response is vital. Evidence of this is the fact that adrenalectomized animals and patients with Addison's disease do poorly when significantly stressed[30]. During stress, cortisol likely diverts glucose utilization from muscle and other tissues to the brain and facilitates the action of, and increases the secretions of, catecholamines, which is thought to aid in maintenance of cardiovascular stability. It is believed that cortisol in increased levels is required for complete restoration of blood volume after hemorrhage. This effect is thought to be related to an osmotic effect of cortisol that causes an increase in extracellular osmolality, leading to a shift of fluid from the intracellular compartment to the interstitial space. This causes an increase in lymphatic transport of protein-rich fluid in the circulation. The mechanism behind this cortisol effect on osmotic pressure is not fully understood but likely relates to cortisol's influence on the hyperglycemic state and substrate mobilization, leading to hyperosmolality. Cortisol's interaction with glucagon and epinephrine is important in modulating the stress response. This interaction will be discussed later in this chapter.

Last, cortisol has direct effects on the immune system that may have profound effects on the organism's ability to handle stress. Increased cortisol levels cause demargination of peripheral neutrophils and decreases eosinophil, lymphocyte, and plasma cell counts[1]. Glucocorticoids cause a reduction in circulating macrophages, sequestration of T cells in the bone marrow, and lysis of immature T cells. They also inhibit interferon and interleukin production.

Glucagon and Insulin

In response to stress—i.e., surgery, burns, trauma—there is a characteristic alteration in the I/G ratio that has significant consequences. Glucagon is increased, possibly due to stimulation of pancreatic cells by cortisol, epinephrine, and/or endorphins. At the same time, there is a relative hypoinsulinemia that may be due to suppression of secretion by catecholamines[31], increase in metabolic clearance[78], or increased urinary insulin loss[79]. This leads to a decrease in the I/G ratio favoring gluconeogenesis, resulting in an increase in hepatic glucose production. Compounding this is the development of insulin resistance. Several mechanisms may be responsible for this phenomenon. Epinephrine has been found to impair tissue sensitivity to increased plasma insulin levels, primarily through β-adrenergic receptors, leading to both peripheral and hepatic resistance to insulin[56]. Rizza et al.[71] simulated moderate stress using cortisol infusions and found that this produced insulin resistance, once again at hepatic as well as extrahepatic sites. Their evidence implicates a postreceptor defect.

The consequence of this increase in glucagon and suppression of insulin secretion, plus insulin resistance, is significant. The result is hyperglycemia and inability of the organism to use substrate at the tissue level, leading to increased nitrogen loss. This may cause serious metabolic consequences at the tissue level in trauma and burn patients, but may also lead to hyperglycemia/hyperosmolality that likely aids in restoration of circulatory volume through earlier mentioned mechanisms.

Growth Hormone

The two primary functions of growth hormone are to regulate somatic growth and to regulate metabolism. These two functions overlap, and the mechanisms for growth hormone's activity are also similar.

Early observations suggested that not all actions of growth hormone were direct. Growth hormone added to the plasma of hypophysectomized animals failed to stimulate in vitro cartilage growth; plasma from pituitary-intact animals, however, did[80]. Thus, it appeared that growth hormone stimulated the elaboration of another substance that produced the growth effects. Subsequently, somatomedins were identified and their function explored[81,82]. Two somatomedins have been identified (A and C) and have been characterized as insulin-like growth factors (IGF-2 and IGF-1)[83]. They are synthesized in the liver and in fibroblasts, and circulate largely bound to carrier proteins whose synthesis is also controlled by growth hormone[2]. These factors have separate receptors, one of which (IGF-1) is similar to insulin receptors, allowing for some degree of shared affinity of the two hormones for each other's receptor.

The metabolic effects of growth hormone are thought to be more direct than the growth effects. These effects are biphasic. Acutely, the effects are insulin-like: enhanced glucose uptake in muscle and adipose tissue, amino acid uptake and protein synthesis in liver and muscle, and inhibition of lipolysis in adipose tissue. These effects are followed within several hours by anti-insulin effects when growth hormone levels are persistently elevated. Glucose uptake and utilization are inhibited and lipolysis is enhanced. These effects are synergistic with those of other hormones (epinephrine, cortisol, glucagon), and identify growth hormone as a counterregulatory hormone.

Increased levels of growth hormone have long been known to be associated with stress[84], surgery[85], trauma[86], and community-acquired lobar pneumonia[87]. It is likely that this elevation contributes to the hyperglycemia of the stress response and is an adaptive addition to the actions of the other counterregulatory hormones.

The theoretical benefit of the protein-sparing effects of growth hormone has led some investigators to use exogenously administered hormone after injury[88] and burns[89], and in sepsis[90]. In all three of these studies, nitrogen wasting was reduced, but administration has also been shown to exacerbate and prolong insulin resistance[91]. Nonetheless, Herndon et al.[92] demonstrated more rapid wound healing in adult burn patients given growth hormone, while similar benefits have been demonstrated in burned children[93], together with reduced length of hospitalization[94]. Finally, growth hormone has been demonstrated to have beneficial effects on preservation of body water compartments in critically ill adult surgical patients[95], though the long-term advantages of this apparent physiologic benefit remain unproven.

The therapeutic use of growth hormone in critical care remains a tantalizing but still largely unproven area ripe for future clinical research. These issues have been well discussed in two excellent reviews[96,97].

Prolactin

Animal studies have demonstrated a short-lived increase in prolactin levels with stress[98], an effect that is attenuated by prior thyroidectomy. Histamine stimulates this release[99], while naloxone[100], an opioid receptor antagonist, blunts stress-induced prolactin release, suggesting a possible role for opioid peptides. Prolactin appears to have a mild diabetogenic effect[101]. Speculation exists based on animal study results about a role for prolactin in maintaining the competence of the immune system[102], though no such role has been demonstrated in humans. Indeed, the pattern of prolactin response to stress in the critically ill patient has not been well characterized, and its role remains unclear, although it probably contributes in a minor way to the hyperglycemia of the stress response.

Thyroid Hormone

The primary role of thyroid hormone is to influence metabolic homeostasis by regulating the synthesis and activity of a variety of proteins. Receptors for T3 are thought to be primarily located in cell nuclei, where their stimulation produces messenger-RNA synthesis. Some important functions modulated or controlled by T3 include adrenergic receptor function, sodium-potassium ATPase, and TRH secretion. Of special interest in the stress response is the interaction between T3 and catecholamines. An inverse relationship exists between serum concentrations of T3 and catecholamines[103]. T3 also increases the numbers of β-adrenergic receptors, while decreasing α-receptors[104–106]. Conversely, sympathetic nervous system stimulation and circulating catecholamines also affect the thyroid and thyroid hormone function. Direct sympathetic stimulation of the thyroid will increase thyroid hormone secretion[107,108] as will infusion of exogenous catecholamines[109,110]. Epinephrine also increases the peripheral deiodination of T4, increasing the amount of active hormone available in the periphery[111].

Although abnormal thyroid hormone levels in nonthyroidal chronic diseases had been previously appreciated, abnormalities in acutely and critically ill patients were first described by McLarty et al.[112] and by Bermudez et al.[113]. Both groups of investigators described low T4 and T3 levels and a relationship between the magnitude of their depression and mortality. McLarty coined the term "sick euthyroid" syndrome and questioned whether administration of exogenous thyroid hormone might alter prognosis.

The observation of decreased thyroid hormone in critically ill patients has been confirmed and elaborated upon by others. The most common pattern of initial decrease in T3, low or normal T4, with a concomitant rise in rT3, has been observed in burn patients[114], those with sepsis[115], trauma patients[115,116], and medical intensive care patients[117]. The degree of T3 and T4 depression correlates with increased morbidity and is usually followed by a recovery toward normal in survivors, which is not seen in nonsurvivors[114–117]. These patients generally have normal TSH levels, although others have shown an 88% incidence of blunted TSH response to TRF stimulation in critically ill adults[118], with a relationship between the magnitude of blunting and lesser survival.

The mechanism of thyroid hormone alterations remains unclear. Some have postulated a role for malnutrition and general catabolic state[119], while others have implicated tumor necrosis factor[120]. Regardless of mechanism, it is of note that most patients with the sick euthyroid syndrome have normal to strikingly increased metabolic rates despite low T3 levels. Some evidence[121] suggests that T3 receptor expression is augmented, allowing this maintenance of clinical euthyroidism. Other alterations in thyroid hormone function have also been described, including altered binding to serum proteins[122] and disruption of the normal circadian pattern of TSH secretion[123].

Zucker et al.[124] investigated thyroid function in critically ill children. Twenty-seven children, both medical and surgical patients, demonstrated significant depression of T3 and T4, with normal TSH levels. All patients who had rT3 measurements also had increases over time, half to levels above normal, suggesting a hormonal pattern identical to that most frequently observed in critically ill adults. However, unlike adult series, there was no relationship between depression of T3 and mortality.

Renin-Angiotensin-Aldosterone

The earlier discussion of the renin-angiotensin-aldosterone system indicated a central role for this system in the maintenance of central hemodynamics and total body water. The system allows for a biphasic response to cardiovascular stresses. An immediate response is mediated by angiotensin II in the form of profound peripheral vasoconstriction. Angiotensin is by no means the sole mediator of this adaptation, but its contributions are important. The longer term conservation of water and sodium, both to maintain and eventually to replenish total body water content is mediated by the angiotensin-stimulated release of aldosterone.

Plasma concentrations of renin, angiotensin, and aldosterone can be shown to be significantly elevated within a short period of time from the onset of numerous forms of stress. Robertson and Michelakis[125] demonstrated a threefold rise in renin activity after various surgical procedures. In an animal burn model, Hilton and Marully[126] showed that plasma angiotensin increases linearly from 15 minutes to 6 hours after burn injury. These investigators implicated these elevations, along with elevations in vasopressin levels, in the postburn myocardial depression that complicates the recovery of these patients[126,127].

Thus, it would appear that like catecholamines, the renin-angiotensin-aldosterone system plays a key adaptive role in the response, both immediate and longer term. Also like catecholamines, some evidence suggests that protracted elevations of these hormones may be detrimental.

Opiate Peptides

Opiate peptides have been shown to cause not only an increase in serum glucose and epinephrine but an inhibition of insulin secretion by pancreatic islet cells. In part, because of these effects, they are believed to play some role in the response to injury or stress. A number of researchers have investigated the role of elevated levels of these compounds in surgical and traumatic stress.

Endogenous opiates have been implicated as a cause of secondary damage after neuronal injury due to evidence from some studies in which improvement in neurologic function was found when opiate antagonists were used. Jiang et al.(128) found elevated levels of β-endorphin in the cerebral spinal fluid of 36 patients with acute head injury. Levels were found to correlate with severity of injury. However, other studies have shown no correlation between β-endorphin levels and severity of illness(129).

Vongsovan et al.(130) found elevated levels of β-endorphin in the serum of patients undergoing dental operations. This rise was attenuated by pretreatment with diazepam. Elevated levels of β-endorphin have also been seen in the cerebral spinal fluid of animals exposed to experimental spinal ischemia(131) and in the plasma of dogs subjected to experimental acute pancreatitis(132). In the pancreatitis study, naloxone improved survival, decreased lactate levels, and reversed cardiovascular compromise, all of which had been associated with increased levels of β-endorphin. They concluded that β-endorphin plays a significant role in the cardiovascular decompensation seen in this model.

Holaday(49), using experimental models of endotoxic, hemorrhagic, and spinal shock, speculated that opiate peptides play a key role in cardiovascular instability. This was based on the findings that naloxone reversed shock and improved survival in each model. However, results of clinical studies have been inconclusive.

In humans, elevation in circulating levels of β-endorphin have been found in response to stress of impending examinations and physical stressors(133). In critically ill children, endorphin levels have been found to be elevated(134,135), especially in those patients who were hyperglycemic and hyperinsulinemic. With recovery, β-endorphin levels decreased, as did insulin levels. While these studies implicate a role for opiate peptides in the stress response, the exact nature of this role is unknown.

Counterregulatory Hormone Interactions

Glucagon, epinephrine, and cortisol are known as counterregulatory hormones because of their opposition to the actions of insulin. Their interactions in response to stressful stimuli have been the subject of much investigation.

In an effort to simulate changes seen in severe stress, Shamoon et al.(136) infused healthy, overnight fasted subjects with epinephrine, glucagon, and cortisol. Simultaneous infusion of the three hormones lead to glucose levels greater than 200 mg/dl despite a 100 to 200% increase in plasma insulin. However, when each hormone was infused singly, the glucose elevation was mild or transient. The elevation in glucose seen with combined infusions was three times higher than the sum of that seen with each hormone infused separately. There was increased glucose production and decreased clearance despite elevated plasma insulin levels, indicating a resistance to insulin, likely due to cortisol or epinephrine. Although insulin levels were increased, they were not of the magnitude expected with the level of hyperglycemia achieved. The relative inhibition of insulin secretion is likely due to an epinephrine effect. These authors concluded that counterregulatory hormones must act synergistically. A possible mechanism for this synergism is based on the fact that glucagon promotes gluconeogenesis by increasing hepatocyte c-AMP by a non-β-receptor mechanism and may, therefore, amplify the β-adrenergic effects of epinephrine. Cortisol has been reported to work synergistically with epinephrine possibly by inhibiting catechol-O-methyl transferase and preventing catecholamine reuptake. It has also been proposed that cortisol may act to increase β-receptor density that would increase the response to catecholamines(31).

Bessey et al.(137) confirmed the findings of Shamoon and associates, finding both an additive and a synergistic effect of infusions of epinephrine, hydrocortisone, and glucagon. However, in their study, doses of infusions were used to simulate moderate injury. In addition to glucose intolerance, hyperinsulinemia, and insulin resistance, their patients exhibited hypermetabolism, negative nitrogen balance, sodium retention, negative potassium balance, and increased white blood cell counts. The levels of cortisol and epinephrine achieved were comparable to those found in patients with moderately severe injury and burns.

Gelfand et al.(69), using glucagon, epinephrine, norepinephrine, and cortisol infusions in different combinations, found similar results but were unable to effect an increase in the metabolic rate. In addition, the sustained nitrogen loss produced by the combination of glucagon, epinephrine, and norepinephrine was no greater than that produced by cortisol alone. However, glucagon, epinephrine, and norepinephrine did transiently augment nitrogen loss. The authors concluded that while counterregulatory hormones play a role in the massive nitrogen loss, muscle proteolysis, and hypermetabolism seen in severe stress, they are not the sole mediators. This conclusion was based on the fact that 3-methylhistidine excretion, an indicator of muscle breakdown, was not significantly increased in these patients. However, in a modification of studies using systemically administered hormone combinations, Gore et al. examined skeletal muscle metabolism in leg muscle of healthy volunteers with femoral arterial infusion of epinephrine, cortisol and glucagon(138). They were able to demonstrate using radiolabeled lysine and vastus lateralis muscle biopsies that protein synthesis increased during infusion by 48.5%, while muscle breakdown increased by 65%, demonstrating a hormonally induced catabolic state.

The infusion of etiocholanolone, an inflammatory agent, in addition to hydrocortisone, glucagon, and epinephrine, caused all of the earlier mentioned changes plus fever, acute phase reactant synthesis, and hypoferremia(137,139). This supports the theory that both endocrine and inflammatory mediators must be active in response to stress and injury.

CONSEQUENCES OF THE STRESS RESPONSE

A first glance at the neuroendocrine response to stress may seem to reveal a jumble of disjointed, rapidly changing hormonal and nervous-system activities which appear to have no pattern or purpose. When one examines the effects of this multipart response, however, and begins to appreciate its adaptive nature, a sense of coordination of the response begins to emerge. These effects are of two types: metabolic effects and water/electrolyte adaptations. We will discuss the first; the second is discussed in detail in Chapters 37 and 38.

Metabolic

The metabolic effects of the neuroendocrine response to stress have generally to do with substrate mobilization and utilization and with energy metabolism.

Carbohydrate Metabolism

One of the most obvious and profound immediate effects of the stress response is the hyperglycemia described earlier. Glucose is the primary and most readily available energy source, and all aspects of the neuroendocrine response act in concert to optimize glucose availability, manifested by the early hyperglycemia seen soon after stress.

The earliest phase of the hyperglycemia results from mobilization of glycogen from the liver[(24)]. The maximal hepatic glycogen store, however, can provide only about 75 g of glucose[(2)], sufficient to meet the glucose needs in a fasting adult for little more than 12 hours but far from sufficient to meet the needs of a stressed or traumatized patient. The hyperglycemic state and continued availability of glucose is thus maintained by other mechanisms.

Gluconeogenesis takes over where glycogenolysis leaves off. Synthesis of new glucose occurs primarily in the liver, and the primary source is amino acids liberated from skeletal muscle breakdown. While skeletal muscle is the primary source of the amino acid glucose precursors, every organ in the body also sustains some degree of protein breakdown. In addition, lactate and pyruvate, as well as glucose, are used by the liver in gluconeogenesis. All of these changes are under the controlled influence of the interacting counterregulatory hormones and the finely tuned ratio of insulin and glucagon secretion.

Protein Metabolism

The most obvious and immediate change in protein metabolism in stress is the acceleration of protein breakdown. This is manifested by negative nitrogen balance and increased serum amino acid levels. Most of the amino acids thus liberated are used for gluconeogenesis, but some are diverted to the increased hepatic synthesis of proteins crucial to the body's immunologic defenses and to wound healing[(24)].

The protein breakdown is thought to have many mediators. Certainly glucagon and cortisol have profound catabolic effects, as discussed earlier. In addition, some studies have suggested a role for certain cytokines and prostaglandins[(140–142)].

Fat Metabolism

The predominant change in fat metabolism, like that of protein, is characterized by breakdown. After stress, both glycerol and free fatty acids are elevated, indicative of lipolysis. The triglycerides thus liberated become a major energy source for the stressed patient[(144)]. This lipolysis is largely under adrenergic control but is also substantially influenced by circulating hormones. In addition, as with proteolysis, there is evidence to suggest a role for cytokines and prostaglandins[(145–147)].

Energy Metabolism

Marked increases in metabolic rate, as measured by indirect calorimetry or radiolabeled substrates, are seen in all forms of stress. Resting energy expenditure is increased after uncomplicated elective surgery[(30)] by 10 to 15%, while in septic patients, increases of up to 140% of normal are not uncommon[(31,148–150)]. The greatest increases in oxygen consumption appear to occur in burn patients. Caloric expenditure increases linearly in uncomplicated burns with the percentage of body surface area burned. This relationship holds true up to about 60% surface area burn, where the caloric expenditure appears to plateau at approximately 200% of normal[(151)]. The increase in metabolic rate is most likely the result of the synergistic influence of cortisol, glucagon, and catecholamines, with the latter playing a primary role[(152)]. In sepsis, other factors may also be operative. Tredget et al.[(153)] have suggested an important role for cytokines.

Energy expenditure in critically ill children is much less well studied, in part because of technical difficulties in making accurate indirect calorimetric measurements of oxygen consumption in the small child and infant. Those studies that have been done, however, suggest degrees and patterns of caloric expenditure in children similar to those seen in adults[(154–156)]. The area of hypermetabolism in the critically ill patient has been recently reviewed by McClave and Snider[(157)].

EFFECTS OF DRUGS ON THE STRESS RESPONSE

As the details of the neuroendocrine response to stress continue to be detailed and our understanding of that response continues to evolve, the potential of harmful drug effects on the response has also begun to be studied. Of the drugs commonly used in critical care, dopamine was the first to be studied extensively.

Devins et al.[(158)] showed 90% reduction in prolactin levels within 4 hours of initiation of dopamine in critically ill adults; this was associated with a transient but significant reduction in T-cell proliferation response to concanavalin A stimulation.

Van den Bergh et al. showed that dopamine infusion suppresses the secretion of leutenizing hormone[159] and of growth hormone[160], and have speculated that this latter effect may play a role in the catabolism of critical illness. Of particular note to the pediatric intensivist are their findings in newborns and children in the first 48 hours after surgery for congenital heart disease[161]. They found that dopamine induced or aggravated a preexisting partial hypopituitarism in these children, that the patterns of suppression differed somewhat from those in critically ill adults, and that the patterns also differ slightly between newborns and nonneonates.

The renal effects of low-dose dopamine have long been appreciated, though these effects may be less clear in infants and children. Moreover, the effects are not always consistent and predictable even in the nonpediatric patient. Duke et al.[162] compared dopamine and dobutamine in comparable low doses to placebo in critically ill, oliguric adults at risk for the development of acute renal failure. Dopamine produced diuresis with no change in creatinine clearance, while dobutamine increased creatinine clearance with no effect on urinary volume. Marik[163] examined the effects of low-dose dopamine on the renin-angiotensin-aldosterone axis in a similar group of patients and found marked increases in plasma renin activity in patients who failed to respond with diuresis to those who did. This leads to speculation that the inconsistency of the diuretic effects of low-dose dopamine may be a result of a previously underappreciated and complex interaction between its endocrine (renin) effects and its direct renal vasodilatory ones.

STRESS RESPONSE IN THE PEDIATRIC PATIENT

It is clear that the adult's response to stress—neurologic and hormonal—and its metabolic and immunologic effects have been fairly well characterized, even if the precise mechanisms and mediators are imperfectly defined. At the other extreme, so few studies have been done in pediatric patients that the pediatrician is left to extrapolate from what is known of adult physiology. Similarly, comparatively little work has been done on neonates; this work has been recently and thoroughly reviewed and summarized by Schmeling and Coran[29]. By comparing the responses known to occur in adults with those seen in infants, it may be possible to make inferences about the nonneonatal pediatric patient **(Tables 44.1 and 44.2).**

Neonates are clearly capable of β-endorphin secretion, as demonstrated by increased levels in cord blood at the time of delivery[29], but further documentation of endorphin response or its role after stress in the neonate are lacking. Similarly, no studies have been done to characterize stress-

Table 44.1. Hormonal Response to Operative Stress in the Adult and Neonate[a]

Hormone	*Adult*	*Neonate*
Endorphins	Increased after stress Actions Modulate ACTH secretion Enhance hypothalamic sympathetic response, increase catecholamine release Modulate insulin and glucagon secretion ? immune modulation	No postoperative data Increased following stress of delivery ? role in septic shock
Pituitary hormones	Increased ACTH, growth hormone, prolactin, vasopressin GH→ Lipolysis Protein synthesis Inhibition of insulin action	No direct data; exogenous ACTH causes increased cortisol levels, suggesting increased ACTH
Catecholamines	Increased epinephrine and norepinephrine; probably responsible for most stress-related catabolic response	Increased epinephrine and norepinephrine with birth stress, perinatal asphyxia, postoperatively Actions Initiates hyperglycemia with decreased insulin and increased glucagon release Increased minute ventilation, cardiac output, heart rate, and blood pressure
Pancreatic hormones	Insulin decreased intraoperatively; conflicting data for postoperative changes Glucagon increased → amino acid mobilization with gluconeogenesis and new protein synthesis	Increased insulin in term neonates; no change in preterm infants
Adrenocorticoids	Increased cortisol → lipolysis and FFA release; amino acid mobilization; glucagon production	Age-dependent increase in cortisol, earlier peak in younger infants
Aldosterone	Increased → sodium and water conservation, volume restoration	No data on stress-induced changes
Renin-angiotensin	Increased renin (3×) postoperatively; increased angiotensin	No data
Vasopressin	No data available on perioperative stress response	Indirect evidence of increase
Thyroid hormone	Decreased T3, increased rT3	No data

[a] *Modified from Schmeling DJ, Coran AG. Hormonal and metabolic response to operative stress in the neonate. JPEN 1991;17:215.*

Table 44.2. Metabolic Response to Operative Stress in the Adult and Neonate[a]

Metabolic Effect	*Adult*	*Neonate*
Metabolic rate and oxygen consumption	Decreased briefly, then increased	Minimal change compared to controls; less than adults
Carbohydrate	Hyperglycemic response, with gluconeogenesis and decreased glucose utilization	Hyperglycemia (2× increased immediately postoperatively), more transient than adults Glycogenolysis more important than in adults than gluconeogenesis
Protein	Negative nitrogen balance, with slight increased protein breakdown proportional to severity of stress; decreased protein synthesis in extrahepatic tissues Increased amino acid utilization for gluconeogenesis, acute-phase reactant synthesis and healing process components	Increased nitrogen excretion, sustained to 5 days Negative nitrogen balance 72–96 hr postoperatively; increased nitrogen loss in neonates compared to older infants Increased muscle protein breakdown, impaired nitrogen utilization Lower serum gluconeogenic amino acid levels than in adults
Fat	Adipose tissue lipolysis with mobilization of nonesterified fatty acids and increased ketone body formation, supplying 75–90% of energy need	Increased lipolysis and ketogenesis→ increased total ketone bodies, increased glycerol and nonesterified fatty acids Postoperative fat utilization exceeds rate of mobilization of free fatty acids

[a] *Modified from Schmeling DJ, Coran AG. Hormonal and metabolic response to operative stress in the neonate. JPEN 1991;17:215.*

related changes in growth hormone, prolactin, and ADH or to elucidate a role for these hormones in the stress response. However, infants are able to mount a cortisol response to operative stress, which, though less than that seen in the adult, suggests that the hypothalamopituitary-adrenal axis is, at least partly, intact and functional[(29)].

Studies of neonates' catecholamine responses to stress, however, are numerous. These studies clearly demonstrate catecholamine increases that are similar, though not identical, to those seen in adults after stress, which are also associated with hyperglycemic response and may be modulated by anesthesia[(165–167)].

Insulin responses to stress in the neonate have also been fairly well studied. Increases in insulin are seen, but are less in magnitude than in the adult, probably reflecting relative immaturity of the neonatal pancreatic islet cells[(164)]. Glucagon responses are less well documented than insulin responses. Anand et al.[(164–167)] have shown that glucose levels remain at baseline during and immediately after stress and fall at 24 hours—a pattern that is strikingly different from that of adults, who experience an immediate and sustained rise in most stress settings. The significance of the reversed glucagon response in the neonate is not understood.

The responses of the renin-angiotensin-aldosterone system, vasopressin, thyroid hormone, and growth hormone have been too incompletely studied to allow conclusive comment. These are clearly important areas ripe for further investigation.

The metabolic responses to the hormonal stimuli in stress in the neonate and the adult are summarized in **Table 44.2**[(29)], while the hormonal changes themselves are described in **Table 44.1**[(29)]. While it is apparent that some of the responses of the pediatric patient are similar to those of the adult, it is also clear that some of the differences are more than subtle. With further investigation, the significance of these differences will become clearer, allowing a more lucid understanding of the neuroendocrine response as a whole, and perhaps leading to more innovative and fruitful interventions in our attempt to facilitate the organism/patient's adaptation to and survival of life-threatening stressors.

References

1. Gann DS, Lilly MP. The neuroendocrine response to multiple trauma. World J Surg 1983;7:101.
2. West JB, ed. Best and Taylor's the physiological basis of medical practice, 12th ed. New York: Williams & Wilkins, 1990.
3. Gordon NH, Scott DB, Robbi WP. Modification of plasma corticosteroid concentration during and after surgery by epidural blockade. Br Med J 1973;1:598.
4. Hume DM, Edgahl RH. The importance of the brain in the endocrine response to injury. Ann Surg 1959;150:697.
5. Kuntscher FR, Galletti PM, Hahn C, et al. Alterations of insulin and glucose metabolism during cardiopulmonary bypass under normothermia. J Thorac Cardiovasc Surg 1987;89:97.
6. Goschke H, Bar E, Girard J, et al. Glucagon, insulin, cortisol and growth hormone levels following major surgery: their relationship to glucose and free fatty acid elevations. Horm Metab Res 1978;10:465.
7. Newsome HH, Rose JC. The response of adrenocorticotrophic hormone and growth hormone to surgical stress. J Clin Endocrinol 1971;33:481.
8. Korpassy A, Stoekel H, Vecses P. Investigations of hydrocortisone secretion and aldosterone excretion in patients with severe prolonged stress. Acta Anaesthesiol Scand 1972;16:161.
9. Cochrane JP, Forsling ML, Gow NM, et al. Arginine vasopressin release following surgical operations. Br J Surg 1981;68:204.
10. Jarek MJ, Legare EJ, McDermott MT, et al. Endocrine profiles for outcome prediction from the intensive care unit. Crit Care Med 1993;21(4):543.
11. Rothwell PM, Lawler PG. Prediction of outcome in intensive care patients using endocrine parameters. Crit Care Med 1995;23(1):78.
12. Maldonado LS, Murata GH, Hershman JM, et al. Do thyroid function tests independently predict survival in the critically ill? Thyroid 1992;2(2):119.
13. Rothwell PM, Udwadia ZF, Lawler PG. Thyrotropin concentration predicts outcome in critical illness. Anaesthesia 1993;48(5):373.
14. Span LF, Hermus AR, Bartelink AK. Adrenocortical function: an indicator of severity of disease and survival in chronic critically ill patients. Intensive Care Med 1992;18(2):93.
15. Gann DS. Parameters of the stimulus initiating the adrenocortical response to hemorrhage. Ann NY Acad Sci 1969;156:740.

16. Yates FE, Russell SM, Dallman MF, et al. Potentiation by vasopressin of corticotropin release induced by corticotropin releasing factor. Endocrinology 1971;88:3.
17. Yasuda N, Greer MA. Studies on the corticotropin-releasing activity of vasopressin, using ACTH secretion by cultured rat adenohypophyseal cells. Endocrinology 1976;98:936.
18. Ramsay DJ, Keil LC, Sharpe MC, et al. Angiotensin II infusion increases vasopressin, ACTH, and 11-hydroxycorticosteroid secretion. Am J Physiol 1978;234:R66.
19. Parker RC, Baxter CR. Divergence in adrenal steroid secretory pattern after thermal injury in adult patients. J Trauma 1987;27:384.
20. Cartensen H, Terner N, Thoren L, et al. Testosterone, luteinizing hormone, and growth hormone in blood following surgical trauma. Acta Chir Scand 1972;138:1.
21. Hamanaka Y, Kurachi K, Aono T, et al. Effects of general anesthesia and severity of surgical stress on serum LH and testosterone in males. Acta Endocrinol 1975;78:258.
22. Wang C, Chan V, Tse TF, et al. Effect of acute myocardial infarction on pituitary-testicular function. Clin Endocrinol 1978;9:249.
23. Woolf PD, Hamill RW, McDonald JV, et al. Transient hypogonadotropic hypogonadism caused by critical illness. J Clin Endocrinol Metab 1985;66:444.
24. Crane-Chartens AC, Odell WB, Thompson JC. Anterior pituitary function during surgical stress and convalescence: radioimmunoassay measurement of blood, TSH, LH, FSH, and growth hormone. J Clin Endocrinol 1969;29:63.
25. Gebhart SSP, Waltt NB, Clark RV, et al. Reversible impairment of gonadotropin secretion in critical illness. Arch Intern Med 1989;149:1637.
26. Spratt DI, Cox P, Orav J, et al. Reproductive axis suppression in acute illness is related to disease severity. J Clin Endocrinol Metab 1993; 76(6):1548.
27. Sato A, Schmidt RF. Somatosympathetic reflexes: afferent fibers, central pathways, discharge characteristics. Physiol Rev 1973;53:916.
28. Greenspan, FS, Forsham PH, eds. Basic & clinical endocrinology, 2nd edition. Los Altos, CA: Lange Medical Publications, 1986.
29. Schmeling DJ, Coran AG. Hormonal and metabolic response to operative stress in the neonate. JPEN 1991;17:215.
30. Weissman C. The metabolic response to stress: an overview and update. Anesthesiology 1990;73:308.
31. Unger RH. Glucagon and the insulin:glucagon ratio in diabetes and other catabolic illnesses. Diabetes 1971;20:834.
32. Hughes JT, Smith W, Kosterlitz HW, et al. Identification of two related pentapeptides from the brain opiate agonist activity. Nature 1975; 258:577.
33. Terenius L. Endorphins—the first three years. Am Heart J 1979;98:681.
34. Snyder S. Opiate receptors and internal opiates. Scientif Am 1977; 236:44.
35. Tseng LL. Intracerebroventricular administration of beta-endorphin releases immunoreactive metenkephalin from spinal cord in cats, guinea pigs and mice. Neuropharmacology 1989;28:1333.
36. Spaziante R, Merola B, Colao A, et al. Beta-endorphin concentrations both in plasma and in cerebrospinal fluid in response to acute painful stimuli. J Neurosurg Sci 1990;39:395.
37. Cahill CA. Beta-endorphin levels during pregnancy and labor: a role in pain modulation? Nurs Res 1989;38:200.
38. Bacigalupo GS, Rosendahl H, et al. Quantitative relationships between pain intensities during labor and beta-endorphin and cortisol concentrations in plasma: decline of the hormone concentrations in the early postpartum period. J Perinat Med 1990;18:289.
39. Herz A, Millan MJ. Opioids and opioid receptors mediating antinociception at various levels of the neuraxis. Physiol Bohemoslov 1990;39:395.
40. Wong CL, Wai MK, Cheng HC, et al. Preliminary study on the antinociceptive effect of elevation in beta-endorphin. Clin Exp Pharmacol Physiol 1990;17:33.
41. Hargreaves KM, Flores CM, Dionne RA, et al. The role of pituitary beta-endorphin in mediating corticotropin-releasing factor-induced antinociception. Am J Physiol 1990;258:235.
42. Radosevich PM, Lacy DB, Brown LL, et al. Central effects of beta-endorphins on glucose homeostasis in the conscious dog. Am J Physiol 1989;256:322.
43. Schleicher RL. Beta-endorphin inhibits insulin secreted pancreatic islets. Endocrinology 1989;124:1254.
44. Ensor DM, Morley JS, Redfern RM, et al. Stimulation of dopamine output from adrenal medullary cells by beta-endorphin and its C-terminal tetrapeptide (MPF). Brain Res 1989;490:196.
45. Volavka J, Cho D, Mallya A. Naloxone increases ACTH and cortisol levels in man. New Engl J Med 1979;300:1056.
46. Boscaro M, Paoletta A, Giacomazzi P, et al. Inhibition of beta-endorphin by ACTH and glucocorticoids. Neuroendocrinology 1990;51:561.
47. Morgan EL, McClurg MR, et al. Suppresion of B-lymphocyte activation by beta-endorphin. 1990;28:209.
48. Kavelaars A, Berkenbosch F, Croiset G, et al. Induction of beta-endorphin secretion by lymphocytes after subcutaneous administration of corticotropin-releasing factor. Endocrinology 1990;126:759.
49. Holaday JW. Cardiovascular effects of opiate opiate systems. Ann Rev Pharmacol Toxicol 1983;23:541.
50. Levick MP, Lovelock M, Smith R, et al. Relation between plasma beta-endorphin and the ventilatory response to hypercapnia in humans. Clin Sci 1989;77:323.
51. DeJong W, Petty MA, Sistsen JM. Role of opioid peptides in brain mechanisms regulating blood pressure. Chest 1983;83:306.
52. Woolf PD, Hamill RW, Lee LA, et al. Free and total catecholamines in critical illness. Am J Physiol 1988;254:E287.
53. Van Loon GR, Sole MJ. Plasma dopamine: source, regulation and significance. Metabolism 1980;29(suppl):1119.
54. Ferreira SH, Vane JR. Half-lives of peptides and amines in the circulation. Nature 1967;215:1237.
55. Felig P, Sherwin RS, Soman V, et al. Hormonal interactions in the regulation of blood glucose. Rec Prog Horm Res 1979;35:501.
56. Deibert DC, DeFronzo RA. Epinephrine-induced insulin resistance in man. J Clin Invest 1980;65:717.
57. Waldhaus WK, Gasic S, Bratusch-Marrain P, et al. Effect of stress hormones on splanchnic substrate and insulin disposal after glucose ingestion in healthy humans. Diabetes 1987;36:127.
58. Bocking JK, Sibbald WJ, Holliday RL, et al. Plasma catecholamine levels and pulmonary dysfunction in sepsis. Surg Gynecol Obstet 1979;148:715.
59. Davies CL, Malyneux SG, Newman RJ. HPLC determination of plasma catecholamines in road accident casualties. Br J Clin Pharmacol 1981;13:P283.
60. Hassett J, Border JR. The metabolic response to trauma and sepsis. World J Surg 1983;7:125.
61. Davies CL, Newman RJ, Malyneux SG, et al. The relationship between plasma catecholamines and severity of injury in man. J Trauma 1984;24:99.
62. Markley K, Smallman ET, Briggs L. Early mortality and temperature regulation in burned mice following administration of catecholamine and adrenergic receptor blocking drugs. J Trauma 1986;19:522.
63. Anand KJ, Hansen DD, Hickey PR. Hormonal-metabolic stress responses in neonates undergoing cardiac surgery. Anesthesiology 1990;73:661–670.
64. Anand KJ, Hickey PR. Halothane-morphine compared with high-dose sufentanil for anesthesia and postoperative analgesia in neonatal cardiac surgery (see comments). N Engl J Med 1992;326:1–9.
65. Wilmore DW, Long JM, Mason AD, et al. Catecholamines: mediator of the hypermetabolic response to thermal injury. Ann Surg 1974; 180:653.
66. Berk JL, Hagen JF, Dunn JM. The role of beta adrenergic blockade in the treatment of septic shock. Surg Gynecol Obstet 1970;130:1025.
67. Breitenstein E, Chiolero RL, Jequier E, et al. Effects of beta-blockade on energy metabolism following burns. Burns 1990;16:259.
68. Lake RB, Gann DS. Dynamic response of the intact canine adrenal to infused ACTH. Ann Biomed Eng 1972;1:56.
69. Gelfand RA, Matthews DE, et al. Role of counterregulatory hormones in the catabolic response to stress. J Clin Invest 1984;74:2238.
70. Yates FE, Marsh DJ, et al. The adrenal cortex. Med Physiol 1980;14:1558.
71. Rizza BA, Mandarino LJ, et al. Cortisol-induced insulin resistance in man: impaired suppression of glucose production and stimulation of glucose utilization due to a postreceptor defect of insulin action. Clin Endocrinol Metab 1982;45:131.
72. Axelrod J, Reisine TC. Stress hormones: their interaction and regulation. Science 1984;224:452.
73. Ganong WF. The stress response—A dynamic overview. Hosp Pract 1988;23:155.
74. Barton RN, Stoner HB, Watson SM. Relationship among plasma cortisol, adrenocorticotropin and severity of injury in recently injured patient. J Trauma 1987;27:384.
75. Baldwin WA, Allo M. Occult hypoadrenalism in critically ill patients. Arch Surg 1993;128(6):673.
76. Kidess AI, Caplan RH, Reynertson RH, et al. Transient corticotropin deficiency in critical illness. Mayo Clin Proc 1993;68(5):435.

77. Reincke M, Allolio B, Wurth G, et al. The hypothalamic-pituitary-adrenal axis in critical illness: response to dexamethasone and corticotropin-releasing hormoone. J Clin Endocrinol Metab 1993; 77(1):151.
78. Black PR, Brooks DC, et al. Mechanisms of insulin resistance following injury. Ann Surg 1982;196:420.
79. Meguid MM, Aun F, et al. The effect of severe trauma on urine loss of insulin. Surgery 1976;79:177.
80. Salmon WD, Daughaday WH. A hormonally controlled serum factor which stimulates sulfate incorporation by cartilage in vitro. J Lab Clin Med 1957;49:825.
81. Van Wyk J, Underwood LE, Hintz RL, et al. The somatomedins: a family of insulin-like hormones under growth hormone control. Res Prog Horm Res 1974;30:259.
82. Phillips LS, Vassilopoulou-Sellin. Somatomedins. N Engl J Med 302:371, 1980;302:438.
83. Svoboda ME, Van Wyk JJ, Knapper DG, et al. Purification of somatomedin C from human plasma: chemical and biological properties, partial sequence analysis and relationship to other somatomedins. Biochemistry 1980;19:790.
84. Meyer V, Knobil E. Growth hormone secretion in the unanesthetized rhesus monkey in response to noxious stimuli. Endocrinology 1967;80:163.
85. Glick SM, Roth J, Yalow RS, et al. The regulation of growth hormone secretion. Rec Prog Horm Res 1965;21:241.
86. Carey LC, Cloutier CT, Lowery BD. Growth hormone and adrenal cortical response to shock and trauma in the human. Ann Surg 1971;174:451.
87. Feldman C, Joffe B, Panz VR, et al. Initial hormonal and metabolic profile in critically ill patients with community-acquired lobar pneumonia. S Afr Med J 1989;76:593.
88. Ziegler TR, Young LS, Ferrari-Baliviera E, et al. Use of human growth hormone combined with nutritional support in a critical care unit. J Parenter Enteral Nutr 1990;14:574.
89. Gore DC, Honeycutt D, Jahoor F, et al. Effect of exogenous growth hormone on whole-body and isolated-limb protein kinetics in burned patients. Arch Surg 1991;126:38.
90. Voerman HJ, van Scihndel RJ, Groeneveld AB, et al. Effects of recombinant human growth hormone in patients with severe sepsis. Ann Surg 1992;216:648.
91. Belcher HJ, Mercer D, Judkins KC, et al. Biosynthetic human growth hormone in burned patients: a pilot study. Burns 1989;15:99.
92. Herndon DN, Hawkins HK, Nguyen TT, et al. Characterization of growth hormone enhanced donor site healing in patients with large cutaneous burns. Ann Surg 1995;221(6):649.
93. Gilpin DA, Barrow RE, Rutan RL, et al. Recombinant human growth hormone accelerates wound healing in children with large cutaneous burns. Ann Surg 1994;220(1):19.
94. Herndon DN, Barrow RE, Kunkel KR, et al. Effects of recombinant human growth hormone on donor-site healing in severely burned children. Ann Surg 1990;212(4):424.
95. Gatzen C, Scheltinga MR, Kimbrouigh TD, et al. Growth hormone attenuates the abnormal distribution of body water in critically ill surgical patients. Surgery 1992; 112(2)181.
96. Ziegler TR. Growth hormone administration during nutritional support: what is to be gained? New Horiz 1994;2(2):244.
97. Voerman HJ, Strack van Schijndel RJ, de Boer H, et al. Growth hormone: secretion and administration in catabolic adult patients, with emphasis on the critically ill patient. Neth J Med 1992;41(5-6):229.
98. Ramalho MJ, Reis LC, Nonaka K, et al. Thyroidectomy significantly reduces prolactin secretion during stress. Brazil J Med Biol Res 1990;23:747.
99. Kjaer A, Knigge U, Olsen L, et al. Mediation of the stress-induced prolactin release by hypothalamic histaminergic neurons and the possible involvement of vasopressin in this response. Endocrinology 1991; 128:103.
100. Onaku T, Yagi K. Differential effects of naloxone on neuroendocrine responses to fear-related emotional stress. Exp Brain Res 1990; 81:53.
101. Delitala G, Tomasi P, Virdis R. Prolactin, growth hormone and thyrotropin-thyroid hormone secretion during stress states in man. Baillieres Clin Endocrinol Metab 1987;1:391.
102. Gala RR. The physiology and mechansims of the stress-induced changes in prolactin secretion in the rat. Life Sci 1990;46:1407.
103. Stoffer SS, Siang NS, Gorman CA, et al. Plasma catecholamines in hypothyroidism and hyperthyroidism. J Clin Endocrinol Metab 1973;33:729.
104. Banerjie SP, King LS. Beta-adrenergic receptors in rat heart: effects of thyroidectomy. Eur J Pharmacol 1981;109:1428.
105. Williams LT, Lefkowitz RJ, Watanabe AM, et al. Thyroid hormone regulation of beta adrenergic receptor number. J Biol Chem 1977;252:2787.
106. Sharma VK, Vannerjee SP. Alpha-adrenergic receptor in rat heart—effects of thyroidectomy. J Biol Chem 1978;253:5277.
107. Melander A, Ericson LE, Ljunggren JG, et al. Sympathetic innervation of the normal thyroid. J Clin Endocrinol Metab 1974;39:713.
108. Melander A, Sundler F. Interactions between catecholamines, 5-hydroxytryptamine and TSH on the secretion of thyroid hormone. Endocrinology 1972;90:959.
109. Ericson LE, Melander A, Owman C, et al. Endocytosis of thyroglobulin and release of thyroid hormone in mice by catecholamines and 5-hydroxytryptamine. Endocrinology 1970;87:915.
110. Kaptein EM, Spencer CA, Kamiel MB, et al. Prolonged dopamine administration and thyroid hormone economy in normal and critically ill subjects. J Clin Endocrinol Metab 1980;51:387.
111. Galton VA. Thyroid hormone-catecholamine interrelationships. Endocrinology 1965;77:278.
112. McLarty DG, Ratcliffe WA, McKoll K, et al. Thyroid hormone levels and prognosis in patients with serious non-thyroidal illness. Lancet 1975;2:275.
113. Bermudez F, Surks M, Oppenheimer J. High incidence of decreased serum triiodothyronine concentration in patients with non-thyroidal disease. J Clin Endocrinol Metab 1975;41:27.
114. Becker RA, Wilmore DW, Goodwin CW. Free T4, free T3 and reverse T3 in critically ill, thermally injured patients. J Trauma 1980;20:713.
115. Baue AE, Gunther B, Hartl W, et al. Altered hormonal activity in severely ill patients after injury or sepsis. Arch Surg 1984;119:1125.
116. Phillips RH, Valente WA, Caplan ES, et al. Circulating thyroid hormone changes in acute trauma: prognostic implications for clinical outcome. J Trauma 1984;24:116.
117. Slag MF, Morley JE, Elson MK, et al. Hypothyroxinemia in critically ill patients as a predictor of high mortality. JAMA 1981;245:43.
118. Sumita S, Ujike Y, Namiki A, et al. Suppression of thyrotropin-releasing hormone and its association with severity of critical illness. Crit Care Med 1994;22(10):1603.
119. Silberman H, Eisenberg D, Ryan J, et al. The relation of thyroid indices in the critically ill patient to prognosis and nutritional factors. Surg Gynecol Obstet 1988;166:223.
120. Van der Poll T, Romijm JA, Wiersinga WM, et al. Tumor necrosis factor: a putative mediator of the sick euthyroid syndrome in man. J Clin Endocrinol Metab 1990;71:1567.
121. Williams GR, Franklyn JA, Neuberger JM, et al. Thyroid hormone receptor expression in the "sick euthyroid" syndrome. Lancet 1990; 335:662.
122. Wilcox RB, Nelson JC, Tomei RT. Heterogeneityin affinities of serum proteins among patients with non-thyroidal illness as indicated by the serum free thyroxine response to serum dilution. Eur J Endocrinol 1994; 131(1):7.
123. Custro N, Scafidi V, Notarbartolo A. Alterations in circadian rhythm of serum thyrotropin in critically ill patients. Acta Endocrinol 1992; 121(1):18.
124. Zucker AR, Chernow B, Fields AI, et al. Thyroid function in critically ill children. J Pediatr 1985;107:552.
125. Robertson D, Michelakis AM. Effect of anesthesia and surgery on plasma renin activity in man. J Clin Endocrinol Metab 1972;34:831.
126. Hilton JG, Marully DS. Trauma induced increases in plasma vasopressin and angiotensin II. Life Sci 1987;41:2195.
127. Hilton JG, McPherson MB, Marullo DS. Effects of blockade of vasopressin V-1 receptors on post-burn myocardial depression. Burns Incl Therm Inj 1987;13:454.
128. Jiang JY, Zhu C, et al. Beta-endorphin-like immunoreactivity in CSF of patients with acute head injury. A clinical report of 36 cases. Chinese Med J 1989;102:137.
129. Zimmerman RS, Hayes RL, et al. Beta-endorphin in cerebrospinal fluid and serum after severe head injury. Neurosurgery 1990;26:764.
130. Vongsavan N, Pavasuthipaisit K, et al. Beta-endorphin, ACTH, and cortisol secretion in man during standardized oral surgical stress and effect of diazepam. J Med Assoc Thai 1990;73:443.
131. De Riu PL, Petruzzi V, et al. Beta-endorphin in experimental canine spinal ischemia. Stroke 1989;20:253.
132. Satake K, Hiura A, et al. Plasma beta-endorphin and the effect of naloxone on hemodynamic changes during experimental acute pancreatitis in dogs. Surg Gynecol Obstet 1989;168:402.
133. Millan MJ. Stress and endogenous opioid peptides: a review. Mod Probl Pharmacopsychiat 1981;17:49.

134. Lloyd DA, Teich S, et al. Serum endorphin levels in injured children. Surg Gynecol Obstet 1991;172:449.
135. Dindar A, Gunoz H, et al. Beta-endorphin levels of children in acute stress. Diabetes Res Clin Prac 1990;9:245.
136. Shamoon L, Hendler R, et al. Synergistic interactions of antiinsulin hormones in man. J Clin Endocrinol Metab 1981;52:1235.
137. Bessey PQ, Watters JM, et al. Combined hormonal infusion simulates the metabolic response to injury. Ann Surg 1984;200:264.
138. Gore DC, Jahoor F, Wolfe RR, et al. Acute response of human muscle protein to catabolic hormones. Ann Surg 1993;218(5):679.
139. Watters JM, Bessey PQ, et al. Both inflammatory and endocrine mediators stimulate host responses to sepsis. Arch Surg 1986;121:179.
140. Baracos V, Rodeman P, Dinarell CA, et al. Stimulation of muscle degradation and prostaglandin E2 release by leukocyte pyrogen. N Engl J Med 1983;308:553.
141. Pomposelli JJ, Flores EA, Bistrian RR. Role of biochemical mediators in clinical nutrition and surgical metabolism. JPEN 1988;12:212.
142. Hasselgren PO, Talamini M, Lafrance R, et al. Effect of indomethacin on proteolysis in septic muscle. Ann Surg 1982;202:557.
143. Hasselgren RO, Warner BW, Hummel R, et al. Further evidence that accelerated muscle protein breakdown during sepsis is not ? mediated by prostaglandin E2. Ann Surg 1988;207:399.
144. Giovanni I, Boldrini G, Castagneto M, et al. Respiratory quotient and patterns of substrate utilization in human sepsis and trauma. JPEN 1983;7:226.
145. Bagby GJ, Croll CB, Thompson JJ, et al. Lipoprotein lipase suppressing mediator in serum of endotoxin-treated rats. Am J Physiol 1986;251:E470.
146. Beutler B, Cerami A. Recombinant interleukin-1 suppresses lipoprotein lipase activity in $3T_3$-L_1 cells. J Immunol 1985;135:3969.
147. Kather H, Biger W, Michel G, et al. Human fat cell lipolysis is primarily regulated by inhibitory modulators acting through distinct mechanisms. J Clin Invest 1985;76:1559.
148. Dickerson RN, Vehe KL, Mullen JL, et al. Resting energy expenditure in patients with pancreatitis. Crit Care Med 1991;19:484.
149. Liggett SB, Renfro AD. Energy expenditures of mechanically ventilated nonsurgical patients. Chest 1990;98:524.
150. Swinamer DL, Grace MG, Hamilton SM, et al. Predictive equation for assessing energy expenditure in mechanically ventilated critically ill patients. Crit Care Med 1990;18:657.
151. Cunningham JJ. Factors contributing to increased energy expenditure in thermal injury: a review of studies employing indirect calorimetry. JPEN 1990;14:649.
152. Turner WW, Ireton CS, Hunt JL, et al. Predicting energy expenditures in burn patients. J Trauma 1985;25:11.
153. Tredget EE, Yu YM, Zhong S, et al. Role of interleukin 1 and tumor necrosis factor on energy metabolism in rabbits. Am J Physiol 1988;255:E760.
154. Cunningham JJ, Lydon MK, Russell WE. Calorie and protein provision for recovery from severe burns in infants and young children. Am J Clin Nutr 1990;51:553.
155. Tilden SJ, Watkins S, Tong TK, et al. Measured energy expenditure in pediatric intensive care patients. Am J Dis Child 1989;143:490.
156. Goran MI, Broemeling L, Herndon DN, et al. Estimating energy requirements in burned children: a new approach derived from measurements of resting energy expenditure. Am J Clin Nutr 1991;54:35.
157. McClave SA, Snider HL. Understanding the metabolic response to critical illness: factors that cause patients to deviate from the expected pattern of hypermetabolism. New Horiz 1994;2(2):139.
158. Devins SS, Miller H, Herndon BL, et al. Effects of dopamine on T-lymphocyte proliferative responses and serum prolactin concentrations in critically ill patients. Crit Care Med 1992; 20(12):1644.
159. Van den Bergh G, de Zegher F, Lauwers P, et al. Leutenizing hormone secretion and hypoandrogeneamia in critically ill men: effect of dopamine. Clin Endocrinol 1994;41(5):563.
160. Van den Bergh G, de Zegher F, Lauwers P, et al. Growth hormone secretion in critical illness: effect of dopamine. J Clin Endocrinol Metab 1994;79(4):1141.
161. Van den Bergh G, de Zegher F, Lauwers P. Dopamine suppresses pituitary function in infants and children. Crit Care Med 1994; 22(11):1747.
162. Duke GJ, Briedis JH, Weaver RA. Renal support in critically ill patients: low-dose dopamine or low-dose dobutamine? Crit Care Med 1994;22(12):1919.
163. Marik PE. Low-dose dopamine in critically ill olliguric patients: the influence of the renin-angiotensin system. Heart Lung 1993;22(2):171.
164. Anand KJS, Brown MJ, Causon JE, et al. Can the human neonate mount an endocrine and metabolic response to surgery? J Pediatr Surg 1985;20:41.
165. Anand KJS, Brown MJ, Bloom SR, et al. Studies on the hormonal regulation of fuel metabolism in the human newborn infant undergoing anesthesia and surgery. Hormone Res 1985;22:115.
166. Anand KJS, Sippell WG, Aynsley-Green A. Randomized trial of fentanyl anaesthesia in preterm babies undergoing surgery: effects on the stress response. Lancet 1987;1(8526):234.
167. Anand KJS, Sippel WG, Schofield NM, et al. Does halothane anaesthesia decrease the metabolic and endocrine stress responses of newborn infants undergoing operation? Br Med J 1988;296:668.

Burns, Inhalational Injury, and Electrical Injury 45

Eva Nozik Grayck
Robert M. Spear
Andrew M. Munster

INTRODUCTION

More than 2 million people receive medical treatment for thermal injury each year. Of the 100,000 patients hospitalized for thermal injuries, 30 to 40% are under the age of 15 years[1]. Despite improvement in survival due to aggressive fluid resuscitation, effective treatment of complications, and improved surgical techniques, burn and inhalational injuries continue to be a major cause of morbidity and mortality in the pediatric population. Further research is required to continue to improve care of the burned patient.

The care of the pediatric burn patient is best managed by a multidisciplinary approach in an experienced center with cooperation of specialists including surgeons, pediatricians, anesthesiologists, psychiatrists, social workers, and nurses.

This chapter covers several important related subjects: burns, inhalation injury, carbon monoxide poisoning, and electrical injury. Emphasis is placed on early management of burns. For further details of long-term care and late surgical reconstruction the reader is referred to more detailed publications available on the subject[2–4].

PATHOPHYSIOLOGY OF THERMAL INJURY

Integument

Thermal injury to tissue results in areas of coagulation necrosis and cell death. The release of vasoactive mediators injure capillary endothelial cells, resulting in increased capillary permeability and edema formation[5]. The mediators responsible for this response include histamine, thromboxane, and cytokines[6]. Large endothelial gaps have been demonstrated by electron microscopy and may persist for several days[7]. Other factors contributing to edema formation include hypoproteinemia and increased osmotic pressure in burned tissue[8]. In areas adjacent to burned tissue, capillary circulation becomes sluggish defining the *zone of stasis.* In the absence of adequate oxygenation and perfusion, this region is susceptible to subsequent ischemia, extending the area of necrosis[9]. Surrounding the zone of stasis is a zone of hyperemia which usually resolves within 10 days.

Edema may occur in tissues distant from the burn wound[7]. A decrease in cell transmembrane potential occurs that leads to a shift of sodium and water from the extracellular to the intracellular space, resulting in cell swelling. A decrease in cell membrane adenosine triphosphatase (ATPase), resulting from hypovolemic ischemia or circulating fatty acids, most likely produces the change in transmembrane potential. With restoration of tissue perfusion, ATPase, transmembrane potential, and capillary integrity are restored 24 to 36 hours after thermal injury. Edema is usually maximal at 24 hours and gradually resolves over the ensuing 3 to 5 days.

Pulmonary

Pulmonary dysfunction associated with thermal injury may be secondary to inhalational injury, aspiration, sepsis, congestive heart failure, shock, or associated trauma. The presence of inhalation injury increases mortality by 20%, while pneumonia increases the risk of mortality by 40% in burn patients[10].

The development of pulmonary insufficiency after burn and inhalation injury can be divided into three phases. In the resuscitation phase (0 to 36 hours), lung injury may result from hypoxia and subsequently reoxygenation, carbon monoxide and cyanide toxicity, upper airway obstruction due to mucosal edema, chemical burns to lower and upper airways, or impaired chest wall compliance due to circumferential third degree burns[11]. Pulmonary hypertension, decreased PaO_2, increased closing volumes, and increased airway resistance have been documented in thermal injury without associated inhalational injury and are attributed to the release of circulating mediators. These mediators include platelet activating factor, thromboxane, serotonin, histamine, leukotrienes C and D, and oxidants[12–14]. Lung injury has not been shown to result from an increase in lung protein permeability[11,15].

In the postresuscitation phase from day 2 to day 6, lung abnormalities result from continued airway obstruction, decreased chest wall compliance, tracheobronchitis, pulmonary edema, and acute respiratory distress syndrome (ARDS). Hypoproteinemia contributes to edema formation[16]. Continued production of inflammatory mediators occurs with surgical excision and contributes to lung injury. In the later phase, from day 7 until wound closure, patients are at risk for wound infections or nosocomial pneumonia, which may lead to ARDS and multisystem organ failure. These processes are associated with high mortality[11].

Cardiovascular

Profound alterations in the cardiovascular system occur in association with thermal injury. Cardiac output is initially decreased largely due to decreased circulating blood volume and an increase in systemic vascular resistance. A serum myocardial depressant factor has been described[17], although in most cases, low cardiac output is secondary to decreased circulating blood volume. Cardiac output usually returns to normal before complete restoration of intravascular volume. Central venous pressure and pulmonary capillary wedge pressure are usually low-normal and may remain so after adequate resuscitation.

Hypertension is a common phenomenon after thermal injury in pediatric patients, occurring in up to 57% of patients[18,19]. Hypertensive encephalopathy has been reported and is characterized by convulsions, marked irritability, extreme lethargy, or disorientation[20]. Popp et al.[18] found hypertensive encephalopathy in 15 of 195 (7%) hypertensive pediatric patients. They noted that 7- to 10-year-old boys with greater than 20% body surface area (BSA) burns had an unusually high incidence of hypertension (57%). Treatment of hypertension with hydralazine and other antihypertensive medications has significantly reduced the incidence of seizures related to hypertension. Besides seizures, no other complication or change in mortality was attributed to hypertension. The mechanism of hypertension is described by Popp et al.[21] and appears to involve hypervolemia associated with elevated systemic vascular resistance. Plasma renin activity and aldosterone were markedly elevated in all patients (hypertensive and normotensive) in the acute phase, and thus appear to be part of the acute systemic response to thermal injury. In the convalescent period, both groups were normotensive, but hypervolemia persisted in the group that was initially hypertensive. The cause of the hypervolemia is unknown.

Szyfelbein and coworkers[22] documented ionized hypocalcemia in the early days after burn injury and noted concomitant hypotension and cardiac electromechanical dissociation during surgery. This ionized hypocalcemia was not predictable from the McLean-Hastings nomogram, although serum protein and total calcium were both decreased. The merits of calcium replacement in burn patients are discussed in their report.

Renal

Renal failure after thermal injury is uncommon but can result from prolonged systemic hypotension, myoglobin released from damaged muscle tissue, or, rarely, hemoglobin released as a result of heat-induced hemolysis. Renal blood flow is decreased immediately after thermal injury[24]. Later, the glomerular filtration rate may increase dramatically, coinciding with the onset of the postburn hypermetabolic state and hyperdynamic circulation. This alteration in renal blood flow becomes important when attempting to achieve therapeutic serum concentrations of antibiotics that are excreted by the kidneys[25]. An intrarenal redistribution of blood flow occurs early in the postburn period, with a reduced ratio of renal outer cortical to inner cortical blood flow occurring independently of resuscitation[26]. The reduction in urinary chloride and sodium concentrations that accompanies this shift in blood flow may be secondary to preferential perfusion of juxtaglomerular nephrons with salt-retaining characteristics.

Hepatic

Hepatic dysfunction is common after burn injury. A decrease in hepatic cellular transmembrane potential difference occurs in experimental burn injury and recovers partially after fluid resuscitation[27]. Failure of active ion transport or changes in relative cell membrane permeability are implicated in the etiology of hepatic dysfunction[27]. The clinical characteristics and the clinical course of hepatic dysfunction are well described in a prospective study of burn patients[28]. Clinical and laboratory evidence of hepatic dysfunction were present in 58% of the patients in the first week. Histologic findings in these patients revealed cytoplasmic vacuolization of centrilobular hepatocytes, congestion of sinusoids and central veins, and centrilobular fatty changes. Canalicular cholestasis was present in patients who were clinically jaundiced. Patients with hepatic injury had a larger surface area burn (58% versus 30%) and greater mortality (74% versus 9%) than patients without evidence of hepatic dysfunction. Clinical jaundice was associated with 90% mortality. Later onset of conjugated hyperbilirubinemia was usually indicative of sepsis. The etiology of hepatic dysfunction remains speculative, although early hemodynamic alterations, hypoxia, and sepsis may be related.

Hematologic

Hematologic changes after burn injury have been reviewed in detail by Eurenius[29].

Platelets

Mild thrombocytopenia occurs during the first several days after burn injury and is followed by thrombocytosis (two to four times normal) by the end of the first week[29]. Thrombocytopenia may persist in the septic patient. In the animal model, chromium-labeled platelet infusions resulted in a significant uptake of label in the burn wound, thus, implicating sequestration into the wound as the cause of early thrombocytopenia[30]. Platelet aggregation may be either depressed or enhanced after burn injury.

Clotting Factors

Prothrombin (PT), partial thromboplastin (PTT), and thrombin times show little change after burn injury. There are, however, significant increases in fibrinogen as well as factors V and VIII[31,32]. Fibrin-fibrinogen split products are usually elevated and tend to parallel fibrinogen levels, although little prognostic value is attributed to these changes. In nonsurvivors, prolongation of prothrombin and partial thromboplastin times has been observed, although the mechanism is unknown[29].

Bleeding and thrombotic complications after thermal injury are usually related to local tissue disease (e.g., gastric or duodenal stress ulcer, thrombophlebitis from venous catheters) rather than to systemic coagulopathy. Congenital coagulation disorders, although rare, may require vigorous therapy in the burn patient[33]. If generalized bleeding occurs, iatrogenic anticoagulation, thrombocytopenia, or disseminated intravascular coagulation (DIC) should be suspected. Persistent thrombocytopenia is associated with poor prognosis, and sepsis should be suspected. Patients with generalized bleeding and thrombocytopenia without evidence of DIC should receive platelet transfusions, as septic bone marrow suppression is likely[29].

DIC with generalized bleeding can occur after thermal injury. DIC is suggested by occurrence of thrombocytopenia, hypofibrinogenemia, prolongation of PT and PTT, and elevation of fibrin-fibrinogen split products. The degree of elevation of fibrin-fibrinogen split products is much greater in the patient with DIC than in the uncomplicated burn patient[29]. Prompt attention to underlying etiology (shock, sepsis, hypoxia), as well as specific treatment of DIC, is critical. Because of the short half-life of transfused platelets in DIC, the transfusion of platelets in this syndrome should be judiciously timed in the event that surgical intervention is required for ongoing problems.

Red Blood Cells

After burn injury, there is a decrease in red cell mass associated with fragmented red cells[29]. Red cell pigment may appear in the plasma and urine. A low hemoglobin is masked in the early stages by hemoconcentration as fluid is lost from the intravascular compartment. There is a decreased deformability of red cells after burn injury, which persists for almost 1 month[34]. In animal models, there is shortened red cell survival in the immediate postburn period, with evidence of intravascular hemolysis[35]. After the first week, red cell survival in patients is not significantly altered, and there is no evidence of continued hemolysis. In severe burns, a refractory anemia is commonly present and persists until wound closure is completed. A decrease in urinary erythropoietin has been demonstrated in major burn injury and when burn injury is associated with sepsis[36]. Surgical blood loss, daily debridement, phlebotomy, and gastric ulcers can also account for significant blood loss in the weeks after burn injury.

Central Nervous System

Central nervous system dysfunction is present in up to 14% of pediatric burn patients[37]. Results of early published reports suggested an unidentified toxin as the cause of *burn encephalopathy,* with a nearly universal fatal outcome[38]. Emery and Reid[39] reported six deaths in patients with minor burns. Convulsions were common and cerebral edema was uniformly found. Warlow and Hinton[40] described six cases of burn encephalopathy with two deaths. Antoon et al.[37] reported 20 cases of burn encephalopathy in a series of 140 children (14%). Unlike previous reports, they found definable causes for the encephalopathy in 19 of 20 patients. Mortality was 50% in their series, and most patients had greater than 50% BSA burns. Only one death was primarily related to the central nervous system insult. In the survivors, neurologic recovery was complete in 9 of 10 patients. Hypoxia occurring in the first 48 hours was the most common cause of encephalopathy and was related to smoke and carbon monoxide inhalation sustained in enclosed area fires. Hypoxia later in the postburn course was related to pulmonary edema and pneumonia. Hypovolemia, hyponatremia, sepsis, cortical vein thrombosis, and gliosis secondary to "water shed" infarct are other entities that produced encephalopathy. Seizures, obtundation, coma, or hallucinations presented neurologic manifestations of the central nervous system dysfunction in that series of patients.

Sepulchre et al.[41] isolated a "neurotoxic factor," a high-molecular-weight lipoprotein that was present in the serum of all patients with greater than 35% BSA burn. When injected into rabbits, this factor caused flattening of the electroencephalogram, followed by trembling and convulsions, with spikes appearing on the electroencephalogram.

Gastrointestinal

Stress ulceration (Curling's ulcer) of the stomach or duodenum is a life-threatening but preventable complication in the burn patient. In patients with severe burns, gastric mucosal abnormalities are found in 90% of patients[42,43]. Prophylaxis with antacids, H_2 antagonists such as cimetidine or ranitidine, or sucralfate is efficacious, and combined therapy is used when bleeding occurs during single agent therapy[44,45].

Major thermal injury is associated with alterations in intestinal permeability. Deitch demonstrated an increased gut permeability to lactulose within 24 hours of injury in patients with moderate to major burn injuries[46]. This effect appears to be more pronounced in burn patients with infection[47]. Studies of thermally injured animals have demonstrated increased translocation of intestinal bacteria that is related to the extent of the burn. Bacterial translocation is further increased in animals whose burn wound is infected[48–50].

Acalculous cholecystitis is reported in patients after thermal injury and is characterized by fever, abdominal distention, and jaundice[51]. Two forms of acalculous cholecystitis are probably seen in burn patients[44]. The first type involves bacterial seeding of the gallbladder in septic patients, whereas the second type occurs in patients with dehydration, ileus, or pancreatitis in whom, characteristically, the gallbladder is distended with sterile fluid[44]. Tube cholecystostomy[52] and cholecystectomy[44] are recommended therapies.

The superior mesenteric artery syndrome is a rare complication of thermal injury, occurring in patients who have lost weight[53]. The third portion of the duodenum, lying between the aorta and superior mesenteric artery, becomes compressed due to loss of retroperitoneal fat. Nausea, vomiting, and abdominal pain are commonly present[54]. Diagnosis is made by fluoroscopy, as barium commonly traverses the duodenum only in the prone or left-side-up position. The patient can be fed in that position, and resolution is common. Rarely, duodenojejunostomy is necessary.

Acute pseudo-obstruction of the colon, characterized by massive colonic dilation without organic obstruction, has been reported in 1% of a large burn population[55]. Significant dilation is evident on plain radiographs of the abdomen.

Metabolic

Thermal injury produces a significant hypermetabolic response that parallels the severity of the burn injury and may approach 200% times normal[56]. A catabolic state occurs that is characterized by skeletal muscle breakdown, increased oxygen consumption, lipolysis, and hepatic gluconeogenesis[57]. Factors that have been implicated in mediating this response include "stress hormones" such as glucagon, catecholamines, and glucocorticoids; cytokines, including interleukin-1, tumor necrosis factor, and interleukin-6; and lipid mediators such as thromboxane B_2 and platelet-activating factor[57]. The escape of bacteria or their products from the burn wound or gut to the circulation may trigger this hypermetabolic response[5,58]. Early enteral feeding immediately after a burn injury has been observed to attenuate the hypermetabolic response, perhaps by preserving the intestinal mucosal barrier and preventing translocation of bacteria or endotoxin[59].

Immunity and Infection

Serious burn injury is associated with immunocompromise, the magnitude of which is directly related to the extent of injury[60]. Thermal injury to the skin causes failure of this local mechanical barrier to bacteria as well as dysfunction of other nonspecific and specific host defense systems. Acquired immunologic defects after burn include changes in concentrations and activities of the components of the complement pathways, reduced circulating fibronectin, depressed serum opsonic activity, impaired macrophage, lymphocyte and neutrophil function, and reduced reticuloendothelial system activity[61]. Decreased antibody levels are associated with increased utilization in the presence of enhanced production[5].

There is ample evidence of depressed immunity in burn-injured patients. Research has focused on identifying the mediators of immunosuppression in these previously healthy individuals. Hypotheses with experimental support include the liberation or generation of immunosuppressive factors that impair cellular immune activity[62]. Nutritional factors[63] and the influences of stress hormones on lymphocytes and neutrophils[61] have also been proposed.

Infection is an important threat to survival in burn patients. Bacteremia is associated with increased mortality after thermal injury. Patients with fatal bacteremia tend to have large burns and inhalational injuries[64]. Burn wound sepsis and pneumonia are major foci of infection; however, in a number of patients with bacteremia no source can be identified[64]. Studies demonstrating increased bacterial translocation in thermally injured animals[48,49] and increased intestinal permeability in burn patients[46,47] lend support to the hypothesis that the gut serves as an important reservoir for invading bacteria. Gut failure may lead to multiple organ failure in patients with burns and other severe injuries[65,5].

ESTIMATION OF BURN SIZE AND DEPTH

Burn size is expressed as a percentage of the total BSA. The contribution made by specific parts of the body to total BSA changes according to the age of the child until adult proportions are reached at 15 years of age. This percentage may be estimated by the "rule of nines" in children over 15 years of age (Fig. 45.1) but requires a more exact measurement in younger children (Fig. 45.2). The size of one side of the child's hand, approximately equal to 1% of the BSA, may be useful in estimating the size of small burns.

Burn depth has been traditionally classified in terms of degrees (first through fourth). Recently, a more useful classification of superficial, superficial partial-thickness, deep partial-thickness, and full-thickness injury has been favored by most clinicians. The descriptions overlap, and both are outlined below. The size and depth of a burn should be estimated at regular intervals during the child's hospital course to assess possible extension of injury and healing.

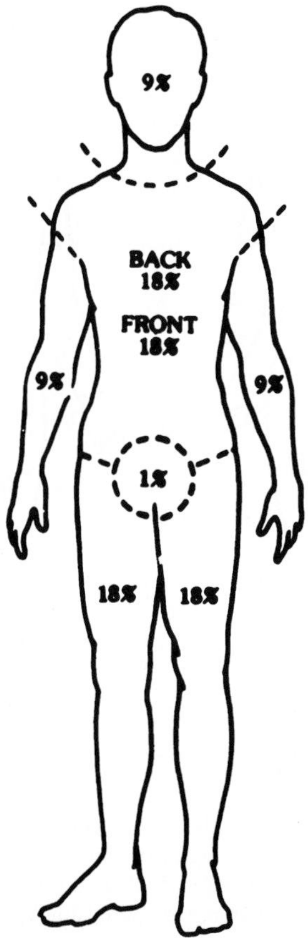

Figure 45.1. An estimate of the percentage of total body surface skin that is burned can be obtained by use of the "rule of nines," whereby the total surface area of skin is divided into areas equaling 9% of the total. (From Demling RH. Fluid and electrolyte management. Crit Care Clin 1985;1:34.)

An accurate assessment of the depth of a burn is difficult in the first few days due to the evolution of the injury.

First-Degree Burn

First-degree burn is a superficial injury, such as a sunburn, which is characterized by erythema and pain and occasionally minor blistering. Tissue loss is restricted to epithelial cells. No treatment is required except for pain relief. Very rarely, an extensive first-degree burn may require intravenous fluid therapy.

Second-Degree Burn

In second-degree burn, tissue death occurs through the epidermis and into a variable portion of the dermis. When damage is superficial partial-thickness, the extent of damage to the dermis is slight. Healing will take place with little or no scarring within 10 to 12 days; if the patient is black, pigment will return to the injured area. A superficial partial-thickness burn is moist, red, and tender. Within a few days, the color becomes pale as a superficial eschar develops, but very often viable dermal papillae can be seen through the thin eschar as tiny red dots separated by intervals of no

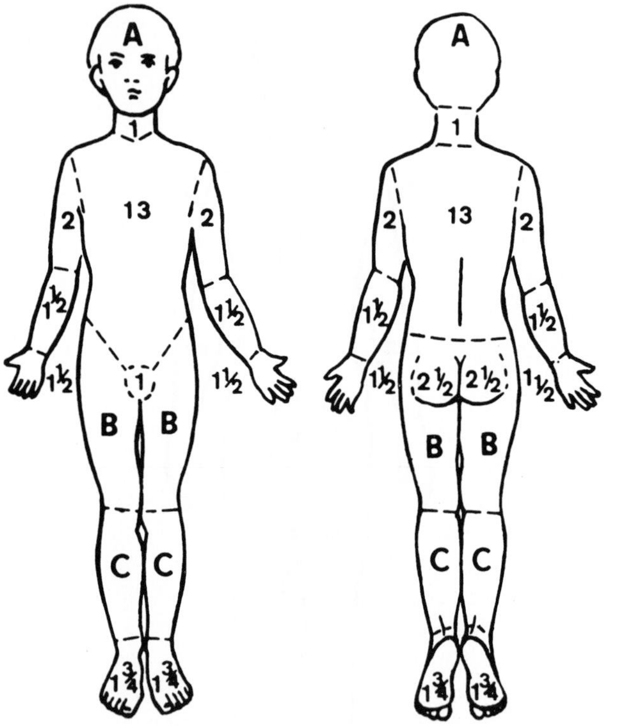

Figure 45.2. This chart of body areas, together with the table showing the percentage of surface area of the head and legs at various ages, can be used to estimate the surface area burned in a child. (From Solomon JR. Pediatric burns. Crit Care Clin 1985;1:161.)

more than 1 mm. When the burn is deep partial-thickness, there is tissue necrosis through most of the dermis, with preservation of the deepest portion of the dermal papillae and the skin appendages. Healing will still occur, but it will take up to 6 weeks and may be accompanied by scarring. If there is infection or nutritional inadequacy, bacterial invasion may convert this to a full-thickness burn. Clinically, a deep partial-thickness burn is also moist and tender, but the developing eschar is whiter and appears thicker. Dermal papillae or "skin buds" either are not visible through the layer or, if visible, are separated by a distance of 2 to 3 mm.

Third-Degree Burn

Third-degree burn refers to full-thickness injury, in which the necrotic area extends through all layers of the skin into the hypodermic fat. This type of burn may heal by contracture if it is very small, but usually surgical closure is indicated. The appearance of such a burn varies from dry and charred to red and nonblanching with pressure. It is not sensitive to touch.

Fourth-Degree Burn

Fourth-degree burn involves deep injury to bone, joint, or muscle, usually occurring secondary to high-voltage electrical injury.

CLASSIFICATION OF BURNS

Minor Burn

In minor burn, the total surface area involved is less than 5%. No significant involvement of hands, feet, face, or perineum is present. No full-thickness component and no other complications are present. Children with these injuries may be treated as outpatients, provided social circumstances permit.

Moderate Burn

Moderate burn is characterized by involvement of 5 to 15% BSA or by the presence of any full-thickness component. Involvement of the hands, feet, face, or perineum or the presence of any complicating factor, such as chemical or electrical injury, also constitutes moderate burn. Patients with these injuries should be admitted to the hospital.

Severe Burn

Severe burns are characterized by a total burn size greater than 15% BSA, by a full-thickness component in excess of 5% BSA, or by the presence of smoke inhalation or carbon monoxide poisoning. The child with this injury should be admitted to a special burn treatment facility or pediatric intensive care unit (PICU) after stabilization.

EPIDEMIOLOGY AND PREVENTION

Burns are a leading cause of death due to injury in young children (1 to 4 years) in the United States, second only to motor vehicle accidents. Burns are the third leading cause of injury associated death in children overall (0 to 19 years of age), after motor vehicle accidents and drowning[64]. There is a similar incidence of burn injury in boys and girls younger than age 6 years, after which males predominate[67].

House fires account for 84% of burn-associated fatalities, the cause of which is most frequently smoke inhalation rather than tissue damage from flames[68]. Scalds are the most common cause of burns in young children, usually occurring in the home[69,70]. Flame injury predominates in older children[71]. Burns by flames normally result in larger surface involvement and therefore represent a greater percentage of severe injuries. The upper extremities, head, and neck are the body areas most frequently burned[71]. **Table 45.1** illustrates the distribution of causal agents and locations of pediatric burns seen at the Baltimore Regional Burn Center from 1979 to 1985. This is similar to national experience.

The mortality associated with burn injury has declined over the past 10 years. The Boston Unit of the Shriners Burn Institute saw a decline from 9% average mortality (1968 to

Table 45.1. Location and Type of Pediatric Burns, Baltimore Regional Burn Center, 1979–1985 (N = 520)

Place of accident	
Home	84.8%
Outside	7.6%
Boat/auto	3.4%
Other	4.0%
Type of burn	
Scald	47.6%
Flame	29.6%
Grease	6.5%
Flash	5.6%
Contact	5.6%
Electrical	3.9%
Chemical	1.1%

1970) to 1% in the 6-year period of 1981 to 1986[67]. In that same institution, burn size had a statistically significant effect on mortality. The mortality for small (less than 15% BSA) burns was 0%, rising steeply for burns of more than 50% BSA and increasing to 65% mortality for burns 90 to 95% BSA. In their pediatric population (11 days to 19 years), age did not show a consistent effect on mortality. Another recent study reported that the burn size resulting in 50% mortality was 95% BSA in a large group of pediatric patients[72]. It appears that young children, including infants, survive burn injury at least as well as young adults.

INITIAL MANAGEMENT

Initial care of the burn victim as recommended by the Committee on Trauma of the American College of Surgeons is directed at assessment for airway compromise, stopping the burning process, and beginning fluid resuscitation. All clothing should be removed, as synthetic fibers may melt into hot plastic residue that continues to burn the patient. Sites of chemical burns should be flushed with copious amounts of water for 20 to 30 minutes.

Traditionally, patients whose history or physical examination suggests thermal injury to the airway have been managed with early, elective tracheal intubation. The approach to patients with inhalation injury has been challenged by some centers whose specialists perform serial bronchoscopy and intubate only for impending respiratory failure[72].

Patients with burns greater than 20% BSA generally require intravenous fluid for replacement of intravascular volume. A large-bore intravenous catheter should be placed in a peripheral vein, through burned tissue if necessary. In adolescents and adults, placement in an upper extremity is desirable because of a high incidence of phlebitis in saphenous veins. Initial fluids are Ringer's lactate. Patients who are treated with intravenous fluid should have a bladder catheter placed for quantitation of urine flow as a guide to fluid requirements. In burns of this magnitude, placement of a nasogastric tube is also warranted. The patient should be weighed to allow calculation of estimated fluid needs. Blood samples for complete blood count (CBC), type and cross-match, carboxyhemoglobin, coagulation, and blood chemistry profiles are indicated. An arterial blood gas measurement may also be appropriate.

Assessment of the degree of injury includes estimation of size and depth of burn, as previously described. A brief history of the mechanism of injury may provide clues to associated trauma or inhalation injury. Exposure to fire in an enclosed space increases the likelihood of significant smoke inhalation. Explosions often propel the victim a distance, resulting in fractures, internal injuries, head trauma, flail chest, and pulmonary contusion. The patient's medical history should be ascertained as well.

Circumferential extremity burns require special care to prevent distal limb ischemia. Remove all jewelry and assess for cyanosis, impaired capillary refill, or neurologic signs such as paresthesias or deep pain. Doppler assessment of pulses is useful. Escharotomy may be necessary if circulatory insufficiency is present.

Narcotic analgesics should be given only after assurance that restlessness and anxiety are caused by pain rather than by hypoxia or hypovolemic shock. Initial wound care should be limited to application of a clean, dry dressing to decrease pain in partial-thickness burns. Blisters should be left intact. Antiseptic solutions are contraindicated, and applying cold water to relieve pain should be avoided in patients with extensive burns.

Tetanus prophylaxis must be addressed in patients with burns. Children over the age of 7 years who have completed their immunization series (three or more doses) should receive intramuscular Td (adult type tetanus and diphtheria toxoids) if it has been more than 5 years since their last dose. Younger children who have not completed three doses should receive diptheria toxoids (DT) (or diptheria and tetanus toxoids and pertussis vaccine (DPT) if appropriate). Patients of any age whose immunization series is uncertain or less than three doses should receive the age-appropriate toxoid and tetanus immune globulin, 250 to 500 units intramuscularly[73].

TRANSPORTING THE BURNED CHILD

Initial stabilization of the burned child may be carried out in the emergency department or pediatric intensive care unit. After the airway is secured and fluid resuscitation and other appropriate measures have been undertaken to ensure tissue perfusion and oxygenation, consideration should be given to referral to a regional burn center. An accurate and complete record of care delivered and patient data should accompany the patient.

In accordance with the recommendations of the American Burn Association, patients with the following injuries usually require referral to a burn center.

1. Partial-thickness and third-degree burns involving more than 10% of the total BSA in patients under 10 years or over 50 years of age
2. Partial-thickness and third-degree burns exceeding 20% of the body surface area in other age groups
3. Partial-thickness and third-degree burns involving the face, eyes, ears, hands, feet, genitalia, perineum, and major joints
4. Third-degree burns greater than 5% of the BSA in any age group
5. Electrical burns, including lightning injury (significant volumes of tissue beneath the surface may be injured and result in acute renal failure and other complications)
6. Chemical burns
7. Burns associated with significant fractures or other major injury in which the burn injury poses the greatest risk of morbidity or mortality
8. Burn injury with inhalation injury
9. Lesser burns in patients with significant preexisting disease

INTRAVENOUS FLUID THERAPY

Restoring intravascular volume with salt-containing fluids has led to improved survival of burn patients. Several useful formulae have been devised that allow one to estimate fluid volumes that are required to replace losses and maintain adequate intravascular hydration. Despite disagreement among authors as to the benefit of isotonic versus hypertonic or crystalloid versus colloid fluid therapy, most agree that tailoring therapy to meet specified endpoints is far better than rigid adherence to any formula. The ultimate goals of fluid resuscitation are to restore and maintain intravascular volume and thus to provide adequate tissue perfusion.

The most useful index of adequate intravascular replacement is urine output. Experimental evidence in the dog model supports the presumption that adequate renal blood flow resulting in acceptable urine output is indicative of adequate perfusion of other organs[74]. A urine output of 0.5 to 1.0 ml/kg/hr is optimal. With rare exceptions, a urine output of less than 0.5 ml/kg/hr is indicative of insufficient intravascular volume. Diuretics are rarely indicated in burn patients, and the induced diuresis obscures the most useful gauge of intravascular volume. Diuretics may be necessary for some patients (electrical injury, soft-tissue injury, muscle burn) with pigmenturia that does not clear with vigorous hydration[44]. Other indices ordinarily useful in assessing volume status have limitations when applied to the burn patient. Massive catecholamine release after thermal injury results in maintenance of systemic arterial blood pressure despite significant hypovolemia, thereby limiting blood pressure as a sensitive gauge of adequate intravascular replacement. Measurements of central venous pressure and pulmonary capillary wedge pressure must be interpreted cautiously in the burn patient, as cardiac output is restored before blood and plasma volumes are[75]. Arbitrary attempts to elevate filling pressures may result in administration of massive volumes of fluid, leading to increased morbidity from edema formation without evidence of clinical improvement related to the higher filling pressures. Cardiac output is usually adequate at low-normal filling pressures. Measurement of cardiac output by thermodilution is infrequently necessary in the pediatric or young adult patient[76].

Children with burns exceeding 15% BSA will require intravenous resuscitation. If the burn size exceeds 30% BSA, placement of a central venous catheter is recommended. If the burn is over 50% BSA, two central venous catheters may be required. In children with large burns (greater than 30% BSA) in whom the need for prolonged intravenous therapy can be anticipated, the initial intravenous catheter can be placed through a burned area while it is still relatively sterile, preserving unburned sites for later use. In smaller burns, the intravenous catheter should be placed in an unburned site. Sterile technique in placing central catheters is of utmost importance because of the high incidence of infectious complications, including bacterial endocarditis, with use of central venous and pulmonary artery catheters in burn patients[77].

Crystalloid resuscitation provides sodium, the principal element necessary to restore circulating plasma volume[78]. Some investigations have advocated the use of hypertonic saline solutions for burn resuscitation in hopes of decreasing fluid administration and tissue edema. Several early studies reported favorable results[79,80]. Horton et al. reported enhanced cardiac contractile function in burned animals resuscitated with hypertonic saline dextran versus lactated Ringer's[81]. However, a prospective randomized study revealed no difference in fluid requirements, weight gain, or tolerance of early enteral feeding in a group of patients (average 23% BSA burn) who received hypertonic sodium lactate versus those who were given lactated Ringer's solution[82]. Controversy continues to exist over the addition of colloid to the resuscitation fluids in the first 24 hours. Increased vascular permeability results in decreased colloid oncotic pressure in the plasma. According to several animal studies, this process occurs primarily during the first 6 to 8 hours after uncomplicated burn injuries[83–85]. These data support the addition of colloid to the fluid during the first 8 to 24 hours of resuscitation. Supplementation with 12.5 g of human serum albumin to each liter of Ringer's lactate will allow maintenance of normal serum albumin levels. There also is a trend toward instituting oral fluids in the first few hours after the burn via a nasogastric or a duodenal tube, decreasing the intravenous fluids to maintain constant fluid intake. The most commonly used formula for estimating fluid requirements is the Parkland formula. This protocol uses crystalloid solutions but may be modified by the addition of colloid or oral fluids. We use the Parkland formula as follows:

First 24 hours—lactated Ringer's solution, 4 ml/kg/%BSA burned is given during the first 24 hours. In infants, maintenance fluid volume (1500 ml/m^2/day) given as lactated Ringer's solution must be added to the Parkland formula. One-half of this volume is given in the initial 8 hours postburn, and the other half is given during the next 16 hours. The rate of resuscitation should be adjusted to maintain a urine output of 0.5 to 1.0 ml/kg/hr. Colloid may be used to improve urinary output and treat hypoalbuminemia.

Second 24 hours—maintenance fluid (1500 ml/m^2/day) is begun with glucose-containing hypotonic fluid. After the completion of the second postburn day, oral feeds should be fully implemented, but if intravenous fluids are still required, they should be chosen to maintain normal sodium, phosphate, calcium, and potassium homeostasis. Because of the intense adrenal response to burn stress, potassium wasting in the urine is common and may reach 200 mEq/liter.

AIRWAY MANAGEMENT

Burn patients may require tracheal intubation for a variety of reasons. As previously noted in the context of initial management, children with evidence of thermal injury to the airway should undergo tracheal intubation early, before edema progresses to airway obstruction and intubation becomes difficult or impossible. Burn-injured patients may need placement of a tracheal tube because of central nervous system dysfunction, inhalation injury of the lung, pneumonia, sepsis, or a surgical procedure with general anesthesia.

Intubating the trachea of a child who has sustained thermal injury may present special problems. Tracheal intubation prior to the onset of edema allows for a standard approach, namely, the use of intravenous anesthetics and a muscle relaxant. A rapid-sequence technique with cricoid pressure is suggested, as aspiration of gastric contents is a significant risk. Other acceptable methods of securing the airway include fiberoptic guided tracheal intubation or intubation without anesthetic or muscle relaxant (awake intubation). The latter techniques may be impractical in a young child, who will most likely be unwilling to cooperate. Burns of the face, lips, pharynx, and hypopharynx can lead to massive edema, making visualization of the larynx extremely difficult or impossible. A most difficult situation exists for the child who has signs of upper airway obstruction. The strategy for securing an airway in this circumstance is similar to that employed in other diseases in which upper airway anatomy is distorted, such as epiglottitis. In these situations, muscle relaxants or sedation is contraindicated prior to successful tracheal intubation. With continuous monitoring and attention to cardiorespiratory status, the child should be transported to the operating room accompanied by an anesthesiologist and a surgeon. Supplies for emergency intubation and tracheotomy should be readily available. Inhalational anesthesia with 100% oxygen should be administered. Spontaneous respiratory effort is maintained, allowing gradual induction of general anesthesia. Direct laryngoscopy can then be performed, allowing tracheal intubation. If this is unsuccessful, oxygen and anesthetic can be resumed with the patient still maintaining spontaneous respiration. If difficulty maintaining a patent airway occurs, discontinuing the inhalational anesthetic should allow for awakening and improvement in airway patency, although tracheotomy or cricothyrotomy may become necessary. In this situation, intubation with a flexible fiberoptic bronchoscope as a guide for the tracheal tube may be successful. Tracheotomy should be avoided when possible in the burn patient, particularly when the tracheotomy would be placed through burned tissue[(86)]. Awake laryngoscopy may be preferred by some in this difficult setting. If adequate visualization of the larynx after initial laryngoscopy is possible, one might then use an anesthetic agent (ketamine or thiopental) and muscle relaxant with cricoid pressure for definitive endotracheal intubation.

Burn-injured patients develop abnormal responses to muscle relaxants that are frequently used to facilitate tracheal intubation and/or maintain neuromuscular blockade. Succinylcholine is contraindicated in burn patients beginning approximately 48 hours postinjury. Hyperkalemia leading to cardiac arrest is a potential complication of succinylcholine in the postburn period[(87)]. Succinylcholine may be an appropriate drug for tracheal intubation during initial resuscitation, as its rapid onset and resolution are useful in the setting of a full stomach or questionable airway. The period of risk for succinylcholine-induced hyperkalemia begins 5 to 15 days postburn and lasts for 3 to 16 months[(88,89)]. The mechanism of the accentuated hyperkalemic response is believed to be increased sensitivity of the muscle membrane to succinylcholine, resulting in potassium exiting and sodium entering the cells[(89)]. In the normal state, the motor endplate alone has altered permeability to sodium and potassium, resulting in mild, insignificant increases in serum potassium concentration (0.5 mEq/liter) after administration of succinylcholine. Pretreatment with nondepolarizing muscle relaxants has been advocated to decrease potassium afflux, but the dose of nondepolarizing relaxant required approaches the full paralyzing dose and thus is impractical[(90)].

Relative resistance to nondepolarizing muscle relaxants in seriously burned patients has been reported[(88,90,91)]. The exact mechanism of this unusual response to depolarizing relaxants is unknown but would appear to be secondary to altered pharmacodynamics in patients with thermal injury[(93,94)]. It is interesting that burn patients and patients with certain neuromuscular diseases have a common response to neuromuscular blockade, namely, a resistance to nondepolarizing agents and a hyperkalemic response to succinylcholine[(88)]. Resistance to nondepolarizing muscle relaxants was seen in one 9-year-old patient 463 days after sustaining serious burns[(88)]. Because of the possibility of a common mechanism for the unusual reactions to both depolarizing and nondepolarizing muscle relaxants, caution is suggested in the use of succinylcholine in patients for long periods of time after burns[(88)], while some specialists advise against the use of succinylcholine for only 3 months after burns[(89)].

WOUND MANAGEMENT

The burn wound should be gently cleansed with saline, and blisters should be debrided. This may be done in the hydrotherapy tub or in bed. After a brief period of drying, a suitable topical agent should be applied to the wound, and the wound is dressed. As previously mentioned, escharotomy or fasciotomy may become necessary within hours of admission to relieve peripheral vascular or nerve compression. Occasionally, thoracic escharotomy is necessary to facilitate chest expansion.

Medications

It is common practice to administer penicillin for 3 days to patients with major burns as antistreptococcal prophylaxis. Penicillin may be given intravenously in doses appropriate for age. Intramuscular or subcutaneous medication should not be given in the early stages of burn therapy until complete cardiovascular stability has been established.

Topical Chemotherapy

The most commonly available agents and their advantages and disadvantages are illustrated in **Table 45.2.** The burn wound becomes colonized with airborne Gram-positive flora and with endogenous Gram-positive flora within the first week of injury. Subsequently, contamination and colonization with Gram-negative organisms is the rule. Multiple organisms can commonly be grown from the wound. Frequent cultures of the burn wound will reveal the changing flora; if facilities exist for quantitative bacteriology of eschar, the likelihood of culturing pathogens rather than colonizing organisms will increase. Organisms from the wound can be cultured and topical therapy adjusted accordingly. Common practice is to use silver sulfadiazine cream as a primary agent. Mafenide cream, because of its rapid penetration and superior spectrum of coverage, is used on high-voltage electrical injuries and on infected burns that had been neglected prior to transfer. Resistance to silver sulfadiazine is almost universal for *Enterobacter cloacae,* common for *Staphylococcus aureus,* and occasional for *Pseudomonas aeruginosa;* all three organisms are usually sensitive to mafenide. Allergy to sulfonamides excludes the use of silver sulfadiazene and mafenide. Iodophors (Efodine cream) and silver nitrate solution are alternatives. In large burns, mafenide therapy may lead to metabolic acidosis because of carbonic anhydrase inhibition. Nitrofurazone has been shown to be useful in treating large burns infected with *E. cloacae* [95]. Complications associated with topical therapy include hypernatremia, hyperosmolality, and metabolic acidosis associated with povidone-iodine therapy[96] and severe hyperosmolality secondary to propylene glycol absorption from silver sulfadiazine cream applied to a large burn[97]. Methemoglobinemia has been reported after the use of silver nitrate solution on burn wounds[98]. Some bacteria are capable of reducing nitrates to nitrites. Methemoglobin is produced if

Table 45.2. Commonly Used Topical Antibacterial Agents

Name	Advantages and disadvantages	Side effects	Dressing orders
Silver sulfadiazine (Silvadene)	Broad antibacterial action; painless; fair penetration of eschar	Sulfonamide sensitivity (rash); absorption into fetal circulation unknown; contraindicated in pregnancy; occasional leukopenia (reversible upon discontinuation)	Apply twice daily; cover with a light layer of dressings on extremities; leave face and chest open
Mafenide (Sulfamylon)	Excellent antibacterial action, particularly against Gram-positives, *Clostridia,* and Gram-negatives; rapid eschar penetration	Painful; sulfonamide sensitivity (rash); carbonic anhydrase inhibition leading to acidosis	Apply twice daily; leave face, chest, and abdomen open; one light layer of dressings elsewhere
Aqueous silver nitrate solution	Universal antibacterial action; poor penetraton of eschar	Leaking of chloride into the dressings with potential hypochloremic alkalosis; strong staining of tissues	Apply twice daily; dress with a light layer of gauze dressings
Iodophors (e.g., Efodine)	Universal antibacterial action; poor penetration of eschar	Strong staining of tissues; iodine absorption	Apply twice daily; dress with a light layer of gauze dressings
Topical bacitracin cream	Limited antibacterial action; poor eschar penetration; cosmetically acceptable, easy to apply; transparent	Rapid development of resistance; conjunctivitis if contacts the conjunctiva	Should only be applied to small areas of cosmetic importance, e.g., second-degree burns of the face; leave open; apply twice daily

sufficient nitrite absorption occurs, converting hemoglobin to methemoglobin.

The clean burn wound is odorless, is free of all but a minimal discharge, and changes appearance little from day to day except for slow eschar separation. Burn wound sepsis is characterized by an unhealthy gray or dark appearance, often with petechial hemorrhages, foul-smelling discharge, and systemic signs of sepsis. In burn wound sepsis, the wound quantitative bacteriologic count is usually higher than 105 organisms per gram of tissue. When the diagnosis of burn wound sepsis is made, systemic antibiotic therapy should be begun based on microbiologic isolates from the wound. However, other sources of sepsis should be carefully sought.

Fever is a common problem in the weeks following burn injury. Blood and urine cultures, chest x-ray, and careful physical examination are mandatory in the evaluation of the febrile patient. Gram-negative septicemia is likely to originate in the wound or lungs, while Gram-positive septicemia may originate in the wound or as a result of intravenous catheter sepsis. If the source cannot be promptly eliminated, empiric antibiotic therapy should be begun. Topical therapy is applied twice daily after cleansing and debridement of the burn wound in a hydrotherapy tub or in bed. Light sterile dressings are applied after use of the topical cream. If silver nitrate solution is used, bulky dressings are necessary.

Biologic Dressings

Xenografts from pigskin and allografts from human cadaver skin are useful when the eschar has separated completely and the wound is clean and awaiting surgical closure[99,3]. Xenografts are used for temporary coverage of large partial-thickness burns during reepithelialization, providing pain control and decreasing evaporative fluid losses. Allografts are most useful for extensive full-thickness burns until permanent grafting with autologous skin can be performed. Synthetic and biosynthetic skin may eventually provide an abundant source of sterile, inexpensive, temporary coverage for burns, although it is currently limited by decreased adherence to wounds[3].

Surgery

Total excision and grafting is indicated for areas of full-thickness injury and for areas of deep partial-thickness burn that would heal with delay and scarring. In patients with massive burns greater than 50% of total BSA, there is urgency in performing surgery and covering the wound to decrease operative bleeding[101] and minimize bacterial colonization. In the remaining children, surgery, if done early, reduces hospitalization time but is not a matter of urgency. Scald burns in children should be observed for 2 weeks before an operative procedure is performed to establish the actual extent of the injury[102].

The principal form of wound coverage is autografting, which creates a donor site. Over the last decade, a technique for culturing autologous and allogenic epithelium for burn wound coverage was developed[99,3]. The technique is particularly applicable in instances of large BSA burn when only a small percentage of skin is available for autografting. In children, the interval between skin biopsy for cell culture and availability of grafts may be as short as 15 days[100]. One multicenter study reported a higher average "take" of the graft (47%) in patients younger than 18 years[100]. Grafting may be performed to a clean burn bed from which all eschar has separated or to a surgically excised burn bed. Ideally, excision and closure of the wound should take place as soon as the child is stable enough for a major general anesthetic, preferably within the first few days of admission. In presurgical care, fluid and electrolyte abnormalities should be corrected, the hematocrit maintained above 30%, and the general condition of the child optimized. After surgery, no dressing changes are necessary for variable periods of time (usually 2 to 3 days), after which dressings may be removed to estimate the percentage take of the graft. Because of the many factors prejudicial to graft take (infection, movement, technical failure), no commitment should be made to the family regarding length of postoperative hospitalization until the graft has been inspected. Future improvements in wound closure may use artificial skin derived from collagen mesh or allodermis and cultured autologous epithelial cells, or full-thickness skin transplantation[3,6,103]. Anesthetic considerations for children with significant burns are discussed in detail elsewhere[104] (see also Chapter 46).

The administration of recombinant human growth hormone (0.2 mg/kg/day) in children accelerates donor-site wound healing, improves nitrogen balance, and decreases protein catabolism[105–107]. These doses of growth hormone raise concentrations of insulin-like growth factor[105]. The use of combination therapy of beta-1 blockade and beta-2 stimulation to decrease oxygen consumption in conjunction with growth hormone and insulin-like growth factor has been suggested as a potentially beneficial strategy which should be addressed in prospective clinical trials[6].

METABOLISM/NUTRITION

The hypermetabolic state produced by a burn injury is characterized by an increased metabolic rate with protein catabolism, lipolysis, and hyperthermia and results in an increased risk of infection and poor wound healing. General measures to control the hypermetabolic response, such as temperature regulation and analgesia, are important.

Appropriate nutrition has a major impact on the outcome of burn victims. In addition to meeting the patient's requirements for macronutrients and micronutrients, the composition, timing, and route of feeding may influence metabolic rate, immune function, and rate of infection. Hence, nutritional support may affect length of hospital stay and mortality in patients with serious burns.

Many formulae for determining energy needs of pediatric burn patients are in use around the country. Several are summarized in **Table 45.3.** Hildreth et al. compared the actual caloric intake (which served to maintain weight) to the caloric requirement predicted by the Curreri Junior For-

Table 45.3. Formulae for Determining Energy Needs of Pediatric Burn Patients

Age (yr)	*Daily Requirement*
Wolfe[98]	
All	Basal metabolic rate × 2
Hildreth and Carvajal[99]	
BSA	
All	1800 kcal/m^2 + 2200 kcal/m^2
Recommended Daily	
0–0.5	kg weight × 115 kcal
Allowance (RDA)[100]	
0.5–1.0	kg weight × 105 kcal
1–3	kg weight × 100 kcal
4–10	kg weight × 85 kcal
M: 11–14	kg weight × 60 kcal
F: 11–14	kg weight × 48 kcal
Curreri Junior[101]	
0–1	Basal cal + 15 kcal/% burn
1–3	Basal cal + 25 kcal/% burn
3–15	Basal cal + 40 kcal/% burn

mula and the Hildreth and Carvajal Formula in 121 children aged 2 months to 15 years. The formulae overestimated the caloric needs by 72 and 22%, respectively[111]. It would appear that the lower range of target calories recommended by Wolfe[108] or the recommended dietary allowance provides a reasonable starting point for pediatric burn patients[112].

Alexander et al. theorized that nutritional support that is adequate to prevent weight loss may not meet the protein requirements of burn patients, as evidenced by low serum albumin, transferrin, and total serum protein[113]. They found that pediatric burn patients who received 23% of calories as protein versus 16.5% had better outcome with regard to advancement of enteral feeding, statistically higher levels of serum proteins, transferrin, C_3, IgG, and opsonic activity and required fewer blood transfusions. Current recommendations for patients with burns of more than 10% BSA are 20% total kilocalories provided from protein, nonprotein kcal/nitrogen ratio 100:1 or 2.5 g/kg/day amino acids[114].

The fat content of the burn patient's diet has also received considerable attention. Dietary lipid content of more than 15% may have an adverse effect on immune function, particularly if it is high in the omega-6 fatty acid series, such as linoleic acid[63]. Gottschlich and coworkers demonstrated a decrease in wound infection and length of stay compared with the percentage of burn in patients fed a modular diet low in fat, high in protein and essential amino acids, low in omega-6 fatty acids, and high in omega-3 fatty acids[115].

Enteral feeding has benefits over the parenteral route in preventing hypermetabolism, catabolism[59], and intestinal translocation of viable organisms[116]. Very early (4 hours postinjury) institution of enteral nutrition may lead to early achievement of positive nitrogen balance[1,118,119]. With appropriate behavioral intervention, a large number of pediatric patients may be capable of consuming adequate calories[113,119], otherwise nighttime or continuous tube feeding should be provided.

PAIN MANAGEMENT

Burn injury is associated with pain that may vary from continuous background pain of moderate intensity to excruciating pain associated with therapeutic procedures such as debridement, physical therapy, and burn dressing change[120]. In addition to alleviating pain, analgesics also decrease metabolic demands, which contributes to improved wound healing. Opioids are commonly administered for burn pain control; however, the dosage range is extremely variable, which may lead to inadequate pain control. Burn patients have described feeling severe pain, especially during therapeutic procedures, and the extent of their pain has been underestimated by care providers[121]. Other factors that may lead to insufficient medication for burn pain include fear of inducing respiratory depression, fear of causing drug addiction, lack of understanding of the pharmacology of analgesics, and patient reticence about expressing feelings of pain. Means of optimizing pain management for burn patients might include systematic and regular use of pain rating scales, education of patients regarding reasonable expectations for pain relief, staff education on pain and the pharmacology of analgesics, and use of continuous infusions or patient-controlled analgesic techniques[122].

Nonopioid analgesics such as acetaminophen may be useful for suppressing mild background pain. Moderate pain may be responsive to orally administered opioids such as oxycodone or morphine, while continuous pain is best managed with a long-acting analgesic such as methadone or sustained release preparations of morphine[120].

Intravenous morphine is widely administered for the treatment of severe pain in burn victims. Initial dosage of 0.1 to 0.2 mg/kg is recommended, recognizing that the effective dose will vary among patients. Frequent small doses (0.02 to 0.04 mg/kg) may be administered every 5 to 10 minutes to achieve adequate analgesia without rigid adherence to a standard dosage. Tolerance can be anticipated when opioids are administered over an extended time, and doses may be adjusted upward. Physical dependence on opioids is likely to occur in burned children treated for prolonged periods but is generally easily managed with a gradual reduction in dosage over days to weeks, once wounds have healed. Addiction and subsequent abuse of opioids introduced during hospitalization is rare[123]. Respiratory depression due to opioid administration is unusual during painful procedures but may be reversed with naloxone should it occur.

Other analgesic drugs may have utility in treating the burn patient. Fentanyl may be useful for a painful intervention of short duration[120]. Lingering sedation is reduced, as its short redistribution half-life results is brief (20 minutes) when administered in doses of 1 to 6 μg/kg. Continuous infusion of methadone has been useful in the control of severe burn pain unresponsive to other methods[124]. Opioid agonist-antagonist analgesics have the theoretical advantage of providing analgesia with less respiratory depression. Nalbuphine compared favorably to morphine with regard to pain control in a study of adult patients[125]. Ketamine has been used successfully in alleviating pain associated with short procedures in burn units[126,127]. Its popularity stems from properties of profound analgesia, respiratory and cardiovascular stimulation, and relative preservation of airway reflexes. Side effects include hypertension, delirium, and hallucinations. Aspiration of gastric contents and laryngospasm, although rare, may occur. Oral ketamine has been reported to result in profound analgesia without loss of consciousness in a 3-year-old patient with burns[128]. Patient-controlled analgesia has been shown to be safe and effective in managing postoperative pain in children and adolescents[129], and a preliminary report suggests efficacy in burn patients[130].

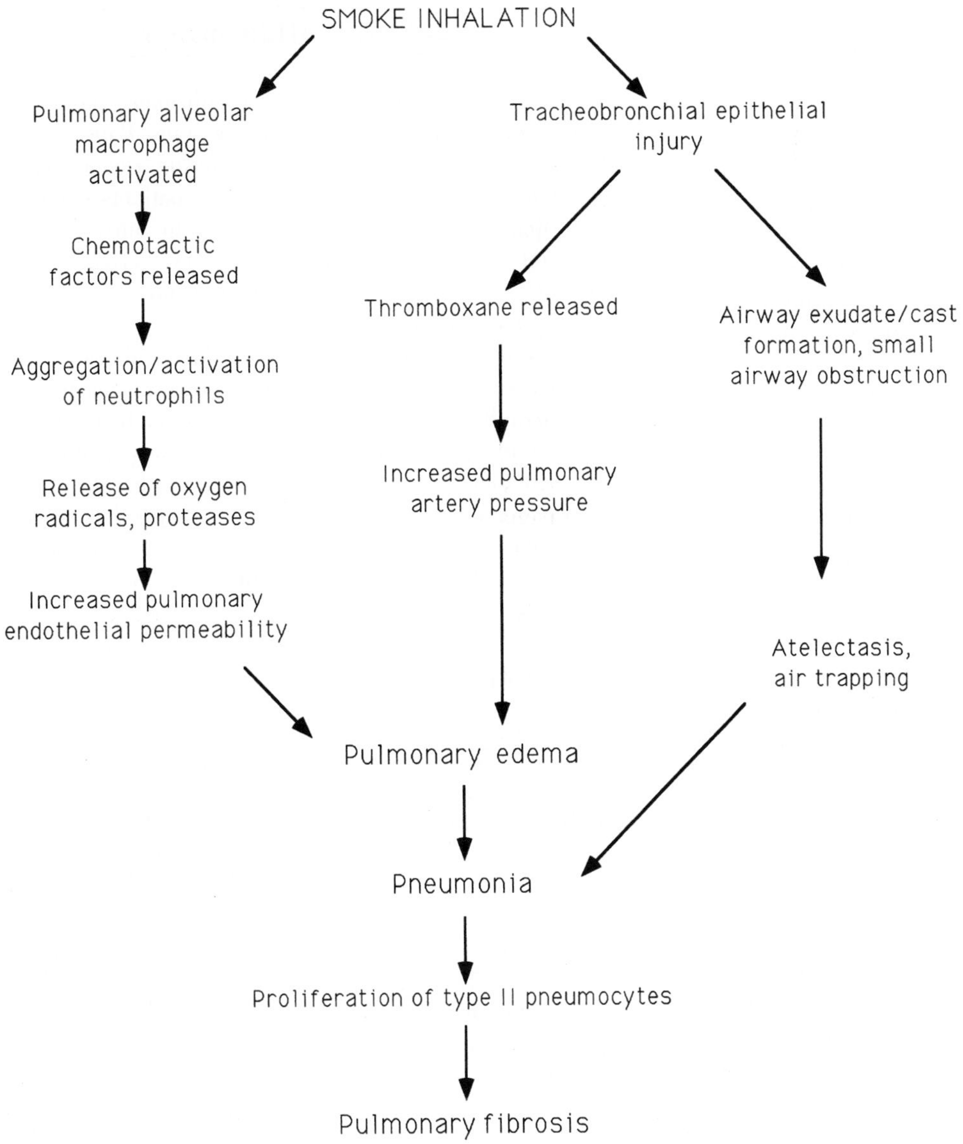

Figure 45.3. Aldehydes and acids produce an inflammatory response that produces lung injury after smoke inhalation. (From Muller MJ and Herndon DN. The challenge of burns. Lancet 1994;343:216.)

INFLAMMATION

Progress may be achieved in the care of the burn patient by the development of strategies to optimize the inflammatory response produced by thermal injury. Severe burns cause impairment of the immune system. A randomized trial with immunoglobulin therapy did not demonstrate improvement in mortality or rate of infections in burn patients[131]. Granulocyte macrophage colony-stimulating factor appears to have beneficial effects in a burn animal model which may prove to be clinically applicable[132]. The complex pathophysiology of burn injury also involves subsequent systemic inflammation and oxidative injury (Fig. 45.3). Potential therapies include the use of topical or systemic inhibitors of prostaglandin synthesis to decrease vascular permeability and attenuate systemic inflammation[6]. Experimental animal models show prevention of burn-induced oxidant injury by fluid resuscitation with defuroxamine[133] and inhibition of hemolysis, renal injury[134], and lipid peroxidation[135] in burned rats by treatment with superoxide dismutase. Antioxidant therapies in human burn victims have not been examined. Understanding the roles of specific cytokines, such as IL-6 and TNF[136,137], and nitric oxide[138] in burn patients may eventually lead to directed therapies in these patients.

PSYCHOSOCIAL ASPECTS OF BURN THERAPY

The care of the severely burned child is an exceedingly stressful experience for the child, family, and staff. Fear, pain, abandonment, and disfigurement contribute to the child's emotional difficulties after injury. There is evidence that the approach taken by nurses to aversive procedures such as burn dressing change influences the child's emotional response to those events and hospitalization in general. Beales found that the use of total physical restraint during dressing changes was associated with feelings of powerlessness and increased fear and anticipation of pain[139]. Beales advocated advance preparation of the child with descriptions and explanations of wound healing, including the value of daily dressing changes and debridement. During the actual conduct of a procedure, discussion of the wound would be minimized and distraction would be employed. Kavanagh proposed an alternative to distraction as a means of enabling the burned child to cope with painful experiences[140]. Her study concluded that encouraging a child to participate in wound care and offering information and explanations of ongoing procedures resulted in less maladaptive responses than conventional distraction technique. The participation method for burn dressing change is well described in an additional study that confirmed its favorable effect[141].

Family members of a burned child are also vulnerable to emotional problems. They often feel guilt, and concerns regarding the child's survival, finances, and disruption of the home may be overwhelming. The patient and family are in need of psychologic support from the outset and may require years of care.

Approximately 80% of children and 60% of mothers experience emotional problems after the child's recovery from severe burns[142,143]. Aspects of the acute injury, including pain and separation, contribute to this high incidence of emotional problems. Some authors emphasize the importance of preexisting psychopathology in the family antedating the burn[144]. Holter and Friedman[145] identify three patterns of burn injury correlating the etiology of the injury to the home situation. First, "accidental injury" occurred when the circumstances were beyond parental control, although poor parental judgment may have contributed. All of these children were well adjusted and had no previous history of accidents. Marital discord was not present, parent-child relationships were good, and all fathers were self-supporting. Second, "situational crisis" involved markedly disturbed family situations with either the child experiencing emotional problems or the mother experiencing emotional difficulties that led to absent or inappropriate supervision of the child. In this group, preexisting stress in the family resulted in a child with an increased propensity to injury. The disturbed mothers in this group were psychotic or depressed or had deserted the family. Third, "child abuse" was suspected in some cases. All mothers in this group had disturbed personalities, and the fathers had serious psychologic problems. Parental response to the child in the hospital was characterized by annoyance and disgust without feelings of grief or guilt. These parents visited the children infrequently.

Evidence of child abuse should be sought at admission of a burned child. Specific patterns of burn injury strongly suggest inflicted injury[146]. Isolated burns of the buttocks or symmetrically scalded hands or feet of full-thickness depth suggest forcible immersion in hot liquid[147].

SMOKE INHALATION INJURY

The association of inhalation injury with major burns significantly effects the outcome of burn victims. Patients with large burns have a high chance of suffering a concomitant inhalation injury (35 to 50%), and these patients make up 50 to 80% of the mortality attributed to burns[148–151]. Smoke inhalation exposes the victims to thermal injury, chemical asphyxiants such as carbon monoxide and cyanide, and mucosal irritants.

Early visualization of the airway by fiberoptic bronchoscopy is a sensitive and specific method of evaluating the airway for inhalation injury[1,152]. Serial bronchcoscopy allows early recognition of changes to the airway mucosa not present on admission, and prompt aggressive therapy of progressive injury[1]. ^{133}Xenon pulmonary scans also provide a definitive diagnosis of inhalation injury. Unfortunately, neither method is able to quantify the extent of the pulmonary injury[5].

Thermal Injury

Thermal injury from smoke inhalation is usually limited to the supraglottic airway. Air is a poor conductor of heat, and efficient heat-dissipating mechanisms of the upper airway cool the smoke before it reaches the lungs. The subglottic airway is also protected by reflex closure of the vocal cords when exposed to heat[153].

Significant thermal injury to the lungs occurs when steam is inhaled, as it has 4000 times the heat-carrying capacity of dry air[151]. Thermal injury due to smoke inhalation may cause life-threatening airway edema very rapidly; therefore, a high index of suspicion and early recognition are paramount. History of enclosed space fire, an unconscious victim, respiratory distress, burns to lips and nose, stridor, hoarseness, and soot in the mouth or nose are clues to significant thermal inhalation injury. If there is evidence of evolving airway obstruction, tracheal intubation should be performed. Fiberoptic examination allows a more thorough inspection of the supraglottic airway for burns and may facilitate intubation. Special considerations regarding tracheal intubation of burn patients have been described earlier in this chapter (see Airway Management).

Asphyxia

Acute asphyxia occurs in an enclosed space when fire rapidly consumes the available oxygen, with ambient oxygen concentration falling to 5% in some circumstances. It is complicated by tissue hypoxia when carbon monoxide and cyanide toxicity decrease oxygen-carrying capacity and oxygen utilization. The cardiodepressant effects of inhaled toxic fumes may further diminish oxygen delivery to the brain and other vital organs. Brain hypoxia disrupts mental and physical capacities and, consequently, the ability of a victim to escape from a burning environment. Acute asphyxia probably accounts for death in most victims who die before reaching the hospital.

Carbon Monoxide Poisoning

Carbon monoxide (CO) intoxication accounts for nearly half of the fatal poisonings in the United States, with 3500 people dying each year from exposure to CO(151). Another 10,000 people seek medical attention because of CO exposure(154). Gormsen et al.(155) found lethal concentrations of carboxyhemoglobin (COHb) in 50% of autopsied fire victims. The higher metabolic rate of the child results in more rapid uptake of CO, placing the pediatric patient at significant risk from CO exposure.

CO is an odorless, colorless, nonirritating gas present in the atmosphere at a concentration of less than 0.001%. CO is produced in humans in insignificant quantities in the metabolism of hemoglobin. The largest source of CO affecting humans is generated from the incomplete combustion of carbon-containing compounds, including automotive fuel, oil, coal gas, and natural gas. Enhanced production of CO occurs during fuel burning when any one of the following are present: (a) incorrect air-fuel mixture, (b) insufficient ventilation of combustion gases, and (c) insufficient intake of fresh air(156). House fires are a major source of CO production and poisoning. Inadequate ventilation, coupled with excessive CO production, was responsible for poisonings associated with indoor charcoal cooking(157), kerosene space heaters(158), Sterno fuel(159), and multiple poisonings in indoor skating rinks(160). Methylene chloride ($CHCl_2$), the main compound present in paint removers, is absorbed by humans and metabolized to CO(161).

Pathophysiology of Carbon Monoxide Poisoning

The mechanism of CO poisoning reversibly binding with hemoglobin to produce tissue hypoxia was described by Bernard in 1857(162). Haldane in 1895(163) described the equilibrium reactions pertaining to CO and hemoglobin. CO toxicity is due, in part, to its tremendous affinity for hemoglobin, binding to hemoglobin with an affinity 240 times greater than oxygen. Haldane's first law states that:

$$(COHb)/(O_2Hb) = MPCO/PO_2$$

where M is the affinity constant of 240, COHb and O_2Hb are concentrations of CO and oxygen bound to hemoglobin, and PCO and PO_2 are partial pressures of CO and oxygen to which the hemoglobin is exposed(164). The hemoglobin molecule is 50% saturated with CO at a partial pressure of only 0.10 mm Hg. In contrast, the hemoglobin molecule is 50% saturated with oxygen (P_{50}) at a partial pressure of 27 mm Hg. CO also causes a leftward shift in the oxyhemoglobin dissociation curve (Fig. 45.4), thereby enhancing oxygen affinity for hemoglobin and impeding oxygen delivery from blood to tissue.

CO also binds to myoglobin and to the intracellular oxygen transport system (cytochrome-oxidases), thereby blocking cellular oxidation, resulting in cellular anoxia(165,166). The importance of the cytochrome-oxidase system in CO poisoning was first discussed by Goldbaum(167). In dogs, it was shown that infusing CO-saturated erythrocytes to obtain COHb concentration of approximately 60% resulted in no symptoms, whereas breathing high concentrations of CO resulted in death, with average COHb concentrations of 65%. Inhalation of CO likely results in high concentrations of dissolved CO in the blood leaving the lungs. Dissolved CO can then cross into the tissues and combine with the cytochrome-oxidase system. Goldbaum concluded that the toxic effect of CO is related to the direct action of CO on the cytochrome-oxidase system and not solely on the reduced oxygen-carrying capacity of the blood.

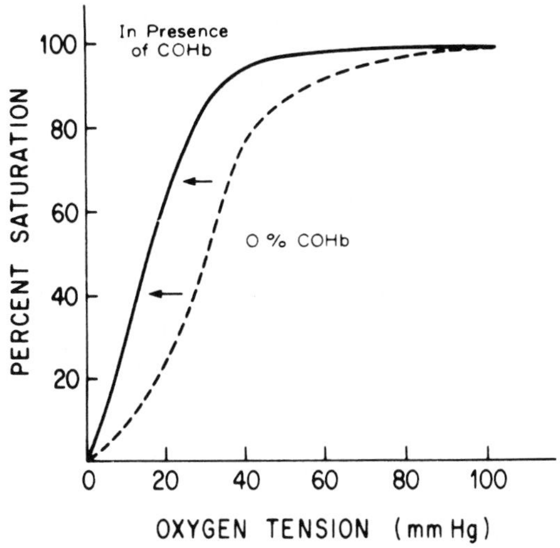

Figure 45.4. Oxygen saturation in carbon monoxide poisoning. (From Zimmerman SS, Truxal B. Carbon monoxide poisoning. Pediatrics 1981;68:218, reproduced by permission of Pediatrics.)

Diagnosis of Carbon Monoxide Poisoning

The diagnosis of CO poisoning is made from history of exposure, physical signs and symptoms, and laboratory data, including measurement of COHb concentration in the blood. COHb in the blood can be measured spectrophotometrically or can be measured from the patient's exhaled air in parts per million by using a CO analyzer and then converting to COHb concentration(168). The spectrophotometric method is most accurate. A COHb value within normal limits does not rule out recent CO poisoning. If significant time has elapsed since exposure to CO, or if supplemental oxygen has been given, the COHb values may have declined by the time the first blood sample was analyzed for COHb concentration.

Clinicians may be misled and rule out CO poisoning when a normal oxygen saturation is reported by the laboratory. Oxygen saturation is usually estimated from nomograms based on measured partial pressures of oxygen. The partial pressure of oxygen is frequently normal in CO poisoning (or greater than normal if oxygen is administered), although the oxygen saturation of hemoglobin is low. Gross error occurs in calculating oxyhemoglobin from partial pressures of oxygen in the presence of a significant COHb concentration. Pulse oximetry is also inaccurate in CO poisoning because COHb absorbs light at the wavelengths used by this device. Therefore, the pulse oximeter represents hemoglobin saturated by both oxygen and CO (SpO_2) and will read falsely elevated. Oximetry is required to measure the actual oxygen saturation (SaO_2) of hemoglobin because the co-oximeter is able to differentiate between hemoglobin bound to oxygen or CO.

Organ System Responses to Carbon Monoxide Poisoning

Cardiovascular

The heart is especially vulnerable to the hypoxic effects of CO poisoning in the child or adult with preexisting cardiac disease. Exposure to CO resulting in COHb concentrations of 5 to 10% led to an increase in coronary blood flow and a decrease in coronary arteriovenous oxygen difference in adult patients(170). The latter effect was due to a decrease in arterial oxygen content without a corresponding decrease in coronary sinus oxygen content. CO exposure causes elevation of heart rate(171,172), while cardiac output increases as COHb concentration exceeds 30%(173).

Anderson et al.(174) found the electrocardiogram (ECG) to be a sensitive measure of determining myocardial insult. Abnormalities include S-T segment and T-wave abnormalities, atrial fibrillation, intraventricular block, extrasystoles, ischemia, and infarction. The pathologic changes associated with cardiac injury in these patients included focal myocardial necrosis, leukocyte infiltration, and punctate hemorrhage. In adults with known cardiac disease, exposure to the Los Angeles freeway for 90 minutes resulted in ECG changes and decreased exercise tolerance at COHb levels of 5%(175).

Pulmonary

Pulmonary injury frequently accompanies CO poisoning, with pulmonary edema occurring in 10 to 30% of cases(176). The mechanism of pulmonary edema associated with CO poisoning remains speculative. Possible causes include tissue hypoxia, toxic effects of CO on alveolar membranes, myocardial damage leading to left ventricular failure, aspiration of gastric contents after loss of consciousness, concomitant smoke inhalation, and neurogenic pulmonary edema(176,177). In the anesthetized and ventilated dog, no increase in extravascular lung water was found after exposure to CO, suggesting that CO uptake and excretion through the lung may occur without causing local tissue injury(178). Sheep exposed to CO maintained normal PaO_2 levels for a 72-hour study period after exposure and lungs showed no discernable histologic changes(179).

Sone et al.(180) reviewed the effects of CO poisoning on the lung and found high morbidity associated with abnormal chest radiographs. Abnormal radiographs were present in 22% of patients upon admission to hospital. Ground-glass appearance was the most common finding. In this series, 42 of 44 patients with normal chest radiographs recovered, while 6 of 18 patients with abnormal chest radiographs survived in a vegetative state.

Arterial oxygen tension (PaO_2) is frequently normal in patients poisoned by CO, although studies have shown that PaO_2 may decrease secondary to augmentation of existing venous admixture(170,181). Minute ventilation is reported to be unchanged(173) or increased(170).

Neurologic

The neurologic manifestations of CO poisoning are protean; some are listed in **Table 45.4.** Disorientation, slurred speech, dizziness, weakness, seizures, and decreased level of consciousness are common in acute poisoning and can be grossly correlated with COHb concentrations. Facial spasms and trismus, mimicking tetanus, have been reported in CO poisoning(182). CO poisoning produces an increase in cerebral blood flow(183,84). Cerebral edema may complicate severe CO poisoning, and aggressive therapy is recommended if evidence of cerebral edema is present(185). Computed tomography (CT) of the head in severe CO poisoning has been studied(186). Symmetrical, low-density areas in the globus pallidus were found in 11 patients; these areas were still present at reevaluation 1 year later. Ventricular enlargement and cortical atrophy were present in all 11 patients at follow-up. Softening and demyelination were confirmed at autopsy in one patient(187). The outcome was poor in all but one of these 11 patients. In contrast, all 10 patients with similar clinical presentation with normal CT scans had a good outcome.

Neurologic sequelae after CO poisoning were found in 12% of patients admitted to hospital with CO poisoning(188). The most frequent symptoms included memory impairment, personality alterations, and signs of parietal lobe dysfunction(189). Little is known about long-term prognosis in chil-

Table 45.4. Clinical Neurologic Symptoms of Carbon Monoxide Poisoning

Headache
Dizziness
Disorientation
Lethargy
Delirium
Altered level of consciousness
Seizures
Depression
Irritability
Akinetic mutism
Amnesia
Dysphasia
Unilateral/bilateral pyramidal signs
Extrapyramidal signs
Hemiplegia
Cortical blindness
Delayed neurologic changes

dren who survive CO poisoning. Three of five children in one series did poorly in school after CO poisoning; two of these children also manifested behavioral difficulties[189]. Recovery after prolonged deficit has been reported[190].

Muscular and Renal

Muscle necrosis leading to myoglobinuria and subsequent acute renal failure may complicate CO poisoning[182]. The mechanisms of myonecrosis include the following: (a) the patient falling unconscious in a position that occludes venous drainage, resulting in swelling and compression of arterial circulation; (b) anoxia as the direct effect of CO poisoning; and (c) associated crush or electrical injury.

Cutaneous

Erythema, edema, and blistering are cutaneous manifestations of CO poisoning and can be mistaken for burns[191,192]. Histologically, skin necrosis is present. The frequently mentioned cherry-red color of skin and mucous membranes is uncommon in CO poisoning.

Ophthalmologic

Blindness (temporary and permanent), visual field deficits secondary to cortical lesions, and retinal findings, including venous congestion, papilledema, retinal hemorrhages, and red retinal veins may occur with CO poisoning[193,194]. Decreased light sensitivity and dark adaptation are reported with low-level CO exposure[195,196]. The similarity of CO retinopathy to the abnormal retinal findings in mountain climbers has suggested hypoxia as the cause of the retinal injury, while Valsalva's maneuver and compression of retinal venous drainage associated with cerebral edema have also been implicated[197,198].

Auditory

Auditory and vestibular injury involving the peripheral organs of hearing and balance, the VIIIth cranial nerve, or brainstem nuclei may occur from CO poisoning[199]. Hearing loss, tinnitus, nystagmus, and ataxia can occur, with vestibular function being affected more frequently than auditory function[199].

Miscellaneous

Hyperamylasemia occurred in 40% of patients admitted to an ICU with CO poisoning[200]. Salivary amylase was responsible for most of the hyperamylasemia. Hyperuricemia has been described in rats poisoned with CO and is related to tissue anoxia[201]. Hepatic and intestinal injury have been reported after CO poisoning[202,203]. A patient with thrombotic thrombocytopenic purpura and microangiopathic hemolytic anemia after CO poisoning has been reported[204]. The unborn child of the pregnant woman is at risk from maternal exposure to CO. In a series of 10 pregnancies complicated by CO poisoning, eight infants developed neurologic sequelae, including mental retardation, cerebral atrophy, microcephaly, seizures, and spasticity[205].

Signs, Symptoms, and Presentation of Carbon Monoxide Poisoning

The signs and symptoms of CO poisoning in the pediatric patient may be subtle and nonspecific, making the diagnosis of CO poisoning difficult when a typical history of exposure is lacking. With COHb concentrations of less than 10%, only shortness of breath with vigorous exertion is seen. With levels of 20%, tightness across the forehead and headache are common. With higher levels (30 to 50%), irritability, nausea, vomiting, weakness, dizziness, dimness of vision, confusion, and fainting on exertion may be present. As COHb concentrations rise above 50%, loss of consciousness and convulsions may appear, with fatalities commonly occurring when COHb concentrations of 60 to 80% are reached **(Table 45.5).** These correlates are only useful as guidelines, as overlap may occur with incongruence existing between signs and symptoms and COHb concentrations.

Therapy in Carbon Monoxide Poisoning

Oxygen therapy (including hyperbaric oxygen), supportive care, and specific therapy of complications are the mainstays in the critical care of the child poisoned with CO[168]. The comatose or hypercapneic child should be intubated. Cerebral edema, if present, should be treated with hyperventilation, hyperosmolar agents (mannitol), diuretics, and fluid restriction. Steroids, contraindicated in major burns, are frequently used, although evidence of efficacy is lacking. Hypothermia, which results in leftward shift of the oxyhemoglobin dissociation curve, and mixtures of 95% oxygen and 5% carbon dioxide (carbogen) are not useful. Mild acidosis should not be pharmacologically corrected, as acidosis results in a rightward shift of the oxyhemoglobin dissociation curve, facilitating release of oxygen to tissues.

The definitive therapy for CO poisoning is oxygen. Oxygen (100%) by tight-fitting, nonrebreathing mask should be

Table 45.5. Symptoms Associated with Varying Concentrations of Carboxyhemoglobin

CO in Atmosphere, %	*COHb in Blood, %*	*Physiologic and Subjective Symptoms*
0.007	10	Shortness of breath on vigorous exertion; possible tightness across the forehead; dilation of cutaneous blood vessels
0.012	20	Shortness of breath on moderate exertion; occasional headache with throbbing in temples
0.022	30	Decided headache; irritable; easily fatigued; judgment disturbed; possible dizziness; dimness of vision
0.035	40–50	Headache; confusion; collapse; fainting on exertion
0.080	60–70	Unconsciousness; intermittent convulsion; respiratory failure; death if exposure is prolonged
0.195	80	Rapidly fatal

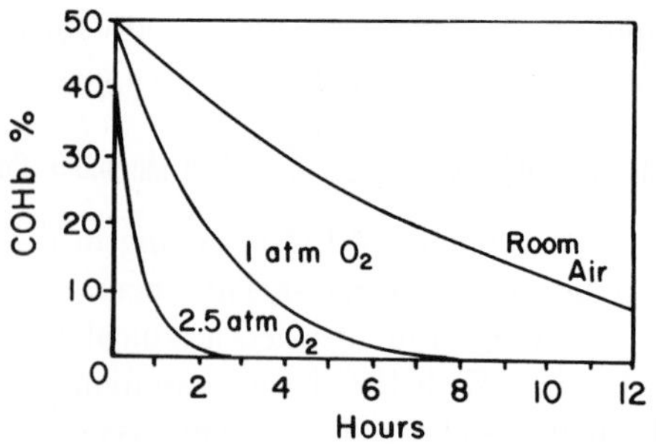

Figure 45.5. Half-life of carboxyhemoglobin at varying inspiratory concentrations of oxygen. Note that half-life is 5 to 6 hours on room air, 90 minutes on 100% oxygen, and 30 minutes on 100% oxygen at 2.5 atmospheres absolute (atm). (Adapted from Winter PM, Miller JN. Carbon monoxide poisoning. JAMA 1976;236:1503.)

given as soon as CO poisoning is suspected and should be maintained until the COHb concentration falls below 5%. It is inappropriate to withhold oxygen therapy until laboratory confirmation of CO poisoning is obtained.

The beneficial effects of oxygen on the patient poisoned by CO are twofold. Oxygen increases arterial oxygen content and accelerates the dissociation of CO from the hemoglobin molecule. During breathing of room air, only small quantities of oxygen are dissolved in plasma, and most oxygen is transported bound to hemoglobin. Breathing 100% oxygen at atmospheric pressure results in a dissolved oxygen content of 2.1 vol% in the plasma, thus supplying one-third of the normal arterial-venous oxygen content difference.

Oxygen is critical in eliminating CO by mass action, significantly reducing the half-life of CO. The half-life of CO is 5 to 6 hours when breathing 21% oxygen, 1½ hours with breathing of 100% oxygen, and less than 30 minutes with breathing of 100% oxygen at 2.5 atmospheres absolute (ATA) pressure (Fig. 45.5). The half-life is related to the degree of hyperoxemia. In the presence of lung disease, the inability to achieve high partial pressures of oxygen in blood will result in a longer half-life than that predicted by the FIO_2. It may be assumed that oxygen acts by this law of mass action to displace CO from other heme protein, such as cytochrome oxidase and myoglobin[206]. The biologic half-life of CO is doubled when poisoning results from methylene chloride, as CO continues to be produced from the metabolism of methylene chloride[123].

Hyperbaric Oxygen Therapy

Hyperbaric oxygen allows for adequate tissue oxygenation by means of oxygen dissolved in plasma rather than oxygen carried by hemoglobin. Wiseman and Grossman clearly define the physiology of hyperbaric oxygen[207] **(Table 45.6).** The arterial PO_2 is 80 to 100 torr in normal people breathing room air at sea level, resulting in a hemoglobin saturation of 95 to 97%. Thus, 19.1 ml of hemoglobin-bound oxygen (15 g of hemoglobin × 95% saturation × 1.34 ml O_2/g of hemoglobin) is carried in every 100 ml of blood. Only 0.3 ml O_2/100 ml of blood is carried in the dissolved form (PaO_2 × 0.003), resulting in total oxygen content of 19.4 ml O_2/100 ml of blood (19.4 vol%). With breathing of 100% oxygen at 1 ATA, the hemoglobin-bound oxygen is 20.1 vol%, resulting in a total oxygen content of 22.1 vol%. During hyperbaric therapy, hemoglobin-bound oxygen is again 20.1 vol%, but dissolved oxygen (1200–1500 torr) is 3.6 to 4.5 vol%, resulting in a total oxygen content of approximately 24 vol%. The dissolved oxygen content alone approaches the amount necessary to supply oxygen requirements.

Hyperbaric oxygen is considered the mainstay of therapy for CO poisoning by most authors[151], while some have suggested cautious skepticism until randomized controlled trials are completed. Hyperbaric oxygen therapy should be instituted when a patient has a COHb concentration above 25%, signs and symptoms of CO poisoning, and a hyperbaric oxygen facility is readily available. Some centers have multiplace chambers in which a physician and nurse can enter the chamber with the patient, thus allowing attention to ongoing problems. Monoplace chambers deny ready access to the patient, thus hyperbaric oxygen therapy is delayed when stabilization of the patient is necessary. Meyers et al.[168] recommend 46 minutes of 100% O_2 at 3 ATA, followed by 2 ATA for 2 hours or until COHb level falls below 10%. Patients who remain unconscious are given a second treatment 6 hours later.

Evidence from case reports suggests that hyperbaric oxygen therapy may be useful even after COHb concentrations have returned to normal[208,209]. Suggested mechanisms of response to hyperbaric oxygen therapy in these cases include a reduction of hypoxia-induced cerebral edema; reduction of hypoxia-induced damaged to the blood-brain barrier; and displacement of CO from tissues, hemoglobin, and

Table 45.6. Body Oxygen Levels on Room Air, 100% Oxygen at 1 Atmosphere Absolute (ATA), and 100% Oxygen at 2 ATA[a]

Body site	*Breathing room air*	*100% oxygen a 1 ATA*	*100% oxygen at 2 ATA*
Inspired PO_2	147 torr	760 torr	1520 torr
Alveolar PO_2	105 torr	660+ torr	1400+ torr
Arterial PO_2	80 to 100 torr	500+ torr	1200+ torr
Hemoglobin oxygen	19.1 ml O_2/100 ml	20.1 ml O_2/100 ml	20.1 ml O_2/100 ml
Dissolved oxygen	+0.3 ml O_2/100 ml	+2.0 ml O_2/100 ml	+4.0 ml O_2/100 ml
Total blood oxygen	19.4 ml O_2/100 ml	22.1 ml O_2/100 ml	24.1 ml O_2/100 ml
Tissue PO_2	40 to 50 torr	50 to 100 torr	300 to 400 torr
Tissue O_2	0.10 ml O_2/100 ml	0.15 to 0.3 ml O_2/100 ml	0.9 to 1.2 ml O_2/100 ml

[a] *Assuming normal lungs and circulation and a hemoglobin level of 15 g/dl.*

the cytochrome-oxidase system[209]. At this time, the benefit of hyperbaric oxygen versus 100% oxygen in CO poisoning remains unknown, although some authors believe that hyperbaric oxygen therapy may lead to a reduction in sequelae and may be useful in the therapy of recurrent symptoms in CO poisoning[208]. Hyperbaric oxygen therapy has also been evaluated and advocated for treatment of thermal burns in addition to CO poisoning. The mechanisms of improved wound healing are not completely understood[210].

Prognosis in Carbon Monoxide Poisoning

Larkin et al.[211] found acidosis on admission to be a poor prognostic sign in CO poisoning, yet Strohl et al.[212] reported three patients with acidosis, including one with a pH of 6.34, who recovered without neurologic sequelae. Bour and Ledingham found reversal of coma within the first 48 hours to be associated with recovery[213]. Correlation between level of consciousness upon admission and later development of neuropsychiatric sequelae has been identified[214]. Abbott[190] reported the case of a teenager who recovered after prolonged presence of disability. Long-term follow-up is necessary to identify and treat the sequelae of CO poisoning. As with all poisonings, prevention should be emphasized.

Cyanide Toxicity

Hydrogen cyanide is present in smoke generated by the combustion of many materials present in household contents. It is a decomposition product of wool, silk, polyvinylchloride, polyurethane, polyester, nylon, and melamin resins[151]. Blood cyanide levels in the lethal range have been detected in victims of house fires and air crashes. Cyanide poisoning from smoke rarely occurs in the absence of CO toxicity, and the two may act synergistically to inhibit oxidative metabolism. Cyanide levels greater than 1.0 mg/liter are associated with cellular injury, although not all laboratories provide ready access to serum levels. The therapy is supportive as well as administration of sodium nitrite and/or thiosulfate. The pathophysiology, diagnosis, and treatment of cyanide intoxication is addressed in detail in Chapter 39.

Pulmonary Inhalation Injury

Smoke is composed of many respiratory irritants produced during combustion of structural materials and home furnishings. It is the effect of these chemicals, rather than heat, which accounts for the lung pathology produced by smoke inhalation. Aldehydes, halogen acids, phosgene, oxides of nitrogen, sulphur compounds, and ammonia are produced by combustion of wood, paper, cotton, wool, silk, rubber, upholstery materials, appliances, carpeting, and other household goods. Water-soluble gases such as ammonia and HCl exert their deleterious effect by reacting with water on mucous membranes to produce strong alkalis and acids, causing an inflammatory effect. Aldehydes cause denaturation of proteins in the tracheobronchial mucosa. The oxides of nitrogen exert local effects via lipid peroxidation in the lung and increased capillary permeability. They cause metabolic derangements as well[151].

There is evidence of both tracheobronchial and pulmonary parenchymal injury due to smoke inhalation. Examination of the former reveals mucosal erythema, edema, and areas of mucosal sloughing in burn victims and experimental animals[215]. Copious quantities of protein-rich exudate, high in polymorphonuclear cells and their degranulation products, have been recovered from the tracheobronchial tree of burn subjects[215]. Thromboxane B_2, a potent smooth-muscle constrictor, is also present in the tracheobronchial exudate of animals subjected to smoke inhalation[215].

Increased pulmonary capillary permeability and increased lung lymph flow have been demonstrated in human and animal studies of smoke inhalation[216]. Extravascular lung water has been shown to be increased in sheep exposed to smoke inhalation compared with those who had burn injury without inhalation injury[217]. Smoke injury decreases ciliary function and destroys pulmonary macrophages[218,219]. Surfactant production is also altered in smoke inhalation[220].

The clinical correlates of this widespread pathophysiology include increased airway resistance[221], airway plugging, bronchorrhea, interstitial edema, atelectasis, decreased pulmonary compliance, bronchitis, pneumonia, and respiratory failure. Stone reported three stages of pulmonary inhalation injury. Victims most severely affected developed respiratory insufficiency early on, with prominence of bronchospasm and lung consolidation. Nine of ten children with early lung consolidation died, most within 48 hours of injury. The development of pulmonary edema characterized a second phase, with onset 6 to 72 hours from the time of injury. Almost all children surviving beyond day 3 developed bronchopneumonia, with a 7% mortality[222].

Patients with pulmonary injury due to smoke inhalation may be asymptomatic and have a normal chest radiograph or minor abnormality on presentation[223]. Inhalation injury may be suspected based on history of smoke exposure in a closed environment. Unconscious patients are at increased risk for serious inhalation injury and respiratory failure. The most common symptoms are dyspnea, coughing, and hoarseness accompanied by signs of wheezing, carbonaceous sputum, perioral burns, singed nasal hairs, stridor, rales, cyanosis, tachypnea, confusion, and anxiety[149]. Arterial blood gases may be normal for 12 to 24 hours, and the earliest abnormality is often a decreased ratio of arterial PO_2 to percentage of inspired oxygen[148].

Bedside fiberoptic bronchoscopy documents inhalation injury by identifying airway edema and inflammation, mucosal necrosis, and the presence of soot and charring in the airway. Xenon lung scanning has also been advocated for the diagnosis of lower respiratory injury in smoke inhalation[5].

The treatment of smoke inhalation respiratory injury is supportive. Humidified oxygen and aggressive pulmonary toilet including incentive spirometry are the mainstay of therapy. Nebulized solutions of heparin (5000 units in 5 ml) and N-acetyl cysteine are used in some centers to mobilize secretions[1]. Mechanical ventilation and positive end-expiratory pressure are necessary in cases of severe injury. Fluid therapy in patients with inhalational injury has been traditionally parsimonious owing to fears of inducing or exacerbating pulmonary edema. Experimental evidence, however, suggests that insufficient fluid resuscitation may cause pulmonary edema[224,225], and fluid requirements in burn patients are actually increased[6]. Prophylactic antibiotics are not indicated, but emperic antibiotics should be administered for documented or suspected infection. Pathogens causing pneumonia include *S. aureus* in the initial days postburn and Gram-negative organisms, particularly *Pseudomonas* species, subsequently[2]. Corticosteroids are controversial in inhalational injury. They have not demonstrated any benefit in lowering morbidity or mortality in randomized prospective studies[226] but may be indicated for refractory bronchospasm[224].

ELECTRICAL INJURY

Since the first fatal electrical accident in 1879, electrical injury has been recognized for its devastating and destructive nature. In 1977, 1183 people died from electrical injury; 22% of these were children[227]. Approximately 3% of admissions to burn centers are for electrical injury[228].

Electrical injury encompasses several different types of injury. These include the severe surface and deep tissue injury associated with heat production as current flows through tissues. High-voltage injury, including lightning injury, results in the most significant damage and is discussed subsequently. Electrical injury also involves pathophysiologic changes that occur as low-voltage electrical current flows through vital structures such as the heart and central nervous system. Multisystem disease with a variety of complications is common in severe electrical injury.

Epidemiology of Electrical Injury

The demographic data in a series (29 patients) of high-tension electrical injury in children were reported by Burke et al.[229]. All of the children were male, ranging in age from 7 to 16 years. Eleven children (38%) suffered only surface burns (average 42% BSA), while 18 (62%) had clear evidence of destruction of deep tissue as well as surface burns (average 18% BSA). Four of these 18 also sustained large surface burns (30 to 60% BSA) from ignition of clothing. Twenty-five (86%) of the children were involved in mischievous activity that involved climbing when they sustained electrical injury. The authors advocate prevention by educating children of the destructive nature of high-tension electrical injury.

Pathophysiology of Electrical Injury

Electrical injury is thought to be primarily a burn resulting from heat produced as current flows through the resistance of tissues. Joule's law states that power (heat) equals amperage squared times resistance ($P = I^2R$). Hunt et al.[230] demonstrated experimentally that electrical injury occurs when electrical current is converted to heat. In their study, tissue damage was maximal adjacent to the contact sites. The anatomic location of injury also was important in determining the amount of tissue damage. In animal limbs of smaller cross-sectional area, the tissue damage was greater because current density was higher and was concentrated in a smaller area; hence, the heat per unit volume of tissue was greater.

In the past, emphasis on varying tissue resistances underscored the belief that once skin resistance was overcome, current traveled preferentially through tissues of low resistance. In high-tension electrical injury, this is not the case. Tissue resistance in decreasing order is as follows: bone, fat, tendon, skin, muscle, blood vessels, and nerves. The work by Hunt et al.[230] in experimental injury refutes the concept of preferential flow of electrical current through low-resistance tissue (blood vessels and nerves). They found a three-phase response of amperage to electrical shock. An initial slow rise in amperage represented a progressive decrease in skin resistance. In the second phase, a rapid increase in amperage coincided with the complete breakdown of skin resistance, allowing unimpeded flow of current through the body. They noted that the body's internal resistance acts as though it is a single, uniform resistance rather than a composite of multiple and varying resistance. In the third phase, amperage fell abruptly, tissue resistance increased as the current arced, and current flow abated as tissue desiccation and carbonization occurred.

Types of Electrical Injury

The amount of tissue damage in electrical injury is dependent on several factors, including voltage. By definition, high-tension electrical injury occurs when voltage is greater than 1000 V. Three types of injury are found in high-tension electrical injury[231]: surface burns, entry and exit wounds, and arc burns. Surface burns result from ignition of clothing or from the heat of the current traveling close to the skin. The entry wound is usually charred and depressed, with swelling occurring proximal to the wound. At the site of grounding, a collection of energy results in extensive tissue necrosis as the current explodes through the skin, creating an exit wound that is usually charred, dry, and circumscribed.

Arc burns are produced by a current that travels external to the body, as an electric arc forms between two objects of opposite charge (usually a highly charged source and the ground)[229]. The arc contains electrons and ionized particles and takes a fusiform course from one pole to the other, with burns occurring when the arc strikes the victim. The temperature of such arcs may reach 3000°C[232].

The surface burns resulting from ignition of clothing or objects in the environment are frequently full-thickness, as the dazed or unconscious victim is unable to escape from the environment.

Type of Current

At low voltages, alternating current is more dangerous than direct current because of its ability to "freeze" the extremity to the source of electricity[(227)]. The slowly alternating current of household sources (60 Hz) results in tetanic muscle contractions. If the victim's hand makes contact with the source, he or she may be unable to release the grasp because the forearm flexors are more powerful than the extensors. Resistance and heat production are increased until carbonization of tissue occurs and the point of contact is broken. At high frequencies, alternating and direct current have a similar effect as the sensitivity of the individual muscle fiber to electrical stimulus is exceeded[(233)].

Electrical Laws and Terminology

Thompson and Ashwal[(227)], in a review of electrical injuries in children, define some basic electrical equations and outline the basic terminology necessary to understand electrical injury. Ohm's law states that current flow (amperes) is equal to potential difference (voltage) divided by resistance (ohms). This is depicted by the equation $V = I \times R$.

Resistance is measured in ohms. The severity of electrical injury is, in part, dependent on the skin resistance. Skin resistance is not constant. Skin resistance in children is lowered by its increased water content and a thinner stratum corneum, compared with that in adults[(234–236)]. Contact with water or saliva lowers skin resistance and thus increases current flow. This accounts for the frequency of severe injuries occurring in children in swimming pools and bathtubs and from biting electrical wires. Internal resistance is estimated to be approximately 500.

Tissue injury is directly proportional to the intensity of the current. The duration of contact is an additional factor important in determining the degree of injury. A longer duration of contact results in more extensive injury.

The concept of grounding is succinctly described by Bruner[(237)]. A ground is a conducting connection, whether intentional or accidental, to earth or some conducting body that serves in place of earth. Ground is whatever is chosen as a reference point in a particular context. The earth is ground for many applications because it is a good conductor and generally available, but ground may be the metal hull of a boat, the frame of an ambulance insulated from earth by rubber tires, the fuselage of an airplane, or a water pipe in a 12th-floor hospital room.

Clinical and Pathologic Findings in Electrical Injury

The hallmark of electrical injury is a deep burn, frequently involving muscle and other structures[(238)]. This type of injury, compared with that of surface burns, necessitates a different therapeutic approach, because the clinical course, complications, and sequelae are unique to this type of thermal injury.

Cardiovascular

Cardiac arrest is common in electrical injury[(239)] and is precipitated by a variety of mechanisms[(240)]. The conducting system of the heart is particularly sensitive to the common frequency of 60 Hz[(233)], with ventricular fibrillation caused by current passing through the chest at 100 mA[(240)]. Ventricular fibrillation most commonly follows an injury in which the path of the current traverses the chest, such as between an arm and a leg or between both arms[(240)]. Asphyxiation can result from tetanic spasm of the respiratory muscles at a current density of 30 mA[(241)]. Respiratory arrest without cardiac arrest may occur after electrical injury and rapidly leads to cardiac arrest if artificial ventilation is not instituted. Death can result from cardiac arrest in electrical injury without demonstrable surface injury[(240)]. Transient arrhythmias are found in 30% of patients with electrical injury[(227)]. Cardiac rupture after electrical injury has been reported[(242)].

Neurologic

Neurologic complications are particularly frequent after electrical injury[(242)] and include loss of consciousness[(243)], seizures[(243)], spinal cord lesions[(242)], deafness[(244)], and mood disturbances[(243)]. Peripheral nerve injury may occur secondary to vascular injury or thermal injury or by a direct effect of the electrical current[(233)]. After electrical injury, peripheral nerve injury is usually transient, unless the injury is a direct result of the burn[(245)].

Renal

Acute renal failure is more common in electrical than surface burns[(233)], occurring, in part, from the massive release of myoglobin from damaged muscle. Renal injury can also result from direct damage by the electrical current[(233)].

Vascular

Vascular complications include delayed hemorrhage from underlying vessels[(238)] and thrombosis resulting from progressive tissue edema[(235)].

Gastrointestinal

Gastrointestinal complications include gastroduodenal ulcerations, ileus, and late development of cholelithiasis.

Treatment of Electrical Injury

Prompt cardiopulmonary resuscitation results in a favorable prognosis for patients incurring cardiac arrest from electrical injury[(235)]. Vigorous and prolonged resuscitation of such victims is indicated[(246,247)].

Fluid therapy is similar to that for burn injury, although larger volumes are usually necessary for a given percentage of surface burn, owing to the large "hidden" component of electrical injury[(248)]. Fluid administration is adjusted to maintain a liberal urine output (2 ml/kg/hr) until gross clearing of myoglobinuria occurs. Mannitol and sodium bicarbonate are advocated by some to prevent acute tubular necrosis from pigment precipitation in the renal tubules[(249)]. Intravenous fluids are adjusted after gross clearing of pigmenturia to maintain a urine output of 0.5 to 1.5 ml/kg/hr.

The full extent of an electrical injury may not be apparent by the surface appearance, and this may delay adequate debridement of necrotic tissue. Technetium-99 pyrophosphate scanning was evaluated in 15 patients as a method to define occult tissue injury. Although this method was sensitive (75%) and specific (100%), it did not decrease the hospital course or surgical procedures in these patients[(250)].

Fasciotomy is frequently necessary after electrical injury. Indications for immediate surgical decompression include extensive limb burns, marked limb edema, decreased distal nerve function, and absent pulses[(235)]. Persistent severe pain is also a common indication for fasciotomy.

Lightning

Lightning is a fascinating, albeit uncommon, form of high-voltage electrical injury. Only 150 to 300 people die each year in the United States secondary to lightning strike, with the highest death rate in adolescents[(251,252)]. Nearly two-thirds of people struck by lightning survive[(253)]. The physics of lightning are well described elsewhere[(253)]. The injury incurred from lightning is often devastating, as temperatures of 60,000°F and current exceeding 1 million V are generated[(253)]. As with other high-voltage injury, survival depends in part on rapid cardiopulmonary resuscitation, as apnea rather than cardiac standstill is the primary event that ultimately leads to arrhythmia and death[(253)]. A broad range of central nervous system and ophthalmologic complications may also occur[(252)].

References

1. Herndon DH, Rutan RL, Rutan TR. Management of the pediatric patient with burns. J Burn Care Rehabil 1993;14:3.
2. Kagan RJ, Warden GD. Management of the burn wound. Clin Dermatol 1994;12:47.
3. Cooper ML, Spielvogel RL. Artificial skin for wound healing. Clin Dermatol 1994;12:183.
4. Demling RH. Burns. N Engl J Med 1985;313:1389.
5. Waywack JP, Rutan RL. Recent advances in burn care. Ann NY Acad Sci 1994;720:230
6. Muller MJ, Herndon DN. The challenge of burns. Lancet 1994; 343:216.
7. Demling RH. Fluid and electrolyte management. Crit Care Clin 1985;1:27.
8. Leape LL. Initial changes in burns: tissue changes in burned and unburned skin of rhesus monkeys. J Trauma 1970;10:488.
9. Zawacki BE. Reversal of capillary stasis and prevention of necrosis in burns. Ann Surg 1974;180:98.
10. Shirani KZ, Pruitt BA, Mason AD. The influence of inhalation injury and pneumonia on burn mortality. Ann Surg 1987;205:82.
11. Demling RH, Chen C. Pulmonary function in the burn patient. Sem Nephrol 1993;13:371.
12. Demling RH, LaLonde C. Systemic lipid peroxidation and inflammation induced by thermal injury persists into the post resuscitation period. J Trauma 1990;30:69.
13. Demling RH, LaLonde C. Identification and modification of the pulmonary and systemic inflammatory and biochemical changes caused by a skin burn. J Trauma 1990;30:57.
14. Friedl HP, Till GO, Trentz O, et al. Role of histamine, complement, and xanthine oxidase in thermal injury of skin. Am J Pathol 1989;135:203.
15. Tranbaugh RF, Lewis FR, Christensen JM, et al. Lung water changes after thermal injury, the effects of crystalloid resuscitation and sepsis. Ann Surg 1980;192:479.
16. Demling RH, et al. Early lung dysfunction after major burns: role of edema and vasoactive mediators. J Trauma 1985;25:959.
17. Baxter CR, Cook WA, Shires GT. Serum myocardial depressant factor of burn shock. Surg Forum 1966;17:1.
18. Popp MB, Friedberg DL, MacMillan BG. Clinical characteristics of hypertension in burned children. Ann Surg 1980;191:473.
19. Falkner B, Roven S, DeClement FA, et al. Hypertension in children with burns. J Trauma 1978;8:213.
20. Lowrey GH. Hypertension in children with burns. J Trauma 1967;7:140.
21. Popp MB, Silberstein EB, Laxmi SS, et al. A pathophysiologic study of the hypertension associated with burn injury in children. Ann Surg 1981;193:817.
22. Szyfelbein SK, Drop LJ, Martyn JA. Persistent ionized hypocalcemia in patients during resuscitation and recovery phases of body burns. Crit Care Med 1981;9:454.
23. Demling RH, Will JA, Belzer FO. Effect of major thermal injury on the pulmonary microcirculation. Surgery 1978;83:746.
24. Ferguson JL, Merrill GF, Miller HI, et al. Regional blood flow redistribution during early burn shock in the guinea pig. Circ Shock 1977;4:317.
25. Boucher BA, Kuhl DA, Hickerson WL. Pharmacokinetics of systemically administered antibiotics in patients with thermal injury. Clin Infect Dis 1992;14:458.
26. Carter JG, Wells CH. Intrarenal redistribution of blood flow in the early postburn period. J Trauma 1975;15:877.
27. Shires GT, Albert SA, Illner H, et al. Hepatocyte dysfunction in thermal injury. J Trauma 1983;23:899.
28. Czaja AJ, Rizzo TA, Smith WR, et al. Acute liver disease after cutaneous thermal injury. J Trauma 1975;15:887.
29. Eurenius K. Hematologic changes in burns. In: Artz CP, Moncrief JA, Pruitt BA Jr, eds. Burns: a team approach. Philadelphia: WB Saunders, 1979:132.
30. Eurenius K, Mortensen RF, Meserol PM, et al. Platelet and megakaryocyte kinetics following thermal injury. J Lab Clin Med 1972;79:247.
31. Fratianne RB. Clotting factors in burn sepsis. RI Med J 1975;58:98.
32. Curreri PW, Katz AJ, Dotin LN, et al. Coagulation abnormalities in the thermally injured patient. Surg Res 1970;2:401.
33. Andes WA, Baron JD, Bowman RP, et al. Thermal injury in von Willebrand disease. Arch Surg 1976;111:280.
34. Schachar NS, Jay AW, Rowlands S, et al. Decreased red cell deformability in burn patients. Can J Surg 1974;17:239.
35. Mortensen RF, Eurenius K. Erythrokinetics and ferrokinetics after thermal injury in the rat. Surg Gynecol Obstet 1974;138:713.
36. Robinson H, Monafo WW, Saver SM, et al. The role of erythropoietin in the anemia of thermal injury. Ann Surg 1973;178:565.
37. Antoon AY, Volpe JJ, Crawford JD. Burn encephalopathy in children. Pediatrics 1972;50:609.
38. Walker J Jr, Shenkin H. Studies on the toxemia syndrome after burns. II: Central nervous system changes as a cause of death. Ann Surg 1945;121:301.
39. Emery JL, Reid DA. Cerebral oedema and spastic hemiplegia following minor burns in young children. Br J Surg 1962;50:53.
40. Warlow CP, Hinton P. Early neurological disturbances following relatively minor burns in children. Lancet 1969;2:978.
41. Sepulchre C, Moati F, Miskulin M, et al. Biochemical and pharmacological properties of a neurotoxic protein isolated from the blood serum of heavily burned patients. J Pathol 1979;127:137.
42. Czaja AJ, McAlhany JC, Pruitt BA Jr. Acute gastroduodenal disease after thermal injury: an endoscopic evaluation of incidence and natural history. N Engl J Med 1974;291:925.
43. Czaja AJ, McAlhany JC, Pruitt BA Jr. Gastric acid secretion and acute gastroduodenal disease after burns. Arch Surg 1976;111:243.
44. Pruitt BA Jr, Goodwin CW. Current treatment of the extensively burned patient. Surg Annu 1983;15:331.
45. Lopez-Herce J, Dorao P, Elola P et al. Frequency and prophylaxis of upper gastrointestinal hemorrhage in critically ill children: a prospective study comparing the efficacy of almagate, ranitidine, and sucralfate. Crit Care Med 1992;20:1082.
46. Deitch EA. Intestinal permeability is increased in burn patients shortly after injury. Surgery 1990;107:411.
47. Ziegler TR, Smith RJ, O'Dwyer ST, Demling RH, Wilmore DW. In-

creased intestinal permeability associated with infection in burn patients. Arch Surg 1988;123:1313.
48. Jones WG, Minei JP, Barber AE, et al. Bacterial translocation and intestinal atrophy after thermal injury and burn wound sepsis. Ann Surg 1990;211:399.
49. Jones WG II, Barber AE, Minei JP, Fahey TJ, Shives GT III, Shires GT. Antibiotic prophylaxis diminishes bacterial translocation but not mortality in experimental burn wound sepsis. J Trauma 1990;30:737.
50. Ryan CM, Bailey SH, Carter EA, Schoenfeld DA, Tompkins RG. Additive effects of thermal injury and infection on gut permeability. Arch Surg 1994;129:325.
51. Munster AM, Goodwin MN, Pruitt BA. Acalculous cholecystitis in burned patients. Am J Surg 1971;122:591.
52. Ternberg JL, Keating JP. Acute acalculous cholecystitis, complication of other illnesses in childhood. Arch Surg 1975;110:543.
53. Reckler JM, Bruck HM, Munster AM, et al. Superior mesenteric artery syndrome as a consequence of burn injury. J Trauma 1972;12:979.
54. Barnett RA. A simple diagnostic sign in the superior mesenteric artery syndrome in a burned patient. Br J Plast Surg 1976;29:322.
55. Lescher TJ, Teegarden DK, Pruitt BA Jr. Acute pseudoobstruction of the colon in thermally injured patients. Dis Colon Rectum 1978;21:618.
56. Wilmore DW, Aulick LH. Metabolic changes in burn patients. Surg Clin North Am 1978;58:1173.
57. Wilmore DW. Pathophysiology of the hypermetabolic response to burn injury. J Trauma 1990;30(Suppl):S4.
58. Deitch EA. The management of burns. N Engl J Med 1990;323:1249.
59. Mochizuki H, Trocki O, Dominioni L, Brackett KA, Joffe SN, Alexander JW. Mechanism of prevention of postburn hypermetabolism and catabolism by early enteral feeding. Ann Surg 1984;200:297.
60. Deitch EA, Gelder F, McDonald JC. Sequential prospective analysis of the nonspecific host defense system after thermal injury. Arch Surg 1984;119:83.
61. Deitch EA. Infection in the compromised host. Surg Clin North Am 1988;68:181.
62. McIrvine AJ, O'Mahony JB, Saporoschetz I, Mannick JA. Depressed immune response in burn patients. Ann Surg 1982;196:297.
63. Alexander JW. Mechanism of immunologic suppression in burn injury. J Trauma 1990;30(Suppl):S70.
64. Sittig K, Deitch EA. Effect of bacteremia on mortality after thermal injury. Arch Surg 1988;123:1367.
65. Deitch EA. Bacterial translocation of the gut flora. J Trauma 1990;30(Suppl):S184.
66. Guyer B, Gallagher SS. An approach to the epidemiology of childhood injuries. Pediatr Clin North Am 1985;32:5.
67. Tompkins RG, Remensnyder JP, Burke JF, et al. Significant reductions in mortality for children with burn injuries through use of prompt eschar excision. Ann Surg 1988;208:577.
68. McLoughlin E, McGuire A. The causes, cost and prevention of childhood burn injuries. Am J Dis Child 1990;144:677.
69. Libber SM, Stayton DJ. Childhood burns reconsidered: the child, the family, and the burn injury. J Trauma 1984;24:245.
70. Banco L, Lapidus G, Zavoski R, Braddock M. Burn injuries among children in an urban emergency department. Ped Emer Care 1994; 10:98.
71. Wachtel TL. Epidemiology, classification, initial care, and administrative considerations for critically burned patients. Crit Care Clin 1985;1:3.
72. Herndon DN, Gore D, Cole M, et al. Determinants of mortality in pediatric patients with greater than 70% full thickness total body surface area thermal injury treated with total excision and grafting. J Trauma 1987;27:208.
73. Committee on Infectious Disease. Tetanus. In: Peter G, ed. Report of the Committee on Infectious Diseases. Elk Grove Village: American Academy of Pediatrics, 1991.
74. Asch MJ, Meserol PM, Mason AD, et al. Regional blood flow in the burned unanesthetized dog. Surg Forum 1971;22:55.
75. Pruitt BA Jr. Fluid and electrolyte replacement in the burned patient. Surg Clin North Am 1978;58:1291.
76. Demling RH. Improved survival after massive burns. J Trauma 1983;23:179.
77. Ehrie M, Morgan AP, Moore FD. Endocarditis with the indwelling balloon-tipped pulmonary artery catheter in burn patients. J Trauma 1978;18:664.
78. Carvajal HF. Fluid resuscitation of pediatric burn victims: a critical appraisal. Pediatr Nephrol 1994;8:357.
79. Monafo WW, Halverson JD, Schechtman K. The role of concentrated sodium solutions in the resuscitation of patients with severe burns. Surgery 1984;95:129.
80. Monafo WW. The treatment of burn shock by the intravenous and oral administration of hypertonic lactated saline solution. J Trauma 1970;10:575.
81. Horton JW, White DJ, Baxter CR. Hypertonic saline dextran resuscitation of thermal injury. Ann Surg 1990;211:301.
82. Gunn ML, Hansbrough JF, Davis JW, Furst SR, Field TO. Prospective, randomized trial of hypertonic sodium lactate versus lactated ringers solution for burn shock resuscitation. J Trauma 1989;29:1261.
83. Brouhard BH, Carvajal HF, Linares HA. Burn edema and protein leakage in the rat. I. Relationship to time of injury. Microvasc Res 1978;15:221.
84. Carvajal HF, Linares HA. Effect of burn depth upon edema formation and albumin extravasation in the rats. Burns 1981;7:79.
85. Carvajal HF, Linares HA, Brouhard BH. Relationship of burn size to vascular permeability changes in rats. Surg Gynecol Obstet 1978;147:161.
86. Eckhauser FE, Billote J, Burke JF, et al. Tracheostomy complicating massive burn injury, a plea for conservatism. Am J Surg 1974;127:418.
87. Tolmie JD, Joyce TH, Mitchell GD. Succinylcholine danger in the burned patient. Anesthesiology 1967;28:467.
88. Martyn JA, Matteo RS, Szyfelbein SK, et al. Unprecedented resistance to neuromuscular blocking effects of metocurine with persistence after complete recovery in a burned patient. Anesth Analg 1982;61:614.
89. Gronert GA, Theye RA. Pathophysiology of hyperkalemia induced by succinylcholine. Anesthesiology 1975;43:89.
90. Choi WW, Gergis SD, Sokoll MD. Controversies in muscle relaxants. Semin Anesth 1985;4:73.
91. Yamashita M, Shiga T, Matsuki A, et al. Unusual resistance to pancuronium in severely burned patients: case reports. Can Anaesth Soc J 1982;29:630.
92. Martyn JA, Szyfelbein SK, Ali HH, et al. Increased *d*-tubocurarine requirements following major thermal injury. Anesthesiology 1980; 52:352.
93. Mills AK, Martyn AJ. Neuromuscular blockade with vecuronium in paediatric patients with burn injury. Br J Clin Pharmacol 1989;28:155.
94. Marathe PH, Dwersteg JF, Pavlin EG, et al. Effect of thermal injury on the pharmacokinetics and pharmacodynamics of atracurium in humans. Anesthesiology 1989;70:752.
95. Munster AM. Treatment of invasive *E. cloacae* burn wound sepsis with topical nitrofurazone. J Trauma 1984;24:524.
96. Scoggin C, McClellan JR, Cary JM. Hypernatraemia and acidosis in association with topical treatment of burns. Lancet 1977;1:959.
97. Fligner CL, Jack R, Twiggs GA, et al. Hyperosmolality induced by propylene glycol, a complication of silver sulfadiazine therapy. JAMA 1985;253:1606.
98. Ternberg JL, Luce E. Methemoglobinemia: a complication of the silver nitrate treatment of burns. Surgery 1968;63:328.
99. Gallico GG III, O'Connor NE, Compton CC, Kehinde O, Green H. Permanent coverage of large burn wounds with autologous cultured human epithelium. N Engl J Med 1984;311:448.
100. DeLuca M, Albanese E, Bondanza S, et al. Multicentre experience in the treatment of burns with autologous and allogenic cultured epithelium, fresh or preserved in a frozen state. Burns 1989;15:303.
101. Desai MH, Herndon DN, Broemeling L, Barrow RE, Nichols RJ Jr., Rutman RL. Early burn wound excision significantly reduces blood loss. Ann Surg 1990;211:753.
102. Desai MH, Rutan RL, Herndon DN. Conservative treatment of scald burns is superior to early excision. J Burn Care Rehabil 1991;12:482.
103. Heinbach D, Luterman A, Burke J, et al. Artificial dermis for major burns. A multi center randomized clinical trial. Ann Surg 1988;208:313.
104. Lamb JD. Anaesthetic considerations for major thermal injury. Can Anaesth Soc J 1985;32:81.
105. Herndon DN, Barrow RE, Kunkel KB, Broemeling L, Rutan RL. Effects of recombinant human growth hormone on donor-site healing in severely burned children. Ann Surg 1990; 212:38.
106. Wilmore DW, Moylan HA, Bristow BF, et al. Anabolic effects of human growth hormone and high caloric feedings following thermal injury. Surg Gynecol Obstet 1974;138:875.
107. Gore DC, Honeycutt D, Jahoor F, et al. Effect of exogenous growth hormone on whole body and isolated-limb protein kinetics in burned patients. Arch Surg 1991;126:38.
108. Wolfe RR. Caloric requirements of the burned patient. J Trauma 1981;21:712.

109. Hildreth M, Carvajal HF. A simple formula to estimate daily caloric requirements in burned children. J Burn Care Rehab 1982;3:78.
110. Day T, Dean P, Adams MC, et al. Nutritional requirements of the burned child: the Curreri junior formula. Proc Am Burn Assoc 1986;18:86.
111. Hildreth MA, Herndon DN, Desai MH, Duke MA. Reassessing caloric requirements in pediatric burn patients. J Burn Care Rehab 1988;9:616.
112. O'Neil CE, Hutsler D, Hildreth MA. Basic nutritional guidelines for pediatric burn patients. J Burn Care Rehab 1989;10:278.
113. Alexander JW, Macmillan BG, Stinnett JD, et al. Beneficial effects of aggressive protein feeding in severely burned children. Ann Surg 1980;192:505.
114. Cunningham JT, Lydon MK, Russell WE. Caloric and protein provision for recovery from severe burns in infants and young children. Am J Clin Nutr 1990;51:553.
115. Gottschlich MM, Jenkins M, Warden GD, et al. Differential effects of three enteral dietary regimens on selected outcome variables in burn patients. JPEN 1990;14:225.
116. Inoue S, Epstein MD, Alexander JW, Trocki O, Jacobs P, Gura P. Prevention of yeast translocation across the gut by a single enteral feeding after burn injury. JPEN 1989;13:565.
117. Chiavelli A, Enzi G, Casadei A, Baggio B, Valeno A, Mazzoleni F. Very early nutrition supplementation in burned patients. Am J Clin Nutr 1990;51:1035.
118. Engelhardt VJ, Clark SM. Early enteral feeding of a severely burned pediatric patient. J Burn Care Rehabil 1994;15:293.
119. White S, Kamples G. Dietary noncompliance in pediatric patients in the burn unit. J Burn Care Rehabil 1990;11:167.
120. Osgood PF, Szyfelbein SK. Management of burn pain in children. Pediatr Clin North Am 1989;36:1001.
121. Perry S, Heidrich G, Ramos E. Assessment of pain by burn patients. J Burn Care Rehabil 1981;2:322.
122. Choiniere M, Melzack R, Girard N, Rondeau J, Paquin M. Comparisons between patients' and nurses' assessment of pain and medication efficacy in severe burn injuries. Pain 1990;40:143.
123. Porter J, Jick H. Addiction rare in patients treated with narcotics. N Engl J Med 1980;302:123.
124. Concilus R, Denson DD, Knarr D, Warden G, Raj PP. Continuous intravenous infusion of methadone for control of burn pain. J Burn Care Rehabil 1989;10:406.
125. Lee JJ, Marvin JA, Heimbach DM. Effectiveness of nalbuphine for relief of burn debridement pain. J Burn Care Rehabil 1989;10:241.
126. Demling RH, Ellerbe S, Jarrett F. Ketamine anesthesia for tangential excision of burn eschar: a burn unit procedure. J Trauma 1978;18:269.
127. Ward CM, Diamond AW. An appraisal of ketamine in the dressing of burns. Postgrad Med J 1976;52:222.
128. Morgan AJ, Dutkiewicz TW. Oral ketamine. Anaesthesia 1983;38:293.
129. Berde CB, Lehn BM, Yee JD, Sethna NF, Russo D. Patient-controlled analgesia in children and adolescents: a randomized, prospective comparison with intramuscular administration of morphine for postoperative analgesia. J Pediatr 1991;118:460.
130. Kinsella J, Glavin R, Reid WH. Patient-controlled analgesia for burn patients: a preliminary report. Burns 1988;14:500.
131. Waywack JP, Jenkins JW, Alexander GD, et al. A prospective trial of prophylactic intraveous immune globin for the prevention of infections in severely burned patients. Burns 1989;15:71.
132. Gennari R, Alexander JW, Gianotti L, Eaves-Pyles T, Hartmann S. Granulocyte macrophage colony-stimulating factor improves survival in two models of gut-derived sepsis by improving gut barrier function and modulationg bacterial clearance. Ann Surg 1994;220:68.
133. Demling R, LaLonde C, Knox J, et al. Fluid resuscitation with deferoxamine prevents systemic burn-induced oxidant injury. J Trauma 1991;31:538.
134. Saitoh D, Kadota T, Senoh A, et al. Superoxide dismutase with prolonged in vivo half-life inhibits intravascular hemolysis and renal injury in burned rats. Am J Emerg Med 1993;11:355.
135. Saitoh D, Okada Y, Ookawara T, et al. Prevention of ongoing lipid peroxidation by wound excision and superoxide dismutase treatment in the burned rat. Am J Emerg Med 1994;12:142
136. Ohxato H, Monden M, Yoshizaki K, et al. Systemic production of interleukin-6 following acute inflammation. Biochem Biophys Res Commun 1993;197:1556.
137. Liu XS, Luo ZH, Yang ZC, Huang WH, Li AN. The significance of changes in serum tumour necrosis factor (TNF) activity in severely burned patients. Burns 1994;20:40.
138. Carter EA, Derojas-Walker T, Tamir S, et al. Nitric oxide production is intensely and persistently increased in tissue by thermal injury. Biochem J 1994;304:201
139. Beales JG. Factors influencing the expectation of pain among patients in a children's burn unit. Burns 1983;9:187.
140. Kavanagh C. A new approach to dressing change in the severely burned child and its effect on burn-related psychopathology. Heart Lung 1983;12:612.
141. Losoff EM, McEttrich MA. Participation versus diversion during dressing change: can nurses' attitudes change? Issues Compre Pediatr Nursing 1986;9:391.
142. Woodward J. Emotional disturbances of burned children. Br Med J 1959;5128:1009.
143. Woodward J, Jackson D. Emotional reactions in burned children and their mothers. Br J Plast Surg 1961;13:316.
144. Long RT, Cope O. Emotional problems of burned children. N Engl J Med 1961;264:1121.
145. Holter JC, Friedman SB. Etiology and management of severely burned children, psychosocial considerations. Am J Dis Child 1969; 118:680.
146. Ellerstein NS. The cutaneous manifestations of child abuse and neglect. Am J Dis Child 1979;133:906.
147. Ayoub C, Pfeifer D. Burns as a manifestation of child abuse and neglect. Am J Dis Child 1979;133:910.
148. Heimbach DM. Inhalation injuries. Ann Emerg Med 1986;17:1316.
149. Young CJ, Moss J. Smoke inhalation: diagnosis and treatment. J Clin Anesth 1989;1:377.
150. Smith DL, Cairns BA, Ramadan F, et al. Effect of inhalation injury, burn size, and age on mortality: a study of 1447 consecutive burn patients. J Trauma 1994;37:655.
151. Weiss SM, and Lakshminarayan S. Acute inhalation injury. Clin Chest Med 1994;15:103.
152. Masanes MJ, Legendre C, Lioret N, et al. Fiberoptic bronchoscopy for the early diagnosis of subglottal inhalation injury: comparative value in the assessment of prognosis. J Trauma 1994;36:59.
153. Moritz AR, Henriques FC, McLean R. The effects of inhaled heat on the air passages and lungs: an experimental investigation. Am J Pathol 1945;21:311.
154. Carbon monoxide intoxication associated with use of a gasoline-powered resurfacing machine at an ice-skating rink—Pennsylvania. MMWR 1984;33:49.
155. Gormsen H, Jeppesen N, Lund A. The causes of death in fire victims. Forensic Sci Int 1984;24:107.
156. Carbon monoxide poisoning—South Dakota. MMWR 1985;34:113.
157. Wilson EF, Rich TH, Messman HC. The hazardous hibachi, carbon monoxide poisoning following use of charcoal. JAMA 1972;221:405.
158. O'Sullivan BP. Carbon monoxide poisoning in an infant exposed to a kerosene heater. J Pediatr 1983;103:249.
159. Murray TJ. Carbon monoxide poisoning from Sterno. Can Med Assoc J 1978;118:800.
160. Johnson CJ, Moran JC, Paine SC, et al. Abatement of toxic levels of carbon monoxide in Seattle ice-skating rinks. Am J Public Health 1975;65:1087.
161. Stewart RD, Hake CL. Paint-remover hazard. JAMA 1976;235:398.
162. Bernard C. Lecons sur les effects des substances toxiques et medicamenteuses. Paris: Bailliere, 1857.
163. Haldane J. The relation of the action of carbonic oxide to oxygen tension. J Physiol (Lond) 1895;18:201.
164. Douglas CG, Haldane JS, Haldane JB. The laws of combination of haemoglobin with carbon monoxide and oxygen. J Physiol (Lond) 1912;44:275.
165. Ball EG, Strittmatter CF, Cooper O. The reaction of cytochrome oxidase with carbon monoxide. J Biol Chem 1951;193:635.
166. Chance B, Erecinska M, Wagner M. Mitochondrial responses to carbon monoxide toxicity. Ann NY Acad Sci 1970;174:193.
167. Goldbaum LR. Is carboxyhemoglobin concentration the indicator of carbon monoxide toxicity? Leg Med Annu 1977;1976:165.
168. Myers RA, Linberg SE, Cowley RA. Carbon monoxide poisoning. The injury and its treatment. J Am Coll Emerg Physician 1979;8:479.
169. Tremper KK, Barker SJ. Pulse oximetry. Anesthesiology 1989;70:98.
170. Ayres SM, Giannelli S Jr, Mueller H. Myocardial and systemic responses to carboxyhemoglobin. Ann NY Acad Sci 1970;174:268.
171. Cramlet SH, Erickson HH, Gorman HA. Ventricular function following acute carbon monoxide exposure. J Appl Physiol 1975;39:482.
172. Adams JD, Erickson HH, Stone HL. Myocardial metabolism during exposure to carbon monoxide in the conscious dog. J Appl Physiol 1973;34:238.
173. Chiodi H, Dill DB, Consolazio F, et al. Respiratory and circulatory responses to acute carbon monoxide poisoning. Am J Physiol 1941;134:683.

174. Anderson RF, Allensworth DC, deGroot WJ. Myocardial toxicity from carbon monoxide poisoning. Ann Intern Med 1967;67:1172.
175. Aronow WS, Harris CN, Isbell MW, et al. Effect of freeway travel on angina pectoris. Ann Intern Med 1972;77:669.
176. Naeije R, Peretz A, Cornil A. Acute pulmonary edema following carbon monoxide poisoning. Intensive Care Med 1980;6:189.
177. Mofenson HC, Caraccio TR, Brody GM. Carbon monoxide poisoning. Am J Emerg Med 1984;2:254.
178. Halebian P, Barie P, Robinson N, et al. Effects of carbon monoxide on pulmonary fluid accumulation. Curr Surg 1984;41:369.
179. Shimazu T, Ikeuchi H, Hubbard GB, Langlinais PC, Masau AD, Pruitt BA Jr. Smoke inhalation injury and the effect of carbon monoxide in the sheep model. J Trauma 1990;30:170.
180. Sone S, Higashihara T, Kotake T, et al. Pulmonary manifestations in acute carbon monoxide poisoning. Am J Roentgenol Radium Ther Nucl Med 1974;120:865.
181. Brody JS, Coburn RF. Carbon monoxide-induced arterial hypoxemia. Science 1969;164:1297.
182. Zimmerman SS, Truxal B. Carbon monoxide poisoning. Pediatrics 1981;68:215.
183. Koehler RC, Jones MD, Traystman RJ. Cerebral circulatory response to carbon monoxide and hypoxic hypoxia in the lamb. Am J Physiol 243 (Heart Circ Physiol) 1982;12:H27.
184. Paulson OB, Parving HH, Olesen J, et al. Influence of carbon monoxide and of hemodilution on cerebral blood flow and blood gases in man. J Appl Physiol 1973;35:111.
185. Boutros AR, Hoyt JL. Management of carbon monoxide poisoning in the absence of hyperbaric oxygenation chamber. Crit Care Med 1976;4:144.
186. Sawada Y, Ohashi N, Maemura K. Computerized tomography as an indication of long-term outcome after acute carbon monoxide poisoning. Lancet 1980;1:783.
187. Sawada Y, Sakamoto T, Nishide K, et al. Correlation of pathological findings with computed tomographic findings after acute carbon monoxide poisoning. N Engl J Med 1983;308:1296 (Letter).
188. Choi HS. Delayed neurologic sequelae in carbon monoxide intoxication. Arch Neurol 1983;40:433.
189. Lacey DJ. Neurologic sequelae of acute carbon monoxide intoxication. Am J Dis Child 1981;135:145.
190. Abbott DF. Slow recovery from carbon monoxide poisoning. Postgrad Med J 1972;48:639.
191. Nagy R, Greer KE, Harman JE Jr. Cutaneous manifestations of acute carbon monoxide poisoning. Cutis 1979;24:381.
192. Long PI. Dermal changes associated with carbon monoxide intoxication. JAMA 1968;205:120.
193. Dempsey LC, O'Donnell JJ, Hoff JT. Carbon monoxide retinopathy. Am J Opthalmol 1976;82:692.
194. Jett GK. Red retinal vein (JETT) sign. Ann Emerg Med 1984;13:644.
195. McFarland RA. The effects of exposure to small quantities of carbon monoxide on vision. Ann NY Acad Sci 1970;174:301.
196. McFarland RA, Roughton FJ, Halperin MH, et al. The effects of carbon monoxide and altitude on visual thresholds. J Aviat Med 1944;15:381.
197. Rennie D, Morrissey J. Retinal changes in Himalayan climbers. Arch Opthalmol 1975;93:395.
198. Shults WT, Swan KC. High altitude retinopathy in mountain climbers. Arch Opthalmol 1975;93:404.
199. Baker SR, Lilly DJ. Hearing loss from acute carbon monoxide intoxication. Ann Otol Rhinol Laryngol 1977;86:323.
200. Takahashi M, Maemura K, Sawada Y, et al. Hyperamylasemia in acute carbon monoxide poisoning. J Trauma 1982;22:311.
201. Katsumata Y, Aoki M, Sato K, et al. Hyperuricemia in rats during acute carbon monoxide poisoning. Forensic Sci Int 1981;18:1.
202. Katsumata Y, Aoki M, Oya M, et al. Liver damage in rats during acute carbon monoxide poisoning. Forensic Sci Int 1980;16:119.
203. Watson A, Williams R. Anoxic hepatic and intestinal injury from carbon monoxide poisoning. Br Med J 1984;289:1113.
204. Stonesifer LD, Bone RC, Hiller FC. Thrombotic thrombocytopenic purpura in carbon monoxide poisoning. Arch Intern Med 1980;140:104.
205. Longo LD. Carbon monoxide in the pregnant mother and fetus and its exchange across the placenta. Ann NY Acad Sci 1970;174:313.
206. Prien T, Traber DL. Toxic smoke compounds and inhalation injury—a review. Burns 1988;14:451.
207. Wiseman DH, Grossman AR. Hyperbaric oxygen in the treatment of burns. Crit Care Clin 1985;1:129.
208. Myers RA, Snyder SK, Emhoff TA. Subacute sequelae of carbon monoxide poisoning. Ann Emerg Med 1985;14:1163.
209. Cianci P, and Sato R. Adjunctive hyperbaric oxygen therapy in the treatment of thermal burns: a review. Burns 1994;20:5.
210. Myers RA, Snyder SK, Linberg S, et al. Value of hyperbaric oxygen in suspected carbon monoxide poisoning. JAMA 1981;246:2478.
211. Larkin JM, Brahos GJ, Moylan JA. Treatment of carbon monoxide poisoning: prognostic factors. J Trauma 1976;16:111.
212. Strohl KP, Feldman NT, Saunders NA, et al. Carbon monoxide poisoning in fire victims: a reappraisal of prognosis. J Trauma 1980; 20:78.
213. Bour H, Ledingham I. Carbon monoxide poisoning. New York: Elsevier Publishing Company, 1967.
214. Smith JS, Brandon S. Morbidity from acute carbon monoxide poisoning at three-year follow-up. Br Med J 1973;1:318.
215. Traber DL, Herndon DN. The pathophysiology of inhalation injury—a review. Burns 1988;14:357.
216. Kinsella J. Smoke inhalation. Burns 1988;14:269.
217. Herndon DN, Barrow RE, Linares HA, et al. Inhalation injury in burned patients: effects and treatment. Burns 1988;14:349.
218. Demarest GB, Hudson LD, Altman LC. Impaired alveolar macrophage chemotaxis in patients with acute smoke inhalation. Am Rev Respir Dis 1979;119:285.
219. Fick RB Jr, Paul E, Reynolds HY, et al. Impaired phagocyte and bactericidal functions of smoke exposed rabbit alveolar macrophages (abstract). Chest 1980;78:516.
220. Nieman GF, Clark WR Jr, Wax SD, et al. The effect of smoke inhalation on pulmonary surfactant. Ann Surg 1980;171:181.
221. Prien T, Traber DL, Richardson JA, Traber LD. Early effects of inhalation injury on lung mechanics and pulmonary perfusion. Intensive Care Med 1988;14:25.
222. Stone HH. Pulmonary burns in children. J Pediatr Surg 1979;14:48.
223. Lee MJ, O'Connell DJ. The plain chest radiograph after acute smoke inhalation. Clin Radiol 1988;39:33.
224. Stone HH. Invited commentary. World J Surg 1978;2:190.
225. Moylan JA, Alexander LG. Diagnosis and treatment of inhalation injury. World J Surg 1978;2:185.
226. Levine BA, Petroff PA, Slade CL, Pruitt BA. Prospective trials of dexamethasone and aerosolized gentamicin in the treatment of inhalation injury in the burned patient. J Trauma 1987;28:188.
227. Thompson JC, Ashwal S. Electrical injuries in children. Am J Dis Child 1983;137:231.
228. Chen CT, Yang JY. Electrical burns associated with head injuries. J Trauma 1994;37:195.
229. Burke JF, Quinby WC Jr, Bondoc C, et al. Patterns of high tension electrical injury in children and adolescents and their management. Am J Surg 1977;133:492.
230. Hunt JL, Mason AD Jr, Masterson TS, et al. The pathophysiology of acute electric injuries. J Trauma 1976;16:335.
231. Baxter CR. Present concepts in the management of major electrical injury. Surg Clin North Am 1970;50:1401.
232. Quinby WC Jr, Burke JF, Trelstad RL, et al. The use of microscopy as a guide to primary excision of high tension electrical burns. J Trauma 1978;18:423.
233. Esses SI, Peters WJ. Electrical burns: pathophysiology and complications. Can J Surg 1981;24:11.
234. Silversides J. The neurologic sequelae of electrical injury. Can Med Assoc J 1964;91:195.
235. Sances A Jr, Larsen S Jr, Myklebust J, et al. Electrical injuries. Surg Gynecol Obstet 1979;149:97.
236. Fish R. Electric shock, Part I: Physics and pathophysiology. J Emerg Med 1993;11:309.
237. Bruner JM. Fundamental concepts of electrical safety. ASA Refresher Course Anesthesiol 1974;2:11.
238. Artz CP. Electrical injury simulates crush injury. Surg Gynecol Obstet 1967;125:1316.
239. Holliman CJ, Saffle JR, Kravitz M, et al. Early surgical decompression in the management of electrical injuries. Am J Surg 1982;144:733.
240. Bernstein T. Effects of electricity and lightning on man and animals. J Forensic Sci 1973;18:3.
241. Hodgkin BC. Some consequences of electric shock. J Maine Med Assoc 1974;65:1.
242. Kirchmer JT Jr, Larson DL, Tyson KR. Cardiac rupture following electrical injury. J Trauma 1977;17:389.
243. Kotagal S, Rawlings CA, Chen S, et al. Neurologic, psychiatric, and cardiovascular complications in children struck by lightning. Pediatrics 1982;70:190.
244. West GB Jr. Lightning as a cause of hearing loss. Laryngoscope 1949;59:1350.

245. Ugland OM. Electrical burns, a clinical and experimental study with special reference to peripheral nerve injury. Scand J Plast Reconstr Surg 1967;2:141.
246. Ravitch MM, Lane R, Safar P, et al. Lightning stroke: report of a case with recovery after prolonged artificial respiration. N Engl J Med 1961;264:36.
247. Taussig HB. "Death" from lightning, and the possibility of living again. Ann Intern Med 1968;68:1345.
248. Rouse RG, Dimick AR. The treatment of electrical injury compared to burn injury: a review of pathophysiology and comparison of patient management protocols. J Trauma 1978;18:43.
249. Hunt JL, Sato RM, Baxter CR. Acute electric burns: current diagnostic and therapeutic approaches to management. Arch Surg 1980;115:434.
250. Hammond J, and Ward CG. The use of Technetium-99 pyrophosphate scanning in management of high voltage electrical injuries. Am Surg 1994;60:886.
251. Apfelberg DB, Masters FW, Robinson DW. Pathophysiology and treatment of lightning injuries. J Trauma 1974;14:453.
252. Volinsky JB, Hanson JB, Lustig JV, Tunnessen WW Jr. Clinical picture. Lightning burns. Arch Fam Med 1994;3:657.
253. Strasser EJ, Davis RM, Menchey MJ. Lightning injuries. J Trauma 1977;17:315.

Pain, Sedation, and Postoperative Anesthetic Management in the Pediatric Intensive Care Unit

46

Myron Yaster
Jolene D. Bean
Scott R. Schulman
Mark C. Rogers

"We must all die. But that I can save (a person) from days of torture, that is what I feel as my great and ever new privilege. Pain is a more terrible lord of mankind than even death itself."—Albert Schweitzer

INTRODUCTION

The treatment and alleviation of pain is a basic human right that exists regardless of age. Unfortunately, even when their pain is obvious, children frequently receive no treatment, or inadequate treatment, for pain and for painful procedures[1–14]. The common "wisdom" that children neither respond to, nor remember, painful experiences to the same degree that adults do is simply false[1,7,8,15–19]. Critically ill children and newborns are particularly vulnerable to undertreatment[17,18,20–22]. In the intensive care unit, pain and sedation management is often ignored and relegated to the lowest rank of therapeutic priorities because of the fear that critically ill patients can neither tolerate potent analgesic drugs nor their side effects. Unfortunately, in its extremes, this policy has resulted in children being pharmacologically paralyzed with muscle relaxants without the concomitant use of analgesics, hypnotics, or amnestics. This occurs despite the fact that muscle relaxants have absolutely no sedative or analgesic properties. What can be more chilling and cruel than to be paralyzed while awake? Is a scream silenced because there is no sound?

Even when physicians decide to treat children in pain, they rarely prescribe potent analgesics or adequate doses, or utilize pharmacologically rational dosing regimens. This tragedy occurs because physicians are very poorly taught about these drugs throughout their medical education and because of their overriding concern that children may be harmed by the use of these drugs[2,3,23–27]. Although the complications of these drugs, such as respiratory depression, cardiovascular collapse, depressed levels of consciousness, and addiction are well known, rarely, if ever, are the adverse physiologic and psychologic effects of acute pain ever discussed[6,11,27–32]. In fact, until very recently, it was difficult to find pain and its medical management mentioned in any of the textbooks of pediatric medicine and surgery[30].

Nurses are taught to be wary of physicians' orders (and patients' requests) as well[8,9,13,29,30,32–35]. The most common prescription order for potent analgesics, "to give as needed" (pro re nata, "prn"), has come to mean "to give as infrequently as possible." The "prn" order also means that either the patient must ask for pain medication or the nurse must identify when a patient is in pain. Neither of these requirements may be met by children in pain, particularly in the intensive care unit.

Even under the best of circumstances, children less than 3 years of age may be unable to verbalize adequately when or where they hurt. Alternatively, they may be afraid to report their pain. Many children will withdraw or deny their pain in an attempt to avoid yet another terrifying and painful experience—the intramuscular injection or "shot"[1,8,11,24–27,29,36]. The alternative of having nurses or physicians assess when children are in pain is even less realistic. Many studies have documented the inability of nurses and physicians to identify and treat pain correctly even in the most obvious situations, such as in postoperative pain[2,3,5,8–10,18,31,32,37–39].

The purpose of this chapter is to highlight (a) pain neurophysiology and its implications in the management of pain; (b) pain assessment, particularly in critically ill patients; (c) recent advances in opioid, local anesthetic, and sedative pharmacology; and (d) appropriate therapeutic uses of these drugs in the management of acute pain.

PAIN NEUROPHYSIOLOGY

Pain is a highly complex and integrated cognitive function that is more than simply the transmission of nociceptive input from peripheral pain receptors to the brain. It is a highly subjective personal experience that is different for every living being and is much akin to other integrated, complex perceptual functions such as sight and sound. When looking at a painting or listening to music, what makes the image beautiful or the sound pleasing? Why do different people experience the same physical phenomenon and attach completely different values and meanings to it? For example, is "rap" music or noise? Even though the physiology of sound transmission is the same regardless of who hears rap music, the interpretation and integration of the physical phenomenon is very different depending on who hears the "music." Similarly, pain is a physical phenomenon that is interpreted uniquely by each person who experiences it.

Operationally, pain is probably best understood in terms of Melzack's and Wall's "gate theory of pain," which can be summarized as follows[40–42]. Following an injury, peripheral pain receptors transmit sensory information to the spinal cord via relatively small diameter (A-δ and C) sensory nerves whose cell bodies are located within the dorsal root ganglia (Figs. 46.1 and 46.2)[40–43]. A-δ fibers are associated with sharp, well-localized pain, whereas C fibers are associated with dull, burning, diffusely localized pain. The C fibers also include efferent sympathetic nerve fibers that increase the sensitivity of peripheral nociceptors to pain. In the periphery, local release of prostaglandins, serotonin, bradykinin, norepinephrine, hydrogen ion, potassium ion, and substance P, a peripheral pain transmitter, can increase the responsiveness of the peripheral nociceptors to painful stimuli (Fig. 46.1)[40–43]. Pharmacologic manipulations of these local factors by prostaglandin inhibitors (e.g., aspirin, acetaminophen, or ibuprofen) can, thereby, blunt pain transmission[26,44].

The nociceptive impulse is transmitted to the dorsal horn of the spinal cord where diverse synapses occur with essentially all incoming sensory input[40–43,45–49]. In the dorsal horn of the spinal cord, interneurons are activated and release substance P, an 11-amino acid peptide pain transmitter that facilitates nociceptive transmission[40,41,46,50]. Interestingly, substance P is depleted by capsaicin, a substance commonly found in hot chili and paprika, and may

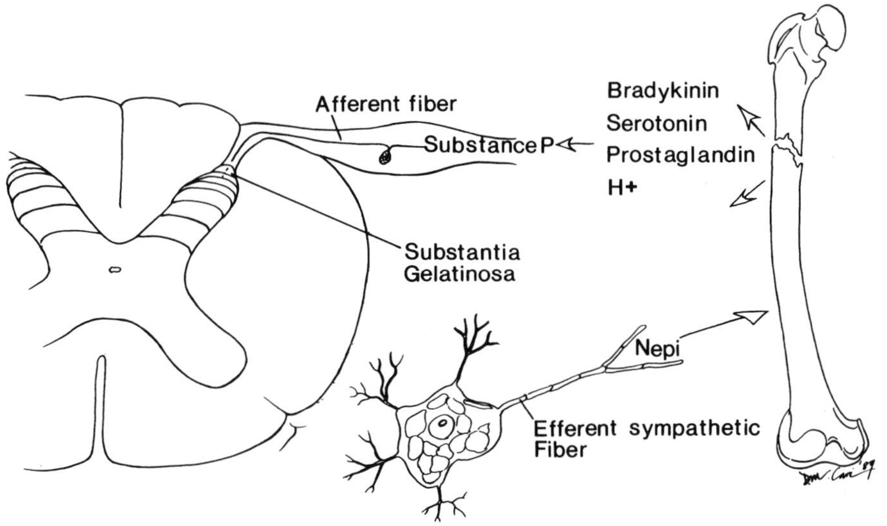

Figure 46.1. Peripheral pain receptors and modulation of their activity are depicted. Note that physical stimuli (e.g., a bone fracture), the chemical environment (pH), adrenergic tone (serotonin level, catecholamine release from sympathetic nerves), and mediator (bradykinin, prostaglandin, etc.) release modify peripheral receptor (afferent fiber) activity. Substance P is one of the peripheral pain transmitters. (Reprinted with permission from Hoekelman RA, ed. Primary pediatric care, 2nd edition.)

explain the taste bud "anesthesia" that follows the initial burning sensation of Mexican or Hungarian food. Alternatively, the nociceptive impulse may be inhibited or completely blocked at the interneurons of the dorsal horn if the interneurons are overwhelmed by innocuous, nonpainful information from other peripheral nerve fibers (Fig. 46.2). Stimulation of large diameter peripheral nerve fibers can, thereby, effectively blockade nociceptive information from the periphery. This is the underlying principle behind transcutaneous electrical nerve stimulation (TENS) (Fig. 46.2)[51–53]. Descending fibers also synapse at the interneurons to inhibit or modulate sensory input about an injury as well, via the release of neuropeptides[40–42,45–46,54–56]. Of these neuropeptides, the opioid peptides (endorphins, enkephalins, etc.) are the best known and most extensively studied (Fig. 46.2).

Indeed, the identification of μ, κ, and to a lesser degree, δ opioid receptors in the dorsal horn of the spinal cord, explains the effects of intrathecal and epidural narcotic administration in the management of pain[50,54,56–66].

If unblocked, nociceptive input is transmitted to the brain via the classic spinothalamic and spinoreticular nerve pathways[40–42,55]. Several areas within the brain may further modulate or abolish pain transmission including the brainstem's medial and lateral reticular formations, the medullary raphe nuclei, the periaqueductal gray, the thalamus, and the cerebral cortex. Binding of either endogenous or pharmacologically administered opiates to receptors in these central locations initiates the modulation of pain transmission. Additionally, it is at this level that other factors such as anxiety, fear, helplessness, affect, cultural background, absence of sleep, previous pain experience, socioeconomic status, and age influence the perception and interpretation of the nociceptive input. Indeed, it is these factors, more than the type and location of surgery or trauma, that determines the perception and intensity of pain.

The gate theory, therefore, depends not only on peripheral stimulation and transmission but also on modulation of the transmission within the spinal cord and higher structures. Thus, pain or the transmission of nociceptive impulses requires intact neuroanatomic pathways from the peripheral pain receptors to the central nervous system. These pathways and receptors develop in early fetal life and are essentially mature and completely developed by birth[17,20]. The development of descending inhibition pathways of no-

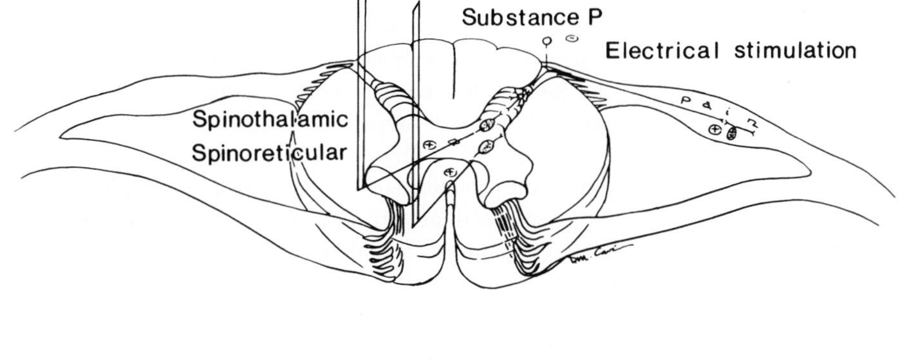

Figure 46.2. Pain transmission within the spinal cord can be modified or completely blocked either endogenously, pharmacologically, or mechanically.

ciceptive neurons and interneurons in the dorsal horn of the spinal cord and within the brainstem occurs during the final third of gestation and is completed during infancy and early childhood.

Pain management can, therefore, be best understood or designed in terms of afferent pain pathways and descending pain modulation. Pain can be relieved (a) by reducing the sensory input from damaged tissue (by prostaglandin inhibitors or local anesthetics administration), (b) by modulating the transmission of the nociceptive input through the central nervous system (by TENS, pharmacologic opioid administration, or by the administration of local anesthetics), and (c) by altering the patient's emotional responses to such actual or perceived sensory input (by antidepressants, hypnotics, amnestics, or stimulants). However, before one can effectively treat pain, one must be able to measure and assess pain and the therapies used in treating it accurately.

Table 46.1. Objective Pain Score[a]

Blood pressure (systolic)	≤10% of control	0
	11–20% of control	1
	>21% of control	2
Crying?	Not crying	0
	Crying but responds to TLC	1
	Crying and does not respond to TLC	2
Movement	None	0
	Restless	1
	Thrashing	2
Agitation	Patient asleep or calm	0
	Mild	1
	Hysterical	2
Verbal evaluation or body language	Asleep or states no pain (preverbal child—no special posture)	0
	Mild pain or cannot localize (preverbal child—flexing extremities)	1
	Moderate pain and can localize (preverbal child—holding location of pain)	2

[a] *A score ≥6 signifies significant pain and should be treated with a potent analgesic.*

PAIN ASSESSMENT

The International Association for the Study of Pain (IASP) defines pain as "an unpleasant and emotional experience associated with actual or potential tissue damage, or described in terms of such damage"[(67)]. Pain is a completely subjective experience; operationally, it can be defined as "what the patient says hurts" and exists "when the patient says it does." Infants, preverbal children, children between the ages of 2 and 7 yr (Piaget's "preoperational thought stage"), and critically ill children may be unable to describe their pain or their subjective experiences. This has led many to conclude that children do not experience pain in the same way that adults do. Clearly, children do not have to know or be able to express the meaning of an experience to have that experience. On the other hand, because pain is essentially a subjective experience, it is becoming increasingly clear that the child's perspective of pain is an indispensable facet of pediatric pain management and an essential element in the specialized study of childhood pain[(6,7,11,35,68–74)]. Indeed, pain assessment and management are interdependent and one is essentially useless without the other. The goal of pain assessment is to provide accurate data about the location and intensity of pain as well as the effectiveness of measures used to alleviate or abolish it.

Validated, reliable instruments currently exist to measure and assess pain in children over the age of 3 years[(7,11,19,49,69,71,75)]. These instruments that measure the quality and intensity of pain are "self-report measures" and make use of pictures or word descriptors to describe pain. Pain intensity or severity can be measured in children as young as 3 years of age by using either the "Oucher" scale (developed by Dr. J. Beyer)—a two part scale with a vertical numerical scale (0–100) on one side and six photographs of a young child on the other—or a visual analog scale—a 10-cm line with a smiling face on one end and a distraught, crying face on the other (Figs. 46.3 and 46.4). Alternatively, color, word-graphic rating scales, and poker chips have been used to assess the intensity of pain in children as well. In infants and critically ill patients who are unable to communicate, pain has been assessed by measuring physiologic responses to nociceptive stimuli, such as blood pressure and heart rate changes or by measuring levels of adrenal stress hormones. Alternatively, behavioral approaches have utilized facial expression, body movements, the presence of tears, and the intensity and quality of crying as indices of response to nociceptive stimuli. The behavioral scoring system we utilize is listed in **Table 46.1** and was developed by Hannallah et al. to assess postoperative pain[(72)]. Finally, it is important to define the location of pain accurately as well. This is readily accomplished by using either dolls or action figures or by using drawings of body outlines, both front and back[(73,74)].

NONOPIOID (OR "WEAKER") ANALGESICS

The "weaker" or "milder" analgesics, of which acetaminophen (Tylenol) and salicylate (aspirin) are the classic examples, comprise a heterogenous group of nonsteroidal anti-inflammatory drugs (NSAID) that provide analgesia primarily by blocking peripheral prostaglandin production[(23,26,75–80)]. These agents are administered enterally via the oral or, on occasion, the rectal route and are particularly useful for inflammatory, bony, or rheumatic pain. One of the newest and most powerful NSAIDs, ketorolac, can be administered parenterally (0.5 mg/kg q 6 hour, maximum dose 30 mg)[(81–85)]. This family of drugs is the most preferred group of analgesics prescribed by pediatricians because they are relatively safe, have few cardiopulmonary side effects, and are nonaddictive[(86–88)]. Unfortunately, re-

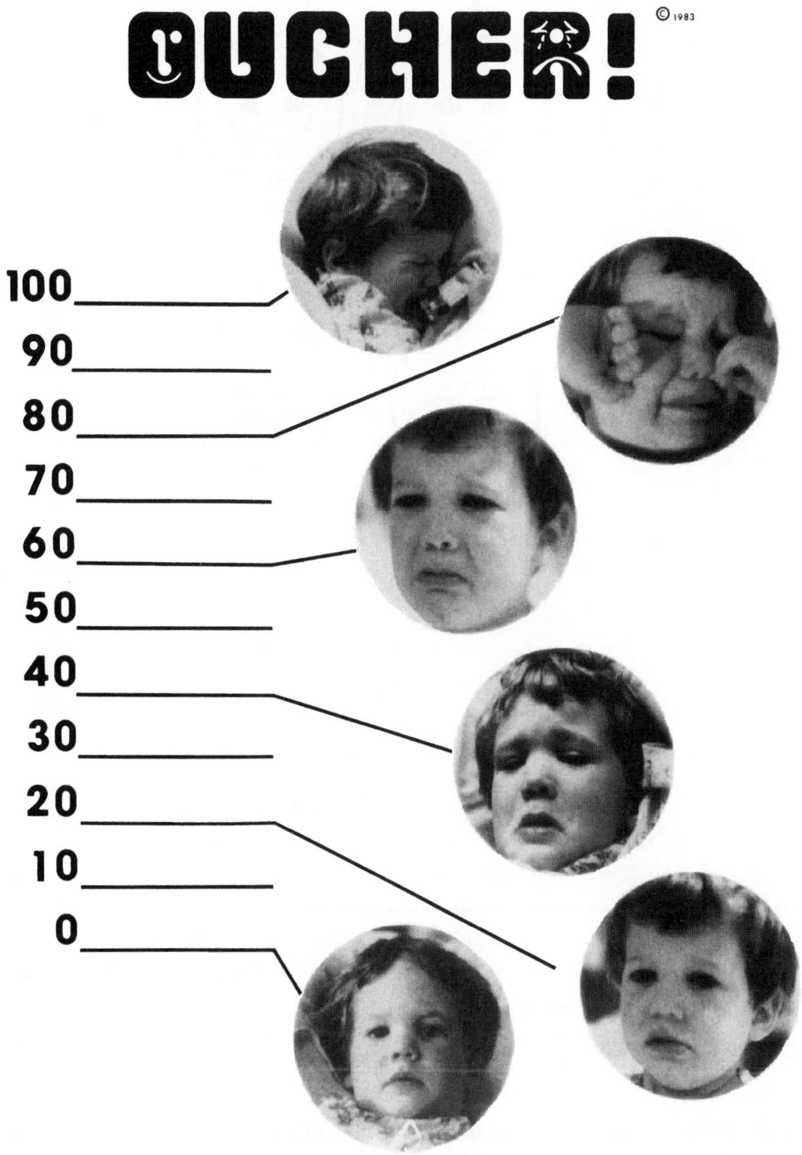

Figure 46.3. The Oucher scale is a visual analog scale used in pain assessment in children. Note that the higher the score, the greater the child's pain. It was developed and copyrighted by Judith E. Beyer, R.N., Ph.D. For more information, contact Dr. Beyer at the University of Colorado Health Sciences Center School of Nursing, Denver, CO. The Oucher scale is reprinted with permission from its author.

gardless of dose, they reach a "ceiling effect" above which pain cannot be relieved by these drugs alone. Indeed, because of this, the nonopioid analgesics are often administered in combination with other more potent agents such as codeine[(89,90)].

There is very little information in the pediatric literature on the use of the newer NSAIDs, such as ibuprofen, naprosyn, tolectin, indomethacin, or ketorolac. Furthermore, because of its possible role in the production of Reye syndrome, aspirin has been largely abandoned in pediatric practice as well. Fortunately, acetaminophen is equally effective and potent as aspirin in the treatment of pain[(86,87)]. When administered in normal doses (10–15 mg/kg-1), it has very few serious side effects. Acute overdosage or poisoning may produce fulminant hepatic failure and death. Fortunately, emergency management with N-acetylcysteine, via the oral or parenteral route, can prevent this tragedy from occurring.

OPIOIDS

Terminology

The terminology used to describe potent analgesic drugs is constantly changing[(23,24,26,91)]. They are commonly referred to as "narcotics" (from the Greek "narco"—to deaden), "opiates" (from the Greek "opi on"—poppy juice, for drugs derived from the poppy plant), "opioids" (for all drugs with morphine-like effects, whether synthetic or naturally occur-

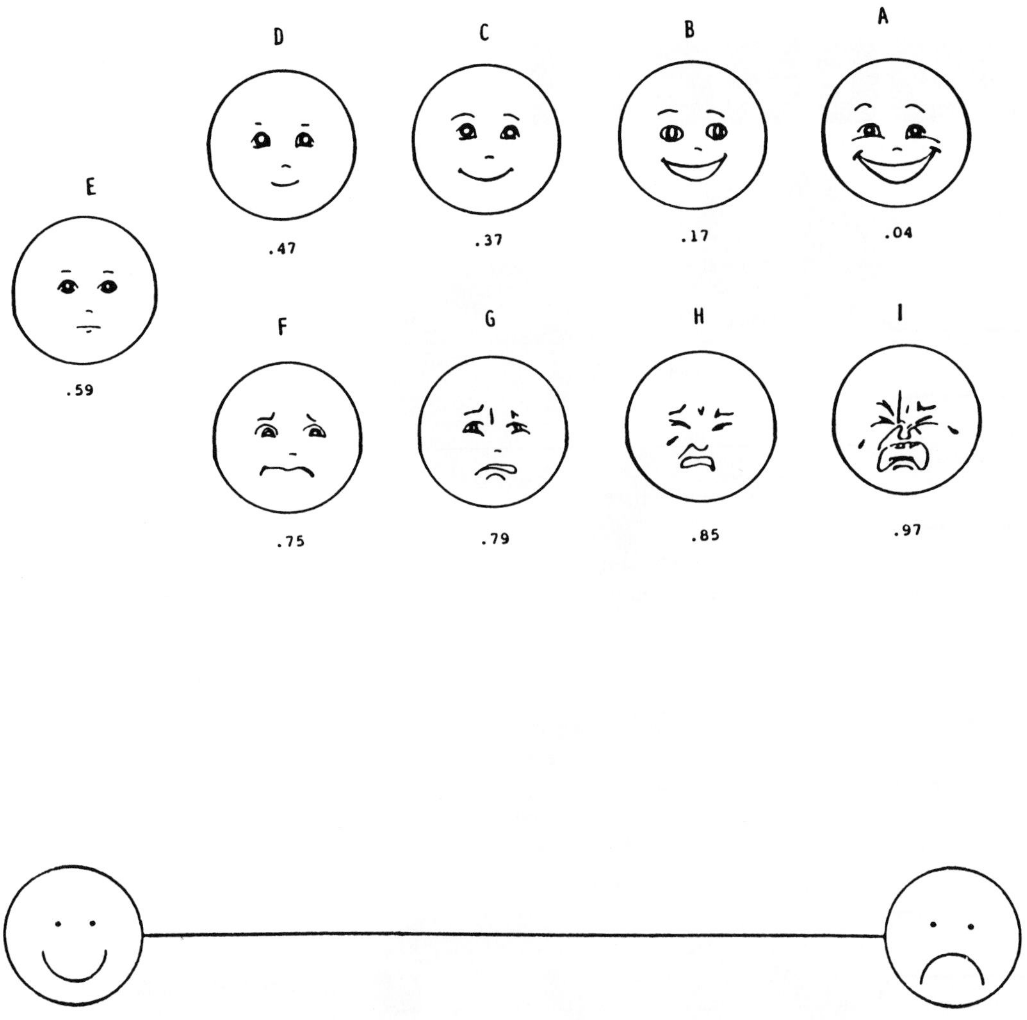

Figure 46.4. Top: A nine-face linear analog scale developed by Patricia McGrath, Ph.D., and reprinted with permission. Bottom: A 10-cm linear scale developed by James W. Varni, Ph.D. (Reprinted with permission from Thompson KL, Varni JW. A developmental cognitive behavioral approach to pediatric pain assessment. Pain 1986;25:283.)

ring), or euphemistically as "strong analgesics" (when the physician is reluctant to tell the patient or the patient's family that narcotics are being used)[27,60,90,91]. Furthermore, the discovery of endogenous endorphins and opioid receptors has necessitated the reclassification of these drugs into agonists, antagonists, and mixed agonist-antagonists based on their receptor-binding properties[27,54,59,60,66,90–97].

Opioid Receptors

Over the past 20 years, multiple opioid receptors and subtypes have been identified and classified **(Table 46.2).** An understanding of the complex nature and organization of these multiple opioid receptors is essential for an adequate understanding of the response to and control of pain. In the central nervous system, there are four primary opioid receptor types, designated mu (μ) (for morphine), kappa (κ), delta (δ), and sigma (σ)[27,48,54,56,59–64,66,90–99]. The receptor is further subdivided into μ1 (supraspinal analgesia) and μ2 (respiratory depression, inhibition of gastrointestinal motility, and spinal analgesia) subtypes. Other receptors and subtypes will surely be discovered as research in this area proceeds.

The differentiation of agonists and antagonists is fundamental to pharmacology. A neurotransmitter is defined as having agonist activity, whereas a drug that blocks the action of a neurotransmitter is an antagonist[54,59,60,62,63,90–99]. By definition, receptor recognition of an agonist is "translated" into other cellular alterations (that is, the agonist initiates a pharmacologic effect), whereas an antagonist occupies the receptor without initiating the transduction step (it has no intrinsic activity or efficacy)[53,59–62,91]. The intrinsic activity of a drug defines the ability of the drug-receptor complex to initiate a pharmacologic effect. Drugs that produce less than a maximal response have a lowered intrinsic activity and are called partial agonists. Partial agonists also have antagonistic properties because, by binding the receptor site, they block access of full agonists to the receptor site. Morphine and related opiates are μ-agonists and drugs that block the effects of opiates at the μ-receptor, such as naloxone, are designated antagonists. The opioids most

Table 46.2. Classificaton of Opioid Receptors

Receptor	Prototype Agonist	CNS Location	Effects
μ	Morphine Fentanyl Meperidine Codeine Methadone Hydromorphone	Brain Laminae III and IV of the cortex, thalamus, periaqueductal gray Spinal cord Substantia gelatinosa	μ^1 supraspinal analgesia, dependence μ^2 respiratory depression, inhibition of gastrointestinal mobility, bradycardia, ++ sedation
κ	Ketocyclazocine Dynorphin ?Butorphanol	Brain Hypothalamus, periaqueductal gray, claustrum Spinal cord Substantia gelatinosa	Spinal analgesia, ++++ sedation, miosis, inhibition of antidiuretic hormone release
δ	Enkephalins DADL	Brain Pontine nucleus, amygdala, olfactory bulbs, deep cortex	Analgesia Euphoria
σ	N-allylnormetazocine Phencyclidine ?Ketamine		Dysphoria, hallucinations, psychomotor stimulation

commonly used in the management of pain are μ-agonists **(Table 46.3).** These include morphine, meperidine, methadone, and the fentanyls. Mixed agonist-antagonist drugs act as agonists or partial agonists at one receptor and antagonists at another receptor. Mixed (opioid) agonist-antagonist drugs include pentazocine, butorphanol, nalorphine, and nalbuphine[99,100]. Most of these drugs are agonists or partial agonists at the κ- and σ-receptors and antagonists at the μ-receptor **(Table 46.4).**

The μ-receptor and its subspecies and the δ-receptor produce analgesia, respiratory depression, euphoria, and physical dependence. Morphine is 50–100 times weaker at the δ than at the μ-receptor. By contrast, the endogenous opiate-like neurotransmitter peptides known as the enkephalins tend to be more potent at δ- and κ- than μ-receptors. The κ-receptor, located primarily in the spinal cord, produces spinal analgesia, miosis, and sedation with minimal associated respiratory depression. Indeed, this may have important clinical significance. As tolerance develops, increasing doses of morphine are required to produce effective analgesia.

It is intriguing to speculate that, at higher doses, the analgesia produced by morphine occurs by its δ and κ effects rather than by its μ-agonist activity. Alternatively, when administered spinally, morphine and other μ-agonists achieve cerebrospinal fluid levels that are log concentrations higher than can be achieved by more conventional routes of drug administration. Indeed, when administered by this route, the concentration of agonists may be high enough to produce analgesia via the κ-receptor. Finally, the σ-receptor is responsible for the psychotomimetic effects observed with some opiate drugs, particularly the mixed agonist-antagonist drugs. These effects include dysphoria and hallucinations. A number of studies suggest that the respiratory depression

Table 46.3. Commonly Used μ-Agonist Drugs

Agonist	Equipotent i.v. Dose (mg/kg)	Duration (hr)	Bioavailability (%)	Comments
Morphine	0.1	3–4	20–40	Seizures in newborns; also in all patients at high doses Histamine release, vasodilation→→avoid in asthmatics and in circulatory compromise MS-contin 8–12 hr duration
Meperidine	1.0	3–4	40–60	Catastrophic interactions with MAO inhibitors Tachycardia; negative inotrope Metabolite produces seizures; not recommended for chronic use
Methadone	0.1	6–24	70–100	Can be given i.v. even though the package insert says s.c. or i.m.
Fentanyl	0.001	0.5–1.0		Bradycardia; minimal hemodynamic alterations Chest, wall rigidity (>5 μg/kg rapid i.v. bolus); Rx naloxone or a succinylcholine, pancuronium
Codeine	1.2	3–4	40–70	PO only Prescribe with acetaminophen
Hydromorphone (Dilaudid)	0.015–0.02	3–4	40–60	< CNS depression than morphine < Itching, nausea than morphine Can be used in i.v. and epidural PCA
Oxycodone (component opioid in Tylox)	0.1	3–4	50–70	Excellent oral bioavailability, much less nausea and vomiting than codeine and is preferred; often prescribed combined with acetaminophen (Tylox)

Table 46.4. Action of Opioids at Receptor Subtypes

Drug/Agent	Receptor Subtype μ	κ	σ
Morphine	Agonist	Agonist	Minimal effect
Naloxone (Narcan)	Antagonist	Antagonist	Antagonist
Naltrexone (Trexan)	Antagonist		
Pentazocine (Talwin)	Antagonist	Agonist	Agonist
Butorphanol (Stadol)	Minimal effect	Agonist	Agonist
Nalbuphine (Nubain)	Antagonist	Partial agonist	Agonist

and analgesia produced by μ-agonists involve different receptor subtypes[94,101,102]. These receptors change in number in an age-related fashion and can be blocked by naloxone. Pasternak et al.[101,102], working with newborn rats, showed that 14-day-old rats are 40 times more sensitive to morphine analgesia than 2-day-old rats[94,101,102]. Nevertheless, morphine depresses the respiratory rate in 2-day-old rats to a greater degree than in 14-day-old rats. Thus, the newborn may be particularly sensitive to the respiratory depressant effects of the commonly administered opioids in what may be an age-related receptor phenomenon. Obviously, this has important clinical implications for the use of narcotics in the newborn.

Morphine

Morphine (from Morpheus, the Greek god of sleep) is the standard for analgesia against which all other opioids are compared. When small doses, 0.1 mg/kg-1 (intravenous, intramuscular), are administered to otherwise unmedicated patients in pain, analgesia usually occurs without loss of consciousness. The relief of tension, anxiety, and pain usually results in drowsiness and sleep as well. Older patients suffering from discomfort and pain usually develop a sense of well-being and/or euphoria following morphine administration. Interestingly, when morphine is given to pain-free adults they may show the opposite effect, namely, dysphoria and increased fear and anxiety. Mental clouding, drowsiness, lethargy, an inability to concentrate and to sleep may occur following morphine administration even in the absence of pain. Less advantageous central nervous system effects of morphine include nausea and vomiting, pruritus, miosis, and at high doses, seizures. Seizures are a particular problem in the newborn because they may occur at commonly prescribed doses (0.1 mg/kg)[103–106]. The nausea and vomiting that are seen with morphine administration is due to stimulation of the chemoreceptor trigger zone in the brainstem **(Table 46.5).**

Although morphine produces peripheral vasodilation and venous pooling, it has minimal hemodynamic effects (e.g., cardiac output, left ventricular stroke work index, pulmonary artery pressure, etc.) in normal, euvolemic, supine patients. The vasodilation associated with morphine is primarily due to its histamine-releasing effects. Significant hypotension may occur if sedatives such as diazepam are concurrently administered with morphine. Otherwise, it produces virtually no cardiovascular effects when used alone. It will cause significant hypotension in hypovolemic patients and its use in trauma patients is, therefore, limited.

Morphine (and all other narcotics at equipotent doses) produces respiratory depression primarily by reducing the

Table 46.5. Physiologic Effects of Opioids by Organ System

Central Nervous System	Respiratory System	Cardiovascular System	Gastrointestinal System	Urinary System
Analgesia	Antitussive	Bradycardia (fentanyl, morphine)	Decreased motility and peristalsis (treatment for diarrhea, constipation common)	Increased tone in ureters, bladder, and detrusor muscles of the bladder
Sedation	Decreased minute ventilation, respiratory rate, and tidal volume	Tachycardia (meperidine)	Increased sphincter tone: sphincter of Oddi, ileocolic	
Nausea and vomiting	Depressed ventilatory response to carbon dioxide and oxygen	Histamine release, venodilation (morphine)		
Miosis		Minimal effects on cardiac output, except meperidine		
Seizures				
Dysphoria				
Euphoria				
Psychotomimetic behaviors, excitation				

sensitivity of the brainstem respiratory centers to hypercarbia and hypoxia. Initially, respiratory rate is affected more than tidal volume, but as the dose of morphine is increased, tidal volume becomes affected as well. The most sensitive means of measuring the respiratory depression produced by any drug is by measuring the reduction in the slope of the carbon dioxide response curve and by the depression of minute ventilation (ml/kg) that occurs at $PCO_2 = 60$ mm Hg. Morphine shifts the carbon dioxide response curve to the right and also reduces its slope. This is demonstrated in Figure 46.5. The combination of any opioid agonist with any sedative produces more respiratory depression than when either drug is administered alone (Fig. 46.5)[(107)]. Clinical signs that predict impending respiratory depression include somnolence, small pupils, and small tidal volumes. Aside from newborns, patients who are at particular risk to opioid-induced respiratory depression include those with an altered mental status, are hemodynamically unstable, have a history of apnea or disordered control of ventilation, have hepatic or renal disease, or who have a known airway problem. Morphine also depresses the cough reflex and the sense of air hunger that occurs when arterial carbon dioxide levels rise. This explains its use as a sedative in terminally ill patients and in critically ill patients who are "fighting the ventilator."

Morphine (and all other narcotics at equipotent doses) inhibits intestinal smooth muscle motility. This decrease in peristalsis and increase in sphincter tone explains the historic use of narcotics in the treatment of diarrhea as well as its "side effect" when treating chronic pain, namely, constipation. In fact, we routinely prescribe laxatives or stool softeners for patients expected to be treated with narcotics for more than 2 or 3 days. Morphine will potentiate biliary colic by causing spasm of the sphincter of Oddi and should be used with caution in patients with, or at risk for, cholelithiasis (e.g., sickle cell disease). Morphine increases tone and contractions in the ureters, bladder, and in the detrusor muscles of the bladder that may make urination difficult. This may also explain the increased occurrence of bladder spasm and pain that occurs when morphine is used to treat postoperative bladder surgery patients **(Table 46.5).**

Pharmacokinetics

To relieve or to prevent pain, the agonist must get to the receptor in the central nervous system (Fig. 46.6). There are essentially two ways that this occurs, either via the bloodstream (following intravenous, intramuscular, oral, nasal, transdermal, or mucosal administration) or by direct application (intrathecal or epidural) into the cerebrospinal fluid (CSF)[(58,59,98)]. Agonists administered via the bloodstream must cross the blood-brain barrier, a lipid membrane interface between the endothelial cells of the brain vasculature and the extracellular fluid of the brain, to reach the receptor. Normally, highly lipid-soluble agonists, such as fentanyl, rapidly diffuse across the blood-brain barrier, whereas agonists with limited lipid solubility, such as morphine, have limited brain uptake[(108–111)]. The blood-brain barrier may be immature at birth and is known to be more permeable to morphine. Indeed, Way et al.[(112,113)] demonstrated that morphine concentrations were two to four times greater in the brains of younger rats than older rats despite equal blood concentrations[(112,113)].

Spinal administration, either intrathecally or epidurally, bypasses the blood and directly places an agonist into the CSF, which bathes the receptor sites in the spinal cord (substantia gelatinosa) and brain. This "back door" to the receptor significantly reduces the amount of agonist needed to relieve pain. After spinal administration, opioids are absorbed by the epidural veins and redistributed to the systemic circulation where they are metabolized and excreted. Hydrophilic agents, such as morphine, cross the dura more slowly than more lipid-soluble agents, such as fentanyl or meperidine[(108–111)]. This physicochemical property is responsible for the more prolonged duration of action of spinal morphine and its very slow onset of action following epidural administration[(57,111,112)].

Although it would be desirable to adjust opioid dosage

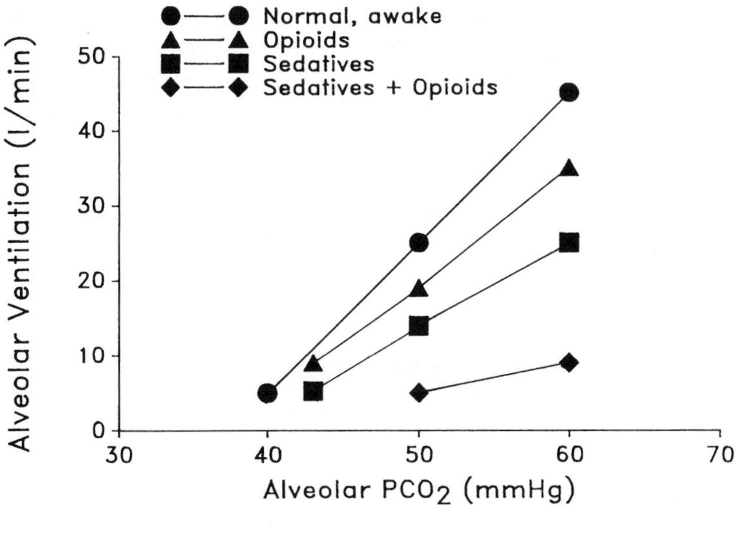

Figure 46.5. The relationship between ventilation and carbon dioxide is represented by a family of curves. Each curve has two parameters—an intercept and slope. Sedatives and opioids shift the position and slope to the right. The combination of drugs produces the most profound effects. (Reprinted with permission from Yaster M, et al. Midazolam-fentanyl intravenous sedation in children: case report of respiratory arrest. Pediatrics 1990;86:463–467.)

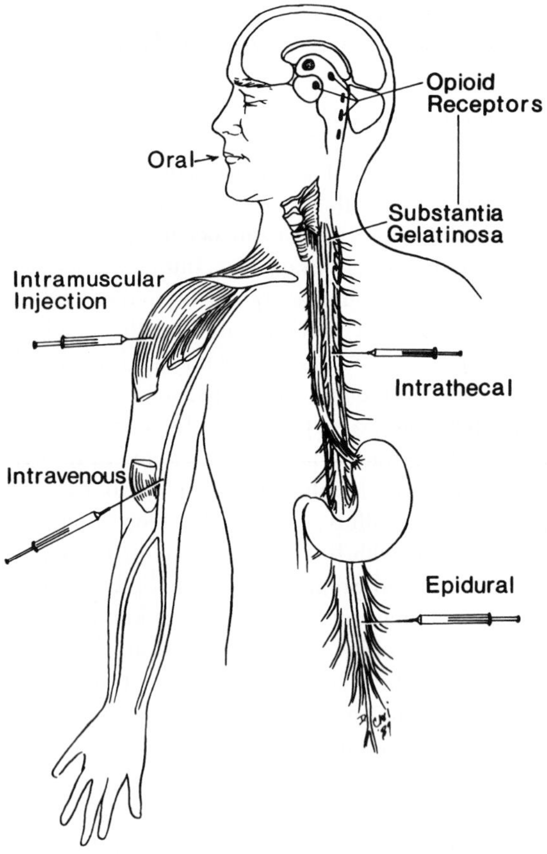

Figure 46.6. Location of opioid receptors within the central nervous system. Opioids reach the receptor following parenteral (i.v., i.m.), spinal (intrathecal, epidural), or enteral (mouth, nose) administration.

based on the concentration of drug achieved at the receptor site, this is rarely feasible. The alternative is to measure blood or plasma concentrations and model how the body handles a drug. Pharmacokinetic studies thereby help the clinician select suitable routes, timing, and dosing of drugs to maximize a drug's dynamic effects.

Following administration, the disposition of a drug is dependent on distribution ($t1/2\alpha$) and elimination. The terminal half-life of elimination ($t1/2\beta$) is directly proportional to the volume of distribution (VD) and inversely proportional to the total body clearance (Cl) by the following formula:

$$t1/2\beta = 0.693 \times (VD/Cl)$$

Thus, a prolongation of the $t1/2\beta$ may be due to either an increase in a drug's volume of distribution or by a decrease in its clearance.

Morphine, meperidine, methadone, and fentanyl are biotransformed in the liver before excretion[58,59,91]. Many of these reactions are catalyzed in the liver by microsomal mixed-function oxidases that require the cytochrome P450 system, NADPH, and oxygen. The cytochrome P450 system is very immature at birth and does not reach adult levels until the first month or two of life. This immaturity of this hepatic enzyme system may explain the prolonged clearance or elimination of some opioids in the first few days to weeks of life. On the other hand, the P450 system can be induced by various drugs (phenobarbital) and substrates and matures regardless of gestational age. Thus, it is the age from birth, and not the duration of gestation, that determines how premature and full-term infants metabolize drugs. Indeed, Greeley et al.[114] have demonstrated that sufentanil is more rapidly metabolized and eliminated in 2- to 3-week-old infants than newborns less than a week of age[114].

The pharmacokinetics of morphine have been extensively studied in adults, older children, and in the premature and full-term newborn[103–106,115–117]. Following an intravenous bolus, 30% of morphine is protein bound in the adult compared with only 20% in the newborn. This increase in unbound ("free") morphine allows a greater proportion of active drug to penetrate the brain. This may explain, in part, the observation of increased brain levels of morphine in the newborn and its more profound respiratory depressant effects by Way et al.[116,117]. The elimination half-life of morphine in adults and older children is 3 to 4 hours and is consistent with its duration of analgesic action **(Table 46.6).** The $t1/2\beta$ is more than twice as long in newborns less than a week of age than older children and adults, and is even longer in premature infants. Clearance is similarly decreased in the newborn compared to the older child and adult **(Table 46.6).** Thus, infants less than 1 month of age will attain higher serum levels that will decline more slowly than older children and adults. This may also account for the increased respiratory depression associated with morphine in this age group.

Interestingly, the half-life of elimination and clearance values of morphine in children older than 2 months of age is similar to adult values. Thus, the hesitancy in prescribing and administering morphine in children less than 1 year of age may not be warranted. On the other hand, the use of any opioid in children less than 2 months of age must be limited to a monitored, intensive care unit setting.

Suggested Dosage

The "unit" dose of intravenously administered morphine is 0.1 mg/kg and is modified based on patient age and disease state **(Table 46.3).** Indeed, to minimize the complications associated with intravenous morphine (or any opioid) administration, we always recommend titration of the dose at the bedside until the desired level of analgesia is achieved. Based on its relatively short half-life (3 to 4 hr), one would expect older children and adults to require morphine supplementation every 2 to 3 hr when being treated for pain, particularly if the morphine is administered intravenously (Fig. 46.7)[23,26]. This has led to the re-

Table 46.6. Morphine Pharmacokinetics

	Premature (<33 weeks)	*Full-term*	*Adult*
$t_{1/2}\beta$	7.4 ± 1.7	6.7 ± 4.6	3.0
Clearance (ml/kg/min)	9.6 ± 4.0	15.5 ± 10.0	3.2
V_D (liter/kg)	5.18 ± 1.6	2.9 ± 2.1	15

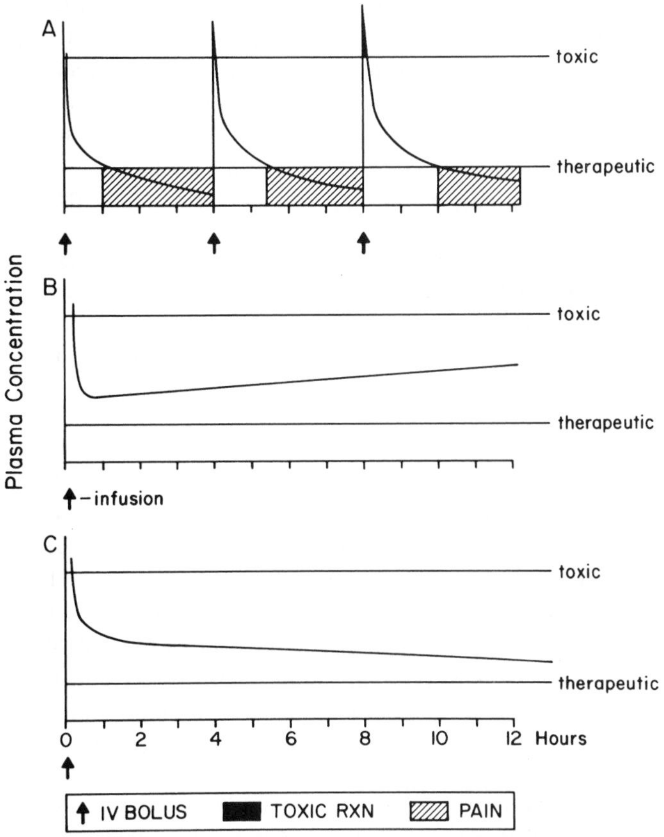

Figure 46.7. Simulated blood concentration-dose relationships for opioids by different administration regimens. A. Intravenous bolus administration (IV bolus) of morphine sulfate (elimination half-life, 4 hr) every 4 hr. B. IV bolus administration of morphine sulfate followed by C an IV bolus administration of methadone (elimination half-life, 19 hr). Note the absence of pain periods in B and C. (Reprinted with permission from Yaster M, et al: The pharmacologic management of pain in children. Comprehens Ther 1989;15:14–26.)

cent use of continuous infusion regimens of morphine (0.02 to 0.03 mg/kg/hr) and patient-controlled analgesia (see below) that maximize pain-free periods(118–122). Alternatively, longer acting agonists, such as methadone, may be used(25,26,124–128). Finally, only about 20 to 30% of an orally administered dose of morphine reaches the systemic circulation(27,36,123,129). When converting a patient's intravenous morphine requirements to oral maintenance, one needs to multiply the intravenous dose by three to five times **(Table 46.3).** Oral morphine is available as a liquid, tablet, and sustained release preparations (MS-contin). MS-contin cannot be crushed and given via a feeding tube.

Fentanyl(s)

Because of its rapid onset and brief duration of action, fentanyl has become a favored analgesic for short procedures, such as bone marrow aspirations, fracture reductions, suturing lacerations, endoscopy, and dental procedures. Fentanyl is approximately 100 times more potent than morphine (the equianalgesic dose is 0.001 mg/kg-1, **Table 46.3**) and is largely devoid of hypnotic or sedative activity. Sufentanil is a potent fentanyl derivative and is approximately 10 times more potent than fentanyl. It is most commonly used as the principal component of cardiac anesthesia and is administered in doses of 1 to 30 μg/kg. Alfentanil is approximately 5 to 10 times less potent than fentanyl and has an extremely short duration of action, usually less than 15 to 20 min.

Fentanyl's ability to block nociceptive stimuli with concomitant hemodynamic stability is excellent and makes it the drug of choice for trauma, cardiac, or intensive care unit patients. Furthermore, in addition to its ability to block the systemic and pulmonary hemodynamic responses to pain, fentanyl also prevents the biochemical and endocrine stress (catabolic) response to painful stimuli that may be so detrimental in the seriously ill patient. Fentanyl does have a serious side effect, namely, the development of chest wall rigidity following rapid infusions of 0.005 mg/kg-1 or greater. This may make ventilation difficult or impossible. Chest wall rigidity can be treated with either muscle relaxants, such as succinylcholine or pancuronium, or with naloxone.

Fentanyl, like morphine, is primarily glucuronidated into inactive forms that are excreted by the kidney. It is highly lipid soluble and is rapidly distributed to tissues that are well perfused, such as the brain and the heart. Normally, the effect of a single dose of fentanyl is terminated by rapid redistribution, rather than by elimination, in a manner very much akin to thiopental. However, following multiple or large doses of fentanyl (e.g., when it is used as a primary anesthetic agent or when used in high dose continuous infusions), prolongation of effect will occur, because elimination and not distribution will determine the duration of effect. This is particularly important in the newborn, where elimination may be further prolonged by abnormal or decreased liver blood flow following acute illness or abdominal surgery(130–134). Additionally, certain conditions that may raise intra-abdominal pressure may further decrease liver blood flow by shunting blood away from the liver via the still patent ductus venosus.

Fentanyl and its structurally related relatives, sufentanil and alfentanil, are highly lipophilic drugs that rapidly penetrate all membranes including the blood-brain barrier. Following an intravenous bolus, fentanyl is rapidly eliminated from plasma as the result of its extensive uptake by body tissues. The fentanyls are highly bound to α-1 acid glycoproteins in the plasma, which are reduced in the newborn. The fraction of free unbound sufentanil is significantly increased in neonates and in children less than a year of age (19.5 ± 2.7% and 11.5 ± 3.2%, respectively) compared with older children and adults (8.1 ± 1.4% and 7.8 ± 1.5%, respectively) and this correlates to levels of α-1 acid glycoproteins in the blood.

Fentanyl pharmacokinetics differ among newborn infants, children, and adults. The total body clearance of fentanyl is greater in infants 3 to 12 months of age than in children older than 1 yr of age or adults (18.1 ± 1.4, 11.5 ± 4.2, and 10.0 ± 1.7 ml/kg-1/min-1, respectively) and the half-life of elimination is longer (233 ± 137, 244 ± 79, and 129 ± 42 min, respectively)(133–136). The prolonged elimination half-life of fentanyl from plasma has important clinical implications. Repeated doses of fentanyl for maintenance of analgesic effects will lead to accumulation of fentanyl and its ventilatory depressant effects[131,132,134–137]. Very large doses (0.05 to 0.10 mg/kg-1, as used in anesthesia) may be expected to induce long-lasting effects because plasma fentanyl levels will not fall below the threshold level at which spontaneous ventilation occurs during the distribution phases. On the other hand, the greater clearance of fentanyl in infants greater than 3 months of age produces lower plasma concentrations of the drug and may allow these children to tolerate more drug without respiratory depression[131,132,134].

Suggested Dosage

When used to provide analgesia for short procedures, fentanyl is often administered intravenously in doses of 2 to 3 μg/kg. However, if any sedative (e.g., midazolam or chloral hydrate) is administered concomitantly, respiratory depression is potentiated and the dose of both drugs must be reduced (Fig. 46.3)[107]. Fentanyl can also be used in the intensive care unit or the operating room to provide virtually complete anesthesia in doses of 10 to 50 μg/kg[139,140]. The lower dose is often used to provide anesthesia for intubation, particularly in the newborn and in head trauma, cardiac, and hemodynamically unstable patients. Continuous infusions of fentanyl are often used to provide analgesia and sedation in intubated and mechanically ventilated patients, particularly those on ECMO. Following a loading dose of 10 μg/kg, an infusion is begun of 2 to 5 μg/kg/hr. Rapid tolerance develops and an increasing dose of fentanyl is required to provide satisfactory analgesia and sedation.

Sufentanil, which is five to ten times more potent than fentanyl, can be administered intranasally in doses of 1.5 to 3.0 μg/kg and produces effective analgesia and sedation within 10 min of administration[141]. Higher doses (4.5 μg/kg) produce untoward side effects including chest wall rigidity, convulsions, respiratory depression, and increased postoperative vomiting[141]. Another exciting alternative to intravenous or intramuscular injection is the fentanyl lollipop or "oral transmucosal fentanyl citrate" (Oralet®)[142–146]. In doses of 15 to 20 μg/kg, this is an effective, nontraumatic method of premedication that is self-administered and extremely well accepted by children. Side effects include facial pruritus (90%), slow onset time (25 to 45 min to peak effect), and an increase in gastric volume compared to unpremedicated patients (15.9 ± 10.8 ml compared with 9.0 ± 6.2 ml [mean + SD])[142–146].

Meperidine

Meperidine (Demerol) is a synthetic narcotic that is most commonly used in children as either a premedicant for anesthesia (or sedation) or as a treatment for postoperative pain. It is ten times less potent than morphine and has pharmacokinetic properties that are very similar. Meperidine is a narcotic agonist that binds to opioid receptors in the central nervous system and can produce analgesia, sedation, euphoria, dysphoria, miosis, and respiratory depression. At equianalgesic doses **(Table 46.3),** there is little quantitative difference between meperidine and morphine in producing these effects. It is unique among all of the opioids in that it prevents or stops shivering. Indeed, it is frequently used for this purpose in patients who shiver following amphotericin administration, blood product (particularly platelet) transfusions, general anesthesia, or who are hypothermic. Meperidine stimulates the chemoreceptor trigger zone in the brainstem to the same degree that morphine does and may, thereby, produce either nausea or vomiting or both. Meperidine differs from morphine in that large doses (toxic levels) may produce slow waves on the electroencephalogram. Additionally, high levels of meperidine's principal metabolite, normeperidine, may produce tremors, muscle twitches, hyperactive reflexes, and convulsions. Indeed, because of the accumulation of this metabolite, the prolonged use of meperidine should be discouraged, if not avoided completely.

At equipotent doses (1.0 mg/kg) **(Table 46.3),** meperidine's effects on respiration and on gastrointestinal motility are similar to the other opioid analgesics. Meperidine is a potent respiratory depressant and antitussive. Unlike morphine, meperidine depresses minute ventilation through a primary reduction in tidal volume rather than a reduction in respiratory rate. It depresses intestinal smooth muscle motility and exerts a spasmogenic effect on intestinal smooth muscle. Thus, gastric motility is decreased and the gastric emptying time of the stomach is increased. Some studies suggest that meperidine exerts less of an effect on the biliary tract, including the common bile duct, than morphine. Specifically, at equianalgesic doses, biliary tract pressure rises to a lesser extent following meperidine than morphine administration making it a preferred agent for biliary colic. This point is often disputed in the literature. Finally, meperidine, unlike the other opioids, depresses cardiac output by approximately 20% and produces a tachycardia when it is administered intravenously.

Pharmacokinetics

Meperidine, like morphine and fentanyl, is nearly completely metabolized in the liver with a plasma half-life of elimination of approximately 3 hr. Unlike morphine and fentanyl, the principal metabolic pathways involved in meperidine metabolism are hydrolysis and N-demethylation. The latter process produces normeperidine that is principally responsible for the sedative and convulsive effects of meperidine. Normeperidine is about one-half as active as meperidine as an analgesic, but twice as active a convulsant. The levels of normeperidine may be increased by ingestion of large doses or because of enzyme induction. Urinary excretion of the metabolites is responsible for final elimination of the drug, whereas approximately one-third of meperidine is demethylated into normeperidine, a metabolite that is half as active as meperidine as an analgesic but twice as active as a convulsant. Because of the propensity of normeperidine to produce seizures, we believe that meperidine should not be prescribed for chronic pain management.

Suggested Dosage

Meperidine is effective whether administered orally or parenterally. The drug is extremely well absorbed from the gastrointestinal tract, and has a bioavailability of approximately 50%, making it among the most popularly prescribed oral narcotics. It is available in both liquid (syrup) and tablet forms **(Table 46.3).** Typically, meperidine, 1 to 3 mg/kg, can exert analgesic effects within 15 to 30 min of oral administration and achieves peak plasma concentrations within 1 to 2 hr of ingestion. Intramuscular injection, 1 mg/kg, which we believe is an unacceptable route of routine drug administration, provides a more rapid onset of analgesia (approximately 10 min) and reaches a peak effect within 60 min of administration. Obviously, plasma concentrations may show marked variability following intramuscular injection based on an individual patient's state of peripheral perfusion.

Meperidine is commonly administered intramuscularly for moderate to severe pain or as part of a "lytic" (sedative) cocktail (meperidine, promethazine, and chlorpromazine) in a dose of 1 to 2 mg/kg-1 **(Table 46.7).** We do not recommend intramuscular administration of analgesics (or any drug) in children nor do we advocate the use of the lytic cocktail. In fact, we consider the lytic cocktail to be an archaic and frankly dangerous sedative combination. We mention this "Darwinian" approach to sedation only to condemn its continued use! Although an intramuscular injection will result in higher sustained plasma levels of meperidine and lengthen the patient's pain-free intervals, it is clear that children will often "suffer in silence" to avoid yet another pain, namely, the "shot." When administered intravenously (1 mg/kg-1) for pain control, meperidine offers few advantages over morphine and must be given cautiously and by titration at the bedside. A much smaller intravenous dose (0.25 to 0.5 mg/kg) effectively prevents or stops shivering. Based on meperidine's plasma half-life of elimination, the frequency of administration ranges between 3 and 4 hr.

Methadone

Primarily thought of as a drug to treat or wean opioid-addicted or -dependent patients, methadone is increasingly being used for postoperative pain relief and for the treatment of intractable pain[25,26,123–128]. It is noted for its slow elimination, very long duration of effective analgesia, and high oral bioavailability **(Table 46.3).** Methadone is metabolized extremely slowly and has a very prolonged duration of action, based in part on the fact that its principal metabolite is morphine. The $t1/2\beta$ of methadone averages 19 hr and clearance averages 5.4 ml/min-1/kg-1 in children 1 to 18 yr of age[128].

Methadone has the longest $t1/2\beta$ of any of the commonly available opiates and may provide 12 to 36 hr of analgesia following a single intravenous or oral dose[123–128]. Pharmacokinetically, children are indistinguishable from young adults. Because a single dose of methadone can achieve and sustain a high drug plasma level, it is a convenient way to provide prolonged analgesia without requiring an intramuscular injection (Fig. 46.7). Indeed, when administered either orally or intravenously, it may be viewed as an alternative to the use of continuous intravenous opioid infusions (a "poor man's" PCA). Berde recommend loading patients with an initial dose of intravenous methadone, 0.1 to 0.2 mg/kg-1, and then titrating in 0.05 mg/kg-1 increments every 10 to 15 min until analgesia is achieved[25,26]. Supplemental methadone can be administered in 0.05 to 0.1 mg/kg-1-increments administered by slow intravenous infusion every 4 to 12 hr as needed. Berde has also reported the use of small incremental doses administered by "sliding scale"[25,26]. "Small increments of methadone are administered intravenously over 20 min every 4 hr via a 'sliding' scale on a 'reverse prn' (the nurse asks the patient) basis: 0.07 to 0.08 mg/kg for severe pain; 0.05 to 0.06 mg/kg for moderate pain; 0.03 mg/kg for little or no pain, if the patient is alert; and no drug if the patient has little pain and is somnolent"[25,26].

The influence of pathophysiology on the pharmacokinetics and pharmacodynamics of methadone are unknown primarily because its use as an analgesic is a relatively recent phenomenon. Dosing decisions in the very young and in patients with various end-organ diseases must be made conservatively.

Additionally, we are using methadone and sustained-relief morphine (MS-contin) to wean patients who have become opioid dependent following prolonged analgesic therapy. When used to treat dependence and withdrawal symptoms, clonidine, an $\alpha 2$-agonist can be concomitantly administered in doses of 2 to 5 μg/kg to reduce withdrawal symptomatology significantly. Finally, because methadone is extremely well absorbed from the gastrointestinal tract and has a bioavailability of 80 to 90%, it is extremely easy to convert intravenous dosing regimens to oral ones.

Hydromorphone

Hydromorphone, a derivative of morphine, is an opioid with appreciable selectivity for μ opioid receptors[59,91]. It is noted for its rapid onset and 4- to 6-hr duration of action. It differs from its parent compound morphine in that it is six to seven times more potent and ten times more lipid soluble. Its half-life of elimination is 3 to 4 hr and, like morphine and meperidine, shows very wide intrasubject pharmacokinetic variability. Hydromorphone is far less sedating than morphine and is thought by many to be associated with fewer systemic side effects. Indeed, it is often used as an alternative to morphine when the latter produces too much sedation or nausea. Additionally, hydromorphone is receiving renewed attention as an alternative morphine for treatment of prolonged cancer-related pain because it can be prepared in more concentrated aqueous solutions than morphine.

Hydromorphone is effective when administered intravenously, subcutaneously, epidurally, and orally(59,91,152,153). The intravenous route of administration is the most commonly used technique in the intensive care unit. Following a loading dose of 0.005 to 0.015 mg/kg, a continuous infusion ranging between 0.003 to 0.005 mg/kg/hr is started. Supplemental boluses of 0.003 to 0.005 mg/kg are administered either by the nurse or by the patient as needed. When administered epidurally, one can use either continuous infusions, 0.001 to 0.003 mg/ kg/hr (the adult dose is 0.15 to 0.3 mg/hr), or continuous infusions with patient-controlled boluses, 0.001 to 0.003 mg/kg/bolus (the adult dose is 0.15 to 0.3 mg/bolus).

Patient-Controlled Analgesia

Because of the enormous individual variations in pain perception and opioid metabolism, fixed ("Harriet Lane") doses

Table 46.7. Commonly Used Sedatives

Drug	*Route of Administration*	*Dose (mg/kg)*	*Comments*
Diazepam (Valium)	p.o.	0.2–0.5	Sedation, anxiolysis, and amnesia
	i.v.	0.05–0.2	No analgesic properties
	i.m.	NR	Painful on injection, poorly absorbed following i.m. injection
Midazolam (Versed)	p.o.	0.5	See diazepam
	i.v.	0.05–0.1	3–4 times more potent than diazepam
	i.m.	0.05–0.15	Painless on injection, well absorbed following i.m. injection or p.o. or p.r.
	p.r.	0.3–1.0	i.v. preparation can be given p.o., very bitter; disguise with concentrated grape-flavored Kool-aid
Pentobarbital (Nembutal)	p.o.	2–4	Hypnotic
	i.m.	2–4	No analgesic properties
	p.r.	2–4	Maximum dose 150 mg
Droperidol (Inapsine)	i.m.	0.01–0.075	Sedation, occasionally dysphoria
	i.v.		Antiemetic
			α and dopaminergic blocker
Promethazine (Phenergan)	i.m.	0.5–1.0	Sedation
			Antiemetic
Chloral hydrate	p.o.	25–100	Hypnotic, no analgesic properties
	p.r.		Maximum dose 2.0 g
			Minimal respiratory depression
Hydroxyzine (Vistaril)	i.m.	0.5–1.0	Sedation
			Antiemetic
Meperidine (Demerol)	p.o.	1–2	This drug combination, developed at The Children's Hospital of Philadelphia is effective p.o. or i.m.
+			
	i.m.		
Diazepam (Valium)		0.2	Must be given at least 30 min before the procedure
+			
Atropine		0.02	
Midazolam (Versed)	i.v.	0.05–0.1	Primarily used to minimize procedure-related pain, this combination can rapidly produce apnea and hypoxemia
+			
Fentanyl		0.001–0.002	Titrate midazolam 0.05 mg/kg very slowly, the peak effect occurs 4–5 min after administration
Meperidine (Demerol)	i.m.	2	The classic "Lytic cocktail" is associated with respiratory depression, hypotension, and hypothermia
+			
Promethazine (Phenergan)		1	Dose should be reduced by 2/3 in cyanotic heart disease
+			
Chlorpromazine (Thorazine)		1	No longer recommended, mentioned only for historical importance
+			
Ketamine	i.v.	0.025–2.0	Very potent analgesic, amnestic; "dissociative anesthetic," hearalded by nystagmus; hallucinogen
	i.m.	3–10	
	p.o.	6–8	Useful in rapid sequence intubations to induce unconsciousness, particularly asthma
			Releases endogenous catecholamines, effective in asthma and ? hypotension
			OK in congenital heart disease, including right-to-left shunt, e.g., tetrology of Fallot
			Potent sialogogue, always give with atropine
			Nightmares (5–10% of patients) can be prevented or treated with benzodiazepines
			Contraindicated with elevated intracranial pressure or with preexisting psychosis
			Protective airway reflexes are blunted

and time intervals make little sense (Fig. 46.7). Based on the pharmacokinetics of the opioids, it should be clear that intravenous boluses of morphine or meperidine may need to be given at intervals of 1 to 2 hr to avoid marked fluctuations in plasma drug levels[23,25–27,153]. Continuous intravenous infusions can provide steady analgesic levels and are preferable to intramuscular injections; they are not a panacea, however, because the perception and intensity of pain is not constant. Indeed, the most common method of opioid administration in adults and children is intramuscular injection. It is well known that children will suffer in silence and underreport their level of pain rather than ask for yet another painful stimulus, namely, the shot[1,8,11,24–27,29,36]. Thus, rational pain management requires some form of titration to effect whenever an opioid is administered. To give patients some measure of control over their pain therapy, demand analgesia or patient-controlled analgesia (PCA) devices have been developed[154–164]. These are microprocessor driven pumps with a button that the patient presses to self-administer a small dose of opioid. This treatment modality may be particularly suitable for adolescent patients, or patients in acute pain such as patients with cancer or sickle cell anemia who present in vaso-occlusive crisis[154,160]. We use this modality extensively in postoperative patients as well.

Demand-analgesia devices allow patients to administer small amounts of an analgesic whenever they feel a need for more pain relief. The opioid, usually morphine, is administered either intravenously or subcutaneously. The dosage of opioid, number of boluses per hour, and the time interval between boluses (the "lock-out period") are programmed into the equipment by the pain service physician to allow maximum patient flexibility and sense of control with minimal risk of overdosage[122,154–164]. Generally, because patients know that if they have severe pain they can obtain relief immediately, many prefer dosing regimens that result in mild to moderate pain in exchange for fewer side effects such as nausea or pruritus. Typically, we initially prescribe morphine, 20 μg/kg/bolus, at a rate of 6 boluses/hr, with an 8- to 10-min lock-out interval between each bolus. Variations include larger boluses (30 to 50 μg/kg), shorter time intervals (5 min), etc. The PCA pump computer stores within its memory how many boluses the patient has received as well as how many attempts the patient has made at receiving boluses. This allows the physician to evaluate how well the patient understands the use of the pump and provides information to program the pump more efficiently. Many PCA units allow low "background" continuous infusions (morphine, 20 to 30 μg/kg/ hr) in addition to self-administered boluses. This is sometimes called "PCA-Plus." A continuous background infusion is particularly useful at night and often provides more restful sleep by preventing the patient from awakening in pain. It also increases the potential for overdosage.

PCA requires a patient with enough intelligence and manual dexterity and strength to operate the pump. Thus, it was initially limited to adolescents and teenagers, but the lower age limit in whom this treatment modality can be used continues to fall. In fact, it has been our experience that any child able to play Nintendo can operate a PCA pump. Extensive studies in adult and adolescent patients reveal that patients are extremely satisfied with this mode of therapy. Difficulties with PCA include its increased costs, patient age limitations, and the bureaucratic (physician, nursing, and pharmacy) obstacles (protocols, education, storage arrangements) that must be overcome prior to its implementation. Contraindications include inability to push the bolus button (weakness, arm restraints), inability to understand how to use the machine, and a patient's desire not to assume responsibility for his or her own care. Whether nurses can or should be allowed to initiate a bolus is controversial. It is our practice to empower intensive care unit nurses with the ability to initiate a "clinician" bolus, particularly since they already have this ability when more conventional opiate administration is in use. However, when we do this, we limit the number of allowable boluses to 1 to 2/hr.

Intrathecal/Epidural Opioid Analgesia

The presence of high concentrations of opioid receptors in the spinal cord makes it possible to achieve analgesia, in both acute and chronic pain, with small doses of opioids administered in either the subarachnoid or epidural spaces (Fig. 46.6)[56,57,63,64,92,94,165,166]. By bypassing the blood and the blood-brain barrier, small doses of agonist are effective because they can reach the receptor by the "backdoor" approach. Indeed, CSF opioid levels, particularly for morphine, are several thousand times greater than those achieved by the parenteral route (see below)[110,138]. It is these high levels that produce the profound and prolonged analgesia that accompanies intrathecal/epidural opioid administration.

Yaksh and others demonstrated, in unanesthetized rats, that intrathecal narcotics produced profound segmental analgesia that is dose dependent and reversible with naloxone[61–64,92,94,165,166]. However, after 1 hr, rostral spread was evident, especially at higher doses. The passage of epidurally administered agonists across the dura into the CSF is dependent on the lipid solubility of the drug. Additionally, once in the CSF, opioids must pass from the water phase of the CSF into the lipid phase of the underlying neuraxis to reach the receptor. This too is dependent on lipid solubility. Hydrophilic agents such as morphine will have a greater latency and duration of action than more lipid-soluble agents, such as fentanyl[109,110]. On the other hand, the lipid-soluble agonists produce more segmental analgesia with less rostral spread than the less lipid-soluble agonists.

Even when administered via the caudal route, epidural morphine has been shown to provide effective postoperative analgesia following abdominal, thoracic, and cardiac surgery[167–171]. Krane et al.[168] recently reported that 0.03 mg/kg of caudal-epidural morphine is equally effective as

0.1 mg/kg in providing post operative analgesia, although the higher dose provides a significantly longer duration of analgesia (13.3 ± 4.7 compared with 10.0 ± 3.3 hr, respectively)[170]. The incidence of side effects was the same in both groups, although one patient receiving 0.1 mg/kg developed late respiratory depression. Therefore, these investigators suggest starting with the lower dose when using this technique. Whether even lower doses would be effective is unknown.

Spinal opiates produce analgesia without altering autonomic or neuromuscular function. Additionally, both light touch and proprioception are preserved. Thus, unlike local anesthetics, spinal opioids allow patients to ambulate without orthostatic hypotension. Common side effects of intrathecal/epidural narcotics include facial or segmental pruritus, urinary retention, nausea and vomiting, and respiratory depression[111,172–177]. These side effects occur with greater frequency when opioids are administered intrathecally as opposed to epidurally. Except for urinary retention, reversal of adverse side effects, with maintenance of adequate analgesia, can be achieved through the use of a low-dose (0.001 to 0.002 mg/kg-1) naloxone infusion. Pruritus and nausea can also be treated with intravenous or oral diphenhydramine (Benadryl), 0.5 to 1.0 mg/kg or hydroxyzine (Vistaril, Atarax). Urinary retention is common following spinally administered opiates. Indeed, the lower one's threshold, 4, 6, 8, or more hours without voiding, the more common it is. Bladder catheterization relieves this problem.

Although rare, respiratory depression is a major risk when utilizing intrathecal/epidural opioids[111,172–177]. Attia et al.[172] demonstrated that the ventilatory response to CO_2 is depressed for as long as 22 hr following the administration of 0.05 mg/kg-1 of morphine epidurally[174]. Following intrathecal morphine administration (0.02 mg/kg), Nichols et al.[138] demonstrated significant depression of the ventilatory response to carbon dioxide for up to 18 hr in children varying between 3 months and 15 yr[138]. The greatest respiratory depression correlated with the highest CSF morphine levels (2863 ± 542 ng/ml), which occurred 6 hr after administration. This depression persisted despite a fall in CSF morphine levels 12 (641 ± 219 ng/ml) to 18 (223 ± 152 ng/ml) hr later. This confirms the clinical impression that respiratory depression usually occurs within the first 6 hr after the administration of epidural or intrathecal morphine but may occur as long as 18 hr afterward.

In clinical practice, respiratory depression most commonly occurs when intravenous or intramuscular narcotics have been administered to supplement the intrathecal opioid. The risk of respiratory depression can be minimized if smaller doses of supplemental narcotics are used, or through the epidural use of shorter-acting, more lipid-soluble agents (fentanyl, sufentanil), which produce more segmental analgesia, with little rostral spread. On the other hand, because of its shorter duration of action, fentanyl and sufentanil are increasingly being administered by continuous epidural infusion, either alone or in combination with very dilute (1/16%, [0.0625 mg/ml] or 0.1% [1.0 mg/ml]) bupivacaine concentrations. Typically, the epidural solution contains 1 to 2 μg/ml of fentanyl, with or without bupivacaine, and is administered at rates ranging between 0.2 and 1.0 ml/kg/hr. This provides effective analgesia for both postoperative and chronic cancer pain. Sufentanil (0.1 to 0.2 μg/kg), the only drug approved for epidural use by the FDA, has been shown to provide effective analgesia in children ranging between 4 and 12 yr for about 2 hr.

Regardless of the opioid prescribed and its route of administration, a regular system of monitoring for respiratory depression is mandatory for safe use[172,177]. Clinical signs that predict impending respiratory depression include somnolence, small pupils, and small tidal volumes. In addition, we insist on the use of oxyhemoglobin saturation monitoring ("pulse oximetry") when instituting this therapy.

Opioid Antagonists

Naloxone

A discussion of opioid analgesics would be incomplete without mentioning the opioid antagonists. Naloxone is a pure opioid antagonist with virtually no agonist activity. It antagonizes the effects of pure agonist drugs, such as morphine, as well as the effects of mixed agonist-antagonist drugs such as butorphanol. In fact, it is the most commonly used opioid antagonist in clinical practice today.

Naloxone is extremely potent and nonselective in its opioid reversal effects **(Table 46.4).** It not only antagonizes the sedation, respiratory depression, and GI effects of the opioid agonists, but it reverses the analgesia as well. Indeed, the antagonism of narcotic agonist effects must be accomplished with great caution, particularly in patients who have been receiving prolonged opioid therapy, who exhibit opioid dependence, or who are in extreme pain, because it may be accompanied by overt withdrawal symptoms. Occasionally, a life-threatening "overshoot" phenomenon may occur in these patients, with the development of tachypnea, tachycardia, hypertension, nausea and vomiting, and sudden death. Obviously, the magnitude of the withdrawal syndrome depends on the dose of naloxone administered, as well as on the degree of the patient's physical dependence. It is our routine practice to employ mechanical ventilation as a safer alternative to using naloxone for treating narcotic-induced respiratory depression in dependent patients or in patients with severe pain. Occasionally, as an alternative, we use very low doses of naloxone in an attempt to antagonize only the undesired side effects of the opioids, such as respiratory depression, pruritus, or nausea, while leaving the analgesia intact. This is done by administering 0.001 mg/kg of naloxone as an intravenous bolus and then starting an infusion of 0.001 mg/kg/hr. When naloxone is administered to patients who have not received opioids, it produces minimal to no effects (except in patients in shock) and has no inherent properties that induce physical dependence or tolerance.

Naloxone is rapidly metabolized (by conjugation with

glucuronic acid) in the liver and is best given parenterally because of its rapid first-pass extraction through the liver following oral administration. Following intravenous administration, it reverses the effects of opioids virtually instantaneously. Unfortunately, it has a plasma elimination half-life of only 60 min and a duration of action that is much shorter than the agonists that it is used to reverse. Therefore, when naloxone is used to reverse narcotic-induced respiratory depression, patients must be monitored for the return of the depression, based on the half-life of the opiate agonist. This may require repeat intravenous doses, intramuscular (depot) injection, or a continuous intravenous infusion.

Naloxone is supplied as a parenteral solution (0.4 mg/ml or 0.02 mg/ml). The standard initial dose for children and adults is 0.01 mg/kg given intravenously. If this dose does not result in the desired degree of clinical improvement, subsequent doses of 0.02, 0.04, 0.08, and 0.1 mg/kg may be administered in a stepwise manner. However, one must remember that this dose of naloxone will also antagonize the analgesic effects of most opioids. When used to reverse neonatal respiratory depression (caused by narcotics administered to the mother during labor), the usual initial resuscitation dose is the same as used for older children (0.01 mg/kg of the 0.02-mg/ml solution). If an intravenous route is not available, naloxone may be administered intramuscularly or subcutaneously.

KETAMINE

Ketamine is a phencyclidine derivative that was introduced with great fanfare as a "foolproof" method of providing anesthesia and analgesia to adults and children in the early 1970s[178,179]. Indeed, initially, it was hoped that ketamine would become the "Swiss army knife" of analgesia and anesthesia and that it could be administered by nonanesthesiologists[179]. Unfortunately, this, like many other claims about new drugs turned out to be more hype and advertising than true.

Ketamine is an outstanding sedative, amnestic, and analgesic that is particularly useful in the treatment of procedure-related pain (e.g., catheterization, tracheal intubation, chest tube insertion, lumbar puncture, fracture reduction, and others) and as an agent to induce anesthesia in patients with congenital heart disease, particularly those with right-to-left shunts[180,181]. It is also an outstanding anesthetic agent in critically ill patients because it produces its effects with minimal perturbations of the cardiovascular or respiratory systems. Unfortunately, it has not gained widespread clinical acceptance, despite its many useful properties, because of the many adverse side effects associated with its use.

When administered intravenously, 2 mg/kg, ketamine rapidly (30 sec) produces a state of hypnosis and amnesia that lasts only 10 to 15 min. The resulting anesthetic state is distinctly unusual in that patients appear "awake," even though they are unconscious[179]. Loss of consciousness is heralded by the appearance of vertical or horizontal nystagmus. Patients become cataleptic with their eyes open in a fixed gaze and with their corneal and papillary reactions intact. Furthermore, depending on dose and route of administration, patients may continue to verbalize and respond to external stimuli. However, they often cannot connect or "associate" the stimulus actually being applied to their internal perceptions of what is happening. For example, a patient who has received ketamine for a kidney biopsy may complain during the insertion of the biopsy needle that his leg hurts or that he is hungry. Indeed, because of this, the anesthesia produced by ketamine is often called "dissociative anesthesia." The mechanism by which ketamine anesthesia occurs is unknown, although recent investigations suggest that the mechanism of action is antagonism of N-methyl-D-aspartate (NMDA)[182].

Ketamine anesthesia has an hallucinatory quality; in fact, patients often describe vivid dreams, auditory and visual illusions, and extracorporeal experiences (a sense of floating outside one's body). These hallucinations may persist for hours or may recur ("flashback"), particularly on the nights ("nightmares" or night terrors) following ketamine administration. Nightmares are much more common in adults than in children. They have been reported in as many as 10% of adult patients, but in less than 5% of children. Indeed, nightmares and flashbacks are one of the most important reasons that ketamine's clinical use has been limited. Fortunately, the incidence of night terrors can be reduced, or eliminated, by the concomitant administration of virtually any benzodiazepine[183].

Ketamine is contraindicated in patients with increased intracranial pressure because it significantly increases cerebral blood flow and blood volume[178,184]. Most anesthetic agents, such as the barbiturates (see below), produce unconsciousness and thereby decrease the cerebral metabolic rate[185,186]. This has the effect of reducing cerebral oxygen consumption, cerebral blood flow, and cerebral blood volume. This decrease in cerebral blood flow and volume decreases intracranial pressure, particularly in injured brains in which intracranial compliance is reduced. Ketamine, on the other hand, is an excitatory hallucinogen that produces a coupled increase in both cerebral metabolism and blood flow. This has the effect of increasing intracranial pressure[179,184]. Obviously, this may be catastrophic in patients with poor intracranial compliance. Additionally, ketamine depresses ventilation and may thereby cause an increase in arterial carbon dioxide concentrations[187,188]. This will further exacerbate ketamine's effects on intracranial pressure because hypercarbia is one of the most potent stimuli to raise cerebral blood flow and intracranial pressure.

Regardless of its route of administration, ketamine significantly increases mean arterial blood pressure, heart rate, and cardiac output and is, therefore, commonly used in patients who are in shock or who are cardiovascularly unstable[179]. At first glance this is surprising, because ketamine is a negative inotrope. However, its negative inotropy is more than counterbalanced by the fact that ketamine administration is associated with dramatic increases in sympathetic outflow and plasma catecholamine levels. Indeed, it is the increase in plasma catecholamines that accompany its administration that accounts for ketamine's ability to raise blood pressure and cardiac output. This also means that if a patient is catecholamine depleted or blocked, ketamine administration may result in profound hypotension and even death.

Ketamine's effects on pulmonary vascular resistance are controversial[191]. Morray et al.[181] demonstrated a significant rise in pulmonary vascular resistance following ketamine administration in spontaneously breathing children undergoing cardiac catheterization. On the other hand, Hickey et al.[191] found no change in pulmonary vascular resistance following intravenous ketamine (2 mg/kg) administration in 14 children who had undergone cardiac surgery[191]. These later investigators concluded that cardiovascular hemodynamics, especially the pulmonary vascular resistance index (PVRI), are minimally affected by ketamine in mildly sedated infants with congenital heart disease. This was true regardless of baseline PVRI, as long as the airway was patent and ventilation was normal. Furthermore, these investigators believed that partial airway obstruction, hypoventilation, or possible catecholamine depletion was responsible for the rise in PVR that was previously reported with ketamine use. This is further supported by the work of Greeley et al.[192], who demonstrated reversal of a right-to-left shunt during a tetralogy of Fallot "spell," following ketamine administration.

Ketamine is a ventilatory depressant[193–195]. It reduces the ventilatory response to carbon dioxide administration, even though resting respiratory rate, tidal volume, end-tidal carbon dioxide concentration, and minute ventilation are unchanged. In fact, a continuous ketamine infusion of 40 μg/kg/min has been shown to shift the carbon dioxide response curve to the right, without altering its slope. This perturbation of ventilatory control is most marked in former preterm neonates[194]. Welborn et al.[195], studying spinal anesthesia in premature neonates who were less than 51 weeks postconceptual age, found that a sedating dose of 1 to 2 mg/kg ketamine given intramuscularly led to prolonged apnea and bradycardia in eight of nine infants studied (89%). None of the eleven infants receiving spinal anesthesia without sedation experienced similar problems[195].

Laryngeal reflexes remain relatively intact during ketamine anesthesia, but airway protection should not be presumed unless the airway is secured with an endotracheal tube. Indeed, there are many reports in the literature of patients who aspirated following ketamine administration. This should not be at all surprising. Any anesthetic agent that induces unconsciousness should be presumed to result in pulmonary aspiration of stomach contents when consciousness is lost. Patients should have no solids by mouth for at least 8 hr prior to ketamine administration and, if this is not possible, "full stomach" precautions (i.e., cricoid pressure, rapid-acting paralytics, tracheal intubation) should always be taken.

Ketamine is a potent bronchial smooth muscle relaxant, making it the ideal anesthetic and analgesic agent in patients with asthma. It increases pulmonary compliance both by direct action on the bronchial smooth muscles and by its ability to increase plasma catecholamine levels. In the rare occasion that asthmatics require intubation, ketamine is the best agent to use to induce anesthesia and to maintain sedation while the patient is being ventilated. Additionally, low doses may be used when invasive, painful procedures, such as arterial catheterization, must be performed in asthmatics in whom reason and distraction techniques fail.

Finally, ketamine increases salivary and bronchial mucous gland secretions, possibly through central cholinergic receptor stimulation. We have seen patients literally drown in their secretions and obstruct their airways following ketamine administration. We, therefore, recommend that whenever ketamine is given, a potent antisialogogue, such as atropine, 0.02 mg/kg, or glycopyrrolate, 0.01 mg/kg, be given concomitantly.

Pharmacokinetics

Ketamine is highly lipid soluble and, following a single intravenous bolus, swiftly crosses the blood brain to produce a loss of consciousness rapidly. Its uptake, distribution, and elimination from the body are remarkably similar to thiopental[198–200]. Redistribution, rather than biotransformation and elimination is responsible for ketamine's short duration of action. Its $t1/2\alpha$ is only 11 to 16 min and its half-life of elimination is 2.5 to 3.0 hr **(Table 46.8)** [196–198]. Indeed, its 2- to 3-hr half-life of elimination may explain why protracted emergence from ketamine anesthesia may occur.

Ketamine is N-demethylated by the liver's microsomal enzyme system to norketamine. This is followed by hydroxylation and conjugation to a glucuronide, which is a nonactive water-soluble metabolite. Clearance is high at 20 ml/min/kg, and closely approximates total liver blood flow, giving ketamine a short elimination half-life of approximately 2 to 3 hr **(Table 46.8).** Reduction in liver blood flow by drugs such as cimetidine, or by immaturity or intra-abdominal pathology, may significantly prolong ketamine's terminal half-life of elimination ($t1/2\beta$) and, therefore, its effects.

Dosage and Route of Administration

Ketamine is effective whether administered intravenously or intramuscularly. Enteral routes, either oral, rectal, or

Table 46.8. Ketamine Pharmacokinetics[a]

Age	$T_{1/2}\beta$ *(min)*	*VDSS (l/kg)*	*Cl (ml/min/kg)*
<3 months	184.7	3.46	12.9
4–12 months	65.1	3.03	35.0
4 years	31.6	1.18	25.1
Adult	107.3	0.75	20.0

[a] *From Lake CH. Pediatric cardiac anesthesia. New York: Appleton & Lange, 1988.*

transmucosal are increasingly being used[199,200]. When administered in small doses (0.25 to 0.5 mg/kg intravenously, 2 to 3 mg/kg intramuscularly, or 4 to 8 mg/kg enterally), ketamine provides very adequate sedation and analgesia for short painful procedures such as dressing changes in burn patients, fracture reductions, central line placement, and others[201,202]. This dose does not completely ablate unconsciousness and can be considered a "stun" dose. When administered intravenously in higher doses, 2 to 4 mg/kg, it will induce general anesthesia and a complete loss of consciousness within 60 sec of administration. Thus, ketamine is particularly useful when intubating asthmatics, children with congenital heart disease, and following trauma[203]. Obviously, the dosage of ketamine should be reduced in the presence of hypovolemia or catecholamine exhaustion.

Regardless of how it is administered, or for what purpose, we strongly recommend that a benzodiazepine (midazolam, 0.05 mg/kg intravenously, 0.1 mg/kg intra muscularly) and an antisialagogue (atropine, 0.02 mg/kg intravenously or intramuscularly) be administered concomitantly. This is necessary to reduce the incidence of emergence delirium, nightmares, and increased salivation that are associated with ketamine use.

Ketamine may also be administered by continuous infusion in subanesthetic doses to provide continuous analgesia and sedation[204,205]. Recently, five children were given ketamine via a bolus dose of 0.5 to 1.0 mg/kg followed by a continuous infusion of 10 to 15 μg/kg/min for up to 4 days[205]. This provided very effective sedation and analgesia and suggests its possible use in asthmatics and children with complex congenital heart disease. The common adverse effects of hypersalivation and emergence delirium and night terrors can be prevented by the concomitant use of antisialogogues and benzodiazepines.

LOCAL ANESTHETICS

The use of local anesthetics in pediatric practice has undergone a revolution[25,170,171,206–211]. For decades, children were considered poor candidates for regional anesthetic techniques because of their overwhelming fear of needles. However, once it was recognized that regional anesthesia could be used as an alternative to systemic opioids and as an adjunct, and not a replacement for general anesthesia, its use has increased exponentially. In the intensive care unit, local anesthetics are increasingly being used to provide continuous postoperative and posttraumatic pain relief utilizing indwelling catheters placed in either the epidural, pleural, or other spaces. To be used safely, a working knowledge of the differences in how local anesthetics are metabolized in infants and children is necessary.

Pharmacology and Pharmacokinetics of Local Anesthetics

The local anesthetics are tertiary amines and are of two types: either "esters" (e.g., tetracaine [Pontocaine], procaine [Novocain], chloroprocaine [Nesacaine], cocaine) or "amides" (lidocaine [Xylocaine], prilocaine, bupivacaine [Marcaine, Sensorcaine]) **(Table 46.9)** [212–218]. Both the ester and amide local anesthetics are weak bases that block nerve conduction primarily at the sodium channel when they are in their ionized (cation) form. To reach the sodium channel, the local anesthetic must cross the nerve membrane and it is only the nonionized (base) form of the drug that can do this. How much drug is available to cross the nerve membrane depends on the pKa of the drug and the pH of the fluid surrounding the nerve. The lower the pKa of the drug, the more nonionized drug is available to cross the nerve membrane at physiologic pH. For example, 28% of lidocaine exists in the base form at pH 7.4 compared with only 2.5% for chloroprocaine because the pKa of these drugs are 7.9 and 9.0, respectively[214–216,219]. Acidosis and hypercapnia, by significantly affecting tissue drug levels, also increase the toxicity of local anesthetics.

The minimum concentration of local anesthetic necessary to block impulse conduction along a given nerve fiber is called the Cm[214–219]. A variety of factors affect Cm, including: fiber size and degree of myelination of the nerve to be blocked, pH, local calcium concentration, and the rate at which a nerve is stimulated[206–219]. Relatively unmyelinated fibers, such as the A-δ and C fibers carry nociceptive information and have a lower Cm than heavily myelinated fibers that control muscle contraction. Because of the lower Cm, less local anesthetic is necessary to block the transmission of pain than is necessary to produce

Table 46.9. Local Anesthetics

	Maximum Dose of Local Anesthetic (mg/kg)[a]		
Drug (Concentration)	*Caudal/Lumbar Epidural*	*Peripheral Nerve*	*Duration of Action*
Lidocaine (Xylocaine) (0.5–2.0%)	5–7[b]	5–7[b]	Intermediate
Bupivacaine (Marcaine) (0.25–0.50%)	2–3[b]	2–3[b]	Long
Tetracaine (Pontocaine) (0.1–0.2%)	2	2	Long
Procaine (Novocain) (0.5–10%)	10–15[b]	10–15[b]	Short
Cocaine (4–10%)	NR[c]	1–2[d]	Intermediate
Prilocaine (Citanest) (1–2%)	NR[c]	5–7[b,e]	Intermediate

[a] *These are suggested safe upper limits for local anesthetic administration. Accidental intravenous or intra-arterial injection of even a fraction of these amounts may result in systemic toxicity.*
[b] *The higher dose is recommended only with the concomitant use of epinephrine 1#200,000.*
[c] *NR = not recommended.*
[d] *For topical use only, maximum adult dose is 200 mg.*
[e] *Maximum dose 600 mg, is not recommended in children less than 6 months of age.*

muscle paralysis. Thus, one can block pain sensation and not motor function by using dilute concentrations of local anesthetics. In fact, concentrated local anesthetic solutions (e.g., 2% lidocaine versus 1.0%) increase the quality of sensory blockade only minimally. On the other hand, a concentrated local anesthetic will increase the incidence of motor blockade and systemic toxicity! Concentrated solutions of local anesthetics can be diluted with preservative-free normal saline. Furthermore, since the process of myelinization of the central nervous system is not completed until approximately 18 months following birth, Cm may be reduced in younger children[(17,20,220,221)]. Thus, newborns and infants may develop complete analgesia and even motor blockade when even dilute concentrations of local anesthetics are used.

Other factors also influence the quality and duration of a nerve block, such as the addition of a vasoconstrictor to the anesthetic mixture, the use of mixtures of local anesthetics, and the site of drug administration. Vasoconstrictors, particularly epinephrine, are frequently added to local anesthetic solutions[(222–226)]. Epinephrine decreases the rate of vascular reabsorption of local anesthetic from the site of administration and thereby lengthens the duration of sensory blockade and decreases peak plasma local anesthetic concentrations. By causing local vasoconstriction, epinephrine also reduces bleeding at sites of injury. Interestingly, epinephrine also improves the intensity of anesthesia achieved and increases the effectiveness of dilute concentration of local anesthetics. Epinephrine-containing solutions should never be injected into areas supplied by end arteries, such as the penis or digits. Injection of epinephrine-containing solutions into these areas may lead to tissue ischemia or necrosis. Epinephrine is usually added to local anesthetic solutions in concentrations of 5 μg/ml (1:200,000). Higher concentrations offer no advantage in further reducing peak plasma local anesthetic concentrations and may, in fact, produce adverse systemic hemodynamic effects.

The onset and duration of a local anesthetic is also affected by using mixtures of different local anesthetics as well as by the site of injection. Mixtures of local anesthetics allow the practitioner to combine drugs with rapid onset but short duration of action, like chloroprocaine or lidocaine, with drugs with longer latencies and duration of action, such as bupivacaine or tetracaine.

The site of an injection also alters the duration of a nerve block based on the nerve's anatomy, differences in the rate of drug absorption, and in the amount of drug deposited. Bupivacaine, for example, has a 4-hr duration when injected epidurally, but a 10-hr duration when injected into the brachial plexus.

Toxicity

The systemic effects of local anesthetics are determined by the total dose of drug administered and by the rapidity of absorption into the blood. This belies the idea of accepted "maximum" doses of these drugs, since even small fractions of the accepted maximum dosages of local anesthetics will produce toxic systemic effects if the local anesthetic is injected intra-arterially, intravenously, or into any highly vascular location. In general, peak absorption of local anesthetic is dependent on the site of the block. The order of absorption from highest to lowest is[(216,217,219,226–239)]:

intercostal, intratracheal > caudal/epidural > brachial plexus > distal peripheral > subcutaneous.

Peak local anesthetic blood levels are directly related to the total dosage of drug administered, regardless of the injection site or the volume of solution used. Thus, the most dilute concentration of a local anesthetic should be used.

At recommended clinical dosages **(Table 46.9),** local anesthetic plasma levels usually remain well below recognized toxic concentrations[(217,238,240,241)]. A continuum of toxic effects exists and is dependent on the rapidity of rise and the total plasma concentration achieved following drug administration. Mild side effects (tinnitus, lightheadedness, visual and auditory disturbances, restlessness, muscular twitching) occur at low plasma concentrations and severe side effects (seizures, arrhythmias, coma, cardiovascular collapse, respiratory arrest) occur as plasma levels increase. Interestingly, cardiovascular and central nervous system toxicity have rarely been observed in children following local anesthetic administration[(170,171,206,242)]. Indeed, the hemodynamic response to regional anesthesia, even after fairly extensive epidural blockade (cutaneous analgesia below T4-T5), is minimal in children compared with adults[(243)]. Furthermore, convulsions have rarely been reported in children even though there are no significant differences in the sensitivity to the toxic effects of local anesthetics between newborn and adult animals[(244–246)]. This may be due to the concomitant use of sedatives, particularly the benzodiazepines, when performing nerve blocks in children[(247)]. The benzodiazepines raise the seizure threshold and may mask or prevent the development of convulsions.

All local anesthetic agents, except for cocaine, are potent peripheral vasodilators. At toxic concentrations, local anesthetics also directly depress the myocardium and its conduction system. These combined effects rapidly produce cardiovascular collapse and cardiac arrest. The treatment of toxic responses to local anesthetics is the same as for any emergency, namely, maintaining a patent Airway, ensuring adequate Breathing, and supporting Circulation; in other words, the ABCs[(240,248,249)]. Patients who are seizing for even brief periods of time become acidotic and have ineffective ventilation[(238,239,246–249)]. Thus, emergency airway and resuscitative equipment must be available for immediate use prior to the administration of any local anesthetic agent[(246,247,250)]. Although true for all local anesthetic agents, bupivacaine-induced cardiovascular depression has been particularly difficult to treat and it is considered more cardiac toxic than other local anesthetics[(251–255)]. Bupivacaine toxicity has been frequently reported following intravenous regional anesthetic techniques (Bier blocks) and during anesthesia for labor and delivery, particularly when 0.75% (7.5 mg/ml) concentrations of bupivacaine were utilized. The ventricular arrhythmias that precede the cardiovascular collapse seen following bupivacaine toxicity are more responsive to treatment with intravenous bretylium than with lidocaine[(254)]. Additionally, we have successfully treated two cases of bupivacaine-induced cardiac arrhythmias with intravenous phenytoin (Dilantin). Drug allergy is very uncommon with amide local anesthetics but does occur with the ester family of drugs[(214–217)]. Usually, a previous history of allergies to local anesthetics or to suntan lotions that contain PABA can be obtained. In our experience, local anesthetic allergy is rare and is often mistakenly attributed to adverse experiences occurring during dental anesthesia. In the dentist's office, many patients experience tachycardia and a sense of flushing and dizziness following nerve root infiltration with procaine and epinephrine. This is usually caused by direct intravascular injection of epinephrine and does not mean that the patient is allergic to local anesthetics.

Pharmacokinetics

The ester local anesthetics are metabolized by plasma cholinesterase. Neonates and infants up to 6 months of age have less than half of the adult levels of this plasma enzyme[(256)]. Clearance may, thereby, be reduced and the effects of ester local anesthetics prolonged. Amides, on the other hand, are metabolized in the liver and bound by plasma proteins. Neonates and young infants (less than 3 months of age) have reduced liver blood flow and immature metabolic degradation pathways[(257,258)]. Thus, larger fractions of local anesthetics are unmetabolized and remain active in the plasma than in the adult. More local anesthetic is excreted in the urine unchanged. Furthermore, neonates and infants may be at increased risk for the toxic effects of amide local anesthetics because of lower levels of albumin and $\alpha 1$-acid glycoproteins, which are proteins essential for drug binding[(259–264)]. This leads to increased concentrations of free drug and potential toxicity, particularly with bupivacaine. On the other hand, the larger volume of distribution at steady-state seen in the neonate for these (and other) drugs may confer some clinical protection by lowering plasma drug levels. The metabolism of the amide local anesthetic prilocaine is unique in that it results in the production of oxidants that can lead to the development of methemoglobinemia. This occurs in adults with doses of prilocaine greater than 600 mg. Because premature and full-term infants have decreased levels of methemoglobin reductase, they are more susceptible to developing methemoglobinemia[(265)]. An additional factor rendering newborns more susceptible to methemoglobinemia is the relative ease by which fetal hemoglobin is oxidized compared to adult hemoglobin[(265)]. Because of this, prilocaine cannot be recommended for use in neonates. Unfortunately, this may limit the use of an exciting new topical local anesthetic, EMLA (eutectic mixture of local anesthetics), in the newborn.

Finholt et al.[(266)] found that the volume of distribution, clearance, and elimination half-life of an intravenous bolus of lidocaine, 1 to 2 mg/kg, used to facilitate tracheal intubation[(267)] or to treat arrhythmias[(268)], is similar in children older than 6 months of age and adults. They recommend that lidocaine doses need not be altered based on age alone when lidocaine is administered intravenously. The elimination half-life of intravenously administered lidocaine in infants less than 6 months of age is prolonged, however. Since neonates have reduced protein binding, repeated administration of lidocaine may predispose these patients to toxic concentrations of drug. The routine administration of intravenous lidocaine in children with right-to-left intracardiac shunts may produce systemic toxicity[(269)]. Normally, approximately 60 to 80% of an intravenous lidocaine bolus is absorbed on the first pass through the lungs, then subsequently released over time[(270)]. In patients with right-to-left intracardiac shunts, venous blood enters directly into the systemic circulation through the intracardiac defect, bypassing the lungs. Peak arterial concentrations of lidocaine would be expected to be higher and to occur more rapidly. In fact, in lambs with right-to-left intracardiac shunts, lidocaine levels were double those of normal controls[(269)].

REGIONAL ANESTHETIC TECHNIQUES

Regional anesthetic techniques are increasingly being used in the management of acute pain in children. Many critically ill and injured patients can benefit from regional anesthetic use even when other analgesic therapies may be harmful or ineffective.

Subcutaneous Injection

Subcutaneous infiltration of the skin with a local anesthetic solution is the most commonly performed regional ("local") anesthetic technique in pediatric practice. Local anesthetics, particularly lidocaine, are commonly injected subcutaneously prior to the performance of many painful medical and surgical procedures to minimize procedure-related pain. Examples of procedures that benefit from prior local anesthetic infiltration include repair of minor surgical wounds (traumatic lacerations or deliberate incisions, e.g., prior to a cutdown for venous access), insertion of an arterial or an intravenous catheter (e.g., routine percutaneous intravenous access or cardiac catheterization), bone marrow aspiration, thoracostomy tube placement, and lumbar puncture. When used in this way, the local anesthetic agent blocks nerve conduction at the most terminal branches of the sensory nerves (Fig. 46.1).

Local anesthetic infiltration of traumatic lacerations requires special attention. Commonly, the wound is dirty and requires extensive scrubbing and irrigation. Should the local anesthetic be administered prior to the cleansing, which would make it painless, or after, to avoid introducing dirt and bacteria into the surrounding tissue? It is our practice to inject the local anesthetic through intact skin adjacent to the wound before the wound is cleaned. Alternatively, we block the peripheral nerve supplying the injured area more proximally because smaller amounts of local anesthetic are used and it requires fewer injections.

Because local anesthetics are manufactured at a pH of 4 to 5 and are administered by injection, they are in and of themselves painful. This pain can be minimized by using buffered anesthetic solutions and small needles[(14)]. Buffering a local anesthetic solution, such as lidocaine, with sodium bicarbonate (9 ml of lidocaine combined with 1 ml of bicarbonate, a 10:1 solution), may make the injection painless and shorten the onset of analgesia[(271)]. Local anesthetics are not manufactured with buffer because the buffering affects the shelf life of the drug. Obviously, using small-gauge needles will affect the amount of pain produced when infiltrating local anesthetics. We use either 26- or 30-gauge needles and inject the local anesthetic immediately as the needle punctures the skin. We do not aspirate first! Rather, we inject local anesthetics as the needle is advanced forward. Aspirating first is unnecessary because the amount of local anesthetic injected is so small (0.1 to 0.2 ml) that even an intravascular injection would be inconsequential.

EMLA Cream

EMLA (eutectic mixture of local anesthetics) cream, a topical emulsion composed of prilocaine and lidocaine, produces complete anesthesia of intact skin following application[(272–278)]. Unfortunately, for best effect, EMLA cream must be applied and covered with an occlusive dressing (such as Saran wrap) for 60 min before a procedure is performed. This limits its use unless the site is prepared well in advance of anticipated use. Furthermore, if the procedure is a venipuncture, multiple sites must be prepared, in case one's initial attempt is unsuccessful.

Unfortunately, the effectiveness of EMLA cream (like all other methods) at reducing pain is dependent on who makes the assessment. Soliman et al.[(272)] studied the efficacy of EMLA cream compared to injected lidocaine at reducing the pain associated with venipuncture. Both an observer and a physician performing the procedure judged pain relief to be virtually complete in both groups. The children involved in the study were not so sanguine and were equally dissatisfied with both methods, particularly if the needle used for venipuncture was visible to them. Thus, despite the fact that two observers thought that the child was pain free, the child's cooperation with venipuncture did not improve. Therefore, it is not clear whether the delay that is involved in the use of EMLA (60-min wait for effect) is justified. On the other hand, EMLA may be more effective in children accustomed to frequent medical procedures (e.g., oncology patients) or for procedures in which the child cannot see the needle such as lumbar puncture or bone marrow aspiration[(278)].

Epidural Anesthesia/Analgesia

The epidural space lies between the spinal dura mater and the spinal periosteum (the ligamentum flavum) and contains large epidural veins and lobulated fat (Fig. 46.8). The epidural space is not as voluminous as the subarachnoid space and extends from the base of the skull to the sacrococcygeal ligament. When the epidural space is entered at the level of the sacrococcygeal ligament, a "caudal" block is produced. When entered at the lumbar or thoracic level, a "lumbar" or "thoracic" epidural is produced. Caudal epidural blockade is much easier to perform than a lumbar epidural and has a lower risk of accidental dural puncture[(170,171,207,210,279–282)]. On the other hand, larger volumes of local anesthetic are required to produce blockade, and the risk of infection, particularly with indwelling catheters, may be greater. The epidural space has complicated direct communications with the paravertebral space and indirect communications with the CSF. The administration of local anesthetics, opioids, and α2-agonists to the epidural

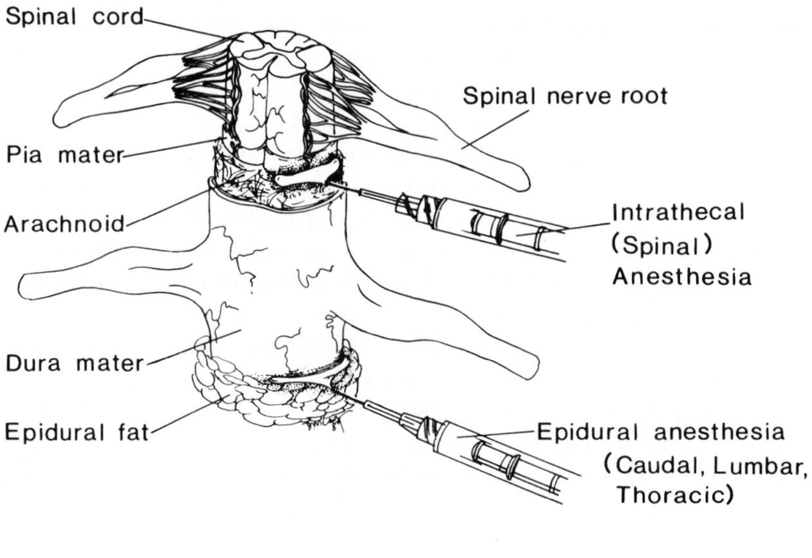

Figure 46.8. The relationship between the spinal cord and its coverings, namely the pia mater, arachnoid, and dura mater are demonstrated. In an intrathecal or "spinal" injection, the needle passes through the dura and arachnoid into the subarachnoid space, which contains cerebrospinal fluid. In an epidural injection, the needle passes through the ligamentum flavum but remains above the dura mater.

space, at any level, provides remarkably effective analgesia with minimal side effects. Local anesthetic administration is noted for its versatility and safety. Depending on the agent and concentration of agent used, sensory, motor, and/or sympathetic nerves can be blocked. Because of its effectiveness and ease of administration, epidural blockade has become the most commonly performed regional anesthetic technique for intraoperative anesthesia and postoperative analgesia in children undergoing urologic, orthopedic, and general surgical procedures below the diaphragm. Furthermore, continuous or long-term analgesia (e.g., terminal cancer) is now possible when indwelling epidural catheters are utilized. Finally, epidural local anesthetics have been recently used to provide continuous sympathetic blockade in children with vascular insufficiency secondary to intense vasoconstriction (e.g., purpura fulminans)[(284)].

Complications are rare. Unlike epidural blockade in adult patients, hypotension is almost unheard of in children less than 8 yr of age, even when high thoracic blockade is achieved[(281,282)]. In adults, hypotension is very common following high epidural blockade because of both sympathetic blockade and systemic absorption of local anesthetic into the bloodstream. Aside from the potential of local anesthetic accumulation following continuous infusion or by a direct intravascular local anesthetic injection, urinary retention and infection at the sight of injection are among the few complications that have been reported with this technique to date. Epidural insertion is contraindicated in patients with a coagulation disorder and if there is an infection at the site of insertion.

In clinical practice, when local anesthetics are utilized, assessment of the height of neural blockade is tested by the ability of the patient to perceive whether a pinprick to the skin is sharp or dull **(Table 46.10).**

Unfortunately, children, particularly those less than 5 yr of age, lose their ability or "desire to participate" in the assessment process once they see a needle. An alternative technique is to use a nerve stimulator set at the low range of tetanic stimulation. Another alternative is to measure the level of sympathetic blockade using either skin temperature changes or galvanic skin responses, since cutaneous sensory blockade is assumed to be analogous to the same level of sympathetic blockade **(Table 46.10).**

Table 46.10. Assessment of Dermatomal Blockade

Landmark	*Segmental Level*	*Significance*
Pinky, ring finger	C8	All cardioaccelerator fibers (T1–T4) are blocked Potential for diaphragmatic paralysis (C3–C5) and apnea is great
Nipple line	T4	Possibility of cardioaccelerator blockade Effective analgesia for upper abdominal procedures
Tip of the xyphoid	T6	Splanchnic (T5–L1) innervation blocked
Umbilicus	T10	Sympathetic blockade of lower extremeties, uterus, bladder, ureters
Inguinal ligament	T12	
Outer aspect of foot	S1	L5–S1 nerve roots are the most difficult nerves to block with an epidural approach

Local Anesthetic Dosage

Bupivacaine and lidocaine are the most commonly used local anesthetic agents used in epidural analgesia. There are multiple dosage schemes based on patient age, height, weight, and level of analgesia required. We typically use a loading dose of 1 ml/kg of either 0.125 to 0.25% bupivacaine, and follow this 1 hr later with a continuous infusion of either a 0.0625 or a 0.125% solution, at a dose not to exceed 0.5 mg/kg/hr. Lidocaine, in concentrations of 0.5 to 1%, can be used as an alternative. Following a loading dose of 1 ml/kg, a continuous infusion not to exceed 2.5 mg/kg/hr is started 1 hr after the loading dose was administered. We prefer to use lidocaine because it is less toxic and, unlike bupivacaine, lidocaine plasma levels can be measured in the chemistry laboratories of virtually every hospital in the country. Indeed, to minimize the risk of toxic accumulations of lidocaine, we routinely monitor plasma levels over the course of an infusion. On the other hand, tachyphylaxis may occur when lidocaine is chronically infused.

Opioid Dosage

The presence of high concentrations of opioid receptors in the spinal cord makes it possible to achieve analgesia, in both acute and chronic pain, with small doses of opioids administered in either the subarachnoid or epidural spaces (Fig. 46.6)[(56,57,63,64,94,166)]. By bypassing the blood and the blood-brain barrier, small doses of agonist are effective because they can reach the receptor by the back-door approach. Indeed, CSF opioid levels, particularly for morphine, are several thousand times greater than those achieved by the parenteral route[(138)]. It is these high levels that produce the profound and prolonged analgesia that accompanies intrathecal/epidural opioid administration. Even when administered via the caudal route, epidural morphine has been shown to provide effective postoperative analgesia following abdominal, thoracic, and cardiac surgery[(169–173)]. Krane et al. recently reported that 0.03 mg/kg of caudal-epidural morphine is equally effective as 0.1 mg/kg in providing postoperative analgesia, although the higher dose provides a significantly longer duration of analgesia (13.3 ± 4.7 versus 10.0 ± 3.3 hr, respectively)[(168)]. The incidence of side effects was the same in both groups, although one patient receiving 0.1 mg/kg developed late respiratory depression. Whether even lower doses would be effective is unknown.

Spinal opiates produce analgesia without altering autonomic or neuromuscular function. Additionally, both light touch and proprioception are preserved. Thus, unlike local anesthetics, spinal opioids allow patients to ambulate without orthostatic hypotension. Common side effects of intrathecal/epidural narcotics include facial or segmental pruritus, urinary retention, nausea and vomiting, and respiratory depression. These side effects occur with greater frequency when opioids are administered intrathecally as opposed to epidurally. Except for urinary retention, reversal of adverse side effects, with maintenance of adequate analgesia, can be achieved through the use of a low-dose (0.001 to 0.002 mg/kg-1) naloxone infusion. Pruritus and nausea can also be treated with intravenous diphenhydramine (Benadryl), 0.5 to 1.0 mg/kg.

Although rare, respiratory depression is a major risk when utilizing intrathecal/epidural opioids[172–177]. Attia et al.[172] demonstrated that the ventilatory response to CO_2 is depressed for as long as 22 hr following the administration of 0.05 mg/kg-1 of morphine epidurally. Following intrathecal morphine administration (0.02 mg/kg), Nichols et al.[138] demonstrated, in children varying between 3 months and 15 yr, significant depression of the ventilatory response to carbon dioxide for up to 18 hr[138]. The greatest respiratory depression correlated with the highest CSF morphine levels (2863 ± 542 ng/ml), which occurred 6 hr after administration. This depression persisted despite a fall in CSF morphine levels 12 (641 ± 219 ng/ml) to 18 (223 ± 152 ng/ml) hr later. This confirms the clinical impression that respiratory depression usually occurs within the first 6 hr after the administration of epidural or intrathecal morphine but late respiratory depression (up to 18 hr) has been reported. The risk of respiratory depression can be minimized through the epidural use of shorter acting, more lipid-soluble agents (fentanyl, sufentanil), which produce more segmental analgesia and less rostral spread. On the other hand, because of its shorter duration of action, fentanyl and sufentanil are increasingly being administered by continuous epidural infusion, either alone or in combination with very dilute (1/16%, 0.0625 mg/ml) bupivacaine concentrations. Typically, the epidural solution contains 1 to 2 μg/ml of fentanyl, with or without bupivacaine, and is administered in concentrations of 10 to 20 μg/ml, at rates ranging between 0.2 and 1.0 ml/kg/hr. This provides an effective algesia for both postoperative and chronic cancer pain. Several studies in children and adults have demonstrated that there is little advantage to adding local anesthetics to epidural fentanyl infusions. The analgesia produced by fentanyl alone is virtually identical to the analgesia produced by the combination of drugs, and omitting the local anesthetic reduces the possibility of local anesthetic systemic toxicity. Although sufentanil is the only member of the "fentanyl" family of drugs approved for epidural use by the FDA, we routinely use generic fentanyl instead because it is a fraction of sufentanil's cost.

Regardless of the opioid and route of administration, a regular system of monitoring for respiratory depression is required. Clinical signs that predict impending respiratory depression include somnolence, small pupils, and small tidal volumes. We also recommend using oxyhemoglobin saturation monitoring, particularly in the first 24 hr of instituting this therapy.

Technique

Although placement of an indwelling epidural catheter is a technical responsibility reserved to anesthesiologists, their management is within the purview of the intensivist. In children older than 6 yr of age (25 to 30 kg), standard adult (19- or 20-gauge) epidural catheters are used. Smaller diameter catheters (21- to 24-gauge) have recently been developed for younger children. However, these catheters kink at the insertion site, are difficult to inject through, and can almost never be aspirated through.

How much catheter to insert depends on the pain site and the child's age. Ideally, the tip of the catheter should lay in close approximation to the dermatomes that need to be blocked. Because the epidural space of young children is filled with loosely packed fat and blood vessels, it is possible to advance even a caudally placed catheter as far as the thorax. Indeed, Bosenberg et al. reported the use of the caudal approach for thoracic placement of an epidural catheter in children less than 2 yr of age. We have used this technique extensively in newborns and in many older children as well (e.g., Nissen fundoplication).

Because epidural catheters may be kept in place for many days at a time, they must be securely fastened both at the skin and at the connection (usually a Touhy-Borst "O" ring) to the infusion pump. Indeed, accidental withdrawal of the catheter or disconnection is the most common cause of failure when using this analgesic technique. We recommend using a transparent wound dressing (OpSite) over the catheter insertion site, which is further secured around its edges with paper tape. The transparent dressing allows visual inspection of the insertion site for evidence of infection as well as for migration of the catheter. The catheter and its connector should also be firmly taped together with paper tape once the "O" ring has been firmly cinched down. Epidural catheters also have depth and tip markers to help assess movement and placement of the catheter. Inspection for the tip marker is essential when an epidural catheter is removed because this is the only way to verify that the catheter has not been sheared on removal.

Prevention of infection is of paramount importance. Experience with intravenous therapy suggests that the epidural solutions and the delivery tubing proximal to the catheter should be changed every 24 to 48 hr. How long catheters can be left in place is unknown. We routinely remove them within 5 days of insertion. If a longer duration of therapy is needed, say for terminal cancer pain, we believe that the catheter should be tunneled subcutaneously. In the intensive care unit, the catheter site should be inspected daily for evidence of infection and by seeking a history of localized back pain or neck stiffness. We also remove epidural catheters whenever a patient has an unexplained fever.

SPECIFIC NERVE BLOCKS

Although a detailed description of all nerve blocks is not within the scope of this textbook, we will discuss techniques that have the widest applications in the intensive care unit in the next section. Fortunately many of these nerve blocks are easy to perform and require much less manual dexterity than is generally appreciated. Obviously, if one is to perform a nerve block, one needs to know which nerves are to be blocked and must have a rudimentary knowledge of the nerve's location and depth. The most effective blocks are those in which a paresthesia can be obtained as the needle approaches the nerve. If this cannot be done, a nerve stimulator may be a helpful adjunct. Emergency airway and resuscitative equipment, as well as individuals trained in using it, must be available for use prior to the performance of a peripheral nerve block. Additionally, if a patient is to be sedated during the performance of a nerve block, one member of the health care team must assume the responsibility of patient monitoring. This person is responsible for monitoring vital signs, assessing the adequacy of the airway, and alerting other members of the health care team if a problem is occurring. This person should not be performing the procedure itself!

Nerve Stimulators

A nerve stimulator can be used for accurate location of peripheral nerves with motor fiber components[286–289]. Since the use of a nerve stimulator does not require cooperation on the part of the patient, upper and lower extremity blocks can be performed with great success on children who are heavily sedated or obtunded. Obviously, children cannot be paralyzed when utilizing a nerve stimulator. Important design characteristics for a nerve stimulator include a constant current output, clearly marked polarity, with high and low output ranges, and a short stimulation pulse (Fig. 46.9). Despite these "ideal" requirements, virtually any peripheral nerve stimulator used to measure neuromuscular blockade will work[287]. When using a nerve stimulator, the nerve block is performed using either a standard, unsheathed steel needle or an insulated needle[289]. In either case, the needle is connected via an alligator clamp to the negative pole of the stimulator (Fig. 46.9). The positive pole is connected via an alligator clamp to an electrode on the skin well clear of the block site. The needle is inserted using standard landmarks and is attached to extension tubing and a syringe of local anesthetic solution. As the needle approaches the depth at which the nerve is expected to be located, the stimulator is turned on to the low range. The area of nerve's motor innervation is observed for muscle contraction. With a sheathed needle, muscle contractions will increase as the needle approaches the nerve and then decrease as the needle passes the nerve. With unsheathed needles, which we use exclusively, the maximum muscle contraction occurs when the needle is past the nerve. Once the nerve is identified, the needle is fixed, and 1 to 2 ml of local anesthetic is injected. This should abolish the muscle contraction completely. If it does not, the needle should be withdrawn and the process should be repeated.

Axillary Block

The axillary nerve block is an ideal block for upper extremity procedures and is our preferred approach to the brachial plexus because of its simplicity[170,171,290–295]. It carries little risk of pneumothorax, phrenic nerve block, or subarachnoid injection. It is particularly useful for fracture reductions and repair of lacerations of the hand and forearm. Because the axillary artery lies within the fascial sheath of the brachial plexus and the spread of local anesthetic solutions within a fascial sheath results in nerve block, local anesthetic solutions deposited anywhere near the axillary artery will usually produce an adequate nerve block.

Performance of the Axillary Nerve Block

The patient's arm is abducted at a right angle, with the forearm and hand supinated; the elbow is flexed with the hand under the head or in a "saluting position" (Fig. 46.10). The

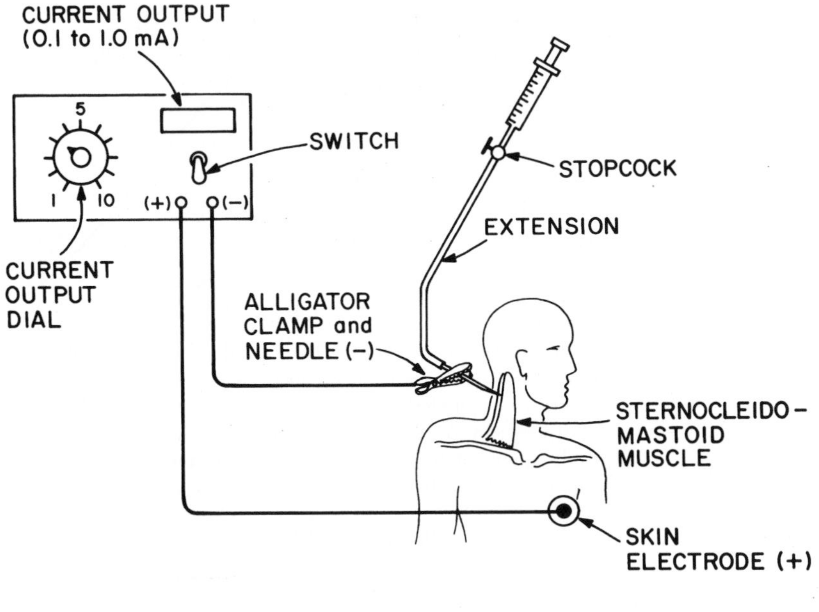

Figure 46.9. A peripheral nerve stimulator for use in locating peripheral nerves with motor fiber components is demonstrated. Note that the negative electrode is attached to the needle. (Reprinted with permission from Yaster M, Maxwell LG. Pediatric regional anesthesia. Anesthesiology 1989; 70:324–338.)

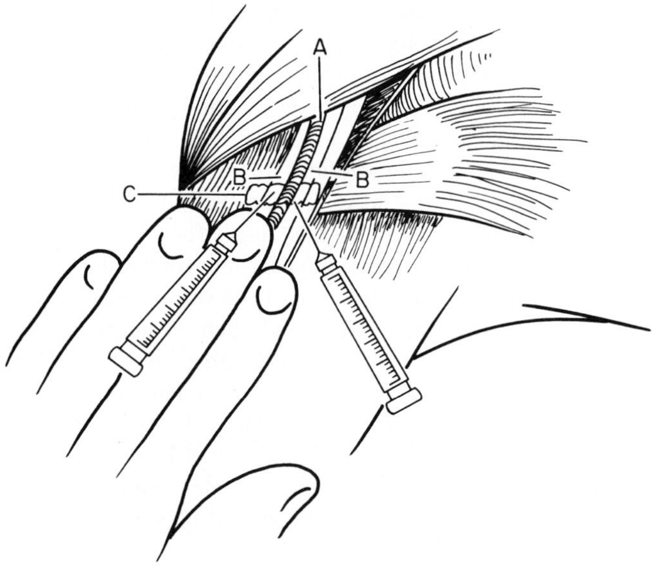

Figure 46.10. The axillary block is depicted. The nonoperative hand is positioned such that the middle finger lies directly over the brachial artery (A) compressing the brachial plexus (B) against the humerus. Following placement of a skin wheal (C), directly over the artery, fan-like injections of local anesthesia are made on each side of the artery as close as possible to the lateral border of the artery. Approximately five sweeps are made on each side of the artery, and 1 ml of local anesthetic is injected on each sweep. (Reprinted with permission from Yaster M, Maxwell LG. Pediatric regional anesthesia. Anesthesiology 1989;70:324–338.)

axillary artery and brachial plexus are very superficial and the artery is used as the landmark. Following aseptic preparation of the skin, the physician's nonoperative hand is positioned such that the middle finger lies directly over the artery and compresses it and the brachial plexus against the humerus. A weal of local anesthetic is deposited directly over the pulsating artery. Using a 25-gauge needle, local anesthetic is deposited on each side of the artery staying as close as possible to the border of the axillary artery. On the initial pass on each side of the artery, the needle is inserted at a depth of approximately 1/2 inch, aspirating constantly. As the needle is withdrawn, 1 ml of local anesthetic is injected. Then, in a fan-like manner, 1 ml of local anesthetic is injected on each sweep. We use 5 ml of local anesthetic (either 1% lidocaine with 1:200,000 epinephrine or 0.25% bupivacaine with 1:200,000 epinephrine) on each side of the artery for a total dose of 10 ml. An alternative approach is a modification of the Winnie block, in which the axillary artery is deliberately transfixed with the needle. Drug is injected deep and superficial to the artery at the point where active blood return, as demonstrated by aspiration through the needle, ceases.

Femoral Nerve Block

The femoral nerve block (L2, L3, L4) is the quickest, easiest, and most effective technique of relieving the pain of a femoral shaft fracture[170,171,296–298]. Rhonchi et al.[298], using bupivacaine without epinephrine in a femoral nerve block, provided fracture patients with adequate anesthesia for the application of traction as well as for the necessary (and usually painful) manipulations that occur during radiologic examinations. The duration of analgesia was 3 hr and peak plasma levels of bupivacaine averaged less than 1 μg/ml-1.

Performance of the Block

Following aseptic preparation of the skin, a 25-gauge needle is inserted perpendicularly, approximately 3 to 5 mm lateral to the pulsation of the femoral artery at the level of the inguinal ligament (Fig. 46.11). The needle is inserted to a depth that is clearly deeper than the artery. The feeling of penetration of the fascia over the nerve (a distinct "pop") helps one judge the depth of penetration. Following a negative aspiration for blood, one injects 5 to 10 ml of local anesthetic solution (0.25% bupivacaine with 1:200,000 epinephrine). Local anesthetic solution is then injected in a fan-like manner lateral and deep to the femoral artery. The maximum dosage of 0.25% bupivacaine used is 1 ml/kg **(Table 46.9).**

Intrapleural Bupivacaine Analgesia

Intrapleural infusions of bupivacaine and epinephrine have been shown to provide postoperative analgesia following chest, kidney, and gallbladder surgery in both children and adults. It is also effective for rib fractures and chronic pancreatitis. Unfortunately, we have not had as much success with this technique as has been reported in the literature, particularly if a chest tube is in place. Additionally, the very

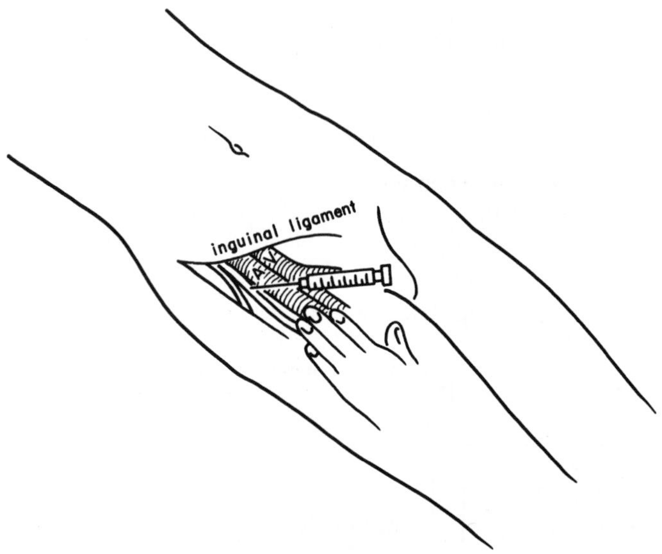

Figure 46.11. The femoral nerve block is depicted. After placing a skin wheal, the nonoperative hand compresses the femoral artery and nerve against the underlying tissue and bone immediately below the inguinal ligament. A 22- or 25-gauge needle is then inserted perpendicularly, approximately 1/2–1 cm lateral to the pulsation of the femoral artery (A) in the femoral nerve's fascial sheath. (Reprinted with permission from Yaster M, Maxwell LG. Pediatric regional anesthesia. Anesthesiology 1989;70:324–338.)

high plasma levels that have been reported with this technique have, quite frankly, frightened us. Finally, like the epidural, this block should be performed only by an anesthesiologist.

Anesthetic Dosage

McIlvaine et al.[299] recommend loading a patient with 0.5 ml/kg of 0.25% bupivacaine with epinephrine (5 μg/ml) at a rate of 1 ml/min. This is followed by a continuous infusion of 0.1 to 0.5 ml/kg/hr. Although no toxicity was seen in their study, plasma bupivacaine levels approached or exceeded toxic levels, particularly in patients undergoing anterior spinal fusion.

Intercostal Nerve Block

The intercostal nerve block is one of the safest and most versatile blocks that can be used in the intensive care unit[237]. It can provide complete sensory analgesia of the chest and abdominal walls and is remarkably easy to perform. It is particularly useful when used prior to chest tube insertion and when treating patients with broken ribs. Indeed, when used for rib fractures, the analgesia produced is nothing short of remarkable. Patients can sit up, take deep breaths, cough, and ambulate almost as soon as the needle is removed. Furthermore, continuous blockade is possible with indwelling intercostal catheters. Unfortunately, this technique is greatly underutilized because misconceptions abound about the risk of pneumothorax and the time and effort required to perform these blocks.

Performance of the Block

With the patient lying on the opposite side and with the upper arm extended forward over the chest, the skin is aseptically prepared. Alternatively, the block may be performed in a patient sitting on the edge of the bed with the legs dangling or with the patient prone. The posterior approach (either sitting or lying) is preferable to the side approach because the risk of pneumothorax is reduced. However, in most situations in the intensive care unit, the mid- or postaxillary line is most accessible for this block. A 25-gauge needle is used in children less than 10 to 15 kg and a 22-gauge, short beveled needle is used in larger children. The skin over the rib to be blocked is rolled superiorly and the needle is inserted to contact the rib. The skin and needle are then allowed to roll inferiorly until the needle slips off the rib. It is then advanced 2 to 4 mm. After aspirating for blood, 1 to 3 ml of local anesthetic solution, usually bupivacaine, 0.25 to 0.5%, with 1:200,000 (5 μg/ml), is injected. This block provides 4 to 10 hr of pain relief. Continuous analgesia with indwelling intercostal catheters is also possible. Finally, if more than one rib is to be blocked, the maximum bupivacaine dosage that can be used is 2.5 mg/kg.

SEDATION AND SLEEP IN THE INTENSIVE CARE UNIT

Anxiety, fear, and lack of sleep will potentiate pain and, if left untreated, can lead to psychosis in critically ill patients. Indeed, "intensive care unit induced psychosis" is a well-described phenomenon in adult patients that typically occurs 3 to 5 days after admission to the intensive care unit. This syndrome is caused by a combination of factors including the patient's premorbid personality (attitude toward illness, age, and defense mechanisms), psychologic disturbances, and the environment (frightening atmosphere, lack of sleep, unusual and disturbing sounds, lack of windows, deprivation of day-night cycles, and others).

A variety of factors prevent sleep in critically ill patients. Patients are subjected to constant light, noise, rounds, visitors, anxious family, pain, procedures, blood letting, and more often than not, an endotracheal tube. Children are frightened by the machines in the intensive care unit and usually misinterpret staff conversations heard from around the bed as well. Although there are some situations in which sedation, anxiolysis, and sleep are undesirable, patients will benefit by the promotion of sleep and by the relief of anxiety in most cases. In the next section, we will review several pharmacologic approaches to accomplish this.

Benzodiazepines

The benzodiazepines comprise a family of drugs that are the most important sedative/hypnotic/anxiolytic drugs currently used in clinical practice. Although there are scores of benzodiazepines, such as diazepam (Valium), midazolam (Versed), triazolam (Halcion), lorazepam (Ativan), and others, they have many more similarities than differences[300–309]. These drugs are extremely potent amnestics, anticonvulsants, sedatives, hypnotics, and skeletal muscle relaxants. They are effective whether given parenterally or enterally and work by augmenting γ-amminobutyric acid (GABA) and glycine transmission. GABA is the major inhibitory neurotransmitter within the brain whereas glycine is an inhibitory neurotransmitter in the spinal cord and brainstem. The GABA receptor has two α and two β subunits. Binding of benzodiazepines to the α subunits of the GABA receptors facilitates GABA binding to the β sites and promotes membrane hyperpolarization and resistance to neuronal excitation[302]. This produces sedation, anxiolysis, muscle relaxation, and anticonvulsant activity. These are receptor-specific effects and suggest that benzodiazepines will be discovered that have either agonist, antagonist, or agonist-antagonist properties, or all three. An agonist-antagonist binds to the α subunit and reduces the efficiency of GABA transmission. This produces central nervous system stimulation. Alternatively, antagonists, such as flumazenil, a newly discovered antagonist, bind to the α subunit and do not alter GABA synaptic transmission efficiency, but competitively block the actions of both agonists and agonist-antagonists[306]. This has the clinical effect of reversing benzodiazepine-induced sedation and respiratory depression.

Within the central nervous system, the benzodiazepines reduce cerebral metabolism and blood flow when they produce sleep. They alter consciousness along a dose-dependent continuum ranging from anxiolysis to sedation to sleep to general anesthesia. It is not known how these different effects are mediated but, probably, absolute receptor occupancy is reflected. It has been estimated that a benzodiazepine receptor occupancy of less than 20% produces anxiolysis, 30 to 50% sedation, and more than 60% unconsciousness[308]. This family is also anti-convulsant drugs and is frequently used as first-line drugs in the treatment of seizures. Finally, benzodiazepines markedly impair the acquisition of new information ("anterograde amnesia") whereas stored information ("retrograde amnesia") is unaffected[309]. In fact, this latter attribute is often used by the intensivist when treating critically ill children. There are occasions in which pain management may be impossible because of the hemodynamic instability of a patient's condition. Examples include cardioversion, intubation in hemodynamically unstable patients, emergency endoscopy, and others. Benzodiazepines provide an alternative mode of therapy. Although they have no intrinsic analgesic properties, they can prevent a patient from remembering a painful experience.

Similarly, the benzodiazepines produce a dose-dependent depression in breathing[310–312]. In small doses, the benzodiazepines minimally affect minute ventilation. In higher doses, however, they can blunt or abolish the respiratory responses to both hypercarbia and hypoxia. Drug-induced respiratory depression is quantified by the ventilatory response to inhaled or rebreathed carbon dioxide (Fig. 46.3). The depressant drug may either reduce the slope of the CO_2 response curve or shift the x-intercept to the right. A reduced slope implies a diminished ventilatory response at any given arterial $PaCO_2$ level. The x-intercept of the curve, known as the apneic threshold, indicates relative position of the curve and is defined as that $PaCO_2$ required to stimulate spontaneous respiration. The benzodiazepines produce hypoventilation primarily by decreasing tidal volume. This is manifested by a reduction of the slope of the CO_2 response curve without a change in the x-intercept (Fig. 46.3). The depressant effect of the benzodiazepines begins within 1 to 4 min of an intravenous injection and lasts for at least 30 min[310–312].

The benzodiazepine-induced decrease in the ventilatory response to hypoxia is particularly dangerous, since the hypoxic drive is the "backup" system in the control of ventilation. Drug-induced hypoventilation rapidly decreases alveolar and arterial oxygen saturation. In unmedicated persons, the hypoxic ventilatory drive provides some protection from hypoventilation-induced hypoxia. If both the hypoxic and hypercarbic drive to breathe are blunted or blocked by the benzodiazepines, apnea and death may result in their use. Furthermore, the respiratory depression seen with the benzodiazepines is potentiated with the concomitant administration of any opioid. This requires a reduction in the dose of both drugs when these drugs are administered together and underscores the need for very close observation and monitoring of patients who receive these drugs. The risk of using these drugs may be significantly increased in children with chronic CO_2 retention, who are less than 1 to 2 months of age, are chronically dependent on the hypoxic drive to ventilate, and who are receiving opioids concomitantly. Finally, the respiratory depression produced by the benzodiazepine agonists can be antagonized by flumazenil.

The benzodiazepines produce minimal cardiovascular effects[313–316]. They reduce both preload and afterload. Arterial blood pressure and cardiac output are minimally affected. However, in the presence of hypovolemia or catecholamine depletion, the benzodiazepines may produce significant hypotension, and must, therefore, be administered with great caution[315]. Benzodiazepines significantly affect blood pressure and cardiac output when combined with opioids and great caution must be exercised when these drugs are combined. Interestingly, diazepam has been reported to decrease coronary vascular resistance and have a nitroglycerin-like effect[315]. Midazolam, on the other hand, decreases coronary sinus blood flow and myocardial oxygen consumption, but does not change coronary vascular resistance.

Midazolam

Midazolam is a water-soluble benzodiazepine that is four times more potent than diazepam and is well absorbed via intramuscular, oral, rectal, or transmucosal routes of administration[317–322]. Unlike diazepam, midazolam can be painlessly administered intravenously and rarely causes thrombophlebitis. Although manufactured as an acid to make it water soluble, at physiologic pH, midazolam becomes highly lipophilic and rapidly crosses the blood-brain barrier to gain access to the benzodiazepine receptors in the central nervous system. This accounts for its dramatic clinical effect. It has a relatively large volume of distribution, short elimination half-life, high clearance, and is hydroxylated in the liver into inactive metabolites **(Table 46.11).** It is characterized by rapid onset and short duration of action following a single parenteral dose and by little accumulation following repeated or continuous infusion dosing[303,304]. When administered orally or rectally, less than 50% of the

Table 46.11. Benzodiazepine Pharmacokinetics

Drug	$T_{1/2}\beta$ *(min)*	V_DSS *(liter/kg)*	*Cl (ml/min/kg)*	$T_{1/2}\beta$ *(hr)*
Diazepam	30–60	0.7–1.7	0.2–0.5	20–50
Midazolam	6–15	1.1–1.7	6.4–11	1.7–2.6
Lorazepam	2–7	0.8–1.3	0.8–1.2	11–22

administered dose is bioavailable because of extraction by the liver ("first-pass liver effects").

Dosage and Route of Administration

Midazolam was initially marketed in an extremely concentrated solution, 5 mg/ml. It was, therefore, very easy to administer toxic doses of the drug when it was administered to patients at the extremes of age. To add to the confusion, a less concentrated form, 1 mg/ml, is now also available from the manufacturer in a vial that is indistinguishable from the more concentrated variety. We recommend that the drug should always be diluted to a 1 mg/ml concentration prior to administration to avoid toxic overdoses.

When used for sedation prior to procedures or as a premedication, midazolam can be administered intravenously (0.05 to 0.08 mg/kg), intramuscularly (0.1 to 0.15 mg/kg), rectally (0.3 to 1.0 mg/kg), orally (0.5 to 1.0 mg/kg), nasally (0.3 to 0.5 mg/kg), or transmucosally (0.5 to 0.75 mg/kg)[317–322]. Obviously, intravenous administration produces the most rapid onset of effect and, therefore, must always be titrated with continuous cardiorespiratory monitoring. It also produces the shortest duration of effect as well. When administered rectally, midazolam takes approximately 10 min to produce its effect, whereas when administered orally, it takes 30 to 60 min to achieve adequate sedation. There have been no reported incidences, to date, of cardiorespiratory problems with midazolam when it is administered via an enteral route[317]. However, this does not mean that there will not be, and patient safety must always be the physician's primary concern when prescribing this, or any, drug. Finally, there is no enteral preparation manufactured by the drug's pharmaceutical company. Rather, the parenteral form is administered enterally. This presents some problems when midazolam is administered orally, nasally, or transmucosally because of its extremely bitter taste. Fortunately, its taste can be disguised with either Coke syrup, concentrated (sugared) Kool-Aid, or flavored gelatin[321,322].

Midazolam can also provide very effective continuous sedation by a constant intravenous infusion[323]. This is true whether it is administered alone or in combination with an opioid, usually morphine or fentanyl. There are several dosing regimens available. Silvasi and Rosen[323] recommend loading a patient with 0.2 mg/kg midazolam, to be followed with a continuous infusion of 0.4 to 0.6 μg/kg/min. On the other hand, Booker et al.[324] required 2 to 6 μg/kg/min to achieve adequate sedation in postoperative cardiac patients, despite using the same loading dose as Silvasi and Rosen[323]. When using midazolam, or an opioid, for continuous sedation over a prolonged period of time, usually more than a week, dependence and withdrawal symptoms may occur when the drug is stopped. Benzodiazepine-induced withdrawal symptoms are similar to withdrawal symptoms of opioids and alcohol. Clonidine, 3 to 5 μg/kg, administered by transdermal patch may be helpful in treating many of the withdrawal symptoms. Alternatively, patients should be gradually tapered from their drugs rather than being abruptly cut off ("cold turkey").

Finally, midazolam can be used to induce general anesthesia when it is administered intravenously[325,326]. In doses of 0.2 to 0.3 mg/kg, midazolam induces general anesthesia within 2 to 3 min of administration. Although, not as rapid in onset as thiopental or ketamine, midazolam produces similar degrees of apnea. General anesthesia is usually an accident of midazolam overdosage rather than a desired effect.

Diazepam

At one time the most commonly used benzodiazepine, diazepam has been largely replaced in clinical practice by midazolam. It is poorly water soluble and the solvent vehicle for parenteral administration contains several organic solvents, such as propylene glycol and sodium benzoate, that are very dangerous in the newborn. Its poor water solubility makes absorption from an intramuscular site erratic and incomplete. Thus, the oral or intravenous route of administration is preferred. Unfortunately, even the intravenous route is problematic because diazepam is painful when administered intravenously and causes thrombophlebitis.

Following absorption, diazepam is very slowly N-demethylated in the liver into two active metabolites, desmethyldiazepam and oxazepam. Desmethyldiazepam is metabolized even more slowly than diazepam and has a half-life of elimination of 48 to 96 hr. Oxazepam is rapidly glucuronidated and excreted in the urine. The presence of these active metabolites explains, in part, the very long duration of action of diazepam and why it has largely been replaced by midazolam.

Dosage and Route of Administration

Diazepam is an effective sedative, anxiolytic, and amnestic when administered orally or intravenously. When administered intravenously, 0.05 to 0.1 mg/kg, it rapidly allays anxiety and apprehension and should be titrated to effect. Additionally, this same dose can be used as an anticonvulsant to stop seizure activity temporarily. The oral dose is two to three times the intravenous dose and takes 30 to 90 min to produce similar hypnotic effects.

Barbiturates

The barbiturates have been greatly supplanted by the benzodiazepines for the treatment of insomnia both in and out of the intensive care unit. These drugs are neither anxiolytics nor analgesics, rather, they globally depress the central nervous system to various degrees, and produce effects ranging from sedation to general anesthesia. In fact, when dealing with patients in pain, caution must be exercised in the use of barbiturates because, in small doses, they increase the perception of pain and cause excitement rather than sedation ("antanalgesic"). However, when barbiturates are given in doses that are high enough to produce general anesthesia, pain perception, in addition to consciousness, is obliterated. A dose-dependent continuum of central nervous system effects exists following barbiturate administration. At lower doses, barbiturates produce sleep and, at higher doses, they produce general anesthesia. Infrequently, barbiturates produce an idiosyncratic, hyperkinetic reaction in children characterized by agitation, incoherence, disorientation, and tantrums. All but methohexital are potent anticonvulsants and can be used acutely and chronically for this purpose. Additionally, they reduce cerebral blood flow and cerebral metabolism in proportion to their degree of cerebral depression and are often used for this purpose following head injury in the intensive care unit[185,186]. Thus, thiopental, for example, is often used to treat spikes of intracranial pressure by producing unconsciousness and thereby reducing cerebral blood flow. However, these drugs are of no prophylactic value in preventing or minimizing secondary brain injury in patients with elevated intracranial pressure. Indeed, the use of barbiturate-induced coma for this purpose has largely been abandoned.

Barbiturates have significant effects on the cardiovascular system[327]. They must be given with great caution in hemodynamically unstable patients. All of the barbiturates directly depress the myocardium and the arterial vascular tree and cause significant hypotension. If the baroreceptor compensatory system is intact, hypotension results in a reflex tachycardia that restores blood pressure. When barbiturates are given to patients with minimal compensatory reserves, such as patients who are catecholamine- or volume-depleted, profound hypotension and even cardiac arrest can occur. Indeed, the dose of ultra-short-acting barbiturates to induce unconsciousness in hypovolemic patients should be reduced by 75% or eliminated in entirety.

Dosage and Route of Administration

The barbiturates are generally classified into long, medium, and ultra-short-acting agents based on their pharmacokinetic and pharmacodynamic profiles. Phenobarbital is a long-acting barbiturate with a half-life of elimination of 24 to 96 hr. It is most commonly used as an anticonvulsant in doses of 10 to 20 mg/kg. Rarely is it used to produce sleep. In fact, its very long duration of action and very slow onset time make it an inappropriate hypnotic agent in any medical setting. Pentobarbital (Nembutal) and secobarbital are medium acting barbiturates with half-lives of elimination ranging between 20 and 45 hr. Sleep is induced within 10 to 15 min of an intravenous or intramuscular bolus injection and will last approximately 2 to 6 hr. It may also be administered orally or rectally. Pentobarbital is generally used to produce sleep, immobility for diagnostic imaging, and long lasting sedation and is administered in doses ranging between 2 and 6 mg/kg, with a maximum dose of 150 mg. Intravenous thiopental (Pentothal), 4 to 7 mg/kg, and methohexital (Brevital), 1 to 2 mg/kg, are ultra-short-acting agents that have half-lives of elimination of 4 to 24 hr, but therapeutic actions that last for less than 10 min[328–330]. Recovery from the effects of intravenous thiopental and methohexital have nothing to do with their biotransformation and elimination from the body. Rather, their effects are terminated by redistribution from the brain to other body tissue compartments. This has very important clinical implications. If thiopental, for example, is given by repeated intermittent doses or by a prolonged intravenous infusion (e.g., in head trauma), prolongation of effect will occur, because elimination and not distribution will determine the duration of the drug's effect[304,305]. The ultra-short-acting agents are generally used to induce general anesthesia intravenously, particularly prior to tracheal intubation. The dose of thiopental, for example, is reduced to 1 to 2 mg/kg rather than 4 to 7 mg/kg when it is given to hemodynamically unstable patients. Because it has a pH greater than 10, thiopental can produce catastrophic damage if it is injected intra-arterially or subcutaneously[331]. Thus, one must be certain of the functionality of an intravenous catheter before this drug is injected. Thiopental and methohexital may also be administered rectally (20 to 30 mg/kg), primarily to produce sleep and immobility that lasts for 60 to 90, rather than 10, min. Methohexital is commonly used in this way in healthy children to provide immobility for diagnostic imaging studies[332–334].

Chloral Hydrate

Chloral hydrate was and continues to be the "gold standard" hypnotic used in pediatric practice. It is a short-acting (6 to 8 hr), relatively safe, short-term agent, that is useful in treating insomnia. In therapeutic doses it has little, if any, effect on respiration or blood pressure. Toxic doses, however, produce apnea and hypotension. Unfortunately, chloral hydrate, like the barbiturates, has absolutely no analgesic properties and excitement and delirium may be initiated if it is given to patients in pain. It is commonly used for producing immobility for painless procedures such as computerized tomography or magnetic resonance imaging. In our experience, it fails when used for this purpose 30 to 40% of the time.

Dosage and Route of Administration

Chloral hydrate is very irritating to the skin and mucous membranes and gastric necrosis has been reported following toxic doses. Because it has a ghastly taste and often causes nausea and vomiting when given orally, chloral hydrate is often administered rectally. It is typically given in doses of 25 to 100 mg/kg, with a maximum dose of 2.0 g.

POSTANESTHETIC MANAGEMENT

A large number of the patients admitted to the pediatric intensive care unit are surgical patients admitted for continuous perioperative monitoring and support. The purpose of the remainder of this chapter is to provide an overview of common perioperative problems and how they impact patient management in the intensive care unit.

ANESTHETIC RISK

In 1961, Rackow et al.[335] reported the incidence of cardiac arrest associated with anesthesia as 1:600 and 1:700 in infants and children, respectively, compared with 1:2500 in the adult population. Perioperative mortality has significantly improved since then and the risk of an anesthetic-related death in a healthy patient is now less than 1:10,000. Factors that increase anesthetic risk include the need for emergency surgery, the presence of organ system failure, anemia, and extremes of age. Risk, however, is not only limited by the patient's medical condition. Obviously, the type of surgery also significantly affects the perioperative mortality and morbidity. The risk of anesthesia and surgery can never be reduced to zero. Factors such as loss of a patient's airway, inability to ventilate and oxygenate, uncontrolled blood loss, anesthetic drug overdosage, equipment failure, and physician error all contribute to this. However, it is gratifying to note that Downes (personal communication) has recently reported an overall anesthetic mortality of only 0.2:10,000 at the Children's Hospital of Philadelphia.

Many, but not all, complications following surgery are related to the anesthetic regimen used to anesthetize a patient. Indeed, in most cases, the risk of surgery is very small compared to the risk of general anesthesia. Many critically ill patients may have to undergo minor surgical procedures, such as a tracheostomy, central line placement, or gastrostomy, for which there is minimal, if any, surgical risk. However, the risk of complications in transporting a critically ill patient to and from the operating room and subjugating that child to general anesthesia may be enormous. In the next section, we will review some of the more common problems seen in pediatric practice and their anesthetic implications.

Preoperative Assessment of Anesthetic Risk

The preoperative evaluation is of paramount importance in optimizing any patient for surgery, including critically ill ones. The past medical history and physical examination provides clues to the presence of significant physiologic derangements that may decrease the margin of safety of anesthesia, or place the patient at an increased risk of postoperative complications. A classification of patients according to physical status, has been outlined by the American Society of Anesthesiologists (ASA) **(Table 46.12).** This physical status score consolidates the accumulated data of a history and physical examination and defines the estimated perioperative risk. It is a shorthand description used by virtually all anesthesiologists. A thorough history of the present illness and a summary of significant physical findings should be made available to the anesthesiologist prior to surgery **(Table 46.13).** Of prime importance are issues related to cardiorespiratory reserve and the integrity of the autonomic nervous system. Disease states that compromise the cardiovascular and respiratory systems or alter the function of the autonomic nervous system greatly increase perioperative risk because virtually all anesthetic agents and techniques depress them. A patient with little reserve can very rapidly deteriorate or arrest on the induction of anesthesia. For example, a patient with an anterior mediastinal mass with mild or no respiratory distress can arrest and be unventilatable on the induction of general anesthesia. Similarly, a patient who is maintaining his or her blood pressure via vasoconstriction and a high circulating level of endogenous catecholamines can become acutely hypotensive and even arrest when anesthetic or sedative agents are given.

Table 46.12. ASA Physical Status Classifications

Class 1
No organic, physiologic, biochemical, or psychiatric disturbance
The pathologic process for which operation is to be performed is localized and not a systemic disturbance
Class 2
Mild-to-moderate systemic disturbance caused either by the condition to be treated surgically or by other pathophysiologic processes
Class 3
Severe systemic disturbance or disease from whatever cause
Class 4
Severe systemic disorder that is already life-threatening and not always correctable by the operative procedure
Class 5
The moribund patient who has little chance of survival but is submitted to operation in desperation

Because anesthesia is a drug-induced alteration in perception and consciousness, anything that impairs drug pharmacokinetics or pharmacodynamics will significantly affect the course of an anesthetic. Thus, it is crucial to know of any disease or drug interactions that may impair renal or hepatic function because of their effects on the bioavailability and excretion of most of the pharmacologic agents employed in the operating room. Similarly, it is important to obtain a detailed history of allergy prior to sending a patient to the operating room. Many drugs administered in the operating room may produce life-threatening anaphylaxis. Histamine-releasing drugs such as morphine, protamine, and barbiturates were considered the most important potential allergens until very recently. In the last few years, however, latex allergy and latex-induced anaphylaxis has become the prime intraoperative allergy concern. This is particularly true in children who require frequent bladder catheterization (e.g., meningomyelocele patients).

In the operating room, blood loss even with minor procedures is to be expected. Preoperative anemia, whether unrecognized or underestimated, has been cited by numerous authors as a primary etiologic event in circulatory arrest associated with surgery. Most healthy patients have normal hematocrits and the need for routine hematocrit testing in them is controversial. However, in critically ill patients, this is vital preoperative information. Anemia results in a reduction in oxygen-carrying capacity and content of the blood and in a shift of the oxygen dissociation curve to the right. Oxygen delivery is dependent on cardiac output and the ability of the hemoglobin to release oxygen to the tissues. If the hematocrit falls below 30%, oxygen delivery is rarely compromised because the heart can compensate by

Table 46.13. Details of Components of Anesthetic History

Preoperative Evaluation
- I. General information
  - A. Name
  - B. Age
  - C. Preoperative diagnosis
  - D. Surgeon
  - E. Proposed operation
  - F. Time, quantity, description of last oral intake
- II. History of present illness
- III. Past medical history
  - A. Surgery
  - B. Anesthesia: date, type, complications
  - C. Allergy/drug reaction
  - D. Medications, street drug use = alter anesthetic plan
  - E. Recent immunizations = possible postoperative febrile course
- IV. Family history
  - A. Anesthetic complications, especially the possibility of malignant hyperthermia
  - B. Inheritable diseases, to include the possibility of pseudocholinesterese deficiency
- V. Review of systems
  - A. Central nervous system (CNS)
    - 1. Seizures = influence choice of anesthetic agents
    - 2. Retardation
    - 3. Apnea = influence time of extubation
  - B. Respiratory
    - 1. Nasal obstruction secondary to secretions or adrenal hypertrophy
    - 2. Loose teeth = aspiration
    - 3. Asthma/bronchiolitis = possibility of wheezing on induction
    - 4. Frequent or current pneumonia
  - C. Cardiovascular
    - 1. Arrhythmias = anesthetic and muscle relaxant exacerbation
    - 2. Congenital heart disease = complication, anesthetic inductions
    - 3. Acquired heart disease (drugs, trauma) = heart failure
  - D. Gastrointestinal
    - 1. Hepatitis/jaundice = altered drug metabolism
    - 2. Intestinal obstruction = regurgitation and aspiration
    - 3. Gastrointestinal reflux = intubations problems with aspiration
  - E. Renal
    - 1. Electrolyte abnormalities
    - 2. Renal failure
    - 3. Dialysis data, if appropriate
  - F. Endocrine
    - 1. Diabetes mellitus = fluid and electrolyte management; coma
    - 2. History of steroid use = adrenal suppression and shock
    - 3. Abnormalities of electrolytes, such as calcium
  - G. Hematologic
    - 1. History of bleeding and/or bruising
    - 2. Hemoglobin; hematocrit; sickle preparation in black patient
    - 3. Oncology patients: note drug therapies and side effects
  - H. Musculoskeletal
    - 1. Severe kyphoscoliosis = intubation and ventilation problems
    - 2. Marked short stature = intubation difficulties
- VI. Special anesthetic problems of acute injuries and illnesses
  - A. Burns = muscle relaxant interactions and electrolytes
  - B. Musculoskeletal trauma = muscle relaxant interactions involving electrolytes as well as bone displacements
  - C. Spinal cord injury = muscle relaxant interactions
  - D. Head trauma = anesthetic induction and increased intracranial pressure; possibility of basilar skull fracture and placement of oral rather than nasal tubes
  - E. Eye injury with open globe = vitreous extrusion during anesthetic induction
  - F. Drug overdose = anesthetic interactions

increasing cardiac output and oxygen delivery to the tissues. This may fail in critically ill children, in whom cardiovascular reserves may be limited. Once the hematocrit falls below 20%, tissues must extract more oxygen to meet their demands. Increased extraction may not be possible for organs such as the brain and heart, which maximally extract oxygen even at rest. Thus, all patients, except for those with a chronic anemia, for example, those in renal failure, should be transfused preoperatively for hematocrits less than 20 to 24%. On the other hand, patients suffering from chronic anemia, which has been compensated for by an increase in total plasma volume, may not require preoperative transfusions. Finally, preoperative correction of any coagulopathy is of paramount importance in patients about to undergo surgery.

Information regarding adverse reactions to previous anesthetics involving the patient, or his or her family, is also essential. Examples of important familial diseases associated with increased anesthetic mortality and morbidity include malignant hyperthermia, familial periodic paralysis, porphyria, and pseudocholinesterase deficiency. There are specific problems associated with well-known pediatric syndromes that have important anesthetic implications[336,337]. It is obvious that special attention must be paid to detecting the patient with a difficult airway. Classically, patients with the Pierre Robin, the Hunter-Hurler, the Goldenhar, or the Treacher Collins syndromes and diastrophic dwarfism have extremely difficult airways to manage **(Table 46.14).** Obviously, patients with an airway lesion such as hemangioma, lymphangioma, or with tumors or masses encroaching on the airway require special care during instrumentation of the airway. It is the patient with an unsuspected difficult airway, however, who is at greatest risk when presenting in an obtunded state or for emergency surgery. Identifying these patients early allows for better planning and greater available expertise. The ability to displace the tongue and to visualize the larynx is not an "all-or-none" phenomenon but varies in degree, depending on the size of the mandible, tongue, and neck and on the flexibility of the cervical vertebrae and temporomandibular joint. In the preoperative evaluation, the child should be asked to extend the neck and open the mouth to determine the presence of limitations. As mandibular hypoplasia results in a marked reduction of the potential space wherein the normal-sized tongue can be displaced, patients with a small jaw frequently have airways difficult to visualize. During evaluation, a lateral view of the patient is mandatory, because the presence and degree of mandibular hypoplasia otherwise are frequently underestimated.

A number of other conditions and syndromes familiar to the pediatrician have great impact on the perioperative course. One example is the association of Trisomy 21 (Down's syndrome) and subluxation of the C1-C2 vertebrae. Another example is the potential for prolonged postoperative muscle weakness in patients suffering from various myopathies. Many of these special problems are reviewed in **Table 46.14.** Two conditions that significantly affect postoperative management, namely, former premature infants and children with a history of sleep apnea will also be discussed.

Premature infants undergoing even minor surgery may require intensive postoperative monitoring due to their far greater incidence of airway-related postoperative complications, e.g., apnea, periodic breathing, atelectasis, stridor, and cyanosis. Postanesthesia-induced apnea may occur in graduates of the premature nursery until they are 60 postconceptual weeks of age[195,338–342]. Similarly, patients with a history of obstructive sleep apnea frequently undergo tonsillectomy and adenoidectomy. These patients should be admitted to the intensive care unit following anesthesia because their control of breathing may be seriously impaired in the presence of residual anesthetics and sedatives may cause apnea.

POSTOPERATIVE COMPLICATIONS OF ANESTHESIA AND SURGERY

There exists a wide spectrum of postoperative complications following anesthesia and surgery. Those involved in the postoperative care of patients need to acquaint themselves with the more common of these problems **(Table 46.15).**

Failure to Awaken

Residual Anesthetic Effect

The patient returning from the operating room who fails to awaken poses a diagnostic dilemma to the clinician. The first consideration in the differential diagnosis must be whether the patient is still anesthetized. Anesthesia is a state of induced sleep in which the response to, and recall of, painful stimulation is attenuated or abolished. This state is produced by a variety of agents, e.g., volatile inhalational agents, opioids, neuroleptics, sedatives, and barbiturates, all of which have in common the ability to depress various functions of the CNS. When determining whether a patient's failure to awaken is secondary to prolonged anesthesia, it is important to seek physical evidence suggestive of anesthetic effects and to review the predicted duration of action of the anesthetics employed. The most common anesthetic techniques employed in pediatric patients incorporate volatile inhalational agents such as halothane, enflurane, and isoflurane, usually in conjunction with an oxygen/nitrous oxide mixture[343–346]. As the anesthetic vapors are inhaled by the patient, they are delivered to the body tissues by the bloodstream according to the alveolar partial pressure of the gas, its solubility in blood and the tissues, and the regional distribution of blood flow[346]. Tissue groups that are richly perfused, e.g., brain, heart, kidney, and splanchnic bed, receive a relatively greater proportion of a given anesthetic per unit time and achieve a state approaching saturation

Text continued on page 1583.

Table 46.14. Conditions and Syndromes That Impact on the Perioperative Course

Name	*Description*	*Anesthetic Implications*
Acrocephalopolysyndactyly	See Carpenter's syndrome	
Acrocephalosyndactyly	See Apert's syndrome	
Adrenogenital syndrome	Inability to synthesize hydrocortisone; virilization of female	All need hyrocortisone, even if not salt-losing; check electrolytes preoperatively
Albers-Schöunberg disease (marble-stone disease)	Brittle bones; pathologic fractures, anemia from marrow sclerosis; hepatosplenomegaly	Care in positioning and use of restraints
Albright-Butler syndrome	Renal tubular acidosis, hypokalemia, renal calculi	Renal impairment; correct electrolytes to within normal limits
Albright's hereditary osteodystrophy	Ectopic bone formation, mental retardation Hypocalcemia: possible electrocardiogram (ECG) conduction defects, neuromuscular problems, convulsions	Check electrolytes, monitor ECG; altered response to muscle relaxants; risk of fat embolism; after osteotomy, fracture or minor trauma
Alport's syndrome	Nephritis and nerve deafness; renal pathology variable; renal failure in second to third decade	Altered renal excretion
Amyotonia congenita (infantile muscular atrophy)	Degeneration of motor neurons	Administration of succinylcholine results in hyperkalemia and cardiac arrest; use minimal doses of thiopental and curare; avoid respiratory depressants
Analbuminemia	Extremely low level of serum albumin (4–100 mg/dl)	Very sensitive to drugs that bind to protein (e.g., thiopental, curare, pancuronium)
Andersen's disease (glycogen storage disease type IV)	Deficiency of glucosyltransferase (brancher enzyme); early severe hepatic cirrhosis; liver failure; splenomegaly; hemmorrhagic tendency	Check coagulation factors preoperatively; treat excessive bleeding with fresh frozen plasma; possibility of hypoglycemia under anesthesia
	Severe midfacial hypoplasia, relative mandibular prognathism; abnormal structure and angle of mandible (triangular facies), kyphoscoliosis	Possible airway problems, and intubation may be difficult; assess respiratory status
Angioedema	Episodic brawny edema of extremities, face, trunk airway, and abdominal viscera; usually for 24–72 hr (4 hr to 1 week); onset in childhood differentiates this from idiopathic form; etiology: abnormal levels of C1 and C4 esterase inhibitor accumulation of vasoactive substances, increased vascular permeability, edema; usually painless: may have prodromal focal tingling or "tightness"; often induced by trauma or vibration; may have bouts of abdominal pain, diarrhea; hemoconcentration, resulting in hypotension, shock, pharyngeal edema (usually develops slowly); most deaths from layngeal edema; mortality rate up to 33%; long-term treat is with antifibrinolytic and hormonal agents; note well the adverse side effects of long-term use of ϵ-aminoca proic (EACA)	Check results of complement assay, hemoatocrit, fluid status, treatment history, previous drug reactions; observe for voice change or dysphasia; prophylaxis (especially in cases for dental or oropharyngeal manipulation): EACA for 2–3 days and/or fresh frozen plasma for 1 day, preoperatively; continue EACA i.v., preoperatively and postoperatively; danazol (androgen) may be useful; acute attack: give epinephrine, steroids, antihistamine; possibly fresh frozen plasma; if pharyngeal edema is imminent or develops, perform endotracheal or nasotracheal intubation (leave in place for 24–72 hr); if this is not possible, perform tracheotomy; Anesthesia: regional when possible; otherwise, use extreme care when instrumenting airway; preoperatively and postoperatively, monitor vital signs closely;
Apert's syndrome (arocephalosyndactyly)	Hypoplastic maxilla and exophthalmos; cranio synostosis, possibly with increased intracranial pressure (ICP), mental retardation, and syndactyly; congenital heart disease (CHD) may be present	If CHD is present, use antibiotic prophylaxis preoperatively; intubation may be difficult
Beckwith's syndrome (Beckwith-Wiedemann syndrome; "infantile gigantism")	Birth weight >4000 g; macroglossia and exophthalmos; visceromegaly and umbilical hernia are common; persistent severe neonatal hypoglycemia due to herinsulinism (see also neonatal hypoglycemia)	Airway problems due to large tongue; monitor blood glucose carefully and treat hypoglycemia
Behcet's syndrome	Gross ulceration of mouth (usually first sign; may extend to esophagus) and genital area; uveitis, iritis, conjunctivitis, skin lesions, nonerosive arthritis; may have vasculitis and myocardial and CNS involvement; risk of sepsis at sites of skin punctures, etc.	Use sterile technique; may have history of steroid therapy; nutritional status may be very poor; intubation may be very difficult due to scarring in pharynx
Carpenter's syndrome (acrocephalopolysyndactly)	Mental retardation, oxycephaly, peculiar facies, syndactly, deformed extremities, CHD, hypogenitalism	If CHD is present, use antibiotic prophylaxis preoperatively; hypoplastic mandible may make intubation difficult

Table 46.14. Conditions and Syndromes That Impact on the Perioperative Course (continued)

Name	*Description*	*Anesthetic Implications*
Central core disease	Muscular dystrophy; hypotonia, without muscle wasting; increased risk of malignant hyperpyrexia	Preoperatively, assess respiratory status carefully; sensitive to thiopental and respiratory depressants: avoid muscle relaxants (postoperative ventilation may be required); high risk for malignant hyperpyrexia
Chediak-Higashi syndrome	Partial albinism, immunodeficiency, hepatosplenomegaly, recurrent infections	Use reverse isolation; supplemental steroid therapy; thrombocytopenia—may require platelet
Cherubism	Fibrous dysplasia of mandibles and maxilae, with intraoral masses, may cause respiratory distress	Intubation may be extremely difficult; if there is acute respiratory distress, tracheotomy may be required
Collagen disease: dermatomyositis; polyarteritis nodosa; rheumatoid arthritis; systemic lupus erythematosus	Systemic connective tissue diseases with variable systemic involvement; osteoporosis, fatty infiltration of muscle, anemia, pulmonary infiltration, or fibrosis	Temporomandibular or cricoarytenoid arthritis may cause airway and intubation difficulties; risk of fat embolism after osteotomy, fracture, or minor trauma; supplement steroid therapy
Crouzon's disease	Craniosynostosis, hypertelorism, parrot-beak nose, hypoplastic maxilla	Intubation may be difficult
Duchenne's muscular dystrophy	Progressive pseudohypertrophy of muscles, with cardiac muscle involvement in many cases; most die in second decade	Narrow margin of safety with anesthetic agents; high risk of malignant hyperthermia (MH) susceptibility; avoid muscle relaxants
Gorlin-Chaudhry-Moss syndrome	Craniofacial dysostosis, patent ductus arteriosus (PDA), hypertrichosis, hypoplasia of labia majora, dental and eye anomalies; normal intelligence	Assymetry of head—difficult airway Problems associated with PDA
Gorlin-Goltz syndrome (basal cell nevus syndrome)	Multiple nevoid basal cell carcinomas, hypertelorism, mandibular prognathism, multiple jaw cysts and fibrosarcomas, kyphoscoliosis, incomplete segmentation of cervical and thoracic vertebrae; congenital hydrocephalus, mental retardation, etc.	Extreme care in positioning and intubating—cervical movement may be limited; increased ICP may be unrecognized
Guillain-Barré syndrome (acute idiopathic polyneuritis)	Acute polyneuropathy: progressive peripheral neuritis, usually involving cranial nerves; bulbar palsy, with hypoventilation and hypoventilation and hypotension; may require tracheotomy and intermittent positive-pressure ventilation (IPPV)	Try not to use succinylcholine for at least 3 months after onset of polyneuritis; if needed, use pretreatment with nondepolarizing drugs
Holt-Oram syndrome (heart-hand syndrome)	Upper limb abnormalities: usually atrial septal defect, possibility of sudden death from pulmonary embolus, coronary occlusion	Antibiotic prophylaxis preoperatively; problems of cardiac defect; no other anesthetic problem
Homocystinuria	Thromboembolic phenomena due to intimal thickening; extopia lentis, osteoporosis kyphoscoliosis; angiography may precipitate thrombosis, especially cerebral	Give fluids to maintain urine output; give dextran 40, to reduce viscosity and platelet adhesiveness and increase peripheral perfusion Antibiotic prophylaxis and chest physiotherapy preoperatively; give large dose of atropine preoperatively; upper airway obstruction and difficult intubation, due to infiltration of lymphoid tissue and larynx and profuse thick secretions; give adequate fluids preoperatively and humidify anesthetic gases
I cell disease (mucolipidosis)	Mental retardation, Hurler-type bone changes, severe joint limitation, chronic pulmonary disease; valvar insufficiency common; death in early childhood (most by 1 yr of age)	Intubation and airway maintenance difficult—limited jaw movement, stiffness of neck and rib cage
Klippel-Feil syndrome	Congenital fusion of two or more cervical vertebrae causing neck rigidity	Intubation may be difficult; should be performed with the patient awake; if possible; otherwise, inhalation induction without muscle relaxant should be performed; do not extubate until patient is fully awake
Maple syrup urine disease (branched-chain ketonuria)	Inability to metabolize leucine, isoleucine, and valine; severe neurologic damage and respiratory disturbances; episodes of hypoglycemia; treated by diet only, from birth; many die within 2 months; acute, life-threatening episodes may require peritoneal dialysis or exchange transfusion	Check acid-base balance and plasma amino acids preoperatively; check serum glucose preoperatively, perioperatively, and postoperatively; state glucose infusion (at least 10–15 mg/kg/min) preoperatively and continue until diet is reestablished

Table 46.14. Conditions and Syndromes That Impact on the Perioperative Course (continued)

Name	*Description*	*Anesthetic Implications*
Marfan's syndrome (arachnodactyly)	Connective tissue disorder; dilation and possible dissection of aortic root, resulting in aortic insufficiency; aortic, thoracic, or abdominal aneurysm; kyphoscoliosis, pectus excavatum; lung cysts; joint instability and dislocation	Antibiotic prophylaxis preoperatively; intubation may be difficult; position carefully to avoid dislocations; avoid hypertension due to aortic dissection; controlled ventilation may result in pneumothorax
Myasthenia congenita	Similar to myasthenia gravis in adults	Do not use respiratory depressants or muscle relaxants; IPPV may be required postoperatively; possibility of cholinergic crisis with anticholinesterase therapy
Myositis ossificans (Fibrodysplasia ossificans progressiva)	Bony infiltration of tendons, fascia, aponeuroses, and muscle; thoracic involvement greatly reduces thoracic compliance; progressive respiratory failure	Check respiratory function and history of steroid therapy; airway and intubation problems if neck is rigid and mouth is fixed
Myotonia congenita	Decreased ability to relax muscles after contraction; diffuse hypertrophy of muscle	Do not use muscle relaxants or respiratory depressants; MH susceptible Check respiratory function; do not use succinylcholine (which cause myotonia in 50%); nondepolarizing drugs do not produce good relaxation; neostigmine induces myotonia; halothane may cause shivering and myotonia postoperatively; extremely sensitive to respiratory depressants—use regional or inhalational agents, with IPPV postoperatively, if necessary; monitor ECG carefully; anticipate postoperative pulmonary complications
Osteogenesis imperfecta	Pathologic fractures, blue sclera, deafness; kyphoscoliosis; fragility of vessels; dentin deficiency results in carious, fragile teeth	Use extreme care in positioning and intubating; teeth are easily broken; hypothermic response to atropine
Phenylketonuria	Phenylalanine hydroxylase deficiency; vomiting, CNS irritability, mental retardation, hypertonia, and convulsions; phenylalanine-deficient diet must be maintained	Induction and maintenance by inhalation technique; control ventilation; give 10% dextrose infusion (tendency to hypoglycemia); hypersensitive to narcotics and other CNS depressants; do not use ketamine or enflurane; monitor body temperature carefully; if epileptic, continue drugs
Pierre Robin syndrome	Cleft palate, micrognathia, glossoptosis; CHD in some; neonates: respiratory obstruction may occur; maintain airway and require tongue suture, intubation, or tracheotomy	Intubation may be very difficult; use awake technique; patient should be fully awake before extubation
Progeria (Hutchinson-Gilford syndrome)	Premature aging starts at 6 months to 3 yrs; cardiac disease—ischemia, hypertension, cardiomegaly; death from coronary artery disease may occur before 10 yr of age	Anesthesia as for adults with myocardial ischemia
Prune belly syndrome	Agenesis of abdominal musculature, with renal anomalies (respiration requires use of accessory muscles); poor cough mechanism, respiratory infections; may have renal insufficiency.	Check renal status; treat as for full stomach; minimize use of muscle relaxants
Riley-Day syndrome (familial dysautonomia)	Deficiency of dopamine β-hydroxylase; hypertensive and hypotensive attacks, emotional lability, absent lacrimation, abnormal sweating, insensitivity to pain, and poor sucking and swallowing; recurrent aspiration pneumonia and chronic lung disease	Labile blood pressure hypersensitive to adrenergic and cholinergic drugs; respiratory center insensitive to CO_2—IPPV is necessary; beware of aspiration potential during postoperative period (see text)
Scleroderma	Diffuse cutaneous stiffening; may have hemifacial atrophy; plastic surgery is required for contractures and constrictions; may have cardiac fibrosis or corpulmonale	Scarring of face and mouth—difficult airway and intubation; chest restriction—poor compliance; diffuse pulmonary fibrosis— hypoxia; venous access limited; check history of steroid therapy
Treacher Collins syndrome (mandibulofacial dysostosis)	Micrognathia, aplastic zygomatic arches, microstomia, choanal atresia; CHD may be present	Possible airway and intubation difficulties (less severe than with Pierre Robin deformity)
von Hippel-Lindau disease	Retinal angiomas and cerebellar hemangioblastomas; pheochromocytoma in some; may have pulmonary, pancreatic, hepatic, adrenal, or renal cysts; paroxysmal hypertension, due to cerebellar tumor or pheochromocytoma	Assess renal and hepatic function and investigate for pheochromocytoma (urinary vanillyl mandelic acid [VMA]); hypertensive crises may occur

Table 46.14. Conditions and Syndromes That Impact on the Perioperative Course (continued)

Name	*Description*	*Anesthetic Implications*
von Recklinghausen's disease (neurofibromatosis)	Café-au-lait spots; tumors, all parts of the CNS (and may be in larynx and right ventricular outflow tract): peripheral tumors associated with nerve trunks; kyphoscoliosis in 50%; may have "honeycomb (cystic) lung"; pheochromocytoma and renal artery dysplasia (hypertension) are common	All these patients should be investigated for pheochromocytoma (urinary VMA); test response to neuromuscular drugs—effects of depolarizing and nondepolarizing muscle relaxants may be prolonged; check pulmonary and renal function; if kidneys are affected, treat with drugs excreted by kidneys
von Willebrand disease (pseudohemophilia)	Prolonged bleeding time (decreased factor VIII activity, resulting in defective platelet adhesiveness) and capillary abnormality	Bleeding can be controlled by transfusions of fresh blood or fresh frozen plasma and/or cryoprecipitate; do not use salicylates
Werdnig-Hoffmann disease (infantile muscular atrophy)	Earlier onset and more severe than Welander's muscular atrophy; feeding difficulties: aspiration of stomach contents; chronic respiratory problems; most die before puberty	Minimal anesthesia is required; do not use muscle relaxants or respiratory depressant drugs; and weaning from this may be difficult; ventilatory support may be required

steady-state in about 20 min. The partial pressure in the brain tissue determines the depth of anesthesia and correlates to the alveolar partial pressure of the agent. By adjustment of the inspired concentration of the gas, the partial pressure of the agent in the alveolus, and thus, the brain concentration, is altered, since only minute amounts of anesthetic enter the lesser perfused tissues during the maintenance of anesthesia. The rapidity with which an inhalational induction proceeds is determined by two factors: (a) the rate of delivery of the agent to the alveolus, which is a function of minute ventilation and inspired concentration; and (b) the rate of removal of the agent from the alveolus, which is determined by cardiac output and agent solubility[346]. Nitrous oxide, a relatively insoluble anesthetic, achieves steady-state within 5 to 10 min. Conversely, halothane, with a solubility coefficient greater than threefold that of nitrous oxide, requires 15 to 20 min to approach a steady state. Emergence or awakening from inhalational anesthesia entails the reversal of these processes. That is, the agent leaves the tissue compartment according to partial pressure gradients and solubility to enter the alveolus for subsequent elimination. The rate of egress is dependent on the alveolar partial pressure creating the gradient and, hence, the minute ventilation, the cardiac output, and the solubility of the agent. In addition, the depth and duration of the anesthetic plays a role in the rate of emergences. In the case of a brief anesthetic, where vessel-poor tissues remain unsaturated owing to their continuing uptake, the speed of recovery is enhanced. The converse is also true. Halothane undergoes hepatic metabolism to a considerable degree once hepatic maturation is attained. Enflurane undergoes far less hepatic metabolism, and along with nitrous oxide and isoflurane, the contribution to reawakening is considered negligible. Factors that depress minute ventilation or cardiac output slow the rate of emergence from anesthesia and should be ruled out in the unarousable postoperative patient. In the presence of a normal minute ventilation and cardiac output, emergence from inhalational anesthesia is usually complete within 15 to 30 min. Recovery from nitrous oxide, due to its low solubility, is complete within 3 to 10 min.

Persistent opioid effect following anesthesia also renders the patient apneic and unresponsive. Generally, this occurs when very large doses of opioids are given for relatively short procedures or when a sedative agent has been administered concomitantly. If the patient fails to initiate respiratory efforts while artificially ventilated, an adequate arterial carbon dioxide pressure ($PaCO_2$) must be ensured, as the carbon dioxide response curve is shifted to the right by both opioids and volatile agents. It is not uncommon to be able to stimulate the narcotized patient to breathe but to find that, without stimulation, apnea ensues despite increasing hypercarbia and hypoxemia. Extremely high levels of PCO_2 may be achieved and may result in hypercarbic narcosis and alterations in acid/base homeostasis. When confronted with this situation, then, it is advisable to maintain a high normal PCO_2 to ensure that residual volatile anesthetics are excreted and narcosis secondary to hypercarbia is avoided. Finally, if excessive opioid administration is thought to be the cause of failure to awaken, great caution must be exercised in antagonizing these effects with naloxone. As discussed above, naloxone antagonizes all of the agonist effects of opioids including analgesia. In many postoperative situations, it is far kinder to ventilate a patient than to remove analgesia.

Table 46.15. Etiology of Postoperative Failure to Awaken

I. Residual anesthetic effect
II. Neuromuscular blockade
III. Metabolic and electrolyte disorders
  A. Hypernatremia or hyponatremia
  B. Diabetic ketoacidosis
  C. Severe hypokalemia
  D. Hypercarbia
IV. CNS event
  A. Postictal
  B. Pneumocephalus
  C. Embolic event
    1. Air embolism
    2. Cardioarterial thromboembolism
  D. Hypoxic CNS injury
  E. Intracranial mass lesion and/or intracranial hypertension

Neuromuscular Blockade

Once the likelihood of residual anesthetic effect is assessed to be remote, the possibility of residual neuromuscular blockade, which can render the patient unable to breathe or to demonstrate a motor response to stimulation despite autonomic and ocular reactivity, must be considered. Neuromuscular blocking agents are widely employed in pediatric anesthesia to facilitate intubation, to provide surgically indicated muscle relaxation, and to reduce the requirement for volatile agents, the therapeutic index of which is reduced in infancy and childhood.

Currently employed neuromuscular blocking agents can be divided into two types, depolarizing and nondepolarizing agents **(Table 46.16)** [347–360]. Of the depolarizing agents decamethonium and succinylcholine, only the latter finds clinical application. Succinylcholine mimics acetylcholine in its structure, binding to the acetylcholine receptor at the motor endplate in a noncompetitive fashion, resulting in depolarization. This is manifest in older children and adults by a phase of muscular fasciculation. Muscle fasiculations increase intragastric, intraocular, and intracranial pressure. They may also be associated with the development of the myalgias that are so common after succinylcholine administration. Interestingly, children under the age of 4 yr may not fasciculate.

The disappearance of muscle fasciculation heralds the onset of a brief period of profound neuromuscular paralysis as succinylcholine continues to occupy the receptor. Succinylcholine subsequently diffuses off the receptor and is metabolized by plasma and hepatic pseudocholinesterase. Newborn infants are relatively resistant to the effects of succinylcholine when dose requirements are compared with adults on a milligram-to-kilogram basis[360]. This is probably due to their increased volume of distribution. In fact, the neonate requires about twice as much succinylcholine (expressed in milligrams per kilogram) as does the adult to produce a 50% neuromuscular blockade. Compared with adults, the dose responsiveness for infants and children is fairly constant when the dose is expressed in milligrams per square meter, reflecting the nearly linear relationship throughout life of body surface area and extracellular fluid volume.

Table 46.16. Neuromuscular Blocking Agents

Agents	*Intubation Dose (mg/kg)*	*Maintenance Dose (mg/kg)*	*Estimated Duration of Action (min)*
Nondepolarizing			
Pancuronium (Pavulon)	0.06–0.1	0.04–0.06	45–60
Rocuronium (Zemuron)	0.6–1.2	0.3–0.6	30–60
d-Tubocurarine (curare)	0.5–0.6	0.3–0.4	45–50
Mivacurium (Mivacron)	0.2–0.4	0.1–0.2	10–15
Atracurium (Tracrium)	0.4–0.5	0.08–0.10	20–35
Vecuronium[a] (Norcuron)	0.08–0.1	0.01–0.015	25–30
Depolarizing			
Succinylcholine	1.0–2.0	Not generally given	5–7

[a] *Infants 7 weeks to 1 yr are more sensitive to vecuronium than are others and require about 1 1/2 times as long to recover.*

Redistribution and metabolism of succinylcholine determine the duration of its neuromuscular blockade. Despite a lower plasma concentration of pseudocholinesterase in infancy, the redistribution of succinylcholine from a relatively small muscle mass to a large extracellular fluid compartment quickly terminates the neuromuscular blocking effects. With prolonged or repeated exposure to succinylcholine, the membrane repolarizes but remains refractory to subsequent depolarization by acetylcholine. A so-called "phase II block" results, the clinical characteristics of which resemble a nondepolarizing block blockade. The exact mechanism of this blockade has not been elucidated.

The neuromuscular blockade following succinylcholine can be prolonged if the patient has an abnormal, genetically derived variant of pseudocholinesterase **(Table 46.17).** The diagnosis of this disorder relies on clinical history of prolonged neuromuscular blockade following standard doses of succinylcholine and may be substantiated by assaying the plasma pseudocholinesterase inhibition by dibucaine. A positive family history is supportive evidence for the diagnosis. Management should consist of controlled ventilation with sedation until the block spontaneously dissipates. Although the administration of blood or plasma has been advocated for the treatment of this disorder, it cannot be recommended because of the inherent risks involved with this approach. Hepatic dysfunction, hypermagnesemia, and pregnancy are also associated with a prolonged blockade following succinylcholine administration.

Because a variety of side effects accompanies the administration of succinylcholine, many pediatric anesthesiologists have condemned its continued use for routine intubation. Succinylcholine stimulates all cholinergic autonomic receptors: nicotinic receptors of both sympathetic and parasympathetic ganglia and muscarinic receptors in the sinus node of the heart. This results in a negative inotropic and chronotropic effect following an initial dose. In children, in whom the parasympathetic tone predominates, severe bradycardia and even sinus arrest may occur. The bradycardia occurs with greater frequency and severity following a second dose of succinylcholine in older children and adults. It can be effectively blocked by pretreatment with atropine (0.02 mg/kg, minimum dose 0.15 mg) or glycopyrrolate (0.01 mg/kg). Succinylcholine, under stable anesthetic conditions, lowers the threshold of ventricular stimulation by catecholamines. Other autonomic stimuli, such as hypoxia, hypercarbia, endotracheal intubation, and surgical stress, are additive to this effect of succinylcholine and commonly yield a wide variety of ventricular dysrhythmias.

A rise in potassium (0.5 mEq/liter) generally accompanies succinylcholine administration, even in normal pa-

Table 46.17. Factors Prolonging Neuromuscular Blockade

Depolarizing Blockade	*Nondepolarizing Blockade*
Deficient pseudocholinesterase	Hypothermia
Genetically derived abnormal variant	Respiratory acidosis
Pregnancy	Hypermagnesemia
Anticholinesterase-containing medication	Hypokalemia
Hepatic dysfunction	Antibiotic administration
Hypermagnesemia	Aminoglycosides
	Tetracyclines
	Lincomycins
	Polymyxins

tients. In the presence of crush injuries, burns, paralysis, neuromuscular disease, or preexisting hyperkalemia, the succinylcholine-induced rise in potassium may be catastrophic and must be avoided. Increases in intraocular pressure following intramuscular or intravenous administration of succinylcholine may result in extrusion of the vitreous and permanent loss of vision in patients with open globe injuries. This effect is not eliminated by pretreatment with small doses of nondepolarizing muscle relaxants. Additionally, Ryan et al. noted a 40% incidence of myoglobinemia in prepubertal patients following the administration of standard doses of succinylcholine with the concomitant use of halothane. The clinical significance of this observation remains to be demonstrated. Cook et al.[359] reported an episode of acute fulminate pulmonary edema following the administration of 4 mg succinylcholine per kilogram intramuscularly, which was attributed to an acute elevation of pulmonary vascular resistance. The occurrence of this complication must be extremely rare, considering the widespread usage of this agent and the paucity of reports. Finally, succinylcholine is associated with the development of severe myalgias in 10 to 30 of patients who receive the drug. The incidence of this pain is reduced in children and may be further reduced by pretreatment with calcium gluconate or with a small dose of a nondepolarizing muscle relaxant.

Succinylcholine is unique in that it produces muscle paralysis virtually instantaneously whether it is administered intravenously (1 to 2 mg/kg) or intramuscularly (4 to 5 mg/kg). Typically, a paralyzing dose of succinylcholine produces paralysis within a minute of administration. This makes it the most ideal agent, despite its many known side effects, for rapid sequence intubations when the risk of pulmonary aspiration of stomach contents is high.

Nondepolarizing neuromuscular blockade results from the administration of pancuronium, d-tubocurare, rocuronium, mivacarium, atracurium, and vecuronium. They represent false transmitters that combine in a competitive fashion with the presynaptic and postsynaptic acetylcholine receptors, resulting in muscular relaxation without producing depolarization. Because of the large margin of safety in the design of neuromuscular transmission, 75 to 80% of the acetylcholine receptors must be occupied before the response to a single 0.1-Hz impulse, the twitch response, becomes apparent. Once 90 to 95% of the receptors are occupied, neuromuscular transmission fails. At birth, neuromuscular transmission is immature, resulting in an altered sensitivity to neuromuscular blocking agents and a heightened risk of respiratory inadequacy in the presence of residual neuromuscular blockade. Dose-response curves for pancuronium, metocurine, and atracurium fail to reveal significant differences among infants, children, and adults. Infants appear to be more sensitive to the effects of d-tubocurare; however, owing to the larger volume of distribution, dosage requirements are unaltered. Vecuronium, an intermediate-acting nondepolarizing neuromuscular blocker in children and adults, demonstrates longer duration of action in infants less than 2 months of age.

The presence of residual neuromuscular blockade can be evaluated by using a peripheral nerve stimulator. The poles of the stimulator are placed over the peripheral nerve as depicted in Figure 46.9, usually the ulnar nerve at the wrist or elbow, and an impulse is applied. The twitch response of the adductor pollicis and flexor digitorum muscles to specific types of electrical stimulation give clues to the presence or absence of blockade. The nondepolarizing neuromuscular blockade is characterized by (a) decreased contraction to a single impulse, (b) unsustained response to tetanic stimulation of 50 Hz at 2.5 sec, (c) diminution of the fourth twitch response compared with the first twitch response, of greater than 70% following four 2-Hz stimuli (train of four), (d) facilitation of the contractile response following tetanic stimulation, and (e) antagonism by acetylcholinesterase inhibitors. Abolition of the fourth twitch response of the train of four correlates with a 75% reduction in standard twitch tension. It must be remembered, however, that magnitude and duration of the impulse influence the twitch response and that twitch response is not altered until greater than 75% of the receptors are blocked. Minute ventilation is generally adequate when less than 75% blockade is present in adults. In the pediatric patient, there is a diminished functional residual capacity and muscle mass and a higher incidence of postextubation airway obstruction. As a result, additional evidence of adequate reversal should be sought to ensure their ability to maintain adequate ventilation, e.g., the ability to sustain leg raise or a hand grip and the ability to sustain a head lift for more than 5 sec.

In the presence of persistent nondepolarizing neuromuscular blockade, antagonism can usually be achieved once a twitch response becomes apparent. Reversal involves inhibition of acetylcholinesterase degradation of acetylcholine, allowing its concentration to rise and displace the neuromuscular blocking agent competitively from the receptor. Agents commonly employed include neostigmine (0.07 mg/kg), edrophonium (1 mg/kg), and pyridostigmine (0.2 mg/kg) administered intravenously[361–364]. Because significant muscarinic effects are exerted by these agents, they should always be combined with atropine (0.02 mg/kg) or glycopyrrolate (0.01 mg/ kg). The effect of edrophonium is very prompt, reaching a maximum within 1 min following intravenous administration. Neostigmine and pyridostigmine have a slower onset of action beginning 3 min after injection and achieving their maximal effect at 10 to 15 min.

The presence of hypokalemia, respiratory acidosis, hypermagnesemia, and hypothermia and the administration of many antibiotics can result in failure of reversal, or the recurrence of blockade **(Table 46.17)** [365–367]. This is sometimes referred to as "recurarization," and follows what was perceived to be adequate reversal **(Table 46.17).** Hypothermia, per se, may result in respiratory insufficiency in infants. The more common antibiotic interactions occur following aminoglycosides, tetracyclines, lincomycins, and polymyxins; however, it does not occur with penicillin. Numerous other pharmacologic agents potentiate the nondepolarizing neuromuscular blockade: local anesthetics (e.g., quinidine), calcium channel blockers, trimethaphan, nitroglycerine, high-dose corticosteroids, and alkylating cytotoxic agents. Patients with myasthenia gravis, any of the muscular dystrophies, myotonia, renal insufficiency, and hypoproteinemia demonstrate increased sensitivity to neuromuscular blocking agents.

If the presence of residual neuromuscular blockade has been established and attempts to reverse the blockade have failed, prudent management dictates continued ventilatory support and sedation until such time as the block spontaneously resolves.

Metabolic and Electrolyte Disorders

Once the presence of residual anesthetic or neuromuscular blockade is excluded, other causes of failure to awaken postoperatively must be evaluated. Disorders in fluid and electrolyte homeostasis, such as hypernatremia or hyponatremia, diabetic ketoacidosis, hyperosmolar nonketotic coma, and hypoglycemia, must be excluded. Hypokalemia may result in marked muscular weakness, mimicking a state of neuromuscular blockade. Profound hypercarbia with $PaCO_2$ levels in excess of 80 to 90 mm Hg may render the patient unarousable. In this situation, sufficient fresh gas flow to prevent rebreathing must be ensured. Rapid normalization of the hypercarbic state occasionally results in arrhythmias in elderly patients suffering from myocardial impairment. This complication is exceedingly rare in pediatric patients. However, rapid assessment of the major cations, glucose, $Pa0_2$, and $PaCO_2$ should be obtained in the case of an unarousable postoperative patient.

Hyponatremia deserves special attention. Hyponatremia, particularly following urologic endoscopy, is a common postoperative anesthetic problem. During cystoscopy, the cystoscope is continuously irrigated with water. Absorption of free water through the bladder or through a perforation is very possible. Similarly, overzealous fluid replacement during any surgery with salt poor crystalloid solutions (D5.2NS) can result in dilutional hyponatremia. Children who are hyponatremic may be agitated, confused, or unarousable. When serum sodium levels acutely fall below 110 to 120 mEq/liter, seizures may occur. Indeed, if hyponatremic seizures do occur, they should be treated with hypertonic (3%) saline emergently.

Central Nervous System Events

Ultimately, the possibility of a perioperative CNS event must be entertained. A wide variety of such events may alter the postoperative state of consciousness. In the presence of a positive history of a seizure disorder, head trauma, or intracranial surgery, the possibility exists that a seizure has occurred in the course of surgery, masked by the use of neuromuscular blocking agents. The patient is then comatose because he or she is postictal. Transient paresis may become apparent as the patient awakens. The clinical course and electroencephalographic data are the major diagnostic aids.

Pneumocephalus may occur in the course of a craniotomy or with a malfunctioning ventricular drain, particularly if nitrous oxide is used during anesthesia. Pneumocephalus has been documented to produce a state of unarousability, particularly when tension results in brainstem traction. It generally resolves over the subsequent 24 to 72 hr, usually without residual. Skull films permit the diagnosis of intracranial air. A computerized axial tomography (CAT) scan may be necessary to allow exclusion of tension pneumocephalus.

All patients undergoing open-heart surgery with extracorporeal circulation and patients with known intracardiac shunts, regardless of the predominant flow direction, are at increased risk for systemic air embolism. Because of the high incidence (10 to 20%) of a probe patent foramen ovale in the pediatric population, great care to avoid intravascular air injection must be taken in every child. Air embolism affects primarily the myocardium and the CNS, resulting in an acute anoxic event. Ventricular electrical instability and electrocardiographic changes consistent with an ischemic insult are the most frequently encountered myocardial effects. Neurologic deficits, as with any embolic phenomenon, depend on the location of the occluded vessel(s) and the extent of embolization. Cardioarterial thromboembolism most frequently occurs in the presence of damaged or prosthetic valves, aneurysmal dilatation, and atrial fibrillation. The majority of these thrombi lodge distally at the bifurcation of the major vessels supplying the extremities, kidneys, or splanchnic bed. About 20 to 25%, however, do lodge in the cerebral circulation, most commonly at the middle cerebral artery, resulting in an altered state of consciousness, seizures, and variable focal deficits. Fat emboli result primarily from bone trauma and are generally filtered by the pulmonary circulation. In the presence of an intracardiac septal defect or a massive embolic load, right ventricular failure and/or systemic embolization involving the myocardium, brain, and kidneys may occur.

The presence of an intracranial mass lesion, hemorrhage, or global brain edema must be included in the differential evaluation of an unarousable patient, particularly following trauma or intracranial surgery. Patients who have presented to the operating room with intracranial hypertension of whatever etiology are at significant risk of developing intracranial pressure elevations resulting in herniation or cerebral hypoperfusion during transport to the operating room, induction of anesthesia, and endotracheal intubation. For the patient suspected of having intracranial hypertension, therefore, appropriate intracranial pressure and systemic arterial pressure monitoring should be initiated prior to these maneuvers whenever clinically feasible. Continuous recording of mean systemic arterial pressure and intracranial pressure affords the best opportunity to ensure an adequate cerebral perfusion pressure by aggressively treating intracranial pressure elevation and maintaining systemic arterial and cerebral perfusion pressures.

Many safeguarding mechanisms have been developed to prevent the delivery of hypoxic gas mixtures to patients receiving anesthesia. Hypoxic brain injury secondary to hypoxic gas mixtures, to inappropriate ventilation, or to inadequate cerebral perfusion remains nevertheless an important differential diagnostic consideration in any patient who fails to awaken. In the absence of residual anesthetics, careful serial neurologic examinations, CAT scan, and evoked potentials may support the diagnosis. In the absence of clear-cut evidence of such an event, the diagnosis remains one of exclusion.

In summary, the patient who fails to awaken postoperatively requires assessment of the anesthetic agents employed, the anesthetic course, and the degree of neuromuscular blockade. Once the contribution of these factors to the altered state of consciousness is judged to be negligible, immediate chemical analyses and neurologic assessment are indicated while respiratory and hemodynamic stability are maintained.

References

1. Owens ME. Pain in infancy: conceptual and methodological issues. Pain 1984;20:213–230.
2. Schechter NL. The undertreatment of pain in children: an overview. Pediatr Clin North Am 1989;36:781–794.
3. Schechter NL, Allen D. Physicians' attitudes toward pain in children. J Dev Behav Pediatr 1986;7:350–354.
4. Schechter NL, Allen DA, Hanson K. Status of pediatric pain control: a comparison of hospital analgesic usage in children and adults. Pediatrics 1986;77:11–15.
5. Pigeon HM, McGrath PJ, Lawrence J, MacMurray SB. Nurses' perceptions of pain in the neonatal intensive care unit. J Pain Symptom Manage 1989;4:179–183.
6. McGrath PJ, Craig KD. Developmental and psychological factors in children's pain. Pediatr Clin North Am 1989; 36:823–836.
7. Beyer JE, Wells N. The assessment of pain in children. Pediatr Clin North Am 1989;36:837–854.
8. Beyer JE, Bournaki MC. Assessment and management of postoperative pain in children. Pediatrician 1989;16:30–38.
9. Beyer JE, Ashley LC, Russell GA, DeGood DE. Pediatric pain after cardiac surgery: pharmacologic management. Dimens Crit Care Nurs 1984;3:326–334.
10. Beyer JE, DeGood DE, Ashley LC, Russell GA. Patterns of postoperative analgesic use with adults and children following cardiac surgery. Pain 1983;17:71–81.
11. McGrath PJ, Unruh AM. Pain in children and adolescents. Amsterdam: Elsevier, 1987:1–351.
12. Ross DM, Ross SA. Childhood pain: the school-aged child's viewpoint. Pain 1984;20:179–191.
13. Kehlet H. Pain relief and modification of the stress response. In: Cousins MJ, Phillips GD, eds. Acute pain management. New York: Churchill Livingstone, 1986:49–76.
14. Yaster M, Maxwell LG. The management of acute pain in children. In: Hoekelman RA, Friedman SB, Nelson NM, Seidel HM, eds. Primary pediatric care. St. Louis: Mosby Year Book, 1992:302–317.
15. Anand KJ. Neonatal stress responses to anesthesia and surgery. Clin Perinatol 1990;17:207–214.
16. Platt MP, Anand KJ, Aynsley Green A. The ontogeny of the metabolic and endocrine stress response in the human fetus, neonate and child. Intensive Care Med 1989;15:S44–S45.
17. Anand KJ, Hickey PR. Pain and its effects in the human neonate and fetus. N Engl J Med 1987;317:1321–1329.
18. Mather L, Mackie J. The incidence of postoperative pain in children. Pain 1983;15:271–282.
19. McGrath PJ, Craig KD. Developmental and psychological factors in children's pain. Pediatr Clin North Am 1989; 36:823–836.
20. Anand KJ, Carr DB. The neuroanatomy, neurophysiology, and neurochemistry of pain, stress, and analgesia in newborns and children. Pediatr Clin North Am 1989;36:795–822.
21. Yaster M. Analgesia and anesthesia in neonates. J Pediatr 1987; 111:394–396.
22. Truog R, Anand KJ. Management of pain in the postoperative neonate. Clin Perinatol 1989;16:61–78.
23. Yaster M, Deshpande JK, Maxwell LG. The pharmacologic management of pain in children. Compr Ther 1989;15:14–26.
24. Yaster M, Deshpande JK. Management of pediatric pain with opioid analgesics. J Pediatr 1988;113:421–429.
25. Berde CB. Pediatric postoperative pain management. Pediatr Clin North Am 1989;36:921–940.
26. Shannon M, Berde CB. Pharmacologic management of pain in children and adolescents. Pediatr Clin North Am 1989;36:855–871.
27. Mather LE, Phillips GD. Opioids and adjuvants: principles of use. In: Cousins MJ, Phillips GD, eds. Acute pain management. New York: Churchill Livingstone, 1986:77–104.
28. McGrath PJ, Johnson GG. Pain management in children. Can J Anaesth 1988;35:107–110.
29. Eland JM. Pharmacologic management of acute and chronic pediatric pain. Issues Compr Pediatr Nurs 1988;11:93–111.
30. Rana SR. Pain: a subject ignored. Pediatrics 1987;79:309–310.
31. Weis OF, Sriwatanakul K, Alloza JL, Weintraub M, Lasagna L. Attitudes of patients, housestaff, and nurses toward postoperative analgesic care. Anesth Analg 1983;62:70–74.
32. Cohen FL. Postsurgical pain relief: patient's status and nurse's medication choices. Pain 1980;9:265–274.
33. Beyer JE, Levin CR. Issues and advances in pain control in children. Nurs Clin North Am 1987;22:661–676.
34. Eland JM. The child who is hurting. Semin Oncol Nurs 1985; 1:116–122.
35. Ross DM, Ross SA. Assessment of pediatric pain: an overview. Issues Compr Pediatr Nurs 1988;11:73–91.
36. OHara M, McGrath PJ, DAstous J, Vair CA. Oral morphine versus injected meperidine (Demerol) for pain relief in children after orthopedic surgery. J Pediatr Orthop 1987;7:78–82.
37. Caswell LJ, Eland JM. "Don't bump my bed, don't touch my feet!" J Pediatr Oncol Nurs 1989;6:111–120.
38. Burokas L. Factors affecting nurses' decisions to medicate pediatric patients after surgery. Heart Lung 1985;14:373–379.
39. Marks RM, Sacher EJ. Under treatment of medical inpatients with narcotic analgesics. Ann Intern Med 1973;78:173–181.
40. Phillips GD, Cousins MJ. Neurological mechanisms of pain and the relationship of pain, anxiety, and sleep. In: Cousins MJ, Phillips GD, eds. Acute pain management. New York: Churchill Livingstone, 1986:21–48.
41. Behbehani M. Physiology of pain. In: Raj PP, ed. Practical management of pain. Chicago: Year Book, 1986:61–77.
42. Strichartz GR. Neural physiology and local anesthetic action. In: Cousins MJ, Bridenbaugh PO, eds. Neural blockade in clinical anesthesia and management of pain. Philadelphia: JB Lippincott, 1988:25–46.
43. Lynn B. The detection of injury and tissue damage. In: Wall PD, Melzack R, eds. Textbook of pain. New York: Churchill Livingstone, 1985:19–33.
44. Amadio P, Jr. Peripherally acting analgesics. Am J Med 1984; 77:17–26.
45. Cuello AC, Matthews MR. Peptides in peripheral sensory nerve fibres. In: Wall PD, Melzack R, eds. Management of pain. New York: Churchill Livingstone, 1985:65–79.
46. Wall PD. The dorsal horn. In: Wall PD, Melzack R, eds. Management of pain. New York: Churchill Livingstone, 1985:80–87.
47. Fitzgerald M. The course and termination of primary afferent fibres. In: Wall PD, Melzack R, eds. Textbook of pain. New York: Churchill Livingstone, 1985:34–48.
48. McGrath PJ, Unruh AM. The nature of pain. In: McGrath PJ, Unruh AM, eds. Pain in children and adolescents. Amsterdam: Elsevier, 1987:47–72.

49. Hammond DL, Yaksh TL. Peripheral and central pathways in pain. Pharmacol Ther 1983;12:33–49.
50. Issenman J, Nolan MF, Rowley J, Hobby R. Transcutaneous electrical nerve stimulation for pain control after spinal fusion with Harrington rods. A clinical report. Phys Ther 1985;65:1517–1520.
51. Carman D, Roach JW. Transcutaneous electrical nerve stimulation for the relief of postoperative pain in children. Spine 1988;13:109–110.
52. Wang WC, George SL, Williams JA. Transcutaneous electrical nerve stimulation treatment of sickle cell pain crises. Acta Haematol (Basel) 1988;80:99–102.
53. Millan MJ. Multiple opioid systems and pain. Pain 1986;27:303–347.
54. Willis WD. The origin and destination of pathways involved in pain transmission. In: Wall PD, Melzack R, eds. Management of pain. New York: Churchill Livingstone, 1985:88–99.
55. Terenius L. The endogenous opioids and other central peptides. In: Wall PD, Melzack R, eds. Management of pain. New York: Churchill Livingstone, 1985:133–141.
56. Cousins MJ, Mather LE. Intrathecal and epidural administration of opioids. Anesthesiology 1984;61:276–310.
57. Cousins MJ, Bridenbaugh PO. Spinal opioids and pain relief in acute care. In: Cousins MJ, Phillips GD, eds. Acute pain management. New York: Churchill Livingstone, 1986:151–186.
58. Wood PL. Multiple opiate receptors: support for unique μ, δ, and κ sites. Neuropharmacology 1982;21:487–497.
59. Jaffe JH, Martin WR. Opioid analgesics and antagonists. In: Gillman AG, Goodman LS, Rall TW, Murad F, eds. The pharmacologic basis of therapeutics. New York: Macmillan, 1985:495–534.
60. Snyder SH. Drug and neurotransmitter receptors in the brain. Science 1984;224:22–31.
61. Yaksh TL, Al Rodhan NR, Jensen TS. Sites of action of opiates in production of analgesia. Prog Brain Res 1988;77:371–394.
62. Yaksh TL. CNS mechanisms of pain and analgesia. Cancer Surv 1988;7:5–28.
63. Yaksh TL. Spinal opiates: a review of their effect on spinal function with emphasis on pain processing. Acta Anaesthesiol Scand Suppl 1987;85:25–37.
64. Yaksh TL. Multiple opioid receptor systems in brain and spinal cord: Part 2. Eur J Anaesthesiol 1984;1:201–243.
65. Mersky H. Pain terms: a list with definitions and notes on usage. Recommended by the IASP subcommittee on taxonomy. Pain 1979; 6:249–252.
66. Aradine CR, Beyer JE, Tompkins JM. Children's pain perception before and after analgesia: a study of instrument construct validity and related issues. J Pediatr Nurs 1988;3:11–23.
67. Beyer JE, Aradine CR. Content validity of an instrument to measure young children's perceptions of the intensity of their pain. J Pediatr Nurs 1986;1:386–395.
68. Varni JW, Walco GA, Katz ER. Assessment and management of chronic and recurrent pain in children with chronic diseases. Pediatrician 1989;16:56–63.
69. Elliott CH, Jay SM, Woody P. An observation scale for measuring children's distress during medical procedures. J Pediatr Psychol 1987;12:543–551.
70. Katz ER, Varni JW, Jay SM. Behavioral assessment and management of pediatric pain. Prog Behav Modif 1984;18:163–193.
71. Ross DM, Ross SA. Childhood pain: the school-aged child's viewpoint. Pain 1984;20:179–191.
72. Norden J, Hannallah R, Getson P, O'Donnell R, Kelliher G, Walker N. Concurrent validation of an objective pain scale for infants and children (abstract). Anesthesiology 1991;75:A933.
73. Unruh A, McGrath P, Cunningham SJ, Humphreys P. Children's drawings of their pain. Pain 1983;17:385–392.
74. Lovell DJ, Walco GA. Pain associated with juvenile rheumatoid arthritis. Pediatr Clin North Am 1989;36:1015–1027.
75. Baum C, Kennedy DL, Forbes MB. Utilization of nonsteroidal anti-inflammatory drugs. Arthritis Rheum 1985;28:686–692.
76. Stiehm ER. Nonsteroidal anti-inflammatory drugs in pediatric patients (editorial). Am J Dis Child 1988;142:1281–1282.
77. Mortenson ME, Rennebohm RM. Clinical pharmacology and use of nonsteroidal anti-inflammatory drugs. Pediatr Clin North Am 1989; 36:1113–1139.
78. Mather LE, Denson DE. Clinical pharmacokinetics of analgesic drug. In: Raj PP, ed. Practical management of pain. Chicago: Year Book, 1986:503–520.
79. Mroszczak EJ, Jung D, Yee J, Bynum L, Sevelius H, Massey I. Ketorolac tromethamine pharmacokinetics and metabolism after intravenous, intramuscular, and oral administration in humans and animals. Pharmacotherapy 1990;10:33S–39S.
80. Litvak KM, McEvoy GK. Ketorolac, an injectable nonnarcotic analgesic (see comments). Clin Pharm 1990;9:921–935.
81. Resman Targoff BH. Ketorolac: a parenteral nonsteroidal antiinflammatory drug. DICP 1990;24:1098–1104.
82. DiPalma JR. Ketorolac: an injectable NSAID. Am Fam Physician 1991;43:207–210.
83. Buckley MM, Brogden RN. Ketorolac. A review of its pharmacodynamic and pharmacokinetic properties, and therapeutic potential. Drugs 1990;39:86–109.
84. Cooper SA. Comparative analgesic efficiencies of aspirin and acetaminophen. Arch Intern Med 1981;141:282–285.
85. Peterson RG. Antipyretics and analgesics in children. Dev Pharmacol Ther 1985;8:68–84.
86. Rumack BH, Peterson RG. Acetaminophen overdose: incidence, diagnosis, and management in 416 patients. Pediatrics 1978;62(suppl): 898–903.
87. Beaver WT. Aspirin and acetaminophen as constitutents of analgesic combinations. Arch Intern Med 1981;141:293–300.
88. Beaver WT. Combination analgesics. Am J Med 1984;77:38–53.
89. Berde CB, Warfield CA. Pediatric pain management. Hosp Pract [Off] 1988;23:83–84, 89, 93.
90. Mather LE. Pharmacology of opioids. Part 1. Basic aspects. Med J Aust 1986;144:424–427.
91. Wood M. Opioid agonists and antagonists. In: Wood M, Wood AJJ, eds. Drugs and anesthesia: pharmacology for anesthesiologists. Baltimore, Williams & Wilkins, 1990;129–178.
92. Yaksh TL. Multiple opioid receptor systems in brain and spinal cord: Part I. Eur J Anaesthesiol 1984;1:171–199.
93. Pasternack GW. Multiple morphine and enkephalin receptors and the relief of pain. JAMA 1988;259:1362–1367.
94. Lord JAH, Waterfield AA, Hughes J, Kosterlitz HW. Endogenous opioid peptides: multiple agonists and receptors. Nature 1977;267: 495–499.
95. Vaught JL, Rotham RB, Westfall TC. Mu and delta receptors: their role in analgesia and in the differential effects of opioid peptides on analgesia. Life Sci 1982;30:1433–1455.
96. Gebhart GF. Opiate and opioid peptide effects on brainstem neurones: relevance to nociception and antinociceptive mechanisms. Pain 1982;12:93–140.
97. Maurer R, Cortes R, Probst A, Palacios JM. Multiple opiate receptors in human brain: an autoradiographic investigation. Life Sci 1983; 33(Suppl I.):231–234.
98. Cousins MJ, Cherry DA, Gourlay GK. Acute and chronic pain: use of spinal opioids. In: Cousins MJ, Bridenbaugh PO, eds. Neural blockade in clinical anesthesia and management of pain. Philadelphia: JB Lippincott, 1988:955–1030.
99. Rita L, Seleny FL, Levin RM. A comparison of pentazocine and morphine for pediatric premedication. Anesth Analg 1970;49:377–382.
100. Rita L, Seleny F, Goodarzi M. Comparison of the calming and sedative effects of nalbuphine and pentazocine for paediatric premedication. Can Anaesth Soc J 1980;27:546–549.
101. Zhang AZ, Pasternak GW. Ontogeny of opioid pharmacology and receptors: high and low affinity site difference. Eur J Pharmacol 1981;73:29–40.
102. Pasternak GW, Zhang AZ, Tecott L. Developmental differences between high and low affinity opiate binding sites: their relationship to analgesia and respiratory depression. Life Sci 1980;27:1185–1190.
103. Lynn AM, Slattery JT. Morphine pharmacokinetics in early infancy. Anesthesiology 1987;66:136–139.
104. Lynn AM, Opheim KE, Tyler DC. Morphine infusion after pediatric cardiac surgery. Crit Care Med 1984;12:863–866.
105. Koren G, Butt W, Pape K, Chinyanga H. Morphine-induced seizures in newborn infants. Vet Hum Toxicol 1985;27:519–520.
106. Koren G, Butt W, Chinyanga H, Soldin S, Tan YK, Pape K. Postoperative morphine infusion in newborn infants: assessment of disposition characteristics and safety. J Pediatr 1985;107:963–967.
107. Yaster M, Nichols DG, Deshpande JK, Wetzel RC. Midazol am-fentanyl intravenous sedation in children: case report of respiratory arrest. Pediatrics 1990;86:463–467.
108. Greene RF, Miser AW, Lester CM, Balis FM, Poplack DG. Cerebrospinal fluid and plasma pharmacokinetics of morphine infusions in pediatric cancer patients and rhesus monkeys. Pain 1987;30:339–348.
109. Gourlay GK, Cherry DA, Plummer JL, Armstrong PJ, Cousins MJ. The influence of drug polarity on the absorption of opioid drugs into CSF

and subsequent cephalad migration following lumbar epidural administration: application to morphine and pethidine. Pain 1987; 31:297–305.
110. Gourlay GK, Cherry DA, Cousins MJ. Cephalad migration of morphine in CSF following lumbar epidural administration in patients with cancer pain. Pain 1985;23:317–326.
111. Etches RC, Sandler AN, Daley MD. Respiratory depression and spinal opioids. Can J Anaesth 1989;36:165–185.
112. Kupferberg HJ, Way EL. Pharmacologic basis for the increased sensitivity of the newborn rat to morphine. J Pharmacol Exp Ther 1963; 141:105–112.
113. Way WL, Costley EC, Way EL. Respiratory sensitivity of the newborn infant to meperidine and morphine. Clin Pharmacol Ther 1965; 6:454–461.
114. Greeley WJ, de Bruijn NP. Changes in sufentanil pharmacokinetics within the neonatal period. Anesth Analg 1988;67:86–90.
115. Bhat R, Chori G, Gulati A, Aldana O, Velamati R, Bhargava H. Pharmacokinetics of a single dose of morphine in preterm infants during the first week of life. J Pediatr 1990;117:477–481.
116. Kupferberg HJ, Way EL. Pharmacologic basis for the increased sensitivity of the newborn rat to morphine. J Pharmacol Exp Ther 1963;141:105–112.
117. Way WL, Costley EC, Way EL. Respiratory sensitivity of the newborn infant to meperidine and morphine. Clin Pharmacol Ther 1965;6:454–461.
118. Dothage JA, Arndt C, Miser AW. Use of a continuous intravenous morphine infusion for pain control in an infant with terminal malignancy. J Assoc Pediatr Oncol Nurses 1986;3:22–24.
119. Owen H, Plummer JL, Armstrong I, Mather LE, Cousins MJ. Variables of patient-controlled analgesia. 1. Bolus size. Anaesthesia 1989;44:7–10.
120. Lawrie SC, Forbes DW, Akhtar TM, Morton NS. Patient-controlled analgesia in children. Anaesthesia 1990;45:1074–1076.
121. Urquhart ML, Klapp K, White PF. Patient-controlled analgesia: a comparison of intravenous versus subcutaneous hydromorphone. Anesthesiology 1988;69:428–432.
122. White PF. Use of patient-controlled analgesia for management of acute pain. JAMA 1988;259:243–247.
123. Gourlay GK, Cherry DA, Cousins MJ. A comparative study of the efficacy and pharmacokinetics of oral methadone and morphine in the treatment of severe pain in patients with cancer. Pain 1986;25:297–312.
124. Plummer JL, Gourlay GK, Cherry DA, Cousins MJ. Estimation of methadone clearance: application in the management of cancer pain. Pain 1988;33:313–322.
125. Gourlay GK, Wilson PR, Glynn CJ. Pharmacodynamics and pharmacokinetics of methadone during the perioperative period. Anesthesiology 1982;57:458–467.
126. Gourlay GK, Willis RJ, Lamberty J. A double-blind comparison of the efficacy of methadone and morphine in postoperative pain control. Anesthesiology 1986;64:322–327.
127. Gourlay GK, Willis RJ, Wilson PR. Postoperative pain control with methadone: influence of supplementary methadone doses and blood-concentration-response relationships. Anesthesiology 1984;61:19–26.
128. Berde CB, Holzman RS, Sethna NF, Dickerson RB, Brustowicz RM. A comparison of methadone and morphine for postoperative analgesia in children and adolescents. Anesthesiology 1988;69(suppl):A768.
129. Gourlay GK, Plummer JL, Cherry DA, Foate JA, Cousins MJ. Influence of a high-fat meal on the absorption of morphine from oral solutions. Clin Pharmacol Ther 1989;46:463–468.
130. Koehntop DE, Rodman JH, Brundage DM, Hegland MG, Buckley JJ. Pharmacokinetics of fentanyl in neonates. Anesth Analg 1986;65: 227–232.
131. Hertzka RE, Gauntlett IS, Fisher DM, Spellman MJ. Fentanyl-induced ventilatory depression: effects of age. Anesthesiology 1989;70:213–218.
132. Gauntlett IS, Fisher DM, Hertzka RE, Kuhls E, Spellman MJ, Rudolph C. Pharmacokinetics of fentanyl in neonatal humans and lambs: effects of age. Anesthesiology 1988;69:683–687.
133. Singleton MA, Rosen JI, Fisher DM. Pharmacokinetics of fentanyl in the elderly. Br J Anaesth 1988;60:619–622.
134. Singleton MA, Rosen JI, Fisher DM. Plasma concentrations of fentanyl in infants, children and adults. Can J Anaesth 1987;34:152–155.
135. McClain DA, Hug CC. Intravenous fentanyl kinetics. Clin Pharmacol Ther 1980;28:106–114.
136. Cartwright P, Prys-Roberts C, Gill K, Dye A, Stafford M, Gray A. Ventilatory depression related to plasma fentanyl concentrations during and after anesthesia in humans. Anesth Analg 1983;62:966–974.
137. Hess R, Herz A, Friedel K. Pharmacokinetics of fentanyl in rabbits in view of the importance for limiting the effect. J Pharmacol Exp Ther 1971;179:474–484.
138. Nichols DG, Yaster M, Deshpande JK, Helfaer M, Lynn AM, Bezman M, Tobias J. Disposition and respiratory effects of intrathecal morphine in children. Anesthesiology 1990;73(suppl):A1135.
139. Robinson S, Gregory GA. Fentanyl-air-oxygen anesthesia for patent ductus arteriosus in preterm infants. Anesth Analg 1981;60:331–334.
140. Yaster M. The dose response of fentanyl in neonatal anesthesia. Anesthesiology 1987;66:433–435.
141. Henderson JM, Brodsky DA, Fisher DM, Brett CM, Hertzka RE. Preinduction of anesthesia in pediatric patients with nasally administered sufentanil. Anesthesiology 1988;68:671–675.
142. Feld LH, Champeau MW, van Steennis CA, Scott JC. Preanesthetic medication in children: a comparison of oral transmucosal fentanyl citrate versus placebo. Anesthesiology 1989;71:374–377.
143. Stanley TH, Leiman BC, Rawal N, Marcus MA, van den Nieuwenhuyzen M, Walford A, Cronau LH, Pace NL. The effects of oral transmucosal fentanyl citrate premedication on preoperative behavioral responses and gastric volume and acidity in children. Anesth Analg 1989;69: 328–335.
144. Streisand JB, Stanley TH, Hague B, van Vreeswijk H, Ho GH, Pace NL. Oral transmucosal fentanyl citrate premedication in children. Anesth Analg 1989;69:28–34.
145. Stanley TH, Hague B, Mock DL, Streisand JB, Bubbers S, Dzelzkalns RR, Bailey PL, Pace NL, East KA, Ashburn MA. Oral transmucosal fentanyl citrate (lollipop) premedication in human volunteers. Anesth Analg 1989;69:21–27.
146. Nelson PS, Streisand JB, Mulder SM, Pace NL, Stanley TH. Comparison of oral transmucosal fentanyl citrate and an oral solution of meperidine, diazepam, and atropine for premedication in children. Anesthesiology 1989;70:616–621.
147. Kerr IG, Sone M, DeAngelis C, Iscoe N, MacKenzie R, Schueller T. Continuous narcotic infusion with patient-controlled analgesia for chronic cancer pain in outpatients. Ann Intern Med 1988;108:554–557.
148. Portenoy RK, Foley KM, Inturrisi CE. The nature of opioid responsiveness and its implications for neuropathic pain: new hypotheses derived from studies of opioid infusions. Pain 1990;43:273–286.
149. Hill HF, Coda BA, Tanaka A, Schaffer R. Multiple-dose evaluation of intravenous hydromorphone pharmacokinetics in normal human subjects. Anesth Analg 1991;72:330–336.
150. Moulin DE, Kreeft JH, Murray-Parsons N, Bouquillon AI. Comparison of continuous subcutaneous and intravenous hydromorphone infusions for management of cancer pain. Clin Pract 1991;337:465–468.
151. Marlowe S, Engstrom R, White PF. Epidural patient-controlled analgesia (PCA): an alternative to continuous epidural infusions. Pain 1989;37:97–101.
152. Urquhart ML, Klapp K, White PF. Patient-controlled analgesia: a comparison of intravenous versus subcutaneous hydromorphone. Anesthesiology 1988;69:428–432.
153. Mather LE, Cousins MJ. Pharmacology of opioids. Part 2. Clinical aspects. Med J Aust 1986;144:475–481.
154. Schechter NL, Berrien FB, Katz SM. The use of patient-controlled analgesia in adolescents with sickle cell pain crisis: a preliminary report. J Pain Symptom Manage 1988;3:109–113.
155. Tyler DC. Patient-controlled analgesia in adolescents. J Adolesc Health Care 1990;11:154–158.
156. Gaukroger PB, Tomkins DP, van der WaltJH. Patient-controlled analgesia in children. Anaesth Intensive Care 1989;17:264–268.
157. Webb CJ, Stergios DA, Rodgers BM. Patient-controlled analgesia as postoperative pain treatment for children. J Pediatr Nurs 1989; 4:162–171.
158. Rodgers BM, Webb CJ, Stergios D, Newman BM. Patient-controlled analgesia in pediatric surgery. J Pediatr Surg 1988;23:259–262.
159. Hill HF, Chapman CR, Kornell JA, Sullivan KM, Saeger LC, Benedetti C. Self-administration of morphine in bone marrow transplant patients reduces drug requirement. Pain 1990;40:121–129.
160. Shapiro BS. The management of pain in sickle cell disease. Pediatr Clin North Am 1989;36:1029–1045.
161. Owen H, Szekely SM, Plummer JL, Cushnie JM, Mather LE. Variables of patient-controlled analgesia. 2. Concurrent infusion. Anaesthesia 1989;44:11–13.
162. Owen H, Mather LE, Rowley K. The development and clinical use of patient-controlled analgesia. Anaesth Intensive Care 1988;16:437–447.
163. Mather LE, Owen H. The scientific basis of patient controlled analgesia. Anaesth Intensive Care 1988;16:427–436.

164. Owen H, Brose WG, Plummer JL, Mather LE. Variables of patient-controlled analgesia. 3: Test of an infusion-demand system using alfentanil. Anaesthesia 1990;45:452–455.
165. Yaksh TL. Spinal pharmacology of pain and its modulation. Clin Neurosurg 1983;31:291–303.
166. Yaksh TL, Rudy TA. Analgesia mediated by a direct spinal action of narcotics. Science 1976;192:1357–1358.
167. Krane EJ, Jacobson LE, Lynn AM, Parrot C, Tyler DC. Caudal morphine for postoperative analgesia in children: a comparison with caudal bupivacaine and intravenous morphine. Anesth Analg 1987;66:647–653.
168. Krane EJ, Tyler DC, Jacobson LE. The dose response of caudal morphine in children. Anesthesiology 1989;71:48–52.
169. Tyler DC, Krane EJ. Epidural opioids in children. J Pediatr Surg 1989;24:469–473.
170. Dalens B. Regional anesthesia in children. Anesth Analg 1989;68:654–672.
171. Yaster M, Maxwell LG. Pediatric regional anesthesia. Anesthesiology 1989;70:324–338.
172. Attia J, Ecoffey C, Sandouk P, Gross JB, Samii K. Epidural morphine in children: pharmacokinetics and CO_2 sensitivity. Anesthesiology 1986;65:590–594.
173. Penon C, Negre I, Ecoffey C, Gross JB, Levron JC, Samii K. Analgesia and ventilatory response to carbon dioxide after intramuscular and epidural alfentanil. Anesth Analg 1988;67:313–317.
174. Benlabed M, Ecoffey C, Levron JC, Flaisler B, Gross JB. Analgesia and ventilatory response to CO_2 following epidural sufentanil in children. Anesthesiology 1987;67:948–951.
175. Negre I, Gueneron JP, Ecoffey C, Penon C, Gross JB, Levron JC, Samii K. Ventilatory response to carbon dioxide after intramuscular and epidural fentanyl. Anesth Analg 1987;66:707–710.
176. Labaille T, Clergue F, Samii K, Ecoffey C, Berdeaux A. Ventilatory response to CO_2 following intravenous and epidural lidocaine. Anesthesiology 1985;63:179–183.
177. Krane EJ. Delayed respiratory depression in a child after caudal epidural morphine. Anesth Analg 1988;67:79–82.
178. Clements JA, Nimmo WS. The pharmacokinetics and analgesic effects of ketamine in man. Br J Anaesth 1981;53:27–30.
179. White PF, Way WL, Trevor AJ. Ketamine—its pharmacology and therapeutic uses. Anesthesiology 1982;56:260–263.
180. Hickey PR, Hansen DD, Cramolini GM, Vincent RN, Lang P. Pulmonary and systemic hemodynamic responses to ketamine in infants with normal and elevated pulmonary vascular resistance. Anesthesiology 1985;62:287–293.
181. Morray JP, Lynn AM, Stamm SJ, Herndon PS, Kawabori I, Stevenson JG. Hemodynamic effects of ketamine in children with congenital heart disease. Anesth Analg 1984;63:895–899.
182. Yamamura T, Horanda K, Okamura A, Kommotsu O. Is the site of action of ketamine the N-methyl-D-aspartate receptor? Anesthesiology 1990;72:704–710.
183. Rita L, Seleny FL. Ketamine hydrochloride for pediatric premedication. II. Prevention of postanesthetic excitement. Anesth Analg 1974;53:380–382.
184. Takeshita H, Okuda Y, Sari A. The effects of ketamine on cerebral circulation and metabolism in man. Anesthesiology 1983;59:294–300.
185. Stanski DR, Mihm FG, Rosenthal MH, Kalman SM. Pharmacokinetics of high-dose thiopental used in cerebral resuscitation. Anesthesiology 1980;53:169–171.
186. Michenfelder JD, Theye RA. Cerebral protection by thiopental during hypoxia. Anesthesiology 1985;39:510–517.
187. Hamza J, Ecoffey E, Gross JB. Ventilatory response to CO_2 following intravenous ketamine in children. Anesthesiology 1989;70:422–425.
188. Welborn LG, Rice LJ, Hannallah RS, Broddman LM, Ruttimann UE, Fink R. Postoperative apnea in former preterm infants: prospective comparison of spinal and general anesthesia. Anesthesiology 1990;72:838–842.
189. Friesen RH, Henry DB. Cardiovascular changes in preterm neonates receiving isoflurane, halothane, fentanyl, and ketamine. Anesthesiology 1986;64:238–242.
190. Wolfe RR, Loehr JP, Schaffer MS, Wiggins JW Jr. Hemodynamic effects of ketamine, hypoxia and hyperoxia in children with surgically treated congenital heart disease residing greater than or equal to 1,200 meters above sea level. Am J Cardiol 1991;67:84–87.
191. Hickey PR, Hansen DD, Cramolini GM, Vincent RN, Lang P. Pulmonary and systemic hemodynamic responses to ketamine in infants with normal and elevated pulmonary vascular resistance. Anesthesiology 1985;62:287–293.
192. Greeley WJ, Stanley TE 3d, Ungerleider RM, Kisslo JA. Intraoperative hypoxemic spells in tetralogy of Fallot. An echocardiographic analysis of diagnosis and treatment. Anesth Analg 1989;68:815–819.
193. Hamza J, Ecoffey C, Gross JB. Ventilatory response to CO_2 following intravenous ketamine in children. Anesthesiology 1989;70:422–425.
194. Tashiro C, Matsui Y, Nakano S, Ueyama H, Nishimura M, Oka N. Respiratory outcome in extremely premature infants following ketamine anaesthesia. Can J Anaesth 1991;38:287–291.
195. Welborn LG, Rice LJ, Hannallah RS, Broadman LM, Ruttimann UE, Fink R. Postoperative apnea in former preterm infants: prospective comparison of spinal and general anesthesia. Anesthesiology 1990;72:838–842.
196. Domino EF, Domino SE, Smith RE, Domino LE, Goulet JR, Domino KE, Zsigmond EK. Ketamine kinetics in unmedicated and diazepam-premedicated subjects. Clin Pharmacol Ther 1984;36:645–653.
197. Grant IS, Nimmo WS, Clements JA. Pharmacokinetics and analgesics effect of IM and oral ketamine. Br J Anaesth 1981;53:805–810.
198. Grant IS, Nimmo WS, McNichol LR, Clements JA. Ketamine disposition in children and adults. Br J Anaesth 1983;55:1107–1111.
199. Stewart KG, Rowbottom SJ, Aitken AW, Rajendram S, Sudhaman DA. Oral ketamine premedication for paediatric cardiac surgery—a comparison with intramuscular morphine (both after oral trimeprazine). Anaesth Intensive Care 1990;18:11–14.
200. Pedraz JL, Calvo MB, Lanao JM, Muriel C, Santos Lamas J, Dominguez Gil A. Pharmacokinetics of rectal ketamine in children. Br J Anaesth 1989;63:671–674.
201. Green SM, Johnson NE. Ketamine sedation for pediatric procedures: Part 2, Review and implications. Ann Emerg Med 1990;19:1033–1046.
202. Green SM, Nakamura R, Johnson NE. Ketamine sedation for pediatric procedures: Part 1, A prospective series. Ann Emerg Med 1990;19:1024–1032.
203. Jankiewicz AM, Nowakowski P. Ketamine and succinylcholine for emergency intubation of pediatric patients. DICP 1991;25:475–476.
204. Cederholm I, Bengtsson M, Bjorkman S, Choonara I, Rane A. Long term high dose morphine, ketamine and midazolam infusion in a child with burns. Br J Clin Pharmacol 1990;30:901–905.
205. Tobias JD, Martin LD, Wetzel RC. Ketamine by continuous infusion for sedation in the pediatric intensive care unit. Crit Care Med 1990;18:819–821.
206. Rice LJ, Hannallah RS. Local and regional anesthesia. In: Motoyama EK, Davis PJ, eds. Smith's anesthesia for infants and children. St. Louis: CV Mosby, 1990:393–426.
207. Yaster M, Maxwell LG. The management of acute pain in children. In: Hoekelman RA, Friedman SB, Nelson NM, Seidel HS, eds. Primary pediatric care. St. Louis: MosbyYear Book, 1992.
208. Dalens BJ. Pediatric regional anesthesia. Boca Raton, FL: CRC Press, 1990.
209. Deleted in proof.
210. Brown TCK, Shulte-Steinberg O. Neural blockade for pediatric surgery. In: Cousins MJ, Bridenbaugh PO, eds. Neural blockade in clinical anesthesia and management of pain. Philadelphia: Lippincott, 1988:669–692.
211. Saint-Maurice C, Steinberg OS. Regional anaesthesia in children. Fribourg 1, Switzerland, Mediglobe SA, 1990.
212. Covino BG. Clinical pharmacology of local anesthetic agents. In: Cousins MJ, Bridenbaugh PO, eds. Neural blockade in clinical anesthesia and management of pain. Philadelphia: JB Lippincott, 1988:111–144.
213. Savaresse JJ, Covino BG. Basic and clinical pharmacology of local anesthetic agents. In: Miller RD, ed. Anesthesia. New York: Churchill Livingstone, 1986:985–1014.
214. Covino BG. Pharmacology of local anesthetic agents. Br J Anaesth 1986;58:701–716.
215. Tucker GT. Pharmacokinetics of local anaesthetics. Br J Anaesth 1986;58:717–731.
216. Wood M. Local anesthetic agents. In: Wood M, Wood AJJ, eds. Drugs and anesthesia: pharmacology for anesthesiologists. Baltimore: Williams and Wilkins, 1990:319–346.
217. Tucker GT, Mather LE. Properties, absorption, and disposition of local anesthetic agents. In: Cousins MJ, Bridenbaugh PO, eds. Neural blockade in clinical anesthesia and management of pain. Philadelphia: JB Lippincott, 1988:47–110.
218. Wildsmith JAW. Peripheral nerve and local anesthetic drugs. Br J Anaesth 1986;56:692–700.
219. Wildsmith JA, Gissen AJ, Takman B, Covino BG. Differential nerve blockade: esters v. amides and the influence of pKa. Br J Anaesth 1987;59:379–384.
220. Murat I, Walker J, Esteve C, Nahoul K, Saint-Maurice C. Effect of lum-

bar epidural anaesthesia on plasma cortisol levels in children. Can J Anaesth 1988;35:20–24.
221. Murat I, Delleur MM, Esteve C, Egu JF, Raynaud P, Saint-Maurice C. Continuous extradural anaesthesia in children. Clinical and haemodynamic implications. Br J Anaesth 1987;59:1441–1450.
222. Murat I, Walker J, Esteve C, Nahoul K, Saint-Maurice C. The effects of age and the addition of adrenalin to bupivacaine for continuous lumbar epidural anesthesia in children. Anesthesiology 1986;65:A428.
223. Warner MA, Kunkel SE, Offord KO, Atchison SR, Dawson B. The effects of age, epinephrine, and operative site on duration of caudal analgesia in pediatric patients. Anesth Analg 1987;66:995–998.
224. Mather LE, Tucker GT, Murphy TM, Stanton-Hicks M'd A, Bonica JJ. The effects of adding adrenaline to etidocaine and lignocaine in extradural anaesthesia. II: pharmacokinetics. Br J Anaesth 1976; 48:989–994.
225. Concepcion M, Maddi R, Francis D, Rocco AG, Murray E, Covino BG. Vasoconstrictors in spinal anesthesia with tetracaine—A comparison of epinephrine and phenylephrine. Anesth Analg 1984;63:134–138.
226. Moore DC, Batra MS. The components of an effective test dose prior to epidural block. Anesthesiology 1981;55:693–696.
227. Moore DC, Bridenbaugh LD, Thompson GE. Factors determining dosages of amide type local anesthetic drugs. Anesthesiology 1977; 47:263–268.
228. deJong RH. Local anesthetics. In: Raj PP, ed. Practical management of pain. Chicago: Year Book, 1986:539–556.
229. Desparmet J, Meistelman C, Barre J, Saint-Maurice C. Continuous epidural infusion of bupivacaine for postoperative pain relief in children. Anesthesiology 1987;67:108–110.
230. Ecoffey C, Desparmet J, Maury M, Berdeaux A, Giudicelli JF, Saint-Maurice C. Bupivacaine in children: pharmacokinetics following caudal anesthesia. Anesthesiology 1985;63:447–448.
231. Ecoffey C, Desparmet J, Berdeaux A, Maury M, Giudicelli JF, Saint-Maurice C. Pharmacokinetics of lignocaine in children following caudal anaesthesia. Br J Anaesth 1984;56:1399–1402.
232. Hastings CL, Brown TC, Eyres RL, Oppenheim RC. The influence of age on plasma lignocaine levels following tracheal spray in young dogs. Anaesth Intensive Care 1985;13:392–394.
233. Eyres RL, Brown TC, Hastings C. Plasma level of bupivacaine during convulsions (letter). Anaesth Intensive Care 1983;11:385–385.
234. Eyres RL, Bishop W, Oppenheim RC, Brown TC. Plasma lignocaine concentrations following topical laryngeal application. Anaesth Intensive Care 1983;11:23–26.
235. Eyres RL, Bishop W, Oppenheim RC, Brown TC. Plasma bupivacaine concentrations in children during caudal epidural analgesia. Anaesth Intensive Care 1983;11:20–22.
236. Eyres RL, Kidd J, Oppenheim R, Brown TCK. Local anaesthetic plasma levels in children. Anaesth Intensive Care 1978;6:243–247.
237. Rothstein P, Arthur GR, Feldman HS, Kopf GS, Covino BG. Bupivacaine for intercostal nerve blocks in children: blood concentrations and pharmacokinetics. Anesth Analg 1986;65:625–632.
238. Moore DC, Thompson GE, Crawford RD. Long-acting local anesthetic drugs and convulsions with hypoxia and acidosis. Anesthesiology 1982;56:230–232.
239. Moore DC. Systemic toxic reactions to high blood levels of local anesthetic drugs. In: Moore DC, ed. Regional block. Springfield, IL: Charles C Thomas, 1979:19–31.
240. Dalens B, Hasnaoui A. Caudal anesthesia in pediatric surgery: success rate and adverse effects in 750 consecutive patients. Anesth Analg 1989;68:83–89.
241. Dohi S, Naito H, Takahashi T. Age related changes in blood pressure and duration of motor block in spinal anesthesia. Anesthesiology 1979;50:319–323.
242. Feldman HS, Arthur GR, Covino BG. Comparative systemic toxicity of convulsant and supraconvulsant doses of intravenous ropivacaine, bupivacaine, and lidocaine in the conscious dog. Anesth Analg 1989; 69:794–801.
243. Horishima HO, Pederson H, Finster M, Sakuma K, Bruce SL, Gutsche B, Stark RI, Covino BG. Toxicity of lidocaine in adult, newborn and fetal sheep. Anesthesiology 1981;55:57–61.
244. Liu PL, Covino BM, Feldman HS. Effect of age on local anesthetic central nervous system toxicity in mice. Regional Anesth 1983;8:57–60.
245. deJong RH, Heavner JE. Diazepam prevents local anesthetics seizures. Anesthesiology 1979;34:523–531.
246. Moore DC, Crawford RD, Scurlock JE. Severe hypoxia and acidosis following local anesthetic induced convulsions. Anesthesiology 1980; 53:259–260.
247. Moore DC, Bonica JJ. Convulsions and ventricular tachycardia from bupivacaine with epinephrine. Successful resuscitation—congratulations. Anesth Analg 1985;64:844–846.
248. American Academy of Pediatrics Committee on Drugs Section on Anesthesiology. Guidelines for the elective use of conscious sedation, deep sedation, and general anesthesia in pediatric anesthesia. Pediatrics 1985;76:317–321.
249. Nancarrow C, Rutten AJ, Runciman WB, Mather LE, Carapetis RJ, McLean CF, Hipkins SF. Myocardial and cerebral drug concentrations and the mechanisms of death after fatal intravenous doses of lidocaine, bupivacaine, and ropivacaine in the sheep. Anesth Analg 1989; 69:276–283.
250. Nancarrow C, Runciman WB, Mather LE, Upton RN, Plummer JL. The influence of acidosis on the distribution of lidocaine and bupivacaine into the myocardium and brain of the sheep. Anesth Analg 1987; 66:925–935.
251. Moller RA, Covino BG. Cardiac electrophysiologic effects of lidocaine and bupivacaine. Anesth Analg 1988;67:107–114.
252. Sage DJ, Feldman HS, Arthur GR, Datta S, Ferretti AM, Norway SB, Covino BG. Influence of lidocaine and bupivacaine on isolated guinea pig atria in the presence of acidosis and hypoxia. Anesth Analg 1984;63:1–7.
253. Badgwell JM, Heavner JE, Kytta J. Bupivacaine toxicity in young pigs is age-dependent and is affected by volatile anesthetics. Anesthesiology 1990;73:297–303.
254. Kasten GW, Martin ST. Successful cardiovascular resuscitation after massive intravenous bupivacaine overdosage in anesthetized dogs. Anesth Analg 1985;64:491–497.
255. Mather LE, Cousins MJ. Local anesthetics: principles of use. In: Cousins MJ, Phillips GD, eds. Acute pain management. New York: Churchill Livingstone, 1986:105–132.
256. Zsigmond EK, Downs JR. Plasma cholinesterase activity in newborns and infants. Can Anaesth Soc J 1989;18:278–285.
257. Mihaly GW, Moore RG, Thomas J, Triggs EJ, Thomas D, Shanks CA. The pharmacokinetics and metabolism of the anilide local anaesthetics in neonates. Eur J Clin Pharmacol 1978;13:143–152.
258. Meffin P, Long GJ, Thomas J. Clearance and metabolism of mepivicaine in the human neonate. Clin Pharmacol Ther 1973;14: 218–225.
259. Lerman J, Strong HA, LeDez KM, Swartz J, Rieder MJ, Burrows FA. Effects of age on the serum concentration of α1-acid glycoprotein and the binding of lidocaine in pediatric patients. Clin Pharmacol Ther 1989;46:219–225.
260. Burrows FA, Lerman J, LeDez KM, Strong HA. α1-Acid glycoprotein and the binding of lidocaine in children with congenital heart disease. Can J Anaesth 1990;37:883–888.
261. LeDez KM, Swartz J, Strong A, Burrows FA, Lerman J. The effect of age on the serum concentration of α1-acid glycoprotein in newborns, infants and children. Anesthesiology 1986;65:A421.
262. Wood M, Wood AJJ. Changes in plasma drug binding and α1-acid glycoprotein in mother and newborn infant. Clin Pharmacol Ther 1973;14:218–225.
263. Morselli PL, Franco-Morselli R, Borsi L. Clinical pharmacokinetics in newborns and infants. Age related differences and therapeutic implications. Clin Pharmacokinet 1980;5:485–527.
264. Shand DG. α1-Acid glycoprotein and plasma lidocaine binding. Clin Pharmacokinet 1984;9:27–31.
265. Feig SA. Methemoglobinemia. In: Nathan DG, Oski FA, eds. Hematology of infancy and childhood. Philadelphia: WB Saunders, 1974: 378–389.
266. Finholt DA, Stirt JA, DiFazio CA, Moscicki JC. Lidocaine pharmacokinetics in children during general anesthesia. Anesth Analg 1986; 65:279–282.
267. Abou-Madi MN, Keszler H, Yacoub JM. Cardiovascular reactions to laryngoscopy and tracheal intubation following small and large intravenous doses of lidocaine. Can Anaesth Soc J 1977;24:12–19.
268. Gelband H, Rosen MR. Pharmacologic basis for the treatment of cardiac arrhythmias. Pediatrics 1975;55:59–69.
269. Bokesch PM, Castaneda AR, Ziemer G, Wilson JM. The influence of a right-to-left cardiac shunt on lidocaine pharmacokinetics. Anesthesiology 1987;67:739–744.
270. Jorfeldt L, Lewis DH, Lofstrom JB, Post C. Lung uptake of lidocaine in healthy volunteers. Acta Anaesthesiol Scand 1979;23:567–574.
271. McKay W, Morris R, Mushlin P. Sodium bicarbonate attenuates pain on skin infiltration with lidocaine, with or without epinephrine. Anesth Analg 1987;66:572–574.
272. Soliman IE, Broadman LM, Hannallah RS, McGill WA. Comparison of the analgesic effects of EMLA (eutectic mixture of local anesthetics) to

intradermal lidocaine in filtration prior to venous cannulation in unpremedicated children. Anesthesiology 1988;68:804–806.
273. Hopkins CS, Buckley CJ, Bush GH. Pain-free injection in infants. Use of a lignocaine-prilocaine cream to prevent pain at intravenous induction of general anaesthesia in 1–5-year-old children. Anaesthesia 1988;43:198–201.
274. Manner T, Kanto J, Iisalo E, Lindberg R, Viinamaki O, Scheinin M. Reduction of pain at venous cannulation in children with a eutectic mixture of lidocaine and prilocaine (EMLA cream): comparison with placebo cream and no local premedication. Acta Anaesthesiol Scand 1987;31:735–739.
275. Engberg G, Danielson K, Henneberg S, Nilsson A. Plasma concentrations of prilocaine and lidocaine and methemoglobin formation in infants after epicutaneous application of a 5% lidocaine-prilocaine (EMLA). Acta Anaesthesiol Scand 1987;31:624–628.
276. Maunuksela EL, Korpela R. Double-blind evaluation of a lignocaine-prilocaine cream (EMLA) in children. Effect on the pain associated with venous cannulation. Br J Anaesth 1986;58:1242–1245.
277. Hallen B, Olsson GL, Uppfeldt A. Pain-free venipuncture. Effect of timing of application of local anaesthetic cream. Anaesthesia 1984; 39:969–972.
278. Price HV. Lignocaine-prilocaine cream for lumbar puncture in children (letter). Lancet 1988;1:1174–1174.
279. Murat I, Montay G, Delleur MM, Esteve C, Saint-Maurice C. Bupivacaine pharmacokinetics during epidural anaesthesia in children. Eur J Anaesthesiol 1988;5:113–120.
280. Murat I, Delleur MM, Levy J, Esteve C, Saint-Maurice C. Continuous epidural anaesthesia for major abdominal surgery in young children. Eur J Anaesthesiol 1987;4:327–335.
281. Murat I, Esteve C, Montay G, Delleur MM, Gaudiche O, Saint-Maurice C. Pharmacokinetics and cardiovascular effects of bupivacaine during epidural anesthesia in children with Duchenne muscular dystrophy. Anesthesiology 1987;67:249–252.
282. Dalens B, Tanguy A, Haberer JP. Lumbar epidural anesthesia for operative and postoperative pain relief in infants and young children. Anesth Analg 1986;65:1069–1073.
283. Rice LJ, Pudimat MA, Hannallah RS. Timing of caudal block placement in relation to surgery does not affect duration of postoperative analgesia in paediatric ambulatory patients. Can J Anaesth 1990; 37:429–431.
284. Anderson CTM, Berde CB, Sethna NF, Pribaz JJ. Meningococcal purpura fulminans: treatment of vascular insufficiency in a 2-yr-old child with lumbar epidural sympathetic blockade. Anesthesiology 1989; 71:463–464.
285. Eyres RL, Hastings C, Brown TC, Oppenheim RC. Plasma bupivacaine concentrations following lumbar epidural anaesthesia in children. Anaesth Intensive Care 1986;14:131–134.
286. Bridenbaugh PO. Patient management for neural blockade: selection, management, premedication, and supplementation. In: Cousins MJ, Bridenbaugh PO, eds. Neural blockade in clinical anesthesia and management of pain. Philadelphia: JB Lippincott, 1988:191–210.
287. Wright B. A new use for the Block-Aid Monitor. Anesthesiology 1969;30:236–237.
288. Bashein G, Haschke RH, Ready LB. Electrical nerve stimulation: numerical and electrophoretic comparison of insulated uv uninsulated needles. Anesth Analg 1984;63:919–924.
289. Ford DJ, Pither C, Raj PP. Comparison of insulated and uninsulated needles for locating peripheral nerves with a peripheral nerve stimulator. Anesth Analg 1984;63:925–928.
290. Winnie AP, Radonjic R, Akkineni SR, Durrani Z. Factors influencing distribution of local anesthetic injected into the brachial plexus sheath. Anesth Analg 1979;58:225–234.
291. Goldberg ME, Gregg C, Larijani GE, Norris MC, Marr AT, Seltzer JL. A comparison of three methods of axillary approach to brachial plexus blockade for upper extremity surgery. Anesthesiology 1987;66:814–816.
292. Selander D. Axillary plexus block: paresthetic or perivascular. Anesthesiology 1987;66:726–728.
293. de Pablo JS, Diez-Mallo J. Experience with three thousand cases of brachial plexus block: its dangers. Report of fatal case. Ann Surg 1948;128:956–964.
294. Winnie AP, Radonjic R, Akkineni SR, Durrani Z. Factors influencing distribution of local anesthetic injected into the brachial plexus sheath. Anesth Analg 1979;58:225–234.
295. Partridge BL, Benirschke K. Functional anatomy of the brachial plexus sheath: implications for anesthesia. Anesthesiology 1987;66:743–747.
296. Berry FR. Analgesia in patients with fractured shaft of femur. Anaesthesia 1977;32:576–577.
297. Grossbard GD, Love BR. Femoral nerve block: a simple and safe method of instant analgesia for femoral shaft fractures in children. Aust NZ J Surg 1979;49:592–594.
298. Rhonchi L, Rosenbaum D, Lenorman Y, Lemaitre JL, Guillet JC. Femoral nerve block with bupivacaine in children. Anesthesiology 1986; 65:A430.
299. McIlvaine WB, Chang JH, Jones M. The effective use of intrapleural bupivacaine for analgesia after thoracic and subcostal incisions in children. J Pediatr Surg 1988;23:1184–1187.
300. Mohler H, Richards JG. The benzodiazepine receptor: a pharmacologic control element of brain function. Eur J Anesthesiol 1988;2:15–24.
301. Reves JG. Benzodiazepines. In: Prys-Roberts C, Hug CC, eds. Pharmacokinetics of anesthesia. Chicago: Blackwell Scientific Publications, 1984:157–186.
302. Reves JG, Fragen RJ, Vinik R, Greenblatt DJ. Midazolam: pharmacology and uses. Anesthesiology 1985;62:310–324.
303. Dundee JW, Haslett WHK. The benzodiazepines—a review of their actions and uses relative to anesthetic practice. Br J Anaesth 1983;55:985–989.
304. Wood M. Intravenous anesthetic agents. In: Wood M, Wood AJJ, eds. Drugs and anesthesia: pharmacology for anesthesiologists. Baltimore: Williams & Wilkins, 1990:179–224.
305. Harvey SC. Hypnotics and sedatives. In: Gilman AG, Goodman LS, Gilman A, eds. The pharmacological basis of therapeutics. New York: Macmillan, 1980:339–375.
306. Amrein R, Hetzel W, Harmann D, Lorscheid T. Clinical pharmacology of flumazenil. Eur J Anesthesiol 1988;2:65.
307. Deleted in proof.
308. Greenblatt DJ, Shader RI, Abernethy DR. Current status of benzodiazepines (two parts). N Engl J Med 1983;309:410–416.
309. Ghoneim M, Mewaldt SP. Benzodiazepines and human memory: a review. Anesthesiology 1990;72:926–938.
310. Gross JB, Smith L, Smith TC. Time course of ventilatory response to carbon dioxide after intravenous diazepam. Anesthesiology 1982; 57:18–21.
311. Alexander CM, Gross JB. Sedative doses of midazolam depress hypoxic ventilatory responses in humans. Anesth Analg 1988;67:377–382.
312. Gross JB, Zebrowski ME, Carel WD, Gardner S, Smith TC. Time course of ventilatory depression after thiopental and midazolam in normal subjects and in patients with chronic obstructive pulmonary disease. Anesthesiology 1983;58:540–544.
313. Samuelson PN, Lell WA, Kouchoukos NT, et al. Hemodynamic responses to anesthetic induction with midazolam or diazepam in patients with ischemic heart disease. Anesth Analg 1981;60:802–809.
314. Rao S, Sherraniuk RW, Prasad K. Cardiopulmonary effects of diazepam. Clin Pharmacol Ther 1973;14:182.
315. Cote P, Gueret P, Courassa MG. Systemic and hemodynamic effects of diazepam in patients with normal and diseased coronary arteries. Circulation 1974;50:1210.
316. Adams P, Gelman S, Reves JG, Greenblatt DJ, et al. Midazolam pharmacodynamics and pharmacokinetics during acute hypovolemia. Anesthesiology 1985;63:140–146.
317. Spear RM, Yaster M, Berkowitz ID, Maxwell LG, Bender KS, Naclerio R, Manolio TA, Nichols DG. Preinduction of anesthesia in children with rectally administered midazolam. Anesthesiology 1991;74:670–674.
318. Rita L, Seleny FL, Mazurek A, Rabins SY. Intramuscular midazolam for pediatric preanesthetic sedation: a double blind controlled study with morphine. Anesthesiology 1985;63.528–531.
319. Wilton NC, Leigh J, Rosen DR, Pandit UA. Preanesthetic sedation of preschool children using intranasal midazolam. Anesthesiology 1988;69:972–975.
320. Saint-Maurice C, Meistelman C, Rey E, et al. The pharmacokinetics of rectal midazolam for premedication in children. Anesthesiology 1987;65:536–538.
321. Rosen DA, Rosen KR. A palatable gelatin vehicle for midazolam and ketamine. Anesthesiology 1991;75:914–915.
322. Peterson MD. Making oral midazolam palatable for children. Anesthesiology 1990;73:1053.
323. Silvasi DL, Rosen DA, Rosen KR. Continuous intravenous midazolam infusion for sedation in the pediatric intensive care unit. Anesth Analg 1988;67:286–288.
324. Booker PD, Beechey A, Lloyd-Thomas AR. Sedation of children requiring artificial ventilation using an infusion of midazolam. Br J Anaesth 1986;58:1104–1108.
325. Salonen M, Kanto J, Iisalo E. Midazolam as our induction agent in children: a pharmacokinetic and clinical study. Anesth Analg 1987; 66:625–628.

326. Gross JB, Caldwell CB, Edwards MW. Induction dose-response curves for midazolam and ketamine in premedicated ASA class III and IV patients. Anesth Analg 1985;64:795–800.
327. Chamberlain JH, Seed RGFL, Chung DC. Effect of thiopental on myocardial function. Br J Anaesth 1977;49:865–870.
328. Brett CM, Fisher DM. Thiopental, dose-response relations in unpremedicated infants, children, and adults. Anesth Analg 1987;66: 1024–1027.
329. Carlon GC, Kahn RC, Goldiner PI, Howland WS, Turnball A. Long-term infusion of sodium thiopental: hemodynamic and respiratory effects. Crit Care Med 1978;6:311–316.
330. Hudson RJ, Stanski DR, Burch PG. Pharmacokinetics of methohexitol and thiopental in surgical patients. Anesthesiology 1983;59: 215–219.
331. Stone HH, Donnelly CC. Then accidental intra-arterial injection of thiopental. Anesthesiology 1961;22:995–1006.
332. Varner PD, Ebert JP, McKay RD, Nail CS, Whitlock TM. Methohexital sedation of children undergoing CT scan. Anesth Analg 1985;64: 643–645.
333. Liu LM, Gaudreault P, Friedman PA, Goudsouzian NG, Liu PL. Methohexital plasma concentrations in children following rectal administration. Anesthesiology 1985;62:567–570.
334. Liu LM, Goudsouzian NG, Liu PL. Rectal methohexital premedication in children, a dose-comparison study. Anesthesiology 1980;53: 343–345.
335. Rackow IH, et al. Frequency of cardiac arrest associated with anesthesia in infants and children. Pediatrics 1961;28:697.
336. Jones AE, Pelton DA. An index of syndromes and their anesthetic implications. Can Anaesth Soc J 1976;23:207.
337. Stehling LC, Zaunder HL, eds. Anesthetic implications of congenital anomalies in children. New York: Appleton Century-Crofts, 1980, 1991.
338. Welborn LG, Hannallah RS, Fink R, Ruttimann UE, Hicks JM. High-dose caffeine suppresses postoperative apnea in former preterm infants. Anesthesiology 1989;71:347–349.
339. Welborn LG, de Soto H, Hannallah RS, Fink R, Ruttimann UE, Boeckx R. The use of caffeine in the control of postanesthetic apnea in former premature infants. Anesthesiology 1988;68:796–798.
340. Kurth CD, Hutchison AA, Caton DC, Davenport PW. Maturational and anesthetic effects on apneic thresholds in lambs. J Appl Physiol 1989;67:643–647.
341. Kurth CD, Spitzer AR, Broennle AM, Downes JJ. Postoperative apnea in preterm infants. Anesthesiology 1987;66:483–488.
342. Liu LM, Cote CJ, Goudsouzian NG, Ryan JF, Firestone S, Dedrick DF, Liu PL, Todres ID. Life-threatening apnea in infants recovering from anesthesia. Anesthesiology 1983;59:506–510.
343. Lerman J, Robinson S, Willis MM, Gregory GA. Anesthetic requirements for halothane in young children 0–1 month and 1–6 months of age. Anesthesiology 1983;59:424–424.
344. Lerman J, Schmitt Bantel BI, Gregory GA, Willis MM 2d. Effect of age on the solubility of volatile anesthetics in human tissues. Anesthesiology 1986;65:307–311.
345. Gregory GA, Eger EI 2d, Munson ES. The relationship between age and halothane requirement in man. Anesthesiology 1969;30:488–491.
346. Eger EI. Anesthetic uptake and action. Baltimore: Williams & Wilkins, 1974:1–371.
347. Fisher DM, OKeeffe C, Stanski DR, Cronnelly R, Miller RD, Gregory GA. Pharmacokinetics and pharmacodynamics of d-tubocurarine in infants, children, and adults. Anesthesiology 1982;57:203–208.
348. Fisher DM, Canfell PC, Spellman MJ, Miller RD. Pharmacokinetics and pharmacodynamics of atracurium in infants and children. Anesthesiology 1990;73:33–37.
349. Rupp SM, Castagnoli KP, Fisher DM, Miller RD. Pancuronium and vecuronium pharmacokinetics and pharmacodynamics in younger and elderly adults. Anesthesiology 1987;67:45–49.
350. Miller RD, Rupp SM, Fisher DM, Cronnelly R, Fahey MR, Sohn YJ. Clinical pharmacology of vecuronium and atracurium. Anesthesiology 1984;61:444–453.
351. Cook DR. Muscle relaxants in infants and children. Anesth Analg 1981;60:335–343.
352. Brandom BW, Stiller RL, Cook DR, Woelfel SK, Chakravorti S, Lai A. Pharmacokinetics of atracurium in anaesthetized infants and children. Br J Anaesth 1986;58:1210–1213.
353. Martyn J, Goldhill DR, Goudsouzian NG. Clinical pharmacology of muscle relaxants in patients with burns. J Clin Pharmacol 1986;26: 680–685.
354. Goudsouzian NG. Muscle relaxants in infants and children. Can Anaesth Soc J 1985;32:S27–S31.
355. Goudsouzian NG, Martyn JJ, Liu LM, Ali HH. The dose response effect of long-acting nondepolarizing neuromuscular blocking agents in children. Can Anaesth Soc J 1984;31:246–250.
356. Goudsouzian NG, Liu LM, Cote CJ. Comparison of equipotent doses of non-depolarizing muscle relaxants in children. Anesth Analg 1981; 60:862–866.
357. Liu LM, DeCook TH, Goudsouzian NG, Ryan JF, Liu PL. Dose response to intramuscular succinylcholine in children. Anesthesiology 1981;55:599–602.
358. Cook DR, Marcy JH. Pediatric anesthetic pharmacology. In: Cook DR, Marcy JH, eds. Neonatal anesthesia. Pasadena: Appleton Davies, 1988:87–126.
359. Cook DR, Westman HR, Rosenfeld L, Hendershot RJ. Pulmonary edema in infants: possible association with intramuscular succinylcholine. Anesth Analg 1981;60:220–223.
360. Goudsouzian NG, Standaert FG. The infant and the myoneural junction. Anesth Analg 1986;65:1208–1217.
361. Rupp SM, McChristian JW, Miller RD, Taboada JA, Cronnelly R. Neostigmine and edrophonium antagonism of varying intensity neuromuscular blockade induced by atracurium, pancuronium, or vecuronium. Anesthesiology 1986;64:711–717.
362. Engbaek J, Ostergaard D, Skovgaard LT, Viby-Mogensen J. Reversal of intense neuromuscular blockade following infusion of atracurium. Anesthesiology 1990;72:803–806.
363. Fisher DM, Cronnelly R, Miller RD, Sharma M. The neuromuscular pharmacology of neostigmine in infants and children. Anesthesiology 1983;59:220–225.
364. Fisher DM, Cronnelly R, Sharma M, Miller RD. Clinical pharmacology of edrophonium in infants and children. Anesthesiology 1984; 61:428–433.
365. Howardy-Hansen P, Rasmussen JA, Jensen BN. Residual curarization in the recovery room: atracurium versus gallamine. Acta Anaesthesiol Scand 1989;33:167–169.
366. Bevan DR, Smith CE, Donati F. Postoperative neuromuscular blockade: a comparison between atracurium, vecuronium, and pancuronium. Anesthesiology 1988;69:272–276.
367. Pavlin EG, Holle RH, Schoene RB. Recovery of airway protection compared with ventilation in humans after paralysis with curare. Anesthesiology 1989;70:381–385.

PICU Administration

Section Ten

Section Editor

Mark C. Rogers

Pediatric Intensive Care Nursing

47

Dorothy G. Lappe

INTRODUCTION

This chapter describes pediatric intensive care unit (PICU) nursing from an organizational viewpoint. A systems approach will be used to discuss the responsibilities and contributions of the nursing staff in this specialty. The physical environment and its impacts on the delivery of care will be discussed. The delivery of nursing care through primary nursing, case management, and family-centered care, will be examined. Multiple system components influence the delivery of care in the PICU. Discussion of nursing education, documentation, clinical quality improvement, and collaborative practice will define these processes and their influence on the unit. The educational needs of the nurses will be discussed, including initial preparation of the new nurse in the PICU and ongoing activities to meet the learning needs of the nursing staff. Examples of PICU quality improvement activities that fulfill the requirements of governing regulatory bodies will provide a framework to design and implement a clinical quality improvement program. An interdisciplinary approach to quality improvement will be cited. The nursing hierarchy and roles within it will be explained. Discussions throughout the chapter will provide a basis on which to establish and maintain an effective pediatric intensive care nursing staff.

SYSTEMS THEORY

The nursing staff of the PICU works within, among, and upon a variety of systems. Systems theory, therefore, provides a useful theoretical framework for the organization of the nursing staff of the PICU and will be used to organize the contents of this chapter. A system can be defined as a set of interacting, interrelated, or interdependent elements[1].

The critical care environment has an impact on all of the lives it touches. A systems perspective of the critical care unit recognizes that an individual functions as a whole, but that the person is more than the sum of his or her parts. One part of the system influences the other parts of the system, which includes individuals, the unit function, and the organization. Each of these parts influences the role and function of the professional nurse in the PICU. The environment in which the nurses work is a structural system. The nursing care delivery, through case management, primary nursing and family-centered care, is a service system. The ability to provide care in the PICU setting is accomplished through the information and work systems of education, documentation, and clinical quality improvement. Collaborative practice forms a social system promoting shared responsibility and decision making by the members of the organization. In each of its positions, the nursing staff is part of an individual personality and a group social system. The many people who are influenced by the PICU include the children, families, and staff who provide this high-technology care. The role of the nursing staff to provide high-quality professional care to critically ill and injured children and their families is integral to the practice of pediatric intensive care. The success of the nursing practice is dependent on each of the parts that influence this outcome.

PHYSICAL ENVIRONMENT

Throughout this book, it has been demonstrated that the PICU provides advanced, high-technology care to children. The physical environment influences the physical, physiological, and psychological needs of critically ill children, their families, and the staff caring for them. Attention must be given to these elements and their effects on the delivery of care by the PICU staff members. The topics of unit design and equipment will be discussed in this portion of the chapter.

The designing and planning process must be comprehensive in an effort to comply with timetables and to achieve a successful outcome. A needs assessment provides information regarding the number of beds, the types of patients to be admitted to the PICU, and the personnel and equipment required for this care. Recommendations from local, state, and federal governing bodies and professional organizations serve as guidelines during the planning phase of establishing a PICU. The Committee on Hospital Care and the Pediatric Section of the Society of Critical Care Medicine have established specific guidelines for PICUs[2,3].

The number of beds required in the PICU is determined by the types of services to be provided, the number of children in need of critical care services, other demographic studies, existing patient information such as census, length of stay, emergency facilities, regional medical services offered, and financial resources. The planning phase of any ICU spans a several-year period. Therefore, decisions are based on current needs as well as projected decline or growth.

The health care environment is one of dynamic change. An institutional strategic plan should consider the current environment, future needs, projected changes in length of stay, reimbursement methodologies, and staffing requirements. The integration of an intermediate care unit with an ICU provides a model that allows flexible responses to changes in patient census, acuity levels, and staffing needs. The planning committee should include representatives from the nursing and medical staff, administrative staff (including the financial managers), and the hospital planning committee.

The hospital's design, size, and space should be considered when decisions are made about the physical facilities. The geographic location of the PICU is important to the daily operations of the unit. The PICU should be in close proximity to the operating rooms, the recovery room, the emergency room, the heliport, the pediatric general care units of the hospital, and the pharmacy, laboratory, and radiology departments. Access to these areas will provide safe, prompt transport of and services to critically ill children.

The physical design of the PICU must accommodate the needs of the children, their families, and the staff. The ICU is a crowded, noisy place filled with activity at all hours. Constant noise, alarms, lighting, and traffic make differentiation between day and night difficult in the PICU. It is surmised that these features contribute to the phenomenon of "ICU psychosis" and staff burn-out[4]. Therefore, the flow of traffic through the unit should be considered in the planning phase in an attempt to minimize the negative effects to children, their families, and the staff. The entrance of the unit should be controlled to regulate traffic and to promote infection control. The decision to design a large, open unit versus a unit comprising smaller rooms depends, in part, on the expected patient population. More critically ill patients may be better served in an open unit that affords maximum flexibility in the movement of patients, equipment, and staff. This open atmosphere allows better patient visibility and improved staff use. The disadvantages include increased noise and traffic and decreased patient and family privacy. The closed-room design is more suitable for the population of less acutely ill patients. While providing privacy and individuality for the child and family, there is decreased visibility of the patient; less interaction among the staff members, resulting in a sense of isolation; and less sharing of resources. While a design that allows a combination of both types of units may be more expensive, it offers greater flexibility. A closed unit designed with break-away doors would meet the needs of children and the staff caring for them.

Certain elements must be present in patient care areas, allowing constant observation of the children, isolation facilities, clean and dirty supply areas, storage space for equipment, radiology viewing areas, and pharmacy and nutrition services space. Individual patient care areas must be large enough to accommodate the patient, the array of equipment, performance of procedures, access for personnel to perform bedside tasks, and enough room for families at the bedside. Plans for this space should take into account the maximum amount of equipment necessary to care for the most seriously ill child. Electrical power, oxygen, compressed air, and vacuum must be sufficient to supply all necessary equipment used at the child's bedside. Emergency back-up supplies of electrical power and gas are required. Local, state, and federal regulations that monitor safety should be investigated during initial planning phases of ICU design.

Space to accommodate family amenities is essential in the design of the PICU because family involvement is integral to the care of the pediatric patient. Necessary areas for parents and other visitors include a waiting lounge, sleep space, and areas to provide activities of daily living. A space designated for private consultation is important for the families and the staff to communicate information effectively.

Necessary areas for staff use include conference rooms for nursing shift reports, nursing and physician educational rounds, and places for staff relief, including sleep areas for physicians, eating areas, and lavatory facilities. Office space for PICU administrative staff located near or in the unit facilitates the interactions of the involved staffs.

EQUIPMENT

A wide variety of equipment is available to monitor and treat the critically ill pediatric patient. While all equipment will not be necessary for use with all children, the equipment must be available for those whose conditions warrant it. The Joint Commission on Accreditation of Healthcare Organizations' (JCAHO) provision of patient care charges that the goal for patient care is to provide individualized, planned, and appropriate care in settings that support the patient's care, treatment, and rehabilitation goals and specific needs. Specialized equipment and supplies need to be available in ICUs to support the plan for treatment and ensure positive patient outcomes **(Table 47.1).** Sophisticated equipment does not take the place of, but rather augments, the assessment and practice of the health care team. It is necessary that individuals acquire a working knowledge of the equipment. This section will review the equipment necessary at each patient's bedside and in the unit.

Monitors provide detailed physiologic information used in the care of all children in the PICU. The minimum monitoring requirements in the PICU include electrocardiography, respiratory rates with apnea detectors, pulse oximetry, blood pressure by sphygmomanometer or noninvasive blood pressure cuff, and temperature. The use of invasive monitoring depends on the child's condition and can include arterial, intracranial, central venous, pulmonary artery, and left and right atrial pressure parameters. End-tidal carbon dioxide monitoring is required in certain patient care situations. The information gained via these monitors is only as useful as the people who interpret the data; therefore, ongoing education by the staff education committee and evaluation of use by the clinical practice committee is essential.

Bedside information systems facilitate the delivery of patient care. The benefits of information systems may outweigh the costs of acquisition and maintenance, depending on the size and complement of the specific unit. A dominant advantage of bedside information systems includes centralized and accurate data collection of patient information. This feature reveals trends in patients' physiological condition and responses to treatment. The information guides the delivery of care. The use of information systems decreases nursing time used for documentation. The ability to perform clinical research is enhanced through ease of data collection through bedside information systems. Cost data are also available through the system. The uses for bedside information systems in a critical care unit will expand as the technology continues to develop.

Other equipment necessary at the bedside of each child includes a manual resuscitation bag with an appropriately sized mask, an oxygen source with tubing, a suction source with appropriately sized catheters, emergency drug calculation chart, sterile water and saline, gloves, and a needle disposal container. Accurate calculation of fluid maintenance and infusion of drugs substantiates the need for infusion pumps, including those capable of microinfusions. Mechanical ventilators and oscillators fitted for use in patients of all sizes are required in the PICU. Other respiratory equipment needed includes air-oxygen blenders, air compressors, and gas humidifiers.

The determination for equipment acquisition depends on the type of patients cared for, recommendations from governing bodies, and financial considerations. A list of emergency equipment needed in a PICU is presented in **Table 47.2.** This equipment is checked each shift for availability and functioning by the charge nurse or designee. If equipment is replaced, cleaned, or repaired in a timely fashion, this list will be adequate to meet any emergency encountered in the pediatric critical care setting.

Table 47.1. Equipment Suggested by the Joint Commission on Accreditation of Healthcare Organizations in Special Care Units

A special care unit has specialized equipment and supplies available to assist in providing patient care and treatment. A sample of such supplies includes the following:

1. Oxygen and compressed air and the means of administration
2. Mechanical ventilatory assistance equipment, including airways, manual breathing bags, and ventilators
3. Cardiac defibrillator with synchronization capability
4. Respiratory and cardiac monitoring equipment
5. Thoracentesis and closed thoracotomy sets
6. Tracheostomy set
7. Tourniquets
8. Vascular cutdown sets
9. Infusion pumps
10. Laryngoscopes and endotracheal tubes
11. Tracheobronchial and gastric suction equipment
12. Portable x-ray
13. Device for weighing bed patients

DELIVERY OF CARE

The nursing staff of the PICU is responsible for the physical, physiological, and psychosocial care of children and their families in the PICU. The nursing care must be delivered in an organized, comprehensive fashion that meets the needs of the child and family, the nursing staff, the medical staff, and the hospital. The child and family need consistent care from a person who is concerned about the welfare of all members of the family, is familiar with the needs and problems of the family, and coordinates the efforts of all health care personnel. The nurse desires direct contact in the delivery of patient and family care. The medical staff depends on reliable, current information regarding the child's condition, progress, and responses. The hospital relies on effective professionals to deliver care according to organizational guidelines and policies. These desirable outcomes are achieved in the PICU through primary nursing, case management, and family-centered care.

Primary Nursing

Primary nursing is an effective system for care delivery in the PICU. The primary nurse, by providing the 24-hour plan of care of the child's biophysical and psychosocial needs during hospitalization, plays the role of advocate for the child and family from admission to discharge. The primary nurse provides consistency of care and fosters growth and development as well as normalcy in this foreign environment by planning interventions. The primary nurse assumes

Table 47.2. Contents of Emergency Cart in the Pediatric Intensive Care Unit

First Drawer	2 Laryngoscope handles (minimum)
	2 Small laryngoscope handles (minimum)
	Laryngoscope blades—sizes 0, 1, 2, 3 (several of each)
	1 Adult Magill forceps
	1 Pediatric Magill forceps
	Extra batteries for laryngoscope handles
	Small laryngoscope lights
	Large laryngoscope lights
	Airways
	Adult no. 5
	Child no. 2
	Infant no. 1, 0, 00, 000
	Medication labels
Second Drawer	Stylets for endotracheal tubes
	8 Yankauer suction catheters
	Oxygen tank handles
	Xylocaine spray and jelly
Third Drawer	Endotracheal tubes (at least two of each)
	2.5 Uncuffed
	3.0 Uncuffed
	3.5 Uncuffed
	4.0 Uncuffed
	4.5 Uncuffed
	5.0 Cuffed and uncuffed
	5.5 Cuffed and uncuffed
	6.0 Cuffed
	7.0 Cuffed
	8.0 Cuffed
	9.0 Cuffed
	2 Adult tracheal dilators
	2 Pediatric tracheal dilators
Bottom Shelf	Pediatric tracheostomy tray
	Adult tracheostomy tray
	Mapleson anesthesia bag
	Cricothyrotomy equipment
Other Emergency Equipment	6 Drug boxes
	ECG machine
	Defibrillator with five sets of paddles
	Adult external
	Pediatric external
	Adult internal
	Pediatric internal
	Neonatal
	Cardiac board
	Intracranial pressure monitoring devices
	Pediatric cutdown trays
	2 Thoracotomy trays
	2 Chest catheter insertion sets
	Chest tubes
	2 Pairs of wire cutters
	1 Large chest stylet
	1 Small chest stylet
	2 Infant rib spreaders
	1 Adult thoracentesis set
	1 Pediatric thoracentesis set
	5 Pacemakers
	3 Disposable sternal/iliac aspiration needles
	2 Transthoracic pacer kits
	2 Transvenous pacer kits
	2 Embolectomy catheters—sizes 2, 3, 5
	Fiberoptic intracranial pressure monitor
	A-V sequential pacemaker
	2 Transport monitors
	Military antishock trousers
	1 Adult pair
	1 Pediatric pair

responsibility for teaching the child and family and for obtaining necessary resources for optimal health care. Acknowledging that each child is unique, the plan of care is individualized by the primary nurse.

For this primary nursing system to work effectively, guidelines are developed, approved, and accepted by the nursing staff. Each nurse is expected to support and practice primary nursing on a regular basis. The nurse who admits a patient assumes responsibility for the assignment of the primary nurse. The admitting nurse can accept this role or find another nurse to assume it. The concept of primary nursing requires consistency of care and frequent interactions with other members of the health care team. Nurses' schedules will influence the selection of a primary nurse. Nurses will also assume the role of the associate nurse. The primary and associate nurses are identified on a designated staff board, on the care plan, and in a file system to be used for records for readmission of patients and evaluation purposes.

The many responsibilities of the primary nurse focus on coordination of care and the communication of this care to the child, family, nursing staff, and other health care professionals. The use of critical pathways guides the primary nurse to deliver efficient, thorough care to children in the PICU. The primary nurse is responsible for the correct use of nursing documentation tools, including the initial assessment screen, nursing care plan, teaching/learning flow sheet, standards of care, and critical pathways. The nursing care plan is reviewed and revised as necessary. The primary nurse ensures contact with the appropriate family members and initiates and coordinates meetings with personnel as indicated. Transfer or discharge plans are coordinated by the primary nurse. Communication of plans of care to the associate nurses and other staff members is the responsibility of this nurse. The associate nurse assumes these patient care responsibilities during the absence of the primary nurse. The system of primary nursing facilitates the coordination and delivery of complex care to patients in the PICU.

Case Management and Critical Pathways

A critical pathway is a patient-centered tool that guides the delivery of patient care. In response to changes in the health care environment, critical pathways provide a means to control costs, decrease length of stay, and maintain quality of care. A critical pathway is an optimal sequencing and timing of interventions by physicians, nurses, and other professionals for care of a child with a specific diagnosis or procedure designed to minimize delays and resource use and to maximize quality patient care. The critical pathway promotes collaborative practice while enhancing beneficial patient outcomes. Critical pathways are typically developed for high-volume, high-risk, and high-cost diagnoses and procedures. The plan of care is designed by a multidisciplinary team of physicians, nurses, social workers, discharge coordinators or case managers, and other health care providers as required by the specific diagnosis or procedure. Children and family members may be included in the development of critical pathways. The critical pathway includes all aspects of the care delivery to the specific patient population, including (but not limited to) assessments, medications, laboratory and radiologic tests, treatments, nutrition, activities, patient and family teaching, discharge planning. Other sections specific to a particular diagnosis or procedure are included. The critical pathway represents a typical or expected progression of interventions for the child admitted to the PICU with a specific illness or injury. It must be adjusted to meet the child's individual needs.

The initiation of critical pathways into the PICU requires education, acceptance, and support from all staff members. A successful plan for the integration involves staff participation in the design phase, education of all staff members, and identification of specific patient groups whose care will favorably fit on a critical pathway. Children with surgical diagnoses who are having procedures performed provide a good population for the introduction of critical pathways. Examples of these include craniotomy for tumor removal, tracheostomy, liver and renal transplantation, and spinal fusion.

The initiation of critical pathways for standardizing practice should involve high volume, high resource utilization, and high variability patients. Critical pathways for patients who require high use of resources will provide opportunities to decrease variability in practice. Defining outcomes for these patients will guide the care. Children with medical conditions produce the greatest variability and resource utilization in care delivery in the PICU. Defining phases of care rather than specific care in these critical pathways meets the needs of children with difficult, unpredictable courses. Phases of care may be defined as evaluation, stabilization, and recovery to discharge. This method will eliminate many variabilities in care delivery while focusing on use of resources in the PICU.

A critical pathway defines a generalized plan of care for a specific diagnosis. The pathway is a flexible tool to facilitate and direct the comprehensive, multidisciplinary plan of care that is individualized to meet the needs of the child and family. The primary goal of the critical pathway is to optimize patient care. The challenge of critical pathways in the pediatric critical care setting encourages a collaborative approach to clinical care, promoting the highest quality of care while focusing on patient outcomes and resource utilization.

Family-Centered Care in the PICU

Medical and surgical problems encountered by the child in the PICU have been addressed in detail throughout this book. In addition to delivering high technology, the PICU staff must consider the emotional and psychological responses of the child and the family and deliver care to meet these needs. The illness and hospitalization of a child results in disruption of family lifestyles. It is necessary to view the pediatric patient both as an individual and as a member of a family unit. When illness afflicts one family member, other family members are affected. Therefore, the care of the pediatric patient must extend to include care of all family members. Family-centered care is essential to the recovery of the child who is cared for in the PICU. In its efforts to define family-centered care, the Association for the Care of Children's Health has identified eight elements to be used as the basis of care delivery for children and their families in all health care settings **(Table 47.3)**[5]. This section of the chapter will address the emotional impact of the PICU on the child and family and will offer suggestions for nursing interventions.

When admission to the PICU is scheduled, the child and family can receive advanced preparation for the child's stay. When planning preparation sessions, the nurse should consider the child's age, developmental level, cognitive level, diagnosis, previous hospital experiences, and planned medical or surgical interventions. Preoperative tours allow the child and family to become familiar with the PICU environment. Same-day surgical admissions require creative scheduling of preoperative tours. Tours of the PICU can coincide with the day of preoperative surgical screening or surgical appointments. When possible, the nurse who conducts the tour should care for the child in the postoperative period. The nursing staff can facilitate this process by listing the children they have taken on tour in one place as a reference for making nursing assignments. This procedure allows the child to see a familiar face when admitted to the PICU. For the parents, meeting and knowing the nurse prior to the admission may relieve their anxiety. If the nurse has not met the family prior to day of admission, introduction on the day of surgery is essential. Meeting the family in the operating waiting area is a means to this introduction. This meeting allows the family to meet the nursing staff and ask questions before the child's admission to the PICU.

Table 47.3. Elements of Family-Centered Care[a]

1. Recognition that the family is the constant in the child's life while the service systems and personnel within those systems fluctuate
2. Facilitation of parent/professional collaboration at all levels of health care
3. Sharing of unbiased and complete information with parents about their child's care on an ongoing basis in an appropriate and supportive manner
4. Implementation of appropriate policies and procedures that are comprehensive and provide emotional and financial support to meet the needs of families
5. Recognition of family strengths and individuality and respect for different methods of coping
6. Understanding and incorporating the developmental and emotional needs of infants, children, and adolescents and their families into health care delivery systems
7. Encouragement and facilitation of parent-to-parent support
8. Assurance that the design of health-care delivery systems is flexible, accessible, and responsive to family needs

[a]Data from Shelton T, Jeppson E, Johnson B. Family-centered care for children with special health care needs. Washington, DC: Association for Care of Children's Health, 1987.

Individual consideration of the child's needs and responses during the tour set the pace for the content of the tour. Some children may wish only to stand in the hallway to look at other children in the PICU. Others will eagerly go directly to another child's bedside. Children as young as 4 or 5 years of age tend to be eager, active participants on their tours, while adolescents seem to stand back and assume a passive role.

The nurse conducting the tour takes cues from the child and offers the amount and type of information the child wants to hear. Information should include why the child will be in the PICU and what will happen to the child while there. The child needs to know what he or she will see and hear, and, most importantly, what he or she will feel. An honest approach to the subject of pain and hurt will gain the child's trust and cooperation[6].

The surgical patient arrives in the PICU directly from the operating room. Often, the child is still under the effects of anesthesia. This allows the nurse time to complete admission procedures before the child is fully awake. As the child awakens, the nurse is present to reorient the child, providing reassurance that the surgery is completed, that the child is all right, and that his or her parents are nearby.

Parents may visit their child as soon as admission procedures are complete and the child has achieved hemodynamic stability. It is important that the parents see their child as soon as possible. During this initial visit, the nurse will reinforce information given during the preoperative tour and will explain the presence and purpose of equipment in use.

The initial visit can be very emotional for the parents. A combination of emotions may be displayed, including (but not limited to) relief, anxiety, protectiveness, fear, and caring. The parents are encouraged to ask questions and to express their fears. Fears often result from confusion or misinterpretation of information. The nurse plays an important role in identifying and alleviating parental fears. Care should be given to the parents' physical needs at this time to offset the emotional impact of seeing their child lying in a bed surrounded by complex technological equipment.

Unplanned PICU admissions are usually urgent. These children are admitted from the pediatric general care units within the hospital, from other hospitals, from the scene of an accident, or from home. Children requiring emergency admission to the PICU have various types of medical problems, surgical emergencies, or injuries. The child who is awake is usually overwhelmed by the foreign nature of the PICU and frightened by the separation from his or her parents. As concerned as the nurse must be about physical assessment, the emotional needs of the child cannot be ignored. With insight and care, the nurse should be able to complete an accurate physical examination while alleviating some of the emotional stress the child is experiencing. A gentle, quiet manner and simple, unhurried explanations of what is happening and why it is happening will help the child use his or her resources to cope with the sudden change in normal life events. The semiconscious or unconscious child is treated the same way as the child recovering in the postanesthesia phase. As the child awakens, information is provided about current location, what has happened, reason for admission to the PICU, and location of parents. The pediatric intensive care nurse is the one consistent care giver, remaining at the child's bedside hour after hour, day after day. This nurse is responsible for delivering technological care as well as psychological and emotional support to the child and family. The ultimate goal in providing emotional support to the pediatric patient is to minimize stress and to enhance feelings of self-confidence and trust in parents and care givers. The goals of nursing care are to restore physiological function and to discharge the child with minimal feelings of anxiety related to the experience.

Since children will react differently to their stay in the PICU, nurses must assess each child individually to plan care that will meet individual needs. The following general guidelines should be used as a foundation to meet the child's emotional needs.

A child of any age needs honest communication about what is going to happen. There should be no surprises. The child should expect and be ready for any procedures that will take place. The nurse should be honest in describing what will hurt and what will not hurt. More time should be allowed to prepare the older child for a painful procedure. Any child needs to know how long the pain will last. The degree of pain is not relevant to the child. Descriptions of the degree of pain should be avoided since the child lacks the capabilities to differentiate these. In each situation, the child should be encouraged to express feelings of pain and should be given permission to cry when something hurts.

However, limits should also be set. Once the parents are able to cope with the stresses of the PICU, they should be encouraged to resume parental roles. They may enforce some restrictions to extremes in the child's behavior. These restrictions should conform with the child's normal methods of coping with pain and disappointment. Although it is acceptable for the child to cry when something hurts or he or she is sad, it would be inappropriate for the child to cry 24 hours a day in the PICU. Providing comfort and diversion during low stress periods helps normalize the child's PICU experience.

Choices, appropriate to developmental level, about his or her care should be given to the child. While it would be inappropriate to allow the child the choice in having blood drawn, it is appropriate for the child to choose from which finger the blood should be drawn. Allowing the child some participation in decision making increases his or her feelings of control.

A sense of security for the child in this foreign environment needs to be maintained. The child should be aware that there is always a nurse present in the room. He or she should know that nothing will happen without someone first explaining the event. The nurse must enforce this practice among the many other health care providers. The nurse should know where the parents are going and when they will return, in order to reassure the child in their absence.

The child gains a sense of security by having special toys or other belongings from home. Pictures of family members around the child's bed promote these feelings of security. For the unconscious child, parents are encouraged to make tapes of happenings from home to be played when the parents are not there. The telephone should be used to enable the child to have contact with family members who cannot visit. These actions will reinforce the child's sense of home.

The PICU nurse must help maintain the child's sense of dignity. While it is important to observe the child's physical state, care must be given to protect the child from needless exposure. The use of hospital gowns or clothes from home can eliminate this problem.

The child in the PICU is subject to sleep deprivation. The nurse is in the position to decrease this phenomenon. Scheduling care to allow periods of uninterrupted sleep at night will give the child energy to face the stresses of the day.

Parental Support

The planned or unplanned admission of the child to the PICU is stressful to parents. Investments to minimize parental stress and promote coping abilities must be made by the PICU staff.

As soon as possible after the child's admission, the primary physician and the primary nurse should be relieved from the child's bedside to meet the parents and to provide information about the child's condition and the PICU. This meeting should take place in an area that provides privacy for the parents to ask questions, grieve, and support each other. Information given at the time of impact of the crisis may be misunderstood or simply not heard. Therefore, this information will need to be repeated often enough for the parents to assimilate it and gain an understanding of their child's problem and treatment. The use of visual aids, such as anatomical drawings and pictures, is helpful when explaining to parents the specific nature of their child's health problem. An anatomical drawing provides the parents with information to which they may refer to begin to understand what is happening to their child.

The nurse's contact with the parents at this time is crucial because it is at the time of impact of stress when parents are most accepting of assistance. They depend upon the nurse, at this time and in later interactions, to clarify and to interpret the information given by the physician. An assessment of the parents' perception of their child's illness and how they have coped with other stressful events are key factors in determining the support measures that will help them cope at this time. The first meeting with the parents should be just long enough to share information, to make a quick assessment of support needs, and to prepare the parents to see their child. The parents must see their child as soon as possible after admission. This first visit may be brief as some parents find it difficult to do more than glance at their child. The importance of the parents' first visit to their child's bedside cannot be overemphasized and should be given high priority in the total plan of the medical admission procedure. Parental preparation prior to the initial visit should include descriptions of the PICU and how their child will look. Seeing their child surrounded with tubes and machinery is devastating and confirms parents' earlier feelings of shock and disbelief. Provisions should be made for the parents to sit down at the bedside while questions about their child's appearance and condition and about equipment are answered. If the child is unconscious, parents need to be encouraged to touch and talk to their child. Some parents will focus attention on the monitor screens and become frightened as those numbers change or when alarms sound. Explanations about monitor alarms and other sounds will make it easier for parents to concentrate on their child. Parents are comforted by knowing that constant nursing attention is being provided to their child.

Parental Orientation

Once the initial visit has taken place, the second phase of parental orientation begins. Usually, parents want to be nearby at all times. An orientation to the physical environment is essential. Parents need to know where to find waiting areas, rest rooms, and privacy areas; where to eat, sleep, and bathe; and where to receive and place telephone calls. A comfortable, convenient physical environment reinforces to parents that their presence is important and that their physical and emotional needs have been considered as a part of the total care of their child.

Although the PICU may not accommodate a parent living at the child's bedside, provisions should be made for parents to sleep nearby. Private parent rooms are ideal for sleep arrangements near the PICU. As the child's condition improves or stabilizes, parents often begin to go home at night or take a room nearby. Although parents find it difficult to sleep when their child is ill, sleep is essential for them as they begin to participate in their child's care.

Often, parents of critically ill children have little or no desire to eat, sleep, or pay attention to their personal-hygiene needs[7]. Parents may feel guilty taking time away from their child's bedside to meet some of these needs. It is important that the parents receive the staff's approval about their choices to seek rest outside of the hospital. When the parents' daily living needs are discussed as part of the overall orientation to the intensive care environment, the message about the staff's concern for them as well as for their child is delivered. Emphasis needs to be placed on the parents taking care of themselves to be better able to cope with their stress.

A comprehensive assessment of the family is essential to develop an individualized care plan for the child and parents[8]. Learning about the events leading to the child's admission helps identify any feelings of guilt and self-blame the parents may have. Resources such as child psychiatry, clinical social work, and clergy services can help parents adapt to their crisis situation. Knowledge of the family composition provides a way to initiate discussion with the parents about how the other members of the family are coping. Often, parents are so preoccupied with the illness of their hospitalized child that it is difficult for them to concentrate on the continuing needs of their other children. Children at home may experience separation anxiety. Finding solutions to separation from other children is easier when the parents reside near the hospital. Parents sometimes call upon adult family members, friends, neighbors, or other members of their community to assist in child care. Relieving each other at the hospital allows some continuity at home. Keeping in touch with children at home is more difficult for those families who live a long distance from the hospital. Suggestions to bolster family unity include telephone calls, sending cards with pictures of the hospital, taped messages, and, when possible, a visit home. Parents sometimes choose to bring other children to the hospital for overnight stays.

The subject of separation anxiety cannot be discussed without describing sibling visiting, which should be an option to families. Careful consideration is given to the individual needs of the siblings, including their age, previous experience with hospitals and seriously ill family members, awareness of this particular brother's or sister's health problem, and the overall strength of the family. The primary nurse and the physician work together with the parents in preparing the visiting siblings. Choosing the most appropriate time for the visit is helpful. A time when the room is less active and staff members are available to give explanations and answer questions without interruption is best. One should take into account the availability of the parents to spend time with the visiting child after the visit. With thoughtful preparation, therapeutic visits can take place at the bedside of the seriously ill or injured or dying child with their sibling.

SYSTEM COMPONENTS

The delivery of high-quality patient and family care in the PICU depends on the existence and function of certain structural systems. The care delivered in the PICU is greatly influenced by the knowledge of the nursing staff. Educational programs that meet initial and ongoing needs will directly affect the delivery of care. The use of documentation tools will facilitate the gathering and sharing of information needed to assess, plan, implement, and evaluate patient care. Clinical quality improvement mechanisms will provide a basis for monitoring and evaluating the care delivered by the staffs in the PICU. The concept of collaborative practice demonstrates a means for successful working relationships for the nursing and medical staffs. Each of these components influences the ability to deliver quality care in the PICU.

Education

The educational needs of the nursing staff in the PICU can be divided into two phases: orientation and continuing education. This section will discuss specific approaches to meet these educational requirements and the design of a unit-based staff education program.

Formal orientation programs are common in hospitals. A formal orientation program provides a more protected environment for the new employee to receive and understand key information and to be integrated into a new workplace and work group. The advantages of a successful orientation program include enhanced recruitment efforts, increased job satisfaction, and successful adjustment to the PICU nursing role, resulting in retention of the nursing staff. The benefits of a formal orientation program outweigh the costs incurred by the program.

Different groups of nurses seek employment in the PICU. These include nurses with previous PICU experience, nurses with adult critical care experience, nurses with general care experience, and recent graduates. The current job market offers selective decision making about recruitment activities. The staff of the individual unit must make a philosophical decision regarding the experience level of prospective employees.

Orientation of an experienced nurse takes place over an 8-week period, under the direct supervision of a preceptor. In addition to the clinical teaching that occurs at the bedside, there are 24 hours of classroom instruction and other self-learning activities. The orientation of a nurse with PICU experience focuses on assessment of the nurse's level of skills and the education of the norms, policies, and procedures of the new unit. A new nurse without previous PICU experience must learn about the care of the critically ill pediatric patient. The orientation of this individual is guided toward assessment, planning, implementation, and evaluation of the pediatric critically ill child. Decision-making and problem-solving skills are integrated into this orientation. After orientation, patient assignments will depend on individual performance of the nurse.

Traditionally, nurse academicians have encouraged and nurse managers have accepted that general care nursing experience benefits graduate nurses before they enter the critical care environment. The commitment by the entire PICU staff to the recruitment, development, and retention of new graduates is the key to their success in critical care nursing. There are benefits, as well as concerns, for the use of new graduates in the critical care setting. As a result of their recent completion of formal academic education, the possible benefits of graduates in the PICU include greater enthusiasm to face the challenge of critical care nursing, the ability to identify learning needs and use appropriate resources readily, and the capability to develop sound clinical skills and professional attitudes that contribute to retention. Some concerns related to nursing graduates in critical care include the need for a more extensive orientation program; limited academic clinical experience, resulting in deficiencies in critical-thinking skills, problem-solving, and priority setting capabilities; and resistance by staff members to accept new graduates in the work environment[(10)].

The orientation program for graduate nurses is designed to apply theoretical concepts learned in a classroom to clinical practice in the PICU. It provides opportunity and time for the graduate to develop psychomotor and technical skills not encountered in a basic nursing program. This goal is achieved through a 16-week internship, divided into two 8-week phases. The first part provides 24 hours per week of structured clinical experience with a preceptor and 16 hours per week of basic classroom instruction. The focus of the first 8 weeks of the program is to expose the graduate nurse to the critical care setting and to teach fundamental ICU tasks and concepts. The second 8 weeks is spent primarily in the clinical setting, supervised by a preceptor. Classroom sessions in this phase focus on advanced instruction dealing with care of specific PICU patient groups. Other course requirements include completion of tests, nursing care plans, patient care presentation, and participation in a support group led by an outside member of the nursing department. The expectation of the graduate nurse at the completion of the 16-week program is to possess the skills needed to care for the moderately ill patient in the PICU. Development continues through staff education programs once the individual graduates from the internship program.

The success of an orientation program relies on the dedication and skills of the preceptor, who plays roles: role model, socializer, and educator[(11)]. The preceptor plans learning activities and evaluates the performance and progress of the new employee. A consistent one-to-one relationship provides the most effective means of learning. The preceptor role is viewed as an advanced role for the staff nurse. The role provides the opportunity for the PICU nurse to develop teaching skills, to invest in the development of another nurse, and to refine clinical skills by attaining new knowledge and affirming existing knowledge. Staff nurses who choose to advance to the preceptor role are offered continuing education to prepare for this experience and ongoing guidance and support as they practice in this role.

Learning does not end with the orientation program. Instead, the philosophy in the PICU is that orientation provides the foundation for the continued learning that will occur throughout the PICU nurse's career. Formal and informal learning occurs to meet the educational needs of the nurses.

The routine continuing education activities are coordinated by the unit-based clinical nurse specialist (CNS) and the unit-based staff education committee. This committee, composed of interested staff members, is chaired by a senior staff nurse. The goals of the committee include ongoing assessment of the educational needs of the PICU nursing staff, planning programs to meet the identified needs, evaluation of the programs, and accurate record keeping of all unit-based activities. The committee is also responsible for compliance with mandatory educational programs as cited by the JCAHO[12]. These include cardiopulmonary resuscitation, fire and safety, infection control, risk management, and sessions related to knowledge of hazardous materials.

The subject matter for the education of the nursing staff is derived from the annual needs assessment, personnel requests, and information from the unit-based clinical quality improvement committee. The clinical quality improvement committee, discussed later in this chapter, presents monitoring results to the staff education committee when corrective actions through education are required.

The staff education committee makes preliminary plans for the year using a body systems approach. Each month the focus is on one body system, and multiple forms of education include formal presentations by staff members or guest speakers, self-learning programs including posters, slide tape/video presentations, review of journal articles, and skills stations. An example of the month's educational programs for the cardiovascular system is presented in **Table 47.4.**

Table 47.4. Examples of Topics for Staff Education on the Cardiovascular System

Lectures
Post-operative care of the patient after undergoing the Fontan procedure
Review of protocol for pulmonary hypertension in the postoperative cardiac surgical patient
Posters
Review of ECG strips
Actions and effects of vasoactive drugs
Self-Learning Packet
Emergency pharmacology
Skills Stations
Use of pacemaker
How to set up vasoactive infusions
Lead placement for 12-lead ECG

Other educational forums are available for the education of the PICU nursing staff. Informal nurse-to-nurse education occurs at the bedside. The charge nurse formally assumes this responsibility, but all staff members are expected to teach each other. Policies and procedures are reinforced during this bedside education. Primary nurse presentations represent another educational forum for PICU nurses. These short sessions allow 15 minutes for the patient presentation and 10 minutes for questions and discussion. The information included may be a review of complicated anatomy, pathophysiology of the disease process, review of a new drug agent, discussion of a complicated discharge plan, presentation of an innovative nursing care plan developed to care for a child with special needs, or discussion of any psychosocial issues related to the patient. The goal of the primary patient presentation is to provide useful information to the PICU nursing staff and to promote interaction and education among staff members.

Another regularly scheduled informal patient conference takes place between the nursing staff and the attending PICU physician. The agenda for this conference is developed by the nursing staff and includes a short patient presentation and discussion of pathophysiology of the disease process, treatment plans, unusual drug therapy, and concerns related to family adjustment and coping. In this forum, open discussions about ethical issues usually arise. As a result of this pattern, a member of the ethics committee may be invited to attend this conference to lead ethical discussions.

Specific certification programs are also used in the PICU, including the topics of intravenous insertion and blood drawing and pediatric arrest and trauma. The purpose of these educational tools is to ensure the acquisition of highly technical skills and advanced theoretical knowledge in certain areas.

Education is a strategy for reducing stress related to the unexpected. The education of the PICU nurse is an ongoing process that begins with orientation and must continue throughout the nurse's career in the critical care unit. Continuing education is essential in maintaining highly technical skills in an area that involves a wide variety of illnesses and levels of acuity where change occurs rapidly.

Documentation

Nursing documentation validates the use of the nursing process in the delivery of patient care. The components of assessment, planning, intervention, and evaluation of patient outcomes are required by the JCAHO to be part of the patient's permanent record. Recording and reporting clinical assessments, treatments, protocols, and patient responses is an essential component of nursing practice in the critical care unit. This section of the chapter includes the description of daily documentation used in the PICU.

Policies are mandatory, nonnegotiable aspects of care directed at the system in which care is delivered. Policies state what can and cannot be done in a particular organization. There is no attempt to discuss how or why some-

Table 47.5. Nursing Policy

Topic: Admission, transfer, discharge: pediatric intensive care unit (PICU)

I. Admission criteria/indicators—patients in the following categories will be admitted to the PICU:
  A. Patients who undergo the following surgical procedures:
    1. Neurosurgical service
      a. Craniotomy for tumor removal
      b. Posterior fossa exploration
      c. Arteriovenous malformation resection
      d. Repair of aneurysm
      e. Hemispherectomy
    2. Ear, nose, and throat service
      a. Tracheostomy
      b. Radical neck dissection
      c. Maxillary/mandibular osteotomy
      d. Total thyroidectomy
    3. Cardiovascular service
      a. Open heart procedures
      b. Closed heart procedures
      c. Heart, lung, and heart-lung transplantation
    4. General pediatric surgery service
      a. Pneumonectomy
      b. Tumor resection
      c. Tracheobronchial reconstruction
      d. Liver transplantation
      e. Renal transplantation
    5. Orthopedic service
      a. Spinal rod placement
      b. Spinal fusion
      c. Cervical laminectomy
    6. Any elective surgical procedure after which respiratory or cardiovascular stability is not ensured
  B. Patients whose condition necessitates the use of the following monitors or equipment:
    1. Intracranial pressure monitoring
    2. Arterial pressure monitoring
    3. Pulmonary artery monitoring
    4. Endotracheal tube
    5. Military antishock trousers
  C. Patients with any of the following conditions:
    1. Shock (hemorrhagic, cardiogenic, or septic)
    2. Hemodynamic instability
    3. Life-threatening arrhythmia
    4. Cardiac arrest
    5. Respiratory insufficiency or arrest requiring intubation and use of a mechanical ventilator
    6. Prolonged or frequent apnea
    7. Obstructive airway
    8. Acute intracranial hypertension
    9. Acutely decreasing level of consciousness
    10. Unstable seizure disorder
    11. Acute renal failure with metabolic complications
    12. Severe electrolyte disorder
    13. Severe acidosis/alkalosis
    14. Any patient at risk for a precipitous, life-threatening event
  D. Patients whose clinical status requires the following nursing care measures or treatments:
    1. Continuous monitoring of physiologic parameters as an adjunct to preventing life-threatening emergencies
    2. Frequent vital signs measurement (more often than every hour for more than 2 hours)
    3. Intracranial pressure monitoring
    4. Constant infusion and regulation of vasoactive drugs or antiarrhythmic agents
    5. Endotracheal tube
    6. Frequent arterial blood gases
    7. Concentrated nursing care in excess of that available on the general care units
  E. Certain patients transported urgently to the hospital as defined below:
    1. Pediatric trauma patients who are transferred by air or land are evaluated in the emergency room and triaged to the appropriate unit.
    2. Critically ill medical or surgical patients transferred by ambulance between hospitals may be directly admitted to the PICU.

II. Transfers from the PICU to other units
  A. Transfer orders are written prior to the transfer of a patient from the PICU to the receiving unit; the attending physician and resident staffs and charge nurses are informed of the transfer.

Table 47.5. Nursing Policy (continued)

B. A transfer note must be written by the transferring physician staff summarizing the hospital course, current therapy, and current problems; the nursing staff completes a written transfer summary and verbal report.
C. Parents are informed at the time of transfer.
D. Patients from the PICU will be considered ready for transfer based on the following criteria:
  1. Stable hemodynamic parameters
  2. Extubated with adequate blood gases
  3. Cardiac arrhythmia controlled for 24 hours
  4. Stable neurologic status
  5. Renal status maintained with dialysis routine
  6. Stable acid/base and electrolyte status
  7. Removal of hemodynamic monitoring lines
  8. Need for medical and nursing is predictable
  9. Patient's need for medical and nursing care can be met by personnel on the general care pediatric floors

III. Discharge home from the PICU
A. Patients may be discharged from the PICU to home if:
  1. The child requires no more general medical or surgical attention, or such care as required will be provided at home under medical direction
  2. The family has an appointment for a follow-up visit with the appropriate physician/clinic
  3. The family demonstrates understanding of all care required at home
B. The child who requires constant or frequent nursing care and/or monitoring may be discharged to home if:
  1. The family desires to care for the child at home
  2. Medical personnel believe there would be no benefit in keeping the child hospitalized
  3. The family can demonstrate and verbalize complete capability and understanding of the child's care
  4. Required equipment is obtained and in the home prior to discharge
  5. The parents understand the risks involved in caring for the child at home
  6. The child has a primary care physician willing to assume responsibility for following the child at home
  7. Payment mechanisms are available to ensure adequate maintenance of equipment and supplies in the home
  8. The physical environment of the home is suitable for the child and the necessary equipment
C. Teaching to be accomplished prior to discharge from the PICU is done on an individual basis by a multidisciplinary team under the direction of the primary nurse.

thing must be done as directed. Policies focus on human issues such as staffing patterns; administrative issues such as admission, discharge, and transfer criteria; material issues such as supplies and equipment needs; and environmental issues such as safety, infection control, and visiting provisions. Policies are effective in maintaining the goals that protect the patient from unsafe practices and limit administrative conflicts. Some policies are mandated by the JCAHO. An example of a nursing policy for PICU admission, discharge, and transfer criteria is depicted in **Table 47.5.**

Standards of care define the level of care a patient can expect to receive. Standards reflect both outcomes and processes of care and include procedures and protocols. Procedures, used as references for infrequently performed tasks, provide step-by-step instruction to perform a psychomotor skill **(Table 47.6).** Protocols define routines for the

Table 47.6. Nursing Procedure

Topic: Obtaining blood cultures

Policy: Blood cultures may be drawn by venipuncture and/or through an existing central line catheter as part of a sepsis work-up. Peripheral cultures can be obtained by a registered nurse certified in venipuncture. Central line cultures can be obtained by registered nurses who have completed central line instruction. A physician order must be written for any blood culture.

Equipment:
1. Gloves
2. Aerobic blood culture bottle
3. Anaerobic blood culture bottle
4. Aerobic resin bottle (if ordered)
5. 1:1 inorganic iodine or 10% povidone-iodine
6. Alcohol swabs
7. 3-cc syringe
8. 23- or 25-gauge butterfly needle (if drawing cultures by venipuncture)
9. 22-gauge needle
10. Saline flush (if drawing culture from a central line)
11. Tourniquet

Procedure:
1. Wash hands.
2. Wear gloves.
3. Remove caps from culture bottles.
4. Wipe bottle surfaces with alcohol.
5. If drawing a peripheral culture, wipe the site with 10% povidone-iodine and allow site to dry for 1 minute.
6. Wipe site with alcohol one time.
7. If drawing blood from a central line, follow steps outlined in the central line procedure. It is preferred that discard blood not be used for cultures.
8. Obtain blood sample (3 to 5 ml per bottle is preferred).
9. Change the needle used for the phlebotomy and inoculate at least 1 ml into each bottle; if only a small amount of blood is obtained, inoculate the aerobic bottle first. A resin bottle must also be inoculated if the patient is on antibiotics, with a negative blood culture, but is persistently febrile.
10. Clean the site with alcohol to remove excess iodine.
11. Fill out bacteriology lab slips, label bottles with patient's name and history number, and send to the lab. Specify catheter lumen if drawn from a central line.
12. Document on the daily flow sheet that cultures were drawn.

PROTOCOLS

CHEST TUBES/MEDIASTINAL TUBES, Nursing management of a patient with a chest tube

I. INDICATIONS FOR USE
   A. Protocol is instituted for patients with chest tubes/mediastinal tubes.

II. RESPONSIBILITY
   A. Chest tube drainage systems are changed only by registered nurses who have demonstrated competency and by physicians.

III. ASSESSMENT
   A. At the beginning of each shift and at least every 12 hr, assess for the following:
      1. Presence/absence of adventitious breath sounds and respiratory rate.
      2. Amount, color, and consistency of drainage in the chest tube drainage system.
      3. Presence of crepitus.
      4. Type and amount of drainage on dressing at insertion site.
      5. Presence of gentle bubbling in the suction control chamber, if suction is ordered.
      6. Fluctuation in water seal chamber with each breath.
      7. All connections are secure and taped.
      8. Chest tube drainage system is below chest level.
      9. Clamp(s) and Xeroform gauze are available at bedside.
   B. During dressing change, observe site for signs of infection.

IV. INTERVENTION
   A. Assess the water level of the suction control chamber and water seal chamber at least once a shift for water evaporation. Add more sterile water, if needed.
      1. Suction control chamber is read with suction turned off.
   B. Change dressing when soiled, or as indicated by physician order.
   C. If crepitus is present, outline area with marking pen.
   D. Strip chest tube only with physician order or per unit protocol.
   E. If a pleural chest tube becomes disconnected:
      1. Do not clamp unless physician order exists.
      2. Reconnect to drainage system as soon as possible after cleaning connections.
      3. If unable to reconnect immediately, submerge the chest tube 1–2 inches below the surface of a 250-ml bottle of sterile water or saline.
   F. If a mediastinal tube becomes disconnected:
      1. Clamp the mediastinal tube.
      2. Set up a new drainage system.
      3. Reconnect drainage system and remove clamp.
   G. If chest tube comes out:
      1. Place sterile Xeroform gauze over the entry site and apply pressure.
      2. Prepare for a new tube insertion.

Figure 47.1. Nursing protocol. Care of the patient with chest tubes.

H. When transporting a patient:
  1. Discontinue the suction per physician order.
  2. Keep chest tube drainage system upright and below chest level.
  3. Do not clamp chest tube.
  4. Sterile gauze and Xeroform must accompany the patient.

I. When changing the chest tube drainage system, follow manufacturer's specific procedure.

V. REPORTABLE CONDITIONS

A. The following conditions should be reported to the physician immediately:
  1. Air leak as noted by presence of bubbling in water seal chamber.
  2. Crepitus or increase in crepitus at the insertion site.
  3. Sudden change in drainage > 100 ml/hr, 10 ml/kg/hr, or sudden cessation of drainage.
  4. Signs and symptoms of infection at the insertion site.
  5. Diminished or absent breath sounds.
  6. Presence of a friction rub.
  7. Dislodged/disconnected chest tube.

VI. DOCUMENTATION

A. Document respiratory assessment every 8 hr.

B. Complete I and O every 24 hr.

C. Document reportable conditions on flowsheet.

Figure 47.1 (continued)

management of common patient care interventions. Protocols establish nursing care to ensure that quality and continuity are achieved. This tool can teach the staff about responsibilities for a specific situation and provide a quick reference for infrequent aspects of care. Examples of protocols include diagnostic, therapeutic, or prophylactic interventions requiring nursing care and use of invasive and noninvasive equipment (Fig. 47–1).

Critical pathways are used to map the plan of care for a patient with a specific diagnosis or undergoing a particular procedure. The critical pathway defines the nursing care, diagnostic and therapeutic interventions, and progress toward these goals. The pediatric critical care nurse assesses the child's progress on the pathway and delivers care accordingly. Variations from the pathway are identified. Variances can be defined as patient variances caused by clinical complications or system variances resulting from work environment issues. Nursing care, using critical pathways, focuses on patient outcomes. The nurse identifies the patient's position on the pathway and identifies the outcomes that will be achieved in the next time period. Patient and family involvement in critical pathways provides an individualized and efficient plan of care.

The high-frequency observation record facilitates collection of pertinent patient data in one place. The flow sheet also reflects integration of unit policies, procedures, protocols, and standards of care with the delivery of patient care. It is designed to streamline nursing documentation, allowing the nurse more time for direct patient care activities. The flow sheet is divided into sections that may include high-frequency graphics chart, assessment sections by system, anecdotal notes, intake and output information, laboratory data, treatments and protocols, response to interventions, and evaluation of patient and family outcomes. A high-frequency observation record is designed to capture all assessment, intervention, and evaluation data comprehensively that are obtained by the nurse while caring for the patient. The design will be determined by the individual unit and department. The flow sheet is maintained at the patient's bedside and is available at all times for review and use by all members of the health care team. Bedside information systems incorporate high-frequency observation records onto computer screens. Interfaces between the bedside system and monitors, infusion pumps, and care plans eliminate manual data entry. Additional information is entered by keyboard and computer programs. Hard copies of this chart are inserted into the permanent record every 24 hours.

Clinical Quality Improvement

Health care personnel who provide direct care to the critically ill or injured child must focus their attention on the delivery of appropriate care in addition to ensuring that the care delivered is of the highest possible quality. This section of the chapter will focus on clinical quality improvement in the PICU.

The initial phase in developing a clinical quality improvement program is the identification of clinical indicators. An indicator is a quantitative measure used to assess the performance of critical care, management, clinical, and support functions that affect patient outcomes. The clinical indicator directs attention to performance issues that may require review within a unit or organization. A rate-based indicator measures an event for which a certain proportion of the events that occur are expected when state-of-the-art care is provided. Additional assessment is required when the rate at which the event occurs crosses a threshold or data suggest opportunities for improvement. An example of a rate-based indicator in the PICU includes the number of patients who encounter an unplanned extubation within the total number of patients who were intubated and moved to planned extubation. A sentinel event indicator measures a serious patient care event that requires further investigation of that specific event each time the event occurs. An example of a sentinel event indicator is readmission to the PICU within 24 hours of transfer. Rate-based and sentinel event indicators measure either process or outcome. Important process indicators assess events or activities that are closely linked to patient outcomes. Measurement of the activities in the process allows an assessment of improvements that can be made. Outcome indicators assess what happens or does not happen after a process is or is not performed. An example of an outcome indicator involves assessment that a parent is able to manage his/her child's respiratory and tracheostomy care as a result of effective patient teaching.

Improvements in quality care can be achieved when steps involved in developing indicators are followed. This plan includes identification of important processes of care and identification of key functions. Key functions are the important parts of care delivery that have the greatest potential to affect patient outcomes and provide important information about improvement opportunities. Key functions reflect high-volume, high-risk, high-cost patient care functions. Identification of clinical indicators is best achieved through a multidisciplinary process and involves brainstorming, input from regulatory bodies, input from other institutions, patient and family surveys, and report of occurrences. This dialogue provides a rationale for the usefulness of the indicator. Dimensions of performance measurements are then identified. Examples of dimensions of performance include availability, appropriateness, effectiveness, efficacy, efficiency, and timeliness of care; respect and caring; and safety in the work environment. Identification of the indicator population and sample is the next step. A population consists of all of the patients, processes, or outcomes that could be measured. A sample may then be identified from the population at a later time. Data collection methodology is defined and includes data sources, method, sample, frequency, analysis, and reporting. A tool is developed that defines the data elements to be collected. An indicator rate is specified by defining the data elements that will represent the numerator and denominator data. The final step in developing the indicator is to determine the trigger for evaluation. Trigger points should be reevaluated periodically. The data retrieved for each indicator do not lead to a conclusion about the quality of care delivered on its own. Trends may require a more in-depth evaluation of the services or processes delivered to identify the cause of a variation. This process will identify opportunities for improvement in the care delivered to children and families in the PICU[12]. A sample of a pediatric critical care clinical quality improvement activity is illustrated in **Table 47.7.**

Table 47.7. Pediatric Intensive Care Clinical Quality Improvement Activity

Aspect of care: endotracheal intubation	
Indicator:	
1. The patient will remain intubated with proper tube placement.	
2. The patient will be adequately sedated while intubated.	
3. Endotracheal tube placement will be confirmed and documented.	
4. The endotracheal tube will be securely and correctly taped in place.	
Threshold for evaluation: 99%	
Results:	99.4% (data collected over a 6-month period; results from number of extubation divided by the number of intubated patient-days).
Conclusions:	At the time of this monitoring activity, there were not excessive accidental extubation.
Corrective Actions:	None at this time.
Follow-up:	Remonitor if more than five unplanned extubations per month occur.

The focus of this model is on the clinical and service aspects of patient care. The JCAHO guidelines require a multidisciplinary approach to quality improvement activities. This multidisciplinary committee is responsible for developing a system to ensure that monitoring and evaluation activities are planned, systematic, comprehensive, and ongoing. The process is based on clinical indicators and thresholds determined acceptable for practice. Routine data collection and evaluation should occur. Appropriate corrective actions should be defined to resolve identified problems. A mechanism to report all activities to a hospital-wide program is necessary.

The multidisciplinary clinical quality improvement program in the PICU meets biweekly or monthly and includes as its members the PICU attending and fellow medical staff and representatives of the nursing, respiratory therapy, radiology, and pathology staffs. The agenda for this meeting includes all clinical indicators and mortality and morbidity occurrences. The mortalities are discussed, including a clinical presentation, events that led to the death, and pathology findings. This discussion concludes with the identification of any aspects of care that should have been modified. Events of morbidity are derived from hospital occurrence forms or from medical, nursing, or respiratory therapy patient event forms. The patient event form is used to identify any event that requires discussion about changes in clinical practice in the ICU. After presentation of the event, discussion occurs regarding clinical practice and existing policies. An outcome is achieved for each account that may be either a change or no change in practice. Minutes of the meeting are forwarded to the department and hospital clinical quality improvement committees.

This multidisciplinary committee is linked to the nursing unit-based clinical quality improvement committee by the nurse manager's participation on the committee. The unit-based committee, chaired by a senior nursing staff member, meets monthly; its membership consists of approximately 10 staff nurses. The goal of the unit-based nursing clinical quality improvement committee is delegation of the nursing quality improvement activities to the staff nurses, thereby empowering them to make decisions about the quality of care. The major benefit of the unit-based program results as the nurses feel more committed to solving a problem they have identified. In addition, nurses quickly learn what constitutes high-quality nursing care and how they affect the quality of care delivered. Nursing and physician monitoring of outcomes is essential in the critical care unit to guarantee the delivery of the highest possible quality of patient care.

Collaborative Practice

The concept of collaboration is not new to clinical practice in the critical care setting. Studies have shown that collaboration positively influences patient outcomes(15) and critical care nurse satisfaction(16). The importance of collaboration has been acknowledged by the American Association of Critical-Care Nurses and the Society of Critical Care Medicine in their joint publication of the Collaborative Practice Model(17). This document promotes collaboration in the management of the critical care unit with shared authority and responsibility by the medical director and the nurse manager for the functioning of the unit. This requires joint planning, goal-setting, problem solving, and decision making. The essential factors in the collaborative model include effective communication, trust, accountability, competence, and administrative support(18).

The medical director and the nurse manager play key roles in the development and acceptance of the collaborative model in the PICU. As these individuals are role models for collaborative practice, this practice becomes an accepted philosophy of the unit and is evidenced in the behaviors of the personnel caring for the patients. The development of collaboration begins with acknowledgment of the concept, acceptance of this as a goal for the individuals and the unit, and a plan to implement the practice. Establishment of communication forums will provide the structure for collaborative practice. Multiple forums enhance this process, including clinical meetings, such as patient care conferences and joint educational sessions; administrative meetings, such as joint clinical quality improvement meetings; and planning meetings for the unit, department, and hospital.

NURSING HIERARCHY

The nursing staff of the PICU provides a critical link in the organizational goals of providing care to critically ill and injured children. Multiple nursing roles are established to impact clinical practice and enhance professional development. These nursing roles will be discussed individually to define the pediatric critical care nursing organization.

Role of the Nurse Manager

The American Association of Critical-Care Nurses' scope of practice advocates that the role of the manager is to provide a supportive environment for patients and nurses(19). The nurse manager assumes the responsibility of translating the organizational goals into action. The individual should possess goal-setting, planning, decision-making, communication, and leadership skills. Personal characteristics necessary for this individual include (but are not limited to) creative insight, versatility, patience, and the ability to be visionary and to focus on the needs of the unit as they are now and will be in the future(20). The nurse manager is viewed as a link connecting the patient, the nurse, and the environment, thereby assuming an influential organizational role.

The general categories of the nurse manager's responsibilities include patient care management, personnel management and development, and management of unit operations. A leader and role model for professional nursing practice, the nurse manager is accountable for defining and maintaining the standard of nursing care and practice, assuming 24-hour responsibility for quality patient care delivery for the nursing unit. Specific performance tasks that ensure the delivery of the highest quality of care must have high priority for the nurse manager. These include participation in the formulation of policies and standards of care and the initiation of a clinical quality improvement program to measure nursing care according to the standards. The nurse manager ensures that clinical practice is evaluated by current clinical knowledge, standards of care, regulatory guidelines, and the results of monitoring activities. By employing the roles of patient and family advocate, clinical resource to the nursing staff, and liaison with the medical staff, the nurse manager uses resources to gather information about the delivery of nursing care.

Personnel management by the PICU nurse manager is pivotal to the development of the staff. Included in these responsibilities are recruitment and retention activities; development, evaluation, and mentoring of staff members; and scheduling and staffing determinations. Each of these parts influences the nursing and unit environment and impacts the overall function and operation of the PICU.

Recruitment and retention strategies influence the functional capabilities of the pediatric intensive care environment. The nurse manager recruits, interviews, and selects staff for the patient care unit. Successful recruitment must be employed by health care organizations to ensure an adequate supply of nurses. The nurse manager plays an important role in the organization's recruitment plan by participating in recruitment activities, developing programs to recruit nurses and student nurses, promoting affiliations with community and professional organizations, and creating and supporting a work climate conducive to the professional development of the nursing staff.

Successful recruitment strategies do not ensure adequate staffing requirements. The loss of nurses through turnover impacts the nursing staff, the delivery of quality care, and the organization's fiscal requirements. The nurse manager plays a role in nurses' job satisfaction, resulting in the retention of qualified personnel. The nurse manager must create a professionally enhancing environment in which each nurse is aware of and committed to the goals of the unit and the nursing staff. By setting high yet achievable expectations, the nurse manager promotes the professional development of staff members that contributes to the successful function of individuals and the staff as a whole. Aware of the expectations, the critical care nurse must then be supported in an autonomous practice, given full accountability for patient care.

The nurse manager plays a crucial role in the development of the nursing staff. This begins with the staff's acquisition of critical care nursing skills and expands to the professional development of the nurse. The nurse manager ensures that an educational system is in place to meet the needs of the nurse new to the critical care unit as well as to the more sophisticated needs of the experienced nurse. Other developmental strategies the nurse manager can plan with the individual staff member include exposure to professional activities and organizations; participation in hospital committees; development of managerial, teaching, or publishing skills; and other career counseling opportunities.

Staffing of the unit is the nurse manager's responsibility. Challenging factors to be considered in the determination of staffing needs include census, acuity, and level of nursing ability. The nurse manager adjusts staffing levels to provide for variable acuity levels with adherence to the budgeted nursing hours of care. Specific scheduling of the nursing staff may be accomplished through self-scheduling or a scheduling committee.

Management of unit operations includes maintenance of an environment that encourages quality patient care and staff satisfaction. This area includes sound fiscal management; efficient use of resources, supplies, and equipment; and effective communication with support services personnel and other departmental or hospital divisions that provide service to the patient care area.

The role of the nurse manager has evolved to one of 24-hour accountability and total responsibility for patient care, nurse performance, and fiscal management of the unit. These three general categories of management provide the structure necessary for optimal functioning of the PICU.

Role of the Clinical Nurse Specialist

The unit-based CNS interfaces with individuals in a variety of roles and services. This individual represents the unit in situations where an extensive clinical knowledge base combined with an organizational perspective is required. This is accomplished through the roles of clinical expert, educator, consultant, researcher, manager, and change agent[20].

The clinical expert role is achieved by the CNS's awareness and knowledge of new clinical trends and treatments. Acting as a role model in delivering nursing care to the complex patient allows the CNS to work with the nursing staff at the bedside. One-on-one interactions with staff nurses facilitates the development of their nursing skills. This individual promotes the concept of critical care when describing care to others outside the PICU setting.

The role of the educator is accomplished through individual teaching, group seminars, and program development. The initiation of new programs, treatments, equipment, and personnel entails continuous education in the pediatric critical care setting. The CNS coordinates the orientation programs for new staff members. Responsibilities include instruction about teaching strategies for staff members new to the preceptor role; assignment of preceptors to the orientee; consultation with both preceptors and orientees regarding progress toward a successful outcome; coordination of activities including schedules, room assignments, and teaching tools; and involvement in the evaluation process. The CNS serves as a liaison with the staff education committee through a consultant role. Demonstrating expertise in the role of education, the CNS guides the committee members through their responsibilities of needs assessments, program development and evaluation, and development of their teaching skills. Staying up to date with the latest clinical developments, the CNS communicates with company representatives to facilitate staff education about new equipment and procedures. Community education provides a further dimension to the CNS's educational role component. One advantage of this forum is public exposure of services, professional activities, and organizational goals. Instruction in an academic setting also enhances the exposure of the role of the CNS while providing the students an arena for practical preparation.

The consultant role of the CNS is achieved by interfacing with many people in the health care setting. The CNS provides unit-to-unit communication when providing the exchange of clinical expertise in other unit settings. Nurse-physician dialogue about patient, unit, or system matters assists in the achievement of improved patient outcomes. The verbal exchanges between bedside nurses and the CNS promote education, development, and collaboration in these roles.

The CNS's role in research will vary depending on the environment and the individual's experience in the role. At a minimum, the CNS disseminates and promotes the use of current research findings pertinent to the PICU setting. This may be accomplished by meetings of a journal club, where the nursing staff reviews and discusses articles pertaining to their practice. Participation by the CNS in interdisciplinary research is another avenue to the achievement of the researcher role. These forums provide a mechanism that allows the CNS to promote research-based practice. The CNS may also direct a unit-based nursing research project.

The CNS's role as manager promotes achievement of the organizational goals through the demonstration of clinical leadership. Awareness of unit resources such as personnel, equipment, and budget allows the CNS to identify organizational attributes and barriers and to plan effectively with and around these to achieve the desired outcome. As described in the other roles, the clinical specialist has frequent contact with the nursing staff. This involvement will add an additional resource for the evaluation of staff members.

The CNS is a change agent. Incorporating aspects of the roles described above to facilitate the integration of the most current knowledge to deliver state-of-the-art care accomplishes this task. Successfully functioning in this advanced position, the PICU CNS meets the role definitions and contributes to positive accomplishments for patients, the nursing staff, and the organization.

Career Ladders

Clinical ladders are used to guide and promote professional growth. Behaviors are defined at different levels of the advancement tool. Achievement of the behaviors allows the nurse to advance through the clinical ladder. The clinical ladder positively influences staff satisfaction, retention of the nursing staff, and individualized performance. The levels and classifications in a clinical ladder are determined by the individual nursing institution. The following sections describe the roles of different clinical nursing positions in the organization.

Role of the Senior Nurse

A position achieved by promotion, the senior staff nurse adds a broader perspective of unit management to professional practice. This PICU nurse, who demonstrates expertise in clinical care, assumes a leadership role for a specific aspect of care delivered in the unit. Recognized as an expert in the given area, the senior nurse is responsible for the development of standards of care, presentation of educational activities, and assurance of quality care in the PICU. Aware of clinical advances in the assigned focus, the senior nurse coordinates the integration of these changes into clinical practice. The diverse range of illnesses and disease entities in the PICU patients promotes this model of accountability and responsibility for a specific clinical area. Examples of role delineations for the senior nurses in the PICU include the respiratory, cardiovascular, neurologic/neurosurgical, trauma, gastrointestinal and nutrition, and renal systems. Other individuals in the senior nurse role may assume leadership responsibilities for unit-related activities such as the primary nursing, scheduling, staff education, clinical practice, and clinical quality improvement committees. The environment of the unit will determine the specific areas that require leadership positions.

The senior staff nurse actively participates in the individual and group development of the nursing staff. The roles of educator, mentor, and evaluator aid in the maturing process of other PICU nurses. The senior nurse is responsible for the clinical and professional development of a group of clinical nurses. This relationship begins when a nurse completes orientation. Regularly scheduled meetings occur between the two individuals. The purposes of the meetings are to define mutual goals, develop a work plan to meet the goals, and evaluate progress toward these goals. The advantages of this relationship for the clinical nurse include the one-to-one attention of a mentor to career development, the mutual attention to achieve clinical experiences, and objective input into the individual's evaluation. The senior nurse is provided with experiences and opportunities to develop management skills, including communication, role development, and evaluation abilities. This structure is useful to provide ongoing feedback, individualized developmental plans, and personnel management experience to a large staff.

Role of the Charge Nurse

The charge nurse is an integral person whose performance affects the daily operations of the PICU. This individual performs multiple tasks; however, he or she does not assume direct patient care responsibilities. Expectations of the role include awareness and knowledge of the condition and status of each patient, the medical plans for the patients, including diagnostic testing, procedures, and surgical interventions; the status of impending admissions to the PICU; and the availability of beds and other resources in the PICU. The charge nurse coordinates daily PICU patient care activities. As a resource to other nurses, this individual provides educational information related to equipment, patient conditions, and anticipation of complications or signs reflective of these complications. The charge nurse provides the second pair of hands needed for patient care. This is particularly important during the admission of the patient and during emergency situations. The charge nurse assumes the nursing leadership role during resuscitative situations. In these instances, communication occurs from the physician in charge to the charge nurse who supervises and delegates tasks to other nursing personnel.

The charge nurse should possess a sound clinical knowledge base, excellent communication skills, and refined teaching skills. The charge nurse brings patient-care-related problem-solving and decision-making abilities to the role. Experiences in this position will further develop these skills in management scenarios. The charge nurse role is beneficial to the daily function of the unit and to the nurse's professional role development.

Role of the Bedside Nurse

The bedside nurse is responsible for the nursing care of the critically ill patient. The medical staff and the nursing staff operate from different bodies of knowledge and practice, yet the integration of both promotes the well-being of the child and family and contributes to the professional development of both disciplines. These disciplines must work closely together to achieve the best outcomes in patient care. This requires close, ongoing communication between the nursing and medical staffs, which develops from the unit's internal philosophy of collaborative practice.

An essential role of the bedside nurse is to provide the continuity necessary in patient care management. Pediatric critical care nurses are the ones who remain at the patient's bedside for 24 hours a day throughout the child's stay in the PICU. This continuity favorably affects patient care,

Table 47–8. Pediatric Intensive Care Unit Nursing Care Guidelines

Bedside Equipment

The following equipment must be available and in working order at each patient's bedside:

1. Oxygen
2. Mask of appropriate size
3. Blood pressure cuff
4. Suction source and appropriately sized suction catheters
5. Manual resuscitation bag
6. Arrest drug calculations
7. Sterile water and sterile saline
8. Gloves
9. Sharps container

Vital Signs

Routine vital signs (temperature, heart rate, respiratory rate, blood pressure) are taken every 1 to 2 hours depending on patient's stability. Newly admitted patients (postoperative, transfer, new admission): every 15 min for 1 hour, every 30 min for 1 hour, then advance to routine vital signs depending on patient's stability. Hemodynamically unstable patients requiring vasoactive therapy: every 15 min for heart rate and blood pressure until 1 hour after therapy discontinued

Monitors

All PICU patients must be on cardiopulmonary monitors at all times. Alarms must be on at all times with appropriate limits set.

IV Fluids

IV bag/bottle is changed every 24 hours on the day shift; IV tubing is changed every 72 hours. Pressure fluid bags are changed every 24 hours. IV fluids are checked against the physician's order and the Medication Administration Record with the off-going nurse and initialed by the oncoming nurse at the beginning of each shift. Peripheral IV dressings are changed daily; central line dressings are changed every 72 hours or more often if the dressing is soiled, is leaking, or has become loose.

Calculate and record the hourly intake of IV fluids every hour. Keep a running total for 24 hours (12:00 midnight to 12:00 midnight). Fluids administered in the operating room or prior to admission to the PICU are not included in the running totals. Replacement fluids are recorded separately from IV fluids. All patients weighing less than 10 kg will have pressure line fluids regulated by an infusion pump.

Chest Tubes

Measure and record drainage every hour. The chest tube system is observed for the presence of an air leak every hour and documented.

Urinary Output

Record urinary output at least every 2 hours, every 1 hour on hemodynamically unstable patients. Check specific gravity and Bilistix every 4 hours unless ordered otherwise.

Nasogastric Tubes

Record nasogastric drainage every 4 hours. Check and record pH and guaiac every 12 hours.

Weights

Obtain admission weight. Daily weights are done on all cardiac and renal patients and children less than 2 years of age.

Blood Drawing

Record the amount of blood drawn from children who weigh less than 10 kg.

Routine Nursing Care

Position Changes

Turn patients every 2 hours during the day and every 4 hours during the night as indicated. Contraindications include patients with labile intracranial pressure and hemodynamics. Perform passive range of motion every 4 hours according to patient's mobility.

Dressing Changes

First postoperative dressing change is performed by the surgeon, then every day by the nurse.

Daily suture line care.

Nasogastric Tubes

Placed in all intubated patients with few exceptions: patients with basilar skull fractures and low platelet counts. Maintain patency by irrigating with 5 to 15 ml of air or sterile saline every 2 hours.

Eye Care

Instill lubricate ointment every 2 hours in the eyes of any child without a normal blink.

Mouth Care

Perform mouth care every 4 hours.

family responses and coping mechanisms, communication with the physician staff, and performance following the unit's determined standards for quality care. General nursing care responsibilities include implementation of medical plans of care, performance of ongoing assessment indicating changes in the patient's condition from physiologic causes or responses to treatment, assumption of the role of the patient's advocate, and assessment and development of plans to meet the family's needs. Generic nursing care guidelines performed in the PICU are listed in **Table 47.8.**

The nursing staff assumes various other roles that promote the organizational goals of the unit. These include education, representation of the PICU to the hospital and community, and the enhancement of professional activities. The PICU nursing staff, by virtue of their critical care skills, are viewed as experts in the areas of physical assessment, emergency procedures, and crisis intervention. Opportunities to further develop these teaching skills are provided through the education of others. The education of new PICU nurses is discussed in the section on orientation. Other recipients of teaching by the PICU nurses are general care unit nurses, prehospital care students, and graduate and undergraduate nursing students. Nurses have been instrumental in the development of an arrest management program through which nurses from the hospital are taught about airway management, emergency pharmacology, and special procedures in didactic and skills stations. As part of their curriculum, paramedic students fulfill the pediatric component of their course work standing side by side with the PICU nurse performing basic care such as suctioning, manual ventilation, taking vital signs, and communicating with children. Nursing students at undergraduate and graduate levels complete their clinical objectives by caring for PICU patients with a PICU nurse preceptor. The results of these educational interactions are multifaceted in meeting the educational needs of the student and developing the teaching skills of the PICU nurse as well as promoting optimal care for the child in a variety of settings.

Projecting a positive image of the PICU is the responsibility of all staff members working in the unit. This goal affects the delivery of care and the development of the staff and the unit. The bedside nurse is influential in promoting the unit's image to the family through the delivery of quality care, recognition of areas in need of improvement, and open communication with all members of the health care team. Effective communication with the many people who interface with the PICU promotes optimal functioning of the unit. This is necessary with persons within the hospital, including support services personnel and staff from other units, and people affiliated with the care of the child prior to admission to or after discharge from the PICU, such as prehospital care givers, private pediatricians, and staff from referring hospitals.

Professional activities are important for individual staff nurse, group, unit, and organizational development. Exposing the nursing staff to professional issues and opportunities influences the delivery of care, the work environment, and the personal accomplishments of the staff. Participation in professional organizations allows the staff to contribute to a larger sphere, affecting their personal lives and professional careers.

The nursing staff of the PICU plays an integral role in the delivery of care to critically ill and injured children. Many systems influence the delivery of this care. Established organizational structures enhance the professional development of the nursing staff and facilitate high-quality patient care that promotes the well-being of the child and family, the ultimate goal of pediatric critical care nursing.

References

1. Gillies DA. Nursing management—a systems approach. Philadelphia: WB Saunders, 1989:71–93.
2. Committee on Hospital Care and Pediatric Section of the Society of Critical Care Medicine. Guidelines for pediatric intensive care units. Pediatrics 1983,72:364–372.
3. Committee on Hospital Care and the Pediatric Section of the Society of Critical Care Medicine. Guidelines for pediatric intensive care units. Critical Care Medicine 1983,11:753–760.
4. Fein IA. Critical care unit design: environmental and psychosocial considerations. In: Fein IA, Strasbourg MA, eds. Managing the critical care unit. Rockville, MD: Aspen Publishers, 1987:113–126.
5. Shelton T, Jeppson E, Johnson B. Family-centered care for children with special health care needs. Washington, DC: Association for the care of children's health, 1987.
6. Petrillo M, Sanger S. Emotional care of hospitalized children. Philadelphia: JB Lippincott, 1972.
7. Broome ME. Working with the family of a critically ill child. Heart Lung 14:368, 1985.
8. Azaronoff PM, Hardgrove C. The family in child health care. New York: John Wiley & Sons, 1981.
9. Haggard A. Hospital orientation handbook for nurses and allied health professionals. Rockville, MD: Aspen Systems Corporation, 1984.
10. American Association of Critical-Care Nurses Management Special Interest Group. Integration of new graduates into critical care. Laguna, CA: AACN, 1988.
11. Alspach JG. From staff to preceptor: a preceptor training program instructor's Manual. Secaucus, NJ: Hospital Publications Inc., 1988.
12. Joint Commission on Accreditation of Healthcare Organizations. Accreditation Manual for Hospitals Oakbrook Terrace, IL: Oakbrook Terrace, 1995:67–68.
13. Schroeder P, Marbusch R. Nursing quality assurance: a unit-based approach. Rockville, MD: Aspen Publication, 1984.
14. American Association of Critical-Care Nurses. Outcome standards for nursing care of the critically ill. Laguna Niguel, CA: AACN, 1990.
15. Baggs JG. Intensive care unit use and collaboration between nurses and physicians. Heart Lung 1989;18:332–338.
16. Baggs JG, Ryan SA. ICU nurse-physician collaboration and nursing satisfaction. Nurse Econ 1990;8:386–392.
17. American Association of Critical-Care Nurses. Collaborative practice model: the organization of human resources in critical care units. Laguna Niguel, CA: AACN, 1982.
18. Devereux PM. Essential elements of nurse-physician collaboration: nursing practice considerations. J Nursing Admin 11:37–39.
19. American Association of Critical-Care Nurses. Scope of critical care nursing practice. Laguna Niguel, CA: AACN, 1986.
20. Ward CR, Cardin S. Selecting competent critical care nurse managers. In: Cardin S, Ward CR, eds. Personnel management in critical care nursing. Baltimore: Williams & Wilkins, 1989:2–10.
21. Hamric AB, Spross JA. History and overview of the CNS role. In: Hamric AB, Spross JA, eds. The clinical nurse specialist—in theory and practice. Philadelphia: WB Saunders, 1989:3–18.

Continuous Quality Improvement in the Pediatric Intensive Care Unit

48

Katherine A. Welkie
J. Michael Dean

INTRODUCTION

The determined, sequential reader of this textbook will have arrived at this chapter after having read nearly two volumes of detailed, highly technical medical information about pediatric critical care. That reader may justifiably ask, Why do I need to know about continuous quality improvement in the pediatric intensive care unit (PICU), or anywhere else, for that matter? Our answer to that question may be surprisingly appealing to a critical care physician or nurse who has a strong scientific bias. This textbook contains nearly 2000 pages of clinical, pathological, and physiological data that have been accrued by careful scientific enterprise in some instances and by widespread anecdotal experience in other instances. Entire journals are devoted to the subject of cerebral metabolism, and careers have been made in determining whether certain classes of drugs can exert particularly beneficial effects in various conditions. What we should all find surprising, nearly to the point of absurdity, is that we have rarely turned the scientific microscope toward the operational aspects of health care. That is, we are believers in the scientific method as long as the object of that methodology is a molecule, cell, or perhaps even an entire patient. However, when it comes to the subject of how we deliver care in the intensive care unit, we have traditionally thrown scientific method out the window. The essence of this chapter, therefore, is to convey the notion that a self-critical, scientifically conducted analysis of our operational aspects of delivering health care, in and out of the intensive care unit, will yield improvements in outcomes, both for the patient as well as for the providers of that care[1–17]. This is particularly pertinent as we enter an increasingly constrained economic environment, because the dollar resources will no longer be as forgiving of variation as has been true in the past.

This chapter contains few, if any, profound concepts. Indeed, we find one of Augustine's laws to be particularly pertinent in this respect:

> Profound concepts are often characterized by their difficulty of being understood; therefore persons unfamiliar with Greek or Latin should give intellectual depth to their ideas by utilizing acronyms to a degree more or less proportionate with the lack of sophistication of the ideas being presented. Q.E.D. (18, page 33).

To many readers, quality assurance or improvement relates to accreditation by the Joint Commission for Accreditation of Healthcare Organizations[19–22]. The hospital-based clinician, whether nurse or physician, has been barraged by quality assurance[23–70], quality improvement, risk management[33,49,71–83], case review, process improvement, total quality management[61,84], total quality improvement, continuous quality improvement, clinical process improvement, and clinical practice improvement[85]. Each of these terminologies has been accompanied by an appropriate set of abbreviations, and a visit to the local bookstore will always reveal an entire shelf of self-help books for business, concentrating on one or more of these various subjects. Both authors of this chapter were busy clinicians in a pediatric intensive care unit for nearly a decade before becoming interested in this subject, and we approached the subject with a great deal of healthy perspective. The major impediment to becoming enthusiastic about this subject, indeed, may have been the terminology and the religious zeal with which each of these buzz-worded subjects was introduced to business. In addition, it has often been confusing to understand how manufacturing concepts could or ought to be applied to the health care system.

Many readers will probably comment quietly to themselves, or perhaps not too quietly, that they did not enter medicine or nursing in order to be part of a business. Indeed, their motivations for entering this field were nearly purely humanitarian, though they recognized that certain benefits accrue to professionals in the health care system. However, clinical medicine is a business. Indeed, clinical medicine is our business. Historically, health care administration has been considered to be the administrators who are in charge of financial matters, quite separate from the deeds or misdeeds of clinicians, who have operated as independent agents within the system. Whether the lack of competition in the medical care system has led to our current health care expenditures is a matter for debate. However, increased management of health care is inevitable, as our society attempts to reign in the escalating costs of medical care in the United States. Increasingly, this means that providers will be at risk for financial loss, dependent upon their performance within the system. While in the past this risk has been assumed nearly solely by hospitals, it is clear that this risk will begin to be assumed increasingly by all physicians. While managed care has often been nicknamed "mangled care," we would suggest that managed care should be interpreted as having the right information in the hands of clinicians in order that they can better deliver the care they desire to provide. Close collaboration with hospitals and payers will be important, otherwise clinicians will not have access to critical data that will allow them to better assess the outcomes of their care. There should be no shame in identifying medicine as a business, as nearly all of us are willing to accept a paycheck in return for our services. Nearly all of us send bills to patients and insurance companies for our services. Nearly all of those patients read their bills, often in excruciating detail. To deny the business aspects of our careers, often in a moral huff, is merely burying one's head in the sand. Medicine is a business. There have been improvements to the way businesses have been managed over the last 30 years, and we would ask the reader to consider the possibility that some of those improvements may in fact be applicable to the health care system.

Many books are available to introduce the concepts of quality improvement in the health care industry[11,77,85–97]. The purpose of this chapter is to convince the reader that continuous quality improvement in the pediatric intensive care unit is crucial to our future survival[98] in the health care system in the United States and elsewhere. The pediatric intensive care unit represents a significant cost center in today's hospitals, and it will become increasingly difficult, if not impossible, to deflect the criticisms of nonclinicians about the way resources are used in the intensive care setting. We must seek to answer several questions, and we must attempt to answer these questions in a relatively scientific manner. First, are we doing the right thing to individual patients? Second, are we identifying the right time at which to do the right thing to such patients? Third, are we doing the right thing in the correct manner? Fourth, what was the final outcome for the patient, after our "doing the right thing at the right time in the correct way" for this individual? The reader should keep these four questions in mind as he or she reads this chapter, as the human patient should provide the focus for all discussions of improvement of a health care system.

TRADITIONAL QUALITY ASSURANCE

For many years quality assurance efforts have focused on the performance of individual clinicians, and most of these activities have been driven by review of specific incidents. There are several flaws in this approach. It is necessary to consider the types of variations that are seen in everyday life and to understand concepts of random and assignable variation, and it is necessary to consider the nature of errors in any field. Traditional quality assurance fails to acknowledge errors as anything but directly assignable problems relating to specific clinicians. Berwick et al. have stated it well: "Elegant in its own way as a descriptive science, academic quality assurance has one other serious flaw: *It lacks a general theory of the sources of hazard in the complex processes of care.* On the whole, to the extent that quality measurement tools have been developed at all, they tend to unveil the *fact* of flaw, not its *cause*." (11, page 11)

For many years case review has been the primary mechanism of determining events that have gone wrong and attempting to ensure that such events do not occur again. For example, when the surgeon performs the incorrect operation, that surgery is reviewed by members of a quality assurance committee, who conclude that indeed the surgeon performed the wrong operation. If such an event occurs frequently enough, then the hospital may sanction the surgeon or decide to remove him or her from the medical staff. Errors in the administration of medications may be noticed because of the resulting complications, and when these patient cases are reviewed, once again the quality assurance committee attempts to assign the cause of the mishap, and by providing feedback to the cause, hopefully the recurrence of such events is reduced.

This approach to quality assurance results in an unsurprising reaction. When individual physicians, nurses, or other health care professionals receive a performance review from a quality assurance committee, indicating perhaps that they did an unfortunate deed, there are several possible reactions, none of which are particularly useful. The first reaction may be denial, in which case the clinician simply tells the quality assurance committee that it does not know what it is talking about. In many cases, the clinician may in fact be correct. A second reaction is anger, as the clinician may indicate to the committee that he or she already understood that the result was unfortunate and was fully aware of the issues surrounding the case. In this instance the quality assurance committee has added nothing to the clinician's ability to change his or her behavior. Third, and perhaps most important, while the quality assurance committee may lay blame at the feet of a specific clinician, it is a fact that as clinicians we oversee a massively complex process of health care, and it is often unclear in what manner a clinician ought to change his or her behavior in order to avoid recurrence of an untoward event or incident. Thus, despite the fact that the quality assurance committee says that a clinician needs to change his or her practice in order to avoid specific recurrence of the specific event, the validity of attribution of the event to a specific clinician may be weak, and the clinician is faced with the difficulty of trying to change something just for the sake of changing something. One can summarize the situation as follows. Traditional quality assurance emphasizes sorting the clinicians by capability and shooting those individuals who are sufficiently bad to exceed some specific threshold value of poor performance. This results in a fear on the part of the clinicians that quality assurance activities may be vindictive, and often results in the clinician "killing the messenger" rather than facing any possibilities of self-improvement. Finally, despite the fact that the clinician may not have done something that he or she can identify as the cause of the mishap, he or she may be tempted to then micro-manage their own process of care, doing almost anything to fix it (whether right or wrong).

An understanding of variation is the key to changing this approach. Let us take two examples of variation from our everyday lives. Consider first the variation of your commuting time to work every morning. Perhaps the average time for you is 20 minutes. You probably leave your home within a predictable window of time, and you arrive at work at a predictable time. It is no surprise that you sometimes have an arrival time of 19 minutes, while other times you may arrive 21 minutes after you leave the house. Such variations are what we would normally call random, and it would have little effect on the actual travel time for the driver to be sent a letter indicating that it had been noticed that on one day he or she had arrived 1 minute off the average. In real life, we take such random variation into account, as normally we leave our houses early enough that even with random variation, we arrive at work during a predictable window of time. We have thus defined a *process* for getting to work on time; the output of this process is satisfactory even in the context of random variation.

For a second example, however, consider the fact that at a particular time of year, construction began on the highway that you normally use to commute. Rather suddenly, there is a 20-minute increment in your travel time, and you now require 40 minutes. If you continued to use your original process of getting to work, you would fail to get there on time. Indeed, you would almost always be late. This failure of process is not related to random variation, but rather is *assignable* to the construction on the freeway. Your only solution is to change the process by which you get to work on time, either by changing routes or by leaving earlier and allowing the extra time of commuting. In the parlance of continuous quality improvement, variation is thus divided into two categories: random and assignable.

Let us return to the medical field, and for the sake of discussion consider several medication errors. In the neonatal ICU a physician has ordered the incorrect medication in one unit of the hospital, while on another day in the same month, an incorrect dosage of a different medication was ordered by a different clinician in the emergency department. In still another corner of the hospital, a particular patient has an idiopathic reaction to a drug, and suffers a serious side effect. Review of these incidents confirms that none of the incidents were related to each other, none of the clinicians were the same in any of the instances, and a thorough review of the third case indicated that there was no sign that would have warned the clinician of the idiosyncratic reaction in advance. The quality assurance committee has reviewed these three events, noted that they have occurred within a few days of each other, and is alarmed. The essential question is, Are these events random variations or assignable variations?

What are the implications of calling these events random? In this instance, it may be useful to generically remind nurses and physicians to be careful with medication ordering and dispensing, but detailed analysis of the events and prolonged discussion with the involved individuals are largely a waste of time. The hospital, the committee, and the involved individuals will be better occupied pursuing other activities than trying to investigate these three drug events. In the instance that we call these events assignable, the implication is that there is a root cause that can be identified and then fixed. In this case, it is worthwhile for the organization to investigate and analyze the events so that the root cause of the errors can be eradicated. This investigation will have real costs (time and money, some anguish) but will hopefully yield a meaningful result (fewer future incidents).

We would classify these three errors as random variation, not assignable variation. In the first instance, the incorrect drug was ordered by the physician. This may in fact be a systematic problem with that individual physician, and he or she may in fact not have sufficient knowledge to practice medicine safely. On the other hand, if the clinician has written 50,000 prescriptions over the previous 5 years, and this is the only medication error that he or she has made, then he or she is functioning in a remarkably accurate manner. It is dubious that one can assign the specific cause of that physician's error on that particular day, hence we term it random. In the second case, a drug dosage calculation error was made, and the same argument applies. Namely, the physician did not decide specifically to order the wrong dose of a drug, and in fact, in the long view, this physician has been highly accurate in his or her ordering behavior.

Finally, in the third case, it is more obvious that this is random. If there was no possibility of warning the clinician (perhaps by history of problems with the same drug), then it is obviously random that this occurred with his or her patient.

Consider, however, a hospital that reviews its drug medication practices on a regular basis and has discovered that a specific physician is responsible for 25% of the drug errors occurring in the hospital. While individual errors by individual physicians may appear to be random, when significant patterns appear in the data, this becomes an assignable form of variation. It becomes clear at this point that the specific physician needs to use more care with medication prescribing, and in the extreme situation, the hospital may elect to rid itself of such a physician.

The danger of treating random variation as assignable variation is that this view fails to acknowledge the reality of random variation in everyday life. Much effort can be expended on pointless "tampering" with processes as one attempts to "chase after" events that are inherently random and not remediable to simple fixes. As noted above, this results in a waste of time for many people and is associated with real costs for little result. In fact, it can be statistically proven that interfering with processes based on random variation will increase the variation with which those processes function, thus causing harm to the organization. Instead, if quality improvement efforts are aimed at variation that is clearly assignable, there is more likely to be benefit from the activity.

How do we separate random variation from assignable variation? In this regard, we are helped by the statistical methods that many of us apply to our research activities. Events that are truly random will behave as random events and are susceptible to statistical analyses. Thus, in a traditional sense, the null hypothesis will apply to such events, while with assignable variations, the null hypothesis will not apply. Later in this chapter, we will discuss some graphical methods for applying statistics in order to separate random from assignable variation. At this point, it is sufficient to state that continuous quality improvement activities need to be focused on assignable variation, not on random variation.

The other major flaw of traditional quality assurance has been its failure to cope with or provide a general theory for the occurrence of errors. Errors are indeed remediable to study[39,99–110], and Leape recently reviewed the subject of error in medicine[107]. Even more recently, a published study examined the causes of human errors in the intensive care environment, with some rather fascinating results[101]. There were significant differences in the numbers of errors committed by physicians versus nurses, there was a diurnal pattern to the frequency of errors, and there were different levels of errors based on body systems of the patients, types of diseases, and complexity of the care of the patients. There were common themes relating to communication or lack thereof between nurses and physicians, and there were human factors that were identified as predisposing to intensive care unit errors. For example, the congestion of intravenous tubing and instrumentation that is commonly seen at the bedside is a human-factors nightmare, and nurses and physicians are expected to interact with this mess of technology without committing any errors. Recognition that errors are, in and of themselves, worthy of study, and recognition that the processes of care rendered in an intensive care unit are the crucial units of analysis, may be the two most important paradigm shifts in continuous quality improvement.

CONTINUOUS QUALITY IMPROVEMENT

It is a given that we need to ensure quality and continually strive to deliver the best health care we can possibly provide to our patients. If traditional quality assurance has largely failed to accomplish this, how are we to proceed? We believe that continuous quality improvement, often called CQI, represents a paradigm shift that is constructive, permitting a more realistic and effective approach to health care quality issues. We begin by discussing the components of quality and factors that affect quality. Then we discuss processes and variation. Finally, we consider the very important issue of customer satisfaction.

Defining Quality

What is quality? What is value? How does quality relate to cost? What do we value in society with respect to health care? What contributes to quality? These are only a few of the questions that muddy the waters when one discusses quality. In this section, we discuss (1) quality and costs, (2) elements of cost, (3) forces driving cost, and (4) costs of poor quality.

Quality and Costs

If one asks, What is the relationship between quality and cost?, one may expect to hear the answer that reduction of cost will reduce quality, and vice versa. Indeed, a reduction of investment often seems to be equated with reduction of quality. However, this is by no means uniformly true. Experience in other industries would suggest, in fact, that increased quality is associated with reduced cost[18].

What do we value in the health care industry? As one approaches continuous quality improvement, he or she must pay constant attention to maintaining the medical care that we all value. Excellence in medical care is often equated with doing everything possible for an individual patient, but we would suggest that this needs to be balanced by recognition of the economic impact of those actions. This does not mean that we should withhold therapies or available services because of economics, but we merely suggest that we use economics as part of our decision making. For example, if two treatments have identical outcomes for patients with a specific disease, but one treatment is notably less expensive than the other, it is of increasing value to our society to use the cheaper therapy. On the other hand, if a therapy that is more expensive also has a better outcome, then this should be the overriding priority rather than the economic cost. Eventually, of course, if economic resources become extremely constrained, even the latter decision will have to have an economic component. We would suggest that "value" of our health care delivery services will relate to delivering the best possible quality of medical care at the lowest possible economic price.

Elements of Cost

Health care costs have become an overriding topic at nearly all levels of our society, ranging from the national level of political debate down to the individual patient level. As we pursue the subject of quality improvement, it is important to understand the components of costs, and how these might relate to quality.

Cost is more complex than at first glance it might appear. One must define what is included in costs[111]. For example, when we total the costs of a hospitalization of a 5-year-old child in the intensive care unit, should we include the lost labor costs that accrued to the father who had to skip work for 2 weeks? Should we include the costs of baby-sitting for the patient's siblings? Should we include the economic value of a 12 year old skipping school, similar to the manner in which economic costs are often ascribed to adults who miss work? Not only are the costs that are included an important issue, but it is important to understand the costs to whom? We need to separate the concepts of costs to the patient, to the family, to the insurance companies, to Medicaid and Medicare, and to ourselves as providers. Finally, we need to understand the denominator of time over which costs are accounted. In general, costs are accounted on an inpatient admission basis, but this is obviously an unsatisfactory manner in which to assess overall health care costs. Indeed, costs ought to be assessed over the continuum of care for the entire duration of an illness. For example, the cost of care of a child who is injured in a motor vehicle crash, is admitted to the intensive care unit for 10 days and the rehabilitation unit for 5 days, may also include costs relating to his disability for the following 6 months. All of these costs would need to be captured in order to obtain an accurate picture of the cost of the motor vehicle crash for that particular child. We tend to focus on the acute medical costs because they are more easily quantified, but the reader should recognize that the magnitude of cost far exceeds the boundaries of the inpatient or outpatient acute management.

Forces Driving Cost

Numerous forces have been driving medical costs up over the past several decades. These forces include demographic changes, epidemiologic events, new technology, changes in scope of services, higher acuity of patients, higher labor and administrative costs, and the costs associated with increasing amounts of regulation. It is worthwhile to consider each of these forces separately.

The demographic changes associated with the end of World War II are well known to all, and it is clear that as the baby-boomer generation ages, societal health care costs will continue to rise. This is to a degree a failure relating to our successes. The average longevity of a man or woman in the United States is considerably greater today than 50 years ago, and the costs of maintaining an increasingly elderly population are high. On the pediatric side, we need point only at the neonatal intensive care unit to identify the major sources of bronchopulmonary dysplasia patients, children who might otherwise have died from respiratory distress. Cardiac and hepatic transplantation are also successes of great scale, but are associated with ongoing high costs. Bone marrow transplantation represents a major breakthrough for a small number of patients, but once again, at a significant economic cost. Therapies for chronic renal failure, such as dialysis, are of a similar nature, representing a medical/clinical success with associated high costs. Increased longevity and the survival of children and adults who would otherwise have died do not by any means represent failures or weaknesses in our system. However, such medical progress provides unrelenting pressure to increase health care costs as we maintain the health of these people.

The most obvious epidemiologic factor of the last decade and a half has been acquired immunodeficiency syndrome (AIDS), caused by the HIV organism. Because of its chronic nature, and slow speed, the precise scope of AIDS in this country and the rest of the world remains unclear. However, its effect on health care costs in this country are unquestionable. Other epidemiologic examples include influenza epidemics, outbreaks in the 1970s of Reye's syndrome, or, going back a few more years, the polio epidemics of the 1930s and 1940s. As these natural disasters drive costs up, we retaliate with efforts at immunizations and other mechanisms of driving the costs down. It is clear that overall health care costs could be driven down quite dramatically if our efforts became increasingly preventive, as effective education of the population could reduce traumatic injuries (use of seat belts), stroke (controlling blood pressure), and heart disease (proper exercise and diet). Once again, we have no sage advice with respect to the epidemiology of new viruses or the habits of the population, but we point these out as examples of epidemiologic factors that will continue to drive health care costs upward.

New technology is often blamed for higher health care costs. Indeed, 20 years ago it was fashionable for states to have a certificate-of-need program, which subjected new technologies and purchases to review by various regulatory committees. By 1995, very few states continued to have a certificate of need program, as these programs failed to contain health care costs and merely added regulatory burdens to an already costly system. Close examination of new technology reveals that costs are often decreased by proper use of such technologies. In addition, there is an obvious quality gain for a patient if a new procedure or technology is less painful than an old procedure. For example, very few trainees today have ever seen a pneumoencephalogram. Computerized tomography (CT) replaced this relatively crude technique, and magnetic resonance imaging (MRI) has provided even further anatomic detail, making the diagnosis of central nervous system diseases more accurate and less invasive. Digital subtraction angiography, a relatively new technology dependent on sophisticated computerization techniques, decreases the amount of dye that is required in angiography and potentially allows visualization of structures without arterial access. The availability of certain types of interventional radiology has permitted patients to have outpatient procedures for patent ductus arteriosus, various valvar stenoses, and a host of other vascular anomalies. Doppler ultrasound has revolutionized the ultrasonographic evaluation of congenital heart disease. Indeed, the number of children who are subjected to cardiac catheterization for diagnostic purposes has dwindled drastically over the last two decades. In summary, while new technology often costs a great deal, there are many applications of such technology that represent true progress, with higher quality and lesser costs.

Having said that, we must point out that the medical profession has not subjected new technology to particularly critical review. For example, the imaging study of choice for a specific condition often relates to the specific training of the radiologist or other clinicians, and may even relate to the recent purchase of new technological equipment. This is almost an inevitable cost of progress, as clinicians need to become more familiar with the limitations of new techniques. Thus, one may see a radiologist preferring to attempt visualization of the cerebral arterial tree by using magnetic resonance angiography rather than more traditional carotid angiography. The question is, how many such technologies have actually been subjected to critical study and comparison? On a topic more related to intensive care, consider one's choice of sedatives and muscle relaxants. After nearly two decades of using pancuronium and diazepam for sedation and muscle relaxation in the pediatric intensive care unit, more recent drugs have become available in the last 5 years and have become popular. Only in the last 1 to 2 years have many clinicians begun to look at these choices, recognizing that these newer drugs do not represent major improvements but yield much higher costs to the system. Thus, while the authors do not blame new technology or new drugs for most of the increase in health care costs over the last several decades, it is clear that we need to increasingly pay attention to a critical assessment of such newer technologies.

Another factor that drives apparent health care costs upward relates to the scope of activities or services that are provided. For example, interventional radiology now permits stenotic cardiac valves to be balloon dilated, avoiding the need for hospitalization or use of the operating room. If one examines the cost of performing a balloon dilation, one finds that the fees are relatively high. A short-sighted review of such costs might make one consider those costs to be exhorbitant, while the longsighted review will recognize that techniques such as balloon dilation have markedly decreased the costs associated with improving the outcome of patients with cardiac valve stenosis by avoiding the costs of the operating room, intensive care unit, and subsequent days in the hospital. Home health care of ventilator-dependent children represents another example of a high cost outpatient endeavor that is cost-efficient when compared to traditional inpatient care. As we have seen home health care costs escalate over the last decade, we must recognize that these represent a redistribution of health care activities and services, with an increased scope of activities on the outpatient side and a reduced scope of activity on the inpatient side.

Such redistribution occurs throughout pediatrics. Indeed, examination of a children's hospital today will reveal a much higher acuity of patients than the children's hospital of 20 years ago, or even perhaps of 10 years ago. It is not unusual for a child to complete an intravenous course of antibiotics at home, with an IV placed by a nurse from a home health care agency. It is no longer unusual for a ventilator patient to be at home. It is inevitable that the health care providers will attempt to identify cheaper locations for providing health care services than inpatient hospital locations, and the result of this will be that hospitals will accrue higher and higher fixed costs for a patient population with increasingly high acuities. This is particularly pertinent for children's hospitals, which already suffer from adverse patient selection. Finally, it would be naive in a discussion about costs to ignore the fact that labor and administrative costs are higher today than they were in the past. Many of the professionals in the health care industry were traditionally paid inadequate wages, and the past 15 years have seen an increase of nursing and respiratory therapy salaries to levels that are more appropriate than in the past. It is clear that different mixes of providers will need to be used at several levels. For example, it is possible to use nurse practitioners or physician's assistants in various inpatient settings, including the pediatric intensive care unit[112,113]. It is also possible to use nursing assistants to increase the scope of activity that a registered nurse can accomplish on a given shift, even in the intensive care unit setting. Innovative and imaginative methods of staffing these units will be required as market pressures continue to force a decrease in reimbursement. Administrative costs have increased as the complexity of reimbursement has increased. There is often literal warfare between providers and payers, relating to the nuances of when and where signatures were obtained for a particular patient. For instance, it is possible for the costs of an entire admission to be denied by state Medicaid agencies, because federal law requires that the certification of the necessity of an inpatient admission be signed on the day of admission. While the patient can be on a ventilator in the pediatric intensive care unit, the absence of such a signature at the time of inspection by Medicaid can result in nonpayment for the entire hospitalization. Other regulatory costs include the approval costs associated with new technology and drugs. It needs no reiteration here that the cost of obtaining approval from the U.S. Food and Drug Administration is exorbitant in this country, and most such drugs and technologies are available outside of the United States for a prolonged period of time before they are available in the United States. We offer no commentary on this issue but merely point out that this is another contributor to the costs of our health care system.

Costs of Poor Quality

Poor quality increases costs. This statement may seem counterintuitive to the reader, but in this section, we hope to demonstrate this. Factors that increase costs because of poor quality include quality waste and rework, increased complexity, low productivity and efficiency, customer replacement costs, warranty costs, ripple effect and fire fighting, and employee turnover and training costs. These costs are not always accurately accounted, and it is perhaps for that reason that most people perceive that high quality requires high cost. As Augustine points out, however, in his Law of Undiminished Expectations:

> It is very expensive to achieve high degrees of unreliability. It is not uncommon to increase the cost of an item by a factor of ten for each factor of ten degradation accomplished (18, page 69).

To paraphrase, it costs a lot of money to build an unreliable product, because an unreliable product costs more money to maintain. We would submit that the health care industry in general delivers an unreliable product, and improvements in our product reliability will decrease health care costs.

As an example of quality waste and rework in the medical field, consider the instance in which a laboratory test is sent to the laboratory as a screening examination for an ICU admission. For example, consider the batteries of chemical tests that are available in laboratories today, often including as many as twenty or more measurements. Perhaps several of these measurements are not clinically indicated, but at least 5% of the time some of those clinically unindicated laboratory results will be outside of the range that we normally construe as normal. (This assumes that we are defining normal with ± 2 standard deviations.) As a result of this laboratory test coming back abnormal, the house officer who sent the original screening examination may be forced to repeat this examination (if it is elective to do so), or may be forced to act upon the laboratory test (if the abnormality is urgent). In the nonurgent circumstance, the repeat laboratory test may come back normal. At that point, the clinician faces the quandary of deciding which of the two results was correct. He or she may even need to send a third laboratory test, perhaps several hours later, to verify by a nearly democratic process whether the patient has this laboratory abnormality at all. In the urgent case, the clinician may send a repeat laboratory test and then act upon the original result. It will be to the clinician's dismay when the repeat laboratory test comes back normal. These same arguments apply whether the laboratory test is abnormal originally because it simply falls outside of two standard deviations of normal, or whether an error occurred in the machinery of the laboratory. In either instance, the resultant frenzied activities that have been described in this paragraph are examples of quality waste. All would have been avoided had the original testing been determined by clinical indication, and particularly if the laboratory test result was simply an error, all of the effort described in this paragraph was completely wasted.

As another example, consider the situation of a drug manufacturer that inspects each of its vials of drugs for bacterial contamination. This hypothetical company then ships only the sterile vials and rejects the vials that have bacterial contamination. Suppose, for the sake of this discussion, that 10% of the vials have bacterial contamination, and the other 90% are sent through for shipment. The company could proudly advertise that by careful inspection, it rejects 10% of its output in order to bring you, the customer, only the very best of quality. Unfortunately, the advertisement will not include the fact that the customer had to pay for the 10% of vials that were rejected, as this rejection process was part of the fixed costs of manufacturing the good (i.e., sterile) drug. In fact, if the company changed its manufacturing process so that the bacterial contamination rate was 0.001%, the costs of inspection and rejection would be avoided. This example may seem far-fetched, but several years ago, a spark plug manufacturer actually placed an advertisement in a national magazine that showed a huge pile of spark plugs that were rejected in order to bring the single, relatively fantastic and perfect, spark plug that was held in the hand of the individual in the advertisement. This advertisement did not run for long, as competitors were quick to point out that the customer had to pay for all the rejected spark plugs when he or she purchased a good spark plug. Again, these are demonstrations of quality waste.

We face further difficulties because of the high complexity of the tasks that we undertake. Consider for example, the work-up of a patient with an acute cerebrovascular accident or stroke. A typical approach might include a CT scan in the emergency department, followed by admission to the pediatric intensive care unit. After a respectable amount of time and several consultations, it may be decided to either repeat the CT scan or perhaps to obtain an MRI imaging study to determine whether there are abnormal areas of the cerebrum to correspond with the clinical physical examination. Subsequently, often at a decent interval following the MRI, the patient may return to the MRI suite to have magnetic resonance angiography performed in order to visualize the vasculature. After the equivocal or even the nonequivocal results of this imaging study are reviewed, the patient may return to the angiography suite on the following day to have the definitive angiogram performed. Subsequently, there may or may not be a 1- or 2-day discussion about whether to anticoagulate the patient, and of course there will be discussions of whether or not surgical intervention is required. Each of the decision points in the management of this patient is relatively complex on one level, and yet upon reflection, one might determine that there is a simpler approach. For example, one might ask whether a patient with an acute change in neurological status consistent with a stroke will ever, in fact, avoid having an angiogram. One might prospectively decide that the approach to future stroke patients would be to obtain a CT scan to rule out a disastrous bleed, followed within 12 to 24 hours by an angiogram. By prospectively attempting to decide what the decision points are, it is possible to reduce the complexity of the process by which we deliver care to patients such as a stroke victim. By reducing this complexity, it is possible to skip various parts of the process that were unnecessary. Those unnecessary parts of the process are another form of quality waste.

Another contributor of poor quality to cost relates to impaired efficiency. To take an earlier example, if the laboratory tests are relatively unreliable in a hospital, the ability of the clinician to efficiently interpret laboratory tests will decrease. In addition, because laboratory results will have to be repeated on a regular basis in order to determine errors and nonerrors, the efficiency of the laboratory will be impaired, and the time required for laboratory tests to be finished and reported back to the clinician will increase. Failure to computerize laboratory data management may lead to inefficient communication of laboratory results to the clinical staff. This will have an adverse effect upon the efficiency of the intensive care units and other areas of the hospital. Indeed, the hospital may need to increase its staff in order to accomplish all of the laboratory testing and reporting that is necessary. In essence, reducing the tasks necessary to deliver a specific health care product to a patient to the absolute minimum will minimize quality waste and maximize efficiency.

Sometimes a complete rearrangement of a process will increase the efficiency of the process. Recently, our medical records department made a change in the manner in which it identified missing signatures on charts. Instead of waiting until the chart was returned to the medical records department and then flagging the signatures for attending physicians, the department sent its workers to the wards, where they flagged those charts contemporaneously with care. As a result, attending physicians sign the charts when they come on rounds, and almost all of the signatures are obtained before the chart is returned to the medical records department. As a result, despite the cost of sending staff to the wards, the overall costs were sharply reduced because the charts were not delayed for nearly as long after they arrived in medical records. Indeed, for relatively the same amount of personnel cost, a marked improvement was made in the process.

Another well-described cost of poor quality relates to customer replacement costs. The authors suggest an experiment for the reader. At the next staff meeting in your intensive care unit, ask how many individuals have gone out of their way to describe the excellent service that they received from a grocery store, hotel, airline, physician, or hospital? Specifically, ask them how many times they have spontaneously told others about the excellent service that they received from any of these types of entities. Then ask how many individuals have specifically and spontaneously complained to others about service that they received in one of these areas. Again, you're interested in unsolicited information that they volunteered to their friends and acquaintances about bad service. If the results of your experiment are comparable to those obtained in other industries and in the authors' experience, there will be a negligible number of people who have spontaneously provided positive information about industries, with a relatively large number of people who have provided negative perceptions to their friends and acquaintances. Estimates in industry range as high as 15 complaints for every positive comment.

Why is this important? Consider a hospital that admits 100 patients and completely satisfies 95% of them. The other 5% are distinctively unsatisfied. On average, the 95 people who were satisfied will tell one or fewer of their acquaintances about their wonderful experience in the hospital. Thus, there will be approximately 95 positive comments, while at the same time, the five individuals will tell an average of 10 to 15 of their acquaintances about their experience, resulting in as many as 75 negative comments. It is striking that despite an overall satisfaction rate of 95%, this hospital will be subject to nearly as many negative comments as positive comments, given our assumptions.

In order to keep a customer or a patient loyal to a hospital, it is necessary to provide good service every time. It is really only necessary to slip once or twice before customer loyalty will switch to another provider of the service. The cost of replacing this patient or customer is called customer replacement cost. Customer replacement costs are considerable. Consider, for example, the same hospital as described in the previous paragraph. Although they are satisfying 95% of their patients, they are permanently losing 5% of the patients that they see from their customer pool. If that hospital expects to maintain its current level of business, which most hospitals attempt to do, they will need to replace these 5% of customers with new customers. The cost of replacing customers is much higher than the cost of maintaining loyal customers, and by maintaining satisfaction at a higher level (perhaps 99.9%), that hospital would avoid the costs of customer replacement.

Another major category of cost relating to poor quality is termed warranty cost. For example, when a manufacturer produces a tape recorder that requires frequent repairs during the first year after manufacture, the warranty costs will be high. The cost of the tape recorder will need to be high enough to compensate for the warranty costs, since customers will normally expect such devices to work for the guaranteed period of the warranty. On the other hand, if the manufacturer makes a tape recorder that is so reliable that the expectation of having to repair it is extremely low, its warranty costs will be negligible. That company will be able to reduce the price of its tape recorders but will make an increased profit because of its low warranty costs. What does this mean in terms of health care costs? Consider the child who receives an incorrect medication, attendant with its adverse side effects, and requires 2 days in the intensive care unit on a mechanical ventilator to make up for this mishap. In our previous and current (not for long) system of fee for service, this has been forgiven, with adequate reimbursement not only for the original mishap but for the repair of the mishap. In prospective reimbursement systems and capitation agreements, such mistakes will represent very real warranty costs to the provider. That is, iatrogenic complications will require repair costs. As clinical processes are improved and complications decrease, the warranty costs drop proportionately, and the overall cost of health care can be decreased. This is brought home by simple arithmetic. In our hospital, a ruptured appendix costs $5000 more than an unruptured appendix in a patient with appendicitis. It has been estimated that a urinary tract infection adds approximately $10,000 to the inpatient admission costs of adults, controlling for all other factors. To the degree that processes can be improved so that these initial events do not occur, the provider will be spared the warranty costs associated with the complications.

Finally, we need to consider the costs of employee turnover and training. If an organization pays poor attention to the morale of its employees or neglects to provide them with ongoing education, that organization will increasingly face the issue of new employees and retraining. Orientation periods for nurses entering the pediatric ICU last as long as 6 months, and most people will concede that it takes 1 to 2 years for a nurse to become a competent intensive care nurse. We have a number of nurse practitioners working in our pediatric intensive care unit, and their value as employees increases everyday. When one allows (or causes) employee turnover, one replaces knowledgeable employees who have a vast fundamental knowledge of their jobs with naive employees who have little knowledge of the jobs they are about to undertake. The costs of this turnover extend far beyond the budgeted training costs, as new employees and clinicians will be less productive and less efficient in all clinical care they render. Thus, as a hospital decides to eliminate lucrative bonus plans for nursing staff who have been there for 20 years, it must consider in balance the retraining costs that may occur when those older staff members retire and are replaced by new graduates from nursing school.

In this section we have tried to describe various aspects of costs that are related to poor quality. While it may in fact be true that more expensive items carry higher quality, in general, we hope the reader will accept the premise that reliable, high quality delivery of health care will ultimately lower costs. If quality and costs can be viewed as two sides of the same coin, it becomes readily apparent that we can increase quality while decreasing costs. Going back to our original premise about value, increased quality at lower cost will increase the value of what we deliver within the health care industry.

Emphasis on Processes

While traditional quality assurance has tended to emphasize the performance of individual clinicians, particularly physicians, an important paradigm shift in continuous quality improvement is its emphasis on processes rather than individuals. Rather than assume that an error is due to an individual cold-bloodedly deciding to commit an error, one would instead take the view that the process in which that individual works permitted an error to occur, despite that individual's best efforts to perform in a correct manner. This emphasis on process may be the fundamental shift that separates traditional quality assurance from continuous quality improvement.

A process is a series of linked steps designed to cause a set of outcomes from a set of inputs. On a very broad level, one can view the inpatient health care process as having a set of inputs (ill patients) and a set of outputs (well patients). Something occurs between the inputs and the outputs: the process of care (Figure 48.1). Obviously, health care represents an incredibly complex series and set of processes, with interrelationships and complexities that make many people wonder how quality improvement techniques from manufacturing can be applied to the health care industry. However, the paradigm of thinking about processes, attempting to define and understand them, and improving them by reducing unintended variation has been relatively successful when applied within the health care industry.

Consider two clinical examples. In the first example, a nurse receives a container of enteral formula that is intended to be administered to the patient by connecting it to a feeding tube. The nurse inadvertently connects this container to the intravenous line stopcock. She opens the stopcock, but several minutes later realizes her error and immediately turns off the formula. In the second example, a

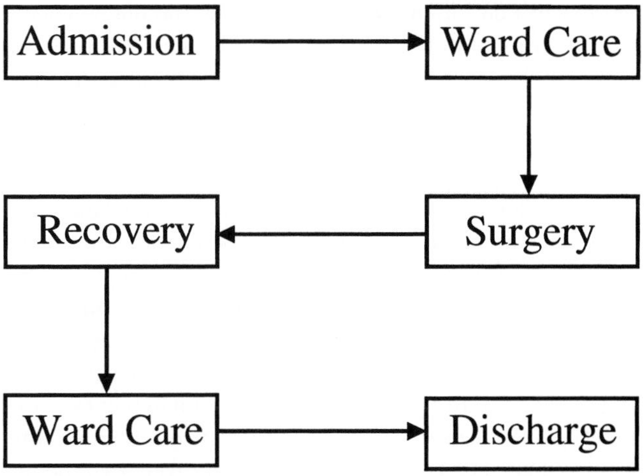

Figure 48.1. Broad process of inpatient health care.

nurse receives a unit of whole blood to transfuse into a patient, and connects it to the stopcock in the patient's intraventricular drainage system (intracranial pressure monitor). This error was detected by the nurse before blood reached the head, since the blood was being transfused by gravity, and the child happened to have somewhat increased intracranial pressure to impede the flow of blood, even from a transfusion bag.

There is a common theme between these two errors. In both instances, the intensive care nurse was an experienced clinician, respected by all her peers. In neither instance did the nurse intend harm, and in both instances the nurse was skilled enough to pick up the error within a few moments. The flaw was not the nurse, but rather the process of care within which she was working. By making the connector of a feeding tube incompatible with the stopcock used in intravenous systems, one can make it physically impossible to connect an enteral feeding tube to an IV catheter. Similarly, as there is no purpose to having a side port for infusion into an intraventricular drain, removing three-way stopcocks from intraventricular drain systems eliminates the possibility that a nurse might accidently connect blood or any other intravenous infusions to that system. In essence, by examining the process and understanding the root of the error, it is possible to build a system in which a well-motivated clinician will be less able to commit errors.

Consider an example of the following pharmaceutical mishap. A child receives a prescription for a drug that is not palatable, and this drug has been mixed in soda pop and placed in a 50-cc hypodermic syringe. The syringe is appropriately labeled by the pharmacy and sent to the inpatient ward where the patient is residing. The nurse mistakenly injects the contents of the syringe into the child's central line. Once again, this nurse did not decide that she was going to inject soda pop into a child when she went to work, but rather committed an error that the process of care allowed her to commit. The solution, of course, is to never use an intravenous device or hypodermic syringe to contain any solution that is not designed to be injected into the bloodstream. In the event that a syringe is desirable for administration into the mouth of a child, the pharmacy can select syringes which are incompatible with vascular systems, such as syringes used for suction from nasogastric tubes.

As a final example, one of the authors had the opportunity to see a patient who had drainage from an enterostomy, and in order to prevent severe electrolyte imbalance, this drainage was being returned to the patient via a nasojejunal tube. It was being administered by placement in a hypodermic syringe mounted in an infusion pump to control the rate of reinfusion into the jejunum. In this case, there was no mishap, but this type of situation is obviously a ticking time bomb. Immediate steps were taken to point out that nothing should ever find its way into an intravenous infusion system that is not intended for intravenous infusion, as it is nearly inevitable that at some point a well-meaning individual will make a mistake and inadvertently connect that pump to an intravenous line, hence injecting the enterostomy drainage into the vascular space.

The purpose of these examples, all of which were real, is to illustrate the subtle distinction between errors of clinicians and flaws in the clinical process. While in each of the above instances the involved individual may have been chastised, it is unlikely that chastisement would affect the future frequency of such errors, particularly because each of these errors was committed by a different individual. The real solution to reducing errors of this type is to understand the process that is involved and improve the process so that such errors are impossible to commit.

In an environment as complex as an intensive care unit or a hospital, it is useful to attempt to identify key processes. One approach is to ask the managers of different areas of a hospital to identify all of the tasks they perform in their area and to prioritize these tasks in order of importance. These may in fact be very broad-stroke processes, but this technique allows one to focus on the important issues. **Tables 48.1–48.6** show key processes obtained in our hospital from various functional areas. By identifying these various processes and collating them into a single document, it is possible to give to each of the managers of the entire hospital an overview of the key processes that occur in the hospital, often allowing coordination of improvement projects.

After identification, we can use various approaches to improve these key processes. In general, four elements are necessary to improve processes: teams, data, tools, and methods. It is worthwhile to discuss each of these elements in some detail.

The first necessary element for improving processes is a team of individuals who have the fundamental knowledge necessary to completely understand the process. It is often very difficult for a single health care professional to understand the activities of another health care professional, and it is virtually hopeless to approach complex processes such as those in the hospital setting without a fairly multidisciplinary group of individuals. At the same time, it is important not to increase these groups beyond a useful size. We again turn to Augustine's laws[18] for several useful comments. The Law of Rampant Committeemanship (page 166) states, "The optimum committee has no members." The Second Law of Averages (page 117) states, "One tenth of the participants produce at least one third of the output, and increasing the number of participants merely reduces the

Table 48.1. Key Processes for Pediatric Critical Care Services

- Ventilation management
- Nutritional support
- Emotional support/intervention
- Admission/transfer/discharge
- Muscular paralysis
- Pain management
- Circulatory support
- Intracranial pressure/neurologic management
- Infectious disease management

Table 48.2. Key Processes for Respiratory Care Services

- Mechanical ventilator management
- Appropriate use of respiratory care interventions
- Continuing staff education
- Chest physiotherapy
- Delivery of aerosolized medication
- Producing an accurate bill

average output." Perhaps most importantly, however, is the Law of the Nest (page 121), which states, "It is better to be the reorganizer than the reorganizee."

Optimum team sizes vary, but in our experience, teams of five to eight individuals are optimum. Larger teams tend to become groups of active participants (usually five to eight or even fewer) and inactive participants. While acknowledging that many individuals on a team may not be as productive as other individuals, it has been our experience that the Law of the Nest (above) may be the most important reason for including individuals who are clearly going to have to live with the solution that is developed by the team. This increases the likelihood of those individuals accepting such a solution and reduces the political problems that may accompany the solution.

The second and most important element for improving processes is the provision of accurate data regarding those processes[114]. While we use data to drive nearly everything else we do in medicine, whether in our reading of the medical literature or measuring the blood pressure in the intensive care unit, data have been sparsely applied to quality improvement or other aspects of operational health care delivery. Instead of using anecdotes, it is necessary to systematically look at health care delivery, collect accurate data with respect to that delivery, and analyze and interpret the data carefully. Nearly every reader of this book will already have been exposed to a somewhat shoddy quality assurance data collection effort. The authors' current approach in the intensive care unit has been to inform people that if they believe the data they are collecting are not of sufficient validity and reliability to make the project potentially worthy of publication in the medical literature, then they should not bother to analyze (or even collect) that data. Similarly, we have adopted the stance that any major continuous quality improvement projects that do not seem worthy of peer review and potential publication in the medical literature should not be undertaken. In essence, we should require of quality improvement activities the same standards of excellence that we require of other aspects of medicine.

Given the provision of data, it is important that people have the tools with which to analyze the data. There are

Table 48.3. Key Processes for Pediatric Transport Services

- Safe transport environment for crew members and patients
- Follow-up to referring health care providers
- Cost-effectiveness
- Integration of neonatal and pediatric transport teams
- Response to teams within 5 minutes

Table 48.4. Key Processes for Regular Inpatient Pediatric Ward

- Discharge planning
- Patient education
- Admitting patients
- Medication administration
- Multidisciplinary plan of care for individual patients
- Continuing education of nurses
- Patient care delivery

various approaches to data analysis in the CQI literature, many of which are aimed at diverting the reader from understanding that he or she is actually dealing with relatively simple statistics. Thus, many graduate school textbooks concerning quality improvement processes have complicated tables for looking up constants that can be used in simple arithmetic equations rather than informing the readers that they simply need to understand the concept of standard deviation. Later in this chapter, we will discuss some of the tools that are commonly used in continuous quality improvement, but we stress at this point that none of these tools are particularly sophisticated for readers of this textbook.

Finally, some method (or philosophy?) is necessary as one attempts to improve processes. The most commonly publicized method is called the Plan-Do-Check-Act, or PDCA cycle. The authors are not particularly fond of the emphasis given to discussing various types of methods such as the PDCA cycle, noting that the scientific method familiar to all readers of this textbook is, in fact, what is being taught or emulated in each instance. In essence, one begins with a hypothesis about an operational aspect of health care delivery. By developing flowcharts and other diagrams relating to the original process of care, one is simply focusing his or her hypothesis. Then one needs to collect some data about this hypothesis, analyze the data, arrive at an interpretation about the hypothesis, and then implement any appropriate operational changes. As with more traditional scientific endeavors, this usually leads to another hypothesis and a repetition of the process. In this manner, we consider continuous quality improvement to be much more of a sound scientific methodology rather than a management philosophy, though a visit by the reader to the local bookstore will confirm the authors' opinion that many writers concerned with CQI consider it to be a management philosophy.

In addition to these four important elements for improving processes, we would be remiss if we did not point out

Table 48.5. Key Processes for Finance and Accounting Department

- Operating budget preparation
- Capital budget preparation
- Monthly statement generation and analysis
- Contracting with payers
- Maintenance of systems (charge and cost files, payroll, general ledger)
- Strategic financial planning and analysis (special projects and reports, benchmarking, market evolution evaluation, cost structure analysis and planning)

Table 48.6. Key Processes for Hospital Charitable Foundation

- Raising money
- Donor relations and record keeping
- Responsiveness to requests and cooperation with others
- External communications
- Management and investment of funds

the need for managers to empower individuals to carry out some of the improvements that they identify. When a team is assembled to study a specific process, and it collects the data and provides the analysis of those data, it is often perfectly permissible for a manager to allow that team to institute that change. In many organizations, however, there is a perceived need for management to approve such changes, and in the authors' opinion, this has a damaging effect on the morale of the individuals who made up the team in the first place. Many papers and even textbooks have been written on this subject, and the authors will not discuss it further in this chapter. We leave this topic with another of Augustine's laws, the Law of Propagation of Misery: "If a sufficient number of management layers are superimposed on top of each other, it can be assured that disaster is not left to chance" (18, page 86).

Customer Satisfaction

Customer satisfaction is a concept that has received lip service from most industries, but only in the past two decades have we begun to examine this concept in greater detail. It is perhaps unfortunate that the health care system of this country has not addressed customer satisfaction in a more aggressive manner, as this would undoubtedly have changed the political climate from which we are often viewed (hostilely). It is helpful for discussion of customer satisfaction to divide the concept of quality into two categories: *quality in fact,* which refers to the quality of the delivered product in its essence, and *quality in perception,* which relates primarily to the service and the delivery quality. The first category is often called production or content quality, while the second is called service or delivery quality. The distinctions between these are quite important in understanding the psychology of customer satisfaction.

To illustrate these concepts, some examples of quality in fact are the employment of good nurses and doctors, the administration of correct medications, having a functioning CT scanner that generates high-quality images, or even the ability to deliver a safe helicopter transport. Examples of quality in perception are visiting hours, whether the furniture in the room is clean and comfortable, whether the food is excellent, and whether people in the hospital setting are friendly. The combination of these two facets of quality make up the total quality picture of the organization (Figure 48.2).

It may be worthwhile to consider two examples from outside of medicine before coming back to the health care industry. For the first example, consider the use of frequent-flier programs by the various airlines. First, the identification of quality in fact is easy. The product delivered by airlines is moving a customer safely from one location to another in relative comfort. From the narrow viewpoint of quality in fact, customer satisfaction should be assumed as long as the airplane does not crash. One might extend the concept by indicating that the travel should be schedulable, and the flight should depart and arrive on time, but otherwise there is little to separate one airline from another airline with regard to the content of its service. Quality in perception is another matter entirely. Frequent travelers will choose an airline based on their ability to concentrate travel and accrue frequent-flier miles. These miles are then used to purchase various degrees of upgrades of service, for instance from coach class to first class. The effectiveness of this strategy is incredible, and it is entirely based on perception, not reality. For example, the difference in price between the meal in first class and coach on a domestic flight in the United States is approximately $2. While liquor is complimentary in the first class cabin, realistically, a determined alcoholic individual could only consume a quantity of alcohol worth less than $20. The complimentary movie is worth $3, and the headphone is of minimally better quality than in the coach cabin. When travelers arrive in the first-class cabin, an attendant offers to take their coat, while in the coach cabin, passengers must stow their own garments. In the first-class cabin, the attendant reads your name from a list before asking what you would like for dinner, while in the coach cabin they simply offer no choices. Finally, but clearly most importantly, the first-class cabin seats offer you approximately 6 inches of added width on each side, and approximately 6 inches of extra leg room in front.

While this description of first-class service on an airline may seem meager, it is a nearly comprehensive description of the differences between first-class and coach travel. The airplane arrives at the same airport with both cabins intact under normal circumstances, and from the standpoint of quality in fact, the first-class passenger has purchased nothing that the coach passenger did not also receive (travel). Despite the objective evidence that there is little to be gained by being in the first-class cabin, passengers have been known to delay flights for up to 3 or 4 hours in order to be on a flight with first-class availability, even when the total length of the flight was only 1 hour. Passengers, including the authors, are often willing to pay $60 to upgrade each direction of a transcontinental flight, despite the fact that flight is less than 4 hours long, and the economic value of the upgrade is far less than the amount requested. Most importantly, the airlines realize that by providing these frequent-flier motivations, they are able to capture the vast bulk of an individual traveler's flying business. All for what? Quality in fact is not the issue; quality in perception determines the market almost entirely.

Other examples of customer satisfaction abound. For instance, when one checks into a Ritz-Carlton hotel, the front desk personnel are almost uniformly more friendly than in

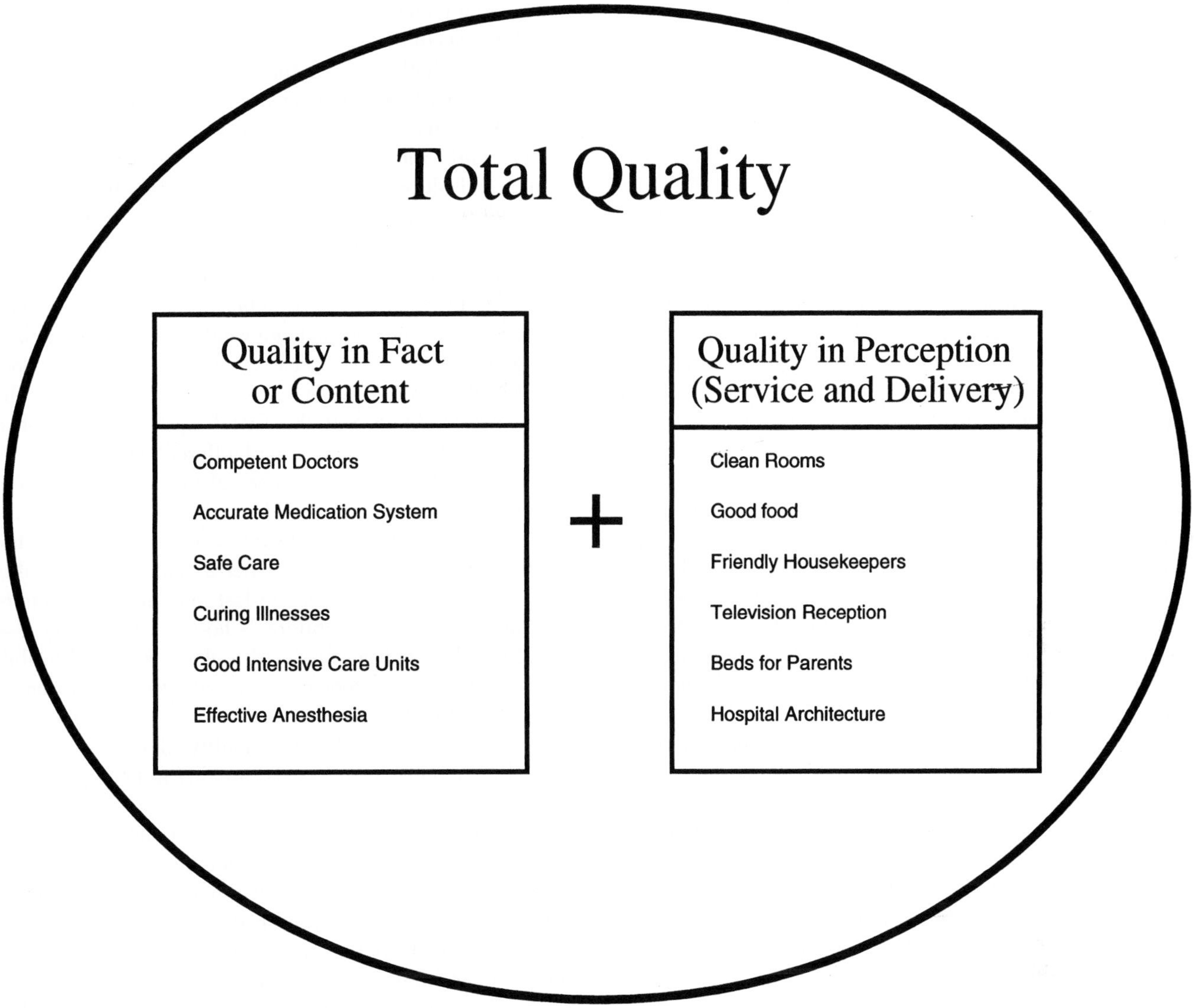
Total Quality
Quality in Fact or Content
Competent Doctors
Accurate Medication System
Safe Care
Curing Illnesses
Good Intensive Care Units
Effective Anesthesia
+
Quality in Perception (Service and Delivery)
Clean Rooms
Good food
Friendly Housekeepers
Television Reception
Beds for Parents
Hospital Architecture

Figure 48.2. Components of quality include content quality and delivery or service quality. The distinction between these two components is important for understanding customer satisfaction.

any other chain of hotels in the world. When a customer comes off of the elevator 30 feet away from the front desk, and the lobby is empty, the individual at the front desk will say "Good morning" to that customer. When a customer calls the front desk and asks to be awakened at 7:30 in the morning, the person at the front desk will uniformly say, "It will be my pleasure, sir/madam." Indeed, this expression is nearly a trademark of the Ritz-Carlton hotels. An anecdotal story has been told that at some of these hotels the staff have been authorized to repaint hotel rooms to meet the satisfaction of a specific customer. Such efforts to satisfy customers did not require particular authorization, but were rather an expected part of everyday activity.

As a final non-health-care industry example, consider for a moment the luxury cruise. Once again, the quality in fact is simple. One flies on an airplane to a location that one does not care about visiting, boards the slowest mode of transportation existent today, and spends 5 to 10 days floating to another destination that the traveler also did not wish to visit. On each of the intervening days, the passenger gets off the floating hotel and visits areas that he or she may indeed have wished to visit, but would never have made a trip to visit in isolation. For the privilege of taking the slowest mode of transportation from one location to another, neither of which the traveler was interested in visiting primarily, passengers pay prices that range from $1000 to $10,000 per person per week. The accommodations are "luxuriant," measuring from 8 feet by 8 feet to perhaps as large as 12 feet by 12 feet. Yet most passengers who have experienced a luxury cruise look forward to repeating the experience, at considerable expense. Given the delivered product in terms of quality in fact, what is the attraction of the luxury cruise? The answer lies entirely in the concept of quality in perception. For example, once a passenger has introduced himself or herself to a staff member in the bar, that staff member will remember that passenger's name without fail for the remainder of the cruise. In the dining room, a casual conversation with an assistant waiter of a dining table about a meal that is perhaps not on the future menu will result in that assistant waiter personally cooking that meal the next afternoon for that passenger. Even the staffing of the dining room is remarkable. Individual tables have an assistant waiter for each pair of customers, with only six customers per table, and each group of three assistant waiters is supervised by the main waiter of that table. The 30 to 80 tables in the room are "super-supervised" by the maitre d'. All members of the staff know the names of the passengers at their tables, and of course one should not forget the sommelier, who guides the passenger with respect to choice of wines, etc. This individual will ensure that the bottle of wine is preserved between meals and has been properly uncorked and aired for the proper amount of time before each meal. That the food is of high quality is obviously an assumption, as in any fine restaurant. The reader should be convinced that the reasons customers will choose to be passengers on cruises relates to the way they are treated on those cruises, not to the delivery of any specific, objective product.

Let's return to the health care industry. Consider the choice that a pregnant woman makes with respect to obstetric services. There are two choices to be made: the obstetrician and the hospital. First, what is the quality in fact? The product of obstetric services is the delivery of a healthy baby from a healthy mother. Quality in fact also includes a reasonable price, a low amount of morbidity, and an infinitesimally low mortality rate for both the infant and the mother. The quality in perception relates to the color of the bedspread, whether the mother is allowed to have the father in the room, and whether the room looks more like a bedroom than a delivery suite. Other aspects of quality in perception relate to the ease with which the patient (customer) gets into the room, the friendliness of the nursing and physician staff, and even the meal that is served after the delivery of the baby. For instance, it is not uncommon in some hospitals to permit the mother to upgrade her meal to lobster or order a bottle of wine with her first postpartum meal. That the mother has to pay an additional $20 to $30 for this upgrade is no surprise; perhaps the surprise is that so many mothers make the purchase.

Having stated the qualities in fact and perception of obstetric services, consider how mothers actually choose obstetric services. We would be deluding ourselves if we believed that anyone choosing an obstetric service questioned the ability of that service to deliver babies. It is in fact assumed by the public that all obstetric services can safely and competently deliver babies, with low morbidity and low mortality. It is uniformly assumed by mothers that deliveries will not be medically problematic at any particular site of delivery. Given that the public generally believes that all obstetric services can equally well deliver babies, we leave it to the reader to consider the factors that enter into the decision about which obstetric service will be selected by a patient.

We are aware of a pediatric intensive care unit where a specific incident occurred that is illustrative of the crossover between quality in fact and quality in perception. A 15-year-old patient was taken to the angiography suite from the outpatient area of one hospital and underwent an embolic procedure for a cerebral arteriovenous malformation. The patient suffered the disastrous complication of having healthy brain embolized and was transferred to the pediatric intensive care unit at a nearby children's hospital. The child was critically ill, developed severe cerebral edema, and ultimately died 2 or 3 days into her intensive care stay. Several weeks after her death, the mother wrote an angry letter to the children's hospital administrator, stating that she considered the medical and nursing care rendered at the children's hospital to have been excellent. However, she indicated that she would never come back to this particular hospital because she had received poor service. She went on to detail the fact that in the outpatient department at the first hospital, the staff had been friendly, and a nurse had offered her a pillow to place behind her head while she sat in the chair adjacent to her daughter's bedside. When she came to the children's hospital in the intensive care environment, the nursing staff did not even offer her a chair. It was for this reason that the mother, who had lost her daughter, wrote to the administrator of the children's hospital. It was because a staff member had not provided a chair or offered to fluff a pillow that this customer was dissatisfied. The example serves to bring home to us the lesson that we are in a service industry, and that the quality of our services is generally appreciated in terms of quality in perception, not quality in fact.

How should we summarize this discussion of customer satisfaction? The essential lesson for the reader to understand is that the delivery of health care is an assumed fact, regardless of the setting of delivery. It is unrealistic to expect that the public will understand that a pediatric intensive care unit is more suitable for a 7 year old than a medical intensive care unit, because they will assume that if a patient is in an intensive care unit, then that unit is capable of rendering the care. It is unrealistic to expect the public to understand the difference between children's hospitals and adult hospitals. We are deluding ourselves to believe that academic university hospitals have an advantage in the eye of the public with respect to their delivery of health care, because if one's personal physician says you can be cared for at St. Somewhere, most of the American public will believe their physician is telling them the truth. For us to truly satisfy our customers, we must pay attention to the concept of quality in perception. We must become much more aligned with the activities that are carried out at high-class hotels and fine restaurants, and we must make satisfaction of the customer (patient and family) our top priority[(88)].

Finally, we must consider our target with regard to customer satisfaction. If our patients and families are satisfied, should we be finished? We have other customers, such as payers and society at large. We need to strive to continually improve. This can be assisted by measuring ourselves against others, a technique known as benchmarking[(90,93,115)]. In this manner, we can compare ourselves with the best and strive to continually improve our delivery of care.

CQI TOOLS

Like other fields of endeavor, quality improvement has spawned its own set of methodologies, including, for example, brainstorming, nominal group techniques, cause and effect diagrams, Pareto diagrams, and control charts[11,85,87,91,94–96,116]. We have already discussed the fact that instead of embracing the scientific method, we have developed entirely new terminologies. At the beginning of this discussion about CQI tools, we wish to emphasize that most readers of this textbook are exceptionally well equipped to collect and analyze data, and none of the methodologies used in quality improvement are particularly difficult or sophisticated.

Brainstorming refers to a method of obtaining ideas from a group. For example, a discussion leader may say, "Please give me examples of improvements that could be made in your intensive care unit." Subsequently, individuals in the group would simply raise their hands and announce examples of improvements they think are needed, and the group would refrain from any judgmental comments about those ideas. The leader would simply place the ideas on the board, without prioritization or judgment. After conducting this exercise for 20 to 30 minutes, one can usually fill a wall with ideas. This activity is called brainstorming. Nominal group techniques are then used to define which of those ideas are most important to the group. We do not intend to explore these techniques but point out that multiple textbooks are available that handle this subject ably[11,96]. The result of nominal group techniques is the identification of a project in which the group is interested.

Cause and effect diagrams (sometimes called Ishikawa diagrams) are useful for identifying causes that lead to various effects or outcomes. Figure 48.3 shows a cause-and-effect diagram relating to the outcome of asthma care in the emergency department. Factors relating to the outcome of asthma care have been divided into four categories: patient, physician, treatment, and nursing factors. Within each of these factor categories, a variety of other details are provided. This diagram can help a group understand the factors that enter into the process they are about to analyze.

Another commonly used CQI tool is flowcharting. Flowcharts should not be new to any reader of this textbook, but it is often more difficult to make a flowchart of a health care process than one would believe. Figure 48.1 shows a flowchart at a simple level. It is not useful to have a flowchart like this, so one needs to get to a level of detail that is clinically applicable. Figures 48.4 and 48.5 show a more realistic pair of flowcharts; Figure 48.4 refers to the existing process of care for asthmatics in the emergency department, and Figure 48.5 shows a reengineered process of

Text continued on page 1641

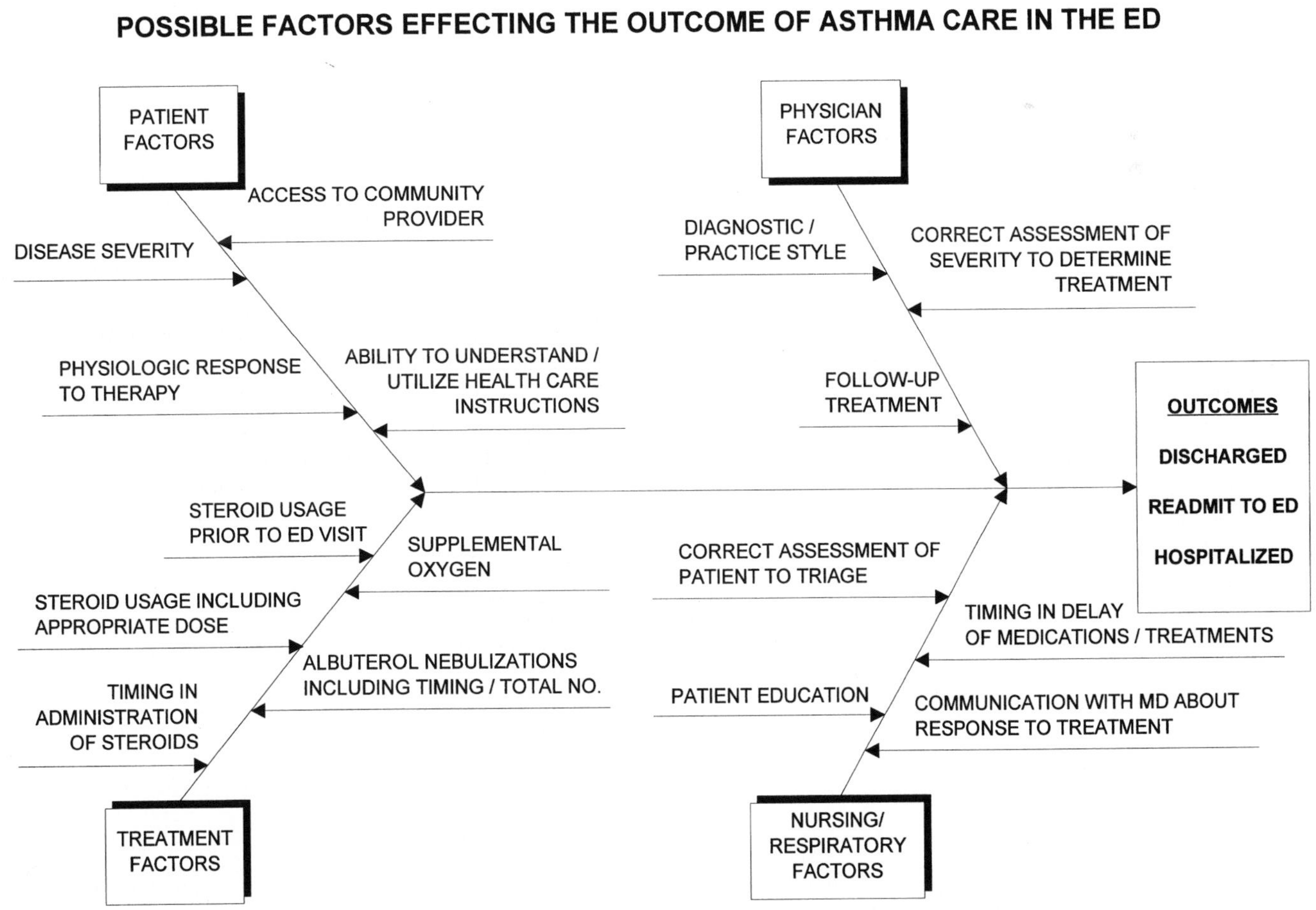

Figure 48.3. Cause-and-effect diagram for the outcome of asthma in the emergency department. Courtesy of Debra Taylor, Department of Quality Management, Primary Children's Medical Center, Salt Lake City.

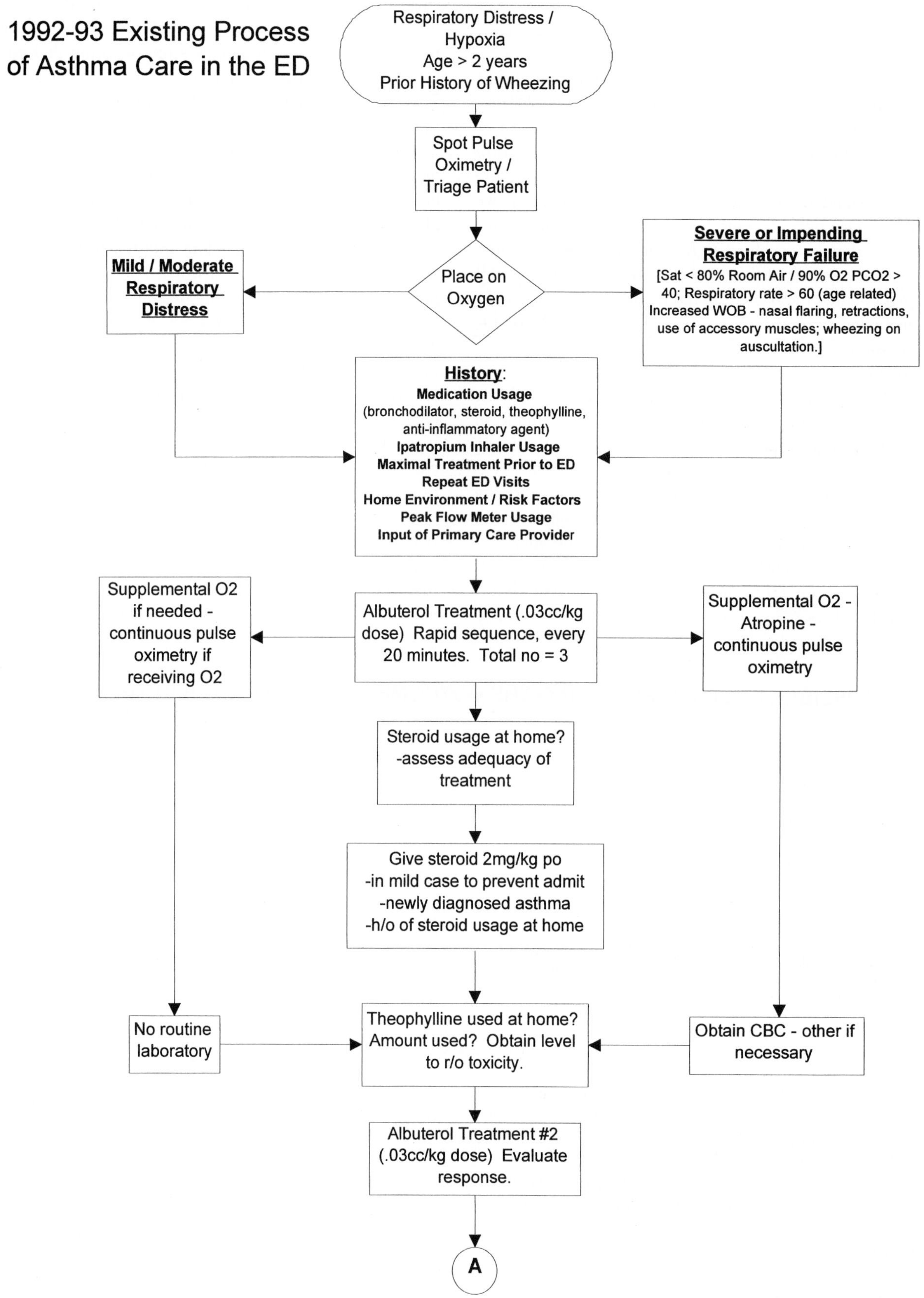

A

Figure 48.4. Flowchart showing the process of care for asthmatics in the emergency department before reengineering the process. Courtesy of Debra Taylor, Department of Quality Management, Primary Children's Medical Center, Salt Lake City.

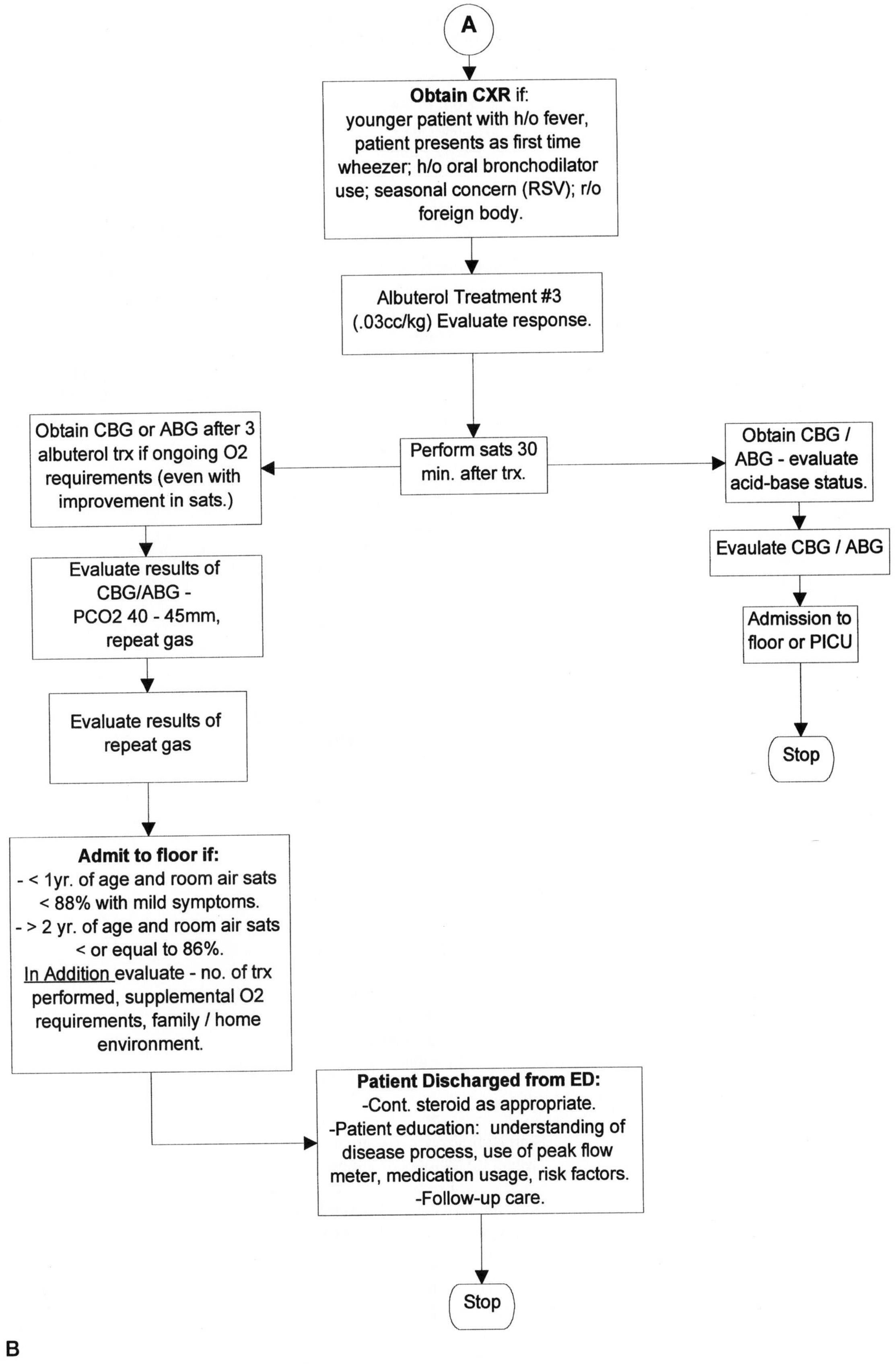

Figure 48.4. Continued.

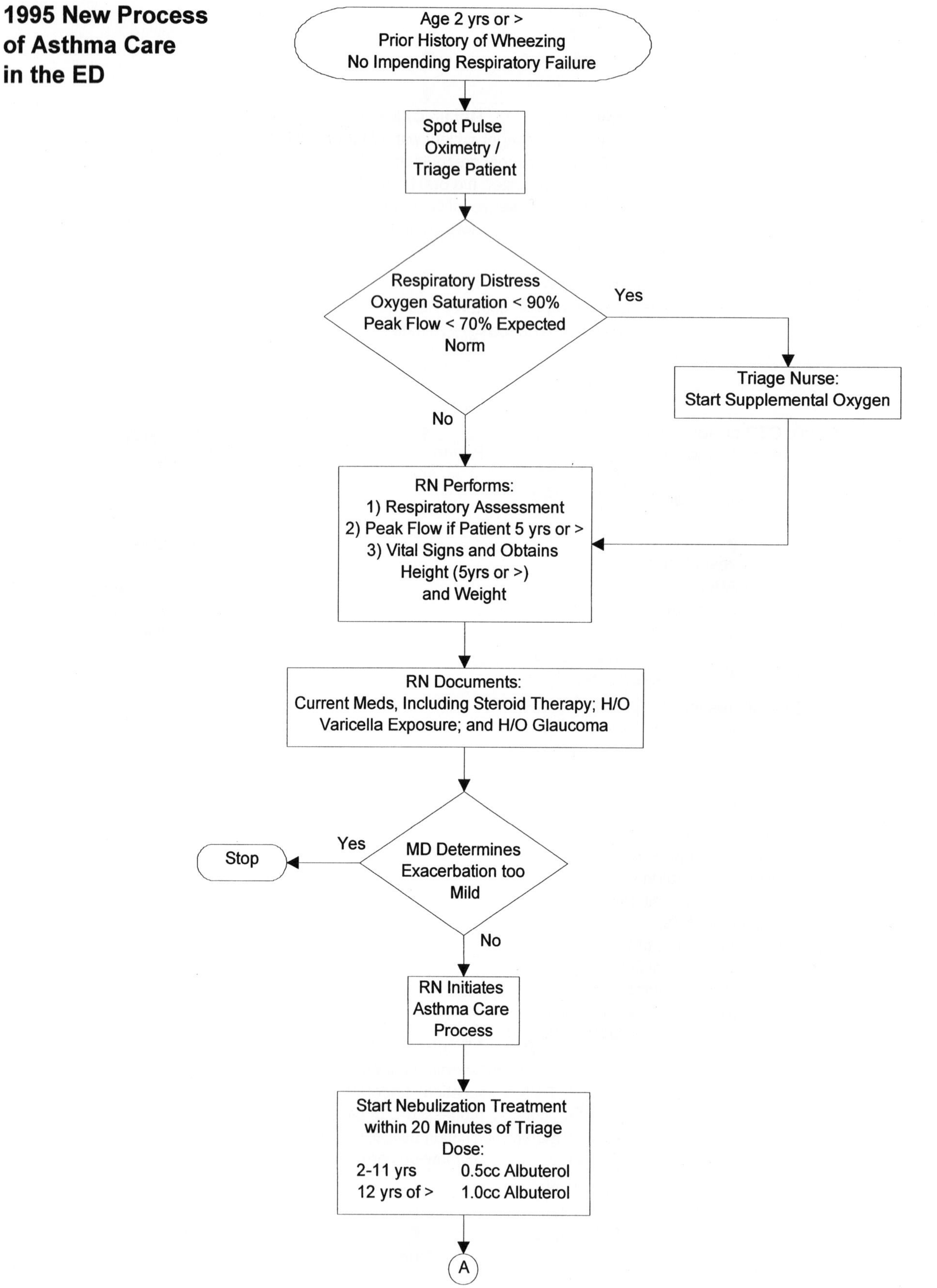

A

Figure 48.5. Flowchart showing the revised process of care for asthmatic patients in the emergency department after a continuous quality improvement project. Courtesy of Debra Taylor, Department of Quality Management, Primary Children's Medical Center, Salt Lake City.

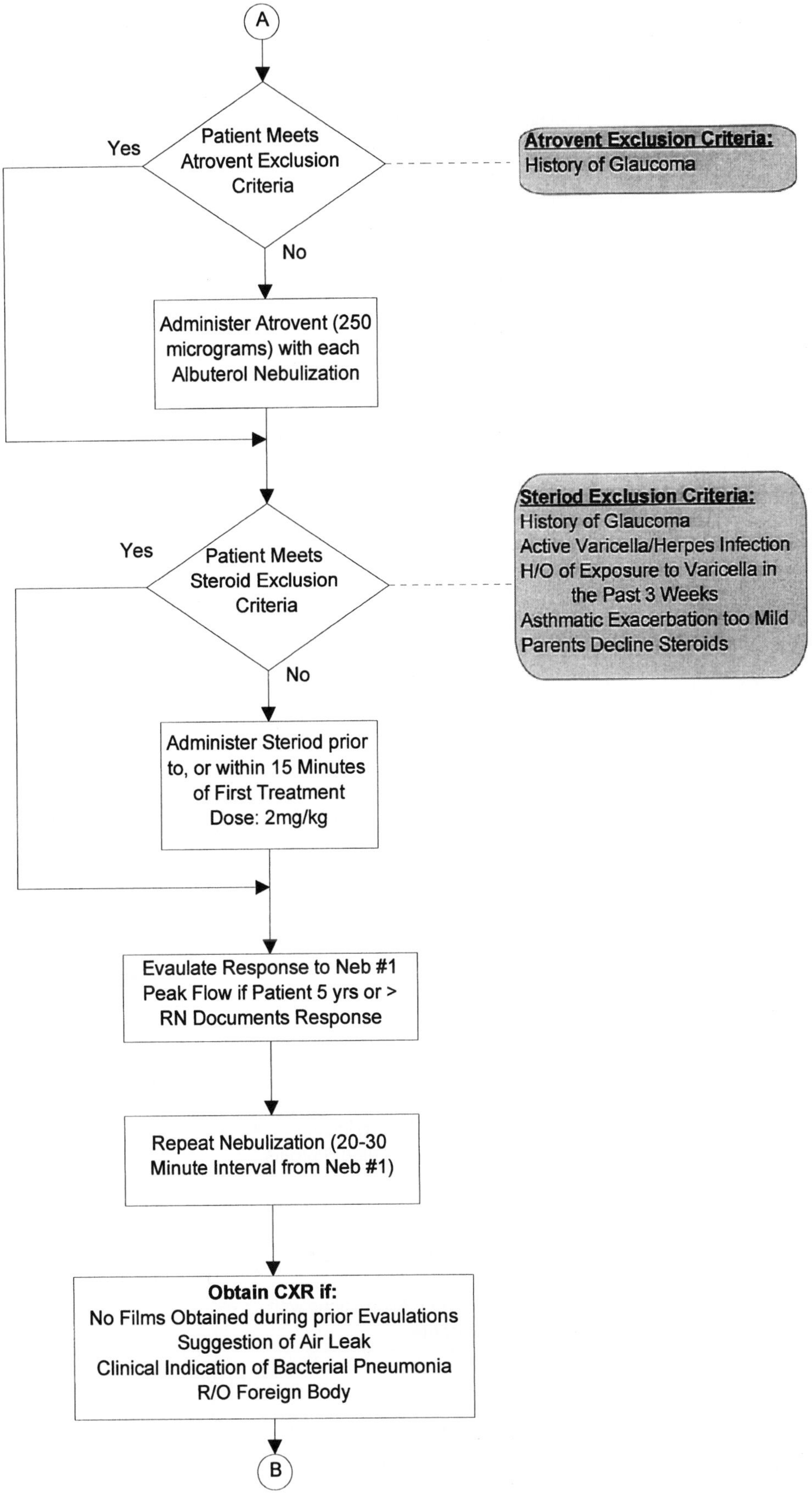

B

Figure 48.5. Continued.

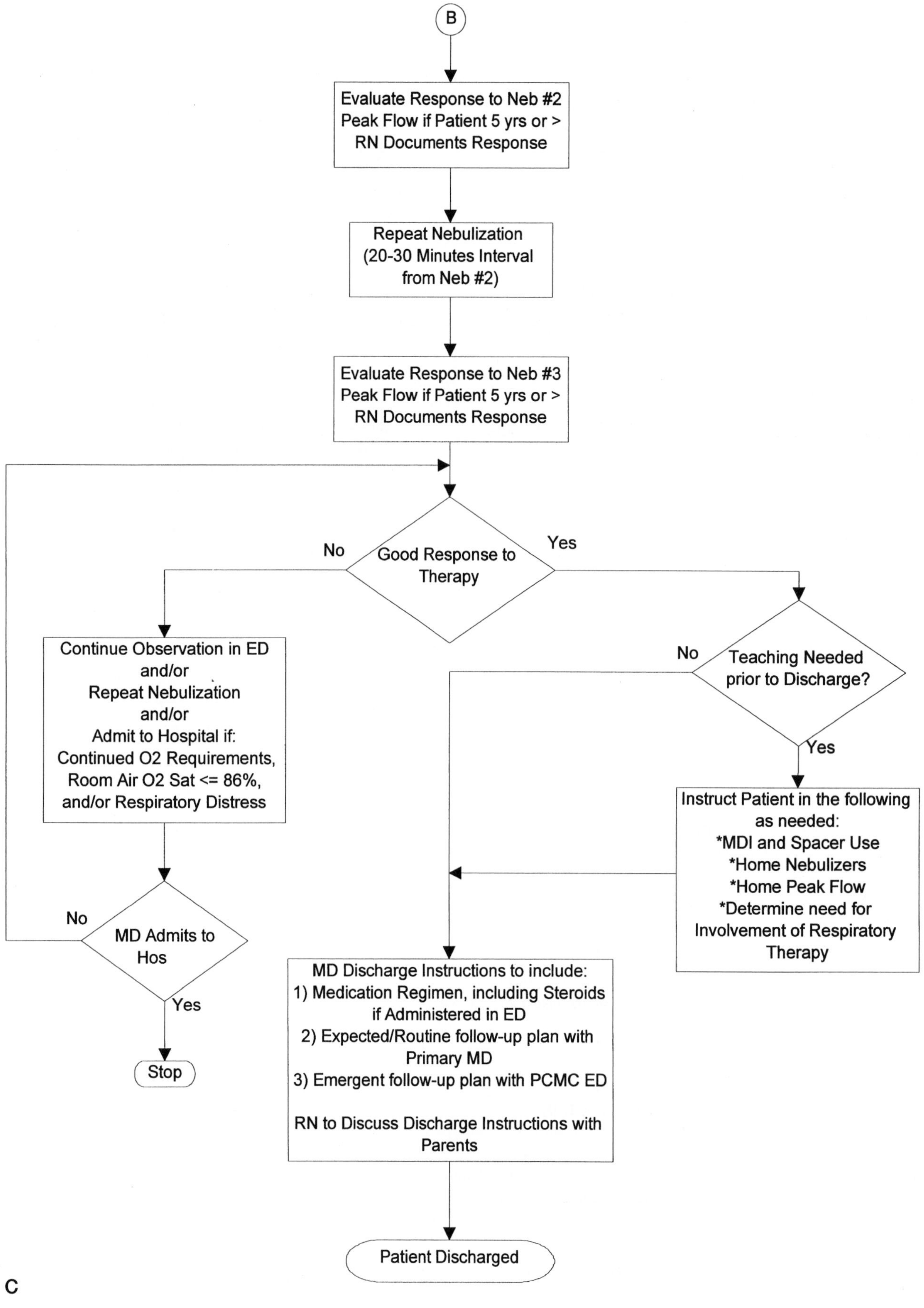

Figure 48.5. Continued.

asthma care in the emergency department. It should be emphasized that the purpose of flowcharts is to allow the group analyzing the process to thoroughly understand the process, and the effort devoted to the flowcharts should be restricted to the effort necessary to achieve that understanding. By generating an appropriate flowchart that analyzes a process, a group can often define what types of data it needs to collect in order to understand the current functioning of the process.

Once data have been collected, the usual methods of statistics and graphics are employed. These include scatterplots, histograms, regression methods, and so forth. Figures 48.6 and 48.7 show scatterplots with a regression line; regression is probably familiar to most readers. Figure 48.8 shows a box plot relating the length of stay in the hospital with the maximum computerized severity index (CSI) score of children on admission to the pediatric intensive care unit. The figure shows the anatomy of a box plot, and such figures are easily drawn on an automatic basis by using computers. Any graphical or statistical technique that the reader has used for a scientific project may be applicable to continuous quality improvement projects.

One type of chart frequently used in quality improvement is the statistical process control chart. While the statistics that underlie this chart are not sophisticated, this is a sufficiently useful chart that we will spend some detail describing it. Consider first a normal distribution of values, as in Figure 48.9. This figure is a frequency histogram of random data with a mean of 1200 and a standard deviation of 200. Lines represent the mean ±1 or 2 standard deviations. The reader will of course understand that approximately 95% of the data points lie between ±2 standard deviations from the mean.

We have already discussed variation in everyday life and have indicated the need to separate random variation from assignable variation. By arbitrarily making a decision that random variation will be whatever occurs between ±2 standard deviations from the mean, one will declare a variation assignable only 5% of the time. If one used some sort of graphical technique to determine when the variation was

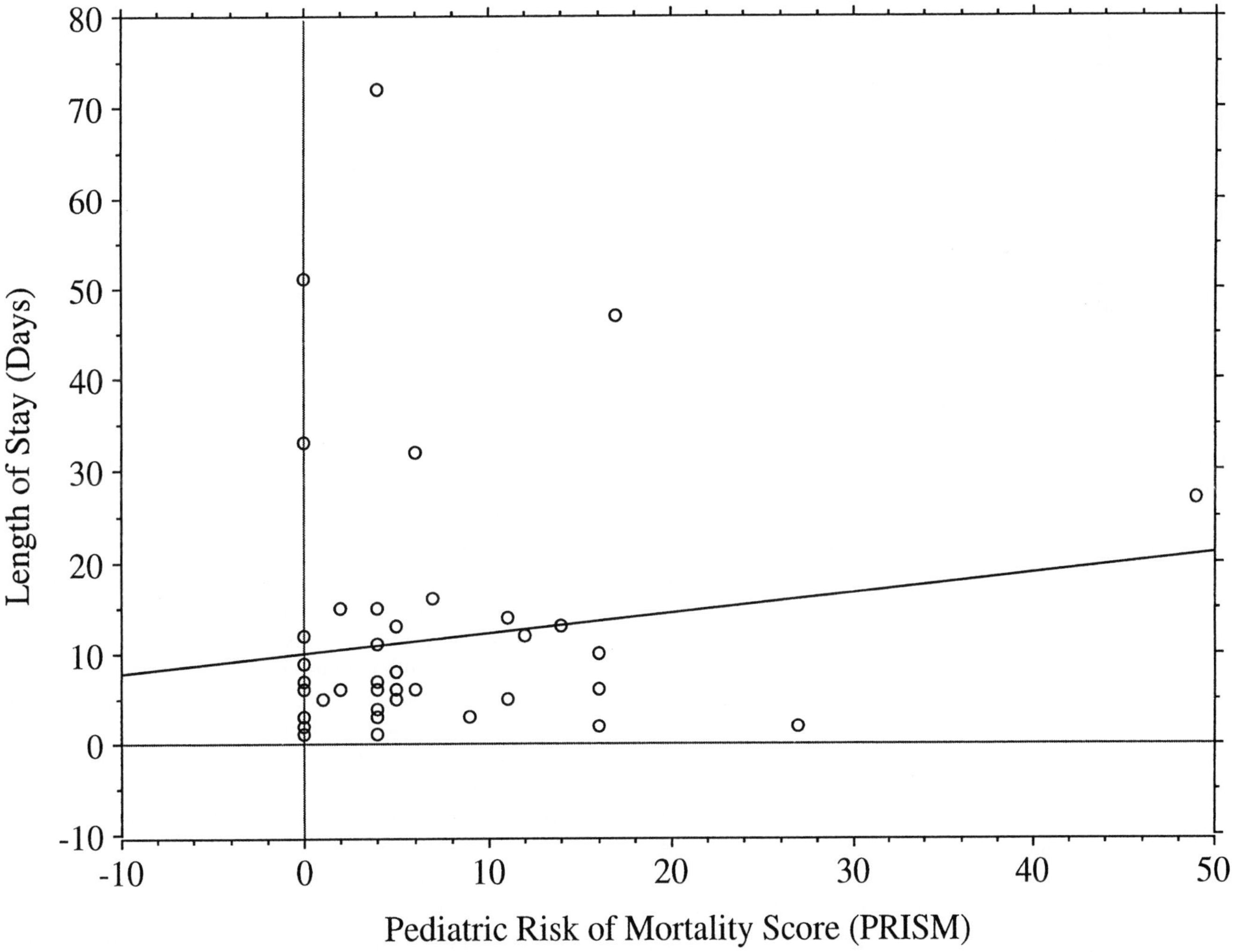

Figure 48.6. Scatterplot of length of stay versus Pediatric Risk of Mortality Score (PRISM) for 50 consecutive patients in the pediatric intensive care unit. A linear regression line is also shown. Courtesy of Susan Horn, Ph.D., Isis Inc., Salt Lake City.

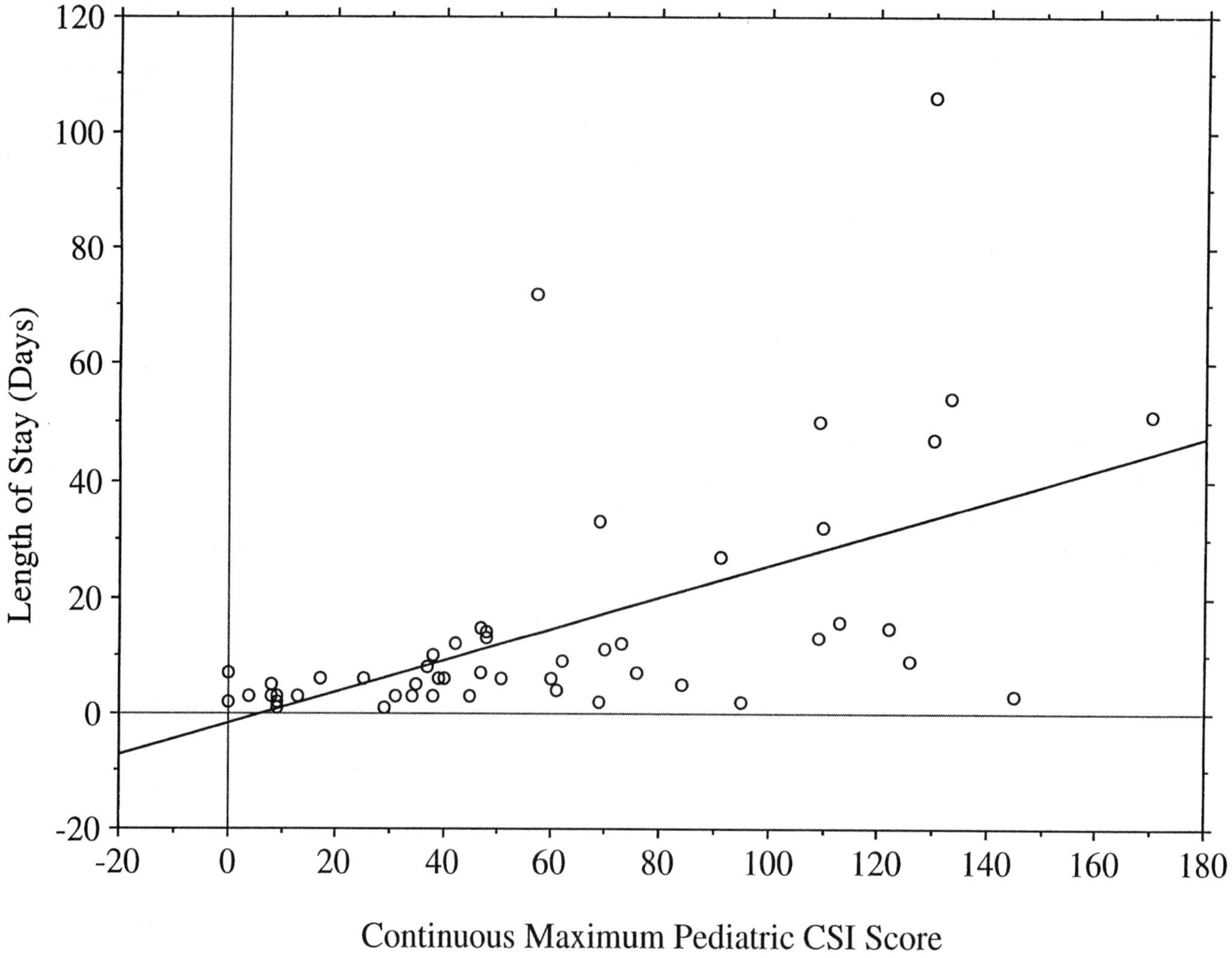

Figure 48.7. Scatterplot of length of stay versus the maximum continuous pediatric computerized severity index for 50 consecutive patients in the pediatric intensive care unit (the same patients as in Figure 48.6). A linear regression line is also shown. Courtesy of Susan Horn, Ph.D.

outside of ±2 standard deviations from the mean, this technique would be useful. In Figure 48.10, we have taken two normal distributions with different means and standard deviations and turned them on their side. One could envision that the left side of this figure represents the frequency of some sort of event associated with an original process. For the sake of discussion, consider the Y axis to be the number of dollars per day spent on medications. After reengineering the process, the distribution of drug charges per day is as seen in the right side of the figure. If the reader visualizes the three lines on each panel as the mean ±2 standard deviations, and then subtracts in his or her mind the underlying normal distribution of values, then the reader will be looking at a skeleton of a statistical control chart. Figure 48.11 shows an actual statistical control chart for medication incidents occurring in the children's hospital over a 5-year-period. On the Y axis is seen the proportion for incidents, which is simply the number of drug errors divided by the total number of drug doses dispensed during the month. In essence, if a data point falls outside the upper or lower control limit, this indicates that it is outside of two standard deviations of the mean. By constructing such control charts, organizations can quickly identify variations that are outside of the expected, allowing them to focus on variations which are assignable.

The astute reader will recognize that it is quite arbitrary where we decide to assign upper and lower control limits. In most non-health-care industries, three standard deviations are routinely used, as inspecting 5% of a manufacturing process would be exhorbitantly expensive. However, most people in health care use two standard deviations, reasoning that it is more important to investigate health care adverse events than manufacturing defects on a factory floor. This represents a trade-off between resources that one can devote toward investigating events and the risk of allowing an assignable variation to go unnoticed. Individual organizations will have to determine what level to use for upper and lower control limits for individual projects.

Finally, it should be noted that all of these techniques are readily applied by using computers. Software for flowcharting, statistics, and graphics are available on all major microcomputer platforms. In our opinion, nearly none of

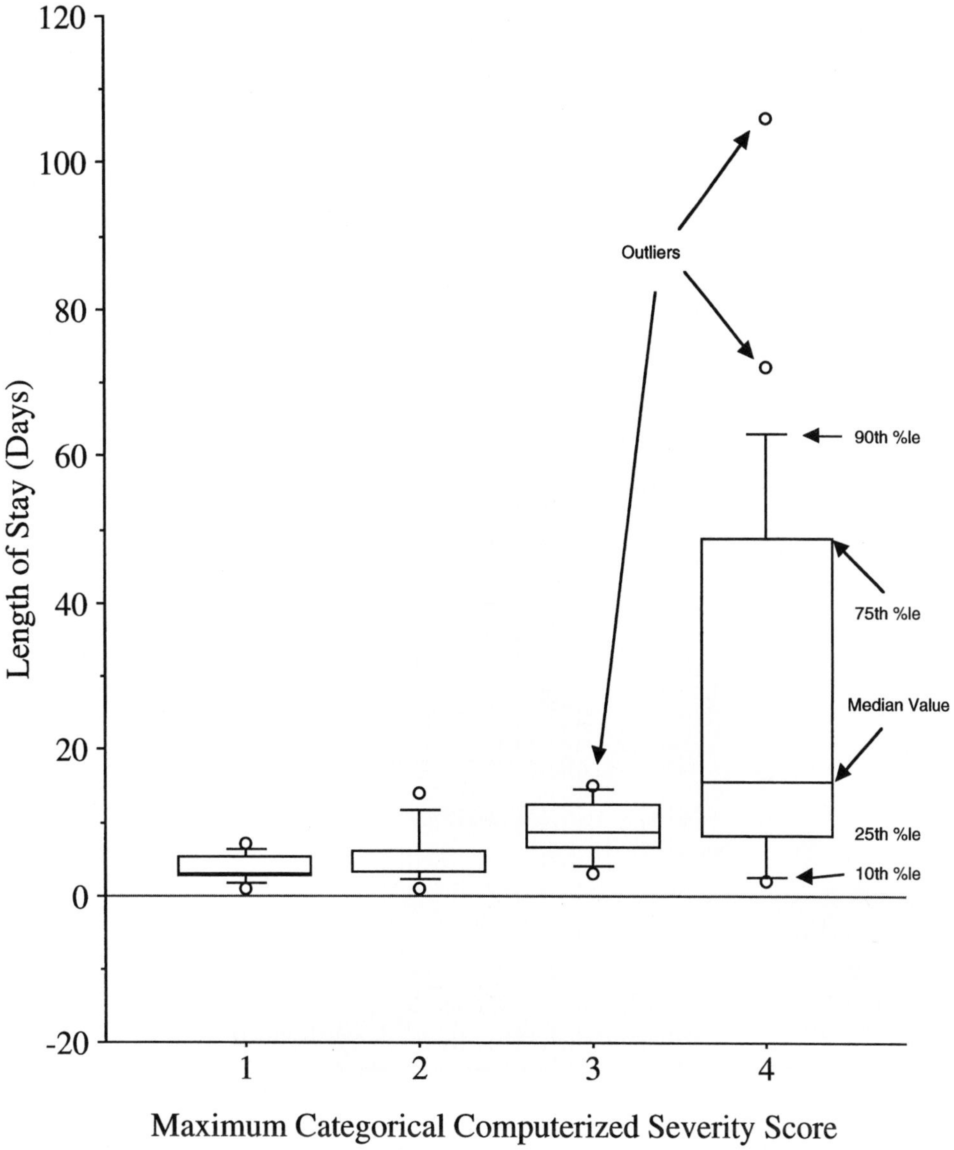

Figure 48.8. Box plot relating length of stay to the maximum categorical computerized severity score (the same patients as in Figures 48.6 and 48.7).

these statistical methods or graphics should be attempted by hand, as the costs of analyzing data for quality improvement must be absorbed by the organization.

SOURCES OF DATA

There are several existing sources of data with which clinicians should be familiar. First, of course, is the medical record itself. The primary difficulty with use of the medical record as a data source for continuous quality improvement relates to its variability and the fact that few data elements are predefined or reliably captured. It should, however, be recognized that with increasing computerization of the medical record, there will be more predefinition of terms, and it is highly likely that the medical record will increase in its value for people who are interested in operational health care research. Second, most hospitals maintain highly elaborate case-mix systems that include demographic information on patients as well as nearly all of the transactions for which there are financial implications. While traditionally physicians have had little use for this type of data, upon reflection one will realize, for example, that any drug that was administered resulted in a cost, and that cost is reflected somewhere in a financial computer program. Until better medical records systems are computerized, these transactional computer systems can be used to try to define the clinical interventions given to specific types of patients.

It is clearly nontrivial to try to implement a continuous quality improvement process that requires an enormous expenditure of effort to make measurements, plot the measured data, and reach reliable conclusions. However, many of these data are already available in the financial systems referred to above, enabling the data collection to be an automatic part of the existing financial process of the hospital. For example, it is highly likely that your hospital knows how many ventilator days there were in your ICU last month and probably knows the number of patients who were on

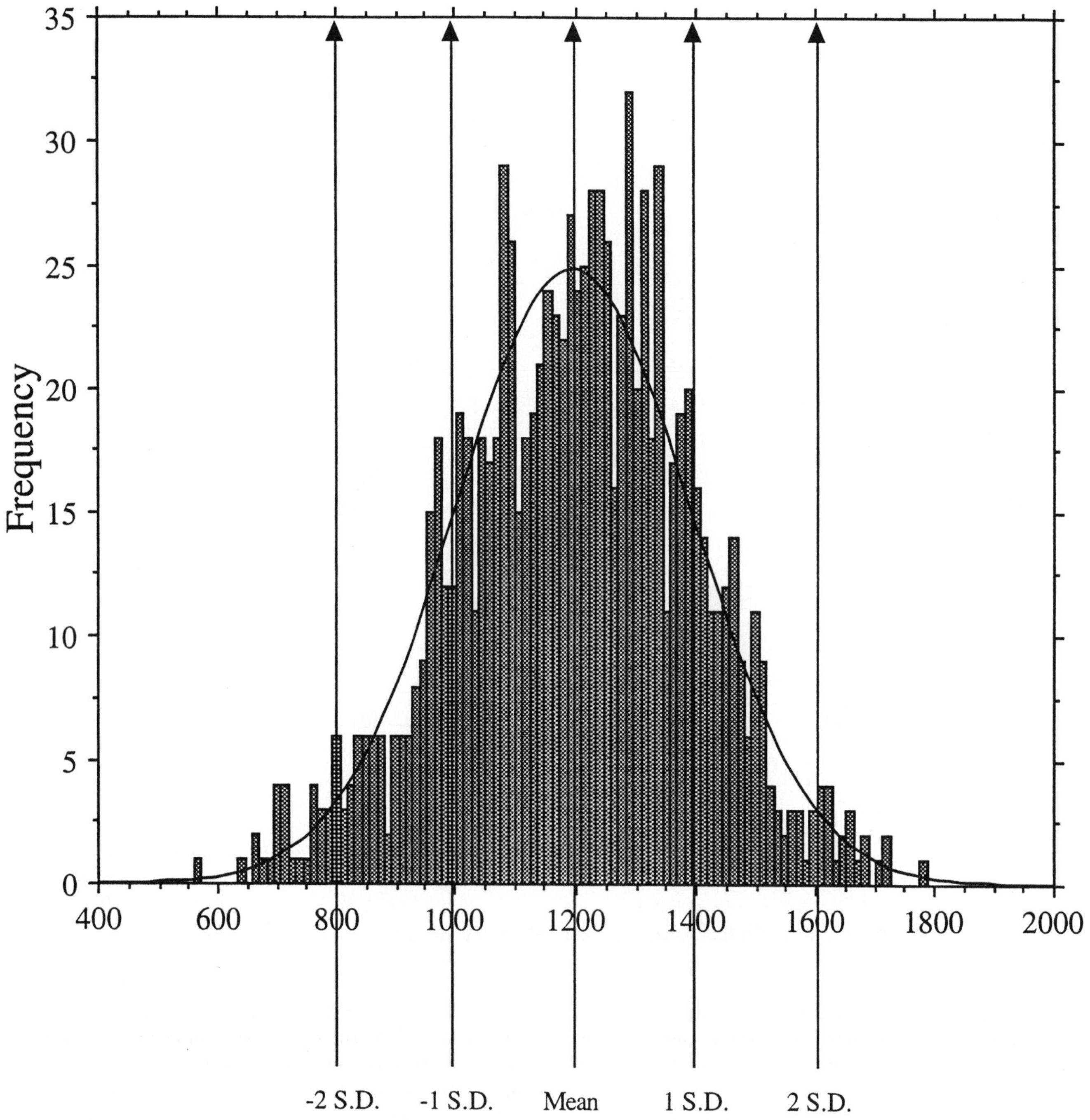

Figure 48.9. Hypothetical frequency histogram of normally distributed random data, with a mean of 1200 and a standard deviation of 200.

ventilators each day of the week. The hospital also knows how many chest x-rays were obtained per day and how many vials of pancuronium were expended. And, if you were to search the case-mix file to find all patients with respiratory distress syndrome, you could figure out which antibiotics were used on which patients by examining the financial-transaction file of the hospital. In our experience, these case-mix file data are often more complete than the data contained in the medical records, and for population studies involving hundreds or thousands of patients, using this computerized data is clearly more efficient.

As an example, our hospital recently has made a significant effort to obtain data on nearly 1200 patients with bronchiolitis. Rather than attempt to review 1200 medical records, the case-mix file was examined to determine which patients had bronchiolitis; the financial-transaction file was then searched for all of the account numbers relating to those patients. Every transaction type that is available in our hospital was examined by one of the authors, working with an outcomes specialist in our hospital, and all transactions were collapsed into one of approximately 40 categories. The result was that for each patient admission, one

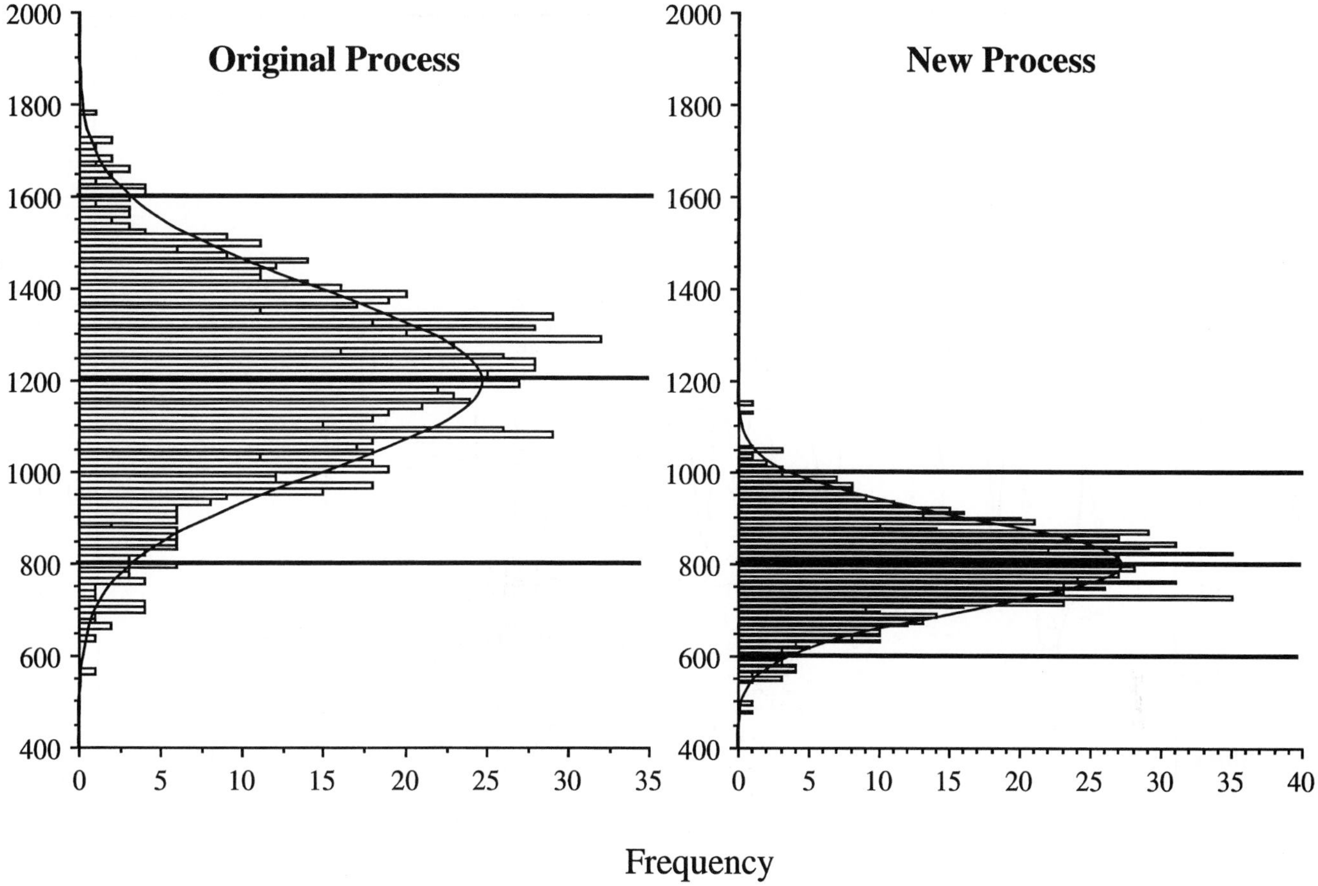

Figure 48.10. Sideways normal distributions form the skeleton of statistical process control charts. The middle lines represent the means, and the top and bottom lines represent 95% confidence limits.

could tell how many dollars in cost and charge were related to paralysis, aerosol therapy, nursing therapy, intensive care, and 35 other categories of transaction. These data on nearly 1200 patients are being used to guide clinicians as they try to improve processes of care rendered to bronchiolitis patients. While eventually we will certainly refer to the medical records of many of these patients to understand the detailed rationale for some of the things that were done, the ability to screen and prepare a database of nearly 1200 patients as a background to a continuous quality improvement project is clearly an advantage of the computerized databases.

ADJUSTMENT FOR RISK SEVERITY

When comparing the care and the outcomes of patients, it is obviously necessary to have some method to adjust for the severity of illness for each patient[117–121]. Such severity adjustment systems in general fall into two categories. The first category includes so-called modeling methods, by which the investigator derives an equation, usually a logistic regression[122,123] equation, based on an initial population of patients. Then the investigator uses that equation to predict the outcome of a validation set of patients, enabling one to assess the accuracy with which the equation predicts some behavior of the subsequent population. Numerous systems such as this exist in adult medicine, the best known of which is the Acute Physiology and Chronic Health Evaluation (APACHE) II system[124–138]. This system has been controversial as it has been applied in a large number of instances[139–154]. The most well-known such system in pediatrics is the Pediatric Risk of Mortality System (PRISM) developed by Pollack et al.[155–158]. The PRISM score enables the clinician to obtain an estimate of the probability of mortality, hence the name of the scoring system. This score has been used in a large number of studies for stratification and was recently validated outside the United States[159–161]. Notably, the PRISM score has raised some of the same controversies as the APACHE system[162–164]. The second category of severity adjustment systems involves defining clinical criteria for severity, based not on statistical modeling but rather on clinical instinct. For example, clinicians might agree that sinus bradycardia is a relatively unimportant rhythm disturbance, while ventricular tachycardia is life threatening. Thus, if one had a possible score of 1 to 4 for a specific symptom, one might score sinus bradycardia as 1 and ventricular tachycardia as 4 (life threat-

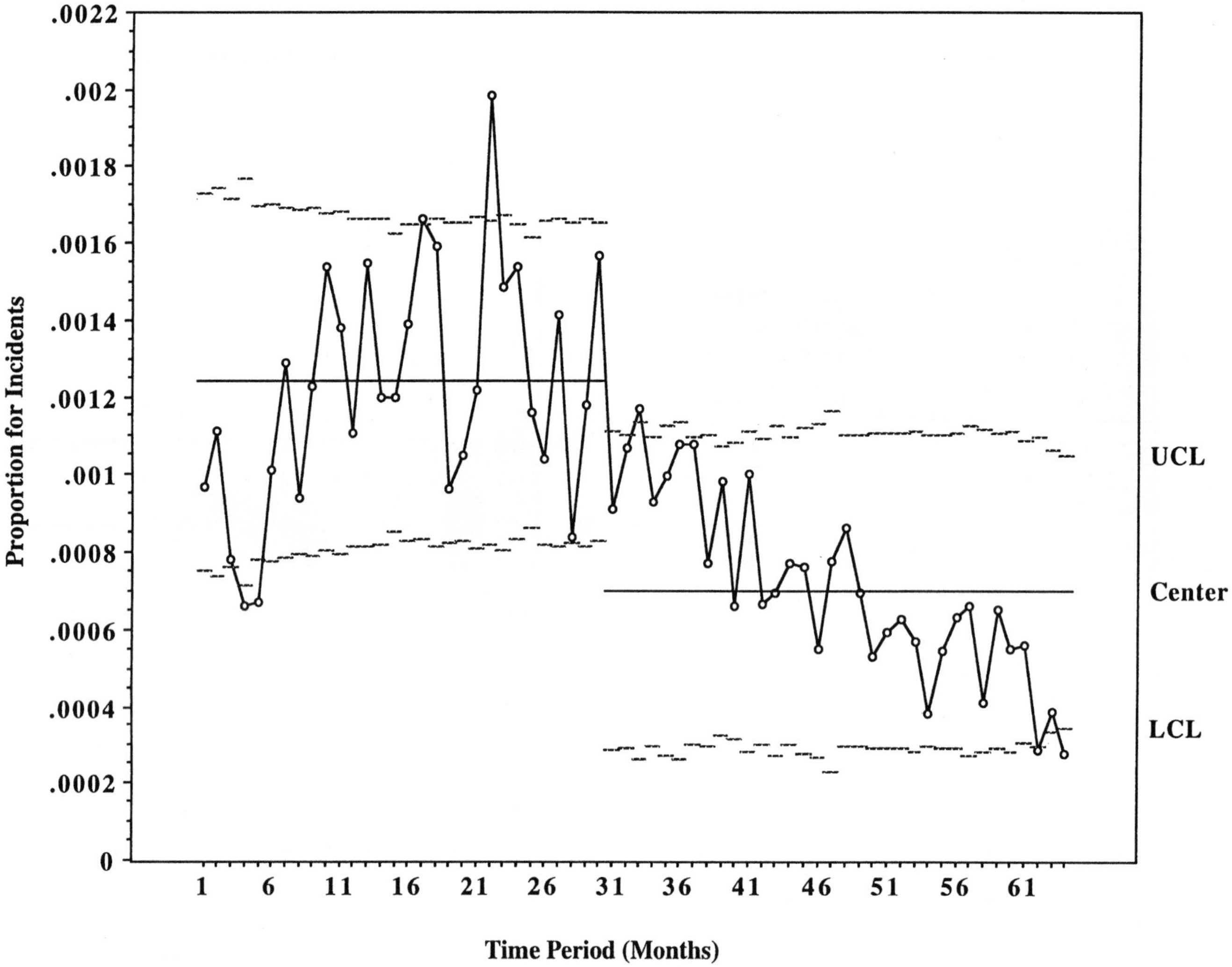

Figure 48.11. Statistical process control chart showing the number of medication incidents occurring over a 5-year period. A significant decline in incidents is evident. Courtesy of Susan Adams, Department of Quality Management, Primary Children's Medical Center, Salt Lake City.

ening). Such systems are often difficult to implement and are inherently more disease-specific. An example of this type of scoring system is the CSI[85,165–167], which is being adapted for pediatric use. In 1994, Iezzoni published an entire textbook on risk adjustment systems[86].

It is important to understand the methodology behind these two categories of severity systems. One commonly reads medical papers in which the APACHE II or PRISM scoring systems are used to compare two populations of patients who are in a clinical trial of some sort. This is intended to provide some sort of stratification, but it must be recognized that the PRISM score is intended to predict mortality and nothing else. Its application to the prediction of resource utilization, length of stay, charges, or any other parameter other than death is dangerous and probably not warranted. Figure 48.6 shows the correlation between the PRISM score and the length of stay of 50 ICU patients. The correlation is very poor (overall model $F = 0.826$, $p = 0.3682$, $R^2 = 0.018$), and this should not be surprising, as length of stay may or may not correlate with mortality probability. If one desires to stratify patients with respect to utilization risks, then one must derive a model that explicitly predicts utilization or use a system that is intrinsically based on the severity of illnesses, not on modeling of a particular parameter. Figure 48.7 shows the correlation between the maximum continuous pediatric CSI score and length of stay. This figure involves the same 50 patients that were scored in Figure 48.6, and the correlation is better than that seen with the PRISM score (overall model $F = 24.28$, $p < .0001$, $R^2 = 0.327$). This comparison is not intended to endorse one system over another but to help make the reader understand the important implications of the underlying methodology for the applicability of various scoring systems that are available today.

In summary, when one uses a scoring system such as PRISM, one must recognize that this scoring system is useful only for predicting one dependent variable; in the case of PRISM, that variable is mortality. On the other hand, a system based entirely on clinical parameters may be useful for predicting a wide variety of dependent variables, as long as none of those variables were used in modeling the behavior of the scoring system. Regardless of what type of scoring system is used, stratification of severity will be necessary for people to conduct meaningful health care outcomes research.

APPLICATION IN THE PEDIATRIC ICU

In late 1992, the authors of this chapter initiated a widescale rollout of continuous quality improvement in the Pediatric Intensive Care Unit at Primary Children's Medical Center and the University of Utah School of Medicine. This was started with a 3-day retreat during which speakers from Intermountain Health Care, Inc., were invited to provide basic information about continuous quality improvement to medical and nursing leadership staff in the intensive care unit. Following this retreat, individuals were asked to assume responsibility for continuous quality improvement projects in the intensive care unit, but little further guidance was initially provided by the authors. After several months, an individual was hired on a full-time basis to nurture continued efforts at continuous quality improvement in the intensive care unit, and this individual was crucial to the ongoing success of the enterprise. Several months later, an additional retreat was held, during which 40 additional nurses and physicians from the intensive care unit were trained.

Several lessons have emerged from our experience. First, many clinicians at the bedside will have ideas about projects that managers would never have considered. Thus, it is useful to teach a broad base of physicians and nurses about quality improvement and to allow them a reasonable amount of flexibility in determining the types of areas that need improvement. However, it is also clear that some guidance needs to be provided in order that crucial projects are actually carried out and resources are available for projects that require a financial investment. Thus, we have attempted to meld these two approaches, enabling individual clinicians and groups of clinicians to conceive their own projects, while simultaneously pointing out project areas that are crucial to the pediatric intensive care unit. Examples of these projects are shown in **Table 48.7.**

Table 48.7. Continuous Quality Improvement Projects for the Pediatric Intensive Care Unit

- Bedside nasojejunal tube placement with early enteral feeding
- Plasmanate/albumin supplies lost charges
- Switch from vecuronium to pancuronium
- Drip changes on postoperative cardiac patients
- NASA (Nursing Assignment Satisfaction Association)
- Reduction in daily morning chest x-rays
- Improving arterial blood gas orders
- Skin care, occipital ulcers, and air-bed use
- Fecal impaction
- Blood wastage
- Utilization patterns of tracheal aspirates
- Bacterial blood cultures: should indications be changed?
- Designing clinical care maps for simple postoperative heart procedures

Some of these projects are straightforward and obvious. For example, numerous muscle relaxants are available today, some of them costing significantly more than others. Realistically, all muscle relaxants accomplish roughly the same goal, and while there are differences in side effects, those differences are relatively minor. Thus, the shift away from pancuronium to other more expensive agents over the last decade has been based on a different spectrum of side effects, but the initial side effects of pancuronium are not particularly severe. Thus, one may decide to examine the costs of paralysis in the intensive care unit, conclude that pancuronium is a reasonable drug to continue to use, and simply stop using the more expensive drug. If the same quality of medical care is rendered at a lower cost, this represents an increase in value to the patient and to society. Another relatively straightforward example concerns morning chest x-rays obtained for the proper indication. Ensuring that morning chest x-rays obtained for purposes of endotracheal tube positioning are taken with the head in the midline is another straightforward example.

As an example of a project that did not arise from management but in fact came from some innovative clinicians in the intensive care unit, consider the use of nasojejunal feeding tubes. The nurse practitioners in the Pediatric Intensive Care Unit at Primary Children's Medical Center were made aware that it was possible to place nasojejunal tubes at the bedside without the use of fluoroscopy. After receiving training in this technique, they began to use it successfully in infants and children. Now, several years later, the use of nasojejunal feeding is widespread in our intensive care unit, even in patients who previously would have been considered too unstable to travel to the radiology suite to undergo fluoroscopic placement of such tubes. As a result, the use of total parenteral nutrition has decreased dramatically over the last 2 years, and the frequency of central line infection has decreased. Many aspects of this project have been reported elsewhere[168–170].

TRAINING ISSUES IN CQI

An organization can spend a great deal of money preparing its employees to engineer CQI projects. A variety of consultants and institutes are available, and it is certainly controversial whether one should attempt to train the entire staff of an intensive care unit or concentrate on a small portion of the staff. In this section we will describe the training method we have used in our hospital.

We decided to train groups of individuals in the hospital who come from the same functional areas, such as the intensive care unit, social work department, or operating room. Groups of approximately 25 to 35 are convened at one time, and the format is a 2- to 3-day retreat.

The retreat begins with approximately 2 hours of introductory material concerning quality and quality improvement, and an attempt is made in this lecture to use examples related to the group of individuals attending the retreat.

Thus, different examples are used for the pharmacy staff than for rehabilitation or nutrition staff. Following this introductory material, the faculty of the retreat lead a brainstorming session, during which ideas about improvement of the functional area attending the retreat are thrown out and placed on the blackboard. Rather than explain to the attendees the definition of brainstorming, the activity is simply carried out, resulting in a list of potential areas of improvement. After spending some time doing this, the attendees are told that what they just did was called brainstorming, and then the retreat moves on to the next stage. The attendees are divided into small groups of five to eight individuals. Each group chooses from the ideas obtained and decides on a project to use for the remainder of the retreat as an educational project.

The faculty members then discuss mission statements (i.e., a hypothesis), explaining the purpose of a mission statement, how to write a mission statement, and other relevant issues. After approximately 10 minutes of discussion, the groups are then asked to write the mission statements for their projects. They are allowed approximately 20 minutes; then the mission statements that are written are discussed by the overall group. Then a faculty member provides approximately 10 minutes of discussion about flowcharting, and the groups are asked to make a flowchart of their projects. After discussions about cause-and-effect diagrams and other tools used in the analysis of processes, the groups actually carry these out. By the end of the first day, data collection has been discussed, and each of the groups submits to the faculty the list of data they will need for their improvement project.

During the evening of the first day, the faculty use computers to create data formatted to meet the requirements of each group. The next morning each of the groups is provided with the data they requested. The faculty make efforts to place patterns in the data to make them interesting, but the groups are given precisely the type of data they wanted, even when the faculty realized that the groups asked for the wrong data. During the second day, statistical and graphical methods are discussed, and the groups use their data to exercise those methods. Finally, in the afternoon of the second day, the groups present their projects as if they had been real, and each project is discussed.

The advantage of using this type of method is that all of the projects that arise in the course of such retreats are based on real problems. After spending 2 days considering the problems, these groups are ready to go back to the hospital and possibly initiate similar projects on a real scale, using real data. In the last 2 years, the authors have helped train nearly 600 individuals in the hospital, and more than 50 projects are currently active.

SUMMARY

The purpose of this chapter has been to acquaint the reader with the potential for CQI activities in the pediatric intensive care unit. As a microcosm of the health care system, the intensive care unit is an excellent site in which to consider improvements in health care delivery.

References

1. Chessare JB, Berwick DM. Variation in clinical practice in the management of febrile seizures. Pediatr Emerg Care 1985;1(1):19–21.
2. McFadden DM, Berwick DM, Feldstein ML, Marter SS. Age-specific patterns of diagnosis of acute otitis media. Clin Pediatr (Phila) 1985;24(10):571–5.
3. Berwick DM. Screening in health fairs. A critical review of benefits, risks, and costs. JAMA 1985;254(11):1492–8.
4. Berwick DM, Coltin KL. Feedback reduces test use in a health maintenance organization. JAMA 1986;255(11):1450–4.
5. Berwick DM, Gorss E, Macone AB, O'Rourke EJ, Goldmann DA. Impact of rapid antigen tests for group A streptococcal pharyngitis on physician use of antibiotics and throat cultures. Pediatr Infect Dis J 1987;6(12):1095–102.
6. Berwick DM. Measuring health care quality. Pediatr Rev 1988; 10(1):11–6.
7. Berwick DM. Continuous improvement as an ideal in health care. N Engl J Med 1989;320(1):53–6.
8. Berwick DM, Hiatt HH. Who pays? [editorial; comment]. N Engl J Med 1989;321(8):541–2.
9. Perrin JM, Homer CJ, Berwick DM, Woolf AD, Freeman JL, Wennberg JE. Variations in rates of hospitalization of children in three urban communities. N Engl J Med 1989;320(18):1183–7.
10. Pantell RH, Berwick DM. Cost-effectiveness analysis in pediatric practice [comment]. Pediatrics 1990;85(3):361–4.
11. Berwick DM, Godfrey AB, Roessner J. Curing Health Care: New Strategies for Quality Improvement. San Francisco, California: Jossey-Bass Publishers, 1990.
12. Berwick DM. The double edge of knowledge [editorial]. JAMA 1991; 266(6):841–2.
13. Berwick DM, Enthoven A, Bunker JP. Quality management in the NHS: the doctor's role II. Brit Med J 1992;304(6822):304–8.
14. Berwick DM, Enthoven A, Bunker JP. Quality management in the NHS: the doctor's role I. Brit Med J 1992;304(6821):235–9.
15. Laffel G, Berwick DM. Quality in health care. JAMA 1992; 268(3):407–9.
16. Laffel GL, Berwick DM. Quality health care. JAMA 1993;270(2):254–5.
17. Berwick DM. Eleven worthy aims for clinical leadership of health system reform. JAMA 1994;272(10):797–802.
18. Augustine NR. Augustine's Laws and Major System Development Programs. New York, New York: American Institute of Aeronautics and Astronautics, Inc., 1983.
19. O'Leary DS. The Joint Commission looks to the future [editorial]. JAMA 1987;258(7):951–2.
20. O'Leary DS, O'Leary MR. From quality assurance to quality improvement. The Joint Commission on Accreditation of Healthcare Organizations and Emergency Care. Emerg Med Clin North Am 1992;10(3): 477–92.
21. Roberts JS, Coale JG, Redman RR. A history of the Joint Commission on Accreditation of Hospitals. JAMA 1987;258(7):936–40.
22. Skolnick AA. Joint Commission will collect, publicize outcomes [news]. JAMA 1993;270(2):165, 168, 171.
23. AMA initiative on quality of medical care and professional self-regulation. JAMA 1986;256(8):1036–7.
24. Quality assurance for office laboratories [letter]. JAMA 1986; 256(2):211–2.
25. Guidelines for quality assurance. Council on Medical Service. JAMA 1988;259(17):2572–3.
26. Quality assurance in cervical cytology. The Papanicolaou smear. Council on Scientific Affairs. JAMA 1989;262(12):1672–9.
27. Quality assurance and dialysis services [editorial]. Lancet 1990; 336(8724):1160–1.
28. Quality assurance in Medicare [letter; comment]. N Engl J Med 1990;323(4):278–9.
29. Bauman TW, Bauman DH. Quality assurance for the radiology-emergency interface. Emerg Med Clin North Am 1991;9(4):881–4.
30. Bennett MJ, Tershakovec AM, Cortner JA, Shannon BM. A quality assurance program for the measurement of capillary blood cholesterol levels in private pediatric practices. The Children's Health Project. Am J Dis Child 1993;147(3):340–5.
31. Bergman DA. Quality improvement: buzz words or boon? Pediatr Rev 1993;14(6):208–13.
32. Bouchard RE, Tufo HM, Beaty HN. The impact of a quality assurance

program on postgraduate training in internal medicine. JAMA 1985;253(8):1146–50.
33. Brennan TA, Localio AR, Leape LL, et al. Identification of adverse events occurring during hospitalization. A cross-sectional study of litigation, quality assurance, and medical records at two teaching hospitals. Ann Intern Med 1990;112(3):221–6.
34. Casamassimo PS. Who defines quality in health care? [editorial]. Pediatr Dent 1994;16(1):8–9.
35. Chassin MR, McCue SM. A randomized trial of medical quality assurance. Improving physicians' use of pelvimetry. JAMA 1986; 256(8):1012–6.
36. Chassin MR. Quality of care. Time to act [editorial; comment]. JAMA 1991;266(24):3472–3.
37. Cohen NA. Quality of care for youths in group homes. Child Welfare 1986;65(5):481–94.
38. Dans PE, Weiner JP, Otter SE. Peer review organizations. Promises and potential pitfalls. N Engl J Med 1985;313(18):1131–7.
39. Davis JW, Hoyt DB, McArdle MS, et al. An analysis of errors causing morbidity and mortality in a trauma system: a guide for quality improvement. J Trauma 1992;32(5):660–5.
40. Fehrsen GS, Henbest RJ. In search of excellence. Expanding the patient-centred clinical method: a three-stage assessment. Fam Pract 1993;10(1):49–54.
41. Fink A, Siu AL, Brook RH, Park RE, Solomon DH. Assuring the quality of health care for older persons. An expert panel's priorities. JAMA 1987;258(14):1905–8.
42. Flint LS, Hammett WH, Martens K. Quality assurance in the emergency department. Ann Emerg Med 1985;14(2):134–8.
43. Goldman RL. The reliability of peer assessments of quality of care. JAMA 1992;267(7):958–60.
44. Graff LG. Utilization review. Emergency medicine implications. Emerg Med Clin North Am 1992;10(3):583–96.
45. Greene CS. Quality assurance in the teaching hospital. Emerg Med Clin North Am 1992;10(3):611–25.
46. Hopkins A, Maxwell R. Contracts and quality of care. Brit Med J 1990;300(6729):919–22.
47. Jencks SF. Quality assurance. JAMA 1990;263(19):2679–81.
48. Kibbe DC, Bentz E, McLaughlin CP. Continuous quality improvement for continuity of care. J Fam Pract 1993;36(3):304–8.
49. Little N. The quality assurance-risk management interface. Emerg Med Clin North Am 1992;10(3):573–81.
50. Kuhn M, Morgan MT, Hoffman JR. Quality assurance in the emergency department: evaluation of the ECG review process. Ann Emerg Med 1992;21(1):10–5.
51. Laffel G, Blumenthal D. The case for using industrial quality management science in health care organizations. JAMA 1989;262(20): 2869–73.
52. Nakayama DK, Saitz EW, Gardner MJ, Kompare E, Guzik E, Rowe MI. Quality assessment in the pediatric trauma care system. J Pediatr Surg 1989;24(2):159–62.
53. Mishriki SF. Quality assurance: monitoring lithotriptor output and its clinical implications. J Urol 1994;152(1):57–61.
54. Mayer TA. Industrial models of continuous quality improvement. Implications for emergency medicine. Emerg Med Clin North Am 1992;10(3):523–47.
55. Overton DT, Delene LM. The cost of quality in health care. Emerg Med Clin North Am 1992;10(3):549–55.
56. Polsky SS, Weigand JV. Quality assurance in emergency medical service systems. Emerg Med Clin North Am 1990;8(1):75–84.
57. Shackford SR, Hollingsworth-Fridlund P, McArdle M, Eastman AB. Assuring quality in a trauma system the Medical Audit Committee: composition, cost, and results. J Trauma 1987;27(8):866–75.
58. Schwartz ML, Sharkey PW, Andersen JA. Quality assurance for patients with head injuries admitted to a regional trauma unit. J Trauma 1991;31(7):962–7.
59. Stair TO. Quality assurance. Emerg Med Clin North Am 1987; 5(1):41–50.
60. Swor RA. Quality assurance in EMS systems. Emerg Med Clin North Am 1992;10(3):597–610.
61. Vikell JH. The process of quality management. Pediatr Nurs 1991;17(6):618–9.
62. Van der Voort E. Outcome and quality assurance standards. Crit Care Med 1993;21(9 Suppl):S402–3.
63. Vuori H. Quality assurance in Finland. Brit Med J 1992;304 (6820):162–4.
64. Waskerwitz S, Unfer SM. Quality assurance in emergency pediatrics. Pediatr Emerg Care 1987;3(2):121–6.
65. Wearmouth EM, Lambert P, Morland R. Quality assurance in preschool surveillance. Arch Dis Child 1994;70(6):505–11.
66. Wenzel RP, Pfaller MA. Infection control: the premier quality assessment program in United States hospitals. Am J Med 1991;91(3B): 27S–31S.
67. Wissow LS, Warshow M, Box J, Baker D. Case management and quality assurance to improve care of inner-city children with asthma. Am J Dis Child 1988;142(7):748–52.
68. Williams RM. Health policy and quality: an ethical dilemma. J Emerg Med 1993;11(3):345–9.
69. Williams SM, Parry BR, Schlup MM. Quality control: an application of the cusum. Brit Med J 1992;304(6838):1359–61.
70. Wiltse BJ, Spooner SH. Hospital policies as they affect quality in the 1990s: a case for change? J Perinat Neonatal Nurs 1993;7(2):10–7.
71. Burke MC, Aghababian RV, Blackbourne B. Use of autopsy results in the emergency department quality assurance plan. Ann Emerg Med 1990;19(4):363–6.
72. Eichelman B. Proactive violence reduction: successful quality assurance [editorial]. JAMA 1989;261(17):2546.
73. George JE, Espinosa JA, Quattrone MS. Legal issues in emergency radiology. Practical strategies to reduce risk. Emerg Med Clin North Am 1992;10(1):179–203.
74. Goldmann DA. Contemporary challenges for hospital epidemiology. Am J Med 1991;91(3B):8S–15S.
75. Holroyd BR, Knopp R, Kallsen G. Medical control. Quality assurance in prehospital care. JAMA 1986;256(8):1027–31.
76. Holt AA, Sibbald WJ, Calvin JE. A survey of charting in critical care units. Crit Care Med 1993;21(1):144–50.
77. Maley RA, Epstein AL, eds. High Technology in Health Care: Risk Management Perspectives. Chicago, Illinois: American Hospital Publishing, Inc., 1993.
78. Nathan JE. Management of the difficult child: a survey of pediatric dentists' use of restraints, sedation and general anesthesia. ASDC J Dent Child 1989;56(4):293–301.
79. Pointer JE, Osur MA. EMS quality assurance: a computerized incident reporting system. J Emerg Med 1987;5(6):513–7.
80. Raines E. Hospital risk management for perinatal care: theory and practice. J Perinatol 1988;8(2):96–100.
81. Sanazaro PJ, Mills DH. A critique of the use of generic screening in quality assessment. JAMA 1991;265(15):1977–81.
82. Valenzuela TD, Criss EA, Spaite DW, Meislin HW. Evaluation of EMS management training offered during emergency medicine residency training. Ann Emerg Med 1989;18(8):812–4.
83. Whitcomb JE, Stueven H, Tonsfeldt D, Kastenson G. Quality assurance in the emergency department. Ann Emerg Med 1985;14(12): 1199–204.
84. Blumenthal D. Total quality management and physicians' clinical decisions. JAMA 1993;269(21):2775–8.
85. Horn SD, Hopkins DSP, eds. Clinical Practice Improvement: A New Technology for Developing Cost-Effective Quality Health Care. Washington, D.C.: Faulkner and Gray, Inc., 1994. Faulkner & Gray's Medical Outcomes and Practice Guidelines Library; vol I.
86. Iezzoni LI, ed. Risk Adjustment for Measuring Health Care Outcomes. Ann Arbor, Michigan: Health Administration Press, 1994.
87. Chambers JM, Cleveland WS, Kleiner B, Tukey PA. Graphical Methods for Data Analysis. Boston: Duxbury Press, 1983. Bickel PJ, Cleveland WS, Dudley RM, eds.
88. Leebov W, Scott G. Service Quality Improvement: The Customer Satisfaction Strategy for Health Care. Chicago, Illinois: American Hospital Publishing, Inc., 1994.
89. Becker-Deems ED. Self-Managed Work Teams in Health Care Organizations. Chicago, Illinois: American Hospital Publishing, Inc., 1994.
90. Gift RG, Mosel D. Benchmarking in Health Care: A Collaborative Approach. Chicago, Illinois: American Hospital Publishing, Inc., 1994.
91. Spath PL, ed. Clinical Paths: Tools for Outcomes Management. Chicago, Illinois: American Hospital Publishing, Inc., 1994.
92. Leebov W, Ersoz CJ. The Health Care Manager's Guide to Continuous Quality Improvement. Chicago, Illinois: American Hospital Publishing, Inc., 1991.
93. Camp RC. Benchmarking: The Search for Industry Best Practices that Lead to Superior Performance. Milwaukee, Wisconsin: Quality Press, 1989.
94. Sloan MD, Chmel M. The Quality Revolution and Health Care: A Primer for Purchasers and Providers. Milwaukee, Wisconsin: ASQC Quality Press, 1991.
95. Cleveland WS. The Elements of Graphing Data. Pacific Grove, California: Wadsworth Advanced Book Program, 1985.

96. Gaucher EJ, Coffey RJ. Total Quality in Healthcare. San Francisco, California: Jossey-Bass Inc., 1993.
97. Marszalek-Gaucher E, Coffey RJ. Transforming Healthcare Organizations: How to Achieve and Sustain Organizational Excellence. San Francisco, California: Jossey-Bass Inc., 1991.
98. Coalition for Critical Care Excellence. ICU Cost Reduction: Practical Suggestions and Future Considerations. Anaheim, California: Society of Critical Care Medicine, 1994.
99. Barry PW, Ralston C. Adverse events occurring during interhospital transfer of the critically ill. Arch Dis Child 1994;71(1):8–11.
100. Corchia C. "Errors" in perinatal medicine: an epidemiological perspective. Paediatr Perinat Epidemiol 1992;6(3):381–4.
101. Donchin Y, Gopher D, Olin M, et al. A look into the nature and causes of human errors in the intensive care unit. Critical Care Medicine 1995;23(2):294–300.
102. Folli HL, Poole RL, Benitz WE, Russo JC. Medication error prevention by clinical pharmacists in two children's hospitals. Pediatrics 1987;79(5):718–22.
103. Hammond JS, Ward CG. Transfers from emergency room to burn center: errors in burn size estimate. J Trauma 1987;27(10):1161–5.
104. Holliman CJ, Wuerz RC, Meador SA. Medical command errors in an urban advanced life support system. Ann Emerg Med 1992;21(4): 347–50.
105. Holliman CJ, Wuerz RC, Meador SA. Decrease in medical command errors with use of a "standing orders" protocol system. Am J Emerg Med 1994;12(3):279–83.
106. Leape LL, Brennan TA, Laird N, et al. The nature of adverse events in hospitalized patients. Results of the Harvard Medical Practice Study II. N Engl J Med 1991;324(6):377–84.
107. Leape LL. Error in medicine. JAMA 1994;272(23):1851–1857.
108. Neale G. Clinical analysis of 100 medicolegal cases. Brit Med J 1993;307(6917):1483–7.
109. Raju TN, Kecskes S, Thornton JP, Perry M, Feldman S. Medication errors in neonatal and paediatric intensive-care units. Lancet 1989;2(8659):374–6.
110. Vincer MJ, Murray JM, Yuill A, Allen AC, Evans JR, Stinson DA. Drug errors and incidents in a neonatal intensive care unit. A quality assurance activity. Am J Dis Child 1989;143(6):737–40.
111. Rice DP, MacKenzie EJ. Cost of Injury in the United States: A Report to Congress. Atlanta, Georgia: Centers for Disease Control, 1989.
112. DeNicola L, Kleid D, Brink L, et al. Use of pediatric physician extenders in pediatric and neonatal intensive care units. Critical Care Medicine 1994;22(11):1856–1864.
113. Pollack MM. Physician extenders. Critical Care Medicine 1994; 22(11):1717–1718.
114. McDonald RC, Martin II WJ. Health-care reform and pulmonary/critical care medicine: a revolution with or without data. Chest 1995; 107(5):1190–1192.
115. Gross PA. Striving for benchmark infection rates: progress in control for patient mix. Am J Med 1991;91(3B):16S–20S.
116. Scherkenbach WW. The Deming route to quality and productivity: road maps and roadblocks. Washington, D.C.: CEEPress Books, 1991.
117. Iezzoni LI. "Black box" medical information systems. A technology needing assessment [editorial; comment]. JAMA 1991;265(22):3006–7.
118. Iezzoni LI, Foley SM, Daley J, Hughes J, Fisher ES, Heeren T. Comorbidities, complications, and coding bias. Does the number of diagnosis codes matter in predicting in-hospital mortality? JAMA 1992; 267(16):2197–203.
119. Iezzoni LI, Shwartz M, Moskowitz MA, Ash AS, Sawitz E, Burnside S. Illness severity and costs of admissions at teaching and nonteaching hospitals. JAMA 1990;264(11):1426–31.
120. Iezzoni LI, Moskowitz MA. A clinical assessment of MedisGroups. JAMA 1988;260(21):3159–63.
121. Iezzoni LI, Moskowitz MA. Clinical overlap among medical diagnosis-related groups. JAMA 1986;255(7):927–9.
122. Afifi AA, Clark V. Computer-aided multivariate analysis. (2 ed.) New York: Van Nostrand Reinhold Company, 1990.
123. Hosmer DW, Lemeshow S. Applied logistic regression. (1 ed.) New York: John Wiley & Sons, 1989. Wiley Series in Probability and Mathematical Statistics.
124. Knaus WA, Draper EA, Wagner DP, Zimmerman JE. APACHE II: a severity of disease classification system. Crit Care Med 1985; 13(10):818–29.
125. Knaus W, Wagner D, Draper E. APACHE III study design: analytic plan for evaluation of severity and outcome in intensive care unit patients. Development of APACHE. Crit Care Med 1989;17(12 Pt 2):S181–5.
126. Knaus W, Wagner D, Draper E. APACHE III study design: analytic plan for evaluation of severity and outcome in intensive care unit patients. Implications. Crit Care Med 1989;17(12 Pt 2):S219–21.
127. Knaus W, Wagner D. APACHE III study design: analytic plan for evaluation of severity and outcome in intensive care unit patients. Individual patient decisions. Crit Care Med 1989;17(12 Pt 2):S204–9.
128. Knaus W, Draper E, Wagner D. APACHE III study design: analytic plan for evaluation of severity and outcome in intensive care unit patients. Introduction. Crit Care Med 1989;17(12 Pt 2):S176–80.
129. Knaus WA, Wagner DP. APACHE: a nonproprietary measure of severity of illness [letter]. Ann Intern Med 1989;110(4):327–8.
130. Draper E, Russo M, Wagner D. APACHE III study design: analytic plan for evaluation of severity and outcome in intensive care unit patients. Efficiency and nurse staff. Crit Care Med 1989;17(12 Pt 2):S217–8.
131. Draper E, Wagner D, Russo M, et al. APACHE III study design: analytic plan for evaluation of severity and outcome in intensive care unit patients. Study design data collection. Crit Care Med 1989;17(12 Pt 2):S186–93.
132. Wagner D, Draper E, Knaus W. APACHE III study design: analytic plan for evaluation of severity and outcome in intensive care unit patients. Development of APACHE III. Crit Care Med 1989;17(12 Pt 2):S199–203.
133. Wagner D, Draper E, Knaus W. APACHE III study design: analytic plan for evaluation of severity and outcome in intensive care unit patients. Analysis: quality of care. Crit Care Med 1989;17(12 Pt 2):S210–2.
134. Wagner D, Knaus W, Bergner M. APACHE III study design: analytic plan for evaluation of severity and outcome in intensive care unit patients. Statistical methods. Crit Care Med 1989;17(12 Pt 2):S194–8.
135. Shortell S, Rousseau D, Gillies R. APACHE III study design: analytic plan for evaluation of severity and outcome in intensive care unit patients. Analysis of process. Crit Care Med 1989;17(12 Pt 2):S213–6.
136. Rowan KM, Kerr JH, Major E, McPherson K, Short A, Vessey MP. Intensive Care Society's APACHE II study in Britain and Ireland II: outcome comparisons of intensive care units after adjustment for case mix by the American APACHE II method. Brit Med J 1993;307(6910): 977–81.
137. Rowan KM, Kerr JH, Major E, McPherson K, Short A, Vessey MP. Intensive Care Society's APACHE II study in Britain and Ireland I: variations in case mix of adult admissions to general intensive care units and impact on outcome. Brit Med J 1993;307(6910):972–7.
138. Rowan KM, Kerr JH, Major E, McPherson K, Short A, Vessey MP. Intensive Care Society's Acute Physiology and Chronic Health Evaluation (APACHE II) study in Britain and Ireland: a prospective, multicenter, cohort study comparing two methods for predicting outcome for adult intensive care patients. Crit Care Med 1994;22(9):1392–401.
139. Berger MM, Marazzi A, Freeman J, Chiolero R. Evaluation of the consistency of Acute Physiology and Chronic Health Evaluation (APACHE II) scoring in a surgical intensive care unit. Crit Care Med 1992;20(12):1681–7.
140. Chang RW, Jacobs S, Lee B. Use of APACHE II severity of disease classification to identify intensive-care-unit patients who would not benefit from total parenteral nutrition. Lancet 1986;1(8496):1483–7.
141. Escarce JJ, Kelley MA. Admission source to the medical intensive care unit predicts hospital death independent of APACHE II score. JAMA 1990;264(18):2389–94.
142. Fedullo AJ, Swinburne AJ, Wahl GW, Bixby KR. APACHE II score and mortality in respiratory failure due to cardiogenic pulmonary edema. Crit Care Med 1988;16(12):1218–21.
143. Franklin C, Layon AJ. On computers and building blocks, APACHE II and HIV, and dark clouds [editorial]. Critical Care Medicine 1995;23(5):797–798.
144. Hopefl AW, Taaffe CL, Herrmann VM. Failure of APACHE II alone as a predictor of mortality in patients receiving total parenteral nutrition. Crit Care Med 1989;17(5):414–7.
145. Johnson MH, Gordon PW, Fitzgerald FT. Stratification of prognosis in granulocytopenic patients with hematologic malignancies using the APACHE-II severity of illness score. Crit Care Med 1986;14(8):693–7.
146. McAnena OJ, Moore FA, Moore EE, Mattox KL, Marx JA, Pepe P. Invalidation of the APACHE II scoring system for patients with acute trauma. J Trauma 1992;33(4):504–6.
147. Meyer AA, Messick WJ, Young P, et al. Prospective comparison of clinical judgment and APACHE II score in predicting the outcome in critically ill surgical patients. J Trauma 1992;32(6):747–53.
148. Moreau R, Soupison T, Vauquelin P, Derrida S, Beaucour H, Sicot C. Comparison of two simplified severity scores (SAPS and APACHE II)

for patients with acute myocardial infarction. Crit Care Med 1989;17(5):409–13.
149. Niskanen M, Kari A, Nikki P, et al. Acute physiology and chronic health evaluation (APACHE II) and Glasgow coma scores as predictors of outcome from intensive care after cardiac arrest. Crit Care Med 1991;19(12):1465–73.
150. Pollak AJ, Strong RM, Gribbon R, Shah H. Lack of predictive value of the APACHE II score in hypoalbuminemic patients. J Parenter Enteral Nutr 1991;15(3):313–5.
151. Rhee KJ, Baxt WG, Mackenzie JR, et al. APACHE II scoring in the injured patient. Crit Care Med 1990;18(8):827–30.
152. Schafer JH, Maurer A, Jochimsen F, et al. Outcome prediction models on admission in a medical intensive care unit: do they predict individual outcome? Crit Care Med 1990;18(10):1111–8.
153. Vassar MJ, Wilkerson CL, Duran PJ, Perry CA, Holcroft JW. Comparison of APACHE II, TRISS, and a proposed 24-hour ICU point system for prediction of outcome in ICU trauma patients. J Trauma 1992;32(4):490–9.
154. Teres D. Peer review, publication policy, and APACHE. Crit Care Med 1989;17(12 Pt 2):S169–72.
155. Pollack MM, Ruttimann UE, Getson PR. Accurate prediction of the outcome of pediatric intensive care. A new quantitative method. N Engl J Med 1987;316(3):134–9.
156. Pollack MM, Ruttimann UE, Getson PR. Pediatric risk of mortality (PRISM) score. Crit Care Med 1988;16(11):1110–6.
157. Pollack MM, Alexander SR, Clarke N, Ruttimann UE, Tesselaar HM, Bachulis AC. Improved outcomes from tertiary center pediatric intensive care: a statewide comparison of tertiary and nontertiary care facilities. Crit Care Med 1991;19(2):150–9.
158. Ruttimann UE, Pollack MM. Objective assessment of changing mortality risks in pediatric intensive care unit patients. Crit Care Med 1991;19(4):474–83.
159. Balakrishnan G, Aitchison T, Hallworth D, Morton NS. Prospective evaluation of the Paediatric Risk of Mortality (PRISM) score. Arch Dis Child 1992;67(2):196–200.
160. Gemke RJ, Bonsel GJ, van Vught AJ. Effectiveness and efficiency of a Dutch pediatric intensive care unit: validity and application of the Pediatric Risk of Mortality score. Crit Care Med 1994;22(9):1477–84.
161. Pollack MM, Patel KM, Ruttimann UE. A look at pediatric intensive care—Dutch style [editorial]. Critical Care Medicine 1995;23(2): 221–222.
162. Fargason CA, Langman CB. Limitations of the pediatric risk of mortality score in assessing children with acute renal failure. Pediatr Nephrol 1993;7(6):703–7.
163. Pollock E, Ford-Jones EL, Corey M, et al. Use of the Pediatric Risk of Mortality score to predict nosocomial infection in a pediatric intensive care unit. Crit Care Med 1991;19(2):160–5.
164. Algren JT, Lal S, Cutliff SA, Richman BJ. Predictors of outcome in acute meningococcal infection in children. Crit Care Med 1993;21(3):447–52.
165. Horn SD, Bulkley G, Sharkey PD, Chambers AF, Horn RA, Schramm CJ. Interhospital differences in severity of illness. Problems for prospective payment based on diagnosis-related groups (DRGs). N Engl J Med 1985;313(1):20–4.
166. Horn SD, Horn RA, Sharkey PD, Beall RJ, Hoff JS, Rosenstein BJ. Misclassification problems in diagnosis-related groups. Cystic fibrosis as an example. N Engl J Med 1986;314(8):484–7.
167. Buckle JM, Horn SD, Oates VM, Abbey H. Severity of illness and resource use differences among white and black hospitalized elderly. Arch Intern Med 1992;152(8):1596–603.
168. Chellis MJ, Sanders SV, Webster H, Dean JM, Jackson D. Early enteral feeding in the pediatric intensive care unit. J Parenter Enteral Nutr (in press).
169. Chellis MJ, Sanders SV, Dean JM, Jackson D. Bedside transpyloric tube placement in the pediatric intensive care unit. J Parenter Enteral Nutr (in press).
170. Price M, Chellis MJ, Welkie K, Dean JM. Cost savings associated with bedside placement of enteral feeding tubes. In: Horn SD, Hopkins DSP, eds. Clinical Practice Improvement: A New Technology for Developing Cost-Effective Quality Health Care. Washington, D.C.: Faulkner & Gray, Inc., 1994:201–208. vol I.

Ethics 49

Robert Truog
Jeffrey Burns

INTRODUCTION

The competent practice of critical care medicine today requires more than a knowledge of the relevant medical science. At least some understanding of medical ethics and related law is required, and perhaps in no area of medicine is this more true than in the care of critically ill patients. During the past century dramatic changes have occurred in physicians' ability to prolong life. The ethical dilemmas associated with the advances in medical technology and the evolution of the physician-patient relationship have become the subject of wide public concern. As we enter into an era of medicine where the cost of care and the utilization of limited resources are increasingly debated, critical care physicians, with expertise in life and death decisions and with responsibility for caring for patients who require life-sustaining treatments, must possess a clear ethical framework for decision making. This chapter focuses on the key foundations of medical ethics and practical approaches to ethical decision making in the pediatric intensive care unit.

THE DEVELOPMENT OF MEDICAL ETHICS

The terms "ethics" and "morality" are often used interchangeably, but most philosophers draw a subtle distinction between the two. Morality consists of social norms of behavior, and often varies dramatically between cultures. The discipline of ethics, on the other hand, involves the development of philosophical reasons for or against a set of moral judgments. Usually the latter effort attempts to articulate and justify principles which form the foundation for rules of conduct and decision making for competing moral claims.

Medical ethics is the discipline devoted to the identification, analysis, and resolution of problems which arise in the care of patients. It is a special kind of ethics only insofar as it relates to the peculiar dilemmas that arise in medicine, and not because it embodies or appeals to some special moral principles or methodology. The term "bioethics" is often used interchangeably with "medical ethics," although the former has a slightly broader meaning, including ethical problems that arise outside the area of medicine (such as issues surrounding research on animals, for example). In summary, the practice of medical ethics seeks to identify and resolve competing moral claims among patients, their families, health care professionals, health care institutions, and society at large.

Concern for ethical issues in medicine dates back at least to the time of Hippocrates. Nevertheless, until the middle of this century, little additional thought was given to the unique problems that arise in the context of clinical practice and medical research. The exposure of the Nazi atrocities after World War II lead to the reaffirmation of the importance of ethics in medicine and research, and was directly responsible for the formulation of codes of ethics pertaining to research on human subjects (e.g., the Nuremberg Code in the late 1940s, followed by the declaration of Helsinki in 1964)[1,2].

In the decades following World War II, the introduction of antibiotics, vaccines and effective diagnostic therapeutic technologies transformed medicine from a profession focused on caring to one focused on curing. The expectations of physicians and patients have grown considerably, yet, medical advances have brought with them ethical dilemmas that increasingly find their way into public and professional consciousness.

A 1962 *Life* magazine article entitled "They Decide Who Lives, Who Dies" marked such an event[3]. The article described the efforts of a committee of ordinary citizens in Seattle, not physicians, charged with the task of allocating access to hemodialysis, then a scarce resource, for critically ill patients who would die without this therapy. The committee disbanded itself after it realized that its selection process was influenced by its own middle class values, rather than by an objectively fair allocation procedure. Public and then Congressional outrage at the reality of scarce but effective medical technology lead to passage in 1973 of the end stage renal disease program. Under this legislation, the Federal Medicare Program assumed responsibility for anyone in need of chronic dialysis, regardless of socioeconomic status. Like many federal initiatives in the 1960s and 1970s, this program has proven to be far more costly than initially expected[4].

The medical profession's attention to these issues was further heightened by a 1973 article in the *New England Journal of Medicine* which described the decision by physicians and parents to withhold treatment from 43 critically ill infants in the neonatal intensive care unit at Yale-New Haven Hospital[5]. This account was among the first to bring attention to the fact that medical technology had reached a point where the decision to end life had to be taken deliberately by physicians and families.

But perhaps no event captured public and professional attention to these difficult issues more than the 1976 New Jersey Supreme Court Decision on patient Karen Ann Quinlan. On the night of April 15, 1973, this 21-year-old woman experienced a respiratory arrest that left her in a persistent vegetative state. Her father petitioned the court for authority to be named her guardian and for permission to discontinue the ventilator. His request was opposed by her doctors, the hospital, and prosecutors for the local county and the State of New Jersey. The New Jersey Supreme Court ruled that she had a constitutional "right to privacy" to be removed from the ventilator if the family, the physicians, and the hospital ethics committee agreed. Despite the prevailing opinion of her doctors, she did not die when removed from the ventilator, but lived for almost another decade. This was the first of many cases that helped to shape our current views about the withdrawal of life-sustaining treatments.

ETHICAL THEORY

Broadly speaking, two dominant ethical theories have developed in the Western intellectual tradition. Both attempt to provide a set of "first principles" for approaching ethical conflict.

The Utilitarian Theory

The first theory is the Utilitarian Philosophy, as developed by English philosophers Jeremy Bentham and John Stuart Mill[6]. Utilitarianism is rooted in the thesis that an action or practice is right (when compared to any alternative action or practice) if it leads to the greatest possible balance of good consequences or the least possible balance of bad consequences, in the world as a whole. According to this view, moral codes and traditions are designed to promote human welfare by maximizing benefits and minimizing harms.

The other dominant ethical theory, deontology, was heavily influenced by the writings of philosopher Immanuel Kant[7]. According to this approach, certain actions or practices are always wrong, regardless of the consequences.

The current debate about euthanasia illustrates the differences between these approaches. Utilitarians may argue, for example, that when a terminally ill patient requests to be killed, the consequences of complying with that request are favorable for everyone concerned. The patient's desires are satisfied, the physician can rest assured that the act was in the patient's best interest (as defined by the patient), and even society may benefit by not incurring the expenses associated with a prolonged dying process. Deontologists, on the other hand, feel differently. For a deontologist, the prohibition against killing should stop us from taking the life of another, regardless of the consequences. Under this approach, euthanasia is always wrong, even if we are convinced that doing so does not harm anyone's interest. Some deontologists base their beliefs upon a religious perspective (the Ten Commandments are a typical list of deontologic principles), whereas others derive a set of duties and obligations by theoretical analysis. Even utilitarians often agree that rules have an important place in ethics, if only because of the inherent difficulties involved in predicting the consequences of our actions. To use the euthanasia example again, a deontologist might claim that even when performing euthanasia does not *appear* to harm anyone's interest, the long-term consequences of permitting this act might be to diminish our respect for human life, and could eventually work to erode the core values of the medical profession. This would be a reason to oppose euthanasia, even by the utilitarian standard.

Ethical Principles

In reality, few people are pure deontologists or utilitarians. Most of us blend these two perspectives in our reasoning about ethical issues. In the search for practical guidance to moral dilemmas, therefore, leading ethical theorists over the last twenty years have turned instead to the so called "principles approach" to moral reasoning. For example, in what is widely regarded as the classic textbook on modern medical ethics, Tom Beauchamp and James Childress advocate four principles on which to ground ethical analysis[8]. These principles are: respect for autonomy (self-determination), beneficence (doing good), nonmaleficence (avoiding harm), and justice (fair distribution).

Beauchamp and Childress have outlined the process of moral justification using the principles approach in terms of three levels:

Principles

—

Rules

—

Particular Judgments

When one is faced with a moral dilemma, the task is to identify the relevant ethical principles that should be brought to bear on the case. These principles will suggest a set of rules that are pertinent to the situation. From these rules, one should be able to discern the proper judgment regarding the particular case.

The obvious problem with this approach is that different principles will give rise to different sets of rules, which will in turn produce conflicting judgments. Assigning priority to one moral principle over another depends on the situation, since none of the principles always trumps any of the others. Analysis of ethical dilemmas in terms of these four principles is therefore seldom sufficient for determining the "correct" answer, but is often useful in helping to identify the salient issues that are at stake.

Criticisms of Principles

More recently, several alternatives to the principle-based mode of analysis have been proposed and developed. Proponents of "case-based reasoning," or casuistic analysis, argue that the four principles of Beauchamp and Childress are too indeterminate and abstract to be of much help with real-life dilemmas[9,10]. They advocate instead the use of "paradigmatic cases," that is, real cases about which there is currently a consensus. As new cases arise, they are analyzed in terms of the ways that they are similar to, or different from, the paradigmatic cases. This has been referred to as "moral triangulation." For example, since the "Baby Doe" episode in 1984, there is general agreement in medicine, law, and ethics that babies with Down syndrome and correctable surgical anomalies should undergo surgical repair of their conditions, and not be allowed to die from them[11]. Similarly, there is also general agreement that babies with Trisomy 13 or 18 who have potentially lethal congenital defects need not be offered life-prolonging therapies, but may ethically be treated with only comfort care. When faced with the problem of how to treat a newborn with congenital anomalies intermediate between those of Trisomy 21 and 13/18, a proponent of the case-based approach might attempt to address the question by first exploring the ways in which the child is more like an infant with Down syndrome, or more like an infant with Trisomy 13/18. In combination with factors such as the severity of the defects and the preferences of the family, this approach would attempt to "triangulate" toward the most reasonable solution.

As the field of bioethics has continued to develop, still other ways of thinking about difficult cases have emerged. An alternative that has arisen from the feminist movement is an approach based upon the primacy of "caring"[12]. In its more radical form, this perspective minimizes the importance of ethical theory and principles, and seeks resolutions to difficult cases that best preserve the relationships involved. As opposed to a principle-based approach, this perspective is less concerned with maintaining internal consistency and with the observance of formal rules. When confronted with a case about whether to allow a small child to donate a kidney to a sibling, for example, a proponent of the "caring" approach would ask which of the alternative options would best promote the well-being of the relationships between the family and others involved.

Finally, a perspective that has developed within the fields of literature and the humanities focuses on the value of "narrative"[13]. Unlike the terse case-histories that tend to be favored in the busy hospital setting, this approach emphasizes the importance of understanding cases in all of their detail and complexity. Rather than attempting to "shrink" cases to their essential elements, and then applying a specific "rule" or "principle," the proponent of the narrative approach will insist that only by analyzing cases in all of their richness and texture can we hope to arrive at solutions that are sufficiently nuanced and sophisticated. Indeed, this approach hearkens back to the admonitions of many of the great medical clinicians who emphasized the overriding importance of careful history taking. These giants of medicine would undoubtedly be just as critical of our over-reliance on invasive technology and imaging studies as the proponent of narrative is critical of "principles."

Ethics and the Law

Physicians generally have one of two attitudes toward the law. Either they claim to be unconcerned about legal precedent and only interested in practicing "good medicine," or they are fearful of making any decision or taking any action without first finding out if it is "legal." Both extreme views could lead to naive or imprudent decisions about difficult ethical dilemmas in clinical practice.

First, when considering legal precedents in ethical decision making it is important to keep in mind that there is no single, monolithic statement that can be made about the "law" in most ethical controversies. The body of law supporting the American legal system is actually the product of many factors. For example, legislative mandates or court decisions in one state do not hold as precedent or law in any other state. Superimposed on state law and legislation is the federal system with its own jurisdictions, which can also disagree over key points.

Second, while both ethics and the law are concerned with identifying which actions are acceptable within a given society, they remain fundamentally distinct. Acting in accordance with the law is no guarantee that one is acting ethically, as emphasized by the Nuremberg Court in evaluating the actions of the Nazi concentration camp guards. Law, as it relates to morality, usually represents the minimum requirements regarding moral duties and rights for a given society. Law represents the floor, and not the ceiling, for standards about morality.

ETHICS AND INFORMED CONSENT

Ethical and Legal Basis of Consent

One of the fundamental tenets of contemporary medical ethics and American law is that a competent adult is the master of his or her own body, and that a physician must obtain the free and informed consent of a patient, or a patient's surrogate if the patient is incompetent, before medical care is provided.

For thousands of years this was not the case in medical decision-making. Dating from the age of Hippocrates until the recent past, most decisions were the sole prerogative of the physician. This approach to medical care can no longer be justified, however, since it fails to respect the fundamental importance of the patient's values and goals by placing the clinician's value structure ahead of that of the patient[14].

The ascendancy of respect for patient autonomy and the right to self-determination has become paramount only in the last several decades, yet the roots of this transformation are much deeper. The philosophical and ethical basis for self-determination can be found in the Medieval and Renaissance thinkers who so greatly influenced the framers of the American Constitution and Bill of Rights. Philosophers such as John Locke, Edmund Burke, and Immanuel Kant, among others, articulated the intellectual foundation for the notion that it is not the State but the individual who is sovereign.

The legal basis for an individual's right to self-determination arose from a series of landmark cases[15]. In an early case from 1914, Justice Cardozo made his celebrated observation that "Every human being of adult years and sound mind has a right to determine what shall be done with his own body, and a surgeon who performs an operation without his patient's consent commits an assault, for which he is liable in damages." For many years, courts held physicians to what is known as the "professional standard" of informed consent, where physicians are expected to disclose only that information which is customarily disclosed by their colleagues. In the 1972 case of *Canterbury v. Spence,* however, the Federal Appeals Court in Washington broke away from the traditional application of a professional standard in favor of a patient-oriented standard that required physicians to disclose all information that might be relevant to the patient in making an informed decision, regardless of whether such information is "customarily" provided by other physicians in the community.

Exceptions to Informed Consent

Two exceptions to "informed consent" have traditionally been recognized. The first, and least controversial, is the emergency exception, which allows a physician to treat a patient when significant harm is imminent, when the patient is incapable of consenting, and when no surrogate is immediately available.

More controversial is the second traditional exception to informed consent, the therapeutic privilege exception. Under this exception, physicians may forego attempts to obtain informed consent when they believe that the patient will experience more harm than benefit from the disclosure. Recently, there has been a tendency in law and ethics to constrain this exception because it assumes that the physician knows what is best for the patient. This assumption violates the general view that patients themselves provide the most reliable information about what is in their best interest, as well as a body of empirical evidence indicating that physicians systematically underestimate the desire of patients to know their diagnosis and to be involved in decision-making[16,17].

Consent for Research on Human Subjects

Informed consent is especially important when patients are given innovative therapies or are recruited for research. Intensivists are often tempted to try new therapies on critically ill patients who are desperate for a cure. Despite the perceived urgency of the situation, physicians must respect the safeguards that have been developed to protect patients from therapies that are potentially harmful. Physicians who skirt the requirements for approval by institutional review boards and informed consent under the guise of being "compassionate" threaten the very future of the innovation they are trying to promote. Finally, children should never receive innovative therapies solely because future patients might benefit from them. In keeping with the fiduciary relationship between doctor and patients, there must be some reasonable expectation that the patient may benefit, regardless of the potential for benefit to future patients[18].

Consent for Practicing Procedures on Newly Deceased Patients

The use of dead patients to teach procedures has been a source of controversy dating at least to the Middle Ages. Some have argued that it is ethically justifiable to perform practice procedures on the newly dead without permission from the family because these procedures cannot harm the deceased, there is substantial social benefit to be gained, and families could not realistically be expected to discuss consent at such a difficult time[19]. Indeed, a recent study showed that 39% of training programs in emergency and critical care medicine use newly dead patients to teach various resuscitation procedures (for example, endotracheal intubation, central line placement, and pericardiocentesis). Few of these programs obtain either verbal or written consent from the families[20].

Despite the frequency of this practice without consent, some have argued that teaching procedures on newly deceased patients is ethical only when permission is first obtained from the family. In addition, given its sensitive nature, this teaching technique should be reserved only for those who truly need to master the skills and only as the culmination of a structured learning sequence, and not a haphazard event[20].

Informed Consent: Inducement for a Therapeutic Alliance

Although the doctrine of informed consent has become standard medical practice, many physicians still view it as a burden imposed by lawyers. In this context, the communication process is reduced to the physicians' effort to avoid a lawsuit. A more constructive view is that the informed consent process can actually help strengthen the communication in the patient-physician relationship. As noted by Gutheil and colleagues, "Informed consent is not an empty gesture toward liability reduction, but an interaction between physician and patient, a dialogue intended not only to satisfy their legal requirements, but to do more as well. The real clinical opportunity offered by informed consent is that of transforming uncertainty from a threat into the very basis on which an alliance can be formed"[21].

MEDICAL DECISION-MAKING

Competency and Decision-Making Capacity

The distinction between competency and decision-making capacity is often misunderstood. All adults over the age of majority (18 years in most states) are presumed to be legally competent. This legal presumption can only be overridden in a court of law. A separate concept is "decision-making capacity." A person can be legally competent and yet not have the capacity to make decisions on his or her own behalf (an acute trauma victim, for example). Conversely, even patients who are considered legally incompetent may have the decision-making capacity to determine whether they want certain medical interventions (most adolescents, for example). As a President's Commission observed, "Determining whether a patient lacks capacity to make a particular health care decision requires assessing the patient's capability to understand information relevant to the decision, to communicate with care givers about it, and to reason about relevant alternatives against a background of reasonably stable personal values and life goals"[22]. Patients with decisional capacity have the right to direct their medical therapy, while those without decisional capacity do not.

Advance Directives

Several mechanisms exist to enable patients to retain some control over health care decisions after they have lost the capacity to participate directly in decision making. Most states now have legislation which recognizes the legality of certain advanced directives. Written and oral instructions, usually called a "living will," contain treatment directives to be followed if and when a patient becomes incapable of making treatment decisions[23]. These documents have been criticized as being too ambiguous in many critical decisions, for no one could possibly anticipate every potential occurrence that might confront them[24].

Over the last decade, the health care durable power of attorney, or "proxy," has emerged as another form of advance directive designed to overcome the limitations presented by living wills. Unlike living wills, which specify treatment decisions in advance, the health care proxy establishes a decision making process. Health care proxy laws permit patients to delegate the authority to make medical treatment decisions for them in the event of incapacity. The Patient Self Determination Act, passed by Congress in 1991, requires that all Medicare-participating institutions inform patients of their rights to formulate advance directives upon admission[25].

In making decisions for patients who no longer have decisional capacity, surrogate decision-makers should base their decisions, in descending order of preference, on the subjective standard, the substituted judgment standard, and the best interests standard[26,27]. The subjective standard is the preferred guide for decision making. This requires that any relevant statements made by the patient while decisionally capable should guide all decisions. If there is not any firm evidence of what the patient specifically desired, then the surrogate should apply the substituted judgment standard. This requires the surrogate to apply the patient's own values, religious beliefs, and preferences in arriving at the treatment decision. When this information is not available, or when the patient never obtained the capacity to espouse such preferences, the next step in the decision-making hierarchy is the best interests standard. Unlike the substituted judgment standard, which focuses on the patient's known preferences to guide decision making, the best interests standard attempts to rely on "objectively" weighing the benefits and burdens of the proposed treatment alternatives.

The Role of Parents in Decision-Making

There is broad societal consensus that parents are the preferred decision makers for their children[27,28]. When a child is too young to have formed any clear preferences regarding treatment, it is left to the parents, most of whom unquestionably have a profound love and commitment to their children, to decide what is in the best interests of the child based on an assessment of the benefits and burdens of proposed treatment.

Although parents will bear much of the hardship of future therapies, and therefore have legitimate concerns about the effect of treatment decisions on themselves and their other children, these concerns cannot be used exclusively to justify the denial of clearly beneficial therapy. To quote a recent expert panel of pediatricians, "When a child would clearly benefit from available treatment, such as appendectomy for appendicitis, or chemotherapy for acute lymphoblastic leukemia, his or her interests must be given precedence"[29].

When parents deny treatment that is *not* clearly beneficial, however, the burden shifts to the health care team to justify the need to override the parents' wishes. For example, in a 1991 Delaware case, Christian Science parents were permitted the right to refuse treatment for their child suffering from Burkitt's lymphoma after expert testimony was introduced stating that the proposed therapy had the potential for significant risk and offered only a 40% chance of success[30]. As in all cases of conflict over medical decision making between patients, families, and providers, resort to legal mechanisms should always be a last step after exhausting all other avenues of resolution, including the use of consultants and institutional ethics committees.

Special Considerations for the Adolescent

While parents generally take full responsibility for decision-making for newborns and young children, this should not be the case for older children and adolescents. The legal age of majority is an oversimplification of the maturational and developmental process in children. Children as young as six or seven are often able to have reasoned opinions about certain aspects of their care, and most adolescents have views and perspectives that deserve serious consideration. The fact that parents must give legal consent for medical treatments performed on minor children does not mean that the opinions of the children and adolescents should be considered irrelevant or ignored.

Many states have recognized this developmental continuum in the form of emancipated minor or mature minor statutes. An emancipated minor, in most jurisdictions, is someone under the age of majority who lives independent from their parents, is the parent of a child, or is in the military. In most states, these patients can legally consent to their own medical treatment[31].

Recognizing that some adolescents do not meet the criteria for emancipated minor and yet are mature enough to make decisions about medical therapy for themselves, many jurisdictions now recognize the concept of a "mature minor"[32]. While the legal requirements may vary, a generally accepted ethical principle is that children should always, at the least, be evaluated for their ability to "assent" to treatment. In other words, while children may not have the cognitive or emotional skills to fully understand all of the implications of various treatment choices, even young children will often have the capacity for a general understanding of the proposed course of treatment and what they should expect. Furthermore, children should be given the opportunity to "assent" to this treatment ("consent" being reserved for those situations in which the patient can fully understand the benefits, risks, and alternatives for the proposed treatment). If the child refuses to assent, considerable effort should be made to explore the child's feelings and to seek strategies for accommodating these views and preferences. Only in unusual circumstances should children not be apprised of a proposed plan of treatment, or should their refusal to assent be categorically overridden.

Religious Beliefs in the Decision-Making Process

While the courts have acknowledged the virtually unlimited right of competent adults to refuse medical treatments, they have been much more protective of children. The threshold for overriding the parents' wishes depends upon an objective assessment of the risks to the child. In general, if the circumstances do not involve life-threatening choices, and there are no certain risks of substantial harm to the child, physicians are obligated to respect the decisions of the parents, even when the physicians strongly disagree with the choice. In some jurisdictions, for example, parents are permitted the right to refuse standard immunizations for religious reasons[28].

It is only as the threat to the child increases, and the benefits of treatment are more certain, that actions to override parental choices are not only legally supportable, but in most jurisdictions required. Numerous court opinions have upheld the notion, first articulated in the famous 1944 case of *Prince v. Massachusetts,* that a parent may make a martyr of himself because of religious convictions, "but he is not free to make a martyr of his child"[33]. In numerous decisions since then, courts have upheld the right of physicians to override parental refusal of transfusions or other accepted therapy when the child's life is at risk[28].

LIMITATIONS OF LIFE-SUSTAINING TREATMENTS

The concept of doing anything less than everything possible to preserve the life of the patient is both old and new. The Hippocratic corpus admonishes physicians "to refuse to treat those who are overmastered by their diseases, realizing that in such cases medicine is powerless"(34). Nevertheless, as the specialty of critical care medicine developed and as the capability to prolong life evolved, the mere ability to use life-sustaining technology was transformed into a virtual imperative. Beginning with the Cruzan case in the mid-1970s, the pendulum has begun to swing back toward a more rational use of this technology. Over the past twenty years, clinicians, ethicists, lawyers, theologians and others have sought to articulate and define the conditions under which limitations in life-sustaining treatments are legitimate and justified.

Do-Not-Resuscitate Orders

Until 1976, no hospital in the United States publicly acknowledged that they ever provided care that was not solely intended to prolong and preserve life. In that year, both the Massachusetts General Hospital and Boston's Beth Israel Hospital acknowledged their use of "do-not-resuscitate" orders in the *New England Journal of Medicine*(35,36). Over the past 20 years, DNR orders have become increasingly accepted and have undergone numerous modifications. More recently, however, there is evidence that the complexity of decision-making around terminally ill patients has progressed to the point where the philosophy behind DNR orders is no longer sufficient. Alternatives to the traditional DNR order will be discussed below.

Procedure-Specific DNR Orders

In most hospitals, DNR orders are written by the attending physician in the Doctor's Orders Sheets. These orders are often vague, and may leave substantial opportunity for miscommunication and error. Does "resuscitation" refer to treatment of an acute cardiac arrest (intubation and ventilation, chest compressions, cardioversion, and medications), or does it also mean "do-not-intubate" for conditions like respiratory failure from a pneumonia? Should patients with DNR orders receive suctioning for airway secretions, be treated with antibiotics, or be given tube feedings? Should they be excluded from the ICU, or denied palliative surgery? The answers to these questions are almost never clear in the interpretation of a simple "DNR order."

In response to these concerns, many institutions have now adopted "procedure-specific DNR orders." This approach is intended to reduce much of the ambiguity surrounding these orders. The form currently used at the Children's Hospital in Boston in shown in Figure 49.1. This page appears at the beginning of the "Doctor's Orders" section of the patient's chart, so that it is readily available at all times in a place easily identified by physicians and other caregivers who may not be familiar with the details of the patient's care at the time of an arrest. The form first specifies whether a "code blue" should be called in the event of a cardiorespiratory arrest, and then provides a checklist of exactly which procedures are to be performed or withheld. There is a section for identifying special instructions, and then lines for the signatures of both the attending physician and the bedside nurse, with a requirement for renewal every 7 days. Finally, there is a section to be completed if the patient or family rescinds the DNR order. A recent study showed that use of procedure-specific DNR forms reduces the uncertainty and confusion that often accompanies the decision not to resuscitate(37).

"CPR-Not-Indicated" Orders

Is it necessary for the patient or family to consent to a DNR order(38–42)? Some states (e.g., New York) have laws that generally require the consent of the patient or family before a DNR order is written, and many hospitals have this requirement in their internal policies(43). Recently, however, some hospitals have adopted policies that permit physicians to write DNR orders without the permission (or sometimes, without even the knowledge) of the patient or family. The presumption behind this approach is the view that CPR is a medical therapy, and that physicians are uniquely qualified to determine whether and when a medical therapy is indicated. These policies are therefore often referred to as "CPR-not-indicated" policies(44).

The belief of many physicians that they should have the authority to determine when CPR is appropriate is understandable. Many patients and families are unable to accept the fact that they or a loved one is terminally ill and about to die. In these situations, patients or families may maintain an irrational belief that CPR can offer them a meaningful extension in the quality or duration of their life. Under these circumstances, caregivers often feel that they are doing CPR to "treat the family," and that performing this procedure when it can offer no real benefit to the patient is a violation of their professional integrity.

On the other hand, this development in DNR orders should be viewed with great caution. As noted in the discussion of informed consent, physicians have a long history of seeing complex situations from a uniquely medical perspective, ignoring important factors related to the patient's values and preferences. Rarely is the question of whether or not to do CPR purely a medical issue. Often the patient's or family's denial of impending death can be overcome by proper counseling, whereas simply using the physician's authority to overrule the family's wishes can be profoundly destructive to the patient/physician relationship. While this debate over the legitimacy of "CPR-not-indicated" orders is far from resolved, there is little doubt that this approach should be used only under the most conservative and well-defined circumstances(44).

Redirection of Care/Comfort Policies

DNR orders are unique. They are the only physician's order that is focused exclusively upon what will *not* be done, rather than what *will* be done. Not surprisingly, patients with DNR orders often feel that they have been abandoned by their caregivers. Indeed, studies have shown that physicians do in fact spend less time caring for patients who have DNR orders. This is not always appropriate, because patients with DNR orders often need more attention in terms of aggres-

Children's Hospital

PHYSICIAN'S ORDERS: DO-NOT-RESUSCITATE

USE PLATE OR PRINT

MR. NO. ____________ DATE ____________

PT. NAME ____________

DATE OF BIRTH ____________

This order sheet will appear first in the Physician's Orders Section. Do-Not-Resuscitate Orders must be renewed weekly. See the House Officer's Manual for additional information.

In case of cardiopulmonary arrest: Call a code ☐ Yes ☐ No

Regarding the following interventions (mark all that apply)

____ No supplemental oxygen
____ No oral airway
____ No intubation
____ No needle thoracentesis
____ No venipuncture
____ No arterial puncture
____ No arrest medications (epi, atropine, $NaHCO_3$, calcium, fluid boluses)
____ No deep suctioning
____ No bag and mask ventilation
____ No chest compressions
____ No chest tube
____ No electrical cardioversion

Additional Instructions:

Attending Physician Signature ____ Date/Time ____ RN Signature ____ Date/Time

Attending Physician ____ (Print Name)

Renewal: Attending Signature ____ Date/Time ____ RN Signature ____ Date/Time

Attending Physician ____ (Print Name)

Renewal: Attending Signature ____ Date/Time ____ RN Signature ____ Date/Time

Attending Physician ____ (Print Name)

Renewal: Attending Signature ____ Date/Time ____ RN Signature ____ Date/Time

Attending Physician ____ (Print Name)

Discontinuation: Specify date and time this order is rescinded:

Attending Physician Signature ____ Date/Time ____ RN Signature ____ Date/Time

Children's Hospital, 300 Longwood Ave., Boston, MA 02115

03287 7/93

Figure 49.1. The Do-Not-Resuscitate Form used at Children's Hospital in Boston.

sive palliative care than patients who are not imminently dying.

In addition, DNR orders tend to be concerned with only a small fraction of the issues that arise with dying patients. Often the question of whether or not a patient should be resuscitated is actually peripheral to the more important questions surrounding the use of less dramatic interventions. Should the patient be intubated and ventilated for the next episode of pneumonia? Should he receive antibiotics? Should he receive opioids to relieve the sensation of dyspnea, even though the respiratory depression from the opioids could hasten his death? Should the patient be fed only as much as he wants, realizing that this could lead to death from gradual dehydration and malnutrition, or should he be given a gastrostomy tube to optimize nutrition and hydration?

These questions are not adequately addressed by the traditional DNR order. Hospitals are therefore increasingly developing more global policies that are more responsive to the variety of issues posed by end-of-life decision-making than narrow DNR policies. The Joint Commission on Accreditation of Hospitals Organization (JCAHO) has indicated that it will soon require hospitals to have policies of this type.

Withdrawing Life-Sustaining Treatments

There is a clear ethical and legal consensus in the United States which supports the right of patients or their surrogates to refuse or remove unwanted medical treatment, even if such a decision involves life-sustaining therapy. This right has been supported by the United States Supreme Court, a special Presidential Commission, and in policy statements by the American Medical Association, the Society for Critical Care Medicine, and the American Thoracic Society[22,45–49].

In discussions about whether or not to provide life-sustaining therapies, several issues arise commonly. Among them are the distinction between ordinary and extraordinary treatments, the distinction between withholding a treatment and withdrawing a treatment, the appropriate role of sedatives and analgesics in the care of the dying, and whether artificial nutrition and hydration ("tube" feedings) may ever be forgone. These issues are discussed below.

The Ordinary/Extraordinary Distinction

One of the most commonly used justifications for withholding "high-tech" therapy from patients is the belief that "extraordinary" treatments are not ethically mandatory. For example, a recent survey showed that 74% of physicians and nurses think that the ordinary/extraordinary distinction is helpful in resolving ethical dilemmas[50]. Although this terminology is still used in the writings of some religious traditions, clinicians should understand that the distinction between ordinary and extraordinary treatments is not considered to be helpful when trying to reason about the ethical aspects of difficult decisions.

To illustrate why this is so, consider two alternative interpretations of the ordinary/extraordinary distinction. One interpretation would be that ordinary treatments are customarily performed, whereas extraordinary treatments are not. Clearly, however, a simple appeal to what is customary cannot suffice as a justification for what is morally required. In addition, from a legal perspective, the courts have explicitly rejected the view that there is any relationship between what is "customary" and what is "legal."

Another interpretation of the ordinary/extraordinary distinction would hold that ordinary treatments are morally required, whereas extraordinary treatments are morally optional. But this is essentially a circular argument, since it claims that ordinary treatments are morally required because they are ordinary, and extraordinary treatments are morally optional because they are extraordinary. Words cannot substitute for moral reasoning.

As an example of this fallacy in the literature, pediatricians were asked about their views on repair of duodenal atresia in healthy babies and in babies with Down syndrome[51]. Most pediatricians said that duodenal atresia was an "ordinary" procedure in the case of healthy infants, but an "extraordinary" procedure in the case of babies with Down syndrome. Since the procedure was the same in each case, the use of the terms "ordinary" and "extraordinary" served to mask the ethical judgments that were being made about the nature of the clinical condition.

A much more legitimate and useful approach to thinking about whether a procedure is ethically required is to inquire about the balance of the benefits versus the burdens for a particular procedure in a particular patient. In other words, instead of relying on terminology like ordinary and extraordinary to decide whether a treatment should be offered, consider instead whether the proposed benefits exceed the burdens. If, for example, a child with a malignancy is unlikely to survive even with the administration of highly toxic chemotherapy, then the burdens of that therapy clearly exceed the benefits. On the other hand, physicians and society now generally agree that the benefits of repairing duodenal atresia in patients with Down syndrome exceed the burdens, and thus the procedure is morally required.

The Withholding/Withdrawing Distinction

Is there a difference between stopping a treatment once it is started, and not starting it in the first place? In other words, is there an ethical difference between deciding not to intubate a patient because we do not think that he will recover, and extubating a patient who has failed to recover despite a period of ventilation? Surveys have repeatedly shown that physicians do believe there is a difference. For example, one recent study reported that 66% of physicians and nurses think that there is an ethical difference between withdrawing and withholding a treatment, and nearly half agreed with the statement "there is an emerging consensus that withdrawing a treatment is ethically different from withholding or not starting it"[50]. In another survey of 360 attendings, housestaff, and medical students, 73% felt that withdrawing is different from withholding[52]. These reports all indicate that physicians are much more comfortable in withholding treatments than in withdrawing them.

This issue is particularly interesting in light of the fact that this opinion among clinicians is strikingly at odds with the prevailing views among ethicists and lawyers. Legal scholars and ethicists have been consistent in expressing the opinion that doctors should not differentiate between decisions to withhold or withdraw medical treatments. In the landmark *Cruzan* case, for example, justices from the US Supreme Court wrote that doctors should consider decisions to withhold and withdraw as equivalent in order to assure that patients receive adequate trials of therapy [45,53,54]. A typical example occurs in the delivery room, when the viability of premature babies is often difficult to assess in the moments immediately after birth. The Supreme Court's decision implies that physicians should deal with this uncertainty by proceeding with the resuscitation, but that the physicians should be willing to withdraw the life-sustaining treatment if, after a trial of therapy, further support is no longer justified.

Despite these opinions from law and philosophy, clinicians persist in believing that there is a difference between these two actions. Part of the reason is clearly psychological. Physicians feel more responsible for the death of a patient when it results from the withdrawal of a therapy than they do when it results from the withholding of a therapy. This psychological distinction is important, and cannot be made to disappear by legal or philosophical reasoning, no matter how persuasive. Nevertheless, when confronted with these situations, physicians should consider the perspectives from law and philosophy, since in many cases adoption of these views will lead to better clinical decision-making.

Another reason clinicians are reluctant to withdraw life-sustaining therapy is their fear of legal liability, both civil and criminal. In this case, however, many clinicians are simply misinformed. In a review by David Orentlicher from the American Medical Association's Council on Judicial and Ethical Affairs, he concludes that "No person has ever been found liable for withdrawing life sustaining treatment without court permission"[53]. This is a strong statement, and should be reassuring to physicians who are concerned about this issue.

On the other hand, physicians often believe that they have no legal liability if they refuse to terminate life-sustaining treatments at the request of a patient or family, as long as they always act to preserve life. This is also a serious misconception. Orentlicher notes that "The risk of liability may be significant when a physician refuses to honor a request to have life-sustaining treatment withdrawn"[53]. He cites two successful suits against physicians who refused to withdraw care at the request of a patient or surrogate. In other words, the commonly held view among physicians that they may be at legal risk if they withdraw life-support but are legally immune if they always act to prolong life can be seen to be exactly backwards!

Sedatives and Analgesics in the Care of the Dying

Unfortunately, physicians who care for patients in a pediatric intensive care unit will frequently be called upon to discontinue life-support from a dying patient. In these often tragic circumstances, the question then becomes how best to manage the patient during the dying process. Some erroneously believe that no sedatives or analgesics should be given in these situations, since they believe that it is important both ethically and legally that the patient die from her underlying disease, without any contribution from the respiratory or cardiac depression that are frequent side effects of these medications.

This reluctance of many physicians to aggressively treat the pain and suffering often experienced by the terminally ill has been one of the most powerful forces driving the movement in favor of euthanasia and physician-assisted suicide over the last several years [55–57]. Individuals who have watched loved ones die without adequate pain relief have spearheaded this movement with the belief that patients should have the opportunity to commit suicide if their suffering is unbearable, particularly since physicians seem unwilling to do whatever is necessary to control that suffering. This is unfortunate, particularly since there is nothing in the law, ethics, or any of the major religious traditions that should preclude physicians from aggressively treating the pain and suffering of the terminally ill, even when such treatment may hasten a patient's demise. Nevertheless, a recent survey showed that as many as 40% of doctors and nurses give inadequate pain medication most often out of fear of hastening a patient's death[50].

The ethical principle that is relevant to this question is the Doctrine of Double Effect, originally developed within the Catholic tradition but now widely acknowledged in other religious traditions as well as in law and philosophy[8]. The doctrine states that when an action has two effects, one of which is inherently good and the other of which is inherently bad, it can be justified if certain conditions are met. For example, the administration of morphine to a dying patient has both a good effect (relief of pain and suffering) and the potential for a bad effect (hastening the patient's death through respiratory depression). The conditions which must be satisfied in order for the action to be justified are:

1. *The action in itself must be good or at least morally indifferent.* (Administration of the morphine itself is morally indifferent.)
2. *The agent must intend only the good effect and not the evil effect. The evil effect is foreseen, not intended. It is allowed, not sought.* (In the case of administering morphine to a terminally ill patient, the physician must intend only the relief of the patient's pain and suffering. Respiratory depression and the potential for an earlier death is a foreseen complication, but is not sought.)

3. *The evil effect cannot be a means to the good effect.* (If the physician administers a bolus of potassium chloride instead of morphine, this condition would be violated. By administering potassium chloride, the evil effect [death] becomes the means to the good effect [relief from suffering]. By contrast, morphine does not depend upon the side effect of death in order to effectively relieve pain.)
4. *The good intended must outweigh the evil permitted.* (In the case of an imminently dying patient, the benefit of pain relief clearly outweighs the risk of death. This would not be true if the patient were not terminally ill. For example, if an otherwise healthy patient required so much morphine for pain control that he developed serious respiratory depression, he should be placed on a ventilator, not allowed to die.)

In summary, despite the beliefs of many clinicians, there are no moral, legal, or religious reasons for withholding adequate pain relief from dying patients. Pain and suffering should always be adequately treated, even if the treatment results in a foreseen but unintended hastening of death.

What is the difference between currently accepted practice and the performance of euthanasia? The key difference lies in the *intention* of the physician. As long as the physician's intention is treatment of the patient's pain and suffering, the administration of analgesics and sedatives is noncontroversial. When the physician's intention is to kill the patient, then the line between accepted practice and euthanasia has been crossed. This distinction is observed within the law as well as within ethics. Physicians should be reassured that as long as they act with the intention of relieving a patient's pain and suffering, the risk of legal liability is exceedingly small. In a recent review by Larry Gostin, then the Executive Director of the American Society of Law and Medicine, he wrote that "In a search of reported decisions, *no case* was found in which a health care professional was convicted of causing, inducing, or assisting in the death of her patient"[58].

Medical Nutrition and Hydration

Should techniques for providing medical nutrition and hydration (IV fluids, parenteral nutrition, tube feedings, etc.) be considered medical treatments? If so, can they then be ethically withdrawn by the same process and criteria that are used for other types of medical treatment? In other words, if it is ethically acceptable to withdraw a ventilator from a terminally ill patient, is it also ethically acceptable to withdraw medically provided nutrition and hydration? (Note that this question does not propose withholding oral feedings from patients who want to eat or drink.)

The last decade has seen a gradually emerging consensus in both law and ethics that answers the questions posed above in the affirmative [59,60]. A large number of court decisions, including the decision of the US Supreme Court in *Cruzan*, have now concluded that medically provided nutrition and hydration should be considered medical treatments, and that patients or their surrogates should have the right to refuse them [45,53,54]. The decision of whether or not to administer this therapy should be based upon the same criteria outlined above for other treatments, that is, an analysis of the balance between the benefits and burdens of providing the therapy.

Many clinicians have been reluctant to accept this approach, at least in part because "feeding" seems to be such a basic and fundamental aspect of the care they provide to their patients. In the terminology of the distinction discussed above, it seems so "ordinary." This provides yet another example of the inadequacies of the ordinary/extraordinary distinction, however, since for certain patients, particularly those who are permanently unconscious or imminently dying, medically administered feedings can no longer provide any benefit.

Pediatricians have been particularly slow to acknowledge this emerging consensus[61]. The reasons for this reluctance are several. First, prognoses are often more uncertain in children, given their remarkable ability to recover from injury. Second, even normal newborns need assistance with feedings, so pediatricians are less likely to see artificial feedings as a "medical" treatment. Third, whereas the hospice experience shows that refusal of food and water is frequently seen in elderly patients dying a natural death, the death of a child is never a "natural" event, and there is a reluctance to accept it with apparent passivity. Nevertheless, the principles that have evolved governing the administration or withdrawal of medically provided feedings in adults are equally applicable in children, and there is no justifiable reason to treat the pediatric population any differently.

How Are Decisions Made?

Relatively little is known about the manner, reasons, and circumstances under which life support is withheld or withdrawn in the intensive care unit. Much of what is known comes from observational studies or surveys of practices. Despite the wide agreement on the principles discussed above, many studies have noted considerable variation in the practices of critical care physicians[62–66]. Faber-Langendoen noted that among 308 randomly selected intensivists responding to a survey, 15% almost never withdrew ventilators from patients[67]. Asch found that among adult intensivists responding to survey, 34% reported continuing life-sustaining treatment despite patient or surrogate wishes that it be discontinued, while approximately 80% admitted to unilaterally withholding or withdrawing life-sustaining treatment they judged to be futile[68].

Descriptive studies of the practices of pediatric intensivists are also limited. Levetown and colleagues reported that 38% of all deaths in 16 PICUs had some form of limitation of life-sustaining treatment[69]. Among those patients with some "restriction" in medical care, the precipitating event was most often an acute illness, and the most common justification for the restriction was the imminent death of the patient (not poor quality of life or excessive burden). Ryan and colleagues examined the modes of death in a neonatal and pediatric intensive care unit in Alberta, Canada and found that the majority of deaths in both units occurred either as a result of withdrawal of treatment or after a no-CPR decision[70].

Finally, a recent study by Cook et al. found that while ICU health care workers identified common factors important to decision making in withdrawing care (likelihood of long-term survival, premorbid cognitive function, and age of the patient), there was extreme variability in the level of care that was chosen for various patient scenarios[71]. This study suggests that ICU providers demonstrate wide variability in values and belief systems in how they approach such decisions.

Breaking Bad News

Doctors receive limited training in learning to talk easily with patients. The difficulties of physicians' problems with communication are especially exposed when dealing with critically ill patients and their families. Studies show that patients, their families, nurses, social workers, and chaplains often complain of the brevity and poor choice of words doctors use in these settings[72–74].

Obviously, patients and their families will react differently to bad news depending on their preparedness, culture, and coping skills. There are several strategies, however, that may prove helpful for the pediatric intensivist:

1. Prepare in advance. Know who will be in the meeting and their relationship to the patient before entering the room. Anticipate questions and prepare answers that will be clear, direct, and understandable from the family's viewpoint.
2. Have everyone be seated. Studies show that families like to be seated near the door when receiving bad news so as to reduce the feeling of being trapped. Do not stand during the conversation. Families find this particularly offensive and studies show that people consistently think the doctor spent less time with them when the physician was standing during the conversation. Introduce yourself and all your colleagues by title and name. Although many families cannot remember anyone's name after hearing tragic news, they appreciate the personal connection the formal introduction establishes.
3. Avoid jargon. Doctors and nurses easily slip into the jargon associated with the intensive care culture, but these loose terms only confuse families or lead to misconceptions that can be difficult to retract.
4. Show caring. Although most physicians believe they really care, families consistently believe the opposite after these events. Many want to hear an expression of sorrow by the healthcare team as an affirmation of their grief. They also wish time to talk and express their feelings.
5. Avoid distractions. As far as possible, make a real effort to establish a therapeutic environment for the sensitive information to be shared. Leave the beeper outside the room, position someone near the door to avoid interruptions, ensure follow-up both immediately and in the days and weeks thereafter with appropriate counselors[75–79].

These are important issues; and physicians, especially critical care physicians, need to spend as much time mastering these skills as they do some of the more technical aspects of the practice. The damage borne by families when this is done poorly can last a lifetime.

REFERENCES

1. The Nuremberg Code. In Beauchamp TL, Walters L, eds. Contemporary issues in bioethics. Belmont, California: Wadsworth Publishing Company, 1989:420.
2. World Medical Association. Declaration of Helsinki. In Beauchamp TL, Walters L, eds. Contemporary issues in bioethics. Belmont, California: Wadsworth Publishing Company, 1989:421–423.
3. Alexander S. They decide who lives, who dies. In Hunt R, Arras J, eds. Ethical issues in modern medicine. Palo Alto, California: Mayfield, 1977:409–424.
4. Iglehart JK. The American health care system. The End Stage Renal Disease Program [see comments]. N Engl J Med 1993;328:366–371.
5. Duff RS, Campbell AG. Moral and ethical dilemmas in the special-care nursery. N Engl J Med 1973;289:890–894.
6. Mill and Utilitarian Theories. In Beauchamp TL, ed. Philosophical ethics: an introduction to moral philosophy. New York: McGraw-Hill, Inc., 1991:127–168.
7. Kant and Deontological Theories. In Beauchamp TL, ed. Philosophical ethics: an introduction to moral philosophy. New York: McGraw-Hill, Inc., 1991:169–208.
8. Beauchamp TL, Childress JF. Principles of biomedical ethics. New York: Oxford University Press, 1994.
9. Jonsen AR, Toulmin S. The abuse of casuistry. University of California Press, Los Angeles: 1988.
10. Toulmin S. The tyranny of principles. Hastings Cent Rep 1981;11: 31–39.
11. Lantos JD. Baby Doe five years later. Implications for child health. N Engl J Med 1987;317:444–447.
12. Carse AL. The "voice of care": implications for bioethical education. J Med Philos 1991;16:5–28.
13. Coles R. The call of stories: teaching and the moral imagination. Boston: Houghton Mifflin, 1989.
14. Katz J. The silent world of doctor and patient. New York: Free Press, 1984.
15. Faden RR, Beauchamp TL. A history and theory of informed consent. New York: Oxford University Press, 1986.
16. Novack DH, et al. Changes in physician's attitudes toward telling the cancer patient. JAMA 1979;241:897.
17. Annas GJ. Informed consent, cancer, and truth in prognosis. N Engl J Med 1994;330:223–225.
18. Abramson NS, Meisel A, Safar P. Informed consent in resuscitation research. JAMA 1981;246:2828–2830.
19. Orlowski JP, Kanoti GA, Mehlman MJ. The ethics of using newly dead patients for teaching and practicing intubation techniques. N Engl J Med 1988;319:439–441.
20. Burns JP, Reardon FE, Truog RD. Using newly deceased patients to teach resuscitation procedures. N Engl J Med 1994;331:1652–1655.
21. Gutheil TG, Bursztajn H, Brodsky A. Malpractice prevention through the sharing of uncertainty. Informed consent and the therapeutic alliance. N Engl J Med 1984;311:49–51.
22. President's Commission for the Study of Ethical Problems in Medicine and Biomedical and Behavioral Research. Deciding to Forego Life-Sustaining Treatment: Ethical, Medical, and Legal Issues in Treatment Decisions. Washington, D.C: U.S. Government Printing Office, 1983:121.
23. Emanuel LL, Emanuel EJ. The medical directive. A new comprehensive advance care document [see comments]. JAMA 1989;261:3288–3293.

24. Brett AS. Limitations of listing specific medical interventions in advance directives. JAMA 1991;266:825–828.
25. La Puma J, Orentlicher D, Moss RJ. Advance directives on admission. Clinical implications and analysis of the Patient Self-Determination Act of 1990 [see comments]. [Review]. JAMA 1991;266:402–405.
26. Steinbrook R, Lo B. Decision making for incompetent patients by designated proxy. California's new law. N Engl J Med 1984;310: 1598–1601.
27. Buchanan AE, Brock DW. Deciding for others: the ethics of surrogate decision making. Cambridge: Cambridge University Press, 1989.
28. Holder AR. Legal issues in pediatrics and adolescent medicine. New Haven: Yale University Press, 1985.
29. Fleischman AR, Nolan K, Dubler NN, et al. Caring for gravely ill children. Pediatrics 1994;94:433–439.
30. Newark v. Williams. 588 A.2d. 1108 (Del.1991).
31. Holder AR. Minors' rights to consent to medical care. JAMA 1987;257:3400–3402.
32. Sigman GS, O'Connor C. Exploration for physicians of the mature minor doctrine. J Pediatr 1991;119:520–525.
33. Prince v. Commonwealth of Massachusetts. 321 U.S. 158 (1944).
34. Hippocrates: art. In Reiser SJ, Dyck AJ, Curran WJ, eds. Ethics in medicine: historical perspectives and contemporary concerns. Cambridge, MA: MIT Press, 1977:6.
35. Rabkin MT, Gillerman G, Rice NR. Orders not to resuscitate. N Engl J Med 1976;295:364–366.
36. Optimum care for hopelessly ill patients. A report of the Clinical Care Committee of the Massachusetts General Hospital. N Engl J Med 1976;295:362–364.
37. Mittelberger JA, Lo B, Martin D, Uhlmann RF. Impact of a procedure-specific do not resuscitate order form on documentation of do not resuscitate orders. Arch Intern Med 1993;153:228–232.
38. Murphy DJ, Finucane TE. New do-not-resuscitate policies: a first step in cost control. Arch Intern Med 1993;153:1641–1648.
39. Snider GL. The do-not-resuscitate order: Ethical and legal imperative or medical decision. Am Rev Respir Dis 1991;143:665–674.
40. Hackler JC, Hiller FC. Family consent to orders not to resuscitate: reconsidering hospital policy. JAMA 1990;264:1281–1283.
41. Tomlinson T, Brody H. Futility and the ethics of resuscitation. JAMA 1990;264:1276–1280.
42. Blackhall LJ. Must we always use CPR? N Engl J Med 1987;317:1281–1285.
43. McClung JA, Kamer RS. Legislating ethics: implications of New York's do-not-resuscitate law. N Engl J Med 1990;323:270–272.
44. Waisel DB, Truog RD. The cardiopulmonary resuscitation-not-indicated order: futility revisited. Ann Intern Med 1995;122:304–308.
45. Annas GJ. Nancy Cruzan and the right to die. N Engl J Med 1990;323:670–673.
46. Orentlicher D. The right to die after Cruzan. JAMA 1990;264:2444–2446.
47. Council on Ethical and Judicial Affairs. American Medical Association. Decisions near the end of life. JAMA 1992;267:2229–2233.
48. Society of Critical Care Medicine Ethics Committee. Consensus report on the ethics of foregoing life-sustaining treatments in the critically ill. Crit Care Med 1990;18:1435–1439.
49. American Thoracic Society. Withholding and withdrawing life-sustaining therapy. Ann Intern Med 1991;115:478–485.
50. Solomon MZ, O'Donnell L, Jennings B, et al. Decisions near the end of life: professional views on life-sustaining treatments [see comments]. Am J Public Health 1993;83:14–23.
51. Shaw A, Randolph JG, Manard B. Ethical issues in pediatric surgery: a national survey of pediatricians and pediatric surgeons. Pediatrics 1977;60:588–599.
52. Caralis PV, Hammond JS. Attitudes of medical students, housestaff, and faculty physicians toward euthanasia and termination of life-sustaining treatment. Crit Care Med 1992;20:683–690.
53. Orentlicher D. From the Office of the General Counsel. Cruzan v Director of Missouri Department of Health: an ethical and legal perspective. JAMA 1989;262:2928–2930.
54. Bioethicists' statement on the U.S. Supreme Court's Cruzan decision. N Engl J Med 1990;323:686–687.
55. Angell M. The quality of mercy. N Engl J Med 1982;306:98–99.
56. Foley KM. The relationship of pain and symptom management to patient requests for physician-assisted suicide. J Pain Symptom Manage 1991;6:289–297.
57. Truog RD, Berde CB. Pain, euthanasia, and anesthesiologists. Anesthesiology 1993;78:353–360.
58. Gostin LO. Drawing a line between killing and letting die: the law, and law reform, on medically assisted dying. Journal of Law, Medicine, and Ethics 1993;21:94–101.
59. McCann RM, Hall WJ, Groth-Juncker A. Comfort care for terminally ill patients: the appropriate use of nutrition and hydration. JAMA 1994;272:1263–1266.
60. Lynn J, ed. By no extraordinary means: the choice to forego life-sustaining food and water. Bloomington, Indiana: University Press, 1989.
61. Frader J. Forgoing life-sustaining food and water: newborns. In: Lynn J, ed. By no extraordinary means: the choice to forgo life-sustaining food and water. Bloomington, Indiana: University Press, 1989:180–185.
62. Smedira NG, Evans BH, Grais LS, et al. Withholding and withdrawal of life support from the critically ill. N Engl J Med 1990;322:309–315.
63. Wilson WC, Smedira NG, Fink C, McDowell JA, Luce JM. Ordering and administration of sedatives and analgesics during the withholding and withdrawal of life support from critically ill patients. JAMA 1992;267:949–953.
64. Lee DKP, Swinburne AJ, Fedullo AJ, Wahl GW. Withdrawing care: experience in a medical intensive care unit. JAMA 1994;271:1358–1361.
65. Jayes RL, Zimmerman JE, Wagner DP, Draper EA, Knaus WA. Do-not-resuscitate orders in intensive care units: current practices and recent changes. JAMA 1993;270:2213–2217.
66. Christakis NA, Asch DA. Biases in how physicians choose to withdraw life support. Lancet 1993;342:642–646.
67. Faber Langendoen K. The clinical management of dying patients receiving mechanical ventilation: a survey of physician practice. Chest 1994;106:880–888.
68. Asch DA, Hansen-Flaschen J, Lanken PN. Decisions to limit or continue life-sustaining treatment by critical care physicians in the United States: conflicts between physicians' practices and patients' wishes [see comments]. American Journal of Respiratory & Critical Care Medicine 1995;151:288–292.
69. Levetown M, Pollack MM, Cuerdon TT, Ruttimann UE, Glover JJ. Limitations and withdrawals of medical intervention in pediatric critical care. JAMA 1994;272:1271–1275.
70. Ryan CA, Byrne P, Kuhn S, Tyebkhan J. No resuscitation and withdrawal of therapy in a neonatal and a pediatric intensive care unit in Canada [see comments]. J Pediatr 1993;123:534–538.
71. Cook DJ, Guyatt GH, Jaeschke R, et al. Determinants in Canadian health care workers of the decision to withdraw life support from the critically ill. Canadian Critical Care Trials Group [see comments]. JAMA 1995;273:703–708.
72. Cassileth BR, Zupkis RV, Sutton-Smith K, March V. Information and participation preferences among cancer patients. Ann Intern Med 1980;92:832–836.
73. Greenberg LW, Jewett LS, Gluck RS, et al. Giving information for a life-threatening diagnosis. Parents' and oncologists' perceptions. American Journal of Diseases of Children 1984;138:649–653.
74. Tolle SW, Elliot DL, Hickam DH. Physician attitudes and practices at the time of patient death. Arch Intern Med 1984;144:2389–2391.
75. Sharp MC, Strauss RP, Lorch SC. Communicating medical bad news: parents' experiences and preferences. J Pediatr 1992;121:539–546.
76. Krahn GL, Hallum A, Kime C. Are there good ways to give "bad news"? Pediatrics 1993;91:578–582.
77. Campbell ML. Breaking bad news to patients. JAMA 1994;271:1052.
78. Quill TE, Townsend P. Bad news: delivery, dialogue, and dilemmas. Arch Intern Med 1991;151:463–468.
79. Lindemann E. Symptomatology and management of acute grief [classical article]. American Journal of Psychiatry 1994;151:155–160.

Outcomes Analysis

50

Debra H. Fiser

INTRODUCTION

Recent focus on health care reform has accelerated the demand for valid and reliable information on the relative effectiveness of health care provided by institutions and physicians. Groups of providers often use risk-adjusted outcomes analysis for "health care report cards" to describe the outcomes of the care that they render[1,2]. Such reports to patients and purchasers of health care have become commonplace in the managed care industry. Unfortunately, the General Accounting Office recently reviewed a national sample of report card projects and concluded that no evaluative studies have been conducted to determine the validity or reliability or these report cards[3]. Meaningful analysis of outcomes remains very challenging[4].

The most straightforward application of outcomes data is epidemiologic or descriptive. Access to pooled outcomes data from many clinicians greatly expands the experience base of individual practitioners, especially for more unusual conditions[5,6]. This information is useful for prognostication and counseling, for development of clinical practice guidelines, and to undergird health policy[1,2,5,7,8].

Outcomes analysis also forms the cornerstone of the continuous quality improvement (CQI) process[9]. Rather than attempting to identify providers who produce poor outcomes, as in more traditional quality assurance methods, CQI identifies faulty processes that produce poor outcomes and corrects those processes[1,10–13].

Professor and Chief, Pediatric Critical Care Medicine and Health Services Research & Epidemiology
University of Arkansas for Medical Sciences and Arkansas Children's Hospital
Little Rock, AR

DOMAINS OF OUTCOME

There are several ways to classify health outcomes. Elinson's classification, that of the 5 Ds, is often cited: death, disease, disability, discomfort, and dissatisfaction[14]. To this schema, some would add a sixth D, destitution, to capture the economic hardship imposed by poor health.

Alternatively, one may consider the range of factors that contribute to quality of life[15]. For most adults, factors that are not amenable to change through health service delivery, such as social support, marital satisfaction, job satisfaction, housing, and socioeconomic circumstances, have greater influence on quality of life than does physical wellbeing[16,17]. Undoubtedly, comparable factors impact quality of life for children as well. As a result, the more specific outcome, health-related quality of life, is often considered[16,18]. The various domains of health-related quality of life include: physical, encompassing functional limitations, pain, and vitality; cognitive; emotional and mental health; social integration and relationships; roles, including employment and economic self-sufficiency in adults and school attendance in children; and self-perceived and subjective health status[16,18].

Across domains, the degree of impairment may vary. The Institute of Medicine has proposed a classification of disabling conditions, based on World Health Organization definitions and the work of Nagi, which considers a continuum of impairment from the presence of an undetectable biologic abnormality through the inability to perform socially expected activities and roles **(Table 50.1)**[18–20]. The underlying assumption is that each person has a certain functional capacity, and that external influences may enhance or thwart functional performance[5]. The classification is often used to assess achievement of the rehabilitation goals of greater independence and decreased requirement for

Table 50.1. The Institute of Medicine Classification of Disabling Conditions Considers a Continuum of Impairment from the Presence of an Undetectable Biologic Abnormality Through the Inability to Perform Socially Expected Activities and Roles.[a]

Pathology	*Impairment*	*Functional Limitation*	*Disability*
Interruption or interference of normal bodily processes or structures	Loss and/or abnormality of mental, emotional, physiological, or anatomical structure or function; includes all losses or abnormalities not just those attributable to active pathology; also includes pain	Restriction or lack of ability to perform an action or activity in the manner or within the range considered normal that results from impairment	Inability or limitation in performing socially defined activities and roles expected of individuals within a social and physical environment
Level of reference			
Cells and tissues	Organs and organ systems	Organism- action or activity performance (consistent with the purpose or function of the organ or organ system)	Society- task performance within the social and cultural context
Example			
Denervated muscle in arm as a result of trauma	Atrophy of muscle	Cannot pull with arm	Change of job; can no longer swim recreationally

[a]*(Reprinted with permission from Pope AM, Tarlov AR. Disability in America. Toward a National Agenda for Prevention. (Copyright 1991 by the National Academy of Sciences. Courtesy of National Academy Press, Washington, D.C.)*

caregiver assistance. It is also useful for considering critical care outcomes[5].

Determining which of the multidimensional outcomes of health care should be evaluated depends on both the context and the purpose of the assessment[21,22]. The context largely determines whose perspective should be evaluated[21]. A growing body of literature acknowledges the degree of incongruity between physician and patient perspectives; it is ideal to measure outcomes both from the perspective of patients and from that of their families, including satisfaction with care and self-perceived general well-being[5,10,23–30].

METHODOLOGY

Classification of Instruments

Instruments for health status measurement may be classified as discriminative or evaluative, generic or condition-specific. The appropriate type of instrument depends on the purpose of the assessment[31]. Discriminative measures determine only whether the outcome is better or worse while evaluative measures quantify the change[31]. Generic instruments apply to a broad range of patients across age, disease, severity, treatment, or service groups[7,27] as opposed to instruments which may be applicable only for certain specific conditions or groups[16,32].

Different instruments also produce different types of scores. Utility measures assess patient preferences for certain health states and weight those preferences relative to the patient's preference for death[31]. These outcome measures are used for deriving "quality-adjusted life year" figures for economic (cost-utility) analyses[14,16]. Health profiles consist of a single instrument and produce a score for each of their composite dimensions[16]. Alternatively, health batteries consist of several instruments or scales aggregated to provide a comprehensive assessment[16]. A third variety, the health index, is a single instrument that produces one score by weighting and aggregating scores on several different dimensions[16]. Although the concept of a single score may be attractive for decision making, it is difficult to interpret summary scores involving disparate dimensions since summary scores may obscure important findings on individual scales[16,24,33].

Pediatric Outcome Instruments

Although a number of health status and quality of life instruments have been developed to assess outcomes in adults, there are very few for children. Of those that have been validated in children, a few are disease-specific, rather than generic, and therefore of limited applicability in a broad evaluation of pediatric critical care services. Others are quality of life or health status measures useful in long range follow-up, but which have limited applicability as outcome measures in clinical settings, especially for acute settings such as intensive care. These include the Dartmouth COOP charts, the Child Health and Illness Profile (CHIP), the Quality of Well-Being Scale, and the Functional Status Measure II-R[34–37]. A pediatric version of the SF-36 from the Medical Outcome Study by Ware et al. (Jeanne Landgraf, personal communication) should soon be generally available.

Most of the instruments which are presently available evaluate level of disability and were developed for use in rehabilitation or development settings. Haley et al. have published an excellent review of these measures[5]. Unfortunately, none of these instruments is particularly well-suited for assessing outcome in the acute care setting owing to the requirement for an extended period of observation of the child after returning to his or her home environment. Two of the most commonly used include the Vineland Adaptive Behavior Scale[38] and the Functional Independence

Measure for Children[39]. The Vineland Adaptive Behavior Scale is a parent-report measure used to assess adaptive behavior: communication, daily living skills, socialization, motor skills, adaptive behavior composite, and maladaptive behavior[38]. The Vineland was validated in 4,800 handicapped and nonhandicapped individuals (birth through adult) in a national sample standardization group. This test produces standard scores with a normal mean of 100 and standard deviation of 15. It has been validated against the original version of the Vineland, the Adaptive Behavior Inventory for Children, and the American Association on Mental Deficiency Adaptive Behavior Scale. Inter-rater reliability ranges from 0.62 to 0.78 for the various domains and is 0.88 for maladaptive behavior. Test-retest reliability is 0.81 to 0.88. Internal consistency is 0.83 to 0.94 for the major domains and 0.69 to 0.84 for the subdomains. The test has been demonstrated to be responsive to change over time. The time required for administration of the instrument is from 20 to 60 minutes.

The Functional Independence Measure (FIM) is a seven-level scale developed to assess "burden of care" for the disabled in 6 realms: self care, sphincter management, mobility, locomotion, communication, and social cognition[39]. Face validity and reliability have been established in over 50 centers. The Functional Independence Measure for Children (WeeFIM) is a modification of the FIM developed for use with children younger than 7 years[40]. Scoring and interpretation are comparable. Administration time for the measure is from 20 to 40 minutes.

To fill the need for a simple generic measure suitable for assessing outcomes of pediatric intensive care, the author adapted the Glasgow Outcome Scales for adults[41] to create the Pediatric Cerebral Performance Category (PCPC) and the Pediatric Overall Performance Category (POPC) Scales **(Tables 50.2 and 50.3)**[42]. Each scale is a six-point scale ranging from a score of 1 to 6 with each interim point representing progressively greater functional impairment. Each scale category is accompanied by age-appropriate operational definitions.

The development of these scales was undertaken with the belief that death was too rare and too insensitive an occurrence in pediatric intensive care to be the sole criterion for quality of care evaluations. A more sensitive measure would decrease the sample size requirement for evaluation. In addition, mortality is often affected by factors other than quality of care, such as patient and family preference. It was also assumed that a need existed for both a measure of cognitive performance for certain applications and an index of more global functional performance for others, hence the development of two scales. Another assumption was that morbidity could be predicted by risk adjustment in much the same way as mortality[43]. In addition, it was clear that for PICU patients, many of whom have pre-existing chronic or debilitating conditions, the functional status at discharge would be highly associated with the functional status prior to the index illness or injury for which the patient was admitted. Therefore, the scales were developed to allow assignment of baseline and discharge functional status scores to perform adequate case-mix adjustment. The difference between the scores, the delta score, was defined as the change in function attributable to the index illness or injury and the care received for it.

The PCPC and POPC scales were initially validated in a sample that included 1539 PICU admissions from Arkansas Children's Hospital[42]. Face and content validity assessment were described in this report. Lacking a gold standard for criterion validity, construct validity was established with this sample. The hypothesized associations between the delta POPC and PCPC scale scores and other related constructs were proven to exist, including association with length of stay, hospital charges, discharge disposition, and PRISM risk of mortality. Responsiveness was established

Table 50.2. Pediatric Cerebral Performance Category Scale (PCPC). The Worst Level of Performance for Any Single Criteria Is Used for Categorizing. Deficits Are Scored Only if They Result from a Neurological Disorder.

Category	*Description*
1. Normal	Age-appropriate level of functioning; pre-school child developmentally appropriate; school age child attends regular classroom at school.
2. Mild Disability	Able to interact at an age-appropriate level[a]; minor neurologic disease that is controlled and does not interfere with daily functioning (e.g. seizure disorder); pre-school child may have minor developmental delays but over 75% of all activity of daily living developmental milestones are above the 10th percentile; school age child attends regular school but grade is not appropriate for age or is failing appropriate grade because of cognitive difficulties.
3. Moderate Disability	Below age-appropriate functioning; neurologic disease that is not controlled and severely limits activities; pre-school child has most activities of daily living developmental milestones that are below the 10th percentile; school age child can perform activities of daily living but attends special classroom because of cognitive difficulties and/or has learning deficit.
4. Severe Disability	Pre-school child has activities of daily living milestones that are below the 10th percentile and has excessive dependence on others for provision of activities of daily living; school age child may be so impaired as to be unable to attend school; school age child is dependent on others for provision of activities of daily living; abnormal motor movements for both pre-school and school age child may include nonpurposeful, decorticate, or decerebrate responses to pain.
5. Coma/vegetative	coma; unawareness
6. Death	

[a]*Frankenburg WK, Dodds J, Archer P, et al. The Denver II: a major revision and restandardization of the Denver Developmental Screening Test. Pediatrics 1992; 89:91–7.*

Table 50.3. Pediatric Overall Performance Category Scale (POPC). The Worst Level of Performance for Any Single Criteria Is Used for Categorizing. Deficits Are Scored if They Result from a Neurologic Disorder (PCPC Scale) or from Other Diseases or Conditions. Age Appropriate Activities of Daily Living Include Those That All but the Lowest 10th Percentile of Children at That Age Can Perform.[a]

Category	*Description*
1. Normal	PCPC = normal; normal age-appropriate activities. Medical and physical problems do not interfere with normal activity.
2. Mild Disability	PCPC = mild; minor chronic physical or medical problems present minor limitations but are compatible with normal life (e.g. asthma); pre-school child has physical disability consistent with future independent functioning (e.g. single amputation) and is able to perform over 75% of age-appropriate activities of daily living[a]; school age child is able to perform age appropriate activities of daily living.
3. Moderate Disability	PCPC = moderate; medical and physical conditions are limiting as described below; pre-school child can not perform most of the age appropriate activities of daily living[a]; school children can perform most activities of daily living but are physically disabled (e.g. cannot participate in competitive physical activities).
4. Severe Disability	PCPC = severe; pre-school child can not perform age appropriate activities of daily living; school age child is dependent on others for most activities of daily living.
5. Coma/vegetative	PCPC = coma/vegetative
6. Death	

[a]*Frankenburg WK, Dodds J, Archer P, et al. The Denver II: a major revision and restandardization of the Denver Developmental Screening Test. Pediatrics 1992; 89:91–7.*

by looking at transition across categories. A change in POPC score from admission to discharge was noted in 34% of cases and in PCPC score in 11%. Inter-rater reliability for rater pairs was excellent with intra-class correlation coefficients ranging from 0.88 to 0.96. These findings have recently been corroborated in a multi-institutional study involving 16 PICUs and over 10,000 patients. At the time of this writing, additional construct validation and evaluation of the test-retest reliability of the instrument are being conducted in a longitudinal study.

Risk Adjustment

Without risk adjustment, outcomes are uninterpretable. Case-mix adjustments must account for the prognostic significance of the burden of illness which the patient brings to the hospital[(44,45)]. Contributing factors often included in case-mix adjustments are demographic factors,[(44)] the patient's social and financial condition,[(21)] health risk factors,[(44)] and admitting and comorbid diagnoses[(21,44,46)]. The validity of risk-adjusted outcomes as a measure of quality depends on the adequacy of the statistical model to quantify accurately baseline differences in case mix among health care providers[(4)]. The predictive model should also explain a substantial portion of the variance in outcomes.

Severity of illness may be described in terms of disease stage classifications or using physiologic scores[(21,44)]. Physiologic scores assigned at the time of ICU admission, such as the Pediatric Risk of Mortality Score (PRISM) are preferred, however[(43)]. In multiple regression models, demographic characteristics such as race or payor status do not independently predict outcome after controlling for the PRISM score (Fiser DH, unpublished work). Presumably, the negative prognostic influence of certain demographic factors has been exerted prior to admission to exacerbate the severity of physiologic instability and is thus measurable with the PRISM at admission.

Another important contribution to the burden of illness is the patient's baseline or pre-existing health or functional status including the impact of comorbid conditions[(21,25,42,44–46)]. Baseline health status is strongly associated with outcome measures[(42,44,47)]. In addition, the reason for admission (e.g., diagnostic or terminal care), or patient preferences and the ultimate goal of therapy (full heroic care vs. withdrawing or withholding some measures) must be assessed[(21,27,42,44)].

Data Quality

Potential origins of measurement error include the source and quality of the data. It is common for outcomes researchers to acquire and analyze large databases for purposes other than that for which they were originally developed. This practice may lead to erroneous conclusions; for example, analysis of diagnosis fields in claims databases may be misleading because providers often list the most "reimbursable" diagnosis code in preference to more appropriate, but less reimbursable diagnoses[(48)]. In addition, coding and data entry errors occur frequently in clinical data sources[(48)]. Nonrandom, systematic sampling bias also occurs in settings with incomplete ascertainment[(4,44)].

Furthermore, standardization of data collection and verification of the reliability of the data are important. Inaccuracies in coding of important risk factors can significantly change interpretation of the data. For example, after implementation of the Cardiac Surgery Reporting System in New York, the prevalence of reported risk factors has increased dramatically each year[(4)]. Hence, physicians have fluctuated widely in rank from one year to the next. In fact, in one year, 46% of the surgeons moved from one half of the ranked list to the other[(4)]. Poor data are worse than no data at all.

Timing of Assessments

The timing of measurement must also be appropriate[(4,7,21)]. There is increasing interest in assessing outcomes longitudinally across providers and organizational boundaries[(7,21)]. However, to evaluate and improve the quality of the care delivered, it is necessary to measure outcomes with attribution to processes. Therefore, in addition to longer range follow-up, assessment across more discrete time frames is desirable for some purposes[12]. This is particularly true in the pediatric intensive care unit setting where multiple disciplines provide care in many units of an integrated system (e.g., emergency medical services, emergency department care, intensive care, rehabilitation and so forth). Evaluating the function of the integrated system requires the longer range perspective while judging performance of the respective units requires more discrete and focused assessment.

Analysis and Interpretation

It is important to identify the unit for outcomes analysis, whether individuals or institutions[21]. In addition, normative data for the measure is essential for interpretation[7,31,33].

OUTCOMES RESEARCH

Outcomes analysis as a research tool has some inherent strengths and weaknesses. For one thing, outcomes analysis allows study of some conditions and patient groups that will never be practical to study using randomized controlled trials (RCTs). Because of the large number of patients whose outcomes may be included in clinical or administrative databases, results of "natural experiments" may have greater generalizability than the results of RCTs which may be limited to certain highly specific populations in somewhat artificial circumstances. However, this strength is also a source of weakness. Because natural variations in practices are not randomly assigned, there is often inherent bias in patient selection and incomparability of treatment groups. For example, sicker patients may be consistently treated with one therapy and less sick patients with another. Hence, case-mix adjustment is *extremely* important in interpreting the results. The potential for additional error when claims data are used for analysis was discussed previously.

A new technique, cross design synthesis, utilizes both outcomes research and RCTs to study the same condition[49]. Outcomes, treatment information, and patient characteristics are extracted from databases of patient records. If the findings from RCTs mirror the findings in comparable patient subgroups in the database, then estimation of treatment effectiveness is possible from the database for additional subgroups of patients which were not originally studied in the RCT[49].

As the availability of computerized clinical networks and databases increases and research dollars for classic RCTs decline, applications and methodologies for the evaluative sciences will inevitably grow. Although it is very unlikely that outcomes research will ever supplant clinical trials, outcomes research may help to focus RCTs by identifying conditions for which there is variability in practice and associated morbidity and excess cost.

References

1. Ellwood PM. The future: clinical outcomes management. Couch JB, ed. Health care quality management in the 21st century. American College of Physician Executives, 1991:465–83.
2. Thier SO. Forces motivating the use of health status assessment measures in clinical settings and related clinical research. Med Care 1992; 30:MS15–22.
3. Health care reform: "report cards" are useful but significant issues that need to be addressed. Washington, D.C.: General Accounting Office, 1994 (GAO/HEHS-94-219).
4. Green J, Wintfeld N. Report cards on cardiac surgeons. Assessing New York State's approach. N Engl J Med 1995;332:1229–32.
5. Haley SM, Coster WJ, Ludlow LH. Pediatric functional outcome measures. Physical Med Rehab Clin NA 1991; 2:689–723.
6. Shortell SM, Zimmerman JE, Gillies RR, et al. Continuously improving patient care: practical lessons in an assessment tool from the national ICU study. QRB 1992; 18:150–5.
7. Lansky D, Butler JBV, Waller FT. Using health status measures in the hospital setting: from acute care to "outcomes management". Med Care 1992; 30:MS57–73.
8. Murray LS, Teasdale GM, Murray GD, et al. Does prediction of outcome alter patient management? Lancet 1993; 341:1487–91.
9. Fiser DH. Outcome evaluations as measures of quality in pediatric intensive care. Pediatr Clin NA 1994;41:1423–38.
10. Berwick DM. Controlling variation in health care: a consultation from Walter Shewhart. Med Care 1991; 29:1212–25.
11. Donabedian A. The role of outcomes in quality assessment and assurance. QRB 1992; 18:356–60.
12. Reinertsen JL. Outcomes management and continuous quality improvement: the compass and the rudder. QRB 1993; 19:5–7.
13. Williams RM. Health policy and quality: an ethical dilemma. J Emerg Med 1993; 11:345–9.
14. Eisenberg JM. Clinical economics: a guide to the economic analysis of clinical practices. JAMA 1989; 262:2879–86.
15. Lohr KN. Impact of Medicare prospective payment on the quality of medical care: a research agenda. Santa Monica: The RAND Corporation, 1985.
16. MacKeigan LD, Pathak DS. Overview of health-related quality-of-life measures. Am J Hosp Pharm 1992; 49:2236–45.
17. Molzahn AE. Should quality of life measures be used to assess quality of care? ANNA Journal 1992; 19:88.
18. Pope AM, Tarlov AR, eds. Disability in America. Toward a national agenda for prevention. Washington, DC: National Academy Press, 1991:76–95, 309–327.
19. Nagi SZ. Some conceptual issues in disability and rehabilitation. In Sussman MB, ed. Sociology and rehabilitation. Washington, DC: American Sociological Association, 1965.
20. International Classification of Impairments, Disabilities and Handicaps: A Manual of Classification Relating to the Consequences of Disease. Geneva: World Health Organization, 1980.
21. Jones JR. Outcomes analysis: methods and issues. Nurs Econ 1993; 11:145–52.
22. Lohr KN, ed. Medicare. A strategy for quality assurance, vol I. Washington, DC, Institute of Medicine: National Academy Press, 1990.
23. Ervin NE, Walcott-McQuigg J, Chen SC, et al. Measuring patients' perceptions of care quality. J Nurs Care Qual 1992; 6:25–32.
24. Fitzpatrick R, Fletcher A, Gore S, et al. Quality of life measures in health care. I: Applications and issues in assessment. Br Med J 1992; 305:1074–7.
25. Greenfield S, Nelson EC. Recent developments and future issues in the use of health status assessment measures in clinical settings. Med Care 1992; 30:MS2-MS41.
26. Hegyvary ST. Issues in outcomes research. J Nurs Qual Assur 1991; 5:1–6.
27. Iezzoni LI. Monitoring quality of care: what do we need to know? Inquiry 1993; 30:112–114.
28. Megivern K, Halm MA, Jones G. Measuring patient satisfaction as an outcome of nursing care. J Nurs Care Qual 1992; 6:9–24.
29. Reiser SJ. The era of the patient. Using the experience of illness in shaping the missions of health care. JAMA 1993; 269:1012–7.
30. Tarlov AR. Call for instruments. Medical Outcomes Trust Bulletin 1994; 2:1.

31. Guyatt GH, Feeny DH, Patrick DL. Measuring health-related quality of life. Ann Intern Med 1993; 118:622–9.
32. Fletcher A, Gore S, Jones D, et al. Quality of life measures in health care. II: Design, analysis, and interpretation. Br Med J 1991; 305:1145–8.
33. Fries JF. The hierarchy of outcome assessment. J Rheumatol 1993; 20:546–7.
34. Kaplan RM, McCutchan JA, Navarro AM, et al. Quality adjusted survival analysis: a neglected application of the Quality of Well-Being Scale. Psychol Health 1994; 9:131–41.
35. Lewis CC, Pantell RH, Kieckhefer GM. Assessment of children's health status. Field test of new approaches. Med Care 1989; 27:S54-S65.
36. Starfield B, Bergner M, Ensminger M, et al. Adolescent health status measurement: Development of the Child Health and Illness Profile. Pediatr 1993; 91:430–5.
37. Wasson J, Walsh TB, Rompkins RK, et al. The common symptom guide: a guide to the evaluation of common adult and pediatric symptoms. New York: McGraw-Hill, 1992.
38. Sparrow SS, Balla DA, Cicchetti DV. Vineland Adaptive Behavior Scales: interview edition—survey form manual. Circle Pines, MN: American Guidance Service, 1984.
39. Center for Functional Assessment Research, Uniform Data System for Medical Rehabilitation for UDS Data Management Service, U.B. Foundation Activities, Inc. Guide for Use of the Uniform Data Set for Medical Rehabilitation Including the Functional Independence Measure (FIM). Buffalo, NY: Research Foundation, State University of New York, 1990.
40. Center for Functional Assessment Research, Uniform Data System for Medical Rehabilitation for UDS Data Management Service, U.B. Foundation Activities, Inc. Guide for Use of the Uniform Data Set for Medical Rehabilitation Including the Functional Independence Measure for Children (WeeFIM). Buffalo, NY: Research Foundation, State University of New York, 1991.
41. Jennett B, Bond M. Assessment of outcome after severe brain damage: a practical scale. Lancet 1975;1:480–4.
42. Fiser DH. Assessing the outcome of pediatric intensive care. J Pediatr 1992; 121:68–74.
43. Pollack MM, Ruttimann UE, Getson PR. Pediatric risk of mortality (PRISM) score. Crit Care Med 1988; 16:1110–6.
44. Deyo RA, Carter WB. Strategies for improving and expanding the application of health status measures in clinical settings: a researcher-developer viewpoint. Med Care 1992; 30:MS176–186.
45. Kahn KL. How well does the patient's burden of illness explain differences in outcome? (editorial) Mayo Clin Proc 1992; 67:1203–5.
46. Dodds TA, Martin DP, Stolov WC, et al. A validation of the functional independence measurement and its performance among rehabilitation inpatients. Arch Phys Med Rehabil 1993; 74:531–6.
47. Falconer JA, Roth EJ, Sutin JA, et al. The critical path method in stroke rehabilitation: lessons from an experiment in cost containment and outcome improvement. QRB 1993; 19:8–16.
48. Green J, Wintfeld N. How accurate are hospital discharge data for evaluating effectiveness of care? Med Care 1993; 31:719–31.
49. Anonymous. Cross design synthesis: a new strategy for studying medical outcomes. Lancet 1992; 340:944–6.

Index

Note: Page numbers in *italics* indicate figures; page numbers followed by t indicate tables.